KT-371-355

Oxford Textbook of
Rheumatology

FOURTH EDITION

Edited by

Richard A. Watts

Philip G. Conaghan

Christopher Denton

Helen Foster

John Isaacs

Ulf Müller-Ladner

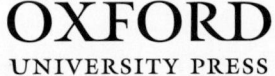

OXFORD

UNIVERSITY PRESS

OXFORD
UNIVERSITY PRESS

Great Clarendon Street, Oxford, OX2 6DP,
United Kingdom

Oxford University Press is a department of the University of Oxford.
It furthers the University's objective of excellence in research, scholarship,
and education by publishing worldwide. Oxford is a registered trade mark of
Oxford University Press in the UK and in certain other countries

© Oxford University Press 2013

The moral rights of the authors have been asserted

First Edition published in 1993

Second Edition published in 1998

Third Edition published in 2004

Fourth Edition published in 2013

Impression: 1

All rights reserved. No part of this publication may be reproduced, stored in
a retrieval system, or transmitted, in any form or by any means, without the
prior permission in writing of Oxford University Press, or as expressly permitted
by law, by licence or under terms agreed with the appropriate reprographics
rights organization. Enquiries concerning reproduction outside the scope of the
above should be sent to the Rights Department, Oxford University Press, at the
address above

You must not circulate this work in any other form
and you must impose this same condition on any acquirer

Published in the United States of America by Oxford University Press
198 Madison Avenue, New York, NY 10016, United States of America

British Library Cataloguing in Publication Data

Data available

Library of Congress Control Number: 2013946780

ISBN 978–0–19–964248–9

Printed and bound in China by
C&C Offset Printing Co. Ltd

Oxford University press makes no representation, express or implied, that the
drug dosages in this book are correct. Readers must therefore always check
the product information and clinical procedures with the most up-to-date
published product information and data sheets provided by the manufacturers
and the most recent codes of conduct and safety regulations. The authors and
the publishers do not accept responsibility or legal liability for any errors in the
text or for the misuse or misapplication of material in this work. Except where
otherwise stated, drug dosages and recommendations are for the non-pregnant
adult who is not breast-feeding.

Links to third party websites are provided by Oxford in good faith and
for information only. Oxford disclaims any responsibility for the materials
contained in any third party website referenced in this work.

WE 544 WAT

369 0291586

DATE DUE

GAYLORD

PRINTED IN U.S.A.

NHS Ayrshire & Arran
Libraries
Crosshouse Hospital

Oxford Textbook of

Rheumatology

Preface

The science of rheumatology has progressed enormously since the third edition of the *Oxford Textbook of Rheumatology* was published in 2004. There have been major developments in all the major subspecialities of rheumatology and rheumatologists are enjoying the fruits of the biotechnology revolution, with a cornucopia of biological agents in routine clinical practice or in development.

In keeping with a new editorial team the content of the book has been thoroughly revised, while retaining the broad structure of the previous editions which were a distinctive feature of the book. The number of chapters has increased from 126 to 173, reflecting the increasing breadth of knowledge. New chapters have been written reflecting the changing face of rheumatology. We have expanded the imaging section to include separate chapters on each of the main modalities, and chapters on therapeutics cover the new biologic agents including areas that we foresee becoming mainstream during the life of the book.

Textbooks of this size are often viewed in the modern electronic age of rapid revision as being ossified and out of date before publication. We, however, believe, as do our publishers Oxford University Press, that textbooks still have a valuable place. Much of the corpus of knowledge contained within textbooks changes quite slowly; principles and practice of examination, clinical features of disease and assessment. Chapters on pathogenesis and treatment become outdated more quickly and we are planning a regular cycle of updates. In addition to completely revising text, we have introduced colour throughout the book.

Electronic books have become widespread since the last edition and in addition to a print edition we are producing an online version, which is not merely the print version reproduced but has enhanced functionality with direct links to references, video images, and links between relevant sections. The ability to use video enables use of multislice MR and CT to be available and real time ultrasound.

We owe a huge debt to the editors of the previous editions—David Isenberg, Peter Maddision, Patricia Woo, David Glass, and Ferdinand Breedveld—who assembled and produced three splendid editions. They felt that the time had come, nearly a decade after the writing of the third edition, that a fresh editorial team was needed.

Richard A. Watts
Ipswich, UK
Philip G. Conaghan
Leeds, UK
Christopher Denton
London, UK
Helen Foster
Newcastle upon Tyne, UK
John Isaacs
Newcastle upon Tyne, UK
Ulf Müller-Ladner
Bad Nauheim, Germany

Acknowledgements

We wish to thank all at Oxford University Press who have contributed to bringing this book to fruition, especially Helen Liepman who has commissioned the *Oxford Textbook of Rheumatology* for four editions, Peter Stevenson who is the senior recommissioning editor for this edition, Carol Maxwell who has ably organized the editorial team and ensured that the contributors produced their work, and Eloise Moir-Ford who took the book through production. Our contributors deserve our thanks for writing outstanding chapters. Finally, we gratefully acknowledge our long-suffering families for putting up with the editors.

Brief contents

Contents

Contributors

Engy Abdelattif
Department of Osteoarticular Pathology
Manchester Medical School
Manchester

Rita Abdulkader
Norfolk and Norwich University NHS Foundation Trust
Norwich

Shazia Abdullah
Department of Rheumatology
Hinchingbrooke Hospital
Hinchingbrooke Park
Huntingdon

Abhishek Abhishek
Department of Rheumatology
Queen Elizabeth Hospital
University Hospital Birmingham NHS Trust
Birmingham

Mario Abinun
Children's BMT Unit
Newcastle General Hospital
Newcastle upon Tyne

Jo Adams
Faculty of Health Sciences
University of Southampton
Highfield
Southampton

Ade Adebajo
Academic Rheumatology Group
University of Sheffield Medical School
Sheffield

Tehseen Ahmed
Royal National Hospital for Rheumatic Diseases
NHS Foundation Trust
Upper Borough Walls
Bath

Jonathan D. Akikusa
Rheumatology Service
Department of General Medicine
Royal Children's Hospital
Parkville, Victoria
Australia

Daniel Aletaha
Division of Rheumatology
Department of Internal Medicine 3
Medical University Vienna
Vienna
Austria

Adil Al-Nahhas
Imperial College Healthcare Trust
Hammersmith Hospital
London

Ismael Atchia
North Tyneside General Hospital
North Shields
Tyne and Wear

Eileen Baildam
Alder Hey Children's NHS Foundation Trust
Eaton Road
Alder Hey
Liverpool

Jyoti Bakshi
Rheumatology Department
Royal Berkshire Hospital
Reading

S. Balamoody
Biomedical Imaging Institute
University of Manchester
Manchester

Thomas Bardin
Université Paris VII
Service de Rhumatologie
Hopital Lariboisière
Paris
France

Anne Barton
Arthritis Research UK Epidemiology Unit
University of Manchester
Manchester

Nuno Batista
Department of Spinal Disorders
Nuffield Orthopaedic Centre
Oxford

Thomas Beckingsale
North of England Bone and Soft Tissue Tumour Service
Freeman Hospital
Newcastle Upon Tyne

David Bending
Rheumatology Unit
UCL Institute of Child Health
London

Mike Benjamin
Emeritus Professor
School of Biosciences
University of Cardiff
Cardiff

Michael W. Beresford
Department of Women's and Children's Health
Institute of Translational Medicine, University of Liverpool
Department of Paediatric Rheumatology
Alder Hey Children's NHS Hospital Foundation Trust
Liverpool

Jessica Bertrand
Institute of Experimental Musculoskeletal Medicine
University Hospital Munster
Munster
Germany

Ashok K. Bhalla
Royal National Hospital for Rheumatic Diseases
NHS Foundation Trust
Upper Borough Walls
Bath

Kuljeet Bhamra
Rheumatology Department
Nuffield Orthopaedic Centre
Oxford

Marc Bijl
Department of Internal Medicine and Rheumatology
Martini Hospital
Groningen
The Netherlands

Johannes W. J. Bijlsma
Department of Rheumatology and Clinical Immunology
University Medical Centre Utrecht
Utrecht
The Netherlands

Fraser Birrell
Institute of Cellular Medicine
Musculoskeletal Research Group
The Medical School
Newcastle University
Newcastle upon Tyne

Nick Bishop
Academic Unit of Child Health
Department of Human Metabolism
University of Sheffield
Sheffield Children's Hospital
Sheffield

Julian Blake
Department of Clinical Neurophysiology
Norfolk and Norwich University Hospital
Norwich

David A. Bong
Instituto Poal de Reumatologia
Barcelona
Spain

Simon Bowman
Rheumatology Department
Queen Elizabeth Hospital
Birmingham B15 2TH, UK

William H. Breidahl
Royal Perth Hospital
Perth
Western Australia
Australia

Paul A. Brogan
University College London
Institute of Child Health and Great Ormond
Street Hospital NHS Trust
London

Barbara M. Bröker
Ernst-Moritz-Arndt-Universität Greifswald
Institut für Immunologie und Transfusionsmedizin
Abteilung Immunologie
Greifswald
Germany

Matthew Brown
University of Queensland Diamantina Institute
Translational Research Institute Princess Alexandra Hospital
Woolloongabba, Brisbane
Queensland
Australia

Philip M. Brown
Musculoskeletal Research Group
Institute of Cellular Medicine
Newcastle University
Newcastle upon Tyne

Kay Brune
Department of Experimental and Clinical Pharmacology and Toxicology
FAU Erlangen-Nuremberg
Erlangen
Germany

Hermine I. Brunner
Division of Rheumatology
Children's Hospital Medical Center
Cincinnati
Ohio

Christopher Buckley
Rheumatology Research Group
Centre for Translational Inflammation Research
School of Immunity & Infection
College of Medical & Dental Sciences
University of Birmingham Research Laboratories
Queen Elizabeth Hospital Birmingham

Gerd-R. Burmester
Department of Rheumatology and Clinical Immunology
Charité-Universitätsmedizin Berlin
Free University and Humboldt University Berlin
Berlin
Germany

Frank Buttgereit
Clinic for Rheumatology and Clinical Immunology
Charité-Universitätsmedizin Berlin
Berlin
Germany

Loreto Carmona
Universidad Camilo Jose Cela
Villafranca del Castillo
Madrid
Spain

Graeme J. Carroll
School of Medicine
University of Notre Dame Australia; and
Fremantle Hospital
Western Australia

Hector Chinoy
The University of Manchester
Manchester Academic Health Science Centre
Salford Royal NHS Foundation Trust
Salford

Alvina D. Chu
Division of Immunology and Rheumatology
Stanford University School of Medicine
Stanford
CA

Julia Clark
Paediatric Infectious Diseases
Infection Management and Prevention Service
Royal Children's Hospital Brisbane Australia

Sophie Cleanthous
Centre for Rheumatology Research
Division of Medicine
University College London
London

Jacqui Clinch
Bristol Royal Hospital for Children
Bristol

Laura C. Coates
Leeds Institute of Rheumatic and Musculoskeletal Medicine
University of Leeds and Leeds NIHR Musculoskeletal Biomedical Research Unit
Leeds Teaching Hospitals NHS Trust
Leeds

J. Gerry Coghlan
Cardiology Department
Royal Free Hospital
London

Helen Cohen
Dept of Rheumatology
Royal National Orthopaedic Hospital
Stanmore
Middlesex

Philip G. Conaghan
Leeds Institute of Rheumatic and Musculoskeletal Medicine
University of Leeds and NIHR Leeds Musculoskeletal Biomedical Research Unit
Leeds

Cyrus Cooper
MRC Lifecourse Epidemiology Unit, University of Southampton;
and NIHR Musculoskeletal Biomedical Unit,
University of Oxford, Oxford

Robert G. Cooper
The University of Manchester
Manchester Academic Health Science Centre
Salford Royal NHS Foundation Trust
Salford

Andrew P. Cope
Head, Academic Department of Rheumatology
Centre for Molecular and Cellular Biology of Inflammation
Division of Immunology, Infection and Inflammatory Diseases
King's College School of Medicine
King's College
London

Nicola Dalbeth
Bone and Joint Research Group
Department of Medicine
University of Auckland
Grafton, Auckland
New Zealand

Bhaskar Dasgupta
Department of Rheumatology
Southend University Hospital NHS Foundation Trust
Westcliff-on-Sea
Essex

Cosimo De Bari
Institute of Medical Sciences
University of Aberdeen
Aberdeen

Chris Deighton
Department of Rheumatology
Royal Derby Hospital
Derby

Angelo Del Buono
Department of Rheumatology
University Campus Biomedico
Rome
Italy

Christopher P. Denton
Centre for Rheumatology and Connective Tissue Diseases
Department of Inflammation
Division of Medicine, UCL Medical School
Royal Free Campus
London

Stanley C. Deresinski
Redwood City
California

Ida Dzifa Dey
Rheumatology Department
University College London Hospital
London

Robert Dinser
Justus-Liebig University Giessen
Internal Medicine and Rheumatology
Kerckhoff-Klinik GmbH
Bad Nauheim
Germany

Michael Doherty
Academic Rheumatology
University of Nottingham
Nottingham, UK

Radboud Dolhain
Department of Rheumatology
Erasmus MC
University Medical Centre
Rotterdam
The Netherlands

Thomas Dörner
Med. Klinik m.S. Rheumatologie und Klinische
Immunologie and DRFZ Berlin
Berlin
Germany

Tilman Drüeke
Inserm ERI-12
UFR de Médecine/Pharmacie
Université de Picardie Jules Verne
Amiens
France

Ciarán M. Duffy
Max Keeping Wing
Children's Hospital of Eastern Ontario
Ottawa, Ontario
Canada

Lisa Dunkley
Department of Rheumatology
Royal Hallamshire Hospital
Sheffield

Christopher Edwards
Department of Rheumatology
Southampton University Hospitals NHS Trust
Southampton General Hospital
Southampton

Mark H. Edwards
MRC Lifecourse Epidemiology Unit
University of Southampton
Southampton General Hospital
Southampton

Hermann Einsele
University Hospital Würzburg
Internal Medicine II
Würzburg
Germany

Despina Eleftheriou
Institute of Child Health
London

Assia Eljaafari
Department of Clinical Immunology and Rheumatology
Hôpital Edouard Herriot
University of Lyon
Lyon
France

Benjamin Ellis
Department of Rheumatology
King's College Hospital
Denmark Hill
London

Edzard Ernst
Complementary Medicine
Peninsula Medical School
Exeter
Devon

Steve Eyre
Centre for Musculoskeletal Research
Institute for Inflammation and Repair
Faculty of Medical and Human Sciences
University of Manchester
Manchester

Jeremy Fairbank
Department of Spinal Disorders
Nuffield Department of Orthopaedics, Rheumatology and
Musculoskeletal Sciences
Nuffield Orthopaedic Centre
Oxford

Saul N. Faust
Wellcome Trust Clinical Research Facility
University of Southampton
Southampton

Eugen Feist
Clinic for Rheumatology and Clinical Immunology
Charité-Universitätsmedizin Berlin
Berlin
Germany

Jeremy Field
Consultant in Trauma and Orthopaedics
Cheltenham General Hospital
Cheltenham

Max Field
Wolfson Medical School Building
University of Glasgow
Glasgow

Francisco Figueiredo
Department of Ophthalmology
Royal Victoria Infirmary
Newcastle University
Newcastle upon Tyne

Andrew Filer
School of Immunity and Infection
MRC Centre for Immune Regulation
College of Medical and Dental Sciences
University of Birmingham
Edgbaston
Birmingham

Volker Fingerle
Bavarian Health and Food Safety Authority
Oberschleißheim
Germany

Roy Fleischmann
University of Texas Southwestern Medical Center
Dallas
TX

Joanne Foo
Rheumatology Department
York District Hospital
York

Helen Foster
Musculoskeletal Research Group
Newcastle University
Medical School
Newcastle upon Tyne

Amy Foulkes
The Dermatology Centre
Salford Royal NHS Foundation Trust
Manchester

Anthony J. Freemont
School of Clinical and Laboratory Sciences
University of Manchester
Manchester

Klaus Frommer
Justus-Liebig University Giessen
Internal Medicine and Rheumatology
Kerckhoff-Klinik GmbH
Bad Nauheim
Germany

Karl Gaffney
Department of Rheumatology
The Norfolk & Norwich University Hospital
NHS Foundation Trust
UK

Maria Galindo
Rheumatology Department
Hospital Universitario 12 de Octubre
Madrid
Spain

Clare Galton
Department of Neurology
Ipswich Hospital NHS Trust
Ipswich

J. S. Hill Gaston
Division of Rheumatology
Department of Medicine
University of Cambridge
Cambridge

Steffen Gay
Department of Rheumatology
University Hospital Zurich
Zurich
Switzerland

Paul Genever
Department of Biology
University of York
York

Craig Gerrand
North of England Bone and Soft Tissue Tumour Service
Freeman Hospital
Newcastle Upon Tyne

Helena Gleeson
Department of Endocrinology
Leicester Royal Infirmary
Leicester

Caroline Gordon
School of Immunity and Infection
College of Medical and Dental Sciences
The Medical School
University of Birmingham
Edgbaston
Birmingham

Andrew Graham
Department of Neurology
Ipswich Hospital NHS Trust
Ipswich

Rodney Grahame
Department of Rheumatology
University College Hospital
London

Andrew J. Grainger
Radiology Department and Leeds Musculoskeletal
Biomedical Research Centre
Chapel Allerton Hospital
Leeds Teaching Hospitals
Leeds

Damian Griffin
Clinical Sciences Research Institute
Warwick Orthopaedics
Warwick Medical School
Coventry

Christopher Griffiths
Dermatology Centre
Salford Royal NHS Foundation Trust
University of Manchester
Manchester

Alexei A. Grom
Cincinnati Children's Hospital Medical Center
Division of Rheumatology
Cincinnati
Ohio

Wolfgang L. Gross
Department of Rheumatology and Clinical Immunology
Vasculitis Center
University Hospital Schleswig Holstein
Lübeck
Germany

Monica N. Gupta
Rheumatology Department
Gartnavel General Hospital
Glasgow

Richard Haigh
Dept. of Rheumatology
Royal Devon and Exeter Foundation Trust
Exeter

Alan J. Hakim
Consultant Rheumatologist and Acute Physician
Honorary Senior Lecturer
Barts Health NHS Trust
London

Philip Hamann
Royal National Hospital for Rheumatic Diseases
Upper Borough Walls
Bath

John Hamburger
University of Birmingham School of Dentistry
Birmingham

Jennifer Hamilton
Queen Elizabeth Hospital
Gateshead
Tyne and Wear

Louise Hamilton
Department of Rheumatology
The Norfolk & Norwich University Hospital NHS
Foundation Trust
Norwich

Nicholas C. Harvey
MRC Lifecourse Epidemiology Unit
University of Southampton
Southampton General Hospital
Southampton

Philip N. Hawkins
National Amyloidosis Centre
Division of Medicine
UCL Medical School
Royal Free Campus
London

Marloes Heijstek
University Medical Centre
Wilhelmina Children's Hospital
Department of Paediatric Immunology and Rheumatology
Utrecht
The Netherlands

Marianne Heitzmann
Institute of Experimental Musculoskeletal Medicine
University Hospital Munster
Munster
Germany

Philip S. Helliwell
Leeds Institute of Rheumatic and Musculoskeletal Medicine
University of Leeds, Leeds

Martina Henniger
Agaplesion Frankfurter Diakonie Kliniken gGmbH
Agaplesion Markus Krankenhaus
Akademisches Lehr-KH der Goethe-Universität
Frankfurt
Germany

Ariane Herrick
The University of Manchester
Manchester Academic Health Science Centre
Salford Royal NHS Foundation Trust
Salford

Sarah Hewlett
Department of Nursing and Midwifery
University of the West of England
Bristol

Geoff Hide
Department of Radiology
Freeman Hospital
Newcastle upon Tyne

Anne Hinks
Arthritis Research UK Epidemiology Unit
Manchester Academic Health Science Centre
The University of Manchester
Manchester

Burkhard Hinz
Institute of Toxicology and Pharmacology
University of Rostock
Rostock
Germany

Julia U. Holle
Department of Rheumatology and Clinical Immunology
Vasculitis Center
University Hospital Schleswig Holstein
Lübeck
Germany

Rosemary J. Hollick
Aberdeen Royal Infirmary
Foresterhill
Aberdeen

Kate L. Holliday
Arthritis Research UK Epidemiology Unit
The Medical School
Manchester

Christopher R. Holroyd
MRC Lifecourse Epidemiology Unit
University of Southampton
Southampton General Hospital
Southampton

Lindsey Hooper
Solent NHS Trust
University of Southampton
Faculty of Health Sciences
Southampton

Susan Hopkins
Department of Microbiology
Division of Medicine, UCL Medical School
Royal Free Campus
London

Kristin Houghton
Division of Rheumatology
Department of Pediatrics
University of British Columbia
Vancouver
Canada

Rachel K. Hoyles
Oxford Centre for Respiratory Medicine
Churchill Hospital
Oxford

Graham R. V. Hughes
Head of the Lupus Centre, London Bridge Hospital
London

Frances Humby
Centre for Experimental Medicine and Rheumatology
2nd Floor, John Vane Science Centre
William Harvey Research Institute
Barts and the London School of Medicine and Dentistry
Queen Mary University of London
London

Jennifer Humphries
Department of Radiology
Freeman Hospital
Newcastle upon Tyne

John D. Isaacs
Musculoskeletal Research Group
Institute of Cellular Medicine
Newcastle University
Newcastle upon Tyne

David Isenberg
Department of Inflammation
UCL Division of Medicine
London

Johannes W. G. Jacobs
Department of Rheumatology and Clinical Immunology
University Medical Center Utrecht
Utrecht
The Netherlands

Deepak R. Jadon
Royal National Hospital for Rheumatic Diseases
NHS Foundation Trust
Upper Borough Walls
Bath

Sharmila Jandial
Musculoskeletal Research Group
Newcastle University
Medical School
Newcastle upon Tyne

David Jayne
Vasculitis and Lupus Clinic
Addenbrooke's Hospital
Cambridge

Karl Johnson
Radiology Department
Birmingham Children's Hospital
Birmingham

Maria Juarez
Rheumatology Research Group
School of Immunity and Infection
College of Medical and Dental Science
University of Birmingham
Birmingham

David Kane
Adelaide and Meath Hospital
Dublin
Republic of Ireland

Lesley Kay
Musculoskeletal Services Directorate
The Newcastle upon Tyne Hospitals NHS Foundation Trust and
Musculoskeletal Research Group
Newcastle University

Andrew Keat
Rheumatology Department
Northwick Park Hospital
Harrow
Middlesex

Gregory J. Keir
Interstitial Lung Disease Unit
Royal Brompton Hospital
London

Clive Kelly
Queen Elizabeth Hospital
Gateshead
Tyne and Wear

Carol A. Kemper
Palo Alto Medical Foundation
Mountain View
California

Patrick Kesteven
Department of Haematology
Freeman Hospital
High Heaton
Newcastle upon Tyne

Munther A. Khamashta
Director of Graham Hughes Lupus Research Laboratory
Division of Women's Health
King's College London
London

Yukiko Kimura
Pediatric Rheumatology Division
Joseph M Sanzari Children's Hospital
Hackensack University Medical Center
Hackensack
New Jersey

Stefan Kluzek
Rheumatology Department
Nuffield Orthopaedic Centre
Oxford

Adelheid Korb
Institute of Experimental Musculoskeletal Medicine
University Hospital Munster
Munster
Germany

Andreas Krause
Department of Rheumatology
Immanuel Krankenhaus Berlin
Berlin
Germany

Thomas Krieg
University of Cologne
Cologne
Germany

Anoop Kuttikat
Department for Rheumatology
Addenbrooke's, Cambridge University Hospitals
Cambridge

Helen J. Lachmann
National Amyloidosis Centre
Division of Medicine
UCL Medical School
Royal Free Campus
London

Joanna Ledingham
Department of Rheumatology
Queen Alexandra Hospital
Cosham
Portsmouth

Myles Lewis
Division of Genetics and Molecular Medicine
Kings College London
Guy's Hospital
London

Mark Lillicrap
Department of Rheumatology
Hinchingbrooke Hospital
Huntingdon

Peter E. Lipsky
1545 London Road
Charlottesville
Virginia

Chris Little
Hand & Upper Limb Surgery Unit
Nuffield Orthopaedic Centre
Oxford University Hospitals NHS Trust
Oxford

Mark Little
Trinity Health Kidney Centre
Trinity College Dublin
Tallaght Hospital Dublin

Berenice Lopez
Department of Chemical Pathology
Harrogate District Hospital
Harrogate

Daniel J. Lovell
Cincinnati Children's Hospital Medical Center
Cincinnati
Ohio

Raashid Luqmani
Rheumatology Department
Nuffield Orthopaedic Centre
Oxford

Alex MacGregor
Norwich Medical School
University of East Anglia
Norwich

Peter J. Maddison
Emeritus Professor of Musculoskeletal Medicine
University of Wales, Bangor

Nicola Maffulli
Centre for Sports and Exercise Medicine
Barts and the London School of Medicine and Dentistry
London;

Department of Musculoskeletal Medicine and Surgery,
Salerno University School of Medicine and Surgery,
Salerno, Italy

Bernhard Manger
Department of Medicine III
University Hospital Erlangen
Erlangen
Germany

Tarnya Marshall
Norfolk and Norwich University NHS Foundation Trust
Norwich
Norfolk

Alberto Martini
IRCCS G. Gaslini
Pediatria II, Reumatologia, PRINTO
Genova
Italy

Helena Marzo-Ortega
Leeds Institute of Rheumatic and Musculoskeletal Medicine
University of Leeds and Leeds NIHR Musculoskeletal
Biomedical Research Unit
Leeds Teaching Hospitals NHS Trust
Leeds

Justin Mason
Vascular Sciences
Imperial Centre for Translational and Experimental Medicine
Imperial College London, Hammersmith Hospital
London

Loren A. Matheson
Centre for Practice Changing Research
Children's Hospital of Eastern Ontario
Ottawa, Ontario
Canada

Wilfried Mau
Instituts für Rehabilitationsmedizin
Medizinische Fakultät
Martin-Luther-Universität Halle-Wittenberg
Halle
Germany

Hayley McBain
Centre of Health Services Research
School of Health Sciences
City University London
London

John McBeth
Arthritis Research UK Epidemiology Unit
The Medical School
Manchester

Candy McCabe
Bath Centre for Pain Services
Royal National Hospital for Rheumatic Diseases
Foundation Trust
Upper Borough Walls
Bath

Liza McCann
Alder Hey Children's NHS Foundation Trust
Liverpool

Andrew McCaskie
Trauma and Orthopaedic Surgery
Freeman Hospital
High Heaton
Newcastle upon Tyne

Janet E. McDonagh
Birmingham Children's Hospital NHS Foundation Trust
Birmingham

Dennis McGonagle
Leeds Institute of Rheumatic and Musculoskeletal Medicine
University of Leeds and Leeds NIHR Musculoskeletal
Biomedical Research Unit
Leeds Teaching Hospitals NHS Trust
Leeds
UK

Laura McGregor
Centre for Rheumatic Disease
Glasgow Royal Infirmary
Glasgow

Neil McHugh
Royal National Hospital for Rheumatic Diseases
Upper Borough Walls
Bath

Ian McNab
Hand & Upper Limb Surgery Unit
Nuffield Orthopaedic Centre
Oxford University Hospitals NHS Trust
Oxford

Esperanza Merino
Department of Infectious Diseases
Universidad Miguel Hernandez
Hospital General Universitario de Alicante
Spain

Sonja Merkesdal
Division of Clinical Immunology and Rheumatology
Working Group for Health Economics and
Clinical Epidemiology
Hannover Medical School
Hannover
Germany

Maribel I. Miguel
Human Anatomy and Embryology Unit
Department of Experimental Pathology and Therapeutics
University of Barcelona
L'Hospitalet de Llobregat
Spain

Kirsten Minden
German Rheumatism Research Centre, Berlin
Epidemiology Unit,
Children´s university hospital
Charité-Universitätsmedizin Berlin
Berlin
Germany

Pierre Miossec
Department of Clinical Immunology and Rheumatology
Hôpital Edouard Herriot
University of Lyon
Lyon
France

Anna Mistry
Rheumatology Department
Nuffield Orthopaedic Centre
Oxford

Pia Moinzadeh
Department of Rheumatology
Royal Free Hospital
London

Ingrid Möller
Instituto Poal de Reumatologia
Barcelona
Spain

Ulf Müller-Ladner
Justus-Liebig University Giessen
Kerckhoff Klinik Bad Nauheim
Germany

Joachim Müller-Quernheim
Department of Pneumology
University Medical Centre Freiburg
Freiburg
Germany

Saraswathi Murthy
Department of Infectious Diseases
Division of Medicine, UCL Medical School
Royal Free Campus
London

Stanley J. Naides
Quest Diagnostics Nichols Institute
Immunology
San Juan Capistrano
California

Michel Neidhart
Center of experimental Rheumatology
University Hospital Zurich
Zurich
Switzerland

Elena Neumann
Justus-Liebig University Giessen
Internal Medicine and Rheumatology
Kerckhoff-Klinik GmbH
Bad Nauheim
GERMANY

Stanton Newman
Centre of Health Services Research
School of Health Sciences
City University London
London

Wan-Fai Ng
Musculoskeletal Research Group
Institute of Cellular Medicine
University of Newcastle
Newcastle upon Tyne

Kiran Nistala
Rheumatology Unit
UCL Institute of Child Health
London

Eleana Ntatsaki
Department of Rheumatology
Norfolk and Norwich University Hospital
Norwich

Anne O'Brien
School of Health and Rehabilitation
Keele University
Keele

Janice O'Connell
Sunderland Hospital
Sunderland
Tyne and Wear

Philip J. O'Connor
Department of clinical radiology and Leeds Musculoskeletal
Biomedical Research Unit
Chapel Allerton Hospital
Leeds

Olabambo Ogunbambi
Hull York Medical School
Hull Royal Infirmary
Hull

John K. Olynyk
Department of Gastroenterology
Fremantle Hospital
Fremantle, WA
Australia;

Institute for Immunology & Infectious Diseases
Murdoch University
Murdoch, WA
Australia;

Curtin Health Innovation Research Institute
Curtin University
Bentley, WA
Australia

Cate H. Orteu
Royal Free Hospital
London

Monika Østensen
Department of Rheumatology
Sørlandet Hospital
Kristiansand
Norway

Andrew J. K. Östör
Department of Rheumatology
Cambridge University Hospitals NHS Foundation Tust
Addenbrookes Hospital
Cambridge

Thomas Pap
Institute of Experimental Musculoskeletal Medicine
University Hospital Munster
Munster
Germany

Eliseo Pascual
Department of Rheumatology
Universidad Miguel Hernandez
Hospital General Universitario de Alicante
Spain

Yusuf I. Patel
Hull York Medical School
Hull Royal Infirmary
Hull

Dorothy Pattison
St Mabyn
Cornwall

Harry Petrushkin
Department of Medical and Neuro-Ophthalmology
Medical Eye Unit
St Thomas' Hospital
London

Matthew C. Pickering
Centre for Complement and Inflammation Research
Department of Medicine
Imperial College London
Hammersmith Campus
London

Clarissa Pilkington
Department of Rheumatology
Great Ormond Street Hospital
London

Nicolò Pipitone
Unita di Reumatologia
Ospedale di Reggio Emilia
Reggio Emilia
Italy

Costantino Pitzalis
Centre for Experimental Medicine and Rheumatology
2nd Floor, John Vane Science Centre
William Harvey Research Institute
Barts and the London School of Medicine and Dentistry
Queen Mary University of London
London

Philip Platt
Rheumatology Department
Freeman Hospital
High Heaton
Newcastle-upon-Tyne

Antje Prasse
Department of Pneumology
University Medical Centre Freiburg
Freiburg
Germany

Elizabeth Price
Department of Rheumatology
Great Western Hospitals NHS Foundation Trust
Swindon

Kari Puolakka
Lappeenranta Central Hospital
Lappeenranta
Finland

Helga Radner
Division of Rheumatology
Department of Internal Medicine 3
Medical University Vienna
Vienna
Austria

Stuart H. Ralston
Molecular Medicine Centre
Institute of Genetics and Molecular Medicine
Western General Hospital
Edinburgh

Athimalaipet V. Ramanan
Paediatric Rheumatology
Bristol Royal Hospital for Children
Bristol

Saaeha Rauz
Academic Unit of Ophthalmology
College of Medical and Dental Sciences
University of Birmingham
Birmingham

Angelo Ravelli
Pediatria II, Reumatologia
Istituto G. Gaslini
Genova
Italy

Gerry Rayman
The Diabetes Centre
Ipswich Hospitals NHS Trust
Ipswich

Anthony C. Redmond
Leeds Institute of Rheumatic and Musculoskeletal Medicine
University of Leeds and Leeds NIHR Musculoskeletal
Biomedical Research Unit
Leeds Teaching Hospitals NHS Trust
Leeds

David Rees
Department of Haematological Medicine
King's College London School of Medicine
King's College Hospital NHS Foundation Trust
London

Stefan Rehart
Agaplesion Frankfurter Diakonie Kliniken GmbH
Agaplesion Markus Krankenhaus
Akademisches Lehr-KH der Goethe-Universität
Frankfurt
Germany

David M. Reid
Medical School
University of Aberdeen
Foresterhill
Aberdeen

Luis Requena
Department of Dermatology
Fundación Jiménez Díaz
Madrid
Spain

Graham Riley
School of Biological Sciences
University of East Anglia
Norwich

Mark Roberts
Department of Neurology
Salford Royal Hope Hospital
Salford

Joanna Robson
Rheumatology Department
Nuffield Orthopaedic Centre
Oxford

Edward Roddy
Arthritis Research UK Primary Care Centre
Primary Care Sciences
Keele University
Keele

Gerhard Rogler
Division of Gastroenterology and Hepatology
University Hospital Zurich
Zurich
Switzerland

Emma L. Rowbotham
Radiology Department
Royal United Hospitals
Bath

Martin Rudwaleit
Endokrinologikum Berlin and Charité University Medicine
Berlin
Germany

Guillermo Ruiz-Irastorza
Department of Internal Medicine
Hospital de Cruces
University of the Basque Country
Bilbao
Spain

Nicolino Ruperto
Istituto G. Gaslini
Pediatria II, Reumatologia, PRINTO
Genova
Italy

Sarah Ryan
The Haywood Hospital
Burslem
Stoke on Trent

Alan Salama
UCL Centre for Nephrology
Royal Free Hospital
London

Benazir Saleem
Rheumatology Department
York District Hospital
York

Carlo Salvarani
Unita di Reumatologia
Ospedale di Reggio Emilia
Reggio Emilia
Italy

Hans-Georg Schaible
Department of Physiology
Friedrich-Schiller University of Jena
Jena
Germany

Georg Schett
Department of Internal Medicine 3
University of Erlangen-Nuremburg
Erlangen
Germany

Benjamin E. Schreiber
Rheumatology Department
Royal Free Hampstead NHS Trust
London

David G. I. Scott
Norfolk and Norwich University Hospital NHS Trust
Norwich and Norwich Medical School,
University of East Anglia, Norwich

David L. Scott
Department of Rheumatology
King's College London School of Medicine
Weston Education Centre
London

Michael P. Seed
Medicines Research Group
School of Sport Health and Bioscience
University of East London
London

Emire Seyahi
University Hospital
Cerrahpasa Medical Faculty
University of Istanbul
Aksaray
Istanbul
Turkey

Sanjeev Sharma
Department of Endocrinology and Diabetes
Peterborough and Stamford Hospitals NHS Foundation Trust
Peterborough

Nicholas Shenker
Department for Rheumatology Addenbrooke's, Cambridge
University Hospitals
Cambridge

Joachim Sieper
Department of Rheumatology
Charité—Campus Benjamin Franklin
Berlin
Germany

Tuulikki Sokka
Jyväskylä Central Hospital
Jyväskylä
Finland

Jeremy Sokolove
Internal Medicine and Rheumatology
VA Palo Alto Health Care System
Palo Alto
California

Taunton R. Southwood
Birmingham Children's Hospital
NHS Foundation Trust and the College of Medical
and Dental Sciences
University of Birmingham
Birmingham

Cathy Speed
c/o Cambridge Lea Hospital
Impington
Cambridge

Cornelia M. Spies
Department of Rheumatology and Clinical Immmunology
Charité-Universitätsmedizin Berlin, Campus Mitte
Berlin
Germany

Miles Stanford
Medical Eye Unit
St Thomas's Hospital
London

Andrew Steer
Department of General Medicine
Royal Children's Hospital Melbourne
Parkville, Victoria
Australia

Vibeke Strand
Division of Immunology/Rheumatology
Stanford University School of Medicine
Palo Alto
California

Rainer H. Straub
Department of Internal Medicine 1
University Hospital Regensburg
Regensburg
Germany

Priya Sukhtankar
Wellcome Trust
Southampton General Hospital
Southampton

Cord Sunderkötter
Department of Dermatology
University Hospital of Münster
Münster
Germany

Deborah P. M. Symmons
Centre for Musculoskeletal Research
Institute of Inflammation and Repair
University of Manchester
Manchester

Mark Taylor
Bioengineering Science Research Group
School of Engineering Science
University of Southampton
Highfield
Southampton

Elke Theander
Rheumatology Department
University Hospital Malmö
Lund University
Lund
Sweden

Ranjeny Thomas
UQ Diamantina Institute
Princess Alexandra Hospital
Woolloongabba, Queensland
Australia

Ben Thompson
Freeman Hospital
High Heaton
Newcastle upon Tyne

Paul Thompson
Poole Hospital NHS Foundation Trust
Poole

Wendy Thomson
Arthritis Research UK Epidemiology Unit
Manchester Academic Health Science Centre
The University of Manchester
Manchester

Clare Thornton
Vascular Sciences
Imperial Centre for Translational and Experimental Medicine
Imperial College London, Hammersmith Hospital
London

Linda Troeberg
The Kennedy Institute of Rheumatology
University of Oxford
Oxford

Lori B. Tucker
Division of Rheumatology
Department of Pediatrics
University of British Columbia
Vancouver, BC
Canada

Carl Turesson
Department of Rheumatology
Skåne University Hospital
Malmö
Sweden

Patrick J. Twomey
Clinical Biochemistry
The Ipswich Hospital
Ipswich

Alan Tyndall
Department of Rheumatology
University Hospital Basel
Basel
Switzerland

Neil Upadhyay
Department of Trauma and Orthopaedic Surgery
Bristol Royal Infirmary
Bristol

Ana Valdes
Department of Twin Research
King's College London
London

Sander van Assen
Department of internal medicine, division of infectious diseases
University Medical Center Groningen
Groningen
The Netherlands

Jacob M. van Laar
Musculoskeletal Research Group
Institute of Cellular Medicine
Newcastle University
Newcastle upon Tyne

Piet van Riel
Radboud University Nijmegen Medical Centre
Nijmegen
The Netherlands

Annibale Versari
Unita di Medicina Nucleare
Ospedale di Reggio Emilia
Reggio Emilia
Italy

Tonia L. Vincent
The Kennedy Institute of Rheumatology
University of Oxford

Arjan Vissink
Department of Oral and Maxillofacial Surgery
University of Groningen
University Medical Center Groningen
Groningen
The Netherlands

Reinhard E. Voll
Department of Rheumatology and Clinical Immunology
University of Freiburg
Freiburg
Germany

Tim Vyse
Division of Genetics and Molecular Medicine
Kings College London
Guy's Hospital
London

David Walker
Musculoskeletal Unit
Freeman Hospital
Newcastle upon Tyne

Karen Walker-Bone
MRC Lifecourse Epidemiology Unit
Southampton General Hospital
Tremona Road
Southampton

Peter Wall
Hospital Health Sciences
Warwick Medical School
Clinical Sciences Research Laboratories
Coventry

David A. Walsh
Arthritis Research UK Pain Centre
Academic Rheumatology
University of Nottingham Clinical Sciences Building
City Hospital
Nottingham

Louise Watson
NIHR Academic Clinical Lecturer
Institute of Translational Medicine University of Liverpool

Richard A. Watts
Department of Rheumatology
Ipswich Hospital NHS Trust
Ipswich

Lucy R. Wedderburn
Rheumatology Unit
UCL Institute of Child Health
London

Athol U. Wells
Royal Brompton Hospital
London

Claire Y. J. Wenham
Leeds Institute of Rheumatic and Musculoskeletal Medicine
University of Leeds and Leeds NIHR Musculoskeletal
Biomedical Research Unit
Leeds Teaching Hospitals NHS Trust
Leeds

Sarah Westlake
Rheumatology Department
Poole Hospital NHS Trust
Poole

Ross Wilkie
Arthritis Research UK Primary Care Centre
Primary Care Sciences
Keele University
Keele

Anita Williams
Directorate of Prosthetics, Orthotics and Podiatry
College of Health Science
University of Salford
Salford

Frances M.K. Williams
Department of Twin Research
King's College London
London

Elspeth Wise
Encompass Healthcare
The Galleries Health Centre
Washington
Tyne and Wear

Roger Wolman
Department of Rheumatology and Sport and
Exercise Medicine
Royal National Orthopaedic Hospital
Brockley Hill
Stanmore
Middlesex

B.P. Wordsworth
National Institute for Health Research Oxford Musculoskeletal
Biomedical Research Unit
Nuffield Department of Orthopaedics Rheumatology and
Musculoskeletal Sciences (University of Oxford)
Nuffield Orthopaedic Centre
Oxford

Jane Worthington
Centre for Musculoskeletal Research
Institute for Inflammation and Repair
Faculty of Medical and Human Sciences
University of Manchester
Manchester

Nico Wulffraat
Department of Paediatric Immunology
University Medical Centre Utrecht
Utrecht
The Netherlands

Matthew Wyse
University Hospitals Coventry and Warwickshire University
Hospital
Coventry

Hasan Yazici
University Hospital
Cerrahpasa Medical Faculty
University of Istanbul
Aksaray
Istanbul
Turkey

Kanako Yoshida
Aberdeen Royal Infirmary
Foresterhill
Aberdeen

Sebahattin Yurdakul
University Hospital
Cerrahpasa Medical Faculty
University of Istanbul
Aksaray
Istanbul
Turkey

Imene Zerizer
Department of Nuclear Medicine
The Royal Marsden Hospital
Surrey

Angela Zink
Epidemiology Unit
Deutsches Rheuma-Forschungszentrum
Berlin
Germany

Gernot Zissel
Department of Pneumology
University Medical Centre Freiburg
Freiburg
Germany

Francesco Zulian
Department of Paediatrics
University of Padua
Padua
Italy

Clinical presentations of rheumatic disease in different age groups

CHAPTER 1

The child patient

Lori B. Tucker

Introduction

Musculoskeletal complaints in children are very common, and most are generally inconsequential and self-resolving. However, it is important to differentiate children with minor problems from those who have developed a more serious musculoskeletal problem possibly associated with long-term illness. This is frequently challenging to the clinician, as the differential diagnosis of conditions associated with musculoskeletal complaints is broad and children present special circumstances to consider. The spectrum of childhood rheumatic diseases is shown in Table 1.1. A full discussion of childhood rheumatic diseases is beyond the scope of this chapter; summaries of many of the important diseases are provided in later chapters or other sources.[1]

Table 1.1 The spectrum of childhood rheumatic disease

JIA	
SLE	SLE
	Neonatal LE
Juvenile dermatomyositis	
Scleroderma	Limited or localized: morphea, linear, generalized cutaneous
	Systemic sclerosis
Vasculitides	Kawasaki disease
	Henoch–Schonlein purpura
	Granulomatous polyangiitis
	Takayasu's arteritis
	Polyarteritis nodosa
Granulomatous disease	Sarcoidosis
Acute rheumatic fever	
Autoinflammatory diseases	Periodic fever syndromes
	CRMO

CRMO, chronic recurrent multifocal osteomyelitis; JIA, juvenile idiopathic arthritis; LE, lupus erythematosus; SLE, systemic lupus erythematosus.

Classifications of rheumatic disease in children

The classification of arthritis and other rheumatic diseases in children has posed significant challenges, and until recently, the use of different classification systems for the most common rheumatic condition, arthritis, resulted in inability to compare research around the world.

Classification of childhood arthritis

The classification of childhood arthritis has evolved over the past 10 years since the publication of the International League of Associations for Rheumatology (ILAR) criteria for juvenile idiopathic arthritis (JIA) in 2002.[2] These criteria were developed by an international committee of paediatric rheumatologists, using expert opinion, as well as a consensus process and evidence-based modifications. Before these criteria were developed, children were diagnosed using either the American College of Rheumatology (ACR) criteria for juvenile rheumatoid arthritis[3] or the European League Against Rheumatism (EULAR) criteria for juvenile chronic arthritis;[4] the use of these differing criteria sets led to difficulty in comparing patient cohorts across different countries and publications (Table 1.2).

Table 1.2 Comparison of criteria for chronic arthritis in childhood[2–4]

ILAR criteria (JIA)	ACR criteria (JRA)	EULAR criteria (JCA)
Oligoarthritis	Pauciarticular	Pauciarticular
Persistent		
Extended		
Polyarthritis RF–	Polyarticular	Polyarticular RF–
Polyarthritis RF+		Polyarticular RF+
Systemic arthritis	Systemic	Systemic
Psoriatic arthritis		Psoriatic
Enthesitis-related arthritis		Ankylosing spondylitis
Undefined arthritis		

JCA, juvenile chronic arthritis; JIA, juvenile idiopathic arthritis; JRA, juvenile rheumatoid arthritis; RF, rheumatoid factor.

There is now more widespread adaptation of the ILAR criteria for childhood arthritis worldwide. The overall term juvenile idiopathic arthritis (JIA) is defined as definite arthritis occurring before the 16th birthday, persisting for at least 6 weeks and of unknown cause. There are seven categories of JIA defined by the ILAR criteria (Table 1.3). Of importance, the ILAR criteria include a category of enthesitis-related arthritis (ERA) which encompasses children

Table 1.3 ILAR criteria for the classification of juvenile idiopathic arthritis[2]

Category	Definition	Exclusions
Oligoarthritis	Arthritis in less than 5 joints during the first 6 months of disease Persistent: never more than 4 joints Extended: more than 4 joints after the first 6 months of disease	1, 2, 3, 4, 5
Polyarthritis RF+	Arthritis in 5 or more joints during the first 6 months of disease, with positive RF test (X2)	1, 2, 3, 5
Polyarthritis RF−	Arthritis in 5 or more joints during the first 6 months of disease, with negative RF test	1, 2, 3, 4, 5
Systemic arthritis	Arthritis with fever of >2 weeks' duration, documented to be quotidian for at least 3 days, and accompanied by one or more of: (a) evanescent, non-fixed rash (b) hepatomegaly or splenomegaly (c) serositis (d) generalized lymphadenopathy	1, 2, 3, 4
Psoriatic arthritis	Arthritis and psoriasis, *or* Arthritis with one or more of: (a) dactylitis (b) nail pitting or onycholysis (c) psoriasis in a first degree relative	2, 3, 4, 5
ERA	Arthritis and enthesitis, *or* Arthritis or enthesitis with one or more of: (a) sacroiliac joint tenderness and/or inflammatory lumbosacral spinal pain (b) HLA B27 positivity (c) acute symptomatic uveitis (d) first-degree relative with HLA B27 associated disease (e) onset of arthritis in a boy over the age of 8 years	1, 4, 5
Undefined arthritis	A child with arthritis who meets criteria for more than one category or for no category	

ERA, enthesitis-related arthritis; RF, rheumatoid factor. Exclusions:

1. Psoriasis in the patient or first-degree relative.
2. Arthritis in an HLA B27 positive male with onset after 8 years of age.
3. Anklyosing spondylitis, enthesitis-related arthritis, sacroilitis with inflammatory bowel disease, Reiter's syndrome, or acute anterior uveitis in a first-degree relative.
4. Presence of IgM RF on at least two occasions more than 3 months apart.
5. The presence of systemic JIA.

previously described as having spondyloarthropathy, seronegative enthesitis and arthropathy, and juvenile ankylosing spondylitis. There has been controversy regarding the use of a family history of psoriasis as an exclusion criteria for some subtypes, and some difficulties of classification in the subtypes of psoriatic, ERA, and unclassified JIA.[4]

Classifications of other childhood rheumatic conditions

The only diagnostic criteria which have been developed specifically for classification or diagnosis of childhood rheumatic diseases are those for acute rheumatic fever[5] and for Kawasaki disease.[6] Both of these criteria sets have reasonably high sensitivity but lower specificity. Specifically, strict application of the Kawasaki disease criteria will exclude children who have what is described as 'atypical Kawasaki disease'. These children do not fulfil the published criteria, but are at high risk for development of coronary artery aneurysms and poor outcome.

Criteria for the diagnosis of most other chronic rheumatic diseases of childhood have generally been adopted in whole or part from classification criteria for adults. For example, the classification criteria for systemic lupus erythematosus (SLE)[7,8] and dermatomyositis[9] are used in general practice for the diagnosis of these conditions in children. However, recent work has been done to examine the validity of classification criteria for systemic vasculitides such as Henoch–Schonlein purpura, polyarteritis nodosa, Takayasu arteritis, and granulomatous polyangiitis (formerly known as Wegener's granulomatosis[10]) for children. In 1990, consensus criteria definitions were proposed by a group of expert rheumatologists from the ACR for these vasculitis conditions.[11,12] In 2008, an international paediatric rheumatology consensus conference was convened to validate and finalize paediatric vasculitis diagnostic criteria; using standard consensus formation methodology and patient case data, finalized classification criteria were published which demonstrated high sensitivity and specificity in these exercises.[11,13]

Epidemiology of childhood rheumatic diseases

It is a common misconception that rheumatic diseases are rare in childhood. In fact, chronic arthritis is one of the most common chronic conditions of childhood associated with disability. In addition, a significant percentage of patients with autoimmune diseases such as SLE have developed the onset of disease in childhood. Some rheumatic diseases such as dermatomyositis and localized scleroderma are more frequent in children and adolescents than in adults. Some diseases such as oligoarticular JIA with uveitis, systemic JIA, acute rheumatic fever, Henoch–Schonlein purpura, and Kawasaki disease occur almost exclusively in childhood. Conversely, there are a number of rheumatic diseases that rarely occur in childhood, including gout, calcium pyrophosphate deposition disease, polymyalgia rheumatica, and primary osteoarthritis.

Accurate data demonstrating the incidence and prevalence of childhood arthritis is surprisingly sparse. Much of the data available has come from paediatric rheumatology-based clinic populations or registries, which may result in under-reporting of the true frequency of disease. The most current information suggests that the prevalence of JIA is between 10 and 400 per 100 000 children, depending on geographic location and case definitions.[14] Of interest, a population-based study by Manners and Diepeveen[15] suggests that the prevalence of chronic arthritis in 12-year-old Australian children was actually much higher than expected (400/100 000). Reported incidence of JIA ranges from 1 to 2 per 100 000 children, with most reports coming from clinic-based studies in Europe or North America.[16] A surveillance-based study from Canada done in 2007–2009 found a calculated incidence rate of 4.3 per 100 000 children;[17,18] however this is likely to be an underestimate as cases were reported by paediatricians only.

Accurate frequencies of the other childhood rheumatic diseases, such as SLE, dermatomyositis, scleroderma, and vasculitis, are even more difficult to find. Population-based studies using administrative data have not been done in these populations.

Age and sex distributions of the rheumatic disorders of childhood differ by disease. For example, SLE is more common in girls than in boys, and far more frequent in children over age 10 years. Oligoarticular JIA is more common in girls younger than age 6 years, and ERA more common in boys over age 6 years. However, these 'rules' are not hard and fast, and clinicians need to be aware that rheumatic disease can present in children as young as 1 year of age.

Ethnic variation occurs in some childhood rheumatic diseases. JIA is found around the world, but the distribution of disease subtypes has been reported to differ in different countries. For example, JIA subtype distribution in India is quite different from that in North America.[19,20]

Interaction of growth and development with childhood rheumatic disease

Physical growth

One of the major differences between childhood-onset and adult-onset rheumatic disease is the potential effect of having a chronic inflammatory disease on the normal growth of the affected child. The presence of active inflammation can stunt the linear growth of an affected child. Additionally, treatments used for chronic inflammatory diseases, most notably corticosteroids, have profound negative effects on growth. Careful documentation of the height and weight of a child with rheumatic disease should be made at each medical encounter, and compared to growth curves for healthy children of the same sex and age. It is important to consider the child's genetic background and parental heights in assessing growth rates for an individual child. Serial measurements ensure that growth velocity over time is normal. Growth rates may increase to allow catch-up growth once disease is controlled; for example, a child with poorly controlled JIA may have a growth spurt once disease is controlled using methotrexate. However, some children will have permanent growth stunting from the combination of severe active disease and the requirement for high doses of corticosteroids.

Motor development

Young children who develop a rheumatic disease may have delayed motor development due to their disease. For example, a very young child who develops JIA may not learn to walk or jump at the appropriate times due to pain and inability to move joints normally. Recognition of the range of normal development in young children is essential for interpretation of findings on the physical examination and functional assessment. There is considerable variation in the age at which individual developmental milestones are achieved. The dates in Table 1.4 should be used as a guideline only.

Delay in achieving motor milestones may occur in a child with any chronic disease, but this may be more evident in the child with a disease affecting the musculoskeletal system, the function of which is the basis for the estimation of developmental stages. Although there may be a delay in the chronically ill child, milestones are eventually achieved over time.

Psychosocial development

Chronic illness can have a major impact on the quality of life of the family, as well as the child, throughout their development. A significant number of children with JIA have disability that interferes with full functioning at some times during childhood and adolescence, and children with serious systemic rheumatic conditions such as systemic lupus, vasculitis, or dermatomyositis may have major interference with regular functioning. For children with rheumatic disease, care needs to be family focused, and is best delivered by a multidisciplinary paediatric rheumatology team which often includes social workers and psychologists.

Educational considerations

The school is one of the child's most important environments, and participation in the school environment is a strong influence on healthy development. Attention to school performance, both academic and social, is critical to promoting healthy development. Children with rheumatic disease should be expected to participate fully in school, with modifications if necessary to account for their physical considerations, physician visits, or treatments. An assessment of school attendance, participation, limits and concerns should be a part of every follow-up visit. Direct contact between the medical team and the child's teachers or counsellors is often beneficial in educating school personnel about the child's condition and designing modifications that are appropriate. For example, the use of a laptop computer for taking notes and tests may

Table 1.4 Normal developmental gross motor milestones in children

Age (months)	Milestones achieved by this age
7	Independent sitting
10	Crawling
12	Cruising, walking with one hand held
15	Walking alone, crawling up stairs
18	Running stiffly
24	Running well; walking up and down stairs one step at a time
30	Jumping
36	Walking up stairs alternating feet, rides tricycle
48	Hopping on one foot
60	Standing on one foot; skipping

be important for the child with arthritis involving the hands and wrists. Children with rheumatic disease should be encouraged to participate in physical activity at school, such as physical education, playtime, or sports teams; routine proscription from activity is not helpful for treatment and leads to social isolation and generalized poor conditioning.

As children move into adolescence, the developmental trajectory begins to include issues relating to self-esteem, sexuality, peer relationships, educational and vocational goals, and independence. Having a chronic rheumatic illness offers unique challenges to the adolescent and their parents, and the support and guidance of a knowledgeable subspecialty team is very important through this time. The timing of transition from the paediatric to the adult healthcare setting varies with the patient, family, physician, and healthcare setting. In general, adolescents will be cared for by the paediatric rheumatology team until the time of completion of secondary education, and entering the workforce or post-secondary education. In some settings, transition clinics have been developed to care for youth with rheumatic disease. The goals of these transition programs are to promote youth independence in health care, educate youth about their disease and needs, and prepare them to move to the adult healthcare setting.[21,22]

Sexual maturation

Chronic inflammatory disease can result in a delay in sexual maturation. Complete genital maturity (Tanner 5) may occur before the age of 13 years, but may not occur until age of 18 years.[23] Menarche occurs at an average of 12–13 years in North America and Europe. The onset of menstruation may be delayed in girls with active inflammatory disease; also, menses may become irregular or cease in a girl who has previously had a regular menstrual pattern.

A delay in sexual maturation may be a source of anxiety for adolescents, and often these patients may not be comfortable raising issues of concern regarding sexuality with the medical team, especially in the presence of their parents. It is useful to have some part of the medical visit with the adolescent alone, and the physician or nurse should directly address issues of sexual maturity and functioning at that time, while reassuring the adolescent of the confidentiality of the conversation. Care should be taken to be certain that the adolescent understands the critical aspects of conversations around medications and teratogenicity or impact on fertility. For example, the comment 'You can't get pregnant while taking cyclophosphamide' may be interpreted to mean that the adolescent does not need to use birth control, rather than being extremely careful to avoid pregnancy.

Assessment

History and physical examination

The history and physical examination provide most of the diagnostic information in children with rheumatic diseases; laboratory tests provide little help. The history should be obtained from the child's usual caregiver if possible (parent or other adult), and the child. Even a young child may be able to provide important information relating to the history of their symptoms or the degree of functional difficulty experienced.

Rheumatic diseases are systemic disorders, and therefore a complete physical examination should be performed in every case, during which the child's comfort, modesty, and dignity must be respected. Children should be offered appropriate-size gowns or shorts, and should be given a private space for changing clothes. The approach to the physical examination of the child requires expertise in understanding how to approach children of different ages. Frequently, providing an explanation to the child of what will occur during the examination is helpful, and reassurance that the examination will not continue if it causes pain. In most cases, examination of painful areas should be left to the last. For small children, the examination may begin by observing the child at play or moving around the room. An apprehensive young child may need to have the physical examination performed while sitting on a parent's lap. In most cases, the skilled examiner will be able to perform a complete examination of even the youngest child.

Age-related normal variations in physical examination must be taken into account:

◆ *Position and range of motion:* In full-term newborns, the elbows, knees, and hips do not fully extend. In the young child, or even the adolescent, hyperextension at the knees and elbows is often greater than in years of age. Asymmetry of range at any age should be considered abnormal. Many children have flat feet resulting from the distribution of fat and limited muscle development until the age of 5 or 6 years. In the absence of symptoms, no investigation or treatment is required.

◆ *Muscle strength:* Evaluation of muscle strength in the young child may be difficult due to difficulty in the child's ability to cooperate in the examination of individual muscle groups. A well trained paediatric physiotherapist is often best able to completely assess a child's muscle strength reliably.

◆ *Ambulation:* In order to be able to assess gait in children, it is critical to know the normal developmental trajectory of ambulation (see Table 1.4). Children who develop arthritis during the time they are learning to walk frequently present with a delay in achieving ambulation, regression in motor milestones, or an abnormal ambulation pattern. Specific physiotherapy may be required to correct poor ambulation habits which persist even after active joint disease is well-controlled. A limp (asymmetry of gait) may result from structural asymmetry, pain, muscle weakness, or arthritis. Although it is helpful to differentiate between a painful and a non-painful limp, it is important to note that some children with active arthritis in the lower extremity may not have pain. Some common causes of limp, by age of the child, are listed in Table 1.5.

Diagnosis of childhood rheumatic diseases

The child with musculoskeletal pain

Many children with rheumatic disease will present to the physician with pain; however, it is important to note that not all children with musculoskeletal pain will have a rheumatic disease, and in fact, some children with arthritis and other rheumatic conditions do not have pain. Therefore, the important job of a physician evaluating a child complaining of musculoskeletal pain is to consider the broad differential diagnosis, and use clinical clues and physical examination to come to the appropriate diagnosis.

Localization of pain to the bone, joint, or soft tissues may help in guiding appropriate investigations, particularly in the context of length of time pain has been present, severity of pain, or history of trauma. Very severe pain in the context of an ill child with fever, or

Table 1.5 Common or significant causes of limping according to age[24]

Toddler/preschool
Infection (septic arthritis, osteomyelitis—hip, spine)
Mechanical (trauma and non-accidental injury)
Congenital/developmental problems (e.g. hip dysplasia, talipes)
Neurological disease (e.g. cerebral palsy, hereditary syndromes)
JIA
Malignant disease (e.g. leukaemia, neuroblastoma)
5–10 years
Mechanical (trauma, overuse injuries, sport injuries)
Transient synovitis 'irritable hip'
Legg–Perthes disease
JIA
Tarsal coalition
Complex regional pain syndromes
Malignant disease
10–17 years
Mechanical (trauma, overuse injuries, sport injuries)
Slipped capital femoral epiphysis
JIA
Idiopathic pain syndromes
Osteochonditis dissecans
Tarsal coalition
Complex regional pain syndromes
Malignant disease (leukaemia, lymphoma, primary bone tumour)

JIA, juvenile idiopathic arthritis.

Table 1.6 Pain in children and adolescents

Back pain
Acute trauma
Fracture, dislocation, hematoma
Spondylolysis, spondylolisthesis
Tumour
Benign (osteoid osteoma)
Malignant (sarcoma, metastatic neuroblastoma, leukaemia, lymphoma)
Infection
Discitis
Vertebral osteomyelitis
Osteoporosis
Scheurmann's disease
Diffuse pain syndrome
Pain in the sacroiliac joints
Septic sacroiliitis
Spondyloarthropathy (arthritis)
Pain in the pelvis
Osteomyelitis
Chronic recurrent multifocal osteomyelitis
Tumour (usually osteogenic sarcoma or Ewing's sarcoma)

Table 1.7 Red flags for evaluation of back pain in children and adolescents

Systemic features: fever, night sweat, weight loss
Night pain
Neurologic symptoms or signs
Gait change
Change in bowel or bladder habits
Focal lower extremity muscle weakness
Painful scoliosis

the child who does not allow movement of a joint or limb, should be investigated for fracture, bone or joint infection, or malignancy. Joint pain in a single or multiple joints, more prominent in the mornings, with gradual difficulty in movement, may be more suggestive of arthritis. Pain after sports activities or exacerbated by sport activities may be mechanical or orthopaedic in nature.

Pain in young children may be particularly challenging to assess. Parents may note a child change how they use a limb, and only when an area is stressed or examined carefully will the child complain. Some young children may refuse to use an arm or leg, or regress in motor milestones as a manifestation of musculoskeletal pain. For example, a child who has been walking but stops walking, limps, or holds the foot in an abnormal position may have arthritis or other problems. Young children often localize pain poorly, and the physician must carefully identify the area of discomfort by palpation and observation of the child's behaviour. The child may withdraw the limb or become anxious when the affected area is examined. Some young children are able to use a pain scale utilizing faces to score their pain.

Pain and dysfunction may be a sign of a chronic idiopathic pain syndrome, not a rare condition in adolescents. These adolescents present with either a very localized area of pain and inability to use a limb or a diffuse pain in many areas of the body associated with disability and fatigue. In patients with localized pain syndrome, an arthritis cannot be demonstrated, and often a bone scan may show decreased blood flow to the area; this condition is similar to reflex sympathetic dystrophy and should be

treated aggressively with physiotherapy. Young people with diffuse pain syndrome may have soft tissue tender points similar to those seen in patients with fibromyalgia, as well as fatigue and inability to participate in normal activities. These patients may be challenging to treat, as they require a multidisciplinary team including physiotherapy, occupational therapy, and psychology for treatment.

The child with back pain

Back pain is an uncommon complaint in childhood, particularly in young children, as compared with adults. Persistent complaint of back pain should always be thoroughly investigated, as the underlying cause could be serious and require prompt treatment. When evaluating a child with back pain, one should consider that back pain can be referred from other areas; for example, from the back to the thigh, from the sacroiliac joint to the buttock. Important causes of back pain in children and adolescents are shown in Table 1.6. Red flags which should prompt clinician concern for serious disease are shown in Table 1.7.

The child with monoarticular arthritis

The differential diagnosis of monoarticular arthritis in the child or adolescent is broad. Children with a new presentation of monoarticular arthritis should be evaluated promptly, because potentially serious causes may not present in the 'typical' manner seen in adults. Some of the more common causes of monoarticular arthritis in children are shown in Table 1.8.

The child or adolescent who presents with isolated hip pain often presents a diagnostic challenge from several aspects. First, it is critical to examine all the joints and axial skeleton carefully, with a view to differentiating the hip pain from the possibility of referred pain from other areas. Hip pain as the sole presenting feature of JIA is relatively rare, and therefore the clinician should consider the possible causes of hip pain as listed in Table 1.9.

Chronic asymmetric joint inflammation in the developing child can result in localized growth disturbances. In general, the bones adjacent to an inflamed joint grow more rapidly, and in consequence, the affected digit or limb is longer. If this occurs in a single knee, a measurable inequality of the legs can result. Monitoring for localized growth disturbances is an important part of the assessment

Table 1.8 Monoarticular arthritis in children and adolescents

Acute monoarthritis	Chronic monoarthritis

Infection
   Septic arthritis
   Osteomyelitis
	Infection
	   Osteomyelitis
	   Chronic septic arthritis (i.e. TB)

Trauma: minor, ligament injury, Fracture	JIA
Malignancy	Inflammatory bowel disease
	Orthopaedic: osteochondritis dissecans, loose body
	Synovial chondromatosis
	Pigmented villonodular synovitis
	Osteoid osteoma

JIA, juvenile idiopathic arthritis; TB, tuberculosis.

Table 1.9 Causes of persistent hip pain in children and adolescents

Condition	Age range/considerations
Congenital hip dysplasia	Usually found in infancy but can be missed
Transient synovitis	3–10 years
Legg–Perthes disease	5–10 years; boys>girls
Slipped capital femoral epiphysis	10–15 years; boys>girls
Idiopathic chondrolysis of the hip	10–16 years; girls>boys
Acute chondrolysis of the hip	10–16 years
JIA—ERA	Any age, usually >8 years
Reactive arthritis	Any age
Osteonecrosis	Any age

ERA, enthesitis-related arthritis; JIA, juvenile idiopathic arthritis.

of a child with arthritis, and may indicate need for more aggressive treatment.

The child with muscle weakness

Muscle weakness is common in children with inflammatory musculoskeletal conditions. Some children with JIA may present with apparent muscle weakness as their main symptom, and only a complete physical examination will demonstrate the findings of arthritis. In addition, a number of rheumatic conditions present in childhood or adolescence with weakness; these include juvenile dermatomyositis, mixed connective tissue disease, and SLE.

The evaluation of the child with muscle weakness may be challenging, particularly when the child is young. It may be difficult to do standard manual muscle testing in a young child, because of the child's short attention span or difficulty following instructions. Careful observation of the child at play, the manner in which they get up from sitting or lying or walk in the examination room or hallway, or their ability to stand on tiptoes and heels, or squat, may provide the best information about the child's level of weakness. For example, the child with weakness of trunk and neck muscles, as seen in dermatomyositis, may have to roll over on their side or abdomen to sit from a supine position. The child with weakness of the hip girdle may be unwilling to squat or stand from a squat without showing Gower's sign. Observation of the gait for a wide-based or Trendelenburg sign may suggest weakness of the hip girdle muscles. Assessment of muscle strength should also include a detailed neurological examination. Asymmetric weakness is not likely to result from an inflammatory myositis such as dermatomyositis, or from a primary myopathy. With patience and experience, the physician or physiotherapist can demonstrate muscle weakness by formal testing in the child over 3–4 years of age. The application of a standardized valid muscle scoring scale, the Childhood Myositis Assessment Scale, is helpful in determining the functional level of weakness, and to follow changes over time.

Dermatomyositis is suggested by the presence of symmetrical proximal muscle weakness; the presence of the classical cutaneous changes and elevated serum muscle enzymes will confirm the diagnosis and differentiate it clinically from primary myopathies. Weakness of one limb or muscle may indicate a peripheral neuropathic lesion or inflammation of an adjacent joint or joints. Severe weakness of the hip girdle or thighs can result from inflammatory sacroilitis or greater trochanteric enthesitis.

The child with fever of unknown origin

Determining the cause of fever of unknown origin (FUO) in a child can be challenging, and frequently the assistance of a paediatric rheumatologist is sought. The consultant must first ascertain that the child in fact does have persistent unexplained fever, and then must think broadly across the differential diagnosis. To be certain that there is fever, actual documentation by a medical professional, sometimes in an in-patient setting, may be required. This observation period may be helpful as well to determine the fever pattern, which may give a clue to the ultimate diagnosis.

The most frequent aetiology of FUO is infectious, and overt or occult infection must be sought. A basic work-up including complete blood count, inflammatory markers such as erythrocyte sedimentation rate (ESR) and C-reactive protein (CRP), liver and kidney function testing, chest radiographs, and abdominal ultrasound may be required. Blood, urine, and other bacterial cultures must be performed to rule out occult sepsis or bacterial endocarditis. A technetium bone scan may be indicated. It is also important to consider and exclude malignancy early in the work-up of a child with FUO; this may require a bone marrow biopsy. Fever with weight loss, the presence of erythema nodosum, arthritis or arthralgia, with or without gastrointestinal symptoms, may suggest the possibility of inflammatory bowel disease. In such instances, there may be anaemia, hypoalbuminaemia, and elevation of the ESR. Definitive diagnosis may require endoscopy of the colon or small bowel with biopsies; more recently, MRI of the bowel has been used as a diagnostic test.

Among the rheumatic conditions to be considered in the child with FUO are systemic arthritis, systemic vasculitis, SLE, or autoinflammatory syndromes.

The onset of systemic arthritis may be characterized by fever and rash before the development of joint disease. It is unusual, however, for arthritis to lag more than a few weeks after the onset of the systemic features of the disease; in addition, a diagnosis of systemic JIA in the absence of arthritis should be considered tentative. One should be aware, however, that arthritis may present in somewhat unusual patterns: for example, the child with neck pain and torticollis, fever, and rash may have arthritis in the cervical spine and the diagnosis of systemic JIA. The fever of systemic JIA is specifically quotidian, and the rash is evanescent and macular; the additional presence of systemic inflammatory features of serositis, splenomegaly, anaemia, leucocytosis, and markedly raised ESR are helpful markers of disease.

Children with vasculitis may present with fever and elevated inflammatory markers without objective physical signs. In Takayasu's arteritis, there may be a prolonged phase of disease prior to detection of deficiencies of peripheral pulses, making diagnosis challenging. Kawasaki's disease is usually diagnosed in children early in their fever course (within the first 10 days); however, there may be children in whom this diagnosis is missed. Signs of renal disease, such as hypertension or haematuria, should be sought in children with FUO. In polyarteritis, the presence of painful subcutaneous nodules, characteristically in the calf or sole of the foot, provides the opportunity for excisional biopsy.

Laboratory investigations

The laboratory evaluation of a child with presumed rheumatic disease serves three functions: to provide or exclude evidence of inflammation, to provide diagnostic evidence, and to exclude non-rheumatic diseases.

In screening for evidence of inflammation, the white blood cell count and differential, haemoglobin, platelet count, and ESR or CRP generally suffice. Some clues from this simple battery of tests may be helpful. A low platelet count in the presence of an elevated ESR should prompt consideration of an underlying malignancy. In acute Kawasaki's disease, the platelet count may exceed 10^6; children with very active systemic onset JIA may also have extreme elevations in platelet counts. Decreased serum albumin in a child with arthritis may suggest the possibility of inflammatory bowel disease.

Tests that have diagnostic specificity for rheumatic diseases are few in number. Although anti-nuclear antibody (ANA) is present in many children with a wide variety of rheumatic diseases, it occurs in non-rheumatic disease and healthy children as well.[25] In the context of a child with arthritis or other symptoms strongly suggestive of a rheumatic condition, the antigenic specificity of the ANA should be determined and may be helpful. Antibody to double-stranded DNA or extractable nuclear antigens such as SSA/Ro, SSB/La, and Sm are highly suggestive of a diagnosis of SLE. Antibodies to cardiolipin and other phospholipid antigens can be seen in patients with SLE, but can be found in children with other rheumatic and non-rheumatic conditions as well. Elevated levels of von Willibrand factor antigen often occur in patients with inflammation of blood vessels, such as Takayasu's arteritis, but also are frequently elevated in children with juvenile dermatomyositis when disease is active. Highly elevated serum ferritin can be seen in children with active systemic JIA, and may be a marker of haemophagocytic syndrome, a potentially fatal complication of this disease. Antineutrophil cytoplasmic antibodies (ANCA) are useful markers of vasculitides in children such as granulomatous polyangiitis (formerly called Wegener's granulomatosis), microscropic polyangiitis, and polyarteritis nodosa.

The presence of a rheumatoid factor (RF) in a child with musculoskeletal pain is generally not helpful in making the diagnosis of arthritis. Studies of the sensitivity and specificity of RF in children have shown that it has little value as a diagnostic test.[26]

Some laboratory investigations are useful in excluding rather than diagnosing disease. Normal white blood cell and platelet counts, ESR, and CRP make the possibility of a rheumatic, malignant, or infectious disease less likely. Normal radiographs may be helpful in excluding some conditions; however, recent-onset pathology cannot be excluded. Technetium bone scans can be very useful in this situation, and a normal three-phase bone scan virtually excludes bone or joint disease in a child with undiagnosed musculoskeletal pain.

References

1. Cassidy JT, Petty RE, Laxer RM, Lindsley CB. *Textbook of pediatric rheumatology*, 6th edn. Elsevier Saunders, Philadelphia, PA, 2011.
2. Petty RE, Southwood TR, Manners PJ et al. International League of Associations for Rheumatology classification of juvenile idiopathic arthritis: second revision, Edmonton, 2001. *J Rheumatol* 2004;31(2):390–392.
3. Brewer EJ, Bass J, Baum J et al. Current proposed revision of the JRA criteria. *Arthritis Rheum* 1977;20(Suppl):194–199.
4. Hofer M, Southwood TR. Classification of childhood arthritis. *Best Pract Res Clin Rheumatol* 2002;16(3):379–396.
5. Special Writing Group of the American Heart Association. Guidelines for the diagnosis of rheumatic fever. *JAMA* 1992;268:2069–2073.
6. Yellen ES, Gauvreau K, Takahashi M et al. Performance of 2004 American Heart Association recommendations for treatment of Kawasaki disease. *Pediatrics* 2010;125(2):e234–e241.
7. Hochberg MC. Updating the American College of Rheumatology revised criteria for the classification of systemic lupus erythematosus. *Arthritis Rheum* 1997;40:1725.
8. Tan EM, Cohen AS, Fries JF et al. The 1982 revised criteria for the classification of systemic lupus erythematosus. *Arthritis Rheum* 1982;25:1271–1277.
9. Bohan A, Peter JB. Polymyositis and dermatomyositis. *New Engl J Med* 1975;292:344–347.
10. Falk RJ, Gross WL, Guillevin L et al. Granulomatosis with polyangiitis (Wegener's): an alternative name of Wegener's granulomatosis. *Arthritis Rheum* 2011;63(4):863–864.

11. Ozen S, Pistorio A, Iusan SM et al. EULAR/PRINTO/PRES criteria for Henoch-Schonlein purpura, childhood polyarteritis nodosa, childhood Wegener granulomatosis and childhood Takayasu arteritis: Ankara 2008. Part II: Final Classification criteria. *Ann Rheum Dis* 2010;69:798–806.

12. Hunder GG. Vasculitis: diagnosis and treatment. *Am J Med* 1996;100(suppl A):37–45.

13. Ruperto N, Ozen S, Pistorio A et al. EULAR/PRINTO/PRES criteria for Henoch-Schonlein purpura, childhood polyarteritis nodosa, childhood Wegener granulomatosis and childhood Takayasu arteritis: Ankara 2008. Part I: Overall methodology and clinical characterization. *Ann Rheum Dis* 2010;69:790–797.

14. Manners PJ, Bower C. Worldwide prevalence of juvenile arthritis: why does it vary so much? *J Rheumatol* 2002;29(7):1520–1530.

15. Manners PJ, Diepeveen DA. Prevalence of juvenile chronic arthritis in a population of 12 year old children in urban Australia. *Pediatrics* 1996;98:84–90.

16. Cassidy J, Petty RE. Chronic arthritis in childhood. In: Cassidy J, Petty RE, Laxer R, Lindsley CB (eds) *Textbook of pediatric rheumatology*, 6th edn. Elsevier Saunders, Philadelphia, PA, 2011:211–235.

17. Tucker LB Dancey P, Oen K et al.; Canadian Alliance for Pediatric Rheumatology Investigators. Canadian national surveillance for juvenile idiopathic arthritis. *Arthritis Rheum* 2008;suppl 9.

18. Tucker LB, Dancey P, Huber A, Oen K. Juvenile idiopathic arthritis: final report. Canadian Paediatric Surveillance Program, Annual Report. http://web.www.cps.ca/English/surveillance/CPSP/Studies/2009Results.pdf 2009; 26–29.

19. Chandrasekaran AN, Rajendran CP, Madhavan R. Juvenile rheumatoid arthritis—Madras experience. *Indian J Pediatr* 1996;63:501–510.

20. Seth V, Kabra SK, Semwal OP, Jain Y. Clinico-immunological profile in juvenile rheumatoid arthritis-an Indian experience. *Indian J Pediatr* 1996;63(3):293–300.

21. Tucker LB, Cabral DA. Transition of the adolescent patient with rheumatic disease: issues to consider. *Rheum Dis Clin North Am* 2007;33(3):661–672.

22. Robertson L. When should young people with chronic rheumatic disease move from paediatric to adult-centered care? *Best Pract Res Clin Rheumatol* 2006;20(2):387–397.

23. Marshall B, Tanner JM. Puberty. In: Falkner F, Tanner JM (eds) *Human growth: a comprehensive treatise*, 2nd edn. Plenum, New York, 1986:171–209.

24. Foster H, Tucker LB. Musculoskeletal disorders in children and adolescents. In: Adebajo A (ed) *ABC of rheumatology*, 4th edn.: BMJ Books, London, 2009:98–106.

25. Cabral DA, Petty RE, Fung M, Malleson PN. Persistent anti-nuclear antibodies in children without identifiable inflammatory rheumatic or autoimmune disease. *Pediatrics* 1992;89(441):444.

26. Eichenfield AH, Athreya B, Doughty RA, Cebul RD. Utility of rheumatoid factor in the diagnosis of juvenile rheumatoid arthritis. *Pediatrics* 1986;78:480–484.

CHAPTER 2

Young people and transitional care in rheumatology

Janet E. McDonagh and Helena Gleeson

Introduction

Adolescent rheumatology is increasingly being recognized as a vital bridge between paediatric and adult rheumatology. Advances in neuroscience has revealed ongoing brain development into the mid twenties, further highlighting the need for both paediatric and adult rheumatology professionals to develop adolescent specific expertise. In so doing, we will ensure all young people at this stage of their life course receive developmentally appropriate rheumatology health care irrespective of which setting they are seen in.

Transitional care is an integral part of adolescent rheumatology and has long been recognized as a key quality indicator of health care for young people with childhood onset disease. Despite being listed in guidance documents for many years, the universal implementation and objective evaluation of transitional care remains underdeveloped.[1–4] Furthermore, transitional care should no longer be perceived as a stand-alone process alongside routine rheumatology care but part of the developmentally appropriate care for all young people. The aims of this chapter are to describe the implications of adolescent development on rheumatic disease; present the current evidence base for effective transitional care and highlight the key quality criteria for young person friendly rheumatology health services.

Adolescence and rheumatic conditions

Disease spectrum in adolescent rheumatology

Musculoskeletal symptoms are the third most common presentation of young people to primary care.[5] Adolescence is also the time of onset of many long-term rheumatic conditions including systemic lupus erythematosus (SLE), certain subtypes of juvenile idiopathic arthritis (JIA), and inflammatory bowel-associated arthritis. Other adolescent-onset rheumatic conditions include chronic idiopathic pain syndromes, anterior knee pain syndrome, Scheuermann's, non-specific mechanical back pain, and idiopathic Raynaud's.[6] Greater effects on measures of mental health, health service use, school, work, and home activities have been reported in adolescents with chronic rheumatic conditions compared to individuals without chronic disease or those with other chronic disease.[7]

Outcome of adolescent rheumatic disease into adulthood

In spite of advances in therapy, JIA can continue into adulthood. Approximately a third of adolescents with JIA had an increase in disease activity after transfer to adult care.[8] Only 35% of young people were in remission at mean follow-up of 16.2 years.[9] Skarin et al. reported that 49% of young people with JIA associated uveitis still had active uveitis at 24 years follow-up.[10] Time will tell whether the newer biologics will influence long-term outcomes. The significant burden and cost of JIA in adulthood is recognized in the literature[11] but considering reports of up to 52% loss to follow-up (JIA),[12,13] the true extent of this burden, whether medical, psychosocial, and/or vocational, may not be fully realized.

A shared concern of paediatric and adult rheumatologists is reduced bone mass accrual, leading to osteoporosis and increased risk of fractures.[14–16] French et al. reported adolescent predictors of low bone mineral density in adults with JIA: reduced calcium intake, smoking, functional disability, and lack of participation in sports.[17]

Despite average or above average educational achievement, there are reports of higher levels of unemployment in UK JIA populations[18,19] although studies elsewhere have reported better outcomes, albeit only in early adulthood.[20] One prospective study reported that although young people with a range of chronic conditions were socially successful in adulthood, this was not matched with vocational success compared to their healthy counterparts with lower odds of graduating from college and/or being employed and higher odds of having a lower income and/or being on public assistance.[21]

There are also particular concerns regarding outcome of adolescent-onset disease. For example, adolescent-onset juvenile systemic lupus erythematosus (JSLE) has been reported to have an increased risk of mortality compared to adult SLE.[22] Whether this is related to pubertal changes, adolescent development and/or health care provision is as yet unknown.

Adolescent development

Adolescence is a bio-psycho-social development process (Table 2.1) leading to adult life. Adolescence can be broadly divided into early (10–13 years), mid (14–16 years), and late stages (17–19 years) in keeping with the World Health Organization chronological definition of 10–19 years.[23] An additional phase of 'emerging adulthood' (19–mid twenties) is now also recognized.[24]

Biological development includes sexual maturation, growth, and bone mass accrual. Longitudinal neuroimaging studies demonstrate that the adolescent brain continues to mature into the third decade although empirical evidence linking neurodevelopmental processes and adolescent real-world behaviour remains limited at present.[25]

In contrast to the biological and psychological changes (Table 2.1), which are fairly universal, the social changes of adolescence are culturally determined. In Western cultures, the social 'tasks' of adolescence are concerned with establishing relationships outside the family, achieving independence from parents, and establishing financial (i.e. vocational) independence. Many of these tasks are shifting into the third decade of life and well beyond the usual age criteria of transfer to adult health care, with more young people staying in education before employment and remaining in the parental home for longer.

Impact of chronic rheumatic disease during adolescence

Many of the challenges in the management of rheumatic conditions during adolescence are not unique to rheumatology. Chronic illness and adolescent development have reciprocal effects on each other. A chronic condition may retard adolescent development, producing pubertal and growth delay, delayed social independence, poor body, sexual and self image, and educational and vocational failure. As well as delaying development, a chronic condition can appear to accelerate development. For example, 18–30-year olds with diabetes are more likely to self-classify themselves as adults earlier than their healthy counterparts, with adult self-classification positively related to glycaemic control.[26]

On the other hand, the imperatives of adolescent development (the search for identity and independence, immature abstract thinking, experimentation, etc.) make chronic illness management challenging for young people, their caregivers, and healthcare providers alike. Experimentation can lead to risk behaviours, which have been reported to be more common in adolescents with chronic conditions compared to the general population.[27] such young people have been described as being in a 'double whammy' situation;[28] as well as the risks of such behaviours which face any young person, young people with chronic conditions have additional risks from their condition

Table 2.1 Bio-psycho-social development during adolescence

	Biological	Psychological	Social
Early adolescence	Girls: Breast bud and pubic hair development (Tanner stage II) Initiation of growth spurt Boys: Testicular enlargement, beginning of genital growth (stage II)	Thinking remains concrete but with development of early moral concepts Progression of sexual identity development: Development of sexual orientation, possible homosexual peer interest Reassessment and restructuring of body image in face of rapid growth	Realization of differences from parents Beginning of strong peer identification Early exploratory behaviours (smoking, violence)
Mid adolescence	Girls: Mid to late puberty (stage IV–V) and completion of growth Menarche (stage IV event) Development of female body shape with fat deposition Boys: Mid puberty (stage III–IV) Spermarche and nocturnal emissions Voice breaking Initiation of growth spurt (stage III–IV)	Emergence of abstract thinking although ability to imagine future applies to others rather than self (self seen as 'bullet-proof') Growing verbal abilities; adaptation to increasing educational demands Conventional morality (identification of law with morality) Development of fervently held ideology (religious/political)	Establishment of emotional separation from parents Strong peer group identification Increased health risk behaviours Heterosexual peer interests develop Early vocational plans Development of an educational trajectory; early notions of vocational future
Late adolescence	Boys: Completion of pubertal development (stage V) Continued androgenic effects on muscle bulk and body hair	Complex abstract thinking Post-conventional morality (ability to recognize difference between law and morality) Increased impulse control Further completion of personal identity Further development or rejection of ideology and religion—often fervently	Further separation from parents and development of social autonomy Development of intimate relationships—initially within peer group, then separation of couples from peer group Development of vocational capability, potential

and/or therapy. An awareness of these inter-relationships between adolescent development and the chronic condition is vital for their appropriate management of these young people.

Transitional care in rheumatology

Principles of transition

Transition is most usefully defined, as 'a multi-faceted, active process that attends to the medical, psychosocial and educational/vocational needs of adolescents as they move from child to adult centred care'.[29]

The aims of transition are to:

♦ provide high quality, coordinated, uninterrupted health care that is patient-centred, age and developmentally appropriate, culturally competent, flexible, responsive and comprehensive with respect to all persons involved

♦ promote skills in communication, decision-making, assertiveness and self-care, self-determination and self-advocacy

♦ enhance the young person's sense of control and interdependence

♦ provide support for the parent(s)/guardian(s) of the young person during this process

♦ maximize lifelong functioning and potential.[30]

It is important to acknowledge that transition is a process, whereas transfer is only one event within the much longer process of transition. Timing of events within transition (including transfer) will depend on many variables and must be individualized to the young person concerned (Box 2.1).

Evidence base for transitional care

The evidence base for transitional care has evolved significantly since the last edition of this textbook.[1,31,32] A multicentre study involving 10 UK paediatric rheumatology centres was the first objective evaluation of an evidence-based transitional care programme in any chronic illness.[33] In this study, significant short-term improvements were reported in health-related quality of life, patient and parent satisfaction, disease knowledge,

vocational readiness, and documentation of adolescent health issues.[33,34]

The content of the rheumatology programme cited in the previous paragraph has since been further validated by subsequent research elsewhere.[31,32] Lugasi et al. reported that the following aspects determined successful transition:

♦ the meaning given to transition by patients

♦ their expectations about transition and adult care

♦ their level of knowledge and skills

♦ transition planning and environment.[31]

In a systematic review, the most commonly used strategies in successful programmes were reported to be (1) patient education and skills training and (2) specific clinics such as combined paediatric and adult clinics and/or dedicated young adult clinics within adult services.[32]

Key elements of a transitional care programme in rheumatology

In spite of the advances in research and publication of national standards for transition,[4,35,36] implementation in clinical practice is not yet universal.[4,37] Various models for transition have been reported,[32,38] including a young adult clinic[32,39,40] which particularly addresses the developmental needs of late adolescence and emerging adulthood.[39] Irrespective of which model is employed, there are key elements common to all (Box 2.2).

Intrinsic to effective transitional care is planning, which should actively involve the young person and their parents and start ideally by early adolescence at the latest.[2,4,33,35,37] Lack of planning has been reported as a major reason for failure of successful transition.[41] The unpredictability of many chronic illnesses can further

---

Box 2.1 Factors to consider in the timing of transition and transfer

♦ Chronological age

♦ Physical maturity

♦ Cognitive maturity

♦ Current medical status

♦ Adherence to therapy

♦ Independence in healthcare

♦ Preparation

♦ Readiness of the young person

♦ Readiness of the parent/caregiver

♦ Availability of an appropriate adult rheumatologist

♦ Readiness of adult rheumatology service

♦ Adolescent expertise within adult rheumatology team

Box 2.2 Key elements of a transitional care programme in rheumatology

♦ Written transition policy agreed by all members of the multidisciplinary team and target adult rheumatology services

♦ Individualized patient-centred planning

♦ A preparation period and education programme, involving knowledge and skills training for patient and parents, starting in early adolescence

♦ Informational resources of transition process and of the adult service

♦ Flexible policy on timing of events

♦ Network of relevant local agencies

♦ Primary health care and social care involvement

♦ Interested and capable adult services

♦ Liaison personnel in paediatric and/or adult teams

♦ Key person identified for each individual patient

♦ Staff training in transitional care and core principles of adolescent health care

♦ Administrative support

accentuate the negative effects of deficient planning. If transition is 'forced' at a time when the young person is ill prepared, their perceived lack of control and choices is further accentuated.

The role of a transition coordinator is well established in the literature,[42] and their potential in determining successful transition is highlighted in a systematic review.[32] In the rheumatology multicentre study ,the local coordinator role was considered better than paper-based resources by the adolescents themselves.[43] A key role for such personnel is that of bridging the gap between the paediatric and adult service, both for the patient and for the multidisciplinary teams. Their other major role is preparing the young person and their family for the many differences between paediatric and adult care.[44]

Effective links with local adult rheumatologists are vital.[44] In several studies of different chronic diseases, including JIA, young people have reported a preference for meeting adult doctors prior to transfer,[45–47] which in turn is associated with positive outcomes.[47]

Adequate administrative support for transitional care must not be underestimated, facilitating effective communication between all the many professionals involved. Young people and their parents have expressed specific fears regarding the actual transfer of information to adult services.[46] A medical summary was considered to one of the top five aspects of transition, according to adult gastroenterologists.[48] In view of the concerns regarding lapse of care at transfer,[13,14] a mechanism to track young people into adult care is a further aspect of administrative support but not yet universally available.[49,50]

Parents of young people with chronic rheumatic conditions

One of the basic tenets of transitional care is that it is inclusive of the family. Parental issues have been reported to be significant during transition,[46,51,52] including some reports that transition is more difficult for parents than for the young people themselves.[51]

Parents can be helped to encourage involvement of their son/daughter in decision-making from early age, to ensure attainment of functional living skills and development of autonomy and self-advocacy skills similar to their peers. A shared leadership approach should be encouraged with the parent moving from providing all the care in early childhood, to managing it with the young person participating during late childhood and, as their son/daughter becomes competent, for the parent to take the role of supervisor as the young person takes over the management, eventually becoming their own supervisor with the parental role evolving into that of consultant.[53]

Knowledge and skills for young people

Knowledge and skills were one of five factors associated with successful transition in a metasummary of the qualitative research literature.[31] Stinson et al. reported that young people with JIA describe a desire to acquire appropriate knowledge and skills to manage their disease including listening to and challenging care providers, communicating with doctors, pain management and managing emotions.[54] The wide range of skills required of a young person to take over the care of their condition is detailed in Box 2.3.

Knowledge deficits, inaccuracies, and misunderstandings have been reported in young people with JIA[55] as in many other conditions.[56–58] Berry et al. also reported that adolescents with JIA were still at the concrete operational stage of cognitive development rather than the more adult abstract stage,[55] a factor which

---

Box 2.3 Key skills to address in adolescent rheumatology clinics

Health

- Seeing health professionals independent of their parents
- Effective health information-seeking behaviours, including cybersafety issues
- Accessing healthcare independently, including booking own appointments, contacting medical team for advice, refilling prescriptions, registering with a new doctor, etc.
- Awareness of own health: recognition of a flare, taking temperatures
- Self-management of their condition
- Adherence to therapy, appointments
- Pain management skills, including procedural pain management
- Fatigue management skills, including pacing
- Emergency strategies
- Practical skills, e.g. urine/blood testing

Psychosocial

- Independent living skills:
  - Chores
  - Meal preparation
  - Self-care
  - Mobility, including travel away from home
  - Driving
  - Hobbies and leisure activities
- Peer support, including independent social life
- Social competencies

Education/vocational

- Communication skills
- Work experience
- Part-time job
- Disclosure of condition to others including teachers, employers

---

must be considered by professionals providing disease education. Young people have also expressed the wish that there should be no gate-keeping of information.[46] In a study of young people with congenital heart disease, Clarizia et al. reported a positive impact of knowledge acquisition during transition, with more knowledgeable young people being more likely to independently respond to the health professional's questions and more likely to understand implications of transition.[59] Multiple methods for health literacy education need to be developed,[46,60] and technologies including the internet and SMS text messaging have great potential in this area.[61–64]

Skills training in addition to health literacy is also core to transition. Independent visits and self-medication practices were reported as baseline predictors of improvement in health-related quality of life after 6 months and 12 months respectively of participation in a transitional care programme.[34] Similarly, in a larger study including young people with JIA, independence during consultations was identified as an important predictor of transition readiness.[65]

A core skill for any individual with a long-term health condition is adherence. Data shows that in JIA populations adherence to medication and physiotherapy varies from 55–95% and 46–86% respectively.[66]

In any discussion regarding adherence, it is important to reflect on what young people with rheumatic conditions face day-to-day. They often have long-term therapeutic regimens which require regular monitoring. The benefit of therapy is not immediately apparent and they have to continue therapy even when they feel well. All of these factors potentially lead to restrictions on leisure time, spontaneity and peer interactions. Non-adherent behaviour may be the only control mechanism open to the young person and be a simple wish to be heard and to take an active role in the decision-making process.

Addressing adherence in the clinic setting should never be about identifying 'poor' adherence. The most important strategy is to decriminalize non-adherence and giving the young person opportunity to disclose difficulties that they are experiencing. 'When was the last time you forgot to take …' Is a much more effective question than 'Do you remember to take …. every day?'. Adherence is multifactorial and assessed as such in terms of health beliefs, previous experiences (first- or second-hand), disease duration, reality factors in terms of inter-relationships with the rheumatology team members, maturity, etc.[66] One of the common misunderstandings in dealing with non-adherence is that explanation about the rationale of therapy will suffice. Demonstrating how the young person can become an active partner in self-management is imperative. Finally, the quality of the relationship between the health professional and the young person—the therapeutic alliance—is an important, yet often underestimated, determinant of adherence.

New technologies offer potential for addressing self-management needs in a youth friendly manner. Several such programmes have already been reported in the rheumatology literature, e.g. Teens Taking Charge: Managing Arthritis Online,[61] Rheumtogrow. org.[62] Other generic tools are similarly useful, such as 'My Health Passport'.[66] There however remain many unanswered questions regarding the efficacy of such interventions.[64]

Adolescent healthcare in transitional care programmes

Developmentally appropriate communication skills, verbal and nonverbal, are integral to adolescent health.[67] Adolescents are reported to be worse at reading facial expressions and body language, than children or adults.[68] Clinical encounters with adolescents are opportunities to nurture their communication, negotiation, problem solving, decision-making, information-seeking, and disclosure skills.

Motivational interviewing techniques are ideal for use with adolescents as they address resistance and/or ambivalence as well as emphasizing self-responsibility in changing or modifying one's behaviour.[69] Brief intervention strategies are useful in time constrained clinics. The 5As of brief intervention strategies are Ask, Assess, Advise, Assist, and Arrange.[70] However, in a study of

rheumatology professionals, 45% did not assess the young person's understanding of units of alcohol when discussing the risks of alcohol and methotrexate use.[71] In a study of paediatricians, only 44% assessed the adolescent's readiness to quit and only 16% assisted them in quit strategies.[70] Very low or low perceived skill in addressing sexual health, drugs, smoking, and alcohol issues was reported by 27%, 45%, 18%, and 18% respectively of rheumatology professionals.[72]

Barriers to appropriate counselling amongst adolescents with JIA have been described and include availability of time, discomfort, and ambivalence of the rheumatologist and the perceived lack of applicability.[73] The importance of the act of simply asking the right questions should not be underestimated, even when the young person is reluctant to answer. Brown et al. reported that if consultations included discussion of a sensitive health topic, young people involved were more likely to have a positive perception of the provider, have their worries eased, be allowed to make decisions, and report taking responsibility for treatment.[74]

Specific needs of young people with rheumatic disease and a learning disability should also be acknowledged and addressed.[75] Although the developmental milestones are likely to be delayed, assessment during adolescence remains important in order to ensure they meet their full potential. A proactive, anticipatory approach to adolescents with or without learning disabilities is required. Psychosocial screening tools such as HEADSS (see Table 2.2) are useful in this regard: as well as acting as a risk assessment for behaviours, they also assist in engaging the young person, identify protective and resilient factors, and provide information useful in future interventions and management.[76] They can be readily integrated into adolescent rheumatology consultations.[21,33,34,46,69,70,71,73,77–92]

Key criteria for young person friendly rheumatology services

Adolescent rheumatology services should provide age and developmentally appropriate health care for young people with rheumatic conditions.[93] In the UK, the 'You're Welcome' quality criteria for services friendly to young people have been developed and endorsed by the World Health Organization (Box 2.4).[94] The task now is that of implementation. Criteria not previously discussed in this chapter will now be considered.

Accessibility

Young people are in effect 'new users' of rheumatology services that were previously accessed on their behalf by their parents. It is important that young people have the confidence and skills to see professionals independently if they so choose. Only 21% of young people were seen independently of their parents by doctors in rheumatology clinics,[95] although young people report valuing such opportunities.[46] Such opportunities were considered best practice and feasible in most UK hospitals by rheumatology professionals, young people, and their parents.[96] Furthermore, such autonomy has been reported to be the key determinant of attendance at the first adult cardiology clinic appointment,[97] and associated with improved health-related quality of life in adolescents with JIA.[33] In a large study of 954 adolescents with chronic conditions, 48% of total variance in transition readiness was explained by their perceived self-efficacy in skills for independent hospital visits and

Table 2.2 Adolescent HEADS for adolescent rheumatology clinics

		Evidence of importance to adolescent rheumatology	Strategies for use in adolescent rheumatology clinics
H	Home	Early incorporation of a child with disabilities into household chores is key for fostering competence and responsibility[77]	Ask questions regarding home life, e.g: – who they live with – who they talk to about what – what they do to help around the home
E	Education	School absence is reported to predict health-related quality of life in JIA[78] Although social success is now being reported in young people with long-term conditions, vocational success is still concerning[21] Improved vocational readiness with transitional care programmes[33]	Address information needs of teachers, particularly head of year and physical education Explore the impact of a long-term condition in specific areas with respect to the school day: – education – environmental considerations – medical needs and – activities of daily living[79] Assessment particularly important at transfer from junior to high school and from high school to further education or employment. Assess vocational readiness in terms of – educational achievement – prior work experience – knowledge of resources – psychological aspects including self-esteem – expectations of the young person, their family, their teachers
E	Exercise	Inactivity in young people with rheumatic disease can lead to – deconditioning – disability – decreased bone mass – reduced quality of life – increased mortality in adulthood[80,81]	Normalize exercise regimes into typical day, e.g. weekly visit to local gym with peers rather than the physiotherapy department Consider less traditional exercise opportunities, e.g. dance, martial arts
A	Activities and peers	Factors which disrupt peer support networks[46,82,83] include Intrinsic: – pain, fatigue – poor self-esteem, reduced self-confidence, impaired body image – limited knowledge and/or inaccurate beliefs about their condition Extrinsic: – hospitalization and clinic appointments – overprotection by family members, bullying – limited transport	Explore interests, hobbies and leisure activities with young person—important considerations when planning management regimens and interventions in order to ensure adherence Ask about friends, both in and out of school Enquire about teasing and/or bullying, particularly with young people with visible impairments or growth restriction[84] Ask about participation in extracurricular activities at school, particularly trips away—excellent opportunities to foster independent skills including self-medication Ask about use of public transport and/or driving—key skills to support an independent social life
D	Drugs	Neglected area in adolescent rheumatology clinics[34,71,73,85] Reported association of substance misuse with non-adherence[86] Smoking is specifically important for young people with lung disease, Raynaud's, SLE, vasculitides or on long-term steroid therapy[85,87]	Ideally young person should be seen independently of parents for such discussions with appropriate assurances of confidentiality to facilitate disclosure Ask whether friends are using substances in order to assess risk, even if young person denies substance use Consider the use of brief intervention, motivational interviewing, and harm reduction strategies[69,70]

(continued)

Table 2.2 (Continued)

		Evidence of importance to adolescent rheumatology	Strategies for use in adolescent rheumatology clinics
S	Sexual health	Many young people are sexually active before transfer to adult rheumatology care[88]	Ideally young person should be seen independently of parents for such discussions with appropriate assurances of confidentiality to facilitate disclosure.
			Use of gender-neutral language should always be advocated[89] and cultural and religious beliefs respected.
			Discussions regarding potential teratogenicity of disease-modifying drugs should emphasize protection against sexually transmitted infections as well as avoidance of pregnancy
S	Suicide and emotional well-being	Frustration and depression were rated by adolescents with JIA as their biggest psychological problems[90]	Useful questions include:
			How do you feel in yourself at the moment on a scale of 1 to 10?
			What sort of things do you do if you are feeling sad/angry/hurt?
			Is there anyone you can talk to? Do you feel this way often?
S	Sleep	Sleep disturbance and fatigue are prevalent among young people with rheumatic diseases[91]	Enquire about sleep routine
S	Safety	Young people with disabilities who engage in risky behaviours experience are at increased risk for medically attended injury[92]	Assess safety strategies, e.g. around substance use, sexual health, internet use

---

Box 2.4 'You're Welcome' quality criteria for youth-friendly health services[108]

- Accessibility
- Publicity
- Confidentiality and consent
- The environment
- Effective interdisciplinary and interagency working
- Health issues for adolescents
- Sexual and reproductive health services
- Mental health services
- Staff training, skills, attitudes and values
- Monitoring and evaluation and involvement of young people

independence during consultations, their attitude towards transition, and their involvement in discussions about transition.[65]

Accessibility issues have important implications for all members of the multidisciplinary team. This includes secretarial and reception staff who are frequently the first point of contact. Accessing advice from the rheumatology team using forms of communication familiar to this age group, including text messaging and email, can also help foster healthcare utilization skill development.[98]

An important aspect of accessibility is timing of clinics. Late afternoon and early evening clinics enable young people to avoid missing school, college, or the first year in their first ever job. Drop-in clinics are another solution to facilitate open access for times of relapse and/or concern.

Publicity

Information regarding the rheumatology service is important to provide in formats suitable for young people as well as for parents. The opportunity to be seen and to access the service independently of parents should be detailed for a young person before their first visit to the service and reiterated the first time they visit the clinic.

The first encounter with the rheumatology service may be the letter informing the patient of their first appointment. However, often this letter is addressed to the parents and fails to include the young person as an addressee—a missed opportunity for respect and engagement of the young person. The copying of clinic letters for young people can help engagement and facilitate disease education and self-management skills training. The implications of sending copies of clinic letters direct to young people need to be carefully considered, however, with particular reference to confidentiality and comprehension.

Confidentiality

Confidentiality is an important attribute of any adolescent-friendly practice.[93,94] Confidentiality, including its limits, needs to be routinely explained to every young person (and their parents). Posters detailing the policy should be clear in the waiting room and included in the service's informational resources.

Clinic environment

Adolescent-focused clinics, wards, and waiting areas have been called for by young people in rheumatology who report finding paediatric environments 'patronizing', adult environments 'distressing', and both isolating.[46] Dedicated adolescent environments were one of three components of transitional care considered to be best practice but feasible in only a few UK centres.[96]

Waiting times are a concern of patients of all ages. Prolonged waiting can be perceived as a lack of respect, and also increases anxiety and boredom.[46] Ensuring there are age-appropriate activities within the waiting area can deflect some of these negative feelings. The waiting area is an opportunity for peer support activities, and is optimized if there is a separate waiting area for young people distinct from their parents and younger children.

Staff training, skills, attitudes, and values

Lack of training in transitional care and/or adolescent health has been reported as a major barrier for service delivery by several authors.[99–101] In a national survey, 43% of rheumatology professionals reported unmet training needs.[99] Rheumatology professionals knowledgeable in transitional care were considered best practice but only feasible in a few hospitals in a UK Delphi study.[96] Provider characteristics were more important determinants of adolescent satisfaction with transitional care in rheumatology than process and/or environmental characteristics.[102]

There is evidence that training in adolescent health is beneficial. Sustainable, improvements in knowledge, skill, and self-perceived competency were reported in a randomized controlled trial,[103] and in rheumatology, screening for risk behaviours improved with training.[73]

Transitional care is an excellent model to use in problem-based learning to highlight such aspects of health care as triadic consultations, cross-boundary and multidisciplinary working, ethics of consent and confidentiality, or holistic care. There are online resources to support teachers (www.euteach.com) and online transition modules which can be accessed individually or used in small group work (www.e-lfh.org.uk).

Joined-up working

Adolescent rheumatology and transitional care is multidisciplinary. In a UK-based Delphi study, consultant rheumatologists (paediatric and adult) considered delivery of transitional care by a multidisciplinary team as less feasible than their allied health professional counterparts, reflecting the challenges of commissioning such services currently.[96]

Adolescent rheumatology clinics require a minimum of two trained health professionals to facilitate concurrent visits for parents and young person in addition to chaperone availability. Continuity of these professionals is of importance both to young people[46,104,105] and to their parents[46] in the building of a therapeutic alliance, vital for confidentiality and engagement.

An integral aspect of joined-up working is effective communication, including written communication. Unfortunately, in a national audit of case notes of recently transferred young people to adult care, there was limited documentation of key transitional care issues. Documentation significantly improved following centre participation in a transitional care research project.[34] Effective communication with other teams such as ophthalmology, orthopaedic surgery, nephrology, and primary care, is important to ensure coordination. Poor intra-agency and interagency coordination was reported by rheumatology professionals in a UK survey of transitional care needs for young people with JIA.[99]

Monitoring and evaluation and involvement of young people

Research has identified differences between the views of young people and the adults close to them, suggesting that adults cannot be used as proxies.[105] Actively involving young people in decision-making promotes citizenship and social inclusion, important for the health of the community. Moreover, strategies for enhancing participation will develop self-esteem and personal development. Guidance on strategies that rheumatology teams can use to involve young people in service delivery, development, evaluation, and research is now available.[106]

Conclusion

Adolescent rheumatology and transitional care have come far since the last edition of this textbook. On reflection, perhaps identifying transitional care as a defined entity was a mistake and it is now time to redefine it as an integral component of the wider concept of adolescent rheumatology. Once we consider the interdependence of adolescent medicine, chronic disease self-management, and the structure of rheumatology service provision and training, we will have a real chance of getting transitional care right.[107] There is now a growing evidence base to support further development of adolescent rheumatology. However in these times of financial restraint, developments will also require professionals to be as imaginative and creative as the young people in their care and to start looking beyond the limits of rheumatology to areas of potential sharing in adolescent health, both interspecialty and interagency. They are, after all, young people first and foremost who happen to be living in the 21st century with a chronic condition. As one young person in the original rheumatology research states 'It's not about arthritis, it's about living with it'.[46]

References

1. McDonagh JE, Kelly D. The challenges and opportunities for transitional care research. *Pediatr Transplant* 2010;14(6):688–700.
2. Gleeson H, Turner G. Transition to adult services. *Arch Disc Child Pract Ed* 2012;97(3):86–92.
3. Department of Health. *Getting it right for children and young people: overcoming cultural barriers in the NHS so as to meet their needs*. Department of Health Publications, London, 2010 (www.dh.gov.uk last accessed 4 November 2011)
4. American Academy of Pediatrics, American Academy of Family Physicians, and American College of Physicians, Transitions Clinical Report Authoring Group. Supporting the health care transition from adolescence to adulthood in the medical home. *Pediatrics* 2011;128(1):182–200.
5. Haller DM, Sanci LA, Patton GC, Sawyer SM. Toward youth friendly services: a survey of young people in primary care. *J Gen Intern Med* 2007;22(6):775–781.
6. Cassidy JT, Petty RE, Laxer R, Lindsley C. *Textbook of pediatric rheumatology*;6th edn. Elsevier Saunders, Philadelphia. PA, 2011.
7. Adam V, St-Pierre Y, Fautrel B et al. What is the impact of adolescent arthritis and rheumatism? Evidence from a national sample of Canadians. *J Rheumatol* 2005;32(2):354–361.
8. Hersh AO, Pang S, Curran ML, Milojevic DS, von Scheven E. The challenges of transferring chronic illness patients to adult care: reflections from pediatric and adult rheumatology at a US academic center. *Pediatr Rheumatol Online J* 2009;7:13.

9. Arkela-Kautiainen M, Haapasaari J, Kautiainen H et al. Functioning and preferences for improvement of health among patients with juvenile idiopathic arthritis in early adulthood using the WHO ICF model. *J Rheumatol* 2006;33(7):1369–1376.

10. Skarin A, Elborgh R, Edlund E, Bengtsson-Stigmar E. Long-term follow-up of patients with uveitis associated with juvenile idiopathic arthritis: a cohort study. *Ocul Immunol Inflamm* 2009;17(2):104–108.

11. Minden K, Niewerth M, Listing J et al. Burden and cost of illness in patients with juvenile idiopathic arthritis. *Ann Rheum Dis* 2004;63:836–842.

12. Hazel E, Zhang X, Duffy CM, Campillo S. High rates of unsuccessful transfer to adult care among young adults with juvenile idiopathic arthritis. *Pediatr Rheumatol Online J* 2010; 8(2) (www.ped-rheum.com/content/8/1/2 last accessed 4 November 2011)

13. Hilderson D, Corstjens F, Moons P, Wouters C, Rene W. Adolescents with juvenile idiopathic arthritis: who cares after the age of 16? *Clin Exp Rheumatol* 2010;28(5):790–797.

14. Stagi S, Masi L, Capannini S et al. Cross-sectional and longitudinal evaluation of bone mass in children and young adults with juvenile idiopathic arthritis: the role of bone mass determinants in a large cohort of patients. *J Rheumatol* 2010;37(9):1935–1943.

15. Thornton J, Pye SR, O'Neill TW et al. Bone health in adult men and women with a history of juvenile idiopathic arthritis. *J Rheumatol* 2011;38(8):1689–1693.

16. Toiviainen-Salo S, Markula-Patjas K, Kerttula L et al. The thoracic and lumbar spine in severe juvenile idiopathic arthritis: magnetic resonance imaging analysis in 50 children. *J Pediatr* 2012;160(1):140–146.

17. French AR, Mason T, Nelson AM et al. Osteopenia in adults with a history of juvenile rheumatoid arthritis. A population based study. *J Rheumatol* 2002;29(5):1065–1070.

18. Foster HE, Marshall N, Myers A, Dunkley P, Griffiths ID. Outcome in adults with juvenile idiopathic arthritis. *Arthritis Rheum* 2003;48:767–775.

19. Packham JC, Hall MA. Long-term follow-up of 246 adults with juvenile idiopathic arthritis: education and employment. *Rheumatology* (Oxford) 2002; 41:1436–1439.

20. Gerhardt CA, McGoron KD, Vannatta K et al. Educational and occupational outcomes among young adults with juvenile idiopathic arthritis. *Arthritis Rheum* 2008;59(10):1385–1391.

21. Maslow GR, Haydon A, McRee AL, Ford CA, Halpern CT. Growing up with a chronic illness: social success, educational/vocational distress. *J Adolesc Health* 2011;49(2):206–212.

22. Tucker LB, Uribe AG, Fernandez M et al. Adolescent onset of lupus results in more aggressive disease and worse outcomes: results of a nested case-control study within LUMINA, a multiethnic US cohort (LUMINA LVII) *Lupus* 2008;17:314–322.

23. WHO. *The health of young people.* World Health Organization, Geneva, 1993.

24. Arnett JJ. Emerging adulthood: a theory of development from the late teens through the twenties. *Am Psychol* 2000;55:469–480.

25. Steinberg L. A behavioral scientist looks at the science of adolescent brain development. *Brain Cogn* 2010;72(1):160–164.

26. Luyckx K, Moons P, Weets I. Self-classification as an adult in patients with type 1 diabetes: Relationships with glycemic control and illness coping. *Patient Educ Couns* 2011;85(2):245–250.

27. Suris JC, Michaud PA, Akre C, Sawyer SM. Health risk behaviors in adolescents with chronic conditions. *Paediatrics* 2008;122:e1113–e1118.

28. Sawyer SM, Drew S, Yeo MS, Britto MT. Adolescents with a chronic condition: challenges living, challenges treating. *Lancet* 2007;369:1481–1489.

29. Blum RW. Garell D, Hodgman CH et al. Transition from child-centred to adult health-care systems for adolescents with chronic conditions. A position paper of the Society for Adolescent Medicine. *J Adolesc Health* 1993;14(7):570–576.

30. McDonagh JE. Young people first—JIA second. *Arthritis Care Res* 2008;59:1162–1170.

31. Lugasi T, Achille M, Stevenson M. Patients' perspective on factors that facilitate transition from child-centred to adult-centred health care: a theory integrated metasummary of quantitative and qualitative studies. *J Adolesc Health* 2011;48:429–440.

32. Crowley R, Wolfe I, Lock K, McKee M. Improving the transition between paediatric and adult healthcare: a systematic review. *Arch Dis Child* 2011;96(6):548–553.

33. McDonagh JE, Southwood TR, Shaw KL. The impact of a coordinated transitional care programme on adolescents with juvenile idiopathic arthritis. *Rheumatology* 2007;46(1):161–168.

34. Robertson LP, McDonagh JE, Southwood TR, Shaw KL. Growing up and moving on. A multicentre UK audit of the transfer of adolescents with juvenile idiopathic arthritis (JIA) from paediatric to adult centred care. *Ann Rheum Dis* 2006;65:74–80.

35. Department of Health. *Transition: getting it right for young people. Improving the transition of young people with long-term conditions from children's to adult health services.* Department of Health Publications, London, 2006.

36. Canadian Paediatric Society. Transition to adult care for youth with special health care needs. *Paediatr Child Health* 2007;12(9):785–788.

37. Scal P, Horvath K, Garwick A. Preparing for adulthood: healthcare transition counselling for youth with arthritis. *Arthritis Rheum* 2009;30:52–57.

38. While A, Forbes A, Ullman R et al. Good practices that address continuity during transition from child to adult care: syntheses of the evidence. *Child Care Health Dev* 2004;30(5):439–452.

39. Jordan A, McDonagh JE. Recognition of emerging adulthood in UK rheumatology: the case for young adult rheumatology service developments. *Rheumatology* 2007;46(2):188–191.

40. Tucker LB, Cabral DA. Transition of the adolescent patient with rheumatic disease: issues to consider. *Pediatr Clin North Am* 2005;52(2):641–652.

41. Lam P-Y, Fitzgerald BB, Sawyer SM. Young adults in children's hospitals: what are they there? *Med J Australia* 2005;182:381–384.

42. Betz CL, Redcay G. Dimensions of the transition service coordinator role. *J Spec Pediatr Nurs* 2005;10(2):49–59.

43. McDonagh JE, Southwood TR, Shaw KL. Growing up and moving on in rheumatology: development and preliminary evaluation of a transitional care programme for a multicentre cohort of adolescents with juvenile idiopathic arthritis. *J Child Health Care* 2006;10(1):22–42.

44. Tattersall R, McDonagh JE. Transition: a rheumatology perspective. *Br J Hosp Med* 2010;71:315–319.

45. Tuchman LK, Slap GB, Britto MT. Transition to adult care: experiences and expectations of adolescents with a chronic illness. *Child Care Health Dev* 2008;34(5):557–563.

46. Shaw KL, Southwood TR, McDonagh JE on behalf of the British Paediatric Rheumatology Group. User perspectives of transitional care for adolescents with juvenile idiopathic arthritis. *Rheumatology* (Oxford) 2004;43(6):770–778.

47. Kipps S, Bahu T, Ong, K, et al. Current methods of transfer of young people with type 1 diabetes to adult services. *Diabet Med* 2002;19:649–654.

48. Barendse RM, aan de Kerk DJ, Fishman LN et al. Transition of adolescents with inflammatory bowel disease from pediatric to adult care: a survey of Dutch adult gastroenterologists' perspectives. *Int J Child Adolesc Health* 2010;3(4):609–616.

49. McLaughlin SM, Diener-West M, Indurkhya A et al. Improving transition from paediatric to adult cystic fibrosis care: lessons from a national survey of current practice. *Pediatrics* 2008; 121:e1160–e1166.

50. De Beaufort C, Jarosz-Chobot P, Frank M, de Bart J, Deja G. Transition from pediatric to adult diabetes care: smooth or slippery? *Pediatr Diabet* 2010;11:24–27.

51. Geerts E, van de Wiel H, Tamminga R. A pilot study on the effects of the transition of paediatric to adult health care in patients with haemophilia and in their parents: patient and parent worries, parental illness-related distress and health-related quality of life. *Haemophilia* 2008;14(5):1007–1013.

52. Brodie L, Crisp J, McCormack B, Wilson V, Bergin P, Fulham C. Journeying from nirvana with mega-mums and broken hearts: the complex dynamics of transition from paediatric to adult settings. *Int J Child Adol Health* 2010;3(4):517–526.

53. Kieckhefer GM, Trahms CM. Supporting development of children with chronic conditions: from compliance toward shared management. *Pediatr Nurs* 2000;26:354–363.

54. Stinson JN, Toomey PC, Stevens BJ et al. Asking the experts: exploring the self-management needs of adolescents with arthritis. *Arthritis Rheum* 2008;59:65–72.

55. Berry SL, Hayford JR, Ross CK, Pachman LM, Lavaigne JV. Conceptions of illness by children with juvenile rheumatoid arthritis: a cognitive developmental approach. *J Pediatr Psychol* 1993;18(1):83–97.

56. Fredericks EM, Dore-Stites D, Well A et al. Assessment of transition readiness skills and adherence in pediatric liver transplant recipients. *Pediatr Transplant* 2010;4(8):944–953.

57. Kadan-Lottick NS, Robison LL, Gurney JG et al. Childhood cancer survivors' knowledge about their past diagnosis and treatment. Childhood Cancer Survivor Study. *JAMA* 2002;287:1832–1839.

58. Dore A, de Guise P, Mercier LA. Transition of care to adult congenital heart centres: what do patients know about their heart condition? *Can J Cardiol* 2002;18:141–146.

59. Clarizia NA, Chalan N, Manlhiot C et al. Transition to adult health care for adolescents and young adults with congenital heart disease: perspectives of the patient, parent and health care provider. *Can J Cardiol* 2009;25(9):e317–e322.

60. Ullrich G, Mattussek S, Dressler F, Thon A. How do adolescents with juvenile chronic arthritis consider their disease related knowledge, their unmet service needs and the attractiveness of various services? *Eur J Med Res* 2002;7:8–18.

61. Stinson JN, McGrath PJ, Hodnett ED et al. Usability testing of an online self-management program for adolescents with juvenile idiopathic arthritis. *J Rheumatol* 2010;37(9):1944–1952.

62. Scal P, Garwick A, Horvath KJ. Making rheum to grow: The rationale and framework for an internet based health carte transition intervention. *Int J Child Adolesc Health* 2010;3(4):451–461.

63. Wolfstadt J, Kaufman A, Levitin J, Kaufman M. The use and usefulness of My Health Passport: an online tool for the creation of a portable health summary. *Int J Child Adolesc Health* 2010;3(4):499–506.

64. Stinson J, Wilson R, Gill N, Yamada J, Holt J. A systematic review of internet-based self-management interventions for youth with health conditions. *J Pediat Psychol* 2009;34:495–510.

65. van Staa A, van der Stege HA, Jedeloo S, Moll HA, Hilberink SR. Readiness to transfer to adult care of adolescents with chronic conditions: exploration of associated factors. *J Adolesc Health* 2011;48(3):295–302.

66. Shaw KL, Dobbels F. When I remember … adherence and chronic rheumatic diseases. In: McDonagh JE, White PH (eds) *Adolescent rheumatology*. Informa Healthcare, New York, 2008:85–105.

67. McDonagh JE, Kaufman M. The challenging adolescent. *Rheumatology* (Oxford) 2009;48(8):872–825.

68. Peng D, Yang M, Yang L. Role of situational and facial clues in expression judgement. *Inf Psychol Sci* 1985;2:26–32.

69. Naar-King S, Suarez M. *Motivational interviewing with adolescents and young adults*. Guildford Press, New York, 2011.

70. Milne B, Towns S. Do paediatricians provide brief intervention for adolescents who smoke? *J Paediatr Child Health* 2007;43(6):464–468.

71. Jackson G, McDonagh JE. Who tells what! An audit of advice regarding alcohol in paediatric rheumatology clinics. *Rheumatology* 2005;44(suppl):i93.

72. McDonagh JE, Southwood TR Shaw KL. Unmet education and training needs of rheumatology health professionals in adolescent health and transitional care. *Rheumatology* (Oxford) 2004;43(6):737–743.

73. Britto MT, Rosenthal SL, Taylor J, Passo MH. Improving rheumatologists screening for alcohol use and sexual activity. *Arch Pediatr Adolesc Med* 2000;154:478–483.

74. Brown JD, Wissow LS. Discussion of sensitive health topics with youth during primary care visits: relationship to youth perceptions of care. *J Adolesc Health* 2009;44:48–54.

75. Kaufman M. Transition of cognitively delayed adolescent organ transplant recipients to adult care. *Pediatr Transplant* 2006;10:413–417.

76. Goldenring JM, Rosen DS. Getting into adolescent heads: an essential update. *Contemp Pediatr* 2004;21(1):64–90.

77. Werner EE, Smith RS. *Overcoming the odds: high risk children from birth to adulthood*. Cornell University Press, Ithaca, NY, 1992.

78. Haverman L, Grootenhuis MA, van den Berg JM et al. Predictors of health-related quality of life in children and adolescents with juvenile idiopathic arthritis: Results from a web-based survey. *Arthritis Care Res* (Hoboken) 2012; 64(5):694–703.

79. McDonagh JE, Hackett J. Growing up in a school with chronic condition. *Br J School Nurs* 2008;3:385–392.

80. Lelieveld OT, Armbrust W, van Leeuwen MA et al. Physical activity in adolescents with juvenile idiopathic arthritis. *Arthritis Rheum* 2008;59(10):1379–1384.

81. Long AR, Rouster-Stevens KA. The role of exercise therapy in the management of juvenile idiopathic arthritis. *Curr Opin Rheumatol* 2010;22(2):213–217.

82. La Greca AM, Bearman KJ, Moore H. Peer relations of youth with pediatric conditions and health risks: promoting social support and healthy lifestyles. *Dev Behav Pediatr* 2002;23:271–280.

83. Sentenac M, Gavin A, Arnaud C, Molcho M, Godeau E, Nic Gabhainn S. Victims of bullying among students with a disability or chronic illness and their peers: a cross-national study between Ireland and France. *J Adolesc Health* 2011;48(5):461–466.

84. Voss LD, Mulligan J. Bullying in school: are short pupils at risk? Questionnaire study in a cohort. *BMJ* 2000;320:612–613.

85. Bidwell C, Bolt I, McDonagh JE. Pertinence of cardiovascular disease risk awareness in adolescent patients with systemic lupus erythematosus patients: comment on the article by Scalzi et al. *Arthritis Rheum* 2008;58(12):3971–3972.

86. Lurie S, Shemesh E, Sheiner PA et al. Nonadherence in pediatric liver transplant recipients—an assessment of risk factors and natural history. *Pediatr Transplant* 2000;4:200–206.

87. Schanberg LE, Sandborg C. Dyslipoproteinaemia and premature atherosclerosis in paediatric systemic lupus erythematosus. *Curr Rheumatol Rep* 2004;6(6):425–433.

88. Packham JC, Hall MA. Long-term follow-up of 246 adults with juvenile idiopathic arthritis: social function, relationships and sexual activity. *Rheumatology* (Oxford) 2002;41:1440–1443.

89. Canadian Paediatric Society. Adolescent sexual orientation. *Paediatr Child Health* 2008;13:619–623.

90. Shaw KL, Southwood TR, Duffy CM, McDonagh JE. Health related quality of life in adolescents with juvenile idiopathic arthritis. *Arthritis Rheum* 2006;55:199–207.

91. Butbul Aviel Y, Stremler R, Benseler SM et al. Sleep and fatigue and the relationship to pain, disease activity and quality of life in juvenile idiopathic arthritis and juvenile dermatomyositis. *Rheumatology* (Oxford) 2011;50(11):2051–2060.

92. Raman SR, Boyce WF, Pickett W. Associations between adolescent risk behaviours and injury: the modifying role of disability. *J Sch Health* 2009;79(1):8–16.

93. McDonagh JE. The importance of developing rheumatology services for adolescents. *Future Rheumatol* 2008;3:133–141.

94. Department of Health. *You're Welcome quality criteria. Making health services young people friendly.* London, 2011 (www.dh.gov.uk last accessed 4 November 2011)

95. Shaw KL, Southwood TR and McDonagh JE on behalf of the British Society of Paediatric and Adolescent Rheumatology. Growing up and moving on in rheumatology: a multicentre cohort of adolescents with juvenile idiopathic arthritis. *Rheumatology* 2005;44:806–812.

96. Shaw KL, Southwood TR, McDonagh JE. Transitional care for adolescents with juvenile idiopathic arthritis: results of a Delphi study. *Rheumatology* 2004;43:1000–1006.

97. Reid GJ, Irvine MJ, McCrindle BW, Sananes R, Ritvo PG, Sui SC, Webb GD. Prevalence and correlates of successful transfer from pediatric to adult health care among a cohort of young adults with complex congenital heart defects. *Pediatrics* 2004;113(3):197–205.

98. Franklin VL, Greene A, Waller A, Greene SA, Pagliari C. Patients' engagement with 'Sweet Talk'—a text messaging support system for young people with diabetes. *J Med Internet Res* 2008;10(2):e20.

99. Shaw KL, Southwood TR, McDonagh JE. Developing a programme of transitional care for adolescents with juvenile idiopathic arthritis: results of a postal survey. *Rheumatology* 2004;43:211–219.

100. McDonagh JE, Southwood TR, Shaw KL. Unmet adolescent health training needs for rheumatology health professionals. *Rheumatology* 2004;43:737–743.

101. Geenen SJ, Powers LE, Sells W. Understanding the role of health care providers during transition of adolescents with disabilities and special health care needs. *J Adolesc Health* 2003;32:225–233.

102. Shaw KL, Southwood TR, McDonagh JE. Young people's satisfaction of transitional care in adolescent rheumatology in the UK. *Child Care Health Dev* 2007;33:368–379.

103. Sanci L, Coffey C, Patton G, Bowes G. Sustainability of change with quality general practitioner education in adolescent health: a five year follow-up. *Med Ed* 2005;39:557–560.

104. Beresford B, Sloper P. Chronically ill adolescents' experiences of communicating with doctors: a qualitative study. *J Adolesc Health* 2003;33:172–179.

105. Shaw KL, Southwood TR, McDonagh JE. Growing up and moving on in rheumatology: parents as proxies of adolescents with juvenile idiopathic arthritis. *Arthritis Care Res* 2006;55(2):189–198.

106. Royal College of Paediatrics and Child Health and Young Persons Health Special Interest Group. *Not just a phase. A guide to the participation of children and young people in health services.* London, 2010. (www.rchcp.ac.uk last accessed 4 November 2011)

107. Kennedy A, Sawyer S. Transition from pediatric to adult services: are we getting it right? *Curr Opin Pediatr* 2008;20:403–409.

CHAPTER 3

The adult patient

Paul Thompson

Introduction

This chapter is for the rheumatologist in training. While inevitably coloured by the author's experience and bias, the text will be evidence-based and refer to published reviews as much as possible. Clinical vignettes will be used to stimulate thought and discussions. In the age of the internet, YouTube and Twitter reference will be made to relevant sites, although it should be noted that in a rapidly changing world new and important sites may be missed. The reader is encouraged to surf the net for additional material.

Rheumatic diseases constitute a wide range of conditions and an inclusive approach is taken here. While many rheumatologists will concentrate their practice on the inflammatory arthritides, others will see patients with regional and widespread pain syndromes. A knowledge of the complex interaction of physical and psychological factors in, for example, patients with chronic disabling back pain, will serve the clinician well in any aspect of practice.

The International Statistical Classification of Diseases and Related Health Problems 10th Revision (ICD-10) lists those conditions considered to be diseases of the musculoskeletal system and connective tissues.[1] Not all the conditions will be covered here, but the chapter will concentrate on patients presenting with arthritis, regional pain syndromes, polymyalgia, and connective tissue diseases.

Principles

Some consideration of how to collect the relevant information to help make a diagnosis and, perhaps more importantly, to understand the person's problem in the context of their beliefs, social, and economic environment, is pertinent.

Recommendations for taking a history and performing a clinical examination relevant to musculoskeletal problems are available (see Woolf and Akesson[2] for a recent review), but it is assumed that the reader has the basic competencies of a trainee specialist.

There are a number of ways in which to approach a patient but in practice physicians use a combination of pattern recognition and hypothetical-deductive methods for most decision-making and extract elements of the full history and examination in selected ways.[3] The rheumatologist makes use of all clues—from the referral letter and the appearance and behaviour of patient and carers, to the formal examination—making hypotheses and testing them with direct questions and specific examination techniques.[4] Use of the 'GALS' locomotor screen, as a brief musculoskeletal

assessment, is recommended and can be incorporated into a systemic review.[5]

Arthritis

For the purposes of this section three separate presentations of arthritis (mono-, oligo-, and polyarthritis) are considered. It will be seen that a specific diagnosis may present in more than one way, or evolve from monoarticular to oligoarticular or oligoarticular to polyarticular, but rarely from more to less joints. Of particular note is that many patients presenting in any of the categories never fulfil the criteria for a specific diagnosis. These 'undifferentiated arthritis' conditions frequently resolve spontaneously.

Monoarthritis

> **Case history**
>
> Early in the evening, a 50-year-old man presents to the Emergency Department with a 24-hour history of pain and swelling in his right knee. He denies recent trauma. He has no prior history of joint disease or joint surgery and has no history of arthritis. His medical history includes hypertension, for which he takes hydrochlorthiazide and metopralol. He drinks three beers per day.[6]
>
> What is the differential diagnosis? What questions would you ask him? What clinical signs would you look for? What initial investigations would you perform? How would you manage this case?

In a review of four studies of monoarthritis, Ma and colleagues[6] listed gout (15–27%), septic arthritis (8–20%), osteoarthritis (5–17%), rheumatoid arthritis (11–16%) and reactive arthritis (0–19%) as the most common diagnoses, but pointed out that the cause was not ascertained in a significant number of patients (16–36%). Other rare causes included pseudogout, psoriatic arthritis, tuberculosis, and spontaneous haemarthrosis.

Although there are no specific studies to ascertain the most useful clinical features, experienced rheumatologists have published the points summarized in Box 3.1.[7,8]

Some presentations are pathognomic of conditions such as podagra, acute gout of the great toe, or a sausage digit in patients with reactive arthritis, but acute monoarthritis is often non-specific

Box 3.1 Recommendations made by experienced rheumatologists to ascertain the most useful clinical features from a patient presenting with arthritis

♦ The history should include the mode and time course of presentation, trauma, previous history of joint disease, family history, prodromal and concurrent illnesses, medications, sexual history, tick bites, alcohol and intravenous drug use, occupation, and recent travel.

♦ In particular, a family history of gout; recent diarrhoea and vomiting; symptoms of urethritis in the patient or their sexual contacts indicating possible reactive arthritis (or rarely gonococcal arthritis); prolonged use of thiazide diuretics in elderly women predisposing to tophaceous gout; intravenous drug use in septic arthritis; tick bites suggesting Lyme disease; and fevers, rigors, and malaise in septic arthritis.

♦ Examination should focus on the involved and contralateral joints, and surrounding areas, examination of other joints (the GALS method is useful as a quick and reliable screen test), looking for systemic manifestations of disease.[7]

and clinical evaluation alone is usually not enough to make a diagnosis.

The most important investigation is arthrocentesis. Observation of the fluid may be enough to differential a non-inflammatory condition (clear viscid fluid), acute haemarthrosis (heavily blood stained), and infection (frank pus), but crystal arthopathies and reactive arthritis fluid can look the same as sepsis. Urgent Gram stain, examination of the fluid under polarized light for uric acid or pyrophosphate (a skill which every rheumatologist should acquire) will help with the acute management. Subsequent culture and additional tests such as rheumatoid factor and anti-citrullinated peptide (anti-CCP) antibodies will be helpful in a few cases. It should be noted that despite these diagnostic assessments a definitive diagnosis is reached in only two-thirds of patients[9] and a significant number of those not diagnosed will have a benign outcome.

Oligoarthritis

Case history

A 45-year-old male born in Suriname was admitted with relapsing fever for one and a half weeks, muscle weakness, and fatigue. Physical examination revealed temperature of 38.8°C, arthritis of the second metacarpophalangeal joint of the right hand, right knee, and both ankles, and erythema nodosum on both lower legs.[10]

What is the most likely diagnosis? What tests would you order?

Laboratory testing showed leucocytes of 13.8×10^9/Litre and an erythrocyte sedimentation rate (ESR) of 128 mm/h. IgM-RF and anti-CCP antibodies were negative. On a chest radiograph, infiltration of the lingula of the left lung was observed. Radiographs of the ankles, hands, and feet showed no abnormalities.

What is the significance of the infiltration of the lingula?

Standard cultures and cultures for tuberculosis (TB) in blood and mucus were negative. Analysis of synovial fluid of the right knee and both ankles revealed leucocytes between 4.0 and 8.2×10^9/Litre and no crystals. Standard and cultures for TB of all obtained synovial fluid samples were negative.

What treatment would you give?

Because of the infiltration of the lingula, treatment with clarithromycin and amoxicillin/clavulanic acid was started. The general condition improved but the arthritis persisted. A radiograph performed 8 weeks after admission showed that the infiltration had not changed. Additional investigations were performed including bronchoscopy to obtain specimens for histology and culture. After 4 weeks one culture of bronchial mucous revealed *Mycobacterium tuberculosis*, and Poncet's disease was diagnosed. Therapy with isoniazid, ethamutol, pyrazinamide, and rifampicin was started, after which the arthritis resolved in a few days.

Oligoarthritis is characterized by observed swelling of only a few joints. Definitions are varied and range from two to four joints or less than six and can be considered acute, subacute, or chronic. The term encompasses a group of diseases including reactive arthritis, psoriatic arthritis, and undifferentiated arthritis in addition to rheumatoid arthritis in evolution.[11] The incidence in adults below 60 years of age is at least of the same magnitude as rheumatoid arthritis. Data on outcome in these patients demonstrate a variable rate of persistence. Longitudinal cohort studies have shown that a surprisingly large proportion of patients do not develop into a recognizable condition (Figure 3.1) with those patients with undifferentiated arthritis either resolving spontaneously after a few months or going

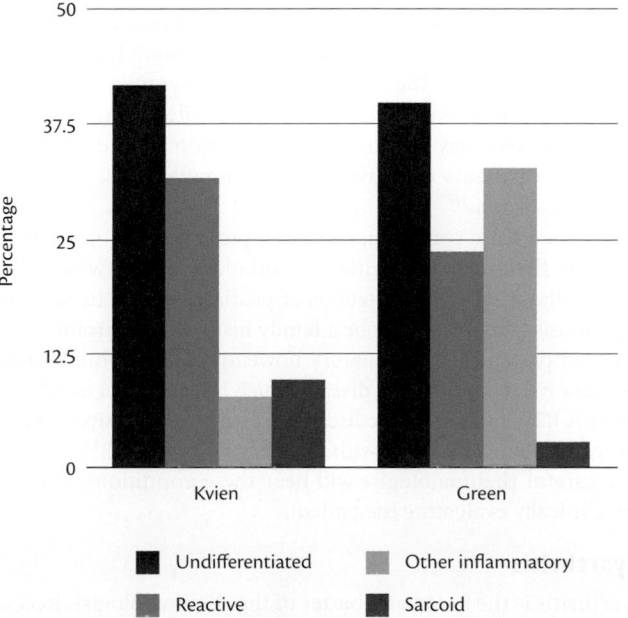

Fig. 3.1 The incidence of four diagnoses made in two longitudinal cohorts of patients presenting with oligoarthritis.

on to a more persistent arthritis after 24 weeks, not fulfilling the case definitions of reactive arthritis or any other clinical rheumatic diagnosis[12] despite treatment with intra-articular corticosteroids.[13] Many of these patients have evidence of subclinical synovitis when examined by ultrasound and might be better classified as having polyarthritis.[11]

Reactive arthritis is so called because many cases follow shortly after an identified infection although the joint inflammation is aseptic. The clinical picture of a systemic illness associated with inflammation of a few, usually large joints, is typical but a proportion of patients will have minimal symptoms of infection so careful questioning and appropriate testing should be carried out. In general there are two subtypes with a number of rare conditions such as in our case history here. Reactive arthritis occurring after a proceeding infection of the urogenital tract with *Chlamydia trachomatis* or after an infection of the gut with enterobacteria are considered to be part of the spondyloarthropathies.[14] Patients carry the HLA B27 antigen in about 50% of cases and some have features of enthestitis, sacroileitis, and uveitis. Affected joints have a dusky appearance and are extremely painful, warm, and swollen. The synovial inflammation may be intense and mimic sepsis or acute gout/pseudogout. Synovial fluid looks turbid and is packed with polymorphonuclear leucocytes but Gram stain is negative and crystals are absent on polaroid light microscopy (essential investigations in the Emergency Department). Sausage digits are not unusual, reminding us of the overlap with psoriatic arthritis.

Poststreptococcal reactive arthritis is often considered to be a condition of children but the age distribution is bimodal with peaks in early teens and late twenties.[15] The clinical presentation is heterogeneous but appears different from rheumatic fever and the HLA B27-associated reactive arthritides. In most cases arthritis is non-migratory, involves one or a few joints, and resolves within a few weeks, although it may recur with further infections.[15]

Sarcoidosis is a heterogeneous multisystem granulomatous disease that primarily affects the lungs and lymphatic system, which is characterized by its pathological hallmark, the non-caseating granuloma. Arthritis is found in 15–25% of patients and is usually acute and transient. Löfgren described the triad of arthritis, bilateral hilar lymphadenopathy, and erythema nodosum but the latter is not always present. The arthritis is usually symmetrical in the large joints of the lower limbs. The ankles are affected in almost all patients and there may be a dusky discolouration around the ankle. One-third of patients will have evidence of enthestitis, usually of the achilles tendon.[16]

Other rheumatic conditions that may present as an oligoarthritis include rheumatoid arthritis or psoriatic arthritis (which may present without skin manifestations of psoriasis—psoriatic arthritis sine psoriasis—but there may be a family history),[17] gastrointestinal disease, in particular inflammatory bowel disease (Crohn's disease and ulcerative colitis), coeliac disease which is usually not associated with HLA B27, and Whipple's disease (probably an infective arthritis a part of a systemic infection with *Tropheryma whippelii*).[18]

The careful rheumatologist will bear these conditions in mind when clinically evaluating the patient.

Polyarthritis

Polyarthritis is the bread and butter of the rheumatologist. Recent major advances in the diagnosis, prediction of outcome, and drug therapies linked to new ways of managing patients (systematic monitoring using outcome targets and escalation protocols leading to tight control) of rheumatoid and psoriatic arthritis have revolutionized the management of these conditions and the achievement of remission is in many patients a realistic goal. However, it is clear from cohort studies of early synovitis clinics that not all patients with polyarthralgias have rheumatoid or psoriatic arthritis and perhaps one-third of these patients will resolve without long-term sequelae. So how will the rheumatologist manage patients who may present in a very similar way but have very different outcomes?

> ### Case history
>
> A 45-year-old white woman was referred to the early synovitis clinic by her GP. She had gradually developed painful wrists over 2 months and consulted her doctor when the pain and early morning stiffness stopped her from doing the housework. The pain spread into her fingers and knees, and she developed some discomfort in her toes on walking. She was taking paracetamol and ibuprofen but her symptoms had prevented her working and she was becoming tearful and depressed (Thompson, personal communication).
>
> **What is the differential diagnosis? What questions would you ask her? What clinical signs would you look for? What initial investigations would you perform? How would you manage this case?**
>
> The hands shown in Figure 3.2 appear to show swelling of all the small joints and a possible nail dystrophy on the left ring finger. Swelling of the metacarpophalangeal joints (MCPs) and proximal interphalangeal joints (PIPs) is typical of rheumatoid arthritis while swelling of the distal interphalangeal joints (DIPs) is more suggestive of nodal osteoarthritis or psoriatic arthritis. This patient had early rheumatoid arthritis (RA).[19]

RA is a chronic inflammatory disease characterized by joint swelling, joint tenderness, and destruction of synovial joints, leading to severe disability and premature mortality. Given the presence of autoantibodies, such as rheumatoid factor (RF) and anti-CCP antibody, which can precede the clinical manifestation of RA by many years, RA is considered an autoimmune disease. The accepted means of defining RA is by use of classification criteria to provide the basis for a common approach to disease definition that can be used to compare across studies and centres and recruit to clinical trials. The most widely used classification criteria are those published by the American Rheumatism Association in 1988.[20] These used seven criteria: morning stiffness, arthritis of more than three areas, arthritis of the hands, symmetrical arthritis, rheumatoid nodules, serum RF, and radiographic change. A patient is said to have RA if at least four of the criteria have been present for at least 6 weeks.

However, these criteria are limited because they were derived to discriminate patients with established RA from those with a combination of other definite rheumatological diagnoses. They are not helpful in identifying patients who would benefit from early effective intervention to prevent them from reaching the chronic, erosive disease state. In view of this a joint working group from the American College of Rheumatology and the European League Against Rheumatism developed a new

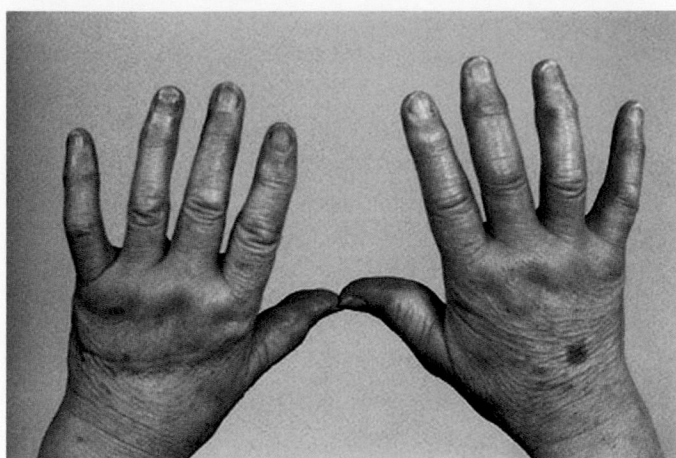

Fig. 3.2 Hands and wrists of a patient presenting with polyarthritis. Note that all joints appear to be swollen and there is a possible nail dystrophy on the left ring finger.
Reproduced with permission from Chappell H (2006) *Essential of Clinical Immunology*, 5th edn. Blackwell Publishing, Oxford. © John Wiley and Sons 2006.

approach to classifying RA.[21] The work focused on identifying, among patients newly presenting with undifferentiated inflammatory synovitis, factors that best discriminated between those who were and those who were not at high risk for persistent and/or erosive disease. In the new criteria set, classification as 'definite RA' is based on the confirmed presence of synovitis in at least one joint, absence of an alternative diagnosis better explaining the synovitis, and achievement of a total score of 6 or greater (of a possible 10) from the individual scores in four domains: number and site of involved joints (range 0–5), serological abnormality (range 0–3), elevated acute-phase response (range 0–1), and symptom duration (two levels; range 0–1) (Box 3.2) and a classification tree can be used.

The classification criteria can be applied to any patient as long as two mandatory requirements are met. First, there must be evidence of currently active clinical synovitis defined as 'swelling' in at least one joint as determined by an expert assessor. All joints of a full joint count may be assessed for this purpose with the exception of the DIPs, the first metatarsophalangeal (MTP) joint and the carpometacarpal (CMC) joint of the thumb, since these joints are typically involved in osteoarthritis. Second, the criteria may be applied only to those patients in whom the observed synovitis is not better explained by another diagnosis. For example, conditions that should be considered and excluded include systemic lupus erythematosus, psoriatic arthritis, and gout.

It should be noted that joint involvement, as used for the determination of the pattern of joint distribution, differs from the definition of synovitis in one joint needed for eligibility in that it refers to any joint with swelling or tenderness on examination that is indicative of active synovitis. Tenderness is included as an equally important feature as swelling for the determination of joint involvement, particularly for the second to fifth MTP joints. Furthermore, any joints with known recent injury that could contribute to swelling or tenderness should not be considered. Additional evidence of joint activity from other imaging techniques (such as MRI or ultrasound) may be used for confirmation of the clinical findings.

Psoriatic arthritis may present in a polyarticular pattern which may mimic RA in addition to an oligoarthritis or axial disease.

Box 3.2 The 2010 American College of Rheumatology/European League against Rheumatism classification criteria for RA

Target population (Who should be tested?): Patients who

1. have at least one joint with definite clinical synovitis (swelling)

2. with the synovitis not better explained by another disease

Classification criteria for RA (score-based algorithm: add score of categories A–D; a score of ≥6/10 is needed for classification of a patient as having definite RA)

A.	Joint involvement	
	1 large joint	0
	2–10 large joints	1
	1–3 small joints (with or without involvement of large joints)	2
	4–10 small joints (with or without involvement of large joints)	3
	>10 joints (at least 1 small joint)	5
B.	Serology (at least 1 test is needed for classification)	
	Negative RF *and* negative ACPA	0
	Low positive RF *or* low positive ACPA	2
	High-positive RF *or* high-positive ACPA	3
C.	Acute-phase reactants (at least 1 test is needed for classification)	
	Normal CRP and normal ESR	0
	Abnormal CRP or normal ESR	1
D.	Duration of symptoms	
	<6 weeks	0
	≥6 weeks	1

Nail dystrophy is usual and psoriatic plaques on the elbows may indicate the diagnosis. For a review of the clinical features see Cantini et al.[22]

Nodal osteoarthritis is one of several clinical presentations of osteoarthritis, typically occurring after 40 years of age in women and affecting the DIPs, PIPs, and thumb base although the MCPs are not infrequently affected. Inflammatory forms may mimic RA or psoriatic arthritis. For a recent consensus report on diagnosis see Zhang et al.[23]

Regional soft tissue and myofascial pain

In the evaluation of the patient with regional pain, the prudent rheumatologist will appreciate the difference between the specific soft tissue conditions such as tennis elbow and frozen shoulder, the myofascial syndromes with local trigger points, and the nonspecific disorders often related to occupational factors.

Two examples will be used here to illustrate the approach to these multifaceted problems: back pain and shoulder/arm pain.

Back pain

Low back pain will be studied in more detail but the principles may be applied to patients presenting with neck pain, and have many features in common with regional myofascial pain syndromes. Isolated thoracic pain is less common and has a greater chance of reflecting more serious pathology (see 'Red flags').

Case history

Mr JT, a 52-year-old drayman, was referred to the rheumatology services with back pain. He said that he often had low backache. 'We all get back pain from time to time because of lifting those barrels, it's part of the job.' While he was being investigated for an unrelated gastrointestinal problem by his GP an abdominal radiograph was reported as showing, 'degenerative changes in the discs and facet joints at several levels'. The GP told Mr T that he had severe arthritis of his spine and should not lift. He turned from a person with a manageable problem to a patient with a disease and never worked again (Thompson, personal communication).

Back pain ranks second only to upper respiratory tract infections as a symptomatic reason to visit a GP. About 70% of adults have back pain at some time but only 14% have an episode that lasts more than 2 weeks and about 2% of these have features of sciatica. Most cases of back pain respond to symptomatic and physical treatments but some are surgically remedial and some are systemic diseases such as cancer, infection, or spondloarthropathies requiring specific therapy, so careful diagnostic evaluation is essential. Furthermore, psychosocial factors are important in chronic back pain disability.

Since a specific cause frequently cannot be identified, diagnostic efforts are often disappointing. Instead of seeking a precise cause in every case of back pain it is more useful to answer three basic questions. (1) Is there a serious systemic disease causing the pain? (2) Is there neurological compromise that may require surgery? (3) Is there social or psychological distress that may amplify or prolong pain? These questions can generally be answered on the basis of history and examination alone, a minority of patients requiring further diagnostic testing.[24]

Red flags

The initial clinical history taking should aim at identifying 'red flags' of possible serious spinal pathology.[25] Red flags are risk factors detected in low back pain patients' past medical history and symptomatology and are associated with a higher risk of serious disorders causing low back pain compared to patients without these characteristics. If any of these are present, further investigation (according to the suspected underlying pathology) may be required to exclude a serious underlying condition, e.g. infection, inflammatory rheumatic disease, or cancer. Red flags are features in addition to low back pain (Box 3.3).

Cauda equina syndrome is likely to be present when patients describe bladder dysfunction (usually urinary retention, occasionally overflow incontinence), sphincter disturbance, saddle anaesthesia, global or progressive weakness in the lower limbs, or gait disturbance. This requires urgent referral.

Yellow flags

Psychosocial 'yellow flags' are factors that increase the risk of developing, or perpetuating chronic pain and long-term disability,

---

Box 3.3 Red flags: risk factors in patients with low back pain associated with an increased chance of underlying systemic disease

- Age of onset less than 20 years or more than 55 years
- Recent history of violent trauma
- Constant progressive, non-mechanical pain (no relief with bed rest)
- Thoracic pain
- Past medical history of malignant tumour
- Prolonged use of corticosteroids
- Drug abuse, immunosuppression, HIV
- Systemically unwell
- Unexplained weight loss
- Widespread neurological symptoms (including cauda equina syndrome)
- Structural deformity
- Fever

---

including work loss, associated with low back pain.[26] Identification of yellow flags should lead to appropriate cognitive and behavioural management. However, there is no evidence on the effectiveness of psychosocial assessment or intervention in acute low back pain.

Examples of yellow flags are:

- Inappropriate attitudes and beliefs about back pain (e.g. belief that back pain is harmful or potentially severely disabling, or high expectation of passive treatments rather than a belief that active participation will help)
- Inappropriate pain behaviour (e.g. fear avoidance behaviour and reduced activity levels)
- Work-related problems or compensation issues (e.g. poor work satisfaction),
- Emotional problems (e.g. depression, anxiety, stress, tendency to low mood, withdrawal from social interaction).

For an in-depth discussion about the assessment of the back pain patient with the available evidence base see the European guidelines for the management of acute non-specific low back pain in primary care.[27]

Shoulder/arm pain

Shoulder pain is a significant cause of morbidity; the prevalence is estimated to be between 16% and 26% and it is the third most common cause of musculoskeletal consultations in primary care. The cause can be difficult to diagnose because of the complex anatomy, the wide spectrum of organic pathologies, and the overlap with regional myofascial pain. Clinical evaluation by specialists can rule out the presence of a rotator cuff tear but more detailed investigations including MRI and ultrasound are often needed to arrive at a firm diagnosis.[28]

A recent review of the literature described over 100 tests for examining the shoulder. The authors concluded that the key steps are as follows: (1) rule out stiffness by checking passive external rotation; (2) evaluate external rotation and supraspinatus power and impingement signs for rotator cuff tears; (3) O'Brien's sign for superior labral anterior posterior lesions; (4) modified cross arm sign/modified O'Brien's sign for acromioclavicular pain; and (5) instability tests if there is a positive history.[29]

Soft tissue musculoskeletal disorders of the neck and upper limb comprise a heterogeneous group of conditions. At one end of the spectrum are relatively clear-cut specific upper limb conditions such as de Quervain's tenosynovitis, lateral epicondylitis, rotator cuff tendonitis, and carpal tunnel syndrome, but at the other end of the spectrum are non-specific regional pain syndromes, e.g. forearm pain, with few objective physical findings and little in the way of demonstrable pathology.

Many of these upper extremity disorders are attributed to occupational factors but, despite a substantial body of epidemiological and scientific publications, this is a field beset by controversy. For a detailed discussion of the problems see Walker-Bone and Cooper[30] and Harald et al.[31]

Myofascial pain syndrome

Myofascial pain is characterized by local areas of muscle tension and spasm which can often be felt as tender nodules forming the basis of the condition long described as 'fibrositis'. It occurs commonly around the shoulder girdle with pain felt in the neck, shoulder blade, axilla, and upper chest. Myofascial pain may occur as a primary phenomenon or complicate other soft tissue conditions. It is associated with psychological factors such as depression, stress, fatigue, and anxiety. Trigger points (irritable foci within skeletal muscles and their ligamentous junctions that produce characteristic referred pain when palpated) are considered important in the diagnosis of the syndrome, although the reliability of detection has been questioned.[32]

Although myofascial pain syndromes have been described in the medical literature for over a century they are often overlooked as a cause of a patient's symptoms, leading to unnecessary investigations and inappropriate treatments. Myofascial pain can be a useful explanation for a patient's symptoms and a diagnosis on which to logically introduce exercise and other self-management strategies. The utility of other treatment techniques such as trigger and tender point injection remains controversial. The clinician will understand the complex interactions between soma and psyche and make a diagnosis of myofascial pain a positive one, rather than just the absence of organic pathology. For a history see Wikipedia and reviews by Bennett, Gerwin, and Delago et al.[33–35]

Polymyalgia

Case history

Ms HG, aged 72 years, went to her GP complaining of generalized pain and stiffness for 6 months but in particular around her shoulders and thighs. She said the symptoms came on gradually over a few weeks and were eased by taking ibuprofen. The symptoms were bad at night with morning stiffness and her sleep was disturbed. She felt tired, weak and generally unwell. On examination her body mass index (BMI) was 34. She had difficulty rising from a chair without using her arms. There were diffuse tender points around her neck and lower back. Cervical and lumbar movements were full but uncomfortable. Temporal arteries appeared normal and there was no obvious muscle wasting or fasciculation. General examination was normal. Her ESR was 44 mm/h with normal blood count (Thompson, personal communication).

What is your diagnosis? What further tests would you perform? How do you think she would respond to a trial of glucocorticosteroids?

The main differential diagnoses are polymyalgia rheumatica (PMR), fibromyalgia (FMS), and polymyositis (PM) with lymphoma, metastatic disease, and hypothyroidism important disorders needing consideration.

Polymyalgia rheumatica

The British Society of Rheumatology guidelines on the management of PMR recommend evaluating four core inclusion criteria: (1) age over 50 years, duration greater than 2 weeks, (2) bilateral shoulder or pelvic girdle aching, or both, (3) morning stiffness duration of greater than 45 min and, (4) evidence of an acute-phase response. They recommend further investigations and a trial of glucocorticosteroid treatment as the response to treatment is an important part of the diagnostic triage.[36]

In Ms G's case she fulfils the first two criteria but we are unsure of the duration of morning stiffness. How reliable is this as a symptom? Finally, does she have evidence of an acute-phase response? At first sight an ESR of 44 mm/h seems pathological and would be reported as such in the author's hospital where the upper limit of normal is 12 mm/h. However, the ESR is a composite measure affected by circulating acute-phase proteins, paraproteins, fibrinogen, and red cell size and shape. The ESR is higher in women than in men, and goes up linearly with age. A formula has been suggested:[37]

$$ESR = [age + 10 (women)]/2.$$

For our patient this means an ESR of up to 41mm/h would be considered within the normal range. In addition to age changes, obesity is associated with an increased ESR. Differences of up to 20% have been reported, making an ESR of 41 mm/h in our case an unreliable marker of an acute-phase response.

A trial of modest doses of oral or intramuscular glucocorticosteroids would be expected to result in a dramatic and sustained improvement in symptoms within a few days, helping to confirm the diagnosis.

Fibromyalgia

Chronic, widespread pain is the defining feature of FMS, but patients may also exhibit a range of other symptoms, including sleep disturbance, fatigue, irritable bowel syndrome, headache, and mood disorders.

The introduction of the American College of Rheumatology (ACR) fibromyalgia classification criteria 20 years ago began an era of increased recognition of the syndrome. The criteria required tenderness on pressure (tender points) in at least 11 of 18 specified sites and the presence of widespread pain for diagnosis. A major revision of the criteria for diagnosis has turned the disorder into one of symptoms. The new criteria are based on patient-reported pain, the widespread pain index, and a symptom severity index consisting of self-reported fatigue and unrefreshed waking, and a wide range of cognitive and systemic symptoms all scored 0 to 3. Patients no longer need to be examined or investigated to make the diagnosis, although a caveat that 'the patient does not have a disorder that would otherwise explain the pain', has been introduced.[38]

In the recent European League Against Rheumatism (EULAR) recommendations for the treatment of FMS there was a negative recommendation for the use of glucocorticosteroids, based on expert opinion that appears to rely on the lack of evidence rather than the evidence of lack of efficacy.[39]

In Ms G's case, while we do not have the detailed self-reported severity scale, it seems likely that she would fulfil the diagnostic criteria, provided we did not consider that her symptoms were caused by PMR. A response to glucocorticosteroids would not be expected although a partial, non-specific improvement, particularly to intramuscular injection, is not uncommon in the author's experience.

Polymyositis

The diagnostic criteria for the autoimmune inflammatory myopathies were formulated by Bohan and Peter in 1975. Their system was (1) primary idiopathic polymyositis (PM), (2) primary idiopathic dermatomyositis (DM), (3) PM or DM with malignancy, (4) juvenile DM (or PM) associated with vasculitis and (5) PM or DM with associated collagen vascular diseases. However, they did not recognize inclusion body myositis or other inflammatory myopathies, such as granulomatous and eosinophilic myositis. While new histological techniques have introduced great potential for a classification that helps in management and prognosis, no consensus has yet been reached as to an alternative. The International Myositis Assessment and Clinical Studies Group is currently coordinating a project to produce a new classification that distinguishes inflammatory myositis from other major mimicking conditions and separates the subtypes from each other.[40]

In Ms G's case further investigations will be needed to make the diagnosis and a response to glucocorticosteroid therapy anticipated, although at much higher doses than that needed to control PMR.

Connective tissue diseases

Case history

Mrs CM, a 23-year-old white woman, presented to her doctor with a 3 year history of joint pains and fatigue. She said that the pains were particularly bad in the mornings and were now interfering with her work as a nursery nurse. On direct questioning she said her hands were always cold and white and she developed chilblains on her toes in the winter. Examination revealed a livido reticularis rash on her thighs but no joint swelling or nail fold abnormalities. Her antinuclear factor was weakly positive but her anti-dsDNA antibodies and extractible nuclear antibody screen was negative (Thompson, personal communication).

How would you classify this patient's condition? Are there other tests that might be helpful? How would you treat her? What prognosis would you offer her?

The term connective tissue disease (CTD) refers to a group of autoimmune disorders that are classified among the systemic rheumatic diseases and include systemic lupus erythematosus (SLE), systemic

Table 3.1 Clinical manifestations of connective tissue diseases associated with autoantibody reactivities

Clinical manifestations	Autoantibody reactivities
Malar rash	Anti-dsDNA
Subacute discoid LE	Anti-Sm
Chronic discoid LE	Anti-P protein
Skin sclerosis	Anti-Scl70
Heliotrope rash	Anti-centromere
Gottron's papules	Anti-La/SSB
Erosive arthritis	Anti-Jo1
	Anti-Mi2

LE, lupus erythematosus.

sclerosis (SSc), polymyositis-dermatomyositis (PM-DM), primary Sjögren's syndrome (pSS), primary anti-phospholipid syndrome (APS), and mixed connective tissue disease (MCTD). Classification of CTDs depends on a patient developing some disease-specific manifestations, e.g. Gottron's papules in DM, or a cluster of non-specific but characteristic findings associated with autoantibody reactivities considered to be specific for a definite CTD (Table 3.1).

The sharing of immunogenic features in these conditions may be why patients present with common clinical features. Taken together they can often represent the onset of a classifiable CTD; remain 'undifferentiated' but associated with a positive anti-nuclear antibody (ANA) suggesting a true autoimmune condition; or remain unclassifiable—for example, many patients presenting with arthralgias and primary Raynaud's phenomenon will have no other features of a CTD and be autoantibody negative. There is considerable debate as to whether those patients have an incomplete or undifferentiated CTD or have more in common with pain syndromes such as fibromyalgia. For a more detailed discussion see Doria et al.[41]

References

1. www.who.int/classification/icd/en/
2. Woolf AD, Akesson K. Primer: history and examination in the assessment of musculoskeletal problems. *Nat Clin Pract* 2008;4:26–33.
3. Sackett DL, Haynes RB, Tugwell P. *Clinical epidemiology: a basic science for clinical medicine*. Little, Brown, MA, 1985.
4. Elstein AS, Schwarz A. Clinical problem solving and decision making: selective review of the cognitive literature. *BMJ* 2002;324:729–732.
5. Doherty M, Dacre J, Dieppe P, Snaith M. The 'GALS' locomotor screen. *Ann Rheum Dis* 1992;51:1165–1169.
6. Ma L, Cranney A, Holroyd-Leduc JM. Acute monoarthritis: What is the cause of my patient's painful swollen joint? *Can Med Ass J* 2009;180:59–65.
7. Baker DG, Schumacher HR. Acute monoarthritis. *N Eng J Med* 1993;329:1013–1020.
8. Siva C, Velazquez C, Mody A et al. Diagnosing acute monoarthritis in adults.: a practical approach for the family physician. *Am Fam Physician* 2003;68:83–90.
9. Freed JF, Nies KM, Boyer RS et al. Acute monoarticular arthritis. A diagnostic approach. *JAMA* 1980;243:2314–2316.
10. Kroot EJA, Hazes JMW, Colin EM, Dolhain RJEM. Poncet's disease: reactive arthritis accompanying tuberculosis. Two case reports and a review of the literature. *Rheumatology* 2007;46:484–489.

11. Wakefield RJ, Green MJ, Marzo-Oretega H et al. Should oligoarthritis be reclassified? Ultrasound reveals a high prevalence of subclinical disease. *Ann Rheum Dis* 2004;63:382–385.

12. Kvien TK, Glennas A, Melby K. Prediction of diagnosis in acute and subacute oligoarthritis of unknown origin. *Br J Rheumatol* 1996;35:359–363.

13. Green M, Marzo-Ortega M, Wakefield RJ et al. Predictors of outcome in patients with oligoarthritis. Results of a protocol of intraarticular corticosteroids to all clinically active joints. *Arthritis Rheum* 2001;44:1177–1183.

14. Sieper J, Rudwaleit M, Braun J, van der Heijde D. Diagnosing reactive arthritis. *Role of clinical setting in the value of serological and microbiologic assays. Arthritis Rheum* 2002;46:319–327.

15. Mackie SL, Keat A. Poststeptococcal reactive arthritis: what is it and how do we know? *Rheumatology* 2004;43:949–954.

16. Visser H, Vos K, Zanelli E et al. Sarcoid arthritis: clinical characteristics, diagnostic aspects, and risk factors. *Ann Rheum Dis* 2002;61:499–504.

17. Helliwell PS, Taylor WJ. Classification and diagnostic criteria for psoriatic arthritis. *Ann Rheum Dis* 2005;64(Suppl II):ii3–ii18.

18. Alghafeer IS, Sigal LH. Rheumatic manifestations of gastrointestinal diseases. *Bull Rheum Dis* 2002 51(2).

19. Chappell H, Haeney M, Misbah S, Snowden N. *Essentials of clinical immunology*, 5th edn. Blackwell, Oxford, 2006.

20. Arnett FC, Edworthy E, Bloch DA et al. The American Rheumatism Association 1987 revised criteria for the classification of rheumatoid arthritis. *Arthritis Rheum* 1988;31:315–324.

21. Aletaha D, Neogi T, Silman AJ. Rheumatoid arthritis classification criteria: an American College of Rheumatology/European League Against Rheumatism collaborative initiative. *Ann Rheum Dis* 2010;69:1580–1588.

22. Cantini F, Niccoli L, Nannini C et al. Psoriatic arthritis: a systematic review. *Int J Rheum Dis* 201013:300–317.

23. Zhang W, Doherty M, Leeb BF et al. EULAR evidence-based recommendations for the diagnosis of hand osteoarthritis: report of a task force of ESCISIT. *Ann Rheum Dis* 2009;68:8–17.

24. Deyo RA, Rainville J, Kent DL. What can the history and physical examination tell us about low back pain? *JAMA* 1992;268:760–765.

25. Royal College of General Practitioners. *Clinical guidelines for the management of acute low back pain*. Royal College of General Practitioners, London, 1996 and 1999.

26. Kendall NAS, Linton SJ, Main CJ. *Guide to assessing psychosocial yellow flags in acute low back pain: risk factors for long-term disability and work loss*. Accident Rehabilitation & Compensation Insurance Corporation of New Zealand and the National Health Committee, Wellington, New Zealand, 1997.

27. van Tulder M, Becker A, Bekkering T et al. European guidelines for the management of acute non-specific low back pain in primary care. *Eur Spine J* 2006;15(Suppl 2):S169–S191.

28. Dinnes J, Loveman E, McIntyre L, Waugh N. The effectiveness of diagnostic tests for the assessment of shoulder pain due to soft tissues disorders: a systematic review. *Health Technol Assess* 2003;7:29.

29. Ronquillo JC, Szomor Z, Murrell G. Examination of the shoulder. *Tech Shoulder Elbow Surg* 2011;12:116–125.

30. Walker-Bone K, Cooper C. Hard work never hurt anyone: or did it? A review of occupational associations with soft tissue musculoskeletal disorders of the neck and upper limb. *Ann Rheum Dis* 2005;64:1391–1396.

31. Harald S. Miedema, Bionka M. Huisstede. A framework for the classification and diagnosis of work related upper extremity conditions: systematic review. *Semin Arthritis Rheum* 2009;38:407–408.

32. Lucas N, Macaskill P, Irwig L, Moran R, Bogduk N. Reliability of physical examination for diagnosis of myofascial trigger points: a systematic review of the literature. *Clin J Pain* 2009;25(1):80–89.

33. Bennett R. Myofascial pain syndromes and their evaluation. *Best Pract Res Clin Rheumatol* 2007;21(3):427-445.

34. Gerwin RD. Classification, epidemiology and natural history of myofascial pain syndrome. *Curr Pain Headache Rep* 2001;5:412–420.

35. Delgado EV, Romero JC, Escoda CG. Myofascial pain syndromes associated with trigger points: a literature review. (i): epidemiology, clinical treatment and etiopathogeny. *Med Oral Patol Cir Bucal* 2009;14:e494–498.

36. Dasgupta B, Borg FA, Hassan N et al. BSR and BHPR guidelines for the management of polymyalgia rheumatica. *Rheumatology* 2009;49(1):186–190.

37. Hamilton PL, Dawson AA, Ogston DD, Douglas AS. The effect of age on the fibrinolytic enzyme system. *J Clin Pathol* 1974;27:326–329.

38. Wolfe K, Clauw D, Fitzcharles M-A et al. The American College of Rheumatology Preliminary Diagnostic Criteria for Fibromyalgia and Measurement of Symptom Severity. *Arthritis Care Res* 2010;62:600–610.

39. Carville SF, Arent-Nielsen S, Bliddal H et al. EULAR evidence-based recommendations for the management of fibromyalgia syndrome. *Ann Rheum Dis* 2008;67:536–541.

40. Sultan SM, Isenberg DA. Re-classifying myositis. 30 years on from Bohan and Peter. *Rheumatology* 2010;49:831–833.

41. Doria A, Mosca M, Franca Gambari P, Bombardieri S. Defining unclassifiable connective tissue diseases: incomplete, undifferentiated or both? *J Rheumatol* 2005;32:213–215.

CHAPTER 4

The elderly patient

Fraser Birrell and Janice O'Connell

Introduction

Rheumatological diseases are among the most common causes of disability in older people.[1] In the most recent United States National Health Interview Survey (2007–9), 50% of adults 65 years or older reported an arthritis diagnosis, of whom 42% had activity limitation attributable to the arthritis.[2] The prevalence continues to rise with age, even in the elderly population: by the age of 85, the lifetime prevalence of arthritis diagnosed by the GP in the UK is 65%.[3] Preservation of motor function is key to the maintenance of independent living in old age, with loss or decline in the ability to walk often being the deciding factor in determining the need for supportive or institutional care. It is clear, therefore, that the rheumatologist has a vital role to play in terms of diagnosis and management of musculoskeletal problems in older people.

Rheumatological practice in old age brings with it a number of challenges that set it apart from the treatment of middle-aged adults, not least the paucity of evidence as old age is often an exclusion from clinical trials.[4] Although some conditions are seen in adults of all ages, the clinical presentation and treatment goals will differ in the frail older person with complex comorbidities. Furthermore, there are some specific conditions that are seen mainly in old age, such as polymyalgia rheumatica.

Epidemiology

The prevalence of degenerative and some inflammatory musculoskeletal diseases increase with age. Osteoarthritis is the most common joint disorder seen in Europe and North America.[5,6] The prevalence varies depending on the definition and joint(s) that are considered. A recent cohort study performed in the Netherlands found that 67% of women and 55% of men aged over 55 years had radiographic evidence of osteoarthritis of their hands.[7] However, not all patients with radiographic changes of arthritis are symptomatic and this may result in discrepancies between different studies of the prevalence of osteoarthritis in various joints. While osteoarthritis is the most common form, affecting women more than men (GP notes diagnosis: knee 33%, hip 20%, hand 9% in women vs. knee 27%, hip 13%, hand 5% in men who reach 85 years[3]). Soft tissue problems, including shoulder problems (adhesive capsulitis, rotator cuff disease, bicipital tendonitis), greater trochanter pain syndrome (the equivalent 'rotator cuff disease of the hip' previously thought to be trochanteric bursitis) and axial disease (including neck and back syndromes) are also more common. Back pain has different implications in this age group, with age itself being a key 'red flag' triggering investigation to rule out a differential diagnosis which includes osteoporotic collapse and malignancy.

Rheumatoid arthritis (RA) also becomes more common from middle age onwards, reaching a prevalence of 5% in females at 85, compared to 0.5% of males. This is a key learning point, as RA is often wrongly stated to be most common in middle age. The rising age-specific incidence and rare occurrence of remission determines that prevalence increases progressively with age.

Crystal arthritis is also more common, with incident gout in 4.4 men vs. 1.3 women per 1000 patient-years in the UK, with the highest rate in those over 80 years.[8] Over a 52-year follow up of the Framingham cohort, 200 men (period prevalence 10%) and 104 of women (4%) developed gout, with similar predictors in men and women: increasing age, obesity, alcohol consumption, hypertension, and diuretic use.[9] Calcium pyrophosphate deposition (CPPD) now has agreed terminology and diagnostic recommendations,[10] with risk factors including ageing, osteoarthritis, and metabolic conditions such as primary hyperparathyroidism, haemochromatosis and hypomagnesaemia. The prevalence of CPPD is 7–10% in those aged 60 years—equal in men and women.[11]

The Hordaland Health Study in Norway reported that the prevalence of primary Sjögren's syndrome was approximately seven times higher in the elderly population (age 71–74 years) compared with individuals aged 40–44 years.[12] Reported prevalence rates vary from 0.1% to 2.7%, depending on the population studied and the classification criteria used.[13] Increased survival and higher incidence rates of systemic lupus erythematosus (SLE) contribute to an increasing prevalence of SLE in the elderly population. Most estimates vary from 0.15% to 0.51%, although some based on self-report diagnosis are as high as 1.2%.

Definitions, classification criteria and diagnostic criteria where appropriate

Frailty

The syndrome of physical frailty in old age is easy to recognize, but perhaps more difficult to define. Various definitions of 'frailty' have been proposed, ranging from the social model focusing on functional dependence to descriptions based on medical comorbidities.[14] Frailty certainly encompasses loss of independence in one's activities of daily living. However, this is a simplistic notion and fails to acknowledge that frailty in the older person is probably a dynamic rather than a static concept. For any individual, there will be a number of different factors that determine if they can still live independently in their own home. This dynamic model of frailty was first described by Brocklehurst,[15] and describes the assets and deficits that help an older person retain their independence in the community. These assets and deficits include a mixture of socio-economic and medical factors. This concept of the dynamic model of frailty is useful to the clinician. In a fit elderly person, their assets will clearly outweigh any concurrent deficits. However, in someone who is more frail, there will be a fine balance between the positive and negative factors that affect independent living. Only a small change in their condition will be required in order to tip the balance in favour of deficits, resulting in loss of independence. This tipping point could be a relatively minor insult that would cause only inconvenience to a younger patient, e.g. a urinary tract infection or monoarticular flare of arthritis.

This view of frailty as a dynamic process is consistent with the decline in physiological reserve that can be recognized with ageing. Ageing is probably best considered as a continuum. The function of most organ systems reaches a peak in the mid-twenties and thereafter a gradual decline may be observed. The process of ageing occurs at a variable rate in different people, influenced by a number of intrinsic (genetic) and extrinsic (environmental and lifestyle) factors. In younger people, organ systems have considerable reserve capacity that is superfluous to normal daily requirements, but is available to respond to any severe physiological stress placed on the individual. Involutional changes with ageing lead to a gradual reduction in this reserve capacity and thus the older person may be unable to mount an adequate response to the additional physiological stresses imposed by acute illness or injury. This rapid decline in functional ability is often witnessed in clinical practice, for example following osteoporotic femoral neck fractures.

Sarcopenia

Changes in the musculoskeletal system with the advancing years are among the most obvious signs of age-related physiological decline. Most people achieve their peak muscle strength in their mid-twenties and in healthy individuals this remains fairly constant up to their fifth decade, at which time decline tends to occur. This age-related loss of muscle mass and strength is termed sarcopenia and is seen in more than 50% of people aged over 80 years. A recent large meta-analysis examined the patterns of loss of muscle strength seen in the general population, confirming the functional decline with age and the acceleration seen after the age of 50 years (0.37kg/yr for hand grip).[16] Sarcopenia is likely to be multifactorial in aetiology, with potential contributory causes including level of physical activity, metabolic, endocrine, and nutritional factors. Moreover, muscle strength is also adversely affected by the presence and duration of inflammatory conditions such as RA.

Age-related changes in bone structure and density are covered in detail elsewhere in this book. However, any discussion of the musculoskeletal system in the older patient must include some consideration of the impact of osteoporosis. Patients with RA, osteoarthritis, and the other conditions mentioned in this chapter are at increased risk of osteoporosis, not only due to their relative immobility but also because many of their prescribed medications can contribute to bone loss. Thus, the role of the rheumatologist

includes consideration of the need for anti-resorptive therapy in all older patients, especially those receiving long-term corticosteroid therapy. This would generally be done after calculation of the 10-year fracture risk using the FRAX website (www.sheffield.ac.uk/FRAX/) or downloadable freestanding app, and linking to the treatment recommendation according to the National Osteoporosis Guideline Group recommendations,[17] in view of ongoing controversy with respect to the NICE technology appraisals[18,19] and in the continued absence of a NICE Clinical Guideline in this area (see Chapter 151).

Clinical features

General principles of disease presentation in old age

Clinical diagnosis in older patients is often fraught with difficulty. Patients may minimize, discount, or ignore relevant symptoms, assuming that these are simply part of the normal ageing process. Furthermore, atypical or non-specific disease presentation is frequent in elderly people. The late Professor Bernard Isaacs first coined the phrase 'geriatric giants' to describe the common clinical presentations seen in older people.[20] The original giants as described by Isaacs were the '4 I s' of Incontinence, Immobility, Impaired intellect (delirium), and Instability (falls). He claimed that, if the physician looked closely enough, all common problems with older people could be related back to one of these giants. In the case of rheumatological disease, there is no doubt that musculoskeletal disease is a major contributor to the risk of immobility and falls in the older person. While the relevance of the other geriatric giants may be initially less obvious, immobility resulting from osteoarthritis could contribute to urinary incontinence and opioid analgesics prescribed for the same condition could cause acute confusion. Indeed, to the original 4 Is described by Isaacs, we should probably add another two: Iatrogenic disease and Inability to look after oneself. The former recognizes the increased likelihood of adverse reactions to medications in older people and the latter the functional decline that often accompanies illness in old age, akin to the syndrome of failure to thrive in children.

Multiple comorbidities

The presence of multiple comorbid illnesses is the norm rather than the exception in older patients. As noted above, disease presentation in old age is often non-specific, with one or more of the geriatric giants. Furthermore, many of the symptoms of rheumatological disease are themselves quite non-specific, for example fatigue, aches, and pains. Patients may find it difficult to describe their current symptoms, especially if they accustomed to some degree of chronic discomfort relating to pre-existing conditions. Diagnosis of musculoskeletal complaints in older individuals with chronic health problems is thus more challenging than in younger patients with symptoms due to a single condition. In the elderly, it is not uncommon for more than one rheumatological illness to coexist in the same person, for example polymyalgia rheumatica and degenerative disease of the cervical spine. In such cases, it may be difficult for the physician to determine the relative contribution of each condition to the patient's overall symptom burden and treatment decisions can be challenging. Moreover, some non-rheumatic conditions that are common in older age groups can present with musculoskeletal symptoms. An example of this is statin-induced myopathy, which can develop after prolonged treatment with HMG CoA reductase inhibitors for hypercholesterolaemia and may mimic polymyositis.[21] In addition, treatments prescribed for chronic illnesses in other body systems can themselves lead to the development of musculoskeletal conditions. Acute gout is not uncommon in patients given large doses of loop diuretics for congestive heart failure.

Case history

A 72-year-old retired miner with a 7-year history of seropositive (titre 1:320) RA and mild generalized osteoarthritis developed haemoptysis, anorexia, and weight loss. He had a 6-year history of diet controlled, non-insulin dependent diabetes mellitus, hypercholesterolaemia, ischaemic heart disease (myocardial infarction 1978, triple coronary artery bypass grafting 1978 and 1982). He had had right carpal tunnel decompression in 2000 and been diagnosed with emphysema and coal workers pneumoconiosis by the respiratory team 5 years previously. His wife also had RA and they lived in a bungalow with good support from family and friends. He was an ex-smoker of 50 packet-years. Both he and his wife were involved in undergraduate teaching of third-year medical students.

He was taking subcutaneous methotrexate 35 mg weekly, with oral folate, aspirin, omeprazole, paracetamol, iron, simvastatin; and beclomethasone and salbutamol inhalers.

A chest radiograph showed a mass at the right hilum with peripheral consolidation. This was confirmed on bronchoscopy to be a squamous cell carcinoma, but did not respond to radiotherapy and he died 6 months later with metastatic disease of the liver and bones.

Functional and social problems

The presence of multiple comorbidities, together with the propensity of acute illness to manifest in non-specific ways, means that older people often present to healthcare services as a result of a decline in their functional abilities. Terms such as 'social admission' should always be avoided, since in the vast majority of cases underlying illness, injury, drug toxicity, or withdrawal will be diagnosed after appropriate investigation. As mentioned above, relatively minor insults such as constipation, urinary infection, or new joint pain can be sufficient to precipitate a rapid functional decline in a frail older person. Indeed, it is often the combination of several small physiological insults that results in the crisis admission to secondary care.

It is evident that clinical assessment of any older person with a musculoskeletal problem is incomplete without due consideration of the impact of their symptoms on their functional abilities. Evaluation of the patient by history and examination should incorporate inspection of their gait, as is routine in rheumatological practice. However, in the frail older person it is also advisable to assess the safety of their transfers and this can be combined with observation of their gait in the 'get up and go test'.[22] The challenge for the rheumatologist may be to determine the relative contribution of several coexisting problems to the patient's current immobility, for example antalgic gait in an older person with kyphosis, low back pain, and arthritic knees. Clinical assessment of the patient can be supplemented by the use of standardized scales, which quantify the ability of the patient to carry out common everyday tasks or activities of daily living (ADL). The Barthel Index is used commonly in UK clinical practice and assesses the most basic personal ADL such as feeding, dressing, bathing, and toileting.[23] Patients who are dependent in one or more of these ADLs are likely to require daily support from others.

The term 'comprehensive geriatric assessment' is often used to describe the multidisciplinary team approach to the management of the frail older person presenting with a recent functional decline. This assessment should encompass social and functional problems as well as medical and psychiatric issues and the resulting management plan should usually include rehabilitation in addition to medical treatments. The functional issues arising from musculoskeletal illness are not restricted to older patients, as many younger people with rheumatological conditions may also experience difficulties with personal or extended ADLs. Rheumatologists are well placed to recognize such disability in their older patients and are likely to work within established multidisciplinary teams with considerable experience in musculoskeletal rehabilitation. In the older patient, the social and psychological aspects of their condition may be especially challenging. The former may include social isolation, recent bereavement or change in accommodation; the latter is discussed in more detail below.

Depression, delirium, and dementia

Depression is a common accompaniment to many chronic diseases, including musculoskeletal conditions. The aetiology of depression in patients with chronic illness is not well understood, but is likely to be multifactorial; contributory factors may include the patient's emotional response to the diagnosis, the functional limitations imposed by the illness and, especially in the case of many rheumatological problems, the effects of chronic pain. Moreover, the relationship between depression and the coexisting chronic physical illness can complicate the clinical presentation, diagnosis, and management of both conditions. Depression in older people can lead to concordance issues with the treatments prescribed for other illnesses. This can be of particular concern with the use of drugs that require strict adherence to a dosage and monitoring schedule, for example disease-modifying anti-rheumatic drugs (DMARDs) in patients with inflammatory arthropathies. A recent systematic review examined 14 studies of varying interventions in older people with osteoarthritis and depression. Strategies such as cognitive behavioural therapy, integrated depression care management, and exercise therapy were associated with a short-term reduction in depressive symptoms. The long-term benefits of depression management in patients with osteoarthritis are unclear.[24] However, physicians must be alert to the possibility that depression may be contributing to the clinical picture in older patients presenting with musculoskeletal problems, especially when symptoms fail to respond as anticipated to usual treatments. Standardized assessment tools such as the Geriatric Depression Scale[25] may be useful in screening for low mood when there is clinical suspicion.

Delirium or 'acute confusional state' is one of the four geriatric giants originally described by Isaacs. The clinical features include disturbances in consciousness, cognition, and perception. The onset is acute, developing over one or two days, and there is often a pronounced diurnal fluctuation in symptoms. Delirium can be difficult to distinguish from dementia when the time course of symptoms is unclear, particularly since elderly people and those with pre-existing cognitive problems are at increased risk of developing delirium. The prevalence of delirium amongst hospital in-patients is estimated to be 20–30% on general medical wards and 10–50% on surgical wards.[26] The consequences of delirium are significant both for the individuals affected and for health and social care services. Delirium is associated with longer length of stay in hospital, more frequent complications, higher mortality rates, and increased likelihood of discharge to institutional care. Delirium may be precipitated by acute illness, injury, systemic insult, drug toxicity or withdrawal, and often by a combination of several of these factors. It is particularly common after fractures of the femoral neck in frail older people, who often have an underlying acute illness that contributed to their fall and then require emergency orthopaedic surgery. However, delirium may also occur after elective surgery such as joint replacement and it is important that any preoperative consultation between physician, patient, and carers should include discussion of the possibility of postoperative confusion.[27] A detailed description of the management of delirium is beyond the scope of this chapter. However, rheumatologists need to be aware of the risks of delirium in any of their older patients, particularly when hospitalized with acute illness and including exacerbations of their joint disease. NICE recommends screening all patients aged over 65 years for risk of delirium, and standardized tools such as the Confusion Assessment Method (CAM) can be helpful in this regard. Interventions such as medication review and management of treatable symptoms such as pain, constipation, and dehydration can be helpful in both the prevention and management of delirium in the older patient. In difficult cases, advice may be sought from colleagues in geriatric medicine.

As with musculoskeletal disorders, the risk of developing dementia increases with age. The rheumatologist is therefore likely to encounter patients with coexisting musculoskeletal and cognitive problems. The prevalence of dementia is estimated to be around 10% in people aged over 65 years, rising to more than 20% of those over 80. Alzheimer's disease is the most common form of dementia, accounting for about two-thirds of cases, with other frequent causes being vascular dementia and dementia with Lewy bodies. All types of dementia lead to progressive cognitive deficits, with a resulting decline in functional abilities. Patients with dementia lose the ability to handle new information and may also develop loss of executive function, with difficulties in organization, planning, and sequencing. This will be of concern to clinicians who wish to initiate complex treatment regimens for newly diagnosed illnesses such as RA, but are worried about the patient's ability to adhere to the prescribed treatment. Disorders of speech and language such as dysphasia are not confined to patients with cerebrovascular cognitive impairment, but may also be seen in other forms of dementia. Diagnosis of musculoskeletal complaints may be challenging in patients who have such word-finding difficulties and are unable to provide a clear description of their symptoms. Non-verbal cues to the presence of symptoms like pain assume more importance, and the observations of the patient's carers regarding their recent behaviour can be invaluable. Behavioural changes such as agitation, aggression, and wandering become more prevalent with advancing dementia. Although pain is not the only possible explanation for agitation in a person with dementia, physicians should ensure that adequate analgesia is prescribed for patients with known or suspected musculoskeletal complaints. A recent cluster randomized controlled trial has in fact shown that a systematic approach to the management of pain, using a stepwise protocol starting with paracetamol, resulted in a significant reduction in agitation in nursing home residents with moderate to severe dementia.[28] In the later stages of dementia, the patient may become physically dependent on others and develop dysphagia, leading to difficulties swallowing food, fluids, and medication. In such cases, pragmatic decisions regarding symptomatic treatment of coexisting musculoskeletal complaints should be made in conjunction with the patient's family and general practitioner. In such cases a palliative approach to end-of-life care may be appropriate.

Case history

Edward was a retired teacher with a 10-year history of seronegative RA. His symptoms responded initially to treatment with methotrexate 15 mg weekly, but he could not tolerate a higher dose, which gave him gastrointestinal upset, despite folate supplementation on the other days of the week. This had to be stepped up to triple therapy (adding sulfasalazine and hydroxychloroquine) following a polyarticular flare of his disease that required a short period of in-patient treatment.

There followed a year of clinical stability on his new drug regime, which was monitored with monthly blood tests at the GP's surgery and annual review at the rheumatology nurse clinic. At this appointment Edward's wife reported to the nurse that her husband was becoming forgetful and often needed to be reminded to take his arthritis medication.

Three days after his 75th birthday, Edward was admitted to the acute geriatric assessment unit with delirium and urinary incontinence. His inflammatory markers are raised and he was noted to have a swollen, painful right knee. Joint aspiration excludes septic arthritis and a rheumatology consult confirmed an exacerbation of his inflammatory arthritis. Analgesia was prescribed and his triple therapy continued.

Edward's daughter reported that his wife died 2 months before this admission to hospital and the family were concerned that he had been failing to cope at home because of his poor memory. A full multidisciplinary assessment was undertaken before Edward was discharged from hospital, including supply of a medication dosette box from the community pharmacy. He was also referred to the memory clinic, where a diagnosis of Alzheimer's disease was confirmed.

Three months later, Edward was readmitted to hospital after being found on the floor by his carer. He had fractured his right neck of femur, which required internal fixation under general anaesthesia. After a prolonged period of postoperative delirium, he was transferred to the orthogeriatric ward for rehabilitation. He remained confused, did not regain his previous level of mobility, and could only walk a few metres with a frame. He was discharged to a nursing home. Over the next few months, Edward's condition deteriorated gradually and his verbal output diminished. He had difficulty expressing his needs. The care staff reported to his GP that he sometimes refused his medication. After consulting Edward's daughter and his rheumatologist, the GP stopped the triple therapy and prescribed regular non-oral analgesia and as required intramuscular corticosteroid. Edward was commenced on the Liverpool Care Pathway (LCP) and died peacefully 3 weeks later.

Differences in disease in the elderly

It is worth considering the relevance of new classification criteria and guidelines to musculoskeletal disease in the elderly. These include the new EULAR/ACR classification criteria for RA,[29] which have not yet been validated in any elderly population, but have similar discrimination to previous criteria in younger populations (e.g. Britsemmer et al.[30]). Subtypes of disease have been described, for example benign RA of the elderly[31–33] and remitting seronegative symmetrical synovitis with pitting oedema (RS3PE),[34] both of which have an excellent prognosis. It would be useful for these subtypes to be investigated using current imaging modalities—especially musculoskeletal ultrasound to confirm that synovitis is present, as polymyalgia rheumatica is an important differential diagnosis in the this age group. There are particular challenges for implementing the clinical guidance for RA[35] in this age group, who may not wish to attend hospital so frequently and may be reluctant to start combination regimes of disease-modifying drugs, especially if they are already taking several medications for comorbid conditions.

Osteoarthritis has clear clinical guidance,[36] which explicitly flags that age is no barrier to key non-pharmacological interventions: education, aerobic and strengthening exercise, and weight loss advice. However, there are increased risks drugs such as non-steroidal anti-inflammatories, including cardiovascular and cerebrovascular risks. There is also new data showing that over-the-counter medications like paracetamol are not without risk and have very modest efficacy: 20% of those taking 3 g of paracetamol for knee pain over 3 months had a drop in haemoglobin of 1 g/dL or more.[10,37]

Drugs in older people

Elderly people have a higher frequency of chronic renal impairment of varying degrees, so dose adjustment will often be necessary for drugs like methotrexate, where clearance is by the kidneys. A typical patient with RA might start on methotrexate monotherapy and escalate to 15 or 20 mg orally per week, depending on renal function, compared to the usual target dose of 25 mg (although there are exceptions—see case history). Similarly, colchicine doses should be reduced, so that acute gout attacks, or the introduction of prophylactic therapy can be covered with 500 micrograms once a day, or even alternate days, rather than usual regime of two to three times a day.

The coexistence of cardio- and/or cerebrovascular disease also warrants extreme caution in the prescribing of non-steroidal anti-inflammatory drugs in this age group and preference for naproxen in those who need them. Coprescription of a proton pump inhibitor is even more cost effective than in younger patients in mitigating the upper gastrointestinal risks.

In contrast, dose reduction of leflunomide is not recommended. However, interactions are more common in view of polypharmacy, including consideration of agents such as warfarin, with the potential for life threatening bleeds; or inducers of the cytochrome P450 system, which can have effects on the clearance of many drugs.

References

1. Urwin M, Symmons D, Allison T et al. Estimating the burden of musculoskeletal disorders in the community: the comparative prevalence of symptoms at different anatomical sites, and the relation to social deprivation. *Ann Rheum Dis* 1998;57(11):649–655.

2. Centers for Disease Control and Prevention. Prevalence of doctor-diagnosed arthritis and arthritis-attributable activity limitation—United States, 2007–2009. *MMWR Morb Mortal Wkly Rep* 2010;59(39):1261–1265.

3. Duncan R, Francis RM, Collerton J et al. Prevalence of arthritis and joint pain in the oldest old: findings from the Newcastle 85+ Study. *Age Ageing* 2011;40(6):752–725.

4. Peat G, Birrell F, Cumming J et al. Arthritis Research UK Clinical Studies Group for Osteoarthritis and Crystal Diseases. Under-representation of the elderly in osteoarthritis clinical trials. *Rheumatology (Oxford)* 2011;50(7):1184–1186.

5. Lane NE. Clinical practice. Osteoarthritis of the hip. *N Engl J Med* 2007;357(14):1413–1421.

6. Bijlsma JW, Berenbaum F, Lafeber FP. Osteoarthritis: an update with relevance for clinical practice. *Lancet* 2011;377(9783):2115–2126.

7. Dahaghin S, Bierma-Zeinstra SM, Ginai AZ et al. Prevalence and pattern of radiographic hand osteoarthritis and association with pain and disability (the Rotterdam study). *Ann Rheum Dis*. 2005;64(5):682–687. Erratum in: Ann Rheum Dis 2005;64(8):1248.

8. Cea Soriano L, Rothenbacher D, Choi HK, García Rodríguez LA. Contemporary epidemiology of gout in the UK general population. *Arthritis Res Ther* 2011;13(2):R39.

9. Bhole V, de Vera M, Rahman MM, Krishnan E, Choi H. Epidemiology of gout in women: Fifty-two-year follow-up of a prospective cohort. *Arthritis Rheum* 2010;62(4):1069–1076.

10. Zhang W, Nuki G, Moskowitz RW et al. OARSI recommendations for the management of hip and knee osteoarthritis: part III: Changes in evidence following systematic cumulative update of research published through January 2009. *Osteoarthritis Cartilage* 2010;18(4):476–499.

11. Richette P, Bardin T, Doherty M. An update on the epidemiology of calcium pyrophosphate dihydrate crystal deposition disease. *Rheumatology (Oxford)*. 2009;48(7):711–715.

12. Haugen AJ, Peen E, Hultén B et al. Estimation of the prevalence of primary Sjögren's syndrome in two age-different community-based populations using two sets of classification criteria: the Hordaland Health Study. *Scand J Rheumatol* 2008;37(1):30–34.

13. Gabriel SE, Michaud K. Epidemiological studies in incidence, prevalence, mortality, and comorbidity of the rheumatic diseases. *Arthritis Res Ther* 2009;11(3):229.

14. Rockwood K, Fox RA, Stolee P, Robertson D, Beattie BL. Frailty in elderly people: an evolving concept. *Can Med Assoc J* 1994; 150:489–495.

15. Brocklehurst JC (ed.) The day hospital. In: *Textbook of* geriatric medicine and geron*tology*, 3rd edn. Churchill Livingstone, London, 1985: 982–995.

16. Beenakker KGM, Ling CH, Meskers CGM et al. Patterns of muscle strength loss with age in the general population and patients with a chronic inflammatory state. *Ageing Res Rev* 2010;9:431–436.

17. Compston J, Cooper A, Cooper C et al. National Osteoporosis Guideline Group (NOGG). Guidelines for the diagnosis and management of osteoporosis in postmenopausal women and men from the age of 50 years in the UK. *Maturitas* 2009;62(2):105–108.

18. NICE. *Alendronate, etidronate, risedronate, raloxifene and strontium ranelate for the primary prevention of osteoporotic fragility fractures in postmenopausal women (TA 160)*. National Institute for Health and Clinical Excellence, London, 2011.

19. NICE. *Alendronate, etidronate, risedronate, raloxifene, strontium ranelate and teriparatide for the secondary prevention of osteoporotic fragility fractures in postmenopausal women (TA 161)*. National Institute for Health and Clinical Excellence, London, 2011.

20. Isaacs B. *The challenge of geriatric medicine*. Oxford University Press, Oxford, 1992.

21. Fernandez G, Spatz ES, Jabliecki C, Phillips PS. Statin myopathy: a common dilemma not reflected in clinical trials. *Cleve Clin J Med* 2011;78:393–403.

22. Quinn TJ, McArthur K, Ellis G, Stott DJ. Functional assessment in older people. *BMJ* 2011;343:d4681.

23. Mahoney FI, Barthel D. Functional evaluation; the Barthel Index. *Maryland State Med J* 1965;14:61–65.

24. Yohannes AM, Caton S. Management of depression in older people with osteoarthritis: a systematic review. *Aging Mental Health* 2010;6:637–651.

25. Yesavage JA, Brink TL, Rose TL et al. Development and validation of a geriatric depression rating scale: a preliminary report. *J Psych Res* 1983;17:27.

26. NICE. *Delirium: diagnosis, prevention and management (CG103)*. National Institute for Health and Clinical Excellence, London, 2010.

27. Ramaiah R, Lam AM. Postoperative cognitive dysfunction in the elderly. *Anesthesiology Clin* 2009;27:485–496.

28. Husebo BS, Ballard C, Sandvik R, Nilsen OB, Aarsland D. Efficacy of treating pain to reduce behavioural disturbances in residents of nursing homes with dementia: cluster randomised clinical trial. *BMJ* 2011;343:d4065.

29. Aletaha D, Neogi T, Silman AJ et al. 2010 Rheumatoid arthritis classification criteria: an American College of Rheumatology/European League Against Rheumatism collaborative initiative. *Ann Rheum Dis* 2010;69:1580–1588.

30. Britsemmer K, Ursum J, Gerritsen M, van Tuyl L, van Schaardenburg D. Validation of the 2010 ACR/EULAR classification criteria for rheumatoid arthritis: slight improvement over the 1987 ACR criteria. *Ann Rheum Dis* 2011;70(8):1468–1470.

31. Kinsella RA. Proceedings of the Interstate Postgraduate Medical Assembly of North America. 1942:13.

32. Porsmann VA. *Proceedings of the Congress of European Rheumatology, vol 2*. Editorial Scienta, Barcelona, Spain, 1951:479.

33. Corrigan AB, Robinson RG, Terenty TR, Dick-Smith JB, Walters D. Benign rheumatoid arthritis of the aged. *Br Med J* 1974;1(5905):444–446.

34. McCarty DJ, O'Duffy JD, Pearson L, Hunter JB. Remitting seronegative symmetrical synovitis with pitting edema. RS3PE syndrome. *JAMA* 1985;254(19):2763–2767.

35. NICE. *Rheumatoid arthritis: the management of rheumatoid arthritis in adults (CG79)*. National Institute for Health and Clinical Excellence, London, 2009.

36. NICE. *Osteoarthritis—The care and management of osteoarthritis in adults (CG59)*. National Institute for Health and Clinical Excellence, London, 2009.

37. Doherty M, Hawkey C, Goulder M et al. A randomised controlled trial of ibuprofen, paracetamol or a combination tablet of ibuprofen/paracetamol in community-derived people with knee pain. *Ann Rheum Dis* 2011;70(9):1534–1541.

Further reading

Bowker L, Price J, Smith S. *Oxford handbook of geriatric medicine*, 2nd edn. Oxford University Press, Oxford, 2012.

Grimley Evans J, Franklin Williams T, Michel J-P, Beattie L. *Oxford textbook of geriatric medicine*, 2nd edn. Oxford University Press, Oxford, 2000.

NICE. *Osteoporosis: assessing the risk of fragility fracture (CG146)*. National Institute for Health and Clinical Excellence, London, 2012.

CHAPTER 5

Principles of clinical examination in children

Sharmila Jandial and Helen Foster

Background

Musculoskeletal (MSK) presentations in childhood are common and rank highly in the self-reported health problems amongst adolescents.[1] MSK presentations result from a spectrum of causes (Table 5.1),[2] and the majority are benign and self-limiting although it is important to note that MSK symptoms can be presenting features of potentially life-threatening conditions such as malignancy, sepsis, vasculitis and non-accidental injury. Furthermore, MSK features often have associations with many chronic paediatric conditions such as inflammatory bowel disease, cystic fibrosis and psoriasis. Referral pathways for children with MSK problems are often complex, depending on local health care provision and organization. Adult rheumatologists play an important part in the triage of children, are integral to referral to specialist paediatric services, and in many areas of the world continue to have a direct role in management of children and young people with rheumatic disease.

It is increasingly apparent that prompt, accurate diagnosis and specialist management are important to optimize outcomes in many MSK conditions in children and young people. This is especially important with acute conditions such as septic arthritis, osteomyelitis or malignancy (e.g. leukaemia or bone tumour) where delay can incur significant morbidity and indeed mortality, but also applies to orthopaedic conditions (such as slipped upper femoral epiphysis or Perthes' disease) or inflammatory arthritis such as juvenile idiopathic arthritis (JIA) where delay increases the risk of significant joint damage and functional disability. With inflammatory arthritis such as JIA, there has been a marked trend towards early and aggressive management in recent decades, with increasingly effective treatments such as methotrexate and biologicals. The importance of early diagnosis and prompt referral to specialist teams is therefore increasingly relevant.[3–6]

The reported global delay in access to care for JIA and other conditions with MSK presentations such as muscular dystrophy and cancer[7,8], is likely multifactorial but evidence clearly highlights the need to improve MSK clinical skills amongst healthcare professionals to whom children may present. Invariably, children do not present directly to paediatric rheumatologists or paediatric orthopaedic surgeons, but to primary care or paediatricians, who will through their assessment, determine subsequent management and referral pathways to specialist services. Within clinical practice poor documentation of MSK assessment

Table 5.1 Differential diagnosis of musculoskeletal pain in children and adolescents

Life-threatening conditions	Malignancy (leukaemia, lymphoma, bone tumour)
	Sepsis (septic arthritis, osteomyelitis)
	Non-accidental injury
Joint pain with minimal or no swelling	Hypermobility syndromes
	Orthopaedic syndromes (e.g. Osgood–Schlatter disease, Perthes' disease)
	Idiopathic pain syndromes (reflex sympathetic dystrophy, fibromyalgia)
	Metabolic (e.g. hypothyroidism, lysosomal storage diseases)
	Tumour (benign and malignant)
Joint pain with swelling	Trauma (haemarthrosis)
	Infection
	Septic arthritis and osteomyelitis (viral, bacterial, mycobacterial)
	Reactive arthritis (postenteric, sexually acquired)
	Infection-related (rheumatic fever, post-vaccination)
	JIA
	Arthritis related to inflammatory bowel disease
	Connective tissue diseases (SLE, scleroderma, dermatomyositis, vasculitis)
	Metabolic (e.g. osteomalacia/rickets, cystic fibrosis)
	Haematological (e.g. haemophilia, haemoglobinopathy)
	Tumour (benign and malignant)
	Chromosomal (e.g. Down's-related arthritis)
	Auto-inflammatory syndromes (e.g. periodic syndromes, chronic recurrent multifocal osteomyelitis)
	Sarcoidosis
	Developmental/congenital (e.g. achondroplasia)

JIA, juvenile idiopathic arthritis; SLE, systemic lupus erythematosus.

Adapted from Foster H, Tucker LB. Musculoskeletal disorders in children and adolescents. In: Adebajo A (ed.) *ABC of rheumatology*, 4th edn. BMJ Books, London, 2009:98–106).

has been observed in general paediatric medical clerking, even in those children presenting with MSK symptoms,[9] and many doctors in primary and secondary care (including paediatrics, emergency medicine, and even orthopaedics) report poor self confidence in their paediatric MSK (pMSK) clinical skills;[10] such observations may be explained by pMSK clinical skills not being 'core' teaching in medical schools[11] or postgraduate programmes.[12]

Appropriate triage of children requires MSK clinical skills and knowledge to manage patients appropriately, and prompt referral. Acquisition of such 'core' pMSK clinical skills needs to start within undergraduate education as the foundation for further postgraduate training, with MSK assessment being integral to the assessment of all children and especially when a child presents with muscle, joint, or bone pain (with or without fever), limp, functional disability, delayed or regression of motor milestones, and in children with chronic conditions where MSK involvement is well recognized and can cause significant morbidity. Box 5.1 lists themes that are regarded as 'core' for all medical students to acquire by the time of graduation from medical school (S. Jandial, personal communication); this list was derived from using consensus methodology involving paediatricians and primary care doctors as well as specialists in paediatric rheumatology and orthopaedics and comprises generic skills (e.g. knowledge of 'red flags') as well as specific MSK (e.g. knowledge of normal development and indicators of pathology). The evidence-based approach to pMSK clinical examination includes a basic examination (pGALS) and a more detailed regional MSK examination (pREMS) which are described later in this chapter. Interpretation of pMSK assessment must be interpreted in the context of general assessment of the child, especially in the unwell child or in the context of red flags. A comprehensive account of detailed joint examination techniques in children and young people is not given here but suggested texts are provided as further reading.

'Children are not small adults' ... the approach to musculoskeletal clinical assessment in children and young people

The approach to pMSK assessment is quite different from that of adults,[13] needing awareness of age-related growth and development (as described in Chapter 1); this includes normal lower limb alignment, major motor milestones, and gait (Table 5.2), and knowledge and recognition of normal variants (Table 5.3). Indeed, many parental concerns arise from observations that may well be normal, e.g. flat feet in a preschool child. It is important to know that the spectrum of pathology varies with age, such as with the limping child (Table 5.4) and the child must be assessed carefully in the context of knowledge of normal development, and awareness of red flags (such as fever, malaise, anorexia, weight loss, bone pain, persistent night waking, or raised inflammatory markers) suggestive

---

Box 5.1 Core themes of undergraduate learning outcomes for pMSK medicine

Core paediatric skills

◆ Use appropriate behaviour and language, and modify history-taking and examination according to child's developmental stage

◆ Demonstrate an understanding of ways to engage children when examining to maintain cooperation and minimize discomfort.

◆ Outline the principles of managing children with chronic disease (e.g. considering impact on school, play, and family; need for medications and monitoring; and the role of healthcare professionals)

Attainment of clinical skills for pMSK medicine

◆ Recognize the need for extended musculoskeletal history in certain presentations (e.g. limp, pain, rashes, refusing to walk)

◆ Recognize features in the history that may distinguish mechanical from inflammatory musculoskeletal pathology

◆ Perform a basic examination of the musculoskeletal system (e.g. pGALS) understanding that positive findings should lead to more detailed examination incorporating a 'look, feel, move' approach.

Recognition of red flag conditions such as malignancy, infection, or inflammatory disease

◆ Recognize clinical features suggestive of a septic joint and the place of appropriate investigations and referral.

◆ Identify the role of blood tests such as full blood count or acute-phase reactants, and discuss these results in context of musculoskeletal presentations and potential implications (e.g. raised white cell count and possible sepsis)

◆ Describe musculoskeletal presentations of malignancy such as nocturnal bone pain, swelling, systemic features such as weight loss

Understand normal pMSK findings

◆ Recognize that normal children have increased joint flexibility compared to adults and may be hypermobile

◆ Observe and describe principles of gait patterns (e.g. symmetry, leg alignment, presence of pain, limp)

◆ Demonstrate awareness that leg alignment and foot posture changes with age and normal variants within these—knock knees, bow legs, flat feet, intoeing

Table 5.2 Normal variants of lower limb development

	Indications for concern and referral to physiotherapy or paediatric orthopaedics unless specified	Comments
Tiptoe walking Common in healthy young children	Toe walking is persistent or asymmetrical Associated developmental delay Child unable to squat or stand with heels on the floor (tightness of calf muscles) Child >3 years old, and unable to stand from floor-sitting without using hands	Can associate with clubfoot or neurological disease (e.g. muscular dystrophy, cerebral palsy, poliomyelitis). Careful neuromuscular/ assessment required. Check for gastrocnemius contracture and shoes for sole wear. Physiotherapy may help mild cases but surgery may be required
Flat feet Common and normal for babies and toddlers, resolves with development of longitudinal arch usually by 4–6 years of age	Signs of pressure on the foot, e.g. blistering Longitudinal arch does not form normally when the child stands on tiptoe Foot is stiff (i.e. the normal arch does not form when the child stands on tiptoe or the big toe is passively extended)	Persistence often familial, more common in hypermobility Insoles may help but should not be worn all the time—walking in bare feet helps promote foot development A non-flexible flat foot may indicate tarsal coalition (often teens) In newborn, exclude vertical talus
Pes cavus Not common—the opposite of flat feet; the arch is extremely pronounced	Often associated with toe clawing, calluses, heel varus, and pain, with footwear difficult to fit May be physiological (familial—so check parents' feet!), residual from clubfoot abnormality, or associated with neurological abnormalities—paediatric neurology/ orthopaedics referral usually needed	Careful neuromuscular/ musculoskeletal assessment required. Neurological conditions to consider include spina bifida, spinal dysraphism, poliomyelitis, Charcot–Marie–Tooth, Friedrich's ataxia Insoles may help and surgery may be required
Curly toes Most resolve by 4 years of age	Surgery rarely needed	Check shoes are well fitting
Knock knees Usually resolve by 6 years of age	Associated with pain or asymmetrical Extreme (>6 cm intermalleolar distance at ankles) or persistent (>6 years)	A gap of 6–7 cm between the ankles is normal (between 2–4 years) Late feature of arthritis of knee (e.g. JIA)
Bow legs Common and normally seen in children until the age of 2 years	Associated with pain or asymmetrical, or the child is short in stature or has other medical problems Extreme (>6 cm intercondylar distance at knees) or persistent (>6 years)	Conditions to exclude include rickets, skeletal dysplasias, syndromes associated with dwarfism (e.g. achondroplasia), Blount's disease Late feature of arthritis of knee (e.g. JIA)
Out-toeing Feet point outwards; usually resolves by 4 years	Recent onset in a teenager—check hips for a slipped upper femoral epiphysis	
Intoeing Feet turning inwards—'pigeon toed' Normal development for many toddlers when just learning to walk, usually resolved by 10 years	Persistence (>10 years) Affecting mobility and function (clumsy, prone to falling) Femoral anteversion and medial tibial torsion; usually resolve by 10 years of age Metatarsus adductus; usually resolve by 5 years of age	Check child's leg alignment when standing Femoral anteversion (90% of cases), patellae pointing inwards Medial tibial torsion (patellae point straight forward) Metatarsus adductus (forefoot abnormal only) Insoles and exercises will not help. Surgery rarely required

JIA, juvenile idiopathic arthritis.

of serious potentially life-threatening conditions such as sepsis or malignancy (see Chapters 13 and 14). Orthopaedic conditions at the hip are commonly present with the well child who is limping, often acutely, and include slipped upper femoral epiphysis (usually the older, often overweight child) and Perthes' disease which may follow a transient synovitis or 'irritable hip' in the younger child. Life-threatening conditions such as acute leukaemia may present with non-specific joint or muscle pain, and in a child with pyrexia of no apparent focus, MSK assessment is important to exclude bone or joint infection. The concept of referred pain from the hip or thigh, for example, must be sought in situations where the child has knee pain but there is no evidence of localized disease at the knee. The patterns of joint involvement in JIA differ from that of adult rheumatoid arthritis (e.g. oligoarticular JIA most commonly affects a single knee or ankle). A delay in major motor milestones may indicate MSK problems as well as neurological disease. However, *regression* of achieved motor milestones is more likely in acquired MSK disease, such as muscle or joint disease; for example, the child who was happy to walk unaided but has recently refused to walk or resorted to crawling again.

Young children may have difficulty in localizing or describing pain and the history is often given by the parent or carer, based

Table 5.3 Normal gait and musculoskeletal development

Sit without support	6–8 months
Creep on hands and knees	9–11 months
Cruise or bottom shuffle	11–12 months
Walk independently	12–14 months
Climb up stairs on hands and knees	~15 months
Run stiffly	~16 months
Walk down steps (non-reciprocal)	20–24 months
Walk up steps, alternate feet	3 years
Hop on one foot, broad jump	4 years
Skipping	5 years
Balance on one foot for 20 seconds	6–7 years
Adult gait and posture	8 years

Comments:

◆ There is considerable variation in the way normal gait patterns develop—such variation may be familial (e.g. 'bottom-shufflers' often walk later) and subject to racial variation (e.g. African black children tend to walk sooner and Asian children later than average.

◆ The normal toddler has a broad base gait for support, and appears to be high stepped and flat footed with arms outstretched for balance. The legs are externally rotated with a degree of bowing. Heel strike develops around 15–18 months with reciprocal arm swing.

◆ Running and change of direction occur after the age of 2 years, although this is often accompanied by frequent falls until the child acquires balance and coordination. In the school-age child, the step length increases and step frequency slows.

on observations from others (e.g. teacher) and may be rather vague with non-specific complaints such as 'my child is limping'. Symptoms such as pain, stiffness, decreasing ability (e.g. hand skills, handwriting, or sport), and reduced or altered interest in play activities may be observed and caregivers may have concerns about deterioration in behaviour (e.g. irritability, poor sleeping). Assessment of pain is important and may be conveyed through non-verbal signs such as withdrawal, crying, or distress (see Chapter 161).

The key features in the history-taking are described in Table 5.5. It is important to ask open questions and to enquire about mode of onset, site, distribution and nature of the symptoms and observations, features suggestive of multisystem involvement (e.g. rash, abdominal pain, headaches, Raynaud's, fatigue), and red flags that warrant concern. Distinguishing mechanical from inflammatory problems is similar to that in adults: for example, locking and instability of a joint may suggest internal derangement (e.g. meniscal injury) or osteochondritis disssecans (see Chapter 158). It is often necessary to probe for symptoms of inflammatory joint or muscle disease (e.g. asking about the child's mood, 'gelling' after periods of rest such as long car journeys, regression of achieved motor milestones, intermittent limping); a child will often adapt their activities to compensate for joint stiffness, pain, or weakness, and a change in the child's play or reluctance to participate in activities may signify inflammatory joint or muscle disease. It is important to ask about school, as MSK problems such as pain, stiffness, or weakness may create difficulties with school work, physical activity, and socialization; a change in academic performance, bullying, or school refusal can result and impact markedly on the child's global well-being, and enquiry about school and feedback from teachers or school nurse can therefore be revealing.

Table 5.4 Significant causes of limp, by age

	0–3 years	4–10 years	11–16 years
Most common	Trauma (including toddler's fracture)	Trauma Transient synovitis Perthes' disease	Trauma Osgood–Schlatter disease
Conditions requiring urgent intervention	Osteomyelitis Septic arthritis	Osteomyelitis Septic arthritis	Osteomyelitis Septic arthritis
	Non-accidental injury Malignancy (e.g. neuroblastoma)	Non-accidental injury Malignant disease (e.g. acute lymphocytic leukaemia)	Slipped upper femoral epiphysis Malignancy (e.g. bone tumours)
	Testicular torsion Inguinal hernia	Testicular torsion Appendicitis Inguinal hernia	Testicular torsion Appendicitis Inguinal hernia
Other important conditions to consider	Developmental dysplasia of the hip JIA	JIA	JIA
	Metabolic (e.g. rickets) Haematological disease (e.g. sickle cell anaemia) Reactive arthritis Lyme arthritis		

JIA, juvenile idiopathic arthritis.

Table 5.5 Key questions to ask when taking a musculoskeletal history

Questions to parent/ carer (and to the child as appropriate)	Points to check for	Comments
What have you or anyone else noticed?	Behaviour, mood, joint swelling, limping, bruising History of trauma	*Limping,* whether intermittent or persistent *always* warrants further assessment. Deterioration in school performance (e.g. sport, handwriting) or avoidance of previously enjoyed activities is always significant. *Joint swelling* is always significant but can be subtle and easily overlooked by the parent (and even healthcare professionals!), especially if the changes are symmetrical. Rather than describing stiffness, the parents may notice the child is reluctant to weight bear, or limps in the mornings, or 'gels' after periods of immobility (e.g. after long car rides or sitting in a classroom). *Trauma*—can be misleading as trauma is a common event in the lives of young children and not necessarily the appropriate explanation for a child's MSK symptoms. Conversely, not all trauma is witnessed by a parent or carer. Repeated episodes of trauma, pattern of injury, or incongruous circumstances or explanation raises concerns about *non-accidental injury*
What is the child like in him/ herself?	Irritability, grumpy, 'clingy', reluctant to play, systemic features (e.g. fever, anorexia, weight loss)	Young children in pain may not verbalize pain but may present with behavioural changes or avoidance of activities previously enjoyed. *Systemic features* including red flags to suggest malignancy or infection
Where is the pain? (ask the child to point) and what is it like?	Take a pain history and focus on locality, exacerbating/relieving factors, timescale, pattern	*Asymmetrical persistent site of pain* is invariably a cause for concern *Referred pain* from the hip may present with non-specific pain in the thigh or knee
How is he/she in the mornings and during the day?	Diurnal variation and daytime symptoms (e.g. limping, difficulty walking, dressing, toileting, stairs?)	*Pain on waking or daytime* symptoms suggestive of *stiffness or gelling* (after periods of inactivity), are indicative of inflammatory joint (or muscle) disease
What is he/she like with walking and running? Has there been any change in his activities?	Motor milestones and suggestion of delay or regression of achieved milestone, including speech and language. Avoidance of activities previously enjoyed (e.g. sport, play) are noteworthy. Mechanical problems may be suggested by *locking or giving way*	*Regression of achieved motor milestones,* functional impairment or avoidance of activity (including play, sport, or writing), are more suggestive of acquired joint or muscle disease (and especially inflammatory causes). An assessment of global neurodevelopment is indicated with delay or regression in speech, language or motor skills. *'Clumsiness'* is a non-specific term but may mask significant musculoskeletal or neurological disease
How is he/she at school or nursery?	School attendance (any suggestion of school avoidance, bullying)	*Behavioural problems* in the young child may manifest as non-specific pains (headaches, tummyaches, or leg pains). Sensitive questioning and may reveal stressful events at home or school
Does he/she wake at night with pain?	Pattern of night waking	*Night waking* is a common feature of growing pains (usually intermittent, and often predictable). Conversely, persistent night waking, especially if there are other concerns (such as unilaterality, limping, unusual location, or systemic features) are of concern and invariably necessitate further investigation
Can you predict when the pains may occur?	Relationship to physical activity (including during or after sporting activities)	Mechanical pains tend to be worse later in the day, evenings and often after busy days. Growing pains often follow busy days and are often predictable in their occurrence
What do you do when he/she is in pain?	Response to analgesics, anti-inflammatory medication, massages, and reaction of parent	Lack of response to simple analgesia is a concern. Vicious circle of reinforced behaviour can occur
What is your main concern?	Sleep disturbance, cosmesis, anxiety about serious disease (arthritis, cancer, family history), pain control	*A family history of muscle disease, arthritis, or autoimmune disease* may indicate a predisposition to muscle or joint disease. Observed 'abnormalities' (such as flat feet, curly toes) may be part of normal development. The parent or carer will undoubtedly have anxieties and concerns about the child, may often fear severe illness and both child and parent have an expectation of investigations (e.g. blood tests)

The full medical history with systematic enquiry into family and past history may be helpful, as many chronic conditions will have MSK associations: for example, inflammatory bowel disease can present initially with joint problems, which may be suggested by intolerance to NSAIDS, poor growth, or pattern of joint involvement such as isolated arthritis of the hip. A recent travel history (e.g. travel to an endemic area for Lyme disease) may be informative and a sexual history is important in the adolescent (e.g. reactive arthritis) although this needs to be explored sensitively and with acknowledgment of safeguarding concerns in the young and the need for privacy and confidentiality in the case of an adolescent patient. A medication history (e.g. response to NSAIDS, potential for drug-induced lupus), family history (e.g. autoimmune disease, muscle disease), and social history and family changes may be revealing. The approach proposed by Malleson and Beauchamp[14] incorporates potential diagnoses according to whether pain is localized or diffuse, whether the child is 'well' or not, and the presence of red flags.

It is notable that MSK history-taking in children, especially the very young, can be misleading; even when taken by experienced clinicians, the history alone may not identify sites of joint involvement.[15] It is important, therefore, that in all cases where MSK disease is suspected, physical examination is performed including an MSK basic examination as a minimum to assess all joints (see 'A musculoskeletal basic examination for children: pGALS'). This is exemplified in JIA, where the most common presenting features are joint swelling, limp, and reduced mobility, rather than pain;[16] notably, *the lack of reported pain does not exclude arthritis*. Swelling is the cardinal diagnostic feature of JIA but this can be subtle and easily overlooked by parents and carers and indeed may be missed in clinical examination, especially if the changes are symmetrical (e.g. swollen ankles in the young child) or the assessor is inexperienced. Children with learning disabilities can be more difficult to assess, and joint problems can easily be overlooked in the child with complex needs. There is an association of inflammatory joint disease with chromosomal disorders (such as Down's syndrome or di George syndrome),[17] and many children with complex genetic conditions (such as mucopolysaccharidoses) may present with or develop joint problems.

Non-specific MSK pain in children is common and often labelled as 'growing pains'; a confident diagnosis can be made when applying the 'rules of growing pains' (Table 5.6). Many children with non-specific aches and pains, including growing pains, are often found to have joint hypermobility, although not all hypermobile children are symptomatic.[18,19] It is important in the child with hypermobility to exclude rare but important syndromes (e.g. Marfan's, Stickler's, and Ehlers–Danlos syndromes), as these children are at risk of retinal and cardiac complications. Non-specific aches and pains may be a presenting feature of metabolic bone disease (such as osteomalacia) and in young children, may result in a waddling gait, leg bowing, irritability, and poor growth (see Chapter 150). Similarly, non-specific aches and pains are a feature of idiopathic pain syndromes, albeit typically, but not exclusively seen in older female children or adolescents, often in stressful social environments. Such patients are often markedly debilitated by their pain and fatigue; the pain can be incapacitating, although the child or adolescent is otherwise well and physical examination is normal (see Chapter 161).

The clinical assessment encompasses general evaluation including bodily systems, growth, and development especially if the child

Table 5.6 Growing pains

'Rules' of growing pains	Pains *never* present at the start of the day after waking
	Child does not limp
	Physical activities not limited by symptoms
	Pains symmetrical in lower limbs and not limited to joints
	Physical examination normal (joint hypermobility may or may not be detected)
	Systemically well and major motor milestones normal
	Age range 3–12 years
Indications for concern	Systemic upset (red flags to suggest sepsis or malignancy)
	Abnormal growth (height and weight)
	Abnormal developmental milestones: ◆ *Delay* (especially major motor skills) suggestive of neurological disease or metabolic bone disease, OR ◆ *Regression* of achieved motor milestones (consider inflammatory joint or muscle disease)
	Impaired functional ability (ask about play, sport, schoolwork, 'clumsiness')
	Limping (intermittent or persistent)
	Morning symptoms (other than tiredness after disturbed sleep) or mood changes may suggest inflammatory arthritis
	Widespread pain (such as upper limbs and back)
	School absenteeism

has complex needs or other comorbidities. Table 1.7 summarizes important features of rheumatic disease that can be elicited through a review of the systems. It is always important to assess the parent–child interaction and check for clues that may raise safeguarding concerns. Height and weight and general growth velocity can be assessed from review of growth charts in the parent-held record,[20] if available. Disproportionate limb and trunk growth may suggest dwarfism syndromes, and dysmorphism raises the suspicion of chromosomal or genetic conditions. Indolent presentations of chronic MSK disease can impact on growth (either localized or generalized) and stature, and may be compounded by use of corticosteroids or protracted disease activity from suboptimal treatment. Additional clinical skills that may be required, pending the clinical scenario, include nailfold capillaroscopy or muscle strength testing in suspected connective tissue or muscle disease and musculoskeletal ultrasound, which is increasingly used as an adjunct to clinical examination; these techniques are described elsewhere in the textbook.

A musculoskeletal basic examination for children: pGALS

The paediatric Gait, Arms, Legs, Spine (pGALS) assessment (Figure 5.1) is a simple evidence-based approach to musculoskeletal

pGALS – A basic musculoskeletal assessment for school-aged children

SCREENING QUESTIONS
- Do you have any pain or stiffness in your joints, muscles or your back?
- Do you have any difficulty getting yourself dressed without any help?
- Do you have any difficulty going up and down stairs?

GAIT
- Observe the child walking
- "Walk on your tip-toes / walk on your heels"

ARMS
- "Put your hands out in front of you"
- "Turn your hands over and make a fist"
- "Pinch your index finger and thumb together"
- "Touch the tips of your fingers with your thumb"
- Squeeze the metacarpophalangeal joints
- "Put your hands together / put your hands back to back"
- "Reach up and touch the sky"
- "Look at the ceiling"
- "Put your hands behind your neck"

LEGS
- Feel for effusion at the knee
- "Bend and then straighten your knee" (Active movement of knees and examiner feels for crepitus)
- Passive flexion (90 degrees) with internal rotation of hip

SPINE
- "Open your mouth and put 3 of your (child's own) fingers in your mouth"
- Lateral flexion of cervical spine – "Try and touch your shoulder with your ear"
- Observe the spine from behind
- "Can you bend and touch your toes?" Observe curve of the spine from side and behind

Fig. 5.1 The components of the pGALS musculoskeletal assessment (Table taken with permission, from *Hands On* pGALS—a paediatric musculoskeletal screening examination for children. www.arthritisresearchuk.org/~/media/Files/Education/Hands-On/HO15-June-2008.ashx).

Box 5.2 pGALS: practical tips

When performing the pGALS examination

- Check that the child is comfortable, ask about pain, and explain what you intend to do
- Observe the child walking in the room, getting undressed, at play
- Check that the child is adequately exposed (socks, shoes, and exposure of limbs)
- Get the child to copy you doing the manoeuvres
- Look for verbal and non-verbal clues of discomfort (e.g. facial expression, withdrawal) while they get undressed or perform manoeuvres
- Do the full screen, as extent of joint involvement may not be obvious from the history
- Look for asymmetry (e.g. muscle bulk, joint swelling, range of joint movement)
- Consider clinical patterns (e.g. non-benign hypermobility and marfanoid habitus or skin elasticity, and association of leg length discrepancy and scoliosis)

When to perform pGALS in the assessment

- Child with muscle, joint, or bone pain
- Unwell child with pyrexia
- Child with limp
- Delay or regression of motor milestones
- The 'clumsy' child in the absence of neurological disease
- Child with chronic disease and known association with musculoskeletal presentations

assessment based on the adult GALS (Gait, Arms, Legs, Spine) screen,[21] and has been shown to have high sensitivity in distinguishing abnormal from normal and detecting significant abnormalities.[22] The pGALS examination is aimed at non-specialists in paediatric rheumatology and is increasingly taught at medical schools in the UK and further afield; a full demonstration of pGALS and supportive documents are available as a web-based free resource: (www.arthritisresearchuk.org/health-professionals-and-students/video-resources/pgals.aspx)

pGALS was developed following testing of adult GALS in children which missed significant abnormalities especially at the foot, ankle, and wrist.[22] pGALS incorporates a series of simple manoeuvres, commonly used in clinical practice. pGALS takes an average of 2 minutes to perform and, although validated in the school-aged child, is often useful in younger children, who will often comply—especially if they copy the examiner and see this as a game. Box 5.2 lists simple practical tips to facilitate the examination and it is recommended that, as a minimum, pGALS should be done in all clinical scenarios where MSK disease is a concern. Overt MSK complaints, or a positive response to any of the three pGALS screening questions (Figure 5.1), necessitates a complete detailed MSK history and subsequent physical examination. However, a negative response to these questions in the context of a MSK complaint does *not* exclude significant MSK disease as in children, especially the very young, it is not uncommon to find joint involvement that has not been mentioned[15] as part of the presenting complaint. In other clinical contexts, the pGALS screening questions may be not be socio-culturally relevant (e.g. walking up

and down stairs in environments without steps, or getting dressed and undressed in hot countries where few clothes are worn)[23] and in such circumstances modification of the questions is required (e.g. rise from a squat position).

Key to appropriate interpretation of pGALS is knowledge of ranges of movement in different ethnicity and age groups[24], looking for asymmetry and careful examination for subtle changes. It is essential to perform all parts of pGALS as joint involvement may be apparently 'asymptomatic', symptoms may not be localized, and it is important to check for verbal and non-verbal clues of joint discomfort such as facial expression or withdrawal of limb. It has been shown that pGALS is practical and helpful in acute paediatric practice,[25] but needs to be interpreted in the context of the physical examination elsewhere (e.g. chest, abdomen, neurological examinations). pGALS was developed in the context of detecting inflammatory joint disease in children but has been shown to be useful in identifying other joint problems (e.g. orthopaedic problems at the hip, scoliosis, hypermobility).

Performing pGALS starts with observing the child coming into the room, interaction with the parent or carer, and their interest in play or activities such as using pencils or crayons. The child should ideally be undressed but compromise, patience, and opportunistic examination is often needed as many children are reluctant to undress—prior request to bring along shorts and T-shirt and provision of privacy to change will facilitate the assessment. As a minimum, the child should be barefoot, the legs exposed to include the knee and thigh and arms to include the elbows. The torso can be exposed to assess the spine in due course.

Observation with the child standing should be done from the front, from behind the child, and from the side. The examination of the upper limbs and neck is best done with the child sitting on an examination couch facing the examiner. The child can copy the various manoeuvres as they are performed by the examiner. The child should then lie supine to allow the legs to be examined and then stand again for spine assessment. Throughout pGALS, the sequence of 'look, feel, move' is followed and it is important to check carefully for symmetry as the changes can be subtle (skin changes, joint swelling and deformity, muscle bulk, and ranges of joint movement) (Figures 5.3 and 5.4).The features of inflammatory arthritis include joint swelling, warmth, loss of movement and tenderness on examination—an isolated hot red joint warrants mandatory investigation to exclude sepsis—however, in a well child with a monoarthritis, in the absence of trauma and sepsis, JIA is the most likely diagnosis.

From the front and back, leg alignment problems such as valgus and varus deformities can be observed. Scoliosis may be suggested by unequal shoulder height or asymmetrical skin creases on the trunk and may be more obvious on forward flexion (Figure 5.2). Subtle abnormalities at the ankle (such as swelling, valgus deformity) are often more obvious from behind the child (Figure 5.3). Leg length inequality may be more obvious from the side and suggested by a flexed posture at the knee; if found, then careful observation of the spine is important to exclude a secondary scoliosis.

Gait is assessed in the context of normal development (Table 5.3). Normal gait follows 'swing', 'stance', and 'toe-off' phases; a painful or antalgic gait leads to shortening of the stance phase on the affected limb, and therefore lengthening of the swing phase. Inability to walk on heels or on tiptoe is a good screening manoeuvre for the ankle and foot, especially as foot or ankle involvement is common in JIA, and enthesitis is a feature of

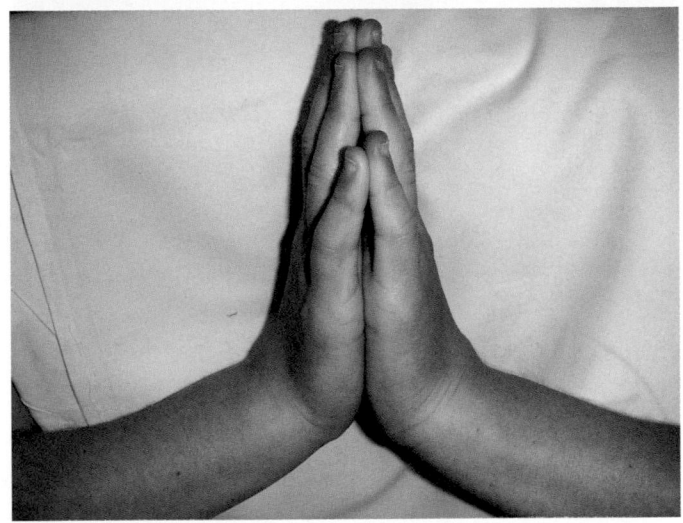

Fig. 5.3 Limited wrist extension and finger extension on pGALS.

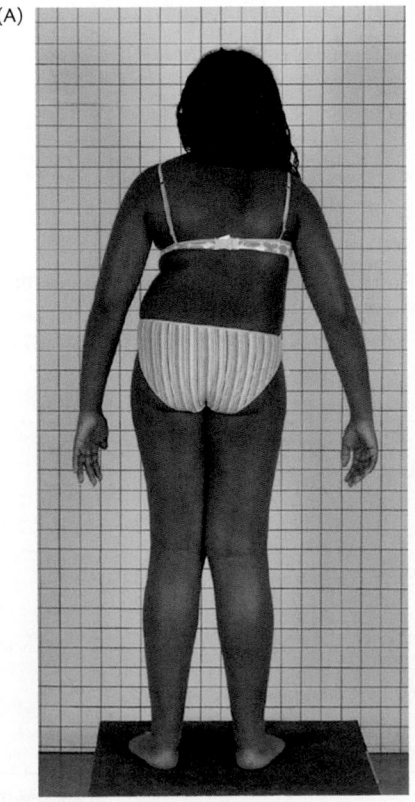
(A)

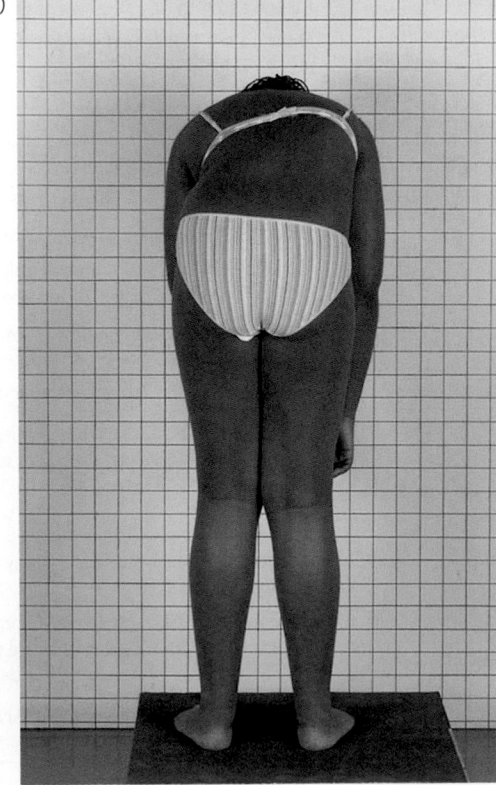
(B)

Fig. 5.2 Scoliosis.

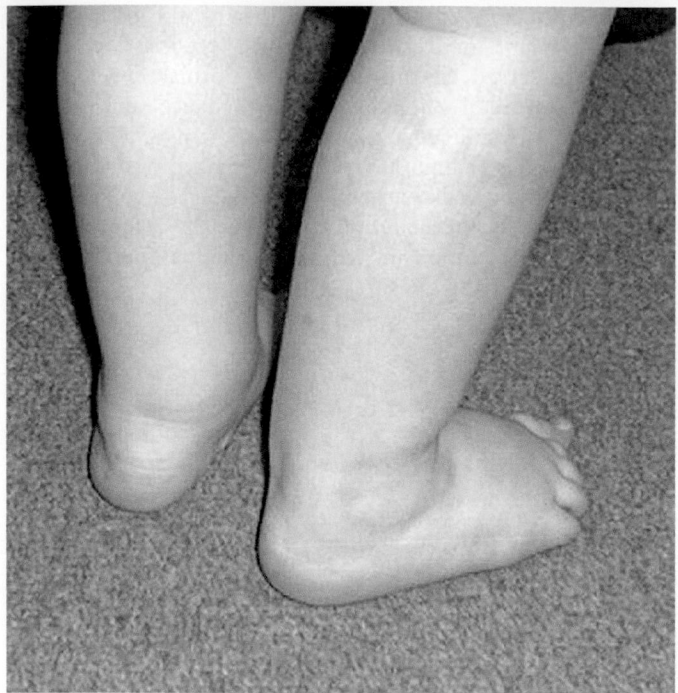

Fig. 5.4 Swelling of ankles, seen from behind.

enthesitis-related arthritis (ERA; a subtype of JIA). Sever's disease (an osteochondritis of the calcaneum) may also present with a painful heel but the site of tenderness is distal to the enthesis. Flat feet are common as a feature of normal development. Standing on tiptoe should create a normal medial longitudinal arch; inability to do so warrants further investigation (e.g. to exclude tarsal coalition). High fixed arches, pes cavus, and persistent toe walking may suggest neurological disease, but the latter has been reported as a feature of JIA.[26]

The pGALS assessment of the arms examines several joints together with each composite movement (Figure 5.1). The pGALS assessment of the legs with the child supine includes observing for leg length (check that the pelvis is straight to avoid false positives), symmetry of muscle bulk (quadriceps wasting is common with JIA involving the knee), and alignment (looking for valgus or varus deformity). Knowledge of characteristic patterns among the JIA subsets is helpful. For example, in a child with juvenile psoriatic arthritis, there may be asymmetrical joint involvement involving small and large joints, and this may include dactylitis or 'sausage digit' (due to arthritis and associated tenosynovitis). It is important to check the nails and skin for psoriasis as the rash of psoriasis can be subtle and typically follows the onset of the arthritis by several years, in contrast to adults with psoriatic arthritis. Isolated hip joint involvement is unusual as a presentation of JIA

Table 5.7 General examination in the context of musculoskeletal disease

	Features	Context and comments
General observations	Overall impression of the child's well-being Child's appearance, demeanour and interaction with parent or carer Features of dysmorphism (including facies and limbs) Height and weight plotted on a growth chart	An unwell child will require prompt admission and assessment for malignancy or sepsis Local safeguarding policies should be followed if concerned about non-accidental injury or neglect Faltering growth may be a sign of systemic or chronic disease Short stature or localized growth problems are features of chronic untreated disease or dwarfism syndromes
Skin inspection	Look for rashes including scalp and hair Overall feel of skin, including colour and texture	Skin psoriasis often presents on the extensor surfaces, or the natal cleft Malar butterfly rash—observed in JJSLE or JDMS Violaceous heliotrope rash or Gottron's papules on the hands—JDMS Evanescent macular salmon pink rash may be seen in systemic-onset JIA (often occurs with spikes of fever) and may demonstrate Koebner phenomenon Localized scleroderma may present with an isolated patch of pigmented skin (morphoea)—systemic sclerosis is rare in childhood Vasculitis or livedo rash may occur in connective tissue disease (including JSLE or JDMS)
Nail examination	Nail pitting (psoriasis) Nail beds and capillaroscopy—can be aided by magnification using a gel and ophthalmoscope or dermascope	Nail change of psoriasis may be subtle, and the only manifestation of psoriasis in children Dilated, tortuous nail bed capillaries suggests active inflammation in the context of connective tissue disease
Ear, nose, and throat examination	Cervical lymphadenopathy Oral mucosa, gums, and teeth Ears and nose (bridge and mucosa) Parotid swelling if sicca features or suspicion of connective tissue disease or sarcoidosis	Significant cervical lymphadenopathy may occur in malignancy or multisystem disease (such as Kawasaki's disease) Mouth ulcers—JSLE and Behçet's disease. Sjögren's syndrome is rare in childhood but may be a feature within mixed connective tissue disease Poor dental hygiene is a concern, particularly in the immunosuppressed child ENT abnormalities are common in ANCA +ve vasculitis, e.g. saddle nose (Wegener's granulomatosis) and sinusitis (Churg–Strauss syndrome)

(Continued)

Table 5.7 (Continued)

	Features	Context and comments
Cardiovascular	Blood pressure and pulses Presence of bruits Heart sounds	Hypertension in the context of rheumatic disease may signify renal involvement (e.g. vasculitic disease) Pericarditis is a feature of systemic-onset JIA and vasculitic disease in childhood Cardiac abnormalities are a feature of non-benign hypermobility syndromes (e.g. Marfan's and Ehlers–Danlos)
Respiratory	Lung fields Pulmonary function testing	Restrictive lung disease may be seen in connective tissue disease
Abdominal	Presence of guarding Hepatosplenomegaly	Abdominal pain may be a non-specific presenting feature of musculoskeletal disease and examination is often needed to exclude other pathology, e.g. limping child with psoas abscess or pyelonephritis. Similarly, a child with hip disease may localize this poorly to the lower abdomen
Neurological	Full neurological examination of the lower limbs is always indicated in children presenting with back pain Cranial nerve assessment in context of headache Peripheral nerve involvement Muscle power	Abnormal neurological examination (such as altered sensation or hyper-reflexia) in a child with back pain should lead to urgent imaging and expert assessment MRI ± angiography may be needed if cerebral vasculitis is suspected Reduced muscle strength is seen in JDMS and mixed connective tissue disease
Eye	Reduced visual acuity Fundoscopy Slit lamp examination	In JIA, uveitis may be asymptomatic and routine eye screening should be a mandatory part of management Multisystem disease (e.g. sarcoidosis, vasculitis) may manifest with ocular involvement
Renal	Blood pressure Urinalysis	Haematuria is a feature of renal disease associated with ANCA +ve vasculitis (i.e. Wegener's granulomatosis) JSLE-associated nephritis may present with hypertension and proteinuria Exclusion of UTI is important in a febrile child, particularly if immunosuppressed

ANCA, anti-neutrophil cytoplasmic antibodies; ENT, ear, nose, and throat; JDMS, juvenile dermatomyositis; JIA, juvenile idiopathic arthritis; JSLE, juvenile systemic lupus erythematosus; UTI, urinary tract infection.

(with the exception of ERA), and in isolation, other pathologies including orthopaedic conditions (dysplasia, slipped upper femoral epiphysis) and sepsis (including mycobacterial infection) need to be excluded. Referred pain such as from the hip or thigh as a cause of knee pain in the absence of physical signs (at the knee) must be considered.

Benign hypermobility is suggested within pGALS by symmetrical hyperextension at the fingers, wrists, elbows, knees, and flat pronated feet, with normal arches on tiptoe. It is important to consider 'non-benign' causes of hypermobility—checking body habitus, skin and sclerae may suggest marfanoid features or other syndromes associated with hypermobility. Conversely, lack of joint mobility, especially if asymmetrical, is always significant—for example, the loss of hyperextension at the knee, as an isolated finding is very suggestive of previous inflammatory arthritis at that joint and corroborates a diagnosis of previous JIA.

Documentation of pGALS

Documentation of pGALS within a standard medical clerking is important. A simple proforma is proposed in Table 5.8 using the example of a child with a short leg, calf wasting, and antalgic gait (Figure 5.5).

Table 5.8 Documentation of pGALS—example (see Figure 5.5)

The pGALS screening questions	
Pain	Right leg
Dressing	No difficulty
Walking	Some difficulty

	Appearance	Movement
Gait		✗
Arms	✓	✓
Legs	✗	✗
Spine	✓	✓

Paediatric regional examination of the musculoskeletal system (pREMS)

Following pGALS as a basic assessment, the observer is directed to a more detailed examination of the relevant area(s). A consensus approach to paediatric regional examination of the musculoskeletal system (called pREMS) has been developed from observation

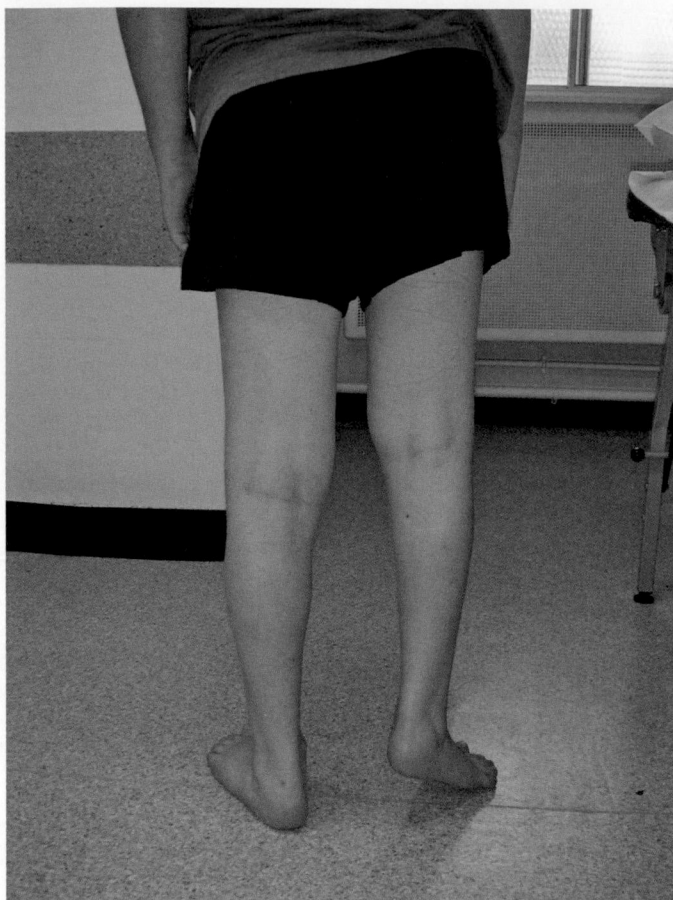

Fig. 5.5 Shortened right leg with resultant toe walking and muscle wasting.

of doctors and allied health professionals working in pMSK medicine.[27] pREMS is based on the 'look, feel, move, function' principle similar to that of adult REMS[28] (see Chapter 6) for each joint or anatomical region, with the same general principles, although it differs by anatomical region, reflecting different pathologies from those observed in adults. pREMS involves active movements performed first and then passively by the examiner and includes the addition of 'measure' for some joints and options pending the clinical scenario (Box 5.3). Details of the examination techniques for each joint are not included in this chapter and the reader is directed

---

Box 5.3 The paediatric regional examination of the musculoskeletal system (pREMS)

pREMS—general principles

Introduction

- Introduce yourself to child and parent/carer

- Explain what you want to examine, gain verbal consent to examine

- Be aware of normal variants in leg alignment, joint range, gait, developmental milestones

---

Box 5.3 (Continued)

Look for

- Swellings, rashes (e.g. psoriasis/vasculitis), muscle wasting, scars, leg length discrepancy

- Deformity, dysmorphism, 'disproportions', discomfort (non-verbal signals)

Feel for

- Temperature, swelling, tenderness (along bones and joint line)

Move

- Full range of movement—active and passive (note any asymmetry)

- Restriction—mild, moderate, or severe

Function and measure

- Functional assessment of joint/anatomic region to include power of muscles and stability

- Measurement of height/leg length

pREMS—Examination schedules by anatomical region[a]

Examination of the hand and wrist

- Inspect hands (palms and backs) for muscle wasting, skin and nail changes

- Feel for radial pulse, tendon thickening, and bulk of thenar and hypothenar eminences

- Feel for skin temperature

- Squeeze metacarpophalangeal joints

- Bimanually palpate swollen or painful joints, including wrists

- Look and feel along ulnar border

- Assess full finger extension and full finger tuck

- Assess wrist flexion and extension, abduction and adduction—active and passive

- Assess function: grip and pinch, picking up small object, writing/drawing

- Options[b]—assess for hypermobility syndromes, muscle power, capillaroscopy, peripheral neuropathy

Examination of the elbow

- Look for carrying angle, scars, swellings or rashes, deformity

- Feel for skin temperature

- Palpate over head of radius, joint line, medial and lateral epicondyles

- Assess full flexion and extension, pronation and supination—actively and passively

- Assess function—e.g. hand to nose or mouth, hands behind head

- Options[b]—assess for hypermobility syndromes, muscle power, instability tests, entheses

(Continued)

Box 5.3 (*Continued*)

Examination of the shoulder

With patient standing or sitting

◆ Inspect shoulders, clavicles, and sternoclavicular joints from the front, side, and behind, and assess shoulder height

◆ Inspect skin in axillae and palpate for lymphadenopathy

◆ Assess skin temperature

◆ Palpate bony landmarks and surrounding muscles

◆ Assess movement and function: hands behind head, hands behind back

◆ Assess (actively and passively) external rotation, flexion, extension and abduction

◆ Observe scapular movement

◆ Options[b]—assess for hypermobility syndromes, muscle power, instability

Examination of the hip

With patient lying supine on couch

◆ Look for flexion deformity and leg length disparity

◆ Check for scars, rashes

◆ Feel the greater trochanter for tenderness

◆ Assess full hip flexion, internal and external rotation, abduction and adduction

◆ Perform the Thomas test

◆ Hip abduction (lying on side)

With patient lying prone on couch

◆ Sacroiliac joint palpation

◆ Hip internal (and external) rotation

With patient standing

◆ Assess posture and leg alignment

◆ Look for gluteal muscle bulk

◆ Perform the Trendelenburg test

◆ Assess function (gait with turning and running, ancillary movements)

◆ Options[b]—assess for hypermobility, muscle power, enthesitis, thigh–foot angle (child with intoeing)

Examination of the knee

With patient standing

◆ Look for varus/valgus deformity, hyperextension, and popliteal swellings

◆ Inspect skin for pattern of bruising and rashes

◆ Assess gait (see hip)

With patient lying on couch

◆ Look from the end of the couch for varus/valgus deformity, muscle wasting, scars, and swellings

◆ Look from the side for fixed flexion deformity

◆ Check for passive hyperextension and leg length discrepancy

◆ Feel skin temperature

◆ With the knee slightly flexed, palpate the joint line and the borders of the patella

◆ Feel the popliteal fossa

◆ Perform a patellar tap and cross-fluctuation (bulge sign)

◆ Assess full flexion and extension (actively and passively)

◆ Options[b]—assess stability of knee ligaments—medial and lateral collateral—and perform anterior draw test

◆ Options[b]—tests for anterior knee pain/patellar maltracking/apprehension/patella glide

◆ Options[b]—assess for hypermobility, enthesitis, hamstring tightness, iliotibial band tightness/thigh–foot angle

Examination of the foot and ankle

With patient lying supine on couch

◆ Look at dorsal and plantar surfaces of the foot

◆ Feel the skin temperature

◆ Palpate for peripheral pulses

◆ Squeeze the metatarsophalangeal joints

◆ Palpate the midfoot, ankle joint line, and subtalar joint

◆ Assess movement (actively and passively) at the subtalar joint (inversion and eversion), the big toe (dorsi- and plantar flexion), the ankle joint (dorsi- and plantar flexion), and midtarsal joints (passive rotation)

◆ Look at the patient's footwear

◆ Options[b]—assess for hypermobility, thigh–foot angle, enthesitis, muscle power, capillaroscopy

With patient standing

◆ Look at the forefoot, midfoot (foot arch), and hindfoot

◆ Assess gait cycle (heel strike, stance, toe-off), running and turning, ancillary movement

◆ Assess muscle bulk (calves)

Examination of the spine

With patient standing

◆ Inspect from the side and from behind

◆ Inspect skin and natal cleft

◆ Inspect limb/trunk proportions

◆ Inspect facial and jaw profile

◆ Palpate the spinal processes and paraspinal muscles and temporomandibular joints (TMJs)

◆ Assess movement: lumbar flexion and extension and lateral flexion; cervical flexion, extension, rotation and lateral flexion, thoracic rotation

(*Continued*)

Box 5.3 (*Continued*)

- Assess TMJ opening
- Options[b]—Schober's test, stork test[c]

With patient sitting on couch (standing, for a younger child)

- Assess thoracic rotation

  With patient lying on couch

- Perform straight leg raising and dorsiflexion of the big toe
- Assess limb reflexes
- Options[b]—assess for leg length discrepancy, hypermobility, sacroiliac joint irritation on palpation

[a]Details of the examination techniques used are available (see Further Reading).

[b]The options refer to additional manoeuvres suggested pending common clinical scenarios.

[c]Stork test—standing on one leg and extension of spine causes pain (suggestive of spondylolysis).

to the Further Reading section. pREMS, in contrast to adult REMS, is primarily aimed at postgraduate medical training in paediatric rheumatology although clearly many of the components are relevant to paediatric orthopaedics as well as to allied health professionals working in pMSK medicine.

References

1. Yeo M, Sawyer S. Chronic illness and disability. *BMJ* 2005;330(7493):721–723.
2. Goodman JE, McGrath PJ. The epidemiology of pain in children and adolescents—a review. *Pain* 1991;46(3):247–264.
3. Flato B, Aasland A, Vinje O, Forre O. Outcome and predictive factors in juvenile rheumatoid arthritis and juvenile spondyloarthropathy. *J Rheumatol.* 1998;25(2):366–375.
4. Sherry DD, Stein LD, Reed AM, Schanberg LE, Kredich DW. Prevention of leg length discrepancy in young children with pauciarticular juvenile rheumatoid arthritis by treatment with intraarticular steroids. *Arthritis Rheum* 1999;42(11):2330–2334.
5. Ravelli A, Martini A. Early predictors of outcome in juvenile idiopathic arthritis. *Clin Exp Rheumatol* 2003;21(5 Suppl 31):S89–S93.
6. Cabral DA, Petty RE, Malleson PN et al. Visual prognosis in children with chronic anterior uveitis and arthritis. *J Rheumatol.* 1994;21(12):2370–2375.
7. Dang-Tan T, Franco EL. Diagnosis delays in childhood cancer: a review. *Cancer* 2007;110(4):703–713.
8. Mohamed K, Appleton R, Nicolaides P. Delayed diagnosis of Duchenne muscular dystrophy. *Eur J Paediatr Neurol* 2000;4(5):219–223.
9. Myers A, McDonagh JE, Hull R et al. More 'cries from the joints': assessment of the musculoskeletal system is poorly documented in routine paediatric clerking. *Rheumatology (Oxford)* 2004;43(8):1045–1049.
10. Jandial S, Myers A, Wise E, Foster HE. Doctors likely to encounter children with musculoskeletal complaints have low confidence in their clinical skills. *J Pediatr* 2009;154(2):267–271.
11. Kay LJ, Deighton CM, Walker DJ, Hay EM. Undergraduate rheumatology teaching in the UK: a survey of current practice and changes since 1990. *Rheumatology* 2000;39(7):800–803.
12. Mayer ML, Brogan L, Sandborg CI. Availability of pediatric rheumatology training in United States pediatric residencies. *Arthritis Rheum* 2006;55(6):836–842.
13. Foster HE, Cabral DA. Is musculoskeletal history and examination so different in paediatrics? *Best Pract Res Clin Rheumatol.* 2006;20(2):241–262.
14. Malleson PN, Beauchamp RD. Rheumatology: 16. Diagnosing musculoskeletal pain in children. *CMAJ* 2001;165(2):183–188.
15. Goff I, Rowan A, Bateman B, Foster HE. Poor sensitivity of musculoskeletal history taking in children. *Arch Dis Child* 2012;97(7):644–646.
16. McGhee J, Burks F, Sheckels J, Jarvis J. Identifying children with chronic arthritis based on chief complaints. Absence of musculoskeletal pain as a predictor of chronic arthritis in children. *Pediatrics* 2002;110:354–359.
17. Cruikshank MC, Gardner-Medwin J. Chromosomal disorders and associated musculoskeletal morbidity. In: Foster HE Brogan PA, ed. *Paediatric rheumatology*. Oxford University Press, Oxford, 2012:318–322.
18. Gedalia A, Press J. Joint hypermobility and musculoskeletal pain. *J Rheumatol* 1998;25(5):1031–1032.
19. Leone V, Tornese G, Zerial M et al. Joint hypermobility and its relationship to musculoskeletal pain in schoolchildren: a cross-sectional study. *Arch Dis Child.* 2009;94(8):627–632.
20. Macfarlane A. 'Personal child health records' held by parents. *Arch Dis Child* 1992;67(5):571–572.
21. Doherty M, Dacre J, Dieppe P, Snaith M. The 'GALS' locomotor screen. *Ann Rheum Dis* 1992;51(10):1165–1169.
22. Foster HE, Kay LJ, Friswell M, Coady D, Myers A. Musculoskeletal screening examination (pGALS) for school-age children based on the adult GALS screen. *Arthritis Rheum* 2006;55(5):709–716.
23. Smith E, Molyneux E, Heikens GT, Foster H. Acceptability and practicality of pGALS in screening for rheumatic disease in Malawian children. *Clin Rheumatol* 2012;31(4):647–653.
24. Cassidy JT PR, Laxer RM, Lindsley CB. *Textbook of paediatric rheumatology*, 5th edn. Elsevier Saunders, Philadelphia, 2005.
25. Goff I, Bateman B, Myers A, Foster H. Acceptability and practicality of musculoskeletal examination in acute general pediatric assessment. *J Pediatr* 2010;156(4):657–662.
26. Dyet L, Pilkington C, Raffles A. A novel presentation of juvenile idiopathic arthropathy. *Arch Dis Child* 2003;88(11):1015–1016.
27. Foster H, Kay L, May C, Rapley T. Pediatric regional examination of the musculoskeletal system: a practice- and consensus-based approach. *Arthritis Care Res* 2011;63(11):1503–1510.
28. Coady D, Walker D, Kay L. Regional Examination of the Musculoskeletal System (REMS): a core set of clinical skills for medical students. *Rheumatology* 2004;43(5):633–639.

Further reading and resources

Houghton KM. Review for the generalist: evaluation of anterior knee. *Pediatr Rheumatol* 2007;5:8 www.ped-rheum.com/content/pdf/1546-0096-5-8.pdf

Houghton KM. Review for the generalist: evaluation of pediatric foot and ankle pain. *Pediatr Rheumatol* 2008;6:6 www.ped-rheum.com/content/pdf/1546-0096-6-6.pdf

Houghton KM. Review for the generalist: evaluation of pediatric hip pain. *Pediatr Rheumatol* 2009;7:10 www.ped-rheum.com/content/pdf/1546-0096-7-10.pdf

Houghton KM. Review for the generalist: evaluation of low back pain in children and adolescents. *Pediatr Rheumatol* 2010;8:28 www.ped-rheum.com/content/pdf/1546-0096-8-28.pdf

Staheli LT. *Fundamentals of pediatric orthopedics*. Lippincott Williams & Wilkins, Philadelphia, PA, 2008.

Szer I. Clinical skills in the evaluation of arthritis. In: Szer I, Kimura Y, Malleson P, Southwood T (eds.) *Arthritis in children and adolescents*. Oxford University Press, Oxford, 2006:3–18.

Free educational resources to demonstrate pGALS and the manoeuvres are available from the Arthritis Research UK website: www.arthritisresearchuk.org/health-professionals-and-students.aspx

CHAPTER 6

Principles of clinical examination in adults

Lesley Kay

Introduction

There is a paradox at the heart of this chapter: clinical examination of the musculoskeletal system is upheld as being of fundamental importance, and yet it is generally poorly performed, and individual clinical examination tests have a scanty evidence base.

This chapter covers the importance of musculoskeletal examination skills, evidence that such skills have been poorly taught and performed, the efforts made to address and improve this situation and describes in particular two programmes of examination. These are the Gait, Arms, Legs and Spine (GALS)[1] screening examination, and the Regional Examination of the Musculoskeletal System (REMS)[2] core set of examination skills for medical students. Rheumatologists and others using this textbook will be in key positions to address the training and competence of doctors and other practitioners working with patients with musculoskeletal conditions in their normal working lives as well as in formal teaching situations.

The importance of musculoskeletal clinical examination skills

Clinical examination is one of the fundamental, core skills of the rheumatologist.[3,4] Evidence shows that the history can establish the correct diagnosis in 56% of cases, rising to 73% when patients have been examined[5,6] in general medicine. Arguably, for musculoskeletal conditions the figures are likely to be even higher. Careful examination limits the number of unnecessary investigations, leading to more rapid and accurate diagnoses,[7] and prompt treatment: advances in diagnostic investigations do not diminish the importance of clinical assessment.[8] In this context it is surprising that there has traditionally been little emphasis within rheumatology on the description of the required skills or the understanding of the validity of individual components of the examination itself. Although recommendations for undergraduate and other curricula emphasize the importance of clinical examination skills, they have not until recent years been specific in their recommendation of which examination tests are important for students and practitioners to learn.[9–14] Musculoskeletal examination skills are recognized as important not only for rheumatologists,[15] orthopaedic surgeons,[16] and other musculoskeletal practitioners,[17,18] but particularly for those working in primary care,[19–21] internal medicine,[22–24] and elderly medicine.[24]

Poor performance and confidence in musculoskeletal examination skills

The literature on the performance of musculoskeletal examination shows unfortunately consistent results. These studies are largely surveys and in some cases formal assessments, but each shows poor confidence in use of clinical skills, poorly rated training, and poor performance. This has been shown at different clinical levels including medical students in Germany,[25] foundation doctors in the UK,[26] and residents in Australia.[27] In general internal medicine (GIM) in the UK and Australia musculoskeletal examination is infrequently performed and recorded.[23,28,29] There is some evidence of use of GALS and other examinations but still low percentage recording and confidence as self-rated by doctors.[30] Despite the high incidence of musculoskeletal complaints presenting to primary care, the findings are no better in general practice in Germany,[31] the UK,[20,32] or the USA,[19,33] where family physicians are less confident in musculoskeletal examination than in other body systems.[34] Even those whose primary work is with patients with musculoskeletal conditions—orthopaedic surgeons[16,22] and rheumatologists[35] in training as well as osteopaths[17]—are found to have less good skills than one might expect. There is little work looking at the practice of trained orthopaedic surgeons or rheumatologists, but it is established that formal joint counts are not undertaken in the majority of consultations with patients with established rheumatoid arthritis,[36] which could suggest that examination is not performed to a high standard or completeness. A similar pattern is found in paediatric rheumatology practice, dealt with elsewhere (Chapter 5).

What are the barriers to performance of adequate musculoskeletal examination?

Irish hospital doctors think that examination of the musculoskeletal system is too difficult to be undertaken routinely,[37] and it is likely that they are not atypical. Performance and confidence in musculoskeletal examination are affected predominantly by undergraduate teaching. Both content and duration of rotations have been proposed as having an effect, but there is also the influential effect of role modelling by other specialists. If senior doctors do not themselves routinely conduct such examinations, or enquire into the results on ward rounds, junior doctors will naturally concentrate on other matters. Low expectations, therefore, are important. At undergraduate level, teachers identify the main barriers to the delivery of effective clinical teaching as including the lack of agreement on what to teach, lack of confidence in teaching amongst non-musculoskeletal specialities, and poor communication between specialties. Students cite similar concerns.[38,39] Eponymous names for tests are thought to add to confusion.[40] The fact that musculoskeletal examination rarely appeared in important examinations may also have been a factor in its low status at medical school.[11]

Clinical examination tests have little demonstrated evidence base

In the past, examination was taught by tradition, relying on expert descriptions and respected textbooks. Available textbooks have, however, been shown to be generally inadequate for musculoskeletal examination in children[41] and adults.[42] Coverage is poor, and in general examination texts the musculoskeletal section is generally short, and positioned last, after the other body systems.[42] There has, however, been a sea change in the view taken of the role of clinical examination. Examination interventions are considered on the same basis as diagnostic tests. Examination should be understood as an evidence-based procedure whose sensitivity and specificity can be determined, to allow the clinician to understand the change in likelihood of a particular diagnosis depending on the results of the test.[43] This leads to the importance of studying examination tests for their performance[44] in terms of their validity, reliability, reproducibility, sensitivity and specificity, and likelihood ratio, as well as the normal range in a given population. Some normal ranges have been established, for example ranges of movement of the cervical and lumbar spine, for generalized hypermobility, and for differences with age and gender. Few examination tests have been well studied in this way, but good examples include systematic reviews of examination tests for meniscal tears[45] and of shoulder special examination tests.[46]

What has been done about it?

Curriculum and course design

The first and most important step has been the recognition of the need to agree and set standards for teaching, learning, and assessment. In one example, medical students at one university reported that even within the same course, delivered at different sites, the content of the course and their experience varied widely.[47] Agreement between specialties may be particularly important,[48] as conflicts are confusing and off-putting for learners, and should be resolved in course design. Recommendations for minimum length of course modules have been made, based on evidence that increasing the duration can improve knowledge outcomes,[49] but other evidence suggests that factors such as agreement about the content and delivery of rotation may be more important.[47] The emphasis has been on the development of courses which are appropriate for particular specialty groups or levels of training,[50] and it has been shown that teaching skills in defined modules improves confidence[33] and performance in musculoskeletal knowledge[49] and examination skills,[51] and in the skills and confidence of those used as tutors or models.[51]

Assessment drives learning

Students' learning, performance and confidence, at whatever level, is improved by clarity about the goals of the teaching, relevance of the material taught, and a clear link between the course content and its assessment. It is a truism in education that 'assessment drives learning' and therefore, rightly, much emphasis has been on the need to ensure that the musculoskeletal system is included in routine assessments of clinical skills, whether at medical school or in postgraduate settings.[48,51–54] There has been a clear increase in teaching and assessment of clinical skills in UK medical schools.[11]

Delivering improved skills training in real-life environments

In busy clinical practice, intensive courses designed to deliver high-quality musculoskeletal skills training can be labour-intensive and expensive.[47,55] Courses must be feasible in the settings in which they are taught,[56] so it is important to find ways of delivering good clinical skills teaching in the changing clinical environment even if it means taking teaching away from the bedside.[57,58] Some less resource-intensive ways of delivering teaching have been shown to be effective, such as using more senior students,[59,60] nurses,[55] or trained patient educators as tutors, and the use of assessment tools which reduce the need for expensive clinical examiners to assess confidence[61] and competence.[62] Curricula and assessments are traditionally derived separately for each institution, but it may be in future that work can be saved by sharing best practice to reduce workload.[63]

Streamlining, consistency, and standardization

The establishment of standardized examination regimes has been the biggest advance in musculoskeletal skills training in the last two decades.[12] The advantages of a standardized programme are: that learners and students are clear about what is to be learned; teaching and learning materials can be developed to support it; and assessment can be designed to test the agreed learning outcomes. It can additionally be tested for fitness-for-purpose, and revised in the light of further evidence. Systematized examination may help to make the best use of the limited time available in a consultation.[64]

GALS screening examination

The first, and most well-known, standardized examination regimen was the 'Gait, Arms, Legs, Spine' screening examination (GALS).[1] GALS is a rapid, simple, choreographed screening examination, which aims to distinguish between a patient with a normal musculoskeletal system and one with a musculoskeletal problem. It does not aim to describe or diagnose the problem, but is a tool that can guide subsequent examination and investigation.

Comparison of the musculoskeletal findings in patients admitted to general medical wards with the musculoskeletal problems and findings recorded in their case notes revealed a large deficiency.[28] Patients were further examined and a 'minimalist screening examination' was devised and validated.[65] This was subsequently published as GALS, as a scripted sequence, with short history questions and suggested notation, recommended for use in all patients by undergraduates, junior hospital doctors, and perhaps primary care (Box 6.1). Medical schools in the UK and Ireland now use GALS routinely in their teaching and it is incorporated into the

---

Box 6.1 Gait, Arms, Legs, Spine (GALS): a screening examination

Screening questions in the routine history

These should be incorporated into the routine systemic enquiry of every patient:

◆ 'Do you suffer from any pain or stiffness in your muscles, joints, or back?'

◆ 'Do you have any difficulty dressing yourself?'

◆ 'Do you have any difficulty walking up and down stairs?'

Gait

◆ Gait is observed for symmetry and smoothness as well as the ability to turn quickly.

◆ With the patient then standing in the anatomical position observe from behind, from the side, and in front of the patient for muscle bulk and symmetry, limb alignment, straight spine, level iliac crests, and the ability to fully extend elbows and knees.

Arms

◆ Asking the patient to put their hands behind their head, assess shoulder abduction and external rotation as well as elbow flexion.

◆ Joint swelling and deformity are then looked for, by observing the back of the patient's hands and wrists with the fingers outstretched.

◆ Ask the patient to turn their hands over. Look at the palms for muscle bulk.

◆ Assess power grip by asking the patient to make a fist

◆ Squeezing the examiner's fingers assesses grip strength.

◆ Assess fine precision pinch which is important functionally.

◆ Squeeze across the metacarpal-phalangeal joints for tenderness—be sure to watch the patient's face while doing this.

Legs

◆ With the patient lying on a couch or bed, assess full flexion and extension of both knees while feeling each knee for crepitus.

◆ Assess internal rotation of both hips by having the hip and knee flexed to 90, while gently guiding the patient's movement by holding their knee and ankle.

◆ Perform a patella tap checks for an effusion of the knee.

◆ Finally, inspect the feet for swelling and deformity as well as callosities on the soles, and squeeze across the metatarsal-phalangeal joints to detect inflammatory joint disease.

Spine

◆ With the patient standing, inspect the spine from behind for evidence of scoliosis and from the side for abnormal lordosis or kyphosis.

◆ Lateral flexion of the neck, is assessed by asking the patient to touch each ear to their shoulder in turn.

◆ Lumbar spine is assessed, by asking the patient to touch their toes. Normal movement of the spinal vertebrae is palpated for during this manoeuvre.

Recording the findings from the screening examination

It is important to record the positive and negative findings in the notes. A simple note of the presence or absence of any changes in the appearance or movement in the gait, arms, legs or spine should be recorded as follows:

	Appearance	Movement
Gait	✓	✓
Arms	✓	✓
Legs	✓	✓
Spine	✓	✓

The sequence is described and illustrated in *Clinical assessment of the musculoskeletal system*, a handbook[66] and DVD[67] available from Arthritis Research UK.

Arthritis Research UK handbook intended for medical students and others,[66] available as a DVD or online.[67]

Evaluation of GALS has been relatively limited,[68] but its widespread uptake shows its face validity and acceptability to teachers. Acceptability to students has not been formally assessed, but a jokey revision version has been recorded,[69] the makers of which describe GALS as 'the Big One' for musculoskeletal examination on their website. Students can learn it in a relatively short time.[70] Such learning improves examination of the musculoskeletal system by graduating medical students,[71] and in the detection of rheumatoid arthritis by physiotherapists.[72] The GALS screen is valid against measures of disability.[73] Its teaching improves confidence in junior doctors[23,30] and it is in limited use in clinical practice.[24,30]

REMS

The next step was to define the examination skills required to examine the patient where a problem had been identified via GALS, to localize and describe it further. The point of reference taken was that of the medical student at the point of qualification: skills should therefore be those relevant to all doctors in whichever specialty they go on to practise. The approach involved a literature review and focus groups with clinicians[40] and students[38] to identify potential examination manoeuvres. These were then listed for prioritization and assessment of relevance in a national survey of rheumatologists, orthopaedic surgeons, geriatricians, and general practitioners. The findings from both parts of the study were then moderated via a group nominative process. This derived 50 musculoskeletal examination skills considered essential for medical students at the point of qualification, and therefore, by implication, all doctors. (Box 6.2).[2] Following the model of GALS, these were then choreographed into a logical sequence of examination manoeuvres

---

Box 6.2 Core set of regional musculoskeletal examination skills appropriate for a medical student at the point of qualification, derived from the REMS project[2]

A student at the point of qualification should be able to:

1. Detect the difference between bony and soft tissue swelling.

2. Elicit tenderness around a joint.

3. Elicit temperature around a joint.

4. Detect synovitis.

5. Have an awareness of the difference between active and passive movements.

6. Perform passive and active movements at all relevant joints.

7. Detect a loss of full extension and a loss of full flexion.

8. Assess gait.

9. Correctly use the terms 'varus' and 'valgus'.

10. Assess limb reflexes routinely, when examining the spine and in other relevant circumstances.

11. Have an understanding of the term 'subluxation'.

12. Where appropriate, examine neurological and vascular systems when assessing a problematic joint (check for intact sensation and peripheral pulses).

13. Assess leg length with a tape measure when assessing for a real leg length discrepancy.

14. Make a qualitative assessment of movement (not joint end feel but features such as cog-wheeling).

15. Assess the median and ulnar nerves.

16. Be able to localize tenderness within the joints of the hand (palpate each small joint of the hand if necessary).

17. Assess power grip.

18. Assess pincer grip in the hand.

19. Make a functional assessment of the hand such as holding a cup.

20. Correctly use the term 'Heberden's nodes'.

21. Be able to perform Phalen's test.

22. Detect a painful arc and frozen shoulder.

23. Make a functional assessment of the shoulder (can the patient put their hands behind their head and their back?).

24. Perform external and internal rotation of the shoulder with the elbow flexed to 90° and held in against the patient's side.

25. Examine a patient's shoulder from behind for scapular movement.

26. Assess the acromioclavicular joint (by palpation alone).

27. Palpate for tenderness over the epicondyles of the elbow.

28. Palpate for tenderness over the greater trochanter of the hip.

29. Perform internal and external rotation of the hip with it flexed to 90°.

30. Perform Trendelenberg's test.

31. Perform Thomas' test.

32. Detect an effusion at the knee.

33. Perform a patellar tap.

34. Demonstrate cross-fluctuation or the bulge sign when looking for a knee effusion.

35. Test for collateral ligament stability in the knee.

36. Use the anterior draw test to assess anterior cruciate ligament stability in the knee.

37. Examine the sole of a patient's feet.

38. Recognize hallux valgus, claw and hammer toes.

39. Assess a patient's feet with them standing.

40. Assess for flat feet (including the patient standing on tip toes).

41. Recognize hindfoot/heel pathologies.

42. Assess plantar flexion and dorsiflexion of the ankle.

43. Assess movements of inversion and eversion of the foot.

(Continued)

Box 6.2 (Continued)

44. Assess the subtalar joint.

45. Perform a lateral squeeze across the metatarso-phalangeal joints.

46. Assess flexion/extension of the big toe.

47. Examine a patient's footwear.

48. Palpate the spinous processes.

49. Assess lateral and forward flexion of the lumbar spine (using fingers, not tape measure).

50. Assess thoracic rotation with the patient sitting.

---

using the Apley structure of 'look, feel, move' and adding 'function', to form a fluent examination series (Box 6.3). This is known as the Regional Examination of the Musculoskeletal System (REMS). REMS has been ratified by the British Orthopaedic Association education committee, the Education and Training committee of the British Society for Rheumatology, the Primary Care Rheumatology Society, and Arthritis Research UK, and incorporated into the Arthritis Research UK handbook and DVD, 'Clinical Assessment of the Musculoskeletal System'.[10,66] REMS has also undergone very limited evaluation. It was found to be acceptable to teachers and to learners, and to give a sustained increase in students' confidence over 6 months.[74] A similar approach has been taken for undergraduate core skills competencies in Canada.[75]

Examination skills required at postgraduate level

GALS and REMS are largely used in the training of medical students, in the hope that skills acquisition at that stage will provide a sound foundation for future practice. GALS and REMS are considered to contain the range of skills that is necessary for the generalist, or for a specialist in another field. Little work has been done to describe, codify, or standardize the range of skills, necessarily much larger, for those practising in specialist musculoskeletal fields, particularly rheumatology and orthopaedics. pREMS,[76] the equivalent of REMS for children, does identify some skills as needed in more specialist practice, and there has been an exercise describing the

---

Box 6.3 Regional examination of the musculoskeletal system (REMS)[2]

General principles

♦ It is important to introduce yourself, ensure that the patient is comfortable, explain what you are going to do, gain verbal consent, and ask the patient to let you know if you cause them any pain or discomfort at any time.

Look

♦ The examination should always start with visual inspection of the exposed area at rest, and a comparison of sides looking for symmetry.

♦ You should look specifically for skin changes, muscle bulk and swelling in and around the joint.

♦ Also look for deformity in terms of alignment and posture of the joint.

Feel

♦ Feel for skin temperature using the back of your hand, across the joint line, and at other relevant sites.

♦ Any swellings should be assessed for fluctuance and mobility. The hard, bony swellings of osteoarthritis should be distinguished from the soft, rubbery swelling of inflammatory joint disease.

♦ Tenderness is an important clinical sign to elicit, in and around the joint.

♦ As a general principle students should be able to elicit synovitis, which relies on detecting the triad of warmth, swelling, and tenderness.

Move

♦ The full range of movement of a joint should be assessed. Both sides should be compared.

♦ As a general rule both active (where the patient moves the joint themselves) and passive (where the examiner moves the joint) movements should be performed.

♦ You should be able to detect a loss of full flexion and a loss of full extension.

♦ A restriction in the range of movement should be recorded as mild, moderate or severe.

♦ The quality of movement should also be recorded, with reference to abnormalities such as the presence of crepitus or cog-wheeling (in Parkinson's disease).

♦ It is not considered necessary for medical students to perform resisted movements.

(Continued)

Box 6.3 (*Continued*)

Function

◆ It is important to make a functional assessment of the joint. For example, in the case of limited elbow flexion, does this limit them getting their hand to their mouth?

Examination of the hands and wrists

◆ This should normally take place with the patient's hands resting on a pillow.

Look

◆ With the patient's hands palm down observe for obvious swelling, deformity, posture, muscle wasting, and scars.

◆ Look at the skin for thinning, and bruising (signs of long-term steroid use) or rashes.

◆ Look for nail changes (for psoriasis) or evidence of nailfold vasculitis.

◆ Decide if changes are symmetrical or asymmetrical.

◆ Do changes mainly involve the distal small joints: PIP and DIPs or MCPs?

◆ Ask them to turn their hands over (do they have problems with this due to elbow and wrist involvement?)

◆ Look again for muscle wasting—is this both thenar and hypothenar eminences? (if thenar alone then perhaps they have carpal tunnel syndrome).

◆ Look at the wrist for a carpal tunnel release scar.

Feel

◆ Assess for the presence of a radial pulse.

◆ Assess for skin temperature using the back of your hand at the patient's forearm, wrist, and MCPs.

◆ Feel the bulk of the thenar and hypothenar eminences.

◆ Test median and ulnar nerve sensation (the thenar and hypothenar eminences).

◆ Assess radial nerve sensation—over the web space of the thumb and index finger.

◆ Gently squeeze across the row of MCP joints while watching the patient's face for signs of tenderness.

◆ Bimanually palpate any MCP joints and any PIP or DIP joints that appear swollen or painful.

◆ Is there evidence of active synovitis? (The joints are warm, swollen, and tender and may have a 'rubbery' feel, or you may even detect effusions).

◆ Bimanually palpate the patient's wrists.

◆ Finally run your hand up their arm to their elbow to look and feel for rheumatoid nodules or psoriatic plaques on the extensor surfaces

Move

◆ Ask the patient to straighten their fingers fully (against gravity).

◆ Ask the patient to make a fist—can they tuck their fingers into their palm?

◆ Assess wrist flexion/extension actively (e.g. by making the 'prayer' sign) then passively.

◆ Assess the median and ulnar nerves for power (abduction of the thumb and finger spread respectively).

◆ In patients where history and examination suggest a diagnosis of carpal tunnel syndrome, perform Phalen's test (forced flexion of the wrists for 30 seconds, looking for reproduction of pain, tingling, or numbness in the median nerve distribution).

Function

◆ Ask them to grip your two fingers. This assesses power grip—very important in function.

◆ Ask them to pinch your finger. This assesses pincer grip.

◆ Ask them to pick a small object such as a coin out of your hand.

(Continued)

Box 6.3 (*Continued*)

Examination of the elbow

Look

♦ Look for scars, muscle wasting, nodules, psoriasis, and swelling.

Feel

♦ Feel the temperature with the back of your hand.

♦ Hold their forearm with one hand and with the elbow flexed to 90° palpate the elbow, feeling head of the radius and joint line with your thumb. If there is swelling, is it fluctuant?

♦ Palpate the medial and lateral epicondyles (golfers' and tennis elbow) and olecranon process for tenderness and evidence of bursitis.

Move

♦ Does the elbow fully extend and fully flex (actively and passively)?

♦ Compare one side to another.

♦ Assess pronation and supination (actively and passively).

Function

♦ An important function of the elbow is to allow the patient's hand to reach their mouth. Other functions dependent on 'hands behind head', 'hands behind back' will have been assessed during the GALS screening examination.

Examination of the shoulder

Look

♦ With the shoulder fully exposed, inspect the patient from in front, the side, and then behind.

♦ Look for muscle wasting (compare sides) and look for scars.

♦ Is their posture normal? Are both shoulders symmetrical?

Feel

♦ Assess the temperature.

♦ Identify any tenderness. Palpate the muscle bulk of supraspinatus, infraspinatus, and deltoid.

♦ Palpate the bony landmarks starting at the sternoclavicular joint, the clavicle, acromioclavicular joint, acromion process, the joint line, and around the scapula.

Move

♦ Ask the patient to put their hands behind their head and then behind their back.

♦ With the elbow flexed at 90° and tucked into the patient's side assess external rotation of the shoulder—compare both sides.

♦ Assess flexion and extension.

♦ Ask the patient to abduct the arm to assess for a painful arc.

♦ Observe scapular movement.

Function

♦ Function of the shoulder includes reaching the hands behind the head and the back.

Examination of the hip

Look

♦ Observe the legs, comparing both sides: Is there an obvious flexion deformity of the hip with the patient lying flat?

♦ If there is a suggestion of a leg length disparity, assess true leg lengths using a tape measure.

♦ Check for scars overlying the hip.

♦ With the patient standing, assess for muscle wasting (gluteal muscle bulk in particular).

(Continued)

Box 6.3 (*Continued*)

Feel

◆ Palpate over the greater trochanter for tenderness.

Move

◆ Assess full hip flexion with the knee flexed at 90°—watch the patients face. Is full flexion painful? Compare both sides.

◆ Assess for a fixed flexion deformity of the hip by performing Thomas's test.

◆ Assess internal and external rotation of both hips with the hip and knee flexed at 90°. This is often limited in hip disease.

◆ A Trendelenburg test should also be performed.

Function

◆ Ask the patient to walk: Do they have an antalgic or Trendelenburg gait?

Examination of the knee

Look

◆ Observe the knee from the end of the bed, comparing both sides. Is the posture of the knee normal?

◆ Look for valgus and varus deformity.

◆ Is there muscle wasting or scars? Is the knee red (inflammation or infection) Is there obvious swelling? Is there a rash (e.g. psoriasis)?

Feel

◆ Feel the temperature using the back of your hand.

◆ Palpate for tenderness along the borders of the patella.

◆ With the knee flexed, palpate the joint line from both femoral condyles to the inferior pole of the patella, then down the inferior patellar tendon to the tibial tuberosity.

◆ Feel behind the knee for a popliteal (Baker's) cyst.

◆ Assess for an effusion by patellar tap

◆ Assess for a fluid bulge if there is no distinct patellar tap.

Move

◆ Do the knees fully extend? (making sure the patient is fully relaxed).

◆ Assess active and passive movement.

◆ Test the stability of the knee ligaments:

• anterior draw test.

• medial and lateral collateral ligament stability.

Function

◆ Ask the patient to stand to look again for varus/valgus deformity.

◆ Ask the patient to walk.

Examination of the foot and ankle

◆ With the patient sitting on a bed and their feet overhanging the end of it:

Look

◆ Observe the feet, comparing both sides for symmetry.

◆ Look specifically at the forefoot for nail changes or skin rashes.

◆ Look at alignment of the toes and evidence of hallux valgus of the great toe.

◆ Look for clawing of the toes, joint swelling and callus formation.

(*Continued*)

Box 6.3 (*Continued*)

◆ Look at the underside or plantar surface for callus formation.

◆ Finally, look at the patient's footwear.

Feel

◆ Assess the temperature over the foot and ankle and check for the presence of peripheral pulses.

◆ Gently squeeze across the MTP joints while watching the patient's face.

◆ Palpate the midfoot, the ankle and the subtalar joint for tenderness.

Move

◆ Movements of inversion and eversion at the subtalar joint, plus dorsiflexion and plantar flexion at the big toe and ankle should be assessed both actively and passively.

◆ Movement of the midtarsal joints are performed by fixing the heel with one hand, then passively inverting/everting the forefoot with the other hand.

◆ With the patient weightbearing:

   • Look again at the forefoot for toe alignment and the mid foot for foot arch position.

   • Look at the hind foot from behind the patient: Achilles tendon thickening or swelling may be seen. There should be normal alignment of the hindfoot.

Function

◆ Assessment of gait should be performed if not already done, observing for the normal cycle of heel strike and toe off.

Examination of the spine

Look

◆ Observe the patient standing. Look initially from behind the patient for any scars, muscle wasting, asymmetry, or scoliosis.

◆ Look from the side for the normal cervical lordosis, thoracic kyphosis, and lumbar lordosis.

Feel

◆ Feel down the spine starting at the occiput and palpating down the spinous processes to the sacrum and also down the paraspinal muscles for tenderness.

Move

◆ Assess lumbar flexion and extension and lateral flexion.

◆ Next, assess the cervical spine movements, which include lateral flexion, rotation, flexion, and extension.

◆ With the patient sitting on the edge of the couch, assess thoracic rotation is.

◆ With the patient lying as flat as possible, perform straight leg raise with the foot at right angles at the ankle.

◆ Finally, assess limb reflexes (upper and lower) and dorsiflexion of the big toe.

◆ If there has been any indication of an abnormality from the history, a full neurological and vascular assessment should be made.

* The sequence is described and illustrated in the 'Clinical Assessment of the Musculoskeletal System' handbook[66] and DVD[67] available from Arthritis Research UK.

examination skills appropriate for higher trainees in general hospital specialities[75] and in orthopaedics in Canada, derived in a similar way to REMS.[77] The European League against Rheumatism (EULAR) has a syllabus for specialist training in rheumatology,[78] and recommendations for continuing professional development:[79] neither mentions clinical examination skills, let alone defining which are needed. A survey of European centres[80] about the competencies needed for rheumatology again does not specifically mention musculoskeletal examination. The most recent UK curriculum for rheumatology higher training acknowledges that 'rheumatology has a very strong reliance on sound clinical skills'[81] and specifies that trainees should be able to perform GALS and REMS, as well as being able to identify, by examination:

◆ The normal musculoskeletal system and its variations, including at extremes of age

◆ The surface anatomical features of the shoulder girdle, elbow, hand/wrist, hip/pelvis, knee, ankle/foot, spine

◆ The normal range of movement (active and passive) of these joints

+ The actions of major muscles/tendons acting on these joints

+ The clinical signs associated with inflammation or structural damage of joints and periarticular structures (muscles, tendons, entheses, bursae, and bone)

+ Non-articular, systemic, and other features of rheumatic disease

+ General medical complications of rheumatological disease

+ Diffuse or regional pain disorders or somatization disorders

It may be that many of the 'special tests' long associated with musculoskeletal examination are more within the domain of orthopaedics than rheumatology, but it is not clear from this curriculum whether they are expected to be part of the rheumatologist's repertoire. Each rheumatologist will have their own subset of such tests that they find useful but for each, it is important to remember that many are unvalidated, and of those that are, they are valid only providing the test is undertaken as originally described and in the situation in which it was evaluated. Original descriptions are not always easy to find in the literature.

A recent trend has been for clinical tests, originally intended for use as outcome measures in clinical trials, to be used in routine clinical practice. Examples include the DAS28 score in rheumatoid arthritis, the BASMI in ankylosing spondylitis, and the Rodnan skin score in scleroderma. As with special tests, it is important that the practitioner understands the validity of the test in the situation in which it is used and interprets the results with caution.

Relationship between clinical examination and imaging

The importance of detection of even quite subtle synovitis has led to a re-evaluation of the role of imaging to improve on examination findings. Ultrasound scanning may improve and augment clinical examination: for example, it can detect synovitis in patients clinically in remission and can detect more Heberden's nodes. MRI also detects more synovitis and can enhance clinical examination, but there are situations where dynamic imaging has advantages.[51] Clinical examination, particularly using the screening and regional approaches advocated in this chapter, is essential to target use of such imaging techniques appropriately, and in their interpretation.

References

1. Doherty M, Dacre J, Dieppe P, Snaith M. The 'GALS' locomotor screen. Ann Rheum Dis 1992;51(10):1165–1169.
2. Coady D, Walker D, Kay L. Regional Examination of the Musculoskeletal System (REMS): a core set of clinical skills for medical students. Rheumatology (Oxford) 2004;43(5):633–639.
3. Dequeker J, Esselens G, Westhovens R. Educational issues in rheumatology. The musculoskeletal examination: a neglected skill. Clin Rheumatol 2007;26(1):5–7.
4. Woolf AD, Akesson K. Primer: history and examination in the assessment of musculoskeletal problems. Nat Clin Pract Rheumatol 2008;4(1):26–33.
5. Sandler G. The importance of the history in the medical clinic and the cost of unnecessary tests. Am Heart J 1980;100(6 Pt 1):928–931.
6. Sandler G. Costs of unnecessary tests. Br Med J 1979;2(6181):21–24.
7. Almoallim H, Khojah E, Allehebi R, Noorwali A. Delayed diagnosis of systemic lupus erythematosus due to lack of competency skills in musculoskeletal examination. Clinical Rheumatol 2007;26(1):131–133.
8. Khan KM, Tress BW, Hare WS, Wark JD. Treat the patient, not the x-ray: advances in diagnostic imaging do not replace the need for clinical interpretation. Clin J Sport Med 1998;8(1):1–4.
9. Doherty M, Dawes P. Guidelines on undergraduate curriculum in the UK. Education Committees of Arthritis and Rheumatism Council and British Society for Rheumatology. Br J Rheumatol 1992;31(6):409–412.
10. Doherty M, Woolf A. Guidelines for rheumatology undergraduate core curriculum. EULAR Standing Committee on Education and Training. Ann Rheum Dis 1999;58(3):133–135.
11. Kay LJ, Deighton CM, Walker DJ, Hay EM. Undergraduate rheumatology teaching in the UK: a survey of current practice and changes since 1990. Arthritis Research Campaign Undergraduate Working Party of the ARC Education Sub-committee. Rheumatology (Oxford) 2000;39(7):800–803.
12. Woolf AD, Walsh NE, Akesson K. Global core recommendations for a musculoskeletal undergraduate curriculum. Ann Rheum Dis 2004;63(5):517–524.
13. Akesson K, Dreinhofer KE, Woolf AD. Improved education in musculoskeletal conditions is necessary for all doctors. Bulletin World Health Org 2003;81(9):677–683.
14. Hewlett S, Clarke B, O'Brien A et al. Rheumatology education for undergraduate nursing, physiotherapy and occupational therapy students in the UK: standards, challenges and solutions. Rheumatology (Oxford) 2008;47(7):1025–1030.
15. Kahn KL, Maclean CH, Wong AL et al. Assessment of American College of Rheumatology quality criteria for rheumatoid arthritis in a pre-quality criteria patient cohort. Arthritis Rheum 2007;57(5):707–715.
16. Freedman KB, Bernstein J. The adequacy of medical school education in musculoskeletal medicine. J Bone Joint Surg 1998;A80(10):1421–1427.
17. Stockard AR, Allen TW. Competence levels in musculoskeletal medicine: comparison of osteopathic and allopathic medical graduates. J Am Osteopath Assoc 2006;106(6):350–355.
18. Ward MJ. Family nurse practitioners: perceived competencies and recommendations. Nursing Res 1979;28(6):343–347.
19. Lynch JR, Gardner GC, Parsons RR. Musculoskeletal workload versus musculoskeletal clinical confidence among primary care physicians in rural practice. Am J Orthop (Belle Mead NJ) 2005;34(10):487–491, discussion 91–92.
20. Raissi GR, Mansoori K, Madani P, Rayegani SM. Survey of general practitioners' attitudes toward physical medicine and rehabilitation. Int J Rehab Res 2006;29(2):167–170.
21. de Jong J, Visser MR, Mohrs J, Wieringa-de Waard M. Opening the black box: the patient mix of GP trainees. Br J Gen Pract 2011;61(591):e650–e657.
22. Freedman KB, Bernstein J. Educational deficiencies in musculoskeletal medicine. J Bone Joint Surg 2002; A84(4):604–608.
23. Lillicrap MS, Byrne E, Speed CA. Musculoskeletal assessment of general medical in-patients—joints still crying out for attention. Rheumatology (Oxford) 2003;42(8):951–954.
24. Marshall RW, Hull RG. For crying out loud: musculoskeletal assessment of inpatients referred to rheumatology. Rheumatology (Oxford) 2004;43(11):1447.
25. Keysser G, Zacher J, Zeidler H. Rheumatologie: Integration in die studentische Ausbildung--die RISA-Studie. Ergebnisse einer Datenerhebung zum aktuellen Stand der studentischen Ausbildung im Fach Rheumatologie an den deutschen Universitaten. [Rheumatology: Integration into student training—the RISA Study. Results of a survey exploring the scale of education and training in rheumatology at German universities.] Z Rheumatol 2004;63(2):160–166.
26. Al-Nammari SS, James BK, Ramachandran M. The inadequacy of musculoskeletal knowledge after foundation training in the United Kingdom. J Bone Joint Surg 2009;B91(11):1413–1418.

27. Crotty M, Ahern MJ, McFarlane AC, Brooks PM. Clinical rheumatology training of Australian medical students. A national survey of 1991 graduates. *Med J Aust* 1993;158(2):119–120.

28. Doherty M, Abawi J, Pattrick M. Audit of medical inpatient examination: a cry from the joint. *J R Coll Physicians Lond* 1990;24(2):115–118.

29. Ahern MJ, Soden M, Schultz D, Clark M. The musculo-skeletal examination: a neglected clinical skill. *Aust NZ J Med* 1991;21(3):303–306.

30. Sirisena D, Begum H, Selvarajah M, Chakravarty K. Musculoskeletal examination—an ignored aspect. Why are we still failing the patients? *Clin Rheumatol* 2011;30(3):403–407.

31. Abou-Raya A, Abou-Raya S. The inadequacies of musculoskeletal education. *Clin Rheumatol* 2010;29(10):1121–1126.

32. Lanyon P, Pope D, Croft P. Rheumatology education and management skills in general practice: a national study of trainees. *Ann Rheum Dis* 1995;54(9):735–739.

33. Lynch JR, Schmale GA, Schaad DC, Leopold SS. Important demographic variables impact the musculoskeletal knowledge and confidence of academic primary care physicians. *J Bone Joint Surg* 2006;A88(7):1589–1595.

34. Matheny JM, Brinker MR, Elliott MN, Blake R, Rowane MP. Confidence of graduating family practice residents in their management of musculoskeletal conditions. *Am J Orthop* (Belle Mead NJ) 2000;29(12):945–952.

35. Mistlin A. Joint examination skills: are rheumatology specialist registrars adequately trained? *Rheumatology* (Oxford) 2004;43(3):387.

36. Pincus T, Segurado OG. Most visits of most patients with rheumatoid arthritis to most rheumatologists do not include a formal quantitative joint count. *Ann Rheum Dis* 2006;65(6):820–822.

37. McCarthy EM, Sheane BJ, Cunnane G. Greater focus on clinical rheumatology is required for training in internal medicine. *Clin Rheumatol* 2009;28(2):139–143.

38. Coady D, Kay L, Walker D. Regional musculoskeletal examination: what the students say. *J Clin Rheumatol* 2003;9(2):67–71.

39. Coady DA, Walker DJ, Kay LJ. Teaching medical students musculoskeletal examination skills: identifying barriers to learning and ways of overcoming them. *Scand J Rheumatol* 2004;33(1):47–51.

40. Coady D, Walker D, Kay L. The attitudes and beliefs of clinicians involved in teaching undergraduate musculoskeletal clinical examination skills. *Med Teacher* 2003;25(6):617–620.

41. Kay LJ, Baggott G, Coady DA, Foster HE. Musculoskeletal examination for children and adolescents: do standard textbooks contain enough information? *Rheumatology* (Oxford) 2003;42(11):1423–1425.

42. Kay LJ, Coady DA, Walker DJ. Joints: if relevant. Do available textbooks contain adequate information about musculoskeletal examination skills for medical students? *Med Teacher* 2001;23(6):585–590.

43. Sackett DL. The rational clinical examination. A primer on the precision and accuracy of the clinical examination. *JAMA* 1992;267(19):2638–2644.

44. McAlister FA, Straus SE, Sackett DL. Why we need large, simple studies of the clinical examination: the problem and a proposed solution. CARE-COAD1 group. Clinical Assessment of the Reliability of the Examination-Chronic Obstructive Airways Disease Group. *Lancet* 1999;354(9191):1721–1724.

45. Solomon DH, Simel DL, Bates DW, Katz JN, Schaffer JL. The rational clinical examination. Does this patient have a torn meniscus or ligament of the knee? Value of the physical examination. *JAMA* 2001;286(13):1610–1620.

46. Tennent TD, Beach WR, Meyers JF. A review of the special tests associated with shoulder examination. Part I: the rotator cuff tests. *Am J Sports Med* 2003;31(1):154–160.

47. Kay L, Walker D. Improving musculoskeletal clinical skills teaching. A regionwide audit and intervention study. *Ann Rheum Dis* 1998;57(11):656–659.

48. Woolf AD, Akesson K. Education in musculoskeletal health—how can it be improved to meet growing needs? *J Rheumatol* 2007;34(3):455–457.

49. Williams SC, Gulihar A, Dias JJ, Harper WM. A new musculoskeletal curriculum: has it made a difference? *J Bone Joint Surg* 2010;B92(1):7–11.

50. Alvarado LI. The development of a course in basic physical examination skills. *Bol Asoc Med Puerto Rico* 1998;90(1–3):45–50.

51. Dacre J, Haq I. Assessing competencies in rheumatology. *Ann Rheum Dis* 2005;64(1):3–6.

52. Dacre J, Besser M, White P. MRCP(UK) PART 2 Clinical Examination (PACES): a review of the first four examination sessions (June 2001–July 2002). *Clin Med* 2003;3(5):452–459.

53. Elder A, McAlpine L, Bateman N et al. Changing PACES: developments to the examination in 2009. *Clin Med* 2011;11(3):231–234.

54. Elder A, McManus C, McAlpine L, Dacre J. What skills are tested in the new PACES examination? *Ann Acad Med Singapore* 2011;40(3):119–125.

55. Badcock LJ, Raj N, Gadsby K, Deighton CM. Meeting the needs of increasing numbers of medical students—a best practice approach. Rheumatology (Oxford) 2006;45(7):799–803.

56. Coady D, Walker D, Kay L. Teaching in the clinical context. *Med Ed* 2003;37(7):663–664.

57. Dacre J, Nicol M, Holroyd D, Ingram D. The development of a clinical skills centre. *J R Coll Physicians Lon* 1996;30(4):318–324.

58. Smith MD, Walker JG, Schultz D et al. Teaching clinical skills in musculoskeletal medicine: the use of structured clinical instruction modules. *J Rheumatol* 2002;29(4):813–817.

59. Perry ME, Burke JM, Friel L, Field M. Can training in musculoskeletal examination skills be effectively delivered by undergraduate students as part of the standard curriculum? *Rheumatology* (Oxford) 2010;49(9):1756–1761.

60. Burke J, Fayaz S, Graham K, Matthew R, Field M. Peer-assisted learning in the acquisition of clinical skills: a supplementary approach to musculoskeletal system training. *Med Teacher* 2007;29(6):577–582.

61. Vivekananda-Schmidt P, Lewis M et al. Validation of MSAT: an instrument to measure medical students' self-assessed confidence in musculoskeletal examination skills. *Med Ed* 2007;41(4):402–410.

62. Vivekananda-Schmidt P, Lewis M et al. Exploring the use of videotaped objective structured clinical examination in the assessment of joint examination skills of medical students. *Arthritis Rheum* 2007;57(5):869–876.

63. Smith J, Laskowski ER, Noll SR. Development of a musculoskeletal examination skills course for a physical medicine and rehabilitation residency program. *Am J Phys Med Rehab* 2001;80(10):747–753.

64. O'Neill J, Williams JR, Kay LJ. Doctor-patient communication in a musculoskeletal unit: relationship between an observer-rated structured scoring system and patient opinion. *Rheumatology* (Oxford) 2003;42(12):1518–1522.

65. Jones A, Ledingham J, Regan M, Doherty M. A proposed minimal rheumatological screening history and examination. The joint answers back. *J R Coll Physicians Lond* 1991;25(2):111–1115.

66. Arthritis Research UK. Clinical assessment of the musculoskeletal system. Arthritis Research UK, 2010 (cited 2011). Available from: www. arthritisresearchuk.org/health-professionals-and-students/student-handbook.aspx.

67. Arthritis Research UK. Clinical assessment of the musculoskeletal system (video) 2010 (cited 2011); Available from: www.arthritisresearchuk.org/health-professionals-and-students/video-resources/rems. aspx.

68. Lee MA. What is the evidence that utilizing the GALS assessment while teaching medical students improves their skills at examining the musculoskeletal system? Rheumatology (Oxford) 2010;49(9):1783–1784.

69. MedRevise.co.uk. The one minute GALS examination. MedRevise.co.uk, 2010 (cited 2011); Available from: http://youtu.be/u4azNJ1HYJQ

70. Fox R MJ, McLure C, Dacre J. Can students learn a locomotor screening examination (the GALS screen)? A comparative study (abstract). *EULAR Congress Abstracts* 1999;84:321.

71. Fox RA, Dacre JE, Clark CL, Scotland AD. Impact on medical students of incorporating GALS screen teaching into the medical school curriculum. *Ann Rheum Dis* 2000;59(9):668–6671.

72. Beattie KA, Macintyre NJ, Pierobon J et al. The sensitivity, specificity and reliability of the GALS (gait, arms, legs and spine) examination when

used by physiotherapists and physiotherapy students to detect rheumatoid arthritis. Physiotherapy 2011;97(3):196–202.

73. Plant MJ, Linton S, Dodd E, Jones PW, Dawes PT. The GALS locomotor screen and disability. *Ann Rheum Dis* 1993;52(12):886–890.

74. Smith AMM, Walker DJ, Coady DA, Kay LJ. Impact of introduction of 'REMS' to medical student clinical skills teaching. *Rheumatology* (Oxford) 2005;44(S1):i78.

75. Wadey VM, Tang ET, Abelseth G et al. Canadian multidisciplinary core curriculum for musculoskeletal health. *J Rheumatol* 2007;34(3):567–580.

76. Foster H, Kay L, May C, Rapley T. Pediatric regional examination of the musculoskeletal system: a practice- and consensus-based approach. *Arthritis Care Res* 2011;63(11):1503–1510.

77. Wadey VM, Dev P, Buckley R, Walker D, Hedden D. Competencies for a Canadian orthopaedic surgery core curriculum. *J Bone Joint Surg* 2009;B91(12):1618–1622.

78. EULAR. *European Curriculum for Rheumatology*. EULAR, 2003 (cited 2011); Available from: www.eular.org/documents/uems_rheumatology_specialist_core_ curriculum_2003.pdf.

79. EULAR. Core curriculum for continuing medical education and professional development. EULAR, 2000 (cited 2011); Available from: www.eular.org/documents/uems_rheumatology_CME_curriculum_2000.pdf.

80. Armour B. What competence does a rheumatologist need? An international perspective. *Ann Rheum Dis* 2000;59:662–667.

81. Joint Royal Colleges of Physicians' Training Board (JRCPTB). *Curriculum for Rheumatology* 2010 (cited 2011); Available from: www.jrcptb.org.uk/specialties/ST3-SpR/Pages/Rheumatology.aspx.

Recommended resources

Apley GA, Solomon L. *Physical examination in orthopaedics*. Hodder Arnold, London, 1997.

Arthritis Research UK. Clinical assessment of the musculoskeletal system, issue 11.2. Available from: www.arthritisresearchuk.org/health-professionals-and-students/student-handbook.aspx

Doherty M, Hazelman BL, Hutton CW, Maddison PJ, Perry JD. *Rheumatology examination and injection techniques*, 2nd edn. W.B. Saunders, London, 1998.

Douglas G, Nicol F, Robertson C. *Macleod's clinical examination*, 12th edn (with DVD). Churchill Livingstone, London, 2009.

MacKinnon PCB, Morris JF. *Oxford textbook of functional anatomy: musculoskeletal system*. Oxford University Press, Oxford, 1994.

SECTION 2

Common clinical presentations of rheumatic disease

CHAPTER 7

Monoarticular disease

Mark Lillicrap and Shazia Abdullah

Introduction

Monoarticular joint pain (joint pain affecting a single joint) is a common presentation both in primary care and in hospital emergency departments. The assessment and management of trauma-associated monoarticular joint pain is beyond the scope of this text. The remainder of this chapter will assume that trauma-associated causes of pain (fracture, avulsion injury, etc.) have been excluded (usually through history, examination, and radiographic imaging).

Atraumatic monoarticular joint pain can occur because of processes occurring in any of the component structures around the joint, as well as being referred from sources of pain at other sites. Inflammatory pain can be caused by microcrystals (gout and pseudogout), microorganisms (septic arthritis), and autoinflammatory diseases (rheumatoid arthritis (RA), reactive arthritis, spondyloarthritis). Mechanical pain can be caused by cartilage degeneration and associated bony reaction (osteoarthritis/osteoarthrosis) or by local effects on ligaments, tendons, and bursae. A more extensive list of the possible causes of monoarticular joint pain is shown in Table 7.1.

Epidemiology

Studies suggest that inflammatory monoarthritis affects men more commonly than women[1] (largely because gout is more common in men) and the most commonly affected joints are the lower limb weight-bearing, joints (particularly the knee).[2] The underlying diagnosis of a transient self-resolving inflammatory monoarthritis may remain unknown, but crystal arthritis is the most common diagnosis; followed by reactive arthritis, RA, and then septic arthritis.[3] Undoubtedly the most important diagnosis to exclude is septic arthritis since, even with current antimicrobial management, it is associated with high levels of morbidity and mortality (approximately 10% case fatality rate).[4] Accurate information on the epidemiology of septic arthritis is lacking, for several reasons. First, the data is derived mainly from retrospective studies; secondly, there is a lack of clarity of case definition. The incidence of proven and probable septic arthritis in western Europe is 4–10 per 100 000 patient-years per year.[4] Various risk factors increase the likelihood of developing septic arthritis, including RA, osteoarthritis, prosthetic joints, low socioeconomic status, intravenous drug abuse, alcoholism, diabetes, previous intra-articular corticosteroid injection, and cutaneous ulcers.[5,6] The incidence of septic arthritis is also significantly higher in HIV infected patients than in the general population.[7] Across all age groups the most common aetiological organism of septic arthritis is *Staphylococcus aureus* followed by *Streptococcus pyogenes*.[5,8] In the young, sexually active population (particularly women) gonococcus remains an important cause, although its prevalence in developed countries is declining.[9] Immunocompromised patients may also develop septic arthritis from more unusual organisms.

Clinical features

General approach to history and examination

When approaching a patient presenting with monoarticular joint pain a number of key questions should be borne in mind:

- Is this inflammatory or non-inflammatory pain?
- Is this an acute or chronic problem?
- Is this a problem within the joint or arising from surrounding tissues?

Inflammatory versus non-inflammatory pain

From the perspective of patient management, the first key division is into those presentations caused by mechanical joint problems and those caused by inflammatory diseases. The patient's history is the key factor in addressing this question. In general, inflammatory joint diseases are associated with early morning stiffness of the affected joint, which will often last for several hours. Patients may spontaneously mention the joint feeling stiff as well as painful. In severe acute inflammatory arthritis this pain and stiffness may be so severe as to limit any movement and, when the lower limbs are involved, may restrict weight bearing. Mechanical joint problems tend to be associated with more short-lived stiffness (a few minutes in duration) and patients tend to identify activity-associated pain (rather than stiffness), which improves with rest, as their major concern.

A history of joint swelling can be an additional indicator of inflammatory joint disease, although this is less reliable when the affected joint is a knee (can occur in osteoarthritis) or an ankle (often due to oedema).

A symptomatic response to treatment with non-steroidal anti-inflammatory drugs (NSAIDs), particularly if the symptoms respond dramatically, can be supportive evidence of an inflammatory rather than a non-inflammatory process.

Table 7.1 Possible causes of monoarticular joint pain

	Inflammatory	Non-inflammatory
Common	Crystal arthritis:	Osteoarthritis
	monosodium urate	Trauma
	monophosphate	Avascular necrosis
	calcium pyrophosphate dihydrate	
	hydroxyapatite	
	calcium oxalate	
	Reactive arthritis	
	Spondyloarthritis:	
	psoriatic arthritis	
	enteropathic inflammatory arthritis	
	Sarcoidosis/Lofgren's syndrome	
	Lyme disease	
	Juvenile idiopathic arthritis	
	Septic arthritis:	
	bacteria (Staphylococcus aureus, streptococcus, enterococcus, E. coli, gonococcus)	
	fungi	
	mycobacteria	
	Haemarthrosis	
	coagulopathy	
	Monoarticular presentations of polyarticular synovitis:	
	rheumatoid arthritis	
	vasculitides	
	connective tissue diseases	
	Idiopathic/self-resolving	
Uncommon	Pigmented villonodular synovitis (PVNS)	Malignancy:
	Foreign body synovitis	synovial metastasis
		bone tumours
		Hypertrophic pulmonary osteoarthropathy
		Synovial chondromatosis
		Synovioma
		Charcot's arthropathy

A history of redness of the skin overlying the joint is highly suggestive of either crystal arthritis (gout or pseudogout) or septic arthritis. This is probably due to the acute neutrophil-driven inflammatory pathology in these diseases. Other causes of monoarthritis are not generally associated with overlying redness.

In patients with pre-existing inflammatory joint disease, such as RA, a clinical suspicion of additional septic arthritis should be considered if the symptoms in a single affected joint are significantly out of proportion to the disease activity reported in other joints.

Acute or chronic

Gout and pseudogout are characterized by a very acute onset of symptoms (usually over hours to days). Symptoms in septic arthritis are usually present for 1–2 weeks, but the onset can be slower,

especially with low-virulence organisms, mycobacterial infection, and prosthesis infection. The other inflammatory arthritides all tend to be associated with a slower onset of symptoms (usually over several weeks).

A monoarthritis is generally considered acute if it has been present for less than 4 weeks,[10] although some have proposed a 2 week cut-off.[1] A joint problem which has persisted for more than 6 weeks is generally categorized as chronic. Although gout, pseudogout, and septic arthritis can occasionally be associated with a chronic monoarthritis, this is unusual. A chronic course would be more suggestive of conditions such as reactive arthritis, spondyloarthritis, chronic mycobacterial or fungal infection (if inflammatory), or osteoarthritis/osteoarthrosis (if non-inflammatory). A migratory monoarthritis, where several different joints are serially affected over time, can also be seen with a chronic autoinflammatory arthritis. However, this pattern is also recognized as a presentation of gonococcal septic arthritis.[9]

Localization of symptoms

It is important to ascertain whether the source of the pain is the joint or other surrounding structures. Joint pain is characteristically a deep-seated pain that may be localized to the joint or may be felt distal to the joint itself. The pain from surrounding structures is often a more superficial pain that the patient can clearly localize to one of the periarticular structures. It is important for the clinician to bear in mind that the common causes of monoarthritis can also affect other surrounding joint structures. Involvement of these areas can help guide diagnosis. Patients with reactive arthritis or other spondylarthritides may describe associated enthesitis, both of the affected joint and at other sites (e.g. plantar fasciitis, Achilles tendonitis)[11]; patients with gout may describe associated bursitis and inflammation of local tendon sheaths, as may patients with gonococcal septic arthritis.[9]

Additional information

Additional risk factors for septic arthritis should be sought in the history. Risk factors for septic arthritis include diabetes, prior RA, previous joint replacement, recent intra-articular corticosteroid injection, HIV infection, intravenous drug usage, or immunosuppression.[5,12] (Margaretten et al.[12] is a key reference here—a systematic review of the evidence base for diagnosis of non-gonococcal septic arthritis.) Other factors of relevance to alternative differential diagnoses that should be considered in the history are recent urethritis (reactive arthritis or gonococcal arthritis); conjunctivitis or diarrhoea (reactive arthritis); a history of cutaneous/nail psoriasis or inflammatory back pain (spondyloarthritis); history of tick bites (Lyme disease); dietary factors or features of the metabolic syndrome (gout); history of erythema nodosum (Lofgren's syndrome/acute sarcoid).

Examination

A screening examination of the musculoskeletal system (such as the GALS screen[13]) should be undertaken in any patient presenting with a monoarthritis.

Examination of the affected area, with an understanding of the relevant functional anatomy, is key to the localization of the problem. A discussion of the relevant regional examination routines can be found in other chapters, and detailed regional musculoskeletal examination routines have been published elsewhere.[6]

The key factors to consider when examining the affected joint of a patient with monoarthritis are:

♦ Is this a true joint problem or a peri-articular problem arising from the bursae or tendons?

♦ Is there evidence of inflammatory changes (a joint effusion, warmth, joint line tenderness)?

♦ Is there evidence of overlying erythema (suggestive of septic arthritis or crystal arthritis)?

General examination

Although the finding of an elevated temperature in conjunction with a hot, red, swollen joint should alert any clinician to a likely diagnosis of septic arthritis, the absence of any of these features does not exclude the diagnosis. In one prospective study of septic arthritis fever was only present in about one-half of the cases.[14] Furthermore crystal arthritis is not uncommonly associated with a low-grade elevation of the temperature[15] as well as swelling and frequently redness of the joint. It is therefore extremely difficult for a clinician to differentiate sepsis, as a cause of monoarthritis, from crystal arthritis, solely on the basis of examination findings.[16]

For other differential diagnoses, additional examination features may guide the diagnostic reasoning process. For example: evidence of relevant skin rashes (psoriasis or nail dystrophy (psoriatic monoarthritis), erythema nodosum (sarcoid/Lofgren's syndrome), keratoderma blenorrhagica (reactive arthritis), erythema chronicum migrans (Lyme disease); additional joint involvement (small joints of the hands (rheumatoid), sacroiliac joints (spondyloarthritis), distal interphalangeal joints (Heberden's nodes (both pseudogout and osteoarthritis)); conjunctivitis (reactive arthritis); anterior uveitis (spondyloarthritis) and cutaneous tophi (gout).

Management

An approach to investigations

The most common causes of an acute monoarthritis are crystal arthritis, reactive arthritis, rheumatoid arthritis, septic arthritis, and osteoarthritis.[3] The primary clinical concern, when assessing any patient with acute monoarthritis, is the exclusion of septic arthritis, because of its attendant morbidity and mortality.[4] For the purposes of diagnosis, all patients presenting with an acute non-traumatic inflammatory monoarthritis should therefore have a plain radiograph and arthrocentesis/synovial fluid analysis. These two investigations, combined with the history and examination, will result in a definitive diagnosis within 2–3 days in approximately three-quarters of cases.[1] Synovial fluid analysis is the most important investigation, facilitating immediate diagnosis in approximately one-third of cases.[1] In addition, synovial fluid analysis enables exclusion of most (but not all) cases of septic arthritis. In a systematic review of the clinical evaluation of septic arthritis, synovial fluid analysis was shown to be the most powerful laboratory test employed.[10]

An algorithm for the approach to a patient presenting with an acute monoarthritis (based in part on the British Society for Rheumatology guidelines 2006[17]) is shown in Figure 7.1. These guidelines, developed by a national working group reviewing the evidence base, give useful practical guidance for clinicians on how to assess and manage a patient presenting with an acute monoarthritis.

Other laboratory investigations can be contributory to diagnosis and management. In most patients a full blood count (to assess both the total white cell count and the neutrophil count), systemic inflammatory markers (C-reactive protein (CRP) or erythrocyte sedimentation rate (ESR)), electrolytes and liver function (important in management decisions) should be checked.[11] The total white cell count is not infrequently normal in patients with septic arthritis at initial presentation; the CRP is a more reliable predictor of septic arthritis in this context.[14] If they are raised, both the total white cell count and the CRP can be used to monitor response to treatment. In suspected septic arthritis blood should always be cultured before the initiation of antibiotic therapy, to increase the chances of identifying the causative organisms.[3–6,7] Sometimes blood cultures can be the only source of a positive microbiological diagnosis.[5] Although frequently checked, the serum uric acid levels are often non-contributory since these levels characteristically fall during an acute systemic inflammatory response. If the levels are found to be elevated the result can be helpful, but if the levels are normal during an acute attack it is not possible to exclude gout as the cause.[18]

If there are features in the history and examination that suggest other differential diagnoses, other appropriate laboratory studies should be undertaken. The relevant investigations for the assessment of other differential diagnoses are highlighted in the other relevant chapters of this book.

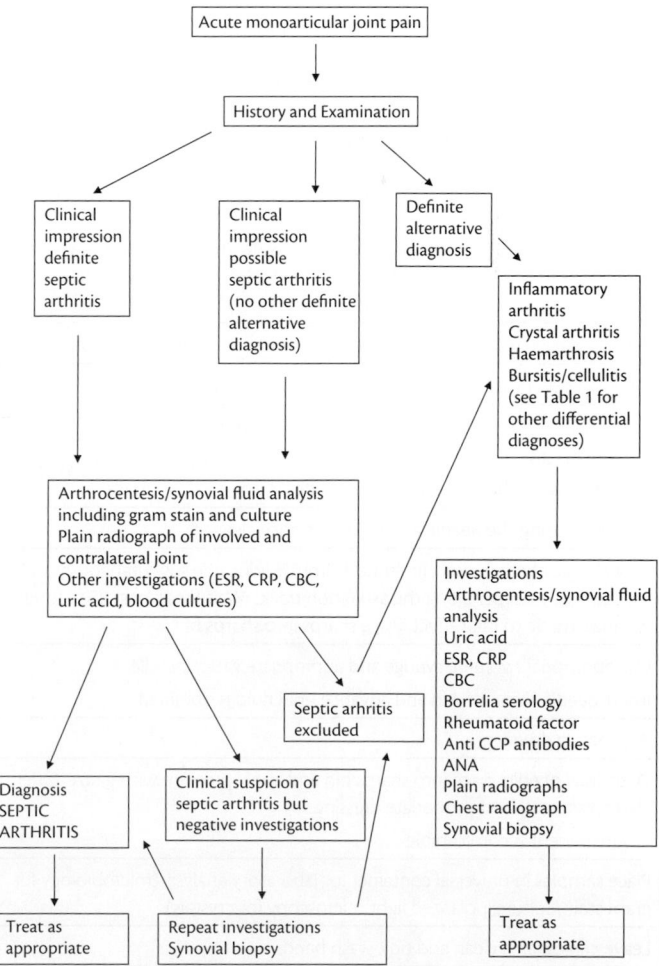

Fig. 7.1 Algorithm for the investigation of acute monoarticular joint pain.

Arthrocentesis

Arthrocentesis and prompt synovial fluid analysis (with Gram staining, culture, and assessment under compensated polarized light) are the key tools in making a diagnosis in patients presenting with acute monoarthritis. In patients with septic arthritis the Gram stain is positive in approximately 50% of cases, and cultures can be positive in approximately 90% of patients.[10,19,20] A negative synovial fluid culture does not exclude the diagnosis of septic arthritis, and the causative organism can sometimes be isolated from other sites (e.g. blood or urine). Where the clinical suspicion is high for septic arthritis, patients should be treated even in the absence of positive cultures.[14]

A structured approach to joint arthrocentesis is shown in Figure 7.2. It is a safe technique that is easily undertaken provided the clinician is aware of the relevant functional anatomy and has had appropriate training.

For skin preparation before aspiration, an aseptic no-touch technique using handwashing, non-sterile gloves, and alcohol swabbing prior to the procedure (also known as a clean technique) is as effective as a sterile technique (with sterile gloves/drapes and iodine swabs).[21]

The initial appearance of aspirated synovial fluid can itself guide the diagnosis. It is useful to document the gross appearance of

AN APPROACH TO ARTHROCENTESIS (JOINT ASPIRATION)
Introduce self; explain reason and nature of procedure.   Gain verbal consent.
Prepare tray including: 10-20ml syringe, 21G (green) needle, some chlorhexidine swabs , gauze, sterile universal containers   NB: If septic arthritis is suspected a wider bore 19G white needle may be used instead.   If local anaesthetic is to be administered, draw up 2ml of 1% lignocaine, using a blue needle and then put a clean 25G (orange) needle on the syringe. (remember to check drug name, dose, route and expiry)
Roll up sleeves, remove watch, wash hands and put on gloves (non sterile).
Identify appropriate surface landmarks for joint to be aspirated
Check skin at the proposed aspiration site is lesion-free.   Clean skin with alcohol or chlorhexidine wipe in circular motion from injection point outwards then wait until cleaned area is dry.
Avoid touching the needle at entry point once cleaned.
If local anaesthetic is used, infiltrate 1-2ml 1% lidocaine subcutaneously and subsequently deeper along the aspiration track. Wait for at least 30 seconds for anaesthetic to take effect. Place sharps into sharps bin
Use appropriate volume syringe and appropriate gauge needle   Insert needle through skin and advance until fluid is obtained.
Aspirate to dryness
Withdraw needle, place into sharps bin and apply pressure with gauze. Offer elastoplast or other appropriate dressing   Ensure patient is comfortable
Place samples in universal container for laboratory analysis (microbiology for gram stain/culture; polarized light microscopy for crystals).
Leave clinical area clean and tidy, wash hands.

Fig. 7.2 An approach to joint aspiration (arthrocentesis).

synovial fluid, describing the colour, clarity, and viscosity. Clear, straw-coloured, viscous synovial fluid is usually indicative of normal or osteoarthrotic synovial fluid. Heavily blood-stained fluid may indicate an underlying traumatic cause or a haemarthrosis secondary to a coagulopathy. As the fluid becomes inflammatory it becomes less viscous and loses clarity due to the accumulation of white blood cells. Mildly cloudy synovial fluid (indicative of a mild or moderately elevated synovial fluid white cell count) is seen in autoinflammatory diseases such as RA and spondyloarthritis as well as crystal arthritis (and some septic arthritis). Turbid synovial fluid, indicative of a high synovial fluid white cell count (usually predominantly neutrophilic), is more commonly seen in septic arthritis.[22] Although synovial fluid white cell count can be measured, it is not a reliable measure to exclude or confirm a diagnosis of septic arthritis.[23]

Polarized light microscopy

In addition to microbiological assessment of aspirated synovial fluid, synovial fluid microscopy under compensated polarized light should also be undertaken. The demonstration of microcrystals within the synovial fluid remains the gold standard for the diagnosis of crystal arthritis. Synovial fluid analysis for monosodium urate monophosphate (uric acid) has a sensitivity of 69% and a specificity of 93%[24,25] (figures for calcium pyrophosphate dihydrate microcrystals are lower). Synovial microcrystals can occasionally coexist with septic arthritis, and the finding of crystals does not entirely exclude septic arthritis. Aspirated synovial fluid should therefore also be Gram stained and cultured if there is any clinical suspicion of sepsis.[25] (Zhang et al.[25] is a key reference—a report of a European task force which identifies 10 key recommendations for the diagnosis of gout.)

Radiology

A study of adult patients with acute non-traumatic monoarthritis[1] demonstrated the benefits of plain radiographs in the diagnostic approach. In their study, radiographs of the involved and the contralateral joint were undertaken and this is advantageous for the purposes of comparison. Radiographs can be diagnostically helpful if they demonstrate chondrocalcinosis (in patients with calcium pyrophosphate dihydrate (CPPD) arthritis/pseudogout). Characteristic radiographic changes can also be seen in other conditions (e.g. osteoarthritis, RA, psoriatic arthritis). Radiographs are rarely adequate to exclude septic arthritis, particularly when these other conditions present with monoarthritis—diseases like RA are a risk factor for the development of septic arthritis.[3] The radiographic changes of gout (e.g. gouty erosions) are occasionally demonstrable, although plain radiographs only have a sensitivity of about 30% for gout.[26] Plain radiographs can also be diagnostic of rarer conditions, e.g. Charcot joint, avascular osteonecrosis, and hypertrophic pulmonary osteoarthropathy.

Other imaging modalities can be helpful in the diagnostic work-up of monoarthritis. Ultrasound can be used both for guiding arthrocentesis and can also be helpful diagnostically. Ultrasound has a much greater sensitivity for gout (96%),[26] detecting stippled foci of uric acid deposition and hyperechoic soft tissue areas which are not seen on plain radiographs. However the specificity of ultrasound for gout is lower (73%).[26]

CT scanning and MRI can also be helpful in the identification of other causes of acute monoarthritis. For example, avascular necrosis, haemochromatosis, pigmented villonodular synovitis, and synovial chondromatosis all have characteristic appearances on MRI. MRI may also allow identification of a foreign body (e.g. a plant thorn) in foreign body synovitis.[27] Where the underlying diagnosis remains unclear despite initial investigations, such additional imaging should be considered to help guide further intervention.

Supplementary investigations

A proportion of patients with acute inflammatory monoarthritis cannot be diagnosed in the first few weeks. Some of these have a spontaneously resolving idiopathic inflammatory arthritis. If monoarthritic symptoms persist for several weeks, consideration should be given to arthroscopic biopsy of the synovium. Certain infections, such as mycobacterial and fungal infections, can present with a more chronic picture. A synovial biopsy can be subjected to prolonged culture and may also show characteristic histological changes such as granulomatous synovitis (suggestive of mycobacterial infection). PCR (of either synovial fluid or synovial tissue) is a further supplementary investigation that can be useful in the diagnosis of atypical infections.[28]

Characteristic histological changes are also seen in pigmented villonodular synovitis and other rarer synovial tumours that can again present with a more chronic indolent course.

Case history

A 75 year old woman, with a history of nodal osteoarthritis (OA) and a previous right total hip replacement, was admitted to hospital with a community-acquired pneumonia. Having been on appropriate intravenous antibiotic treatment for 48 hours she developed an acute monoarthritis of her left wrist. On general examination she had a pyrexia (temperature 37.8 °C) and changes on respiratory examination in keeping with pneumonia. On musculoskeletal examination she had nodal osteoarthritis changes of the distal interphalangeal joints and a scar from her previous total hip replacement. The left wrist itself was erythematous, warm, and tender with a markedly restricted range of movement. There was a palpable effusion with associated boggy synovial swelling.

What is the likely diagnosis and how should this be managed?

The first concern, in this clinical context, is septic arthritis and this diagnosis must be excluded. As highlighted in this chapter, pre-existing osteoarthritis is a recognized risk factor for septic arthritis and the presence of a coexisting infectious source would increase the likelihood of this. However, it is also possible that this is a crystal arthritis. In fact the most likely diagnosis, in this clinical setting, is pseudogout. As highlighted in the chapter on crystal arthritis (Chapter 151), pseudogout commonly occurs on a background of nodal osteoarthritis, can be triggered by intercurrent infection, and affects medium/large joints including, quite commonly, the wrist.

Reviewing the appropriate management in the algorithm illustrated in Figure 7.1, this patient would be described as having possible septic arthritis (although pseudogout/crystal arthritis is possible, it is not a definite diagnosis).

In this case the following investigations were initiated:

◆ joint aspiration/synovial fluid analysis (undertaken by the on-call rheumatologist)

◆ blood tests including CBC, CRP. and ESR and blood cultures

◆ plain radiograph of both wrists.

The following initial results were obtained:

◆ synovial fluid: turbid, inflammatory, blood-stained aspirate obtained

◆ Gram stain negative

◆ blood and synovial fluid cultures negative after 3 days

◆ weakly positively birefringent rhomboid crystals identified on polarized light microscopy

◆ chondrocalcinosis of triangular fibrocartilage complex on radiography.

Septic arthritis was therefore excluded and the patient was managed as having pseudogout. The pain was initially managed with NSAIDs but due to ongoing symptoms (when the culture results were known) the wrist joint itself was injected with hydrocortisone, resulting in a resolution of the patient's symptoms.

References

1. Freed JF, Nies KM, Boyer RS, Louie JS. Acute monoarticular arthritis. A diagnostic approach. *JAMA* 1980;243(22):2314–2316.

2. Mjaavatten HD, Haugen AJ, Helgetveit K et al. Pattern of joint involvement and other disease characteristics in 634 patients with arthritis of less than 16 weeks duration. *J Rheumatol* 2009;36(7):1401–1406.

3. Ma L, Cranney A, Holroyd-Leduc JM. Acute monoarthritis: What is the cause of my patient's painful swollen joint? *CMAJ* 2009; 180(1):59–65.

4. Mathews CJ, Weston VC, Jones A, Field M, Coakley G. Bacterial septic arthritis in adults. *Lancet* 2010;375(9717):846–855.

5. Weston VC, Jones AC, Bradbury N, Fawthorp F, Doherty M. Clinical features and outcome of septic arthritis in a single UK Health District 1982-1991. *Ann Rheum Dis* 1999;58:214–219.

6. Arthritis Research UK. *Clinical assessment of the musculoskeletal system.* Available at: www.arthritisresearchuk.org/health-professionals-and-students/student-handbook.aspx

7. Kaandorp CJ, Van Schaardenburg D, Krijnen P, Habbema JD, van de Laar MA. Risk factors for septic arthritis in patients with joint disease. A prospective study. *Arthritis Rheum* 1995;38:1819–1825.

8. Morgan DS, Fisher D, Merianos A, Currie BJ. An 18 year clinical review of septic arthritis from tropical Australia. *Epidemiol Infect* 1996;117(3):423–428.

9. Bardin T. Gonococcal arthritis. *Best Pract Res Clin Rheumatol* 2003;17(2): 201–208.

10. Parker JD, Capell HA, An acute arthritis clinic—one year's experience. *Br J Rheumatol* 1986;25(3):293–295.

11. Turan Y, Durouz MT, Cerrahoglu L. Relationship between enthesitis, clinical parameters and quality of life in spondyloarthritis. *Joint Bone Spine* 2009;76(6):642–647.

12. Margaretten ME, Kohlwes J, Moore D, Bent S. Does this adult patient have septic arthritis? *JAMA* 2007;297(13):1478–1488.

13. Arthritis Research UK. Musculoskeletal screening examination: GALS video. www.arthritisresearchuk.org/health-professionals-and-students/video-resources/rems.aspx

14. Gupta MN, Sturrock RD, Field M. A prospective 2-year study of 75 patients with adult-onset septic arthritis. *Ann Rheum Dis* 2001;40(1):24–30.

15. Ho G Jr, DeNuccio M. Gout and pseudogout in hospitalized patients. *Arch Intern Med* 1993;153(24):2787–2790.

16. Gupta MN, Sturrock RD, Field M. Prospective comparative study of patients with culture proven and high suspicion of adult onset septic arthritis. *Ann Rheum Dis* 2003;62(4):327–331.

17. Coakley G, Mathews C, Field M et al. BSR & BHPR, BOA, RCGP and BSAC guidelines for the management of the hot swollen joint in adults. *Rheumatology* 2006;45:1039–1041.

18. Logan JA, Morrison E, McGill PE. Serum uric acid in acute gout. *Ann Rheum Dis* 1997;56:696–697.

19. Swan A, Amer H, Dieppe P. The value of synovial fluid assays in the diagnosis of joint disease: a literature survey. *Ann Rheum Dis* 2002;61:493–498.

20. Ryan MJ, Kavanagh R, Wall PG, Hazleman BL. Bacterial joint infections in England and Wales: analysis of bacterial isolates over a four year period. *Br J Rheumatol.*1997;36:370–373.

21. Baima J, Isaac Z. Clean versus sterile technique for common joint injections: a review from the physiatry perspective. *Curr Rev Musculoskeletal Med* 2008;1(2):88–89.

22. Shmerling RH, Delbanco TL, Tosteson AN, Trentham DE. Synovial fluid tests. What should be ordered? *JAMA* 1990;264(8):1009–1014.

23. Mathews CJ, Kingsley G, Field M et al. Management of septic arthritis: a systematic review. *Ann Rheum Dis* 2007;66:440–445.

24. Gordon C, Swan A, Dieppe P. Detection of crystals in synovial fluid by light microscopy: sensitivity and reliability. *Ann Rheum Dis* 1989;48:737–742.

25. Zhang W, Doherty M, Pascual E et al. EULAR evidence based recommendations for gout. Part 1: Diagnosis. *Ann Rheum Dis* 2006;65:1301–1311.

26. Rettenbacher T, Ennemoser S, Weirich H et al. Diagnostic imaging of gout: comparison of high-resolution US versus conventional X-ray. *Eur Radiol* 2008;18(3):621–630.

27. Stevens KJ, Theologis T, McNally EG. Imaging of plant-thorn synovitis. *Skeletal Radiol* 2000;29(10);605–608.

28. Van der Heijden IM, Wilbrink B et al. Rheumatology 2008;38(6): 547–553.

CHAPTER 8

Oligoarticular disease

Andrew Keat

Introduction

The definition of oligoarthritis as involving four or fewer joints over the first 6 months of the course of disease arises from childhood arthritis studies.[1] The term pauciarticular arthritis is also used with the same meaning and, in children, evolution of persistent arthritis to involve more than four joints is often referred to as 'extended oligoarthritis'. In adults the term is also sometimes used to apply to five or fewer joints.[2]

Involvement of a few joints is as characteristic a pattern of rheumatic disease as the monoarthritis of gout or sepsis and the symmetrical polyarthritis of rheumatoid arthritis. Typically, large joints such as the knee and ankle are primarily involved, though forefoot and toe joints may also be affected; upper limb joints are affected less commonly, unless psoriasis is present. In a few cases oligoarticular onset of disease in adulthood evolves into characteristic polyarticular or even monoarticular syndromes, but most cases either remain as undifferentiated oligoarthritis or differentiate into a more typical form of spondyloarthritis (SpA). The most common diagnoses to be made in patients presenting with oligoarticular arthritis are reactive arthritis and sarcoidosis,[2] but most patients defy convenient labelling. Most of these may be said to have undifferentiated peripheral SpA.

As the major diagnostic group of oligoarthritides, peripheral SpA requires some clarification before the diagnostic approach is considered. SpA currently defies tight diagnostic criteria. Initial criteria built on the description of 'seronegative polyarthritis' by Moll, Wright, and colleagues[3,4] were introduced by Amor and colleagues in 1990[5] and by the European Spondyloarthritis Study Group (ESSG) in 1991.[6] Both use a scoring system to identify SpA and the ESSG criteria specifically allow differentiation into principally spinal or peripheral disease. However, neither set of criteria works well as potential diagnostic criteria across a range of patients considered to have SpA. More recently the Assessment of Spondyloarthritis International Society (ASAS) has published further criteria for classification of spondyloarthritis[7] and these new criteria for classification of peripheral SpA are shown in Figure 8.1. Although the sensitivity of these criteria for diagnostic purposes remains modest at 77.8%, specificity exceeds that of the Amor and ESSG criteria;[7] these criteria are often used for diagnosis.

The classification of peripheral SpA overlaps with the diagnosis of the individual syndromes of psoriatic arthritis, enteropathic arthritis, and reactive arthritis and may accompany axial disease. The extent to which oligoarthritis associated with these

ASAS Classification Criteria for Peripheral Spondyloarthritis (SpA)

Arthritis or enthesitis or dactylitis plus

≥ 1 SpA feature
- uveitis
- psoriasis
- Crohn's/colitis
- preceding infection
- HLA-B27
- sacroiliitis on imaging

OR

≥ 2 Other SpA feature
- arthritis
- enthesitis
- dactylitis
- inflammatory back pain (ever)
- family history for SpA

Sensitivity: 77.8%, Specificity: 82.2%; n=266

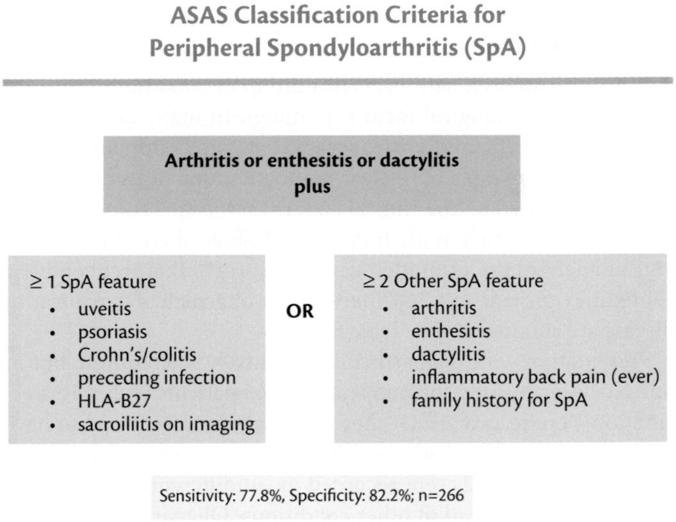

Fig. 8.1 Assessment of Spondyloarthritis International Society (ASAS) classification criteria for peripheral spondyloarthritis.
Reproduced from *Annals of the Rheumatic Diseases*, M Rudwaleit et al., 70 (1), with permission from BMJ Publishing Group Ltd.

conditions actually represents a single condition is unresolved, so that at present both the individual syndromes and the over-arching 'peripheral SpA' concept are widely used.

The characteristic features of peripheral SpA and other conditions considered in this chapter are described elsewhere in this volume.

Epidemiology

Measuring or estimating the prevalence of oligoarthritis, including peripheral SpA, is fraught with difficulties. Epidemiologically it is pertinent and pragmatic to consider peripheral SpA as a surrogate for oligoarthritis, as this diagnosis accounts for the majority of patients. However, although data on prevalence of SpA as a group—including axial SpA—are available, it is strongly influenced by the prevalence of HLA B27 and the ethnic mix of the population under study. The prevalence of peripheral SpA may be assumed to be lower than the true figure for SpA overall. Moreover, it is clear that recognition of the various subtypes of peripheral SpA varies, so that psoriatic arthritis is generally under-recognized and many cases of reactive arthritis resolve. In the absence of clear diagnostic criteria or long-term outcome studies to establish which cases evolve into another disease, designation of the patients is also difficult, especially in undifferentiated SpA.

Bearing in mind these difficulties, Haglund and colleagues[8] estimated the prevalence of SpA (not including chronic reactive arthritis) as 0.45% (95% CI 0.44%–0.47%) in Sweden; this included prevalences of psoriatic arthritis (0.25%), ankylosing spondylitis with peripheral involvement (0.12%), undifferentiated SpA (0.10%), and arthritis associated with inflammatory bowel disease (0.015%). The prevalence of SpA overall was similar in men and women. Reveille[9] estimated the prevalence of SpA in the United States at 0.2–0.5% for ankylosing spondylitis, 0.1% for psoriatic arthritis, 0.065% for enteropathic peripheral arthritis, and 0.05–0.25% for enteropathic axial arthritis. This review concluded that the overall prevalence of SpA was likely to be around 1%, a prevalence figure similar to that of rheumatoid arthritis.[10] Prevalence figures for individual SpA syndromes are given in the relevant chapters.

Aetiology

As oligoarthritis is a heterogeneous group of conditions there are no common aetiological factors, although in many cases a combination of genetic and environmental factors is implicated. Few oligoarticular diseases have clear pathognomonic features, so that diagnosis is based on the clinical pattern, associated comorbidities, and a few laboratory tests. Immunopathological and histopathological analyses are of limited value. Disorders that frequently or sometimes present in adult life with an oligoarticular pattern of disease are summarized in Table 8.1.

Presentation with oligoarthritis is relatively uncommon, but in one Norwegian study the outcomes of 146 patients with this presentation were recorded.[2] Of these, 46 patients were found to have reactive arthritis, 15 had sarcoidosis, 15 had non-inflammatory joint disease, and 62 were recorded as 'undifferentiated arthritis' with 8 having a spread of other conditions. Oligoarticular presentations of disseminated gonococcal and meningococcal infection are unusual but well recognized,[11,12] and this pattern is characteristic of Lyme disease.[13] Septic arthritis is usually monoarticular though multifocal joint sepsis may occur, especially in the case of tuberculosis. Oligoarticular involvement is typical of Behçet's syndrome,[14] and evolution of oligoarthritis to rheumatoid arthritis or Sjögren's syndrome is not rare. In Kvien et al.'s study[2] the diagnosis of oligoarthritis was made in some patients with osteoarthritis; in older patients an inflammatory element with joint swelling is often present with osteoarthritis, so that the diagnosis may not be straightforward.

The features of sarcoidosis and spondyloarthritis are considered elsewhere. However, the term 'peripheral SpA' covers a large spectrum of rheumatology without absolute clarity of meaning. Under the terms of the ASAS classification criteria[7] this term covers peripheral forms of psoriatic arthritis, reactive arthritis, enteropathic arthritis, and the arthritis associated with axial SpA. In many patients, however, the disease does not meet the strict criteria and yet the arthritis has characteristic features of asymmetrical lower limb oligoarthritis and the HLA B27 gene may be present. Clinical studies have generally focused on the 'polar' forms of disease such as psoriatic arthritis, for which clear criteria exist (CASPAR),[15] and reactive arthritis; relatively little work provides evidence of the assumed homogeneity of peripheral SpA. Based on the likely role of initiating infections in reactive arthritis[16,17] and the high frequency of HLA B27 throughout the SpA,[18,19] it remains likely that there is a range of initiating triggers with some commonality of pathogenetic mechanisms. Potential initiating events are discussed in appropriate chapters (see Chapter 123, Psoriatic arthritis; Chapter 124, Reactive arthritis and enteropathic arthropathy).

Exploration of potential synovial characteristics which might allow differentiation of peripheral SpA from other inflammatory joint diseases and of individual SpA syndromes have not led to identification of any reliable histological differentiators.[20] Nonetheless, evidence of increased synovial mast cell numbers and of increased expression of IL-17 by mast cell in SpA synovium may offer both mechanistic clues and a degree of differentiation from other forms of arthritis including RA.[21] Increased IL-17 production has also been noted in specific CD4 T-cell lines from patients with SpA.[22] The known link between spondyloarthritis and IL-23 receptor polymorphisms[23] may underpin increased IL-17 production and this might be both an important element of pathogenesis and a potential target for treatment.

In the absence of hard diagnostic criteria, it is unclear whether oligoarticular psoriatic arthritis really represents the same condition as polyarticular disease or whether some cases of the latter are more closely allied to rheumatoid arthritis.[24,25]

The approach to diagnosis

It is not uncommon for symptoms suggestive of oligoarthritis to reflect non-inflammatory lesions, so care should be taken to discriminate between true synovitis and arthralgia, regional pain syndromes, and other painful lesions. Similarly, presentation may be with a single symptomatic joint but with additional inflamed joints being identified by thorough examination. An early element of the diagnostic approach is, therefore, the objective demonstration of the presence and extent of inflammatory synovitis by clinical joint assessment, ultrasound, or MRI. As in other aspects of rheumatic

Table 8.1 Disorders that frequently or sometimes present in adult life with oligoarticular arthritis

Spondyloarthritis	Infective	Miscellaneous	Atypical rheumatic
Reactive arthritis	Gonococcal arthritis	Sarcoidosis	Rheumatoid arthritis
Psoriatic arthritis	Meningococcal arthritis	Paraneoplastic arthritis	Sjögren's syndrome
Enteropathic arthritis	Lyme disease	Behçet's syndrome	Crystal arthritis
Juvenile SpA	HIV infection	Haemoglobinopathies	Osteoarthritis
Axial SpA with peripheral arthritis	Whipple's disease		Polymyalgia rheumatica
Undifferentiated SpA	Septic arthritis		

SpA, spondyloarthritis.

Table 8.2 Three layers of diagnostic information in oligoarthritis

Layer	Elements	Examples
1	Age, gender, ethnicity	Reactive arthritis, sickle cell disease in young adults
		Polymyalgic or paraneoplastic arthritis in elderly people
2	Personal and family history	Previous monoarthritis at knee or hip suggests SpA
		Family history of comorbidities suggests SpA or atypical RA
3	SpA-associated features	Eye, skin, bowel, enthesis spine lesions suggest SpA

RA, rheumatoid arthritis; SpA, spondyloarthritis.

disease, diagnosis is heavily dependent on three 'layers' of diagnostic information (Table 8.2).

The first layer consists of age, gender, and ethnicity. Infection-related arthritides and episodic arthritis associated with haemoglobinopathies[26] particularly affect the young; atypical connective tissue diseases and sarcoidosis may be suggested by oriental or Afro-Caribbean origins while, in elderly people, joint disease associated with polymyalgia rheumatica,[27] paraneoplastic syndromes,[28] and atypical crystal synovitis may be suspected.

The second layer includes personal and family history. Occurrence of an idiopathic monoarthritis at the knee or hip in childhood or teenage is a frequent precursor or early feature of SpA; a family history of ankylosing spondylitis, psoriasis, iritis, inflammatory bowel disease, or multiple joint replacements in early adult life suggests peripheral SpA.

The third layer pertains to comorbidities present in the patient, including a personal history of inflammatory eye disease, possible inflammatory bowel disease, spinal pain, genitourinary or gut infection, and psoriasis. The use of comorbidities as signposts to the diagnosis of oligoarthritis is illustrated in Figure 8.2 and the case histories.

A methodical approach to reaching a diagnosis in the case of an adult patient presenting with oligoarthritis based on comorbidities is suggested in Figure 8.2A and developed in Figure 8.2B–F.

The diagnostic approach is exemplified by the following illustrative case histories.

Consideration of diagnoses according to confirmed or potential comorbidities is a sensitive part of the diagnostic process. The

Case history 1

A 32-year-old white woman presents with a 3-week history of pain and swelling at the right knee. She has been previously well, but over the preceding few days had noticed discomfort at the right forefoot and ankle. She felt systemically well.

She worked as a bank cashier and had last travelled abroad some 7 months ago.

The family history was notable but non-specific. She was single, but both parents were alive and she had four siblings. Her

father suffered from some back pain attributed to his work as a builder; one sister had an undiagnosed skin rash, and another was said to suffer from 'colitis'. The maternal grandmother was said to have rheumatoid arthritis but this was unconfirmed.

Enquiry into the past history did not disclose any significant illnesses apart from intermittent abdominal discomfort with alternating diarrhoea and constipation ascribed to irritable bowel syndrome.

The patient's general health was reportedly good with steady weight (BMI 27.3), bowel symptoms as above but without passage of blood per rectum. Specific enquiry revealed some 'scalp dryness' but no eye symptoms, skin rashes, dysuria, vaginal discharge, or breathlessness.

Physical examination confirmed the presence of synovitis with effusion at the right knee and soft tissue swelling and tenderness at the right second and third metatarsophalangeal (MTP) joints. The remainder of the physical examination was normal.

In this instance the age of the woman raises several diagnostic possibilities, as indicated in Table 8.1. As is often the case, the personal and family history raise issues that may well be non-contributory but raise suspicions about possible links with inflammatory bowel disease, psoriasis, and ankylosing spondylitis.

diagnostic pathways are summarized in Figure 8.2B and C. In the first instance establishment of a comorbid lesion or symptom leads on to further analysis of the possibilities. In the case cited, intestinal inflammation and skin lesions are indicated as possible comorbid lesions although the history would be consistent with unrelated irritable bowel syndrome and non-specific skin dryness. Figure 8.2B sets out possible gut-associated disorders and suggests a pathway for investigation; similarly, Figure 8.2c sets out the various skin lesions which should be sought and their potential diagnostic implications.

Enquiry about genital tract symptoms and possibility of recent genital tract infection should be made in all patients with

Case history 2

A 37-year-old Afro-Caribbean man presents with a 3-week history of painful ankles. He works in an office and runs regularly; he initially ascribed the ankle pain to a possible running injury. Over the previous 2 months he has felt tired but attributed this to working long hours. There is no history of skin rash, back pain, recent infections, cough, fever, diarrhoeaor eye symptoms. There was no weight loss. In the past he has been well and the family history was non-contributory.

He appeared unwell. Examination revealed soft tissue swelling with some induration of the skin over both ankles but no other clinical features. In particular, there was no lymphadenopathy and the chest was clinically clear.

The diagnostic algorithm in this case of a systemically unwell patient with no apparent comorbidities is described in Figure 8.2D. In a man of this age the most likely diagnosis is sarcoidosis.

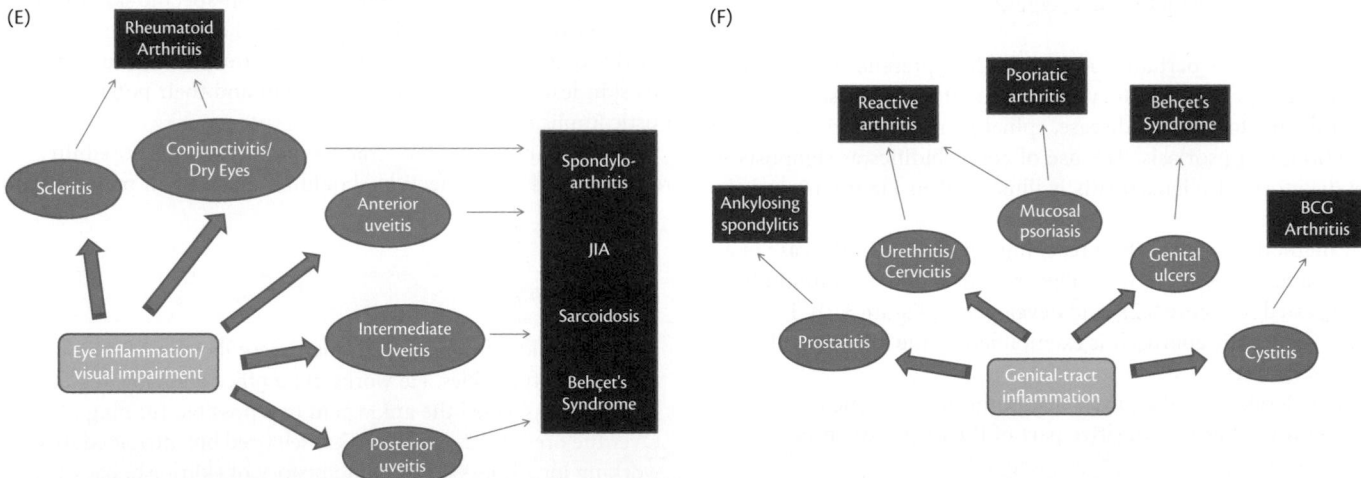

Fig. 8.2 Approach to investigation of a patient with oligoarthritis: (A) key diagnostic comorbidities; (B) oligoarthritis with diarrhoea and/or abdominal pain; (C) oligoarthritis with skin lesions; (D) oligoarthritis in a systemically unwell patient with no apparent comorbidities; (E) oligoarthritis with eye lesions; (F) oligoarthritis with genital tract lesions.

oligoarthritis, especially in young adults. The personal history may also have disclosed previous infections or high-risk behaviour, though urethritis and genital lesions may occur in their absence and ongoing infection, especially in women and passive homosexual men, may be asymptomatic or unrecognized by the patient. Key genital tract lesions of diagnostic significance are indicated in Figure 8.2F.

Case history 3

A 23-year-old man presents with pain at the right foot. Symptoms have been present for 7 weeks in spite of taking ibuprofen prescribed by his primary care physician. In other respects he is well, though walking is now difficult because of pain and work is interrupted. There is no family history of note and he feels generally well. On questioning he described an episode of a painful red eye at the age of 18 years for which he consulted an ophthalmologist and which settled over 2–3 weeks with topical treatment. There was no other history offered. Enquiry about possible diarrhoea or genital tract symptoms revealed no symptoms, but he acknowledged several recent new sexual contacts.

Examination revealed a well man with marked synovitis at the second, third, and fourth MTP joints of the right foot. There was also tenderness but not swelling at the attachment of the right Achilles tendon and a small right knee effusion. The combination of oligoarthritis and previous probable inflammatory eye disease prompted referral to a genitourinary physician who identified non-gonococcal urethritis. History obtained subsequently from the general practitioner confirmed the diagnosis of acute anterior uveitis in the past.

A history of an episode (or episodes) of painful red eye is always important. Acute anterior uveitis is seldom synchronous with episodes of arthritis, though may occur episodically during persistent arthritis and, because of its intensity in adults, the diagnosis may be known. It is usually impossible for non-ophthalmologists to distinguish the various causes of 'painful red eye', so every opportunity should be taken to arrange ophthalmological assessment when symptoms or signs are present. Visual disturbance may also be associated with all forms of uveitis, so careful expert assessment of both the anterior and posterior elements of the eyes is important in establishing the diagnosis. Key diagnostic possibilities are outlined in Figure 8.2e.

References

1. Petty RE, Southwood TR, Manners P et al. International League of Associations for Rheumatology International League of Associations for Rheumatology classification of juvenile idiopathic arthritis: second revision, Edmonton, 2001. *J Rheumatol* 2004;31(2):390–392.
2. Kvien TK, Glennas A, Melby K. Prediction of diagnosis in acute and subacute oligoarthritis of unknown origin. *Br J Rheumatol* 1996;35:359–363.
3. Moll JM, Haslock I, Macrae IF, Wright V. Associations between ankylosing spondylitis, psoriatic arthritis, Reiter's disease, the intestinal arthropathies and Behçet's syndrome. *Medicine* (Baltimore) 1974;53:343–364.
4. Wright V, Moll JMH. *Seronegative polyarthritis*. North-Holland, Amsterdam, 1996.
5. Amor B, Dougados M, Mijiyawa M. Criteria for the classification of spondylarthropathies. *Rev Rhum Mal Osteoartic* 1990;57:85–89.
6. Dougados M, van der Linden S, Juhlin R et al. The European Spondylarthropathy Study Group preliminary criteria for the classification of spondylarthropathy. *Arthritis Rheum* 1991;34(10):1218–1227.
7. Rudwaleit M, van der Heijde D, Landewé R et al. The Assessment of Spondyloarthritis International Society classification criteria for peripheral spondyloarthritis and for spondyloarthritis in general. *Ann Rheum Dis* 2011;70:25–31.
8. Haglund B, Bremander AB, Petersson IF et al. Prevalence of spondyloarthritis and its subtypes in southern Sweden. *Ann Rheum Dis* 2011;70:943–948.
9. Reveille JD. Epidemiology of spondyloarthritis in North America. *Am J Med Sci* 2011;34:284–286.
10. Abdel-Nasser AM, Rasker JJ, Valkenburg HA. Epidemiological and clinical aspects relating to the variability of rheumatoid arthritis. *Semin Arthritis Rheum* 1997;27(2):123–140.
11. Bardin T. Gonococcal arthritis. *Best Pract Res Clin Rheumatol* 2003;17:201–208.
12. Cabellos C, Nolla JM, Verdaguer R et al. Arthritis related to systemic meningococcal disease: 34 years' experience. *Eur J Clin Microbiol Infect Dis* 2012;31(10):2661–2666.
13. Steere AC , Glickstein L. Elucidation of Lyme arthritis. *Nat Rev Immunol.* 2004;4(2):143–152.
14. Yurdakul S, Yazici H. Behçet's syndrome. *Best Pract Res Clin Rheumatol* 2008;22(5):793–809.
15. Taylor W, Gladman D, Helliwell P et al.; CASPAR Study Group. Classification criteria for psoriatic arthritis: development of new criteria from a large international study. *Arthritis Rheum* 2006;54(8): 2665–2673.
16. Keat A. Reiter's syndrome and reactive arthritis in perspective. *N Engl J Med* 1983; 29;309(26):1606–1615.
17. Hannu T. Reactive arthritis. *Best Pract Res Clin Rheumatol* 2011;25(3):347–357.
18. Reveille JD. A genetic basis of spondyloarthritis. *Ann Rheum Dis* 2011;70 Suppl 1: i44–i50.
19. Evans DM, Reveille JD, Brown MA et al. The genetic basis of spondyloarthritis: SPARTAN/IGAS 2009. *J Rheumatol.* 2010;37(12):2626–2631.
20. Thevison K, Vercoutere W, Bombardier C, Landewe RB. Diagnostic and prognostic value of synovial biopsy in adult undifferentiated peripheral inflammatory arthritis: A systematic review. *J Rheumatol Suppl* 2011;87:45–47.
21. Noondenbos T, Yeremenko M, Gofito I et al. IL-17-positive mast cells attributed to synovial inflammation in spondyloarthritis. *Arthr Rheum* 2012;64(1):99–109.
22. Bowness P, Ridley A, Shaw J et al. TH-17 cells expressing KIR3DL2+ and responsive to HLA-B27 homodimers are increased in ankylosing spondylitis. *J Immunol* 2011;186:2672–2680.
23. Duvallet E, Semeramo L, Assie RE, Falgarone G, Boissier MC. Interleukin-23: A key cytokine in inflammatory diseases. *Ann Med* 2011;47:503–511.
24. Helliwell PS, Taylor WJ. Classification and diagnostic criteria for psoriatic arthritis. *Ann Rheum Dis* 2005;64 (Supple 2):ii308.
25. Van Kuijk AWR, Tak PP. Synovitis in psoriatic arthritis: Immunohistochemistry comparisons with rheumatoid arthritis and effects of therapy. *Curr Rheum Rep* 2011;13:353–359.
26. de Ceulaer K, Forbes M, Roper D, Serjeant GR. Non-gouty arthritis in sickle cell disease: report of 37 consecutive cases. *Ann Rheum Dis* 1984;43(4):599–603.
27. Narvaez J, Nolla-Sole JM, Narvaez JM et al. Musculoskeletal manifestations in polymyalgia rheumatica and temporal arteritis. *Ann Rheum Dis* 2001;60:1060–1063.
28. Butler RC, Thompson JM, Keat AC. Paraneoplastic rheumatic disorders: a review. *J R Soc Med* 1987;80(3):168–172.

CHAPTER 9

Polyarticular disease

Ade Adebajo and Lisa Dunkley

Introduction

When presented with a patient who has joint disease, it is important to have a clinical strategy for making a diagnosis and effecting an appropriate management plan. The first question that the clinician should ask is 'Is this a joint problem?', as one needs to make sure the patient does not have bony pain, muscle pain/weakness, or a tendon or other soft tissue problem (Table 9.1). If it is a joint problem, one should ask, 'Does this affect one joint (monoarthritis), a few joints (oligoarthritis), or multiple joints (polyarthritis)'? With these basic first steps, the clinician is already beginning to formulate a differential diagnosis.

The presentation of monoarthritides is considered elsewhere (Chapter 7). Here we consider a clinical approach to polyarticular disease.

General information from clinical history and examination

All clinical assessment begins with a clinical history and examination. Specific information relating to individual diagnoses will be considered in later sections, but the following are useful generic points to consider when assessing a patient with polyarticular disease.

Age

Inflammatory joint disease may occur at any age from childhood to very old age, but degenerative disease is much more common as we get older. Gout is uncommon before the fifth decade and calcium pyrophosphate disease typically develops from the seventh decade.

Gender

Gout is more common in men, but the autoimmune diseases are more common in women with female: male ratios of 3–5:1 (rheumatoid arthritis, RA) and 9:1 (systemic lupus erythematosus, SLE).

Table 9.1 Examples of mimics of joint disease

Symptom	Possible causes
Bone pain	Osteomalacia, Paget's, bony metastases, hypertrophic pulmonary osteoarthropathy (HPOA)
Muscle pain/weakness	Polymyalgia rheumatica, vitamin D deficiency, polymyositis

Lifestyle factors

Smoking is associated with RA, which is three times more common in smokers than in non-smokers. Alcohol is associated with gout and psoriasis. Obesity is associated with osteoarthritis (OA) of the knees and feet, but equally, patients with a history of high-level sports activity are also at risk of early OA (e.g. in the knees of footballers or the shoulders of cricketers or racquet sports players). Occupational history is also important; physical jobs can similarly lead to early OA, e.g. of the knee in plumbers, and classically of the hip in farmers. High-risk behaviour for contraction of blood-borne diseases raises the possibility of arthritis related to chronic infections, such as hepatitis B and C.

Family history/personal medical history

Patients with one autoimmune disease often develop another, or have family members with autoimmunity. Ask about thyroid disorders, vitiligo, and pernicious anaemia. Also ask about underlying conditions that might be directly associated with joint disease—Crohn's disease. ulcerative colitis, skin psoriasis, uveitis. Patients with the 'metabolic syndrome' (central obesity, type 2 diabetes, hypertriglyceridaemia, and hypertension) are at high risk of developing gout (or vice versa) and there is often a positive family history. Patients with renal impairment are also at risk of gout. Metabolic conditions can be associated with calcium pyrophosphate disease (CPPD), most commonly primary hyperparathyroidism, but rarer associations include hypomagnesaemia, Wilson's disease, and acromegaly.

Honing the diagnosis: inflammatory versus non-inflammatory disease

There are many approaches to formulating a differential diagnosis. Considering whether a patient presents with inflammatory or non-inflammatory symptoms is often helpful (see Table 9.2).

Inflammatory joint pain

Patients typically describe pain and *stiffness* within the affected joints, that is often worst first thing in the morning (after the inactivity of being asleep all night) and again after a period of rest (often later in the evening as they relax before bed). Moderate movement typically eases this stiffness and pain—'Once I get going again I'm fine'. Generally early morning stiffness is considered significant and indicative of inflammatory pathology, if it lasts at least

Table 9.2 Comparison of inflammatory and degenerative joint symptoms

Symptoms	Inflammatory	Degenerative
Pain	Eases with use	Increases with use Often clicks/clunks heard
Stiffness	Significant (>60 min) Early morning/at rest (evening)	Not prolonged (<30 min) Morning/evening
Swelling	Synovial ± bony	None or bony
Inflammation	Hot and red?	Not clinically inflamed
Patient demographics	E.g. young, psoriasis, family history	E.g. older, prior occupation/sport
Joint distribution	E.g. hands and feet	E.g. 1st CMCJ, DIPJ, knees
Responds to NSAIDs	Positive response	Less convincing response

CMCJ, carpometacarpophalangeal joint; DIPJ, distal interphalangeal joint; NSAIDs, non-steroidal anti-inflammatory drugs.

30–60 minutes. Non-steroidal anti-inflammatory drugs (NSAIDs) may be of significant benefit, more so than paracetamol or codeine-based simple analgesia, but this is not ubiquitously true. If steroids have been administered, usually either orally or intramuscularly, these would be expected to bring about a substantial but temporary relief of symptoms.

Non-inflammatory joint pain

Patients also describe pain and stiffness, but the stiffness is usually less persistent than in inflammatory disease. Both of these symptoms are at their worst in the evenings, and typically movement of a joint makes the pain worse. Early morning stiffness may be present, especially in osteoarthritis of the hands, but the duration and intensity of stiffness is not as marked as in inflammatory disease.

NSAIDs are often of no additional benefit to simple codeine/paracetamol-based analgesia.

Joint distribution

The distribution of affected joints can help differentiate not only between inflammatory and non-inflammatory disease, but also between specific types of inflammatory disease (Figure 9.1).

Involvement of the first carpometacarpal (CMC) joint is almost always due to osteoarthritis; RA rarely involves the distal interphalangeal (DIP) joints of the hands, and never in isolation. The commonest joints to be affected by gout are the first metatarsophalangeal (MTP) joints (classical podagra), ankles, and knees.

Appearance of the joints

A red, hot, swollen joint classically occurs with the very acute history of gout/pseuogout. A septic joint can also present in this way. Both may present with systemic fever. The chronic inflammatory arthritides of RA and psoriatic arthritis typically present with a more subacute picture of swelling and warmth, but not classically markedly erythematous joints.

Chronicity of symptoms

Typical timelines of various polyarticular conditions are illustrated in Figure 9.2. Crystal disease and infection are usually acute conditions; RA and psoriatic arthritis may evolve slowly over many months, waxing and waning in that time frame, but for a small proportion of patients, these too can be 'explosive' and rapidly progressive.

Inflammatory versus non-inflammatory disease

The clinician has now established whether the patient has inflammatory or non-inflammatory joint symptoms. Considering the joint pain paradigm as shown in Figure 9.3, it is now possible to explore the non-inflammatory versus the inflammatory arms and begin to work towards a specific diagnosis.

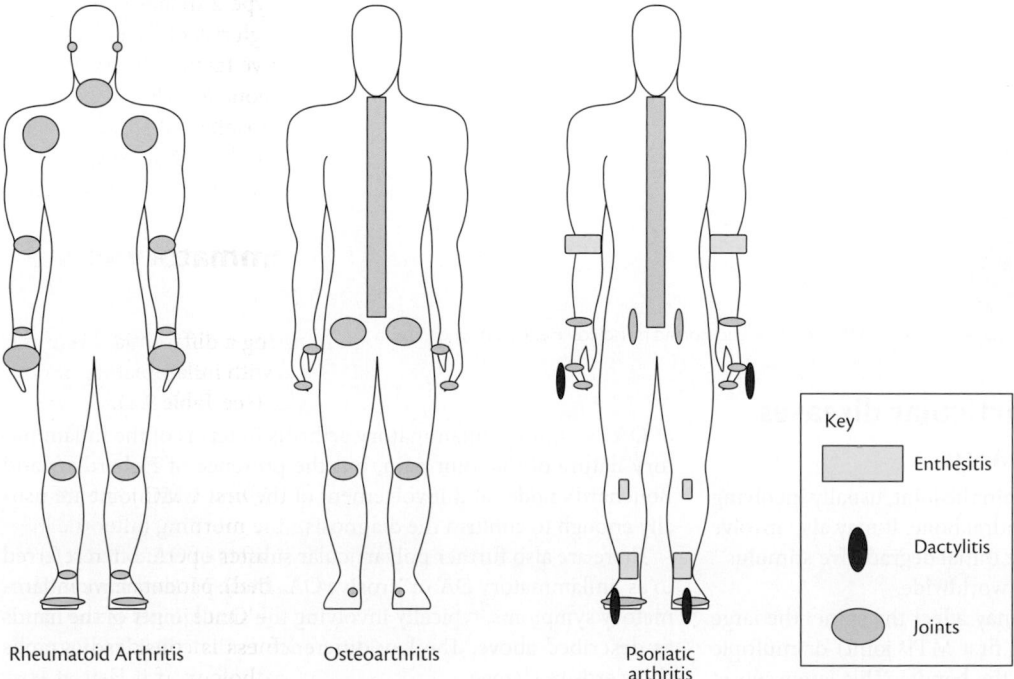

Rheumatoid Arthritis   Osteoarthritis   Psoriatic arthritis

Key
Enthesitis
Dactylitis
Joints

Fig. 9.1 Usual joint distribution of common arthritides.

Chronicity of joint symptoms

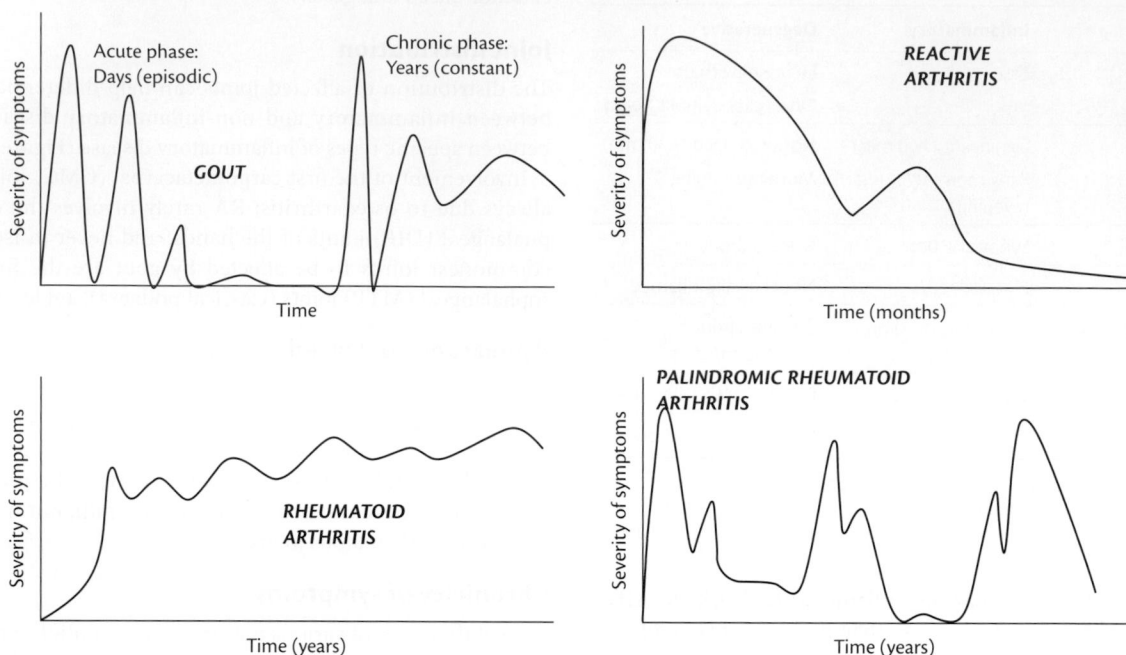

Fig. 9.2 Typical chronicity of symptoms in common arthritides.

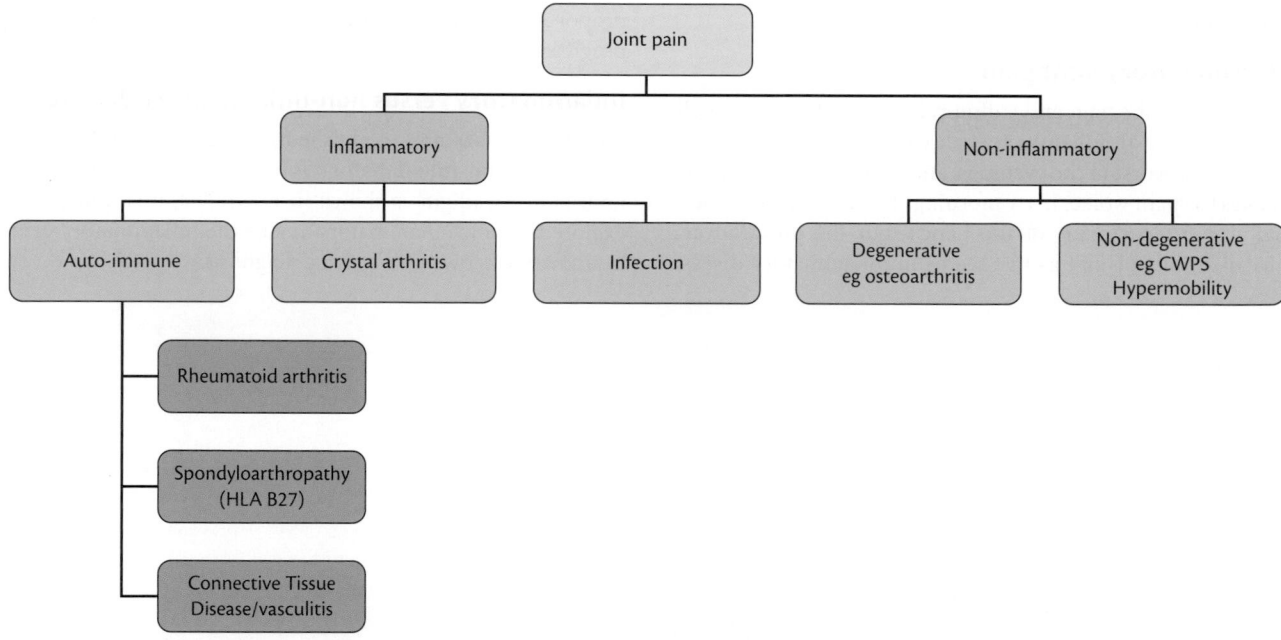

Fig. 9.3 A paradigm for diagnosis of polyarticular joint pain. CWPS = chronic widespread musculoskeletal pain syndrome.

Non-inflammatory polyarticular diseases

Degenerative disease: osteoarthritis

OA is a condition of degradation within the joint, usually involving cartilage loss and damage to subchondral bone. It may also involve an exaggerated repair response to the initial degradative stimulus.[1] It is the commonest form of arthritis worldwide.

Different patterns of OA exist. It may affect the spine, the large joints, isolated small joints (e.g. the first MTP joint) or multiple small joints (typically 'nodal OA' of the hands). This latter subset of OA can mimic inflammatory arthritis in terms of the inflammatory nature of the joint pain, but the presence of Heberden's and Bouchard's nodes and involvement of the first CMC joint are usually enough to confirm the diagnosis.

There are also further polyarticular subsets of OA, often referred to as 'inflammatory OA' or 'erosive OA'. These patients have inflammatory symptoms, typically involving the small joints of the hands as described above. The key difference is that their radiographs show erosive change.

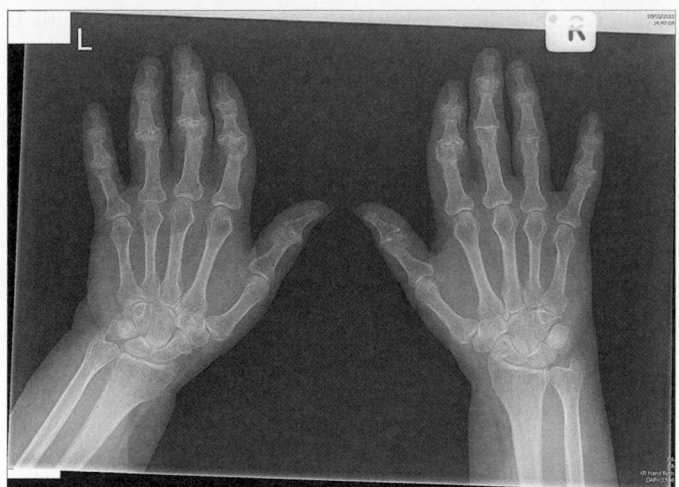

Fig. 9.4 Erosive osteoarthritis involving proximal and distal interphalangeal joints.

In one subset, patients have erosive disease of the proximal and distal interphalangeal joints of the fingers, and symptoms are often poorly responsive to conventional treatments. Typical radiographs are shown in Figure 9.4.

The second subset of patients are those who have arthritis associated with CPPD. This is also often referred to as 'inflammatory OA' but has a propensity to involve the second and third MCP joints in isolation. Secondary causes of CPPD, such as haemochromatosis, diabetes, hypomagnesaemia, and hyperparathyroidism show this same pattern of joint involvement (see also section 'Pseudogout: calcium pyrophosphate disease').

Non-degenerative disorders

Benign joint hypermobility syndrome

Approximately 10% of the adult population are hypermobile.[2] Joint hypermobility in itself is not pathological, but may be considered so if associated with persistent pain and joint dysfunction. Diagnosis of benign joint hypermobility syndrome (BJHS) is made using the Brighton criteria[3] which identify the combination of joint hypermobility *and* patient symptoms. Joint hypermobility may be associated with chronic non-inflammatory joint pain. The pain might be restricted to one or two (often weight-bearing) joints, but can present as a symmetrical polyarticular condition. The clue to diagnosis is often the initial examination.

Chronic widespread musculoskeletal pain

Chronic widespread musculoskeletal pain syndrome (CWPS) is also referred to by many as 'fibromyalgia'. These overarching terms encompass a syndrome of widespread joint and muscle pain that is accompanied by multiple associated symptoms, including fatigue, poor sleep, and mood disturbance. Taking a careful history to elicit these associated symptoms, and establishing the presence of widespread but non-inflammatory pain, helps confirm the diagnosis.

Inflammatory polyarticular diseases

Autoimmune conditions

Rheumatoid arthritis

RA is a symmetrical, erosive polyarthritis that typically affects the small joints of the hands and feet. The key features of the history are inflammatory pain and stiffness, usually progressive over several months, and a description of joint swelling. Patients may also describe fatigue or general malaise. As described above, there may often be a family history of RA or other autoimmune disease. Symptoms and signs can be quite subtle, but some patients present with rapidly progressive synovitis and grossly swollen 'boxing glove' hands.

Examination typically demonstrates swelling and/or tenderness in the wrists, MCP and PIP joints of the hands and MTP joints of the feet. Look for callus on the soles of the feet, and rheumatoid nodules which typically occur on the extensor surfaces of the elbow, hands, and the Achilles tendon. Some patients, however, have large joint predominant disease, so it is important to examine these joints too.

Spondyloarthropathy

The 'spondyloarthropathies' encompass a broad range of related arthritides that are variously associated with the tissue type HLA B27 (see Table 9.3). The clinical presentation varies widely between and within them. As well as inflammatory arthritis, the hallmark of these conditions is the presence of an enthesopathy. The arthritis itself may be a symmetrical small joint polyarthropathy (typically psoriatic arthritis) but may be restricted to the spine only (ankylosing spondylitis), or present as a peripheral large joint oligoarthritis (psoriatic arthritis, reactive arthritis, enteropathic arthritis). There is much overlap between the individual spondyloarthropathies, and a patient may evolve between diagnoses over time.

Spinal involvement is indicated by inflammatory back pain—stiffness after a period of rest, pain directly over the sacroiliac joints (i.e. mid-buttock), thoracic and anterior chest wall pain, and significant early morning stiffness in the spine. A patient may not know that he/she has psoriasis. It is worth asking for a history of itchy, scaly skin patches, remembering the 'hidden' sites for psoriasis—the scalp, behind the ears, umbilicus, natal cleft, palms and soles, nails. Dystrophic toenails may be psoriatic rather than fungal, and nail clippings are worth sending if in doubt. The patient may not have psoriasis (yet) but there may be a family history.

Enquire about bowel symptoms and uveitis—both current and historical. Take a sexual history, but be sure to make the relevance of this clear 'some arthritis conditions can be triggered by sexually transmitted infections'. This may require a second visit, a telephone call, or a discreet question in a separate examination room if the patient is accompanied by a partner. Even if the history is 'negative', if reactive arthritis is a possibility, invite the patient to self-refer to the genitourinary medicine clinic.

Examine for peripheral arthritis, enthesitis (commonly Achilles tendon with associated plantar fasciitis, and/or epicondylitis at the

Table 9.3 The HLA association of spondyloarthropathies[4]

Diagnosis	HLA B27 positivity (% of patients)
Ankylosing spondylitis	90–95%
Psoriatic arthritis	50% overall (10–20% peripheral disease; 60–70% if spinal involvement)
Reactive arthritis	70–85%
Enteropathic arthritis	50%
Isolated anterior uveitis	50%

Table 9.4 ILAR classification of juvenile idiopathic arthritis (JIA)[5]

JIA subtype	Key features
Systemic onset (SOJIA)	10–20% patients; usually polyarticular, quotidian (daily) fever, evanescent rash, lymphadenopathy. Differential diagnosis includes infection/malignancy
Oligoarthritis	Most common form of JIA. 1–4 joints in 1st 6 months; age usually <6 yrs. May 'extend' to >4 joints—'extended oligoarticular'—after 1st 6 months; **worst prognosis and often missed at onset**
Polyarticular RF (−)	Typically young children, girls > boys, ANA(+) = high risk of anterior uveitis
Polyarticular RF (+)	Typically teenage girls; much like adult RA
Psoriatic arthritis	Dactylitis common
Enthesitis-related	Often boys >6 yrs. Resembles adult AS, but peripheral involvement greater
Undifferentiated	Does not fit into any of the categories above

For all the above, arthritis of unknown aetiology occurring before the 16th birthday and persisting for >6 weeks. All other known conditions excluded.

elbow), chest wall involvement (sternoclavicular joint, costochondral joints) and spinal restriction.

Juvenile idiopathic arthritis

The above sections address inflammatory joint disease in adults. Children and young people may also develop inflammatory arthritides, but the clinical presentation, natural disease history, and management can be very different. A separate classification of diseases is used (Table 9.4) and it is critical that these patients are managed by multidisciplinary, multiagency teams that have specific expertise in managing all aspects of their care. 30–50% continue with their arthritis into adulthood so it is important that clinical pathways exist to manage this transition properly.

All patients with juvenile idiopathic arthritis (JIA), particularly those under the age of 11 and those with positive anti-nuclear antibodies, must have ophthalmic screening. Anterior uveitis is common; it is an important reversible cause of childhood blindness in the UK, and is often asymptomatic in children.

Connective tissue disease/vasculitis

Connective tissue diseases and vasculitides originally became the domain of the rheumatologist as they can present with arthritis (and latterly because they are also immunologically driven). These conditions can be associated with life-threatening organ involvement, so remember that what might appear to be a 'simple (unclassified) inflammatory arthritis' may herald a more severe systemic disease.

Remember too that connective tissue diseases may occur as overlap syndromes: a patient with limited cutaneous systemic sclerosis may have true erosive RA alongside the scleroderma.

A selection of diagnoses is considered in Table 9.5.

Crystal arthritis

Both gout and pseudogout show acute and chronic forms. In general, the acute disease is a mono- or oligoarthritis, whilst the chronic disease is polyarticular.

Gout

Gout is painful. Patients often describe waking in the early hours with joint pain, and by the morning being unable to put their foot to the floor. The affected joint is typically hot, red, and swollen. The patient may be systemically unwell. Joint distribution has been described earlier (first MTP joint, knees, ankles). Diffuse involvement of the midfoot is also common. It can also present as a truly polyarticular disease, especially if there is a more chronic history of joint pain. In this latter scenario, when you explore the patient's history you will usually elicit the typical acute monoarthritis history of gout from several years or even decades earlier. In this situation, examine for gouty tophi—if present, these will help confirm the diagnosis.

Serum uric acid may be elevated, but can be normal or low during an acute attack. The gold standard for diagnosis is polarized microscopy of synovial fluid from an acutely affected joint, demonstrating the classical negatively birefringent needle-shaped crystals of uric acid. Radiographs may show 'punched out' periarticular erosions.

Table 9.5 Clinical presentations of common connective tissue diseases/vasculitides

Diagnosis	Associated arthritis	Non-articular features
SLE	'Jaccoud's arthritis'—symmetrical, correctible polyarthritis—phenotypically like RA but typically non-erosive	Photosensitivity, malar rash, mouth ulcers, hair fall, fatigue, abnormal nailfold capillaries
MCTD	Arthralgia/symmetrical erosive arthritis—75% of patients have true RA overlap	Raynaud's, sclerodactyly, myositis, pulmonary hypertension, pleuritis/pericarditis
PSS	Non-erosive inflammatory arthralgia/arthritis	Sicca complex (dry eyes/dry mouth and mucous membranes), fatigue, peripheral and central nervous system involvement. Risk of lymphoma (NHL)
Large-vessel vasculitis	Myalgia and stiffness (polymyalgia rheumatica); not typically true arthralgia	Temporal arteritis/vascular bruits/systemic malaise/jaw, tongue, calf claudication
ANCA-associated vasculitis	Inflammatory, erosive (true RA?) or non-erosive	Respiratory/renal/cardiac/ENT/neurological involvement of vasculitis + systemic malaise

ANCA, anti-neutrophil cytoplasmic antibodies; MCTD, mixed connective tissue disease; NHL, non-Hodgkin's lymphoma; PSS, primary Sjögren's syndrome; RA, rheumatoid arthritis; SLE, systemic lupus erythematosus.

Pseudogout: calcium pyrophosphate disease

Pseudogout or calcium pyrophosphate disease is common in elderly people. It often occurs during or following an intercurrent illness and presents, like gout, with a hot, swollen, red joint. Wrists and knees are classically affected in acute disease. Synovial fluid examination reveals positively birefringent rhomboid crystals of calcium pyrophosphate. Radiographs may show chondrocalcinosis (linear calcification of the cartilage), typically in the menisci of the knees or the triangular ligament of the wrist. If looked for, chondrocalcinosis may also be present in the symphysis pubis.

The more chronic polyarticular form of calcium pyrophosphate disease can affect any joint, but often the second and third MCP joints, wrists, elbows, shoulders, and knees. This clinical picture is often described synonymously with 'inflammatory OA' and is alluded to in the earlier section on OA. Radiographs may show hook osteophytes, usually at the second and third MCP joints (Figure 9.5).

Other crystal deposition diseases

Calcium hydroxyapatite and calcium oxalate crystals may also cause crystal-associated arthritis. As with gout and pseudogout, presentation may be acute/mono- or oligoarticular, or chronic/polyarticular. Patients may have associated renal stone disease.

Infection

The classical history of joint sepsis is that of a single hot, red swollen joint in a patient who may be systemically unwell. Joint sepsis can, however, be polyarticular in up to 20% of cases[6,7] and may involve the spine/intervertebral discs/sacroiliac joints as well as peripheral joints. Mortality is much higher, at 30% compared with 4–8% for monarticular sepsis. Risk factors for polyarticular disease include RA, diabetes, SLE, malignancy, alcoholism, and immunosuppression, but it can occur in patients with none of these. The clinician must maintain a high index of suspicion for sepsis in polyarticular presentations. Diagnosis is confirmed by joint aspiration, and if necessary radiologically guided aspiration should be undertaken.

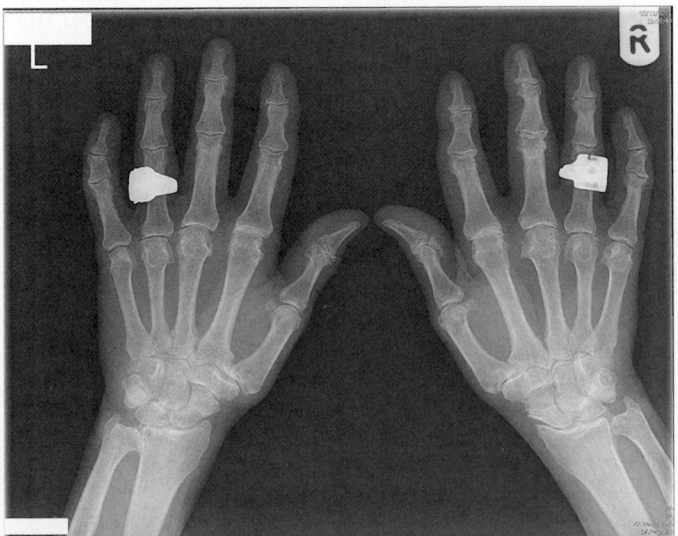

Fig. 9.5 Typical hook osteophytes and narrowing at MCPJ 2&3 in CPPD—in this case associated with haemochromatosis.

> **Box 9.1** Systemic conditions known to be associated with inflammatory joint symptoms
>
> - Coeliac disease
> - Whipple's disease
> - Lymphocytic colitis
> - Primary biliary cirrhosis/chronic active hepatitis
> - Infectious hepatitis/HIV
> - Sarcoidosis
> - SAPHO (synovitis, acne, pustolosis, hyperostosis, osteitis)
> - Infections—post strep/post viral/parvovirus/Lyme disease/tropical arthritis
> - Inflammatory—Behçet's, familial Mediterranean fever

Rarities

This chapter has deliberately concentrated on common clinical presentations. There are, however, rarer causes of polyarticular joint disease. Most of these are systemic conditions associated with inflammatory joint pain but, with the exception of sarcoidosis and SAPHO syndrome, usually cause a non-erosive arthritis. Some examples are listed in Box 9.1.

Generic management of polyarticular disease

Confirming the diagnosis

The first step, after clinical assessment of the patient, is to confirm the diagnosis. For some conditions this will rely on the clinical assessment alone, but often we can supplement this with additional investigations.

Blood tests may confirm inflammation (or sepsis) with raised white cell count, thrombocytosis, elevated inflammatory markers (ESR and CRP) and often elevated alkaline phosphatase too. Specific autoimmune diagnoses may be supported by the presence of antibodies such as rheumatoid factor, anti-CCP, ANA, and ENA. Elevated uric acid may be present in gout. Synovial fluid examination for crystals or infection may be important. Imaging with plain films, ultrasound, and MRI is often useful. Isotope bone scanning is used less these days.

Response to a one-off dose of intramuscular steroid (usually depomedrone or triamcinolone) is often used to confirm the presence of inflammatory vs non-inflammatory pathology. Relief of symptoms is indicative of underlying inflammatory disease.

Managing the 'non-inflammatory' patient

Management of non-inflammatory joint pain is often supportive; to reduce pain and optimize function whilst attempting to minimize future joint damage. This requires the input of a multidisciplinary team.

Medical management includes simple analgesia and anti-inflammatories (NSAIDs) if required,[8] with all the usual precautions about prescription of the latter. For selected patients with OA, intra-articular injection of steroids may be appropriate.

Patients with 'inflammatory OA' associated with calcium pyrophosphate deposition may benefit from NSAIDs, low-dose colchicine, low-dose oral steroid or even methotrexate and hydroxychloroquine.[9]

Input from other members of the multidisciplinary team should include physiotherapy, occupational therapy, podiatry, and often pain management specialists. Principles of therapy include maintenance of appropriate muscle strength and flexibility, maximizing function despite joint disease/pain, joint protection, pacing of activities, and consideration of the impact of occupational and recreational activities on joints and vice versa.

Surgical management is reserved for patients where medical and conservative therapy has failed. The usual indication for joint surgery is intractable pain and/or instability.

Managing the 'inflammatory' patient

The generic multidisciplinary management described for 'non-inflammatory' joint pain applies equally to patients with inflammatory disease. In addition, these patients require specific therapy to treat the underlying inflammatory process.

Management of individual conditions will be addressed in detail in later chapters of this book. What follows is an overview of the principles of treatment.

Erosive/organ-threatening disease

In most cases, where joint disease is driven by inflammation, the earlier we treat, the better the outcome. Modern management of erosive/organ-threatening disease takes a zero tolerance approach to inflammation. Treat early and treat hard, using combinations of drugs where appropriate to induce disease remission. Maintenance of disease remission may be achieved at a later date with less aggressive therapy.

Non-erosive disease

In the case of non-erosive disease, we still want to control inflammation but can use the patient's symptoms as an indicator of severity, rather than worrying about underlying joint/organ damage. In certain conditions, treatment of the underlying disease, e.g. a gluten-free diet in coeliac disease or viral eradication therapy in hepatitis B/C, will be the most helpful strategy in controlling joint symptoms.

Managing the chronic disease

Most of our patients with inflammatory disease have chronic disease. We need to manage not only their acute presentations/relapses but their ongoing disease, even when it is well controlled. We use drugs that require monitoring as they can cause toxicity and complications. We now know that patients with chronic inflammatory disease are at higher risk of cardiovascular events and osteoporosis.

Box 9.2 describes the components required for chronic disease management, and gives a generic checklist of topics to cover in a routine patient review.

The future

With the advent of biological drugs, the last decade has seen a period of immense change in the management of rheumatological disease. In future we may well see more targeted therapy, hopefully guided by individual patient biomarkers/genetic predictors, so that the most aggressive therapy is appropriately targeted to the patients that really need it. Regardless, we believe that the need for a comprehensive history, thorough clinical examination, and appropriate investigations will continue to be precursors to an accurate diagnosis and an effective management of polyarticular disease.

Box 9.2 Management principles for chronic inflammatory joint disease

Management of chronic polyarticular disease[10–12]

- Assessment of disease activity (DAS, PsARC, BASDAI, SLEDAI, etc.)
- Drug toxicity? (bloods, CXR/PFTs, blood pressure)
- Multidisciplinary team accessible to patient
- Helpline/counselling/rapid access for flares
- Shared care with GP
- Patient information and education/modification lifestyle factors/acceptance of chronic disease

Checklist for routine review

- Disease activity
- Drug monitoring
- Extra-articular features disease/new symptoms
- Osteoporosis assessment/DEXA
- Cardiovascular risk factors
- Vaccinations (in patients on immunosuppressive drugs)
- Special considerations, e.g. pregnancy

References

1. Martel-Pelletier J. Pathophysiology of osteoarthritis. *Osteoarthritis Cartilage* 1999;7:371–373.
2. Grahame R. Joint hypermobility and genetic collagen disorders: are they related? *Arch Dis Childhood* 1999;80:188–191.
3. Grahame R, Bird HA, Child A. The revised (Brighton 1998) criteria for the diagnosis of benign joint hypermobility syndrome (BJHS). *J Rheumatol* 2000;27:1777–1779.
4. Gran JT, Husby G. HLA-B27 and spondyloarthropathy: value for early diagnosis? *J Med Genet* 1995;32:497–501.
5. ILAR: International League of Associations for Rheumatology: Classification of Juvenile Idiopathic Arthritis. *J Rheumatol* 2004;31(2): 390–392.
6. Dubost JJ, Fis I, Denis P et al. Polyarticular septic arthritis. *Medicine* 1993;72:296–310.
7. Christodoulou C, Gordon P, Coakley G. Polyarticular septic arthritis. *BMJ* 2006;333:1107–1108.
8. Zhang W, Doherty M, Leeb BF et al. EULAR evidence base recommendations for the management of hand osteoarthritis: Report of a Task Force of the EULAR Standing Committee for International Clinical Studies Including Therapeutics (ESCISIT). *Ann Rheum Dis* 2007;66:377–388.
9. Zhang W, Doherty M, Pascual E et al. EULAR recommendations for calcium pyrophosphate deposition . Part II: management. *Ann Rheum Dis* 2011;70:896–904.
10. National Ankylosing Spondylitis Society (NASS). *Looking ahead: Best practice for the care of people with ankylosing spondylitis (AS)*. April 2010. Available from: http://nass.co.uk/download/4cceacf2c1d0a
11. National Institute for Health and Clinical Excellence (NICE). *Rheumatoid arthritis: the management of rheumatoid arthritis in adults (CG79)*. February 2009. Available from: www.nice.org.uk/CG79.
12. Arthritis & Musculoskeletal Alliance (ARMA). *Standards of care for people with inflammatory arthritis*. November 2004. Available from: www.arma.uk.net.

CHAPTER 10

The systemically ill patient

Joanna Robson, Anna Mistry, Kuljeet Bhamra, Stefan Kluzek, and Raashid Luqmani

Introduction

Diagnosis of the systemically unwell patient is a very common rheumatological problem. The patient may present with seemingly disparate problems in different organ systems; the challenge is to identify whether there is a unifying underlying disease process, such as infection, malignancy, an autoimmune inflammatory condition, or an autoinflammatory disease, or if different disease processes are coincidentally occurring within the same patient. Table 10.1 lists the differential diagnoses of the systemically unwell patient. A systematic approach requires a thorough history, examination, and appropriate baseline investigations, before the use of potentially more invasive and specialist tests—because common things are common. With practice, the diagnostic process should also be one of pattern recognition; examining each feature and asking: does this fit—or is there something we are missing? This caution to ensure the correct diagnosis before starting treatment is appropriate; for example, gaining biopsy evidence of systemic vasculitis before starting therapy with steroids or immunosuppressants is important, to avoid inappropriate treatment which may mask or worsen an underlying condition such as tuberculosis or lymphoma. In individual cases, though, delays brought about through waiting for further investigations to conclusively prove the diagnosis, will be less acceptable in the case of a patient with rapidly worsening organ or life-threatening disease. In this chapter we propose a stepwise approach to the systemically unwell patient; the outline of this is shown in Figure 10.1.

First line assessments—history, examination, and baseline investigations

Constitutional features

Of patients presenting with unintentional weight loss, a quarter have malignant disease; a third a non-malignant gastrointestinal tract disorder; and only 2–3% have an underlying rheumatological disorder.[1] Sixteen to 30% of patients with a fever of unknown origin (FUO) have an underlying infection; 7–10% a malignancy; 22–33% a non-infectious inflammatory condition; and no cause is found in 20–51% of cases.[2] The pattern of constitutional features may be informative; for example, patients with adult-onset Still's disease present with spiking fevers and evanescent rashes occurring in a quotidian pattern. The significance of night sweats is not well defined because they are reported in up to 40% of adult in-patients within 3 months prior to admission.[3] Night sweats are a presenting feature in 40% of cases of lymphoma[4] and 50% of cases of tuberculosis.[5] It is usual to perform three sets of blood cultures in patients with FUO; without a clinical suspicion of endocarditis, however, continuing to culture beyond this is unlikely to be diagnostic.[2]

Initial investigations

Inflammation, infection, and malignancy can all result in similar abnormalities on the full blood count, namely anaemia of chronic disease, thrombocythaemia, lymphocytosis, and neutrophilia.[6] Eosinophilia is seen in lymphomatous diseases,[4] parasitic infestations,[7] cholesterol emboli, or eosinophilic granulomatosis with polyangiitis (formerly termed Churg–Strauss syndrome).[8] Pancytopenia may be secondary to bone marrow infiltration from malignancy or infection[9] or marrow suppression due to medications such as methotrexate or azathioprine.[10] Systemic lupus erythematosus (SLE) can present with immune-mediated haemolytic anaemia, thrombocytopenia, lymphopenia, or neutropenia.[10] Baseline investigations should include parvovirus serology, a peripheral blood film, serum and urine electrophoresis, haematinics, direct Coomb's test, and lactate dehydrogenase (LDH).[10]

Respiratory system

A focused respiratory history, including symptoms of breathlessness, hoarseness, wheeze, cough, and haemoptysis may help to delineate between infection,[11] malignancy,[12] and inflammatory conditions.[13] Haemoptysis, for example, is caused by infection in 60–70% of cases, especially tuberculosis in people from developing countries[14]; and is rarely caused by pulmonary embolic disease or a small-vessel vasculitis such as granulomatosis with polyangiitis (Wegener's), which account for only 1.4% of cases.[15] In patients with FUO, a baseline chest radiograph has a high specificity of 87% but a lower sensitivity of 60%, so may need to be supplemented with further investigations.[2]

Cardiovascular system

Patients with systemic inflammatory diseases may develop a spectrum of cardiovascular manifestations; for example, pericarditis in SLE; cardiac amyloid or sarcoidosis causing conduction defects; pulmonary hypertension in systemic sclerosis or SLE; valvular

Table 10.1 Differential diagnosis of the systemically unwell adult patient

Infection	Drugs and environment	Systemic connective tissue diseases	Paraneoplastic
Infective endocarditis Viral infections: 　Hepatitis B and C virus 　HIV 　Human T cell lymphotropic virus type 1 　Parvovirus B19 　Herpes simplex and varicella zoster virus 　Cytomegalovirus and Epstein–Barr virus 　Alpha-viruses Bacterial infections: 　Mycobacterium tuberculosis 　Neisseria meningitidis 　Streptococcus pneumonia 　Salmonella 　Chlamydia pneumonia 　Treponema pallidum Parasitic infections 　Plasmodium spp. 　Giardia 　Toxoplasma gondii 　Shistosoma Fungal infections 　Aspergillus spp. 　Cryptococcus neoformans 　Histoplasma capsulatum 　Pneumocystis jirovecii Systemic inflammatory disease secondary to infection: 　Borrelia burgdorferi—Lyme disease 　Tropheryma whippelii—Whipple's 　Group A streptococcus—rheumatic fever	Acute poisoning: 　Paracetamol 　EtOH 　Ethylene glycol and methanol 　Cyanide 　Organophosphates 　Heavy metals and solvents 　Lead Drug-induced SLE: 　Procainamide 　Hydralazine 　Quinidine 　Isoniazid 　Methyldopa 　Chlorpromazine 　Minocycline Drugs associated with ANCA-positive vasculitis: 　Hydralazine 　Propylthiouracil 　Leukotriene inhibitors 　Sulfasalazine 　Minocycline 　D-Penicillamine 　Ciprofloxacin 　Phenytoin 　Clozapine 　Allopurinol Drug-induced vasospasm: 　Methysergide 　Ergot derivatives	Rheumatoid arthritis SLE Primary Sjögren's syndrome Systemic sclerosis Mixed connective tissue disease Dermatomyositis/polymyositis Adult-onset Still's disease Anti-phospholipid syndrome Eosinophilic fasciitis IgG4 related systemic disease Macrophage activation syndrome	Myelodysplastic syndrome Lymphoid malignancies: 　Non-Hodgkin's lymphoma 　Hodgkin's disease 　Chronic lymphocytic leukaemia 　Multiple myeloma Solid tumours: 　Lung cancers 　Gynaecological and genitourinary cancers 　Breast cancers 　Mesothelioma

		Systemic vasculitides	Other
		Small-vessel vasculitis (ANCA-associated): 　Granulomatosis with polyangiitis (Wegener's) 　Microscopic polyangiitis 　Eosinophilic granulomatosis with polyangiitis (Churg Strauss) Medium vessel vasculitis: 　Polyarteritis nodosa Large-vessel vasculitis: 　Giant cell arteritis 　Takayasu's arteritis Other: 　IgA Vasculitis 　Cryoglobulinaemic vasculitis 　Behçet's disease 　Relapsing polychondritis 　Cogan's and Berger's disease	Autoinflammatory syndromes e.g.: 　Familial Mediterranean fever (FMF) 　Pyogenic arthritis, pyoderma gangrenosum, and acne (PAPA) syndrome 　TNF receptor associated periodic syndrome 　Deficiency of IL-1 receptor antagonist 　Cryopyrin-associated periodic fever syndromes 　Hyper IgD syndrome Hypersensitivity syndromes Atherosclerosis/embolic disease Venous thromboembolic disease Haematological: 　Thrombotic thrombocytopenic purpura 　Haemolytic uraemic syndrome 　Sickle cell disease

disease secondary to inflammatory aortitis; and peripheral arterial disease through primary or secondary vasculitis.[16] Absent pulses, asymmetrical blood pressure readings, and peripheral bruits are important clues. Peripheral stigmata of infective endocarditis include splinter haemorrhages. Inflammation is a risk factor for accelerated atherosclerosis in patients with rheumatological diseases;[16] an assessment of their classical risk factors, such as smoking, hypertension, and hypercholesterolaemia, is therefore important.

Gastrointestinal system

Intra-abdominal infection should always be considered in patients with a FUO, particularly patients who are immunosuppressed, have had previous surgery, or have a reduced mental state or spinal cord injury.[17] Diarrhoea may be secondary to small bowel inflammation and malabsorption; cancer or inflammation of the colon; pancreatic insufficiency; motility problems; or functional disorders.[18] Common causes of acute liver failure include drug-induced, viral hepatitis, autoimmune liver disease, and shock or hypoperfusion;

in 20% of cases there is no discernible cause.[19] Medications that are associated with acute liver abnormalities are listed in Table 10.2. Seventy-five per cent of patients who present with ascites will have cirrhosis; other causes include malignancy in 10%, heart failure in 3%, tuberculosis in 2%, and pancreatitis in 1%.[20]

Renal system

Acute renal failure is characterized by a rise in the serum creatinine and urea, often associated with oliguria or anuria.[21] Acute tubular necrosis secondary to multiple nephrotoxic insults such as sepsis, hypotension, and nephrotoxic drugs (e.g. NSAIDs, antibiotics, diuretics, or contrast agents used for radiological imaging) is the most common cause of in-hospital acute renal failure, especially in elderly people and patients with pre-existing comorbidities.[21] On urine dipstick testing, the presence of haematuria should prompt a search for red cell casts which are seen in glomerulonephritis (can be postinfective or related to medications, or secondary to an underlying systemic vasculitis or connective tissue disease); any proteinuria should be quantified by sending a sample for a

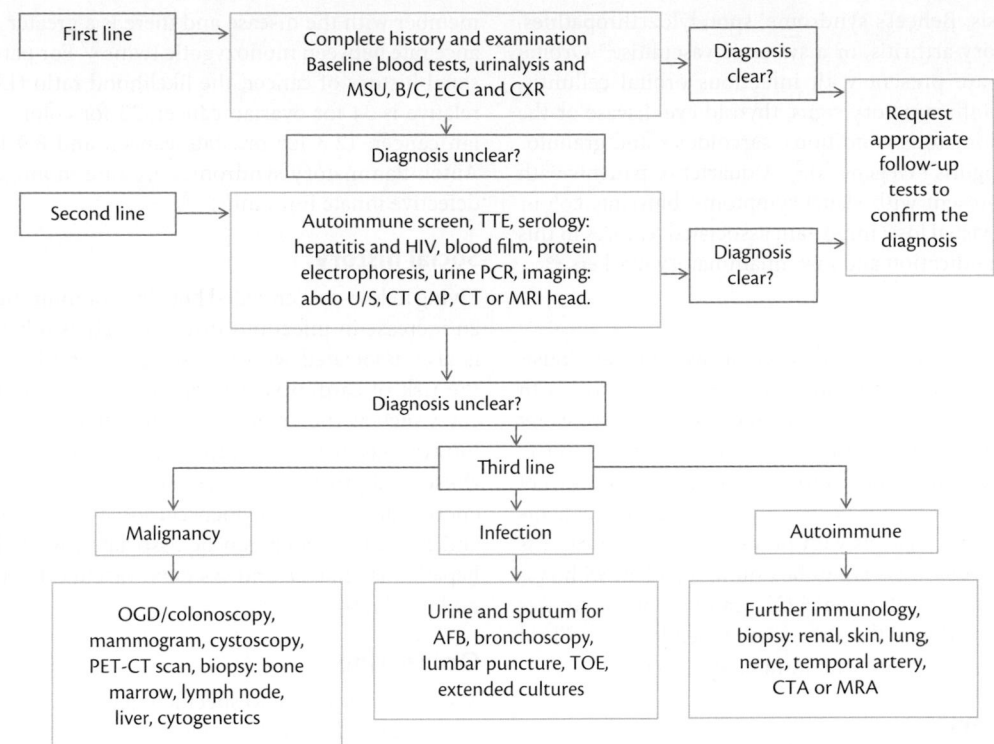

Fig. 10.1 Approach to the investigating the systemically unwell patient. AFB, acid-fast bacilli; B/C, blood culture; CT CAP, CT of chest, abdomen, and pelvis; CTA, CT angiography; CXR, chest radiograph; ECG, electrocardiography; MRA, magnetic resonance angiography; MSU, mid-stream urine; OGD, oesophagogastroduodenoscopy; PET-CT, positron emission tomography–CT; TOE, transoesophageal echocardiography; TTE, transthoracic echocardiography; U/S, ultrasound; urine PCR, urine protein:creatinine ratio.

Table 10.2 Drugs capable of causing clinical syndromes similar to SLE and vasculitis, and drugs that can induce hepatitis

Drug-induced vasculitis	Drug-induced lupus	Drug-induced hepatitis
Propylthiouracil	Hydralazine	Diclofenac
Allopurinol	Procainamide	Antibiotics, e.g. sulphonamides, isoniazid, dapsone
Hydralazine	Isoniazid	
Colony stimulating factors	Minocycline	Antihypertensives, e.g. lisinopril, methyldopa
	Pyrazinamide	
Ceflacor	Quinidine	Antiepileptics, e.g. phenytoin, sodium valproate
Minocycline	D-penicillamine	
D-penicillamine	Carbamazepine	Antiarrhythmics, e.g. amiodarone
Phenytoin	Phenytoin	Statins
Isoretinoin	Propefone	Propylthiouracil
Methotrexate		Halothane
Sulfasalazine		Amphetamines/ecstasy
Quinolones		Herbals medications
Carbimazole		Antivirals, e.g. efavirenz
Cocaine		Antifungals, e.g. ketoconazole
Levamisole		Allopurinol
		Diabetic medications, e.g. metformin, tioglitazone

protein:creatinine ratio and a sample should also be sent for culture.[21] In those without red cell casts, other causes of haematuria such as bladder cancer or infections such as schistosomiasis should be considered, especially in those with a travel history or risk factors such as smoking, exposure to aniline dyes, or cyclophosphamide treatment. However, it is important to remember that unless urine is carefully examined soon after the sample is provided, red cell casts may not be seen.

Nervous system

Chronic non-pathological headache affects up to 70% of all adults, but atypical presentations should raise concern.[22] The presence of photophobia, neck stiffness, or altered mental state suggest meningoencephalitis;[23] a thunderclap headache confers an increased likelihood of a subarachnoid haemorrhage (SAH); a sudden severe unilateral headache radiating into the neck with a Horner's syndrome may be due to arterial dissection.[22] There is an increased rate of intracranial haemorrhage in younger (40–50%) rather than older patients (15–20%) presenting with stroke, although cerebral infarction is still the most common cause.[24] In younger patients, the following conditions should be considered: anti-phospholipid syndrome; connective tissue disease such as SLE or Sjögren's; cardiac embolization secondary to rheumatic heart disease or infective endocarditis; Behçet's syndrome (specifically venous sinus thrombosis); primary cerebral vasculitis; HIV; sarcoidosis or one of the systemic vasculitides (from small to large vessel).[24] Neuropsychiatric symptoms associated with systemic inflammatory diseases also include diffuse symptoms, such as depression and cognitive impairment, through to distinct entities such as transverse myelitis or peripheral neuropathy.

Ophthalmic features

Infectious causes of uveitis include toxoplasmosis, herpes, tuberculosis, , syphilis, and, in those with a travel history, West Nile virus, Rift Valley fever, dengue, and chikungunya.[25] Forty per cent of patients with uveitis will have an underlying autoimmune disease including sarcoidosis, Behçet's syndrome, spondyloarthropathies, juvenile inflammatory arthritis, or a systemic vasculitis.[26] Orbital pain and swelling are present with infectious orbital cellulitis, tumour with acute inflammatory signs, thyroid eye disease or the multisystem granulomatous conditions: sarcoidosis and granulomatosis with polyangiitis (Wegener's).[27] A quarter of patients with giant cell arteritis present with visual symptoms: blurring, colour fading, or complete visual loss; important associated features in this subgroup are jaw claudication and low inflammatory markers.[28]

ENT features

Patients with chronic rhinosinusitis, cocaine use, fungal sinusitis, lymphoma, sarcoidosis, tuberculosis, and granulomatosis with polyangiitis (Wegener's) may describe nasal crusting and recurrent sinusitis; in a proportion there may also be a depression of the overlying skin secondary to underlying necrosis of the septum or adjacent structures.[8] A history of nasal polyposis is reported in 50% of patients with eosinophilic granulomatosis with polyangiitis (Churg–Strauss syndrome).[8] Sinus radiographs are unhelpful in a patient with systemic disease and sinus involvement;[2] CT scanning of the sinuses can identify any destruction of the sinuses and nasendoscopy will aid visualization and biopsy in those with intranasal lesions.[8]

Musculoskeletal system

Septic arthritis is the most serious type of monoarthritis, with a mortality rate of 11%; other causes of monoarthritis include crystal arthropathies, reactive arthritis, or a limited form of a polyarthritis: all should be investigated with urgent joint aspiration if there are no contraindications.[29] Inflammatory polyarthritis secondary to viruses such as parvovirus B19, rubella, mumps, and acute hepatitis B usually resolve within 6 weeks; beyond this time point inflammatory arthropathies such as rheumatoid arthritis become more likely, particularly in the presence of rheumatoid factor or anti-citrullinated peptide antibodies. Inflammatory arthritis is discussed extensively elsewhere in this book.

Dermatological features

Drug reactions can cause many skin manifestations; ranging from mild transient erythema through to toxic epidermal necrolysis, which has a mortality of 25%.[30] Common culprits include antibiotics and antiepileptics.[30] Rashes in the systemically unwell patient may be secondary to an underlying condition: for example, infections such as herpes simplex or mycoplasma cause erythema multiforme;[31] inflammatory conditions such as sarcoidosis or Behçet's syndrome are associated with erythema nodosum[32] or small-vessel vasculitis (leucocytoclastic vasculitis).[33] The presence of finger clubbing, splinter haemorrhages, and abnormal capillary loops can indicate cancer, endocarditis, or connective tissue disease respectively.[34]

Drug history

All medication and recreational drugs taken by the patient should be recorded, with careful attention to the time frame between drug and onset of illness. Drugs that can mimic or precipitate vasculitis,[35] SLE,[36] or hepatitis[19] are shown in Table 10.2.

Family history

A family history of autoimmune disease is important to elicit; for example, up to 10% of patients with SLE have another family member with the disease and there is a greater than 20% concordance rate between monozygotic twins.[37] For patients without a personal history of cancer, the likelihood ratio (LR) in a first-degree relative is 34 for ovarian cancer, 23 for colon cancer, 14 for ovarian cancer, 12.3 for prostate cancer, and 8.9 for breast cancer.[38] Autoinflammatory syndromes are rare monogenic disorders with defective innate immunity.

Social history

Living in low-cost crowded housing communities is associated with an increase in infectious diseases such as tuberculosis.[39] Smoking is also associated with low socio-economic status and increases the risk of cardiovascular disease, cancer, and autoimmune diseases such as rheumatoid arthritis. Higher risk behaviours such as intravenous drug use, tattoos, unprotected sexual activity, alcohol abuse, and prostitution predispose to bacterial infections, such as endocarditis and staphylococcal abscesses, and viruses such as HIV and hepatitis, which can be associated with the development of hepatic malignancy and systemic vasculitides such as polyarteritis nodosa (PAN).[40]

Occupation

The risk of exposure to specific infectious diseases differs between occupations. Hepatitis, tuberculosis, and MRSA occur in healthcare workers; *Brucella* spp., *Borrelia* spp., *Clostridium tetani*, *Strongyloides sercoralis*, and *Toxoplasma gondii* are seen in farmers and veterinarians; and *Brucella spp.*, hepatitis, and *Toxoplasma gondii* occur in refuse collectors.[41] Baking, farming, and occupational exposure to silica may predispose to granulomatosis with polyangiitis (Wegener's)[42]; farming and insecticide exposure may increase the risk of developing SLE or rheumatoid arthritis (RA)[43]; and asbestos, silica, and coal mining all predispose to lung cancer.[44]

Travel history

A detailed history is important, documenting geographical location, urban vs rural dwelling, exposure to bites, daily activities, sexual contacts. and prior vaccination and chemoprophylaxis.[7] Arboviruses are the most common viral infections in the returning traveller; chikungunya, West Nile virus, and Japanese encephalitis present with fever, myalgia and headache, and a maculopapular rash.[7] Intermittent or periodic fever, headache, myalgia, and abdominal pain suggest malaria, while a slow, grumbling, increasing fever with abdominal pain is characteristic of *Salmonella typhi*.[7] HIV seroconversion should be considered in a patient with fever, pharyngitis, lymphadenopathy, rash, myalgia, oral ulceration, headache, and general malaise. A viral serology screen is helpful but the results need expert interpretation in distinguishing a current from a past infection.[7]

Second line investigations

Further haematological tests

Bone marrow aspirate and biopsy can be useful; in patients with prolonged fever, it has been shown to result in a definitive diagnosis in one-fifth of patients, specifically detecting haematological malignancy, infection, systemic mastocytosis, or granulomatous disease.[45] Lymph node biopsies may be considered; a core needle or excisional node biopsy is preferable to a fine needle aspiration because of increased diagnostic yield.[46,47] Granulomas are present in lymph node biopsies in tuberculosis, sarcoidosis, or granulomatosis with polyangiitis (Wegener's).[46]

Autoimmune screen

Autoantibodies are common in the normal population, particularly with increasing age; the pre-test likelihood of a positive autoantibody in normal females aged 60 and above is 20%.[9] Serological testing should only be considered when the clinical features suggest an autoimmune process is present and results should be carefully interpreted, bearing in mind that a generally unwell patient with overwhelming infection or malignancy can have non-specifically positive serology.[9] The range of autoantibodies and their potential associations with infectious diseases, malignancies, and rheumatological conditions are outlined in Table 10.3; a practical approach to the stepwise use of autoantibodies is summarized by Stinton and Fritzler (2007).[9]

Further imaging

In patients with FUO, abdominal ultrasound has a sensitivity of 86% and a specificity of 65%, CT scanning of the chest has a sensitivity of 82% and a specificity of 77%, and CT scanning of the abdomen has a sensitivity of 92% and a specificity of 63% for correctly identifying the underlying diagnosis.[2] FDG-PET scans have a sensitivity of 92% and a specificity of 78% in patients with FUO[2]; they can be diagnostic for large-vessel vasculitis, and identify the site of infection or malignancy to allow further targeted investigation and biopsy.[2]

Biopsy

Histology is key to establishing the diagnosis in a patient presenting with multisystem disease; the use of a focused history, examination, and investigations increases the diagnostic yield by identifying a specific target organ to biopsy,[2] for example the lung, gut, kidney, skin, or nerve. Temporal artery biopsy is the current but imperfect gold standard for diagnosis of giant cell arteritis; the presence of skip lesions can lead to false-negative results.[48] Due to the risk of blindness in giant cell arteritis, steroid treatment should be initiated on clinical suspicion before a biopsy; these will in any case remain positive for up to 1–2 weeks following steroid therapy.[48]

Cardiovascular investigations

Angiography of the arterial tree is still the gold standard test for the presence of arterial stenosis or aneurysm in patients with suspected medium- or large-vessel vasculitis (such as polyarteritis nodosa or Takayasu's arteritis); however, non-invasive techniques such as CT or MR angiography (MRA) and cardiac MRI are now more widely available.[16] The negative predictive value of a normal transthoracic echocardiogram in a patient with normal heart valves is 90% or more;[49] it therefore sensitive enough to be a screening test for native valve infective endocarditis, although complex cases may be aided by a transoesophageal echocardiogram. Ultrasonography of the temporal artery is currently undergoing validation for use in the diagnosis of giant cell arteritis.[48]

Neurological investigations

Infection, inflammation, tumours, haemorrhage, or ischaemia can all result in neurological symptoms; a stepwise approach to investigation, starting with CT or MRI head, then lumbar puncture for

Table 10.3 An overview of autoantibodies and potential associated medical conditions

Test	Association
ANA	SLE, MCTD, SSc, PM, DM, SjS, RA, older age
ACPA	RA, PsA, TB
dsDNA, Sm	SLE
Centromere	lcSSc, PBC
Scl 70/topo-I, fibrillarin	dcSSc
Jo-1	PM, DM
C1q antibodies	HUV
C-ANCA (PR3 positive)	GPA, MPA, EGPA
aCL, β2GI and LA	APS
RF	RA, SLE, SSc, MCTD, SjS, PM, sarcoid, chronic hepatic and pulmonary diseases, chronic infections (subacute bacterial endocarditis, tuberculosis, parasitic infections, HIV, parasitic infections), cryoglobulinaemia, and malignancies
PL-7	PM/DM with ILD
Ro(SS-A) and La (SS-B)	SjS, SLE
U1-RNP	Mixed connective tissue disease
Low C3, C4	SLE, urticarial vasculitis, cryoglobulinaemia, RA, infectious diseases (subacute bacterial endocarditis, pneumococcal or Gram-negative sepsis, hepatitis B, parasitaemias), glomerulonephritis (membranoproliferative or post-streptococcal)
PM/Scl	PM-SSc overlap
Cryoglobulins	Cryoglobulinaemia (types I,II and III)
P-ANCA (MPO positive)	MPA, EGPA, GPA, drug-induced syndromes
P-ANCA (MPO negative)	UC, autoimmune liver disease, RA, SLE, HIV infection, other chronic infections or malignancies

aCL, anti-cardiolipin antibodies; ACPA, anti-citrullinated protein antibody; ANA, anti-nuclear antibodies; APS, anti-phospholipid antibodies; β2GI, β2-glycoprotein I; C-ANCA, anti-neutrophil cytoplasm antibodies; dcSSC, diffuse systemic sclerosis; DM, dermatomyositis; dsDNA, double-stranded DNA; EGPA, eosinophilic granulomatosis with polyangiitis (Churg–Strauss syndrome); HIV, human immunodeficiency virus; HUV, hypocomplementaemic urticarial vasculitis; ILD, interstitial lung disease; Jo-1, histidyl tRNA synthetase; LA, lupus anticoagulant; lcSSc, limited systemic sclerosis; MCTD, mixed connective tissue disease; MPA, microscopic polyangiitis; MPO, myeloperoxidase; P-ANCA, anti-neutrophil cytoplasm antibodies; PL7, threonyl-tRNA;PM, polymyositis; PR3, proteinase 3; PsA, psoriatic arthritis; RA, rheumatoid arthritis; SjS, Sjögren's syndrome; SLE, systemic lupus erthematosus; TB, tuberculosis.

Gram stain and culture of cerebrospinal fluid for bacteria, fungi, and viruses is indicated as first line;[6] MRA and MR venography are second line investigations to look for abnormalities in the blood vessels of the brain as seen in cerebral vasculitis or venous sinus thrombosis in Behçet's syndrome.

Respiratory investigation

Sputum cultures, specifically for acid-fast bacilli (AFB), and early morning urine specimens should be sent in patients with risk factors for tuberculosis and serological tests such as the Elispot or interferon-gamma release assays should be performed. Bronchoscopy in patients with FUO can allow direct visualization, bronchial washings, and biopsies of suspicious lesions for histology and microbiology.[2]

References

1. Lankisch P, Gerzmann M, Gerzmann JF, Lehnick D. Unintentional weight loss: diagnosis and prognosis. The first prospective follow-up study from a secondary referral centre. *J Intern Med* 2001;249(1):41–46.

2. Bleeker-Rovers CP, Vos FJ, de Kleijn EM et al. A prospective multicenter study on fever of unknown origin: the yield of a structured diagnostic protocol. *Medicine* (Baltimore) 2007;86(1):26–38.

3. Lea MJ, Aber RC. Descriptive epidemiology of night sweats upon admission to a university hospital. *South Med J* 1985;78(9):1065–1067.

4. Anderson T, Chabner BA, Young RC et al. Malignant lymphoma. 1. The histology and staging of 473 patients at the National Cancer Institute. *Cancer* 1982;50(12):2699–2707.

5. Miller LG, Asch SM, Yu EI et al. A population-based survey of tuberculosis symptoms: how atypical are atypical presentations? *Clin Infect Dis* 2000;30(2):293–299.

6. Varghese GM, Trowbridge P, Doherty T. Investigating and managing pyrexia of unknown origin in adults. *BMJ* 2010;341:C5470.

7. Spira AM. Assessment of travellers who return home ill. *Lancet* 2003;361(9367):1459–1469.

8. Fuchs HA, Tanner SB. Granulomatous disorders of the nose and paranasal sinuses. *Curr Opin Otolaryngol Head Neck Surg* 2009;17(1):23–27.

9. Stinton LM, Fritzler MJ. A clinical approach to autoantibody testing in systemic autoimmune rheumatic disorders. *Autoimmun Rev* 2007;7(1):77–84.

10. Hepburn AL, Narat S, Mason JC. The management of peripheral blood cytopenias in systemic lupus erythematosus. *Rheumatology (Oxford)* 2010;49(12):2243–2254.

11. (a) Lenner R, Schilero G, Lesser M. Hemoptysis: diagnosis and management. *Compr Ther* 2002;28(1):7–14;
    (b) Santiago S, Tobias J, Williams AJ. A reappraisal of the causes of hemoptysis. *Arch Intern Med* 1991;151(12):2449–2451.

12. Hamilton W, Peters TJ, Round A, Sharp D. What are the clinical features of lung cancer before the diagnosis is made? A population based case-control study. *Thorax* 2005;60(12):1059–1065.

13. Jennette JC, Falk RJ. Small-vessel vasculitis. *New Engl J Med* 1997; 337(21):1512–1523.

14. Mourad O, Palda V, Detsky AS. A comprehensive evidence-based approach to fever of unknown origin. *Arch Intern Med* 2003;163(5): 545–551.

15. Soares Pires F, Teixeira N, Coelho F, Damas C. Hemoptysis—etiology, evaluation and treatment in a university hospital. *Rev Port Pneumol* 2011;17(1):7–14.

16. Sitia S, Atzeni F, Sarzi-Puttini P et al. Cardiovascular involvement in systemic autoimmune diseases. *Autoimmun Rev* 2009;8(4):281–286.

17. Solomkin JS, Mazuski JE, Bradley JS et al. Diagnosis and management of complicated intra-abdominal infection in adults and children: guidelines by the Surgical Infection Society and the Infectious Diseases Society of America. *Clin Infect Dis* 2010;50(2):133–164.

18. Thomas PD, Forbes A, Green J et al. Guidelines for the investigation of chronic diarrhoea, 2nd edition. *Gut* 2003;52 Suppl 5, v1–v15.

19. Polson J, Lee WM. AASLD position paper: the management of acute liver failure. *Hepatology* 2005;41(5):1179–1197.

20. Moore KP, Aithal GP. Guidelines on the management of ascites in cirrhosis. *Gut* 2006;55 Suppl 6, vi1–vi12.

21. Hilton R. Acute renal failure. *BMJ* 2006;333(7572):786–790.

22. Jordan JE. Headache. *AJNR Am J Neuroradiol* 2007;28(9):1824–1826.

23. Durand ML, Calderwood SB, Weber DJ et al. Acute bacterial meningitis in adults—a review of 493 episodes. *New Engl J Med* 1993;328(1):21–28.

24. Griffiths D, Sturm J. Epidemiology and etiology of young stroke. *Stroke Res Treat* 2011;209–370.

25. Khairallah M, Chee SP, Rathinam SR, Attia S, Nadella V. Novel infectious agents causing uveitis. *Int Ophthalmol* 2010;30(5):465–483.

26. Pras E, Neumann R, Zandman-Goddard G et al. Intraocular inflammation in autoimmune diseases. *Semin Arthritis Rheum* 2004;34(3):602–609.

27. Gordon LK. Orbital inflammatory disease: a diagnostic and therapeutic challenge. *Eye (London)* 2006;20(10):1196–1206.

28. Borg FA, Salter VL, Dasgupta B. Neuro-ophthalmic complications in giant cell arteritis. *Curr Allergy Asthma Rep* 2008;8(4):323–330.

29. Coakley G, Mathews C, Field M et al. BSR & BHPR, BOA, RCGP and BSAC guidelines for management of the hot swollen joint in adults. *Rheumatology (Oxford)* 2006;45(8):1039–1041.

30. Roujeau JC. Clinical heterogeneity of drug hypersensitivity. *Toxicology* 2005;209(2):123–129.

31. Hughey LC. Approach to the hospitalized patient with targetoid lesions. *Dermatol Ther* 2011;24(2):196–206.

32. Kisacik B, Onat AM, Pehlivan Y. Multiclinical experiences in erythema nodosum: rheumatology clinics versus dermatology and infection diseases clinics. *Rheumatol Int* 2013;33(2):315–318.

33. Sunderkotter C, Bonsmann G, Sindrilaru A, Luger T. Management of leukocytoclastic vasculitis. *J Dermatolog Treat* 2005;16(4):193–206.

34. Fawcett RS, Linford S, Stulberg DL. Nail abnormalities: clues to systemic disease. *Am Fam Physician* 2004;69(6):1417–1424.

35. Radic M, Martinovic Kaliterna D, Radic J. Drug-induced vasculitis: a clinical and pathological review. *Neth J Med* 2012;70(1):12–17.

36. Vasoo S. Drug-induced lupus: an update. *Lupus* 2006;15(11):757–761.

37. Kelly JA, Moser KL, Harley JB. The genetics of systemic lupus erythematosus: putting the pieces together. *Genes Immun* 2002;3 Suppl 1, S71–S85.

38. Murff HJ, Spigel DR, Syngal S. Does this patient have a family history of cancer? An evidence-based analysis of the accuracy of family cancer history. *JAMA* 2004;292(12):1480–1489.

39. Govender T, Barnes JM, Pieper CH. Living in low-cost housing settlements in Cape Town, South Africa—the epidemiological characteristics associated with increased health vulnerability. *J Urban Health* 2010;87(6):899–911.

40. Patel N, Khan T, Espinoza LR. HIV infection and clinical spectrum of associated vasculitides. *Curr Rheumatol Rep* 2011;13(6):506–512.

41. Haagsma JA, Tariq L, Heederik DJ, Havelaar AH. Infectious disease risks associated with occupational exposure: a systematic review of the literature. *Occup Environ Med* 2012;69(2):140–146.

42. Knight A, Sandin S, Askling J. Occupational risk factors for Wegener's granulomatosis: a case-control study. *Ann Rheum Dis* 2010;69(4): 737–740.

43. Parks CG, Walitt BT, Pettinger M et al. Insecticide use and risk of rheumatoid arthritis and systemic lupus erythematosus in the Women's Health Initiative Observational Study. *Arthritis Care Res (Hoboken)* 2011;63(2):184–194.

44. Algranti E, Buschinelli JT, De Capitani EM. Occupational lung cancer. *J Bras Pneumol* 2010;36(6):784–794.

45. Hot A, Jaisson I, Girard C et al. Yield of bone marrow examination in diagnosing the source of fever of unknown origin. *Arch Intern Med* 2009;169(21):2018–2023.

46. Cunha BA. Fever of unknown origin: focused diagnostic approach based on clinical clues from the history, physical examination, and laboratory tests. *Infect Dis Clin North Am* 2007;21(4):1137–1187, xi.

47. McNamara C, Davies J, Dyer M et al. Guidelines on the investigation and management of follicular lymphoma. *Br J Haematol* 2012; 156(4):446–467.

48. Mukhtyar C, Guillevin L, Cid MC et al. EULAR recommendations for the management of large vessel vasculitis. *Ann Rheum Dis* 2009; 68(3):318–323.

49. McDermott BP, Cunha BA, Choi D, Cohen J, Hage J. Transthoracic echocardiography (TTE): sufficiently sensitive screening test for native valve infective endocarditis (IE). *Heart Lung* 2011;40(4):358–360.

CHAPTER 11

Spinal pain

Karl Gaffney and Louise Hamilton

Introduction

Spinal pain is so common that it could be considered, like the common cold, a normal part of life. Yet it is also the second commonest cause of both long-term disability and chronic work-related absence in the UK, costing at least £10 billion annually.[1] It has a similar impact in other developed countries, with the yearly cost to the US economy exceeding $100 billion.[2]

Around a third of the UK adult population annually complains of low back pain.[3] For most people episodes are short-lived and self-limiting. Only a fifth of those with pain will consult their GP,[4] and by 3 months 90% of patients will have stopped consulting.[5] However, it is a mistake to assume that they are therefore symptom-free. At 12 months a majority still have pain, with 60% reporting relapsing symptoms.[6]

Despite huge advances in musculoskeletal medicine and a reduction in heavy manual labour in the last half-century, the prevalence of musculoskeletal pain in general has increased since the 1950s, with a doubling of low back pain prevalence in one UK study.[7] However, it is the exponential rise in chronic disability that has led to claims of an epidemic of back pain, and this is as much a social and cultural problem as a medical one. The point prevalence of back pain is similar throughout the world, but associated disability seems to be a phenomenon of the developed world.

For the rheumatologist, the art in assessing patients with spinal pain is to identify those with a serious underlying cause for their symptoms without over-medicalizing the vast majority with non-specific pain.

Some definitions

Terminology relating to spinal pain is varied. We define pain as acute when the duration is less than 6 weeks, subacute if 6–12 weeks and chronic if more than 12 weeks, while recognizing that symptoms are often recurrent. Non-specific back pain is diagnosed in the absence of a clear pathological cause.

Sciatica means different things to different people and is therefore a term best avoided. Instead we use 'leg pain' if the pain radiates and 'nerve root pain' for neuropathic pain caused by nerve root impingement.

Overview of anatomy

The spine is an articulated column supporting the body and protecting the spinal cord (Figure 11.1). The two areas of natural curvature (or lordosis) in the cervical and lumbar regions develop after birth, once a child starts to mobilize. Vertebrae articulate anteriorly through the intervertebral discs and posteriorly through the facet joints. These are synovial joints, innervated by medial branches of the dorsal rami, which protect the intervertebral discs from axial shear forces. The intervertebral disc comprises a gel-like collagen and proteoglycan core (nucleus pulposus) surrounded by concentric sheets of collagen fibres (annulus fibrosus). It acts as a shock absorber and allows some movement in the sagittal plane. Disc degeneration is common with age and often asymptomatic. The nucleus pulposus can also herniate through the annulus fibrosus, narrowing the spinal canal and impinging on the cauda equina or traversing nerve roots.

The spinal cord is housed in the spinal canal and terminates at the conus medullaris between the T12 and L2 vertebrae. Distal to this the lumbar and spinal nerve roots form the cauda equina, exiting the spinal canal through their respective foramina.

Pain can arise from any of the structures in the spine, which are manifold. There are 24 articulating vertebrae; 9 fused sacral and

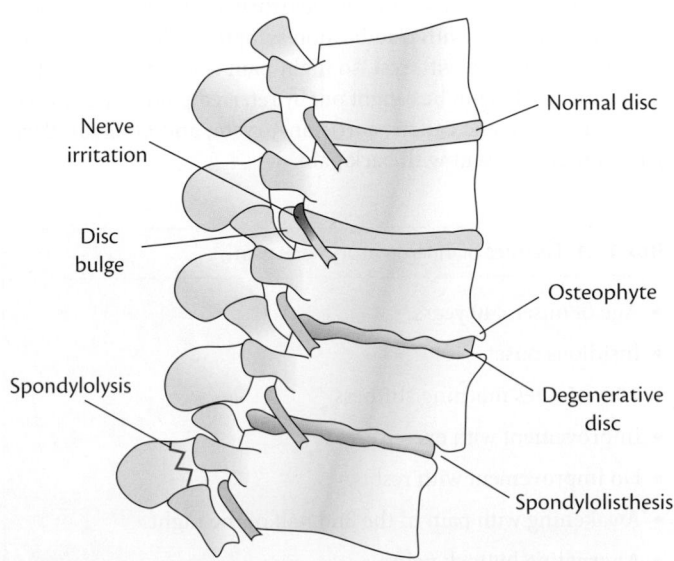

Fig. 11.1 Schematic diagram of the spine showing a normal vertebral unit with examples of structural abnormalities.

coccygeal vertebrae; 24 intervertebral discs; 139 joints; ligaments, bursae, and muscles, together with the spinal cord and nerve roots. However, correlation between symptoms and imaging findings is weak and in as many as 85% of patients with low back pain a specific diagnosis cannot be made.

Most patients describe some referred pain in the legs, and this too can arise from any structure in the back. Referred pain tends to be a diffuse dull ache which does not extend below the knee. Nerve root pain, on the other hand, has a neuropathic quality (burning, associated with paraesthesia), conforms to a dermatomal distribution, and usually radiates to the foot. It is also uncommon, with a lifetime prevalence around 5%.[8]

Approaching the patient with spinal pain

History

A thorough history is key when evaluating spinal pain, enabling decisions to be made about imaging and further management. The aim should be to answer three questions:[9]

- Is there serious underlying pathology?
- Is there an indication for surgery?
- Are there psychosocial factors which may impede recovery?

Age does not affect the overall prevalence of back pain,[10] but does change the likely underlying cause of new-onset pain. Think about axial spondyloarthropathy (SpA) in young adults, disc disease in the middle-aged, and osteoporosis and malignancy in the elderly. Reassess symptoms each time a patient presents with an exacerbation; having a blinkered approach to a patient with a label of chronic back pain risks missing their vertebral fracture or malignancy.

The pain

Ask about onset, radiation, and duration. Remember that osteoporotic fractures may occur in the absence of trauma. Radiation of pain into the leg is common and not specific for nerve root compression; radiculopathy is more likely if the leg pain is worse than the back pain. Are there features of inflammatory back pain (Box 11.1)? Is pain provoked by straining (disc herniation) or lumbar spine extension? (facet joint osteoarthritis). Patients with spinal stenosis can present with claudication symptoms. Mechanical pain will tend to improve with rest, so night pain is a red flag symptom (see Box 11.2). Do not be caught out by referred pain; conditions as diverse as pancreatic cancer, aortic aneurysm, and Guillain–Barré syndrome can present with back pain.

Box 11.1 Features of inflammatory back pain

- Age of onset <40 years
- Insidious onset
- >30 minutes morning stiffness
- Improvement with exercise
- No improvement with rest
- Awakening with pain in the 2nd half of the night
- Alternating buttock pain
- Improvement with NSAIDs

Box 11.2 Red flags—features suggestive of serious spinal pathology

- Age of onset <20 or >55 years
- Thoracic pain
- Nocturnal pain disturbing sleep
- Fever and unexplained weight loss
- Bladder or bowel dysfunction
- History of malignancy
- History of osteoporosis (or prolonged steroid use)
- Progressive neurological deficit
- Saddle anaesthesia

Other symptoms

Ask specifically about paraesthesiae and weakness in the limbs, saddle anaesthesia, and loss of sphincter control (cauda equina syndrome). Fevers, weight loss, and malaise suggest infection or malignancy and would be a definite indication for imaging.

Past medical history

Prior history of malignancy (especially breast, lung, and prostate) raises the possibility of spinal metastases. Spinal tuberculosis (TB) is rare in the developed world but should be considered in those with risk factors such as HIV infection. Ask about conditions associated with axial SpA: psoriasis, inflammatory bowel disease, iritis, and peripheral arthritis.

Social history

There may be diagnostic clues; intravenous drug abuse is a risk factor for discitis. Psychosocial factors are also an important determinant of outcome in non-specific low back pain. The development of chronic pain is associated with so-called 'yellow flags' (see Box 11.3) and early identification allows these risk factors to be modified.

Examination

The general physical examination may be expanded to include breast and prostate examination if malignancy is a concern. Examine the

---

Box 11.3 Yellow flags—psychosocial factors leading to chronic back pain

- Attitudes—believing that pain and activity are harmful, catastrophizing, passive attitude towards treatment.
- Behaviours—extended rest, increased alcohol use, avoiding normal activities
- Compensation issues—previous claims
- Diagnostic and treatment issues—lack of satisfaction with treatment, inappropriate expectations, conflicting diagnoses
- Emotions—depression, anxiety, stress, fear of making pain worse
- Family—either overprotective or lack of support
- Work—manual work, unhappy at work, shift work, job dissatisfaction, no opportunity for gradual return to work

spine for deformity: kyphosis (convex-posterior curvature), scoliosis (lateral curvature), and spondylolisthesis (a step may be palpable). An apparent scoliosis due to muscle spasm will generally correct when the patient lies prone. Localized vertebral tenderness suggests infection or a fracture. Examine the hips—buttock pain is frequently due to hip osteoarthritis.

Perform a straight leg raise in patients with leg symptoms. Passively raise the leg with the knee fully extended until the patient complains of pain. The test is positive if leg pain is elicited at an angle of 30–70°. Pain on straight leg raise can be due to hamstring tightness or ischial bursitis; only increased pain on dorsiflexing the foot confirms L5/S1 nerve root irritation. Pain provoked by raising the contralateral leg implies the presence of a central disc prolapse. Pain on femoral stretch (extending the affected leg while the patient is prone) is pathognomonic of an L4/5 disc protrusion. Focus the neurological examination on the L5 and S1 nerve roots by checking extensor hallucis longus power and ankle jerks, though bilateral loss of ankle reflexes can occur with age.

Range of motion testing is not helpful in differential diagnosis, though a reduced Schober's test does at least indicate organic pathology. Signs of a behavioural component to a patient's pain include non-dermatomal weakness and sensory disturbance, pain on axial loading, and a discrepancy in the degree of straight leg raise when the patient is supine and sitting.[11]

Investigations

For the great majority of patients a diagnosis of uncomplicated low back pain can be made at this stage without the need for any further investigation.

If further tests are indicated, avoid a scatter-gun approach. The low pre-test probability of serious spinal pathology means that untargeted investigations risk a high false-positive rate.

A number of blood tests have been suggested in evaluating red flag patients (Box 11.4), but in only a handful is the predictive value known.[12]

Radiography is readily available and useful when osteoporotic vertebral fractures are suspected. Otherwise it is of limited benefit in assessing acute low back pain. Lateral lumbar spine radiographs will only reveal bony destruction once 50% of a vertebra is destroyed, so abnormalities may take weeks to develop. The bottom line is that a normal radiograph does not exclude serious pathology.

Box 11.4 Blood tests in spinal pain

- ESR and CRP—↑ in malignancy, infection, (axial SpA)
- White cell count—↑ in infection
- Haemoglobin—normocytic anaemia with chronic inflammation/ infection/myeloma
- Serum protein electrophoresis—paraprotein in multiple myeloma
- Serum calcium—↑ in myeloma, bony metastases
- Alkaline phosphatase—↑ in metastatic disease, Paget's (and also as acute-phase protein)
- HLA B27—only useful if axial SpA suspected clinically

An MRI scan should be performed immediately if cauda equina syndrome is suspected, and urgently if malignancy or spinal infection is likely. Although patients with non-specific pain report higher levels of satisfaction if they are offered immediate lumbar spine imaging (radiography or MRI) there is no clinical benefit in terms of pain and disability.[13] Radiological investigations should therefore be avoided at the outset unless serious underlying pathology is suspected. Patients' expectations about investigations may need to be managed, but education can be helpful in this respect.[14]

MRI can be considered after 4–6 weeks in patients with ongoing nerve root pain severe enough to warrant surgery, or features of spinal stenosis where surgery is considered an option. For non-specific low back pain MRI should only be offered if a referral is being made for spinal fusion.[3] Clinicians must be alert to the high prevalence of abnormal radiological findings in asymptomatic patients, and resist the urge to pronounce an incidental finding the source of pain. The majority of people aged over 40 have facet joint osteoarthritis on CT scanning; this does not correlate with symptoms.[15] Over half of asymptomatic adults have bulging discs on MRI and 28% have disc herniation.[16] Spondylolysis (a stress fracture of the pars interarticularis) causes no pain in 50% of cases.[17] The most clinically significant findings on MRI scanning are disc extrusions, nerve root compression, and at least moderate spinal stenosis.[18]

An isotope bone scan can be useful in the detection of spinal metastases and occult infection, but has a lower sensitivity and specificity than MRI.

Specific disease processes

'Red flag' pain

Cauda equina syndrome

Compression of the caudal nerve roots is a true surgical emergency necessitating immediate investigation and treatment. The usual cause is a massive disc prolapse into the spinal canal, but any space-occupying lesion (e.g. tumour, abscess, haematoma) can have a similar effect. The syndrome presents with severe back and bilateral leg pain, perineal numbness, and eventually an inability to void (due to involvement of the sacral nerve roots). A rectal examination will reveal reduced tone. It often manifests on a background of less severe back and leg pain, so patients presenting with nerve root signs should be instructed to report the development of perineal numbness and sphincter disturbance immediately.

Osteoporotic fracture

Most vertebral fractures are asymptomatic and diagnosed incidentally on a chest radiograph, or once a patient has developed a kyphotic deformity. When symptomatic, the pain can be severe, and may last for up to 6 months. The pain will start acutely, often after minimal or no trauma (coughing or twisting is sufficient), and may radiate in a dermatomal pattern bilaterally. Most fractures occur in the mid-thoracic or thoracolumbar vertebrae. Have a high index of suspicion in patients with risk factors (chronic steroid use, early menopause, family history, alcohol abuse). The pain may be severe enough to need opiates initially and some patients, particularly elderly people, may need hospital admission. Intravenous pamidronate and calcitonin can help intractable acute pain, but vertebroplasty is not usually recommended in the acute setting. Patients will need to start appropriate treatment for osteoporosis, usually with a bisphosphonate and calcium and vitamin D supplement.

Malignancy

Spinal tumours typically present with unremitting back pain, though neurological involvement including spinal cord compression may be the first indication of pathology. Almost three-quarters are due to metastatic spread, with prostate, breast, and lung cancers having a particular predilection for the spine. Spinal metastases should be suspected in anyone with a prior history of malignancy, or features of systemic disease (weight loss, night sweats, etc.). An erythrocyte sedimentation rate (ESR) over 20 is 78% sensitive and 67% specific in identifying occult malignancy presenting as back pain.[12] Most primary spinal tumours are benign, though even benign tumours can have aggressive features and therefore management usually involves surgical excision.

Infection

The terms vertebral osteomyelitis and discitis are used interchangeably to describe localized spinal infection. Spread is usually haematogenous but can be a complication of injection or instrumentation. Think about underlying infective endocarditis, particularly in patients with valvular heart disease. *Staphylococcus aureus* is the causative organism in over half of cases, but pseudomonas and candida are seen in IV drug users and brucella is important in the Middle East. Pain starts insidiously and early on there may be no suspicious features. Well-localized spinal tenderness is a reliable sign but only half of patients have a fever. Positive blood cultures are seen in 70% of patients[19] and elevated inflammatory markers in 80%.[20] Most patients respond to intravenous antibiotics, though vertebral instability or abscess formation may necessitate surgery.

Spinal involvement is seen in 1–2% of cases of TB. In the developed world it is a late manifestation associated with reactivation, but in endemic areas it is a disease of the young. Diagnostic delay is common, as is neurological compromise at presentation.[21] Constitutional symptoms and an abnormal chest radiograph are seen in fewer than half of cases, so a high index of suspicion is needed. Over 90% of patients with spinal tuberculosis have a positive tuberculin test,[22] but the diagnosis should be confirmed by biopsy. A 6 month course of therapy including rifampicin should be sufficient, but as with pyogenic osteomyelitis surgical stabilization or debridement may be required.

Axial spondyloarthropathy

Ankylosing spondylitis is the prototypical spondyloarthropathy. It usually presents in early adulthood with inflammatory back pain. Radiographic changes occur late, so MRI scanning of the whole spine and sacroiliac joints is the radiological investigation of choice to avoid the diagnostic delay sadly typical of this condition (see Chapter 122).

Diffuse idiopathic skeletal hyperostosis

Diffuse idiopathic skeletal hyperostosis (DISH) is a non-inflammatory disease characterized by widespread ossification of the spinal ligaments and entheses, and can be confused with ankylosing spondylitis. Patients present with back pain, often with associated morning stiffness, but may also complain of dysphagia (due to oesophageal compression by large anterior osteophytes), recurrent Achilles tendonitis, and palpable bony spurs. Radiographs show flowing calcification, typically in the thoracic region, likened to wax dripping down a candle. Treatment is symptomatic with analgesia, and rarely surgery (when osteophytes are large enough to cause dysphagia or myelopathy).

Crystal arthritis

Both gout and pseudogout can involve the spine. The usual presentation is with pain, fever and raised inflammatory markers, but large tophi can cause nerve root symptoms or spontaneous fractures. Atlanto-axial disease is typical of pseudogout. Because of the associated systemic upset crystal arthritis is frequently mistaken for infection or malignancy, and only diagnosed at the time of surgery.

Lumbar radiculopathy

Acute nerve root irritation is usually due to a herniated disc. Although the pain may be severe enough to warrant bed rest (which is usually discouraged) at the start, most episodes resolve without surgery. MRI scanning is only indicated in those whose symptoms have not improved after 6 weeks or those with progressive neurological signs. Only 10% of patients ultimately require surgery. Epidural steroid injections can improve pain in the short term, but do not reduce the rate of subsequent surgery.[23]

Spinal stenosis

Narrowing of the central canal by a number of pathologies can cause compression or ischaemia of the nerve roots. Degenerative arthritis is the commonest cause, but disc herniation, space-occupying lesions, and bony hypertrophy (e.g. in DISH, Paget's, ankylosing spondylitis) may also play a role. Patients typically present with bilateral leg pain, worse on walking or standing (neurogenic claudication) and relieved by sitting or bending forward. Neurological examination is usually normal, with a negative straight leg raise test. MRI is the investigation of choice although, as always, results should be interpreted with caution; at least a fifth of asymptomatic adults over 60 have radiological spinal stenosis.[24] In most patients the course is benign, and conservative treatment options (physiotherapy, analgesia) should be exhausted before surgery is contemplated.

Degenerative disease

The classical medical model of low back pain would dictate further sections here on facet joint arthritis, degenerative disc disease, and spondylolisthesis. We have deliberately avoided this approach as the 20th century's focus on a structural cause for back pain has not helped to reduce its prevalence and has not improved treatment. There is no good evidence to support the use of facet joint injections[25] or intradiscal therapy[26] in managing low back pain, and many 'abnormalities' are normal features of ageing not correlated with symptoms.[27] That said, it would be equally wrong to lump all patients with degenerative changes into the 'non-specific low back pain' group. There are undoubtedly individual patients who benefit from facet joint blocks, and the following management guidelines are just that—evidence-based guidelines, not dogma.

Managing non-specific low back pain

This is an overview of management. For more details, including comprehensive literature reviews, see the current UK[3,28] and European[10,29] guidelines.

Acute pain

Education

Reassure the patient that there is unlikely to be a serious underlying cause for their pain, that they do not need radiographs or scans, and that they will get better rapidly. Warn them that recurrence is possible, but is not a sign of ongoing damage. Use neutral terms like 'sprain' or 'strain' when explaining the pain, and avoid at all costs 'crumbling discs'. Encourage them to take responsibility for their recovery. Written information for patients such as *The Back Book*[30] can be helpful.

Activity

Encourage normal activity and warn against bed rest. There is no evidence that a back-specific exercise programme is helpful in acute pain—general aerobic exercise to avoid deconditioning is adequate. Try hard to keep the patient at work—a patient off work for a month has a 20% chance of still being off at a year, and by 2 years they are unlikely to work again.[31] A return to full duties may be slower if a patient has a very physically demanding job, but there is no good evidence that occupational factors cause back pain or delay recovery.[32]

Medication

Start with regular paracetamol and add a non-steroidal anti-inflammatory drug (NSAID) and/or a weak opioid if necessary. Strong opioids may be needed in the short term for patients with severe pain, but benzodiazepines are best avoided. Tricyclic antidepressants can be helpful for patients who remain symptomatic at this stage, especially if there is nerve root pain, but selective serotonin reuptake inhibitors should not be used for this purpose.

Physical methods

Spinal manipulation is safe in acute back pain without radiculopathy.

Most patients will have recovered by 6 weeks. For those with ongoing symptoms consider:

- *Physical therapies:* Depending on patient preference offer a structured exercise programme (group or one-on-one), a course of acupuncture, or spinal manipulation. Injections are not indicated for non-specific pain.

- *Rehabilitation programme:* A combined physical and psychological treatment programme should be offered to patients who have tried at least one of the physical therapies and have ongoing pain with either high disability levels or psychological distress.

Surgery

A referral for spinal fusion can be considered when patients have completed a rehabilitation programme but still have severe pain. Surgery before this point is inappropriate as neither spinal fusion[33] nor disc replacement surgery[34] is clinically more effective than intensive rehabilitation. Non-surgical interventions such as radiofrequency facet joint denervation[35] and intradiscal therapy[35] are not indicated for those with non-specific chronic low back pain.

Is prevention better than cure?

The identification of risk factors for non-specific low back pain has not translated easily into evidence-based interventions. Primary prevention studies are difficult because of the high lifetime prevalence of back pain, and only exercise has been shown to be protective. Obesity[36] and smoking[37] are associated with low back pain but the effect is modest and there is no evidence that interventions are beneficial in primary prevention. Manual handling is seen as an important preventive measure but there is no evidence that training workers to lift 'correctly' or use mechanical aids prevents back pain.[38]

In patients who have already had pain, physical activity is beneficial in preventing relapses and work absence[39] and weight loss programmes can improve disability[40] and pain.[41] However, encouraging patients to engage with lifestyle changes may be difficult. One Australian study showed that while 68% of respondents to an online survey were overweight or obese, only 8% were actively trying to lose weight and only 19% of all patients were trying to exercise.[42]

Perhaps the most important goal is preventing long-term disability and unemployment in patients with back pain. Interventions should be timely, as the prognosis is determined by levels of pain and disability in the first 3 months of symptoms.[43] Temporary job modifications can help with an early return to work,[39] and cognitive behavioural therapy can reduce absenteeism at 1 year.[44] At the societal level successful return to work is more likely in countries in which there is an emphasis on reintegration without loss of partial benefits, rather than a need for patients to adopt a sick role and demonstrate their disability to doctors in order to qualify for compensation.[45] Ultimately the cure for disabling back pain is social, not medical.

References

1. Maniadakis N, Gray A. The economic burden of back pain in the UK. *Pain* 2000;84.(1):95–103.
2. Katz JN. Lumbar disc disorders and low-back pain: socioeconomic factors and consequences. *J Bone Joint Surg Am* 2006;88 Suppl 2:21–24.
3. Savigny P KS, Watson P, Underwood M et al. *Low back pain: early management of persistent non-specific low back pain.* National Collaborating Centre for Primary Care and Royal College of General Practitioners, London, 2009.
4. Macfarlane GJ, Jones GT, Hannaford PC. Managing low back pain presenting to primary care: where do we go from here? *Pain* 2006; 122(3):219–222.
5. Croft PR, Macfarlane GJ, Papageorgiou AC, Thomas E, Silman AJ. Outcome of low back pain in general practice: a prospective study. *BMJ* 1998;316(7141):1356–1359.
6. Hestbaek L, Leboeuf-Yde C, Manniche C. Low back pain: what is the long-term course? A review of studies of general patient populations. *Eur Spine J* 2003;12(2):149–165.
7. Harkness EF, Macfarlane GJ, Silman AJ, McBeth J. Is musculoskeletal pain more common now than 40 years ago? Two population-based cross-sectional studies. *Rheumatology (Oxford)* 2005;44(7):890–895.
8. Heliovaara M, Impivaara O, Sievers K et al. Lumbar disc syndrome in Finland. *J Epidemiol Community Health* 1987;41(3):251–258.
9. Deyo RA. Early diagnostic evaluation of low back pain. *J Gen Intern Med* 1986;1(5):328–338.
10. Airaksinen O, Brox JI, Cedraschi C et al. Chapter 4. European guidelines for the management of chronic nonspecific low back pain. *Eur Spine J* 2006;15 Suppl 2:S192–S300.
11. Waddell G, McCulloch JA, Kummel E, Venner RM. Nonorganic physical signs in low-back pain. *Spine* ((Phila Pa 1976) 1976) 1980;5(2):117–125.
12. Deyo RA, Diehl AK. Cancer as a cause of back pain: frequency, clinical presentation, and diagnostic strategies. *J Gen Intern Med* 1988;3(3): 230–238.
13. Chou R, Fu R, Carrino JA, Deyo RA. Imaging strategies for low-back pain: systematic review and meta-analysis. *Lancet* 2009;373(9662):463–472.

14. Deyo RA, Diehl AK, Rosenthal M. Reducing roentgenography use. Can patient expectations be altered? *Arch Intern Med* 1987;147(1):141–145.

15. Kalichman L, Li L, Kim DH et al. Facet joint osteoarthritis and low back pain in the community-based population. *Spine* ((Phila Pa 1976) 1976) 2008;33(23):2560–2565.

16. Jensen MC, Brant-Zawadzki MN, Obuchowski N et al. Magnetic resonance imaging of the lumbar spine in people without back pain. *New Engl J Med* 1994;331(2):69–73.

17. Magora A, Schwartz A. Relation between low back pain and X-ray changes. 4. Lysis and olisthesis. *Scand J Rehabil Med* 1980;12(2):47–52.

18. Jarvik JJ, Hollingworth W, Heagerty P, Haynor DR, Deyo RA. The Longitudinal Assessment of Imaging and Disability of the Back (LAIDBack) Study: baseline data. *Spine* ((Phila Pa 1976) 1976) 2001;26(10):1158–1166.

19. Nolla JM, Ariza J, Gomez-Vaquero C et al. Spontaneous pyogenic vertebral osteomyelitis in nondrug users. *Semin Arthritis Rheum* 2002;31(4):271–278.

20. Beronius M, Bergman B, Andersson R. Vertebral osteomyelitis in Goteborg, Sweden: a retrospective study of patients during 1990–95. *Scand J Infect Dis* 2001;33(7):527–532.

21. Nussbaum ES, Rockswold GL, Bergman TA, Erickson DL, Seljeskog EL. Spinal tuberculosis: a diagnostic and management challenge. *J Neurosurg* 1995;83(2):243–247.

22. Berney S, Goldstein M, Bishko F. Clinical and diagnostic features of tuberculous arthritis. *Am J Med* 1972;53(1):36–42.

23. Wilson-MacDonald J, Burt G, Griffin D, Glynn C. Epidural steroid injection for nerve root compression. A randomised, controlled trial. *J Bone Joint Surg Br* 2005;87(3):352–355.

24. Boden SD, Davis DO, Dina TS, Patronas NJ, Wiesel SW. Abnormal magnetic-resonance scans of the lumbar spine in asymptomatic subjects. A prospective investigation. *J Bone Joint Surg Am* 1990;72(3):403–408.

25. Staal JB dBR, de Vet HCW, Hildebrandt J, Nelemans P. Injection therapy for subacute and chronic low-back pain. *Cochrane Database Syst Rev* 2008:CD001824.

26. Urrutia G, Kovacs F, Nishishinya MB, Olabe J. Percutaneous thermo-coagulation intradiscal techniques for discogenic low back pain. *Spine* ((Phila Pa 1976)) 2007;32(10):1146–1154.

27. van Tulder MW, Assendelft WJ, Koes BW, Bouter LM. Spinal radiographic findings and nonspecific low back pain. A systematic review of observational studies. *Spine* ((Phila Pa 1976)) 1997;22(4):427–434.

28. Waddell GMA, Hutchinson A, Feder G, Lewis M. *Low back pain evidence review*. Royal College of General Practitioners, London, 1999.

29. van Tulder MB, Bekkering A, Breen T et al. on behalf of the COST B13 Working Group on Guidelines for the Management of Acute Low Back Pain in Primary Care. European guidelines for the management of acute nonspecific low back pain in primary care. 2004 (cited 2011) Available from: www.backpaineurope.org/web/files/WG1_Guidelines.pdf

30. Royal College of General Practitioners. *The Back Book*, 2nd edn. The Stationery Office, London, 2002.

31. Waddell G. *The back pain revolution*.: Churchill Livingstone, Edinburgh, 1999.

32. Kwon BK, Roffey DM, Bishop PB, Dagenais S, Wai EK. Systematic review: occupational physical activity and low back pain. *Occup Med (Lond)* 2011;61(8):541–548.

33. Fairbank J, Frost H, Wilson-MacDonald J et al. Randomised controlled trial to compare surgical stabilisation of the lumbar spine with an intensive rehabilitation programme for patients with chronic low back pain: the MRC spine stabilisation trial. *BMJ* 2005;330(7502):1233.

34. Hellum C, Johnsen LG, Storheim K et al. Surgery with disc prosthesis versus rehabilitation in patients with low back pain and degenerative disc: two year follow-up of randomised study. *BMJ*;342:d2786.

35. Chou R, Atlas SJ, Stanos SP, Rosenquist RW. Nonsurgical interventional therapies for low back pain: a review of the evidence for an American Pain Society clinical practice guideline. *Spine* (Phila Pa 1976) 2009;34(10):1078–1093.

36. Shiri R, Karppinen J, Leino-Arjas P, Solovieva S, Viikari-Juntura E. The association between obesity and low back pain: a meta-analysis. *Am J Epidemiol* 2010;171(2):135–154.

37. Shiri R, Karppinen J, Leino-Arjas P, Solovieva S, Viikari-Juntura E. The association between smoking and low back pain: a meta-analysis. *Am J Med* 2010;123(1):87 e7–35.

38. Verbeek JH MK-P, Karppinen J, Kuijer PPFM, Viikari-Juntura E, Takala E-P. Manual material handling advice and assistive devices for preventing and treating back pain in workers. *Cochrane Database Syst Rev* 2011;6:CD005958.

39. Burton AK, Balague F, Cardon G et al. Chapter 2. European guidelines for prevention in low back pain: November 2004. *Eur Spine J* 2006;15 Suppl 2:S136–S168.

40. Roffey DM, Ashdown LC et al. Pilot evaluation of a multidisciplinary, medically supervised, nonsurgical weight loss program on the severity of low back pain in obese adults. *Spine J* 2011;11(3):197–204.

41. Kotowski SE, Davis KG. Influence of weight loss on musculoskeletal pain: Potential short-term relevance. *Work* 2010;36(3):295–304.

42. Wilk V, Palmer HD, Stosic RG, McLachlan AJ. Evidence and practice in the self-management of low back pain: findings from an Australian internet-based survey. *Clin J Pain* 2010;26(6):533–540.

43. Heymans MW, van Buuren S, Knol DL et al. The prognosis of chronic low back pain is determined by changes in pain and disability in the initial period. *Spine J* 2010;10(10):847–856.

44. Linton SJ, Andersson T. Can chronic disability be prevented? A randomized trial of a cognitive-behavior intervention and two forms of information for patients with spinal pain. *Spine* (Phila Pa 1976) 2000;25(21):2825–2831; discussion 2824.

45. Anema JR, Schellart AJ, Cassidy JD et al. Can cross country differences in return-to-work after chronic occupational back pain be explained? An exploratory analysis on disability policies in a six country cohort study. *J Occup Rehabil* 2009;19(4):419–426.

CHAPTER 12

Pain and fatigue

Candy McCabe, Richard Haigh,
Helen Cohen, and Sarah Hewlett

Introduction

Pain and fatigue are cardinal symptoms of the rheumatic diseases. The majority of patients will experience them over the course of their disease, though the intensity and quality of them may vary over the time course. This chapter focuses on the identification and management of pain and fatigue in the clinical setting and provides a broad overview of the mechanisms that drive these symptoms and their incidence. In each section pain is discussed first, followed by fatigue.

Epidemiology

Pain

In both developed and developing countries, 25–30% of the total adult population, and approximately 8% of children, may be affected by musculoskeletal pain.[1,2] As the mean age of the global population rises, it is likely that these percentages will increase. Joint pain is estimated to affect 12.9–57.0% of those over 85 years of age, with the lower limb most commonly involved.

The financial burden of musculoskeletal pain is also high. UK data for chronic low back pain alone has estimated direct healthcare costs of £1632 million per year with indirect costs of £10 668 million.[3] In the US, common pain conditions account for a loss of 13% of the total workforce at any one time and 6.2% of this group report some form of arthritis or musculoskeletal pain.[4]

Fatigue

Fatigue is experienced by over 90% of people with a rheumatic condition, who often rate their fatigue as more severe than their pain,[5] with severity levels as severe as those seen in chronic fatigue syndrome.[6] People without a long-term condition report mean fatigue scores of 20.5 on a visual analogue scale of 0–100, while in rheumatic conditions fatigue ranges from 40.8 (psoriatic arthritis) to 74.4 (primary Sjögren's syndrome), with fatigue scores for people with rheumatoid arthritis (RA), osteoarthritis (OA), lupus, ankylosing spondylitis, and fibromyalgia lying between those two extremes.[7] The financial burden of fatigue in rheumatic disease is not readily identifiable, but people with inflammatory arthritis consider fatigue the primary cause of days lost from paid work.[8]

Definitions of pain and fatigue

Pain

Pain is defined by the International Association for the Study of Pain (IASP) as:

> An unpleasant sensory and emotional experience associated with actual or potential tissue damage, or described in terms of such damage.

For those with a rheumatic disease pain is usually chronic (≥12 weeks duration) and most commonly falls within one or more of the following classifications: musculoskeletal, inflammatory, neuropathic, or a dysfunctional state.

Musculoskeletal pain

Musculoskeletal pain is pain that arises from any structures within the musculoskeletal system such as bone, muscles, tendons, and/or ligaments. Pain may arise from mechanical dysfunction within a joint, as in advanced OA, or from the bone, as in Paget's disease or malignancy. Pain that arises from the muscles alone is commonly referred to as 'myofascial pain'.

Inflammatory pain

Inflammatory pain arises from tissue-damaged associated inflammation that is usually accompanied by oedema, redness, heat, and a possible reduction in function. When present in the joints it is commonly associated with a perception of stiffness.

Neuropathic pain

Neuropathic pain may be central or peripheral in origin and is defined as 'pain caused by a lesion or disease of the (central/peripheral) somatosensory system'.[9] Clinical signs of neuropathic pain may include evidence of **allodynia** (pain to a stimulus that is not normally painful) and **hyperalagesia** (increased pain to a stimulus that normally evokes pain) (see IASP Taxonomy[10]).

Dysfunctional state

This is the term given to conditions where there is a lack of structural cause for the persistent pain experienced, such as fibromyalgia and complex regional pain syndrome.[11] People with these conditions may present with the clinical signs and symptoms of other pain states, such as neuropathic and myofascial pain, but there is no evidence of an underlying pathology.

Fatigue

Fatigue has been defined and classified in a number of ways, yet there is no overall consensus. In terms of the fatigue that is related to musculoskeletal conditions, a broad conceptual definition appears the most appropriate:

> Fatigue is a subjective, unpleasant symptom which incorporates total body feelings ranging from tiredness to exhaustion, creating an unrelenting overall condition which interferes with individuals' ability to function in their normal capacity.[12]

Here, the term 'function' should be assumed to include physical and/or cognitive function. The term 'tiredness' might be disputed, as people with RA consider tiredness to be the phenomenon experienced by healthy people, and believe the terms 'fatigue' or 'exhaustion' are necessary to encapsulate the intensity of the symptoms experienced within chronic illness.[13,14]

Aetiopathogenesis

Pain mechanisms

The pain pathway describes the anatomical route that a peripheral stimulus takes to the brain, via peripheral nerves, dorsal horn, and spinal cord, to register as a painful perception. Central projections of the pain pathway from the thalamic nuclei include somatosensory cortex and the limbic system. Although the pain pathway is a credible neuroanatomical concept, multiple brain areas are activated during a pain experience in addition to the classic lateral sensory–discriminative and medial emotional–affective areas involved in pain processing. Melzack and others have proposed that this extensive network of brain regions activated during pain perception, represents a specific cerebral signature, a pain neuromatrix.[15] A pain experience can be modified by dysfunction at multiple levels along this pathway, ranging from changes in the molecular constituents of the peripheral inflammatory milieu to alterations in the complex circuitry of cortical representation. Disease states, psychosocial factors, and medical interventions can influence the activity of the pathway.

Despite the elaborate multifaceted system of pain perception, broad types can be identified which correlate with known pain mechanisms (see 'Pain'). It should be noted that much of the research that underpins our knowledge of the neurobiology of pain is undertaken in animal models.

Nociceptive pain is caused by stimulation of peripheral nerve fibres (Aδ and C fibres) via tissue pathology such as inflammation, ischaemia, and mechanical stimuli such as pressure and heat. C fibres can release local peptides to induce neurogenic inflammation via neuropeptides such as substance P and calcitonin gene-related peptide (CGRP), which induce vasodilatation, plasma extravasation, and interaction with immune cells.

Neuropathic pain (see 'Pain') arises via nerve signalling from ectopic discharges of damaged neurons or those induced by adjacent healthy nerves, including sympathetic system fibres. Both nociceptive and neuropathic signals can be modified along the pain pathway, so that a given stimulus is amplified—this is sensitization. At the site of tissue damage and inflammation, a large number of mediators can cause the reduction in excitation thresholds of peripheral nociceptors, thereby increasing signalling to the spinal cord dorsal horn. These alterations to the properties of ion channels can be short lived, as in the case of prostaglandins or bradykinins, or much longer lasting such as the effects of cytokines, including tumour necrosis factor alpha (TNFα) and nerve growth factor. There are also important inhibitory mechanisms present in peripheral tissues, and the balance between proinflammatory/excitatory mechanisms and the inhibitory cytokines, cannabinoid, and opioid systems play an important role. The peripheral nerve message can be amplified on a molecular level by complex intracellular mechanisms which modulate gene transcription via second messenger systems.

Central sensitization is considered the main pathophysiological mechanism responsible for neuropathic pain and contributes significantly to nociceptive pain. Peripheral nociceptor hyperactivity causes major secondary changes in the spinal cord dorsal horn, such as enhanced AMP acid (AMPA) N-methyl-D-aspartate (NMDA) receptor activation in the dorsal horn, mediated by protein kinases, and upregulation of the signalling cascade that modulates gene transcription (e.g. c-*fos*, c-*jun*). In addition, changes in the descending modulatory systems and functional changes in spinal cord microglial cells and astrocytes contribute to the enhanced signal transmission of central sensitization.

Specific joint and musculoskeletal pain mechanisms

Features that reflect local joint pathology and characteristics such as mood, social circumstances, and central pain processing mechanisms determine pain report in arthritis. Both peripheral and central mechanisms contribute to chronic arthritis pain.[16] Peripheral mechanisms such as inflammation, oxidative stress, and ischaemia may be more important in the early disease, with central mechanisms having a greater influence on pain report and disability in later stages. Patients with arthritis often describe a 'neuropathic pain' pattern, but whether this reflects true neuropathic pathology or the complex pain experience derived from multiple dysfunctional systems is unclear.

Joints are well innervated by sensory, sympathetic, and nociceptive fibres, though large proportions of them are usually insensitive to normal stimuli. These normally quiescent nerve fibres, the 'silent nociceptors', can be sensitized by peripheral joint pathology and respond to mechanical stress such as (normal) movement. Joint effusion, especially in chronic arthritis where the synovium and capsule are less compliant, causes significant increases in intraarticular pressure that can activate joint nociceptors.

Rheumatoid arthritis

Despite modern treatment approaches, a majority of patients with RA still describe chronic pain. Some of the abnormal pain processing can revert to normal after prolonged periods, as evidenced by restoration of pain threshold and descending pain analgesic pathways, following joint replacement. There may be differences in chronic pain due to OA and RA; for example, RA patients have lower pain thresholds than controls.[17] This may reflect subtle differences in joint innervation in chronic synovitis, combined with altered pain processing, endogenous opioid systems, and descending control.

Osteoarthritis

Why an osteoarthritic joint is painful is not clear. Multiple joint structures are abnormal in established OA. It is likely that combinations of peripheral inflammation, synovitis, bone marrow lesions (seen with MRI scanning), and mechanical stress on periarticular structures, along with peripheral and central sensitization, are responsible. Whether clinical examination and readily available imaging can predict which of these is the dominant pathway and therefore guide treatment is debatable. Poor outcome from joint replacement may be related to preoperative pain experience, such as rest pain, night pain, and low pain threshold which may be construed as neuropathic.

Fibromyalgia

The chronic widespread pain of fibromyalgia is a common presentation to rheumatologists. Extensive clinical observation, quantitative sensory testing, and functional neuroimaging studies all point towards significant abnormalities in pain perception; widespread multisystem pain report, diffusely lower pressure pain thresholds, temporal summation, deficiencies in descending pain modulation, and cognitive disturbance. This evidence suggests a global amplification of central pain processing. The relative contributions of aberrant descending analgesic serotonergic–noradrenergic system activity, and peripheral and central sensitization is unclear. Further imaging studies have suggested that spontaneous pain is related to enhanced activity in multiple brain networks—additional evidence of a disseminated pain processing problem.[18]

Fatigue mechanisms

The causal mechanism for fatigue in musculoskeletal disorders remains an issue of debate fuelled by poor study design and conflicting results from studies that are largely cross-sectional using small or biased samples (e.g. patients in flare). Although some studies show that fatigue may be causally linked to inflammatory processes, mood, disability, sleep, pain behaviours, and beliefs, the evidence is inconsistent[19] and associations vary across musculoskeletal conditions.[20] In inflammatory musculoskeletal conditions, it has been suggested that interleukins IL-1 and IL-6 might provide a partial explanatory mechanism.[21]

It is proposed there are three main elements driving fatigue in musculoskeletal conditions (Figure 12.1).[22] Disease processes including inflammation and pain may affect fatigue directly, or indirectly through poor sleep, disability, and deconditioning. Cognitions, feelings, and behaviours may interact to produce over- or under-exertion in physical activities, such as 'boom and bust' behaviours. These three elements interact to form a multicausal pathway, where for each patient, different factors are present in different strengths and interact to produce fatigue, with different combinations on each occasion.[22] Such an aetiology would account for a symptom that occurs across the whole spectrum of musculoskeletal conditions, disease durations, and levels of inflammation, and also allows for fatigue as both cause and effect (e.g. sometimes fatigue may be driven by low mood, and at other times low mood may be driven by fatigue).

Clinical features

Pain

Pain may be intermittent or continuous and vary in nature depending on the cause and course of the disease.

Pain arising from inflammation, such as in RA, will be accompanied by the other classical signs (see 'Inflammatory pain') and is commonly described as throbbing in nature, at rest and on movement, and exacerbated by use of the affected part. The descriptions that patients with RA use to describe their pain may alter depending on the time of day, the duration of their disease, the joints that are involved, and whether those joints are moving or at rest.[23] Diurnal variation of pain and stiffness is common, with patients describing an increase in intensity of these symptoms at the start and end of the day.

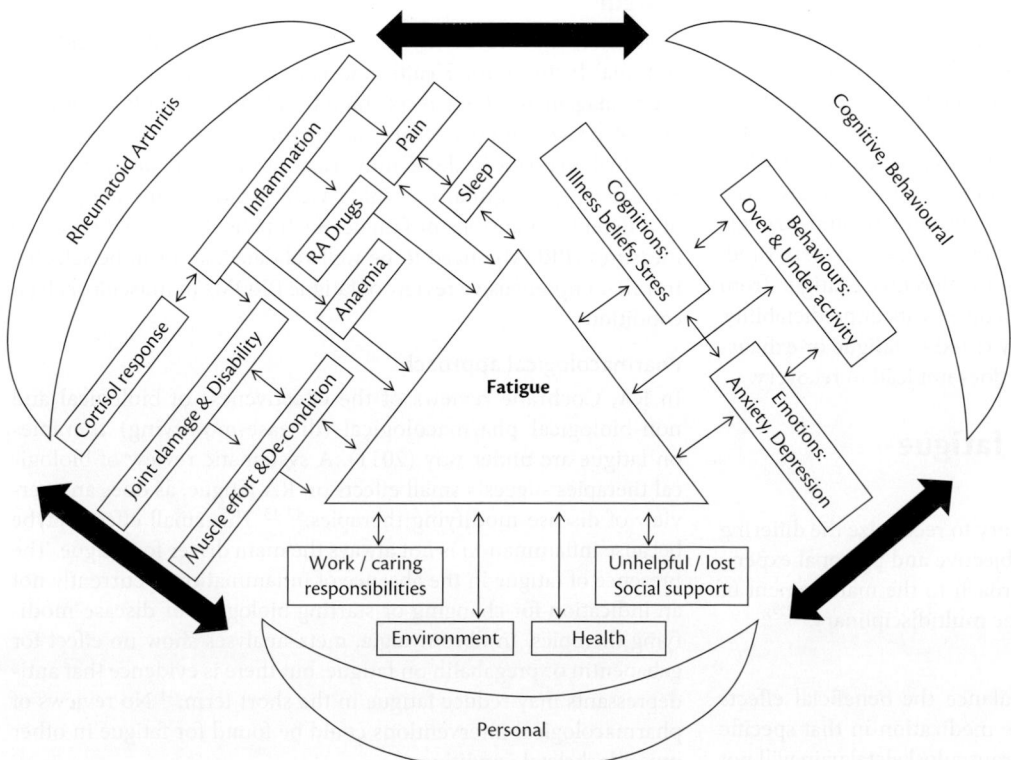

Fig. 12.1 Conceptual model of RA fatigue (by kind permission of Rheumatology).

Myofascial pain may be diffuse and poorly localized with reports of a cramp-like, dull aching pain either at rest or in motion.[24] Other musculoskeletal pains, such as osteoarthritic joint pain, is typified by the sufferer describing stiffness on initial movement, increasing pain with prolonged movement and disturbed sleep due to pain.[25] There is a reduction in the range of movement in the affected joint and associated muscle weakness.

Neuropathic pain is typically burning in quality and commonly associated with allodynia (see 'Neuropathic pain'). Decreased (hypoaesthesia) and increased (hyperaesthesia) sensitivity to stimulation may coexist in the affected region, and itchiness may also be present. The patient may avoid touch to the affected part by themselves and others. They may prefer to keep allodynic areas free from clothing during the day and from the bedclothes at night.

People with fibromyalgia report more widespread chronic pain that is commonly associated with fatigue and psychological distress.[26] Although hyperalgesia and allodynia are commonly reported at specific trigger points these sensations often spread far beyond these areas, with sufferers describing generalized sensitivity.[27]

Fatigue

Fatigue has a very similar picture across RA, lupus, OA, and fibromyalgia, with numerous qualitative research studies evidencing common perceptions of the nature, consequences and attitudes toward fatigue (e.g.[13,28,29]). Fatigue is the physical feeling of a heavy body that seems hard to move ('paralysed') and has run out of energy. Fatigue also has a cognitive element, with descriptions of 'foggy-headedness', with difficulty concentrating or focusing, a feeling of an 'absent presence'. The extremes of this physical and mental fatigue are akin to being 'wiped out' with exhaustion or 'overwhelmed'. Fatigue occurs on most days for many people and varies in intensity, with duration ranging from hours to weeks.

Fatigue threatens people's normal roles. It reduces or even stops their ability to perform everyday activities and chores, social and leisure activities, voluntary and paid work, because of either physical or cognitive exhaustion. It has emotional consequences from frustration, leading to anger and depression, and may cause difficulties with relationships when social arrangements are cancelled. This is compounded by a reluctance to discuss fatigue as it is invisible, therefore people feel disbelieved or fraudulent, and struggle with the society's general perception that everybody gets tired. People with musculoskeletal conditions differentiate fatigue from the tiredness experienced by healthy people by its unpredictability, lack of causality ('unearned'), intensity (tired vs fatigue or exhaustion), constancy, and the fact that rest does not lead to recovery.

Management of pain and fatigue

Pain

To manage pain effectively, it is necessary to recognize the differing components that contribute to the subjective and personal experience termed 'pain'. Therefore the approach to the management of chronic musculoskeletal pain should be multidisciplinary.[30–38]

Pharmacological approach

The use of oral analgesics should balance the beneficial effects on pain against the risk profile of the medication in that specific patient.[39] Many patients with chronic musculoskeletal pain will not achieve a pain-free state. Referral to a pain clinician should be considered when; a patient is gaining medications or increasing doses for little further impact on pain but accruing short and long-term adverse effects, or is on high dose strong opioids. Patients with concurrent chronic pain states or neuropathic pain may also need neuromodulatory agents and specialist pain advice. The pharmacological approach to management of patients with chronic musculoskeletal pain is summarized in Figure 12.2.

Non-pharmacological treatment—multidisciplinary approach in chronic pain

Exercise should be a core treatment irrespective of age, comorbidity, pain severity, and disability, and should include local muscle strengthening and general aerobic fitness.[30] Physiotherapy will play a key role in initiating and advising how a patient can safely exercise. Weight reduction is beneficial, and patients may need encouragement and advice. Many patients may have significant psychosocial comorbidity including depression and anxiety, which if left untreated will hamper pain management. Psychological support such as counselling and cognitive behavioural approaches should be considered.[30,31] Orthotics, podiatry, physiotherapy, and occupational therapy can provide advice on appropriate braces, splints, assistive devices, and walking aids. Assessment of footwear and provision of insoles may relieve pain, improve gait and posture, and help to reduce falls.

Pain management approach

Patients with chronic musculoskeletal pain who have exhausted medical and surgical management options and continue to struggle in coping with their symptoms should be considered for a multidisciplinary pain management approach.[40,41] Pain management programmes can be outpatient or in-patient based, and are usually accessed through the pain clinic.[41]

Fatigue

Guidelines by the British Society for Rheumatology and the National Institute for Health and Clinical Excellence (NICE) on the management of RA recommend that fatigue is addressed, but do not provide guidance on management. Assessment could be by visual analogue scale or numerical rating scale, or by multidimensional questionnaires, which yield a more complete picture of different dimensions of fatigue. Such patient-reported outcome measures (PROMs) need to be well validated, and can be selected from a comprehensive review of fatigue PROMs in musculoskeletal conditions.[7]

Pharmacological approach

In RA, Cochrane reviews of the effectiveness of biological and non-biological pharmacological (disease-modifying) therapies on fatigue are under way (2011). A systematic review of biological therapies suggests small effects on RA fatigue, as does an overview of disease-modifying therapies.[42,43] This small effect maybe because inflammation is not always the main driver for fatigue. The presence of fatigue in the absence of inflammation is currently not an indication for changing or starting biological or disease-modifying therapies. In fibromyalgia, meta-analyses show no effect for gabapentin or pregabalin on fatigue, but there is evidence that antidepressants may reduce fatigue in the short term.[44] No reviews of pharmacological interventions could be found for fatigue in other musculoskeletal conditions.

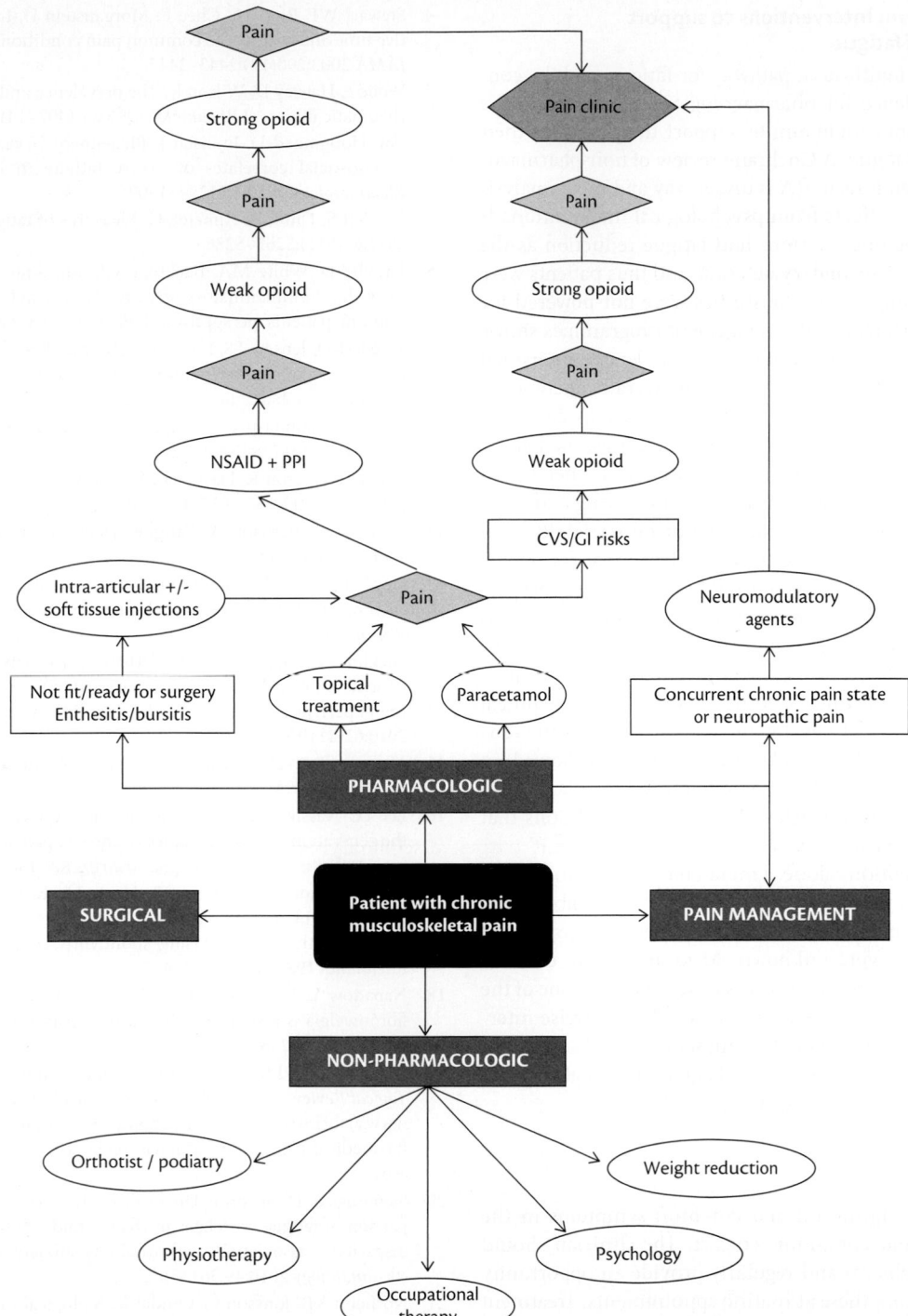

Fig. 12.2 An approach to the management to the patient with chronic musculoskeletal pain. The flow diagram is based on the references cited in the text. Each step is additive.

◆ When considering use of an oral NSAID, the potential adverse cardiovascular risks (any NSAID, especially COX II), adverse effect upon the cardioprotective action of low-dose aspirin, adverse renal effects, and gastrointestinal ulceration risks (especially COX I) need to be assessed for the individual patient.

◆ Intra-articular injections: both corticosteroid and hyaluronic acid injections are used, although the evidence base for efficacy is difficult to interpret.[3]

◆ Surgical options may include arthroplasty or spinal surgery such as discectomy. Pain clinics may offer additional interventional procedures such as nerve root blocks or epidurals for chronic back pain.

CVS, cardiovascular; GI, gastrointestinal; NSAID, non-steroidal anti-inflammatory drug; PPI, proton pump inhibitor.

Multidisciplinary team interventions to support self-management of fatigue

Given the presumed multicausal pathway for fatigue, and the consequent limited evidence for pharmacological interventions, the multidisciplinary team should aim to support the patient in their self-management of fatigue. A Cochrane review of non-pharmacological fatigue interventions in RA is under way and meta-analysis currently shows small effects from psychological interventions.[45] However, none of the interventions had fatigue reduction as the main aim: fatigue was a secondary outcome and thus patients were not recruited with fatigue, and the studies were not powered for fatigue. A review of arthritis self-management programmes shows courses that aim to enhance self-efficacy (confidence in personal ability to undertake a task) result in better overall outcomes.[46] Self-efficacy can be enhanced by approaches such as cognitive behavioural therapy (CBT)—linking thoughts, feelings, and behaviours—or social cognition (groups and peer role models), and include teaching patients skills such as problem-solving and goal-setting. Subsequently, a single randomized controlled trial (RCT) of group CBT that specifically aimed to reduce the impact of fatigue in RA has shown benefit, and this utilized high/low energy activity monitoring, pacing, sleep, and stress management and assertiveness skills, using a goal-setting approach over 6 weeks.[47] However, the intervention was facilitated by a clinical psychologist—a resource most rheumatology departments do not have—therefore clinical teams need to find ways of developing skills to deliver interventions using these approaches. In fibromyalgia, reviews showed no effects on fatigue from either CBT or acupuncture, but a short-term effect was seen with educational/psychological interventions that included exercise.[48]

For exercise interventions alone, a meta-analysis in fibromyalgia showed a small effect on fatigue.[49] A Cochrane review of fibromyalgia exercise interventions in which fatigue was reported concluded that effects on fatigue were unknown. Meta-analysis of exercise interventions in RA showed small effects on fatigue, but none of the interventions had fatigue as their main aim.[45] Few exercise interventions have been performed in other musculoskeletal conditions that either specifically target or report fatigue, but single studies suggest exercise may be useful (e.g. in lupus).[50]

Conclusion

Pain and fatigue are significant and common symptoms in the rheumatic diseases and commonly coexist. The clinician should be aware of these problems and regularly provide an opportunity for the patient to discuss these at routine appointments. Treatment strategies should be informed by clinical presentation and knowledge of mechanistic pathways. A multidisciplinary approach to care is important for optimum outcome. Regular review of pain and fatigue throughout the disease trajectory is required to accommodate changes driven by disease activity and patient lifestyle.

References

1. White KP, Harth M. The occurrence and impact of generalized pain. *Baillières Clin Rheumatol* 1999;13(3):379–389.
2. Woolf AD, Pfleger B. Burden of major musculoskeletal conditions. *Bull. World Health Org.* 2003;81(9):646–656.
3. Maniadakis N, Gray A. The economic burden of back pain in the UK. *Pain* 2000;84(1):95–103.
4. Stewart WF, Ricci JA, Chee E, Morganstein D, Lipton R. Lost productive time and cost due to common pain conditions in the US workforce. *JAMA* 2003;290(18):2443–2445.
5. Wolfe F, Hawley D, Wilson K. The prevalence and meaning of fatigue in rheumatic disease. *J Rheumatol* 1996;23:1407–1417.
6. Van Hoogmoed D, Fransen J, Bleijenberg G van Riel P. Physical and psychosocial correlates of severe fatigue in rheumatoid arthritis. *Rheumatology* 2010;49:1294–1302.
7. Hewlett S, Dures E, Almeida C. Measures of fatigue. *Arthritis Care Res* 2011;63(S11):S263–S286.
8. Lacaille D, White MA, Backman CL, Monique A. Problems faced at work due to inflammatory arthritis: New insights gained from understanding patients' perspective. *Arthritis Care Res* 2007;57:1269–1279.
9. Treede RD, Jensen TS, Campbell JN et al. Redefinition of neuropathic pain and a grading system for clinical use: consensus statement on clinical and research diagnostic criteria. *Neurology* 2008;70:1630–1635.
10. www.iasp-pain.org/AM/Template.cfm?Section=Pain_Defi...isplay.cfm&ContentID=1728#Neuropathicpain
11. Jensen TS, Baron R, Haanpää M et al. A new definition of neuropathic pain. *Pain* 2011;152(10):2204–2205.
12. Ream E, Richardson A. Fatigue: a concept analysis. *Int J Nurs Stud* 1996;33(5)519–529.
13. Hewlett S, Cockshott Z, Byron M et al. Patients' perceptions of fatigue in rheumatoid arthritis: Overwhelming, uncontrollable, ignored. *Arthritis Rheum* 2005;53:697–702.
14. Nicklin J, Cramp F, Kirwan J, Urban M, Hewlett S. Collaboration with patients in the design of patient reported outcome measures: Capturing the experience of fatigue in rheumatoid arthritis. *Arthritis Care Res* 2010:62(11):1552–1558.
15. Melzack R. Evolution of the neuromatrix theory of pain. *Pain Pract* 2005;5(2):85–94.
16. Lee YC, Nassikas NJ, Clauw DJ The role of the central nervous system in the generation and maintenance of chronic pain in rheumatoid arthritis, osteoarthritis and fibromyalgia. *Arthritis Res Ther* 2011;13(2):211.
17. Gerecz-Simon EM, Tunks ER, Heale JA, Kean WF, Buchanan WW. Measurement of pain threshold in patients with rheumatoid arthritis, osteoarthritis, ankylosing spondylitis, and healthy controls. *Clin Rheumatol* 1989;8(4):467–474.
18. Napadow V, LaCount L, Park K et al. Intrinsic brain connectivity in fibromyalgia is associated with chronic pain intensity. *Arthritis Rheum* 2010;62:2545–2555.
19. Hewlett S, Nicklin J, Treharne GJ. Fatigue in musculoskeletal conditions. *Topical Reviews Series* 2008; 6(1). Arthritis Research UK. Available from www.arthritisresearchuk.org/shop/products/publications/information-for-medical-professionals/topical-reviews/series-6-x-stock/tr1-series-6.aspx
20. Stebbings S, Herbison P, Doyle TCH, Treharne GJ, Highton J. A comparison of fatigue correlates in rheumatoid arthritis and osteoarthritis: disparity in associations with disability, anxiety and sleep disturbance. *Rheumatology* 2010;49:361–367.
21. Norheim KB, Jonsson G, Omdal R. Biological mechanisms of chronic fatigue. *Rheumatology* 2011;50:1009–1018.
22. Hewlett S, Chalder T, Choy E et al. Fatigue in rheumatoid arthritis: time for a conceptual model. *Rheumatology* 2011;50;1004–1006.
23. Papageorgiou AC, Badley EM. The quality of pain in arthritis: the words patients use to describe overall pain and pain in individual joints at rest and on movement. *Rheumatology* 1989;16(1):106–112.
24. Arendt-Nielsen L, Svensson P. Referred muscle pain: basic and clinical findings. *Clin J Pain* 2001;17(1):11–19.
25. Dieppe PA, Lohmander LS. Pathogenesis and management of pain in osteoarthritis. *Lancet* 2005;365:965–973.
26. Wolfe F, Smythe HA, Yunus MB et al. The American College of Rheumatology 1990 criteria for the classification of fibromyalgia. Report of the multicenter Criteria Committee. *Arthritis Rheum* 1990;33:160–172.

27. Staud R, Vierck CJ, Cannon RL, Mauderli AP, Price DD. Abnormal sensitisation and temporal summation of second pain (wind up) in patients with fibromyalgia syndrome. Pain 2001;91:165–175.

28. Pettersson S, Möller S, Svenungsson E, Gunnarsson I, Henriksson EW. Women's experience of SLE-related fatigue: a focus group interview study. Rheumatology 2010;49:1935–1942.

29. Söderberg S, Lundman B, Norberg A. The meaning of fatigue and tiredness as narrated by women with fibromyalgia and healthy women. J Clin Nurs 2002;11:247–2455.

30. NICE. Osteoarthritis: national clinical guideline for care and management in adults (CG59). National Institute for Health and Clinical Excellence, London, 2008. Available at: www.nice.org.uk/CG059 (accessed 27 November 2011).

31. NICE. Low back pain: Early management of persistent non-specific low back pain (CG588). National Institute for Health and Clinical Excellence, London, 2009. Available at: www.nice.org.uk/CG0588 (accessed 27 November 2011).

32. Zhang W, Nuki G, Moskowitz RW et al. OARSI recommendations for the management of hip and knee osteoarthritis Part III: changes in evidence following systematic cumulative update of research published through January 2009. Osteoarthritis Cartilage 2010;18(4):476–499.

33. Porcheret M, Healey E, Dziedzic K, et al. Osteoarthritis: a modern approach to diagnosis and management. Reports on the Rheumatic Diseases (Series 6), Hands On 10. Arthritis Research UK, Chesterfield, 2011. Available at: www.arthritisresearchuk.org/health-professionals-and-students/reports/hands-on/hands-on-autumn-2011.aspx (accessed 6 December 2012).

34. Jordan KM, Arden NK, Doherty M et al. EULAR recommendations 2003: an evidence-based approach to the management of knee osteoarthritis [Report of a task force of the Standing Committee for International Clinical Studies Including Therapeutic Trials (ESCISIT)]. Ann Rheum Dis 2003;62:1145–1155.

35. Zhang W, Doherty M, Arden N et al. EULAR evidence based recommendations for the management of hip osteoarthritis: report of a task force of the EULAR Standing Committee for International Clinical Studies Including Therapeutics (ESCISIT). Ann Rheum Dis 2005;64:669–681.

36. Zhang W, Doherty M, Leeb BF et al. EULAR evidence based recommendations for the management of hand osteoarthritis: Report of a Task Force of the EULAR Standing Committee for International Clinical Studies Including Therapeutics (ESCISIT). Ann Rheum Dis 2007;66:377–388.

37. American College of Rheumatology Subcommittee on Osteoarthritis Guidelines, Recommendations for the Medical Management of Osteoarthritis of the Hip and Knee. Arthritis Rheum 2000;43(9):1905–1915.

38. Simon LS, Lipman AG, Jacox AK et al. Pain in osteoarthritis, rheumatoid arthritis and juvenile chronic arthritis. American Pain Society, Glenview, IL, 2002:179.

39. Schnitzer TJ. Update in the guidelines for the treatment of chronic musculoskeletal pain. Clin Rheumatol 2006;25(S1):S22–S29.

40. Main CJ, Williams AC. ABC of psychological medicine: musculoskeletal pain. BMJ 2002;325(7363):534–537.

41. BPS. Recommended guidelines for pain management programmes for adults. British Pain Society, London, 2007. Available at: www.britishpainsociety.org/pub_professional.htm#pmp (accessed 6 December 2012)

42. Chauffier K, Salliot C, Berenbaum F, Sellam J. Effect of biotherapies on fatigue in rheumatoid arthritis: a systematic review of the literature and meta-analysis. Rheumatology (Oxford) 2012;51(1):60–68.

43. Strand V, Singh JA. Improved health-related quality of life with effective disease-modifying anti-rheumatic drugs: Evidence from randomized controlled trials. Am J Manag Care 2007;13(S9):S237–S251.

44. Üçeyler N, Häuser W, Sommer C. A systematic review on the effectiveness of treatment with antidepressants in fibromyalgia syndrome. Arthritis Rheum 2008;59(9):1279–1298.

45. Cramp F, Hewlett S, Almeida C et al: Non-pharmacological interventions for fatigue in rheumatoid arthritis: a Cochrane review. Arthritis Rheum 2011;63(S10):1557.

46. Iversen MD, Hammond A, Betteridge N. Self-management of rheumatic diseases: state of the art and future perspectives. Ann Rheum Dis 2010;69:955–963.

47. Hewlett S, Ambler N, Cliss A et al. Self-management of fatigue in Rheumatoid Arthritis: a randomised controlled trial of group cognitive-behavioural therapy. Ann Rheum Dis 2011;70:1060–1067.

48. Häuser W, Bernardy K, Arnold B, Offenbächer M, Schiltenwolf M. Efficacy of multicomponent treatment in fibromyalgia syndrome: a meta-analysis of randomized controlled clinical trials. Arthritis Rheum 2009;61(2):216–224.

49. Häuser W, Klose P, Langhorst J et al. Efficacy of different types of aerobic exercise in fibromyalgia syndrome: a systematic review and meta-analysis of randomised controlled trials. Arthritis Res Therapy 2010;12:R79.

50. Tench CM, McCarthy M, McCurdie I, White PD, D'Cruz DP. Fatigue in systemic lupus erythematosus: A randomized controlled trial of exercise. Rheumatology 2003;42(9):1050–1054.

Sources of patient information

There are several professional websites providing good information for patients with chronic musculoskeletal pain or fatigue. The following links to the British Pain Society and Arthritis Research UK provide some examples. Opioid medications for chronic pain Available at: www.britishpainsociety.org/book_opioid_patient.pdf (accessed 27 November 2011).

Understanding chronic pain Available at: www.britishpainsociety.org/book_understanding_pain.pdf (accessed 12 December 2012).

Pain management programmes for adults: information for patients Available at: www.britishpainsociety.org/book_pmp_patients.pdf (accessed 12 December 2012).

Pain and arthritis Available at: www.arthritisresearchuk.org/arthritis-information/arthritis-and-daily-life/pain-and-arthritis.aspx (accessed 12 December 2012).

Fatigue and arthritis Available at: www.arthritisresearchuk.org/arthritis-information/arthritis-and-daily-life/fatigue.aspx (accessed 12 December 2012).

CHAPTER 13

The limping child

Yukiko Kimura and Taunton R. Southwood

Introduction

Musculoskeletal pain with or without dysfunction is a very common complaints in children and adolescents which frequently requires medical evaluation. Being able to effectively triage such patients and formulate a differential diagnosis is therefore an important skill for generalists and specialists alike.[1] Some diagnoses may require more rapid treatment than others (e.g. sepsis, non-accidental injury, leukaemia, localized neoplasia, vasculitis, Kawasaki's disease) or may require referral to different subspecialists. Being able to identify specific abnormalities in gait and recognizing symptom patterns in children who are limping will enable clinicians to triage effectively and make more accurate diagnoses. The evaluation should start with a thorough history and physical examination, supplemented by laboratory studies and imaging studies if necessary.[2]

History

Although a multitude of conditions can cause limping in children, a thorough and systematic history and physical examination will enable the practitioner to narrow the differential diagnoses and prioritize conditions based on likelihood. There are many factors that must be considered in this process, but the three key initial differentiating factors are (1) the presence or absence of fever, (2) the location of the pain (whether it affects one joint or one location or is more generalized), and (3) the age of the patient. These factors dictate the urgency of the investigation, and also greatly assist in prioritizing the differential diagnoses. This process is highlighted in the following sections 'Fever and the child with a limp,' and 'Differential diagnosis based on age'. In addition to these key factors, essential elements for taking the history in any child with a limp or musculoskeletal pain are outlined in Table 13.1.

Fever and the child with a limp

When a child presents with limping or joint pain along with fever, and especially when the pain is localized to one area, an immediate concern should be whether there could be a bacterial infection of the bone or joint (septic arthritis or osteomyelitis).[3] This likelihood is greater if the pain and limitation are severe, and if it is accompanied by warmth, redness, and inability to bear weight completely. If bacterial infection seems likely, an urgent evaluation consisting of blood tests (complete blood count, ESR with or without C-reactive protein, blood culture) and arthrocentesis or aspiration of the possible affected bone or joint for culture should be done before any treatment with antibiotics in order to identify the suspected organism. If a bacterial infection is ruled out or seems extremely unlikely, then a work-up for a suspected inflammatory or other cause should begin.

If more than one joint or location are involved, the likelihood of an inflammatory disorder increases.[4] However, red flags such as inability to bear weight with or without an ill appearance are suggestive of malignancy, especially if accompanied by lymphadenopathy, or hepatosplenomegaly and abnormal laboratory tests (such as abnormal blood cell counts or a highly elevated lactate dehydrogenase), even in the absence of lymphoblasts on the blood film.[5–7] A complete review of systems and a thorough physical examination are both essential to localize the pain and to assess for other signs and symptoms which can be clues to the diagnosis.

Figures 13.1 and 13.2 present an algorithmic approach to the diagnosis of the child with a limp, based on the presence or absence of fever in the child as the primary differentiating point. It is also important to take the child's age into account in considering the range of differential diagnoses that may account for a limping gait (Table 13.1).

Physical examination of the limping child

The astute clinician begins the physical evaluation of any child or young person as soon as they lay eyes on them, even from a distance. Relatively 'covert' surveillance may be the only opportunity for the clinician to assess unguarded musculoskeletal movement, and this should continue during the history taking, to provide important diagnostic clues (Table 13.2). The posture of the child may reveal subtle favouring of a limb which the child may compensate for, or even disguise, with more formal examination. This is particularly true for the limping child, as the child may self-consciously alter their gait patterns during clinical gait analysis.

The general appearance and behaviour of the child may highlight disturbed conscious states such as drowsiness, listlessness, or irritability suggesting fever, infection, pain, inanition or exhaustion (Table 13.3). The interaction between the carer and the patient may also be informative, ranging from parental hypervigilance of an apparently well child, to parental indifference to an apparently sick child. The opinion of an experienced and observant clinic nurse is often helpful, particularly if they have assessed the child's general

Table 13.1 Age-based differential diagnosis of the limping child

	Infants and toddlers	School-age children	Adolescents
Developmental	Congenital dislocation hip Coxa vara Cerebral palsy Skeletal dysplasia	Avascular necrosis of the hip Osteochondroses Osteochondritis dissecans Discoid meniscus Tarsal coalition Inherited connective tissue disease (Marfan's, Ehlers–Danlos)	Slipped upper femoral epiphysis Osteochondroses Osteochondritis dissecans Inherited connective tissue disease (Marfan's, Ehlers–Danlos)
Trauma	Toddler's fracture Non-accidental injury	Sport-related injuries Hypermobility	Sport-related injuries Hypermobility

Infection-related	Septic arthritis
	Osteomyelitis
	Discitis
		Reactive arthritis:
		  Rheumatic fever
		  Gastrointestinal related
			Reactive arthritis:
			  Gastrointestinal related
			  STD related

Neoplasia	Neuroblastoma ALL	ALL Lymphoma	Lymphoma Local bone tumours
Myopathy	Dermatomyositis Muscular dystrophies	Dermatomyositis Muscular dystrophies	Dermatomyositis
JIA	Oligoarthritis Systemic arthritis Polyarthritis (RF negative)	Oligoarthritis Systemic arthritis Polyarthritis (RF negative) ERA	Polyarthritis (RF positive) ERA
Chronic pain	Nocturnal idiopathic pain	Nocturnal idiopathic pain	Complex regional pain Fibromyalgia
Other	Kawasaki's disease Coeliac disease	Henoch–Schonlein purpura IBD-related arthritis SLE	SLE Systemic vasculitis

ALL, acute lymphoblastic leukaemia; ERA, enthesitis-related arthritis; IBD, inflammatory bowel disease; RF, rheumatoid factor; SLE, systemic lupus erythematosus; STD, sexually transmitted disease.

appearance of health and their cooperation with measuring vital signs and anthropometry.

General physical examination

Every limping child requires a thorough general physical examination and a detailed musculoskeletal assessment. The most common misdiagnoses in a limping child are made because the clinician limits their physical examination to the feet and legs only. Examples of diseases outside the musculoskeletal system that can cause limping can include testicular torsion, inguinal hernia, and intra-abdominal pathology (such as appendicitis, intussusception, or psoas infection). In addition, even if the primary complaint is knee pain and arthritis is discovered, it can be present in other locations as well, which would impact the diagnosis and treatment. Lastly, it is important to examine extra-articular systems, as musculoskeletal dysfunction is common in many multisystemic diseases (see 'Vital signs and examination of extra-articular systems').

Growth

Anthropometric measures are of relevance to the diagnosis of a limping child. The patient's current height and weight should be recorded on appropriate percentile charts, as well as growth records

for the previous few years. The combination of short stature and abnormal gait may be found in skeletal dysplasias (achondroplasia, multiple epiphyseal dysplasia, spondyloepiphyseal dysplasia) and chromosomal abnormalities (Turner's and Down's syndromes). Any indication of growth failure or a decline from the child's normal growth trajectory could signal a systemic illness, such as inflammatory bowel disease, malignancy, severe juvenile idiopathic arthritis (JIA), or systemic lupus erythematosus (SLE), among others. Abnormally rapid growth (e.g. Marfan's syndrome, Marshall–Weaver syndrome, hyperthyroidism) may also be associated with musculoskeletal pain and limping in a child.

Vital signs and examination of extra-articular systems

Every child should have temperature, pulse and respiratory rate, and blood pressure documented by the clinic nurse before review by the doctor. In a child or young person who is limping, abnormal findings in these parameters are always relevant. A systematic general examination is also mandatory, as a wide range of primarily extra-articular diseases may present with gait disturbance or musculoskeletal pain (Table 13.4). A general physical examination may also highlight many systemic manifestations of diseases in which musculoskeletal involvement is well recognized. Thorough skin

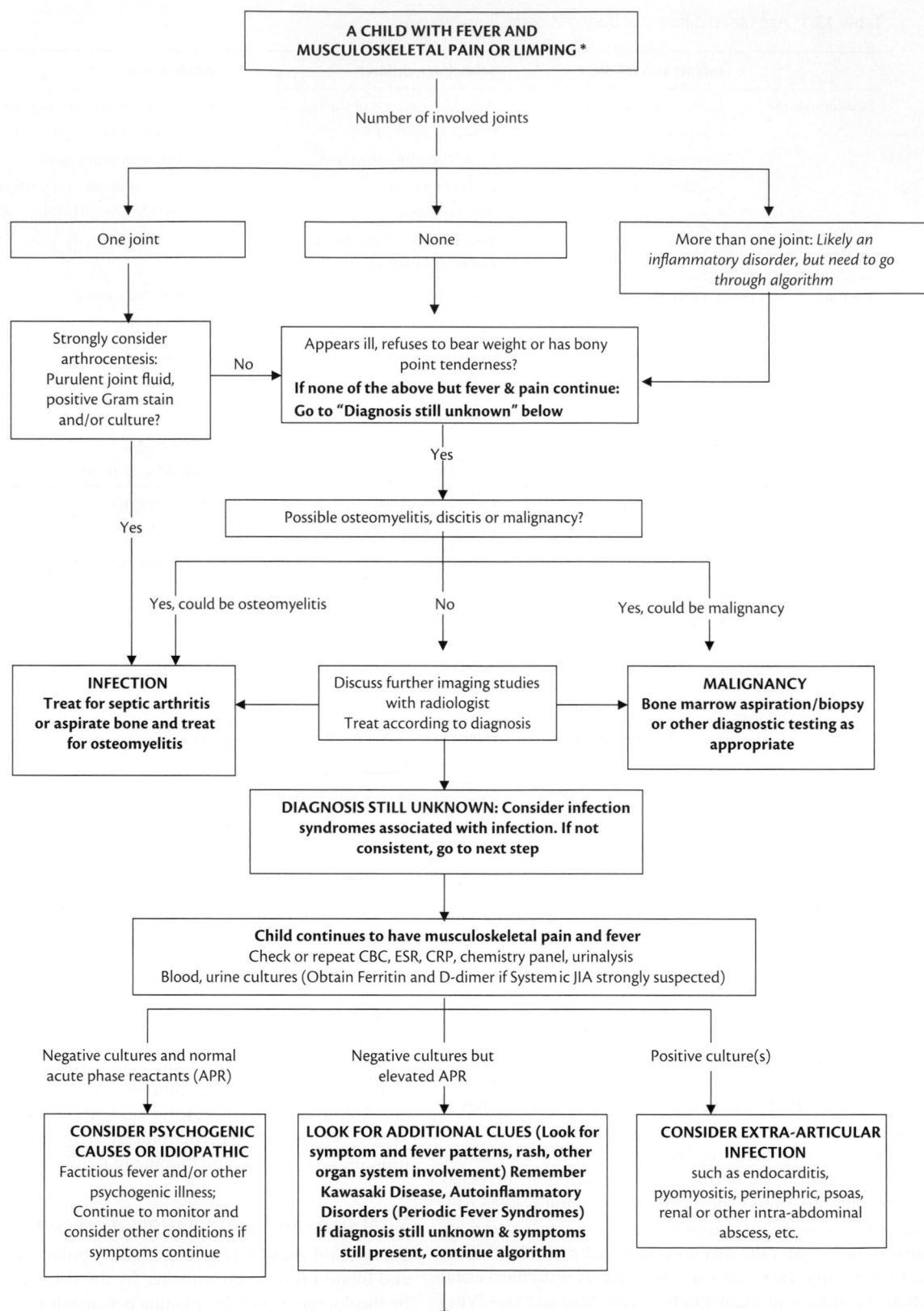

Fig. 13.1 Algorithm: the child with fever and musculoskeletal pain.

Reproduced with permission from Oxford University Press in 2012 Y Kimura. "Common Presenting Problems," in IS Szer, Y Kimura, PN Malleson and TR Southwood, eds., Arthritis in Children and Adolescents. Oxford, UK: Oxford University Press 2006.

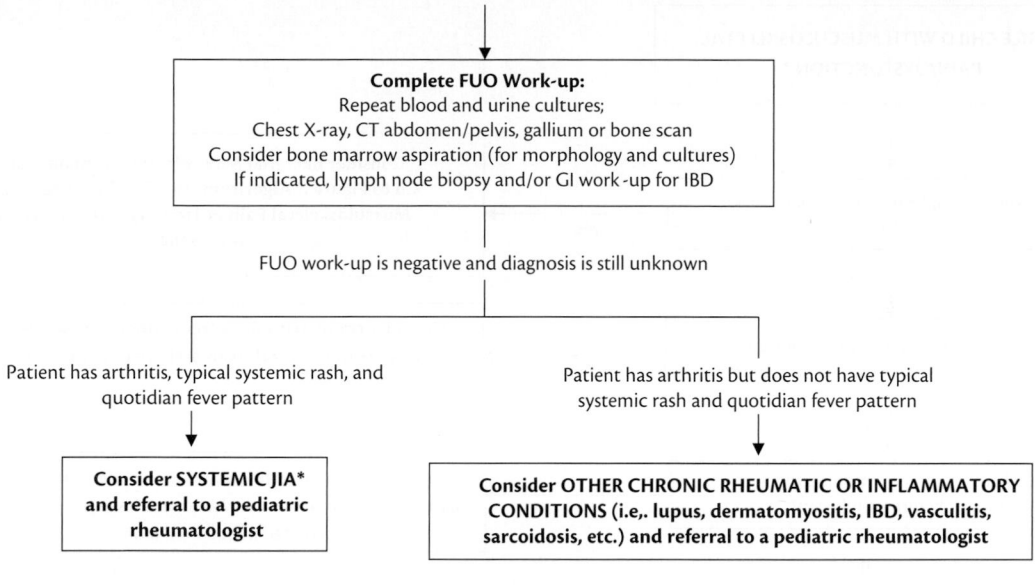

Complete FUO Work-up:
Repeat blood and urine cultures;
Chest X-ray, CT abdomen/pelvis, gallium or bone scan
Consider bone marrow aspiration (for morphology and cultures)
If indicated, lymph node biopsy and/or GI work-up for IBD

FUO work-up is negative and diagnosis is still unknown

Patient has arthritis, typical systemic rash, and quotidian fever pattern

Patient has arthritis but does not have typical systemic rash and quotidian fever pattern

Consider SYSTEMIC JIA* and referral to a pediatric rheumatologist

Consider OTHER CHRONIC RHEUMATIC OR INFLAMMATORY CONDITIONS (i.e,. lupus, dermatomyositis, IBD, vasculitis, sarcoidosis, etc.) and referral to a pediatric rheumatologist

*IMPORTANT NOTES:

Children with significant continued fever and musculoskeletal pain should have the following during the work-up:

- Complete blood count with differential
- Acute phase reactants (ESR, C-reactive protein)
- Routine serum chemistries (including creatinine, muscle and liver enzymes)
- Urinalysis
- ASO titre
- Cultures as appropriate (blood, urine, throat); if considering endocarditis, obtain at least 2 blood cultures from separate sites (remember that endocarditis can present with polyarthritis and fever)
- Testing for mycobacterial infection
- Imaging studies of involved area (plain X-rays, other tests as indicated in algorithm)
- Immunoglobulins and other immunodeficiency studies as appropriate

Fig. 13.1 (Continued)

examination skin is of particular relevance: a wide variety of rashes (e.g. scaling, purpuric, erythematous, nodular, infected) are part of the typical patterns of rheumatic disease (e.g. JIA, systemic arthritis, psoriatic arthritis, enthesitis-related arthritis, rheumatic fever, Henoch–Schonlein purpura, Kawasaki's disease and other forms of vasculitis, SLE, dermatomyositis).

The musculoskeletal examination

pGALS screening musculoskeletal examination

The paediatric Gait, Arms, Legs, Spine (pGALS) is a simple and systematic method to screen for musculoskeletal problems in children that allows busy practitioners to quickly assess the musculoskeletal system[8]. The pGALS assessment is covered in more detail in Chapter 5.

Gait

Gait is the first part of the pGALS, and an important element of the musculoskeletal examination that is often overlooked. It is easier to observe a child's gait when they are wearing shorts, barefoot, and walking repeatedly up and down a long hallway. Further clues may be gained by asking the child to walk on tiptoes (away from the examiner, to facilitate comparison of heel height off the ground), and on heels (towards the examiner, to facilitate comparison of toe height off the ground).

Abnormal gaits
Antalgic gait

The most commonly seen abnormal gait is the antalgic gait, which displays a shortened stance (weight bearing) on the affected leg because of pain in the hip, knee, and/or ankle and foot.

Hypermobile gait

Hypermobility is commonly seen and can present with multiple musculoskeletal complaints. Key features to note are pes planus, foot overpronation at the subtalar joint (subtalar valgus), and knee valgus and recurvatum on standing. There may also be increased lumbar lordosis. If the child is asked to walk on their toes, the foot arch will be restored unless there is a neuropathy or a structural disorder such as tarsal coalition.

Trendelenburg gait

The Trendelenburg gait is characterized by a lateral trunk lean toward the supported limb during the stance phase. The trunk will bend toward the affected side to keep the centre of gravity directly over the hip joint. When viewed from behind as the foot lifts off the ground, it is clear that the unsupported side of the pelvis (the non-stance side) will drop and the sagittal plane of the pelvis will tilt laterally towards that side. This is due to weakened core stability muscles (hip abductors especially). It is usually seen in diseases of the hip joint, and also in muscle weakness.

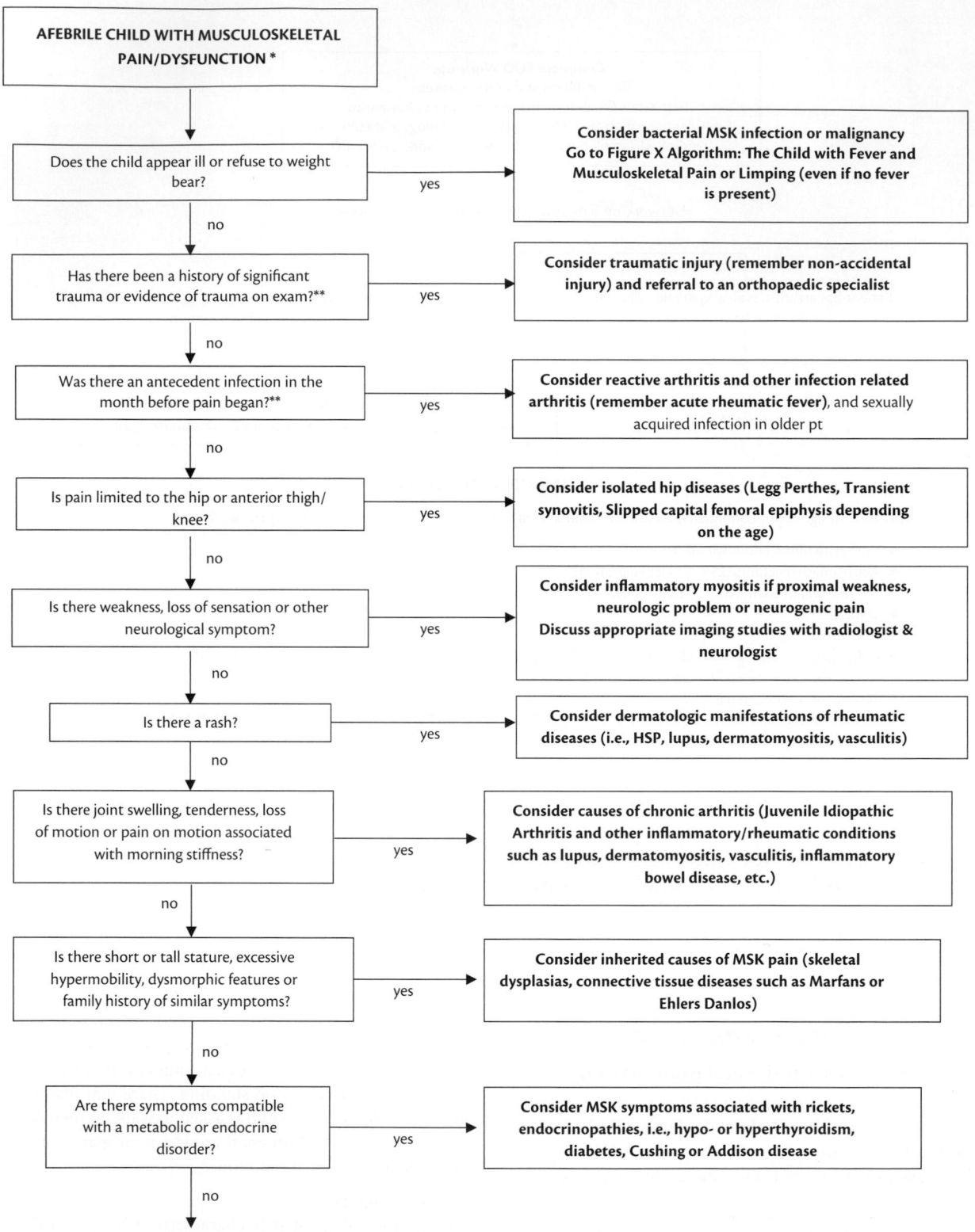

Fig. 13.2 Algorithm: the child with musculoskeletal pain or limping (without fever).

Reproduced with permission from Oxford University Press Y Kimura. "Common Presenting Problems," in IS Szer, Y Kimura, PN Malleson and TR Southwood, eds., Arthritis in Children and Adolescents. Oxford, UK: Oxford University Press 2006.

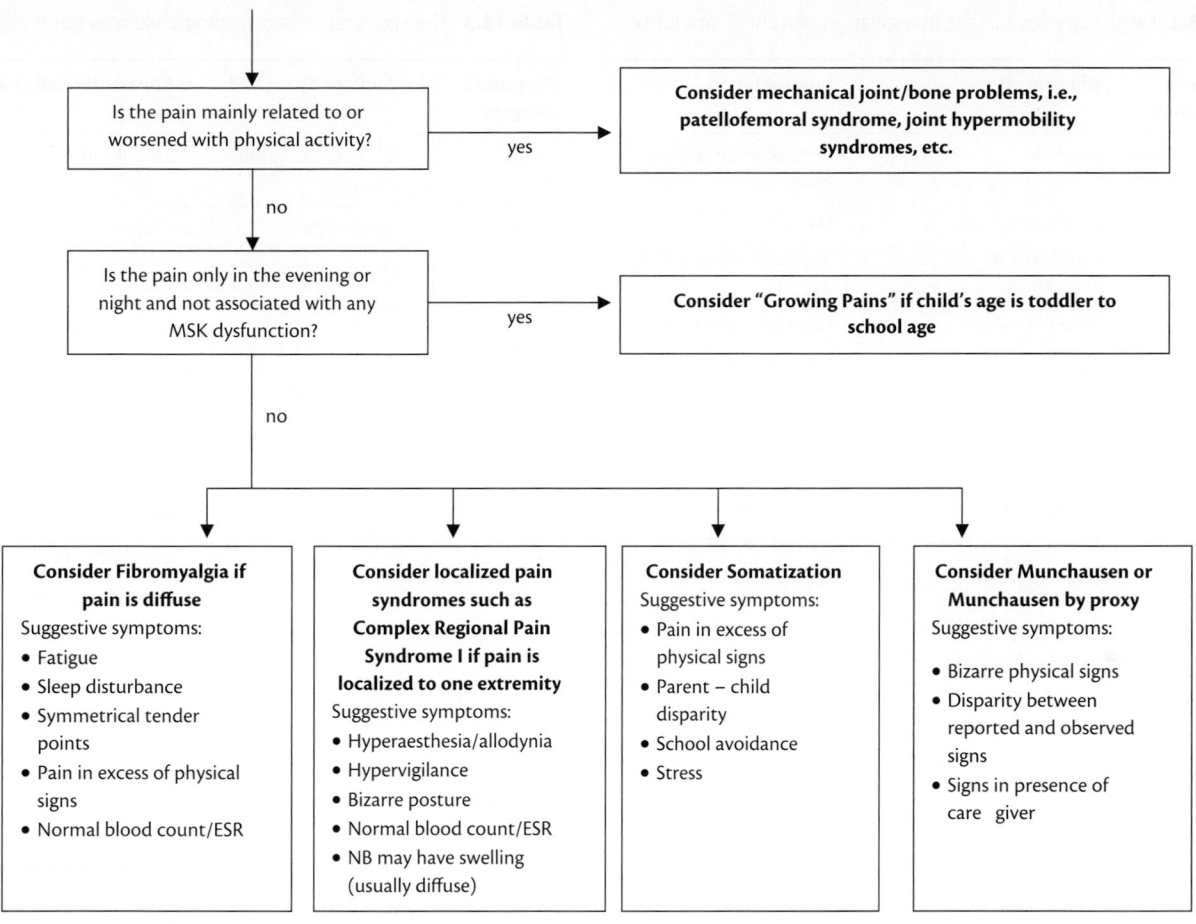

Is the pain mainly related to or worsened with physical activity?

— yes → **Consider mechanical joint/bone problems, i.e., patellofemoral syndrome, joint hypermobility syndromes, etc.**

no

Is the pain only in the evening or night and not associated with any MSK dysfunction?

— yes → **Consider "Growing Pains" if child's age is toddler to school age**

no

Consider Fibromyalgia if pain is diffuse
Suggestive symptoms:
- Fatigue
- Sleep disturbance
- Symmetrical tender points
- Pain in excess of physical signs
- Normal blood count/ESR

Consider localized pain syndromes such as Complex Regional Pain Syndrome I if pain is localized to one extremity
Suggestive symptoms:
- Hyperaesthesia/allodynia
- Hypervigilance
- Bizarre posture
- Normal blood count/ESR
- NB may have swelling (usually diffuse)

Consider Somatization
Suggestive symptoms:
- Pain in excess of physical signs
- Parent – child disparity
- School avoidance
- Stress

Consider Munchausen or Munchausen by proxy
Suggestive symptoms:
- Bizarre physical signs
- Disparity between reported and observed signs
- Signs in presence of care giver

*IMPORTANT NOTES:

Children with persistent musculoskeletal pain should have the following work-up considered:

- Complete/full blood count with differential
- Acute phase reactants (ESR, C-reactive protein)
- Routine serum chemistries (including creatinine, liver and muscle enzymes)
- Urinalysis
- Imaging studies (plain X-rays of involved area, other studies as indicated in the algorithm(s))
- Testing for mycobacterial infection

**CAVEATS:

- Minor trauma and infections are common in children and may not necessarily be related to the diagnosis
- Remember infection, malignancy and non-accidental injury (child abuse) at each stage

Fig. 13.2 (Continued)

Weak gait

The weak gait is characterized by poor lateral stability and a tendency to waddle. There is a tendency to walk with a toe–toe pattern and exhibit bilateral drop-foot through the swing phase. Increased lumbar lordosis, due to weak abdominal muscles, and an exaggerated arm swing to aid in forward propulsion will often be noted. A Gower sign, a series of manoeuvres necessary to achieve an upright position in the presence of pelvic and trunk weakness, is a hallmark of muscle weakness. This is most often seen in myopathies such as Duchenne muscular dystrophy and dermatomyositis.

Leg-length discrepancy

Any condition which increases the length of one leg over the other will tend to result in a circumduction gait. The longer leg is swung laterally to avoid catching the big toe on the ground. This is typically seen in JIA, especially if there is asymmetrical knee involvement, other idiopathic conditions such as Blount's disease, and in any disease associated with hemihypertrophy. An effective leg-length discrepancy type gait can also be seen in peripheral neuropathy with foot drop, when the functional length of the leg is increased due to the lack of toe clearance. Leg shortening (e.g. in Perthes' disease) may also result in a leg-length discrepancy and a similar gait pattern.

Spasticity

Spasticity can also cause abnormal gaits. Patients with spastic diplegia may have a waddling gait due to the upper motor neuron lesion of the lower limbs; waddling, plantar grade foot deformities, and poor coordination are observed. Patients with hemiplegia often

Table 13.2 Laboratory tests in the investigation of a child with limp

Laboratory investigation	Abnormalities	Interpretation
Full blood count	Anaemia	Chronic inflammation, blood loss
	Leukopaenia	SLE, MAS
	Leukocytosis	Sepsis, JIA, systemic arthritis
	Thrombocytopaenia	ALL, SLE
	Thrombocytosis	Kawasaki's disease, JIA
Acute-phase reactants	ESR, CRP	Inflammation
		ALL
Biochemistry	Disordered renal function	SLE
	Elevated liver enzymes	MAS
	Elevated LDH	Malignancy
	Elevated muscle enzymes	Dermatomyositis
Urinalysis	Haematuria, proteinuria	SLE, vasculitis
Autoantibodies	Anti-nuclear antibody	SLE
	Double-stranded DNA	SLE
	Extractable nuclear antigens	SLE
	Rheumatoid factor	JIA (only for classification)
Microbiology	Bacterial sepsis	Septic arthritis, osteomyelitis
	Antistreptolysin O titres	Reactive arthritis
	Elevated mycoplasma titres	Reactive arthritis
	Elevated viral titres	Reactive arthritis
	Borrelia titres, antigen tests	Lyme arthritis

ALL, acute lymphoblastic leukaemia; CRP, C-reactive protein; ESR, erythrocyte sedimentation rate; JIA, juvenile idiopathic arthritis; LDH, lactate dehydrogenase; MAS, macrophage activation syndrome; SLE, systemic lupus erythematosus.

Table 13.3 The appearance of a limping child may guide diagnosis

Diagnostic category	Apparently ill child	Apparently well child
Idiopathic inflammation	JIA: systemic arthritis Vasculitis	JIA: oligoarthritis
Infection	Septic arthritis Osteomyelitis	Reactive arthritis
	Rheumatic fever	
Neoplasia	Leukaemia, lymphoma	
	Neuroblastoma	
Pain syndromes		Regional
		Generalized
Mechanical		Non-accidental injury
		Hypermobility
Other		Osteochondroses and avascular necroses
		Slipped capital femoral epiphysis

Table 13.4 Primarily extra-articular diseases which may have limping and other musculoskeletal manifestations

Disease	Musculoskeletal manifestation
Acute lymphoblastic leukaemia	Bone pain, joint swelling
Lymphoma	Bone pain
Neuroblastoma	Bone metastases
Haemophilia and bleeding diatheses	Haemarthrosis, muscle haematoma
Haemoglobinopathies	Avascular necrosis, bone infarction
Cystic fibrosis	Small- and large-joint arthropathy
Diabetes	Cheiroarthropathy
Thyroid disease (hyper or hypo)	Bone pain
Pancreatitis	Osteolytic lesions
Inflammatory bowel disease	Arthritis, sacroiliitis, enthesitis, spondylitis, erythema nodosum
Coeliac disease	Arthritis, bone pain
Down's syndrome	Arthritis, carpal osteolysis
Cyanotic congenital heart disease	Hypertrophic osteoarthopathy
Non-accidental injury	Periostitis, fractures
Autistic spectrum disorder	Musculoskeletal pain

have flexed posturing of the affected upper extremity, a supinated and inverted affected foot through the swing phase, and retraction of the hemipelvis on the involved side.

Range-of-motion assessment of the lower limb

It is important to perform the range-of-motion examination in the lower extremities with the patient supine. **Passive range of motion** refers to the amount of movement that a joint displays when the examiner manipulates the joint. **Active range of motion** refers to the motion of the joint when the patient performs the movement. Significant weakness in a muscle group may result in a decrease in the active motion of a joint without a decrease in passive motion. A contracture in a joint will result in loss of motion of the joint in the active and passive modes. Tendinitis may cause loss of active motion in a joint without loss of passive motion.

When assessing passive range of motion, it is important to push the joint to the full endpoint of motion to accurately assess the full mobility of the joint and not just to see if the joint moved. It is important to always examine at least one joint above and at least one joint below the symptomatic joint, because joint pain can be referred proximally and distally, which can lead to the patient complaining of pain in a particular joint although the abnormality is in the joint proximal or distal to the symptomatic joint. A

common example of this phenomenon is when a child complains of knee pain but may in fact have a hip problem such as transient synovitis with pain referred to the knee. Another example is that sometimes patients experiencing pain around the hip, especially down the buttocks, may actually have a spinal injury. It is equally important to always compare the affected limb with the non-affected limb.

It is important for paediatricians to understand that there is a relatively wide range of normal passive and active motion for all body joints. The inability of a joint to achieve full motion in the plane of flexion or extension is a joint contracture, which can be due to arthritis, postsurgical arthrofibrosis, skeletal dysplasias, and other conditions.

It must be remembered that decreased mobility can also be due to **spasticity**. Spasticity manifests as an increase in tone that occurs in a muscle or muscle group when forcefully stretched. Once the muscle relaxes, the tone decreases and the muscle will stretch further.

Joint laxity is usually due to a ligamentous abnormality, not to a muscular or tendinous problem. Laxity can be acute when it occurs after a complete rupture or tear of the anterior cruciate ligament. Chronic laxity that occurs with **hypermobility syndromes** can range from benign hypermobility syndrome to more extreme examples, such as Ehlers–Danlos syndrome.

Laboratory studies and imaging

Laboratory tests should be requested in most cases of a limping child unless there is a history of significant trauma (Table 13.2).

Plain radiographs of affected area(s) can assist in excluding occult traumatic injury, tumours, bone dysplasias, and other bony lesions, and should be performed in most cases. However, a normal radiograph does not rule out many conditions, such as inflammatory arthritis (unless there has been damage from long-standing disease), early osteomyelitis (radiographic changes such as periostitis take 10–14 days to develop), non-displaced fractures, septic arthritis, or sprains. Beyond plain radiographs, other imaging tests (MRI, CT scan, bone scan) may be helpful depending on the clinical situation. MRI is useful for detecting osteomyelitis, anatomical abnormalities, and joint effusions but should be obtained with contrast (gadolinium) if an inflammatory disorder,

such as arthritis, or tumour is suspected. A bone scan can also help in situations where symptoms are poorly localized in a child with a limp.

Conclusion

Many conditions with a wide range of medical urgency can present as a child with a limp. This chapter presents a systematic process of evaluation that will allow the busy practitioner to first assess the urgency of the problem, and then proceed through logical steps in order to make the correct diagnosis.

References

1. Foster H, Kimura Y. Ensuring that all paediatricians and rheumatologists recognise significant rheumatic diseases. *Best Pract Res Clin Rheumatol* 2009;23(5):625–642.
2. Kimura Y, Southwood TR. Evaluation of the child with joint pain or swelling. www.uptodate.com/contents/evaluation-of-the-child-with-joint-pain-or-swelling
3. Kimura Y. Acute and chronic infections of bones and joints. In: Szer IS, Kimura Y, Malleson PN, Southwood TR (eds) *Arthritis in Children and Adolescents*. Oxford University Press, Oxford, 2006:63–85.
4. Kimura Y. Common presenting problems. In: Szer IS, Kimura Y, Malleson PN, Southwood TR (eds) *Arthritis in Children and Adolescents*. Oxford University Press, Oxford, 2006:24–48.
5. Wallendal M, Stork L, Hollister JR. The discriminating value of serum lactate dehydrogenase levels in children with malignant neoplasms presenting as joint pain. *Arch Pediatr Adolesc Med* 1996;150(1):70–73.
6. Jones OY, Spencer CH, Bowyer SL et al. A multicenter case-control study on predictive factors distinguishing childhood leukemia from juvenile rheumatoid arthritis. *Pediatrics* 2006;117(5):e840–e844.
7. Cabral DA, Tucker LB. Malignancies in children who initially present with rheumatic complaints. *J Pediatr* 1999;134(1):53–57.
8. Foster HE, Kay LJ, Friswell M, Coady D, Myers A. Musculoskeletal screening examination (pGALS) for school-age children based on the adult GALS screen. *Arthritis Rheum* 2006;55(5):709–716.

CHAPTER 14

The systemically unwell child

Athimalaipet V. Ramanan and
Jonathan D. Akikusa

Introduction

The systemically unwell child is a common clinical problem in paediatrics. For the purposes of this chapter, the term systemically unwell refers to the presence of fever, with or without associated non-specific symptoms such as lethargy and weight loss. In the majority of cases a cause is found following a round of simple investigations. This will usually be infection, and depending on the causative agent, the child will improve spontaneously or following appropriate antimicrobial therapy. When routine investigations fail to reveal an aetiology and the child remains unwell, the differential diagnoses should be broadened to include, among others, paediatric rheumatic diseases. Figure 14.1 presents the important rheumatologic differentials of systemic illness in children according to the age at which they typically occur.[1-14] Table 14.1 provides a summary of the key clinical and laboratory features of these conditions. Once rheumatologic differentials relevant to the age of the child under evaluation are identified, they can be refined based on knowledge of the incidence and clinical and laboratory features of the diseases concerned. This chapter provides a brief overview of these conditions focusing on key clinical features, common diagnostic pitfalls, and investigations important in their diagnosis.

Kawasaki's disease

Kawasaki's disease (KD) is a self-limiting primary systemic vasculitis with a peak incidence in pre-school-aged children and a propensity to cause arterial aneurysms, particularly of the coronary vessels. It is the most common cause of acquired paediatric heart disease in developed countries. Of all the recognized paediatric primary systemic vasculitides (Box 14.1), KD is the one that most commonly presents with fever. The diagnosis is made in the presence of fever for more than 5 days with at least four of five defined clinical features: mucocutaneous changes, polymorphic rash, changes in the extremities, non-purulent conjunctivitis, and cervical lymphadenopathy (see Chapter 130 for more details). Some children with KD may lack the number of clinical features required to satisfy diagnostic criteria and are considered to have an 'incomplete' form. Although KD is usually seen in children between 6 months and 5 years of age, it is recognized in children outside this age range; these children are more likely to present with the incomplete form, which may lead to a significant delay in diagnosis. Infants under 6 months of age, in particular, have a high risk of incomplete disease and coronary artery aneurysms, mandating a high index of suspicion and low threshold for treatment in this age group.[15] There is a higher risk of KD in children of Asian origin (including children from the Indian subcontinent),[16,17] and it is being increasingly recognized in the developing world where infectious conditions are prevalent.

Key clinical features

Fever is the predominant symptom and is required for diagnosis although it is important to remember that not all the other diagnostic features need to be present at the same time. This is a common misconception that may lead to the diagnosis being missed.

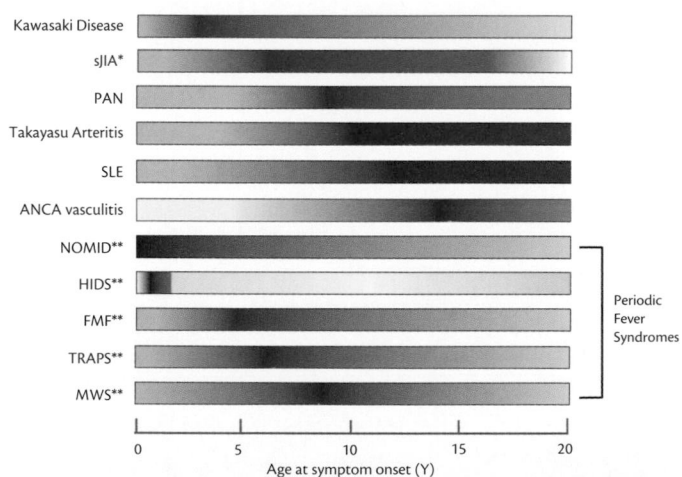

sJIA – Systemic Juvenile Idiopathic Arthritis; PAN – Polyarteritis Nodosa; SLE – Systemic Lupus Erythematosus; ANCA- Anti-neutrophil Cytoplasmic Antibodies; NOMID – Neonatal Onset Multisystem Inflammatory disease; HIDS – Hyper IgD syndrome; FMF – Familial Mediterranean Fever, TRAPS- Tumor Necrosis Factor Receptor Associated Periodic Syndrome; MWS – Muckle-Wells Syndrome
* By definition cannot occur >16yrs, similar syndrome may occur after this age as Adult Onset Still's Disease.
** Refers to age at onset of symptoms. Diagnostic delay common in these syndromes.
Fig. 14.1 Average age (peak shading) and age range at diagnosis of important rheumatologic conditions associated with fever in children.

Table 14.1 Summary of key clinical and laboratory features of these paediatric rheumatic diseases

Condition	Key clinical features	Typical results of important laboratory investigations
KD	Fever ≥ 5 days Combination of ocular, mucosal, cutaneous, peripheral and lymph node changes per KD criteria Flare at BCG scar site in Asian children GI symptoms in older children	Increased ESR/CRP Increased WCC, PLT (subacutely) Mild increase in LFTs Decreased albumin Sterile pyuria
sJIA	Fever- 1–2 spikes per day (quotidian) Evanescent, salmon-pink rash Hepatosplenomegaly, lymphadenopathy Arthritis not always present initially	Increased ESR/CRP Increased WCC, PLT Decreased Hb Increased ferritin (typically >1000 µg/L) Increased CD163 staining of bone marrow
Vasculitis (AAV/TA/PAN)		
All	Non-specific constitutional symptoms	Increased ESR/CRP Decreased Hb Serum creatinine may be abnormal
ANCA-associated	Skin—palpable purpura (leukocytoclastic) Dyspnoea, cough, haemoptysis Symptoms of uraemia Sinusitis Scleritis/episcleritis	ANCA positive >80% (usually specific for PR3 or MPO) Urinalysis may be abnormal
Takayasu's arteritis	Hypertension, claudication, bruits	Large-vessel imaging—wall thickening with stenosis or aneurysms
Polyarteritis nodosa	Skin—livedo, tender nodules Myalgia Mono/polyneuropathy	Medium-vessel imaging—aneurysms
SLE	Rash—malar/discoid Photosensitivity Oral/nasal ulcers—typically painless Polyarthritis—typically painful Oedema if nephrotic, symptoms of uraemia. Behaviour/cognitive changes; headache; seizures	Positive ANA May have positive anti-ENA, dsDNA and phospholipid antibodies Increased ESR (CRP typically normal unless infection/arthritis/serositis) May have haemolytic anaemia, thrombocytopenia May have renal impairment, decreased albumin, increased LFTs
MAS	Persistent fever Purpuric rash Multiorgan failure Features of underlying rheumatic disease	Pancytopenia Increased ferritin >10 000 µg/L Abnormal LFTs
Periodic fever syndromes		
All	Well between febrile periods NB: NOMID patients typically have persistent rash and other non-fever-related manifestations	ESR/CRP elevated during fever, normal between episodes NB: NOMID patients usually have chronic elevation of acute-phase reactants
FMF	Fever usually <72 h Serositis Monoarthritis Erysipeloid rash	Elevated serum amyloid A Mutation testing of *MEFV* (≥1 identifiable mutation in 70–80%)
HIDS	Fever typically 4–6 days Cervical lymphadenopathy Maculopapular rash Abdominal pain	Urine mevalonic acid elevated during febrile episodes Elevated IgD Mutation testing of *MVK* (≥1 mutation in >50%)

(Continued)

Table 14.1 (Continued)

Condition	Key clinical features	Typical results of important laboratory investigations
TRAPS	Fever frequently >1 week Migratory rash Periorbital oedema Arthralgia/ myalgia	Mutation testing of *TNFRSF1A* (detectable mutation in 10–50%)
FCAS/MWS	Fever usually <24 h Urticarial rash	Mutation testing of *CIAS1* (detectable mutation in 70–90%)
NOMID	Fever—non-remitting Urticarial rash from birth Lymphadenopathy Aseptic meningitis Arthropathy	Mutation testing of *CIAS1* (detectable mutation in 50%)

ANA, antinuclear antibodies; ANCA, anti-neutrophil cytoplasmic antibody; BCG, bacille Calmette–Guérin; CRP, C-reactive protein; ENA, extractible nuclear antigens; ESR, erythrocyte sedimentation rate; GI, gastrointestinal; Hb, haemoglobin; KD, Kawasaki's disease; LFT, liver function tests; MAS, macrophage activation syndrome; MPO, myeloperoxidase; PLT, platelet; PR3, proteinase 3; SLE, systemic lupus erythematosus; WCC, white cell count. For other abbreviations see text.

Box 14.1 Overview of main forms of primary systemic vasculitis in children

Predominantly affecting large vessels

◆ Takayasu's arteritis

Predominantly affecting medium vessels

◆ Childhood polyarteritis nodosa

◆ Cutaneous polyarteritis

◆ Kawasaki's disease

Predominantly affecting small vessels

◆ Wegener's granulomatosis (now granulomatosis with polyangiitis) } ANCA - associated vasculitides

◆ Microscopic polyangiitis

◆ Churg–Strauss syndrome

◆ Henoch-Schönlein Purpura (HSP)

◆ Isolated cutaneous leukocytoclastic vasculitis

◆ Hypocomplementaemic urticarial vasculitis

Adapted from Ozen S et al., *Ann Rheum Dis* 2006;**65**:936–941, with permission from BMJ Publishing Group Limited.

Apart from the clinical features required for diagnosis, another useful clinical clue is a flare of the BCG scar site, particularly in children of Japanese or Indian origin.[18]

Older children tend to present with more gastrointestinal symptoms compared to children under 5 years of age.[19] Abdominal symptoms such as diarrhoea and vomiting are seen in up to 25% of younger children with KD. This figure increases to more than 50% in those older than 5 years.

A change in the extremities with redness of palms and soles is a characteristic feature of KD. Common pitfalls/atypical presentations which result in a delay in, or not making, the diagnosis include: presence of just prolonged fever with/without cervical lymphadenopathy; sterile pyuria in child with fever; diagnosis of

meningitis/encephalitis in a young child presenting with irritability; and rash in a child with fever being wrongly attributed to antibiotics.[18]

KD should be considered in any child with fever for more than 5 days. Clinical and laboratory features that might potentially help make the diagnosis should then be actively looked for to avoid missing KD and the risk of future poor coronary outcome that may result.

Useful investigations

Although there is no laboratory finding diagnostic of KD, there are patterns of abnormality that aid the diagnosis. These include elevated erthrocyte sedimentation rate (ESR) and C-reactive protein (CRP), high white cell count, transient mild elevation of liver enzymes, low albumin, and eosinophilia.[20] Hypoalbuminaemia and hyponatraemia are associated with more severe and prolonged acute disease.[18,21] There are important caveats to the above. An elevated platelet count is characteristically seen in the second week of illness, but a low platelet count in the first week of illness does not exclude the diagnosis and is potentially a marker of poor prognosis.

Systemic juvenile idiopathic arthritis

Systemic juvenile idiopathic arthritis (sJIA) is characterized by fever, rash, and arthritis. The diagnostic criteria include fever of at least 2 weeks' duration with arthritis and one or more of the following: evanescent, erythematous rash; serositis; generalized lymphadenopathy or hepatomegaly and/or splenomegaly. sJIA is an important and common rheumatological diagnosis to consider in a child of any age presenting with fever. Case series from the literature highlight the significant prevalence of this condition in children with fever of unknown origin.[22–25] More detail about sJIA is given in Chapter 116.

Key clinical features

There are several characteristic clinical features of sJIA which can be useful pointers to the diagnosis. The fever pattern is quotidian, with one or two daily spikes of variable duration, in between which

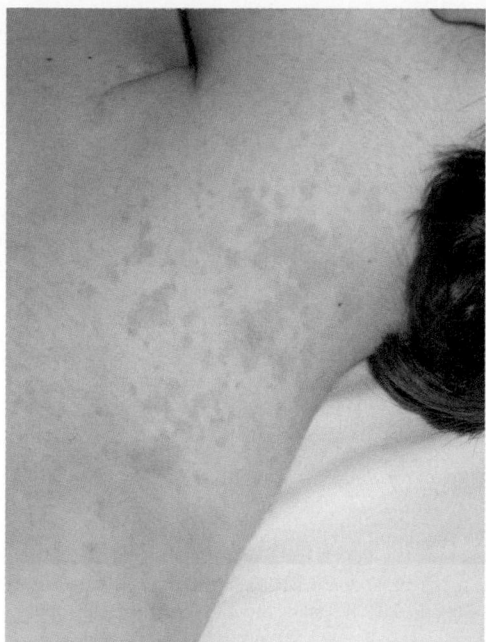

Fig. 14.2 The typical salmon pink macular rash of sJIA.

the temperature returns to normal. During periods of fever the children appear ill and a 'Still's rash' typically appears. In contrast, during periods without fever, the child often appears well and the rash is absent. The rash consists of salmon pink macules, typically on the proximal limbs and torso (Figure 14.2) with demonstrates the Koebner phenomenon. The rash can be hard to identify in dark-skinned individuals.

Arthritis may not always be present initially and there are reports of 'formes frustes' of this disease without arthritis.[26] It can be difficult to exclude malignancy in these children and a formal work-up, including a bone marrow aspirate and trephine, may be required. Systemic JIA can also present with macrophage activation syndrome (MAS) at onset (see Chapter 168). In this situation the children are more likely to be very ill with coagulopathy, raised transaminases, and very high ferritin (>10 000μg/L). It is important to diagnose and treat these children quickly as MAS may be fatal if appropriate therapy is delayed.

Useful investigations

The characteristic laboratory picture is of anaemia, leukocytosis, thrombocytosis, and raised inflammatory markers (CRP and ESR), but this picture is not unique to sJIA. Autoantibodies are not helpful as they are usually negative in these children. A markedly elevated serum ferritin is characteristic of sJIA—typically reaching levels higher than 1000 μg/L. However, again this is not unique to sJIA as other processes, including infection and malignancy, may result in hyperferritinaemia.[27,28] If a bone marrow biopsy is performed then staining for CD163 (a marker for macrophages) might help in the diagnosis of sJIA.[29]

Primary systemic vasculitis

The primary systemic vasculitides (PSVs) are a heterogeneous group of disorders characterized by inflammation of vascular walls and distinguished by the size and pathologic appearance of affected vessels and associated clinical and laboratory features (see Chapter 136). Box 14.1 summarizes the main types of primary systemic vasculitis in children based on recent consensus criteria.[30]

Some PSVs, such as Henoch–Schonlein purpura (HSP) and isolated cutaneous leukocytoclastic vasculitis, are rarely associated with systemic illness. Others, in particular Takayasu's arteritis, polyarteritis nodosa, and the anti-neutrophil cytoplasmic antibody (ANCA)-associated vasculitides (AAV), may be associated with a prolonged period of non-specific constitutional symptoms before the diagnosis becomes apparent.[1,3,31] KD is discussed earlier in this chapter (see section 'Kawasaki's disease').

Key clinical features

ANCA-associated vasculitides

The commonest types of AAV in the paediatric population are granulomatosis with polyangiitis (GPA) and microscopic polyangiitis (MPA). Constitutional symptoms, such as fever, weight loss, and fatigue, are the most frequent symptoms at presentation of GPA.[1,3] Symptoms related to pulmonary, renal, ear, nose and throat disease, and skin, are the next most common and typically manifest as dyspnoea, haemoptysis/pulmonary haemorrhage, pulmonary nodules, fixed pulmonary infiltrates, active urinary sediment, sinusitis, upper airway mucosal ulceration, and skin purpura.[1,3] The symptom complex and frequency of organ involvement in MPA is similar to GPA with the exception that ear, nose and throat involvement is not seen and lung involvement occurs primarily as pulmonary haemorrhage.[12,32,33]

Takayasu arteritis

Common symptoms of Takayasu arteritis (TA) include headache (reported in up to 64% of patients), arthralgia (43%), weight loss (36%), and fever (29%).[31] Hypertension is the most common clinical sign, reported in more than 80% of patients.[31,34] In this context, signs of vessel stenosis including bruits, reduced or absent peripheral pulses, and differential blood pressure between limbs are an important clue to the presence of large-vessel disease.

Polyarteritis nodosa

The commonest clinical features of polyarteritis nodosa (PAN) involve the skin, muscles, gastrointestinal system and nervous system.[12] They include livedo reticularis, tender subcutaneous nodules, significant myalgia and associated muscle tenderness, abdominal pain, and a mono- or polyneuropathy, which represent many of the recently validated classification criteria for this condition in children.[30]

Useful investigations

Acute-phase reactants, such as CRP and ESR, are typically elevated in these forms of vasculitis. Anaemia and thrombocytosis may also occur, and provide further evidence of underlying systemic inflammation. The absence of abnormalities in at least one of these parameters makes the diagnosis of active TA, PAN, or AAV unlikely. Other useful routine investigations include urinalysis and a chest radiograph, which may reveal an active urine sediment or pulmonary changes suggestive of AAV, respectively. Tests for ANCA, with specificity for either proteinase 3 (PR3) or myeloperoxidase (MPO), will be positive in more than 80% of patients with AAV.[1,3,12,32]

An important objective in the diagnosis of any of the vasculitides is confirming inflammation within the vascular tree. In

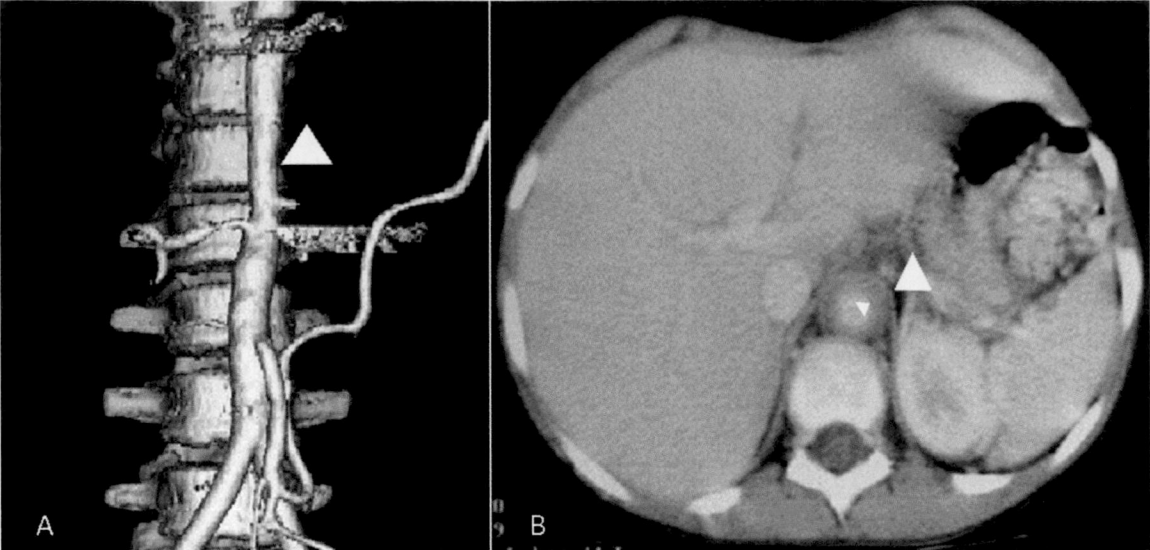

Fig. 14.3 (A) Three-dimensional reconstruction of a CT angiogram demonstrating narrowing of the suprarenal abdominal aorta (white arrow) in a patient with Takayasu arteritis. (B) Axial CT image from the same patient demonstrating luminal narrowing secondary to significant wall thickening (between small and large white arrows).

TA, ultrasound, CT, or MRI may be used to detect large-vessel wall abnormalities; typically thickening with consequent stenosis (Figure 14.3), but occasionally aneurysmal dilation.[35] In PAN, medium-vessel vasculitis may be demonstrated in biopsies of skin lesions, or typical aneurysmal dilatation of medium-sized vessels may be seen on abdominal angiography.[36] Although the AAV may occasionally involve medium-sized vessels, small-vessel involvement is the hallmark of this group of diseases. This may be demonstrated in biopsies of the skin, upper respiratory tract, and other involved organs. Vasculitis is rarely demonstrated in renal tissue in AAV; however, pauci-immune necrotizing glomerulonephritis is typical.[1]

Connective tissue disease

The term 'connective tissue disease' encompasses the clinical entities of juvenile systemic lupus erythematosus (JSLE), scleroderma, juvenile dermatomyositis, mixed connective tissue disease, and overlap/undifferentiated connective tissue disease, which are covered in detail in other chapters. Of these, JSLE is the most likely to present with systemic illness such as malaise, fatigue, and fever. Although fever may occur at presentation in other forms of connective tissue disease, it is not usually a prominent feature.[37–40] The diagnosis of JSLE is requires the presence of at least four of the clinical and laboratory features listed in the current American College of Rheumatology classification criteria for SLE,[41,42] which function as diagnostic criteria in both adults and children. Although it is found in all ethnic groups, SLE has a higher incidence in non-white populations.

Key clinical features

Skin and joint disease are frequent features of JSLE in children at presentation, seen in 44–70% and around 65% of children, respectively.[6,7,43] Skin involvement occurs typically as a photosensitive malar rash which characteristically spares the nasolabial folds. Less commonly, a non-photosensitive discoid rash may be seen. Mucous membrane involvement may occur as oral or nasal

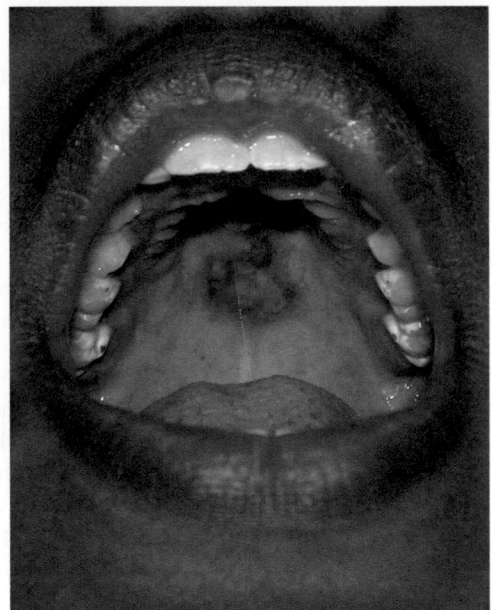

Fig. 14.4 Oral ulceration in SLE, demonstrating the typical appearance and location on the hard palate.

ulceration. The ulceration is usually painless and in the mouth typically occurs on the hard palate, which may be missed if not specifically examined (Figure 14.4). The arthritis of SLE tends to be a painful peripheral polyarthritis. Renal and haematological disease are also common at presentation, seen in 20–47% and 55% of patients, respectively.[6,7] Other clinical features which may occur at presentation include serositis, as pleural or pericardial effusions, and central nervous system disease, such as headache, psychosis, and cognitive dysfunction.

Useful investigations

The most useful investigation in the work-up for SLE is an assay for anti-nuclear antibodies (ANA), which are found in most, if not all, patients.[7] Their absence virtually excludes the diagnosis. If ANA are found to be present, further testing should be done for antibodies against double-stranded DNA, extractable nuclear antigens (e.g. anti-Smith, -Ro, and -La antibodies) and phospholipids (i.e. anti-cardiolipin and lupus anticoagulant). A urinalysis should be performed looking for active urine sediment, suggestive of glomerulonephritis. A full blood count may reveal anaemia, leukopenia (particularly lymphopenia), and thrombocytopenia. If haemolysis is suspected a Coombs test should be performed to confirm an immune basis.

Macrophage activation syndrome

Haemophagocytic lymphohistiocytosis (HLH) is a clinical syndrome of hyperinflammation resulting from immune dysregulation. It may occur as a primary phenomenon, in which immune the dysregulation has a genetic basis, or as a secondary phenomenon in the context of infection, malignancy and autoimmune diseases.[44] HLH complicating rheumatic disease is termed macrophage activation syndrome (MAS). sJIA is the rheumatic disease most commonly associated with MAS, although it may also be seen in JSLE and KD. Children with this condition are usually very unwell, with cytopenias, coagulopathy resembling disseminated intravascular coagulation (DIC), and multiorgan failure.

Key clinical features

The clinical presentation of HLH can vary depending on the underlying trigger. Children may present with prolonged fever and gradually worsening clinical status, or acutely unwell with fever and multiorgan failure. The diagnostic criteria for HLH/MAS are usually met only in the late stages of the disease. Patients may have signs of expansion of the reticuloendothelial system, such as lymphadenopathy and hepatosplenomegaly, and evidence of capillary leak in the form of oedema. A purpuric rash may occur in those with significant coagulopathy. In children with sJIA, the fever associated with MAS is more likely to be sustained or have several spikes as opposed to the one or two spikes seen with active systemic disease.

Useful investigations

The diagnosis of HLH should be considered in any febrile child with the combination of pancytopenia (or two cell line cytopenia), raised liver enzymes, and coagulopathy. A falling ESR, secondary to low fibrinogen, can also be a useful clue to the diagnosis. Serum ferritin is perhaps the most useful 'routine' investigation in the work-up for HLH; a serum ferritin of more than 10 000 μg/L has a specificity of 96% and a sensitivity of 90% for the diagnosis.[45]

The current HLH diagnostic criteria have some limitations when applied to everyday practice, as they include tests for sCD25 and NK cell function, which are not available at all centres. The criteria are also limited in their applicability to MAS. The requirement for significant cytopenias may not be met in those with significant pre-existing elevated counts, such as children with sJIA. In these children, a fall in previously elevated cell counts in the setting of ongoing fever is concerning for MAS, even though the counts may still be within the 'normal' range. These children will also have low ESR in spite of inflammation, due to the low fibrinogen associated with a consumptive process.

Periodic fever syndromes

The periodic fever syndromes come under the category of autoinflammatory disease. They result from defects in the pathways which initiate and regulate the inflammatory response and are characterized by recurrent episodes of inflammation, stereotypical for each condition. They have a strong genetic basis; mutations in specific genes have been identified for many of these conditions. Although the prevalence of some of these disorders is strongly influenced by ethnicity (e.g. familial Mediterranean fever (FMF) in those from the Mediterranean region), sporadic mutations occur. Further detail for each of the conditions is given in Chapter 164.

Key clinical features

The onset of symptoms in most of these syndromes is in early childhood (Figure 14.1) with recurrent episodes of fever and associated symptoms and signs. A good clinical history, paying attention to the features typical of each condition, is essential (see Chapter 5). The duration of attacks, in particular, may help in distinguishing between the various syndromes. The use of a symptom diary assists in the documentation the specific features of the episodes, their duration and frequency. Affected children are well between attacks, demonstrating normal growth patterns. This is a useful distinguishing feature from autoimmune disease.[46,47]

- **FMF** typically causes episodes lasting less than 72 hours. Associated features include abdominal and chest pain as a result of sersositis, joint pain, and erysipeloid rash. The abdominal pain may be severe, and in the context of fever a surgical cause may be mistakenly suspected.
- **TNF receptor associated periodic fever syndrome (TRAPS)** causes attacks of fever lasting longer than a week with skin manifestations in most. Conjunctivitis, abdominal pain, arthralgia, myalgia, and periorbital oedema may also occur.
- **Hyper IgD syndrome (HIDS)** is characterized by fever with cervical lymphadenopathy, arthralgias, skin lesions, and abdominal pain. The fevers usually last for 4–6 days and attacks are classically seen every 4–6 weeks.
- **Cryopyrin associated periodic fever syndromes (CAPS)** are usually characterized by an urticarial rash. Some of the CAPS conditions also have low grade fever, headaches, blurred vision, and arthralgia during attacks.

Useful investigations

Most children with periodic fever syndromes have elevated acute-phase reactants during an episode of fever. The diagnosis is usually made by identifying the underlying genetic mutation.[47]

The acute-phase reactants are usually normal in between attacks, which helps to distinguish them from chronic infectious and autoimmune diseases. Urine mevalonic acid can be raised during attacks in children with HIDS.

Other conditions

Sarcoidosis

Early onset sarcoidosis (EOS) is a distinct clinical entity quite different from the sarcoidosis seen in adults and older children. It is increasingly recognized that most children with early-onset sarcoidosis possibly have a form of Blau's syndrome with underlying mutations in the *NOD2* gene.[48]

Key clinical features

The characteristic triad of manifestations is rash, arthritis, and uveitis. Many children will also have low-grade fever.[49] The presence of low-grade fever, rash, and arthritis may lead to confusion with sJIA.[50] The presence of uveitis, unusual in sJIA, is a clue to the correct diagnosis. A slit lamp examination of the eyes should therefore be obtained in children under 5 years with fever and arthritis.

The rash of sarcoidosis is different from the sJIA rash. In sJIA there is an evanescent macular rash, whereas the rash in EOS is more likely to be papular or occur as plaques with scaling (Figure 14.5). The arthritis seen with EOS is also more likely to be painless, boggy, synovial thickening without much restriction in the range of movement.

Useful investigations

Anaemia, leucopenia, and eosinophilia are common. Angiotensin converting enzyme (ACE) levels are increased in more than 50% of those with late-onset sarcoidosis. Genetic testing in the EOS patients looking for mutations in the *NOD2* gene is helpful where feasible.

Kikuchi's disease

Kikuchi's disease is a necrotizing lymphadenitis which typically presents in adolescents or young adults with fever and lymphadenopathy.[51] Less frequent symptoms include night sweats, weight loss, nausea and vomiting. Although self-limiting, it can evolve into lupus in some.[52,53] These children typically have raised inflammatory markers and elevation of lactate dehydrogenase (LDH), and almost half will have leukopenia. The diagnosis is usually made on the histological appearances of the lymph node.

Castlemans's disease

Castleman's disease is characterized by lymph node hyperplasia. It can present as unicentric or multicentric variants. Although uncommon in children, it may occur during adolescence. The unicentric variant is more likely to present with lymph node swelling, with systemic features in some. The multicentric variant almost always presents with significant systemic symptoms. Laboratory tests may reveal anaemia, thrombocytopenia, and significantly elevated CRP. The condition is secondary to high levels of IL-6, of which the CRP can be a useful surrogate marker. The diagnosis is usually made on lymph node histology.[54]

Malignancy

An important aspect of the rheumatologic evaluation of the systemically unwell child is consideration of mimics, especially malignancy. Three malignancies in particular—acute leukaemia, neuroblastoma, and lymphoma—may present with clinical and investigational features, such as arthritis and elevation of acute-phase reactants, that overlap with those of the rheumatic diseases discussed in this chapter.[55] A high index of suspicion should therefore be maintained during the evaluation. Many children with rheumatic diseases who are systemically unwell will ultimately require steroid therapy. It is essential to be certain that malignancy is not the cause of symptoms before such treatment is begun, as in many cases this will result in partial treatment and make subsequent diagnosis on tissue samples difficult. At times it is not possible to be certain that malignancy is not present, and investigations such as a bone marrow aspirate and trephine are required to rule it out. Leukaemia and lymphoma may present at any age whereas neuroblastoma typically presents in children under 6 years. Important clues to the possible presence of malignancy are pain and disability in excess of physical signs, bone pain, pain that wakes the child from sleep, cytopenias, elevated ESR in the face of a low-normal platelet count, and a significantly elevated serum LDH.[55–57]

References

1. Akikusa JD, Schneider R, Harvey EA et al. Clinical features and outcome of pediatric Wegener's granulomatosis. *Arthritis Rheum* 2007;57(5):837–844.
2. Brik R, Shinawi M, Kepten I, Berant M, Gershoni-Baruch R. Familial Mediterranean fever: clinical and genetic characterization in a mixed pediatric population of Jewish and Arab patients. *Pediatrics* 1999;103(5):e70.
3. Cabral DA, Uribe AG, Benseler S et al. Classification, presentation, and initial treatment of Wegener's granulomatosis in childhood. *Arthritis Rheum* 2009;60(11):3413–3424.
4. Caroli F, Pontillo A, D'Osualdo A et al. Clinical and genetic characterization of Italian patients affected by CINCA syndrome. *Rheumatology (Oxford)* 2007;46(3):473–478.
5. Dode C, Andre M, Bienvenu T et al. The enlarging clinical, genetic, and population spectrum of tumor necrosis factor receptor-associated periodic syndrome. *Arthritis Rheum* 2002;46(8):2181–2188.
6. Font J, Cervera R, Espinosa G et al. Systemic lupus erythematosus (SLE) in childhood: analysis of clinical and immunological findings in 34 patients and comparison with SLE characteristics in adults. *Ann Rheum Dis* 1998;57(8):456–459.
7. Hiraki LT, Benseler SM, Tyrrell PN et al. Clinical and laboratory characteristics and long-term outcome of pediatric systemic lupus erythematosus: a longitudinal study. *J Pediatr* 2008;152(4):550–556.
8. Holman RC, Belay ED, Christensen KY et al. Hospitalizations for Kawasaki syndrome among children in the United States, 1997–2007. *Pediatr Infect Dis J* 2010;29(6):483–488.
9. Kummerle-Deschner JB, Tyrrell PN, Reess F et al. Risk factors for severe Muckle-Wells syndrome. *Arthritis Rheum* 2010;62(12):3783–3791.
10. Muranjan MN, Bavdekar SB, More V et al. Study of Takayasu's arteritis in children: clinical profile and management. *J Postgrad Med* 2000; 46(1):3–8.
11. Oen K, Duffy CM, Tse SM et al. Early outcomes and improvement of patients with juvenile idiopathic arthritis enrolled in a Canadian

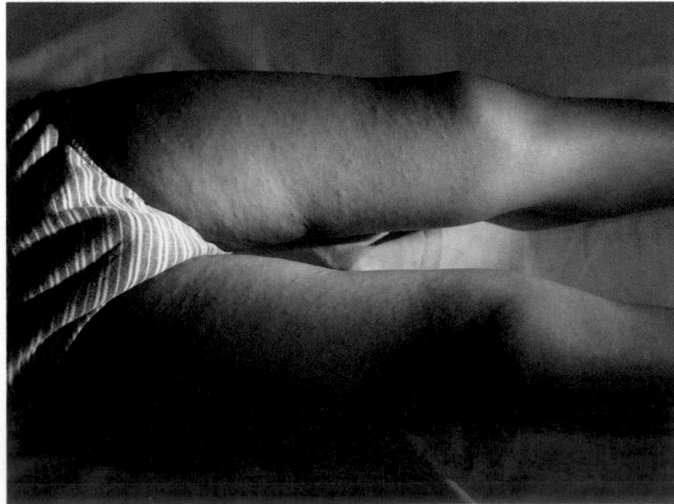

Fig. 14.5 The scaly papular rash of sarcoidosis.

multicenter inception cohort. *Arthritis Care Res* (Hoboken) 2010;62(4): 527–536.

12. Ozen S, Anton J, Arisoy N et al. Juvenile polyarteritis: results of a multicenter survey of 110 children. *J Pediatr* 2004;145(4):517–522.

13. Singh-Grewal D, Schneider R, Bayer N, Feldman BM. Predictors of disease course and remission in systemic juvenile idiopathic arthritis: significance of early clinical and laboratory features. *Arthritis Rheum* 2006;54(5):1595–1601.

14. van der Hilst JC, Bodar EJ et al. Long-term follow-up, clinical features, and quality of life in a series of 103 patients with hyperimmunoglobulinemia D syndrome. *Medicine* (Baltimore) 2008;87(6):301–310.

15. Minich LL, Sleeper LA, Atz AM et al. Delayed diagnosis of Kawasaki disease: what are the risk factors? *Pediatrics* 2007;120(6):e1434–e1440.

16. Kushner HI, Macnee RP, Burns JC. Kawasaki disease in India: increasing awareness or increased incidence? *Perspect Biol Med* 2009;52(1):17–29.

17. Singh S, Aulakh R, Bhalla AK et al. Is Kawasaki disease incidence rising in Chandigarh, North India? *Arch Dis Child* 2011;96(2):137–140.

18. Newburger JW, Takahashi M, Gerber MA et al. Diagnosis, treatment, and long-term management of Kawasaki disease: a statement for health professionals from the Committee on Rheumatic Fever, Endocarditis, and Kawasaki Disease, Council on Cardiovascular Disease in the Young, American Heart Association. *Pediatrics* 2004;114(6):1708–1733.

19. Stockheim JA, Innocentini N, Shulman ST. Kawasaki disease in older children and adolescents. *J Pediatr* 2000;137(2):250–252.

20. Tremoulet AH, Jain S, Chandrasekar D et al. Evolution of laboratory values in patients with kawasaki disease. *Pediatr Infect Dis J* 2011; 30(12):1022–1026.

21. Watanabe T, Abe Y, Sato S et al. Hyponatremia in Kawasaki disease. *Pediatr Nephrol* 2006;21(6):778–781.

22. Lohr JA, Hendley JO. Prolonged fever of unknown origin: a record of experiences with 54 childhood patients. *Clin Pediatr* (Phila) 1977;16(9): 768–773.

23. McClung HJ. Prolonged fever of unknown origin in children. *Am J Dis Child* 1972;124(4):544–550.

24. Pizzo PA, Lovejoy FH, Jr., Smith DH. Prolonged fever in children: review of 100 cases. *Pediatrics* 1975;55(4):468–473.

25. Steele RW, Jones SM, Lowe BA, Glasier CM. Usefulness of scanning procedures for diagnosis of fever of unknown origin in children. *J Pediatr* 1991;119(4):526–530.

26. Prendiville JS, Tucker LB, Cabral DA, Crawford RI. A pruritic linear urticarial rash, fever, and systemic inflammatory disease in five adolescents: adult-onset still disease or systemic juvenile idiopathic arthritis sine arthritis? *Pediatr Dermatol* 2004;21(5):580–588.

27. Fautrel B, Le Moel G, Saint-Marcoux B et al. Diagnostic value of ferritin and glycosylated ferritin in adult onset Still's disease. *J Rheumatol* 2001;28(2):322–329.

28. Ota T, Higashi S, Suzuki H, Eto S. Increased serum ferritin levels in adult Still's disease. *Lancet* 1987;i(8532):562–563.

29. Behrens EM, Beukelman T, Paessler M, Cron RQ. Occult macrophage activation syndrome in patients with systemic juvenile idiopathic arthritis. *J Rheumatol* 2007;34(5):1133–1138.

30. Ozen S, Ruperto N, Dillon MJ et al. EULAR/PReS endorsed consensus criteria for the classification of childhood vasculitides. *Ann Rheum Dis* 2006;65(7):936–941.

31. Zhu WH, Shen LG, Neubauer H. Clinical characteristics, interdisciplinary treatment and follow-up of 14 children with Takayasu arteritis. *World J Pediatr* 2010;6(4):342–347.

32. Peco-Antic A, Bonaci-Nikolic B, Basta-Jovanovic G et al. Childhood microscopic polyangiitis associated with MPO-ANCA. *Pediatr Nephrol* 2006;21(1):46–53.

33. Yu F, Huang JP, Zou WZ, Zhao MH. The clinical features of anti-neutrophil cytoplasmic antibody-associated systemic vasculitis in Chinese children. *Pediatr Nephrol* 2006;21(4):497–502.

34. Jain S, Sharma N, Singh S et al. Takayasu arteritis in children and young Indians. *Int J Cardiol* 2000;75 Suppl 1:S153–S157.

35. Kothari SS. Takayasu's arteritis in children—a review. *Images Paediatr Cardiol* 2002(2):4–23.

36. Brogan PA, Davies R, Gordon I, Dillon MJ. Renal angiography in children with polyarteritis nodosa. *Pediatr Nephrol* 2002;17(4):277–283.

37. Martini G, Foeldvari I, Russo R et al. Systemic sclerosis in childhood: clinical and immunologic features of 153 patients in an international database. *Arthritis Rheum* 2006;54(12):3971–3978.

38. Ramanan AV, Feldman BM. Clinical features and outcomes of juvenile dermatomyositis and other childhood onset myositis syndromes. *Rheum Dis Clin North Am* 2002;28(4):833–857.

39. Tsai YY, Yang YH, Yu HH et al. Fifteen-year experience of pediatric-onset mixed connective tissue disease. *Clin Rheumatol* 2010;29(1):53–58.

40. Vaz CC, Couto M, Medeiros D et al. Undifferentiated connective tissue disease: a seven-center cross-sectional study of 184 patients. *Clin Rheumatol* 2009;28(8):915–921.

41. Hochberg MC. Updating the American College of Rheumatology revised criteria for the classification of systemic lupus erythematosus. *Arthritis Rheum* 1997;40(9):1725.

42. Tan EM, Cohen AS, Fries JF et al. The 1982 revised criteria for the classification of systemic lupus erythematosus. *Arthritis Rheum* 1982;25(11):1271–1277.

43. Hoffman IE, Lauwerys BR, De Keyser F et al. Juvenile-onset systemic lupus erythematosus: different clinical and serological pattern than adult-onset systemic lupus erythematosus. *Ann Rheum Dis* 2009;68(3):412–415.

44. Freeman HR, Ramanan AV. Review of haemophagocytic lymphohistiocytosis. *Arch Dis Child* 2011;96(7):688–693.

45. Allen CE, Yu X, Kozinetz CA, McClain KL. Highly elevated ferritin levels and the diagnosis of hemophagocytic lymphohistiocytosis. *Pediatr Blood Cancer* 2008;50(6):1227–1235.

46. Grateau G, Duruoz MT. Autoinflammatory conditions: when to suspect? How to treat? *Best Pract Res Clin Rheumatol* 2010;24(3):401–411.

47. Kastner DL, Aksentijevich I, Goldbach-Mansky R. Autoinflammatory disease reloaded: a clinical perspective. *Cell* 2010;140(6):784–790.

48. Rose CD, Martin TM, Wouters CH. Blau syndrome revisited. *Curr Opin Rheumatol* 2011;23(5):411–418.

49. Shetty AK, Gedalia A. Childhood sarcoidosis: a rare but fascinating disorder. *Pediatr Rheumatol Online J* 2008;6:16.

50. Sharma SM, Martin TM, Rose CD, Dick AD, Ramanan AV. Distinguishing between the innate immune response due to ocular inflammation and infection in a child with juvenile systemic granulomatous disease treated with anti-TNFalpha monoclonal antibodies. *Rheumatology (Oxford)* 2011;50(5):990–992.

51. Hutchinson CB, Wang E. Kikuchi-Fujimoto disease. *Arch Pathol Lab Med* 2010;134(2):289–293.

52. Cheng CY, Sheng WH, Lo YC et al. Clinical presentations, laboratory results and outcomes of patients with Kikuchi's disease: emphasis on the association between recurrent Kikuchi's disease and autoimmune diseases. *J Microbiol Immunol Infect* 2010;43(5):366–371.

53. Goldblatt F, Andrews J, Russell A, Isenberg D. Association of Kikuchi-Fujimoto's disease with SLE. *Rheumatology (Oxford)* 2008;47(4): 553–554.

54. Roca B. Castleman's disease. a review. *AIDS Rev* 2009;11(1):3–7.

55. Cabral DA, Tucker LB. Malignancies in children who initially present with rheumatic complaints. *J Pediatr* 1999;134(1):53–57.

56. Jones OY, Spencer CH, Bowyer SL et al. A multicenter case-control study on predictive factors distinguishing childhood leukemia from juvenile rheumatoid arthritis. *Pediatrics* 2006;117(5):e840–e844.

57. Wallendal M, Stork L, Hollister JR. The discriminating value of serum lactate dehydrogenase levels in children with malignant neoplasms presenting as joint pain. *Arch Pediatr Adolesc Med* 1996;150(1):70–73.

CHAPTER 15

Primary care presentation

Elspeth Wise

Primary care

Primary care physicians, also known as family practitioners or general practitioners (GPs), perform a unique role within the United Kingdom National Health Service (NHS). They are generally the first healthcare professional that patients access, and act as the gatekeeper to other services, including secondary care. Primary care doctors manage 90% of the conditions that they see, along with the help of the primary healthcare team.[1]

The roles of a primary care doctor (adapted from WONCA[2]) are:

♦ The provision of comprehensive and continuing care to every individual seeking medical care, irrespective of age, sex, and illness.

♦ Caring for individuals in the context of their family, their community, and their culture.

♦ Management plans, which should be holistic and utilize the knowledge and trust engendered by repeated contacts.

♦ Health promotion/disease prevention.

Primary care in the United Kingdom has changed over recent years. At the inception of the NHS in the mid-20th century, patients used to register to be on a specific doctor's list and this was the doctor they saw if they were unwell. Group practices and health centres began to develop after the introduction of a new contract in 1966, but even then the patient still had to register with a particular doctor.[3] This was referred to as a 'personal list'. In more recent years this idea of a personal list has disappeared. Most GPs work in group practices or health centres, the patient registers with a particular surgery and they can see any doctor they choose. This allows both patients and doctors to benefit from the different skills that individual primary care physicians may have. Many doctors now develop a special interest in a particular area and so there can be internal referring of patients between them, e.g. for contraceptive advice, joint injections, or minor surgery.

Consultation patterns have also changed over recent years. The length of a general practice consultation has increased to around 10 minutes per patient.[4] The number of telephone consultations has increased, and nurses have a more involved role in patient care. Specially trained practice nurses now coordinate care and perform disease monitoring for chronic illnesses, particularly those specified in the Department of Health's Quality and Outcomes Framework. There are also more salaried doctors, who often work part time, which can have implications on continuity of care.

Patients still appreciate the role of the primary care physician as being 'their doctor' who has looked after them and also members of their family for a number of years. The idea of a GP looking after a patient from 'cradle to grave' remains, and is a cherished part of their identity.

Prevalence of musculoskeletal conditions

Musculoskeletal conditions are common in primary care in the United Kingdom. There are varying estimates suggesting that they form 15–30% of a GP's workload, i.e. in their average surgery most GPs will see one or two patients presenting with a musculoskeletal condition.[5,6] Their musculoskeletal complaint may often be an aside—'while I'm here, doctor' or may be the main reason for their presentation. Primary care physicians may also find themselves having to deal with other associated problems in addition to the musculoskeletal complaint, e.g. the effect on the patient's working life, their mental health, and their family. The focus of the consultation may therefore be on other things rather than the complaint itself, which can become secondary. The prevalence of musculoskeletal conditions is expected to rise as the proportion of elderly people in the population rises, as do other causative factors such as obesity.[7]

The prevalence data for musculoskeletal conditions in the United Kingdom is variable in quality. Different sources have to be used with some being more up to date than others.[8] Table 15.1 shows the prevalence of different musculoskeletal conditions in the United Kingdom. The third column uses the prevalence data to show, as an estimate, how many patients a GP may expect to have on their list with the conditions mentioned, using a suggested list size of 1800 patients per GP. This table highlights how few patients a GP may see with conditions that are considered to be reasonably common in secondary care, and who may form the majority of some specialist's workload.

Accurate data for the prevalence of conditions in primary care is not available, partly for reasons already documented. GPs are encouraged to give a problem code to every consultation they have, but doctors often work with symptoms and do not make a formal diagnosis when dealing with a patient. For example, primary care doctors may treat a patient as having 'knee pain' rather than osteoarthritis of the knee. This is evidenced in studies that have looked at the different general practice databases available.[10,11] There are a number of putative reasons as to why this may occur, including not making a definitive diagnosis until investigations/secondary care

Table 15.1 Prevalence of different musculoskeletal conditions in the United Kingdom

Condition	Prevalence	Estimated no of patients per GP
Rheumatoid arthritis (England)[a]	0.8%	14
JIA (UK)[a]	0.07%	1
Ankylosing spondylitis[a] (consulting annual period prevalence in the UK)	0.04%	0.7
Gout[b]	1.4%	25
SLE	0.03%	0.5
Scleroderma	0.003%	0.05
Back pain	?5%	90

JIA, juvenile idiopathic arthritis; SLE, systemic lupus erythematosus.
[a] Data from Parsons et al.[8]
[b] Data from Annemans et al.[9]

opinion is available, or that the doctor is not confident in making a definitive diagnosis. In many cases it may be difficult to make a definitive diagnosis early in the course of the condition, as symptoms may be vague and not fit a recognized pattern. In these cases primary care doctors may use time as part of their treatment to see how the condition develops.

Patient presentation

As already discussed, many of the musculoskeletal conditions that form the focus of textbooks and teaching are not commonly seen in primary care. Back pain is the most frequent presenting complaint and can account for about 20% of all musculoskeletal consultations, although very little time is focused on it during medical school training.[11]

A consultation in primary care is generally around 10 minutes in length. During this time the doctor must take a history, examine their patient, formulate a diagnosis, create a management plan, and then act on this plan. GPs are encouraged to allow patients to say their piece. It has been shown that if patients are left to talk, their initial opening statement lasts, on average, 92 seconds, and 78% of people will finish their initial statement in 2 minutes.[12] This limits the amount of time the doctor has to complete the rest of the consultation. Patients often save up their problems before coming to see a doctor, and can cite struggling to get an appointment as a reason for this. Their musculoskeletal problem may be the last one on their list and may be mentioned just before they leave, as their 10 minutes is drawing to a close. This can mean that little time is spent discussing it, or the patient may be asked to come back at a later date—which they may fail to do.

Patients present to doctors with symptoms such as back pain or knee pain, whereas textbooks are generally ordered/categorized by diagnoses. Many primary care doctors have limited experience at managing musculoskeletal conditions before starting in primary care, and may struggle to find a suitable diagnosis that fits with the constellation of symptoms and signs that their patient has.[13] This could be a reason why GPs work with vague diagnoses such as shoulder pain or hip pain. Another reason could be that the early signs of a condition can be non-specific. One area where this may

be detrimental to the patient's health is when diagnosing inflammatory arthritis. It is recognized that the early signs of inflammatory arthritis can be non-specific and that it can take time for the characteristic symptoms and signs described in textbooks to develop. This, coupled with the fact that primary care doctors have very little musculoskeletal experience and may only see a new case of rheumatoid arthritis (the second most common inflammatory arthritis after gout) every other year, means that patients can often be referred later than desired.[8,14,15]

One way to try to improve the management of conditions in primary care is to create guidelines. Many interested parties develop guidelines, with primary care as one of their target audiences, but they may not disseminate them appropriately and so they are not even read, let alone followed. Primary care doctors receive a large number of guidelines each year and can receive different recommendations from different sources for the same condition,[16,17] causing some confusion as to which is best to follow. Other areas exist where the flow of information from secondary to primary care is not ideal. Examples of these which are highlighted in the literature include educating primary care doctors about new medications and their side effects (e.g. anti-tumour necrosis factor medication) and the requirement for annual influenza vaccination in patients with inflammatory joint diseases.[18,19]

Primary care doctors play a pivotal role in the management of musculoskeletal diseases, as they are the first point of call for patients in many healthcare systems. The majority of patients in these systems are looked after in primary care and it is only the tip of the iceberg that is seen by specialists. Education of primary care physicians is essential, improving both patient management and their confidence.

References

1. JCPTGP. *Training for general practice*. Joint Committee on Postgraduate Training for General Practice, London, 1992.
2. WONCA Europe. *The European definition of general practice/family medicine—edition 2011*. Available at: www.woncaeurope.org/content/european-definition-general-practice-family-medicine-edition-2011 (Accessed 6 December 2012).
3. Kmietowicz Z. A century of general practice. *BMJ* 2006;332(7532):39–40.
4. The Information Centre. *2006/07 UK general practice workload survey*, 2007. Available at: www.ic.nhs.uk/webfiles/publications/gp/GP%20Workload%20Report.pdf
5. Office of Population Censuses and Surveys. *Morbidity statistics from general practice—fourth national study 1991/92*. HMSO, London, 1995.
6. Department of Health. *The musculoskeletal services framework*. The Stationery Office, London, 2006.
7. Khaw KT. How many, how old, how soon? *BMJ* 1999;319:1350–1352.
8. Parsons S, Ingram M, Clarke-Cornwell A M, Symmons DPM. *A heavy burden. The occurrence and impact of musculoskeletal conditions in the United Kingdom today*. Arthritis Research UK Epidemiology Unit, Manchester, 2011.
9. Annemans L, Spaepen E, Gaskin M et al. Gout in the UK and Germany: prevalence, comorbidities and management in general practice 2000–2005. *Ann Rheum Dis* 2008;67:960–966.
10. Linsell L, Dawson J, Zondervan K et al. Prevalence and incidence of adults consulting for shoulder conditions in UK primary care; patterns of diagnosis and referral. *Rheumatology* 2006;45(2):215–221.
11. Arthritis Research UK National Primary Care Centre, Keele University. Consultations for selected diagnoses and regional problems. *Musculoskeletal Matters. Bulletin* 2;2010. Available at www.keele.ac.uk/media/keeleuniversity/ri/primarycare/bulletins/Musculoskeletal Matters2.pdf (Accessed on 6 December 2012).

12. Langewitz W, Denz M, Keller A et al. Spontaneous talking time at start of consultation in outpatient clinic: cohort study. *BMJ* 2002;325:682–683.

13. Lanyon P, Pope D, Croft P. Rheumatology education and management skills in general practice: a national study of trainees. *Ann Rheum Dis* 1995;54:735–739.

14. Foster HE, Eltringham MS, Kay LJ et al. Delay in access to appropriate care for children presenting with musculoskeletal symptoms and ultimately diagnosed with juvenile idiopathic arthritis. *Arthritis Rheum* 2007;57:921–927.

15. Irvine S, Munro R, Porter D, et al. Early referral, diagnosis, and treatment of rheumatoid arthritis: evidence for changing medical practice. *Ann Rheum Dis* 1999;58:510–513.

16. Hibble A, Kanka D, Pencheon D, Pooles F. Guidelines in general practice: the new Tower of Babel? *BMJ* 1998;317:862–863.

17. Cornwall PL, Scott J. Which clinical practice guidelines for depression? An overview for busy practitioners. *Br J Gen Pract* 2000;50: 908–911.

18. Wise EM, Burdon ACJ, Nicholl K et al. Documentation of anti-TNF therapy in primary care health records. *Rheumatology* 2007; 46(suppl 1):i105.

19. Doe S, Pathare S, Kelly CA et al. Uptake of influenza vaccination in patients on immunosuppressant agents for rheumatological diseases: a follow-up audit of the influence of secondary care. *Rheumatology* 2007;46(4):715–716.

Clinical presentations: views from different perspectives

SECTION 3

Clinical presentations: views from different perspectives

CHAPTER 16

Obstetrics and pregnancy

Monika Østensen, Radboud Dolhain,
and Guillermo Ruiz-Irastorza

Fertility

Rheumatic diseases can impair fertility and fecundity (time to achieving pregnancy) in several ways. Factors involved are active disease, fetotoxic therapy, autoimmunity, hormonal imbalance, and periods with impaired sexual functioning.[1] The influence of biological factors is often impossible to separate from other reasons such as a decrease in the frequency of intercourse relating to pain and functional disability from arthritis. Several studies have shown reduced fertility in patients with rheumatoid arthritis (RA), other inflammatory chronic arthritis, and juvenile idiopathic arthritis (JIA).[2] Compared to healthy women, patients have fewer children, need a longer time to conceive, and have prolonged interpregnancy intervals.[3] Reduced family size in spite of normal fertility and fecundity can be a result of pregnancy loss either as miscarriage or stillbirth, or can be due to perinatal deaths as in connective tissue diseases (CTD) and vasculitis. Smaller family size need not necessarily be attributed to lower fertility; it may also reflect the choice of rheumatic patients to limit their family size.[4]

Pregnancy and rheumatic disease

Rheumatoid arthritis

RA remits during pregnancy and flares after delivery. Since the first description of this phenomenon by Hench in 1938, this finding has been reconfirmed in several studies.[5] In the earlier studies, predominantly of retrospective study design and relying upon patient's self-report, remission rates of up to 90% were demonstrated.[5]

More recently, two large prospective studies have been published.[6,7] In the first study, from late pregnancy until 6 months after delivery, 63% of women retrospectively reported improvement of disease activity during pregnancy, whereas 16% of women were in total remission during the third trimester, which was defined as having no swollen joints and receiving no antirheumatic therapy. In this study 66% of women experienced a flare after delivery.[5]

In the second study, disease activity was prospectively assessed from pre-pregnancy until 6 months after delivery, using the disease activity score for 28 joints (DAS28). In this study it was shown that remission (as defined by DAS28 <2.6) increased from 17% during the first trimester to 27% during the third trimester. According to the DAS28-based EULAR response criteria, 48% of patients had at least a moderate response during pregnancy.[7] Despite the improvement of disease activity during pregnancy, functionality as determined by the health assessment questionnaire (HAQ) worsened.[8] This phenomenon is not specific for RA, however, but can also be observed in healthy pregnant women due to pregnancy itself. After pregnancy almost 40% of patients experienced a flare, despite restarting medication.[7] A prospective study with a 12 year follow up found no significant influence of pregnancy on long-term RA outcome, but found a trend for patients with multiple pregnancies to have less radiographic joint damage and a better functional level.[9]

The disease response during previous pregnancies seems predictive for the disease response in subsequent pregnancies.[5] Furthermore, RA patients who are negative for rheumatoid factor (RF) and anti-citrullinated protein antibodies (ACPA) are more likely to improve during pregnancy.[10] In the Dutch prospective study of 118 patients, 75% of patients negative for RF and cyclic citrullinated peptide (CCP) antibodies improved compared to only 39% of those positive for RF and CCP antibodies. Breastfeeding has been associated with the occurrence of the postpartum flare in RA patients.[5] The interpretation of this association is difficult, however, since women who breastfeed are in general not receiving medication and hence are more likely to flare.

Several theories have been put forward to explain the improvement of RA during pregnancy. The basis of all these theories is that profound changes of the maternal immune system take place during pregnancy, in order to accommodate the fetal allograft.[11] Because of the small sample size of most studies, it often cannot be concluded whether the observed changes only represent a general adaptation of the immune system during pregnancy or whether these changes are also responsible for the ameliorating effect of pregnancy on RA.

New studies have shown that pregnancy outcome is less favourable in RA than previously thought.[12,13] Several studies report a small but increased risk for small for gestational age infants, intrauterine growth restriction, hypertensive disorders, preterm delivery, and caesarean sections.[12,13] Adverse pregnancy outcomes, particularly lower birthweight, seem to be associated with disease activity in RA.[12] Lower birth weight, even within the normal range, has been associated with increased risk of future developmental delay, metabolic syndrome, and cardiovascular disease. Whether the same holds true for the lower birth weight of children born to women with active RA is not known.

New data have questioned the general medical opinion about a prevailing beneficial effect of pregnancy on RA. Although RA improves during pregnancy, the effect is less impressive than previously thought and a high percentage of women still have considerable disease activity.[6,7] Furthermore, despite improvement of disease activity, functionality worsens. Tight disease control, if necessary with sulfasalazine, hydroxychloroquine, and low-dose prednisone during pregnancy, is essential to secure good maternal and fetal outcomes.

Other chronic inflammatory arthritides: ankylosing spondylitis, psoriatic arthritis, and juvenile idiopathic arthritis

Inflammatory arthritis in peripheral joints and/or the spine characterizes ankylosing spondylitis (AS), psoriatic arthritis (PsA), and JIA. Increased B cell activity with autoantibody production or extensive organ involvement is, with the exception of some subtypes of JIA, not a feature of these diseases. Interactions between pregnancy and AS, JIA, and PsA have been much less investigated than in RA. AS and JIA share an aggravation of disease within the first 6 months after delivery, occurring in 52–90% of cases, particularly in patients with active disease at conception.[14,17–18]

The few reports on PsA and pregnancy do not allow any definite statement,[15] but in the absence of reports to the contrary, no major influence of pregnancy on PsA may be anticipated.

Ankylosing spondylitis

Both retrospective and prospective studies of AS have shown that disease activity is not substantially altered during pregnancy.[14,16] The typical pattern is active disease during the first and early second trimester, sometimes accompanied by a flare around week 20, and some mitigation of symptoms in the third trimester. Though some AS patients experience improvement of peripheral joint disease during pregnancy, complete subsidence of spinal symptoms has not been observed. The frequency of acute peripheral arthritis or anterior uveitis is reduced 1.5–3 times during pregnancy compared to postpartum.[14]

Juvenile idiopathic arthritis

For 40–50% of JIA patients the disease persists into adulthood with ongoing disease activity and need for therapy. Patients with onset of JIA in early childhood and severe involvement may suffer as adults from sequelae such as growth retardation, osteoporosis, hip joint replacement, and functional disability interfering with reproductive performance.

Retrospective studies have shown that subsets of JIA differ in their response to pregnancy. Improvement occurs in about two-thirds of patients with polyarticular and oligoarticular JIA, whereas only 29% with systemic disease improve during pregnancy.[17] Patients in complete remission at the start of pregnancy seldom suffer a relapse of arthritis during pregnancy. Chronic uveitis remains unchanged during pregnancy.[18] Most patients with inactive JIA in adulthood, and those with monoarticular JIA, will have uneventful pregnancies and deliver healthy children of normal birth weight.[17,18]

Outcome of pregnancy

An increase in miscarriage or pre-eclampsia has not been documented for AS, PsA, or JIA. A large population-based case-control study of women with chronic inflammatory arthritides including RA, AS, PsA, and JIA found an increase in the rate of caesarean section, and premature and small for gestational age infants.[13] The children had also lower mean birth weight (P = 0.01) and higher perinatal mortality (OR 3.26 [95% CI 1.04–10.24]).

Connective tissue diseases

Systemic lupus erythematosus and antiphospholipid syndrome

No systemic autoimmune diseases are so closely related with pregnancy complications as systemic lupus erythematosus (SLE) and anti-phospholipid syndrome (APS).

Maternal complications

SLE activity can increase during pregnancy and the puerperium in more than 50% of patients.[19] Women with current or recent activity at the time of conception and those who withdraw hydroxychloroquine are more likely to suffer a disease flare.[20,21] Although most flares are mild, severe renal involvement has been reported in some series.[22] Pregnancy can be especially harmful for women with a high degree of irreversible organ damage. The progressive increase of plasma volume during pregnancy demands adaption to higher load from the kidneys, heart, and lungs. Women with severe renal failure, cardiac insufficiency, pulmonary hypertension, or severe restrictive pulmonary disease are at a high risk for deteriorating organ dysfunction and even for maternal death. Women with baseline serum creatinine levels higher than 2.5–2.8 mg mg/dL (220–250 µmol/L) are most likely to suffer postpartum renal function decline.[23] A modest increase in global irreversible damage postpartum, determined by disease activity and the presence of damage before conception, has been found in women with SLE.[24]

APS is a well-known cause of arterial and venous thrombosis. Women with previous thrombotic events, especially those with stroke, can suffer recurrent thrombosis during pregnancy.[25] This risk seems to be lower for women with only obstetric manifestations of APS and for asymptomatic carriers of antiphospholipid antibodies (aPL).[26]

Obstetric complications

Women with high lupus activity during pregnancy have a two- to fourfold higher chance of suffering prematurity and perinatal death and have a lower frequency of live births.[20] Increasing doses of prednisone used to treat flares may contribute, at least in part, to such complications.

A recently published systematic review and meta-analysis has found a higher likelihood of suffering hypertension and prematurity in lupus women with active nephritis, whilst those with past lupus nephritis had a higher risk for hypertension and pre-eclampsia.[27]

The presence of aPL is one of the most important predictors of adverse pregnancy outcomes, in women with and without SLE. Women with aPL are at a higher risk for hypertension, pre-eclampsia, fetal death, placental insufficiency with growth restriction, and prematurity.[28,29] Combined positivity for lupus anticoagulant (LA), anticardiolipin antibodies (aCL), and anti-β_2-glycoprotein I, as well as a history of maternal thrombosis, multiplies the risk for obstetric complications.[30,31] Treatment of obstetric APS is still subject to debate. Aspirin and heparin are the drugs of choice, but there is still controversy regarding the specific role of each of these, alone or in combination, especially in women with recurrent early miscarriages.[26]

Primary Sjögren's syndrome

Most patients with primary Sjögren's syndrome (pSS) have completed their families before disease onset. The few studies that have investigated pregnancy outcome in pSS found no major changes of sicca symptoms during pregnancy.[32,33]

Recent studies have not shown an increase in adverse outcomes and concluded that neither pSS itself nor the presence of anti-SSA and anti-SSB antibodies influenced the outcome of pregnancy.[32] However, transmission of maternal anti-Ro/SSA or anti-La/SSB antibodies during pregnancy can cause neonatal lupus syndromes in neonates.

Neonatal lupus and congenital heart block

Neonatal lupus syndrome (NNLS) is a rare complication closely related to the presence of maternal anti-Ro/SSA and anti-La/SSB antibodies, affecting children born to mothers with lupus, Sjögren's syndrome, other autoimmune diseases or asymptomatic carriers of those antibodies.[34] Anti-Ro/SSA and anti-La/SSB gain access to the fetal circulation during the physiological active transport of IgG across the placenta, starting from early second trimester and increasing throughout gestation. The most serious form of presentation is congenital heart block (CHB), but skin rashes, thrombocytopenia, and elevated liver enzymes may also occur. The risk of CHB among newborns of anti-Ro/SSA-positive women is around 2%,[35] but this risk increases to around 20% in younger siblings of an infant with CHB or other forms of NNLS.[34,36] Most children affected with CHB will need a permanent pacemaker and around 20% may die in the perinatal period.[34]

In case of incomplete heart block, myocarditis, ascites, or hydrops therapy with fluorinated steroids—dexamethasone or betamethasone, which cross the placenta—is recommended since there is a chance for reversibility (total or partial).[37] Recently, two clinical trials have failed to reduce the expected rate of recurrent CHB (20%) in women treated with intravenous immunoglobulin (IVIG) during pregnancy.[38,39] On the other hand, a recent case-control study has suggested a protective effect of hydroxychloroquine on the development of cardiac manifestations in children with NNLS born to mothers with lupus and anti-Ro/anti-La antibodies.[40] Noncardiac postnatal manifestations of NNLS subside spontaneously as maternal antibodies are cleared from the baby's circulation.

Systemic sclerosis

Early case reports and small series described adverse, sometimes fatal maternal outcomes in pregnant patients with systemic sclerosis (SSc). Large retrospective case-control studies and one prospective study showed that pregnancy does not profoundly alter the disease.[41] In a study of 133 pregnancies in 69 patients no change in disease-related symptoms was found in 88%, improvement in 5%, and aggravation in 7% of pregnancies.[42] Cutaneous disease did not change much and progression of skin disease was uncommon during pregnancy or postpartum in any of the studies. Usually, Raynaud's phenomenon improved and arthralgias and reflux worsened during pregnancy, whereas cardiopulmonary problems essentially remained unchanged in women with SSc.[41,42]

Serious organ manifestations of SSc such as renal disease or pulmonary hypertension (PHT) can threaten the outcome of pregnancy. A fourfold increase in hypertensive disorders, including pre-eclampsia, was found in a retrospective study of 504 pregnancies in women with SSc.[43] Risk factors for renal crisis are early diffuse systemic sclerosis and rapidly progressing skin disease. Treatment with high dose prednisolone may be an additional risk factor. Case-control studies have shown that renal crisis does not occur more frequently in pregnant compared to non-pregnant SSc patients. Pulmonary hypertension has still a poor survival rate of about 2.8 years, with a 25–50% risk of maternal mortality in case of pregnancy. Fortunately, a multidisciplinary team approach has now improved pregnancy outcome even in these high-risk pregnancies.[43]

The rate of miscarriage is not increased in patients with SSc, except for women with long-standing diffuse scleroderma.[41] The most prominent adverse outcome in SSc is prematurity and an increased rate of full-term small infants.[41–43] The risk of adverse pregnancy outcome is greater in patients with the diffuse form than with the limited form of SSc. Women with early diffuse and rapidly progressing disease should postpone conception until SSc is less active. Patients with severe organ involvement such as cardiomyopathy, severe restrictive lung disease, pulmonary hypertension, malabsorption, or severe renal insufficiency should probably be discouraged from becoming pregnant.

Polymyositis and dermatomyositis

The few data from case reports and small series indicate that most women with polymyositis (PM) or dermatomyositis (DM) with inactive disease at conception have normal pregnancies with a good outcome.[44–46] Relapses at a quiescent stage of PM/DM seem rather infrequent during pregnancy. In contrast, women with active disease at conception or disease onset during pregnancy are at high risk of pregnancy loss, intrauterine growth restriction, preterm delivery, and neonatal death. It is important to control the disease before pregnancy and promptly treat a disease flare if it occurs during pregnancy.[46]

Vasculitis and pregnancy

With the exception of Takayasu's arteritis (TAK), which preferentially affects young women of childbearing age, systemic vasculitides (SV) are rare diseases in women in general and particularly those under the age of 40 years. As a consequence, pregnancy experience in polyarteritis nodosa (PAN), granulomatosis with polyangiitis (Wegener's) (GPA), eosinophilic granulomatosis with polyangiitis (Churg–Strauss syndrome, EGPA), and microscopic polyangiitis (MPA) consists altogether of less than 100 pregnancies described in case reports and small series collected over several decades with variance in patient characteristics and management.[46,47]

Takayasu's arteritis during pregnancy

Reports of more than 150 pregnancies in women with TAK show that disease activity is not influenced by pregnancy.[46,48] Complications during pregnancy and the outcome are related to whether the extent of arteritis is confined to the aortic arch or extends to the descending and abdominal aorta and its branches. The risk of TAK associated with pregnancy is mainly due to arterial hypertension and/or pre-eclampsia, with a greater risk in more severe and extensive cases of large-vessel arteritis.[48] Complications occurred preferentially in the third trimester, during delivery, or in the immediate postpartum period. No case of maternal death has been reported. Patients with complications such as hypertension, retinopathy, aortic incompetence, or aneurysm must be regarded as high risk, with need for close monitoring and therapy during pregnancy and delivery. Patients with severe aortic valvular disease or aortic aneurysm should be discouraged from pregnancy because of the risk of maternal morbidity and mortality.

In spite of a moderate increase in miscarriage and prematurity, the outcome of pregnancy was favourable in 70–85% of cases. Neonatal outcome has been good in most studies, but in mothers with one severe or several complications of TAK the birthweight of neonates was slightly reduced.[48]

Vasculitis of medium and small vessels

The most common manifestations of necrotizing vasculitides (PAN, GPA, EGPA, and MPA) are in the respiratory tract and the kidneys. Old case reports tend to describe more adverse pregnancy outcomes than recent ones, due to less developed obstetric medicine and fewer available treatment modalities. The extent of vasculitis, type of organs involved and resulting organ damage as well as disease activity at conception influence maternal and fetal outcome. However, a state of remission before conception does not guarantee the absence of a relapse, which occurs in 20–25% of pregnancies. In recent publications, reported global pregnancy outcomes were good; there were no maternal deaths and all live-born infants were healthy.[46,49,50] In most cases SV required only minor adjustments of immunosuppressive therapy during pregnancy. However, the rate of miscarriage and of prematurity is increased, and life-threatening complications can occur in the mother.[46] Whether pregnancy increases or decreases the activity or the relapse rate of necrotizing vasculitis compared to the non-pregnant state has not been investigated. Disease onset of PAN, EGPA, CSS, and MPA during pregnancy or active disease during pregnancy limit the option for effective therapy, particularly with cyclophosphamide. New onset or aggravation of renal disease during the second and third trimesters of pregnancy render diagnosis of pre-eclampsia difficult. Prematurity and pre-eclampsia are the most common complications in pregnancies with renal involvement.

Behçet's disease

Available data suggest that pregnancy does not aggravate maternal disease, though a relapse may occur in about 20% of Behçet's disease (BD) pregnancies. Three retrospective series reporting on 25, 44, and 77 pregnancies of women with BD respectively showed improvement or even remission in 53–80%.[46] Flares consisted of oral or genital ulcers, arthritis, and eye inflammation. Serious maternal complications were rare.

A case-control study comparing 77 pregnancies in BD patients and 288 pregnancies in healthy controls showed a significantly higher rate of adverse outcome in BD patients than in the control group (26% vs 2%). Miscarriage occurred in 21% of BD patients compared to 5.2% in healthy women.[51] Surgical delivery was more frequent in women with BD (15% vs 5%). Hypertension and gestational diabetes mellitus occurred more often in pregnant BD patients. No difference was found in regard to neonatal health or birthweight.

Preconception counselling and monitoring during pregnancy

Pregnancy in patients with CTD requires preconception counselling. The task of the physician is to discuss disease-related problems, identify maternal and fetal risks, and organize the adequate monitoring during pregnancy and postpartum. In general, a higher

risk for the mother and the fetus is marked by an early stage of disease, an active disease at conception, the presence of aPL or anti-Ro/SS-A and/or anti-La/SS-B, and some types of drugs before or at certain stages of pregnancy (Box 16.1). An early stage of disease implies that the pattern of disease severity is not yet apparent and complications could still develop in the near future. A patient with active rheumatic disease should postpone pregnancy until remission or stable disease is achieved and has persisted for at least 6 months. A review of the previous obstetric history of the patient reveals past adverse events during pregnancy which are highly predictive of complications during subsequent pregnancies. Also, a high degree of damage in vital organs, such as the heart, lung, or kidneys, markedly increases the probability of further maternal deterioration and decreases the likelihood of a term live birth. A suggested list of items to be checked in the preconception visit is given in Box 16.1.

Before pregnancy, access to familial and social support should be evaluated, so it is advantageous to include the patient's partner or a family member in the preconception counselling. In order for the patient with impaired function to prepare for the task of childcare after delivery, consulting an occupational therapist is advisable. All patients should be informed about the influence of lifestyle factors, and be advised to stop smoking and to take supplementary folic acid before conception.

At the start of pregnancy a complete clinical and laboratory assessment is necessary in order to monitor disease activity. High-risk pregnancies are best monitored by an interdisciplinary specialist team including the obstetrician and the rheumatologist/internist, and, occasionally, the paediatrician. The frequency of visits depends on disease severity, type of therapy, and stage of pregnancy. Regular assessment of fetal growth can predict whether the fetus is at risk. Doppler flow techniques allow evaluation of the uteroplacental and umbilical circulation, and help predict complications such as pre-eclampsia and intrauterine growth restriction. The negative predictive value of Doppler studies is very high, so a normal examination is reassuring. Women with a previous history

---

Box 16.1 Preconception visit checklist

- Age
- Any previous pregnancy?
- Previous pregnancy complications (pre-eclampsia, prematurity, intrauterine growth restriction)?
- Presence of severe irreversible organ damage (kidney, lung, heart)?
- Recent or current disease activity?
- Presence of antiphospholipid antibodies/syndrome?
- Positivity of anti-Ro/anti-La?
- Current treatment with fetotoxic drugs (including cyclophosphamide, methotrexate, mycophenolate, angiotensin-converting enzyme inhibitors, angiotensin II receptor blockers, diuretics, and statins?)
- Other chronic medical conditions? (hypertension, diabetes, etc.)
- Smoking?

Table 16.1 Drug therapy of complications of rheumatic diseases during pregnancy

Disease	Complication	Drugs compatible in case of pregnancy complication	Time of treatment during pregnancy	Drugs to be discontinued before pregnancy
Rheumatoid arthritis, ankylosing spondylitis, JIA, psoriatic arthritis	Active arthritis during pregnancy	NSAIDs	1st + 2nd trimester, discontinue at week 32	Rituximab, abatacept, tocilizumab, anakinra methotrexate, leflunomide, misoprostol
		Paracetamol	Throughout pregnancy	
		Antimalarials, salazopyrine	Throughout pregnancy	
		Prednisone	Throughout pregnancy	
		Intra-articular corticosteroids	Throughout pregnancy	
		TNF inhibitors	1st trimester	
Systemic lupus erythematosus	Active disease during pregnancy	Antimalarials, prednisone	Throughout pregnancy	MMF, cyclophosphamide, rituximab, belimumab
		Azathioprine	Throughout pregnancy	
	Lupus nephritis	Ciclosporin, tacrolimus	Throughout pregnancy	
		IVIG	Throughout pregnancy	
Antiphospholipid syndrome	Prevention of fetal loss	Low dose aspirin alone or plus LMWH*	Throughout pregnancy at prophylactic dose LMWH	
	Prevention of thrombosis	Low dose aspirin + LMWH	Throughout pregnancy at therapeutic dose LMWH	Coumarin derivatives
Systemic sclerosis	Renal crisis	Antihypertensives, e.g. methyldopa, nifedipine, atenolol	Throughout pregnancy	ACE inhibitors, endothelin receptor antagonists, coumarin derivatives
	Pulmonary hypertension Restrictive lung disease	Prostaglandin analogues, sildenafil, LMWH	Throughout pregnancy	
Polymyositis/dermatomyositis	Active disease during pregnancy	Prednisone, azathioprine, IVIG	Throughout pregnancy	Methotrexate, cyclophosphamide, MMF
Systemic vasculitis	Active vasculitis	Prednisone, azathioprine, IVIG	Throughout pregnancy	Cyclophosphamide, rituximab
Neonatal lupus syndromes	1st or 2nd degree AV block Myocarditis, ascites, hydrops fetalis	Preferentially betamethasone, dexamethasone (more side effects on child)	2nd and 3rd trimester	

AV, atrioventricular; IVIG, intravenous immunoglobulin; LMWH, low molecular weight heparin; MMF, mycophenolate mofetil; NSAIDs, non-steroidal anti-inflammatory drugs.

of pre-eclampsia, placental insufficiency, hypertension, renal disease (even if in remission and with normal renal function), and aPL, as well as those with multiple pregnancies, are candidates for Doppler studies starting at week 20. Serial fetal echocardiography between weeks 18 and 28 is important for detecting early incomplete heart block and myocarditis in a fetus with anti-Ro/SS-A and/or anti-La/SS-B-positive mother, since both conditions have the potential for improvement after treatment.

Specific therapy of the different rheumatic diseases during pregnancy should be guided by disease severity and fetal safety (Table 16.1). Prophylactic withdrawal of safe drugs must be avoided, since the risk of a disease flare, with harmful consequences for both the mother and the fetus, is high.

References

1. Østensen M. New insights into sexual functioning and fertility in rheumatic diseases. *Best Pract Res Clin Rheumatol* 2004;18:219–232.

2. Wallenius M, Skomsvoll JF, Irgens LM, et al. Fertility in women with chronic inflammatory arthritides. *Rheumatology (Oxford)* 2011;50: 1162–1167.

3. Skomsvoll JF, Østensen M, Baste V, Irgens LM. Number of births, inter-pregnancy interval, and subsequent pregnancy rate after a diagnosis of inflammatory rheumatic disease in Norwegian women. *J Rheumatol* 2001;28:2310–2314.

4. Katz PP. Childbearing decisions and family size among women with rheumatoid arthritis. *Arthritis Rheum* 2006;55(2):217–223.

5. Nelson JL, Ostensen M. Pregnancy and rheumatoid arthritis. *Rheum Dis Clin North Am* 1997;23(1):195–212.

6. Barrett JH, Brennan P, Fiddler M, Silman AJ. Does rheumatoid arthritis remit during pregnancy and relapse postpartum? Results from a nation-wide study in the United Kingdom performed prospectively from late pregnancy. *Arthritis Rheum* 1999;42(6):1219–1227.

7. de Man YA, Dolhain RJ, van de Geijn FE, Willemsen SP, Hazes JM. Disease activity of rheumatoid arthritis during pregnancy: results from a nationwide prospective study. *Arthritis Rheum* 2008;59(9): 1241–1248.

8. de Man YA, Hazes JM, van de Geijn FE, Krommenhoek C, Dolhain RJ. Measuring disease activity and functionality during pregnancy in patients with rheumatoid arthritis. *Arthritis Rheum* 2007;57(5):716–722.

9. Drossaers-Bakker KW, Zwinderman AH, van Zeben D, Breedveld FC, Hazes JM. Pregnancy and oral contraceptive use do not significantly influence outcome in long-term rheumatoid arthritis. *Ann Rheum Dis* 2002;61:405–408.

10. de Man YA, Bakker-Jonges LE, Goorbergh CM, et al. Women with rheumatoid arthritis negative for anti-cyclic citrullinated peptide and rheumatoid factor are more likely to improve during pregnancy, whereas in autoantibody-positive women autoantibody levels are not influenced by pregnancy. *Ann Rheum Dis* 2010;69(2):420–423.

11. Østensen M, Villiger PM. The remission of rheumatoid arthritis during pregnancy. *Semin Immunopathol* 2007;29(2):185–191.

12. Hazes JM, van der Heide H, Willemsen SP et al. Association of higher rheumatoid arthritis disease activity during pregnancy with lower birth weight: results of a national prospective study. *Arthritis Rheum* 2009; 60(11):3196–3206.

13. Wallenius M, Skomsvoll JF, Irgens LM et al. Pregnancy and delivery in women with chronic inflammatory arthritides with a specific focus on first birth. *Arthritis Rheum* 2011;63(6):1534–1542.

14. Østensen M, Østensen H. Ankylosing spondylitis—the female aspect. *J Rheumatol* 1998;25(1):120–124.

15. Østensen M. Pregnancy in psoriatic arthritis. *Scand J Rheumatol* 1988;17:67–70.

16. Østensen M, Fuhrer L, Mathieu R, Seitz M, Villiger PM. A prospective study of pregnant patients with rheumatoid arthritis and ankylosing spondylitis using validated clinical instruments. *Ann Rheum Dis* 2004;63(10):1212–1217.

17. Østensen M. Pregnancy in patients with a history of juvenile rheumatoid arthritis. *Arthritis Rheum* 1991;34:881–887.

18. Musiej-Nowakowska E, Ploski R. Pregnancy and early onset pauciarticular juvenile chronic arthritis. *Ann Rheum Dis* 1999;58:475–480.

19. Ruiz-Irastorza G, Lima F, Alves JD et al. Increased rate of lupus flare during pregnancy and the puerperium: a prospective study of 78 pregnancies. *Br J Rheumatol* 1996;35:133–138.

20. Clowse MEB, Magder LS, Witter F, Petri MA. The impact of increased lupus activity on obstetric outcomes. *Arthritis Rheum* 2005;52:514–521.

21. Clowse MEB, Magder L, Witter F, Petri MA. Hydroxychloroquine in lupus pregnancy. *Arthritis Rheum* 2006;54:3640–3467.

22. Petri M. The Hopkins Lupus Pregnancy Center: ten key issues in management. *Rheum Dis Clin N Am* 2007;33:27–35.

23. Germain S, Nelson-Piercy C. Lupus nephritis and renal disease in pregnancy. *Lupus* 2006;15:148–155.

24. Andrade RM, McGwin Jr G, Alarcon GS et al. Predictors of post-partum damage accrual in systemic lupus erythematosus: data from LUMINA, a multiethnic US cohort (XXXVIII). *Rheumatology* 2006;45:1380–1384.

25. Cuadrado MJ, Mendonça LLF, Khamashta MA et al. Maternal and fetal outcome in antiphospholipid syndrome pregnancies with a history of previous cerebral ischemia. *Arthritis Rheum* 1999;42:S265.

26. Ruiz-Irastorza G, Crowther MA, Branch W, Khamashta MA. Antiphospholipid syndrome. *Lancet* 2010;376:1498–1509.

27. Smyth A, Oliveira GHM, Lahr BD et al. A systematic review and meta-analysis of pregnancy outcomes in patients with systemic lupus erythematosus and lupus nephritis. *Clin J Am Soc Nephrol* 2010;5(11):1–9.

28. Nodler J, Moolamalla SR, Ledger EM, Nuwayhid BS, Mulla ZD. Elevated antiphospholipid antibody titers and adverse pregnancy outcomes: analysis of a population-based hospital dataset. *BMC Preg Childbirth* 2009;9:11.

29. Yamada H, Atsumi T, Kobashi G et al. Antiphospholipid antibodies increase the risk of pregnancy-induced hypertension and adverse pregnancy outcomes. *J Reprod Immunol* 2009;79:188–195.

30. Ruffatti A, Calligaro A, Hoxha A et al.| Laboratory and clinical features of pregnant women with antiphospholipid syndrome and neonatal outcome. *Arthritis Care Res* 2010;62: 302–307.

31. Bramham K, Hunt BJ, Germain S et al. Pregnancy outcome in different clinical phenotypes of antiphospholipid syndrome. *Lupus* 2010;9:58–64.

32. Takaya M, Ichikawa Y, Shimizu H et al. Sjögren's syndrome and pregnancy. *Tokai J Exp Clin Med* 1991;16:83–88.

33. Haga HJ, Gjesdal CG, Koksvik HS et al. Pregnancy outcome in patients with primary Sjögren's syndrome. *J Rheumatol* 2005;32:1734–1736.

34. Izmirly PM, Rivera TL, Buyon JP Neonatal lupus syndromes. *Rheum Dis Clin N Am* 2007;33: 267–285.

35. Brucato A, Frassi M, Franceschini F et al. Risk of congenital complete heart block in newborns of mothers with anti-Ro/SSA antibodies detected by counterimmunoelectrophoresis: a prospective study of 100 women. *Arthritis Rheum* 2001;44:1832–1835.

36. Izmirly PM, Llanos C, Lee LA et al. Cutaneous manifestations of neonatal lupus and risk of subsequent congenital heart block. *Arthritis Rheum* 2010;62:1153–1157.

37. Ostensen M, Khamashta M, Lockshin M et al. Anti-inflammatory and immunosuppressive drugs and reproduction. *Arthritis Res Ther* 2006;8:209–227.

38. Friedman D, Llanos C, Izmirly PM et al. Evaluation of fetuses in a study of intravenous immunoglobulin as preventive therapy for congenital heart block: Results of a multicenter, prospective, open-label clinical trial. *Arthritis Rheum* 2010;62:1138–1146.

39. Pisoni C, Brucato A, Ruffatti A et al. Failure of intravenous immunoglobulin to prevent congenital heart block: Findings of a multicenter, prospective, observational study. *Arthritis Rheum* 2010;62:1147–1152.

40. Izmirly PM, Kim MY, Llanos C et al. Evaluation of the risk of anti-SSA/Ro-SSB/La antibody-associated cardiac manifestations of neonatal lupus in fetuses of mothers with systemic lupus erythematosus exposed to hydroxychloroquine. *Ann Rheum Dis* 2010;69:1827–1830.

41. Steen VD. Scleroderma and pregnancy. *Rheum Dis Clin North Am* 2007;33:345–358.

42. Østensen M, Brucato A, Carp H et al. Pregnancy and reproduction in autoimmune rheumatic diseases. *Rheumatology (Oxford)* 2011;50(4): 657–664.

43. Chakravarty EF, Khanna D, Chung L. Pregnancy outcomes in systemic sclerosis, primary pulmonary hypertension, and sickle cell disease. *Obstet Gynecol* 2008;111:927–934.

44. Silva CA, Sultan SM, Isenberg DA. Pregnancy outcome in adult-onset idiopathic inflammatory myopathy. *Rheumatology* 2003;42:1168–1172.

45. Vancsa A, Ponyi A, Constantin T et al. Pregnancy outcome in idiopathic inflammatory myopathy. *Rheumatol Int* 2007;27:435–439.

46. Doria A, Iaccarino L, Ghirardello A et al. Pregnancy in rare autoimmune rheumatic diseases: UCTD, MCTD, myositis, systemic vasculitis and Behçet disease. *Lupus* 2004;13:690–695.

47. Pagnoux C, Le Guern V, Goffinet F et al. Pregnancies in systemic necrotizing vasculitides: report on 12 women and their 20 pregnancies. *Rheumatology (Oxford)* 2011;50(5):953–961.

48. Iscovich A, Gislason R, Fadev A, Grisaru-Granovsky S, Halpern S. Peripartum anesthetic management of patients with Takayasu's arteritis: case series and review. *Int J Obstet Anesth* 2008;17:358–364.

49. Koukoura O, Mantas N, Linardakis H, Hajioannou J, Sifakis S. Successful term pregnancy in a patient with Wegener's granulomatosis: case report and literature review. *Fertil Steril* 2008;89:457, e1–e5.

50. Corradi D, Maestri R, Facchetti F. Postpartum Churg-Strauss syndrome with severe cardiac involvement: Description of a case and review of the literature. *Clin Rheumatol* 2009;28(6);739–742.

51. Uzun S, Alpsoy E, Durdu M, Akman A. The clinical course of Behçet's disease in pregnancy: a retrospective analysis and review of the literature. *J Dermatol* 2003;30:499–502.

CHAPTER 17

Skin

Christopher Griffiths and Amy Foulkes

How to approach the patient with a rash

Background

Structure and function of skin

A basic overview of the structure and function of skin allows a greater understanding of the morphology of skin disease. Skin is composed of three layers: epidermis, dermis, and subcutis (Figure 17.1). Epidermis, the outermost avascular layer, is composed primarily of keratinocytes. Pathology affecting the epidermis leads to a change in the texture of the skin, such as scaling or erosion. Other important epidermal cells are melanin-synthesizing melanocytes and antigen-presenting Langerhans cells.

The dermis is vascular and less cellular than the epidermis. Fibroblasts predominate; the main extracellular matrix constituents are collagen and elastin. Pathology affecting the dermis may alter skin morphology, e.g. swelling/lump with a normal skin surface. Below the dermis is the subcutaneous layer, the subcutis. This layer is composed primarily of adipose tissue, blood vessels, nerves, and the base of hair follicles and sweat glands.

The primary functions of the skin are its barrier function, immune surveillance, prevention of desiccation, temperature control, and sensory function.

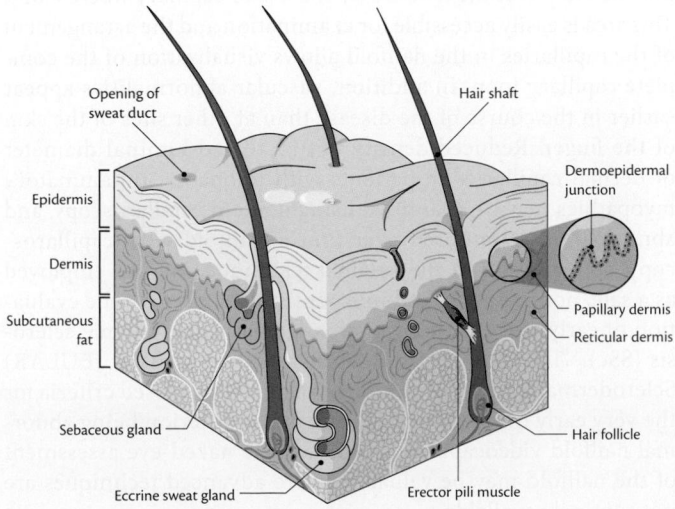

Fig. 17.1 Structure of skin.

History taking

Taking a history from a dermatology patient requires asking specific questions in order to elucidate the relevant details. Questions are divided into consideration of site/distribution, and morphology of the rash.

Site

◆ Where is the rash at present?

◆ Where did the rash start?

◆ How has the rash changed since it started?

◆ Did each lesion progress or were they stationary?

◆ Was the rash transient (e.g. urticarial wheals lasting less than 24 hours)?

Distribution

Many diseases have a characteristic pattern, e.g. psoriasis vulgaris over extensor surfaces, chronic cutaneous lupus erythematosus at photoexposed sites (scalp, face, anterior chest, dorsa of hands).

◆ Did the rash cover all areas of the body equally or are there areas of sparing?

◆ Did the rash migrate?

◆ Does the rash vary with season and/or exposure to sunlight?

Morphology

◆ What is the appearance of each area of affected skin?

◆ Is the rash painful?

◆ Does it itch?

◆ Did the rash ever bleed/weep/crust over?

Other questions

◆ Is there anything that provokes the rash or helps it resolve such as antihistamines?

◆ Drug history: For dermatology this should include use of topical agents, treatment with phototherapy, and systemic agents as well as the use of over-the-counter preparations

◆ Family history of skin disease.

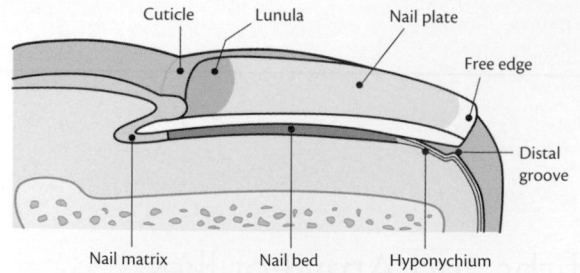

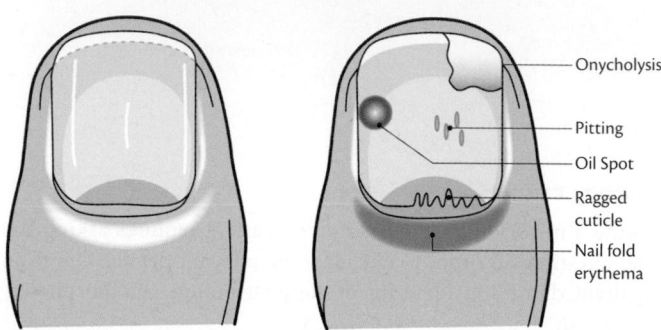

Fig. 17.2 Normal nail anatomy and pathology.

How to examine the skin

Before examining the skin, the set-up of a room and the positioning of the patient are important.

Site and distribution

The examination room should be well lit (ideally with natural light) with a couch that can accommodate the patient lying down and be raised in order to view lesions on the back or feet. The patient must be adequately undressed to view the rash.

Specific areas are frequently missed, for example scalp, nails, and mucous membranes. Nail structure and nail pathology seen in rheumatological disease are illustrated in Figure 17.2.

Patients frequently photograph their rashes and these may provide valuable clinical clues. The distribution of a rash can only be evaluated if the whole of the skin is examined.

Morphology

Description of a rash

An accurate description of the rash may allow diagnosis or gain a swift referral diagnosis perhaps by telephone. For example a papular, pruritic erythematous eruption affecting the trunk and limbs sparing the face, palms, and soles would be a typical description of a classic drug eruption. Similarly, accurate detailed description may aid diagnosis, e.g. the distribution of dermatomyositis over the extensor surfaces of the fingers. Dermatological descriptors are listed in Figure 17.3. The colour of a rash is important. Pigmentation is variable and not merely brown or black. 'Erythematous' means redness, but rashes may also appear purple or violaceous, e.g. lichen planus (rashes that have similar histology and phenotypically appear purple are termed 'lichenoid', e.g. dermatomyositis).

Skin lesions may have a characteristic or diagnostic appearance, e.g. targetoid with erythema multiforme (Figure 17.4).

Investigations

Where clinical morphology is insufficient for a firm diagnosis, investigative techniques may be employed. In dermatology these include:

- Blood tests
  - Autoantibodies
  - Indirect immunofluorescence
- Histology
  - Haematoxylin and eosin (H&E)
  - Direct immunofluorescence
- Other
  - Nailfold capillary microscopy/videocapillaroscopy

Although a skin biopsy is a commonly performed minor procedure, we recommend that all diagnostic biopsies be taken by a dermatologist, or a by healthcare professional adequately trained in the technique with expert dermatopathology support available.

Clinico-pathological correlation is required, with dermato-histopathology support in order to facilitate accurate diagnosis. Where possible, a link provided to a clinical photograph or a sketch of the initial distribution or eruption may be of assistance to the pathologist.

Histology may not always yield a diagnosis. Immunohistological techniques allow for the detection of antigens, antibodies and other tissue components to aid a specific diagnosis.[1] Immunofluorescence (IMF) utilizes an antibody to bind to a required antigen and a fluorochrome dye to detect the position of the antibody. Direct IMF is used on skin biopsy samples and indirect IMF may be used on blood samples. The primary application in dermatology is the recognition of autoimmune bullous disorders, where autoantibodies are directed against adhesive proteins such as desmogleins in the epidermis and basement membrane. Another example is the detection of IgA in dermal vessels in Henoch–Schonlein purpura.

In connective tissue disease, distortion in capillary architecture may be viewed at the nailfold by the use of capillary microscopy. This area is easily accessible for examination and the arrangement of the capillaries in the nailfold allows visualization of the complete capillary loop. In addition, vascular abnormalities appear earlier in the course of the disease than at other sites of the skin of the finger. Reduced density but increased luminal diameter of dermal capillaries in patients with idiopathic inflammatory myopathies may be quantified using nailfold capillaroscopy, and abnormalities monitored over time.[2] Nailfold videocapillaroscopy, an extension of the original technique, may be employed as a safe, non-invasive, and inexpensive technique in the evaluation of early and advanced microangiopathy in systemic sclerosis (SSc).[3] The European League against Rheumatism (EULAR) Scleroderma Trial and Research Group have proposed criteria for the very early diagnosis of SSc, one major criterion being abnormal nailfold videocapillaroscopy.[4] Simple naked-eye assessment of the nailfold may be valuable where advanced techniques are not routinely available.

Lesion	Definition	Morphology	Examples
Primary skin lesions			
Macule	A flat impalpable area of altered skin pigmentation	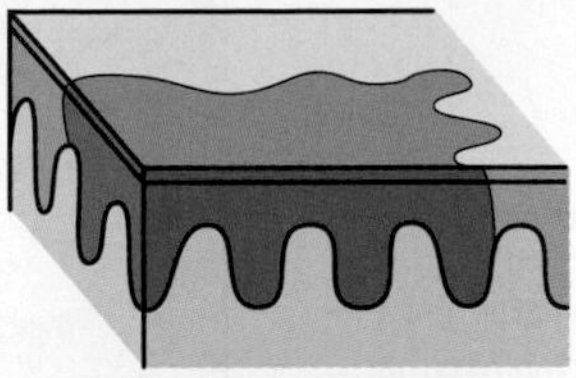	Ephelides (freckle) Lentigo ('liver spot') Café au lait macule
Papule	A palpable (raised) area under 0.5cm in diameter	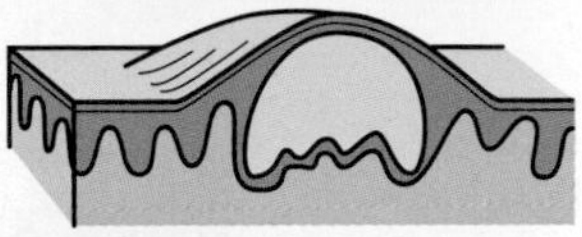	Acrochordon (skin tag), viral wart, lesion of widespread eruption
Nodule	A large papule 0.5–1cm in diameter	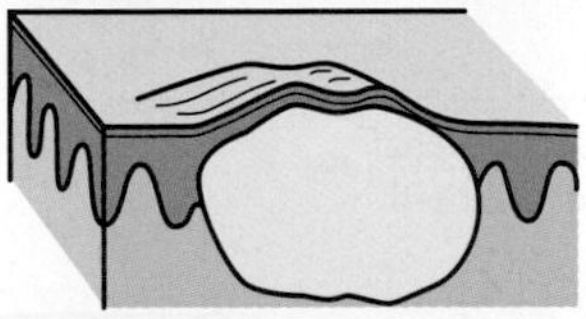	Basal cell carcinoma
Plaque	Raised area of over 1cm diameter	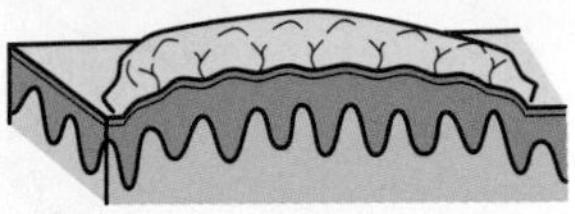	Plaque of psoriasis
Vesicle	A small blister (fluid-filled lesion) >0.5cm in diameter	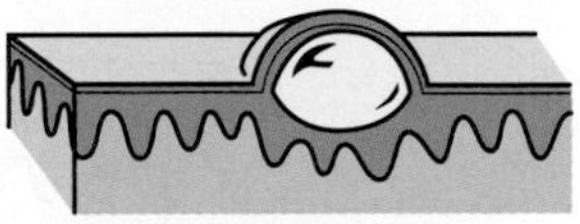	Herpes simplex
Bulla	A blister >0.5cm in diameter	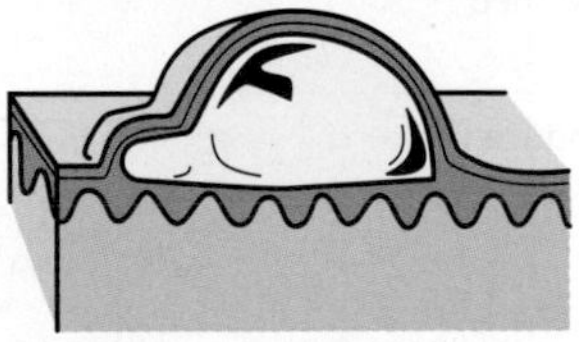	Oedema blister, blister of bullous pemphigoid
Pustule	Pus filled papule	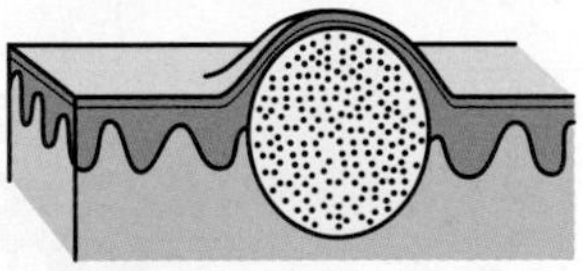	Acne, impetigo, folliculitis, pustular psoriasis
Secondary skin lesion			
Crust	Collection of cellular debris, dried serum and blood—a scab. Usually follows a vesicle, bulla or pustule	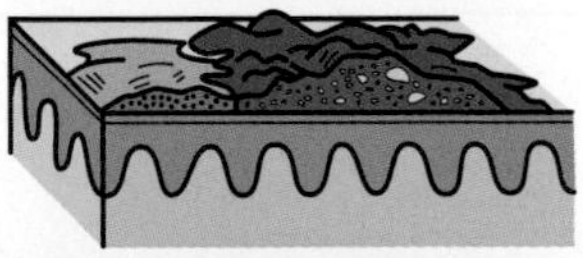	
Erosion	Partial focal loss of epidermis. May heal without scarring. A linear erosion produced by scratching is an excoriation.	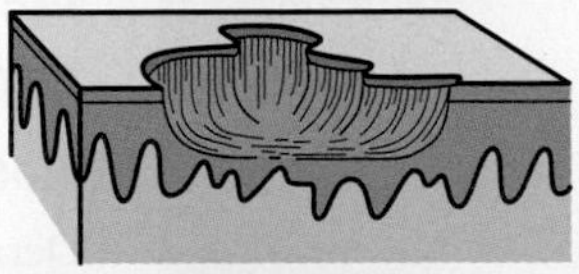	
Ulcer	Loss of epidermis and dermis 'full-thickness' heals with scarring	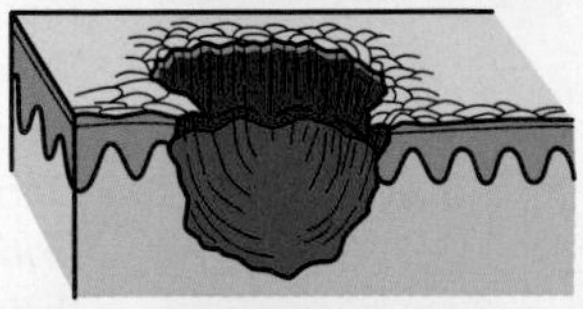	Pyoderma gangrenosum
Fissure/crack	Vertical loss of epidermis +/– dermis with sharply defined walls	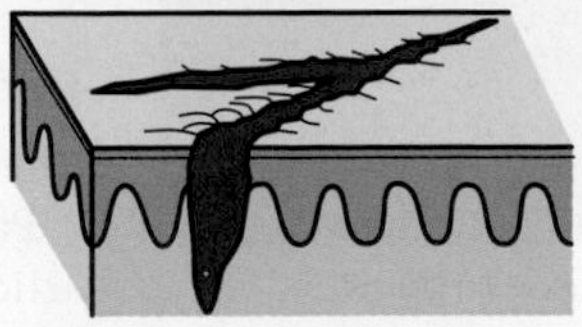	Complicates palmo-plantar pustulosis or hand and foot eczema

Fig. 17.3 Dermatological descriptors.

Cyst	Fluid filled nodule	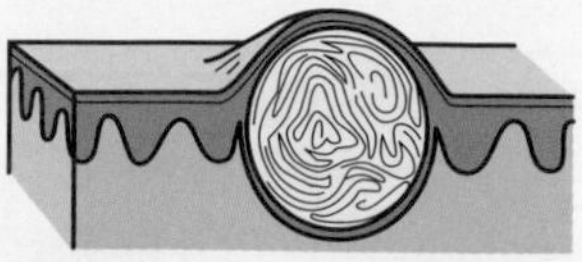	Acne, epidermal cyst
Scar	A collection of new connective tissue; may be raised (hypertrophic) or indented (atrophic). Proceeded by epidermal/dermal damage.	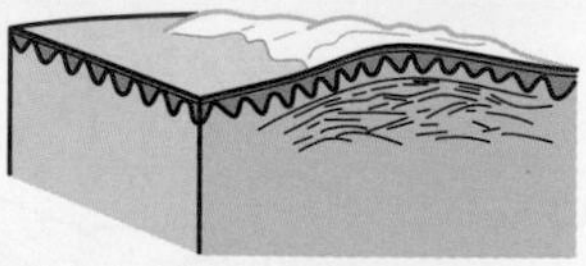	
Scale	Thick stratum corneum that results from hyperproliferation or increased cohesion of keratinocytes	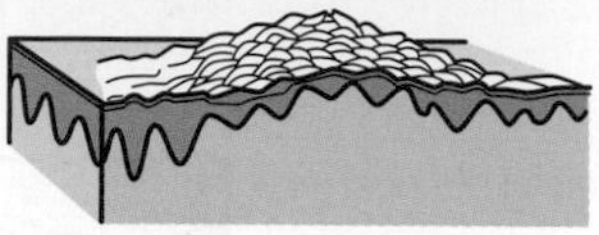	Psoriasis, chronic cutaneous lupus erythematosus
Comedo	Collection of sebum & keratin around a hair follicle. May be open 'blackhead' or closed 'whitehead'	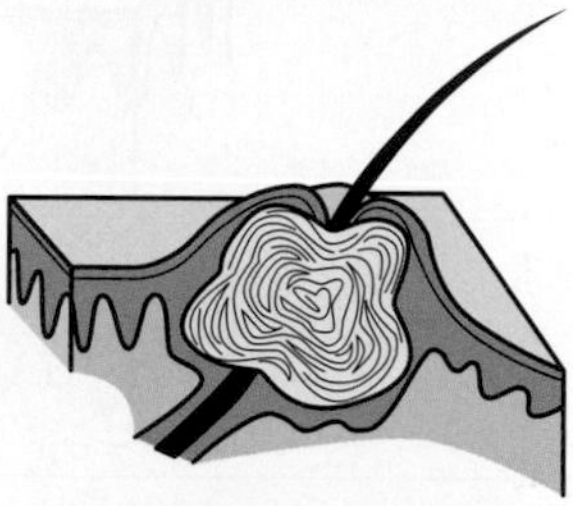	Acne
Atrophy	Thinning of the epidermis, dermis or subcutis. Epidermal atrophy may lead to wrinkled appearance. Atrophy with telangiectasia is termed poikiloderma.	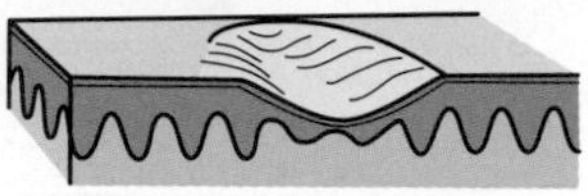	Steroid atrophy in patient with chronic cutaneous lupus erythematosus
Lichenification	Focal area of thickened skin produced by scratching/rubbing.	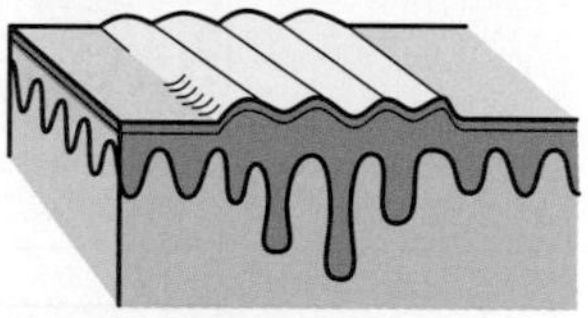	
Telangiectasia	Small dilated superficial blood vessels that disappear with pressure	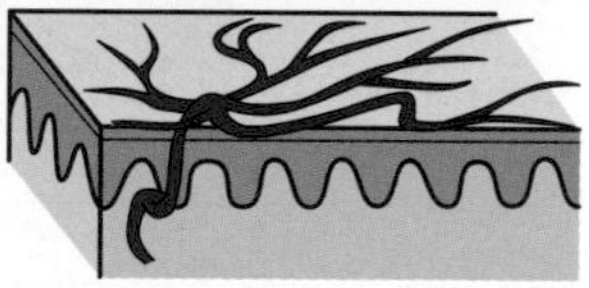	Dermatomyositis

Fig. 17.3 (Continued)

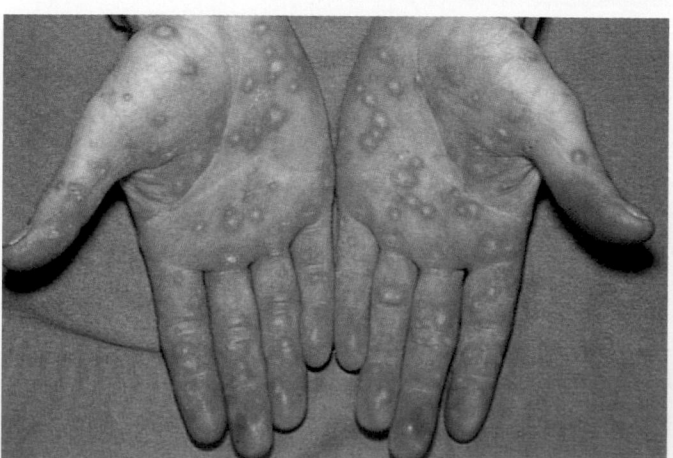

Fig. 17.4 Erythema multiforme; characteristic 'target lesions' on palms.

Dermatological manifestations of rheumatological disease

Note on treatment modalities in dermatology

Dermatological therapies can be broadly divided into three groups: topical therapy, phototherapy, and systemic/biological therapy. Therapeutic agents from each group may be combined to form the optimum management for an individual patient. The British Association of Dermatologists has published a number of clinical guidelines in the *British Journal of Dermatology*.[5,6] Up-to-date versions are available via their website www.bad.org.uk/site/622/default.aspx.[7]

Rheumatoid arthritis

Rheumatoid arthritis (RA) is discussed in Chapters 109–112.

Patients with RA may have general or specific cutaneous extra-articular manifestations of their disease The possible cutaneous manifestations of RA have been well reviewed,[8,9] and a comprehensive overview of individual manifestations may be found elsewhere.[10]

General cutaneous extra-articular manifestations of RA include palmar erythema (a general reddening of the palms) skin fragility with atrophy, easy bruising, and pseudo-sclerodermatous changes, particularly of the hands. Nail changes include longitudinal ridging (onychorrhexis) and clubbing.[9]

Specific cutaneous extra-articular manifestations are described in the following sections.

Rheumatoid vasculitis

Vasculitis refers to inflammation of blood vessels (arteries and/or veins). Rheumatologists may encounter vasculitis as a component of systemic disease including RA, systemic lupus erythematosus (SLE), Sjögren's syndrome, dermatomyositis, and mixed connective tissue disease, amongst others. Rheumatoid vasculitis refers to the spectrum of inflammation of blood vessels seen in RA. Vasculitis may be local or systemic, primary or secondary, and any size of vessel may be affected. Many vasculitides have a cutaneous component and classification is confusing. For a comprehensive review of cutaneous vasculitides, see Cox et al.[11]

The mounting evidence for vascular pathology in RA, with the occurrence of large-vessel atherosclerosis, is discussed in Chapter 109.

Demographics

Rheumatoid vasculitis occurs in less than 1% of patients with RA.[12] Livido reticularis, a condition where dilatation of capillaries leads to mottled reticular discolouration of the skin, may also occur, most frequently on the extremities (Figure 17.5).

Cutaneous small-vessel vasculitis (otherwise known as leucocytoclastic or hypersentivity vasculitis) is the most common cutaneous vasculitis, affecting both children and adults, more commonly in women.

Key clinical features

Palpable purpura of the distal extremities (Figure 17.6). Purpura may coalesce, leading to erosion or ulceration, and bullae may occur (Figure 17.7). Other cutaneous lesions may include digital infarcts. Associated features may include peripheral neuropathy.

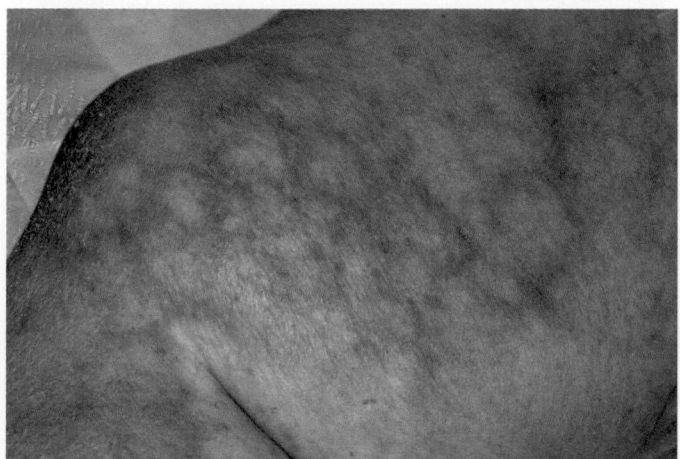

Fig. 17.5 Livedo reticularis; right thigh of hospitalized patient.

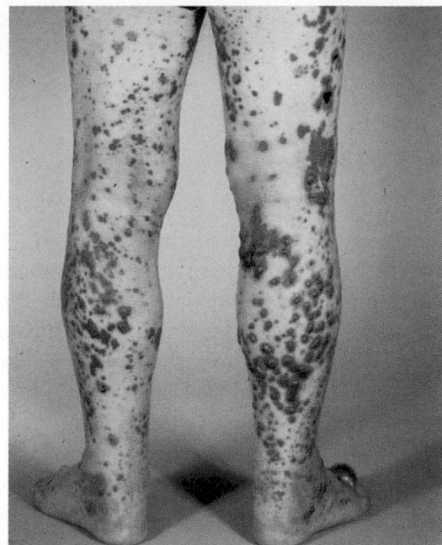

Fig. 17.6 Cutaneous small-vessel vasculitis; symmetrically distributed across lower legs.

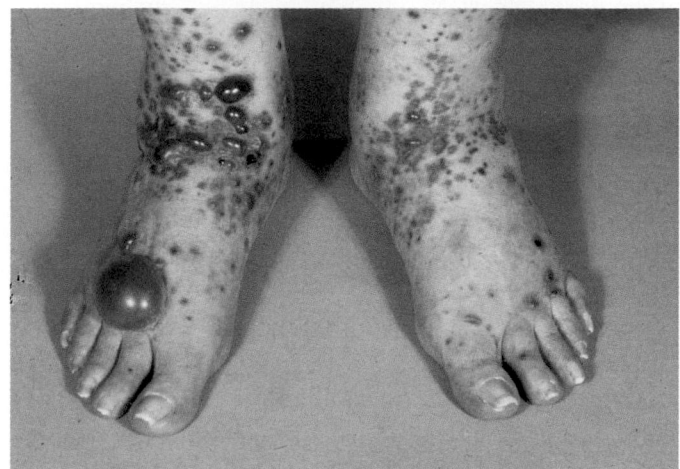

Fig. 17.7 Cutaneous small-vessel vasculitis; bullae forming across oedematous feet.

Rheumatoid vasculitis must be considered where leg ulcers develop in a patient with RA.

Investigations   The evaluation of a patient with suspected vasculitis should include clinical evaluation to examine the extent of disease with regard to skin and internal organ involvement, an attempt to discern the aetiology, and histopathological correlation of the clinical diagnosis. Although extensive investigations may fail to elucidate an underlying cause, blood pressure measurement and urinalysis are essential initial investigations.

Biopsy of an affected area may confirm the clinical diagnosis as vasculitis but provide few clues to the underlying cause, and should be carefully considered where the affected limb is swollen, as poor healing may occur. Classic histology of cutaneous small-vessel vasculitis would demonstrate endothelial swelling, fibrinoid necrosis of vessel walls, extravasation of erythrocytes, and an infiltrate of neutrophils with fragmentation of nuclei (leucocytoclasia).

Management   Overall, cutaneous small-vessel vasculitis has a benign course. Rest with elevation of the affected limbs is essential, as is expert meticulous topical skin care of purpuric lesions/erosions or ulceration to prevent trauma and secondary infection.

Nailfold infarction has no specific treatment.

Rheumatoid nodule

This is discussed in Chapter 111.

Demographics

Classic rheumatoid nodules occur in approximately 25% of cases of RA and are the most common extra-articular manifestation.[9] Although most common on the ulnar border of the forearm, they may be found elsewhere, including dorsa of the hands, ears, and over the scapulae.[10] They may also appear in other organs, including the lungs. Classically firm in consistency, with a propensity to ulcerate with trauma, they may also demonstrate overlying skin changes such as violaceous discolouration. Rheumatoid nodules are more likely to be associated with severe disease, positive rheumatoid factor,[9] and anti-nuclear factor.[10] Histologically, rheumatoid nodules show palisading fibroblasts and histiocytes, with foci of fibrinoid necrosis.

Differential diagnoses

Rheumatic fever, Still's disease, erythema elevatum diutinum.

Investigations

Unlikely to require investigation, unless there is either superadded infection—staphylococcal secondary infection can lead to septic arthritis, or diagnostic uncertainty, where histopathology may distinguish from the aforementioned differential diagnoses.

Management

Patient advice and topical treatment of ulceration may be required.

Felty's syndrome

The triad of RA, leucopenia, and splenomegaly is discussed in Chapter 111.

Demographics

The incidence of Felty's disease in RA is approximately 1%.[13]

Key clinical features

Cutaneous manifestations include rheumatoid nodules, hyperpigmentation and leg ulcers.[14] Patients may also be at an increased risk of malignant melanoma.[15]

Differential diagnoses

Rheumatoid nodules, hyperpigmentation, and leg ulcers may also be seen in RA.

Management

Treatment of the RA.

Rheumatoid neutrophilic dermatosis

Demographics

Rheumatoid neutrophilic dermatosis is a rare condition, occurring in patients with severe, active RA.

Key clinical features

Typically asymptomatic, characterized by symmetrically distributed erythematous papules, plaques and/or vesicles over the extensor surfaces.

Differential diagnosis

Sweet's syndrome (another form of neutrophilic dermatosis, Figure 17.8), pyoderma gangrenosum associated with RA.

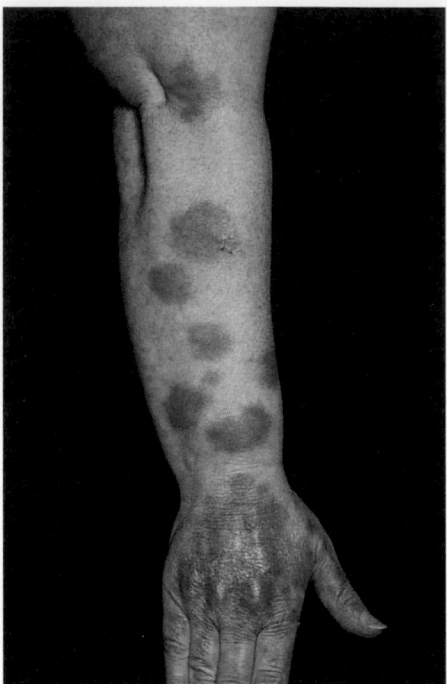

Fig. 17.8 Sweet's syndrome: plaques on forearm and dorsa of hand.

Investigations

Diagnostic skin biopsy will demonstrate dense dermal neutrophilic infiltration that may extend upwards into the epidermis and/or deeply into the subcutaneous fat.

Management

Immunosuppression of the active RA may lead to resolution of the associated condition. Topical corticosteroid, dapsone or hydroxychloroquine may be effective.[10]

Pyoderma gangrenosum

Pyoderma gangrenosum is an uncommon chronic ulcerative condition, part of the spectrum of neutrophilic dermatoses.

Demographics

Commonest in women over the age of 50 years.[16] More than 50% of patients have associated systemic disease, classically inflammatory bowel disease.

Key clinical features

Painful ulceration rapidly develops, with a characteristic overhanging purple/blue edge. Ulceration may commence at a site of recent trauma known as 'pathergy' (Figure 17.9).

Differential diagnoses

Can be difficult to distinguish clinically from infective causes of ulceration, malignancy, and venous ulceration.

Investigations

Diagnosis is made on clinical features and exclusion of other ulcerative conditions. Histology is variable and non-specific but should always be performed to exclude malignancy, specifically squamous cell carcinoma.

Management

Potent immunosuppression; if the ulcer is small this could be local high potency topical corticosteroid or systemic therapy with

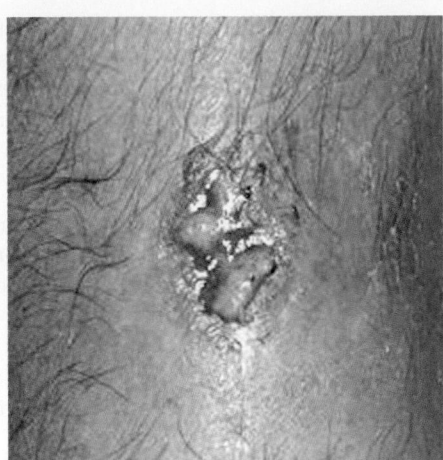

Fig. 17.9 Pyoderma gangrenosum; ulceration developing at site of needle entry (pathergy response).

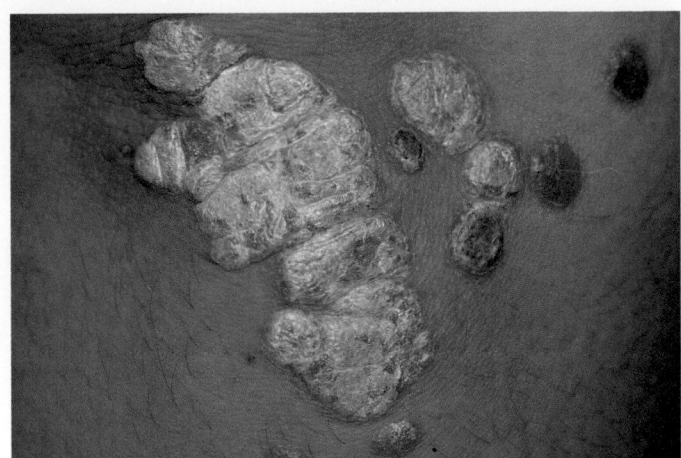

Fig. 17.10 Psoriasis vulgaris; characteristic scaly plaque.

prednisolone, ciclosporin, or a TNF-antagonist biologic such as infliximab.

Psoriasis

Demographics

Psoriasis is a common chronic inflammatory skin disease affecting 1.5–3% of the population.[17] Often dismissed as simply 'a skin disorder', psoriasis is associated with a significant reduction in a patient's quality of life[18] comparable to that of cancer or diabetes.[19] It is associated with a seronegative inflammatory arthritis (psoriatic arthritis) in 7–26% of patients.[20] Patients suffer reduced employment and income[21] and serious comorbidities such as cardiovascular disease[22] and depression.[23] The pathogenesis of psoriasis is incompletely understood. There exists a complex interplay of genetic and environmental factors, leading to a disease-predisposing environment. Most cases of chronic plaque psoriasis present prior to the age of 40 years and are classified as early-onset or type I psoriasis. Late-onset disease, after the age of 40 years, may be classified as type II disease.[24]

Key clinical features

The most common type of psoriasis, psoriasis vulgaris, has a characteristic phenotype; well-delineated erythematous plaques with overlying silvery scale develop symmetrically, with a predominance for the extensor surfaces (Figures 17.10 and 17.11).[17] Where psoriasis covers more than 90% of the body surface area, it is termed erythrodermic (Figure 17.12). Common nail changes include pitting, onycholysis (where nail plate has lifted from nail bed, seen as white patches at distal nail) and translucent yellow/red nail bed discolouration, termed 'salmon patches' or 'oil drops' (Figures 17.2 and 17.13–17.15). Emerging evidence associated the nail changes more closely with enthesitis rather than the accompanying skin disease.

Differential diagnoses

Due to the variety of presentations and clinical manifestations of psoriasis, it may resemble numerous other dermatological conditions such as facial psoriasis and the common inflammatory skin condition seborrhoeic dermatitis, and psoriasis vulgaris may resemble pityriasis rubra pilaris, a rare skin condition characterized by orange/red scaly plaques.

Investigations

Histologically, plaques of psoriasis demonstrate; hyperplasia, increased vascularity in the dermis and a dermal and epidermal

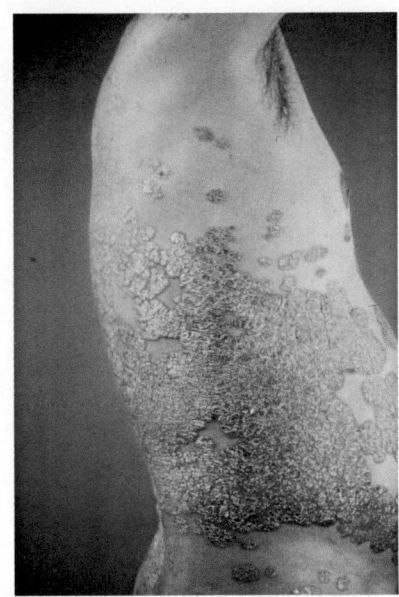

Fig. 17.11 Psoriasis vulgaris; severe disease with small plaques across trunk.

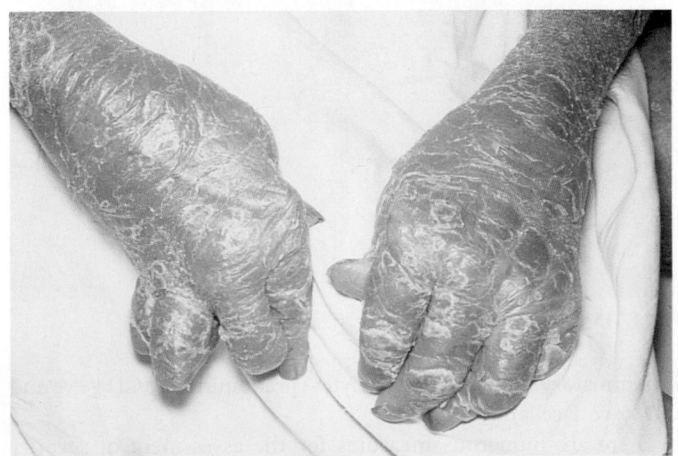

Fig. 17.12 Erythrodermic psoriasis involving the hands in an elderly man with psoriatic arthritis.

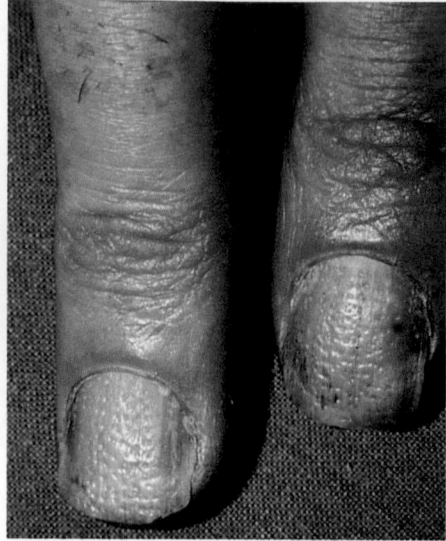

Fig. 17.13 Psoriasis: nail pits with early onycholysis.

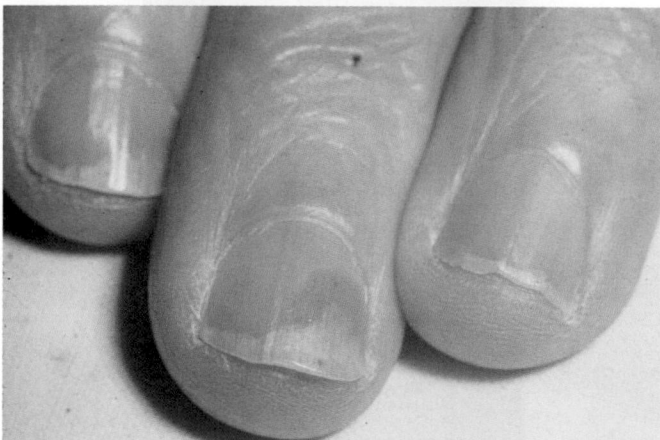

Fig. 17.14 Psoriasis: onycholysis with 'salmon patch'.

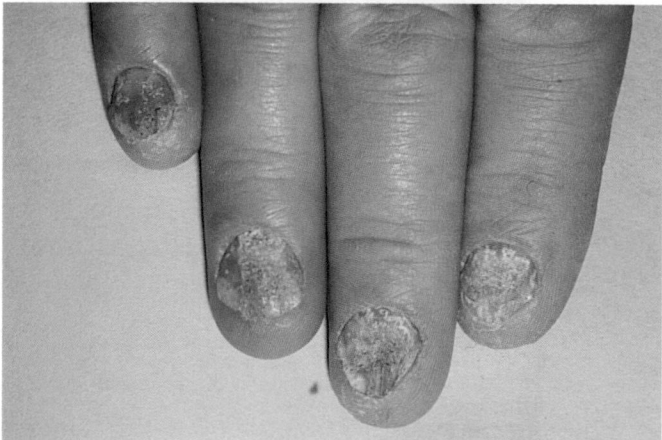

Fig. 17.15 Psoriasis: onycholysis, gross pitting, and nail deformity.

inflammatory infiltrate of leucocytes (predominantly CD4 +ve and CD8 +ve T cells).[17]

There are numerous measures for the assessment of severity of psoriasis and its effect on quality of life indices. The psoriasis area and severity index (PASI) was introduced in the 1970s by Fredriksson and Pettersson and is the most extensively studied psoriasis clinical severity score,[25] although it has limitations, including low responsiveness in mild disease.[26] To calculate a PASI, the erythema, induration, and desquamation at body areas are recorded to form a score between 0 and 72, where 72 is the most severe.

Management

The British Association of Dermatologists has published clear guidelines on the use of biologic therapies in severe psoriasis.[6]

Of note, both the use of potent topical corticosteroids and systemic corticosteroids may lead to severe recurrence of chronic plaque psoriasis (rebound psoriasis) on withdrawal of therapy or the serious complication of generalized pustular Von Zumbusch psoriasis, a variant with appreciable morbidity and mortality.

Connective tissue disorders

Lupus

Lupus erythematosus comprises a group of autoimmune multisystem disorders associated with antibodies against components of the cell nucleus.

Lupus may be divided into two main forms; SLE, which is covered in Chapters 118–119, and chronic cutaneous lupus erythematosus (CCLE) or discoid lupus erythematosus.

Demographics

Discoid lupus is the most common form of cutaneous lupus.[27] The disease typically occurs in adults, with a preponderance for women over the age of 40 years;[28] 80% of patients with CCLE are smokers.[29]

Key clinical features

Clinically, CCLE leads to erythematous scaled, inflamed patches, which heal with scarring and frequently hypopigmentation, thus are cosmetically unsightly (Figure 17.16 and 17.17). The rash tends to occur in a photosensitive distribution. Prominent adherent scale is seen at the hair follicles, with keratotic spikes projecting and resembling carpet tacks, thus the 'carpet tack sign'. CCLE in the scalp is a cause of scarring alopecia (Figure 17.18).

Differential diagnoses

Psoriasis, pityriasis rosea (a self-limiting scaly erythematous rash typically preceded by a 'herald patch').

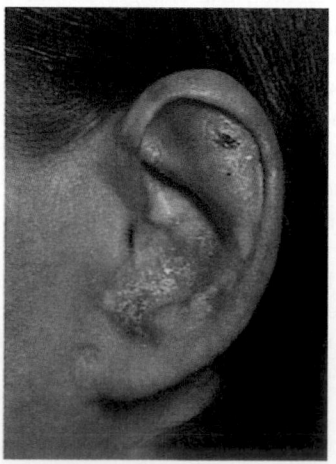

Fig. 17.16 Discoid lupus erythematosus affecting the external ear.

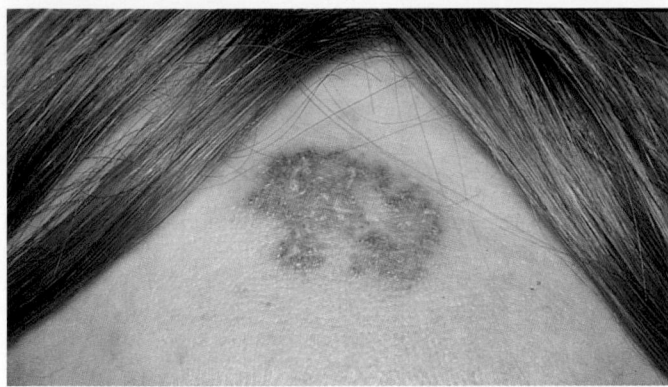

Fig. 17.17 Scaling plaque of discoid lupus erythematosus on a light-exposed area of forehead.

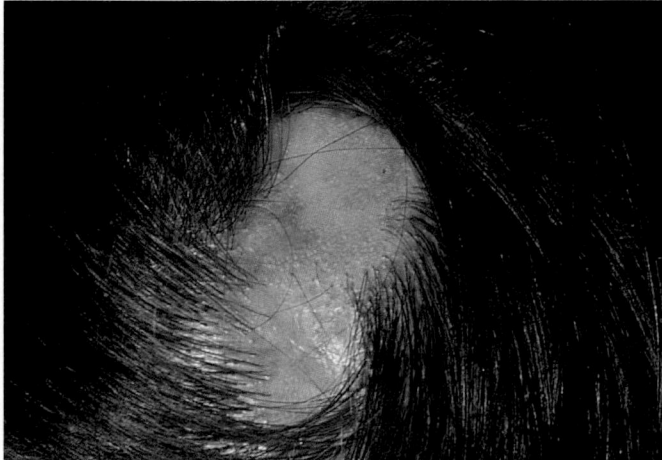

Fig. 17.18 Scarring alopecia of the scalp in discoid lupus erythematosus.

Investigations

Histopathological evaluation reveals degeneration of the basal layer of the epidermis and connective tissue and an intradermal infiltrate of lymphocytes. Epidermal atrophy with plugging of the hair follicles may also occur.[10]

Management

Hydroxychloroquine is the treatment of choice. Factors affecting response to hydroxychloroquine therapy are unclear, and whilst cigarette smoking has been suggested to be associated with poor outcome, a multicentre observational pharmacogenetic study demonstrated that neither cigarette smoking nor cytochrome P450 polymorphisms are associated with clinical outcome of therapy.[30]

Photoprotection with a high-factor sunscreen is advised and patients may benefit from cosmetic camouflage.

Sarcoid

Sarcoidosis is a multisystem granulomatous disease discussed in detail in Chapter 167.

Demographics

Discussed in Chapter 167.

Key clinical features

The clinical morphology of cutaneous sarcoidosis is variable, with the disease being termed 'the great imitator'. Cutaneous sarcoid may appear as plaques occurring on the extremities, buttocks, and trunk with a brown-yellow 'apple jelly' colour on diascopy. Lupus pernio refers to purple plaques occurring on the nose and face (Figure 17.19). In young women persistent erythema in the nasolabial region should raise the possibility of sarcoid or lupus. Sarcoid is a cause of scarring alopecia.

Sarcoid exhibits the Koebner phenomenon, where skin lesions form in areas of trauma, e.g. a surgical wound or an excoriation. Other diseases that exhibit the Koebner phenomenon are listed in Table 17.1.

Investigations

Histopathological examination is not diagnostic, as several skin diseases are associated with granuloma formation.

Management

Many lesions are asymptomatic and may remain under observation alone. Potent topical corticosteroids or injected corticosteroids may be beneficial for limited plaques. For widespread disease, oral corticosteroids, hydroxychloroquine, methotrexate or azathioprine may be used.

Dermatomyositis

Dermatomyositis (DM) is an acquired autoimmune disease comprising inflammation of skeletal muscles and skin, part of the group of idiopathic inflammatory myopathies.

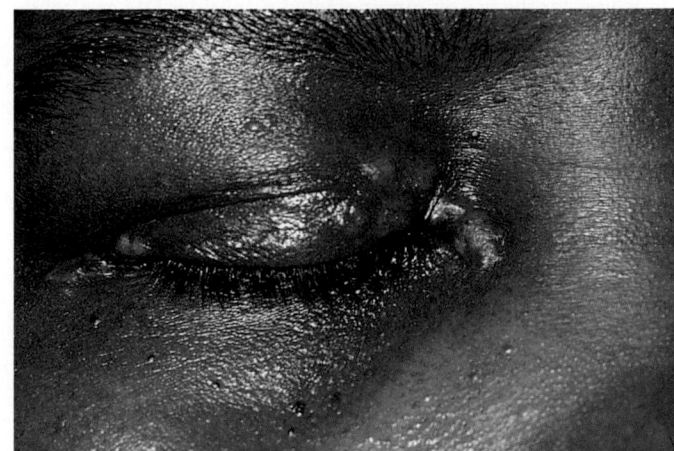

Fig. 17.19 Cutaneous sarcoid in an Afro-Caribbean patient: yellowish papules around the eyelids.

Table 17.1 Conditions that exhibit the Koebner phenomenon

Psoriasis	See 'Psoriasis' section
Sarcoid	See 'Sarcoid' section
Lichen planus	Lichen-like appearance to skin rash of this chronic condition affecting skin and mucosal surfaces; purple polygonal pruritus papules
Lichen nitidis	Chronic disease of pruritic small, uniform, red-brown papules
Vitiligo	Autoimmune skin depigmentation
Viral warts	Skin lesions caused by HPV infection
Lichen sclerosus	Chronic condition with purple polygonal pruritic papules

HPV, human papillomavirus.

Demographics

DM is discussed in detail in Chapter 124.

Key clinical features

Cutaneous features of DM may occur in the absence of musculoskeletal changes: dermatomyositis sine myositis. Characteristically, the lichenoid (purple-ish) eruption is recognized by prominent periocular involvement, termed a heliotrope rash, as it is the same colour as the alpine flower of that name. Involvement of the dorsa of the hands has a characteristic pattern, referred to as Gottron's papules and plaques (Figure 17.20). The key clinical feature is prominent nailfold telangiectasia (Figure 17.21). The rash is photosensitive and may occur in a shawl-like photosensitive distribution (across neck and back). Patients can progress to erythroderma. The rash may remain prominent despite treatment, and where it is associated with malignancy it may persist despite treatment of the underlying neoplasm.

Investigations

See Chapter 124.

Management

Corticosteroids remain the mainstay of therapy for control of both skin and muscle disease. Biologic therapies have been added to the traditional therapeutic options of immunosuppressive agents such as methotrexate, ciclosporin, azathioprine, and the cytotoxic agent cyclophosphamide. In the United Kingdom, Department of Health guidelines for the use of immunoglobulin consider DM as a condition for which treatment is considered highest priority.[31]

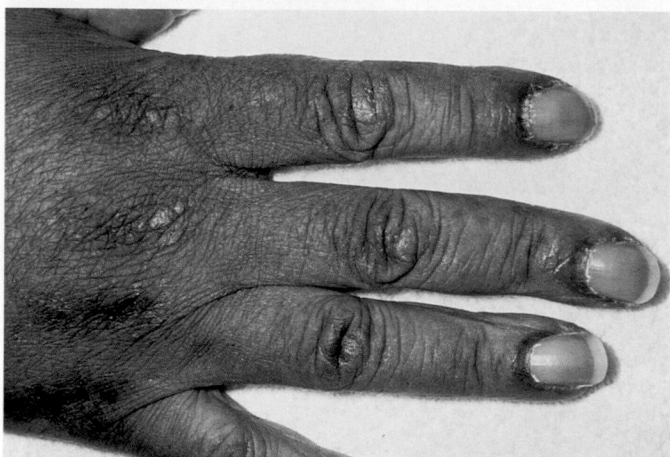

Fig. 17.20 Dermatomyositis: 'Gottron's papules', purple papules, and plaques across bony prominences of dorsa of hand. Prominent nailfold telangiectasia also seen.

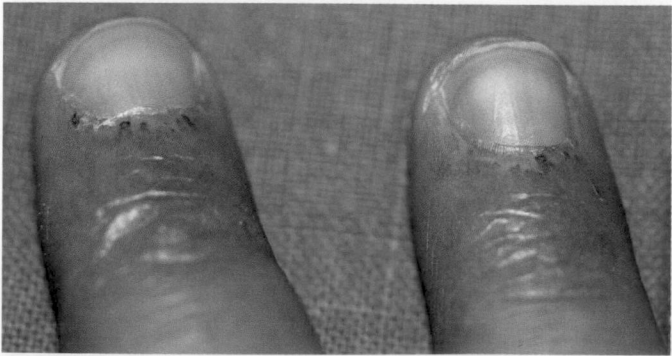

Fig. 17.21 Dermatomyositis: nailfold telangiectasia.

Dermatological guidelines for the management of DM were last published in 1996,[32] and highlighted the use of additional measures for the control of skin disease, such as photoprotection and potent topical corticosteroid for pruritus.

Scleroderma

Systemic sclerosis (SSc), a multisystem connective tissue disease characterized by fibrosis and ischaemic atrophy, is discussed in Chapter 121. The term scleroderma should strictly refer to sclerosis of the skin, either localized or generalized. Morphoea is a condition of unknown cause characterized by localized cutaneous sclerosis.

Demographics

The incidence of systemic sclerosis is 1 and 6 per million in males and females respectively.[33] Morphoea may occur at any age, with peak incidence between the ages of 20–40 years and a female to male ratio of 3:1.

Key clinical features

There are five distinct phenotypic variants of scleroderma: plaque, generalized, bullous, linear, and deep. Rare variants include a nodular or keloidal scleroderma.[34]

Along with the hallmark skin features, vascular changes such as Raynaud's phenomenon and multiple cutaneous telangiectases may be seen.[35] Digital ulcers, vasculitis, and pruritus may occur.

Clinical subtypes of morphea include plaque type, profunda, bullous, and linear morphea where occurrence on the forehead is termed 'en coup de sabre'. Plaque type morphoea presents as smooth indurated plaques, initially purplish in colour, subsequently pale with a purplish edge.

Differential diagnoses

Lichen sclerosus.

Investigations

See Chapter 121.

Management

For SSc, see Chapter 121. Plaque morphoea improves with time, often with post-inflammatory hyperpigmentation, so intervention may be avoided in uncomplicated cases. Potent topical or intralesional corticosteroids may be useful.

Panniculitis

Subcutaneous fat has many important roles, such as provision of padding and a role in thermoregulation. It also has a cosmetic function, contributing to the contours of the face and body that are characteristic of youth. Their loss may have profound social consequences. Panniculitis refers to a group of conditions characterized by inflammation of the fat.

Key clinical features

Clinically, skin over an area of panniculitis feels thickened or 'woody' and is often red and tender (Figure 17.22). Resolution with atrophy of the involved fat may lead to normal-looking skin tethered to an overlying area of inflammation. Septal panniculitides include erythema nodosum (EN), where inflammation also affects the overlying dermis. Sudden-onset painful symmetrical erythematous plaques develop typically on the lower legs (although they may occur at any site). The diagnosis of EN should be clinical and resolution usually occurs without treatment. Lupus panniculitis is a rare condition often associated with overlying chronic cutaneous lupus (Figure 17.23).

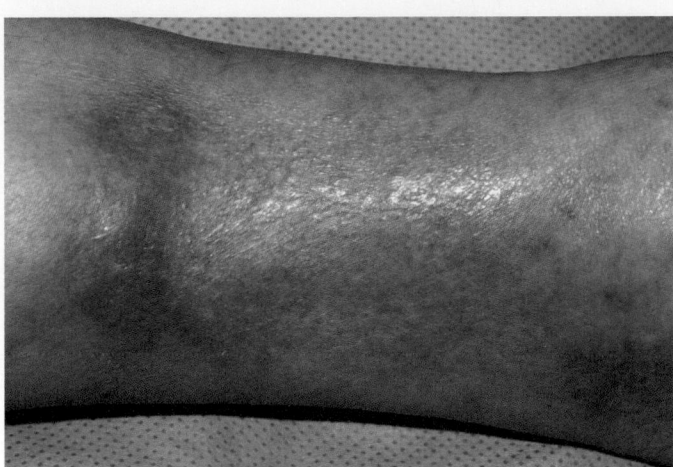

Fig. 17.22 Panniculitis of arm.

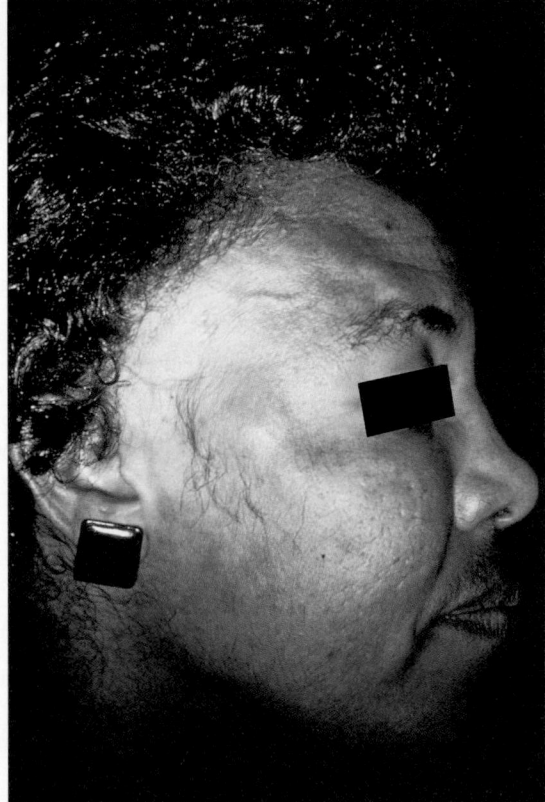

Fig. 17.23 Facial panniculitis in patient with systemic lupus erythematosus.

Differential diagnoses

Malignancy, including lymphoma.

Investigations

Diagnosis relies on adequate biopsy (deep enough to obtain a sufficient sample of affected fat), which cannot be done with a conventional punch technique. Panniculitis may be classified histologically as septal, lobular or mixed, with or without vasculitis

Management

Management should begin with treatment of the underlying disease. Conservative management with rest, elevation, compression, and analgesia are key. Therapy common to multiple forms of panniculitis includes potent topical corticosteroid, which may be delivered topically under occlusive dressings to increase potency or by intralesional injection.

Drug eruptions

Overview

Drug eruptions are a significant cause of morbidity and mortality. There are no reliable estimates of the incidence of drug eruptions. Sources of information are sparse; the British National Formulary is poor at separating skin diseases due to drugs (often simply listed as 'rash').

Diagnosis

Although definitive treatment for any drug eruption is discontinuation of the offending agent, this may not always be possible. Identification of the culprit drug may be difficult due to polypharmacy. In this instance, referral to dermatology, with biopsy of the eruption as necessary, may be vital. Clinicopathological correlation is required, as drug eruptions do not always have diagnostic histological appearances. Often a diagnosis remains uncertain despite discontinuation of the putative agent and rechallenge with a suspected offending agent may be an unavoidable clinical scenario. The dermatology team may be able to provide supportive measures for any ensuing eruption.

Individual drugs can cause several patterns of cutaneous eruption, and diagnosis is aided by clinicopathological correlation from a skin biopsy. The eruption may persist beyond clearance of the putative agent and cutaneous signs such as pigmentation may be permanent.

Types of drug eruption

Common and serious forms of drug eruption seen with rheumatological treatments are described in Figure 17.24.

Anti-tumour necrosis factor alpha

Anti-tumour necrosis factor alpha-induced psoriasis

Specific mention should be made of the phenomenon of induction and exacerbation of psoriasis in arthritis patients treated with anti-tumour necrosis factor alpha (TNFα) biologic therapies. An association is supported by data from the British Society for Rheumatology Biologics Register (BSRBR) indicating an increased incidence of psoriasis in patients treated with anti-TNFα therapy.[36] Two scenarios have been seen: a true psoriasis vulgaris picture or palmoplantar pustulosis (PPP), which is now believed to be genetically distinct from chronic plaque psoriasis.[37]

A proposed mechanism for the development of PPP or psoriasis during TNF blockade is dysregulation of interferon-α. It is thought that in some cases TNFα is a modulating cytokine in psoriasis and its blockade allows breakthrough of interferon-α driven disease.

The outcome of reported cases is varied. The largest case series to date reported resolution in 15.4% cases where anti-TNFα agent was switched,[38] suggesting a class effect. Management of mild or moderate cases may be conducted with topical agents or phototherapy, whereas in severe cases treatment may involve discontinuation of the anti-TNF agent and provision of systemic treatment such as ciclosporin.

Eruption	Illustration	Description	Possible drug precipitants	Treatment/comment
Morbilliform drug eruption		Most common form of drug eruption. Erythematous macules or papules seen across trunk and limbs, classically sparing the face, mucous membranes, palms and soles. May resemble viral rash.	Antibiotics, non-steroidal anti-inflammatory agents (NSAIDs) Penicillamine, gold	Withdrawal of offending agent. Supportive measures with emollient for pruritus and anti-pyretic if associated fever.
Fixed drug eruption	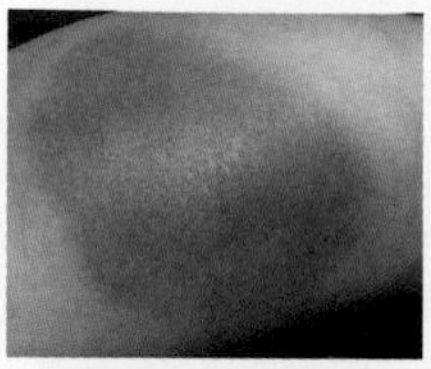	Well-delineated lesions develop rapidly after drug ingestion. Lesions vary in morphology, may be erythematous macules or bullae, more commonly occurring on limbs than trunk. Frequently resolve with hyperpigmentation.	NSAIDs	Mechanism of eruption unknown. Re-challenging key to confirmation of the diagnosis.
Bullous eruptions	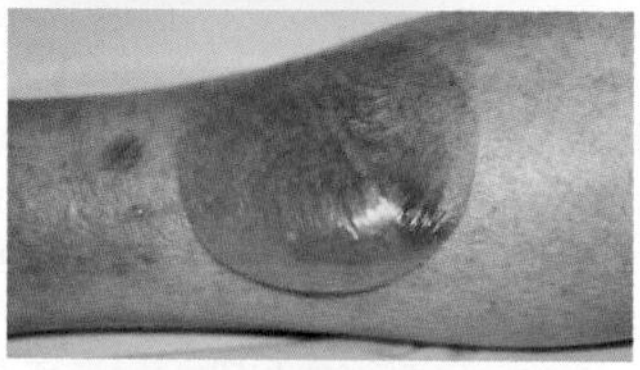	Bullous drug eruptions include fixed drug eruptions with bullae, porphyria cutanea tarda, erythropoeitc protoporphyria and pseudoporphyria. Pseudoporphyria may be seen with NSAIDs. Drug eruptions may mimic immunobullous disorders such as variants of pemphigus or pemphgoid.		Direct (from skin) and indirect (from blood) immunohistochemistry are required to establish a diagnosis.
Urticaria		Mast cell degranulation leads to pale urticarial weals, surrounded by an erythematous flare. Accompanied by intense pruritus.	NSAIDs	5% of population will exhibit dermographism, where stroking skin provokes an urticarial weal. Oral antihistamines treatment of choice for uncomplicated urticaria.
Pigmentation change	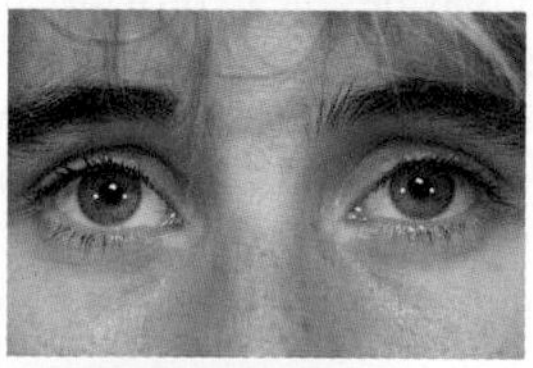	Many pigmentary disturbances are possible as drug adverse events. Antimalarials may lead to a deep slate-grey pigmentation. As with fixed drug eruptions (see above), eruptions often leave darker 'postinflammatory hyperpigmentation' following resolution. Pigmentation may or may not be associated with photosensitivity.		Pigmentary disturbances are often lasting or permanent due to only slow possible resolution with macrophage clearance of deposited pigment. Postinflammatory pigmentation often lasts 3–6 months. Ochronosis is often permanent.
Photosensitivity	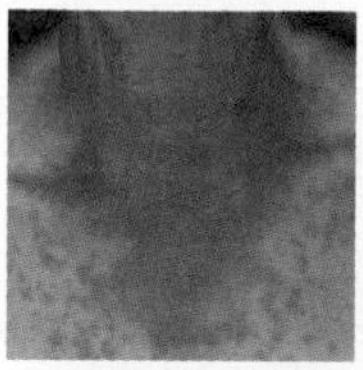	Reactions may be phototoxic, where UV activates a photosensitising agent, or photoallergic, an immune response in which the antigen is the UV activated photosensitising agent.	Sulphasalazine, tetracyclines, quinine	Photo-drug testing possible at some specialist centres to allow identification and thereafter avoidance.
Stevens Johnson syndrome (SJS) and toxic epidermal necrolysis (TEN) suggest splitting these two and the diagnostic test is skin biopsy which will demonstrate keratinocyte necrosis in TEN they are different conditions	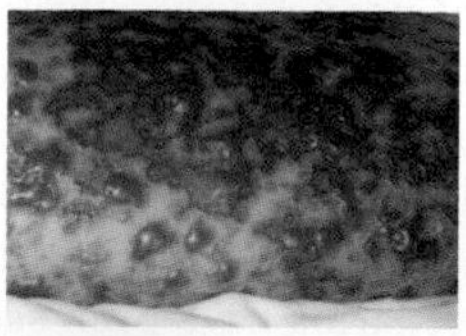 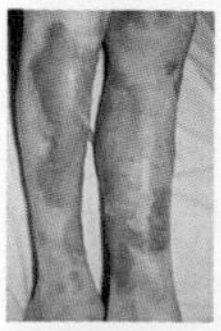	Rare severe drug eruptions. Prodromal phase often precedes acute onset painful erythematous eruption with varying morphology e.g. targetoid or macular. Painful mucous membrane involvement and less than 10% skin surface involvement features of SJS whereas with TEN patient tends to have >10% skin surface involved and can be erythrodermic. Sheets of skin slough on minor pressure 'Nikolsky sign'.	Sulphasalazine Allopurinol Diclofenac	Emergency dermatological conditions requiring specialist care. Early diagnosis and withdrawal of culprit drug essential.
Erythema multiforme	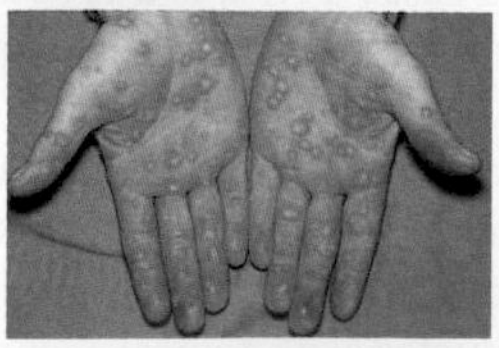	Polymorphic eruption with targetoid lesions composed of erythematous/ dusky centre, pale pink swollen (dermal oedema) ring then outer bright erythematous ring.	Allopurinol, NSAIDs, anticonvulsants	Most commonly triggered by herpes viruses, drug causes are uncommon
Acute generalised exanthematous pustulosis		Acute development of multiple widespread small pustules, often with associated fever and malaise	Hydroxychloroquine	Skin peeling seen with resolution.

Fig. 17.24 Common and serious forms of drug eruption seen with rheumatological therapy.

Drug hypersensitivity syndrome	Severe drug eruption, known also as Drug Reaction with Eosinophilia and Systemic Symptoms (DRESS)	Allopurinol, sulphonamides, anticonvulsants
Pruritus	Pruritus/itch can lead to excoriations and lichenification as well as sleep disturbance and depression	Gold

Fig. 17.24 *(Continued)*

References

1. Calonje E. Histopathology of the skin: general principles. In: Burns T, Breathnach S, Cox N, Griffiths CE (eds) *Rook's textbook of dermatology*, 8th edn. Wiley-Blackwell, Oxford, 2010:251.

2. Mercer LK, Moore TL, Chinoy H et al. Quantitative nailfold video capillaroscopy in patients with idiopathic inflammatory myopathy. *Rheumatology (Oxford)* 2010;49(9):1699–1705.

3. Herrick AL, Cutolo M. Clinical implications from capillaroscopic analysis in patients with Raynaud's phenomenon and systemic sclerosis. *Arthritis Rheum* 2010;62(9):2595–2604.

4. Matucci-Cerinic M, Allanore Y et al. The challenge of early systemic sclerosis for the EULAR Scleroderma Trial and Research group (EUSTAR) community. It is time to cut the Gordian knot and develop a prevention or rescue strategy. *Ann Rheum Dis* 2009;68(9):1377–1380.

5. Meggitt SJ, Anstey AV, Mohd Mustapa MF, Reynolds NJ, Wakelin S. British Association of Dermatologists' guidelines for the safe and effective prescribing of azathioprine 2011. *Br J Dermatol* 2011;165(4):711–734.

6. Smith CH, Anstey AV, Barker JNWN et al. British Association of Dermatologists' guidelines for biologic interventions for psoriasis 2009. *Br J Dermatol* 2009;161(5):987–1019.

7. *British Association of Dermatologists Clinical Guidelines*. British Association of Dermatologists, London, 2008.

8. Jorizzo JL, Daniels JC. Dermatologic conditions reported in patients with rheumatoid arthritis. *J Am Acad Dermatol* 1983;8(4):439–457.

9. Sayah A, English JC, 3rd. Rheumatoid arthritis: a review of the cutaneous manifestations. *J Am Acad Dermatol* 2005;53(2):191–209; quiz 10–12.

10. Goodfield M, Jones S, Veal D. The connective tissue diseases. In: Burns T, Breathnach S, Cox N, Griffiths CE (eds) *Rook's textbook of dermatology*, 8th edn. Wiley-Blackwell, Oxford, 2010:2604–2608.

11. Cox NH, Jorizzo JL, Bourke JF, Savage COS. Vasculitis, neutrophilic dermatoses and related disorders. In: Burns T, Breathnach S, Cox N, Griffiths CE (eds) *Rook's textbook of dermatology*, 8th edn. Wiley-Blackwell, Oxford, 2010:2379–2474.

12. Panush RS, Katz P, Longley S et al. Rheumatoid vasculitis: diagnostic and therapeutic decisions. *Clin Rheumatol* 1983;2(4):321–330.

13. Goldberg J, Pinals RS. Felty syndrome. *Semin Arthritis Rheum* 1980;10(1):52–65.

14. Sienknecht CW, Urowitz MB, Pruzanski W, Stein HB. Felty's syndrome. Clinical and serological analysis of 34 cases. *Ann Rheum Dis* 1977;36(6):500–507.

15. Gridley G, Klippel JH, Hoover RN, Fraumeni JF, Jr. Incidence of cancer among men with the Felty syndrome. *Ann Intern Med* 1994;120(1):35–39.

16. von den Driesch P. Pyoderma gangrenosum: a report of 44 cases with follow-up. *Br J Dermatol* 1997;137(6):1000–1005.

17. Griffiths CEM, Barker JNWN. Pathogenesis and clinical features of psoriasis. *Lancet* 2007;370(9583):263–271.

18. Finlay AY, Kelly SE. Psoriasis-an index of disability. *Clin Exp Dermatol* 1987;12(1):8–11.

19. Rapp SR, Feldman SR, Exum ML, Fleischer AB, Jr., Reboussin DM. Psoriasis causes as much disability as other major medical diseases. *J Am Acad Dermatol* 1999;41(3 Pt 1):401–407.

20. Prey S, Paul C, Bronsard V et al. Assessment of risk of psoriatic arthritis in patients with plaque psoriasis: a systematic review of the literature. *J Eur Acad Dermatol Venereol* 2010;24 Suppl 2:31–35.

21. Horn EJ, Fox KM, Patel V et al. Association of patient-reported psoriasis severity with income and employment. *J Am Acad Dermatol* 2007;57(6):963–971.

22. McDonald CJ, Calabresi P. Psoriasis and occlusive vascular disease. *Br J Dermatol* 1978;99(5):469–475.

23. Gupta MA, Schork NJ, Gupta AK, Kirkby S, Ellis CN. Suicidal ideation in psoriasis. *Int J Dermatol* 1993;32(3):188–190.

24. Henseler T, Christophers E. Psoriasis of early and late onset: characterization of two types of psoriasis vulgaris. *J Am Acad Dermatol* 1985;13(3):450–456.

25. Puzenat E, Bronsard V, Prey S et al. What are the best outcome measures for assessing plaque psoriasis severity? A systematic review of the literature. *J Eur Acad Dermatol Venereol* 2010;24 Sup(2):10–16.

26. Spuls PI, Lecluse LLA, Poulsen M-LNF et al. How good are clinical severity and outcome measures for psoriasis?: quantitative evaluation in a systematic review. *J Invest Dermatol* 2010;130(4):933–943.

27. Tebbe B, Orfanos CE. Epidemiology and socioeconomic impact of skin disease in lupus erythematosus. *Lupus* 1997;6(2):96–104.

28. Kyriakis KP, Michailides C, Palamaras I et al. Lifetime prevalence distribution of chronic discoid lupus erythematosus. *J Eur Acad Dermatol Venereol* 2007;21(8):1108–1109.

29. Miot HA, Bartoli Miot LD, Haddad GR. Association between discoid lupus erythematosus and cigarette smoking. *Dermatology* 2005;211(2):118–122.

30. Wahie S, Daly AK, Cordell HJ et al. Clinical and pharmacogenetic influences on response to hydroxychloroquine in discoid lupus erythematosus: a retrospective cohort study. *J Invest Dermatol* 2011;131(10):1981–1986.

31. Provan D, Chapel HM, Sewell WAC, O'Shaughnessy D; UK Immunoglobulin Expert Working Group. Prescribing intravenous immunoglobulin: summary of Department of Health guidelines. *BMJ* 2008;337:a1831.

32. Drake LA, Dinehart SM, Farmer ER et al. Guidelines of care for dermatomyositis. American Academy of Dermatology. *J Am Acad Dermatol* 1996;34(5 Pt 1):824–829.

33. Silman A, Jannini S, Symmons D, Bacon P. An epidemiological study of scleroderma in the West Midlands. *Br J Rheumatol* 1988;27(4):286–290.

34. Ling TC, Herrick AL, Andrew SM, Brammah T, Griffiths CEM. Keloidal scleroderma. *Clin Exp Dermatol* 2003;28(2):171–173.

35. Murray A, Moore T, Herrick A. Clinical images: systemic sclerosis-related telangiectases. *Arthritis Rheum* 2011;63(2):572.

36. Harrison MJ, Dixon WG, Watson KD et al. Rates of new-onset psoriasis in patients with rheumatoid arthritis receiving anti-tumour necrosis factor alpha therapy: results from the British Society for Rheumatology Biologics Register. *Ann Rheum Dis* 2009;68(2):209–215.

37. Asumalahti K, Ameen M, Suomela S et al. Genetic analysis of PSORS1 distinguishes guttate psoriasis and palmoplantar pustulosis. *J Invest Dermatol* 2003;120(4):627–632.

38. Ko JM, Gottlieb AB, Kerbleski JF. Induction and exacerbation of psoriasis with TNF-blockade therapy: a review and analysis of 127 cases. *J Dermatol Treat* 2009;20(2):100–108.

Information sources

British Association of Dermatologists(www.bad.org.uk). Resource includes excellent patient information leaflets: www.bad.org.uk/site/792/default.aspx

New Zealand Dermatological Society Incorporated (http://dermnetnz.org/)

CHAPTER 18

Nervous system

Andrew Graham and Clare Galton

Introduction

Many rheumatological disorders may be complicated by nervous system involvement; either as a direct or indirect consequence of the underlying disease process or occasionally as an adverse effect of treatment. Sometimes neurological symptoms may be the presenting feature of an underlying rheumatological condition—e.g. systemic lupus erythematosus (SLE) presenting with seizures, or a systemic vasculitis presenting with multiple mononeuropathies—but more commonly neurological complications arise on the background of an already established rheumatological diagnosis. As in all branches of medicine, the recognition and accurate diagnosis of neurological disorder depends primarily on careful clinical assessment, but this evaluation can be challenging (even to an experienced neurologist) in the face of significant rheumatological disease. Pain and joint stiffness, swelling and deformity can cloud the assessment and sometimes a final diagnosis will only be reached through investigations, primarily imaging with MRI and/or CT for central nervous system (CNS) syndromes and neurophysiology for the peripheral nervous system (PNS).

Principles

The most crucial skill in neurological assessment is the ability to take and appropriately organize the history.[1] Evaluation has three main aspects:

◆ **Organization**. Neurological symptoms such as headache and tingling are ubiquitous even in the normal population and are not necessarily an indicator of underlying disease. All potentially neurological symptoms must be accurately defined, arranged in chronological order, and grouped into coherent clusters. Not every symptom is relevant, and symptoms such as fatigue are very non-specific.

◆ **Localization**. Each cluster of neurological symptoms may suggest either a process (e.g. syncope or seizure), or an anatomical localization. For an intermittent process such as seizures, examination is often uninformative and the diagnosis is typically made from the history alone. For symptoms that localize well, the anatomy can often be specified precisely from the history alone (e.g. tingling and numbness of both legs rising to a level on the trunk, difficulty in walking, and urinary hesitancy all suggest spinal cord disease), but sometimes there is a differential (e.g. with a foot drop it may not be evident from the symptoms alone whether

this is due to a peripheral nerve or root lesion). Structured examination then helps to define the localization further.

◆ **Causation**. Having established the source of symptoms, their onset and time course often give a clue to causation. For example, in a patient with myelopathy an acute onset may suggest a vascular event (e.g. spinal cord stroke); subacute onset may suggest inflammation or demyelination (e.g. transverse myelitis); and a chronic course suggests a structural or degenerative process (e.g. compressive myelopathy). The point here is that the signs on examination may be similar in all three cases; it is the history that tells them apart.

Clinical reasoning

Rheumatological disorders may involve almost any aspect of the nervous system. A brief guide to neurological localization is given in Table 18.1 and a sample case history is given to exemplify clinical reasoning, but for further details readers are advised to consult one of the classic texts.[2,3]

Case history

A 47 year old woman with a 2 year history of primary Sjögren's syndrome (persistent ocular and oral dryness, positive anti-Ro antibodies, and a positive Schirmer test) complains of left facial numbness and numbness and weakness of both legs, with dragging of the right leg on walking.

The symptoms sound neurological; it is difficult to explain the facial and leg symptoms on the basis of a single anatomical lesion, so they will be treated separately. The facial numbness suggests a trigeminal sensory neuropathy. For the legs the differential in localization is between cervical/thoracic spinal cord and a polyneuropathy. The next step is to define the symptoms further. Does the numbness extend up onto the trunk, indicating spinal cord disease, or follow a glove and stocking distribution, indicating a polyneuropathy? Are there symptoms of bladder dysfunction, usually indicating a myelopathy but also seen with a conus/cauda equina lesion in association with saddle numbness? What has been the time course of each symptom?

(Continued)

(Case history)

Numbness extends to a vague level on the trunk. She complains of pain and tingling in the right hand at night but no fixed numbness in the hands, and mild urinary hesitancy. The facial numbness has evolved over 6 months but the leg symptoms over a fortnight.

The distribution of numbness and the bladder symptoms suggest a myelopathy rather than a polyneuropathy. The right hand symptoms could be significant, but may equally represent a separate peripheral nerve lesion. The difference in time courses supports the idea that there is more than one process at work. The next step is to examine the patient. Is there evidence of upper or lower motor neuron weakness in the legs, are reflexes brisk or depressed, and what is the distribution of sensory loss?

Numbness of the left face extends back to the vertex. There are no signs in the arms. In the legs, tone is increased with a spastic character; there is a mild asymmetric pyramidal weakness (right more so than left); reflexes are generally brisk but absent at both ankles; the right plantar is extensor; and sensation is reduced to joint position in the right leg and to pinprick on the left, extending to an uncertain level on the abdomen.

The facial numbness is consistent with a trigeminal sensory neuropathy. The lack of signs in the right hand suggests that symptoms here are most likely due to carpal tunnel syndrome. The signs in the legs confirm a spinal cord lesion, specifically a predominantly right-sided thoracic myelopathy (a Brown–Séquard syndrome). From the history this is subacute and likely inflammatory/demyelinating. The next step is to investigate, with imaging of the spinal cord and other tests as appropriate.

An MRI of the cervical and thoracic spine shows a longitudinally extensive high signal cord lesion from approximately T1 to T5. An MRI brain scan is normal, with no evidence of any trigeminal lesion. Anti-aquaporin antibodies are positive. Cerebrospinal fluid (CSF) is not examined. Nerve conduction studies confirm a mild median neuropathy at the right wrist but also a mild predominantly sensory axonal polyneuropathy

The longitudinally extensive transverse myelitis due to anti-aquaporin disease may be treated acutely with steroids and/or plasma exchange, with consideration of a second line immunosuppressant to prevent recurrence. No treatment is currently indicated for the trigeminal neuropathy. The mild carpal tunnel syndrome can be treated conservatively with neutral wrist splints or a local steroid injection if it worsens. The incidental polyneuropathy does not need attention, although most neurologists would probably check blood glucose and protein electrophoresis as screening tests for a secondary cause.

Rheumatoid arthritis

The most common neurological complication of rheumatoid arthritis (RA) is entrapment neuropathy, particularly carpal tunnel syndrome in patients with active hand flexor tenosynovitis. Wrist splints at night or a steroid injection may afford some relief, but the

definitive treatment is surgical decompression. A generalized, typically mild, length-dependent sensory polyneuropathy may be seen in patients with longstanding or severe disease, but rarely requires specific treatment. Systemic (as opposed to cutaneous) rheumatoid vasculitis is rare, affecting less than 1% of patients,[4,5] but when present may be associated with multiple mononeuropathies and require immunosuppression. Direct CNS involvement is also rare, but occasional patients develop a chronic pachymeningitis with thickening and enhancement of meninges on MRI. Treatment here is speculative.

Otherwise, the most significant neurological complication of RA is cervical myelopathy due to anterior atlantoaxial subluxation and compression by soft tissue pannus. Subluxation is rare in early disease but present in more than 25% of patients with disease duration of more than 15 years.[6] Early subluxation is usually asymptomatic, but 1 in 50 patients with RA will eventually develop a clinically significant compressive cervical myelopathy.[4] This is usually chronic but may present acutely or be unmasked by provocation, e.g. following neck trauma or injudicious manipulation. Surgical stabilization of anterior subluxation can prevent further neurological deterioration but will not usually improve existing symptoms. With disease progression subluxation may be succeeded by vertical atlantoaxial impaction, in which the skull descends and the odontoid process passes superiorly through the foramen magnum, causing lower brainstem compression. Surgical treatment of atlantoaxial impaction is challenging and may involve both odontoid process resection (transorally) and posterior fusion (e.g. of the occiput to C2).

Connective tissue diseases

Systemic lupus erythematosus

SLE may be associated with a bewildering variety of neurological disorder; in 1999 the American College of Rheumatology proposed case criteria for 19 separate CNS and PNS syndromes,[7] often collectively referred to as neuropsychiatric SLE (NPSLE; see Box 18.1).

Estimates of the prevalence of the various NPSLE syndromes vary widely depending on study size, population, focus, and ascertainment methods. A recent meta-analysis of 17 studies involving a total of 5057 patients with SLE found an overall prevalence of 28.2% for all NPSLE syndromes, rising to 56.3% (95% confidence intervals 42.5% 74.7%) when only the highest-quality prospective studies were considered.[8]

However, many syndromes reported are of minimal clinical significance and in any case not all symptoms can be directly attributed to SLE disease activity. First, neurological disorder in patients with SLE may result both from direct nervous system involvement (e.g. due to vasculopathy, antibody-mediated effects, and inflammation) and as a secondary consequence of other factors (e.g. hypertension, renal failure, infections, and drug toxicity). In one series, more than 40% of neurological syndromes in patients with SLE were due to indirect causes.[9] Second, some neurological symptoms are so common that they are bound to be seen in patients with any chronic disease. Although headache is often listed as a common neuropsychiatric manifestation of SLE, a meta-analysis of 7 controlled studies involving 478 patients found that the prevalence of all headache types, including migraine, was not different from controls, with no evidence to support a separate entity of 'lupus headache'.[10]

A reasonable conclusion is that while up to half of all patients with SLE may experience neurological symptoms at some stage in their illness, the cumulative incidence of neurological disorder is

Table 18.1 Common localizations in neurology

Localization	Symptoms	Signs	Common causes
Median nerve	Sensory > motor; pain and tingling in the lateral hand, particularly at night	Tinel's and Phalen's tests are notoriously unreliable; thenar wasting and weakness of APB or opponens pollicis generally only seen in severe cases	Entrapment at the wrist, e.g. carpal tunnel syndrome in RA
Ulnar nerve	Sensory = motor; pain and tingling in the medial hand with weakness of grip	Sensory loss classically involving the little finger and splitting the ring finger; wasting and weakness of FDI and all intrinsic hand muscles except for those supplied by the median nerve	Vasculitic mononeuropathy, e.g. in Churg–Strauss syndrome
Radial nerve	Sensory < motor; wrist drop	Weakness of wrist and finger extensors plus brachioradialis; triceps also weak in proximal lesions, brachioradialis spared in distal lesions (posterior interosseous nerve palsy); minimal sensory loss	Compression in the spiral groove, i.e. Saturday night palsy—causes a classic radial nerve palsy sparing triceps
Peroneal nerve	Sensory < motor; foot drop	Weakness of ankle dorsiflexion plus inversion and eversion; minimal sensory loss over dorsum of foot	Vasculitic mononeuropathy, e.g. in Churg–Strauss syndrome
Spinal cord	Sensory, motor and sphincters; tingling and numbness of both legs rising to a level on the trunk, difficulty in walking and urinary hesitancy	Spastic increase in tone; pyramidal weakness (flexors weaker than extensors in lower limbs, converse in upper limbs), brisk reflexes, extensor plantars, sensory level on trunk	Transverse myelitis, e.g. LETM in SLE
Polyneuropathy	Sensory and motor; distal numbness, tingling, and weakness, typically legs > arms in a length-dependent manner	Distal weakness, reduced or absent reflexes, glove and stocking sensory loss	Distal symmetric polyneuropathy, e.g. in Sjögren's syndrome

APB, abductor pollicis brevis (thumb abduction); FDI, first dorsal interosseous (index finger abduction); LETM, longitudinally extensive transverse myelitis; RA, rheumatoid arthritis; SLE, systemic lupus erythematosus.

probably less than 20% when syndromes such as headache, minor cognitive dysfunction, anxiety, mood disorder, and symptoms of polyneuropathy with negative neurophysiology are excluded.[11,12] Significant neuropsychiatric events may precede, coincide, or follow the diagnosis of SLE but commonly occur within the first year after SLE diagnosis and in the presence of generalized disease activity. The most common manifestations (cumulative incidence 5–15%) are stroke and seizures, while serious cognitive dysfunction, delirium, and PNS disorders are uncommon (1–5%) and myelitis, aseptic meningitis, cranial neuropathies, and movement disorders are all well recognized but rare (<1%).[11] The spectrum of psychiatric and psychological disorder in rheumatic diseases is wide and forms the subject of a separate chapter (see Chapter 26).

Stroke

Patients with SLE are at increased risk of ischaemic stroke and transient ischaemic attack (TIA) due to a variety of mechanisms; haemorrhagic stroke is rare. Atherosclerosis is accelerated in SLE,[13] and patients often require aggressive management of conventional vascular risk factors such as smoking, hypertension, hyperlipidaemia, and diabetes. Patients with SLE have a five- to sixfold increased risk of ischaemic heart disease overall (in younger women the excess risk may be 50-fold) and are at risk of cardioembolism due to rhythm disorder or structural heart disease. In addition, SLE is closely associated with the presence of antiphospholipid antibodies (APAs), an important risk factor for both venous and arterial thrombosis.

Acute stroke or TIA management is similar to that in the general population, consisting of immediate clinical evaluation, imaging with CT and/or MRI, thrombolysis where indicated or antiplatelet treatment unless contraindicated, and then full secondary prevention measures including carotid endarterectomy where appropriate. For ischaemic stroke in association with positive APAs the usual consensus is also to anticoagulate with warfarin, although in trials the benefits of warfarin over aspirin have not been clearly established[14] and for most patients there is no clear advantage of high-intensity over low-intensity anticoagulation.[15,16] However, patients with APAs are a heterogeneous group and data specifically relating to antiphospholipid syndrome in association with SLE is lacking. For a younger patient with SLE and a first ischaemic stroke in association with persistent high-titre anti-cardiolipin/anti-β_2-microglobulin antibodies and a positive lupus anticoagulant test, most physicians would have no hesitation in anticoagulating long-term, quite possibly aiming for a higher target INR of 3–4; whereas for an older patient with weakly positive anticardiolipin antibodies not meeting full criteria for antiphospholipid syndrome, aspirin alone and attention to conventional risk factors may be more appropriate. Stroke due to cerebral vasculitis is very rare in SLE and immunosuppression post stroke is not usually indicated unless it is to control accompanying generalized disease activity.

Seizures

Seizures are common in SLE, again due to a variety of mechanisms. Sporadic seizures may be provoked by metabolic derangement or intercurrent infection, while for recurrent seizures the most important pathology is probably underlying vascular disease (particularly in association with APAs). In some patients with negative brain

Box 18.1 (Neuropsychiatric SLE syndromes)

Central nervous system

- Aseptic meningitis
- Cerebrovascular disease
- Demyelinating syndromes
- Headache (including migraine and idiopathic intracranial hypertension)
- Movement disorder (chorea)
- Myelopathy
- Seizure disorder
- Acute confusional state
- Anxiety disorder
- Cognitive dysfunction
- Mood disorder
- Psychosis

Peripheral nervous system

- Acute inflammatory demyelinating polyradiculopathy (Guillain–Barré syndrome)
- Autonomic disorder
- Mononeuropathy, single or multiplex
- Myasthenia gravis
- Cranial neuropathy
- Plexopathy
- Polyneuropathy

Source: ACR (1999).

imaging a more specific antibody-mediated mechanism may be suspected, but of the many non-APA autoantibodies reported in NPSLE none has proven diagnostic or therapeutic utility in seizure disorders.

The general management of seizures in SLE is similar to that in the general population. Brain imaging, ideally with MRI, is required to exclude any structural lesion and to assess the extent of any vascular disease. EEG is not usually helpful in diagnosis but may help to specify the epilepsy syndrome and can add information about the risk of further seizures. In the United Kingdom antiepileptic drug treatment is not usually given following a single or provoked seizure unless there are risk factors for recurrence such as a structural lesion on MRI or clear continuing epileptiform activity on the EEG; in such cases, or if seizures are already recurrent, treatment is symptomatic with the usual range of antiepileptic medications. Fulminating seizures may require further investigation, for example an MR venogram to exclude dural sinus thrombosis (requiring anticoagulation, particularly in association with the antiphospholipid syndrome) or CSF examination to exclude infection (requiring antiviral or antibacterial treatment). Immunosuppression is rarely indicated unless it is to control accompanying generalized disease activity; lupus 'encephalitis' or 'cerebritis' is not an ACR-defined neuropsychiatric syndrome and in patients who are unwell with

encephalopathy and seizures it is usually worth investigating for a more specific (primary or secondary) cause.

Myelitis

Myelitis is an uncommon neurological complication in SLE but deserves mention because it may be associated with particular underlying pathology and requires specific treatment. In recent years the investigation and management of inflammatory spinal cord disease has been reshaped by the identification of a specific antibody to the aquaporin-4 (AQP4) water channel in patients with the demyelinating condition of neuromyelitis optica (NMO) or Devic's syndrome, consisting of so-called longitudinally extensive transverse myelitis (LETM—myelitis extending over three or more spinal segments) and optic neuritis.[17] Studies show that a positive anti-AQP4 antibody test is strongly associated with the NMO phenotype, but not typical multiple sclerosis (MS),[18] and is a predictor of a severe disease course with a high likelihood of future relapses.[19] However, unlike in MS, relapse rates in patients with anti-AQP4-positive NMO can be reduced by aggressive treatment with steroids, second line immunosuppressants such as azathioprine and mycophenolate mofetil, and antibody-directed treatment such as rituximab. Accurate diagnosis of NMO spectrum disorders is therefore very important, and anti-APQ4 antibodies are increasingly recognized in patients with SLE and either myelitis or recurrent optic neuritis. One recent study of 28 patients with NPSLE found positive anti-APQ4 antibodies in 6/6 patients with LETM and 2/2 patients with recurrent optic neuritis; testing was negative in patients with all other neuropsychiatric syndromes including chorea, psychosis, seizure disorders, and polyneuropathy.[20] Conversely, non-organ-specific autoantibodies are frequently found in NMO spectrum disorders, with at least some patients meeting clinical criteria for SLE.[21]

A reasonable conclusion is that anti-aquaporin disease should be excluded in any patient with SLE and LETM or recurrent optic neuritis, and that when NMO is diagnosed it should be regarded as a coexisting disorder rather than a direct complication of SLE, often requiring separate treatment. Neurologists are now very familiar with this condition, but where local advice is not available a national service has recently been established in the United Kingdom, offering anti-AQP4 antibody testing and guidance on management for all National Health Service patients with NMO (www.nmouk.nhs.uk).

Sjögren's syndrome

Sjögren's syndrome is associated with a wide spectrum of PNS syndromes.[22] The hallmark complication is sensory ataxic neuronopathy, usually subacute but occasionally acute and dramatic. Patients develop gait and limb ataxia with severe loss of posterior column sensation (vibration and joint position), often leading to significant disability. Treatment is speculative but the syndrome may occasionally respond to steroids, intravenous immunoglobulin (IVIG), or other immunosuppressants. Sensory trigeminal neuropathy and an autonomic neuropathy are also seen: individual patients may present with symptoms of more than one syndrome or an unclassifiable overlap syndrome. Neuropathy may sometimes be the presenting feature of underlying Sjögren's syndrome, in which case patients are more likely to present to a neurologist than a rheumatologist.

CNS involvement in Sjögren's is less common but just as in SLE LETM has historically been well described, responding to treatment with steroids and azathioprine.[23,24] The current view is that, similarly to SLE, many if not all of these cases are due to coexisting anti-aquaporin disease.[20,21]

Systemic sclerosis

As in Sjögren's syndrome, systemic sclerosis is more often associated with PNS than CNS manifestations. Up to a quarter of patients develop carpal tunnel syndrome, and trigeminal sensory neuropathy and a mild autonomic neuropathy are also seen. More significant polyneuropathy or multiple mononeuropathies are rare. Basal ganglia calcification is a common finding on brain imaging but is not usually of clinical significance.

Mixed connective tissue disease

Mixed connective tissue disease (MCTD) may be associated with both CNS and PNS disease; the pattern of central involvement is similar to that seen in SLE, while peripheral involvement mirrors that seen in systemic sclerosis, particularly trigeminal sensory neuropathy. In addition, inflammatory muscle disease histologically resembling dermatomyositis is a common complication of MCTD.

Spondyloarthropathies

Neurological involvement in ankylosing spondylitis is usually due to mechanical cord or root compression. The spectrum of neurological involvement in reactive arthritis is much wider, including aseptic meningoencephalitis, seizures, psychosis, cranial neuropathies, radiculopathy, and polyneuropathy. Neurological involvement in psoriatic arthropathy is rare.

Vasculitis

Nervous system involvement in systemic vasculitis is common, with differing patterns according to the specific vasculitis syndrome.[25]

ANCA-associated vasculitis

The syndromes of ANCA-associated vasculitis (Churg–Strauss syndrome, Wegener's granulomatosis, microscopic polyangiitis and classical polyarteritis nodosa [PAN]) are associated with PNS complications in up to 40% of patients, most notably in Churg–Strauss syndrome where neurological manifestations are the first symptoms of vasculitis in up to 25% of patients and presentation is almost as likely to be to a neurologist as a rheumatologist.[25] CNS manifestations are less common, but still relatively frequent: stroke, seizures, and altered mental status occur in up to 10% of patients.

PNS involvement in Churg–Strauss syndrome, microscopic polyangiitis and classical PAN typically takes the form of acute or subacute single or multiple mononeuropathies, usually sensorimotor and painful. The commonest nerves affected are the peroneal nerve in the lower limb (causing foot drop) and the ulnar nerve in the upper limb (causing intrinsic hand weakness);[26] when sufficient individual peripheral nerves are involved the end result may be indistinguishable from a generalized sensorimotor axonal polyneuropathy. Although pain, swelling, and asymmetry of symptoms and signs should all alert the clinician to the possibility of underlying vasculitis, stepwise progression is not always seen and a significant minority of patients present with a distal symmetric polyneuropathy from the outset.[26] PNS involvement is less common in Wegener's granulomatosis and is rarely the presenting feature. However, Wegener's is associated with a range of other neurological syndromes related to orbital mass formation and granulomatous infiltration originating from the ear, nose, and throat (ENT) tract, including multiple cranial nerve palsies (most commonly optic

neuropathy), pachymeningitis, and pituitary gland involvement. The treatment of primary ANCA-associated vasculitis is discussed elsewhere in this volume but generally involves steroids and pulsed IV cyclophosphamide for induction and then a second line agent such as methotrexate. For refractory granulomatous disease, anti-CD20 therapy such as rituximab has been used with some success (see Chapter 141).

Large-vessel vasculitis

Takayasu's arteritis is associated with carotid or vertebral artery inflammation, stenosis, or occlusion, with a predilection for the anterior circulation. Extracranial artery involvement is often asymptomatic but may be complicated by ischaemic stroke in up to 10% of patients. Takayasu's arteritis does not usually affect the intracranial vessels or the PNS. Temporal arteritis is classically associated with occlusion of the posterior ciliary artery causing anterior ischaemic optic neuropathy, but may also involve the vertebral arteries, leading to posterior circulation stroke in up to 5% of patients. When treating temporal arteritis, low-dose antiplatelet therapy as stroke prophylaxis is recommended in addition to steroids.[27]

Behçet's disease

Behçet's disease is associated with significant neurological complications in perhaps 10% of patients, with two main patterns of involvement.[28,29] First, parenchymal neuro-Behçet's disease, in which CNS inflammation (typically affecting the upper brainstem and basal ganglia but sometimes extending more diffusely through brain and spinal cord) results in a range of corresponding manifestations including ophthalmoplegia, pyramidal and extrapyramidal dysfunction, seizures, and behavioural change. Symptoms usually evolve over a few days or weeks, often associated with headache; MRI shows a varying distribution of inflammatory lesions, occasionally with contrast enhancement, while CSF generally shows a pleiocytosis and raised protein with absent oligoclonal bands. Steroids are the mainstay of management, but second line treatment is speculative.[29] The second main pattern is non-parenchymal or vasculo-Behçet's disease, usually manifesting with dural sinus thrombosis and raised intracranial pressure. In this situation parenchymal lesions are absent on MRI but sinus thrombosis may be seen on MR venography; CSF examination shows raised pressure but is usually otherwise unremarkable. Dural sinus thrombosis is typically treated with anticoagulation unless there is an obvious contraindication.

Drug effects

Many of the medications used to treat rheumatological disease have potential for neurological side effects. Non-steroidal anti-inflammatory drugs (NSAIDs), commonly prescribed as symptomatic therapy, may be associated with an aseptic meningitis (which must be borne in mind when examining CSF in patients on long-term NSAIDs). The associations of older disease-modifying drugs such as gold (with neuropathy) and penicillamine (with myasthenia gravis) are well known. Modern first line disease-modifying therapies such as low-dose methotrexate are not often associated with neurological complications, but newer second line agents have been reported to cause a number of central and peripheral nervous system syndromes. Leflunomide may be associated with a distal sensory or sensorimotor axonal polyneuropathy;[30] in some patients symptoms improve with discontinuation, but in others symptoms persist (suggesting irreversible axonal loss). The TNFα inhibitors etanercept, infliximab, and adalumimab may be associated with both CNS[31] and PNS[32] demyelinating disease. Centrally, TNFα inhibitors are associated with an increased relapse rate in already established MS;[33] it is uncertain whether their use in rheumatic conditions induces CNS demyelination *de novo* or simply exposes latent disease.[34] Peripherally, TNFα inhibitors can also induce chronic inflammatory demyelinating polyradiculoneuropathy (CIDP) with positive anti-ganglioside antibodies, or multifocal motor neuropathy (MMN). Discontinuation of TNFα inhibitor therapy is typically associated with improvement of CNS and PNS inflammation, without the need for more specific treatment, but recovery may be slow and incomplete. In rare cases a leukoencephalopathy has been described that may continue to progress despite withdrawal of treatment.

References

1. Compston DAS. Introduction and approach to the patient with neurological disease. In: Warrell DA, Firth JD, Cox TM (eds) *Oxford Textbook of Medicine*, 5th edn. Oxford University Press, Oxford, 2010.

2. O'Brien M. *Aids to the examination of the peripheral nervous system*, 5th edn. : Saunders Elsevier, Edinburgh, 2010.

3. Patten J. *Neurological differential diagnosis*, 2nd edn. Springer, New York, 1996.

4. Turesson C, O'Fallon WM, Crowson CS, Gabriel SE, Matteson EL. Extra-articular disease manifestations in rheumatoid arthritis: incidence trends and risk factors over 46 years. *Ann Rheum Dis* 2003;62(8):722–727.

5. Watts RA, Lane SE, Bentham G, Scott DG. Epidemiology of systemic vasculitis: a ten-year study in the United Kingdom. *Arthritis Rheum* 2000;43(2):414–419.

6. Naranjo A, Carmona L, Gavrila D et al. Prevalence and associated factors of anterior atlantoaxial luxation in a nation-wide sample of rheumatoid arthritis patients. *Clin Exp Rheumatol* 2004;22(4):427–432.

7. The American College of Rheumatology nomenclature and case definitions for neuropsychiatric lupus syndromes. *Arthritis Rheum* 1999;42(4):599–608.

8. Unterman A, Nolte JES, Boaz M et al. Neuropsychiatric syndromes in systemic lupus erythematosus: a meta-analysis. *Semin Arthritis Rheum* 2011;41(1):1–11.

9. Hanly JG, McCurdy G, Fougere L, Douglas JA, Thompson K. Neuropsychiatric events in systemic lupus erythematosus: attribution and clinical significance. *J Rheumatol* 2004;31(11):2156–2162.

10. Mitsikostas DD, Sfikakis PP, Goadsby PJ. A meta-analysis for headache in systemic lupus erythematosus: the evidence and the myth. *Brain* 2004;127(Pt 5):1200–1209.

11. Bertsias GK, Ioannidis JP, Aringer M et al. EULAR recommendations for the management of systemic lupus erythematosus with neuropsychiatric manifestations: report of a task force of the EULAR standing committee for clinical affairs. *Ann Rheum Dis* 2010;69(12):2074–2082.

12. Hanly JG, Urowitz MB, Su L et al. Prospective analysis of neuropsychiatric events in an international disease inception cohort of patients with systemic lupus erythematosus. *Ann Rheum Dis* 2010;69(3):529–535.

13. Bruce IN. 'Not only…but also': factors that contribute to accelerated atherosclerosis and premature coronary heart disease in systemic lupus erythematosus. *Rheumatology (Oxford)* 2005;44(12):1492–1502.

14. Levine SR, Brey RL, Tilley BC et al. Antiphospholipid antibodies and subsequent thrombo-occlusive events in patients with ischemic stroke. *JAMA* 2004;291(5):576–584.

15. Crowther MA, Ginsberg JS, Julian J et al. A comparison of two intensities of warfarin for the prevention of recurrent thrombosis in patients with the antiphospholipid antibody syndrome. *N Engl J Med* 2003;349(12):1133–1138.

16. Finazzi G, Marchioli R, Brancaccio V et al. A randomized clinical trial of high-intensity warfarin vs. conventional antithrombotic therapy for the prevention of recurrent thrombosis in patients with the antiphospholipid syndrome (WAPS). *J Thromb Haemost* 2005;3(5):848–853.

17. Wingerchuk DM, Lennon VA, Pittock SJ, Lucchinetti CF, Weinshenker BG. Revised diagnostic criteria for neuromyelitis optica. *Neurology* 2006;66(10):1485–1489.

18. Lennon VA, Wingerchuk DM, Kryzer TJ et al. A serum autoantibody marker of neuromyelitis optica: distinction from multiple sclerosis. *Lancet* 2004;364(9451):2106–2112.

19. Weinshenker BG, Wingerchuk DM, Vukusic S et al. Neuromyelitis optica IgG predicts relapse after longitudinally extensive transverse myelitis. *Ann Neurol* 2006;59(3):566–569.

20. Wandinger KP, Stangel M, Witte T et al. Autoantibodies against aquaporin-4 in patients with neuropsychiatric systemic lupus erythematosus and primary Sjogren's syndrome. *Arthritis Rheum* 2010;62(4):1198–1200.

21. Pittock SJ, Lennon VA, de Seze J et al. Neuromyelitis optica and non-organ-specific autoimmunity. *Arch Neurol* 2008;65(1):78–83.

22. Mori K, Iijima M, Koike H et al. The wide spectrum of clinical manifestations in Sjogren's syndrome-associated neuropathy. *Brain* 2005;128(Pt 11):2518–2534.

23. Mochizuki A, Hayashi A, Hisahara S, Shoji S. Steroid-responsive Devic's variant in Sjogren's syndrome. *Neurology* 2000;54(6):1391–1392.

24. Hawley RJ, Hendricks WT. Treatment of Sjogren syndrome myelopathy with azathioprine and steroids. *Arch Neurol* 2002;59(5):875; author reply 6.

25. Lane SE, Watts RA, Shepstone L, Scott DG. Primary systemic vasculitis: clinical features and mortality. *QJM* 2005;98(2):97–111.

26. Said G, Lacroix C. Primary and secondary vasculitic neuropathy. *J Neurol* 2005;252(6):633–641.

27. Mukhtyar C, Guillevin L, Cid MC et al. EULAR recommendations for the management of large vessel vasculitis. *Ann Rheum Dis* 2009;68(3):318–323.

28. Akman-Demir G, Serdaroglu P, Tasci B. Clinical patterns of neurological involvement in Behcet's disease: evaluation of 200 patients. The Neuro-Behcet Study Group. *Brain* 1999;122 (Pt 11):2171–2182.

29. Al-Araji A, Kidd DP. Neuro-Behcet's disease: epidemiology, clinical characteristics, and management. *Lancet Neurol* 2009;8(2):192–204.

30. Metzler C, Arlt AC, Gross WL, Brandt J. Peripheral neuropathy in patients with systemic rheumatic diseases treated with leflunomide. *Ann Rheum Dis* 2005;64(12):1798–1800.

31. Mohan N, Edwards ET, Cupps TR et al. Demyelination occurring during anti-tumor necrosis factor alpha therapy for inflammatory arthritides. *Arthritis Rheum* 2001;44(12):2862–2869.

32. Shin IS, Baer AN, Kwon HJ, Papadopoulos EJ, Siegel JN. Guillain-Barre and Miller Fisher syndromes occurring with tumor necrosis factor alpha antagonist therapy. *Arthritis Rheum* 2006;54(5):1429–1434.

33. The Lenercept Multiple Sclerosis Study Group and The University of British Columbia MS/MRI Analysis Group. TNF neutralization in MS: results of a randomized, placebo-controlled multicenter study. *Neurology* 1999;53(3):457–465.

34. Fernandez-Espartero MC, Perez-Zafrilla B, Naranjo A et al. Demyelinating disease in patients treated with TNF antagonists in rheumatology: data from BIOBADASER, a pharmacovigilance database, and a systematic review. *Semin Arthritis Rheum* 2011;40(4):330–337.

CHAPTER 19

Cardiovascular system

J. Gerry Coghlan and Benjamin E. Schreiber

Introduction

Rheumatologists face a huge task in identifying potentially highly lethal multisystem diseases, often hidden among large numbers of patients with painful but non-threatening conditions like fibromyalgia and osteoarthritis. In addition, they must provide chronic care for relapsing remitting conditions, while monitoring for adverse effects of increasingly toxic therapeutic regimens. Given the exercise limitation that is common to virtually all such patients and the fact that most cardiac patients notice symptoms only on effort, particular skill is required to identify cardiac complaints among this population.

Yet cardiac problems are prevalent in the average rheumatological clinic, whether simply fortuitously (those with osteoarthritis are often elderly) or due to a generic increase in cardiac risk associated with inflammation[1] and metabolic syndrome[2] or a recognized complication of specific rheumatological conditions.[3] In this chapter we address the general problem of identifying cardiac conditions among rheumatological patients and the generic association between inflammation and cardiac disease, explore in particular the relationship between rheumatological disease and coronary heart disease, and finally provide an overview of cardiac conditions thought to be associated with rheumatological conditions in tabular form (Table 19.1).

Identifying cardiac disease in rheumatology patients

Cardiac symptoms

Coronary artery disease progresses asymptomatically for a variable period of time and may in a significant minority present abruptly with myocardial infarction or sudden death. However, more usually it presents with stable effort limitation due to chest discomfort or progressive reduction in effort tolerance over days to weeks preceding myocardial infarction.[4] In many patients with rheumatological disease exercise ability is already limited either in terms of magnitude of task performed or the ease with which such tasks are performed, thus masking the symptoms of coexisting coronary artery disease.

Dyspnoea on effort is another common cardiac symptom typically due to systolic and diastolic myocardial dysfunction, valvular heart disease, tachycardia myopathies, and pulmonary hypertension. Syncope on significant effort may occur in conditions that limit cardiac output such as aortic stenosis, hypertrophic cardiomyopathy, and pulmonary hypertension. Arrhythmias usually present with palpitations, or alterations in consciousness, but may present as sudden death. Finally, fatigue may limit effort in constrictive pericarditis and slowly progressive cardiac conditions such as mitral stenosis.

Presentation of cardiac disease in rheumatological conditions

Rheumatological conditions may not only mask cardiac symptoms through chronic effort limitation; they may also mimic them, being a known cause similar of symptoms (fatigue, dyspnoea), resulting in failure to explore possible cardiac pathology. Finally, expert patients may filter their symptoms to fit preconceptions as to the most desirable consult outcome. Difficulty in diagnosing cardiac conditions is compounded by an increase prevalence of cardiac disease as exemplified in rheumatoid arthritis (RA),[5] lupus,[3] and systemic sclerosis.[6]

Diagnosing cardiac disease in rheumatology clinics

Improved access to highly discriminatory diagnostic tools, coupled with a heightened index of suspicion, is required in the average rheumatological clinic. Patients should be assessed annually for traditional cardiac risk factors and their additional cardiac risk level associated with their rheumatological diagnosis considered. For example, patients with RA have a doubling of coronary risk,[5] those with systemic sclerosis a thousandfold increased risk for pulmonary hypertension[7] (Figure 19.1). Young women with systemic lupus erythematosus (SLE) have a fiftyfold increased coronary risk,[8] and patients with gout, and indeed all others with elevated urate, may exhibit increased cardiovascular risk.[9] In patients whose effort tolerance changes over a short period of time, consideration should always be given to whether the change is adequately explained by manifest change in the activity of their rheumatological condition or whether detailed investigation is required. Finally, probing of the patient's symptoms may be particularly revealing—patients often offer explanations for symptoms that seem sensible and fit with their disease profile, but gentle probing often reveals that the symptom pattern does not hold and suggests alternate causes. Of particular note, chronic obesity tends to limit effort tolerance through pain rather than dyspnoea,[10] and advancing age does not cause rapid deterioration in effort tolerance.[11]

A simple blood test (N-terminal proBNP or BNP) will identify most patients with systolic or diastolic heart failure[12]; thus, wherever such a differential exists this test should be requested. Coronary calcification

Table 19.1 Cardiovascular risks associated with rheumatological conditions

Disease	Associations	Comment
RA	Pericarditis	Effusions are common but clinical episodes are uncommon, and are associated with seropositive disease, active synovitis
	Myocarditis	Rare as a clinical manifestation, though subclinical abnormalities common at autopsy, can be granulomatous or interstitial
	Valvular disease	Rare as a clinical manifestation, rheumatoid granulomata on 3–5% of autopsies, minor valvular abnormalities in over 10% on echo
	Coronary disease	See discussion above, may also cause a small-vessel arteritis
	Conduction	First degree heart block up to 10%, bifasicular block more common. High grade block rare. Rheumatoid nodules may affect conduction system
	Aortitis	Previously found in 5% of autopsy series, may now be recognized more frequently with PET scanning. Aneurysm formation rare
	Iatrogenic	Hydroxychloroquine (cardiac toxicity) NSAIDs may unmask heart failure
	Amyloidoisis	Patients with longstanding active disease are at risk of AA amyloidosis causing an infiltrative cardiomyopathy
SLE	Coronary disease	See discussion above. Note: was rare in pre-steroid era
	Valvular disease	Asymptomatic verrucous valvular lesions are common (up to 75%). More severe form, Libman–Sacks endocarditis, associated with mitral regurgitation (much less common with effective therapy)
	Pericardial disease	Clinical pericarditis is the most common cardiac manifestation (up to 30% with active disease). Treatment of lupus resolves it, though effusions may persist
	Myocarditis	Clinically uncommon, subclinical involvement in up to 40%
	Conduction	Congenital heart block associated with anti-Ro/SSA and anti-La/SSB antibodies. Atrial and more rarely ventricular arrhythmias may accompany myocarditis, pericarditis and coronary disease.
	Thrombotic	Typically associated with APS, venous and arterial thrombosis, including leading to stroke and myocardial infarction
	Pulmonary hypertension	PAH in approximately 1%, may have vasculitis component and respond to immunosupression. Also PH secondary to lung disease may occur
Systemic sclerosis	Pulmonary hypertension	7–12% develop PAH associated with a very poor prognosis requiring aggressive treatment. Approximately 3% develop postcapillary PH (due to left heart disease) and another 3% lung disease associated PH
	Coronary disease	No definite association; however, small-vessel disease purported to underlie myocardial scarring in this condition
	Pericardial disease	Symptomatic disease uncommon, fibrinous pericarditis especially during active early phase. Later transudates secondary to pulmonary hypertension or heart failure
	Myocarditis	Myocardial scarring in a non-coronary distribution is common and may lead to heart failure or arrhythmias. Whether due to microvasculopathy or myocarditis is unresolved
	Conduction	All types of heart block, septal infarction pattern, atrial and ventricular arrhythmias described. ECG abnormal in 50% slightly more than in age-matched population
Osteoarthritis	Increased cardiovascular mortality[61]	Possible confounders include exercise, obesity, use of NSAIDs
Gout	Coronary heart disease[62]	Hyperuricemia is also associated with obesity, hypertension, and diabetes[63]
Sjögren's syndrome	Pericarditis	Acute pericarditis is rare, but effusions are common
Takayasu's arteritis	Aorta and major branches	Granulomatous arteritis progressing to intimal hyperplasia and adventitial sclerosis. Coarctation and major vessel stenoses cause most complications – including hypertension (renal artery) and heart failure (hypertensive and aortic regurgitation). Pressure differential between limbs is a major clinical sign
	Coronary disease	Involvement of the coronaries occurs in ~10% causing angina, infarction. and heart failure
Giant cell arteritis	Aortic aneurysm, aortic dissection, large-artery stenosis[64]	Medium-vessel arteritis dominates clinical course, larger head and neck vessel involvement leads to stenotic lesions. Aortic involvement may produce no cardiovascular symptoms unless aneurysm formation results
Churg–Strauss	Endomyocarditis and heart failure[65]	Involvement of pericardium, myocardium, endocardium, and coronaries all described and in total affect over half of patients. Patients with marked eosinophilia at particular risk

(Continued)

Table 19.1 (*Continued*)

Disease	Associations	Comment
Polyarteritisnodosa	Coronary disease	Coronary arteritis affecting small subepicardial vessels, modest aneurysm formation. Infarction may result as may pericarditis
Behçet's	Inflammatory vasculopathy	Previously Behçet's was thought to be associated with frequent cardiac involvement. More recent data suggests dominant involvement of the pulmonary arteries, large aortic branch vessels, and large veins, leading to aneurysm formation and occlusion
Spondyloarthropathies	Aorta	Adventitial scarring with intimal proliferation and scarring typically seen in ankylosing spondylitis, less common in Reiter's and rare in psoriasis. Aortic root dilation and aortic regurgitation due to leaflet shortening and distortion are characteristic
	Conduction	Fibrosis of the AV node associated with all degrees of heart block in Ankylosing Spondylitis. In Reiter's responsiveness to immunosupression suggests inflammatory component
	Coronary disease	Rare involvement of the coronary ostia may cause angina

scoring (Figure 19.2) requires minimal radiation exposure and will reliably exclude prognostically significant coronary disease[13]; further, where positive this test identifies individuals at increased risk of coronary events and in need of secondary prevention and investigation for ischaemia. The recent National Institute for Health and Clinical Excellence (NICE) guidance on chest pain[14] should result in widespread availability of this technique in the next few years.

Symptom profile may be altered: in patients with RA and coronary disease, as in patients with diabetes mellitus, chest pain may not be experienced.[15] Thus changes in dyspnoea burden should lead to consideration of atypical angina in the differential.

Failure to recognize symptoms of cardiac disease may occur for many reasons: breathlessness may already be present from associated parenchymal lung disease, chest wall arthritis, and respiratory muscle weakness or reflux oesophagitis, thus changes in dyspnoea may never even be reported. Chest wall discomfort and reflux may also mask cardiac pain.

Other cardiac conditions may appear abruptly without pre-existing abnormalities to detect: thus coronary thrombosis in normal arteries occur in lupus; stroke and pulmonary emboli typically in antiphospholipid syndrome (APS)[16]; and major vessel thrombosis or aneurysms in Behçet's syndrome.[17] Subtle myocardial fibrosis or microvascular disease in lupus[3] or systemic sclerosis[6] (Figure 19.3) may manifest as tachyarrhythmia, sudden death, or conduction disorders without prodrome.

Inflammation and cardiac disease

Although some cardiac diseases are obviously inflammatory in nature (pericarditis, myocarditis) and inflammation plays a pivotal

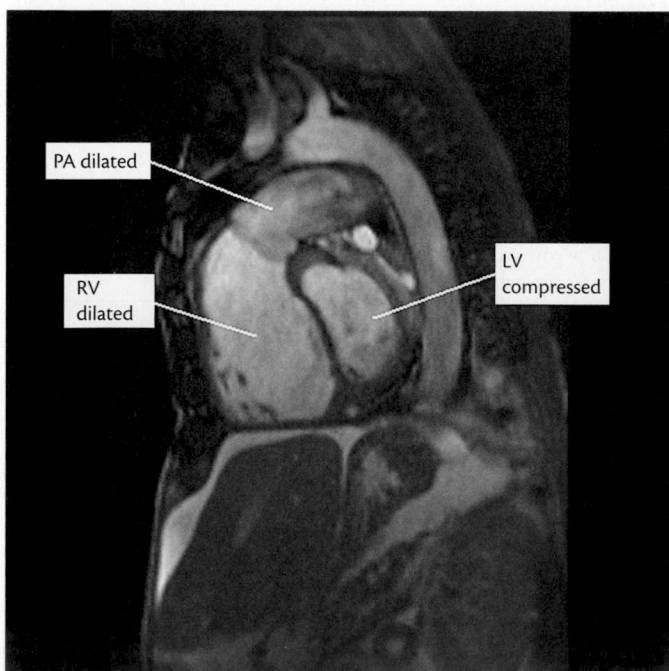

Fig. 19.1 MRI showing grossly dilated pulmonary artery (PA) and right ventricle (RV) secondary to pulmonary arterial hypertension in a patient with systemic sclerosis. The left ventricle (LV) is compressed by the pressure overloaded RV.

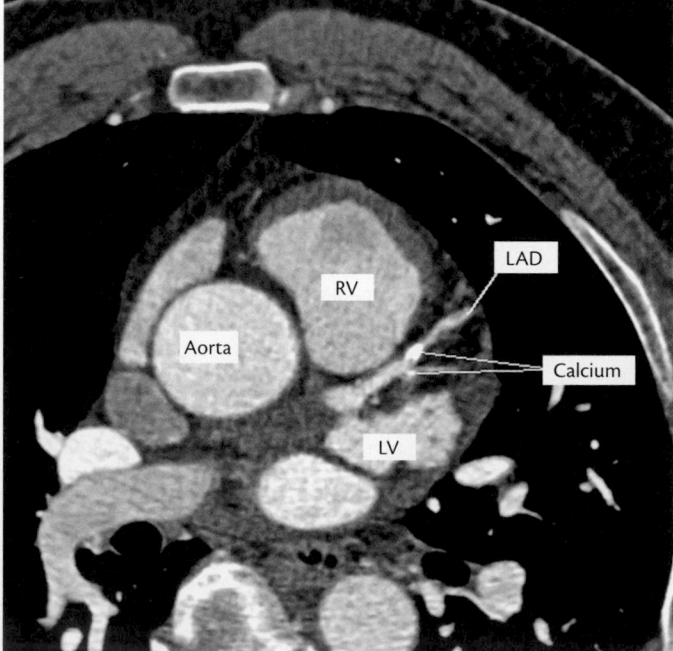

Fig. 19.2 CT coronary angiogram showing heavy calcification of the anterior descending artery–first diagonal bifurcation, indicative of the presence of significant coronary disease at this location. RV, right ventricle; LV, left ventricle.

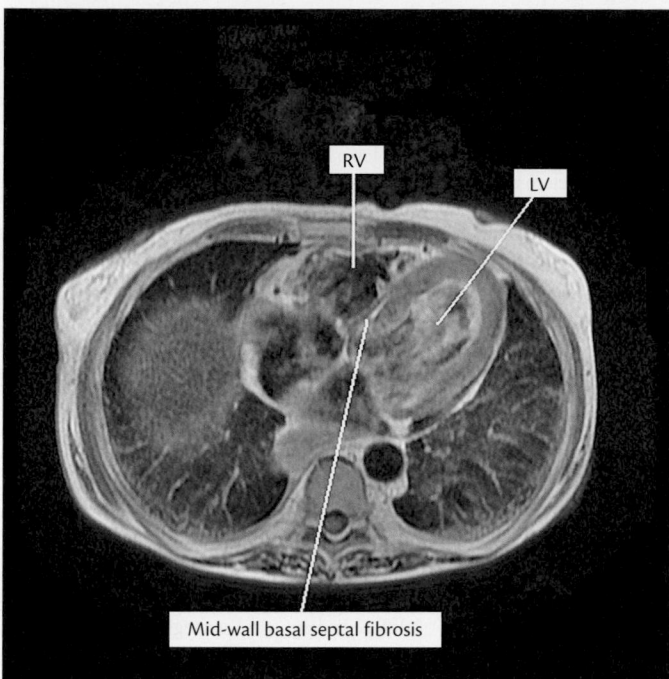

Fig. 19.3 Late gadolinium MRI of a patient with systemic sclerosis and myocardial fibrosis. Gadolinium sequesters in the interstitial space in collagen, clearing very slowly, remaining enhanced on delayed imaging. RV, right ventricle; LV, left ventricle.

role in the evolution of myocardial infarction and heart failure, it has become increasingly evident that inflammation is pathogenic in atherosclerosis and hypertension as well. How precisely this relates to systemic inflammatory conditions is as yet unclear, though it is apparent that rheumatological conditions are strongly associated with increased cardiac event rates. One link between inflammation and accelerated atherosclerosis which has been elucidated is the increased myeloperoxidase-catalysed lipoprotein carbamylation which accelerates atherosclerosis.[18]

While studies of C-reactive protein (CRP) as a risk factor[19] provide strong support for inflammation being an important contributor to in cardiovascular disease, they tell us little of the mechanism and do not give insight into the possible mechanisms by which rheumatological conditions might lead to heart disease. Likewise, elevated urate levels associate with cardiovascular mortality but, other than speculation about the role of intracellular oxidative stress, provide little illumination.[20]

The first specific proinflammatory cytokine to be associated with heart failure was tumour necrosis factor alpha (TNFα.[21] Unfortunately anti-TNF therapy has not proved successful.[22] It is presently postulated that physiological levels of TNFα may be required for remodelling and repair.[23] Although the early promise has not materialized, it is still held that improved understanding of the role of TNFα, dosing of anti-TNF agents, and exploration of the different actions of available agents may yet lead to a therapeutic role for anti-TNFα agents in heart failure.[24]

Monocyte chemoattractive protein-1 (MCP-1) levels are predictive of acute and chronic outcome in acute coronary syndromes[25] and heart failure.[26] The monocyte response to myocardial infarction is complex, however, with inflammatory monocytes peaking at day 3 and reparative monocytes at day 5.[27] While in theory it would be attractive to downregulate the inflammatory response and upregulate

the reparative response, the protean roles of cytokines make the outcome difficult to predict. Thus fractalkine appears to promote reparative monocyte response but may also enhance atherosclerosis.[28]

Chronically elevated IL-6 levels were found to be associated with a doubling of risk for fatal and non-fatal myocardial infarction in a large United Kingdom population-based study.[29] More recent data suggests that IL-6 may explain the association between markers of inflammation (serum viscosity, fibrinogen, leucocyte count, CRP) and coronary disease as well as ischaemic stroke, as IL-6—unlike other inflammatory markers—retains significance when corrected for traditional risk factors.[30] Elevated IL-6 levels have also been associated with adverse outcomes in heart failure[31] and with an increased incidence of sudden death.[32] Circulating Il-6 levels are increased after myocardial infarction and associated with an adverse prognosis.[33] However, discrepant findings in animal models (a protective effect of gp130 activation) suggest that disruption of downstream effects in the setting of infarction may reset the balance of effects toward inflammation rather than protection.[34]

Thus the precise relationship between circulating and tissue levels of IL-6 and variable downstream effects make predictions of the possible therapeutic impact of IL-6 antagonist therapy difficult to predict. This is of course of immediate relevance in RA where tocilizumab (an IL-6 receptor inhibitor) is in use. The impact on myocardial inflammation and repair is not well understood; in addition, adverse effects on lipid profile have been observed.[35]

Systemic hypertension is associated with inflammation via the metabolic syndrome. In addition, in experimental studies there is some supportive evidence for a direct relationship between hypertension and inflammation. The role of angiotensin II (ATII) in hypertension is not doubted: ATII has proinflammatory effects mediated via NF-κB, IL-6, and IL-1β.[36] ATII infusions in humans have been shown to increase IL-6,[37] but as yet there is no clear evidence that hypertension can be directly caused by inflammation.

Inflammation may also play a significant role in pulmonary hypertension (PAH), as reviewed recently.[38] The strong association between PAH and rheumatological conditions, the reversal of PAH in some patients with immunosuppressive therapy, the frequent autoimmune abnormalities in idiopathic PAH, the histological findings of inflammatory cell infiltrates and the monocrotaline models all argue for a pivotal role of inflammation in PAH, the precise nature of which has yet to be defined.

Not only can one point to immunological perturbations associated with cardiovascular disease, but also the increased incidence and prevalence of cardiac disease in virtually all rheumatological conditions.

Coronary disease in rheumatoid arthritis and lupus

Rheumatoid arthritis

A recent meta-analysis of 24 observational studies including 111 758 patients found that cardiovascular disease mortality is increased by approximately 50% in RA patients compared to the general population.[5] Possible explanations include traditional cardiovascular risk factors, novel risk factors associated with inflammation, and therapies such as glucocorticoids and non-steroidal anti-inflammatory drugs (NSAIDs). An analysis of the Nurses' Health Study compared women with RA to those without, and found no difference in the prevalence of diabetes, hypertension, current smoking, or dyslipidaemia.[39] As expected, CRP levels were significantly higher in patients with RA.

Several other novel risk factors, whose significance is not clear, are associated with RA.[40] It is speculated that active inflammation in RA may accelerate atherosclerosis. Although high CRP is highly associated with ischaemic heart disease,[41] recent studies have shown that the association is not likely to be causal.[42]

A study from the British Society of Rheumatology Biologics Register compared the rate of myocardial infarction in 8670 patients with active RA treated with anti-TNF inhibitors to the rate in 2170 patients treated with traditional disease-modifying antirheumatic drugs (DMARDs). Following adjustment for baseline cardiovascular risk factors, they found no significant difference between the two groups. However, myocardial infarction rates were lower in patients who responded to anti-TNF therapy compared to those who did not (adjusted incidence rate ratio 0.36, 0.16–0.69).[43]

Glucocorticoid use is associated with an increased risk of ischaemic heart disease, in patients with RA[44] as well as in the general population.[45] However, this has not been shown to be causal. The effect of glucocorticoids on the lipid profile is also not clear.[46]

NSAIDs are associated with increased risk of cardiovascular disease. Of all NSAIDs, including COX-2 selective NSAIDs, naproxen is associated with least harm.[47]

SLE is associated with a substantial increase in the risk of stroke and coronary events.[48] The association with atherosclerosis is supported not just by evidence of much higher rates of clinical events such as angina and myocardial infarction,[49,50] but also much greater prevalence of coronary calcification,[51,52] carotid intimal thickening,[53] and disordered endothelial function.[54] Despite the impressive excess of atherosclerosis and atherosclerotic events shown in many studies, all cohorts are small and only one has a truly rigorous control cohort of adequate size.[52]

From the available studies it is evident that traditional risk factors in part explain the excess observed[51]; other factors such as the age at onset of disease,[53] duration of disease,[53] renal involvement,[55] and nature of immunosuppressive therapy used[56] also play a role. In addition, genetic variants such as homozygosity for mannose-binding lectin variant alleles are associated with an increased risk of arterial thrombotic events in SLE.[57] Nevertheless, the failure to recruit to treatment trials[58] means that one cannot assert that managing patients differently will alter outcome. It follows that for the moment optimal assessment of and management of traditional risk factors is the goal,[59] and this goal is not presently being met.[60]

Conclusion

Rheumatologists require a heightened index of suspicion and access to the latest investigational strategies to diagnose cardiac diseases prevalent in their patients. The population provides immense opportunities for research into the links between inflammation, autoimmunity, and heart disease.

References

1. Ridker PM, Cannon CP, Morrow D et al. C-reactive protein levels and outcomes after statin therapy. *N Engl J Med* 2005;352(1):20–28.
2. Onat A. Metabolicsyndrome: nature, therapeutic solutions and options. *Expert Opin Pharmacother* 2011;12(12):1887–1900.
3. McMahon M, Hahn B, Skaggs B. Systemic lupus erythematosus and cardiovascular disease: prediction and potential for therapeutic intervention. *Expert Rev Clin Immunol* 2011;7(2):227–241.
4. Pryor DB, Shaw L, McCants CB et al. Value of the history and physical in identifying patients at increased risk for coronary artery disease. *Ann Intern Med* 1993;118(2):81–90.
5. Aviña-Zubieta JA, Choi HK, Sadatsafavi M et al. Risk of cardiovascular mortality in patients with rheumatoid arthritis: a meta-analysis of observational studies. *Arthritis Rheum* 2008;59(12):1690–1697.
6. Kahan A, Coghlan G, McLaughlin V. Cardiac complications of systemic sclerosis. *Rheumatology* 2009;48:iii45–iii48.
7. Mukerjee D, St.George D, Coleiro B et al. Prevalence and outcome in systemic sclerosis associated pulmonary arterial hypertension: Application of a registry approach. *Ann Rheum Dis* 2003;62:1088–1093.
8. Manzi S, Meilahn EN, Rairie JE et al. Age-specific incidence rates of myocardial infarction and angina in women with systemic lupus erythematosus. *Am J Epidemiol* 1997;145:408–415.
9. Kim SY, Guevara JP, Kim KM et al. Hyperuricemia and coronary heart disease: a systematic review and meta-analysis. *Arthritis Care Res (Hoboken)* 2010;62(2):170–180.
10. Hulens M, Vansant G, Claessens AL et al. Predictors of 6-minute walk test results in lean, obese and morbidly obese women. *Scand J Med Sci Sports* 2003;13(2):98–105.
11. Fitzgerald MD, Tanaka H, Tran ZV et al. Age-related declines in maximal aerobic capacity in regularly exercising vs. sedentary women: a meta-analysis. *J Appl Physiol* 1997;83(1):160–165.
12. Mant J, Doust J, Roalfe A, Barton P et al. Systematic review and individual patient data meta-analysis of diagnosis of heart failure, with modelling of implications of different diagnostic strategies in primary care. *Health Technol Assess* 2009;13(32):1–207, iii.
13. Sarwar A, Shaw LJ, Shapiro MD et al. Diagnostic and prognostic value of absence of coronary artery calcification. *JACC Cardiovasc Imaging* 2009;2(6):675–688.
14. *Chest pain of recent onset: assessment and diagnosis of recent onset chest pain or discomfort of suspected cardiac origin.* http://guidance.nice.org.uk/CG95
15. Maradit-Kremers H, Crowson CS, Nicola PJ et al. Increased unrecognized coronary heart disease and sudden deaths in rheumatoid arthritis: a population-based cohort study. *Arthritis Rheum* 2005;52(2):402–411.
16. Cervera R, Khamashta MA, Shoenfeld Y et al. Morbidity and mortality in the antiphospholipid syndrome during a 5-year period: a multicentre prospective study of 1000 patients. *Ann Rheum Dis* 2009;68(9):1428–1432.
17. Aguiar de Sousa D, Mestre T et al. Major vessel involvement in Behçet's disease: an update. *J Neurol* 2011;258(5):719–727.
18. Wang Z, Nicholls SJ, Rodriguez ER et al. Protein carbamylation links inflammation, smoking, uremia and atherogenesis. *Nat Med* 2007;13(10):1176–1184.
19. Lavie CJ, Milani RV, Verma A et al. C-reactive protein and cardiovascular diseases—is it ready for primetime? *Am J Med Sci* 2009; 338:486–492.
20. Yu M-A, Sanches-Lozada L, Johnson RJ et al. Oxidative stress with an activation of the renin-angiotensin system in human vascular endothelial cells as a novel mechanism of uric acid-induced endothelial dysfunction. *J Hypertens* 2010;28:1234–1242.
21. Dutka DP, Elborn JS, Delamere F, Shale DJ, Morris GK. Tumour necrosis factor alpha in severe congestive cardiac failure. *Br Heart J* 1993;70(2):141–143.
22. Chung ES, Packer M, Lo KH et al. Randomized, double-blind, placebo-controlled, pilot trial of infliximab, a chimeric monoclonal antibody to tumor necrosis factor-alpha, in patients with moderate-to-severe heart failure: results of the anti-TNF Therapy Against Congestive Heart Failure (ATTACH) trial. *Circulation* 2003;107(25):3133–3140.
23. Mann DL. Inflammatory mediators and the failing heart: past, present, and the foreseeable future. *Circ Res* 2002; 91:988–998.
24. Heymans S, Hirsch E, Anker SD et al. Inflammation as a therapeutic target in heart failure? A scientific statement from the Translational Research Committee of the Heart Failure Association of the European Society of Cardiology. *Eur J Heart Fail* 2009;11:119–129.
25. De Lemos JA, Morrow DA, Blazing MA et al. Serial measurement of monocyte chemoattractant protein-1 after acute coronary syndromes: results from the A to Z trial. *J Am Coll Cardiol* 2007;50:2117–2124.
26. Hohensinner PJ, Rychli K, Zorn G et al. Macrophage-modulating cytokines predict adverse outcome in heart failure. *Thromb Haemost* 2010;103:435–441.

27. Tsujioka H, Imanishi T, Ikejima H et al. Impact of heterogeneity of human peripheral blood monocyte subsets on myocardial salvage in patients with primary acute myocardial infarction. *J Am Coll Cardiol* 2009;54:130–138.

28. White GE, Tan TC, John AE et al. Fractalkine has antiapoptotic and pro-liferative effects on human vascular smooth muscle cells via epidermal growth factor receptor signaling. *Cardiovasc Res* 2010;85:825–835.

29. Danesh J, Kaptoge S, Mann AG et al. Long-term interleukin-6 levels and subsequent risk of coronary heart disease: two new prospective studies and a systematic review. *PLoS Med* 2008;5:e78.

30. Patterson CC, Smith AE, Yarnell JW et al. The associations of interleukin-6 (IL-6) and downstream inflammatory markers with risk of cardiovascular disease: the Caerphilly Study. *Atherosclerosis* 2010;209: 551–557.

31. Jug B, Salobir BG, Vene N et al. Interleukin-6 is a stronger prognostic predictor than high-sensitive C-reactive protein in patients with chronic stable heart failure. *Heart Vessels* 2009;24:271–276.

32. Empana JP, Jouven X, Canoui-Poitrine F et al. C-reactive protein, interleukin 6, fibrinogen and risk of sudden death in European middle-aged men: the PRIME study. *Arterioscler Thromb Vasc Biol* 2010;30:2047–2052.

33. Ikeda U, Ohkawa F, Seino Y et al. Serum interleukin 6 levels become elevated in acute myocardial infarction. *J Mol Cell Cardiol* 1992;24:579–584.

34. Hilfiker-Kleiner D, Shukla P, Klein G et al. Continuous glycoprotein-130 -mediated signal transducer and activator of transcription-3 activation promotes inflammation, left ventricular rupture, and adverse outcome in subacute myocardial infarction. *Circulation* 2010;122:145.

35. Smolen JS, Beaulieu A, Rubbert-Roth A et al. Effect of interleukin-6 receptor inhibition with tocilizumab in patients with rheumatoid arthritis (OPTION study): a double-blind, placebo-controlled, randomised trial. *Lancet* 2008;371:987–997.

36. Fanz-Rosa D, Oubiña MP, Cediel E et al. Effect of AT1 receptor antagonism on vascular and circulating inflammatory mediators in SHR: role of NF-kappaB/IkappaB system. *Am J Physiol Heart Circ Physiol* 2005;288:H111–H115.

37. Chamarthi B, Williams GH, Ricchiuti V et al. Inflammation and hypertension: the interplay of interleukin-6, dietary sodium, and the renin–angiotensin system in humans. *Am J Hypertens* 2011;24:1143–1148.

38. Kherbeck N, Tamby MC, Bussone G et al. The role of inflammation and autoimmunity in the pathophysiology of pulmonary arterial hypertension. *Clin Rev Allergy Immunol* 2011 Mar 11. [Epub ahead of print] PMID: 21394427.

39. Solomon DH, Curhan GC, Rimm EB, Cannuscio CC, Karlson EW. Cardiovascular risk factors in women with and without rheumatoid arthritis. *Arthritis Rheum* 2004;50(11):3444–3449.

40. De Pablo P, Dietrich T, Karlson EW. Antioxidants and other novel cardiovascular risk factors in subjects with rheumatoid arthritis in a large population sample. *Arthritis Rheum* 2007;57(6):953–962.

41. Sabatine MS, Morrow DA, Jablonski KA et al.; PEACE Investigators. Prognostic significance of the Centers for Disease Control/American Heart Association high-sensitivity C-reactive protein cut points for cardiovascular and other outcomes in patients with stable coronary artery disease. *Circulation* 2007;115(12):1528–1536.

42. C-Reactive Protein Coronary Heart Disease Genetics Collaboration (CCGC), Wensley F, Gao P, Burgess S et al. Association between C reactive protein and coronary heart disease: mendelianrandomisation analysis based on individual participant data. *BMJ* 2011;342:d548.

43. Dixon WG, Watson KD, Lunt M et al. Reduction in the incidence of myocardial infarction in patients with rheumatoid arthritis who respond to anti-tumor necrosis factor alpha therapy: results from the British Society for Rheumatology Biologics Register. *Arthritis Rheum* 2007;56(9):2905–2912.

44. Davis JM 3rd, Maradit Kremers H, Crowson CS et al. Glucocorticoids and cardiovascular events in rheumatoid arthritis: a population-based cohort study. *Arthritis Rheum* 2007;56(3):820–830.

45. Wei L, MacDonald TM, Walker BR. Taking glucocorticoids by prescription is associated with subsequent cardiovascular disease. *Ann Intern Med* 2004;141(10):764–770.

46. Svenson KL, Lithell H, Hällgren R, Vessby B. Serum lipoprotein in active rheumatoid arthritis and other chronic inflammatory arthritides. II. Effects of anti-inflammatory and disease-modifying drug treatment. *Arch Intern Med* 1987;147(11):1917–1920.

47. Trelle S, Reichenbach S, Wandel S et al. Cardiovascular safety of non-steroidal anti-inflammatory drugs: network meta-analysis. *BMJ* 2011;342:c7086.

48. Bessant R, Hingorani A, Patel L et al. Risk of coronary heart disease and stroke in a large British cohort of patients with systemic lupus erythematosus. *Rheumatology (Oxford)* 2004;43(7):924–929.

49. Manzi S, Meilahn EN, Rairie JE et al. Age-specific incidence rates of myocardial infarction and angina in women with systemic lupus erythematosus: comparison with the Framingham Study. *Am J Epidemiol* 1997;145(5):408–415.

50. Petri M, Perez-Gutthann S, Spence D, Hochberg MC. Risk factors for coronary artery disease in patients with systemic lupus erythematosus. *Am J Med* 1992;93(5):513–519.

51. Asanuma Y, Oeser A, Shintani AK et al. Premature coronary-artery atherosclerosis in systemic lupus erythematosus. *N Engl J Med* 2003;349(25):2407–2415.

52. Von Feldt JM, Scalzi LV, Cucchiara AJ et al. Homocysteine levels and disease duration independently correlate with coronary artery calcification in patients with systemic lupus erythematosus. *Arthritis Rheum* 2006;54(7):2220–2227.

53. Roman MJ, Shanker BA, Davis A et al. Prevalence and correlates of accelerated atherosclerosis in systemic lupus erythematosus. *N Engl J Med* 2003;349(25):2399–2406.

54. El-Magadmi M, Bodill H, Ahmad Y et al. Systemic lupus erythematosus: an independent risk factor for endothelial dysfunction in women. *Circulation* 2004;110(4):399–404.

55. Manger K, Kusus M, Forster C *et al.* Factors associated with coronary artery calcification in young female patients with SLE. *Ann Rheum Dis* 2003;62(9):846–850.

56. McMahon M, Grossman J, Skaggs B et al. Dysfunctional proinflammatory high- density lipoproteins confer increased risk of atherosclerosis in women with systemic lupus erythematosus. *Arthritis Rheum* 2009;60(8): 2428–2437.

57. Øhlenschlaeger T, Garred P, Madsen HO, Jacobsen S. Mannose-binding lectin variant alleles and the risk of arterial thrombosis in systemic lupus erythematosus. *N Engl J Med* 2004;351(3):260–267.

58. Costenbader KH, Karlson EW, Gall V et al. Barriers to a trial of atherosclerosis prevention in systemic lupus erythematosus. *Arthritis Rheum* 2005;53(5):718–723.

59. Yazdany J, Panopalis P, Gillis JZ et al. A quality indicator set for systemic lupus erythematosus. *Arthritis Rheum* 2009;61(3):370–377.

60. Demas KL, Keenan BT, Solomon DH, Yazdany J, Costenbader KH. Osteoporosis and cardiovascular disease care in systemic lupus erythematosus according to new quality indicators. *Semin Arthritis Rheum* 2010;40(3):193–200.

61. Nüesch E, Dieppe P, Reichenbach S et al. All cause and disease specific mortality in patients with knee or hip osteoarthritis: population based cohort study. *BMJ* 2011;342:d1165.

62. Choi HK, Curhan G. Independent impact of gout on mortality and risk for coronary heart disease. *Circulation* 2007;116(8):894–900.

63. Feig DI, Kang DH, Johnson RJ. Uric acid and cardiovascular risk. *N Engl J Med* 2008;359(17):1811–1821.

64. Nuenninghoff DM, Hunder GG, Christianson TJ, McClelland RL, Matteson EL. Incidence and predictors of large-artery complication (aortic aneurysm, aortic dissection, and/or large-artery stenosis) in patients with giant cell arteritis: a population-based study over 50 years. *Arthritis Rheum* 2003;48(12):3522–3531.

65. Neumann T, Manger B, Schmid M et al. Cardiac involvement in Churg-Strauss syndrome: impact of endomyocarditis. *Medicine (Baltimore)* 2009;88(4):236–243.

CHAPTER 20

Respiratory system

Rachel K. Hoyles and Athol U. Wells

Introduction

Pulmonary involvement is common in the connective tissue diseases (CTDs) and is associated with significant morbidity and mortality. Improved management of systemic disease has led to increasing numbers of surviving patients with clinically significant pulmonary disease. Screening for pulmonary complications highlights the frequency of subclinical involvement. In this chapter, the pulmonary manifestations of the more common CTDs are detailed, including rheumatoid arthritis (RA), systemic sclerosis (SSc), systemic lupus erythematosus (SLE), polymyositis/dermatomyositis (PM/DM), Sjögren's syndrome (SS) and, more briefly, ankylosing spondylitis (AS); the discussion is stratified by pulmonary complication. A broad spectrum of pulmonary disorders are seen in association with the CTDs or the drugs used to treat the underlying disorder. In many cases, two or more pulmonary manifestations of CTD coexist or there are other concurrent diseases such as asthma and lung cancer, resulting in potentially confusing mixed imaging and pulmonary function abnormalities.

Respiratory symptoms

Exertional dyspnoea is non-specific and common, especially in SSc, but is an unreliable marker of lung involvement, as it may result from an increased work of locomotion (arthritis, myositis); moreover, in severe systemic disease, patients may be unable to exercise sufficiently to experience dyspnoea, despite significant lung function impairment. Wheeze more specifically localizes pathology to large or small airways, including asthma, chronic obstructive pulmonary disease (COPD), bronchiolitis, or bronchiectasis. Cough is a common symptom, which is often nocturnal in asthma and reflux, is associated with purulent sputum in bronchiectasis or pneumonia, is typically dry and unrelenting in the interstitial lung diseases, and is common in SS, due to tracheobronchial involvement. Pleuritic pain is a common initial manifestation of RA and SLE. Digital clubbing is common in patients with advanced rheumatoid lung but is extremely rare in the other CTDs. The rate of onset of respiratory symptoms, or temporal association with disease-modifying therapies, often provide clues to the underlying aetiology. There is increasing recognition that lung involvement often precedes the systemic manifestations of CTDs.

Spectrum of lung disease in the connective tissue diseases

Pulmonary complications of connective tissue diseases (CTDs) potentially involve the entire respiratory tract, including large and small airways, lung parenchyma, pulmonary vasculature, pleura, and respiratory muscles. In this chapter, considerable focus is placed on the interstitial lung diseases (ILD), as these disorders provide the most significant diagnostic and management challenges.

Interstitial lung disease

Prevalence

Pulmonary fibrosis (PF) is most prevalent in SSc, forming part of the American Rheumatism Association minor diagnostic criteria for SSc.[1] Lung function impairment is seen in up to 90%, chest radiography abnormalities in 25–65%, with high-resolution CT (HRCT) identifying many patients with subclinical disease.[2] Estimates of clinically significant SSc-PF approximate 30%, with many patients experiencing disabling breathlessness. ILD is also frequent in PM/DM, with at least 30% of patients having clinically overt disease.[3] Clinically important ILD is uncommon in RA, although lung diffusing capacity (DL_{CO}) is reduced in 40%. Less than 5% of SLE patients have clinical or chest radiographic evidence of ILD at presentation and a further 5% develop progressive ILD during follow-up. Clinically overt ILD approximates 10% in primary SS, although 35% have CT abnormalities, and there is a high prevalence of respiratory symptoms, especially cough.[4] AS is frequently associated with limited non-specific CT abnormalities, but clinically significant upper zone fibrobullous disease is rare. In summary, clinically significant PF occurs in approximately 30% of patients with SSc and PM/DM, in 10% with SS, and in less than 5% with SLE or RA, with a much higher prevalence of subclinical disease in all of these disorders.

Aetiology and predisposing factors

There are genetic associations with ILD in SSc (HLA DR3, 52a) and RA (HLA-B8 and HLA-Dw3). Genetic predilections are amplified by the autoantibody status. In PM/DM, significant ILD is often seen with the anti-synthetase syndrome, associated with aminoacyl tRNA synthetases including Jo-1. In RA, ILD is associated with high rheumatoid factor titres. In SSc, titres of anti-topoisomerase (ATA) and anti-centromere (ACA) antibodies are a strong determinant of lung and pulmonary vascular disease respectively.[5] Smoking is a risk factor for the development of overt ILD in RA. Other extrinsic triggers, such as rapeseed cooking oil denatured with aniline in SSc, may be cofactors for the development of pulmonary disease.

Pathogenesis

The pathogenesis of PF has been most extensively studied in SSc; a widely accepted model is that the accumulation of connective tissue in the lung is autoimmune, with environmental factors triggering initial alveolar epithelial cell injury and a subsequent amplification of the immune and inflammatory response in genetically susceptible individuals.[6] Mediators including transforming growth factor beta, tumour necrosis factor alpha (TNFα), connective tissue growth factor, and a T-helper cell 1 (Th1) to Th2 cytokine shift, promote a profibrotic microenvironment. The ATA antibody may have an immunopathogenetic role.

Pathology

Histological appearances can be broadly subdivided into fibrotic and inflammatory abnormalities. The fibrotic histological patterns of ILD in the CTDs are usual interstitial pneumonia (UIP) and non-specific interstitial pneumonia (NSIP). UIP is characterized by heterogeneous thickening of alveolar walls by inflammatory and connective tissue matrix cells, type II pneumocyte proliferation, and vascular obliteration; the disease is maximal subpleurally and basally with evolution to honeycombing in advanced disease. In NSIP, there is a more homogeneous distribution of septal inflammation and fibrosis, with a basal predominance. In SSc, fibrosing NSIP and, less frequently, cellular NSIP predominate. There is no difference in survival between NSIP or UIP subgroups, in contrast to outcome differences in idiopathic disease.[7] In RA, UIP is slightly more prevalent than NSIP, with prominent peribronchiolar lymphoid follicles a frequent finding. Fibrotic disease in PM/DM and SS almost always has a pattern of fibrotic NSIP. Clinically significant chronic irreversible disease is rare in SLE with anecdotal reports suggesting that fibrotic NSIP predominates.

In RA and PM/DM, inflammatory lung disease most often takes the form of organizing pneumonia (OP), consisting histologically of plugs of granulation tissue in the air spaces distal to and including the terminal bronchioles, associated with lymphocytic infiltration. OP presents with multifocal consolidation, a restrictive functional defect, and is usually responsive to corticosteroids. However, the good prognosis with treatment seen in cryptogenic OP is not invariable in the CTDs as supervening fibrosis is not infrequent.

Other forms of inflammatory interstitial disease are less frequent. Lymphocytic interstitial pneumonitis (LIP) is reported in RA and PM/DM, but is more prevalent in SS. In general, in SS, lymphocytic interstitial infiltration is the usual form of interstitial inflammation, ranging from LIP (characterized by a diffuse lymphocytic infiltrate, prominent around bronchioles), through pseudolymphoma (with the formation of lymphoid follicles) to pulmonary lymphoma.

Rare but clinically important histological patterns exist in CTD lung disease. Acute interstitial pneumonia (AIP), an accelerated course of ILD, with the histological features of diffuse alveolar damage, is seen most often in PM/DM. Diffuse alveolar damage may also contribute to the poor outcomes seen in some patients with the entity of 'acute lupus pneumonitis', occurring in up to 2% of SLE patients. In AS, histological appearances consist of a variable admixture of lymphocytic infiltration, fibrosis and bullous change.

Prognosis

In SSc and PM/DM, pulmonary disease (including ILD, aspiration pneumonitis, and pulmonary vascular disease) is now the most common cause of death. In SSc, ILD is associated with a 30% 10 year mortality rate, and is usually most progressive within 4 years of the onset of systemic disease: however, a significant subgroup of patients with subclinical or mild lung involvement remain stable during prolonged follow-up. In PM/DM, ILD carries a 5 year survival of 60–85%; the clinical course of these patients tends to be dominated by pulmonary disease.[8] AIP has a mortality of over 50%, once respiratory failure has supervened. In general, severe pulmonary involvement identifies progressive disease with a poor outcome; for example, in RA with PF requiring hospitalization, the 5 year survival is less than 50%.

Fibrobullous disease

Although rare, ILD confined to the upper zones is a well-described feature of AS. Cavities within distorted fibrotic apical tissue may be colonized by mycobacteria or fungi. An increased prevalence of pneumothorax probably reflects subpleural bullous degeneration. Apical fibrosis is rarely seen in RA and MS, but localized apical bulla formation and emphysema is a more prevalent and striking finding in MS, associated with a high (5–10%) prevalence of pneumothoraces.[9]

Pulmonary infection

The CTDs have an increased prevalence of pulmonary infection, due to lowering of host defences both by the presence of the systemic disease, and by immunosuppressive treatments. Bronchopneumonia is a common terminal event in RA and PM/DM, accounting for 15–20% of deaths in RA.

Gram-negative bacterial infections, including *Klebsiella pneumoniae*, *Escherichia coli*, and *Pseudomonas aeruginosa*, are more frequent in the CTDs, and infection with *Legionella* spp. is more frequent in the immunosuppressed patient. Fungal colonization, especially *Aspergillus fumigatus*, is common in fibrocavitary lung disease. Mycetoma are often asymptomatic and do not require specific therapy, but life-threatening haemoptysis may require bronchial artery embolization. Surgical resection is generally contraindicated, as the postoperative complication rate is very high. Mycobacterial infections are seen in patients with CTDs, and are characterized by lung infiltrates, multifocal nodularity, and small airways exudates on CT, and often require bronchoscopy for diagnosis. New widespread ground-glass opacification in an immunosuppressed patient should raise the possibility of *Pneumocystis jirovecii* or viral infection.

Aspiration pneumonia is seen most frequently in PM/DM and is associated with a marked increase in mortality. It occurs in 20% of patients and should always be suspected when pneumonia occurs in a patient with dysphagia due to pharyngeal muscle weakness.

The high prevalence of pneumothorax in MS of 5–10%, which are often recurrent and bilateral, is ascribable to the rupture of subpleural bullae; emphysema is evident on chest radiography in the majority of Marfan's patients with pneumothoraces.

Pulmonary nodules

Pulmonary nodules may be associated with underlying CTD, but malignant disease must always be considered. Pulmonary rheumatoid nodules, present in over 20% of patients with RA, may be single or multiple, are often peripheral, are usually associated with extrapulmonary rheumatoid nodules, and vary in size depending on RA activity (sometimes simulating a malignant growth pattern). Complications include nodule cavitation and pneumothorax. In Caplan's syndrome, single or multiple variably cavitating nodules are associated with coal miner's pneumoconiosis.

DM is associated with an increased prevalence of malignancy, with systemic disease rsometimes representing a paraneoplastic phenomenon; recent studies have indicate that the prevalence of lung malignancy was previously overstated.[10] However, there is undoubtedly an increased risk of lung malignancy in association with PF, first described in idiopathic ILD, independent of the risk conferred by smoking. The likelihood of malignancy is increased if nodule diameter is greater than 10 mm.

Pseudolymphoma masses may arise in primary SS patients with prominent lymphocytic infiltration and often responds well to corticosteroid therapy; however, progression to pulmonary lymphoma occurs with a prevalence of 1–2%.

Wegener's granulomatosis is often associated with pulmonary nodules, which may be multiple, rapidly enlarge, and cavitate. The differential diagnosis for cavitating pulmonary nodules includes malignancy and pulmonary abscesses.

Bronchiectasis and large-airway disease

Bronchiectasis, characterized by bronchial wall inflammation and dilatation, is most prevalent in RA (and unusual in other CTDs), and may precede the development of systemic disease. It is often clinically silent, and usually less disabling than idiopathic bronchiectasis. However, in a minority of RA patients, bronchiectasis is associated with progressive airflow obstruction and recurrent infective exacerbations. The prescription of immunomodulatory drugs for systemic disease further complicates management.

Xerotrachea occurs in 25–50% of patients with primary SS and consists of atrophy of tracheobronchial mucous glands in association with a lymphoplasmocytic infiltrate, manifesting clinically as a relentless dry cough, and may be associated with bronchial hyperresponsiveness, to be differentiated from asthma. Relapsing polychondritis is associated with thickening of the tracheal rings and tracheal or airway collapse on inspiration, best appreciated on a flow–volume loop or dynamic CT. Approximately 10% of deaths are respiratory, generally resulting from airway stricture, collapse and distal infection.

Bronchiolitis

Bronchiolitis may be classified as obliterative (OB) or follicular (FB). The cardinal features of OB are infiltration of the bronchiolar wall by granulation tissue, effacement of the lumen, and eventual replacement of the bronchiole by fibrous tissue. Most cases of OB in CTDs occur in RA, although the prevalence of OB in RA is low. Small-airway disease tends to be clinically silent until advanced, and is often admixed with interstitial lung disease. OB may be associated with rapidly progressive airflow obstruction which is often unresponsive to corticosteroid treatment.

FB is a rare disorder, characterized by external compression of bronchioles by hyperplastic lymphoid follicles, and variable lymphocytic infiltration of the bronchiolar wall, occurring most frequently in SS. Clinically significant isolated FB is rare in RA but its recognition is important because a response to corticosteroid therapy is more likely than in other forms of bronchiolitis.

Pleural disease

Pleural disease is common in RA and SLE. Pleural effusions (representing a serositis) are the most common pulmonary complication in RA, and are often asymptomatic, although pleuritic pain is present at some time in at least 20% of patients.[11] Aspiration is often required to exclude infection or malignancy. The pleural fluid is exudative, with reduced glucose levels and pH and a lymphocytosis, therefore if empyema is clinically suspected, management often relies upon microbiology as traditional fluid markers are less discriminatory for infection.

Overt pleural involvement is present in 20% of patients with newly diagnosed SLE; pleural abnormalities are found at autopsy in 50–100%. The fluid is usually serosanguinous, exudative, and neutrophilic during acute pleurisy, and lymphocytic in chronic effusions. The histological appearance of fibrinous pleuritis is nonspecific.

Chest wall disease

In SLE, the 'shrinking lung' syndrome, characterized by elevation of the hemidiaphragms and basal atelectasis, results from extrapulmonic restriction,[12] with exertional dyspnoea and a restrictive ventilatory defect associated with relative preservation of DL_{CO} and elevation of the transfer coefficient (K_{CO}). The shrinking lung syndrome is usually self-limited. By contrast, respiratory muscle weakness resulting from myositis may progress to hypercapnic respiratory failure, although this is seen in less than 5% of PM/DM patients. Immobilization of the chest wall is common in AS, but is often clinically silent, with surprisingly preserved pulmonary function. Chest wall deformities may be striking in MS, although isolated pectus excavatum is usually asymptomatic. Extrapulmonic restriction in SSc may be due to severe scleroderma of the chest wall, leading to respiratory failure.

Pulmonary vascular disease

Pulmonary vascular disease in the CTDs may take the form of isolated pulmonary arterial disease, pulmonary vasculitis, thromboembolism, or pulmonary artery aneurysms (in Beçhet's syndrome) and may also result from vascular ablation due to extensive interstitial lung disease.

Pulmonary arteriolar hypertension occurs most commonly in SSc, with concentric arteriolar fibrosis with ablation of the intima and media, and clusters with limited cutaneous SSc and the ACA antibody. It is associated with a high mortality, accounting for a 5 year survival of less than 10% in patients with DL_{CO} levels of less than 40% of predicted.

Pulmonary hypertension was once regarded as rare in SLE but is now increasingly recognized. Vasoconstriction is likely to play a greater pathogenetic role than pulmonary vasculitis, together with recurrent thromboembolism in patients with anti-phospholipid antibodies.

Pulmonary capillaritis resulting in diffuse alveolar haemorrhage (DAH) is seen much more frequently in SLE than in other CTDs; it occurs in only 2% of SLE patients, but is responsible for over 20% of SLE hospital admissions, and is often life-threatening, with a mortality of over 50%.

Drug-induced pulmonary toxicity

Methotrexate-induced interstitial pneumonitis is the most frequently encountered drug-induced pulmonopathy encountered in the CTDs, with a prevalence of approximately 5%, in treated RA patients.[13] Methotrexate pneumonitis is potentially life-threatening with a mortality of 15–20%, presenting with cough, dyspnoea, fever, widespread crackles, a restrictive functional defect, and pulmonary infiltrates, and should always be suspected in the treated patient presenting with progressive lung disease. Peripheral eosinophilia is seen in 50%. Although sometimes explosive, the onset is more often subacute over many weeks, and the majority of cases are diagnosed within 4 months of starting methotrexate. The clinical, radiological, and histological findings are not diagnostic, although features of a hypersensitivity pneumonitis with lymphocytic infiltration are common. Whether pre-existing lung disease predisposes to methotrexate lung is uncertain; conflicting published data suggests that functional impairment is a relative but not an absolute contraindication to the use of methotrexate. Particular caution is warranted when pulmonary reserve is grossly compromised, and patients with previous methotrexate toxicity should not be rechallenged.

Pulmonary toxicity has also been documented with non-steroidal anti-inflammatory agents (NSAIDs), sulfasalazine, gold therapy, penicillamine, and anti-TNF agents. OP associated with sulfasalazine is rare and occurs most commonly in the upper lobes. Lung infiltrates induced by gold are often associated with fever or skin rash, and a bronchoalveolar lavage (BAL) lymphocytosis. Penicillamine has been implicated in the development of OB in RA, and has also induced hypersensitivity pneumonitis as well as a pulmonary–renal syndrome manifesting most commonly as DAH. Most patients with pulmonary toxicity respond well to withdrawal of the agent and corticosteroid therapy.

Investigation of lung disease

Pulmonary function tests

Spirometric measures of FEV_1 (forced expiratory volume in 1s) and FVC (forced vital capacity) are simple screening tools; an FEV_1/FVC ratio of less than 70% reflects obstructive airways disease, whereas a ratio of more than 80% reflects restrictive lung pathology including interstitial and chest wall disorders. The carbon monoxide gas transfer (DL_{CO}) is reduced in disorders that impede the efficacy of transfer of soluble gases from alveolus to capillary, including interstitial fibrosis, pulmonary hypertension, pulmonary embolic disease, emphysema, and anaemia. The most typical patterns of functional impairment in unselected patients with connective tissue disease are an isolated depression of gas transfer (reflecting subclinical interstitial involvement or pulmonary vascular disease) and, less frequently, a restrictive defect, due to overt PF.

ILD is characterized by a restrictive ventilatory defect and a reduction in DL_{CO}; in SSc, baseline DL_{CO} of less than 50% or FVC of less than 55% is unequivocally significant in the ILDs.[14] DL_{CO} alone does not discriminate between ILD severity and the presence of pulmonary hypertension, but the combined assessment of DL_{CO} and FVC can discriminate: in isolated pulmonary hypertension, a very low DL_{CO} is often associated with a normal FVC.

Airflow obstruction may denote smoking-related lung damage, bronchiectasis, or bronchiolitis. Extrapulmonic restriction, due to pleural or chest wall disease, often mimics the functional consequences of ILD, but there is relative preservation of DL_{CO}. Respiratory muscle weakness may be assessed by lying and standing FVC, although mouth pressures are more sensitive. Marked elevation of both DL_{CO} and K_{CO} is a pathognomonic finding in DAH if measured within 36 hours.

Serial pulmonary function tests are central to monitoring progression of disease, defined as a fall of more than 10% in predicted FVC or more than 15% in DL_{CO} from baseline values. In SSc-associated ILD, serial DL_{CO} assessment over 3 years appears to be predictive of survival.[7]

Chest radiology

Plain chest radiograph (CXR) confidently diagnoses consolidation, large pulmonary nodules, and pleural effusions, but often underestimates the ILD severity. An apparently normal chest radiograph should not inhibit the further investigation of symptomatic patients.

High-resolution CT (HRCT) has revolutionized the approach to ILD, owing to its high sensitivity and good correlation with the underlying histological appearance.[15] In fibrotic NSIP (common in SSc and PM/DM; Figure 20.1A), lower zone ground-glass

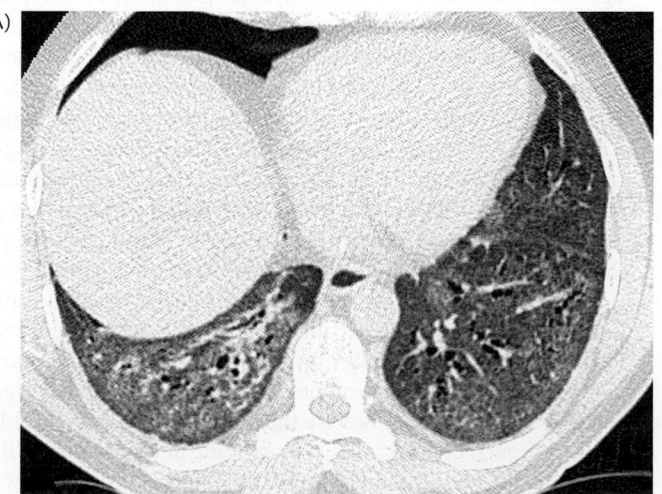
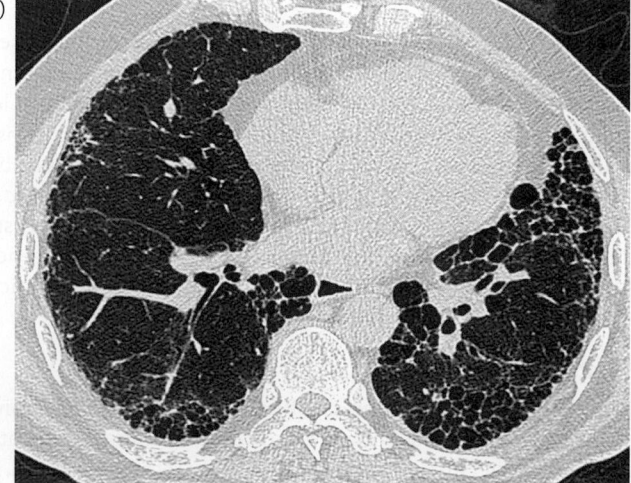

Fig. 20.1 CT images in CTD associated interstitial lung disease: (A) A fibrosing non-specific interstitial pneumonia (NSIP) pattern is commonly seen in SSc, with evidence of ground-glass and traction bronchiolar dilatation. (B) A usual interstitial pneumonia (UIP) pattern is more prevalent in RA, with basal subpleural honeycombing on CT.

attenuation is associated with reticulation and traction bronchiectasis, indicating fine intralobular fibrosis. In a minority of patients with cellular NSIP, ground-glass attenuation without traction bronchiectasis may predominate. A UIP pattern, common in RA, is characterized by peripheral, basal reticulation and honeycombing, without substantial ground-glass attenuation (Figure 20.1B). An admixture of OP and fibrosis is commonly seen in PM/DM, and other disease processes are often evident, especially bronchiolitis and bronchiectasis (in RA) and pleural disease (in RA and SLE).[16] The cardinal CT feature of OP is patchy bilateral airspace consolidation, which is often subpleural but occasionally bronchovascular. By contrast, OB is characterized by areas of mosaic attenuation, due to both bronchiolitis and regional hypoxic vasoconstriction. In SS, subclinical abnormalities are commonly evident on CT, including airways disease, ground-glass attenuation, reticular abnormalities, and patchy consolidation.

A simple CT staging system for ILD in SSc determines the overall disease extent as greater or less than 20%, and this is highly discriminatory of outcome, with extensive disease (>20%) predictive of mortality. When HRCT findings are difficult to classify using this approach, an FVC threshold of 70% of predicted normal values is used to classify disease as extensive or mild. This simple system aids the selection of a higher-risk patient for potentially toxic therapies.[17]

Nuclear medicine techniques

The clearance of radiolabelled diethylene triamine pentacetate clearance($^{99\,m}$Tc-DTPA) detects subclinical ILD and may be used to evaluate prognosis in SSc, but it is not available in many centres. In SSc, rapid $^{99\,m}$Tc-DTPA clearance denotes loss of epithelial cell integrity; persistently rapid clearance identifies an increased risk of subsequent deterioration.[18]

Bronchoalveolar lavage

BAL is invaluable in the exclusion of infection, particularly opportunistic pathogens, in an immunosuppressed patient with lung infiltrates. However, recent data have failed to validate the historical observation that a BAL neutrophilia in SSc is associated with a much worse outcome. Thus, BAL has only a limited role in routine prognostic evaluation.[19]

Lung biopsy

Transbronchial lung biopsy is often used to confirm the presence of OP but cannot reliably discriminate between fibrotic patterns of disease. CT guided biopsy is often used to sample peripheral lung nodules, particularly to exclude malignancy. Surgical lung biopsy is seldom required in the investigation of ILD in the CTDs, as distinctions between patterns of fibrotic disease carry little prognostic significance in SSc[7]—although there are inconclusive data suggesting that UIP may have a worse outcome than NSIP in RA. In general, surgical biopsy should be considered only when disease is clinically significant and HRCT appearances are atypical.

Vascular studies

Doppler echocardiography is often used to detect pulmonary hypertension; estimated pressures correlate with measurements of pulmonary artery pressures made at right heart catheterization, and right ventricular dilatation or hypertrophy may suggest pulmonary hypertension in the absence of a tricuspid regurgitant jet.

Screening for pulmonary disease

Screening for lung disease has an important role in the CTDs, both to identify early disease, and to assess the impact of potentially pneumotoxic immunosuppression. In general, those CTDs with a high prevalence of PF (SSc, PM/DM) should be screened with lung function and CXR at diagnosis, with a low threshold for CT if abnormalities are detected. Screening with PFTs in CTDs with a low prevalence of ILD (SLE, SS, AS) should probably be reserved for those with respiratory symptoms or CXR abnormalities. Screening in RA is more difficult to define, as there is a relatively low prevalence of clinically significant ILD. However, many therapies used in RA cause pulmonary toxicity and we therefore advocate a screening regimen akin to that of SSc. Knowledge of baseline PFT levels allows earlier detection of significant functional decline due to drug-induced lung disease.

Treatment decisions in relation to prognostic evaluation

The prediction of likely natural history is particularly relevant in ILD associated with CTDs. Many patients with ILD have limited disease with minor functional impairment, and remain stable without treatment, whereas a smaller group deteriorate more rapidly and should be treated as early as possible. Predictors of decline are often extrapolated from studies of SSc-associated ILD, where extensive disease on CT or pulmonary function tests, deteriorating pulmonary function tests, and a short duration of systemic disease are major indicators for treatment.[20] The extent of cutaneous disease, the pattern of fibrotic abnormalities on HRCT and biopsy, and BAL cell counts are less useful in determining prognosis or in treatment selection. Pending disease specific analyses, these principles can be applied to treatment decisions in lung disease associated with other CTDs.

Treatment options

Interstitial lung disease in the connective tissue diseases

There is limited trial evidence in the treatment of ILD in the CTDs; trial recruitment has been particularly problematic, because of disease heterogeneity, and variations in the severity and progressiveness of disease. In many studies, there is no clear distinction between regression of disease and prevention of progression, now accepted to be a positive outcome in predominantly fibrotic disease. The treatment of ILD in SSc has been most widely evaluated. High-dose corticosteroid therapy is not efficacious and may trigger scleroderma renal crisis.[21] Daily treatment with oral cyclophosphamide(2 mg/kg per day) for 1 year was associated with a small statistically significant benefit in FVC in a placebo-controlled randomized controlled trial (RCT),[22] but this effect was short-lived, suggesting that prolonged treatment is required.[23] In a smaller RCT, intravenous cyclophosphamide (600 mg/m^2 monthly), followed by oral azathioprine (2.5 mg/kg per day), in combination with low-dose prednisolone (e.g. 10 mg/day), conferred marginal FVC benefits at 1 year.[24] Taken together, these studies provide conceptual support for the widespread use of immunosuppressive therapy in clinically significant SSc-associated ILD, despite the relatively small effect on FVC levels. However, the low average magnitude of effect in these RCTs underlines the need to validate other treatment approaches, including the use of novel antifibrotic agents. Small retrospective studies of mycophenolate mofetil suggest a possible role but prospective evaluation is required.[25] Autologous haematopoietic cell transplantation following immunoablative high-dose immunosuppression is being evaluated in European and US trials.[26] CD20-positive B-cell depletion with rituximab had a positive impact on lung function in an open-label RCT,[27] and our experience suggests that it is useful in rapidly progressive lung disease in CTD. A recent RCT evaluation established that endothelin antagonism did not influence the likelihood of clinically significant worsening.[28]

Interstitial lung disease associated with polymyositis/dermatomyositis

Uncontrolled reports suggest that high-dose corticosteroid therapy is more efficacious in PM/DM-associated ILD, reflecting the greater prevalence of OP, even when fibrotic disease is present. If the ILD is of moderate severity, a second-line agent (usually azathioprine, mycophenolate mofetil, or methotrexate) is often added to steroid therapy. However, disease is fulminant in a minority of cases with a mixture of OP and diffuse alveolar damage and high-dose intravenous methylprednisolone (1 g/day for 3 days) and cyclophosphamide may be required, with variable efficacy.[29] Retrospective studies have suggested a favourable outcome with rituximab in the anti-synthetase syndrome.[30]

Interstitial lung disease in rheumatoid arthritis

The treatment of ILD in RA suffers from an extreme paucity of outcome data. Historically, high doses of oral corticosteroids have been used, with the addition of an immunosuppressive agent (in particular azathioprine) as steroid therapy is reduced in selected patients, based upon disease severity and progressiveness.[31] The impact of T- and B-cell modifying therapies on rheumatoid-associated ILD is currently unclear.

Organizing pneumonia and drug-induced lung disease

High-dose corticosteroid therapy is usual in OP and drug-induced lung disease. However, especially in patients with OP, supervening fibrotic disease is not uncommon, with second line agents not infrequently required to prevent disease progression. Similarly, in LIP with SS, a good response to corticosteroid therapy is frequent but not invariable and there are no definitive therapeutic trials. In explosive ILD (diffuse alveolar damage, acute lupus pneumonitis, DAH, severe non-haemorrhagic vasculitis), there is no option but to intervene aggressively after infection has been rigorously excluded, usually with intravenous methylprednisolone and early use of cyclophosphamide; however, this empirical approach is based solely upon anecdotal responses. Pneumonitis due to drug toxicity generally responds well to withdrawal of the offending agent and corticosteroids, provided that fibrosis has not supervened.

Bronchiolitis

Regression of disease rarely occurs in OB with corticosteroid or immunosuppressive therapy; whereas disease stabilization or regression with therapy is seen in FB. A trial of corticosteroids is warranted in symptomatic pleural disease in RA or SLE: some patients with rheumatoid effusions respond well and a good outcome is seen in SLE, although prolonged treatment may be required. Somewhat surprisingly, steroid responsiveness has been documented in the shrinking lung syndrome of SLE.

Pulmonary vascular disease

Intervention in pulmonary vascular disease is complicated by the multiplicity of possible pathogenetic mechanisms. Treatment of SSc-associated pulmonary arteriolar hypertension includes anticoagulants, diuretics, supplemental oxygen, synthetic prostacyclins, endothelin-1 antagonism, and phosphodiesterase inhibitors, and is reviewed elsewhere.[32] In other CTDs, especially in SLE and mixed connective tissue disease, PAH may respond to corticosteroid or immunosuppressive therapy.

Bronchiectasis

The management of bronchiectasis mirrors that in the general population, namely regular sputum clearance with physiotherapy, and aggressive (microbiology guided) treatment of infective exacerbations (10–14 days). Inhaled bronchodilators and corticosteroids may be useful in alleviating airflow obstruction in bronchiectasis.

Lung transplantation in endstage interstitial lung disease

In endstage ILD, lung transplantation for systemic disease remains controversial. A recent series reports transplant outcomes to be similar in SSc and idiopathic ILD, although increased acute rejection rates were seen in SSc.[33] In many centres, aggressive connective tissue disease is regarded as an absolute contraindication to transplantation. In terminal disease, the need for regular oxygen therapy and treatment of supervening heart failure and infection are the primary therapeutic considerations.

In summary, the decision to treat many pulmonary complications of the CTDs is multifaceted and difficult, and requires a multidisciplinary approach with close interaction between the rheumatologist and respiratory physician.

Conclusion

Lung involvement occurs frequently in the CTDs, but in many patients pathological processes are self-limited and subclinical. Clinically significant lung disease often consists of an admixture of interstitial, airway-centred, vascular, or pleural processes. Careful evaluation allows the clinician to identify the predominant pathophysiological process, stage disease severity, estimate the likely prognosis, select treatments most likely to be efficacious, and choose the most appropriate investigations to monitor disease progression.

References

1. Preliminary criteria for the classification of systemic sclerosis (scleroderma). Subcommittee for scleroderma criteria of the American Rheumatism Association Diagnostic and Therapeutic Criteria Committee. *Arthritis Rheum* 1980;23(5):581–590.
2. Wells AU, Steen V, Valentini G. Pulmonary complications: one of the most challenging complications of systemic sclerosis. *Rheumatology (Oxford)* 2009;48 Suppl 3:iii40–iii44.
3. Schwarz MI. The lung in polymyositis. *Clin Chest Med* 1998;19(4): 701–712, viii.
4. Ito I, Nagai S, Kitaichi M et al. Pulmonary manifestations of primary Sjögren's syndrome: a clinical, radiologic, and pathologic study. *Am J Respir Crit Care Med* 2005;171(6):632–638.
5. Wells AU, Steen V, Valentini G. Pulmonary complications: one of the most challenging complications of systemic sclerosis. *Rheumatology (Oxford)* 2009;48 Suppl 3:iii40–iii44.
6. Yamamoto T. Autoimmune mechanisms of scleroderma and a role of oxidative stress. *Self Nonself* 2011;2(1):4–10.
7. Bouros D, Wells AU, Nicholson AG et al. Histopathologic subsets of fibrosing alveolitis in patients with systemic sclerosis and their relationship to outcome. *Am J Respir Crit Care Med* 2002;165(12):1581–1586.

8. Marie I, Hachulla E, Cherin P et al. Interstitial lung disease in polymyositis and dermatomyositis. *Arthritis Rheum* 2002;47(6):614–622.

9. Karpman C, Aughenbaugh GL, Ryu JH. Pneumothorax and bullae in Marfan syndrome. *Respiration* 2011;82(3):219–224.

10. Zahr ZA, Baer AN. Malignancy in myositis. *Curr Rheumatol Rep* 2011;13(3):208–215.

11. Amital A, Shitrit D, Adir Y. The lung in rheumatoid arthritis. *Presse Med* 2011;40(1 Pt 2):e31–e48.

12. Carmier D, Diot E, Diot P. Shrinking lung syndrome: recognition, pathophysiology and therapeutic strategy. *Expert Rev Respir Med* 2011;5(1):33–39.

13. Lateef O, Shakoor N, Balk RA. Methotrexate pulmonary toxicity. *Expert Opin Drug Safety* 2005;4(4):723–730.

14. Assassi S, del Junco D, Sutter K et al. Clinical and genetic factors predictive of mortality in early systemic sclerosis. *Arthritis Rheum* 2009;61(10):1403–1411.

15. Woodhead F, Wells AU, Desai SR. Pulmonary complications of connective tissue diseases. *Clin Chest Med* 2008;29(1):149–164, vii.

16. Tanaka N, Kim JS, Newell JD et al. Rheumatoid arthritis-related lung diseases: CT findings. *Radiology* 2004;232(1):81–91.

17. Goh NS, Desai SR, Veeraraghavan S et al. Interstitial lung disease in systemic sclerosis: a simple staging system. *Am J Respir Crit Care Med* 2008;177(11):1248–1254.

18. Wells AU, Hansell DM, Harrison NK et al. Clearance of inhaled 99 mTc-DTPA predicts the clinical course of fibrosing alveolitis. *Eur Respir J* 1993;6(6):797–802.

19. Goh NS, Veeraraghavan S, Desai SR et al. Bronchoalveolar lavage cellular profiles in patients with systemic sclerosis-associated interstitial lung disease are not predictive of disease progression. *Arthritis Rheum* 2007;56(6):2005–2012.

20. Latsi PI, Wells AU. Evaluation and management of alveolitis and interstitial lung disease in scleroderma. *Curr Opin Rheumatol* 2003;15(6):748–755.

21. DeMarco PJ, Weisman MH, Seibold JR et al. Predictors and outcomes of scleroderma renal crisis: the high-dose versus low-dose D-penicillamine in early diffuse systemic sclerosis trial. *Arthritis Rheum* 2002;46(11):2983–2989.

22. Tashkin DP, Elashoff R, Clements PJ et al. Cyclophosphamide versus placebo in scleroderma lung disease. *N Engl J Med* 2006;354(25):2655–2666.

23. Tashkin DP, Elashoff R, Clements PJ et al. Effects of 1-year treatment with cyclophosphamide on outcomes at 2 years in scleroderma lung disease. *Am J Respir Crit Care Med* 2007;176(10):1026–1034.

24. Hoyles RK, Ellis RW, Wellsbury J et al. A multicenter, prospective, randomized, double-blind, placebo-controlled trial of corticosteroids and intravenous cyclophosphamide followed by oral azathioprine for the treatment of pulmonary fibrosis in scleroderma. *Arthritis Rheum* 2006;54(12):3962–3970.

25. Koutroumpas A, Ziogas A, Alexiou I, Barouta G, Sakkas LI. Mycophenolate mofetil in systemic sclerosis-associated interstitial lung disease. *Clin Rheumatol* 2010;29(10):1167–1168.

26. van Laar JM, Farge D, Tyndall A. Autologous Stem cell Transplantation International Scleroderma (ASTIS) trial: hope on the horizon for patients with severe systemic sclerosis. *Ann Rheum Dis* 2005;64(10):1515.

27. Daoussis D, Liossis SN, Tsamandas AC et al. Experience with rituximab in scleroderma: results from a 1-year, proof-of-principle study. *Rheumatology (Oxford)* 2010;49(2):271–280.

28. Seibold JR, Denton CP, Furst DE et al. Randomized, prospective, placebo-controlled trial of bosentan in interstitial lung disease secondary to systemic sclerosis. *Arthritis Rheum* 2010;62(7):2101–2108.

29. Yamasaki Y, Yamada H, Yamasaki M et al. Intravenous cyclophosphamide therapy for progressive interstitial pneumonia in patients with polymyositis/dermatomyositis. *Rheumatology (Oxford)* 2007;46(1):124–130.

30. Sem M, Molberg O, Lund MB, Gran JT. Rituximab treatment of the antisynthetase syndrome: a retrospective case series. *Rheumatology (Oxford)* 2009;48(8):968–771.

31. Nannini C, Ryu JH, Matteson EL. Lung disease in rheumatoid arthritis. *Curr Opin Rheumatol* 2008;20(3):340–346.

32. McLaughlin V, Humbert M, Coghlan G, Nash P, Steen V. Pulmonary arterial hypertension: the most devastating vascular complication of systemic sclerosis. *Rheumatology (Oxford)* 2009;48 Suppl 3:iii25–iii31.

33. Saggar R, Khanna D, Furst DE et al. Systemic sclerosis and bilateral lung transplantation: a single centre experience. *Eur Respir J* 2010;36(4):893–900.

CHAPTER 21

Gastrointestinal system

Gerhard Rogler

Intestinal mucosa as an immune organ

The gastrointestinal (GI) tract represents the largest barrier between the human body and the environment, with a surface area of up to 400 m^2. Its lining is an epithelial monolayer, representing a very thin physical barrier. Below this epithelial layer, separated by a basal membrane, the lamina propria contains antigen-presenting cells (APCs) as well as lymphocytes.[1] The lamina propria substantially contributes to the barrier function of the intestinal mucosa.[2] APCs from the lamina propria form podocytes reaching through the basal membrane to the epithelial cells and even into the gut lumen.[3]

Under normal conditions the intestinal immune system mediates tolerance to our commensal flora. In inflammatory bowel disease (IBD), this tolerance is broken.[4] Genetic factors have been identified in 30–40% of IBD patients causing susceptibility for these diseases. Many of the susceptibility factors play an important role in the recognition of bacterial antigens (pattern recognition receptors, PRRs) and have functions in innate immune defence.[5]

The adaptive immunity in the GI tract is mediated by gut-associated lymphoid tissue (GALT). Morphologically this is composed of the Peyer's patches (PP), the lymphoid aggregates and lymph follicles of the intestinal wall and the mesenteric lymph nodes. In addition, B and T cells are scattered throughout the mucosa.[6] The mucosa-associated lymphoid cells can be divided into two phenotypic and functionally different cell populations: lamina propria lymphocytes (LPL) and intraepithelial lymphocytes (IEL).

The LPL constitute the largest portion of lymphocytes in the intestinal mucosa. In the lamina propria T lymphocytes clearly outweigh B lymphocytes and plasma cells. They consist to 95% of $\alpha\beta$ T cells, which can be subdivided into CD4+ and CD8+ T cells. CD4 cells are two to four times as frequent as CD8 cells.[6] In contrast, IEL consist mainly of $\gamma\delta$ CD8+ T cells, which differ morphologically and functionally from the LPL. They suppress inflammatory reactions and are tolerogenic.

In mouse models it is possible to discriminate clearly between Th1 cells, secreting proinflammatory cytokines such as IL-12, and Th2 cells, secreting a more anti-inflammatory pattern such as IL-4 or IL-10, but this much harder in human mucosa. None of the human inflammatory intestinal diseases can be described as a pure Th1- or Th2-mediated inflammation.

Regulatory T cells can also be found in the intestinal mucosa. The anti-inflammatory, 'regulatory' effect of those cells is attributed to the high production of IL-10. Regulatory T cells are in principle able to control or prevent intestinal inflammation, due to their immunosuppressive characteristics.[7]

Since its discovery, the Th17 cell population has attracted the attention of gastroenterologists.[8] This subgroup of T cells, which expresses the cytokine IL-17 in large amounts, plays an important role for the chronification of intestinal inflammation. Th17 cells may induce and maintain a chronic colitis independent of Th1 cells.[8] In animal models IL-17 secretion in the intestine is followed by production and secretion of chemokines, which recruit further inflammatory cells. The induction of Th17 cells is induced by several recently described interleukins such as IL-23, which therefore also can be regarded as pathophysiological relevant factors. IL-23 is secreted by APCs in the mucosa.[8] Interestingly, polymorphisms in the IL-23 receptor are associated with the risk of developing IBD.[9]

The GI tract contains three times as much immunoglobulin-producing plasma as the spleen, lymph nodes, and bone marrow combined.[10] In addition, mucosal mast cells have been shown to play an important role in chronic intestinal inflammation.

IEL are normally found in the epithelial layer, in a ratio of 5 lymphocytes to 100 enterocytes. They have regulatory functions. However, in coeliac disease IEL are a histological hallmark of inflammation and a diagnostic marker; they contribute to disease pathogenesis and epithelial damage.

T-cell-mediated and humoral immunity are controlled and regulated by GI hormones and the innate immune system. In turn, they affect physiological GI functions such as transport, permeability, and contractility. APCs in the GI mucosa activate the lymphatic cells via the secretion of cytokines such as tumor necrosis factor (TNF), tissue growth factor beta (TGFβ), interferon gamma (IFNγ), IL-23, and IL-10.[11]

In the intestine IgA is the dominant immunoglobulin secreted into the gut lumen. The secretory IgA differs from serum IgA.[10] The oral uptake of soluble antigens may induce an inability to produce systemic antibody or a T-cell-mediated reaction to parenteral stimulation with the same antigen, a phenomenon called oral tolerance.[7] An important aspect of oral tolerance is the suppression of immunological reactions against food antigens.[7] Secretory IgA and IgM are bound via cysteine residues to the mucus secreted on the apical side by epithelial cells to form a so-called 'unstirred layer' which is a part of the GI barrier. The penetration of potentially dangerous antigens into the organism is prevented by binding them on the surface of the mucus layer.

Immunomediated gastrointestinal diseases with rheumatological manifestations

Inflammatory bowel diseases

The IBDs can be divided into Crohn's disease (CD) and ulcerative colitis (UC) as well as a non-classifiable colitis (indeterminate colitis or 'colitis not classified'). Other forms of chronic mucosal inflammation such as lymphocytic, eosinophilic, and collagenous colitis are relatively rare but with increasing incidence in recent years. IBD is most frequently diagnosed between 20 and 30 years of age.[12]

CD may affect the entire intestinal tract, with a clear preference for the terminal ileum and/or the large intestine. CD is a transmural, partially granulomatous inflammation, which may involve the serosa and regional lymph nodes. Affected gut segments are discontinuous, and distant parts of the mucosa may be involved. UC is limited to the mucosa of the large intestine. It always involves the rectum and shows variable extension to the left-sided or entire colon. If only the rectum is involved the disease is called ulcerative proctitis; if the whole colon is involved, it is termed pancolitis. Typical histological changes may be found, but are not obligatory for diagnosis. For both types of IBD the diagnosis is made by clinical criteria integrating histological, biochemical, clinical, endoscopic, and radiological findings.

The prevalence of IBD in Europe is around 40–50 cases per 100 000 inhabitants; the incidence is 4–6 new cases per year per 100 000 inhabitants.[12] In most epidemiological studies UC is found more frequently than CD.[12] Gender distribution is largely balanced. In Europe a north–south gradient has been reported; both diseases are more frequent in northern Europe than in southern Europe.[13] IBD is clearly more frequent in countries with a 'Western' lifestyle than in other regions of the world.[12]

The aetiology of IBD is still only partially understood. There is no doubt that genetic susceptibility is an important factor. About 20–30% of IBD patients have a positive family history, and monozygotic twins more frequently develop IBD than heterozygotes.[12] The pathogenesis of CD and UC involves a complex interaction of genetic risk factors (polygenic aetiology) with immunological and environmental factors. In 2001 the first risk gene for CD was identified: 20–30% of all patients with CD carry one of three single nucleotide polymorphisms (SNPs) in a CAspase Recruitment Domain (CARD)-containing protein called NOD2. Muramyl dipeptide (MDP), a component of the bacterial cell wall, is the ligand for Nod2. Many genome-wide association studies (GWAS) have been performed, increasing the number of further genetic susceptibility factors to up more than 70 in CD and more than 30 in UC.[14] Relevant genetic risk factors were identified in components of the autophagosome, which processes intracellular bacteria and contributes to their recognition and destruction by the proteins ATG16L1 and IRGM.[14] A number of risk genes are shared between IBD and rheumatologic diseases, such as *PTPN2* or *PTPN22*.[15]

Epidemiological data support an important pathogenic role of environmental factors. People with a higher socio-economic status are at higher risk of developing IBD. A number of studies point to the fact that an increased risk of suffering from IBD is associated with higher hygiene standards.[16] An increased risk for CD and a worse disease course is found in smokers. In contrast, smoking appears to be 'protective' for UC.[16]

Genetic and environmental factors induce a defect of the mucosal barrier function.[7] In the phase of chronification of the inflammation, excessive activation of the intestinal immune system occurs.[7] In a cascade-like reaction, via secretion of cytokines as well as chemotactic factors, migration of neutrophils, monocytes/macrophages, and T cells into the mucosa is induced.

The most important symptoms of CD are chronic diarrhoea with or without bloody bowel movements, weight loss, abdominal pain, fever, fatigue, and perianal fistula.[17] They vary according to the extent and site of intestinal involvement. CD is characterized by a fluctuating natural disease activity; the frequency of flares and recurrence is unpredictable and varies markedly in different patients.[17]

The main symptom of UC is bloody diarrhea, frequently associated with abdominal pain. 70% of the UC patients exhibit only a proctitis/proctosigmoiditis or left-sided colitis, and only 30% will have extended disease.[17] Fever and weight loss are less frequent as compared to CD, and are always a sign of severe disease.

Extraintestinal manifestations are frequent in both CD and UC. Rheumatological manifestations are joint involvement (arthralgia or arthritis in up to one-third of patients), oligoarthritis, spondylarthritis, erythema nodosum, pyoderma gangraenosum, uveitis, and iritis.[18] The frequency of peripheral arthritis in IBD has been reported to range between 17% and 20%. Enthesitis has been reported in up to 7% of patients.[19] Two types of peripheral arthritis associated with IBD are discriminated: The type I or pauciarticular form usually is acute and associated with intestinal IBD activity.[20] The joint involvement is asymmetric and both large and small joints may be affected. The arthropathy may even appear before the diagnosis of IBD is made. On the other hand the type II or polyarticular form has a more chronic course, is independent of intestinal IBD activity, and involves mainly small joints in a more symmetric pattern.[20]

Ankylosing spondylitis (AS) and other forms of axial involvement also are frequently found in patients with IBD. AS it is more common in CD (5%–22%) as compared to UC (2%–6%).[19] The prevalence is 10%–20% for sacroiliitis and 7%–12% for AS.[19] Up to 30% of the patients with IBD have inflammatory low back pain, 33% have abnormal Schober index, and 30% have unilateral or bilateral grade I or II sacroiliitis.[19] Axial symptoms may precede gut symptoms. The clinical course of the extraintestinal IBD manifestation is independent of the intestinal disease activity. AS associated with IBD can develop at any age.[19]

In UC patients there is an increased risk for the development of a colorectal carcinoma which depends on the long-term activity and extent of the disease. UC may also be associated with the occurrence of primary sclerosing cholangitis—an autoimmune inflammation of small and large bile ducts which puts patients at a risk of cholangiocarcinoma and increases colonic carcinoma risk.

Investigation and diagnosis

A detailed medical history and physical examinations are of high value for the diagnosis of IBD. The most important diagnostic tool, however, is ileocolonoscopy. In UC it will always result in pathological findings, and a diagnosis can also be made in CD with involvement of the colon and/or the terminal ileum. Usually biopsies are taken during endoscopy, and may reveal typical histological results.

In CD patients, if only the jejunum or the proximal ileum is affected diagnosis may only be possible by MRI, CT, or capsule endoscopy. Ultrasound is a very valuable diagnostic tool; bowel wall thickening is an objective sign of inflammatory activity.

Treatment

During mild or moderate flares of UC, 5-aminosalicylic acid (5-ASA) is the treatment of choice.[21] In distal and left-sided UC topical treatment with suppositories, foam preparations, or enemas has been shown to be more effective than oral (systemic) treatment. If left-sided colitis does not respond to 5-ASA application, steroid therapy should be used.[21] In more extended disease, oral therapy with 5-ASA is the treatment of choice. Sulfasalazine, which is well known in rheumatology and also useful in the presence of joint manifestations, is used less frequently these days mainly because of its side effects such as fatigue, abdominal pain, and gastroesophageal reflux disease (GERD).

In more severe disease courses, or in case of a lack of response to first line therapy, oral or intravenous administration of steroids, e.g. 40–100 mg prednisolone equivalent, with consecutive dose tapering is necessary.[21] In steroid-refractory cases the administration of ciclosporin or anti-TNF antibodies has been proven to be effective. Thus colectomy can be avoided in the long term in approximately 50% of these severely ill patients.[21] Long-term immunosuppression with azathioprine or anti-TNF antibodies must be discussed with respect to the option of colectomy, which in many centres can be done laparoscopically.

After remission is achieved it can be maintained by administration of 5-ASA. In more severe cases, and after induction of remission by steroids, azathioprine may be useful (2–2.5 mg/kg bw).

Several studies have confirmed that administration of oral steroids during acute flares of CD can induce remission. The response rate to steroid therapy is around 70–80%.[22] In chronically active and steroid-refractory patients, azathioprine (2–2.5 mg/kg per day) is effective. The administration of methotrexate induces remission in more than 40% of patients. Anti-TNF antibodies are very effective in refractory and more severe CD.[22] Infliximab, adalimumab, and certolizumab pegol have similar efficacy.[22] Azathioprine is also able to maintain remission.

Gluten-sensitive enteropathy (coeliac disease)

Gluten-sensitive enteropathy or coeliac disease is characterized by an atrophy of the duodenal and small intestinal villi, which is accompanied by the typical symptoms of malabsorption.[23] Characteristically the clinical and histological changes disappear under a gluten-free diet and typically recur within 2 years of re-exposure to gluten.[23] An important pathogenic factor for this disease is a 31-amino-acid peptide of gluten that cannot be digested or degraded by the proteases of the human GI tract. It is presented to T cells via a specific MHC II molecule (HLA-DQ 2/8); this HLA type is present in a quarter to a third of the European population. The prevalence of coeliac disease is up to 1% of the population in European countries.

Coeliac disease is frequently found in familial clusters. An IgA deficiency predisposes for its occurrence.[23] Very different prevalence and incidence rates have been reported, with the highest incidence in northern Europe (e.g. Finland). With the help of serum markers, which may be more sensitive than the clinical activity, a prevalence ranging from 1:250 to 1:100 was found in Europe.[23]

Although there is a clear familial predisposition for coeliac disease, the inheritance pattern does not follow a mendelian pattern, so multigenetic or multifactorial pathogenesis has been assumed.[23] The concordance in monozygotic twins is 75%, and in HLA-identical siblings it is 30%. Genetic risk factors induce an increased susceptibility for sensitization by gliadin. In a next step the formation of auto-antibodies against the enzyme tissue transglutaminase (tTG2) occurs.[23] tTG2 deaminates certain gluten peptides, increasing their affinity for HLA-DQ2 and HLA-DQ8 is. This leads to CD4 Th1 activation, which then initiates mucosal inflammation. Gluten can also activate the innate immune system. γδ T-cell-receptor positive lymphocytes are found in increased number in the periphery.[23]

Coeliac disease and dermatitis herpetiformis are parts of the spectrum of gluten-sensitive enteropathy. The symptoms often begin between the first and third year of life, when the child's nutrition is changed. A second peak of incidence is found in the third decade. The most prominent clinical symptoms are diarrhoea, meteorism, weight loss, fatigue, and symptoms due to deficiency of vitamins or minerals. Several diseases may be associated, such as IgA nephropathy, primary biliary cirrhosis, and sclerosing cholangitis.[23]

Connective tissue diseases are found in 7.2% of patients with coeliac disease, Sjögren's syndrome in 3.3%. Autoimmune thyroid diseases are also reported to be associated.[23]

Because the clinical presentation is frequently uncharacteristic, the histology of duodenal biopsies is important for diagnosis. In several guidelines the determination of IgA antibodies against human tissue transglutaminase is recommended as initial screening test.[24] It is important to quantify total IgA in parallel, as coeliac disease is more frequent in IgA deficiency syndrome.

A completely gluten-free diet is the only and most important therapeutic measure; this means a diet free of wheat, rye, and barley. On such a diet clinical complaints improve within days, and histological normalization occurs within weeks or months.

Chronic atrophic gastritis type A and pernicious anaemia

Chronic atrophic gastritis type A, which involves the gastric corpus and fundus, is followed by a complete atrophy of the gastric glands. Basal neuroendocrine cell complexes and an increase of glandular endocrine cells may be found, as well as autoantibodies against parietal cells and intrinsic factor.[25] A lack of intrinsic factor finally results in vitamin B_{12} malabsorption (pernicious anaemia).[25] Both genetic influences and environmental factors have been found to play a role in the pathogenesis: familiar accumulation and associations with HLA A-3, B-7 and also DR-2 and DR-4 were observed. A discordance in monozygotic twins indicates additional environmental factors.

Gastritis is one of the most frequent diseases of the human stomach: signs of chronic gastritis can be found in 60–70% of the adult population. However, mild forms are usually found and a progression to atrophic gastritis is unlikely.[25] The prevalence of pernicious anaemia in the Western world is about 0.1%.

In chronic atrophic gastritis there is no general disturbance of humoral or cellular immune functions. Circulating autoantibodies against intrinsic factor, parietal cells, and gastrin receptor are detected only if pernicious anaemia develops.[25] Chronic atrophic gastritis type A is not associated with serious symptoms, but associated vitamin B_{12} deficiency as consequence may lead to haematological (macrocytic anaemia) and neurological symptoms (funicular myelosis). Diagnosis is only possible by endoscopy and subsequent histology. Reduced vitamin B_{12} levels add to the diagnosis. The detection of autoantibodies is not sufficient for the diagnosis, as they can also be found in type 1 diabetes, Hashimoto's thyroiditis, and Addison's disease. Cytotoxic autoantibodies against cell surface antigens of parietal cells have a high disease specificity, but they are not part of routine diagnostics. The therapy of pernicious anaemia consists of parenteral vitamin B_{12} substitution.

Collagenous colitis and lymphocytic colitis

In both forms of microscopic colitis, collagenous colitis and lymphocytic colitis, endoscopic appearance of the colonic mucosa is normal. The diagnosis is based on histological findings and clinical symptoms. In specimens from patients with collagenous colitis a linear layer of collagen is found beneath the epithelium, which consists of type 1 and type 3 collagen.[26] The standard treatment of collagenous colitis is the administration of 5-ASA (3 g/day) or budesonide (3 × 3 mg/day). The time interval from start of therapy to symptom improvement may vary markedly.[26]

In patients with lymphocytic colitis, usually in the entire large bowel, an increased number of intraepithelial lymphocytes in a somewhat flattened epithelial surface can be found histologically, as well as an infiltration with neutrophils and other inflammatory cells.[27] The first line therapy also is based on 5-ASA, but it may be necessary to apply topical or systemic steroids or immunosuppressants if the disease appears to be refractory to steroids.[27] The annual incidence of microscopic colitis seems to be higher than was assumed in the past: incidence rates have been found that are similar to those of Crohn's disease (CD).

The pathogenesis of both forms of microscopic colitis is unknown.[27] Clinically, both forms present with watery diarrhoea in all patients, and more than 80% also have arthritis. The prognosis in general is good. A transformation to ulcerative pancolitis has been reported.

Autoimmune pancreatic diseases

Autoantibodies against antigens of the exocrine pancreas are found in patients with IBD and in patients with Sjögren's syndrome as well as in primary sclerosing pancreatitis (which is very rare).

In addition, a new pancreatitis entity has been described recently: autoimmune pancreatitis.[28] The clinical symptoms are very variable. Severe abdominal or other signs of acute pancreatitis are rare. In two-thirds of cases a 'painless jaundice' occurs. An exocrine dysfunction may be found as well as secondary diabetes. The exocrine dysfunction usually improves or resolves completely after the start of adequate therapy. Imaging may support the diagnosis and can include CT, MRI, endoscopic retrograde cholangiopancreatography (ERCP), and endosonography.[28]

In autoimmune pancreatitis, segmental or relatively long strictures of the pancreatic duct with prestenotic dilatations are typical. Strictures of the common bile duct may also occur. Hypergammaglobulinemia and elevated IgG4 immunoglobulins are very characteristic, although cases without IgG4 elevation have also been described.[28] Symptoms usually rapidly improve upon systemic steroid therapy. Almost all pancreatic changes of can completely resolve under this therapy. A IgG4-associated cholangitis has also been described. An overlap with autoimmune pancreatitis can occur and the two diseases may be hard to discriminate in certain cases.

Rheumatic diseases with intestinal manifestations

Behçet's disease

In 1937 Behçet first described a syndrome with repeated occurrence of oral and genital aphthous lesions together with eye inflammation and occasionally intestinal ulcerations.[29] A familiar accumulation pattern can be found, and an association with certain HLA antigens and with specific unusual immune reactions. Behçet's syndrome is more frequently found in the Mediterranean area.

Therapy includes administration of steroids or, thalidomide (2 × 100–200 mg/day). Colchicine (1 × 0.6 mg/day) and ciclosporin A (5 mg/kg per day) have also been reported to be effective.

The involvement of the gastrointestinal tract is frequently not obvious and only rarely important for diagnosis; only 10% of all patients with Behçet's syndrome are severely affected by gastrointestinal manifestations.[29]

Vasculitis and intestinal inflammation

During the course of vasculitis or rheumatoid arthritis (RA), involvement of the intestinal tract is frequently reported. Ileitis and colitis have been described in the context of SLE, polyarteriitis nodosa, or Henoch–Schönlein purpura, and are occasionally observed with Churg–Strauss syndrome.

Abdominal pain is the most common symptom of gastrointestinal involvement during Henoch–Schönlein purpura. Other symptoms may include nausea or melena. These symptoms are secondary to vasculitis involving the splanchnic circulation (mesenteric vasculitis),[30] and may be confused with typical IBD symptoms. Usually, skin manifestations precede gastrointestinal manifestations, but in one-fourth of cases skin lesions occur after gastrointestinal manifestations.[30] Endoscopic findings are not typical and only histology is diagnostic. Joint involvement is found in about two-thirds of patients. Typically, non-migratory, non-destructive polyarthralgias occur which are symmetrical in distribution and mostly involve the knees and ankles.[30]

Gastrointestinal and hepatic manifestations of rheumatoid arthritis

An enteric origin for various arthritides has frequently been discussed. Similar molecular signatures have been found in intestinal bacteria and synovium or cartilage. Intestinal infections caused by typical pathogens such as *Salmonella* and *Campylobacter jejuni* may be accompanied by joint involvement such as arthritis or arthralgia. However, a clear pathophysiological link has never been established and generally acknowledged.

Non-steroidal anti-inflammatory drugs (NSAIDs), frequently used for the treatment of joint pain in arthritis, may impair the intestinal barrier function. NSAIDS are well known to cause damage to the intestinal mucosa. Diclofenac, ibuprofen, or naproxen may cause flares of IBD within 2 weeks of therapy in up to 25% of treated patients.

In patients with RA undergoing colonoscopy, an inflammation of the terminal ileum is found in up to 11% of cases. When 54 patients with RA underwent ileocolonoscopy and biopsies were taken, 15% of the RA patients had histological signs of inflammation.[31] 20–25%

of RA patients have increased levels of serum IgA correlating with extra-articular symptoms and intestinal abnormalities.[32]

Rheumatoid vasculitis occurs in about 1–5% of patients with RA and up to one-third of those patients will suffer from intestinal involvement.[33] In severe cases patients may suffer from multiple ischemic ulcers and perforations or segmental extensive bowel infarction, sometimes complicated by intraperitoneal haemorrhage.[33]

Gastrointestinal and hepatic manifestations of systemic lupus erythematous

SLE can involve the entire GI tract and the liver. GI symptoms may occur in up to 50% of patients with SLE; they are usually mild.[34] Intestinal pseudo-obstruction is a rare complication and only found with active lupus serology. It preferentially involves the small bowel.[34] Another rare condition, protein-losing enteropathy, characterized by diarrhoea, oedema, and hypoalbuminaemia, may even be the initial presentation of SLE. Associated with coeliac disease, a malabsorption may occur in 9.5%. Pancreatitis appears with an annual incidence of 0.4–1 in 1000. About 10% of patients with autoimmune hepatitis have SLE. On the other hand, 4.7% of patients with SLE have chronic active hepatitis correlating with the presence of antibody to ribosomal P protein.[34]

References

1. Brandtzaeg P. Mucosal immunity: induction, dissemination, and effector functions. *Scand J Immunol* 2009;70(6):505–515.
2. Kelsall BL, Rescigno M. Mucosal dendritic cells in immunity and inflammation. *Nat Immunol* 2004;5(11):1091–1095.
3. Niess JH, Brand S, Gu X et al. CX3CR1-mediated dendritic cell access to the intestinal lumen and bacterial clearance. *Science* 2005;307(5707):254–258.
4. Duchmann R, Schmitt E, Knolle P et al. Tolerance towards resident intestinal flora in mice is abrogated in experimental colitis and restored by treatment with interleukin-10 or antibodies to interleukin-12. *Eur J Immunol* 1996;26(4):934–938.
5. Pierik M, De Hertogh G, Vermeire S et al. Epithelioid granulomas, pattern recognition receptors, and phenotypes of Crohn's disease. *Gut* 2005;54(2):223–227.
6. Brandtzaeg P, Kiyono H, Pabst R, Russell MW. Terminology: nomenclature of mucosa-associated lymphoid tissue. *Mucosal Immunol* 2008:1(1):31–37.
7. Xavier RJ, Podolsky DK. Unravelling the pathogenesis of inflammatory bowel disease. *Nature* 2007;448(7152):427–434.
8. Abraham C, Cho J. Interleukin-23/Th17 pathways and inflammatory bowel disease. *Inflamm Bowel Dis* 2009;15(7):1090–1100.
9. Duerr RH, Taylor KD, Brant SR et al. A genome-wide association study identifies IL23R as an inflammatory bowel disease gene. *Science* 2006;314(5804):1461–1463.
10. Macpherson AJ, McCoy KD, Johansen FE, Brandtzaeg P. The immune geography of IgA induction and function. *Mucosal Immunol* 2008;1(1):11–22.
11. Hausmann M, Rogler G. Immune-non immune networks in intestinal inflammation. *Curr Drug Targets* 2008;9(5):388–394.
12. Shanahan F, Bernstein CN. The evolving epidemiology of inflammatory bowel disease. *Curr Opin Gastroenterol* 2009;25(4):301–305.
13. Shivananda S, Lennard-Jones J, Logan R et al. Incidence of inflammatory bowel disease across Europe: is there a difference between north and south? Results of the European Collaborative Study on Inflammatory Bowel Disease (EC-IBD). *Gut* 1996;39(5):690–697.
14. Marks DJ. Defective innate immunity in inflammatory bowel disease: a Crohn's disease exclusivity? *Curr Opin Gastroenterol* 2011;27(4):328–334.
15. Scharl M, McCole DF, Weber A et al. Protein tyrosine phosphatase N2 regulates TNFalpha-induced signalling and cytokine secretion in human intestinal epithelial cells. *Gut* 2011;60(2):189–197.
16. Baumgart DC, Carding SR. Inflammatory bowel disease: cause and immunobiology. *Lancet* 2007;369(9573):1627–1640.
17. Herfarth H, Rogler G. Inflammatory bowel disease. *Endoscopy* 2005;37(1):42–47.
18. Larsen S, Bendtzen K, Nielsen OH. Extraintestinal manifestations of inflammatory bowel disease: epidemiology, diagnosis, and management. *Ann Med* 2010;42(2):97–114.
19. Rodriguez-Reyna TS, Martinez-Reyes C, Yamamoto-Furusho JK. Rheumatic manifestations of inflammatory bowel disease. *World J Gastroenterol* 2009;15(44):5517–5524.
20. Orchard TR, Wordsworth BP, Jewell DP. Peripheral arthropathies in inflammatory bowel disease: their articular distribution and natural history. *Gut* 1998;42(3):387–391.
21. Meier J, Sturm A. Current treatment of ulcerative colitis. *World J Gastroenterol* 2011;17(27):3204–3212.
22. Vavricka SR, Rogler G. Recent advances in the aetiology and treatment of Crohn's disease. *Minerva Gastroenterol Dietol* 2010;56(2):203–211.
23. Schuppan D, Junker Y, Barisani D. Coeliac disease: from pathogenesis to novel therapies. *Gastroenterology* 2009;137(6):1912–1933.
24. Hill PG, Forsyth JM, Semeraro D, Holmes GK. IgA antibodies to human tissue transglutaminase: audit of routine practice confirms high diagnostic accuracy. *Scand J Gastroenterol* 2004;39(11):1078–1082.
25. Adamu MA, Weck MN, Gao L, Brenner H. Incidence of chronic atrophic gastritis: systematic review and meta-analysis of follow-up studies. *Eur J Epidemiol* 2010;25(7):439–448.
26. Ung KA, Kilander A, Nilsson O, Abrahamsson H. Long-term course in collagenous colitis and the impact of bile acid malabsorption and bile acid sequestrants on histopathology and clinical features. *Scand J Gastroenterol* 2001;36(6):601–609.
27. Datta I, Brar SS, Andrews CN. Microscopic colitis: a review for the surgical endoscopist. *Can J Surg* 2009;52(5):E167–E172.
28. Webster GJ, Pereira SP, Chapman RW. Autoimmune pancreatitis/IgG4-associated cholangitis and primary sclerosing cholangitis—overlapping or separate diseases? *J Hepatol* 2009;51(2):398–402.
29. Hatemi G, Silman A, Bang D et al. Management of Behcet disease: a systematic literature review for the European League Against Rheumatism evidence-based recommendations for the management of Behcet disease. *Ann Rheum Dis* 2009;68(10):1528–1534.
30. Sohagia AB, Gunturu SG, Tong TR, Hertan HI. Henoch-Schonlein purpura—a case report and review of the literature. *Gastroenterol Res Pract* 2010;2010:597648.
31. Porzio V, Biasi G, Corrado A et al. Intestinal histological and ultrastructural inflammatory changes in spondyloarthropathy and rheumatoid arthritis. *Scand J Rheumatol* 1997;26(2):92–98.
32. Pillemer SR, Reynolds WJ, Yoon SJ, Perera M, Newkirk M, Klein M. IgA related disorders in rheumatoid arthritis. *J Rheumatol* 1987;14(5):880–886.
33. Ebert EC, Hagspiel KD. Gastrointestinal and hepatic manifestations of rheumatoid arthritis. *Dig Dis Sci* 2011;56(2):295–302.
34. Ebert EC, Hagspiel KD. Gastrointestinal and hepatic manifestations of systemic lupus erythematosus. *J Clin Gastroenterol* 2011;45(5):436–441.

CHAPTER 22

Neuroendocrine system

Rainer H. Straub

Introduction

Endocrine abnormalities in chronic autoimmune rheumatic diseases (CARDs) are based on an altered systemic neuroendocrine response stimulated by inflammatory stimuli or by direct autoimmune involvement of endocrine glands (the latter is not considered in this chapter). The neuroendocrine–immune interplay serves regulation of energy homeostasis and metabolism. These programmes have not been positively selected for CARDs due to negative selection pressure or lack of selection pressure (Box 22.1).[1]

Evolutionary theory says that genes, signalling pathways, and networks have been positively selected for normal physiology or

---

Box 22.1 Three major reasons for missing positive selection of disease-modifying genes after outbreak of a chronic autoimmune rheumatic disease (CARD)

- **High negative selection pressure**: CARDs lead to loss of reproducibility because affected individuals are at a disadvantage: excluded or impaired in the competition for food, positions in the group, and sexual partners. In addition, the long-term high inflammatory activity inhibits the hypothalamic–pituitary–gonadal (HPG) axis, leading to impairment of fertility (see below).

- **Absence of selection pressure**. At present, many CARDs only become manifest in patients at older ages. Due to the short life expectancy in the past, our ancestors did not suffer from the CARDs we know today.

- **There has been no time for natural selection**. This situation would occur if various CARDs did not exist some 100–200 years ago. Indeed, there is a suggestion that RA, for example, is a relatively new disease.

Genes whose products operate in the symptomatic phase of CARDs will not be positively selected, because of the negative influence of the disease. Nevertheless, genes can be transmitted before the outbreak of a CARD and persist among descendants. Transmitted genes may confer an increased risk for a CARD, but most probably, these genes were positively selected for fitness in reproduction and survival at younger ages independent of the CARD (antagonistic pleiotropy[2]). A perfect example is HLA DR4 (DRB1*04) because this genetic variant protects from dengue haemorrhagic fever. This has been summarized elsewhere.[1]

---

transient serious, albeit non-life-threatening, inflammatory episodes such as infection, foreign body reactions, wound healing, or similar.[1] Likewise, mechanisms for energy regulation have been positively selected for normal physiology and transient inflammatory episodes but not for CARDs.[3] Energy regulation involves many endocrine and neuronal pathways, which are summarized in Figure 22.1. In short-lived inflammatory episodes, there is a transient reallocation programme that redirects energy-rich fuels like glucose, amino acids (alanine, glutamine), and free fatty acids from classical stores such as liver, muscle, and fat tissue to the activated immune system (Figure 22.1).[3] This adaptive redirection programme is active as long as inflammation persists. In CARDs, the continuous use of these programmes leads to a permanent energy appeal reaction that leads to multiple systemic neuroendocrine abnormalities, as discussed in this chapter (Box 22.2).

Mild activation of the hypothalamic–pituitary–adrenal axis

Altered cortisol regulation in patients with CARDs has been intensively discussed for years. To summarize:

- Cortisol serum levels are somewhat elevated in untreated patients with CARDs.

- The hypothalamic–pituitary–adrenal (HPA) axis is visibly disturbed when subtle stress tests are applied.[4]

- Cortisol levels are low in relation to inflammation (see next section).

In addition, the HPA-axis-related adrenal androgen production is almost switched off at the expense of cortisol production.[5]

As a result of the allocation of energy-rich fuels to the immune system, mildly elevated levels of cortisol and severely downregulated anabolic androgens support gluconeogenesis by stimulating glucogenic enzymes in the liver and, concomitantly, muscle protein breakdown (provision of glucogenic amino acids). The cortisol-to-androgen preponderance supports cachectic obesity.[6] As cortisol and adrenaline support each other's signalling pathways, the concomitant increase in both hormones potentiates gluconeogenesis (sympathetic activation, see 'Mild activation of the sympathetic nervous system'). Growth hormone stimulates lipolysis by cortisol at physiological levels, and in this way provides the

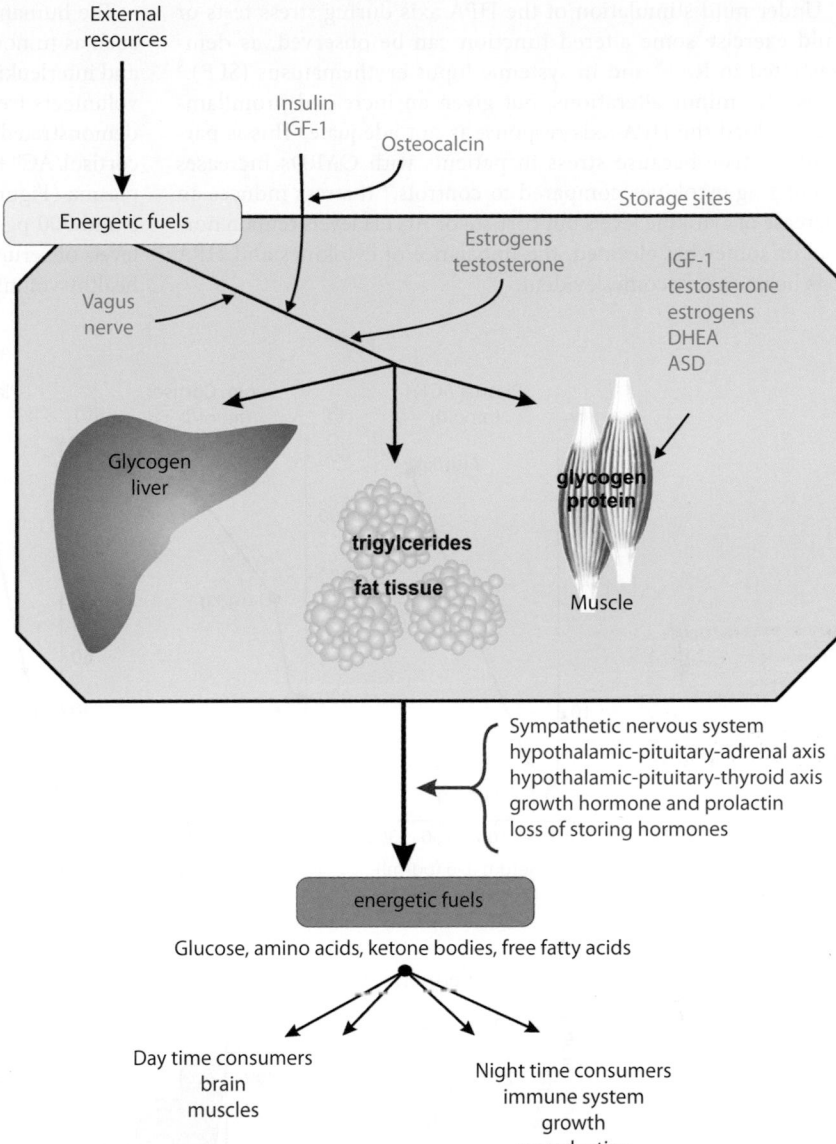

Fig. 22.1 Energy regulation involves many endocrine and neuronal pathways. Energy-rich fuels are taken up and stored if there is no actual need for higher energy resources. During systemic inflammation, cytokines induce an energy appeal reaction in order to redirect fuels to the activated immune system. Under normal conditions, a circadian rhythm of allocation of energy-rich substrates exists to serve daytime and night-time consumers. Factors shown in green are typically storage factors, while factors in red release energy-rich substrates from storage sites. ASD, androstenedione; DHEA, dehydroepiandrosterone; IGF-1, insulin-like growth factor 1.

Box 22.2 Systemic neuroendocrine abnormalities linked to a continuous energy appeal reaction of the activated immune system

- Endocrine abnormality
- Mild activation of the HPA axis
- Inadequate secretion of ACTH and cortisol relative to inflammation (disproportion principle)
- Mild activation of the SNS
- High serum levels of oestrogens relative to androgens (androgen drain)
- Inhibition of the HPG axis and consequences for fertility
- Fat deposits adjacent to inflamed tissue
- Increase of serum prolactin and immunostimulation
- Hyperinsulinemia, insulin resistance, and the metabolic syndrome
- Circadian rhythms of hormones, cytokines, and symptoms

immune system with energy-rich fuels. However, mild hypercortisolemia is not high enough to suppress the inflammatory process.

Inadequate secretion of ACTH and cortisol relative to inflammation—the disproportion principle

In humans, severe HPA axis alterations have not been found; only smaller changes were observed.[7] There are no big differences in basal blood levels of ACTH and cortisol in CARDs compared to healthy controls. Even with strong stimulation such as insulin hypoglycaemia these hormone levels showed no significant alterations.[7] This outcome was expected, because life-threatening situations need counteraction, which is obviously possible in medically treated CARD patients. Similarly, injection of corticotropin-releasing hormone (CRH) or adrenocorticotropin (ACTH) did not reveal marked alterations of the HPA axis, as summarized earlier.[7] It seems that some patients with CARDs demonstrate an escape in the dexamethasone/CRH test as substantiated in rheumatoid arthritis (RA) and multiple sclerosis.[7]

Under mild stimulation of the HPA axis during stress tests or mild exercise some altered function can be observed, as demonstrated in RA[4,8] and in systemic lupus erythematosus (SLE).[8] These are minor alterations, but given an increased proinflammatory load the HPA axis response is not adequate. This is particularly true because stress in patients with CARDs increases circulating cytokines compared to controls.[9] If stress induces an increase of cytokine levels but cortisol or ACTH levels remain normal or somewhat elevated, the imbalance of cytokines and HPA axis hormones becomes evident.

The human HPA axis response is activated by single cytokines such as tumour necrosis factor (TNF), interferon (IFN)-α, IFN-γ, and interleukin (IL)-6.[10] A fivefold elevation is observed in human volunteers treated with IL-6.[10] A dose–response relationship was demonstrated with a high linearity between serum IL-6 levels and cortisol/ACTH levels in a range of 3 to 300 pg IL-6 per mL serum/plasma (Figure 22.2).[10] Since patients with CARDs have between 3 and 300 pg/mL of IL-6, one would expect them to have similar levels of serum cortisol or plasma ACTH as found in this study in healthy volunteers. If patients have cytokine levels in this range, the

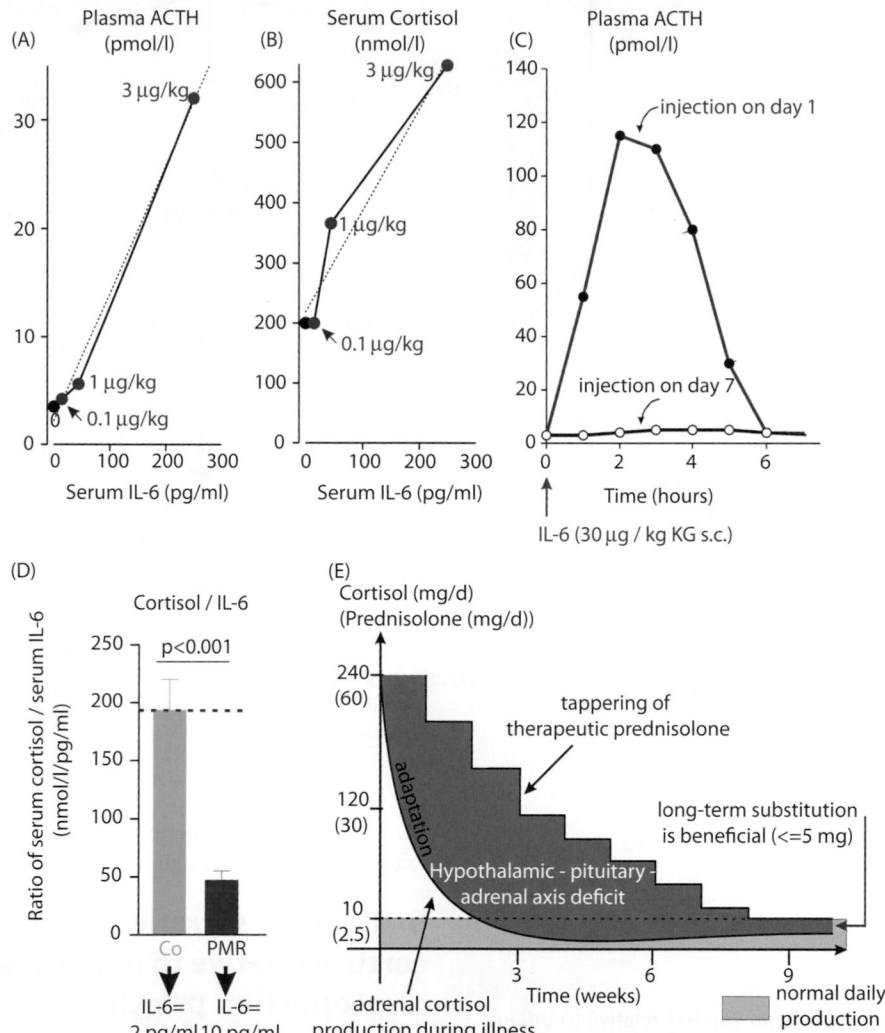

Fig. 22.2 Disproportion principle. (A-C): Adaptive downregulation of hypothalamic–pituitary–adrenal (HPA) axis activity upon repeated inflammatory stimuli. (A) Positive correlation between serum IL-6 levels and plasma ACTH after injection of indicated doses of IL-6 (red numbers) to healthy volunteers.[10] (B) Positive correlation between serum IL-6 levels and serum cortisol after injection of IL-6.[10] (C) Blunted ACTH response after repeated daily injection of IL-6 (red: day 1; black: day 7).[49] Panel C demonstrates the adaptive downregulation of HPA axis activity (here ACTH) during long-term elevation of serum IL-6. Adaptive downregulation is a cause for inadequate secretion of HPA axis hormones relative to inflammation. (D–E): Inadequate cortisol secretion in relation to inflammation. (D) Relatively low levels of cortisol in relation to IL-6 in patients with polymyalgia rheumatica (PMR). The original raw data were taken from a previous study.[50] In the given range of 2–10 pg IL-6/mL, the ratio of serum cortisol divided by serum IL-6 should be constant according to panel B. Controls show approximately 180 nmol/L cortisol in relation to 1 pg/mL of serum cytokine. This is different in patients with PMR who demonstrated approximately 50 nmol/L cortisol per 1 pg IL-6/mL. (E) The HPA axis deficit. An immediate increase of cortisol production can be observed after acute inflammatory stimulation such as an outbreak of an inflammatory disease (up to 240 mg/day), but this production rate is not maintained for a long period of time due to rapid adaptation of the HPA axis (see panel C). To control the disease a higher amount of daily glucocorticoids is needed, and the physician is providing high-dose prednisolone therapy starting at 60 mg/day (tapering down regimen). The orange area between the adrenal production rate and the exogenous prednisolone amount per day demonstrates the HPA axis deficit. The HPA axis is not able to produce the necessary amount. Importantly, the adrenal production rate can arrive at lower production rates compared to baseline, requiring long-standing substitution, e.g. in patients with PMR. The substitution therapy of 2.5 mg prednisolone per day reflects the basal adrenal production rate of cortisol.

hormone/cytokine ratio should be similar in healthy controls and in patients with CARDs (Figure 22.2). However, in patients with polymyalgia rheumatica, RA, and reactive arthritis, hormone levels were much lower in relation to IL-6 (Figure 22.2D).[11] This is known as the **disproportion principle**: inadequately low secretion of cortisol/ACTH in relation to stimulating cytokines such as IL-6 and TNF (Figure 22.2).

But what is the teleological significance of this? Persistently elevated glucocorticoid levels would lead to aggravation of systemic infectious illness, because cortisol inhibits essential defence reactions of the body. A brisk rise and fall of ACTH/cortisol has been positively selected by evolution in order to support an immediate response, thus preventing inhibitory influence on the immune system.[1] In short, the HPA axis response is defective precisely because it is normal.[7] One can hypothesize that such an inadequate response can even lead to disease perpetuation in CARDs, because secretion is somewhat elevated, supporting gluconeogenesis and lipolysis, but anti-inflammatory effects are absent.

High serum levels of oestrogens relative to androgens—the androgen drain

An increased conversion of androgen precursors to downstream oestrogens (independent of gender) was found in inflamed tissue and inflammatory cells of patients with CARDs.[12] It can be observed in immune cells by directly studying the conversion of androgen to oestrogen.[13] TNF is able to activate the aromatase in peripheral cells, thus leading to high local oestrogen levels.[14] This proinflammatory cytokine blocks the activation of biologically inactive androgen precursors in synovial cells of RA patients, such as the conversion of dehydroepiandrosterone sulphate (DHEAS) to bioactive dehydroepiandrosterone (DHEA).[14] In consequence, TNF leads to androgen loss by stopping supplies and by increasing the downstream drainage to oestrogens. This is supported by the inhibition of adrenal production of DHEAS and DHEA, as observed in CARDs.[15] A cytokine-induced block of androgen production in the adrenal and gonadal glands leads to low serum levels of androgens,[14] which in older subjects is responsible for the decline of adrenal androgen secretion also.

Another important proinflammatory pathway of steroid hormone conversion exists for DHEA. Stimulated by TNF, this hormone is converted into 7α-DHEA in synovial fibroblasts of patients with RA and in experimental arthritis in mice.[16] Since 7α-DHEA has proinflammatory activities, this steroid hormone conversion is unfavourable. Downstream of androgens, 17β-oestradiol is converted to proinflammatory and proproliferative 16α-hydroxylated oestrogens but not to anti-inflammatory 2- or 4-hydroxylated oestrogens.[17] The 16α-hydroxylated estrogens can stimulate the female type of subcutaneous lipid accumulation.[18] Increased levels of oestrogens (also in men) relative to androgens can support female-type fat distribution, cachectic obesity, and even generation of regional fat depots in the proximity of inflamed tissue (see 'Fat deposits adjacent to inflamed tissue'). In addition, the increase of oestrogens relative to androgens aggravates muscle wasting, as seen in transsexuals.[18]

Those alterations of the homeostatic steroid axes evolved to cope with short-lasting inflammatory episodes, but their long-term occurrence in CARDs is deleterious because they support allocation of energy-rich fuels to the immune system and lead to disease sequelae such as cachectic obesity and muscle wasting.

Inhibition of the hypothalamic–pituitary–gonadal axis and consequences for fertility

Inflammation-induced alteration of the hypothalamic–pituitary–gonadal (HPG) axis has been extensively studied in animals.[19] In humans, similar overall HPG axis abnormalities appear, especially in male RA patients, in whom follicle-stimulating hormone (FSH) and luteinizing hormone (LH) are elevated compared to controls.[20] This was confirmed in postpubertal boys and girls with SLE,[21] in male patients with ankylosing spondylitis and SLE,[22] in juvenile dermatomyositis,[23] and by a luteinizing hormone releasing hormone (LHRH) function test in patients with Sjögren's syndrome.[24] Elevated FSH and LH imply peripheral gonadal dysfunction, whereas lower levels of these hormones are an indicator of central abnormalities. Lower levels of LH were also found in patients with RA and SLE, probably demonstrating central involvement.[25]

Because of these alterations of the HPG axis and peripheral sex hormones, one would expect fertility problems in patients with CARDs. Indeed, the testicular Sertoli cell function and testicular volume are markedly altered in male SLE patients,[22,26] and patients with ankylosing spondylitis demonstrate sperm abnormalities that are ameliorated by anti-TNF therapy.[27] Similarly, women with SLE often demonstrate amenorrhea and abnormalities of FSH and LH,[25] and patients with juvenile dermatomyositis presented delayed menarche.[23] A recent population-based study demonstrated that RA patients were more often nulliparous compared to a control group.[28] Although, rheumatologists try to treat their patients to the best of current knowledge, these studies clearly demonstrate the negative impact of inflammation (not only of disease-modifying anti-rheumatic drugs, DMARDs) on HPG axis function in CARDs, leading to negative selection pressure.

Aberrant function of the HPG axis is not restricted to rheumatic diseases; it has been described in patients with filarial infections, leprosy, urinary bilharziasis, and HIV infection. Acute hantavirus infections or toxoplasmosis can induce acute hypogonadism. Keeping this in mind, the question arises why these alterations appear with such a uniform expression in many systemic inflammatory diseases.

With regard to energy regulation, inflammation leads to a diversion of energy-rich substrates to the activated immune system. Since courtship behaviour and reproduction are extremely energy-consuming, HPG axis activities and reproduction are switched off at the expense of the HPA axis stress response. This adaptive programme is highly favourable for short-lived inflammatory disease, to supply the immune system with energy-rich substrates.

Fat deposits adjacent to inflamed tissue

Nearly all lymph nodes are embedded in adipose tissue,[29] and most smaller adipose depots enclose one or more lymph nodes. Lipolysis and release of glycerol from perinodal fat depots was increased through activation of lymph nodes by proinflammatory stimuli.[29] As fatty acids can be used by immune cells, it is obvious that lymph node-associated adipose tissue is needed as a local source of energy-rich fuels.[29]

Selective hypertrophy of adipose depots in the proximity of inflammatory lesions is common in several CARDs including RA, osteoarthritis, Crohn's disease, mesenteric panniculitis, and Graves' ophthalmopathy.[30] Along with energy-rich fuels (fatty acids), adipocytes produce proinflammatory adipokines, such as leptin, high-molecular weight isoforms of adiponectin, TNF, IL-1β, monocyte chemotactic protein-1 (MCP-1), or IL-6, as well as anti-inflammatory factors such as trimeric adiponectin.[30,31] Thus, the finely tuned balance of pro- and anti-inflammatory factors supports processes in neighbouring lymph nodes such as clonal expansion of antigen-specific lymphocytes.

It is very likely that fat tissue in the proximity of inflamed tissue keeps the local inflammation going. Adipocytes differentiate from pluripotent mesenchymal stem cells, which readily enter chronically inflamed tissue.[30] If stimuli for adipocyte differentiation are available, adipose tissue adjacent to inflammatory lesions can develop locally. Regional adipose tissue is a store of energy-rich substrates fuelling the neighbouring inflammatory process.

Increase of serum prolactin

Prolactin levels typically increase with the start of sleep, and this has been linked to the night-time increase in proinflammatory cytokines.[32] In this respect, it has a similar role to that of melatonin and growth hormone. In addition, prolactin is a classical stress hormone that increases during inflammatory episodes.[10]

In CARDs, serum levels of prolactin were found to be normal or slightly elevated (by a factor of 2) reaching serum levels of approximately 15–25 ng/mL.[33,34] Increased values were demonstrated in RA, SLE, multiple sclerosis, Sjögren's syndrome, Hashimoto's thyroiditis, polymyalgia rheumatica, systemic sclerosis, and others.[33,34] A further link between CARDs and prolactin has recently been discovered: The PRL-1149 G/T polymorphism (rs1341239) in the prolactin gene decreases prolactin expression, and this is associated with a decreased risk of developing RA.[35]

Prolactin has many immunostimulatory (T helper type 1 favouring) and proinflammatory activities.[33,34] Therapeutic inhibition of pituitary prolactin secretion has been studied using bromocriptine or other dopamine agonists in some small studies.[33,34] The therapeutic effect was not strong, but some patients might profit.[33,34] No randomized placebo-controlled clinical trials have been performed with these agents. In addition, since prolactin can be secreted from immune cells and other local tissue cells such as lymphocytes and fibroblasts,[33] the modulation of pituitary prolactin secretion seems to be a doubtful strategy because it would only block the dopamine-dependent pituitary production of this hormone.

In the context of energy regulation in systemic inflammation, prolactin has three major roles:

♦ It decreases lipogenesis in white adipose tissue by inhibiting important lipogenic enzymes (inhibition of triglyceride storage, thus, provision to the immune system).[36]

♦ It increases insulin secretion from pancreatic β-cells, leading to higher insulin levels (support of immune cells, see 'Hyperinsulinaemia and insulin resistance').[36]

♦ It stimulates immune cells.

All three effects support the reallocation of energy-rich substrates to the immune system and activation of inflammatory cells.

Hyperinsulinaemia and insulin resistance

Using an early version of the glucose tolerance test, endocrine imbalances with unresponsiveness to hyperglycaemia, insulin

resistance, and increased gluconeogenesis in patients with RA and ankylosing spondylitis were demonstrated about 60 years ago.[37] These results were supported by the finding that basal serum insulin levels and the maximum insulin response to glucose loading were significantly higher in patients with RA than in control subjects.[38] It was concluded that impaired glucose handling in RA is due to peripheral insulin resistance mediated by the inflammatory process.[38] This was supported by the euglycaemic hyperinsulinaemic glucose clamp technique.[38] In other studies it was shown that serum levels of C-reactive protein (CRP) and disease activity negatively correlated with insulin sensitivity in RA.[39] Insulin resistance is not a phenomenon of RA alone but is a general principle in CARDs.

Energy-rich fuels are needed to feed the immune system (mainly glucose and glutamine, other glucogenic amino acids, ketone bodies, and free fatty acids; see Figure 22.1). During activation of the immune system, muscle proteins are degraded and glucogenic amino acids are used for gluconeogenesis. In the presence of elevated activity of the sympathetic nervous system (SNS; see 'Mild activation of the sympathetic nervous system') and slightly increased activity of the HPA axis (albeit relatively low in relation to inflammation, see 'Mild activation of the hypothalamic–pituitary–adrenal axis'), gluconeogenesis results in somewhat higher circulating glucose levels (as tested by increased fructosamine and pentosidine levels in CARDs), and increased levels of free fatty acids (such as the 20:3ω6 and 20:4ω6 fatty acids). Free fatty acids induce insulin resistance and, in parallel, proinflammatory cytokines such as TNF can disturb insulin receptor signalling.[40] This has been shown by the improvement of insulin resistance and IGF-1 resistance associated with TNF neutralizing therapies.[14,41] Most probably, the increased proinflammatory load with elevated circulating cytokines is the main contributor to insulin resistance in CARDs. The important question appears to be whether immune cells become insulin resistant.

Immune cells take up glucose via the GLUT1, GLUT3, and GLUT4 transporters that are activated by specific immune stimuli such as lipopolysaccharides, anti-CD3 antibodies, cytokines (e.g. IL-7, IL-4), hormones (e.g. leptin), and also by insulin.[42] In addition, glycolysis and pentose phosphate pathways are switched on in activated immune cells[42] and they do not become insulin resistant. In contrast, insulin is important for glucose uptake, cytokine synthesis, and activation of immune cells.

In summary, the energy appeal reaction increases the insulin resistance of liver, muscle, and adipose tissue in order to deflect energy-rich fuels to the activated immune system. The activated immune cells themselves do not become insulin resistant.

Circadian rhythms of hormones and cytokines and pathophysiology link to symptoms

In CARDs, symptoms follow a circadian rhythm leading to an early morning peak in symptoms such as stiffness, functional disability, and pain.[32] These symptoms are a consequence of the nightly increase of proinflammatory cytokines such as IL-6 and TNF whose function is tightly linked to plasma extravasation, stimulation of sensory nerve fibres, and activation of central nervous microglia. The increase of TNF and IL-6 stimulates the morning rise of endogenous ACTH, cortisol, adrenaline, and noradrenaline showing a lag phase of 30–60 minutes between cytokine and later hormone increase.[43] When hormones reach the peak level in the early morning they are able to suppress cytokines, leading to spontaneous reduction of cytokine serum levels and symptoms during the later morning.

With the start of sleep, proinflammatory hormones such as prolactin, melatonin, and growth hormone activate the nocturnal immune system. In parallel, a decrease in catecholamines and cortisol leads to the rise of cytokines until the next morning. This self-regulating interacting fluctuation of hormones and cytokines serves energy regulation.[3]

The allocation of energy-rich fuels follows circadian rhythms because the uptake of energy resources is limited (the upper threshold of uptake is approximately 20 000 kJ). Energy-rich substrates need to be partitioned between brain, muscles, and immune system (and body growth).[3] Since brain and muscle need these fuels during the day (daytime consumers) and the immune system and growth-associated pathways request energetic substrates during the night (night-time consumers), circadian rhythms are a positively selected adaptive programme to overcome possible fuel shortage.[3] These circadian rhythms are controlled by higher-order neuroendocrine centres in the brain that regulate peripheral immune function and, hence, disease outcome.

Recent therapeutic developments are based on an understanding of the circadian rhythm because night-time release of therapeutic glucocorticoids has intriguing advantages over classical morning glucocorticoids.[44]

Mild activation of the sympathetic nervous system

An increased activity of the SNS can be found in different diseases.[45] Decreased levels of serum cortisol lead to increased basal sympathetic tone in relation to the degree of inflammation since there is a certain cooperativity of cortisol and noradrenaline on a molecular level via the β-adrenergic receptor signalling cascade. Functional loss of one factor (mainly cortisol in relation to inflammation) probably upregulates the other factor in order to maintain common functions such as blood glucose homeostasis (glycogenolysis, gluconeogenesis), lipolysis, blood pressure control, and regulation of the bronchial lumen. Such anti-inflammatory cooperativity of cortisol and noradrenaline can be found in synovial inflammation in RA.[46]

The SNS with its two effector arms, the adrenal medulla and peripheral sympathetic nerve fibres, is the main regulator of glycogenolysis, gluconeogenesis, and lipolysis. Although the adrenal medulla generally stimulates the splanchnic organs, sympathetic nerve fibres can stimulate distinct adipose tissue regions in the body. Provision of energy-rich fuels by the SNS depends on β_2-adrenergic receptor signalling. For example, catecholamines via β_2-adrenoceptors activate hormone-sensitive lipase in order to breakdown triglycerides into glycerol and fatty acids. The α_2-adrenergic receptor exerts antilipolytic, so-called lipogenic, effects.[47] Thus, elevated systemic SNS activity supports lipolysis, gluconeogenesis, and glycogenolysis. In addition, a high firing rate of sympathetic nerve fibres to adipose tissue supports local lipolysis.

Many CARDs are accompanied by increased levels of circulating proinflammatory cytokines and elevated SNS activity, which can be a substantial risk factor for cardiovascular disease. The circulating cytokines directly stimulate the SNS in the hypothalamus but also the local proinflammatory process in vascular lesions. In addition, hyperinsulinaemia accompanying CARDs is related to increased SNS activity because insulin stimulates the SNS.

From an energy regulation perspective, somewhat higher SNS activity is important to sustain allocation of energy-rich fuels to the immune system and, at the same time, maintain systemic circulation. Indeed, denervation of the SNS largely decreased early inflammation in animal models.[48] In conclusion, we can postulate that elevated systemic SNS activity as a consequence of an energy appeal reaction and local retraction of sympathetic nerve fibres are important for the activated immune system.

Conclusion

Neuroendocrine abnormalities are manifold and are a consequence of systemic inflammation. Systemic inflammation induces a neuroendocrine immune energy appeal reaction that redirects energy-rich substrates from stores such as liver (glucose, triglycerides), adipose tissue (triglycerides), or muscle (amino acids) to activated immune cells in primary/secondary lymphoid organs or locally inflamed tissue. Orchestrated energy regulation on the systemic and local cellular level has been positively selected for normal physiology and for transient serious, albeit non-life-threatening, inflammatory episodes, but these mechanisms have not been positively selected for CARDs. In transient inflammatory processes, the increase and decrease of immune responses (e.g. in infection) are part of a coordinated and highly regulated process. In CARDs, due to the chronic course of the disease, a similar coordinated regulation does not exist. Rather, the long-standing energy appeal reaction induces many neuroendocrine abnormalities, which are perpetuating and aggravating the course of CARDs. Hopefully, recognition of the importance of energy fluxes and related neuroendocrine alterations during both acute and chronic inflammation can provide a new perspective of disease pathogenesis and lead to better approaches for diagnosis and treatment.

References

1. Straub RH, Besedovsky HO. Integrated evolutionary, immunological, and neuroendocrine framework for the pathogenesis of chronic disabling inflammatory diseases. *FASEB J* 2003;17:2176–2183.
2. Williams GC. Pleiotropy, natural selection, and the evolution of senescence. *Evolution* 1957;11:398–411.
3. Straub RH, Cutolo M, Buttgereit F, Pongratz G. Energy regulation and neuroendocrine-immune control in chronic inflammatory diseases. *J Intern Med* 2010;267:543–560.
4. Dekkers JC, Geenen R, Godaert GL et al. Experimentally challenged reactivity of the hypothalamic pituitary adrenal axis in patients with recently diagnosed rheumatoid arthritis. *J Rheumatol* 2001;28:1496–1504.
5. Masi AT, Aldag JC, Jacobs JW. Rheumatoid arthritis: neuroendocrine immune integrated physiopathogenetic perspectives and therapy. *Rheum Dis Clin North Am* 2005;31:131–160.
6. Roubenoff R, Roubenoff RA, Cannon JG et al. Rheumatoid cachexia: cytokine-driven hypermetabolism accompanying reduced body cell mass in chronic inflammation. *J Clin Invest* 1994;93:2379–2386.
7. Jessop DS, Harbuz MS. A defect in cortisol production in rheumatoid arthritis: why are we still looking? *Rheumatology (Oxford)* 2005;44:1097–1100.

8. Pool AJ, Whipp BJ, Skasick AJ et al. Serum cortisol reduction and abnormal prolactin and CD4+/CD8+ T-cell response as a result of controlled exercise in patients with rheumatoid arthritis and systemic lupus erythematosus despite unaltered muscle energetics. *Rheumatology (Oxford)* 2004;43:43–48.

9. Straub RH, Kalden JR. Stress of different types increases the proinflammatory load in rheumatoid arthritis. *Arthritis Res Ther* 2009;11:114.

10. Tsigos C, Papanicolaou DA, Defensor R et al. Dose effects of recombinant human interleukin-6 on pituitary hormone secretion and energy expenditure. *Neuroendocrinology* 1997;66:54–62.

11. Straub RH, Paimela L, Peltomaa R, Schölmerich J, Leirisalo-Repo M. Inadequately low serum levels of steroid hormones in relation to IL-6 and TNF in untreated patients with early rheumatoid arthritis and reactive arthritis. *Arthritis Rheum* 2002;46:654–662.

12. Castagnetta LA, Carruba G, Granata OM et al. Increased estrogen formation and estrogen to androgen ratio in the synovial fluid of patients with rheumatoid arthritis. *J Rheumatol* 2003;30:2597–2605.

13. Schmidt M, Weidler C, Naumann H, Schölmerich J, Straub RH. Androgen conversion in osteoarthritis and rheumatoid arthritis synoviocytes —androstenedione and testosterone inhibit estrogen formation and favor production of more potent 5alpha-reduced androgens. *Arthritis Res Ther* 2005;7:R938–R948.

14. Straub RH, Härle P, Sarzi-Puttini P, Cutolo M. Tumor necrosis factor-neutralizing therapies improve altered hormone axes: an alternative mode of antiinflammatory action. *Arthritis Rheum* 2006;54:2039–2046.

15. Lahita RG, Bradlow HL, Ginzler E, Pang S, New M. Low plasma androgens in women with systemic lupus erythematosus. *Arthritis Rheum* 1987;30:241–248.

16. Dulos J, van der Vleuten MA, Kavelaars A, Heijnen CJ, Boots AM. CYP7B expression and activity in fibroblast-like synoviocytes from patients with rheumatoid arthritis: regulation by proinflammatory cytokines. *Arthritis Rheum* 2005;52:770–778.

17. Schmidt M, Hartung R, Capellino S et al. Estrone/17beta-estradiol conversion to, and tumor necrosis factor inhibition by, estrogen metabolites in synovial cells of patients with rheumatoid arthritis and patients with osteoarthritis. *Arthritis Rheum* 2009;60:2913–2922.

18. Elbers JM, Asscheman H, Seidell JC, Gooren LJ. Effects of sex steroid hormones on regional fat depots as assessed by magnetic resonance imaging in transsexuals. *Am J Physiol* 1999;276:E317–E325.

19. Rivier C. Role of endotoxin and interleukin-1 in modulating ACTH, LH and sex steroid secretion. *Adv Exp Med Biol* 1990;274:295–301.

20. Gordon D, Beastall GH, Thomson JA, Sturrock RD. Androgenic status and sexual function in males with rheumatoid arthritis and ankylosing spondylitis. *Q J Med* 1986;60:671–679.

21. Athreya BH, Rafferty JH, Sehgal GS, Lahita RG. Adenohypophyseal and sex hormones in pediatric rheumatic diseases. *J Rheumatol* 1993;20:725–730.

22. Suehiro RM, Borba EF, Bonfa E et al. Testicular Sertoli cell function in male systemic lupus erythematosus. *Rheumatology (Oxford)* 2008;47:1692–1697.

23. Aikawa NE, Sallum AM, Leal MM et al. Menstrual and hormonal alterations in juvenile dermatomyositis. *Clin Exp Rheumatol* 2010;28:571–575.

24. Johnson EO, Moutsopoulos HM. Neuroendocrine manifestations in Sjogren's syndrome. Relation to the neurobiology of stress. *Ann N Y Acad Sci* 2000;917:797–808.

25. Silva CA, Deen ME, Febronio MV et al. Hormone profile in juvenile systemic lupus erythematosus with previous or current amenorrhea. *Rheumatol Int* 2011;31(8):1037–1043.

26. Soares PM, Borba EF, Bonfa E et al. Gonad evaluation in male systemic lupus erythematosus. *Arthritis Rheum* 2007;56:2352–2361.

27. Villiger PM, Caliezi G, Cottin V et al. Effects of TNF antagonists on sperm characteristics in patients with spondyloarthritis. *Ann Rheum Dis* 2010;69:1842–1844.

28. Wallenius M, Skomsvoll JF, Irgens LM et al. Fertility in women with chronic inflammatory arthritides. *Rheumatology (Oxford)* 2011;50:1162–1167.

29. Pond CM. Paracrine relationships between adipose and lymphoid tissues: implications for the mechanism of HIV-associated adipose redistribution syndrome. *Trends Immunol* 2003;24:13–18.

30. Schäffler A, Müller-Ladner U, Schölmerich J, Büchler C. Role of adipose tissue as an inflammatory organ in human diseases. *Endocr Rev* 2006;27:449–467.

31. Neumann E, Frommer KW, Vasile M, Muller-Ladner U. Adipocytokines as driving forces in rheumatoid arthritis and related inflammatory diseases? *Arthritis Rheum* 2011;63:1159–1169.

32. Straub RH, Cutolo M. Circadian rhythms in rheumatoid arthritis: implications for pathophysiology and therapeutic management. *Arthritis Rheum* 2007;56:399–408.

33. Walker SE, Jacobson JD. Roles of prolactin and gonadotropin-releasing hormone in rheumatic diseases. *Rheum Dis Clin North Am* 2000;26:713–736.

34. Jara LJ, Medina G, Saavedra MA, Vera-Lastra O, Navarro C. Prolactin and autoimmunity. *Clin Rev Allergy Immunol* 2011;40:50–59.

35. Lee YC, Raychaudhuri S, Cui J et al. The PRL -1149 G/T polymorphism and rheumatoid arthritis susceptibility. *Arthritis Rheum* 2009;60:1250–1254.

36. Ben-Jonathan N, Hugo ER, Brandebourg TD, LaPensee CR. Focus on prolactin as a metabolic hormone. *Trends Endocrinol Metab* 2006;17:110–116.

37. Liefmann R. Endocrine imbalance in rheumatoid arthritis and rheumatoid spondylitis; hyperglycemia unresponsiveness, insulin resistance, increased gluconeogenesis and mesenchymal tissue degeneration; preliminary report. *Acta Med Scand* 1949;136:226–232.

38. Svenson KL, Lundqvist G, Wide L, Hallgren R. Impaired glucose handling in active rheumatoid arthritis: relationship to the secretion of insulin and counter-regulatory hormones. *Metabolism* 1987;36:940–943.

39. Dessein PH, Stanwix AE, Joffe BI. Cardiovascular risk in rheumatoid arthritis versus osteoarthritis: acute phase response related decreased insulin sensitivity and high-density lipoprotein cholesterol as well as clustering of metabolic syndrome features in rheumatoid arthritis. *Arthritis Res* 2002;4:R5.

40. Hotamisligil GS, Peraldi P, Budavari A et al. IRS-1-mediated inhibition of insulin receptor tyrosine kinase activity in TNF-alpha—and obesity-induced insulin resistance. *Science* 1996;271:665–668.

41. Gonzalez-Gay MA, De Matias JM, Gonzalez-Juanatey C et al. Anti-tumor necrosis factor-alpha blockade improves insulin resistance in patients with rheumatoid arthritis. *Clin Exp Rheumatol* 2006;24:83–86.

42. Frauwirth KA, Thompson CB. Regulation of T lymphocyte metabolism. *J Immunol* 2004;172:4661–4665.

43. Crofford LJ, Kalogeras KT, Mastorakos G et al. Circadian relationships between interleukin (IL)-6 and hypothalamic—pituitary-adrenal axis hormones: failure of IL-6 to cause sustained hypercortisolism in patients with early untreated rheumatoid arthritis. *J Clin Endocrinol Metab* 1997;82:1279–1283.

44. Buttgereit F, Doering G, Schaeffler A et al. Efficacy of modified-release versus standard prednisone to reduce duration of morning stiffness of the joints in rheumatoid arthritis (CAPRA-1): a double-blind, randomised controlled trial. *Lancet* 2008;371:205–214.

45. Dekkers JC, Geenen R, Godaert GL, Bijlsma JW, van Doornen LJ. Elevated sympathetic nervous system activity in patients with recently diagnosed rheumatoid arthritis with active disease. *Clin Exp Rheumatol* 2004;22:63–70.

46. Straub RH, Günzler C, Miller LE et al. Anti-inflammatory cooperativity of corticosteroids and norepinephrine in rheumatoid arthritis synovial tissue in vivo and in vitro. *FASEB J* 2002;16:993–1000.

47. Pedersen SB, Kristensen K, Hermann PA, Katzenellenbogen JA, Richelsen B. Estrogen controls lipolysis by up-regulating

alpha2A-adrenergic receptors directly in human adipose tissue through the estrogen receptor alpha. Implications for the female fat distribution. *J Clin Endocrinol Metab* 2004;89:1869–1878.

48. Levine JD, Dardick SJ, Roizen MF, Helms C, Basbaum AI. Contribution of sensory afferents and sympathetic efferents to joint injury in experimental arthritis. *J Neurosci* 1986;6:3423–3429.

49. Mastorakos G, Chrousos GP, Weber JS. Recombinant interleukin-6 activates the hypothalamic-pituitary-adrenal axis in humans. *J Clin Endocrinol Metab* 1993;77:1690–1694.

50. Straub RH, Glück T, Cutolo M et al. The adrenal steroid status in relation to inflammatory cytokines (interleukin-6 and tumour necrosis factor) in polymyalgia rheumatica. *Rheumatology* 2000;39:624–631.

CHAPTER 23

Malignancy

Jennifer Hamilton and Clive Kelly

Rheumatic disorders with an increased risk of malignancy

Rheumatoid arthritis

Although the overall incidence of malignancy in rheumatoid arthritis (RA) is not increased, an association between RA and lymphoma was suspected nearly 50 years ago[1] and confirmed 20 years later.[2] Duration rather than severity of RA was initially felt to be the main risk factor.[3] One year later, a large cohort study reported an increased incidence of myeloma in patients with RA.[4] The presence of a paraprotein was found to increase the probability of developing myeloma or lymphoma in RA.[5] More recent work has confirmed a twofold increase in both the prevalence and the incidence of lymphoma in RA.[6] The risk of leukaemia is similarly doubled, but no association of myeloma was found. This appears to be a consequence of the chronic inflammatory nature of RA and associated immunosuppression, rather than the consequence of treatment.[7] The risk of lymphoma in patients treated with anti-tumour necrosis factor (TNF) was also similar when corrected for disease duration.[6] Similar data from the British Society for Rheumatology Register (BSRBR) has also been reported recently.[8]

The standardized incidence ratio (SIR) of cancers at certain other sites are also influenced by the presence of RA. Colon and rectal cancer is reduced (SIR 0.77), probably as a result of the use of non-steroidal anti-inflammatory drugs (NSAIDs), while lung cancer is increased (SIR 1.63), perhaps due to smoking and the increased prevalence of interstitial lung disease.[9] Skin and prostate cancers are also reportedly more common in RA.[10] Age-adjusted mortality from cancer has been shown to be increased in patients with RA,[11] perhaps as a result of later detection, with patients hospitalized as a result of RA having a hazard ratio for overall survival of 1.31.[12]

Sjögren's syndrome

Lymphoma is strongly associated with primary Sjögren's syndrome (pSS) with a SIR of around 40.[13] Diffuse large B-cell lymphoma and salivary marginal zone B-cell lymphomas (MALTomas) are seen in up to 5% of pSS patients,[14] and relate to disease activity and severity.[15] The incidence of second malignancy is increased in patients with pSS and lymphoma.[16] Other malignancies are not significantly associated with pSS.[16]

Scleroderma

Population-based studies initially gave conflicting results on the association of scleroderma with malignancy.[17,18] There is now good evidence that lung cancer (especially alveolar cell and adenocarcinoma) is increased in diffuse disease, and is often associated with pulmonary fibrosis.[19] Breast cancer, B-cell lymphoma, and tongue cancer are also commoner in scleroderma.[20,21] There is now evidence to show that some patients develop scleroderma as a consequence of RNA polymerase antibodies expressed by cancer,[22] suggesting that scleroderma may sometimes be a paraneoplastic phenomenon.

Dermatomyositis

Myositis is associated with an increased risk of malignancy, and this is much greater in patients with dermatomyositis, where up to 25% of patients may develop a malignancy.[23] It is associated with severe skin and/or muscle involvement, but less likely in those with renal or lung disease. Careful investigation of all new or recurrent presentations with myositis is recommended. This should include a chest radiograph and often an upper gastrointestinal endoscopy and pelvic ultrasound. Malignancies of the lung, oesophagus, and ovary are most frequently associated with dermatomyositis.[23,24] Anti-p 155/140 antibodies appear to predict malignancy, and the skin and muscle inflammation may result from an immune response to antigenic material expressed by the underlying neoplasm.[24]

Systemic lupus erythematosus

There is a small overall increase in cancer (SIR 1.15) in patients with systemic lupus erythematosus (SLE).[25] The incidence of cancer is especially increased in patients under the age of 40. There is a three-fold increased risk of non-Hodgkin's lymphoma (NHL), and it is unclear whether this relates to the disease or its treatment. The risk of lung cancer and other lymphomas are increased to a lesser degree. Vulvovaginal and cervical cancers are also increased in SLE,[26] possibly as a result of delayed clearance of human papillomavirus. Table 23.1 summarizes the SIRs of specific cancers associated with rheumatic disorders.

Cancer associated with therapy of rheumatic disease

Immunosuppressive drugs used in the treatment of rheumatic disease increase the likelihood of certain types of neoplasia. It can be

Table 23.1 Standardized incidence ratios (SIR) of specific cancers associated with rheumatic disorders

Disease	Cancer	SIR	References
Rheumatoid arthritis	NHL	2.1	6–8
	Leukaemia	2.0	6
	Lung cancer	1.63	9
	Prostate	N/A	10
	Colorectal	0.77	9
Primary Sjögren's syndrome	NHL	40 (approx)	13–16
Scleroderma	Lung	23.0	19–21
	Oesophagus	15.9	19–21
	Tongue	9.6	19–21
	NHL	N/A	19–21
	Breast	N/A	19–21
Dermatomyositis Polymyositis	Lung	N/A	23–24
	Oesophagus	N/A	23–24
	Ovary	N/A	23–24
Systemic lupus erythematosus	NHL	3.0	25
	Lung	N/A	25
	Vulvovaginal	N/A	25
	Cervical	N/A	25

NHL, non-Hodgkin's lymphoma.

difficult to assess the degree of risk from clinical studies as many of the rheumatic diseases also carry an increased risk of cancer.

Methotrexate

Methotrexate is most commonly used disease-modifying antirheumatic drug (DMARD). A 3 year prospective French study suggested that overall the risk of NHL was not significantly increased in RA patients treated with methotrexate. However the incidence of Hodgkin's disease (HD) was significantly increased in comparison to the French population (SMR 7.4 [3.0–15.3; $p < 0.001$]). Of the 7 cases of HD, 5 were associated with Epstein–Barr virus (EBV).[27] Another study demonstrated the presence of latent EBV in 7/13 lymphomas arising during methotrexate treatment, versus only 2 out of 11 in patients not treated with methotrexate. This suggests that EBV-related transformation is important in the pathogenesis of lymphomas in patients on methotrexate treatment.[28] This is important, as some tumours will regress within 4 weeks of methotrexate cessation.[29]

Cyclophosphamide and azathioprine

High-dose cyclophosphamide and azathioprine have also been linked with an increased risk of haematological malignancy. Overall the relative risk for all types of cancer when azathioprine is used in RA is 1.4–8.7. Up to 16% of patients with Wegener's granulomatosis will have bladder cancer by 15 years when treated with prolonged courses of cyclophosphamide. Use of drugs such as cyclophosphamide has led to a significant reduction in mortality from diseases such as SLE and granulomatosis with polyangiitis (Wegener's). Recent studies have shown that lower total doses of

cyclophosphamide are as effective as the old high-dose regimens, but carry with them improved morbidity.[30] The decision to treat with immunosuppressive drugs is always a balance of risk versus potential benefit. High levels of vigilance for development of cancer must be maintained, often for many years after the drug is discontinued. The commonest types of cancer in this cohort of patients are skin, haematological, and bladder cancer in cyclophosphamide-treated patients. It therefore makes sense to advise patients to wear high-factor sun block, ensure GPs have a low threshold for investigating persistent lymphadenopathy and B-cell symptoms in patients with rheumatic disease, and continuing to regularly dip urine of patients treated with cyclophosphamide for many years after discontinuation of treatment. In the future more tailored use of biologics such as rituximab in patients with connective tissue disease will decrease this risk still further.

Ciclosporin and mycophenolate

Both these agents carry an increased risk of inducing malignancy, especially skin cancer and lymphoma. Most of the available data is derived from the transplantation literature.[31,32] The risk increases with increased dose and duration of use.[33]

Biologic agents

Theoretically the inhibition of anti-TNF may potentiate the risk of malignancy in humans as a result of the activity of anti-TNF against tumours in laboratory models. Although results from biologic registries have been reassuring, this conflicts with reports from metanalyses. Data from the South Swedish Arthritis Treatment Group showed that although the SIR for all types of malignancy was no different between patients treated with etanercept or infliximab and patients treated with conventional DMARDs, the relative risk of lymphoma in the TNF inhibitor group was 11.5 (95% CI 3.7–26.9) compared with 1.3 (95% CK 0.2–4.5) for the DMARD group. However, other studies have shown no increase in risk. There is more evidence to support a link between biologic agents and non-melanoma skin cancer in patients treated with TNF inhibitors. It should be remembered that biologics are contraindicated in patients with a history of cancer within the preceding 10 years.[34–37]

Cancer drugs causing rheumatic symptoms

Many of the drugs used to treat cancer have been associated with rheumatological side effects (Table 22.2). The agents associated with the most significant joint and muscle symptoms are those that inhibit microtubular function, and these side effects are often dose related. In general the symptoms will develop within 48–72 hours of chemotherapy and will last for 4–7 days. Risk factors for acute musculoskeletal side effects include antecedent peripheral neuropathy, diabetes, alcohol use, age, prior neurotoxic chemotherapy, and history of arthritis or neuromuscular disorder. Where rest, simple analgesics and NSAIDs fail to improve symptoms, corticosteroids and opiates may be tried.[38]

Taxanes are widely used in female pelvic, breast, respiratory, and genitourinary malignancy. Up to 75% of patients will experience significant joint or muscle morbidity. This usually develops within 24–48 hours and may persist for 3–5 days. Premedication with dexamethasone may decrease this.

In addition, a 'postchemotherapy rheumatism syndrome' may occur in patients receiving adjuvant chemotherapy for breast cancer.

Table 23.2 Rheumatological side effects of anti-cancer drugs

Drug	Rheumatic complaint
Aromatase inhibitors, interferon, topotecan, bryostatin, fludarabine, dacarbazine, altretamine, vinorelbine, gemcitabine, procarbazine, isotretenoin	Arthralgia Osteoporosis
Bleomycin	Scleroderma Raynaud's
Taxanes	Myalgia and arthritis
Glucocorticoids	Osteonecrosis
Bisphosphonates	Musculoskeletal pain and osteonecrosis
Radiotherapy	Myalgia and stiffness
Taxols	Scleroderma like syndrome Joint pain, acute myalgia and arthralgia
Intravesical BCG	Reactive arthritis, septic arthritis
High-dose methotrexate	Increased bone resorption and inhibition of bone formation leading to osteoporosis and fracture

BCG, bacille Calmette–Guérin.

Serological tests, autoimmune markers, and imaging are all unremarkable although patients may have mild periarticular swelling. NSAIDs are usually ineffective but some patients may respond to low-dose steroids.

Additionally, aromatase inhibitors are associated with an increased risk of osteoporosis as a result of accelerated bone loss.[39] This is particularly accelerated in premenopausal females and has led to recent guidelines on the use of prophylactic bisphosphonates and regular surveillance of bone density in such patients.[40]

Intravesical bacillus Calmette–Guérin (BCG)

Intravesical BCG is used for prophylaxis and treatment of superficial bladder cancer. Arthritis or arthralgia occur in approximately 0.5–1% of patients.[41]

A reactive arthritis may develop in the lower limbs within 2 weeks of BCG instillation. Up to 53% may be HLA B27 positive and a small proportion of these may go on to develop chronic symptoms. The majority will settle with discontinuation of treatment and NSAIDs. If symptoms fail to settle after a couple of weeks, glucocorticoids may be appropriate. Septic arthritis is rare but must be considered in patients presenting with an effusion especially if it only affects one joint.[42–43]

Gout

In addition to polyarthritis patients undergoing treatment for malignancy, especially lymphoproliferative disorders, can develop acute gout as a result of release of nucleic acids from killed tumour cells and formation of uric acid. Patients at risk from the tumour lysis syndrome should receive aggressive rehydration and urate-lowering agents prior to receiving chemotherapy.

Rheumatological presentations of malignancy

The first manifestation of malignancy may be rheumatological. Skeletal metastases may present as either bone pain or a vertebral crush fracture. Patients can however present with polyarthritis, features suggestive of polymyalgia rheumatica, vasculitis, regional limb pain and symptoms suggestive of connective tissue disease. In one retrospective study 23.1% of patients admitted to a general medical ward with previously unclarified rheumatic disorders were found to have an occult malignancy.[4,44] In 9 of the 25 cases long term remission of neoplasia was achieved, and this was associated with an improvement in rheumatic symptoms.

In the majority of patients evidence of malignancy will be found on routine examination or laboratory tests. However, rheumatologists should maintain a high level of suspicion and consider more extensive investigation for malignancy in patients presenting with seronegative disease, abrupt onset of symptoms, atypical features, significant weight loss or other systemic symptoms, and where either degree of symptoms or inflammatory markers are disproportionate to the physical signs. Breast examination should always be

Table 23.3 Conditions that may present to rheumatologists and could suggest malignancy

Condition	Associated cancer	Features that should raise suspicion
Erythema nodosum	Hodgkin's lymphoma T-cell lymphoma with direct skin infiltration	Recurrent rashes Atypical mediastinal lymphadenopathy
Sweet's syndrome (20–25% have associated malignancy)	Mainly acute myelogenous leukaemia, other lymphoproliferative disorders. 15% of tumours are solid affecting GU tract, breast and GI tract	Should be considered in all patients presenting with Sweet's syndrome
Pyoderma gangrenosum	Usually lymphoproliferative. Most commonly associated with IBD	Should be considered in all patients especially where no underlying IBD
Cancer-associated fasciitis panniculitis syndrome	May present with symptoms suggestive of scleroderma	Should be considered in autoantibody-negative scleroderma especially if atypical or systemic features
Pancreatic panniculitis	Pancreatic; presents with tender erythematosus nodules which may ulcerate	
Vasculitis	Usually haematological malignancy	Risk of underlying cancer small; further investigations should be guided by other features in history and examination

GI, gastrointestinal; GU, genitourinary; IBD, inflammatory bowel disease.

considered in patients who do not regularly self-examine or attend for screening. Pancoast tumours should enter the differential diagnosis in patients presenting with shoulder pain. Shoulder pain is present in up to 96% of patients and treatment for other disorders may lead to a delay in diagnosis. The tumour may not always be apparent on plain film so a CT scan of chest should be considered where there is marked muscle wasting, extreme pain, and/or night waking. Because of the location of the tumour, respiratory features may not present until later in the disease.[45–47]

There are certain rheumatological presentations that are strongly suggestive of malignancy, e.g. hypertrophic pulmonary osteoarthropathy (HPOA). In one Japanesese study of 2625 patients with lung cancer, HPOA was present in 0.7% of patients and was strongly associated with adenocarcinoma of the lung. It is characterized by abnormal proliferation of skin and osseous tissue at the distal extremities and leads to digital clubbing and periostosis in the long bones, and can also be associated with joint effusion. Arthropathy can sometimes develop before the finger clubbing. Treatment of the lung cancer normally causes the clinical manifestations to regress but is not always effective. If NSAIDs or other analgesics fail to relieve symptoms, treatment with IV bisphosphonates has been found to be effective in case reports.[48,49]

Other rheumatic presentations of malignancy are shown in Table 23.3.

References

1. Lea AJ. An association between the rheumatic diseases and the reticuloses. *Ann Rheum Dis* 1964;23:480–482.
2. Prior P, Symmons DPM, Hawkins CF et al. Cancer morbidity in rheumatoid arthritis. *Ann Rheum Dis* 1984;43:128–131.
3. Symmons DPM, Ahern B, Bacon PA et al. Lymphoproliferative malignancies in rheumatoid arthritis. *Ann Rheum Dis* 1984;43(2).132 135.
4. Katusic S, Beard CM, Kurland LT et al. Occurrence of malignant neoplasms in the Rochester Minnesota rheumatoid arthritis cohort. *Am J Med* 1985;78:50–55.
5. Kelly CA, Griffiths ID. The prognostic significance of paraproteinaemia in rheumatoid arthritis. *Intern Med* 1998;6:145–148.
6. Askling J, Fared CM, Baecklund E et al. Haematopoetic malignancy in rheumatoid arthritis: lymphoma risk and characteristics after exposure to TNF antagonists. *Ann Rheum Dis* 2005;64:1414–1420.
7. Baecklund E, Iliadou A, Askling J, et al: Association of chronic inflammation, not its treatment, with increased lymphoma risk in rheumatoid arthritis. *Arthritis Rheum* 2006;54:692–701.
8. Mercer LK, Dixon WG. Looking beyond incidence in the relationship between anti-tumor necrosis factor therapy and malignancy. *Arthritis Rheum* 2011;63,1773–1775.
9. Smitten AL, Simon TA, Hochberg MC, Suissa S. A meta-analysis of the incidence of malignancy in adult patients with rheumatoid arthritis. *Arthritis Res Ther* 2008;10:R45.
10. Hemminki K, Li X, Sundquist K, Sundquist J. Cancer risk in hospitalised rheumatoid arthritis patients. *Rheumatology* 2008;47:698–701.
11. Franklin J, Lunt M, Bunn D, Symmons D, Silman A. Influence of inflammatory polyarthritis on cancer incidence and survival: results from a community based prospective survey. *Arthritis Rheum* 2007;56:790–798.
12. Ji J, Liu X, Sundquist K, Sundquist J. Survival of cancer in patients with rheumatoid arthritis: a follow up study in Sweden of patients hopsitalised with rheumatoid arthritis 1 year before diagnosis of cancer. *Rheumatology* 2011;50:1513–1518.
13. Voulgarelis M, Skopouli FN. Clinical, immunologic, and molecular factors predicting lymphoma development in Sjogren's syndrome patients. *Clin Rev Allergy Immunol* 2007;32:265–274.
14. Tzioufas AG, Voulgarelis M. Update on Sjögren's syndrome autoimmune epithelitis: from classification to increased neoplasias. *Best Pract Res Clin Rheumatol* 2007;21:989–1010.
15. Smedby KE, Baecklund E, Askling J. Malignant lymphomas in autoimmunity and inflammation: a review of risks, risk factors, and lymphoma characteristics. *Cancer Epidemiol Biomarkers Prev* 2006;15:2069–2077.
16. Lazarus MN, Robinson P, Mak V, Moller H, Isenberg DA. Incidence of cancer in a cohort of patients with primary Sjögren's syndrome. *Rheumatology* 2006;45:1012–1015.
17. Rosenthal A, McLaughlin J, Linet M, Persson I. Scleroderma and malignancy: an epidemiological study. *Ann Rheum Dis.* 1993;52:531–533.
18. Chatterjee S, Dombi G, Severson RK, Mayes MD. Risk of malignancy in scleroderma: a population-based cohort study. *Arthritis Rheum* 2005;52:2415–2424.
19. Wooten M. Systemic sclerosis and malignancy: a review of the literature. *South Med J* 2008;101:59–62.
20. Dark CT, Rasheed M, Artlett CM, Jimenez SA. A cohort study of cancer incidence in systemic sclerosis. *J Rheumatol* 2006;33:113–116.
21. Marasini B, Conciato L, Belloli L, Massaratti M. Systemic sclerosis and cancer. *Int J Immunopathol Pharmacol* 2009;22:533–538.
22. Shah A, Rosen A, Hummers L, Wigley F, Casciola-Rosen L. Close temporal relationship between onset of cancer and scleroderma in patients with RNA polymerase I/III antibodies. *Arthritis Rheum* 2010;62:2787–2795.
23. Chen Y-J, Wu C-Y, Huang Y-L et al. Cancer risks of dermatomyositis and polymyositis: a nationwide cohort study in Taiwan. *Arthritis Res Ther* 2010;12(2):R70.
24. Zahr ZA, Baer AN. Malignancy in myositis. *Curr Rheumatol Rep* 2011;13:208–215.
25. Bernatsky A, Ramsey-Goldman R, Clarke AE. Malignancy in systemic lupus erythematosus: what have we learned? *Best Pract Res Clin Rheumatol* 2009;23:639–647.
26. Gayed M, Bernatsky S, Ramsey-Goldman R, Clarke AE, Gordon C. Lupus and cancer. *Lupus* 2009;18:479–485.
27. Mariette X, Cazals-Hatem D, Warszawki J et al. Lymphomas in rheumatoid arthritis patients treated with methotrexate: a 3 year prospective study in France. *Blood* 2002;99:3909–3912.
28. Menke DM, Griesser H, Moder KG et al. Lymphomas in patients with connective tissue disease. Comparison of p 53 protein expression and latent EBV infection in patients immunosupressed and not immunosupressed with methotrexate. *Am J Clin Pathol* 2000;113:212–215.
29. Kamel OW, vande Rijn M, Weiss LM et al. Brief report: reversible lymphomas associated with Epstein-Barr virus occurring during methotrexate therapy for rheumatoid arthritis and dermatomyositis. *New Engl J Med* 1993;328:1317–1321.
30. Silman AJ, Petrie J, Hazleman B, Evans SJ. Lymphoproliferative cancer and other malignancy in patients with RA treated with azathioprine: a 20 year follow up study. *Ann Rheum Dis* 1988;47:988–994.
31. Mithoefer AB, Supran S, Freeman RB. Risk factors associated with skin cancer after liver transplantation. *Liver Transpl* 2002;8(10):939–942.
32. Glover MT, Deeks JJ, Raftery MJ, Cunningham J, Leigh IM. Immunosuppression and risk of non-melanoma skin cancer in renal transplant recipients. *Lancet* 1997;349:398–402.
33. Dantal J, Hourmant M, Catarovich D et al. Effect of long term immunosuppression in kidney graft recipients on cancer incidence: randomised comparison of 2 cyclosporin regimens. *Lancet* 1998;351:623–628.
34. Askling J, van Vollenhoven RF, Granath F et al. Cancer risk in patients with rheumatoid arthritis treated with anti-tumor necrosis factor alpha therapies: does the risk change with the time since start of treatment? *Arthritis Rheum* 2009;60:3180–3187.
35. Bongartz T, Sutton AJ, Sweeting MJ et al. Anti-TNF antibody therapy in rheumatoid arthritis and the risk of serious infections and malignancies: systematic review and meta-analysis of rare harmful effects in randomized controlled trials. *JAMA* 2006;295:2275–2279.

36. Geborek P, Bladstrom A, Turesson C et al. Tumour necrosis factor blockers do not increase overall tumour risk in patients with rheumatoid arthritis but may be associated with an increased risk of lymphomas. *Ann Rheum Dis* 2005;64:699–701.

37. Wolfe F, Michaud K. Biologic treatment of rheumatoid arthritis and the risk of malignancy: analysis from a large US observational study *Arthritis Rheum* 2007;56:2886–2890.

38. Yarbro CH, Frogge MH, Goodman M. *Cancer symptom management*, 3rd edn. Jones and Bartlett Publishers, Boston, MA.

39. Confavreux CB, Fontana A, Guastalla JP et al. Estrogen-dependent increase in bone turnover and bone loss in postmenopausal women with breast cancer treated with anastrozole. Prevention with bisphosphonates. *Bone* 2007;41:346–349.

40. Reid DM, Doughty J, Eastell R et al. Guidance for the management of breast cancer treatment-induced bone loss: a consensus position statement from a UK Expert Group. *Cancer Treat Rev.* 2008;34 Suppl 1:S3.

41. Tinazzi E, Ficarra V, Simeoni S, Artibani W, Lunardi C. Reactive arthritis following BCG immunotherapy for urinary bladder carcinoma: a systematic review. *Rheumatol Int* 2006;26:481–482.

42. Clavel G, Grados F, Lefauveau P, Fardellone P. Osteoarticular side effects of BCG therapy. *Joint Bone Spine* 2006;73(1):24–26.

43. Lamm DL, Stogdill VD, Stogdill BJ, Crispen RG. Complications of bacillus Calmette-Guerin immunotherapy in 1,278 patients with bladder cancer. *J Urol* 1986;135:272–275.

44. Naschitz JE, Yeshurun D, Rosner I. The rheumatic manifestations of occult cancer. *Cancer* 1995;75:2954–2957.

45. Van Houtte P, Maclennan I, Poulter C, Rubin P. External radiation in management of superior sulcus tumour. *Cancer* 1984, 54:223–227

46. Miller JI, Mansour KA, Hatcher CR. Carcinoma of the superior pulmonary sulcus. *Ann Thorac Surg* 1979;28:44–47.

47. Shahian DM, Neptune WB, Ellis FH. Pancoast tumours: Improved survival with preoperative and post operative radiotherapy. *Ann Thorac Surg* 1987;43:32–38.

48. Ito T, Goto K, Yoh K et al. Hypertrophic pulmonary osteoarthropathy as a paraneoplastic manifestation of lung cancer. *J Thorac Oncol* 2010; 5:976–979.

49. King MM, Nelson DA. Hypertrophic osteoarthropathy effectively treated with zoledronic acid. *Clin Lung Cancer* 2008;9:179–181.

CHAPTER 24

The eye

Harry Petrushkin and Miles Stanford

Introduction

Most rheumatological diseases have ocular complications, many of which are specific to the disease, and consequently the ophthalmologist has an important diagnostic role. Many ophthalmic complications require specific therapy and in some cases may actually dictate the systemic therapy for the disease. Furthermore, rheumatological diseases require a wide range of drugs and several of these have important ocular side effects; the ophthalmologist therefore has a role in monitoring the eye and preventing complications.

In general, diseases that involve the uvea, sclera, or cornea cause painful red eyes with preserved vision, whereas involvement of the retina or optic nerve causes profound visual loss without pain or redness. Fortunately, with the particular exception of juvenile idiopathic arthritis (JIA), most of the ocular complications that affect sight are symptomatic, so the rheumatologist can easily notice these when taking a focused history.

The more common eye symptoms encountered in patients with rheumatological diseases are dry, gritty eyes; photophobia; watering; redness; pain; floaters; and, most importantly, blurring or actual loss of vision. The differential diagnosis of the painful red eye and of sudden loss of vision is outlined in Tables 24.1 and 24.2.

Common eye disorders encountered in rheumatological disease

Dry eyes

Patients with dry eyes may complain of a foreign-body sensation, redness, grittiness, and excessive mucus secretion. Keratoconjunctivitis sicca occurs when the secretory function of the lacrimal and accessory lacrimal glands are of insufficient quality or quantity to maintain an adequate tear film and stable ocular surface.

Reduction in secretion, usually secondary to destruction of the lacrimal gland is associated primarily with autoimmune diseases such as Sjögren's syndrome,[1] systemic lupus erythematosus (SLE),[2] rheumatoid arthritis (RA),[3] and systemic sclerosis.[4] Infiltrative conditions such as lymphoma, sarcoidosis,[5] and amyloidosis[6] can also cause a reduction in lacrimal gland secretion.

Staining the cornea with fluorescein can help diagnose a dry eye. In early cases of keratoconjunctivitis sicca the stain may be limited to the conjunctiva and in severe cases can be seen all over the cornea.

Frequent ocular lubricants are the mainstay of treatments and these range from thin, watery preparations, which need to be instilled regularly, to more viscous gels and ointments which last longer, but tend to cause more blurring of vision. Occasionally

Table 24.1 Differential diagnosis of the painful red eye

Ocular pathology	Vision	Pain	Distribution of redness	Extra signs	Likely systemic disease
Conjunctivitis	Good	Mild	Diffuse	Purulent, sticky exudate	Reiter's syndrome
Dry eyes	Good	Gritty	Mild diffuse	Schirmer's test Reduced tear film break-up time	Rheumatoid arthritis Systemic vasculitis Sjögren's syndrome (primary and secondary)
Episcleritis	Good	Irritation or 'bruised' sensation	Diffuse or nodular	Mobile nodules	Rheumatoid arthtitis Systemic vasculitis
Scleritis	May be reduced	Very severe	Diffuse or nodular	Keratitis	Rheumatoid arthritis
Anterior uveitis	Reduced	Mild to severe	Circumcorneal or diffuse	Small or irregular pupil Photophobia	Seronegative spondyloarthropathies Sarcoidosis Behçet's disease

Table 24.2 Differential diagnosis of sudden loss of vision

Cause of visual loss	History of visual loss	Field	Pupil reaction	Media	Fundus	Likely systemic disease
Vitreous haemorrhage	Sudden	Generalized constriction	Normal	Hazy	Not usually visible New vessels or venous occlusion may be visible	Systemic vasculitis Behçet's disease Diabetes Trauma
Macular oedema	Gradual, with distortion	Small, relatively central scotoma	Normal	Hazy	Swollen disc	Behçet's disease Sarcoidosis Seronegative arthropathies Intermediate uveitis
Central retinal artery occlusion	Sudden	Dense, large, central scotoma	Afferent pupillary defect	Clear	Normal or pale optic disc Pale retina Cherry red spot	Systemic vasculitis Polyarteritis nodosa Cardiovascular disease
Ischaemic optic neuropathy	Sudden	Dense, altitudinal scotoma	Afferent pupillary defect	Clear	Pale or swollen optic disc	Systemic vasculitis Giant cell arteritis Cardiovascular disease
Inflammatory optic neuropathy	Progressive	Central, or centro-caecal scotoma	Afferent pupillary defect	Clear or hazy	Pale or swollen optic disc	Sarcoidosis Wegener's granulomatosis Demyelinating disease

punctal plugs can be inserted into the lacrimal punctae to block the drainage of what few tears there are.

Episcleritis

The episclera is a thin layer of transparent tissue lying between the conjunctiva and the sclera. Episcleritis is a benign, self-limiting condition, reported to be associated with systemic inflammatory disease in 3–5% of patients; it can also be the presenting feature of gout.[7]

Scleritis

Scleritis is a serious, potentially sight-threatening condition which, in contrast to episcleritis, is almost always painful and does not subside spontaneously. Pain is often described as 'deep or boring' and may be excruciating. Characteristically, patients report that the pain wakes them from sleep. The inflamed area is red and can be in a nodular, diffuse, or necrotizing in its pattern (Figure 24.1). Spread to the cornea produces peripheral ulceration, keratitis, and photophobia, whereas involvement of the posterior sclera causes retinal folds, serous retinal detachment, and optic disc swelling.

An unusual variant of scleritis is scleromalacia perforans (Figure 24.2), which occurs in elderly women with severe RA. This is characteristically painless and the affected sclera becomes chalky-white because of the underlying arteritic infarction.[8] Eventually the sclera becomes atrophic and the blue of the underlying choroid can be seen bulging through it. Actual perforation of the globe is very rare, despite the name.

Autoimmune diseases are present in up to 50% of patients with scleritis,[9] and include RA, systemic vasculitis (particularly Wegener's granulomatosis), SLE, inflammatory bowel disease (IBD), and relapsing polychondritis. Patients with scleritis tend to have more aggressive systemic disease than those without scleritis.

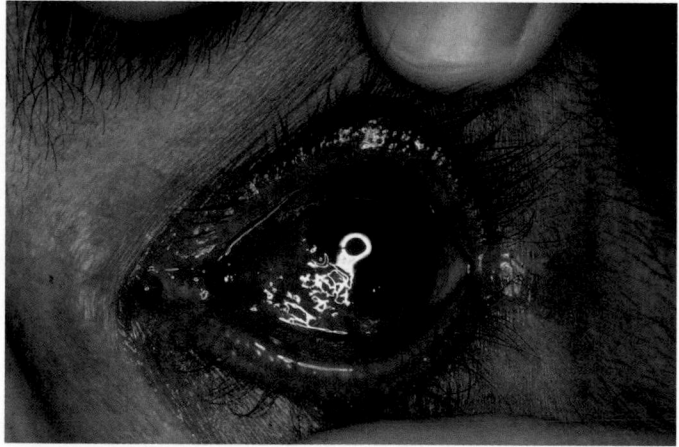

Fig. 24.1 Scleritis. A 35 year old man presents with severe pain in his left eye. He is unable to sleep as the pain is so severe. The eye is tender to touch and the sclera is a dusky red colour, typical of scleritis.

Scleritis can also occur in SLE and is most common when the disease is poorly controlled.[10] These patients usually require aggressive medical treatment. A recent case series found that 5% of patients with scleritis had IBD, although the most common ocular manifestation of IBD is uveitis.[11] Relapsing polychondritis can often present with scleritis, which is characterized by recurrent inflammation of type II collagen fibres present in the sclera.[12]

Acute anterior uveitis

Acute anterior uveitis (AAU) is inflammation within the anterior chamber of the eye. The patient complains of an acutely painful, red

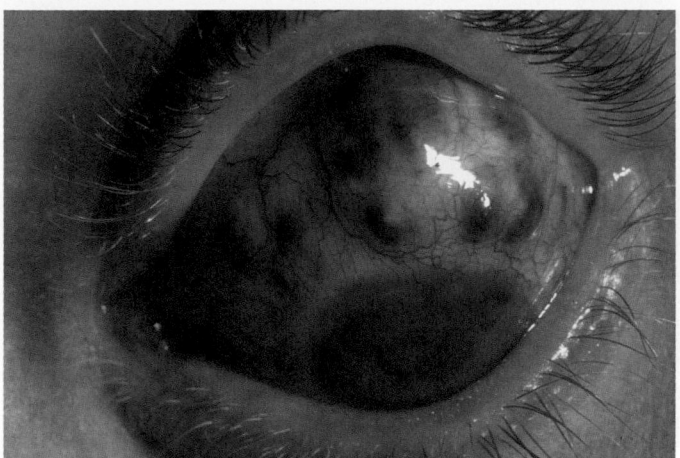

Fig. 24.2 Scleromalacia perforans. A 50 year old woman with severe rheumatoid arthritis has suffered from relapsing scleritis for over 20 years. She now has a very thin superior sclera with underlying choroid bulging through.

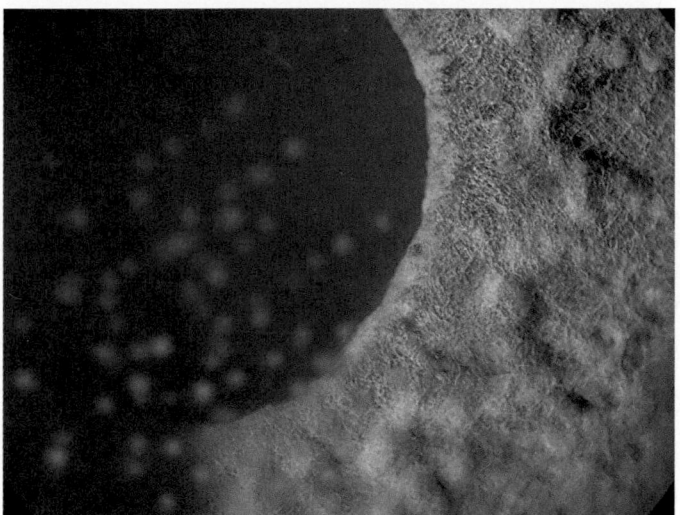

Fig. 24.3 Granulomatous uveitis. A 40 year old woman presented with photophobia and decreased visual acuity. She has had symptoms for 3 weeks and has developed keratic precipitates and Koeppe nodules on her iris.

eye with photophobia, sometimes associated with blurred vision. The condition is generally unilateral and frequently recurrent. The ophthalmological signs consist of circumcorneal redness and keratic precipitates on the endothelial surface of the cornea. Flare (protein) and cells (white blood cells) in the anterior chamber resemble 'a shaft of light with specks of dust' when viewed through the slit lamp. Koeppe and Busacca nodules can form on the iris in cases of granulomatous uveitis (Figure 24.3) and cells can gravitate to form a fluid level called a hypopyon. The pupil is small and poorly reactive and the intraocular pressure can be either low, due to ciliary body inflammation, or high, due to blockage or inflammation of the trabecular meshwork.

The lifetime cumulative incidence of AAU in the general population has been calculated to be about 0.2%, which increases to 1% in HLA B27-positive subjects.[13] Patients who are HLA B27 positive tend to be younger at the time of their first attack, have more severe ocular inflammation, and a longer recovery period than those who are HLA B27 negative.[14]

Retinal vasculitis and posterior uveitis

In patients with seronegative arthropathies and Behçet's disease there may be inflammation in the posterior chamber of the eye. Patients may complain of floaters and blurred or distorted central vision secondary to macular oedema. In mild to moderate cases, fundoscopy reveals focal or diffuse white sheathing of the retinal veins; in severe cases there are also scattered haemorrhages. Occlusion of the retinal veins leading to neovascularization of the optic disc or peripheral retina may also develop. The new vessels, similar to those in diabetes mellitus, generally develop as a consequence of retinal ischaemia, but may also appear as a reaction to the intraocular inflammatory process. Their walls are fragile and they frequently bleed, leading to vitreous haemorrhages, which are an important cause of visual morbidity in these patients.

In contrast, patients with systemic vasculitis do not usually develop inflammation within the eye but the vasculitic process affects the retinal capillaries and arterioles to produce retinal or choroidal ischaemia.

Optic neuropathy

Diseases of the optic nerve invariably cause profound visual loss. Symptoms range from blurred central vision and difficulty differentiating colours to complete blindness. The cardinal ophthalmological signs of optic nerve disease are reduced visual acuity, impaired or absent colour vision, a central or altitudinal visual field defect and a relative afferent pupillary defect (RAPD). The optic disc may look swollen, pale, or even normal depending on where the inflammation has occurred along the optic nerve.

The pattern of visual loss can vary from sudden and complete to slow and progressive. This depends on whether the optic nerve has undergone infarction, such as in giant cell arteritis, or slow compression from a granuloma. All patients who develop disease of the optic nerve require urgent investigation.

Specific ocular manifestations of systemic inflammatory diseases

The ocular manifestations of systemic inflammatory disease varies according to the size and type of vessel predominantly affected by the disease process. As a general rule, diseases that affect arterioles involve the cornea, episclera, sclera, and retinal arterioles, whereas those affecting the venules produce uveitis, macular oedema, and retinal venous disease.

Giant cell arteritis

Giant cell arteritis is an ophthalmic emergency and an important cause of preventable blindness in elderly people. Twenty-five per cent of patients develop ocular disease and the majority experience sudden loss of vision in one eye, with a dense, central field defect.[15] The cause of blindness is usually infarction of the optic nerve, causing an ischaemic optic neuropathy and/or occlusion of the central retinal artery (Figure 24.4). About 12% of patients may also present with a cranial nerve palsy, giving rise to diplopia. Treatment is with immediate, high-dose systemic steroids (e.g. intravenous methylprednisolone 1–2 mg/kg daily or oral prednisolone 60–80 mg daily) to produce symptomatic relief of the headache and, most importantly, to prevent blindness in the other eye. Recovery of vision in the affected eye is rare.

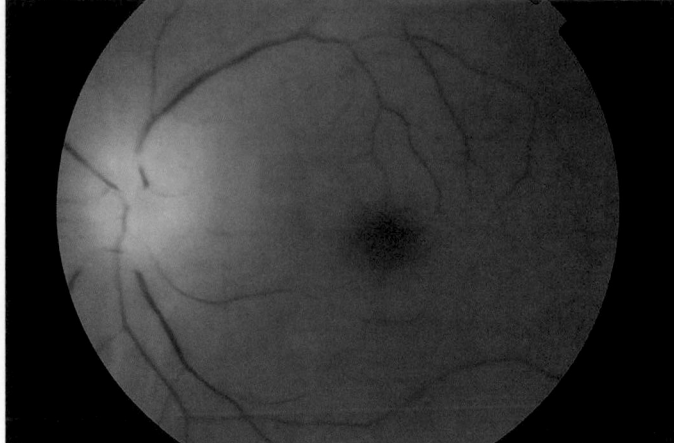

Fig. 24.4 Giant cell arteritis. An 80 year old man with scalp tenderness, weight loss, and jaw claudication presents to casualty with recent loss of vision in his left eye. The optic disc is swollen and pale, indicating an anterior ischaemic optic neuropathy (AION). There is also a secondary central retinal artery occlusion.

Unusual neuro-ophthalmological complications of giant, cell arteritis include Horner's syndrome, cortical blindness (due to embolization from affected vertebral arteries), internuclear ophthalmoplegia, and visual hallucinations.[16]

Systemic lupus erythematosus

Eye symptoms are common in patients with SLE and range from minor external problems to severe retinopathy.[17] Five per cent of patients will develop scleritis at some time during the course of their disease, and this is occasionally seen at presentation. Scleritis indicates active systemic disease and may require adjustment of systemic therapy. Uveitis is very rare in SLE and only occurs in association with severe scleritis.[18]

The most important ophthalmic manifestation is retinopathy consisting of cotton-wool spots, retinal haemorrhages, and central or branch retinal artery occlusions.[19] Retinal vascular occlusion in SLE is due to deposition of immune complexes within the vessels, rather than vasculitis; however, vasculitis can occur in the choroid, leading to choroidal infarcts (Figure 24.5).[20] The presence of anti-cardiolipin antibodies may be a marker for the development of retinal vascular occlusion (Figure 24.6).[21]

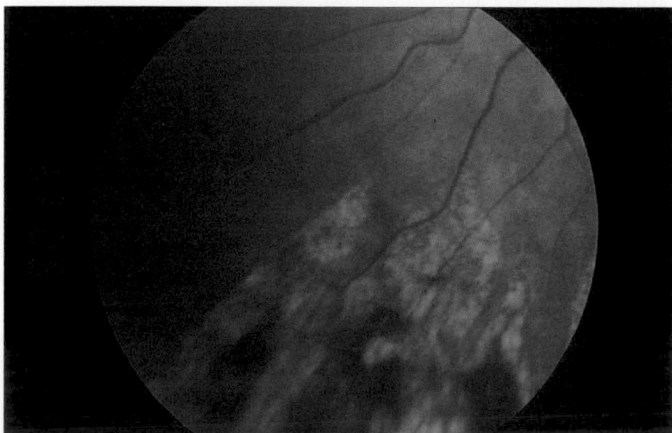

Fig. 24.5 Choroidal infarcts in systemic lupus erythematosus.

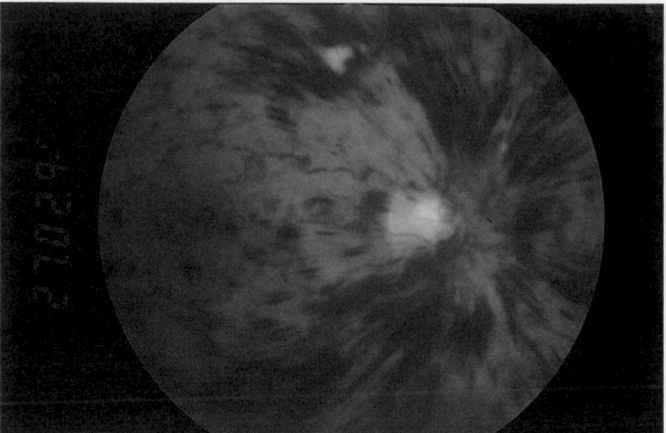

Fig. 24.6 Central retinal vein occlusion in a woman who suffers from systemic lupus erythematosus.

Polyarteritis nodosa

Ocular involvement is present in 10–20% of patients with polyarteritis nodosa.[22] The most common manifestation is choroidal and retinal vasculitis, which is secondary to accelerated hypertension. It can be characterized by arteriovenous nipping, cotton-wool spots, and flame shaped haemorrhages.

Patients can also develop conjunctival infarction, keratoconjunctivitis sicca, episcleritis, scleritis, and necrotizing scleritis associated with peripheral ulcerative keratitis. Choroidal infarcts and exudative serous retinal detachments can occur due to involvement of the posterior ciliary arteries and choroidal vessels.

The development of scleritis or retinal vascular disease in the absence of hypertension warrants investigation of the systemic disease.

Wegener's granulomatosis

Eye problems develop in 29–52% of patients with Wegener's granulomatosis, with 8% of patients suffering disease-related vision loss.[23,24] It is the only systemic inflammatory disease that commonly presents with orbital disease due to infiltration of the orbit with granulomatous tissue. Patients may complain of proptosis, caused by the orbital mass; red eyes caused by scleritis; or blurred vision from compression of the optic nerve by the granulomatous tissue (Figure 24.7). They may also develop swollen optic discs and choroidal folds. Many patients also suffer from epiphora (watering eyes) due to destruction of the nasolacrimal duct in sinus disease. Of these conditions, scleritis usually occurs first, with nasolacrimal and orbital disease occurring after years of disease activity. A similar disease pattern can be seen in eosinophilic granulomatosis with polyangiitis (Churg–Strauss) and IgG4 disease.

Systemic sclerosis

The most common eye complaint in systemic sclerosis is dry eye, a loss of eyelid elasticity, and eyelid telangiectasia, which can occur in approximately 50% of patients.[25] Lid changes are thought to be due to sclerosis of the eyelid connective tissue, resulting in a 'woody' feeling and leading to difficulty everting the upper eyelids during examination. These changes tend to occur most commonly in patients who have more extensive skin involvement (i.e. diffuse cutaneous systemic sclerosis).

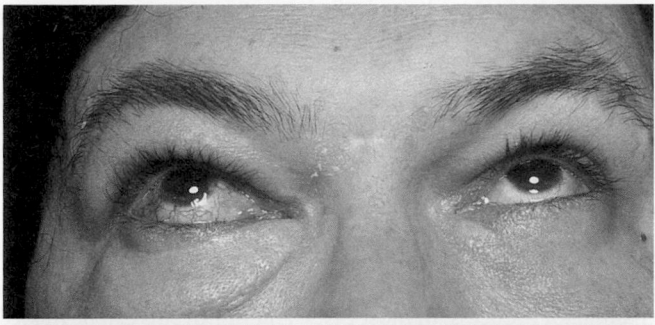

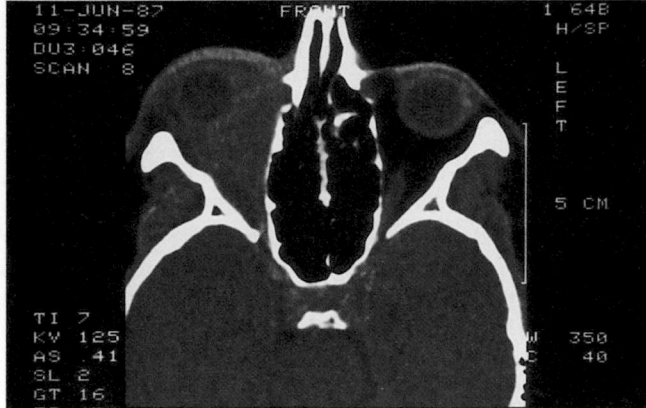

Fig 24.7 Orbital disease in Wegener's Granulomatosis.

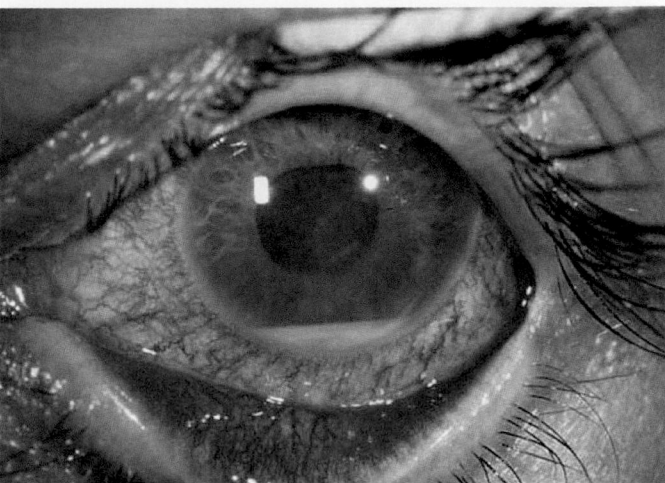

Fig. 24.8 Hypopyon in Behçet's disease. A 20 year old man with known Behçet's disease presented with a red eye, decreased visual acuity, and a visible hypopyon associated with a fibrinous uveitis.

A minority of patients develop retinopathy similar to that seen in the other systemic vasculitides, with cotton-wool spots, haemorrhages and occlusion of retinal arteries.

Recent studies have suggested that patients with systemic sclerosis have an increased incidence of normal-tension glaucoma (NTG).[26] There is also evidence that the disease can lead to increased central corneal thickness, an important factor in the interpretation of intraocular pressure.[27]

Rheumatoid arthritis

A third of patients with RA suffer from dry eyes and in 10% this is combined with a dry mouth (Sjögren's syndrome). Five per cent of patients presenting with episcleritis and 30% presenting with isolated scleritis have RA. Bilateral scleritis, while still rare, is more common when associated with RA.[28]

Scleromalacia perforans (see Figure 24.2) affects elderly women predominantly. Advancing scleral disease in these patients almost always heralds a flare-up of their systemic disease (particularly the vasculitic complications).

Ankylosing spondylitis and the seronegative arthropathies

AAU is the most important ocular disease in this group of patients. It occurs in 33% of patients with ankylosing spondylitis and in 10–15% of patients with other associated seronegative arthropathies.[29] The clinical symptoms and signs are similar, regardless of the accompanying disease. Attacks are usually unilateral but both eyes can become affected during the course of the disease. Severe cases can develop a fibrinous uveitis with posterior synechiae (adhesions between the iris and the lens capsule) and raised intraocular pressure.[30]

Posterior segment disease is less common in this group of diseases. Ten per cent of these patients develop vitritis and a retinal vasculitis affecting predominantly the capillaries and postcapillary venules.

Behçet's disease

Ocular manifestations in Behçet's disease occur in up to 60% of patients.[31] Severe anterior uveitis, often in a painless eye, is common and a hypopyon may form (Figure 24.8). The anterior uveitis is typically recurrent but can resolve spontaneously.

Internationally, approximately a quarter of patients with Behçet's disease go blind as a result of their uveitis.[32,33] The pathognomonic features are sequential occlusions of branch retinal veins and retinal infiltrates. The nature of the venous occlusions results in progressive ischaemia and eventually the entire retinal vasculature is obliterated and results in optic disc atrophy.

Ocular involvement in rheumatic conditions of childhood

Uveitis occurring before the age of 16 years is approximately three times less common than uveitis in the general population.[34] In two reviews of uveitis in childhood, systemic illnesses such as sarcoidosis, Behçet's disease, and vasculitis accounted for less than 8% of patients.[35]

The most common associated disorder is seronegative JIA.

Juvenile idiopathic arthritis

The chronic anterior uveitis that occurs in association with JIA deserves special mention, particularly as it does not occur in adults. Affected children are mostly girls, and are usually young at onset of arthritis (mean age 3 years). Joint involvement is usually pauciarticular, although it may spread to become polyarticular.[36] Most patients have associated anti-nuclear antibodies (ANA) in their serum. Arthritis generally predates the eye involvement by 1–3 years or sometimes much longer, but 5–10% of cases present with uveitis and the ophthalmologist should therefore ask for a rheumatological opinion in any young child with chronic anterior uveitis. Similarly, because the eye disease is usually asymptomatic until complications occur, the rheumatologist must arrange for an early slit lamp examination on all children. Regular follow up will be arranged by the ophthalmologist depending on the age of the child, their ANA status, and their age (Box 24.1).

The non-granulomatous iridocyclitis runs an uncomplicated course in one-third of affected children. The majority of untreated cases develop numerous complications such as band keratopathy, posterior synechiae, cataracts, or glaucoma. Early onset of uveitis, either symptomatic or when picked up in routine screening within the first year of arthritis, and particularly if associated with posterior synechiae at this first examination, are associated with a significantly worse prognosis for vision. Most eye involvement develops for the first time 4–5 years after of the onset of arthritis, and after this the risk is much lower. This is unlike the acute symptomatic anterior uveitis in ankylosing spondylitis, which may occur for the first time very many years later than the original musculoskeletal symptoms.

Treatment of ocular manifestations of systemic disease

Mild anterior segment inflammation such as dry eye, conjunctivitis, and episcleritis will invariably respond to local treatment. This can often be with simple ocular lubricants, but occasionally a mild topical steroid may be indicated.

Scleritis

Scleritis is an indication for systemic treatment. Adequate doses of non-steroidal anti-inflammatory drugs (NSAIDs) can often control pain and help reduce ocular inflammation (e.g. flurbiprofen 50 mg three times a day). If NSAIDs do not help to control symptoms,

systemic steroids are indicated. Occasionally, steroid-sparing agents are necessary (e.g. cyclophosphamide, azathioprine, ciclosporin, or mycophenolate mofetil).

Biological agents have been used successfully in the management of scleritis. Rituximab, an anti-CD20 B-cell monoclonal antibody, has been shown to be of use in scleritis refractory to multiple other agents.

Uveitis

The treatment for uveitis depends primarily on the site of the inflammatory process. In most cases, anterior uveitis can be treated topically with steroid eye drops to reduce the inflammation and a dilating agent such as cyclopentolate 1% to prevent posterior synechiae.

If the vision drops due to occlusion of the retinal vasculature, or involvement of the optic nerve, systemic immunosuppressants are indicated. Corticosteroids are usually sufficient in the first instance, but they may also be used in conjunction with ciclosporin, azathioprine, mycophenolate mofetil, or methotrexate.

Recently trials of biologic agents such the tumour necrosis factor alpha (TNF-α) inhibitor infliximab[37–39] and interferon alpha[40–42] have been used with good results, particularly in Behçet's disease and JIA.

Other biologic agents have been used to treat the ocular complications of various rheumatological diseases. Etanercept[43] and adalimumab[44] have been used successfully to treat JIA and Behçet's disease uveitis as well as macular oedema associated with uveitis. Rituximab has had good responses in JIA patients who have failed to respond to corticosteroids, methotrexate, etanercept, or infliximab.[45]

Daclizumab is a monoclonal antibody that targets interleukin 2 (IL-2), it has had promising results in patients with JIA, non-infective intermediate, posterior, and panuveitis.[46]

Small trials have used intravenous immunoglobulin (IVIG) to treat uveitis. The use of this has been limited due to the severe side effects (thromboembolism, aseptic uveitis) and high cost.[47]

Antirheumatic therapy with ocular side effects

Hydroxychloroquine is a commonly used drug in the treatment of RA and SLE. It has a high affinity for melanin-containing tissue in the eye, such as the retinal pigment epithelium. The pathophysiology of retinal damage is related to a malfunction of phagolysosomes, resulting in faulty clearance of ageing photoreceptor membranes.[48,49] Hydroxychloroquine has a better ocular side-effect profile than chloroquine, possibly because it does not cross the blood–retina barrier as easily.

Corneal deposits occasionally occur in patients taking quinolones, as the drug is deposited within the epithelium. The deposits, which can appear as punctate changes or whorl-like patterns, usually resolve on discontinuation of the drug.

The features of hydroxychloroquine retinopathy begin with a fine stippling of the macula and loss of the foveal light reflex. This can then produce a 'bull's eye' maculopathy made up of pigmented and depigmented rings centred on the fovea, resulting in loss of visual acuity and visual field loss. Even if treatment is stopped, atrophy of the retinal pigment epithelium can continue for a time before stabilizing.

Box 24.1 Current UK screening guidelines for anterior uveitis in juvenile idiopathic arthritis

The first screening visit should be carried out within 6 weeks of referral. This should be followed by a review every 2 months **from onset of arthritis** for 6 months, then 3–4 monthly screening for time outlined below:

Age at onset	Screening period
Oligoarticular involvement irrespective of ANA status and onset <11 years of age	
<3 years	8 years
3–4 years	6 years
5–8 years	3 years
9–10 years	1 year
Polyarticular involvement, ANA positive, onset <10 years of age	
<6 years	5 years
6–9 years	2 years
Polyarticular involvement, ANA negative, onset <7 years of age	
All children need 5 years screening	

Royal College of Ophthalmologists. *Guidelines for screening for uveitis in juvenile idiopathic arthritis*, 2009.

The most recent (2009) guidelines from the Royal College of Ophthalmologists[50] recommend that regular screening for hydroxychloroquine toxicity is **not** carried out. This is a significant change from the previous guidelines and is based on the following:

- The incidence of clinically significant hydroxychloroquine retinopathy is very low—in a large prospective study of patients taking the maximum dose of hydroxychloroquine (6.5 mg/kg) only 2 of the 400 patients developed irreversible toxicity and both of the patients affected had been taking the drug for over 6 years.

- There is no reliable method for detecting retinal toxicity at a reversible stage—visual fields, Amsler charts, distance and near visual acuity, autofluorescence, and multifocal electroretinography are all used to detect macular changes, but none provides a definite endpoint at which the toxicity level becomes irreversible.

Recommendations for rheumatologists are given in Box 24.2.

Corticosteroids

Both oral and topical corticosteroids may cause a variety of ophthalmic side effects[51]:

- Cataracts commonly develop after high doses of systemic steroids, but these can usually be easily dealt with surgically when the patients become symptomatic.

- Raised intraocular pressure. Five per cent of the population are termed 'steroid responders' because of a significant, but asymptomatic increase in pressure. The frequency, duration, and strength of oral or topical steroid all influence this effect. Where possible, steroid-sparing agents should ideally be used in these patients.

- Patients on steroids are more prone to infections and their use can also worsen underlying ocular infections such as herpes simplex. A full slit lamp examination should be carried out on all patients with a red eye before starting topical steroids to rule out an infectious cause.

Immunosuppressives

Patients on long-term immunosuppressives are at risk of developing opportunistic infections such as cytomegalovirus retinitis or

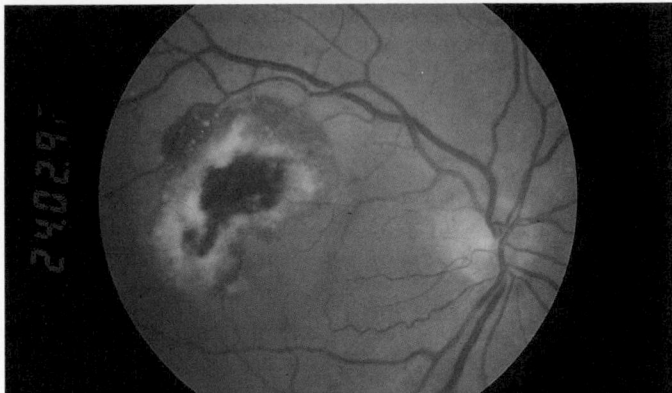

Fig. 24.10 Cytomegalovirus retinitis.

acute retinal necrosis (herpes simplex and zoster) (Figure 24.10). Any patient presenting with a new onset of floaters, red eye, visual field defect, or decreased visual acuity should have a dilated slit lamp examination.

References

1. Whitcher JP, Shiboski CH, Shiboski SC et al. A simplified quantitative method for assessing keratoconjunctivitis sicca from the Sjogren's Syndrome International Registry. *Am J Ophthalmol* 2010;149(3):405–415.
2. Gilboe IM, Kvien TK, Uhlig T, Husby G. Sicca symptoms and secondary Sjogren's syndrome in systemic lupus erythematosus: comparison with rheumatoid arthritis and correlation with disease variables. *Ann Rheum Dis* 2001;60(12):1103–1109.
3. Lemp MA. Dry eye (keratoconjunctivitis sicca), rheumatoid arthritis, and Sjogren's syndrome. *Am J Ophthalmol* 2005;140(5):898–899.
4. Avouac J, Sordet C, Depinay C et al. Systemic sclerosis-associated Sjogren's syndrome and relationship to the limited cutaneous subtype: results of a prospective study of sicca syndrome in 133 consecutive patients. *Arthritis Rheum* 2006;54(7):2243–2249.
5. Mavrikakis I, Rootman J. Diverse clinical presentations of orbital sarcoid. *Am J Ophthalmol* 2007;144(5):769–775.
6. Prabhakaran VC, Babu K, Mahadevan A, Murthy SR. Amyloidosis of lacrimal gland. *Indian J Ophthalmol* 2009;57(6):461–463.
7. Singh J, Sallam A, Lightman S, Taylor S. Episcleritis and scleritis in rheumatic disease. *Curr Rheumatol Rev* 2011;7(1):15–23.
8. Smith JR, Mackensen F, Rosenbaum JT. Therapy insight: scleritis and its relationship to systemic autoimmune disease. *Nat Clin Pract Rheum* 2007;3(4):219–226.
9. Okhravi N, Odufuwa B, McCluskey P, Lightman S. Scleritis. *Surv Ophthalmol* 2005;50(4):351–363.
10. Taylor SR, McCluskey P, Lightman S. The ocular manifestations of inflammatory bowel disease. *Curr Opin Ophthalmol* 2006;17(6):538–544.
11. Watts RA, Scott DGI. Relapsing polychondritis. In: Watts RA, Scott DGI (eds) *Vasculitis in clinical practice*. Springer, London, 2010:173–179.
12. Stanford MR, Graham EM. Systemic associations of retinal vasculitis. *Int Ophthalmol Clin* 1991;31(3):23–33.
13. Linssen A, Rothova A, Valkenburg HA et al. The lifetime cumulative incidence of acute anterior uveitis in a normal population and its relation to ankylosing spondylitis and histocompatibility antigen HLA-B27. *Invest Ophthalmol Vis Sci* 1991;32:2568–2578.
14. Chen C-H, Lin K-C, Chen H-A et al. Association of acute anterior uveitis with disease activity, functional ability and physical mobility in patients with ankylosing spondylitis: a cross-sectional study of Chinese patients in Taiwan. *Clin Rheumatol* 2007;26(6):953–957.
15. Hayreh SS, Zimmerman B. Management of giant cell arteritis. Our 27-year clinical study: new light on old controversies. *Ophthalmologica* 2003;217(4):239–259.

Box 24.2 Hydroxychloroquine: recommendations for rheumatologists

- Do not exceed the maximum dose of 6.5 mg/kg (200–400 mg/day) of hydroxychloroquine.

- Establish renal and liver function before starting treatment.

- Enquire about any visual impairment not correctable with glasses before starting treatment and at yearly review.

- Before starting treatment, test the patient's reading vision with their reading glasses, (using a near vision chart or newspaper).

- If visual impairment is suspected the patient should be advised to consult an optometrist in the first instance. Any abnormality would then be referred to an ophthalmologist in the usual way.

16. Watts RA, Scott DGI. Giant cell arteritis. In: Watts RA, Scott DGI (eds) *Vasculitis in clinical practice*. Springer, London, 2010:35–45.

17. Peponis V, Kyttaris VC, Tyradellis C, Vergados I, Sitaras NM. Ocular manifestations of systemic lupus erythematosus: a clinical review. *Lupus* 2006;15(1):3–12.

18. Davies JB, Rao PK. Ocular manifestations of systemic lupus erythematosus. *Curr Opin Ophthalmol* 2008;19(6):512–518.

19. Au A, O'Day J. Review of severe vaso-occlusive retinopathy in systemic lupus erythematosus and the antiphospholipid syndrome: associations, visual outcomes, complications and treatment. *Clin Experiment Ophthalmol*. 2004;32(1):87–100.

20. Carbone J, Sanchez-Ramon S, Cobo-Soriano R, et al. Antiphospholipid antibodies: a risk factor for occlusive retinal vascular disorders. Comparison with ocular inflammatory diseases. *J Rheumatol* 2001;28(11):2437–2441.

21. Cobo-Soriano R, Sanchez-Ramon S, Aparicio MJ, et al. Antiphospholipid antibodies and retinal thrombosis in patients without risk factors: a prospective case-control study. *Am J Ophthalmol* 1999;128(6):725–732.

22. Perez VL, Chavala SH, Ahmed M, et al. Ocular manifestations and concepts of systemic vasculitides. *Surv Ophthalmol* 2004;49(4):399–418.

23. Hoffman GS, Kerr GS, Leavitt RY. Wegener's granulomatosis: an analysis of 158 patients. *Ann Intern Med* 1992;116:488–498.

24. Bullen CL, Liesegang TJ, McDonald TJ. Ocular complications of Wegener's granulomatosis. *Ophthalmology* 1983;90:279–290.

25. Gomes Bde A, Santhiago MR, Magalhaes P et al. Ocular findings in patients with systemic sclerosis. *Clinics (Sao Paulo)*. 2011;66(3):379–385.

26. Kitsos G, Tsifetaki N, Gorezis S, Drosos AA. Glaucomatous type abnormalities in patients with systemic sclerosis. *Clin Exp Rheumatol* 2007;25(2):341.

27. Serup L, Serup J, Hagdrup HK. Increased central cornea thickness in systemic sclerosis. *Acta Ophthalmol* (Copenh) 1984;62(1):69–74.

28. Stone JH, Matteson EL. Rheumatoid vasculitis. In: Stone JH (ed.) *A clinician's pearls and myths in rheumatology*. Springer, London, 2010:15–22.

29. Gran JT, Skomsvoll JF. The outcome of ankylosing spondylitis: a study of 100 patients. *Rheumatology* 1997;36(7):766–771.

30. Chudomirova K, Abadjieva T, Yankova R. Clinical tetrad of arthritis, urethritis, conjunctivitis, and mucocutaneous lesions (HLA-B27-associated spondyloarthropathy, Reiter syndrome): report of a case. *Dermatol Online J* 2008;14(12):4.

31. Sungur G, Hazirolan D, Hekimoglu E, Kasim R, Duman S. Late-onset Behçet's disease: demographic, clinical, and ocular features. *Graefes Arch Clin Exp Ophthalmol* 2010;248(9):1325–1330.

32. Kitaichi N, Miyazaki A, Iwata D et al. Ocular features of Behçet's disease: an international collaborative study. *Br J Ophthalmol* 2007;91(12):1579–1582.

33. Mendes D, Correia M, Barbedo M et al. Behçet's disease—a contemporary review. *J Autoimmun* 2009;32(3–4):178–188.

34. Kump LI, Cervantes-Castañeda RA, Androudi SN, Foster CS. Analysis of pediatric uveitis cases at a tertiary referral center. *Ophthalmology* 2005;112(7):1287–1292.

35. Cunningham Jr ET, Suhler EB. Childhood uveitis—young patients, old problems, new perspectives. *J AAPOS* 2008;12(6):537–538.

36. Julian K, Terrada C, Quartier P, LeHoang P, Bodaghi B. Uveitis related to juvenile idiopathic arthritis: familial cases and possible genetic implication in the pathogenesis. *Ocul Immunol Inflamm* 2010;18(3):172–177.

37. Tynjala P, Lindahl P, Honkanen V, Lahdenne P, Kotaniemi K. Infliximab and etanercept in the treatment of chronic uveitis associated with refractory juvenile idiopathic arthritis. *Ann Rheum Dis* 2007;66(4):548–550.

38. Suhler EB, Smith JR, Giles TR et al. Infliximab therapy for refractory uveitis: 2-year results of a prospective trial. *Arch Ophthalmol* 2009;127(6):819–822.

39. Sugita S, Yamada Y, Mochizuki M. Relationship between serum infliximab levels and acute uveitis attacks in patients with Behcet disease. *Br J Ophthalmol* 2011;95(4):549–552.

40. Plskova J, Greiner K, Forrester JV. Interferon-alpha as an effective treatment for noninfectious posterior uveitis and panuveitis. *Am J Ophthalmol* 2007;144(1):55–61.

41. Onal S, Kazokoglu H, Koc A et al. Low dose and dose escalating therapy of interferon alfa-2a in the treatment of refractory and sight-threatening Behçet's uveitis. *Clin Exp Rheumatol* 2009;27(2 Suppl 53):S113–S114.

42. Onal S, Kazokoglu H, Koc A, et al.. Long-term efficacy and safety of low-dose and dose-escalating interferon alfa-2a therapy in refractory Behcet uveitis. *Arch Ophthalmol* 2011;129(3):288–294.

43. Wang F, Wang NS. Etanercept therapy-associated acute uveitis: a case report and literature review. *Clin Exp Rheumatol* 2009;27(5):838–839.

44. Tynjala P, Kotaniemi K, Lindahl P, et al. Adalimumab in juvenile idiopathic arthritis-associated chronic anterior uveitis. *Rheumatology* 2008;47(3):339–344.

45. Miserocchi E, Pontikaki I, Modorati G et al. Rituximab for uveitis. *Ophthalmology* 2011;118(1):223–224.

46. Sen HN, Levy-Clarke G, Faia LJ et al. High-dose daclizumab for the treatment of juvenile idiopathic arthritis-associated active anterior uveitis. *Am J Ophthalmol* 2009;148(5):696–703e1.

47. Rosenbaum JT, George RK, Gordon C. The treatment of refractory uveitis with intravenous immunoglobulin. *Am J Ophthalmol* 1999;127(5):545–549.

48. Payne JF, Hubbard GB, 3rd, Aaberg TM, Sr, Yan J. Clinical characteristics of hydroxychloroquine retinopathy. *Br J Ophthalmol*. 2011;95(2):245–250.

49. Semmer AE, Lee MS, Harrison AR, Olsen TW. Hydroxychloroquine retinopathy screening. *Br J Ophthalmol*. 2008;92(12):1653–1655.

50. Royal College of Ophthalmologists. *Hydroxychloroquine and ocular toxicity: recommendations on screening*. Royal College of Ophthalmologists, London, 2009. Available from: www.rcophth.ac.uk

50. Carnahan MC, Goldstein DA.. Ocular complications of topical, peri-ocular, and systemic corticosteroids. *Curr Opin Ophthalmol* 2000;11(6):478–483.

CHAPTER 25

The kidney

Mark Little and Alan Salama

Introduction

Kidney involvement in the setting of rheumatology practice is frequently associated with increased mortality and considerable morbidity.[1] It may arise as part of the underlying rheumatic disease or may be a complication of its treatment. As with many other causes of kidney disease, early diagnosis allows timely intervention which is associated with an increased chance of recovery and prevention of chronic renal dysfunction. It is therefore of considerable importance that rheumatologists have a clear understanding of the causes and signs of renal disease. Relying solely on serum creatinine as a measure of renal dysfunction will result in a late appreciation of established kidney disease, and represents a missed opportunity for early detection of renal abnormalities.

The kidney is a complex organ that can be affected by abnormalities predominantly affecting its vasculature (such as in scleroderma), its filtration compartment (in glomerulonephritis secondary to systemic conditions such as systemic lupus erythematosus, SLE) or its concentrating and reabsorptive compartment (in tubulointerstitial nephritis secondary to non-steroidal anti-inflammatory drugs, NSAIDs). Although all three compartments may be affected simultaneously, particular disease patterns may arise due to individual compartments being predominantly affected. This can often be deduced from basic investigations, which may provide strong clues as to the likely aetiology of the renal dysfunction. Moreover, some changes may precede the elevation in serum creatinine, or decline in glomerular filtration rate (GFR), making them important early markers of kidney involvement.

Assessment of renal function

The serum creatinine is a reliable marker of changes in GFR if its limitations are understood. The urea level is a less reliable marker of changes in renal function, primarily because it may be elevated in several conditions where renal function is stable, such as gastrointestinal bleeding and steroid administration. As a result, rises in urea are best interpreted in relation to changes in the serum creatinine.

Approximately 20% of urinary creatinine excretion under physiological conditions is due to tubular secretion. Therefore, as glomerular filtration declines and tubular secretion of creatinine contributes a greater fraction of creatinine excretion, increases in the serum creatinine and a fall in the creatinine clearance tend to underestimate the true decrease in GFR that has occurred.[2]

Some medications, such as trimethoprim, competitively inhibit tubular creatinine secretion, leading to an increase in serum creatinine in the absence of any changes in GFR.

It is important to note that one can only infer GFR from a relatively stable creatinine level as the creatinine rise in acute kidney injury (AKI), which is dependent on the ongoing production of creatinine by muscle, lags behind the abrupt decline in GFR. For example, it is quite possible to have a GFR of 1 mL/min with a creatinine level of, say, 140 μmol/L if the GFR reduction occurred within the previous 24 hours. In this setting of zero or near-zero excretory kidney function the creatinine level will usually rise by about 80–100 μmol/L per day.

Finally, because the serum creatinine is roughly inversely proportional to creatinine clearance or GFR at relatively normal levels of renal function, changes in the serum creatinine tend to be a relatively insensitive biomarker of falling GFR. For example, an increase in the serum creatinine from 80 μmol/L to 160 μmol/L would represent a 50% decline in GFR. Once such a change has occurred, substantial renal function has been lost, despite what appears to be only a modest increase in the serum creatinine. An increase in the serum creatinine from 80 μmol/L to 90 μmol/L, if real, represents a 9% decline in GFR, also potentially significant. However, the standard laboratory assay for serum creatinine has a variation of about 10%, meaning that any change of 10 μmol/L in the serum creatinine level could (correctly or incorrectly) be attributed to laboratory variation. Therefore, it is important that even seemingly small changes in the serum creatinine should not be discounted and that particular attention should be made to temporal changes. If a major doubt persists, GFR should be measured by radionuclide methods. Novel biomarkers, such as neutrophil gelatinase-associated lipocalin (NGAL) and kidney injury molecule-1 (KIM-1),[3–5] show promise as sensitive early markers of renal injury but are not yet in general clinical practice. To overcome the problems of using serum creatinine alone to estimate renal GFR, physicians have used estimated GFRs based on equations which take into account the variables of production by including age, sex, and ethnicity in their derivations (see www.renal.org/eGFRcalc/GFR.pl and [6]). Some form of estimated GFR is now frequently provided by biochemistry laboratories and reported with the patients' serum creatinine. However, these equations are not intended for use when the renal function is normal or changing rapidly (as in AKI), or in patients with non-standard body morphology who may have greater or lesser muscle mass than average for their age.

Other important biomarkers of kidney disease are to be found in the urine, in particular in the form of proteinuria and haematuria. Proteinuria is a marker of renal inflammation and of irreversible injury. It may develop much earlier in the course of renal dysfunction than elevation in serum creatinine or decline in estimated GFR and in those patients with persistent protein leaks, is generally regarded as one of the most important predictors of future decline in renal function. Identification of proteinuria is generally by means of a dipstick test, but its quantification is also important in helping predict the source of leak and potential underlying disease process as well as monitoring response to treatment.

Proteinuria

Following validation of the technique, protein estimations on spot urine corrected for urine creatinine have become more commonplace and in many centres have replaced the 24 hour collections. When both protein and creatinine are quantified in mg/dL the urine protein:creatinine ratio is equivalent to the daily rate of protein excretion in grams.[7] These spot assessments are more convenient for patients, are processed more rapidly, and are reported in the form of a spot protein:creatinine ratio.

It is important to consider the nature of the protein excreted as this varies depending on the renal compartment affected. In health, urine has a low protein content, up to 80 mg/day, consisting of roughly half glomerular (filtered plasma) proteins and half tubular proteins. Glomerular protein loss (seen in active or chronic glomerulonephritis) consists mostly of albumin which is actively excluded in the urine by the glomerular filtration barrier, while tubular protein loss (seen in tubulointerstitial disease) is due to the failure of tubular resorption of filtered or secreted proteins, and consists of low molecular weight proteins such as retinol binding protein and β_2-microglobulin (Table 25.1). Under certain circumstances it is therefore important to measure both the albumin:creatinine and protein:creatinine ratio (which will pick up both albumin and low molecular weight proteins).

Haematuria

Haematuria is defined by the abnormal finding of red blood cells in the urine. It may be of renal origin or arise from lower down in the urinary tract (Table 25.2); it may be detected only on dipstick or microscopy (microhaematuria) or be visible to the naked eye (macrohaematuria). False-positive haematuria may arise when certain drugs, dyes, or pigments discolour the urine, giving the impression of blood, or when myoglobin or haemoglobin is present due to processes such as rhabdomyolysis or intravascular haemolysis, respectively. It is therefore important to confirm all dipstick positive haematuria with urine microscopy. In health, only a few red cells

Table 25.1 Glomerular and tubular proteinuria

Glomerular proteinuria	Tubular proteinuria
Albumin	Low molecular weight proteins
Microalbuminuria (>2.5–3.5<30 mg/mmol)	Usually about 1 g/day or PCR 100 mg/mmol
Macroalbuminuria (>30 mg/mmol)	
Nephrotic range (>3 g/day or PCR >300 mg/mmol): nephrotic syndrome	

PCR, protein/creatinine ratio.

Table 25.2 Causes of haematuria

Intrinsic renal bleeding	Lower tract bleeding
Glomerulonephritis	Infection
Thrombotic microangiopathy	Prostatic hypertrophy/ malignancy
Tubulointerstitial nephritis	
Pyelonephritis	Ureteric/bladder malignancy
Structural abnormalities, e.g. thin glomerular basement membrane lesion, Alport's syndrome, Fabry's disease	Haemorrhagic cystitis
	Renal/bladder stones
Renal tumour	Anticoagulant therapy
Renal vein/arterial thrombosis	Trauma
Papillary necrosis	Vascular malformations
Polycystic kidneys	Factitious
Trauma	

(up to 3 per high power field) are found in the urine, the majority being excluded by the glomerular basement membrane. Under pathological conditions those red cells that traverse the glomerulus may become deformed and dysmorphic, while any bleeding from the lower urinary tract leaves the cells intact. Therefore urine microscopy can, in experienced hands, provide clues as to the origin of the haematuria, by careful examination for dysmorphic red cells. Haematuria always needs investigation and whether this starts with renal or lower tract investigation will depend on the age of the patient and the clinical setting. Urine cytology may provide important clues as to the nature of the red cells and other diagnostic cells in the sample. Examination of the lower urinary tract with cystoscopy, and imaging with ultrasound or CT, are important tools in investigating haematuria.

Urine dipstick testing

The urine dipstick is one of the most useful tools available to detect renal disease. Not only does it detect proteinuria and haematuria, it also allows detection of leucocyturia (suggesting inflammation or infection), and can provide important information regarding tubular dysfunction causing changes in concentrating ability, glucose leak, and acidification abnormalities. These are often overlooked but represent an early and sensitive marker of renal dysfunction. The main protein detected by urine dipsticks is albumin and it is important to remember that dipsticks are insensitive to globulins, including Bence Jones protein, making them an inadequate tool for assessing renal involvement in plasma cell dyscrasias.

Tubular damage occurs consequent to interstitial inflammation leading to a number of functional tubular defects, the pattern of which is dependent on the predominant region of the tubule affected (Table 25.2). Urine dipstick testing may also reveal glycosuria which, if the blood glucose level is normal, suggests a renal glucose leak; a low urine specific gravity (indicating a potential concentrating defect); and an alkaline pH (suggesting a defect in urine acidification).

Renal failure: acute

Definitions

Acute renal failure is defined as a sudden decline in renal function, usually measured by an increase in serum creatinine and blood urea, or a decrease in GFR. For most of the first part of the 21st century, an acute decline in kidney function was defined according to the Acute Dialysis Quality Initiative (ADQI) 'RIFLE' criteria. These definitions had many limitations, leading to the introduction of the Acute Kidney Injury Network (AKIN) criteria:

◆ an abrupt (within 48 hours) absolute increase in the serum creatinine concentration of ≥0.3 mg/dL (26.4 μmol/L) from baseline, or

◆ a percentage increase in the serum creatinine concentration of ≥50%, or

◆ oliguria of <0.5 mL/kg per hour for more than 6 hours.[8]

The term 'acute kidney injury (AKI)' is now used in place of 'acute renal failure'. It remains controversial as to whether prerenal and postrenal acute declines in GFR should be included in the AKI definition; for the purposes of this discussion, we shall assume that they are included and that AKI refers to any abrupt rise in creatinine level.

Diagnostic approach to the patient with acute kidney injury

The commonest cause of an acute rise in serum creatinine level is a prerenal insult, and the initial assessment should focus on assessment and correction of the extracellular fluid volume status (assessed clinically: dependent oedema, status of neck vein filling, and postural blood pressure), use of NSAIDs, angiotensin-converting enzyme (ACE) inhibitors and angiotensin receptor blockers (ARBs), or other factors that could reduce effective renal perfusion.

Once prerenal issues have been addressed, the key questions that one should consider when faced with persisting AKI are:

1. Is this truly acute, or is there an element of chronic (presumed irreversible) kidney disease (CKD) at play?

2. Are the kidneys obstructed (hydronephrotic)?

3. Is there a severe immunologically mediated intrinsic renal disease present?

An estimate of the disease duration and tempo (acute, subacute, or chronic) can be derived from the history, an early telephone call to the patient's family doctor for information on historic creatinine values, and urgent imaging of the kidneys. A recent clinical syndrome of defined onset, such as general malaise, joint pains, rash, or change in urine colour, suggests that there is at least an acute element to the decline in GFR, although it does not exclude the possibility that this is occurring on a background of CKD. This is an important issue as it determines what will be achievable in terms of renal function recovery. Therefore, the most important piece of data to obtain in a patient with an elevated serum creatinine level is a recent creatinine value in the normal range; all efforts should thus be made to identify a clinical scenario within the previous 6 months where a creatinine level may have been measured.

The key investigation that will help one decide whether the kidneys are acutely injured (and therefore potentially recoverable) or obstructed is a renal ultrasound scan, which should be performed as soon as possible in AKI. This will provide reliable information on the presence or absence of lower urinary tract obstruction (in which case hydronephrosis will be present), and on renal size and asymmetry. In the setting of established CKD the kidneys are usually, but not always, reduced in size and echogenic. A skilled ultrasonographer will comment on the thickness of the renal cortex, which is also reduced in CKD. The presence of normal-sized kidneys with a normal cortical thickness in the context of AKI is often the start of a pathway towards diagnostic renal biopsy. The kidneys may occasionally be large (>13 cm) on ultrasound; in the setting of AKI this usually indicates an infiltrative process, such as amyloidosis or lymphoma. If one kidney is more than1.5 cm smaller than the other, this suggests longstanding severe renal artery stenosis to the small kidney (and by inference possible renal artery stenosis to the larger kidney also), which is of particular relevance in the setting of ACE inhibitor and ARB use. One should also note that, while unilateral hydronephrosis generally does not cause a significant rise in serum creatinine, if the other kidney is atrophic then urinary tract obstruction can be implicated as the sole cause of AKI, as the small kidney may not be providing any excretory renal function.

In the rheumatology setting, the next major question that needs to be considered is whether the kidneys are severely injured by an intrarenal process that would respond to a specific therapy, such as rapidly progressive glomerulonephritis (RPGN), haemolytic uraemic syndrome (HUS), acute interstitial nephritis, or myeloma cast nephropathy. These conditions are discussed in more detail below (see 'Diagnostic approach to the patient with acute kidney injury'). If the creatinine level is rising day by day and the ultrasound demonstrates normal-sized unobstructed kidneys, the diagnosis will most often be acute tubular necrosis (ATN), especially in the hospital setting, but one must always consider whether an acute glomerular or other tubulointerstitial process is present. Most helpful in this setting is careful urinalysis of urine which is freshly obtained and not catheter derived. If there is blood and protein present on dipstick testing, and especially if red cell casts are seen on urine microscopy, it is likely that the patient has RPGN. It must be emphasized that appropriate immunosuppressive treatment of RPGN often results in marked improvement in renal function and that, without it, glomerular destruction progresses relentlessly to the point where the patient develops irreversible dialysis-dependent renal failure. Therefore, urgent appropriate serological testing and early referral to a nephrologist for consideration of kidney biopsy are essential. The probability of RPGN being the cause of AKI is highest if certain underlying rheumatological conditions are present, in particular ANCA vasculitis, SLE, Henoch–Schönlein purpura (HSP), and cryoglobulinemia, and/or if there is a coexistent pulmonary syndrome, such as lung haemorrhage or a new lung infiltrate.

If the kidneys are unobstructed and of normal size, and the patient has AKI with a normal urine dipstick test, important diagnoses to consider are HUS[9] and other causes of thrombotic microangiopathy, and myeloma cast nephropathy.[10] In the former there is reduction in glomerular blood flow because of intraglomerular capillary thrombosis; in the latter there is tubular obstruction and damage by complexed Tamm–Horsfall protein and light chains. The focus in this clinical scenario should be on looking for features of the systemic disease: hypertension, thrombocytopenia, and microangiopathic haemolytic anaemia in HUS; hypercalcaemia, anaemia, lytic bone lesions, serum paraprotein/free light chains, and urine Bence Jones protein in multiple myeloma. If the AKI occurs in the setting of systemic sclerosis (SSc), early consideration must be given to scleroderma renal crisis, which is also associated with a relatively normal urinalysis. The key feature of scleroderma renal crisis is severe and progressive hypertension which may be characterized by features of malignant hypertension, such as papilloedema. Note that occasionally there may be minimal skin changes of scleroderma and that a renal crisis may be the presenting feature of SSc.

If there is persisting AKI, but no evidence of RPGN, HUS, or myeloma, and the urine dipstick demonstrates proteinuria and leucocytes, the diagnosis may be acute interstitial nephritis, an often overlooked condition. Traditionally, if interstitial nephritis is suspected, one is taught to look for systemic evidence of hypersensitivity, such as rash, eosinophilia, and eosinophiluria. In practice these findings are rarely helpful and the diagnosis can only be made on renal biopsy.

The next step in the assessment of the patient with AKI is diagnostic blood testing. The priority here is to liaise with the laboratory to ensure that serological tests are run urgently if RPGN is suspected. Of the serological tests available, the ANCA test has greatest utility in this setting. When ethanol-fixed neutrophils are exposed to patient serum and antibody binding is detected using fluorescently labelled antibodies, two patterns of indirect immunofluorescent staining may be identified: fine granular cytoplasmic (c-ANCA) and perinuclear (p-ANCA). Proteinase 3 (PR3) and myeloperoxidase (MPO) are the most commonly identified autoantigens leading to the c-ANCA and p-ANCA appearances, respectively, and therefore the terms PR3-ANCA and MPO-ANCA are frequently used. A positive PR3-ANCA ELISA test, when combined with a positive immunofluorescence test, is highly sensitive and specific for active granulomatosis with polyangiitis (GPA; previously Wegener's). Of note, immunofluorescence testing alone is not sufficiently specific and should always be combined with an ELISA looking for the specific antibody.[11,12] The overall sensitivity is estimated to be 66%, those with limited upper airway disease often being ANCA negative, and the overall specificity for the combined test is 99%.[12,13] One potential pitfall to bear in mind is chronic cocaine use, which may mimic the nasal and sinus features of GPA, and is occasionally associated with anti-PR3 antibodies; in addition, there is strong evidence to support an association between levamisole-tainted cocaine and ANCA- vasculitis.[14] During active GPA, the pooled sensitivity increases to 91% and the pooled specificity rises to 99%. Whether titres of ANCA correlate directly with disease activity remains controversial.[15,16]

It is worth mentioning that a positive ANA test may be confused with a positive p-ANCA staining pattern, reinforcing the importance of combining the immunofluorescence test with the ELISA. The sensitivity of a positive p-ANCA plus anti-MPO antibody test for MPA is 67%, and the allied specificity (when the test is performed in the appropriate clinical context) is 99%.[12,13] Among those with positive ANCA serologies (both immunofluorescence and ELISA) and a clinical presentation of RPGN, the positive predictive value of finding a pauci-immune crescentic glomerulonephritis on renal biopsy is at least 98% in all age groups.[17,18] Of note, classical polyarteritis nodosa (which is not characterized by crescentic glomerulonephritis) is not associated with the presence of ANCA.

In rheumatological settings other than systemic vasculitis, the following antibody tests also have specific utility:

+ In patients with SLE, anti-C1q antibodies are associated with renal involvement and may be associated with renal flares.[19]

+ In patients with SSc, fibrillarin (U3-RNP) and anti-RNA polymerases (I and III) are associated with the development of scleroderma renal crisis.[20,21]

In addition to antibody testing, it is useful in the setting of AKI to measure serum levels of complement components C3 and C4. If depressed, this strongly suggests a renal disorder characterized by glomerular deposition or serum consumption of complement: lupus nephritis, cryoglobulinemic glomerulonephritis (C4 is often depressed in isolation), or HUS.

Potential causes of acute kidney injury in rheumatological practice

Prerenal acute kidney injury

Probably the most frequently encountered cause of acute prerenal AKI in rheumatological practice is an NSAID-induced reduction in renal perfusion by diversion of eicosanoid synthesis away from prostacyclin (these agents are also instrumental in causing acute interstitial nephritis, discussed below; see 'Acute interstitial nephritis'). Volume depletion, hepatic disease, and lupus nephritis predispose to the adverse renal haemodynamic changes associated with the NSAIDs. The alterations in renal function are reversed upon discontinuation of the offending drug. The ACE inhibitors and ARBs can also induce decreased renal perfusion and an acute decline in renal function through dilatation of intrarenal efferent arterioles. Such alterations in renal function are enhanced when there is underlying volume depletion, renal vascular disease, or pre-existing glomerular disease.[22–24] In addition to being the preferred treatment for kidney disease characterized by proteinuria, these antihypertensives have been particularly efficacious in the treatment of malignant hypertension associated with scleroderma renal crisis and the microangiopathies. When using these medications, renal function and serum electrolytes must be monitored closely because of the risk of AKI and electrolyte abnormalities, such as hyperkalaemia. Having said that, most nephrologists would expect (and tolerate) a 10% rise in creatinine level after starting an ACE inhibitor or ARB.

Postrenal acute kidney injury

Postrenal AKI is characterized by oliguria caused by an intrarenal or extrarenal obstruction to urine flow. Intrarenal obstruction may be due to crystallization of a substance within the renal tubules. This might be endogenous, such as uric acid or a calcium salt, or exogenous, such as crystals of methotrexate or aciclovir. However, the most important cause of intrarenal postrenal AKI is obstruction and destruction of tubules by casts composed of light chains and Tamm–Horsfall mucoprotein in the context of multiple myeloma. Light chains have a molecular weight of approximately 22 000 and are freely filtered by the glomerulus. Normally, the daily filtered quantity of 30 mg/day is reabsorbed in the proximal tubule; with vastly excessive overproduction (up to 20 g/day) by a malignant plasma cell clone, this reabsorptive capacity is overwhelmed with consequent precipitation in complex with Tamm–Horsfall mucoprotein in the loop of Henle. Any patient with AKI and a negative urine dipstick test should undergo formal quantification of urine protein excretion rate and a screen for multiple myeloma. Volume depletion (especially when induced by loop diuretics), radiocontrast administration, and increased urinary calcium excretion (e.g. in hypercalcemia) greatly increase the risk of AKI in multiple myeloma. Traditionally, advanced renal insufficiency caused by myeloma cast nephropathy was considered largely irreversible. However, recent advances in myeloma therapy (e.g. bortezomib therapy) and serum light chain removal (with high-flux, extended-hours dialysis) may allow recovery of kidney function.[25] Therefore, early referral is essential for patients with AKI in the context of myeloma, even if the creatinine level is only mildly elevated.

Clinically apparent extrarenal obstruction to urinary flow most commonly involves the lower urinary tract because the obstruction of only one of two functioning kidneys will allow the non-affected kidney to continue to make urine, so oliguria and a reduction in GFR will not result. The characteristic feature of AKI secondary to extrarenal obstruction is marked reduction in urine output, often to the extent of anuria: acute anuria should be considered due to obstructive uropathy until proven otherwise by ultrasound scanning; if the ultrasound scan is normal, consideration should be given to whether there is bilateral renal infarction due to an acute occlusion of arterial blood supply.

By far the commonest causes of extrarenal obstruction causing AKI are prostatic disease (in which case the bladder will be markedly distended clinically) and locally advanced pelvic cancer (in particular, cervical and bladder). Bilateral papillary necrosis could lead to obstruction of the upper urinary tract through occlusion of both ureters, but this would be a most unusual event. Postrenal failure can be reversed if the obstruction is relieved before onset of renal parenchymal damage.

Intrinsic acute kidney injury: key relevant pathologies

Rapidly progressive glomerulonephritis

The pathological hallmark of RPGN is the glomerular crescent, which is a non-specific pathophysiological response to severe glomerular injury, and is observed as the result of a variety of insults which are classified according to the presence or absence of glomerular deposition of immunoproteins:

◆ Linear deposition of IgG along the glomerular basement membrane (GBM) is seen in conjunction with circulating anti-GBM antibodies in Goodpasture's disease. This is the rarest form of RPGN, but tends to be the most severe. It is relatively unusual for patients with this condition to recover kidney function if they present requiring dialysis.

◆ Widespread deposition of immunoproteins (immunoglobulins, complement components) throughout the glomerulus. In a rheumatological setting this is most often seen in SLE, but may also be a feature of severe HSP (IgA deposits), postinfectious glomerulonephritis and cryoglobulinaemia.

◆ Relative absence of immunoprotein deposition: so-called pauciimmune crescentic glomerulonephritis. In this case the glomerular injury occurs secondary to inflammatory necrosis of the glomerular tuft due to vasculitis of the afferent arteriole, and is pathognomonic of systemic small-vessel vasculitis, usually in association with circulating anti-PR3 or anti-MPO antibodies. The clinical term applied to this condition is determined by the nature of the extrarenal manifestations. If necrotizing granulomatous inflammation of the nasal passages, sinuses, and upper airways is present, or there are granulomata evident on chest imaging, this is termed GPA. If the there is no granulomatous inflammation and the predominant extrarenal manifestation is 'vasculitic' (i.e. alveolar haemorrhage, leukocytoclastic skin vasculitis, iritis, mononeuritis multiplex), this is termed MPA. Of note, small-vessel vasculitis limited to the kidney is now

considered 'single organ vasculitis'. The renal lesion of MPA and GPA is pathologically indistinguishable and is generally treated in the same way, although patients with MPA tend to have more chronic lesions and more extensive glomerular scarring at diagnosis.

Crescentic glomerulonephritis is usually treated with high-dose corticosteroids and cyclophosphamide and, when sufficient immunosuppression is given, appreciable recovery of renal function often follows (except in cases of advanced anti-GBM disease). A delicate balance needs to be struck between the adverse effects of such intense immunosuppression and the consequences of advanced irreversible renal failure. It is worth appreciating in this regard that chronic dialysis therapy is tolerated poorly in elderly people and that the equation usually falls on the side of giving immunosuppression if the kidney biopsy shows acute, potentially reversible, glomerular lesions. In ANCA vasculitis there is now strong clinical trial evidence to support the use of the anti-CD20 monoclonal antibody rituximab in place of cyclophosphamide in severe glomerular disease, especially when there is a perceived risk of infection or desire to preserve fertility.[26,27] In addition, plasma exchange is often used in anti-GBM disease and in severe ANCA-associated vasculitis (creatinine level >500 μm).[28]

Thrombotic microangiopathy

In some cases of intrinsic AKI the lesion is confined to the microvessels of the glomerulus, with evidence of acute thrombosis but no inflammatory infiltrate or glomerulonephritis. In these cases of thrombotic microangiopathy, two important diagnoses must be considered and differentiated:

Scleroderma renal crisis

The presence of microscopic renal lesions in patients with systemic sclerosis may occur in up to 80% of individuals, although only 40–50% will present with clinical renal involvement, including hypertension, proteinuria, or renal impairment. In 15–20% of patients who develop hypertension in the setting of diffuse cutaneous SSc, the onset is abrupt with severe elevation of diastolic blood pressure, often associated with cardiac failure, retinopathy and rapid deterioration of renal function: so-called scleroderma renal crisis. This severe complication of SSc almost invariably occurs within 5 years of diagnosis, and usually within 2 years. Prior use of high-dose glucocorticoids appears to be a risk factor. In some patients, scleroderma renal crisis may be the presenting feature of SSc, with little involvement of skin, peripheral vessels, or joints, in which case differentiation from thrombotic thrombocytopaenic purpura (TTP) and HUS may become difficult. Histologically, the small arterioles of the kidney in patients with the malignant form of hypertension in SSc show extensive fibrinoid necrosis and microthrombus formation, with 'onion-skin' intimal hypertrophy. Glomerular changes show varying degrees of thrombosis and necrosis secondary to ischaemia. The accelerated hypertension and rapidly progressive renal failure are life threatening and demand prompt, intensive intervention. The initial priority is to bring the blood pressure under control, and ACE inhibitors are the mainstay of therapy in this regard. Even if oliguria and progressive renal failure supervene despite control of blood pressure, antihypertensive therapy should be continued because it will protect other organs from the damaging effects of severe hypertension and renal function may return after months of dialysis support.[20,29]

Thrombotic thrombocytopenic purpura and haemolytic uraemic syndrome

TTP and HUS are classical examples of microangiopathic haemolytic anaemia and have many features in common, including anaemia, thrombocytopenia, and renal involvement. The two syndromes are similar in most of their clinical and laboratory findings, although patients with prominent neurological features are generally considered as having classical TTP, and those with dominant renal features are considered as having HUS. Many cases of HUS are associated with a diarrhoeal illness; those that are not are termed 'atypical' or 'D-' HUS. Mutations in the genes for complement proteins including C3, factors H, B, and I, and CD46 are associated with approximately 50% of cases of atypical HUS. Recent work has sought to classify TTP based on the level of ADAMTS13 (**A D**isintegrin-like **A**nd **M**etalloprotease with **T**hrombo**S**pondin type 1 repeats), deficiency of which leads to accumulation of unusually large Von Willebrand factor multimers, which in turn promote platelet aggregation.[30] Although useful, the exact link with TTP remains controversial, and reduced levels of this protease are also observed in other conditions such as sepsis.[31] The classical pathological finding in the kidney in both syndromes is occlusive lesions of arterioles and glomerular capillaries with fibrin, platelets, and red blood cells. The features of TTP and HUS may be seen in patients with SLE, and it is also seen in the setting of severe disseminated intravascular coagulation, sepsis, quinine therapy, allogeneic bone marrow transplantation and systemic vasculitides. Plasma exchange has become the mainstay of therapy in TTP and HUS.

Acute interstitial nephritis

Tubulointerstitial nephritis (TIN) is an inflammatory renal condition in which the damage is focused on the tubules and interstitium. It is of considerable importance, since tubulointerstitial damage correlates more closely with impairment of renal function than the degree of glomerular damage. Interstitial inflammation may be secondary to glomerular injury, renovascular or metabolic disease, or may be initiated primarily within the interstitial compartment. The commoner causes of TIN are drug reactions, but infections and certain rheumatological diseases may have predominant impact on the tubulointerstitium (Box 25.1). Many drugs commonly used in rheumatological practice, such as NSAIDs, proton pump inhibitors, or antibiotics, may induce TIN, and these do not always manifest with other allergic manifestations, making the diagnosis difficult unless a renal biopsy is obtained.

TIN may result in AKI, accounting for up to 27% of cases presenting with renal failure and normal-sized kidneys on ultrasound.[32,33] Many clinical features are common to TIN irrespective of its

Box 25.1 Rheumatological conditions associated with tubulointerstitial nephritis

- ◆ Systemic lupus erythematosus
- ◆ Mixed connective tissue disease
- ◆ Sjögren's syndrome
- ◆ Sarcoidosis
- ◆ Tubulointerstitial nephritis and uveitis (TINU)
- ◆ Primary systemic vasculitis
- ◆ Relapsing polychondritis

Table 25.3 Sites of injury and patterns of tubular dysfunction in tubulointerstitial nephritis

Site of injury	Tubular dysfunction	Clinical features
Proximal tubule	Decreased reabsorption of Na^+, glucose, HCO_3^-, urate, PO_4^-, amino acids	Glycosuria, hypouricaemia, hypophosphataemia, aminoaciduria, alkaline urine, acidaemia[a]
Distal tubule	Decreased secretion of Na^+, H^+	Alkaline urine, acidaemia,[b] hyperkalaemia, inability to preserve Na^+
Medulla and papilla	Decreased reabsorption of Na^+ Decreased concentrating ability	Polyuria, nocturia, inability to preserve free water[c]

[a]Proximal renal tubular acidosis.
[b]Distal renal tubular acidosis.
[c]Nephrogenic diabetes insipidus.

aetiology (Table 25.3). However, since suggestive clinical features can be absent or the diagnosis may not be suspected, renal biopsy is required to confirm the diagnosis. There may be evidence of systemic acidaemia, hypo- or hyper-kalaemia, hypophosphatemia, or hypouricaemia. Immunological tests should be performed in all cases and may be helpful in the diagnosis of systemic disorders associated with TIN.

Interstitial nephritis induced by NSAIDs appears to be unique among the drug-induced tubular interstitial nephritides in its association with heavy proteinuria. The propionic acid derivatives—fenoprofen, ibuprofen, and naproxen—have accounted for three-quarters of the cases reported, with fenoprofen alone accounting for over one-half of the incidence of tubulo-interstitial disease induced by NSAIDs.[34] The lesions have also been found after the self-administration of over-the-counter ibuprofen and may recur after exposure to different NSAIDs of the same group or upon re-exposure to the same agent. Renal function improves within days of discontinuing the offending agent, although proteinuria may persist for weeks to months and the GFR may remain permanently reduced in 40% of cases.[35] Alternative agents infrequently associated with nephrotoxicity include meclofenamate and sulindac. The issue of corticosteroid treatment of TIN remains controversial and there are no trial data to guide their use. However, most nephrologists would advocate treatment with up to 6 weeks of corticosteroids in patients who do not demonstrate improvement in kidney function within 1 week of withdrawal of the offending agent.

Drug-induced acute tubular injury

Nephrotoxic agents generally cause injury to the tubular components of the nephrons, particularly the highly metabolically active proximal tubule. A large range of agents can cause nephrotoxicity and AKI; we consider in detail several of relevance to rheumatological practice:

Radiocontrast agents

These agents, particularly older high-osmolality contrast agents, are a common cause of acute tubular injury, probably mediated by intrarenal vasoconstriction. By far the biggest risk factor is pre-existing renal dysfunction, with diabetes mellitus providing additive risk. Congestive cardiac failure and multiple myeloma also increase the risk. The induced renal dysfunction is generally mild, non-oliguric, and reversible within 3–5 days, suggesting that overt tubular necrosis does not generally occur.

Aminoglycosides

Aminoglycosides cause non-oliguric AKI in approximately 10% of treated individuals, which is usually mild and reversible upon stopping the agent. The main injury is to the proximal tubule, where the drug is concentrated, giving very high intracellular levels; dysfunction of proximal tubular cells may give rise to a Fanconi-type syndrome, with glycosuria, aminoaciduria, and phosphate wasting. Distal tubular damage may also result and is manifested as polyuria and renal magnesium wasting. There is a close relationship between drug exposure and risk of injury, so long treatment courses with high trough drug levels are the main risk factor. Advanced age, sepsis, and pre-existing renal disease (mainly due to the increased risk of overdosing) are the other main risk factors. Use of infrequent dosing schedules (every 24–48 hours) reduces the risk of toxicity.[36]

Calcineurin inhibitors

Calcineurin inhibitor (CNI, ciclosporin and tacrolimus) nephrotoxicity causes AKI (which is largely reversible after reducing the dose), or chronic progressive irreversible renal disease. The acute effect is dose dependent and mediated by endothelial injury resulting in intense vasoconstriction of intrarenal arterioles. Occasionally, thrombotic microangiopathy occurs with features of microangiopathic haemolytic anaemia. Because of the tight association of AKI with blood levels of the drug, it is important to measure levels at regular intervals in all patients treated with a CNI.

The clinical features of AKI are summarized in Table 25.4.

Table 25.4 Features of acute kidney injury

Type of acute kidney injury	Characteristic features
Prerenal acute kidney injury (reduced renal perfusion)	
Volume depletion (over-diuresis, vomiting, diarrhoea)	◆ Oliguria
Hypotension	◆ Concentrated urine
Congestive cardiac failure	◆ No intrinsic renal damage
Cirrhosis (hepatorenal syndrome)	◆ Reversible upon correction of underlying problem
ACE inhibitors/ARBs/NSAIDs	
Hypercalcaemia	
Postrenal acute kidney injury (obstructive uropathy)	
Prostate hypertrophy or cancer	◆ Anuria
Ureteric obstruction by tumour at the base of the bladder (cervical, bladder, ovarian)	◆ Obstruction must be bilateral to cause significant reduction in GFR
Ureteric obstruction by retroperitoneal fibrosis	◆ Hydronephrosis
Intraureteric obstruction (bilateral calculus, bilateral papillary necrosis, bilateral blood clot)	◆ Causes irreversible intrinsic renal damage if prolonged
Intrarenal tubular obstruction (myeloma casts, oxalate crystals (e.g. ethylene glycol ingestion, aciclovir crystals)	◆ Bland urine sediment
	◆ Elevated PCR with negative urine dipstick (Bence Jones proteinuria)
Intrinsic acute kidney injury	
Crescentic glomerulonephritis (ANCA-associated vasculitis, class III/IV lupus nephritis, anti-GBM disease, IgA nephropathy (HSP), cryoglobulinemia)	◆ Glomerular haematuria
	◆ Red cell casts
Glomerular microangiopathy (haemolytic uraemic syndrome)	◆ Bland urine
	◆ Red cell fragments on blood film
	◆ Hypertension
Vascular causes (scleroderma renal crisis, malignant hypertension, atheroemboli, renal vein thrombosis)	◆ Hypertension
	◆ Red cell fragments on blood film
	◆ Relatively bland urine sediment
Ischemic tubular injury (prolonged prerenal state, sepsis syndrome)	◆ Clear preceding factors
Toxic tubular injury (aminoglycosides, myoglobin, antiretrovirals)	◆ High urinary sodium excretion
	◆ Tubular dysfunction (renal glucose and phosphate wasting)
Tubulointerstitial nephritis (penicillins, NSAIDs, PPI, sacroidosis)	◆ Non-nephrotic range proteinuria
	◆ Preserved urine output
	◆ Leukocyturia

ACE, angiotensin-converting enzyme; ARBs, angiotensin receptor blockers; GFR, glomerular filtration rate; HSP, Henoch–Schönlein purpura; NSAIDs, non-steroidal anti-inflammatory drugs; PPI, proton pump inhibitor; PCR, protein/creatinine ratio.

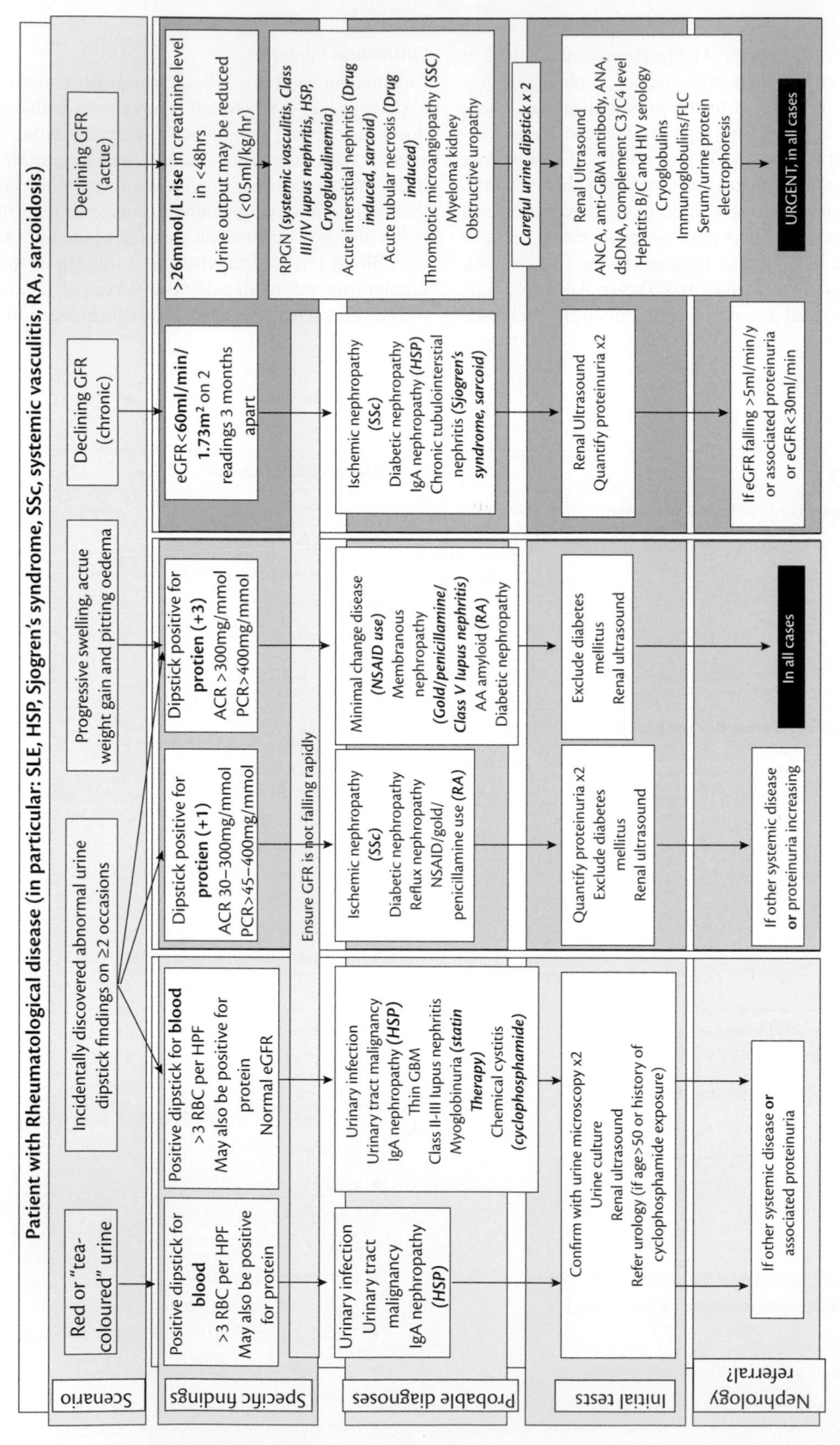

Patient with Rheumatological disease (in particular: SLE, HSP, Sjogren's syndrome, SSc, systemic vasculitis, RA, sarcoidosis)

Scenario	Red or "tea-coloured" urine	Incidentally discovered abnormal urine dipstick findings on ≥2 occasions	Progressive swelling, actue weight gain and pitting oedema	Declining GFR (chronic)	Declining GFR (actue)

Specific findings

- Positive dipstick for **blood** >3 RBC per HPF May also be positive for protein
- Positive dipstick for **blood** >3 RBC per HPF May also be positive for protein Normal eGFR
- Dipstick positive for **protien (+1)** ACR 30–300mg/mmol PCR>45–400mg/mmol
- Dipstick positive for **protien (+3)** ACR >300mg/mmol PCR>400mg/mmol
- eGFR<60ml/min/ 1.73m² on 2 readings 3 months apart
- >26mmol/L rise in creatinine level in <48hrs Urine output may be reduced (<0.5ml/kg/hr)

Ensure GFR is not falling rapidly

Probable diagnoses

- Urinary infection Urinary tract malignancy IgA nephropathy (HSP)
- Urinary infection Urinary tract malignancy IgA nephropathy (*HSP*) Thin GBM Class II–III lupus nephritis Myoglobinuria (*statin Therapy*) Chemical cystitis (*cyclophosphamide*)
- Ischemic nephropathy (*SSc*) Diabetic nephropathy Reflux nephropathy NSAID/gold/ penicillamine use (*RA*)
- Minimal change disease (*NSAID use*) Membranous nephropathy (*Gold/penicillamine/ Class V lupus nephritis*) AA amyloid (*RA*) Diabetic nephropathy
- Ischemic nephropathy (*SSc*) Diabetic nephropathy IgA nephropathy (*HSP*) Chronic tubulointerstial nephritis (*Sjogren's syndrome, sarcoid*)
- RPGN (*systemic vasculitis, Class III/IV lupus nephritis, HSP, Cryoglubulinemia*) Acute interstitial nephritis (*Drug induced, sarcoid*) Acute tubular necrosis (*Drug induced*) Thrombotic microangiopathy (*SSC*) Myeloma kidney Obstructive uropathy

Initial tests

- Confirm with urine microscopy x2 Urine culture Renal ultrasound Refer urology (if age>50 or history of cyclophosphamide exposure)
- Quantify proteinuria x2 Exclude diabetes mellitus Renal ultrasound
- Exclude diabetes mellitus Renal ultrasound
- Renal Ultrasound Quantify proteinuria x2
- *Careful urine dipstick x 2* Renal Ultrasound ANCA, anti-GBM antibody, ANA, dsDNA, complement C3/C4 level Hepatits B/C and HIV serology Cryoglobulins Immunoglobulins/FLC Serum/urine protein electrophoresis

Nephrology referral?

- If other systemic disease **or** associated proteinuria
- If other systemic disease **or** proteinuria increasing
- In all cases
- If eGFR falling >5ml/min/y or associated proteinuria or eGFR<30ml/min
- **URGENT, in all cases**

Fig. 25.1 Algorithm depicting typical diagnostic pathways following various clinical scenarios. Acute kidney injury and nephrotic syndrome should lead to timely nephrology referral.

General principles of management of acute kidney injury

The prognosis of AKI is determined both by the underlying disease and by the quality of medical management. Individuals with renal dysfunction complicating a rheumatic disorder should be followed up jointly by a rheumatologist and a nephrologist (see Figure 25.1). Early consultation with a nephrologist is advisable in order to rapidly diagnose the underlying aetiology of AKI. In many situations, prompt resolution of the inciting factors can lead to a rapid return of renal function. In cases where deterioration cannot be halted, nephrologic support by means of renal replacement therapy can be initiated in a timely manner. The chief cause of complications in the setting of AKI is not azotaemia, but associated fluid and electrolyte abnormalities. In the acutely ill, highly catabolic patient with systemic illness, early and frequent dialysis may be required. The rheumatologist and nephrologist should review the prescribed medications critically as soon as AKI is recognized. The dosage schedule for potentially nephrotoxic agents such as NSAIDs, aminoglycosides, and amphotericin B should be adjusted for the level of renal failure or discontinued if possible. Intravascular radiocontrast procedures should be avoided during AKI. If it is necessary to use a diagnostic procedure requiring contrast, a minimal dose should be employed and the patient intensively hydrated before, during, and after the procedure to promote excretion of the radiocontrast agent. The presence of a highly catabolic state caused by corticosteroid therapy, gastrointestinal bleeding, parenteral nutrition, or septicaemia can induce a rise in the blood urea by as much as 30 mM/day in the setting of AKI. Such levels of azotaemia are detrimental to platelet and neutrophil function, and may potentiate a bleeding diathesis or further compromise host defences. Therefore, daily or continuous dialysis may be warranted.

Kidney failure: chronic

Definitions

Chronic kidney disease (CKD) is much commoner than AKI; it is estimated that approximately 8% of the population has renal disease resulting in a chronic reduction in eGFR to less than 60 mL/min. The internationally accepted definition of CKD consists of:

♦ the presence of markers of kidney damage for ≥3 months, as defined by structural or functional abnormalities of the kidney with or without decreased GFR, that can lead to decreased GFR, manifested by either pathological abnormalities or other markers of kidney damage (such as haematuria or proteinuria), or abnormalities in imaging tests, or

♦ the presence of GFR <60 mL/min/1.73 m^2 for ≥3 months, with or without other signs of kidney damage as described above.[37]

Irrespective of the cause, and even in those in whom the renal injury has been effectively treated, there is a tendency for ongoing loss of GFR over time, an observation related to hyperfiltration and overload of the remaining nephrons. The rate of progression is dependent on many factors, including persistence of the inciting renal disease, carriage of certain genetic polymorphisms, ethnicity, degree of hypertension, and presence of comorbid conditions. The strongest predictor of progressive loss of GFR is the degree of proteinuria (Table 25.5).

Diagnostic approach to the patient with chronic kidney disease

In rheumatological practice, the presence of CKD is usually suggested by the anecdotal finding of an elevated serum creatinine level or abnormal urine dipstick result. The reduction in GFR is well tolerated clinically until the patient reaches stage IV–V CKD and the GFR drops below 20 mL/min. The vast majority of patients with CKD are thus asymptomatic, although they may manifest features of the underlying disease. If the renal dysfunction is very severe (stage V CKD) the patient may display clinical features of the 'uraemic syndrome': mental dullness, anorexia, and vomiting, usually associated with progressive swelling, itching, and shortness of breath.

The principal causes of CKD 3 or greater in the United Kingdom are diabetic nephropathy, glomerulonephritis, hypertension, ischemic nephropathy (secondary to renovascular disease), reflux nephropathy, and monogenetic renal disease (particularly adult polycystic kidney disease). Diagnostic clues include the following:

♦ Diabetic nephropathy is typically associated with albuminuria, which may exceed protein/creatinine ratio (PCR) >300 mg/mmol. Indeed, diabetic nephropathy is the commonest cause of nephrotic syndrome.

♦ Chronic glomerulonephritis may be associated with dipstick haematuria or features of a systemic disease such as SLE, HSP, or SSc.

♦ Renovascular disease is characterized by hypertension, asymmetric kidneys on ultrasound, and a bland urine dipstick.

♦ Reflux nephropathy is a commoner cause of CKD in younger patients and is characterized by renal scarring on DMSA renography and low grade (non-nephrotic) proteinuria.

♦ The presence of bilateral enlarged kidneys with cysts on ultrasound is diagnostic of adult polycystic kidney disease and mandates nephrologist referral.

The initial priority is to identify and reverse superimposed AKI, as detailed above. Thereafter, most cases of mild–moderate CKD are managed in primary care. Indications for referral to a nephrologist include relatively rapid decline of GFR (>5 mL/min per year), associated proteinuria (PCR>100) or presence of CKD stage IV or greater (GFR<30 mL/min). Such cases of advanced CKD are generally managed in a dedicated clinic where the emphasis is on management of CKD complications (anaemia, volume overload, hypertension, hyperkalemia, acidosis, and renal bone disease) and preparation for dialysis or transplantation.

Table 25.5 Stages of chronic kidney disease (the numbers in parentheses indicate the prevalence in the general population)[38]

Stage 1	Normal GFR (>90 mL/min per 1.73 m^2) and persistent albuminuria (1.8%)
Stage 2	GFR 60–89 mL/min per 1.73 m^2 and persistent albuminuria (3.2%)
Stage 3	GFR 30–59 mL/min per 1.73 m^2 (7.7%)
Stage 4	GFR 15–29 mL/min per 1.73 m^2 (0.35%)
Stage 5	GFR <15 mL/min per 1.73 m^2 or endstage renal disease (0.24%)

References

1. Collins AJ, Foley RN, Chavers B et al. United States Renal Data System 2011 Annual Data Report: Atlas of chronic kidney disease & end-stage renal disease in the United States. *Am J Kidney Dis* 2012;59(1 Suppl 1): A7, e1–420.

2. Shemesh O, Golbetz H, Kriss JP, Myers BD. Limitations of creatinine as a filtration marker in glomerulopathic patients. *Kidney Int* 1985;28(5):830–838.

3. Mishra J, Dent C, Tarabishi R et al. Neutrophil gelatinase-associated lipocalin (NGAL) as a biomarker for acute renal injury after cardiac surgery. *Lancet* 2005;365(9466):1231–1238.

4. Bennett M, Dent CL, Ma Q et al. Urine NGAL predicts severity of acute kidney injury after cardiac surgery: a prospective study. *Clin J Am Soc Nephrol* 2008;3(3):665–673.

5. Han WK, Waikar SS, Johnson A et al. Urinary biomarkers in the early diagnosis of acute kidney injury. *Kidney Int* 2008;73(7):863–869.

6. Levey AS, Bosch JP, Lewis JB et al. A more accurate method to estimate glomerular filtration rate from serum creatinine: a new prediction equation. Modification of Diet in Renal Disease Study Group. *Ann Intern Med* 1999;130(6):461–470.

7. Schwab SJ, Christensen RL, Dougherty K, Klahr S. Quantitation of proteinuria by the use of protein-to-creatinine ratios in single urine samples. *Arch Intern Med* 1987;147(5):943–944.

8. Mehta RL, Kellum JA, Shah SV et al. Acute Kidney Injury Network: report of an initiative to improve outcomes in acute kidney injury. *Crit Care* 2007;11(2):R31.

9. Remuzzi G. HUS and TTP: variable expression of a single entity. *Kidney Int* 1987;32(2):292–308.

10. Sakhuja V, Jha V, Varma S et al. Renal involvement in multiple myeloma: a 10-year study. *Ren Fail* 2000;22(4):465–477.

11. Rao JK, Allen NB, Feussner JR, Weinberger M. A prospective study of antineutrophil cytoplasmic antibody (c-ANCA) and clinical criteria in diagnosing Wegener's granulomatosis. *Lancet* 1995;346(8980):926–931.

12. Stone JH, Talor M, Stebbing J et al. Test characteristics of immunofluorescence and ELISA tests in 856 consecutive patients with possible ANCA-associated conditions. *Arthritis Care Res* 2000;13(6):424–434.

13. Hagen EC, Daha MR, Hermans J et al. Diagnostic value of standardized assays for anti-neutrophil cytoplasmic antibodies in idiopathic systemic vasculitis. EC/BCR Project for ANCA Assay Standardization. *Kidney Int* 1998;53(3):743–753.

14. McGrath MM, Isakova T, Rennke HG et al. Contaminated cocaine and antineutrophil cytoplasmic antibody-associated disease. *Clin J Am Soc Nephrol* 2011;6(12):2799–2805.

15. Boomsma MM, Stegeman CA, van der Leij MJ et al. Prediction of relapses in Wegener's granulomatosis by measurement of antineutrophil cytoplasmic antibody levels: a prospective study. *Arthritis Rheum* 2000;43(9):2025–2033.

16. Nowack R, Grab I, Flores-Suarez LF et al. ANCA titres, even of IgG subclasses, and soluble CD14 fail to predict relapses in patients with ANCA-associated vasculitis. *Nephrol Dial Transplant* 2001;16(8):1631–1637.

17. Jennette JC, Wilkman AS, Falk RJ. Diagnostic predictive value of ANCA serology. *Kidney Int* 1998;53(3):796–798.

18. Rao JK, Weinberger M, Oddone EZ et al. The role of antineutrophil cytoplasmic antibody (c-ANCA) testing in the diagnosis of Wegener granulomatosis. A literature review and meta-analysis. *Ann Intern Med* 1995;123(12):925–932.

19. Moura CG, Mangueira CL, Cruz LA, Cruz CM. Negative anti-C1q antibody titers may influence therapeutic decisions and reduce the number of renal biopsies in systemic lupus erythematosus. *Nephron Clin Pract* 2011;118(4):c355–C360.

20. Penn H, Howie AJ, Kingdon EJ et al. Scleroderma renal crisis: patient characteristics and long-term outcomes. *QJM* 2007;100(8):485–494.

21. Nguyen B, Mayes MD, Arnett FC et al. HLA-DRB1*0407 and *1304 are risk factors for scleroderma renal crisis. *Arthritis Rheum* 2011;63(2):530–534.

22. MacDowall P, Kalra PA, O'Donoghue DJ et al. Risk of morbidity from renovascular disease in elderly patients with congestive cardiac failure. *Lancet* 1998;352(9121):13–16.

23. Ljungman S, Kjekshus J, Swedberg K. Renal function in severe congestive heart failure during treatment with enalapril (the Cooperative North Scandinavian Enalapril Survival Study (CONSENSUS) Trial). *Am J Cardiol* 1992;70(4):479–487.

24. Stirling C, Houston J, Robertson S et al. Diarrhoea, vomiting and ACE inhibitors—an important cause of acute renal failure. *J Hum Hypertens* 2003;17(6):419–423.

25. Hutchison CA, Cockwell P, Stringer S et al. Early reduction of serum-free light chains associates with renal recovery in myeloma kidney. *J Am Soc Nephrol* 2011;22(6):1129–1136.

26. Stone JH, Merkel PA, Spiera R et al. Rituximab versus cyclophosphamide for ANCA-associated vasculitis. *N Engl J Med* 2010;363(3):221–232.

27. Jones RB, Tervaert JW, Hauser T et al. Rituximab versus cyclophosphamide in ANCA-associated renal vasculitis. *N Engl J Med* 2010;363(3):211–220.

28. Jayne DR, Gaskin G, Rasmussen N et al. Randomized trial of plasma exchange or high-dosage methylprednisolone as adjunctive therapy for severe renal vasculitis. *J Am Soc Nephrol* 2007;18(7):2180–2188.

29. Steen VD, Medsger TA, Jr. Long-term outcomes of scleroderma renal crisis. *Ann Intern Med* 2000;133(8):600–603.

30. Hovinga JA, Vesely SK, Terrell DR, Lammle B, George JN. Survival and relapse in patients with thrombotic thrombocytopenic purpura. *Blood* 2010;115(8):1500–1511; quiz 662.

31. Booth KK, Terrell DR, Vesely SK, George JN. Systemic infections mimicking thrombotic thrombocytopenic purpura. *Am J Hematol* 2011;86(9):743–751.

32. Haas M, Spargo BH, Wit EJ, Meehan SM. Etiologies and outcome of acute renal insufficiency in older adults: a renal biopsy study of 259 cases. *Am J Kidney Dis* 2000;35(3):433–447.

33. Farrington K, Levison DA, Greenwood RN, Cattell WR, Baker LR. Renal biopsy in patients with unexplained renal impairment and normal kidney size. *QJM* 1989;70(263):221–233.

34. Clive DM, Stoff JS. Renal syndromes associated with nonsteroidal anti-inflammatory drugs. *N Engl J Med* 1984;310(9):563–572.

35. Baker RJ, Pusey CD. The changing profile of acute tubulointerstitial nephritis. *Nephrol Dial Transplant* 2004;19(1):8–11.

36. Munckhof WJ, Grayson ML, Turnidge JD. A meta-analysis of studies on the safety and efficacy of aminoglycosides given either once daily or as divided doses. *J Antimicrob Chemother* 1996;37(4):645–663.

37. K/DOQI clinical practice guidelines for chronic kidney disease: evaluation, classification, and stratification. *Am J Kidney Dis* 2002;39(2 Suppl 1): S1–266.

38. Levey AS, de Jong PE, Coresh J et al. The definition, classification, and prognosis of chronic kidney disease: a KDIGO Controversies Conference report. *Kidney Int* 2011;80(1):17–28.

CHAPTER 26

Psychology

Hayley McBain, Sophie Cleanthous, and Stanton Newman

Impact of rheumatic disease on the individual

Symptoms

Pain

Arthritis is one of the most common causes of pain, and this is customarily ranked as the most important symptom by people with arthritis. The majority rate their pain as being severe and this can lead to limitations in daily activities and difficulties in leading a 'normal' life. The impact of pain also extends to more frequent use of medications and health services, and time off work.

Descriptions of pain vary between different rheumatic conditions. For example, people with fibromyalgia describe their pain as aching, exhausting, and nagging while those with rheumatoid arthritis (RA) use the word 'stiff' more frequently. Pain quality also appears to relate to activity, with pain at rest described as throbbing or aching, and pain on movement described as shooting and spreading.

Physiological models have been unable to explain variations in the reports of pain. Identical conditions or injuries do not predict the severity, intensity, or quality of self-reported pain, therefore other intervening psychological and social factors must play a role. In this chapter pain will be linked with a number of psychological outcomes including depression and anxiety as well as adaptive and maladaptive coping strategies and cognitions.

It is not surprising that pain, which can persist for months and years, will influence all aspects of a person's functioning and in particular psychological well-being. There is a vast amount of literature demonstrating a bidirectional relationship between pain and depression.[1] In addition feelings of anxiety, in particular fear in relation to completing tasks which may exacerbate pain, can lead a patient to avoid activities and situations that involve movement. Research suggests that it is this fear of movement and re-injury which better predicts disability than biological factors and even pain severity and duration.

Stiffness

Stiffness has been the subject of less research and although it has been described in the literature as a slowness and difficulty in moving the joints, its qualities are poorly understood. Because of its temporal nature, individuals who are able to adjust their timetable to accommodate early-morning stiffness and those who can be more flexible in their work patterns are often more able to deal with stiffness. But despite morning stiffness being a part of the classification criteria for RA and potentially leading to early withdrawal from work,[2] more research is needed to better understand and define this symptom.

Fatigue

Fatigue is a primary and debilitating symptom of rheumatic disease. The experience of fatigue is complex, comprising both physical and cognitive features with an associated impact on functional and emotional outcomes. The prevalence of significant fatigue varies from 41% in RA and osteoarthritis (OA)[3] to 90% in systemic lupus erythematosus (SLE).[4] Despite the prevalence of fatigue and the importance patients place on this symptom, the mechanisms which cause or exacerbate the condition are not well understood. Fatigue has been related not only to the arthritis itself but to the medications used to treat the condition. Arthritis-related fatigue has also been associated with sleep difficulties, reduced physical activity,[5] greater pain, anxiety,[6] greater functional disability,[7] and depression.[8]

Sleep difficulties

Poor sleep quality is a very common complaint in arthritis. Sleep complaints and related daytime symptoms are reported by up to 80% of patients with arthritis. Complaints include difficulties in falling asleep, poor quality sleep, non-restorative sleep, numerous awakenings during the night, early morning awakening, and excessive daytime sleepiness. Poor sleep and restlessness in SLE have been associated with pain, fatigue, and depressed mood.[5,9,10] Sleep disorders are also more common including, sleep apnoea, and restless leg syndrome.

Physical functioning

Disability

Epidemiological surveys of disability estimate that activity limitations affect approximately 8% of people with arthritis and this is set to grow as the population ages. Individuals with a rheumatic disease, despite appearing similar on clinical criteria, differ in self-reported physical function. Along with clinical variables, psychosocial factors appear to be important in predicting disability. An example of the importance of psychosocial variables is in a study examining 155 patients with RA.[11] Clinical and psychosocial variables combined accounted for 54% of the variance in disability at baseline and 35% at a 12-month follow-up. Feelings of helplessness added significantly to the prediction of disability, independent of disease severity, suggesting that patients who feel powerless in their ability to control the course of their illness and its impact report greater limitations on their ability to perform day-to-day activities. The importance of mood has also been demonstrated, with depressed RA patients being more impaired in their daily functioning than non-depressed patients.[12] Levels of disability tend to increase over time and predictors of this increase include older age, female, of a lower socio-economic status, being rheumatoid factor (RF) positive, greater pain, fatigue, depression, and functional and radiological damage, particularly in late RA.[13]

Social functioning

Employment and work

Rheumatic diseases are often associated with an inability to work. Work disability (WD) can effect up to 50% of the arthritis population even in the early stages of the disease, and this only increases with disease duration. WD not only constitutes a financial burden for patients and their families and an economic burden for society but it has a negative impact on self-esteem and opportunities to socialize, and is associated with poorer quality of life (QoL).

Determinants of WD are relatively consistent between different conditions. Disease activity, pain, and physical functioning along with age, socio-economic status, and lower education are all associated with WD. The nature of work also appears to be an important predictor of retaining employment. The association between educational level and WD is often attributed to the type of work performed, with physically demanding jobs linked with increased WD.

Relationships

The challenges of rheumatic disease are thought to burden relationships, as they may lead to increased levels of irritability, bad temper, dependency and isolation, and decreasing interest in sexual activity. Sexual functioning has important implications on personal relationships, and overall QoL and 50% of arthritis patients report sexual dysfunction. Physical limitations due to rheumatic stiffness and limited mobility are the principal predictors of sexual disability, but diminished desire and satisfaction are also reported across rheumatic conditions with psychosocial variables such as depression, anxiety, and body image all playing a role.

In contrast to the above, it is important to note that a large number of patients with RA report experiencing interpersonal benefits after their diagnosis, such as an appreciation of the support offered by loved ones. Thus, interpersonal relationships can not only be negatively affected by a diagnosis of arthritis but can also be strengthened at a time of increased stress and uncertainly.

Social support

Social support is the process by which interpersonal relationships promote well-being by buffering stress and protecting people from a decline in health. Social support involves family, friends, healthcare professionals, and patient groups, who offer emotional as well as practical support. Social support has been conceptualised as structural (the number of people in a person's network) and functional (a person's evaluation of the quality of the support they receive). Research suggests it is the quality rather than quantity of social support which is important to well-being. The provision of support implies a shared understanding of need, what is required, when, and an ability to negotiate the provision of support at a time when the provider is ready to offer it.

Support can not only be positive but also potentially problematic, when it may be perceived as non-supportive. Problematic support has been linked with increased depression and when patients experience greater problematic support in association with low positive support they may report more arthritis-related symptoms. Problematic support has also been found to predict depression and is linked with lower family functioning and life satisfaction in RA.[14] In fact, spousal criticism in RA has been associated with both depression and anxiety. Conversely, satisfaction with social support has been associated with promoting adaptive coping strategies where greater use of cognitive reframing, emotional expression, and problem-solving in association with arthritis-related pain are used.

Psychosocial well-being

Quality of life

QoL refers to the physical, psychological, and social impact of a chronic illness on a patients' life. Recommendations now state that QoL should be systematically assessed within routine clinic time to establish the impact of the rheumatic disease on the patient's daily life. Impaired QoL in physical, mental, and social domains has been reported for those with arthritis when compared to both the general population and other chronic conditions.[15,16]

It is important to recognize that QoL is not associated with disease activity or damage but has been linked with age and gender as well as a number of psychosocial variables. Physical QoL has been associated consistently with symptoms such as pain and physical function, whereas mental health QoL has been linked with increased levels of depression, anxiety, and poor social support.[17] The measurement of QoL in clinical practice is important as it acknowledges the impact arthritis is having from the patient's perspective.

Mood

We have already noted the impact that arthritis symptoms, as well as the physical and social consequences of arthritis, can have on depressed mood. Depression is of particular concern in arthritis as research suggests that the presence of clinical depression increases the risk of mortality.[18] Depression affects 15–66% of the arthritis population and anxiety 13–70%. However, the occurrence of depression in SLE is more complex due to the presence of neurological symptoms in almost half of patients. This co-occurrence has led some to suggest that it is difficult to distinguish whether depression in SLE is indicative of central nervous system involvement or whether it reflects the psychological impact of a long-term condition.

The prevalence of depression in RA is greater than in the general population but similar to other chronic conditions, thus reflecting the general effects of living with a chronic illness. Research has shown that soon after diagnosis RA is characterized by more anxiety and established RA with depression.[19] This may be because early on patients are dealing with the shock of diagnosis and uncertainty about the future, while over time the increased levels of disability and pain provoke higher levels of depression.

Besides the impact physical and symptomatic changes have upon mood in arthritis, the beliefs and cognitions a patient holds about their disease also play a role. For example, those who see more negative consequences to their arthritis tend to be more depressed.[20] Conversely, depression also appears to have an impact on beliefs. For example, those suffering from depression are less likely to believe in medication effectiveness and importance, thus suggesting that depression may impact upon medication adherence. Depressed mood is generally associated with dramatically reduced perceptions of QoL and physical functioning, and individuals with high levels of depression may restrict their social activities and become isolated as a result of this. Taken together, these findings illustrate the difficulty in establishing causal relations between mood and other measures in arthritis as the effects are likely to be bidirectional.

Impact of psychological variables on health status and well-being

Research suggests that the consequences of arthritis are dependent upon how individuals interpret their illness, how others respond to their needs, and aspects of their environment. A number of psychological concepts have been used in attempting to account for the mediation between disease and its consequences, and it is to these that we now turn (see Figure 26.1).

Coping

There are many stressors for someone with arthritis. These include accepting the diagnosis, adjusting to the medical treatment and consequences of the condition, and uncertainty about the future. People with arthritis use different coping strategies in an attempt to reduce the impact of these stressors. Research on the ways in

which individuals cope with arthritis has been growing in recent years and there are many classification systems and ways of measuring this concept.

One classification has been between active and passive coping strategies. Active coping involves taking action or exerting efforts to remove or circumvent the stressor. In contrast, passive strategies focus on withdrawing or passing control on to something or someone else. In RA the literature suggests that passive coping strategies are linked to increased levels of pain, depression, and anxiety. Similarly, avoidant coping—another maladaptive strategy—tends to have negative outcomes in both cross-sectional and longitudinal studies.[21] In contrast, active coping has been associated with increased social support[22] and less pain, disability, and depression.[23]

Taken together these studies suggest that coping strategies in arthritis are important determinants of health status. However, as with most chronic diseases, rheumatological conditions are not static and change over time. This requires a continual adjustment to new demands if coping is to remain successful.

Beliefs

Beliefs about the disease, its treatments, and what one can do about it also have an impact on outcomes. These beliefs act as a mediator between the disease and adaptation, and are important in the management of arthritis.

Self-efficacy

Self-efficacy is one such belief and concerns an individual's belief in their ability to undertake a task. In a condition such as arthritis, which involves the patient managing aspects of the disease and its treatment, this concept is fundamental to good health and well-being. Measures of self-efficacy can be general, as to how one behaves in the world, or specific to arthritis.

In a 2-year longitudinal study low self-efficacy was related to increased RA-related pain, fatigue, disability, and poor QoL. In fact high self-efficacy at the start of the study was related to improved health status at follow-up.[24] Patients who report greater self-efficacy also experience less depression, are more physically active, and adhere more closely to medication regimes.

Beliefs about arthritis

How people perceive their illness and the beliefs they hold in relation to their condition has been termed illness perceptions. As part of the self-regulation or common sense model,[25] cognitions are said to provide patients with a framework for coping with and understanding their illness. Overall the perceptions patients have about their arthritis tend not to be related to clinical measures but do correlate significantly with the impact of the condition on psychological well-being, disability, depression, and QoL.[26]

Viewing the consequences of arthritis as being more serious, feeling less control over the illness, and believing that it can be cured has been associated with increased levels of disability and poorer physical and social functioning[26,27] as well as future levels of depression, anxiety and pain.[20,28] Not only are the beliefs a patient holds important, but when they are in agreement with a partner this results in better adjustment in the future,[29] thus acknowledging the importance of the social environment as an influence on the impact of arthritis.

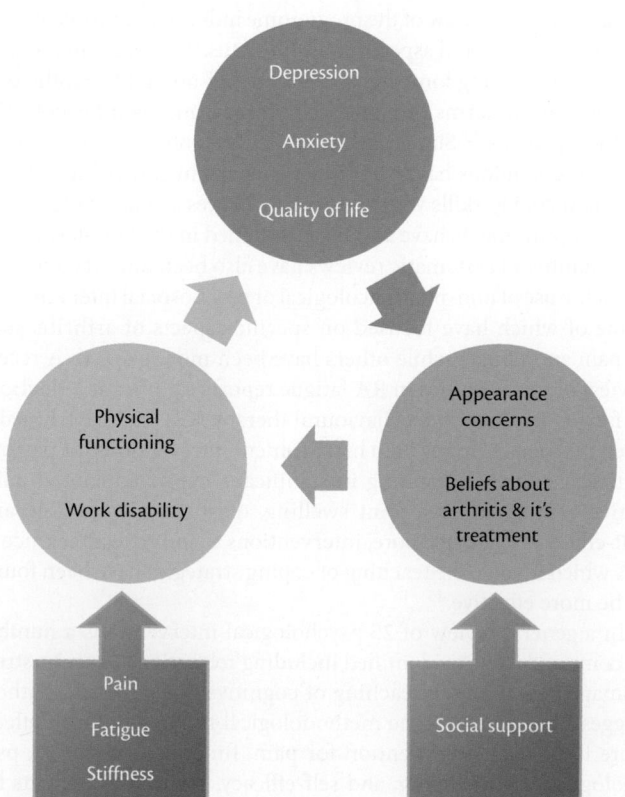

Fig. 26.1 Representation of the impact of clinical, social, and psychosocial factors on psychological well-being.

Appearance concerns

It is not surprising that patients with arthritis can have concerns about their appearance, as many rheumatic conditions are characterized by inflammation which can cause disability and disfigurement. Disfigurement of the hands and feet is common and these changes can impact upon not only psychological well-being but also social interactions. In fact, how a person perceives their appearance contributes to levels of depression in patients with RA and SLE.[30]

Patients with arthritis often speak of embarrassment, self-consciousness, and distress about their appearance and this tends to be in relation to their joints. The hands are of particular concern, with reports of anger, shyness, disgust, and shame, suggesting that feelings of stigmatization may be related to the visible and public nature of RA.[31] These feelings can often lead to the avoidance of social situations and an increased desire for surgical intervention.[32,33] Similarly, changes to the appearance of the feet are also of concern, particularly for women, who describe a loss of femininity and sexuality as a result of prescribed footwear. The choices available to these women, as well as the associated disfigurement, may force them to take on an altered body image and hence change their social behaviour by either covering themselves or avoiding social interaction.

Adherence and beliefs about treatment

Approximately 60% of patients with arthritis are at some point non-adherent to medications. Non-adherence is complex; it can be either unintentional (e.g. memory failure) or intentional (i.e. making a deliberate choice). The most frequently cited reasons tend to be unintentional and include changes in daily routines and not being able to obtain a refill. Intentional reasons for non-adherence are much more complicated and include the beliefs the patient holds about a specific medication and their overall attitude towards taking medications in general. Broadly speaking, lower adherence has been associated with negative beliefs about the potential side effects of medications such as non-steroidal anti-inflammatory drugs (NSAIDs) and disease-modifying anti-rheumatic drugs (DMARDs), lower perceived efficacy of the treatment,[34] a belief that the medication is unnecessary, that medications in general are overused,[35,36] and fear of addiction.[37]

Adherence to lifestyle recommendations such as changes to diet, exercise, physical therapy, clinic appointments, and the use of assistive devices makes the regimen complex for many patients. Adherence to these behaviours is also suboptimal. Patient beliefs about the causes of RA, flare-ups, and whether the treatment advice is compatible with the patient's coping system and feelings of self-efficacy have been shown to predict adherence to some of these behaviours.[38]

Psychosocial interventions

As there is clear evidence for the role of psychological variables in arthritis and because these factors are potentially modifiable, a number of psychosocial interventions have been developed. These attempt to modify the individuals' understanding, beliefs, coping style, and social support in order to influence psychological well-being and health status. Many of these interventions include disease information and a range of skills to help enhance their ability to manage the disease.

Providing information is a small but significant component that appears integral to most interventions. Education-based interventions have found to increase knowledge among participants,[39] and in some studies to produce small short-term effects on disability, joint count, patient global assessment, psychological status, and depression. There is, however, no evidence for long-term benefits in adults with RA.[40] The behavioural and cognitive techniques taught to participants are therefore vital.

Most psychosocial interventions are derived, at least in part, from theories and this will determine the components incorporated in the intervention. For example, those that are based on social learning theory aim to enhance patients' self-efficacy to manage their disease. Others attempt to influence beliefs about symptoms and disability and use a cognitive behavioural framework. Some focus on the social environment and aim to improve a patients' ability to enlist social support. These interventions may include training in cognitive pain management, joint protection, exercise, communication skills, and problem-solving, among other techniques.

Interventions can be delivered by healthcare professionals to either individuals or groups and usually take place in a hospital setting, although some have been delivered by telephone or using a self-instruction manual or computer program.

The best-known psychosocial intervention is the Arthritis Self-Management Programme (ASMP). The intervention, set within a self-efficacy framework, aims to enhance a patient's perceived ability to control various aspects of their arthritis through skills mastery, modelling, reinterpretation of symptoms, and persuasion. This programme differs from many others in that it is community based and delivered by trained lay leaders who themselves have arthritis. Groups can include people with different types of arthritis and it has broadened further to include people with a variety of chronic conditions. A 12-year review of the programme indicated improved behaviour, self-efficacy, and aspects of health status.[41] Subsequent research in the United Kingdom suggests benefits of up of 12 months post intervention in terms of mood, self-efficacy, and pain for both OA and RA patients.[42] Similar self-management interventions in other arthritic conditions have also been beneficial in enhancing self-efficacy and coping skills while decreasing depression and fatigue, and these improvements have also been sustained in the long-term.

A number of systematic reviews have also been undertaken looking at the use of non-pharmacological or psychosocial interventions, some of which have focused on specific aspects of arthritis such as pain and fatigue while others have been more general. A recent review of seven studies in RA fatigue reports significant reductions in fatigue for cognitive behavioural therapy (CBT).[43] CBT has also been the focus of many pain management interventions for patients with RA and OA, resulting in significant improvements in pain, active coping, anxiety, joint swelling, disability, depression, and self-efficacy.[44] Furthermore, interventions to improve adherence in RA which involve the teaching of coping strategies have been found to be more effective.[45]

In a general review of 25 psychological interventions a number of components were identified including relaxation, imagery, stress management, and the teaching of cognitive coping skills. Authors suggest that despite some methodological flaws, significant effects were found post intervention for pain, functional disability, psychological status, coping, and self-efficacy. Long-term benefits for tender joints, psychological status, and coping were also found. However, no clear or consistent patterns emerged as to which types of interventions were more beneficial. Findings do however, suggest that these psychological interventions may be more effective for patients who have had the illness for a shorter period of time.[46]

Conclusion

Research on the psychological factors associated with rheumatic disease has shown that attempts to predict disability and psychological well-being need to incorporate how individuals perceive their disease, how they try to deal with the stresses it creates, and factors in their social environments. This has spawned a number of non-pharmacological interventions where there now exists some evidence for efficacy.

References

1. Dickens C, McGowan L, Clark-Carter D, Creed F. Depression in rheumatoid arthritis: a systematic review of the literature with meta-analysis. *Psychosomat Med* 2002;64(1):52–60.

2. Westhoff G, Buttgereit F, Gromnica-Ihle E, Zink A. Morning stiffness and its influence on early retirement in patients with recent onset rheumatoid arthritis. *Rheumatology* 2008;47(7):980–984.

3. Wolfe F, Hawley DJ, Wilson K. The prevalence and meaning of fatigue in rheumatic disease. *J Rheumatol* 1996;23(8):1407–1417.

4. Ad Hoc Committee on Systemic Lupus Erythematosus Response Criteria for Fatigue. Measurement of fatigue in systemic lupus erythematosus: A systematic review. *Arthritis Care Res* 2007;57(8):1348–1357.

5. Da Costa D, Dritsa M, Bernatsky S et al. Dimensions of fatigue in systemic lupus erythematosus: relationship to disease status and behavioral and psychosocial factors. *J Rheumatol* 2006;33(7):1282–1288.

6. Mancuso CA, Rincon M, Sayles W, Paget SA. Psychosocial variables and fatigue: a longitudinal study comparing individuals with rheumatoid arthritis and healthy controls. *J Rheumatol* 2006;33(8):1496–1502.

7. Repping-Wuts H, Fransen J, Van Achterberg T, Bleijenberg G, Van Riel P. Persistent severe fatigue in patients with rheumatoid arthritis. *J Clin Nurs* 2007;16(11c):377–383.

8. Omdal R, Waterloo K, Koldingsnes W, Husby G, Mellgren SI. Fatigue in patients with systemic lupus erythematosus: the psychosocial aspects. *J Rheumatol* 2003;30[2]:283–287.

9. Mckinley PS, Ouellette SC, Winkel GH. The contributions of disease activity, sleep patterns, and depression to fatigue in systemic lupus erythematosus. *Arthritis Rheum* 1995;38(6):826–834.

10. Jump RL, Robinson ME, Armstrong AE et al. Fatigue in systemic lupus erythematosus: contributions of disease activity, pain, depression, and perceived social support. *J Rheumatol* 2005;32(9):1699–1705.

11. Lorish C, Abraham N, Austin J. Disease and psychosocial factors related to physical functioning in rheumatoid arthritis. *J Rheumatol* 1991;18(8):1150–1157.

12. Katz P, Yelin E. Prevalence and correlates of depressive symptoms among persons with rheumatoid arthritis. *J Rheumatol* 1993;20(5):790–796.

13. Scott D, Smith C, Kingsley G. Joint damage and disability in rheumatoid arthritis: an updated systematic review. *Clin Exp Rheumatol* 2003;21(Suppl 31):S20–S27.

14. Coty MB, Wallston KA. Problematic social support, family functioning, and subjective well-being in women with rheumatoid arthritis. *Women Health* 2010;50(1):53–70.

15. Jolly M. How does quality of life of patients with systemic lupus erythematosus compare with that of other common chronic illnesses? *J Rheumatol* 2005;32(9):1706–1708.

16. Jakobsson U, Allberg I. Pain and quality of life among older people with rheumatoid arthritis and/or osteoarthritis: a literature review. *J Clin Nurs* 2002;11(4):430–443.

17. Kojima M, Kojima T, Ishiguro N et al. Psychosocial factors, disease status, and quality of life in patients with rheumatoid arthritis. *J Psychosomat Res* 2009;67(5):425–431.

18. Ang DC, Choi H, Kroenke K, Wolfe F. Comorbid depression is an independent risk factor for mortality in patients with rheumatoid arthritis. *J Rheumatol* 2005;32(6):1013–1019.

19. Isik A, Koca S, Ozturk A, Mermi O. Anxiety and depression in patients with rheumatoid arthritis. *Clin Rheumatol* 2007;26(6):872–878.

20. Sharpe L, Sensky T, Allard S. The course of depression in recent onset rheumatoid arthritis: The predictive role of disability, illness perceptions, pain and coping. *J Psychosomat Res* 2001;51(6):713–719.

21. Ramjeet J, Smith J, Adams M. The relationship between coping and psychological and physical adjustment in rheumatoid arthritis: a literature review. *J Clin Nurs* 2008;17(11c):418–428.

22. Zyrianova Y, Kelly B, Sheehan J, McCarthy C, Dinan T. The psychological impact of arthritis: the effects of illness perception and coping. *Irish J Med Sci* 2011;180[1]:203–210.

23. Brown GK, Nicassio PM. Development of a questionnaire for the assessment of active and passive coping strategies in chronic pain patients. *Pain* 1987;31(1):53–64.

24. Brekke M, Hjortdahl P, Kvien TK. Self-efficacy and health status in rheumatoid arthritis: a two-year longitudinal observational study. *Rheumatology* 2001;40(4):387–392.

25. Leventhal H, Brissette I, Leventhal EA. The common-sense model of self-regulation of health and illness. In: Cameron LD, Leventhal H (eds) *The self-regulation of health and illness behaviour.* Routledge, New York, 2003:42–65.

26. Graves H, Scott DL, Lempp H, Weinman J. Illness beliefs predict disability in rheumatoid arthritis. *J Psychosomat Res* 2009;67(5):417–423.

27. Scharloo M, Kaptein AA, Weinman J et al. Illness perceptions, coping and functioning in patients with rheumatoid arthritis, chronic obstructive pulmonary disease and psoriasis. *J Psychosomat Res* 1998;44(5):573–585.

28. Groarke A, Curtis R, Coughlan R, Gsel A. The impact of illness representations and disease activity on adjustment in women with rheumatoid arthritis: A longitudinal study. *Psychol Health* 2005;20(5):597–613.

29. Sterba KR, DeVellis RF, Lewis MA et al. Effect of couple illness perception congruence on psychological adjustment in women with rheumatoid arthritis. *Health Psychol* 2008;27(2):221–229.

30. Monaghan SM, Sharpe L, Denton F et al. Relationship between appearance and psychological distress in rheumatic diseases. *Arthritis Care Res* 2007;57(2):303–309.

31. Lempp H, Scott D, Kingsley G. The personal impact of rheumatoid arthritis on patients' identity: a qualitative study. *Chronic Illn* 2006;2(2):109–120.

32. Bogoch ER, Judd MGP. The hand: a second face? *J Rheumatol* 2002; 29(12):2477–2483.

33. Vamos M. *Body image in rheumatoid arthritis: The relevance of hand appearance to desire for surgery.* Br J Med Psychol 1990;63(3):267–277.

34. Garcia-Gonzalez A, Richardson M et al. Treatment adherence in patients with rheumatoid arthritis and systemic lupus erythematosus. *Clin Rheumatol* 2008;27(7):883–889.

35. Treharne GJ, Lyons AC, Kitas GD. Medication adherence in rheumatoid arthritis: effects of psychosocial factors. *Psychol Health Med* 2004;9(3):337–349.

36. de Thurah A, Norgaard M, Harder I, Stengaard-Pedersen K. Compliance with methotrexate treatment in patients with rheumatoid arthritis: influence of patients' beliefs about the medicine. A prospective cohort study. *Rheumatol Int* 2010;30(11):1441–1448.

37. Sale JEM, Gignac M, Hawker G. How bad does the pain have to be? A qualitative study examining adherence to pain medication in older adults with osteoarthritis. *Arthritis Care Res* 2006;55(2):272–278.

38. Brus H, van de Laar M, Taal E, Rasker J, Wiegman O. Determinants of compliance with medication in patients with rheumatoid arthritis: the importance of self-efficacy expectations. *Patient Educ Couns* 1999; 36(1):57–64.

39. Hirano PC, Laurent DD, Lorig K. Arthritis patient education studies, 1987–1991: a review of the literature. *Patient Educ Couns* 1994;24(1):9–54.

40. Riemsma RP, Kirwan JR, Taal E, Rasker JJ. Patient education for adults with rheumatoid arthritis. *Cochrane Database Syst Rev* 2003;2:CD003688.

41. Lorig K, Holman H. Arthritis self-management studies: a twelve-year review. *Health Educ Q* 1993;20(1):17–28.

42. Barlow JH, Turner AP, Wright CC. A randomized controlled study of the Arthritis Self-Management Programme in the UK. *Health Educ Res* 2000;15(6):665–680.

43. Neill J, Belan I, Ried K. Effectiveness of non-pharmacological interventions for fatigue in adults with multiple sclerosis, rheumatoid arthritis, or systemic lupus erythematosus: a systematic review. *J Adv Nurs* 2006;56(6):617–635.

44. Dixon KE, Keefe FJ, Scipio CD, Perri LM, Abernethy AP. Psychological interventions for arthritis pain management in adults: a meta-analysis. *Health Psychol* 2007;26(3):241–250.

45. Elliott R. Poor adherence to medication in adults with rheumatoid arthritis: reasons and solutions. *Dis Manag Health Outcomes* 2008;16(1):13–29.

46. Astin JA, Beckner W, Soeken K, Hochberg MC, Berman B. Psychological interventions for rheumatoid arthritis: A meta-analysis of randomized controlled trials. *Arthritis Care Res* 2002;47(3):291–302.

The impact of rheumatic disease

CHAPTER 27

Epidemiology and the rheumatic diseases

Deborah P. M. Symmons

Introduction

Epidemiology is the study of the distribution and determinants of disease in populations. Clinical epidemiology is the study of the distribution and determinants of outcomes in populations with a specific disease. Understanding the epidemiology of disease is important from a number of perspectives. First, it is important for those planning and paying for health services at any level to know the likely burden of disease (i.e. the number of cases and the spectrum of severity) in their locality. Secondly, it is the starting point of the diagnostic process for any clinician. Diagnosis is an iterative process based on likelihoods of specific diseases or conditions.[1] Thus, as a patient with joint pain arrives for their first rheumatology consultation, the 'preconsultation' likelihood of osteoarthritis (OA) or systemic lupus erythematosus (SLE) varies according to the age, gender, and ethnicity of the patient. As the consultation proceeds and more information is elicited (e.g. on additional symptoms and signs, weight, or occupation) the likelihood of each diagnosis changes and further investigations and so on are directed towards the most likely diagnoses.

Whereas assessing the distribution of disease is largely a descriptive process; assessing the determinants of disease requires a comparison group. For example, only by comparing the occurrence of disease in smokers and non-smokers can one conclude whether or not smoking is likely to be a determinant of that disease.

This chapter addresses the basic concepts of epidemiology and epidemiological study design with specific reference to being able to apply these to the diagnosis and care of the patient with a musculoskeletal disorder. The epidemiology of specific musculoskeletal conditions is covered in the relevant chapters of this book, but this chapter includes templates of the age- and sex-specific incidence and prevalence of the most common musculoskeletal disorders taken, as far as possible, from the single perspective of primary care in the United Kingdom, in order to give some indication of their relative frequency in different age groups. The chapter also includes a summary of identified risk factors for the development of the more common musculoskeletal disorders.

Case definition

The first step in describing the occurrence of disease is to decide on a case definition. Comparison between studies is facilitated by the use of a widely accepted and validated case definition.

Unfortunately the vast majority of rheumatic diseases do not have a single pathognomic feature, such as characteristic histology or a biomarker that is found uniquely in that disease and no other. Thus case definitions have to be based on combinations of clinical, laboratory, and imaging characteristics. The methodology for developing and validating case definitions has been progressively refined over the decades, leading to the need to revisit case definitions at regular intervals. In the past, case definitions have generally used the 'physician's opinion' as the gold standard. However, the most recent case definition for rheumatoid arthritis (RA)[2] is based on the 'physician's decision to start methotrexate' in a patient with recent-onset inflammatory arthritis. The development of an acceptable case definition comprises a series of steps in which a list of variables likely to discriminate, in combination, between the disease in question and other similar diseases is assembled, tested, and refined[3]; then a large series of cases (according to the gold standard) and controls (who have similar diseases) is collected from a wide variety of sources, together with information on the list of variables. Then statistical modelling is used to develop algorithms which discriminate between the cases and controls with the greatest accuracy. Finally the algorithms are tested in a wide range of settings (e.g. different countries, different stages of disease, patients with a variety of comorbidities). Generally speaking, even when the process has been very rigorous, the accuracy of the algorithm is not sufficient for it to be used to diagnose disease in the individual patient. This is particularly the situation for diseases which have a wide variety of manifestations, not all of which can be encompassed within the criteria set. Thus generally the case definitions are referred to as 'classification' rather than 'diagnostic' criteria. Classification criteria are useful to ensure that homogenous groups of patients are being compared in studies of disease occurrence and as entry criteria for clinical trials and other clinical research studies. This ensures that the results of such studies can be generalized from one population to another. Many of the case definitions in current use have been developed by the American College of Rheumatology (www.rheumatology.org/practice/clinical/classification) and European League against Rheumatism (www.eular.org/) and can be accessed via their websites.

Disease classification

Most of the sources discussed in this chapter classify musculoskeletal conditions in accordance with the International Classification

Table 27.1 ICD codes for musculoskeletal disorders

Condition	ICD7	ICD8	ICD9	ICD10
	1955	1965	1975	1992
Rheumatoid arthritis	722.0[a]	712.1, 712.3	714.0–714.2	M05, M06
Juvenile idiopathic arthritis	722.0[a]	712.0	714.3	M08, M09
Ankylosing spondylitis	722.1	712.4	720.2–720.9	M45
Gout	288	274	712.0*274.0†	M10
Polymyalgia rheumatica	726.3	446.3	725	M35.3
Osteoarthritis	723.0	713.0	715	M15-M19
Systemic lupus erythematosus	456[a]	734.1	710.0	M32
Scleroderma	710.0[a]	734.0	710.1	M34
Psoriatic arthritis	706.0	696.0	696.0	M07.0–M07.3
Osteoporosis	733[a]	723.0	733.0	M80, M81
Fracture of neck of femur	N820	N820	820	S72.0
Fractured vertebra	733[a]	723.9[a]	733.1	S32.0

[a]Includes other conditions.

of Diseases (ICD).[4] This international agreed system of nomenclature and terminology is now in its 10th revision,[5] and the 11th revision is in an advanced state of preparation. The ICD codes for various musculoskeletal conditions are shown in Table 27.1. The changing codes reflect the evolving understanding of the nature of these disorders over the past half century. For example, ankylosing spondylitis was originally thought to be a variant of RA (until ICD9).

Describing the occurrence of disease (disease distribution)

The occurrence of disease is generally described in terms of incidence and prevalence.

Incidence

The *incidence* of disease should be expressed as a rate, i.e. the number of new cases occurring in the population at risk in a given time period (usually 1 year). In order to study incidence it is important to be able to determine the date of onset of symptoms. Sometimes the date of diagnosis is used as the incidence date, but this is influenced by many factors such as access to appropriate clinicians and the diagnostic acumen of those clinicians. Incidence can be studied by performing two cross-sectional studies 1 year apart and identifying those who have the disease at the second time point who did not have it at the first. However, more commonly new cases are ascertained as they present in either primary or secondary care, often, these days, from computerized records of the reason for consultation. It is difficult to keep the same population of people under surveillance for a year or longer—people move into or out of an area, some people may die. Thus it is better to express the denominator as person-years of observation with each person contributing the appropriate proportion of a person-year according to the proportion of the year that they spent within the sampling

frame for new cases (which might be a particular geographical area or on the list of a particular primary care physician). Individuals should only be included in the numerator of a study of incidence if they are also in the denominator.

Incidence can be expressed as the number of people who experience a disease or condition for the first time during that year or the number of new episodes of a disease or condition there are during the year (called *episode incidence*—in which individuals may contribute more than one episode to the numerator). For health service planners it may be more useful to know the number of new episodes, for example of back pain in a year, than the number of people who experience back pain for the first time. On the other hand, researchers interested in the aetiology of back pain may wish to study people who are experiencing their first ever attack of back pain or those who are experiencing recurrent attacks, so it may be important to be able to distinguish these. *Cumulative incidence* is the number of people who have ever had an episode of the disease in question (e.g. neck pain) divided by the number of people in the population at risk.

Prevalence

The *prevalence* of disease is the proportion of the population who have the disease in question at a particular point in time. In the case of chronic, non-resolving, and non-fatal conditions cumulative incidence and prevalence may be the same or very similar. Prevalence may be established in a cross-sectional population survey or, again more often these days, from computerized records of primary care physicians or health maintenance organizations. This may require adapting the case definition into a suitable format for use with computerized data, in which the completeness of information on some variables may be rather poor. As with studies of incidence, it is important that individuals should only be included in the numerator if they are also in the denominator. The denominator should only include those at risk of developing the disease.

Thus studies of the prevalence of childhood arthritis should define the upper age limit for the study and only include those below that age limit in the numerator and the denominator. It is a very common error to take studies of the prevalence of a musculoskeletal condition in the adult population and then apply the figures to the whole population. For example, the prevalence of rheumatoid arthritis (RA) is around 0.8–1% of the adult population.[6] However, many publications estimate the number of individuals with RA in a given population by applying the figure of 0.8–1% to the whole population, thus assuming that the prevalence of RA is the same in children as in adults. This leads to massive overestimation of the number of cases.

Disease duration

Incidence and prevalence are related by the equation:

incidence × disease duration = prevalence

Disease duration is influenced by recovery and death. Conditions with a similar incidence rate may have very different prevalences if one has a short duration (e.g. gout) and another a long duration (e.g. RA); or one a high case fatality rate and another a low one. Treatments which prolong life, for example renal dialysis for patients with scleroderma and renal failure, may increase prevalence without any change in incidence.

Studies of incidence and prevalence

There are several available methods of measuring disease occurrence. In the past this was done predominantly using cross-sectional surveys. This is still the most appropriate method for common conditions such as back pain, for which sufferers do not always seek medical attention. Such surveys may either be specifically designed for the purpose or may be incorporated into government-sponsored national or regional health interview or health examination surveys which can study several medical conditions and lifestyle factors simultaneously. Examples of musculoskeletal health surveys include the COPCORD programme which has conducted surveys in a wide range of countries.[7] Examples of government-sponsored health surveys include the Health Survey for England which has been conducted annually since 1991 (www.dh.gov.uk/en/Publicationsandstatistics/PublishedSurvey/HealthSurvey For England /Healthsurveybackground/index.htm) and the National Health and Nutrition Examination Surveys (NHANES) in the United States (www.cdc.gov/nchs/nhanes/about_nhanes.htm).

For less common conditions—or for conditions where patients generally seek medical attention—studies of disease occurrence can take place in the primary or secondary care setting. As might be expected, the incidence and prevalence of conditions measured by attendance at primary care is lower than the prevalence of self-reported symptoms. Examples of primary care databases that can be interrogated for the incidence and prevalence of musculoskeletal disorders include the General Practice Research Database (GPRD) (www.gprd.com/) in the United Kingdom and health administration databases such as Kaiser Permanente in the United States. The GPRD is a computerized database based on the consultation records of approximately 630 practices. Data are currently being collected on around 5 million people, which is just under 10% of the entire United Kingdom population.

Much information on the incidence and prevalence of common musculoskeletal conditions has come from the Rochester Epidemiology project.[8] The Mayo Clinic in Rochester, Minnesota, together with the Olmsted medical practice, provides the only source of medical care to the local population (which is predominantly of Scandinavian extraction) of around 100 000 residents. These two organizations maintain a single medical record for all medical contacts for each resident. These records have been indexed by diagnosis and procedure since 1910 and can be retrieved with considerable accuracy.

The occurrence of disease may be described in terms of person (by age, sex, occupation, and ethnicity), place (e.g. country or region) and time (looking for secular changes or birth cohort effects). Studies of incidence and prevalence which present their results only for the whole population or the whole adult population are of limited value beyond the local situation. Ideally studies should be large enough to present their results by age and gender. Thus, by a process known as standardization, it is then possible to apply the results from one study population to a different population in order to estimate the likely number of cases in the second population. Also it is possible to compare age- and sex-specific incidence and prevalence between populations, whereas any differences in disease frequency for the whole population may simply be due to differences in population structure. Over the next decades the age and sex structure of the population of most countries will change substantially—predominantly with an increased number of elderly people, particularly those aged over 80. This will have dramatic effects on the burden of musculoskeletal conditions, most of which increase in incidence and prevalence with age.

Mortality

Mortality is clearly an important outcome measure for many musculoskeletal disorders. Mortality may be expressed in a variety of ways. *Case fatality* is the probability of death among diagnosed cases of disease during a particular time period. It is calculated by dividing the number of deaths due to the disease in the specified time period by the number of cases of the disease alive at the beginning of the time period. For musculoskeletal disorders the 1 year or 5 year mortality of some connective tissue diseases or vasculitis may be of relevance. Similar figures can be used to discuss and present the 1 year or 5 year survival. More often it is of relevance to compare the all-cause (or cause-specific) mortality in a disease population with that of the local general population. These results are presented as *standardized mortality ratios* (SMRs). SMRs are calculated by a process called indirect standardization. The disease population (who must all be alive at the beginning of the period of the study) is divided into a number of age and gender groups (e.g. 10 year bands) and each death that occurs during the period of observation is assigned to one of these groups. The total time of observation for each patient is assigned to one or more of these age bands (as the patient ages they may contribute observation time to different age bands). Then the total time of observation for each band is calculated. The expected number of deaths for each age band for the person-time of observation may be estimated using published data (most countries and/or regions publish mortality rates for the general population). The SMR is the number of observed deaths divided by the number of expected deaths multiplied by 100. An SMR of 100 indicates that the disease population has the same mortality as would be expected from the general population.

SMRs cannot be directly compared between studies for a number of reasons: first, the background population may not be the same (in terms of geography, calendar time, age, and gender make-up); secondly, the period of observation may not be the same (the longer the period of observation the more the SMR is likely to approach 100 as, in the end, everyone dies and is expected to die).

Practical examples of relative disease frequency

Tables 27.2–27.5 show the estimated incidence and prevalence of the most common musculoskeletal disorders for men and women in the United Kingdom. These figures were assembled by conducting a literature search up to the end of 2010. To be eligible, studies had to include age- and sex-specific rates and be based on attendance in primary care in the United Kingdom. Where more than one relevant study was identified we selected the one which was based on the GPRD or the most recent one. For some diseases (SLE, scleroderma) only data from secondary care were available and for a few diseases (e.g. ankylosing spondylitis) data had to be taken from overseas. Until 1991 the Royal College of General Practitioners (RCGP) in the UK conducted a 10 yearly morbidity survey in the year of the national census.[9–12] A representative sample of GPs recorded the reason for every consultation and whether this was the first time that the patient had consulted with that complaint. The last RCGP morbidity survey

Table 27.2 Incidence of common musculoskeletal disorders in men

Incident cases per 100 000 males							
Condition (reference)	**Age 0–14**	**Age 15–24**	**Age 25–44**	**Age 45–64**	**Age 65–74**	**Age 75+**	**All ages[a]**
Inflammatory arthritis[13]	=Childhood arthritis	13	25	45	49	64	32
Childhood arthritis[14]	4	–	–	–	–	–	–
Ankylosing spondylitis[15]	1	16	23	8	4	4	12
Gout[14]	0	0	170	402	692	772	302
SLE[16]	0	0	1	1	1	2	1
Scleroderma[17]	–	–	–	–	–	–	0.1
Polymyalgia rheumatica[14]	0	0	4	17	118	301	37
Osteoarthritis[14]	0	11	103	1021	2194	2890	746
Back pain[12]	290	1860	3680	4550	3940	4220	3680
Hip fracture[b] [18]	–	–	–	42	140	491	17

[a]'All ages' rates apply to the adult population (i.e. 15+ years), with the exception of hip fracture (55+ years), inflammatory arthritis (16+ years), AS (16+ years), and back pain (16+ years).
[b]Age bands for incident hip fracture are 55–64, 65–74, 75+ years. 'All ages' is for 55+ years.

Table 27.3 Incidence of common musculoskeletal disorders in women

Incident cases per 100 000 females							
Condition (reference)	**Age 0–14**	**Age 15–24**	**Age 25–44**	**Age 45–64**	**Age 65–74**	**Age 75+**	**All ages[a]**
Inflammatory arthritis[13]	=Childhood arthritis	33	53	93	97	49	71
Childhood arthritis[14]	15	–	–	–	–	–	–
Ankylosing spondylitis[15]	1	4	5	3	1	0	3
Gout[14]	0	0	18	58	173	275	70
SLE[16]	3	3	6	8	6	2	6
Scleroderma[17]	0	–	–	–	–	–	0.6
Polymyalgia rheumatica[14]	0	0	5	75	255	405	91
Osteoarthritis[14]	–	6	122	1562	3226	3572	1197
Back pain[12]	460	2900	4610	5660	5000	4720	4670
Hip fracture[b] [18]	–	–	–	50	244	1573	578

[a]'All ages' rates apply to the adult population (i.e. 15+ years), with the exception of hip fracture (55+ years), inflammatory arthritis (16+ years), AS (16+ years), and back pain (16+ years).
[b]Age bands for incident hip fracture are 55–64, 65–74, 75+ years. 'All ages' is for 55+ years.

Table 27.4 Prevalence of common musculoskeletal disorders in men

Prevalent cases per 100,000 males

Condition (reference)	Age 0–14	Age 15–24	Age 25–44	Age 45–64	Age 65–74	Age 75+	All ages[a]
Rheumatoid arthritis[6]	= Childhood arthritis	10	20	580	1140	2180	440
Childhood arthritis [14]	30	10	8	5	4	3	–
Ankylosing spondylitis[12]	0	30	70	120	20	25	70
Gout[14]	0	20	400	1240	2080	2550	873
SLE[b] [19]	0	5	5	7	7	7	6
Scleroderma[20]	–	0	2	8	2	0	4
Polymyalgia rheumatica[14]	0	0	0	50	530	1330	140
Osteoarthritis[14]	0	10	170	2420	5780	8680	1830
Back pain[12]	350	2170	4710	6240	5340	5380	4810
Osteoporosis (of hip only)[21]	–	–	–	3490	5180	15640	5800
Disablement (mHAQ >0.5 + pain)[22]	–	1710	7920	16725	12010	18470	13830

[a]'All ages' rates apply to the adult population (i.e. 15+ years), with the exception of osteoporosis (50+ years), RA (16+ years), AS (16+ years), and back pain (16+ years).

[b]Age bands for prevalent SLE are 0–18, 15–24, 25–44, 45–59, 60–74, 75–84. 'All ages' is for 18+ years.

Table 27.5 Prevalence of common musculoskeletal disorders in women

Prevalent cases per 100 000 females

Condition (reference)	Age 0–14	Age 15–24	Age 25–44	Age 45–64	Age 65–74	Age 75+	All ages[a]
Rheumatoid arthritis[6]	= Childhood arthritis	63	160	1670	2330	2740	1110
Childhood arthritis [14]	40	13	11	7	5	4	–
Ankylosing spondylitis[12]	0	0	20	20	10	0	14
Gout[14]	0	0	30	160	450	940	192
SLE[b] [19]	2	30	70	88	71	12	63
Scleroderma [20]	0	0	9	35	28	14	22
Polymyalgia rheumatica[14]	0	0	10	160	930	1770	311
Osteoarthritis[14]	0	20	270	3770	9010	11780	3207
Back pain[12]	510	3300	5670	7360	6580	6260	5890
Osteoporosis (of hip only)[21]	–	–	–	7660	24350	49360	22500
Disablement (mHAQ >0.5 + pain)[22]	–	2420	9140	14380	18340	30740	17800

[a]'All ages' rates apply to the adult population (i.e. 15+ years), with the exception of osteoporosis (50+ years), RA (16+ years), AS (16+ years), and back pain (16+ years).

[b]Age bands for prevalent SLE are 0–18, 15–24, 25–44, 45–59, 60–74, 75–84 years. 'All ages' is for 18+ years.

was conducted in 1991. Since then a smaller sample of GPs (collectively termed the RCGP Research and Surveillance Centre) has continued to record the reason for every consultation. Where no published data from the GPRD were available, this was used as the source of the incidence and prevalence estimates. However, this source only records the reason for consultation to three digits of the ICD (which is adequate for some musculoskeletal disorders but not others). Some smoothing of figures has been done to provide internal consistency. As the published studies used were conducted at different time points and with varying definitions of the background population at risk they are not directly comparable and should be used as a guide to the relative frequency and burden of disease rather than an absolute indication of the number of cases.

These data show that, amongst these musculoskeletal conditions, back pain is the most frequent reason for consultation. The incidence of most musculoskeletal conditions in higher in women than in men, with the exception of ankylosing spondylitis, gout, and back pain. The incidence of most musculoskeletal conditions increases with age, with the exception of ankylosing spondylitis which peaks at age 25–44 and back pain which peaks at age 45–64.

These data show that the prevalence of most musculoskeletal conditions rises with age. The exceptions are scleroderma (possibly due to premature mortality), ankylosing spondylitis (possibly because patients cease to consult for this in older age), and back pain (reflecting the episodic nature of this complaint and the peak age of onset in middle age). Overall, 1 in 6 males and 1 in 5 females consults with a prevalent musculoskeletal condition each year.[14]

Describing the determinants of disease

Diseases do not occur at random. Although a few rheumatic diseases are the result of, for example, a single gene mutation or a single environmental trigger, most occur as a consequence of a complex interaction of genetic factors and environmental triggers. Although the basic structure of genes is constant throughout life, genes may be modified by, for example, methylation, or the gene product (protein) may be modified by, for example, citrullination. Thus the influence of a person's genetic make-up on disease susceptibility changes during the lifespan. Environmental risk factors are also very diverse and include lifestyle factors (e.g. smoking, diet, alcohol), occupational factors, infections, other medical conditions and their therapy, hormones, and air pollution among others. Some environmental factors may exert their influence many years before disease development and some quite close to the onset of symptoms. A variety of epidemiological study designs is available to investigate the associations between genetic and environmental risk factors and the subsequent development of disease. All involve the use of a comparison cohort (usually individuals without disease) so that exposure status may be compared between those with and without the disorder. This is known as analytical epidemiology, and is hypothesis testing as opposed to hypothesis generating. Increasingly complex statistical methodology and increasing computing power mean that it is possible to explore multiple risk factors and their interactions simultaneously.

Study designs for assessing determinants of disease or disease outcome

To be a determinant of disease or outcome, a risk factor must operate before the onset of disease or the outcome of interest. Thus study design should ideally incorporate the perspective of time. There are essentially three types of study design in epidemiology: cross-sectional, cohort, and case-control studies.[23] The reporting of observational studies in epidemiology is covered by the STROBE statement (STrengthening the Reporting of OBservational studies in Epidemiology).[24]

Cross-sectional studies

Cross-sectional studies collect information about disease and exposure status simultaneously. They can be used to demonstrate associations between, for example, obesity and osteoarthritis (OA), but they cannot determine the direction of association. In other words, they cannot discern between the hypothesis that obesity is associated with an increased risk of OA, and the hypothesis that OA is associated with an increased risk of obesity. There are now statistical methods to test whether a confounder such as physical activity acts as a 'mediator' of the link between obesity and OA in the context of a cross-sectional study. However, this still does not provide information on the direction of the association between obesity and OA.

Cohort studies

In cohort studies individuals are usually recruited before the onset of disease and then followed prospectively. The cohort can be divided into those with and without the exposure of interest and the relative incidence (relative risk) of disease in the two groups compared. Sometimes two separate cohorts are assembled—one with and one without the exposure of interest (which might be exposure to a particular drug or occupation). Cohort studies have the advantage that information about exposure status is collected at the start of the study and so they are not subject to recall bias. However, they have the disadvantage that individuals may have to be followed for long periods of time before the disease of interest develops and so a robust system of case ascertainment and follow-up is necessary.[25] They are thus expensive and often not as efficient as case-control studies in addressing a specific question. However, sometimes cohorts can be identified retrospectively. For example, the databases of health maintenance organizations and the GPRD already exist and may include information on some exposures, such as smoking, weight, and occupation as well as the subsequent medical history of millions of individuals. Such studies tend to suffer from large amounts of missing data on either or both of the exposure status or outcome, as the data were not collected with this purpose in mind. The investigator must establish the extent and degree of bias in missing data before deciding whether this is a viable setting to test the study hypothesis, and whether and how missing data should be imputed. Most computerized multivariable models can only include subjects with complete sets of data. Thus the more variables that are included in the analysis, the more critical becomes the issue of missing data.

Case-control studies

Like cohort studies, case-control studies include the perspective of time. In case-control studies subjects (cases) are selected on the basis that they have recently developed the disease or outcome of interest.[26] Information about exposure status is then collected retrospectively, perhaps by administering a questionnaire to the participants or searching their medical records.[27] The selection of an appropriate control group is often challenging. The controls should be subjects who would have been eligible to be cases if they had developed the disease. In matched case-control studies, the controls are matched to the cases for items that are not the immediate subject under study—such as age and sex. This makes the study design more efficient. However, if the study has a matched case-control design then the matching must be maintained during the analysis (i.e. the case and their control(s) are analysed as a unit according to whether they are concordant or discordant for the outcome of interest). If the number of available cases is limited (perhaps because the disease is rare) then the power of the study may be increased by recruiting more than one control per case. Results from case-control studies are expressed as odds ratios.

Some environmental predictive and protective factors for musculoskeletal conditions are listed in Table 27.6. For genetic risk factors for these diseases, readers are referred to the individual chapters.

Table 27.6 Some examples of environmental predictive and protective factors for musculoskeletal conditions

Musculoskeletal condition	Environmental risk factor	Protective factor	Risk factors for a poor prognosis
RA[28]	Female gender Smoking Obesity Silica exposure Nulliparity	Oral contraceptive use High fruit intake Moderate alcohol intake	Rheumatoid factor and anti-citrullinated peptide antibodies
Ankylosing spondylitis	Male gender Certain infections	Smoking	
Psoriatic arthritis[29,30]	Psoriasis Trauma		
Gout[31]	Alcohol (especially beer and spirits) Dietary factors (e.g. meat, seafood, sugary drinks, fructose) Early menopause Thiazide and loop diuretics Chemotherapy for cancer Components of the metabolic syndrome	Dietary factors (e.g. dairy produce, cherries, coffee)	
SLE[32]	Female gender Ethnicity[33,34] Current smoking Silica exposure Female hormones Some drugs	Moderate alcohol intake	Ethnicity Lower socio-economic status[35]
Scleroderma[36]	Female gender Ethnicity Silica exposure Organic solvents Some drugs (e.g. bleomycin)		
Polymyalgia rheumatica[37]	Female gender Age >50 Northern latitude		
Osteoarthritis of the hip[38]	Obesity (bilateral disease) Childhood hip disease (e.g. Perthes) Hip dysplasia High bone mass Certain occupations (e.g. farming)	Frequent squatting	
Osteoarthritis of the knee[38]	Obesity High bone mass Joint laxity Certain sports (e.g. football) and occupations	Smoking	Obesity Quadriceps muscle weakness Low vitamin C or D intake
Back pain[39]	Smoking Anatomical factors Psychosocial factors Certain occupations and activities Driving		Psychosocial factors
Osteoporosis[40]	Smoking Excess alcohol Low body mass index Reproductive factors: e.g. late menarche, early menopause Inflammatory disorders: e.g. RA, SLE Endocrine disorders: e.g. thyrotoxicosis, Cushing's, type 1 diabetes Malignancy Immobilization Drugs: e.g. corticosteroids, anticonvulsants, heparin	Obesity African origin	Conditions predisposing to falls [41]

RA, rheumatoid arthritis; SLE, systemic lupus erythematosus.

Clinical trials

Treatment is one of the major determinants of disease outcome. The role of treatment in disease outcome should be formally assessed in clinical trials. A clinical trial is an example of an epidemiological cohort study in which the exposure (treatment or placebo) is assigned to the patient by the investigator. In phase I and II trials there may be no comparison group and the trial is analysed as a descriptive, or hypothesis-generating study. In phase III trials the patient will be assigned (usually randomly) to receive either the study treatment or an active comparison or a placebo. The primary outcome measure must be specified in advance. Phase III trials are thus hypothesis testing and should be analysed like any other longitudinal cohort study comparing the outcome of interest in the two or more groups.[42] Clinical trial design is addressed in Chapter 30.

Pharmacoepidemiology

Pharmacoepidemiology is a relatively new discipline which studies the use of and the effects of drugs in large numbers of people.[43] Generally speaking pharmacoepidemiology studies focus on drug safety. Whereas treatment efficacy can be assessed in clinical trials (controlled epidemiological experiments), trials are usually too small to study any but the most common side effects. In addition, clinical trials often have strict inclusion criteria which mean that many patients who are prescribed a new medication after licensing would not have been eligible for inclusion in the trials—usually because of comorbidity. Thus studies of drug safety are usually conducted either by setting up registries specifically for the purpose or in the context of existing large administrative databases such as the GPRD or health maintenance organizations in the United States. Such databases provide many methodological challenges including their size, the large number of potential covariates and often also large amounts of missing data, the fact that the data were not collected for the purpose that they are now being used (and so terminology may not map), and individual patients may be followed in them for very varying and non-overlapping lengths of time.

Expressing the results of epidemiological studies—uses and abuses

As described above, the results of analytical epidemiological studies are usually expressed as either *relative risks* or as *odds ratios*. In both cases this describes the risk associated with a particular determinant in multiples of the background risk. The higher the multiple, the more likely the association is to be biologically important and statistically significant. However, from the patient's and clinician's perspective such figures are not easy to interpret—and can sound very alarmist. What matters to the patient is not, for example, by how many times a particular drug increases their risk of skin cancer, but what their *absolute risk* of skin cancer would be if they were to take the drug and if they were not. This difference is known as the *attributable risk* and should be expressed as a rate, e.g. 1 per 100 patient years of exposure. This can be interpreted as saying that, for every 100 patients treated with this drug for a year, one additional skin cancer will occur. In the case of a patient with RA treated with an anti-TNF agent it is more meaningful to be told that their absolute risk of admission to hospital in the next year with a serious infection is 1 in 20 than to be told that their risk of infection is increased by 60% compared to the background rate in patients with RA not treated with anti-TNF. Another meaningful way of looking at such data is in terms of number needed to treat or number needed to harm.[44] How many additional patients with RA would need to be treated with anti-TNF for a year in order to see one additional infection? Or, in the context of a clinical trial, how many patients would need to be treated with a new drug to, for example, prevent one patient from developing radiological erosions?

Much is often made of the high relative risk of myocardial infarction (MI) in young women with SLE. In the University of Pittsburgh lupus cohort, women with SLE aged 35–44 were more than 50 times as likely to have an MI as women without SLE in the Framingham Offspring study (RR 52.43; 95% CI 21.6–98.5).[45] And yet the background rate of MI in young women is so low that, even with this much higher relative risk, both the absolute rate and the rate of MI attributable to SLE is much higher in older than in younger women with SLE. Failure to appreciate this may lead to preventive strategies being targeted exclusively at the young.

The *population attributable risk fraction* is the proportion of cases of the disease in the population that can be attributed to the risk factor. This is a useful figure for those concerned with population health. So, for example, it would indicate what proportion of cases of RA would be prevented if no one smoked; or what proportion of cases of OA of the knee can be attributed to obesity.

Conclusion

In summary, the study of epidemiology in general and the epidemiology of specific musculoskeletal conditions in particular is the starting point in terms of understanding disease aetiology and making a diagnosis. All physicians need to know the relative frequency of the conditions which they see in the clinic, and their distribution by age and gender. An understanding of the environmental risk factors enables the likely diagnosis to be refined after taking a detailed history and may enable public health physicians to formulate preventive strategies. Patients look to their healthcare team to be able to predict their prognosis and to choose therapies accordingly. Epidemiology provides the methods for studying treatment interventions and evaluating their safety. An ability to interpret basic disease statistics and expressions of risk will enable the healthcare professional to explain to others the results of studies and also to rationalize sensational reports of disease cures or treatment harms which may appear in the popular press.

Acknowledgements

I would like to thank Sarah Parsons and Mary Ingram for their help in compiling the data for Tables 27.2–27.5.

References

1. Hennekens CH, Buring JE. Measures of disease frequency and association. In: Mayrent SL (ed.) *Epidemiology in medicine*. Little Brown, Boston, 1987:54–98.
2. Aletaha D, Neogi T, Silman AJ et al. 2010 rheumatoid arthritis classification criteria: an American College of Rheumatology/European League Against Rheumatism collaborative initiative. *Ann Rheum Dis* 2010;69(9):1580–1588.
3. Funovits J, Aletaha D, Bykerk V et al. The 2010 American College of Rheumatology/European League Against Rheumatism classification criteria for rheumatoid arthritis: methodological report phase I. *Ann Rheum Dis* 2010;69(9):1589–1595.

4. Israel RA. The history of the International Classification of Diseases. *Health Bull* (Edinb) 1991;49(1):62–66.

5. World Health Organization. *International statistical classification of diseases and related health problems*, 10th revision. WHO, Geneva, 1992.

6. Symmons D, Turner G, Webb R et al. The prevalence of rheumatoid arthritis in the United Kingdom: new estimates for a new century. *Rheumatology* (Oxford) 2002;41(7):793–800.

7. Haq SA, Rasker JJ, Darmawan J, Chopra A. WHO-ILAR-COPCORD in the Asia-Pacific: the past, present and future. *Int J Rheum Dis* 2008;11(1):4–10.

8. Maradit KH, Crowson CS, Gabriel SE. Rochester Epidemiology Project: a unique resource for research in the rheumatic diseases. *Rheum Dis Clin North Am* 2004;30(4):819–834, vii.

9. Logan WPD, Cushion AA. *Morbidity statistics from general practice.* H.M.S.O., London, 1958.

10. Office of Population Censuses and Surveys, Great Britain. Department of Health and Social Security, Royal College of General Practitioners. *Morbidity statistics from general practice.* H.M.S.O., London, 1979.

11. Royal College of General Practitioners, Office of Population Censuses and Surveys, Department of Health and Social Security. *Morbidity statistics from general practice: third national study 1981–1982.* HMSO, London, 1986.

12. McCormick A, Fleming D, Charlton J, et al. *Morbidity statistics from general practice: fourth national study 1991–92.* HMSO, London, 1995.

13. Wiles N, Symmons DP, Harrison B et al. Estimating the incidence of rheumatoid arthritis: trying to hit a moving target? *Arthritis Rheum* 1999;42(7):1339–1346.

14. Incidence and prevalence of diseases: unpublished data provided by the RCGP Research and Surveillance Centre (formerly the Birmingham Research Unit) during the period October 2005–June 2009.

15. Carbone LD, Cooper C, Michet CJ et al. Ankylosing spondylitis in Rochester, Minnesota, 1935–1989. Is the epidemiology changing? *Arthritis Rheum* 1992;35(12):1476–1482.

16. Nightingale AL, Farmer RD, de Vries CS. Incidence of clinically diagnosed systemic lupus erythematosus 1992–1998 using the UK General Practice Research Database. *Pharmacoepidemiol Drug Saf* 2006;15(9):656–661.

17. Silman A, Jannini S, Symmons D, Bacon P. An epidemiological study of scleroderma in the West Midlands. *Br J Rheumatol* 1988;27(4):286–290.

18. Lawrence TM, Wenn R, Boulton CT, Moran CG. Age-specific incidence of first and second fractures of the hip. *J Bone Joint Surg Br* 2010;B92(2):258–261.

19. Gourley IS, Patterson CC, Bell AL. The prevalence of systemic lupus erythematosus in Northern Ireland. *Lupus* 1997;6(4):399–403.

20. Allcock RJ, Forrest I, Corris PA, Crook PR, Griffiths ID. A study of the prevalence of systemic sclerosis in northeast England. *Rheumatology* (Oxford) 2004;43(5):596–602.

21. Kanis JA, Melton LJ, III, Christiansen C, Johnston CC, Khaltaev N. The diagnosis of osteoporosis. *J Bone Mineral Res* 1994;9(8):1137–1141.

22. Urwin M, Symmons D, Allison T et al. Estimating the burden of musculoskeletal disorders in the community: the comparative prevalence of symptoms at different anatomical sites, and the relation to social deprivation. *Ann Rheum Dis* 1998;57(11):649–655.

23. MacMahon B, Trichopoulos D. *Epidemiology : principles and methods.* Little, Brown, Boston, 1996.

24. Vandenbroucke JP, von Elm E, Altman DG et al. Strengthening the Reporting of Observational Studies in Epidemiology (STROBE): explanation and elaboration. *PLoS Med* 2007;4(10):e297.

25. Hunt JR, White E. Retaining and tracking cohort study members. *Epidemiol Rev* 1998;20(1):57–70.

26. Miettinen OS. The 'case-control' study: valid selection of subjects. *J Chronic Dis* 1985;38(7):543–548.

27. Correa A, Stewart WF, Yeh HC, Santos-Burgoa C. Exposure measurement in case-control studies: reported methods and recommendations. *Epidemiol Rev* 1994;16(1):18–32.

28. Lahiri M, Morgan C, Symmons DP, Bruce IN. Modifiable risk factors for RA: prevention, better than cure? *Rheumatology* (Oxford) 2012;51(3):499–512.

29. Pattison E, Harrison BJ, Griffiths CE, Silman AJ, Bruce IN. Environmental risk factors for the development of psoriatic arthritis: results from a case-control study. *Ann Rheum Dis* 2008;67(5):672–676.

30. Eder L, Law T, Chandran V et al. Association between environmental factors and onset of psoriatic arthritis in patients with psoriasis. *Arthritis Care Res* (Hoboken) 2011;63(8):1091–1097.

31. Singh JA, Reddy SG, Kundukulam J. Risk factors for gout and prevention: a systematic review of the literature. *Curr Opin Rheumatol* 2011;23(2):192–202.

32. Simard JF, Costenbader KH. What can epidemiology tell us about systemic lupus erythematosus? *Int J Clin Pract* 2007;61(7):1170–1180.

33. Danchenko N, Satia JA, Anthony MS. Epidemiology of systemic lupus erythematosus: a comparison of worldwide disease burden. *Lupus* 2006;15(5):308–318.

34. Bae SC, Fraser P, Liang MH. The epidemiology of systemic lupus erythematosus in populations of African ancestry: a critical review of the 'prevalence gradient hypothesis'. *Arthritis Rheum* 1998;41(12):2091–2099.

35. Sutcliffe N, Clarke AE, Gordon C, Farewell V, Isenberg DA. The association between socio-economic status, race, psychosocial factors and outcome in patients with systemic lupus erythematosus. *Rheumatology* (Oxford) 1999;38(11):1130–1137.

36. Mayes MD. Scleroderma epidemiology. *Rheum Dis Clin North Am* 2003;29(2):239–254.

37. Salvarani C, Cantini F, Boiardi L, Hunder GG. Polymyalgia rheumatica and giant-cell arteritis. *N Engl J Med* 2002;347(4):261–271.

38. Felson DT, Lawrence RC, Dieppe PA et al. Osteoarthritis: new insights. Part 1: the disease and its risk factors. *Ann Intern Med* 2000;133(8):635–646.

39. Manek NJ, MacGregor AJ. Epidemiology of back disorders: prevalence, risk factors, and prognosis. *Curr Opin Rheumatol* 2005;17(2):134–140.

40. Holroyd C, Dennison E, Cooper C. Epidemiology and classification of metabolic bone disease. In: Hochberg MC, Silman A, Smolen J, Weinblatt M, Weisman M (eds) *Rheumatology*, 5th edn. Mosby/Elsevier, Philadelphia, 2011:1937–1944.

41. Cooper C. Osteoporosis: disease severity and consequent fracture management. *Osteoporos Int* 2010;21(Suppl 2):S425–429.

42. Hackshaw AK. *A concise guide to clinical trials.* Wiley-Blackwell, Oxford, 2009.

43. Strom BL. *Pharmacoepidemiology*, 4th edn. Wiley, Chichester, 2005.

44. Cook RJ, Sackett DL. The number needed to treat: a clinically useful measure of treatment effect. *BMJ* 1995;310(6977):452–454.

45. Manzi S, Meilahn EN, Rairie JE et al. Age-specific incidence rates of myocardial infarction and angina in women with systemic lupus erythematosus: comparison with the Framingham Study. *Am J Epidemiol* 1997;145(5):408–415.

CHAPTER 28

Assessment of rheumatic disease

Piet van Riel

Introduction

The examination of the musculoskeletal system can be considered under two headings: (1) the systematic screening of virtually all the accessible joints of the body to identify abnormalities such as signs of inflammation, destruction, or abnormal function, and establish their distribution; (2) the more detailed analysis of an abnormal joint or group of joints, trying to quantify inflammation and loss of function. The screening is intended to be brief but comprehensive and efficient. It can be accomplished in a few minutes and should be part of the routine examination taught to all medical students (see Chapter 6).

The patient is best examined lying comfortably on a couch or bed for most of the examination, but sitting up for the shoulders and neck, and standing for the final stages of examining the feet and the movements of the back. Walking should be observed, either at the start when the patient comes into the room or at the end of the examination if the patient is already undressed. For a very young patient, much of the examination can be carried out while the child sits on the parent's lap.

The examination starts most logically with the hands, the calling cards of many of the rheumatic diseases, then moves up the arms to the joints of the shoulder girdle and the jaw, down the spine from the neck to the coccyx and on to the legs, finishing with the toes. The same basic pattern governs the examination of the most of the joints: inspection, palpation, and establishing the range of movement. This pattern is altered for some parts— the back, for example—in the interests of efficiency. It is important to realize that sometimes pain in a certain joint is being caused by a process outside the musculoskeletal system. For instance, a patient with a malignant tumour in the lung can have complains of severe pain in the shoulder. This is also called 'referred pain'; in this case no abnormalities will be found by examining the painful joint.

Inspection

Where a joint is paired, both should be exposed to allow comparison of the two sides. Redness overlying a joint is an important indicator of acute, severe inflammation, as in gout or septic arthritis. Any skin rash, subcutaneous nodules, cysts, scars, or evidence of local infection are noted. Muscle wasting is often associated with joint disease, but may be masked by joint swelling. Swelling or deformity should be sought. Discrepancies in limb or digit length may indicate growth problems secondary to inflammation, as in juvenile idiopathic arthritis.

Palpation

Temperature change is assessed relative to the same joint on the other side, or to surrounding normal skin. The back of the hand is rapidly moved between the areas to be compared. Errors may occur if one side has been kept warmer by a bandage, glove, or splint. Tenderness is elicited with firm pressure along the joint margins, and over tendons and ligaments. This should be carried out with the examiner's eyes on those of the patient, rather than on the joint, so as to pick up the first signs of discomfort. Swelling noted on inspection is palpated, to answer the question: 'Is this swelling bone, soft tissue, or fluid?' Bony swelling is especially a feature of osteoarthritis. Other causes are new bone formation with psoriatic arthritis, Charcot's joints, and callus formation after a fracture. Soft tissue swelling about a joint is most often synovial. The consistency of synovial swelling is more doughy than bouncy, like foam rubber. Where synovial fluid and synovial swelling coexist, the fluid can be pushed away or aspirated, allowing the synovium to be palpated. Fluid is recognizable for its compressibility; palpating a lax effusion is easy, because the fluid can be pushed from one part of the joint to another (fluctuation). A tense effusion can be recognized by its bouncy quality, like a firm rubber ball. Joint noises are frequently better felt than heard. Loud cracks and snaps, particularly on pulling the fingers or rotating the ankles, may be quite normal. Pulling the fingers creates a vacuum and the popping sound represents the sudden development of a gas cavity in the joint fluid. The snap on rotating an ankle is related to the slipping of one tendon over another. Similar, harmless snapping and crunching noises occur when the head is extended and rotated from side to side, or the shoulders are braced back and rotated. Velvet crepitations are too soft to be audible, but may be felt. They occur when the joint contains small particles of proteinaceous material, most typically in rheumatoid arthritis (RA). Crepitus in the joint of a patient with osteoarthritis feels like a dull, coarse crunching, and is caused by irregularities in the cartilage.

Eburnation crepitus is both heard and felt, occurring when the cartilage has been destroyed and the two bony surfaces are in contact. The name means 'turning to ivory' and the sound is thought to be similar to that of ivory grinding on ivory. Most often it emanates from the hip or the knee, and then care is needed to work out which is the affected joint as the vibrations are well transmitted up or down the femur. To demonstrate eburnation crepitus, the examiner lays a hand on the joint and asks the patient to move it. Passive movement may fail to elicit the sign because the joint surfaces are not so closely opposed when the muscles are relaxed.

Range of movement

The patient is usually first asked to move the joint actively. If a full range of active movement can be carried out without discomfort, there is rarely any need to proceed to passive movement. If the patient is unable to carry out the full range of active movement, then the passive movements will be most informative. In general, where active and passive restriction are the same, limitation of movement will reflect one of the following: inflammation of a joint; contracture of the tendons or ligaments surrounding the joint; destruction of bone or cartilage in the joint. Restriction of active but not passive movement indicates rupture or inflammation of a tendon, muscle weakness, or failure of the nerve supply to the muscle. The 'normal' range of movement must be interpreted with caution. There is much variation in joint mobility with age and race, and from individual to individual. An excessive range of movement in otherwise normal joints is referred to as hypermobility. An excessive range in diseased joints reflects damage to the articular surfaces or the capsule and ligaments, leading to instability.

Systematic survey

Rheumatic diseases are often multisystem in their effects, and many systemic diseases will present with rheumatic complaints. The discussion of the examination of the other systems in the body is outside the scope of this chapter, but it should be remembered that the examination of the musculoskeletal system is only one aspect of the careful and comprehensive history-taking and general physical examination that makes up the assessment of the patient with rheumatic symptoms.

Hands

Inspection
This is summarized in Box 28.1.

Nails
The nails may show the pitting or lifting from the nail bed (onycholysis) typical of psoriasis, nailfold infarcts typical of vasculitis, or the shaggy cuticles and periungual erythema of dermatomyositis (Figure 28.1). Dilated capillary loops in the nailfold can be seen with the naked eye, though more easily with a magnifying glass or with a capillary scope, and tend to accompany certain rheumatic diseases, for example systemic sclerosis and dermatomyositis.

Skin
A rash on the backs of the hands may be due to psoriasis or to dermatomyositis, best distinguished from each other by the distribution. Dermatomyositis tends to affect the extensor surfaces of the joints in a neat and symmetrical fashion, while psoriasis is more likely to be distributed at random across the hand. Palmar erythema is common in patients with connective tissue diseases, and is frequently different in nature from the palmar erythema of pregnancy or liver disease, looking more mottled and indeed more like

palmar livedo reticularis than erythema. This appearance seems to be associated with systemic vasculitis.

Muscle wasting
This is common whenever joints are inflamed, but attention should be paid to any significant patterns of muscle wasting, such as the wasting of the thenar eminence in carpal tunnel syndrome, which spares only the adductor pollicis, visible as a band parallel to the wrist. Wasting of opponens pollicis commonly accompanies osteoarthritis of the first carpometacarpal joint (see Box 28.1).

Tendon involvement
Tenosynovitis of the flexor tendons may be seen as a fullness in the palm. It differs from contracture by the absence of skin tethering over the surface, and the presence of crepitus on flexing the fingers. To detect crepitus of the flexor tendon, the examiner places

Box 28.1 Inspecting the hands

Nails
- Pitting
- Onycholysis
- Splinter haemorrhages
- Shaggy cuticles
- Nailfold infarcts
- Periungual erythema
- Dilated capillary loops

Skin
- Rash of psoriasis, dermatomyositis
- Vitiligo
- Purpura
- Raynaud's colour changes
- Infarcts
- Tophi
- Calcinosis
- Waxy thickening
- Nodules
- Palmar erythema

Muscles
- Wasting

Tendons
- Swelling of sheath
- Rupture
- Displacement

Joints
- Swelling
- Deformity

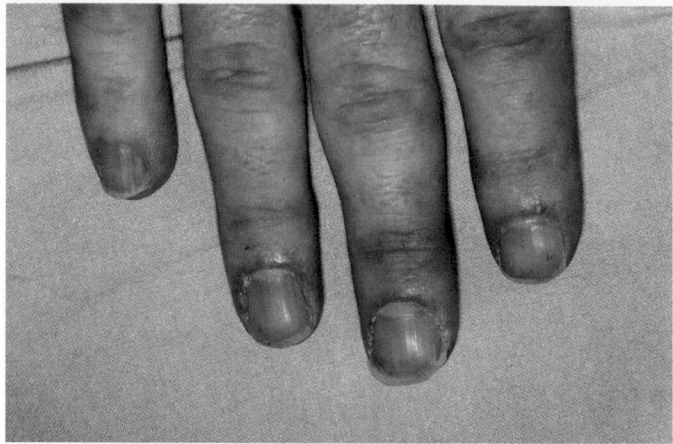

Fig. 28.1 The shaggy cuticles and periungual erythema seen in connective tissue diseases, especially mixed connective tissue disease or dermatomyositis.

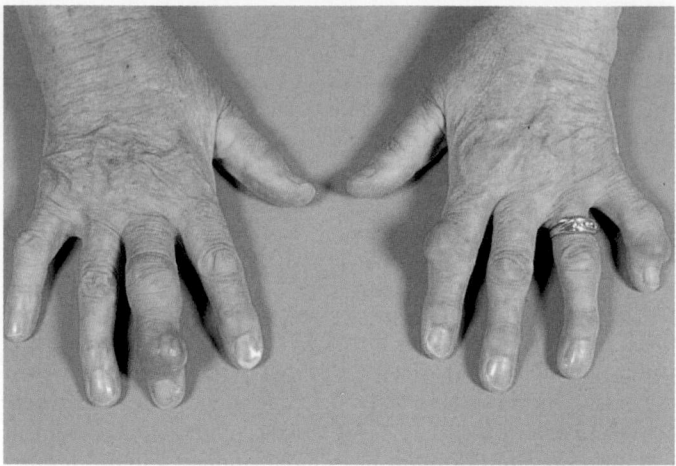

Fig. 28.2 Polyarticular gout affecting the hand, with visible tophi.

the index and middle fingers over the course of the tendon, with the thumb on the back of the hand exerting firm pressure. The patient is then asked to make a fist, and crepitus or nodularity may be felt as the tendon moves within its sheath. The procedure is repeated for each of the flexor tendons in turn. Trigger finger occurs when the finger locks in flexion, but can be passively (albeit painfully) straightened. This is caused by a nodule on the tendon passing through a stricture in the tendon sheath. The weaker extensor muscles are unable to pull the nodule back through the same obstruction. The nodule is usually to be found in the palm just proximal to the metacarpal head, but will only be detected during active movement of the affected digit.

Swelling

The hands may look generally puffy with no localization of this over joints. This is especially common in mixed connective tissue disease or early systemic sclerosis, where the hands may resemble a bunch of sausages, and also occurs with systemic lupus erythematosus (SLE), dermatomyositis, polymyalgia rheumatica, reflex sympathetic dystrophy, and early RA.

Where only one or two fingers have a diffuse, cylindrical swelling, not centred on a joint, we speak of a 'sausage' digit. These may represent swelling of the flexor tendon, as in the seronegative spondyloarthropathies (particularly in psoriatic arthritis), diffuse soft tissue inflammation as in gout (Figure 28.2), or infection as in leprosy or tuberculosis.

Synovial swelling in the proximal interphalangeal (PIP) joints is sometimes called spindling because of the fusiform appearance. Osteoarthritis causes a swelling of these joints that is bony and irregular, occasionally with effusions.

Distribution

The distribution of joint swelling gives an immediate clue to the diagnosis. Swelling predominantly of the terminal (distal) interphalangeal joints indicates osteoarthritis, psoriatic arthritis (Figure 28.3), or occasionally gout. Osteoarthritis also predominantly affects the first carpometacarpal joint, an articulation spared by most other arthropathies. The carpus looks to be squared, because of osteophyte formation, wasting of the surrounding muscles, and adduction of the thumb. RA has a predilection for the metacarpophalangeal joints, as well as the proximal interphalangeal joints.

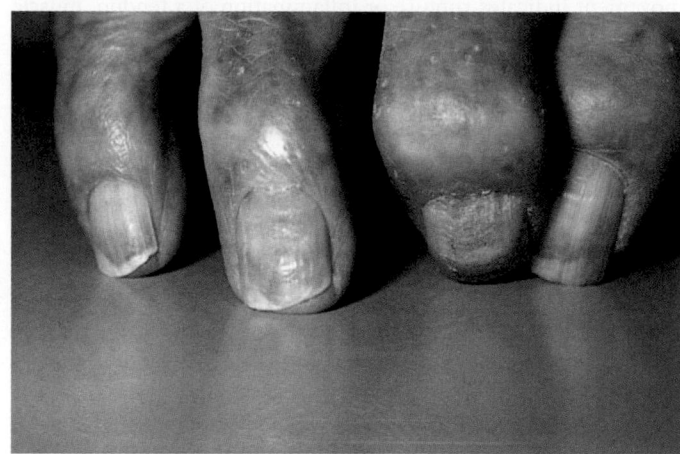

Fig. 28.3 Psoriatic arthritis with typical distal interphalangeal (DIP) joint involvement and nail dystrophy with pitting.

Deformities

Note deformities such as swan neck, boutonnière, ulnar drift, and Z thumbs. Palmar subluxation of the metacarpophalangeal joints is often mistaken for synovial swelling, but the exposed metacarpal heads are rounded and bony on palpation. Palmar subluxation is easily confirmed by running a finger along the back of the patient's hand and fingers to assess whether the phalanges are on the same plane as the metacarpals.

Range of movement

The patient should be able to make a fist, burying the fingertips in the palm, a movement that requires 90° of flexion in each of the three phalangeal joints. Hypermobility is indicated by more than 90° extension in the metacarpophalangeal joints and ability to approximate thumb to forearm, passively.

Wrist

Swelling

In RA, exuberant soft tissue swelling may be seen, originating either from the wrist joint itself or from the synovial tendon sheaths, and spreading both sides of the extensor pollucis retinaculum. An undulating swelling of the ulnar border of the wrist is a particular feature of RA. The undulations are the result of synovial swelling pushing its way through the fibres of the extensor retinaculum. This appearance is associated with an increased risk of rupture of the fourth and fifth extensor digitis tendons.

Swelling of the wrist joint is associated with compression of the median nerve in the carpal tunnel. Particular attention should be paid to looking for evidence of this complication. Inflammation of the abductor pollicis longus tendon at the wrist (de Quervain's tenosynovitis) is best diagnosed by inspecting the wrists from the radial side, with the palms together and any watches or bracelets removed. Unilateral swelling may then easily be seen, extending from the first carpometacarpal joint proximally. The diagnosis can be confirmed using Finkelstein's test. In this the patient is asked to bring the thumb across the palm and clasp the fingers around it. The examiner holds the clenched fist and tweaks it sharply in an ulnar direction, putting a sudden but not excessive pull on the inflamed tendon. This elicits a sharp pain, and should be done with care, watching the patient's face for signs of discomfort.

Deformity

Deformity of the wrist joint usually takes the form of radial deviation (with ulnar deviation of the fingers in the metacarpophalangeal joints) and palmar subluxation, owing to the stronger pull of the flexor than the extensor muscles of the forearm. Prominence of the lower end of the ulna is also common, because synovial proliferation at the inferior radioulnar joint weakens the ligaments and allows the bone to ride up in a deformity that may be either fixed or mobile. When the bone is mobile it is often painful, giving rise to the 'piano-key' sign, whereby pressure on the bone leads to the production of an audible protest from the patient.

Range of movement

The 'prayer position' normally allows 90° of passive palmar and dorsiflexion (Figure 28.4). The active range is 20° less in each direction.

Elbow

Inspection

Inspecting the elbows is a fruitful source of clues to the diagnosis in many rheumatic diseases. Rheumatoid nodules, gouty tophi, tendon xanthomata, olecranon bursitis, and the rash of psoriasis or

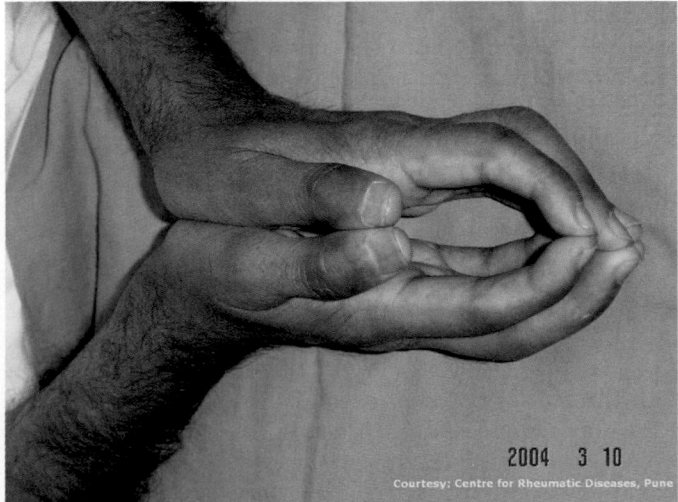

Fig. 28.4 The reversed 'prayer position', demonstrating wrist palmar flexion.

of dermatomyositis may all be detected by a glance at the extensor surface of the elbow, just distal to the olecranon. The joints are most easily compared with the elbows flexed and the arms folded.

Palpation

Palpation for synovial proliferation or joint effusion is best done in the groove between the lateral epicondyle and the olecranon process. The radioulnar joints are frequently involved in RA, leading to loss of pronation and supination. The examiner places one thumb on the radial head and the other on the inferior radioulnar joint at the wrist, then passively pronates and supinates the patient's forearm, feeling for crepitus in one or both joints.

Tenderness of the lateral or medial epicondyles and the muscles inserting into them is found in 'tennis elbow' or 'golfer's elbow', respectively. To confirm, the patient is asked to clench the fist and to extend or flex the wrist against resistance. These manoeuvres should cause pain at the affected muscle insertion.

Range of movement

Flexion is usually limited by the interposition of soft tissues, and should be about 150°. Extension beyond 10° implies hypermobility. Pronation and supination take place at the superior and inferior radioulnar joints and must be done with the elbows flexed to exclude movement at the shoulder joint. The hands can normally be fully supinated and pronated.

Shoulder girdle

The three shoulder girdle joints are best considered together, as all three work together in movements of the shoulder, and pain from all three is felt around the shoulder and upper arm. Acromioclavicular pain is usually felt at the tip of the shoulder. Pain in the glenohumeral joints is most often felt over the deltoid muscle and midhumerus. The manubriosternal joint is often swollen and sometimes painful in RA and in seronegative spondyloarthritis.

Sternoclavicular joint

The sternoclavicular joint is often neglected, despite the fact that it is frequently affected in a variety of arthropathies, including polymyalgia rheumatica, RA, the seronegative spondyloarthropathies, and septic arthritis. Pain is rarely localized to the joint, even when there is obvious swelling and redness, but is referred to the upper arm. Palpation should include the inner end of the clavicle and the articular surface of the manubrium, directly below it. Pain can best be elicited by asking the patient to brace the shoulders forward and back, or to shrug the shoulders up and down, movements which do not involve the glenohumeral joint. If these movements are painful but external rotation of the shoulder is not, there is strong evidence of sternoclavicular disease.

Acromioclavicular joint

The acromioclavicular joint is near the surface and can easily be seen and palpated if swollen. Passive adduction of the arm across the chest will often cause pain if the joint is inflamed. There may be a painful arc on abduction above 90°.

Shoulder (glenohumeral) joint

Inspection

Wasting of muscles should be noted both from the front and the back. Swelling of the shoulder joint is not always obvious. A shoulder effusion in a patient with RA may give that shoulder a more normal-looking contour. Rupture of the shoulder capsule may lead to fluid tracking down to the upper arm. A dislocated shoulder may appear square and dropped, while in RA the shoulders appear both square (due to muscle wasting) and raised, owing to upward subluxation of the humeral heads as a result of dysfunction of the rotator cuff and muscle contracture.

Palpation

A shoulder effusion is best felt by placing the thumb in front and the fingers behind the joint and fluctuating the fluid back and forth across the shoulder. Tenderness may be elicited over the whole line of the joint in capsulitis or inflammatory arthritis, or may be localized where there is an isolated lesion of the tendon. Inflammation of the long head of biceps gives tenderness in the bicipital groove anteriorly, while supraspinatus tendinitis causes tenderness in the subacromial bursa. Rupture of the long head of biceps is best appreciated by asking the patient to contract the muscle against resistance. The affected muscle will form a ball (the 'Popeye sign').

Movements of the shoulder girdle

Although individual arcs of movement may be attributed to each of the three joints of the shoulder girdle, in practice they work smoothly together when the arm is raised. The sternoclavicular joint is the single point of bony connection between the arm and the trunk, and allows considerable movement of the clavicle, which in turn acts as a strut to add freedom of movement to the arm. The acromioclavicular joint has less movement, but allows for rotation of the scapula on the thorax. Pure glenohumeral movement can be isolated from movement of the scapula across the thorax by fixing the inferior angle of the scapula with one hand and passively abducting the arm with the other. Normally, the scapula starts to move at 30° of abduction, but if it is fixed at least 90° of glenohumeral movement is possible. Passive external rotation is another reliable measure of pure glenohumeral movement. Restriction of this movement is a first sign of inflammation of the glenohumeral joint. The last few degrees of abduction may be lost in patients with a painful neck lesion. Passive movements should always be checked if the active range is incomplete. Loss of active and passive range in equal measure suggests intracapsular disease such as arthritis or adhesive capsulitis ('frozen shoulder'). Loss of active more than passive movement, accompanied by pain, suggests a lesion of tendon or rotator cuff. Limitation or weakness of active movement with a full and pain-free passive range suggests muscular or neurological disease.

The painful arc

During abduction of the arm, pain may be experienced in an arc, above or below which movement is pain free. The most common cause is supraspinatus tendinitis. In this condition pain occurs somewhere in the arc from 60 to 100° as the greater tuberosity impinges on the acromion, pinching the supraspinatus tendon. The pain may be severe enough to prevent abduction. The patient is often able to elevate the arm fully by forward flexion, but if asked to take it down sideways, will complain of pain as the upper limit of the painful arc is reached. A painful arc above 90° occurs in acromioclavicular disease.

Resisted movements

Specific tendon lesions can be identified by using resisted movements to elicit pain. Pain on resisted abduction suggests a supraspinatus lesion. Pain on resisted external rotation suggests an infraspinatus lesion. Pain on resisted internal rotation suggests a subscapularis lesion.

Range of movement

Movement at the shoulder comprises forward flexion to 180°, abduction to 180°, extension to 45°, and rotation to 70° internally and externally. Movement at the sternoclavicular joint includes protraction and retraction of the clavicle in an arc of 60°, and elevation of the clavicle to 60°.

Temporomandibular joint

Palpate the joints for tenderness or swelling and ask the patient to open the mouth wide. These joints are most frequently involved in RA. The complaint is of pain on chewing or yawning and sometimes of pain in the ear. The joints rarely look abnormal, but there is local tenderness and pain on opening the jaws. Normally, it is possible for the fully open jaws to accommodate the middle three digits of the patient's hand, held vertically between the teeth. Restricted mouth opening from disease of the temporomandibular joints may be differentiated from that caused by scleroderma by inspecting the lips and the skin around the mouth, which will be drawn tight in scleroderma. Micrognathia occurs as a result of temporomandibular joint inflammation in childhood, as in juvenile idiopathic arthritis. Premature closure of the epiphysis leads to failure of normal development of the mandible.

Cervical spine

Inspection

Neck posture may indicate underlying disease. A poking chin with dorsal kyphosis often accompanies cervical spondylosis. Acute torticollis can be recognized as the patient enters the room: one sternocleidomastoid muscle in spasm and the head tilted to the side and slightly rotated. The patient with RA will often have lost neck height and there may be a lateral asymmetry if there has been softening and erosion of bone.

Palpation

Palpation of the neck should include the occipital ridge, the spinous processes, and the paravertebral muscles overlying the facet joints. The occipital ridge is frequently tender in cervical spondylosis, especially over the greater occipital nerve. The spinous processes normally form a lordotic arc, with C2 and C7 being prominent at either end of the curve. Loss of lordosis or even a reversed curve can be appreciated by palpation. Palpation of the paravertebral muscles may reveal spasm in any case of neck pain, but especially after a whiplash injury or in cases of headache and neck pain related to stress. Through the paravertebral muscles, the facet joints can be felt, and tenderness or swelling elicited. Each pair of facet joints should be palpated in turn.

Range of movement

The patient should be able to touch the chin to the chest, tip the head back until the forehead and nose are parallel to the ceiling, and rotate in each direction to 70°. Lateral flexion is normally 45° each side, and this movement is lost early in ankylosing spondylitis. Passive neck movements are not a part of the routine examination, as neck instability is a feature of the rheumatic diseases. Lhermitte's sign is more correctly a symptom. The patient complains of paraesthesia down the body on flexing the neck. It is sometimes present in cases of compression of the cervical cord, especially in RA. The examiner should not attempt to elicit this sign by forcible neck flexion.

Thoracic spine

Inspection

This will reveal postural abnormality such as kyphosis or scoliosis. Destruction or collapse of vertebrae may lead to a sharply angled kyphosis, or angular gibbus, most often seen in tuberculosis. Kyphosis in adolescents suggests Scheuermann's disease or an osteoporotic vertebral fracture. Scoliosis may be developmental, in which case there is usually some rotation of the ribs, which can be exaggerated by asking the patient to bend forward so that the rotation is more easily appreciated. Scoliosis resulting from muscle spasm becomes less obvious on forward flexion.

Palpation

The spinous processes and paravertebral muscles are next palpated, especially for tenderness. Recent collapse of a vertebra, malignant deposits, or vertebral osteomyelitis all produce local or 'point' tenderness. If direct pressure over the spinous process is insufficient to elicit this, it is worth trying percussion, laying two fingers over each process in turn and striking these with the fist, gently at first, then more firmly if no discomfort is elicited. Tenderness of the upper thoracic vertebrae and the paravertebral muscles is a common feature of thoracic spondylosis.

Range of movement

Rotation is best assessed with the patient seated to fix the pelvis and is usually 45°. Flexion is most easily measured with a tape measure. Distraction on flexion between marks made at C7 and T12 is normally at least 2.5 cm. Costovertebral movement is measured by chest expansion at the level of the nipples, usually more than 7 cm.

Lumbar spine

Examination

Patient standing

The examiner inspects the back for abnormality of posture or deformity, such as scoliosis or kyphosis, then palpates the paravertebral muscles for evidence of spasm. Palpation for tenderness is best left until the patient is lying down.

Forward flexion and extension are relatively more restricted in the patient with a mechanical back pain, while lateral flexion is the first to be lost in ankylosing spondylitis. Schober's test is a useful method of measuring lumbar flexion, especially in ankylosing spondylitis. Using a tape measure, the examiner makes two marks, one 5 cm below the level of the sacroiliac dimples and one 10 cm above. The patient bends forward and the examiner measures the distance between the marks. Distraction of at least 5 cm is normal. Asking the patient to take a few steps on the heels and toes is a crude but useful test of power in the legs and feet, and at the same time the buttocks can be inspected for any evidence of a Trendelenburg sign (dipping down of the pelvis when the ipsilateral foot is raised from the ground) suggesting muscle weakness.

Patient lying face up

Straight-leg raise (Lasègue's sign): the patient lies supine while the examiner grasps one ankle and raises it from the couch, keeping the knee straight with a hand on the knee, and watching the patient's face for any sign of discomfort. Normally 80–90° can be attained without discomfort, depending on the tightness of the hamstrings. Irritation of the dural sleeve of any of the nerve roots contributing to the sciatic nerve will result in pain when the sciatic nerve is put on the stretch, and a much reduced straight-leg raise on the affected side. The usual cause of this is a prolapsed lumbar disc protruding posterolaterally. Bilateral reduction in straight-leg raising implies a central disc prolapse. To distinguish between sciatic irritation and hip disease, the leg is raised with the knee flexed. This will now be painless in sciatic irritation, but just as uncomfortable in hip disease.

Sciatic stretch test: this may be useful in distinguishing sciatic irritation from tight hamstrings if the straight-leg raise is reduced. Once the limit of straight-leg raising is established, the leg is lowered a fraction until the pain is relieved. Now the examiner dorsiflexes the foot. If the pain was due to sciatic irritation, it returns. After the straight-leg raise, the examiner tests the knee, ankle, and plantar reflexes. Testing power in each of the major muscle groups of the legs, especially the hip muscles, may cause difficulties if the patient is in pain. It may be necessary to reassess the patient after adequate control of the pain. Sensation to light touch and pinprick is next elicited, following a dermatomal pattern over the anterior aspects of both legs and the soles of the feet.

Patient lying face down

It is important to have the couch flat, with pillows removed, to avoid painful hyperextension. A pillow under the patient's abdomen will usually increase comfort and render the examination easier. The examiner palpates each spinous process in turn, gently at first, then increasing the pressure by using one hand laid on the other. Then the examiner palpates for tenderness in the paravertebral muscles, the posterior iliac crests, and over the sacrum and coccyx. Coccygeal tenderness may also be felt by a rectal examination.

Point tenderness is a feature of local infection or malignancy. More diffuse tenderness is common in patients with mechanical back pain. The femoral stretch test is the parallel of the straight-leg raising test, putting the femoral nerve roots on the stretch. The examiner takes the prone patient's ankle in one hand, flexing the knee to 90°, and raising the bent leg to extend the hip. Pain during this manoeuvre may indicate a lesion of a high lumbar disc or hip disease. Loss of sensation around the saddle area is an important clue to the presence of cauda equina lesions and should always be tested for. Buttock tone is assessed by asking the patient to pinch the cheeks of the buttocks together as hard as possible, and palpating the two sides. A rectal examination is helpful where there is any hint of a lesion of the cauda equina, to assess sphincter tone and sensation, in addition to its importance as part of the general assessment of the patient.

Sacroiliac joints

Inspection and palpation

Inspecting the joints from behind may reveal evidence of swelling or deformity, especially in tuberculous infection. Palpation is best done with the four fingers of the hand along the length of the joint. Nodules of tender fibrofatty tissue often overlie the joints, and are of no significance except that they are often found in patients with chronic back pain. Bony fusion of the joints in ankylosing spondylitis obliterates the joint line. The synovial portion of the joint lies too deep to be felt under normal circumstances.

Range of movement

Moving the sacroiliac joints is not easy, as there is only a small amount of rotational glide, but they may be stressed by a variety of manoeuvres. The simplest method is to press firmly on the sacrum while the patient lies prone, then on the pelvic brim as the patient lies supine and on one side. If the sacroiliac joints are inflamed, these manoeuvres may elicit pain. Instability of the sacroiliac joints, especially postpartum, may cause pain, which is aggravated when the patient is asked to stand on one leg. Sometimes the excessive movement can be appreciated by placing one finger on each side of the joint as the patient makes the manoeuvre.

Hip

Screening

Inspection

The gait is particularly important in the assessment of the lower limb joints. The patient with a fixed flexion deformity of the hips throws the spine into an exaggerated lordosis to compensate. The patient with weak hip muscles walks with a waddle, and one with a painful hip walks in such a way as to spend the least possible time on the painful leg, leaning to the opposite side, often with a walking stick. This is called the antalgic gait. Inspection of the hips should always include comparison of leg lengths and attention to the position of the leg. The leg that is short and externally rotated suggests a fractured neck of femur, or a legacy of juvenile idiopathic arthritis. Failure to observe the back of the hips may mean that the evidence of previous surgery is missed.

Palpation

Palpation of the hip is difficult because the joint is so deep, although occasionally an effusion can be detected by fluctuation just beneath the inguinal ligament. A psoas abscess may cause a very painful, stiff hip with spasm that cannot be overcome without anaesthesia. The psoas abscess will eventually point as a mass below the inguinal ligament. The greater trochanteric bursa lies over the greater trochanter and if it is inflamed, tenderness can easily be elicited with the patient lying on the unaffected side.

Range of movement: flexion, 110°; extension, 30°; abduction, 50°; adduction, 30°; internal and external rotation, each 45°.

A fixed flexion deformity can be demonstrated with Thomas's test. The patient lies supine and one knee and hip are flexed until any lumbar lordosis has been obliterated. Flexion of the other hip during this manoeuvre indicates a fixed flexion deformity of that hip. A catch for the inexperienced is the patient with a painful knee that is held in flexion. Attempts to straighten the knee in the bed are unsuccessful because of pain, and yet no other abnormality is seen in the knee. This patient probably has disease of the hip, with a fixed flexion deformity and pain referred to the knee. If the examiner were to straighten the knee while maintaining a flexed hip, a full range of movement would be found in most cases. Rotation may also be tested in extension, by rolling the leg. Where both hips have a limited range of abduction, it is useful to record the maximum distance between the two medial malleoli. Extension of the hip is best measured with the patient lying on the side or prone.

Knee

Inspection

Knee swellings can be recognized by fullness of the suprapatellar pouch and obliteration of the hollows either side of the patella.

Quadriceps wasting may be masked by swelling of the knee and measurement of quadriceps bulk should be made above the upper limit of the suprapatellar bursa. Deformities may be varus or valgus, forward or backward slip.

Palpation

Tenderness of the medial collateral ligaments occurs early in osteoarthritis, followed by the development of a tender bony ridge as osteophytes develop. A knee effusion can be demonstrated in one of three ways, depending on the quantity of fluid present, as follows:

- A small effusion can be milked from one side of the patella to the other in the 'bulge sign'. Any fluid in the medial side of the joint is swept firmly laterally and upward into the suprapatellar pouch. Then the back of the hand presses firmly and sharply on the lateral side of the joint. When a small effusion is present, a bulge will appear on the medial side of the joint as the fluid returns.

- A moderate effusion is best detected by eliciting the 'patellar tap'. One hand is placed on the suprapatellar pouch, the finger and thumb exerting side-to-side pressure, squeezing any fluid in the pouch to the retropatellar space. The patella is then sharply depressed with the fingers of the other hand, so that it floats through the fluid to strike the lower end of the femur. This sharp tap will not be felt if the undersurface of the patella is covered with synovial pannus, which acts as a blanket to muffle the impact. A tap may be felt in the absence of fluid if intra-articular fat is squeezed behind the patella.

- A large, tense effusion can be confirmed by fluctuation across the joint, from one side of the patella to the other.

A cyst of the calf or popliteal fossa is often easier to feel than to see, and has the consistency of a firm rubber ball.

Testing stability

To test the cruciate ligaments the examiner grasps the flexed knee just below the knee, with both hands, and exerts pressure first anteriorly, then posteriorly. To test the medial and lateral collaterals the examiner raises the patient's leg, supported with the fingers of one hand under the knee, holding it slightly flexed, and the other under the ankle. Then pressure is exerted with the heel of each hand, producing a stress across the knee joint, centred on the ligament to be tested.

McMurray's sign

This is a test for cartilage tears. The patient lies supine and the examiner grasps the knee in one hand and the ankle in the other. The examiner then flexes the knee fully, internally rotates the lower leg as far as it will go, and slowly straightens the knee. Then the test is repeated with external rotation. If the hand over the knee detects a clunk on straightening, accompanied by wincing or other expression of pain from the patient, the test is positive.

Range of movement: extension, 0°; flexion, 135°. Hyperextension can be tested by holding the knee firmly on the bed and lifting the ankle. Extension beyond 10° is abnormal.

Ankle joint

Inspect for swelling or deformity. Palpate the anterior joint line for tenderness, swelling. Assess dorsiflexion and plantar flexion. Swelling can be detected anteriorly, between the malleoli, where it has the appearance and feeling of a 'spare tyre', quite unlike the diffuse swelling of ankle oedema. Swelling behind the lateral malleolus suggests peroneal tendinitis. Synovitis of the extensor tendons results in swelling both above and below the extensor retinaculum.

Range of movement: dorsiflexion, 20°; plantar flexion, 70°.

Subtalar (talocalcaneal) joint

Inspect for varus or valgus deformity of the hindfoot. Grasp the heel and assess inversion and eversion. Swelling is seen below the malleoli. This joint is prone to symptomless involvement, especially in RA and juvenile chronic arthritis. Talipes valgus deformity usually results, and is best appreciated from behind, with the patient standing.

Range of movement: inversion, 25°; eversion, 15°.

Heel and foot

Inspect both the dorsal and plantar aspects of the foot, and the back of the heel. Palpate the Achilles tendon insertion, the plantar fascia insertion, and the metatarsophalangeal joints. Apply torsion to the midfoot to test movement in the midtarsal joints. Painful feet may be caused by vascular or neurological lesions. The peripheral pulses and sensation should always be assessed, and search made for ulcers, sinuses, or skin infarcts. Occasionally a prolapsed lumbar disc will present with foot pain without back pain or sciatica.

Achilles tendon

This is inspected from behind, either with the patient standing or lying prone. Thickening, tenderness, and rupture can be detected. With rupture, the patient may have difficulty in standing on tiptoe at first, though fibrosis later occurs, rendering the movement possible. The Achilles tendon is a common site for traumatic bursas related to pressure from shoes, rheumatoid nodules, gouty tophi, and tendon xanthomata.

Heel

Heel pain is commonly due to plantar fasciitis. The heel can be inspected from below with the patient lying down. It is unusual to see swelling or discoloration, though the affected side often feels firmer. Tenderness is elicited by pressure directly cranial from the centre of the heel and by pressure from side to side at the level of the anterior margin of the calcaneum.

Midfoot

The naviculocuneiform joint is subject to osteoarthritis and is often found to show bony enlargement.

Sole

Callosities under the metatarsal heads develop when the metatarsophalangeal joints are subluxated. The rash of psoriasis or keratoderma blennorrhagica may be detected on the soles.

Toes

Inspect the toes for deformities such as hallux valgus, clawing, overlapping toes, undersized toes. In RA, fibular drift of the toes is common. Clawed toes press on the uppers of shoes and callosities form over the proximal interphalangeal joints. 'Sausage toes' suggest seronegative spondylarthropathies, gout, or psoriatic arthropathy. A bursa between the joints will spread the toes. Diffuse swelling over the metatarsophalangeal joints may be easier to feel than see; tenderness may be elicited by palpating each joint individually. Beware of squeezing the forefoot, as this can cause severe pain if the joints are inflamed.

Standardized quantification

Standardized instruments are useful and required for the evaluation of disease progress and treatment efficacy in rheumatic patients. Measures that are reproducible, valid, and sensitive to relevant changes are used both in clinical trials and daily clinical practice. Many of these have been reviewed in detail recently.[1]

Several devices have been developed and validated to quantify for instance range of motion, muscle strength, and skin elasticity. Furthermore, indices are developed that combine clinical assessments into a single outcome measure (see Chapter 29).

Objective assessment

Skin

Skin elasticity can be assessed with a cutometer SEM 474 or 575. This cutometer exerts a controlled vacuum force on a skin area using a 2 mm or 8 mm probe. In systemic scleroderma it showed good correlation with the subjective skin score, with better reproducibility. It can assess changes in skin extensibility over time, and may be useful in monitoring the disease and its treatment.[2]

In scleroderma skin thickness can be measured, next to that the maximal oral opening, and the distance between third finger and the distal palmar crease in full flexion respectively extension (flexion/extension index) can be done.

In systemic sclerosis the severity of skin thickness is determined by physical examination of specified sites. Each site is graded on a three-point scale, and to obtain a total skin score all scores are summed (modified Rodnan skin score).[1] Capillaroscopy may be used to assess the extent and severity of nailfold capillary lesions in scleroderma.[3]

The extent of psoriatic lesions in psoriatic arthritis can be assessed using the Psoriasis Area and Severity Index (PASI).[4]

Muscles

Muscle strength—both isometric and isokinetic—can be assessed using dynamometers produced by several manufacturers. RA patients show decreased muscle strength compared to healthy controls. For patient or trial evaluation no standards for muscle strength assessments are recommended. The reliability and validity of the different dynamometers are still to be determined. Grip strength is the most frequently assessed aspect, although the type of instrument used is not standardized. A sphygmomanometer cuff is inflated to 30 mmHg and the patient squeezes it with one hand. The maximum reading achieved in three attempts is recorded. The muscle strength index is the mean score of standardized isometric extension and flexion strength of the knee and elbow joints. The index is reliable and correlates with self-reported functional disability and radiological damage in RA.

Muscle tenderness can be measured, in fibromyalgia for example, using a dolorimeter (or palpometer). The dolorimeter (Fisher or Chatillon) consists of a flat circular rubber probe of varying diameters, attached to a spring-loaded gauge. The probe is placed on a skin area, and the minimum pressure is recorded that provokes tenderness. However, the validity of the dolorimeter compared to a manual tender point examination is disputed. The tender point score is an index of 18 selected points which are frequently tender on pressure in patients with fibromyalgia.[5] The score is moderately reliable as diagnostic criterion, and is moderately responsive to perceived symptomatic change.

Joints

Joint tenderness is usually ascertained by manual pressure on the joint margins, or by passive movement for less palpable joints. These methods show large interobserver variation because the pressure is not standardized. Swelling of superficial joints is mostly assessed by manual palpation.

A goniometer is necessary: for accurate measurement of angles of movement or degrees of deformity in range of motion assessment. It is useful to have a long-armed one for large joints and a smaller one for joints of hands and feet. The arms of the goniometer should be lined up along the long axis of the joint, the hinge on the joint line, and the maximum angles of flexion and extension recorded. The position of the joint in the extended anatomical position is taken as zero, and further extension is recorded as a minus value.

Several joint counts have been developed, counting a varying number of joints that are tender and/or swollen. Examples frequently used in RA are the 28-joint count for pain and for swelling, the 68-joint count for pain, and the 66-joint count for swelling. The Ritchie articular index is a method of recording activity in RA by means of grading the tenderness to firm pressure or pain on movement in 53 joints, divided over 26 units, with a score ranging from 0 to 78. The most widely used is 28-joint count for tenderness (yes/no) and swelling (yes/no), and this is used in the DAS28 (see Chapter 28).

For the spinal and chest mobility several tests are described that are frequently used in ankylosing spondylitis[6]:

- Occiput–wall distance, measured in centimetres with the patient standing as erect as possible with heels and back against the wall.

- Chest expansion, assessed as the difference in centimetres between the circumference of the chest at nipple line on full inspiration and full expiration.

- Schober 10 cm test (measured in centimetres), with the patient erect, mark the skin at the level of the posterior superior iliac spines (dimples of Venus) and another 10 cm above in the midline. Ask the patient to bend maximally forward without bending the knees.

- Fingertip-to-floor-distance, recorded as the distance in centimetres between the third finger and the floor with the patient bending forward maximally, without flexing the knees.

- Lumbar lateral flexion, measured as a percentage of the body height.

Enthesitis

Several enthesitis indices have been developed to assess the extent of inflammation at site of ligament, tendon and joint capsule insertion into bone. These involve standardized palpation and ascertaining the presence of absence of tenderness. They can be used in AS and psoriatic arthritis.[4]

References

1. Katz P. Patient outcomes in rheumatology, 2011. *Arthritis Care Res* 2011;63(suppl iii):S1–S3.
2. Rodnan GP, Lipinski E, Luksick J. Skin thickness and collagen content in progressive systemic sclerosis and localized scleroderma. *Arthritis Rheum* 1979;22(2):130–140.
3. Lambova N, Muller Ladner U. Capillaroscopic pattern in systemic lupus erythematosus and undifferentiated connective tissue disease: What we still have to learn? *Rheumatol Int* 2013 Mar;33(3):689-95.
4. Mease PJ. Measures of psoriatic arthritis. *Arthritis Care Rheum* 2011;63(suppl ii):S64–S85.
5. Wolfe F. The relation between tender points and fibromyalgia symptom variables: evidence that fibromyalgia is not a discrete disorder in the clinic. *Ann Rheum Dis* 1997;56:268–271.
6. Moll J, Wright V. Measurement of spinal movements. In: Jayson MIV (ed.) *The lumbar spine and back pain*, 3rd edn. Churchill Livingstone, Edinburgh, 1987:215–234.

CHAPTER 29

Outcomes

David L. Scott

What are disease outcomes?

Each disease has its own natural history. These histories reflect what would happen without medical interventions. Outcomes assess differences between the overall benefits of medical treatments and the natural histories of untreated disease. Although effective treatment generally improves outcomes, some patients have poor outcomes due to adverse events. Clinical outcomes must therefore focus on groups of patients, with successful management giving substantially more positive than negative outcomes.[1–5]

In short-term diseases with sudden onset it is simple to assess relationships between clinical interventions and disease outcomes. However, in long-term diseases, which include many rheumatic disorders, outcomes reflect a large range of influences in addition to the disease itself and its treatment. These multiple confounding factors create challenges for judging the overall impact of treatment on outcomes.

Types of outcomes

Clinical outcomes can be classified in several ways. First, there is the type of outcome assessed. These fall into several broad areas:

- *Disease measures:* reflecting the presence and severity of the underlying disease, e.g. the presence and severity of joint inflammation in arthritis

- *End-organ damage:* indicating the severity of the unwanted consequences of disease, e.g. the extent and severity of joint damage in arthritis.

- *Quality of life measures:* these more general assessments made by patients indicate the impact of their disease on their lives in general. Some are disease specific; for example, the HAQ assesses disability in arthritis. Others are generic and are applicable in all disease; examples include the Short Form 36 (SF-36) and EuroQol.

Some crucial outcomes are of limited relevance in rheumatic diseases. The best example is death. Mortality rates associated with different medical interventions, though useful guides to the value of treatments, are only relevant in diseases with high mortality rates. In most rheumatic diseases death is uncommon. Another example, the ability to work, is an increasingly important assessment of the overall impact of disease, but is not relevant in diseases affecting elderly patients who will usually have retired.

Another issue is the nature of the outcome assessed. Some outcomes are categorical, which range from binary outcomes, like alive or dead, to longer scales dividing patients into three, four or five categories. Some outcomes have longer numeric scales; examples include joint counts, radiographic scores, and quality of life measures like HAQ scores. Their apparent simplicity hides complex analytical issues. For instance, in measures like the HAQ, increments in scores along the scale from 0–3, although numerically similar, may not equate to identical changes in the disability.

The final domain is time. Outcomes can be short term—weeks and months—or long term, extending over years and decades. Short-term outcomes, though readily related to treatment, are often less relevant to patients. Clinical trials focus on short-term outcomes whereas observational studies explore longer-term outcomes.

Interrelationships between outcomes

Different clinical outcomes are closely interrelated. Patients with arthritis who have good clinical outcomes usually have reduced joint counts, less joint damage and better quality of life. The converse is equally true. As a consequence there is no need to measure all outcomes; a few carefully chosen outcomes can capture the overall response to treatment. Reducing the number of outcomes measured has some limitations. Several other factors are involved in determining individual outcomes. For example, in patients with rheumatoid arthritis the presence of rheumatoid factor increases the likelihood of erosive joint damage irrespective of the response to treatment. Similarly, the presence of comorbidities worsens patients' quality of life irrespective of their responses to treatment.

One crucial issue is whether some outcomes provide more useful information than others. Outcomes which capture issues of direct importance to patients are preferable to overtly medical outcomes. For instance, most experts believe it is more important to assess quality of life than laboratory measures like the erythrocyte sedimentation rate (ESR) or erosive damage on radiographs. However, these patient-related outcomes have drawbacks: they can be highly subjective, they may showed marked variations between patients, and their accuracy and reproducibility may be limited.

An associated issue is the generalizability of outcome measurements. Generic measures like the SF-36 and EuroQol can be applied across a wide range of diseases, including arthritis, connective tissue diseases and non-rheumatological disorders. They provide comparable measures of the benefits of medical treatment in many patients. Such broad comparability is offset by reductions in sensitivity to changes in arthritis and a lack of specificity in detecting treatment effects.

Confounding factors

Clinical outcomes attempt to capture the impact of treating rheumatic diseases. However, many other factors, often not directly related to the disease itself, are of equal importance. These confounding factors can make it challenging to compare outcomes between centres, because they may have very different confounding factors, which may not be unravelled by attempts to correct for them. Key confounding factors are:

◆ *Demography*: age, gender, ethnicity, and disease duration are all relevant, with worse outcomes anticipated in elderly patients from ethnic minority groups who have long disease durations.

◆ *Deprivation*: poverty shortens life and invariably worsens outcomes.

◆ *Comorbidities*: patients with multiple comorbid conditions usually have worse quality of life and their outcomes are poorer for all diseases.

These multiple confounding factors mean that comparing outcomes across units without adjustment will invariably show major differences. Given the difficulties making appropriate adjustments, it appears inevitable that all comparisons will be flawed. In addition, treatment probably ought to vary across units as they will see very different patients. Within the United Kingdom there has been concern about 'postcode' prescribing, with treatments varying depending on where patients live. However, such concerns are based on mistaken assumptions; variations between centres make postcode prescribing inevitable.

Outcomes in arthritis—rheumatoid arthritis as model

It is impractical to outline outcome assessments in all rheumatic diseases. Instead it is best to use one major disorder as an exemplar for outcomes in rheumatology. The obvious example is rheumatoid arthritis.

The rheumatoid arthritis outcome matrix spans five domains (Table 29.1). Outcomes include symptoms and assessments of disease activity,[6] damage and quality of life, the overall result—remission—and end results like joint replacement and death. There is no need to record all outcomes. A few measures can capture the impact of treatment. Joint counts and acute-phase measures like the ESR

are most useful in short-term studies whereas joint replacement and death are more relevant in long-term studies.

Disability and quality of life

Patients assess their disability, function, and quality of life. Consequently these measures are termed 'patient-related outcome measures' (PROMs).[7] In the United Kingdom National Health Service (NHS), PROMs have assumed central positions. One reason is that they are easily measured. In addition, treatment should result in improvements noticed by patients.

The main limitation of PROMs is that they are highly subjective. If patients believe they are disabled or have major health problems, their scores will reflect these health beliefs. In addition, generic outcome measures were not designed for patients with arthritis and therefore are relatively insensitive in detecting improvements in health status. The various measures may not give identical findings. Patients may record poor outcomes in some scores but not in others. Finally, the various PROMs have scales of differing lengths with views on how to describe normal. Some consider normal function should be scored as zero, with limitations of quality of life giving higher scores. The HAQ and the Nottingham Health Profile (NHP) are examples of such positive scoring. Others consider normal function should be classified as scoring 100% or 1 (on a 0–1 scale), with limitations of quality of life giving lower scores. The Short Form 36 (SF-36) and EuroQol are examples of such negative scoring.

Patient-related outcome measures

There are three dominant measures—HAQ, SF-36, and EuroQol—which are summarized in Table 29.2. There are also many other measures which are less commonly used.

Health Assessment Questionnaire

HAQ scores, also termed the HAQ Disability Index (HAQ-DI), assesses function by asking questions across eight categories—dressing, rising, eating, walking, hygiene, reach, grip, and usual activities.[8] Patients respond on four-point scales, ranging from 0 (no disability) to 3 (completely disabled). These are added to give the HAQ score on a 0–3 scale. The smallest increment is 0.125. It is a disease-specific measure, designed for patients with arthritis, and is used mainly in rheumatoid arthritis. The HAQ has been widely translated into many different languages.

Short Form 36

The SF-36 gives eight scaled scores based on patients' responses to 36 questions. Each domain is transformed into 0–100 scales.

Table 29.1 Outcome matrix for rheumatoid arthritis

Symptoms	Damage	Quality of life	Overall	End result
Joint counts	New erosions	HAQ	Remission	Joint replacement
ESR	Sharp scores	AIMS2	Work disability	Death
C-reactive protein	Larsen scores	SF-36		
DAS28 scores		EuroQol		
		NHP		

AIMS2, Arthritis Impact Measurement Scale 2; ESR, erythrocyte sedimentation rate; HAQ, Health Assessment Questionnaire; NHP, Nottingham Health Profile; SF-36, Short Form 36.

Table 29.2 Patient-related outcome measures for function and quality of life

Measure	Health Assessment Questionnaire	Short Form 36	EuroQol
Abbreviation	HAQ	SF-36	EQ-5D
Use	Disease specific	Generic	Generic
Components	Function	Function, pain, general health, vitality, social role, mental health	Mobility, self-care, usual activities, pain, mental health

The eight domains are physical function, physical role, bodily pain, general health, vitality, social role, emotional role, and mental health.[9] The first four can be combined into a physical component summary score and the latter four into a mental component summary score. There are also shorter similar scores, such as the SF-12, which are brief but less sensitive to changing health. The SF-36 is a generic measure, designed to capture health status in many different conditions. Like the HAQ, the SF-36 has been widely translated. There are many datasets available for SF-36 scores in healthy control groups.

EuroQol

The EuroQol or EQ-5D consists of the EQ-5D descriptive system and the EQ visual analogue scale. The EQ-5D descriptive system has five dimensions: mobility, self-care, usual activities, pain/discomfort, and anxiety/depression.[10] Each dimension has three levels: no problems, some problems, extreme problems. EQ-5D can be presented for each dimension. Usually they are combined in an index which ranges from 1 (completely healthy) to 0 (no health at all, which can be viewed as being equivalent to death); for technical reasons some patients have scores below 0. The EQ visual analogue score assesses patients' current health as a 100 mm visual analogue score. The EuroQol is another generic measure which has been widely translated. Scores for normal healthy controls are widely available.

Others

There are many other disease-specific and generic PROMs. Examples include the Arthritis Impact Measurement Scale (AIMs-2),[11] the Nottingham Health Profile (NHP)[12] and the Rheumatoid Arthritis Quality of Life (RAQoL) questionnaire.[13] All have strong points and are useful and valid. However, for a variety of reasons, they are less widely used.

Health economics

PROMs inform health economic assessments. They are useful in the first steps of such analyses, which involve identifying the impact of an intervention on patients' quality of life. Utility scores (on scales of 0–1, like EuroQol) when combined with information about time, can generate quality-adjusted life years (QALY). These are based on the number of years of life added by treatment based on the concept of perfect health being assigned the value of 1.0 down to a value of 0.0 for death.[14] Multiplying the average utility score by the time spent in this health state generates QALYs. Health economic analyses then compare the difference in QALYs attributable to treatment. The EuroQol can be used to directly measure QALYs, the SF-36 and

SF-12 scores can be used to generate utility data, and HAQ scores can be used in modelling studies to provide data on QALYs. The potential role of these PROMs in judging the cost-effectiveness of treatments is an important part of their role in assessing health.

Outcomes in inflammatory arthritis

The multiplicity of outcome measures and rheumatic diseases make it impractical to provide detailed information on all outcomes in all diseases. Rheumatoid arthritis provides a good as an example for what happens to outcomes over time with treatment. Findings in rheumatoid arthritis are broadly similar in other forms of inflammatory arthritis, including early undifferentiated arthritis and psoriatic arthritis.

HAQ scores

Early rheumatoid arthritis

HAQ scores are often relatively high at disease onset and improve over the next 6–12 months due to the impact of treatment. Thereafter they gradually increase over time. This has been termed the 'J-shaped' curve (Figure 29.1a).[15] There is some evidence that the nature of rheumatoid arthritis is changing over time. Although the pattern of change is similar, more recent patients have lower mean HAQ scores, which may reflect changes in the disease itself, better treatment, and differences in referral patterns.

Established rheumatoid arthritis

After the initial treatment has been completed, mean HAQ scores in established rheumatoid arthritis gradually increase over time (Figure 29.1b).[16,17] The rate of increase varies between studies: it reflects the severity of disease, the extent of erosive damage, the effectiveness of treatment and the presence of comorbidities. The annual rate of increase in HAQ scores is in the region of 0.03 per year. This equates to an average 1% increase.[18] In groups of patients with rheumatoid arthritis a change in HAQ scores of more than 0.22 is considered clinically important.[19]

Mean changes in HAQ scores do not show individual variation over short time periods, which can be marked. Mean changes hides the marked fluctuation in HAQ scores over months in individual patients.[20]

HAQ scores fall with effective treatment, particularly with disease modifying antirheumatic drugs (DMARDs) and biologics. The changes are maximal by 6 months and thereafter stabilize. Systematic reviews show broadly similar falls with both simple treatment with DMARD monotherapy and intensive treatments with combination DMARDs and tumour necrosis factor (TNF) inhibitors in more severe disease (Figure 29.2).[21]

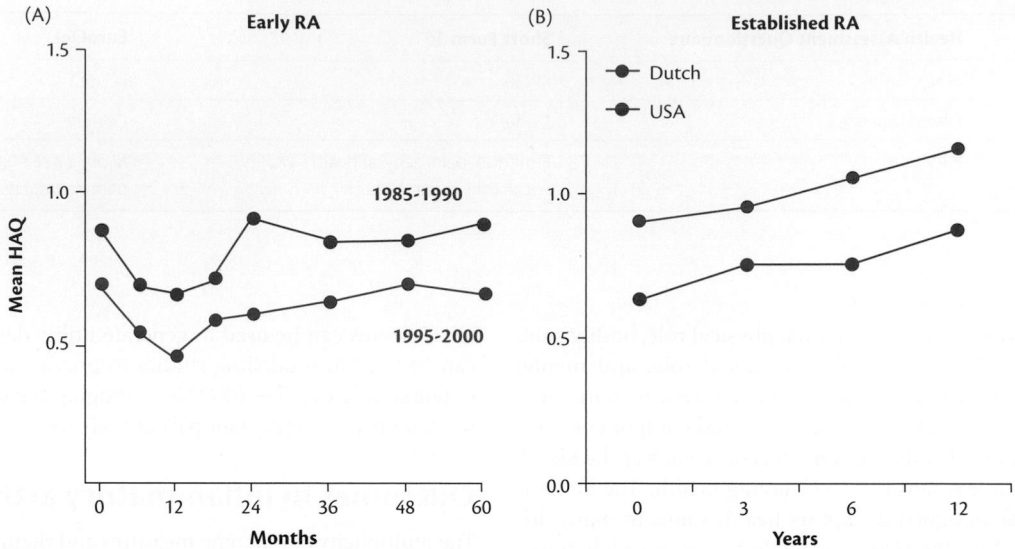

Fig. 29.1 Changes in health assessment questionnaire scores in rheumatoid arthritis: (A) early disease (Welsing et al. 2005).[15] (B) established disease (Drossaers-Bakker et al. 1999; Wolfe, 2000).[16,17]

Welsing PM, Fransen J, van Riel PL. Is the disease course of rheumatoid arthritis becoming milder? Time trends since 1985 in an inception cohort of early rheumatoid arthritis. Arthritis Rheum 2005; 52: 2616–24.

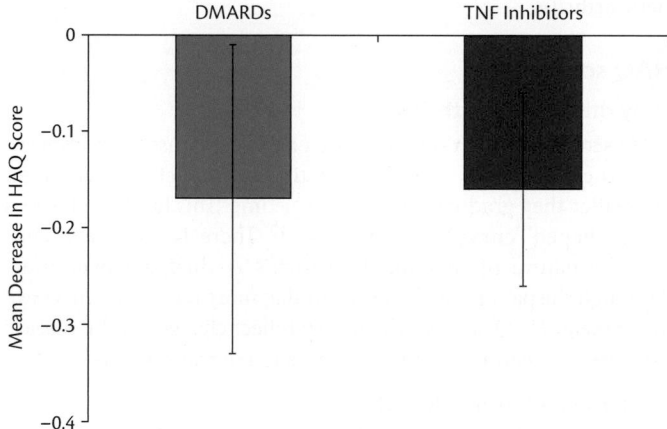

Fig. 29.2 Changes in Health Assessment Questionnaire (HAQ) scores in trials of combination disease modifying anti-rheumatic drugs (DMARDs) and tumour necrosis factor (TNF) inhibitors (from Ma et al. 2010).[21] Mean differences and 95% confidence intervals are shown.

Ma MH, Kingsley GH, Scott DL. A systematic comparison of combination DMARD therapy and tumour necrosis inhibitor therapy with methotrexate in patients with early rheumatoid arthritis. Rheumatology 2010; 49: 91–8.

SF-36 scores in rheumatoid arthritis

SF-36 shows a complex profile of outcomes in rheumatoid arthritis, and this is shown in Figure 29.3.[22] Functional domains show marked changes, with very low scores. Mental health domains show less severe changes, though these are reduced compared to healthy individuals. There is some evidence that mental health domains show similar changes to those seen in major treated psychological diseases like depression.

Treatment with disease modifying drugs and biologics improves SF-36 scores. This can be seen both in individual domains and in summary scores. Interestingly, there is some evidence that biologics improve both physical and mental components of

health whereas conventional treatments only improve physical components.[23]

EuroQol

This is a different type of measure and has very different properties from assessments such as HAQ. The nature of the three-point scoring system means that the way patients complete the assessments impacts on the measurements. This is shown by comparison to HAQ scores in a cross-sectional study of rheumatoid arthritis.[24] HAQ scores have a Gaussian distribution, albeit with a tail towards normal. In contrast EuroQol scores have two peaks; most patients cluster around the midpoint, but a few patients have very low scores, with some being below zero. This means it is difficult to transpose HAQ scores directly into EuroQol scores.

Successful treatment increases EuroQol scores, although the changes can be relatively small as the scale is very compressed. Changes of 0.1–0.2 are clinically relevant. The impact of biologics on EuroQol scores is shown in an observational study from Sweden, which indicates that there are greater changes with the first TNF inhibitor compared to second and third inhibitors.[25]

Integrated outcomes

Ideally outcomes should be captured using a single score or profile. This would have the benefits of simplicity and speed and would also allow comparisons to be made across units and countries. However, simple assessments may be inadequate and superficial and there is a complex balance between straightforward, easy approaches and oversimplifying complex problems.

One new measure, which may achieve wide use, is the Rheumatoid Arthritis Impact of Disease (RAID) score, which is a patient-derived composite measure of the impact of rheumatoid arthritis. RAID uses a simple questionnaire which has individual numeric rating scales that record seven key outcomes—pain, functional capacity,

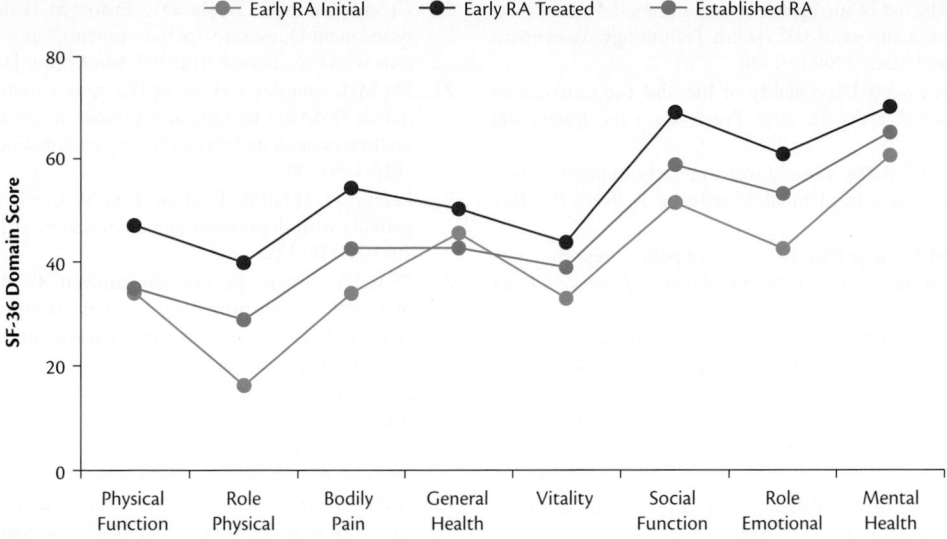

Fig. 29.3 Mean SF-36 domain scores in early rheumatoid arthritis (RA)—initial and treated—and established treated RA (after Lempp et al. 2011).[22]
Reproduced with permission from Lempp H, Ibrahim F, Shaw T, Hofmann D, Graves H, Thornicroft G, Scott I, Kendrick T, Scott DL. Comparative quality of life in patients with depression and rheumatoid arthritis. Int Rev Psychiatry 2011; 23: 118–24. © Informa Healthcare, 2011.

Table 29.3 Outcome matrix for inflammatory myositis

Clinical features	Damage	Quality of Life	Overall	End result
Manual muscle testing CPK Myositis disease activity assessment tool	Muscle biopsy score Myositis damage index	Myositis Functional index SF-36 EuroQol	Remission Work disability	Death

CPK, creatine phosphokinase; SF-36, Short Form 36.

fatigue, physical well-being, emotional well-being, sleep, and coping. Values in each domain are weighted by patients' assessments of their relative importance. They are then combined in a single score. Its proponents believe it will give clear and reliable data on overall outcomes.[26] However, it is premature to draw firm conclusions about its likely value.[27]

Outcomes in connective tissue diseases—inflammatory myositis as another model

Just as rheumatoid arthritis can act as a model for outcomes in arthritis, inflammatory myositis—polymyositis and dermatomyositis—can provide a comparable guide to outcomes in connective tissue diseases.[28] The myositis outcome matrix can also be divided into five domains, which are shown in Table 29.3. Key outcomes include clinical features like muscle weakness, overall activity from measures like the myositis disease activity assessment tool,[29] and biochemical measures like creatine phosphokinase levels. Damage can be assessed by muscle biopsies or end-organ failure assessed by the myositis damage index.[30] Quality of life can be assessed by specific measures like the myositis functional index,[31] generic assessments of quality of life like the SF-36, the overall result—remission—and end results like death.

The general approach to assessing outcomes is similar in myositis and rheumatoid arthritis, though the specific clinical measures used varies considerably. There are also differences in responses to treatment and in the frequency of different types of outcome. Other connective tissue disease, such as systemic lupus erythematosus, involve comparable outcome assessments.[32]

Conclusions

Measuring disease outcomes is an essential for good medical care, which can only improve when clinicians know the results of their treatments and involves patients' views.[33] Rheumatologists need to appreciate who they are seeing as patients and what happens as a consequence of their treatments. These sentiments are widely held but rarely followed. However, change seems inevitable with the widespread use of electronic records and the linking of records within and between institutions.

It is tempting to use outcome assessments to compare individual clinicians or units. However, this approach may be inappropriate and misleading. The diversity of patients and resources means heterogeneity is inevitable between and even within units. Rather than comparing absolute outcomes, we should focus on changes in outcomes. Despite the heterogeneity between units, clinicians should all be showing improved outcomes over time. The real cause of concern is not variations in absolute outcomes but differences in the direction of change. Poor performance is not having bad outcomes so much as having worsening outcomes over time.

References

1. Scott DL, Smith C, Kingsley G. What are the consequences of early rheumatoid arthritis for the individual? *Best Pract Res Clin Rheumatol* 2005;19:117–136.
2. Fransen J, van Riel PL. Outcome measures in inflammatory rheumatic diseases. *Arthritis Res Ther* 2009;11:244.
3. Wells GA. Patient-driven outcomes in rheumatoid arthritis. *J Rheumatol Suppl* 2009;82:33–38.

4. Taylor RS, Elston J. The use of surrogate outcomes in model-based cost-effectiveness analyses: a survey of UK Health Technology Assessment reports. *Health Technol Assess* 2009;13:1–50.

5. Kingsley G, Scott IC, Scott DL. Quality of life and the outcome of established rheumatoid arthritis. *Best Pract Res Clin Rheumatol* 2011;25:585–606.

6. van Riel PL, Fransen J. DAS28: a useful instrument to monitor infliximab treatment in patients with rheumatoid arthritis. *Arthritis Res Ther* 2005;7:189–190.

7. Marshall S, Haywood K, Fitzpatrick R. Impact of patient-reported outcome measures on routine practice: a structured review. *J Eval Clin Pract* 2006;12:559–568.

8. Fries JF, Spitz PW, Young DY. The dimensions of health outcomes: the health assessment questionnaire, disability and pain scales. *J Rheumatol* 1982;9:789–793.

9. Ware JE, Sherbourne CD. The MOS 36-Item Short-Form Health Survey (SF-36). I. Conceptual framework and item selection. *Med Care* 1992;30:473–483.

10. Rabin R, de Charro F. EQ-5D: a measure of health status from the EuroQol Group. *Ann Med* 2001;33:337–343.

11. Meenan RF, Mason JH, Anderson JJ, Guccione AA, Kazis LE. AIMS2. The content and properties of a revised and expanded Arthritis Impact Measurement Scales Health Status Questionnaire. Arthritis Rheum 1992;35:1–10.

12. Hunt SM, McEwen J, McKenna SP. Measuring health status: a new tool for clinicians and epidemiologists. *J R Coll Gen Pract* 1985;35:185–188.

13. de Jong Z, van der Heijde D, McKenna SP, Whalley D. The reliability and construct validity of the RAQoL: a rheumatoid arthritis-specific quality of life instrument. *Br J Rheumatol* 1997;36:878–883.

14. La Puma J, Lawlor EF. Quality-adjusted life-years. Ethical implications for physicians and policymakers. *JAMA* 1990;263:2917–2921.

15. Welsing PM, Fransen J, van Riel PL. Is the disease course of rheumatoid arthritis becoming milder? Time trends since 1985 in an inception cohort of early rheumatoid arthritis. *Arthritis Rheum* 2005;52:2616–2624.

16. Drossaers-Bakker KW, de Buck M, van Zeben D et al. Long-term course and outcome of functional capacity in rheumatoid arthritis: the effect of disease activity and radiologic damage over time. *Arthritis Rheum* 1999;42:1854–1860.

17. Wolfe F. A reappraisal of HAQ disability in rheumatoid arthritis. *Arthritis Rheum* 2000;43:2751–2761.

18. Scott DL, Garrood T. Quality of life measures: use and abuse. *Baillieres Best Pract Res Clin Rheumatol* 2000;14:663–687.

19. Wolfe F, Michaud K, Strand V. Expanding the definition of clinical differences: from minimally clinically important differences to really important differences. Analyses in 8931 patients with rheumatoid arthritis. *J Rheumatol* 2005;32:583–589.

20. Greenwood MC, Doyle DV, Ensor M. Does the Stanford Health Assessment Questionnaire have potential as a monitoring tool for subjects with rheumatoid arthritis? *Ann Rheum Dis* 2001;60:344–348.

21. Ma MH, Kingsley GH, Scott DL. A systematic comparison of combination DMARD therapy and tumour necrosis inhibitor therapy with methotrexate in patients with early rheumatoid arthritis. *Rheumatology* 2010;49:91–98.

22. Lempp H, Ibrahim F, Shaw T et al. Comparative quality of life in patients with depression and rheumatoid arthritis. *Int Rev Psychiatry* 2011;23:118–124.

23. Strand V, Smolen JS, van Vollenhoven RF et al. Certolizumab pegol plus methotrexate provides broad relief from the burden of rheumatoid arthritis: analysis of patient-reported outcomes from the RAPID 2 trial. *Ann Rheum Dis* 2011;70:996–1002.

24. Scott DL, Khoshaba B, Choy EH, Kingsley GH. Limited correlation between the Health Assessment Questionnaire (HAQ) and EuroQol in rheumatoid arthritis: questionable validity of deriving quality adjusted life years from HAQ. *Ann Rheum Dis* 2007;66:1534–1537.

25. Gülfe A, Kristensen LE, Saxne T et al. Utility-based outcomes made easy: the number needed per quality-adjusted life year gained. An observational cohort study of tumor necrosis factor blockade in inflammatory arthritis from Southern Sweden. *Arthritis Care Res* 2010;62:1399–1406.

26. Heiberg T, Austad C, Kvien TK, Uhlig T. Performance of the Rheumatoid Arthritis Impact of Disease (RAID) score in relation to other patient-reported outcomes in a register of patients with rheumatoid arthritis. *Ann Rheum Dis* 2011;70:1080–1082.

27. Gullick NJ, Scott DL. Rheumatoid arthritis: clinical utility of the RAID (RA impact of disease) score. *Nat Rev Rheumatol* 2011;7:499–500.

28. Oddis CV. Outcomes and disease activity measures for assessing treatments in the idiopathic inflammatory myopathies. *Curr Rheumatol Rep* 2005;7:87–93.

29. Sultan SM, Allen E, Oddis CV et al. Reliability and validity of the myositis disease activity assessment tool. *Arthritis Rheum* 2008;58:3593–3599.

30. Sultan SM, Allen E, Cooper RG et al. Interrater reliability and aspects of validity of the myositis damage index. *Ann Rheum Dis* 2011;70:1272–1276.

31. Alexanderson H, Broman L, Tollbäck A et al. Functional index-2: Validity and reliability of a disease-specific measure of impairment in patients with polymyositis and dermatomyositis. *Arthritis Rheum* 2006;55:114–122.

32. Strand V, Chu AD. Measuring outcomes in systemic lupus erythematosus clinical trials. *Expert Rev Pharmacoecon Outcomes Res* 2011;11:455–468.

33. Higginson IJ, Carr AJ. Measuring quality of life: Using quality of life measures in the clinical setting. *BMJ* 2001;322:1297–1300.

CHAPTER 30

Design of clinical trials in rheumatology

Vibeke Strand, Jeremy Sokolove, and Alvina D. Chu

Introduction

Randomized controlled trials (RCTs) in the rheumatic diseases have undergone a rapid evolution since 1998, driven by approval of 11 new disease-modifying anti-rheumatic drugs (DMARDs) for treatment of rheumatoid arthritis (RA), 9 of which are biologic agents. In addition to many detailed reviews on clinical trials in rheumatic diseases,[1-6] guidelines for development of new agents for treatment of RA, osteoarthritis (OA), and systemic lupus erythematosus (SLE) have been issued by the United States Food and Drug Administration (FDA)[7] and the European Medicines Agency (EMA)[8] as well as by the International Conference on Harmonisation (ICH) for use by worldwide regulatory agencies.[9] This chapter is intended to provide a basic overview of clinical trial design and terminology while also providing some important lessons specific to clinical development in individual rheumatic diseases.

Phases in development of new therapeutic agents

Phase 1

Phase 1 trials are intended to demonstrate the initial safety and pharmacokinetics (PK) and/or pharmacodynamics (PD) of a new agent in humans, based on extensive preclinical data in animal models of disease, toxicology, absorption, distribution, metabolism, and excretion (ADME) studies and pharmacokinetics data in mice, rats, and primates as well as dogs, rabbits, and pigs.[10] 'First in human' studies are first single ascending dose (SAD) followed by multiple ascending dose (MAD) escalation studies to confirm successful delivery of the product and initial PK/PD data. They may be performed in healthy volunteers or in subjects with the disease in question—especially if the agent is immunologically active, as are most biologic agents. Ideally the goal of phase 1 is to determine the maximum tolerated dose (MTD) as well as the minimally effective dose, and characterize pharmacokinetics: half-life ($t_{1/2}$), maximal and minimal achieved concentration (C_{max}, C_{min}), and average concentration over time known as area under the curve (AUC). Sometimes a smaller phase 1A study is performed to assess safety with a longer phase 1B study performed subsequently for additional PK/PD and dose-finding data. As these may differ between healthy

volunteers and subjects with disease, due to differing immunologic processes in play, typically only healthy volunteers are utilized in phase 1A trials. However, if phase 1A or 1B studies are performed in subjects with disease then they may provide preliminary signs of efficacy, especially if a specific biomarker or early marker of 'response' can be measured.

Phase 2

Phase 2 studies are designed to provide additional PK/PD data and to establish proof of concept, e.g. that an agent has activity in the disease in question. Proof-of-concept trials in RA generally require at least 12 weeks' treatment duration to prove benefit for a sufficient duration of time that longer-term trials as well as 'rescue' with the experimental agent are warranted. It must be emphasized that careful and thorough conduct of phase 2 trials will result in a more efficient phase 3 programme and significantly increase the probability of success. By the conclusion of phase 2 studies, the pharmacokinetics of the agent should be well characterized, including MTD and minimal effective dose, and one or at most two doses and/or dosing regimens should have been selected for study in phase 3 trials. Additionally, clinical data generated in phase 2 should allow sample size calculations for phase 3 trials by estimating the effect size of the experimental agent. This is especially important given the size and cost of phase 3 trials designed to support regulatory approval of a new therapy.

Phase 3

Phase 3 RCTs are designed to support approval of a new therapy, and must be studied in an adequate number of subjects with the disease in question to support its safety, and in replicate (but not identical) trials to confirm its efficacy. Though regulatory agencies require two studies to confirm statistical superiority, it is risky to conduct an identical study twice as it is highly unlikely one will obtain the same results, especially in heterogeneous rheumatic diseases. This is well illustrated by the phase 3 RCTs comparing leflunomide and MTX, equivalent DMARDs where in one trial (US301) leflunomide was statistically superior and in the other, (MN302) MTX was superior.[11,12] Ideally the same question, efficacy in a certain disease indication, can be confirmed with two complementary but not identical patient populations, such as DMARD-failure and DMARD-naive subjects, or by comparing induction with maintenance therapy.

Issues common to randomized controlled trials

Treatment allocation and rescue

Allocation refers to assignment of subjects to specific treatment groups. To enrol any subject into a well-controlled trial there must exist equipoise, or genuine uncertainty on the part of the investigator (or evaluator) of the benefit of an intervention. If proof-of-concept studies have already indicated a positive effect for a promising therapy then equipoise may be maintained if there is an imbalance in randomization, such as a 2:1 assignment of subjects to active vs control therapy. This can result in loss of power and offers the opportunity for more adverse events to accrue in active than in control therapy. Another strategy is adaptive randomization in which the next randomization depends on previous responses. This works best with proof-of-concept studies utilizing biomarkers and/or early markers of response, typically in phase 2. Adaptive studies are not generally accepted for phase 3 RCTs.

'Treatment rescue' is another means to maintain equipoise whereby subjects are offered rescue with active therapy after documented non-response after 3–6 months of enrolment. If there exists a positive proof-of-concept study, then subjects may be rescued with the new therapy in an open-label continuation protocol designed to accrue safety data over longer-term exposure. Otherwise, subjects may be considered 'treatment failures' and exit the protocol for active therapy, having met a predefined protocol endpoint for statistical analysis. Alternatively, they may continue protocol participation but be considered 'non-responders', provided they have not experienced an adverse event that would require treatment withdrawal.

Blinding and bias

Blinding is a critical, if imperfect, tool to prevent bias in RCTs. The ability to balance randomization such that significant covariates do not interfere with trial results is critical. In most cases 'perfect' balance is impossible and thus most trials are subjected to analyses of covariance (ANCOVA).

There are well-known confounding characteristics to be considered when studying biologic agents in RCTs. Parenteral administration may result in first dose reactions (injection site or infusion reactions) and or rapid onset of effect leading to unblinding. Expectation bias on the part of subjects and physicians may result in higher placebo responses.[13] Concomitant effects of background therapy, immunogenicity, and use of 'industrial strength' rather than pharmacological or physiological doses may confound results.[10] For this reason regulatory agencies frequently require different treating and evaluating physicians.

Statistical analyses

Size/power

Statistical significance is *always* predefined, referred to as the alpha (α) level and often set by convention to be p <0.05, thus representing a less than 5% risk that the difference observed is due to chance (or the alternative, more than 95% confidence that the observed effect is real.) The power of a study refers to the ability of trial results

to reject a false null hypothesis, thus identifying a true treatment effect. Mathematically, power can be represented by the expression 1-β, where β is the risk of a false-negative decision (type 2 error). Thus, the lower the risk of a type 2 error, the greater the power. Calculating power is not difficult, but rather, factors entering into the assumptions of a power calculation require extensive understanding of estimated effect sizes as well as standard deviations of the observations. Typically these are generated from earlier phase 2 studies which also demonstrate the variability of responses around both active and control treatments. Phase 3 trials must account for heterogeneity among subjects enrolled and disease characteristics at baseline, geographical and site variability, and other potential influential factors such as presence or absence of biomarkers. Thus, all phase 3 analyses make use of a 'model' which takes into account those covariates that are statistically significant when assessed by univariate analyses.

Analysis populations

No trial is likely to have all enrolled subjects complete the trial. Thus, investigators must plan in advance for dropouts, and typically increase sample sizes to accommodate expected dropout rates. The 'intention to treat' (ITT) population refers to all subjects who were randomized, and in the case of biologic agents, received at least one dose of study drug. The 'per protocol' (PP) population includes only those subjects without major protocol violations and may be used as supportive analyses in phase 2 trials and as the primary analysis population in an active controlled trial that does not include a placebo group. The 'safety' population includes all patients randomized, whether or not they receive treatment. Although some therapies may have a delayed onset of benefit, it is expected that use of adequate sample sizes will allow sufficient randomization that there will be equal numbers of early dropouts in both active and control arms.

Missing data

'Last observation carried forward' (LOCF) has been the typical means for accounting for missing data whereby the last value available for a subject is brought forward for endpoint analyses. Although a well-accepted statistical analysis, it imputes the 'best value' for a subject who may be a responder but is forced to discontinue early due to an intolerable adverse event. This analysis can be used to assess responses over time (e.g. American College of Rheumatology (ACR) responses over time) but will falsely elevate responses if an agent displays early efficacy yet ultimately has a poor safety or tolerability profile. A more conservative statistical approach to account for dropouts is use of the non-responder imputation (NRI), where 'all cause' dropouts, due either to lack of efficacy, adverse events, or other reasons are considered non-responders, regardless of their response status at time of dropout. These subjects remain in the denominator as the ITT population, but only those who complete the trial are eligible for consideration as responders. Another more conservative approach, popular for use in analgesic trials, is 'baseline carried forward' (BOCF), where changes from baseline in early dropouts are set to zero. In a sense this is a measure of 'effectiveness' in that a therapy that cannot be tolerated over 3–6 months would not be considered effective in the relief of chronic pain.

Another option is use of regression models to impute missing data such as radiographic results at 12 months in subjects who discontinue treatment or are rescued at 6 months (or earlier). To test the validity of such modelling sensitivity analyses are performed, substituting the worst data in the control population (placebo) for missing data in the active arm until statistical significance is lost, and vice versa.[14]

Interim analyses

Although not generally performed in phase 3 RCTs, other phases of clinical development may employ interim analyses, prespecified for safety or to ascertain the need to adjust sample sizes. A major risk of an interim analysis is that it will alter the conduct of the study or even unblind the results. In very large RCTs, an interim analysis based on an early marker of response may allow ascertainment of potential success with little loss of p value, but in general they put the final statistical analyses at risk. A preferred method is to utilize data safety monitoring boards (DSMBs) who review trial data on an ongoing basis for safety and efficacy and advise the sponsor to discontinue a treatment group without revealing specific results.

Non-inferiority vs superiority analyses

Classic regulatory trials are designed to demonstrate superiority of an experimental therapy over the control, be it placebo+failed background therapy or placebo+standard of care. Active controlled RCTs which lack a control arm are often performed post approval, as phase 3B or 4 studies; these include 'treat to target' and other trials designed to reflect clinical practice. As drug development is generally an iterative process, most regulatory trials are designed to demonstrate superiority to a control therapy, with or without 'non-inferiority' to an active comparator. If non-inferiority is satisfied, then an agent may be tested for superiority. Two major caveats apply: (1) that demonstration of true 'superiority' requires replicate results in separate RCTs, and (2) results in RCTs in RA and other rheumatic diseases differ across protocol populations, reflecting the heterogeneity of disease characteristics and demographics at baseline such that responses by accepted outcome criteria vary widely even with the same active, and approved, product. Thus, it is risky to conduct an active controlled trial for regulatory purposes without a control group to prove that the active comparator is, in fact, efficacious. And to demonstrate superiority frequently would require enrolment of an impractically large number of subjects. Thus, many trials are now designed to show non-inferiority or equivalence to an existing therapy.

Choice of outcome measures

A primary endpoint must be prespecified, with iterative analyses of secondary, 'supportive' outcome measures. Phase 2 RCTs are designed for data mining and even 'post hoc' or subgroup analyses may be employed to better define responsive populations and/or derive evidence-based responder analyses. However, in phase 3 studies, secondary analyses must be strictly prespecified, including the order in which they are analysed until such time as statistical significance is lost. If the outcomes are independent of each other, such that they do not closely correlate and are separated in time, then the order of their analyses may be prespecified without statistical corrections for multiple comparisons—the 'Hochberg principle'.[15,16] As examples, the US301 RCT comparing leflunomide vs methotrexate vs placebo utilized three co-primary endpoints: the first two at 6 and 12 months for improvement in signs and symptoms of RA and inhibition of radiographic progression, and maintenance of physical function and health-related quality of life (HRQoL) at 24 months.[11] Similarly, the first phase 3 trial

of a biologic agent, infliximab, in ATTRACT (Anti-TNF Trial in Rheumatoid Arthritis with Concomitant Therapy), had a primary endpoint at 30 weeks for signs and symptoms,[17] radiography at 52 weeks,[18] and physical function and HRQoL at 104 weeks.[19]

Types of analyses

Unlike cardiovascular or cancer studies which utilize dichotomous outcomes such as mortality, rheumatic studies have required development of reliable composite indexes to define responses to therapy. Responder analyses are now standard in rheumatology, in part due to the efforts of the international consensus effort, Outcome Measures in Rheumatology (OMERACT) in collaboration with ACR and European Leagues Against Rheumatism (EULAR). Figure 30.1 demonstrates a model of the core (required), secondary (nice but not necessary), and ancillary (research agenda) outcome measures recommended for use in several rheumatic disease trials. In general, responder indices decrease sample sizes by including parameters which do not directly correlate with each other. An example is the ACR 20/50/70 response criteria for RA, which includes tender and swollen joint counts, physician and patient global assessments of disease activity, patient-reported pain, and a measure of physical function, generally the Health Assessment Questionnaire, as well as an acute-phase reactant, either C-reactive protein (CRP) or erythrocyte sedimentation rate (ESR). Improvement of 20% or more in five of seven criteria, including joint count, is required for responses. Of the seven criteria, only tender and swollen joint counts are moderately correlated with a coefficient of approximately 0.4—thereby indicating the breadth of improvement necessary across multiple independent measures to achieve a response. Validated responder indices across a wide variety of rheumatic diseases are presented in Table 30.1. All were proposed based on evidence-based data mining and have been prospectively validated in RCTs.

External validity of randomized controlled trials

External validity reflects the ability of the results of a RCT to be extrapolated to the real-world patient population. It is well recognized that subjects enrolled in RCTs tend to be healthier with fewer comorbidities than 'wild type' populations, because exclusion criteria rule out patients with significant concomitant diseases that could affect both safety and efficacy, and inclusion criteria requiring active disease exclude many patients 'typically' seen in practice. Several series have demonstrated that most patients followed in practice and enrolled in RA registries would not be eligible for RCTs.[20,21]

The ICH Guidelines (ICH E9, Section 2.2.1) clearly acknowledge that no individual RCT can be expected to be representative of future users. This is due to the possible influences of geographical location and variability in medical practice. Especially for rheumatic diseases with their heterogeneity and extended natural history, disease duration and timing of the trial with respect to the course of disease progression pose challenges when extrapolating results from trials to individual subjects, well illustrated by results of therapies in subjects with early vs longstanding RA.

Increasingly trials must be multinational and multicultural to enrol adequate numbers of subjects to demonstrate a treatment response—this is certainly true in RA and SLE, and raises concerns about variability in clinical practice, definitions of 'treatment

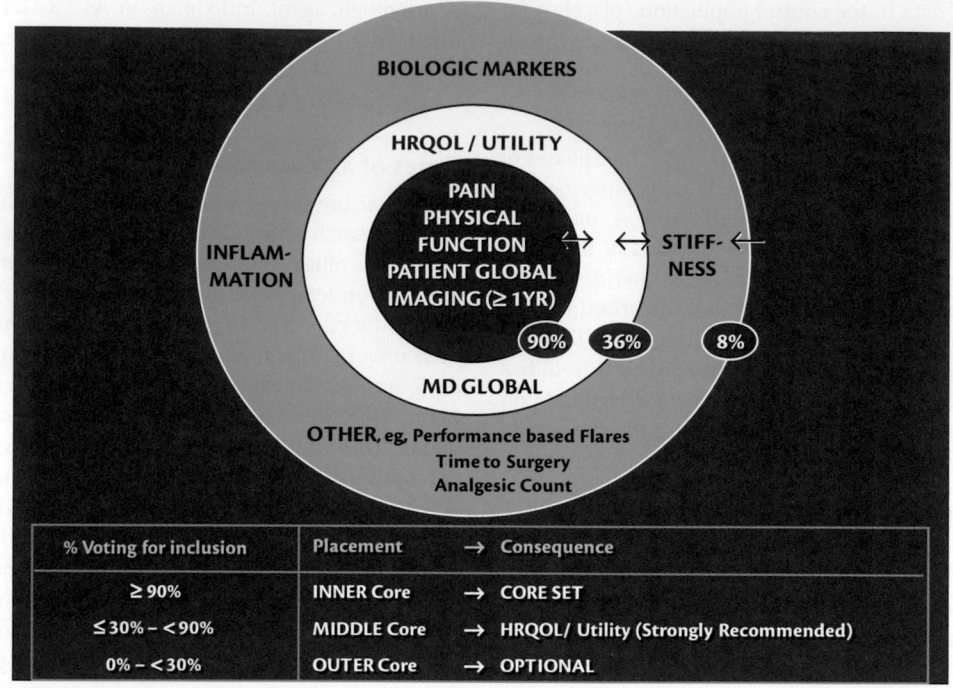

Fig. 30.1 Domains recommended by OMERACT for inclusion in RCTs in osteoarthritis: inner core: required; intermediate ring: nice but not necessary; outer ring: research agenda.

Table 30.1 Rheumatic diseases and outcome measures

	Rheumatoid arthritis	**Osteoarthritis**	**Systemic lupus erythematosus**	**Psoriatic arthritis**	**Ankylosing spondylitis**	**Gout**
Clinical development activity	10 new therapies approved since 1998	No disease-modifying drugs approved; only symptomatic relief	1 new therapy approved in 2011	4 new therapies approved since 2002	4 new therapies approved since 2003	2 new therapies approved since 2009
Patient populations tested	◆ DMARD-naive ◆ Failed DMARD ◆ Biologic-naive RA ◆ Failed biologic	◆ Knee OA ◆ Hip OA ◆ Hand OA	◆ Active SLE receiving SOC therapy ◆ Active lupus nephritis ◆ Induction vs maintenance	◆ DMARD-naive ◆ Biologic naive ◆ Failed TNFi	◆ DMARD-naive ◆ Failed TNFi	◆ Chronic gout ◆ Acute gout
Common outcome measurements	◆ Composite responder indices: ACR, DAS/EULAR responses ◆ Radiography ◆ Physical Fxn/HRQoL	◆ Composite responder index: OMERACT-OARSI ◆ WOMAC ◆ Structure modification (radiography, MRI)	◆ Composite responder indices: SRI, BICLA ◆ Changes in corticosteroid doses ◆ Time to flare and incidence of flares	◆ Composite responder indices: ACR, PsARC ◆ GRAPPA scoring system in progress	◆ Composite responder indices: ASDAS, ASAS	◆ Serum uric acid level ◆ Acute flares ◆ Tophus burden
Patient-reported outcome measurements	◆ Pt global VAS ◆ pain VAS ◆ HAQ ◆ SF-36 ◆ FACIT fatigue ◆ WPS-RA ◆ WIS	◆ Pt global VAS ◆ WOMAC ◆ SF-36	◆ Pt global VAS ◆ SF-36 ◆ FACIT fatigue	◆ Pt global VAS ◆ pain VAS ◆ HAQ ◆ SF-36	◆ Pt global VAS ◆ BASDAI ◆ BASFI	◆ Pt global VAS ◆ pain VAS ◆ HAQ ◆ SF-36

(Continued)

Table 30.1 *(Continued)*

	Rheumatoid arthritis	Osteoarthritis	Systemic lupus erythematosus	Psoriatic arthritis	Ankylosing spondylitis	Gout
Composite responder indices?	Yes	Yes	Yes	Yes	Yes	No
Biomarkers/PD marker of response	Only as component of composite scores	Cartilage breakdown products	◆ ANA, dsDNA antibodies ◆ C3/C4 complement ◆ circulating B-cell subsets	None specific	None specific	◆ Serum uric acid <6.1
Approximate sample size of recent pivotal studies	200–800	200–400	800–900	200–400	200–400	100–1000
Duration of pivotal studies to primary endpoint	3–6 months for signs/symptoms 6–12 months for radiographic changes	3 months for symptoms 12–24 months for structure	12 months	3–6 months	3–6 months	6 months

DMARD, disease-modifying anti-rheumatic drug; HRQoL, health-related quality of life; OA, osteoarthritis; PD, pharmacodynamic; RA, rheumatoid arthritis; SLE, systemic lupus erythematosus; SOC, standard of care; TNFi, tumour necrosis factor inhibitor.

failure', and generalizability to populations with less disease activity and/or more comorbid conditions.

Beyond statistics, what is clinically meaningful?

Regardless of statistical significance, patients and their physicians want to interpret results of RCTs in the context of the individual subject. These are defined improvements (and/or deteriorations) in patient-reported outcomes (PRO) perceptible to patients, as well as degrees of change and/or attainment of a state that feels acceptable: a patient-acceptable state (PASS).[22] The minimum clinically important difference (MCID) reflects that amount of improvement that is detectable to patients, and the number of subjects who report improvements meeting or exceeding MCID in a given PRO or multiple PROs can be considered 'responders' and used to derive a 'number needed to treat' (NNT) to gain the defined benefit. Similarly, larger improvements, or 'really important differences' (RID) or attainment of defined levels of PASS offer higher goals for treatment. Finally with the use of generic measures such as the Health Assessment Questionnaire (HAQ) or the Medical Outcomes Survey Short Form 36 (SF-36), patient-reported data may be compared to normative values to better understand the impact of disease on physical function and/or HRQoL, offering goals for attainment when evaluating treatment associated improvements.

'Number needed to harm' (NNH), or the number of subjects potentially at risk for a bad outcome, can similarly be calculated based on the incidence of serious adverse events (SAEs) of interest, reflecting the effects of the experimental treatment and/or the underlying disease. Although they are estimates only, NNT vs NNH comparisons are increasingly utilized to understand better the potential benefits of a new therapy.

Disease-specific trial design

Rheumatoid arthritis

The development of the ACR response criteria[23,24] and EULAR 'good and moderate' responses[24] has contributed to the introduction of 10 new DMARDs since 1998; significant progress from the two 6-month studies in 126 subjects which supported the approval of methotrexate in 1986.[25,26] Trials in RA are now expected to be at least 3–6 months in duration for improvement in signs and symptoms, with radiographic progression assessed at 6 and 12 months. Seminal RCTs in RA tested primary endpoints at no earlier than 1 year.[11] The time required for assessment of the primary endpoint of signs and symptoms has been shortened over the years to 3 months, based on concerns over duration of placebo exposure and with the precedent of 10 approved products in RA since 1998.

Background therapy

The clear benefit of early DMARD therapy in RA has made use of pure placebo difficult for ethical reasons. With current evidence for rapid progression of irreversible damage as manifest by worsening in HAQ scores and progression in structural damage even over 3–6 months of placebo treatment,[27,28] the standard has become to perform step-up trials in which patients are randomized to experimental therapy or placebo added to failed background DMARD therapy. This poses challenges: (1) variability in responses due to background therapy in both placebo and active treatment arms, and (2) inability to assess directly the effect of the new therapy as monotherapy, thus essentially 'wedding' a new molecule to its background therapy.[28,29] Active controlled trials are another alternative, the challenge being documented variability in responses of the active comparators. For example,

ACR20 response rates in methotrexate control arms have ranged from 46% to 72% with nearly as wide variability among trials of biologic monotherapy. Thus, the requirement for an abbreviated placebo arm as was utilized in the relatively recent AMBITION trial[30] investigating the efficacy of tocilizumab compared with methotrexate. This assured that both active monotherapies were efficacious.

Additionally, step-up designs have led to concerns that results may be confounded by the background therapy, even if patients were no longer responsive to it. It is clear that the duration of the failed therapy prior to study enrolment as well as how long it was administered at stable doses have influenced overall placebo response rates—not to mention issues regarding definitions of 'treatment failure'. Patients may still be accruing responses to methotrexate as a background therapy if they have not received at least 3 months' treatment at maximally tolerated doses. Further, background therapy, even if failed, may offer benefit when coadministered with a biologic agent, such as prolongation of half-life and decreased immunogenicity.[10] Because of these issues, it has been advocated that phase 3 include a three-arm RCT in DMARD-naive subjects comparing either monotherapy or DMARD vs experimental agent; vs combination of the two.

Treatment to target

Although RCTs remain the gold standard for evaluation of therapeutic efficacy, protocols designed for regulatory approval clearly do not mimic clinical practice. Lack of flexibility to adjust treatment over time limits extrapolation of the results to 'real-world' use. The advent of 'treatment to target' studies, although not designed for regulatory approval, provides an opportunity to study therapeutic regimens with predefined changes based on responses/nonresponses, including their effect on patient expectations[3] which might occur with any perceived change in therapy. These trials are particularly helpful in comparing recently approved therapies as well as understanding responses in more heterogeneous disease populations.

Other inflammatory arthritides

Specific challenges in RCT design have accompanied clinical development of therapeutics for psoriatic arthritis (PsA), ankylosing spondylitis (AS), and gout, different from those in RA. Although RA-specific outcome measures have been adapted and validated for use in PsA trials, they most accurately reflect changes in polyarticular disease.[31,32] The Disease Activity Index for Reactive Arthritis (DAREA) has been utilized in PsA studies, which combines patient pain and global assessments, joint counts, and CRP, but this index also emphasizes peripheral arthritis.[33,34] Because PsA includes skin disease and spondyloarthropathy as well as enthesitis and dactylitis, a PsA-specific disease severity and responder index is being developed by the Group for Research and Assessment of Psoriasis and Psoriatic Arthritis (GRAPPA) to assess skin as well as different articular manifestations (Figure 30.2).[31]

Studies in AS have utilized disease-specific outcome measurements, but have not been successful to date in demonstrating benefit on progression of structural damage. The Spondylitis Disease Activity Index (BASDAI) does not correlate with structural damage and may not accurately reflect the full spectrum of disease where both axial and peripheral joints are involved.[31] The Assessment of SpondyloArthritis international Society (ASAS)

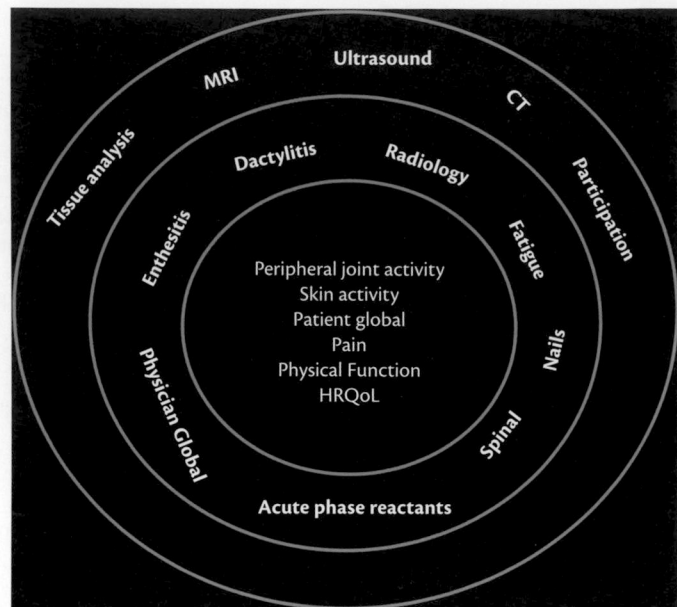

Fig. 30.2 Domains recommended by OMERACT for inclusion in RCTs in psoriatic arthritis: inner core: required; intermediate ring: nice but not necessary; outer ring: research agenda.

disease activity score (ASDAS), which incorporates components of pain, inflammation, peripheral signs, and PRO, has been recently validated, and discriminates between high and low disease activity states.[35]

In gout, different challenges are posed by trials in acute vs chronic gout.[36] Two recent product approvals, febuxostat and pegloticase, have facilitated trial designs in chronic gout. The lowering of serum urate levels to less than 6.0 mg/dL has been accepted as a pharmacodynamic measure of efficacy in chronic gout, as well as objective measures for assessing tophus size and PRO of pain, physical function, and HRQoL.[36,37] Efforts continue to define flare and accurately measure its duration in acute gout (Figure 30.3).

Osteoarthritis

To date no agent has been shown to have disease-modifying effects on structural progression of OA. Many have been demonstrated to offer symptomatic relief including non-steroidal anti-inflammatory drugs (NSAIDs), cyclooxygenase-2 selective agents (COX-2s), intra-articular hyaluronic acid (IA-HA) injections and opioids. FDA[7] and European Medicines Agency (EMA)[8] guidelines for evaluation of new therapeutic agents for symptomatic relief of OA recommend measures of patient pain and function and for structural modification measurement of joint space width (JSW) by radiography and/or MRI, currently the best-accepted methodology.

Major challenges for development of disease-modifying OA drugs (DMOADs) include the need for improved measures of structural damage (beyond use of radiography) as well as improved understanding of the appropriate population and/or disease stage for intervention. OA is a final common pathway following many predisposing factors and thus therapeutics may have limited, if any, efficacy in those with pre-existing joint damage, biomechanical predisposition, and/or obesity.[38]

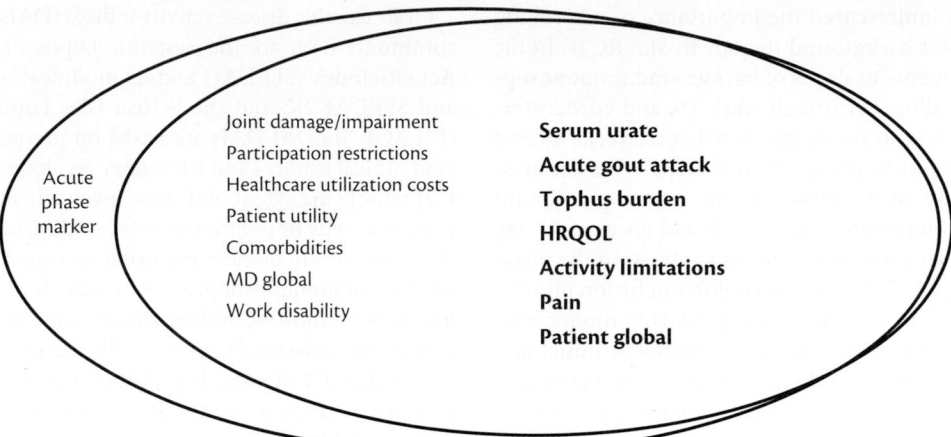

Fig. 30.3 Domains for inclusion in RCTs in acute and chronic gout: those in bold type are required; within the inner ring nice but not necessary; acute-phase marker part of the research agenda.

Measures of pain and function

Historically, the most widely used metric for outcome in OA trials has been the Western Ontario and McMaster University OA Index (WOMAC), consisting of three subscales: pain (5 questions), physical function (17 questions), and stiffness (2 questions).[39] Extensive evaluation of the WOMAC pain subscale compared to the McGill Pain Questionnaire and a single 10 cm visual analogue (VAS) pain scale has been performed. Although all scales correlated well, the severity of anxiety, depression, and fatigue correlated with McGill and not the WOMAC pain score. Similarly, total osteophyte score by joint radiography correlated well with WOMAC but not McGill pain score,[40] further indicating that responses in evaluation of treatment of OA should include physical function as well as pain. More recently the OMERACT/Osteoarthritis Research Society International (OARSI) responder definition has been validated and adopted. This index defines responders by improvements from baseline in WOMAC pain or physical function subscores by 50% or more with absolute changes 20 mm or more (termed 'strict responders'), or 20% or more with absolute changes of at least 10 mm in two of three measures: pain, physical function, and/or patient global assessment of disease,[41] again demonstrating the value of a composite metric in identifying response.

Measures of structure modification

To be defined as a DMOAD, an agent must be demonstrated to retard, arrest, or reverse the degenerative processes seen in OA. Although conventional radiography cannot directly visualize articular cartilage, the use of JSW on plane radiographs has been validated to follow progression of OA. However, measuring JSW by radiography in RCTs is limited by variability in (1) technique including positioning of the joint, (2) location of disease and rate of progression among individuals, and (3) duration of time over which loss of cartilage can occur.[4] Recent trials have attempted to use MRI to directly delineate structure and preservation of cartilage volume. Whole-organ scoring systems to provide semiquantitative assessments of structural damage over time (WORMS),[42] and to assess changes in signal intensity considered to represent degrees of inflammation or joint synovitis, will hopefully improve sensitivity and specificity of JSW determinations.[43]

Other outcome measures in OA RCTs have ranged from direct arthroscopic visualization[44] to use of surrogate markers for cartilage turnover[45] to the more pragmatic, but highly variable, measurement of time to joint replacement,[46] which is influenced by multiple factors such as standard of practice, economics, and healthcare practices beyond the impact of OA itself.

Systemic lupus erythematosus

The variety of different RCT designs to date in SLE reflects the heterogeneity of disease manifestations and a relapsing/remitting disease course. FDA guidance documents for new products for treatment of SLE and SLE nephritis have provided recommendations for trial designs and outcome measures.[47,48] A regulatory precedent was set in 2011 when the first therapy after 40 years was approved for treatment of SLE in the United States and the European Union after completion of two pivotal RCTs (BLISS-76 and BLISS-52) of belimumab, a monoclonal antibody against B-cell activating factor (BLyS/BAFF).[49,50] As the regulatory history of approved products in SLE has been brief, trial design will likely evolve as lessons are learned with successive RCTs.

Study duration

The recommended period of time to conduct an RCT in SLE is at least 1 year to evaluate the following endpoints: reduction in disease activity, complete clinical response or remission, reduction in flare or increase in time to flare, and maintenance of response.[47] A trial should be of sufficient length to measure durability of response as well as safety. Nonetheless 'induction' regimens or treatment of acute flares may be evaluated at earlier time points, such as 6 months, provided there is evidence of 'maintenance' of effect over 12–24 months.

Superiority over standard-of-care therapy

As in RA, most trials in SLE have been parallel, randomized, controlled superiority RCTs. These are typically add-on trials in which either the experimental agent or placebo are added to standard-of-care (SOC) therapy, as denial of active therapy could potentially lead to irreversible harm. In comparison to failed background therapy in RA, SOC has been active, e.g. the 'best that we can do', including antimalarials, immunosuppressive agents, and corticosteroids. The phase 3 belimumab trials (BLISS-76 and BLISS-52) demonstrated superiority of belimumab+SOC compared with SOC alone.[49,50] The practice of adding experimental therapies to SOC has underscored the importance of controlling changes in concomitant background therapy in SLE RCTs. In the phase 3 RCTs, adjustments to doses of background immunosuppressive agents were allowed through week 16, and corticosteroids through week 24, with no increases between weeks 44 and 52.[49,50] These restrictions in background therapy were designed to decrease variability in responses as the primary endpoint approached, when achievement of corticosteroid doses of 7.5 mg or less per day was a goal for treatment. In contrast, in the phase 2b study of abatacept, a CTLA-4-immunoglobulin fusion protein, and the phase 2/3 trial of rituximab, an anti-CD20 monoclonal antibody, high doses of prednisone were required at initial and retreatment time points with prolonged tapering regimens over 6–9 months.[51,52] Together these may have confounded the ability to distinguish treatment responses from SOC.

In SLE nephritis trials, the experimental agents have been compared to a single SOC medication for superiority. The Aspreva Lupus Management Study (ALMS) included a 6 month induction phase followed by a 36 month maintenance phase. While the primary endpoint was not achieved in the induction phase,[53] superiority of mycophenolate mofetil (MMF) over azathioprine was demonstrated in the maintenance phase by prolongation of time to treatment failure and fewer treatment failures.[54]

In contrast to the ALMS study, the phase 3 trial of rituximab in patients with active SLE nephritis examined the addition of rituximab vs placebo to background with MMF and corticosteroids.[55] The primary endpoint at week 52 was not achieved; again, high doses of corticosteroids may have confounded treatment differences. Similarly, a phase 2/3 study of abatacept in patients with SLE nephritis showed no significant improvement in renal outcomes when abatacept was added to background therapy of MMF and high-dose corticosteroids compared with background therapy alone.[56]

Predefinition of 'treatment failure'

The definition of 'treatment failure' in a protocol allows patients to exit the trial to receive necessary therapy, having met a statistical endpoint for analysis in the RCT. This is important whether 'treatment failure' is the primary efficacy variable, such as in the ALMS study,[54] or as a component of a responder index, and allows equipoise to be maintained, thereby permitting close adherence to protocol mandated restrictions regarding changes in background therapy, yet enabling flexibility for appropriate treatment of a disease manifestation.

Patient population

Selection of the patient population to include in the RCT has been important to recent success of trials in SLE. Identification of biomarkers associated with the mechanism of action of an experimental therapy may help to enrich for a responsive population. Post-hoc analyses of the phase 2 belimumab RCT revealed that 71.5% of patients were seropositive by anti-nuclear (ANA) and/or anti-double-stranded DNA (dsDNA) antibody, associated with higher BLyS/BAFF levels, disease activity, renal involvement, and hypocomplementaemia.[57,58]

Outcome measures used in systemic lupus erythematosus trials

A variety of outcome measures have been used to assess disease activity, damage, HRQoL, and adverse events in SLE, as recommended by OMERACT.[6,59]

Of six existing disease activity indices (DAIs) in SLE, the two most commonly used are the Systemic Lupus Erythematosus Disease Activity Index (SLEDAI) and its modifications: SELENA-SLEDAI and SLEDAI-2K; and the British Isles Lupus Assessment Group (BILAG). SLEDAI DAIs are based on presence or absence of specific clinical features and laboratory results, and yield a global score that reflects the extent of disease involvement.[60] The BILAG scores disease activity by organ systems according to need for therapy; e.g., 'A' reflects severe disease, requiring increases in prednisone and/or addition of immunosuppressive agents, 'B' active disease, requiring low-dose prednisone and/or symptomatic treatment with NSAIDs and/or antimalarials.[61] An A or 2Bs are indicative of severe flares, C reflects mild disease, D reflects previous but no current organ system involvement, and E an organ system never involved. It is the only DAI that captures improving, unchanged, or worsening features of disease activity.[6]

No disease-specific HRQoL measures have been validated for use in multinational SLE RCTs; the generic Medical Outcomes Survey Short Form 36 (SF-36) is validated and has been most commonly used.[59] SF-36 includes 'physical' domains: physical functioning, role physical, bodily pain, and general health perceptions; and 'mental' domains: vitality (which includes fatigue, energy, and pep), social functioning, role emotional, and mental health impact.[6] Domain scores generally better reflect the impact of SLE and its treatment than exclusively using the physical and mental component summary (PCS and MCS) scores, and can be compared with population norms.[62] Two measures of fatigue, Krupp Fatigue Severity Scale and Functional Assessment of Chronic Illness Therapy (FACIT) Fatigue scale, have been utilized in RCTs, although the vitality domain of SF-36 may be more sensitive to treatment effects.[6] Finally the transition question of SF-36: 'Compared to one year ago, how are you today?' can offer valuable information as to whether patients consider themselves 'somewhat better' or 'much better' following treatment.[63]

Recently, composite responder indices have been developed that are evidence based, derived from data-mining phase 2 trials. The SLE Responder Index (SRI) is a composite index used as the primary outcome in the phase 3 BLISS trials.[49,50,57] An SRI response was defined as a reduction of 4 points or more in SELENA-SLEDAI score, no new BILAG A or 2B domain scores, and no deterioration from baseline in physician's global assessment (MDGA) by 0.3 or more on a 3.0 point scale, provided a patient is not a 'treatment failure,' defined by increased or new use of prohibited medications or early withdrawal from the study. A BILAG-based composite index (BICLA) is the primary endpoint variable for the ongoing phase 3 trials with epratuzumab, an anti-CD22 monoclonal antibody.[64,65] Components include reduction of all baseline As to B/C/D and Bs to C/D in all organ systems, no worsening in other organ systems, and no deterioration in SLEDAI or MDGA. An enhanced BILAG responder index is defined as resolution of all As and Bs to C/D in all organ systems.[64]

Other multisystem rheumatic diseases

Many of the challenges faced in trial design in SLE are also present in heterogeneous multisystem diseases such as systemic sclerosis and vasculitis. A recent approval for rituximab for treatment of ANCA-associated vasculitis offers encouragement,[66,67] while RCTs in systemic sclerosis remain limited by variability in natural history of skin, lung, and other internal organ disease, thus limiting reliability of standardized outcome measures.[68]

Conclusion

Considerable progress has been made in trial design over the last 10–15 years in rheumatology, largely facilitated by the development of composite responder indices—important when evaluating treatment effects in multisystem, heterogeneous diseases. Based on the work accomplished so far, it is fair to expect that trial design will continue to evolve as promising therapies are introduced to the clinic.

References

1. Strand V, Simon LS. Randomized controlled trials. Chapter 40 in: Smolen JS, Lipsky PE (eds) *Targeted therapies in rheumatology*. Martin Dunitz, London, 2003:653–666.

2. Simon LS, Boers M. Design of trials for new therapies in patients with RA. Chapter 11a in: Hochberg MC, Silman AJ, Smolen JS, Weinblatt MS, Weisman M (eds) *Rheumatoid arthritis*, Mosby Elsevier, Philadelphia, PA, 2009:387–393.

3. Strand V, Sokolove J. Randomized controlled trial design in rheumatoid arthritis: the past decade. *Arthritis Res Ther* 2009;11(1):205.

4. Strand V, Hochberg MC. Study design and outcome measures in osteoarthritis clinical trials, Chapter 18 in: Moskowitz RW, Altman RD, Hochberg MC, Buckwalter JA, Goldberg VM (eds) *Osteoarthritis*, 4th edn. Lippincott, Williams & Wilkins, Philadelphia, PA, 2007:313–325.

5. Strand V. Issues in drug development in SLE: clinical trial design, outcome measures & biomarkers. In Wallace DJ, Hahn BH (eds) *Dubois' lupus erythematosus*, 7th edn. Lippincott, Williams & Wilkins, Philadelphia, PA, 2007:1317–1332.

6. Strand V, Chu AD. Measuring outcomes in systemic lupus erythematosus clinical trials. *Exp Rev Pharmacoecon Outcomes Res* 2011;11(4):455–468.

7. www.fda.gov

8. www.ema.europa.eu

9. www.ich.org

10. Strand V, Kimberly R, Isaacs JD. Biologic therapies in rheumatology: lessons learned, future directions. *Nat Rev Drug Discov* 2007;6(1):75–92.

11. Strand V, Cohen S, Schiff M et al. Treatment of active rheumatoid arthritis with leflunomide compared with placebo and methotrexate. Leflunomide Rheumatoid Arthritis Investigators Group. *Arch Intern Med* 1999;159(21):2542–2550.

12. Emery P, Breedveld FC, Lemmel EM et al. A comparison of the efficacy and safety of leflunomide and methotrexate for the treatment of rheumatoid arthritis. *Rheumatology (Oxford)* 2000;39(6):655–665.

13. Epstein WV. Expectation bias in rheumatoid arthritis clinical trials. The anti-CD4 monoclonal antibody experience. *Arthritis Rheum* 1996;39(11):1773–1780.

14. Leung H, Hurley F, Strand V. Issues involved in a metaanalysis of rheumatoid arthritis radiographic progression. Analysis issues. *J Rheumatol* 2000;27(2):544–8; discussion 52.

15. Simes J. An improved Bonferroni procedure for multiple tests of significance. *Biometrika* 1986;73:751–754.

16. Hochberg Y. A sharper Bonferroni procedure for multiple tests of significance. *Biometrika* 1988;75:800–802.

17. Maini R, St Clair EW, Breedveld F et al. Infliximab (chimeric anti-tumour necrosis factor alpha monoclonal antibody) versus placebo in rheumatoid arthritis patients receiving concomitant methotrexate: a randomised phase III trial. ATTRACT Study Group. *Lancet* 1999;354(9194):1932–1939.

18. Lipsky PE, van der Heijde DM, St Clair EW et al. Infliximab and methotrexate in the treatment of rheumatoid arthritis. Anti-Tumor Necrosis Factor Trial in Rheumatoid Arthritis with Concomitant Therapy Study Group. *N Engl J Med* 2000;343(22):1594–1602.

19. Maini RN, Feldmann M. How does infliximab work in rheumatoid arthritis? *Arthritis Res* 2002;4 Suppl 2:S22–S28.

20. Sokka T, Pincus T. Most patients receiving routine care for rheumatoid arthritis in 2001 did not meet inclusion criteria for most recent clinical trials or American College of Rheumatology criteria for remission. *J Rheumatol* 2003;30(6):1138–1146.

21. Greenberg JD, Kishimoto M, Strand V et al. Tumor necrosis factor antagonist responsiveness in a United States rheumatoid arthritis cohort. *Am J Med* 2008;121(6):532–538.

22. Strand V, Boers M, Idzerda L et al. It's good to feel better but it's better to feel good and even better to feel good as soon as possible for as long as possible. Response criteria and the importance of change at OMERACT 10. *J Rheumatol* 2011;38(8):1720–1727.

23. Felson DT, Anderson JJ, Boers M et al. The American College of Rheumatology preliminary core set of disease activity measures for rheumatoid arthritis clinical trials. The Committee on Outcome Measures in Rheumatoid Arthritis Clinical Trials. *Arthritis Rheum* 1993;36(6):729–740.

24. van Gestel AM, Prevoo ML, van 't Hof MA et al. Development and validation of the European League Against Rheumatism response criteria for rheumatoid arthritis. Comparison with the preliminary American College of Rheumatology and the World Health Organization/International League Against Rheumatism Criteria. *Arthritis Rheum* 1996;39(1):34–40.

25. Weinblatt ME, Coblyn JS, Fox DA et al. Efficacy of low-dose methotrexate in rheumatoid arthritis. *N Engl J Med* 1985;312(13):818–822.

26. Williams HJ, Willkens RF, Samuelson CO, Jr et al. Comparison of low-dose oral pulse methotrexate and placebo in the treatment of rheumatoid arthritis. A controlled clinical trial. *Arthritis Rheum* 1985;28(7):721–730.

27. Olsen N SM, Strand V. Alternate therapy with leflunomide (LEF) or methotrexate (MTX) after switch from initial treatment in patients with active rheumatoid arthritis (RA) [abstract]. *Arthritis Rheum* 1999;42 (suppl):S241.

28. Strand V. Counterpoint from the trenches: a pragmatic approach to therapeutic trials in rheumatoid arthritis. *Arthritis Rheum* 2004;50(4):1344–1347.

29. Boers M. Add-on or step-up trials for new drug development in rheumatoid arthritis: a new standard? *Arthritis Rheum* 2003;48(6):1481–1483.

30. Jones G, Sebba A, Gu J et al. Comparison of tocilizumab monotherapy versus methotrexate monotherapy in patients with moderate to severe rheumatoid arthritis: the AMBITION study. *Ann Rheum Dis* 2010;69(1):88–96.

31. Helliwell PS, Fitzgerald O, Strand CV, Mease PJ. Composite measures in psoriatic arthritis: a report from the GRAPPA 2009 annual meeting. *J Rheumatol* 2011;38(3):540–545.

32. Coates LC, Mumtaz A, Helliwell PS et al. Development of a disease severity and responder index for psoriatic arthritis (PsA)—report of the OMERACT 10 PsA special interest group. *J Rheumatol* 2011;38(7):1496–1501.

33. Schoels M, Aletaha D, Funovits J et al. Application of the DAREA/DAPSA score for assessment of disease activity in psoriatic arthritis. *Ann Rheum Dis* 2010;69(8):1441–1447.

34. Nell-Duxneuner VP, Stamm TA, Machold KP et al. Evaluation of the appropriateness of composite disease activity measures for assessment of psoriatic arthritis. *Ann Rheum Dis* 2010;69(3):546–549.

35. Lukas C, Landewe R, Sieper J et al. Development of an ASAS-endorsed disease activity score (ASDAS) in patients with ankylosing spondylitis. *Ann Rheum Dis* 2009;68(1):18–24.

36. Schumacher HR, Taylor W, Edwards L et al. Outcome domains for studies of acute and chronic gout. *J Rheumatol* 2009;36(10):2342–2345.

37. Singh JA. Discordance between self-report of physician diagnosis and administrative database diagnosis of arthritis and its predictors. *J Rheumatol* 2009;36(9):2000–2008.

38. Felson DT, Kim YJ. The futility of current approaches to chondroprotection. *Arthritis Rheum* 2007;56(5):1378–1383.

39. Bellamy N. Pain assessment in osteoarthritis: experience with the WOMAC osteoarthritis index. *Semin Arthritis Rheum* 1989;18(4 Suppl 2):14–17.

40. Creamer P, Lethbridge-Cejku M, Hochberg MC. Determinants of pain severity in knee osteoarthritis: effect of demographic and psychosocial variables using 3 pain measures. *J Rheumatol* 1999;26(8):1785–1792.

41. Pham T, Van Der Heijde D, Lassere M et al. Outcome variables for osteoarthritis clinical trials: The OMERACT-OARSI set of responder criteria. *J Rheumatol* 2003;30(7):1648–1654.

42. Peterfy CG, Guermazi A, Zaim S et al. Whole-Organ Magnetic Resonance Imaging Score (WORMS) of the knee in osteoarthritis. *Osteoarthritis Cartilage* 2004;12(3):177–190.

43. Guermazi A, Roemer FW, Hayashi D. Imaging of osteoarthritis: update from a radiological perspective. *Curr Opin Rheumatol* 2011;23(5):484–491.

44. Ayral X, Dougados M. Viability of chondroscopy as a means of cartilage assessment. *Ann Rheum Dis* 1995;54(8):613–614.

45. Lohmander LS, Felson DT. Defining the role of molecular markers to monitor disease, intervention, and cartilage breakdown in osteoarthritis. *J Rheumatol* 1997;24(4):782–785.

46. Maillefert JF, Dougados M. Is time to joint replacement a valid outcome measure in clinical trials of drugs for osteoarthritis? *Rheum Dis Clin North Am* 2003;29(4):831–845.

47. Center for Drug Evaluation and Research, Center for Biologics Evaluation and Research, Center for Devices and Radiological Health. *Guidance for industry: systemic lupus erythematosus—developing medical products for treatment.* U.S. Department of Health and Human Services, Food and Drug Authority, Washington, DC, 2010.

48. Center for Drug Evaluation and Research, Center for Biologics Evaluation and Research, Center for Devices and Radiological Health. *Guidance for industry: lupus nephritis caused by systemic lupus erythematosus—developing medical products for treatment.* U.S. Department of Health and Human Services, Food and Drug Authority, Washington, DC, 2010.

49. Van Vollenhoven RF, Zamani O, Wallace DJ et al. Belimumab, a BLyS-specific inhibitor, reduces disease activity and severe flares in seropositive SLE patients: BLISS-76 study. *Ann Rheum Dis* 2010;69(Suppl3):74.

50. Navarra SV, Guzman RM, Gallacher AE et al. Efficacy and safety of belimumab in patients with active systemic lupus erythematosus: a randomised, placebo-controlled, phase 3 trial. *Lancet* 2011;377(9767):721–731.

51. Merrill JT, Burgos-Vargas R, Westhovens R et al. The efficacy and safety of abatacept in patients with non-life-threatening manifestations of SLE: Results of A 12-month exploratory study. *Arthritis Rheum* 2010;62(10):3077–3087.

52. Merrill JT, Neuwelt CM, Wallace DJ et al. Efficacy and safety of rituximab in moderately-to-severely active systemic lupus erythematosus: the randomized, double-blind, phase II/III systemic lupus erythematosus evaluation of rituximab trial. *Arthritis Rheum* 2010;62(1):222–233.

53. Appel GB, Contreras G, Dooley MA et al. Mycophenolate mofetil versus cyclophosphamide for induction treatment of lupus nephritis. *J Am Soc Nephrol* 2009;20(5):1103–1112.

54. Wofsy D, Appel GB, Dooley MA et al. Aspreva Lupus Management Study maintenance results. *Lupus* 2010;19:27 [abstract CS12.5].

55. Furie R, Looney RJ, Rovin B et al. Efficacy and safety of rituximab in subjects with active proliferative lupus nephritis (LN): Results from the randomized, double-blind phase III LUNAR study. *Arthritis Rheum* 2009;60:S429.

56. Furie R NK, Cheng T, Houssiau F et al. Efficacy and safety of abatacept over 12 months in patients with lupus nephritis: results from a multicenter, randomized, double-blind, placebo-controlled Phase II/III study. *Arthritis Rheum* 2011;63:S962.

57. Furie RA, Petri MA, Wallace DJ et al. Novel evidence-based systemic lupus erythematosus responder index. *Arthritis Rheum* 2009;61(9):1143–1151.

58. Wallace DJ, Stohl W, Furie RA et al. A phase II, randomized, double-blind, placebo-controlled, dose-ranging study of belimumab in patients with active systemic lupus erythematosus. *Arthritis Rheum* 2009;61(9):1168–1178.

59. Strand V, Chu AD. Generic versus disease-specific measures of health-related quality of life in systemic lupus erythematosus. *J Rheumatol* 2011;38(9):1821–1823.

60. Bombardier C, Gladman DD, Urowitz MB, Caron D, Chang CH. Derivation of the SLEDAI. A disease activity index for lupus patients. The Committee on Prognosis Studies in SLE. *Arthritis Rheum* 1992;35(6):630–640.

61. Hay EM, Bacon PA, Gordon C et al. The BILAG index: a reliable and valid instrument for measuring clinical disease activity in systemic lupus erythematosus. *Q J Med* 1993;86(7):447–458.

62. Strand V, Crawford B, Singh J, Choy E, Smolen JS, Khanna D. Use of 'spydergrams' to present and interpret SF-36 health-related quality of life data across rheumatic diseases. *Ann Rheum Dis* 2009;68(12):1800–1804.

63. Strand V, Levy RA, Cervera R et al. Belimumab, a BLyS-specific inhibitor, improved fatigue and SF-36 Physical and Mental Component Summary scores in patients with SLE: BLISS-76 and -52 studies. *Arthritis Rheum* 2010;62:S773.

64. Wallace D, Kalunian K, Petri M et al. Epratuzumab demonstrates clinically meaningful improvements in patients with moderate to severe systemic lupus erythematosus (SLE): Results from EMBLEM, a Phase IIB study. *Ann Rheum Dis* 2010;69(Suppl3):558.

65. Kalunian K, Wallace D, Petri M et al. BILAG-measured improvement in moderately and severely affected body systems in patients with systemic lupus erythematosus (SLE) by Epratuzumab: Results from EMBLEM, a Phase IIB study. *Ann Rheum Dis* 2010;69(Suppl3):553.

66. Stone JH, Merkel PA, Spiera R et al. Rituximab versus cyclophosphamide for ANCA-associated vasculitis. *N Engl J Med* 2010;363(3):221–232.

67. Jones RB, Tervaert JW, Hauser T et al. Rituximab versus cyclophosphamide in ANCA-associated renal vasculitis. *N Engl J Med* 2010;363(3):211–220.

68. Furst D, Khanna D, Matucci-Cerinic M et al. Systemic sclerosis—continuing progress in developing clinical measures of response. *J Rheumatol* 2007;34(5):1194–1200.

CHAPTER 31

Health economics

Sonja Merkesdal and Wilfried Mau

Cost of illness in rheumatic diseases

Low back pain, osteoarthritis, and inflammatory diseases account for substantial proportions of the overall costs of musculoskeletal diseases, and have been scientifically recognized as important targets for cost-of-illness analyses.[1,2]

Cost-of-illness studies are used to describe the health-economic impact of a disease due to costs incurred by (1) direct healthcare-related resource consumption, (2) non-medical disease-related resource consumption, and (3) productivity losses. Depending on the perspective chosen, patients' out-of-pocket expenses or intangible costs (e.g. quality of life) may also be incorporated. This costing data is useful for a comparison of disease entities (see Table 31.1 for the diagnoses included) but also enables us to learn more about the cost-structure of a disease and to generate input data for health-economic models.

Low back pain

The costs of low back pain have been addressed by some European studies in the last decade showing annual estimates of €211 (Sweden),[3] €260 (United Kingdom),[4] and €1322 (Germany)[5] per person. The huge impact of this condition on healthcare costs results from its high prevalence (15–30%).[6–8]

A more recent cost evaluation has been carried out as an economic piggy-back study accompanying a randomized controlled guideline implementation study in primary care (Germany).[9] Acute low back pain incurred mean overall costs of €1002 and chronic low back pain as much as €1790 during a 6 month study period. These costs are clearly higher than in other studies and might partly be explained by different study settings but also by an increasing use of imaging and surgical procedures.

All costing studies identified productivity costs as the main cost contributor, representing more than 50% of overall costs. Direct costs are mainly driven by in-patient treatment (acute or rehabilitation facilities) and therapeutic procedures.[9] The identification of subgroups with increased costs should be an important focus of further health-economic evaluations, in order to assign resources to tailored cost-limiting procedures in these patients.

Osteoarthritis

There is some evidence on disease-related costs in osteoarthritis, although the types are mostly not differentiated and the term 'general osteoarthritis' is used. Estimates of direct costs (adjusted to 2005 US dollars) range from $345 in France, $1272 in Italy, and $2878 in Canada, to $4792 in the United States; productivity losses range from $864 in Hong Kong, $1210 in the United States, and $1683 in Italy to more than $9000 in Canada.[10] This review demonstrates that there are major differences in cost assessment in the cited studies. The most important source of these observed variations seems to be the choice of cost components included in the cost-of-illness studies, but the nature of the underlying database and specific features of the respective healthcare systems also contribute. There is still a lack of standardized cost-of-illness data that will have to be addressed in future economic studies of osteoarthritis.

Rheumatoid arthritis

Of the inflammatory rheumatic diseases, rheumatoid arthritis (RA) has attracted most attention from the health-economic viewpoint. Many studies have addressed cost assessment in RA and a recent review summarizes the results of all evaluations presenting original costing data.[11] Mean costs of 26 studies were calculated by converting to 2006 euros. Overall average direct cost estimates amount to €4170 per year. Depending on the methodology use, productivity costs ranged from €1441 (friction cost method; see 'Methodological aspects of cost-of-illness evaluation' for details of methods) to €8452 (human capital approach). Mean patient- and family-related costs account for €2284, underlining the importance of costs from the patient's perspective. Medication and hospitalization costs are the most important contributors to direct costs, amounting to €1567 and €1243, respectively.

Although these results provide a sound basis for cost estimation in RA, it has to be kept in mind that costing structures might change over time. Since the introduction of biologicals in the treatment of RA the medication costs have risen markedly, whereas hospitalization and productivity costs appear to have decreased.[12] The economic impact of these changes has to be explored in detail in order to capture the potential economic benefits of expensive treatments from the societal perspective.

Ankylosing spondylitis

Ankylosing spondylitis (AS) has a high prevalence of about 0.5%,[13,14] creating substantial societal costs caused by productivity losses from patients at a relatively young age. The review by Franke et al.[11] also addressed the literature relating to cost-of-illness evaluation

Table 31.1 Average cost estimates or cost estimate ranges derived from the literature converted to 2011€ for back pain, osteoarthritis, rheumatoid arthritis, ankylosing spondylitis, psoriasis arthritis, and systemic lupus erythematosus

Indication	Direct annual costs	Indirect annual costs	Ratio (direct:indirect costs)
Back pain	249–3831[3–9]		n.a.
Osteoarthritis	417–10, 890[10]	1047–10,890[10]	1:1–1:2.5
Rheumatoid arthritis	4900[11]	1693 (FC)[11] 9931 (HC)[11]	1:0.3–1:2
Ankylosing spondylitis	234 + 1297 (OOPE) = 1531[11]	2668 (FC)[11] 7377 (HC)[11]	1:1.7–1:4.8
Psoriasis arthritis	1858–4150[15]	2873–3174 (HC)[15]	1:0.7–1:1.7
Systemic lupus erythematosus	3302–6404[19] 11 762–12 738[19a]	966–3781 (FC)[19] 3702–12919 (HC)[19]	1:0.3–1:1.2

FC, friction cost approach; HC, human capital approach; n.a., not applicable; OOPE, out-of-pocket-expenses.

[a] Three studies with longer disease duration (<10 years).

of AS. Their estimation of average costs is based on seven studies providing original costing data. The direct annual costs are lower than in RA, amounting to €1992 per patient, and patient and family costs account for €1104 per patient. When it comes to productivity losses, however, it becomes obvious that they are comparably high, ranging from €2271 (friction cost method) to €6278 (human capital approach). Productivity costs are shown to be even more important in AS (mean proportion of overall costs 66%) than in RA (57%). Outstanding cost components of direct costing are medication (€628), hospitalization costs (€592), and non-physician service utilization (€428, mainly physiotherapy). Future economic research should also focus on the assessment of long-term productivity costs in AS using incidence-based cost-of-illness studies, since the lifetime costs might even be higher than in RA because of the younger age at onset.

Psoriatic arthritis

Some cost-of-illness studies for psoriatic arthritis (PsA) have been conducted in Hong Kong, Hungary, Italy, and Germany.[15] These studies show similar costs to those reported for AS. In the Hong Kong cost-of-illness study,[15] direct costs were estimated to be $4141 (in 2006 US dollars) for all patients, and a separate description of peripheral and axial disease showed costs for patients with axial manifestation to be substantially higher (peripheral $3530, axial $6711). The main contributors of direct costing were physician visits, in-patient treatment, and patient costs (out-of-pocket expenses). Indirect costs were also remarkable: $3127 for all patients and $2604 and $5199 for patients with peripheral or axial disease, respectively. A Hungarian study[16] reported figures of €1681 for direct costs and €2600 for indirect costs. This sample included no patients on biological therapy, possibly explaining the lower direct costs, but described high costs of non-medical services. An Italian cohort of patients failing usual care[17] incurred direct costs of €943 in 6 months. Higher costs were reported in a study of German data for 2002[18]: €3156 direct and €2414 indirect costs (friction cost method). This substantial economic burden of PsA is mainly related to pain and physical function;[15] further studies will have to address the impact of cost-saving measures.

Systemic lupus erythematosus

The evidence regarding systemic lupus erythematosus (SLE) is not so wide-ranging: a recent summary of cost-of-illness studies identifies 11 evaluations reporting on original data.[19] Direct cost estimates range from $3735 to $7244 (in 2008 US dollars) and three studies identify even much higher costs ($13 305–14 410). The reason might be the older age and longer disease durations of these cohorts. As with to the other inflammatory diseases, in-patient costs and medication costs are the outstanding contributors to overall costs. However, in SLE subsets with longstanding disease, the costs for diagnostic procedures become similarly important.

Most of the studies did not report on patient costs or non-medical costs. Indirect costs exceed direct costs in almost all studies, but the range of estimates is wide because of the use of different assessment methods ($1093–4277 for the friction cost method and $4188–14 614 for the human capital approach).

In contrast to other inflammatory diseases where costing is mainly associated with physical functioning, in SLE costs are, to a substantial extent, independently associated with the occurrence of disease flares. This makes the development of novel expensive biological therapies for the prevention of flares a challenging health-economic target. In order to identify patient subsets who bear most of the costs, it would be important to learn more about lifetime costing data while the disease progresses.

Methodological aspects of cost-of-illness evaluation

Summarizing disease-related cost components for a specific disease entity is often used to point out its health-economic relevance, and the cost estimates are subsequently compared between diseases that are competing for resources to be allocated. While doing this, we have to keep some methodological confounders in mind. The choice of cost components to be included is very important for the completeness of cost description and the perspective of the cost study carried out. Standardization of this procedure has been achieved for RA,[20] for example, by developing and structuring a matrix of cost domains. Based on this subset of defined cost components, all domains that are relevant from a certain perspective are chosen for cost-of-illness assessment. To avoid double counting, it is crucial to consider the perspective of the evaluation. For example, from the patient's perspective, indirect costs are represented by lost wages; productivity losses at work must not be counted in addition, since this would be double counting of the same costing aspect.

Another methodological issue is the aggregation level of cost assessment. The level of detail that can be achieved and the accuracy of the information are dependent on the data source. In addition to insurance data, questionnaires may be employed for the additional assessment of domains such as non-medical costs, or patient and family costs. The breakdown of medical costs may also include detailed information on therapeutic and diagnostic procedures, but the accuracy with which patients can report these facts is limited. In RA it has been shown that the major domains such as physician visits, hospitalization, medication, non-physician service utilization, and therapeutic and diagnostic procedures can be reported accurately by the patient[21] when highly aggregated items are used.

The strong influence of methodological approaches on the costing results can be seen in the evaluation of productivity costs.[22] In early cost-of-illness studies the *human capital approach* was generally used to describe the value of lost productivity. In this approach all times of lost or impaired productivity at work (short and long term) are summarized and subsequently evaluated using the average gross hourly income of an employed worker. This approach was subsequently altered because it is now recognized that there is underemployment in most economic systems and the lost productivity of an impaired worker will be replaced after a period defined, for example, by the mean duration of job vacancies. This is the *friction cost method*. The difference between these approaches is striking,[18,22] and the results cannot directly be compared between studies. The valuation of lost productivity is subject to similar limitations. The recommended method of valuation is to use the average income, but alternatively the individual income of the patient can be employed. Because there is a tendency for patients with lower income to have more productivity losses and vice versa, valuation with individual incomes leads to substantially lower costs than valuation with average incomes.

These examples of methodological variations illustrate the general need to develop standardized assessment methods for cost-of-illness evaluations. In RA all of these standardization issues have been addressed by recommendations and guidelines[23,24] and the evidence regarding cost of illness is quite broad and consistent.

Cost-effectiveness of biologicals in rheumatic diseases

The assessment of cost-effectiveness in cost-effectiveness analysis (CEA) or cost-utility analysis (CUA) yields some kind of relation between economic input (costs) and clinical output—e.g. response in in terms of American College of Rheumatology outcome measures ('ACR response') or quality of life (QoL) improvement. In CUA this relationship is generally transformed to the monetary outcome (e.g. in euros) per quality-adjusted life-year (QALY). A QALY represents 1 year at perfect health. Results showing costs lower than €50 000/QALY are usually found to be cost-effective in the countries of the euro zone. According to the United Kingdom National Institute for Health and Clinical Excellence (NICE) the threshold is

about £20, 000–30,000/QALY. Results about 50% above this frontier are often called 'conditionally cost-effective' in the current literature. The QALY construct is used to create comparability between the respective main clinical outcomes in different diseases (e.g. ACR response and reduction of blood pressure in mmHg). Since the assessment of QALYs often requires mathematical transformation and mapping processes, the validity of this construct is still under discussion. More recent CEAs have also employed stricter outcomes such as clinical remission. The obvious advantage of these clear-cut outcomes is that they are far more meaningful to a rheumatologist.

For rheumatic disease, a special health-economic focus has been placed on biological therapies, which are all characterized by high treatment costs and comparably high effectiveness compared to traditional therapeutic options. There is already a comprehensive body of evidence with contradictory results, especially for RA.

Rheumatoid arthritis

The first health technology assessment (HTA) performed for TNF-inhibiting drugs in RA rendered discouraging results.[25] In the following years it became obvious that it is crucial to differentiate subsets of RA patients according to disease duration and prior treatment, leading to more favourable results in a subsequent HTA.[26]

For modelling purposes the term 'early RA' is used for patients with a disease duration of less than 2 years and either no prior treatment with disease-modifying anti-rheumatic drugs (DMARDs) or monotherapy with methotrexate or sulfasalazine. The results of CEAs in this field[26–28] show concordantly that TNF inhibitors are cost-effective if used according to guidelines[29] after two consecutive unsuccessful DMARD therapies. When TNF inhibitors were employed as initial therapy results were less favourable and were judged as conditionally cost-effective with incremental cost-effectiveness ratios (ICERs) ranging from €50 000 to €75 000/QALY. Cost-effective results were also reported by Davies et al.[28] comparing a defined DMARD sequence with adalimumab and methotrexate combination therapy followed by the same DMARD sequence in early RA (see also Table 31.2, showing a summary of cost-effectiveness results).

All RA patients with disease durations of more than 2 years are classified as having advanced disease in the cost-effectiveness models. In TNF-inhibitor-naive patients with advanced RA treated according to current guidelines, two CEAs[26,30] report on cost-effective results for the use of etanercept and adalimumab in combination with methotrexate (ICER <€50 000/QALY). In both of these studies, infliximab proved not to be cost-effective (ICER >€50 000/QALY).

Regarding RA patients with advanced disease who have discontinued one TNF-inhibiting therapy due to either lack of efficacy or side effects, the most prominent health-economic issue is whether another TNF inhibitor should be employed, or an alternative biological treatment such as rituximab or abatacept. There are three CEAs investigating this issue,[31–33] regarding rituximab in comparison to a change of TNF inhibitor. These studies agree that rituximab is more cost-effective used in TNF-inhibitor-refractory patients (ICER <€15 000/QALY). In a recent HTA[34] for the use of biologics in patients with TNF failure these results are emphasized and cost-effective ICERs for all biological options (infliximab, etanercept, adalimumab, abatacept, and

Table 31.2 Evidence for the cost-effectiveness of biological treatment in patients with rheumatoid arthritis, ankylosing spondylitis, psoriasis arthritis, and systemic lupus erythematosus, derived from the current literature

Indication	Evidence for cost-effectiveness of biological compounds
Rheumatoid arthritis Disease duration <2 yrs	As initial therapy: ◆ ETN and ADA conditionally cost-effective (ICERs €50 000–70 000/QALY) vs MTX[26,27] ◆ ADA cost-effective[28] compared to a prior DMARD sequence After 2 DMARDs (according to recommendations): ◆ IFX, ETN, and ADA cost-effective vs DMARDs[26]
Rheumatoid arthritis Disease duration >2 yrs	After 2 DMARDs (according to recommendations): ◆ ETN and ADA (+MTX) cost-effective versus MTX[26,30] ◆ IFX (+MTX) versus MTX not cost-effective[26] ◆ TNF inhibitors cost-effective based on registry data vs DMARDs[35] After failure of a standard DMARD sequence: ◆ ETN, IFX, and ADA cost-effective versus DMARDs[26] After failure of a prior TNF inhibitor: ◆ change from TNF inhibitor (IFX, ETN, ADA) to ABA, and RTX cost-effective compared to another TNF inhibitor[34] ◆ RTX dominates TNF inhibitors (more effective and less costly)[34] ◆ RTX economically more favourable than ABA[34]
Ankylosing spondylitis	In active NSAID-refractory disease: ◆ ETN and ADA cost-effective vs NSAIDs[41–44]
Psoriatic arthritis	In moderate to severe active disease: ◆ ETN cost-effective vs DMARDs[46–49] ◆ ADA, IFX, GOL cost-effective vs DMARDs[48,49]
Systemic lupus erythematosus	◆ No evidence on cost-effectiveness ◆ Preliminary report on belimumab shows conditionally cost-effective ICERs well above €50 000/QALY[50]

ABA, abatacept; ADA, adalimumab; DMARD, disease-modifying anti-rheumatic drug; ETN, etanercept; GOL, golimumab; IFX, infliximab; NSAID, non-steroidal anti-inflammatory drug; RTX, rituximab.

rituximab) are reported. However, rituximab and abatacept have better cost-effectiveness than TNF inhibitors and the comparison of rituximab and abatacept reveals even more favourable results for rituximab.

The employment of biological therapies in RA patients with advanced disease who have been treated with all conventional DMARD options available is defined as a last resort. Chen et al.[26] have compared the cost-effectiveness of the TNF inhibitors infliximab, adalimumab, and etanercept given as a final option in patients with advanced RA. For this indication, all TNF inhibitors investigated appear to be cost-effective with ICERs of about €38 000/QALY for infliximab, €30 000/QALY for adalimumab, and €24 000€/QALY for etanercept. Other biological therapies have not been economically assessed in this patient subset.

In summary, the use of TNF inhibitors in biologic-naive patients seems to be cost-effective in most subsets with the exception of early RA when TNF inhibitors are employed as initial therapy. However, these models should be re-run with observational data and a longer time horizon in order to capture the real-life effectiveness. A model using registry data has further underlined the cost-effective use of the TNF inhibitors as a class compared to DMARDs according to the current recommendations in RA.[35] Regarding TNF-inhibitor-resistant RA, the summarized evidence shows that a change of TNF inhibitor as well as the use of another biological

(rituximab, abatacept) is cost-effective. The most favourable results in this group are found for rituximab.

Ankylosing spondylitis

Current cost-effectiveness data on the biological treatment of AS is restricted to the TNF inhibitors infliximab, etanercept, and adalimumab. There are five CEAs reporting on infliximab,[36–40] of which four report on cost-effective results in comparison to usual care in different settings (United Kingdom, Canada, Spain). All studies present data from the societal perspective, and two of them additionally adopt the insurance perspective, where cost-effective results were also found. The study by Boonen et al.[40] compares infliximab and etanercept and finds more favourable results for etanercept.

Two further CEAs investigate etanercept alone vs usual care. In a United Kingdom setting[41] etanercept was cost-effective from the insurance perspective, employing both a short- and a long-term horizon. A recent German CEA study[42] reproduced these results using the societal perspective, but from the insurance perspective the results were not cost-effective. This contradictory finding was explained by the different pricing of etanercept in the United Kingdom and Germany.

There is only one cost-effectiveness study for adalimumab.[43] This CEA is from the United Kingdom and compares adalimumab to usual care adopting the insurance perspective. Employed according to current guidelines, adalimumab proves to be cost-effective in the short and long run. This data is partially contradicted by the NICE appraisal,[44] with CEAs for infliximab, etanercept, and adalimumab all showing ICERs well above £50 000/QALY. However, due to marked differences from the manufacturers' model a decision support unit revised this model and came to the conclusion that etanercept and adalimumab are cost-effective in active AS with ICERs of £20 000–30 000/QALY. Infliximab was considered not to be cost-effective as its ICER was clearly less favourable.

In summary, all economic models developed according to current recommendations report on cost-effective results of TNF inhibition in active AS refractory to non-steroidal anti-inflammatory drugs (NSAIDs) from the societal viewpoint. Adherence to ASAS guidelines (i.e. discontinuation of TNF inhibition in non-responders after 12 weeks) reduces the costs remarkably. Two comparative models propose that the cost-effectiveness of infliximab is potentially less favourable, but this finding has to be interpreted cautiously (e.g. different dosing regimens). In AS these results have to be seen within the context that TNF inhibitors are the only option available for patients refractory to usual care.

Psoriatic arthritis

In PsA three approved biologicals—infliximab, etanercept, and adalimumab—are used. A current CEA[45] incorporates all biological options into the model and reports that for PsA patients with mild to moderate skin disease etanercept is the most cost-effective option (ICER vs palliative care, £16 000/QALY). In comparison to etanercept, infliximab proved not to be cost-effective (ICER £54 000/QALY). Adalimumab is also found not to be cost-effective in this model compared to etanercept. The superior ICER of etanercept compared to infliximab was supported by a UK-based analysis,[46] whereas Cummins et al. show comparable and cost-effective results for all TNF inhibitors with the most favourable ICER for infliximab.[47] A current CEA on golimumab[48] also reports cost-effective results. The updated HTA[49] and the current CEAs by Cummins et al. support the evidence that all biologicals are cost-effective in patients with moderate to severe psoriasis.

Systemic lupus erythematosus

The only targeted biological therapy option for SLE, belimumab, has recently been approved. Up to now there is no evidence on cost-effectiveness in the published literature. Some preliminary information is given on the NHS HTA programme website,[50] developing a base case scenario with costs of £64 410/QALY. No information on cost-effectiveness is available for other biologicals that are investigated in SLE or that are used off-label in patient subgroups, such as rituximab, infliximab, or tocilizumab.

Limitations of cost-effectiveness studies

Regarding the summary of evidence on cost-effectiveness of biologicals for different diseases, some common limitations have to be pointed out. The comparability of CEAs is generally limited, for several reasons. An outstanding issue is the 'QALY problem'—every CEA uses its own more-or-less complex construct to transform (for instance) ACR responses or BASDAI improvements into QALYs. Even the same outcome parameter might be mapped onto the QALY scale by different approaches. Furthermore, there are also relevant variations in the assessment of disease-related costs (see

'Methodological aspects of cost-of-illness evaluation') and in many CEAs the cost components included and the valuation methods employed are not broken down. Especially in chronic inflammatory disorders, the disease progression rate under treatment is important and in many CEAs it represents a sensitive parameter that can influence results considerably. The certainty of these estimates can be improved by long-term results provided by registries and observational studies. This is true also for other sensitive variables such as the continuation rates of biologicals. Still, the health-economic evidence already collected helps to inform health-political decision-making by showing how the high costs of medication might be partially offset. Most of the CEAs demonstrate that biologicals can be employed in different indications in a cost-effective way.

References

1. Fautrel B, Guillemin F. Cost of illness studies in rheumatic diseases. *Curr Opin Rheumatol* 2002;14:121–126.
2. Statistisches Bundesamt. Krankheitskosten je Einwohner in € (Costs of illness per resident in €). www.destatis.de
3. Ekman M, Johnell O, Lidgren L. The economic cost of low back pain in Sweden in 2001. *Acta Orthop* 2005;76:275–284.
4. Maniadakis N, Gray A. The economic burden of back pain in the United Kingdom. *Pain* 2000;84:95–103.
5. Wenig CM, Schmidt CO, Kohlmann T et al. costs of back pain in Germany. *Eur J Pain* 2009;13:280–286.
6. Cassidy JD, Carroll LJ, Cote P. The Saskatchewan health and back pain survey. The prevalence of low back pain and related disability in Saskatchewan adults. *Spine* 1998;23:1860–1866.
7. Raspe HH, Kohlmann T. [The current backache epidemic]. *Ther Umsch* 1994;51:367–374.
8. Papageorgiou AC, Croft PR, Ferry S et al. Estimating the prevalence of low back pain in the general population. Evidence from the South Manchester Back Pain Survey. *Spine* 1995;20:1889–1894.
9. Becker A, Held H, Redaelli M, et al. Low back pain in primary care: costs of care and prediction of future health care utilization. *Spine* 2010;35:1714–1720.
10. Xie F, Thumboo J, Li S. True difference or something else? Problems in cost of osteoarthritis studies. *Semin Arthritis Rheum* 2007;37:127–132.
11. Franke LC, Ament AJHA, van de Laar MAFJ, Boonen A, Severens JL. Cost-of-illness of rheumatoid arthritis and ankylosing spondylitis. *Clin Exp Rheumatol* 2009;27:S118–S123.
12. Kirchhoff T, Ruof J, Mittendorf T et al. Cost of illness in rheumatoid arthritis in Germany in 1997–98 and 2002: cost drivers and cost savings. *Rheumatology (Oxford)*. 2011;50:756–761.
13. Braun J, Bollow M, Remlinger G et al. Prevalence of spondylarthropathies in HLA-B27 positive and negative blood donors. *Arthritis Rheum* 1998;41:58–67.
14. Saraux A, Guedes C, Allain J et al. Prevalence of rheumatoid arthritis and spondyloarthropathy in Brittany, France. Société de Rhumatologie de l'Ouest. *J Rheumatol* 1999;26:2622–2627.
15. Zhu TY, Tam L, Leung Y et al. Socioeconomic burden of psoriatic arthritis in Hong Kong: direct and indirect costs and the influence of disease pattern. *J Rheumatol* 2010;37:1214–1220.
16. Brodszky V, Balint P, Geher P et al. Disease burden of psoriatic arthritis compared to rheumatoid arthritis. Hungarian experiment. *Rheumatol Int* 2009;30:199–205.
17. Olivieri I, de Portu S, Salvarani C et al.; PACE working group. The psoriatic arthritis cost evaluation study: a cost-of-illness study on tumour necrosis factor inhibitors in psoriatic arthritis patients with inadequate response to conventional therapy. *Rheumatology* 2008;47:1664–1670.
18. Huscher D, Merkesdal S, Thiele K et al.; German Collaborative Arthritis Centres. Cost of illness in rheumatoid arthritis, ankylosing spondylitis,

psoriatic arthritis and systemic lupus erythematosus in Germany. *Ann Rheum Dis* 2006;65:1175–1183.

19. Zhu TY, Tam LS, Li EK. Cost-of-illness studies in systemic lupus erythematosus: a systematic review. *Arthritis Care Res* 2011;63:751–760.

20. Merkesdal S, Ruof J, Huelsemann JL et al. Development of a matrix of cost domains in economic evaluation of rheumatoid arthritis. *J Rheumatol* 2001;28:657–661.

21. Ruof J, Huelsemann JL, Mittendorf T et al. Patient-reported health care utilization in rheumatoid arthritis: what level of detail is required? *Arthritis Rheum* 2004;51:774–781.

22. Merkesdal S, Ruof J, Mittendorf T, Zeidler H, Mau W. Indirect medical costs in the first three years of rheumatoid arthritis: comparison of current methodological approaches. *Expert Rev Pharmacoecon Outcomes Res* 2002;2:89–94.

23. Maetzel A, Tugwell P, Boers M et al.; OMERACT 6 Economics Research Group. Economic evaluation of programs or interventions in the management of rheumatoid arthritis: defining a consensus-based reference case. *J Rheumatol* 2003;30:891–896.

24. Graf von der Schulenburg JM, Greiner W, Jost F et al.; Hanover Consensus Group. German recommendations on health economic evaluation: third and updated version of the Hanover Consensus. *Value Health* 2008;11:539–544.

25. Kulp W, Greiner W, Graf von der Schulenburg JM. [Cost-effectiveness of pharmaceutical interventions. Health economic aspects of rheumatoid arthritis treatment with TNF-alpha antagonists.] *Pharm Unserer Zeit* 2003;32:420–425.

26. Chen YF, Jobanputra P, Barton P et al. A systematic review of the effectiveness of adalimumab, etanercept and infliximab for the treatment of rheumatoid arthritis in adults and an economic evaluation of their cost-effectiveness. *Health Technol Assess* 2006;10:iii–iv, xi–xiii, 1–229.

27. Spalding JR, Hay J: Cost effectiveness of tumour necrosis factor-alpha inhibitors as first-line agents in rheumatoid arthritis. *PharmacoEconomics* 2006;24(12):1221–1232.

28. Davies A, Cifaldi MA, Sigurado OG, Weisman MH. Cost-effectiveness of sequential therapy with tumor necrosis factor antagonists in early rheumatoid arthritis. *J Rheumatol* 2009;36:16–26.

29. Smolen JS, Landewe R, Breedveld FC et al. EULAR recommendations for the management of rheumatoid arthritis with synthetic and biological disease-modifying antirheumatic drugs. *Ann Rheum Dis* 2010;69:964–975.

30. Wailoo AJ, Bansback N, Brennan A et al. Biologic drugs for rheumatoid arthritis in the Medicare program: a cost-effectiveness analysis. *Arthritis Rheum* 2008;58:939–946.

31. Merkesdal S, Kirchhoff T, Wolka D, et al. Cost-effectiveness analysis of rituximab treatment in patients in Germany with rheumatoid arthritis after etanercept-failure. *Eur J Health Econ* 2010;11:95–104.

32. Kielhorn A, Porter D, Diamantopoulos A, Lewis G. UK cost-utility analysis of rituximab in patients with rheumatoid arthritis that failed to respond adequately to a biologic disease-modifying antirheumatic drug. *Curr Med Res Opin* 2008;24:2639–2650.

33. Lindgren P, Geborek P, Kobelt G. Modeling the cost-effectiveness of treatment of rheumatoid arthritis with rituximab using registry data from Southern Sweden. *Int J Technol Assess Health Care* 2009;25:181–189.

34. Malotti K, Barton P, Tsourapas A et al. Adalimumab, etanercept, infliximab, rituximab and abatacept for the treatment of rheumatoid arthritis

after the failure of a tumor necrosis factor inhibitor: a systematic review. *Health Technol Assess* 2011;15:1–278.

35. Brennan A, Bansback N, Nixon R et al. Modelling the cost effectiveness of TNF-alpha antagonists in the management of rheumatoid arthritis: results from the British Society for Rheumatology Biologics Registry. *Rheumatology* 2007;46:1345–1354.

36. Kobelt G, Andlin-Sobocki P, Brophy S et al. The burden of ankylosing spondylitis and the cost-effectiveness of treatment with infliximab (Remicade). *Rheumatology (Oxford)* 2004;43:1158–1166.

37. Kobelt G, Andlin-Sobocki P, Maksymowych WP: The cost-effectiveness of infliximab (Remicade) in the treatment of ankylosing spondylitis in Canada. *J Rheumatol* 2006;33:732–740.

38. Kobelt G, Sobocki P, Sieper J, Braun J: Comparison of the cost-effectiveness of infliximab in the treatment of ankylosing spondylitis in the United Kingdom based on two different clinical trials. *Int J Technol Assess Health Care* 2007;23:368–375.

39. Kobelt G, Sobocki P, Mulero J et al. The cost-effectiveness of infliximab in the treatment of ankylosing spondylitis in Spain. Comparison of clinical trial and clinical practice data. *Scand J Rheumatol* 2008;37:62–71.

40. Boonen A, van der Heijde D, Severns JL et al. Markov model into the cost-utility over five years of etanercept and infliximab compared with usual care in patients with active ankylosing spondylitis. *Ann Rheum Dis* 2006;65:201–208.

41. Ara RM, Reynolds AV, Conway P: The cost-effectiveness of etanercept in patients with severe ankylosing spondylitis in the UK. *Rheumatology (Oxford)* 2007;46:1338–1344.

42. Neilson AR, Sieper J, Deeg M: Cost-effectiveness of etanercept in patients with severe ankylosing spondylitis in Germany. *Rheumatology (Oxford)* 2010;49:2122–2134.

43. Botteman MF, Hay JW, Luo MP, Curry AS, Wong RL, van Hout BA: Cost-effectiveness of adalimumab for the treatment of ankylosing spondylitis in the United Kingdom. *Rheumatology (Oxford)* 2007;46:1320–1328.

44. National Institute for Health and Clinical Excellence. *TA 143 Adalimumab, etanercept and infliximab for ankylosing spondylitis*, May 2008. www.nice.org.uk/nicemedia/live/11992/40761/40761.pdf

45. Bojke L, Epstein D, Craig D et al. Modelling the cost-effectiveness of biologic treatments for psoriatic arthritis. *Rheumatology* 2011;50(suppl 4):iv39–iv47.

46. Bravo Vergel Y, Hawkins NS, Claxton K et al. The cost-effectiveness of etanercept and infliximab for the treatment of patients with psoriatic arthritis. *Rheumatology* 2007;46:1729–1735.

47. Cummins E, Asseburg C, Punekar YS et al. Cost-effectiveness of infliximab for the treatment of active and progressive psoriatic arthritis. *Value Health* 2011;14:15–23.

48. Cummins E, Asseburg C, Prasad M, Buchanan J, Punekar YS. Cost-effectiveness of golimumab for the treatment of active psoriatic arthritis. *Eur J Health Econ* 2012;13(6):801–809.

49. Rodgers M, Epstein D, Bojke L et al. Etanercept, infliximab and adalimumab for the treatment of psoriatic arthritis: a systematic review and economic evaluation. *Health Technol Assess* 2011;15:i–xxi,1–329.

50. Warwick Evidence Review Group. Belimumab for the treatment of active autoantibody-positive systemic lupus erythematosus. www.hta.ac.uk/2527

CHAPTER 32

Comorbidities of rheumatic disease

Tuulikki Sokka, Kari Puolakka, and Carl Turesson

Introduction

In this chapter, we discuss the impact of comorbidities in rheumatic diseases. We address the challenge that common comorbidities bring to daily rheumatology care. We also discuss practical strategies against comorbidities, to improve patients' outcomes. We use rheumatoid arthritis (RA) as an example of a prototype of inflammatory rheumatic diseases.

Comorbidities—impact in patient care

All other diseases that coexist with a disease of interest are called comorbidities.[1,2] Comorbidities in inflammatory rheumatic diseases may be associated with persistent inflammatory activity or disease-related organ damage, or may be related to medications. Lifestyle choices such as smoking or physical inactivity contribute to comorbidity. Patients with rheumatic diseases meet health professionals regularly and are more often tested for osteoporosis or cholesterol levels than individuals without rheumatic disease, which may contribute to a higher prevalence of some comorbidities in patients with rheumatic diseases. Comorbidities can also be unrelated to rheumatic diseases or their treatments.

Comorbidity indices such as the Charlson Comorbidity Index[3] or the Index of Coexistent Diseases[4] estimate the frequency and severity of comorbidities and are used in clinical studies. Higher scores for these and other comorbidity indices predict morbidity, mortality, costs, and hospitalization in rheumatic diseases. In clinical care, comorbidities are reviewed and recorded by a health professional by indicating whether a medical condition exists or not. In surveys, patients select from a list comorbidities that apply and a plain number of comorbidities is calculated without an indication of severity.

The impact of comorbidities in rheumatic diseases is multidimensional. Some comorbidities, such as cardiovascular disease, lymphoma, renal and pulmonary diseases, and infections are associated with premature mortality. As inflammation is the common pathophysiology in rheumatic diseases and in many comorbidities, suppression of inflammatory activity is essential. This emphasizes timely and active treatment of every patient with early

RA to bring the disease to sustained remission in order to diminish the risk of these comorbidities. Furthermore, careful monitoring of patients at high risk of comorbidities, in particular those with severe, treatment-refractory disease, is necessary. This may require close collaboration between rheumatologists and other specialists. Education of the medical community on these issues is of major importance.

In addition to the risk that is caused by inflammation, patients with rheumatic diseases are at least as likely as the general population to have traditional cardiovascular risk factors such as hypertension, diabetes, and hyperlipidaemia. Furthermore, patients with RA are more likely to smoke and be physically inactive than the general population. Therefore, traditional risk factors for cardiovascular disease need to be reviewed and addressed on a regular basis, and interventions against adverse lifestyle factors and other important predictors should be initiated when indicated.

Depression and fibromyalgia are comorbidities that increase the risk of work disability, which is the most costly consequence of RA. A review of patients' psychological well-being should be routine practice at rheumatology visits. A multidisciplinary team including nurses, physiotherapists, social workers, and psychologists facilitates the management of patients with these comorbidities. It is particularly important to differentiate such problems from complications driven directly by inflammation, as the management is completely different.

Osteoporosis is a prevalent comorbidity in rheumatic diseases. Patients need to be screened and treated for osteoporosis. Patients at high risk, in particular those who are treated with long-term corticosteroid treatment, should preferably be started on preventive treatment before osteoporosis develops.

Some comorbidities are drug-related, e.g. gastrointestinal ulcers with perforation or bleeding, and in the past these were often seen in patients who made heavy use of non-steroidal anti-inflammatory drugs (NSAIDs). Serious infections and pulmonary diseases are rare but potentially life-threatening side effects of current antirheumatic medications. However, it is worth to remember that 'side effects' of untreated or poorly treated RA overall are worse than the side effects of current antirheumatic drugs.[5] It is also important to communicate this to patients.

Rheumatoid arthritis and comorbidities—burden in daily life

Active and severe RA causes a burden in daily life, which is heavier in older than in younger people. In general, women experience a heavier burden from RA than men do.[6] On the other hand, patients who reach early clinical remission may live a normal life, including fully preserved work capacity.[7]

As with the effects of RA itself, the burden from comorbidities may vary. Asymptomatic conditions that are kept under control with simple medications, such as hypertension or thyroid disease, may not cause any significant burden. However, in general, individuals with several comorbidities have higher scores for functional disability, pain, and global health assessment compared to those who have fewer or no comorbidities (Figure 32.1).[8]

Mortality as a consequence of comorbidities

According to an old saying, 'the way to live a long life is to acquire rheumatism'.[9] There was a period when RA was regarded in the majority of patients as a disease with a good prognosis. The traditional teaching was that RA could be controlled in most patients with aspirin and later alternative NSAIDs. However, data from RA cohorts and epidemiological studies revealed that patients with RA on average died many years earlier than the general population. The traditional view reflected the previous lack of systematic follow-up data and the lack of available potent interventions. Over time, the interest in long-term outcomes, including mortality, as well as preventive measures, has increased considerably.

Cardiovascular disease is the most common acute cause of death in patients with RA, similarly to the general population.[10] (Table 32.1). In a review of 50 reports of patients with RA in the United States and western European countries in 1953–2008, cardiovascular disease was the acute attributed cause of death in 40.5% of patients. It appears that infection and renal, respiratory, and gastrointestinal diseases are over-represented as an immediate cause of death in patients with RA.

It may be tempting to try to classify causes of death in patients with RA as 'related to RA' or 'not related to RA'. However, this classification may be artificial as inflammation appears to be part of the underlying pathophysiology for many comorbidities such as infectious, pulmonary, renal, and cardiovascular diseases. When an individual with RA (or any inflammatory rheumatic disease) dies of any cause 5–15 years earlier than expected according to that person's age and sex, the death appears in some way to be related to the inflammatory disease.

The most significant predictors of premature mortality in patients with RA are older age, male sex, comorbidities, patient's and physician's global estimates, severe extra-articular manifestations, and poor functional status assessed by physical measures and patient questionnaires.

Poor physical function and low muscle strength are significant predictors of mortality in RA and other chronic diseases, in ageing individuals, and in the general population.[11] Poor physical function predicts earlier mortality in diseased and normal populations as well or better than most known biomedical predictors, such as laboratory tests. In the Quantitative Monitoring of Patients with RA (QUEST-RA) study, which reviews patients who receive usual care in several countries, only 13.8% of 5,235 patients in 21 countries reported physical exercise 3 times a week or more.[12] A majority of the patients were physically inactive: more than 80% of patients in seven countries, 60–80% in 12 countries, and 45% and 29% of patients in two other countries reported no regular weekly exercise. Physical function is a modifiable risk factor for mortality, regardless of underlying health condition. The importance of regular exercise should be communicated to all individuals with rheumatic diseases whether or not they have comorbidities, to promote general health and longevity.

Some therapies for RA, including gold salts,[13] methotrexate,[14,15] and tumour necrosis factor (TNF) inhibitors,[16] have been reported to be associated with reduced mortality rates in patients with RA. This is to be expected, as these therapies are associated with improved values for quantitative prognostic indicators of premature mortality. Mortality in RA that is attributable to therapies occurs in fewer than 2% of deaths, although therapies for RA can sometimes lead to fatal consequences. As with any potent, long-standing treatment, risks and benefits need to be balanced in treatment decisions for every individual patient.

Cardiovascular disease

During past decades, cardiovascular events have been found to occur approximately a decade earlier in RA than in the general population, suggesting that RA, similarly to diabetes mellitus, is an independent risk factor for premature ischemic heart disease. Nontraditional risk factors, in particular RA disease activity/severity measures, including inflammatory markers, disease activity scores, seropositivity, physical disability, destructive changes on joint radiographs, extra-articular manifestations, and corticosteroid use, have repeatedly shown significant associations with increased cardiovascular risk.[17,18] Taken together, this suggests that disease severity, in particular systemic inflammation, is a major predictor of cardiovascular comorbidity in patients with RA.

Scores that have been developed to estimate cardiovascular risk for the general population based on traditional cardiovascular risk factors alone are unlikely to accurately estimate cardiovascular risk in patients with active RA. In addition to targeting remission in RA, evaluation, care, and patient education concerning cardiovascular risk factors should be routine in every rheumatology

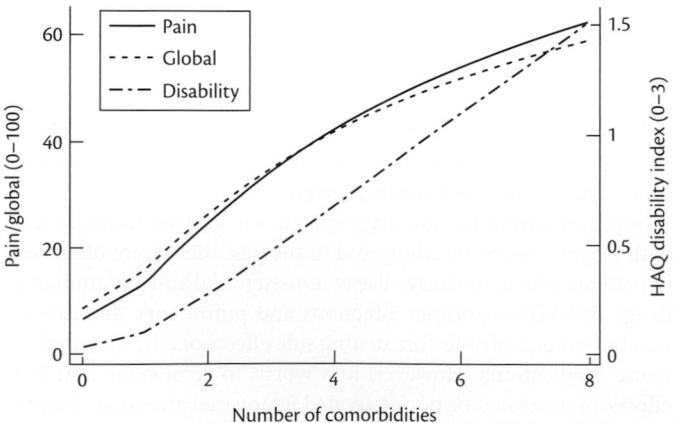

Fig. 32.1 Self-reported pain, global health assessment, and functional disability scores increase (deteriorate) with an increasing number of disease conditions.[8] Reproduced from Annals of the Rheumatic Diseases Krishnan E, Hakkinen A, Sokka T, Hannonen P. 2005;64(9):1350–2. with permission from the BMJ.

Table 32.1 Summary of causes of death in patients with RA in the United States population in 1977 and 2005: percentages of deaths due to various causes according to period and type of study[10]

	1953–1989	1990–2000	2001–2008	Special studies	Population studies	Total	U.S. averages 1977	U.S. averages 2005
No. of reports (cohorts)	14(14)	9(9)	10(11)	10(13)	7(7)	50(54)	—	—
Patient population	5 696	5 986	3 083	6 163	70 690	91 618	—	—
Total no. of deaths	1 779	1 589	619	2 039	27 224	33 250	—	—
Cause of death								
Cardiovascular	39.6	46.7	38.6	33.5	43.5	39.6	41.0	38.3*
Cancer	13.4	19.8	18.7	17.1	16.3	16.8	20.4	22.8
Renal	8.3	3.2	7.5	4.8	4.3	5.8	1.1	1.8
Respiratory	7.2	6.5	12.9	11.8	7.8	9.0	3.9	5.3
Infection	18.5	6.5	17.1	17.0	5.8	14.3	1.0	4.4
Gastrointestinal	5.1	5.8	5.2	4.2	5.8	5.1	2.4	1.1
Sudden death	—	2.9	3.3	0.0	—	3.1	—	—
Accidents or intoxication	1.5	5.4	4.4	6.3	5.2	4.2	5.4	6.9
RA/musculoskeletal diseases	12.9	8.3	6.5	4.1	9.2	9.4	—	—
Other	8.9	9.5	20.5	13.0	14.4	12.9	24.8	21.4

clinic. Current guidelines recommend that the method for calculating the risk score and/or the algorithm for intervening against traditional risk factors should be adapted in order to take into account the increased risk associated with severe RA itself.[19]

The risk of myocardial infarction is increased in patients who use NSAIDs and cyclooxygenase-2 inhibitors. On the other hand, treatment with methotrexate and other disease-modifying antirheumatic drugs (DMARDs) is associated with a lower risk for cardiovascular events in RA patients compared to patients who had never used DMARDs. In the QUEST-RA study, longer use of biologic agents and DMARDs such as methotrexate, leflunomide, and sulfasalazine was associated with a decreased risk of cardiovascular disease (Table 32.2).[20]

Many patients with RA are informed and worried about an increased risk of cardiovascular comorbidity. It is worth noting that studies that indicate an increased risk were conducted before the era of active treatment strategies for RA. Although a majority of RA patients worldwide still suffer from active disease,[21] remission is a realistic goal in the management of RA and can be achieved in the majority of patients with early and active treatment. In the NEO-RACo trial, more than 80% of all patients with early active RA were in DAS28 remission at 2 years—a comparator arm involved a triple therapy (methotrexate, sulfasalazine, hydroxychloroquine) plus prednisolone and the active arm was intensified with half-a-year initial infliximab therapy.[22] A Dutch pilot study (intensified COBRA) involved a triple therapy plus high-dose prednisolone. Infliximab was started in 6 of 21 patients who did not reach a treatment target.[23] At 40 weeks, 90% of the patients were in DAS28 remission. In a recent cross-sectional analysis, up to 40–50% of patients in clinics with active treatment strategies were in remission.[24,25]

Improved outcomes have been documented for many severe outcomes in RA, as will be discussed later. It can be anticipated that

cardiovascular comorbidity will become less prominent over the years, with active treatment strategies for RA and routine evaluation and care of traditional cardiovascular risk factors. Signals indicating such a development are already present, as discussed later.

Pulmonary disease

Pulmonary disease has recently attracted a lot of attention in RA for several reasons. Pulmonary disease, especially pneumonia, has been a major cause of death in RA for decades (Table 32.1). Pulmonary fibrosis—rheumatoid lung disease, 'RA lung', or RA-associated interstitial lung disease (RA-ILD)—is still one the of the most feared manifestations of RA as its treatment options are limited and it is associated with high mortality.[26] Fear of RA-ILD is not diminished by the fact that idiopathic pulmonary fibrosis (without rheumatic disease) has even worse prognosis and the clinical effectiveness of newly available anti-fibrotic drugs remains questionable.

In the QUEST-RA study, 4.5% of 9448 patients with a clinical diagnosis of RA in 34 countries were reported to have pulmonary fibrosis. However, symptomatic RA-ILD appears to constitute only a fraction of truly existing lung disease in RA. The availability of techniques such as high-resolution CT (HRCT) has revealed that interstitial lung disease may be found in 20–40% of patients with RA and was found in 19% in consecutive patients with RA in the United Kingdom in the late 1990s.[27] A 13–15 year follow-up of the cohort indicated that extensive interstitial involvement in HRCT, which was seen in 3.3% (5 of 150) cases, was associated with a poor prognosis and was leading to respiratory failure and death in 4 of 5 cases. However, in those who had borderline or limited HRCT involvement, lung disease remained silent and possibly would have needed no more intervention than smoking cessation.[28] This

Table 32.2 Years of exposure to disease-modifying anti-rheumatic drugs and cardiovascular morbidity in patients with rheumatoid arthritis in the QUEST-RA study[20]

	HR[a] (95% CI) CV all types	HR[b] (95% CI) CV all types	HR[c] (95% CI)		
			CV all types	Myocardial infarction	Stroke
Methotrexate	0.82 (0.79–0.86)[d]	0.84 (0.80–0.87)[d]	0.85 (0.81–0.89)[d]	0.82 (0.74–0.91)[d]	0.89 (0.82–0.98)[e]
Glucocorticoids	0.94 (0.92–0.97)[d]	0.95 (0.93–0.97)[d]	0.95 (0.92–0.98)[d]	0.96 (0.91–1.00)	0.98 (0.93–1.03)
Antimalarials	0.94 (0.91–0.98)[f]	0.95 (0.91–0.99)[f]	0.98 (0.94–1.02)	0.94 (0.85–1.03)	0.87 (0.76–1.01)
Sulfasalazine	0.91 (0.87–0.96)[d]	0.92 (0.88–0.97)[f]	0.92 (0.87–0.98)[f]	0.82 (0.69–0.98)[e]	0.90 (0.79–1.03)
Gold	0.96 (0.92–1.00)[e]	0.96 (0.92–1.00)[e]	0.99 (0.95–1.03)	1.04 (0.98–1.10)	0.98 (0.89–1.07)
Leflunomide	0.52 (0.38–0.72)[d]	0.55 (0.41–0.75)[d]	0.59 (0.43–0.79)[f]	0.52 (0.26–1.06)	0.91 (0.65–1.28)
TNFα blockers	0.67 (0.53–0.85)[f]	0.71 (0.56–0.89)[f]	0.64 (0.49–0.83)[f]	0.42 (0.21–0.81)[e]	0.64 (0.39–1.05)

[a]Crude hazard ratio.

[b]Adjusted hazard ratio by age and gender.

[c]Adjusted hazard ratio by age, gender, disease activity/severity (DAS 28 [disease activity score using 28 joint counts] and Health Assessment Questionnaire), rheumatoid arthritis characteristics (rheumatoid factor-positive and extra-articular manifestations), and traditional cardiovascular risk factors (hypertension, hyperlipidemia, diabetes, smoking ever, and obesity).

[d]$P <0.001$.

[e]$P <0.05$.

[f]$P <0.01$.

CI, confidence interval; CV, cardiovascular; QUEST-RA, Questionnaires in Standard Monitoring of Patients with Rheumatoid Arthritis; TNFα, tumor necrosis factor alpha.

suggests that evaluation of the extent of lung involvement with HRCT is a useful prognostic tool.

Respiratory symptoms reflecting an idiosyncratic drug-induced pneumonitis are sometimes seen in patients who receive methotrexate or leflunomide. Treatment with TNF inhibitors may lead to worsening of pre-existing RA-ILD, although the magnitude of this risk and the risk/benefit ratio in patients with RA-ILD remains to be defined. Therefore, a common practice before initiating these medications is to take baseline chest radiographs in all patients and pulmonary function tests in patients who are at higher risk for lung disease, as well as to advise patients to quit smoking.

Cancer

An association between long-lasting RA and haematological malignancies was first documented in the 1970s.[29] Later, it was demonstrated that continuous inflammatory activity is strongly associated with the risk of lymphoma.[30] The incidence of lung cancer is increased in RA,[31] possibly related in part to smoking, while the incidence of colorectal cancer is lower than in the general population.[32] It is presently unclear whether there is an association between skin cancer and RA.

In clinical practice, many patients and healthcare providers are concerned about whether medications for RA increase the risk of cancer. Such a risk was not found in a recent review of methotrexate monotherapy for RA.[33] Concerning biologic agents, the current understanding, based on extensive observational studies, is that these drugs do not increase cancer risk.[34]

Infections

Active inflammation in RA increases the risk of infections, including bacterial, tubercular, fungal, opportunistic, and viral infections. High doses of oral corticosteroids contribute to the likelihood of infections, as documented in observational series.[35] Anti-TNF therapy increases the risk of the activation of latent tuberculosis.

In order to prevent infections, patient education should include general advice to be cautious about infections. In particular, patients must be reminded about oral hygiene and regular dental check-ups. Feet with deformities and fragile skin need special attention, including consultation with a podiatrist. Patients who are planned to start biologic agents should be screened for latent tuberculosis. Such patients, and other patients with a complicated disease course, should also be considered for vaccination against *Streptococcus pneumoniae* and influenza. Current guidelines recommend that patients are vaccinated during a stable phase of their disease.[36] General vaccination programmes should also be followed.

Infection is the acute cause of death with the highest relative excess mortality in RA patients compared to the general population (Table 32.1): 14.3% in patients with RA compared to 1.0% in the United States population in 1977 and 4.4% in 2005 (suggesting an older population and/or more accurate reporting in 2005). It is worth to note that the proportion of deaths attributed to infection has not changed substantially over the years, being much the same in recent years as in the era before treatment with methotrexate and biologic agents.[10] In population-based studies from Olmsted County, Minnesota, conducted before the era of biologics, the risk of serious infections was increased compared to the general population,[37] and measures of disease severity were major predictors of comorbidity from infections.[38]

Osteoporosis

Patients with RA are at increased risk of developing osteoporosis compared to the general population. The development of osteopenia is associated with the extent of erosive changes in joints. Rheumatoid inflammation appears to be involved in the pathophysiology of both general and local bone loss in RA.[39] Treatment of corticosteroids is a well-known risk factor for osteoporosis; physical inactivity and smoking contribute to the risk.

Osteoporosis is a comorbid condition that can be prevented. Routine patient education includes advice concerning physical exercise to prevent osteoporosis; smokers are advised to quit smoking. Patients should be given advice concerning calcium and vitamin D supplementation according to national guidelines. Adults should get 500–1000 g calcium every day, from food or calcium supplements. In countries that have long periods without sunshine, all elderly women are advised to consume a minimum of 800 IU (20 μg) vitamin D every day. If this amount is not received from food, vitamin D supplementation is advised, with a maximum of 2000 IU (50 μg) a day.

Patients with RA should be monitored for bone mass by dual-energy X-ray absorptiometry (DXA). It is worth remembering that corticosteroid therapy also has direct deleterious impact on bone and increases fracture risk even at osteopenic DXA values. Therefore, such patients should be considered for preventive treatment with bisphosponates. Parathyroid hormone may be considered in patients with refractory osteoporosis, or those who do not tolerate bisphosphonates.

Outcomes of RA are improving—does this apply to comorbidities?

Concomitantly with an increasing use of early and active treatment strategies, overall clinical outcomes in patients with RA have improved compared to previous decades. Even before the era of biologic treatments, improvements were seen in patients' clinical status according to disease activity,[40,41] functional capacity,[41–43] radiographic scores,[41,44] and other clinical measures.[41] Furthermore, lower mortality rates were reported in patients who responded to gold,[13] methotrexate,[15,45] and biologic agents,[16] and lower work disability rates were seen in patients who responded to anti-rheumatic drugs.[7] More recently, studies from Western countries and Japan suggest that rates of total joint replacement and other RA-related surgeries have been stable or even decreased in patients with RA in the last decade.[46] In addition, the health status of the general population in Western countries is currently better than in previous decades in many respects.

The improving health of patients with RA and the general population suggests that the prevalence and impact of comorbidities in patients with RA should also improve (i.e. become more like that of the general population); patterns of causes of death should become more similar to the background population; and, finally, the lifespan of patients with RA should increase to the population level.

In 2007, a mailed survey was conducted to study self-reported lifestyle, health status, and morbidities in patients with RA and in the general population. All RA patients from a hospital district of 275 000 people were included in a rheumatology clinic RA database. For each RA patient, three age-, sex-, and habitat-matched control subjects were randomly sampled from the population register. An extended health assessment questionnaire was mailed to patients and control subjects. The response rate was 70%. Table 32.3 presents the self-reported prevalence of selected health conditions in 1635 patients with RA and 4264 control subjects (in both groups, mean age was 65 years and 73% were women),

Table 32.3 Percentage of individuals with a self-reported health condition

	General population	RA	P
Coronary artery disease	13	12	0.42
Smoking now	10	11	0.22
Hypertension	47	44	0.011
Diabetes	11	8	0.001
Stroke	4.3	4.3	0.99
Peptic ulcer	5	5	0.81
Asthma	13	15	0.008
Chronic bronchitis	1.5	2.5	0.014
Thyroid disease	11	10	0.36
Cancer	8	5.5	0.001
Chronic back pain	26	22	0.001
Musculoskeletal trauma	13	11	0.007
Fibromyalgia	6	8	0.002
Psychiatric disease	3.6	2.8	0.15
Alcohol abuse	1.4	1.1	0.35
Osteoarthritis	30	32	0.15
Osteoporosis	6.5	18	<0.001
Cataracts	15	18	0.014

matched for sex, age, and location, in the Central Finland Health Care district in 2007.[47]

The prevalence estimates of cardiovascular diseases and traditional cardiovascular risk factors were similar between groups or more favourable in patients with RA. Lung diseases, fibromyalgia, osteoporosis, and cataracts were more frequent in RA patients, likely related to RA and/or its treatments. More frequent diagnostic tests in patients with RA may influence the detection and reported prevalence of osteoporosis and fibromyalgia. The prevalence of cancer, chronic back pain, and musculoskeletal trauma was higher in the background population. RA may lead to changes in lifestyle that reduce the risk of these comorbidities. The data on cardiovascular disease and its risk factors indicates favourable changes in this comorbidity compared to historical data. On the other hand, studies on self-reported prevalent diseases may not reflect the full burden of fatal comorbidities. In a study with long-term follow-up of patients with RA enrolled in 1978 and 1995, the incidence of fatal and non-fatal cardiovascular events remained increased compared to the general population in the year 1995, with similar risk ratios in both cohorts.[48] Further studies of this issue are necessary, and efforts to reduce the burden of comorbidities should remain a high priority for rheumatologists.

Reviewing and managing comorbidities: clinic infrastructure

Quantitative monitoring of RA as part of daily clinical practice may have improved since Dr Wright's observation in 1983 that 'clinicians may all too easily spend years writing "doing well" in the notes of a patient who has become progressively crippled before their eyes…'.[49] Standard quantitative monitoring with a treatment goal has been shown to be beneficial to patient outcomes in randomized clinical trials. Quantitative monitoring has also contributed to improved long-term outcomes for RA seen in clinical care.

The QUEST-RA programme was established in 2005[50] to promote quantitative assessment in rheumatology, and by end of 2011 it had expanded to 34 countries involving 9000 patients. In this programme, the patient completes an expanded health assessment questionnaire including questions about functional capacity, psychological well-being, symptoms, lifestyle, life environment, and work status. The rheumatologist completes a

Table 32.4 Electronically available clinical evaluation of an example patient with RA. Data collected using GoTreatIT, DiaGraphITas, Kristiansand, Norway

Date	25.01.2012
ID	xxxxxxxxxx
Name	XXXXXXXXX
Age, gender	77, female
Work status	Retired
Diagnosis	Rheumatoid Arthritis
Diagnosis criteria	◆ Symptoms (ACR RA): Polyarticular 1.2011
	◆ Clinical diagnosis (ACR RA): 6.2011
Highest RF (IgM)	Negative (8) 9.2010
Highest (aCCP)	Positive (60) 5.2011
Erosions	Negative 6.2011
Drug (now)	Sulfasalazine 12.2011
	◆ 2000.00 mg per oral every day
	Hydroxychloroquine 12.2011
	◆ 300.00 mg per oral every day
	Prednisolone 6.2011
	◆ 2.50 mg per oral every day
	Methotrexate 6.2011
	◆ 20,00 mg Peroral Once a week
Comorbidity	Osteopenia by bone density 9.2011
	◆ Info: After rheuma diagnosis
	Cerebral infarction
	◆ Info: Before rheuma diagnosis
	Heart rhythm disorder
	◆ Info: Before rheuma diagnosis
	Mitral insufficiency
	◆ Info: Before rheuma diagnosis
Data confirmed	12.12.2011, miina_l

Table 32.4 (Continued)

Latest scores				
Date	20.06.2011	30.06.2011	27.09.2011	12.12.2011
Health status				
Pain (0–100)	90	16	0	4
Fatigue (0–100)	87	7	8	0
Patient global (0–100)	61	3	5	0
Morning stiffness (h)	3.00	0.08	0.00	0.00
Rheumatic activity (0–100)	70	4	0	1
Physical exercise	≥3/week	≥ 3/week	≥3/week	≥3/week
M-HAQ (0–3)	1	0.13	0	0
PS-HAQ (0–3)	1	0	0	0
HAQ (0–3)	1.75	0.63	0	0
Disease activity				
Dr Global (0–100)	60		0	14
ESR	48		10	7
CRP	16		2	2
TJC 28/32	10/10		0/0	0/0
SJC 28/32	9/9		0/0	1/1
DAS28	6.2		1.7	1.6
CDAI	31.1		0.5	2.4
Anthropometric data				
Weight	61	61	62	62
BMI	23	23	24.2	24.2

structured clinical evaluation including a checklist of past and current comorbidities, extra-articular RA manifestations, and current clinical status.

The idea of a structured patient evaluation was developed further, and currently many clinics use software that collects real-time data from each patient, to assist clinical decision-making and improve the quality of clinical care. The patient self-report clinical status and its changes, history of RA and medications, comorbidities, and surgeries are readily available as a flowsheet (Table 32.4) or a graph (Figure 32.2). Time is saved for a focused discussion, as reviewing dozens of pages of patient's medical records or numerous screens of electronic medical records is not necessary. Easily available data enables better adherence to a 'treat to target' approach, which is a preventive strategy against many comorbidities in RA. A structured electronic evaluation saves time for review and advice concerning clinically important comorbidities such as risk factors for cardiovascular disease and osteoporosis.

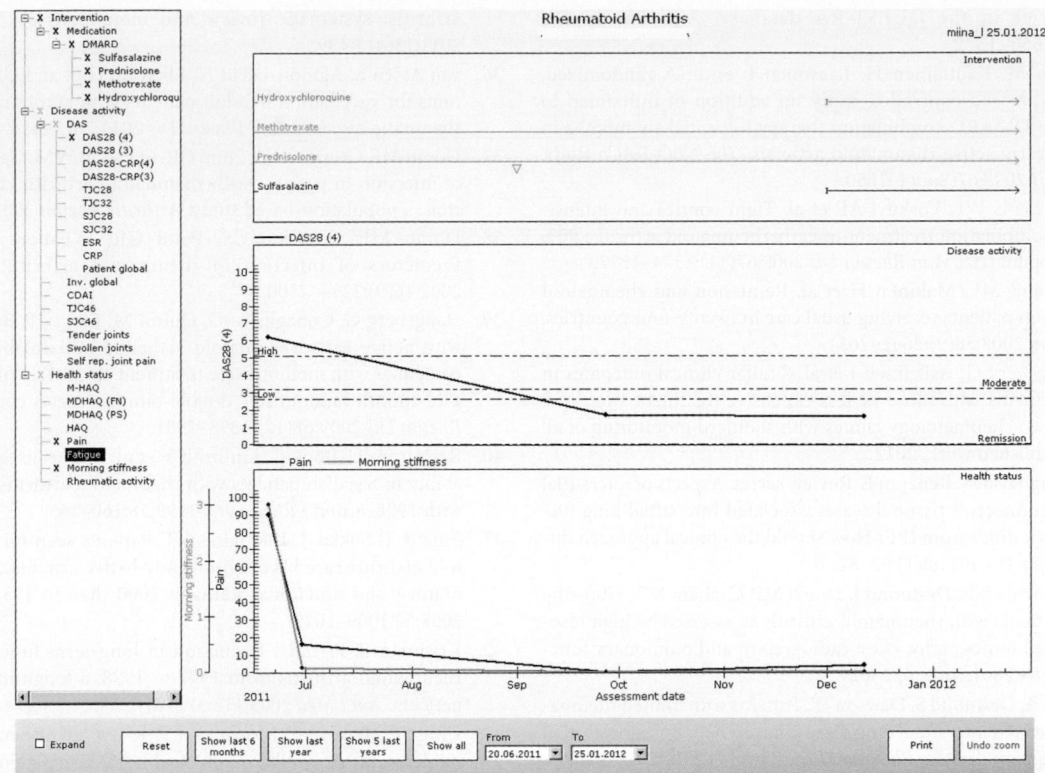

Fig. 32.2 Electronically available clinical evaluation of an example patient with RA: a graphical presentation. Data collected using GoTreatIT, DiaGraphITas, Kristiansand, Norway.

References

1. Michaud K, Wolfe F. Comorbidities in rheumatoid arthritis. *Best Pract Res Clin Rheumatol* 2007;21(5):885–906.

2. Gabriel SE, Michaud K. Epidemiological studies in incidence, prevalence, mortality, and comorbidity of the rheumatic diseases. *Arthritis Res Ther* 2009;11(3):229.

3. Charlson ME, Pompei P, Ales KL, MacKenzie CR. A new method of classifying prognostic comorbidity in longitudinal studies: development and validation. *J Chronic Dis* 1987;40:373–383.

4. Gabriel SE, Crowson CS, O'Fallon WM. A comparison of two comorbidity instruments in arthritis. *J Clin Epidemiol* 1999;52(12):1137–1142.

5. Pincus T, Kavanaugh A, Sokka T. Benefit/risk of therapies for rheumatoid arthritis: underestimation of the 'side effects' or risks of RA leads to underestimation of the benefit/risk of therapies. *Clin Exp Rheumatol* 2004;22(Suppl 35):S2–S11.

6. Sokka T, Toloza S, Cutolo M et al. Women, men, and rheumatoid arthritis: analyses of disease activity, disease characteristics, and treatments in the QUEST-RA Study. *Arthritis Res Ther* 2009;11(1):R7.

7. Puolakka K, Kautiainen H, Möttönen T et al. Early suppression of disease activity is essential for maintenance of work capacity in patients with recent-onset rheumatoid arthritis: five-year experience from the FIN-RACo trial. *Arthritis Rheum* 2005;52(1):36–41.

8. Krishnan E, Hakkinen A, Sokka T, Hannonen P. Impact of age and comorbidities on the criteria for remission and response in rheumatoid arthritis. *Ann Rheum Dis* 2005;64(9):1350–1352.

9. Cobb S, Anderson F, Bauer W. Length of life and cause of death in rheumatoid arthritis. *N Engl J Med* 1953;249:553–556.

10. Sokka T, Abelson B, Pincus T. Mortality in rheumatoid arthritis: 2008 update. *Clin Exp Rheumatol* 2008;26(5 Suppl 51):S35–61.

11. Sokka T, Hakkinen A. Poor physical fitness and performance as predictors of mortality in normal populations and patients with rheumatic and other diseases. *Clin Exp Rheumatol* 2008,26(5 Suppl 5):14–20.

12. Sokka T, Hakkinen A, Kautiainen H et al. Physical inactivity in patients with rheumatoid arthritis: data from twenty-one countries in a cross-sectional, international study. *Arthritis Rheum* 2008;59(1):42–50.

13. Lehtinen K, Isomäki H. Intramuscular gold therapy is associated with long survival in patients with rheumatoid arthritis. *J Rheumatol* 1991;18(4):524–529.

14. Alarcon GS. Response to methotrexate and reduced mortality in patients with rheumatoid arthritis: comment on the article by Krause et al. *Arthritis Rheum* 2000;43(8):1902–1903.

15. Choi HK, Hernán MA, Seeger JD, Robins JM, Wolfe F. Methotrexate and mortality in patients with rheumatoid arthritis: a prospective study. *Lancet* 2002;359:1173–1177.

16. Jacobsson LTH, Turesson C, Nilsson JA et al. Treatment with TNF blockers and mortality risk in patients with rheumatoid arthritis. *Ann Rheum Dis* 2007;66(5):670–675.

17. Turesson C, Jacobsson LT, Matteson EL. Cardiovascular co-morbidity in rheumatic diseases. *Vasc Health Risk Manag* 2008;4(3):605–614.

18. Gabriel SE, Crowson CS. Risk factors for cardiovascular disease in rheumatoid arthritis. *Curr Opin Rheumatol* 2012;24(2):171–176.

19. Peters MJ, Symmons DP, McCarey D et al. EULAR evidence-based recommendations for cardiovascular risk management in patients with rheumatoid arthritis and other forms of inflammatory arthritis. *Ann Rheum Dis* 2010;69(2):325–331.

20. Naranjo A, Sokka T, Descalzo MA et al. Cardiovascular disease in patients with rheumatoid arthritis: results from the QUEST-RA study. *Arthritis Res Ther* 2008;10(2):R30.

21. Sokka T, Kautiainen H, Pincus T et al. Disparities in rheumatoid arthritis disease activity according to gross domestic product

in 25 countries in the QUEST-RA database. *Ann Rheum Dis* 2009;68(11):1666–1672.

22. Leirisalo-Repo M, Kautiainen H, Laasonen L et al. A randomized, double-blind, placebo-controlled study on addition of infliximab to the FIN-RACo DMARD combination therapy for initial six months in patients with early active rheumatoid arthritis. *The NEO-RACo study. Ann Rheum Dis* 2008;67(Suppl II):50.

23. van Tuyl LH, Lems WF, Voskuyl AE et al. Tight control and intensified COBRA combination treatment in early rheumatoid arthritis: 90% remission in a pilot trial. *Ann Rheum Dis* 2008;67(11):1574–1577.

24. Sokka T, Hetland ML, Makinen H et al. Remission and rheumatoid arthritis: Data on patients receiving usual care in twenty-four countries. *Arthritis Rheum* 2008;58(9):2642–2651.

25. Sokka T, Haugeberg G, Asikainen J et al. Similar clinical outcomes in rheumatoid arthritis with more vs. less expensive treatment strategies. Results from two rheumatology clinics with standard monitoring of all patients. Unpublished work, 2012.

26. de LA, Veeraraghavan S, Renzoni E. Review series: Aspects of interstitial lung disease: connective tissue disease-associated interstitial lung disease: how does it differ from IPF? How should the clinical approach differ? *Chron Respir Dis* 2011;8(1):53–82.

27. Dawson JK, Fewins HE, Desmond J, Lynch MP, Graham DR. Fibrosing alveolitis in patients with rheumatoid arthritis as assessed by high resolution computed tomography, chest radiography, and pulmonary function tests. *Thorax* 2001;56(8):622–627.

28. Sathi N, Urwin T, Desmond S, Dawson JK. Patients with limited rheumatoid arthritis-related interstitial lung disease have a better prognosis than those with extensive disease. *Rheumatology (Oxford)* 2011;50(3):620.

29. Isomäki HA, Hakulinen T, Joutsenlahti U. Excess risk of lymphomas, leukemia and myeloma in patients with rheumatoid arthritis. *J Chronic Dis* 1978;31:691–696.

30. Baecklund E, Sundstrom C, Ekbom A et al. Lymphoma subtypes in patients with rheumatoid arthritis: increased proportion of diffuse large B cell lymphoma. *Arthritis Rheum* 2003;48(6):1543–1550.

31. Kauppi M, Pukkala E, Isomaki H. Excess risk of lung cancer in patients with rheumatoid arthritis. *J Rheumatol* 1996;23(8):1484–1485.

32. Kauppi M, Pukkala E, Isomaki H. Low incidence of colorectal cancer in patients with rheumatoid arthritis. *Clin Exp Rheumatol* 1996;14(5):551–553.

33. Salliot C, van der Heijde D. Long-term safety of methotrexate monotherapy in patients with rheumatoid arthritis: a systematic literature research. *Ann Rheum Dis* 2009;68(7):1100–1104.

34. Solomon DH, Mercer E, Kavanaugh A. Observational studies on the risk of cancer associated with tumor necrosis factor inhibitors in rheumatoid arthritis: a review of their methodologies and results. *Arthritis Rheum* 2012;64(1):21–32.

35. Dixon WG, Suissa S, Hudson M. The association between systemic glucocorticoid therapy and the risk of infection in patients with rheumatoid arthritis: systematic review and meta-analyses. *Arthritis Res Ther* 2011;13(4):R139.

36. van Assen S, Agmon-Levin N, Elkayam O et al. EULAR recommendations for vaccination in adult patients with autoimmune inflammatory rheumatic diseases. *Ann Rheum Dis* 2011;70(3):414–422.

37. Doran MF, Crowson CS, Pond GR, O'Fallon WM, Gabriel SE. Frequency of infection in patients with rheumatoid arthritis compared with controls: a population-based study. *Arthritis Rheum* 2002;46(9):2287–2293.

38. Doran MF, Crowson CS, Pond GR, O'Fallon WM, Gabriel SE. Predictors of infection in rheumatoid arthritis. *Arthritis Rheum* 2002;46(9):2294–2300.

39. Haugeberg G, Conaghan PG, Quinn M, Emery P. Bone loss in patients with active early rheumatoid arthritis: infliximab and methotrexate compared with methotrexate treatment alone. Explorative analysis from a 12-month randomised, double-blind, placebo-controlled study. *Ann Rheum Dis* 2009;68(12):1898–1901.

40. Bergstrom U, Book C, Lindroth Y et al. Lower disease activity and disability in Swedish patients with rheumatoid arthritis in 1995 compared with 1978. *Scand J Rheumatol* 1999;28:160–165.

41. Pincus T, Sokka T, Kautiainen H. Patients seen for standard rheumatoid arthritis care have significantly better articular, radiographic, laboratory, and functional status in 2000 than in 1985. *Arthritis Rheum* 2005;52:1009–1019.

42. Krishnan E, Fries JF. Reduction in long-term functional disability in rheumatoid arthritis from 1977 to 1998: a longitudinal study of 3035 patients. *Am J Med* 2003;115:371–376.

43. Uhlig T, Heiberg T, Mowinckel P, Kvien TK. Rheumatoid arthritis is milder in the new millennium: health status in patients with rheumatoid arthritis 1994–2004. *Ann Rheum Dis* 2008;67(12):1710–1715.

44. Sokka T, Kautiainen H, Häkkinen K, Hannonen P. Radiographic progression is getting milder in patients with early rheumatoid arthritis. Results of 3 cohorts over 5 years. *J Rheumatol* 2004;31:1073–1082.

45. Krause D, Schleusser B, Herborn G, Rau R. Response to methotrexate treatment is associated with reduced mortality in patients with severe rheumatoid arthritis. *Arthritis Rheum* 2000;43:14–21.

46. Khan NA, Sokka T. Declining needs for total joint replacements for rheumatoid arthritis. *Arthritis Res Ther* 2011;13(5):130.

47. Sokka T, Kautiainen H. Current profile of comorbidities in patients with rheumatoid arthritis (RA) in comparison to community controls. Unpublished work, 2012.

48. Bergstrom U, Jacobsson LT, Turesson C. Cardiovascular morbidity and mortality remain similar in two cohorts of patients with long-standing rheumatoid arthritis seen in 1978 and 1995 in Malmo, Sweden. *Rheumatology (Oxford)* 2009;48(12):1600–1605.

49. Smith T. Questions on clinical trials (editorial). *BMJ* 1983;287:569.

50. Sokka T, Kautiainen H, Toloza S et al. QUEST-RA: quantitative clinical assessment of patients with rheumatoid arthritis seen in standard rheumatology care in 15 countries. *Ann Rheum Dis* 2007;66:1491–1496.

CHAPTER 33

Social aspects (work)

Ross Wilkie

Introduction

Rheumatic conditions are the most frequently cited reason for absence from work.[1] In recent years, the impact of rheumatic diseases on work has demanded more attention from all stakeholders, including clinicians and policy-makers. Work participation is important to individuals with rheumatic conditions and society. Reduced work participation affects the quality of life of patients and their families, and has major financial consequences for the individual and society. The ability to manage rheumatic diseases in order to continue in paid work has always been important for clinicians. This chapter outlines key aspects supporting increased interest in improving work participation for those with rheumatic diseases. It then draws on the results of empirical studies to highlight potential targets and strategies to reduce work restriction.

Why are we increasingly interested in the impact of rheumatic conditions on work?

The following sections highlight three of the key reasons for the increased interest in the impact of rheumatic conditions on work.

Impact on the individual

There is now greater acknowledgement of the benefits of work participation for the individual. A number of reviews have highlighted the benefits of work participation and the importance of 'good work' to health and well-being.[1-3] Extensive background evidence suggests that work is generally good for physical health, mental health and well-being; it is beneficial to an individual's prosperity and is important to psychosocial needs in societies where employment is the norm. It is central to identity, social roles, and social status, and employment and social status are the main drivers of social gradients in physical and mental health and mortality.[2] In contrast, not being in employment is associated with significantly poorer overall self-rated health, more depressive symptoms, and a greater decline in health status (although these are also reasons for being out of work).[4] The general view of work being positive for individuals has encouraged clinicians and policy-makers to focus on improving work participation through preventing premature work cessation (i.e. prior to retirement age) and encouraging return to work. Improving or maintaining work participation is encouraged as a target for working age adults with rheumatic conditions.

Size of the burden

There is considerable evidence of the size of the adverse impact of rheumatic conditions on work. Impact can be described in terms of:

- *work disability:* ceasing to work before retirement age
- *absenteeism:* missing part or whole days from work (e.g. number of days/hours off work)
- *presenteeism:* an individual remains in work but with difficulty or reduced efficiency/productivity.

Absenteeism and presenteeism contribute to the indirect costs of rheumatic diseases, which are far higher than for other diseases but are not considered as much by policy-makers, who usually focus primarily on direct costs based on healthcare usage and long-term disability directly attributed to rheumatic conditions. Work productivity loss is estimated to be far greater due to presenteeism than absenteeism.[5] Estimates of presenteeism vary and are dependent on the measuring tool. A challenge is to measure productivity accurately to provide a clear and meaningful understanding of rheumatic diseases on productivity. The following sections are not exhaustive but provide an outline of the extent to which rheumatic conditions impact on work, taking rheumatoid arthritis (RA, the most common autoimmune disease), low back pain (the most common musculoskeletal condition affecting working age adults), and osteoarthritis (OA, the most common form of arthritis) as examples.

Rheumatoid arthritis

The impact of autoimmune disease on work for individuals is high. Taking RA (where 60–75% of people are of working age at diagnosis) to illustrate this, the annual prevalence of sick leave for those with RA who remain in work is 53–82%.[6] On average patients take 46 days off per year compared to a population average of 11 days.[6] Numbers of days of sick leave is strongly associated with work disability (i.e. ceasing to work prior to retirement age).[7] One in four people (23%) who are diagnosed with RA stop working in the 3 years following diagnosis.[8] This increases to one in three (35%) by 10 years and more than half (51%) of those with duration longer than 25 years will have stopped working before retirement age.

The annual incidence of work disability is 10%.[8] Once out of work, most people with RA never return to work, and RA is thus linked to unemployment and underemployment.[9] However, the prevalence of work disability is decreasing; previously, 50% of newly diagnosed RA cases had work disability within 10 years of diagnosis. This is indicative of improved treatment, changes in the nature of employment, and perhaps improved conditions in the workplace, which is also evidenced by an increasing rate of return to work.[8] The reduction in the proportion of those with RA taking sick leave may result in an increase in presenteeism, if individuals are more likely to remain in work but with limited capabilities. Currently, 34% of workers with RA report a decrease in productivity due to their condition, although comparable data is not available over the past decade to determine whether this is an increasing trend.[10]

Non-inflammatory conditions—low back pain

Although the impact on the individual is often much greater, the cumulative burden of non-inflammatory arthropathies and disorders such as back pain, OA, and limb pain as a whole results in a much greater economic and human cost to society than autoimmune disease. Low back pain illustrates this point. The prevalence of RA in the United Kingdom is 0.81%, but low back pain affects over one-third of adults at any one time, and each year approximately 3.5 million people in the United Kingdom develop back pain.[11] It is the most common reason for middle-aged people to visit primary care, with approximately 6–9% of adults consulting for this condition each year.[12] Although many back pain patients stop consulting their GP within 3 months, 60–80% of people still report pain or disability a year later, and up to 40% of those who have taken time off work will have future episodes of work absence.[13–14] In the United Kingdom, the annual cost of absenteeism due to low back pain is estimated at 1% of gross domestic product.[15] The impact of presenteeism due to low back pain may be 7.5 times this due to lost productivity.

Non-inflammatory conditions—osteoarthritis/joint pain

OA is associated with work limitation, sick leave, being out of work (unemployment), and early retirement.[16–18] On average those with OA take 9.6 days sick leave per year.[19] Although the effect on work for individuals tends to be smaller than that for RA,[20] the sheer number of people with OA means that it has a larger impact on work. Like low back pain, OA and its main symptom (joint pain) is common in adults aged 50 years and over (i.e. annual prevalence of knee pain is 46% in those over the age of 50).[21] The effect of OA is more on presenteeism than on absenteeism.[18] In those with knee pain, around one in five indicate problems at work.[22] Reduced productivity is 3–5 times more likely in those with OA than in those without.[16,23,24] Three-quarters of working adults with OA make some changes to their work situation to maintain their participation in work.[25]

Extensions to working life

Policies to extend working life have become a central response to the development of ageing populations. Delaying retirement is viewed as a means to mitigate the effects of worsening demographic ratios while increasing financial resources for later life. Such policies are important from a fiscal and social point of view. Many governments have raised pension ages along with a range of other measures such as anti-age discrimination legislation. It is in this context that our ability to maintain the capacity of individuals with rheumatic conditions to remain in work, or return to work, is increasingly under the spotlight. More than three-quarters of the population do not have disability-free life expectancy as long as 68 years, much of which is attributable to rheumatic conditions.[3] As the prevalence of rheumatic conditions increases with age and as working lives extend, there will be many more employees with musculoskeletal problems in years to come; there will be more people in work coping with rheumatic conditions which compromise their work ability and productivity. The challenge is to keep individuals with rheumatic conditions in work, reduce the size of the impact of rheumatic conditions on work and contribute to the health and well-being of individuals.

Targets and strategies to improve work participation

New approaches impose the view that work loss does not need to be a consequence of a musculoskeletal disorder or disability.[1] It is clear that the impact of rheumatic diseases on an individual's ability to remain in work depends on complex interactions between biological, psychological, social and occupational factors. This underlines the importance of a biopsychosocial and interdisciplinary approach involving interaction between those with a musculoskeletal condition, employers, clinicians, and policy-makers.

Factors that reduce work participation

The starting point for managing rheumatic conditions and work is to gain an understanding of the predictors of work loss and the potential targets for interventions. There are numerous predictors (not all are listed here) which can be considered in the following categories.

Condition-specific factors

Notably, disease duration and symptom severity are linked to poor work participation. However, clinical factors add little to models of work disability.[26] This is because clinical factors tend to be associated with poor work outcomes through their impact on physical function.

Comorbidity

Comorbidity contributes to work problems in those with joint pain.[2] More notably, the co-occurrence of mental health problems with rheumatic conditions has a big impact. For example, many patients with musculoskeletal pain also suffer from depression,[27] which is a key factor for developing chronic disabling pain.[28] This combination is associated with increased absence from work,[29] and return to work is increased by interventions that reduce the severity of depression in those with chronic pain.[30]

Socio-economic and environmental factors

Low socio-economic status, in terms of low income and low education, is linked to working patterns through links with pain and health behaviour.[3] Low socio-economic status is also linked to more physical occupations and poorer working conditions which have an impact on rheumatic conditions and work participation. Living in areas of higher socio-economic deprivation and low work opportunities is linked to increased work disability.[23]

Psychological factors

In addition to mental health problems, psychological factors are a major obstacle to maintaining work participation and return to work. Examples of key psychological factors that impact on work are catastrophizing, negative illness beliefs (false beliefs and pervasive thoughts about personal illness), low self-efficacy, and lack of self-esteem.[31]

Occupational and workplace factors

Physically and mentally demanding or high-paced jobs have a negative impact on work participation for those with rheumatic conditions.[26,32] A non-supportive work environment is a key factor; the lack of work accommodations (e.g. flexibility and changes to working hours, adaptations to working practice and environment, use of aids and appliances), negative work culture, and a lack of support from colleagues and managers is linked to absence and reduced productivity.[33]

Models for organizing predictors of work disability

Psychological and occupational factors are increasingly recognized as the key reasons for reduced work participation. A framework to organize and understand the psychological, occupation and workplace influences is offered by the 'flags' concept, which has been developed in the fields of occupational medicine and psychology.[34] This system links with the clinical use of 'red flags' to highlight the existence of serious pathology (e.g. malignancy) and the need for immediate medical input. Three additional flags (yellow, blue, and black) are warning signals that psychosocial factors in or around the individual are acting as obstacles to full recovery and return to work, and each flag points to specific reasons for work disability:

- *Yellow flags* relate to the individual and to their thoughts, beliefs, behaviours, and emotional responses that are important predictors for the development of long-term problems. Many of these can be considered as the response of the individual to their rheumatic condition. These include beliefs about pain and injury, pessimism, catastrophizing, poor coping strategies, and low self-efficacy.

- *Blue flags* refer to perceptions of work and working conditions at an individual level. Examples of negative perceptions of work are fear of exacerbation of symptoms or disease induced by the job, high perceived physical job demand, job-related stress, low expectation of return to work. Poor working conditions are lack of job accommodations/modified work, and lack of employer communication with employees.

- *Black flags* are objective work characteristics and contextual conditions which may be specific to the individual's organization. Examples are unhelpful policies/procedures used by employers, such as the absence of a mechanism to provide alternate duty for employees returning from sickness absence. These are environmental factors that perhaps clinicians can do little about but must be aware of when managing patients' work participation, as they can communicate with employers about the importance of addressing these issues.

The flags approach directs a broad approach to the reasons for work problems and opens up different interventions and management strategies that can be adopted to improve work participation. The emphasis of this approach is to systematically identify and then categorize obstacles to returning to or staying at work, and then identify appropriate strategies for their removal or resolution. The different flags highlight the heterogeneity of issues with adults with rheumatic conditions leading to work problems. Taking this approach further, identifying common clusters or subgroups of people with similar characteristics may lead to efficiency in delivering common but tailored interventions to groups of workers. Based on a review of risk factors for work disability that can be identified early on in the course of a low back pain episode,[35,36] four distinct groups of workers have been identified:

- A group at *low risk* for prolonged work absence and disability.

- A *high risk-immobilized* group: key characteristics included fear avoidance, pain catastrophizing, physical dysfunction, and poor expectations for resuming activity.

- A *high risk-disemployed* group: key characteristics are workplace problems including having a job with high physical demands, poor employer responses to the report of injury, no modified duties available, and short job tenure.

- A *high risk-overwhelmed* group, characterized by multiple issues: depressive symptoms and otherwise negative mood symptoms, life adversity, high levels of work stress experienced, and high levels of fear and worry.

These subgroups have different propensities for absenteeism and presenteeism and different intervention strategies are indicated. The success of this approach is based on early identification of modifiable factors and requires an understanding of the barriers that prevent work participation.

Managing musculoskeletal disorders and work

The approach to managing musculoskeletal conditions and work is evolving. A coherent and effective response to the worker's need for support in continuing to work or returning to work is necessary. A greater emphasis on a 'joined-up' approach to the sick worker's problems involving the worker, the multidisciplinary team (e.g. rheumatologist, physiotherapist, occupational therapist, psychologist, occupational health professional, and/or employer advisor) and the employer is required. Improving work capability in older adults with rheumatic conditions requires a multifactorial approach which addresses physical, psychological, social, and occupational factors and focuses on managing the condition and associated comorbidities rather than all taking a narrow focus on treating or 'curing' the condition.[37] This is important as most people with musculoskeletal disorders have the potential to continue to work despite the persistence of symptoms.

Role of health professionals

Greater emphasis is now placed on early intervention, which is essential if a short-term problem is not to be translated into long-term sickness absence. Early diagnosis and treatment are key and a medical approach has a crucial role to play with autoimmune conditions. There is increasing evidence that aggressive treatment of autoimmune conditions leads to improved work participation. Aggressive treatment of RA with a combination of disease-modifying anti-rheumatic drugs (DMARDs) compared to a single DMARD significantly reduced the extent of sick leave and work disability.[38] Early treatment with a combination of a biologic therapy and methotrexate reduced absenteeism and presenteeism through a reduction in work cessation, number of sick days and improved work productivity.[39,40]

Increased involvement of allied health professionals may be required to enhance patient care; for example, a physiotherapist could make a functional assessment and initiate treatment to maintain or improve key functional abilities related to work.[41] Early physiotherapy intervention is linked with improved health and well-being in workers with rheumatic conditions.[42] Competencies in ergonomic job accommodation, communication, and conflict resolution could be even more important for success at work than physical treatments of the condition.[43] Ergonomic changes (restructuring work tasks, aids and appliances, workplace adaptations, work station redesign) are linked to maintaining work participation and return to work.[32] Patients with rheumatoid arthritis who have had received workplace ergonomic changes are 2.5 times more likely to remain in work.[26]

Identifying work-related problems may be as simple as directly asking about work absence and performance, but may require more systematic approaches, using already existing tools which allow patients or workers to report work performance, ability and barriers. The Work Instability Scale,[44] Workplace Activity Limitations Scale[45] and the Work Experience Survey-Rheumatic Conditions (WES-RC)[46] have been developed to aid clinicians to identify work limitation and the barriers that may impede resolution. These could potentially become part of routine information gathering before, during, or after the consultation; or may simply outline questions that will help the clinician and patient explore work issues together during consultation. A more thorough approach to identifying work problems and barriers to return to work is outlined in the following website—www.lni.wa.gov/IPUB/200-002-000.pdf). http://www.lni.wa.gov/IPUB/200-002-000.pdf

Role of the employer

Maintaining some people with rheumatic conditions in work rests on the ability to adapt the workplace and work requirements to the physical limitations of the worker. This highlights the need for clinicians to communicate with the workplace and become involved in managing occupational, as well as social and psychological factors for work problems (i.e. areas where clinicians have been reluctant to get involved[47]). The role of line managers, return to work coordinators, and human resource departments, and their interaction with health care professions, will become increasingly important and crucial to reducing absenteeism and presenteeism. Focusing on line managers is important because they provide support in the workplace and play a mediating role within organizations. Line managers need to consider the symptoms and functional limitations of such workers to optimize their performance. If they are deficient in relevant skills and knowledge in advising and supporting people with these conditions, there may be barriers to return to work and excessive work loss.

It is also important to recognize that individuals with musculoskeletal and work problems often identify and arrange their own accommodations or do so in concert with fellow employees, and there may be a role for training workers and coworkers to facilitate the accommodations process. Improving individuals ability to self-manage musculoskeletal conditions and work problems is extremely important and should be an important target for clinical interventions.[48] Indeed, the vast majority of people with short-term work disability should be able to return without involvement of any specialized services such as occupational health or vocational

rehabilitation. The most important interaction is between the employee and employer, and only in the occasional instance where this is problematic might a return-to-work coordinator be helpful.[49]

At an organizational level, the provision of in-house health care will also be beneficial and links with the vocational rehabilitation approach described above. Good examples are available of the positive influence of vocational rehabilitation and linkage between health professionals and managers.[50] But occupational health services must engage with all stakeholders (particularly line managers and clinicians) to be effective in improving return to work. Large employers may be better placed to act in line with positive policies to prevent absence and encourage return to work. Smaller and medium-sized employees may not have the capacity to offer these accommodations in the same way, and for these employees, health professionals become even more important.

Further considerations

Prevention of the impact of rheumatic diseases on work

The sheer size of the current burden of rheumatic diseases on work, and the potential for this to increase, signals the need for preventive strategies to prevent work disability and aid return to work. Prevention will need to target both the impact of the musculoskeletal disorder and work disability. Current models of care to reduce the impact of musculoskeletal disorders on work will need to move towards more proactive preventive health policies related to the workplace, in similar ways to those which have emerged in primary care, which has moved from exclusive concern with sickness to being concerned with prevention of disease and reduction of disability, through health promotion and screening programmes. This requires a shift towards promoting health in the worker and in the workplace as distinct from an exclusive concern with avoiding injury or dealing with sickness when it arises.

Following this, there is a need to explore the cost-effectiveness of accommodations and support programmes in the workplace and the community that can maintain work participation. Timing of interventions is important; although we know that being off work for a longer period increases the risk of long-term absence, more information is needed about the timing of interventions to ensure optimal outcomes. Much is known about ergonomic factors and the role of types of work and workplace environment in predisposing to musculoskeletal disorders, but there are many unanswered questions about prevention, causation, treatment, and prognosis which must be addressed to ensure that the needs of those in work are being met. In particular there is a lack of good quality evidence to guide the preventive, therapeutic and rehabilitative arms of the response to the whole problem of musculoskeletal disorders and work in older adults.

Further research

The major concern with demographic change is the increasing number of older workers and the impact they will have. Most research on work and musculoskeletal conditions has not focused on older workers. Further work is required to assess if extended working life is good for all older workers who have musculoskeletal disorders. How will extensions to working life affect musculoskeletal disorders? Will this exacerbate their development? What will be the impact of prolonged working life on future health and well-being? What are the best methods to maximize opportunities for making employment-related choices, which promote health, safety, and life satisfaction in later years? If staying in work exacerbates musculoskeletal disorders, what is the additional cost to society in terms of health and social care costs? Investigation of the health and economic impact is required to provide further direction for policy on older workers.

Conclusion

Musculoskeletal disorders are the most frequently cited reason for absence from work and there is a need for new approaches and attitudes to assess and reduce the burden. The cumulative burden of non-inflammatory arthropathies and disorders such as back pain, OA, and limb pain as a whole, results in a much greater economic and human cost to society than autoimmune disease. As the incidence of these conditions increases with age and as working lives extend, there will be many more employees with musculoskeletal problems in years to come. Significantly, new approaches impose the view that work loss does not need to be a consequence of a musculoskeletal disorder or disability. There are many opportunities to improve work participation; it presents an achievable challenge to everyone and underlines the importance of a biopsychosocial and interdisciplinary approach involving interaction between those with a musculoskeletal condition, clinicians, employers, and policy-makers.

References

1. Black C. *Working for a healthier tomorrow*. The Stationery Office, London, 2008.
2. Waddell G, Burton AK. *Is work good for your health and well-being?* The Stationery Office, London, 2006.
3. Marmot M, Allen J, Goldblatt P et al. *Fair society, healthy lives: the Marmot review. Strategic review of health inequalities in England post-2010*. Department of Health, London, 2010.
4. Burgard SA, Brand JE, House JS. Toward a better estimation of the effect of job loss on health. *J Health Soc Behav* 2007;48:369–384.
5. Stewart WF, Ricci JA, Chee E, Morganstein D, Lipton R. Lost productive time and cost due to common pain conditions in the US workforce. *JAMA* 2003;290(18):2443–2454.
6. Geuskens GA, Burdorf A, Hazes JM. Consequences of rheumatoid arthritis for performance of social roles—a literature review. *J Rheumatol* 2007;34:1248–1260.
7. de Buck PD, de Bock GH, van Dijk F et al. Sick leave as a predictor of job loss in patients with chronic arthritis. *Int Arch Occup Environ Health* 2006;80:160–170.
8. Allaire S, Wolfe F, Niu J, Lavalley MP. Contemporary prevalence and incidence of work disability associated with rheumatoid arthritis in the US. *Arthritis Rheum*. 2008;59(4):474–480.
9. Verstappen SM, Bijlsma JW, Verkleij H et al.; Utrecht Rheumatoid Arthritis Cohort Study Group. Overview of work disability in rheumatoid arthritis patients as observed in cross-sectional and longitudinal surveys. *Arthritis Rheum* 2004;51(3):488–497.
10. Björk M, Thyberg I, Rikner K, Balogh I, Gerdle B. Sick leave before and after diagnosis of rheumatoid arthritis--a report from the Swedish TIRA project. *J Rheumatol* 2009;36(6):1170–1179.
11. Maniadakis N, Gray A. The economic burden of back pain in the UK. *Pain* 2000; 84:95–103.
12. Dunn KM, Croft PR. Classification of low back pain in primary care: using 'bothersomeness' to identify the most severe cases. *Spine* 2005;30:1887–1892.
13. Croft PR, Macfarlane GJ, Papageorgiou AC, Thomas E, Silman AJ. The outcome of low back pain in general practice: a prospective study. *BMJ* 1998;316:1356–1359.
14. Hestbaek L, Leboeuf YC, Manniche C. Low back pain: what is the long-term course? A review of studies of general patient populations. *Eur Spine J* 2003;12:149–165.
15. Chatterji M, Tilley C. Sickness, absenteeism, presenteeism, and sick pay. *Oxford Economic Papers* 2002;54(4):669–687.
16. Mäkelä M, Heliovaara M, Sievers K et al. Musculoskeletal disorders as determinants of disability in Finns aged 30 years or more. *J Clin Epidemiol* 1993;46:549–559.
17. Grotle M, Hagen KB, Natvig B, Dahl FA, Kvien TK. Prevalence and burden of osteoarthritis: results from a population survey in Norway. *J Rheumatol* 2008;35:677–684.
18. Bieleman HJ, Bierma-Zeinstra SM, Oosterveld FG, Reneman MF, Verhagen AP, Groothoff JW. The effect of osteoarthritis of the hip or knee on work participation. *J Rheumatol* 2011;38(9):1835–1843.
19. Rabenda V, Manette C, Lemmens R et al. Direct and indirect costs attributable to osteoarthritis in active subjects. *J Rheumatol* 2006;33:1152–1158.
20. Maetzel A, Li LC, Pencharz J, Tomlinson G, Bombardier C. The economic burden associated with osteoarthritis, rheumatoid arthritis, and hypertension: a comparative study. *Ann Rheum Dis* 2004;63:395–401.
21. Jinks C, Jordan K, Ong BN, Croft P. A brief screening tool for knee pain in primary care (KNEST). 2. Results from a survey in the general population aged 50 and over. *Rheumatology* 2004;43(1):55–61.
22. Wilkie R, Jordan K, Blagojevic, M, Croft P. What will happen if state pension age rises for people with joint pain? Impact and individual and area-level factors associated with work limitation;n in adults aged 50 to 75 with knee pain. *Rheumatology* 2008;47(suppl 2):ii11.
23. Lerner D, Reed JI, Massarotti E, Wester LM, Burke TA. The Work Limitations Questionnaire's validity and reliability among patients with osteoarthritis. *J Clin Epidemiol* 2002;55:197–208.
24. Fautrel B, Hilliquin P, Rozenberg S et al. Impact of osteoarthritis: results of a nationwide survey of 10,000 patients consulting for OA. *Joint Bone Spine* 2005;72:235–240.
25. Gignac MA, Cao X, Lacaille D, Anis AH, Badley EM. Arthritis-related work transitions: a prospective analysis of reported productivity losses, work changes, and leaving the labor force. *Arthritis Rheum* 2008;59:1805–1813.
26. Lacaille D, Sheps S, Spinelli JJ, Chalmers A, Esdaile JM. Identification of modifiable work-related factors that influence the risk of work disability in rheumatoid arthritis. *Arthritis Rheum*. 2004 Oct 15;51(5):843–852.
27. Druss BG, Rosenheck RA, Sledge WH. Health and disability costs of depressive illness in a major US corporation. *Am J Psychiatry* 2000;157:1274–1278.
28. Linton SJ, Andersson T. Can chronic disability be prevented? A randomized trial of a cognitive-behavior intervention and two forms of information for patients with spinal pain. *Spine* 2000;25:2825–2831.
29. Currie SR, Wang JL. Chronic back pain and major depression in the general Canadian population. *Pain* 2004;107:54–60.
30. Sullivan MJL, Adams H, Tripp, D, Stanish WD. Stage of chronicity and treatment response in patients with musculoskeletal injuries and concurrent symptoms of depression. *Pain* 2008;135:151–159.
31. Franche RL, Cullen K, Clarke J et al.; Institute for Work & Health (IWH) Workplace-Based RTW Intervention Literature Review Research Team. Workplace-based return-to-work interventions: a systematic review of the quantitative literature. *J Occup Rehabil* 2005;15:607–631.
32. Main CJ, Sullivan MJL, Watson PJ. *Pain Management*, 2nd edn. Churchill-Livingstone, Edinburgh, 2007.
33. Wilkie R, Cifuentes M, Pransky G. Exploring extensions to working life: job lock and predictors of decreasing work function in older workers. *Disabil Rehabil* 2011;33:1719–1727.

34. Kendall N, Burton K, Main C, Watson P. *Tackling musculoskeletal problems: a guide for clinic and workplace identifying obstacles using the psychosocial flags framework.* The Stationery Office, London, 2009.

35. Shaw WS, Means-Christensen A, Slater MA et al. Shared and independent associations of psychosocial factors on work status among men with subacute low back pain. *Clin J Pain* 2007;23:409–416.

36. Steenstra IA, Ibrahim SA, Franche RL et al. Validation of a risk factor-based intervention strategy model using data from the readiness for return to work cohort study. *J Occup Rehabil* 2010;20(3):394–405.

37. Waddell G. Preventing incapacity in people with musculoskeletal disorders. *Br Med Bull* 77 2006;78:55–69.

38. Puolakka K, Kautiainen H, Möttönen T et al. Impact of initial aggressive drug treatment with a combination of disease-modifying antirheumatic drugs on the development of work disability in early rheumatoid arthritis: a five-year randomized follow up trial. *Arthritis Rheum* 2004;50:55–62.

39. Bejarano V, Quinn M, Conaghan PG et al.; Yorkshire Early Arthritis Register Consortium. Effect of the early use of the anti-tumor necrosis factor adalimumab on the prevention of job loss in patients with early rheumatoid arthritis. *Arthritis Rheum* 2008;59:1467–1474.

40. Anis A, Zhang W, Emery P et al. The effect of etanercept on work productivity in patients with early active rheumatoid arthritis: results from the COMET study. *Rheumatology* 2009;48(10):1283–1289.

41. Campbell J, Wright C, Moseley A et al. Avoiding long-term incapacity for work: Developing an early intervention in primary care, 2007. www.dwp.gov.uk/docs/hwwb-developing-an-early-intervention-in-primary-care.pdf

42. Boorman S. NHS Health & Well-being Review, Final report, 2009. www.nhshealthandwellbeing.org/FinalReport.html

43. Shaw WS, Pransky G, Winters T. The Back Disability Risk Questionnaire for work-related, acute back pain: prediction of unresolved problems at 3-month follow-up. *J Occup Environ Med* 2009;51:185–194

44. Gilworth G, Chamberlain MA, Harvey A et al. Development of a work instability scale for rheumatoid arthritis. *Arthritis Rheum* 2003;49:349–354.

45. Gignac MA, Badley EM, Lacaille D et al. Managing arthritis and employment:making arthritis-related work changes as a means of adaptation. *Arthritis Rheum* 2004;51(6):909–916.

46. Allaire S, Keysor JJ. Development of a structured interview tool to help patients identify and solve rheumatic condition-related work barriers. *Arthritis Care Res* 2009;61(7):988–995.

47. Pincus T, Woodcock A, Vogel S. Returning back pain patients to work: how private musculoskeletal practitioners outside the national health service perceive their role (an interview study). *J Occup Rehabil* 2010;20:322–330.

48. Shaw WS, Tveito TH, Geehern-Lavoie M et al. Adapting principles of chronic pain self-management to the workplace. *Disabil Rehabil* 2012;34(8):694–703.

49. Pransky G, Shaw W, Franche RL, Clarke A. Disability prevention and communication among workers, physicians, employers, and insurers—current models and opportunities for improvement. *Disabil Rehabil* 2004; 26(11):625–634.

50. Waddell G, Burton AK, Kendall NAS. *Vocational rehabilitation evidence review: what works, for whom, and when?* The Stationery Office, London, 2008.

CHAPTER 34

Biologics registries

David Isenberg and Angela Zink

Introduction

Periodically a new treatment emerges for human diseases that carries the prospect of radically improving the outcome of a variety of conditions. Examples include the development of dialysis, transplantation, antibiotics and, most impressively for those with inflammatory musculoskeletal diseases, corticosteroids. Sixty years on from the introduction of corticosteroids it is very hard for today's rheumatologists to imagine what life was like without the availability of, say, low-dose oral steroids to manage polymyalgia rheumatica, high-dose oral steroids to treat giant cell arteritis and vasculitis, intramuscular or intravenous steroids to manage acute rheumatoid flares, or intra-articular steroids to help resolve localized knee inflammation.

The modern equivalent of the introduction of corticosteroids is of course the advent of the era of biologic therapy. There are significant lessons to be learnt from the introduction of corticosteroids. Too little attention was paid initially to the potentially serious side effects of steroids, especially when given for long periods in doses exceeding 10 mg/day. It took a long time before the major problems of osteoporosis, increased risk of infection, diabetes, and hypertension were linked unequivocally to steroid use. It is at least arguable that these problems would have been appreciated far sooner had today's warning systems and instruments such as drug registries been developed 60 years ago.

A registry is invariably prospective in nature, enrolling patients to capture the full side-effect profile of a particular drug (or other therapeutic intervention). Most registries will also assess the effectiveness of a new drug, since safety and effectiveness are often interrelated. Registries reflect the experience of 'real life' patients, which is not the case even in large double-blind controlled trials. Such trials invariably 'cherry pick' patients deemed most suitable by virtue of their having more straightforward disease without confounding comorbidities and often excluding the more serious manifestations of a given disease.

The establishment of many European and some North American registries in rheumatic diseases has been a success story in the past decade, as several recent reviews attest.[1-3] In this chapter we briefly describe how registries are established and run, and summarize the most important findings on effectiveness and safety. We focus on registries for patients with rheumatoid arthritis (RA). Some countries have also established registries for ankylosing spondylitis,

psoriatic arthritis, and more recently systemic lupus erythematosus, but there are little published data.

Establishment and management of biologic registries

Ideally a wholly independent funding source, such as a national Department of Health, should fund a register in order to obviate any accusation of bias (which would inevitably be the concern were the register solely to be funded by a major pharmaceutical company) and to ensure academic independence. We are unaware of any such arrangement or of its likely development. On the other hand, since it is the companies' responsibility to ensure the safety of their products, it is reasonable for them to support independent, well-managed registries. In order to ensure unbiased assessment of risks and benefits, all drugs of a certain class (such as biologic agents) should be observed in parallel and all companies producing these drugs should jointly support the register. Independence is crucial and can be ensured by setting a filter and/or by appropriate contracts.

The funding of the British Society for Rheumatology Rheumatoid Arthritis Register (BSRBR-RA) is a case is in point. In the United Kingdom those companies whose drugs are being studied provide substantial funds to the British Society for Rheumatology who pass the vast majority of this support to the Arthritis Research UK Epidemiology Unit based at the University of Manchester. In this model (which is strongly supported by the National Institute of Health and Clinical Excellence) pharmaceutical companies receive long-term safety data both on their own product and from a contemporary control group with active RA not being treated with a biological agent. The group in Manchester is free to design its own research agenda and to publish what it wishes. There are, however, two caveats. Firstly, the British Society for Rheumatology has established a Biologics Register Committee whose function is to oversee and approve the arrangements both with the pharmaceutical companies and with the University of Manchester. Secondly, before submission, any papers or abstracts are sent (approximately 2 weeks for an abstract and a month for a full manuscript) both to the Committee and to nominated individuals within the pharmaceutical companies. Any comments are passed back to the Epidemiology Unit by the Chairman of the Biologics Register Committee. Although in theory these comments may be ignored, the researchers often find the questions helpful and will often amend their abstract or manuscript accordingly. This system provides a necessary set of checks and balances and works principally because it provides an arrangement in which each party derives benefit.

Registries in other countries are funded and organized in a variety of ways, but a general principle is that long-term funding is provided jointly by several companies and that conduct, analysis, and publication of results remain in the hands of academia. In Germany, the state-owned Rheumatism Research Centre has one single seven-sided contract with all companies who own licensed biologics for the treatment of RA. Full academic freedom is guaranteed for the principal investigators running the register, which includes a procedure of feedback on publications similar to that described for the BSRBR. The contract ensures that funds are provided for long-term observation, i.e. for at least 6 years after the last patient has been enrolled. In Sweden, in addition to private money, it has been possible to get funds from public sources.

In some countries, registries specific to individual drugs have been set up in the last few years. Although it is still possible that these registries are independent of company influence, it is much more difficult to guarantee their independence. Thus we strongly recommend joint funding concepts with different companies involved.

Day-to-day management of registries

Invariably each registry employs a varying number of permanent staff to collect, monitor, analyse, and publish the data. Most registries started with the goal of collecting data over a minimum period of 5 years, and equally most have come to accept that a much longer period of time is necessary partly to help establish the really long-term benefit of biologic drugs and partly to capture the long-term side effects they may have (by analogy, even heavy smoking may take many years before its serious deleterious effects become evident). Most of the registries started by collecting paper-based information both from physicians and patients. With the passage of time electronic capture of data has become much more popular and in some instances, for example in Denmark, the amount of data entered via the internet now greatly exceeds that captured on paper.

Registries—similarities and difference

Much information on this topic has, as alluded to above, been published elsewhere but a summary of some of the main European and United States registries is shown in Table 34.1. It is vital when making comparisons between results obtained from registries to appreciate that there are some quite significant differences in terms of which patients may be prescribed biological agents in different countries. For example, in the United Kingdom biologic therapies may only be prescribed to patients with RA with a DAS28 score greater than 5.1 who are deemed to have failed two previously prescribed disease-modifying anti-rheumatic disease agents (DMARDs), one of which is invariably methotrexate. In Germany, although there are no strict guidelines about the use of biological agents, it is generally recommended that they will not be started until patients have demonstrated high disease activity with the failure of least one conventional DMARD. In Sweden the authorities do not restrict the use of biologics and this probably explains why around 20% of patients with RA on the population level are prescribed these drugs, probably close to twice as many as in the United Kingdom and Germany.

Although, as explained above, some differences exist in terms of when patients with RA (or other diseases) are started on biological agents, it clearly makes sense for biologics registries to standardize their data collection methods, observation periods, and types of analysis as far as possible. It is particularly important to help establish the real prevalence of less common adverse events and, eventually, to ascertain whether the prevalence of side effects varies significantly with respect to e.g. age of onset, gender, disease duration, ethnicity, comorbidity and comedication and, increasingly importantly, with the use of multiple biologic agents.

The European registries, in particular those run in the United Kingdom, Sweden, and Germany have worked closely together during the past decade and, as detailed elsewhere,[1,3] share a number of features. They include all biological agents given to patients with RA from the day of first licensing. They provide each funding company with regular, usually semi-annual, reports on adverse events that have occurred in patients treated with this company's drug (or in the comparator group), which helps the companies to fulfil the requirements of their periodical safety update reporting to the European Medicines Agency. In order to coordinate reporting and data analysis and interpretation, the registries have held regular meetings which were either open to all registries or held only among those with reporting commitments. All registries use comparator cohorts to put the results into perspective. These cohorts vary from register to register. In the United Kingdom the comparator cohort consists of patients with active RA whose DAS28 score at inclusion exceeds 4.2 but who are not taking a biologic therapy and are treated in the many collaborating rheumatologic units. In contrast, in Germany previous DMARD failure and the start of a new DMARD therapy is an inclusion criterion for the control group which is observed under the same protocol and in the same rheumatology units as the patients on biologics. Switching of therapies can then be followed easily. In other counties historical cohorts are used as comparators (e.g. the EMECAR cohort in Spain). Some countries, like Sweden, Denmark, and the United Kingdom, can link the data from their biologic cohorts to national population databases recording deaths, hospitalizations, and/or cancer. There are also some differences in the coding of adverse events. Whereas the British, Spanish, and German registries utilize the coding system known as MedDRA, the Swedish registry uses ICD-10 in order to be comparable to the national registries.

Do the biologic registries prove that biologic drugs work?

Given the careful selection of cases entered into double-blind controlled trials it was always likely that 'real life' results using tumour necrosis factor alpha (TNFα) blockade in RA would not be as impressive. Two studies comparing the effectiveness of TNFα blocking treatment from biologic registries with results of major clinical trials have confirmed that this is the case. However, if the strict inclusion criteria of the major trials had applied to the patients followed up in the registries, a very similar clinical response would have been found.[4,5]

The south Swedish registry, which contributes to the national biologics registry ARTIS, reported that 45% of patients treated with etanercept and 40% treated with infliximab had sustained ACR 50 responses at 12 months.[6] Encouragingly, the national Danish registry reporting ACR 20/50/70 response rates in their 2000/2001

Table 34.1 Overview of European registries with published data used in this chapter

Acronym	Country	Year established	Comparator group	Key features
ARTIS	Sweden	1999	No true comparator group but linkage with national registries for mortality, cancer, inpatient and outpatient care	Patients are documented at routine clinical visits, registry is part of clinical care
Biobadaser	Spain	2000	Contemporary cohort of non-biologic treated RA patients has been used (EMECAR)	Initially (2000–2006) ~50% of all musculoskeletal patients on biologics were included. Subsequently fewer patients have been studied, but with greater intensity
BSRBR	UK	2001	A contemporary group of just under 4000 patients with RA on DMARDs	4000 patients each with RA on Enbrel, infliximab, and adalimumab recruited; minimum follow-up was 5 yrs, now planned to increase to 10 yrs. Plus 1100 on rituximab recruited and aiming to collect 2000 on certolizumab and 1000 on tocilizumab. Data collection has been paper based
DANBIO	Denmark		Contemporary control groups (early RA and RA on DMARDs) now established	All 26 rheumatology units contribute. Patients with RA (>4500), AS, psoriatic arthritis and other diseases are included
DREAM	Netherlands	2003	Use of contemporary inception cohort of early RA not given DMARDs (Nijmegen)	11 collaborating rheumatology centres, >1000 patients enrolled
RABBIT	Germany	2001	Patients at onset of DMARD therapy after failure of at least one other	7000 patients enrolled at start of a biologic, 3000 controls. Patients are followed at 3, 6, and 12 months after commencing treatment and bi-annually thereafter
RATIO	France	2004–2006	No comparator group	National registry for lymphomas and opportunistic infections, event-based, now closed
SCQM	Switzerland	1997	Controls are taken from the quality management database	Not originally a biologics registry. Patients are enrolled at regular visits, at least once a year
SSATG	South Sweden	1999	See ARTIS	90% of all prescriptions of biologics in South Sweden are included, regular follow-up

AS, ankylosing spondylitis; DMARD, disease-modifying anti-rheumatic drug; RA, rheumatoid arthritis.

cohort compared to the 2005 cohort showed an increase from 53%/31%/13% to 69%/51%/30% respectively.[7]

Another way of judging the effectiveness of TNFα therapies is determining the percentage of patients who remain on these drugs over time. As detailed elsewhere,[2] approximately 70% of patients on etanercept, infliximab, or adalimumab being treated for RA will remain on these drugs a year after starting though several analyses have shown that adding methotrexate (or another DMARD) tends to increase treatment continuation.[8–12] Thus the BSRBR[8] reported that a combination of etanercept and methotrexate was still being used in 84% of patients 6 months after starting treatment, compared to 78% on the etanercept treatment only. The comparative figures for infliximab were 79% vs 70%. In the RABBIT register[11] at 12 months the survival rates for etanercept and methotrexate were 82% compared to 71% for etanercept-only therapy, with comparable figures for infliximab being 77% and 67%.

Switching biologic therapies

Given the increasing availability of biologic drugs including those blocking TNFα, CD20, and the interleukin (IL)-6 receptor (among others) and as significant numbers of patients stop their first such agent because of side effects or lack of efficacy, the desire to try a second (or even third or fourth) biologic agent is increasing. Reports from the British registry have indicated that the likely survival of a second agent was broadly comparable to the first. The reasons for stopping a second TNF inhibitor (lack of efficacy or adverse events) were related to those for stopping the first one, indicating that there are patients more prone to adverse events or to ineffectiveness.[12] It could be further shown that patients who switched to a second TNF inhibitor had better functional outcomes after 1 year than those who continued anti-TNF treatment despite non-response.[13]

The Spanish BIOBADASER register showed higher age to be a risk factor for discontinuation due to adverse events whereas switching because of inefficacy was more frequent in younger patients. Patients with ankylosing spondylitis had longer retention rates than those with RA.[14]

In the Swiss Clinical Quality Management Cohort, the major cause of switching was adverse events, with 56% of cases.[15] Data from the same register showed that switching to rituximab after failure of a first anti-TNF treatment was more successful than trying a second anti-TNF agent if the reason for switching was ineffectiveness. In other cases of switching there was no difference in response to the second treatment.[16,17]

Adverse events associated with TNFα blockage

Cancer risk

Given that the initial estimates for the numbers of patients that were studied in biologic registries were predicated on the risk of cancer, specifically lymphoma, links between TNFα blockade and neoplasia are being carefully scrutinized. A potential confounding factor is that in patients with RA the risk of non-Hodgkin's lymphoma is increased (reviewed in detail recently[18]). The French RATIO registry,[19] which is different from the other registries described so far, was designed to collect cases with lymphoma or tuberculosis in patients receiving anti-TNF treatment between 2004 and 2006 on a national basis. The denominator can therefore only be estimated. RATIO reported a two- to threefold increase of lymphoma in patients receiving anti-TNF therapy but also confirmed that this is similar to that expected for such patients with severe inflammatory diseases. Furthermore, a study linking data from the Swedish biologics registry, the Swedish RA registry, and the Swedish cancer registry identified and analysed cancer in a national cohort of 6366 patients with RA who started their TNF therapy between 1999 and 2006.[20] As a comparative cohorts they used a national biologics-naive RA cohort (n = 61 160), a cohort of patients with RA newly starting methotrexate (n = 5999), a cohort of patients with RA newly starting DMARD combination therapy (n = 1838), and the general population of Sweden. The conclusion was that during the first 6 years following the start of anti-TNFα therapy in routine care no overall increase of cancer risk was noted.

In the RABBIT registry, the risk of incident malignancies was assessed with a nested case-control study in 5120 RA patients. The incidence was 6.0 per 1000 patient-years, and there was no difference between patients exposed or not to anti-TNF agents.[21] In the Spanish BIOBADASER registry the age- and sex-adjusted incidence rate for cancer was 3.0 per 1000 patient-years in patients exposed to biologics and 5.6 in those unexposed (EMECAR cohort), compared to 4.6 in the general population.[22]

Recently the BSRBR[23] as well as the RABBIT registry[24] considered the question of whether patients with previous malignancies were at increased risk of having a recurrence if they were treated with TNFα blockade. In the BSRBR, 177 patients treated with anti-TNFα and 117 patients treated with DMARDs had a history of malignancy: 13 recurrent tumours occurred in the anti-TNF group and 9 in the DMARD group. This resulted in a recurrence rate of 25.3/1000 person years and 38.3/1000 patient-years, respectively. In RABBIT 14 recurrent tumours were observed in 122 patients, resulting in a recurrence rate of 45.5 per 1000 patient-years in patients treated with anti-TNF agents and 31.4 in those treated with conventional DMARDs. The recurrence rate ratios between anti-TNF and DMARD were thus 0.6 in the BSRBR and 1.4 in RABBIT, neither of which is significant. However, reasons for the discrepant results may be that the DMARD group in the BSRBR had a shorter observation time and shorter time since the last tumour than the anti-TNF group. In addition the British rheumatologists had waited significantly longer than those in Germany before starting an anti-TNF treatment after a previous tumour (58% of anti-TNF treated patients in the BSRBR but only 23% in RABBIT had gone more than 10 years since the last tumour at the start of anti-TNF treatment). Therefore, further observation and comparison with data from other countries are needed.

By linking data from the Swedish biologics register ARTIS and clinical RA registries with national registries on cancer, hospitalization, and outpatient care it was shown that cancers occurring in patients treated with TNF inhibitors had a similar stage at cancer diagnosis and similar post-cancer survival rates to biologics-naive patients.[24]

To summarize the evidence, the data available so far are reassuring concerning the overall risk of cancer. However, it must be emphasized that site-specific increases in risk (especially skin cancer) cannot be ruled out yet.[25]

Further observation should also consider potentially increased risks in subgroups of patients such as older patients or those undergoing specific additional treatments.

Infections

Because of its mode of action, the risk of serious infections was a major concern at initiation of anti-TNF therapy. An increased incidence of tuberculosis reactivation is well established, in particular for the monoclonal antibodies,[22,26,27] and systematic screening has turned out to be an effective method of prevention.[28] Further, there seems to be an increased risk of viral infection, in particular herpes zoster, in patients treated with monoclonal antibodies.[29] An increased risk of septic arthritis in anti-TNF treatment was found in the BSRBR.[30]

Several registries have addressed the important question of whether TNFα blockade is linked to an overall increased risk of serious bacterial infection. Compared to conventionally treated patients, odds ratios ranging from 1.3 to 2.1 were reported.[31–33] The overall risk of serious infection under TNF blockade has been reported as between 4 and 6 per 100 patient-years.

There was a consistent observation that the risk of serious infection was highest in the first 3–6 months after start of treatment and declined thereafter.[30,34,35] The question is whether this decline on the cohort level is equivalent to a risk reduction in the individual patient. The German registry recently showed that about two-thirds of this decline in risk can be explained by 'depletion of susceptibles' (patients who experience an infection early on are taken off the drug, leaving those less susceptible on treatment), whereas about one-third of the decline can be attributed to improvement of the disease and reduction in the glucocorticoid dosage over time.[36] Taking all these factors into account, the incidence rate ratio for anti-TNF treatment compared to conventional DMARDs was 1.8. The data allow a calculation of individual patients' risk of experiencing a serious infection in the light of their risk profile. Thus, according to these data, a patient without any further risk factors has a very low 12-month risk of serious infection of 1% under conventional DMARDs and 2% under TNF inhibition. However, if a patient is older than 60 years, has a chronic renal disease, and is treated with glucocorticoids at 15 mg/day or above, the expected risk is 12% for conventional DMARDs and 21% for TNF inhibition. Switching such a patient from conventional DMARDs to anti-TNF and simultaneously reducing the glucocorticoid dose to less than 7.5 mg/day results in an overall risk of 5%. Thus, the infection risk conferred by anti-TNF treatment must be seen in the light of a patient's overall risk profile and must be balanced against the risks of alternative treatments and the clinical benefits.

Cardiovascular events and mortality

RA patients have a twofold increased risk of having a myocardial infarct.[37,38] The reasons for this seem to be linked to the role of inflammation in the development of atherosclerosis. The encouraging news from the BSRBR-RA treated with anti-TNFα therapy was that those who responded to the treatment within 6 months had a significantly lower rate of myocardial infarct compared to those who did not. Results from the Spanish registry supported this useful role for TNFα blockade,[39] reporting a decrease in mortality from cardiovascular events in TNFα-treated patients compared to that of a clinical cohort of conventionally treated patients. They also noted that the mortality of patients treated with these biologic agents was similar to that in the general population when matched for age and gender. No increase in overall mortality was also found in the BSRBR when comparing 12 672 patients on biologics and 3,522 DMARD-continue patients with a total of more than 60 000 patient-years of observation.[40]

Pregnancy

The BSRBR reported on 120 pregnancies with exposure to anti-TNF treatment at or prior to conception and 10 in women never exposed.[41] The rates of spontaneous abortion were higher in patients exposed to anti-TNF (with or without further DMARDs) at conception compared to those never exposed or exposed before conception. There was no further difference in the rates of pregnancy complications or the proportion of live births. Four congenital malformations were observed, two in both of the groups with exposure at or prior to conception. The German RABBIT registry has published a preliminary report on 42 pregnancies in 31 women.[2] In 24 pregnancies the mother was exposed to anti-TNF treatment during the first trimester. There was no difference in the rates of spontaneous abortion between women exposed or unexposed to anti-TNF at conception. No congenital malformation was reported. However, a large proportion of those women who had stopped anti-TNF treatment at conception or shortly thereafter experienced severe flares of the disease during pregnancy. These results are still too limited to allow firm conclusions. There is more information from inflammatory bowel disease suggesting that TNF blockers are safe during the first trimester of pregnancy and can be used in patients with highly active disease.[42]

The future for biologic registries—thoughts and expectations

There is no doubt that the development of biologic registries has been enormously helpful in our attempts to understand the long-term benefits and adverse effects of this new therapeutic modality. We know about the increased risk of serious infection, and we are able to act on it clinically. Concerns regarding incident skin cancer and recurrence of melanoma remain. The only unexpected adverse event reported so far was the development of psoriasis in some rheumatoid patients treated with TNFα blockade.[43] Some initial concerns about an increase in the development of diseases such as lupus or demyelinization have not materialized. However, it is essential to remember that it is still relatively early days with these drugs and we simply have no idea whether continuous immunosuppression by cytokine blockade or depletion of cells for 10, 20, or 30 years will not be followed by a host of serious or unpleasant side effects or simply failure of these drugs to work effectively

beyond a finite period. On the other hand, it is likely that further positive long-term effects of anti-TNF blockade will be detected. As shown for myocardial infarction and bacterial infections, the risk for comorbidity resulting from the disease itself or from current comedication may be reduced by effective control of the disease activity.

As more new registries are set up in various countries with various indications, it is vital to ensure that the best scientific benefit is gained from them. The European League against Rheumatism (EULAR) has recently decided to set up a Subcommittee on Biologics Registries within its Standing Committee on Epidemiology, which builds upon the work of a previous task force.[44] The aim is to coordinate the efforts throughout Europe, to ensure a high quality of conduct by exchange of methodologies and to further enhance our knowledge by making use of all available evidence.

References

1. Zink A, Askling J, Dixon WG et al. European biologicals registers: methodology, selected results and perspectives. *Ann Rheum Dis* 2009;68:1240–1246.
2. Zink A, European biologic registers. In: Hochberg MC, Silman AJ, Weinblatt ME, Weisman MH (eds) *Textbook of rheumatology*. Mosby Elsevier, Philadelphia, PA, 2009:419–426.
3. Curtis JR, Jain A, Askling J et al. A comparison of patient characteristics and outcomes in selected European and U.S. rheumatoid arthritis registries. *Semin Arthritis Rheum* 2010;40:2–14.
4. Zink A, Strangfeld A, Schneider M et al. Effectiveness of tumor necrosis factor inhibitors in rheumatoid arthritis in an observational cohort study: comparison of patients according to their eligibility for major randomized clinical trials. *Arthritis Rheum* 2006;54:3399–3407.
5. Kievit W, Fransen J, Oerlemans AJ et al. The efficacy of anti-TNF in rheumatoid arthritis, a comparison between randomised controlled trials and clinical practice. *Ann Rheum Dis* 2007;66:1473–1478.
6. Geborek P, Crnkic M, Petersson IF, Saxne T; South Swedish Arthritis Treatment Group. Etanercept, infliximab, and leflunomide in established rheumatoid arthritis: clinical experience using a structured follow up programme in southern Sweden. *Ann Rheum Dis* 2002;61:793–798.
7. Hetland ML, Lindegaard HM, Hansen A et al. Do changes in prescription practice in patients with rheumatoid arthritis treated with biological agents affect treatment response and adherence to therapy? Results from the nationwide Danish DANBIO Registry. *Ann Rheum Dis* 2008;67:1023–1026.
8. Hyrich, KL, Symmons DP, Watson KD, Silman AJ, British Society for Rheumatology Biologics Register. Comparison of the response to infliximab or etanercept monotherapy with the response to co-therapy with methotrexate or antother disease modifying anti-rheumatic drug in patients with rheumatoid arthritis: results from the British Society for Rheumatology Biologics Register. *Athritis Rheum* 2006;54:1786–1794.
9. Zink A, Listing J, Kary S et al. Treatment continuation in patients receiving biological agents or conventional DMARD therapy. *Ann Rheum Dis* 2005;64:1274–1279.
10. Hyrich KL, Watson KD, Silman AJ, Symmons DP; Predictors of response to anti-TNF-alpha therapy among patients with rheumatoid arthritis: results from the British Society for Rheumatology Biologics Register. *Rheumatology* 2006;45:1558–1565.
11. Strangfeld A, Hierse F, Kekow J et al. Comparable effectiveness of tumour necrosis factor alpha inhibitors in combination with either methotrexate or lefluonomide. *Ann Rheum Dis* 209;68:1856–1862.
12. Hyrich KL, Lunt M, Watson KD, Symmons DP, Silman AJ. British Society for Rheumatology Biologics Register. Outcomes after switching from one anti-tumor necrosis factor alpha agent to a second anti-tumor necrosis factor alpha agent in patients with rheumatoid arthritis: results from a large UK national cohort study. *Arthritis Rheum* 2007;56:13–20.

13. Hyrich KL, Lunt M, Dixon WG, Watson KD, Symmons DP; BSR Biologics Register. Effects of switching between anti-TNF therapies on HAQ response in patients who do not respond to their first anti-TNF drug. *Rheumatology (Oxford)* 2008; 47(7):1000–1005.

14. Busquets N, Tomero E, Descalzo MA et al.; on behalf of the BIOBADASER 2.0 Study Group. Age at treatment predicts reason for discontinuation of TNF antagonists: data from the BIOBADASER 2.0 registry. *Rheumatology (Oxford)* 2011;50(11):1999–2004.

15. Du Pan SM, Dehler S, Ciurea A et al.; Swiss Clinical Quality Management Physicians. Comparison of drug retention rates and causes of drug discontinuation between anti-tumor necrosis factor agents in rheumatoid arthritis. *Arthritis Rheum* 2009;61(5):560–568.

16. Finckh A, Ciurea A, Brulhart L et al.; on the behalf of the doctors of the Swiss Clinical Quality Management Programme for Rheumatoid Arthritis. Which subgroup of patients with rheumatoid arthritis benefits from switching to rituximab versus alternative anti-tumour necrosis factor (TNF) agents after previous failure of an anti-TNF agent? *Ann Rheum Dis* 2010;69(2):387–393.

17. Finckh A, Ciurea A, Brulhart L et al.; Physicians of the Swiss Clinical Quality Management Program for Rheumatoid Arthritis. B cell depletion may be more effective than switching to an alternative anti-tumor necrosis factor agent in rheumatoid arthritis patients with inadequate response to anti-tumor necrosis factor agents. *Arthritis Rheum* 2007;56(5):1417–1423.

18. Dias C, Isenberg DA. Susceptibility of patients with rheumatic diseases to B-cell non-Hodgkin lymphoma. *Nat Rev Rheumatol* 2011;6:3608.

19. Mariette X, Tubach F, Bagheri H et al. Lymphoma in patients treated with anti-TNF: results of the 3-year prospective French RATIO registry. *Ann Rheum Dis.* 2010;69:400–408.

20. Askling J, van Vollenhoven R, Granath F et al. Cancer risk in patients with rheumatoid arthritis treated with anti-tumour necrosis factor alpha therapies. Does the risk change with the time since start of treatment? *Arthritis Rheum* 2009;60:3180–3189.

21. Strangfeld A, Hierse F, Rau R et al. Risk of incident or recurrent malignancies among patients with rheumatoid arthritis exposed to biologic therapy in the German biologics register RABBIT. *Arthritis Res Ther* 2010;12(1):R5.

22. Carmona L, Abasolo L, Descalzo MA et al.; BIOBADASER Study Group; EMECAR Study Group. Cancer in patients with rheumatic diseases exposed to TNF antagonists. *Semin Arthritis Rheum.* 2011;41(1):71–80.

23. Dixon WG, Watson KD, Lunt M et al.; British Society For Rheumatology Biologics Register Control Centre Consortium; British Society for Rheumatology Biologics Register. Influence of anti-tumor necrosis factor therapy on cancer incidence in patients with rheumatoid arthritis who have had a prior malignancy: results from the British Society for Rheumatology Biologics Register. *Arthritis Care Res* 2010;62:755–763.

24. Raaschou P, Simard JF, Neovius M, Askling J; Anti-Rheumatic Therapy in Sweden Study Group. Does cancer that occurs during or after anti-tumor necrosis factor therapy have a worse prognosis? A national assessment of overall and site-specific cancer survival in rheumatoid arthritis patients treated with biologic agents. *Arthritis Rheum* 2011;63(7):1812–1822.

25. Mercer LK, Galloway JB, Lunt M, Dixon WG, Watson KD, BSRBR Control Centre Consortium, Symmons, DP, Hyrich KL, on behalf of the BSRBR. The influence of anti-TNF therapy upon incidence of non-melanoma skin cancer (NMSC) in patients with rheumatoid arthritis (RA): Results from the BSR Biologics Register (BSRBR). *Arthritis Rheum* 2009;60(10 Suppl):S772.

26. Dixon WG, Hyrich KL, Watson KD et al.; BSRBR Control Centre Consortium, Symmons DP; BSR Biologics Register. Drug-specific risk of tuberculosis in patients with rheumatoid arthritis treated with anti-TNF therapy: results from the British Society for Rheumatology Biologics Register (BSRBR). *Ann Rheum Dis* 2010;69(3):522–528.

27. Solovic I, Sester M, Gomez-Reino JJ et al. The risk of tuberculosis related to tumour necrosis factor antagonist therapies: a TBNET consensus statement. *Eur Respir J* 2010;36(5):1185–1206.

28. Carmona L, Gómez-Reino JJ, Rodríguez-Valverde V et al.; BIOBADASER Group. Effectiveness of recommendations to prevent reactivation of latent tuberculosis infection in patients treated with tumor necrosis factor antagonists. *Arthritis Rheum* 2005;52(6):1766–1772.

29. Strangfeld A, Listing J, Herzer P et al. Risk of herpes zoster in patients with rheumatoid arthritis treated with anti-TNF-alpha agents. *JAMA* 2009;301(7):737–744.

30. Galloway JB, Hyrich KL, Mercer LK et al.; on behalf of the BSR Biologics Register. Risk of septic arthritis in patients with rheumatoid arthritis and the effect of anti-TNF therapy: results from the British Society for Rheumatology Biologics Register. *Ann Rheum Dis* 2011;70(10):1810–1814.

31. Listing J, Strangfeld A, Kary S et al. Infections in patients with rheumatoid arthritis treated with biologic agents. *Arthritis Rheum* 2005;52:3403–3412.

32. Dixon WG, Watson K, Lunt M et al.; British Society for Rheumatology Biologics Register. Rates of serious infection, including site-specific and bacterial intracellular infection, in rheumatoid arthritis patients receiving anti-tumor necrosis factor therapy: results from the British Society for Rheumatology Biologics Register. *Arthritis Rheum* 2006;54(23):68–76.

33. Askling J, Fored CM, Brandt L et al. Time-dependent increase in risk of hospitalisation with infection among Swedish RA patients treated with TNF antagonists. *Ann Rheum Dis* 2007;66:1339–1344.

34. Dixon WG, Symmons DP, Lunt M, Watson KD, Hyrich KL; British Society for Rheumatology Biologics Register Control Centre Consortium, Silman AJ; British Society for Rheumatology Biologics Register. Serious infection following anti-tumor necrosis factor alpha therapy in patients with rheumatoid arthritis: lessons from interpreting data from observational studies. *Arthritis Rheum* 2007;56(9):2896–2904.

35. Galloway JB, Hyrich KL, Mercer LK et al.; BSRBR Control Centre Consortium; British Society for Rheumatology Biologics Register.Anti-TNF therapy is associated with an increased risk of serious infections in patients with rheumatoid arthritis especially in the first 6 months of treatment: updated results from the British Society for Rheumatology Biologics Register with special emphasis on risks in the elderly. *Rheumatology (Oxford)* 2011;50(1):124–131.

36. Strangfeld A, Eveslage M, Schneider M et al. Treatment benefit or survival of the fittest: what drives the time-dependent decrease in serious infection rates under TNF inhibition and what does this imply for the individual patient? *Ann Rheum Dis* 2011;70(11):1914–1920.

37. Dixon WG, Symmons DP. What effects might anti-TNFalpha treatment be expected to have on cardiovascular morbidity and mortality in rheumatoid arthritis? A review of the role of TNFalpha in cardiovascular pathophysiology. *Ann Rheum Dis* 2007;66:1132–1136.

38. Dixon WG, Watson KD, Lunt M, Hyrich KL, British Society for Rheumatology Biologics Register Control Centre Consortium, Silman AJ. Reduction in the incidence of myocardial infarction in patients with rheumatoid arthritis who respond to anti-tumor necrosis factor alpha therapy: results from the British Society for Rheumatology Biologics Register. *Arthritis Rheum* 2007;56:2905–2912.

39. Carmona L, Descalzo MA, Perez-Pampin E et al.; BIOBADASER and EMECAR Groups. All-cause and cause-specific mortality in rheumatoid arthritis are not greater than expected when treated with tumour necrosis factor antagonists. *Ann Rheum Dis* 2007;66:880–885.

40. Lunt M, Watson KD, Dixon WG; British Society for Rheumatology Biologics Register Control Centre Consortium, Symmons DP, Hyrich KL; British Society for Rheumatology Biologics Register. No evidence of association between anti-tumor necrosis factor treatment and mortality in patients with rheumatoid arthritis: results from the British Society for Rheumatology Biologics Register. *Arthritis Rheum* 2010;62(11):3145–3153.

41. Verstappen SM, King Y, Watson KD, Symmons DP, Hyrich KL; BSRBR Control Centre Consortium, BSR Biologics Register. Anti-TNF therapies

and pregnancy: outcome of 130 pregnancies in the British Society for Rheumatology Biologics Register. *Ann Rheum Dis* 2011;70(5):823–826.

42. Hazes JM, Coulie PG, Geenen V et al. Rheumatoid arthritis and pregnancy: evolution of disease activity and pathophysiological considerations for drug use. *Rheumatology (Oxford)* 2011;50(11):1955–1968.

43. Harrison MJ, Dixon WG, Watson KD et al.; British Society for Rheumatology Biologics Register Control Centre Consortium; BSRBR.

Rates of new-onset psoriasis in patients with rheumatoid arthritis receiving anti-tumour necrosis factor alpha therapy: results from the British Society for Rheumatology Biologics Register. *Ann Rheum Dis* 2009;68(2):209–215.

44. Dixon WG, Carmona L, Finckh A et al. EULAR points to consider when establishing, analysing and reporting safety data of biologics registers in rheumatology. *Ann Rheum Dis* 2010;69(9):1596–1602.

CHAPTER 35

Outcomes of paediatric rheumatic disease

Kirsten Minden

Introduction

Paediatric rheumatic diseases (PRD) influence all aspects of a child's and their family's life, and may have multidimensional consequences. This chapter describes the instruments that have been developed to assess these consequences and the outcomes that have been reported for patients with PRD, with an emphasis on measures and outcomes in juvenile idiopathic arthritis (JIA), juvenile systemic lupus erythematosus (JSLE), and juvenile dermatomyositis (JDM).

Outcome measures

A methodology and standardization is required for measuring and valuing the range of health states associated with PRD.

Therapeutic response measures

A variety of instruments are available for measuring disease activity in JIA, JSLE, and JDM. However, due to the high variability in the clinical presentation and outcome of PRD, no single measure can reliably capture disease activity in all patients. To achieve a standardized approach, core sets of variables have been established (Table 35.1).[1,2] Beyond the core sets, there are other parameters that have yet to be incorporated into standard outcome assessment, but allow for a more sensitive assessment of disease activity, such as biomarkers (e.g. serum cytokine profiles, S100 proteins) or new imaging modalities (e.g. ultrasound coupled with power Doppler [USPW], MRI).

Using the core sets of disease activity measures, response criteria for use in therapeutic trials and in standard clinical care in JIA, JSLE, and JDM have been created.[1,3,4] These criteria enable determination of whether individual patients demonstrate clinically important improvement at a defined point in time. In JIA the definition of improvement is equivalent to the so-called American College of Rheumatology (ACR) paediatric 30 response (Box 35.1). Given the increasing demand of higher response levels, ACR paediatric 50, 70, 90, and 100 levels of response were defined. The ACR paediatric response criteria do not make it possible to quantify the absolute level of disease activity. For this, a composite disease activity score for JIA, the Juvenile Arthritis Disease Activity Score (JADAS) is available, which is also based on the core set criteria (Box 35.2). In addition, criteria were developed by Wallace et al. in order to define a state of inactive disease or remission (Box 35.2).

Disease status measures

Physician-reported outcomes

Traditional disease status measures comprise clinically measurable signs or symptoms of the disease assessed by the physician, such as current disease activity and organ system damage. Standardized definitions of disease activity states (e.g. inactive disease, clinical remission, and minimal disease activity state) have been developed for JIA (Box 35.2).[5,6]

Validated, standardized, clinical measures aimed at assessing damage or permanent alterations in joint structures or extra-articular organ/systems as a result of disease or its treatment are available for JIA, JSLE, and JDM.[7–9] These instruments differ somewhat from damage instruments applied in adult-onset diseases, because they also consider the potential reversibility of some damage items in children and include assessment of growth retardation and pubertal delay.

In JIA, imaging has been of particular importance to assess structural joint damage. The reference standard method for assessing joint damage is plane radiography. Several radiographic scoring systems have been developed that allow for a standardized quantification of radiographic joint changes (e.g. Poznanski score, Dijkstra composite score, adapted Sharp/van der Heijde score, Childhood Arthritis Radiographic Score of the Hip). The newer imaging methods, MRI and USPD, for which corresponding scoring systems are in development, are even more sensitive for joint damage assessment.[10]

Patient-reported outcomes

The patients' perspective on outcome is equally important as the physician-based outcomes. This includes the direct effect of illness with subjectively perceived signs and symptoms: pain, fatigue, adverse effects from therapy, and disability. Given the current inability to prevent or cure rheumatic diseases, the primary aim of care is to ensure the best possible lifelong functioning and quality of life. This necessitates formal methods for measuring patient's experience

Table 35.1 Core sets of disease activity measures for juvenile idiopathic arthritis (JIA), juvenile systemic lupus erythematosus (JSLE), and juvenile dermatomyositis (JDM)

	JIA	JSLE	JDM
Generic domains			
Global assessment by physician	Physician global assessment of disease activity (VAS, NRS)	Physician global assessment of disease activity (VAS, NRS)	Physician global assessment (VAS, NRS)
Global assessment by parents/patients	Patient/parent global assessment of overall well-being (VAS, NRS)	Patient/parent global assessment of overall well-being (VAS, NRS)	Patient/parent global assessment of overall well-being (VAS, NRS)
Disability or health-related quality of life	Functional ability (e.g. CHAQ)	Health-related quality of life (e.g., CHQ-Physical summary score)	Functional ability (e.g. CHAQ) Health-related quality of life (e.g. CHQ-Physical summary score)
Disease-specific domains			
Disease-specific measures	Active joint count Restricted joint count		Muscle strength (e.g. MMT, CMAS)
Global disease activity		Global disease activity tool (e.g. ECLAM, SLEDAI, BILAG, SLAM)	Global disease activity tool (e.g. DAS, MDAA)
Laboratory measures	Acute-phase reactant (ESR or CRP)	Renal involvement (urine protein: creatinine ratio, 24-hour proteinuria)	Muscle enzymes (CK, LDH, ALT, AST, aldolase)
Additional	Spiking fever (to be used for systemic JIA)		

ALT, alanine aminotransferase; AST, aspartate aminotransferase; BILAG, British Isles Lupus Assessment Group; CHAQ, Childhood Health Assessment Questionnaire; CHQ, child health questionnaire; CK, creatine kinase; CMAS, childhood myositis assessment scale; CRP, C-reactive protein; DAS, disease activity score; ECLAM, European consensus lupus activity measurement; ESR, erythrocyte sedimentation ratio; LDH, lactate dehydrogenase; MDAA, myositis disease activity assessment tool; MMT, manual muscle testing; NRS, numeric rating scale; SLAM, systemic lupus activity measure; SLEDAI, SLE disease activity index; VAS, visual analogue scale.

Box 35.1 Definition of improvement in JIA

◆ **ACR paediatric 30 response:** 3 of any 6 of the core set variables (see Table 35.1) improved by ≥30%, with no more than 1 of the remaining variables worsening by >30%. For systemic JIA, absence of spiking fever (≤38 °C during the week preceding the evaluation) is also required.

◆ **ACR paediatric 50/70/90 response:** 3 of any 6 of the core set variables improved by ≥50/70/90%, with no more than 1 of the remaining variables worsening by >30%.

Box 35.2 Criteria for defining clinical inactive disease and remission in selected categories of juvenile idiopathic arthritis (JIA)—persistent and extended oligoarthritis, rheumatoid factor positive and negative polyarthritis, and systemic JIA[5]

All of the following criteria must be met in order to consider a patient to be in a state of inactive disease:

◆ No joints with active arthritis.

◆ No fever, rash, serositis, splenomegaly, or generalized lymphadenopathy attributable to JIA.

◆ No active uveitis (according to the SUN Working Group: 'grade zero cells,' indicating <1 cell in field sizes of 1 mm by a 1 mm slit beam).

◆ ESR or CRP level within normal limits in the laboratory where tested or, if elevated, not attributable to JIA.

◆ Physician's global assessment of disease activity score of best possible on the scale used.

◆ Duration of morning stiffness of ≤15 minutes.

Clinical remission on medication: the criteria for inactive disease must be met for a minimum of 6 continuous months while the patient is on medication.

Clinical remission off medication: the criteria for inactive disease must be met for a minimum of 12 continuous months while off all anti-arthritis and anti-uveitis medications.

CRP, C-reactive protein, ESR, erythrocyte sedimentation rate.

---

of disease. An accepted means of describing the health and functioning of an individual is the WHO International Classification of Functioning, Disability and Health (ICF). According to the ICF, 'functioning' comprises all different aspects of the way in which a specific health condition affects life and thus includes body functions and structures, activities, and participation related to environmental and personal factors.[11]

Instruments developed to measure patients' functioning and health are summarized in Table 35.2. Of the function-oriented health status measures, the Childhood Health Assessment Questionnaire (CHAQ) in childhood or the Health Assessment Questionnaire (HAQ) in adulthood are the most widely used, mainly because of their ease of use and their validation in long-term outcome studies. Health-related quality of life (HRQoL) can be measured by different approaches. So-called generic measures allow for the valuation and

Table 35.2 Patient-reported outcomes in juvenile idiopathic arthritis (JIA), juvenile systemic lupus erythematosus (JSLE), and juvenile dermatomyositis (JDM)

	JIA	JSLE	JDM
Function-oriented health status measures	Childhood Health Assessment Questionnaire (CHAQ) in childhood or Health Assessment Questionnaire (HAQ) in adulthood Juvenile Arthritis Functionality Scale (JAFS) Juvenile Arthritis Functional Assessment Report (JAFAR) Juvenile Arthritis Self-Report Index (JASI) Childhood Arthritis Impact Measurement Scales (CHAIMS)		
Health-related quality of life	Child Health Questionnaire (CHQ) in childhood or Medical Outcomes Short-Form 36 (SF-36) in adulthood Pediatrics Quality of Life Inventory (PedsQL) Generic Core Module PedsQL Rheumatology Module Quality of My Life Questionnaire (QoMLQ) Paediatric Rheumatology Quality of Life Scale (PRQL)		
	Juvenile Arthritis Quality of Life Questionnaire (JAQQ) Childhood Arthritis Health Profile (CAHP)	Simple Measure of the Impact of Lupus Erythematosus in Youngsters (SMILEY)	
Overall well-being	Visual analogue scale (VAS) / numerical rating scale (NRS)		
Pain	VAS/NRS		
Fatigue	PedsQL Multidimensional Fatigue Scale		
Composite scores	Juvenile Arthritis Multidimensional Assessment Report (JAMAR) Juvenile Arthritis Parent Assessment Index (JAPAI), Juvenile Arthritis Child Assessment Index (JACAI)		

comparisons of HRQoL of healthy people versus that of patients with different diagnoses. Conversely, disease-specific measures value the health of patients with a specific disease and are therefore thought to better capture changes in the degree of health.

Health outcomes

Given the substantial improvement in outcomes for patients with PRD over the past several decades, there has been a shift from measuring short-term mortality and morbidity to examining long-term outcomes and preventing the adult consequences of childhood-onset disease. However, many of the long-term outcome studies published have inconsistent case definitions. Studies often include patients from tertiary referral clinics, meaning they may reflect only those who have a disease severe enough to come to and remain at special healthcare facilities. Studies also vary substantially in years of follow-up and in whether they are prospective or retrospective. These factors help to explain both the variability and the limitations associated with outcome studies which are presented in the following. Yet, further variability is likely to be seen in future estimates associated with variations in availability and uptake of new treatments.

Physical consequences of juvenile rheumatic diseases for the individual

Mortality

Juvenile-onset inflammatory rheumatic diseases are associated with increased mortality rates compared with the general population.

However, mortality rates have considerably decreased over the past decades. Mortality rates among children with chronic arthritis were 4–7% in the 1970s, which represented a 10-fold increase over the general population. In 2010, Hashkes reported a global mortality rate of 0.2 for children with JIA, which did not differ significantly from the mortality rate of the general population.[12] JIA patients are still at increased risk of mortality in their young adult years.[13,14] Two population-based studies demonstrated that adult patients with childhood-onset arthritis have a roughly fourfold higher overall mortality than the general population. Elaine Thomas and colleagues estimated standardized mortality ratios (SMR) of 5 for women and 3 for men with childhood-onset arthritis, twice as high as those calculated for men and women with rheumatoid arthritis.

Children with systemic connective tissue diseases, such as JSLE and JDM, and primary vasculitis (except for Kawasaki's disease and Henoch–Schönlein purpura) still have a significantly higher mortality risk than the general population. Patients with primary vasculitis carry the highest risk, with a mortality rate of 1.9% and a SMR of 4.71 according to the study by Hashkes.[12] Patients with JSLE follow, with a rate of 1.2% and a SMR of 3.06. A cohort study from the United States noted a particularly high SMR of 20 for JSLE in the age category 19–34 years.[15] Of course, the lifespan of JSLE patients has improved dramatically. While global survival at 5 and 10 years follow-up was 42–72% and 40–70% for the patients studied in the 1980s, respectively, these values reached 88–100% at 5 years and 86–90% at 10 years follow-up in the studies published after the year 2000.[12,15–18] A marked improvement in prognosis was also demonstrated for patients with JDM, for whom mortality rates of almost

40% were reported in the presteroid era as compared to 0.8%–3.1% in the year 2010.[12,19]

Knowledge about specific causes of death in the various PRD is very limited. In the 1970s, the major causes of death in patients with childhood-onset chronic arthritis were renal failure (in one-half of the cases due to amyloidosis) and infections. Amyloidosis accounted for more than 40% of all causes of death, but is no longer a relevant cause of death in these patients. Systemic-onset JIA still accounts for two-thirds of the mortality seen in JIA, with macrophage activation syndrome (MAS) being the leading cause for mortality. Approximately 10% of patients with systemic-onset JIA are diagnosed with MAS which has a mortality of 8–22%.[20] To what extent cardiovascular diseases, infections, or even hematopoietic malignancies attribute to the increase in SMR, especially later in life, is unidentified. With regard to the risk of cancer occurrence, preliminary data point to an increased risk of malignancies (particularly of the lymphoproliferative type) in patients with JIA which cannot be explained by the introduction of biological therapies.[21] The relevance of this for early mortality seems insignificant. Causes

of death later in life among JSLE patients are better known. They include cardiovascular disease or infection, which account for approximately one-half of the deaths in adulthood.[15] Death in JDM most often results from respiratory insufficiency or interstitial lung disease, myocarditis, or from gastrointestinal ulceration with intestinal perforation and bleeding. Information about causes of death in adult JDM is missing.

Disease activity

Persisting disease activity is a significant consequence of disease for patients because it is closely linked to important symptoms such as pain, fatigue, and functional limitations. Outcome studies published since the year 2000 show that rheumatic diseases beginning in childhood frequently continue into adulthood (Table 35.3).

In JIA most remissions occur in the first 5 years after disease onset. After more than 10 years of disease duration 40–60% of the patients still have an active arthritis. The probability of remission varies significantly with disease-onset type, being best for oligoarticular JIA,

Table 35.3 Outcome studies of juvenile idiopathic arthritis (JIA), juvenile systemic lupus erythematosus (JSLE), and juvenile dermatomyositis (JDM) which comprised at least 20 patients with a specific disease, had a follow-up of at least 10 years, published since the year 2000

Study (year, country)	Number of patients assessed	Median or mean disease duration (years)	Patients (in %) with		
			Active disease	Functional limitations (Steinbrocker Class > I or HAQ > 0)	Erosive joint changes
JIA—systemic onset					
Lomater et al. (2000, Italy)[22]	80	11	43	57	n.g.
Minden et al. (2002, Germany)[23]	30	17	46	45	n.g.
Packham et al. (2002, UK)[24]	52	29	n.g.	63[a]	75[b]
Lurati et al. (2009, Italy)[25]	98	10[c]	66	n.g.	n.g.
JIA—Oligoarthritis					
Minden et al. (2002, Germany)[23]	85	17	41	28	n.g.
Arkela-Kautiainen et al. (2005, Finland)[26]	78	16[c]	58	n.g.	n.g.
Flato et al. (2009, Norway)[27]	137	15	30	30	13
JIA—RF-negative polyarthritis					
Foster et al. (2002, UK)[28]	20	21[c]	65	n.g.[d]	n.g.
Minden et al. (2002, Germany)[23]	27	16	59	52	n.g.
Packham et al. (2002, UK)[24]	41	30	n.g.	50[a]	56[b]
Lurati et al. (2009, Italy)[25]	94	10[c]	78	n.g.	n.g.
JIA—RF-positive polyarthritis					
Packham et al. (2002, UK)[24]	41	29	n.g.	53[a]	60[b]
Lurati et al. (2009, Italy)[25]	26	10[c]	100	n.g.	n.g.
JIA—enthesitis-related arthritis					
Minden et al. (2002, Germany)[23]	33	15	79	45	39[e]
Packham et al. (2002, U.K.)[24]	32	27	n.g.	16[a]	34[b]
Flato et al. (2006, Norway)[29]	55	15	56	51	35[e]/26[f]

(Continued)

Table 35.3 (Continued)

Study (year, country)	Number of patients assessed	Median or mean disease duration (years)	Patients (in %) with		
			Active disease	Functional limitations (Steinbrocker Class > I or HAQ > 0)	Erosive joint changes
JIA—psoriatic arthritis					
Flato et al. (2009, Norway)[27]	31	15	35	45	23
JSLE					
Candell Chalom et al. (2004, USA)[17]	29	13	52[g]	n.g.	46
Hersh et al. (2009, USA)[30]	90	17	68[h]	n.g.	31[i]
JDM					muscle damage
Sanner et al. (2009, Norway)[31]	39	17	61[j]	36	52

DAS, disease activity score; HAQ, Health Assessment Questionnaire; n.g., not given.

[a]HAQ > 1.5; [b]patients with joints replaced; [c]disease duration of the whole group; [d]mean HAQ = 1.36; [e]radiographic sacroiliitis; [f]peripheral joint erosions; [g]SLEDAI score > 4; [h]receiving prednisone therapy; [i]dialysis or renal transplant; [j]DAS≥3.

at approximately 50%, and worst for polyarticular JIA, in which it approaches 15%.[25,32] The probability of remission decreases progressively after 10 years. If remission does not occur within 10 years of disease onset, it is unlikely to occur at all.

Similar results have been reported in JSLE, with over one-half of patients having active disease after a mean follow-up period of 13 years.[17] and over two-thirds of patients receiving oral corticosteroids at a mean follow-up of 16.5 years.[30] The median time to remission in JDM was estimated to be 4.7 years. In other words, one-half of patients with JDM will have achieved remission 4.5 years after diagnosis.[33] A similar percentage was found in studies with a follow-up of 8 and 17 years.[19,31]

Organ system damage

Cumulative disease activity over time has been shown to be a highly significant predictor of disease damage in children with inflammatory rheumatic diseases.[34] Five years after disease onset, damage has occurred in approximately one-half of the patients. Table 35.4 summarizes those studies on damage in JIA, JSLE, and JDM which used standardized damage instruments. In JIA, articular damage is the most important component of global damage, representing almost 80% of the total JADI (juvenile arthritis damage index) score in the study by Russo.[35] Ocular damage, growth failure, and muscle atrophy are the most frequent extra-articular damage components in JIA. Renal, neuropsychiatric, musculoskeletal, and ocular systems are the most commonly damaged organ systems in JSLE. In JDM, the skin leads the list of the most frequently affected organs, followed by the musculoskeletal and endocrine organ systems.

Articular damage

In JIA, articular damage is most common in hip, wrist, and temporomandibular joints.[35] Ten years after disease onset, at least one in four JIA patients has developed radiographic joint changes with erosions, joint space narrowing, or even destruction (Figure 35.1). Depending on the patient collective studied, between 2% and 50% of the 20–35 year old JIA patients have already been supplied with

endoprostheses.[23,24,28,32] Patients with systemic-onset show the highest frequency of joint replacements, and the hip is the most frequently replaced joint. As a result of change in treatment strategies, i.e. the early use of intra-articular steroids and immunomodulatory drugs, such as methotrexate and biological agents, joint damage is decreasing. In JSLE and JDM articular damage is rarely seen; however, joint contractures are seen in about 20% of JDM patients.

Extra-articular damage

Linear growth failure occurs in about 10% of children with PRD, with a decreasing trend over the past decades. Total body inflammation and corticosteroid therapy are strongly implicated as causes of growth failure. In view of the whole JIA group, growth failure is therefore more likely to develop in patients with systemic and polyarticular JIA. Simon and colleagues.[43] found a mean final height standard deviation score of −2.0 in 24 patients with systemic JIA, with 41% of subjects' height more than 2 SD below the mean. The prevalence of short stature (final height below the 3rd percentile) in 65 adult JIA patients was reported to be nearly 11% in a long-term follow-up study from Denmark, with all of the severely growth-retarded patients having polyarticular JIA.[44]

Local growth disturbances

In JIA local growth disturbances mainly occur at sites of inflammation and can take the form of overgrowth or undergrowth (Figure 35.2). There is a tendency to accelerated maturation of epiphyses, leading for example to increased leg length, or overcrowding and fusion of the joint in wrists and ankles. Limb length discrepancies and micrognathia (Figure 35.3) are the most frequently observed local growth disturbances in up to one-quarter of adult patients.[23,24]

Abnormal body composition

Abnormalities in body composition, i.e. a decreased lean body mass, an increased fat mass, and a reduced bone mineral density have been documented in patients with PRD. Up to 50% of adolescents and young adults with JIA, JSLE, and JDM experience

Table 35.4 Summary of studies on cumulative organ damage after more than 5 years of disease, assessed by JADI in juvenile idiopathic arthritis (JIA), SDI in juvenile systemic lupus erythematosus (JSLE), and MDI in juvenile dermatomyositis (JDM)

	JIA			JSLE					JDM		
	Viola et al. (2005, Italy)[7]	Russo et al. (2008, Argentina)[35]	Sarma et al. (2008, India)[36]	Ravelli et al. (2003, Italy)[37]	Miettunen et al. (2004, Canada)[18]	Lilleby et al. (2005, Norway)[38]	Descloux et al. (2008, France)[39]	Tucker et al. (2008, Canada)[40]	Rider et al. (2009, USA)[41]	Ravelli et al. (2010, multicentre)[19]	Mathiesen et al. (2011, Denmark)[42]
Patients (n)	158	43 (sJIA)	49 (ERA)	387	51	71	55	31	143	490	53
Mean/median disease duration, years	7.3	6	6.0	5.7	7.2	10.8	7.1	5.1	6.8	7.7	13.9
Patients in % with DI ≥1		43		51	59	61		65	79	69	60
Patients with damage by organ/system in %											
Articular damage	47	38	35			3					
Extra-articular	37	19	10								
Ocular	6–10[a]	2	0	11	12	4	11	10	7	2	
Musculoskeletal				12	27	13	13	19			
Muscle atrophy	9	8	6			11				24	34
Leg-length discrepancy		6									
Avascular necrosis of bone	0	8			20						
Skin		2		10	12	3	13	10	49	53	40
Calcinosis									26	24	20
Endocrine									27	18	
Growth failure	11	13	8						14	8	
Pubertal delay		2	4						4		
Premature gonadal failure				4	2	4	2	13	n.a.		
Diabetes	0	0		1	0	1	2	3	1		

(Continued)

Table 35.4 (*Continued*)

	JIA			JSLE					JDM		
	Viola et al. (2005, Italy)[7]	Russo et al. (2008, Argentina)[35]	Sarma et al. (2008, India)[36]	Ravelli et al. (2003, Italy)[37]	Miettunen et al., (2004, Canada)[18]	Lilleby et al. (2005, Norway)[38]	Descloux et al. (2008, France)[39]	Tucker et al. (2008, Canada)[40]	Rider et al. (2009, USA)[41]	Ravelli et al. (2010, multicentre)[19]	Mathiesen et al. (2011, Denmark)[42]
Neuropsychiatric				16	14	28	15	29			
Renal				22	10	13	20	45			
Pulmonary				2	4	4	0	3	15	6	
Cardiovascular				3	12	6	4	7	4	3	
Peripheral vascular				6	12	9	0	0	3	2	
Gastrointestinal				4	4	4	7	3	17	9	
Secondary amyloidosis	0	0	2								
Malignancy	0			0	0	1	0	3	0	0	

JADI, Juvenile Arthritis Damage Index; MDI, Myositis Damage Index; n.a., not applicable; SDI, Systemic Lupus International Collaborative Clinics/American College of Rheumatology Damage Index.

[a]right and left eye; [b]joint contractures.

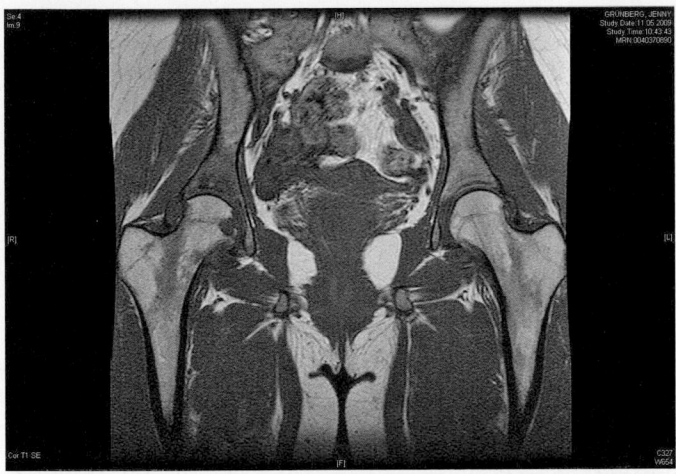

Fig. 35.1 An 18-year-old girl with extended oligoarthritis and pronounced destructive changes in the right hip (MRI, coronary T1-weighted SE).

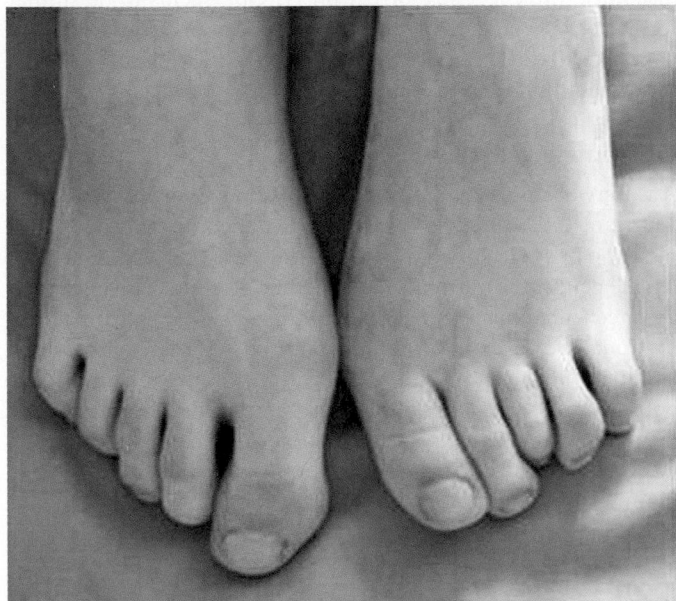

Fig. 35.2 Shortening of the left third toe in a child with polyarticular JIA.

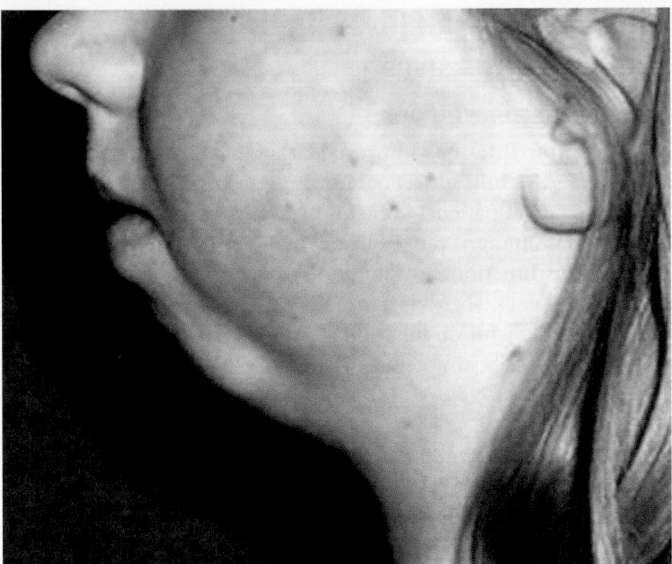

Fig. 35.3 Girl with rheumatoid-factor-negative polyarthritis since early childhood and micrognathia due to temporomandibular joint arthritis.

decreased bone mass at lumbar spine or femoral neck, and up to 10% osteoporosis.[45,46] The abnormalities in the amount and the geometric distribution of bone mass are of concern as both determine bone strength and the fracture threshold and put the patients at increased risk of osteoporosis and fractures later in life.

Muscle loss

Muscle loss, which is critically responsible for the bone loss, occurs in all forms of PRD. Muscle mass and force are reduced in JIA patients; about 10% demonstrate persistent muscle atrophy on clinical examination. In patients with longstanding JDM muscle weakness has been found in 31–42% of patients in three series after more than 10 years of follow-up, whereas MRI-detected muscular damage was found in one-half of the patients.[31]

Ocular sequelae

Apart from musculoskeletal system damage, ocular sequelae are of major concern in JIA. They develop as consequences of uveitis in at least one-third of affected patients within the first 7 years of disease, and most frequently consist of cataract, posterior synechiae, glaucoma, and band keratopathy. The ocular complications result in a permanent, significant visual loss (<0.5) in 10–20% of patients. Blindness (20/200 or worse) due to uveitis in at least one eye still occurs in 5–10% of uveitis patients.[47] Most complications and reduction of visual acuity occur within the first 7 years of disease, but their prevalence increases with longer follow-up. More than 15 years after disease onset, uveitis is still active in almost one-half of the patients.

Atherosclerosis and cardiovascular disease

Patients with chronic inflammatory rheumatic diseases are probably at increased risk of premature atherosclerosis and early-onset cardiovascular disease. The aetiology may be multifactorial, attributable to manifestations of the disease itself (such as chronic inflammation, chronic hypertension, renal disease, or abnormal lipid profiles), adverse effects of medication (such as steroids and non-steroidal anti-inflammatory drugs) and lifestyle issues (such as decreased physical activity due to disease-related disability). Impaired vascular function has been shown in JIA and carotid intima-media thickness in JSLE, but the exact extent of the increased cardiovascular risk is unknown.

Fertility problems

Fertility disorder is of particular concern to patients. Fertility is not impaired in females with JIA, but fecundity was found to be reduced.[48] Also, pregnancy outcome was less successful in these women, with a significantly increased rate of miscarriage. Patients with systemic connective tissue disorders or vasculitides may even be at higher risk for decreased reproductive fitness than JIA patients as a consequence of their chronic inflammatory condition or the medications used to treat it (e.g. alkylating agents such as cyclophosphamide). Their true risk of infertility or low follicular/ovarian reserve is not known, however.

Consequences of juvenile rheumatic diseases

Functional consequences

Treatment for PRD has improved dramatically, accompanied by a steady and significant reduction in disability rates. In the 1970s the frequency of patients in Steinbrocker functional class I (i.e. no functional limitation) ranged from 25% to 40% and that of patients with serious functional disability (corresponding to Steinbrocker functional classes III and IV) from 17% to 22%, but higher frequencies of patients with no functional limitation (60%) and lower frequencies of patients in Steinbrocker classes III and IV (10%) were recorded in the 1990s. Most recent outcome studies used a more sensitive functional measure, the HAQ, for the assessment of the patients' physical disability. According to the HAQ, approximately 40% of patients with PRD are somehow limited in their functional capacity in their young adult years (see Table 35.3). Approximately 10% of them are in need of assistance and/or aids in order to manage their activities of daily living, which corresponds well with the percentage of patients being in Steinbrocker functional class III or IV. Severe disability is most frequently seen in patients with rheumatoid factor positive polyarthritis and systemic onset of JIA, followed by patients with rheumatoid factor-negative polyarthritis and extended oligoarthritis. In contrast, patients with persistent oligoarthritis hardly ever report functional disability in early adulthood.[23,32,49]

Societal consequences

Symptoms associated with PRD, such as fatigue, pain, stiffness, and physical disability, may lead to reduced participation in daily school and social activities. However, children and adolescents with PRD more frequently cut back on participation in social activities rather than school activities. Patients with PRD miss on average 1–2 days of school per month due to their illness. Nevertheless, their academic achievement is comparable to that of the general population, or even better. However, entering the labour force is difficult for young people with PRD. JIA patients have lower employment rates compared to age-matched local controls.[23,24,28,49] The lower employment rates result from significantly higher rates of unemployment in JIA patients in comparison with controls, extended training periods, or early retirement. As compared to JIA patients, young adults with JSLE have an even lower employment rate. At a mean age of 24 years, only 40% worked full time.[17]

PRD have consequences not only for the individual, but also for their friends and family and for the whole of society. Parents may miss days at work and experience financial burdens. Klein-Gitelman and colleagues reported that one in five guardians of children with JIA, JSLE, and JDM reported having taken time off work, and 3% had stopped work in order to care for problems related to their child's rheumatic disease. Of families queried, 24% reported having lost income, with 14% having lost over $500 within the survey period of 3 or 6 months.[50] The economic burden of PRD is difficult to measure. The total costs of illness (both medical and societal costs) depend on the patient collective studied and the medical care delivery system. The few estimated direct costs of JIA range from €1800 to €27 700 per patient per year.[50] The main cost driver in JIA is medication, in particular biological agents. However, costs incurred in childhood have to be seen in view of lifetime pain, disability, and patient impairment. In adulthood, indirect costs due to work disability and sick leave account for most of the total cost in the active JIA population. Those costs incurred in adulthood might decline in the future as a result of new treatment strategies which have improved the prognosis of PRD. Long-term cost effectiveness studies are needed to prove this.

Quality of life

The impact of disease and its treatment on bodily, functional, and social level is reflected in impairments of patient's health status or perceived quality of life. How adolescents and young adults with PRD value their health has been repeatedly analysed using quality of life measures, such as the SF-36. Controlled outcome studies showed that patients with PRD judge their quality of life lower than age- and sex-matched controls.[17,19,28] They feel particularly impaired in their physical health (e.g. physical functioning, vitality, and bodily pain). Worse HRQoL is related to greater pain, fatigue, disease activity, damage, and functional disability. The effect size of JIA on HRQoL seems to be similar to that of JSLE and JDM. In general, a very high percentage of patients with PRD classify themselves as having a high quality of life in adulthood.

Outcome prediction

A variety of studies have investigated factors that will predict the course of PRD, to guide a risk-adapted and cost-effective treatment. Some indicators of poor health were identified, e.g. for JIA female gender, polyarticular and symmetrical joint involvement, elevated inflammatory markers, and rheumatoid factor positivity. Today, however, it cannot be predicted at disease onset which children will go on to have an unremitting disease and experience poor outcome or quality of life. Most interesting so far has been the prediction of prognosis based upon early treatment response, with outcomes at 3–12 months predicting response at later points in time.

Conclusion

The recent outcome studies are a testament that rheumatic diseases beginning in childhood are not benign. After 5–10 years of disease duration, approximately one-half of patients will have active disease, and will have developed damage due to the disease itself or to the adverse effects of treatment. Patients face a considerable morbidity in adulthood and lower life expectancy compared to their peers. Control of disease activity is important in order to decrease the damage. Owing to improved management, including early recognition and more-sophisticated treatment options, the outlook for children with juvenile rheumatic diseases has dramatically improved. In particular, functional outcomes have improved tremendously, with most patients exhibiting no or mild disability and able to lead a normal life.

Recently established large inception-cohort studies, with follow-up into adulthood, are expected to better characterize the multidimensional outcomes of patients with PRD. The data from these studies will lead to a better understanding of the disease prognosis, and could potentially form the basis of tailor-made treatment strategies for these illnesses presenting during childhood.

References

1. Giannini EH, Ruperto N, Ravelli A et al. Preliminary definition of improvement in juvenile arthritis. *Arthritis Rheum* 1997;40:1202–1209.

2. Ruperto N, Ravelli A, Murray KJ et al.; Paediatric Rheumatology International Trials Organization (PRINTO); Pediatric Rheumatology Collaborative Study Group (PRCSG). Preliminary core sets of measures for disease activity and damage assessment in juvenile systemic lupus erythematosus and juvenile dermatomyositis. *Rheumatology* (Oxford) 2003;42:1452–1459.

3. Brunner HI, Higgins GC, Wiers K et al. Prospective validation of the provisional criteria for the evaluation of response to therapy in childhood-onset systemic lupus erythematosus. *Arthritis Care Res* (Hoboken) 2010;62:335–344.

4. Ruperto N, Pistorio A, Ravelli A et al.; Paediatric Rheumatology International Trials Organization (PRINTO); Pediatric Rheumatology Collaborative Study Group (PRCSG). The Paediatric Rheumatology International Trials Organization provisional criteria for the evaluation of response to therapy in juvenile dermatomyositis. *Arthritis Care Res* (Hoboken) 2010;62:1533–1541.

5. Wallace CA, Giannini EH, Huang B, Itert L, Ruperto N; Childhood Arthritis Rheumatology Research Alliance; Pediatric Rheumatology Collaborative Study Group; Paediatric Rheumatology International Trials Organization. American College of Rheumatology provisional criteria for defining clinical inactive disease in select categories of juvenile idiopathic arthritis. *Arthritis Care Res* (Hoboken) 2011;63:929–936.

6. Magni-Manzoni S, Ruperto N, Pistorio A et al. Development and validation of a preliminary definition of minimal disease activity in patients with juvenile idiopathic arthritis. *Arthritis Rheum* 2008;59:1120–1127.

7. Viola S, Felici E, Magni-Manzoni S et al. Development and validation of a clinical index for assessment of long-term damage in juvenile idiopathic arthritis. *Arthritis Rheum* 2005;52:2092–2102.

8. Gutiérrez-Suárez R, Ruperto N, Gastaldi R et al. A proposal for a pediatric version of the Systemic Lupus International Collaborating Clinics/American College of Rheumatology Damage Index based on the analysis of 1,015 patients with juvenile-onset systemic lupus erythematosus. *Arthritis Rheum* 2006;54:2989–2996.

9. Rider LG, Lachenbruch PA, Monroe JB et al.; IMACS Group. Damage extent and predictors in adult and juvenile dermatomyositis and polymyositis as determined with the myositis damage index. *Arthritis Rheum* 2009;60:3425–3435.

10. Breton S, Jousse-Joulin S, Finel E et al. Approaches for evaluating peripheral joint abnormalities in juvenile idiopathic arthritis. *Semin Arthritis Rheum* 2012;41(5):698–711.

11. WHO International Classification of functioning, disability and health (ICF). Available at: http://www3.who.int/icf/icftemplate.cfm

12. Hashkes PJ, Wright BM, Lauer MS et al. Mortality outcomes in pediatric rheumatology in the US. *Arthritis Rheum* 2010;62:599–608.

13. French AR, Mason T, Nelson AM, O'Fallon WM, Gabriel SE. Increased mortality in adults with a history of juvenile rheumatoid arthritis: a population-based study. *Arthritis Rheum* 2001;44:523–527.

14. Thomas E, Symmons DP, Brewster DH et al. National study of cause-specific mortality in rheumatoid arthritis, juvenile chronic arthritis, and other rheumatic conditions: a 20 year follow-up study. *J Rheumatol* 2003;30:958–965.

15. Hersh AO, Trupin L, Yazdany J et al. Childhood-onset disease as a predictor of mortality in an adult cohort of patients with systemic lupus erythematosus. *Arthritis Care Res* (Hoboken) 2010;62:1152–1159.

16. Gonzalez B, Hernández P, Olguín H et al. Changes in the survival of patients with systemic lupus erythematosus in childhood: 30 years experience in Chile. *Lupus* 2005;14:918–923.

17. Candell Chalom E, Periera B, Rettig P et al. Educational, vocational and socioeconomic status and quality of life in adults with childhood-onset systemic lupus erythematosus. *Pediatr Rheumatol Online J* 2004;2:207–226.

18. Miettunen, PM, Ortiz-Alvarez, O, Petty, RE et al. Gender and ethnic origin have no effect on long-term outcome of childhood-onset systemic lupus erythematosus. *J Rheumatol* 2004;31:1650–1654.

19. Ravelli A, Trail L, Ferrari C et al. Long-term outcome and prognostic factors of juvenile dermatomyositis: a multinational, multicenter study of 490 patients. *Arthritis Care Res* (Hoboken) 2010;62:63–72.

20. Sawhney S, Woo P, Murray KJ. Macrophage activation syndrome: a potentially fatal complication of rheumatic disorders. *Arch Dis Child* 2001;85:421–426.

21. Simard JF, Neovius M, Hagelberg S, Askling J. Juvenile idiopathic arthritis and risk of cancer: a nationwide cohort study. *Arthritis Rheum* 2010;62:3776–3782.

22. Lomater C, Gerloni V, Gattinara M et al. Systemic onset juvenile idiopathic arthritis: a retrospective study of 80 consecutive patients followed for 10 years. *J Rheumatol* 2000;27:491–496.

23. Minden K, Niewerth M, Listing J et al. Long-term outcome in patients with juvenile idiopathic arthritis. *Arthritis Rheum* 2002;46:2392–2401.

24. Packham JC, Hall MA. Long-term follow-up of 246 adults with juvenile idiopathic arthritis: functional outcome. *Rheumatology* (Oxford) 2002;41:1428–1435.

25. Lurati A, Salmaso A, Gerloni V, Gattinara M, Fantini F. Accuracy of Wallace criteria for clinical remission in juvenile idiopathic arthritis: a cohort study of 761 consecutive cases. *J Rheumatol* 2009;36:1532–1535.

26. Arkela-Kautiainen M, Haapasaari J, Kautiainen H et al. Favourable social functioning and health related quality of life of patients with JIA in early adulthood. *Ann Rheum Dis* 2005;64:875–880.

27. Flatø B, Lien G, Smerdel-Ramoya A, Vinje O. Juvenile psoriatic arthritis: long-term outcome and differentiation from other subtypes of juvenile idiopathic arthritis. *J Rheumatol* 2009;36:642–650.

28. Foster HE, Marshall N, Myers A, Dunkley P, Griffiths ID. Outcome in adults with juvenile idiopathic arthritis: a quality of life study. *Arthritis Rheum* 2003;48:767–775.

29. Flatø B, Hoffmann-Vold AM, Reiff A et al. Long-term outcome and prognostic factors in enthesitis-related arthritis: a case-control study. *Arthritis Rheum* 2006;54:3573–3582.

30. Hersh AO, von Scheven E, Yazdany J et al. Differences in long-term disease activity and treatment of adult patients with childhood- and adult-onset systemic lupus erythematosus. *Arthritis Rheum* 2009;61:13–20.

31. Sanner H, Kirkhus E, Merckoll E et al. Long-term muscular outcome and predisposing and prognostic factors in juvenile dermatomyositis: A case-control study. *Arthritis Care Res* (Hoboken) 2010;62:1103–1111.

32. Oen K, Malleson PN, Cabral DA et al. Disease course and outcome of juvenile rheumatoid arthritis in a multicenter cohort. *J Rheumatol* 2002;29:1989–1999.

33. Stringer E, Singh-Grewal D, Feldman BM. Predicting the course of juvenile dermatomyositis: significance of early clinical and laboratory features. *Arthritis Rheum* 2008;58:3585–3592.

34. Magnani A, Pistorio A, Magni-Manzoni S et al. Achievement of a state of inactive disease at least once in the first 5 years predicts better outcome of patients with polyarticular juvenile idiopathic arthritis. *J Rheumatol* 2009;36:628–634.

35. Russo RA, Katsicas MM. Global damage in systemic juvenile idiopathic arthritis: preliminary early predictors. *J Rheumatol* 2008;35:1151–1156.

36. Sarma PK, Misra R, Aggarwal A. Outcome in patients with enthesitis-related arthritis (ERA): juvenile arthritis damage index (JADI) and functional status. *Pediatr Rheumatol Online J* 2008 Oct 22;6:18.

37. Ravelli A, Duarte-Salazar C, Buratti S et al. Assessment of damage in juvenile-onset systemic lupus erythematosus: a multicenter cohort study. *Arthritis Rheum* 2003;49:501–507.

38. Lilleby V, Flato B, Forre O. Disease duration, hypertension and medication requirements are associated with organ damage in childhood-onset systemic lupus erythematosus. *Clin Exp Rheumatol* 2005;23:261–269.

39. Descloux E, Durieu I, Cochat P et al. Paediatric systemic lupus erythematosus: prognostic impact of antiphospholipid antibodies. *Rheumatology* (Oxford) 2008;47:183–187.

40. Tucker LB, Uribe AG, Fernández M et al. Adolescent onset of lupus results in more aggressive disease and worse outcomes: results of a nested matched case-control study within LUMINA, a multiethnic US cohort (LUMINA LVII). *Lupus* 2008;17:314–322.

41. Rider LG, Lachenbruch PA, Monroe JB et al.; IMACS Group. Damage extent and predictors in adult and juvenile dermatomyositis and polymyositis as determined with the myositis damage index. *Arthritis Rheum* 2009;60:3425–3435.

42. Mathiesen P, Hegaard H, Herlin T et al. Long-term outcome in patients with juvenile dermatomyositis: a cross-sectional follow-up study. *Scand J Rheumatol* 2012;41(1):50–58.

43. Simon D, Fernando C, Czernichow P, Prieur AM. Linear growth and final height in patients with systemic juvenile idiopathic arthritis treated with long-term glucocorticoids. *J Rheumatol* 2002;29:1296–1300.

44. Zak M, Müller J, Karup Pedersen F. Final height, armspan, subischial leg length and body proportions in juvenile chronic arthritis. A long-term follow-up study. *Horm Res* 1999;52:80–85.

45. Zak M, Hassager C, Lovell DJ et al. Assessment of bone mineral density in adults with a history of juvenile chronic arthritis: a cross-sectional long-term follow-up study. *Arthritis Rheum* 1999;42:790–798.

46. Lilleby V, Lien G, Frey Frøslie K et al. Frequency of osteopenia in children and young adults with childhood-onset systemic lupus erythematosus. *Arthritis Rheum* 2005;52:2051–2059.

47. Skarin A, Elborgh R, Edlund E et al. Long-term follow-up of patients with uveitis associated with juvenile idiopathic arthritis: a cohort study. *Ocul Immunol Inflamm* 2009;17:104–108.

48. Ostensen M, Almberg K, Koksvik HS. Sex, reproduction, and gynecological disease in young adults with a history of juvenile chronic arthritis. *J Rheumatol* 2000;27:1783–1787.

49. Flato B, Lien G, Smerdel A et al. Prognostic factors in juvenile rheumatoid arthritis: a case-control study revealing early predictors and outcome after 14.9 years. *J Rheumatol* 2003;30:386–393.

50. Minden K. What are the costs of childhood-onset rheumatic disease? *Best Pract Res Clin Rheumatol* 2006;20:223–240.

CHAPTER 36

Assessment of paediatric rheumatic disease

Loren A. Matheson and Ciarán M. Duffy

Outcome measures: rationale and development

Today, most paediatric rheumatic diseases are not life threatening. However, they impact children and their families by interfering with normal health, and they may negatively influence a child's happiness. Generally, the goals of paediatric rheumatology interventions are to alleviate the patient's subjective disease symptoms and minimize inflammation in order to avoid permanent damage and ameliorate their overall quality of life (QoL). Improvements in functional outcomes have heightened QoL expectations, which in turn have become increasingly important to assess. QoL outcome measures are of direct interest and importance to patients because they provide effective measurements of patient status. Not only are QoL assessments predictive of patient functional outcome, they also produce reliable and effective measures of treatment impact, side effects, and comorbidities.[1]

The development and validation approaches for outcome measures that are used to assess the state of health-related (HR) QoL in the paediatric rheumatic diseases have been well established.[2] The development of a new instrument requires a number of lengthy steps including rationale justification, item generation, and reduction, and a description of the instrument in terms of reproducibility, consistency (reliability), and validity (accuracy). The process used to develop and validate health outcome measurement instruments, specifically focused on children with rheumatic diseases, has been detailed elsewhere.[2] This chapter describes a number of these instruments and provides an overview of relevant information around usage and popularity.

Instruments for juvenile idiopathic arthritis

Many tools have been developed for the assessment of children with juvenile idiopathic arthritis, including disease-specific measures of functional status and HRQoL. In addition, there are a number of generic instruments used to assess HRQoL in children with juvenile idiopathic arthritis (JIA) that have received widespread use. A number of the most popular instruments are discussed briefly here. Table 36.1 summarizes these instruments and provides details relating to usage, age range, and applicability. A relative comparison of the tools, including functional properties and QoL measures is presented in Table 36.2.

Childhood Health Assessment Questionnaire (CHAQ)

The adult Health Assessment Questionnaire formed the basis for the CHAQ (reviewed in [3]). The Disability Index within CHAQ assesses function in eight areas: dressing and grooming, arising, eating, walking, hygiene, reach, grip, and activities, for a total of 30 items. Discomfort is determined by the presence of pain, as measured by a visual analogue scale (VAS). In addition, a VAS measures patient or parent global assessment of arthritis. In the original validation study, reliability and convergent validity were very good, with excellent correlations with Steinbrocker functional class, active joint count, disease activity index, and degree of morning stiffness (reviewed in [3]). CHAQ has been successfully used for outcome evaluation in longitudinal studies.[4,5] It has also been used in a variety of settings, translated into many different languages, and undergone modifications in attempts to improve it while still maintaining excellent reliability and validity. Although many studies report good parent–child correlations, one study indicates that proxy and adolescent dyads who completed the CHAQ are more likely to disagree in those with severe disease as well as in those adolescents who report depressive symptoms.[6] Good responsiveness has been shown in other studies, including several longitudinal studies of etanercept.[7,8] Several studies have shown its usefulness in the evaluation of rehabilitative interventions.[9,10] It has also been suggested that the CHAQ is predictive of the presence of significant pain, as well as short-term outcomes, in a large cohort of Canadian children.[11] A digital form of the CHAQ has been developed and validated.[12] Although it took longer to complete than the paper version, the digital form was preferred by the majority of patients.

A recent study examined whether the CHAQ Disability Index scoring system and its responsiveness to change differed when calculated with and without the aids/devices and help sections of the questionnaire.[13] These components have been questioned because of their possible misinterpretation by the parent or child. The aids/devices and help items should only be completed if the need is

Table 36.1 Commonly used instruments for assessing juvenile idiopathic arthritis outcomes

Instrument	Usage	Age range	Proxy report	Applicability
JADAS	New	Children of all ages	No	Clinical and research
CHAQ	Widespread	Children of all ages	Yes	Research
JAQQ	Moderate	Children of all ages	Yes	Research
PedsQL	Widespread	2–18 years	Yes, 2–18 years	Research
PRQL	New	7–18 years	Yes, 7–18 years	Clinical
JAMAR	New	7–18 years	Yes, 2–18 years	Clinical and research
KIDSCREEN	Moderate	8–18 years	Yes, 8–18 years	Research
CHQ	Widespread	5–18 years	Yes	Research

Child Health Questionnaire (CHQ); Childhood Health Assessment Questionnaire (CHAQ); Juvenile Arthritis Disease Activity Score (JADAS); Juvenile Arthritis Multidimensional Assessment Report (JAMAR); Juvenile Arthritis Quality of Life Questionnaire (JAQQ); Pediatric Quality of Life Inventory (Peds QL); Rheumatology Quality of Life Scale (PRQL).

Table 36.2 Validation parameters for instruments commonly used for assessing outcomes in juvenile idiopathic arthritis

Parameter	JADAS	CHAQ	JAQQ	PedsQL	PRQL	JAMAR	KIDSCREEN
Clinical evaluation	Very strong	No	No		No	Very strong	No
Physical function measure	No	Moderate	Strong	Moderate	No	Very strong	Strong
Quality of Life measure	No	No	Strong	Strong	Strong	Very strong	Very strong
Pain measurement	Moderate	Moderate	Strong	Moderate	No	Very strong	No
Reliability	Strong	Strong	Strong	Strong	TBD	TBD	Strong
Validity	Strong	Strong	Strong	Strong	Strong	Strong	Strong
Responsiveness	Very strong	Moderate	Very strong	Strong	TBD	TBD	TBD
Discriminative ability	Strong	Very Strong	Strong	Strong	TBD	TBD	TBD
Applicable to a wide range	Strong	Very strong	Very strong	Very strong	Very strong	Strong	Very strong
Applicable to a heterogenous population	Strong	Very strong	Very strong	Strong	Very strong	Strong	Very strong
Tested widely	Moderate	Very strong	Strong	Strong	No	No	Strong
Easy to use	Strong	Strong	Strong	Strong	Very strong	Strong	Strong

Child Health Questionnaire (CHQ); Childhood Health Assessment Questionnaire (CHAQ); Juvenile Arthritis Disease Activity Score (JADAS); Juvenile Arthritis Multidimensional Assessment Report (JAMAR); Juvenile Arthritis Quality of Life Questionnaire (JAQQ); Pediatric Quality of Life Inventory (Peds QL); Rheumatology Quality of Life Scale (PRQL); TBD, to be determined.

due to the disease and not age-related limitations. The Paediatric Rheumatology International Trials Organization suggests that the removal of the aids/devices and help from the CHAQ does not alter the interpretation of the Disability Index. They report that the simplified questionnaire is a more effective alternative when assessing disability in patients with JIA.

Both with and without modifications, CHAQ has excellent reliability and validity and reasonable responsiveness. It also has good discriminative properties, can be administered to children of all ages, and is of great use in the clinical setting for long-term follow-up of children with JIA. It is valuable for longitudinal studies and clinical trials and has become the preferred measure in both settings. For these reasons, the CHAQ is the functional status measure most used as one of the six core variables for the assessment of change in JIA.

Juvenile Arthritis Quality of Life Questionnaire (JAQQ)

The JAQQ was designed to measure physical and psychosocial function as well as an array of general symptoms (reviewed in[3]). The instrument contained items across four dimensions: gross motor function, fine motor function, psychosocial function, and general symptoms. The initial validation study demonstrated good construct validity, moderate correlations with measures of disease activity and excellent correlations with pain. Responsiveness was shown by correlations of change scores, as well as by the ability of JAQQ to discriminate among patients based on physician global assessment of change.

A second iteration of the JAQQ saw the item number reduced to 74. A pain dimension, added as a supplement to JAQQ, included a VAS, a five-point ordinal scale, and, for children younger than

10 years, a five-point happy/sad face model. Twenty paediatric rheumatologists and therapists confirmed face and content validity of this version. Construct validity and responsiveness were established. Responsiveness was also shown to be maintained over time and to be at least as good as responsiveness of CHAQ, CHQ, or Peds QL. Enhancement of responsiveness was shown by a reduction in the number of items scored.

JAQQ has been translated into different languages and used in different cultural settings while maintaining its measurement properties (reviewed in[3]). A Canadian study showed that JAQQ was highly predictive of several short-term outcomes in a large cohort of children with JIA.[11] JAQQ has been developed in a detailed fashion, resulting in excellent reliability, validity, and responsiveness. It can be administered to children of all ages and disease onset types in a reasonable time with minimal assistance, and it can be scored quickly by hand; this makes it practical for use in both clinical and research settings.

Quality of My Life Questionnaire (QoMLQ)

The QoMLQ was developed to measure overall quality of life separate from health status or HRQoL. The instrument is made up of two separate 100 mm VAS, with the descriptors 'worst' and 'best,' that direct respondents to indicate their QoL. This is meant to assess problems caused by the disease itself and those caused by overall difficulties not directly related to the disease. This approach demonstrated clear differences between the scales, indicating that separation of the two factors is important. The QoMLQ demonstrated fair parent–child agreement and good convergent construct validity.[14] The minimal clinically important difference for improvement in QoL and HRQoL were given scores that enables clinicians to interpret QoMLQ results in a clinically meaningful way. QoMLQ is a short and easy-to-use generic instrument that is highly reliable and valid.

In further work from the same group, a novel approach was used in an attempt to measure the gap between one's current situation and one's expectations. The Gap Study quantified these gaps for a whole series of domains in children with rheumatic diseases.[15] The result was the development of a measure with 72 items distributed among five-gap scales (GapS). The GapS is currently undergoing further development.

Child Health Questionnaire (CHQ)

The CHQ is a family of generic quality-of-life instruments that have been designed for children 5–18 years of age. The CHQ measures 14 unique physical and psychosocial concepts. The parent form is available in two lengths (50 or 28 items) distributed in several dimensions: global health, physical activities, everyday activities, pain, behaviour, well-being, self-esteem, general health, and family. Scores can be analysed separately, the CHQ Profile Scores, or combined to derive an overall physical and psychosocial score, the CHQ Summary Scores.

The Paediatric Rheumatology International Trials Organization (PRINTO) has validated CHQ for use in 32 countries (reviewed in [3]). In one study that included 6639 participants (one-half had JIA, and one-half were healthy), mean scores for physical and psychosocial summary scores were significantly lower for JIA patients relative to controls. In a further study that included three distinct geographical regions (eastern Europe, western Europe, and Latin America), determinants of poor HRQoL were similar across all regions, with physical well-being affected by the level of disability and psychosocial well-being affected by the intensity of pain.[16] A study on improvements in HRQoL with abatacept used the CHQ to demonstrate tangible benefits of the drug.[17] CHQ was used in combination with CHAQ in a trial of etanercept, where it was shown to be highly responsive[7]; a comparable trial of methotrexate came to the same conclusion.[18] It has been suggested that JAQQ may be at least as responsive as CHQ for studies in JIA,[1] although CHQ has become the preferred measure of QoL for JIA trials because of its general nature.

Paediatric Quality of Life Inventory (PedsQL)

PedsQL is a modular instrument, containing generic and disease-specific cores, designed to measure HRQoL in children and adolescents 2–18 years old. Since 1999, the generic core has undergone various iterations and translations, the most recent of which, the PedsQL 4.0 Generic Core Scales, contains 23 items distributed in four scales: physical, emotional, social, and school functioning. A Rheumatology Module was developed for the PedsQL and it contains 22 disease-specific items distributed over five scales: pain, daily activities, treatment, worry, and communication.[19] It is completed by children and their parents and consists of versions appropriate for either children or teenagers and parents of children or teenagers. When it is completed separately, parent–child concordance has been good. This instrument was shown to have excellent reliability, validity, and responsiveness in a study of 271 children with various rheumatic diseases, 91 of whom had JIA, and their parents. Reliability varied with the age of the child, being less for younger children. In addition, a PedsQL Multidimensional Fatigue Scale was developed and validated in conjunction with the core scales and rheumatology modules.[20] The results of that initial study confirmed the initial reliability and validity of the PedsQL Multidimensional Fatigue Scale in paediatric rheumatology.

PedsQL remains an instrument that is in widespread use[21,22] and has been an important addition to the outcome measures available for use in JIA.

KIDSCREEN

The KIDSCREEN project set out to develop and validate the first European cross-cultural family of HRQoL instruments for children and adolescents, including self-reported and proxy-rated versions. The 10 dimensions examined on the KIDSCREEN instrument are: physical well-being, psychological well-being, mood and emotions, social support and peers relation, parents relation and home life, self-perception, autonomy, cognitive and school functioning, bullying and social rejection, and perceived financial opportunities. In the initial validation study, 2526 child/proxy pairs (aged 8–18 years) from 7 different European countries completed the questionnaire. The results demonstrated that the initial 52 item KIDSCREEN instrument proved to be a valid measure to assess relationships between youth and proxy reports.[23]

Since its initial validation, KIDSCREEN-52 has undergone psychometric property assessment. The questionnaire was administered to 22 827 children and adolescents in 13 European countries, which demonstrated acceptable levels of sensitivity and validity.[24] The instrument has also been shortened to 27 and 10 items and translated into many languages, with accompanying validation studies for each version. This is a promising tool for use in clinical and epidemiological studies. Of particular interest is a study that used the KIDSCREEN-52 questionnaire to measure the outcome effectiveness of a psychosocial rehabilitation programme by assessing HRQoL of children living with different chronic diseases, including JIA.[21]

Paediatric Rheumatology Quality of Life Scale (PRQL)

The PRQL is a recently developed, simple, 10-item questionnaire that focuses on HRQoL in both physical health and psychosocial health.[25] Although there are a number of HRQoL scales available for use in children with JIA, it has been suggested that there is a need for an instrument that is simple, easy to administer, quick, and can be used in patients across different paediatric rheumatic diseases. The PRQL aims to fill that void by targeting incorporation into regular clinical care. The short questionnaire is intended for use as a proxy and self-report with a proposed age range of 7–18 years. The PRQL underwent preliminary validation in approximately 470 children with JIA and 800 healthy children in one study at one Italian centre.[25]

The PRQL was found to have good measurement properties and is reported as a valid instrument for clinical and research assessments of HRQoL in children with JIA. Further study with this instrument is needed to determine if the validity holds across multiple rheumatological diseases and in different cultural environments.

Juvenile Arthritis Multidimensional Assessment Report (JAMAR)

JAMAR was recently developed as an instrument that combines the traditional patient-reported outcomes used in clinical evaluation of children with JIA with other outcomes measures not addressed by conventional instruments.[26] There are a total of 15 measurements on the JAMAR, including assessments of overall well-being, pain, functional ability and HRQoL, as well as an evaluation of morning stiffness, overall level of disease activity, rating of disease activity and course, proxy or self-assessment of joint involvement and extra-articular symptoms, description of side effects from medications, and assessment of therapeutic compliance and satisfaction with the outcome of the illness. The JAMAR is proposed for use as both a proxy report for parents of patients aged 2–18 and a patient self-report with the suggested age range of 7–18 years old. The JAMAR is the first questionnaire to include a proxy or self-report assessment of articular symptoms.

In a validation study of 332 children and 618 parents of children with JIA over 2563 visits, the JAMAR was found to be feasible and to possess face and content validity.[26] The report indicates that parents and patients found that the JAMAR was user-friendly, easy to understand, and quick to complete (<15 minutes). Scoring of the various elements can be achieved in less than 5 minutes. The JAMAR was designed to be completed in a clinical setting and focuses on information needed for care, therefore only two straightforward measures were selected for assessment of physical function and HRQoL. The VAS for pain, well-being, and disease activity are presented as 21 numbered circles, instead of the conventional 10 cm horizontal line, to facilitate scoring without a ruler. A study by the same group determined that the simpler 21 numbered circles increases the precision of the parent/patient ratings.[27]

The main limitation to the validation study of the JAMAR is that the instrument was tested in Italian parents and patients at only one centre. In addition, the JAMAR may not provide sufficient detail regarding patient-reported outcomes of sleep disturbances, fatigue, coping, and family life, because of the short nature of the questionnaire. Research with this report is ongoing and will be followed with interest given its multidisciplinary nature.

Composite disease activity scores for juvenile idiopathic arthritis

The paediatric response criteria and American College of Rheumatology (ACR) JIA core set focus on change in disease state and assess improvement or worsening of disease activity. Currently, the ACR Pedi 30, representing a 30% change from baseline, is the measure of disease activity used to demonstrate efficacy of biologic therapy in JIA.[28] The Juvenile Arthritis Disease Activity Score (JADAS) was recently developed as a composite disease activity score for JIA. This instrument includes four of the measures from the core set: active joint count, physician's global assessment of disease activity, patient and parent global assessment of overall well-being, and erythrocyte sedimentation rate(ESR). Joint count is modified based on evaluation of 10, 27, or 71 joints in three different versions of the instrument. JADAS has been shown to have good measurement properties, including reliability and responsiveness to clinical change; however, a recent study has shown that there are properties of the JADAS-27 that may hamper its feasibility.[29] In addition, JADAS cut-off values for remission, minimal disease activity, and parent- and child-acceptable symptom state in JIA have been developed.[30] In cross-validation analyses, the JADAS proved to have good construct and discriminant validity and ability to predict disease outcome; however, misclassification of active disease versus inactive disease by JADAS scores was not uncommon.[31] A number of recent research studies have used the JADAS-27 and JADAS-71 as their disease activity measurement.[32,33]

Instruments for use in other rheumatic diseases

In recent years, rheumatic diseases other than JIA have been brought to international attention where a number of instruments have been developed and validated for use in both adults and children. Specifically, both juvenile dermatomyositis (JDM) and juvenile systemic lupus erythematosus (JSLE) have measures of disease activity and damage for both adult- and childhood-onset disease.

Two different groups developed similar core sets of measures for the juvenile idiopathic inflammatory myopathies. The International Myositis Assessment Clinical Studies Group (IMACS) used consensus methods to develop a core set that is applicable to both adult and paediatric idiopathic inflammatory myopathy. The PRINTO and the Paediatric Rheumatology Collaborative Study Group (PRCSG) also developed core set measures for JDM and JSLE. There are elements of each core that are common to both sets: the physician and patient global assessments, muscle strength, physical function, and muscle enzymes. PRINTO and PRCSG recently provided a definition of JDM improvement that reflects the consensus rating of experienced clinicians. They have incorporated clinically meaningful change in core set variables for the evaluation of global response to therapy in JDM.[34] The IMACS group has also published their efforts to provide a definition of improvement in the juvenile idiopathic inflammatory myopathies.[35] The agreed-upon improvement definition involves three of the six core set measures bettered by more than 25%; however, this definition awaits further validation.

There are three validated tools for the assessment of strength, physical function, and endurance in children with JDM.[36] First, muscle strength has been assessed with the Manual Muscle Testing (MMT), where several variations exist depending on the number of muscles assessed and how muscle strength is scored.[37] Although the 8-muscle MMT performed similarly to the 26-muscle MMT score and demonstrated good reliability, construct validity and responsiveness, there are concerns about inter-rater reliability and application standardization. At least one study has made use of this test in conjunction with additional tools to demonstrate a greater severity of proximal weakness in polymyositis in comparison with dermatomyositis.[38]

CHAQ has also been validated for use in children with JDM in two separate studies where construct validity, reliability and responsiveness were demonstrated (reviewed in[3]). The Childhood Myositis Assessment Scale (CMAS) is an alternate assessment of physical function. This instrument is a 14-item observational performance-based tool that includes assessment of proximal, distal, and axial strength and upper and lower extremity strength and also includes timed endurance items. This instrument has good inter-rater reliability, construct validity and responsiveness. In addition, age-related norms have been published.[39] The drawback to the CMAS is that it is therapist administered and requires significant time to complete. One long-term outcomes study in JDM has determined that chronic course was the strongest predictor of poor prognosis.[40] This report makes good use of a combination of the three available instruments to study JDM: MMT, CHAQ, and CMAS.

As discussed earlier, the development of disease activity measures for JSLE was undertaken at the same time as the JDM initiative. Ultimately, the measures for JSLE included specific immunologic tests and renal function measures, as well as physician and parent global assessments, a measure of growth and development and a measure of HRQoL. The Systemic Lupus Erythematosus Disease Activity Index (SLEDAI), British Isles Lupus Assessment Group Index (BILAG), and Systemic Lupus Activity Measure (SLAM) were tested in the assessment of JSLE and were all shown to be highly sensitive to clinical change. The same group showed the responsiveness of European Consensus Lupus Activity Measurement (ECLAM) for juvenile SLE and suggested that it might be more sensitive than SLEDAI in this population. A recent study has described preliminary criteria for global flares in juvenile SLE and are based around absolute changes in the SLEDAI and BILAG.[41]

The CHQ, PedsQL, and CHAQ have been used as HRQoL measures in juvenile SLE patients[42–44]; however, there was a need for a new HRQoL instrument designed specifically for JSLE. The Simple Measure of Impact of Lupus Erythematosus in Youngsters (SMILEY) is a brief questionnaire that includes parallel child and parent versions with a 5-faces scale for responses. It includes four domains: effect on self, limitations, social, and burden of SLE. A multicentre validation study demonstrated face, content, construct, and concurrent validity, test–retest reliability, and internal consistency.[45] Further work with this instrument has been an international effort to provide a cross-cultural adaptation with translation to 13 different languages.[46] Studies to validate the translated and adapted versions of SMILEY are ongoing and will be of interest to achieve widespread use. There have been recent reports of studies on SLE patients that make use of the English version of SMILEY.[47]

Instrument usage and applicability

The majority of instruments discussed here, and HRQoL assessments in general, have been used mainly within a clinical research setting. However, the use of patient-reported outcomes in daily clinical practice has been the topic of much discussion in recent years. This encompasses self-assessment of functional status, as well as symptoms or other concerns, such as patient needs and satisfaction with care. The use of these instruments in a clinical setting may be of use in the early detection of HRQoL problems and may allow for a tailored intervention prior to an escalation of the issue. In particular, children with a chronic disease are at greater risk of HRQoL problems than their healthy peers.[48] For example, the effects of childhood disease and its treatment often increase the child's dependence on adults and decrease the child's participation in peer- and school-based activities. This could have an adverse effect on the accomplishment of developmental tasks, resulting in an impaired QoL. A questionnaire designed to capture pertinent information given to the clinician prior to or at the time of consultation might be of use to identify, monitor, and discuss particular HRQoL issues faced by children with JIA.

The choice of instrument is dependent upon the extent, impact, and type of paediatric rheumatic disease. For example, there are some instruments that focus on measuring the impact of physical function alone and others that assess physical function as a part of overall health status or QoL.

A survey conducted by one of us in 2005 determined that while paediatric rheumatologists are aware of this form of measurement and have participated in studies that have included such measures, in general, clinicians tend not to use them in clinical practice (unpublished data). It is possible that these instruments have been slow to infiltrate the clinical picture as a result of logistical issues around completing the forms and having the information available to the clinician in a timely fashion. New technology and the availability of web-based platforms (see 'Electronic applications') may facilitate the usage of HRQoL assessments in clinical practice by allowing the clinician to access the data at the time of a clinic visit. In the future, these instruments could potentially become an integral part of complete patient care.

Electronic applications

The concept of using technology to make clinical assessment of HRQoL more efficient is expected to gain momentum across all fields in the coming years. For example, the general HRQoL survey, KIDSCREEN-27, was recently translated into an online version, and consistency as well as reliability scores were comparable to those reported in the literature for the paper version.[49]

To overcome the practical issues around completing HRQoL forms in the clinic for clinical assessment, a group based in the Netherlands has developed a novel and innovative web-based application (KLIK PROfile) for patient-reported outcome measures. This program is tailored to general daily paediatric clinical practice, and specifically targets children with chronic diseases.[50] The authors envision parents and children completing the HRQoL at home up to 3 days before the consultation, and clinicians retrieving the patient-reported outcomes directly from the website. It will be of interest to follow the KLIK PROfile and its evaluation for ease of implementation and use. This type of program may promote the widespread use of HRQoL instruments in daily clinical practice, as well as facilitating collaborative research between centres.

Conclusion

QoL, HRQoL, physical function, and health status instruments are often used as outcome measures in children with significant musculoskeletal involvement, but mostly for research purposes. These tools allow healthcare providers and researchers to account for varying degrees of patient-perceived states of ability as well as the impact of disability on overall well-being. When used at regular intervals during a disease course, the instruments are also able to account for changes in HRQoL perceptions, and many longitudinal research studies take patient -reported outcome measurements every 6 months. There are now many instruments available and it is important that when one is determining which instrument to use that the specific purpose of measurement be considered. If one is considering a measurement of physical function, the CHAQ is adequate for most purposes for most diseases. If one is considering a measurement of HRQoL in children with JIA, the JAQQ or Peds QL would be appropriate. The JADAS is an excellent measure of disease activity and could be adopted as an instrument to help plan disease management. Several newer measures including the KIDSCREEN and JAMAR are now available and it will be interesting to monitor their use over time. In addition, the SMILEY looks like an excellent tool for the assessment of HRQoL in childhood SLE.

Despite a broad range of available instruments, concern persists around the utility of these measures for clinical practice. However, availability of electronic and web-based versions of these instruments will, in all likelihood, enhance their use in the clinical setting. Whether this proves to be the case in practice remains to be determined.

References

1. Duffy CM. Measurement of health status, functional status, and quality of life in children with juvenile idiopathic arthritis: clinical science for the pediatrician. *Rheum Dis Clin N Am* 2007;33(3):389–402.
2. Brunner HI, Ravelli A. Developing outcome measures for paediatric rheumatic diseases. *Best Pract Res Clin Rheumatol* 2009;23(5):609–624.
3. Duffy CM, Feldman BM. Assessment of health status, function, and quality of life outcomes. In: Cassidy J, Laxer R, Petty R, Lindsley C (eds) *Textbook of pediatric rheumatology*. Elsevier Saunders, Philadelphia, PA, 2012:157–167.
4. Susic GZ, Stojanovic RM, Pejnovic NN et al. Analysis of disease activity, functional disability and articular damage in patients with juvenile idiopathic arthritis: a prospective outcome study. *Clin Exp Rheumatol* 2011;29(2):337–344.
5. Thastum M, Herlin T. Pain-specific beliefs and pain experience in children with juvenile idiopathic arthritis: a longitudinal study. *J Rheumatol* 2011;38(1):155–160.
6. Lal SD, McDonagh J, Baildam E et al. Agreement between proxy and adolescent assessment of disability, pain, and well-being in juvenile idiopathic arthritis. *J Pediatrics* 2011;158(2):307–312.
7. Prince FHM, Geerdink LM, Borsboom GJJM et al. Major improvements in health-related quality of life during the use of etanercept in patients with previously refractory juvenile idiopathic arthritis. *Ann Rheum Dis* 2010;69(1):138–142.

8. Halbig M, Horneff G. Improvement of functional ability in children with juvenile idiopathic arthritis by treatment with etanercept. *Rheumatol Int* 2009;30(2):229–238.
9. Miller ML, Kress AM, Berry CA. Decreased physical function in juvenile rheumatoid arthritis. *Arthritis Care Res* 1999;12(5):309–313.
10. Wessel J, Kaup C, Fan J et al. Isometric strength measurements in children with arthritis: reliability and relation to function. *Arthritis Care Res* 1999;12(4):238–246.
11. Oen K, Tucker L, Huber AM et al. Predictors of early inactive disease in a juvenile idiopathic arthritis cohort: results of a Canadian multicenter, prospective inception cohort study. *Arthritis Rheum* 2009;61(8):1077–1086.
12. Geerdink LM, Prince FHM, Looman CWN, van Suijlekom-Smit LWA. Development of a digital Childhood Health Assessment Questionnaire for systematic monitoring of disease activity in daily practice. *Rheumatology* (Oxford) 2009;48(8):958–963.
13. Saad-Magalhães C, Pistorio A, Ravelli A et al. Does removal of aids/devices and help make a difference in the Childhood Health Assessment Questionnaire disability index? *Ann Rheum Dis* 2010;69(1):82–87.
14. Gong GWK, Young NL, Dempster H, Porepa M, Feldman BM. The Quality of My Life questionnaire: the minimal clinically important difference for pediatric rheumatology patients. *J Rheumatol* 2007;34(3):581–587.
15. Gong GWK, Barrera M, Beyene J et al. The Gap Study (GapS) interview—developing a process to determine the meaning and determinants of quality of life in children with arthritis and rheumatic disease. *Clin Exp Rheumatol* 2007;25(3):486–493.
16. Gutiérrez-Suárez R, Pistorio A, Céspedes Cruz A et al. Health-related quality of life of patients with juvenile idiopathic arthritis coming from 3 different geographic areas. The PRINTO multinational quality of life cohort study. *Rheumatology* (Oxford) 2007;46(2):314–320.
17. Ruperto N, Lovell DJ, Li T et al. Abatacept improves health-related quality of life, pain, sleep quality, and daily participation in subjects with juvenile idiopathic arthritis. *Arthritis Care Res* 2010;62(11):1542–1551.
18. Céspedes-Cruz A, Gutiérrez-Suárez R, Pistorio A et al. Methotrexate improves the health-related quality of life of children with juvenile idiopathic arthritis. *Ann Rheum Dis* 2008;67(3):309–314.
19. Varni JW, Burwinkle TM, Limbers CA, Szer IS. The PedsQL as a patient-reported outcome in children and adolescents with fibromyalgia: an analysis of OMERACT domains. *Health Qual Life Outcomes* 2007;5:9.
20. Varni JW, Burwinkle TM, Szer IS. The PedsQL Multidimensional Fatigue Scale in pediatric rheumatology: reliability and validity. *J Rheumatol* 2004;31(12):2494–2500.
21. Békési A, Török S, Kökönyei G et al. Health-related quality of life changes of children and adolescents with chronic disease after participation in therapeutic recreation camping program. *Health Qual Life Outcomes* 2011;9:43.
22. Butbul Aviel Y, Stremler R, Benseler SM et al. Sleep and fatigue and the relationship to pain, disease activity and quality of life in juvenile idiopathic arthritis and juvenile dermatomyositis. *Rheumatology (Oxford)* 2011;50(11):2051–2060.
23. Robitail S, Simeoni M-C, Erhart M et al. Validation of the European proxy KIDSCREEN-52 pilot test health-related quality of life questionnaire: first results. *J Adolesc Health* 2006;39(4):596.e1–10.
24. Ravens-Sieberer U, Gosch A, Rajmil L et al. The KIDSCREEN-52 quality of life measure for children and adolescents: psychometric results from a cross-cultural survey in 13 European countries. *Value Health* 2008;11(4):645–658.
25. Filocamo G, Schiappapietra B, Bertamino M et al. A new short and simple health-related quality of life measurement for paediatric rheumatic diseases: initial validation in juvenile idiopathic arthritis. *Rheumatology (Oxford)* 2010;49(7):1272–1280.
26. Filocamo G, Consolaro A, Schiappapietra B et al. A new approach to clinical care of juvenile idiopathic arthritis: the Juvenile Arthritis Multidimensional Assessment Report. *J Rheumatol* 2011;38(5):938–953.

27. Filocamo G, Davì S, Pistorio A et al. Evaluation of 21-numbered circle and 10-centimeter horizontal line visual analog scales for physician and parent subjective ratings in juvenile idiopathic arthritis. *J Rheumatol* 2010;37(7):1534–1541.

28. Lovell DJ, Giannini EH, Reiff A et al. Etanercept in children with polyarticular juvenile rheumatoid arthritis. Pediatric Rheumatology Collaborative Study Group. *New Engl J Med* 2000;342(11):763–769.

29. de Vries L, Heijstek M, Groot N, Bulatović M, Wulffaat N. Validation of the juvenile arthritis disease activity score in 1124 patient visits. *Pediatr Rheumatol* 2011;14;9(Suppl 1):154.

30. Consolaro A, Bracciolini G, Ruperto N et al. Remission, minimal disease activity and acceptable symptom state in juvenile idiopathic arthritis. *Arthritis Rheum* 2012;64(7):2366–2374.

31. Ringold S, Wallace CA, Rivara FP. Health-related quality of life, physical function, fatigue, and disease activity in children with established polyarticular juvenile idiopathic arthritis. *J Rheumatol* 2009;36(6):1330–1336.

32. Pelajo CF, Lopez-Benitez JM, Kent DM et al. 25-Hydroxyvitamin D levels and juvenile idiopathic arthritis: Is there an association with disease activity? *Rheumatol Int* 2012;32(12):3923–3929.

33. Gheita T, Kamel S, Helmy N, El-Laithy N, Monir A. Omega-3 fatty acids in juvenile idiopathic arthritis: effect on cytokines (IL-1 and TNF-α): disease activity and response criteria. *Clin Rheumatol* 2012;31(2):363–366.

34. Ruperto N, Pistorio A, Ravelli A et al. The Paediatric Rheumatology International Trials Organization provisional criteria for the evaluation of response to therapy in juvenile dermatomyositis. *Arthritis Care Res* 2010;62(11):1533–1541.

35. Oddis CV, Rider LG, Reed AM et al. International consensus guidelines for trials of therapies in the idiopathic inflammatory myopathies. *Arthritis Rheum* 2005;52(9):2607–2615.

36. Huber AM. Update on the assessment of children with juvenile idiopathic inflammatory myopathy. *Curr Rheumatol Rep* 2010;12(3):204–212.

37. Rider LG, Koziol D, Giannini EH et al. Validation of manual muscle testing and a subset of eight muscles for adult and juvenile idiopathic inflammatory myopathies. *Arthritis Care Res* 2010;62(4):465–472.

38. Harris-Love MO, Shrader JA, Koziol D et al. Distribution and severity of weakness among patients with polymyositis, dermatomyositis and juvenile dermatomyositis. *Rheumatology (Oxford)* 2009;48(2):134–139.

39. Rennebohm RM, Jones K, Huber AM et al. Normal scores for nine maneuvers of the Childhood Myositis Assessment Scale. *Arthritis Rheum* 2004;51(3):365–370.

40. Ravelli A, Trail L, Ferrari C et al. Long-term outcome and prognostic factors of juvenile dermatomyositis: a multinational, multicenter study of 490 patients. *Arthritis Care Res* 2010;62(1):63–72.

41. Brunner HI, Mina R, Pilkington C et al. Preliminary criteria for global flares in childhood-onset systemic lupus erythematosus. *Arthritis Care Res* 2011;63(9):1213–1223.

42. Moorthy LN, Harrison MJ, Peterson M, Onel KB, Lehman TJA. Relationship of quality of life and physical function measures with disease activity in children with systemic lupus erythematosus. *Lupus* 2005;14(4):280–287.

43. Houghton KM, Tucker LB, Potts JE, McKenzie DC. Fitness, fatigue, disease activity, and quality of life in pediatric lupus. *Arthritis Rheum* 2008;59(4):537–545.

44. Meiorin S, Pistorio A, Ravelli A et al. Validation of the Childhood Health Assessment Questionnaire in active juvenile systemic lupus erythematosus. *Arthritis Rheum* 2008;59(8):1112–1119.

45. Moorthy LN, Peterson MGE, Baratelli M et al. Multicenter validation of a new quality of life measure in pediatric lupus. *Arthritis Rheum* 2007;57(7):1165–1173.

46. Moorthy LN, Peterson MGE, Baratelli MJ, Hassett AL, Lehman TJA. Preliminary cross-cultural adaptation of a new pediatric health-related quality of life scale in children with systemic lupus erythematosus: an international effort. *Lupus* 2010;19(1):83–88.

47. Moorthy LN, Peterson MGE, Hassett A, Baratelli M, Lehman TJA. Impact of lupus on school attendance and performance. *Lupus* 2010;19(5):620–627.

48. Grootenhuis MA, Koopman HM, Verrips EGH, Vogels AGC, Last BF. Health-related quality of life problems of children aged 8–11 years with a chronic disease. *Dev Neurorehabil* 2007;10(1):27–33.

49. Lloyd K. Kids' Life and Times: using an Internet survey to measure children's health-related quality of life. *Qual Life Res* 2011;20(1):37–44.

50. Haverman L, Engelen V, van Rossum MAJ, Heymans HSA, Grootenhuis MA. Monitoring health-related quality of life in paediatric practice: development of an innovative web-based application. *BMC Pediatrics* 2011;11:3.

Genetics and environment

SECTION 5

Genetics and
environment

CHAPTER 37

Basics of genetics

Anne Barton

Why should we be interested in genetics?

Human beings are more than 99% genetically identical to one another but it is the differences in the genetic code between individuals that account for differences in characteristics such as hair colour, eye colour, and height. These genetic differences also contribute to the risk of developing many diseases, including musculoskeletal diseases. An individual's genetic make-up does not change during life; therefore, the genetic changes exist before disease onset and may *cause* disease as opposed to being a *result* of disease. Thus, understanding which genetic changes are involved in disease has the potential to identify important biological pathways that could be targeted by the development of new drugs. Patients vary in the severity of their disease and response to treatment; again, genetic variation may be important and could be used to select the best drugs to use in particular patient groups.

How do we know if a disease has a genetic component?

Twin, family, migration, and adoption studies can all be used to determine whether there is a strong contribution from genetic factors to a particular disease. Twin studies assume that monozygotic (MZ) twins are genetically identical, whereas dizygotic (DZ) twins share only 50% of their genetic code. If a disease is more common in MZ than DZ twins, that is strong supporting evidence for a genetic component to risk. For rarer diseases, where it is more difficult to identify MZ and DZ twins, family studies can provide support for a role for genetics. The **sibling recurrence risk ratio**, λ_s, measures the ratio of disease in the siblings of patients with disease compared to the general population:

$$\text{Sibling Recurrence risk } (\lambda_s) = \frac{\text{risk of disease in sibling}}{\text{risk of disease in general population}}$$

The higher the value of λ_s, the stronger the genetic contribution to disease. Table 37.1 shows the estimated λ_s values for a number of autoimmune and musculoskeletal diseases.

What is genetics?

Genetic information is carried by DNA, which is located within the nucleus of cells. The total genetic code for an individual is called

Table 37.1 The sibling recurrence risk (λ_s) for a number of common musculoskeletal diseases

Disease	Estimated λ_s
Rheumatoid arthritis	2–11
Systemic lupus erythematosus	20–40
Psoriatic arthritis	20–40
Juvenile idiopathic arthritis	10–20
Systemic sclerosis	10–150
Osteoarthritis	1–9
Ankylosing spondylitis	30–40

the genome and can be thought of as a book. Within this book, the information is divided into chapters (chromosomes). Each cell carries all the genetic information but not all of it is used in every cell. For example, genes that code for enzymes important in the processing of alcohol, are only used (expressed) in liver cells. This is analogous to highlighting sections of a book pertinent to different readers. DNA is made up of four nucleotides: adenine (A), guanine (G), cytosine (C), and thymidine (T), similar to letters in our alphabet. Different combinations of three nucleotides result in amino acids, which are arranged into **exons**, and these exons can be thought of as words. As in language, different words make up different sentences and in this analogy, it is the sentence that is the equivalent of a gene. Different genes code for different protein products. The spaces in between the exons are the **introns** and, although they are not involved in the structure of the final protein product, a sentence would not make sense without these spaces.

Genetic variation

Many books contain typographical errors and the same is true of the genome. The simplest type of variation is where one nucleotide is replaced by another and this is called a **single nucleotide polymorphism (SNP)** (Figure 37.1). As we inherit two copies of the genome (one from our mother and one from our father), the change in the DNA sequence may be present on none, one, or both strands of DNA. Each version of the DNA sequence at that point is called an **allele**. For example, suppose that at a given point in the

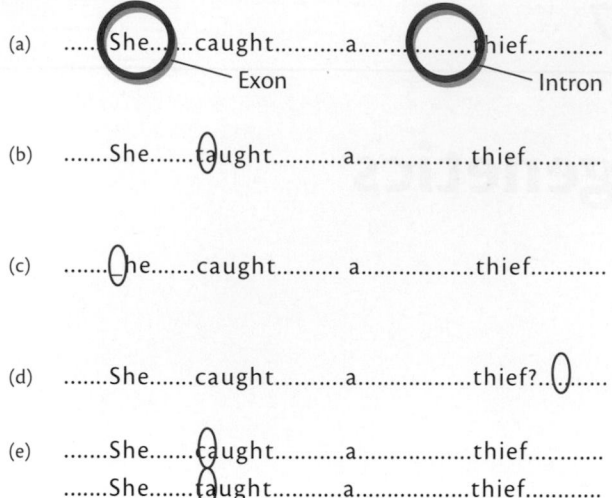

Fig. 37.1 Variation in the DNA sequence is analogous to typographical errors in a book. (a) Genes are like sentences with the words being exons and the spaces between being introns. Note that the introns in a gene are larger than the spaces between words in a sentence. Note also that in the genome sequence, introns are also letters but do not make words. There are more letters in the English alphabet than in the genetic alphabet, which consists of just A, C, G, and T. (b) A change in a single letter (equivalent to a C to T single nucleotide polymorphism (SNP)) in an exon can change the meaning of the sentence. This is analogous to a non-synonymous amino acid substitution that changes the function of a protein. (c) An example of a deletion that changes the meaning of the sentence/protein. (d) In the genome, most changes occur in introns or in the DNA between genes but this can still affect the function of the protein. (e) Individuals inherit two copies of each gene. If a C/T SNP occurs at the position shown, for an individual, the genotype could be CC, CT, or TT depending on whether the nucleotide is changed in none, one or both versions of the gene.

DNA sequence, some people in the population carry an A nucleotide but some people carry a G, the A version is called the **A allele** and vice versa. The allele that is less common in the population is called the **minor allele**. International efforts have resulted in a catalogue of these variants being made; each is assigned an **rs number** so that researchers across the world will know what variant is being analysed if it is called by its rs number. It is like saying Chapter 3, page 4, paragraph 2, line 7, letter 18. If the SNP occurs in an exon, it may result in a change in the amino acid coded for, which may in turn affect the function of the protein. However, most SNPs occur in the introns of genes and in the DNA between genes. Other types of variation occur in the genome such as insertions or deletions, copy number variants, and other types of repeat sequences. However, SNPs are the most abundant type of variation and are easy to accurately genotype using modern technologies, so they have become the marker of choice for testing in genetic studies.

Linkage disequilibrium

Linkage disequilibrium (LD) is the non-random inheritance of alleles. During meiosis, recombination occurs on average once per chromosome arm. Therefore, variants that are close together on a chromosome are unlikely to become separated by recombination and are said to be in LD (Figure 37.2). In the general population, a lot of meiotic events separate individuals but, as recombination tends to occur at specific points in the genome (recombination hot spots), there are still blocks of DNA which are always inherited together and the variants within those blocks will always be in LD

with each other. This means that it is not necessary to genotype every variant across the genome to find which occur more frequently in people with a disease; because of LD, genotyping one variant will provide information on the other variants that segregate with it. The r^2 value measures the degree of correlation between variants. An r^2 value of 1 between two variants means that the genotype at one will perfectly predict the genotype at the second variant. For two variants to be perfectly correlated, they must have identical allele frequencies. If the allele frequencies are different, the r^2 value will be less than 1. The down side of LD is that if a genetic variant is found to occur more frequently in cases with disease, it may be acting as a marker for another variant which is the one causing disease, rather than being the causal variant itself.

Association studies

The most common study design in genetic studies is the **case–control association study**. The frequency of alleles at different locations across the genome is compared between cases with disease and those without (controls). The observed genotype and/or allele frequency in cases is compared with the expected frequency seen in controls using a basic χ^2 test, which can be translated into a significance (p) value. Alleles that occur at significantly different frequencies between cases and controls are said to be associated with disease. A common study design is the **candidate gene** approach in which variants in particular genes or genetic regions are selected for investigation. This approach requires a prior hypothesis about the role of the locus in disease, based on knowledge about the disease or results of previous studies of the same locus. There are approximately 30 000 genes and 10 million SNPs in the genome, so selecting the right variants in the right gene requires considerable luck. In recent years, a more systematic, hypothesis-free approach has been adopted in which hundreds of thousands of SNPs spanning the genome are tested for association, the **genome-wide association study** (GWAS). This has proved to be more successful in identifying variants associated with many musculoskeletal diseases.

Genome-wide association study: basic principles

As technology has improved, chip-based genotyping methods have developed and evolved to allow genotyping of ever-increasing numbers of SNPs, ranging from hundreds of thousands to millions of variants, dependent on the type of chip purchased. Allele frequencies of the SNPs are compared between cases and controls and if significant differences are found, the locus is said to be associated with disease. However, this simply provides an indication that the region is important. Given that there are estimated to be 10 million SNPs in the genome, the chance that the causal variant for a particular disease has been included on the SNP chip is low and association more commonly arises due to LD with the causal variant. Hence, fine mapping of the region and, ultimately, functional studies are required to identify the variant that causes the disease.

'Common disease, common variant' hypothesis

Common musculoskeletal diseases are complex; that is, both genetic and environmental factors contribute to susceptibility. In different individuals with disease, different combinations of genetic and environmental factors cause the same disease, so identifying the effect of a single genetic variant is diluted because not all cases will carry that variant. The 'common disease, common variant'

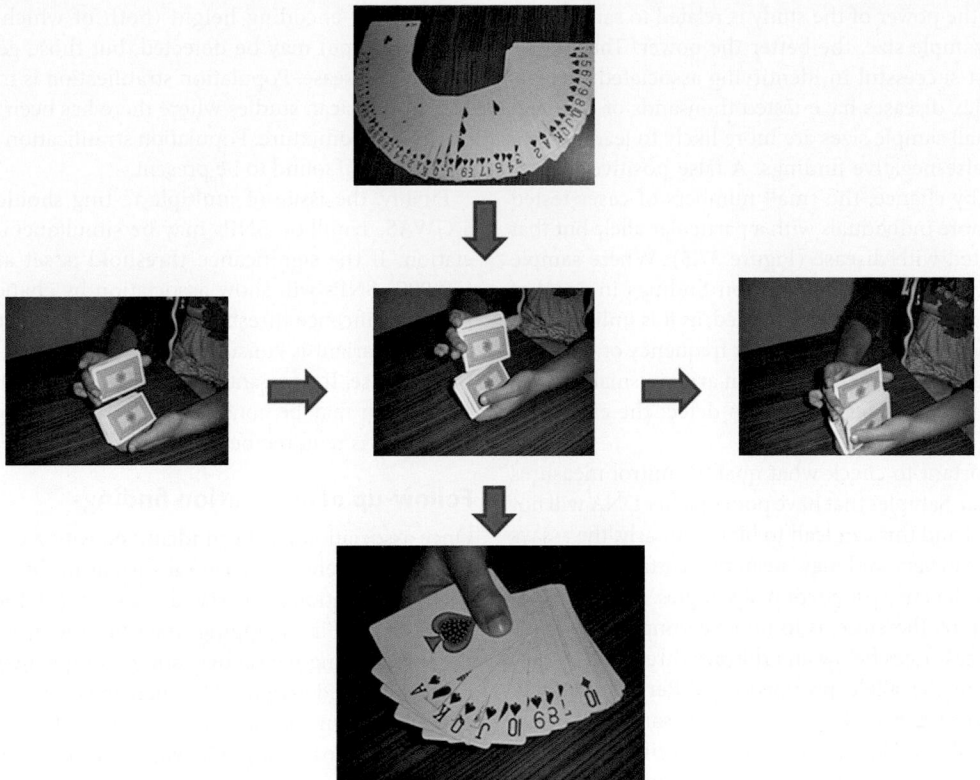

Fig. 37.2 Linkage disequilibrium (LD) is like shuffling a pack of cards. If a new pack of cards is shuffled, there will still be runs of the same suit that occur together because shuffling has not separated them. This is analogous to LD where chunks of DNA are inherited together so the genotype at one position can predict the genotype at another. Shuffling occurs during meisosis in the genome by recombination. Two unrelated individuals from the same ethnic group are likely to have been descended from a few common ancestors. Therefore, even though many generations has passed and many shuffling opportunities have occurred, there are still runs of nucleotides in the genome that are inherited together and are similar between individuals.

hypothesis assumes that complex diseases, particularly those that present later in life, will be caused by variants that are common in the population. Thus, if a mutation occurs in the DNA sequence that has a major effect on health, that individual will be unlikely to reproduce and the mutation will die out with the individual. However, if the variant produces only a small detrimental effect on health, the individual will be able to reproduce and the mutation will be passed on through successive generations until the allele is common in the population. For late-onset diseases, disease-causing alleles will not affect reproductive health and so it is expected that they will be common in the population and individually will have modest effects on disease risk. Indeed, this has proved to be true for many of the variants found to be associated with musculoskeletal diseases.

Effect sizes and power

The effect size of a variant refers to its contribution to disease risk; for diseases that are relatively uncommon in the population, such as most of the inflammatory musculoskeletal diseases, the effect size is equivalent to the odds ratio (OR) from a case–control study. For example, an OR of 3 (equivalent to the largest genetic effect contributing to rheumatoid arthritis (RA)) means that an individual is three times more likely to develop disease compared to the general population. This must be set into the context of the risk of disease in a population. Thus, if the risk of RA in the general population is 1%, then carrying the major risk allele only increases the risk

to 3%. For complex diseases, many genetic variants contribute to risk but each has only a modest effect. For example, many of the risk variants have OR of 1.1 to 1.2, equating to a 10–20% increased risk of developing disease. The **power** of the study relates to the ability to detect these effect sizes at a given significance threshold. Power is directly related to sample size; the bigger the sample size, the greater the power to detect associated variants. The power is also influenced by the allele frequency of associated variants; if the minor allele is uncommon in the population (<5%, for example) even larger sample sizes are required to have sufficient power to detect the effect. It is conventional to describe the test statistics in relation to the minor allele. Thus, an OR of 0.8 with confidence intervals that do not include 1 means that the minor allele protects against disease, or that the more common major allele increases risk. Whereas alleles contributing to the risk of diseases may only have modest effect sizes, side effects from drugs can be caused by alleles with very large effect sizes. For example, the OR of developing liver toxicity after using the antibiotic flucloxacillin is increased over 80-fold if patients carry the HLA-B*5701 allele. The sample size required to detect such effects is much lower because power is also determined by the effect size that is expected.

Assessing the quality of a case–control association study

When reading articles reporting findings of case–control association studies, there are several points worth bearing in mind. First, as described above, the power of the study is related to sample size and the larger the sample size, the better the power. The studies that have been most successful in identifying associated variants for common, complex diseases have tested thousands of case and control samples. Small sample sizes are more likely to lead to both false-positive and false-negative findings. A false-positive finding may arise because, by chance, the small numbers of cases tested happen to contain more individuals with a particular allele but that allele is not associated with disease (Figure 37.3). Where sample sizes are small, validation of the association findings in another case control sample is therefore recommended, as it is unlikely that the second set of cases will also have a higher frequency of the allele simply by chance. False-negative findings can arise in small sample sizes because the study is underpowered to detect the effect size expected.

Second, it is important to check what quality control measures have been undertaken. Samples that have poor-quality DNA will not be reliably genotyped and this can lead to bias. Similarly, the assays for SNP genotyping can vary and may mean that certain SNPs only produce high quality data in a proportion of samples. An important quality control measure, therefore, is to remove samples and SNPs with genotyping success rates below an arbitrary threshold.

Third, SNPs where the allele proportions differ significantly from Hardy–Weinberg expectations in control samples should be removed from analysis. **Hardy–Weinberg equilibrium** occurs when two alleles (p and q) in a population that is randomly mating result in frequencies that satisfy the formula:

$$p^2 + q^2 + 2pq = 1$$

The most common reason for deviation from Hardy–Weinberg equilibrium is genotyping error. However, it is possible that disease is only caused in cases if two copies of the minor allele are present and, in that situation, Hardy–Weinberg expectations would not be met in the cases. For that reason, exclusion of SNPs from analysis is generally based on the Hardy–Weinberg results in the control sample.

Fourth, it is important to consider whether population stratification could have resulted in a false-positive finding. Population stratification refers to populations of different ancestral or ethnic backgrounds being included in the case and/or control samples. For example, if all the cases are recruited from Scotland and all the controls from Italy, associations with the gene encoding red hair

H H T H H H H T T H   T H H H T T T T H T
1st attempt   2nd attempt
7 H, 3 T   4H, 6T

Fig. 37.3 The influence of chance on results from case–control studies when sample sizes are small. I flicked a 2p coin 10 times and the results are shown, where H = heads and tails = T. If I did this a large number of times, I would expect 50% H and 50% T. Indeed, overall, there were 11H and 9T, almost 50:50. In this small sample, however, by chance, there were 7 H and 3 T at the first attempt but more T than H the second time. If the first attempt was cases and the second attempt controls, one might conclude that H is more common in cases and T more common in controls, i.e. that H is associated with being a case rather than a control. Although this is an extreme example and such small sample sizes would never be published for a genetic association study, it illustrates the point that small sample sizes can bias findings; the larger the sample size, the more robust the estimates of true allele frequency are.

or the gene encoding height (both of which differ significantly across Europe) may be detected, but those genes are not associated with disease. Population stratification is more of a problem in North American studies where there has been Hispanic and Afro-Caribbean admixture. Population stratification can be corrected for statistically, if found to be present.

Finally, the issue of multiple testing should be considered. In a GWAS, 1 million SNPs may be simultaneously tested for association. If the significance threshold is set at p = 0.05, 1 in 20 (50 000) SNPs will show association by chance alone. Therefore, strict significance thresholds of $p < 5 \times 10^{-8}$ are generally required before a variant is considered to be confirmed as being associated with disease. If a variant is associated at $p < 0.05$ but $>5 \times 10^{-8}$, the association may be considered possible or suggestive but further validation is required before it can be confirmed.

Follow-up of association findings

Once association has been identified with a disease, the next stage is to try to identify the causal variant in the region. As described above, association may arise due to LD with the true causal variant at the locus. Fine mapping describes the process of interrogating the surrounding region by testing multiple markers to identify the most associated variant. Resequencing of the surrounding region is emerging as an alternative approach as the cost of the technology reduces. In most cases, this will still leave a group of variants with equal evidence for association, but bioinformatics approaches can be used to determine which are most likely to affect the function of the DNA and, therefore, which are most likely to play a role in disease causation. Ultimately, proof that a particular variant causes disease requires functional studies to explore how and why that particular genetic variation predisposes to disease.

Other study designs

In the early part of this century, linkage studies remained a popular choice of study design for investigating complex diseases. Linkage studies are performed in families and, for late-onset diseases like the musculoskeletal diseases, families in which two affected siblings were identified were studied. At a particular marker in the genome with two alleles, *A* and *a*, the siblings have a 25% chance of both having the genotype *AA*, a 50% chance of *Aa*, and a 25% chance of *aa*. If both siblings have the disease and the marker is linked with disease, then the siblings will show a deviation from the expected allele sharing so that they share the allele linked with disease more often. Linkage studies in complex diseases have been largely disappointing and so genetic researchers now undertake association studies. Although the focus in this chapter has been on case control association studies, the **transmission disequilibrium test (TDT)** is an alternative association study design that can be undertaken in families. The test assesses the inheritance of alleles from heterozygous parents (for example, genotype *Aa*) to offspring affected with disease. For a locus not linked or associated with disease, the *A* allele would be expected to be transmitted to the offspring 50% of the time and the *a* allele 50%. The TDT examines large number of families and tests for a deviation from the expected 50:50 transmission of alleles. An allele that is transmitted more than 50% of the time is linked and associated with disease. For equivalent power, more samples need to be tested in a TDT (2 parents and 1 offspring) compared with a case control study (1 case and 1 control) so most researchers now undertake case–control association studies.

Case–control association studies remain the most popular and effective way of identifying loci that increase susceptibility to musculoskeletal diseases, but other designs are required to address important clinical questions. For example, patients vary in their response to treatment and, in extreme cases, can develop serious side effects. **Nested case control** or **cohort study** designs can be used to identify genetic contributions. For example, if response to therapy is measured using a continuous scale such as the 28 joint count disease activity score (DAS28) used in RA, then the sample will consist only of cases with RA treated with the drug of interest and on whom the DAS28 at specific time points is recorded. Logistic regression analysis can be used to correlate changes in the DAS28 over time with genotype. Similarly, investigation of genetic variants influencing other outcome measures, such as the development of erosions in RA, require prospectively recruited cohorts of patients in which some will develop erosions and others will not, by specified time points.

Clinical applications of genetics

Currently, the only routine genetic test performed in musculoskeletal settings is testing of thiopurine *S*-methyltransferase (TPMT) polymorphisms in patients starting azathioprine. Variations in the gene have a large effect on the activity of the enzyme and metabolism of azathioprine. Hence, knowledge about the genotype can inform clinical decisions about whether to start azathioprine and at what dose. Although a huge number of genetic associations have been discovered in the past 5 years for a range of musculoskeletal diseases, it is too soon for these breakthroughs to translate into the development of new drugs, but that aim is actively being pursued by many research groups. In coming years, the breakthroughs in identifying genetic variations increasing the risk of common musculoskeletal conditions should lead to a better understanding of how these diseases occur and how they can be better treated or prevented.

Further reading

Anderson CA, Pettersson FH, Clarke GM et al. Data quality control in genetic case-control association studies. *Nat Protoc* 2010;5:1564–1573.

Cardon LR, Palmer LJ. Population stratification and spurious allelic association. *Lancet* 2003;361:598–604.

Clarke GM, Anderson CA, Pettersson FH et al. Basic statistical analysis in genetic case-control studies. *Nat Protoc* 2011;6:121–133.

Palmer LJ, Cardon LR. Shaking the tree: mapping complex disease genes with linkage disequilibrium. *Lancet* 2005;366:1223–1234.

CHAPTER 38

Environment

Christopher R. Holroyd, Nicholas C. Harvey, Mark H. Edwards, and Cyrus Cooper

Introduction

Musculoskeletal disease covers a broad spectrum of conditions, the aetiology of many of which remains poorly understood. It is generally accepted that most chronic diseases result from both genetic predisposition and environmental exposures, and there is increasing evidence that the interaction between the two plays a major role. Recent attention has focused primarily on identifying possible genetic risk factors, and although this has provided clues regarding disease pathogenesis, it is becoming clear from genome-wide association studies (GWAS) that fixed genetic variation leaves a substantial part of disease variability unexplained. Environmental factors and their interaction with the genome may account for a greater proportion of chronic disease risk than previously thought, and thus represent a large missing piece of the puzzle. Attention might sensibly be focused on developing methods to assess an individual's environmental exposure with the same precision currently employed in the characterization of fixed genetic variation.

In this chapter we discuss the importance of evaluating environmental exposure and describe the evidence that disease pathogenesis may be partly determined by the interplay of environment and genotype, through mechanisms such epigenetics. We then describe the environmental influences on musculoskeletal disease across the whole life course, using three examples: osteoarthritis (OA), osteoporosis, and rheumatoid arthritis (RA).

Gene–environment interactions

It has long been proposed that many musculoskeletal diseases have a large genetic component. Advances in genotyping technologies over recent years, such as the introduction of the polymerase chain reaction and the completion of the Human Genome project, have made it possible to perform association studies on a genome-wide basis by analysing large numbers of single nucleotide polymorphisms (SNPs) spread at close intervals across the genome, rather than focusing in on one gene at a time. These GWAS have been applied to many rheumatic diseases, and have identified numerous potential genes involved in their pathogenesis. Interestingly, the effect size of most of the polymorphic variants identified has been small and variants identified in one study may not be consistently reproduced in others.

Although future studies employing more detailed assessment of the genome may yet delineate a substantial fixed genetic component of disease pathogenesis, it is likely that non-genetic 'environmental factors' and subsequent gene–environment interaction contributes to a substantial proportion of risk. Gene–environment interactions are thought to be involved in most complex diseases and explain how a specific genotype may result in several different phenotypes depending on environmental factors. This concept underlies the phenomenon of developmental plasticity, ubiquitous in the natural world.

If the interplay of complex environmental and genetic factors is to be elucidated, it is important that both genetic variation and environmental exposures are reliably measured. While GWAS techniques continue to be refined, there has been a relative paucity in the effort to accurately assess the other half of the gene–environment equation. It is essential that modern methods are developed to assess an individual's environmental exposure with the same precision as is possible for the individual's genome.

The exposome

The concept of the 'exposome' was first proposed in a 2005 editorial.[1] It is defined as a record of all environmental exposures, both internal and external, that an individual receives over their lifetime, from conception through to childhood, early and late adulthood, and finally death. These exposures are numerous and include environmental chemicals, radiation, diet, drugs, behaviour and lifestyle, infections, and psychological stress (Figure 38.1). Unlike the genome, which is fixed at conception, an individual's chemical environment is dynamic and varies over the life course due to changes in internal and external exposures. Thus, characterizing the human exposome is likely to be extremely challenging and would require longitudinal sampling, especially during critical time points such as fetal development, puberty, and early adulthood. Generally long-term exposures are not assessed and often any environmental exposure data that is collected in studies is via questionnaire-based methods which may be limited in their capacity to capture comprehensive and accurate data. This is particularly common in dietary assessment, which is particularly prone to measurement error, and highlights the need to improve the tools used for quantitative exposure assessment.

Two approaches have been suggested by epidemiologists to characterize the exposome: a 'bottom-up' or 'top-down' strategy (Figure 38.2).[2] A top-down approach measures both exogenous and endogenous chemicals such as protein adducts, metals, and metabolites as well as gene expression using repeated blood samples collected during the life of an individual. This would identify all potentially important exposures, but would provide no information regarding source. The bottom-up approach would involve sampling water, dietary sources, and air, with subsequent quantification of chemicals in the samples. This would identify potential exogenous exposures and their sources, but would miss any endogenous exposures such as gender, obesity, and psychological stress. It is currently not possible to measure all chemicals in blood, so it has been suggested that the focus should be on classes of substances that are known to be biologically active.[2] Although challenging, the exposome could promote discovery of key exposures responsible for chronic disease and potentially pave the way for personalized medicine.

Epigenetic mechanisms

Key times in the potential influence of the exposome on adult chronic disease are the period in utero and early infancy. There is increasing evidence that epigenetic mechanisms are central to the process by which early environmental exposure affects health and disease in later life. Epigenetics literally means 'above genes' and refers to changes in phenotype, usually mediated by altered gene expression, caused by mechanisms other than changes in the underlying DNA sequence. These changes are stable and heritable, and may last through multiple generations.[3] The most studied epigenetic mechanism is DNA methylation, which involves the addition of a methyl group to DNA mainly at CpG sites. Methylation within the promoter area of genes generally leads to gene repression. Thus, there is usually an inverse relationship between the extent of CpG methylation and gene expression. At the single-cell level, a gene is either methylated or not (i.e. 0 or 100%), but across a tissue, some cells will contain a methylated gene and some an unmethylated gene. This balance of methylation and non-methylation across the whole tissue allows a continuous range of methylation (0–100%) at the tissue level, and thus a graded relationship between environment and gene expression.

Histone modification is a second epigenetic pathway and involves post-translational changes of the amino acids that make up histones. Histones are small proteins involved in packaging of DNA into chromatin. If the amino acids in the chain are changed, the shape of the histone will be modified and consequently the way that DNA is wrapped around the histones may also change, leading to

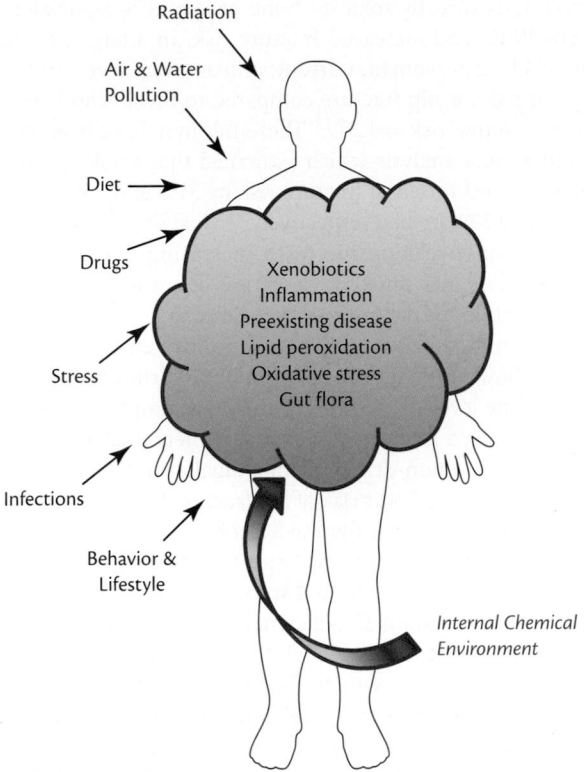

Fig. 38.1 The exposome represents the combined exposures from all sources that reach the internal chemical environment.

Reprinted by permission from Macmillan Publishers: Rappaport SM. Implications of the exposome for exposure science. Journal of Exposure Science and Environmental Epidemiology 2011;21:5–9.

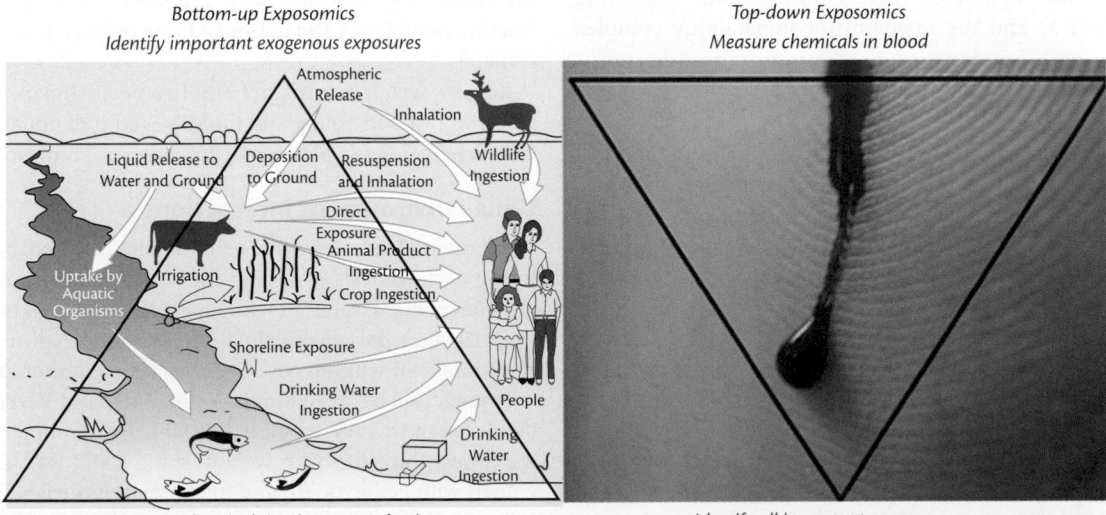

Fig. 38.2 Two strategies for characterizing the exposome.

Reprinted by permission from Macmillan Publishers: Rappaport SM. Implications of the exposome for exposure science. Journal of Exposure Science and Environmental Epidemiology 2011;21:5–9.

alterations in gene expression. The two types of epigenetic modification are mechanistically linked and work together to determine which gene or gene set is transcribed.

DNA methylation is an essential process for normal development in higher organisms. Patterns of methylation differ through the phases of development: after conception, and with the exception of imprinted genes, gamete methylation patterns are erased during early blastocyst formation. During embryonic and fetal development, maternal or environmental factors can disrupt the patterns of DNA methylation; examples of this process have been shown in animal models. Abnormal DNA methylation during development may permit specific genes to undergo inappropriate expression during adult life, resulting in disease development.[4]

The first example of an association between a periconceptional exposure and DNA methylation in humans was shown in Dutch subjects prenatally exposed to famine during the Dutch Hunger Winter in 1944–1945.[5] Exposed subjects showed persistent epigenetic differences in a variety of genes compared to their unexposed, same-sex siblings. Epigenetic mechanisms are now well established in the development and progression of a variety of cancer types,[6] and there is increasing evidence that they may have a role in the development of musculoskeletal disease.

The remainder of this chapter focuses on the environmental influences on three musculoskeletal diseases: osteoporosis, RA, and OA.

Osteoporosis

Genetic factors

Although it has been estimated that between 50% and 85% of the variance in bone mineral density (BMD) is genetically determined,[7] genes identified by over 10 GWAS only account for 4–5% of the genetic variance in BMD. Genetic regulation of bone mass is likely to be determined by numerous genes, all with a small effect size.[8] Of the genes identified, many encode proteins known to influence bone mass, such as oestrogen receptor 1 (ESR1), vitamin D receptor (VDR), lipoprotein receptor-related protein 5 (LRP5), and the tumour necrosis factor (TNF) receptor superfamily (TNFSF). The mechanisms by which other identified genes affect bone mass remains unknown. Examples include microtubule-regulating kinase 3 (MARK3) and the major histocompatability complex (MHC).

Early environmental factors

There is evidence that the risk of osteoporosis might be modified by early environmental factors. Retrospective studies of adults aged 60–75 years have shown that there is a significant relationship between low weight at 1 year and reduced adult bone mineral content (BMC) at the spine and hip in late adulthood.[9] Similarly, poor growth in utero and during the first year of life, using the same cohort, was associated with alterations in bone architecture, cortical size and geometry, with a reduction in BMC, resulting in increased fracture in later life.

Prospective studies of mother–offspring cohorts have shown that certain maternal lifestyle factors during pregnancy and body composition are associated with offspring bone mass at birth and in later childhood.[10–12] Independent predictors of greater neonatal BMC include greater maternal birth weight, height, parity, fat stores (triceps skinfold thickness), and lower physical activity in late pregnancy. Maternal smoking is associated with lower neonatal bone mass. Maternal serum 25(OH)-vitamin D concentration has also been associated with reduced offspring bone mass at birth and in later childhood.[12]

Late environmental factors

Lifestyle factors associated with low bone mass include excess alcohol, smoking, low calcium intake, low body weight, physical inactivity, and vitamin D deficiency.

Smoking is directly toxic to bone cells and is associated with reduced BMD and increased fracture risk. In a large prospective study of 116 229 women, current smokers were seen to have an increased risk for hip fracture compared to those who have never smoked (relative risk = 1.3).[13] These findings have been consolidated in a meta-analysis which estimated that smoking increases lifetime hip and vertebral fracture risk by 31% and 13% in women and 40% and 32% in men respectively.[14] Most studies have reported a dose–response relationship, with increasing fracture risk with increasing amounts smoked. Cessation of smoking is associated with a reduction in fracture risk over time.

Alcohol in moderation may have a positive effect on BMD and has been shown to reduce markers of bone turnover and parathyroid hormone levels.[15] However, excess consumption is associated with an increased fracture risk. A recent meta-analysis concluded that compared to non-drinkers, individuals who consume up to 1 drink per day have a lower risk of hip fracture (relative risk 0.8) and those who consume more than two alcoholic drinks per day have a higher risk.[16] There is some evidence that drinking beer increases fracture risk more than wine and spirits.

Calcium and vitamin D deficiencies are associated with bone loss. In the United States NHANES III survey, greater calcium intake was associated with higher BMD in women but not in men.[17] Supplementation with calcium alone has been associated with gains in BMD compared with placebo, but may be insufficient to prevent postmenopausal bone loss and fracture. Combining calcium supplementation with vitamin D may be more effective; a recent systematic review of randomized trials in which calcium or calcium in combination with vitamin D supplementation was administered to adults aged over 50 year concluded that supplementation was associated with a modest (12%) risk reduction for fracture of all types and a reduced rate of bone loss at the hip and spine.[18]

Regular weightbearing activity has been shown to increase or preserve BMD in young and middle-aged individuals, but appears insufficient alone to prevent postmenopausal bone loss.[19]

Gene–environment interactions

Two potential gene–environment interactions have been described in the pathogenesis of osteoporosis. Polymorphisms in the IL-6 gene have been associated with hip BMD in women who were more than 15 years post menopause and in those with inadequate calcium intake or without oestrogen replacement therapy.[20] Similarly, the interaction between lumbar spine BMD and VDR genotype has been shown to vary with birthweight.[21,22] Among individuals in the lowest third for birth weight, spine BMD was higher in individuals with genotype *BB* and in contrast, spine BMD was reduced in individuals with the same genotype in the upper third of birth weight distribution. This suggests that genetic effects on BMD may be modified by the uterine environment.

Epigenetic mechanisms

Epigenetic mechanisms may play a role in the pathogenesis of osteoporosis, although exact mechanisms remain to be elucidated. Epigenetic modifications may underlie the association between low maternal vitamin D, low umbilical cord calcium concentration, and reduced offspring bone mass. Vitamin D mediates its effects by acting upon vitamin D response elements in the promoter region of target genes, and in animal studies has been shown to influence genes encoding calcium transporters.[23] One study has demonstrated that the expression of the placental calcium transporter PMCA3 gene predicts neonatal BMC.[24] Modified expression of the genes encoding placental calcium transporters, by epigenetic regulation, might represent the means whereby maternal vitamin D status could influence neonatal bone mineral accrual.

Epigenetic modulation of the hypothalamic–pituitary–adrenal (HPA) axis may represent a second mechanism whereby poor maternal environment can impair offspring bone mineral accrual. Elevated levels of circulating cortisol in adult life have been associated with reduced BMD and increased rates of bone loss.[25] Animal studies have confirmed that protein restriction during pregnancy is associated with reduced methylation of key CpG-rich islands in the promoter region of the glucocorticoid receptor (GR) gene, and this results in elevated GR expression and features of hypercortisolism.[26]

Rheumatoid arthritis

Genetic factors

Candidate gene analysis and GWAS have identified numerous genes implicated in the pathogenesis of RA. Although the shared epitope of HLA DRB1 remains the strongest genetic risk factor, polymorphisms in other genes have been identified and replicated in different populations, such as the protein tyrosine phosphatase gene (PTPN22), which has a role in B- and T-cell regulation. The peptidyl arginine gene (PAD14) has also been implicated, but findings have not been consistently replicated across different populations. Recent work has focused on other genes such as CTLA4, FCRL3, and the major histocompatability complex 2A (MHC2A), and the possibility that certain polymorphisms may predict a patient's response to treatment.

Early environmental factors

There is limited evidence regarding the developmental origins of RA or the effect of exposures during early life. Data from the prospective Nurses' Health Study of 87 077 white women has suggested that increased birthweight may be associated with a twofold increase in the risk of adult onset RA, compared with those of average birthweight, even after adjustment for confounders and other potential risk factors.[27] One explanation for this finding is that individuals with a higher birthweight have lower serum cortisol levels, as do patients with RA, and may be unable to increase cortisol production in response to chronic inflammation and stress. These findings need replication before any firm conclusions can be made.

Late environmental factors

Most studies investigating potential environmental factors in the development of RA have focused on smoking, hormonal factors, and diet. Caffeine intake has also been investigated in some studies,

yielding mixed and often inconclusive results.[28,29] Smoking has been consistently linked with RA, in terms of both disease risk and severity. Current smokers and those who have quit within 10 years appear to have a moderately increased risk of RA especially if the individual is male or seropositive.[30,31] Both duration of smoking and intensity appear to be risk factors, with heavy smokers having over a 13-fold increased risk.[30] After 10 years post-cessation of smoking, risk of RA appears to return to that of the normal population. Some studies have not implicated smoking as a risk factor for seronegative RA.[32]

High consumption of olive oil, fruit and vegetables, oily fish, or vitamin D (a 'Mediterranean diet')[33,34] have been suggested as playing a possible protective role in the development of RA. Red meat consumption has been implicated as moderately increasing the risk of inflammatory arthritis,[35] but this has not been confirmed in a more recent study.[36]

Other environmental factors that have been associated with RA include exposure to viruses (Epstein–Barr and parvovirus), blood transfusion, stress, and obesity; alcohol consumption and breast-feeding may have a protective role.

Gene–environment interactions

There is increasing evidence highlighting potential gene-environmental interactions in RA. A recent population-based case control study of 858 RA cases and 1048 controls suggested a potential interaction between smoking and the HLA DRB1 shared isotope.[37] The risk of developing seropositive RA was increased in individuals who smoked and carried double copies of the HLA DRB1 isotope compared to smokers with no copies of HLA DRB1. There is also evidence to suggest an interaction between smoking and the PTPN22 gene.

Epigenetics

RA patients are generally considered to have a Th1-based phenotype; histone modification, particularly histone deacetylation, has been implicated in epigenetically regulating T helper cell differentiation.[38,39] Similarly smoking, which is associated with an increased risk for RA and a more severe disease outcome, has been shown to reduce the expression of the histone deacetylases (HDAC) SIRT1 and 2 in the lungs of rats.[40] Furthermore, pretreatment of macrophages with the SIRT1 activator significantly inhibited the smoke-induced production on proinflammatory cytokines. This has led to the development of HDAC inhibitors as therapeutic agents, which have been used with beneficial effects in vitro or in experimental models of RA.[41]

DNA methylation may represent a second epigenetic pathway. For example, methylation of genomic DNA of T cells derived from RA patients has been shown to be globally lower than that of T cells from healthy controls.[42] Areas of hypomethylation in the IL-6 gene have been identified in the peripheral blood mononuclear cells in RA patients compared to healthy donors.[43] It has been postulated that this hypomethylation may lead to increased expression of the proinflammatory cytokine IL-6.

Osteoarthritis

Genetic factors

It has been estimated from studies in twins that 58% of OA is genetic and it appears that different genes may influence the development of

OA at different sites. For example, the IL-1 gene cluster may confer susceptibility for knee OA but not hip OA.[44] Other potential genetic influences for the development of knee OA include the oestrogen receptor-alpha (*ESR1*) gene, the metalloproteinase gene (*ADAM12*), *GDF5*, and *PTGS2*, which encodes the enzyme cyclooxygenase 2. The frizzled-related protein-3 (*FRZB*) gene has been associated with hip OA in females. There appears to be greater genetic effects on OA of the hand compared to other sites, possibly due to the relatively weaker environmental role in the pathogenesis of hand OA. There is a moderately increased risk of familial clustering of hand OA, especially amongst sisters of women severely affected by hand OA. Genes associated with hand OA include *VDR* and *MATN3*, which encodes the extracellular matrix protein, matrilin-3.

Early environmental factors

A few studies have described a relationship between birthweight and the development of OA. In the MRC National Study of Health and Development, a prospective study of 2986 men and women, low weight at birth was associated with the development of hand OA in men, but not in women, at age 53 years.[45] Similarly, in a separate United Kingdom cohort, the Hertfordshire Cohort, low birthweight and weight at 1 year was associated with an increased prevalence of lumbar spine OA in men aged 65 years.[22]

Late environmental factors

Major cohort studies of OA, such as the Framingham Study,[46] the Chingford 1000 Women Study,[47] and the Bristol OA500 Study[48] have identified several environmental risk factors associated with OA. Of these, obesity, prior joint surgery, and physical activity are most frequently reported. Obesity, which is the main preventable risk factor, has been repeatedly shown to significantly increase the risk of knee OA in both sexes. In addition, high body mass index (BMI) is more strongly associated with bilateral rather than unilateral knee osteoarthritis. Results from the Framingham Osteoarthritis Study and other cohorts suggest that weight loss reduces the risk of developing knee OA. Individuals who lost weight in the 10-year period prior to their baseline radiograph had a 50% reduction in the odds of having radiographic knee OA for every 2 kg/m^2 decrease in BMI.[49] There is also a positive association between obesity and hip OA; however, this appears to be of lower strength than that observed with knee OA. Some authors have reported an association between obesity and hand OA but results have been conflicting and the relationship remains controversial.

Individuals with a history of regular sports participation or who have abnormal or injured joints are also at an increased risk of OA. Data again from the Framingham cohort have shown that the number of hours per day of heavy physical activity was associated with the risk of incident radiographic knee osteoarthritis (odds ratio = 1.3 per hour) after adjustments were made for confounding factors.[50] Risk was greatest among individuals in the upper tertile of BMI who performed more than 3 hours/day of heavy physical activity. No association was seen from moderate and light physical activity, number of blocks walked, or number of flights of stairs climbed daily.

Gene–environment interactions

There is some evidence of a gene–environment interaction in the development of OA. Prevalence of lumbar spine OA has been shown to vary according to VDR genotype and birthweight.[21,22]

Among individuals in the lowest third for birth weight, individuals with genotype 'BB' had an increased prevalence of vertebral osteophytes; in contrast, prevalence of osteophytes was reduced in individuals of the same genotype in the highest third of birthweight distribution.

Epigenetics

Despite a relative paucity of data, early evidence points to a possible role of epigenetics in OA. Differences in the promoter methylation status of genes associated with OA have been observed in a few small studies. For example, 8 out of 9 patients with OA had at least one unmethylated site in the promoter region of the *MMP9* gene, whose expression is increased in OA, compared to 1 out of 5 controls. Further studies have reported differences in the methylation status in the MMP-3 and ADAM-TS4 gene promoter regions in chondrocytes from patients with OA compared to patients without OA. Although these studies have shown an association, there was considerable variation between patients and further work is needed to prove that hypomethylation results in the activation of degradative enzymes involved in OA.

Conclusion

It is likely that most chronic musculoskeletal disease results from a combination of genes, environmental factors, and an interaction between the two. There is increasing evidence for the role of the environment in early life, in addition to later environmental influences in osteoporosis, RA, and OA pathogenesis. Lifelong environmental influences (the exposome) are difficult to capture; however, addressing gene–environment interactions, with better assessment of the exposome, may lead to novel strategies to reduce the burden of chronic musculoskeletal disease in future generations.

Acknowledgements

This work was supported by grants from the Medical Research Council, Arthritis Research UK, National Osteoporosis Society, and the International Osteoporosis Foundation.

References

1. Wild CP. Complementing the genome with an 'exposome': the outstanding challenge of environmental exposure measurement in molecular epidemiology. *Cancer Epidemiol Biomarkers Prev* 2005;14(8):1847–1850.
2. Rappaport SM. Implications of the exposome for exposure science. *J Expo Sci Environ Epidemiol* 2011;21(1):5–9.
3. Jaenisch R, Bird A. Epigenetic regulation of gene expression: how the genome integrates intrinsic and environmental signals. *Nat Genet* 2003;33(Suppl):245–254.
4. Tang WY, Ho SM. Epigenetic reprogramming and imprinting in origins of disease. *Rev Endocr Metab Disord* 2007;8(2):173–182.
5. Heijmans BT, Tobi EW, Stein AD et al. Persistent epigenetic differences associated with prenatal exposure to famine in humans. *Proc Natl Acad Sci U S A* 2008;105(44):17046–17049.
6. Gronbaek K, Hother C, Jones PA. Epigenetic changes in cancer. *APMIS* 2007;115(10):1039–1059.
7. Pocock NA, Eisman JA, Hopper JL et al. Genetic determinants of bone mass in adults. A twin study. *J Clin Invest* 1987;80(3):706–710.
8. Ralston SH, Uitterlinden AG. Genetics of osteoporosis. *Endocr Rev* 2010;31(5):629–662.
9. Dennison EM, Syddall HE, Sayer AA, Gilbody HJ, Cooper C. Birth weight and weight at 1 year are independent determinants of bone mass in the seventh decade: the Hertfordshire cohort study. *Pediatr Res* 2005;57(4):582–586.

10. Harvey NC, Poole JR, Javaid MK et al. Parental determinants of neonatal body composition. *J Clin Endocrinol Metab* 2007;92(2):523–526.

11. Godfrey K, Walker-Bone K, Robinson S et al. Neonatal bone mass: influence of parental birthweight, maternal smoking, body composition, and activity during pregnancy. *J Bone Miner Res 2001*;16(9):1694–1703.

12. Javaid MK, Crozier SR, Harvey NC et al. Maternal vitamin D status during pregnancy and childhood bone mass at age 9 years: a longitudinal study. *Lancet* 2006;367(9504):36–43.

13. Cornuz J, Feskanich D, Willett WC, Colditz GA. Smoking, smoking cessation, and risk of hip fracture in women. *Am J Med* 1999;106(3):311–314.

14. Ward KD, Klesges RC. A meta-analysis of the effects of cigarette smoking on bone mineral density. *Calcif Tissue Int* 2001;68(5):259–270.

15. Rapuri PB, Gallagher JC, Balhorn KE, Ryschon KL. Alcohol intake and bone metabolism in elderly women. *Am J Clin Nutr* 2000;72(5):1206–1213.

16. Berg KM, Kunins HV, Jackson JL et al. Association between alcohol consumption and both osteoporotic fracture and bone density. *Am J Med* 2008;121(5):406–418.

17. Bischoff-Ferrari HA, Kiel DP, Dawson-Hughes B et al. Dietary calcium and serum 25-hydroxyvitamin D status in relation to BMD among U.S. adults. *J Bone Miner Res* 2009;24(5):935–942.

18. Tang BM, Eslick GD, Nowson C, Smith C, Bensoussan A. Use of calcium or calcium in combination with vitamin D supplementation to prevent fractures and bone loss in people aged 50 years and older: a meta-analysis. *Lancet* 2007;370(9588):657–666.

19. Prince RL, Smith M, Dick IM et al. Prevention of postmenopausal osteoporosis. A comparative study of exercise, calcium supplementation, and hormone-replacement therapy. *N Engl J Med* 1991;325(17):1189–1195.

20. Ferrari SL, Karasik D, Liu J et al. Interactions of interleukin-6 promoter polymorphisms with dietary and lifestyle factors and their association with bone mass in men and women from the Framingham Osteoporosis Study. *J Bone Miner Res* 2004;19(4):552–559.

21. Dennison EM, Arden NK, Keen RW et al. Birthweight, vitamin D receptor genotype and the programming of osteoporosis. *Paediatr Perinat Epidemiol* 2001;15(3):211–219.

22. Jordan KM, Syddall H, Dennison EM, Cooper C, Arden NK. Birthweight, vitamin D receptor gene polymorphism, and risk of lumbar spine osteoarthritis. *J Rheumatol* 2005;32(4):678–683.

23. Kimball S, Fuleihan G, Vieth R. Vitamin D: a growing perspective. *Crit Rev Clin Lab Sci* 2008;45(4):339–414.

24. Martin R, Harvey NC, Crozier SR et al. Placental calcium transporter (PMCA3] gene expression predicts intrauterine bone mineral accrual. *Bone* 2007;40(5):1203–1208.

25. Dennison E, Hindmarsh P, Fall C et al. Profiles of endogenous circulating cortisol and bone mineral density in healthy elderly men. *J Clin Endocrinol Metab* 1999;84(9):3058–3063.

26. Weaver IC, Cervoni N, Champagne FA et al. Epigenetic programming by maternal behavior. *Nat Neurosci* 2004;7(8):847–854.

27. Mandl LA, Costenbader KH, Simard JF, Karlson EW. Is birthweight associated with risk of rheumatoid arthritis? Data from a large cohort study. *Ann Rheum Dis* 2009;68(4):514–518.

28. Karlson EW, Mandl LA, Aweh GN, Grodstein F. Coffee consumption and risk of rheumatoid arthritis. *Arthritis Rheum* 2003;48(11):3055–3060.

29. Heliovaara M, Aho K, Knekt P et al. Coffee consumption, rheumatoid factor, and the risk of rheumatoid arthritis. *Ann Rheum Dis* 2000 Aug;59(8):631–635.

30. Hutchinson D, Shepstone L, Moots R, Lear JT, Lynch MP. Heavy cigarette smoking is strongly associated with rheumatoid arthritis (RA), particularly in patients without a family history of RA. *Ann Rheum Dis* 2001;60(3):223–227.

31. Uhlig T, Hagen KB, Kvien TK. Current tobacco smoking, formal education, and the risk of rheumatoid arthritis. *J Rheumatol* 1999; 26(1):47–54.

32. Stolt P, Bengtsson C, Nordmark B et al. Quantification of the influence of cigarette smoking on rheumatoid arthritis: results from a population based case-control study, using incident cases. *Ann Rheum Dis* 2003;62(9):835–841.

33. Linos A, Kaklamani VG, Kaklamani E et al. Dietary factors in relation to rheumatoid arthritis: a role for olive oil and cooked vegetables? *Am J Clin Nutr* 1999;70(6):1077–1082.

34. Merlino LA, Curtis J, Mikuls TR et al. Vitamin D intake is inversely associated with rheumatoid arthritis: results from the Iowa Women's Health Study. *Arthritis Rheum* 2004;50(1):72–77.

35. Pattison DJ, Symmons DP, Lunt M et al. Dietary risk factors for the development of inflammatory polyarthritis: evidence for a role of high level of red meat consumption. *Arthritis Rheum* 2004;50(12):3804–3812.

36. Benito-Garcia E, Feskanich D, Hu FB, Mandl LA, Karlson EW. Protein, iron, and meat consumption and risk for rheumatoid arthritis: a prospective cohort study. *Arthritis Res Ther* 2007;9(1):R16.

37. Padyukov L, Silva C, Stolt P, Alfredsson L, Klareskog L. A gene-environment interaction between smoking and shared epitope genes in HLA-DR provides a high risk of seropositive rheumatoid arthritis. *Arthritis Rheum* 2004;50(10):3085–3092.

38. Chang S, Aune TM. Dynamic changes in histone-methylation 'marks' across the locus encoding interferon-gamma during the differentiation of T helper type 2 cells. *Nat Immunol* 2007;8(7):723–731.

39. Raza K, Falciani F, Curnow SJ et al. Early rheumatoid arthritis is characterized by a distinct and transient synovial fluid cytokine profile of T cell and stromal cell origin. *Arthritis Res Ther* 2005;7(4):R784–R795.

40. Yang SR, Wright J, Bauter M et al. Sirtuin regulates cigarette smoke-induced proinflammatory mediator release via RelA/p65 NF-kappaB in macrophages in vitro and in rat lungs in vivo: implications for chronic inflammation and aging. *Am J Physiol Lung Cell Mol Physiol* 2007;292(2): L567–L576.

41. Grabiec AM, Tak PP, Reedquist KA. Targeting histone deacetylase activity in rheumatoid arthritis and asthma as prototypes of inflammatory disease: should we keep our HATs on? *Arthritis Res Ther* 2008;10(5):226.

42. Richardson B, Scheinbart L, Strahler J et al. Evidence for impaired T cell DNA methylation in systemic lupus erythematosus and rheumatoid arthritis. *Arthritis Rheum* 1990;33(11):1665–1673.

43. Nile CJ, Read RC, Akil M, Duff GW, Wilson AG. Methylation status of a single CpG site in the IL6 promoter is related to IL6 messenger RNA levels and rheumatoid arthritis. *Arthritis Rheum* 2008;58(9): 2686–2693.

44. Loughlin J, Dowling B, Mustafa Z, Chapman K. Association of the interleukin-1 gene cluster on chromosome 2q13 with knee osteoarthritis. *Arthritis Rheum* 2002;46(6):1519–1527.

45. Poole J, Sayer AA, Cox V et al. Birth weight, osteoarthritis of the hand, and cardiovascular disease in men. *Ann Rheum Dis* 2003;62(10):1029.

46. Felson DT, Zhang Y, Hannan MT et al. Risk factors for incident radiographic knee osteoarthritis in the elderly: the Framingham Study. *Arthritis Rheum* 1997;40(4):728–733.

47. Hart DJ, Doyle DV, Spector TD. Incidence and risk factors for radiographic knee osteoarthritis in middle-aged women: the Chingford Study. *Arthritis Rheum* 1999;42(1):17–24.

48. Dieppe P, Cushnaghan J, Tucker M, Browning S, Shepstone L. The Bristol 'OA500 study': progression and impact of the disease after 8 years. *Osteoarthritis Cartilage* 2000;8(2):63–68.

49. Felson DT, Zhang Y, Anthony JM, Naimark A, Anderson JJ. Weight loss reduces the risk for symptomatic knee osteoarthritis in women. The Framingham Study. *Ann Intern Med* 1992;116(7):535–539.

50. McAlindon TE, Wilson PW, Aliabadi P, Weissman B, Felson DT. Level of physical activity and the risk of radiographic and symptomatic knee osteoarthritis in the elderly: the Framingham study. *Am J Med* 1999; 106(2):151–157.

CHAPTER 39

Epigenetics

Steffen Gay and Michel Neidhart

Introduction

Epigenetics is defined as the study of heritable changes in gene expression that are not due to changes in DNA sequences. The importance of environmental influences and epigenetic changes in the development of cancer and other diseases is increasingly being noticed. The involvement of factors such as drugs, UV light, infection, and diet, is reflected by the facts that the frequency of the consequential abnormalities differs from country to country and that geographic segregation of patients suffering from a given autoimmune disease has been identified.[1] The perplexing observation that concordance with respect to rheumatoid arthritis (RA) or systemic lupus erythematosus (SLE) is never 100% in monozygotic twins[2] raises the question as to what happens to the transcription and translation machineries between the genotype upstream and the phenotype downstream. The discordance results, at least in part, from epigenetics, which has been cited as a mechanism by which cells with as few as 30 000 genes differentiate into so many different cell types and vary so extensively at different developmental and functional stages. Epigenetics also plays a key role in the development of diseases associated with ageing. The molecular basis for epigenetics is in great part elucidated (Figure 39.1), involving chemical modifications of the DNA itself or to histones, which are proteins closely associated with DNA. In addition, a prominent role for microRNAs is also emerging.

Molecular basis of epigenetics

DNA methylation

DNA methylation is a crucial epigenetic modification of the genome that is involved in regulating many cellular processes (Figure 39.2). These include embryonic development, transcription, chromatin structure, X chromosome inactivation, genomic imprinting, and chromosome stability. The only known epigenetic modification of DNA in mammals is the methylation of cytosine at position C5 in CpG dinucleotides.[1,3] The most efficient way to silence gene transcription is to prevent the binding of transcription factors to DNA. To achieve this, DNA methyltransferases (DNMTs) convey a methyl group to the 5′ carbon position of cytosines of CpG dinucleotides. The mammalian DNA methylation machinery is composed of two components: the DNMTs, which establish and maintain DNA methylation patterns, and the methyl-CpG binding proteins (MBDs), which are involved in 'reading' methylation marks.

Methylation of CpG dinucleotides

The methylation process is catalysed by the protein family of DNMTs, which uses the methyl donor S-adenosylmethionine (SAM) to specifically methylate the fifth carbon atom of the cytosine ring. In normal cells, DNA methylation occurs predominantly in repetitive genomic regions, including satellite DNA and parasitic elements such as long interspersed transposable elements (LINES), short interspersed transposable elements (SINES), and endogenous retroviruses.[3] DNA methylation is a potent mechanism for silencing gene expression and maintaining genome stability in the face of a vast quantity of repetitive DNA, which can otherwise mediate illegitimate recombination events and cause transcriptional deregulation of nearby genes. The silencing of genes allows cell differentiation and explains how, for example, a neuronal cell can be different form a muscle cell in spite of the same genetic background.[4] The methylation of CpG dinucleotides represses transcription directly, by inhibiting the binding of specific transcription factors, and indirectly, by recruiting MBDs.

DNA methyltransferases

DNA methylation is catalysed by a group of enzymes in mammals called DNMT1, DNMT3a, and DNMT3b. DNMT1, known as the 'maintenance methyltransferase', has been shown to have a 10-fold preference for hemimethylated DNA (only one of the two DNA strands is methylated) compared with an unmethylated strand, and is used mostly by the cell to maintain the DNA methylation status in a stable fashion through cell division.[5] DNMT3a and DNMT3b, known as 'de-novo' methyltransferases, are used by the mammalian cell to methylate previously unmethylated DNA.

In somatic cells, DNMT1 is the predominant DNA methyltransferase.[6,7] The direct interaction between DNMT1 and proliferating cell nuclear antigen ensures that patterns of methylation are faithfully preserved in DNA synthesis.[8,9] Reduction of DNMT1 levels leads to hypomethylation, genomic instability, and tumorigenesis.[10]

Methyl-CpG binding proteins

DNA methylation leads to silencing by direct inhibition of transcription factor binding to their relative sites and by recruitment

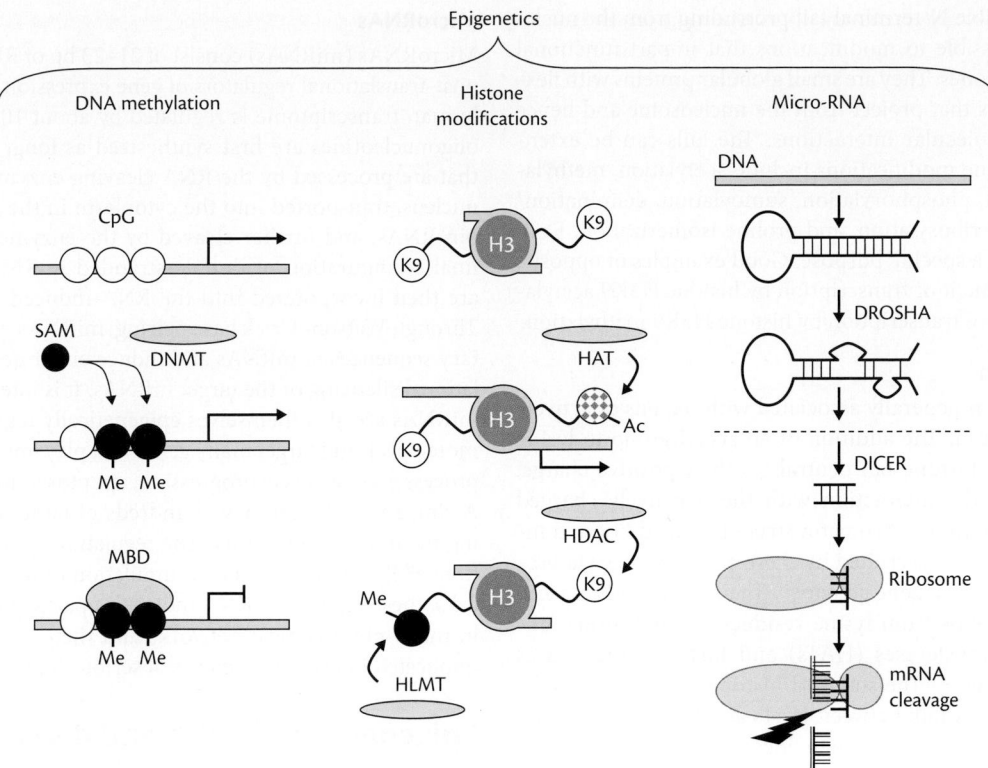

Fig. 39.1 Epigenetic mechanisms.

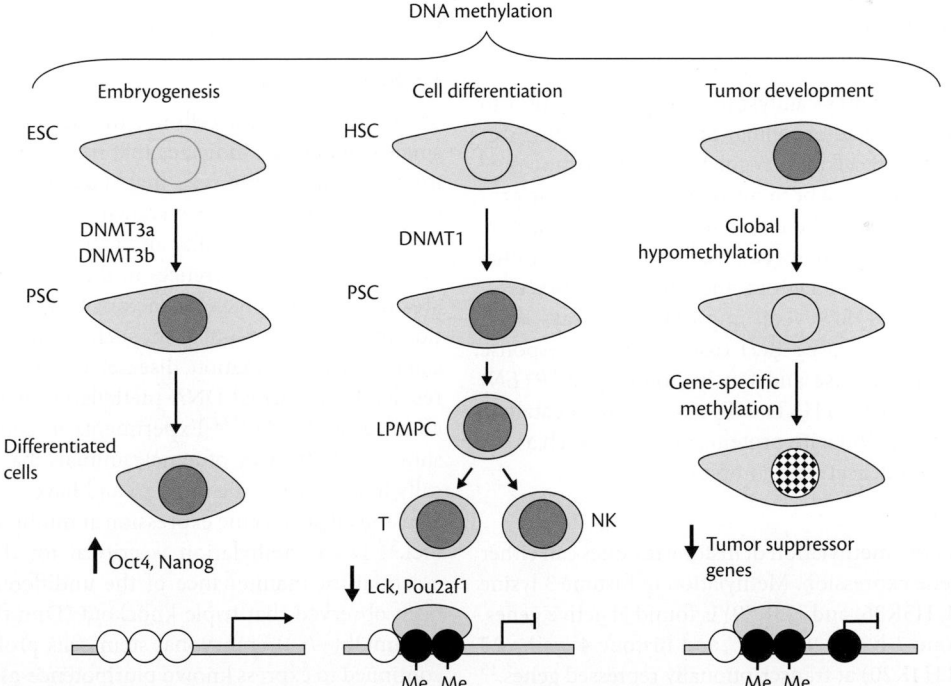

Fig. 39.2 Biological processes involving DNA methylation.

of methyl-binding domain proteins (MBDs),[11] for example MDB1, MeCP2, MBD3, and MBD4. These MBDs are present in transcription corepressor complexes involving several other members of the epigenetic machinery such as histone deacetylases and histone methyltransferases, resulting in chromatin reconfiguration and gene silencing.[12,13] The deletion of MeCP2 causes the neurodevelopmental disorder called Rett's syndrome.[14]

Histone modifications

The nucleosome is the basic subunit of chromatin. It consists of 146 base pairs (bp) of DNA wrapped around an octamer of two copies each of H2A, H2B, H3, and H4 classes of histones. Nucleosomes, of which there are an estimated 10 million per cell, are organized into regular arrays.[1] These structures present as small glomerular proteins with a flexible N-terminal tail protruding from the nucleosome that is accessible to modifications that impart functional capacities to the histones. They are small globular proteins with flexible N-terminal tails that project from the nucleosome and hence are available for molecular interactions. The tails can be extensively modified.[15] The modifications include acetylation, methylation, ubiquitination, phosphorylation, sumoylation, deimination/citrullination, ADP-ribosylation, and proline isomerization. Each modification serves a specific purpose. Good examples of opposite effects are enhancement of transcription by histone H3K9 acetylation and repression of transcription by histone H3K9 methylation.

Histone acetylation

Histone acetylation is generally associated with regions of actively transcribed chromatin. The addition of an acetyl group to lysine residues within the histone tail neutralizes their positive charge, thereby disrupting the interaction with the negatively charged DNA which loosens up the chromatin structure. In addition, transcriptional activators are recruited by these acetyl-lysines via bromodomains and enhance gene activity.[16] The enzymes adding and removing acetyl groups from lysine residues in the histone tails are histone acetyltransferases (HATs) and histone deacetylases (HDACs), respectively.[17] The status of histone acetylation results from an intricate cross-talk between HATs and HDACs. HATs are separated according to their cellular location and function into two distinct groups: the cytoplasmic B-type HATs and the nuclear A-type HATs.[18] The latter are presumed to have more impact on gene transcription, whereas cytoplasmic HATs can catalyse acetylation of non-histone proteins.

Histone deacetylation

HDACs are a class of enzymes catalysing the opposite action to HATs. They influence a myriad of cellular processes including signal transduction, apoptosis, cell cycle regulation, and cell growth.[19] HDACs catalyse deacetylation of both histone and nonhistone proteins and, similar to HATs, can be either nuclear or cytoplasmic. This cytoplasmic deacetylase activity can lead to post-translational modifications of transcription factors and chaperone proteins, and can have major effects on several important pathways, such as the NF-κB pathway,[20] the APE1-Ref1 oxidative stress response pathway,[21] and the phosphatase and tensin homologue (*PTEN*) phosphatase gene.[22] Similarly to HATs, HDACs exert their catalytic activity through an association with protein complexes, such as the sirtuin 1 (SIRT1) protein deacetylase complex.[23]

Histone methylation

In contrast to acetylation, methylation of histone residues can either activate or repress gene expression. Methylation of histone 3 lysine 4, 36, and 79 (H3K4, H3K36, and H3K79) is found at active genes, methylation of histone 3 lysine 9 and 27 and histone 4 lysine 20 (H3K9, H3K27, and H4K20) at transcriptionally repressed genes.[15] Histone lysine methyltransferases catalyse the addition of up to three methyl groups in a site-specific manner, i.e. these enzymes can only recognize lysine residues within a very specific sequence of amino acids. Accordingly, also histone lysine demethylases act site-specific. The methylation of arginines is catalysed by protein arginine methyltransferases. Up to now there is only one report of a histone arginine demethylase.[24] Removal of the methyl group can also occur by demethylimination by peptidylarginine deiminase 4 (PAD4). The residue is thereby converted to citrulline.[25]

MicroRNAs

MicroRNAs (miRNAs) consist of 21–23 bp of RNA and function as post-translational regulators of gene expression.[26] One-third of the human transcriptome is regulated by about 1000 miRNAs. These oligonucleotides are first synthesized as long, non-coding RNAs that are processed by the RNA cleaving enzyme DROSHA in the nucleus, transported into the cytoplasm in the form of short hairpin RNAs, and further cleaved by the enzyme DICER into their final configuration of double-stranded miRNAs.[27] The miRNAs are then incorporated into the RNA-induced silencing complex. Through Watson–Crick base pairing, miRNAs bind to complementary sequences of mRNAs and induce either degradation or translational silencing of the target mRNAs. It is interesting to note that miRNAs are also themselves epigenetically regulated at their promoter level, and target many genes that play important roles in such processes as cell cycle progression, apoptosis, and differentiation.[28] A single miRNA can have hundreds of target mRNAs, highlighting the implication of this gene regulation system in cellular functions.[29] By controlling the accumulation of the target protein(s) in cells, these regulatory RNA molecules participate in key functions in many physiological networks and their deregulation has been implicated in the pathogenesis of serious human disorders.[30]

Epigenetics in health and disease

Epigenetics play a fundamental role in biological diversity such as phenotypic variation among genetically identical individuals.[31] It could also explain the phenotypic differences between monozotic twins, especially regarding the susceptibility to certain diseases.

Embryogenesis

The fact that all of the cells in a multicellular organism arise from a single original cell indicates that tremendous phenotypic variability can occur among cells that share a common genome. On the organism level, it has been shown that monozygotic twins can differ in disease susceptibility and many anthropomorphic features.[32] These phenotypic differences in the context of a common genome are attributed to epigenetic factors. During embryogenesis, disruption in epigenetic regulation, such as aberrant DNA methylation, can lead to malformation, disease, or death.[3,33] Embryonic lethality results if the normal DNA methylation patterns are disrupted by absence of DNMT1.[34] Experiments in conditional mutants have shown that offspring of female animals that lack DNMT3a specifically in germ cells, die in utero and have disrupted DNA methylation and allele-specific expression at multiple maternally imprinted loci.[35] DNA methylation is critical for differentiation, but not essential for maintenance of the undifferentiated state, as it has been observed that triple knockout (Dnmt1(−/−) / Dnmt3a(−/−) / Dnmt3b(−/−)) embryonal stem cells proliferated normally and continued to express known pluripotence-associated markers, such as Oct4 and Nanog.[36] These cells only showed evidence of impaired proliferation when they were induced to differentiate.

Cell differentiation

Haematopoeitic progenitor cells can differentiate into lymphoid-primed multipotent progenitor cells, and the common lymphoid progenitors derived from these cells give rise to lymphocytes and NK cells. They have a reduced ability to develop into cells of the megakaryocytic or erythroid lineages. The dynamic generation of blood cells in the adult seems to be designed in a manner that allows each sub-branch of the system to operate autonomously.[37]

Many genes that are initially methylated in stem or precursor cells are found to undergo selective demethylation in a tissue- or lineage-specific manner. These genes include *Lck*, which undergoes demethylation in T cells and encodes a SRC family kinase that is responsible for initiating signalling downstream of the T-cell receptor, as well as POU domain class 2-associating factor 1 (*Pou2af1*), which encodes a B-cell-specific coactivator and undergoes demethylation in B cells.

Tumour development

Cancer cells have genome-wide aberrations at the epigenetic level, including global hypomethylation, promoter-specific hypermethylation, histone deacetylation, global down-regulation of miRNAs, and upregulation of certain actors of the epigenetic machinery such as EZH2. These aberrations confer a selective growth advantage to neoplastic cells. In various cancers, the 5-methylcytosine content was found to decrease by an average of 10%,[38] leading to apoptotic deficiency, uninhibited cellular proliferation, and tumorigenicity.[39]

Hypomethylation in cancer

Global DNA hypomethylation was the first epigenetic alteration noted in cancer cells.[40] Hypomethylation in tumor cells is primarily due to the loss of methylation from repetitive regions of the genome (LINE-1 and Alu),[41] and the resulting genomic instability is a hallmark of tumour cells.[42] This chromosomal instability can be associated with rearrangements and reactivation of transposon promoters.[43–49] Loss of genomic methylation correlates with disease severity and metastatic potential in many tumour types. This leads to the disruption of normal gene expression and potential activation of growth-promoting and anti-apoptotic pathways. Furthermore, promoter hypomethylation can lead to reactivation of miRNAs embedded in the coding regions of certain genes, resulting in silencing or aberrant expression of the corresponding protein.[28] Hypomethylation by genetic disruption of DNMT1 is protective against carcinogenesis in some models,[50] but can also promote tumour formation in others.[43]

Promoter-specific methylation in cancer

DNA methylation is an alternative way of silencing tumour suppressor genes, in a manner equivalent to genetic mutations.[44,45] Examples of this mechanism of tumorigenesis are numerous, notably methylation of the mismatch repair gene human mutL homologue 1 (*MLH1*) in colorectal cancer, the DNA repair gene O-6-methylguanine-DNA methyltransferase (*MGMT*) in gliomas and colorectal cancer, and the cell cycle regulator *p16* (cyclin-dependent kinase inhibitor 2A, *CDKN2A*) in colorectal and other malignancies.[46] Similar to mutations, silencing of tumour suppressor genes confers a selective proliferative advantage to corresponding cells, mediates invasiveness, and facilitates metastasis.

Non-neoplastic diseases

Diseases such as cardiovascular, metabolic, musculoskeletal, and haematopoietic disorders, which can be attributed to the interaction between genetic and environmental factors as well as to processes of ageing, are highly prevalent in industrialized nations and can be associated with a large burden on healthcare resources.[47,48] They are influenced by environmental factors, as in the contribution of smoking to the development of rheumatic diseases and atherosclerosis.[49] Metabolic disorders (e.g. obesity and diabetes)[50] and neurodegenerative disorders such as Alzheimer's disease and dementia[51] can also have an epigenetic component (Figure 39.3).

Metabolic and cardiovascular diseases

Obesity results from interactions between environmental and genetic factors. Known susceptibility variants do not fully explain the heritability of obesity and therefore other forms of variation, such as epigenetic marks, have been considered.[52] Failures in imprinting are known to cause extreme forms of obesity (e.g. Prader–Willi syndrome), but have also been associated with susceptibility to obesity. It

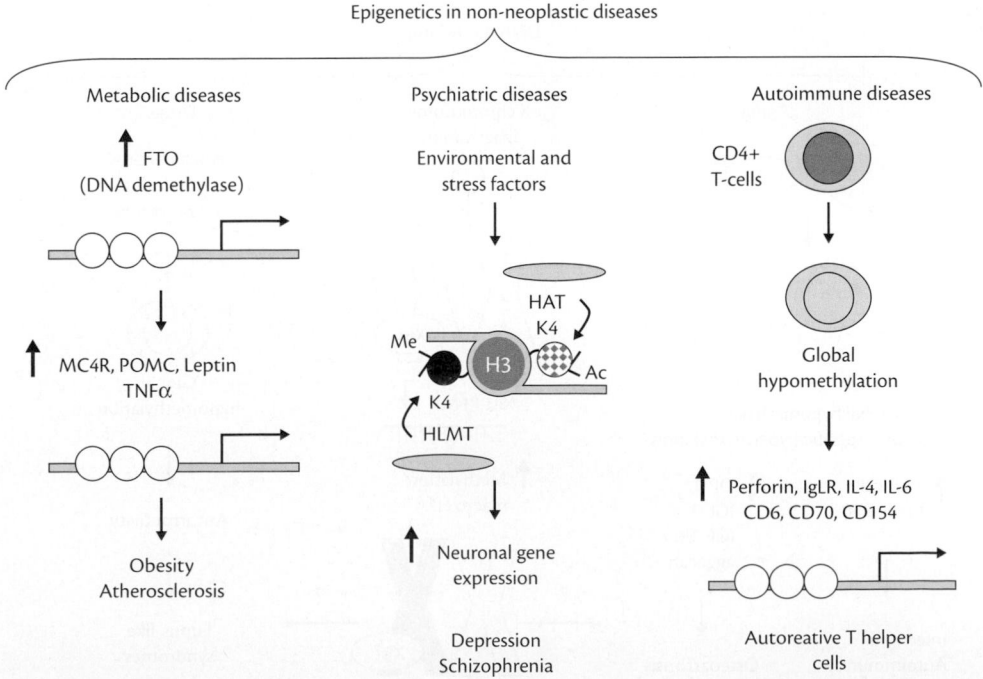

Fig. 39.3 Epigenetic imbalance in non-neoplastic diseases.

has been shown that obese mothers tend to have obese children and that clinical interventions causing maternal weight loss reduced risk of obesity in the offspring. Evidences indicate that the establishment of the epigenome can be affected by environmental factors during critical development periods. Possible disturbances of methylation may arise during fetal development due to a lack of availability of dietary methyl donors.[53] Potential interactions between the environment and DNA methylation mediating the expression of genes associated with increased body mass index and adiposity also has been suggested for the following loci: *FTO*,[5,53] *MC4R*,[54] *POMC*,[61] and leptin.[55] Interestingly, the *FTO* locus encodes for a DNA-demethylase enzyme,[59] and polymorphisms of this gene were associated with obesity in Pima Indians,[63] a population with increased incidence of RA.[56] Polymorphism in the *MC4R* gene also has been associated with RA.[57] In rats, hypermethylation of the proopiomelanocortin (POMC) promoter leading to decreased hypothalamic–adrenocortical activity has been associated with obesity.[61] Furthermore, in obese patients, tumour necrosis factor alpha (TNFα) promoter methylation is a predictive biomarker of hypocaloric diet-induced weight loss.[58] Thus, great similarities are found between metabolic and inflammatory diseases. Adiposity is a predisposing condition to atherosclerosis and RA accelerates the process. Endothelial dysfunction and carotid intima–media thickness, early preclinical markers of atherosclerosis which are the main determinants of cardiovascular morbidity and mortality, occur early on in RA.

Psychiatric diseases

Environmental factors signal to the neural stem cell genome to regulate cell fate decisions and neurogenesis.[59] Sequence-specific transcription factors work in concert with the chromatin machinery to direct the neuronal lineage programme within neural stem cells. In the stem cell state, repressive chromatin remodelling machinery maintains neuronal gene repression through one set of histone modifications, such as H3K9 methylation and DNA methylation. Stimulation by environmental factors and/or stress signals (during

disease) can induce adult neurogenesis and survival/maturation of newborn neurons by derepressing or activating neuronal gene expression through the hyperacetylation and/or switch in histone modification to H3K4 methylation. Epigenetic modifications in various brain regions were linked to neuropsychiatric disorders, including depression[60] and schizophrenia.[73] In addition, a wealth of information is known to date about epigenetic modifications with regards to hippocampal function and dysfunction.[74–77]

Autoimmune diseases

Accumulation of autoreactive lymphocytes and production of antibodies against a wide range of self-antigens are the hallmarks of autoimmune diseases that damage kidneys, skin, lung, and other organs.[61] The role of genetics has been suggested by the observation that the incidence of SLE is fivefold higher in monozygotic twins than in dizygotic twins. However, the concordance rate between monozygotic twins can range from 5% to 75%, and these variations suggest the involvement of additional triggers from the environment.[61] The CD4+ lymphocytes of patients with SLE, but not their CD8+ T lymphocytes, manifest a defective capacity to methylate their DNA; the degree of this inhibition correlates with disease activity.[79] The consequence of this fault is that several methylation-sensitive autoreactivity-promoting genes are overexpressed in CD4+ T cells, including those for perforin, immunoglobulin (Ig)-like receptor, interleukin (IL)-4, IL-6, and the B-cell costimulatory molecules CD70, CD6, and CD154.[80–84]

Variations have also been described in histones of CD4+ T cells from patients with SLE.[85] In particular, H3 and H4 acetylation levels have been shown to correlate negatively with disease activity.

Ageing

In peripheral blood lymphocytes, the pattern of DNA methylation of the two members of a pair of monozygotic twins, as well as their H3 and H4 acetylation profile, diversifies increasingly with ageing (Figure 39.4).[32] One reason for this is that the total genomic

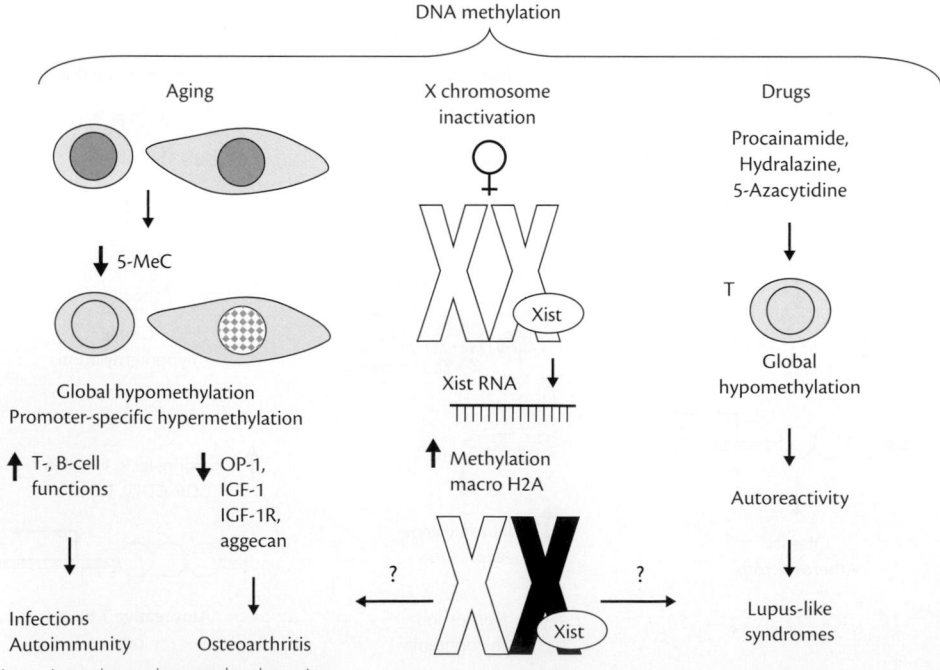

Fig. 39.4 Variables influencing epigenetics: ageing, gender, therapies.

5-methylcytosine content decreases with age, but at different rates in each twin. Similarly, in tissue culture, genomic DNA is demethylated in the long term, particularly DNA of those genes involved in cell differentiation.[62] A supplementary reason for increased diversity of H3/H4 acetylation with age is that environmental exposure is cumulative, so that there is every likelihood that small initial differences will become substantial with time.

Although DNA methylation patterns in adult cells are relatively stable, important changes have been described in ageing tissues. A global decrease in 5-methylcytosine content was reported in cultured human fibroblasts[63] and promoter-specific hypermethylation was observed in epithelial tissues.[88,89] Global profiling demonstrated several hundreds of gene promoters to acquire methylation in intestinal mucosae of ageing mice, whereas hundreds of others were found to have a parallel loss of DNA methylation.[64] This linear change of 5-methylcytosine content with ageing has a strong tissue specificity and has been shown to be common across mammals. Indeed, both the amount and pattern of DNA methylation have been found to diverge between human monozygotic twins as they age.[32] An age-related decline in chondrocyte production of osteogenic protein-1 (OP-1) (Bone Morphogenetic Protein-7) may contribute to cartilage loss in osteoarthritis. Age-related methylation of the OP-1 promoter may contribute to a decrease in OP-1 production in cartilage and a decrease in expression of OP-1 responsive genes such as IGF-1, the IGF-1R, and aggrecan.[65]

Gender

Autoimmune diseases demonstrate a gender bias and represent the fifth leading cause of death by disease among females of reproductive age.[66] Studies in SLE and systemic sclerosis indeed point to a skewed X inactivation.[67,68] Clinical and murine experimental studies indicate that the gender bias in autoimmunity may be influenced by sex hormones.[69] RA is more common in women than in men, whereas atherosclerosis shows the reverse pattern.[70] With ageing, these sex-related differences become less obvious. An interesting question is whether sex differences in disease prevalences in middle-aged adults could be associated with differential imprinting of the X chromosome—an epigenetic process—since one X chromosome in women should always be inactivated by DNA methylation. In women, *Xist*, a large regulatory RNA transcribed from the X inactivation centre (XiC) is produced by the future inactivated X chromosome (Xi) and initiates the silencing process.[71] In the Xi chromosome, DNA methylation at gene promoter CpG islands (CGIs) has been correlated with permanent expression silencing.[11] The recent observation that demethylation of the inactivated X chromosome in CD4+ T cells from female SLE patients is associated with overexpression of the B-cell-stimulating CD40 ligand points to a potential reason for the female sex predominance in this autoimmune disease.[67]

Drugs

A number of drugs have been suspected of causing SLE, most notably procainamide, hydralazine, and 5-azacytidine. There is evidence that these drugs inhibit DNA methylation.[72,73] The same group have reported data supporting an increase in lymphocyte function-associated antigen expression and the ensuing proliferation of autoreactive T cells in patients with SLE.[74]

Epigenetics in rheumatoid arthritis

RA is a chronic inflammatory disease of the joints affecting around 1% of the population worldwide.[75] One of the main characteristics of this autoimmune-related disorder is the hyperplastic synovial lining composed of infiltrating inflammatory cells and synovial fibroblasts (Figure 39.5).[76] Beside cytokines and chemokines that fuel the synovial inflammation, these resident cells produce matrix-degrading enzymes which lead to a progressive destruction of articular cartilage and bone.[77] Although our understanding of the cause of RA remains patchy it is generally accepted that it arises from an interplay of genetic predisposition (in particular HLA-DR allele subtypes and specific gene polymorphisms), immunological

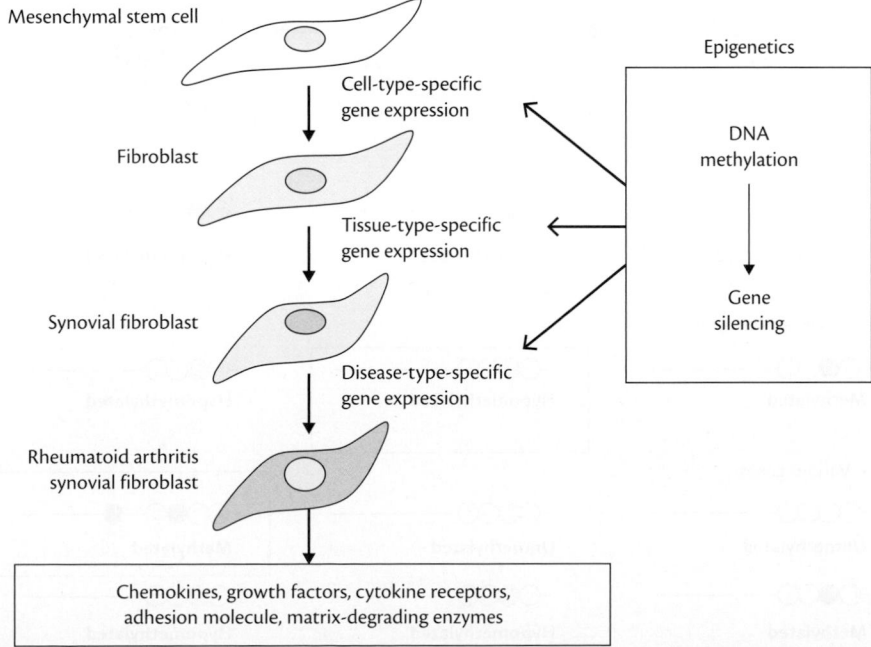

Fig. 39.5 Differentiation of fibroblasts and development of the activated phenotype in rheumatoid arthritis is controlled by epigenetics.

deregulation (e.g. autoantibody production), and environmental factors (such as nutrition, smocking, or exposure to infectious agents).[78,79]

TNFα derived from monocytes/macrophages is involved in the pathogenesis of RA, as shown by the beneficial effect of anti-TNF therapies.[80] Interestingly, the expression of TNFα is regulated by epigenetic mechanisms.[81] Thus, a positive correlation has been reported between high expression levels of TNFα and low methylation status. In non-responders to the TNF blockade (these represent up to one-third of the patients receiving TNFα blockers), inhibiting of a single cytokine does not seem to be enough to alleviate the symptoms. Furthermore, in many cases the symptoms return when therapy is stopped. This could be due to inflammation-independent processes or an epigenetically imprinted disease phenotype.[79]

Autoreactive T cells

T-cell development

RA patients are considered to have a Th1-biased phenotype.[75] Paradoxically, in synovial fluid, high levels of IL-4 and IL-13 can be measured in patients with early RA and very low expression in established disease;[80] this would implicate a temporary Th2 disposition in early RA. However, it should be noted here that RA is an infiltrating disease and that paradox patterns of T-cell subpopulations are often observed in the periphery during active disease.[82]

DNA hypomethylation

T cells of patients with RA exhibit an aberrant DNA methylation pattern (Figure 39.6).[74] The global methylation of genomic DNA of T cells derived from patients is reduced, compared to T cells from healthy donors. CD4+ T cells treated with the DNMT1 inhibitor 5-azacytidine respond to autologous antigen-presenting cells and induce autologous B-cell differentiation without exogenous antigen or mitogen.[83] T cells treated with DNMT1 inhibitors and ERK

pathway inhibitors overexpress CD70,[84] a costimulatory molecule for B cells. DNMT1 inhibitors also cause LFA-1 overexpression directly by demethylating the CD11a promoter.[85] Taken together, these mechanisms could contribute to T-cell autoreactivity, and potentially to autoimmunity.

Aggressive synovial fibroblasts

Mesenchymal stem cell development

Mesenchymal stem cells are undifferentiated, multipotent cells that reside in various human tissues and have the potential to differentiate into osteoblasts, chondrocytes, adipocytes, fibroblasts, and other cells of mesenchymal origin. In the human body they can be regarded as readily available reservoirs of reparative cells that are capable of mobilizing, proliferating, and differentiating into the appropriate cell type in response to certain environmental signals.[86] During the normal differentiation of mesenchymal stem cells into fibroblasts, two key transition points are regulated by epigenetic processes: first, the development of mesenchymal stem cells into a transient fibroblastic phenotype, and, second, the termination of lineage expansion. Both of these transition points are tightly regulated in space and time.[87] The hypothesis is that synovial fibroblasts emerge from mesenchymal stem cells and develop into tissue-specific cells under the influence of the microenvironment and under epigenetic control.[88]

Fibroblasts and phenotypic plasticity

Fibroblasts are thought to develop specific characteristics in response to their microenvironment; for example, fibroblasts in the skin, spleen, kidney, lung, or synovium exhibit different patterns of growth factor release. To produce such characteristics, certain genes are silenced in fibroblasts in some tissues but expressed in those in other tissues. Specific patterns of gene expression are, in great part, under epigenetic control. Many diseases are associated

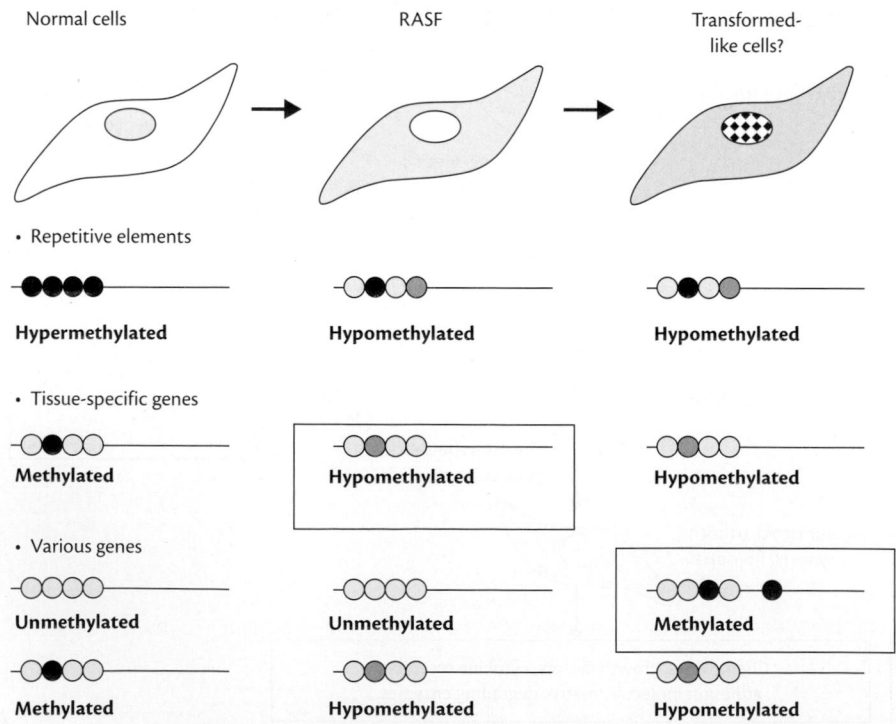

Fig. 39.6 Methylation in rheumatoid arthritis synovial fibroblasts (RASF).

with deregulation of the injury-repair response and fibroblast function, which leads to an increase or decrease in the deposition of extracellular matrix proteins, altered tissue architecture, impaired function, and, in some cases, substantial morbidity and mortality. In such cases, the fibroblasts are hypothesized to either not react or overreact to a given stimulus; this incorrect response can have different causes that include deregulated epigenetic controls.[78,88]

Rheumatoid arthritis synovial fibroblasts

In RA, a cytokine-independent pathway seems to be responsible for the ongoing joint destruction mediated by synovial fibroblasts.[78] The pathological changes associated with this process include excessive hyperplasia of the synovial tissue and an infiltration of inflammatory cells into it. The activated phenotype of RA synovial fibroblasts could be an intrinsic property of these cells, since these cells coimplanted with human cartilage into severe combined immunodeficient (SCID) mice are invasive even in the absence of other cells of the human immune system.[76] This concept is reflected in vitro by, for example, the increased production of matrix-degrading enzymes and adhesion molecules by these cells.[77] In contrast to normal synovial fibroblasts or those from patients with osteoarthritis, synovial fibroblasts from patients with RA show 'spontaneous' activities that are associated with an aggressive phenotype. For example, these cells show upregulated expression of proto-oncogenes,[76] specific matrix-degrading enzymes,[77] adhesion molecules,[89] and cytokines.[90] Histone acetylation is increased in RA synovial fibroblasts[88] and levels of specific miRNAs are changed,[91] suggesting that multiple epigenetic pathways in addition to genomic methylation[92] are altered.

DNA hypomethylation

The endogenous retroviral element LINE-1 is reactivated in the RA synovial lining and at sites of cartilage and bone invasion.[92-93] Most LINE-1 elements are retrotransposition-defective. The expression of LINE-1 proteins in RA synovial fibroblasts is associated with a partially hypomethylated promoter region.[92] The incorrect methylation patterns induce either cellular dedifferentiation or a completely new phenotype.[88] Genes normally silenced by methylation might contribute to the activated phenotype of rheumatoid arthritis synovial fibroblasts. For example, IL-6 could be upregulated due to demethylation of a single CpG site in the *IL6* promoter region.[94]

CXCL12 (SDF-1α) is differentially expressed in RA and osteoarthritis synovial tissues and isolated fibroblasts. Recently, the methylation status of the CXCL12 promoter has been examined.[95] A lower percentage of CpG methylation was found in the CXCL12 promoter of RA synovial fibroblasts.

Proinflammatory cytokines such as TNF, IL-1β, and IL-6

These proinflammatory molecules have multiple influences on the pathogenesis of RA; IL-1β and IL-6[96] can also affect genomic methylation. IL-6 stimulates translocation of DNMT1 to the nucleus. An important point to note is that proinflammatory cytokines and growth factors accelerate the cell cycle. During DNA replication, normal synovial fibroblasts recruit DNMT1,[93] which has been shown to interact with proliferating cell nuclear antigen at the DNA replication fork to ensure the correct setting of methylation markers.[9] In RA synovial fibroblasts, then, a relative deficiency of DNMT1could lead to loss of methylation markers in daughter cells, and induce the irreversible differentiation into an aggressive phenotype.

Histone modification

Studies of histone modifications in RA have mostly concentrated on histone acetylation and particularly on the use of histone deacetylase inhibitors as therapeutic agents. Paradoxically, in whole synovial tissue of patients with RA, the balance of HAT and HDAC activity is already shifted towards a loss of HDAC activity as compared to osteoarthritis and normal synovium.[88] In particular, the expression of HDAC1 and 2 was significantly reduced. Smoking is associated with an increased risk for developing RA and a more severe disease outcome.[97] Chronic exposure to cigarette smoke led to strongly reduced expression of the histone deacetylases SIRT1 and 2 in the lungs of rats. Pretreatment of macrophage cells with the SIRT1 activator resveratrol significantly inhibited the smoke-induced production of proinflammatory cytokines.

MicroRNA

Recent studies have uncovered dysregulated microRNA (MiR) expression in patients with RA, suggesting that abnormalities in MiR expression may contribute to the molecular mechanisms of the disease. The following MiRs are upregulated in peripheral blood mononuclear cells of patients with RA: MiR-16, MiR-132, MiR-146a, MiR-1555, and MiR-363.[98] In RA synovial fibroblasts, MiR-146a and MiR155 are also upregulated,[91] in addition to MiR-124a, MiR-203, MiR-223, and MiR-346.[91] The implication of miRNAs in immune-mediated disorders such as RA has recently emerged, suggesting that miRNA-based therapeutic approaches may have a promising potential in these diseases.[98]

Epigenetic therapies

Nutrients and epigenetics

Nutrients play essential roles in the following epigenetic events. First, folate, vitamin B$_{12}$, and methionine participate in the generation of SAM, which acts as a methyl donor in the methylation of cytosines in DNA. Second, covalent attachment of biotin to histones plays a role in gene silencing and in the cellular response to DNA damage.[99] Epigenetic mechanisms have recently been recognized as major contributors to nutrition-related longevity and ageing control. Studies of the comparison of DNA methylation levels in pancreatic acinar cells between caloric restriction-fed rats and control rats fed ad libitum suggest that it increases the methylation level of proto-oncogenes such as Ras.[100] Caloric restriction also induces a DNA hypermethylation of the p16INK4a promoter, blocking the access of E2F-1.[101] DNMT1 activity is significantly elevated in response to caloric restriction to correct the decreased methylation level during ageing.

The best-characterized of all animal models in which an epigenetic change in a gene is inherited and leads to well-defined pathological outcomes is the Avy mouse. The coat colour of these mice is governed by the expression of the *agouti* gene.[102] The agouti coat colour of wild-type mice results from a band of yellow pigmentation in the middle of the hair follicle, which is otherwise darkly pigmented. The expression of the *agouti* gene is under control of a promoter in the long terminal repeat (LTR) of an intracisternal A particle (IAP) proximal to the gene, whose ability to drive expression is correlated with the degree of IAP methylation. Most intriguingly, the addition of nutrients likely to enrich the pool of methyl donors and vitamin cofactors required for methylation to the diet of mothers increases methylation of the IAP promoter site, such that more offspring are pseudoagouti and less prone to the yellow-obese syndrome.[53,103,104] Such experiments have made viable yellow mice a powerful model to study the relationship between epigenetics, maternal diet, the so-called metabolic syndrome, and disease prevention.[105]

DNA methylation is governed by a variety of dietary factors, including folate, vitamin B_2 (riboflavin), vitamin B_{12} (cobalamin), vitamin B_6 (pyridoxine), methionine, choline, and alcohol, that mediate one-carbon metabolism and thereby increase the amount of available SAM.[106] SAM serves as the primary donor to add methyl groups to a wide range of acceptors, including DNA, RNA, and histone proteins. The end result of this reaction is the production of S-adenosylhomocysteine (SAH) as a by-product of the reaction. SAM was effective in a dog model of osteoarthritis[107] and in human depression.[108]

Histone deacetylase inhibitors

There have been a number of reports of beneficial effects from the use of histone deacetylase (HDAC) inhibitors (HDI) in experimental models of RA or in in-vitro studies.[109] In a mouse model of autoantibody-mediated arthritis intravenous application of the HDI FK-228 rapidly reduced the symptoms of arthritis with a marked decrease in the expression of TNFα and IL-1β in the synovium. The expression of the cell cycle inhibitors p16[INK4a] and p21[WAF1/Cip1] was increased, which could be linked to an increased protein acetylation at the p16INK4a promoter after incubation of RA-FLS with the HDI in vitro.

Modulators of microRNAs

The function of most miRNA genes is still awaiting gain- and loss-of-function studies. Unfortunately, creating genetic knockouts to determine miRNA function through homologous recombination in murine models is difficult. Additionally, paralogous miRNA genes are often expressed from multiple genomic loci, posing redundant function that further hampers knockout studies. Presently, loss-of-function studies rely on introduction of chemically modified antisense oligonucleotides, which act as competitive inhibitors of miRNAs. To increase the stability of the antisense oligo backbone, a methyl group is added to the $2'o$ position on the nucleic acid.[110] Similarly, locked nucleic acid modifications are also commonly used. An effective miRNA inhibitor that has been demonstrated to spontaneously spread into organs, even in the context of whole organisms, is based on a cholesterol conjugate. This was originally developed by the Tuschl and Stoffel laboratories in collaboration with Rajewsky and Alnylam Pharmaceuticals Inc. and was dubbed antagomir.[111] Currently, these modified miRNAs are under investigation in cardiovascular[112] and chronic liver diseases.[113]

Conclusion

The RA synovium contains cells of various types that exhibit hypomethylated DNA. Among these, T cells[74] and synovial fibroblasts[92] contain fewer 5-methyl-cytosine residues than normal cells and in the case of RA synovial fibroblasts this difference is conserved over long-term culture in vitro. Furthermore, expression of LINE-1 mRNA and proteins are associated with hypomethylated promoters.[92,113] This characteristic reflects a global state of DNA hypomethylation, which has important consequences for RA synovial fibroblasts, since an important mechanism of epigenetic control seems to be defective. As a demonstration of the consequences of this loss of epigenetic control, inhibition of DNMT1 expression in normal synovial fibroblasts is sufficient to produce an aggressive phenotype that includes upregulated expression of matrix-degrading enzymes and adhesion molecules. Indeed, the level of DNMT1 protein in proliferating RA synovial fibroblasts is lower than that in normal synovial fibroblasts. Thus, during DNA replication in RA synovial fibroblasts, the correct methylation patterns are not transmitted, or incorrect patterns could be transmitted, from mother cells to daughter cells. Consequently, genes in the daughter cells that should be silenced are expressed. This mechanism explains in great part the high number of transcripts that are upregulated in RA synovial fibroblasts. Several mechanisms can lead to the upregulation of gene transcripts as a consequence of DNA hypomethylation, either directly, through the loss of methylation markers in gene promoter regions, or indirectly, through the action of transcription factors or signalling pathways that are modulated by methylation. Since DNA methylation interacts with histone modifications and miRNA activity, these other epigenetic mechanisms could also be affected and could contribute to development of the aggressive phenotype. Two major questions remains: what is the cause of the DNA demethylation in RA (e.g. enhanced recycling of polyamines[114]) and how to interfere in this mechanism to render RA synovial fibroblasts less aggressive.

References

1. Renaudineau Y, Youinou P. Epigenetics and autoimmunity, with special emphasis on methylation. *Keio J Med* 2011;60(1):10–16.
2. Jarvinen P, Aho K. Twin studies in rheumatic diseases. *Semin Arthritis Rheum* 1994;24(1):19–28.
3. Robertson KD. DNA methylation and human disease. *Nat Rev Genet* 2005;6(8):597–610.
4. Lu Q, Ray D, Gutsch D, Richardson B. Effect of DNA methylation and chromatin structure on ITGAL expression. *Blood* 2002;99(12): 4503–4508.
5. Jones PA, Liang G. Rethinking how DNA methylation patterns are maintained. *Nat Rev Genet* 2009;10(11):805–811.
6. Jair KW, Bachman KE, Suzuki H et al. De novo CpG island methylation in human cancer cells. *Cancer Res* 2006;66(2):682–692.
7. Bestor TH, Verdine GL. DNA methyltransferases. *Curr Opin Cell Biol* 1994;6(3):380–389.
8. Turek-Plewa J, Jagodzinski PP. The role of mammalian DNA methyltransferases in the regulation of gene expression. *Cell Mol Biol Lett* 2005; 10(4):631–647.
9. Chuang LS, Ian HL, Koh TW et al. Human DNA-(cytosine-5) methyltransferase-PCNA complex as a target for p21WAF1. *Science* 1997; 277(5334):1996–2000.
10. Kimura F, Seifert HH, Florl AR et al. Decrease of DNA methyltransferase 1 expression relative to cell proliferation in transitional cell carcinoma. *Int J Cancer* 2003;104(5):568–578.
11. Klose RJ, Bird A.P. Genomic DNA methylation: the mark and its mediators. *Trends Biochem Sci* 2006;31(2):89–97.
12. Nan X, Ng HH, Johnson CA et al. Transcriptional repression by the methyl-CpG-binding protein MeCP2 involves a histone deacetylase complex. *Nature* 1998;393(6683):386–389.
13. Ballestar E, Esteller M. Methyl-CpG-binding proteins in cancer: blaming the DNA methylation messenger. *Biochem Cell Biol* 2005;83(3): 374–384.
14. Zoghbi HY. Rett syndrome: what do we know for sure? *Nat Neurosci* 2009;12(3):239–240.
15. Kouzarides T, Chromatin modifications and their function. *Cell* 2007; 128(4):693–705.
16. Haberland M, Montgomery RL, Olson EN. The many roles of histone deacetylases in development and physiology: implications for disease and therapy. *Nat Rev Genet* 2009;10(1):32–42.

17. Smith BC, Denu J.M. Chemical mechanisms of histone lysine and arginine modifications. *Biochim Biophys Acta* 2009;1789(1):45–57.

18. Yang XJ, The diverse superfamily of lysine acetyltransferases and their roles in leukemia and other diseases. *Nucleic Acids Res* 2004;32(3):959–976.

19. Yang XJ, Seto E. HATs and HDACs: from structure, function and regulation to novel strategies for therapy and prevention. *Oncogene* 2007;26(37):5310–5318.

20. Ashburner BP, Westerheide SD, Baldwin AS Jr. The p65 (RelA) subunit of NF-kappaB interacts with the histone deacetylase (HDAC) corepressors HDAC1 and HDAC2 to negatively regulate gene expression. *Mol Cell Biol* 2001;21(20):7065–7077.

21. Tell G, Quadrifoglio F, Tiribelli C, Kelley MR The many functions of APE1/Ref-1: not only a DNA repair enzyme. *Antioxid Redox Signal* 2009;11(3):601–620.

22. Ikenoue T, Inoki K, Zhao B, Guan KL. PTEN acetylation modulates its interaction with PDZ domain. *Cancer Res* 2008;68(17):6908–6912.

23. Vaziri H, Dessain SK, Ng Eaton E et al. hSIR2(SIRT1) functions as an NAD-dependent p53 deacetylase. *Cell* 2001;107(2):149–159.

24. Chang B, Cheng Y, Zhao Y, Bruick RK. JMJD6 is a histone arginine demethylase. *Science* 2007;318(5849):444–447.

25. Wang Y, Wysoka J, Sayegh T, Hashimoto H et al. Human PAD4 regulates histone arginine methylation levels via demethylimination. *Science* 2004;306(5694):279–283.

26. Lindsay MA. microRNAs and the immune response. *Trends Immunol* 2008;29(7):343–351.

27. Ghildiyal M, Zamore PD. Small silencing RNAs: an expanding universe. *Nat Rev Genet* 2009;10(2):94–108.

28. Davalos V, Esteller M. MicroRNAs and cancer epigenetics: a macrorevolution. *Curr Opin Oncol* 2010;22(1):35–45.

29. Lim LP, Lau NC, Garett-Engele P, Grimson A et al. Microarray analysis shows that some microRNAs downregulate large numbers of target mRNAs. *Nature* 2005;433(7027):769–773.

30. Schickel R, Boyerinas B, Park SM, Peter ME. MicroRNAs: key players in the immune system, differentiation, tumorigenesis and cell death. *Oncogene* 2008;27(45):5959–5974.

31. Morgan HD, Sutherland HG, Martin DI, Whitelaw E. Epigenetic inheritance at the agouti locus in the mouse. *Nat Genet* 1999;23(3):314–318.

32. Fraga MF, Ballestar E, Paz MF et al. Epigenetic differences arise during the lifetime of monozygotic twins. *Proc Natl Acad Sci* U S A 2005;102(30):10604–10609.

33. Costello JF, Frühwald MC, Smiraglia DJ et al. Aberrant CpG-island methylation has non-random and tumour-type-specific patterns. *Nat Genet* 2000;24(2):132–138.

34. Li E, Beard C, Jaenisch R. Role for DNA methylation in genomic imprinting. *Nature* 1993;366(6453):362–365.

35. Kaneda M, Okano M, Haka K et al. Essential role for de novo DNA methyltransferase Dnmt3a in paternal and maternal imprinting. *Nature* 2004;429(6994):900–903.

36. Tsumura A, Hayakawa T, Kumaki Y et al. Maintenance of self-renewal ability of mouse embryonic stem cells in the absence of DNA methyltransferases Dnmt1, Dnmt3a and Dnmt3b. *Genes Cells* 2006;11(7): 805–814.

37. Cedar H, Bergman Y. Epigenetics of haematopoietic cell development. *Nat Rev Immunol* 2011;11(7):478–488.

38. Feinberg AP, Gehrke CW, Kuo KC, Ehrlich M. Reduced genomic 5-methylcytosine content in human colonic neoplasia. *Cancer Res* 1988;48(5):1159–1161.

39. Taby R, Issa JP. Cancer epigenetics. *CA Cancer J Clin* 2010;60(6):376–92.

40. Lapeyre JN, Becker FF. 5-Methylcytosine content of nuclear DNA during chemical hepatocarcinogenesis and in carcinomas which result. *Biochem Biophys Res Commun* 1979;87(3):698–705.

41. Estecio MR, Gharibyan V, Shen L et al. LINE-1 hypomethylation in cancer is highly variable and inversely correlated with microsatellite instability. *PLoS One* 2007;2(5): p. e399.

42. Chen RZ, Pettersson U, Beard C et al. DNA hypomethylation leads to elevated mutation rates. *Nature* 1998;395(6697):89–93.

43. Eden A, Gaudet F, Whagmare A, Jaenisch R. Chromosomal instability and tumors promoted by DNA hypomethylation. *Science* 2003;300(5618):455.

44. Jones PA, Baylin SB. The epigenomics of cancer. *Cell* 2007;128(4):683–692.

45. Issa JP, Ottaviano YL, Celano P et al. Methylation of the oestrogen receptor CpG island links ageing and neoplasia in human colon. *Nat Genet* 1994;7(4):536–540.

46. Herman JG, Baylin SB. Gene silencing in cancer in association with promoter hypermethylation. *N Engl J Med* 2003;349(21):2042–2054.

47. Eggermann T, Meyer E, Caglayan AO et al. ICR1 epimutations in llp15 are restricted to patients with Silver-Russell syndrome features. *J Pediatr Endocrinol Metab* 2008;21(1):59–62.

48. Hauke J, Riessland M, Lunke S et al. Survival motor neuron gene 2 silencing by DNA methylation correlates with spinal muscular atrophy disease severity and can be bypassed by histone deacetylase inhibition. *Hum Mol Genet* 2009;18(2):304–317.

49. Gerli R, Sherer Y, Bocci EB et al. Precocious atherosclerosis in rheumatoid arthritis: role of traditional and disease-related cardiovascular risk factors. *Ann N Y Acad Sci* 2007;1108:372–381.

50. Stoger R, Epigenetics and obesity. *Pharmacogenomics* 2008;9(12):1851–1860.

51. Chiang PK, Lam MA, Luo Y. The many faces of amyloid beta in Alzheimer's disease. *Curr Mol Med* 2008;8(6):580–584.

52. Herrera BM, Keildson S, Lindgren CM. Genetics and epigenetics of obesity. *Maturitas* 2011;69(1):41–49.

53. Waterland RA, Jirtle RL. Early nutrition, epigenetic changes at transposons and imprinted genes, and enhanced susceptibility to adult chronic diseases. *Nutrition* 2004;20(1):63–68.

54. Widiker S, Karst S, Wagener A et al. High-fat diet leads to a decreased methylation of the Mc4r gene in the obese BFMI and the lean B6 mouse lines. *J Appl Genet* 2010;51(2):193–197.

55. Milagro FI, Campion J, Garcia-Diaz DF et al. High fat diet-induced obesity modifies the methylation pattern of leptin promoter in rats. *J Physiol Biochem* 2009;65(1):1–9.

56. Ferucci ED, Templin DW, Lanier AP. Rheumatoid arthritis in American Indians and Alaska Natives: a review of the literature. *Semin Arthritis Rheum* 2005;34(4):662–667.

57. Ziegler A, Ewhida A, Bendel M, Kleensang A. More powerful haplotype sharing by accounting for the mode of inheritance. *Genet Epidemiol* 2009;33(3):228–236.

58. Campion J, Milagro FI, Goyenecha E, Martinez JA. TNF-alpha promoter methylation as a predictive biomarker for weight-loss response. *Obesity* (Silver Spring) 2009;17(6):1293–1297.

59. Hsieh J, Eisch AJ. Epigenetics, hippocampal neurogenesis, and neuropsychiatric disorders: unraveling the genome to understand the mind. *Neurobiol Dis* 2010;39(1):73–84.

60. Renthal W, Nestler EJ. Epigenetic mechanisms in drug addiction. *Trends Mol Med* 2008;14(8):341–350.

61. Lleo A, Inverzinni P, Gao B et al. Definition of human autoimmunity—autoantibodies versus autoimmune disease. *Autoimmun Rev* 2010;9(5): p. A259–A266.

62. Bork S, Pfister S, Witt H et al. DNA methylation pattern changes upon long-term culture and aging of human mesenchymal stromal cells. *Aging Cell* 2010;9(1):54–63.

63. Wilson VL, Jones PA. DNA methylation decreases in aging but not in immortal cells. *Science* 1983;220(4601):1055–1057.

64. Maegawa S, Hinkai G, Kim HS et al. Widespread and tissue specific age-related DNA methylation changes in mice. *Genome Res* 2010; 20(3):332–340.

65. Loeser RF, Im HJ, Richardson B, Chubinskaya S. Methylation of the OP-1 promoter: potential role in the age-related decline in OP-1 expression in cartilage. *Osteoarthritis Cartilage* 2009;17(4):513–517.

66. Ozcelik T. X chromosome inactivation and female predisposition to autoimmunity. *Clin Rev Allergy Immunol* 2008;34(3):348–351.

67. Lu Q, Wu A, Tesmer L et al. Demethylation of CD40LG on the inactive X in T cells from women with lupus. *J Immunol* 2007;179(9):6352–6358.

68. Uz E, Loubiere LS, Gadi VK et al. Skewed X-chromosome inactivation in scleroderma. *Clin Rev Allergy Immunol* 2008;34(3):352–355.

69. Zandman-Goddard G, Peeva E, Shoenfeld Y. Gender and autoimmunity. *Autoimmun Rev* 2007;6(6):366–372.

70. Sokka T, Toloza S, Cutolo M et al. Women, men, and rheumatoid arthritis: analyses of disease activity, disease characteristics, and treatments in the QUEST-RA study. *Arthritis Res Ther* 2009;11(1): p. R7.

71. Wutz A. Xist function: bridging chromatin and stem cells. *Trends Genet* 2007;23(9):457–464.

72. Cornacchia E, Golbus J, Maybaum J et al. Hydralazine and procainamide inhibit T cell DNA methylation and induce autoreactivity. *J Immunol* 1988;140(7):2197–2200.

73. Richardson B, Cornacchia E, Golbus J et al. N-acetylprocainamide is a less potent inducer of T cell autoreactivity than procainamide. *Arthritis Rheum* 1988;31(8):995–999.

74. Richardson B, Scheinbart L, Srtrahler J et al. Evidence for impaired T cell DNA methylation in systemic lupus erythematosus and rheumatoid arthritis. *Arthritis Rheum* 1990;33(11):1665–1673.

75. Firestein GS, Evolving concepts of rheumatoid arthritis. *Nature* 2003; 423(6937):356–361.

76. Muller-Ladner U, Pap T, Gay RE, Neidhart M, Gay S Mechanisms of disease: the molecular and cellular basis of joint destruction in rheumatoid arthritis. *Nat Clin Pract Rheumatol* 2005;1(2):102–110.

77. Konttinen YT, Ainola M, Valleala H et al. Analysis of 16 different matrix metalloproteinases (MMP-1 to MMP-20) in the synovial membrane: different profiles in trauma and rheumatoid arthritis. *Ann Rheum Dis* 1999;58(11):691–697.

78. Karouzakis E, Neidhart M, Gay RE, Gay S. Molecular and cellular basis of rheumatoid joint destruction. *Immunol Lett* 2006;106(1):8–13.

79. Trenkmann M, Brock M, Ospelt C, Gay S. Epigenetics in rheumatoid arthritis. *Clin Rev Allergy Immunol* 2010;39(1):10–19.

80. McInnes IB, Schett G. Cytokines in the pathogenesis of rheumatoid arthritis. *Nat Rev Immunol* 2007;7(6):429–442.

81. Sullivan KE, Reddy AB, Dietzmann K et al. Epigenetic regulation of tumor necrosis factor alpha. *Mol Cell Biol* 2007;27(14):5147–5160.

82. Neidhart M, Pataki F, Schönbächler J, Brühlmann P. Flow cytometric characterisation of the 'false naive' (CD45RA+, CD45RO-, CD29 bright+) peripheral blood T-lymphocytes in health and in rheumatoid arthritis. *Rheumatol Int* 1996;16(2):77–87.

83. Richardson BC, Liebling MR, Hudson JL. CD4+ cells treated with DNA methylation inhibitors induce autologous B cell differentiation. *Clin Immunol Immunopathol* 1990;55(3):368–381.

84. Oelke K, Lu Q, Richardson B et al. Overexpression of CD70 and overstimulation of IgG synthesis by lupus T cells and T cells treated with DNA methylation inhibitors. *Arthritis Rheum* 2004;50(6): 1850–1860.

85. Kaplan MJ, deng C, Yang J, Richardson B. DNA methylation in the regulation of T cell LFA-1 expression. *Immunol Invest* 2000; 29(4):411–425.

86. Pountos I, Corscadden D, Emery P, Giannoudis PV. Mesenchymal stem cell tissue engineering: techniques for isolation, expansion and application. *Injury* 2007;38 Suppl 4: p. S23–S33.

87. Boquest AC, Noer A, Collas P. Epigenetic programming of mesenchymal stem cells from human adipose tissue. *Stem Cell Rev* 2006;2(4):319–329.

88. Karouzakis E, Gay RE, Gay S, Neidhart M. Epigenetic control in rheumatoid arthritis synovial fibroblasts. *Nat Rev Rheumatol* 2009; 5(5):266–272.

89. Rinaldi N, Weis D, Brado B et al. Differential expression and functional behaviour of the alpha v and beta 3 integrin subunits in cytokine stimulated fibroblast-like cells derived from synovial tissue of rheumatoid arthritis and osteoarthritis in vitro. *Ann Rheum Dis* 1997; 56(12):729–736.

90. Firestein GS, Alvaro-Gracia JM, Maki R. Quantitative analysis of cytokine gene expression in rheumatoid arthritis. *J Immunol* 1990; 144(9):3347–3353.

91. Stanczyk J, Pedrioli PM, Brentano F et al. Altered expression of MicroRNA in synovial fibroblasts and synovial tissue in rheumatoid arthritis. *Arthritis Rheum* 2008;58(4):1001–1009.

92. Neidhart M, Rethage J, Kuchen S et al. Retrotransposable L1 elements expressed in rheumatoid arthritis synovial tissue: association with genomic DNA hypomethylation and influence on gene expression. *Arthritis Rheum* 2000;43(12):2634–2647.

93. Karouzakis E, Gay RE, Michel BA, Gay S, Neidhart M. DNA hypomethylation in rheumatoid arthritis synovial fibroblasts. *Arthritis Rheum* 2009;60(12):3613–3622.

94. Nile CJ, Read RC, Akii M et al. Methylation status of a single CpG site in the IL6 promoter is related to IL6 messenger RNA levels and rheumatoid arthritis. *Arthritis Rheum* 2008;58(9):2686–2693.

95. Karouzakis E, Rengel Y, Jüngel A et al. DNA methylation regulates the expression of CXCL12 in rheumatoid arthritis synovial fibroblasts. *Genes Immun* 2011;12(8):643–652.

96. Wehbe H, Henson R, Meng F et al. Interleukin-6 contributes to growth in cholangiocarcinoma cells by aberrant promoter methylation and gene expression. *Cancer Res* 2006;66(21):10517–10524.

97. Vittecoq O, Lequerré T, Göeb V et al. Smoking and inflammatory diseases. *Best Pract Res Clin Rheumatol* 2008;22(5):923–935.

98. Duroux-Richard I, Presumey J, Courties G et al. MicroRNAs as new player in rheumatoid arthritis. *Joint Bone Spine* 2011;78(1): 17–22.

99. Oommen AM, Griffin JB, Sarath G, Zempleni J. Roles for nutrients in epigenetic events. *J Nutr Biochem* 2005;16(2):74–77.

100. Hass BS, Hart RW, Lu MH, Lynn-Cook BD. Effects of caloric restriction in animals on cellular function, oncogene expression, and DNA methylation in vitro. *Mutat Res* 1993;295(4–6):281–289.

101. Li Y, Liu L, Tollefsbol TO. Glucose restriction can extend normal cell lifespan and impair precancerous cell growth through epigenetic control of hTERT and p16 expression. *FASEB J* 2010;24(5):1442–1453.

102. Duhl DM, Vrieling H, Miller KA et al. Neomorphic agouti mutations in obese yellow mice. *Nat Genet* 1994;8(1):59–65.

103. Cooney CA, Dave AA, Wolff GL. Maternal methyl supplements in mice affect epigenetic variation and DNA methylation of offspring. *J Nutr* 2002;132(8 Suppl):2393S–2400S.

104. Waterland RA, Jirtle RL. Transposable elements: targets for early nutritional effects on epigenetic gene regulation. *Mol Cell Biol* 2003;23(15): 5293–5300.

105. Dolinoy DC, Weidman JR, Waterland RA, Jirtl RL. Maternal genistein alters coat color and protects Avy mouse offspring from obesity by modifying the fetal epigenome. *Environ Health Perspect* 2006;114(4): 567–572.

106. Niculescu MD, Zeisel SH. Diet, methyl donors and DNA methylation: interactions between dietary folate, methionine and choline. *J Nutr* 2002;132(8 Suppl):2333S–2335S.

107. Imhoff DJ, Gordon-Evans WJ, Evans RB et al. Evaluation of S-adenosyl l-methionine in a double-blinded, randomized, placebo-controlled, clinical trial for treatment of presumptive osteoarthritis in the dog. *Vet Surg* 2011;40(2):228–232.

108. Levkovitz Y, Alpert JE, Brintz CE, Mischoulon D, Papakostas GI. Effects of S-adenosylmethionine augmentation of serotonin-reuptake inhibitor

antidepressants on cognitive symptoms of major depressive disorder. *Eur Psychiatry* 2012;27(7):518–521.

109. Grabiec AM, Tak PP, Reedquist KA. Targeting histone deacetylase activity in rheumatoid arthritis and asthma as prototypes of inflammatory disease: should we keep our HATs on? *Arthritis Res Ther* 2008;10(5):226.

110. Tuschl T, Zamore PD, Lehman R et al. Targeted mRNA degradation by double-stranded RNA in vitro. *Genes Dev* 1999;13(24):3191–3197.

111. Krutzfeldt J, Rajewsky N, Braich R et al. Silencing of microRNAs in vivo with 'antagomirs'. *Nature* 2005;438(7068):685–689.

112. Hinkel R, Trenkwalder T, Kupatt C. Gene therapy for ischemic heart disease. *Expert Opin Biol Ther* 2011;11(6):723–737.

113. Lorenzen JM, Haller H, Thum T. MicroRNAs as mediators and therapeutic targets in chronic kidney disease. *Nat Rev Nephrol* 2011;7(5):286–294.

114. Karouzakis E, Gay RE, Gay S, Neidhart M. Increased recycling of polyamines is associated with global DNA hypomethylation in rheumatoid arthritis synovial fibroblasts. *Arthritis Rheum.* 2012; 64(6):1809–1817.

CHAPTER 40

Genetics of rheumatoid arthritis

Steve Eyre and Jane Worthington

Genetic contribution to rheumatoid arthritis

The observation of clustering of cases of rheumatoid arthritis (RA) within families provided the first evidence for a genetic basis to the disease. The increased risk to the sibling of a proband compared to the population prevalence, known as the sibling relative risk or λ_s, is estimated to be between 2 and 10. Studies in twins can also be used to quantify genetic risk. The concordance rates for monozygotic twins and dizygotic twins of 15% and 3.6% respectively indicates that both genetic and non-genetic factors determine susceptibility, and on the basis of these observations the heritability of RA is estimated to be about 60%. RA is thus defined as a complex disease in which both genetic and environmental risk factors determine susceptibility (Figure 40.1). The various attempts to quantify the size of the genetic component of susceptibility must be viewed as estimates, as they fail to account for the effect of the shared environmental exposures of those living together or for any interactions between genetic variants or between genetic and environmental risk factors.

RA is a heterogeneous disease with a range of clinical presentations, variable degrees of severity, rates of progression, and responses to therapies. It is now thought that the particular disease course followed by an individual patient is influenced at various stages by both genetic and environmental risk factors.

Most studies to date have focused on determining the risk factors for susceptibility to RA defined by the 1987 ACR criteria, failing to include in analyses milder cases with an inflammatory arthritis that may in fact satisfy the newly revised criteria for disease. Indeed the vast majority of data emerging in the postgenomic era is based on the analysis of autoantibody-positive cases. More refined investigations are now required, using carefully ascertained and longitudinally followed patient cohorts in well-powered studies to determine (1) whether there are genetically distinct subgroups of disease and (2) whether genetic markers can be used to classify patients at symptom onset in order to identify those likely to have the more severe phenotypes. Pharmacogenetic studies are also under way to identify genetic markers for the prediction of the efficacy of therapies and of risk of adverse events.

HLA and the shared epitope hypothesis

The association of RA with genes from within the major histocompatibility complex (MHC), along with the detection of autoantibodies (rheumatoid factor) in the serum of RA patients led to the classification of RA as an autoimmune condition. In 1976 Stastny[1] first reported association of the MHC class II antigen HLA DRw4 with RA. The introduction of DNA molecular typing methods, used in many studies across numerous populations, revealed

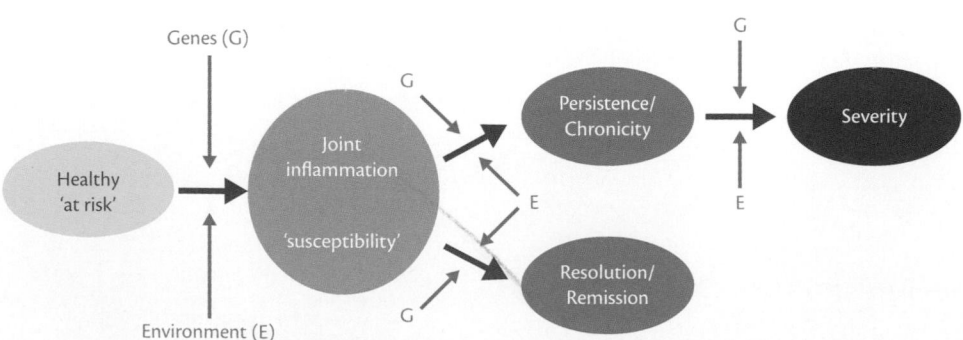

Fig. 40.1 Combinations of genetic and environmental risk factors act together over time to determine initial susceptibility to inflammatory arthritis and the subsequent disease course followed by an individual patient, leading to a spectrum of outcomes from natural remission through to rapidly progressing, treatment-resistant rheumatoid arthritis.

a complex picture with multiple *HLA DRB1* alleles associated with RA. In 1987 Gregersen et al.[2] described a unifying hypothesis based on the observation that all associated alleles had in common a 5-amino-acid sequence within the third hypervariable region of the *HLADRB1* gene. The so-called 'shared epitope' (SE) at positions 70–74 (amino acid sequence QRRAA) forms a critical part of the binding groove of the HLA DRB1 protein in which peptides are held and presented to the immune system. Although many of the RA-associated *HLA DRB1* alleles share the identical amino acid sequence at the SE there appears to be a hierarchy in terms of the risk they confer such that the association of *HLA DRB1*0401* is greater than *HLA DRB1*0101* and the genotype *0401/*0404* is associated with by far the highest risk for OR. The SE hypothesis has recently been refined by employing SNP genotyping in large cohorts of cases and controls and the statistical imputation of HLA alleles. These analyses suggest that the genetic association signal from the SE can be simplified to the amino acid at position 11, at the bottom of the DRB1 binding groove, and to amino acids at positions 71 and 74, also in the antigen-binding groove. The addition of two further independent genetic associations, for a single amino acid in HLA-B and one in HLA-DPB1, again both in the antigen-binding groove, explain fully the genetic association signal over the MHC region.[3]

The role of the HLA DRB1 protein is to present short peptides to T cells; a key step in the shaping of the immune response through deletion or positive selection of T-cell clones. The position of amino acids 11, 71, and 74 within the peptide-binding groove is assumed to have an influence on the nature and orientation of presented peptides, although the pathogenic mechanism, whether this is the presentation of self or foreign peptide, remains unknown. A number of alleles negatively associated with RA share a different amino acid region at positions 70–74 (DERAA) and have a very different shaped peptide-binding groove.

The effect size reported for the SE and RA varies considerably. The effect size is much greater in autoantibody-positive compared to autoantibody-negative disease. It is highest in patients with the most severe forms of RA such as those with erosive disease and extra-articular manifestations such as Felty's disease and lowest in cohorts with a broad spectrum of disease, such as those to be found in primary-based care. The question as to whether the SE determines susceptibly or persistence/severity remains a subject of debate.

Despite many unanswered questions, the importance of the HLA region in RA is undisputed. Estimated to account for between 40–60% of the genetic component of susceptibility, this locus is the major genetic influence on susceptibility to RA. This means that approximately one-half of the genetic susceptibility is determined by loci outside the MHC and in recent years much effort has focused on defining the non-HLA component of susceptibility, with the aim of gaining greater insight into the aetiology of disease, on the assumption that an understanding of genetic susceptibility is dependent on knowledge of *all* significant risk loci.

Protein tyrosine phosphatase N22 (PTPN22)

Even before the advent of genome-wide association studies (GWAS), major advances in technology facilitated the discovery of the second risk locus for RA. The first large-scale SNP-based candidate gene study, led by Begovich,[4] tested 16 000 potentially functional SNPs from immune-related genes. Large sample sizes and the use of both test and replication stages were strengths of the study which identified an association to the minor allele (C) of a SNP at position 1858 which resulted in an arginine to tryptophan change (R620W). In a parallel candidate gene study in type 1 diabetes targeting genes on T-cell signalling pathways, the same association was observed. Subsequently these results have been replicated many times and the same variant has been associated with many other autoimmune diseases.[5] This variant does not exist in Asian populations and no other associations within PTPN22 have been found in non-whites, providing strong evidence of genetic heterogeneity between populations for RA. The *PTPN22* gene encodes the protein Lyp and the disease-associated variant is thought to disrupt binding to Csk in the TCR-mediated negative regulatory signalling pathway. Recent studies indicate that the associated variant not only decreases binding to Csk, but may also increase binding to proteolytic enzymes, increasing degradation of the PTPN22 protein.[6] This could explain the reduction in PTPN22-mediated T-cell control, with a reduced amount of a less effective protein. Some studies suggest the association is restricted to autoantibody-positive RA, but in the largest study to date association was detected in seronegative RA, albeit with a lower effect size.

STAT4

The first hypothesis-free approach to searching the genome for susceptibility loci was non-parametric linkage analysis based on the analysis of polymorphic microsatellite markers in affected sibling pair families. A series of studies, each individually underpowered, largely served to confirm the importance of the MHC region. The exception was a SNP-based fine mapping study of one of the linkage peaks detected in a United States cohort, where 13 candidate genes were targeted in a well-powered study using over 7500 samples and significant association to a SNP in the gene *STAT4* was detected. The effect of *STAT4* (odds ratio = 1.2) is more modest than that of SE or *PTPN22*, but interestingly the strength of association is same in seronegative and seropositive RA and is also seen in other autoimmune diseases. Although the biological effect of the associated variant has not been determined, *STAT4* is a highly plausible candidate gene for RA as it encodes a transcription factor involved in cytokine-mediated signalling in T cells.

PADI4

Strong evidence of association to SNPs within the *PADI4* gene first emerged from studies in Asian populations.[7] Various hypotheses have emerged as to why RA patients develop antibodies to citrullinated peptides. To test the possibility of genetic variants influencing this process, a Japanese group investigated 100 SNPs in a region encoding a series of enzymes involved in citrullination. They found risk of RA associated with SNPs in non-coding regions of *PADI4*. This association has been replicated in a number of Asian populations and seems to represent the major non-MHC locus in these populations (odds ratio = 1.3). Association to this locus in white populations has subsequently been confirmed.

Genome-wide association studies

The impact of genome-wide associations on the identification of risk variants for a range of complex diseases, not least RA, has been enormous. RA was one of seven diseases studied in the United Kingdom's Wellcome Trust Case Control Consortium (WTCCC) which performed a groundbreaking proof-of-principle study demonstrating that high-throughput genotyping of 500 000 SNPs in 2000 cases for each of 7 common diseases and a shared set of 3000 controls could detect associations to known and novel loci.[8] Although for RA, only associations to HLA and PTPN22 exceeded genome-wide levels of significance ($p < 5 \times 10^{-8}$), targeting nine loci ($p = 1 \times 10^{-5}$ to 5×10^{-7}) in a validation study led to the identification of the third-largest effect size locus for white RA at 6q23 (rs6920220, odds ratio = 1.2).[9]

In the same year, two additional GWAS for RA were published. The first was a small-scale study using an early-generation Affymetrix chip with just 100 000 SNPs and a two-stage study design with relatively small sample sizes. Only one SNP reached genome-wide significance, with the minor allele of rs13207033, at the same 6q23 locus identified in the United Kingdom study, being associated with protection from RA. Interestingly, both associated SNPs map over 180 kb from the nearest gene, lying between OLIG3 and TNFAIP3. A fine mapping study of this region of the 6q23 region in United Kingdom samples has revealed further complexity, with a third independent association detected within intron 2 of the TNFAIP3 gene (rs5029937).[10] This raises the possibility that effect sizes for a locus, based on the initial GWAS association, may be underestimates. The risk to an individual of carrying at least one risk allele at rs6920220 and rs5029937 and no protective allele at rs13207033 rises (odds ratio = 1.5). TNFAIP3 is an attractive candidate gene for RA; the A20 (murine protein product of TNFAIP3) knockout mouse develops cachexia and systemic and joint inflammation. Recent studies in myeloid-specific A20 knockout mice resulted in the development of a phenotype including spontaneous erosive polyarthritis with many features of RA. TNFAIP3 is on the signalling pathway for tumour necrosis factor (TNF), the central cytokine driving inflammation in RA. It acts as a potent inhibitor of NFκB and is therefore a potent anti-inflammatory protein. Markers at the 6q23 locus have now been associated with RA in a number of populations and with other autoimmune diseases including systemic lupus erythematosus (SLE), coeliac disease and type 1 diabetes. Across these studies multiple SNPs have been implicated and further fine mapping studies will be required for each disease to discover whether the aetiological variants are the same for each disease.

The third GWAS of 2007 combined data from United States and Swedish studies (1500 seropositive cases and 1800 controls genotyped for 300 000 SNPs). After HLA and PTPN22, the strongest association in this study was to markers in the TRAF-C5 locus. The association was validated within the original publication and subsequently in multiple independent studies.

Validation studies and meta-analyses

Initial results from GWAS in RA and other complex diseases revealed that the new and yet to be discovered loci were almost certainly numerous, but of small effect sizes (odds ratio <1.2). In turn this confirmed that a GWAS of 1000–2000 cases and similar numbers of controls had limited power to detect such effects. The GWAS data therefore harboured many genuine associations that did not reach statistical significance, and the challenge was to separate those from potential false-positive associations. One way to do this is to increase the power of studies by increasing the sample size

used. By this method, further loci (PRKCQ, AFF3, KIF5A) from the WTCCC were confirmed at genome-wide significance by expanding the number of controls to include the non-autoimmune disease cases.

As an increasing number of confirmed susceptibility loci were reported across autoimmune and chronic inflammatory diseases the overlap in terms of genetic susceptibility between these conditions became increasingly apparent. Replication studies in independent RA cohorts targeting loci from SLE, type 1 diabetes, and coeliac disease was highly successful in adding AFF3, IL2/IL21, TAGAP, CTLA-4, UBE2L3, and BLK as confirmed RA susceptibility loci.

Meta-analysis of GWAS data offers an attractive and relatively low-cost solution to increasing the power to detect small effects. Although each of the first three major GWAS studies used different SNP chips and hence generated genotypes for different sets of SNPs, the introduction of methods to impute the genotypes of missing SNPs, means that combination of the three studies was possible. The first RA meta-analysis, of 3929 cases and 5807 controls, led to the identification of association with rs4810485 in intron 2 of the CD40 gene. To facilitate the selection of SNPs from GWAS to be targeted in validation studies, Raychaudhuri developed a bioinformatics programme (GRAIL) which screens potential loci against confirmed loci. This was used with great effect on the meta-GWAS data to prioritize 22 SNPs from 179 regions, from which 7 (TAGAP, CD28, TRAF6, PTPRC, FCGR2A, PRDM1, CD2-CD58) were confirmed as novel RA susceptibility loci through an international collaboration to genotype large validation sample sets.

In the United States a further independent RA GWAS identified REL as a novel RA susceptibility locus. Most recently, combination of this GWAS data with new data from United States and Canadian samples culminated in a meta-analysis of 5539 autoantibody-positive RA cases and 20 169 controls.[11] Following the use of GRAIL and findings from other autoimmune diseases, genotyping of 34 SNPs in a further 6768 cases and 8806 controls confirmed 10 additional novel associations, taking the number of RA susceptibility loci confirmed at genome-wide significance to 31.

More recently advantage was taken of the great overlap in the genetic association findings in autoimmune diseases to design a common genotyping array, Immunochip, containing over 200 000 SNPs across 186 associated loci. The RA community formed a consortium, RACI, to test over 11 000 RA cases and 15 000 controls with this array. Data from this experiment has increased the number of confirmed RA loci in white populations to over 45. Newly identified loci include IL6R, the target for a therapeutic intervention, IRAK1, the first locus located on the X chromosome associated with RA, and IKZF3, a region previously robustly associated with asthma. The fine mapping experiment also highlighted a number of potentially aetiologically causal, exonic variants and focused the signal in around half of the associated regions to encompass just a single, candidate gene.[12]

The current state of knowledge of RA susceptibility loci is summarized in Figure 40.2. GWAS have revolutionized our knowledge of non-HLA disease susceptibility loci, resulting in the identification of large numbers of risk loci with small effect sizes. Many challenges and questions remain. Despite this apparent success, the RA loci are estimated to explain only around 55% of the genetic heritability, with the majority of that accounted for by the SE.

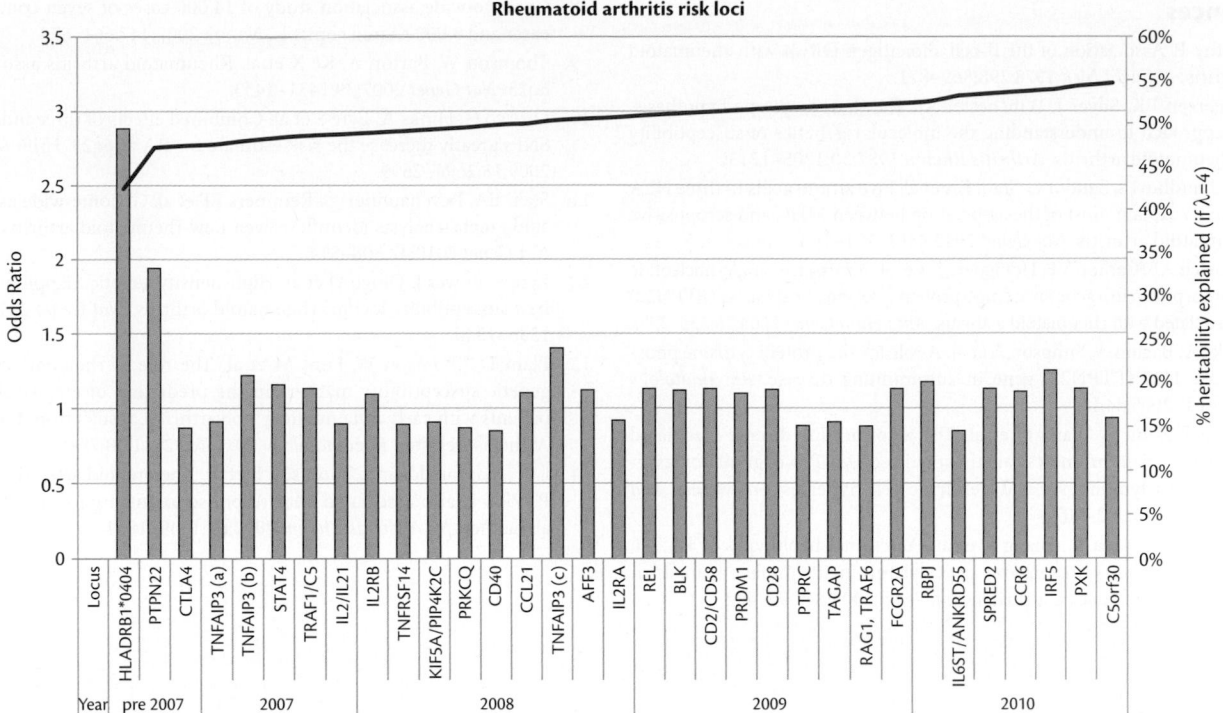

Fig. 40.2 Current rheumatoid arthritis genetic risk loci, plotted in order of discovery. Odds ratio and confidence interval on the y-axis (left) and increase heritability explained on the y-axis (right), assuming $\lambda_s = 4$.

The same situation is seen in other complex diseases and has a fuelled a debate; the so-called 'missing heritability question'. Possible explanations to account for why GWAS have failed to capture the missing heritability include the following:

- Multiple additional loci remain to be identified: it is highly likely that analysis of sample sets of increasing size will continue to reveal new associations.

- Inaccurate estimate of odds ratios for individual loci from GWAS: fine mapping may reveal multiple effects, better identify the causal SNP, and produce more accurate estimates of odds ratios.

- Rare variants: these have not been well captured on the current generation of SNP chips. The challenge here will be assembling sufficiently powered studies to detect the associations.

- Structural variants such as copy number variations (CNVs) and insertion/deletions: A CNV GWAS failed to detect any significant associations with RA, it did however conclude that most simple CNV's are well captured by SNP chips, reducing the likelihood of this being a valid explanation.

- Gene–gene and gene–environment interactions: these have largely not been addressed due to lack of data (environmental risks) or lack of power.

Insights into pathogenesis

Although our understanding of the genetic basis of susceptibility to RA is far from complete, the new knowledge of genetic susceptibility loci gained in the post-GWAS era can add to our understanding of pathogenesis. One proviso that should be born in mind is that many of the associations arising from GWAS are to markers outside the traditionally defined boundaries of any genes,

or within gene-rich regions. Although loci tend to be 'named' according to the nearest recognizable relevant gene, fine mapping and functional studies will be required to more accurately map associations, before we can be certain of the genes implicated in the disease process.

With these limitations in mind, it is still tempting to look for clues about pathogenesis amongst the loci identified so far. Genetic studies have confirmed the central role that T cells play in the susceptibility to RA, which can be clearly seen in the associated genes highlighted in a T-cell priming pathway. In addition, most of the genes implicated are enriched in pathways associated with antigen processing and presentation or with the regulation of T-cell activation, regulation, and proliferation. It will be informative to determine whether these pathways, or a subset, need to be perturbed in all patients and whether genetic variants within specific pathways can predict the observed disease heterogeneity. Indeed, there is already preliminary evidence that certain genes associated with disease onset are also involved in the eventual outcome: for example, the same variants in *TRAF1* associated with susceptibility are also associated with the development of erosions.[13]

Ongoing work is also highlighting genes that may play a role in treatment response. Early studies indicate that *PTPRC*,[14] implicated in the susceptibility to RA, may also be involved in how well a patient responds to treatment. Well-powered GWAS, similar to the studies performed for susceptibility loci, will be needed to determine whether any novel loci are associated with response to treatment, in terms of disease outcome or adverse side effects. Genetic profiling of a patient at presentation in order to determine their probable disease course and make informed choices about the treatments is a goal for the future.

References

1. Stastny P. Association of the B-cell alloantigen DRw4 with rheumatoid arthritis. *N Engl J Med* 1978;298:869–871.

2. Gregersen PK, Silver J, Winchester RJ. The shared epitope hypothesis. An approach to understanding the molecular genetics of susceptibility to rheumatoid arthritis. *Arthritis Rheum* 1987;30:1205–1213.

3. Raychaudhuri S, Sandor C, Stahl EA et al. Five amino acids in three HLA proteins explain most of the association between MHC and seropositive rheumatoid arthritis. *Nat Genet* 2012;44(3):291–296.

4. Begovich AB, Carlton VE, Honigberg LA et al. A missense single-nucleotide polymorphism in a gene encoding a protein tyrosine phosphatase (PTPN22) is associated with rheumatoid arthritis. *Am J Hum Genet* 2004;75:330–337.

5. Hinks A, Barton A, Simpson A et al. A role for the protein tyrosine phosphatase N22 (PTPN22) gene in autoimmune disease. *Rheumatology* (Oxford) 2005;44:I5.

6. Zhang J, Zahir N, Jiang Q et al. The autoimmune disease-associated PTPN22 variant promotes calpain-mediated Lyp/Pep degradation associated with lymphocyte and dendritic cell hyperresponsiveness. *Nat Genet* 2011;43:902–907.

7. Suzuki A, Yamada R, Chang X et al. Functional haplotypes of PADI4, encoding citrullinating enzyme peptidylarginine deiminase 4, are associated with rheumatoid arthritis. *Nat Genet* 2003;34:395–402.

8. Genome-wide association study of 14,000 cases of seven common diseases and 3,000 shared controls. *Nature* 2007;447:661–678.

9. Thomson W, Barton A, Ke X et al. Rheumatoid arthritis association at 6q23. *Nat Genet* 2007;39:1431–1433.

10. Orozco G, Hinks A, Eyre S et al. Combined effects of three independent SNPs greatly increase the risk estimate for RA at 6q23. *Hum Mol Genet* 2009;18:2693–2699.

11. Stahl EA, Raychaudhuri S, Remmers EF et al. Genome-wide association study meta-analysis identifies seven new rheumatoid arthritis risk loci. *Nat Genet* 2010;42:508–514.

12. Eyre S, Bowes J, Diogo D et al. High-density genetic mapping identifies new susceptibility loci for rheumatoid arthritis. *Nat Genet* 2012;44(12): 1336–1340.

13. Plant D, Thomson W, Lunt M et al. The role of rheumatoid arthritis genetic susceptibility markers in the prediction of erosive disease in patients with early inflammatory polyarthritis: results from the Norfolk Arthritis Register. *Rheumatology* (Oxford) 2011;50:78–84.

14. Cui J, Saevarsdottir S, Thomson B et al. Rheumatoid arthritis risk allele PTPRC is also associated with response to anti-tumor necrosis factor alpha therapy. *Arthritis Rheum* 2010;62:1849–1861.

CHAPTER 41

Genetics of spondyloarthropathies

Matthew Brown

Introduction

The spondyloarthropathies (SpA) are a group of clinically and aetiologically related forms of inflammatory arthritis that include ankylosing spondylitis (AS); psoriatic arthritis (PsA); colitic arthritis, complicating inflammatory bowel disease (IBD); and reactive arthritis. AS is the prototypic disease. All are characterized histopathologically by the presence of enthesitis, and to a varying degree, all share genetic associations, notably with HLA B27. An increasing number of other genetic associations have been reported with these diseases, providing further information as to the immunopathogenic mechanisms underlying them.

Genetic epidemiology

As a group the spondyloarthropathies are very common; up to 2.4 million Americans suffer from SpA, compared with 1.3 million suffering from rheumatoid arthritis (RA).[1] The prevalence of AS is around 0.5% in people of white European ancestry. The disease has a global distribution, with the exception that it is uncommon in people of African or Australian Aboriginal descent, as HLA B27 is rare in these ethnicities. Psoriasis is even more common, with a prevalence of 2–3% in people of white European ancestry, with the disease being less common in people of Asian and African ancestry.[2,3]

The typical age of onset is in the early 20s, and onset over 45 years of age is uncommon. AS has a moderate male predominance (~2–3:1), whereas colitic arthritis and axial spondyloarthritis have a more balanced gender distribution.[4,5] Psoriatic spondyloarthritis, as with AS itself, has a strong male predominance.[6] The reason for the male predominance of AS and psoriatic spondyloarthritis is unknown.

AS runs very strongly in families, and most of the risk of developing AS is inherited, with heritability in excess of 90%.[7,8] Siblings or children of AS patients have about 12% likelihood of developing AS, and the likelihood of recurrent disease in more distant relatives is much lower (≤1%).[9,10] The recurrence risks of AS in relatives of AS patients are reported in Table 41.1. A major role for genetic factors in the risk of developing AS is supported by this strongly familiality, and by twin studies. These studies, although not large,

suggest that the heritability of the risk of developing the disease is over 90%.[7,8] Twin and family studies also indicate that the severity of AS is highly heritable, with the heritability of radiographic severity measures being 62%,[11] and family studies indicating significant heritability of disease activity and severity measures such as the Bath Ankylosing Spondylitis Disease Activity Index (BASDAI) and Bath Ankylosing Spondylitis Functional Index (BASFI), as well as age of symptom onset.[12,13]

Psoriasis is also known to be highly heritable; the concordance rate in monozygotic (MZ) twins is significantly higher than in dizygotic (DZ) twins (35–72% vs 12–23%), indicating greater sharing of risk factors, most probably genetic (estimated heritability 80%).[14] PsA also runs strongly in families; sibling of a first-degree relative with PsA are 12–49 times more likely to develop the condition themselves than relatives of individuals without PsA, though only 4 times more frequently than in spouse controls, suggesting that there is a significant environmental component to PsA risk.[15,16] Concordance of pattern of PsA within families does not appear to be strong, suggesting that in psoriasis there is an underlying predisposition for synovitis/enthesitis rather than for a specific disease pattern.[15]

Histocompatibility antigen associations

The association of AS with HLA B27, the major gene involved in the disease, was made in the early 1970s,[17–19] yet it is still unclear as to how it causes the condition. Theories range from differences in its capacity to present antigens, to problems caused by the formation of homodimers of B27 itself, or by its propensity to misfold in the endoplasmic reticulum. The latter theory proposes that

Table 41.1 Risk of ankylosing spondylitis in relatives of cases, given HLA B27 status[9]

	B27 status unknown	B27-positive	B27-negative
Grandparent	1%	5%	0%
Parent/sibling	10%	15%	0%
Identical twin	60%	60%	—

accumulation of misfolded HLA B27 induces an endoplasmic reticulum stress response,[20] leading to secretion of proinflammatory cytokines such as interleukin (IL)-23,[21] which is considered a major driver of inflammation in the disease. It remains unclear exactly how HLA B27 induces AS, although recent genetic findings indicate that the mechanism involves aberrant peptide handling, narrowing the potential range of mechanisms significantly.[22]

There are now over 65 known subtypes of HLA B27 which are thought to have evolved from the common ancestor HLA B27 allele, *HLA B*2705*. Most subtypes are very rare, and in most populations worldwide, variation within HLA B27 makes no difference to the likelihood of these individuals developing the condition. In white European populations the two most common subtypes, *HLA B*2702* and *B*2705*, are equally disease associated.[23] Two other subtypes, *HLA B*2706* which is found in Asians[24] and *HLA B*2709* which is found in Sardinians,[25] appear to be protective or neutrally associated with disease. HLA B27 is rare in most African populations, where the development of seronegative arthritis such as AS appears more closely related to HIV infection than genetic risk factors. In Scandinavian countries and amongst the Inuit HLA B27 has a much higher prevalence(10–37%),[26] suggesting that either HLA B27 provides a survival advantage (perhaps through protection against an infectious disease) or that the high prevalence is due to a founder effect or genetic drift.

The strength of the association of HLA B27 with reactive arthritis is considerably lower than with primary AS, with most series reporting B27-carriage rates of 20–60%. In case series with axial spondyloarthritis, the prevalence of HLA B27 varies substantially, reflecting the lower specificity of the diagnostic criteria for axial spondyloarthritis compared with AS. There is no HLA B27 association with psoriasis (which is associated with HLA Cw6), but in patients with psoriatic spondyloarthritis there is a strong association with HLA B27. HLA B27 appears to act primarily as a dominant gene in AS, although there is some evidence that individuals carrying two copies of the gene have higher risk of AS, and may develop more severe AS, than heterozygotes.[27] HLA B27-negative patients have a later age of disease onset by about a decade than HLA B27-positive patients.[27,28]

There has been considerable research into the influence of HLA alleles other than HLA B27 with AS. Association of HLA B60 with AS is well established, having first been reported by Robinson et al. in 1989,[29] and subsequently confirmed in white Europeans[23] and in east Asians.[30] Considering the non-B27 alleles only in cases and controls, the association of HLA B60 carries an odds ratio of 3.5–3.6 in HLA B27-positive and -negative cases.[23] Whether this association is specifically due to HLA B60 or due to linkage disequilibrium with a nearby genetic variant is unclear, and to date no other major histocompatibility complex (MHC) genetic associations have been reported and confirmed with definitive statistical confidence.

Other genetic associations of spondyloarthropathies

Ankylosing spondylitis

Although *HLA B27* is clearly the major gene in AS, twin and family studies indicate that other genes must be involved. Rapid advances are being made in identifying further genetic loci associated with the disease (Table 41.2).[22,31]

Table 41.2 Genes with confirmed associations with ankylosing spondylitis

Gene	Locus	Likely function
HLA B27	6p21.3	Presentation of peptides to T cells, or misfolding leading to endoplasmic reticulum stress reaction
21q22	21q22	Unknown
2p15	2p15	Unknown
ANTXR2	4q21	Unknown
CARD9	9q34	Th17 activation after β-glucan exposure
ERAP1	5q15	Peptide trimming prior to HLA class I presentation
IL12B	5q33	Activation/differentiation of IL-23R expressing cells
IL1R2	2q11	Influence on IL-1 cytokine response
IL23R	1p31	Activation/differentiation of IL-23R expressing cells
KIF21B	1q32	Unknown
PTGER4	5p13	Induction of IL23 expression, in turn driving activation/differentiation of IL-23R expressing cells; bone anabolism
RUNX3	1p36	Reduction in CD8 lymphocyte counts
TBKBP1	17q21	TNF signalling
TNFR1/LTBR	12p13	TNF signalling

The first two genes identified as being associated with AS other than *HLA B27* are *ERAP1* (*ARTS-1*) and *IL23R*.[31] *ERAP1* encodes an aminopeptidase which is expressed in the endoplasmic reticulum, and which is involved in preparing peptides for HLA class I presentation to immune effector cells. Its association with AS is restricted to *HLA B27*-positive cases, the first confirmed human example of gene–gene interaction in any common human disease.[22] *ERAP1* has also recently been shown to be associated with psoriasis, and in this condition the association is restricted to *HLA Cw6*-positive cases.[32] This suggests that HLA B27 and HLA Cw6 operate in AS and psoriasis by similar mechanisms. The protective *ERAP1* variants prevent conformational changes in ERAP1 which are thought to be required for peptide cleavage,[33] and lead to less peptide presentation in the endoplasmic reticulum to HLA class I molecules. The restriction of the association of *ERAP1* with HLA B27-positive AS indicates that HLA B27 must operate in AS by a mechanism involving ERAP1, and thus through aberrant peptide handling.

IL23R encodes the receptor for the cytokine IL-23, which is involved in activation of a range of proinflammatory cells including Th17 lymphocytes, gamma-delta cells, mast cells, and others. Stimulated by the discovery of the association of *IL23R* with AS, trials of IL-17 blockade have been initiated in AS, and in a phase 2 study strong beneficial effects similar to those observed with TNF-antagonist medications have been reported.[34]

Other genetic associations with AS with effects on the IL-23 pathway include *IL12B*, *CARD9*, *PTGER4*, and *IL1R2*. *PTGER4* is of particular interest as it forms part of the mechanostat, linking physical stress at entheses with induction of IL-23 production and anabolic bone formation signals, thus identifying a mechanism by which inflammation leads to bone formation in AS. *IL12B* encodes IL-12p40, the shared subunit of IL-12 and IL-23. *CARD9* encodes a protein involved in signalling between the innate immunity receptor dectin-1 and the nucleus, leading to IL-23 production. This is of particular interest given the recent demonstration in the Skg mouse model that dectin-1 stimulation by the fungal cell wall component beta-glucan induces spondyloarthritis, episodic unilateral uveitis, and colitis resembling Crohn's disease.[35] This shows a mechanism by which spondyloarthritis can develop in the absence of HLA B27 through innate immune pathways.

Psoriatic arthritis

Although there have been many large studies of psoriasis genetics, psoriatic arthritis is less well understood and fewer studies have been published. Distinguishing between associations of psoriasis and the arthritis complicating psoriasis is also challenging. It seems likely that genes will contribute to the development of arthritis in psoriasis cases. However, with the exception of the association of HLA B27 with axial psoriatic arthritis, no gene has been convincingly shown to be associated with psoriatic arthritis independently of the skin disease.

Psoriasis is strongly associated with HLA Cw6.[36] The mechanism for this association is unknown but is presumed to relate to a predisposition to present particular antigenic peptides, in turn leading to an immune reaction in the skin. As mentioned above, the association of psoriasis with the same ERAP1 haplotypes associated with AS, and the restriction of this association to HLA Cw6-positive psoriasis[32], suggests that HLA Cw6 operates in psoriasis by a similar mechanism to that by which HLA B27 operates in AS. This most likely involves aberrant peptide presentation.

Genome-wide association studies (GWAS) have recently identified several genetic associations with psoriasis (see Table 41.3),

Table 41.3 Genetic associations of psoriasis

Gene	Locus	Likely function
HLA Cw6	6p21.3	Uncertain. ?Presentation of peptides to T cells
ERAP1	5q15	Peptide trimming prior to HLA class I presentation
IL12B	5q33	Activation/differentiation of IL-23R expressing cells
IL23R	1p31	Activation/differentiation of IL-23R expressing cells
LCE3B/C	1q21	Barrier protection
DEFB4	8p23.1	Barrier protection
IFIH1	2q24	Interferon signalling
IL28RA	1p36	Interferon signalling
IL4/IL13	5q31	Cytokine signalling, modulates Th2 lymphocyte activation
IL23A	12q13	Activation/differentiation of IL-23R expressing cells
TYK2	19p13	IL-23R signalling
NFKB1A	14q13	NFκB1 pathway
TNFAIP3	6q23	NFκB1 pathway
TNIP1	5q33	NFκB1 pathway
REL	2p16	NFκB1 pathway
RNF114	20q13	Unknown
FBXL19	16p11.2	? through NFκB1 pathway effects
NOS2	17q11.2	Inducible nitric oxide synthetase? Involved in microbial defence

many of which overlap with both AS and IBD. As with AS and IBD, genes involved in the IL-23R pathway are over-represented in psoriasis associations, and include IL23R, IL12B, TYK2, and IL23A.[32,37] These findings have been important in stimulating clinical trials in psoriasis of cytokine-inhibition therapy targeting this pathway, with clear beneficial effects. For example, ustekinumab, an antibody treatment targeting IL-12p40, is now a licensed treatment for psoriasis in many countries, and is effective for both psoriatic skin and joint disease.[38] Anti-IL-17A antibody treatment has also been shown to be effective for both psoriasis and PsA.[39]

Several genes which can broadly be said to act through NFκB1 show association with psoriasis, something which is more a feature of seropositive diseases such as RA, perhaps explaining the clinical overlap of psoriatic arthritis with RA. These include NFKB1A, REL, TRAF3IP2, and TNIP1.[32,40]

A surprise finding from genetic studies has been the association of genes involved in interferon signalling pathways and psoriasis. IL28RA encodes a type III interferon receptor subunit. IFIH1 encodes an innate immunity receptor, stimulation of which by microbes leads to a type 1 interferon response. TYK2 encodes a tyrosine kinase involved in signalling from various cytokine receptors including IL-23R and interferon receptors. This suggests that interferon signalling induced by microbial infection may be important in psoriasis pathogenesis.

Conclusion

Genetic studies have confirmed significant overlaps between the genetic architecture of AS and psoriasis, particularly involving IL-23 signalling pathways, but also significant differences in HLA and other associations, which are likely to be important in determining the phenotype of spondyloarthritis that occurs in genetically predisposed individuals. These findings have greatly advanced research into the causes of spondyloarthritis and have already led to translational advances with new treatments entering clinical practice for these common conditions. Only a minority of the genetic risk of these conditions has yet been explained though, and many more genetic associations with these conditions remain to be discovered.

References

1. Helmick CG, Felson DT, Lawrence RC et al. Estimates of the prevalence of arthritis and other rheumatic conditions in the United States: Part I. *Arthritis Rheum* 2008;58(1):15–25.
2. Gelfand JM, Stern RS, Nijsten T et al. The prevalence of psoriasis in African Americans: results from a population-based study. *J Am Acad Dermatol* 2005;52(1):23–26.
3. Yip SY. The prevalence of psoriasis in the Mongoloid race. *J Am Acad Dermatol* 1984;10(6):965–968.
4. Kennedy LG, Will R, Calin A. Sex ratio in the spondyloarthropathies and its relationship to phenotypic expression, mode of inheritance and age at onset. *J Rheumatol* 1993;20(11):1900–1904.
5. Rudwaleit M, van der Heijde D, Landewe R et al. The development of Assessment of SpondyloArthritis international Society classification criteria for axial spondyloarthritis (part II): validation and final selection. *Ann Rheum Dis* 2009;68(6):777–783.
6. Edmunds L, Elswood J, Kennedy LG, Calin A. Primary ankylosing spondylitis, psoriatic and enteropathic spondyloarthropathy: a controlled analysis. *J Rheumatol* 1991;18(5):696–698.
7. Brown MA, Kennedy LG, MacGregor AJ et al. Susceptibility to ankylosing spondylitis in twins: the role of genes, HLA, and the environment. *Arthritis Rheum* 1997 Oct;40(10):1823–1828.

8. Pedersen OB, Svendsen AJ, Ejstrup L et al. Ankylosing spondylitis in Danish and Norwegian twins: occurrence and the relative importance of genetic vs. environmental effectors in disease causation. *Scand J Rheumatol* 2008;37(2):120–126.

9. Brown MA, Laval SH, Brophy S, Calin A. Recurrence risk modelling of the genetic susceptibility to ankylosing spondylitis. *Ann Rheum Dis* 2000;59(11):883–886.

10. Thjodleifsson B, Geirsson AJ, Bjornsson S, Bjarnason I. A common genetic background for inflammatory bowel disease and ankylosing spondylitis: a genealogic study in Iceland. *Arthritis Rheum* 2007;56(8):2633–2639.

11. Brophy S, Hickey S, Menon A et al. Concordance of disease severity among family members with ankylosing spondylitis? *J Rheumatol* 2004;31(9):1775–1778.

12. Brown MA, Brophy S, Bradbury L et al. Identification of major loci controlling clinical manifestations of ankylosing spondylitis. *Arthritis Rheum* 2003;48(8):2234–2239.

13. Hamersma J, Cardon LR, Bradbury L et al. Is disease severity in ankylosing spondylitis genetically determined? *Arthritis Rheum* 2001;44(6):1396–1400.

14. Duffy DL, Spelman LS, Martin NG. Psoriasis in Australian twins. *J Am Acad Dermatol* 1993;29(3):428–434.

15. Myers A, Kay LJ, Lynch SA, Walker DJ. Recurrence risk for psoriasis and psoriatic arthritis within sibships. *Rheumatology* 2005;44(6):773–776.

16. Moll JM, Wright V. Familial occurrence of psoriatic arthritis. *Ann Rheum Dis* 1973;32(3):181–201.

17. Brewerton DA, Hart FD, Nicholls A et al. Ankylosing spondylitis and HL-A 27. *Lancet* 1973;1(7809):904–907.

18. Caffrey MF, James DC. Human lymphocyte antigen association with ankylosing spondylitis. *Nature* 1973;9(242):121.

19. Schlosstein L, Terasaki PI, Bluestone R, Pearson CM. High association of an HL-A antigen, W27, with ankylosing spondylitis. *N Engl J Med* 1973;288(14):704–706.

20. Turner MJ, Sowders DP, DeLay ML et al. HLA B27 misfolding in transgenic rats is associated with activation of the unfolded protein response. *J Immunol* 2005;175(4):2438–2448.

21. DeLay ML, Turner MJ, Klenk EI et al. HLA B27 misfolding and the unfolded protein response augment interleukin-23 production and are associated with Th17 activation in transgenic rats. *Arthritis Rheum* 2009;60(9):2633–2643.

22. Evans DM, Spencer CC, Pointon JJ, Su Z, Harvey D, Kochan G, et al. Interaction between ERAP1 and HLA B27 in ankylosing spondylitis implicates peptide handling in the mechanism for HLA B27 in disease susceptibility. *Nat Genet* 2011;43(8):761–767.

23. Brown MA, Pile KD, Kennedy LG et al. HLA class I associations of ankylosing spondylitis in the white population in the United Kingdom. *Ann Rheum Dis* 1996;55(4):268–270.

24. Gonzalez-Roces S, Alvarez MV, Gonzalez S et al. HLA B27 polymorphism and worldwide susceptibility to ankylosing spondylitis. *Tissue Antigens* 1997;49(2):116–123.

25. D'Amato M, Fiorillo MT, Galeazzi M et al. Frequency of the new HLA B*2709 allele in ankylosing spondylitis patients and healthy individuals. *Dis Markers* 1995;12(3):215–217.

26. Oen K, Postl B, Chalmers IM, Ling N et al. Rheumatic diseases in an Inuit population. *Arthritis Rheum* 1986;29(1):65–74.

27. Jaakkola E, Herzberg I, Laiho K et al. Finnish HLA studies confirm the increased risk conferred by HLA B27 homozygosity in ankylosing spondylitis. *Ann Rheum Dis* 2006;65(6):775–780.

28. Feldtkeller E, Khan MA, van der Heijde D, van der Linden S, Braun J. Age at disease onset and diagnosis delay in HLA B27 negative vs. positive patients with ankylosing spondylitis. *Rheumatol Int* 2003;23(2):61–66.

29. Robinson WP, van der Linden SM, Khan MA et al. HLA Bw60 increases susceptibility to ankylosing spondylitis in HLA B27+ patients. *Arthritis Rheum* 1989;32(9):1135–1141.

30. Wei JC, Tsai WC, Lin HS, Tsai CY, Chou CT. HLA B60 and B61 are strongly associated with ankylosing spondylitis in HLA B27-negative Taiwan Chinese patients. *Rheumatology* (Oxford) 2004;43(7):839–842.

31. Burton PR, Clayton DG, Cardon LR et al. Association scan of 14,500 nonsynonymous SNPs in four diseases identifies autoimmunity variants. *Nat Genet* 2007;39(11):1329–1337.

32. Strange A, Capon F, Spencer CC, Knight J et al. A genome-wide association study identifies new psoriasis susceptibility loci and an interaction between HLA C and ERAP1. *Nat Genet* 2010;42(11):985–990.

33. Kochan G, Krojer T, Harvey D et al. Crystal structures of the endoplasmic reticulum aminopeptidase-1 (ERAP1) reveal the molecular basis for N-terminal peptide trimming. *Proc Nat Acad Sci U S A* 2011;108(19):7745–7750.

34. Baraliakos X, Braun J, Laurent DD et al. Interleukin-17A blockade with secukinumab reduces spinal inflammation in patients with ankylosing spondylitis as early as week 6, as detected by magnetic resonance imaging. *Arthritis Rheum* 2011;63(10):S972.

35. Ruutu M, Thomas G, Steck R et al. Beta-glucan triggers spondyloarthropathy and Crohn's-like ileitis in SKG mice. *Arthritis Rheum* 2012;64(7):2211–2222.

36. Tsuji K, Inouye H, Nose Y et al. Further study on HLA A, B, C, D, DR and haplotype antigen frequencies in psoriasis vulgaris. *Acta Derm Venereol Suppl* (Stockh) 1979;87:107–108.

37. Nair RP, Ruether A, Stuart PE et al. Polymorphisms of the IL12B and IL23R genes are associated with psoriasis. *J Invest Dermatol* 2008;128(7):1653–1661.

38. Gottlieb A, Menter A, Mendelsohn A et al. Ustekinumab, a human interleukin 12/23 monoclonal antibody, for psoriatic arthritis: randomised, double-blind, placebo-controlled, crossover trial. *Lancet* 2009;373(9664):633–640.

39. McInnes I, Sieper J, Braun J et al. Anti-interleukin 17a monoclonal antibody secukinumab reduces signs and symptoms of psoriatic arthritis in a 24-week multicenter, double-blind, randomized, placebo-controlled trial. *Arthritis Rheum* 2011;63(10):S306.

40. Nair RP, Duffin KC, Helms C et al. Genome-wide scan reveals association of psoriasis with IL-23 and NF-kappaB pathways. *Nat Genet* 2009;41(2):199–204.

CHAPTER 42

Genetics of connective tissue diseases

Myles Lewis and Tim Vyse

Genome-wide association scans in connective tissue diseases

The scale of genetics projects has increased dramatically in recent years. Technological advances mean that millions of single nucleotide polymorphisms (SNPs) and other genetic variants such as copy number variation (CNV) can be tested on a single chip. The realization that much larger cohorts are required to increase the power of genetic studies has meant that thousands rather than hundreds of patients are now recruited through international collaboration, even in uncommon diseases such as systemic sclerosis (SSc). Only recently has this begun to increase our understanding of disease pathogenesis. Early evidence of a genetic contribution to connective tissue diseases came from twin and familial studies in systemic lupus erythematosus (SLE): the concordance in monozygotic twins was 24% compared to 2% in dizygotic twins. The sibling recurrence risk ratio (λ_s) for SLE is estimated to be 29-fold higher than in the general population, compared to 5.3 for RA.[1]

To date, five genome-wide association studies (GWAS) have been conducted in SLE, two in SSc and two in Behçet's disease. In SLE, three GWAS[2-4] and a large replication study[5] of individuals of European ancestry, and two GWAS in East Asian populations[6,7] have provided convincing evidence for 31 susceptibility genes, which have reached genome-wide significance (p $<5\times10^{-8}$; Table 42.1). There is suggestive evidence for a further 10 loci, which require confirmation. In systemic sclerosis, a total of nine loci have been found with good evidence at the genome-wide level of significance, with a further four loci implicated (Table 42.2).[8-10] Two GWAS of Behçet's disease have confirmed an extremely strong association with *HLA B*51:01* and identified *IL10* and *IL23R-IL12RB2* regions as genetic risk loci.[11,12] Examining these lists of genes, it is clear that a substantial amount of overlap is seen between SLE and systemic sclerosis, and many of these genes also overlap with rheumatoid arthritis (RA). As ever more genes are identified, they can be functionally grouped into known pathogenic pathways, to help elucidate the links between the risk variants and disease itself.

Major histocompatibility complex

The importance of the MHC in human immunological responses has long been appreciated, but the strong association with MHC haplotypes and autoimmune diseases has been difficult to dissect because of (1) long-range linkage disequilibrium (LD) and (2) duplication of regions leading to CNV and pseudogenes. The strongest genetic associations identified in GWAS of SLE, systemic sclerosis, and Behçet's all lie within the MHC, although it is clear now that this is due to multiple genetic effects. The MHC is an extremely gene-dense region, with at least 250 genes across 3.6 Mb of the classical MHC, with linkage disequilibrium extending the region to 7.6 Mb in size.[13] Whereas gene clusters in other areas of the genome are inherited in clusters of the order of 20 kb long, at the MHC, LD can extend up to 2 Mb. This is a major confounding factor in MHC genetic association studies. Prior to the advent of more detailed mapping of the MHC region, the 8.1 MHC haplotype was associated with a strikingly large number of diverse autoimmune diseases (Table 42.3). The 8.1 haplotype extends to include *HLA-A1*, *B8*, *C4AQ0*, *C4B1*, *DRB1*03:01* and *DQA1*05:01*, *DQB1*02:01* (DQ2), encompassing two significant class III genes, complement C4A null as well as the *TNF-308A* allele. Only recently have genetic studies developed sufficient statistical power or employed techniques such as transancestral mapping to dissect which genes within the MHC are responsible for disease association, rather than merely find associations with the block as a whole. The IMAGEN study[14] examined 1472 tag SNPs in multiple autoimmune diseases including SLE, Crohn's disease, ulcerative colitis, and RA. It resolved three separate signals in class III loci: *SKIV2L*, a locus in between *TNXB-CREBL1* and *NOTCH4*. The highest HLA risk in IMAGEN was observed for *HLA-DRB1*03:01*, with a weaker effect observed for *HLA-DRB1*15:01*. The HLA region has not yet been fine-mapped in other CTD, but HLA typing has confirmed that the *HLA-DRB1*03-DQA1*05* haplotype is the strongest HLA association in the idiopathic inflammatory myopathies (IIM), including dermatomyositis, polymyositis, and CTD-overlap myositis.[15] The *DRB1*03/DPB1*01:01* haplotype was associated with anti-Jo-1 positive cases, predominantly due to *DRB1*03*. The strongest genetic effect so

Table 42.1 SLE susceptibility loci identified in GWAS, replication, and large-scale association studies

Likely causal genes at locus	Chr	OR	P value	Ref	Confirmed by
Good evidence					
MHC	6p21.32	1.98	2.0×10^{-60}	5	3,4,7,21
TNXB-CREBL1	6p21.32	2.4	5.63×10^{-29}	14	
HLA-DRB1*03:01	6p21.32	2.1	1.06×10^{-23}	14	
HLA-DRB1*15:01	6p21.32	1.3	1.46×10^{-5}	14	
STAT4	2q32.2	1.51	5.17×10^{-42}	6	2–5,7,21
TNFSF4	1q25.1	1.46	2.53×10^{-32}	6	5,21
ETS1	11q24	1.37	1.77×10^{-25}	6	7
BLK	8p23.1	0.69	2.09×10^{-24}	6	2–5,7,21
IRF5	7q32.1	1.88	5.8×10^{-24}	5	3,4,6,21
ITGAM	16p11.2	1.62	1.6×10^{-23}	3	2,4,5,21
IKZF1	7p12	0.72	2.75×10^{-23}	6	5
TNFAIP3	6q23.3	1.72	1.37×10^{-17}	6	2,5,7
UBE2L3	22q11.2	0.78	1.48×10^{-16}	6	3,5,21
RASGRP3	2p22.3	0.7	1.25×10^{-15}	5	
TNIP1	5q33	1.27	3.8×10^{-13}	5	6,21
PTPN22	1p13.2	1.35	3.4×10^{-12}	5	3,21
PRDM1-ATG5	6q21	1.25	5.18×10^{-12}	6	3,5,21
WDFY4-LRRC18	10q11	1.24	7.22×10^{-12}	6	7
SLC15A4	12q24.32	1.26	1.77×10^{-11}	6	5
NCF2	1q25	1.19	2.87×10^{-11}	5	
PHRF1-IRF7	11p15.5	0.78	3.0×10^{-10}	3	5
BANK1	4q24	1.38	3.7×10^{-10}	20	
JAZF1	7p15.2	1.19	1.5×10^{-9}	5	
UHRF1BP1	6p21	1.28	5.3×10^{-9}	21	5
LYN	8q12.1	0.77	5.40×10^{-9}	3	
PXK	3p14.3	1.25	7.1×10^{-9}	3	5
IRF8	16q24.1	1.16	1.24×10^{-8}	5	
IFIH1	2q24	1.15	1.63×10^{-8}		
FCGR3B copies	1q23	2.21*	2.7×10^{-8}	29	
TYK2	19p13.2	1.17	3.88×10^{-8}	5	
IL10	1q24	1.19	4.0×10^{-8}	5	21
FCGR2A	1q23.3	0.82	5.6×10^{-7}	21	3
IRAK1-MECP2	Xq28	1.11	7.5×10^{-7}	5	21
Suggestive evidence					
NMNAT2	1q25.3	0.85	1.08×10^{-7}	3	
SCUBE1	22q13.2	0.78	1.21×10^{-7}	3	
ICA1	7p21.3	1.32	1.90×10^{-7}	3	
ARMC3	10p12.31	1.18	2.0×10^{-7}	5	
IL12RB2	1p31.3	1.18	3.4×10^{-7}	5	
LYST	1q42.1	1.18	4.6×10^{-7}	5	

Table 42.1 (*Continued*)

Likely causal genes at locus	Chr	OR	P value	Ref	Confirmed by
MLF1IP	4q35.1	1.23	7.6×10^{-7}	5	
TAOK3	12q	1.18	7.7×10^{-7}	5	
SPPL3	12q24.31	1.14	8.2×10^{-7}	5	
PTTG1	5q33.3	1.15	1.6×10^{-6}	5	21

*OR for <2 vs ≥2 copies.

Table 42.2 Susceptibility genes identified in systemic sclerosis

Gene locus	Chr	OR	P	Ref	Confirmed
Good evidence—GWAS					
HLA-DQB1	6p21	0.62	2.3×10^{-37}	8	9,10
HLA-DPA1/DPB1 (ATA+)	6p21	2.67	1.4×10^{-22}	9	
MHC/ PSORS1C1	6p21	1.25	5.7×10^{-10}	8	
IRF5	7q32	1.50	1.9×10^{-13}	10	8
STAT4	2q32	1.38	2.3×10^{-13}	8	10
CD247	1q22	0.82	2.1×10^{-7}	10	8
CDH7	18q22	1.53	2.3×10^{-7}	10	
EXOC2-IRF4	6p25	0.82	1.2×10^{-8}	10	
RHOB	2p24	1.20	4.7×10^{-6}	8	
TNIP1	5q33	1.31	4.7×10^{-9}	8	
IRF8 (lcSSc)	16q24.1	0.75	2.3×10^{-12}	9	
IL12RB2	1p31	1.17	2.8×10^{-9}		
Suggestive evidence—GWAS					
RPL41/ESYT1 (dcSSc)	12q13.2	1.23	6.0×10^{-8}	9	
SOX5 (ACA+)	12p12.1	1.36	1.4×10^{-7}	9	
GRB10 (lcSSc)	7p12.1	1.15	1.3×10^{-6}	9	
MHC/ NOTCH4 (ATA+)	6p21	0.64	1.2×10^{-4}	9	
Candidate gene studies					
TBX21	17q21.32	3.37	1.4×10^{-15}	23	
BLK	8p23.1	1.2	1.69×10^{-5}		
BANK1 (dcSSc)	4q24	0.70	3.39×10^{-4}	19	
CTGF	6q23.1	2.2	$<1 \times 10^{-3}$		
TNFSF4	1q25.1	0.88	2.3×10^{-3}		
FAS	10q24.1	1.23	4×10^{-3}		

ACA+, anti-centromere positive; ATA+, anti-topoisomerase I positive; dcSSc, diffuse cutaneous systemic sclerosis; lcSSc, limited cutaneous systemic sclerosis.

far identified in Wegener's granulomatosis is from the MHC, with tagging SNPs identifying *HLA-DPB1* alleles, particularly *04:01*.[16] A possible second signal lies in the neighbouring *RXRB-RING1* locus, but finer mapping is required for confirmation. Evaluating the relationship between HLA associations and SNP associations at the MHC is a complex and challenging question: thus far, no firm conclusion can be reached, although it is likely that both HLA

Table 42.3 Autoimmune diseases associated with HLA 8.1 haplotype

Connective tissue diseases	Systemic lupus erythematosus
	Systemic sclerosis
	Polymyositis/dermatomyositis
	Sjögren's syndrome
	Wegener's granulomatosis
Gastrointestinal	Autoimmune hepatitis
	Primary biliary cirrhosis
	Primary sclerosing cholangitis
Other	Sarcoidosis
	Myasthenia gravis
	Inclusion body myositis
	Grave's disease
	Addison's disease
	Idiopathic thrombocytopenic purpura
	Common variable immunodeficiency
	IgA deficiency

molecules and non-HLA genes contribute to the genetics of the MHC associations in SLE and other CTD.

Interferon response genes

High levels of type I interferon have been linked to autoimmune pathogenesis in several connective tissues including SLE, systemic sclerosis, and inflammatory myopathies. Several genes along the interferon pathway are associated with increased risk of CTD, including *IRF5*, *STAT4*, *IRAK1*, and possibly *IRF7*. Interferon regulatory factor 5 (IRF5) is a transcription factor which plays a central role in induction of the type I interferon (IFN) response, downstream of Toll-like receptor (TLR) signalling and antiviral pathways. Candidate gene studies had already discovered a splice variant in exon 1B, but resequencing of SLE patients identified novel rare variants including a 30 bp insertion in exon 6 and a 3′ untranslated region (UTR) variant, which increased mRNA stability, strongly increasing IRF5 protein expression.[17] Combining all three variants showed the strongest risk of SLE and the highest levels of serum IFN-α activity in SLE patients. Signal transducer and activators of transcription-4 (STAT4) is a key transcription factor activated in response to type I IFN, and appears to act downstream of IRF5. The *STAT4* risk alleles increased sensitivity to IFN-α in peripheral blood mononuclear cells (PBMC) from SLE patients,[18] and in a combined genetic analysis of *IRF5* and *STAT4* four or more risk alleles were linked to a substantial risk of SLE (odds ratio = 5.83), suggesting a genetic interaction. STAT4 is activated in response to IL-12 and IL-23, and may be involved in other pathways such as directing Th1 and Th17 responses, and production of IFN-γ in antigen-presenting cells. The same *IRF5* and *STAT4* risk haplotypes are associated with systemic sclerosis.[19] Other interferon pathway genes with good evidence for their involvement in autoimmune diseases include *IFIH1*, *TYK2*, *IRF8*, while further confirmation is required for *IRF7*, *TRAF6*, and *IKBKE*.

Genes specific to lymphocyte function

Three key genes involved in B-cell receptor (BCR) signalling have been associated with SLE in GWAS: B-lymphoid tyrosine kinase (*BLK*), B-cell scaffold protein with ankyrin repeats (*BANK1*), and *LYN*, which phosphorylates Igα/β as a key signalling event following BCR stimulation.[3,4,20] Three SNPs with potential functional effects were identified in *BANK1*: the strongest evidence is for a branch point SNP (rs17266594), which affects transcription of different splice variants, increasing the level of the main transcript.[20] The same three SNPs in *BANK1* associated with SLE are also associated with diffuse SSc, particularly anti-topoisomerase I antibody positive individuals.[19] SNPs in the *BLK* promoter region were identified in the first SLE GWAS, and shown to reduce BLK expression.[4] BLK is a Src family tyrosine kinase, like Lyn. Although the B-cell functions of BLK are not understood, the genetic association with SLE has been reproduced across multiple studies,[2–5,7,21] while a weak association was seen in a meta-analysis of SSc patients.

Two well-replicated disease susceptibility genes in SLE affect T lymphocyte function: *PTPN22* and *TNFSF4*. *PTPN22* encodes lymphoid tyrosine phosphatase, with dual B- and T-cell functions. The non-synonymous SNP rs2476601 encodes an Arg620Trp substitution, leading to a more potent phosphatase, with impaired B-cell tolerance checkpoints and increased numbers of autoreactive B cells. The same variant is associated with RA, SLE, SSc, Crohn's disease, and type 1 diabetes, with less strong evidence that it may be associated with the inflammatory myopathies and ANCA-positive Wegener's granulomatosis. In addition to its B-cell effects, the 620Trp substitution has a paradoxical effect on T cells, leading to reduced T-cell receptor signalling. TNF ligand superfamily member 4 (*TNFSF4*) encodes OX40L, a costimulation cell surface ligand involved in T-cell activation during antigen presentation. Cross-linking of OX40L causes B-cell proliferation and increased immunoglobulin secretion. The risk haplotype identified in both SLE and SSc increases OX40L expression.[22]

An interesting gene found in both SSc GWAS is *CD247*, which encodes the T-cell receptor subunit zeta (CD3ζ).[8,10] An earlier candidate gene study in SLE suggested that SNPs in the 3′ UTR, which lowered CD3ζ expression, predisposed to SLE. The *TBX21* gene, which has so far only been found in association with SSc,[23] encodes T-bet, a major transcription factor critical for Th1 development and suppression of Th17 differentiation. T-bet deficiency increased skin fibrosis in a bleomycin-induced skin fibrosis mouse model.

Regulators of the NFκB inflammatory pathway

The protein encoded by *TNFAIP3* (TNFα induced protein 3) is better known as the deubiquitinating enzyme A20, which is involved in deactivating a number of NFκB pathway intermediates and preventing TNF-induced apoptosis, downstream of TLR signals. A20 deficiency in mice leads to a profound autoinflammatory phenotype with cachexia and early mortality due to hypersensitivity to TNF. A coding SNP (rs2230926) associated with SLE and RA has been shown to reduce A20-mediated inhibition of TNFα. Sequencing of A20 exons shows that the main genetic effect is on control of A20 expression through variants in the 5′ and 3′ UTR. Association with *TNIP1*, which interacts with A20, has been confirmed in GWAS of SLE, SSc, and psoriasis[5,6,8] Studies using *Tnip1*-deficient mice suggest that, unlike A20, *TNIP1* does not control NFκB activation, but is still critical for preventing TNF-induced apoptosis.

Genetics of complement deficiency in systemic lupus erythematosus

Homozygous deficiency of complement C1q, C2, and C4 is associated with the development of a SLE-like disease with surprisingly high penetrance. There is evidence of a hierarchy, with higher risk conferred by earlier components of the classical pathway: 93% of case reports of C1q deficiency were associated with a lupus-like illness,[24] 57% for C1r and C1s, 75% for C4, while for C2 deficiency the risk is estimated to be 10–30%. With C3 deficiency the most prominent clinical features are recurrent pyogenic infections and membranoproliferative glomerulonephritis, and around 13% of cases develop SLE. Attempts to explain the association between complement deficiencies and SLE have concentrated on key functions of complement: transport and processing of immune complexes via the liver and spleen; phagocytosis of apoptotic cells; and generation of tolerance signals during antigen presentation. The 'waste disposal hypothesis' proposes that complement deficiency leads to failed clearance of organ-damaging immune complexes, as well as overexposure of autoantigens due to impaired clearance of apoptotic cells. This theory is supported by evidence from C1q-deficient mice, which developed lupus autoantibodies and nephritis associated with defective phagocytosis of apoptotic cells.[25] However, the development of autoimmunity in these mice is critically dependent on the mixed 129×C57BL/6 genetic background,[26] although the phagocytic defect due to C1q deficiency is unaffected by these genetic factors. It must be remembered that inherited complete deficiencies of classical pathway complement components are extremely rare: only 41 cases of C1q deficiency have been reported. As part of a commonly duplicated RCCX module in the MHC class III region, the C4A and C4B genes are affected by CNV, which directly correlates with serum levels of C4. Recent evidence suggests that partial deficiency of C4 may not act as a susceptibility factor in SLE.[27]

Other genes involved in phagocytosis and immune complex processing

ITGAM has consistently appeared with strong association in recent GWAS. ITGAM encodes alpha-chain integrin α_M, which is part of the complement receptor 3 (CR3) cell surface receptor, also known as CD11b or Mac-1. CR3 is expressed on a wide variety of immune cells and is involved in uptake of immune complexes by binding iC3b or cell surface signalling through ligands such as intercellular adhesion molecule-1 (ICAM-1) and ICAM-2. Evidence is accumulating that the main functional variant in ITGAM is a non-synonymous rs1143679 polymorphism strongly associated with SLE,[28] but interestingly is not associated with RA or SSc. This variant causes a R77H substitution, whose functional effect is to severely reduce neutrophil adhesion via ICAM-1 and -2, and impair iC3b-mediated phagocytosis.

The low-affinity Fc receptor genes FCGR2A, FCGR2B, FCGR3A, and FCGR3B suffer from extensive sequence homology due to duplication of genetic segments. The non-synonymous SNP rs1801274 associated with SLE[3] causes a missense His131Arg substitution in the ligand binding domain of FcγRIIa, leading to inhibition of phagocytosis via reduced affinity for IgG2. Duplication of a segment between FCGR3B and FCGR2C is common, resulting in between zero and six copies in a typical diploid human genome. Low FCGR3B CNV (less than two copies) is a major predisposing factor to SLE, microscopic polyangiitis, and Wegener's granulomatosis,[29] and predisposes to immune-mediated nephritis in rats. Expression of FcγRIIIb, which is restricted to neutrophils, correlates with copy number of FCGR3B, and the low CNV of FCGR3B seen in SLE is associated with decreased immune complex adhesion and uptake by neutrophils.[30] Another variant found in South-east Asian and white European SLE patients, whose function has been investigated, is the Ile232Thr substitution in the inhibitory Fc receptor FcγRIIb. This substitution leads to exclusion of FcγRIIb from signalling lipid rafts, preventing its inhibitory action on other activatory Fc receptors in B cells.[31]

Other important genes

In Behçet's disease, SNPs in the promoter region of the suppressive cytokine IL10 have been confirmed in two GWAS, with evidence in stimulated monocytes that these variants cause reduced IL-10 production.[12] A different SNP downstream of IL10 (rs3024505, which was not associated with Behçet's disease), has been found in association studies in SLE, Crohn's, and autoimmune diabetes. Genetic association with Behçet's disease in the IL23R-IL12RB2 region showed greater overlap with the IL-23 receptor, consistent with findings in other diseases such as ankylosing spondylitis, psoriasis, and IBD. If the IL23R association is confirmed it would be of considerable importance, because it would implicate the Th17 axis in the pathogenesis of Behçet's disease. On the other hand, a recent study in SSc confirmed an intronic signal at the centre of IL12RB2, independent of IL23R. The IL-12 pathway may be important in scleroderma, since it promotes proinflammatory Th1 responses and signals through STAT4, which is another SSc susceptibility gene.

Genetics of autoimmune diseases in mouse models

Although mouse models have been very useful for studying specific immunological pathways in rheumatic diseases, a surprisingly large number of genetic manipulations led to a lupus-like illness in mice. However, these results must be interpreted with caution. Until very recently the techniques used for gene targeting ('knockout mice') always led to incorporation of sections of genome from two different mouse strains: 129 and C57BL/6. Interaction between various loci of 129 and C57BL/6 genomes commonly leads to lupus autoantibodies and in some cases organ involvement including nephritis.[26] As a demonstration of this issue, until recently it was thought that deficiency of Fcgr2b in mice led to lupus-like autoimmunity. However, Fcgr2b-deficient mice generated on a pure C57BL/6 genetic background failed to develop lupus.[32]

Researchers have identified genes responsible for certain lupus-predisposing genetic loci in inbred strains commonly used as mouse models of SLE. The key locus in BXSB mice, Yaa, is a duplication of TLR7 caused by Y chromosome translocation, since TLR7 is normally only present on the mouse X chromosome.[33] In MRL/lpr mice, the key locus lpr is a non-functional mutation of the apoptosis signalling receptor Fas. Notably, the human equivalent is Canale–Smith syndrome, a lymphoproliferative disorder,[34] and lpr mice on a C57BL/6 background only show mild autoimmunity, confirming the necessity of the MRL background in lpr-induced fatal lupus nephritis and organ damage. In (NZB×NZW)F1 mice, several loci have been identified including Sle1 (subdivided a–d) on chromosome 1, analogous to a region of multiple SLE susceptibility loci on human chromosome 1.[35] The *Sle1b* locus corresponds to polymorphisms in *Slamf6*, encoding the SLAM receptor Ly108, which regulates lymphocyte interactions and B-cell tolerance.

Mouse models of SSc have highlighted the importance of several pathogenic genes in causing systemic fibrosis.[36] In Tight Skin-1 (TSK-1) mice there is a duplication of the fibrillin-1 gene (*Fbn1*), which leads to skin fibrosis and evidence of autoimmunity. Excessive activation of TGF-β pathways in fibroblasts using a transgenic mouse with conditional expression of TGF-β receptor type I (TGFβRI) also mimicked SSc.

Environmental factors associated with connective tissue disease

Even if the complexity of genetic factors and how they interact could be fully understood, the evidence from twin studies suggests that other factors are needed to explain the predisposition to connective tissue diseases. The key groups of environmental factors for which there is at least some supportive evidence includes infectious agents, particularly in SLE and vasculitis, airborne exposure, especially smoking and silica, as well as certain toxins which cause syndromes mimicking CTD (summarized in Table 42.4).

Table 42.4 Environmental factors with reasonable evidence of causal association with connective tissue diseases

Exposure	Disease
Infections	
EBV	Systemic lupus erythematosus
Staph. aureus	Wegener's granulomatosis
Hepatitis C	Cryoglobulinaemia
Hepatitis B	PAN
Environment	
Sunlight/UV	Cutaneous lupus
Low vitamin D	Systemic lupus erythematosus
Airborne	
Smoking	Systemic lupus erythematosus, but not systemic sclerosis
Silica dust	Rheumatoid arthritis, systemic sclerosis
Drugs	
Hydralazine, procainamide and many others	Drug-induced lupus
TNF inhibitors, interferon-α	Lupus autoantibodies, occasional autoimmune phenomena
Propylthiouracil	ANCA-type vasculitis
Gadolinium	Nephrogenic systemic fibrosis
Toxins	
Rapeseed oil denatured with aniline	Toxic oil syndrome
Contaminated L-tryptophan supplements	Eosinophilic myalgic syndrome
Vinyl chloride	Scleroderma-like syndrome

Infections and connective tissue disease

Several infections have been shown to be critical pathogenic induction agents, particularly for the vasculitides. Hepatitis C virus is the causative agent for mixed cryoglobulinaemia, and hepatitis B is associated with polyarteritis nodosa (discussed in more detail in the relevant clinical chapters). Nasal carriage of *Staphylococcus aureus* is associated with relapse in ANCA-associated vasculitis, and hence antibiotic prophylaxis with septrin has been shown to reduce relapse.

There is a strong story for involvement of Epstein–Barr virus (EBV) in SLE pathogenesis. EBV is a human herpesvirus which infects 90% of all adults and is linked to several cancers, particular B-cell lymphomas (Hodgkin's and Burkitt's) and nasopharyngeal carcinoma. A study of children and young adults with SLE found virtually all (99%) had seroconverted against EBV compared to only 70% of controls.[37] SLE patients exhibit a 15-fold increase in EBV viral load.[38] The humoral response to EBV in 90% of healthy EBV-infected adults involves the generation of antibodies against Epstein–Barr nuclear antigen 1 (EBNA-1), one of several key EBV proteins which mark its latent cycle. Several groups have shown that antibodies against lupus autoantigens Sm B′ and Sm D1 cross-react with EBNA-1.[39] The suggestion is that epitope spreading against EBNA-1 and perhaps other EBV proteins including EBNA-2 may be central to propagation of lupus autoantibody responses.

Exposure to sunlight and ultraviolet light

Studies have consistently shown that 60–70% of SLE patients have abnormally low levels of 25-hydroxyvitamin D. There is limited evidence that serum levels of 25-hydroxyvitamin D may have an inverse relationship to disease activity, and that low vitamin D is associated with ANA positivity, even in healthy individuals.[40] However, longitudinal studies have not been done, nor have studies to determine whether vitamin D supplementation will have any impact on disease activity. An increasing body of literature has focused on the effects of the biologically active form 1,25-dihydroxyvitamin D on innate and adaptive immune responses, and found that 1,25-dihydroxyvitamin D and vitamin D receptor agonists have potent anti-inflammatory effects on B and T cells, including induction of regulatory T cells. A recent GWAS in multiple sclerosis, a disease known to have a north–south geographical distribution, identified two key genes in vitamin D metabolism (*CYP27B1* and *CYP24A1*), which encode 25-hydroxyvitamin D_3-1-alpha hydroxylase and 1,25-dihydroxyvitamin D 24-hydroxylase respectively. A study searching for SNPs with functional effects on serum vitamin D levels identified several which also showed an overlap with risk of type 1 diabetes.

Although photosensitive skin rashes are a widely recognized clinical feature of SLE, as evidenced by their inclusion in the diagnostic criteria for SLE, the mechanism is unclear. It is universally agreed that lupus skin manifestations can be induced and augmented by UV-B (280–320 nm), but there is less agreement over UV-A (320–400 nm). Some studies suggest that UV-A can also induce pathogenic skin lesions at slightly lower rates to UV-B.[41] One small controlled study suggested that low levels of longer wavelength UV-A1 (340–400 nm) can actually improve systemic disease activity in SLE. Anti-Ro and anti-La antibodies are associated with cutaneous lupus manifestations. Although some studies found that anti-Ro or anti-La positive patients were more likely to show pathological photoprovocation reactions, this is not a consistent finding.[41]

Airborne environmental factors

Of occupational environmental factors, exposure to silica, especially due to mining, has consistently strong evidence for a link to development of multiple different connective tissue diseases. A meta-analysis of epidemiological surveys confined to SSc estimated the relative risk (RR) due to silica exposure in men to be 3.02 (95% CI 1.24–7.35).[42] This is largely derived from a German cohort study of 50 000 male uranium miners, which found a RR of 7.41 for development of SSc. Population studies which failed to find an association were usually based on occupation derived from death certificates, and may have miscategorized individuals with low or moderate silica exposure. A recent study looking at almost 800 confirmed cases of silicosis found a high proportion of patients with connective tissue disorders, especially RA and ANCA-associated vasculitis. However, a large Swedish case-control study with over 2200 Wegener's granulomatosis patients and 22 000 controls found no evidence of increased risk with any occupation.[43]

While there is good evidence for a link between cigarette smoking and increased risk of RA, this evidence has been harder to find for other connective tissue disorders. A large meta-analysis found that smoking modestly increased the risk of SLE, with an odds ratio of 1.5 (95% CI 1.09–2.08).[44] Smoking is specifically linked to increased lupus skin manifestations and subsequent scarring. Within SLE patients, presence of anti-dsDNA antibodies is more common in smokers and smoking may increase disease activity, revealing a parallel between the association of smoking and development of anti-CCP antibodies in the pathogenesis of RA. Unlike RA, smoking is not associated with increased risk of development of SSc.[45] Smoking substantially increases the risk of giant cell arteritis (sixfold) with a 17-fold increased risk with heavy smoking.[46]

Drugs

Drugs are a well-recognized cause of some connective tissue diseases, especially drug-induced lupus (DIL) and propylthiouracil in ANCA-associated vasculitis. Many drugs have been implicated in DIL (reviewed in ref. 47), and their chemical structures typically contain aromatic amines, hydrazines, or a phenol ring with or without sulfhydryl groups. The two commonest inducing agents are hydralazine and procainamide. The clinical features of DIL are covered in more detail in Chapter 126. Antibodies against DNA-binding histones are typically seen in DIL, but can also be seen in non-drug-related SLE. Drug–DNA interactions may be a pathogenic factor, since both procainamide and hydralazine are able to bind polynucleotide chains. However, hydralazine has also been shown to interact with DNA–histone complexes. In contrast to idiopathic lupus, HLA-DR4 (*DRB1*04*) has been associated with hydralazine-induced lupus, but it is difficult to draw any firm conclusions because of the small numbers of patients studied.

TNF inhibitors are well recognized to cause an increase in the development of ANA (range 23–57%) and to a lesser extent anti-dsDNA antibodies (9–33%).[47] However, induction of lupus-like features attributed to TNF blockade is rare, and the majority of patients with new lupus autoantibodies show no clinical signs. Only a few definite cases of new onset SLE have been reported. Similarly other

biological agents, particularly IFN-α, are associated with autoimmune phenomena and autoantibody development, but only rarely cause full SLE.

Toxins

Although many studies have looked at chemical exposure and risk of various connective tissue disorders, the vast majority of these cases are not systematically linked to exposure to any particular group of chemicals or toxins. However, several syndromes with similarities to connective tissue disorders, particularly scleroderma, can be attributed to exposure to certain chemicals. Toxic oil syndrome occurred in Spain in 1981, and affected nearly 20 000 individuals, causing over 300 deaths. It was characterized by the development of acute pneumonitis, followed by a chronic illness affecting the skin, peripheral nerves, and muscles, with scleroderma-like skin thickening and neuromyopathy. The syndrome was attributed to ingestion of contaminated rapeseed oil, denatured by aniline. Individuals developed eosinophilia, elevated IgE, and in some cases autoantibodies. A few years later, peaking in 1989, at least 1500 individuals were affected by a second disease with similar features, named eosinophilia–myalgia syndrome (EMS).[48] Although the chemical exposure was traced in nearly all cases to dietary supplements containing L-tryptophan, an essential amino acid, it remains uncertain whether the true culprit was excessive doses of L-tryptophan itself, or other contaminants or chemical by-products. Vinyl chloride, a gas used to manufacture plastics, also caused another scleroderma-like illness in over 50 factory workers. Clinical features included pulmonary fibrosis, acro-osteolysis, and cryoglobulin formation. A previous controversy suggesting a link between silicone gel used in breast implants and scleroderma has since been disproven by several large studies and meta-analysis, which have found no association between silicone breast implants and risk of connective tissue disorders.[49]

Conclusion

GWAS have identified a large number of novel genes in SLE, SSc and Behçet's disease, and further studies are in progress in ANCA-associated vasculitis and inflammatory myopathies. These rewritten genetic susceptibility maps highlight the major overlap in genes predisposing to autoimmune diseases, but are also beginning to explain differences in genetic susceptibility between specific connective tissue diseases. Key environmental triggers to CTD include infections particularly viruses (EBV, HBV, and HCV), and airborne toxins, especially cigarette smoke and silica. Increasing evidence points to low vitamin D, which has genetic as well as environmental causes, as a risk factor for the development of autoimmune diseases.

References

1. Alarcon-Segovia D, Alarcon-Riquelme ME, Cardiel MH et al. Familial aggregation of systemic lupus erythematosus, rheumatoid arthritis, and other autoimmune diseases in 1,177 lupus patients from the GLADEL cohort. *Arthritis Rheum* 2005;52(4):1138–1147.
2. Graham RR, Cotsapas C, Davies L et al. Genetic variants near TNFAIP3 on 6q23 are associated with systemic lupus erythematosus. *Nat Genet* 2008;40(9):1059–1061.
3. Harley JB, Alarcon-Riquelme ME, Criswell LA, et al. Genome-wide association scan in women with systemic lupus erythematosus identifies susceptibility variants in ITGAM, PXK, KIAA1542 and other loci. *Nat Genet* 2008;40(2):204–210.

4. Hom G, Graham RR, Modrek B et al. Association of systemic lupus erythematosus with C8orf13-BLK and ITGAM-ITGAX. *N Engl J Med* 2008;358(9):900–909.

5. Gateva V, Sandling JK, Hom G et al. A large-scale replication study identifies TNIP1, PRDM1, JAZF1, UHRF1BP1 and IL10 as risk loci for systemic lupus erythematosus. *Nat Genet* 2009;41(11):1228–1233.

6. Han JW, Zheng HF, Cui Y et al. Genome-wide association study in a Chinese Han population identifies nine new susceptibility loci for systemic lupus erythematosus. *Nat Genet* 2009;41(11):1234–1237.

7. Yang W, Shen N, Ye DQ et al. Genome-wide association study in Asian populations identifies variants in ETS1 and WDFY4 associated with systemic lupus erythematosus. *PLoS Genet* 2010;6(2):e1000841.

8. Allanore Y, Saad M, Dieude P et al. Genome-wide scan identifies TNIP1, PSORS1C1, and RHOB as novel risk loci for systemic sclerosis. *PLoS Genet* 2011;7(7):e1002091.

9. Gorlova O, Martin JE, Rueda B et al. Identification of novel genetic markers associated with clinical phenotypes of systemic sclerosis through a genome-wide association strategy. *PLoS Genet* 2011;7(7): e1002178.

10. Radstake TR, Gorlova O, Rueda B et al. Genome-wide association study of systemic sclerosis identifies CD247 as a new susceptibility locus. *Nat Genet* 2010;42(5):426–429.

11. Mizuki N, Meguro A, Ota M et al. Genome-wide association studies identify IL23R-IL12RB2 and IL10 as Behcet's disease susceptibility loci. *Nat Genet* 2010;42(8):703–706.

12. Remmers EF, Cosan F, Kirino Y et al. Genome-wide association study identifies variants in the MHC class I, IL10, and IL23R-IL12RB2 regions associated with Behcet's disease. *Nat Genet* 2010;42(8):698–702.

13. Horton R, Wilming L, Rand V et al. Gene map of the extended human MHC. *Nat Rev Genet* 2004;5(12):889–899.

14. Rioux JD, Goyette P, Vyse TJ et al. Mapping of multiple susceptibility variants within the MHC region for 7 immune-mediated diseases. *Proc Natl Acad Sci U S A* 2009;106(44):18680–18685.

15. Chinoy H, Payne D, Poulton KV et al. HLA-DPB1 associations differ between DRB1*03 positive anti-Jo-1 and anti-PM-Scl antibody positive idiopathic inflammatory myopathy. *Rheumatology* (Oxford) 2009;48(10):1213–1217.

16. Heckmann M, Holle JU, Arning L et al. The Wegener's granulomatosis quantitative trait locus on chromosome 6p21.3 as characterised by tag-SNP genotyping. *Ann Rheum Dis* 2008;67(7):972–979.

17. Graham RR, Kyogoku C, Sigurdsson S et al. Three functional variants of IFN regulatory factor 5 (IRF5) define risk and protective haplotypes for human lupus. *Proc Natl Acad Sci U S A* 2007;104(16):6758–6763.

18. Kariuki SN, Kirou KA, MacDermott EJ et al. Cutting edge: autoimmune disease risk variant of STAT4 confers increased sensitivity to IFN-alpha in lupus patients in vivo. *J Immunol* 2009;182(1):34–38.

19. Dieude P, Wipff J, Guedj A et al. BANK1 Is a genetic risk factor for diffuse cutaneous systemic sclerosis and has additive effects with IRF5 and STAT4. *Arthritis Rheum* 2009;60(11):3447–3454.

20. Kozyrev SV, Abelson AK, Wojcik J et al. Functional variants in the B-cell gene BANK1 are associated with systemic lupus erythematosus. *Nat Genet* 2008;40(2):211–216.

21. Taylor KE, Chung SA, Graham RR et al. Risk alleles for systemic lupus erythematosus in a large case-control collection and associations with clinical subphenotypes. *PLoS Genet* 2011;7(2):e1001311.

22. Cunninghame Graham DS, Graham RR, Manku H et al. Polymorphism at the TNF superfamily gene TNFSF4 confers susceptibility to systemic lupus erythematosus. *Nat Genet* 2008;40(1):83–89.

23. Gourh P, Agarwal SK, Divecha D et al. Polymorphisms in TBX21 and STAT4 increase the risk of systemic sclerosis: evidence of possible gene-gene interaction and alterations in Th1/Th2 cytokines. *Arthritis Rheum* 2009;60(12):3794–3806.

24. Pickering MC, Botto M, Taylor PR, Lachmann PJ, Walport MJ. Systemic lupus erythematosus, complement deficiency, and apoptosis. *Adv Immunol* 2000;76:227–324.

25. Botto M, Dell'Agnola C, Bygrave AE et al. Homozygous C1q deficiency causes glomerulonephritis associated with multiple apoptotic bodies. *Nat Genet* 1998;19(1):56–59.

26. Bygrave AE, Rose KL, Cortes-Hernandez J et al. Spontaneous autoimmunity in 129 and C57BL/6 mice-implications for autoimmunity described in gene-targeted mice. *PLoS Biol* 2004;2(8):E243.

27. Boteva L, Morris DL, Cortes-Hernandez J et al. Genetically determined partial complement c4 deficiency states are not independent risk factors for SLE in UK and Spanish populations. *Am J Hum Genet* 2012;90(3): 445–456.

28. Nath SK, Han S, Kim-Howard X et al. A nonsynonymous functional variant in integrin-alpha(M) (encoded by ITGAM) is associated with systemic lupus erythematosus. *Nat Genet* 2008;40(2):152–154.

29. Fanciulli M, Norsworthy PJ, Petretto E et al. FCGR3B copy number variation is associated with susceptibility to systemic, but not organ-specific, autoimmunity. *Nat Genet* 2007;39(6):721–723.

30. Willcocks LC, Lyons PA, Clatworthy MR et al. Copy number of FCGR3B, which is associated with systemic lupus erythematosus, correlates with protein expression and immune complex uptake. *J Exp Med* 2008;205(7): 1573–1582.

31. Floto RA, Clatworthy MR, Heilbronn KR et al. Loss of function of a lupus-associated FcgammaRIIb polymorphism through exclusion from lipid rafts. *Nat Med* 2005;11(10):1056–1058.

32. Boross P, Arandhara VL, Martin-Ramirez J et al. The inhibiting Fc receptor for IgG, FcgammaRIIB, is a modifier of autoimmune susceptibility. *J Immunol* 2011;187(3):1304–1313.

33. Pisitkun P, Deane JA, Difilippantonio MJ. Autoreactive B cell responses to RNA-related antigens due to TLR7 gene duplication. *Science* 2006;312(5780):1669–1672.

34. Drappa J, Vaishnaw AK, Sullivan KE, Chu JL, Elkon KB. Fas gene mutations in the Canale-Smith syndrome, an inherited lymphoproliferative disorder associated with autoimmunity. *N Engl J Med* 1996;335(22): 1643–1649.

35. Morel L. Genetics of SLE: evidence from mouse models. *Nat Rev Rheumatol* 2010;6(6):348–357.

36. Beyer C, Schett G, Distler O, Distler JH. Animal models of systemic sclerosis: prospects and limitations. *Arthritis Rheum* 2010;62(10):2831–2844.

37. James JA, Kaufman KM, Farris AD et al. An increased prevalence of Epstein-Barr virus infection in young patients suggests a possible etiology for systemic lupus erythematosus. *J Clin Invest.* 1997;100(12): 3019–3026.

38. Moon UY, Park SJ, Oh ST et al. Patients with systemic lupus erythematosus have abnormally elevated Epstein-Barr virus load in blood. *Arthritis Res Ther* 2004;6(4):R295–R302.

39. James JA, Harley JB. Linear epitope mapping of an Sm B/B' polypeptide. *J Immunol* 1992;148(7):2074–2079.

40. Ritterhouse LL, Crowe SR, Niewold TB et al. Vitamin D deficiency is associated with an increased autoimmune response in healthy individuals and in patients with systemic lupus erythematosus. *Ann Rheum Dis* 2011;70(9):1569–1574.

41. Sanders CJ, Van Weelden H, Kazzaz GA et al. Photosensitivity in patients with lupus erythematosus: a clinical and photobiological study of 100 patients using a prolonged phototest protocol. *Br J Dermatol* 2003;149(1):131–137.

42. McCormic ZD, Khuder SS, Aryal BK, Ames AL, Khuder SA. Occupational silica exposure as a risk factor for scleroderma: a meta-analysis. *Int Arch Occup Environ Health* 2010;83(7):763–769.

43. Knight A, Sandin S, Askling J. Occupational risk factors for Wegener's granulomatosis: a case-control study. *Ann Rheum Dis* 2010;69(4): 737–740.

44. Costenbader KH, Kim DJ, Peerzada J et al. Cigarette smoking and the risk of systemic lupus erythematosus: a meta-analysis. *Arthritis Rheum* 2004;50(3):849–857.

45. Chaudhary P, Chen X, Assassi S et al. Cigarette smoking is not a risk factor for systemic sclerosis. *Arthritis Rheum* 2011;63(10):3098–3102.

46. Duhaut P, Pinede L, Demolombe-Rague S et al. Giant cell arteritis and cardiovascular risk factors: a multicenter, prospective case-control study. Groupe de Recherche sur l'Arterite a Cellules Geantes. *Arthritis Rheum* 1998;41(11):1960–1965.

47. Mongey AB, Hess EV. Drug insight: autoimmune effects of medications—what's new? *Nat Clin Pract Rheumatol* 2008;4(3):136–144.

48. Silver RM. Eosinophilia-myalgia syndrome, toxic-oil syndrome, and diffuse fasciitis with eosinophilia. *Curr Opin Rheumatol*. 1993;5(6):802–808.

49. Janowsky EC, Kupper LL, Hulka BS. Meta-analyses of the relation between silicone breast implants and the risk of connective-tissue diseases. *N Engl J Med* 2000;342(11):781–790.

Table 43.1 Juvenile idiopathic arthritis: non-HLA genetic susceptibility loci validated in more than one independent cohort

Gene	SNP	Reference	Study population	Subtypes tested[a]	Association (yes/no)
PTPN22	rs2476601	11	UK	All	Y
	rs2476601	12	Norway	All	Y
	rs2476601	13	Finland	PO and RF-P	N not in total dataset
	rs2476601	14	US and German	PO, EO and RF-P	Y
IL2RA	rs2104286	21	UK	All	Y
	rs2104286	21	US	PO, EO, and RF-P	Y
	rs2104286	16	US	All	N
IL2	rs6822844	23	Dutch	PO, EO, RF-P, and SO	Y
	rs6822844	22	UK	All	Y
	rs17388568	14	US and German	PO, EO, and RF-P	Y
STAT4	rs7574865	15	UK	All	Y
	rs7574865	16	US	All	Y
	rs7574865	14	US and German	PO, EO, and RF-P	Y
TRAF1/C5	rs10818488	36	Dutch	PO, EO, RF-P, RF+P, and SO	N not in total dataset Association in the polyarticular subset
	rs3761847	35	US	All	Y
	rs2900180	15	UK	All	Y
	rs3761847	16	US	All	N
	rs3761847 rs2900180	14	US	PO, EO, and RF-P	N
TNFAIP3	rs6920220 rs13207033	15	UK	All	Y
	rs6920220 rs10499194	16	US	All	Y
	rs6920220 rs13207033 rs10499194	14	US and German	PO, EO, and RF-P	N
CCR5	CCR5Δ32	28	US	PO, EO, RF-P, RF+P, and SO	Y
	CCR5Δ32	30	Norway	All	N
	CCR5Δ32	29	UK	All	Y
C12orf30/SH2B3/ATXN2	rs17696736	16	US	All	Y
	rs653178	31	UK	All	Y
	rs17696736	14	US and German	PO, EO, and RF-P	Y
PTPN2	rs7234029	14	US and German	PO, EO, and RF-P	Y
	rs7234029	47	UK	All	Y
COG6	rs7993214	14	US and German	PO, EO, and RF-P	Y
ANGPT1	rs1010824	14	US and German	PO, EO, and RF-P	Y

[a]ILAR subtypes investigated: EO, extended oligoarthritis; PO, persistent oligoarthritis; RF-P, rheumatoid factor negative polyarthritis; RF+P, rheumatoid factor positive polyarthritis; SO, systemic onset.

within the gene have recently been found to be associated with JIA in a United States cohort and replicated in an independent cohort of United States and German cases.[14] PTPN2 encodes a protein tyrosine phosphatase, similar to PTPN22, which also plays a role in activation and regulation of T and B cells.

COG6 and ANGPT1

A recent study in a United States cohort found two novel associations with JIA in the COG6 and ANGPT1 genes; these were validated in an independent cohort of United States and German cases and controls.[14]

Other potential loci

There are a number of loci which show association with JIA in just one study which require validation in independent cohorts or with meta-analysis. These include associations in the C-type lectin domain family 16, member A (*CLEC16A*) gene,[34] cytotoxic T lymphocyte antigen 4 (*CTLA4*), AF4/FMR2 family member 3 (*AFF3*), protein kinase C, theta (*PRKCQ*), and the lim domain containing preferred translocation partner in lipoma (*LPP*) genes.

The candidate gene approach has been successful in the search for JIA genetic susceptibility risk factors, but is obviously limited by prior knowledge of a disease.

Genome-wide association studies in juvenile idiopathic arthritis

Genetic studies of complex autoimmune diseases have been transformed by the development of the genome-wide association study (GWAS) in the mid 1990s following a number of advances, the identification of millions of SNPs across the genome, and the technical ability to genotype these SNPs rapidly and cheaply. This approach has proved highly successful in identifying novel risk factors for many complex diseases. It would be fair to say that the difficulty in collecting large sample sizes for JIA has hindered progress in the search for genetic risk factors for JIA using GWAS approaches, but these are now being published. The first two were performed on very modest sample sizes. The first identified association with the *TRAF1/C5* locus on chromosome 9[35]; different SNPS in this region have also been associated with JIA in independent candidate gene studies.[15,36] The second identified association of the *VTCN1* (B7-homolog4 (*B7-H4*)) gene with JIA, which was validated in an independent dataset.[37] More recently a larger study has been reported investigating United States and European JIA cases and controls. It identified two novel JIA susceptibility loci, *c3orf1*, IL-15 (*IL15*), and the jumanji domain containing 1C (*JMJD1C*) region,[38] which show replication in United Kingdom and German cohorts. Further JIA GWAS are in progress; combined meta-analyses of the studies to date will validate previous findings, and the increased power should enable the discovery of additional novel loci.

Fine mapping and identification of causal variants

There is now a growing list of SNPs associated with JIA. In most cases these SNPs will not be the actual disease-causing variant but will be correlated with nearby variants that cause a functional change to the gene and thus cause disease. The next stage of analysis is challenging: in some cases there may be obvious candidate genes in the region and candidate SNPs such as exonic SNPs or SNPs which affect the expression of the gene. But in most cases a large study investigating all possible variation in the region by resequencing, followed by fine mapping to identify the most likely causal variant, is required. This will then be followed by appropriate functional studies to show how the variant alters the gene function (e.g. protein expression level or differences in cellular function).

For JIA the fine mapping stage is being facilitated by involvement in the Immunochip consortium which was initiated by the Wellcome Trust Case-Control consortium (WTCCC) of leading investigators of a number of different autoimmune diseases.[39] The Immunochip is an Illumina Infinium custom genotyping chip designed for fine mapping of established genes associated with autoimmune diseases, many of which also confer susceptibility to JIA. It enables cost-effective fine mapping and the potential for identification of novel JIA loci. Large cohorts of JIA cases from the United Kingdom, the United States, and Germany have been genotyped and the consortium are sharing control data, thereby increasing power for the individual studies.

Subtype-specific associations

Power issues in JIA are compounded by the fact that JIA is a clinically heterogeneous disease and can be classified into more homogeneous subtypes by the ILAR classification criteria.[2] Thus the search for genetic risk factors for JIA to date has been across all JIA subtypes or just the most common subtypes, oligoarthritis and RF-negative polyarthritis. But it is likely that there will be subtype-specific effects, as there may be distinct pathogenic pathways for these clinically diverse subtypes. Any stratified genetic analysis by ILAR subtype leads to small sample sizes and the subsequent loss in power that this entails, as well as multiple testing issues.

A number of potential subtype-specific associations have been identified but it is clear that large collaborative efforts are required to confirm or refute these findings.

The systemic JIA (sJIA) subtype is now more often thought of as an autoinflammatory disease rather than an autoimmune disease like the other JIA subtypes.[40] There is some emerging data that the subtype also differs genetically: for example, there is no evidence that sJIA is associated with *PTPN22*[41] and the HLA associations identified to date are weak. There is evidence for validated association of SNPs in the IL-1 ligand and receptor cluster with sJIA.[42]

The enthesitis-related arthritis (ERA) subtype of JIA is characterized by arthritis and enthesitis which may widen to affect the sacroiliac and spinal joints. The children may develop symptoms similar to ankylosing spondylitis (AS) and it mainly affects male, *HLA B27* positive, children. A non-synonymous SNP in the endoplasmic reticulum aminopeptidase 1 (*ERAP1*) gene is a well-established susceptibility gene for AS and a recent study found that this SNP was also associated with the ERA subtype of JIA.[43] Likewise the *IL23R* gene is a confirmed psoriasis susceptibility gene and a SNP in this gene shows association with the juvenile-onset psoriatic arthritis subtype.[43] Both these findings require validation in independent datasets for confirmation, but suggest distinct pathogenic pathways for these subtypes.

It is hoped that a greater understanding of the genetic basis of JIA as a whole may help clinically in defining the different subtypes of JIA and aid in the classification of this heterogeneous disease.

Prediction of disease risk and outcome

One of the original goals in genetic studies was that the identification of genetic risk factors would enable the prediction of individual disease risk for patients. But the evidence emerging from these genetic studies of complex diseases is that there will be multiple genetic risk factors (possibly hundreds), each conferring a very small effect, and we are yet to understand how these may interact with each other.

It is proposed that the knowledge of genetic susceptibility factors may be more useful in the prediction of disease outcome in children with JIA. The identification of children with a poorer prognosis would enable potentially more targeted or aggressive treatment which is especially important in children to prevent future joint damage and disability. These investigations rely on large long-term prospective outcome studies such as the Childhood Arthritis Prospective Study (CAPS)[44] and Childhood Arthritis Response to Medication study.[45,46]

Conclusions

The last few years have seen great progress in the understanding of the genetic basis of JIA with new loci identified and confirmed in independent cohorts. There are now 12 JIA susceptibility loci with evidence for association in more than one study, but further advances will emerge in the next few years following large scale GWAS, meta-analyses, and fine mapping strategies. Many of the loci identified to date confer susceptibility to multiple autoimmune diseases and play a role in the immune response. It is hoped that this knowledge will lead not only to a better understanding of disease pathogenesis for JIA and its subtypes but also aid in the classification of this heterogeneous disease. It may identify new pathways for potential therapeutic targets and help in the prediction of disease outcome.

References

1. Chinoy H, Lamb JA, Ollier WE, et al. Recent advances in the immunogenetics of idiopathic inflammatory myopathy. *Arthritis Res Ther* 2011;13:216.
2. Petty RE, Southwood TR, Manners P et al. International League of Associations for Rheumatology classification of juvenile idiopathic arthritis: second revision, Edmonton, 2001. *J Rheumatol* 2004;31:390–392.
3. Savolainen A, Saila H, Kotaniemi K et al. Magnitude of the genetic component in juvenile idiopathic arthritis. *Ann Rheum Dis* 2000;59:1001.
4. Ansell BM, Bywaters EG, Lawrence JS. Familial aggregation and twin studies in Still's disease. Juvenile chronic polyarthritis. *Rheumatology* 1969;2:37–61.
5. Glass DN, Giannini EH. Juvenile rheumatoid arthritis as a complex genetic trait. *Arthritis Rheum* 1999;42:2261–2268.
6. Prahalad S, O'Brien E, Fraser AM et al. Familial aggregation of juvenile idiopathic arthritis. *Arthritis Rheum* 2004;50:4022–4027.
7. Prahalad S, Zeft AS, Pimentel R et al. Quantification of the familial contribution to juvenile idiopathic arthritis. *Arthritis Rheum* 2010;62:2525–2529.
8. Thomson W, Barrett JH, Donn R et al. Juvenile idiopathic arthritis classified by the ILAR criteria: HLA associations in UK patients. *Rheumatology* (Oxford) 2002;41:1183–1189.
9. Prahalad S, Ryan MH, Shear ES et al. Juvenile rheumatoid arthritis: linkage to HLA demonstrated by allele sharing in affected sibpairs. *Arthritis Rheum* 2000;43:2335–2338.
10. Burn GL, Svensson L, Sanchez-Blanco C, Saini M, Cope AP. Why is PTPN22 a good candidate susceptibility gene for autoimmune disease? *FEBS Lett* 2011;585(23):3689–3698.
11. Hinks A, Barton A, John S et al. Association between the PTPN22 gene and rheumatoid arthritis and juvenile idiopathic arthritis in a UK population: Further support that PTPN22 is an autoimmunity gene. *Arthritis Rheum* 2005;52:1694–1699.
12. Viken MK, Amundsen SS, Kvien TK et al. Association analysis of the 1858C>T polymorphism in the PTPN22 gene in juvenile idiopathic arthritis and other autoimmune diseases. *Genes Immun* 2005;6:271–273.
13. Seldin MF, Shigeta R, Laiho K et al. Finnish case-control and family studies support PTPN22 R620W polymorphism as a risk factor in rheumatoid arthritis, but suggest only minimal or no effect in juvenile idiopathic arthritis. *Genes Immun* 2005;6:720–722.
14. Thompson SD, Sudman M, Ramos PS et al. The susceptibility loci juvenile idiopathic arthritis shares with other autoimmune diseases extend to PTPN2, COG6, and ANGPT1. *Arthritis Rheum* 2010;62:3265–3276.
15. Hinks A, Eyre S, Ke X et al. Overlap of disease susceptibility loci for rheumatoid arthritis and juvenile idiopathic arthritis. *Ann Rheum Dis* 2010;69:1049–1053.
16. Prahalad S, Hansen S, Whiting A et al. Variants in TNFAIP3, STAT4, and C12orf30 loci associated with multiple autoimmune diseases are also associated with juvenile idiopathic arthritis. *Arthritis Rheum* 2009;60:2124–2130.
17. Remmers EF, Plenge RM, Lee AT et al. STAT4 and the risk of rheumatoid arthritis and systemic lupus erythematosus. *N Engl J Med* 2007;357:977–986.
18. Vella A, Cooper JD, Lowe CE et al. Localization of a type 1 diabetes locus in the IL2RA/CD25 region by use of tag single-nucleotide polymorphisms. *Am J Hum Genet* 2005;76:773–779.
19. Hafler DA, Compston A, Sawcer S et al. Risk alleles for multiple sclerosis identified by a genomewide study. *N Engl J Med* 2007;357:851–862.
20. Maier LM, Lowe CE, Cooper J et al. IL2RA genetic heterogeneity in multiple sclerosis and type 1 diabetes susceptibility and soluble interleukin-2 receptor production. *PLoS Genet* 2009;5:e1000322.
21. Hinks A, Ke X, Barton A et al. Association of the IL2RA/CD25 gene with juvenile idiopathic arthritis. *Arthritis Rheum* 2009;60:251–257.
22. Hinks A, Eyre S, Ke X et al. Association of the AFF3 gene and IL2/IL21 gene region with juvenile idiopathic arthritis. *Genes Immun* 2010;11:194–198.
23. Albers HM, Kurreeman FA, Stoeken-Rijsbergen G et al. Association of the autoimmunity locus 4q27 with juvenile idiopathic arthritis. *Arthritis Rheum* 2009;60:901–904.
24. Barton A, Eyre S, Ke X et al. Identification of AF4/FMR2 family, member 3 (AFF3) as a novel rheumatoid arthritis susceptibility locus and confirmation of two further pan-autoimmune susceptibility genes. *Hum Mol Genet* 2009;18:2518–2522.
25. Zhernakova A, Alizadeh BZ, Bevova M et al. Novel association in chromosome 4q27 region with rheumatoid arthritis and confirmation of type 1 diabetes point to a general risk locus for autoimmune diseases. *Am J Hum Genet* 2007;81:1284–1288.
26. van Heel DA, Franke L, Hunt KA et al. A genome-wide association study for celiac disease identifies risk variants in the region harboring IL2 and IL21. *Nat Genet* 2007;39:827–829.
27. Orozco G, Hinks A, Eyre S et al. Combined effects of three independent SNPs greatly increase the risk estimate for RA at 6q23. *Hum Mol Genet* 2009;18:2693–2699.
28. Prahalad S, Bohnsack JF, Jorde LB et al. Association of two functional polymorphisms in the CCR5 gene with juvenile rheumatoid arthritis. *Genes Immun* 2006;7:468–475.
29. Hinks A, Martin P, Flynn E et al. Association of the CCR5 gene with juvenile idiopathic arthritis. *Genes Immun* 2010;11:584–589.
30. Lindner E, Nordang GB, Melum E et al. Lack of association between the chemokine receptor 5 polymorphism CCR5delta32 in rheumatoid arthritis and juvenile idiopathic arthritis. *BMC Med Genet* 2007;8:33.
31. Hinks A, Martin P, Flynn E et al. Investigation of type 1 diabetes and coeliac disease susceptibility loci for association with juvenile idiopathic arthritis. *Ann Rheum Dis* 2010;69:2169–2172.
32. Coenen MJ, Trynka G, Heskamp S et al. Common and different genetic background for rheumatoid arthritis and coeliac disease. *Hum Mol Genet* 2009;18:4195–4203.
33. Dubois PC, Trynka G, Franke L et al. Multiple common variants for celiac disease influencing immune gene expression. *Nat Genet* 2010;42:295–302.
34. Skinningsrud B, Lie BA, Husebye ES et al. A CLEC16A variant confers risk for juvenile idiopathic arthritis and anti-CCP negative rheumatoid arthritis. *Ann Rheum Dis* 2010;69(8):1471–1474.
35. Behrens EM, Finkel TH, Bradfield JP et al. Association of the TRAF1-C5 locus on chromosome 9 with juvenile idiopathic arthritis. *Arthritis Rheum* 2008;58:2206–2207.
36. Albers HM, Kurreeman FA, Houwing-Duistermaat JJ et al. The TRAF1/C5 region is a risk factor for polyarthritis in juvenile idiopathic arthritis. *Ann Rheum Dis* 2008;67:1578–1580.
37. Hinks A, Barton A, Shephard N et al. Identification of a novel susceptibility locus for juvenile idiopathic arthritis by genome-wide association analysis. *Arthritis Rheum* 2009;60:258–263.

38. Thompson SD, Marion MC, Sudman M et al. Genome-wide association analysis of juvenile idiopathic arthritis identifies a new susceptibility locus at chromosomal region 3q13. *Arthritis Rheum* 2012;64: 2781–2791.

39. Cortes A, Brown MA. Promise and pitfalls of the Immunochip. *Arthritis Res Ther* 2011;13:101.

40. Ramanan AV, Grom AA. Does systemic-onset juvenile idiopathic arthritis belong under juvenile idiopathic arthritis? *Rheumatology* (Oxford) 2005;44:1350–1353.

41. Hinks A, Worthington J, Thomson W. The association of PTPN22 with rheumatoid arthritis and juvenile idiopathic arthritis. *Rheumatology* (Oxford) 2006;45:365–368.

42. Stock CJ, Ogilvie EM, Samuel JM et al. Comprehensive association study of genetic variants in the IL-1 gene family in systemic juvenile idiopathic arthritis. *Genes Immun* 2008;9:349–357.

43. Hinks A, Martin P, Flynn E et al. Subtype specific genetic associations for juvenile idiopathic arthritis: ERAP1 with the enthesitis related arthritis subtype and IL23R with juvenile psoriatic arthritis. *Arthritis Res Ther* 2011;13:R12.

44. Adib N, Hyrich K, Thornton J et al. Association between duration of symptoms and severity of disease at first presentation to paediatric rheumatology: results from the Childhood Arthritis Prospective Study. *Rheumatology* (Oxford) 2008;47:991–995.

45. Hinks A, Moncrieffe H, Martin P et al. Association of the 5-aminoimidazole-4-carboxamide ribonucleotide transformylase gene with response to methotrexate in juvenile idiopathic arthritis. *Ann Rheum Dis* 2011;70:1395–1400.

46. Moncrieffe H, Hinks A, Ursu S et al. Generation of novel pharmacogenomic candidates in response to methotrexate in juvenile idiopathic arthritis: correlation between gene expression and genotype. *Pharmacogenet Genomics* 2010;20:665–676.

47. Hinks A, Cobb J, Sudman M et al. Investigation of rheumatoid arthritis susceptibility loci in juvenile idiopathic arthritis confirms high degree of overlap. *Ann Rheum Dis* 2012;71:1117–1121.

CHAPTER 44

Genetics of osteoarthritis

Alex MacGregor, Ana Valdes,
and Frances M. K. Williams

Introduction

Charcot is credited with first recognizing the hereditary nature of osteoarthritis (OA) of the hands in his description of this condition in 1881.[1] The 1940s saw the first formal study of familial clustering of the disease when Stecher showed a two- to threefold increased risk of the disease among the mothers and sisters of cases with Heberden's nodes.[2] Stecher's work was confirmed and extended by Kellgren et al, in epidemiological studies conducted in the United Kingdom in the 1950s and 1960s,[3] which showed that 'generalized OA' (co-occurrence of hand and knee OA) conferred a twofold risk of disease to first-degree relatives of affected cases compared with population controls.

Modern era twin and family studies

Limitations of these early family studies include their methods for case selection, the lack of standard methods for case definition (including a lack of distinction between clinical and radiographic disease), and the lack of age matching among relatives, all of which might potentially upwardly bias the assessment of genetic influence. However, with the advances in knowledge of the biology and clinical characteristics of OA, greater standardization of radiological and clinical definitions, and the emergence and maturation of large, genetically informative cohorts of twins and families, a more comprehensive picture of the genetic influence on OA has emerged.

In 1996, the St Thomas' UK Adult Twin Registry reported evidence that radiographic OA at the hand and knee has a substantial heritable component.[4] This was followed by two studies published in the 1998 (the Baltimore Longitudinal Study of Aging[5] and the Framingham Offspring Study[6]) that showed significant familial clustering for hand and knee OA. Both family studies used unselected population samples; a particular strength of the Framingham Offspring Study design was that all the subjects were assessed at adult ages. A genetic influence on hip OA was suggested in two studies[7,8] that showed a higher than expected prevalence of hip OA among relatives of probands with total hip replacement. These observations were confirmed using data from Nottingham.[9] Through to 2010, further studies conducted in the TwinsUK Registry confirmed a genetic contribution to radiological disease at the hip.[10]

Twin studies may be used to derive quantitative estimates of heritability, a measure of the proportion of variation of a trait attributable to population-level genetic variation. For hand, hip, and knee OA reported heritability estimates in the range 40–75% are evidence that individual genes have a causal role in the disease. Family studies also offer further insight into the mode of action of genes. Modelling segregation patterns based on the distribution of hand and knee OA in the Framingham Offspring Study[6] has provided evidence of a polygenic mode of inheritance, in which the disease is accounted for by multiple genetic variants each having small effect on risk. These studies have provided the justification for the more detailed search for individual genes that has escalated in recent years through major advances in genetic technology.

Insights from inherited osteoarthritis

While segregation studies indicate that classical mendelian inheritance does not explain the population occurrence of the disease, insight into the mechanisms by which individual genes might have a direct influence on the occurrence and expression of OA emerges from studies of inherited diseases in which OA is a feature (Table 44.1).[11] These inherited diseases illustrate that a range of genetically determined features have a bearing on the OA phenotype. They also highlight the depth of penetrance of gene action by showing that single gene defects can have ramifications through the disease phenotype. In addition, they provide a framework for the systematic search for the gene variants responsible for the occurrence of OA in the general population.

Linkage, candidate gene, and genome-wide association studies

Advances in understanding the role of individual genes in OA need to be interpreted against a backdrop of rapid progress in genotyping technology and analytical techniques applied to increasingly extensive and detailed clinical collections of people with OA; and population samples of both symptomatic and radiographic disease. With this continuing exponential rise in genetic information, any account of the gene variants implicated must be qualified by an appreciation of the rate at which new pathways are continuing to emerge. Online tools, including for example the Human Gene

Epidemiology Navigator,[12] provide a continuously updated account of this rapidly evolving picture.

For more than a decade researchers have been engaged in comprehensively screening the genome to detect gene variants implicated in OA. The first approaches involved studies designed to detect genetic linkage using methods that examine whether chromosomal regions are coinherited among related individuals with the disease. Several regions have been implicated in OA through linkage. This information was brought together most recently in a meta-analysis conducted by Lee et al.[13] which combined the results of three whole-genome linkage scans[14-16] using the Genome Scan Meta-Analysis (GMSA) method.[17] Five regions provided combined evidence of linkage with a probability <0.05: 7q34–7q36.3, 11p12–11p13.4, 6p21.1–6q15, 2q31.3–2q34, 15q21.3–15q26.1. These findings have generated considerable interest, and have concentrated attention on specific genes harboured within linked regions. including the interleukin (IL)-1 gene cluster, *FRZB*, and matrillin-3 located on chromosome 2, and the IL-4 receptor gene on chromosome 16.[18]

Candidate gene studies that focus on identifying the risk of disease associated with genetic variants among individuals in the population provide an additional approach to linkage analysis. Typically these studies target genes for which there is biological evidence to support a potential role in disease. They are therefore limited by knowledge of disease pathways in the tissues involved in OA, for which there remains considerable uncertainty. It is difficult to know how much importance to attach to candidate gene findings. However, for some time there has been the capability to conduct genome-wide association studies (GWAS), and screen for genetic associations agnostically. Technological advances continue to extend screening to a greater depth, allowing the detection of rare variants.[19]

The vast potential of genetic association studies to screen for large numbers of associations brings with it a substantial risk of false discovery. Interpretation needs attention to both the statistical veracity of reported associations and their reproducibility in different settings and in different population groups. With these caveats, a number of genes have emerged that merit more detailed attention.[20] For a number of the strongest and most consistent associations, functional genetic studies have begun to provide further evidence of their role in disease pathogenesis.

Collagen-related genes

Collagen genes have been considered as candidates of interest given their role in inherited diseases in which OA is a feature. Numerous studies have reported associations with genes encoding collagen I, II, IV,, and XI variously at the hip, knee, and spine.[21] However, there has been remarkable inconsistency between studies and a failure to replicate. In GWAS, the collagen type VI alpha 4 pseudogene 1 gene (*COL6A4P*; previously named dual von Willebrand factor A (*DVWA*)) emerged as the strongest association in a 2008 study conducted among Asian populations.[22] Most recently, *COL11A1* was reported as one of the strongest signals to emerge in association with hip OA in the United Kingdom arcOGEN study.[23] This gene codes for the alpha-1 polypeptide chain of type XI collagen, penetrant mutations of which are responsible for Stickler's syndrome (Table 44.1).

Growth and differentiation factor 5 gene (*GDF5*)

Associations with genes encoding GDF5 are some of the most consistently reported in OA.[20] GDF5 is an extracellular signalling molecule (member of the transforming growth factor beta (TGF-β) superfamily) and is intimately involved in bone formation and in

the maintenance and repair of joint tissue. Functional studies of OA-associated single nucleotide polymorphisms (SNPs) in *GDF5* alleles have revealed allele-dependent differences in gene transcription—an effect that is seen in all joint tissue and not confined to cartilage alone.[24] This gives strong support for an aetiological role of *GDF5* variants in OA.

Asporin gene (*ASPN*)

Asporins are components of extracellular matrix, bind TGF-β, and are negative regulators of chondrogenesis. Overexpression of *ASPN*, the gene encoding asporin, leads to a decrease in TGF-β1 mediated chondrogenesis. Associations between *ASPN* with knee OA have been reported in Japanese, Korean, and Chinese populations,[25] although they have been either weak or absent in European populations.[26]

SMAD family member 3 (*SMAD3*)

The SMAD proteins are downstream mediators of TGF-β signals. SMAD3 acts to maintain articular cartilage in the quiescent state by repressing chondrocyte hypertrophic differentiation and regulating matrix molecule synthesis. The gene has been associated with OA in independent European hip and knee cohorts.[27]

Acidic leucine-rich nuclear phosphoroprotein 32 family member A gene (*ANP32A*)

Chondrocyte apoptosis is evident in OA when compared with age-matched controls.[28] *ANP32A* encodes a tumour suppressor molecule that has a regulatory role in apoptosis and interferes with Wnt signalling. It has been associated with hip OA in white women.[29]

Type II iodothyronine deiodinase gene (*DOI2*)

The gene encoding type II iodothyronine deiodinase (*DOI2*) is responsible for the bioavailability of thyroid hormone in a number of tissues including growth plate, and has a role in chondrocyte proliferation and differentiation. This was one of the few genes to be identified in both GWAS and linkage studies.[20] The association with OA may be mediated though an influence on hip geometry.[30]

Interleukin genes

Associations with interleukins are of interest given the contribution of inflammation to the pathogenesis of OA. Variants in *IL1*, *IL6*, and *IL10* have been reported to be associated with OA, with some variants in *IL1* reported to be associated with OA severity.[20]

Frizzled related protein gene (*FRZB*)

Frizzled related protein is involved in bone formation and in regulation of the Wnt receptor signalling pathway that has a central role in skeletal development and is involved in the maintenance of the structure and function of bone and cartilage. Variants of *FRZB* have been reported in a number of studies to be associated with hip OA and knee OA.[31,32]

Oestrogen receptor gene (*ESR1*)

The oestrogen receptor is an important mediator of signal transduction and is expressed in human chondrocytes. Associations with OA have been reported in some white and Asian populations, although the differences in variants examined and the overall inconsistency of these associations make the data hard to interpret.[20]

Vitamin D receptor gene (*VDR*)

The role of vitamin D in OA is of interest because of its established role of bone metabolism and inflammation. *VDR* has been of the

Table 44.1 Inherited diseases in which osteoarthritis is a feature

Condition	Features	Mode of inheritance	Gene/protein implicated
Spondyloepithelial dysplasia	Heterogeneous group of disorders characterized by abnormal development of axial skeleton; dwarfism. Generalized OA in early teens. Disc herniation been reported in spondyloepithelial dysplasia tarda	AD, AR, and XL	COL2A1
Familial calcium pyrophosphate disease	Chondrocalcinosis of knees symphysis pubis and wrist	AD and AR	Linkages in humans reported to chromosome 5p and 8q in one family; *ank* gene implicated in mice
Familial hydroxyapatite deposition disease	Teninitis, bursitis, and articular OA commonly involving the shoulders wrists and hips	AD	
Stickler's syndrome	Myopia, hearing loss, epiphyseal dysplasia. Mandibular dysplasia. Severe OA develops in the third and fourth decades	AD	COL2A1, COL11A2, COL11A1
Kniest dysplasia	Shortening of trunk and limbs, flattening of the face. Articular cartilage soft with low resilience. Severe premature OA of the hips and knees	AD	COL2A1
Multiple epiphyseal dysplasia	Heterogeneous group of disorders characterized by alteration in epiphyseal growth, irregularity, and fragmentation of epiphyses of long bones. Premature OA in weight bearing and non-weightbearing joints in childhood or early adulthood	AD and AR	COMP, MATN3, COL9A1,COL9A2. COL9A3, DTDST
Metaphyseal chondrodysplasia	Group of disorders characterized by metaphyseal dysplasia. Short stature, short limbs. Bowed legs. Premature OA of the hips and knees	AD	COL10A1. PTH/PTHrP
Achondroplasia	Short limb dwarfism. OA and spinal stenosis in adulthood	AD	fibroblast growth factor
Blount's disease	Disturbance in growth of medial aspect of the proximal tibial epiphysis. Premature OA of the knees	AD	
Alkaptonuria	Inborn metabolic defect leading to deposition of homogentisic acid. Results in premature OA involving the shoulders and the lateral compartments of the knees. High frequency of intervertebral disc disease	AR	HGD
Familial lumbar stenosis	Case report of familial lumbar stenosis with disc herniation	AD	
Kyphoscoliosis	3-dimensional deformity of spinal growth ; disc lesions common	AD and XL	Genome-wide microsatellite screen identified areas suggestive of linkage on 9q31.2-q34.2, and 17q25.3
Camptodactyly– arthropathy– coxa vara– pericarditis syndrome	Rare familial disorder characterized by flexion contractures of the fingers, coxa vara deformity, and a non-inflammatory arthropathy with synovial hyperplasia, features of and non-inflammatory pericardial effusion	AR	Defects secreted proteoglycan (superficial zone protein)

AD, autosomal dominant; AR, autosomal recessive; XL, X-linked.

Full references can be found at Online Mendelian Inheritance in Man (www.ncbi.nlm.nih.gov/omim).

most extensively studied candidate genes in OA, with associations demonstrated at the knee and spine.[21] However, reports of association have been inconsistent and *VDR* has notably failed to emerge strongly in GWAS studies as associated with OA.

Disease heterogeneity

While OA is characterized by common pathological features and disease mechanisms, it also shows considerable clinical heterogeneity. Epidemiologically there is variation in the contribution of risk factors for disease, for example in males and females, at different ages, and for different joints. It would be naive to assume that the genetic influences in OA are constant across all affected individuals and all clinical disease features.

Twin studies indicate that the strength of the genetic influences differs among individual disease features even within the same body site. For example at the hip, while joint space narrowing is strongly heritable, sclerotic changes in bone associated with OA and osteophytes show significantly less genetic influence.[10] Genetic influences also differ across body sites. In an analysis of monozygotic and dizygotic twin participants in the TwinsUK Registry assessed radiographically for OA at the hand (DIP, PIP, and CMC joints), knee, and hip joints, genetic influences were strongly correlated among joints in the hand; however, there was little evidence of common genetic pathways to account for the co-occurrence of OA at the hand, knee, and hip.[33] This work showed no evidence that common or shared genetic factors determine the occurrence of disease across all these skeletal sites.

The findings suggest that there are important aetiological differences in the genetic contribution to disease at different skeletal sites. This observation helps explain some of the inconsistency in results of linkage and association studies that has emerged.

The extended OA phenotype including musculoskeletal pain

Genetic influences on OA extend beyond measures of radiographic change. Joint shape, itself a potential predictor of disease, is strongly genetically determined. For example, acetabular dimensions including acetabular depth and centre edge angle have been shown to have a heritability of 60%.[34] COMP, a biomarker of cartilage degeneration, is also genetically determined.[35] C-reactive protein (CRP) levels are also recognized to be influenced genetically.[36] Thus the genetic influence on OA acts on collagen structure and cartilage metabolism, and on the pro-inflammatory cytokine cascades that influence the inflammatory component of the disease.

There is an increasing awareness of a genetic influence on pain, including joint pain in OA. Studies conducted among twins have shown that reported pain has a heritability between 28–39% at a range of peripheral sites including the knee, thigh, hand, and foot.[37] In the same dataset, pain reporting at different sites was modestly but uniformly correlated, with a single factor accounting for 95% of the overall variance in pain reporting. This common pain reporting factor itself has a heritability of 46%. The observations in twins support the notion that a single genetic factor underlies a general propensity for individuals to report joint pain. This is in stark contrast with radiographic OA which is determined by genetic factors specific to each anatomical site and suggests that the genetic influence on radiographic OA and the pain related to OA are quite distinct. The genetic architecture of OA thus mirrors the clinical observation that pain and the extent of radiographic disease are poorly correlated.

Genes implanted in pain in osteoarthritis

As with the study of radiographic OA, the capacity to identify individual genes that might be implicated in pain in OA continues to expand rapidly.[38] A number of genes have emerged that are of particular relevance.

Catechol-O-methytransferase gene (COMT)

Catechol-O-methytransferase is involved in the regulation of catecholamine and encephalin levels. Polymorphic variation in the COMT gene has been associated with clinical pain processing. Functional variants of COMT have been associated with hip pain in OA.[39]

Sodium channel protein type 9 gene (SCN9A)

This gene encodes a voltage-gated sodium channel which plays a significant role in nociception signalling. When present in OA it is associated with higher pain scores than in controls.[40]

Sparteine/debrisoquine oxidase gene (CYP2D6)

Sparteine/debrisoquine oxidase is one of the hepatic cytochrome p450 enzymes and is involved in the activation of codeine by O-demethylation to morphine. Poor metabolizer status occurs in 10% of white people and 2% of Asians and African Americans. In both clinical and experimental pain, poor metabolizers show reduced analgesic efficacy to codeine.[41] Basal pain thresholds are also influenced by CYP2D6 status.[42]

Paired amino acid converting enzyme 4 gene (PACE4)

A single nucleotide polymorphism in the gene that encodes PACE4 has been shown to protect against pain in subjects with knee OA.[43]

Mice carrying a null mutant of this gene are resistant to acute pain. PACE4 is expressed in peripheral and central nervous system tissues involved in nociception, including dorsal root ganglia, amygdalae, and spinal cord.

Transient receptor potential cation channel subfamily V member 1 gene (TRPV1)

TRPV1 encodes the capsaicin receptor and is responsible for mediating the sensation to scalding heat. A study of seven cohorts from the United Kingdom, the United States, and Australia showed an association between low thermal pain sensitivity TRPV1 genotype and a lower risk of symptomatic knee OA.[44] TRPV1 is an excellent target for pharmacological intervention: capsaicinoids are used widely in the treatment of pain and there are several new molecules acting on this receptor under investigation at present.[45]

Epigenetic influences on osteoarthritis

Epigenetic effects are the heritable changes in gene expression that occur without changes in primary DNA sequence. They include DNA methylation, histone modification, and non-coding RNAs. These effects can arise from environmental influences and act either at the level of gene transcription or post-transcriptionally. There is accumulating evidence of epigenetic processes operating in OA.[46] Altered methylation patterns have been associated with the promoter of genes encoding metalloproteinase including MMP13 and ADAMTS4; histone methylation has been associated with increased COX-2 and iNOS transcription; non-coding microRNAs are differentially expressed in normal and OA cartilage and may induce the expression of matrix-degrading enzymes.

Epigenetic effects may have an impact on the penetrance of disease susceptibility genes. For example, the imbalance in allele expression of GDF5 has been shown to be influenced significantly by DNA methylation.[47] These findings serve to emphasize that studies of allelic association alone are unlikely fully to explain the heritability of OA, and that knowledge of the epigenetic status of genetically associated disease genes will be a vital part of understanding their contribution to disease.

Conclusion

A genetic influence of OA is firmly established and rapid technological advances in molecular genetics are providing a more detailed picture of the role of individual gene variants in determining the diverse phenotypic manifestations of the condition. While the genetic contribution to OA is manifestly complex, knowledge of the genetic influence on all aspects of the OA phenotype provides insight into disease mechanisms and potential therapeutic targets. The increasing understanding of OA genetics also raises the realistic possibility of developing tools for detecting susceptible groups, and for targeting individualized treatments.

References

1. Charcot JM. *Clinical lectures on senile and chronic diseases*. The New Sydenham Society, London, 1881.
2. Stecher RM. Heberden's nodes: heredity in hypertrophic arthritis of the finger joints. *Am J Med Sc* 1941;210:801–809.
3. Kellgren JH, Lawrence JS, Bier F. Genetic factors in generalised osteoarthritis. *Ann Rheum Dis* 1963;22:237–255.
4. Spector TD, Cicuttini F, Baker J, Loughlin J, Hart D. Genetic influences on osteoarthritis in women: a twin study. *BMJ* 1996;312(7036):940–943.

5. Hirsch R, Lethbridge-Cejku M, Hanson R et al. Familial aggregation of osteoarthritis: data from the Baltimore longitudinal study on aging. *Arthritis Rheum* 1998;41(7):1227–1232.

6. Felson DT, Couropmitree NN, Chaisson E et al. Evidence for a Mendelian gene in a segregation analysis of generalised radiographic osteoarthritis. *Arthritis Rheum* 1998;41(6):1064–1071.

7. Lindberg H. Prevalence of primary coxarthrosis in siblings of patients with primary coxarthrosis. *Clin Orthop Relat Res* 1986;203:273–275.

8. Chitnavis J, Sinsheimer JS, Clipsham K et al. Genetic influences in end-stage osteoarthritis. Sibling risks of hip and knee replacement for idiopathic osteoarthritis. *J Bone Joint Surg Br* 1997;79(4):660–664.

9. Lanyon P, Doherty S, Muir K, Doherty M. Strong genetic predisposition to hip osteoarthritis. *Arthritis Rheum* 1998;41(9):S351.

10. MacGregor AJ, Antoniades L, Matson M, Andrew T, Spector TD. The genetic contribution to radiographic hip osteoarthritis in women: results of a classic twin study. *Arthritis Rheum* 2000;43(11):2410–2416.

11. Smith R, Wordsworth BP. *Clinical and biochemical disorders of the skeleton*.: Oxford University Press, Oxford, 2005.

12. HuGE Navigator (version 2.0) HuGE Literature Finder 2012. Available from: www.hugenavigator.net/HuGENavigator/startPagePubLit.do.

13. Lee YH, Rho YH, Choi SJ, Ji JD, Song GG. Osteoarthritis susceptibility loci defined by genome scan meta-analysis. *Rheumatol Int* 2006;26(11):959–63; 996–1000.

14. Chapman K, Mustafa Z, Irven C et al. Osteoarthritis-susceptibility locus on chromosome 11q, detected by linkage. *Am J Hum Genet* 1999;65(1):167–174.

15. Stefansson SE, Jonsson H, Ingvarsson T et al. Genomewide scan for hand osteoarthritis: a novel mutation in matrilin-3. *Am J Hum Genet* 2003;72(6):1448–1459.

16. Hunter DJ, Demissie S, Cupples LA, Aliabadi P, Felson DT. A genome scan for joint-specific hand osteoarthritis susceptibility: The Framingham Study. *Arthritis Rheum* 2004;50(8):2489–2496.

17. Levinson DF, Levinson MD, Segurado R, Lewis CM. Genome scan meta-analysis of schizophrenia and bipolar disorder, part I: Methods and power analysis. *Am J Hum Genet* 2003;73(1):17–33.

18. Peach CA, Carr AJ, Loughlin J. Recent advances in the genetic investigation of osteoarthritis. *Trends Mol Med* 2005;11(4):186–191.

19. Valdes AM, Spector TD. The genetic epidemiology of osteoarthritis. *Curr Opin Rheumatol* 2010;22(2):139–143.

20. Valdes AM, Spector TD. Genetic epidemiology of hip and knee osteoarthritis. *Nat Rev Rheumatol* 2011;7(1):23–32.

21. Ryder JJ, Garrison K, Song F et al. Genetic associations in peripheral joint osteoarthritis and spinal degenerative disease: a systematic review. *Ann Rheum Dis* 2008;67(5):584–591.

22. Miyamoto Y, Shi D, Nakajima M et al. Common variants in DVWA on chromosome 3p24.3 are associated with susceptibility to knee osteoarthritis. *Nat Genet* 2008;40(8):994–998.

23. Panoutsopoulou K, Southam L, Elliott KS et al. Insights into the genetic architecture of osteoarthritis from stage 1 of the arcOGEN study. *Ann Rheum Dis* 2011;70(5):864–867.

24. Egli RJ, Southam L, Wilkins JM et al. Functional analysis of the osteoarthritis susceptibility-associated GDF5 regulatory polymorphism. *Arthritis Rheum* 2009;60(7):2055–2064.

25. Kizawa H, Kou I, Iida A et al. An aspartic acid repeat polymorphism in asporin inhibits chondrogenesis and increases susceptibility to osteoarthritis. *Nat Genet* 2005;37(2):138–144.

26. Atif U, Philip A, Aponte J et al. Absence of association of asporin polymorphisms and osteoarthritis susceptibility in US Caucasians. *Osteoarthritis Cartilage* 2008;16(10):1174–1177.

27. Valdes AM, Spector TD, Tamm A et al. Genetic variation in the SMAD3 gene is associated with hip and knee osteoarthritis. *Arthritis Rheum* 2010;62(8):2347–2352.

28. Kim HA, Blanco FJ. Cell death and apoptosis in osteoarthritic cartilage. *Curr Drug Targets* 2007;8(2):333–345.

29. Valdes AM, Lories RJ, van Meurs JB et al. Variation at the ANP32A gene is associated with risk of hip osteoarthritis in women. *Arthritis Rheum* 2009;60(7):2046–2054.

30. Waarsing JH, Kloppenburg M, Slagboom PE et al. Osteoarthritis susceptibility genes influence the association between hip morphology and osteoarthritis. *Arthritis Rheum* 2011;63(5):1349–1354.

31. Lane NE, Lian K, Nevitt MC et al. Frizzled-related protein variants are risk factors for hip osteoarthritis. *Arthritis Rheum* 2006;54(4):1246–1254.

32. Valdes AM, Loughlin J, Oene MV et al. Sex and ethnic differences in the association of ASPN, CALM1, COL2A1, COMP, and FRZB with genetic susceptibility to osteoarthritis of the knee. *Arthritis Rheum* 2007;56(1):137–146.

33. MacGregor AJ, Li Q, Spector TD, Williams FM. The genetic influence on radiographic osteoarthritis is site specific at the hand, hip and knee. *Rheumatology* (Oxford) 2009;48(3):277–280.

34. Antoniades L, Spector TD, Macgregor AJ. The genetic contribution to hip joint morphometry and relationship to hip cartilage thickness. *Osteoarthritis Cartilage* 2001;9(6):593–595.

35. Williams FM, Andrew T, Saxne T et al. The heritable determinants of cartilage oligomeric matrix protein. *Arthritis Rheum* 2006;54(7):2147–2151.

36. MacGregor AJ, Gallimore JR, Spector TD, Pepys MB. Genetic effects on baseline values of C-reactive protein and serum amyloid A protein: a comparison of monozygotic and dizygotic twins. *Clin Chem* 2004;50(1):130–134.

37. Williams FM, Spector TD, MacGregor AJ. Pain reporting at different body sites is explained by a single underlying genetic factor. *Rheumatology* (Oxford) 2010;49(9):1753–1755.

38. Mogil JS. Pain genetics: past, present and future. *Trends Genet* 2012;28(6):258–266.

39. van Meurs JB, Uitterlinden AG, Stolk L et al. A functional polymorphism in the catechol-O-methyltransferase gene is associated with osteoarthritis-related pain. *Arthritis Rheum* 2009;60(2):628–629.

40. Reimann F, Cox JJ, Belfer I et al. Pain perception is altered by a nucleotide polymorphism in SCN9A. *Proc Natl Acad Sci U S A* 2010;107(11):5148–5153.

41. Poulsen L, Brosen K, Arendt-Nielsen L et al. Codeine and morphine in extensive and poor metabolizers of sparteine: pharmacokinetics, analgesic effect and side effects. *Eur J Clin Pharmacol* 1996;51(3–4):289–295.

42. Sindrup SH, Poulsen L, Brosen K, Arendt-Nielsen L, Gram LF. Are poor metabolisers of sparteine/debrisoquine less pain tolerant than extensive metabolisers? *Pain* 1993;53(3):335–339.

43. Malfait AM, Seymour AB, Gao F et al. A role for PACE4 in osteoarthritis pain: evidence from human genetic association and null mutant phenotype. *Ann Rheum Dis* 2012;71(6):1042–1048.

44. Valdes AM, De Wilde G, Doherty SA et al. The Ile585Val TRPV1 variant is involved in risk of painful knee osteoarthritis. *Ann Rheum Dis* 2011;70(9):1556–1561.

45. Bevan S, Andersson DA. TRP channel antagonists for pain—opportunities beyond TRPV1. *Curr Opin Investig Drugs* 2009;10(7):655–663.

46. Reynard LN, Loughlin J. Genetics and epigenetics of osteoarthritis. *Maturitas* 2012;71(3):200–204.

47. Reynard LN, Bui C, Canty-Laird EG, Young DA, Loughlin J. Expression of the osteoarthritis-associated gene GDF5 is modulated epigenetically by DNA methylation. *Hum Mol Genet* 2011;20(17):3450–3460.

CHAPTER 45

Genetics of chronic musculoskeletal pain

Kate L. Holliday, Wendy Thomson, and John McBeth

Introduction

Regional and widespread musculoskeletal pain disorders are common in the general population, with 33% reporting low back pain (LBP) and 11% chronic widespread pain (CWP), the defining feature of fibromyalgia (FM), in any one month.[1] For most pain disorders prevalence increases almost linearly with age, plateauing around the sixth decade, and women are more likely to report symptoms at all ages.[2]

Aetiology is poorly understood and current treatments lack efficacy. Twin studies suggest a genetic basis; however, research has been hampered by small sample sizes and phenotypic complexity,[3] since gastrointestinal disorders, fatigue, sleep disturbance, cognitive dysfunction, and psychological distress, among others, are common comorbidities. Elucidating the genetic susceptibility could identify the biological mechanisms involved, phenotypic subgroups, and novel therapeutic targets for use in personalized medicine. Additionally, other rheumatic diseases may benefit from this research as it could, for example, help to explain the common discordance in structural damage and pain severity observed in osteoarthritis (OA) or why FM is prevalent in rheumatoid arthritis (RA) patients. This chapter presents a state-of-the-art summary of current research in the field of pain genetics and highlights some of the methodological challenges in this field.

Heritability

Family studies have suggested a genetic component to FM; relatives of FM patients were eight times more likely to have FM than relatives of RA patients.[4] The extent of variance explained by additive genetic effects compared to shared environment was estimated in a study of Finnish twins with possible FM (based on a number of symptoms including tenderness, stiffness, and neck pain) to be approximately 50%.[5] A similar estimate of heritability (h^2) was reported for CWP in a study of Swedish twins (Table 45.1).[6]

The majority of twin studies have been conducted on LBP and neck pain, and h^2 estimates vary widely.[7–18] In a cohort of United Kingdom twins a common factor explained 95% of the variance in pain reporting at seven bodily sites for which h^2 = 46% (95% confidence interval 0.40, 0.52), suggesting that the genetic component to pain reporting did not differ by pain site. It may, however, differ by the extent and severity of pain reported. Higher h^2 has been reported for multisite than single-site pain,[15,17] and severe disabling and/or radiating pain results in higher h^2 estimates compared to ever reporting LBP or neck pain.[10]

Age also appears to influence h^2, with low estimates reported for widespread and LBP in 11 year old Finnish twins.[19,20] Similarly, a study of Danish twins found that h^2 was low in under 16s; however, h^2 increased dramatically in 16–18 year olds and then decreased to age 40.[8] Other studies have also suggested a decline in h^2 with age. Among subjects aged over 70 years in a Danish cohort there was no evidence of h^2 for LBP in females but h^2 = 27% in men, while h^2 was negligible for neck pain for both sexes.[11] Despite the increased prevalence of chronic musculoskeletal pain in females, h^2 estimates have not significantly differed between genders in most studies.[6,15,21]

These twin studies have mainly relied on self-reported pain and in some cases a simple question such as 'Have you ever had back pain?' has been used to classify subjects. This may be problematic, particularly in elderly populations where pain may be explained by structural damage or disease. Despite a strong correlation between lumbar disc degeneration (LDD) and LBP, only a limited amount of h^2 for LBP was explained by LDD[13,18] in twin studies that have undertaken clinical assessments and used MRI to assess pathology.

What genes are likely to be involved?

Heritability studies point to genes that may be involved in chronic pain susceptibility. A common heritable component to chronic pain, anxiety, depression, and psychological distress has been reported,[7,10,22] suggesting that susceptibility genes for mood disorders may also be involved in chronic pain susceptibility. A common heritable component to CWP and other functional pain syndromes independent of mood disorders has also been reported,[22] suggesting that genes influencing pain processing and perception may be

Table 45.1 Twin studies of chronic musculoskeletal pain

Reference	Population	N pairs	Age	Sex	Pain phenotype	h(2)
Mikkelsson et al., 2001 (19)	FinnTwin12	1789	11	M/F	Widespread	7%
Reichborn-Kjennerud et al., 2002 (7)	Norwegian Medical Birth Cohort	2135	18–25	M/F	LBP or neck	30% (20–39)
Hestbaek et al., 2004 (8)	Danish Registry	8287	16 to 41	M/F	LBP	44% (37–50) in males, 40% (34–46) in females
Hartvigsen et al., 2004 (9)	Longitudinal Study of Aging Danish Twins	1033	≥70	M/F	Back	27% (3–51) in males, no h(2) in females
Macgregor et al., 2004 (10)	TwinsUK	532	45–79	F	LBP	52% (33–72)
					Neck	48% (29–67)
Hartvigsen et al., 2005 (11)	Longitudinal Study of Aging Danish Twins	1054	≥70	M/F	Neck	Negligible
Fejer et al., 2006 (12)	Danish Registry	10938	20–71	M/F	Neck	45% (40–49)
Kato et al., 2006 (6)	Swedish Registry	15806	59.8±11.1	M/F	CWP	48% (0–67) in males, 54% (23, 66) in females
Battie et al., 2007 (13)	Finnish cohort	300	35–70	M	Back	Frequency 30% (14, 47)
						Intensity 34% (16–52)
El-Metwally et al., 2008 (14)	FinnTwin12	1790	11	M/F	LBP	<10%
Markkula et al., 2009 (5)	Finnish Twin Cohort	5304	43.4±7.6	M/F	FM	51% (45–56)
Hartvigsen et al., 2009 (15)	Danish Twin Registry	7764	20–71	M/F	LBP	38% (33–42)
					Mid-back	32% (26–39)
					Neck	39% (34–43)
Williams et al., 2010 (16)	TwinsUK	2065	18–82	M/F	Neck	44% (35–53)
					Back	34% (25–43)
					Elbow	38% (28–49)
					Knee	28% (19–37)
					Thigh	36% (25–48)
					Hand	44% (34–53)
					Foot	39% (29–50)
					All sites	46% (40–52)
Nyman et al., 2010 (17)	Swedish cohort (STAGE)	6903	21–47	M/F	LBP	30% (20–39)
					NSP	24% (16–31)
					LBP & NSP	60% (51–68)
Livshits et al., 2011 (18)	TwinsUK	1069	18–84	F	LBP	44%

CWP, chronic widespread pain; h^2, heritability; LBP, low back pain; NSP, neck–shoulder pain.

involved. The susceptibility genes may differ in accordance with subphenotypes. Some individuals report pain but not psychological disturbance while others have severe psychological distress. Chronic pain is a heterogeneous phenotype and its genetic makeup is likely to reflect this.

Mendelian-inherited pain disorders have identified a number of genes which are important in pain perception, particularly in ion channels. *SCN9A* encodes the alpha subunit of the voltage-gated sodium channel Na$_v$1.7. Multiple mutations in *SCN9A* resulting in either a severe pain disorder or congenital insensitivity to pain

Table 45.2 Genetic association studies of chronic musculoskeletal pain

Gene	Polymorphism(s)	Phenotype(s)	Findings	Reference
ADRB2	rs1042713 (R16G), rs1042714 (Q27E)	FM	Haplotype of rs1042713 (R allele) and rs1042714 (Q allele) associated with increased risk of FM	Vargas-Alarcon et al., 2009 (35)
	Multiple SNPs including rs1042713 (R16G)	Chronic pain, CWP	R allele of rs1042713 associated with reduced risk of CWP	Hocking et al., 2010 (31)
COMT	rs4680 (V158M)	Symptomatic hip OA	M allele of rs4680 associated with increased risk of hip pain in women	van Meurs et al., 2009 (33)
	Multiple SNPs including rs4680 (V158M)	Chronic pain, CWP	No association	Hocking et al., 2010 (31)
	rs4633, rs4680 (V158M), rs6269, rs4818	CWP	No association	Nicholl et al., 2010 (32)
GCH1	rs10483639, rs3783641, rs8007267	CWP	No association.	Holliday et al., 2009 (37)
HTR2A	Tag SNPs including rs6313 (T102C)	CWP and number of pain sites reported	Evidence of association between SNPs and CWP and the number of pain sites reported	Nicholl et al., 2010 (40)
OPRM1	rs1799971 (N40D), rs563649	CWP	No association	Holliday et al., 2009 (37)
SCN9A	rs6746030 (R1150W)	WOMAC pain score	W allele associated with increased pain scores	Reimann et al., 2010 (23)
	rs6746030 (R1150W)	WOMAC pain score, widespread pain	W allele not associated with WOMAC pain score but associated with increased risk of widespread pain	Valdes et al., 2010 (47)
SLC6A4	44bp indel (5HTTLPR)	FM	No association	Potvin et al., 2010 (42)
TRPV1	rs8065080 (I585V)	Symptomatic knee OA	II genotype associated with reduced risk of symptomatic knee OA	Valdes et al., 2011 (27)

CWP, chronic widespread pain; FM, fibromyalgia; OA, osteoarthritis; WOMAC, Western Ontario and McMaster Universities Arthritis Index.

have been reported in families.[23] Susceptibility loci for common complex diseases commonly occur in genes causing phenotypically similar mendelian disorders, therefore, as well as adding to the understanding of the biological mechanisms underlying pain perception, these studies highlight candidate genes for chronic pain susceptibility.

Candidate gene studies

Candidate gene genetic association studies of chronic musculoskeletal pain phenotypes have been undertaken to identify susceptibility genes. The main findings of these studies are summarized below and in Table 45.2.

Voltage-gated sodium channel, Na$_v$1.7 alpha subunit (SCN9A)

Reimann et al. identified a non-synonymous SNP, R1150W (rs6746030), in SCN9A associated with pain perception in OA and replicated this finding in other cohorts with different types of clinical pain.[23] The variant W allele, which was associated with increased pain scores, increases excitability of nociceptive neurons in the dorsal root ganglion.[24] Valdes et al. subsequently disputed the finding of Reimann et al. as they observed no association with pain scores in OA but they did observe an association with widespread pain in population-based cohorts.[25]

Transient receptor potential vanilloid receptor 1 (TRPV1)

TRPV1 is an ion channel gene which encodes a thermosensitive channel expressed in primary afferent neurons. Valdes et al.[27] observed that the II genotype of the non-synonymous SNP I585V

(rs8065080) in TRPV1, which has been associated with reduced cold pain sensitivity,[26] was associated with reduced risk of knee OA in 4368 cases compared to 3852 controls from seven United Kingdom cohorts. The effect was much larger when comparing symptomatic to asymptomatic knee OA cases or controls, implicating the SNP in peripheral pain sensitivity in OA.[27]

Catechol-O-methyltransferase (COMT)

COMT is an enzyme which degrades catecholamines, such as dopamine and adrenaline (epinephrine). COMT is the most widely studied pain susceptibility gene, largely due to a non-synonymous SNP (V158M) affecting enzymatic activity,[28] and a study found the M allele to be associated with increased pain sensitivity as a result of reduced μ-opioid activity in the brain in response to a painful stimulus.[29] V158M is located in a haplotype shown to distinguish pain sensitivity levels in healthy females and to be associated with incident temporomandibular joint disorder (TMD).[30] V158M has also been investigated in multiple small scale candidate gene studies of FM but with equivocal findings.[3]

More recently, COMT has been investigated in larger population-based cohorts. No association was observed between V158M or 10 other SNPs in COMT and CWP in a United Kingdom birth cohort.[31] Nor was an association observed between the pain sensitivity haplotype and CWP in United Kingdom and European cohorts.[32] In contrast, in a Dutch population-based cohort, the M allele of V158M was associated with an increased risk of hip pain in women with radiographic hip osteoarthritis.[33]

β₂ adrenergic receptor (ADRB2)

The catecholamines target the adrenergic receptors, one of which has been implicated as a chronic pain gene. An *ADRB2* haplotype including the variant alleles of two common non-synonymous SNPs (rs1042713 and rs1042714) has been associated with incident TMD and reporting somatic symptoms in 202 United States females.[34] and increased risk of FM in 156 FM cases and 119 controls from Mexico and Spain.[35] In contrast in a United Kingdom birth cohort, the minor A allele of rs1042713 was associated with a reduced risk of having CWP (n = 846) compared to a pain-free control group (n = 3310).[31]

μ-opioid receptor (OPRM1)

OPRM1 encodes the μ-opioid receptor which binds exogenous and endogenous opiates. A non-synonymous polymorphism, N40D (rs1799971) known to influence receptor binding affinity has received a lot of attention. The largest study to date to examine N40D was a comprehensive study of the variation across *OPRM1* with pain sensitivity. Although N40D did not associate, an additional potentially functional SNP (rs563649) was associated with increased pain sensitivity.[36] However, rs563549 and N40D did not associate with CWP in two population-based cohorts.[37]

GTP cyclohydrolase (GCH1)

GCH1, which encodes GTP cyclohydrolase, an enzyme involved in the production of BH4, which is essential in synthesis of neurotransmitters, has also been implicated in influencing pain sensitivity. A low pain sensitivity haplotype in *GCH1*, also shown to protect against persistent pain, has been reported and is associated with reduced expression of *GCH1*,[38] but findings in subsequent studies of pain sensitivity have been conflicting. The low pain sensitivity haplotype was found to be more common in individuals with persistent CWP (19%) compared to pain-free individuals (15%) in a UK population-based cohort, but the difference was not statistically significant.[37]

Serotonergic system

Because of the strong link between psychological distress and incident chronic pain, pathways that may mediate this relationship have also been investigated in candidate gene studies. One such pathway is the serotonergic system, abnormalities in which have been reported in FM.[39]

A synonymous SNP, S34S (rs6313, also known as T102C) in a serotonin (5HT) receptor gene (*HTR2A*) has been investigated in a number of small studies of clinic-based FM patients and healthy controls, with equivocal findings.[3] A recent study comprehensively assessed the role of SNPs across *HTR2A* in CWP cases compared to pain-free controls and with a quantitative measure of pain reporting (measured by the number of painful sites reported). A region of moderate to high linkage disequilibrium around rs6313 showed association with both phenotypes in two population-based cohorts, implicating this region as a pain susceptibility locus. Comorbid mood disorder is common in subjects with pain disorders and serotonin also has a role in depression, therefore the findings were adjusted for depressive symptoms. This attenuated the effects but associations persisted, suggesting that this region may have pleiotrophic effects on pain and mood disorders as proposed by twin studies.[40]

A 44 bp insertion or deletion (indel) in the promoter of a 5HT transporter gene, *SLC6A4,* known as 5HTTLPR, has been widely studied with psychological and psychiatric disorders due to its effect on expression.[41] Studies investigating the role of the indel in chronic musculoskeletal pain have been limited to small groups of clinic-based FM patients and healthy controls, which have yielded equivocal findings.[3,42]

The candidate gene studies of chronic musculoskeletal pain phenotypes conducted to date have yielded conflicting findings. There are a number of factors which may have contributed to this. Differing phenotypes assessed in different ways have been studied for the same genes/SNPs. For example, FM clinic patients may not be directly comparable to community subjects with CWP. However, the predominant limitation in these studies is sample size, particularly in clinic-based studies. Larger population-based studies are emerging but are most likely still underpowered to detect the anticipated modest genetic effects. Compared to other complex traits pain research is in its relative infancy, and therefore the known study design challenges of genetic association studies have largely not been addressed.[3]

Genome-wide association studies

Despite an extensive list of potential candidates only a small number of genes have been investigated and a limited number of polymorphisms within those genes studied. Genome-wide association studies (GWAS) can address both these limitations but have not yet been utilized. GWAS studies of migraine have been conducted and have demonstrated that susceptibility loci can be identified and validated with large sample sizes and well-defined phenotypes.[43,44]

Challenges

Pain is a subjective experience that is largely dependent on self-report. The genes underlying the psychological factors that influence how people report pain may prove as important as the genes involved in pain processing pathways. Pain is also episodic and will resolve in some individuals and persist in others, and assessing pain at a single time-point may not be informative. Genetic factors may have a key role in determining whether pain is transient or persistent and longitudinal studies could be used to address this question.

Pain is heterogeneous, and defining the phenotype for use in genetic studies is challenging. for example, in studies of fm the acr 1990[45] criteria are commonly used; however, these criteria only incorporate widespread pain (pain above and below the waist on both sides of the body and in the axial skeleton) and tenderness (11 or more of 18 tender-points), ignoring other common features such as fatigue, somatization, sleep disturbance, and cognitive dysfunction. New criteria for FM have recently been proposed that incorporate these characteristics[46]; however, subjects identified using these new criteria are also likely to be a heterogeneous group.

Likewise, identifying suitable controls is challenging. Some studies have used pain-free groups as controls; however, they are not representative of the general population as experiencing some pain is normal. Using large population-based cohorts as controls is now common place in GWAS, but owing to the relatively high prevalence of chronic pain disorders this approach will reduce power to detect modest genetic effects.

Future prospects

In order for genetic studies of chronic musculoskeletal pain to be fruitful, large well-phenotyped cohorts are required. More sophisticated approaches could be utilized to elucidate the genetic component. One such approach may be to use intermediate phenotypes, which are quantifiable phenotypes related to the outcome that have a simpler genetic basis. Alternatively, subgroups with different phenotypic characteristics could be identified, reducing heterogeneity and increasing the ability to detect subtle effects. Dissecting cohorts in this way means that much larger sample sizes will be required.

Genetic architecture varies by phenotype and the contribution of common genetic variation to chronic pain susceptibility may be limited. Other types of variation such as rare variants, structural variation (e.g. copy number variation or epigenetic modification) as well as gene–gene (epistasis) and gene–environment interactions may contribute to the heritability of chronic musculoskeletal pain and should be considered in future research.

Conclusion

Twin studies strongly suggest musculoskeletal pain is heritable. Genes involved in psychological distress and pain processing pathways may be important. Genes that influence pain perception have been identified in families. Attempts to elucidate the genes involved, however, have been limited with underpowered studies yielding equivocal findings. Current methodologies such as GWAS and next-generation sequencing have yet to be utilized, most likely due to limited availability of suitable cohorts. To move this research forward, phenotypes need to be refined and sample sizes increased.

References

1. McBeth J, Jones K. Epidemiology of chronic musculoskeletal pain. *Best Pract Res Clin Rheumatol* 2007;21(3):403–425.
2. Macfarlane GJ, Jones GT, McBeth J. Epidemiology of pain. In: McMahon S, Koltzenburg M (eds) Wall and Melzack's textbook of pain. Churchill Livingstone, London, 2005.
3. Limer KL, Nicholl BI, Thomson W, McBeth J. Exploring the genetic susceptibility of chronic widespread pain: the tender points in genetic association studies. *Rheumatology (Oxford)* 2008;47(5):572–577.
4. Arnold LM, Hudson JI, Hess EV et al. Family study of fibromyalgia. *Arthritis Rheum* 2004;50(3):944–952.
5. Markkula R, Jarvinen P, Leino-Arjas P et al. Clustering of symptoms associated with fibromyalgia in a Finnish Twin Cohort. *Eur J Pain* 2009;13(7):744–750.
6. Kato K, Sullivan PF, Evengard B, Pedersen NL. Importance of genetic influences on chronic widespread pain. *Arthritis Rheum* 2006;54(5):1682–1686.
7. Reichborn-Kjennerud T, Stoltenberg C, Tambs K et al. Back-neck pain and symptoms of anxiety and depression: a population-based twin study. *Psychol Med* 2002;32(6):1009–1020.
8. Hestbaek L, Iachine IA, Leboeuf-Yde C, Kyvik KO, Manniche C. Heredity of low back pain in a young population: a classical twin study. *Twin Res* 2004;7(1):16–26.
9. Hartvigsen J, Christensen K, Frederiksen H, Petersen HC. Genetic and environmental contributions to back pain in old age: a study of 2,108 Danish twins aged 70 and older. *Spine* 2004;29(8):897–901.
10. MacGregor AJ, Andrew T, Sambrook PN, Spector TD. Structural, psychological, and genetic influences on low back and neck pain: a study of adult female twins. *Arthritis Rheum* 2004;51(2):160–167.
11. Hartvigsen J, Petersen HC, Frederiksen H, Christensen K. Small effect of genetic factors on neck pain in old age: a study of 2,108 Danish twins 70 years of age and older. *Spine* 2005;30(2):206–208.
12. Fejer R, Hartvigsen J, Kyvik KO. Heritability of neck pain: a population-based study of 33,794 Danish twins. *Rheumatology* (Oxford) 2006;45(5):589–594.
13. Battie MC, Videman T, Levalahti E, Gill K, Kaprio J. Heritability of low back pain and the role of disc degeneration. *Pain* 2007;131(3):272–280.
14. El-Metwally A, Mikkelsson M, Stahl M et al. Genetic and environmental influences on non-specific low back pain in children: a twin study. *Eur Spine J* 2008;17(4):502–508.
15. Hartvigsen J, Nielsen J, Kyvik KO et al. Heritability of spinal pain and consequences of spinal pain: a comprehensive genetic epidemiologic analysis using a population-based sample of 15,328 twins ages 20–71 years. *Arthritis Rheum* 2009;61(10):1343–1351.
16. Williams FM, Spector TD, MacGregor AJ. Pain reporting at different body sites is explained by a single underlying genetic factor. *Rheumatology* (Oxford) 2010;49(9):1753–1755.
17. Nyman T, Mulder M, Iliadou A, Svartengren M, Wiktorin C. High heritability for concurrent low back and neck-shoulder pain—a study of twins. *Spine* (Phila Pa 1976] 2011;36(22):E1469–1476.
18. Livshits G, Popham M, Malkin I et al. Lumbar disc degeneration and genetic factors are the main risk factors for low back pain in women: the UK Twin Spine Study. *Ann Rheum Dis* 2011;70(10):1740–1745.
19. Mikkelsson M, Kaprio J, Salminen JJ, Pulkkinen L, Rose RJ. Widespread pain among 11-year-old Finnish twin pairs. *Arthritis Rheum* 2010;44(2):481–485.
20. Mikkelsson M, El-Metwally A, Kautiainen H et al. Onset, prognosis and risk factors for widespread pain in schoolchildren: a prospective 4-year follow-up study. *Pain* 2008;138(3):681–687.
21. Fejer R, Hartvigsen J, Kyvik KO. Sex differences in heritability of neck pain. *Twin Res Hum Genet* 2006;9(2):198–204.
22. Kato K, Sullivan PF, Evengard B, Pedersen NL. A population-based twin study of functional somatic syndromes. *Psychol Med* 2009;39(3):497–505.
23. Reimann F, Cox JJ, Belfer I et al. Pain perception is altered by a nucleotide polymorphism in SCN9A. *Proc Natl Acad Sci U S A* 2010;107(11):5148–5153.
24. Estacion M, Harty TP, Choi JS et al. A sodium channel gene SCN9A polymorphism that increases nociceptor excitability. *Ann Neurol* 2009;66(6):862–866.
25. Valdes AM, Arden NK, Vaughn FL et al. Role of the Na(V)1.7 R1150W amino acid change in susceptibility to symptomatic knee osteoarthritis and multiple regional pain. *Arthritis Care Res* (Hoboken) 2011;63(3):440–444.
26. Kim H, Mittal DP, Iadarola MJ, Dionne RA. Genetic predictors for acute experimental cold and heat pain sensitivity in humans. *J Med Genet* 2006;43(8):e40.
27. Valdes AM, De WG, Doherty SA et al. The Ile585Val TRPV1 variant is involved in risk of painful knee osteoarthritis. *Ann Rheum Dis* 2011;70(9):1556–1561.
28. Syvanen AC, Tilgmann C, Rinne J, Ulmanen I. Genetic polymorphism of catechol-O-methyltransferase (COMT): correlation of genotype with individual variation of S-COMT activity and comparison of the allele frequencies in the normal population and parkinsonian patients in Finland. *Pharmacogenetics* 1997;7(1):65–71.
29. Zubieta JK, Heitzeg MM, Smith YR et al. COMT val158 met genotype affects mu-opioid neurotransmitter responses to a pain stressor. *Science* 2003;299(5610):1240–1243.
30. Diatchenko L, Slade GD, Nackley AG et al. Genetic basis for individual variations in pain perception and the development of a chronic pain condition. *Hum Mol Genet* 2005;14(1):135–143.
31. Hocking LJ, Smith BH, Jones GT et al. Genetic variation in the beta2-adrenergic receptor but not catecholamine-O-methyltransferase predisposes to chronic pain: results from the 1958 British Birth Cohort Study. *Pain* 2010;149(1):143–151.
32. Nicholl BI, Holliday KL, Macfarlane GJ et al. No evidence for a role of the catechol-O-methyltransferase (COMT) pain sensitivity haplotype in chronic widespread pain. *Ann Rheum Dis* 2010;69(11):2009–2012.
33. van Meurs JB, Uitterlinden AG, Stolk L et al. A functional polymorphism in the catechol-O-methyltransferase gene is associated with osteoarthritis-related pain. *Arthritis Rheum* 2009;60(2):628–629.

34. Diatchenko L, Anderson AD, Slade GD et al. Three major haplotypes of the beta2 adrenergic receptor define psychological profile, blood pressure, and the risk for development of a common musculoskeletal pain disorder. *Am J Med Genet B Neuropsychiatr Genet* 2006;141(5):449–462.

35. Vargas-Alarcon G, Fragoso JM, Cruz-Robles D et al. Association of adrenergic receptor gene polymorphisms with different fibromyalgia syndrome domains. *Arthritis Rheum* 2009;60(7):2169–2173.

36. Shabalina SA, Zaykin DV, Gris P et al. Expansion of the human mu-opioid receptor gene architecture: novel functional variants. *Hum Mol Genet* 2009;18(6):1037–1051.

37. Holliday KL, Nicholl BI, Macfarlane GJ, Thomson W, Davies KA & McBeth J. Do genetic predictors of pain sensitivity associate with persistent widespread pain? *Mol Pain* 2009;5(1):56.

38. Tegeder I, Costigan M, Griffin RS et al. GTP cyclohydrolase and tetrahydrobiopterin regulate pain sensitivity and persistence. *Nat Med* 2006;12(11):1269–1277.

39. Gupta A, Silman AJ. Psychological stress and fibromyalgia: a review of the evidence suggesting a neuroendocrine link. *Arthritis Res Ther* 2004;6(3):98–106.

40. Nicholl BI, Holliday KL, Macfarlane GJ et al. HTR2A polymorphisms are associated with chronic widespread pain and the extent of musculoskeletal pain: results from two population-based cohorts. *Arthritis Rheum* 2011;63(3):810–818.

41. Lesch KP, Bengel D, Heils A et al. Association of anxiety-related traits with a polymorphism in the serotonin transporter gene regulatory region. *Science* 1996;274(5292):1527–1531.

42. Potvin S, Larouche A, Normand E et al. No relationship between the ins del polymorphism of the serotonin transporter promoter and pain perception in fibromyalgia patients and healthy controls. *Eur J Pain* 2010;14(7):742–746.

43. Anttila V, Stefansson H, Kallela M et al. Genome-wide association study of migraine implicates a common susceptibility variant on 8q22.1. *Nat Genet* 2010;42(10):869–873.

44. Chasman DI, Schurks M, Anttila V et al. Genome-wide association study reveals three susceptibility loci for common migraine in the general population. *Nat Genet* 2011;43(7):695–698.

45. Wolfe F, Smythe HA, Yunus MB, Bennett R, Bombardier C. The American College of Rheumatology 1990 Criteria for the Classification of fibromyalgia. *Arthritis Rheum* 1990;33(2):160–172.

46. Wolfe F, Clauw DJ, Fitzcharles MA et al. The American College of Rheumatology preliminary diagnostic criteria for fibromyalgia and measurement of symptom severity. *Arthritis Care Res* (Hoboken) 2010;62(5):600–610.

47. Valdes AM, Arden NK, Vaughn FL et al. Role of the Na(V)1.7 R1150W amino acid change in susceptibility to symptomatic knee osteoarthritis and multiple regional pain. *Arthritis Care Res* 2011;63(3):440–444.

Tissues in health and disease

CHAPTER 46

Normal functional anatomy of joints

Mike Benjamin and Dennis McGonagle

Introduction and basic definitions

Joints occur where skeletal elements meet and they can be classified in different ways (Box 46.1). From a functional stance, joints can be distinguished according to the amount of movement allowed as diarthrodial (highly moveable), amphiarthrodial (slightly moveable), and synarthrodial (immoveable) joints. However, a functional classification is less common than an anatomical one. According to such a scheme, the major joints recognized are synovial, secondary cartilaginous and fibrous joints. Synovial joints are typical of the limbs and their defining feature is the presence of a synovial cavity containing fluid secreted by a synovial membrane. It is the lubricated cavity between the skeletal elements that promotes the free movement that characterizes these joints. The functional integration between synovium and cartilage is well recognized, with the cartilage deriving its nutrition and lubrication from the synovium via the fluid—a plasma ultrafiltrate. The synovial membrane also contains a population of resident macrophages that are likely to remove microdebris from the joint cavity and help to maintain the rheological properties of the fluid. This arrangement underlies normal cartilage homeostasis but is delicately poised, with any disruption of synovial or cartilage homeostasis rapidly culminating in joint inflammation that can exacerbate cycles of joint damage, irrespective of the trigger.

Fibrous and fibrocartilaginous joints lack synovium, and disease at the latter is especially associated with the seronegative spondyloarthopathies.[1] The cartilage of fibrocartilaginous joints is referred to as 'secondary cartilage' as it appears relatively late in development and *after* ossification has commenced in the contributing skeletal elements. Thus, a secondary cartilaginous joint (like a primary one—see next paragraph) is one where cartilage unites the bones. However, whereas in a primary joint the formation of cartilage precedes that of bone, in a secondary joint it is the other way around. Secondary cartilaginous joints may be called fibrocartilaginous joints, because the tissue uniting the bones is fibrocartilage, rather than hyaline cartilage. They are also called symphyses. Examples of such joints include the manubriosternal joints, the pubic symphysis, and the joints between adjacent vertebral bodies. From a functional standpoint, they can be regarded as amphiarthroses. Finally, fibrous joints are those where the skeletal elements are linked by pure fibrous tissue. Some fibrous joints completely preclude any movement (i.e. are synarthroses, like the sutures between the bones of the cranium), but others allow slight movement (syndesmoses—such as the inferior tibiofibular joint). Whether movement is completely or partly prevented depends on the quantity of fibrous tissue that holds the bones together. There is more fibrous tissue in a syndesmosis and it spans a greater distance across the bones.

In all the older anatomy texts, the site at which a long bone epiphysis meets the shaft early in development is regarded as a joint. The

---

Box 46.1 The classification of joints

Functional

- Diarthrodial (highly moveable—e.g. synovial)
- Amphiarthrodial (slightly moveable—secondary cartilaginous)
- Synarthrodial (immoveable—e.g. sutures)

Structural (anatomical)

Fibrous

- Suture (e.g. between skull flat bones)
- Syndesmosis (e.g. inferior tibiofibular)

Cartilaginous

- Primary (e.g. a long-bone growth plate)
- Secondary (e.g. manubriosternal)

Synovial

- Plane (e.g. facet)
- Hinge (e.g. interphalangeal)
- Pivot (e.g. superior radioulnar)
- Condyloid (e.g knee)
- Ellipsoid (e.g. wrist)
- Ball and socket (e.g. glenohumeral or hip)
- Saddle (sellar) (e.g. 1st carpometacarpal)

site of union is marked by a plate of hyaline cartilage that is a temporarily persisting part of the cartilaginous anlagen that preceded any bone formation. Specifically, such a structure is referred to as a *primary cartilaginous joint*. However, in the view of Rogers,[2] such a 'joint' is better known by its alternative name of 'growth plate' or 'epiphysial plate' and should not be regarded as a joint at all, for it is simply a temporary feature of a single skeletal element. Wood Jones,[3] on the other hand, regards epiphyses as 'separate ossifications developed in joint cavities as specializations of articular cartilage'. He regarded them as quite distinct bones that unite with the limb bones at a fused junction called a *synchondrosis*. Nevertheless, whatever standpoint is adopted, the term 'joint' most typically refers to permanent features of the skeleton. With respect to the rheumatic diseases, the epiphyseal plate regions are rarely recognized as being the primary drivers, or indeed being involved in the pathogenesis of the rheumatic diseases, and as such support the concept that these regions are not joints from the pathophysiological functional standpoint. However, thus far, one possible exception has been recognized. In the Muckle–Wells syndrome, a hereditary autoinflammatory disease, epiphyseal hyperplasia in association with joint inflammation is well recognized.[4] This raises the question of whether epiphyseal plate cartilaginous tissue could indeed be of more widespread relevance for understanding joint inflammation, especially in paediatric inflammatory disease.

Synovial joints

General features

Although a synovial joint permits free movement between bones, the plane of movement (i.e. the joint cavity) is actually between two layers of cartilage that cover or line the ends of the bones and not

directly between bone tissue (Figure 46.1). This is because cartilage is better suited to withstanding compression than bone. In most instances, the cartilage is hyaline cartilage, though occasionally it is fibrocartilage (e.g. in the temporomandibular joint).

The reason that cartilage can withstand compression is because it has a high water content and is avascular. Blood vessels are absent because they would collapse under pressure. This also explains why there is no perichondrium on the surface of articular cartilage. The high water content of cartilage relates largely to the presence of aggrecan. This is a large proteoglycan that attracts tissue fluid into the cartilage by capillarity. The collagen fibrils within the articular cartilage hold the aggrecan molecules in place, thus maintaining the capillary channels and ensuring that the tissue fluid is not readily squeezed out. Some inevitably is lost during the daytime, but it seeps back at night. The high tissue fluid content of articular cartilage not only enables the tissue to withstand compression, but contributes along with the synovial fluid (see next paragraph) to ensuring that chondrocytes can survive without blood vessels. Not only is articular cartilage avascular, it is also aneural. This contributes to the lateness with which osteoarthritis (OA) is often detected. There is an absence of pain until the cartilage is completely eroded and the underlying (highly innervated) bone is exposed.

The other striking feature of a synovial joint is the synovial cavity that contains a thin film of slightly viscous fluid, secreted by a synovial membrane. This membrane lines all non-articular surfaces of the joint (i.e. it is not found on the surface of the articular cartilage, because of the vascularity of the cartilage) and has two layers—a surface or intimal layer that is highly cellular and a vascular subintima that contains connective tissue. Its surface area can be significantly increased by folds (synovial villi)—a proliferation of which is a characteristic feature of synovitis. In some joints, the cavity extends through and

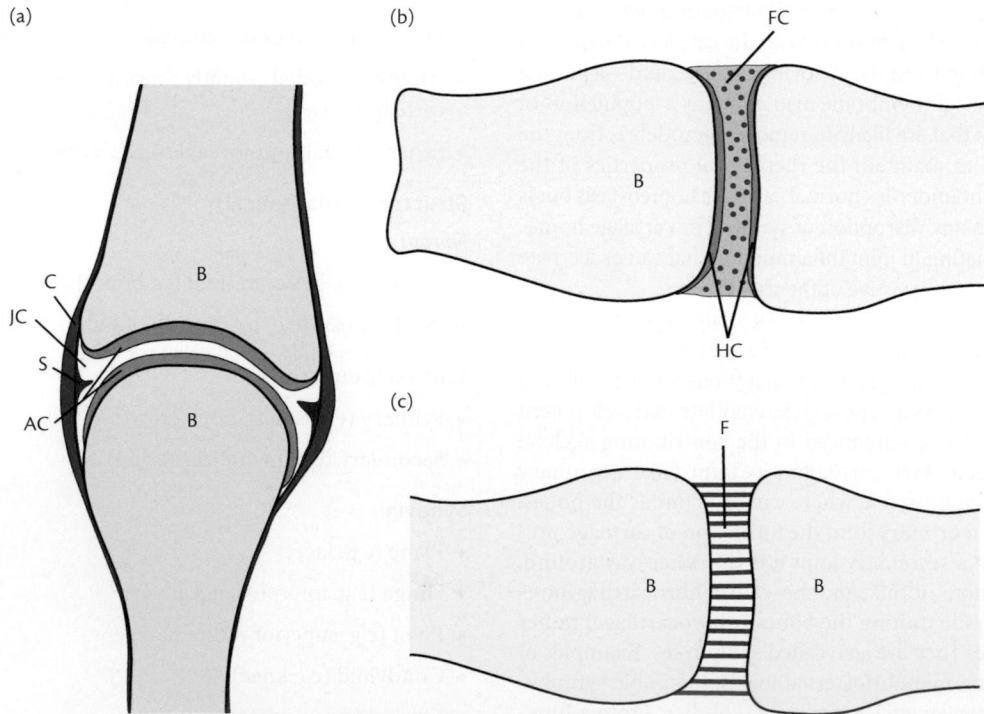

Fig. 46.1 Diagrammatic representation of the three types of joints included in a basic anatomical classification: (a) A synovial joint. The articulating bones (B) are (typically) covered with hyaline articular cartilage (AC) and separated by a joint cavity (JC) containing fluid secreted by a lining synovial membrane (S). This lines the non-articular parts of the joint, including the joint capsule (C). (b) A cartilaginous joint, exemplified by a secondary cartilaginous joint. The bones are covered with a thin layer of hyaline cartilage, but joined by fibrocartilage (FC). (c) A fibrous joint, exemplified by a suture. Here the bones are joined by dense fibrous connective tissue (F).

thus beyond the joint capsule to become continuous with associated bursae. This is the case with the subdeltoid bursa at the shoulder that serves to reduce friction between the joint and the deep surface of the deltoid muscle. However, there are other bursae close to joints that are not in direct communication with joint cavities.

The lubricating molecule that is secreted by the synovial membrane and reduces the frictional forces between the bones is lubrican. This, together with hyaluronan, is produced by fibroblasts (type B synoviocytes) within the intimal layer. The other common intimal cell type is the macrophage (type A synoviocyte)—cells that can phagocytose debris within the synovial cavity and which are also act as antigen-presenting cells. The water content of the synovial fluid represents an exudate from blood vessels in the subintima and its presence aids the access of nutrient and metabolites to and from the cartilage cells. The subintima is a connective tissue layer of variable character. It may be fibrous, loose connective (areolar), or adipose (fatty) tissue. Sometimes the fat in synovial joints is so striking that it merits a specific name, e.g. Hoffa's fat pad in the knee. It seems that adipose tissue is a particular feature of joints that bear significant pressure and absent in those that do not.[3] Thus, fat is not seen in large quantities in the shoulder, wrist, or hand. It is always present where a non-articular part of a bone lies within the joint capsule.[3] The tissue is likely to be implicated in joint pain, for it contains nociceptive nerve fibres[5] and it promotes the efficient spread of synovial fluid. The nerve fibres contain mediators including substance P that can induce an inflammatory response within the knee joint and trigger vasodilation and associated oedema.[5]

Clearly, with the presence of a complete cavity between the articulating bone, there must also be strong, fibrous bonds between the bones. The linkage is created by a fibrous capsule and associated ligaments (Figure 46.1). The capsule develops from the same population of mesenchymal cells as those that are present around the developing bones and give rise to the periosteum. Wood Jones[3] regards this sleeve of tissue as a specialized part of the deep fascia—called 'periosteum' around the bones and 'capsule' around the joints. The ligaments may be local thickenings of the capsule (e.g. the medial collateral ligament of the knee) or independent structures outside (e.g. the lateral collateral ligament of the knee) or inside (e.g. the cruciate ligaments) the joint cavity. Tendons can also reinforce or replace the joint capsule (see below), or can pass through the joint cavity. This is particularly so where their associated muscle has undergone phylogenetic shifting: i.e. with postural changes during evolution, there has been a migration of the origin or insertion of the tendon.[3] As a generalization, ligaments serve to guide and limit joint movements: i.e. because of the way in which they are arranged around the joint periphery, they allow some movements, but prohibit others. They resist stretch (i.e. have a high tensile strength) and thus have a high content of type I collagen and a sparse population of cells. The cells are usually fibroblasts, but if the ligament also needs to resist compression (e.g. in the annular ligament of the superior radioulnar joint), fibrocartilage cells may be evident. The relatively low numbers of cells and the paucity of blood vessels are significant factors accounting for the slow healing of ligaments following injury.

Tendons that fuse with or replace joint capsules include those of the rotator cuff and the extensor tendons that cross the interphalangeal joints. Here, the tendons not only replace the joint capsule dorsally, but also form an articular surface for the neighbouring bone. It is thus worth noting that when a finger is flexed, the head of its proximal phalanx articulates with the deep surface of the extensor tendon in addition to the base of the intermediate phalanx.[1] It is intriguing that the articular fibrocartilage of the tendon (referred to as a sesamoid fibrocartilage[1]) is the region clearly perforated in a boutonnière deformity of the finger and is where a signal change in MRI can be evident in dactylitis.[6]

Some synovial joints contain menisci. They are generally fibrocartilaginous discs but their function is sometimes unclear. It has been suggested that they serve as shock absorbers, that they increase joint congruity and make for a more efficient distribution of weight across a joint surface. That they aid load distribution is a widely accepted view of their function in the knee joint, and doubtless relates to the observation that there is a significant increase in the incidence of OA after meniscectomy.[7] Prominent though knee joint menisci are, they do not create two separate compartments within the joint as they can do elsewhere, e.g. in the sternoclavicular and temporomandibular joints (TMJ). Here it is suggested that they allow for different movements in the two compartments on either side of the disc. Thus, it is often proposed that the superior joint compartment in the TMJ facilitates gliding movements and the inferior compartment allows for hinge-like movements. However, as Wood Jones[3] points out, the disc in the sternoclavicular joint is very similar to that in the TMJ, but no one has ever suggested that it has a similar functional role. Wood Jones favours the idea that the disc is present in both joints because all moving bones are membrane bones and thus the bearing surfaces must develop from the mesoblasts of the primitive joint cavity.[3]

Different types of synovial joint

The subclasses of synovial joint include plane, hinge, pivot, condyloid, ellipsoid, ball and socket, and saddle (sellar) joints.[8]

Plane synovial joints

In a plane synovial joint, the articular surfaces are flat, as in the intercarpal joints, and such joints promote only a slight gliding movement between the bones. The movement allowed by the other joints is more obvious and can be uniaxial (hinge or pivot joints), biaxial (condyloid and ellipsoid joints), or multiaxial (ball and socket and saddle joints).

Hinge joints

Hinge joints are exemplified by the elbow, ankle, and interphalangeal joints. The movements are simple flexion and extension movements, restricted to one plane only.

Pivot joints

Pivot joints are represented by the atlanto-axial joint, where the head, supported by the atlas, pivots around the dens, within the confines of a restraining transverse ligament. The rotatory movements between atlas and axis allow the head to move from side to side. The only other pivot joint is the superior radioulnar joint, where the rounded head of the radius pivots around the ulna within the confines of the restraining annular ligament. As Sinclair[9] points out, the 'pivot' of each joint lies vertically when the body is in the anatomical position.

Condyloid joints

Condyloid joints are those in which the articular surfaces form distinct condyles—as in the knee, but also in the metacarpophalangeal joints.

Ellipsoid joints

In ellipsoid joints, one articular surface is again in the form of a socket, but the other forms an ovoid, rather than spherical, articular surface. The wrist joint is the classic example.

Ball and socket joints

Ball and socket joints include those of the hip and shoulder, but also the talocalcaneonavicular joint. They are multiaxial joints permitting a wide range of movement. One articular surface is spherical and fits into a cup-shaped socket. The socket is deeper in the hip joint to promote greater stability and shallower in the glenohumeral joint to promote a free range of movement. Such is the complexity of movements in a ball and socket joint that, for descriptive purposes, they are referred to as flexion, extension, abduction, adduction, medial rotation, and lateral rotation.

Saddle (sellar) joints

A saddle joint is only found in the thumb and is the joint between the trapezium and the first metacarpal bone. As the name suggests, the articular surfaces are reciprocally saddle shaped. It is important for the dexterity of the thumb.

Biomechanical/functional considerations

The position at which the contact area between the contributing bones of a synovial joint is maximal is the most stable position of the joint and is known as the close-packed position. It effectively converts the bones into a unified lever and is the most efficient weight-bearing and/or stress-reducing position.[9] Close packing usually occurs towards the end of the range of movement of a joint when the capsule and the ligament are tense.[2] Thus, at the knee joint, the close-packed position more or less corresponds to full extension. According to Sinclair,[9] close packing is rarely maintained for long because it is less conducive to efficient joint lubrication. He argues that even when standing upright, there are subtle movements of the lower limb joints that encourage the spread of synovial fluid within the joint. In contrast to the close-packed position, where ligaments are tense, there is also a 'position of rest' where the ligaments are slack and the surrounding muscles relaxed. Wood Jones[3] gives a good account of the position of rest of the hand.

Although joint stability is clearly an issue greatly influenced by the shape of the articulating bones and the restraining action of the capsule and ligaments, another key factor is surrounding muscles. This is clearly explained by Sinclair.[9] Briefly, the simplistic view of an antagonistic muscle relaxing while a prime mover contracts to enable the movement is misleading. What generally happens is that the antagonists continue to generate tension in order to prevent any dangerous overcontraction of the prime movers. Thus, the antagonists actually lengthen as they generate tension—a movement known as 'eccentric contraction'. Sinclair[9] refers to muscles acting in such a manner as 'extensile ligaments' and points out that they are common in highly mobile joints such as the glenohumeral joint. Here, the shallow glenoid cavity and the slack capsule promote dislocation, but the efficiency of the rotator cuff muscles reduces the risk.

When rapid movement occurs in a joint, there may be a tendency for the two sides of the joint to come apart. Muscles that cross the joint and run along the long axis of one of the bones play a key role in preventing this, e.g. brachioradialis. This is an example of a 'shunt muscle' because it shunts one bone into another.[10] It crosses the elbow joint, spanning between the inferior part of the humerus and the lower end of the radius. As the elbow is straightened by a rapid contraction of triceps, brachioradialis contracts to help maintain joint integrity. The fact that brachioradialis inserts at such a distance from the elbow adds to the efficiency with which it can act as a shunt muscle. Triceps, however, is acting as a 'spurt muscle' in this example, for it allows for a fast movement. Its insertion immediately beyond the joint on which it acts (to the olecranon) is conducive to a fast movement.

Movement at a synovial joint may be 'active' if it is actioned by skeletal muscles that cross the joint and act on it, or 'passive' if it is the consequence of an external force. (including gravity). The range of passive movement is nearly always greater than that of active movement.[9] This is easily exemplified by using one hand to bend the fingers of the other passively beyond the limits that can be achieved by contraction of the extensor muscles. Passive movements can also occur at joints that cannot be matched by the active movement of muscles—e.g. the slight rotation that can be achieved passively at the metacarpophalangeal joints, where there are no muscles that can promote active rotation.

Particularly in highly mobile synovial joints, there is often a complex network of blood vessels in the vicinity. These 'anastomoses' offer alternative routes for blood flow if some vessels are temporarily occluded because of joint position.

Fibrocartilaginous joints

In a fibrocartilaginous joint, the ends of the bones are covered with a thin layer of hyaline cartilage (which in the symphysial joints of the vertebral bodies is represented by the vertebral endplate) and joined by a plug of fibrocartilage. Although there is no synovial joint cavity, a cavity may develop in the middle of the tissue. Intriguingly, all fibrocartilaginous joints lie in the sagittal plane of the body. Their clinical significance relates strongly to their involvement in the seronegative spondyloarthropathies and we have conceptualized this in relationship to simultaneous tension and compression forces contributing to the triggering of an osteitis at sites of bony microdamage.[11]

Fibrous joints

Fibrous joints are those where the bones are united by pure dense fibrous connective tissue (i.e. with no cartilaginous phenotype). They include the sutures of the skull and the syndesmotic inferior tibiofibular joint. Only a small amount of movement is possible, but is nevertheless important. Thus, it allows the mortise created by the malleoli of the ankle to widen slightly during dorsiflexion—which is necessary because of the shape of the trochlear surface of the talus. It is also important that skull sutures can allow some movement, so that the infant's head can be moulded during childbirth.[12]

Structures related to joints—bursae

Bursae are thin sacs lined partly or completely by synovial membrane and containing a film of synovial fluid that facilitates movement between adjacent structures. They are common near synovial joints because the movement promoted between the bones means that other tissues may also have to move relative to each other during joint movement. For example, when the knee is flexed, the skin over the patella must move freely over the bone, or it will be torn; hence the need for a 'prepatellar bursa'. A further example is given by the deep infrapatellar bursa which occupies the angle between the patellar tendon and the tibia at the insertion site of the tendon. This allows the insertional angle of the patellar tendon to change during flexion and extension of the knee and is a specific example of a general class of bursae known as 'subtendinous bursae' that characterize insertion sites that lie close to synovial joints.[13]

Recent advances in understanding functional anatomy and predicting disease

Historically, the link between cartilage and synovium has focused on the relationship between articular surfaces and synovium in synovial joints such as the knee, hips, and small joints. The functional anatomy of this interlink is described above. However, we have recently drawn attention to the intimate link between synovium and the cartilage of numerous enthesis organs, including that of the Achilles tendon.[14] We have termed such functional units 'synovio-entheseal complexes' and have highlighted their importance for understanding mechanisms of synovitis in spondyloarthritis (SpA) and OA.[14] e complexes are also conspicuous at sites within the midsubstance of joint capsules (e.g. in the proximal interphalangeal joints) and also where tendons wrap around bony prominences. Thus, the functional integration of synovium and cartilage is much wider than previously appreciated and this may have far reaching consequences for understanding perturbed tissue homeostasis and joint inflammation in different settings.

Conclusion

In the last decade it has emerged that the functional anatomy of joints is highly relevant for a better understanding of why it is that different rheumatic disorders localize to different sites. With the availability of modern imaging, site-specific derangements of these tissues and structures can now be appreciated. This is important for diagnosis and for the development of a better understanding of joint disease.

References

1. Benjamin M, McGonagle D. The anatomical basis for disease localisation in seronegative spondyloarthropathy at entheses and related sites. *J Anat* 2001;199(Pt 5):503–526.
2. Rogers AW. *Textbook of anatomy.* Churchill Livingstone, Edinburgh, 1992.
3. Wood Jones F. *The principles of anatomy as seen in the hand.* Churchill, London, 1920.
4. Granel B, Philip N, Serratrice J et al. CIAS1 mutation in a patient with overlap between Muckle-Wells and chronic infantile neurological cutaneous and articular syndromes. *Dermatology* (Basel, Switzerland) 2003;206(3):257–259.
5. Clockaerts S, Bastiaansen-Jenniskens YM, Runhaar J et al. The infrapatellar fat pad should be considered as an active osteoarthritic joint tissue: a narrative review. *Osteoarthritis Cartilage* 2010;18(7):876–882.
6. McGonagle D, Benjamin M, Marzo-Ortega H, Emery P. Advances in the understanding of entheseal inflammation. *Curr Rheumatol Rep* 2002;4(6):500–506.
7. Rangger C, Kathrein A, Klestil T, Glotzer W. Partial meniscectomy and osteoarthritis. Implications for treatment of athletes. *Sports Med* 1997;23(1):61–68.
8. Basmajian JV. *Grant's method of anatomy,* 9th edn. Williams & Wilkins, Baltimore, 1975.
9. Sinclair D. *An introduction to functional anatomy,* 4th edn. Blackwell, Oxford, 1970.
10. Standring S. *Gray's anatomy: the anatomical basis of clinical practice,* 38th edn. Churchill Livingstone, Edinburgh, 2004.
11. Benjamin M, H T, Suzuki D, Redman S, Emery P, McGonagle D. Microdamage and altered vascularity at the enthesis-bone interface provides an anatomic explanation for bone involvement in the HLA-B27 associated spondyloarthrides and allied disorders. *Arthritis Rheum* 2007;56:224–233.
12. Joseph J. Locomotor system. In: Hamilton WJ (ed.) *Textbook of human anatomy.* Macmillan, London, 1976:19–200.
13. Benjamin M, Moriggl B, Brenner E et al. The 'enthesis organ' concept: Why enthesopathies may not present as focal insertional disorders. *Arthritis Rheum* 2004;50(10):3306–3313.
14. McGonagle D, Lories RJ, Tan AL, Benjamin M. The concept of a 'synovio-entheseal complex' and its implications for understanding joint inflammation and damage in psoriatic arthritis and beyond. *Arthritis Rheum* 2007;56(8):2482–2491.

CHAPTER 47

Measuring movement and gait

Lindsey Hooper, Mark Taylor, and Christopher Edwards

Introduction

Measuring movement and gait is an important part of assessing the effect of rheumatological disorders on a patient's ability to perform tasks of daily living. In order to do this, clinicians need to understand how the biomechanical properties of joints are influenced by anatomy, physiology, and pathology. This can be a complex challenge that requires the sharing of ideas between the disciplines of mechanical engineering and medicine.

New technology has made the collection and analysis of biomechanical information much easier and a realistic possibility in many clinics (Figure 47.1). Clinicians of the future may well find themselves engaging with technology-assisted gait assessment, which synthesizes three-dimensional (3D) motion capture and joint imaging. With this in mind we aim to introduce the rheumatologist to the basic principles of measuring movement and gait, in both healthy and pathological joints and tissues. The clinical application of mechanical theory is discussed and the knee is considered as an example throughout.

Key definitions and phases of gait

There are three main planes of motion that describe movement. The sagittal plane passes through the body, front to back, dividing it into left and right halves. Movement in this plane is described as flexion or extension. The frontal (or coronal) plane passes through the body left to right, dividing it into front and back halves. Movement in this plane is described as adduction or abduction. The transverse plane passes through the middle of the body dividing it into upper and lower halves. Movement in this plane is described as internal or external rotation.

Gait, the motion of bipedal walking, is a coordinated repeated sequence of movements that occur simultaneously in a number of joints of the lower limb, in multiple planes. This repeated pattern of movement is termed the gait cycle and can be divided into two further phases; the stance phase, when the foot is in contact with the ground (40–60% of cycle), and the swing phase, when the foot

is above the ground. A further period during the gait cycle is that of double support, where both feet are in contact with the ground. The period of double support, occurring at the beginning and end of each stance phase, is particular to a walking gait and is absent during running. The duration of double support depends upon the gait velocity. At a normal velocity (3–4 mph or 5–6 km/h), there will be two double support phases, each lasting 10–12% of the cycle.[1]

The stance phase is divided into four episodes: heel strike, foot flat, heel off, and toe off. Clinical observation of these key events can be used to help identify and evaluate problems in the sequencing, timing or coordination of gait. Abnormalities occurring within the stance phase are considered to be particularly pertinent because of the undue stress exerted upon the joints or soft tissues when loaded.

Evaluating gait

Kinematic analysis

The evaluation of movement, without regard to the forces that cause it, is termed kinematics. Thus, the kinematic evaluation of gait is concerned with observing and describing:

1. In which joints is movement occurring?

2. In what plane of motion is movement occurring?

3. How much movement is occurring?

4. Is the movement occurring in the correct sequence?

A structured observation of these elements provides a basis for systematic analysis. Clinically, assessment of gait can be enhanced with joint-by-joint evaluation of movement against normal ranges of motion (Table 47.1). However, it is rare for a single joint to only move in the primary range of motion, i.e. the desired direction. In fact, a number of accessory movements can occur in perpendicular planes and their clinical effect should be evaluated.

Observation of multiple joints in sequence is the first step in measuring movements associated with gait. Comparing observed

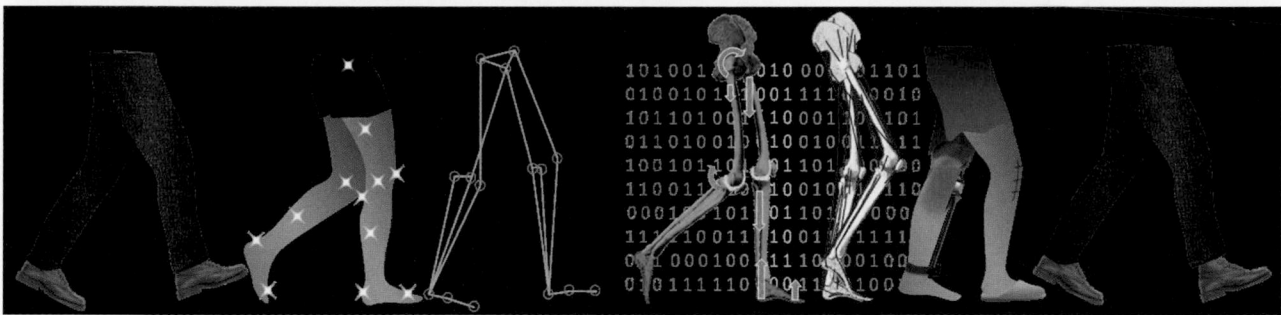

Fig. 47.1 The historical and future application of mechanical analysis within rheumatology.

motion with normal ranges allows the clinician to begin to identify problematic areas. However, it would be unwise to consider only a single joint in isolation. Movement of a single joint may have a consequential effect on neighbouring proximal and distal joints. Therefore, a joint that appears to be functioning abnormally may be doing so in compensation for a damaged neighbouring joint and have no disease itself.

Clinical application: accessory movement at the knee joint

The primary motions of the knee, specific to the tibiofemoral joint, are flexion and extension, along with smaller degrees of anterior–posterior translation and internal–external rotation. Accessory knee motions consist of medial–lateral translation and valgus–varus tilting, although these are considered to be minor in a healthy joint. Nonetheless, this combination of motions leads to a complex movement of rotational gliding and rolling of the bony structures. Such complex movements result in changing orientations of the femur or tibia, which has an effect on the neighbouring proximal hip and distal ankle joint function. The converse is also true, with the knee being affected by movements occurring in the hip or ankle.

For example, excessive pronation at the subtalar joint may result in increased internal rotation of the tibia due to the tightly bound connective tissue ankle mortise. During internal rotation of the tibia, the lateral femoral condyle moves backwards over the lateral tibial condyle while the medial femoral condyle moves forwards over the medial tibial condyle. During external rotation the reverse mechanism takes place. Therefore the bony orientation of each articulation, and the relative degree of motion, will affect the pattern of movement. In this case, the knee may appear excessively inward facing (squinting patella) or have a genu valgum appearance. During gait, increased episodes of medial loading during the stance phase may be evident and become clinically symptomatic. Correction of the foot position, via inhibition of excessive pronation, will reduce the linked-segment rotational effect and help reorient the knee into a more neutral alignment. Conversely, management of the knee in isolation may relieve symptoms in the short term, but would not address the underlying problem.[2]

Evaluating kinematics using technology

The use of technology in gait analysis aims to quantify the movements associated with human walking. This can provide more robust data than that generated by clinical observation alone. The technology used has progressed dramatically since the photogrammetry systems used prior to 1990, because of major advances in computing hardware (camera/sensor and computing devices), and software (engineering algorithms).[3] Previous systems were also labour intensive and therefore mainly restricted to research activity. However, it is increasingly possible to collect, filter, and process digital movement sequences ready for analysis within the period of a clinical appointment. Thus, the use of assistive motion analysis technologies, for the purposes of biomechanical assessment, within the clinical setting, is an increasingly realistic option.

Motion analysis captures information about the relative movement of adjacent structures (indicated by markers positioned on the patient), muscular activity (ascertained via electromyography), and forces exchanged with the environment (typically indicated with a force plate). Multiplanar movements and resultant loads transmitted across body segments are then calculated. The positioning of markers and analysis processes used for gait analysis have been standardized by the use of internationally agreed recommendations.[4] The movement of the markers is recorded by infrared or electromyomagnetic camera systems, which track the orientation of the markers around a known capture area. The use of multiple cameras means that the information from the markers can then be reconstructed using mathematical algorithms to replicate 3D models of the patient. The acquired force information can be added to the model to generate estimations of the dynamic joint forces and moments during the observed movement. Similarly, the acquired elecromyographic (EMG) data can be added to the model to generate estimations of individual muscle function throughout the gait cycle.

Kinetic analysis

The kinematic evaluation of gait can provide a good basis for the evaluation of human walking. However, kinematics does not take into account the forces that cause joint movement, or occur as a consequence of it. Thus, the evaluation of movement, with regard to the forces that cause it, termed kinetics, is important in motion analysis. Kinetics is concerned with both the magnitude and direction of a number of forces which may be applied and generated simultaneously across a joint or the mass of a segment (e.g. the thigh).

External forces are applied to the body as a result of gravity acting upon the body's mass and its interaction with external surfaces. Internal forces are generated by the muscles in order to produce the movement of a body segment (lever) about a joint (pivot) and

Table 47.1 Lower limb joint ranges of motion during gait

Joint	Active movement	Accessory movement	Typical range of motion	Phase of the gait cycle at which movement occurs
Hip	Flexion (anteversion)	Medial glide	120–140°	Stance phase (initial contact—midstance) and swing phase (toe off—midswing)
	Extension (retroversion)	Lateral glide	20–30°	Stance phase (midstance—toe off) and swing phase (midswing—heel strike)
	Internal rotation	–	40°	Midstance—toe off
	External rotation	–	30° (hip extended) 50° (hip flexed)	Loading response after heel strike
	Abduction	–	50° (hip extended) 80° (hip flexed)	Swing phase
	Adduction	–	30° (hip extended) 20° (hip flexed)	Loading response after heel strike
Knee (tibiofemoral)	Flexion	Anterior/ posterior translation, Internal/ external rotation	120–150°	Stance phase (initial contact—midstance) and swing phase (toe off—midswing)
	Extension	Anterior/posterior translation, Internal/ external rotation	5–10°	Stance phase (midstance—toe off) and swing phase (midswing—heel strike)
	Internal rotation	–	10°	Stance phase (initial loading response)
	External rotation	–	30–40°	Midstance and swing phase
Knee (patellofemoral)	Proximal translation	Lateral glide	-	As knee flexion
Ankle	Plantarflexion	–	30°	Loading response, end of stance phase and at terminal swing
	Dorsiflexion	–	0–10°	Midstance and toe off
Subtalar	Pronation	–	5°	Stance phase (heel strike—midstance)
	Supination	–	20°	Stance phase (midstance—toe off)

additional forces are generated by the passive constraints of ligaments and other soft tissues. Thus, in a similar manner to the observation of kinematics discussed in the previous section, it is possible to determine the magnitude and direction of forces acting upon a single joint as a consequence of multiple imputations of complex movements and forces.

Determining joint forces and moments

The net forces and moments, (the sum of segment mass, speed and direction of motion, and force direction and magnitude), acting across a joint can be calculated based upon a simplified anatomical model, termed a link–segment model (Figure 47.2a). The moment calculation is completed using a technique known as inverse dynamics. In order to complete this analysis, three sets of information are required:

◆ kinematic data (the relative positions of segments and their accelerations)

◆ kinetic data (external forces acting upon segments)

◆ anthropometric data (the dimensions and masses of segments).

The link–segment model only accounts for bony anatomy and ignores the action of muscles. Therefore, only the net force and moment acting across a joint is derived. During a particular activity there may be cocontraction of antagonistic muscle pairs. However, using inverse dynamics, only the net moment is calculated. For example, either a net flexion or extension moment, representative of the overall anatomical movement, is derived (Figure 47.2b). Additionally, as with any mathematical model, there are a number of assumptions that impact the predicted output. The following constraints should therefore be considered:

◆ The joints are idealized; for example, the knee is commonly modelled as a simple hinge.

◆ The anthropometric data is usually scaled from standard tables and may not truly represent the patient's anatomy.

◆ The kinematic data may not truly represent the underlying motion of the bony segments, due to motion artefact of the markers placed on the superior skin surface.

While the determination of predicted forces and moments can be highly indicative, the absolute values should be treated with caution. None the less, this assessment method is often reported in clinical gait studies and has been successfully used to identify normal and pathological movement characteristics.

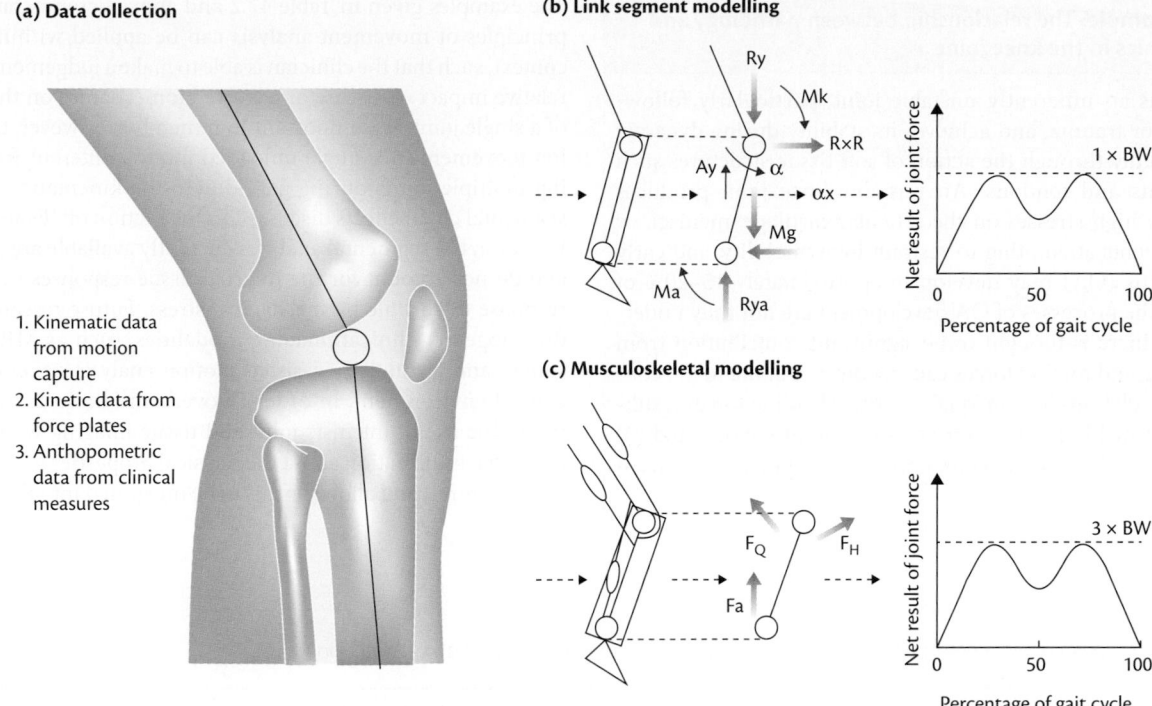

(a) Data collection

1. Kinematic data from motion capture
2. Kinetic data from force plates
3. Anthopometric data from clinical measures

(b) Link segment modelling

(c) Musculoskeletal modelling

Figure 47.2 Determination of knee joint forces and moments.

Clinical application: calculation of internal forces in a knee joint

The knee joint contact forces can be estimated using reconstructed data algorithms (discussed in the section 'Evaluating kinematics using technology').

The link–segment model can be enhanced to include representations of muscles and ligaments. The enhanced models allow the calculation of intersegmental muscle and contact (bone-on-bone) forces. However, because of the number of muscles in the lower limb, the number of unknown parameters usually exceeds the number of equilibrium equations possible, leading to an indeterminate calculation. Therefore mathematical optimization techniques are used.[5] A number of other assumptions, including the line of action, geometry, and cross-sectional area of each muscle, are also assumed to complete the model. During level gait or stair climbing it is estimated that the knee experiences average forces of between 3.1 and 5.4 times body weight. In addition, accessory shear forces of between 0.6 and 1.3 times body weight can occur (Figure 47.2).[5] However, data from in-vivo measurements of joint forces, using telemetric implants, suggests the models overestimate internal forces, particularly at high flexion angles, and more realistic values are between 2.5 and 4 times body weight.[6] Thus, moving from theory to clinical practice remains somewhat constrained. However, modelling techniques are rapidly evolving, particularly with regard to joint replacement surgery or modelling pathology.[8] For patients undergoing total knee replacement surgery, observation of the internal loads generated pre- and postoperatively, to both the surgical and neighbouring joints, may inform the likely long-term outcome. For example, the function of the limb during gait or the stresses exerted on an artificial implant can be calculated. Particular

kinetic changes, e.g. elevated adduction moments in the contralateral knee, can be calculated postoperatively and their effect on the gait cycle determined.[7]

The importance of biomechanics in rheumatological disease

The application of biomechanics to rheumatology requires clinicians to consider (1) biomechanical principles, (2) the anatomy, physiology, and morphology of the patient, and (3) the pathological processes of rheumatological disease. All three components are inherently linked and need to be considered when assessing movement within a patient. In many rheumatological conditions both the internal architecture of the joint (e.g. articular surface congruency, malalignment deformity, synovial fluid viscosity), and the integrity of conjunctive soft tissues, (e.g. ligament laxity, calcification of connective tissues, myopathy), is impacted. Thus, a joint that has deteriorated as a consequence of disease may function in an abnormal manner. Conversely, a joint functioning in an abnormal manner may affect the loading response or mechanical wear of joint tissue and exacerbate a rheumatological condition. Therefore when considering the relationship between rheumatological disease and biomechanical function two questions should be considered:

◆ To what extent is disease activity or progression impacting the biomechanics of gait?

◆ To what extent is the biomechanics of gait impacting disease activity or progression?

These questions should be evaluated in conjunction with the biomechanical analysis approaches discussed earlier (see 'Kinematic analysis'). Clinicians may find a logical structural approach to biomechanical assessment within rheumatology useful, as exemplified in Table 47.2.

Clinical example: The relationship between pathology and biomechanics in the knee joint

The knee is an inherently unstable joint, particularly following injury or trauma, and achieves its stability during dynamic motion mainly through the action of soft tissue structures such as ligaments and tendons. An unstable knee joint produces abnormally high stresses on the articular cartilage, menisci, or other ligaments attempting to restrain hypermobility, and early osteoarthritis (OA) may develop in approximately 15–20% of patients.[9] The processes of OA development are not fully understood, but there is thought to be significant contribution from (1) shearing and torsion forces causing direct trauma to the contacting articulations, (2) unequal repetitive loading forces resulting in abnormal bone turnover at specific joint regions, and (3) immunologically mediated inflammatory responses to microtrauma.[10]

The examples given in Table 47.2 and above demonstrate how the principles of movement analysis can be applied within a clinical context, such that the clinician is able to make a judgement about the relative impact of disease or adverse biomechanics on the function of a single joint. It is important to remember, however, that assessing movement in a single unloaded joint is different from assessing multiple joints during gait, due to the kinematic and kinetic segmental chain effects discussed in the section on 'Evaluating gait'. However, the segmental analyses currently available are not perfect and do not account for the internal tissue responses occurring in response to chronic biomechanical stress. Future research aims to draw together clinical imaging modalities, such as MRI or ultrasound, and technology-assisted motion analysis systems within a clinical environment, in order to overcome these current limitations. The use of intrinsic joint and tissue imaging would provide beneficial information about the physical properties of joint and tissue structures, and allow for this to be integrated into the modelling

Table 47.2 Relationship between rheumatological disease manifestations and biomechanical function

Pathology	Biomechanical action	Common observation in gait
Inflammation	Perpetuates cycle of inflammatory joint destruction, thus further impeding joint congruency, internal joint loading responses and shear stresses affected, proliferation of synovium and other mechanically mediated cellular responses, upregulation of biological responses to tissue stress, perpetuation of inflammation	Pain on movement may inhibit willingness to use full joint ranges of motion; compensatory gait, offloading forces away from the affected area is common
Synovial hypertrophy	Increased internal joint forces; reduced ranges of motion during acute episodes, increased ranges of motion after chronic episodes due to distension of collateral joint architecture; altered kinetic function as tissue loading response is affected, compounded by altered synovial fluid viscosity	If knee affected: increased periods of double support phase If ankle affected: notably reduced ranges of motion
Tendonitis	Altered tensile strength of tissue, particularly with degradation of fibrillar tendon structure; abnormal force transference; altered lever action	Antalgic gait with a tendency to offload the affected region
Tendon rupture	Increased range of motion in the plane of synergist; increased internal and external loading forces; poorly controlled moments of inertia due to reduced muscular inhibition	Failure to produce active movement about the joint, passive movement is increased until inhibited by ligamentous structures; e.g. tibialis posterior tendon rupture results in increased calcaneal eversion until inhibition by the medial collateral ankle ligaments
Tendon equinus	Reduced ranges of motion in the plane of synergist	Commonly affecting the insertion of gastrocnemius; resulting in early heel lift and excessive forefoot loading
Muscle atrophy	Muscular imbalance between concentrically (mobilizers) and eccentrically (stabilizers) acting antagonistic muscle pairs; insufficient force generation to achieve movement	Poor balance, reduced stride length and cadence, tripping and falls in cases of early or rapid onset If peroneal muscle group affected: inability to sufficiently achieve forefoot ground clearance, forefoot abduction, widened base of support, reduced cadence, lateral foot loading If tibialis anterior and intrinsic dorsal extensor muscles affected: lesser digit retraction, reduced forefoot stability and limited ankle dorsiflexion
Ligament laxity	Poorly limited terminal joint ranges of motion, which may exceed those of normative ranges; altered kinetic function, with poorly regulated internal joint loading mechanisms	Increased rotational joint motions; e.g. genu varum/valgum at the knee or excessive subtalar joint pronation may be apparent. Increased accessory movement (beyond active/passive normative end ranges)

(Continued)

Table 47.2 (Continued)

Pathology	Biomechanical action	Common observation in gait
Cartilage damage	Change in articular congruency; quality, range and direction of motion affects kinematic and kinetic joint function; internal joint loading altered; kinetic joint function altered	Locking of the joint in primary ranges of motion; kinematic abnormality may be particularly evident within the frontal plane; kinetic abnormality may result in muscular imbalance
Connective tissue function (elasticity and plasticity)	Internal loading forces are moderated by the deformation rate of surrounding tissues, thus net moments are altered	Typically evidenced via alterations in reported joint stability, notable widened base of support, reductions in stride length, or increased plantar foot pressures

algorithms. Advances such as this will help to make biomechanical assessment a more realistic way to diagnose abnormal movement and direct treatment for patients with rheumatological disease.

References

1. Cappozzo A. Gait analysis methodology. *Hum Mov Sci* 1984;3:27–50.
2. Foroughi N, Smith RM, Lange AK et al. Dynamic alignment and its association with knee adduction moment in medial knee osteoarthritis. *Knee* 2010;17(3):210–216.
3. Holt C, Johnson G. CMBBE special issue on motion analysis and musculoskeletal modelling. *Comput Methods Biomech Biomed Engin* 2008;11(1):1–2.
4. Cavanagh P, Wu G. ISB recommendation on definitions of joint coordinate system of various joints for the reporting of human joint motion—part I: ankle, hip, and spine. *J Biomech* 2002;35:543–548.
5. Taylor WR, Heller MO, Bergmann G, Duda GN. Tibio-femoral loading during human gait and stair climbing. *J Orthop Res* 2004;22(3):625–632.
6. D'Lima DD, Patil S, Steklov N, Colwell CW. The 2011 ABJS Nicolas Andry Award: 'Lab'-in-a-knee: in vivo knee forces, kinematics, and contact analysis. *Clin Orthop Relat Res* 2011;469(10):2953–2970.
7. Alnahdi AH, Zeni JA, Snyder-Mackler L. Gait after unilateral total knee arthroplasty: frontal plane analysis. *J Orthop Res* 2011; 29(5):647–652.
8. Worsley P, Stokes M, Taylor M. Predicted knee kinematics and kinetics during functional activities using motion capture and musculoskeletal modelling in healthy older people. *Gait Posture* 2011; 33(2):268–273.
9. Miyazaki T, Wada M, Kawahara H et al. Dynamic load at baseline can predict radiographic disease progression in medial compartment knee osteoarthritis. *Ann Rheum Dis* 2002;61(7):617–622.
10. Foroughi N, Smith R, Vanwanseele B. The association of external knee adduction moment with biomechanical variables in osteoarthritis: a systematic review. *Knee* 2009;16(5):303–309.

CHAPTER 48

Innate vs acquired immunity

Reinhard E. Voll and Barbara M. Bröker

Introduction

In this chapter we introduce the reader to the basic components, mechanisms, and functions of the innate and the adaptive immune system and highlight the differences in pathogen recognition and elimination employed by the two systems. Also, we elucidate the close interactions of both arms of the immune system in the host response. B and T lymphocytes are described in detail in Chapters 49 and 50. Finally, the basis of autoinflammatory and autoimmune diseases is briefly discussed.

The immune system has evolved during evolution to defend organisms against invasion by pathogens. Moreover, the immune system allows the organism to be colonized by commensals and to live in symbiosis with billions of microorganisms while maintaining the integrity of the border to the inner milieu. The commensals do not only provide enzymes which improve the digestion of food: the residential microflora also competes with pathogens for space and nutrients and may create an uncomfortable micromilieu for many pathogens, for instance low pH generated by lactobacilli.

Host defence mechanisms are not unique to multicellular organisms or eukaryotes. Bacteria have developed mechanisms such as restriction endonucleases, which can cleave the DNA of invading bacteriophages, but preserve their own bacterial genome, which does not contain the respective restriction nuclease recognition sequences. Hence, restriction endonucleases may represent one of the phylogenetically oldest mechanisms of self—non-self discrimination.

Innate immune system

Mechanical barriers, interferons, and soluble antimicrobial factors

In multicellular organisms virtually all cells participate in the host defence. For instance, viral infections lead to production of type I interferons, which protect neighbouring cells and potently activate antigen-presenting cells (APCs). The type I interferons consist of more than 10 different interferon-α molecules and only one interferon-β molecule, which all signal via the interferon-α/β receptor. Depending on the cell type, stimulation of the interferon receptor leads to the expression of antiviral proteins including 2′-5z-oligoadenylate synthase as well as interferons themselves. In addition, major histocompatibility complex (MHC) expression and maturation of dendritic cells is induced.[1-5] Other mechanisms

induce apoptotic cell death of infected cells as an attempt to inhibit viral replication and spreading.[1-4]

Multicellular organisms are protected by specialized surface cells, **epithelial cells**, with tight junctions in between providing a physical barrier. On the mucosa, **mucus** forms an additional mechanical barrier. Moreover, soluble antimicrobial proteins/peptides, also contained within the mucus, are employed to protect the organism's surfaces. Secreted enzymes such as lysozyme and phospholipase A_2 can digest the cell wall of bacteria or lyse membrane lipids, respectively. Antimicrobial peptides such as defensins damage bacterial cell membranes.[1-4] Upon invasion of bacteria the complement system can be directly activated on the pathogen's surface and marks the pathogen for efficient engulfment by complement receptor bearing phagocytes, or may directly kill the microbe by forming the membrane attack complex. During complement activation potent chemoattractants, C3a and C5a, are generated and lead to the invasion of mononuclear and polymorphonuclear phagocytes (see Chapter 64).[1-4,6]

Phagocytes

Even in early multicellular organisms, certain cells began to differentiate into specialized immune cells, phagocytes, recognizing and killing invading pathogens. Eli Metchnikoff was the first to describe phagocytic cells, which he observed in the invertebrate sea star. Mammalians have developed specialized types of phagocytes: rather short-lived polymorphonuclear granulocytes (neutrophils, eosinophils, basophils), dendritic cells (DC), and blood monocytes, which eventually differentiate into tissue macrophages. The extraordinary importance of neutrophils in fighting bacteria and fungi is obvious from neutropenic conditions or functional deficiencies such as chronic granulomatous disease resulting in a defect of oxidative burst. In particular, opsonized pathogens, meaning that they are decorated by antibodies and/or complement, are readily phagocytosed.[7] Neutrophil extracellular traps (NETs) consisting of externalized chromatin and contents of granules contribute to the elimination of bacteria.[8] Increased formation or impaired degradation of NETs can make nuclear antigens accessible to the immune system in a proinflammatory context, and may thereby foster the immunopathogenesis of systemic lupus erythematosus (SLE).[9-11] Monocytes and macrophages are critically involved in the clearance of apoptotic and necrotic cells, and regulate pro- vs anti-inflammatory outcomes.[12-14] Defective clearance of dying cells might predispose to anti-nuclear autoimmunity and SLE.[15] Opsonized bacteria and immune complexes are efficiently taken up by macrophages and antigens can be presented to T cells. Similar to NK cells and neutrophils, monocytes/macrophages can exert antibody-dependent cellular cytotoxicity. Upon activation by interferon γ, macrophages efficiently eliminate intracellular bacteria such as mycobacteria. In rheumatoid arthritis (RA) and other inflammatory diseases, macrophages might on the one hand cause tissue damage, but on the other hand exert immunoregulatory functions.

DC represent the most powerful APCs and can efficiently activate naive T cells.[1-4] Plasmacytoid DC show an appearance similar to plasma cells and might be rather poor APCs due to low expression of MHC class II and costimulatory molecules. Upon TLR7 and TLR9 stimulation, especially with simultaneous Fcγ receptor engagement, plasmacytoid DC release high amounts of interferon α, thereby playing a role in antiviral responses, but may also contribute to the pathogenesis of SLE.[10] Important cell types of the innate immune system, which mostly belong to the myeloid lineage, and their role in the pathogenesis of diseases are summarized in Table 48.1.[1-4,7,16-18]

Pathogen receptors of the innate immune system

The numbers of receptors employed by the innate immune system is limited to a few dozens. These germline-encoded receptors recognize usually highly conserved non-protein structures, called pathogen-associated molecular patterns (PAMPs), that are common to groups of related pathogens. The respective receptors were therefore named pattern recognition receptors (PRRs).[1-4,19-20] Some of these receptors are also stimulated by endogenous molecules indicating necrotic cell death, termed damage associated molecular patterns (DAMPs) or 'alarmins'. Some heat shock proteins (HSPs) and the nuclear protein HMGB1 serve such a function and activate innate immune cells similar to PAMPs.[21] In Table 48.2

general properties of the PRRs of the innate immune system are compared with those of the B- and T-cell receptors of the adaptive immune system. Because PAMPs generally represent molecules which play an important role in the life cycles of pathogens, escape mutants from PRR, if not deadly in the first place, should strongly impair the fitness of the microorganism.

PRRs can be soluble molecules. **Lysozyme** recognizes and cleaves β(1,4) linkages between *N*-acetylglucosamine and *N*-acetylmuramic acids. **Mannose-binding lectin (MBL)** attaches to microbial glycans of many bacteria and fungi, whereas the ficolins bind to acetylated oligosaccharides. The respective oligosaccharides on the surfaces of the eukaryotic host cells are mostly masked by the attachment of sialic acid, so that the aforementioned PRRs cannot bind to them. MBL and ficolins start the complement activation on microbial surfaces (see Chapter 64).[1-4,6] Gut epithelial cells and phagocytes express Toll-like receptors (TLRs), either on the cell surface (TLR1, 2, 4, 5, 6) or in the endosomal compartment (TLR3, 7, 9) (Figure 48.1). The TLRs sense various PAMPs and DAMPs and induce a proinflammatory response within the immune cells by potently activating the transcription factor NFκB.[1-4,19,20]

In order to fight intracellular invaders such as viruses and intracellular bacteria, cytoplasmic surveillance molecules recognizing bacterial or viral components have developed during evolution (Table 48.3). The NOD-like receptor family consists of several subfamilies: the NOD proteins NOD1 and NOD2 recognizing components of bacterial cell walls, AIM2 sensing pathogens containing double-stranded DNA, and the pyrin-domain-containing NLRP subfamily. The NLRP proteins, of which the best investigated is NALP3 as a component of the NALP3-inflammasome, might not directly recognize pathogens; rather, they are activated by cellular stress responses. Upon decrease of intracellular K+ concentrations,

Table 48.1 Cells of the innate immune system

Innate immune cell	Origin	Functions	Relevance in diseases
Neutrophil (granulocyte)	Common myeloid progenitor	Elimination of bacteria and fungi by phagocytosis, content of granules, NET formation	Deficiency results in bacterial and fungal infections; granulomatous disease. Contribution to pathogenesis of gout and RA
Eosinophil (granulocyte)	Common myeloid progenitor	Release of eosinophil cationic protein; eosinophil peroxidase; elimination of antibody-coated helminths	Asthma; Churg–Strauss syndrome*, eosinophilic fasciitis
Basophil (granulocyte)	Common myeloid progenitor	Defence against parasites; histamine and serotonin release upon FcR crosslinking	Induction of allergic inflammatory responses
Mast cell	Common myeloid progenitor	Defence against parasites; histamine and serotonin release upon FcR crosslinking	Induction of allergic inflammatory responses
Monocyte/ macrophage	Common myeloid progenitor	Clearance of apoptotic and necrotic cells; phagocytosis of bacteria, elimination of intracellular bacteria upon IFNγ activation, antigen presentation; ADCC	Overwhelming activation in macrophage activation syndrome
Dendritic cell (lymphoid, myeloid, plasmacytoid, Langerhans cell)	Common myeloid progenitor or common lymphoid progenitor	Uptake of antigen in the periphery and transport to the lymphnodes for antigen presentation to T cells; activation of T cells including naive T cells; immune regulation	T-cell activation by DC in RA and SLE; in SLE IFNα release from plasmacytoid dendritic cells,
NK cell	Common lymphoid progenitor	Killing of virus-infected and otherwise altered (e.g. malignant) cells; ADCC via FcγRIII; inhibitory receptors prevent killing of autologous MHC-expressing cells. IFNγ secretion	

ADCC, antibody-dependent cellular cytotoxicity; DC, dendritic cells; IFN, interferon; NET, neutrophil extracellular trap; RA, rheumatoid arthritis; SLE, systemic lupus erythematosus; *, Eosinophilic granulomatosis with polyangiitis.

Table 48.2 Comparison of pathogen recognition by receptors of the innate and adaptive immune systems

	Receptors of the innate immune system (PRR)	**Receptors of the adaptive immune system**
Genes	Germ line encoded	Somatic gene rearrangement
Diversity	Limited (~100 specificities)	Extremely high (>10^9)
Ligands	Highly conserved molecules essential for the life cycles of a pathogen, usually no proteins	TCR: individual peptides presented in MHC molecules BCR: most kinds of molecules can be recognized
Escape mutants of pathogens	Very rare, usually loss of fitness	Frequent, do not necessarily impair pathogen fitness
Specificity	Recognizing a whole class of pathogens (e.g. Gram +ve bacteria, fungi); no change in receptor specificity	TCR and BCR: usually highly specific for a single pathogen BCR: affinity maturation during infection (germinal centre reaction), isotype switch
Number of receptor bearing cells/memory	Many cells (e.g. all monocytes, neutrophils) express the same set of receptors, no dramtic changes in receptor-expressing cells; no memory	Before pathogen exposure: extremely low numbers of cells bearing the individual receptor; during infection dramatic expansion of antigen-specific clones; memory
Reactivity with self	Certain PRR recognize endogenous 'danger molecules' (alarmins such as HMGB1) causing activation of the innate immune cells and inflammation	Accidentally; may result in autoimmune diseases
Time to response	Immediate	First contact: delayed by some days Repeated contact: immediate

PRR, pattern recognition receptor.

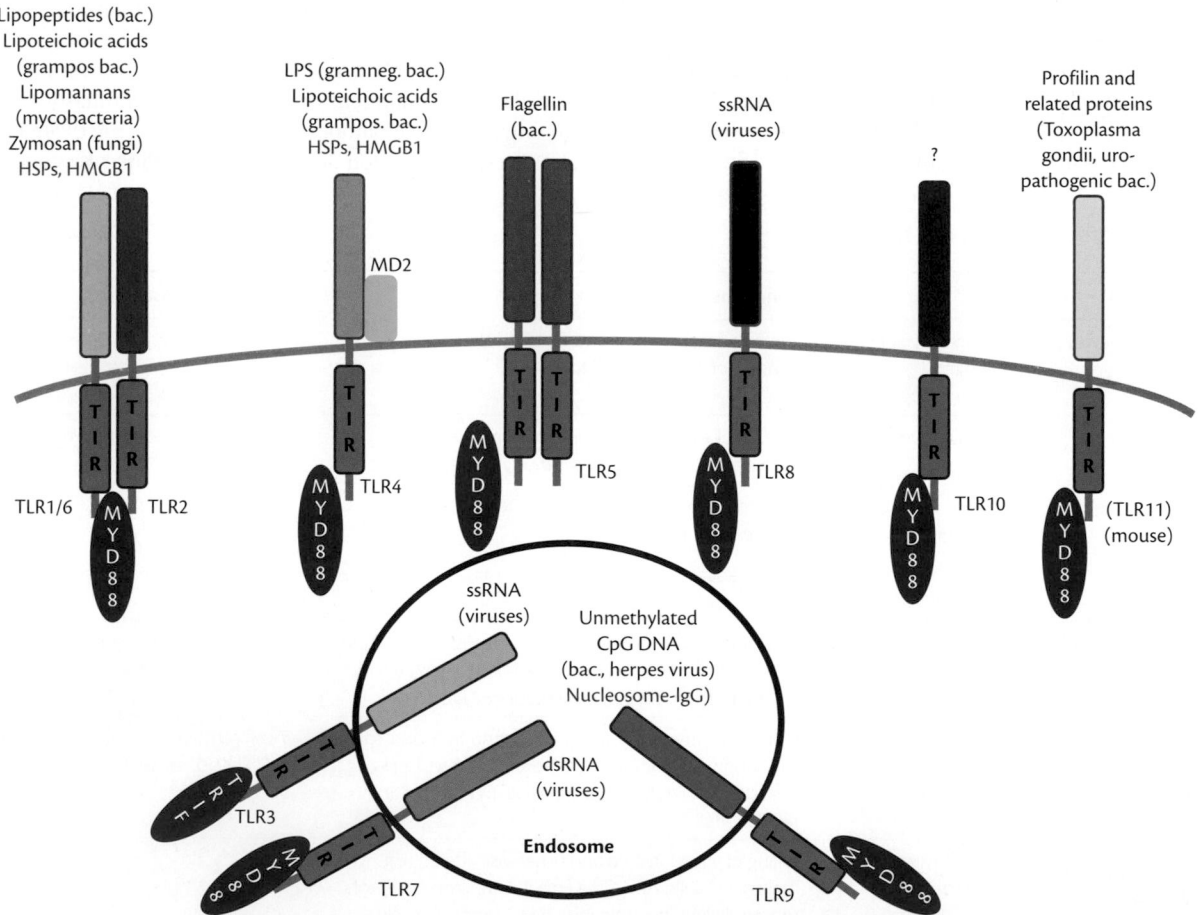

Fig. 48.1 Toll-like receptors and their exogenous and endogenous ligands. HSPs and HMGB1 are endogenous ligands (red). Bac., bacteria; ds, double-stranded; ss, single stranded.

Table 48.3 Cytoplasmic pattern recognition receptors of the innate immune system

Cytoplasmic PRRs (cell types)	Specificity	Function
NOD-like receptors		
NOD1 (macrophages, dendritic cells)	γ-Glutamyl diaminopimelic acid (from Gram ve bacteria)	Activation of the innate immune system upon infection with intracellular bacteria (e.g. listeria, salmonella)
NOD2 (macrophages, dendritic cells, Paneth cells)	Muramyl dipeptide (from peptidoglycan of most bacteria)	Expression of α and β defensins in Paneth cells (NOD2); loss of function associated with Crohn's disease, gain of function mutants with Blau's syndrome
NLRP family (phagocytes)	? Activation upon decrease of intracellular K^+ concentration	
NALP3/cryopyrin		NALP3 is part of the inflammasome, which is activated upon cellular stress/damage (e.g. gout) and leads to IL-1β production; mutations in the NOD domain cause hereditary periodic fever syndromes including Muckle–Wells syndrome
AIM2	Recognition of dsDNA genomes (e.g. vaccinia virus)	IL-1β production in response to vaccinia virus infection; defence against *Francisella tularensis*
RIG-I-like helicases (most cells)		
RIG-I MDA5	'Uncapped' viral ssRNA, dsRNA	Defence against viral infections. Activation of type I interferon production via IRF3; production of proinflammatory cytokines via NFκB activation

dsDNA, double-stranded DNA; PRR, pattern recognition receptor; ssDNA, single stranded DNA.

NALP3 induces caspase 1 activation and interleukin (IL)-1β secretion.[1–4,19–20,22] The RIG-I-like helicases sense cytoplasmic RNAs of viral origin and potently induce interferon regulatory factors (IRFs) leading to type I interferon production with its antiviral activity.[4,5,23]

Adaptive immune system

Higher vertebrates from jawed fish onwards developed an adaptive immune system as an additional powerful level of defence. The cells of the adaptive immune system are lymphocytes and their features are summarized in Table 48.4. Somatic recombination and hypermutation generate such a huge arsenal of receptors that virtually all pathogens can be recognized by at least a few lymphocyte clones. The RAG enzymes enable the recombination of multiple gene segments.[1–4] The addition of variable numbers of nucleotides to the joining ends without a DNA template can introduce new amino acids, thereby further increasing the variability of the antigen binding sites. The basic mechanisms of receptor diversification are homologous in T and B cells.[1–4] In contrast to T cells, the antigen receptor of mature B cells can undergo affinity maturation during the germinal centre reaction.[24] After clonal expansion of the few pathogen-specific lymphocytes out of millions of different specificities, pathogen-specific cells (T lymphocytes) as well as soluble molecules (antibodies derived from B cells, especially plasma cells) mount a highly specific and efficient immune response. Most importantly, the adaptive immune system has a memory function, which can mediate a long-lasting, often lifelong protection ('immunity') against this particular pathogen.[1–4,24–26] Remarkably, this protection can be partially transferred to the offspring via active transport of IgG antibodies through the placenta to the fetus and the transfer of IgA antibodies with the milk to neonates.[1–4] However, these new, effective host defence mechanisms of the adaptive immune system come at a cost: the inherent risk of autoreactivity and autoimmunity.

Table 48.4 Cells of the adaptive immune system

Cell type	Origin	Immunoreceptor	Function
CD4+ T helper cell	Common lymphocyte precursor/thymus	αβTCR	T-cell help, orchestrating the specific immune response
CD4+ T regulatory cell	Common lymphocyte precursor/thymus	αβTCR	Regulation of immune responses; prevention of autoimmunity
CD8+ cytotoxic T cell	Common lymphocyte precursor/thymus	αβTCR	Elimination of virus-infected cells
γδ T cells	Common lymphocyte precursor/thymus	γδTCR	Subepithelial defence line recognizing also non-peptide ligands
B cell/ plasma cells	Common lymphocyte precursor/bone marrow	BCR/IgM, IgG, IgA	Neutralization of viruses, toxins, defence against extracellular bacteria, protection of the neonate

BCR, B-cell receptor; TCR, T-cell receptor.

Immune response: joint effort of the innate and adaptive immune systems

During an immune response the innate and the adaptive immune systems cooperate closely and are connected at multiple layers. On the one hand, the APCs of the innate immune system control activation of the adaptive immune system and guide T-cell differentiation into the direction most appropriate for the invading pathogen. On the other hand, the adaptive immune system often relies on components of the innate immune system for many effector functions, especially elimination of pathogens. For instance, antibodies activate the complement system or engage Fc receptors of phagocytes and NK cells, which eventually kill the invading microbes or the infected cells.

Containment of commensal microorganisms

It has been hypothesized that the immune system has developed in evolution to enable us to house a wealth of commensal bacteria, which colonize the inner and outer surfaces of the body. The composition of the human microbiome is highly complex, and the number of bacteria amounts to around 10^{14}, exceeding that of the eukaryotic cells by a factor of 10. The relationship with our endogenous microflora, the vast majority of which resides in the gut, is usually characterized by mutualism: The microorganisms benefit from the regular food intake and the homeostatic mechanisms of their multicellular eukaryotic host, while providing it with numerous enzymes that are not encoded in the host's genome. These can break down indigestible molecules, and it has been estimated that this allows the eukaryotic host to extract around 14% more calories from food.[27,28] In former times, which were characterized by scarceness of food, this must have conveyed a significant survival advantage. However, the happy balance between the host and its commensals is risky and requires enormous efforts to keep up. It is estimated that 10^{12} cells, i.e. one out of ten eukaryotic cells, belong to the immune system in the strict sense. At least half of them reside in the gut, one of their main tasks being the containment of the endogenous microbial flora. If it fails to control the colonizing microbes, the body immediately becomes prey to the degrading potential of its own commensals.[23,27,28] In fact, in the industrialized world around 80% of bacterial infections are of endogenous origin.

It thus seems to be appropriate to first consider the immune response at the body surfaces, namely the 2 m^2 of skin, and the mucous membranes of the respiratory system (50 m^2) and the gut (200–400 m^2).

Very few microorganisms can withstand the low pH in the stomach to reach the gut. There the mucus forms a barrier which is difficult to penetrate even for flagellated microorganisms, even more so as it is impregnated with high concentrations of antimicrobial peptides, derived from the Paneth cells at the bottom of the crypts. The mucus is continuously produced by goblet cells and then transported out of the body via the bowel movements or the action of ciliated epithelia of the respiratory tract.[1–4,27]

As a second layer of defence, numerous immune cells densely line the epithelial layers and accumulate in the lamina propria and the Peyer's patches, guarding the body's interface with the outside world. Once an adaptive immune response has been established, specific IgA is also found in high concentrations in the mucus and the bodily secretions, where it contributes to the control of the endogenous microflora.

It is fascinating that containment of the microorganisms usually proceeds in a largely non-inflammatory manner. A milieu of immune tolerance is essential for the maintenance of immunological food tolerance in the gastrointestinal system and for efficient gas exchange in the alveoli of the lung.

Reaction to microbial invasion

This peaceful scenario immediately gives way to a vigorous inflammatory response when the barriers are broken and microorganisms invade host cells or tissues. It should be stressed that both commensals and pathogens are equipped with PAMPs and are able to elicit an immune response. The hallmark of pathogens is their invasive behaviour. Upon barrier failure the PAMPs can be sensed by the immune system and trigger an immune response.[23,28] Now the task is to very quickly control and ultimately eliminate the invaders, since these are able to multiply rapidly at the host's cost. It is equally important to minimize damage to the host tissues, an inevitable side effect when the powerful effector mechanisms of the immune system are unleashed. Ideally the system reacts in a fast, focused, and effective manner, utilizing specialized functions to optimally control different types of pathogens. This is achieved by the concerted action of innate and adaptive immune systems. It is essential for health that the immune reaction is terminated and homeostasis is re-established as soon as the microbial invasion has been dealt with.

Innate immune reaction to microbial invasion

Initially, microbial invasion is sensed by the innate immune system via PRRs, which herald 'stranger anddanger', namely microbial factors and substances released upon cell and tissue damage.[23,27,28]

Wherever the attack may happen, sentinel cells—macrophages, dendritic cells, and mast cells—and complement factors are already in place, and they are called into action immediately. Macrophages are professional phagocytes, which take up the microorganisms and kill many of them. Their action is facilitated by the deposition of complement fragments on the microbial surface, since the phagocytes possess complement receptors (opsonization, or opsonophagocytosis). Some microorganisms can be killed by the membrane attack complex formed on their surface by the complement cascade (see Chapter 64).[6]

Inflammation

If the microbial challenge reaches a certain threshold, the immune system will respond with inflammation, which has been diagnosed since antiquity by four cardinal symptoms: rubor, calor, tumor, and dolor. When sensing PAMPs the sentinel cells release inflammatory cytokines, soluble mediators of the immune system, such as TNFα and CXCL8/IL-8.[1–4] These activate the endothelial cells lining the small local blood vessels at the interface between the focus of infection in the tissue and the bloodstream, which connects to the reservoirs of immune cells in the bone marrow and the peripheral lymphatic organs. The blood vessels dilate, the blood stream slows down (rubor and calor), and immune cells intensify their contact with the inner vessel wall, which has become decorated with adhesion molecules in reaction to the inflammatory cytokines.[29] A three-step process termed 'homing' guarantees that the various types of immune cells leave the blood vessels at the right time and in the proper place: (1) Selectins on the endothelium bind to their ligands on the immune cells. These molecular bonds are rapidly formed and dissociated again, so that the cells are gradually slowed down, rolling along the vessel wall. (2) This enables them to bind locally produced chemokines with their chemokine receptors, resulting in (3) conformational changes of cell surface integrin molecules. These permit high-affinity binding to integrin ligands on the activated endothelium. The immune cells now firmly attach to the endothelium and begin to leave the blood vessels by reversibly opening the tight junctions in the endothelial layer. In the tissues they follow concentration gradients of chemokines and/or complement fragments, which guide them to the focus of infection, where they can accumulate in large numbers (tumour). When they perceive the local 'stranger anddanger' signals, the newly recruited immune cells become activated and join in the attack against the invaders.

When the inflammatory cytokines are released in high amounts they cause systemic effects such as fever, and a systemic inflammatory response syndrome (SIRS) develops. IL-6 is a key factor, triggering the liver to change its protein synthesis programme and release increased amounts of defence molecules such as lipopolysaccharide-binding protein, MBL, and components of the complement and coagulation cascades.[1-4]

Adaptive immune reaction to microbial invasion

The adaptive immune response is initiated by activated innate immune cells, and it takes several days to become effective. The complex programme is orchestrated in the peripheral lymphatic organs, which function as 'conference centres' of the immune system. Numerous components need to interact in a highly organized manner to start a primary adaptive immune response.[1-4] Take the lymph node as an example: naive T cells and B cells are recruited from the bloodstream into lymph nodes through specialized high endothelial venules via CCR7 signals. In the lymph node they home to different compartments, the primary B-cell follicles and the T-cell areas. Antigens and antigen-presenting dendritic cells reach the lymph node via the lymphatic vessels, which drain almost all tissues. DC are the sentinels of the adaptive immune system: Through macropinocytosis they sample the antigenic milieu in the tissues, and during homeostasis low numbers of non-activated dendritic cells continuously move with the lymph into the lymph nodes, where they present self-antigens to T cells in a tolerogenic, non-inflammatory fashion, contributing to the maintenance of immunological self-tolerance. Upon microbial invasion and during inflammation, however, the DC become activated by the PAMPs and DAMPs at the site of infection. They now stop the antigen uptake in order to preserve the antigenic spectrum incorporated at the site of danger, and while moving into the lymph nodes in increased numbers, they differentiate into professional APCs, which are characterized by the ability to activate naive T cells and guide their differentiation.

Antigen recognition

The activation of naive T cells is a stringently controlled process requiring the activated DC to give three types of signal: (1) MHC–peptide complexes, which the T cells recognize with their antigen-specific T-cell receptors; (2) costimulatory molecules such as CD80 and CD86 which bind to CD28 on the T-cell surface; and (3) a cytokine cocktail. This corresponds to the first phase of an adaptive immune response: antigen recognition.[1-4]

The first signal for B cells is antigen in its native, unprocessed form as it reaches the lymph nodes via the lymph vessels. The B cells recognize their antigenic epitopes with their B-cell receptors (BCR), which are membrane-anchored antibody molecules.

Clonal expansion and differentiation

Fully activated T cells divide rapidly with a generation time of around 6 hours and form a clone. Importantly, all progeny of an activated T cell express molecularly identical T-cell receptors on their surface, i.e. they are specific for the same antigen. During this process the T cells differentiate into effector T cells (Teff), of which there are different functional types (see 'Immunological tolerance' below and Chapter 49). B lymphocytes behave in a similar way upon antigen recognition, but in most cases they require T-cell help to become fully activated (see below).

Effector phase

While naive T cells can only home to the peripheral lymphoid organs, where they scan the local DC for their antigenic MHC–peptide complexes, activated T cells are able to enter the tissues having left the bloodstream via the capillaries. Upon re-encounter with their antigenic MHC–peptide complexes on local APC they exert their effector functions and contribute to the elimination of the invading microorganisms. Activated B cells differentiate into plasma blasts or plasma cells, whose most prominent effector function is the secretion of antibodies. These are soluble forms of the antigen-specific BCRs which originally triggered the activation and proliferation of the B cell and thus have the same antigen specificity (see Chapter 50).

Clonal contraction

Having eliminated the invasive microorganisms, homeostasis needs to be re-established, and the formerly expanded T-cell and B-cell clones contract again. Apoptosis is the essential mechanism at this stage of an adaptive immune response.

Memory

Having overcome the dangerous situation, not all effector cells die. In the case of T cells, around 10% develop into memory T cells, which divide very slowly once every 1–2 weeks, just enough to compensate cell loss by apoptosis. T-cell memory clones can persist for many years. The next antigenic challenge will thus be met by many more antigen-specific T cells than at the first exposure. Additionally, memory T cells have a lower activation threshold, are less demanding with regard to the second and third signals, can respond much faster than naive T cells, and, importantly, they also memorize and quickly recall their special effector functions (see below).

B cell memory consists of (1) memory B cells, which are able to rapidly respond to antigenic rechallenge with proliferation and differentiation into plasma cells, and in addition, (2) long-lived plasma cells populating special microenvironmental niches in the bone marrow, where they continuously produce antibodies, maintaining high antigen-specific antibody titres. During a secondary or memory immune response the antibodies will immediately bind to their antigen, such as invading microorganisms, and elicit their biological effector functions.[26]

Immune memory is a core competence of the adaptive immune system enabling it to react much faster and more efficiently to a re-encounter with the same antigenic stimulus. All vaccination strategies rely on this feature of the adaptive immune system. Moreover, IgG antibodies are actively transported into the fetus and provide an immediate protection to the neonate during the first weeks after birth.

T-cell help for B cells—the germinal centre reaction

Antibodies are very important effector molecules of the adaptive immune system. Their producers, the plasma cells, appear to be terminally differentiated cells that function largely 'on autopilot', and they can be very long-lived producing high amounts of specific antibodies for decades, possibly lifelong. Consequently, the priming of a B-cell response must be stringently regulated, and this control is exerted by T lymphocytes in the germinal centre reaction. Naive T cells recognize their antigen on DC in the T-cell areas, proliferate, differentiate into effector T cells, and, guided by cytokine gradients, then move towards the edge of the B-cell follicles. Here they meet B cells, which have been activated by antigen binding to their specific BCR, which has stimulated them to migrate into the opposite direction towards the T-cell area. In this way it becomes possible for the very few antigen-specific T cells, not more than 1 out of 10 000 in a primary response, to cooperate with the very few B cells that recognize the same antigen in a process termed **cognate T cell–B cell interaction**. Only if the B cells are able to internalize the correct antigen via their BCR, process it and present it to the T cells, will the latter exert an effector function known as T-cell help. Via cell–cell contact and cytokines the T cells stimulate the B cells to enter a complex programme of (1) proliferation, (2) immunoglobulin class switch, and (3) somatic hypermutation, namely the accumulation of point mutations in the antigen binding sites. A quality control process selects those B cells whose BCR exhibit an increased affinity for the recognized antigen (affinity maturation) and allows them to develop into antibody-secreting plasma cells and memory B cells.[24] Their BCR and the secreted antibodies will have usually switched from IgM, which characterizes naive B cells, to another immunoglobulin class: IgG, IgA, or IgE. The class switch is not a random process, but is guided by the effector cytokines of the T helper cells: IFNγ favours the development of proinflammatory IgG subclasses, which can activate complement and bind to Fcγ-receptors on phagocytes and NK cells. TGFβ promotes the class switch to IgA, and IL-4 is essential for the elaboration of IgE.[1–4]

Microbial habitat and the optimal defence strategy

During coevolution microorganisms and viruses have specialized to persist or multiply in different compartments of the eukaryotic host. They have been most inventive regarding mechanisms of immune evasion, which highlights that the immune system puts them under strong pressure once they have managed to break the barriers. While there are general immune strategies in antimicrobial defence, the control of every microbial species is a story of its own.

Staphylococci, streptococci, and their toxic products, for example, are mainly found in the extracellular compartment, while mycobacteria are specialized to live in intracellular vesicles. Some bacteria—listeria and burkholderia species—have evolved mechanisms to destroy the phagosomal membrane, escape into the cytoplasm, and are even able to move from cell to cell directly. Viruses depend on the metabolism of their host cells for multiplication, and viral particles are assembled in the cytoplasm. After budding, however, they temporarily transit the extracellular space. Clearly, no single immune defence strategy can fit all these situations, and some specialized immune functions are described below. First, it is reassuring that the innate immune system can survey all the mentioned compartments with its repertoire of PRRs. For example, TLRs are found in the outer cell membrane as well as in the intracellular vesicles, while NOD-like receptors and RIG-I-like receptors recognize 'stranger and danger' in the cytoplasm (Figure 48.1, Table 48.3). MBL can be regarded as an extracellular pattern recognition molecule of the complement cascade.

Defence against extracellular microorganisms

Extracellular microorganisms, viruses, and toxins are accessible to antibodies and complement. Thus T-cell help for B cells is important for their control. Antibodies may neutralize the invaders, i.e. prevent their binding to the specific receptors, and thereby interfere with their function or cellular uptake. Neutralization is the essential function of IgA, the most abundant Ig class, which is found in high concentrations in the bodily secretions and on the mucous membranes. Importantly, antigen neutralization by IgA does not trigger inflammation.

This is different in the case of IgG, which can activate complement and bind to Fc receptors on phagocytes, both leading to enhanced phagocytosis and activation of the phagocytes, which then secrete inflammatory cytokines. In synergy with the opsonization by IgG and/or complement, Th17 cells, a T-cell subpopulation discovered only in the 21st century, mobilize neutrophils from the bone marrow and attract them to the focus on inflammation. Here they avidly phagocytose and destroy the marked microorganisms.[1–4]

Defence against intravesicular microorganisms

Some microorganisms have developed strategies to prevent phagocytes from killing them after uptake. In such cases IFNγ, a product of Th1 cells, helps macrophages to overcome this block and direct their aggressive potential, e.g. reactive oxygen and nitrogen mediators as well as proteolytic enzymes, at the invaders. The importance of the Th1 response is underlined by the fact that defects in this function, either inborn or acquired as a consequence of HIV infection, render patients highly susceptible to fulminant tuberculosis.[1–4]

Defence against intracytoplasmic microorganisms

Once microbes have managed to leave the phagosomes, they are out of reach of the effector mechanisms of the phagocytes. Intracytoplasmic PRR (see Table 48.3) can sense cytoplasmic bacteria and viruses and induce mechanisms to mark the infected cells and activate the immune system. Ultimately in case of intracellular bacterial infection, there is only one effective countermeasure: the infected cell has to be eliminated. The same is true for viral infection, which can hit any nucleated cell of the body. The elimination of cells with cytoplasmic infection is the function of NK cells and cytotoxic T lymphocytes (CTLs). These induce a cell death programme called apoptosis in the affected cells, and the apoptotic cells or their fragments are rapidly taken up and digested by macrophages. Obviously, the cytotoxic immune cells are dangerous for the organism itself, and their activation is therefore strictly controlled. Naive CD8+ T cells cannot kill before they have differentiated into CTLs. This becomes possible only after they have recognized their antigen (a complex of MHC-I molecule and antigenic peptide) on a professional APC, and in many cases T-cell help from Th1 cells is necessary in addition.[1–4]

Defence against parasites

Exposure to large numbers of ecto- and endoparasites has been an everyday reality during human evolution, and in large parts of the world it still is. These parasites are usually not immediately life threatening, and there is rarely sterile immunity, but the immune system has evolved mechanisms to reduce parasite density, e.g. by expelling worms from the intestinal tract or preventing ticks from enjoying a full blood meal. IgE, elaborated with the help of Th2 cells, is the key effector molecule of this immune defence mode. IgE binds to high-affinity Igε-receptors on mast cells and basophils even in the absence of antigen, providing the cells with antigen recognition capacity. Multivalent antigens will then bind to the specific binding sites of IgE on the cell surfaces, cross-link the attached Igε-receptors and induce the rapid release of inflammatory mediators. These enhance mucus secretion in the gut and stimulate bowel contractions, facilitating parasite expulsion. In the skin, itching directs the attention of the host to the parasite attack, and a strong oedema limits the parasite's blood meal or makes invasion more difficult. In addition, eosinophil granulocytes are recruited and activated, which enhance this response in a positive feedforward loop.

When they are misdirected at innocuous environmental antigens, the IgE-mediated defence mechanisms just described can drive allergic responses.[1-4,30]

Immunological tolerance

In a healthy individual the powerful inflammatory effector functions of the immune system are balanced by equally strong regulatory mechanisms, which ensure that a non-inflammatory state is dominant during homeostasis. Various negative feedback loops and active tolerance mechanisms stop the inflammation as soon as the microbes have been eliminated. Wound healing processes set in, the damaged tissues are repaired, and the system is reset to its non-inflammatory default status.

In this context, the adaptive immune system merits special attention because its unique capacity to recognize 'virtually everything' by means of its vast receptor repertoire continually challenges immunological self-tolerance. Since the many different receptors are assembled independently of antigen contact, the development of autoreactive T cells and B cells cannot be avoided. Adaptive immune tolerance, mediated by active and passive mechanisms, is thus vitally important. In the first instance, nascent T cells and B cells are filtered in the thymus and bone marrow, and most autoreactive clones are eliminated (central tolerance). The remaining autoreactive clones mature, and they need to be controlled for the lifetime of the organism (peripheral tolerance).

Toward the end of the 20th century it became apparent that a subpopulation of T cells known as regulatory T cells (Tregs) has a crucial role in this process. The so-called 'natural Tregs' develop in the thymus, while 'induced Tregs' differentiate from naive mature T cells under the influence of anti-inflammatory cytokines such as IL-10 and TGFβ. Upon antigen recognition Tregs suppress the activation of neighbouring naive T cells and interfere with their development into Teff cells, but they are also able to inhibit the effector functions of fully differentiated Teff cells, regardless of whether they are Th1, Th2, Th17, or follicular Th cells.[1-4]

Rare monogenetic immune defects, which interfere with the development or function of Tregs, are associated with a very severe autoimmune and allergic phenotype, which can be recapitulated in animal models. The discovery of an active mechanism of immune tolerance—the adoptive transfer of Tregs establishes tolerance in previously non-tolerant animals—has raised hopes that it may be possible to harness this cell type for therapeutic interventions in chronic immune-mediated inflammation. There is now good evidence that in allergy the specific immune therapy (SIT), which consists of the repeated application of minute allergen doses, relies largely on the induction of allergen-specific Tregs.

Autoinflammation, autoimmunity, and autoimmune disease

The inflammatory response serves the host defence and tissue repair; some collateral damage to the host tissues appears to be a necessary trade-off. However, overwhelming or self-perpetuating chronic inflammation can cause major harm to the organism. In certain pathologic conditions release or extracellular accumulation of endogenous molecules may exert a massive inflammatory response. In gout and pseudogout sodium urate or calcium pyrophosphate crystals are phagocytosed by neutrophils and lead to strong inflammasome activation. Autoinflammatory or hereditary periodic fever syndromes can be caused by defective regulatory mechanisms such as defective cleavage of the membrane-bound TNF receptor in TRAPs (TNF receptor associated periodic fever syndrome). Consequently, the natural decoy receptor for TNF is missing and even minor amounts of TNF may cause a systemic inflammatory response. In other autoinflammatory syndromes, e.g. cryopyrine-associated diseases, mutations in components of the inflammasome may lower the activation threshold of the inflammasome, resulting in spontaneous or inadequate IL-1β secretion in response to minor stimulation.[31,32]

Autoimmunity, i.e. the presence B or T cells which can react with autologous structures, is a rather frequent phenomenon. However, the mere presence of such autoreactive lymphocytes, which have escaped from negative selection during development in the bone marrow or thymus respectively, rarely results in clinically relevant autoimmune diseases. Autoreactive lymphocytes are usually well controlled by mechanisms of peripheral tolerance.[1-4] However, in certain conditions, there is an increased risk of breaking tolerance, at least transiently:

♦ During infection or tissue necrosis exogenous or endogenous 'danger signals' (PAMPs or DAMPs) activate APC of the innate immune system. Costimulatory molecules and proinflammatory cytokines are expressed. Presentation of self-peptides by fully activated APC may result in the activation of self reactive T lymphocytes.

♦ Molecular mimicry, i.e. structures of pathogens that closely resemble those of the organism, can cause autoimmunity. However, even fully identical peptide stretches within an endogenous and a microbial protein have only a limited risk of breaking self-tolerance. Only those individuals who can process and present these peptides within their MHC molecules are at risk of developing autoimmunity due to molecular mimicry of T-cell epitopes.

Obviously, the innate immune system essentially contributes to the generation of a protective adaptive immune response as well as to the break of tolerance and autoimmune responses. These and other mechanisms leading to autoimmunity are discussed in the chapters on specific diseases.

References

1. Abbas AK, Lichtman AH, Pillai S. Cellular. *Molecular immunology*, 7th edn. W.B. Saunders, Philadelphia, PA, 2011.
2. Paul WE. *Fundamental immunology*, 6th edn. Lippincott Williams & Wilkins, Philadelphia, PA, 2008.
3. Delves PJ, Martin SJ, Burton DR, Roitt IM. *Roitt's Essential immunology*, 12th edn. Wiley, New York, 2011.

4. Murphy K. *Janeway's immunobiology*, 8th edn. Garland Science, New York, 2011.

5. Taniguchi T, Takaoka A. The interferon alpha/beta system in antiviral responses: a multimodal machinery of gene regulation by the IRF family of transcription factors. *Curr Opin Immunol* 2002;14:111–116.

6. Sturfelt G, Truedsson L. Complement in the immunopathogenesis of rheumatic disease. *Nat Rev Rheumatol* 2012;8(8):458–468.

7. Borregaard, N. Neutrophils, from marrow to microbes. *Immunity* 2010;33:657–670.

8. Brinkmann V, Reichard U, Goosmann C et al. Neutrophil extracellular traps kill bacteria. *Science* 2004;303(5663):1532–1535.

9. Hakkim A, Fürnrohr BG, Amann K et al. Impairment of neutrophil extracellular trap degradation is associated with lupus nephritis. *Proc Natl Acad Sci U S A* 2010;107(21):9813–9818.

10. Lande R, Ganguly D, Facchinetti V et al. Neutrophils activate plasmacytoid dendritic cells by releasing self-DNA-peptide complexes in systemic lupus erythematosus. *Sci Transl Med* 2011;3(73):73ra19.

11. Garcia-Romo GS, Caielli S, Vega B et al. Netting neutrophils are major inducers of type I IFN production in pediatric systemic lupus erythematosus. *Sci Transl Med* 2011;3(73):73ra20.

12. Voll RE, Herrmann M, Roth EA et al. Immunosuppressive effects of apoptotic cells. *Nature* 1997;390(6658):350–351.

13. Green, DR, Ferguson T, Zitvogel L, Kroemer G. Immunogenic and tolerogenic cell death. *Nat Rev Immunol* 2009;9:353–363.

14. Uderhardt S, Herrmann M, Oskolkova OV et al. 12/15-lipoxygenase orchestrates the clearance of apoptotic cells and maintains immunologic tolerance. *Immunity* 2012;36(5):834–846.

15. Kruse K, Janko C, Urbonaviciute V et al. Inefficient clearance of dying cells in patients with SLE: anti-dsDNA autoantibodies, MFG-E8, HMGB-1 and other players. *Apoptosis* 2010;15(9):1098–1113.

16. Karasuyama H, Mukai K, Tsujimura Y, Obata, K. Newly discovered roles for basophils: a neglected minority gains new respect. *Nat Rev Immunol* 2009;9:9–13.

17. Sun JC, Lanier LL. NK cell development, homeostasis and function: parallels with CD8(+) T cells. *Nat Rev Immunol* 2011;11:645–657.

18. Shi C, Pamer EG. Monocyte recruitment during infection and inflammation. *Nat Rev. Immunol* 2011;11:762–774.

19. Coll RC, O'Neill LA. New insights into the regulation of signalling by toll-like receptors and nod-like receptors. *J Innate Immun* 2010;2(5):406–421.

20. Kawai T, Akira S. Toll-like receptors and their crosstalk with other innate receptors in infection and immunity. *Immunity* 2011;34:637–650.

21. Urbonaviciute V, Voll RE. High-mobility group box 1 represents a potential marker of disease activity and novel therapeutic target in systemic lupus erythematosus. *J Intern Med* 2011;270(4):309–318.

22. Schröder K, Tschopp J. The inflammasomes. *Cell* 2010 ;140(6):821–832; Lavelle EC, Murphy C ,O'Neill LA ,Creagh EM. The role of TLRs, NLRs, and RLRs in mucosal innate immunity and homeostasis. *Mucosal Immunol* 2010;3(1):17–28.

23. Shlomchik MJ, Weisel F. Germinal center selection and the development of memory B and plasma cells. *Immunol Rev* 2012;247:52–63.

24. McHeyzer-Williams M, Okitsu S, Wang N, McHeyzer-Williams L. Molecular programming of B cell memory. *Nat Rev Immunol* 2012;12:24–34.

25. Radbruch A, Muehlinghaus G, Luger EO et al. Competence and competition: the challenge of becoming a long-lived plasma cell. *Nat Rev Immunol* 2006;6:741–750.

26. Cerf-Bensussan N, Gaboriau-Routhiau V. The immune system and the gut microbiota: friends or foes? *Nat Rev Immunol* 2010;10: 735–744.

27. Abreu MT. Toll-like receptor signalling in the intestinal epithelium: how bacterial recognition shapes intestinal function. *Nat Rev Immunol* 2010;10:131–144.

28. Pober JS, Sessa WC. Evolving functions of endothelial cells in inflammation. *Nat Rev Immunol* 2007;7:803–815.

29. Allen JE, Maizels RM. Diversity and dialogue in immunity to helminths. *Nat Rev Immunol* 2011;11:375–388.

30. Sakaguchi S, Yamaguchi T, Nomura T, Ono M. Regulatory T cells and immune tolerance. *Cell* 2008;133:775–787.

31. Turner MD, Chaudhry A, Nedjai B. Tumour necrosis factor receptor trafficking dysfunction opens the TRAPS door to pro-inflammatory cytokine secretion. *Biosci Rep* 2012;32(2):105–112.

32. Wurster VM, Carlucci JG, Edwards KM. Periodic fever syndromes. *Pediatr Ann* 2011;40(1):48–54.

CHAPTER 49

Cellular side of acquired immunity (T cells)

Assia Eljaafari and Pierre Miossec

Introduction

Foreign invaders are recognized by cells of the innate immune system, which leads to the activation of adaptive immune responses. However, a crucial prerequisite for defence against external pathogens is the ability to discriminate self from non-self. Otherwise, the immune response can become threatening for the body, leading to autoimmunity and organ damage.

T cells are critical in the adaptive immune response. New subsets have been recently described, allowing a better understanding of the respective contribution in normal life as well as in disease. This understanding has led to new therapeutic approaches, and more options are coming.

The adaptive T-cell immune response

To initiate an adaptative immune response, a T cell has to come into tight contact with an antigen-presenting cell (APC). An immunological synapse is created to allow T cells to receive signals from APCs. Two signals play a preponderant role in T-cell activation. The first signal is provided after interaction with the cognate antigen–MHC ligand complex, through the T-cell receptor (TCR), and this gives specificity to the immune response. The second signal is antigen-independent and is delivered by the interaction of B7-1/CD80 and B7-2/CD86 costimulatory molecules on APC with the CD28 molecule on T cells.[1] This signal promotes T-cell clonal expansion, lymphokine secretion and effector functions. The combination of these two signals determines whether a T cell becomes activated or anergic. CD8/CD4 T-cell coreceptors and CD40 ligand amplify these signals by binding to HLA class I, class II, or CD40 molecules, respectively, on APC. On the other hand, CTLA4 (cytotoxic T lymphocyte antigen), a CD28 homologue, is a negative regulator of the immune response. Its expression is induced in a second step during activation, with the aim of regulating T-cell expansion by competing with the CD28 molecule for binding to B7-1 and B7-2 molecules. Moreover, this molecule was shown to play a key role in regulatory T-cell suppressive function.[2]

Dendritic cells

Dendritic cells (DCs) are the most potent professional APCs and play a critical role in the induction of adaptive immune responses and tolerance. They represent a heterogeneous population where immature DCs rather promote tolerogenic responses and mature DCs immunogenic responses. Peripheral DCs display an 'immature' phenotype characterized by expression of low surface levels of MHC II and of costimulatory molecules and induce suboptimal T-cell priming, resulting in T-cell anergy or tolerance. Immature DCs secrete interleukin (IL)-10, and promote tolerance in vivo by either deleting antigen-specific T cells or expanding regulatory T cells (Tregs). Conversely, upon stimulation, DCs undergo maturation characterized by expression of high levels of MHC class II molecules and costimulatory molecules. They induce robust T-cell activation and effector cell differentiation. Such DCs secrete high levels of IL-12.[3] However, many distinct DC subtypes, related to different routes of DC differentiation from precursors, have recently been discovered. Those DC subsets display specialized functions corresponding to particular locations.[4]

Link between innate and adaptive immunity

Adaptive immune responses depend on the microbial antigens that stimulate APC, and more particularly DC. DC express pattern-recognition receptors (PRRs). Those receptors recognize conserved structures of microbes, known as pathogen-associated molecular patterns (PAMPs). Among the PRRs are the Toll-like receptors (TLRs) and the Nod-like receptors (NLRs). TLRs are a family of 10 receptors in human and of 12 in mouse.[5] Most TLRs are expressed on the plasma membrane of myeloid cells and occasionally lymphoid leucocytes. They recognize various viruses, bacteria, fungi, and parasites. Different TLRs specialize in the recognition of particular PAMP motifs.[6] Their ligand molecules are expressed by different sets of bacteria. For example, TLR1, 2, and 6 detect lipopeptides, TLR5 detects flagelline, while TLR4 recognizes a variety of lipopolysaccharides. Among the various TLRs, TLR3, TLR7, TLR8, and TLR9 are intracellular, localized in endosomes and implicated in nucleic acid recognition. These four TLRs are expressed in leucocytes, such as DCs, macrophages, and B cells. They are involved in response against viruses, except TLR9, which recognizes demethylated CpG oligonucleotides in bacteria.[7,8]

Presentation of PAMPS through TLRs results in the activation of NFκB and interferon regulatory factor (IRF) transcription factors and this leads to increased expression of proinflammatory cytokines.[9] On the other hand, cytosolic NLRs lead to the activation of the IRF3 transcription factor (IRF3), which induces type I interferon (IFN) production and a series of proinflammatory cytokine secretion, like interleukin (IL)-1β, IL-18, or IL-33, through activation of the inflammasome and cleavage of their immature form by caspase-1.[10] This TLR/NLR strategy allows a limited set of receptors to recognize a wide range of pathogens, rapidly inducing local inflammation and providing a link with a specific and memory immune response, i.e. the adaptive immune response (see Chapter 48).

T-cell differentiation and Th subsets

Upon interaction with their cognate antigen, naive CD4+T cells differentiate into a number of different subsets characterized by patterns of cytokines and transcription factors. Naive T cells are circulating cells, but upon encounter with APC in lymphoid tissues, they commit and migrate to inflamed non-lymphoid tissues where antigens are present at high concentrations. There they produce cytokines, proliferate, and/or directly lyse infected cells. A few memory T cells, know as central memory T cells, recirculate like naive T cells in order to rapidly proliferate and produce new T effector memory cells and effector cells, during a secondary response to the same antigen.

Mosmann and Coffman first defined Th1 and Th2 effector cells.[11] Th1 cells play a role in immunity against intracellular pathogens and are involved in delayed-type hypersensitivity responses. Their commitment from naive T cells is related to the secretion of IL-12 by APCs, and subsequent expression of the Tbet transcription factor. This results in the secretion of IFNγ, which activates macrophages and NK cells at the site of inflammation. When IL-10 instead of IL-12 is secreted by APCs, T cells rather commit into IL-4/STAT6-Th2 cells under the control of the GATA3 transcription factor. Th2 cells secrete IL-5/IL-10/IL-13, and play a role in immunity against parasites. They are implicated in allergy and asthma, through induction of IgE production, and activation of eosinophils. Importantly, Th2 cytokines, particularly IL-4, strongly inhibit Th1 differentiation, while IFNγ and IL-12 inhibit Th2 generation, thus leading to a reciprocal counter-regulation.[12]

Along with Th1 and Th2 cells, new subsets have been recently described, such as Th3, Th9, Th17, Th22, follicular helper T cells (TFh), or Tregs. Of these new subsets, Th17, Th22, and Tregs have attracted most attention, due to their implication in chronic inflammation and autoimmune diseases, such as multiple sclerosis, psoriasis, rheumatoid arthritis (RA), and inflammatory bowel disease (Figure 49.1).

Th17 cells

Characterization of the Th17 subset

Th17 cells were first characterized by the ability to secrete IL-17.[13] IL-17 (now IL-17A) is a member of the IL-17 family composed of six cytokines, A–F. IL-17A is the major actor of the Th17 cells, along with IL-17F with which it shares 50% homology. IL-17A and IL-17F signal through the IL-17RA IL-17RC receptor complex which is ubiquitously expressed.[14] IL-17A activates mitogen-activated protein kinases (MAPK) and NFκB via association with Act1 and activation of TNF receptor associated factor 6 (TRAF6).[15]

The Th17 subset was discovered through observations of the experimental autoimmune encephalitis (EAE) model, where IFNγ-deficient mice were unexpectedly found to be more susceptible to disease.[16] IL-12 is the key factor for the differentiation of Th1 cells.

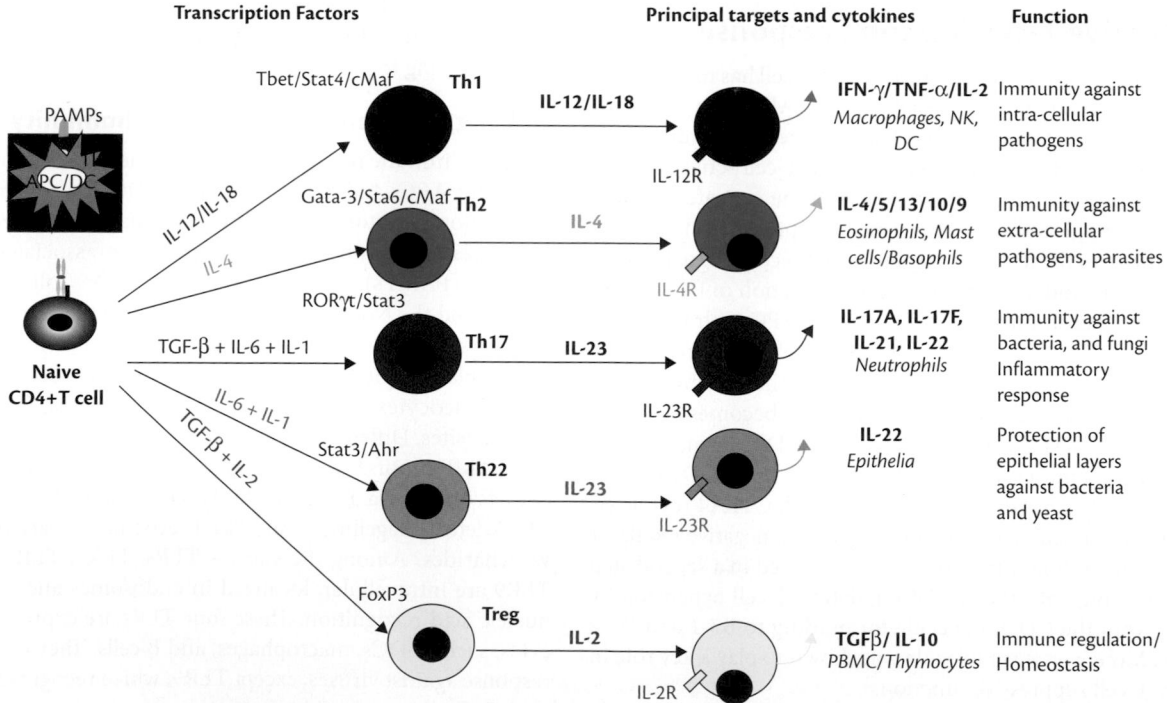

Fig. 49.1 Subsets of T cells. Upon interaction with their cognate antigen, naive CD4+T cells differentiate into a number of different subsets characterized by patterns of cytokines and transcription factors. The cytokines present in the microenvironment drive this differentiation, but the profile of cytokines depends on the microbial antigens that stimulate APC, and more particularly DC which express pattern-recognition receptors (PRRs). Those receptors recognize conserved structures of microbes, named pathogen-associated molecular patterns (PAMPs).

It is made up of two subunits, p35 and p40. The p40 subunit is also one of the components of IL-23, which is a heterodimer consisting of of IL-12p40 and p19.[17] The use of mice deficient for these two molecules clearly demonstrated that IL-23 but not IL-12 was crucial for the development of EAE.[18] The discovery of a unique subset of T cells secreting IL-17 but not IFNγ or IL-4 then led to the description of a new subset, Th17, involved in inflammation and autoimmunity.

However, naive T cells do not express the IL-23 receptor, and therefore cannot be converted into Th17 cells under the sole influence of IL-23. The differentiation of Th17 cells is now seen as a three-step process. In the first step, the combination of TGFβ, IL-1β and IL-6 drives naive T cells towards the Th17 pathway; IL-6 through STAT3 triggers the activation of retinoic acid orphan receptor γ thymus (RORγT) in mouse, or RORC in human, the crucial transcription factor implicated in Th17 development.[19] TGFβ renders naive T cells sensitive to IL-23 by increasing the expression of its receptor.[20] In the second and third steps, IL-21 participates to Th17 expansion, whereas IL-23 stabilizes the Th17 phenotype.[21]

The role of TGFβ was found to be quite intriguing. TGFβ alone is involved in generation of Tregs through FoxP3. However, in the presence of IL-1β and IL-6, this cytokine activates Th17 differentiation. Since IL-6 inhibits FoxP3, this suggests that Tregs and Th17 cells are developmentally regulated.[22] Supporting the existence of such a balance is the recent finding that IL-2, a growth factor important for Treg expansion and activation, inhibits Th17 promotion. Thus Th17 cells are promoted when IL-2 is consumed, notably by Tregs. This inhibition of IL-17A production is related to the competitive inhibition of STAT-3 and STAT-5 for binding to the IL-17-enhancer element (Figure 49.2).[23]

Another balance between Th1 and Th17 cells has also been described. IFNγ inhibits Th17 promotion in different models[24] and, conversely IL-17A inhibits Th1 cells by blocking the expression of the IL-12Rβ chain, the IL-12 specific chain of the IL-12 receptor.[25] In reality, the situation is probably more complex. Th17 cells were shown to produce IFNγ by themselves, particularly in the presence of IL-12, or in the absence of IL-23 and the presence of IL-2 in vitro.[26] Moreover, Th17 cells expressing both Tbet and RORγt were found in the brain of mice with EAE, and were described as more pathogenic.[27] Such plasticity of Th17 cells does not seem to be restricted to the Th1 pathway, with studies demonstrating the ability of Th17 cells to secrete IL-10 in the presence of TGFβ. These TGFβ-induced Th17 cells expressing IL-10 are, however, likely to have limited pathological potential.[28]

Role of Th17 cells in disease
Response to infectious agents
IL-17A and IL-17F induce the recruitment of neutrophils to the site of inflammation, through the release of chemokines, like CXC-chemokine ligand-1 (CXCL1), CXCL2, IL-8, or GCP2/CXCL6.[29] Administration of IL-17A induces accumulation of neutrophils in the br onchoalveolar and joint areas. IL-17A increases neutrophil elastase and myeloperoxydase (MPO) activity and plays an important role in defence against bacteria and fungi that are not cleared by Th1 or Th2 cells, such as *Propionibacterium acnes*, *Klebsiella pneumoniae*, *Citrobacter rodentium*, *Borrelia burgdorferi*, or *Candida albicans*. In the hyper-IgE syndrome, a mutation in *STAT3* results in a defect in Th17 cells with recurrent *C. albicans* and *Staphylococcus aureus* skin and lung infections.[30]

Chronic inflammation and autoimmunity
IL-17A was found to mediate local tissue inflammation by inducing the release of proinflammatory cytokines (such as IL-1, TNFα, and IL-6) and the activation of metalloproteases in fibroblasts or epithelial cells.[31] In addition to neutrophil chemokines, the local release of granulocyte colony-stimulating factor (G-CSF) and granulocyte-macrophage colony-stimulating factor (GM-CSF), monocyte

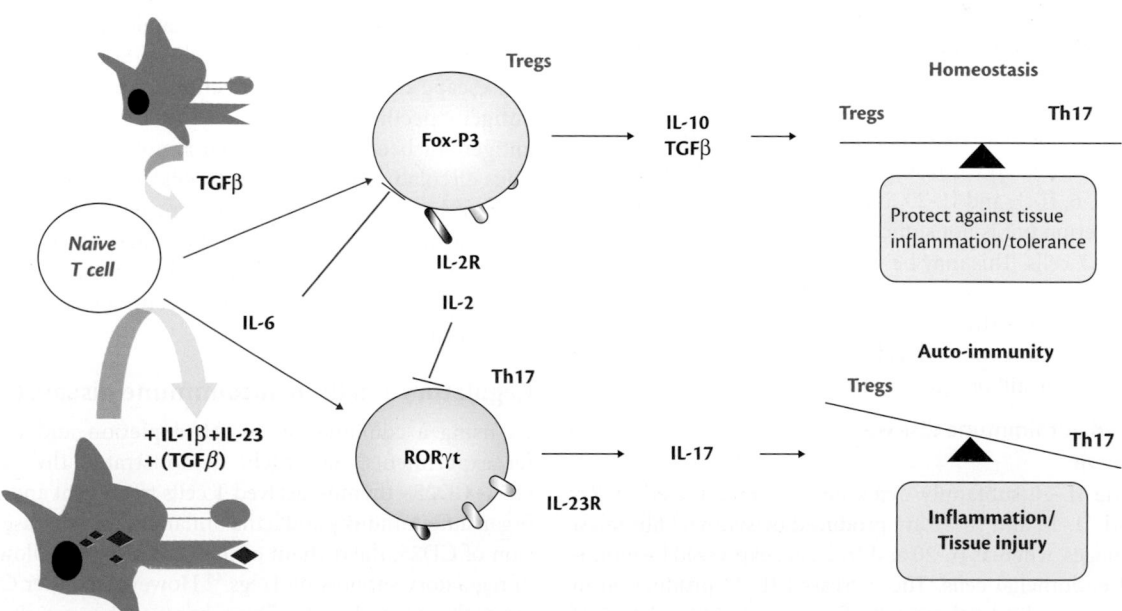

Fig. 49.2 Reciprocal balance between Th17 cells and Tregs. The combination of TGFβ, IL-1β and IL-6 drives naive T cells towards the Th17 pathway; IL-6 triggers the activation of RORγT in mouse, or RORC in human, the crucial Th17 transcription factor. TGFβ alone is involved in Treg generation through FoxP3. But, in the presence of IL-1β and IL-6, TGFβ induces Th17 differentiation. IL-6 inhibits FoxP3 activation, and thus Treg generation. Reciprocally, IL-2, a growth factor important for Treg expansion and activation, inhibits Th17 promotion. Thus Th17 cells are promoted when IL-2 is consumed, notably by Tregs. Tregs and Th17 cells are therefore developmentally regulated. A dysregulation of the Treg/Th17 balance leads to autoimmune diseases.

chemokine protein (MCP-1), or CCL20 attracts mononuclear cells such as monocytes, DCs, or Th17 cells to the site of inflammation. Therefore, Th17 cells were suggested to promote autoimmunity and chronic inflammation. In RA, IL-17A and IL-17F were found to trigger bone resorption, through extracellular matrix destruction, and stimulation of the RANK/RANKL interaction leading to osteoclast activation.[32] TNFα and IL-1β were found to act synergistically with IL-17A, in the release and activation of inflammatory cytokines or enzymes. In addition in RA, Th17 cells were found to accumulate in the tissues of patients suffering from psoriasis, multiple sclerosis, or bowel diseases.[33] IL-17A was found elevated in the serum and synovial fluid of RA patients, or cerebrospinal fluid of multiple sclerosis patients. It was suggested in the latter case that Th17 cells infiltrate the blood brain–barrier as a result of CCL20 attraction through their CCR6 expression.[34]

Th22 cells

Characterization of the Th22 subset

IL-22 is a member of the IL-10 family, which is subdivided into three subgroups. IL-10 is an immunomodulatory and anti-inflammatory cytokine, and IL-22 belongs to the IL-20 subfamily, together with IL-19, IL-20, IL-24, and IL-26. These cytokines, especially IL-22, protect epithelial cells from invasion by extracellular pathogens such as bacteria and yeast and contribute to tissue remodelling and wound healing. This family of cytokines maintains tissue integrity and restores homeostasis of epithelial layers during infection and inflammatory responses. The third group contains IL-28A, and IL-28B and IL-29, which protect epithelial cells from viral infections by synergizing with type I IFN to boost host antiviral response.[35] Stat3 is the key downstream transcription factor used by IL-10 and IL-20 subfamily cytokines, but Stat3 is also critical for Th17 cell differentiation in mouse and human. IL-22 is indeed an effector cytokine of Th17 cells. However, IL-22 and IL-17 are not always coexpressed and their regulation is different. Notably TGFβ, which contributes to IL-17 production, is a potent inhibitor of IL-22 production, while it drives IL-10 production by Th17 cells.[36] Therefore TGFβ controls the production of IL-22 but drives against IL-10 by Th17 cells. Accordingly IL-22 is induced by IL6/IL23/IL1β, while IL-10 is rather induced by TGFβ/IL-6. Thus, IL-10 and IL-22 are rarely expressed by the same cell. Stat3, which is triggered by IL-6, IL-1, and IL-23, is crucial for RORγT expression and IL-17 secretion but is not sufficient alone to lead to IL-22 production in Th17 cells. This may be related to the aryl hydrocarbon receptor (AhR), a transcription factor which plays an essential role in IL-22 expression by Th17 cells. While Stat-3 deficient mice are impaired in IL-22 expression, Th cells from AhR deficient mice fail to secrete IL-22, but still produce IL-17.[37]

Th22 cells and autoimmune diseases

Exacerbating role

IL-10 and the IL-20 subfamily cytokines are upregulated in RA synovial fluid. IL-19 and IL-22 are produced by synovial fibroblast and macrophages, whereas IL-20 and IL-24 are expressed by mononuclear and endothelial cells. The increased IL-22 production in RA synovium may also be the result of increased accumulation of Th17 cells which contribute to IL-22 production. IL-19 increases the production of IL-6 by RA synovium and decreases apoptosis of the synovial cells, whereas IL-22 enhances proliferation of synovial fibroblasts and secretion of chemokines.[35] The implication of IL-22 in RA has been demonstrated in IL-22-deficient mice, which showed a delayed onset of collagen-induced arthritis (CIA) and decreased synovial proinflammatory cytokine expression.[38]

IL-22 has also been implicated in the pathogenesis of psoriasis. Skin overexpression of IL-22 leads to key features of this disease, by increased recruitment of leucocytes through secretion of proinflammatory cytokines and chemokines, and increased keratinocyte proliferation and differentiation.[39] Mice overexpressing IL-22 die within a few days, but exhibit a thickened epidermis with hallmarks of psoriasis. IL-22 injection into the skin of normal mice induces keratinocyte hyperplasia and secretion of defensins.[35]

Protective role

Contrasting with their exacerbating role in RA or psoriasis, Th22 cells appear to play a protective role in some autoimmune diseases such as systemic lupus erythematosus (SLE), where high plasma levels of IL-22 were negatively correlated with disease activity.[40] In inflammatory bowel diseases, IL-22 contributes to protection through the secretion of inflammatory cytokines and chemokines by colonic epithelial cells and myofibroblasts, which leads to the recruitment of leucocytes that control invading pathogens. IL-22 also induces the secretion of antimicrobial peptides such as defensins, or C-type lectins from intestinal epithelial cells. Finally, it also stimulates mucosal wound healing.[35]

Regulatory T cells

Definition and functions

Intrathymic selection of T cells is a central process that ensures deletion of most of the autoreactive T cells. This is a two-step process, where a first positive selection is driven by the interaction of a self-MHC restricted TCR with its antigen presented by thymic stromal cells. The second step is a negative selection of T cells expressing TCR with high affinity for self-antigen.[41] This step is under the control of DC, which give a negative signal to T cells. Therefore negative selection is the major mechanism responsible for deletion of autoreactive T cells.[42] Some aut-reactive T cells can escape from thymus depletion, either because they express antigen-specific TCR with too low affinity for the target self-antigen, or because this antigen is not expressed in the thymus. Thus circulating autoreactive T cells are present in the periphery even of healthy individuals. To prevent autoimmunity, various mechanisms are present in the periphery, such as anergy, clonal deletion, ignorance, or silencing by Tregs. Autoimmunity can develop as the result of a failure of central or peripheral tolerance mechanisms.[43]

Regulatory T cells in autoimmune diseases

By using a combination of self-depletion and adoptive transfer experiments, Sakaguchi demonstrated the crucial role of CD4+CD25+ thymus-derived T cells to prevent and control multiorgan autoimmunity and lethal inflammatory disease. High expression of CD25, the α chain of the IL-2 receptor, allows enrichment of regulatory suppressor Tregs.[44] However, neither CD4 nor CD25 are exclusive markers for Tregs, because they are also expressed by activated T cells. But forkhead domain DNA-binding transcription factor 3 (FoxP3) is specifically expressed in Tregs in mice, and is essential for development and function of Tregs. Genetic mutation of FoxP3 leads to the lethal scurfy disease in mice, demonstrating that this transcription factor is required for the homeostasis of the immune system.[45] In humans, the IPEX syndrome (immunodysregulation, polyendocrinopathy, enteropathy, X-linked) also indicates the crucial role of FoxP3.[46] However, FoxP3 in humans is also expressed after T-cell activation.

The emergence of autoimmune diseases can also be linked to an altered function of Tregs. In RA, although Tregs are identified in the joint, they show functional defects.[47] CTLA-4 is essential for the function of Tregs which constitutively express this molecule.[48] CTLA-4 deficiency in FoxP3+ Tregs impairs their suppressive function. CTLA-4 acts in part through the downregulation of CD80 and CD86 molecules on APC, leading to reduced stable interactions between activated T cells and APCs.[49] Polymorphisms of the *CTLA4* gene have been associated with genetic susceptibility to a variety of autoimmune diseases including RA, and may therefore account for the functional defects.[50]

Conclusion

Foreign invaders are recognized first by cells of the innate immune system. This leads to a rapid and non-specific inflammatory response, followed by induction of the adaptive and specific immune response. Different adaptive responses can be promoted, depending on the predominant effector cells that are involved, which themselves depend on the microbial/antigen stimuli. As examples, Th1 cells contribute to cell-mediated immunity against intracellular pathogens, Th2 cells protect against parasites, Th17 cells against extracellular bacteria and fungi that are not cleared by Th1 and Th2 cells. Among the new subsets, Th22 cells protect against disruption of epithelial layers secondary to invading pathogens, such as bacteria or yeast. Finally these effector subsets are regulated by Tregs. These Th subsets counteract each other to maintain the homeostasis of the immune system.

This balance can be easily disrupted, leading to chronic inflammation or autoimmune diseases. The challenge is to detect early changes in this balance, prior to its clinical expression. New molecular tools such as microarrays could be used to determine the predominant profile of the immune effector cells involved in a disease process. Such understanding should provide better therapeutic tools to counteract dysregulated effector cells.

References

1. Lenschow DJ, Walunas TL, Bluestone JA. CD28/B7 system of T cell costimulation. *Annu Rev Immunol* 1996;14:233–258.
2. Walunas TL, Lenschow DJ, Bakker CY et al. CTLA-4 can function as a negative regulator of T cell activation. *Immunity* 1994;1:405–413.
3. Steinman RM. The dendritic cell system and its role in immunogenicity. *Annu Rev Immunol* 1991;9:271–296.
4. Geissmann F, Manz MG, Jung S et al. Development of monocytes, macrophages and dendritic cells. *Science* 2010;327:656–661.
5. Medzhitov R, Preston-Hurlburt P, Janeway CA Jr. A human homologue of the Drosophila Toll protein signals activation of adaptive immunity. *Nature* 1997;388:394–397.
6. Barbalat R, Ewald S. Nucleic acid recognition by the innate immune system. *Annu Rev Immuno* 2011;29:185–214.
7. Barton GM. Viral recognition by Toll-like receptors. *Semin Immunol* 2007;19(1):33–40.
8. Krieg AM. CpG motifs in bacterial DNA and their immune effects. *Annu Rev Immunol* 2002;20:709–760.
9. Akira S, Takeda K. Toll-like receptor signalling. *Nat Rev Immunol* 2004;4(7):499–511.
10. Mariathasan S, Monack DM. Inflammasome adaptors and sensors:intracellular regulators of infection and inflammation. *Nat Rev Immunol* 2007;7:31–40.
11. Mosmann TR, Coffman RL. TH1 and TH2 cells:different patterns of lymphokine secretion lead to different functional properties. *Annu Rev Immunol* 1989;7:145–173.
12. Murphy KM, Reiner SL. The lineage decisions of helper T cells. *Nat Rev Immunol* 2002;2:933–944.
13. Yao Z, Painter SL, Fanslow WC et al. Human IL-17: a novel cytokine derived from T cells. *J Immunol* 1995;155:5483–5486.
14. Kolls JK, Linden A. Interleukin-17 family members and inflammation. *Immunity* 2004;21:467–476.
15. Chang SH, Park H, Dong C. Act1 adaptor protein is an immediate and essential signaling component of interleukin-17 receptor *J Biol Chem* 2006;281:35603–35607.
16. Ferber IA, Brocke S, Taylor-Edwards C et al. () Mice with a disrupted IFN-gamma gene are susceptible to the induction of experimental autoimmune encephalomyelitis (EAE). *J Immunol* 1996;156:5–7.
17. Oppmann B, Lesley R, Blom B et al. Novel p19 protein engages IL-12p40 to form a cytokine, IL-23, with biological activities similar as well as distinct from IL-12. *Immunity* 2000;13:715–725.
18. Cua DJ, Sherlock J, Chen Y, et al. Interleukin-23 rather than interleukin-12 is the critical cytokine for autoimmune inflammation of the brain. *Nature* 2003;421:744–748.
19. Ivanov II, McKenzie BS, Zhou L, et al. The orphan nuclear receptor RORgammat directs the differentiation program of proinflammatory IL-17(+) T helper cells. *Cell* 2006;126:1121–1133.
20. Veldhoen M, Hocking RJ, Atkins CJ, Locksley RM, Stockinger B. TGFbeta in the context of an inflammatory cytokine milieu supports de novo differentiation of IL-17-producing T cells. *Immunity* 2006;24:179–189.
21. Zhou L, Ivanov II, Spolski R et al.. IL-6 programs T(H)-17 cell differentiation by promoting sequential engagement of the IL-21 and IL-23 pathways. *Nat Immunol* 2007;8:967–974.
22. Bettelli E, Carrier Y, Gao W et al. Reciprocal developmental pathways for the generation of pathogenic effector TH17 and regulatory T cells. *Nature* 2006;441:235–238.
23. Laurence A, Tato CM, Davidson TS et al. Interleukin-2 signaling via STAT5 constrains T helper 17 cell generation. *Immunity* 2007;26:371–381.
24. Harrington LE, Hatton RD, Mangan PR et al. Interleukin 17-producing CD4+ effector T cells develop via a lineage distinct from the T helper type 1 and 2 lineages. *Nat Immunol* 2005;6:1123–1132.
25. Toh ML, Kawashima M, Hot A, Miossec P. Role of IL-17 in the Th1 systemic defects in rheumatoid arthritis through selective IL-12Rbeta2 inhibition. *Ann Rheum Dis* 2010;69:1562–1567.
26. Boniface K, Blumenschein WM, Brovont-Porth K et al. Human Th17 cells comprise heterogeneous subsets including IFN-gamma-producing cells with distinct properties from the Th1 lineage. *J Immunol* 2010;185:679–687.
27. Jäger A, Dardalhon V, Sobel RA, Bettelli E, Kuchroo VK. Th1, Th17, and Th9 effector cells induce experimental autoimmune encephalomyelitis with different pathological phenotypes. *J Immunol* 2009;183:7169–7177.
28. McGeachy MJ, Bak-Jensen KS, Chen Y et al. TGF-b and IL-6 drive the production of IL-17 and IL-10 by T cells and restrain T(H)-17 cell-mediated pathology. *Nat Immunol* 2007;8:1390–1397.
29. Ye P, Rodriguez FH, Kanaly S et al.. Requirement of interleukin 17 receptor signaling for lung CXC chemokine and granulocyte colony-stimulating factor expression, neutrophil recruitment, and host defense. *J Exp Med* 2001;194:519–527.
30. Milner JD, Brenchley JM, Laurence A et al. Impaired T(H)17 cell differentiation in subjects with autosomal dominant hyper-IgE syndrome. *Nature* 2008;452:773–776.
31. Chabaud M, Fossiez F, Taupin JL, Miossec P. Enhancing effect of IL-17 on IL-1-induced IL-6 and leukemia inhibitory factor production by

rheumatoid arthritis synoviocytes and its regulation by Th2 cytokines. *J Immunol* 1998;161:409–414.

32. Page G, Miossec P. RANK and RANKL expression as markers of dendritic cell-T cell interactions in paired samples of rheumatoid synovium and lymph nodes. *Arthritis Rheum* 2005;52:2307–2312.

33. Miossec P, Korn T, Kuchroo VK. Interleukin-17 and type 17 helper T cells. *N Engl J Med* 2009;361:888–898.

34. Kebir H, Kreymborg K, Ifergan I et al. Human T(H)17 lymphocytes promote blood-brain barrier disruption and central nervous system inflammation. *Nat Med* 2007;13:1173–1175.

35. Ouyang W, Rutz S, Crellin N, Valdez P, Hymowitz S. Regulation and functions of the IL-10 family of cytokines in inflammation and disease. *Annu Rev Immunol* 2011;29:71–109.

36. Duhen T, Geiger R, Jarrossay D, Lanzavecchia A, Sallusto F. Production of interleukin 22 but not interleukin 17 by a subset of human skin-homing memory T cells. *Nat Immunol* 2009;10:857–863.

37. Veldhoen M, Hirota K, Westendorf AM et al.. The aryl hydrocarbon receptor links TH17-cell-mediated autoimmunity to environmental toxins. *Nature* 2008;453:106–109.

38. Geboes L, Dumoutier L, Kelchtermans H et al. Proinflammatory role of the Th17 cytokine interleukin-22 in collagen-induced arthritis in C57BL/6 mice. *Arthritis Rheum* 2009;60:390–395.

39. Wolk K, Haugen HS, Xu W et al. IL-22 and IL-20 are key mediators of the epidermal alterations in psoriasis while IL-17 and IFN-γ are not. *J Mol Med* 2009;87:523–536.

40. Cheng F, Guo Z, Xu H, Yan D, Li Q. Decreased plasma IL22 levels, but not increased IL17 and IL23 levels, correlate with disease activity in patients with systemic lupus erythematosus. *Ann Rheum Dis* 2009;68:604–606.

41. Palmer E. Negative selection-clearing out the bad apples from the T-cell repertoire. *Nat Rev Immunol* 2003;3:383–391.

42. Bonasio R, Scimone ML, Schaerli P et al. Clonal deletion of thymocytes by circulating dendritic cells homing to the thymus. *Nat Immunol* 2006;7:1092–1100.

43. Sakaguchi S. Naturally arising CD4_ regulatory T cells for immunologic selftolerance and negative control of immune responses. *Annu Rev Immunol* 2004;22:531–562.

44. Sakaguchi S, Sakaguchi N, Asano M, Itoh M, Toda M. Immunologic self-tolerance maintained by activated T cells expressing IL-2 receptor alpha-chains (CD25] Breakdown of a single mechanism of self-tolerance causes various autoimmune diseases. *J Immunol* 1995;155:1151–1164.

45. Brunkow ME, Jeffery EW, Hjerrild KA, et al. () Disruption of a new forkhead/winged-helix protein, scurfin, results in the fatal lymphoproliferative disorder of the scurfy mouse. *Nat Genet* 2001;27:68–73.

46. Wildin RS, Ramsdell F, Peake J et al. X-linked neonatal diabetes mellitus, enteropathy and endocrinopathy syndrome is the human equivalent of mouse scurfy. *Nat Genet* 2001;27:18–20.

47. Flores-Borja F, Jury EC, Mauri C, Ehrenstein MR. Defects in CTLA-4 are associated with abnormal regulatory T cell function in rheumatoid arthritis. *Proc Natl Acad Sci U S A* 2008;105:396–401.

48. Kolar P, Knieke K, Hegel JK et al. CTLA-4 (CD152] controls homeostasis and suppressive capacity of regulatory T cells in mice. *Arthritis Rheum* 2009;60:123–132.

49. Wing K, Onishi Y, Prieto-Martin P et al. CTLA-4 control over Foxp3+ regulatory T cell function. *Science* 2008;322:271–275.

50. Ueda H, Howson JM, Esposito L et al.. Association of the T-cell regulatory gene CTLA4 with susceptibility to autoimmune disease. *Nature* 2003;423:506–511.

CHAPTER 50

Cellular side of acquired immunity (B cells)

Thomas Dörner and Peter E. Lipsky

Introduction

The traditional model of rheumatoid arthritis (RA) pathogenesis postulated a central role for CD4+ T cells and macrophages.[1] Therefore, early therapeutic trials employed anti-CD4 therapy in RA, which failed to show clinical benefit and raised questions about the central role of CD4+ T cells.[2] However, recently, the successful treatment of RA by blocking T-cell costimulation with CTLA4Ig (abatacept) has again implied a role for CD4+ T cells in RA pathogenesis, although effects of this product on cells expressing CD80/86 have not permitted a firm indication on its primary target of action.

Clinical application of anti-cytokine therapy in RA appears to be closely linked to blocking aspects of innate immunity, leaving unresolved the central role of B cells in RA pathogenesis. Despite this, it has been accepted that autoantibodies play an important amplifying role in joint inflammation and serve as diagnostic, classification, and prognostic markers. More recently, however, the success of B-cell-depleting therapy in ameliorating RA inflammation and inhibiting radiographic progression even after failure of tumour necrosis factor (TNF) blockade[3] has documented a role for B cells in RA pathogenesis. It is clear from these clinical results that CD4+ T cells, B cells, and the innate immune system all may play important roles in the initiation as well as the perpetuation of RA.

Role of B cells in immune responses

B cells are an essential component of normal immune responses and are responsible for the maintenance of humoral protective memory.[4] The nature of the serologic component of protective memory is illustrated by the persisting protective antibody titres against a variety of microorganisms.[5] Interestingly, CD4+ T cells are important in instructing memory B cells to differentiate into long-lived plasma cells, whereas these long-lived non-proliferating antibody-secreting cells survive independent of antigen and further direct interaction with antigen-specific T cells.[6] However, antigen-non-specific interactions with T cells may contribute to the survival of human plasma cells in secondary lymphoid organs.[7,8]

Normal B-cell development in health

In order to understand the role of B cells in RA and also to delineate possible points for therapeutic targeting, it is important to understand the role of these cells under normal conditions. B cells follow a tightly regulated life cycle (Figure 50.1). In the bone marrow, B cells develop from stem cells through a series of precursor stages during which they rearrange their immunoglobulin genes to generate a wide range of unique antigen-binding specificities and emigrate as immature CD20+ B cells expressing surface IgM/IgD into the peripheral blood and differentiate through a series of maturational or transitional cell stages into mature naive B cells. These cells can migrate between blood and secondary lymphoid organs, able to reaction to the combination of specific B-cell-receptor stimulation and T-cell help. A summary of B-cell subsets and origins are shown in Table 50.1.

T-cell-dependent B-cell activation

After encountering their cognate antigen and receiving T-cell help in follicles in secondary lymphoid organs, B cells undergo germinal centre (GC) reactions, during which antigen-specific B cells clonally expand, somatically mutate their Ig genes to achieve avidity maturation, undergo Ig heavy-chain class switch recombination, and mature either into memory B cells or Ig-secreting plasma cells. Because of somatic hypermutation and class switch recombination, the avidity of the B-cell immunglobulin receptor can be increased and the biological function of secreted Ig altered. Important for the interaction with T cells and the generation of GC reactions are a series of ligand–receptor interactions, including those mediated by CD154/CD40 CD28/CD80-CD86, and ICOS-L/ICOS. Defects in these interactions have been shown to lead to hyper-IgM syndrome, resulting in impaired plasma cell and memory B-cell generation and adult onset of common variable hypogammaglobulinemia, respectively.[9] Some B cells can respond to specific antigens in a T-cell-independent manner (TI responses). TI responses largely induce production of IgM antibodies and do not generate post-switch memory B cells. In the mouse, these responses are thought to be restricted to CD1d+/IgM^{high} marginal zone B cells residing in the spleen which recognize polysaccharide antigens.

In addition, B cells are characteristically divided into two major lineages, B1 cells and B2 cells. It is still a matter of debate whether

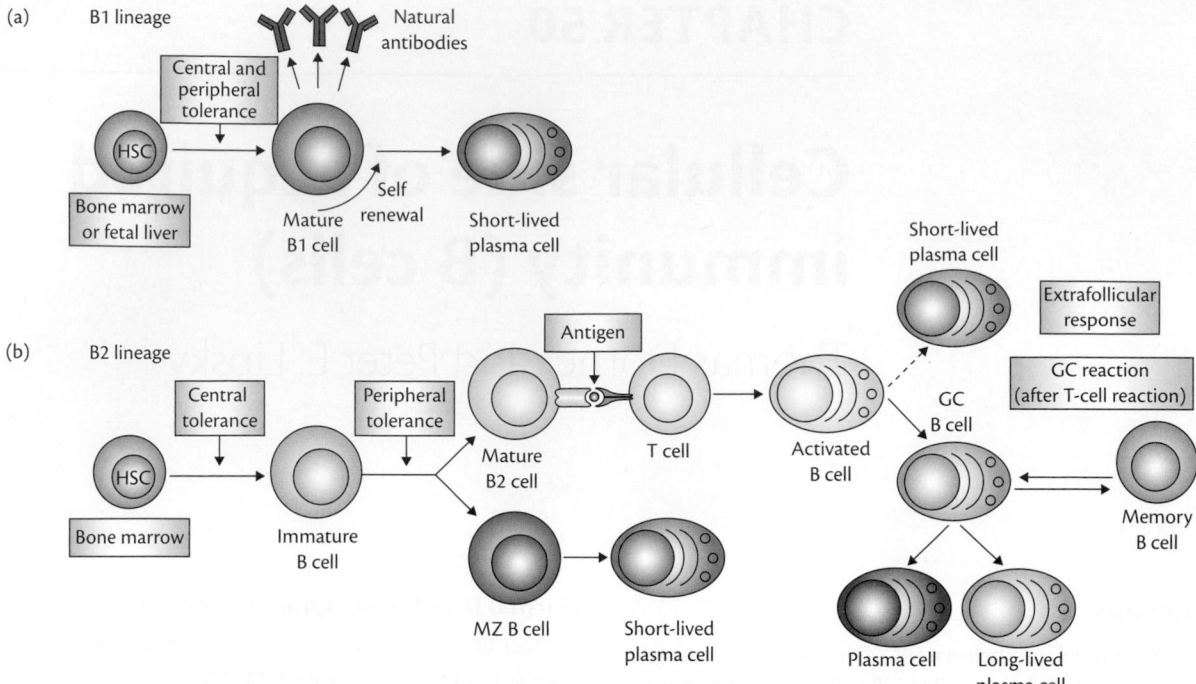

Fig. 50.1 A schematic of B-cell development. B1 and B2 cell lineages seem to be independently regulated and undergo tightly controlled developmental processes. (a) B1 cells develop from haematopoietic stem cells (HSCs) in the bone marrow or fetal liver, are self-renewing, and produce natural antibodies involved in self-defence. (b) B2 cells develop from HSCs in the bone marrow. Following rearrangement of their B-cell-receptor chain genes and removal of autoreactive cells via central tolerance, immature (transitional) B2 cells relocate to the spleen. Those immature B2 cells that escape the processes of peripheral tolerance differentiate into MZ B cells or mature follicular B2 cells, which upon T-cell-dependent activation develop into long-lived plasma cells or memory B cells. B1 cells and MZ B cells are thought to be the main sources of short-lived plasma cells; the contribution of B2 cells to this population has not been delineated (as indicated by the dashed arrow). GC, germinal centre; HSC, haematopoietic stem cell; MZ, marginal zone.
Dorner T, Radbruch A, Burmester GR. B-cell-directed therapies for autoimmune disease. Nature Reviews Rheumatology 2009 Aug;5(8):433–41.

Table 50.1 B-cell subsets: function and origin

B-cell subset	Function	Antibody genes	Origin	Residence	Susceptibility to superantigen-induced death	Rate of healing $(t_{1/2})^a$	Rate of decay $(t_{1/2})^b$
B1a	Natural antibodies	Often canonical without non-templated insertions	Fetal liver	Peritoneal cavity and secrete immunoglobulin in the spleen	Yes	Very slow (permanent defect?)	Very slow
B1b	Natural antibodies	Non-templated insertions ± mutations	Perinatal liver and bone marrow	Peritoneal cavity and secrete immunoglobulin in the spleen	Yes	Unknown	Unknown
Marginal zone	Anti-polysaccharide	Less common mutations	Adult bone marrow	Along the marginal sinus	Yes (early)	21 weeks	Very slow
B2 (follicular)	Protein (conventional)	Hypermutated non-templated insertions and diverse heavy-chain CDR3	Adult bone marrow	Recirculating, spleen, blood and lymph nodes	Yes (late)	13 weeks	18 weeks

[a]Rate of healing refers to studies that evaluated the time taken to replace clones in vivo after B cells were deleted by B-cell superantigen, $t_{1/2}$ represents the time taken to replace or replenish half of the affected pool.
[b]Rate of decay refers to studies in adult mice in which the capacity to generate new antibody gene rearrangements in B-cell precursors was blocked, which prevented new B cells from entering and replenishing peripheral mature B-cell compartments. These studies characterized the normal turnover of these populations when unaffected by specific challenge.
CDR, complementarity-determining regions.
According to Silverman GJ, Goodyear CS. Confounding B-cell defences: lessons from a staphylococcal superantigen. *Nat Rev Immunol* 2006;6:465–475.

B1 and B2 cells are similar in mice and humans.[10] In particular, the expression of CD5 used as a marker of these cells in mice is not reliable in humans since the molecule is expressed during B-cell activation and B-cell maturation.[11] B1 cells are considered to be self-renewing and long-lived, emerging early in development, and residing in the peritoneal and pleural cavities. In mice, B1 cells produce polyreactive IgM antibodies. The natural autoantibodies produced by B1 cells are important in the clearance of apoptotic material, senescent red blood cells and other cellular and subcellular debris. In mice the subset of B1 cells has therefore been considered to be a bridge between innate with adaptive immunity.

B2 cells or conventional B cells comprise the adaptive portion of humoral immune responses. B2 cells participate preferentially in GC reactions, during which they can hypermutate their IgV gene rearrangements, switch Ig classes, and differentiate into memory cells and long-lived plasma cells. However, B2 cells can also be activated during TI responses. B2 cells are generated in the bone marrow where there are checkpoints for removal of autoreactive cells (central tolerance). The immature survivors with functional B-cell receptors leave the marrow where they are thought to be exposed to further negative selection to remove residual autoreactive clones (peripheral tolerance). Although it has not been delineated for humans, in mice, cells at this point are routed into either a mature follicular B cell or a marginal zone B cell (MZ-B) programme.[12] Follicular B cells traffic throughout the secondary lymphoid organs, whereas MZ-B cells are specialized to reside in a compartment in the spleen that samples the bloodstream for pathogens. Both B1 and MZ-B cells are key parts of the adaptive immune system that can be activated rapidly and respond immediately to pathogens in the blood as well as the peritoneal and pleural cavities.[13] Both their responses occur independent of T-cell help and they are thought to be excluded from undergoing GC reactions and undergo Ig switch recombination and somatic hypermutation poorly and do not generate long-lived plasma cells or B-cell memory. In contrast, B2 cells respond to TD antigens, participate in GC responses, undergo extensive class switch recombination and somatic hypermutation, and generate long-lived plasma cells and memory B cells.

Fine regulation of the immune system via inhibitory and activating receptors

In this context, innate immune cells such as monocytes, macrophages, immature DCs, mast cells and neutrophils constitutively express activating and inhibitory Fc receptors that contribute to a finely balanced innate immune response.[14,15] By contrast, T cells upregulate inhibitory receptors (PD-1, CTLA-4 etc.) after activation via antigen-presenting cells (APC).[16] Finally, B cells also express constitutively inhibitory (ICOS-L, FcRIIb, CD22) and activating receptors (FcRIIa, FcRIII, BCR). Although it remains to be further elucidated and translated into clinical application, B cells share a number of receptors expressed by cells of the innate immune system (including TLR, NLR, FcRIIb) and regulatory processes and therefore could be considered as a part of both the innate and adaptive immune systems.[17] This is notable, since at the same time they represent cells with a very sophisticated surface immunoglobulin receptor with the unique capacity to recognize the universe of antigens, including (1) three-dimensional structures and (2) post-translationally modified self-proteins such as glycoproteins and polysaccharides.[13]

Role of GC-dependent B-cell activation

Naive follicular B cells encounter antigens in the secondary lymphoid organs and, after receiving T-cell help, undergo proliferation and differentiation either into plasmablasts, plasma cells, or memory B cells.[18] Newly generated plasma cells emerge after 2–3 days, providing immediate responses to a pathogen[19] which can be detected between days 6–8 in peripheral blood of humans after secondary vaccination.[20] In mice, the initial immune response resulting in activation of antigen-specific B cells, local expansion, and the generation of short-lived plasma cells represents the extrafollicular immune response since the B cells involved migrate from the T cell–B cell interface through the bridging channels into the extrafollicular red pulp of the spleen. Subsequently in the T-cell-dependent (TD) immune response, activated B cells migrate into the B-cell follicle where a well-organized structure or 'immune unit', called a GC, is formed.[21] Establishment of these structures requires a number of precisely timed, fine-tuned cellular and humoral processes, including the action of T-follicular helper cells producing IL-21, the production of chemokines such as CXCL13, and the availability of follicular dendritic cells and antigen-specific T cells. In this regard, provision of CXCL13 by stroma cells and interaction with CXCR5 expressed by B cells and follicular helper T cells are important signals to navigate B cells into GCs where they can undergo clonal expansion and differentiation. These processes do not appear to be restricted to classical lymphoid organs and are also active in ectopic GCs, as shown for the role of CXCL13 for the RA synovium.[18,22] Once established, lymphotoxin β produced by B cells is involved in the differentiation of follicular dendritic cells into secondary lymphoid organs and the organization of an effective lymphoid architecture.

Role of B cells in animal arthritis models

B cells can function as APCs, as has been demonstrated by instructive data from animal models[23] in which a lupus-like disease developed when autoimmune-prone mice were reconstituted with B cells that lacked the ability to secrete Ig but not when they were deprived of B cells completely. Although these studies were performed in a murine lupus model, it provided data on antigen presentation by B cells.

The K/BxN model has raised particular interest for the potential role of humoral immunity in the development of arthritis.[24] In this model, spontaneous arthritis occurs in mice that express both the transgene-encoded KRN T-cell receptor and the IAg[7] MHC class II allele. The transgenic T cells have specificity for glucose-6-phosphate isomerase (G6PI) and are able to break tolerance in the B-cell compartment, resulting in the production of autoantibodies to G6PI. Affinity-purified anti-G6PI Ig from these mice can transfer joint specific inflammation to healthy recipient mice. G6PI bound to the surface of cartilage is the target for anti-G6PI binding and subsequent complement-mediated damage. However, analyses of anti-G6PI antibodies in the serum of RA patients indicate that these autoantibodies apparently do not play a significant role and confirm clearly the limitations of animal data for understanding the details of human disease.

Further involvement of B-cell activation has also been shown for antibody-mediated arthritis by coligation of TLR with the B-cell receptor (BCR) in collagen-induced arthritis with inflammatory joint destruction and CpG-induced TLR9 and BCR activation in adjuvant-induced arthritis.[25] Another model[26] was able to demonstrate the importance of antibodies against citrullinated α- and β-fibrinogen, providing additional evidence for the role of B cells and autoreactive Ig in inducing and maintaining arthritis. However, an additional murine model in which nominal antigen-expressing transgenic mice crossed to a specific T-cell receptor (TCR) developed inflammatory arthritis showed no role for B cells, in that arthritis developed when B cells were genetically absent.[27]

Role of B cells in rheumatoid arthritis

B cells are directly and indirectly involved in the regulation of certain parts of immune activation in RA. They can ultimately differentiate into antibody-producing cells known to produce IgM-rheumatoid factor (IgM-RF) and IgG-anti-CCP antibodies (ACPA) in 60–80% of patients. Higher RF and ACPA levels in synovial fluid vs serum, direct production of autoantibodies by cultured synovial organ cultures,[28] and differentiation of B cells into autoreactive plasma cells indicate that they are locally produced. Ig secretion within the synovium also results in local formation of immune complexes and activation of the complement cascade and the coagulation system with local production of anaphylatoxins and fibrin generation and induction of antibodies against citrullinated fibrin, but apparently requires a genetic predisposition of HLA-DR4 and PADI4,[29] each of which can contribute and amplify local inflammation.

Autoantibodies such IgM-RF and ACPA are the autoantibodies most frequently found in patients with RA and RF. Quantitative expression of these autoantibodies has been considered in the revised classification criteria of RA,[30] reflecting that production of autoantibodies ('humoral imprinting')[31] is associated with severe forms of RA. This emphasizes the role of the activated B-cell system in those patients.

Autoantibodies are usually taken as an indication of the breakdown of immune tolerance. The mechanisms of breaking immune tolerance are very complex, since IgM-RF usually occurs nonspecifically in many active inflammatory diseases and is associated with ageing, and therefore may have a quantitative threshold. ACPA are almost exclusively induced in patients with RA, although citrullination occurs non-specifically in many inflamed tissues,[32] and may therefore represent a qualitative biomarker of disease specific B-cell activation. Importantly, ACPA is directed against a surrogate autoantigen, being a cyclic ring of citrullinated amino acid residues that provides cross-reactivity to citrullinated antigens expressed in inflamed tissues. With regard to the citrullinated antigens expressed in inflamed sites, a central question is whether these are autoantigens or neoantigens that are widely expressed and to which there is no natural tolerance.

It remains unclear whether IgM-RF and IgG ACPA are generated using different forms of T-cell help. Moreover, RA patients also produce IgG-RF and IgA-RF which require class switch and likely are produced from progeny of B2 cells after costimulation by T cells. A substantial number of IgM-RF carries V_H gene rearrangements in germline configuration, which can frequently be found in lymphomas. By contrast, RA-associated RFs usually have somatically mutated V_H gene rearrangements and probably have developed using T-cell help. It is interesting to note that the production of ACPA is linked to the shared epitope of HLA-DR4 and PADI4 alleles, indicating that these autoantibodies are related to a defined MHC class II antigen in European patients.[32,33] Notably, this has not been found in patients in the United States.[34]

Induction of rheumatoid arthritis specific autoantibodies before the onset of disease

RF and/or anti-CCP can be found in about 50–70% of RA patients as much as 6–10 years before the onset of the clinical disease, indicating that the breakdown of immune tolerance in the B-cell system can be a very early step in disease pathogenesis.[35,36]

Seropositivity and diagnostic/therapeutic considerations

In addition to having a poorer prognosis and a greater tendency for erosive disease, it is interesting to note that patients who are positive for IgM-RF and ACPA-IgG have a two- to threefold higher likelihood to respond to B-cell depletion compared to seronegative RA patients.[3] The titre of IgM-RF decreases in about one-third of RA patients treated with B-cell-depleting therapy,[3] over varying time periods. ACPA also decreases with B-cell-depleting therapy,[37] suggesting that a portion of these specific autoantibodies derives from antibody-secreting cells that express CD20 on their surface directly or those plasma cells that require continuous replenishment from CD20+ B cells. It is likely that this subset of antibody-secreting cells is sensitive to a variety of other therapeutic agents, since glucocorticoids, methotrexate, gold,[31] and TNF blockers as well as abatacept have also been reported to reduce autoantibody levels.

Immunopathogenic functions of B cells potentially important in rheumatoid arthritis patients

Antigen presentation

Another important function of B cells is antigen presentation. This activity is especially expressed by memory B cells, and is facilitated by expression of high-avidity BCR and also MHC class II molecules on their surface.[38,39] Despite the efficiency of antigen uptake, memory B cells appear to be most effective at presenting antigen and stimulating memory T cells, whereas dendritic cells are the preferred APCs for initiating responses of naive T cells.

Antigen presentation mediated by MHC class II can be performed by cognate B cells after receiving help by autoreactive T cells that in turn have been activated by mature DCs. Thus, antigen presentation by B cells, in particular by memory B cells, may be important in the amplification and maintenance of autoimmunity after it has been initiated. In this context, enlarged pools of memory B cells have been found in RA patients,[40] and delayed repopulation of pre- and post-switched memory B cells was associated with long-term response after treatment with rituximab.[41] Since normalization of memory B-cell frequencies has also been observed under successful TNF blockade[42,43] and IL-6R inhibition,[44] this subpopulation appears to be an important amplifier of RA immunopathogenesis.

Production of proinflammatory cytokines

B cells also produce proinflammatory cytokines, such as TNF and interleukin (IL)-6, and immunoregulatory cytokines, such as IL-10. The cytokines produced by activated B cells may influence the function of antigen-presenting DCs.[17] Proinflammatory cytokines, such as TNF and IL-6, may activate macrophages, amplifying the proinflammatory signal and resulting in enhanced levels of IL-1, IL-6, and additional TNF. Although IL-6 itself is an important cytokine for B-cell growth, BAFF produced by synovial fibroblasts and regulated by TNF and IFNγ also can maintain RA synovial B cells.[45] Another important cytokine produced by B cells is IL-10, which is able to activate DCs to be more effective APCs, and with the help of T cells, to enhance the differentiation of B cells into plasma cells. The extent to which cytokines produced by B cells contribute to certain steps in immune activation in general, as well as for RA in particular, is unknown.

In addition, B cells are indirectly involved in the production of cytokines, as indicated by the loss of Th17 cells after rituximab treatment.[46] Moreover, there is a close interrelationship between B cells and bone cells. B cells differentiate from haematopoietic stem cells in defined niches of endosteal bone areas where osteoblasts support haematopoietic stem cells (HSC) and B-cell differentiation.[47] A series of transcription factors regulates B-cell differentiation residing in these niches, and the same transcription factors appear also to be involved in maintenance of the bone phenotype based on relationships between macrophage/osteoclast and B cell differentiation. Notably, an important factor connecting B cells and bone cells is the RANKL-RANK system, with a reciprocal effect on their differentiation. It has been found that activated B cells exert a number of bony changes based on their inflammatory roles and therefore at least appear to be involved in radiographic progression in RA.

Dendritic cell differentiation and organization of the lymphatic architecture

B cells also regulate follicular DC differentiation and the organization of the lymphatic architecture. Mice that lack B cells do not develop antigen-presenting M cells in the gut. B cells are also involved in the regulation of T-cell activation, anergy, differentiation, and the expansion of T cells. B cells play an important role in T-cell activation. In humans, this conclusion is supported by recent studies in patients with systemic lupus erythematosus (SLE) that demonstrated a deactivation of T cells after selective B-cell depletion,[48] but it has not yet been shown for RA patients. However, data from experiments in which synovial tissue was transplanted into *scid*/NOD mice[49] showed that B-cell depletion by rituximab caused a substantial downregulation of T-cell activation and reduction in IFNγ occurred. These data suggest that synovial B cells are necessary for T-cell activation.

Formation of ectopic germinal centre

It is known that memory B cells and plasma cells reside in the RA synovium[50] in proximity to ectopic GCs in the affected tissue. Aggregates of CD20+ B cells have been identified in synovial tissue in about one-third of patients with RA,[50] surrounded by T cells and follicular dendritic cells (FDCs) within these GC-like structures. The role of these FDCs has not been intensively studied in the RA synovium. Specifically, it is not known whether they have the full capacity to select antigen-reactive cells appropriately as in typical GCs. Notably, ectopic GCs are detectable in only about 25–35% of RA patients, whereas there is only moderate infiltration or even slight infiltration in the remaining patients.[51] These aggregates have been found in a variety of autoimmune conditions, although it remains to be shown if these structures alone can drive autoimmunity independent of classic GCs. Although it cannot be formally excluded that synovial B and plasma cells have migrated into the site of inflammation, the presence of these cells in RA synovium likely reflects local generation in ectopic GC. Whereas higher RF levels in the synovial fluid than in blood argue for the primary role of GCs in the synovial membrane, detection of various clones of plasma cells and even the presence of anti-tetanus specific plasma

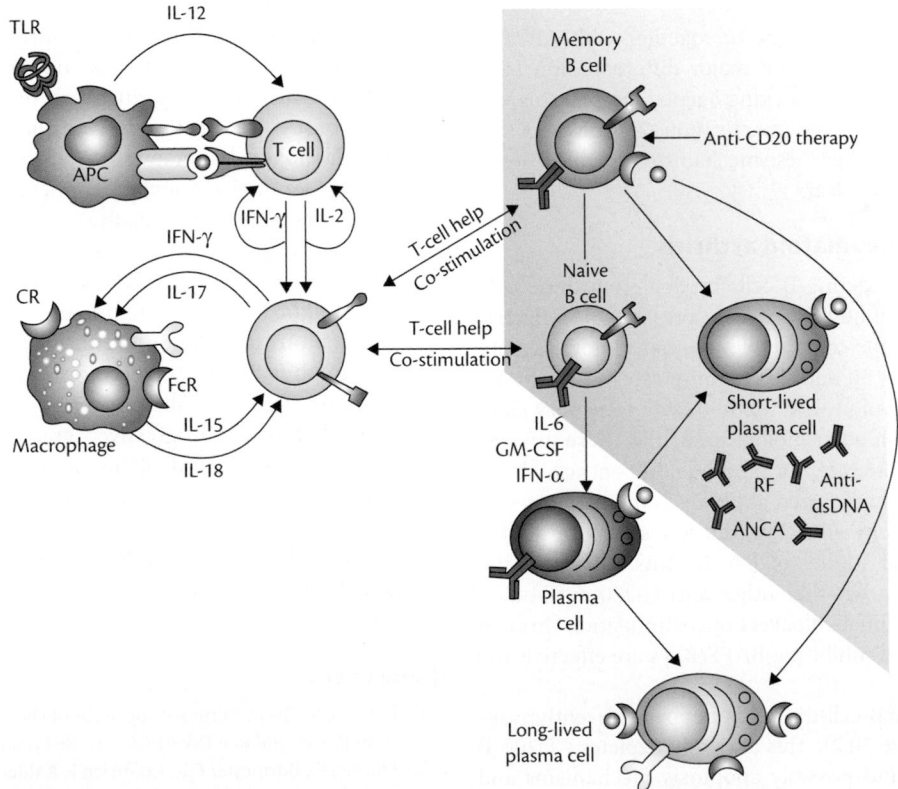

Fig. 50.2 Targets of anti-CD20 antibody therapy. Interactions between APCs and T cells are important during activation of the adaptive immune system, which leads to activation of B2 cells; the resultant memory B cells (reactive memory) and plasma cells (humoral memory) are long-lived and persist independent of the presence of antigen. Anti-CD20 antibody therapy leads to depletion of CD20+ B cells, which thereby affects memory B cells and blocks the generation of short-lived plasma cells (as highlighted by the shading in this figure). ANCA, antineutrophil cytoplasmic antibodies; APC, antigen-presenting cell; CR, complement receptor; dsDNA, double-stranded DNA; FcR, Fc receptor; GM-CSF, granulocyte-macrophage colony-stimulating factor; IL, interleukin; IFN, interferon; RF, rheumatoid factor; Th1, type 1 T helper cell; TLR, Toll-like receptor.
Dorner T, Radbruch A, Burmester GR. B-cell-directed therapies for autoimmune disease. Nature Reviews Rheumatology 2009 Aug;5(8):433–41.

cells after systemic tetanus vaccination[52] suggest that the synovial membrane may be a site of immigration of at least some plasma cells after egress from a distant site of induction, possibly the lymph nodes. Available data indicate that the formation of ectopic GCs in the RA synovium is a typical but not an essential finding of autoimmunity. One possibility is that they represent exaggerated local immune reactions, but whether the presence of these structures correlates with disease activity is not known.

Mechanisms of T-cell-independent B-cell activation and B-cell survival factors in rheumatoid arthritis

BAFF/BLyS and possibly APRIL (a proliferation-inducing ligand) which belong to the TNF family caused increased survival of most B-cell subsets as well as plasma cells. Enhanced BAFF levels could contribute to prolonged survival of autoreactive cells which otherwise would be deleted. BAFF/BLyS and APRIL, therefore, may lead to a vicious cycle of continuous antibody-mediated inflammation and tissue destruction. Fibroblast-like synoviocytes of mesenchymal origin express functional BAFF/BLyS in response to proinflammatory cytokines (TNF, IFNγ) in the synovium of patients with RA.[45] Notably, however, BAFF transgenic mice[53] develop autoimmunity, including Sjögren's-like disease, but they do not develop arthritis. BAFF/BLyS levels in autoimmune diseases, such as Sjögren's syndrome, SLE, and RA were found to be significantly increased and BAFF/BLyS levels in the RA synovial fluid are higher than in the blood.[54] Whether this increase reflects the degree of inflammation or is a primary factor in disease pathogenesis, especially in RA, is not known.

Studies blocking BAFF/BLyS alone or together with APRIL[55] in patients with RA did not show a major differentiation from placebo as with other cytokine blocking agents. Despite this, the degree to which BAFF is involved in activation or survival of certain B-cell subsets, and whether these mechanisms are operative in RA patients, is currently not clear.

Targeting B cells in rheumatoid arthritis

Recent data show that targeting B cells by depleting these cells using an anti-CD20 antibody, rituximab, provides an effective therapy with a safety profile comparable to other biologic agents. Interestingly, the ACR20, 50 and 70 response rates when rituximab was used in combination with methotrexate were very similar to those observed with other biologics, such as those directed toward TNF, IL-1, and IL-6 receptor blockade. In contrast, blocking BAFF/BLyS with the humanized antibody belimumab, as well as blocking BLys/APRIL by atacicept, did not show substantial improvements in clinical studies of RA patients. Other studies are under way, exploring whether other anti-CD20 antibodies, such as TRU015, ofatumumab, blockers of costimulation through CD80/86 by RhuDex, and inhibiting BAFF/BLys are effective and safe in RA treatment.[31]

The broadest data set of B-cell-directed therapy is currently available for rituximab (Figure 50.2). This antibody depletes CD20+ B cells by ADCC, CDC, and possibly apoptosis mechanisms and therefore does not target CD20 pro B cells and subsets of CD20 human plasma cells. With regard to apoptosis, it is notably that it occurs in vitro after binding to CD20, a molecule with a hitherto unknown function. On the other hand, anti-CD20 effects are inhibited in FcR KO mice,[56] which suggests that the 'workhorse' of rituximab is probably ADCC.

Repletion of B cells occurs within 6–8 months, although there is a trend that subsequent courses lead to longer-lasting periods of B-cell depletion, i.e. an increase from 7.5 months after the first cycle to 8.1 months after the second cycle of treatment.[41] Repletion of CD20+ B cells is also characterized by modulation of B-cell subsets with a preferential recurrence of naive B cells and a delay in the recurrence of memory B cells. In particular, the reduction of memory B cells is very striking and may reflect a 'resetting' of the immune system similar to that observed after autologous stem cell transplantation in SLE. It has also been reported that early recurrence of CD27+ memory B cells was associated with a significantly higher likelihood of an early RA flare as compared to patients maintaining predominantly naive B cells.[41] Constant production of IgA plasmablasts during peripheral B-cell depletion has been identified,[57] indicating that their precursors, which likely reside in the lamina propria, are resistant to RTX depletion.

One concern about B-cell depletion has been the consequence of depletion on protective antibody titres. There are a number of reports that have shown that anti-tetanus and anti-pneumococcus antibody titres remain stable although primary responses to pneumococcus are diminished,[37] whereas there is a decline in IgM-RF along with IgG ACPA with rituximab therapy. The difference between the protective antibody titres versus autoantibody titres is very striking. One explanation could be that the responsible plasma cell subsets are different in terms of their half-life, survival conditions, their ability to be mobilized, or their CD20 expression density.

An important consideration not only restricted to anti-CD20 therapy involves appropriate vaccination as recommended.[58,59] Patients with RA receiving rituximab have been investigated for their response to vaccination in two studies.[60,61] Any patient considered for rituximab therapy should receive all indicated vaccines (hepatitis B for at-risk population, pneumococcus, tetanus toxoid every 10 years, influenza annually) before treatment.

In one study,[37] an increase of the autoantibodies was seen before the recurrence of active RA. However, it should be noted that the declines in IgM-RF titres were initially very similar in the control group (methotrexate alone) and the patients treated with rituximab (in combination with methotrexate) likely because of the use of high-dose steroids in the first 17 days,[62] but this decrease was more long lasting and progressively greater in the latter group. The apparent effect of B-cell depletion and methotrexate on RF titres became also apparent in that patients treated with the combination of rituximab and methotrexate compared to rituximab alone[62] had substantially longer periods of RF reduction. This confirms the complexity of RA and indicates the need for effective combination therapy.

References

1. Panayi GS. The immunopathogenesis of rheumatoid arthritis (Reprinted from *Rheumatol Rev* 1992;1:63–74). *Br J Rheumatol* 1993;32:4–14.
2. Horneff G, Burmester GR, Emmrich F, Kalden JR. Treatment of rheumatoid arthritis with an anti-CD4 monoclonal antibody. *Arthritis Rheum* 1991;34(2):129–140.
3. Cohen SB, Emery P, Greenwald MW et al. Rituximab for rheumatoid arthritis refractory to anti-tumor necrosis factor therapy—Results of a multicenter, randomized, double-blind, placebo-controlled, phase III trial evaluating primary efficacy and safety at twenty-four weeks. *Arthritis Rheum* 2006 Sep;54(9):2793–2806.

4. Lipsky PE. Systemic lupus erythematosus: an autoimmune disease of B cell hyperactivity. *Nature Immunol* 2001;2(9):764–766.

5. Hammarlund E, Lewis MW, Hansen SG et al. Duration of antiviral immunity after smallpox vaccination. *Nature Med* 2003;9(9):1131–1137.

6. Manz RA, Thiel A, Radbruch A. Lifetime of plasma cells in the bone marrow. *Nature* 1997;388(6638):133–134.

7. Dorner T, Radbruch A. Antibodies and B cell memory in viral immunity. *Immunity* 2007;27(3):384–392.

8. Withers DR, Fiorini C, Fischer RT et al. T cell-dependent survival of CD20(+) and CD20(-) plasma cells in human secondary lymphoid tissue. *Blood* 2007;109(11):4856–4864.

9. Warnatz K, Peter HH. [Classification and diagnosis of immunodeficiency syndromes]. *Internist* 2004;45(8):868–881.

10. Griffin DG, Holodick NE, Rothstein TL. Human B1 cells in umbilical cord and adult peripheral blood express the novel phenotype CD20+ CD27+ TD43+ CD70. *J Exp Med* 2011;208(1):67–80.

11. Lee J, Kuchen S, Fischer R, Chang S, Lipsky PE. Identification and characterization of a human CD5(+) pre-naive B cell population. *J Immunol* 2009;182(7):4116–4126.

12. Tarlinton D, Radbruch A, Hiepe F, Dorner T. Plasma cell differentiation and survival. *Curr Opin Immunol* 2008;20(2):162–169.

13. Dörner T, Jacobi AM, Lipsky PE. B cells in autoimmunity. *Arthritis Res Ther* 2009;11(5):247.

14. Nimmerjahn F, Ravetch JV. Fc-receptors as regulators of immunity. *Adv Immunol* 2007;96:179–204.

15. Vivier E, Nunes JA, Vely F. Natural killer cell signaling pathways. *Science* 2004;306(5701):1517–1519.

16. Rudd CE, Taylor A, Schneider H. CD28 and CTLA-4 coreceptor expression and signal transduction. *Immunol Rev* 2009;229:12–26.

17. Dorner T, Lipsky PE. B-cell targeting: a novel approach to immune intervention today and tomorrow. *Expert Opin Biol Ther* 2007;7(9):1287–1299.

18. Radbruch A, Muehlinghaus G, Luger EO et al. Competence and competition: the challenge of becoming a long-lived plasma cell. *Nat Rev Immunol* 2006 Oct;6(10):741–750.

19. McHeyzer-Williams LJ, McHeyzer-Williams MG. Antigen-specific memory B cell development. *Annu Rev Immunol* 2005;23:487–513.

20. Odendahl M, Mei H, Hoyer BF et al. Generation of migratory antigen-specific plasma blasts and mobilization of resident plasma cells in a secondary immune response. *Blood* 2005;105(4):1614–1621.

21. Manser T. Textbook germinal centers? *J Immunol* 2004;172(6):3369–3375.

22. Manz RA, Arce S, Cassese G et al. Humoral immunity and long-lived plasma cells. *Curr Opin Immunol* 2002;14(4):517–521.

23. Chan OTM, Hannum LG, Haberman AM, Madaio MP, Shlomchik MJ. A novel mouse with B cells but lacking serum antibody reveals an antibody-independent role for B cells in murine lupus. *J Exp Med* 1999;189(10):1639–1647.

24. Matsumoto I, Staub A, Benoist C, Mathis D. Arthritis provoked by linked T and B cell recognition of a glycolytic enzyme. *Science* 1999;286(5445):1732–1735.

25. Ronaghy A, Prakken BJ, Takabayashi K et al. Immunostimulatory DNA sequences influence the course of adjuvant arthritis. *J Immunol* 2002;168(1):51–56.

26. Ho PP, Lee LY, Zhao XY et al. Autoimmunity against fibrinogen mediates inflammatory arthritis in mice. *J Immunol* 2010;184(1):379–390.

27. Rankin AL, Reed AJ, Oh S et al. CD4(+) T cells recognizing a single self-peptide expressed by APCs induce spontaneous autoimmune arthritis. *J Immunol* 2008;180(10):7047.

28. Wernick R, Merryman P, Jaffe I, Ziff M. IgG and IgM rheumatoid factors in rheumatoid arthritis—quantitative response to penicillamine therapy and relationship to disease activity. *Arthritis Rheum* 1983;26(5):593–598.

29. Delvaeye M, Conway EM. Coagulation and innate immune responses: can we view them separately? *Blood* 2009;114(12):2367–2374.

30. Aletaha D, Neogi T, Silman AJ et al. 2010 Rheumatoid arthritis classification criteria: an American College of Rheumatology/European League Against Rheumatism collaborative initiative. *Ann Rheum Dis* 2010;69(9):1580–1588.

31. Dorner T, Radbruch A, Burmester GR. B-cell-directed therapies for autoimmune disease. *Nat Rev Rheumatol* 2009;5(8):433–441.

32. Klareskog L, Ronnelid J, Lundberg K, Padyukov L, Adfredsson L. Immunity to citrullinated proteins in rheumatoid arthritis. *Annu Rev Immunol* 2008;26:651–675.

33. Klareskog L, Catrina AI, Paget S. Rheumatoid arthritis. *Lancet* 2009;373(9664):659–672.

34. Lee HS, Lee AT, Criswell LA et al. Several regions in the major histocompatibility complex confer risk for anti-CCP-antibody positive rheumatoid arthritis, independent of the DRB1 locus. *Mol Med* 2008;14(5–6):293–300.

35. van Gaalen FA, van Aken J, Huizinga TWJ et al. Association between HLA class II genes and autoantibodies to cyclic citrullinated peptides (CCPs) influences the severity of rheumatoid arthritis. *Arthritis Rheum* 2004;50(7):2113–2121.

36. van Gaalen FA, Linn-Rasker SP, van Venrooij WJ et al. Autoantibodies to cyclic citrullinated peptides predict progression to rheumatoid arthritis in patients with undifferentiated arthritis—a prospective cohort study. *Arthritis Rheum* 2004;50(3):709–715.

37. Cambridge G, Leandro MJ, Edwards JCW et al. Serologic changes following B lymphocyte depletion therapy for rheumatoid arthritis. *Arthritis Rheum* 2003;48(8):2146–2154.

38. Bernasconi NL, Traggiai E, Lanzavecchia A. Maintenance of serological memory by polyclonal activation of human memory B cells. *Science* 2002;298(5601):2199–2202.

39. Bernasconi NL, Onai N, Lanzavecchia A. A role for Toll-like receptors in acquired immunity: up-regulation of TLR9 by BCR triggering in naive B cells and constitutive expression in memory B cells. *Blood* 2003;101(11):4500–4504.

40. Henneken M, Dorner T, Burmester GR, Berek C. Differential expression of chemokine receptors on peripheral blood B cells from patients with rheumatoid arthritis and systemic lupus erythematosus. *Arthritis Res Ther* 2005;7(5):R1001–R1013.

41. Roll P, Dorner T, Tony HP. Anti-CD20 therapy in patients with rheumatoid arthritis—predictors of response and B cell subset regeneration after repeated treatment. *Arthritis Rheum* 2008;58(6):1566–1575.

42. Souto-Carneiro MM, Mahadevan V, Takada K et al. Alterations in peripheral blood memory B cells in patients with active rheumatoid arthritis are dependent on the action of tumour necrosis factor. *Arthritis Res Ther* 2009;11(3):R84.

43. Anolik JH, Ravikumar R, Barnard J et al. Cutting edge: Anti-tumor necrosis factor therapy in rheumatoid arthritis inhibits memory B lymphocytes via effects on lymphoid germinal centers and follicular dendritic cell networks. *J Immunol* 2008;180(2):688–692.

44. Roll P, Muhammad K, Schumann M et al. In vivo effects of the anti-interleukin-6 receptor inhibitor tocilizumab on the B cell compartment. *Arthritis Rheum* 2011;63(5):1255–1264.

45. Ohata J, Zvaifler NJ, Nishio M et al. Fibroblast-like synoviocytes of mesenchymal origin express functional B cell-activating factor of the TNF family in response to proinflammatory cytokines. *J Immunol* 2005;174(2):864–870.

46. van de Veerdonk FL, Lauwerys B, DiPadova F et al. The anti-CD20 antibody rituximab reduces the Th17 response. *Cytokine* 2009;48(1–2):98.

47. Horowitz MC, Fretz JA, Lorenzo JA. How B cells influence bone biology in health and disease. *Bone* 2010;47(3):472–479.

48. Tokunaga M, Saito K, Kawabata D et al. Efficacy of rituximab (anti-CD20] for refractory systemic lupus erythematosus involving the central nervous system. *Ann Rheum Dis* 2007;66(4):470–475.

49. Takemura S, Klimiuk PA, Braun A, Goronzy JJ, Weyand CM. T cell activation in rheumatoid synovium is B cell dependent. *J Immunol* 2001;167(8):4710–4718.

50. Schroder AE, Greiner A, Seyfert C, Berek C. Differentiation of B cells in the nonlymphoid tissue of the synovial membrane of patients with rheumatoid arthritis. *Proc Natl Acad Sci U S A* 1996;93(1):221–225.

51. Krenn V, Souto-Carneiro MM, Kim HJ et al. Histopathology and molecular pathology of synovial B-lymphocytes in rheumatoid arthritis. *Histol Histopathol* 2000;15(3):791–798.

52. Fryauff DJ, Mouzin E, Church LWP et al. Lymphocyte response to tetanus toxin T-cell epitopes: effects of tetanus vaccination and concurrent malaria prophylaxis. *Vaccine* 1999;17(1):59–63.

53. Groom J, Kalled SL, Cutler AH et al. Association of BAFF/BLyS overexpression and altered B cell differentiation with Sjogren's syndrome. *J Clin Invest* 2002;109(1):59–68.

54. Stohl W, Scholz JL, Cancro MP. Targeting BLyS in rheumatic disease: the sometimes-bumpy road from bench to bedside. *Curr Opin Rheumatol* 2011;23(3):305–310.

55. Tak PP, Thurlings RA, Rossier C et al. Atacicept in patients with rheumatoid arthritis. *Arthritis Rheum* 2008;58(1):61–72.

56. Uchida JJ, Hamaguchi Y, Oliver JA et al. The innate mononuclear phagocyte network depletes B lymphocytes through Fc receptor-dependent mechanisms during anti-CD20 antibody immunotherapy. *J Exp Med* 2004;199(12):1659–1669.

57. Mei HE, Frolich D, Giesecke C et al. Steady-state generation of mucosal IgA(+) plasmablasts is not abrogated by B-cell depletion therapy with rituximab. *Blood* 2010;116(24):5181–5190.

58. Buch MH, Smolen JS, Betteridge N et al. Updated consensus statement on the use of rituximab in patients with rheumatoid arthritis. *Ann Rheum Dis* 2011;70(6):909–920.

59. van Assen S, Agmon-Levin N, Elkayam O et al. EULAR recommendations for vaccination in adult patients with autoimmune inflammatory rheumatic diseases. *Ann Rheum Dis* 2011;70(3):414–422.

60. van Assen S, Holvast A, Benne CA et al. Humoral responses after influenza vaccination are severely reduced in patients with rheumatoid arthritis treated with rituximab. *Arthritis Rheum* 2010;62(1):75–81.

61. Bingham CO, Looney RJ, Deodhar A et al. Immunization responses in rheumatoid arthritis patients treated with rituximab results from a controlled clinical trial. *Arthritis Rheum* 2010;62(1):64–74.

62. Edwards JCW, Cambridge G. B-cell targeting in rheumatoid arthritis and other autoimmune diseases. *Nat Rev Immunol* 2006;6(5):394–403.

CHAPTER 51

Fibroblasts and mesenchymal cells

Andrew Filer, Maria Juarez, and
Christopher Buckley

Introduction

Mesenchymal cell precursors, i.e. mesenchymal stem cells (MSC) or mesenchymal progenitor cells (MPC), are spindle-shaped cells connected to other cells in three-dimensional matrices. Mesenchymal precursor cells are able to differentiate into tissue fibroblasts, and also osteoblasts, adipocytes, chondroblasts, or myoblasts, a property termed pluripotentiality. In embryological development MSC migrate regionally, giving rise to specific tissues. The recognition that MSC and fibroblasts share morphological and functional features (including pluripotentiality) has led to the suggestion that they may indeed be the same cell type. Indeed the current definition of MSC suggested by the International Society of Cellular Therapy is incapable of distinguishing such cells from generic fibroblasts (for review see Uccelli et al.[1]).

Origin of fibroblasts

In this chapter we concentrate on the fibroblast as the prototype stromal cell. However, the stroma also consists of blood and lymphatic vessels and a wider definition of stromal cells might include endothelial cells, pericytes, and even tissue resident macrophages.

Origin in tissues

The question of the local origin of fibroblasts is an important one. Both inflammation and wound healing are characterized by formation of new tissue. There is growing evidence that fibroblasts exist as subsets of cells, often with different functions. Novel markers have recently been identified that start to demarcate such subsets with distinct functional roles.

Upon appropriate stimulation, fibroblasts can proliferate locally to regenerate new cells. However, fibroblasts may arise from other sources (Figure 51.1). The first of these is local epithelial–mesenchymal transition (EMT): upon epithelial stress such as inflammation or injury, epithelial cells lose polarity, and rearrange their F-actin fibres, transforming into mobile mesenchymal cells.

Secondly, recent research has confirmed the presence of circulating cells of a mesenchymal phenotype. These cells bear a remarkable resemblance to the synovial fibroblasts isolated from the joints of patients with rheumatoid arthritis (RA), which accumulate in enormous quantities in the inflamed joint despite little evidence of proliferation. Interestingly, Marinova-Mutafchieva and colleagues have shown that an influx of such cells precedes inflammation in a collagen-induced mouse arthritis model, suggesting a role for blood-borne stromal cell precursors in the initiation of inflammatory diseases.[2] Another circulating precursor that could account for accumulation of fibroblasts in disease is the fibrocyte. Fibrocytes elaborate matrix once in tissue, but arise from the CD14+ (monocyte) fraction in peripheral blood, and have been shown to rapidly enter sites of tissue injury and contribute to tissue remodelling in models of inflammatory lung disease.[3]

Fibroblast identity and microenvironments

Until recently, fibroblasts had been thought of as generic cells with a common phenotype. However, there is now evidence that fibroblasts from different organs have unique morphology and unique repertoires of extracellular matrix (ECM) proteins, cytokines, and chemokines. Transcriptional profiling of human fibroblasts has shown large-scale differences related to three anatomical divisions: anterior–posterior, proximal–distal, and dermal–non-dermal.[4] Recent evidence confirms epigenetic changes as effectors of these differing phenotypes. Epigenetic changes are hereditable changes in gene expression that do not result from alteration of the underlying DNA sequence.[5] They are 'switches' that control gene expression determining whether a particular gene is expressed ('on') or not ('off'). In healthy fibroblasts, expression of a non-coding RNA (termed HOTAIR) residing in the HOXC locus results in silencing of genes in the HOXD locus that are responsible for positional identity. This provides proof of epigenetic control of site-specific gene expression in fibroblasts. However there is now increasing evidence for epigenetic regulation of disease phenotypes in many cells, including fibroblasts.

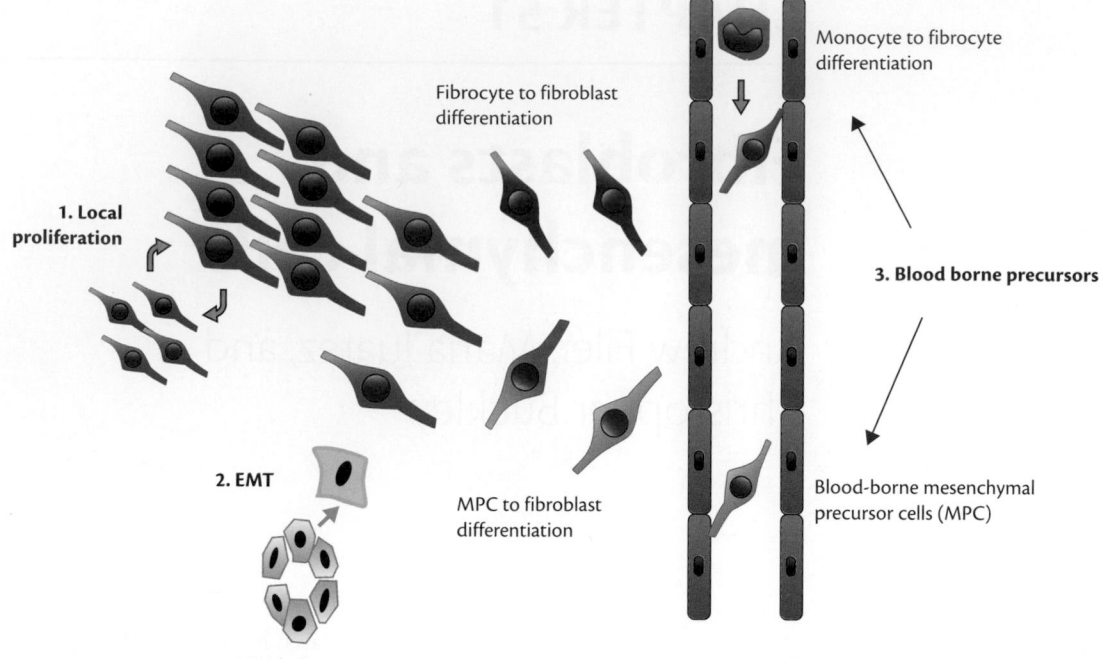

Fig. 51.1 In response to persistent inflammation, increased numbers of fibroblasts accumulate within tissues: (1) Fibroblasts may proliferate locally to regenerate new cells. (2) Epithelial–mesenchymal transition: following stress, epithelial cells lose polarity and rearrange F-actin fibres transforming into mobile mesenchymal cells. (3) Blood-borne mesenchymal precursor cells may be recruited to tissues and undergo local differentiation to fibroblasts. Fibrocytes arise from the monocyte fraction of blood and then differentiate into fibroblasts within tissues.

Fibroblasts in physiology

Production, interaction, and degradation of extracellular matrix

Ensuring ECM homeostasis is one of the primary functions of fibroblasts. To fulfil this role, fibroblasts are able to produce and degrade ECM, as well as adhering to and interacting with ECM components.

Production of extracellular matrix

Fibroblasts produce a number of ECM molecules that are assembled into a 3-dimensional network. This provides a framework through which other cell types can move, a substrate for the deposition of haptotactic chemokine gradients, and stores of growth factors to direct cellular movement and behaviour in a regional fashion.[6] ECM molecular repertoires differ between tissues, reflecting fibroblast diversity. For example, dermal fibroblasts produce significant amounts of type VII collagen while fibroblasts in lung and kidney produce mainly interstitial, fibrillar collagens (types I and III).

Interaction with extracellular matrix

Integrins are key mediators of cell–matrix and cell–cell adhesive interactions. They are the main family of adhesion molecules responsible for the attachment of fibroblasts to collagen, fibronectin and vitronectin. Syndecans allow interaction with a large variety of ligands including fibroblast growth factors, vascular endothelial growth factor (VEGF), transforming growth factor beta (TGFβ), and ECM molecules such as fibronectin.

Degradation of extracellular matrix

Remodelling of the ECM requires fibroblasts to express an extensive repertoire of matrix-degrading enzymes with varying specificity.

These are crucial to tissue maintenance and repair, but inappropriate overexpression can result in joint damage in arthritis. Such enzymes fall into a number of families including matrix metalloproteinases (MMPs), tissue inhibitors of metalloproteinases (TIMPs), cathepsins, and aggrecanases. With the exception of MMP-2 and the membrane-type MMPs (MT-MMPs) which are constitutively expressed, MMP expression is regulated by extracellular signals via transcriptional activation in fibroblasts. The major groups of inducers are proinflammatory cytokines such as interleukin (IL)-1, growth factors such as fibroblast growth factor (FGF) and platelet-derived growth factor (PDGF), and matrix molecules including collagen, fibronectin, and their degradation products.[7]

Wound healing and tissue repair

Tissue injury and wound healing are accompanied by changes in the ECM, serum exposure, mechanical stress. and inflammation. These stimuli activate fibroblasts to become myofibroblasts, with expression of smooth muscle actin and secretion of high levels of ECM proteases (e.g. MMP2, MMP3, and MMP4), leading to increased ECM turnover and modified ECM composition. Growth factors (e.g. hepatocyte growth factor, FGF) that induce proliferative signals within adjacent epithelial cells are also secreted. Myofibroblasts proliferate more than their normal counterparts, but once the wound is repaired their number decreases and the resting phenotype is restored. However, evidence is accumulating that in fibrosis and cancer, fibroblasts abnormally maintain a myofibroblast phenotype resulting in organ damage, with underlying epigenetic changes driving persistence.[8]

Fibroblasts in immunity

Fibroblasts are capable of elaborating a broad repertoire of inflammatory mediators, which fully justifies their classification as immune sentinel cells. Through expression of Toll-like receptors (TLR) 2, 3, and 4, fibroblasts respond to bacterial products such as lipopolysaccharide (LPS) by activating the classical NFκB and AP-1 inflammatory pathways, generating chemokines capable of recruiting inflammatory cells, and MMPs capable of degrading matrix. Furthermore, fibroblasts are capable of bridging innate and adaptive immune responses through expression of the molecule CD40. Engagement of CD40 by its ligand CD40L expressed on a restricted population of immune cells including activated T lymphocytes is critical for the further induction of proinflammatory cytokines and chemokines from fibroblasts during an immune response.

Fibroblast-like synoviocytes in normal synovium

The normal synovium provides an excellent example of fibroblast heterogeneity within tissues. In health, the synovium is a thin structure divided into two layers: the lining and the sublining. The lining layer is a 1–2 cell thick layer formed in roughly equal proportions of CD68+ type A macrophage-like synoviocytes and type B mesenchymal, fibroblast-like synoviocytes. The sublining layer is composed of less densely packed fibroblasts and macrophages in a loose tissue matrix along with blood vessel networks. Fibroblasts of the lining layer express a number of cellular markers, including CD55 (decay accelerating factor, DAF), (vascular cell adhesion molecule-1 (VCAM-1), uridine diphosphoglucose dehydrogenase (UDPGD), and the novel marker GP38 (also expressed in sublining lymphatic cells and pericytes). Sublining fibroblasts express the non-specific cellular marker CD90 (also expressed by endothelial cells) and the recently discovered marker CD248 (also expressed by pericytes). Fibroblasts of the lining layer subserve a barrier function that is unsupported by a basement membrane, conventional tight junctions or desmosomes; instead, the strong homophilic/homotypic adhesion between synoviocytes is mediated by cadherin-11.[9]

Fibroblasts in rheumatoid arthritis

Persistence of inflammation within joints is a hallmark feature of RA. Although it is recognized that in RA persistent inflammation results from complex interactions between haematopoietic and stromal cells, research into the pathogenesis of the disease has traditionally concentrated on cells and cytokines of the immune system, neglecting the role of stromal cells. As a consequence, biological treatments have been developed that have led to a step-change in the management of the disease. Nevertheless, these treatments neither reverse tissue damage nor lead to disease cure. At best they induce a significant clinical response (ACR70) in less than 60% of patients, most of whom will relapse on treatment withdrawal, suggesting that additional therapeutic targets, responsible for persistence of inflammation, remain to be discovered. An increasing body of evidence implicates RA synovial fibroblasts in driving the persistent and destructive characteristics of the disease.

RA synovial fibroblasts exhibit a persistent, activated phenotype that is maintained in the absence of exogenous stimulation and remains stable even after multiple passages in vitro. Activated RA synovial fibroblasts (RASFs) play crucial roles in determining the site at which inflammation occurs, and in the subsequent maintenance of persistent inflammation, and are key mediators of cartilage and bone destruction.

Fibroblasts and the switch to persistent disease

In order for an inflammatory lesion to resolve, dead or redundant cells that were recruited and expanded during the active phases of the response must be removed. The 'switch to resolution' is an important signal that permits tissue repair to take place and enables immune cells to return to draining lymphoid nodes in order for immunological memory to become established. However, in RA, fibroblasts become persistently activated, leading to tissue-specific initiation and subsequent relapse of chronic persistent inflammatory disease; effectively a 'switch to persistence'.

The synovial microenvironment in rheumatoid arthritis

In RA, the synovium undergoes radical change. The lining layer undergoes dramatic hyperplasia, becoming a mass of 'pannus' tissue rich in fibroblasts, macrophages, and osteoclasts, which aggressively invades the adjacent articular cartilage and subchondral bone. The sublining layer also undergoes expansion, with huge infiltrates of inflammatory cells (macrophages, T and B cells, mast cells, plasma cells and dendritic cells). T and B lineage cells may remain in diffuse infiltrates, or may coalesce into aggregates of cells varying from simple perivascular 'cuffs' to structures resembling B-cell follicles in up to 20% of samples (tertiary lymphoid structures).[10] In this abnormal microenvironment, activated RASFs actively maintain chronic inflammation by distorting the homeostatic balance between leukocyte recruitment, proliferation, emigration, and death (Figure 51.2).

Recruitment of inflammatory infiltrates into the joint

Activated RASFs produce inflammatory chemokines implicated in leukocyte recruitment to diseased synovium. Neutrophil attracting chemokines are expressed at high levels by stimulated fibroblasts and include CXCL8 (IL-8), CXCL5, and CXCL1.[11] Monocytes and T cells are recruited by a range of chemokines found at high levels in the synovium; CXCL10 and CXCL9 are highly expressed in synovial tissue and fluid. CXCL16 is also highly expressed in the RA synovium and acts as a potent chemoattractant for T cells. CCL2 is found in synovial fluid and known to be produced by synovial fibroblasts; it is considered to be a pivotal chemokine for the recruitment of monocytes. CCL3, CCL4, and CCL5 (RANTES) are chemotactic for monocytes and lymphocytes, and are products of synovial fibroblasts. CX3CL1 (Fractalkine) is also widely expressed in the rheumatoid synovium. The expression of some chemokine receptors differs between peripheral blood and synovial leucocytes, suggesting enrichment in the synovium either through selective recruitment by chemokines, or following upregulation by the microenvironment after recruitment.

Fibroblast support for leucocyte survival

In RA the resolution phase of inflammation becomes disordered.[12] Failure of synovial T cells to undergo apoptosis contributes to the persistence of the inflammatory infiltrate. Type I interferons (interferons α and β), produced by RASFs and macrophages, promote this prolonged T-cell survival in the rheumatoid joint. Similarly, fibroblast-expressed BAFF, VCAM-1, and CXCL12 promote B-cell survival.[13] Fibroblasts have also been shown to support NK cell and neutrophil survival in the synovium.[14,15]

Fibroblast-mediated leucocyte retention

Inhibition of leucocyte death by stromal cells at sites of chronic inflammation is unlikely to be the only mechanism underlying accumulation, because lymphocytes should also be able to leave

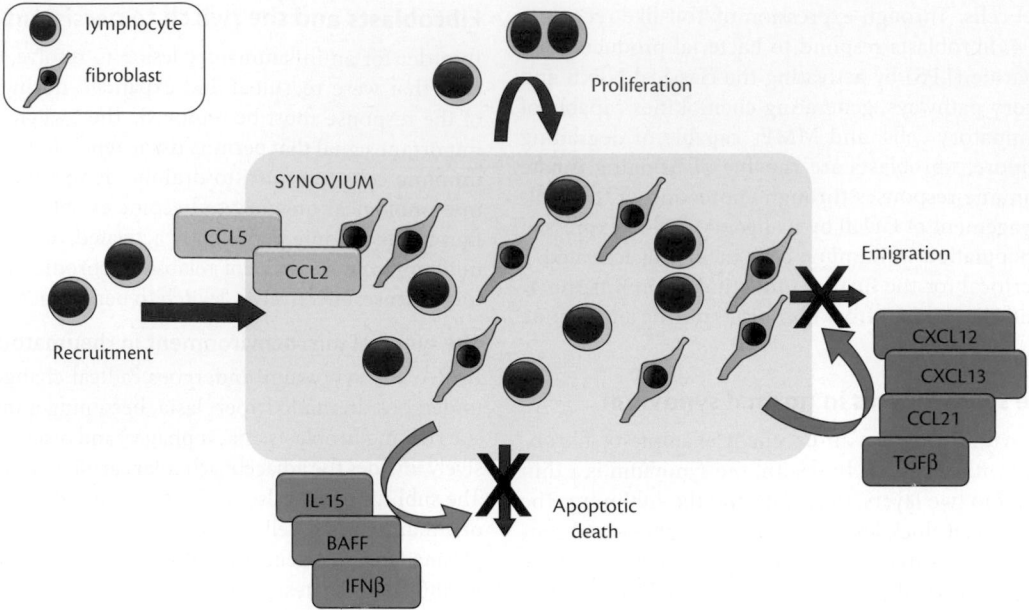

Fig. 51.2 Fibroblasts direct chronic inflammation in rheumatoid arthritis. The maintenance of persistent leukocyte infiltrates results from a distorted homeostatic balance between lymphocyte recruitment, proliferation, emigration and death. Activated RASFs produce inflammatory chemokines (CCL5, CCL2) implicated in lymphocyte recruitment to diseased synovium, survival factors (type I interferon, IL-15, BAFF) and constitutive chemokines (e.g. CXCL12, CCL21). The net result is the chronic accumulation, survival, and retention of lymphocytes at sites of disease.

inflamed tissue, even if their death is inhibited. However, constitutive chemokines that in health regulate the traffic of leucocytes are ectopically expressed by RASF. For example, the constitutive chemokine CXCL12 and its receptor CXCR4 play an important role in the recruitment and retention of haemopoietic cells within the bone marrow. Activated T lymphocytes in the RA synovium express CXCR4 receptors at abnormally high levels as a result of RASF-derived TGFβ,[16] while the ligand CXCL12 is highly expressed on endothelial cells and fibroblasts. The stability of lymphocyte infiltrates is reinforced by a positive feedback loop: tissue CXCL12 promotes CD40 ligand expression on T cells, which in turn stimulates further CXCL12 production by CD40 expressing synovial fibroblasts, further enhanced by T-cell IL-17 production.[17]

Lymphoid neogenesis

The genesis of 'tertiary' lymphoid follicular structures in RA also relies upon ectopic stromal expression of constitutive chemokines such as CCL19, CXCL13, and CCL21, in association with the lymphotoxins alpha and beta (LTα and LTβ) and tumour necrosis factor alpha (TNFα). The degree of lymphoid organization seen in the rheumatoid synovium has been shown to correlate with expression of the chemokines CCL21 and CXCL13, while transgenic mice overexpressing TNFα develop a chronic arthritis similar to RA and display increased formation of focal lymphoid aggregates.[18]

Fibroblasts and cartilage destruction

In addition to their extensive role in the perpetuation of the inflammatory response, activated RASFs are key mediators of joint damage. In the early RA joint, activated RASFs attach to and overgrow the cartilage surface, then invade and destroy cartilage and induce bone resorption. They act both directly via

secretion of multiple MMPs and cathepsins that degrade cartilage and indirectly by regulating monocyte to osteoclast differentiation resulting in bone damage. In-vitro functional assays such as the matrigel invasion assay have demonstrated that the degree of invasion with a given in-vitro cultured fibroblast sample correlates with the degree of radiographic progression seen in the joints of the patient from whose samples the fibroblasts were initially cultured.[19] Active degradation of cartilage in vivo has been elegantly demonstrated in the SCID mouse model of arthritis. Here, cultured fibroblasts with human cartilage are implanted under the kidney capsule forming a tissue construct in mice with no functioning adaptive immune response. RASFs but not normal or osteoarthritis synovial fibroblasts attach to and invade coimplanted healthy human cartilage in the absence of cells of the immune system. This experiment not only confirms that these cells have an invasive phenotype that is responsible for cartilage damage but also that such phenotype is stable after multiple in-vitro passages and disease specific.[20] This model has been used to explore the in-vivo mechanisms governing invasiveness. For instance, targeting MMP1 and cathepsin L using ribozymes was shown to inhibit cartilage destruction.

Fibroblast migration in vivo

Recently, it has been demonstrated that fibroblasts implanted in SCID mice with cartilage will migrate to a contralateral cell-free implant, and that subcutaneously, intraperitoneally, and intravenously injected fibroblasts will also migrate to sections of human cartilage, suggesting a tropism to damaged cartilage tissue.[21] This finding has significant implications for the study of synovial fibroblasts in arthritis, as the nature of systemic disease and the specific patterns of joint disease observed in different diagnostic groups (RA and psoriatic arthritis, for instance), could be partly explained by the trafficking of stromal cells around the body.

Acquisition of the RASF phenotype

One of the key questions arising from these observations is: how do RASFs become persistently activated? It has been proposed that activation could arise from molecular cross-talk between RASFs and other cells of the synovial microenvironment early in disease. Toll-like receptors have been shown to be involved in the initial stages of synovial activation.[22] It is thought that microbial components or endogenous ligands present in the RA synovium activate RASFs through TLR signalling and lead to upregulated expression of proinflammatory cytokines and chemokines which in turn cause attraction and accumulation of immune cells in the synovium and, through a stimulatory loop, lead to persistent inflammation.[23] In RA, synovial fibroblasts exhibit excessive responses to stimuli such as TLR ligands and persistently upregulate expression of adhesion molecules (VLA-3, VLA-4, VLA-5), matrix MMPs (MMP13, MT-MMP) and proto-oncogenes (c-myc) while displaying low expression or mutations of tumour suppressor genes (e.g. PTEN, p53).[24] These persistent changes in transcription are important contributors to their aggressive behaviour.

Epigenetic modifications have been proposed as determinants of this distinctive RASF phenotype. The most studied epigenetic modifications to date are non-coding RNA, DNA methylation, and histone modifications. RASFs display global genomic DNA hypomethylation, an epigenetic change associated with upregulation of gene expression of disease relevant genes (growth factors, adhesion molecules, and MMPs). Notably, treatment of normal synovial fibroblasts with the DNA hypomethylator 5-aza-2′-deoxycytidine resulted in their transformation into cells resembling activated RASFs.[25]

This example illustrates how the epigenetic hypothesis may not only provide a mechanistic explanation for this phenotype but also a tool to modify it. Both the addition and the removal of epigenetic modifications are enzymatically mediated processes and thus present attractive targets for future therapies in RA.[26]

Fibroblasts as therapeutic targets in cancer and arthritis

The importance of the stromal microenvironment in cancer has been recognized for some years (for review see Kalluri and Zeisberg[27]). It is now widely accepted that cancer is a disease that develops as a result of genetic and epigenetic alterations in clonal cells, but that the growth, survival, and metastasis of these cells are regulated by stromal–cancer cell interactions. Studies in human lung, breast, colon, and prostate cancer have demonstrated a key role of stromal cells—termed cancer-associated fibroblasts (CAFs)—in initiation and progression of disease. The term 'cancer stroma' has been coined to refer to macroscopic and functional differences between this and the corresponding normal tissues. Cancer stroma is characterized by a modified ECM composition, increased microvessel density, inflammatory cells, and activated fibroblasts. PDGF and TFGβ are the most important factors in the process of CAF activation.[28,29] In parallel with observations of RASFs, in-vivo studies have demonstrated persistent phenotypes in CAFs: for instance, coimplantation of prostate tumour fibroblasts (but not normal fibroblasts) with normal epithelial prostate cells leads to malignant transformation and proliferation of epithelial cells.[30] Obvious parallels can be drawn between CAFs and RASFs, leading to common therapeutic approaches.

Targeting signals responsible for activation of fibroblasts

Inhibitors of PDGF and TGFβ, which promote activation of CAFs, are being used successfully in the treatment of cancer. Imatinib inhibits tyrosine kinases including the PDGF receptor and is an effective treatment in chronic myeloid leukaemia.[31] TGFβ inhibitors are currently in development (e.g. lerdelimumab, metelimumab).[32] In RA, therapies such as anti-TNF and anti-IL-6 receptor (tocilizumab) have indirectly targeted stromal cells either by targeting cytokines impacting upon fibroblasts or by blocking their significant products respectively. These share the shortcomings of existing biologicals, inhibiting key pleiotropic proinflammatory cytokines leading to significant adverse events while on the other hand failing to address persistence of disease. Cellular MAPKinase and NFκB signalling pathways are heavily implicated in the proinflammatory and cartilage-damaging activities of synovial fibroblasts. Inhibiting such generic pathways carries significant risks of off-target effects.[33] However, imatinib shows promise as a therapy in RA that has been shown to modulate synovial fibroblast proliferation rates.[34,35]

Targeting fibroblast-expressed exoenzymes

Many cells express enzymes bound to the surface plasma membrane which have roles including receptor signalling and ECM engagement. Such enzymes can be initially targeted with antibodies as proof of concept; however, ultimately their enzymatic activity may be pharmacologically inhibited in order to provide more selective inhibition. An example of the first approach is the use a humanized monoclonal antibody (sibrotuzumab) against the fibroblast activation protein (FAP), a membrane-bound glycoprotein with serine protease activity and thus an exoenzyme. It is highly expressed in the tumour stroma and has been shown to enhance tumour growth in vivo. A phase I study using sibrotuzumab in patients with metastatic colorectal and lung cancer demonstrated repeat infusions of sibrotuzumab to be safe and well tolerated,[36] although a phase II study in metastatic colorectal cancer with less dramatic impact has now prompted further research.[37] Similarly, PBEF (visfatin) is an exoenzyme highly expressed on RASF in the lining layer of the pathological rheumatoid joint. Specific inhibitors exist to this molecule, although exploring their use in arthritis is at an early stage.[38,39] PBEF is of particular interest as part of the adipokine family. Serum and synovial fluid concentrations are closely linked to clinical disease activity, and PBEF induces proinflammatory cytokine and MMP production by RASFs in vitro.

Novel fibroblast markers

More specific targeting will result from recent discoveries of novel markers for stromal subpopulations, such as FAP. In RA, cadherin 11 is expressed by synovial fibroblasts of the lining layer. Cadherin 11 knockout mice subjected to models of inflammatory arthritis show less cartilage damage than their wild-type counterparts.[40] Although not a realistic therapeutic target, this provides proof of concept that stromal subset deletion could impact on progression of disease. Further synovial stromal markers have been identified, including the sublining marker CD248, a cell surface protein marker (endosialin) with restricted expression, and important roles in cancer progression. Maia et al. have shown that knockouts of CD248 result in amelioration of murine arthritis induced by anti-collagen antibodies, suggesting potential as a therapeutic target.[41]

Epigenetic therapies

CAFs in human gastric carcinomas have been shown to exhibit global DNA hypomethylation and, more broadly, cancerous epithelial cells are characterized on the one hand by global DNA hypomethylation that promotes chromosomal instability and activates proto-oncogenes, and on the other by regional promoter hypermethylation resulting in downregulation of tumour suppressor genes. Understanding of the molecular basis of these epigenetic mechanisms has led to the development of epigenetic therapies. The DNA methylation inhibitor 5-aza-2′-deoxycytidine is used for the treatment of myelodysplastic syndromes, acting by reversing pathological hypermethylation of the tumour suppressor gene and cell cycle regulator CDKN2B in affected cells, and also shows promise when used in combination with conventional chemotherapy.[42,43] In-vitro and in-vivo studies of the use of epigenetic therapies in arthritis have also started to emerge. Histone acetylation/deacetylation are epigenetic modifications that have a critical role in regulation of gene transcription by altering chromatin structure. Jüngel and colleagues[44] treated RASFs with the histone deacetylase inhibitor trichostatin A (TSA), resulting in inhibition of their proliferation and sensitization to TNF-related apoptosis-inducing ligand (TRAIL)-induced apoptosis. Subsequently, Nasu and colleagues[45] conducted an in-vivo study to analyse the effects of TSA treatment in the collagen antibody-induced arthritis (CAIA) mouse model leading to dose-dependent amelioration of disease. Non-coding RNA species such as microRNAs (miRs) are also becoming recognized as relatively specific controllers of aberrant gene expression and are frequently under epigenetic regulation. One such example in arthritis is miR203. This molecule is under the direct control of DNA methylation, and drives expression of IL-6 and MMP production by synovial fibroblasts.[46] These studies suggest that epigenetic therapies may become a reality for the treatment of arthritis in the near future.

References

1. Uccelli A, Moretta L, Pistoia V. Mesenchymal stem cells in health and disease. *Nat Rev Immunol* 2008;8(9):726–736.

2. Marinova-Mutafchieva L, Williams RO, Funa K, Maini RN, Zvaifler NJ. Inflammation is preceded by tumor necrosis factor-dependent infiltration of mesenchymal cells in experimental arthritis. *Arthritis Rheum* 2002;46(2):507–513.

3. Phillips RJ, Burdick MD, Hong K et al. Circulating fibrocytes traffic to the lungs in response to CXCL12 and mediate fibrosis. *J Clin Invest* 2004;114(3):438–446.

4. Chang HY, Chi JT, Dudoit S et al. Diversity, topographic differentiation, and positional memory in human fibroblasts. *Proc Natl Acad Sci U S A* 2002;99(20):12877–12882.

5. Bird A. DNA methylation patterns and epigenetic memory. *Genes Dev* 2002;16(1):6–21.

6. Kuschert GS, Coulin F, Power CA et al. Glycosaminoglycans interact selectively with chemokines and modulate receptor binding and cellular responses. *Biochemistry* 1999;38(39):12959–12968.

7. Loeser RF, Forsyth CB, Samarel AM, Im HJ. Fibronectin fragment activation of proline-rich tyrosine kinase PYK2 mediates integrin signals regulating collagenase-3 expression by human chondrocytes through a protein kinase C-dependent pathway. *J Biol Chem* 2003;278(27):24577–24585.

8. Bechtel W, McGoohan S, Zeisberg EM et al. Methylation determines fibroblast activation and fibrogenesis in the kidney. *Nat Med* 2010;16(5):544–550.

9. Valencia X, Higgins JM, Kiener HP et al. Cadherin-11 provides specific cellular adhesion between fibroblast-like synoviocytes. *J Exp Med* 2004;200(12):1673–1679.

10. Weyand CM, Goronzy JJ. Ectopic germinal center formation in rheumatoid synovitis. *Ann N Y Acad Sci* 2003;987:140–149.

11. Koch AE, Kunkel SL, Harlow LA et al. Epithelial neutrophil activating peptide-78: a novel chemotactic cytokine for neutrophils in arthritis. *J Clin Invest* 1994;94(3):1012–1018.

12. Buckley CD. Michael Mason prize essay 2003. Why do leucocytes accumulate within chronically inflamed joints? *Rheumatology* (Oxford) 2003;42(12):1433–1444.

13. Bombardieri M, Kam NW, Brentano F et al. A BAFF/APRIL-dependent TLR3-stimulated pathway enhances the capacity of rheumatoid synovial fibroblasts to induce AID expression and Ig class-switching in B cells. *Ann Rheum Dis* 2011;70(10):1857–1865.

14. Chan A, Filer A, Parsonage G et al. Mediation of the proinflammatory cytokine response in rheumatoid arthritis and spondylarthritis by interactions between fibroblast-like synoviocytes and natural killer cells. *Arthritis Rheum* 2008;58(3):707–717.

15. Filer A, Parsonage G, Smith E et al. Differential survival of leukocyte subsets mediated by synovial, bone marrow, and skin fibroblasts: Site-specific versus activation-dependent survival of T cells and neutrophils. *Arthritis Rheum* 2006;54(7):2096–2108.

16. Buckley CD, Amft N, Bradfield PF et al. Persistent induction of the chemokine receptor CXCR4 by TGF-beta 1 on synovial T cells contributes to their accumulation within the rheumatoid synovium. *J Immunol* 2000;165(6):3423–3429.

17. Kim KW, Cho ML, Kim HR et al. Up-regulation of stromal cell-derived factor 1 (CXCL12] production in rheumatoid synovial fibroblasts through interactions with T lymphocytes: role of interleukin-17 and CD40L-CD40 interaction. *Arthritis Rheum* 2007;56(4):1076–1086.

18. Keffer J, Probert L, Cazlaris H et al. Transgenic mice expressing human tumour necrosis factor: a predictive genetic model of arthritis. *EMBO J* 1991;10(13):4025–4031.

19. Tolboom TC, van der Helm-van Mil AH, Nelissen RG et al. Invasiveness of fibroblast-like synoviocytes is an individual patient characteristic associated with the rate of joint destruction in patients with rheumatoid arthritis. *Arthritis Rheum* 2005;52(7):1999–2002.

20. Muller-Ladner U, Kriegsmann J, Franklin BN et al. Synovial fibroblasts of patients with rheumatoid arthritis attach to and invade normal human cartilage when engrafted into SCID mice. *Am J Pathol* 1996;149(5):1607–1615.

21. Lefèvre S, Knedla A, Tennie C et al. Synovial fibroblasts spread rheumatoid arthritis to unaffected joints. *Nat Med* 2009;15(12):1414–1420.

22. Brentano F, Kyburz D, Schorr O, Gay R, Gay S. The role of Toll-like receptor signalling in the pathogenesis of arthritis. *Cell Immunol* 2005;233(2):90–96.

23. Pierer M, Rethage J, Seibl R et al. Chemokine secretion of rheumatoid arthritis synovial fibroblasts stimulated by Toll-like receptor 2 ligands. *J Immunol* 2004;172(2):1256–1265.

24. Pap T, Franz JK, Hummel KM et al. Activation of synovial fibroblasts in rheumatoid arthritis: lack of Expression of the tumour suppressor PTEN at sites of invasive growth and destruction. *Arthritis Res* 2000;2(1):59–64.

25. Karouzakis E, Gay RE, Michel BA, Gay S, Neidhart M. DNA hypomethylation in rheumatoid arthritis synovial fibroblasts. *Arthritis Rheum* 2009;60(12):3613–3622.

26. Filippakopoulos P, Qi J, Picaud S et al. Selective inhibition of BET bromodomains. *Nature* 2010;468(7327):1067–1073.

27. Kalluri R, Zeisberg M. Fibroblasts in cancer. *Nat Rev Cancer* 2006;6(5):392–401.

28. Moustakas A, Souchelnytskyi S, Heldin CH. Smad regulation in TGF-beta signal transduction. *J Cell Sci* 2001;114(Pt 24):4359–4369.

29. Piek E, Heldin CH, Ten DP. Specificity, diversity, and regulation in TGF-beta superfamily signaling. *FASEB J* 1999;13(15):2105–2124.

30. Olumi AF, Grossfeld GD, Hayward SW et al. Carcinoma-associated fibroblasts direct tumor progression of initiated human prostatic epithelium. *Cancer Res* 1999;59(19):5002–5011.

31. Capdeville R, Buchdunger E, Zimmermann J, Matter A. Glivec (STI571, imatinib), a rationally developed, targeted anticancer drug. *Nat Rev Drug Discov* 2002;1(7):493–502.

32. Bonafoux D, Lee WC. Strategies for TGF-beta modulation: a review of recent patents. *Expert Opin Ther Pat* 2009;19(12):1759–1769.

33. Wendling D, Prati C, Toussirot E, Herbein G. Targeting intracellular signaling pathways to treat rheumatoid arthritis: Pandora's box? *Joint Bone Spine* 2010;77(2):96–98.

34. Paniagua RT, Sharpe O, Ho PP et al. Selective tyrosine kinase inhibition by imatinib mesylate for the treatment of autoimmune arthritis. *J Clin Invest* 2006;116(10):2633–2642.

35. Terabe F, Kitano M, Kawai M et al. Imatinib mesylate inhibited rat adjuvant arthritis and PDGF-dependent growth of synovial fibroblast via interference with the Akt signaling pathway. *Mod Rheumatol* 2009;19(5):522–529.

36. Cheng JD, Dunbrack RL, Jr., Valianou M et al. Promotion of tumor growth by murine fibroblast activation protein, a serine protease, in an animal model. *Cancer Res* 2002;62(16):4767–4772.

37. Hofheinz RD, al-Batran SE, Hartmann F et al. Stromal antigen targeting by a humanised monoclonal antibody: an early phase II trial of sibrotuzumab in patients with metastatic colorectal cancer. *Onkologie* 2003;26(1):44–48.

38. Evans L, Williams AS, Hayes AJ, Jones SA, Nowell M. Suppression of leukocyte infiltration and cartilage degradation by selective inhibition of pre-B cell colony-enhancing factor/visfatin/nicotinamide phosphoribosyltransferase: Apo866-mediated therapy in human fibroblasts and murine collagen-induced arthritis. *Arthritis Rheum* 2011;63(7):1866–1877.

39. Ospelt C, Mertens JC, Jungel A et al. Inhibition of fibroblast activation protein and dipeptidylpeptidase 4 increases cartilage invasion by rheumatoid arthritis synovial fibroblasts. *Arthritis Rheum* 2010;62(5):1224–1235.

40. Lee DM, Kiener HP, Agarwal SK et al. Cadherin-11 in synovial lining formation and pathology in arthritis. *Science* 2007;315(5814):1006–1010.

41. Maia M, de Vriese A, Janssens T et al. CD248 and its cytoplasmic domain: a therapeutic target for arthritis. *Arthritis Rheum* 2010;62(12):3595–3606.

42. Raj K, Mufti GJ. Azacytidine (Vidaza(R)) in the treatment of myelodysplastic syndromes. *Ther Clin Risk Manag* 2006;2(4):377–388.

43. Silverman LR, Demakos EP, Peterson BL et al. Randomized controlled trial of azacitidine in patients with the myelodysplastic syndrome: a study of the cancer and leukemia group B. *J Clin Oncol* 2002;20(10):2429–2440.

44. Jungel A, Baresova V, Ospelt C et al. Trichostatin A sensitises rheumatoid arthritis synovial fibroblasts for TRAIL-induced apoptosis. *Ann Rheum Dis* 2006;65(7):910–912.

45. Nasu Y, Nishida K, Miyazawa S et al. Trichostatin A, a histone deacetylase inhibitor, suppresses synovial inflammation and subsequent cartilage destruction in a collagen antibody-induced arthritis mouse model. *Osteoarthritis Cartilage* 2008;16(6):723–732.

46. Stanczyk J, Ospelt C, Karouzakis E et al. Altered expression of miR-203 in rheumatoid arthritis synovial fibroblasts and its role in fibroblast activation. *Arthritis Rheum* 2011;63(2):373–381.

CHAPTER 52

Synovial pathology

Costantino Pitzalis, Frances Humby, and Michael P. Seed

Introduction

The understanding of synovial pathology is becoming considerably more advanced through access to synovial tissues at earlier stages of disease via minimally invasive tissue microsampling and new molecular techniques. Internationally agreed recommendations have been published for the standardization of biopsy techniques for clinical trials[1]: 6–8 samples from within a joint provide data with less than 10% variance for T cells, B cells, macrophages, and activation markers, as well as a twofold difference in gene expression (via PCR). Wrist and knee joints appear comparable, though metacarpal joints may differ. Unfortunately, the availability of therapeutically naive tissues, and patient and tissue heterogeneity, continue to confound.

The synovium is made up of a surface, or lining, layer of overlapping cells. Unlike other serosal surfaces, this intimal lining lacks epithelial cells and basement membrane, and has no tight junctions (reviewed by Edwards[2]; Figure 52.1). The synovial lining layer is 2–3 cells thick and consists of type A (CD14, CD18 macrophage) and type B (uridine diphosphoglucose dehydrogenase, UDPGD-expressing fibroblast) synoviocytes. The macrophages are in the minority, with fibroblasts separating them by 100 μm. The intimal layer overlies a connective tissue stroma, termed the subintima (reviewed by Edwards and Wilkinson[3]). The subintima comprises a network of capillaries, fibroblasts, scattered macrophages, and mast cells. It is innervated, and in large joints contains adipose tissue. The lining contains collagen types III, V, and VI, tenascin, and decorin synthesized by the type B synoviocytes, in addition to hyaluronic acid via UDPGD. Synovial fluid hyaluronan permits free flow of synovium over its own folds as well as the cartilage surface. Synovitis, inflammation of the synovium, is characterized by a thickening of the synovial lining layer from two to up to six cells thick (Figure 52.1). Effusion into the joints occurs through endothelial cell gaps.

In rheumatoid arthritis (RA) this picture can be florid (Figure 52.2), as it can occasionally be with osteoarthritis (OA; see Figure 52.6 below), with neoangiogenesis and a profoundly inflamed soft tissue which develops into a granulomatous tissue of fibroblasts and macrophages invading the joint space as villous fronds, or an invasive tissue that erodes into cartilage and bone. Pannus erodes the joints by encroaching over cartilage, or under

it by eroding through subchondral bone into the medullary space, or both.[4] The tissue is innervated and is thus a significant source of the inflammatory pain experienced by RA sufferers. The cells of the sublining layer can become organized into loose or more structured aggregates termed ectopic lymphoid structures (ELS).

The initiating stimulus for the synovial response in RA remains unknown. Although circulating rheumatoid factor (RF) and/or anti-citrullinated protein antibodies (ACPA) antibodies predicts high risk for disease, synovium from these patients taken before the onset of symptoms does not show subclinical inflammation.[5] A secondary 'hit' of unknown origin, probably inflammatory,[6] is required.

Intimal lining layer

The first responses of the synovium in RA are tissue oedema and fibrin deposition.[4] As the plasma exudes and neutrophil accumulation occurs in the synovial fluid, fibrin is deposited. The synovial lining layer in RA[3] thickens with synoviocytes increasing in depth from two to up to six cells thick (Figure 52.1). Type A macrophage-like cells are derived from bone marrow,[7] and their expansion in synovitis is through cell recruitment from the circulation. Mitotic figures are thus rare, and DNA synthesis does not reflect that of a proliferative tissue. Lining-layer macrophage numbers are increased within the first 2 days of symptoms and in uninvolved joints. Their proportion increases to dominate the subintimal layer, and it becomes stratified with macrophages overlying and underlying the fibroblast-like synoviocytes (FLS). Lining-layer macrophages and FLS interact either through direct molecular interactions such as CD97/C55, or indirectly.

Matrix metalloproteinase-1 (*MMP1*) gene expression is seen within 2 weeks of diagnosis and correlates with CD68 macrophage numbers in the lining and sublining layers. The supporting matrix becomes diffuse, with collagen types II and III and tenascin being more widely distributed.

The invasive tissue originates from the synovial–cartilage junction.[8] This wedge-shaped tissue overlies the cartilage, and is contiguous with the synovium. It is vascular, containing fibroblasts and monocyte (CD14)-derived cells, and it is thought that it is this that migrates over the cartilage to form the erosive front. RA cartilage contains immune complexes, including RF complexes and

(A) 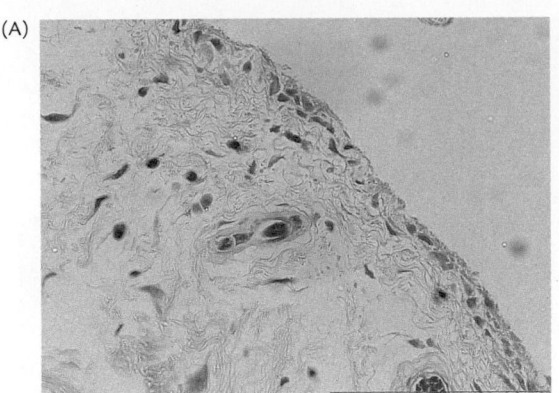 (B)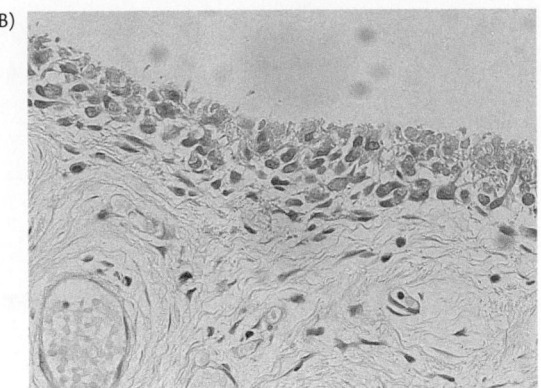

Fig. 52.1 The expansion of the synovial lining layer seen in rheumatoid arthritis from a thin 2–3-cell layer (A) to a thick hypertrophic synovium (B). Note the change in cell morphology into fatter, more rounded cells reflecting the recruitment of type A macrophage-like synoviocytes.
Courtesy of Professor C. Pitzalis and Dr R. Hands, MRC PEAC Database.

fibronectin, all of which are thought to act as a stimulus for cells to migrate and erode the cartilage. Without these, the anionic cartilage surface rejects cell adhesion and is protected from synoviocyte invasion by synovium-derived products such as lubricin, which is deficient in RA. As to which cells are involved in the erosion of cartilage at the cartilage–pannus junction (CPJ), neutrophils, macrophages, mast cells and fibroblast-like cells are all seen at different sites.

Fassbender first described the progression of FLS across the cartilage,[4,9] and they are seen to advance ahead of the pannus.[10] Macrophages follow by migrating between this cell layer and the cartilage-bound fibronectin, and erosion occurs under the macrophage zone. FLS feature prominently in pannus and joint erosion,[11] and are highly proliferative. Fassbender also first noted differences in fibroblast phenotypes in RA pannus, namely the presence of fibrocytes as well as classical fibroblasts. Fibrocytes are bone-marrow-derived myeloid cells involved in angiogenesis and tissue repair. They can function as antigen-presenting cells, or play a similar role to fibroblasts. Fibrocytes provide a role as a tissue scaffold, and are active in inflammatory cell traffic and erosion. There are subtypes, those with a myofibroblast gene pattern in inflammatory pannus and insulin type growth factor (IGF)-regulated fibroblasts in areas of low inflammation.[12] Fibroblast invasiveness *ex vivo* correlates with the rate of joint destruction, and in turn correlates with *MMP-1*, *MMP-3*, *MMP-10*, and *MMP14* expression. Indeed, the fibroblast phenotype appears to be involved in aggressive erosion. Subcutaneous implantation of RA fibroblasts in juxtaposition with RA cartilage in mice results in its erosion, and the fibroblasts can circulate to contralateral implants to form erosive aggregates.

There are two distinct forms of CPJ. Cartilage proteoglycan and chondrocyte depletion occurs under the invasive cellular form of CPJ, unlike under the quiescent or 'indistinct' CPJ (Figure 52.3).[8] These observations correlate with interleukin (IL)-1α and tumour necrosis factor alpha (TNFα)-expressing CD68 macrophages present in the invasive form and transforming growth factor beta (TGFβ) in the indistinct form. Other cells can occasionally be seen in the active cellular form, namely neutrophils, mast cells, dendritic cells, and plasma cells.[13] In mature pannus, there is a correlation between the inflammatory activity of the subintimal layer and the erosive activity of the underlying CPJ.

Synovial sublining layer

The general microscopic view of RA synovitis is one of a frank and vigorous chronic inflammatory tissue made up of monocytes, macrophages, lymphocytes (T and B cells) plasma cells, dendritic cells, and fibroblasts.

Cell recruitment is evidenced by perivascular cell aggregates, and the formation of specialized vasculature with high endothelial venule (HEV) morphology as well as new blood vessels (neo-angiogenesis) driven by high levels of vascular endothelial growth factor (VEGF) and VEGF receptors expressed in the endothelium and pericyte layers. The vessels express adhesion molecules, induced by interstitial macrophage cytokines. The tissue can develop a lymphatic system, with lymphangiogenesis. Thus not only is there active recruitment of monocytes, lymphocytes, and neutrophils, there is a chemokine imbalance between the lymphatic and blood vessel systems that results in the retention of cells once recruited, impairing lymphatic return.

The characterization of migrated cells shows distinct T-cell distribution profiles, with CD4 helper T cells accumulating in perivascular cuffs, and diffuse CD8 cytotoxic T cells. Joint disease activity and systemic inflammation correlate well with the presence of the major inflammatory cell type, the CD68 macrophage.[14,15] CD68 serves as a useful biomarker for synovial macrophages, as Toll-like receptors (TLRs) and Fc IgG receptors may vary between sites. Earlier macrophages reside in the sublining layer, and more mature macrophages are found in the synovial lining layer, suggesting recruitment of monocytes through vasculature of the sublining followed by residence in the lining. The greater the macrophage cellularity of the sublining layer, the greater the cellularity of the lining layer. In turn the degree of erosion and pain scores directly correlates with macrophage density, as opposed to T and B lymphocyte populations.[14] Plasma cells can be widely distributed as well as surrounding aggregates, while B cells, if they are present, are found within ELS aggregates. Neutrophils are sparse, but when they are seen they are seen between blood vessels and the intimal surface and assumed to be *en passant* to the synovial fluid.

Synovitis also comprises of T and B cells which can be seen in aggregates, compartmentalizing into B- and T-cell areas with macrophages and dendritic cells. Myofibroblasts are present and produce cytokines and chemokines that orchestrate the migration and

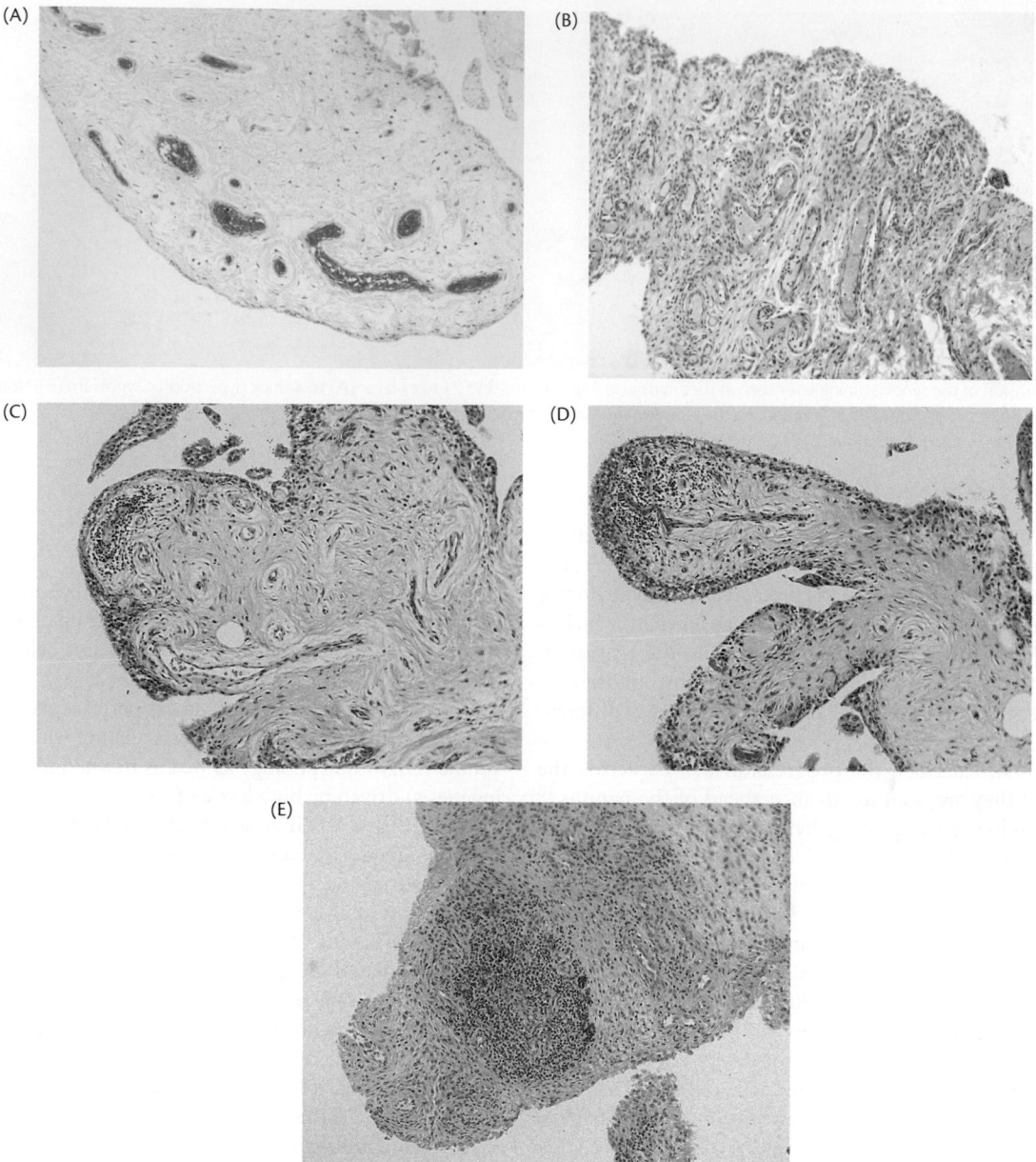

Fig. 52.2 The florid inflammatory nature of rheumatoid synovium, and the formation of ELS: (A) Normal synovium. (B) Rheumatoid picture, showing a profound diffuse inflammatory sublining with neoangiogenesis. The synovia (C–E) have been graded according to the radial cell count taken from the blood vessel to the periphery. The determination is made at the point of widest infiltration and specimens must exhibit a synovial cell lining layer in order to be properly graded. Cell aggregates with a radial cell count of 2–5 cells are classified as grade 1 (C). Grade 2 specimens have a radial count of 6–10 cells (D), while grade 3 specimens have a radial count of more than 10 cells (E). In addition, mixed infiltrates must be predominantly lymphocytic and it must be noted if there is diffuse inflammatory infiltrate present in the tissue. Analysis of over 100 samples shows there is a gradual distribution between ELS naive and highly organized structures. 47% of RA samples exhibit lymphoid structures at some stage of development.
Courtesy of Professor C. Pitzalis and Dr R. Hands, MRC PEAC Database.

positioning of lymphocytes.[16] B cells are almost wholly confined to follicular structures, which could provide the basis for defining specific therapeutic modalities. Thus the inflammatory infiltrate can become organized into various degrees of aggregation (Figure 52.2C–E), leading to the formation of ELS.

Ectopic lymphoid structures

When considering lymphoid aggregates, it must be stressed these are not a purely pathological processes, but may result from a normal chronic immune response. The development of local immunocompetent structures has advantages over the requirement for the development of systemic immunity, not least providing immunocompetent cells at the site of infection and local adaptive response limitation. Originally thought to be a result of chronicity in RA, these structures are found in early as well as chronic RA pannus (Figure 52.4). They may form as a result of chronic antigen drive. Indeed, the cyclic nature of RA erosive activity and antigen exposure may add to the drive for their development. This has been reviewed.[17,18]

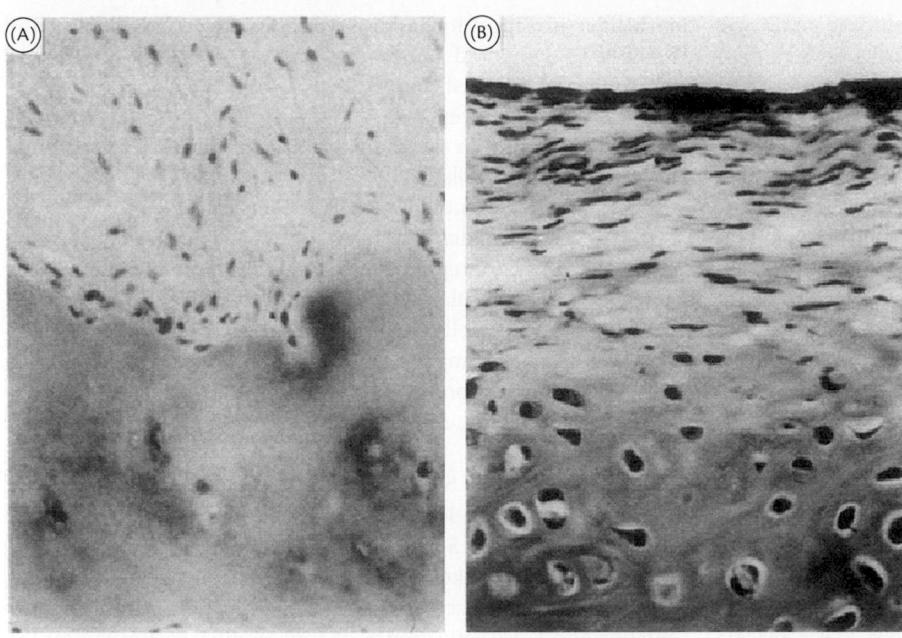

Fig. 52.3 Distinct (A) and Indistinct (B) types of pannus invasion of cartilage at the cartilage–pannus junction.

Reproduced from Annals of the Rheumatic Diseases, S A Allard, K D Muirden, R N Maini, 50 (5), 278–83, 1991 with permission from BMJ Publishing Group Ltd.

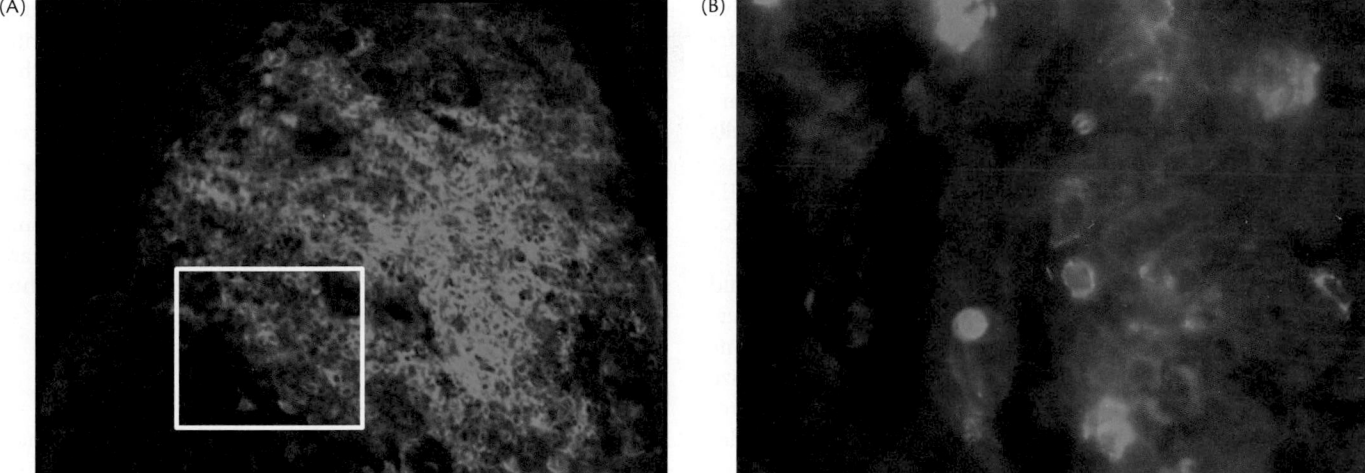

Fig. 52.4 Functional ectopic lymphoid structures in RA pannus. B cells (stained with anti-CD20, green) producing anti-citrullinated protein antibodies (stained with citrullinated fibrin, red) surrounding a B-cell aggregate. A) Low magnification; B) Figure 52.4A selected area magnified.

F. Humby et al., PLoS Med. 2009 Jan 13;6(1):e1.

ELS are inducible non-encapsulated lymphoid structures capable of forming in mucosal or non-mucosal areas as a result of sustained immune infiltration. However, not all lymphoid structures can function as true ELS as they frequently lack the immunological and proliferative properties of secondary lymphoid tissue (SLT). They may reflect two functions, a local adaptive response to limit systemic generation, or the failure of the secondary system to limit the problem such as seen in human kidney and cardiac transplants.

The variability in reporting of aggregates is probably as a result of sampling and laboratory variables. Histomorphometric analysis has now been standardized between laboratories into a grading system (G1–3) (Figure 52.2) to permit the quantification of aggregate organization, molecular mechanisms, and clinical outcomes. G2–3 T–B lymphocyte aggregates are found in 30% of active knees[19,20]

and 44% of samples from late arthritis at arthroplasty.[21] Differences between studies can reflect the historical treatment context, as the modern treatment paradigm is early and aggressive, as well as disease stage and sampling differences.

RA synovial ELS can be functional as they possess HEV, and express peripheral lymph node addressin (PNAd) which is usually associated with SLT for lymphocyte homing, and is colocalized with CCL21 which is produced by lymph node myofibroblasts. Thus the RA ELS has the apparatus required for lymphocyte homing and trafficking. They still retain a less organized morphology than classical SLT, with blurring and even intermixing of the T- and B-cell zones. Despite this, dendritic cells are found, similar to SLT, colocalizing with CCR7-expressing cells, which raises the possibility of functional immunological synapses. Some ELS exhibit large interfollicular activation-induced cytidine deaminase (AID)+ B cells which are usually confined to the ELS T-cell zone with dendritic morphology.[22] Gene transcripts reveal T-cell receptor (TCR) and costimulatory pathway signalling, suggestive of active antigen presentation.

It has been known for some time that RA synovial follicles display oligoclonal immunoglobulins with highly mutated V-regions similar to those found in antigen-driven germinal centres. AID is required for somatic hypermutation and Ig class switch recombination, and is found in the follicular dendritic cell (FDC) network within RA synovial ELS and is associated with the expression of class-switched ACPA.[22] These FDC networks occur in 40% of RA samples,[21] and AID transcripts in CD21L+ samples occur in a further 20%. Like classical germinal centres, the ELS contain antigen-naive, unswitched, and switched memory B cells. Thus RA ELS possess the ability to programme both memory T and B cells. B cells are important to ELS integrity, as rituximab (anti-CD20) treatment of xenograft-coimplanted SCID mice induces dissolution of the synovial architecture, and depletion of T cells and macrophages.[23] Treatment of RA patients with rituximab also reduces the prevalence of T–B-cell lymphoid aggregates, T cells, FDCs, plasma cells, and subintimal macrophages in responders.

ELS probably contribute to RF and ACPA, but the contribution of secondary lymphocyte structures to circulating antibody confounds the interpretation. For example, ACPA can be seen in ELS-negative patients[22] as well as in spondyloarthropathy and OA. ACPA occurs years prior to the development of disease.[24] Local concentrations of RF and ACPA are greater in ELS biopsies, plasma cell numbers are elevated, and IgG1/2 transcripts are greater. Synovial plasma cells in ELS synovia correlate with synovial fluid ACPA and xenotransplantation of functional ELS containing RA synovia into SCID mice results in circulating levels of human ACPA that persists for several weeks.[22]

The enhanced detection of functional ectopic structures could explain the lack of correlation between aggregates and disease severity. One trial shows that joint destruction is increased in patients with lymphoid aggregates.[25], but two others with larger sample size do not show such a correlation.[19,20] Not only this, ELS structures within the same patient can show the coexistence of various grades of ELS structure, suggesting a dynamic process.[19]

Cytokines in the synovium

Cytokine networks reflecting adaptive immune pathways are prominent,[6,26] and the state of synovial organization distinguishes them according to their cytokine profiles.[27] In general, highly granulomatous synovia have high transcription rates for IFNγ, IL-4, IL-1β, and TNFα, while those with diffuse infiltrates are lower. Those with follicular aggregates possess high IFNγ, for example. Macrophage cytokines found in synovium include IL-1, TNF, IL-6, IL-12, IL-15, IL-32, granulocyte-macrophage colony-stimulating factor (GMCSF), as well as chemokines and are seen wherever the macrophages reside. IL-1α is seen primarily in endothelial cells, IL-1β predominantly in macrophages and also fibroblasts. TNFα is found in cells of the lining layer, in scattered macrophages, around blood vessels, and highly expressed at pannus adhered to cartilage[28]; The TNFα receptor is distributed in a similar manner and its receptors are found in on CD3 T cells in lymphoid aggregates. The ubiquitous nature of TNFα, both in cells and through its receptors

with their juxtaposition with each other and positioning at the lining layer, lymphoid aggregates, and CPJ, and its positioning in macrophages, demonstrates the central role this cytokine plays in RA. IL-1α and its receptor IL-1R appear even more predominant than TNFα. Found in the same locations as TNFα, it is seen in a high proportion of cells.[28] The endogenous antagonist on the other hand, IL-1ra, is present in less than 10% of cells.

IL-6 is also abundantly expressed,[29] being localized to some synovial T cells but preponderantly in synovial macrophages in the lining layer, perivascular aggregates, and especially those in juxtaposition to plasma cells. It is also synthesized by FLS and can be considered to be as important to RA as TNFα. IL-6 induces bone resorption, autoantibody production via stimulation of helper T-cell IL-21 synthesis, endothelial cell activation, and T- and B- cell proliferation.

The presence of ELS in synovia manifests in the expression of greater amounts of IL-1, IL-6, IL12, and IL-2 than those with diffuse cellularity. IL-12, IL-15, IL-18, and IL-23 are expressed by synovial myeloid and B-cell like (plasmacytoid) dendritic cells along with HLA class II and the accessory molecules involved in antigen presentation and T-cell activation. IL-12, an essential costimulus for the proliferation of T0 cells into T-helper cells and produced by macrophages and dendritic cells, colocalizes with CD68 macrophages.

The other important cytokine in the adaptive response is IL-17. Although IL-17 is sparsely seen in RA synovitis, when present it is found in T-cell subsets. The abundance of macrophage and dendritic cell TGFβ, IL-1, IL-6, IL-21, and IL-23 is a cytokine environment that will support Th17 differentiation at the cost of T-suppressor cells.

Examination of cytokines at the CPJ shows that cytokine expression follows the different morphological types[28]: TNFα, IL-1α, IL-6, GM-CSF and TGFβ are all found in CD68 macrophages in juxtaposition to the cartilage. However, of the diffuse CPJ subtype, only TGFβ is seen in the fibroblast-like cells. None of these cytokines are seen at other quiescent areas of the CPJ. IL-1β, IFNγ, and lymphotoxin seem not to be in the CPJ.

Bone erosion

Bone is eroded by pannus advancing along the subchondral surface, as well as via the inflamed bone marrow by osteoclasts (Figure 52.5). RA synovitis and pannus play a central role both directly as well as through cytokine expression.[30] Macrophages are a major source of osteoclastogenic cytokines such as TNF, IL-1, IL-6, and IL-17, as well as prostaglandin E$_2$. Macrophages may also serve as osteoclast precursors. Lymphoidneogenic structures can be seen in bone marrow alongside osteoclast activity. However, the presence of such B-cell structures need not mean that such association is entirely destructive. Defective B-cell follicle formation in hTNFα arthritic mice is associated with reduced endosteal bone formation, but with increased pannus activity,[31] so in this scenario it appears B-cell aggregation may be reparative.

Pannus itself secretes TNFα, IL-1a, IL-6, IL-17, macrophage colony-stimulating factor (M-CSF), and RANKL. CD4 T-cells and RA fibroblasts both synthesize RANKL. The heightened expression of RANKL over its decoy receptor osteoprotegerin (OPG) results in the promotion of octeoclastogenesis and matches the observation that osteoclasts are seen at the pannus–bone junction. TNFα induces marrow stromal cells to elaborate RANKL and M-CSF, as does IL-1, and inhibits osteoblast maturation as well as differentiation, thus leaving osteoclasts

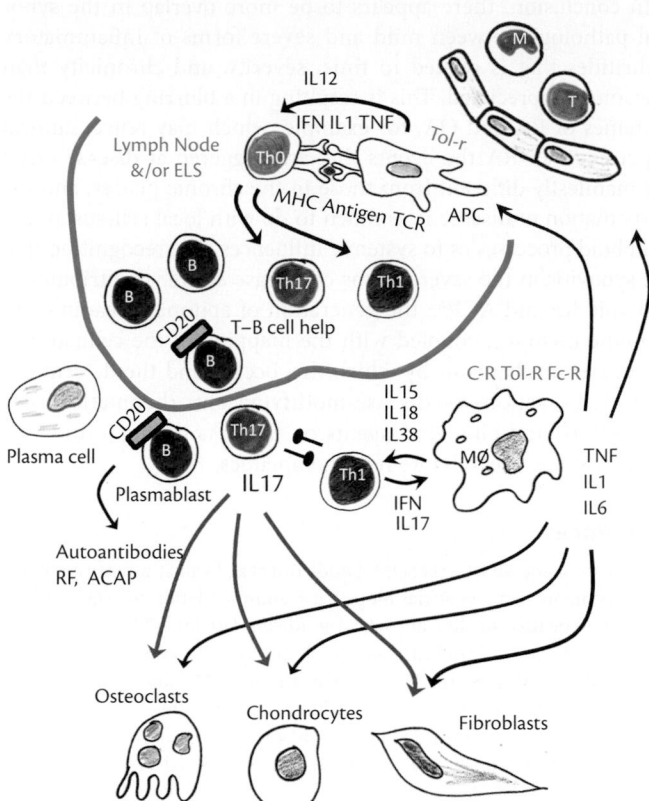

Fig. 52.5 Pannus cytokine pathways and joint destruction in rheumatoid arthritis. Immune processes in the rheumatoid synovium, and the destruction of cartilage and bone, showing the major targets of modern anti-rheumatic biological agents. Central to this process is the presentation of an antigen by antigen-presenting cells (APC) to T cells to produce a T-helper 1 (Th1) and T-helper 17 (Th17) response. This occurs primarily in lymph nodes, but sometimes in synovial ectopic lymphoid structures (ELS) that can develop into a variety of organizational states to produce B-cell (B) and T-cell (T) responses leading to antibody synthesis, T-cell activation, and memory. The production of interferon-γ (IFNγ) aggravates a pathogenic cooperation between Th1 cells and macrophages (MØ), enhanced further by ligation of complement receptors (C-R), Fc receptors (Fc-R), and Toll (T-R) receptors by their ligands to result in the production of pro-inflammatory cytokines, especially TNF, IL-6, and IL-1. These in turn mediate monocyte (M) and T-cell recruitment, angiogenesis, lymphangiogenesis, and joint destruction. Erosion occurs either directly or through synoviocyte stimulation and RANKL, the stimulation of osteoclast differentiation, and bone resorption, as well cartilage destruction through chondrocytes and pannus.
Reproduced by kind permission of the publishers.

unopposed. IL-6 upregulates osteoclast differentiation through the induction of cyclooxygenase 2 and prostaglandin E_2 synthesis which in turn increases the RANKL:OPG ratio through the expression of RANKL. IL-17 is an important bone resorption factor that also acts through RANKL. These data suggest that RA bone erosion should respond to RANKL inhibition as well as anti-cytokine therapies. Indeed this is the case, with anti-TNFα, IL-1, anti-IL-6, anti-IL-17, and anti-RANKL all reducing focal bone erosions in RA, often with a better response when coadministered with methotrexate.[32]

Synovial pathology drug effects

Few clinical trials include synovial biopsies and not as primary clinical endpoints. However, biopsy has allowed the influence of the gold standard methotrexate on synovial cell composition[33] in responsive patients to be observed. T cells (CD3), cytotoxic T cells (CD8), plasma cells (CD38), and macrophages (CD68) are all significantly reduced. Non-significant reductions in helper T cells (CD4), B cells (CD22), IL2-R (CD25), and type B synoviocytes is reported. Functional changes such as reduced mitosis (Ki67), IL-1β, TNFα, E-selectin, ICAM-1, and VCAM are seen. Prednisolone treatment[34] dramatically reduces synovial lining CD68 macrophages, CD5 B and T cells, CD163 macrophages, CD4 T cells, CD38 plasma cells, and CD55 fibroblasts. Similarly affected cytokines are IL-1β and TNFα in the sublining.

Anti-TNFα therapy is not solely associated with reduced CD68 macrophage numbers, but has a wider and dramatic effect on synovial pathology.[35] The neovasculature is severely compromised, and lymphangiogenesis is increased, while lymphatic and chemokine imbalance is corrected. T cells are reduced, along with VCAM-1 and E-selectin, as is synovial TNFα.[36] It has also been demonstrated to have a modulatory effect on synovial lymphoneogenesis.[20]

The summation of both the successful and unsuccessful trials is that CD68 macrophage suppression is a common though not specific feature of response to treatment. DAS28 scores of 88 patients from a variety of trials comprising methotrexate, leflunomide, sulphasalazine (or combinations), and infliximab correlate sublining CD68 macrophage with disease suppression.[37] Furthermore, sublining macrophage number does not change following ineffective therapy[38,39] or placebo,[40] and as such is being increasingly used in early-phase clinical trials to reduce the size and duration of studies.

This predictivity does not hold well for all treatments. Anti-B-cell therapy has variable effects on the CD68 population. It was expected that synovial B-cell depletion would predict outcome, but this is not so and is not explained by fluctuations in circulating antibody levels or the presence of anti-rituximab antibodies.[41] Differences in response are seen between trials, especially with regard to CD68 macrophages and CD3 T cells.[42] Synovial cytokine levels for TNFα, IL-6, and MMP1 also remained unaffected, as do indicators of B-cell activity—APRIL, BAFF, and SDF-1. There is an association with plasma cell depletion,[43] and response is accompanied by reduced synovial IgG and IgM synthesis and local B-cell proliferation, strongly suggesting that interruption of functional synovial B-cell pathways maybe key to clinical response.

Spondyloarthritis

Spondyloarthritis differs from RA in several respects.[44] The synovial lining layer highly expresses αVβ3, involved in fibroblast activation and proliferation, while this is much lower in the sublining layer. Instead, RA synovium expresses abundant αVβ5 in the sublining layer, which may indicate the more erosive, aggressive, nature of this disease when compared to spondyloarthritis. CD20 cells are almost absent and CD3 and CD4 helper T cells are less prevalent. CD68 macrophages, are as prevalent as seen in RA, as are plasma cells and neutrophils. The vascularity is more exaggerated and tortuous, as opposed to being more linear in RA. As the global scores increase, CD168 macrophages and neutrophils become more prevalent. Ectopic structures are also less prevalent.

Psoriatic arthritis

Ectopic lymphoid neogenesis is seen in psoriatic arthritis, and mimics the features of aggregates reported in RA,[45] with T- and

B-cell segregation, with PNAd expressing HEVs associated with CXCL13 and CCL21. As in RA, their presence appears unrelated to time of synovitis. Responsive treatment with anti-TNFα results in regression of the ectopic structures, and ineffective response is accompanied by their persistence. CD68 cells are globally present in psoriatic arthritis, to a similar degree to RA, but CD14 macrophages are fewer, which could be interpreted as reduced monocyte numbers. Mast cells contribute a significant presence and the vasculature is tortuous as opposed to linear in RA. Psoriatic synovia respond to anti-TNFα with reductions in CD3 and CD4 T cells.[46,47] CD68 is reduced as a trend in the first and significantly in the second trial. Anti-IL-1 does not have this activity. It thus seems that CD3 may be the synovial cell biomarker for psoriatic arthritis.

Osteoarthritis

It is now clear that there is significant involvement of the synovium in OA, despite the definition of OA as a non-inflammatory condition. In some patients there is a significant synovitis accompanied by hyperplasia, villous projections (Figure 52.6), and fibrosis. The synovial lining layer is often thickened, with perivascular as well as diffuse lymphocytes, and the presence of plasma cells in one-quarter of specimens. A notable minority exhibit CD4 and CD8 T cells. Samples can contain large follicular aggregates as well as perivascular accumulations,[48] containing CD4 and CD8 cells with the CD80 activation marker, and indications of FDCs. Class II HLA molecules can also be seen, as can mast cells. Cartilage shards in the synovium are associated with synovitis, and the presence of giant cells in some samples shows there is an aspect of frustrated phagocytosis of degradation products.[49]

The severity of synovitis is associated with more severe degradative disease, and also arthroscopy shows that inflammation can be subclinical. The synovitis seen in OA is associated with areas of pathological bone and cartilage damage and produces MMPs and collagenase as well as cytokines such as IL-1α, VEGF, bFGF, prostaglandin E_2, and nitric oxide.[50] VEGF and bFGF both lead to angiogenesis.

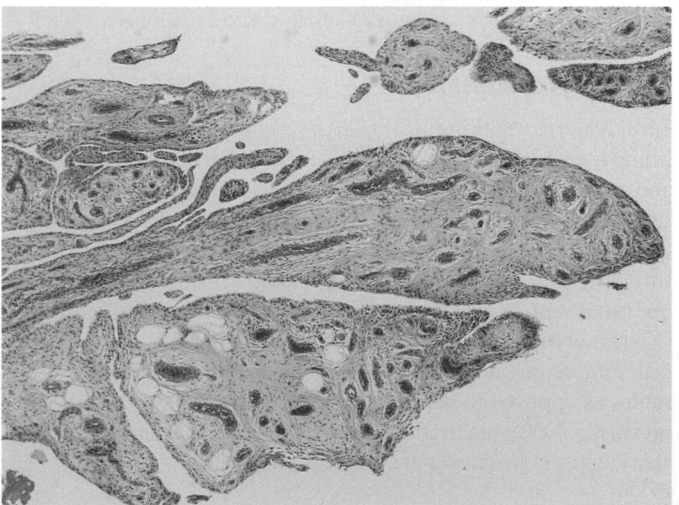

Fig. 52.6 Severe synovitis in osteoarthritis, showing thickening of the intimal layer, subsynovial lining inflammation, and neoangiogenesis, and the villous projections reminiscent of those seen in rheumatoid arthritis.
(Courtesy of Professor C. Pitzalis & Dr R. Hands, MRC PEAC Database.)

In conclusion, there appears to be more overlap in the synovial pathology between mild and severe forms of inflammatory arthritides that is related to time, severity, and chronicity than previously appreciated. This is resulting in a blurring between the extremes of RA and OA, for example, which may reflect clinical experience. In RA the events that are triggered at disease onset are manifestly different from those in the chronic phases, and the perpetuation of disease is as much to do with local self-sustaining lymphoid processes as to systemic influences. The recognition that the synovitis in the severe forms of disease actively contributes to systemic RF and ACPA; the generation of epitope spreading and immune memory; coupled with the mapping of the cellular and molecular mechanisms by which this occurs and the determination of the actions of disease-modifying anti-rheumatic drugs (DMARDs) and biological agents on them, is having a dramatic impact on the research into new therapeutics.

References

1. van de Sande MG, Gerlag DM, Lodde BM et al. Evaluating antirheumatic treatments using synovial biopsy: a recommendation for standardisation to be used in clinical trials. *Ann Rheum Dis* 2011;70(3):423–427.
2. Edwards JC. Fibroblastic synovial lining cells (synoviocytes). In: Henderson B, Edwards JC, Pettipher ER (eds) *Mechanisms and models in rheumatoid arthritis*. Academic Press, London, 1995:153–161.
3. Edwards JC, Wilkinson LS. Immunohistochemistry of rheumatoid synovium. In: Henderson B, Edwards JC, Pettipher ER (eds) *Mechanisms and models in rheumatoid arthritis*. Academic Press, London, 1995:132–152.
4. Fassbender HG, Gay S. Synovial processes in rheumatoid arthritis. *Scand J Rheumatol Suppl* 1988;76:1–7.
5. van de Sande MG, de Hair MJ, van der Leij C et al. Different stages of rheumatoid arthritis: features of the synovium in the preclinical phase. *Ann Rheum Dis* 2011;70(5):772–777.
6. McInnes IB, Schett G. The pathogenesis of rheumatoid arthritis. *N Engl J Med* 2011;365(23):2205–2219.
7. Edwards JC. The origin of type A synovial lining cells. *Immunobiology*. 1982;161(3–4):227–231.
8. Allard SA, Muirden KD, Maini RN. Correlation of histopathological features of pannus with patterns of damage in different joints in rheumatoid arthritis. *Ann Rheum Dis* 1991;50(5):278–283.
9. Fassbender HG. Histomorphological basis of articular cartilage destruction in rheumatoid arthritis. *Coll Relat Res* 1983;3(2):141–155.
10. Shiozawa S, Shiozawa K, Fujita T. Morphologic observations in the early phase of the cartilage-pannus junction. Light and electron microscopic studies of active cellular pannus. *Arthritis Rheum* 1983;26(4):472–478.
11. Neumann E, Lefevre S, Zimmermann B, Gay S, Muller-Ladner U. Rheumatoid arthritis progression mediated by activated synovial fibroblasts. *Trends Mol Med* 2010;16(10):458–468.
12. Kasperkovitz PV, Timmer TC, Smeets TJ et al. Fibroblast-like synoviocytes derived from patients with rheumatoid arthritis show the imprint of synovial tissue heterogeneity: evidence of a link between an increased myofibroblast-like phenotype and high-inflammation synovitis. *Arthritis Rheum* 2005;52(2):430–441.
13. Bromley M, Woolley DE. Histopathology of the rheumatoid lesion. Identification of cell types at sites of cartilage erosion. *Arthritis Rheum* 1984;27(8):857–863.
14. Tak PP, Smeets TJ, Daha MR et al. Analysis of the synovial cell infiltrate in early rheumatoid synovial tissue in relation to local disease activity. *Arthritis Rheum* 1997;40(2):217–225.
15. Baeten D, Demetter P, Cuvelier C et al. Comparative study of the synovial histology in rheumatoid arthritis, spondyloarthropathy, and osteoarthritis: influence of disease duration and activity. *Ann Rheum Dis* 2000;59(12):945–953.

16. Holt AP, Haughton EL, Lalor PF et al. Liver myofibroblasts regulate infiltration and positioning of lymphocytes in human liver. *Gastroenterology* 2009;136(2):705–714.

17. Manzo A, Pitzalis C. Lymphoid tissue reactions in rheumatoid arthritis. *Autoimmun Rev* 2007;7(1):30–34.

18. Manzo A, Bombardieri M, Humby F, Pitzalis C. Secondary and ectopic lymphoid tissue responses in rheumatoid arthritis: from inflammation to autoimmunity and tissue damage/remodeling. *Immunol Rev* 2010; 233(1):267–285.

19. Thurlings RM, Wijbrandts CA, Mebius RE et al. Synovial lymphoid neogenesis does not define a specific clinical rheumatoid arthritis phenotype. *Arthritis Rheum* 2008;58(6):1582–1589.

20. Cañete JD, Celis R, Moll C et al. Clinical significance of synovial lymphoid neogenesis and its reversal after anti-tumour necrosis factor alpha therapy in rheumatoid arthritis. *Ann Rheum Dis* 2009;68(5):751–756.

21. Takemura S, Braun A, Crowson C et al. Lymphoid neogenesis in rheumatoid synovitis. *J Immunol* 2001;167(2):1072–1080.

22. Humby F, Bombardieri M, Manzo A et al. Ectopic lymphoid structures support ongoing production of class-switched autoantibodies in rheumatoid synovium. *PLoS Med* 2009;6(1):e1.

23. Takemura S, Klimiuk PA, Braun A, Goronzy JJ, Weyand CM. T cell activation in rheumatoid synovium is B cell dependent. *J Immunol* 2001; 167(8):4710–4718.

24. Rantapää-Dahlqvist S, de Jong BA, Berglin E et al. Antibodies against cyclic citrullinated peptide and IgA rheumatoid factor predict the development of rheumatoid arthritis. *Arthritis Rheum* 2003;48(10):2741–2749.

25. Klimiuk PA, Sierakowski S, Latosiewicz R et al. Histological patterns of synovitis and serum chemokines in patients with rheumatoid arthritis. *J Rheumatol* 2005;32(9):1666–1672.

26. McInnes IB, Schett G. Cytokines in the pathogenesis of rheumatoid arthritis. *Nat Rev Immunol* 2007;7(6):429–442.

27. Klimiuk PA, Goronzy JJ, Björnsson J, Beckenbaugh RD, Weyand CM. Tissue cytokine patterns distinguish variants of rheumatoid synovitis. *Am J Pathol* 1997;151(5):1311–1319.

28. Chu CQ, Field M, Allard S et al. Detection of cytokines at the cartilage/pannus junction in patients with rheumatoid arthritis: implications for the role of cytokines in cartilage destruction and repair. *Br J Rheumatol* 1992;31(10):653–661.

29. Firestein GS, Alvaro-Gracia JM, Maki R. Quantitative analysis of cytokine gene expression in rheumatoid arthritis. *J Immunol* 1990;144(9): 3347–3353.

30. David JP, Schett G. TNF and bone. *Curr Dir Autoimmun* 2010;11: 135–144.

31. Hayer S, Polzer K, Brandl A et al. B-cell infiltrates induce endosteal bone formation in inflammatory arthritis. *J Bone Miner Res* 2008;23(10): 1650–1660.

32. Karmakar S, Kay J, Gravallese EM. Bone damage in rheumatoid arthritis: mechanistic insights and approaches to prevention. *Rheum Dis Clin North Am* 2010;36(2):385–404.

33. Dolhain RJ, Tak PP, Dijkmans BA et al. Methotrexate reduces inflammatory cell numbers, expression of monokines and of adhesion molecules in synovial tissue of patients with rheumatoid arthritis. *Br J Rheumatol* 1998;37(5):502–508.

34. Gerlag DM, Haringman JJ, Smeets TJ et al. Effects of oral prednisolone on biomarkers in synovial tissue and clinical improvement in rheumatoid arthritis. *Arthritis Rheum* 2004;50(12):3783–3791.

35. Taylor PC, Peters AM, Paleolog E et al. Reduction of chemokine levels and leukocyte traffic to joints by tumor necrosis factor alpha blockade in patients with rheumatoid arthritis. *Arthritis Rheum* 2000;43(1):38–47.

36. Ulfgren AK, Andersson U, Engström M et al. Systemic anti-tumor necrosis factor alpha therapy in rheumatoid arthritis down-regulates synovial tumor necrosis factor alpha synthesis. *Arthritis Rheum* 2000;43(11):2391–2396.

37. Haringman JJ, Gerlag DM, Zwinderman AH et al. Synovial tissue macrophages: a sensitive biomarker for response to treatment in patients with rheumatoid arthritis. *Ann Rheum Dis* 2005;64(6):834–838.

38. Wijbrandts CA, Vergunst CE, Haringman JJ et al. Absence of changes in the number of synovial sublining macrophages after ineffective treatment for rheumatoid arthritis: Implications for use of synovial sublining macrophages as a biomarker. *Arthritis Rheum* 2007;56(11):3869–3871.

39. Bresnihan B, Pontifex E, Thurlings RM et al. Synovial tissue sublining CD68 expression is a biomarker of therapeutic response in rheumatoid arthritis clinical trials: consistency across centers. *J Rheumatol* 2009;36(12):1800–1802.

40. Baeten D, Houbiers J, Kruithof E et al. Synovial inflammation does not change in the absence of effective treatment: implications for the use of synovial histopathology as biomarker in early phase clinical trials in rheumatoid arthritis. *Ann Rheum Dis* 2006;65(8):990–997.

41. Thurlings RM, Teng O, Vos K et al. Clinical response, pharmacokinetics, development of human anti-chimaeric antibodies, and synovial tissue response to rituximab treatment in patients with rheumatoid arthritis. *Ann Rheum Dis* 2010;69(2):409–412.

42. Kavanaugh A, Rosengren S, Lee SJ et al. Assessment of rituximab's immunomodulatory synovial effects (ARISE trial). 1: clinical and synovial biomarker results. *Ann Rheum Dis* 2008;67(3):402–408.

43. Teng YK, Levarht EW, Toes RE, Huizinga TW, van Laar JM. Residual inflammation after rituximab treatment is associated with sustained synovial plasma cell infiltration and enhanced B cell repopulation. *Ann Rheum Dis* 2009;68(6):1011–1016.

44. Baeten D, Kruithof E, De Rycke L et al. Infiltration of the synovial membrane with macrophage subsets and polymorphonuclear cells reflects global disease activity in spondyloarthropathy. *Arthritis Res Ther* 2005;7(2):R359–R369.

45. Cañete JD, Santiago B, Cantaert T et al. Ectopic lymphoid neogenesis in psoriatic arthritis. *Ann Rheum Dis* 2007;66(6):720–726.

46. van Kuijk AW, Gerlag DM, Vos K et al. A prospective, randomised, placebo-controlled study to identify biomarkers associated with active treatment in psoriatic arthritis: effects of adalimumab treatment on synovial tissue. *Ann Rheum Dis* 2009;68(8):1303–1309.

47. Pontifex EK, Gerlag DM, Gogarty M et al. Change in CD3 positive T-cell expression in psoriatic arthritis synovium correlates with change in DAS28 and magnetic resonance imaging synovitis scores following initiation of biologic therapy—a single centre, open-label study. *Arthritis Res Ther* 2011;13(1):R7.

48. Haynes MK, Hume EL, Smith JB. Phenotypic characterization of inflammatory cells from osteoarthritic synovium and synovial fluids. *Clin Immunol* 2002;105(3):315–325.

49. Dodds RA, Connor JR, Drake FH, Gowen M. Expression of cathepsin K messenger RNA in giant cells and their precursors in human osteoarthritic synovial tissues. *Arthritis Rheum* 1999;42(8):1588–1593.

50. Sellam J, Berenbaum F. The role of synovitis in pathophysiology and clinical symptoms of osteoarthritis. *Nat Rev Rheumatol* 2010;6(11): 625–635.

CHAPTER 53

Bone turnover

Georg Schett

Composition of bone

Bone is a specialized connective tissue that serves (1) locomotion by providing the insertion site of the muscles, (2) protection of the internal organs and the bone marrow as well as (3) metabolic function such as storage and provision of calcium to the body. Bone consists of cells and the extracellular matrix, which is composed of type I collagen fibres and a number of non-collagenous proteins. The specific composition of the bone matrix allows its mineralization, which is a specific feature of bone.

There are two major types of bones: the flat bones, which are built by intramembraneous ossification, and the long bones, which emerge from endochondral ossification. Intramembranous bone formation is based on the condensation of mesenchymal stem cells, which directly differentiate in bone-forming osteoblasts. In contrast, during endochondral ossification of the long bones, the mesenchymal stem cells first differentiate into chondrocytes that will further be replaced by osteoblasts. Long bones consist of (1) the epiphyses, which are protrusions at the ends of the long bones, (2) the diaphysis constituting its shaft, and (3) the metaphyses, which are located between the epiphysis and the diaphysis (Figure 53.1). The metaphysis is separated from the epiphysis by the growth plate, a proliferative cartilage layer, which is essential for the longitudinal growth of bones. After finishing growth, this cartilage layer is entirely remodelled into bone.

The external shape of bones is formed by a dense cortical shell (cortical or compact bone), which is particular strong along the diaphysis, where the bone marrow is located. The cortical bone shell becomes progressively thinner towards the metaphyses and epiphyses, where most of the trabecular bone is located. Trabecular

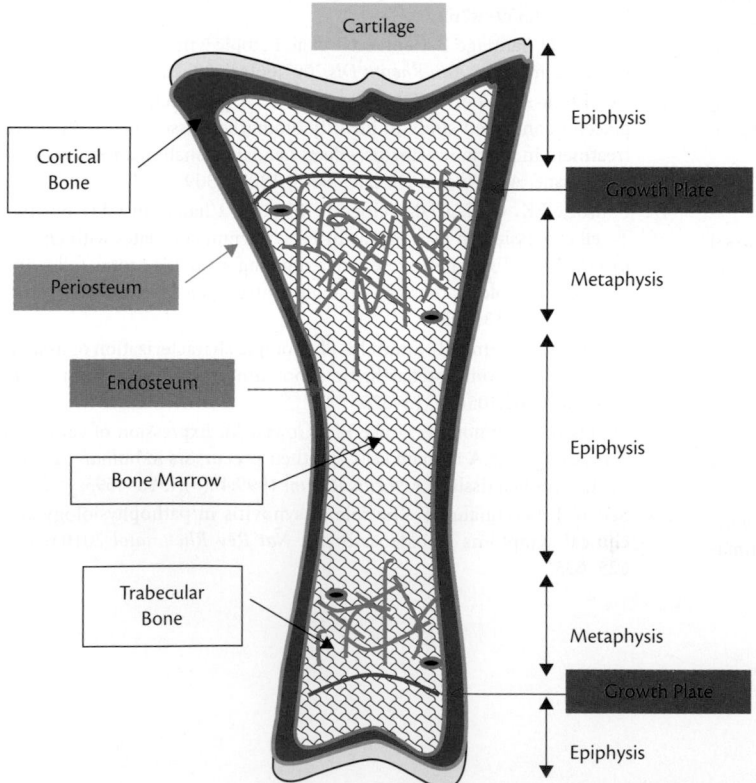

Fig. 53.1 Composition of long bones. Long bones consist of the epiphyses separated by growth plates from the metaphyses, which contain most of the trabecular bone. The outer lining of bone is the dense cortical bone, which is covered by the periosteum (outer surface) and the endosteum (inner surface). The latter connects bone to the bone marrow. The bony endplates are covered by the articular cartilage, consisting of a mineralized deep zone and a non-mineralized surface zone.

bone (also called cancellous bone) is a sponge-like network consisting of myriads of highly interconnected bony trabeculae. The outer and the inner surfaces of cortical bone are covered by layers of osteogenic cells, termed the periosteum and the endosteum, which are involved in the growth of width by bone apposition at the periosteal and bone resorption at the endosteal sites.

Although cortical and trabecular bone is composed of the same cells and same matrix components, there is a substantial difference between these two forms of skeletal tissue. Cortical bone almost exclusively consists of mineralized tissue (up to 90%) allowing it to fulfil its mechanical requirements. In contrast, only 20% of trabecular bone is mineralized tissue, whereas the bone marrow, the blood vessels and a network of mesenchymal stem cells cover the rest. As a consequence, trabecular bone shares a vast surface with the non-mineralized tissue, which is the basis for the metabolic function of bone, requiring a high level of communication between the bone surface and the non-mineralized tissue.

Bone matrix and bone remodelling

The key protein component of bone is collagen type I. Collagen fibres follow specific directions, forming the basis for the lamellar structure of bone. This lamellar structure allows a very dense packaging, resulting in optimal resistance to mechanical load. The lamellar collagen structures can be assembled in parallel (e.g. along the cortical bone surfaces and inside the bony trabeculae) or concentrically around blood vessels embedded in the haversian channels of the cortical bone. In case of rapid deposition of new bone such as during fracture healing, this lamellar structure is missing and the bone is then called woven bone. Woven bone is consecutively

remodelled into lamellar bone, which is also considered as being 'mature' bone. The composition of the collagen backbone also facilitates the deposition of spindle- or plate- shaped hydroxyapatite crystals, which contain calcium phosphate, allowing the calcification of the bone matrix. Apart from collagen type I, other, so called non-collagenous, proteins are found in bone. Some of them, such as osteocalcin, osteopontin, and fetuin, are mineralization inhibitors that make it possible to balance the degree of mineralization of the skeletal tissue. Aside from their intrinsic function in bone, non-collagenous proteins also exert important metabolic functions, such as the control of energy metabolism by osteocalcin.

Bone matrix is subject to a continuous remodelling process (Figure 53.2), which allows developmental bone growth, post-developmental maintenance, and repair of bone. Adults continuously remodel their skeleton, a process that runs even faster in the childhood and adolescence. In adults, it is considered to take 7–10 years to remodel the entire skeleton, indicating that it is fully replaced several times during a human lifetime. Most of the bone remodelling happens in the trabecular bone, which make it possible to build an optimal inner microstructure adapted to the individual mechanical demands. Trabecular bone is the leading structure in the vertebral bodies (up to two-thirds of the bone substance) and in long bones such as the femur (about 50% of the bone substance). Normal physiological circumstances ensure balance between bone formation and bone resorption to maintain skeletal homeostasis. This bone remodelling process requires a tight mutual regulation of bone resorption by osteoclasts and bone formation by osteoblasts, a phenomenon called **coupling**. Coupling is regulated on at least three different levels: (1) by a direct interaction between osteoblasts and osteoclasts; (3) by local interactions between the immune

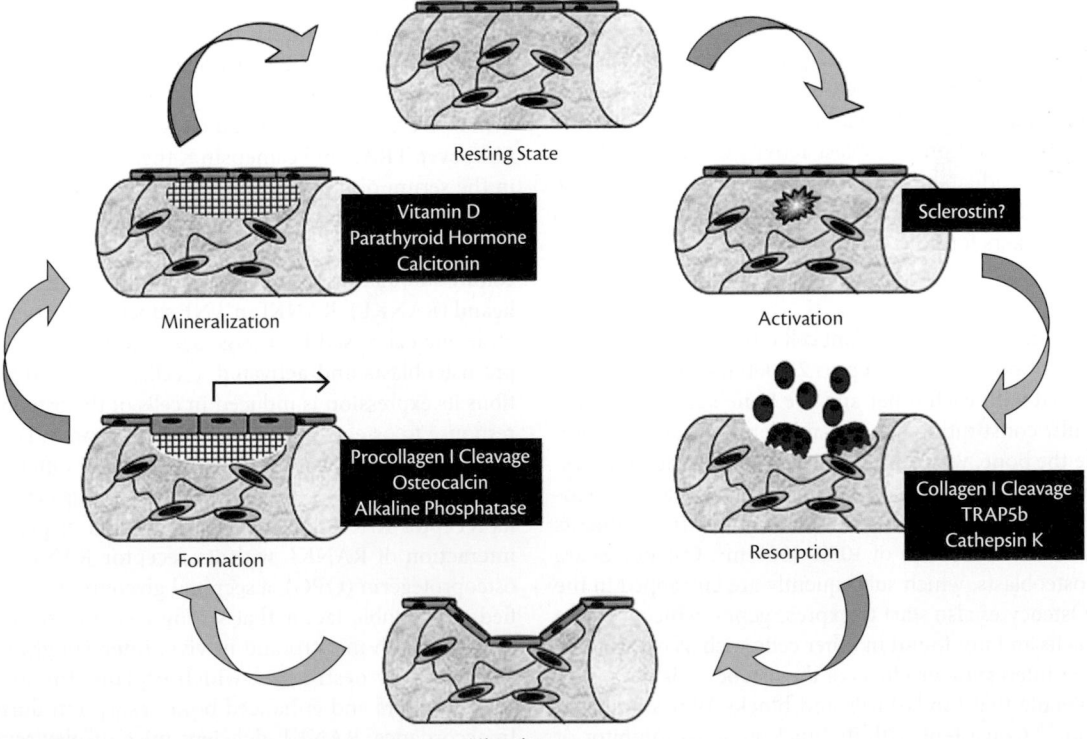

Fig. 53.2 Bone remodelling and markers. Bone remodelling cycle with *activation* characterized by sensing of damage by osteocytes, *resorption* by osteoclast differentiation and removal of bone matrix, *migration* of bone-lining mesenchymal cells into the resorbed area, *formation* of new bone matrix by osteoblasts (cuboid cells), and *mineralization* of the newly synthesized matrix. Biomarkers reflecting the different steps of bone remodelling are indicated by black boxes.

system and bone cells; and (3) by neuroendocrine systemic control of bone metabolism.

The entire bone remodelling process takes about 3–6 months and is controlled by the bone cells. It is initiated by so far unknown factors, which may likely be of mechanical nature and sensed by the osteocytes. Death of osteocytes and the resulting metabolic changes may govern this activation process. It is followed by a resorptive phase dominated by osteoclast-mediated degradation of the bone matrix, resulting in a resorption lacuna. The naked bone surface inside this lacuna is subsequently populated by mesenchymal cells immigrating from the neighbouring bone surface, which start differentiating into osteoblasts and produce the new bone matrix (also termed osteoid). This matrix is then mineralized and the bone returns to its resting state again. Importantly, the activity of bone cells during the remodelling process can be monitored in the peripheral blood of humans, allowing quantifying the activity of bone formation and bone resorption.

Bone cells

Osteoblasts

Osteoblasts are the bone-forming cells that derive from the mesenchymal stem cells of the bone marrow. Osteoblasts are cuboid-shaped cells that form clusters covering the bone surface. They are metabolically highly active, synthesizing the collagenous and non-collagenous bone matrix proteins, which are excreted and then deposited between the osteoblasts and the bone surface. This newly built matrix, which is not yet calcified, is termed the **osteoid**. The lag phase between osteoid deposition and its mineralization is approximately 10 days. Prostaglandin E_2 (PGE2), insulin-like growth factor (IGF)-1, parathyroid hormone (PTH), bone morphogenic proteins (BMPs) as well as Wingless and Int-1 (Wnt) proteins are key stimuli for osteoblast differentiation.[1] Osteoblast activity can be measured in the serum by assessing the production of alkaline phosphatase and osteocalcin, both of which represent specific differentiation markers of the osteoblasts, which are secreted by the differentiated cell. In addition osteoblast activity can be also determines by cleavage products of procollagen type I. These cleavage fragments of procollagen type I can be also measured in the serum and are used as markers for bone formation.

Osteocytes

Osteocytes are by far the most abundant cell type within bone. One cubic millimetre of bone contains up to 25 000 osteocytes, which are well connected with each other and the bone surface by small tubes (canaliculi) constituting a large and dense communication network inside the bone, which has similarities to the nervous system. The surface of this network of lacunae containing the osteocytes and the canaliculi containing the interconnecting filaments of the osteocytes covers an area of 1000–4000 m^2. Osteocytes are derived from osteoblasts, which subsequently are entrapped in the bone matrix. Osteocytes also start to express genes, which are specific for these cells and not found in other cells such as osteoblasts. One of the most interesting products of the osteocyte is sclerostin, a secreted molecule that binds LRPs and blocks Wnt-stimulated bone formation.[2,3] Consistent with its function as an inhibitor of bone formation, overexpression of sclerostin leads to low bone mass, whereas deletion of sclerostin leads to increased bone density and strength. Loss-of-function mutations in the human *SOST* gene

encoding sclerostin entail increased bone mass, a disease termed sclerosteosis. Several local and systemic factors have been suggested as possible regulators of sclerostin expression by osteocytes. For instance, intermittent administrations of PTH, which are associated with strong anabolic effects on the bone, potently inhibits sclerostin expression. No biomarkers for osteocyte function have yet been used in routine settings; however, measurement of sclerostin levels may close this gap in the future.

Osteoclasts

Osteoclasts are multinucleated cells containing up to 20 nuclei and are unique in their ability to resorb bone.[4,5] They are directly attached to the bone surface and build resorption lacunae (Howship lacunae). Apart from their multiple nuclei, another characteristic of the osteoclast is the ruffled border, a highly folded plasma membrane facing the bone matrix and designed to secrete and resorb proteins and ions into the space between the osteoclast and the bone surface. The space between this ruffled border and the bone surface is the place where bone resorption occurs. This area is sealed by a ring of contractible proteins and tight junctions, since it represents one of the few regions of the human body, where a highly acidic milieu is found. Bone degradation by osteoclasts comprises two major steps: (1) demineralization of inorganic bone components, and (2) removal of organic bone matrix. To demineralize bone, osteoclasts secrete hydrochloric acid through proton pumps into the resorption lacunae. This proton pump requires energy, which is provided by an ATPase allowing enriching protons in the resorption compartment, which, in fact, represents an extracellular lysosome. In addition to protons and chloride, osteoclasts release matrix-degrading enzymes, including tartrate-resistant acid phosphatase (TRAP), lysosomal cathepsin K, and other cathepsins. Cathepsin K, for instance, can effectively degrade collagens and other bone matrix proteins. Degradation products of collagen type I are the most widely used markers of bone resorption. The can be measured in the urine as well as in the serum. Both C-terminal cleavage fragments (CTX) and N-terminal cleavage fragments (NTX) are used. Moreover, TRAP and cathepsin K themselves can also be measured in the serum of humans and their level reflects the extent of bone resorption in the body.

Essential signals for osteoclast differentiation are macrophage colony stimulating factor (M-CSF) and receptor activator of NFκB ligand (RANKL). RANKL, a TNF superfamily member, is a surface molecule expressed by a large set of different cell types including pre-osteoblasts and activated T cells.[6] Under steady state conditions its expression is induced in cells of the osteoblastic lineage in response to osteotropic factors such as vitamin D, PTH, and prostaglandins. RANKL is essential for the final differentiation steps of osteoclasts as well as for their bone-resorbing capacity by engaging its receptor RANK on monocytic osteoclast-precursor cells. The interaction of RANKL with its receptor RANK is modulated by osteoprotegerin (OPG), a secreted glycoprotein, which was identified as a soluble factor that strongly suppresses osteoclast differentiation both in vitro and in vivo. Interestingly, OPG expression is induced by oestrogens, which explains the increase in osteoclast numbers and enhanced bone resorption during menopause. In accordance, RANKL-deficient mice display severe osteopetrosis due to the lack of osteoclasts. Regarding the central role of the RANKL–RANK–OPG signalling system in bone resorption, the therapeutic targeting of this system in human disease has drawn increasing interest and recently the potent antiresorptive effect of a neutralizing RANKL antibody (denosumab) has been shown in clinical trials on postmenopausal osteoporosis.[7] Methods measuring RANKL and OPG in the serum of humans have been developed. In particular, the ratio between RANKL and OPG is considered as a marker for the bone remodelling activity in an individual.

Mineralization

Apart from these cell-controlled mechanisms of bone resorption and bone formation, which are of key importance for controlling the bone mass, it is also necessary to mineralize the bones appropriately to allow a maximum strength at certain degree of elasticity. This principle is achieved by mineralization of the bone matrix, which required sufficient supply of calcium ions. Vitamin D metabolites such as 25-hydroxycholecalciferol and its active from 1,25-dihydroxycholecalciferol are essential for maintaining calcium supply to the bone by fostering intestinal calcium uptake. Both vitamin D metabolites can be measured in the blood. Low vitamin D level due to poor UV light exposure or malnutrition is associated with impaired mineralization of the bones and decreased stability, a condition known as rickets.

Hypocalcaemia resulting from low vitamin D level is also the strongest signal for the production of PTH from the parathyroid glands, which is the key hormone in calcium homeostasis. PTH is directly regulated by blood calcium content, with low calcium levels inducing PTH production through calcium receptors.[8] Drugs mimicking calcium and binding to the calcium receptor are called calcimimetics, which are used to suppress enhanced PTH release in the case of chronic renal insufficiency.[9] PTH-mobilized calcium from the bones, by inducing osteoclasts, blocks calcium excretion through the kidneys and induces uptake of calcium in the intestinum via induction of vitamin D. Low PTH level due to impaired parathyroid gland function leads to hypocalcaemia, whereas overfunction due to hyperplasia or ademomata leads to high serum calcium levels. Measurement of PTH levels is a reliable tool to measure parathyroid function and calcium homeostasis in humans. Calcitonin is the natural antagonist of PTH and is also produced in the parathyroid glands.[10] Calcitonin can be seen as the calcium brake, as this hormone fosters the renal excretion of calcium and thus lowers calcium levels. Finally, renal derived fibroblast growth factor (FGF)-23 indirectly influences calcium homeostasis by controlling the excretion of phosphate through the kidneys.[11] Both calcitonin and FGF23 can be reliably measured in human serum and allow a detailed characterization of calcium–phosphate homeostasis in conjunction with PTH and vitamin D.

Conclusion

Bone is continuously remodelled by bone-resorbing osteoclasts and bone-forming osteoblasts. This remodelling process allows best adaptation of the bone architecture to the individual demands and tight control of calcium homeostasis.

References

1. Karsenty G, Kronenberg HM, Settembre C. Genetic control of bone formation. *Annu Rev Cell Dev Biol* 2009;25:629–648.
2. Poole KE, van Bezooijen RL, Loveridge N et al. Sclerostin is a delayed secreted product of osteocytes that inhibits bone formation. *FASEB* 2005;19:1842–1844.
3. Semënov M, Tamai K, He X. SOST is a ligand for LRP5/LRP6 and a Wnt signaling inhibitor. *J Biol Chem* 2005;280:26770–26775.
4. Teitelbaum SL, Ross FP. Genetic regulation of osteoclast development and function. *Nat Rev Genet* 2003;4:638–649.
5. Boyle WJ, Simonet WS, Lacey DL. Osteoclast differentiation and activation. *Nature* 2003;423:337–342.
6. Wada T, Nakashima T, Hiroshi N, Penninger JM. RANKL-RANK signaling in osteoclastogenesis and bone disease. *Trends Mol Med* 2006;12(1):17–25;
7. McClung MR, Lewiecki EM, Cohen SB et al. Denosumab in postmenopausal women with low bone mineral density. *N Engl J Med* 2006;354:821–831.
8. Fraser WD. Hyperparathyroidism. Lancet 2009;374:145–158.
9. Goldsmith DJ, Cunningham J. Mineral metabolism and vitamin D in chronic kidney disease—more questions than answers. *Nat Rev Nephrol* 2011;7:341–346.
10. Austin LA, Heath H 3rd. Calcitonin: physiology and pathophysiology. *N Engl J Med* 1981;304:269–278.
11. Tiosano D. Fibroblast growth factor-23 and phosphorus metabolism. *Endocr Dev* 2011;21:67–77.

CHAPTER 54

Enthesitis

Martin Rudwaleit

Introduction

Entheses are ligaments or tendons connecting either two bones or connecting muscles and bone. Enthesitis refers to an inflammation at the site of the insertion of an enthesis or ligament to bone. Enthesitis is one of the key clinical manifestations of diseases belonging to the spectrum of spondyloarthritis (SpA) and of psoriatic arthritis. Enthesitis may occur in other inflammatory rheumatic diseases as well, such as rheumatoid arthritis (RA) or Behçet's disease, but in these conditions enthesitis is less common. In SpA, other musculoskeletal manifestations are peripheral arthritis, which is typically oligoarticular, asymmetric, and involves the lower limb; dactylitis; and inflammatory back pain. The spectrum of spondyloarthritides includes ankylosing spondylitis (AS), reactive arthritis, SpA associated with psoriasis or with inflammatory bowel disease, undifferentiated SpA, and juvenile SpA. Enthesitis in SpA is a non-infectious inflammatory process in origin, as are arthritis and inflammatory back pain. Flares of all clinical manifestations of SpA including enthesitis can be triggered by a preceding bacterial infection. Principally, enthesitis can occur at any site in the body where entheses are found, yet the most frequently affected peripheral sites in SpA are the heel (insertion of the Achilles tendon and insertion of the plantar fascia at the calcaneal bone) and the knee (patellar ligament, quadriceps ligament). Other characteristic sites in SpA are the anterior chest wall (manubriosternal junction) and the pelvis. MRI studies have revealed the presence of enthesitis also at sites such as the shoulder, sacroiliac joints, and spine.

Epidemiology

Across studies in SpA worldwide the frequency of enthesitis is about 20–50% in adults.[1-3] Similar figures of 15–53% have been reported for psoriatic arthritis.[4,5] Enthesitis in established SpA is usually accompanied by peripheral arthritis or inflammatory back pain (IBP) or both. Isolated enthesitis in SpA without concomitant arthritis or IBP may occur, in particular in the subgroup of undifferentiated SpA which may evolve later into AS or another defined subgroup of SpA.[6] In children, enthesitis is a hallmark of the subgroup of juvenile idiopathic arthritis (JIA) termed 'enthesitis-related arthritis (ERA)', a condition characterized by the presence of both peripheral enthesitis and arthritis, an age of onset of 6–9 years or older, and association with HLA B27.[7] In some children, ERA evolves to AS in adulthood.

Definitions and classification criteria

The term 'enthesitis' refers to an inflammation at the site of the enthesis insertion, whereas the term 'enthesopathy' refers to any kind of pathological abnormality of an enthesis irrespective of whether this is caused by degenerative processes, trauma, or metabolic conditions. Enthesitis of the heel has been considered as an essential and distinct clinical feature of the entire group of SpA, and was therefore included in the European Spondylarthropathy Study Group (ESSG) criteria and the Amor criteria for SpA.[8,9] In the more recent Assessment of SpondyloArthritis international Society (ASAS) criteria for axial SpA, enthesitis of the heel is one of the additional items which are required in addition to the presence of either sacroiliitis on imaging or positivity for HLA B27 in a patient with chronic back pain and age at onset of less than 45 years.[10] In the recent ASAS criteria for peripheral SpA, enthesitis of any site is one of the main entry criteria along with peripheral arthritis (asymmetric, usually involving the lower limb) and dactylitis.[11] Similarly, enthesitis is also one of the major entry criteria in the CASPAR criteria for psoriatic arthritis.[5] A child can be classified as having ERA, a subgroup of JIA best representing SpA in juveniles, if a child has either arthritis and enthesitis or has either of arthritis or enthesitis together with two more SpA features.[12] In all these sets of classification criteria the assessment of enthesitis is done clinically i.e. according to the medical history and physical examination (Table 54.1). This approach has been and still is being criticized, given uncertainties in the clinical assessment of enthesitis and lack of standardization.

Clinical picture

Enthesitis typically presents as pain or tenderness on pressure applied to the affected entheses. Pain is often most prominent after long periods of rest, in particular in the morning, and is relieved to some extent upon movement. Enthesitis in SpA most often affects the lower limb, in particular the knee and the heel. Enthesitis in SpA can also occur at the shoulder, sacroiliac joints, pelvis, and spine. In the spine, ligaments connecting the spinous processes, for example, can be affected. Many of the enthesitic sites are not visible. If visible, however, the affected enthesis can be swollen such as the Achilles tendon (Figure 54.1). Enthesitis may spontaneously resolve after some time or may run a chronic course. Accordingly, the duration of enthesitis is variable and it may last from days to

Table 54.1 Enthesitis in classification criteria

Classification criteria	Description of enthesitis in the criteria	Place of enthesitis in the criteria
ESSG criteria (1991)	Enthesiopathy: past or present spontaneous pain or tenderness at examination of the site of the insertion of the Achilles tendon or plantar fascia	Additional item
Amor criteria (1990)	Heel pain or other enthesiopathy: heel pain (but not pain originating in the Achilles tendon—non-specific) should be taken into account; pain in the anterior tibial tuberosity, midsternum pain, pain in the medial epicondyle	Additional item (2 points)
ASAS criteria for axial SpA (2009)	Enthesitis (heel): past or present spontaneous pain or tenderness at examination of the site of the insertion of the Achilles tendon or plantar fascia at the calcaneus	Additional item
ASAS criteria for peripheral SpA (2011)	Enthesitis: current enthesitis, diagnosed clinically by a physician	Main entry criterion
	Enthesitis: past or present spontaneous pain or tenderness at examination of an enthesis	Additional item (if either arthritis or dactylitis are present and considered as main entry criterion)
CASPAR criteria for psoriatic arthritis (2006)	Inflammatory articular disease (joint, spine, entheseal): no detailed description	Main entry criterion
Juvenile idiopathic arthritis; subgroup of enthesitis-related arthritis (ERA) (2004)	Enthesitis: tenderness at the insertion of a tendon, ligament, joint capsule of fascia to bone	Main entry criterion

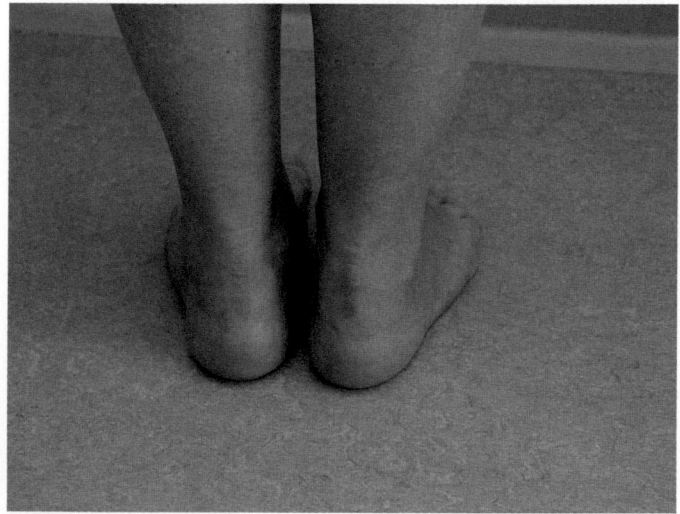

Fig. 54.1 Enthesitis of the left Achilles tendon in a female patient with spondyloarthritis, HLA B27 positive. The tendon is thickened and tender on palpation.

even years. The pain can be mild or very severe and disabling. In longstanding enthesitis a bony spur can arise at the insertion site, referred to as enthesiophyte.[13]

Differential diagnosis

Pain or tenderness upon pressure on bony insertion sites of entheses can result from a variety of conditions including simple mechanical overuse and degenerative changes, trauma, metabolic conditions, and widespread pain syndromes (Box 54.1). Degenerative changes of the Achilles tendon are common and, similar to enthesitis, may lead to thickening and tenderness of the tendon. In Achilles degenerative enthesopathy the pain is often less severe than in Achilles tendon enthesitis. but this finding does not sufficiently discriminate between degeneration and inflammation. In patients with widespread pain syndromes such as fibromyalgia, the established tender points may mimic enthesitic sites upon clinical examination, making it difficult to differentiate between enthesitis and tender sites due to fibromyalgia. The distribution pattern of painful sites may be a diagnostic clue since in enthesitis associated with SpA frequently single entheses are affected, often with an asymmetric distribution, whereas in fibromyalgia multiple sites referred to as 'tender points' are affected, usually in a symmetric distribution. Thus, a careful medical history and a thorough physical examination are of great importance to distinguish these conditions. The absence of other SpA manifestations (i.e. IBP, arthritis, uveitis, limited spinal mobility), and absence of laboratory and imaging findings suggesting SpA including HLA B27, elevated C-reactive protein (CRP), and sacroiliitis on radiographs or MRI helps to rule out SpA and supports the presence of a widespread pain syndrome rather than true enthesitis. A particular diagnostic challenge is posed by secondary fibromyalgia in patients with established SpA, which has been reported to occur in at least 4–10% of patients with SpA.[14] Imaging technology such as ultrasound together with power Doppler revealing hypervascularization at the insertion site of the enthesis or MRI showing an increased signal at the insertion site corresponding to

Box 54.1 Differential diagnoses of entheseal pain

- Enthesitis associated with spondyloarthritis including psoriatic arthritis
- Degenerative enthesiopathy (shoulder, Achilles tendon, iliotibial tract)
- Trauma
- Metabolic
- Acute enthesitis following overuse
- Localized infectious (septic) enthesitis
- Widespread pain syndromes, e.g. fibromyalgia

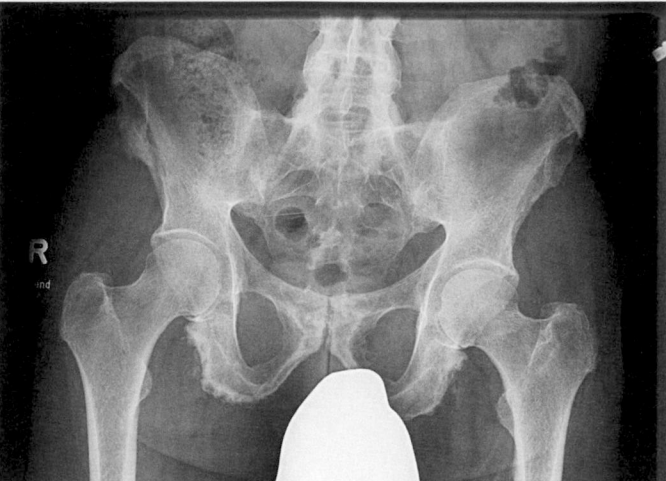

Fig. 54.2 Plain radiographs of a male patient with longstanding ankylosing spondylitis showing widespread enthesitis in the pelvis with formation of fluffy enthesiophytes, particularly at the ischial bone bilaterally. In addition, symphysitis, ankylosed sacroiliac joints, and syndesmopyhtes at the spine can be seen.

enthesitis/osteitis may occasionally be needed for the distinction of true enthesitis from simple tender points.

Pathology and histopathology

The inflammation in enthesitis is anatomically not restricted to the enthesis as such but involves to a variable extent the bone to which the enthesis attaches. Visualization of joints and bone by MRI has revolutionized our understanding of the pathology of SpA and has stimulated research into the anatomical and histopathological characteristics of entheses and enthesitis.[13] Osteitis, a pathological hallmark of SpA, is often detected at the inflamed insertion site of an enthesis, and enthesitis and osteitis often occur together in SpA. It has been speculated that enthesitis is the key pathological element in SpA,[15,16] yet François et al. have demonstrated that in sacroiliitis, synovitis and ankylosis of the sacroiliac joints occur independent of enthesitis.[17,18] Fundamental work has been done by Benjamin, McGonagle and coworkers who studied extensively the anatomical basis of entheses and enthesitis.[19–23] Two major types of entheses can be differentiated, fibrous and fibrocartilaginous entheses. While fibrous entheses are typical for attachment of ligaments/tendons to bone in areas distant from joints, fibrocartilaginous entheses are typically found at the region of joint movement where shear and compression forces take place, such as at the Achilles tendon. At the Achilles tendon sesamoid fibrocartilage, which is found on the inner side of the tendon, protects the Achilles tendon from damage when it is compressed against the calcaneal bone, which itself is covered by periostal fibrocartilage. The subachillae bursa and the Kager fat pad further facilitate smooth movements of the tendon. Since these various anatomical structures function in an orchestrated complex way, Benjamin et al. coined the term 'enthesis organ'.[20] He also coined the terms 'functional enthesis' which refers to tendons which wrap around bony pulleys, and the term 'synovio-entheseal complex' which refers to an enthesis organ that is part of a synovial joint such as the shoulder or the knee.[21] In general, histological data on acute enthesitis is scarce because of the inaccessibility of tissue, in contrast to synovitis, and most data have been obtained from post-mortem studies.[22] In SpA preferentially fibrocartilaginous entheses are affected by the inflammatory process. Histologically, T lymphocytes, bone marrow oedema, and macrophages can be detected close to fibrocartilaginous areas. Bony erosions, entheseal calcification, and bony spurs occur in chronic enthesitis.[13] Ultrasound studies revealed that bone erosion in SpA occurred either at the proximal insertion or the superior tuberosity

of the Achilles tendon, while bony spurs occurred exclusively at the distal enthesis. In one study small bony spurs occurred in both early SpA patients and healthy controls whereas large bony spurs were found only in chronic SpA (9 of 17 patients) but in none of 20 patients with early SpA.[23] Thus, biomechanical factors likely play an important role in the pathophysiology of enthesitis associated with SpA. However, entheseal calcifications and bony spurs also occur frequently in degenerative conditions. Typical sites are the supraspinal tendon (tendinosis calcarea), the ileotibial tract, and very frequently the heel with plantar and dorsal heel spurs. Earlier work using xeroradiography suggested that fluffy and complex spurs occur more often in inflammatory conditions whereas simple spurs occur in degenerative enthesiopathy.[13]

Imaging

Enthesitis can be visualized using plain radiographs, bone scintigraphy, MRI, and ultrasonography. Plain radiographs may show the sequelae of chronic enthesitis such as calcification of tendons and bony spurs. These changes, which can be quite extensive, are often seen in longstanding AS (Figure 54.2). In recent studies, either MRI or ultrasound with power Doppler has been used for visualization of active enthesitis. For the axial skeleton MRI is most useful.[24] MRI is also highly useful for detecting enthesitis and associated osteitis at peripheral sites such as the heel and midfoot, knee, hips, anterior chest wall including the manubriosternal junctions, shoulder, and elbow (Figure 54.3). Whole-body MRI is an ideal tool to visualize widespread enthesitis, but the procedure is not widely available[25,26] and is lengthy, taking at least 45–60 minutes. On MRI, active inflammation is usually characterized by a bright signal on T2 fat-suppressed images or STIR images. Intravenous contrast agents such as gadolinium may add further important information. Furthermore, specific MRI protocols have recently been developed which may even better visualize pathological changes of entheses.[27] If MRI is unavailable bone scintigraphy can provide useful information, but the anatomical resolution is far better with MRI than with bone scans.

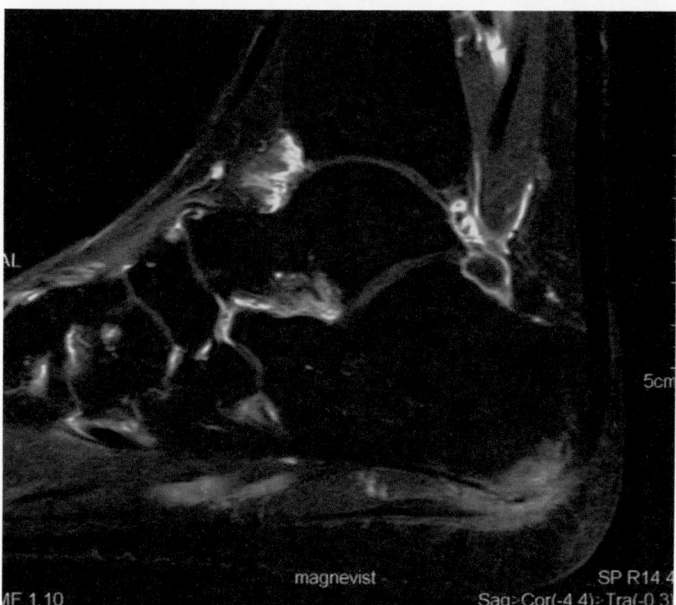

Fig. 54.3 MRI of the right foot of a patient with HLA B27-positive ankylosing spondylitis, peripheral arthritis of the ankle, and enthesitis. Fat-suppressed sequence after intravenous gadolinium administration. Enhanced signals are seen at the calcaneal bone at the insertion site of the plantar fascia. The Achilles tendon is not thickened and the insertion site of the Achilles tendon is normal. Effusion in the ankle joint is also seen.

For peripheral enthesitis ultrasound in conjunction with power Doppler has evolved to be of great clinical use in experienced hands.[28] Using ultrasound, features such as tendon thickening, calcifications, erosions, enlarged bursae as a sign of inflammation of the bursae, and power Doppler are being assessed. Ultrasound scoring systems have been developed for use in clinical practice and in trials.[29–31] In these scoring systems, entheses located at the lower extremity predominate and all scoring systems include the knee with the insertion of the quadriceps tendon at the patella, the patellar ligament insertion at the inferior pole of the patella and distally at the anterior tibial tuberosity, the Achilles tendon insertion, and the plantar fascia insertion at the calcaneus.

In general and across studies, ultrasound is more sensitive than the clinical examination in the detection of enthesitis. Among 18 HLA B27-positive patients with recurrent acute anterior uveitis but no other clinical signs of SpA, enthesitis by ultrasound was found in 55%, suggesting subclinical SpA in these patients.[32] Two recent diagnostic studies revealed ultrasound to be a useful tool. Among the entheseal abnormalities to be detected, the landmark of ultrasound enthesitis in SpA with the highest specificity is an increased vascularization at the insertion site.[33,34] In a study of 118 patients with suspected SpA ultrasound was performed without knowledge of clinical data. At least one vascularized enthesis was found in 76% of 51 SpA patients but in only 19% of 48 patients without SpA, yielding a positive likelihood ratio (LR+) of 4.1.[33] In contrast, entheseal abnormalities on B-mode ultrasound without power Doppler did not sufficiently differentiate between groups (86% in SpA, 60% in non-SpA, LR+ 1.4). Another diagnostic study used the semiquantitative Madrid sonography enthesitis index (MASEI). Patients with SpA (n = 113) had a significantly higher MASEI score than 23 patients without SpA (23.3 vs 16.0). A cut-off score greater than 20 yielded a sensitivity of 56%, a specificity of 89%,

and a LR+ of 5.3. Again, a positive Doppler signal had the greatest discriminative capacity among all ultrasound features.[34] In another recent diagnostic study on 51 SpA patients with or without heel pain and 24 controls, however, neither MRI nor power Doppler differentiated between SpA and control. In particular, power Doppler ultrasound did not show any difference between SpA patients and controls.[35] Thus, some controversy still exists about the exact place of ultrasound as a diagnostic tool. Ultrasound is examiner dependent and interobserver variability in detecting and scoring power Doppler signals can be substantial, as can be the interpretation of findings.[36,37] Advantages of ultrasound are the non-invasive nature of the procedure without radiation exposure. Moreover, ultrasound can visualize several entheses of interest during a single examination in contrast to MRI (except whole-body MRI).

Studies systematically comparing MRI and ultrasound in the detection of enthesitis were scarce until recently and yielded conflicting results. In an earlier study of 32 patients with SpA and clinical heel enthesitis the sensitivity of detecting entheseal abnormalities was greater using B-mode ultrasound without power Doppler (100%) than with MRI (62%; osteitis present in 40%). Inversely, in another study on 14 SpA patients retrocalcaneal bursitis was detected better by MRI (73%) than by ultrasound (only 50% of MRI bursitis was also detected by ultrasound). In recent studies, MRI was superior to ultrasound and power Doppler in the detection of tendon abnormalities.[27,35]

Clinical scoring methods

The first instrument was the Mander enthesitis index.[38] It scores 66 entheses, each in a semiquantitative way from 0–3 for the severity of pain. Since the Mander enthesitis index is complex and time-consuming for clinical use, it was modified in two ways in a data-driven approach. First, the scale from 0–3 for tenderness was reduced to 0 or 1 for each enthesis, and the number of sites was reduced according to the most often affected sides in an observational AS cohort. This modification, also referred to as the Maastricht AS enthesitis score (MASES), assesses 13 entheses: first costochondral joint left/right, seventh costochondral joint left/right, posterior superior iliac spine left/right, anterior superior iliac spine left/right, iliac crest left/right, fifth lumbar spinous process, and proximal insertion of Achilles tendon left/right.[39] The Spondyloarthritis Research Consortium of Canada (SPARCC) developed and validated an enthesitis index based on MRI findings and ultrasound findings.[40] This index includes 16 peripheral entheses located at the shoulder (supraspinatus tendon), the elbow (medial and lateral epicondyles), greater trochanter, knee, and heel (Achilles tendon and plantar fascia). The Leeds enthesitis index has been developed for use in psoriatic arthritis.[41] It scores six sites: lateral epicondyle left/right, medial femoral condyle left/right, and Achilles tendon left/right. Currently, the MASES index is the most frequently used scoring instrument in clinical trials, but none of these indices is used in routine daily practice.

Treatment

Non-steroidal anti-inflammatory drugs (NSAIDs) and physiotherapy are often used for the treatment of enthesitis. In severe or refractory cases local steroid injections can be effective. Radiotherapy has been and still is applied in chronic enthesitis. Sometimes modification of physical activities and the use of orthoses can be helpful.

Several uncontrolled and controlled studies suggest that traditional disease-modifying anti-rheumatic drugs (DMARDs), in particular sulfasalazine, are ineffective for treating enthesitis. In a recent unblinded randomized study comparing etanercept and sulfasalazine in axial spondyloarthritis, improvement in the MASES score occurred in both groups equally after 48 weeks. However, improvement in MASES after 24 weeks was much greater in etanercept-treated patients than in sulfasalazine-treated patients.[42] In double-blind controlled and also in open-label clinical trials of infliximab, etanercept, and adalimumab in AS enthesitis was usually a secondary outcome parameter. In these trials, which often used one of the defined scoring instruments, enthesitis usually responded very well to anti-TNF therapy. Only one placebo-controlled trial focused on enthesitis of the heel as the primary outcome. In this study, 24 patients with heel enthesitis and MRI inflammation of the calcaneal bone at the insertion site were treated for 12 weeks with either etanercept 50 mg per week ssubcutaneously or with placebo. An improvement of at least 50% of the global patient assessment was achieved in 66% of etanercept-treated vs 8% of placebo-treated patients.[43] However, the difference between the groups regarding the reduction of the size of MRI bone marrow oedema at the heel was less impressive after 12 weeks of treatment, suggesting that maybe longer treatment periods are necessary to see significant differences.

ASAS recommends the use of anti-TNF agents in patients with axial SpA for the treatment of resistant enthesitis not responding to conventional treatment including NSAIDs and local treatment.[44,45] Similarly, the European League Against Rheumatism (EULAR) recommendations as well as the Group for Research and Assessment of Psoriasis and Psoriatic Arthritis (GRAPPA) recommendations for the management of psoriatic arthritis consider anti-TNF agents for the treatment of active enthesitis if NSAID treatment or local injections have failed.[46,47] The National Institute for Health and Clinical Excellence (NICE) has published guidance on the use of anti-TNF agents in active AS but without special reference to enthesitis.[48]

Conclusion

Enthesitis is a characteristic muskuloskeletal manifestation of all disorders of the group of SpA including including AS and psoriatic arthritis. Tremendous progress has been made in the anatomical and histological basis of entheses and enthesitis over the last decade. Enthesitis is usually assessed clinically, yet imaging by ultrasound together with power Doppler and MRI has emerged to be very useful for visualizing enthesitis. Both ultrasound and MRI represent an area of active research in enthesitis, in particular their use as diagnostic tools. Local treatment and NSAIDs are the cornerstones of standard therapy, and anti-TNF agents are effective in treatment-resistant enthesitis. Clinical trials in patients with predominant enthesitis are scarce and, apart from psoriatic arthritis, none of the anti-TNF agent has been approved for treatment of enthesitis in peripheral SpA.

References

1. Collantes-Estevez E, Cisnal del Mazo A, Muñoz-Gomariz E. Assessment of 2 systems of spondyloarthropathy diagnostic and classification criteria (Amor and ESSG) by a Spanish multicenter study. European Spondyloarthropathy Study Group. *J Rheumatol* 1995;22(2):246–251.
2. Vander Cruyssen B, Ribbens C, Boonen A et al. The epidemiology of ankylosing spondylitis and the commencement of anti-TNF therapy in daily rheumatology practice. *Ann Rheum Dis* 2007;66(8):1072–1077.
3. Rudwaleit M, Haibel H, Baraliakos X et al. The early disease stage in axial spondylarthritis: results from the German Spondyloarthritis Inception Cohort. *Arthritis Rheum* 2009;60(3):717–727.
4. Gladman DD, Chandran V. Observational cohort studies: lessons learnt from the University of Toronto Psoriatic Arthritis Program. *Rheumatology (Oxford)* 2011;50(1):25–31.
5. Taylor W, Gladman D, Helliwell P et al.; CASPAR Study Group. Classification criteria for psoriatic arthritis: development of new criteria from a large international study. *Arthritis Rheum* 2006;54(8):2665–2673.
6. Olivieri I, Barozzi L, Padula A. Enthesiopathy: clinical manifestations, imaging and treatment. *Baillieres Clin Rheumatol* 1998;12(4):665–681
7. Weiss PF, Klink AJ, Behrens EM et al. Enthesitis in an inception cohort of enthesitis-related arthritis. *Arthritis Care Res (Hoboken)* 2011;63(9):1307–1312.
8. Dougados M, van der Linden S, Juhlin R et al. The European Spondylarthropathy Study Group preliminary criteria for the classification of spondylarthropathy. *Arthritis Rheum* 1991;34(10):1218–1227.
9. Amor B, Dougados M, Mijiyawa M. [Criteria of the classification of spondylarthropathies]. *Rev Rhum Mal Osteoartic* 1990;57(2):85–89.
10. Rudwaleit M, van der Heijde D, Landewé R et al. The development of Assessment of SpondyloArthritis international Society classification criteria for axial spondyloarthritis (part II): validation and final selection. *Ann Rheum Dis* 2009;68(6):777–783.
11. Rudwaleit M, van der Heijde D, Landewé R et al. The Assessment of SpondyloArthritis International Society classification criteria for peripheral spondyloarthritis and for spondyloarthritis in general. *Ann Rheum Dis* 2011;70(1):25–31.
12. Petty RE, Southwood TR, Manners P et al.; International League of Associations for Rheumatology. International League of Associations for Rheumatology classification of juvenile idiopathic arthritis: second revision, Edmonton, 2001. *J Rheumatol* 2004;31(2):390–392.
13. Gerster JC, Vischer TL, Bennani A, Fallet GH. The painful heel. Comparative study in rheumatoid arthritis, ankylosing spondylitis, Reiter's syndrome, and generalized osteoarthrosis. *Ann Rheum Dis* 1977;36(4):343–348.
14. Almodóvar R, Carmona L, Zarco P et al. Fibromyalgia in patients with ankylosing spondylitis: prevalence and utility of the measures of activity, function and radiological damage. *Clin Exp Rheumatol* 2010;28(6 Suppl 63):S33–S39.
15. McGonagle D, Gibbon W, O'Connor P et al. Characteristic magnetic resonance imaging entheseal changes of knee synovitis in spondylarthropathy. *Arthritis Rheum* 1998;41(4):694–700.
16. McGonagle D, Gibbon W, Emery P. Classification of inflammatory arthritis by enthesitis. *Lancet* 1998;352(9134):1137–1140.
17. François RJ, Gardner DL, Degrave EJ, Bywaters EG. Histopathologic evidence that sacroiliitis in ankylosing spondylitis is not merely enthesitis. *Arthritis Rheum* 2000;43(9):2011–2024.
18. François RJ, Braun J, Khan MA. Entheses and enthesitis: a histopathologic review and relevance to spondyloarthritides. *Curr Opin Rheumatol* 2001;13(4):255–264.
19. Benjamin M, McGonagle D. The anatomical basis for disease localisation in seronegative spondyloarthropathy at entheses and related sites. *J Anat* 2001;199(Pt 5):503–526.
20. Benjamin M, Moriggl B, Brenner E et al. The 'enthesis organ' concept: why enthesopathies may not present as focal insertional disorders. *Arthritis Rheum* 2004;50(10):3306–3313.
21. Benjamin M, McGonagle D. Histopathologic changes at 'synovio-entheseal complexes' suggesting a novel mechanism for synovitis in osteoarthritis and spondylarthritis. *Arthritis Rheum* 2007;56(11):3601–3609.
22. McGonagle D, Marzo-Ortega H, O'Connor P et al. Histological assessment of the early enthesitis lesion in spondyloarthropathy. *Ann Rheum Dis* 2002;61(6):534–537.
23. McGonagle D, Wakefield RJ, Tan AL et al. Distinct topography of erosion and new bone formation in achilles tendon enthesitis: implications

for understanding the link between inflammation and bone formation in spondylarthritis. *Arthritis Rheum* 2008;58(9):2694–2699.

24. Muche B, Bollow M, François RJ et al. Anatomic structures involved in early- and late-stage sacroiliitis in spondylarthritis: a detailed analysis by contrast-enhanced magnetic resonance imaging. *Arthritis Rheum* 2003;48(5):1374–1384.

25. Appel H, Hermann KG, Althoff CE, Rudwaleit M, Sieper J. Whole-body magnetic resonance imaging evaluation of widespread inflammatory lesions in a patient with ankylosing spondylitis before and after 1 year of treatment with infliximab. *J Rheumatol.* 2007;34(12):2497–2498.

26. Eshed I, Bollow M, McGonagle DG et al. MRI of enthesitis of the appendicular skeleton in spondyloarthritis. *Ann Rheum Dis* 2007;66(12):1553–1559.

27. Hodgson RJ, Grainger AJ, O'Connor PJ et al. Imaging of the Achilles tendon in spondyloarthritis: a comparison of ultrasound and conventional, short and ultrashort echo time MRI with and without intravenous contrast. *Eur Radiol* 2011;21(6):1144–1152.

28. D'Agostino MA. Ultrasound imaging in spondyloarthropathies. *Best Pract Res Clin Rheumatol* 2010;24(5):693–700.

29. D'Agostino MA, Said-Nahal R, Hacquard-Bouder C et al. Assessment of peripheral enthesitis in the spondylarthropathies by ultrasonography combined with power Doppler: a cross-sectional study. *Arthritis Rheum* 2003;48(2):523–533.

30. Alcalde M, Acebes JC, Cruz M et al. A sonographic enthesitic index of lower limbs is a valuable tool in the assessment of ankylosing spondylitis. *Ann Rheum Dis* 2007;66(8):1015–1019.

31. de Miguel E, Cobo T, Muñoz-Fernández S et al. Validity of enthesis ultrasound assessment in spondyloarthropathy. *Ann Rheum Dis* 2009;68(2):169–174.

32. Muñoz-Fernández S, de Miguel E, Cobo-Ibáñez T et al. Enthesis inflammation in recurrent acute anterior uveitis without spondylarthritis. *Arthritis Rheum* 2009;60(7):1985–1990.

33. D'Agostino MA, Aegerter P, Bechara K et al. How to diagnose spondyloarthritis early? Accuracy of peripheral enthesitis detection by power Doppler ultrasonography. *Ann Rheum Dis* 2011;70(8):1433–1440.

34. de Miguel E, Muñoz-Fernández S, Castillo C et al. Diagnostic accuracy of enthesis ultrasound in the diagnosis of early spondyloarthritis. *Ann Rheum Dis* 2011;70(3):434–439.

35. Feydy A, Lavie-Brion MC, Gossec L et al. Comparative study of MRI and power Doppler ultrasonography of the heel in patients with spondyloarthritis with and without heel pain and in controls. *Ann Rheum Dis* 2012;71(4):498–503.

36. D'agostino MA, Aegerter P, Jousse-Joulin S et al. How to evaluate and improve the reliability of power Doppler ultrasonography for assessing enthesitis in spondylarthritis. *Arthritis Rheum* 2009;61(1):61–69.

37. Gandjbakhch F, Terslev L, Joshua F et al.; Ultrasound Task Force O. Ultrasound in the evaluation of enthesitis: status and perspectives. *Arthritis Res Ther* 2011;13(6):R188.

38. Mander M, Simpson JM, McLellan A et al. Studies with an enthesis index as a method of clinical assessment in ankylosing spondylitis. *Ann Rheum Dis* 1987;46(3):197–202.

39. Heuft-Dorenbosch L, Spoorenberg A, van Tubergen A et al. Assessment of enthesitis in ankylosing spondylitis. *Ann Rheum Dis* 2003;62(2):127–132.

40. Maksymowych WP, Mallon C, Morrow S et al. Development and validation of the Spondyloarthritis Research Consortium of Canada (SPARCC) Enthesitis Index. *Ann Rheum Dis* 2009;68(6):948–953.

41. Healy PJ, Helliwell PS. Measuring clinical enthesitis in psoriatic arthritis: assessment of existing measures and development of an instrument specific to psoriatic arthritis. *Arthritis Rheum* 2008 15;59(5):686–691.

42. Song IH, Hermann K, Haibel H et al. Effects of etanercept versus sulfasalazine in early axial spondyloarthritis on active inflammatory lesions as detected by whole-body MRI (ESTHER): a 48-week randomised controlled trial. *Ann Rheum Dis* 2011;70(4):590–596.

43. Dougados M, Combe B, Braun J et al. A randomised, multicentre, double-blind, placebo-controlled trial of etanercept in adults with refractory heel enthesitis in spondyloarthritis: the HEEL trial. *Ann Rheum Dis* 2010;69(8):1430–1435.

44. van der Heijde D, Sieper J, Maksymowych WP et al.; Assessment of SpondyloArthritis international Society. 2010 Update of the international ASAS recommendations for the use of anti-TNF agents in patients with axial spondyloarthritis. *Ann Rheum Dis* 2011;70(6):905–908.

45. Braun J, van den Berg R, Baraliakos X et al. 2010 update of the ASAS/EULAR recommendations for the management of ankylosing spondylitis. *Ann Rheum Dis* 2011;70(6):896–904.

46. Gossec L, Smolen JS, Gaujoux-Viala C et al. European League Against Rheumatism recommendations for the management of psoriatic arthritis with pharmacological therapies. *Ann Rheum Dis* 2012;71(1):4–12.

47. Ritchlin CT, Kavanaugh A, Gladman DD et al.; Group for Research and Assessment of Psoriasis and Psoriatic Arthritis (GRAPPA). Treatment recommendations for psoriatic arthritis. *Ann Rheum Dis* 2009;68(9):1387–1394.

48. www.nice.org.uk/guidance/index.jsp?action=article&r=true&o=34836

CHAPTER 55

Skeletal muscle physiology and damage

Robert Dinser[†] and Ulf Müller-Ladner

Muscle structure and physiology

Structure and molecular function

Muscle fibres are huge cells formed through the fusion of many separate cells. They contain cylindrical organelles termed myofibrils, consisting of columns of sarcomeres, constituting the contractile unit. In it, thin filaments anchored at the Z-disk overlap with thick filaments (Figure 55.1). Thin filaments are formed by double-stranded helical polymers of actin. The thick filaments are positioned midway between the Z-discs and are formed by three-stranded helical polymers of the dimeric myosin organized in a hexagonal lattice.[1]

Contractions result from a transient cross-bridge between the myosin heads with actin that forms in the presence of ADP, orthophosphate, and Ca^{2+}. Once orthophosphate is released, a conformational change in the myosin heads generates the sliding force. After release of ADP, ATP dissociates myosin from actin. In the absence of Ca^{2+}, a regulatory complex of tropomyosin and troponins blocks the myosin binding site of actin.[1] Many congenital myopathies have been linked to mutations in structural muscle proteins.[2]

Contractile properties are determined by the isoformes of myosin chains and regulatory proteins they contain. Fibres are classified according to their size, speed of contraction and release, and resistance to fatigue. Different fibres may be found within a single muscle. Type I (slow) fibres are characterized by a slow but sustained contraction. Type II (fast) fibres have rapid and brief contraction times and appear whiter due to a lower content of myoglobin. Their oxidative capacity is lower and they have higher stores of glycogen. Muscle fibres are innervated by axonal branches of an α-motorneuron activated in the central nervous system. All fibres depending on one neuron are of the same type; the complex is called the motor unit. One neuron orchestrates the simultanous contraction of its depending fibres. Motor units differ in size, excitability, and patterns of excitation.

The muscle cell membrane is surrounded by a basal membrane along its entire surface. Attachment complexes consist of muscle isoforms of the transmembrane protein integrin and its receptor at the basal lamina, laminin. In addition, a specialized adhesion complex connects actin through intracellular and transmembranous proteins to the basal lamina (Figure 55.2). At the myotendinous

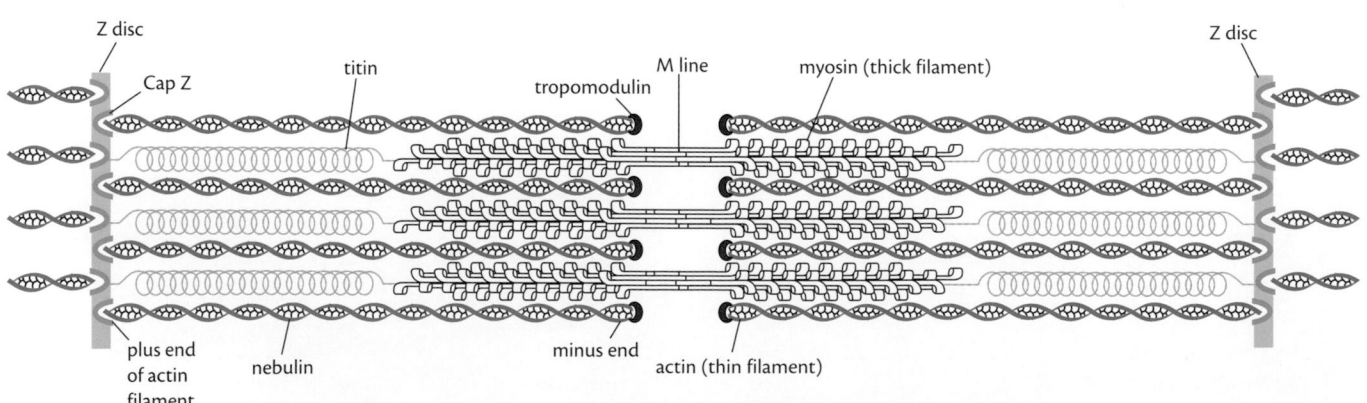

Fig. 55.1 Structure of a sarcomere, including key proteins participating in the stabilization and the contraction of the sarcomere.
Copyright 2008 from *Molecular Biology of the Cell* by Bruce Alberts et al. Reproduced by permission of Garland Science/Taylor & Francis Books, LLC.

† Sadly, Professor Dinser died on 8 May 2012.

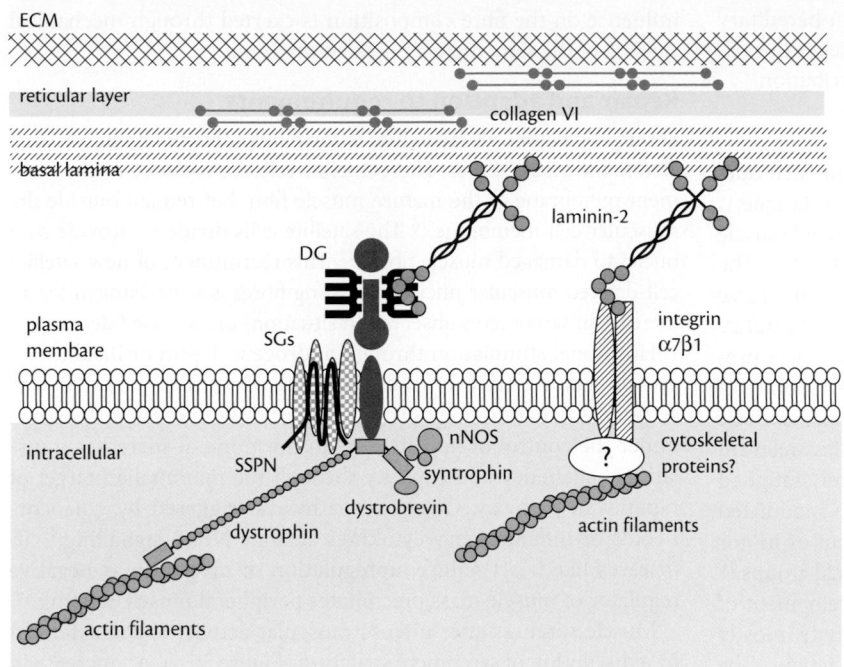

Fig. 55.2 Schematic representation of the organization of molecules involving skeletal muscle cell matrix linkage, including central proteins determining function.
Reproduced from Kanagawa M, Toda T. The genetic and molecular basis of muscular dystrophy: roles of cell-matrix linkage in the pathogenesis. J Hum Genet 2006;51(11):915–26 with permission of Nature Publishing Group.

junction, myofibrils are separated by invaginations of the cell membrane filled with collagen arising from the tendon. The actin filaments insert at an integrin-containing cell membrane complex connected through laminin to the tendinous collagen. Mutations in the proteins involved in the adhesion complex cause destructive myopathies sch as Duchenne-type muscular dystrophy.[3]

Neuromuscular transmission

The myofibrils are separated within the muscle cells by the sarcoplasmatic reticulum (SR). The SR stores and releases Ca^{2+} to the cytosolic myofibrils, depending on the electrical activity of the cell membrane. The cell membrane is invaginated in multiple sites to form a transverse tubular network to conduct action potentials into the interior of the cell. The action potential of the axonal branch is transmitted to the dependent muscle fibre at the neuromuscular junction situated halfway along the length of the fibre. Axon-derived acetylcholine binding to its receptor at the muscular end of the synapse opens Na^+ channels, inducing a depolarization of the cell membrane. The resulting action potential is transmitted through the invaginations of the cell membrane, where dihydropyridine receptors interact with the juxtaposed ryanodine receptors of the SR to allow Ca^{2+} flux from the SR to the cytosolic myofibrils (Figure 55.3). The network of transverse tubules and the multiple sites of interaction with the SR cause an efficient excitation–contraction coupling. Disturbances of the neuromuscular junction lead to characteristic myopathies, such as Lambert–Eaton syndrome or myasthenia gravis.[4] Mutations in the ion channels also lead to muscle weakness and disturbances in excitability, such as periodic paralysis and different myotonias.[2,5]

Energy metabolism

Energy is consumed by the myosin heads cross-bridging to actin filaments, and by the Ca^{2+} pumps of the SR. The intracellular pool of ATP is small, requiring ATP production during contraction. Under

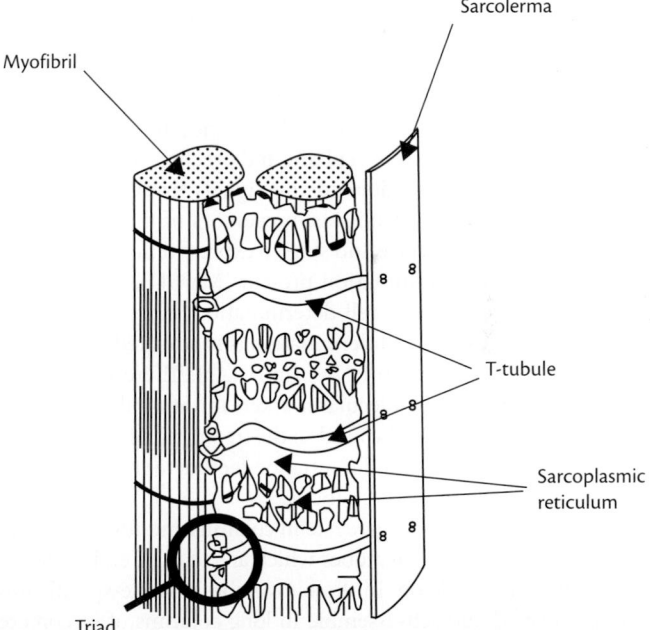

Fig. 55.3 Diagram of the network of T tubules and sarcoplasmic reticulum reaching the proximity of myofibrils to allow electromechanical coupling.
By permission of Oxford University Press.

aerobic conditions, oxidative metabolism of glycogen and triglycerides constitutes the dominant ATP-producing mechanism, generating up to 38 ATP per glucose molecule. In anaerobic settings of maximal exercise, the first source of ATP is the dephosphorylation of phosphocreatine via creatine kinase. As the exercise continues, pyruvate generated through glycolysis is converted to lactic acid, generating 2 ATP per glucose molecule. This process is faster than the aerobic metabolism, but can be sustained only for short periods of time due to the rapid depletion of glycogen stores.[6,7] Mitochondrial dysfunction is not only the basis for muscle disease in hereditary mitochondropathies, but also a pathophysiological correlate in various diseases leading to muscle wasting[8] and fibre redistribution.

Fatigue

Intensive exercise leads to a decline in the strength generated during contraction: muscular fatigue. A key mechanism to fatigue is the failure of ryanodine receptor Ca^{2+} channels on repeated muscle activation, decreasing the availability of intracellular Ca^{2+}.[7,9] The increase in orthophosphate during contraction reduces the force of cross-bridging and Ca^{2+} sensitivity of myofilaments. Entrance of orthophosphate to the SR may lead to calcium phosphate precipitation, reducing the Ca^{2+} available for release.[9] Availability of ATP decreases during high-intensity exercise. Intracellular acidosis and accumulation of lactate in anaerobic exercise are less relevant for muscle fatigue, as the acidosis observed in severely fatigued muscles has little impact on force production. Fatigue is modulated by factors influencing the efficiency of the recruitment of motor units and inhibitory reflexes when using different muscle groups.[10] In addition to these muscle-based reasons for the development of peripheral fatigue, a failure of the motor neuron activity, mostly in situations of low-intensity exercise, is called central fatigue. The relevance of this aspect of fatigue for the decline in muscular performance during exercise is less well understood.

Muscle changes throughout life

Embryology

Skeletal muscles arise at about the sixth week of gestation. The muscles of the trunk and limbs are derived from the paraxial mesoderm, neck and head muscles from cephalic and prechordal mesoderm.[11] Induction of myogenesis depends on signals from neighbouring tissues. The developing myoblasts, precursors of the muscle cells, withdraw from the cell cycle and start to express differentiation factors like myoblast determination protein (MYOD), or myogenin. These factors drive muscle cell determination and differentiation. The process of muscle cell differentiation is modulated through the action of non-coding microRNAs (miRNAs). These miRNAs are beginning to be used as molecular markers for muscular diseases,[12] and may in the future also be used in the treatment of some muscular disorders.[13] The use of differentiation factors to improve muscle repair is an important research focus.[14]

The evolving myoblasts aggregate in columns and fuse to produce multinucleated primary myotubes which are, at their ends, attached to the developing skeleton. In these myotubes, muscle-specific proteins are formed and self-assemble in long columns of sarcomeres on cytoskeletal scaffolding. The myofibrillogenesis proceeds from the periphery to the centre of the evolving muscle fibre so that the nuclei migrate to the border of the syncytium. The number of muscle fibres is more or less constant throughout life. Growth in length is achieved through the addition of sarcomeres at the end of the fibre.[15]

Part of the difference between different muscle fibre types is determined by differing embryological origins of the myogenic precursors, involving different signalling patterns.[14] Once the nervous system begins to interact with the developing muscle at 10 weeks of gestation, the patterns of contractile activity modulate the ensuing fibre type up to the first months of postnatal life. The differences in neural activity lead to differences in intracellular Ca^{2+} levels that are sensed by calcineurin, leading to altered gene expression. Further

influence on the fibre composition is exerted through mechanical sensing of the sarcomere associated myozenins.

Repair and adaption to requirements

Some progenitor cells fail to fuse to form myotubes but remain associated to the muscle fibres. These satellite cells are enclosed by the basement membrane of the mature muscle fibre but remain outside the muscular cell membrane.[16] The satellite cells divide to provide new nuclei to damaged muscle fibres.[11] This recruitment of new satellite cell-derived muscular nuclei to existing fibres is a mechanism for an increase in sarcomeres observed in situations of increased demand.

Hormonal stimulation through androgens, leptin or insulin-like growth factor 1 (IGF-1) leads to increased muscle mass. IGF-1 is secreted as an autocrine hormone in response to mechanical stress under the control of hepatic growth hormone. It increases translational efficiency and capacity through the mammalian target of rapamycin pathway. Catabolic pathways triggered by glucocorticoids or inflammatory cytokines activate NFκB signalling.[17] In diseases like heart failure, upregulation of myostatin as negative regulator of muscle mass precipitates peripheral muscle wasting.[18]

Muscle soreness after intense muscular activity is characterized by a disruption of sarcomere structure (Figure 55.4). An increase in membrane permeability through the activation of stretch-induced ion channels leads to an impairment of excitation–contraction coupling, explaining the reduced strength immediately after damage. The ensuing local inflammatory reaction stimulates the synthesis of new sarcomeres to protect muscles on repeated activity, leading to increased muscle strength.[9]

Although it appears difficult to transform myosin heavy chain isoforms through physical exercise in healthy individuals, imposed inactivity leads to a predominance of type II fibres.[19] Training causes an increase in the number of mitochondria, resulting in an increased oxidative capacity. Exercise increases the use of fatty acids to preserve glycogen stores during prolonged exercise and improves

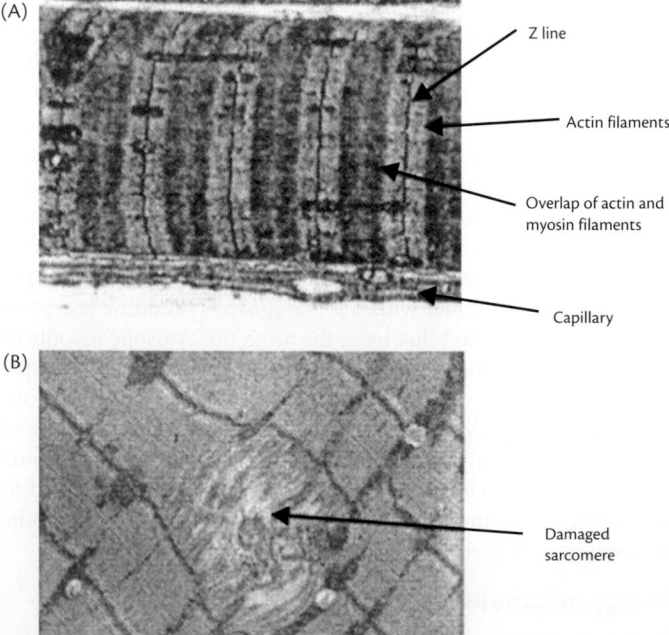

Fig. 55.4 Sarcomere damage caused by overextension during eccentric exercise. By permission of Oxford University Press.

the uptake of glucose. Exercise may stimulate angiogenesis. Stimuli like hypoxia, increases in calcium availability, or changes in concentration of ATP influence the transcription of proteins that are relevant for the efficiency of the oxidative process.[7]

Another mechanism to contain the effects of damage is axon sprouting on denervation. Neighbouring axons grow new branches that connect to denervated muscle fibres. This increases the size of the motor unit and can lead to a switch in fibre type depending on the newly innervating neuron.

Ageing

After a peak of muscle mass in the third decade, muscle strength and bulk decrease physiologically (sarcopenia). As in pathological muscle wasting, lost muscle is replaced by adipose and connective tissue.[20]

While cycles of denervation and reinnervation are normal throughout life, increasing age is associated with a loss of α-motor neurons of type II fibres, accelerating in the seventh decade. Some fibres are reinnervated through axonal sprouting from type I fibres, leading to excessively large motor units. Later, type I fibres are lost in a comparable manner. This loss of reinnervation may be caused by a decline in neural survival factors.[20]

Damage in mitochondrial DNA with ensuing defects in the efficiency of the respiratory chain components precipitates age-related changes in muscle.[8] Part of the mitochondrial dysfunction may be caused by iron accumulation in mitochondria. Iron is central to the function of mitochondrial proteins, so that mitochondria possess their own system of regulatory proteins for iron homeostasis. Mitochondrial dysfunction leads to increased muscle cell apoptosis.

A decline in sex hormones and growth hormones with age leads to a decreased synthesis of muscle proteins and to a decrease in satellite cell proliferation.[16] While relevant signalling pathways regulating skeletal muscle mass[17] have been established, the age-associated imbalance has not been related to these pathways. A decrease in satellite cell number impairs repair capacity. Other age-associated factors not directly related to muscle physiology, such as malnutrition, also affect the loss of muscle tissue.[20]

Clinical approach to muscle disease

Clinical assessment

A useful semiquantitative system for assessing muscle strength in muscle groups and single muscles is the system of the Medical Research Council, grading strength from 0 (no contraction) to 5 (normal power). This method is insensitive but easily applied. Other methods of strength assessment include the measurement of isometric muscle strength or assessments of repetitive muscle function, like the measurement of the time required to stand up and sit down from a chair 10 times. A thorough clinical assessment of other organ systems is of utmost importance in the diagnostic workup.

Laboratory analysis

Testing for intracellular muscular enzymes reveals the extent of muscle damage. Useful are creatine kinase (CK), aldolase, myoglobin, alanine aminotransferase (ALT, GPT), aspartate aminotransferase (AST, GOT), and lactate dehydrogenase (LDH). None of these enzymes is specific for muscle.

A screening test for a suspected metabolic myopathy is the forearm ischaemic exercise test.[21] This test measures lactate as a product of anaerobic glycolysis and ammonia generated through the conversion of AMP to inosine monophosphate by the myoadenylate cyclase, allowing assessment of most glycogen storage diseases (except acid maltase deficiency) and myoadenylate cyclase deficiency. The test is performed after drawing a venous blood sample for lactate and ammonia at rest. Under conditions of suprasystolic arterial compression, the patient exercises his arm with maximal intensity for 2 minutes or until the patient cannot tolerate the discomfort. Two minutes after re-establishing arterial flow, lactate and ammonia are measured. Lactate and ammonia should rise threefold over baseline in a normal response. In the case of a glycogen storage disease, only ammonia increases, whereas in myoadenylate deficiency, only lactate levels increase. The test is valid only if maximal exercise effort has been applied. Any positive result should be confirmed by appropriate further enzyme analysis.

Electrodiagnostic studies and imaging

Electromyography and electroneurography are helpful in differentiating myopathic and neuropathic conditions and in localizing neuropathic changes to the central nervous system, anterior horn of the spinal cord, peripheral nerves, or the neuromuscular junction. Electrodiagnostic studies help in analysing muscle dysfunction but most findings are not specific for defined diseases. Over the time course of a disease, the electrodiagnostic pattern may be altered by increasing muscle fibrosis.

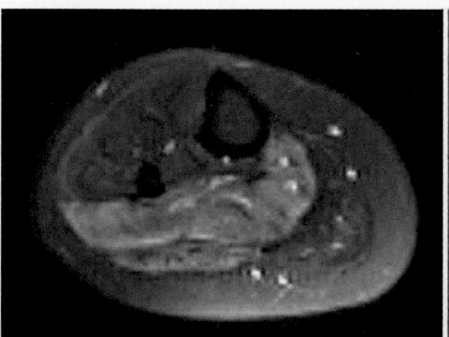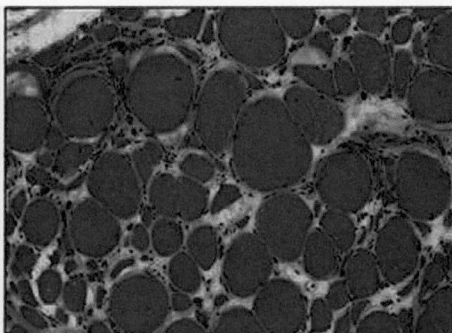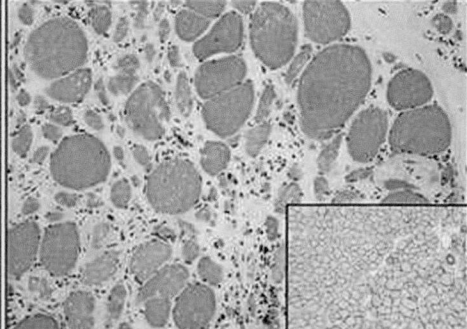

Fig. 55.5 MRI of a 24 year old woman with clinical myositis shows oedematous changes in distinct muscle areas of the calf (left). Haematoxylin–eosin staining characterizes the typical variability in muscle fibre size with some lymphocytic infiltrates (middle), but lacks CD8+ cells (not shown). The immunohistochemistry against dysferlin reveals a complete absence of staining (right), confirming a genetic lack of dysferlin as the origin of myopathy. A positive dysferlin staining is shown in the insert. Courtesy of Dr Anne Schänzer (Marburg).

MRI allows a clear differentiation between normal, inflamed, and atrophic muscle (Figure 55.5). It is used to characterize the distribution of a myopathy and helps determining the localization for a muscle biopsy.[22]

Histology

Histological analysis of muscle tissue is essential to establish a diagnosis. Except for enzyme deficiency diseases, specific diagnoses may not be provided by the histological analysis, but the confirmation of inflammatory disease may be decisive for treatment decisions. Several types of analysis are performed. Conventional histology from paraffin-embedded tissue can describe alterations in fibre arrangement, in the localization of nuclei, scarring, fatty replacement, and infiltrations of lymphocytes or other cells. Histochemical stains on frozen sections allow an assessment of the fibre type, glycogen and lipid stores, and the characterization of infiltrating non-muscular cells (Figure 55.5). Enzyme deficiencies can be ascertained by analysing enzyme activity in a tissue protein extract. Ultrastructural analysis by electron microscopy can identify an altered mitochondrial morphology. Both the surgeon and the pathologist need sufficient information about the suspected clinical problem in order to select an adequate specimen and to allow the correct handling of the biopsy.

References

1. Alberts B, Johnson A, Lewis J et al. The cytoskeleton (subchapter molecular motors). Chapter 16 in *Molecular biology of the cell*, 5th edn. Garland Science, New York, 2007.

2. Laing NG. Congenital myopathies. *Curr Opin Neurol* 2007;20:583–589.

3. Kanagawa M, Toda T. The genetic and molecular basis of muscular dystrophy: roles of cell-matrix linkage in the pathogenesis. *J Hum Genet* 2006;51:915–926.

4. Vincent A. Autoimmune channelopathies: well-established and emerging immunotherapy-responsive diseases of the peripheral and central nervous sytem. *J Clin Immunol* 2010;30(S1):S97–S102.

5. Platt D, Griggs R. Skeletal muscle channelopathies: new insights into the periodic paralyses and nondystrophic myotonias. *Curr Opin Neurol* 2009;22:524–531.

6. Alberts B, Johnson A, Lewis J etal. Energy conversion: mitochondria and chloroplasts (subchapter the mitochondrion). Chapter 14 in *Molecular biology of the cell*, 5th edn. Garland Science, New York, 2007.

7. Westerblad H, Bruton JD, Katz A. Skeletal muscle: energy metabolism, fiber types, fatigue and adaptability. *Exp Cell Res* 2010;316:3093–3099.

8. Marzetti E, Hwang JCY, Lees HA, et al. Mitochondrial death effectors: relevance to sarcopenia and disuse muscle atrophy. *Biochim Biophys Acta* 2010;1800:235–244.

9. Allen DG. Skeletal muscle function: role of ionic changes in fatigue, damage and disease. *Clin Exp Pharmacol Physiol* 2004;31:485–493.

10. Enoka RM, Duchateau J. Muscle fatigue: what, why and how it influences muscle function. *J Physiol* 2008:586:11–23.

11. Braun T, Gautel M. Transcriptional mechanisms regulating skeletal muscle differentiation, growth and homeostasis. *Nature Rev Mol Cell Biol* 2011;12:349–361.

12. Eisenberg I, Eran A, Nishino I, et al. Distinctive patterns of microRNA expression in primary muscular disorders. *Proc Natl Acad Sci U S A* 2007;104:17016–17021.

13. Alexander MS, Casar JC, Motohashi N et al. Regulation of DMD pathology by an ankyrin-encoded miRNA. *Skelet Muscle* 2011;1:27.

14. Meadows E, Flynn JM, Klein WH. Myogenin regulates exercise capacity but is dispensable for skeletal muscle regeneration in adult mdx mice. *PLoS One* 2011;6:e16184.

15. Alberts B, Johnson A, Lewis J et al. Specialized tissues, stem cells and tissue renewal (subchapter genesis, modulation, and regeneration of skeletal muscle). Chapter 23 in *Molecular biology of the cell*, 5th edn. Garland Science, New York, 2007.

16. LeGrand F, Rudnicki MA. Skeletal muscle satellite cells and adult myogenesis. *Curr Opin Cell Biol* 2007;19:628–633.

17. McCarthy JJ, Esser KA. Anabolic and catabolic pathways regulating skeletal muscle mass. *Curr Opin Clin Nutr Metab Care* 2010;13:230–235.

18. Heineke J, Auger-Messier M, Xu J et al. Genetic deletion of myostatin from the heart prevents skeletal muscle atrophy in heart failure. *Circulation* 2010;121:419–425.

19. Schiaffino S. Fiber types in skeletal muscle: a personal account. *Acta Physiol* 2010;199:451–463.

20. Narici MV, Maffulli N. Sarcopenia: characteristics, mechanisms and functional significance. *Br Med Bull* 2010;95:139–159.

21. Valen PA, Nakayma D, Veum JA, Sulaiman AR, Wortmann RL. Myoadenylate deaminase deficiency and forearm ischemic exercise testing. *Arthritis Rheum* 1987;30:661–668.

22. Schweitzer ME, Fort J. Cost-effectiveness of MR imaging in evaluation polymyositis. *Am J Roentgenol* 1995;165:1469–1471.

CHAPTER 56

Joint biochemistry

Thomas Pap, Adelheid Korb, Marianne Heitzmann, and Jessica Bertrand

Introduction

Articular joints are key components of the musculoskeletal system that provide flexible support to neighbouring bone structures and allow for the movement in different parts of our body. This is particularly true for synovial joints that are found mainly at our extremities and constitute the structural basis for key physiological activities such as walking, climbing, and gripping. Synovial joints are composed of different morphological structures, including bone, tendons, cartilage, the synovial membrane, and the synovial space with the synovial fluid. Under physiological conditions they can be well separated, but the close functional relationship of these structures as well as the cellular and molecular interactions between the tissue components of a joint makes it seem advisable to look at synovial joints as at distinct organs. This concept becomes relevant particularly under pathological conditions such as arthritis, which not only affect joints as a whole but which are also based on complex pathological interactions between tissue components of the joints such as cartilage and synovium.

Cartilage development, biology, and metabolism

Cartilage is perhaps the key component of synovial joints. Supported by the synovial fluid, cartilage provides a smooth and low-friction surface that is needed for gliding of both bony ends. At the same time the articular cartilage functions as an elastic and load-absorbing tissue.[1] The biomechanical properties of articular cartilage are achieved by its unique structure. It is characterized by the presence of only one cell type, the chondrocytes, which are loosely embedded into a highly complex and organized extracellular matrix (Figure 56.1).[2] The articular cartilage is organized into at least four distinct zones that differ with respect to the density and orientation of the cartilage fibrils as well as the number and shape of embedded chondrocytes.[3]

Although articular cartilage is usually looked at as a covering tissue that is placed on top of the underlying bone, it actually constitutes a specific part of the cartilaginous template, from which both the joints and the long bones are formed during embryogenesis through endochondral ossification. However, articular cartilage areas are not purely remnants of the bone formation process, in which ossification comes to a halt. Rather, it has been demonstrated that articular cartilage differs from growth plate cartilage and that articular chondrocytes originate from a distinct population of mesenchymal progenitor cells that can be identified very early in limb development.[4] These cells are derived from an area called the interzone and are characterized by a specific molecular pattern including the expression of the growth factor Gdf5.[5,6] Their differentiation appears to be regulated by the concerted action of members of the Wnt family of molecules such as Wnt9a, formerly known as Wnt14, through activation of the Wnt/β-catenin signalling pathway.[7,8]

Those cells of the mesenchymal condensations that are more distant from the interzone also undergo chondrogenic differentiation and then longitudinal growth until the cartilage template is formed. Subsequently, these chondrocytes differentiate further to initiate endochondral ossification, which eventually results in the replacement of the cartilage template with trabecular bone. In addition to the transcription factor Sox-9 that is involved most prominently in chondrocyte differentiation, these steps are controlled by genes of the *Hox* family.[9,10] and regulated by the concerted action of different signalling proteins, particularly sonic hedgehog (shh), indian

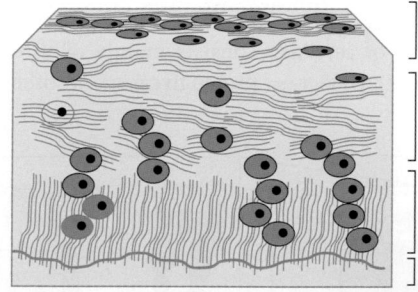

Fig. 56.1 Zonal organization of cartilage. Articular cartilage can be divided into four zones. The superficial zone (also called the tangential zone, because of its structural organization) makes up about 10% of the cartilage thickness. It is in direct contact with the joint cavity. It is characterized by densely packed cartilage fibrils with long-shaped chondrocytes in between. The middle zone makes up about 40% of the articular cartilage and is also called the transitional zone. It has more round-shaped chondrocytes, which are embedded into a less densely packed extracellular matrix. The deep or radial zone is the thickest layer of articular cartilage, and the chondrocytes here are oriented perpendicular to the cartilage surface. The deep radial zone is separated by the tide mark from the calcified zone that is in direct contact with the subchondral bone.

The figure labels read: Superficial zone, Middle zone, Deep or radial zone, Tidemark with calcified zone.

hedgehog (ihh), and growth factors of the fibroblast growth factor (FGF) family.[11-13] Components of the extracellular matrix contribute significantly to chondrogenesis and thus to key properties of cartilage. They serve as a structuring scaffold for limb and joint development and are involved in creating gradients of growth factors. Mutations in genes encoding for heparan sulfate (HS) species such as perlecan,[14,15] or in enzymes that contribute to the assembly of HS side chains, lead to severe skeletal defects.[16,17] As a next step in endochondral ossification, chondrocytes from the middle of the cartilage template start differentiating into hypertrophic chondrocytes, which is associated with fundamental changes in their biochemical profile. Hypertrophic chondrocytes switch their collagen profile to type X collagen and are able to calcify their surrounding matrix. Moreover, hypertrophic differentiation is strongly linked to the increased expression of matrix-degrading enzymes, particularly matrix metalloproteinase (MMP)-13,[18] vascular endothelial growth factor (VEGF),[19] and transglutaminase 2.[20] These changes are controlled prominently by hypoxia, and it has been suggested that HIF-2α is a central transactivator regulating the expression of type X collagen and other catabolic genes critical for endochondral ossification.[21,22] However, this view has been challenged by the observation that endochondral bone formation is only transiently and modestly delayed in mice harbouring a homozygous loss of HIF-2α in limb bud mesenchyme.[23] Thus, while the mechanisms that regulate the differentiation of hypertrophic chondrocytes and subsequent degradation of the extracellular matrix during bone development are only partly understood, an in-depth understanding of these processes helps explain the cellular and biochemical structure of adult joints, and recent data also suggest that joint pathologies such as osteoarthritis are characterized by the (re)activation of certain parts of this embryogenic programme (Figure 56.2).

The primary function of the chondrocytes in the articular cartilage is to maintain the structure of the surrounding matrix through coordinated production and degradation of its components. The exact mechanisms that ensure the homeostatic stability of these resting chondrocytes remain elusive, but it is important to emphasize that the term 'resting chondrocytes' does not mean low metabolic activity. Rather, these cells are characterized by the high-level production of cartilage matrix components, which allows for continuous cartilage remodelling and provides the basis for the regenerative capacity of the cartilage.

The extracellular matrix of cartilage consists mainly of three structural elements: cartilage collagens, proteoglycans, and other non-collagenous proteins. The main collagen of cartilage is type II collagen. It has a triple helical structure and forms fibrillar suprastructures that includes type IX collagen as a fibril-associated collagen with interrupted triple helix (FACIT) as well as type XI collagen.[24] As has been only recently understood, these additional collagens within the collagen II fibrils are important for fibrillogenesis.[25] In addition to collagen types II, IX, and XI, other collagens such as type VI are found in the cartilage.[26] Collagens constitute the backbone of extracellular matrix in the cartilage and their turnover rate is low. Thus, the half-life of type II collagen has been estimated as to more than a human lifetime, which explains why cartilage damage can be considered largely irreversible once the integrity of the collagen network is lost. However, the regenerative capacity of cartilage is considerable, and this is largely due to the constant renewal of other key components of its extracellular matrix, namely the glycosaminoglycans and proteoglycans.

Hyaluronan (HA) is a key glycosaminoglycan in cartilage.[27] It constitutes the structural basis for the formation of large water-binding aggregates with proteoglycans, mainly aggrecan. The amount of hyaluronan in the cartilage, as determined by the rate of synthesis as well as the length of the individual hyaluronan molecules, is therefore an important determinant of the cartilage structure and its functional properties.[28] Other glycosaminoglycans in the cartilage include HS, chondroitin sulfate, and keratan sulfate, which are usually bound to proteins in specific proteoglycans.

Aside from the collagen network, such proteoglycans constitute the most important components of the cartilage matrix, with aggrecan being the most abundant proteoglycan of cartilage.[29] It can be cleaved by different metalloproteinases, including ADAMTS4 (aggrecanase-1) and ADAMTS5 (aggrecanase-2) as well as MMPs such as MMP-3 (stromelysin) and MMP-13 (collagenase-3), and contains a large number of keratan sulfate and chondroitin sulfate side chains. The specific function of the large number of highly sulfated chondroitin sulfate side chains is a matter of intense studies, particularly because several lines of evidence suggest that the sulfation pattern is not only variable but changes significantly during ageing.

Proteoglycans are also found on the surface of chondrocytes (Figure 56.3). These cell-surface proteoglycans include the families of syndecans and glypicans and are anchored to the cell either through a transmembrane domain, as characteristic for the syndecans, or through covalent binding of the C-terminus to glycosylphosphatidylinositol, as found in glypicans. They are endowed with individually characteristic numbers of heparan sulfate or

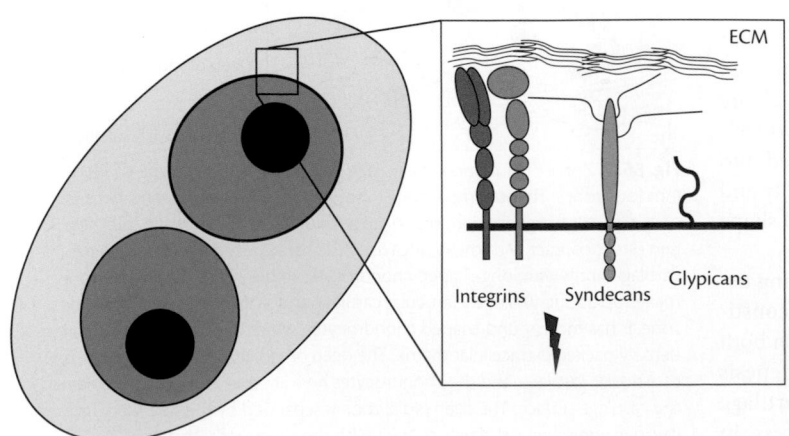

Fig. 56.2 Cell–matrix interactions in cartilage. The interaction of chondrocytes with the extracellular matrix (ECM) plays a critical role in regulating the differentiation of chondrocytes during physiological development, as in embryogenesis, but also under pathological conditions such as degenerative joint diseases (e.g. osteoarthritis) or chronic inflammatory arthritis (e.g. rheumatoid arthritis). Three classes of cell-surface molecules have been identified to contribute most prominently to the interaction of chondrocytes with ECM components: integrins, syndecans, and glypicans. The integrins and syndecans contain intracellular domains and can initiate signalling cascades both independently and in collaboration with one another.

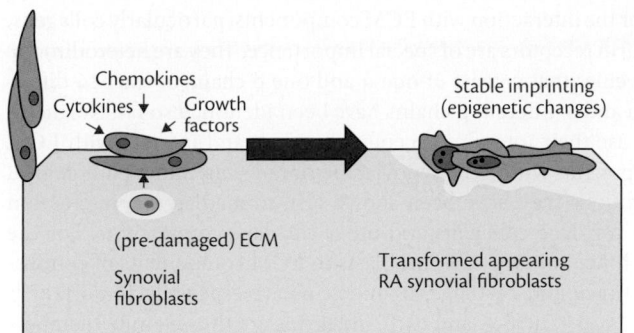

Fig. 56.3 Fibroblast-mediated cartilage destruction in rheumatoid arthritis. Under normal conditions, the physiological function of synovial fibroblasts is to build a lining membrane that secretes lubricants and provides the joint cavity and the adjacent cartilage with nutritive plasma proteins. In addition, synovial fibroblasts are involved in matrix remodelling. In rheumatoid inflammation, cellular alterations following activation through inflammatory stimuli, chemokines, and growth factors result in a tumour-like transformation of these cells. Importantly, several lines of evidence suggest that in addition to these soluble factors, damaged cartilage contains ECM components that contribute to the stable activation of RA synovial fibroblasts. These cells exhibit a special phenotype with unique features such as reduced susceptibility to apoptosis, expression of cartilage adhesion molecules, and the increased production of matrix-degrading enzymes. At a morphological level, RA synovial fibroblasts show a rough endoplasmatic reticulum, large nuclei with prominent nucleoli, and a more rounded shape. The mechanisms that imprint these changes into transformed-looking fibroblasts are not entirely clear, but epigenetic changes have been shown to constitute an important factor in this process.

chondroitin sulfate side chains that can bind a variety of molecules including components of the extracellular matrix such as fibronectin and a growing list of soluble mediators, particularly growth factors but also cytokines and chemokines.[30] Our knowledge about the role of these cell-surface heparan sulfate proteoglycans (HSPG) in the regulation of chondrocyte differentiation and behaviour has increased dramatically in recent years, and it has been shown that the effects of growth factors such as FGF-2,[31] and also cytokines such as osteopontin[32] or chemokines such as CXCL10,[33] are regulated strongly by HSPGs such as syndecan-4. Importantly, cell-surface HSPGs can modulate the effects of soluble factors in different ways, and the role of syndecan-4 in FGF-2 signalling is best investigated in this context. Thus, it has been shown that the clustering of syndecan-4 and initiation of syndecan-4 specific PKCα signals together with altered receptor internalization contribute to syndecan-4-mediated modulation of FGF-2 signalling.[34] Whether similar mechanisms also work for other syndecan ligands and whether such independent and most likely specific signalling function of syndecans can be separated from this non-specific role is a matter of intense research.

Cartilage biochemistry and pathology in arthritis

Osteoarthritis (OA) is the most common joint disease and, at the same time a pathological condition that is most closely linked to changes in cartilage biology. It is a debilitating disorder that is characterized by the progressive destruction of articular cartilage through uncontrolled proteolysis of extracellular matrix and typically leads to a remodelling of affected joints. OA as a disease is discussed in more detail in other chapters of this book, but is

important to note at this point that although the incidence of OA increases with age, it is not a pure ageing phenomenon. Rather, OA is characterized by profound alterations to the biology of chondrocytes that shows important similarities to enchondral ossification as it occurs during embryogenesis, as described above. Recent data suggest that the triggers that initiate and drive the disease process in OA in some respect may be distinct from those in embryonic development and more influenced by inflammation, which is why the term 'osteoarthritis' has been chosen. However, accumulating evidence supports the view that OA constitutes quite a uniform way of how chondrocytes and cartilage as a whole react to stress that they are unable to compensate for. This means that although the triggers that initiate OA and the contribution of individual factors such as genetics, inflammation, mechanical stress, and others may vary considerably from patient to patient, there is an ultimately rather narrow path or programme that characterizes its pathophysiology.

Thus, during OA articular chondrocytes revert to an immature chondrocytic stage and even undergo prehypertrophic to terminal chondrocyte maturation, indicating that their differentiation state, although normally permanent, is not terminal. Losing their differentiated phenotype, the chondrocytes in affected cartilage enter an enchondral ossification-like cascade of proliferation and hypertrophic differentiation.[35] This change is accompanied by marker expression for the overt hypertrophic differentiation stage,[36] such as alkaline phosphatase and type X collagen, with subsequent apoptotic death and mineralization of the diseased cartilage.[37] Therefore, recent studies focus on the mechanisms that either stabilize the articular phenotype or induce chondrocyte dedifferentiation. It has been learnt that osteoarthritic changes are associated with the re-expression of molecules and pathways in articular chondrocytes that are characteristic for different stages of enchondral ossification. The transmembrane HSPGs mentioned earlier, particularly syndecan-4, are a prime example for this concept. Thus, it was demonstrated that syndecan-4 is re-expressed in both in human OA and in animal models of the disease and this correlates with its severity. Interestingly, the loss of synedcan-4 in genetically modified mice or its inhibition by specific antibodies prevented mice from the development of OA-like changes suggesting that, indeed, interrupting the cascade that leads to the completion of the aberrant chondrocyte differentiation programme may be of therapeutic value.[38] Likewise, it was demonstrated that the hypoxia-inducible factor HIF-2α, which (as outlined above) has been implicated strongly in enchondral ossification and in the regulation of genes involved in chondrocyte hypertrophy, also contributes to the development of OA.[39]

It has been well established that matrix-degrading enzymes, mainly metalloproteinases of the ADAMTS and the MMP families, are ultimately responsible for the breakdown of extracellular matrix in OA and, thus, for the progressive loss of articular cartilage. Among the different enzymes, particularly MMP-13 and ADAMTS-5 have been associated with chondrocyte-mediated cartilage damage, and it has been demonstrated in animal models of OA that the loss of these enzymes or inhibition of their activation results in less-severe cartilage damage. However, not only is it likely that the relevance of individual members of the MMP and ADAMTS family varies during different phases of OA, but it may also hypothesized that other MMPs, e.g. MMP-3 or MT1-MMP, which themselves are a critical activators of other MMPs and cathepsins, contribute to the loss of articular cartilage in OA. It needs to be emphasized, however, that cartilage matrix can be degraded by these enzymes not only when they are released from chondrocytes themselves but also when there is an increased and unbalanced expression in neighbouring tissues such as the synovial membrane. The most prominent example of a disease where cartilage destruction is mediated mainly by an invading synovial membrane is rheumatoid arthritis (RA). In RA, the inflamed and hyperplastic synovial membrane that attaches to the articular cartilage grows deeply into the cartilage matrix and destroys it. Data from different animal models including the SCID mouse model of RA-like cartilage destruction and the human TNFα transgenic (hTNFtg) mouse suggest that cartilage destruction by the inflamed and hyperplastic synovium requires the attachment and, thus, the direct contact of the synovial tissue with the cartilage. Also, the early loss of proteoglycans from the cartilage, which is most likely driven by the chondrocytes themselves, appears to constitute an important prerequisite for the pannus tissue to invade. This notion has been derived not only from studying the sequence of destructive events in the hTNFtg mouse but also from experiments in which these hTNFtg mice were crossed with animals that lack interleukin (IL)-1, an important mediator of early proteoglycan loss.[40] The resulting hTNFtg/IL-1 knockout mice do develop inflammatory arthritis with pannus formation, but their cartilage is largely protected, showing no significant loss of proteoglycans and also no attachment and invasion of the pannus tissue.

Composition and biochemistry of the synovial membrane

The synovial membrane is a second specific component of synovial joints. Normally, it is only a few (~4–5) cell layers thick and consists mainly of fibroblast-like cells that through cell–cell contacts form a layer that lines up the synovial membrane against the joint cavity and the synovial fluid. The fibroblast-like synoviocytes (FLS) have a key function in providing the joint cavity and the adjacent cartilage with lubricating molecules such as hyaluronic acid as well as with plasma-derived nutrients. Unlike other bordering membranes, the synovium has no basal membrane, which makes it significantly different from the classical composition of an epithelium. Also, cellular contacts between the FLS lack tight junctions and desmosomes, which together with the absence of a basal membrane, facilitates the efflux of serum components from the small capillaries into the synovial space. However, this means that the most superficial layer of the synovial membrane, the intimal lining layer, has to take over these functions. In this context, the adhesion molecule cadherin-11 has been shown to mediate a strong homophilic adhesion between synoviocytes and to be largely responsible for their organization into a tissue.[41] This most superficial lining layer of the synovium can be separated histologically from the looser network of fibroblasts underneath, which is called the sublining. In addition to the FLS, also termed type B synoviocytes, there are macrophages in the synovial membrane, which are also called type A synoviocytes. In addition to providing the synovial cavity with nutrients and lubricating factors, production of extracellular matrix (ECM) components and cross-linking these into the specific three-dimensional structure is the main function of the cells of the synovial membrane, mainly the FLS. This is an active process in which the fibroblasts have to migrate to sites of tissue remodelling and to interact with ECM molecules through specific surface receptors (Figure 56.3).

For the interaction with ECM components, particularly collagens, integrin receptors are of special importance. They are heterodimeric molecules that consist of one α and one β chain; at least 16 different α and 8 different β chains have been identified so far. Normally, FLS use their integrins receptors to sense and interact with ECM components within the synovial membrane, but under pathological conditions they have been shown also to mediate the interaction with cartilage collagens and other cartilage components. For the attachment of synovial fibroblasts to ECM components of connective tissue and cartilage, β_1-integrins are especially important.[42] $\alpha_1\beta_1$-, $\alpha_2\beta_1$-, $\alpha_{10}\beta_1$-, and $\alpha_{11}\beta_1$-integrins are those family members that are mainly responsible for the attachment of fibroblasts to collagen. Other members of the β_1 integrin family including $\alpha_4\beta_1$- and $\alpha_5\beta_1$-integrins are responsible for the attachment of fibroblasts to fibronectin and its spliced variants. It is important to emphasize that the engagement of integrin receptors on the surface of FLS, just like on other cells, does not merely establish a cell–matrix contact but leads to the formation of adhesive cell structures that are called focal adhesions. As a consequence of their formation, intracellular signalling cascades are being activated that regulate the transcription of genes and thus control cell proliferation and survival, and secretion of certain cytokines and chemokines as well as matrix deposition and resorption. Among the molecules that transmit the signals from integrin clusters to the interior of FLS, the focal adhesion kinase (FAK) plays a central role.[43] However, many signalling pathways can also be activated by FAK-independent signalling mechanisms, particularly through growth factors but also cytokines and chemokines, and the question of how the signals from different sources, including those from focal adhesions, are coordinated into a specific cellular response is a matter of intense research.

The analysis of cell–matrix interactions of FLS is complicated by two observations. First, other and even more complex adhesive and invasive structures have been identified and characterized in recent years and the question of what role such podosome-like structures play in normal and pathological joint remodelling remain unclear. While classical podosomes are found mainly on macrophages and related cells, it has been reported that podosome-like structures such as invadopodia are also found on other cells such as fibroblasts, particularly when they are transformed.[44] The second important observation has been that in addition to integrins, syndecans are involved in the attachment of fibroblasts to ECM components as well as in their response to growth factors and cytokines. In the joint, syndecans are expressed not only on chondrocytes but also on fibroblasts. It could be demonstrated that the response of syndecan-4-deficient fibroblasts to fibronectin attachment is significantly altered[45] and that syndecan-4-deficient fibroblasts have a reduced ability to differentiate into alpha-smooth muscle actin (α-SMA) positive myofibroblasts. The exact mechanisms by which syndecans are involved in the specific functions of different fibroblast populations will soon be elucidated—it appears that syndecans are important cell-surface receptors that, due to their unique properties, integrate signals from ECM components and soluble factors.

The fibroblasts of the synovial membrane are not only responsible for the deposition of ECM molecules and their assembly, but are also prominently involved in their destruction and removal. For the degradation of ECM components, FLS produce a diversity of matrix-degrading enzymes. These include members of the metalloproteinase family, including MMPs and ADAMTS but also different cathepsins. Most MMPs are not expressed constitutively but only upon induction by specific stimuli such as cytokines, growth factors, or ECM molecules. Among the cytokines, IL-1 is perhaps the most potent inducer of a variety of MMPs and has been shown to strongly regulate the expression of MMP-1, -3, -8, -13 and -14. Growth factors such as FGF and platelet-derived growth factor (PDGF) can also induce MMPs in fibroblasts and, thus, act synergistically with cytokines on MMP expression. The third group of MMP inducers are matrix proteins, and especially their degradation products; these activate MMP expression in fibroblasts, providing the possibility for a site-specific MMP activation in regions of matrix breakdown.[46] There are several intracellular signalling pathways that are responsible for the transcriptional activation of MMPs. Thus, bindings sites for the activator protein-1 (AP-1) are present in the promoters of nearly of all MMPs, suggesting that the jun/fos transcription factors contribute prominently to the regulation of these enzymes. Indeed, there is ample evidence that all three mitogen/stress-activated protein kinase (MAPK/SAPK) families, ERK, JNK, and p38 kinase are involved in the regulation of MMP expression by integrating signals upstream of jun/fos. This has been shown particularly for MMP-1, -9 and -13.[47-49] Importantly, the promoter regions of several MMPs that have been shown to be relevant in pathologic tissue destruction also contain binding sites for NFκB,[47-49] STAT,[50] and Ets.[51]

Synovial biochemistry in arthritis

The composition, the molecular pattern, and also the biochemistry of the synovial membrane change dramatically during inflammation. This is true for acute inflammatory episodes where the accumulation of inflammatory cells with subsequent stimulation of the local mesenchyme occurs for a limited period of time, but even more so for chronic inflammation. The mechanisms that regulate the switch from acute to chronic inflammation within the synovium are not very well understood. However, it has been shown that FLS contribute significantly to this process. This has become particularly evident for RA, where these cells are a key part of the local immune system in the joints and integrate signals from different sources into a pathological tissue response. While responding to the stimuli in the chronically inflamed synovium, RA FLS undergo fundamental changes, and multiple lines of evidence suggest that the result is a stable activation, which is maintained even in the absence of continuous stimulation by inflammatory triggers. As a consequence of this stable FLS activation, the disease process is perpetuated and might progress when inflammation ameliorates. The underlying mechanisms are not entirely clear, but the chronic exposure of FLS to inflammatory cytokines, growth factors, and the ECM appears to result in the imprinting of an aggressive phenotype. However, it should be mentioned that due to their general properties, FLS are involved very prominently in regulating and modulating the local immune response in the joints. To this end, they not express a variety of cytokine receptors but also Toll-like receptors (TLRs) through which they can react to damage-associated molecular pattern (DAMP), and Fc-receptors to respond to immunglobulins.

Of note, synovial fibroblasts are not only stimulated by inflammatory and immune cells and their mediators but in turn also contribute to the accumulation of these cells. Thus, the influx of CD4+ T cells into the proliferating synovium is enhanced by RA synovial fibroblasts due to their production of CXCL16 and IL-16. RA FLS are also an important source of cytokines with IL-2-like activity,

IL-15, and IL-7, in RA joints. RA synovial fibroblasts have been shown to contribute to the attraction and accumulation of B cells in inflamed tissue. For example, the secretion of SDF-1 by synovial fibroblasts has been shown to facilitate B-cell migration and activation to the synovium. In summary, the interaction between mesenchymal, immune and inflammatory cells is mediated by a tightly regulated, extremely complex network of cytokines that results in the maintenance of inflammation.

References

1. Pearle AD, Warren RF, Rodeo SA. Basic science of articular cartilage and osteoarthritis. *Clin Sports Med* 2005;24(1):1–12.

2. Poole AR, Kojima T, Yasuda T et al. Composition and structure of articular cartilage: a template for tissue repair. *Clin Orthop Relat Res* 2001(391 Suppl):S26–S33.

3. Hunziker EB, Michel M, Studer D. Ultrastructure of adult human articular cartilage matrix after cryotechnical processing. *Microsc Res Tech* 1997;37(4):271–284.

4. Archer CW, Dowthwaite GP, Francis-West P: Development of synovial joints. *Birth Defects Res C, Embryo Today* 2003;69(2):144–155.

5. Koyama E, Shibukawa Y, Nagayama M et al. A distinct cohort of progenitor cells participates in synovial joint and articular cartilage formation during mouse limb skeletogenesis. *Dev Biol* 2008;316(1):62–73.

6. Francis-West PH, Abdelfattah A, Chen P et al. Mechanisms of GDF-5 action during skeletal development. *Development* 1999;126(6):1305–1315.

7. Hartmann C, Tabin CJ. Wnt-14 plays a pivotal role in inducing synovial joint formation in the developing appendicular skeleton. *Cell* 2001;104(3):341–351.

8. Spater D, Hill TP, O'Sullivan RJ et al. Wnt9a signaling is required for joint integrity and regulation of Ihh during chondrogenesis. *Development* 2006;133(15):3039–3049.

9. Mundlos S, Olsen BR: Heritable diseases of the skeleton. Part I: Molecular insights into skeletal development-transcription factors and signaling pathways. *FASEB J* 1997;11(2):125–132.

10. DeLise AM, Fischer L, Tuan RS. Cellular interactions and signaling in cartilage development. *Osteoarthritis Cartilage* 2000;8(5):309–334.

11. Vortkamp A, Lee K, Lanske B et al. Regulation of rate of cartilage differentiation by Indian hedgehog and PTH-related protein. *Science* 1996;273(5275):613–622.

12. Yang Y, Niswander L. Interaction between the signaling molecules WNT7a and SHH during vertebrate limb development: dorsal signals regulate anteroposterior patterning. *Cell* 1995;80(6):939–947.

13. Ehlen HW, Buelens LA, Vortkamp A. Hedgehog signaling in skeletal development. *Birth Defects Res C Embryo Today* 2006;78(3):267–279.

14. Costell M, Gustafsson E, Aszodi A et al. Perlecan maintains the integrity of cartilage and some basement membranes. *J Cell Biol* 1999;147(5):1109–1122.

15. Arikawa-Hirasawa E, Watanabe H, Takami H, Hassell JR, Yamada Y: Perlecan is essential for cartilage and cephalic development. *Nat Genet* 1999;23(3):354–358.

16. Koziel L, Kunath M, Kelly OG, Vortkamp A. Ext1-dependent heparan sulfate regulates the range of Ihh signaling during endochondral ossification. *Dev Cell* 2004;6(6):801–813.

17. Legeai-Mallet L, Rossi A, Benoist-Lasselin C et al. EXT 1 gene mutation induces chondrocyte cytoskeletal abnormalities and defective collagen expression in the exostoses. *J Bone Miner Res* 2000;15(8):1489–1500.

18. D'Angelo M, Yan Z, Nooreyazdan M et al. MMP-13 is induced during chondrocyte hypertrophy. *J Cell Biochem* 2000;77(4):678–693.

19. Gerber HP, Vu TH, Ryan AM et al. VEGF couples hypertrophic cartilage remodeling, ossification and angiogenesis during endochondral bone formation. *Nat Med* 1999;5(6):623–628.

20. Johnson KA, Terkeltaub RA. External GTP-bound transglutaminase 2 is a molecular switch for chondrocyte hypertrophic differentiation and calcification. *J Biol Chem* 2005;280(15):15004–15012.

21. Saito T, Fukai A, Mabuchi A et al. Transcriptional regulation of endochondral ossification by HIF-2alpha during skeletal growth and osteoarthritis development. *Nat Med* 2010;16(6):678–686.

22. Stewart AJ, Houston B, Farquharson C. Elevated expression of hypoxia inducible factor-2alpha in terminally differentiating growth plate chondrocytes. *J Cell Physiol* 2006;206(2):435–440.

23. Araldi E, Khatri R, Giaccia AJ, Simon MC, Schipani E. Lack of HIF-2alpha in limb bud mesenchyme causes a modest and transient delay of endochondral bone development. *Nat Med* 2011;17(1):25–26; author reply 27–29.

24. Mendler M, Eich-Bender SG, Vaughan L, Winterhalter KH, Bruckner P. Cartilage contains mixed fibrils of collagen types II, IX, and XI. *J Cell Biol* 1989;108(1):191–197.

25. Blaschke UK, Eikenberry EF, Hulmes DJ, Galla HJ, Bruckner P. Collagen XI nucleates self-assembly and limits lateral growth of cartilage fibrils. *J Biol Chem* 2000;275(14):10370–10378.

26. Eyre D: Collagen of articular cartilage. *Arthritis Res* 2002;4(1):30–35.

27. Hascall V, Esco JD. Hyaluronan. In: Varki A, Cummings RD, Esco JD et al. (eds) *Essentials of glycobiology*. Cold Spring Harbor Laboratory Press, Cold Spring Harbor, NY, 2009.

28. Knudson CB, Knudson W. Hyaluronan and CD44: modulators of chondrocyte metabolism. *Clin Orthop Relate Res* 2004;427(Suppl):S152–S162.

29. Knudson CB, Knudson W. Cartilage proteoglycans. *Semin Cell Dev Biol* 2001;12(2):69–78.

30. Tumova S, Woods A, Couchman JR. Heparan sulfate proteoglycans on the cell surface: versatile coordinators of cellular functions. *Int J Biochem Cell Biol* 2000;32(3):269–288.

31. Volk R, Schwartz JJ, Li J, Rosenberg RD, Simons M: The role of syndecan cytoplasmic domain in basic fibroblast growth factor-dependent signal transduction. *J Biol Chem* 1999;274(34):24417–24424.

32. Kon S, Ikesue M, Kimura C et al. Syndecan-4 protects against osteopontin-mediated acute hepatic injury by masking functional domains of osteopontin. *J Exp Med* 2008;205(1):25–33.

33. Jiang D, Liang J, Campanella GS et al. Inhibition of pulmonary fibrosis in mice by CXCL10 requires glycosaminoglycan binding and syndecan-4. *J Clin Invest* 2010;120(6):2049–2057.

34. Horowitz A, Tkachenko E, Simons M. Fibroblast growth factor-specific modulation of cellular response by syndecan-4. *J Cell Biol* 2002;157(4):715–725.

35. Pfander D, Swoboda B, Kirsch T. Expression of early and late differentiation markers (proliferating cell nuclear antigen, syndecan-3, annexin VI, and alkaline phosphatase) by human osteoarthritic chondrocytes. *Am J Pathol* 2001;159(5):1777–1783.

36. Dreier R. Hypertrophic differentiation of chondrocytes in osteoarthritis: the developmental aspect of degenerative joint disorders. *Arthritis Res Ther* 2010;12(5):216.

37. Fuerst M, Bertrand J, Lammers L et al. Calcification of articular cartilage in human osteoarthritis. *Arthritis Rheum* 2009;60(9):2694–2703.

38. Echtermeyer F, Bertrand J, Dreier R et al. Syndecan-4 regulates ADAMTS-5 activation and cartilage breakdown in osteoarthritis. *Nat Med* 2009;15(9):1072–1076.

39. Yang S, Kim J, Ryu JH et al. Hypoxia-inducible factor-2alpha is a catabolic regulator of osteoarthritic cartilage destruction. *Nat Med* 2010;16(6):687–693.

40. Zwerina J, Redlich K, Polzer K et al. TNF-induced structural joint damage is mediated by IL-1. *Proc Natl Acad Sci U S A* 2007;104(28):11742–11747.

41. Valencia X, Higgins JM, Kiener HP et al. Cadherin-11 provides specific cellular adhesion between fibroblast-like synoviocytes. *J Exp Med* 2004;200(12):1673–1679.

42. Rinaldi N, Schwarz EM, Weis D et al. Increased expression of integrins on fibroblast-like synoviocytes from rheumatoid arthritis in vitro correlates with enhanced binding to extracellular matrix proteins. *Ann Rheum Dis* 1997;56(1):45–51.

43. Mitra SK, Hanson DA, Schlaepfer DD. Focal adhesion kinase: in command and control of cell motility. *Nat Rev Mol Cell Biol* 2005;6(1):56–68.

44. Juin A, Billottet C, Moreau V et al. Physiological type I collagen organization induces the formation of a novel class of linear invadosomes. *Mol Biol Cell* 2012;23(2):297–309.

45. Echtermeyer F, Streit M, Wilcox-Adelman S et al. Delayed wound repair and impaired angiogenesis in mice lacking syndecan-4. *J Clin Invest* 2001;107(2):R9–R14.

46. Loeser RF, Forsyth CB, Samarel AM, Im HJ. Fibronectin fragment activation of proline-rich tyrosine kinase PYK2 mediates integrin signals regulating collagenase-3 expression by human chondrocytes through a protein kinase C-dependent pathway. *J Biol Chem* 2003;278(27):24577–24585.

47. Brauchle M, Gluck D, Di Padova F, Han J, Gram H. Independent role of p38 and ERK1/2 mitogen-activated kinases in the upregulation of matrix metalloproteinase-1. *Exp Cell Res* 2000;258(1):135–144.

48. Barchowsky A, Frleta D, Vincenti MP. Integration of the NF-kappaB and mitogen-activated protein kinase/AP-1 pathways at the collagenase-1 promoter: divergence of IL-1 and TNF-dependent signal transduction in rabbit primary synovial fibroblasts. *Cytokine* 2000;12(10):1469–1479.

49. Mengshol JA, Vincenti MP, Coon CI, Barchowsky A, Brinckerhoff CE. Interleukin-1 induction of collagenase 3 (matrix metalloproteinase 13) gene expression in chondrocytes requires p38, c-Jun N-terminal kinase, and nuclear factor kappaB: differential regulation of collagenase 1 and collagenase 3. *Arthritis Rheum* 2000;43(4):801–811.

50. Li WQ, Dehnade F, Zafarullah M. Oncostatin M-induced matrix metalloproteinase and tissue inhibitor of metalloproteinase-3 genes expression in chondrocytes requires Janus kinase/STAT signaling pathway. *J Immunol* 2001:166(5):3491–3498.

51. Westermarck J, Seth A, Kahari VM. Differential regulation of interstitial collagenase (MMP-1) gene expression by ETS transcription factors. *Oncogene* 1997;14(22):2651–2660.

CHAPTER 57

Vascular biology

Clare Thornton and Justin Mason

Introduction

Vascular biology involves the study not only of the physiological functions of the vasculature but also of how the vasculature may itself be a target for disease processes. Although the relevance of vascular biology to the rheumatic diseases has long been recognized, our appreciation and understanding of its importance has developed considerably over the last 15 years. The vasculature can be implicated at various levels. First, the microvasculature provides the portal of entry for leucocytes migrating to the sites of inflammation including the rheumatoid joint. Second, the vasculature may be the direct target for primary disease mechanisms in systemic sclerosis, the anti-phospholipid syndrome, and the vasculitides. The vasculature may also be a secondary target, with chronic systemic inflammation predisposing to endothelial dysfunction and increased arterial stiffness, thus escalating the risk of thrombosis and accelerated atherogenesis. Finally, the vasculature represents an important therapeutic target for disease-modifying drugs, biological therapies, and novel anti-angiogenic approaches, as well as for the deleterious effects of some agents.

Structure of the vasculature and heterogeneity of endothelium

The vasculature, composed of blood vessels, lymphatics, and the heart, originates embryologically from the mesoderm. The systemic and pulmonary circulations have the same basic organization of blood vessels, with large elastic arteries exiting the heart, followed by small muscular arteries, arterioles (the site of autoregulation of vascular tone) and then the capillary bed (the site of nutrient and waste product exchange), which feeds back into postcapillary venules (where the majority of leucocyte-endothelial cell interactions take place), and lastly large veins to return blood to the atria.

Blood vessels have walls composed of three layers (Figure 57.1), although their size and relative composition varies. The tunica intima is comprised of the endothelium, the one-cell-thick inner lining of all blood vessels, and the subendothelial basement membrane to which they are attached. The tunica media is formed from layers of fibroelastic tissue and smooth muscle in elastic arteries, and a thicker layer of smooth muscle in muscular arteries, distinctly separated from the intima by the internal elastic lamina.

Atherosclerotic plaques form between the intima and internal elastic lamina. The adventitia is made up of surrounding layers of connective tissue, through which runs the vasa vasorum: a capillary network supplying the tissues of the arterial wall. The same layers exist in veins, the main differences being a larger lumen and thinner smooth muscle layers. Capillaries consist only of endothelium and a basement membrane, in order to allow the efficient diffusion of nutrients and waste products.

The endothelium forms a continuous monolayer throughout the entire vasculature. The historical view of its function was of an inert tissue layer that maintained vessel wall permeability, but research conducted over the last 30 years reveals a biologically active tissue that carries out diverse functions, acting at the interface between blood constituents and the tissues.

The endothelium within different organs and vessels is heterogeneous. For example, brain endothelial cells (EC) are linked by tight junctions in order to maintain the blood–brain barrier, while the bone marrow has discontinuous EC to facilitate cellular trafficking, and the glomerular capillary tuft contains fenestrations to permit ultrafiltration.

EC heterogeneity may influence the spatial distribution of vascular diseases: atherosclerotic plaques preferentially occur at arterial branch points and sites of turbulent blood flow, suggesting that mechanical forces acting on EC are important in their initiation and development. Thrombus content and formation differs according to the vessel type involved. Lastly, the systemic vasculitides are classified by their predilection for blood vessels of a specific size, suggesting that there are predisposing features peculiar to each type.

The endothelium is the focus of much vascular biology research on account of its diverse functions and because it is the site of initial injury in many vascular diseases. For example, the 'response to injury' hypothesis to explain atherogenesis suggests that this starts with endothelial injury and dysfunction,[1] while angiogenesis begins with vessel destabilization and endothelial migration. Human umbilical vein endothelial cells (HUVEC) are the predominant cell type used in in-vitro vascular biology research, although cell lines are available that represent arterial, pulmonary, and microvascular endothelium. Although it may seem counterintuitive to study the origins of vascular diseases using cells that are venous and of fetal origin, HUVEC have proved a reliable model for the study of endothelial biology as a whole.

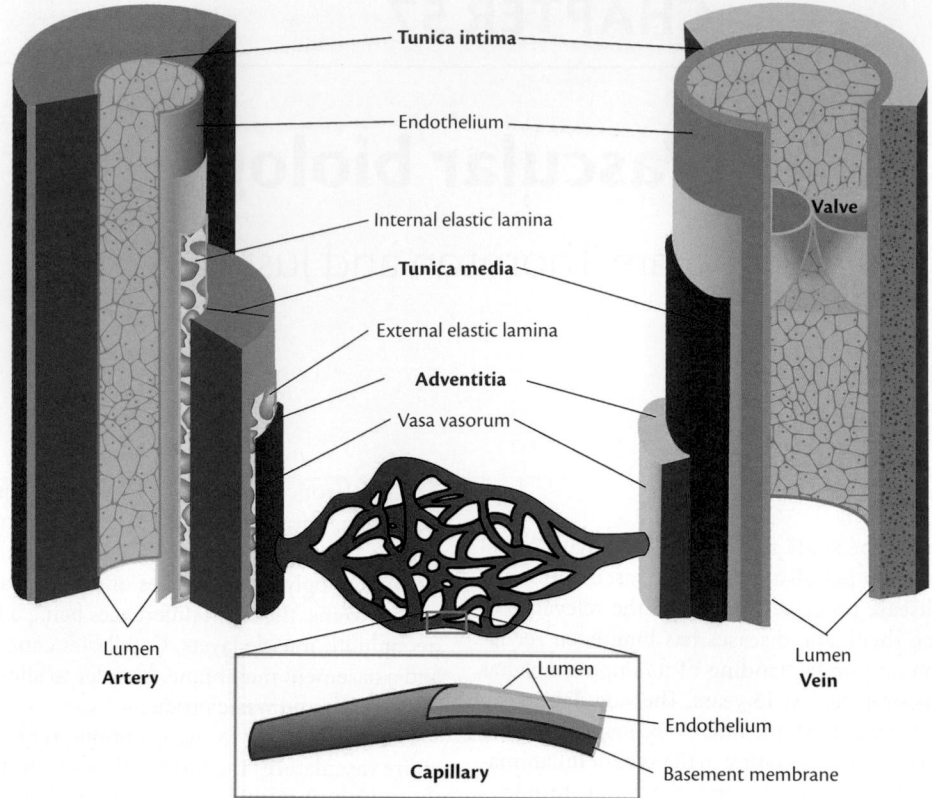

Fig. 57.1 The structure of the vasculature and blood vessel walls.

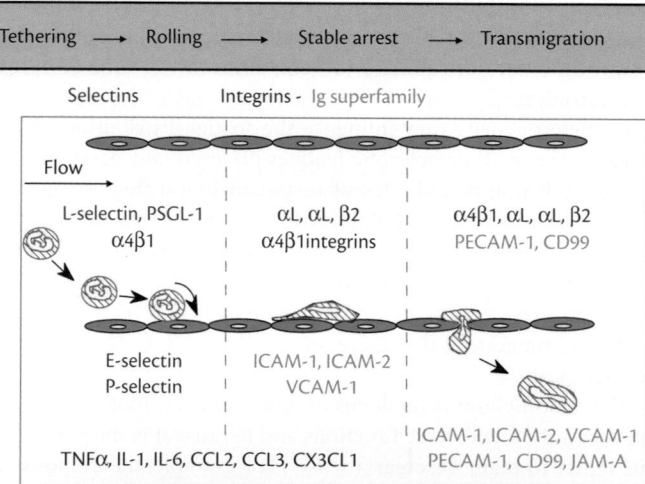

Fig. 57.2 The leucocyte adhesion cascade. Leucocyte recruitment is a multistep process in which initial tethering and rolling of leucocytes is facilitated by low-affinity interactions between selectins and their carbohydrate ligands. Rolling allows leucocytes to sample the microenvironment and following leukocyte integrin activation by chemokines, stable cellular arrest is achieved through the interaction of β₂-integrins and their immunoglobulin superfamily ligands including ICAM-1 and VCAM-1. E-selectin, ICAM-1, and VCAM-1 expression on the endothelial surface is upregulated by proinflammatory cytokines including TNFα and IL-1. Adherent leucocytes migrate to intercellular junctions and transmigrate across the endothelial barrier and underlying basement membrane, following chemokine gradients and utilizing interactions with a variety of junctional proteins such as PECAM-1 and CD99.

Leucocyte trafficking

The vascular endothelium plays a central role in the regulation of leucocyte recruitment to sites of inflammation and infection. The multistep cascades involved in the specific recruitment of neutrophils, monocytes, and lymphocytes are now well-defined (Figure 57.2). Leucocyte recruitment is modulated by molecular interactions with EC, alongside additional direct and indirect influences from pericytes, vascular smooth muscle cells, and the extracellular matrix. The initial step, leucocyte tethering and rolling, is facilitated by the selectins: E-selectin and P-selectin expressed on the surface of cytokine-activated endothelium, and L-selectin present on the leucocyte surface. Selectins bind carbohydrate ligands including sialyl Lewis X and PSGL-1. Interactions between integrins and immunoglobulin superfamily members are principally involved in the arrest and spreading of leucocytes on the endothelial surface, a process dependent upon chemokine-mediated integrin activation. Thus, integrins including LFA-1 and $\alpha_4\beta_1$ interact with ICAM-1 and VCAM-1 respectively.[2] Leucocyte transmigration is promoted by junctional adhesion molecules (JAM) A and C, PECAM-1 (CD31), CD99, and VE-cadherin, with migration directed by a chemokine gradient.[3]

Failure to regulate the inflammatory response is a characteristic feature of chronic arthritis. The endothelium of postcapillary venules at these sites is activated, rich in cellular adhesion molecules, and provides the portal of entry to the synovium for

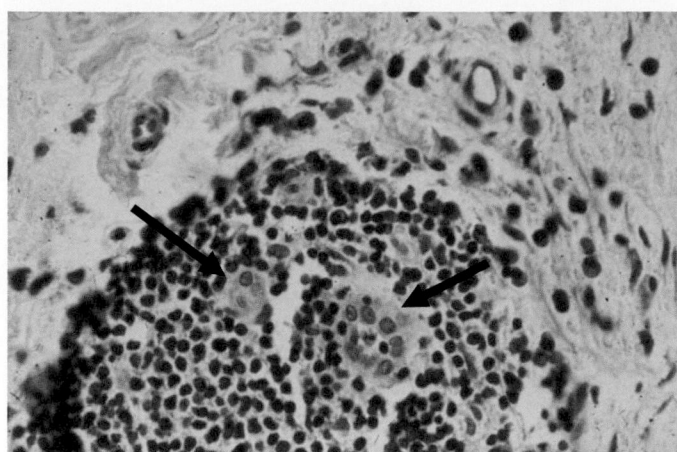

Fig. 57.3 The rheumatoid synovium. Photomicrograph of rheumatoid synovium stained with haematoxylin and eosin. The arrows points to inflamed high endothelial venules which act as the portal of entry for the leucocyte infiltrate.

leucocytes (Figure 57.3). These observations led to clinical trials of monoclonal antibody therapy directed at specific cellular adhesion molecules in rheumatoid arthritis (RA), which proved largely ineffective.[4] Conventional disease-modifying anti-rheumatic drugs (DMARDs) including methotrexate and mycophenolate may modulate adhesion molecule induction by proinflammatory cytokines. However, targeting upstream proinflammatory cytokines has proved particularly effective and relatively safe. This is exemplified by the tumour necrosis factor (TNF)α antagonists, which reverse vascular endothelial activation and suppress cellular adhesion molecules including E and P-selectin, ICAM, and VCAM-1.

Vascular injury

Vascular injury represents an important primary component in a variety of rheumatic diseases including systemic lupus erythematosus (SLE), vasculitides, and the anti-phospholipid syndrome. In ANCA-associated vasculitides (AAV), activated neutrophils are responsible for local disruption of the endothelial monolayer and recent studies suggest a role for complement in AAV-associated vascular injury,[5,6] which can be severe enough to result in life-threatening haemorrhage. The efficacy of B-cell-depleting monoclonal antibody therapy in AAV also suggests a direct role for B cells in pathogenesis, above and beyond their role as plasma cell precursors.[7]

The large-vessel vasculitides, giant cell arteritis (GCA) and Takayasu's arteritis, are characterized by granulomatous inflammation. The vaso vasorum acts as the portal of entry for an inflammatory infiltrate comprising activated dendritic cells, α/β and γ/δ T lymphocytes, B lymphocytes, macrophages, and multinucleated giant cells. Intimal hyperplasia is the consequence of myofibroblast proliferation, driven by growth factors including platelet-derived growth factor (PDGF), and resulting in progressive loss of the arterial lumen. Intriguing recent studies suggest that Toll-like receptors (TLR) influence the pattern of vascular injury in GCA. In a human–murine chimera model, TLR4 ligands induced a panarteritis and TLR5 ligands a periarteritis, a response related to differential dendritic cell responses, chemokine secretion, and T-cell recruitment.[8]

Endothelial dysfunction and accelerated atherosclerosis

Homeostatic mechanisms maintain a quiescent, anti-thrombotic, anti-adhesive vascular endothelium and control vasodilatation and permeability. This requires biosynthesis of nitric oxide (NO) and prostacyclin, expression of thrombomodulin, anti-apoptotic proteins including Bcl-2 and A1, and anti-oxidant/anti-inflammatory enzymes such as superoxide dismutase and haem oxygenase-1. These processes, controlled by intrinsic gene expression and external stimuli, maintain vascular integrity and initiate repair in the face of noxious stimuli including advanced glycation end products, proinflammatory cytokines, activated leucocytes, and oxidatively modified low-density lipoproteins. Prolonged systemic inflammation in RA and SLE is associated with endothelial apoptosis, inducing a local inflammatory response and endothelial dysfunction.[9] The latter, an important precursor to atherosclerosis, is potentially reversible and characterized by reduced NO biosynthesis, oxidative stress, increased permeability, and accumulation of lipoproteins and monocytes in the subintimal space.

RA and SLE are independent risk factors for accelerated atherogenesis.[10,11] Mechanisms include increased levels of oxidative stress and proinflammatory cytokines, resulting in endothelial activation, enhanced leucocyte adhesion, deleterious effects of immune complexes, anti-phospholipid antibodies, homocysteinaemia, and CD4+CD28– T cells.[12,13] Anti- high-density lipoprotein (HDL) antibodies may interfere with anti-atherogenic effects of HDL, as may anti-apolipoprotein A-I (apo A-I), as apo A-I is one of the major constituents of HDL.[14] These antibodies have been associated with reduced activity of HDL paroxonase, an anti-oxidant which prevents oxidation of low-density lipoprotein (LDL), thus contributing to the anti-atherogenic effects of HDL.

Despite the increased risk, only a subset of patients develop premature atherosclerosis and effective means for their early identification are required. Flow-mediated dilatation and pulse-wave velocity demonstrate endothelial dysfunction and aortic stiffness, and improvements with therapy have been reported.[15] High-resolution ultrasound can monitor intima-media thickness, identify early plaque, and predict risk of a cardiovascular event.[16,17] Positron emission tomography (PET) and MRI can identify microvascular dysfunction, arterial inflammation, and early asymptomatic atherogenesis in patients with RA, SLE, and Takayasu's arteritis.[18–22] However, identification of the optimal method(s) for detecting preclinical vascular disease and prospective data to demonstrate the effectiveness of this approach is required.

Thrombosis

Thrombosis is an important pathological process in many rheumatological diseases. Large-vessel thromboses, both venous and arterial, occur in Behçet's syndrome and the anti-phospholipid syndrome (APLS). Thrombosis also occurs in small vessels, principally as the end result of chronic vessel wall hyperplasia or inflammation, in diseases such as systemic sclerosis, vasculitis, and pulmonary arterial hypertension.

Activation of the coagulation cascade, leading to thrombosis, may be caused by abnormalities in the vessel wall, blood constituents, or blood flow, as described by Virchow's triad. Of most relevance to rheumatological disease is thrombosis triggered by abnormalities in the vessel wall, i.e. the endothelium. Endothelial activation leads to expression of tissue factor on the luminal surface, which triggers the extrinsic clotting cascade pathway.

APLS is associated with thrombosis in both arteries and veins.[23] Anti-phospholipid antibodies directed against β_2-glycoprotein-1 activate EC, along with monocytes and platelets. Activated EC express adhesion molecules and upregulate tissue factor production (as do monocytes). Increased tissue factor and thromboxane A2 from platelets leads to a procoagulant state, but for thrombosis to occur, a second hit is needed. This may be provided, for example, by complement cascade activation. Anti-phospholipid antibodies may also interact with other proteins within the coagulation cascade such as prothrombin, factor X, protein C, and plasmin and may therefore adversely affect fibrinolysis.

Thrombosis is also a prominent clinical feature of Behçet's syndrome. The majority are venous, causing superficial thrombophlebitis and deep venous thromboses, including superior vena cava obstruction, cerebral vein thrombosis, and Budd–Chiari syndrome. In a small number of cases, there is a pulmonary arterial vasculitis, leading to in-situ pulmonary arterial thromboses. Although small studies have suggested that thrombosis in Behçet's syndrome is linked to the concurrent presence of a prothrombotic condition such as factor V Leiden or prothrombin mutations, this is not thought to be the cause in the majority of cases.[24] There is indirect evidence to suggest that the procoagulant state arises from an abnormally 'sticky' activated endothelium, as a result of chronic vascular inflammation.[25] Clinically, this is supported by a small trial comparing treatment of thromboses in Behçet's syndrome by anticoagulation, immunosuppression, or both together.[26] A higher proportion of patients treated by anticoagulation alone had recurrent thromboses compared to those given immunosuppression, suggesting that it is the suppression of inflammation, which would be expected to reduce the degree of endothelial activation, that minimizes the tendency to thrombosis, rather than inhibition of the coagulation cascade.

Angiogenesis

Angiogenesis is a carefully regulated multistep process driven by proangiogenic mediators including growth factors, chemokines, and cellular adhesion molecules, acting via specific receptors. In adults, angiogenesis is involved in the menstrual cycle and wound healing. Angiogenesis has been implicated in various rheumatic diseases and most widely studied in RA, with development of neovessels being one of the earliest detectable changes in the rheumatoid synovium.[27–29] In psoriatic arthropathy, angiogenic vessels can be distinguished morphologically from those in RA, with the former described as tortuous and bushy and the latter straight and branching.[30] In the vasculitides, angiogenic neovessels are found in the arterial wall in GCA, while proangiogenic growth factors are increased in the serum of patients with AAV and Kawasaki's syndrome. However, the role of angiogenesis in this setting is poorly understood.

Neovascularization permits the delivery of cells, proinflammatory mediators, and nutrients to the developing rheumatoid pannus and predisposes to joint and tendon damage. Neovessels are inherently unstable with poor EC–pericyte interactions and evidence of oxidative damage and this may contribute to persistent intra-articular

hypoxia.[31] Of note, impaired vasculogenesis may be a contributory factor, with reduced, poorly functioning endothelial progenitor cells reported.[32] Likewise in systemic sclerosis impaired angiogenesis and vasculogenesis have been implicated in pathogenesis.[33]

An array of proangiogenic and angiostatic cytokines are present in the rheumatoid joint. These include vascular endothelial growth factor A (VEGF-A), basic fibroblast growth factor (FGF-2), transforming growth factor beta (TGFβ), PDGF, TNFα and CXCL8/IL-8, CXCL12/stromal-derived growth factor-α, and CXCL1/Gro-α.[34] VEGF-A, which induces EC proliferation and changes in vascular permeability, correlates with joint destruction in inflammatory arthritis.[35] Hypoxia is a key driver of VEGF synthesis, through the stabilization of hypoxia inducible factors (HIF) 1 and 2.[36]

Although there is considerable interest in anti-angiogenic therapies, further work is required to identify the most effective sites for intervention. The efficacy of an anti-angiogenic approach has been demonstrated in rodents. Thus, inhibition of $\alpha V\beta_3$ or VEGF signalling pathways attenuates rabbit and murine inflammatory arthritis respectively.[37–39] Methotrexate, sulphasalazine, and hydroxychloroquine all exert anti-angiogenic effects, at least in vitro,[28] while anti-TNFα therapy reduces proangiogenic mediators and synovial vascularity.[35,40,41] However, while development of more specific anti-angiogenic therapies may be beneficial, progress has been slow. Although anti-VEGF approaches are of interest, the significant side effects associated with the prolonged use of anti-VEGF-A monoclonal antibody (bevacizumab), including hypertension and thrombosis, may preclude its use in chronic diseases.[42,43]

Effect of drugs on the endothelium

Although it is well established that chronic inflammation leads to vascular injury and eventually atherosclerosis, much less is known about whether treating the primary inflammatory condition also reduces the associated cardiovascular disease (CVD) burden. Given that the development of atherosclerosis begins with endothelial dysfunction, an understanding of which drugs influence EC function—whether beneficially or harmfully—would assist the development of treatment regimes designed to delay or prevent vascular damage.

Statins and angiotensin converting enzyme (ACE) inhibitors—drugs commonly used in the treatment of CVD or its associated metabolic precursors—have been demonstrated to have specific beneficial effects on the vascular endothelium, in addition to their established lipid-lowering and vasodilatory actions. Likewise, several disease-modifying or immunosuppressant drugs have been investigated for their effects on endothelial function and in a few cases have been shown to reduce the incidence of CVD in chronic inflammation. Conversely, others may in fact be harmful.

Statins

The principal lipid-lowering mechanism of action of statins is inhibition of 3-hydroxy-3-methylglutaryl-CoA (HMG-CoA) reductase in hepatocytes, leading to reduced cholesterol synthesis and hence a reduction in CVD. However, large primary prevention trials also indicate that they can reduce cardiovascular morbidity and mortality independent of changes in serum cholesterol. This pleiotropic effect arises from the inhibition of HMG-CoA reductase in EC and other cells of the immune system, which appears

Table 57.1 Summary of clinical data regarding the cardiovascular effects of various commonly prescribed immunosuppressants and DMARDs

Drug	CVD mortality	CVD incidence	Endothelial dysfunction	Carotid intima–media thickness
Methotrexate	Reduced in RA[52–54]	Reduced in RA and inflammatory arthritis[52–54]	Improved[55]; improved in responders[56]	No change[57,58]; Reduced in associated with HCQ[59]; and in associated with prednisolone[60]
Anti-TNFα therapy		Reduced[61]; reduced in responders[62]; no effect[63]	Improved[55,58,64]; improved in responders[65]	No change[57,58]
Rituximab			Improved in short term[66]	
Ciclosporin			Worsened in transplant pts[67]; worsened compared to AZA[68] or rapamycin[69]	Improved in LN[70]
Mycophenolate mofetil		Improved cardiac allograft vasculopathy[71]		No change in LN[70] or SLE[72]
Azathioprine		Use associated with CVD events in SLE but disease severity confounding[73,74]	No change in kidney transplant patients[68]	No change in LN[70]; worsened in SLE but disease severity confounding[75]
Sulphasalazine		No effect[52]; improved in combination with MTX[76]		
Hydroxychloroquine		Improved in combination with MTX and SSZ[76]; no effect[52]		Improved in combination with MTX[59]; no change in LN[70]
Glucocorticoid steroids		Increased[63]	Worsened in (juvenile) SLE but confounding disease severity[77]; low dose no change in RA[78]	Improved in combination with MTX in RA[60]; no change in LN[70]
Tocilizumab			Improved in short term[79]	
Leflunomide		Reduced[63] although 6 patients only		

AZA, azathioprine; CVD, cardiovascular disease; HCQ, hydroxychloroquine; jSLE, juvenile SLE; LN, lupus nephritis; MTX, methotrexate; RA, rheumatoid arthritis; SLE, systemic lupus erythematosus; SSZ: sulphasalazine.

to have anti-inflammatory effects. The METEOR trial examined changes in C-reactive protein (CRP) in patients taking rosuvastatin, and showed a 36% reduction,[44] while the JUPITER trial demonstrated that rosuvastatin reduced CV mortality in individuals with normal LDL concentrations but a raised CRP analysed using a high-sensitivity assay.[45] An anti-inflammatory effect was also observed in the TARA trial in which atorvastatin improved RA disease activity.[46]

HMG-CoA reductase inhibition improves EC function in various ways. It prevents synthesis of isoprenoid intermediates such as geranylgeranyl pyrophosphate, important for the activation of small GTP-ase signalling molecules such as Rho and Rac (Figure 57.4).[47,48] Statins inhibit Rho and Rac signalling, and this leads to upregulation of endothelial NO synthase and thus increased NO biosynthesis. NO is both anti-inflammatory and vasodilatory. Disruption of Rho and Rac also modulates signalling pathways which induce cytoprotective genes such as haem oxygenase-1 and the complement inhibitory protein decay-accelerating factor (DAF).[49,50] Lastly, the anti-inflammatory effects of statins on EC also include inhibition of cellular adhesion molecules, so reducing leucocyte trafficking and potentially retarding the development of atherosclerotic plaques.[51]

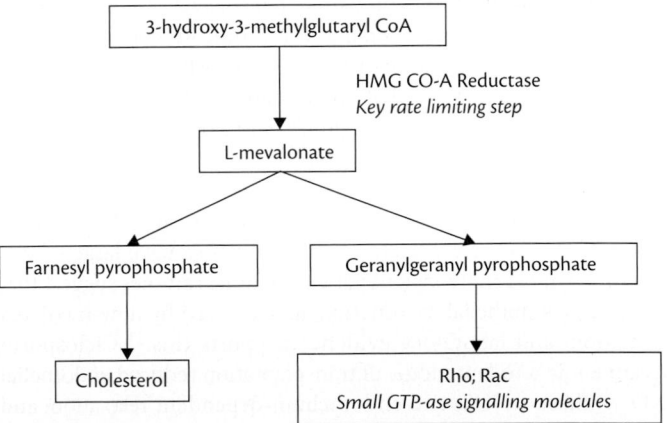

Fig. 57.4 The downstream effects of HMG Co-A reductase inhibition.

Statins also affect other cells of the immune system important for atherogenesis. In macrophages, they can induce expression of the anti-inflammatory transcription factor PPARγ, and prevent IL-6 mediated induction of MCP-1. They also exhibit immunomodulatory and anti-thrombotic effects in T lymphocytes and platelets respectively.

A major caveat, however, when discussing the vasculoprotective properties of statins, is that they have largely been demonstrated using concentrations in vitro and in vivo that exceed 1 μM, several-folds higher than the concentrations achieved in patient sera. Nonetheless, these combined immunomodulatory, anti-inflammatory, and complement inhibitory actions may prove to be important mechanisms underlying the anti-rheumatic and vasculoprotective effect of statins.

DMARDs and immunosuppressant drugs

A number of DMARDs and immunosuppressant drugs have been investigated with respect to their effects on CVD, with some likely to be beneficial (methotrexate and anti-TNFα therapy) and others possibly harmful (ciclosporin). It is unknown whether these effects are due purely to their anti-inflammatory properties, or whether they have additional specific actions on the endothelium. Clinical research to date is summarized in Table 57.1, although it should be noted that some of these studies derive from the transplant literature.

Clinical evidence suggests methotrexate has a beneficial effect on vascular biology when prescribed in RA. Choi et al.[52] demonstrated a relative risk reduction of 70% in cardiovascular mortality in RA patients taking methotrexate compared to those on other DMARDs (hydroxychloroquine, sulphasalazine, gold, D-penicillamine). This has recently been reinforced by a systematic review[53] and meta-analysis,[54] although lesser degrees of relative risk reduction were found. Smaller studies have demonstrated that methotrexate improves endothelial dysfunction in patients with RA.[55,56] In-vitro work indicates that methotrexate has anti-inflammatory effects on EC: it downregulates the TNFα-induced upregulation of ICAM-1 and VCAM-1,[80] as well as increasing adenosine production (as a proportion of total nucleotides).[81] Methotrexate also reduces endothelial cell proliferation in vitro and angiogenesis in vivo[82]; hence, inhibition of synovial neovascularization may contribute to its anti-rheumatic effects.

Although the cumulative experience with anti-TNFα therapy may yet be too short to demonstrate conclusively an effect on RA cardiovascular mortality, small studies indicate it is likely to be improved. Data from the British Society for Rheumatology (BSR) Biologics Register shows that anti-TNFα responders had a lower incidence of myocardial infarction,[62] and reversal of endothelial dysfunction has also been reported.[55,64]

Ciclosporin, an immunosuppressant used in the treatment of connective tissue diseases such as polymyositis, may have deleterious effects on the vasculature, although these have largely been examined in organ transplant patients. Clinical studies suggest that it worsens endothelial dysfunction, as measured by flow-mediated dilatation, and laboratory evidence supports this.[83] Ciclosporin treatment in a rodent model of transplantation reduced endothelial NO synthase (eNOS) and endothelium-dependent relaxation, and increased endothelin-1 expression. However, tacrolimus, a related drug, may preserve endothelial function relative to ciclosporin, and it does not induce endothelin-1. Similarly, rapamycin also exhibits a more favourable vascular profile.[84]

The majority of other DMARDs and biological agents are either too new or not yet prescribed with sufficient frequency for their influence on cardiovascular risk in chronic inflammation to be determined. However, there are a few factors to take into account. Tocilizumab, an inhibitor of IL-6 signalling, might be expected to have a beneficial effect on cardiovascular risk, but this may be mitigated by its adverse effects on lipid profile. Leflunomide, while very effective in treating RA, can worsen hypertension, thus offsetting any beneficial effect on the vasculature. One family of drugs very commonly used in clinical practice, whose effects on the vasculature might be expected to be well known by now, are glucocorticoid steroids. However, they cause such a range of both beneficial and harmful effects, that no conclusive overall picture has yet been reached.

NSAIDs and COX-2 inhibitors

The effects of cyclooxygenase (COX)-2 inhibition on the vasculature has received much attention recently, due to the withdrawal of rofecoxib following concerns that it increased the rate of myocardial infarction (MI).[85] It is now understood that both traditional NSAIDs and COX-2 inhibitors may increase the risk of MI, although establishing the degree of risk and the relative safety profiles between drugs is difficult, owing to trial heterogeneity and a lack of randomized controlled trial data on older NSAIDs. A recent network meta-analysis has suggested that no traditional NSAID or COX-2 inhibitor is entirely safe, but naproxen appears least harmful.[86]

The mechanisms that explain how COX inhibition increases the risk of cardiovascular events relate to its downstream effects on synthesis of prostaglandins and thromboxane A2. COX inhibition reduces prostaglandin synthesis in the kidney, reducing renal medullary blood flow and thereby increasing water and salt retention. This can precipitate heart failure in susceptible individuals. Secondly, it alters the balance between prostacyclin production in EC, which causes vasodilation and platelet inhibition, and thromboxane-A2 production in platelets, which causes vasoconstriction and platelet activation. Perturbation of this balance may underlie the increased incidence of MI seen with most NSAIDs and COX-2 inhibitors.

Nevertheless, many questions remain, including whether COX-1 or COX-2 is the predominant source of endothelial prostacyclin. In addition, there is evidence to suggest that celecoxib may improve vascular endothelial function in men with coronary artery disease.[87] Recent in-vitro work has demonstrated that celecoxib, like atorvastatin, can induce haem oxygenase-1 in EC. This effect was independent of COX inhibition and not seen with other COX-2 inhibitors.[88] These and other reports have led to current interest in the specific COX-independent actions of celecoxib.[89]

Future approaches

In light of the cardiovascular sequelae associated with many chronic inflammatory rheumatic diseases, consideration needs to be given to the design of treatment regimens that maximize benefits to the vascular endothelium. Success can subsequently be measured as a return in cardiovascular mortality towards that seen in the general population. This ambition requires a detailed knowledge of the effects of DMARDs and immunosuppressant drugs on the vasculature, including their effects on protective pathways such as NO synthesis, anti-inflammatory and anti-oxidant gene expression, and on signalling pathways and transcription factors that control vasculoprotective genes. Furthermore, long-term clinical trials of sufficient size and with defined cardiovascular endpoints are required. It will be challenging to achieve this, particularly given the relative rarity of many chronic inflammatory conditions. However, results from clinical trials in RA may reasonably be extrapolated to rarer diseases, so optimizing future protection from vascular injury for our patients.

References

1. Ross R. Atherosclerosis—an inflammatory disease. *N Engl J Med* 1999;340(2):115–126.

2. Rao RM, Yang L, Garcia-Cardena G, Luscinskas FW. Endothelial-dependent mechanisms of leukocyte recruitment to the vascular wall. *Circ Res* 2007;101(3):234–247.

3. Ley K, Laudanna C, Cybulsky MI, Nourshargh S. Getting to the site of inflammation: the leukocyte adhesion cascade updated. *Nat Rev Immunol* 2007;7(9):678–689.

4. Szekanecz Z, Koch AE. Vasculogenesis in rheumatoid arthritis. *Arthritis Res Ther* 2010;12(2):110.

5. Schreiber A, Xiao H, Jennette JC et al. C5a receptor mediates neutrophil activation and ANCA-induced glomerulonephritis. *J Am Soc Nephrol* 2009;20(2):289–298.

6. Xiao H, Schreiber A, Heeringa P, Falk RJ, Jennette JC. Alternative complement pathway in the pathogenesis of disease mediated by anti-neutrophil cytoplasmic autoantibodies. *Am J Pathol* 2007;170(1):52–64.

7. Savage CO. Pathogenesis of anti-neutrophil cytoplasmic autoantibody (ANCA)-associated vasculitis. *Clin Exp Immunol* 2011;164 (Suppl1):23–26.

8. Deng J, Ma-Krupa W, Gewirtz AT et al. Toll-like receptors 4 and 5 induce distinct types of vasculitis. *Circ Res* 2009;104(4):488–495.

9. Le Brocq M, Leslie SJ, Milliken P, Megson IL. Endothelial dysfunction: from molecular mechanisms to measurement, clinical implications, and therapeutic opportunities. *Antioxid Redox Signal* 2008;10(9):1631–1674.

10. del Rincon ID, Williams K, Stern MP, Freeman GL, Escalante A. High incidence of cardiovascular events in a rheumatoid arthritis cohort not explained by traditional cardiac risk factors. *Arthritis Rheum* 2001;44(12):2737–2745.

11. Esdaile JM, Abrahamowicz M, Grodzicky T et al. Traditional Framingham risk factors fail to fully account for accelerated atherosclerosis in systemic lupus erythematosus. *Arthritis Rheum* 2001;44:2331–2337.

12. Haskard DO. Accelerated atherosclerosis in inflammatory rheumatic diseases. *Scand J Rheumatol* 2004;33(5):281–292.

13. Sattar N, McCarey DW, Capell H, McInnes IB. Explaining how 'high-grade' systemic inflammation accelerates vascular risk in rheumatoid arthritis. *Circulation* 2003;108(24):2957–2963.

14. O'Neill SG, Giles I, Lambrianides A et al. Antibodies to apolipoprotein A-I, high-density lipoprotein, and C-reactive protein are associated with disease activity in patients with systemic lupus erythematosus. *Arthritis Rheum* 2010;62(3):845–854.

15. Maki-Petaja KM, Wilkinson IB. Anti-inflammatory drugs and statins for arterial stiffness reduction. *Curr Pharm Des* 2009;15(3):290–303.

16. El-Magadmi M, Bodill H, Ahmad Y et al. Systemic lupus erythematosus: an independent risk factor for endothelial dysfunction in women. *Circulation* 2004;110(4):399–404.

17. Evans MR, Escalante A, Battafarano DF et al. Carotid atherosclerosis predicts incident acute coronary syndromes in rheumatoid arthritis. *Arthritis Rheum* 2011;63(5):1211–1220.

18. Keenan NG, Mason JC, Maceira A et al. Integrated cardiac and vascular assessment in Takayasu arteritis by cardiovascular magnetic resonance. *Arthritis Rheum* 2009;60(11):3501–3509.

19. Mason JC. Takayasu arteritis—advances in diagnosis and management. *Nat Rev Rheumatol* 2010;6(7):406–415.

20. Ng WF, Fantin F, Ng C et al. Takayasu's arteritis: a cause of prolonged arterial stiffness. *Rheumatology* 2006;45(6):741–745.

21. Pugliese F, Gaemperli O, Kinderlerer AR et al. Imaging of vascular inflammation with (11C)-PK11195 and positron emission tomography/computed tomography angiography. *J Am Coll Cardiol* 2010;56(8):653–661.

22. Recio-Mayoral A, Mason JC, Kaski JC et al. Chronic inflammation and coronary microvascular dysfunction in patients without risk factors for coronary artery disease. *Eur Heart J* 2009;30:1837–1843.

23. Ruiz-Irastorza G, Crowther M, Branch W, Khamashta MA. Antiphospholipid syndrome. *Lancet* 2010;376(9751):1498–1509.

24. Leiba M, Seligsohn U, Sidi Y et al. Thrombophilic factors are not the leading cause of thrombosis in Behcet's disease. *Ann Rheum Dis* 2004;63(11):1445–1449.

25. Mehta P, Laffan M, Haskard DO. Thrombosis and Behcet's syndrome in non-endemic regions. *Rheumatology* (Oxford) 2010;49(11):2003–2004.

26. Ahn JK, Lee YS, Jeon CH, Koh EM, Cha HS. Treatment of venous thrombosis associated with Behcet's disease: immunosuppressive therapy alone versus immunosuppressive therapy plus anticoagulation. *Clin Rheumatol* 2008;27(2):201–205.

27. Fassbender HG, Annefeld MS. The potential aggressiveness of synovial tissue in rheumatoid arthritis. *J Pathol* 1981;139:399–406.

28. Koch AE. Angiogenesis. Implications for rheumatoid arthritis. *Arthritis Rheum* 1998;41:951–962.

29. Koch AE. The role of angiogenesis in rheumatoid arthritis: recent developments. *Ann Rheum Dis* 2000;59 (suppl I):i65–i71.

30. Reece RJ, Canete JD, Parsons WJ, Emery P, Veale DJ. Distinct vascular patterns of early synovitis in psoriatic, reactive, and rheumatoid arthritis. *Arthritis Rheum* 1999;42(7):1481–1484.

31. Kennedy A, Ng CT, Biniecka M et al. Angiogenesis and blood vessel stability in inflammatory arthritis. *Arthritis Rheum* 2010;62(3):711–721.

32. Grisar J, Aletaha D, Steiner CW et al. Depletion of endothelial progenitor cells in the peripheral blood of patients with rheumatoid arthritis. *Circulation* 2005;111(2):204–211.

33. Distler JH, Gay S, Distler O. Angiogenesis and vasculogenesis in systemic sclerosis. *Rheumatology (Oxford)* 2006;45 Suppl 3:iii26–iii27.

34. Szekanecz Z, Koch AE. Mechanisms of disease: angiogenesis in inflammatory diseases. *Nat Clin Pract Rheumatol* 2007;3(11):635–643.

35. Ballara S, Taylor PC, Reusch P et al. Raised serum vascular endothelial growth factor levels are associated with destructive change in inflammatory arthritis. *Arthritis Rheum* 2001;44(9):2055–2064.

36. Taylor PC, Sivakumar B. Hypoxia and angiogenesis in rheumatoid arthritis. *Curr Opin Rheumatol* 2005;17(3):293–298.

37. Choi ST, Kim JH, Seok JY, Park YB, Lee SK. Therapeutic effect of anti-vascular endothelial growth factor receptor I antibody in the established collagen-induced arthritis mouse model. *Clin Rheumatol* 2009;28(3):333–337.

38. Miotla J, Maciewicz R, Kendrew J, Feldmann M, Paleolog E. Treatment with soluble VEGF receptor reduces disease severity in murine collagen-induced arthritis. *Lab Invest* 2000;80(8):1195–1205.

39. Storgard CM, Stupack DG, Jonczyk A et al. Decreased angiogenesis and arthritic disease in rabbits treated with an alphavbeta3 antagonist. *J Clin Invest* 1999;103(1):47–54.

40. Goedkoop AY, Kraan MC, Picavet DI et al. Deactivation of endothelium and reduction in angiogenesis in psoriatic skin and synovium by low dose infliximab therapy in combination with stable methotrexate therapy: a prospective single-centre study. *Arthritis Res Ther* 2004;6(4):R326–R334.

41. Paleolog EM, Young S, Stark AC et al. Modulation of angiogenic vascular endothelial growth factor by tumor necrosis factor alpha and interleukin-1 in rheumatoid arthritis. *Arthritis Rheum* 1998;41(7):1258–1265.

42. Eremina V, Jefferson JA, Kowalewska J et al. VEGF inhibition and renal thrombotic microangiopathy. *N Engl J Med* 2008;358:1129–1136.

43. Hurwitz H, Saini S. Bevacizumab in the treatment of metastatic colorectal cancer: safety profile and management of adverse events. *Semin Oncol* 2006;33(5 Suppl 10):S26–S34.

44. Peters SA, Palmer MK, Grobbee DE et al. C-reactive protein lowering with rosuvastatin in the METEOR study. *J Intern Med* 2010;268(2):155–161.

45. Ridker PM, Danielson E, Fonseca FA et al. Rosuvastatin to prevent vascular events in men and women with elevated C-reactive protein. *N Engl J Med* 2008;359(21):2195–2207.

46. McCarey DW, McInnes IB, Madhok R et al. Trial of Atorvastatin in Rheumatoid Arthritis (TARA): double-blind, randomised placebo-controlled trial. *Lancet* 2004;363(9426):2015–2021.

47. Zhou Q, Liao JK. Pleiotropic effects of statins—basic research and clinical perspectives. *Circ J* 2010;74(5):818–826.

48. Greenwood J, Mason JC. Statins and the vascular endothelial inflammatory response. *Trends Immunol* 2007;28(2):88–98.

49. Mason JC, Ahmed Z, Mankoff R et al. Statin-induced expression of decay-accelerating factor protects vascular endothelium against complement-mediated injury. *Circ Res* 2002;91(8):696–703.

50. Ali F, Hamdulay SS, Kinderlerer AR et al. Statin-mediated cytoprotection of human vascular endothelial cells: a role for Kruppel-like factor 2-dependent induction of heme oxygenase-1. *J Thromb Haemost* 2007;5(12):2537–2546.

51. Bu DX, Griffin G, Lichtman AH. Mechanisms for the anti-inflammatory effects of statins. *Curr Opin Lipidol*;22(3):165–170.

52. Choi HK, Hernan MA, Seeger JD, Robins JM, Wolfe F. Methotrexate and mortality in patients with rheumatoid arthritis: a prospective study. *Lancet* 2002;359(9313):1173–1177.

53. Westlake SL, Colebatch AN, Baird J et al. The effect of methotrexate on cardiovascular disease in patients with rheumatoid arthritis: a systematic literature review. *Rheumatology (Oxford)* 2010;49(2):295–307.

54. Micha R, Imamura F, Wyler von Ballmoos M et al. Systematic review and meta-analysis of methotrexate use and risk of cardiovascular disease. *Am J Cardiol* 2011;108(9):1362–1370.

55. Turiel M, Tomasoni L, Sitia S et al. Effects of long-term disease-modifying antirheumatic drugs on endothelial function in patients with early rheumatoid arthritis. *Cardiovasc Ther* 2010;28(5):e53–e64.

56. Galarraga B, Belch JJ, Pullar T, Ogston S, Khan F. Clinical improvement in rheumatoid arthritis is associated with healthier microvascular function in patients who respond to antirheumatic therapy. *J Rheumatol* 2010;37(3):521–528.

57. Ferrante A, Giardina AR, Ciccia F et al. Long-term anti-tumour necrosis factor therapy reverses the progression of carotid intima-media thickness in female patients with active rheumatoid arthritis. *Rheumatol Int* 2009;30(2):193–198.

58. Mazzoccoli G, Notarsanto I, de Pinto GD et al. Anti-tumor necrosis factor-alpha therapy and changes of flow-mediated vasodilatation in psoriatic and rheumatoid arthritis patients. *Intern Emerg Med* 2010;5(6):495–500.

59. Ristic GG, Lepic T, Glisic B et al. Rheumatoid arthritis is an independent risk factor for increased carotid intima-media thickness: impact of anti-inflammatory treatment. *Rheumatology (Oxford)* 2010;49(6):1076–1081.

60. Georgiadis AN, Voulgari PV, Argyropoulou MI et al. Early treatment reduces the cardiovascular risk factors in newly diagnosed rheumatoid arthritis patients. *Semin Arthritis Rheum* 2008;38(1):13–19.

61. Jacobsson LT, Turesson C, Gulfe A et al. Treatment with tumor necrosis factor blockers is associated with a lower incidence of first cardiovascular events in patients with rheumatoid arthritis. *J Rheumatol* 2005;32(7):1213–1218.

62. Dixon WG, Watson KD, Lunt M et al. Reduction in the incidence of myocardial infarction in patients with rheumatoid arthritis who respond to anti-tumour necrosis factor alpha therapy: results from the British Society for Rheumatology Biologics Register. *Arthritis Rheum* 2007;56(9):2905–2912.

63. Suissa S, Bernatsky S, Hudson M. Antirheumatic drug use and the risk of acute myocardial infarction. *Arthritis Rheum* 2006;55(4):531–536.

64. Hurlimann D, Forster A, Noll G et al. Anti-tumor necrosis factor-alpha treatment improves endothelial function in patients with rheumatoid arthritis. *Circulation* 2002;106(17):2184–2187.

65. Sidiropoulos PI, Siakka P, Pagonidis K et al. Sustained improvement of vascular endothelial function during anti-TNFalpha treatment in rheumatoid arthritis patients. *Scand J Rheumatol* 2009;38(1):6–10.

66. Gonzalez-Juanatey C, Llorca J, Vazquez-Rodriguez TR et al. Short-term improvement of endothelial function in rituximab-treated rheumatoid arthritis patients refractory to tumor necrosis factor alpha blocker therapy. *Arthritis Rheum* 2008;59(12):1821–1824.

67. Maamoun H, Esmail E, Soliman A. Vascular endothelial function of sirolimus maintenance regimen in renal transplant recipients. *Transplant Proc* 2011;43(5):1616–1618.

68. Morris ST, McMurray JJ, Rodger RS, Farmer R, Jardine AG. Endothelial dysfunction in renal transplant recipients maintained on cyclosporine. *Kidney Int* 2000;57(3):1100–1106.

69. Joannides R, Etienne I, Iacob M et al. Comparative effects of sirolimus and cyclosporin on conduit arteries endothelial function in kidney recipients. *Transpl Int* 2010;23(11):1135–1143.

70. Sazliyana S, Mohd Shahrir MS, Kong CT et al. Implications of immunosuppressive agents in cardiovascular risks and carotid intima media thickness among lupus nephritis patients. *Lupus* 2011;20(12):1260–1266.

71. Gibson WT, Hayden MR. Mycophenolate mofetil and atherosclerosis: results of animal and human studies. *Ann N Y Acad Sci* 2007;1110:209–221.

72. Kiani AN, Magder LS, Petri M. Mycophenolate mofetil (MMF) does not slow the progression of subclinical atherosclerosis in SLE over 2 years. *Rheumatol Int* 2012;32(9):2701–2705.

73. Ahmad Y, Shelmerdine J, Bodill H et al. Subclinical atherosclerosis in systemic lupus erythematosus (SLE): the relative contribution of classic risk factors and the lupus phenotype. *Rheumatology* (Oxford) 2007;46(6):983–988.

74. Haque S, Gordon C, Isenberg D et al. Risk factors for clinical coronary heart disease in systemic lupus erythematosus: the lupus and atherosclerosis evaluation of risk (LASER) study. *J Rheumatol* 2010;37(2):322–329.

75. Doria A, Shoenfeld Y, Wu R et al. Risk factors for subclinical atherosclerosis in a prospective cohort of patients with systemic lupus erythematosus. *Ann Rheum Dis* 2003;62(11):1071–1077.

76. van Halm VP, Nurmohamed MT, Twisk JW, Dijkmans BA, Voskuyl AE. Disease-modifying antirheumatic drugs are associated with a reduced risk for cardiovascular disease in patients with rheumatoid arthritis: a case control study. *Arthritis Res Ther* 2006;8(5):R151.

77. Schanberg LE, Sandborg C, Barnhart HX et al. Premature atherosclerosis in pediatric systemic lupus erythematosus: risk factors for increased carotid intima-media thickness in the atherosclerosis prevention in pediatric lupus erythematosus cohort. *Arthritis Rheum* 2009;60(5):1496–1507.

78. Hafstrom I, Rohani M, Deneberg S et al. Effects of low-dose prednisolone on endothelial function, atherosclerosis, and traditional risk factors for atherosclerosis in patients with rheumatoid arthritis—a randomized study. *J Rheumatol* 2007;34(9):1810–1816.

79. Protogerou AD, Zampeli E, Fragiadaki K et al. A pilot study of endothelial dysfunction and aortic stiffness after interleukin-6 receptor inhibition in rheumatoid arthritis. *Atherosclerosis* 2011;219(2):734–736.

80. Yamasaki E, Soma Y, Kawa Y, Mizoguchi M. Methotrexate inhibits proliferation and regulation of the expression of intercellular adhesion molecule-1 and vascular cell adhesion molecule-1 by cultured human umbilical vein endothelial cells. *Br J Dermatol* 2003;149(1):30–38.

81. Cronstein BN, Eberle MA, Gruber HE, Levin RI. Methotrexate inhibits neutrophil function by stimulating adenosine release from connective tissue cells. *Proc Natl Acad Sci U S A* 1991;88(6):2441–2445.

82. Hirata S, Matsubara T, Saura R, Tateishi H, Hirohata K. Inhibition of in vitro vascular endothelial cell proliferation and in vivo neovascularization by low-dose methotrexate. *Arthritis Rheum* 1989;32(9):1065–1073.

83. Nickel T, Schlichting CL, Weis M. Drugs modulating endothelial function after transplantation. *Transplantation* 2006;82(1 Suppl):S41–S46.

84. Tepperman E, Ramzy D, Prodger J et al. Surgical biology for the clinician: vascular effects of immunosuppression. *Can J Surg* 2010;53(1):57–63.

85. Bresalier RS, Sandler RS, Quan H et al. Cardiovascular events associated with rofecoxib in a colorectal adenoma chemoprevention trial. *N Engl J Med* 2005;352(11):1092–1102.

86. Trelle S, Reichenbach S, Wandel S et al. Cardiovascular safety of non-steroidal anti-inflammatory drugs: network meta-analysis. *BMJ* 2011;342:c7086.

87. Chenevard R, Hurlimann D, Bechir M et al. Selective COX-2 inhibition improves endothelial function in coronary artery disease. *Circulation* 2003;107(3):405–409.

88. Hamdulay SS, Wang B, Birdsey GM et al. Celecoxib activates PI-3K/Akt and mitochondrial redox signaling to enhance heme oxygenase-1-mediated anti-inflammatory activity in vascular endothelium. *Free Radic Biol Med* 2010;48(8):1013–1023.

89. Zweers MC, de Boer TN, van Roon J et al. Celecoxib: considerations regarding its potential disease-modifying properties in osteoarthritis. *Arthritis Res Ther* 2011;13(5):239.

CHAPTER 58

Acute-phase responses and adipocytokines

Elena Neumann, Klaus Frommer, and Ulf Müller-Ladner

Introduction

Adipose tissue is a structural component of many organs. The central function of adipose tissue in energy metabolism is well known, with adipocytes being the dominant cell type. This cell produces and secretes highly bioactive substances, the adipokines, which are also called adipocytokines, such as adiponectin, resistin, leptin, and visfatin.[1–4] In addition, adipocytes produce several proinflammatory factors including tumour necrosis factor alpha (TNFα), interleukin (IL)-6, and factors of the complement system, growth factors, and adhesion molecules. All of them contribute actively to activation of the innate immune system and modulation of the immune response.[1,3–5] There is increasing knowledge on the various effects of adipokines under different pathophysiological conditions including rheumatic diseases.[3,6] As outlined below, the potency of adipokines to modulate the immune system under healthy and chronic inflammatory pathophysiological conditions is significant and has a substantial part in the initiation and perpetuation of the respective disease entities.

Immunomodulatory adipokines

Adiponectin

Adiponectin is mainly but not exclusively produced by adipocytes and accounts for 0.05% of total serum protein in humans. Adiponectin is a complex molecule which exists in different isoforms with sometimes counteracting functions under pathophysiological conditions including rheumatic diseases.[3] The effects of the respective isoforms are most likely mediated by induction of different signalling cascades and selective receptor affinity binding.[3,7] Oligomerization and the expression levels of its receptors directly influence the effects mediated by adiponectin.[7,8]

The human adiponectin isoforms are well described, in contrast to the murine isoforms. In humans, the isoforms are formed from the adiponectin monomer leading to a 'bouquet of flowers' structure.[7] The adiponectin trimer, the low molecular weight (LMW) adiponectin isoform, is composed of three full-length adiponectin monomers that form a collagen triple helix with a C-terminal globular head domain (gC1q domain).[7] The hexamer isoform is a combination of two adiponectin trimers and called middle molecular weight (MMW) adiponectin. The high molecular weight (HMW) adiponectin consists of 12–18 monomers. The globular adiponectin isoform consists solely of the head domain of trimeric adiponectin and is formed by proteolytic cleavage.

Two adiponectin receptors with signalling function, adipoR1 and adipoR2, have been characterized. AdipoR1 has a higher affinity for globular adiponectin. AdipoR2 has a higher affinity for trimeric adiponectin and most likely the higher molecular weight isoforms.[9] In addition to the known adiponectin receptors, additional potential adiponectin receptors have been described. Among those are progestin and the adipoQ receptor family members III (PAQR3) or X (PAQR10).[3] Their affinity for the individual adiponectin isoforms and their functions are largely unknown. In addition, an integral membrane protein, T-cadherin, binds MMW and HMW adiponectin but not globular or trimeric adiponectin.[10] T-cadherin has no cytosolic signalling domain and may therefore serve as a coreceptor or accessory surface molecule. Furthermore, other surface molecules are able to modulate the function or activity of the adiponectin receptors, such as APPL1,[11] protein kinase CK2,[12] and ERp46.[13]

Besides its metabolic functions, adiponectin is involved in the modulation of several immunomodulatory pathways in different diseases.[1,4,14] Although initially mainly anti-inflammatory and anti-fibrotic effects have been described, there is growing evidence for a proinflammatory and prodestructive role of adiponectin under different pathophysiological conditions. Examples of the heterogeneous role of adiponectin are listed in Table 58.1.

Resistin

Similar to adiponectin, an immunomodulatory potential for resistin has also been described. In contrast to adiponectin, the main effects of resistin in the immune system seem to be proinflammatory.[15] For example, resistin induces proinflammatory cytokines in mouse and human macrophages[3,6,16,17] and activates human endothelial cells.[16] Furthermore, cytokines as well as chemokines are induced in a variety of human cells, including fibroblasts and endothelial

Table 58.1 Examples of the heterogeneous functions of adiponectin

Effect on inflammation and joint destruction	Effect
Pro-inflammatory	Induction of proinflammatory cytokines and chemokines in RA effector cells Induction of NO synthase in chondrocytes
Anti-inflammatory	Mitigates arthritis severity in the collagen-induced arthritis mouse model Inhibition of cell proliferation
Pro-destructive	Induction of RANKL and inhibition of OPG in osteoblasts
Anti-destructive	Inhibition of osteoclast formation, increase of osteoblast mineralization activity
Anti-apoptotic	Suppression of endothelial cell apoptosis by HMW adiponectin

HMW, high molecular weight; NO, nitric oxide; OPG, osteoprotegerin; RA, rheumatoid arthritis.

cells after stimulation with resistin.[3,16] Therefore, resistin seems to be associated with inflammation and exerts proinflammatory effects on the innate and adaptive immune system.[18] Similar to adiponectin, resistin forms multimeric structures. Physiologically, resistin exists as a monomer and a dimer. The resistin monomer is a non-covalent assembly of three protomers, while the dimeric resistin consists of two such monomers joined covalently by disulfide bonds.

Leptin

Leptin is a central adipokine in energy metabolism. Leptin also has immunoregulatory functions similar to adiponectin and resistin. The leptin serum levels are altered under pathophysiological conditions including chronic inflammatory diseases.[2,3,6] Acute as well as initial proinflammatory responses are modulated by leptin.[19,20] Leptin is involved in modulation of T-cell-mediated immune responses.[2] Additionally, other cells involved in inflammation are activated by leptin including monocytes, fibroblasts, and neutrophils.[2,19,20] However, the actual role of leptin in the inflammatory adipokine network is difficult to define because of its central regulatory role in metabolism and energy homeostasis.

Visfatin/PBEF

Visfatin, also known as pre-B cell colony enhancing factor (PBEF) or Nampt because of its nicotinamide phosphoribosyl-transferase (NAmPRTase) activity, is also involved in cell metabolism. Similar to resistin, it has an immunomodulatory potential with mainly proinflammatory effects under pathophysiological conditions.[5] Visfatin/PBEF is positively correlated with serum C-reactive protein (CRP) in different diseases, including rheumatoid arthritis (RA).[3,6] Furthermore, leucocytes are activated by visfatin/PBEF resulting in increased amounts of co-stimulatory molecules on the cell surface. In lymphocytes and monocytes, it induces proinflammatory cytokines in rheumatoid arthritis.[3,5,6] Furthermore, lymphocyte proliferation is stimulated by visfatin/PBEF in RA.[3,5,6] Cells such as neutrophils are protected from

apoptosis by visfatin/PBEF under pathophysiological conditions such as atherosclerosis or sepsis.[21]

Visfatin/PBEF has been shown to be involved in inflammatory processes of different (chronic) inflammatory diseases including RA.[3,5,6,22] Visfatin/PBEF is increased under chronic inflammatory conditions and may be involved in chronification due to its potential to further increase the proinflammatory reactions within the affected tissues.

Other 'new' adipokines

Omentin

Omentin is a recently identified adipokine of the omental adipose tissue.[23,24] It is secreted as a homotrimeric glycoprotein consisting of 313 amino acids with a molecular weight of 34 kDa per monomer.[24] Omentin is differentially expressed in omental adipose tissue under pathophysiological conditions, specifically in patients with Crohn's disease.[24] It is able to mediate metabolic as well as immunological effects.[25,26] Because of functional similarities to lectins, omentin was also called intelectin. Omentin has been also discussed as lactoferrin-binding protein and thought to be a lactoferrin receptor with immunomodulatory potential.[27]

Vaspin

Vaspin, which is similar to omentin, has recently been added to the list of adipokines. It belongs to the serin protease inhibitor family and has insulin-sensitizing effects. It is predominantly expressed in visceral adipose tissue. In addition, a role in inflammation and obesity has been suggested for vaspin.[25,28]

Chemerin

Chemerin was first discovered as a chemokine[29] and was only later added to the group of adipokines.[30–32] Similar to leptin, it is involved in energy metabolism as well as metabolic syndrome.[30–32] Chemerin occurs in different isoforms[33] and is structurally related to cathelicidin precursors (antibacterial peptides). Chemerin circulates as an inactive precursor and is activated by proteolytic cleavage at the C-terminus involving proteases. After activation, it is a strong chemoattractant for immature dendritic cells and macrophages[29] and is involved in inflammatory processes.[34]

Adipokines in inflammatory rheumatic diseases

In inflammation, adipokines are induced locally under different pathophysiological conditions including rheumatic diseases.[3,6] Although an altered expression and secretion of adipokines has been described for several adipokines in rheumatic diseases,[2,3,6] knowledge about the role of the respective adipokines in the disease pathology is limited. However, there is evidence that adipokines are able to induce immunomodulatory responses in different cell types responsible for inflammation as well as tissue remodelling/destruction.[3,6,8,17,22] Interestingly, adipokines are able to induce each other, forming an 'adipokine network' potentially contributing to the early induction of inflammation as well as to chronification of the respective disease.

Adipokines in rheumatoid arthritis

Most information on the role of adipokines in rheumatic diseases is available for RA. Adipokines including adiponectin, visfatin/PBEF, resistin, leptin, chemerin, vaspin, and omentin are increased or decreased in serum and/or synovial fluid of RA patients.[3,6,14,25] Adiponectin, resistin and visfatin serum or plasma levels, respectively, were increased in RA vs controls, although in some adiponectin studies no significant differences could be observed.[2,3,6] These different findings may be due to the increase of adiponectin especially in erosive vs mild RA, which also seems to correlate with joint erosion[2,3,6,14] and, interestingly, with vascular endothelial growth factor (VEGF) levels.[35]

Adipokines are not only produced by adipose tissue but also locally by additional cell types. The possibility of an existing adipokine network influencing the inflammatory response is reflected by the presence of different adipokines in the same compartments within the affected tissue. For example, the adipokines adiponectin, visfatin, and resistin are not only expressed by articular adipose tissue[33] and especially at the synovial lining layer and invasion zone, but also in the perivascular area, lymphocyte infiltrates, and single cells in the sublining.

In these compartments, a major source of adipokines are the RA synovial fibroblasts (RA-SF) as well as macrophages (Figure 58.1).[2,3,6,14] The adipokines produced in the synovium affect different effector cell types especially at sites of joint destruction, synovial angiogenesis, and inflammation. In addition, some knowledge is available about the effects of adipokines on the cell types localized in these areas. With regard to the early initiation of inflammation, the correlation of adipokines with inflammation markers is the first hint showing the link between adipokines and inflammation in RA. For example, CRP and other proinflammatory markers are correlated with systemic resistin and visfatin levels.[2,3,6,15]

Adiponectin has been described as being systemically increased in RA and as being associated with radiographic damage.[3,6,36,37]

A central cell type of cartilage destruction, the RA-SF, produces increased amounts of proinflammatory cytokines, growth factors and especially chemokines in response to adiponectin.[2,3,6,8,38,38a] Furthermore, chemokine production, which enhances further articular inflammation, is induced by adiponectin in endothelial cells, lymphocytes as well as chondrocytes in the synovium.[2,3,14]

However, in contrast to the above-mentioned proinflammatory effects on local synovial cells in vitro, in an in-vivo model of RA, the collagen-induced arthritis (CIA) model, application of adiponectin resulted in reduced severity of arthritis.[3,6] The reasons for the observed differences in the effects mediated by adiponectin are not completely clear. The different effects could be due to different protein (isoform) function in rodents and humans, the differences of the human and murine adiponectin (isoform) proteins, the use of different recombinant proteins with varying isoform compositions in the respective experiments, or systemic effects in vivo that are not visible in single-cell type experiments in vitro.

In contrast to the in part contradictory results on the immunomodulatory effects of adiponectin in RA, resistin and visfatin seem to be solely proinflammatory. Besides the correlation of proinflammatory markers such as CRP, IL-1ra, or TNFα with serum resistin, local resistin concentrations in the synovial fluid are higher than in the serum of the same patients.[3,6,16] Similar to adiponectin, resistin induced proinflammatory cytokines in peripheral blood mononuclear cells (PBMC)[16] and chondrocytes.[39] In turn, resistin is inducible in PBMC by proinflammatory factors showing a proinflammatory feedback loop locally active in the synovium.[16] In addition, a strong proinflammatory effect of resistin was confirmed using an in-vivo model by an intra-articular resistin injection, which led subsequently to rapid joint destruction.[16]

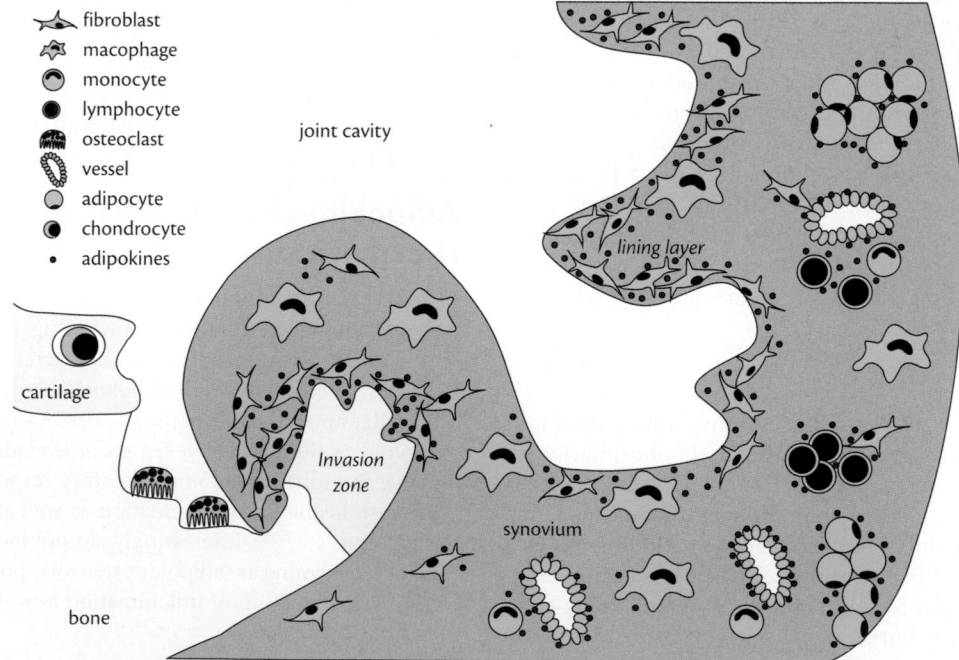

Fig. 58.1 Adipokines in rheumatoid arthritis (RA) synovial tissue. Adipokines such as adiponectin, resistin, visfatin/PBEF, omentin, and chemerin are expressed in the synovial lining layer. Perivascular areas, lymphocyte infiltrates, and adipocytes in the synovium express adipokines as well as single cells in the synovial sublining. Of note, in the invasion zone into cartilage, mainly consisting of invading fibroblasts, adipokines such as adiponectin and visfatin/PBEF are also expressed. Therefore, a variety of cell types involved in RA pathophysiology are exposed to adipokines and, depending on the cell type, in turn respond to these factors by releasing proinflammatory and prodestructive factors. Of note, the presence of adipokines in the synovial fluid and serum is not depicted in this figure.

Table 58.2 Adipokines in rheumatoid arthritis

	Systemic parameters	Local effects	Therapeutic effects
Adiponectin	Systemic adiponectin correlates with disease activity and severity	Proinflammatory and prodestructive factors are induced in RA-SF, chondrocytes Proinflammatory effects are induced in lymphocytes, endothelial cells	Influence of anti-TNF treatment visible but unclear Adiponectin reduces CIA severity
Visfatin	Systemic visfatin is increased in RA patients as well as in synovial fluids. Systemic visfatin correlates with systemic inflammation parameters and disease activity	Visfatin expression by RA-SF is regulated by TLRs and chemokines Visfatin induces proinflammatory and prodestructive factors in RA-SF. Visfatin protects synovial cells from apoptosis	In CIA, visfatin inhibition ameliorates arthritis severity
Resistin	Systemic resistin is increased in RA patients Systemic inflammation markers correlate with systemic resistin. Synovial fluid/serum resistin ratio is increased in RA	Proinflammatory factors are induced in RA-SF and inflammatory cells by resistin	Anti-TNF treatment reduces systemic resistin. Intra-articular resistin injection induces arthritis in rodents
Leptin	Potential association between leptin levels and RA (progression). Synovial fluid/serum ratios correlate with RA progression and activity	In RA-SF and chondrocytes, IL-8 is increased by leptin Leptin influences T cell activity and Treg proliferation	No influence of anti-TNF treatment on systemic leptin levels. Arthritis severity in leptin-deficient ob/ob mice is reduced and zymosan-induced arthritis. Acute inflammation resolution is delayed
Chemerin Omentin Vaspin	Vaspin synovial fluid levels are increased in RA, omentin levels decreased. Omentin levels correlate with serum ACPA and IgM-RF. Chemerin synovial fluid levels are higher than systemic levels	Chemerin has pro-inflammatory effects on RA-SF. Chemerin is induced by IL-1	Not available

ACPA, anti-citrullinated protein antibodies; CIA, collagen-induced arthritis; IL, interleukin; RA, rheumatoid arthritis; RA-SF, rheumatoid arthritis synovial fibroblasts; TLR, Toll-like receptors; TNF, tumour necrosis factor; Treg, regulatory T cell.

Visfatin is also increased locally in the synovial fluid of affected RA joints and in the serum as mentioned above. The proinflammatory effects on leucocytes, synovial fibroblasts, and neutrophils have been shown by different groups,[3,6,22] and seem to have an additional effect on the hyperplasia of the synovium by protection from apoptosis of synovial cells such as fibroblasts and neutrophils.[21] Similar to resistin, inhibition of visfatin results in reduced arthritis severity and anti-inflammatory responses in inflammatory cells in the CIA model, suggesting a proinflammatory role of visfatin in RA.[3,6] Taken together, these findings show that resistin, visfatin, and potentially adiponectin locally contribute to central inflammatory processes operative in RA joints.

In contrast to the findings from the above-mentioned adipokines, the function of leptin on RA inflammation and joint destruction is difficult to elucidate. Systemic levels of leptin seem to be increased in RA. However, leptin levels are influenced by body fat content, body mass index (BMI), treatment, and disease activity and progression, leading to discrepancies in the measured leptin levels in RA patients vs controls.[2,3,6] In the synovial fluid, leptin concentrations seem to be increased in comparison to the systemic leptin levels and to be correlated to joint erosion.[3,6] Interestingly, severity of arthritis in leptin-deficient ob/ob mice was reduced in comparison to controls.[3,6] In addition, detailed data on the effects of leptin on different cell types is limited. Although leptin influences the inflammatory response, especially via T cells,[2,6] and a proinflammatory effect via an increase of IL-8 in RA-SF[6] has been described,

the available information on systemic and local effects of leptin on destructive and inflammatory processes is not sufficient to confirm a clear pro- or anti-inflammatory role.

On a number of proteins recently identified as adipokines, only limited information is available about their role in RA pathophysiology. Vaspin levels in synovial fluid of RA patients were significantly higher than in osteoarthritis (OA) controls[25] as well as in serum.[40] In contrast, omentin levels in synovial fluids were reduced in RA when compared to osteoarthritis in this study. Both factors did not correlate with CRP or synovial fluid leucocyte counts. Of note, omentin but not vaspin correlated with anti-citrullinated protein antibodies (ACPA) and IgM-RF, showing a potential role in chronic RA inflammation.[25]

Interestingly, plasma concentrations of chemerin isoforms chem163S, chem158K, and chem157S are lower than synovial fluid levels in patients with RA, psoriatic arthritis, and OA, although no significant differences could be found for the respective diseases.[41] An increased expression of chemerin in the lining, sublining, and endothelial cells could be detected in RA in comparison to OA.[42,43] In addition, chemerin was identified as proinflammatory activator of RA-SF.[42,43] After proteolytic activation, it is a strong chemoattractant for immature dendritic cells and macrophages[29] but not for synovial fibroblasts,[43] although it does increase cell motility of this cell type.[42] Chemerin is secreted by adipose tissue[32] but also by other cell types including RA-SF[43] and chondrocytes.[44,45] It is found in similar concentrations in synovial fluid of patients with RA, OA, and psoriatic arthritis[43]; however, chemerin activity is increased in synovial fluid of RA patients compared to OA patients.[29] Additionally, chemerin increased TLR4 expression and MCP-1 secretion of synovial fibroblasts,[43] and enhanced the secretion of proinflammatory factors in chondrocytes.[44] These results suggest a role of chemerin in the innate immune system-associated joint inflammation.

In summary, the data suggest a potential proinflammatory local adipokine network active in RA synovial tissue within the affected joints (Table 58.2). However, interaction and comparison of systemic to local effects are still to be evaluated to clarify the in part contradictory data available on the role of adipokines in RA pathophysiology.

Adiponectin in systemic lupus erythematosus

In contrast to RA, the knowledge on the role of adipokines in the pathogenesis of other rheumatic diseases is mainly limited to information on serum levels and correlation to inflammation markers. However, besides the increased plasma and urine adiponectin levels in patients with systemic lupus erythematosus (SLE), especially with glomerulonephritis,[3,6] a proinflammatory role of adiponectin has been identified. Recombinant full-length adiponectin (consisting of all isoforms) but not globular adiponectin induced the chemokines IL-8 and MCP-1 in microvascular endothelial cells and monocytes,[3,6] although these effects may not be completely specific for SLE.

Serum levels of leptin were negatively correlated to androstenedione in SLE as well as RA patients[3] and may be involved in RA and SLE hypoandrogenicity. In addition, leptin and a high-fat diet induced proinflammatory high-density lipoproteins in lupus-prone mice.[6] In contrast, although resistin levels did not differ between SLE patients and controls, resistin was correlated with systemic inflammation in these patients.[46]

Adiponectin in spondyloarthropathies

Although Toussirot and colleagues found no altered adiponectin serum levels detectable in ankylosing spondylitis (AS) patients,[3] Derdemezis and colleagues reported increased adiponectin but not leptin levels in AS.[47] Serum levels of resistin were increased when compared to OA controls.[3,6] In contrast, synovial fluid resistin levels were not as high as in RA or OA in this study. As in RA, the data on systemic leptin levels in AS is not clear, as increased as well as decreased leptin serum levels have been reported.[3] However, systemic leptin levels seem to be correlated with CRP and IL-6,[3] and again adjustment to BMI and other metabolic parameters may be required for these analyses. However, leptin seems to be associated with proinflammatory effects on PBMC in AS patients, due to the increased expression of leptin, IL-6, and TNF in PBMC from AS patients in comparison to healthy controls.[48]

Adiponectin in other inflammatory rheumatic diseases

In systemic sclerosis (SSc), leptin levels seem to be reduced.[3] However, no additional information is available on the effects of adipokines on SSc-related inflammation and fibrosis. Similarly, limited information is available with respect to other rheumatic diseases such as vasculitis. In ANCA-associated vasculitis, leptin levels were significantly lower in comparison to healthy controls and were negatively correlated with disease activity in this study.[49]

In contrast, in Behçet's disease, leptin concentrations during active disease were increased when compared to inactive periods as well as in patients with longer disease duration.[3] Resistin and IL-6 serum levels were significantly higher in these patients in comparison to healthy controls.[50] Although no information on the effects and local expression at sites of pathophysiological alterations are available in these diseases, a link to inflammation is to be expected. However, the anti- and proinflammatory potential of these factors remains to be clarified.

Clinical features of adipokines in rheumatic diseases

The presence of adipokines in the serum, local compartments and tissues is not only affected by the respective pathophysiological condition, it is in part influenced by therapeutic interventions potentially serving as a parameter of treatment efficiency.

For example, in RA patients, systemic adiponectin is altered by treatment with TNF inhibitors showing an increase of adiponectin serum levels after TNF blockade in two studies, although there were also studies showing decreased or unaltered adiponectin serum levels after anti-TNF therapy.[3,6] In contrast, methotrexate seems to increase adiponectin serum levels in RA patients and resistin seems to be downregulated after anti-TNF treatment whereas leptin is not influenced.[3,6] In AS, systemic adiponectin and leptin levels were not altered by anti-TNF treatment.[6]

Conclusion

Adipokines affect the immune system and may be involved in early innate immune responses in addition to processes leading to chronic inflammation. Adipokines also affect matrix remodelling depending on the respective disease in addition to their role in inflammation. Because of the pluripotent functions of adipokines, there are currently many efforts to analyse the role of an adipokine or different adipokines under pathophysiological conditions, especially in chronic inflammatory diseases. However, as adipokines are able to influence each other and show partly contrary effects depending on the tissue, organ, and pathophysiological condition analysed, it is necessary to further characterize the adipokine network before potential therapeutic interventions in central adipokine-dependent pathways can be developed. Adipokine function has to be characterized, especially as adipokines are central effectors of metabolism and systemic therapeutic intervention may lead to strong unknown side effects that are reflected in the data available in animal models. Detailed understanding of the adipokine effects on the innate and adaptive immune system are required to identify specific isoforms, adipokine interactions, or receptors which make it possible to modulate the local response of adipokines without modifying central, vital pathways. The variety of possibilities in this relatively new field of 'immunoendocrinology' offers various possibilities for interesting new insights in adipokine-oriented research for the near future.

References

1. Fantuzzi G. Adipose tissue, adipokines, and inflammation. *J Allergy Clin Immunol* 2005;115(5):911–919.
2. Stofkova A. Leptin and adiponectin: from energy and metabolic dysbalance to inflammation and autoimmunity. *Endocr Regul* 2009;43(4): 157–168.

3. Neumann E, Frommer KW, Vasile M, Müller-Ladner U. Adipocytokines as driving forces in rheumatoid arthritis and related inflammatory diseases? *Arthritis Rheum* 2001;63(5):1159–1169.

4. Schaffler A, Scholmerich J. Innate immunity and adipose tissue biology. *Trends Immunol* 2000;31(6):228–235.

5. Moschen AR, Kaser A, Enrich B et al.. Visfatin, an adipocytokine with proinflammatory and immunomodulating properties. *J Immunol* 2007;178(3):1748–1758.

6. Gomez R, Conde J, Scotece M et al. What's new in our understanding of the role of adipokines in rheumatic diseases? *Nat Rev Rheumatol* 2001;7(9):528–536.

7. Tsao TS, Murrey HE, Hug C, Lee DH, Lodish HF. Oligomerization state-dependent activation of NF-kappa B signaling pathway by adipocyte complement-related protein of 30 kDa (Acrp30] *J Biol Chem* 2002;277.33): 29359–29362.

8. Frommer KW, Zimmermann B, Meier FM et al. Adiponectin-mediated changes in effector cells involved in the pathophysiology of rheumatoid arthritis. *Arthritis Rheum* 2000;62(10):2886–2899.

9. Kadowaki T, Yamauchi T. Adiponectin and adiponectin receptors. *Endocr Rev* 2005;26(3):439–451.

10. Hug C, Wang J, Ahmad NS et al. T-cadherin is a receptor for hexameric and high-molecular-weight forms of Acrp30/adiponectin. *Proc Natl Acad Sci U S A* 2004;101(28):10308–10313.

11. Mao X, Kikani CK, Riojas RA et al. APPL1 binds to adiponectin receptors and mediates adiponectin signalling and function. *Nat Cell Biol* 2006;8(5):516–523.

12. Heiker JT, Wottawah CM, Juhl C et al. Protein kinase CK2 interacts with adiponectin receptor 1 and participates in adiponectin signaling. *Cell Signal* 2000;21(6):936–942.

13. Charlton HK, Webster J, Kruger S et al. ERp46 binds to AdipoR1, but not AdipoR2, and modulates adiponectin signalling. *Biochem Biophys Res Commun* 2001;392(2):234–239.

14. Muller-Ladner U, Neumann E. Rheumatoid arthritis: the multifaceted role of adiponectin in inflammatory joint disease. *Nat Rev Rheumatol* 2009;5(12):659–660.

15. Kontunen P, Vuolteenaho K, Nieminen R et al. Resistin is linked to inflammation, and leptin to metabolic syndrome, in women with inflammatory arthritis. *Scand J Rheumatol* 2001;40(4):256–262.

16. Bokarewa M, Nagaev I, Dahlberg L, Smith U, Tarkowski A. Resistin, an adipokine with potent proinflammatory properties. *J Immunol* 2005;174(9):5789–5795.

17. Bostrom EA, Svensson M, Andersson S et al. Resistin and insulin/insulin-like growth factor signaling in rheumatoid arthritis. *Arthritis Rheum* 2001;63(10):2894–2904.

18. Fargnoli JL, Sun Q, Olenczuk D et al. Resistin is associated with biomarkers of inflammation while total and high-molecular weight adiponectin are associated with biomarkers of inflammation, insulin resistance, and endothelial function. *Eur J Endocrinol* 2000;162(2):281–288.

19. Cai C, Hahn BH, Matarese G, La Cava A. Leptin in non-autoimmune inflammation. *Inflamm Allergy Drug Targets* 2009;8(4):285–291.

20. Maya-Monteiro CM, Bozza PT. Leptin and mTOR: partners in metabolism and inflammation. *Cell Cycle* 2008;7(12):1713–1717.

21. van der Veer E, Ho C, O'Neil C et al.. Extension of human cell lifespan by nicotinamide phosphoribosyltransferase. *J Biol Chem* 2007;282(15):10841–10845.

22. Brentano F, Schorr O, Ospelt C et al. Pre-B cell colony-enhancing factor/visfatin, a new marker of inflammation in rheumatoid arthritis with proinflammatory and matrix-degrading activities. *Arthritis Rheum* 2007;56(9):2829–2839.

23. Wurm S, Neumeier M, Weigert J, Schaffler A, Buechler C. Plasma levels of leptin, omentin, collagenous repeat-containing sequence of 26-kDa protein (CORS-26] and adiponectin before and after oral glucose uptake in slim adults. *Cardiovasc Diabetol* 2007;6:7.

24. Schaffler A, Neumeier M, Herfarth H et al. Genomic structure of human omentin, a new adipocytokine expressed in omental adipose tissue. *Biochim Biophys Acta* 2005;1732(1–3):96–102.

25. Senolt L, Polanska M, Filkova M et al. Vaspin and omentin: new adipokines differentially regulated at the site of inflammation in rheumatoid arthritis. *Ann Rheum Dis* 2000;69(7):1410–1411.

26. Yamawaki H, Kuramoto J, Kameshima S et al. Omentin, a novel adipocytokine inhibits TNF-induced vascular inflammation in human endothelial cells. *Biochem Biophys Res Commun* 2001;408(2):339–343.

27. Shin K, Wakabayashi H, Yamauchi K, Yaeshima T, Iwatsuki K. Recombinant human intelectin binds bovine lactoferrin and its peptides. *Biol Pharm Bull* 2008;31(8):1605–1608.

28. Hida K, Wada J, Eguchi J et al. Visceral adipose tissue-derived serine protease inhibitor: a unique insulin-sensitizing adipocytokine in obesity. *Proc Natl Acad Sci U S A* 2005;102(30):10610–10615.

29. Wittamer V, Franssen JD, Vulcano M et al. Specific recruitment of antigen-presenting cells by chemerin, a novel processed ligand from human inflammatory fluids. *J Exp Med* 2003;198(7):977–985.

30. Bozaoglu K, Bolton K, McMillan J et al. Chemerin is a novel adipokine associated with obesity and metabolic syndrome. *Endocrinology* 2007;148(10):4687–4694.

31. Goralski KB, McCarthy TC, Hanniman EA et al. Chemerin, a novel adipokine that regulates adipogenesis and adipocyte metabolism. *J Biol Chem* 2007;282(38):28175–28188.

32. Roh SG, Song SH, Choi KC et al. Chemerin—a new adipokine that modulates adipogenesis via its own receptor. *Biochem Biophys Res Commun* 2007;362(4):1013–1018.

33. Kontny E, Plebanczyk M, Lisowska B et al. Comparison of rheumatoid articular adipose and synovial tissue reactivity to proinflammatory stimuli: contribution to adipocytokine network. *Ann Rheum Dis* 2012;71(2):262–267.

34. Ernst MC, Sinal CJ. Chemerin: at the crossroads of inflammation and obesity. *Trends Endocrinol Metab* 2010;21(11):660–667.

35. Choi HM, Lee YA, Lee SH et al. Adiponectin may contribute to synovitis and joint destruction in rheumatoid arthritis by stimulating VEGF, matrix metalloproteinase-1, and matrix metalloproteinase-13 expression in fibroblast-like synoviocytes more than proinflammatory mediators. *Arthritis Res Ther* 2009;11(6):R161.

36. Giles JT, van der Heijde DM, Bathon JM. Association of circulating adiponectin levels with progression of radiographic joint destruction in rheumatoid arthritis. *Ann Rheum Dis* 2011;70(9):1562–1568.

37. Klein-Wieringa IR, van der Linden MP, Knevel R et al. Baseline serum adipokine levels predict radiographic progression in early rheumatoid arthritis. *Arthritis Rheum* 2011;63(9):2567–2574.

38. Kusunoki N, Kitahara K, Kojima F et al. Adiponectin stimulates prostaglandin E(2) production in rheumatoid arthritis synovial fibroblasts. *Arthritis Rheum* 2010;62(6):1641–1649.

38a. Frommer KW, Schäffler A, Büchler C et al. Adiponectin isoforms: a potential therapeutic target in rheumatoid arthritis? *Ann Rheum Dis* 2012;71(10):1724–1732.

39. Zhang Z, Xing X, Hensley G et al. Resistin induces expression of pro-inflammatory cytokines and chemokines in human articular chondrocytes via transcription and messenger RNA stabilization. *Arthritis Rheum* 2010;62(7):1993–2003.

40. Ozgen M, Koca SS, Dagli N et al. Serum adiponectin and vaspin levels in rheumatoid arthritis. *Arch Med Res* 2010;41(6):457–463.

41. Zhao L, Yamaguchi Y, Sharif S et al. Chemerin 158K is the dominant chemerin isoform in synovial and cerebrospinal fluids but not in plasma. *J Biol Chem* 2011;286(45):39520–39527.

42. Kaneko K, Miyabe Y, Takayasu A et al. Chemerin activates fibroblast-like synoviocytes in patients with rheumatoid arthritis. *Arthritis Res Ther* 2011;13(5):R158.

43. Eisinger K, Bauer S, Schaffler A et al. Chemerin induces CCL2 and TLR4 in synovial fibroblasts of patients with rheumatoid arthritis and osteoarthritis. *Exp Mol Pathol* 2012;92(1):90–96.

44. Berg V, Sveinbjornsson B, Bendiksen S et al. Human articular chondrocytes express ChemR23 and chemerin;ChemR23 promotes inflammatory signalling upon binding the ligand chemerin(21–157) *Arthritis Res Ther* 2010;12(6):R228.

45. Conde J, Gomez R, Bianco G et al. Expanding the adipokine network in cartilage: identification and regulation of novel factors in human and murine chondrocytes. *Ann Rheum Dis* 2011;70(3):551–559.

46. Almehed K, d'Elia HF, Bokarewa M, Carlsten H. Role of resistin as a marker of inflammation in systemic lupus erythematosus. *Arthritis Res Ther* 2008;10(1):R15.

47. Derdemezis CS, Filippatos TD, Voulgari PV et al. Leptin and adiponectin levels in patients with ankylosing spondylitis. The effect of infliximab treatment. *Clin Exp Rheumatol* 2010;28(6):880–883.

48. Park MC, Chung SJ, Park YB, Lee SK. Pro-inflammatory effect of leptin on peripheral blood mononuclear cells of patients with ankylosing spondylitis. *Joint Bone Spine* 2009;76(2):170–175.

49. Kumpers P, Horn R, Brabant G et al. Serum leptin and ghrelin correlate with disease activity in ANCA-associated vasculitis. *Rheumatology* 2008;47(4):484–487.

50. Yalcindag FN, Yalcindag A, Batioglu F et al. Evaluation of serum resistin levels in patients with ocular and non-ocular Behcet's disease. *Can J Ophthalmol* 2008;43(4):473–475.

CHAPTER 59

Pain neurophysiology

Hans-Georg Schaible and Rainer H. Straub

The nature of pain

- **Physiological nociceptive pain** is evoked by high-energy stimuli acting on healthy tissue which potentially or actually damage the tissue (noxious stimuli). This type of pain is a warning sensation and essential for survival because it triggers adequate protective reactions of the endangered organism. Pain treatment must not impair this type of pain.

- **Pathophysiological nociceptive pain** occurs during inflammation or after injury. It appears as allodynia (occurrence of pain upon an innocuous stimulus of low energy which is normally not painful) and/or hyperalgesia (increased pain during the application of noxious stimuli). Finally, resting pain (in the absence of intentional stimulation) may occur. This pain impairs normal life and requires treatment.

- **Neuropathic pain** is evoked by damage to the neurons of the nociceptive system. Causes are nerve damage, metabolic diseases (e.g. diabetes mellitus), infections such as herpes zoster and others. Neuropathic pain does not primarily signal noxious tissue stimulation, is often felt to be abnormal (burning or electrical character), and can be persistent or occur in short episodes (e.g. trigeminal neuralgia). It may be combined with hyperalgesia and allodynia or with sensory loss.[1]

The nociceptive system

Nociception is the encoding and processing of noxious stimuli. Neurons which encode noxious stimuli (see above) at the different levels of the neuraxis form the nociceptive system (see scheme in Figure 59.1A). It consists of the peripheral nociceptors supplying almost all organs and tissues of the body, nociceptive spinal cord neurons, which are synaptically activated by nociceptors, and nociceptive neurons in the thalamocortical system, which are activated by ascending neural tracts such as the spinothalamic tract. Furthermore, ascending tracts (the spinothalamic and spinoreticular tract) activate nociception-related nuclei in the brain stem. From there further neural projections branch into cerebral structures such as the amygdala. As shown in Figure 59.1B, some brainstem nuclei, the periaqueductal grey (PAG), and the rostral ventral medulla (RVM) and their axons, form descending systems which control the nociceptive processing at the spinal level either in an inhibitory or facilitatory fashion.[2]

Peripheral **nociceptors** are thinly myelinated (Aδ-fibres) or unmyelinated (C-fibres). Their sensory endings are so-called 'free nerve endings', i.e. they are not equipped with corpuscular end organs. Most of the nociceptors are polymodal, responding to noxious mechanical stimuli (painful pressure, squeezing or cutting the tissue), to noxious thermal stimuli (heat or cold), and to chemical stimuli.[3] It is highly important that a proportion of the afferent sensory nerve fibres, the **peptidergic** nociceptors, not only have an afferent function by transmitting nociceptive input to the central nervous system but that they have in addition an efferent function by releasing substance P and other neuropeptides such as calcitonin-related peptide (CGRP) and galanin into the vicinity of the peripheral nerve terminal. Upon trauma with or without infection, these afferent fibres can also induce vasodilation, plasma extravasation, and other pathophysiological effects, e.g. the attraction of macrophages or the degranulation of mast cells. This **neurogenic inflammation** is the first component of an innate inflammatory response that induces a cascade of subsequent mechanisms such as chemotaxis, upregulation of adhesion molecules, and activation of immune cells. In particular substance P is an immunostimulatory neuropeptide that activates macrophages, fibroblasts, neutrophils, lymphocytes, and other immune cells leading to secretion of proinflammatory cytokines.[4] The other subset of nociceptors is **non-peptidergic** (IB4-positive neurons). The skin is innervated by both peptidergic and IB4-positive nociceptive afferents, but the vast majority of afferents in the musculoskeletal system are peptidergic.

A single peripheral nociceptor supplies a specific site of the body such as the skin, skeletal muscle, a joint, or a visceral organ. In contrast, many **nociceptive neurons in the spinal cord** exhibit convergent inputs from nociceptors from different organs/tissues.[5] This is the basis for referred pain, i.e. pain is sometimes felt in a structure other than the stimulated one. In particular, pain originating in the visceral tissues may be felt in the somatic tissue of the same neuronal segment. Nociceptive spinal neurons are either ascending tract neurons (see above) or interneurons that are part of segmental motor or vegetative reflex pathways. However, the spinal cord through sympathetic reflexes and the brain itself through descending influences can influence diverse pathological processes in the affected tissues. This is relevant for the neuronal influences on the course of inflammation.

The conscious sensation of pain is generated in the thalamocortical system (Figure 59.1A). The **lateral thalamocortical system** consists of relay nuclei in the lateral thalamus and the areas SI and

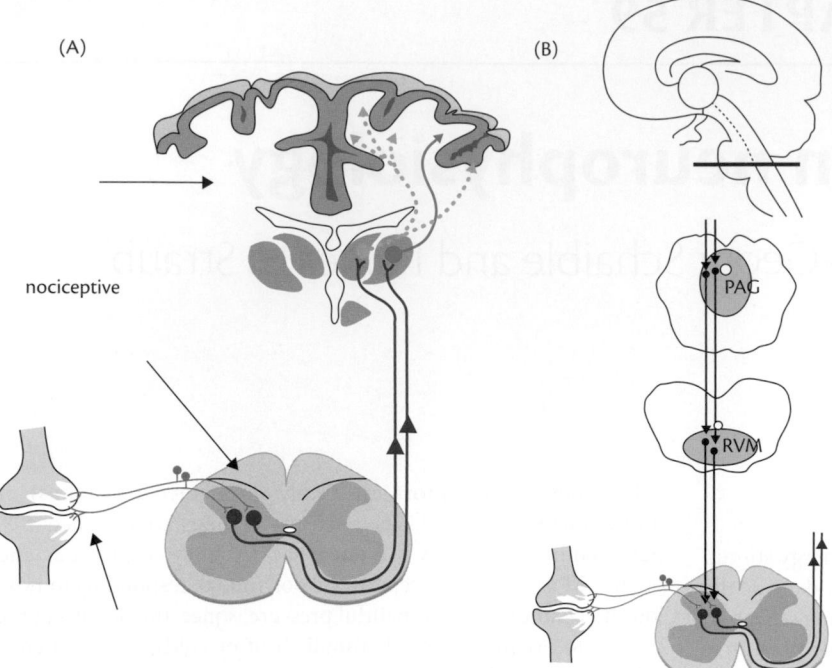

nociceptive

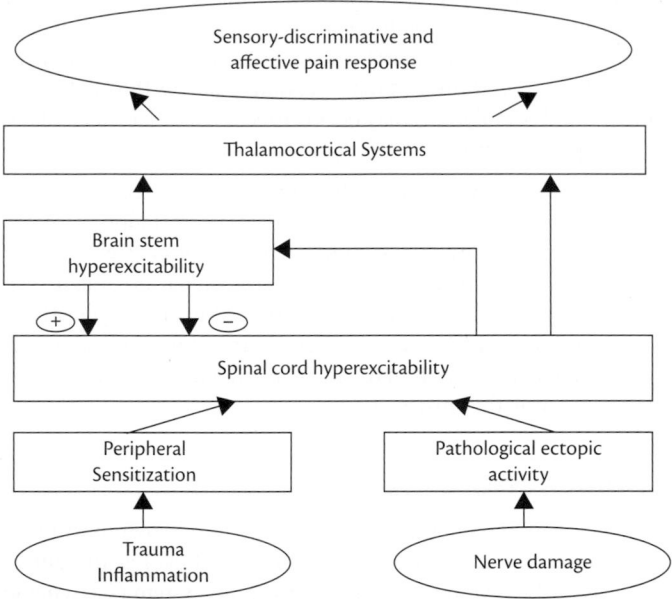

Fig. 59.1 Simplified scheme of the structure of the nociceptive system and major events during inflammatory pain states. (A) Upon inflammation the sensory nociceptive system exhibits sensitization of peripheral nociceptors (peripheral sensitization) and hyperexcitability of nociceptive neurons in the spinal cord (central sensitization). The latter determines the amount of activation of the thalamocortical nociceptive system. (B) Descending systems originating in the brainstem which inhibit or facilitate the nociceptive processing at the spinal level. PAG, periaqueductal grey matter; RVM: rostroventral medulla.

SII in the postcentral gyri. In these areas the noxious stimulus is analysed for its location, duration, and intensity (sensory discriminative aspect). The **medial thalamocortical system** consists of relay nuclei in the central and medial thalamus and the anterior cingulate cortex (ACC), the insula, and the prefrontal cortex. In these structures the affective component of suffering is produced, and in particular the ACC is thought to be involved in the selection of the proper response.[6] In addition these structures contribute to the activation of the inhibitory system which descends from the brainstem to the spinal cord in the dorsolateral funiculus (see Figure 59.1B). This system is thought to be responsible for the powerful analgesic placebo effects.[2,6]

Nociceptive processing under normal and pathological conditions

In the healthy individual, pain is only elicited by stimuli of high intensity which are potentially or actually tissue damaging (physiological nociceptive pain). During inflammation and injury of organs/tissue, the nociceptive system is sensitized (Figure 59.2), which is the neuronal basis of allodynia and hyperalgesia, main features of pathophysiological nociceptive pain. Nociceptive sensitization has a peripheral component (sensitization of nociceptors in the tissue) and a central component (development of hyperexcitability in nociceptive neurons in the central nervous system). Peripheral sensitization reduces the excitation threshold of the nociceptors such that they are excitable by stimuli of light intensity such as palpation. Nociceptors in the muscle and joint are strongly sensitized to mechanical stimuli, whereas cutaneous nociceptors are rather sensitized to thermal stimuli.[3] Furthermore, silent nociceptors, i.e. nociceptors with extremely high thresholds in normal tissue, are then activated by stimuli.[5] These processes cause an enhanced neuronal input into the spinal cord, which further activates and sensitizes spinal cord neurons. **Central**

Fig. 59.2 Schematic display of the activation of the nociceptive system by inflammation/injury and neuropathic events and elicitation of descending inhibition or facilitation of nociception.

Reproduced with permission from BioMed Central from Schaible H-G, Ebersberger A, Natura G (2011). Update on peripheral mechanisms of pain: beyond prostaglandins and cytokines. Arthritis Res Ther, 13, 210.

sensitization describes a state of hyperexcitability, in which central neurons respond more readily to their peripheral inputs. It amplifies the nociceptive input from the periphery.[7]

While physiological and pathophysiological pain is induced by noxious stimulation or inflammatory conditions in the innervated organs/tissues, neuropathic pain is generated by damage or disease of injured nerve fibres themselves. Mechanistically, action potentials in injured nerve fibres are often initiated at the nerve lesion site or in the dorsal root ganglion, i.e. they are not elicited in the sensory endings in the tissue (where this normally takes place) but in the course of the nerve fibre (thus they are called **ectopic discharges**, which may occur regularly or episodically).[1] Episodic discharges are usually not related to noxious stimuli applied to the tissue, and therefore this input is felt abnormal by the individual. Figure 59.2 shows that episodic discharges may also cause central sensitization.

Figure 59.2 also indicates that the brain stem may either reduce or aggravate the nociceptive processing at the spinal level. During short-lasting acute inflammation, the feedback is rather negative, i.e. descending inhibitory systems try to reduce central sensitization. During prolonged inflammation this descending inhibition is attenuated, and studies in pain patients have suggested that some forms of descending inhibition (in particular the descending noxious inhibitory control, DNIC) are even out of order. DNIC is a form of inhibition in which the application of painful stimuli to one site of the body reduces the pain at other sites of the body (DNIC is therefore considered to be one mechanism involved in acupuncture).[2] There is evidence that under neuropathic conditions the brainstem rather facilitates nociception at the spinal level.

Although nociceptive pain and neuropathic pain are different, there may be an overlap under certain clinical conditions. First, surgery may damage tissue and nerve fibres. Bone cancer may evoke an inflammatory component but may also invade nerve branches. In addition, nerve injury is associated with a local inflammatory reaction at the lesion site, and there is some preliminary evidence that chronic lesions such as osteoarthritis may also have a neuropathic component.

Inflammation induces a change of tissue innervation that leads to a sprouting response of sensory nerve fibres and to a parallel loss of sympathetic nerve fibres. The imbalance leads to a preponderance of substance P over sympathetic neurotransmitters, which supports the local inflammatory process but also pain processing.[8]

Molecular mechanisms of peripheral nociception and sensitization

Transduction of stimuli and generation of action potentials

The sensory endings of nociceptors are equipped with numerous ion channels and membrane receptors (Figure 59.3). Sensor molecules in the sensory endings of nociceptors transduce mechanical, thermal, and chemical stimuli into a sensor potential, and when the amplitude of the sensor potential is sufficiently high, action potentials are triggered and conducted by the axon to the dorsal horn of the spinal cord or the brainstem. Some sensor molecules have been identified.[9] The best-known receptor is the transient receptor potential vanilloid 1 (TRPV1) receptor. TRPV1 is a ligand-gated ion channel. Upon opening, cations, in particular Ca^{2+}, flow into the cell and depolarize it. The TRPV1 receptor is expressed in nociceptors but not in other peripheral neurons. It is opened by temperatures higher than 43 °C which are felt as painful heat by humans, by chemicals which elicit burning pain (such as capsaicin and ethanol applied to a wound), by low pH (<5.9) which occurs in inflamed tissue, and it is activated by metabolites of arachidonic acid produced by lipoxygenases such as 12-hydroperoxyeicosaenoic acid (12-HPETE), and by endocannabinoids such as anandamide and

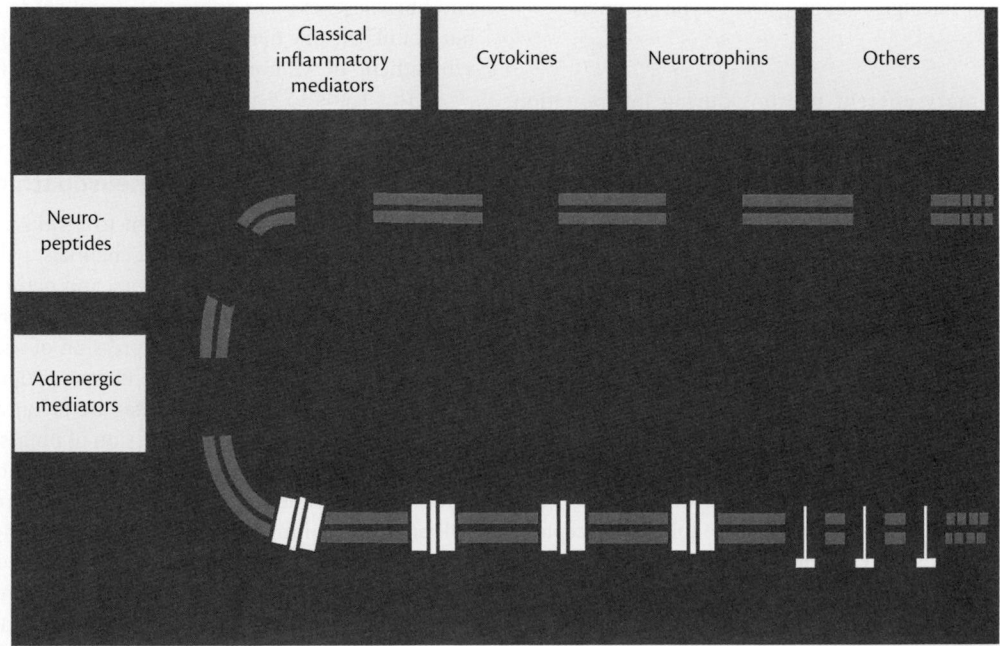

Fig. 59.3 Schematic drawing of a sensory ending of a nociceptor in the tissue. The membrane at the bottom shows ion channels for transduction (which produce a sensor potential), a voltage-gated Na^+ channel for the generation of action potentials (APs), and voltage-gated K^+ and Ca^{2+} channels which control excitability. ASIC, acid sensing ion channel; PTX, purinergic ion channel; TRP, transient receptor potential; TTX, tetrodotoxin. The other part of the membrane displays receptors for mediators which act on different second-messenger systems. Classical inflammatory mediators are bradykinin, prostaglandin E_2, 5-hydroytryptamine, and histamine.

Reproduced from Schaible H-G, Ebersberger A, Natura G. Update on peripheral mechanisms of pain: beyond prostaglandins and cytokines. Arthritis Res Ther 2011;13:210, with permission.

NADA. Furthermore, TRPV1 is indirectly sensitized, via second messengers, by the inflammatory mediators bradykinin, prostaglandin E_2, extracellular ATP, glutamate, proteases, cytokines, and nerve growth factor. It is one transducer of noxious heat, and it is crucial for inflammatory **thermal hyperalgesia**. Thus TRPV1 is considered a key receptor of nociception.

Other TRP channels such as TRPV2, TRPV3, TRPV4, TRPM8, and TRPA1 are also expressed in proportions of primary afferent neurons, and some of them are coexpressed with TRPV1 in one and the same nociceptive neuron, whereas others are expressed in non-nociceptive neurons. For example, TRPM8 is opened by temperatures which are felt as cool—hence TRPM8 is assumed to be the transducer in non-nociceptive cold fibres but in general the role of these other TRP channels is less clear. An open question is whether TRP channels are also involved in the transduction of mechanical stimuli and mechanical hyperalgesia, which is more important than thermal hyperalgesia.[9]

Once the ending is sufficiently depolarized by the influx of cations, voltage-gated Na^+ channels are opened and action potentials are triggered (Figure 59.3). Different types of Na^+ channels exist. Nociceptive afferent neurons express mainly $Na_v1.7$, $Na_v1.8$, and $Na_v1.9$ whereas large-sized non-nociceptive neurons express mainly $Na_v1.1$, $Na_v1.6$, and $Na_v1.7$, and some $Na_v1.8$. These channels differ in their kinetics and their activation threshold, and their presence determines the threshold for opening. While $Na_v1.7$ and $Na_v1.8$ are directly involved in the generation of the action potential, $Na_v1.9$ influences the threshold for action potentials. These channels can be up- or downregulated by second-messenger pathways involving protein kinase A, protein kinase C, sphingomyelinase, calmodulin, and p38 MAP kinase. The excitability of neurons may also be controlled by K^+ channels (e.g. of the KCNQ family) and Ca^{2+} channels. Excitability is increased when voltage-gated K^+ channels are closed (this evokes sustained depolarization of neurons) or when Ca^{2+} flows into the neuron through voltage-gated T-type channels.[3]

Sensitization

Sensitization of primary afferent neurons during inflammation is generated by inflammatory mediators. These inflammatory mediators act on specific membrane receptors (see Figure 59.3). In general, ligand binding of these membrane receptors activates second-messenger systems which then affect both transduction molecules and voltage-gated ion channels such that they are more excitable (e.g. by phosphorylation). In the long term, some of them may also regulate the expression of such molecules in the membrane. In addition, sensory nerve endings possess Toll-like receptors that signal molecular patterns of infectious agents, indicating an important role of the nociceptive nerve fibres in the context of innate immunity.

'Classical' inflammatory mediators such as bradykinin and prostaglandins activate and/or sensitize neurons within minutes. For example, prostaglandin E_2 acts on G-protein-coupled EP receptors which increase cAMP. This activates protein kinase A, which finally leads to a phosphorylation of TRPV1 receptors and voltage-gated Na^+ currents. Upon a single application the effects are quite short (minutes only). By contrast, injection of proinflammatory cytokines such as interleukin (IL)-6 and tumour necrosis factor alpha (TNFα) into the joint leads to a slowly developing but persistent sensitization of nociceptive afferents (i.e. increase of the number of action potentials to a stimulus) lasting at least several hours. In addition, cytokines regulate the expression of receptors (e.g. TNFα upregulates TRPV1 receptors).[5] These cytokine effects can be blocked by anti-cytokine therapy with biological agents, and it is expected that this also inhibits release of proinflammatory substance P and other neuropeptides.

The neuropeptides substance P and CGRP sensitize part of the neurons, whereas opioid peptides and somatostatin inhibit the neurons. The latter two peptides may also be released from sympathetic nerve endings but this may be disturbed due to the loss of sympathetic nerve fibres.

Nerve growth factor (NGF) is an essential neurotrophin for the development of sensory nerve fibres. In the adult, a large proportion of sensory nerve fibres remains dependent on the trophic effect of NGF. These neurons express TrkA receptors (specific receptor for NGF), and NGF is required for their structural and functional integrity. However, substantial amounts of NGF are also produced at inflammatory sites and NGF can act as an inflammatory mediator. It enhances currents through TRPV1 channels and reduces the threshold of thermal excitation. Long-term exposure to NGF increases the expression of TRPV1, bradykinin receptors, P2X receptors, Na^+ channels, and the synthesis of putative nociceptive transmitters such as substance P and CGRP. In addition, NGF stimulates inflammatory cells to release inflammatory compounds. Thus NGF is a key molecule for nociceptor biology, and its neutralization proved to be highly analgesic in humans.[3]

There exist nerve repellent factors that are able to repel peripheral nerve fibres from the innervation site within minutes to hours. These repellent factors are important in guiding nerve fibres during embryological development of the central and peripheral nervous system. In inflamed tissue, repellent factors of the semaphorin group were detected such as semaphorin 3C and 3F.[10] Macrophages and fibroblasts express only nerve repellent factors of sympathetic but not of sensory nerve fibres, thus explaining the specific loss of sympathetic nerve fibres while sensory nerve fibres are not affected.[11] This leads to a preponderance of sensory over sympathetic nerve fibres, called sensory hyperinnervation.

Ectopic discharges and/or 'neuropathic' activation

Different mechanisms are thought to produce ectopic discharges: changes in the expression of ionic channels, pathological activation of axons by inflammatory mediators, and pathological activation of injured nerve fibres by the sympathetic nervous system (α-adrenergic effects). After nerve injury the expression of such sodium channels is increased, which alters the membrane properties of the neuron in such a way that rapid firing rates are favoured (bursting ectopic discharges). Changes in the expression of potassium channels of the neurons were also shown. Inflammatory mediators such as prostaglandins, nitric oxide (NO), and cytokines are produced by Schwann cells and by inflammatory cells which invade the injured nerve, and damaged axons become sensitive to these mediators. The sympathetic nervous system does not activate primary afferent nerve fibres in normal tissue. Injured nerve fibres may, however, become sensitive to adrenergic mediators. This cross-talk may occur at different sites. Adrenergic receptors may be expressed at the sensory nerve fibre ending. A direct connection between afferent and efferent fibres (so-called 'ephapses') is considered. Sympathetic endings are expressed in increased numbers in the dorsal root ganglion after nerve injury. The cell bodies of injured nerve fibres are surrounded by 'baskets' consisting of sympathetic fibres.[1]

Molecular mechanisms of central sensitization

Different neuronal receptor/transmitter systems are involved in the induction and maintenance of central sensitization. Both the release of excitatory/sensitizing mediators from presynaptic neurons and the excitability of postsynaptic neurons are enhanced. In addition, glial cells are involved in the nociceptive processing, at least in neuropathic pain states.

Glutamate is the main transmitter in nociceptors. It activates ionotropic N-methyl-D-aspartate (NMDA) and non-NMDA receptors and metabotropic glutamate receptors in spinal cord neurons. The activation of non-NMDA receptors is the basis for synaptic activation of neurons. The opening of NMDA receptors (this occurs upon strong depolarization as during noxious stimulation) allows a strong calcium influx into the neurons which then triggers cellular mechanisms of increased excitability. This is a key mechanism of the induction and maintenance of central sensitization.[5,7]

Upon noxious stimulation and peripheral inflammation, the neuropeptides substance P, neurokinin A, and CGRP are spinally released from sensitized nociceptors. They act on neuropeptide receptors on spinal cord neurons and support the development of central sensitization, probably by a facilitation of glutamatergic synaptic transmission. Spinal sensitization is also supported by spinal prostaglandins. The latter are synthesized by a proportion of nociceptors and numerous cells in the spinal cord. Further involved are spinal neurotrophins such as brain-derived neurotropic factor (BDNF).[5]

More recently, glial cells have come into the focus. Neuropathic pain states involve the release of proinflammatory cytokines from astroglia and microglia, and suppression of the activation of glial cells can prevent and/or reverse neuropathic pain.[12] Cytokines such as IL-1β, IL-6, and TNF play a dominant role in cytokine-induced hypersensitivity, and these cytokines are also induced in the spinal cord during experimental arthritis. The cellular mechanisms are only incompletely understood but the following signalling pathways have been mentioned: NFκB, protein kinase A, protein kinase C, c-Jun N-terminal kinase, JAK/STAT3 signalling pathway, p38 mitogen-activated protein kinase (MAPK), Src-family kinase, arachidonic acid pathways, and others.

For example, the p38 pathway was demonstrated to be an important proinflammatory signalling cascade in spinal neurons and microglia cells in experimental arthritis. Phosphorylated p38 is increased in microglial and neuronal cells during the course of experimental arthritis. The intrathecal administration of a specific p38 inhibitor led to decreased synovial inflammation but also suppressed articular cytokine and protease expression as well as joint destruction.[13] TNF can be a signalling element upstream of p38 by activating p38-phosphorylating kinases or downstream of phosphorylated p38 that induces TNF secretion. Intrathecal, but not subcutaneous, TNF neutralization with etanercept inhibited p38 phosphorylation and peripheral inflammation,[13,14] along with a pronounced antinociceptive effect.[14] The efferent pathways for these effects have not been unequivocally identified. In a state of

spinal hyperexcitability dorsal root reflexes may be generated in the spinal cord (i.e. action potentials are generated in the spinal terminals of afferent fibres which are conducted retrogradely from the spinal cord to the periphery where neuropeptides are released[15]) and/or sympathetic efferent fibres may be activated.[5,14]

Sensitization may be counteracted by transmitters which inhibit neurons. Such transmitters are GABA, opioid peptides, 5-hydroxytryptamine, and noradrenaline, the latter two being involved in descending inhibition. It has been suggested that such inhibitory mechanism may fail under neuropathic conditions.

Pain and sensitization: evolutionary considerations

Why peripheral and central sensitization have been positively selected during evolution is an important question. Sensitization of pain has a protective role because it warns about potential danger, enables us to remove noxious stimuli, and stimulates wound management. Furthermore, avoidance of painful situations in the future would be highly desirable. This is nicely indicated by the fact that peripheral inflammatory stimulation of sensory neurons can induce central IL-1β release in the hippocampus,[16] a cytokine that is instrumental in hippocampal learning phenomena.[17] Sensitization is an amplification factor which should last as long as painful/noxious stimuli are present (or even a little longer, to stimulate wound management). Thus, sensitization is a supportive factor of innate immunity. It has been positively selected as an evolutionarily conserved learning phenomenon, which will not be stopped until inflammation is terminated, i.e. the noxious stimulus is removed.

References

1. Schaible H-G, Richter F. Pathophysiology of pain. *Langenbeck's Arch Surg* 2004;389:237–243.
2. Ossipov MH, Dussor GO, Porreca F. Central modulation of pain. *J Clin Invest* 2010;120:3779–3787.
3. Schaible H-G, Ebersberger A, Natura G. Update on peripheral mechanisms of pain: beyond prostaglandins and cytokines. *Arthritis Res Ther* 2011;13:210.
4. Straub RH, Cutolo M. Involvement of the hypothalamic-pituitary-adrenal/gonadal axis and the peripheral nervous system in rheumatoid arthritis. *Arthritis Rheum* 2001;44:493–507.
5. Schaible H-G. Joint pain—basic mechanisms. In: McMahon SB, Koltzenburg M (eds) *Wall and Melzack's textbook of pain*, 6th edn. W.B. Saunders, London, 2013.
6. Schweinhardt P, Bushnell MC. Pain imaging in health and disease—how far have we come? *J Clin Invest* 2010;120:3788–3797.
7. Woolf CJ, Salter MW. Neuronal plasticity: increasing the gain in pain. *Science* 2000;288:1765–1768.
8. Straub RH. Autoimmune disease and innervation. *Brain Behav Immun* 2007;21:528–534.
9. Basbaum AI, Bautista DM, Scherrer G, Julius D. Cellular and molecular mechanisms of pain. *Cell* 2009;139:267–284.
10. Fasold A, Falk W, Anders S et al. Soluble neuropilin-2, a nerve repellent receptor, is increased in rheumatoid arthritis synovium and aggravates sympathetic fiber repulsion and arthritis. *Arthritis Rheum* 2009;60:2892–2901.
11. Miller LE, Weidler C, Falk W et al. Increased prevalence of semaphorin 3C, a repellent of sympathetic nerve fibers, in the synovial tissue of patients with rheumatoid arthritis. *Arthritis Rheum* 2004;50:1156–1163.

12. McMahon SB, Malcangio M. Current challenges in glia-pain biology. *Neuron* 2009;64:46–54.

13. Boyle DL, Jones TL, Hammaker D et al. Regulation of peripheral inflammation by spinal p38 MAP kinase in rats. *PLoS Med* 2006;3:e338.

14. Boettger MK, Weber K, Grossmann D et al. Spinal tumor necrosis factor alpha neutralization reduces peripheral inflammation and hyperalgesia and suppresses autonomic responses in experimental arthritis: a role for spinal tumor necrosis factor alpha during induction and maintenance of peripheral inflammation. *Arthritis Rheum* 2010;62:1308–1318.

15. Willis WD Jr. Dorsal root potentials and dorsal root reflexes: a double-edged sword. *Exp Brain Res* 1999;124:395–421.

16. Laye S, Bluthe RM, Kent S et al. Subdiaphragmatic vagotomy blocks induction of IL-1 beta mRNA in mice brain in response to peripheral LPS. *Am J Physiol* 1995;268:R1327–R1331.

17. Goshen I, Yirmiya R. Interleukin-1 (IL-1): a central regulator of stress responses. *Front Neuroendocrinol* 2009;30:30–45.

CHAPTER 60

Pathogenesis of juvenile idiopathic arthritis

David Bending, Kiran Nistala,
and Lucy R. Wedderburn

Introduction

Juvenile idiopathic arthritis (JIA) is the most prevalent form of the chronic rheumatological diseases affecting children. The hallmark of the disease is inflamed synovium, which is thickened, hypervascular, and contains a dense inflammatory infiltrate, of which T cells are typically the most abundant cell type. JIA itself is not one condition (see Chapter 114) but represents a spectrum of conditions with differing degrees of overlap and phenotypes.[1] It is thus unsurprising that the pathogenesis of JIA differs according to subtype, but central themes do emerge—in particular a critical role for the immune system in disease pathogenesis. This chapter therefore seeks to underline common pathological mechanisms involved in disease pathogenesis in JIA, but also extends its reach to highlight subset-specific pathologies where these are thought to be of importance to disease understanding.

Principles in understanding pathogenesis of childhood arthritis

An important principle to understand is that the clinical criteria used to classify JIA into its different subsets (see Chapter 114) may blur the identification of common, underlying pathological mechanisms; in particular, the classification based on the number of joints affected could suggest that such subsets have fundamentally differing pathological mechanisms, when in fact they may have many common features but differ merely in severity (e.g. anti-nuclear antibody positive (ANA+) forms of oligoarticular-(o)-JIA and rheumatoid factor negative (RF−) polyarticular (poly)-JIA.[2]).

Most methods to analyse the pathogenesis of JIA, such as immunological and gene expression profiling, have segregated conditions using criteria that are employed for classification of JIA such as the number of joints affected and/or the presence/absence of psoriasis. However alternative analyses, such as the criteria of the age of onset,[3] may better correlate with gene expression profiles in the peripheral blood of patients than the number of joints affected.[4] Where such data exist, these will be referred to, and their relevance to helping our understanding of JIA discussed.

One subgroup, systemic JIA (sJIA), however, does appear to have a distinct pathogenesis in that it resembles an autoinflammatory-like disorder with central roles for the innate immune system.[5] In particular the cytokines IL-1β, IL-6, and IL-18 are implicated in the pathogenesis of sJIA[5] (see 'Systemic juvenile idiopathic arthritis—a special case of innate dysregulation?'). o-JIA and poly-JIA, on the other hand, are thought to be T-cell-mediated autoimmune conditions, with a key part played by the adaptive immune system, and as will be discussed their pathogenesis is linked to the interplay between T effectors (Teff) and T regulatory (Treg) cells.[6] In this chapter, therefore, we analyse central pathological themes involving the adaptive and innate immune systems and, where appropriate, refer to subset-specific mechanisms of disease. Since o-JIA and poly-JIA account for most cases of JIA, we first address the involvement of the adaptive immune system in these forms of JIA.

Adaptive immune system involvement in the pathogenesis of non-systemic juvenile idiopathic arthritis

It is thought that the autoreactive response in children who develop JIA is initiated by the activation of T and/or B cells. For instance, data from many association studies, recently confirmed by genome-wide association studies, have identified that there exist subtype-specific HLA associations (see Chapter 43),[7] which supports the involvement of the adaptive immune system in disease progression. In particular, the strongest associations exist with alleles at the *HLA DRB1* locus, which codes for the β chain of MHC class II molecules, whose central role is the presentation of peptide antigens to CD4+ T cells. As well as distinct subtype-specific genetic associations, several studies have also shown an age-specific risk conferred by particular *HLA* alleles and haplotypes. For example the *HLA DRB1*1103/*1104* allele, which is strongly associated with o-JIA, is also a risk factor for other clinical types on JIA in younger children (onset <6 years) but not older children.[8] In addition to *HLA* genes, single nucleotide polymorphisms (SNPs) in genes involved in T-cell activation, such as the tyrosine phosphatase *PTPN22*,[9] or T-cell regulation (i.e. the α chain of the IL-2 receptor (CD25),[10] a molecule that is crucially important for Treg), have been reported to be associated, suggesting that T-cell dysregulation is a likely factor in the pathogenesis of JIA. Furthermore, data from mouse models also give insight into this notion: mice with a genetically altered threshold for T-cell activation due to a mutation in the *ZAP70* gene (important for transducing TCR signals) go on to develop arthritis spontaneously[11]; and additionally, T-cell self-reactivity can create a cytokine milieu that can drive the spontaneous development of pathogenic T cells, which can mediate autoimmune arthritis.[12]

What triggers this self-reaction is not clear; however, research from mouse models has suggested that gut-residing bacteria may have a role to play in the generation of Th17 cells that target the joint,[13] and, intriguingly, that self-antigen recognition may not always be necessary for the development of arthritis—local joint injury in mice, such as microbleeding, can lead to an IL-6- and IL-17A-dependent arthritis in the absence of tissue antigen recognition in a genetically prone mouse strain.[14]

B cells are thought to play less prominent roles in the progression of JIA than T cells, but recent data have suggested that their involvement may be underappreciated since an early B cell signature can identify early-onset arthritis independent of the number of joints affected.[3] Autoimmune B cells, or mature plasma cells, are the source of the ANA autoantibody, a risk factor for the complication of uveitis in JIA, although the direct pathogenic role of ANA antibodies remains unproven. One potential function of B cells in contributing to pathogenesis[15] is not their capability to produce autoreactive antibody but to act as antigen-presenting cells (APC) and prime Th1 cell development. It is this Teff development, and immune regulation[6] that appear to be highly influential factors in dictating the outcome of disease progression in non-systemic forms of JIA.

T-cell roles in the pathogenesis of juvenile idiopathic arthritis

As already stated, T cells are thought to play essential roles in non-systemic forms of JIA. In the following section, the relative contribution of Teffs, which are thought to mediate damage, and their interplay with Treg, which act to restrain inflammation, is discussed. The issues of Teff resistance to regulation and Treg function and stability at sites of inflammation will be discussed to generate a conceptual framework in order to help understand disease progression in the joint.

Effector T cells

In the majority of cases of JIA, CD3+ T cells constitute the major population in synovial fluid mononuclear cell (SFMC) compartments. These are almost exclusively of the CD45RO+, highly activated 'memory' population.[16] Of the CD4+ Th cells, both Th1 and Th17 populations have been observed and both are enriched compared to the peripheral blood compartment, with a relative abundance of interferon (IFN)γ+ Th1 cells.[16,17] Despite the high prevalence of IFNγ+ T cells, blockade of IFNγ has not proven beneficial in mouse models or clinical trials in adult inflammatory arthritis. However, it is known that both Th1 and Th17 cells can also make TNFα, and blockade of this cytokine, using biologics, has shown excellent therapeutic benefit.[18]

IL-17A, the signature cytokine of Th17 cells, which are enriched in the joints of o-JIA patients,[17] is increased in synovial fluid[19] and in-vitro modelling has shown that it can drive the production of IL-6, IL-8, and matrix metalloproteinases (MMPs) from synovial fluid fibroblasts,[19] demonstrating that IL-17A can induce many of the immunopathological features of arthritis.

Both Th1 and Th17 cells may become enriched in the joints by a variety of mechanisms. Preferential recruitment of Th1 cells may be an important factor, in part via recruitment mediated by the receptors CCR5 and CXCR3,[16] as, interestingly, individuals expressing a mutant form of CCR5 (CCR5d32) show relative protection from JIA development.[20] Th17 recruitment may occur in response to tissue injury, such as microbleeding,[14] leading to the upregulation of CCL20 and recruitment of CCR6-expressing Th17 cells.[17] In comparison between mild o-JIA (known as persistent o-JIA), and the more severe extended form, the enrichment of Th17 cells is significantly higher in extended o-JIA.[17] Th1 cells may also be enriched due to Th17 conversion to Th1 in the joint,[21] which may be driven by the abundance of IL-12 and absence of TGFα in the synovial fluid environment.[21] This 'functional plasticity' may mask the apparent importance of Th17 cells in disease progression. Supporting this claim is that, in the remitting form of o-JIA (known as persistent o-JIA), a higher turnover of Teffs in the synovial fluid compared to peripheral blood compartment is observed,[22] suggesting constant recruitment and turnover at the inflammatory sites. Many 'snapshot in time' analyses, therefore, are unlikely to reveal the highly dynamic nature of T-cell behaviour in the joints.

For CD8+ T cells, these cells may have an increased importance in the o-JIA subset, since the CD4:CD8 ratio has predictive power in determining the likelihood that children may go on to develop more severe disease.[23] It has been hypothesized that levels of a CD8+ T cell chemo-attractant, CCL5 (RANTES), may be important in recruiting CD8+ T cells to the joints in children who go on to develop extended o-JIA.[23] CCL5 is known to be high in synovial fluid, and is produced by the synovial CD8+ T cells in high amounts compared to peripheral blood CD8 T cells, creating a positive feedback loop.[24]

As well as the production of cytokines and chemokines, activated T cells in the synovium alter the balance of bone deposition and breakdown in neighbouring bone, through the high production of osteoclast-activating factors such as RANKL (a member of the TNF family),[25] and osteopontin,[26] which contribute to local osteoporosis typically seen around actively inflamed joints.

Teff pathology, however, does not go unchecked, and as well as an enrichment of effector cells, FOXP3-expressing Tregs are also enriched in the joints of patients.[17,27,28] In fact, the ratios of Teffs to Tregs may be an important feature in dictating the outcome of the disease process.[17] The next section, therefore, discusses the crucial role that Tregs play in the control of disease pathogenesis.

Regulatory T cells

Since Tregs are also enriched at the sites of inflammation when compared to peripheral blood,[27] it seems plausible that active attempts are made by the immune system to regulate the inflammatory response. In keeping with the importance of regulation in affecting disease outcome, associations with the *IL10* gene itself[29] and IL-10-regulated genes have been made.[4] Both the nature and number of Tregs appear important: in the o-JIA form of disease, preferential recognition of the self-antigens hsp60 and dnaJ by Tregs correlates with the milder form of disease,[30] and an enhanced frequency of Tregs is observed in the synovial compartment of patients with remitting o-JIA compared to those with the more severe extended o-JIA.[17,27] The set-point for regulation may be an opportunity for therapeutic intervention, since patients treated with autologous transplantation displayed increased proportions of Tregs after the procedure.[31]

The increased proportion of Tregs at the sites of inflammation may at first seem paradoxical. This has led to the question of whether Tregs are suboptimal or subfunctional in patients with JIA; on the other hand, Teffs themselves may become less susceptible to regulation due to the inflammatory milieu in the joint. It is the nature of the Treg–Teff interaction that will determine the outcome of disease progression, and it is likely that both extrinsic factors (environment, i.e. cytokine milieu) as well as intrinsic factors (e.g. genetic factors—see Chapter 43) have roles to play.

Teff resistance vs Treg stability and functionality

The programme of synovial fluid Tregs is thought to be as stable as that of peripheral blood Tregs, since epigenetic analysis of the Treg-specific demethylated region in these cells has shown that both types display demethylation at this locus—a hallmark that is associated with stable FOXP3 expression.[32] In addition, work in mice using genetic fate-tracking technology has documented that Tregs maintain stability in inflammatory environments,[33] although such work has not been rigorously assessed in humans (in part because FOXP3, the accepted marker of Tregs, can be promiscuously upregulated in Teffs following their activation).

Although there is still some debate as to whether Treg stability may be an issue in inflammatory environments, the in-vitro functionality of Tregs isolated from the site of inflammation has been assessed. Using Treg suppression assays, the suppressive nature of synovial fluid Tregs has been compared to Tregs isolated from the blood of patients. When these in-vitro assays have been conducted (and similar findings have been demonstrated in animal models of type 1 diabetes[34]), synovial fluid Tregs have been equally suppressive[32] as peripheral blood Tregs (possibly more so[28]); however, neither set of Tregs have been effective in suppressing the proliferation of Teffs that were isolated from synovial fluid.[32] This suggests that the defect might not lie in the biology of Tregs but in the biology that controls the resistance of Teffs to suppression.

Very recently, some insight into the biology of what may drive the resistance of Teffs to regulation has been gained. Studies of Teffs isolated from synovial fluid have shown that activation of the PKB/AKT pathway in Teffs, in part due to inflammatory signals like IL-6 and TNFα, confers resistance of Teffs to TGFα-mediated inhibition of proliferation.[32] Although questions remain as to whether this represents a disease-specific phenomenon, or whether Teffs acquire resistance to regulation as part of their differentiation during chronic immune responses, there is no doubt that this is an intriguing area of research with the potential to open up new therapeutic strategies. It is highly likely, therefore, that the tuning of the biology of Teffs at the sites of inflammation will now become an area of intense investigation.

B cells

Although autoantibodies are common in many types of JIA (although in sJIA there is notable absence of specific autoantibody production), in particular ANA, the presence of mature germinal centres in the inflamed synovia in JIA is rare compared to rheumatoid arthritis patients.[35] Although the pathogenic role of the ANA antibody is unclear, it remains a valuable clinical tool in indicating

risk for autoimmune uveitis.[36] For example in one study of 426 cases of recently diagnosed JIA,[36] uveitis was detected in 24.5% of cases; ANA was present in 66% of patients with uveitis compared to 37% of patients without uveitis (p<0.001). The ANA has also been proposed as a useful biomarker for a homogeneous phenotype of childhood arthritis, namely young-onset disease with risk of uveitis.[2]

One interesting publication has reported that early-onset disease (irrespective of the number of joints affected) had a distinct gene expression signature indicative of immature B cells in the blood of patients.[3] This gene expression profile may be linked to the enrichment of transitional B cells seen in the blood of JIA patients when compared to age-matched controls.[35]

B cells can also function as APC, and it has been reported that activated B cells within the joint, displaying high levels of costimulatory molecules CD80/CD86, may be important in the priming of Th1 responses.[35] Interestingly, an expansion of B cells within the joint has been linked with increased risk of disease extension in oligoarticular forms of JIA.[23]

Innate immune system in the pathogenesis of juvenile idiopathic arthritis

Successful treatments with biologics have implicated innate cytokines in the pathogenesis of JIA—particularly in sJIA, where innate cell dysregulation is thought to be a key factor in disease progression (see 'Systemic JIA—a special case of innate dysregulation?'). It should also be appreciated that the innate immune system is likely to be party to all the immunological events in JIA (Figure 60.1)—e.g. antigen presentation to autoreactive T cells, monocyte infiltration in response to T-cell infiltration, the induction of matrix remodelling and joint erosion, activation of endothelia, and the induction of angiogenesis.

In fact, the activation of cells of the innate immune system and stroma likely contributes many aspects that lead to the clinical symptoms of JIA. Cytokine production and chemokine production drive inflammation and cell recruitment; cytokines may act to induce the production of tissue remodelling enzymes like MMP-1 and MMP-3, leading to tissue destruction; vascular endothelial growth factor (VEGF) production by monocytes and macrophages will drive angiogenesis; and inflammatory mediators will activate endothelia leading to the further recruitment of immune cells, contributing to joint swelling and pain. Targeting innate immune pathways has proven successful, and therefore the contribution of this arm of the immune response to disease pathogenesis will be discussed. Given its unique innate immune system signatures, a separate section is devoted to sJIA.

Monocytes

Whilst proportions are similar between synovial fluid and peripheral blood compartments, these cells are much more highly activated in SF.[23] They can secrete a vast array of cytokines, such as IL-6, IL-1β, and TNFα,[37] and chemokines, such as CCL5, CCL20, IL-8, MCP-1, and CXCL10. Joint hypoxia has been shown to induce CCL20 production from monocytes,[38] which may contribute to the recruitment of CCR6+ Th17 cells.

In o-JIA, a distinct IFNγ signature is present in the monocyte population,[23] which is more severe in those children who go on to develop extended disease. IFNγ can also drive production of

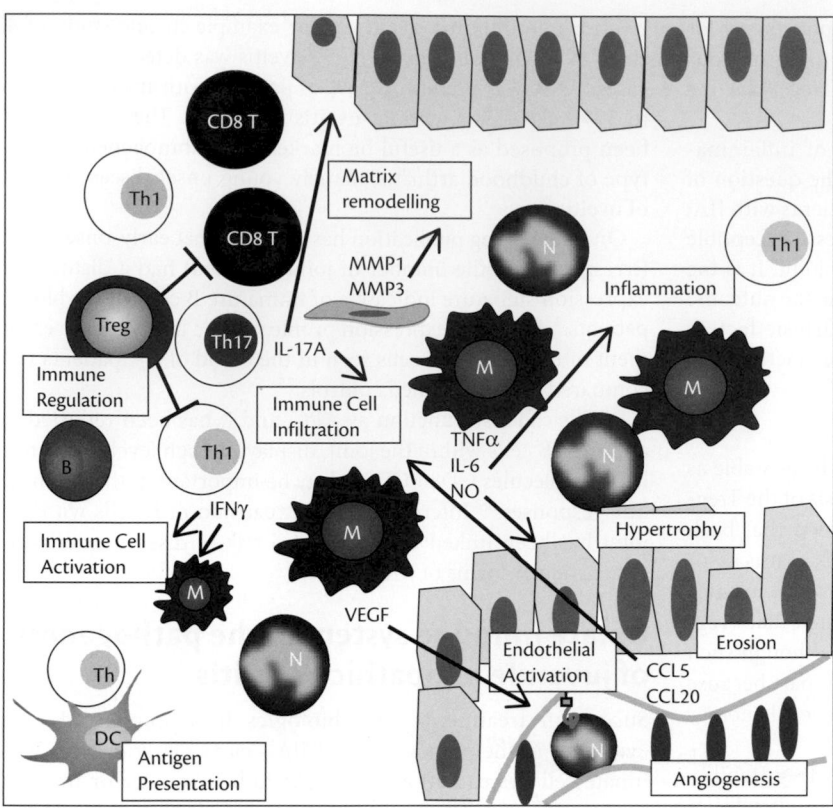

Fig. 60.1 Immune cell involvement in the joints of children with JIA. Cells from all arms of the immune system are involved in the pathogenesis of JIA. B, B cell; DC, dendritic cell; M, monocyte; MMP, matrix metalloproteinase; N, neutrophil; NO, nitric oxide; VEGF, vascular endothelial growth factor.

reactive oxygen species, such as nitric oxide (NO)—and in the joint this is likely to be immune-cell derived since NO production correlates with lymphomononuclear cell frequency.[39] Reactive oxygen species will have direct effects on the stroma and synovium, which in response may produce cytokines and MMP, thus setting in motion an amplification loop of inflammation and tissue destruction. In addition, innate or stromal cytokine production may create a cytokine environment that renders Teffs resistant to regulation,[32] potentiating inflammation.

Neutrophils

Highly elevated levels of myeloid reactive protein (MRP)8/14, secreted by activated monoctyes and neutrophils, are present in sJIA patients,[40] and very elevated MRP levels in synovial fluid are also typical of o-JIA and poly-JIA, where they correlate with disease activity. Such augmented levels of proteins can induce IL-17 production from CD8+ T cells,[41] illustrating how disrupted innate immunity can lead to dysregulated adaptive immunity. MRP8/14 is also elevated in serum of all subtypes of JIA compared to controls, although at lower levels than in the synovium, and serum levels of this protein complex, measured prior to withdrawal of treatment in children who achieve apparent remission, can be used to predict those who are at high risk of flare after drug withdrawal.[42]

Examination of the gene expression patterns of neutrophils between patient and control blood found over 700 genes to be differentially expressed, with gene families linked to IL-8 and IFNγ being prominent amongst them.[43] Interestingly, these gene levels did not revert back to baseline levels after clinical remission, suggesting that remission in patients reflected a state of immunological rebalancing, and not a return to normality.

Systemic juvenile idiopathic arthritis—a special case of innate dysregulation?

Systemic-onset JIA presents with overproduction of IL-1, IL-6, and IL-18. Given the absence of autoantibody and (as yet) no current HLA associations, this strongly suggests that sJIA is a disease of innate dysregulation.[44]

Features of this disease are high serum levels of IL-6[45] and augmented IL-1β—activation of patient peripheral mononuclear blood cells (PBMCs) leads to a release of a large amount of this cytokine.[46] Additionally, IL-18 levels are chronically elevated, which is thought to explain the defect in NK cell cytotoxicity[47] found in this subtype of JIA.

Serum levels of MRP8 and MRP14 are very high in sJIA, and the MRP8/14 complex has recently been shown to be a sensitive indicator of disease activity and likelihood of disease relapse.[48] It is thought that MRP8/14 may drive IL-1β levels, since removal of this complex almost completely attenuates the potential of sJIA serum to induce IL-1β[40]; however, the primacy of IL-1β to disease pathogenesis has been questioned since only one-half of patients respond to blockade of the IL-1β pathway,[49] and this is thought to reflect heterogeneity in the pathological mechanisms driving disease in the group currently classified as sJIA. Disrupting IL-6 with a soluble IL-6 receptor (tocilizumab), on the other hand, has proven much more successful,[50] and given that IL-6 expression is likely to be upregulated by (amongst others) IL-1β, it may act as the final common pathway for inflammation.

Macrophage populations have been analysed and both classical highly inflammatory ('M1 type') and alternatively activated ('M2 type'; in some environments more anti-inflammatory) phenotypes are apparent at the single-cell level.[51] Analyses during inactive

Table 60.1 Subset-specific pathologies

Subtype	General	Innate defects	Adaptive defects
sJIA	Predominantly an innate immune disorder	High levels IL-1b, IL-6, and IL-18 Response to IL-1b can segregate into two groups[49] Individuals with fewer joints affected and higher neutrophil count respond better to IL-1b disruption; MAS	Possible alteration of T-cell subsets[58]
o-JIA	T-cell-driven disease; disease severity dictated by Treg–Teff balance	IFNγ signature in monocyte population in individuals who go on to extend[23] Increased CCL5 in extended-to-be group[23]	Severity of disease correlates with Th17:Treg ratio[17] Higher proportion of CD30+ HSP-specific Tregs favours milder disease[53] Genetic associations differ between mild and severe forms (e.g. MHC alleles at HLA-DRB1 locus[7]; IL-10[29]) Teffs in joint are resistant to suppression[32] CD4:CD8 ratio can be predictive of disease extension[23]
RF+ poly-JIA	More analogous to Rheumatoid arthritis		Shares genetic associations at HLA locus with rheumatoid arthritis, *HLA-DRB1*0101* and *0401*[7]; Antibodies detected against cyclic citrullinated peptides—may be pathological under conditions of low-grade joint inflammation
RF−poly-JIA	Gene expression analysis suggests several separate signatures in patients; ANA+ Poly-JIA may represent a more severe form of o-JIA	A monocyte-related gene signature subset[54] An immediate early genes associated subset [54]; Increased pDC subset [54]	Subset has reduced CD8+ T cells and increased pDC[54]; ANA+ poly-JIA does not fit into one of the three subset signatures[54] and may represent a more severe form of ANA+ o-JIA, as these two cluster together upon expression analysis[2]
ERA/psoriatic arthritis	Some features clinically and genetically shared with adult AS	ERA is associated with inflammatory bowel disorder; MMP-3 serum level correlates with disease activity[55] Membrane TLRs are overexpressed in PB- and SF-MCs, resulting in raised IL-6 and IL-8 production upon TLR ligation[56]	*HLA B27* association—misfolding of molecule in the context of microbial antigens can drive IL-23 production and promote Th17 response[57]; other genes coding for proteins crucial to ER function are also associated, such as ERAP

ANA, anti-nuclear antibody; AS, ankylosing spondylitis; DC, dendritic cell; ERA, enthesitis-related arthritis; ERAP, endoplasmic reticulum-associated peptidase; ER, endoplasmic reticulum; HLA, human leukocyte antigen; HSP, heat-shock protein; IL, interleukin; MAS, macrophage activation syndrome MC, mononuclear cells; MHC, major histocompatiblity complex; MMP, matrix metalloproteinases; o-JIA, oligo-articular juvenile idiopathic arthritis; pDC, plasmacytoid DC; RF, rheumatoid factor; SF, synovial fluid; TLR, toll-like receptor.

phases of disease have lead some authors to conclude that this is due to the manifestation of 'compensated inflammation'.[51]

A pathological feature of sJIA is macrophage activation syndrome (MAS). This potentially life-threatening condition arises as a result of activation of T cells and haemophagocytic macrophages. These macrophages express CD163, a scavenger receptor, which recognizes haptoglobin–haemoglobin complexes. Increased uptake of such complexes can leads to production of ferritin by macrophages, thus providing an explanation for the hyperferritinaemia associated with MAS. In keeping with the phenotype, CD25 and soluble CD163 have been identified as potential biomarkers of this condition.[52] The causes of MAS are unknown; however, defects in genes associated with cell-mediated cytotoxicity, such as the perforin gene and genes involved in its secretory pathway (e.g. *MUNC13-4*), have been associated with some studies in JIA, but not in others.

Subset-specific pathologies

The previous sections have aimed to bring together common pathogenic mechanisms, but each subset has its own specific pathologies; for ease of reference, these are listed in Table 60.1.

Conclusion

In essence, the pathogenesis of JIA is the direct result of disrupted immune regulation, with both genetic (Chapter 43) and environmental factors influencing the course of disease. The major immunopathological distinction in JIA is between the sJIA form, which is thought to represent a disorder of dysregulated innate immunity, and the o-JIA and poly-JIA forms, where the balance between Teffs and Tregs is crucial to disease outcome. It is likely that future research will seek to better understand mechanisms of immune regulation at the sites of inflammation, and how and why these mechanisms may fail to bring about immune homeostasis in the joints of children with JIA. This new information will help identify novel pathways for therapeutic intervention, as well as identify subset-specific biomarkers of disease.

References

1. Petty RE, Southwood TR, Manners P et al. International League of Associations for Rheumatology classification of juvenile idiopathic arthritis: second revision, Edmonton, 2001. *J Rheumatol* 2004;31:390–392.
2. Ravelli A, Felici E, Magni-Manzoni S et al. Patients with antinuclear antibody-positive juvenile idiopathic arthritis constitute a homogeneous

subgroup irrespective of the course of joint disease. *Arthritis Rheum* 2005;52:826–832.

3. Barnes MG, Grom AA, Thompson SD et al. Biologic similarities based on age at onset in oligoarticular and polyarticular subtypes of juvenile idiopathic arthritis. *Arthritis Rheum* 2010;62:3249–3258.

4. Barnes MG, Grom AA, Thompson SD, et al. Subtype-specific peripheral blood gene expression profiles in recent-onset juvenile idiopathic arthritis. *Arthritis Rheum* 2009;60:2102–2112.

5. Mellins ED, Macaubas C, Grom AA. Pathogenesis of systemic juvenile idiopathic arthritis: some answers, more questions. *Nat Rev Rheumatol* 2011;7:416–426.

6. Nistala K, Wedderburn LR. Th17 and regulatory T cells: rebalancing pro- and anti-inflammatory forces in autoimmune arthritis. *Rheumatology (Oxford)* 2009;48:602–606.

7. Thomson W Barrett JH, Donn R et al. Juvenile idiopathic arthritis classified by the ILAR criteria: HLA associations in UK patients. *Rheumatology (Oxford)* 2002;41:1183–1189.

8. Hollenbach JA, Thompson SD, Bugawan TL, et al. Juvenile idiopathic arthritis and HLA class I and class II interactions and age-at-onset effects. *Arthritis Rheum* 2010;62:1781–1791.

9. Hinks A Barton A John S et al. Association between the PTPN22 gene and rheumatoid arthritis and juvenile idiopathic arthritis in a UK population: further support that PTPN22 is an autoimmunity gene. *Arthritis Rheum* 2005;52:1694–1699.

10. Hinks A, Ke X, Barton A et al. Association of the IL2RA/CD25 gene with juvenile idiopathic arthritis. *Arthritis Rheum* 2009;60:251–257.

11. Sakaguchi N, Takahashi T, Hata H et al. Altered thymic T-cell selection due to a mutation of the ZAP-70 gene causes autoimmune arthritis in mice. *Nature* 2003;426:454–460.

12. Hirota K, Hashimoto M, Yoshitomi H et al. T cell self-reactivity forms a cytokine milieu for spontaneous development of IL-17+ Th cells that cause autoimmune arthritis. *J Exp Med* 2007;204:41–47.

13. Wu HJ, Ivanov II, Darce J et al. Gut-residing segmented filamentous bacteria drive autoimmune arthritis via T helper 17 cells. *Immunity* 2010;32:815–827.

14. Murakami M, Okuyama Y, Ogura H et al. Local microbleeding facilitates IL-6- and IL-17-dependent arthritis in the absence of tissue antigen recognition by activated T cells. *J Exp Med* 2011;208:103–114.

15. Morbach H, Wiegering V, Richl P et al. Activated memory B cells may function as antigen-presenting cells in the joints of children with juvenile idiopathic arthritis. *Arthritis Rheum* 2011;63:3458–3466.

16. Wedderburn LR, Robinson N, Patel A, Varsani H, Woo P. Selective recruitment of polarized T cells expressing CCR5 and CXCR3 to the inflamed joints of children with juvenile idiopathic arthritis. *Arthritis Rheum* 2000;43:765–774.

17. Nistala K, Moncrieffe H, Newton KR et al. Interleukin-17-producing T cells are enriched in the joints of children with arthritis, but have a reciprocal relationship to regulatory T cell numbers. *Arthritis Rheum* 2008;58:875–887.

18. Lovell DJ, Giannini EH, Reiff A et al. Etanercept in children with polyarticular juvenile rheumatoid arthritis. Pediatric Rheumatology Collaborative Study Group. *N Engl J Med* 2000;342:763–769.

19. Agarwal S, Misra R, Aggarwal A. Interleukin 17 levels are increased in juvenile idiopathic arthritis synovial fluid and induce synovial fibroblasts to produce proinflammatory cytokines and matrix metalloproteinases. *J Rheumatol* 2008;35:515–519.

20. Hinks A, Martin P, Flynn E et al. Association of the CCR5 gene with juvenile idiopathic arthritis. *Genes Immun* 2010;11:584–589.

21. Nistala K, Adams S, Cambrook H et al. Th17 plasticity in human autoimmune arthritis is driven by the inflammatory environment. *Proc Natl Acad Sci U S A* 2010;107:14751–14756.

22. Brunner J, Herrmann M, Metzler M et al. The turnover of synovial T cells is higher than in T cells in the peripheral blood in persistent oligoarticular juvenile idiopathic arthritis. *Rheumatol Int* 2010;30: 1529–1532.

23. Hunter PJ, Nistala K, Jina N et al. Biologic predictors of extension of oligoarticular juvenile idiopathic arthritis as determined from synovial fluid cellular composition and gene expression. *Arthritis Rheum* 2010;62:896–907.

24. Pharoah DS, Varsani H Tatham RW et al. Expression of the inflammatory chemokines CCL5, CCL3 and CXCL10 in juvenile idiopathic arthritis, and demonstration of CCL5 production by an atypical subset of CD8+ T cells. *Arthritis Res Ther* 2006;8:R50.

25. Varsani H, Patel A, van Kooyk Y, Woo P, Wedderburn LR. Synovial dendritic cells in juvenile idiopathic arthritis (JIA) express receptor activator of NF-kappaB (RANK). *Rheumatology (Oxford)* 2003;42:583–590.

26. Gattorno M, Gregorio A, Ferlito F et al. Synovial expression of osteopontin correlates with angiogenesis in juvenile idiopathic arthritis. *Rheumatology (Oxford)* 2004;43:1091–1096.

27. de Kleer IM, Wedderburn LR, Taams LS et al. CD4+CD25bright regulatory T cells actively regulate inflammation in the joints of patients with the remitting form of juvenile idiopathic arthritis. *J Immunol* 2004;172:6435–6443.

28. Ruprecht CR, Gattorno M, Ferlito F et al. Coexpression of CD25 and CD27 identifies FoxP3+ regulatory T cells in inflamed synovia. *J Exp Med* 2005;201:1793–1803.

29. Crawley E, Kay R, Sillibourne J et al. Polymorphic haplotypes of the interleukin-10 5′ flanking region determine variable interleukin-10 transcription and are associated with particular phenotypes of juvenile rheumatoid arthritis. *Arthritis Rheum* 1999;42:1101–1108.

30. Massa M Passalia M Manzoni SM, et al. Differential recognition of heat-shock protein dnaJ-derived epitopes by effector and Treg cells leads to modulation of inflammation in juvenile idiopathic arthritis. *Arthritis Rheum* 2007;56:1648–1657.

31. de Kleer I, Vastert B, Klein M et al. Autologous stem cell transplantation for autoimmunity induces immunologic self-tolerance by reprogramming autoreactive T cells and restoring the CD4+CD25+ immune regulatory network. *Blood* 2006;107:1696–1702.

32. Wehrens EJ, Mijnheer G, Duurland CL et al. Functional human regulatory T cells fail to control autoimmune inflammation due to PKB/c-akt hyperactivation in effector cells. *Blood* 2011;118:3538–3548.

33. Rubtsov YP, Niec RE, Josefowicz S et al. Stability of the regulatory T cell lineage in vivo. *Science* 2010;329:1667–1671.

34. D'Alise AM, Auyeung V, Feuerer M et al. The defect in T-cell regulation in NOD mice is an effect on the T-cell effectors. *Proc Natl Acad Sci U S A* 2008;105:19857–19862.

35. Corcione A, Ferlito F, Gattorno M et al. Phenotypic and functional characterization of switch memory B cells from patients with oligoarticular juvenile idiopathic arthritis. *Arthritis Res Ther* 2009;11:R150.

36. Kotaniemi K, Kautiainen H, Karma A, Aho K. Occurrence of uveitis in recently diagnosed juvenile chronic arthritis: a prospective study. *Ophthalmology* 2001;108:2071–2075.

37. Saxena N, Aggarwal A, Misra, R. Elevated concentrations of monocyte derived cytokines in synovial fluid of children with enthesitis related arthritis and polyarticular types of juvenile idiopathic arthritis. *J Rheumatol* 2005;32:1349–1353.

38. Bosco MC, Delfino S, Ferlito F et al. Hypoxic synovial environment and expression of macrophage inflammatory protein 3gamma/CCL20 in juvenile idiopathic arthritis. *Arthritis Rheum* 2008;58:1833–1838.

39. Lotito AP, Muscara MN, Kiss MH, et al. Nitric oxide-derived species in synovial fluid from patients with juvenile idiopathic arthritis. *J Rheumatol* 2004;31:992–997.

40. Frosch M, Ahlmann M, Vogl T et al. The myeloid-related proteins 8 and 14 complex, a novel ligand of toll-like receptor 4, and interleukin-1beta form a positive feedback mechanism in systemic-onset juvenile idiopathic arthritis. *Arthritis Rheum* 2009;60:883–891.

41. Loser K, Vogl T, Voskort M et al. The Toll-like receptor 4 ligands Mrp8 and Mrp14 are crucial in the development of autoreactive CD8+ T cells. *Nat Med* 2010;16:713–717.

42. Foell D, Wulffraat N, Wedderburn LR et al. Methotrexate withdrawal at 6 vs 12 months in juvenile idiopathic arthritis in remission: a randomized clinical trial. *JAMA* 2010;303:1266–1273.

43. Jarvis JN, Petty HR, Tang Y et al. Evidence for chronic, peripheral activation of neutrophils in polyarticular juvenile rheumatoid arthritis. *Arthritis Res Ther* 2006;8:R154.

44. Macaubas C, Nguyen K, Deshpande C et al. Distribution of circulating cells in systemic juvenile idiopathic arthritis across disease activity states. *Clin Immunol* 2010;134:206–216.

45. de Benedetti F, Massa M, Robbioni P et al. Correlation of serum interleukin-6 levels with joint involvement and thrombocytosis in systemic juvenile rheumatoid arthritis. *Arthritis Rheum* 1991;34:1158–1163.

46. Pascual V, Allantaz F, Arce E, Punaro M, Banchereau, J. Role of interleukin-1 (IL-1) in the pathogenesis of systemic onset juvenile idiopathic arthritis and clinical response to IL-1 blockade. *J Exp Med* 2005;201:1479–1486.

47. Grom AA, Villanueva J, Lee S et al. Natural killer cell dysfunction in patients with systemic-onset juvenile rheumatoid arthritis and macrophage activation syndrome. *J Pediatr* 2003;142:292–296.

48. Holzinger D, Frosch M, Kastrup A et al. The Toll-like receptor 4 agonist MRP8/14 protein complex is a sensitive indicator for disease activity and predicts relapses in systemic-onset juvenile idiopathic arthritis. *Ann Rheum Dis* 2012;71:974–980.

49. Gattorno M, Piccini A, Lasiglie D et al. The pattern of response to anti-interleukin-1 treatment distinguishes two subsets of patients with systemic-onset juvenile idiopathic arthritis. *Arthritis Rheum* 2008;58:1505–1515.

50. Yokota S, Imagawa T, Mori M et al. Efficacy and safety of tocilizumab in patients with systemic-onset juvenile idiopathic arthritis: a randomised, double-blind, placebo-controlled, withdrawal phase III trial. *Lancet* 2008;371:998–1006.

51. Macaubas C, Nguyen KD, Peck A et al. Alternative activation in systemic juvenile idiopathic arthritis monocytes. *Clin Immunol* 2012;142:362–372.

52. Bleesing J, Prada A, Siegel DM, et al. The diagnostic significance of soluble CD163 and soluble interleukin-2 receptor alpha-chain in macrophage activation syndrome and untreated new-onset systemic juvenile idiopathic arthritis. *Arthritis Rheum* 2007;56:965–971.

53. de Kleer IM, Kamphuis SM, Rijkers GT et al. The spontaneous remission of juvenile idiopathic arthritis is characterized by CD30+ T cells directed to human heat-shock protein 60 capable of producing the regulatory cytokine interleukin-10. *Arthritis Rheum* 2003;48:2001–2010.

54. Griffin TA, Barnes MG, Ilowite NT et al. Gene expression signatures in polyarticular juvenile idiopathic arthritis demonstrate disease heterogeneity and offer a molecular classification of disease subsets. *Arthritis Rheum* 2009;60:2113–2123.

55. Viswanath V, Myles A, Dayal R, Aggarwal A. Levels of serum matrix metalloproteinase-3 correlate with disease activity in the enthesitis-related arthritis category of juvenile idiopathic arthritis. *J Rheumatol* 2011;38:2482–2487.

56. Myles A, Rahman MT, Aggarwal A. Membrane-bound Toll-like receptors are overexpressed in peripheral blood and synovial fluid mononuclear cells of enthesitis-related arthritis category of juvenile idiopathic arthritis (JIA-ERA) patients and lead to secretion of inflammatory mediators. *J Clin Immunol* 2012;32(3):488–496.

57. Goodall JC, Wu C, Zhang Y et al. Endoplasmic reticulum stress-induced transcription factor, CHOP, is crucial for dendritic cell IL-23 expression. *Proc Natl Acad Sci U S A* 2010;107:17698–17703.

58. Omoyinmi E, Hamaoui R, Pesenacker A et al. Th1 and Th17 cell subpopulations are enriched in the peripheral blood of patients with systemic juvenile idiopathic arthritis. *Rheumatology (Oxford)* 2012;51:1881–1886.

Practical investigation of rheumatic disease

CHAPTER 61

Haematology

Patrick Kesteven

Introduction

A wide variety of haematological abnormalities may be found in patients with diverse rheumatic disorders. These are summarized in Box 61.1.

Anaemia

Some degree of anaemia is found frequently in any active rheumatoid condition. In the majority of cases this will be the anaemia of chronic disease (ACD), which may mask the many other, rarer, anaemias associated with these conditions. Diagnosing these requires a thorough understanding of ACD as well as maintaining a healthy level of suspicion should the patient's full blood count parameters not reflect the underlying clinical picture.

Anaemia of chronic disease

This is the commonest anaemia associated with rheumatoid conditions. ACD may occur in response to any activity in the immune system (infective, autoimmune, or malignant). Several mechanisms have been postulated for ACD, acting individually or in combination. Several cytokines, including interleukin(IL)-1, IL-6 and tumour necrosis factor (TNF), have been shown to affect erythropoiesis by inhibition of iron release from gut endothelium, hepatocytes, and macrophages (via induction of hepcidin)[1]; inhibition of marrow stromal growth; and reduced erythropoietin (EPO) production. Although patients with ACD have elevated levels of plasma EPO, levels are not as high as in iron deficiency anaemia with the same haemoglobin level. Furthermore, some improvement in ACD has been noted following administration of EPO. Improved haemoglobin levels in ACD have also been induced by TNFα blockade[2] and by IL-6 receptor blockade with tocilizumab.[3]

When interpreting haematological parameters it is simplest to consider ACD as due to a block in the transfer of iron from reticuloendothelial stores to red cell precursors. This process can be seen in bone marrow biopsies stained for iron. The depth of the anaemia will depend in part on the degree of immune activation—in shorthand, how high the erythrocyte sedimentation rate (ESR) is—and also on the duration of the disease process. In isolated form it is unusual for the haemoglobin to fall below 8 g/dL, while white cell and platelet counts usually remain in the normal range. The mean corpuscular volume (MCV) is usually low–normal, but if the process continues for months, red cells become microcytic. The blood

Box 61.1 Haematological abnormalities in rheumatic disorders

Red cells
- Anaemia of chronic disease
- Iron deficiency
- Vitamin B_{12} and folate deficiency
- Sideroblastic anaemia
- Pure red cell aplasia, especially systemic lupus
- Haemolytic anaemia: immune (especially SLE)/non-immune
- Erythrocytosis

White cells
- Neutrophilia and monocytosis
- Neutropenia (e.g. Felty's syndrome)
- Lymphopenia
- Eosinophilia (polyarteritis nodosa)

Platelets
- Thrombocytosis
- Thrombocytopenia: immune/non-immune
- Platelet dysfunction
- Thrombotic thrombocytopenic purpura

Coagulation
- Lupus anticoagulant
- Acquired coagulation factor deficiencies (immune related)
- Disseminated intravascular coagulation

Others
- Pancytopenia (SLE)
- Myelofibrosis
- Drug-related changes (e.g. aplastic anaemia and pure red cell aplasia)
- Amyloidosis

SLE, systemic lupus erythematosus.

film is unremarkable other than rouleaux formation reflecting the raised ESR, and the reticulocyte count will never be raised.

Iron stores are normal, or increased, due to reduced usage in red cell production and may be measured by serum ferritin or by examining bone marrow aspirate stained for iron (Perl stain). In addition to normal or increased reticuloendothelial stores, the bone marrow will demonstrate absence of stainable iron in the developing red cells (siderotic granulation).

Interpretation of serum iron results may be difficult. The serum iron concentration is low, and similar to levels seen in iron deficiency. But unlike the latter, the serum total iron-binding capacity (sTIBC—mostly made up of transferrin) is also reduced, such that the percentage saturation (serum iron/sTIBC × 1000) remains approximately normal. In iron deficiency, by contrast, the sTIBC is greatly increased so that the percentage saturation tends to be very low (see Table 61.1).

Treatment is only occasionally indicated, and only in the short term, for blood transfusion to prepare a patient for surgery. Suppression of the increased immune activity will result in a climb in haemoglobin levels. The importance in making this diagnosis is the exclusion of other causes of anaemia which may require more active investigation or intervention.

Iron deficiency

Iron deficiency may be difficult to diagnose in patients when ACD is also present. Iron deficiency is an extremely common cause of anaemia in all patients, but in particular, anti-inflammatory medications may cause upper gastrointestinal bleeding. This is an important diagnosis to make as, until proven otherwise, all iron deficiency is due to blood loss which must be stopped; and treatment of the iron deficiency is simple and clinically effective.

As seen in the previous section, laboratory results must be interpreted with care (see Table 61.1). The MCV will tend to be lower than in the ACD, and in severe cases a reactive thrombocytosis (if active bleeding is present) or mild neutropenia may coexist. If it proves impossible to distinguish iron deficiency from ACD on laboratory results, a trial of oral iron supplements may be warranted or, in very complex cases, a bone marrow aspirate stained for iron will establish the diagnosis.

Treatment of the iron deficiency is merely by supplements of iron—either orally, or for those intolerant, intravenously. Because oral iron supplements may themselves cause gastric upset treatment should be started at a very low dose and built up to full dose over a few weeks, as tolerated.

Haemolytic anaemia: immune

Any patient with circulating immune complexes may be found to have a positive Coomb's test. This test merely demonstrates the presence of immunoglobulins on the red cell surface and may be non-specific.

In autoimmune haemolytic anaemia, found in 10% of patients with systemic lupus erythematosus (SLE),[4] it is necessary to demonstrate both a positive Coomb's test and evidence of reduced red cell survival: raised reticulocyte count (reflecting increased red cell production) and hyperbilirubinaemia (reflecting increased red cell destruction). True haemolysis requires the presence of autoantibodies directed against specific red blood cell antigens in the presence of complement component C3.4. Serum haptoglobins are low or absent in the presence of true haemolysis. However, levels will also be reduced in cases with liver dysfunction.

Haematinic deficiency

Deficiency of folic acid or, less frequently, vitamin B_{12}, may occur in any chronically ill patient and could be masked by ACD. The MCV will tend to be higher than expected and both deficiencies can be diagnosed simply by blood tests.

Other causes of anaemia

Causes of anaemia in rheumatoid conditions may be multiple and it is therefore important that minor or rare aetiologies, masked by either ACD or iron deficiency, are not missed. These include sideroblastic anaemia, amyloidosis, drug-induced aplastic anaemia, pure red cell aplasia, and marrow fibrosis. However, a complete list of rare causes of anaemia is extremely long. Diagnosis of these conditions will rely on maintaining a high level of suspicion should the blood results not reflect the clinical state. Warning signs will show if the haemoglobin, MCV, and reticulocyte count are monitored. All can be diagnosed by bone marrow biopsy.

Case history

A 27 year old SLE patient, well maintained on long-term immunosuppressant therapy presented with a gradually worsening pancytopenia. The bone marrow was hypercellular of normal cells, suggesting relapse of her SLE. Despite increased immunosuppression her blood picture worsened, so a second bone marrow biopsy was performed. This showed widespread leishmaniasis. She had been on a 2 week holiday in Africa 6 months earlier.

White cells

Leucocytosis

Any inflammatory process, such as in connective tissue disease (CTD), may be associated with a neutrophilia. Neutrophil counts are rarely greater than 20×10^9/L and these cells are morphologically normal on blood smears or may be mildly left-shifted. Glucocorticoids may have a similar effect. Apart from being markers of underlying disease activity this is of no clinical significance, but needs to be differentiated from an acute infection. Monocytosis may also be noted with any autoimmune disorder.

Neutropenia

Neutropenia may result from drug effects or be a feature of Felty's syndrome—the association of low white cell count (and occasionally reduced platelet count) and splenomegaly in patients with rheumatoid arthritis (RA). The mechanisms involved in Felty's syndrome

Table 61.1 Serum iron and iron-binding capacity in iron deficiency and anaemia of chronic disease

Condition	Serum iron	Total iron-binding capacity	% saturation
Iron deficiency	Low	High (liver produces more transferrin)	Very low
Anaemia of chronic disease	Low (iron retained intracellularly)	Low (transferrin production is reduced)	Normal

are multifactorial and not merely due to a dilutional effect from the enlarged spleen. This is usually only trivial, but may, rarely, be very large. Increased sequestration of neutrophils within the spleen certainly occurs, but reduced marrow production due to immune-complex-mediated and humoral inhibition of granulopoiesis is also involved. Antibodies to mature neutrophils have been reported in SLE, as have functional defects in polymorph and lymphocyte function.

Lymphopenia

Mild lymphopenia occurs in both SLE and RA, and may be a measure of disease activity. If an isolated finding it is of no clinical significance.

Eosinophilia

Eosinophilia may be seen in SLE, RA, polyarteritis nodosa, and Churg–Strauss syndrome. The pathogenesis is unknown, but presumably involves release of cytokines by T lymphocytes.

Platelets

Thrombocytosis

A moderately raised platelet count (up to 1000×10^9/L)—known as a reactive thrombocytosis—is a frequent finding in cases of chronic inflammation or blood loss. These two, of course, will need to be distinguished on clinical grounds and examination of haemoglobin, reticulocyte count, and iron status. The blood cell morphology on a smear will be normal, as will the platelet size (mean platelet volume).

However, it is important to distinguish a reactive thrombocytosis from a primary thrombocythaemia which is one of the myeloproliferative disorders. In the latter there may be abnormalities in the red cell and white cell line; abnormal platelet morphology; or splenomegaly. The JAK2 (Janus kinase 2—available as a blood test) mutation is positive in approximately 50% of cases of primary thrombocythaemia.[5] A bone marrow biopsy may be required to establish the diagnosis.

Thrombocytopenia: immune/non-immune

A mild reduction in platelet count ($100–150 \times 10^9$/L) may be found in any widespread inflammation, due to non-specific activation of coagulation. In RA this may be aggravated by an element of hypersplenism as part of Felty's syndrome.

Platelet counts below 100×10^9/L require investigation as they may represent an immune thrombocytopenia (ITP). This is a common manifestation of SLE and also occurs in mixed CTD, scleroderma, RA, and dermatomyositis. The pathogenesis involves binding of immune complexes to the platelet surface. These are recognized by the reticuloendothelial system and such platelets are sequestered and destroyed, usually in the spleen. ITP needs to be distinguished from failure of platelet production due to a bone marrow disorder. In ITP the bone marrow will be normal or may, in chronic cases, show an increase in megakaryocyte number and activity.

First-line treatment of ITP is suppression of immune activity (steroids or other immune-suppressing drugs) or rituximab (a monoclonal antibody directed against CD20 found primarily on B lymphocytes). Intravenous infusion of immunoglobulin concentrates is usually beneficial in acute cases. The mechanism of action of this treatment is uncertain but may involve swamping of immunoglobulin Fc-binding sites. Other therapies include infusion of anti-D (rhesus), and splenectomy. Trials of thrombopoietin analogues have shown benefit in some cases.[6]

Thrombotic thrombocytopenic purpura

Thrombocytopenia may occasionally be due to thrombotic thrombocytopenic purpura (TTP), a condition associated with any autoimmune condition. Antibodies directed against a vascular endothelial protein (ADAMTS-13) impair cleavage of von Willebrand factor (vWF). When ADAMTS-13 levels are reduced, large vWF multimers proliferate and aggregate platelets. TTP is characterized by the combination of thrombocytopenia and microvascular haemolysis.[7]

Coagulation

A wide range of minor coagulation changes may occur in patients with rheumatic conditions. This can be due to liver and renal disease or to drug effects. Plasma fibrinogen is a very sensitive marker of underlying inflammation and will be raised in parallel with the C-reactive protein (CRP).

Low-grade Disseminated intravascular coagulation (DIC) may be found in patients with high levels of circulating immune complexes and resulting endothelial cell activation. In such cases the plasma fibrinogen level may not be as high as expected (from the CRP) or may be mildly subnormal. D-dimers, a product of both coagulation cascade and fibrinolytic activity, will be raised.

Intra-articular activation of coagulation systems may be found in all cases of arthritis, but especially those due to immune activity. This may result in intra-articular deposition of fibrin and a wash-over effect into the systemic circulation.

Lupus anticoagulant

The lupus anticoagulant (LA) occurs as a complication in about 10% of patients with SLE and is (paradoxically) associated with a thrombotic tendency, thrombocytopenia, recurrent miscarriages, and pulmonary hypertension. This is an in-vitro phenomenon due to antibodies directed against the phospholipid substrate on which coagulation occurs (the thromboplastin in coagulation assays). Although it is named as the 'lupus' anticoagulant after the first group of patients in whom it was identified, LA may occur in a very wide range of clinical conditions and even in normal individuals, and may be transient. It is, however, important to identify, firstly to differentiate from other causes of prolonged clotting assays (which may be associated with a haemorrhagic tendency); and secondly, as an important part of the anti-phospholipid syndrome.

The laboratory diagnosis of LA involves finding a prolonged clotting test—almost invariably the activated partial thromboplastin time (APTT)—which can be corrected by 'swamping' the sample with excess phospholipid substrate, to dilute the antibodies. Commercial thromboplastins are available which are relatively insensitive to the anti-phospholipid antibodies and are useful as screening tests for LA.

During heparin infusions levels of anticoagulation are usually monitored by the ratio of the patient's APTT to the 'normal' APTT. In patients with LA it is important to note that this ratio will not be effective and that the patient's pre-heparin APTT may need to be used as the ratio's denominator.

LA needs to be differentiated from clotting factor inhibitors encountered in patients with CTD (especially SLE) including antibodies to vWF and to factors VIII, VII, and fibrinogen.

References

1. Mehta A, Hoffbrand V. Haematological aspects of systemic disease. Chapter 59 In: Hoffbrand V, Catovsky D, Edward G, Tuddenham E (eds) *Postgraduate haematology*, 5th edn. Blackwell, Oxford, 2005: 965–968.

2. Davis D, Charles P, Potter A et al. anaemia of chronic disease in rheumatoid arthritis: in-vivo effects of tumour necrosis factor α blockade. *Br J Rheum* 1997;36:950–956.

3. Zhang X, Peck R. Clinical pharmacology of tocilizumab for the treatment of patients with rheumatoid arthritis. *Exp Rev Clin Pharm* 2011;4/5: 539–558.

4. Gomard-Mennesson E, Ruivard M, Koenig M et al. Treatment of isolated severe immune haemolytic anaemia associated with systemic lupus erythematosus. *Lupus* 2006;15:223–232.

5. Lussana F, Caberlon S, Pagani C et al. Association of V617F Jak2 mutation with the risk of thrombosis among patients with essential thrombocythaemia or idiopathic myelofibrosis: a systematic review. *Thromb Res* 2009;124:409–417.

6. Elalfy MS, Abdelmaksoud AA, Eltonbary KY. Romiplostim in children with chronic refractory ITP: randomized placebo controlled study. *Ann Hematol* 2011;90:1341–1344.

7. Rottem M, Krause I, Fraser A et al. Autoimmune hemolytic anaemia in the antiphospholipid syndrome. *Lupus* 2006;15:473–477.

CHAPTER 62

Biochemical investigation of rheumatic diseases

Berenice Lopez and Patrick J. Twomey

Introduction: clinical quality of results

Biochemical tests are generally ordered to support a diagnosis, or to detect a complication of a disease or a side effect of therapy. Irrespective of the intended use, it is important for clinicians to have an awareness of the quality of the result i.e. the extent to which they can be relied upon for the clinical purpose in hand. Despite the reporting of absolute numbers, every single quantitative result produced by laboratories has an associated uncertainty. This is largely a consequence of biological variation within and between individuals and the limitations of the measurement technology. In addition, the quality of a test result is affected by the sensitivity of laboratory internal quality control and external quality assurance procedures to detect clinically important errors. Without this understanding, a clinician's ability to determine whether a specific pathological process is occurring in a patient or interpret the implications of a difference between sequential results, particularly when monitoring chronic disease, can be compromised and patients may be misdiagnosed, overinvestigated, or even inappropriately treated.

Although there are currently no clearly defined best practice standards for how to incorporate uncertainty into the reporting of laboratory results, in the future more information about the confidence interval for a result and guidance on the significance of a change between serial results may be provided by laboratories. In the interim, adequate completion of request forms with a statement clarifying the pertinent clinical question as well as direct communication with clinical laboratory consultants can help, particularly in acute or difficult clinical scenarios.

Renal function

Patients with rheumatoid disorders are a high-risk group for kidney disease.[1] This may arise as a part of the pathology of a systemic disease particularly in conditions such as connective tissue diseases and vasculitides. However, renal impairment may also be a consequence of drug treatment, sepsis, and/or coincidental renal pathology as may be seen in rheumatic conditions such as osteoarthritis (OA), which affects large numbers of elderly patients with significant comorbidity.

Patients may present with acute kidney injury (AKI), a nephrological emergency which may lead to endstage renal failure and is associated with high mortality. AKI is most frequently caused by ischaemia, sepsis, and/or nephrotoxic drugs but may also be a consequence of rhabdomyolysis, contrast agents, or systemic diseases such as scleroderma crisis which occurs in 5–10% of patients with systemic sclerosis.[2] However, a more common presentation is slowly progressive chronic kidney disease. A classic example is secondary amyloidosis in rheumatoid arthritis (RA) and other inflammatory rheumatic diseases, although the incidence of endstage renal failure is decreasing with improvements in medical care.[3] Notwithstanding, data indicates a high prevalence of chronic kidney disease in rheumatology outpatient clinics.[4] Renal function should therefore be regularly evaluated in patients with rheumatic diseases to enable the early detection of kidney disease and institution of treatment to prevent or slow down progression to endstage renal failure.

Biochemical assessment of renal function

Glomerular filtration rate (GFR), the sum of the filtration rates in all functioning nephrons, numerically represents residual renal function and is currently widely viewed as the best overall index of kidney health.[5] Serum creatinine and its derivative eGFR are the most readily available surrogate markers of GFR and are used to assess degree of renal impairment and monitor its course. Additional screening for kidney damage is often performed by assessment of glomerular integrity including proteinuria, albuminuria, or haematuria and sometimes by diagnostic imaging for evidence of structural disease including renal scarring.

More subtle renal damage reflecting tubular injury—e.g. mild urinary sediment abnormalities, tubulopathy and acid–base disorders—are, however, frequently unrecognized but may also predict GFR and progression towards renal failure. Detection is important but often delayed until a decrease in renal excretory function as measured by serum creatinine or GFR occurs.

Glomerular filtration

GFR varies according to renal mass and correspondingly to body mass. It is conventionally corrected for body surface area (BSA), which in the average human being is 1.73 m^2, to account for this. When the GFR is corrected for BSA, a reference interval can be derived.[6–8] GFR is difficult to measure directly and as gold standard methods are expensive, time-consuming, technically demanding, and not readily available, other markers are usually used. Serum creatinine, the most widely used marker, may, however, not accurately reflect kidney function as its level also depends on muscle mass and is subject to a number of other non-GFR related influences.[9] In addition, serum creatinine is not linearly related to GFR as a consequence of functional renal reserve, enhanced tubular secretion as levels increase, and other factors.[20–22] A large number of equations have been developed to estimate GFR using age, gender, ethnic origin, and weight as surrogates for muscle mass, in order to improve accuracy. The four-variable Modification of Diet in Kidney Disease study equation is currently in widespread use in the United Kingdom to estimate GFR in adults ≥18 years.[10] It uses serum creatinine, age, ethnic origin, and gender, has been validated in patients with chronic kidney disease, and is reasonably accurate at GFR levels less than 60 mL min^{-1}. However, bias and imprecision may limit its use at higher GFRs.[11] An awareness of other limitations is important. First, equations do not account for all the non-GFR related factors affecting serum creatinine levels such as the effect of drugs,[12,13] diurnal variation,[14] cooked meat consumption,[15] and analytical influences such as time to centrifugation[16,17] and creatinine method.[18] As regards the latter, efforts have been recently made to standardize creatinine measurements across the United Kingdom to ensure that the MDRD formula is appropriately corrected for different local creatinine assays. Second, the coefficients in the equation represent average effects observed in the population used to derive the equation and may not be applicable to other groups, particularly those where creatinine production is atypical or where the volume of distribution of creatinine may be altered. These include muscle wasting states, malnourished or oedematous patients, individuals at the extremes of body size, or pregnant women. Thirdly, a steady state is required and equations should not be used to assess kidney function in acutely unwell patients with AKI or changing renal function.[19]

In most clinical settings, it is sufficient to know whether GFR, and thus disease severity, is changing or stable. A change in serum creatinine of up to ±15% may simply reflect biological and analytical variability.[23] Recent National Institute for Health and Clinical Excellence (NICE) guidelines state that a GFR loss over 1 year of 5 mL min^{-1} or 10 mL min^{-1} L over 5 years may indicate significant progression and should trigger nephrology advice or referral.[10]

Glomerular integrity

Some protein, including small amounts of albumin, low-molecular-weight immunoglobulins, and secreted tubular proteins such as Tamm–Horsfall protein, is normally excreted in the urine. However, urinary protein excretion in the normal adult should be less than 150 mg/day. Higher rates of protein persisting beyond a single measurement may indicate impaired glomerular membrane integrity and kidney damage and must be evaluated.

Glomerular proteinuria is a cardinal sign of kidney disease and carries powerful prognostic information, identifying a subpopulation of chronic kidney disease (CKD) patients at greatly increased risk of kidney disease progression,[24,25] cardiovascular disease,[26,27] and death.[28,29] Although the most common cause of progressive kidney disease with proteinuria in the United Kingdom is diabetes mellitus, in patients with chronic inflammatory diseases, glomerular proteinuria may herald the development of secondary amyloidosis or nephropathy from other causes and this should be regularly

screened for. Other types of proteinuria include overflow, typically the mechanism by which Bence Jones protein is first detected in urine and tubular proteinuria.

Assessment of protein:creatinine (PCR) or albumin: creatinine ratio (ACR) in a spot urine sample is more reproducible and useful than 24 hour collections. Samples should not be collected during acute illness or menstruation. Early morning urine samples correlate best with 24 hour urinary protein and albumin excretion, but random samples are acceptable although subsequent specimens should ideally be collected at about the same time.

Urinary albumin measurement provides a quantitative, relatively standardized measurement of excretion of the single most important protein in most nephropathies but samples with higher urinary albumin concentrations can be technically demanding because commercial urinary albumin assays have limited analytical ranges and manual or automatic dilutions may be required. In addition, there is a risk of antigen excess (prozone) phenomenon with some immunoassay approaches.[29a] Urinary protein measurement on the other hand is relatively non-specific, imprecise at low concentrations, and cannot be standardized, but most of the evidence for intervention thresholds in non-diabetic CKD is based on 24 hour urine protein excretion. In general, as ACR has a far greater sensitivity for the detection of low levels of proteinuria, it should be the test of choice for the initial detection of proteinuria but the PCR may be best used to monitor established proteinuria.

Reagent strips predominantly detect albumin not total protein, are not reliable quantitatively, and should not be used for the detection or monitoring of proteinuria. They may, however, provide a more reliable assessment of haematuria than laboratory testing. Haematuria, together with proteinuria, usually localizes the cause of the proteinuria to a glomerular pathology.

Tubular injury—tubular function and integrity

Tubular function

Renal tubules make up 95% of the renal mass, do the bulk of the metabolic work, and modify the ultrafiltrate in the urine. Considering the spectrum of tubular functions, these disorders result in varied, non-specific manifestations and a high index of suspicion is required. Renal tubular disorders may affect multiple or specific tubular functions and should be considered in adults with potassium and acid–base disturbances, hypophosphataemia, hypomagnesaemia, polyuria, osteomalacia or osteoporosis as well as renal calculi, and nephrocalcinosis.

Tubular integrity

Tubular proteinuria may be due to the increased excretion of several endogenous, freely filtered, low-molecular-weight proteins, including β$_2$-microglobulin and retinol binding protein, or due to failure of reabsorption in proximal tubular disease. Tubular proteinuria may also reflect epithelial cell injury and may be a source of biomarkers for the early detection and risk stratification of AKI. A multimarker panel including urinary neutrophil gelatinase associated lipocalin (NAGL) and kidney injury molecule-1 (KIM-1) may be useful in this context,[30,31] but a large number of other proteins are being assessed.

Liver function testing

Abnormalities of liver function tests (LFTs) and liver function are not uncommon in patients with rheumatic diseases. Systemic inflammation can cause benign fluctuations in serum aminotransferase (alanine aminotransferase (ALT) or aspartate aminotransferase (AST)) and alkaline phosphatase (ALP) levels, but a hepatitic or cholestatic picture may mark the presence of primary, rheumatic disease-associated liver disease or coincidental pathology or infection. Elevations of serum aminotransferases may be seen in conditions such as viral hepatitis or autoimmune hepatitis. Disproportionate elevations of ALP may be seen in infiltrative including granulomatous diseases or early in the course of cholestatic disorders such as primary biliary cirrhosis, although bilirubin often becomes elevated in most patients as the disease progresses and is a poor prognostic sign. Of note, ALP elevations may reflect osteoblastic activity and ALP isoenzyme analysis should be performed where the source of ALP is in doubt, although a normal gamma-glutamyl transferase (GGT) level in this context usually excludes a hepatic source. Hypoalbuminaemia can be an ominous sign in patients with liver involvement, heralding the presence of severe liver damage, but various other conditions may be responsible including systemic inflammation and malnutrition.

The medical management of rheumatic diseases involves medications which are often hepatotoxic and routine monitoring of LFTs is recommended. Hepatotoxicity may also present as either a hepatocellular or cholestatic injury although some patients may present acutely with jaundice with a proportion rapidly developing hepatic failure. Irrespective of cause, chronic liver injury can lead to fibrosis and cirrhosis with the attendant complications of portal hypertension, impaired hepatic function, and hepatocellular carcinoma. A key question is whether monitoring LFTs is sufficient to detect the development of fibrosis—the rheumatology literature would agree.

Elevations of serum aminotransferases have been found to be predictive of abnormal or worsening histological grade on liver biopsy,[32] and for most disease-modifying drugs anti-rheumatic drugs (DMARDs) the current British Society for Rheumatology guidelines recommend withholding treatment when serum aminotransferases—either ALT or AST—exceed twice the upper reference limit (URL).[33] There are a number of problems with this approach, however. First, using multiples of the URL to define action thresholds is problematic because there is no consensus reference interval for aminotransferases and large differences in the URL can exist between laboratories, due mostly to variable reference intervals rather than method-specific biases.[34] The variability may be due to a the application of historical intervals constructed before anti-HCV testing and restrictive behavioural criteria for donor selection were implemented or because reference intervals have been constructed with varying regard for factors known to significantly modulate aminotransferases including gender, age, glucose, cholesterol, triglycerides, and body mass index (BMI).[35,36] In addition, serum aminotransferases have a skewed distribution with a tail to the right, so it is more difficult to be precise about the URL. Recent studies have provided a strong argument for the implementation of lower and more sensitive outcome-based reference intervals for ALT, but this remains controversial.[35,37] Nonetheless, agreeing and adopting common URLs for aminotransferases is highly desirable.

Second, many patients may have aminotransferase elevations from causes other than drugs. Biological variation of ALT, for example, can be significant within any one individual because it is subject to factors such as time of day and exercise,[38] coffee intake,[39] and dietary intake of sugars such as fructose and calories.[40] In addition,

raised ALT may be due to random analytical error. Thus elevations may be a transient or spurious abnormality.[41] Self-resolving liver enzyme abnormalities cannot, however, be distinguished from drug-induced liver injury (DILI) although observation of trends may be helpful. Both AST and to a lesser degree ALT are found in the cytosol of cells other than liver and elevations may also reflect leakage of these enzymes into the bloodstream due to myofibrillar damage as seen in myositis and other muscle diseases.[42] Raised aminotransferases may also be due to liver disease other than DILI.

Thirdly, there is evidence from the hepatology literature that LFTs are insufficiently sensitive or specific for the detection of liver fibrosis and cirrhosis,[43–46] and the potential for serious liver damage may still need to be explored when aminotransferase elevations are less than twice the URL, particularly in patients with other risk factors for liver disease.

Thus it is advisable that before initiation of therapy, a careful history for risk factors is taken with a particular emphasis on alcohol intake, risk factors for blood-borne viruses (e.g. blood transfusions, tattoos, intravenous drug abuse) or non-alcoholic fatty liver disease (NAFLD), e.g. diabetes mellitus and obesity, and any family history of liver disease. Patients should also be assessed for signs of liver disease (spider naevi, hepatomegaly, splenomegaly, jaundice). Those considered to be at risk and/or who have physical signs or abnormalities in baseline LFTs, full blood count (FBC), and prothrombin time (PT) including low platelets, low albumin, raised liver enzymes, raised bilirubin, or prolonged PT should undergo further liver evaluation. A liver screen including serum autoimmune as well as an immunoglobulin profile, hepatitis B and C serology, serum ferritin, serum α_1-antitrypsin, copper, and caeruloplasmin (if age <50 years), plasma glucose and lipid profile, and an ultrasound evaluation of the liver and spleen should be considered. A coeliac disease screen may also be helpful as this may be present in up to 9% of patients with unexplained elevated liver enzymes.[47–49] Most patients with baseline abnormalities in LFTs and a negative liver screen will, however, have either alcohol-related or fat-related liver disease. On this note, a positive diagnosis of NAFLD can be only be currently made on the basis of a negative liver screen, fatty liver on ultrasound, alcohol intake within recommended limits, and the presence of metabolic risk factors.[49] A liver biopsy or other marker or measure of liver fibrosis should be performed in those where the diagnosis is uncertain or the risk of advanced fibrosis and cirrhosis is high. With respect to clinical and routine laboratory variables, older age (>45 years), presence of diabetes, increasing BMI, low platelet counts, low albumin levels, and an AST/ALT ratio of greater than 1, are all predictive of advanced liver disease in NAFLD.[50]

Risk factors should also be assessed in patients who develop raised aminotransferases while on treatment with a DMARD. An enquiry into alcohol intake and exposure to risk of blood-borne viruses by intravenous drug abuse, blood transfusions, or multiple sex partners is pertinent. Opportunistic infections may also have to be ruled out in rheumatic patients.

Assessment of the severity and progression of DILI may be facilitated in the near future by the use of non-invasive quantitative testing for hepatic fibrosis. Although liver biopsy remains the gold standard for the staging of fibrosis, this is a flawed reference standard because of the potential for sampling error as well as inter- and intraobserver variability. It is also costly, invasive, and associated with a mortality risk of 0.01–0.1%. Non-invasive approaches offer a number of advantages including reduced risk of adverse effects as compared with liver biopsy, reduced risk of sampling error, objectivity in interpretation of results, appropriateness for repeated measurements, increased availability, and lower cost. A novel ultrasound technique that measures hepatic elasticity (Fibroscan) has been found to reliably identify advanced fibrosis but its clinical role is still being determined.[51] A range of surrogate serological markers have also been evaluated including indirect markers of liver fibrosis such as platelet counts and AST/ALT ratio as well as more direct measures of liver fibrosis such as procollagen type III N-terminal peptide (P3NP), hyaluronic acid, and type IV collagen. These measure matrix turnover rather than fibrosis per se and are not liver specific, thus levels may be high in acute inflammation in the liver or at other sites such as synovial membrane, limiting their utility.[52–54] A growing number of panels have also been developed using various combinations of these markers. The performance of serological markers and transient elastography and their diagnostic cut-offs vary among different liver diseases, however,[55] and as yet even the more successful markers and panels have only been validated in specific patient groups with utility restricted to the identification of the near-absence or the presence of advanced fibrosis and cirrhosis. The current armoury of non-invasive tests cannot be used to identify intermediate stages or to monitor the progression of fibrosis in an individual patient and liver biopsy continues to be required, at least for the time being.

Calcium and bone biochemistry

Calcium and phosphate homeostasis are coordinated by systemic and local factors that regulate intestinal absorption, influx and efflux from bone, and kidney excretion and reabsorption of these ions. Parathyroid hormone (PTH), secreted by the parathyroid gland in response to hypocalcaemia, maintains normocalcaemia by increasing tubular calcium reabsorption, stimulating the conversion of calcidiol (25-hydroxyvitamin D) to calcitriol (1,25-dihydroxyvitamin D) thereby increasing intestinal calcium and phosphate absorption and, with calcitriol, stimulating osteoclastogenesis, increasing calcium and phosphate efflux from bone. Normal phosphate balance is maintained through phosphaturic effects. In addition to PTH and calcitriol, phosphate homeostasis is also regulated by dietary phosphate intake.[56] Two new proteins, klotho and fibroblast growth factor 23 (FGF23) are also emerging as important players in phosphate and calcium metabolism.[57,58] FGF23, a secreted phosphatonin, induces renal phosphate wasting and inhibits synthesis of calcitriol acting through specific FGF receptors with the important cofactor klotho protein. Klotho also directly modulates renal phosphate excretion and calcium reabsorption through effects on transporters.[59] Both overexpression and deficiency of FGF23 cause several clinical diseases including inherited and acquired forms of hypophosphataemic rickets and hyperphosphataemic familial tumoral calcinosis (HFTC).

Biochemical tests in calcium and bone pathology

At physiological pH, 15% of plasma calcium is bound to organic and inorganic anions, 40% is bound to albumin, and 45% is free or ionized calcium. It is the ionized calcium that is physiologically active and under tight homeostatic control, so this should ideally be measured, but difficulties in accurate analysis, lack of standardization, and strict sampling requirements mean that total calcium is more conveniently measured. Better correlation between total calcium and ionized calcium may be achieved when total calcium is adjusted for the plasma albumin because changes in serum albumin concentration can affect total calcium without affecting ionized calcium. The correction equation applied should be specific for the individual laboratory's albumin method and the local population.[60] It is worth noting, however, that use of correction equations, particularly when albumin is in the normal range or higher, remains controversial.[60a,60b] Acid–base disturbances,[61] hyperparathyroidism,[62] and hyperphosphataemia may also affect ionized calcium without affecting total calcium and in these instances direct measurement of ionized calcium may be useful. The underlying pathology of any calcium abnormality can usually be elucidated by the simultaneous measurement of calcium, renal function, and PTH.

Serum phosphate can also provide an initial indication of the pathology of any calcium abnormality, with calcium and phosphate concentrations usually changing in the same direction unless PTH is inappropriately in excess or deficient or renal failure is present. Isolated hypophosphataemia may be seen in primary or secondary hyperparathyroidism, inherited or acquired hypophosphataemic rickets is typically seen in children, or oncogenic osteomalacia in adults. Prolonged phosphate deficiency is associated with bone demineralization, resulting in rickets and osteomalacia. Hyperphosphataemia is a common and serious complication of chronic renal failure and contributes to secondary hyperparathyroidism. On occasion, hypo- or hyperphosphataemia may be spurious, resulting from analytical interference by a paraprotein.[63]

PTH is a relatively unstable peptide hormone which is broken down in blood after venepuncture but is stable for 48 hours in EDTA.[64] PTH circulates in different molecular forms, including the intact molecule (PTH 1–84) and various truncated forms (e.g. PTH 7–84), which may be differentially recognized by the various antibodies used in PTH immunoassays so that PTH results from different laboratories may not be comparable even though quoted reference intervals may be the same.[65] The biological variability of PTH is high and concentrations must change by more than 50% before they can be assumed to be real.[66]

Calcidiol is the major circulating form of vitamin D, with a half-life of 2–3 weeks. It is the best indicator of nutritional vitamin D status but method-related differences means that the comparability and accuracy of different assays may be a concern.[67] This may improve as uniform standards are widely implemented. Of note, calcidiol varies in a sinusoidal manner with large seasonal differences relative to mean concentration so that a single vitamin D measurement may not capture overall vitamin D status.[68] Measurement of calcitriol is not useful for monitoring vitamin D status because its circulating half-life is only 4 hours; levels are 1000 times lower than calcidiol and do not reflect nutritional vitamin D reserves. Measurement may, however, be useful in acquired and inherited disorders of vitamin D and phosphate including hereditary phosphate wasting disorders, oncogenic osteomalacia, and chronic granulomatous disorders such as sarcoidosis.

FGF23 and Klotho assays are currently not harmonized and do not appear ready for routine clinical use.[69]

Biochemical markers of bone turnover

Bone is constantly being remodelled in adults and bone formation is tightly coupled to bone resorption so that bone mass is preserved. Metabolic bone diseases occur when bone formation and bone resorption are uncoupled. This group of disorders traditionally includes osteomalacia, osteoporosis, and Paget's disease of bone. However, rheumatic diseases, particularly those associated with widespread systemic inflammation, may produce generalized effects on bone remodelling that may affect the entire skeleton.

Changes in the rate of bone turnover are an important determinant of bone disease. Several assays are currently available that measure bone turnover markers (BTM), which are collagen breakdown products and other molecules released from osteoclasts and osteoblasts during the process of bone resorption and formation. Urinary and serum N-terminal telopeptide of collage type 1 (NTX) and C-terminal telopeptide of type 1 collagen (CTX) are the most clinically useful markers of bone resorption, while serum bone specific ALP and procollagen type 1 N-terminal propeptide (PINP) are the most clinically useful markers of bone formation.[70] Their main application is to provide guidance as to whether a patient has a high or low bone turnover, and the impact of therapy.

BTMs are not, currently, widely used in clinical practice because of biological and analytical variability.[71] Bone turnover and BTMs follow a circadian rhythm and are altered by food intake, thus urine should be collected as a second morning fasting sample and blood collected in the morning after an overnight fast. Patients should have all their measurements performed by the same laboratory.

References

1. Niederstadt C, Happ T, Tatsis E et al. Glomerular and tubular proteinuria as markers of nephropathy in rheumatoid arthritis. *Rheumatology* 1999;38(1):28–33.

2. Denton CP, Lapadula G, Mouthon L et al. Renal complications and scleroderma renal crisis. *Rheumatology* 2009;48(3):32–35.

3. Immonen K, Finne P, Gronhagen-Rista C et al. A marked decline in the incidence of renal replacement therapy associated with inflammatory rheumatic diseases—data from nationwide registries in Finland. *Amyloid* 2011;18(1):25–28.

4. Hill AJ, Thompson RJ, Hunter JA, Traynor JP. The prevalence of chronic kidney disease in rheumatology outpatients. *Scott Med J* 2009; 54:(2):9–12.

5. National Kidney Foundation. K/DOQI clinical practice guidelines for chronic kidney disease: evaluation classification and stratification. *Am J Kidney Dis* 2002;39 (suppl 1):S1–S266.

6. Singer MA, Morton AR. Mouse to elephant: biological scaling and Kt/V. *Am J Kidney Dis* 2000;35:306–309.

7. McCance R, Widdowson E. The correct physiological basis on which to compare infant and adult renal function. *Lancet* 1952;2:860–862.

8. Du Bois E, Du Bois D. A formula to estimate the approximate surface area if height and weight be known. *Arch Intern Med* 1916;17: 863–871.

9. Perrone RD, Madias NE, Levey AS. Serum creatinine as an index of renal function: new insights into old concepts. *Clin Chem* 1992;38: 1933–1953.

10. Joint Specialty Committee on Renal Medicine of the Royal College of Physicians and the Renal Association and the Royal College of General Practitioners. *Chronic kidney disease in adults: UK guidelines for identification, management and referral*. Royal College of Physicians, London, 2006.

11. Stevens LA, Coresh J, Feldman HI, et al. Evaluation of the modification of diet in renal disease study equation in a large diverse population. *J Am Soc Nephrol* 2007;18:2749–2757.

12. Berg KJ, Gjellestad A, Nordby G et al. Renal effects of trimethoprim in ciclosporin- and azathioprine-treated kidney-allografted patients. *Nephron* 1989;53(3):218.

13. Hilbrands LB, Artz MA, Wetzels JF et al. Cimetidine improves the reliability of creatinine as a marker of glomerular filtration. *Kidney Int* 1991;40(6):1171.

14. Pasternack A, Kuhlback B. Diurnal variations of serum and urine creatinine and creatinine. *Scand J Clin Lab Invest* 1971;27(1):1–7.

15. Preiss DJ, Godber IM, Lamb EJ et al. The influence of a cooked-meat meal on estimated glomerular filtration rate. *Ann Clin Biochem* 2007;44 (Pt 1):35–42.

16. Shepherd J, Warner M, Kilpatrick E. Stability of creatinine with delayed separation of whole blood and implications for e.GFR. *Ann Clin Biochem* 2007;44(4):384–387.

17. Ford L, Berg J. Delay in separating blood samples affects creatinine measurement using the Roche kinetic Jaffe method. *Ann Clin Biochem* 2008;45(1):83–87.

18. Lawson N, Lang T, Broughton A et al. Creatinine assays: time for action? *Ann Clin Biochem* 2002;39:599–602.

19. Waiker SS, Bonverte JV. Creatinine kinetics and the definition of acute kidney injury. *J Am Soc Nephrol* 2009;20:672–679.

20. Tomlanovich S, Golbertz H, Perloth M, Stinson E, Myers BD. Limitations of creatinine in quantifying the severity of cyclosporine-induced chronic nephropathy. *Am J Kidney Dis* 1986;8:332–337.

21. Baboolal K, Jones GA, Janezic A, Griffiths DR, Jurewicz WA. Molecular and structural consequences of early renal allograft injury. *Kidney Int* 2002;61:686–696.

22. Swedko PJ, Clark HD, Paramsothy K, Akbari A. Serum creatinine is an inadequate screening test for renal failure in elderly patients. *Arch Intern Med* 2003;163: 356–360.

23. Smellie S. What is a significant difference between sequential laboratory results? *J Clin Path* 2006;61:419–425.

24. Ruggenenti P, Perna A, Mosconi L, Pisoni R, Remuzzi G. Urinary protein excretion rate is the best independent predictor of ESRF in non-diabetic proteinuric chronic nephropathies. *Kidney Int* 1998;53(5):1209–1216.

25. Ruggenenti P, Perna A, Mosconi L et al. Proteinuria predicts end-stage renal failure in non-diabetic chronic nephropathies. The 'Gruppo Italiano di Studi Epidemiologici in Nefrologia' (GISEN). *Kidney Int* 1997;63(suppl):S54–S57.

26. Wagener DK, Harris T, Madans JH. Proteinuria as a biomarker: Risk of subsequent morbidity and mortality. *Environ Res* 1994, 66:160–172.

27. Chiu YW, Adler SG, Budoff MJ, et al. Coronary artery calcification and mortality in diabetic patients with proteinuria. *Kidney Int* 2010;77(12):1107–1114.

28. Kannel WB, Stampfer MJ, Castelli WP, Verter J. The prognostic significance of proteinuria: The Framingham Study. *Am Heart J* 1984;108(5):1347–1352.

29. Torffvit O, Agardh C-D. The predictive value of albuminuria for cardiovascular and renal disease. A 5-year follow-up study of 476 patients with Type 1 diabetes mellitus. *J Diab Comp* 1993;7(1):49–56.

29a. Lamb EJ, Mackenzie F, Stevens PE. How should proteinuria be detected? *Ann Clin Biochem* 2009;46:205–217.

30. Parikh C, Lu JC, Coca SG, Devarajan P. Tubular proteinuria in acute kidney injury: a critical evaluation of current status and future promise. *Ann Clin Biochem* 2010;47:301–312.

31. Lock E. Sensitive and early markers of renal injury;where are we and what is the way forward? *Toxicol Sci* 2010;116(1):1–4.

32. Kremer JM, Furst DE, Weinblatt ME et al. Significant changes in serum AST across hepatic histological biopsy grades: prospective analysis of 3 cohorts receiving methotrexate therapy for rheumatoid arthritis. *J Rheumatol* 1996;23(3):459.

33. Chakravarty K, Mc Donald H, Pullar T et al. BSR/BHPR guidelines for disease-modifying anti-rheumatic drug (DMARD) therapy in conjunction with the British Association of Dermatologists. *Rheumatology(Oxford)* 2008; 47(6):924–925.

34. Dutta A, Saha C, Johnson CS et al. Variability in the upper limit of normal for serum alanine aminotransferase levels: a statewide study. *Hepatology* 2009;50:1957.

35. Prati D, Taioli E, Zanella A et al. Updated definitions of healthy ranges for serum alanine aminotransferase levels. *Ann Intern Med* 2002;137:1–9.

36. Kariv R, Lestino M, Beth-or A et al. Re-evaluation of serum aminotransferase upper normal limit and its modulating factors in a large scale population study. *Liver Int* 2006;26(4):445–450.

37. Kim HC, Nam CM, Jee SH et al. Normal serum aminotransferase concentration and risk of mortality from liver diseases: prospective cohort study. *BMJ* 2004;328:983–989.

38. Dufour R, Lott JA, Nolte FS et al. National Academy of Clinical Biochemistry standards of laboratory practice: laboratory guidelines for screening, diagnosis and monitoring of hepatic injury. *Clin Chem* 2000;46(12):2027–2068.

39. Urgert R, Meyboom S, Kuilman M et al. Comparison of effect of cafetière and filtered coffee on serum concentrations of liver aminotransferases and lipids: 6 month randomised controlled trial. *BMJ* 1996;313:V1362–V1366.

40. Kechagias S, Ernersson A, Dahlquist O et al. Fast food based hyperalimentation can induce rapid and profound elevation of serum alanine aminotransferase in healthy subjects. *Gut* 2008;57:649–654.

41. Lazo M, Selvin E, Clark JM et al. Brief communication: clinical implications of short-term variability in liver function test results. *Ann Intern Med* 2008;148:348–352.

42. Edge K, Chinog H, Cooper RG. Serum alanine aminotransferase elevations correlate with serum creatinine phosphokinase levels in myositis. *Rheumatology* 2006;45(4): 487–488.

43. Bacon BR, Farahvash MJ, Janney CG et al. Non-alcoholic steatohepatitis an expanded clinical entity. *Gastroenterology* 1994;107:1103–1109.

44. Mofrad P, Contos MJ, Haque M et al. Clinical and histologic spectrum of non-alcoholic fatty liver disease associated with normal ALT values. *Hepatology* 2003;37:1286–1292.

45. Mc Cullough AJ, The clinical features, diagnosis and natural history of non-alcoholic fatty liver disease associated with normal ALT values. *Clin LiverDis* 2004;40:475–483.

46. Afdhal NH, Nunes D. Evaluation of liver fibrosis: a concise review. *Am J Gastroenterol* 2004;99:1160–1174.

47. Rubio-Tapia A, Murray JA. The liver in coeliac disease. *Hepatology* 2007;46:1650–1658.

48. Volta U, De Franceschi L, Lari F et al. Coeliac disease hidden by cryptogenic hypertransaminasemia. *Lancet* 1998;352:26–29.

49. Bardella MT, Vecchi M, Conte D et al. Chronic unexplained hypertransaminasemia may be caused by occult celiac disease. *Hepatology* 1999;29:654–657.

50. Day C, Adams PC. A chat on fat in the liver. *Can J Gastroenterol* 2006;20(7):461–462.

51. Cohen EB, Afdhal NH. Ultrasound based hepatic elastography: origins, limitations and applications. *J Clin Gastroenterol* 2010:44(9):637–645.

52. Lindsay K, Fraser AD, Layton A et al. Liver fibrosis in patients with psoriatic arthritis on long term cumulative dose methotrexate therapy. *Rheumatology* 2009;48:569–572.

53. Zachariae H, Heickendorff L, Sogaard H. The value of amino-terminal propeptide of type III procollagen in routine screening for methotrexate-induced liver fibrosis: a 10-year follow-up. *Br J Dermatol* 2001;144:100–103.

54. Zachariae H, Aslam HM, Bjerring P et al. Serum aminoterminal propeptide of type III procollagen in psoriasis and psoriatic arthritis: relation to liver fibrosis and arthritis. *J Am Acad Dermatol* 1991;25:50–53.

55. Duarte-Rojo A, Altamirano JT, Field JJ. Non-invasive markers of fibrosis: key concepts for improving accuracy in daily clinical practice. *Ann Hepatol* 2012;11(4): 426–443.

56. Levi M, Lotscher M, Sorribas V et al. Cellular mechanisms of acute and chronic adaptation of rat renal phosphate transporters to alterations in dietary phosphate. *Am J Physiol* 1994;267: F90.

57. Kuro-o M. Overview of the FGF23-Klotho axis. *Pediatr Nephrol* 2010;25:583–590.

58. Prie D, Friedlander G. Reciprocal control of 1,25-dihydroxyvitamin D and FGF23 formation involving the FGF23/Klotho system. *Clin J Am Soc Nephrol* 2010;5:1717–1722.

59. Jeon US. Kidney and calcium homeostasis. *Electrolyte Blood Press* 2008;6:68–76.

60. James MT, Zhang J, Lyon A et al. Derivation and internal validation of an equation for albumin adjusted calcium. *BMC Clin Pathol* 2008;8:12.

60a. Parent X, Spielmann C, Hanser AM. Corrected calcium status underestimation in non-hypoalbuminaemic patients and in hypercalcaemic patients. *Ann Biol Clin (Paris)* 2009;67(4):411–418.

60b. http://www.aacc.org/publications/cln/2011/September/Pages/calcium. aspx?[2/09/2011 11:06:08 AM] last accessed 28th June 2013.

61. Wang S, McDonnell EH, Sedor FA et al. PH effects on measurements of ionised calcium and ionised magnesium in blood. *Arch Pathol Lab* 2002;126(8):947.

62. Ladenson JH, Lewis JW, McDonald JM et al. Relationship of free and total calcium in hypercalcaemic conditions. *J Clin Endocrinol Metab* 1979;48(3):393.

63. Dalal B, Bridgen ML. Factitious biochemical measurements resulting from haematological conditions. *Am J Clin Pathol* 2009;131: 195–204.

64. English E, McFarlane I, Taylor KP et al. The effect of potassium EDTA on the stability of parathyroid hormone in whole blood. *Ann Clin Biochem* 2007;44(3):297–299.

65. Sturgeon CM, Sprague SM, Metcalfe W. Variation in parathyroid hormone immunoassay results: a critical governance issue in the management of chronic kidney disease. *Nephrol Dial Transplant* 2011;26:3440–3445.

66. Gardham C, Stevens P, Delaney M et al. Variability of parathyroid hormone and other markers of bone mineral metabolism in patients receiving haemodialysis. *Clin J Am Soc Nephrol* 2010;5(7):1261–1267.

67. Carter GD. Accuracy of 25 hydroxy-vitamin D assays: confronting the issues. *Curr Drug Targets* 2011;12(1):19–28.

68. Shobes AB, Kestenbaum B, Levin G et al. Seasonal variation in 25 hydroxy-vitamin D concentrations in the Cardiovascular Health Study. *Am J Epidemiol* 2011;174 (12):1363–1372.

69. Wesseling-Perry K. FGF-23: Is it ready for prime time? *Clin Chem* 2011;57(11):1–2.

70. Sandhu SK, Hampson G. The pathogenesis, diagnosis, investigation and management of osteoporosis. *J Clin Pathol* 2011;64:1042–1050.

71. Stokes FJ, Petko I, Bailey LM et al. The effects of sampling procedures and storage conditions on short term stability of blood based biochemical markers of bone metabolism. *Clin Chem* 2011;57:138–140.

CHAPTER 63

Autoimmune serology

Philip Hamann and Neil McHugh

Introduction

The term 'antibody' was first published in 1891 by Paul Ehrlich in an article on experimental studies of immunity. However, the concept of toxic autoantibodies was initially dismissed by Ehrlich's doctrine of the *'horror autotoxicus'*, or the implausibility of pathogenic autoimmunity. Driven largely by the desire to produce new vaccines to infective diseases, further investigations into autoimmunity were largely ignored; it was not until many decades later that the very concept of autoimmunity began to gain acceptance.

With Erik Waaler's, and subsequently Harry Rose's, discovery in the 1940s of rheumatoid factor (RF) from the agglutination of indicator sheep erythrocytes in serum of rheumatoid arthritis (RA) patients tested for syphilis, autoimmune serology found its first diagnostic use in helping to characterize RA. From this discovery, the pathophysiology of RA, and many other autoimmune conditions began to be understood.

Over the past 60 years, autoimmune serology has become central in the characterization of many rheumatic conditions. Indeed, in many cases the presence of an autoantibody may form part of the diagnostic criteria. Interpretation of serological results can be complex, due to varied terms and experimental methods. However, with a thorough understanding of the techniques and terms, as well as the clinico-pathological significance of autoantibodies, autoimmune serology can be extremely helpful in diagnosis and prognosis of many autoimmune conditions.

Serological methods for autoantibody detection

Indirect immunofluorescence

Indirect immunofluorescence (IMF) is a widely used and highly useful technique for screening for the presence of autoantibodies and in some cases for identification of the autoantibody specificity. The type of substrate used for IMF will depend on the autoantibody profile sought. HEp-2 epithelial cells are most commonly used for screening for the presence of an anti-nuclear antibody (ANA), as the individual organelles can be easily visualized and cell-cycle-specific autoantigens detected more readily as the cells are rapidly dividing. Other tissue substrates (e.g. murine liver, kidney, stomach, monkey oesophagus) are sometimes used for screening, but are less sensitive and may miss certain autoantibodies (e.g. anti-centromere

(ACA)) However, tissue substrates may detect other specificities sometimes seen in organ-specific autoimmune disease (e.g. anti-mitochondrial antibody in primary biliary cirrhosis, anti-endomysial antibodies in coeliac disease). Human neutrophils fixed in ethanol are used for screening for the presence of anti-neutrophil cytoplasmic antibodies (ANCA), with the immunofluorescence pattern providing some information on likely specificity. *Crithidia luciliae*, a haemoflagellate, possesses a giant mitochondrion containing a mass of double-stranded DNA (dsDNA), termed a kinetoplast, and is a useful substrate for confirming the presence of anti-dsDNA antibodies. Examples of typical ANA patterns seen on IMF are shown in Figure 63.1. In most cases additional techniques are needed to confirm autoantibody identity. Also, the IMF test is not a perfect screen and may be reported low titre or negative for some specificities (e.g. anti-Ro (-SSA)). Addressable laser bead assays are a more recent advance that provide a platform for simultaneous testing for multiple autoantibody specificities by flow cytometry. Selected antigens are attached to microspheres labelled with different ratios of fluorochromes for each antigen, creating a spectral array that can be quantitated for the reaction with the corresponding autoantibody. It remains uncertain whether the quantitative data obtained by multiplex bead assays yield similar data to other methods. In addition, bead assays rely on the relevant autoantigen being included in the system and therefore may miss the full repertoire of autoreactivity. Other IMF and non-IMF autoantigen microarray systems are under ongoing development.

Immunodiffusion

Gel diffusion techniques (e.g. Ouchterlony, counterimmune electrophoresis) are methods for detecting autoantibodies to autoantigens that can be purified from extracts (e.g. calf or rabbit thymus, human spleen)—hence the term extractable nuclear antigen (ENA). Traditionally autoantibodies to autoantigens such as Ro (-SSA) La (-SSB), U1-RNP, Sm, Jo-1, topoisomease-1 (-Scl-70), and PM-Scl have been identified by this method. However these techniques may be time consuming and relatively insensitive, and are being superseded by solid phase assays.

Enzyme-linked immunosorbent assay techniques

Enzyme-linked immunosorbent assay (ELISA) techniques are popular as they are more automated, less costly, and allow more widespread screening; recombinant proteins for a wide range of

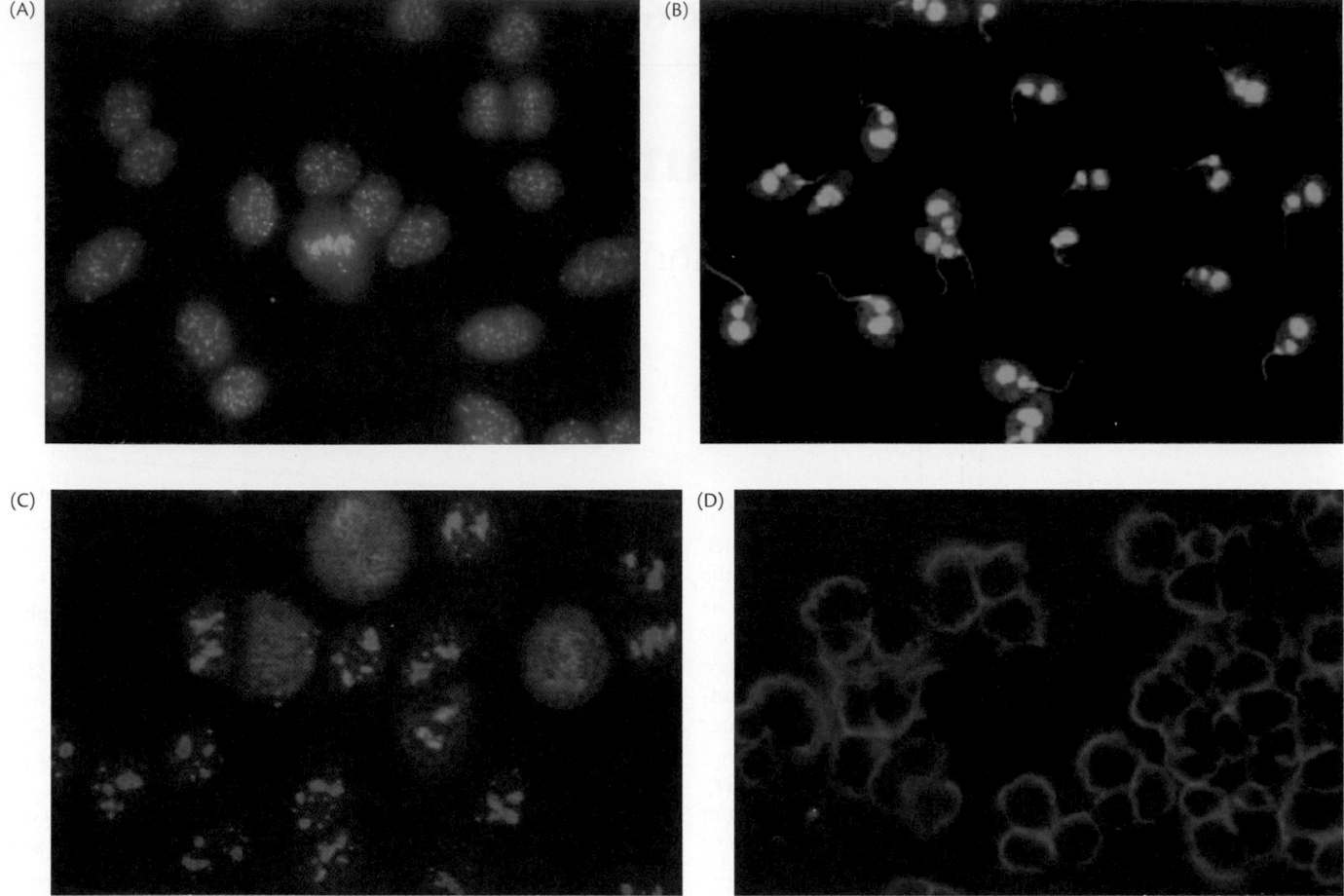

Fig. 63.1 Typical immunofluorescence patterns: (A) anticentromere staining during metaphase in HEp2 cells. (B) dsDNA in the kinetoplast of *Crithidia luciliae*. (C) nucleolar staining in HEp2 cells. (D) Perinuclear ANCA staining in human neutrophils.

autoantigen specificities have become available. ELISA methods may provide more false-positive results usually by non-specific binding of immunoglobulin, but work well for certain autoantibody systems. ELISA may be the sole method for detecting some autoantibody specificities such as anti-cardiolipin (aCL) and anti-β_2-glycoprotein I (anti-β2GPI), anti-citrullinated protein antigens (ACPA), or for confirming autoantibody specificity (e.g. type of ANCA). Also, as ELISA provides semiquantitative results there is the potential for more detailed investigation of how autoantibody levels relate to disease activity—e.g. ANCA levels and vasculitis, anti-dsDNA binding, and systemic lupus erythematosus (SLE).

Immunoblotting

Immunoblotting methods may provide advantages in determining the finer specificity of autoantigen recognition (e.g. the profile of polypeptide determinants within a complex autoantigen that an autoantibody recognizes). Dot-blots or line-blots are derivative methods that contain custom selected profiles of either purified or recombinant autoantigen; they are semiquantitative and gaining increased use.

Immunoprecipitation

Immunoprecipitation (IP) of either protein or RNA from cell lines followed by gel separation is the gold standard for detecting a large range of autoantibody specificities that are difficult to detect by other

means (Figure 63.2). The technique is not widely available, due to constraints from handling radioactivity and the expertise and labour intensity involved. However, certain nucleolar autoantibodies can still only be reliably detected by IP. Also IP may display additional autoantigen targets for which the specificity remains unknown.

Other methods

Agglutination techniques may still be used for detecting RF. The Rose–Waaler test using sheep cells is more specific than the RF latex test using beads. Other methods for detecting RF, including laser nephelometry or ELISA, are more commonly used. There may be the potential for false-positive results by ELISA due to the anti-globulin activity of RF. Fluid-phase radioimmunoassays such as the Farr assay for detecting high-affinity antibodies to dsDNA have been replaced by ELISA and/or the *Crithidiae* test (see above).

Autoantibodies

Antibodies to citrullinated protein antigens

ACPA are the most specific biomarkers in widespread use for detecting RA. Citrullination of peptides occurs during cell apoptosis and is mediated by the peptidyl-arginine deiminases (PADs) class of enzymes. Loss of cell wall integrity during apoptosis in an inflamed joint increases permeability to calcium and the resultant escalation in intracellular calcium levels activates PADs. PADs are present

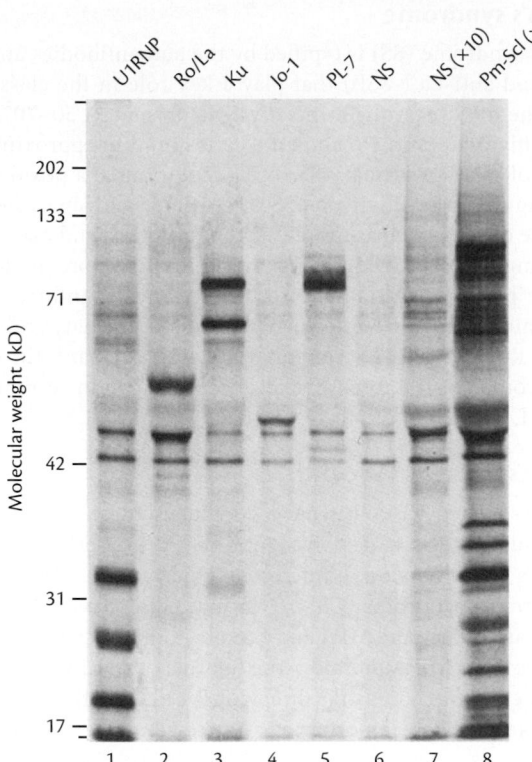

Fig. 63.2 Examples of some autoantibodies detected by the technique of immunoprecipitation. Each lane contains the autoantigen that has been precipitated out from a radiolabelled cell line by serum containing the autoantibody, then separated out on a SDS-PAGE gel and identified following autoradiography and according to its profile and molecular weight. NS, normal serum.

in high concentrations in neutrophils and monocytes, and their activation results in substitution of positively charged arginines by neutrally charged citrullines (citrullination) in autologous peptides. This increased citrullination of peptides in an inflamed joint may lead to the development of ACPA.[1] However the association of cigarette smoking with ACPA, particularly in shared epitope positive individuals, may indicate citrullination of peptides in the lung as the initiating event in ACPA formation (see Chapter 109).

Rheumatoid factor

RF are autoantibodies with specificity against the C-terminal domain of the constant region of the heavy chain in human IgG. Chronic inflammation and oxidative stress play a key role in altering the structure of IgG, which makes the constant region of the IgG more available and may enhance the development of RF.[2] Immune complexes of RF and autologous IgG and subsequent activation of complement and the inflammatory cascade leads to localized tissue damage. IgG RF also have the potential to activate cells via Fc-γ receptor binding.[3] Between 1% and 4% of healthy persons in a white population of European origin will have RF, and titre increases with age. RF can also form an important part of host defence against bacterial and viral pathogens.[2]

Anti-nuclear antibodies and extractable nuclear antibodies

ANA is a general term encompassing the group of antibodies to intranuclear antigens, that is sometimes generalized to include anti-cytoplasmic antibodies that may be detected using the same technique (also some autoantigens are located in both the cell nucleus and the cytoplasm). Although many ANAs are disease specific, positive results can be found in healthy individuals and results need interpretation within the clinical context. Approximately 3–5% of randomly selected healthy individuals in a white population of European origin will have a positive ANA, and the prevalence of healthy individuals with a positive ANA rises with increasing age.

ANA staining pattern on IMF can be grouped broadly into three subclasses: nucleoplasmic, nucleolar, and cytoplasmic.[4] Nucleoplasmic staining antibodies are further subclassified according to the pattern seen on IMF, into homogenous (which includes specificities for dsDNA, histone, chromatin, topoisomerase 1(-Scl70); speckled (Sm, nRNP, Ro (-SSA), La (-SSB), PCA, Ku, RNA polymerase II (RNAP II)); peripheral (Lamin A/B/C, nuclear pores); and centromere (CENP A/B/C). ACA is specific for systemic sclerosis (SSc) and requires no further quantification; however, all other nucleoplasmic antibodies require identification with further techniques.

Nucleolar staining antibodies are most commonly found in SSc and consist of antibodies to fibrillarin (U3-RNP), RNAP I/III, hUBF (-NOR-90), Pm-Scl, and Th(1–7).

Lastly, cytoplasmic staining antibodies seen on IMF comprise most of the myositis-related autoantibodies (aminoacyl tRNA synthetases, anti-SRP), as well as anti-mitochondrial antibodies, anti-ribosomal, anti-Golgi apparatus (Golgin), and anti-Ro (-SS-A).

Anti-neutrophil cytoplasm autoantibodies

ANCA are antibodies directed against the lysosomal compartment of neutrophils and monocytes. The two main subtypes of ANCA, anti-myeloperoxidase (anti-MPO) and anti-proteinase 3 antibodies (anti-PR3) yield a typical staining pattern on IMF that can be used as a screen, but ELISA is necessary for confirmation of specificity. A cytoplasmic ANCA (C-ANCA) pattern on IMF is associated with anti-PR3 antibodies, whereas perinuclear (P-ANCA) staining represents the presence of anti-MPO antibodies.

MPO and PR3 antigens are normally only present on intracellular granules. However, in primed neutrophils, these antigens migrate to the surface and are available for binding by ANCA. This leads to production of reactive oxygen species and release of proteolytic enzymes that cause vascular damage and localized inflammation.[5,6]

Anti-phospholipid antibodies

Anti-phospholipid antibodies refer to a heterogeneous group of antibodies variously directed against phospholipids and phospholipid binding proteins. Currently, aCL and anti-β2GPI are antibodies used in the diagnosis of anti-phospholipid syndrome (APS), although numerous other subsets of anti-phospholipid antibodies have been identified.

The presence of a lupus anticoagulant (LA) is demonstrated in vitro by an increase in clotting time in phospholipid-driven clotting studies (such as APTT, dRVVT, KCT). The lack of reversibility of increased clotting time when control plasma is added indicates the presence of an inhibitor of the reagent used to drive the reaction in vitro, rather than a lack of clotting factor from the original sample.[7] The term 'lupus anticoagulant' is a misnomer as the antibodies that cause a positive LA result may be found in conditions other than lupus and are prothrombotic (see Chapter 61).

Cardiolipin was initially identified as the antigen for aCL antibodies, but in the 1990s β2GPI, a cardiolipin binding protein, was identified as a major antigenic target of aCL antibodies. β2GPI is a phospholipid binding protein which has natural anticoagulant properties. Antibodies to β2GPI interfere with its anticoagulant properties, and alter the homeostatic mechanisms leading to a prothrombotic state.

Rheumatic conditions associated with specific antibodies

Rheumatoid arthritis

Approximately 55–70% of patients with RA are ACPA positive, whereas RF is present in less than 50% of patients with early RA, rising to 60–90% in more advanced disease.[8] ACPA is the most specific test for RA and has a sensitivity of around 67% and specificity of 95% compared with 69% and 85% respectively for RF.[9] ACPA are linked with smoking and are the strongest single predictor of radiographic progression in early RA. ACPA and RF titres are not useful biomarkers to assess response to treatment, and absolute antibody titres do not correlate with disease severity. Approximately 50%[10] of RA patients are dually positive for ACPA and RF and, in a healthy individual, dual positivity has a near 100% positive predictive value for the subsequent development of RA.[11] Although very specific for RA, ACPA may be found in low prevalence in other autoimmune conditions and some infections. RF is commonly found in many other autoimmune and infectious conditions and is a relatively non-specific marker for RA.

Systemic lupus erythematosus

ANA is a useful screening test for systemic lupus erythematosus (SLE) with a sensitivity of 90–95%. It's specificity is limited, however, with a positive predictive value of only 11–13%.[4] Anti-dsDNA titres correlate well with disease activity in SLE and a strongly positive, or rising, anti-dsDNA level often precedes onset of a flare (often lupus nephritis). Anti-Sm antibodies are virtually pathognomonic of SLE; they are present in 5–30% of patients with the condition and are associated with lupus nephritis, although antibody titre does not appear to correlate with disease activity.[12] Anti-U1RNP may coexist with anti-Sm, as they both target ribonuclear proteins on the spliceosome complex, but anti-U1RNP is less specific for SLE (found in 20–40% of cases[4]) and is a marker for mixed connective tissue disease (MCTD) when present in high titres.[12] Anti-ribosomal P antibodies are also highly specific to SLE and, in some studies but not others, linked with neuropsychiatric manifestations of the disease.

Anti-phospholipid syndrome

Due to the relative frequency of thromboses and miscarriage in the general population, the detection of anti-phospholipid antibodies plays a pivotal role in the diagnosis of APS. The presence of anti-phospholipid antibodies is associated with an increased risk of thrombosis.[13] The risk of thrombosis or fetal loss is greatest with high levels of IgG aCL together with the presence of a LA. As anti-β2GPI and aCL can be found often transiently in many other autoimmune conditions, acute infections as well as malignancies,[7] it is essential to confirm positivity with repeat sampling at least 12 weeks later.

Sjögren's syndrome

Sjögren's syndrome (SS) is typified by the autoantibodies anti-Ro (-SSA) and anti-La (-SSB) that play a key role in the classification of the disease. Anti-Ro positivity is present in 50–70% and dual positivity for anti-Ro and anti-La is found in approximately 30–60% of cases of primary SS (pSS). Single anti-La positivity is rarely found. Seropositivity in pSS is associated with an earlier age of disease onset as well as more frequent parotitis, and extraglandular complications. Sialogram abnormalities are more frequently found in patients with anti-Ro positivity and lip infiltration is more common in anti-La positive pSS.[14] Seropositivity and titres for anti-Ro and anti-La remain relatively constant throughout the course of the disease, and do not change in response to treatment.

ANCA-associated vasculitis

ANCA-associated vasculitis (AAV) includes three disease entities: granulomatosis with polyangiitis (GPA, formerly known as Wegener's granulomatosis), microscopic polyangiitis (MPA), and Churg–Strauss syndrome (CSS). Typically, GPA is associated with anti-PR3 antibodies and MPA and CSS are both associated with the presence of anti-MPO antibody. The full role of ANCA in AAVs is yet to be elucidated, but the efficacy of B-cell depletion therapies highlights their likely importance.

Inflammatory myositis and dermatomyositis

Autoantibodies in myositis are grouped into myositis-specific antibodies (MSA) and myositis-associated antibodies (MAA). MSAs include the anti-tRNA synthetases (e.g. anti-Jo-1), anti-SRP, and anti-Mi2, as well as more recently discovered antibodies.[15] The MSAs correlate very closely to disease phenotype and can be useful in directing screening for future complications of the disease.[16] The MAAs include anti-PMScl, anti-Ku, and anti-U1RNP and are found in myositis, but have a significant overlap with other connective tissue disorders, especially SSc. The largest group of MSAs consist of the anti-tRNA synthetases, which are associated with a symptom complex that has become known as the anti-synthetase syndrome. Features include inflammatory muscle disease, Raynaud's phenomenon, interstitial lung disease, characteristic cutaneous manifestations, and arthritis. Both dermatomyositis and myositis are associated with an increased incidence of malignancy,[17] especially in patients with antibodies to transcription intermediate factor-1 gamma (anti-TIF-1γ). Anti-SRP antibodies are associated with immune-mediated necrotizing myositis (IMNM), and antibodies to HMG CoA reductase with IMNM associated with the use of statins.

Systemic sclerosis

Over 90% of patients with SSc are ANA positive and in most cases a disease-specific autoantibody can be detected that is associated with certain clinical features The serotype can be useful in predicting the disease outcome as it does not alter significantly during the disease course.[18]

ACA and anti-topoisomerase-1 (-Scl-70) are the most commonly found antibodies in SSc (30–35% and 20–25% of cases respectively, and they hardly ever coexist). Anti-topoisomerase-1 (-Scl-70) can be found in both diffuse and limited cutaneous SSc and is more closely associated with pulmonary fibrosis, which contributes to a high mortality. Conversely, ACA are associated with a limited SSc (lSSc) phenotype with distal skin thickening, peripheral vascular damage, calcinosis, and isolated pulmonary hypertension (but not pulmonary fibrosis). ACA is generally associated with a better disease prognosis and a more indolent disease course. In patients with isolated Raynaud's, ACA can be predictive of future development of lSSc.[18]

RNAP-III antibodies are associated with diffuse SSc (dSSc) and internal organ involvement, with a renal preponderance. Historically, anti-RNAP III antibodies were associated with the worst prognosis due to their association with renal crises, but the development of angiotensin converting enzyme (ACE) inhibitors and improved medical management of renal disease has reduced mortality from this complication.

The remaining anti-nucleolar antibodies, are less commonly seen, but all have distinct disease phenotypes (see Table 63.1).

Mixed connective tissue disease

MCTD has overlapping clinical features of SLE, SSc, RA, and inflammatory myositis. It is characterized by the presence of anti-U1RNP, which is required to make a diagnosis of MCTD, as well as (less commonly) anti-U1RNA antibodies. A strongly positive speckled staining pattern is usually seen by IMF.[19] Anti-U1RNP can be detected before clinical disease onset, but symptoms usually develop within 1 year of antibody induction.[19] In some studies, anti-phospholipid and anti-endothelial antibodies have been detected with anti-U1RNP and appear to be predictive of pulmonary hypertension. The exact mechanism remains unknown, but could involve the activation of endothelial adhesion factors in the pulmonary vasculature along with the upregulation of cytokines, particularly interleukin (IL)-1 and IL-6.[20]

See Table 63.1 for a summary of antibodies and their associations with rheumatoid diseases.

Table 63.1 Antibodies associated with rheumatic disease

Antibody	Primary disease associations	Clinical association
ACPA	RA	Erosive joint disease
RF	RA	Erosive joint disease
Anti-nuclear antibodies (ANA)		
Anti-dsDNA	SLE	Lupus nephritis
Anti-Sm	SLE	Vasculitis, CNS lupus
Anti-ribosomal P	SLE	Neuropsychiatric manifestations
Anti-histone	Drug induced SLE when found in isolation	Use of: hydralazine, procainamide, isoniazid, methyldopa, chlorpromazine, quinidine, minocycline
Anti-chromatin	SLE, Drug induced lupus	Renal involvement
Anti-lamin A/B/C	SLE, APLS, and autoimmune hepatitis	
Anti-PCNA	SLE	
Anti-CENP A/B/C (Anti-centromere)	SSc	Limited cutaneous SSc, pulmonary hypertension (but not pulmonary fibrosis), female gender
Anti-topoisomerase 1 (Anti-Scl70)	SSc	Pulmonary fibrosis
Anti-U1-RNP	SSc, IM, MCTD	High levels with MCTD
Anti-Ku	SSc, IM and SLE	
Anti-fibrillarin (Anti-U3-RNP)	SSc	Pulmonary hypertension
Anti-PM-Scl	SSc/IM overlap	Myositis overlap
Anti-RNAP I & III	SSc	Renal involvement
Anti-Th (1–7)	SSc	Limited SSc and gastrointestinal complications
Anti-hUBF (Anti-NOR-90)	Non-specific marker of systemic autoimmune conditions including, SSc, SLE, RA, Sjögren's syndrome and malignancies	
Anti-Ro60 & 52 (SSA)	Sjogrens, SLE, myositis, and SSc. Single Anti-Ro52 positivity without Anti-La associated with IM	Sicca symptoms Anti-Ro52 with cardiac conduction abnormalities in neonatal lupus
Anti-La (SSB)	Sjogrens, SLE, IM, and SSc	Sicca symptoms Cardiac conduction abnormalities in neonatal lupus
Anti-aminoacyl tRNA synthetases[a]	IM	Anti-synthetase syndrome

(Continued)

Table 63.1 (*Continued*)

Antibody	Primary disease associations	Clinical association
Anti-SRP	IM	Necrotizing myopathy
Anti-p155/140 (Anti-TIF-1γ)	JDM, DM	JDM: DM and ulceration Adults: DM and malignancy
Anti-HMG CoA reductase	IM	Statin induced necrotizing myopathy
Anti-Mi2	DM	
Anti-nuclear pore	PBC	
Anti-mitochondrial	PBC	
Anti-Golgi apparatus	Non-specific autoimmune conditions	
Anti-neutrophil cytoplasm autoantibodies (ANCA)		
Anti-MPO	MPA, CSS, GPA (in order of association) also drug-induced lupus	Small to medium vessel vasculitis
Anti-PR3	GPA, MPA, CSS (in order of association)	Small to medium vessel vasculitis and granulomata
Anti-phospholipid antibodies (APA)		
aCL	APLS	Thromboembolic disease, pregnancy loss
aβ2GPI	APLS	Thromboembolic disease, pregnancy loss

aCL, anti-cardiolipin; ANA, anti-nuclear antibody; ANCA, anti-neutrophil cytoplasm autoantibody; anti-CENP, anti-centromeric peptide; APS, anti-phospholipid syndrome; aβ2GPI, anti-B2 glycoprotein I; CSS, Churg–Strauss syndrome; DM, dermatomyositis; dsDNA, double-stranded DNA; GPA, granulomatosis with polyangiitis (Wegener's disease); IM, inflammatory myositis; JDM, juvenile dermatomyositis; MCTD, mixed connective tissue disease; MPA, microscopic polyangiitis; PBC, primary biliary cirrhosis; RA, rheumatoid arthritis; RF, rheumatoid factor; SLE, systemic lupus erythmatosus; SSc, systemic sclerosis.

[a]Including: Jo-1 (anti-histidyl), PL-12 (alanyl), PL-7 (threonyl), EJ (glycyl), OJ (isoleucyl), KS (asparginyl), Ha (tyrosyl), Zo (phenylalanyl).

References

1. Demoruelle MK, Deane K. Antibodies to citrullinated protein antigens (ACPAs): clinical and pathophysiologic significance. *Curr Rheumatol Rep* 2011;13(5):421–430.

2. Renaudineau Y, Jamin C, Saraux A, Youinou P. *Rheumatoid factor on a daily basis. Autoimmunity* 2005;38(1):11–16.

3. Edwards JC, Cambridge G, Abrahams VM. Do self-perpetuating B lymphocytes drive human autoimmune disease? *Immunology* 1999;97(2):188–196.

4. Lyons R, Narain S, Nichols C, Satoh M, Reeves WH. Effective use of autoantibody tests in the diagnosis of systemic autoimmune disease. *Ann N Y Acad Sci* 2005;1050(1):217–228.

5. Kallenberg CGM, Heeringa P, Stegeman CA. Mechanisms of disease: pathogenesis and treatment of ANCA-associated vasculitides. *Nat Clin Pract Rheumatol* 2006;2(12):661–670.

6. Kallenberg CGM. Pathogenesis of ANCA-associated vasculitides. *Ann Rheum Dis* 2011;70(Suppl 1):i59–i63.

7. Urbanus RT, de Groot PG. Antiphospholipid antibodies—we are not quite there yet. *Blood Rev* 2011;25(2):97–106.

8. Steiner G. Auto-antibodies and autoreactive T-cells in rheumatoid arthritis: pathogenetic players and diagnostic tools. *Clin Rev Allergy Immunol* 2007;32(1):23–36.

9. Nishimura K, Sugiyama D, Kogata Y et al. Meta-analysis: diagnostic accuracy of anti-cyclic citrullinated peptide antibody and rheumatoid factor for rheumatoid arthritis. *Ann. Intern. Med* 2007;146(11):797–808.

10. Inanc N, Dalkilic E, Kamali S et al. Anti-CCP antibodies in rheumatoid arthritis and psoriatic arthritis. *Clin. Rheumatol* 2007;26(1):17–23.

11. Taylor P, Gartemann J, Hsieh J, Creeden J. A systematic review of serum biomarkers anti-cyclic citrullinated peptide and rheumatoid factor as tests for rheumatoid arthritis. *Autoimmune Dis* 2011; 2011:815038.

12. Migliorini P, Baldini C, Rocchi V, Bombardieri S. Anti-Sm and anti-RNP antibodies. *Autoimmunity* 2005;38(1):47–54.

13. Gershwin ME, Shoenfeld Y, Gershwin ME, Shoenfeld Y, Meroni P-L (eds). *Autoantibodies*, 2nd edn. Elsevier Science, Amsterdam, 2007:733–739.

14. Hernández-Molina G, Leal-Alegre G, Michel-Peregrina M. The meaning of anti-Ro and anti-La antibodies in primary Sjögren's syndrome. *Autoimmun Rev* 2011;10(3):123–125.

15. Betteridge ZE, Gunawardena H, McHugh NJ. Novel autoantibodies and clinical phenotypes in adult and juvenile myositis. *Arthritis Res Ther* 2011;13(2):209.

16. Gunawardena H, Betteridge ZE, McHugh NJ. Myositis-specific autoantibodies: their clinical and pathogenic significance in disease expression. *Rheumatology* 2009;48(6):607–612.

17. Zahr ZA, Baer AN. Malignancy in myositis. *Curr Rheumatol Rep* 2011; 13(3):208–215.

18. Hamaguchi Y. Autoantibody profiles in systemic sclerosis: Predictive value for clinical evaluation and prognosis. *J Dermatol* 2010;37(1):42–53.

19. Hoffman RW, Maldonado ME. Immune pathogenesis of mixed connective tissue disease: a short analytical review. *Clin. Immunol* 2008; 128(1):8–17.

20. Keith MP, Moratz C, Tsokos GC. Anti-RNP immunity: implications for tissue injury and the pathogenesis of connective tissue disease. *Autoimmun Rev* 2007;6(4):232–236.

CHAPTER 64

Complement

Matthew C. Pickering and Jyoti Bakshi

Complement biology

Complement was first identified as a heat-sensitive component in blood that enhanced ('complemented') the ability of antibodies to destroy bacteria. The biological functions of complement are: (1) host defence and the inflammatory response, (2) the physiological removal of immune complexes and dying cells ('waste disposal'), and (3) an accessory role in the induction of immune responses ('natural adjuvant'). Complement can be activated through three pathways (classical, lectin, and alternative pathways, Figure 64.1). All generate complexes that can cleave intact C3 to its active form,

C3b. C3b can be rapidly amplified through a feedback cycle termed the C3b amplification loop, resulting in opsonization of the activating surface. C3b can trigger the activation of complement C5 and the terminal pathway. This results in (1) the generation of the membrane attack complex (MAC), which can damage or lyse the activating surface, and (2) the production of C5a, a cleavage fragment of C5 that is a potent anaphylatoxin. Finally, C3b itself or further proteolytic fragments (sequentially termed iC3b and C3d) can interact with cellular receptors (termed complement receptors, Figure 64.1).

The triggers of the three pathways are distinct. The classical pathway is triggered by an interaction between C1q and antibody bound

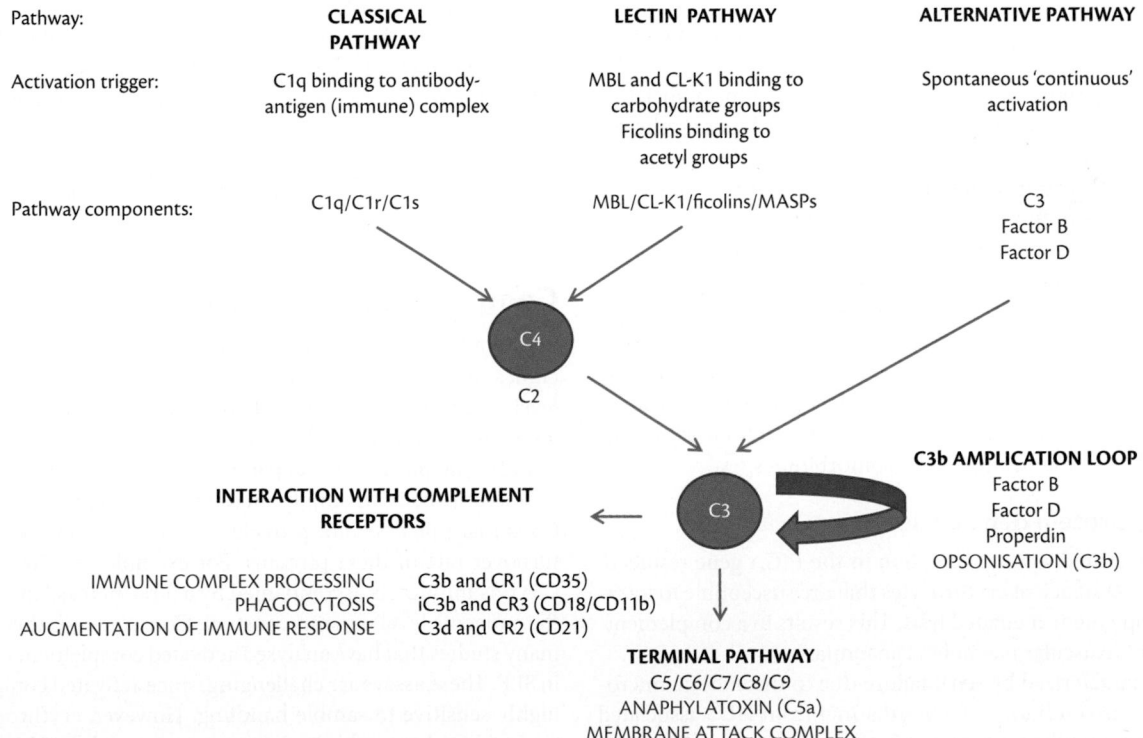

Fig. 64.1 Schematic depiction of the complement system. Complement is activated through three pathways that converge on C3. Each pathway has distinct activating signals. The detailed biochemistry of the activation pathways is not clinically relevant but it is important to note that C4 is one of the activation proteins of the classical pathway. Therefore, in immune complex disease where there is increased classical pathway activation, C4 levels are typically reduced with or without a reduction in C3 levels. Only rarely is isolated reduction in C3 seen and this usually indicates abnormal activation of the alternative pathway. Key complement functions are depicted in red. C4 and C3 are schematically emphasised as these are the most frequently measured activation proteins. The other activation proteins are depicted in blue within their respective pathways. MBL, mannose-binding lectin; MASP, MBL-associated serine protease.

to antigen (immune complex). The lectin pathway is triggered by pattern recognition molecules that recognize carbohydrate or acetyl residues on surfaces. These include mannose-binding lectin (MBL), CL-K1 (CDC (cell division cycle)-like kinase 1) and ficolins.[1] (Degn et al.[1] is a key reference, providing a comprehensive review of complement biology and disease-associated complement mutations). The alternative pathway does not require a specific trigger. It is in a continuous state of activation, constantly generating C3b.

Complement activation is controlled by regulatory proteins that act at multiple steps in the activation pathways. Clinically, key regulators are C1 inhibitor (C1INH), CD59, factor H, and factor I. C1INH prevents classical pathway activation and is defective in hereditary angioedema (HAE). CD59 inhibits the MAC and is deficient on erythrocytes in paroxysmal nocturnal haemoglobinuria (PNH). Factor H and factor I regulate the alternative pathway and deficiencies are associated with C3 glomerulopathy and atypical haemolytic uraemic syndrome (aHUS).

Complement deficiency states

Complement deficiency states can be divided into those due to impaired activation and those due to excessive activation (Table 64.1).

Activation protein deficiencies

Increased susceptibility to childhood pyogenic bacterial infection is frequently seen for many of the homozygous deficiencies, whereas heterozygous deficiency is usually asymptomatic (Table 64.1). Infections become less frequent or even absent during adulthood when the protective antibody repertoire has expanded.[2] Alternative and terminal pathway deficiencies are particularly associated with neisserial infection.[3]

The most important non-infective phenotype is the association between classical pathway deficiency and systemic lupus erythematosus (SLE). Over 95% of homozygous C1q-deficient individuals develop SLE.[4] The reasons for this association are complex and include abnormal immune complex processing and impaired tolerance to autoantigens through defective clearance of apoptotic cells (see Chapter 115). The association between C2 deficiency and SLE is much less strong and is approximately 10%.[4]

Homozygous deficiencies are rare with the exception of C2, MBL and, in Japanese populations, C9 deficiency. C2 deficiency occurs in 1:20 000 individuals and is usually asymptomatic. MBL deficiency occurs in 5–10% of individuals but increased infection risk is only seen if there are immunosuppressive comorbidities.[1,5]

Regulatory protein deficiencies

In PNH an acquired somatic mutation in the *PIGA* gene results in a clone of CD59-deficient erythrocytes that are susceptible to intravascular complement-mediated lysis. This results in a complement-dependent intravascular haemolytic anaemia.

aHUS is characterized by renal failure due to thrombotic microangiopathy. This condition, which is distinct from HUS associated with shigatoxin-producing strains of *E. coli*, is associated with mutations in the alternative pathway. These mutations result in impaired regulation of complement along the renal endothelium. This results in a complement-dependent thrombotic microangiopathy.

C3 glomerulopathy is characterized by isolated accumulation of C3 within glomeruli. This condition is associated with impaired regulation of the alternative pathway in plasma. This results in the accumulation of C3 along the glomerular basement membrane with consequent glomerulonephritis. Examples include dense deposit disease and complement factor H-related protein 5 nephropathy.[6–8]

HAE is associated with heterozygous C1INH deficiency. It is an autosomal dominant condition which may be due to absent (type I) or dysfunctional (type II) C1INH. Rarely, SLE and lymphoproliferative disorders may be associated with C1INH deficiency due to anti-C1INH autoantibodies.[9]

Important features that suggest HAE are: (1) recurrent angioedema, lasting more than 24 hours, non-pruritic and not responsive to anti-histamines, (2) absence of urticaria, (3) unexplained abdominal pain, especially if recurrent and 'colicky' in nature, (4) a family history of any of these features, and (5) low C4 level.[10]

C1INH is a protease inhibitor with multiple biological actions. It is a complement inhibitor (inhibiting the classical and lectin pathways) from which it derives its name. In C1INH deficiency uncontrolled classical pathway activation results in a low C4 level.

To appreciate the pathophysiology of HAE it is critical to understand that C1INH has multiple actions outside of its role as an inhibitor of the complement C1 complex.[11] It inhibits proteases of the contact system (kallikrein and factor XIIa), the coagulation system (thrombin), and the fibrinolytic system (plasmin and tissue plasminogen activator). The pathogenesis of the angioedema in C1INH deficiency relates to its role as an inhibitor of factor XIIa and kallikrein of the contact system. Failure of C1INH to inhibit these enzymes results in uncontrolled bradykinin generation and angioedema.

Mutations in the contact system that result in HAE in the presence of normal C1INH (type III HAE) have been reported.[12–14] Type III hereditary angioedema predominantly affects females and is associated with high oestrogen levels.

The commonest cause of acquired angioedema is angiotensin converting enzyme (ACE) inhibitors which impair the breakdown of bradykinin through the inhibition of kininase II.[15]

Complement investigations

The standard and specialized complement assays typically used in clinical practice are listed in Table 64.2. Most commonly antigenic levels of circulating C3 and C4 are measured in rheumatology clinics as part of the laboratory assessment of SLE activity. Low levels indicate enhanced classical pathway activation and active disease.

One drawback in simply measuring antigenic levels of C3 and C4 is that this does not provide information about the metabolic turnover rate of these proteins. For example, if a 50% increase in C3 consumption is accompanied by a 50% increase in C3 synthesis the antigenic level remains constant. Consequently, there have been many studies that have analysed activated complement components in SLE. These assays are challenging, since activated components are highly sensitive to sample handling. However, erythrocyte-bound C3d and C4d are stable and measurement of these SLE biomarkers may be feasible in clinical practice.[16]

A particular difficulty can arise with interpretation of C4 levels in SLE. The C4 gene locus is extremely complex, with frequent variation in both the number and size of C4 genes. In one study the number of C4 genes in healthy individuals varied between two and

Table 64.1 Complement deficiency and disease

Complement deficiency	Phenotype	Comments
Activation proteins		
Classical pathway deficiency: C1q, C1r, C1s, C2, C4	SLE Recurrent encapsulated bacterial infections	All extremely rare except C2 deficiency where estimated prevalence is 1:20 000 Association with SLE weakest for C2 deficiency
Alternative pathway deficiency: factor B, factor D	Recurrent meningococcal infections Recurrent encapsulated bacterial infections	All extremely rare (factor B deficiency only reported in a single incompletely characterized case)
Lectin pathway deficiency: MBL, ficolins, MASP-1, MASP-2 and MASP-3, CL-K1	Increased infection among immunocompromised individuals (MBL deficiency) H-ficolin deficiency associated with necrotizing enterocolitis Mutations in the genes encoding CL-K1 (*COLEC11*) and MASP-3 and MASP-1 (*MASP1*) associated with an autosomal recessive developmental syndrome termed '3MC syndrome'[a]	All extremely rare except MBL deficiency where estimated prevalence is 5-10% in white populations
Terminal pathway C5, C6, C7, C8 and C9	Recurrent meningococcal infections	All rare except C9 deficiency in Japanese where estimated prevalence is 1:1000
C3	Recurrent encapsulated bacterial infections Membranoproliferative glomerulonephritis (rare) SLE-like illness (rare)	Extremely rare
Regulatory proteins		
C1INH Negative regulator of: ♦ classical and lectin pathways ♦ contact system ♦ coagulation system ♦ fibrinolytic system	Hereditary angioedema	Estimated prevalence 1:50 000 Angioedema results from uncontrolled production of bradykinin due to dysregulation of the contact system, i.e. does not arise from uncontrolled complement activation Associated with low C4 due to uncontrolled classical pathway activation
Factor H, factor I, and CD46 Negative regulators of the alternative pathway and C3b amplification loop	aHUS C3 glomerulopathy	All rare aHUS manifests in heterozygous deficiency states Complete factor H deficiency associated with both aHUS and C3 glomerulopathy
Factor H-related protein 5 Putative modulator of C3 processing within the kidney—biological function incompletely understood	C3 glomerulopathy ('CFHR5 nephropathy')	Rare Predominantly individuals with Cypriot ancestry
CD59 Negative regulator of terminal pathway activation	Paroxysmal nocturnal haemoglobinuria	Rare Acquired somatic mutation Renders CD59-deficient erythrocytes susceptible to complement-mediated intravascular haemolysis
Properdin Positive regulator of C3 activation	Recurrent meningococcal infections	Rare X-linked deficiency

aHUS, atypical haemolytic uraemic syndrome; C1INH, C1 inhibitor; CD46, also known as membrane cofactor protein; CL-K1, also known as collectin-11; HUS, haemolytic uraemic syndrome; MBL, mannose-associated lectin; MASP-2, MBL-associated serine protease; SLE, systemic lupus erythematosus.
[a] 3MC syndrome is a term used to describe clinically identical syndromes that were independently described: the Mingarelli, Malpuech, Michels, and Carnevale syndromes.

five and there was a positive correlation between C4 levels and gene number.[17] C4 null alleles are frequent in SLE patients.[18] Therefore where a low C4 level is detected in healthy individuals or where a C4 level in an SLE patient remains low despite absence of active disease, the cause may be C4 genetic variation not classical pathway activation. The number and size of C4 genes can be measured in specialized complement laboratories, although this is rarely indicated.

C1INH assessment includes both antigenic and functional assays to detect type I and II deficiency.

Screening for activation protein deficiency starts with functional assays that test the integrity of the three activation pathways. These are available in most laboratories, typically as CH100 and AP100, (Table 64.2) with lectin pathway assessed using an ELISA-based assay. If these assays yield abnormal results, referral

Table 64.2 Complement investigations

Standard assays	Comments
Serum C4	Reduced levels usually indicate classical pathway activation or presence of C4 null alleles
	If C4 low with normal C3 this indicates predominant classical pathway activation and typical causes include:
	◆ Active SLE
	◆ HUVS
	◆ C1 inhibitor deficiency
	◆ Mixed essential cryoglobulinaemia
	◆ Rheumatoid vasculitis
	◆ Chronic infections associated with immune complex formation, e.g. subacute bacterial endocarditis
Serum C3	Reduced levels indicate complement activation
	Commonly reduced in active SLE, usually in combination with reduced C4 level, indicating classical pathway activation
	Low C3 with normal C4 indicates predominant alternative pathway activation. This is rare and causes include:
	◆ Poststreptococcal glomerulonephritis
	◆ C3 glomerulopathy, e.g. dense deposit disease
CH100	Functional test in which classical pathway activation is triggered in vitro and terminal pathway activation assessed by measurement of the membrane attack complex either directly (using anti-C5b-9 antibodies) or indirectly (using red cell lysis)
	Normal CH100 requires intact classical pathway, functional C3 and intact terminal pathway
	Important test to screen for complement deficiency
AP100	Functional test in which alternative pathway activation is triggered in vitro and terminal pathway activation assessed by measurement of the membrane attack complex either directly (using anti-C5b-9 antibodies) or indirectly (using red cell lysis)
	Normal AP100 requires intact alternative pathway, functional C3 and intact terminal pathway
	Important test to screen for complement deficiency
C1 inhibitor (C1INH) assays	Standard assays test both antigenic and functional activity of C1INH
	Essential test to detect type I and type II hereditary angioedema
Specialized assays	
Anti-C1q antibodies	Associated with SLE nephritis but not routinely measured in clinical practice
	Indicated in suspected HUVS
C3 nephritic factor	Represents an autoantibody that enhances the C3 convertase of the alternative pathway
	Associated with enhanced alternative pathway activation
	Indicated in C3 glomerulopathy
Anti-factor H autoantibodies	Associated with enhanced alternative pathway activation
	Indicated in atypical HUS and C3 glomerulopathy
Mutation screening for structural and sequence variation in complement genes encoding alternative pathway proteins and regulators	Indicated in patients with atypical HUS prior to renal transplantation

HUS, haemolytic uraemic syndrome; HUVS, hypocomplementaemic urticarial vasculitis; SLE, systemic lupus erythematosus.

to specialized complement laboratories is required to define the specific defect.

Specialized assays include anti-C1q autoantibodies which are strongly associated with the development of glomerulonephritis in SLE (reviewed by Pickering and Botto[19]). In addition they are a defining serological feature of hypocomplementaemic urticarial vasculitis syndrome (HUVS).[19] These antibodies rise prior to lupus nephritis flares,[20] and serial measurements may be helpful in this setting.

In C3 glomerulopathy and aHUS complement genetic screening, in addition to specialized serological assays such as C3 nephritic factor and anti-factor H autoantibodies, may be indicated and are best guided by specialist expertise.

Hypocomplementemic urticarial vasculitis syndrome

HUVS is a rare multisystem disorder first recognized in the early 1970s.[21-23]

Classification criteria and clinical features

Originally patients were identified on the basis of the presence of unexplained urticarial rash with biopsy evidence of leucocytoclastic vasculitis together with evidence of hypocomplementaemia (low C1q, C2, and C4) and anti-C1q antibodies.[22] (Wisnieski et al.[22] is a key reference, outlining the clinical spectrum of HUVS.)

Using these criteria the most frequent clinical manifestations were angioedema, ocular inflammation, mesangial or membranoproliferative glomerulonephritis, and chronic obstructive pulmonary disease (COPD).[22] Typically the urticarial lesions persist for more than 24 hours (distinguishing them from non-vasculitic urticaria). It is important to consider the presence of cardiac valvular abnormalities in these patients, a complication that may accompany Jaccoud's arthropathy.[24,25]

Pathogenesis

Anti-C1q autoantibodies bind to the collagen-like region of C1q. They have been demonstrated in murine models to enhance complement activation triggered by C1q-containing immune complexes in the kidney.[26] Conceptually they can be thought of as acquired factors that augment classical pathway activation by tissue-bound C1q-containing immune complexes.[27] Of course this mechanism would be predicted to apply to immune complex-triggered complement activation at any site and not just within the glomerulus. Whether a similar mechanism could operate at other tissue sites is not known.

Hypocomplementaemia is a defining part of the syndrome. Typically the classical pathway proteins (C1q, C2, and C4) together with C3 are reduced.[23] In common practice C4 and C3 are the most useful tests as, unlike C1q and C2 assays, these are widely available in clinical practice. Levels of alternative and terminal pathway proteins are not affected.

Histologically the cutaneous lesions in HUVS are leucocytoclastic vasculitis. One report has described pulmonary capillaritis and severe panacinar emphysema in an affected individual with progressive COPD.[28] In one report of valvulopathy histological analysis demonstrated acute necrotizing endocarditis and fibrin deposition on the surface of valve leaflets.[24]

Diagnosis

The diagnosis is established by (1) the presence of urticarial vasculitis with biopsy evidence of leucocytoclastic vasculitis, (2) evidence of hypocomplementaemia (low C4 with or without low C3), (3) the presence of anti-C1q autoantibodies, and (4) exclusion of SLE.

Case series have used other criteria such as: the presence of typical urticarial skin lesions and hypocomplementaemia together with two of the following: dermal venulitis, arthritis, glomerulonephritis, episcleritis or uveitis, recurrent abdominal pain, and anti-C1q antibodies.[21] In these studies individuals with positive anti-nuclear and/or anti-dsDNA antibodies were excluded.

Differential diagnosis

SLE and mixed essential cryoglobulinaemia are the important differential diagnoses to consider in patients with hypocomplementaemia and cutaneous vasculitis.

Treatment

HUVS is a rare condition and there are no published controlled trials investigating therapy. Consequently, therapeutic considerations derive from case series. Corticosteroid therapy is effective and usually combined with steroid-sparing agents such as methotrexate, azathioprine, and mycophenolate mofetil. Dapsone[29] and hydroxychloroquine[30] have been used in the treatment of the cutaneous lesions but may be more effective in combination with glucocorticoids or other immunosuppressive therapy.

It is imperative that patients with HUVS are strongly discouraged from smoking as this condition is associated with significant lung involvement which is accelerated by smoking.[21]

Therapeutic manipulation of the complement system

C1 inhibitor

C1INH deficiency can be treated by (1) increasing production of C1INH by the unaffected allele since the condition is due to heterozygous deficiency, (2) preventing C1INH breakdown, and (3) C1INH replacement.[31] The last strategy is most commonly used and there are now three C1INH preparations available for clinical use. Two are derived from plasma, Berinert P[32] and Cinryze,[33] and the third is a recombinant C1INH molecule, named Rhucin.[34] All are administered intravenously so there are inherent practical difficulties with this approach.

Increased production of C1INH through the use of attenuated androgen therapy has been used but side effects are poorly tolerated. Prevention of C1INH consumption with tranexamic acid has also been used but again is limited by side-effect profile.[10]

C1INH is rapidly effective in acute attacks of oedema. In one study of laryngeal oedema, the most feared complication, administration of C1INH reduced the median duration of the attack from 100 ± 26 hours to 15 ± 9 hours.[35] C1INH should be given rapidly at the first sign of an attack and prophylaxis considered if attacks are frequent or patients are undergoing procedures that may trigger an attack, e.g. dental procedures. A detailed consensus document outlining approaches to home therapy has recently been published.[36]

With the knowledge that the pathogenesis of the angioedema results from dysregulated bradykinin production, two other therapeutic approaches have been developed: bradykinin B2 receptor blockade (icatibant, a 10-amino-acid peptide) and inhibition of kallikrein (ecallantide, a 60-amino-acid protein). Both are effective in acute attacks,[37,38] can be administered subcutaneously, and, unlike C1INH preparations, are effective in type III angioedema.

Eculizumab (monoclonal anti-complement C5 antibody)

Eculizumab is a monoclonal antibody that blocks complement C5 activation.[39] It prevents the production of the anaphylatoxin C5a and the generation of the MAC. It is licensed for the treatment of transfusion-dependent haemolytic anaemia in PNH.[40] In this condition MAC-mediated lysis of the abnormal CD59-deficient erythrocytes is prevented and transfusion requirements reduce or cease. It is administered intravenously and has the important side effect of increased susceptibility to neisserial infection. This is a predictable side effect since it is well known that terminal pathway deficiencies are associated with increased susceptibility to neisserial infection and eculizumab induces an acquired C5 (and therefore terminal pathway) deficiency state. Patients receiving this agent are therefore immunized against neisserial strains and, if needed, treated with prophylactic antibiotic therapy.

Recently eculizumab has been shown to be effective in treating patients with aHUS,[41,42] and is now licensed for this indication both in the United States and in Europe. Its efficacy reflects the observation that C5 activation along the renal endothelium is critical for the thrombotic microangiopathy to develop.[43]

References

1. Degn SE, Jensenius JC, Thiel S. Disease-causing mutations in genes of the complement system. *Am J Hum Genet* 2011; 88:689–705.

2. Sjoholm AG, Jonsson G, Braconier JH, Sturfelt G, Truedsson L. Complement deficiency and disease: an update. *Mol Immunol* 2006;43:78–85.

3. Ross SC, Densen P. Complement deficiency states and infection: epidemiology, pathogenesis and consequences of neisserial and other infections in an immune deficiency. *Medicine* (Baltimore) 1984;63:243–273.

4. Pickering MC, Botto M, Taylor PR, Lachmann PJ, Walport MJ. Systemic lupus erythematosus, complement deficiency, and apoptosis. *Adv Immunol* 2000;76:227–324.

5. Botto M, Kirschfink M, Macor P et al. Complement in human diseases: Lessons from complement deficiencies. *Mol Immunol* 2009;46:2774–2783.

6. Gale DP, de Jorge EG, Cook HT et al. Identification of a mutation in complement factor H-related protein 5 in patients of Cypriot origin with glomerulonephritis. *Lancet* 2010;376:794–801.

7. Gale DP, Pickering MC. Regulating complement in the kidney: insights from CFHR5 nephropathy. *Dis Model Mech* 2011;4:721–726.

8. Smith RJ, Harris CL, Pickering MC. Dense deposit disease. *Mol Immunol* 2011;48:1604–1610.

9. Cicardi M, Zingale LC, Pappalardo E, Folcioni A, Agostoni A. Autoantibodies and lymphoproliferative diseases in acquired C1-inhibitor deficiencies. *Medicine* (Baltimore) 2003;82:274–281.

10. Gompels MM, Lock RJ, Abinun M et al. C1 inhibitor deficiency: consensus document. *Clin Exp Immunol* 2005;139:379–394.

11. Cugno M, Zanichelli A, Foieni F, Caccia S, Cicardi M. C1-inhibitor deficiency and angioedema: molecular mechanisms and clinical progress. *Trends Mol Med* 2009;15:69–78.

12. Bork K, Gul D, Hardt J, Dewald G. Hereditary angioedema with normal C1 inhibitor: clinical symptoms and course. *Am J Med* 2007;120: 987–992.

13. Cichon S, Martin L, Hennies HC et al. Increased activity of coagulation factor XII (Hageman factor) causes hereditary angioedema type III. *Am J Hum Genet* 2006;79:1098–1104.

14. Dewald G, Bork K. Missense mutations in the coagulation factor XII (Hageman factor) gene in hereditary angioedema with normal C1 inhibitor. *Biochem Biophys Res Commun* 2006;343:1286–1289.

15. Hoover T, Lippmann M, Grouzmann E, Marceau F, Herscu P. Angiotensin converting enzyme inhibitor induced angio-oedema: a review of the pathophysiology and risk factors. *Clin Exp Allergy* 2009;40:50–61.

16. Kao AH, Navratil JS, Ruffing MJ et al. Erythrocyte C3d and C4d for monitoring disease activity in systemic lupus erythematosus. *Arthritis Rheum* 2010;62:837–844.

17. Yang Y, Chung EK, Zhou B et al. Diversity in intrinsic strengths of the human complement system: serum C4 protein concentrations correlate with C4 gene size and polygenic variations, hemolytic activities, and body mass index. *J Immunol* 2003;171:2734–2745.

18. Pickering MC, Walport MJ. Links between complement abnormalities and systemic lupus erythematosus. *Rheumatology* (Oxford) 2000;39:133–141.

19. Pickering MC, Botto M. Are anti-C1q antibodies different from other SLE autoantibodies? *Nat Rev Rheumatol* 2010;6:490–493.

20. Sinico RA, Rimoldi L, Radice A et al. Anti-C1q autoantibodies in lupus nephritis. *Ann N Y Acad Sci* 2009;1173:47–51.

21. Schwartz HR, McDuffie FC, Black LF, Schroeter AL, Conn DL. Hypocomplementemic urticarial vasculitis: association with chronic obstructive pulmonary disease. *Mayo Clin Proc* 1982;57:231–238.

22. Wisnieski JJ, Baer AN, Christensen J et al. Hypocomplementemic urticarial vasculitis syndrome. Clinical and serologic findings in 18 patients. *Medicine* (Baltimore) 1995;74:24–41.

23. Zeiss CR, Burch FX, Marder RJ et al. A hypocomplementemic vasculitic urticarial syndrome. Report of four new cases and definition of the disease. *Am J Med* 1980;68:867–875.

24. Houser SL, Askenase PW, Palazzo E, Bloch KJ. Valvular heart disease in patients with hypocomplementemic urticarial vasculitis syndrome associated with Jaccoud's arthropathy. *Cardiovasc Pathol* 2002;11: 210–216.

25. Palazzo E, Bourgeois P, Meyer O et al. Hypocomplementemic urticarial vasculitis syndrome, Jaccoud's syndrome, valvulopathy: a new syndromic combination. *J Rheumatol* 1993;20:1236–1240.

26. Trouw LA, Groeneveld TW, Seelen MA et al. Anti-C1q autoantibodies deposit in glomeruli but are only pathogenic in combination with glomerular C1q-containing immune complexes. *J Clin Invest* 2004;114: 679–688.

27. Holers VM. Anti-C1q autoantibodies amplify pathogenic complement activation in systemic lupus erythematosus. *J Clin Invest* 2004;114: 616–619.

28. Hunt DP, Weil R, Nicholson AG et al. Pulmonary capillaritis and its relationship to development of emphysema in hypocomplementaemic urticarial vasculitis syndrome. *Sarcoidosis Vasc Diffuse Lung Dis* 2006;23:70–72.

29. Fortson JS, Zone JJ, Hammond ME, Groggel GC. Hypocomplementemic urticarial vasculitis syndrome responsive to dapsone. *J Am Acad Dermatol* 1986;15:1137–1142.

30. Lopez LR, Davis KC, Kohler PF, Schocket AL. The hypocomplementemic urticarial-vasculitis syndrome: therapeutic response to hydroxychloroquine. *J Allergy Clin Immunol* 1984;73:600–603.

31. Morgan BP. Hereditary angioedema—therapies old and new. *N Engl J Med* 2011;363:581–583.

32. Krassilnikova S, Craig ET, Craig TJ. Summary of the International Multicenter Prospective Angioedema C1-inhibitor Trials 1 and 2 (IMPACT1 and 2). *Expert Rev Clin Immunol* 2010;6:327–334.

33. Zuraw BL, Busse PJ, White M et al. Nanofiltered C1 inhibitor concentrate for treatment of hereditary angioedema. *N Engl J Med* 2010;363: 513–522.

34. Zuraw B, Cicardi M, Levy RJ et al. Recombinant human C1-inhibitor for the treatment of acute angioedema attacks in patients with hereditary angioedema. *J Allergy Clin Immunol* 2010;126:821–827 e814.

35. Bork K, Barnstedt SE. Treatment of 193 episodes of laryngeal edema with C1 inhibitor concentrate in patients with hereditary angioedema. *Arch Intern Med* 2001;161:714–718.

36. Longhurst HJ, Farkas H, Craig T et al. HAE international home therapy consensus document. *Allergy Asthma Clin Immunol* 2010;6:22.

37. Cicardi M, Banerji A, Bracho F et al. Icatibant, a new bradykinin-receptor antagonist, in hereditary angioedema. *N Engl J Med* 2010;363:532–541.

38. Cicardi M, Levy RJ, McNeil DL et al. Ecallantide for the treatment of acute attacks in hereditary angioedema. *N Engl J Med* 2010;363:523–531.

39. Parker CJ, Kar S, Kirkpatrick P. Eculizumab. *Nat Rev Drug Discov* 2007;6:515–516..*KEY REFERENCE Comprehensive review of the first human complement inhibitor to enter clinical practice

40. Hillmen P, Young NS, Schubert J et al. The complement inhibitor eculizumab in paroxysmal nocturnal hemoglobinuria. *N Engl J Med* 2006;355:1233–1243.

41. Gruppo RA, Rother RP. Eculizumab for congenital atypical hemolytic-uremic syndrome. *N Engl J Med* 2009;360:544–546.

42. Nurnberger J, Philipp T, Witzke O et al. Eculizumab for atypical hemolytic-uremic syndrome. *N Engl J Med* 2009;360:542–544.

43. de Jorge EG, Macor P, Paixao-Cavalcante D et al. The development of atypical hemolytic uremic syndrome depends on complement C5. *J Am Soc Nephrol* 2011;22:137–145.

CHAPTER 65

Limb anatomy and medical imaging

Mike Benjamin, Dennis McGonagle,
Maribel I. Miguel, David A. Bong,
and Ingrid Möller

Introduction

In ultrasonography (US) there is clearly a need for identifying and naming specific anatomical structures so that the topography of a limb can be successfully navigated. However, this is comprehensively covered by modern atlases.[1,2] What is more often ignored in writings aimed principally at clinicians is a discussion of basic limb anatomical principles. This is now highly relevant with the widespread availability of high-resolution US, which can routinely distinguish between structures 0.1–0.2 mm apart; the highest-resolution machines can resolve down to 0.04 mm. The resultant superb image definition, along with the ability to examine tissues dynamically and evaluate their vasculature, gives the clinical imager access to the body that was previously limited to anatomists.

Our purpose is to present a more generalized framework for understanding basic principles of limb anatomy and function. The aim is help the clinician to master the anatomic component of image acquisition and interpretation in a way analogous to that of a mathematician applying a series of general formulae to solve a specific problem. This can help the sonographer with this challenging anatomic aspect of image acquisition and interpretation, going beyond the two-dimensional world of the 'semiotic slice' into real three-dimensional anatomy.

Basic design of the limbs

Upper limb

The upper limb is ultimately geared towards enabling the hand to move with ease and precision anywhere in three-dimensional space. This principal is underpinned by the distribution of different types of synovial joints in the limb—e.g. a shoulder ball and socket joint, elbow hinge and pivot joints, and finger hinge joints. It also means that the heaviest part of the limb must be proximal and the lightest distal, so that the limb tapers towards its free end. All this is necessary to economize the effort needed to move the hand and fingers. Consequently, the biggest muscles are proximal

(e.g. pectoralis major, latissimus dorsi, deltoid) but the most numerous and longest tendons are distal (e.g. any of the tendons operating the digits). Many tendons are thus crowded into the wrist region, placing a premium on space in the carpal tunnel, which must also accommodate the median nerve. Anything that reduces space in the tunnel (e.g. synovitis) may compress the nerve and result in neuropathy. Because the hand must be the smallest and lightest of the three segments of the upper limb, it follows that its intrinsic muscles are also the smallest. They promote precise movements of the fingers, whereas the larger forearm muscles facilitate a more powerful, gripping action of the hand. From the imaging perspective, these principles require techniques to be valid in the detection of subtle changes in very small and densely packed structures. This is exemplified by the sonographer's ability to detect changes in the median nerve in the case of carpal tunnel syndrome and its potential aetiology with the evaluation of surrounding structures (Figure 65.1).[3,4]

Lower limb

The lower limb is both an organ of propulsion and a column that supports the body weight. Thus, it must have stronger and more numerous ligaments and more powerful muscles that are securely attached to the axial skeleton, and is longer and heavier than the upper limb. Following the general principle of limb structure, the greater bulk of muscle tissue is proximal and tendons are more evident distally. Unlike the upper limb, the lower limb rotates during embryonic development. This is why muscles extending the knee joint lie on the front of the thigh, whereas those that extend the elbow are on the back of the arm. It also accounts for why the dermatomes of the lower limb follow a spiral course and why the femoral/popliteal artery twists around the femur.

The foot is not a 'lower limb hand'

Upon learning, or relearning, the muscles of the leg, a clinician examining the region may focus on the fact that some muscles are dorsiflexors, plantarflexors, invertors, or evertors. However, such movements occur when the foot is *off* the ground and much of the

(a)

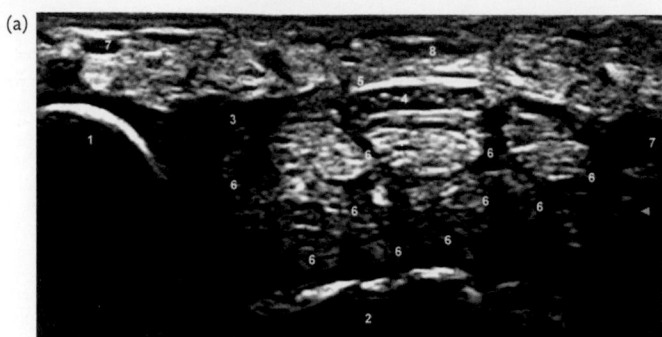

(b)

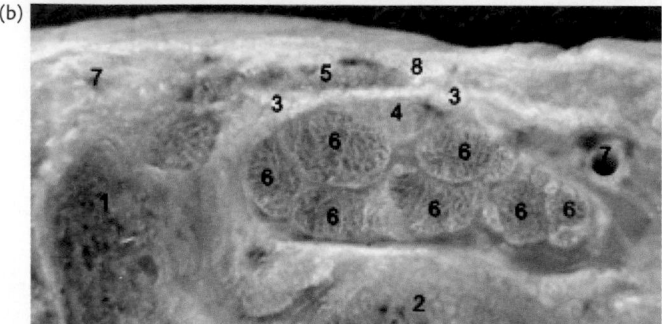

Fig. 65.1 Transverse high-resolution ultrasound (a) and anatomic (b) images of the proximal end of the carpal tunnel distinguishing the numerous structures traversing the wrist at this level. The tunnel is bordered by the scaphoid (1) and capitate (2) bones and the overlying flexor retinaculum (3). Within the tunnel, the median nerve.(4) with its fascicular pattern is located superficially and is surrounded by a bright hyperechogenic perineurium (5). The majority of the tunnel is occupied by the tendons (6) of the extrinsic hand muscles with their characteristic fibrillar pattern. It is also possible to differentiate blood vessels (7) and superficial fascia with intervening fat (8) above carpal tunnel.

time this is not the case. Thus, it is not often realized that a primary role of all of the muscles of the leg (and not just soleus) is postural control. Consider flexor hallucis longus (FHL). It is relatively easy for the skilled medical imager to identify its tendon and muscle belly. Yet a proper appreciation of its function is less common. Most anatomy texts will correctly say that it flexes the terminal phalanx of the big toe, but this movement is not of great consequence.[5] It is much more important to realize that FHL is a postural muscle. Thus, the distal part of the muscle–tendon unit (its insertion on the terminal phalanx of the big toe) becomes the fixed point, while it is the proximal end (its origin from the fibula) that moves. If the centre of gravity of the body shifts to the front of the ankle joint, FHL contracts and draws the leg backwards over the foot to help restore stability.[5] It also contributes (along with the fibularis muscles) to pulling the leg outwards over the foot when the centre of gravity of the body shifts to the medial side of the ankle.[5] It is in a position to do this because the tendon of FHL enters the foot medially. By comparison, flexor pollicis longus (FPL) is obviously concerned with flexing the thumb and such a movement is of great importance to the overall dexterity of the hand. The problem comes when FHL is simply viewed as the functional counterpart of FPL in the foot.[5]

Basic principles of muscle action and design

Muscles are 'pulling engines'

One of the first things that is often learned about muscles is that 'they pull, but do not push'.[6] If muscles pushed rather than pulled,

their tendons would need to be stiff rods rather than flexible sinews—which would obviously not facilitate joint movement and flexibility.

Prime movers, antagonists, synergists and fixators

Muscles may act as prime movers if they promote a movement, antagonists if they oppose a movement, synergists if they remove some unwanted component of muscle action that might otherwise occur in the prime mover, and fixators if they keep a part of the body (typically a bone) from moving.[7] Consider the apparently simple action of abducting the little finger so that it is drawn away from the hand. The prime mover is abductor digiti minimi (located in the hypothenar eminence). In order to act more efficiently in moving the finger in this way, its proximal attachment to the pisiform must be stabilized—i.e. this bone must be prevented from moving by the contraction of a further muscle that is also attached to it, the flexor carpi ulnaris (FCU), but is located in the forearm. FCU acts as a fixator. However, it is also capable of flexing the wrist joint. Hence, muscles on the extensor aspect of the forearm must contract to keep the wrist in a neutral position. In doing so, they act as synergists. Furthermore, FCU can also act as an ulnar deviator of the wrist, so to prevent this unwanted movement from occurring, flexor carpi radialis is further engaged as a synergist. Thus, it is important to think not only of muscles that execute actions as prime movers, but also of the supporting cast of antagonists, synergists, and fixators. Indeed, some muscles rarely act as prime movers at all—e.g. those of the rotator cuff, where the chief purpose is to act as 'extensible ligaments', maintaining shoulder joint stability and adapting their tension according to the joint position.[8] As pointed out, the muscular work involved in performing what seems at first sight to be the tiniest of action (simply moving the little finger!) is out of all proportion to the purely mechanical requirements of the act. As a corollary to this, it should now be obvious that if a muscle is compromised by injury or disease, then its loss will be felt in several actions other than those which it performs as a prime mover. Hence, one should not think of a given muscle just in relation to one definite action.

Several points emerge from the above that are worthy of mention in relation to the above account of muscle actions.

Movements and not muscles are represented in the cerebral cortex

Although limb muscles are described as 'voluntary skeletal muscles', only the action of a prime mover is under voluntary control. This reflects the fact that it is movements and not muscles that are represented in the cerebral cortex.[9] As an example, sneezing is an involuntary action that is determined by the lower centres rather than the cerebral cortex; it involves the contraction of some voluntary muscles that span between the trunk and the upper limb (notably latissimus dorsi). Thus, in a paralysed individual who has suffered motor cortex damage, it is still possible for a voluntary muscle to contract even though it may be paralysed for a voluntary action.

Muscle fibre contraction is 'all or nothing'

Muscles 'go full steam on half-boilers, and not half-steam on all boilers'.[9] Thus for example, the subtle control of the action of a prime mover by its antagonist does not involve the contraction of all its muscle fibres. Those that do contract, contract fully—and if a more powerful muscle action is required, then more motor units are recruited. This is probably clinically relevant in myositis where weakness only manifests when fibre loss is considerable. Furthermore, this principle is particularly relevant for large rather than small muscles, as the latter tend to be used for finesse rather than power e.g. the extrinsic eye muscles.

Gravity has a considerable modifying effect on muscle action

If the act of adducting the arm (so that it is brought back to the side of the body) is resisted, then pectoralis major and latissimus dorsi contract powerfully in an effort to perform the action. However, if the movement is not resisted, these adductors remain relaxed and it is deltoid (an abductor and antagonist in this action) that actually contracts eccentrically (i.e. the muscle lengthens during its action). What it is doing is to control the speed and precision with which the arm is moved—it pays out slack in much the same way as one pays out a length of rope wrapped around a windlass that acts as a pulley. This eccentric contraction mechanism of muscle action is very common in all regions of the body and is widely deployed as a way of controlling the action of a prime mover with smoothness, subtlety, and precision.

Larger muscles are not necessarily more powerful than smaller ones

It seems that the best predictor of the ability of a muscle to generate force is its macroscopic architecture—i.e. the number and orientation of its muscle fibres.[10] Ultrasound can distinguish between parallel-fibred muscles such as sartorius, that have long fibres spanning the length of the muscle, and pennate muscles such as deltoid that have shorter fibres arranged at an angle to the long axis of the muscle. Different subtypes of pennate arrangement are recognized (unipennate, bipennate, multipennate, and circumpennate).[7] In essence, parallel-fibred muscles are well suited to promoting delicate actions where there is a wide range of movement of a joint. Pennate muscles are more powerful, but act over a shorter range. Muscles with coarse fascicles (fascicles are bundles of muscle fibres) are typical of muscles which facilitate relatively gross movements of average strength, but it takes a muscle with finer fascicles to produce delicate movements.[8] While the largest muscle in the lower limb is gluteus maximus, the strongest muscles are vastus lateralis, gluteus medius and soleus.[10] Intriguingly, the strongest individual muscle is soleus—situated in the distal half of the limb—where lightness is at a premium for efficiency of movement.[10]

Fibre architecture and biarticular muscles

The soleus is a muscle that only crosses one joint (the ankle) and its architecture differs strikingly from that of the more proximal biarticular muscles (sartorius, gracilis, and semitendinosus) whose tendons form the pes anserinus complex. All of these muscles, act on both the hip and knee joint and thus need the wide range of excursion that a parallel-fibred architecture can promote.[10] Interestingly, biarticular muscles (e.g. the hamstrings) often exhibit conflicting length changes at either end of the muscle (i.e. shortening at one end and lengthening at the other), that effectively cancel each other out and mean that the muscles act with relatively little overall change in length—i.e. a pseudoisometric or 'econcentric' contraction. Since the movements at either end of the hamstrings occur simultaneously, the overall net length changes are far less than if two separate monoarticular muscles were to control the hip and knee movements.[10] The role of biarticular muscles gets even more subtle, as they can transfer moments to distal joints that they do not actually cross, by combining their activation strategies with other

biarticular muscles that cross one of the same joints, but then go on to cross another more distal joint. This means that the hamstrings (that cross the hip and knee joints) have an influence on the ankle joint via the gastrocnemius muscle that crosses the knee and ankle joints. This makes it difficult to say what the role of any individual muscle is during the gait cycle.[10]

Fibre architecture on opposing side of a limb

A comparison of muscle groups that cross a common lower limb joint (e.g. ankle, knee, or hip) shows that differences in physiological cross-sectional area (PCSA, the total area of all cross-sections that are perpendicular to the fibres in a muscle) correlate with differences in the power with which the movement can be executed. Two examples will suffice:

- Plantar flexion, an anti-gravity movement that is a key to forward propulsion in the gait cycle, is a more powerful action than dorsiflexion. Accordingly, the plantar flexors have a greater total PCSA and shorter muscle fibres.[10]

- The quadriceps femoris muscles have a greater PCSA than the hamstrings and this in the line with the common observation that knee extension is more powerful than knee flexion.[10]

The foregoing discussion highlights how complex muscle action is. It also illustrates how distant muscles are involved in the execution of fine movements and helps one to understand the implication of dysregulation of these processes or 'muscle imbalance' in the causation of pain or aching. This is very poorly understood.

Tendons and ligaments

Tendons are characteristic of limb muscles and can be rounded, oval, or flattened and have a distinctive and well-recognized ultrasound pattern. If the muscle with which a tendon is associated is an extensive flattened sheet (e.g. latissimus dorsi or pectoralis major), then its tendon will probably also be highly flattened. Such tendons are called aponeuroses. Ligaments generally link two different bones across a joint, but occasionally they run from one region of a bone to another part of the same bone and can vary greatly in shape and may be rounded or greatly flattened. It is well known that they guide and limit joint movements, but their proprioceptive potential (stemming from their rich afferent nerve supply) should not be forgotten. Indeed, the loss of this, following ligament rupture, may present as great a challenge to a patient's rehabilitation as the failure of mechanical function. Most ligaments attach close to joints. Some are thickenings of the joint capsule (e.g. the medial collateral ligament of the knee joint), but others form distinctive intra- or extracapsular structures (e.g. the cruciate and lateral collateral ligaments respectively).

Tendons obviously serve to transfer muscle pull to bones. However, they have several other functions as well.[5] Some tendons concentrate the pull of different heads/bellies of a muscle on to a single bony point (e.g. the tendon of triceps brachii). Others dissipate muscle action onto several different bones (e.g. flexor digitorum superficialis and profundus). This will serve to reduce the local stress concentration at the meeting of hard and soft tissues. However, it may have other significance as well. Thus, a tendon that splits into two or more segments may be a way of holding bones in position during muscle action. For example, the tendon of tibialis posterior divides into numerous slips as it approaches its insertional area and these slips attach to all of the tarsal bones except the talus. Such a complex arrangement draws the bones together and helps to maintain the arches of the foot.[5] A tendon that splits into two may allow a single muscle to oppose the action of two muscles on the opposite side of the limb. The tendon of flexor carpi radialis exemplifies this. As the muscle approaches its insertion, it splits into two slips that attach to the bases of the index and middle fingers. This allows the muscle to be an effective antagonist for both extensor carpi radialis longus and brevis. If a muscle has two tendinous insertions, this may allow it to have different point of action in different positions of the joint.[11] Importantly, tendons can economize on muscular effort by their elastic recoil following the release of a stretching force.[12]

Tendons can be very efficient at facilitating the longitudinal excursion that is necessary somewhere in the muscle–tendon unit when a muscle contracts concentrically (i.e. shortens when it contracts). Unlike muscles, their movement can be facilitated by tightly fitted, but lubricated synovial sheaths—muscle bellies must rely on a covering of loose connective tissue to glide over neighbouring structures. The role of such loose connective tissue in inflammation and in skeletal pain has not been defined. The corollary of this, however, is that punctured tendon sheaths offer an easy passage to the spread of infection. Knowing the detail of the topography of these sheaths can thus be highly relevant to a clinician. As an illustration, an infection in the thumb can spread via the tendon sheath of FPL to the palm, but an infection affecting the middle finger stays within the sheath of that digit. It is also useful to know that the typical response of the body to a damaged synovial sheath is to seal up this lubricating space around the tendon. US demonstrates the spectrum of tendon sheath pathology, ranging from effusion or synovial hypertrophy encircling the tendon to dynamic evaluation of tendon motion.

Finally, tendons can alter the direction of muscle pull because they can resist compression in regions where they contain fibrocartilage.[13] Fibrocartilage is avascular and the tendon cells gain their access to tissue fluid by virtue of the water-imbibing properties of aggrecan molecules within the fibrocartilage. The pressure exerted on a tendon as it wraps around a bony pulley (the medial malleolus, for example, in the case of the tibialis posterior tendon) is reduced as the tendon widens locally. A tendon may also be thicker than in adjacent, non-compressed regions, because of the presence of aggrecan and the associated increased water content. Hence in this ankle region, the sonographer may well see a change in shape and/or thickness of tendons and thus should be aware that such features do not necessarily suggest pathology.

The anatomical and biomechanical configuration of tendons where they wrap around the malleoli has been likened to a functional enthesis.[14] This is because mechanically or inflammatory related pathology at such sites is often associated with underlying bone abnormalities. However, unlike a true enthesis, the underlying bone pathology occurs with bone contact alone—i.e. not requiring bone attachment. The role of the underlying bone in the pathophysiology of tendon-related joint pain was not fully appreciated until these abnormalities could be observed on MRI.

The enthesis organ concept

The concept of an enthesis as simply the site of attachment of a tendon, ligament, or joint capsule to a bone has been broadened in recent years to include adjacent structures that are functionally related to the enthesis (primarily because they reduce stress concentration in the area) and which collectively constitute an enthesis organ.[14,15] Ultrasound is useful in evaluating the enthesis organ and its pathologic changes. Many enthesis organs exist in both the upper and lower limbs, but the best example for understanding the fundamentals of the concept is provided by that of the Achilles tendon. The insertion site itself lies at the middle of the posterior surface of the calcaneus. However, the superior tuberosity of that bone creates a raised eminence that presses against the deep surface of the tendon when the foot is dorsiflexed. The larger the tuberosity (its size varies between individuals), the greater the compression. In order for the bone and the deep surface of the tendon at the point of mutual contact to be able to cope with the pressure, both surfaces are fibrocartilaginous.

As the tendon must move relative to the bone (i.e. its 'insertional angle' changes) during dorsiflexion, there is a bursa (retrocalcaneal) at the insertion site that forms a synovio-entheseal complex with the tendon.[16] To minimize pressure changes within the bursa that could occur with foot movements, there is a fat pad (Figure 65.2) that acts like a variable plunger during dorsi- and plantarflexion.[17,18] The fat could also facilitate the spread of synovial fluid, prevent tendon–bone adhesions, and play a key role in proprioception.[19] Thus, retrocalcaneal bursitis should be considered in relation to the whole enthesis organ and it may well be a mistake to regard it as a pathological change in the bursa alone. It is difficult to envisage the bursa being involved without other changes occurring elsewhere in

(a)

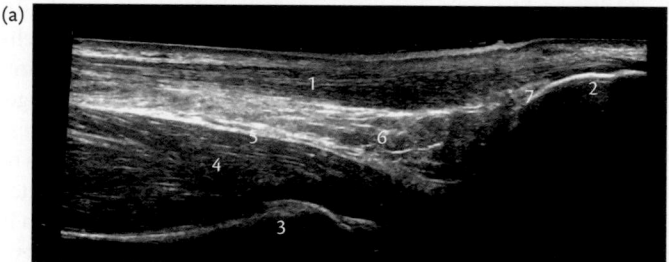

(b)

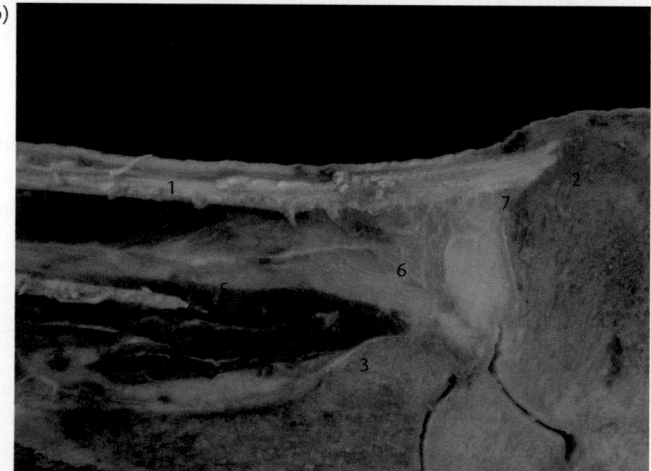

Fig. 65.2 Longitudinal, high-resolution ultrasound (a) and anatomic (b) images of the Achilles tendon (1) and its insertion onto the calcaneus (2). Deep to the tendon and lying above the tibia (3) is the flexor hallucis longus muscle (4). Its fascia (5) separates it from the extensive Kager's fat pad (6). Note the small distal extension of the fat pad (7) into the space occupied by the retrocalcaneal bursa (which is not visualized).

the enthesis organ, for the walls of the bursa are actually constituted of these other parts.

In the upper limb, a good example of an enthesis organ is provided by the insertion of the central slip of the extensor tendon of the fingers on to the base of the intermediate phalanx.[15] Here, the tendon presses on the head of the proximal phalanx when the finger is flexed and thus has a sesamoid fibrocartilage within it signifying the site of compression. The joint cavity itself is the functional equivalent of the retrocalcaneal bursa and the head of the proximal phalanx is the counterpart of the superior tuberosity.

Historically, clinicians have viewed enthesitis as a focal insertional disorder with inflammation confined to a small territory—something that was clinically supported by the pattern of tenderness at inflamed insertions. However, imaging studies of enthesitis have shown that the inflammatory process extends over a large area to involve the adjacent bone and the adjacent soft tissues and synovial cavity. When the microanatomy of entheses was more thoroughly explored,[14,15] it became evident that fibrocartilages were not just confined to attachment points, but also lined the adjacent surfaces of tendons or ligaments, and that the mechanical stress during movement was distributed over a wide area. Therefore, it is important to appreciate that there is a functional integration between the soft tissues of the enthesis and also between the enthesis and the bone around it.[20] The anatomical complexity of entheses and enthesis organs explains why enthesitis-associated pathology may be associated with diffuse pain, osteitis, or immediately adjacent synovitis. It also explains why the sonographer must look over a wider area than the actual point of insertion to appreciate the cause of enthesitis-associated pain. Given that many insertions are clinically inaccessible, MRI is necessary to recognize such pathology.

Nerves

The motor nerves supplying limb muscles generally enter the muscle belly on its deep surface (thus protecting the nerve from damage) and often do so at the geometric centre of the muscle.[8] The number of nerve fibres increases progressively in a motor nerve if the nerve is traced along its course in the limb. This is because of branching of the original fibres, a process that continues within the muscle itself. One motor nerve supplies a group of muscle fibres (i.e. a motor unit) and these motor units are typically large in muscles producing powerful but coarse actions, and small in muscles promoting delicate precise movements. The peripheral nerves supplying muscles also contain afferent nerve fibres (muscle spindles) that play a key role in proprioception. Not surprisingly, muscle spindles are prominent in postural muscles, e.g. in the muscles of all three compartments of the leg.

In gross anatomical dissections and even in MRI and static US imaging, nerves can look like tendons because the tissue that accounts for most of the bulk of a 'nerve' is connective tissue, rather than nervous tissue itself. This connective tissue enables nerves to resist stretch and to provide a conduit for blood vessels. If nerves could not resist stretch, they would be easily torn in limb movements. The key component that resists stretch in tendons is the type I collagen fibre, and it is the same in a nerve. The perineurial sheath in particular is highly collagenous and is often thick and dense. This sheath (which groups nerve fibres into fascicles) creates a special 'microenvironment' around the nerve fibres that is conducive to the conduction of nerve impulses. To the best of our knowledge it has not been adequately considered that neuropathies may actually be primarily linked to dysregulation of intraneuronal fibrous tissue.

The importance of fascia

'Fascia' is a vague term embracing a variety of connective tissue structures that are found throughout all segments of both limbs. Historically, fascia has often been dismissed as an inconsequential packing, wrapping or binding tissue that occupies spaces not filled by 'more important' structures. Fortunately, there is a strong resurgence of interest in fascia that is doing much to dispel this view.[21]

Many of the fascias that are most significant to clinicians are either made of loose (areolar) or dense fibrous connective tissue. The former are exemplified by the superficial fascia that lies beneath the skin or by the films of areolar tissue within muscles. Loose connective tissue is a conduit for blood vessels. Its cellular composition includes occasional fat cells and the native fibroblasts that differentiated in situ from mesenchymal cells. The remaining cells are an immigrant and transitory population of white blood cells that have migrated through the walls of exchange vessels within the connective tissue.

Beneath the skin, loose connective tissue (constituting the papillary layer of the dermis) is essential for its blood supply and, within muscles and nerves, it brings exchange vessels close to muscle cells and nerve fibres. The loose connective tissue can also act as a mechanosensitive signalling system capable of integrating structures in different regions of the limb analogous to that of the nervous system.[22,23] Of central importance here is the network of communication between the native fibroblasts via gap junctions.[22,23] The fascial planes are readily visible in US owing to their bright signal intensity and are the clue that leads the sonographer to discover the important neurovascular structures (Figure 65.3).

Dense connective tissue fascias include the deep fascia of the limbs and its specializations (e.g. intermuscular septa, retinacula, the palmar and plantar fascia, and digital fibrous tunnels). The deep fascia and the intermuscular septa arising from it play a well-documented role in partitioning groups of muscles into functional compartments. This is best illustrated in the leg, where the dorsiflexors are grouped into an anterior compartment, the plantarflexors fill the superficial and deep posterior compartments, and the evertors occupy the lateral compartment.

The deep fascia of the lower limb has been described[5] as forming an 'ectoskeleton' that supports and confines the deeper soft tissues and serves as an important site of tendon and muscle attachment. It enables the lower limb to act as a column supporting the body weight as well as an appendage promoting movement. This means that certain muscles (e.g. gluteus maximus) must attach to the limb as a whole and not just to one particular region of it.[5] Recent attention has been drawn to the fact that force transmission in muscles is not just to tendons but to fascia as well.[24–27] Consequently, it does not follow that in fusiform muscles with tendons at both ends, the forces transmitted to those tendons are equal.[28]

Some diseases such as polymyalgia rheumatica (PMR) are associated with diffuse pain that is hard to explain in terms of synovial-based disease alone. This is accompanied by inflammatory changes within fascial planes that are visible on MRI.[29] Extrasynovial involvement in PMR is well recognized, but to what degree the primary inflammatory reaction targets the fascia has not been defined. With the exception of a few clinicopathological entities fascia has

(a)

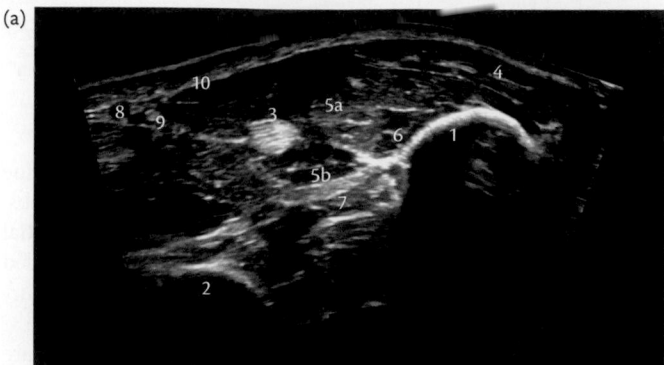

(b)

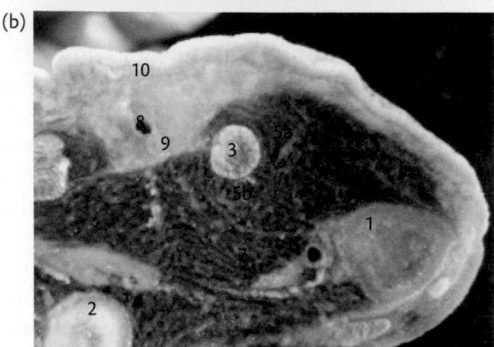

Fig. 65.3 Transverse high-resolution ultrasound (a) and anatomic (b) images of the intrinsic thenar muscles between the first and second metacarpal bones (1 and 2, respectively) and the tendon of the extrinsic flexor pollicis longus muscle (3). The intrinsic muscles include abductor pollicis brevis (4), the superficial and deep heads of flexor pollicis brevis (5a and 5b), opponens pollicis (6), and adductor pollicis (7). Note the vessels (8) and nerve (9) located in the deep fascia (10).

largely been overlooked in the pathogenesis of the rheumatic diseases and is an area that needs further work. Nevertheless, the deep and superficial fascias, their various specializations, and their pathology can readily be identified by US. As an example, the thickened portion of the fascia of the lateral hip region continues distally to insert into the anterolateral aspect of the tibia at Gerdy's tubercle. The location of the mechanical pathology involving its fibrillar structure or an associated bursa can be easily differentiated by US, whether involvement is at its insertion or as it passes over the lateral condyle of the femur. In a similar fashion, US plays an important role in the static and dynamic evaluation of many other fascial structures including the plantar and palmar fascia, the flexor and extensor retinacula of the wrist and ankle, and the annular pulleys of the flexors of the fingers. The US changes not only directly involve the retinacula themselves (changes in echogenicity, vascularization, and tears) but affect the structures which the retinacula support and restrain. This results in distinct clinical problems such as carpal tunnel and tarsal tunnel syndromes.

Adipose tissue

Since adipose tissue is dominated by fat cells, and these in turn are dominated by large lipid droplets, making the tissue pressure-tolerant. Where adipose tissue is particularly important as a cushion, it is often mixed with fibrous tissue that is anchored to adjacent structures. The integrity of both is important for normal function.[30] The copresence of fat and fibrous tissue ensures that the fat is held in

the position where it is needed and is not squeezed out into neighbouring areas.[31] It is also a conduit for blood vessels, thus allowing the adipose tissue itself to be virtually avascular.[32] Among the best-known sites in the limbs where adipose tissue resists pressure are the palms and soles. Pockets of fat, separated by conspicuous strands of fibrous tissue, are a familiar sight in MRI scans beneath the calcaneus or under the heads of the metatarsal bones. Indeed MRI offers considerable potential for exploring the mechanical properties of fat pads, via the continued development of MR elastography techniques.[33,34]

Heel fat pads are readily imaged by US[35] and are resilient structures that return 70% of the energy used to deform them.[36] These pads are involved both in rheumatoid arthritis and in the spondyloarthropathies. In the palm of the hand, the fat that is conspicuous beneath the palmar aponeurosis has a primary role in protecting the underlying vessels and nerves from pressure when the hand is gripping an object.

Blood vessels

The main arteries in the limbs run on the flexor aspects because here they are less likely to be exposed to tension during limb movements.[8] Although branches enter muscles to supply them, the main trunk of the artery that continues distally avoids the muscles and is thus not compressed by muscle contraction. Nevertheless, it is also a general rule that arteries take the shortest routes in the limbs possible; if this means that they pass through a muscle, there is usually a fibrous arch to protect the vessel from compression (e.g. in adductor magnus where the femoral artery becomes continuous with the popliteal artery). In the major joints of the limbs (e.g. the knee and elbow joints), there are characteristic arterial anastomoses that serve to ensure that one route of passage to more distal parts remains open when others are closed by joint movement that compresses vessels. The most distal parts of the limbs (toes and fingers) share the common feature that they receive a blood supply from a vessel(s) that forms a communicating link(s) between two muscular arteries. This is exemplified by the plantar arches in the foot and the palmar arches in the hand. As Sinclair[37] points out, this not only gives alternative routes of blood supply in the event of a local blockage, but could also provide a mechanism for equalizing pressure in the digital branches springing from arch vessels.

Haemodynamic factors tend to dictate the angle at which arterial branches leave the parent vessel, so that the loss of energy in the circulatory system is minimal and so that there are no undue falls in arterial pressure.[8] Hence branches of equal size (e.g. the common iliac arteries arising from the aorta) tend to make equal angles with the main stem and small side branches often leave the parent vessel at a large angle (e.g. the anterior tibial artery branching off the popliteal artery).

Arteries in the limbs tend to be accompanied by veins and commonly there are two veins (venae comitantes) accompanying one medium-sized artery. This, theoretically at least, allows the pulsatile nature of the arteries to aid in pumping the blood back to the heart in the veins. This is most likely when the veins are held close to the artery by numerous cross-connexions.[8] As is well known, muscles (particularly in the leg) also have a key role in milking the veins in this manner and venous return is greatly enhanced by valves. The presence of valves is thus an indication that the vessel is subject to intermittent compression—they are absent in bone marrow veins, because these are protected from all external pressure. Not all veins accompany arteries, of course, and superficial vessels of this type are particularly characteristic of the limbs and are exemplified by the great saphenous and cephalic veins. This reflects the pattern of development of the cardiovascular system whereby superficial marginal veins appear first and deeper routes of venous drainage appear later—presumably when it becomes disadvantageous for venous drainage to occur entirely by subcutaneous routes.[8] This opens the possibility for blood to be transferred between superficial and deep venous systems according to functional requirements, e.g. in the leg when prolonged standing and thus postural control exerted by its muscles occludes the deep vascular channels and forces blood into the superficial veins. Of relevance to power Doppler US is the observation that small nutrient arteries on bone can be misinterpreted as inflammation-related signal and the nutrient foramen can be misdiagnosed as an erosion.

Facilitating movement between adjacent structures in the limbs

Two key points need to be appreciated in understanding how movement is promoted between adjacent structures in the limb.

◆ Where two structures (e.g. muscles) are in contact with each other, loose (areolar) connective tissue is often present to allow movement. This is because its extracellular matrix contains hyaluronan (better known in synovial fluid) secreted by the native fibroblasts. Hence, when a sonographer sees two structures in real time that seem to be in immediate contact with each other, moving relative to each other, the movement is possible because there is actually a sheet of areolar tissue between them. The same explanation also applies to intratendinous movements that can be very obvious in US examinations. One fascicle or group of fascicles moves relative to its neighbours, by sliding in a plane of loose connective tissue. Such partial independence of the subunits of tendon structure reduces the risk of catastrophic failure of the whole tendon. This same tissue is also where infection is evident—and where infection can spread from one region to another.

◆ Adipose tissue (fat), which is easy to recognize in various forms of imaging, can also suggest that movement occurs at this site, as fat is liquid at body temperature. A key difference between fat and areolar connective tissue is the bulk of the two tissues—fat can fill a significant three-dimensional volume, whereas areolar connective tissue is usually in the form of thin (almost two-dimensional) films or sheets of tissue. Two of the constant regions where fat may be seen by the medical imager, and where the tissue facilitates movement, are in the mid palmar space, adjacent to the deep flexor tendons, and on the deep fascia covering pronator quadratus.[38]

All of these anatomical considerations are relevant in understanding anterior cruciate ligament (ACL) function in the knee where three major fibre bundles with multiple fascicles are present and where synovium and fat are interposed between fascicles. All function together to minimize stress at attachment sites, but clearly this fails as the osteoarthritic knee may be ACL-deficient in almost one-quarter of cases.

Conclusion

This chapter was written with the clinical ultrasonographer in mind and covers various aspects of functional musculoskeletal anatomy in order to promote a better understanding of normal anatomy and disease processes. Where possible, we have highlighted some structures visible on ultrasound that have not been previously considered in relationship to the pathogenesis of musculoskeletal disease.

References

1. Weir J, Abrahams PH. *Imaging atlas of human anatomy*. Mosby, Edinburgh, 2003:226.
2. Ryan S, McNicholas M, Eustace S. *Anatomy for diagnostic imaging*, 2nd edn. W.B. Saunders, Edinburgh, 2004:527.
3. Klauser AS, Halpern EJ, De Zordo T et al. Carpal tunnel syndrome assessment with US: value of additional cross-sectional area measurements of the median nerve in patients versus healthy volunteers. *Radiology* 2009;250(1):171–177.
4. Kamolz LP, Schrogendorfer KF, Rab M et al. The precision of ultrasound imaging and its relevance for carpal tunnel syndrome. *Surg Radiol Anat* 2001;23(2):117–121.
5. Wood Jones F. *Structure and function as seen in the foot*. Ballière, Tindall and Cox, London, 1949.
6. Keith A. *The engines of the human body*. Williams and Norgate, London, 1925.
7. Standring S. *Gray's anatomy: the anatomical basis of clinical practice*, 38th edn. Churchill Livingstone, Edinburgh, 2004.
8. Le Gros Clark W. *The tissues of the body*, 2nd edn. Clarendon Press, Oxford, 1949.
9. Wood Jones F. *The principles of anatomy as seen in the hand*. Churchill, London, 1920.
10. Lieber RL, Ward SR. Skeletal muscle design to meet functional demands. *Phil Trans Roy Soc London* 2011;366(1570):1466–1476.
11. Stack H. Muscle function in the fingers. *J Bone Joint Surg* 1962;44B: 899–909.
12. Kurokawa S, Fukunaga T, Fukashiro S. Behavior of fascicles and tendinous structures of human gastrocnemius during vertical jumping. *J Appl Physiol* 2001 90(4):1349–1358.
13. Benjamin M, Qin S, Ralphs JR. Fibrocartilage associated with human tendons and their pulleys. *J Anat* 1995;187(Pt 3):625–633.
14. Benjamin M, McGonagle D. The anatomical basis for disease localisation in seronegative spondyloarthropathy at entheses and related sites. *J Anat* 2001 199(Pt 5):503–526.
15. Benjamin M, Moriggl B, Brenner E et al. The 'enthesis organ' concept: Why enthesopathies may not present as focal insertional disorders. *Arthritis Rheum* 2004;50(10):3306–3313.
16. McGonagle D, Lories RJ, Tan AL, Benjamin M. The concept of a 'synovio-entheseal complex' and its implications for understanding joint inflammation and damage in psoriatic arthritis and beyond. *Arthritis Rheum* 2007;56(8):2482–2491.
17. Theobald P, Bydder G, Dent C et al. The functional anatomy of Kager's fat pad in relation to retrocalcaneal problems and other hindfoot disorders. *J Anat* 2006;208(1):91–97.
18. Canoso JJ. The premiere enthesis. *J Rheumatol* 1998;25(7):1254–1256.
19. Shaw HM, Santer RM, Watson AH, Benjamin M. Adipose tissue at entheses: the innervation and cell composition of the retromalleolar fat pad associated with the rat Achilles tendon. *J Anat* 2007;211(4):436–443.
20. Benjamin M, Tourni H, Suzuki D et al. Microdamage and altered vascularity at the enthesis-bone interface provides an anatomic explanation for bone involvement in the HLA-B27 associated spondyloarthrides and allied disorders. *Arthritis Rheum* 2007;56:224–233.
21. Benjamin M. The fascia of the limbs and back—a review. *J Anat* 2009; 214(1):1–18.

22. Langevin HM, Cornbrooks CJ, Taatjes DJ. Fibroblasts form a body-wide cellular network. *Histochem Cell Biol* 2004;122(1):7–15.

23. Langevin HM. Connective tissue: a body-wide signaling network? *Med Hypotheses* 2006;66(6):1074–1077.

24. Huijing PA. Epimuscular myofascial force transmission: a historical review and implications for new research. International Society of Biomechanics Muybridge Award Lecture, Taipei, 2007. *J Biomech* 2009;42(1):9–21.

25. Huijing PA, Baan GC. Myofascial force transmission causes interaction between adjacent muscles and connective tissue: effects of blunt dissection and compartmental fasciotomy on length force characteristics of rat extensor digitorum longus muscle. *Arch Physiol Biochem* 2001;109(2):97–109.

26. Huijing PA, Baan GC. Extramuscular myofascial force transmission within the rat anterior tibial compartment: proximo-distal differences in muscle force. *Acta Physiol Scand* 2001;173(3):297–311.

27. Huijing PA, Baan GC, Rebel GT. Non-myotendinous force transmission in rat extensor digitorum longus muscle. *J Exp Biol* 1998; 201(Pt 5):683–691.

28. Huijing PA. Epimuscular myofascial force transmission between antagonistic and synergistic muscles can explain movement limitation in spastic paresis. *J Electromyogr Kinesiol* 2007;17(6):708–724.

29. McGonagle D, Stockwin L, Isaacs J, Emery P. An enthesis based model for the pathogenesis of spondyloarthropathy. additive effects of microbial adjuvant and biomechanical factors at disease sites. *J Rheumatol* 2001;28(10):2155–2159.

30. Jahss MH, Kummer F, Michelson JD. Investigations into the fat pads of the sole of the foot: heel pressure studies. *Foot Ankle* 1992;13(5):227–232.

31. Snow SW, Bohne WH. Observations on the fibrous retinacula of the heel pad. *Foot Ankle Int* 2006;27(8):632–635.

32. Cichowitz A, Pan WR, Ashton M. The heel: anatomy, blood supply, and the pathophysiology of pressure ulcers. *Ann Plast Surg* 2009;62(4): 423–429.

33. Cheung YY, Doyley M, Miller TB et al. Magnetic resonance elastography of the plantar fat pads: Preliminary study in diabetic patients and asymptomatic volunteers. *J Comput Assist Tomogr* 2006;30(2):321–326.

34. Weaver JB, Doyley M, Cheung Y et al. Imaging the shear modulus of the heel fat pads. *Clin Biomech* (Bristol, Avon) 2005;20(3):312–319.

35. Uzel M, Cetinus E, Ekerbicer HC, Karaoguz A. Heel pad thickness and athletic activity in healthy young adults: a sonographic study. *J Clin Ultrasound* 2006;34(5):231–236.

36. Bennett MB, Ker RF. The mechanical properties of the human subcalcaneal fat pad in compression. *J Anat* 1990;171:131–138.

37. Sinclair D. *An introduction to functional anatomy*, 4th edn. Blackwell, Oxford, 1970.

38. Reidenbach MM, Schmidt HM. [Clinical anatomy of the fat body in the forearm and in the palm]. *Ann Anat* 1993;175(1):11–20.

CHAPTER 66

Radiographic imaging

Emma L. Rowbotham and Andrew J. Grainger

Introduction

It is recognized that advanced imaging modalities, in particular MRI and ultrasound, are increasingly being used in the assessment of rheumatological conditions. This is due to increased sensitivity of cross-sectional imaging, the ability to image soft tissues and cartilage simultaneously, and the ability of these modalities to make earlier diagnosis when structural abnormalities may still be reversible. However, there is still an important role for conventional plain film imaging, both as a useful screening tool for initial diagnosis and as an adjunct to more complex cross-sectional imaging.

Radiographic assessment

A standard approach using the 'ABCDE' mnemonic is widely employed by radiologists to assess radiographs in patients with an arthropathy; this system of assessment may be utilized to evaluate plain radiographs of any joint in a systematic fashion:

A Alignment

B Bone changes including osteopenia and enthesitis

C Cartilage

D Distribution

E Erosions

F Soft tissue swelling

Alignment

Malalignment of the joints is a feature common to many arthropathic conditions and has a variety of causes including ligament degeneration or disruption, tendon rupture or subluxation, cartilage loss, and bone attrition or erosion. Deformities common to osteoarthritis include varus and valgus angulation at the knee joint caused by asymmetric cartilage loss and ligament laxity. Classic hand deformities in rheumatoid arthritis (RA) include swan-neck and boutonnière changes.

Bone changes

Osteopenia is a common and early finding in patients with inflammatory arthropathy, although subtle osteopenic change may be difficult to detect. It is perhaps more readily identified in cases of monoarticular or pauciarticular disease where changes may be compared with other non-affected joints (Figure 66.1).

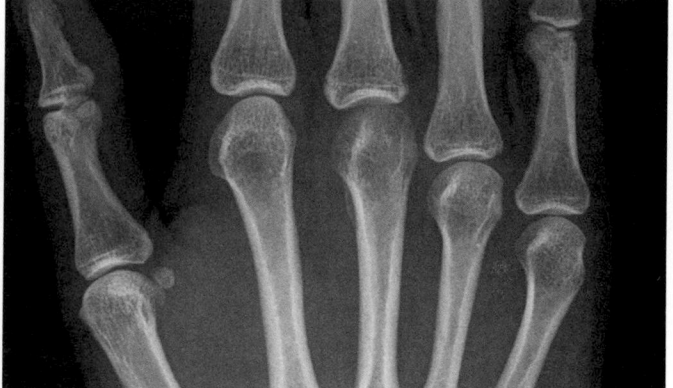

Fig. 66.1 DP radiograph of the right hand showing the metacarpophalangeal (MCP) joints. The patient has an early septic monoarthritis of the middle finger MCP joint. Note the relative osteopenia of the middle finger MCP joint head compared with the adjacent bones.

Enthesitis is a characteristic finding associated with seronegative arthritis. Plain film imaging may be used to identify enthesophyte formation and erosive change. Enthesophytes are seen as areas of bony proliferation at or immediately adjacent to an enthesis. They may appear either as coarse bony spurs with both cortical and medullary bone present or as more 'whisker-like' structures (Figure 66.2). The entheses of the lower limbs are more frequently involved than those of the upper limbs, with calcaneal enthesitis one of the most frequently affected areas. Large, bulky enthesophytes are associated with reactive arthritis, psoriasis, and diffuse idiopathic skeletal hyperostosis (DISH). Fine, more delicate ossification is usually more typical of ankylosing spondylitis (AS).

Cartilage

Destruction of articular cartilage is identified as joint space loss on conventional radiographs; this feature is common to many joint diseases (Figure 66.3). In osteoarthritis (OA) there is typically non-uniform joint space loss, in contrast to inflammatory arthritis where the loss of joint space is more classically uniform across a joint. Once joint space loss is evident there has been irreversible damage caused to the joint in question. Preservation of the joint space is also an important feature to recognize on imaging and is characteristic of gout as well as amyloid arthropathy (Figure 66.4).

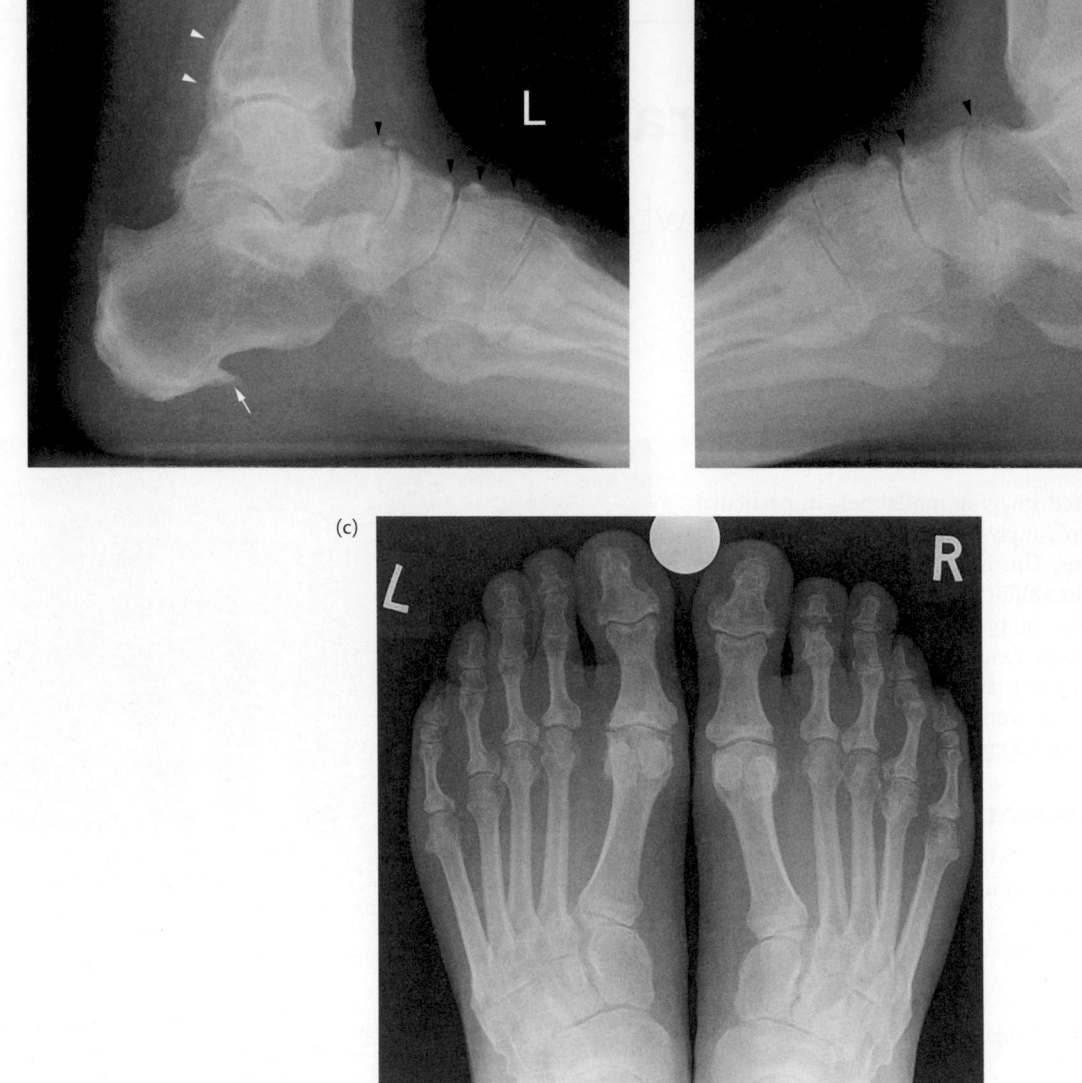

Fig. 66.2 (a, b) Lateral radiographs of the mid- and hindfeet in a patient with reactive arthritis. There is enthesophyte formation seen associated with the intertarsal joints (black arrowheads) and at the plantar fascia origins (white arrow). Note also periosteal new bone associated with the dorsal tibia (white arrowheads) and the erosive change at the Achilles enthesis on the right (black arrow). (c) DP views of the same patient's feet. There is erosive change at the MTP joints and interphalangeal joints with further bone hypertrophy representing enthesophyte formation (seen particularly at the second distal interphalangeal joint).

Distribution

Arthropathy may be monoarticular, oligoarticular, or polyarticular in nature; this distinction alone may help to narrow the differential diagnosis. Infection, pigmented villonodular synovitis (PVNS), crystal deposition, and synovial chondromatosis are more likely to be mono- or oligoarticular in distribution, whereas RA is more likely to be polyarticular.

Typically RA, scleroderma and systemic lupus erythematosus (SLE) all show symmetrical joint involvement. In contrast, the seronegative arthritides will often show a more asymmetric pattern of disease. Sacroiliac joint disease is also seen to be either symmetric in nature (usually suggestive of AS) or asymmetric, seen in reactive and psoriatic arthropathy (PsA) and more rarely in RA.

Distribution of joint involvement in the hands and feet may also be useful, with RA tending to show a proximal distribution (Figure 66.5) whereas PsA usually demonstrates a distal distribution with sparing of the wrists and metacarpophalangeal (MCP) joints. OA typically involves the distal interphalangeal (DIP) and proximal interphalangeal (PIP) joints with characteristic trapezocentric thumb base involvement, while the other wrist joints are preserved (Figure 66.6).

Erosions

Bone erosions are a hallmark of inflammatory arthritis and are a sign of significant joint damage. Proliferative erosions are associated with new bone formation and are classically a feature of

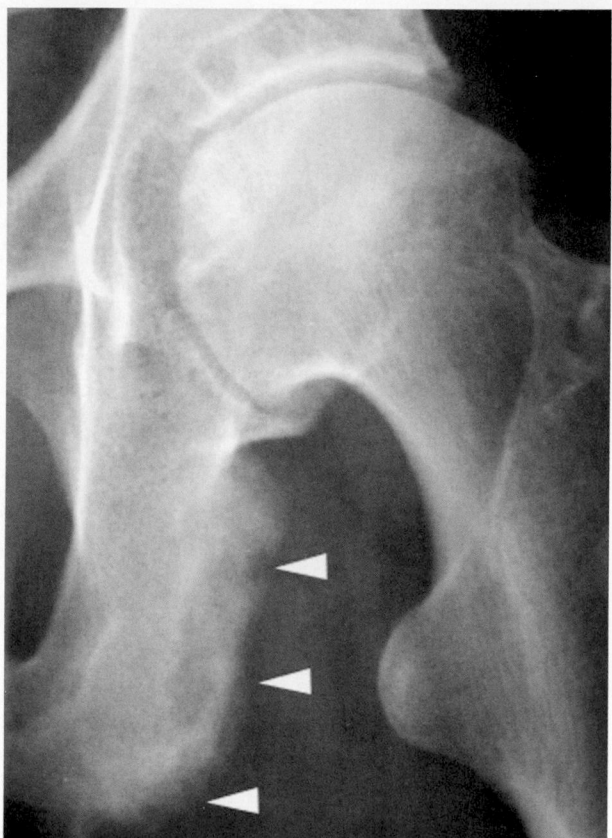

Fig. 66.3 AP view of the left hip in this patient with psoriatic arthritis shows a uniform (symmetrical) joint space loss—a characteristic feature of an inflammatory arthropathy. There is also fluffy new bone and enthesophyte formation along with erosion seen at muscle attachments of the ischium (arrowheads).

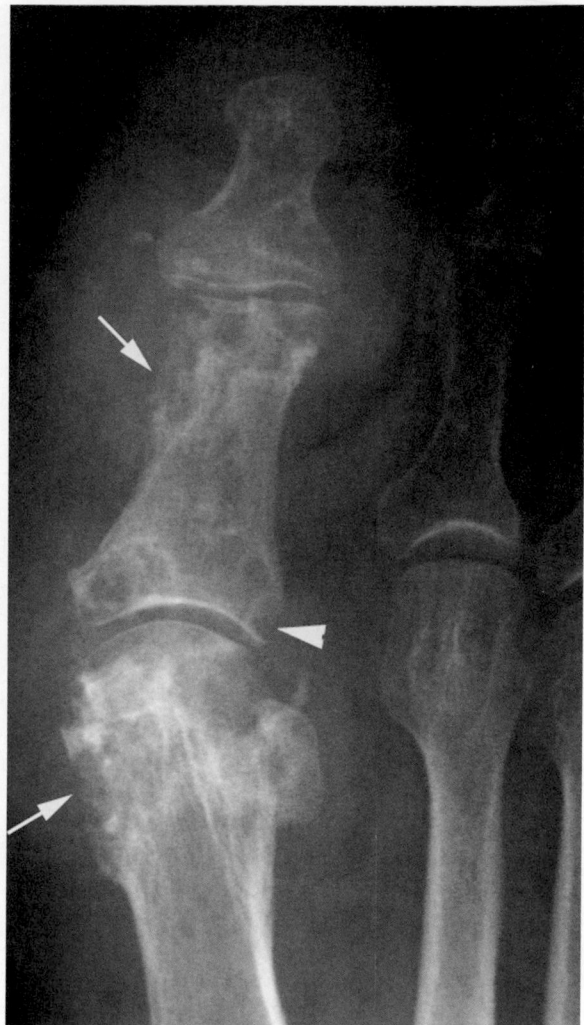

Fig. 66.4 DP radiograph of the left great toe in a patient with gout. There is extensive erosive change to the first toe. Some erosions have the typical overhanging sclerotic margins associated with gout (arrowhead) while others show a typical juxta-articular location some distance from the joint (arrows). Note the marked relatively dense soft tissue swelling. Despite the extensive disease there is preservation of joint space at both the interphalangeal and metatarsophalangeal joints.

entheseal disease; non-proliferative erosions are a feature of seropositive (rheumatoid) arthritis. Erosions are also described in terms of their position relative to the joint and may be central, marginal, or juxta-articular. Marginal erosions occur at the edge of the joint line and involve the exposed bone between the edge of the articular cartilage and the joint capsule (Figure 66.7). They are a typical feature of RA. Central erosions occur, as their name suggests, into bone normally covered by the articular cartilage. Juxta-articular erosions occur further away from the joint and are typically seen in gout (Figure 66.4). Cortical breaks are only seen when erosions lie in a plane perpendicular to the X-ray beam. En-face erosions will be seen as focal lucencies within the bone without associated cortical breach and may be indistinguishable from cysts. The detection of early erosive disease has become increasingly important and it is recognized that ultrasonography and MRI are more sensitive than conventional radiographs for erosive change, largely as a result of their multiplanar capabilities.

Soft tissue swelling

Soft tissue swelling is often the first detectable radiographic change in arthritis. There is inevitably a wide variation in what might be considered to be within the normal range; however, comparison with a previous radiograph or, in the case of an oligoarthritis, the contralateral side or other joints, may be helpful in confidently describing soft tissue swelling (Figure 66.8). Careful evaluation of

the fat planes normally identified adjacent to the joints may help in determining the degree of any pathological soft tissue swelling.

Fusiform swelling of a joint is usually indicative of a joint effusion or inflammatory pannus and is commonly seen in RA and septic arthritis. Diffuse swelling of a digit, often termed 'sausage finger', suggests inflammatory change outside the joint space and is more typically seen in cases of inflammatory arthritis. Typically, tophaceous deposits associated with gout tend to be eccentric to the joint and have an irregular appearance (Figure 66.4).

Calcification may also be seen within the soft tissues.

Osteoarthritis

OA shows characteristic radiographic findings including non-uniform joint space loss, osteophyte formation, subchondral sclerosis, and subchondral cyst formation (Figure 66.9). However, it is well recognized that the degree of radiographic abnormality in this condition does not correlate well with the severity of symptoms experienced by the patient. Two views in orthogonal planes of the

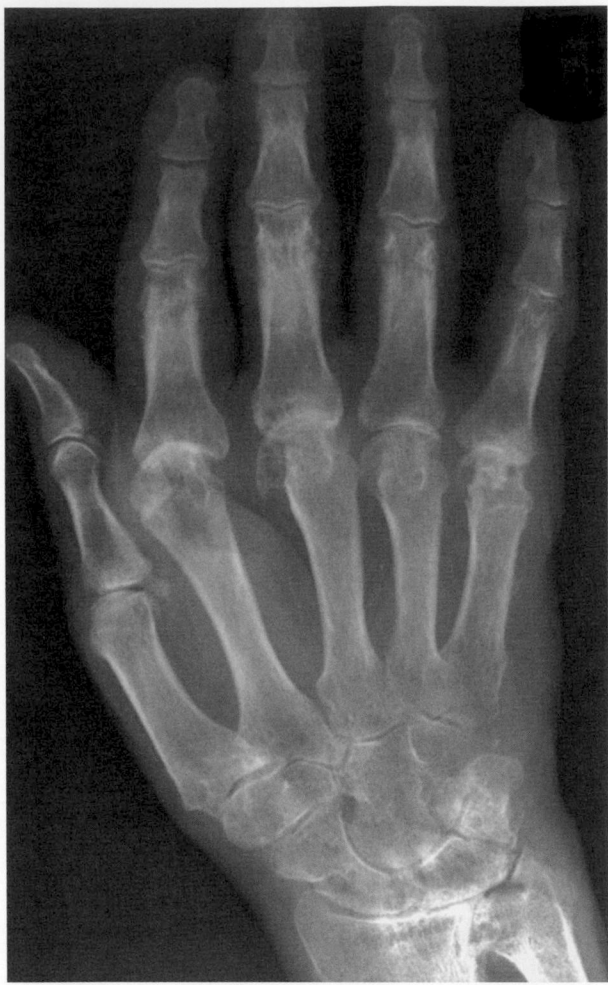

Fig. 66.5 DP radiograph of the right hand of a patient with chronic rheumatoid arthritis showing typical changes of deformity, joint space loss, and erosion. Note the proximal disease distribution involving the wrist (all joints) and metacarpal and proximal interphalangeal joints, with relative sparing of the distal interphalangeal joints.

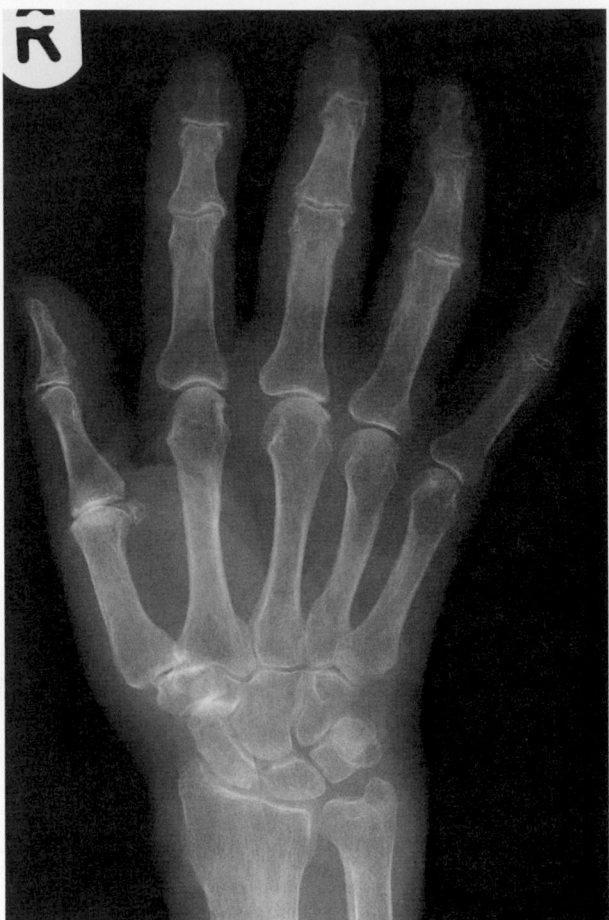

Fig. 66.6 DP radiograph of the right hand of a patient with osteoarthritis showing typical disease distribution. The disease distribution predominantly involves distal and proximal interphalangeal joints with less marked metacarpophalangeal joint involvement. Note that in the wrist the majority of joints are preserved with the exception of the thumb base carpometacarpal and scaphoid–trapezoid–trapezial (STT) joints.

affected joint should be obtained, with additional weightbearing views as necessary. Primary OA most commonly affects the hands, hips, knees, and spine.

Hand and wrist

In the hands the diagnosis of OA may be substantiated by the typical findings of sclerosis, loss of joint space, and marginal osteophyte formation. Typically in the hands and wrists the most common sites to be affected are the first carpometacarpal joint and the scaphoid trapezium trapezoid complex (STT) (trapezocentric disease) along with the interphalangeal joints, with a predilection for the DIP joints (Figure 66.6). Involvement of the PIP joints without DIP involvement is unusual. While all the classic features of OA may be seen at the interphalangeal joints, subchondral cyst formation is particularly prominent. In contrast to many other joints affected by OA the interphalangeal joints also tend to show a more uniform joint space loss. A characteristic 'sawtooth' appearance is used to describe the articular surfaces secondary to areas of eburnation and subchondral collapse (Figure 66.10).

In idiopathic, primary OA wrist involvement is usually confined to the thumb base. Involvement elsewhere suggests the changes

have a secondary cause, most typically trauma. Previous scaphoid fracture predisposes to radiocarpal OA, generally between the distal pole of the scaphoid and the radial styloid; this condition is termed scaphoid non-union advanced collapse (SNAC). Radiocarpal and subsequently midcarpal disease as a consequence of scapholunate dissociation is termed scapholunate advanced collapse (SLAC). Although non-traumatic SLAC wrist has been recognized,[1] the absence of a relevant history of trauma and involvement of the radiocarpal or midcarpal joints would suggest an alternative diagnosis such as pyrophosphate arthropathy.

Osteoarthritis at the ulnocarpal joint secondary to ulnocarpal impaction syndrome is seen in cases of positive ulnar variance due to repetitive loading of the ulnocarpal joint, resultant lunotriquetral disruption, and triangular fibrocartilage complex (TFCC) tears.[2] Radiographic findings will include flattening of the articular surface, subchondral cyst formation, and sclerosis to both the lunate and the distal ulnar (Figure 66.11).

Knee

Knee OA may involve all three joint compartments, but the severity typically varies between compartments, frequently involving the medial tibiofemoral and patellofemoral joints most severely

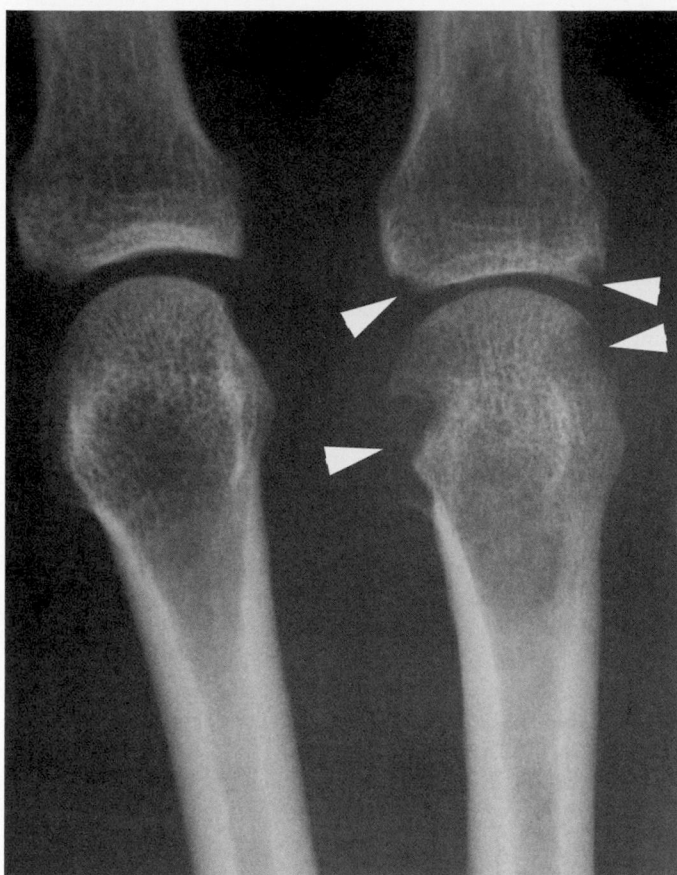

Fig. 66.7 DP radiograph of the right index and middle metacarpophalangeal (MCP) joint of a patient with rheumatoid arthritis. The middle MCP joint shows typical marginal erosions (arrowheads). Note also the joint space loss compared to the adjacent index MCP joint.

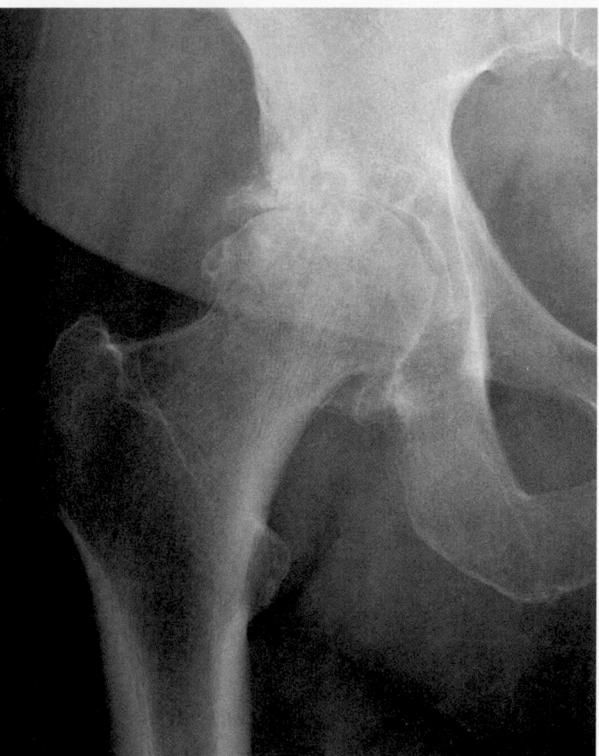

Fig. 66.9 AP radiograph of the right hip showing typical changes of severe osteoarthritis. There is joint space narrowing which is asymmetric, appearing more marked superiorly, along with osteophytosis, subchondral cyst formation, and subchondral sclerosis.

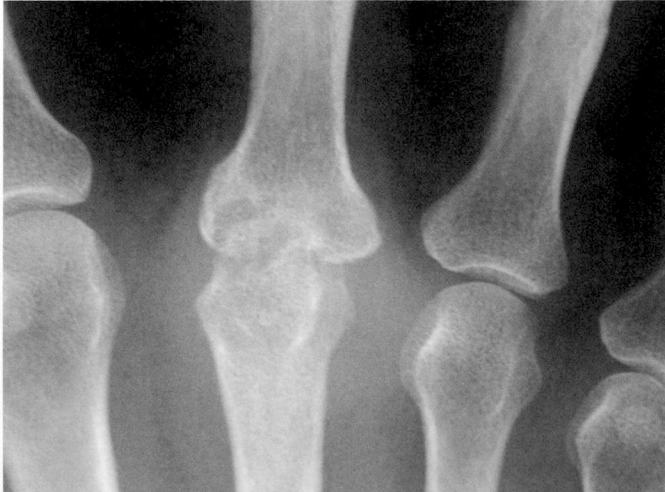

Fig. 66.8 Soft tissue swelling, seen as increased density of the periarticular soft tissues, is seen around the middle finger metacarpophalangeal (MCP) joint in this patient with rheumatoid arthritis. The loss of definition of the surrounding fat planes between the MCP joints can also be appreciated. In this case there is also joint space loss and erosive change.

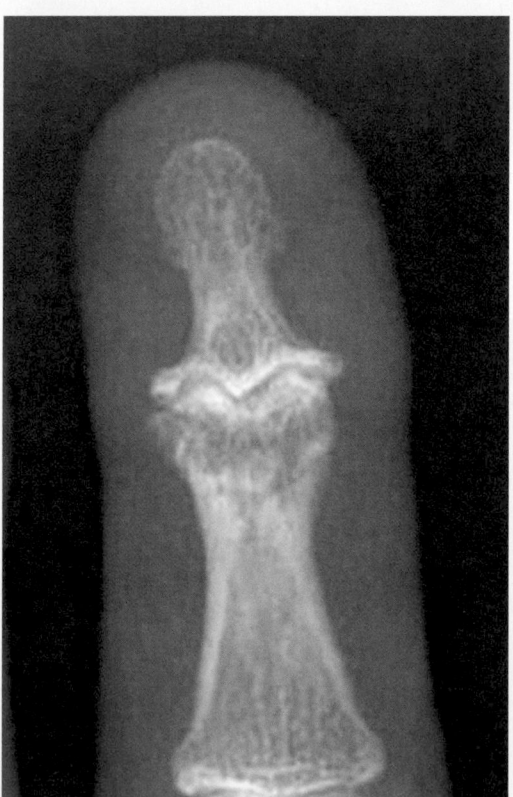

Fig. 66.10 Osteoarthritis affecting the left middle finger distal interphalangeal joint showing the typical 'sawtooth' pattern of joint involvement as a result of subchondral collapse and attrition.

with a corresponding uneven distribution of joint space loss.[3] More marked joint space loss and bone attrition in the medial compartment compared to the lateral compartment is typical and may result in varus deformity, although isolated or more marked lateral changes may also be seen. Where radiographs show uniform arthropathic change in all knee compartments, consideration should be given to alternative diagnoses such as an inflammatory arthritis. Positioning of the knee joint during radiography is important but at present there is no consensus as to the optimal technique. Radiography of the knee joints should ideally be performed in a weightbearing position if joint space is being assessed (Figure 66.12).[4] A recent large study assessing change in joint space width during treatment with disease-modifying OA

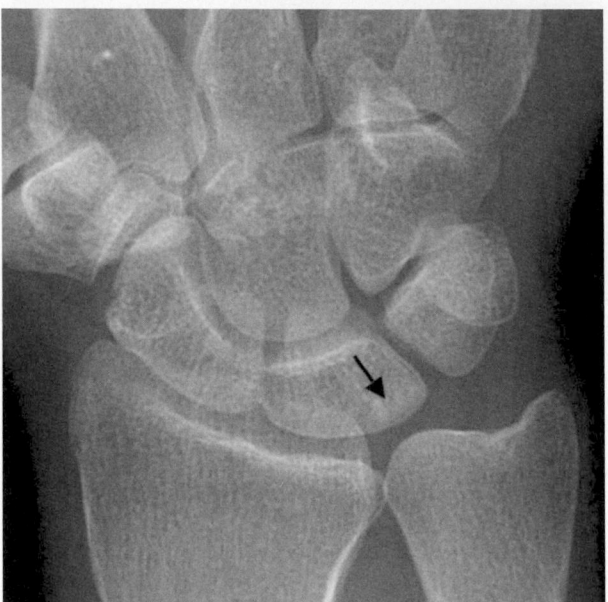

Fig. 66.11 Ulna–lunate impaction syndrome. DP view of the wrist joint in a patient with positive ulnar variance. There is subchondral sclerosis and early cystic change seen within the ulnar aspect of the proximal lunate (black arrow).

drugs has demonstrated that semiflexed views may present advantages over extended views.[5] In this technique the patient stands with the knees in a semiflexed position and in contact with the film cassette, with the feet slightly externally rotated.

Hip

In hip OA cartilage loss typically occurs within the superior weightbearing portion of the joint. However, early cartilage loss may be difficult to detect as pelvic radiographs are not routinely obtained in a weightbearing position.[6] Less commonly, a medial pattern of joint space loss is seen (Figure 66.13). A particular feature of hip OA which appears to be very sensitive to the diagnosis is the formation of new bone along the medial femoral neck of the femur, termed buttressing (Figure 66.13).[7,8]

Inflammatory osteoarthritis

A subgroup of patients with OA are described as having an inflammatory form of disease. Unlike the more common form of OA, erosions may be seen in this group and therefore the terms 'inflammatory OA' and 'erosive OA' have both been used to describe this condition. Inflammatory OA characteristically affects the small joints of the hands, although more rarely large-joint involvement is also seen and has been shown to have a higher clinical burden and worse outcome than non-erosive OA.[9]

The characteristic radiographic findings in inflammatory OA are the presence of subchondral erosion, cortical destruction, and subsequent reparative change which may include bony ankylosis.[10] The distribution of disease within the hands is the same as for generalized primary OA, although erosive change at the thumb base is rarely seen. The erosions are typically central in location leading to the typical 'seagull wing' appearance,[11] a feature which may help distinguish between inflammatory OA and rheumatoid or PsA (Figure 66.14).

Differentiating erosive OA from inflammatory arthropathy can be challenging; in particular, the distinction between erosive OA and PsA may be difficult as both demonstrate bony proliferation and have a distal distribution. More florid periosteal bone formation

(a)

(b)

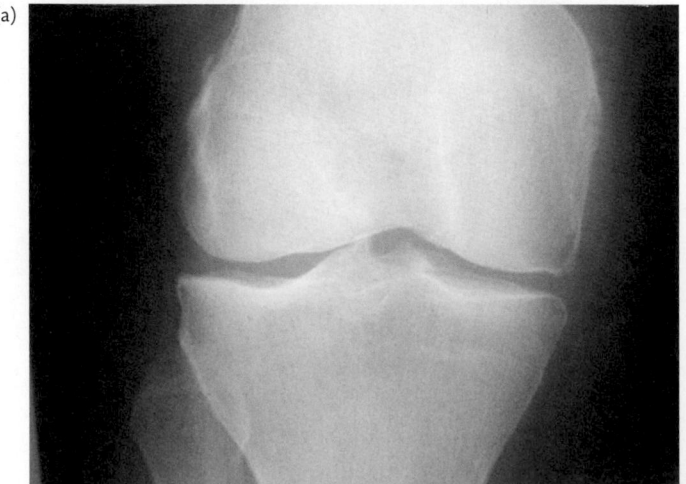
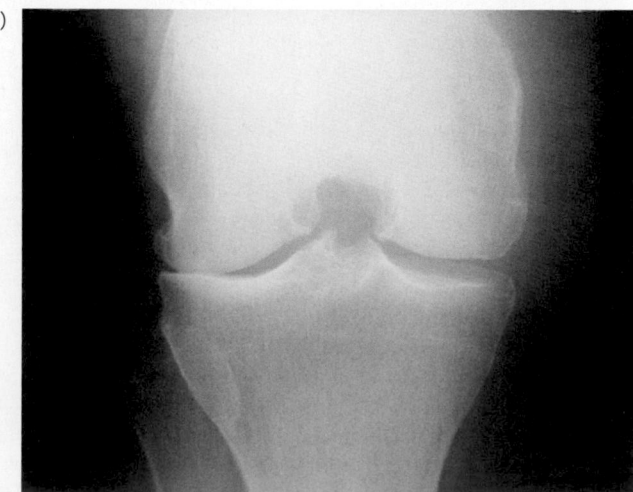

Fig. 66.12 Standing views of the right knee: (a) AP view with the knee in extension. There is mild joint space narrowing in both medial and lateral compartments with subchondral sclerosis and irregularity consistent with osteoarthritis. (b) PA view of the same knee with 45° of flexion (Rosenberg view). This partially flexed view shows marked joint space loss in the lateral joint compartment not appreciated on the standard AP view.

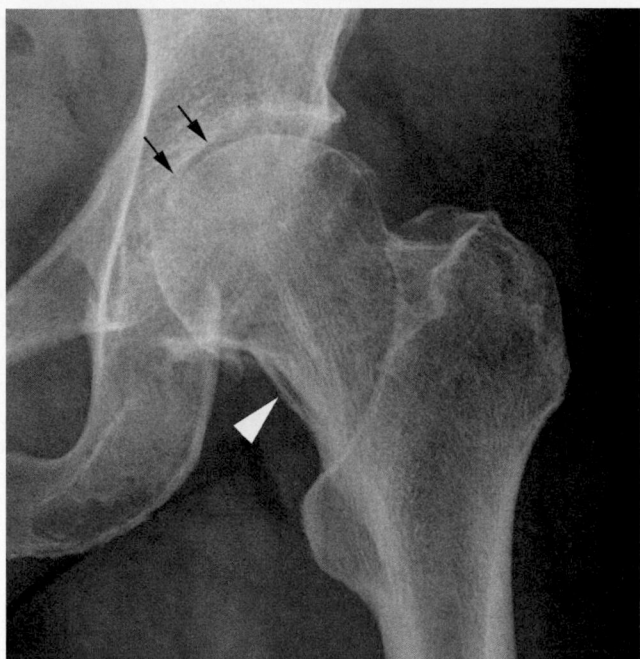

Fig. 66.13 AP hip radiograph showing osteoarthritis with a predominatly central (axial) pattern of joint space loss; compare with Figure 66.9 (arrows). Note also buttressing along the medial femoral neck (arrowhead).

may be seen in PsA and central bone erosions are more characteristic of erosive OA. The presence of OA at additional sites within the hand such as the thumb base may help with the diagnosis.

Diffuse idiopathic skeletal hyperostosis

DISH predominantly results in extensive ossification of the paraspinal ligaments and soft tissues including the anterior longitudinal ligament and the annulus fibrosis. However involvement of extravertebral sites such as the pelvis, calcaneus, ulnar olecranon, and patella have all been frequently described.[12] The criteria for diagnosing DISH on imaging as determined by Resnick and Niwayama are[13]:

♦ flowing ossification along the anterior and anterolateral aspects of at least four contiguous vertebrae of the thoracic spine

♦ preserved intervertebral disc height

♦ absence of apophyseal joint or sacroiliac joint changes.

This last feature allows distinction from AS. Ossification and calcification of the posterior longitudinal ligament has been described in the cervical spine and has been associated with cervical myelopathy.[14] The thoracic spine is most commonly affected, shown to be involved in 100% of patients in one study,[15] followed by the lumbar and more rarely the cervical spine (Figure 66.15).

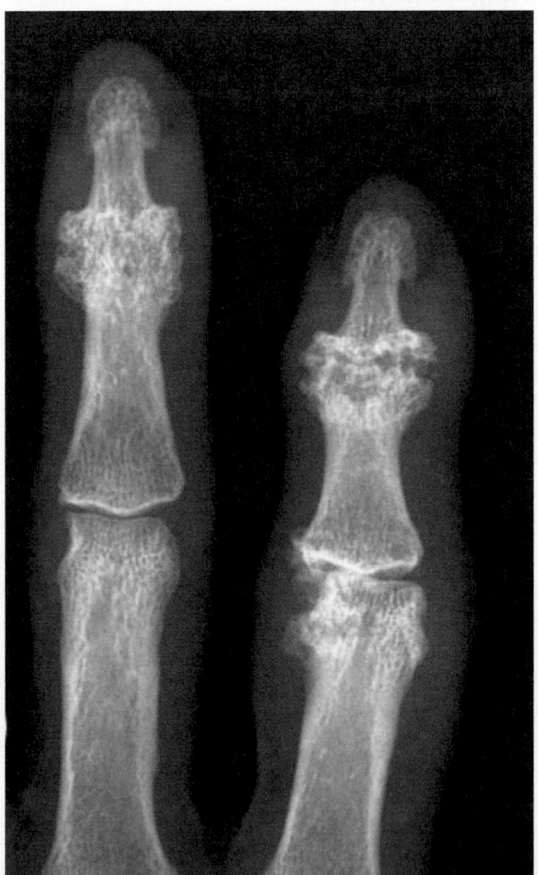

Fig. 66.14 DP radiograph of the ring and middle interphalangeal joints of a patient with erosive osteoarthritis. Note the central erosions in the intermediate phalanx of the index finger. There is also marked joint space loss and associated soft tissue swelling.

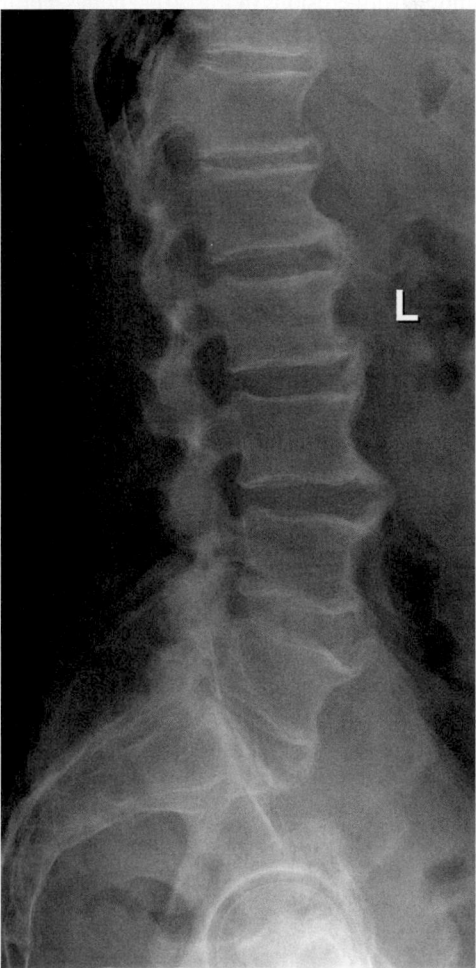

Fig. 66.15 Diffuse idiopathic skeletal hyperostosis. This lateral view of the lumbar spine reveals the classic flowing mature ossification of the anterior longitudinal ligament. Note the preservation of disc spaces.

Extra-axial radiographic findings in DISH include entheseal new bone formation—commonly seen at the tibial spines, calcaneus, superior patella, and olecranon[16]—and ossification of the sacrotuberous ligament and the symphysis pubis.

Inflammatory arthritis

Rheumatoid arthritis

Despite its limitations in the detection of synovitis and bone oedema, and relative insensitivity to early bone changes,[17] plain film imaging of RA remains commonplace. The hallmarks of RA on plain film imaging are soft tissue swelling, periarticular osteopenia, joint space loss, erosion, and malalignment. The earliest change seen in RA on plain film imaging is usually periarticular soft tissue swelling due to the presence of a joint effusion and synovitis. Osteopenia also occurs early in the disease process and is seen initially in a periarticular distribution but progresses in chronic disease to become more generalized, secondary to disuse. Proximal disease is the hallmark of RA in the hand and wrist and the commonest sites for early detection of erosive change are the radial aspects of the metacarpal heads and ulnar aspect of the carpal bones and ulnar styloid. The first appreciable sign of erosion is the so called 'dot–dash' type of deossification associated with localized osteopenia (Figure 66.16). En-face erosions may simulate cysts, a common finding with erosions in the carpal bones. For this reason the Norgaard or 'ballcatcher's' view has been recommended for the assessment of early rheumatoid disease. This modified AP oblique view allows improved visualization of the radial aspect of the base of the proximal phalanges, the first and second carpometacarpal joints and the pisotriquetral joint (Figure 66.17).

In chronic disease ligamentous rupture can lead to instability patterns and deformity including ulnar translocation, scapholunate dissociation, and distal radioulnar subluxation.

The acromioclavicular joint is commonly involved in RA; early changes manifest as erosion of the distal clavicle and erosion of the coracoclavicular ligament insertion (Figure 66.18). The sternomanubrial and sternoclavicular joints may also be involved but are much less frequently imaged.

Involvement of the thoracic and lumbar spine is unusual in RA; however, the cervical spine is commonly involved. In particular the

atlantoaxial region is one of the most common locations for lesions in RA.[18] Erosions of the odontoid peg may be detected on plain film imaging, although this has been shown to be relatively insensitive compared with both MRI and CT.[19] Atlantoaxial subluxation may be seen resulting in malalignment at the C1–2 level with widening of the atlantoaxial distance (Figure 66.19). Normally this distance should not exceed 2.5–3 mm in adults. Multiplanar reconstructive CT imaging of this region is probably the gold standard for diagnosis[20]; however, lateral plain film radiography of the cervical spine is useful in measuring the degree of subluxation, and flexion and extension views may be employed for dynamic assessment of instability.[21]

Atlantoaxial subluxation in the axial plane may also be seen resulting in the tip of the odontoid peg protruding into the foramen magnum and the anterior arch of the atlas aligning with the body of the dens (Figure 66.19). This may be associated with severe neurological complications and MRI assessment is often required.

Seronegative arthritis

Enthesitis is a characteristic feature of the seronegative arthritides. On plain film imaging the important bone changes which may be appreciated in enthesitis are enthesophyte formation and erosion. Enthesophytes which develop either at or immediately adjacent to the site of an enthesis are seen as areas of bone proliferation.

Ankylosing spondylitis

One of the key imaging features of AS is the distribution of disease with symmetric involvement of the sacroiliac (SI) joints a characteristic feature. Early radiographic findings include loss of cortical definition followed by erosions and joint widening. In the more chronic phase of disease there will be sclerosis and ultimately ankylosis of the SI joints (Figure 66.20).

Within the spine early changes of AS are manifest as small erosions at the anterior corners of the vertebral bodies. These are usually surrounded by reactive sclerosis and have been termed Romanus lesions (Figure 66.21). Squaring of the vertebral body is also common, a feature caused by a combination of corner erosions and periosteal new bone formation along the anterior aspect of the vertebral body. This is followed by syndesmophyte formation in which ossification of the outer fibres of the annulus fibrosus form, eventually bridging continuously. In endstage AS there will be ankylosis of the spine leading to the typical 'bamboo' spine of chronic AS with fusion of vertebral bodies and the facet joints along with prominent spinous enthesophytes. The fused and subsequently osteoporotic spine seen in chronic AS is particularly susceptible to fracture (Figure 66.22).[22]

The hip is the most common appendicular site of AS involvement. If protrusion or other radiographic hip abnormalities are found then the sacroiliac joints should be examined.[6] Other joints such as the glenohumeral, sternomanubrial, and costochondral joints are less commonly involved.

Psoriatic arthritis

Typically PsA is seen to affect the small joints of the hands and feet with a distal distribution. Findings are often asymmetric, in contrast to RA which tends to be more symmetric in distribution. Enthesitis is a common feature and typically affects the calcaneus, ischial tuberosity, femoral troachanter, anterior patella, and the

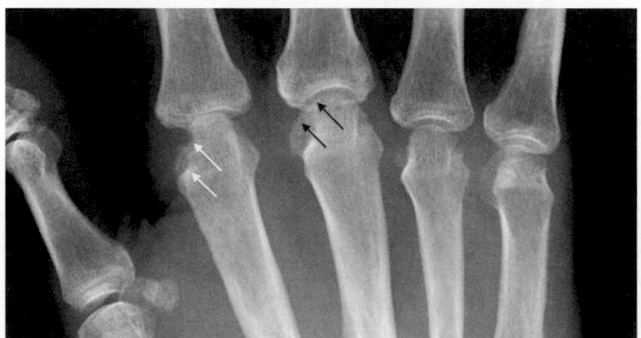

Fig. 66.16 Rheumatoid arthritis (RA). This DP image of the right hand in a patient with RA shows various stages of disease within the metacarpophalangeal (MCP) joints. The little MCP joint is normal with no erosive change and normal joint space. The cortex of the third metacarpal head revels the classic 'dot-dash' pattern associated with early erosive change (black arrows) and there is early joint space loss. The index finger metacarpal head shows frank erosive change on the radial margin and marked joint space loss (white arrows).

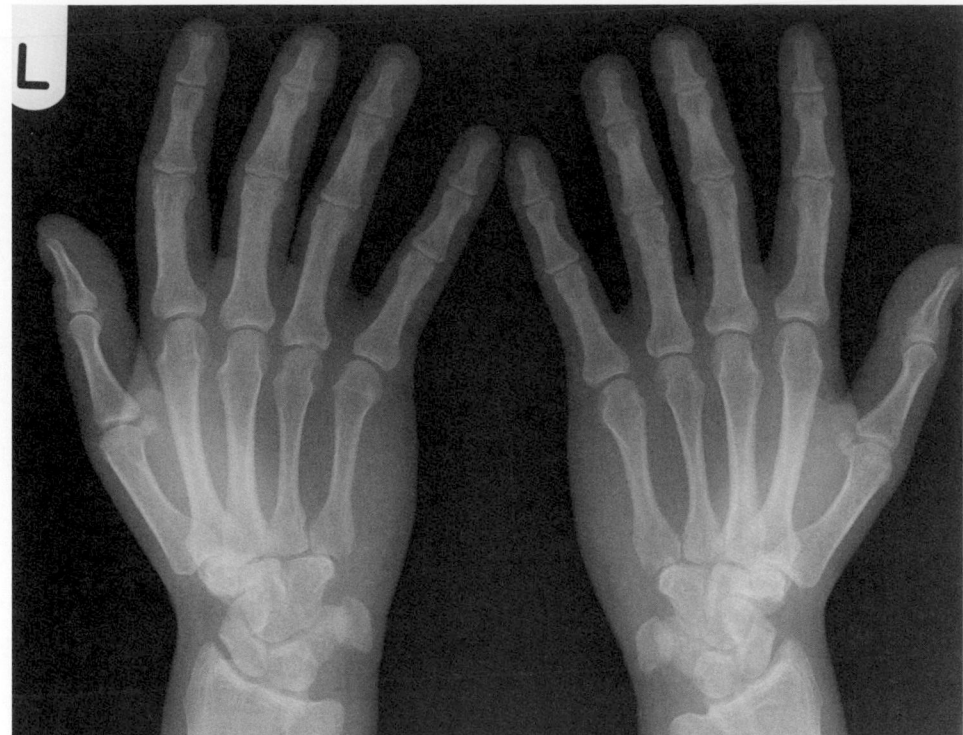

Fig. 66.17 The Norgaard or ballcatcher's projection is optimal for reviewing the radial aspect of the metacarpal heads for early erosive change. The forearms are placed in supination with 45° of obliquity.

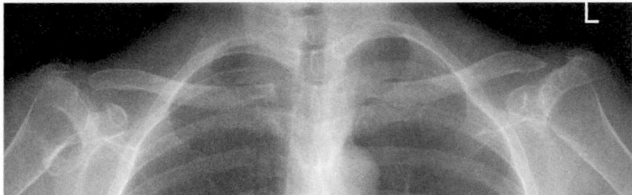

Fig. 66.18 Erosive change is seen affecting the distal end of the clavicles in this patient with long-standing rheumatoid arthritis. There is also erosion and subluxation of the humeral head bilaterally.

olecranon—this is not a feature of RA. Radiographic findings in the hands of patients with PsA are:

♦ **Bone erosion** beginning in a periarticular distribution and progressing to more central areas, and eventually osteolysis leading to the classic 'pencil-in-cup' deformity (Figure 66.23).

♦ **Asymmetrical destruction of the DIP with bony ankylosis**: in contrast, RA preferentially affects the MCP joint and PIP joints.

♦ **Resorption of terminal phalangeal tufts**; occasionally increased density of the terminal phalanges is seen, termed 'ivory phalanx'.

♦ **Periosteal reaction and small enthesophytes** may also be seen within the phalanges.

In the feet interphalangeal and metatarsophalangeal joint erosive change is common and the site of insertion of the Achilles tendon and/or plantar fascia is often affected, with enthesophyte formation and erosive change.

SI joint involvement is often asymmetrical with marginal erosions but fusion is not a feature. Another common site of disease is the spine where there is often bulky asymmetrical non-marginal osteophyte formation. These are commonly seen in the thoracolumbar spine initially and may progress to involve other areas of the spine.

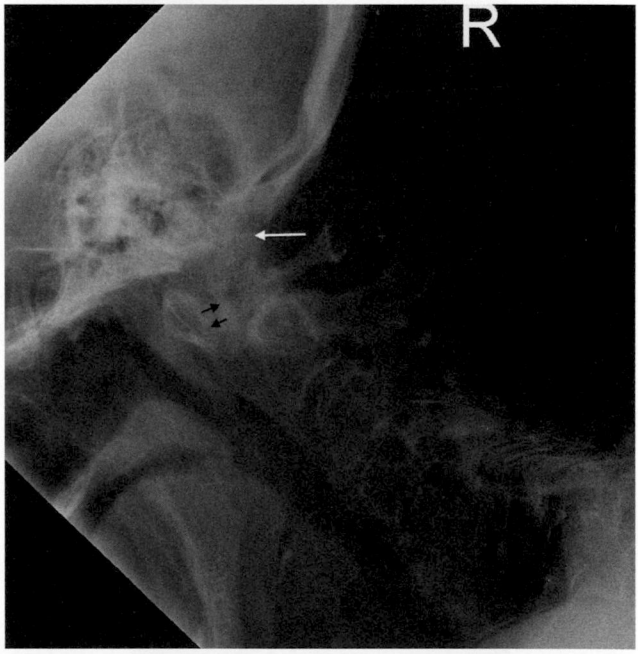

Fig. 66.19 Lateral flexed cervical spine radiograph in a patient with rheumatoid arthritis. There is anterior subluxation of C1 on C2 with widening of the atlantoaxial distance (black arrows). The odontoid peg has migrated in a superior direction, giving rise to basilar invagination (white arrow). Note also that the malalignment is also evident between the spinous processes of C1 and C2.

Reactive arthritis

In the early stage of disease radiographs may be normal. However, in more progressive disease an asymmetrical distribution is seen with predominantly lower limb involvement. Characteristic sites of abnormality include the calcaneus, ankle, knee, and SI joints.

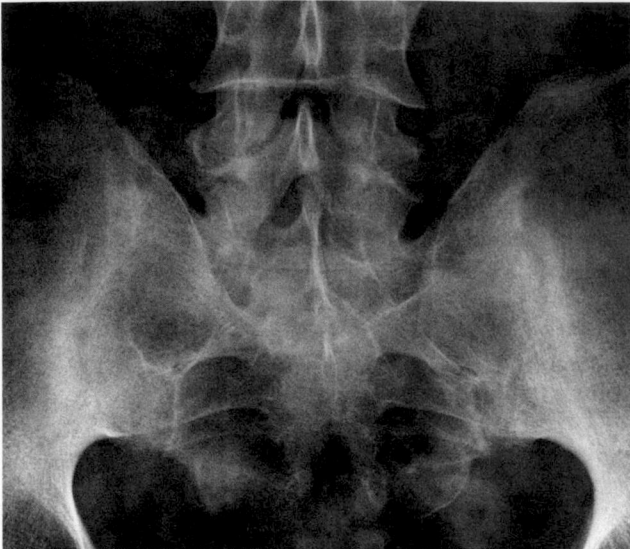

Fig. 66.20 Ankylosing spondylitis (AS) of the sacroiliac joints. AP film of the sacroiliac joints in this patient with long-standing AS shows complete fusion of the superior portion of the joint bilaterally. The lower portions of the joints show irregularity and sclerosis bilaterally but without ankylosis.

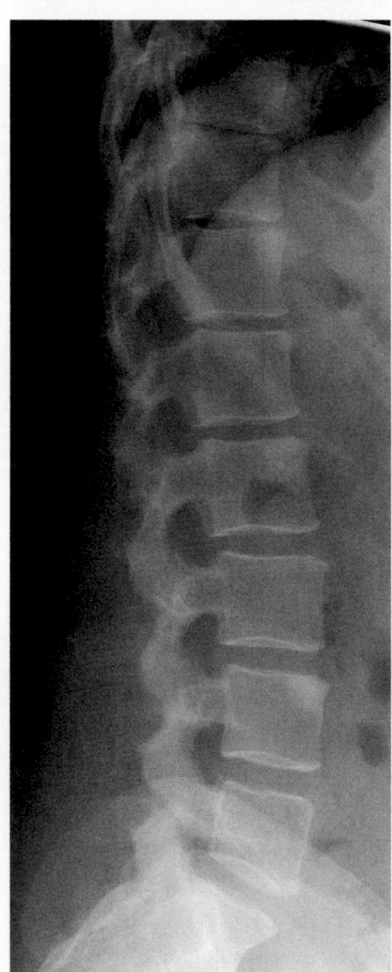

Fig. 66.21 Lateral view of the lumbar spine demonstrating early changes of ankylosing spondylitis. There is squaring of the vertebral bodies with associated sclerosis of the corners (Romanus lesions).

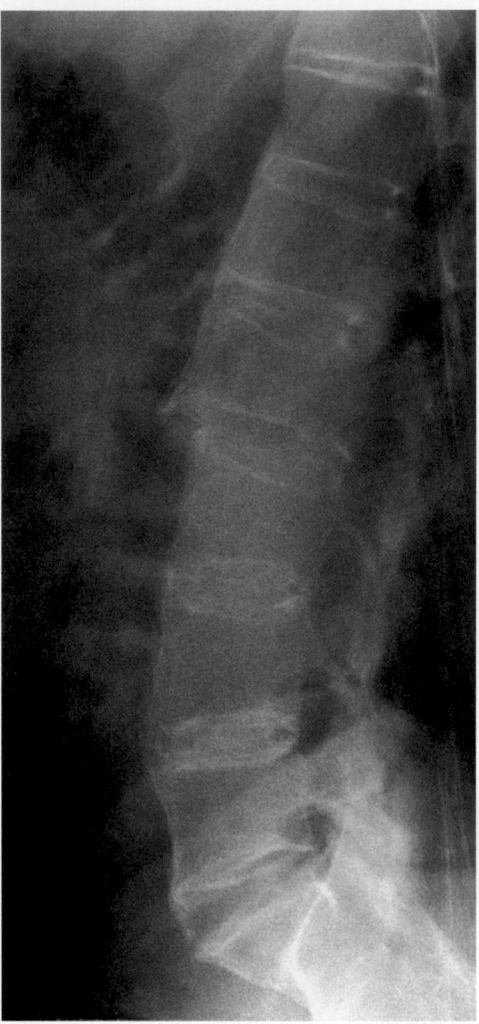

Fig. 66.22 Ankylosing spondylitis with Anderson fracture. Extensive ankylosis is seen in both the thoracic and lumbar spine. In addition there is a fracture through the spine at the L2/L3 level. Fractures of this nature usually extend through the fused posterior elements and are unstable.

Radiographic changes are similar to those seen in PsA with soft tissue swelling, joint space narrowing and marginal erosions with enthesophyte formation (Figure 66.2). In addition there may be sesamoid enlargement secondary to periostitis.[23] Periarticular osteopaenia is often seen with acute exacerbations.

Juvenile idiopathic arthritis

The most common radiographic abnormalities in patients with juvenile idiopathic arthritis (JIA) have been shown to be soft tissue swelling around the affected joint, growth disturbances (thought to be due to hyperaemia), joint space narrowing, and erosions.[24] Plain radiographic evidence of erosive change is also a relatively late and irreversible sign and as with adult inflammatory arthritis, MRI is increasingly being employed to assess for early signs of disease.[25] The wrist has been shown to be the most informative joint to detect bone erosions on plain radiography.[26] The knee is the most common site of involvement and there is often epiphyseal enlargement, overgrowth of the patella, and widening of the intercondylar notch. In the hands changes include boutonnière, flexion, and swan-neck deformities of the fingers alongside widened phalanges and

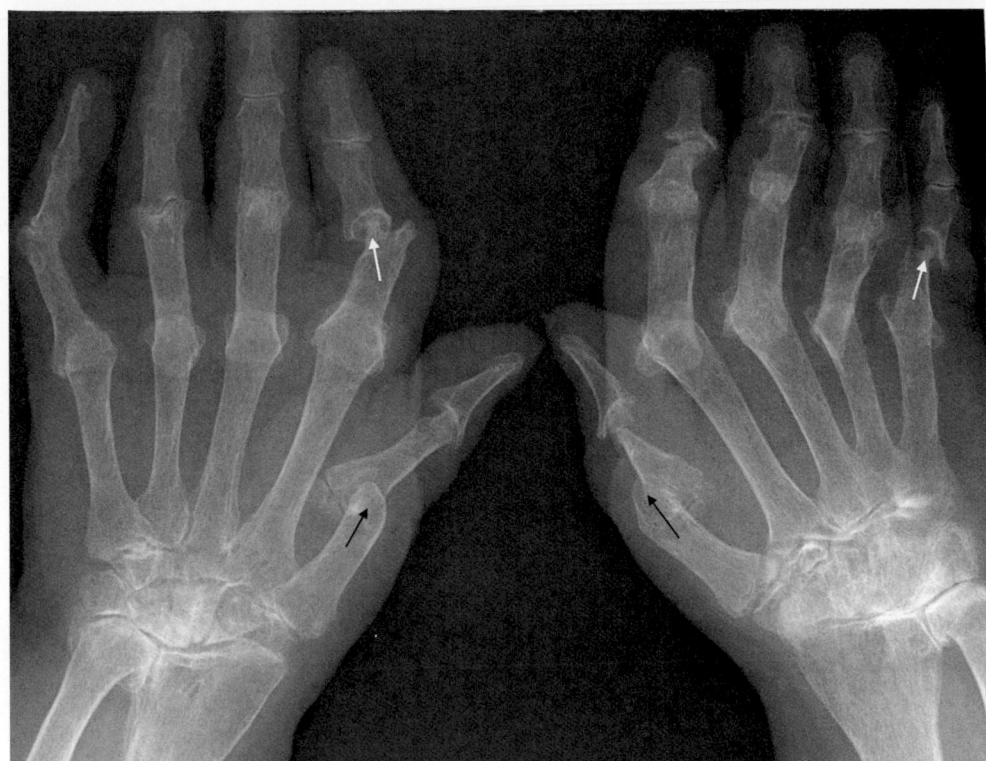

Fig. 66.23 There is a severe mutilating polyarthritis in this patient with psoriatic arthritis with subluxation at the metacarpophalangeal joints and extensive erosive disease. The right index and left little finger proximal interphalangeal joints show developing changes of a pencil-in-cup deformity (white arrows). The thumb metacarpals also show early pencil-in-cup change bilaterally (black arrows).

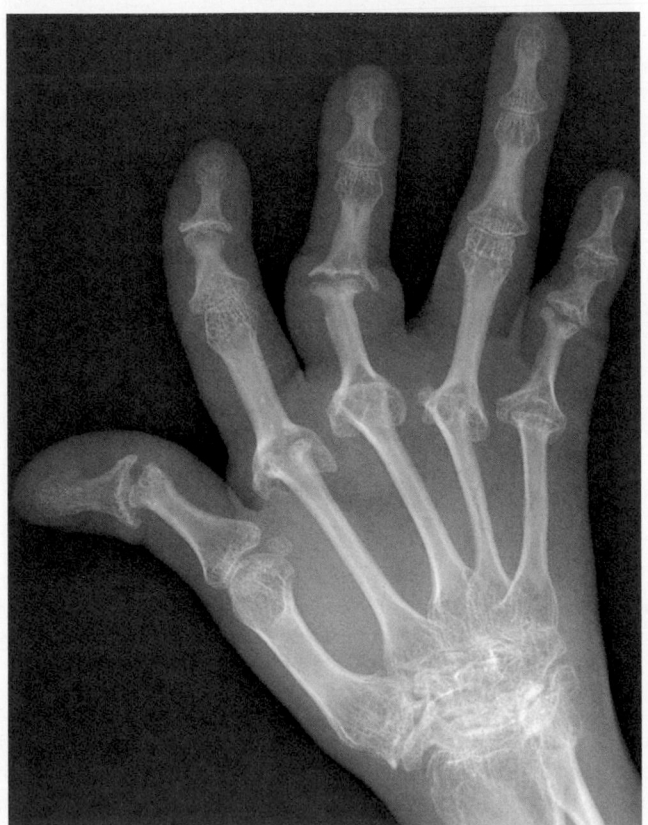

Fig. 66.24 Chronic changes in an adult resulting from juvenile idiopathic arthritis. Severe arthropathic change is seen at the wrist joints and within the carpi with fusion of several of the carpal bones. The joints of the hands are also abnormal, with cupping deformity of the proximal phalangeal bases and metaphyseal overgrowth.

metacarpals as a result of growth disturbance and periosteal new bone formation (Figure 66.24). Ankylosis of the involved joint is also a feature of the condition in its chronic stage and is common at the wrist joint. Osteoporosis associated with the condition may lead to epiphyseal collapse and deformity as a result of compression fractures secondary to abnormal stress on the bone.

Crystal arthritides

The crystal-induced arthritides are characterized by crystal deposition either in or adjacent to an affected joint. This is a heterogeneous group of diseases resulting in a variety of radiographic findings. Common crystals implicated are monosodium urate (producing gout), calcium pyrophosphate dihydrate, and calcium hydroxyapatite.

Gout

Conventional radiographs typically show changes only in advanced chronic gout.[27] However, this modality is still useful in monitoring articular and soft tissue lesions over time, especially in response to urate-lowering therapy.

Radiological features of gout may take 5–10 years to become evident following the first symptomatic episode. In contrast to other arthropathies, joint space and bone density are typically preserved until late in the disease process in gout and articular cartilage remains intact—this is one of the features that may be helpful to distinguish gout from other arthritides (Figure 66.4). Soft tissue swelling is typically irregular and asymmetric. The tophaceous swellings are relatively radio-opaque compared to the surrounding soft tissues, but do not usually show calcification unless there is concomitant renal disease. Late-stage features are typified by progressive erosions, classically with overhanging margins, in a juxta-articular distribution with sclerotic margins and intra-articular deposits (Figure 66.4). Although disuse osteopaenia may occur late in the disease, periarticular osteopaenia is not usually a feature of gout.

Gout typically affects the peripheral joints of the appendicular skeleton and rarely involves the axial joints.[28] The first MTP joint is frequently involved but other MTP joints and interphalangeal joints of the feet may also be affected. Joint disease in the hand most commonly involves the interphalangeal joints in an asymmetrical distribution. The wrist may also be involved and extensive osseous erosion in the wrist is not uncommon. In the knee the patellofemoral compartment is most commonly affected where tophaceous masses are commonly located on the medial aspect of the infrapatellar fat pad and anterior joint recess, while erosions are most commonly seen at the lateral rim of the lateral femoral condyle.[29]

Calcium pyrophosphate crystal deposition disease

Both the radiographic findings and distribution of the arthropathy associated with calcium pyrophosphate crystal deposition (CPPD) are relatively distinctive. Although any joint may be involved, the most commonly affected are the knees, wrists, and hips and the distribution is usually bilaterally symmetric. The characteristic finding is the presence of CPPD crystals in or around the joint. Most commonly this is present as chondrocalcinosis, but crystal deposition may also occur in either synovial or capsular tissue. The presence of these findings does not necessarily imply pyrophosphate arthropathy; this term refers to a pattern of joint damage occurring in CPPD which has similarities to OA with joint space narrowing, subchondral sclerosis, and cyst formation either with or without associated chondrocalcinosis. The distribution of these two conditions differs, however; in the hands CPPD favours the radiocarpal joint as opposed to the typical trapeziocentric pattern seen in OA and tends to affect the MCP joints in preference to the interphalangeal joints. Chondrocalcinosis at the wrist is frequently seen in the triangular fibrocartilage and also in the lunate–triquetral ligament.[30] Chronic disease may be associated with scapholunate dissociation and eventually SLAC.[31] (Figure 66.25). A further feature of the disease in the hand is the presence of hook-like osteophytes seen typically on the radial aspect of the first metacarpal head; this pattern is classically seen in patients with either haemochromotosis or pyrophosphate arthropathy.

At the knee, crystal deposition is seen within the menisci and also within the hyaline cartilage; patellofemoral arthropathy predominates over involvement of the tibiofemoral compartments. Calcium deposition in the gastrocnemius tendon origin is also associated with CPPD disease of the knee.[32] Hip involvement is less common but should be considered where there are large subchondral femoral head cysts present particularly in the presence of chondrocalcinosis.

Calcium hydroxyapatite crystal deposition disease

Calcium hydroxyapatite deposition disease results in either periarticular or intra-articular crystal deposition which may cause either acute or chronic joint symptoms. This condition is most commonly recognized at the shoulder with calcification located either within the rotator cuff tendons, the biceps tendon, or the subacromial–subdeltoid bursa (Figure 66.26). The most common site of calcium deposition at the wrist is the flexor carpi ulnaris tendon, although deposits are occasionally also found in the flexor

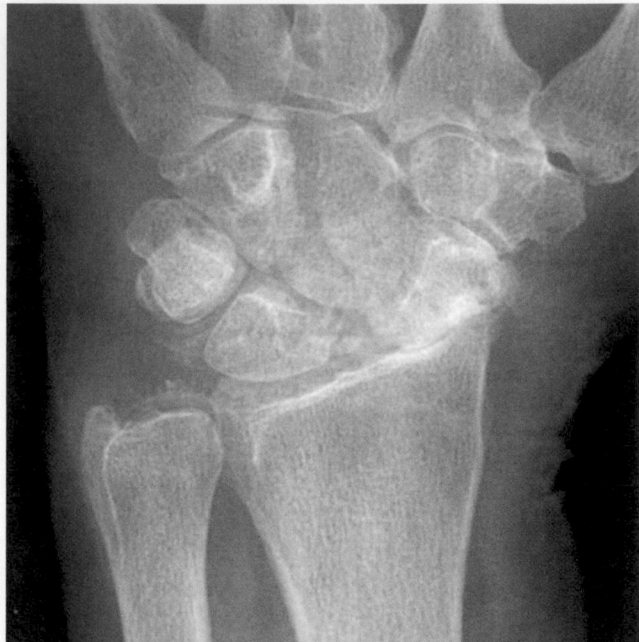

Fig. 66.25 Calcium pyrophosphate arthropathy at the wrist with scapholunate advanced collapse (SLAC). Synovial calcification with chondrocalcinosis is seen at the ulnocarpal joint (note also calcification between the lunate and triquetrum in the lunate-triquetral ligament). This is associated with radiocarpal arthropathy and scapholunate dissociation.

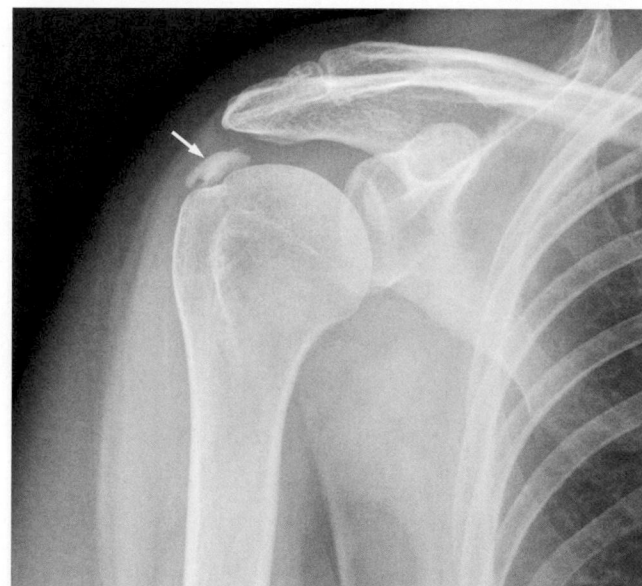

Fig. 66.26 Hydroxyapatite deposition in supraspinatus tendon. The AP shoulder radiograph shows a large deposit of amorphous calcification in the supraspinatus tendon representing hydroxyapatite deposition (arrow).

carpi radialis, abductor pollicis longus, or extensor pollicis brevis tendons.[33] This calcification is usually readily appreciated on plain film imaging and, in contrast to calcium pyrophosphate, has an amorphous appearance without internal trabeculation. Intra-articular hydroxyapatite deposition has also been described, again commonly affecting the shoulder joint and associated with chronic tears of the rotator cuff—this has been termed the Milwaukee shoulder syndrome. On plain radiographs there is glenohumeral joint destruction, narrowing, and sclerosis with occasional cyst formation; osteophyte formation is not prominent. The hands and wrists are also commonly involved.

Although the exact aetiology remains unknown there is some suggestion that hydroxyapatite deposition in soft tissues may be related to repetitive low-grade trauma.[34]

Connective tissue disease

Scleroderma, dermatomyositis, and polymyositis, and SLE all have associated arthropathy as a common feature; they share some similar radiographic findings such as osteoporosis and soft tissue wasting.

Scleroderma

Articular manifestations are common in systemic sclerosis, and joint pain is therefore a common presentation of disease.[35]

In the soft tissues flexion contractures have been shown to be the most common radiographic finding, with soft tissue atrophy over the distal phalanges and soft tissue calcification also both extremely prevalent findings. The soft tissue calcification is dystrophic in origin and amorphous in appearance and is most commonly seen in the digits; however, it may be seen in any location including within the joints either in the presence or the absence of joint destruction (Figure 66.27).

The most common site of bony resorption is the tufts of the terminal phalanges of the hands, but this phenomenon may also be seen at the angle of the mandible, the posterior ribs and diffusely around the wrist.[36] Resorption in the toes is far less common than in the fingers and is usually less severe. In chronic disease patients may develop an erosive arthropathy, which typically affects the DIP and PIP joints with sparing of the wrists.

Dermatomyositis and polymyositis

The most common radiographic change of dermatomyositis is the finding of 'sheet-like' calcification within the subcutaneous soft tissues along muscle or fascial planes. Typically these areas of calcification are diffuse, affecting both the skin and skeletal musculature, with the thigh being the most common site of involvement. Joint disease may also occur clinically but radiographs are usually unremarkable or may demonstrate subtle changes such as periarticular osteopaenia and soft tissue swelling. Other imaging findings such as muscle oedema, fatty infiltration of the muscles, and wasting are more readily appreciated on MRI. Polymyositis has similar radiographic findings but involves only skeletal muscle.

Systemic lupus erythematosus

Articular symptoms are common in SLE and have been reported in 76% of patients with this condition. The hands and wrists are commonly affected, although the feet are also sometimes involved. The most frequent finding is synovitis which will manifest as soft tissue swelling and osteopenia. Classic joint deformities are also seen secondary to ligamentous laxity and include ulnar subluxation of the MCP joints and hyperextension at the thumb interphalangeal joint. The arthropathy associated with SLE is typically non-erosive—a feature which allows distinction between this condition and RA. Osteonecrosis is a well-recognized feature in SLE and may occur in the femoral head, humeral head, knee, and MCP heads. Soft tissue calcification is a less common radiographic feature in some patients and is usually seen in a periarticular distribution.

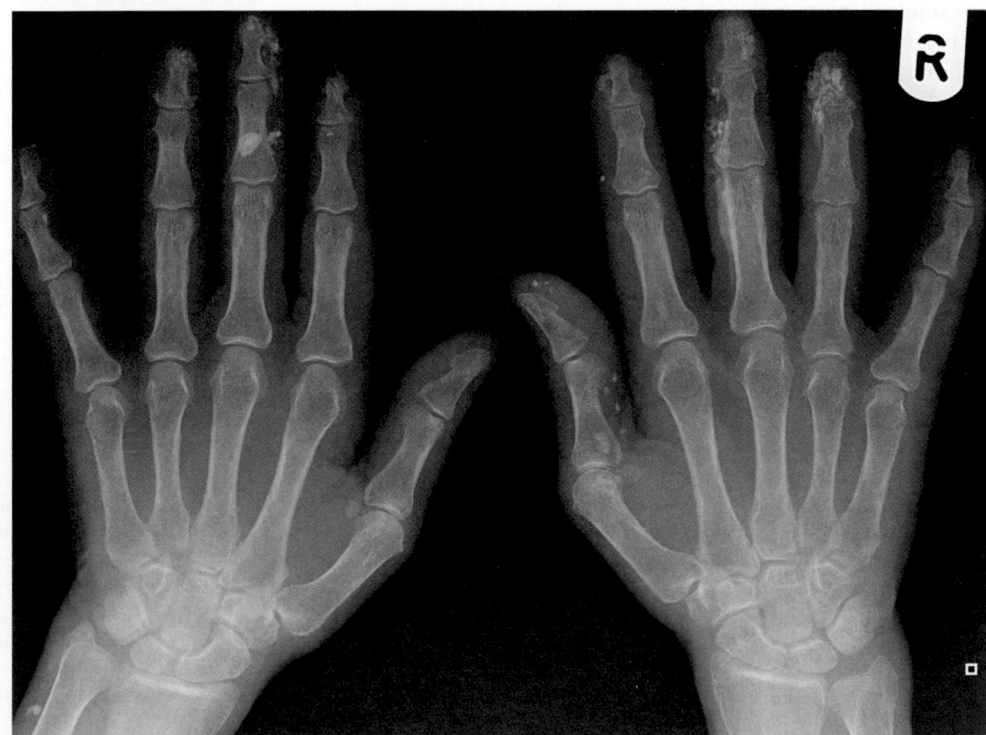

Fig. 66.27 Scleroderma. There is extensive soft tissue calcification seen within the subcutaneous tissues adjacent to the index, middle, and ring fingers bilaterally and the right thumb. There is also soft tissue loss from the distal ends of the fingers. This combination of findings is typical for scleroderma.

Miscellaneous conditions

SAPHO syndrome

The radiological appearances of the skeletal manifestations of the synovitis, acne, pustulosis, hyperostosis, and osteitis (SAPHO) syndrome are crucial in the diagnostic process.[37] The bone changes associated with this condition are thought to be due to an inflammatory process. Many of the manifestations described are appreciable on plain film imaging and studies have shown that although radiographs performed in the first 3 months of the disease course were normal in 80%, all patients had abnormal radiographs at the end of follow-up.[38] The most common site of bony involvement is the anterior chest wall and in particular the sternoclavicular, costochondral, manubriosternal, and costosternal junctions.[39] The distribution and severity of involvement varies from the adult to the paediatric form of chronic recurrent multifocal osteomyelitis (CRMO).

The radiographic findings have been subdivided into three stages: stage 1 is localized to the costoclavicular junction and is characterized by soft tissue swelling, erosion and new bone formation; stage 2 is generalized involvement of the ipsilateral sternocostoclavicular region with sternoclavicular arthropathy and increased sclerosis of the medial end of the clavicle; and stage 3 is further progression of hyperostosis, osteosclerosis and hypertrophy of the medial ends of the clavicle.[39] The spine is the second most common site of involvement with six main radiological manifestations: vertebral body corner lesions, non-specific spondylodiscitis, and osteodestructive lesions all seen in both adults and children, and osteosclerotic vertebral lesions, paravertebral ossification, and sacro-iliitis seen only in adults.[40]

Neuropathic arthropathy

The radiographic findings associated with a neuropathic joint are similar irrespective of the aetiology. Two distinct patterns of arthropathy are described, namely atrophic and hypertrophic neuropathic osteoarthropathy. Atrophic destruction manifests as osteolysis usually affecting the distal ends of tubular bones, usually in non-weightbearing joints, which may be mistaken for surgical amputation. The more common pattern of involvement is hypertrophic and characteristically the findings at an affected joint have been described as increased bone density, debris production, dislocation, disorganization, and destruction (Figure 66.28). Osteophytes are also formed in neuropathic arthropathy and may differ from those seen in osteoarthritis on the basis of ill-defined and rounded margins. Early changes may, however, be difficult to differentiate from OA, infection, or more rarely tumour. Neuropathic changes are much more commonly seen in the lower limbs than in the upper limbs or spine. Fractures associated with neuropathy are common and may be difficult to diagnose due to surrounding destruction and debris.

Haemochromatosis

Arthropathy associated with haemochromatosis is similar in radiographic presentation to the features of CPPD but there are some distinguishing features; haemochromatosis arthropathy typically involves the second and thirrd MCP joints where hook-like osteophytes are seen to the radial aspect of the metacarpal head and the metacarpal heads become flattened. In more chronic disease there

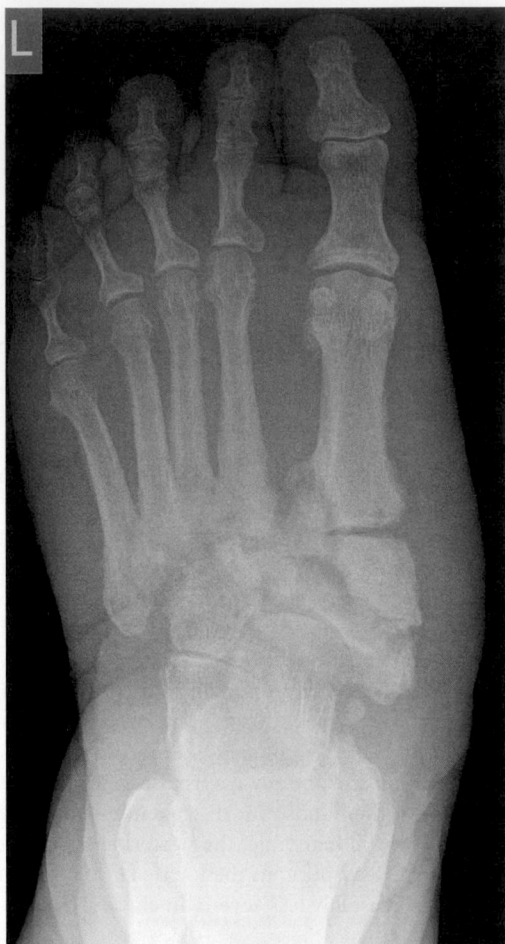

Fig. 66.28 Charcot foot. There is marked disruption of the midfoot in this patient with diabetes. There is a divergent Lis Franc dislocation and fragmentation of the midfoot bones.

may be large-joint involvement, usually of the knees, hips, and shoulders. In these joints there may be multiple subchondral cysts, subchondral sclerosis, and symmetric joint space loss. Disease progression is usually slow.

References

1. Pollock J, Giachino AA, Rakhra K et al. SLAC wrist in the absence of recognised trauma and CPPD. *Hand Surg* 2010;15(3):193–201.
2. Tomaino MM, Elfar J. Ulnar impaction syndrome. *Hand Clin* 2005;21(4):567–575.
3. Boegard T, Jonsson K. Radiography in osteoarthritis of the knee. *Skeletal Radiol* 1999;28(11):605–615.
4. Wolfe F, Lane NE, Buckland-Wright C. Radiographic methods in knee osteoarthritis: a further comparison of semiflexed (MTP), schuss-tunnel, and weight-bearing anteroposterior views for joint space narrowing and osteophytes. *J Rheumatol* 2002;29(12):2597–2601.
5. Gossec L, Jordan JM, Mazzuca SA et al. Comparative evaluation of three semi-quantitative radiographic grading techniques for knee osteoarthritis in terms of validity and reproducibility in 1759 X-rays: report of the OARSI-OMERACT task force. *Osteoarthritis Cartilage* 2008;16(7):742–748.
6. Manaster BJ. From the RSNA Refresher Courses. Radiological Society of North America. Adult chronic hip pain: radiographic evaluation. *Radiographics* 2000;20 Spec No:S3–S25.

7. Altman R, Alarcon G, Appelrouth D et al. The American College of Rheumatology criteria for the classification and reporting of osteoarthritis of the hip. *Arthritis Rheum* 1991;34(5):505–514.

8. Dixon T, Benjamin J, Lund P, Graham A, Krupinski E. Femoral neck buttressing: a radiographic and histologic analysis. *Skeletal Radiol* 2000;29(10):587–592.

9. Kloppenburg M, Kwok WY. Hand osteoarthritis—a heterogeneous disorder. *Nat Rev Rheumatol* 2011;8(1):22–31.

10. Punzi L, Frigato M, Frallonardo P, Ramonda R. Inflammatory osteoarthritis of the hand. *Best Pract Res Clin Rheumatol* 2010;24(3):301–312.

11. Greenspan A. Erosive osteoarthritis. *Semin Musculoskelet Radiol* 2003;7(2):155–159.

12. Cammisa M, De Serio A, Guglielmi G. Diffuse idiopathic skeletal hyperostosis. *Eur J Radiol* 1998;27 Suppl 1:S7–S11.

13. Resnick D, Niwayama G. Radiographic and pathologic features of spinal involvement in diffuse idiopathic skeletal hyperostosis (DISH). *Radiology* 1976;119(3):559–568.

14. Resnick D, Guerra J, Jr., Robinson CA, Vint VC. Association of diffuse idiopathic skeletal hyperostosis (DISH) and calcification and ossification of the posterior longitudinal ligament. *AJR Am J Roentgenol* 1978;131(6):1049–1053.

15. Scutellari PN, Orzincolo C, Princivalle M, Franceschini F. [Diffuse idiopathic skeletal hyperostosis. Review of diagnostic criteria and analysis of 915 cases] *Radiol Med* 1992;83(6):729–736.

16. Littlejohn GO, Urowitz MB. Peripheral enthesopathy in diffuse idiopathic skeletal hyperostosis (DISH): a radiologic study. *J Rheumatol* 1982;9(4):568–572.

17. Narvaez Garcia JA. Evaluation through imaging of early rheumatoid arthritis. *Reumatol Clin* 2010;6(2):111–114.

18. Shimada H, Abematsu M, Ishido Y et al. Classification of odontoid destruction in patients with rheumatoid arthritis using reconstructed computed tomography: reference to vertical migration. *J Rheumatol* 2011;38(5):863–867.

19. Younes M, Belghali S, Kriaa S et al. Compared imaging of the rheumatoid cervical spine: prevalence study and associated factors. *Joint Bone Spine* 2009;76(4):361–368.

20. Nagayoshi R, Ijiri K, Takenouchi T et al. Evaluation of occipitocervical subluxation in rheumatoid arthritis patients, using coronal-view reconstructive computed tomography. *Spine* 2009;34(24):E879–E881.

21. Reynolds H, Carter SW, Murtagh FR, Silbiger M, Rechtine GR. Cervical rheumatoid arthritis: value of flexion and extension views in imaging. *Radiology* 1987;164(1):215–218.

22. Vosse D, Landewe R, van der Heijde D et al. Ankylosing spondylitis and the risk of fracture: results from a large primary care-based nested case-control study. *Ann Rheum Dis* 2009;68(12):1839–1842.

23. Kauppi M, Laiho K, Neva M. Diagnosing atlantoaxial impaction and basilar invagination. *J Bone Joint Surg* 2002;84A(3):491–492.

24. van Rossum MA, Zwinderman AH, Boers M et al. Radiologic features in juvenile idiopathic arthritis: a first step in the development of a standardized assessment method. *Arthritis Rheum* 2003;48(2):507–515.

25. Johnson K, Wittkop B, Haigh F, Ryder C, Gardner-Medwin JM. The early magnetic resonance imaging features of the knee in juvenile idiopathic arthritis. *Clin Radiol* 2002;57(6):466–471.

26. Magni-Manzoni S, Rossi F, Pistorio A et al. Prognostic factors for radiographic progression, radiographic damage, and disability in juvenile idiopathic arthritis. *Arthritis Rheum* 2003;48(12):3509–3517.

27. Perez-Ruiz F, Dalbeth N, Urresola A, de Miguel E, Schlesinger N. Imaging of gout: findings and utility. *Arthritis Res Ther* 2009;11(3):232.

28. Konatalapalli RM, Demarco PJ, Jelinek JS et al. Gout in the axial skeleton. *J Rheumatol* 2009;36(3):609–613.

29. Ko KH, Hsu YC, Lee HS, Lee CH, Huang GS. Tophaceous gout of the knee: revisiting MRI patterns in 30 patients. *J Clin Rheumatol* 2010;16(5):209–214.

30. Yang BY, Sartoris DJ, Djukic S, Resnick D, Clopton P. Distribution of calcification in the triangular fibrocartilage region in 181 patients with calcium pyrophosphate dihydrate crystal deposition disease. *Radiology* 1995;196(2):547–550.

31. Chen C, Chandnani VP, Kang HS et al. Scapholunate advanced collapse: a common wrist abnormality in calcium pyrophosphate dihydrate crystal deposition disease. *Radiology* 1990;177(2):459–461.

32. Yang BY, Sartoris DJ, Resnick D, Clopton P. Calcium pyrophosphate dihydrate crystal deposition disease: frequency of tendon calcification about the knee. *J Rheumatol* 1996;23(5):883–888.

33. Hayes CW, Conway WF. Calcium hydroxyapatite deposition disease. *Radiographics* 1990;10(6):1031–1048.

34. Gandee RW, Harrison RB, Dee PM. Peritendinitis calcarea of flexor carpi ulnaris. *AJR Am J Roentgenol* 1979;133(6):1139–1141.

35. Baron M, Lee P, Keystone EC. The articular manifestations of progressive systemic sclerosis (scleroderma). *Ann Rheum Dis* 1982;41(2):147–152.

36. Bassett LW, Blocka KL, Furst DE, Clements PJ, Gold RH. Skeletal findings in progressive systemic sclerosis (scleroderma). *AJR Am J Roentgenol* 1981;136(6):1121–1126.

37. Boutin RD, Resnick D. The SAPHO syndrome: an evolving concept for unifying several idiopathic disorders of bone and skin. *AJR Am J Roentgenol* 1998;170(3):585–591.

38. Maugars Y, Berthelot JM, Ducloux JM, Prost A. SAPHO syndrome: a followup study of 19 cases with special emphasis on enthesis involvement. *J Rheumatol* 1995;22(11):2135–2141.

39. Earwaker JW, Cotten A. SAPHO: syndrome or concept? Imaging findings. *Skeletal Radiol* 2003;32(6):311–327.

40. Depasquale R, Kumar N, Lalam RK et al. SAPHO: What radiologists should know. *Clin Radiol* 2012;67(3):195–206.

CHAPTER 67

Ultrasound

David Kane and Philip Platt

Use of ultrasound in rheumatology

The inclusion for the first time in this textbook of a chapter on ultrasound indicates the recognition of musculoskeletal ultrasound (MSUS) as a routine part of rheumatological practice. The first report on the use of ultrasound in a rheumatology clinic was published over 30 years ago.[1] Ultrasound assessment of small joints, a particular interest for rheumatologists, only became feasible in the 1990s with the advent of high-frequency transducers.[2] Further technical advances and falling equipment costs have allowed rheumatologists to obtain equipment and begin training, and have facilitated the introduction of ultrasound into routine clinical practice. Training in the use of ultrasound is currently a compulsory part of rheumatology training in some European countries, with training courses and programmes established in most European countries. In 2005 up to 93% of rheumatologists in the United Kingdom reported that they used ultrasound in the management of patients, with 33% performing ultrasound themselves.[3]

The principal advantage of ultrasound over MRI, CT, and scintigraphy is its immediate availability in a clinical setting. It is performed after clinical history and examination, allowing the rheumatologist to focus in on the key joint or joints of interest. The diagnosis can therefore be immediately confirmed or refuted and therapy instigated without delay. Ultrasound allows guidance of aspiration and injection, improving the accuracy rates of procedures. Other advantages are that it is non-invasive, non-radioactive, and has very high patient acceptability with no issues regarding claustrophobia or pregnancy. Soft tissue imaging with ultrasound provides higher definition than other imaging modalities, including MRI. Although there are initial equipment costs, the running costs are low and ultrasonography is largely immune to the metal artefacts that can cause difficulties with MRI and CT.

The disadvantages of ultrasound are that it requires the initial purchase of equipment and a significant commitment to training. Adding an ultrasound scan to your patient assessment will lengthen the initial appointment time, but usually reduces the need to review the patient again for the same complaint, thus saving time overall. Ultrasound cannot image into or beyond bone, which MRI and CT imaging can, and ultrasound has a limited resolution for deeper joints, such as the hip, particularly in obese patients. There are also valid concerns about the standardization of examinations by different sonographers and how best to assess and certify competency in trainee ultrasonographers.

Ultrasound by rheumatologists is complementary to that of musculoskeletal radiologists but it does not replace it completely. Patients who undergo an ultrasound examination by a rheumatologist often have different clinical characteristics and diagnostic targets from those assessed by a radiologist. Formal ultrasound by an experienced musculoskeletal radiologist is still invaluable in cases of diagnostic uncertainty and for the selection and interpretation of other imaging modalities such as MR and CT.

Technical aspects of ultrasound

Equipment

There are a number of important considerations when selecting ultrasound equipment.[4] Cost relates directly to image resolution and quality, but the cost of equipment is falling and the quality is improving. It is a good principle to purchase the best machine that you can afford, particularly for your first ultrasound system. The choice of probe size and frequency depends on the size and depth of the structures you wish to image. A higher-frequency probe (10–20 MHz), ideal for small superficial structures, has a smaller footprint with high resolution, but poor tissue penetration. The reverse is true for lower frequency probes (<7.5 MHz). Linear array transducers are the preferred option for most musculoskeletal scanning. Equipment portability is an advantage for multisite use, but incurs more expense to obtain the equivalent image quality of a larger, less mobile system. Colour and power Doppler options are essential for rheumatology practice.

Ultrasound technology

Ultrasonography uses reflected pulses of high-frequency sound to assess soft tissue, cartilage, bone surfaces, and fluid-containing structures. These pulses are emitted and reflections are received by the same ultrasound transducer. The basic principle of ultrasonography is that the denser the material the sound wave is passing through, the more reflective it is, the stronger the reflected signal received by the transducer, and the whiter (or more echoic) it appears on screen. Water is the least reflective body material. Sound waves pass straight through water with minimal reflection and it appears black (or anechoic). Bone is the most reflective body material and appears as a bright white line (hyperechoic).

Greyscale or B-mode ultrasonography displays the different intensities of echoes in black, white, and shades of grey. Where a tissue has organized into areas of different density and structure there may be multiple reflections, such as occurs in a tendon where reflections from the multiple tendon fibres give a characteristic linear appearance.

Doppler

Doppler ultrasound uses the principle that sound waves increase in frequency when they reflect from objects (such as red blood cells) that are moving towards the transducer (displayed as a red signal) and decrease when they are moving away from the transducer (displayed as a blue signal). Power Doppler ultrasound measures the amplitude of the Doppler signal (which is determined by the volume of blood flow) and superimposes it on the greyscale image, thereby depicting increased microvascular blood flow.

Power Doppler is generally used for assessment of small-vessel blood flow that occurs in inflammatory soft tissues, whereas colour Doppler is used for larger-vessel assessment, as in temporal arteritis. A subjective assessment of the degree of vascularity present in soft tissues can be made by scoring on a semiquantitative scale of 0 to 3, where the score is assigned according to the number of vessels or the percentage area of vascularity within the joint tissue (0, no Doppler signal; 1, signal <10% of the field; 2, signal is 10–50% of the field; 3, signal >50% of the field).

Standard views and artefacts

Ultrasound scans are defined by two views and all examinations should include both planes: transverse or short axis (similar to axial views on CT/MRI) and longitudinal or long axis. The correct probe size and frequency should be selected according to the size and depth of the joint to be examined. Most ultrasound systems used in rheumatology practice now have presets for different joints, allowing the appropriate settings of the ultrasound equipment to be adjusted. A more detailed technical description of ultrasound system technology is outside the scope of this chapter but can be found in all major ultrasonography textbooks.[5]

There are a few ultrasound artefacts to be aware of:

• **Anisotropy**. This is the property of certain tissues to change their reflectivity with changes in the angle of incidence of the ultrasound beam. If the beam is not perpendicular to the tissue being scanned, the sound waves are scattered rather than being reflected back to the transducer. This causes the structure to appear darker than it should and can result in the inaccurate diagnosis of, for example, tendinosis or tendon tears.

• **Edge artefact**. Hypoechoic areas occur at the edge of spherical structures such as tendons or fluid collections, giving an edge artefact or refractile shadow.

• **Acoustic shadowing**. This occurs when the ultrasound beam hits a highly reflective surface such as bone, air, or calcified tissue. The region below (behind) it appears anechoic (black) or hypoechoic (grey) as very few sound waves can reach it.

• **Power Doppler artefacts**. Caution has to be exercised when assessing power Doppler signal. It is extremely operator and machine dependent. Doppler signal is very sensitive to the slightest movement of the transducer and too much pressure on the transducer can occlude small vessels, thus giving a false,negative power Doppler signal.[6]

Variability

A valid concern is the high degree of operator dependence in ultrasonography. In order to minimize variability it is best to use a standard scanning protocol.[7] All images should always be interpreted in light of the clinical history and examination. The OMERACT ultrasound task force has confirmed good levels of inter- and intra-observer variability of ultrasound imaging among expert ultrasonographers and there is good reliability between experts using different types of ultrasound machine.[8]

Ultrasound pathology

Ultrasound has been shown to have many uses in the diagnosis and management of musculoskeletal disorders. MSUS is consistently superior to clinical examination in

• measuring the extent of anatomical damage and inflammation in early arthritis

• assessing inflammatory and non-inflammatory soft tissue diseases

• determining therapy efficacy

• providing guidance for joint and soft tissue injection.[9,10]

Musculoskeletal ultrasound should always complement clinical examination and has the further advantage of improving the operator's knowledge of functional anatomy and pathological processes.[4] The high resolution of today's ultrasound machines means that normal amounts of synovial fluid can often be detected in healthy joints. Standard reference values have been compiled in order to help distinguish between normal and pathological structures.[11] The OMERACT MSUS group published the first definitions of sonographic pathology for rheumatologists in 2005.[12] Specific pathologies are fully described in the relevant disease sections.

Rheumatoid arthritis

The application of ultrasound in the diagnosis of inflammatory arthritis was a key event in positively influencing the uptake of ultrasound performed by rheumatologists. Initial studies in established rheumatoid arthritis (RA) had confirmed the accuracy of ultrasound in detecting joint and soft tissue inflammation.[2] A number of studies then confirmed the increased sensitivity of ultrasound diagnosis of joint inflammation over clinical examination in early RA, facilitating earlier diagnosis and therapeutic intervention.[13–15]

Joint inflammation is detected as joint effusion, an anechoic or hypoechoic appearance, that is compressible and displaceable, or as synovitis (Figure 67.1). Synovitis is diagnosed by the presence of an abnormally thickened hypoechoic tissue around the joint that is partially compressible but not displaceable. Normal synovium is not visualized in healthy joints and the presence of synovitis is closely correlated with the presence of effusion. Ultrasound is more sensitive than clinical examination in the detection of synovitis.[9,16] It has been shown to detect subclinical synovitis, which can predict radiographic progression in both the early and established stages of disease.[17] Tenosynovitis is also detected frequently on ultrasound of RA joints.

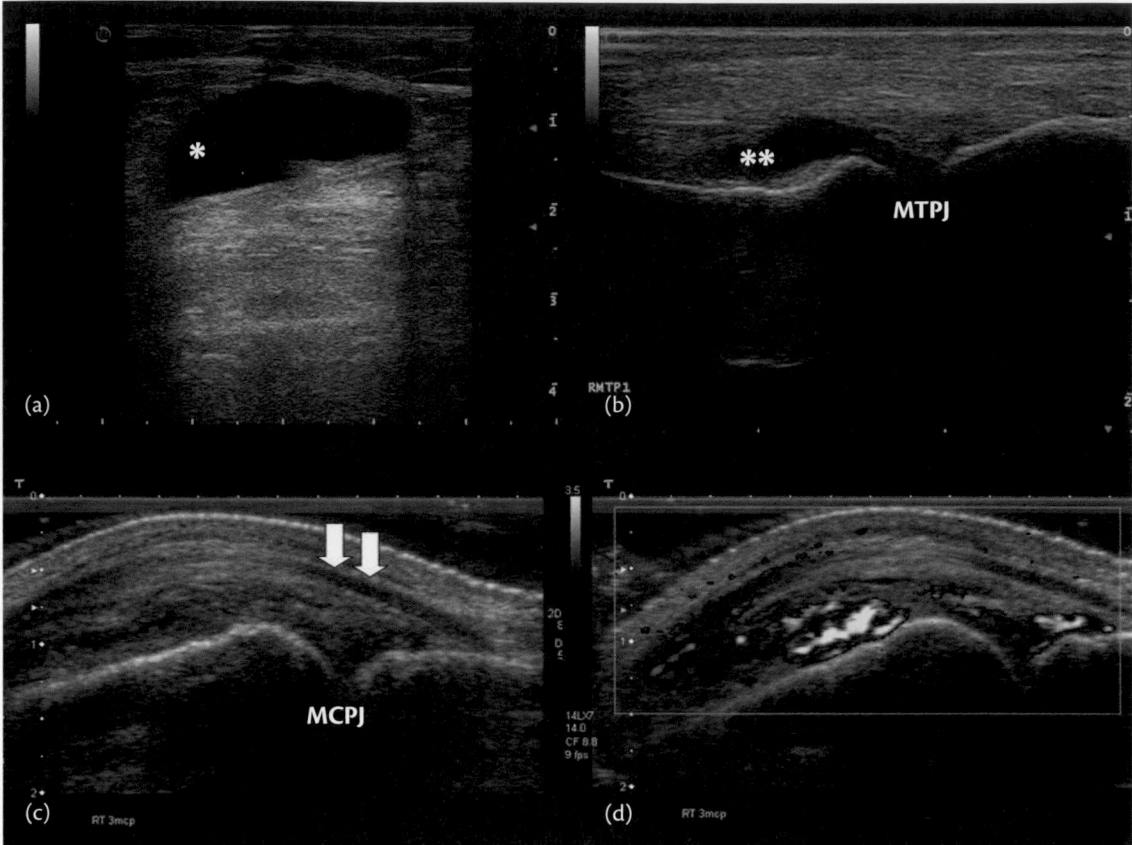

Fig. 67.1 Ultrasound in rheumatoid arthritis: (A) Characteristic anechoic well-circumscribed Baker's cyst (**) in effusion of the knee in rheumatoid arthritis (posterior longitudinal view). (B) Mixed echogenicity with anechoic effusion (*) and hypoechoic synovial thickening in metatarsophalangeal (MTP) joint synovitis (dorsal longitudinal view)—the joint is labelled at the junction of the hyperechoic bony cortex of the metatarsal and phalanx. (C) MCP joint synovitis with hypoechoic synovial thickening causing convex displacement (arrowed) of the extensor tendon (dorsal longitudinal view). (D) MCP joint synovitis with power Doppler signal in the hypoechoic synovial thickening (dorsal longitudinal view).

Power Doppler scanning has become an integral part of the sonographic assessment for synovitis and tenosynovitis (Figure 67.2). Doppler is most sensitive in the superficial joints, such as the hands and feet, and is less sensitive in the deeper joints, such as the hip and shoulder. Joint hyperaemia due to vasodilatation is an early feature of articular inflammation. Angiogenesis is a key feature of synovial pannus formation leading to chronic inflammation and joint destruction. Power Doppler can detect minimal increases in perfusion in the synovium and has comparable sensitivity and specificity to MRI[15] with proven correlation to histological vascular density of the inflamed synovial membrane.[18]

The presence of power Doppler signal in RA implies active tissue inflammation. It can be quantified and has shown better inter- and intra-observer reproducibility than greyscale synovitis across several studies. Advances in ultrasound imaging now produce similar sensitivity for joint inflammation with either colour or power Doppler in most modern ultrasound systems. However, Doppler has the potential for a number of well-recognized artefacts leading to false-positive results, and care must be taken in using appropriate machine settings and minimizing movement and systematic artefact.[19]

MSUS is increasingly being used as a clinical tool to monitor disease activity in RA and to assess response to treatment. Power Doppler has been shown to be a valid method for monitoring

response to anti-TNFα therapy in RA. It is reproducible and sensitive to change and may have predictive value in relation to radiological outcome.[17] Taylor et al.[20] looked at patients with early RA and measured the degree of synovial thickening in 10 metacarpophalangeal (MCP) joints and a Doppler-based vascularity score. There was a marked improvement following treatment with infliximab compared to controls and the vascularity score was more sensitive than the clinical disease activity score (DAS).

Both greyscale and power Doppler ultrasound have validity in assessing changes in articular inflammation and a number of objective scoring systems have been proposed. As these systems have been reported by experienced ultrasonographers assessing large numbers of joints with ultrasound,[21,22] an ultrasound score for RA remains a research tool at present. A recent study looked at a number of these measurement tools and found that ultrasound evaluation was an outcome measure 'at least as relevant as physical examination'.[23] The OMERACT ultrasound task force is currently developing a Global OMERACT Scoring System (GLOSS) for use in RA in addition to sonographic scoring systems for enthesitis and osteoarthritis.[24]

Radiographic bone erosion is a key pathophysiological feature of RA and is one of the American College of Rheumatology (ACR) diagnostic criteria. Radiographic erosions can be scored to allow monitoring of disease progression and outcome. Several studies

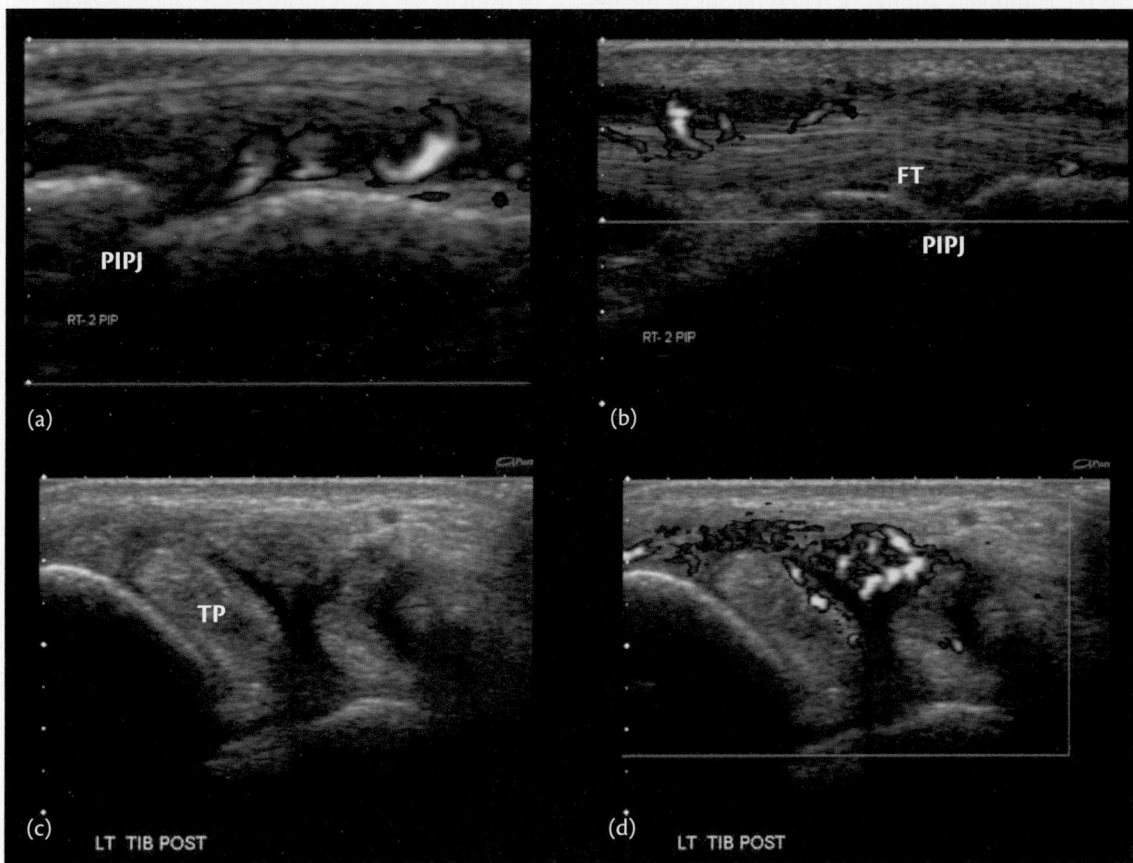

Fig. 67.2 Ultrasound in rheumatoid and seronegative arthritis: (A) Proximal interphalangeal (PIP) joint synovitis in rheumatoid arthritis with hypoechoic synovial thickening and power Doppler signal on the extensor aspect of the joint (dorsal longitudinal view). (B) Flexor tenosynovitis (FT) is seen in the palmar longitudinal view of the PIP joint in panel A with hypoechoic widening of the tendon sheath and power Doppler signal in the tendon and sheath. The presence of tendon inflammation is a common feature in RA and does not differentiate seropositive from seronegative arthritis. (C) Tibialis posterior tenosynovitis in reactive arthritis shows similar hypoechoic widening of the tendon sheath (transverse view over medial ankle). (D) Panel C with power Doppler signal in the tendon sheath and tendon.

have confirmed that MSUS is more sensitive than plain rtadiuography in the detection of bone erosions in patients with RA. Wakefield et al.[14] reported that ultrasound detected 6.5 times more erosions than plain radiography in the MCP joints of patients with early RA and 3.4 times more in established RA. MRI and MSUS correlate well in the detection of bone erosion, though MRI has advantages in less accessible joints, such as the wrist and the third and fourth MCP joints. There is a high level of reliability within and between observers in detecting bone erosion on MSUS.[14,15] The development of an objective ultrasound erosion score to replace radiographic scoring is ongoing.

Spondyloarthropathies

Spondyloarthritis (SpA) is the preferred terminology for a group of diseases characterized by joint synovitis, tendonitis, and enthesitis peripherally in combination with pathognomic axial inflammation particularly at the sacroiliac joints. SpA may occur in association with psoriasis, inflammatory bowel disease, or uveitis, usually in the absence of rheumatoid factor and anti-citrullinated peptide antibodies.

All of the peripheral pathologies in SpA can be readily identified on ultrasound imaging, and initial studies show the potential for ultrasound in imaging sacroiliac joints and psoriasis. The increased sensitivity of ultrasound in the diagnosis of synovitis is well described in RA. There are no consistent qualitative or quantitative features that discriminate synovitis in RA from SpA.

Greyscale and Doppler MSUS are sensitive techniques in the detection of synovitis of the hand and knee in established psoriatic arthritis (PsA) and in the objective monitoring of response of synovitis to therapy.[25,26] MSUS can also detect subclinical PsA in patients with psoriasis.[27] In early seronegative oligoarthritis, the increased sensitivity of MSUS in the diagnosis of synovitis led to 29/80 patients (36%) clinically classified as oligoarticular being reclassified as polyarthritis based on MSUS. The implication of this study is that MSUS may identify patients with SpA who have higher disease activity and who merit more aggressive early therapy.

Inflammation of the enthesis—the tendon, ligament, or capsule junction with bone—is a common feature of SpA and has stimulated much research and debate on the classification and pathophysiology of SpA. But enthesitis is not exclusive to SpA and can occur in gout or secondary to mechanical stress in many rheumatic diseases. MSUS features of enthesitis include hypoechoic entheseal thickening, fibrillar separation of the enthesis due to oedema, presence of power Doppler signal within the enthesis, associated bursitis, and bony insertion erosive change and enthesophyte formation.[28,29]

Tendonitis has similar ultrasound appearances distal to the insertion with the additional features of tenosynovitis of the tendon sheath and paratenonitis. Using MSUS as the gold standard, clinical examination was initially reported to have a low sensitivity (22.6%) and moderate specificity (79.7%) for the detection of enthesitis of the lower limbs.[29,30] Enthesitis can be observed at any enthesis, but is most frequent in the lower limbs particularly at the plantar fascia and Achilles tendon (Figure 67.3).[31] A recent review noted that there are now more than 20 studies of scoring of enthesitis that confirm ultrasound as the most sensitive diagnostic tool.[32] The Glasgow Ultrasound Enthesitis Scoring System (GUESS) is the most commonly used score, though there is no agreement on a standardized ultrasound enthesitis score that incorporates all the ultrasound features of enthesitis.

Dactylitis of the digits and distal interphalangeal (DIP) joint involvement are characteristic clinical features of PsA. MSUS and MRI studies confirm that flexor tenosynovitis and diffuse soft tissue swelling are the principal component features of dactylitis in early SpA,[33,34] while synovitis is also found in patients with dactylitis and established PsA.[35] DIP joint disease is a feature of a number of arthritides and MSUS can differentiate PsA DIP disease from erosive or nodular osteoarthritis, chronic tophaceous gout, calcification in systemic sclerosis, and simple synovial cysts.[36]

MRI is the gold standard for imaging sacroiliitis in SpA, but MSUS with colour Doppler and microbubble contrast agent enhancement has shown excellent correlation with MRI sacroiliitis (sensitivity 94%, specificity 86%)[37] and can be used to monitor the response to anti-TNF therapy.[38] MSUS may be used to detect structural damage such as bony erosion in patients with PsA.[36] Given that the rate of radiological damage in early PsA is modest, more sensitive techniques such as MSUS and MRI have a potential role in future clinical trials.

Osteoarthritis

Ultrasound has emerged as a very promising imaging modality for osteoarthritis (OA) with the ability to reliably detect changes in articular cartilage, both thickness and quality, the presence of effusions, synovial hypertrophy, other soft tissues, and bone surface.[39] Potential OA changes can be evaluated readily in knee hip and finger joints, although research has centred predominantly on knee OA.

Normal articular cartilage is anechoic, whereas degenerative cartilage has increased echogenicity. Ultrasound can demonstrate loss of normal sharpness of chondral surface and chondrosynovial interface with reduction in thickness of the cartilage. Increased echogenicity of the osteochondral interface and sensitive detection of osteophytic change and identification of erosions have been reported.[39] There are some limitations, including difficulty in delineating progressive changes in articular cartilage due to problems with reproducibility, and also the limitation of acoustic windows into some joints.[39]

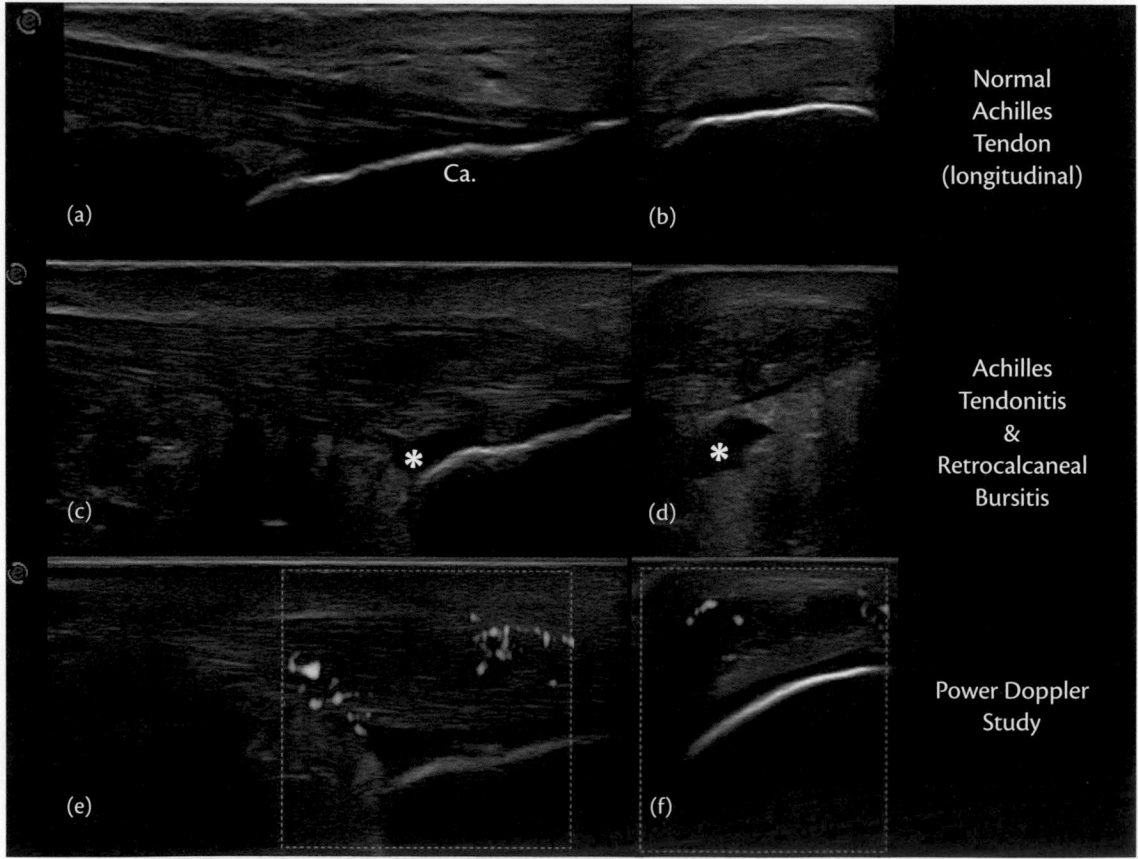

Fig. 67.3 Achilles tendonitis in seronegative spondyloarthritis: (A) Normal longitudinal view of Achilles tendon insertion. (B) Normal transverse view of Achilles tendon insertion. (C) Hypoechoic thickened Achilles tendon at calcaneal insertion (Ca.) with mixed echogenic retrocalcaneal bursal effusion and synovitis (longitudinal view). (D) Transverse view of previous panel. (E, F) Increased power Doppler signal in the thickened Achilles tendon. * marks the site of the retrocalcaneal bursitis.

Ultrasound has demonstrated that synovitis is a common feature of OA. In a study of 600 patients with knee pain, D'Agostino et al.[40] demonstrated effusion and/or synovitis in 46% of knees. Ultrasound has been shown to be more sensitive in detecting effusion and Baker's cyst than clinical examination.[41] However, the detection of hip and knee effusion and synovitis does not predict response to intra-articular steroid injection.[41,42]

Non-inflammatory soft tissue disorders

Ultrasonography is the imaging modality of choice for tendons. The resolution for superficial tendons is greater than for MRI and has the advantage that the real-time imaging allows movement of tendons and hence dynamic assessments. The characteristic appearance is due to low echogenic collagen fibrils surrounded by highly echogenic connective tissue matrix. This gives the tendon a bright, striated, appearance on ultrasonography, when imaged with the probe perpendicular to the long axis of the tendon. When the tendon runs obliquely to the ultrasound beam the echogenicity is reduced and is described as anisotropy.

Tendon pathology in the form of tendinopathy, is characterized on ultrasound by swelling of the tendon with inhomogeneous hypoechoic areas in the tendon substance. This is often accompanied by neovascularization demonstrated by power Doppler ultrasound. Tendon rupture is characterized by the absence of echoes between the free edges of the tear if the gap is filled by fluid, or rather more echogenic material if the gap is filled with haematoma or tissue herniating in to fill the 'gap'. There is also a lack of synchronous movements on dynamic scanning. Tears are frequently accompanied by signs of tendinopathy.

Tendons may be enclosed in a synovial sheath, such as around the wrist and ankle, or a much thinner paratenon of loose vascular connective tissue, as in the case of Achilles and rotator cuff tendons. Tenosynovitis is readily demonstrated on greyscale ultrasound as excessive fluid between the tendon and the synovial sheath or paratenon, and where there is a synovial sheath, synovial hypertrophy. Power Doppler frequently demonstrates significantly increased vascularity in tissues surrounding the tendon. In mild cases of tenosynovitis the most obvious abnormality may be loss of the normal smooth sliding action of affected tendons on movement. Localized thickening of the tendon sheath, often with a Doppler signal in the thickened area of tendon sheath, is seen in De Quervain's. Increased fluid around a tendon does not always indicate tenosynovitis. Fluid around the long head of the biceps tendon may indicate a shoulder effusion and increased amounts of fluid are often seen around the tendons which cross the ankle joint.

Enthesopathy, such as patella tendinopathy or lateral epicondylopathy is characterized by expansion of the tendon at the insertion, inhomogeneous hypoechoic areas, and frequently increased vascularity as demonstrated by power Doppler.

Shoulder

The joint where ultrasonography has made the most significant impact is the shoulder. Rotator cuff tears, tendinopathy, and impingement are common indications for ultrasound examination. Ultrasound is as sensitive and specific at demonstrating rotator cuff pathology as MRI scanning.[43] Although it does not offer the sensitivity of MRI arthrography, it is much more cost effective and is non-invasive.

The complete intra-articular course of the long head of the biceps tendon cannot be visualized, but it can be clearly seen in the bicipital grove as homogeneous, linear, and echogenic. Pathology in the form of tenosynovitis, tears, and subluxation can all be identified. Supraspinatus tendinopathy is common and earliest changes are seen in anterior and distal tendon edges.[44] Tendinopathy is seen as hypoechoic swelling. Tears are seen as a focal area of tendon defect, with the margins separated by fluid or herniated deltoid or subdeltoid bursa.[44] Partial tears may only be identified by a change in the contour of the supraspinatus tendon. Isolated severe subscapularis tendinopathy or tear is uncommon, being more likely to occur as part of a massive rotator cuff tear or previous dislocation. Similarly, isolated infraspinatus pathology is unusual.

Ankle

Normal Achilles tendons are highly echogenic, and anisotropy occurs where fibres curve down to insert into the calcaneum. The superficial nature and lack of any overlying bone make the Achilles tendon an ideal subject for MSUS. A number of pathologies can be readily identified including tendinopathy, enthesopathy and enthesitis, tears, inflamed paratenon, and bursas. Tendinopathy of the Achilles tendon (Figure 67.4) normally affects the mid section of the tendon some 4–6 cm from the calcaneum. The tendon becomes swollen with development of hypoechogenic areas and loss of the normal fibrillary pattern. Power Doppler often shows increased vascularity with new vessels penetrating deep into the tendon. In Achilles tendon tears fluid can be seen between the torn margins; if there is intervening haematoma this can be more difficult to distinguish as the appearance is not dissimilar to tendinopathy (Figure 67.5).

Of the tendons that cross the ankle, the tibialis posterior and the peroneal tendons are most likely to demonstrate pathological changes in the form of tendinopathy, tenosynovitis, or tears. In the case of the tibialis posterior tendinopathic changes are most commonly found close to the medial malleolus and close to its insertion into the navicular bone. Changes of tenosynovitis in the tibial posterior and peroneal tendons are most likely to be found close to the malleoli.

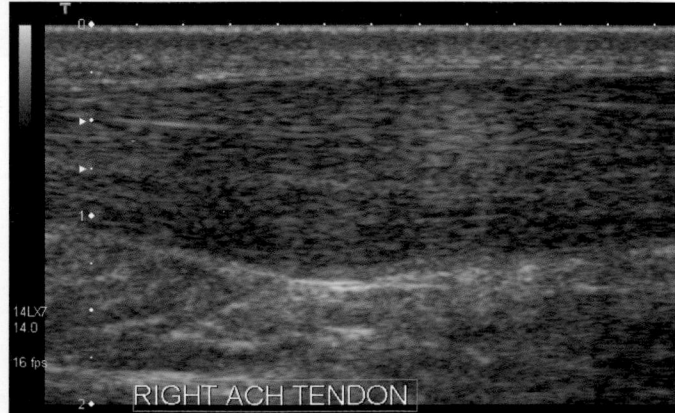

Fig. 67.4 Achilles tendinopathy showing expansion of the mid zone of the tendon, with increased low echogenic areas (longitudinal view).

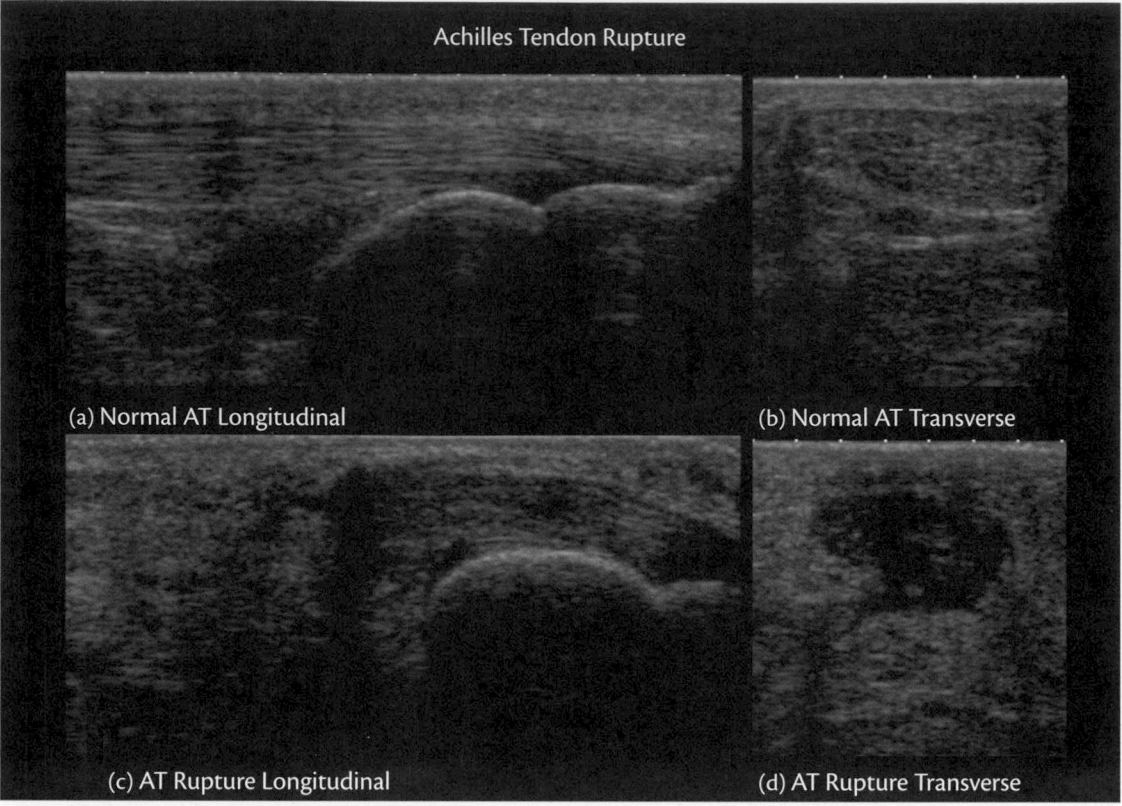

Fig. 67.5 Complete rupture of the Achilles tendon: (A) Normal longitudinal view of Achilles tendon insertion. (B) Normal transverse view of Achilles tendon insertion. (C) Hypoechoic Achilles tendon with complete loss of fibrillar structure (longitudinal view). (D) Transverse view of previous panel.

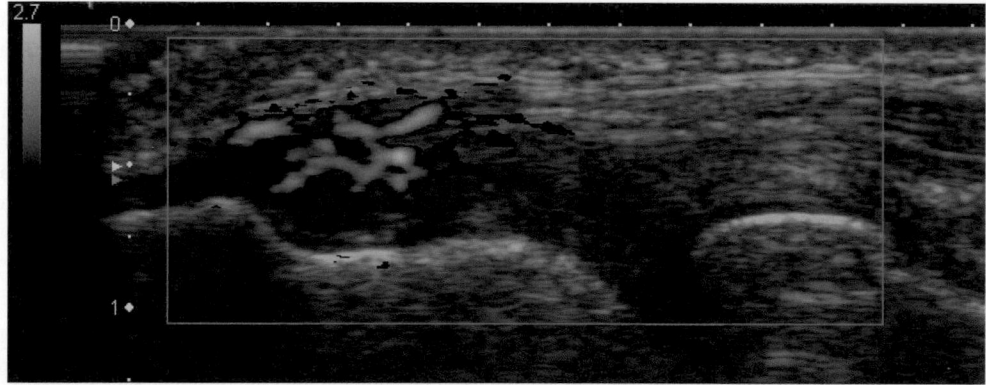

Fig. 67.6 Lateral epicondylopathy (tennis elbow), showing radial head, joint margin of elbow joint and lateral epicondyle. Significant power Doppler signal from hard areas close to insertion.

Enthesopathy or insertional tendinopathy

These include common conditions such as lateral epicondylopathy (Figure 67.6), patellar tendinopathy (Figure 67.7), Achilles enthesopathy (Figure 67.8), and lateral hip pain or so-called trochanteric bursitis. Abnormalities demonstrated on MSUS in all these areas follow the same pattern of expansion of the tendon close to insertion, hypoechogenicity, loss of the normal bright fibrillary pattern, and increased vascularity demonstrated on power Doppler. The degree of vascularity of the lesions can be quite striking and is reversible. The role of the vascularity in terms of symptoms and its correlation with degree of symptoms and their disappearance is still controversial. Dense calcification can be seen in all these areas in chronic conditions together with some irregularity of the underlying bone.

Crystal-induced arthritis

As with other causes of erosive disease, ultrasound is a sensitive method of detecting erosive changes in gout.[45] Gout can also produce characteristic ultrasound appearances, the 'double contour' or 'train track' sign in both clinically affected and unaffected joints due to the deposition of monosodium urate crystals on the surface of the hyaline cartilage (Figures 67.9 and 67.10).[45] Tophi have a range of appearances on ultrasound from hypoechogenic areas (soft tophi), to hyperechoic areas (hard tophi), with areas of calcification (Figure 67.11).

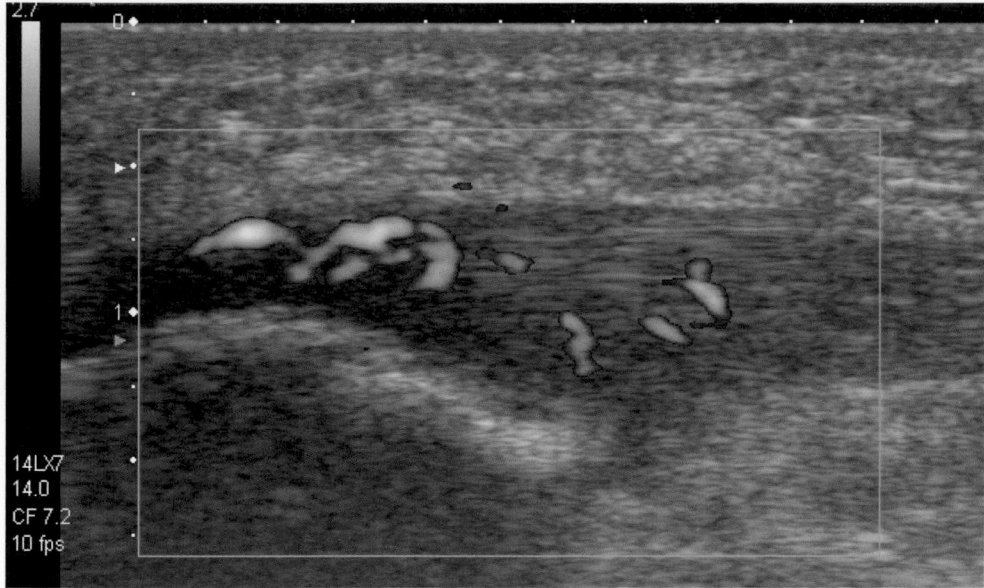

Fig. 67.7 Patellar tendinopathy showing expansion of the patella tendon with hypoechoic areas and power Doppler signal (longitudinal view).

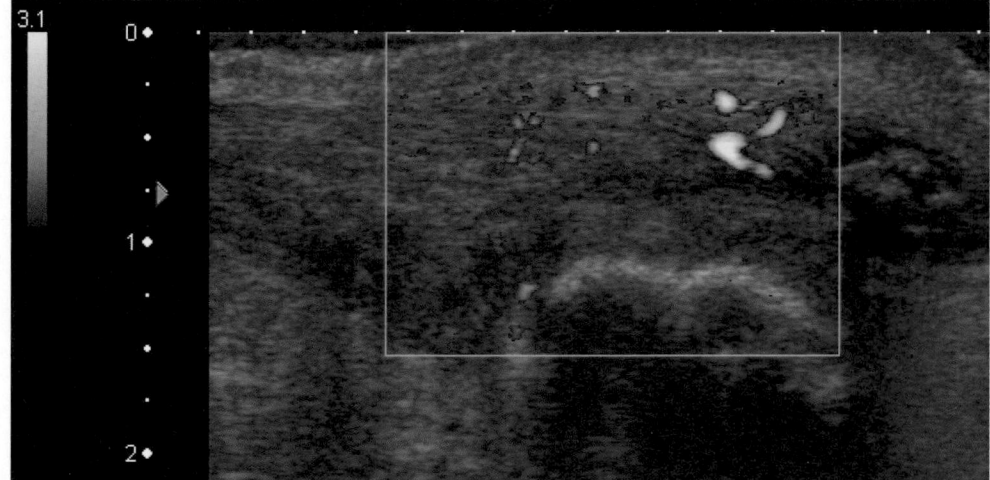

Fig. 67.8 Achilles enthesitis with expansion of the enthesis, power Doppler signal (longitudinal view).

In calcium pyrophosphate deposition disease, the crystals are found within the substance of hyaline cartilage and are seen as linear hyperechoic deposits. They may also be detected in fibrocartilage as hyperechoic deposits that persist even when the gain of the ultrasound beam is markedly reduced.

Connective tissue diseases and vasculitis

Systemic lupus erythematosus

The potential for the use of ultrasound in connective tissue diseases has been relatively neglected compared to RA. Erosive changes in Jaccoud's arthropathy have been demonstrated using ultrasound, which were not detected on plain radiography.[46] Synovitis and/or effusions in wrist and hands are found commonly, being reported in one-half the cases in one study,[47] with tenosynovitis in one-quarter and structural damage in 14%. Significant findings have also been reported in larger joints, including synovitis in 40% and effusion in 20% of knees.[48] Vascular changes in systemic lupus erythematosus

(SLE) have been more fully evaluated, with carotid plaques reported in 18% of SLE patients with nephritis compared to 2% in controls and increased plaque progression and intimal thickening.[49]

Systemic sclerosis

High-frequency ultrasound is reported to be a reliable and reproducible method of measuring digital dermal thickness in patients with systemic sclerosis.[50] Significant dermal thickening was reported in all groups, oedematous being thicker than fibrotic, which in turn was thicker than atrophic, with significant correlation with modified Rodman score. Patients with early disease (<2 years), are characterized by increased skin thickness and low skin echogenicity reflecting oedema, useful to detect patients with diffuse involvement at a very early stage.[51] Ultrasound elastography being evaluated for use in systemic sclerosis in assessing skin involvement, but appears to be limited to areas of thicker dermis and where bone hyper-reflection is minimal, effectively excluding use in hands.[52]

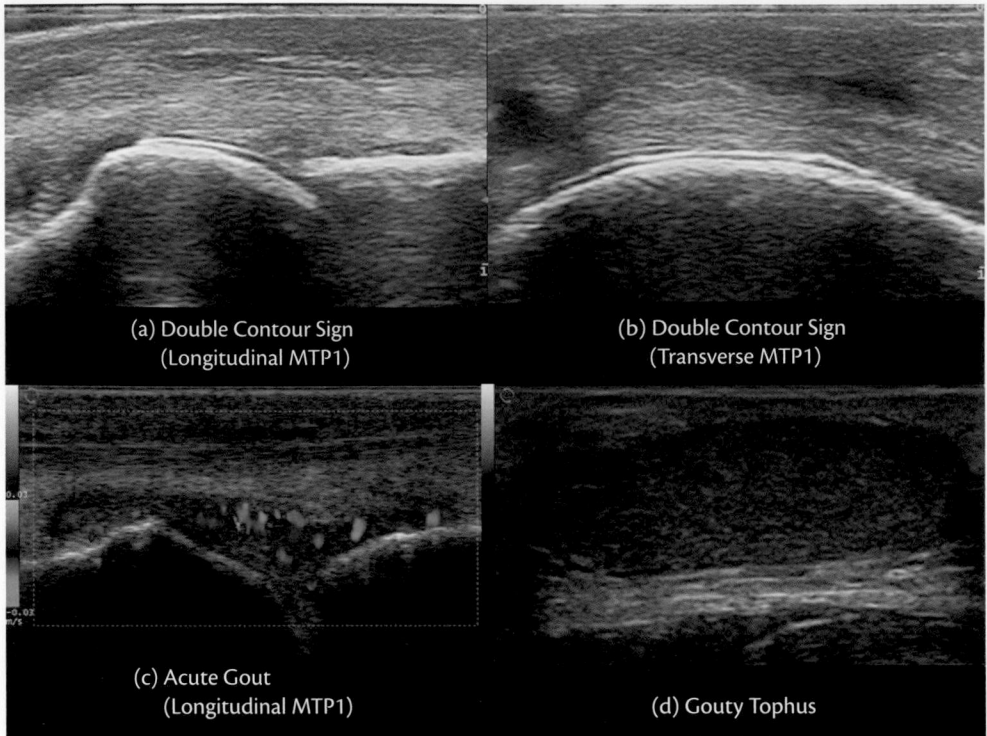

(a) Double Contour Sign
(Longitudinal MTP1)

(b) Double Contour Sign
(Transverse MTP1)

(c) Acute Gout
(Longitudinal MTP1)

(d) Gouty Tophus

Fig. 67.9 (A) Double contour sign in gout of the first metatarsophalangeal (MTP) joint (dorsal longitudinal view). (B) Dorsal transverse view of double contour sign. (C) Hypoechoic synovial thickening and effusion with power Doppler signal in acute gout of the first MTP joint. (D) Gouty tophus.

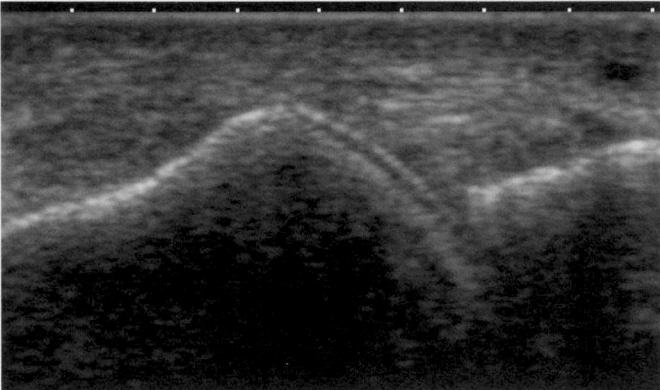

Fig. 67.10 First MTP joint showing double contour or train track sign due to deposition of urate crystals on the surface of the articular cartilage (dorsal longitudinal view).

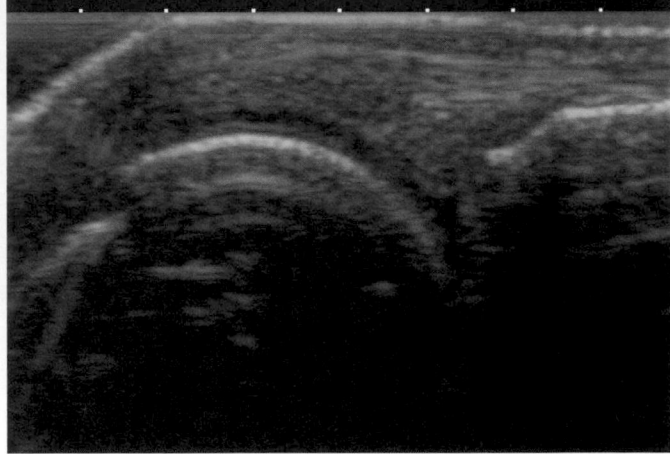

Fig. 67.11 Second metacarpophalangeal (MCP) joint showing line of calcification in the midzone of the articular cartilage.

Sjögren's syndrome

In the early stage the salivary glands on ultrasound may be normal or show diffuse enlargement with normal echogenicity.[53] The late features are more diagnostic: a heterogeneous echo pattern with multiple round hypoechoic areas within the parenchyma, sometimes containing frank cystic changes. In long-standing disease, the involved glands appear small and atrophic with a hypoechoic echotexture or may have a reticulated pattern.[54] It has recently been suggested that submandibular gland sonography might be a practical alternative to sialography in the classification of Sjögren's syndrome.[55]

Vasculitis

The combination of greyscale ultrasound and Doppler in the form of duplex ultrasonography has the potential to make a significant contribution to the diagnosis and monitoring of giant cell arteritis. The use of duplex ultrasound was described by Schmidt et al.,[56] who reported a 'halo' appearance on ultrasound due to hypoechoic oedematous swollen temporal arterial wall in active giant cell arteritis. Recent meta-analyses have reported sensitivity of 69% and specificity 82% compared to biopsy[57] and a sensitivity of 68% and a specificity of 91% when compared to ACR criteria.[58] Schmidt et al.[59] reported that extending ultrasound to

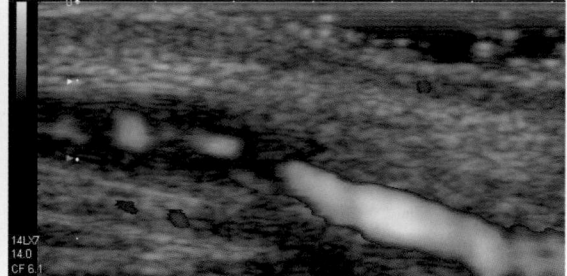

Fig. 67.12 (a) Dark ring of oedematous arterial wall around power Doppler signal on a cross-sectional temporal artery scan. (b) Transition between abnormal arteritis area of the temporal artery with narrowed flow as indicated by power Doppler and a normal area.

the proximal upper extremity arteries significantly increased the diagnostic yield in large-vessel giant cell arteritis. In Takayasu's arteritis ultrasound is capable of localizing areas of arteritis in extracranial vessels (Figure 67.12), although the access is limited in some areas.

Polymyalgia rheumatica (PMR) was previously believed to be an extra-articular disease, but shoulder subdeltoid bursitis has been reported in 55 out of 57 patients.[60] Long head of biceps tenosynovitis and synovitis of glenohumeral and hip joints have also been described and confirmed on MRI. A longitudinal study has shown reduced subdeltoid bursitis with steroid treatment although persistence at low levels was seen in some cases.[61]

Peripheral nerve disease

MSUS is ideal for assessing peripheral nerves and allows superior image definition when compared with MRI or CT. Ultrasound is useful for assessing nerve entrapments, the commonest of which is carpal tunnel syndrome (CTS). Ultrasound of the carpal tunnel can reveal causes of extrinsic compression such as anatomical anomalies, tenosynovitis, or a ganglion. Ultrasonography is certainly more acceptable to patients than nerve conduction studies, which are the current gold standard investigation for diagnosing CTS.

Initial studies by Fornage in 1988[62] reported successful imaging of peripheral nerves; major improvement in image quality have been made since then. Studies have been mainly on CTS, and to a lesser extent cubital tunnel syndrome. Peripheral nerves show uniform changes in compression syndromes irrespective of site: fusiform swelling proximal to the compression site caused by intraneural venous congestion and oedema, decrease in diameter of the nerve at the point of compression with hypoechoic loss of fascicular pattern. Doppler studies have shown increased blood flow patterns due to hyperaemia.[63]

In CTS Buchberger et al.[64] described a diagnostic triad of proximal nerve swelling, bowing of the retinaculum, and distal nerve flattening. Maximal cross-sectional area has since been reported to be the most reliable method for diagnosis of nerve compression.[65] In cubital tunnel syndrome focal nerve swelling with loss of fascicular pattern has been reported.[66]

Morton's neuromas, which are benign masses of perineural fibrosis and may be multiple and bilateral, can be demonstrated as round hypoechoic masses in the intermetatarsal spaces. Fluid in the intermetatarsal bursas is often an associated finding.[67]

Muscle pathology

Ultrasound can be used in sports medicine to localize and define the extent of partial or complete muscle rupture. Dynamic testing at the site of muscle symptoms enhances the sensitivity of ultrasound in the detection of tears. It can also demonstrate features of oedema in inflammatory muscle disease although MRI is more sensitive. The potential of ultrasound for evaluation of inflammatory myopathies was described almost two decades ago,[68] with a sensitivity of 82% in detecting histologically proven cases. Different types of myopathies showed typical but not specific ultrasound features; polymyositis showed atrophy and increased echogenicity.[68] The degree of lipomatous change present had larger effect on echogenicity than muscle fibrosis. In a recent review Adler and Garfalo[69] concluded that it is a viable alternative to MRI and that there were promising results from newer ultrasound techniques including power Doppler, extended field of view, contrast enhanced, and sonoelastography.

Interventional musculoskeletal ultrasound

Corticosteroid joint injections are common practice in rheumatology but there are few well-designed randomized studies that demonstrate their efficacy. Traditionally, joint aspiration, intra-articular injection, and soft tissue injection are performed using palpation of bony landmarks as guidance (Figure 67.13). Palpation-guided injections may result in inaccurate needle placement in up to 50% of cases,[70] and this may have an adverse effect on the clinical outcomes.[70,71] Inaccurate placement of corticosteroid can also contribute to local tissue damage, though this can be difficult to quantify.

Injections using direct ultrasound guidance may be preferable in situations where:

♦ accuracy is imperative such as radioactive synovectomy
♦ the anatomy is distorted by disease process or obesity
♦ the target joint is deep, such as the sacroiliac joint or the hip
♦ there are nearby vital structures such as blood vessels or nerves
♦ palpation-guided injection has already failed
♦ there are no bony landmarks to guide injection—bursa or tendon sheath.

This is covered in more detail in Chapter 87 on joint injections.

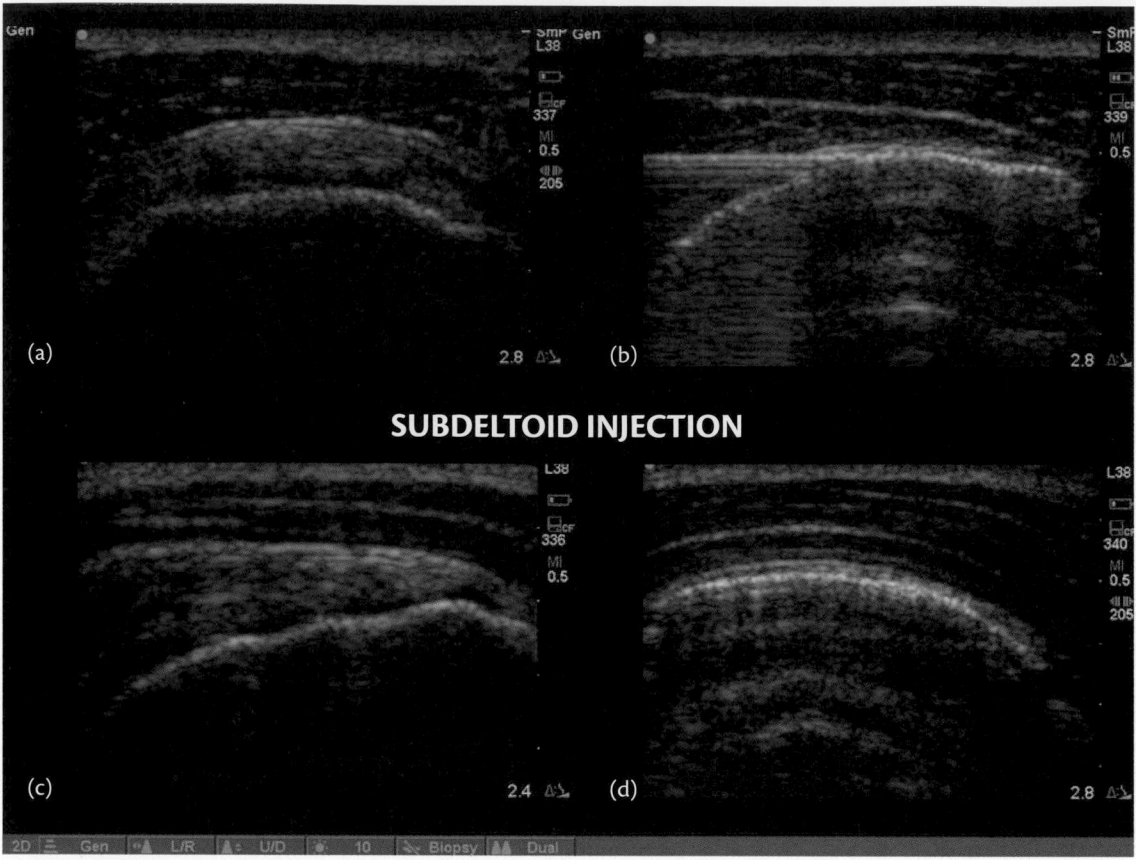

Fig. 67.13 Subdeltoid bursa injection: (A) Transverse view of subdeltoid bursa. (B) Injection of subdeltoid bursa (transverse view). (C) Longitudinal view of supraspinatus tendon and bursa. (D) Following injection the supraspinatus is obscured by the hyperechoic steroid now in the bursa.

Musculoskeletal ultrasound in primary care and professions allied to medicine

Ultrasonography is becoming increasingly popular in the primary care setting. Many general practitioners (GPs) perform obstetric ultrasound, but as yet there have been no publications regarding the use of MSUS in primary care. As in secondary care, the main barriers to progress are the initial cost of the ultrasound equipment and the time that needs to be devoted to training and competency assessment. Some GPs have been fortunate enough to get mentorship from trained sonographers and have gone on to obtain a postgraduate certificate recognized by the Royal College of Radiologists.

Rheumatology specialist nurses have already been trained to perform clinical assessment of disease activity in RA. It has been suggested that they could be trained in the ultrasound assessment of the wrists and hands.[72] Specialist nurses already perform ultrasound assessments in other specialities such as obstetrics, and some physiotherapists and podiatrists use sonography in their everyday clinical practice.[73,74] A training pathway and course structure is under development with both basic and advanced training courses available for physiotherapists. Whatever discipline is using MSUS, it is essential to have access to suitable training and mentorship. At all times, trainees need to be aware of their limitations and ready to refer difficult patients to a more experienced colleague.

Education and training

The single biggest obstacle to performing ultrasound in rheumatology is the length of time required to develop the necessary practical skills. For the last 10 years, both national (BSR) and international (EULAR) rheumatological societies have organized basic, intermediate, and advanced ultrasound courses and these are a useful learning point for the would-be sonographer. Recommendations for the content and conduct of EULAR MSUS courses have been published,[75] and this is a useful step towards the standardization of training. Short courses can be a stimulus to learning and web-based packages can be a useful adjunct to face-to-face teaching.[76] Neither is a substitute for continuous learning with an experienced mentor.

A recent survey has shown that there has been a considerable uptake of MSUS across Europe.[77] There is, however, huge variation in training and practice between different European countries. MSUS training is already integrated into the training curriculum of rheumatologists in a number of European countries including Germany and Italy. There are varying opinions as to what constitutes adequate training and competency. The ACR recommend that their trainees perform 500 supervised scans to achieve an acceptable standard. The Royal College of Radiologists has published guidelines for non-radiologist-operated ultrasound and suggest weekly mentorship by an experienced sonographer with at least 250 scans performed. There is a need for a single consensus on MSUS training in rheumatology in order to promote the international development of ultrasound in rheumatology.

Published scans are available[78] with a complete collection of all images of standard scans online (www.doctor33.it/eular/ultrasound/Guidelines.htm). Using this website an untrained novice was able to obtain acceptable musculoskeletal images after 24 non-consecutive hours of mostly self-directed learning on healthy subjects and patients with arthritis.[79] Certification of competency is desirable and European guidelines for certification are under development. A recent report from Northern Ireland described a modular training programme for rheumatologists that used logbook validation and an exit exam to assess basic competency in ultrasound.[80]

Conclusion

MSUS has revolutionized the practice of many rheumatologists in the past decade, but it comes at a price. The initial investment in equipment and training is substantial and it can be difficult to find time in a busy outpatient clinic to perform ultrasonography. However the application of ultrasound has the potential to deliver more accurate and earlier diagnosis in the clinic to the benefit of our patients. Appropriate training is essential and standardization of training and assessment is well under way. Issues of concern regarding validity and reproducibility are being addressed. MSUS is a continuously expanding field and the advent of increasingly powerful machines and 3D ultrasound are likely to further extend its applications in rheumatology.

References

1. Coperberg PL, Tsang I, Truelove L, Knickerbocker WJ. Gray scale ultrasound in the evaluation of rheumatoid arthritis of the knee. *Radiology* 1978;126(3):759–763.
2. De Flaviis L, Scaglione P, Nessi R, Ventura R, Calori G. Ultrasonography of the hand in rheumatoid arthritis. *Acta Radiol* 1988;29(4)457–460.
3. Cunnington J, Platt PN, Raftery G, Kane D. Attitudes of United Kingdom rheumatologists to musculoskeletal ultrasound practice and training. *Ann Rheum Dis* 2007;66(10):1381–1383.
4. Kane D, Balint PV, Sturrock R, Grassi W. Musculoskeletal ultrasound: state of the art review in rheumatology Part 1: current controversies and issues in the development of musculoskeletal ultrasound in rheumatology. *Rheumatology* 2004;43(7):823–828.
5. Bianchi S, Martinoli C. *Ultrasound of the musculoskeletal system.* Springer, Berlin, 2007.
6. Lee V, Zayat A, Wakefield RJ. The effect of joint position on Doppler flow in finger joint synovitis. *Ann Rheum Dis* 2009;68(4):603–604.
7. Naredo E, Moller I, Moragues C et al. EULAR working group for musculoskeletal ultrasound interobserver reliability in musculoskeletal ultrasonography: results from a 'teach the teachers' rheumatologist course. *Ann Rheum Dis* 2006;65(1):14–19.
8. D'Agostino MA, Wakefield R, Backhaus M et al. Combined evaluation of influence of the sonographer and machine type on the reliability of power Doppler ultrasonography for the detecting, scoring and scanning synovitis in rheumatoid arthritis patients: result of an inter-machine reliability exercise. *Ann Rheum Dis* 2008;67 Suppl 11:421(FR10440).
9. Karim Z, Wakefield RJ, Conaghan PG et al. The impact of ultrasonography on diagnosis and management of patients with musculoskeletal conditions. *Arthritis Rheum* 2001;44(12):2932–2933.
10. Kane D, Balint PV, Sturrock R. Ultrasonography is superior to clinical examination in the detection of and localization of knee joint effusion in rheumatoid arthritis. *J Rheumatol* 2003;30(5):966–971.
11. Schmidt WA, Schmidt H, Schicke B, Gromnica-Ihle B. Standard reference values for musculoskeletal ultrasonography. *Ann Rheum Dis* 2004;63(8):988–994.
12. Wakefield RJ, Balint PV, Szkudlarek M et al. Musculoskeletal ultrasound including definitions for ultrasonographic pathology. *J Rheumatol* 2005;32(12):2485–2487.
13. Backhaus M, Kamradt T, Sandrock D et al. Arthritis of the finger joints: a comprehensive approach comparing conventional radiography, scintigraphy, ultrasound, and contrast-enhanced magnetic resonance imaging. *Arthritis Rheum* 1999;42:1232–1245.
14. Wakefield RJ, Gibbon WW, Conaghan PG et al. The value of sonography in the detection of bone erosions in patients with rheumatoid arthritis: a comparison with conventional radiography. *Arthritis Rheum* 2000;43(12):2762–2770.
15. Szkudlarek M, Court-Payen M, Strandberg C et al. Power Doppler ultrasonography for assessment of synovitis in the metacarpophalangeal joints of patients with rheumatoid arthritis: acomparison with dynamic magnetic resonance imaging. *Arthritis Rheum* 2001;44(9):2018–2023.
16. Grassi W. Clinical evaluation versus ultrasonography: who is the winner? *J Rheumatol* 2003;30(5):908–909.
17. Brown AK, Congahan PG, Karim Z et al. An explanation for the apparent dissociation between clinical remission and continued structural deterioration in rheumatoid arthritis. *Arthritis Rheum* 2008;58(10):2958–2967.
18. Walther M, Harms H, Krenn V et al. Correlation of power Doppler sonography with vascularity of the synovial tissue of the knee joint in patients with osteoarthritis and rheumatoid arthritis. *Arthritis Rheum* 2001;44(2):331–338.
19. Torp-Pedersen ST, Terslev L. Settings and artefacts relevant in colour/power Doppler ultrasound in rheumatology. *Ann Rheum Dis.* 2008;67(2):143–149.
20. Taylor PC, Steuer A, Gruber J et al. Comparison of ultrasonographic assessments of synovitis and joint vascularity with radiographic evaluation in a randomised, placebo controlled study of infliximab therapy in early rheumatoid arthritis. *Arthritis Rheum* 2004;50(4):1107–1116.
21. Naredo E, Rodriguez M, Campos C et al. Ultrasound Group of the Spanish Society of Reumatology. Validity, reproducibility and responsiveness of a twelve joint simplified power Doppler ultrasonographic assessment of joint inflammation. *Arthritis Rheum* 2008;59(4):515–522.
22. Backhaus M, Ohrndorf S, Kellner H et al. Evaluation of a novel 7 joint ultrasound score in daily rheumatologic practice: a pilot project. *Arthritis Rheum* 2009;61(9):1194–1201.
23. Dougados M, Jousse-Joulin S, Mistretta F et al. Evaluation of several ultrasonography scoring systems for synovitis and comparison to clinical examination: results from a prospective multicentre study of rheumatoid arthritis. *Ann Rheum Dis* 2010;69(5):828–833.
24. D'Agostino MA, Conaghan PG, Naredo E et al. The OMERCAT ultrasound task force: advances and priorities. *J Rheumatol* 2010; 36(8):1829–1832.
25. Fraser AD, van Kuijk AW, Westhovens R et al. A randomised, double-blind, placebo controlled, multi- centre trial of combination therapy with methotrexate plus cyclosporin in patients with active psoriatic arthritis. *Ann Rheum Dis* 2005;64(6):859–864.
26. Fiocco U, Cozzi L, Rubaltelli L, Rigon C, De Candia A, Tregnaghi A, et al. Long-term sonographic follow-up of rheumatoid and psoriatic proliferative knee joint synovitis. *Br J Rheumatol* 1996;35(2):155–163.
27. De Simone C, Caldarola G, D'Agostino M et al. Usefulness of ultrasound imaging in detecting psoriatic arthritis of fingers and toes in patients with psoriasis. *Clin Dev Immunol* 2011;2011:390726.
28. Balint PV, Kane D, Wilson H, McInnes IB, Sturrock RD. Ultrasonography of entheseal insertions in the lower limb in spondyloarthropathy. *Ann Rheum Dis* 2002;61(10):905–910.
29. D'Agostino MA, Said-Nahal R, Hacquard-Brouder C et al. Assessment of peripheral enthesitis in the spondyloarthropathies by ultrasound

combined with power Doppler: a cross sectional study. *Arthritis Rheum* 2003;48(2):523–533.

30. Wakefield RJ, Green MJ, Marzo-Ortega H et al. Should oligoarthritis be reclassified? Ultrasound reveals a high prevalence of subclinical disease. *Ann Rheum Dis* 2004;63(4):382–385.

31. Balint PV, Sturrock RD. Inflamed retrocalcaneal bursa and Achilles tendonitis in psoriatic arthritis demonstrated by ultrasonography. *Ann Rheum Dis* 2000;59(12):931–933.

32. Gandjbakhch F, Terslev L, Joshua F et al.; OMERACT Ultrasound Task Force. Ultrasound in the evaluation of enthesitis: status and perspectives. *Arthritis Res Ther* 2011;13:R188.

33. Olivieri I, Barozzi L, Favaro L et al. Dactylitis in patients with seronegative spondylarthropathy. Assessment by ultrasonography and magnetic resonance imaging. *Arthritis Rheum* 1996;39(9):1524–1528..

34. Olivieri I, Barozzi L, Pierro A et al. Toe dactylitis in patients with spondyloarthropathy: assessment by magnetic resonance imaging. *J Rheumatol* 1997;24(5):926–930.

35. Kane D, Greaney T, Bresnihan B, Gibney R, FitzGerald O. Ultrasonography in the diagnosis and management of psoriatic dactylitis. *J Rheumatol* 1999;26(8):1746–1751.

36. Grassi W, Filippucci E, Farina A, Cervini C. Sonographic imaging of the distal phalanx. *Semin Arthritis Rheum* 2000;29(6):379–384.

37. Klauser A, Springer P, Frauscher F et al. Comparison between magnetic resonance imaging, unenhanced and contrast enhanced ultrasound in the diagnosis of active sacroiliitis. *Arthritis Rheum* 2002;46:S426.

38. Unlü E, Pamuk ON, Cakir N. Color and duplex Doppler sonography to detect sacroiliitis and spinal inflammation in ankylosing spondylitis. Can this method reveal response to anti-tumor necrosis factor therapy? *J Rheumatol* 2007;34(1):110–116.

39. Iagnocco A. Imaging the joint in osteoarthritis: a place for ultrasound. *Best Pract Res Clin Rheumatol* 2010;24:27–38.

40. D'Agostino MA, Conaghan P, Le Bars M et al. EULAR report on the use of ultrasonography in painful knee osteoarthritis. Part 1: prevalence of inflammation in osteoarthritis. *Ann Rheum Dis* 2005;64:1703–1709.

41. Pendleton A, Millar A, O'Kane D, et al. Can sonography be used to predict the response to intra-articular corticosteroid injection in primary osteoarthritis of the knee? *Scand J Rheumatol* 2008;37(5):395–397.

42. Atchia I, Kane D, Reed MR, Isaacs JD, Birrell F. Efficacy of a single ultrasound-guided injection for the treatment of hip osteoarthritis. *Ann Rheum Dis* 2011;70:110–116.

43. de Jesus JO, Parker L, Frangos AJ, Nazarian LN. Accuracy of MRI, MR arthrography, and ultrasound in the diagnosis of rotator cuff tears: a meta analysis. *AJR Am J Roentgenol* 2009;192:1701–1707.

44. Ostlere S. Imaging the shoulder. *Imaging* 2003;15:162–173.

45. Wright SA, Filippucci E, McVeigh C et al. High resolution ultrasonography of the first metatarsal phalangeal joint in gout: a controlled study. *Ann Rheum Dis* 2007;66(12):859–864.

46. Saketkoo LA, Quinet R. Revisiting Jaccoud arthropathy as an ultrasound diagnosed erosive arthropathy in systemic lupus erythematosus. *J Clin Rheumatol* 2007;13(6):322–327.

47. Delle Sedie A, Riente L, Scire CA et al. Ultrasound imaging for the rheumatologist, XXIV, Sonographic evaluation of the wrist and hand joint and tendon involvement in systemic lupus erythematosus. *Clin Exp Rheumatol* 2009;27(6):897–901.

48. Ossandon A, Iagnocco A, Alessandri C et al. Ultrasonographic depiction of knee joint alterations in systemic lupus erythematosus. *Clin Exp Rheumatol* 2009;27(2):329–332.

49. Gallelli B, Burdick I, Quaglini S et al. Carotid plaques in patient with long-term lupus nephritis. *Clin Exp Rheumatol* 2010;28(3):386–392.

50. Kaloudi O, Bandinelli F, Fillopucci E, et al. High frequency ultrasound measurement of digital dermal thickness in systemic sclerosis. *Ann Rheum Dis* 2010;69(6):1140–1143.

51. Hesselstrand R, Scheja W, Wildt M, Akesson A. High frequency ultrasound of skin involvement in systemic sclerosis reflects oedema, extension and severity in early disease. *Rheumatology* 2008;47(1)84–87.

52. Iagnoco A, Kaloudi O, Perella C, Bandinelli F et al. Ultrasound elastography assessment of skin involvement in systemic sclerosis; lights and shadows. *J Rheumatol* 2010;37(8):1688–1691.

53. Bradus RJ, Hybarjer P, Gooding GA. Parotid gland: US findings in Sjögren's syndrome. *Radiology* 1988;169:749–751.

54. Ahuja AT, Metreweli C. Ultrasound features of Sjögren's syndrome. *Australas Radiol* 1996;40:10–14.

55. Takagi Y, Kimura Y, Nakamura H et al. Salivary gland ultrasonography: can it be an alternative to sialography as a imaging modality for Sjogren's syndrome? *Ann Rheum Dis* 2010;69(7):1321–1324.

56. Schmidt WA, Kraft HE, Vorphal K, Volker L, Grominica-Ihle EJ. Colour duplex ultrasonography in the diagnosis of temporal arteritis. *N Engl J Med* 1997;337:1336–1342.

57. Karissa FB, Matsagas MI, Schmidt WA, Ioannidis JP. Metanalysis: test performance of ultrasonography for giant cell arteritis. *Ann Intern Med* 2005;142:359–369.

58. Arida A, Kyprianou M, Kanakis M, Sfikakis PP. The diagnostic value of ultrasonography derived edema of the temporal artery wall in giant cell arteritis: a second meta-analysis. *BMC Muscukloskelet Disord* 2010; 11:44–51.

59. Schmidt et al Ultrasound of proximal upper extremity arteries to increase the diagnostic yield in large vessel giant cell arteritis. *Rheum* 2008;47:96–101.

60. Salvarani CF, Olivieri I, Niccoli L et al. Shoulder ultrasonography in the diagnosis ofpolymyalgia rheumatica: a case control study. *J Rheumatol* 2001;28(5):1049–1055.

61. Macchioni P, Catanoso MG, Pipitone N, Boiardi L, Salvarani C. Longitudinal examination with shoulder ultrasound of patients with polymyalgia rheumatica. *Rheumatology* (Oxford) 2009;48(12): 1566–1569.

62. Fornage BD. Peripheral nerves of the extremities:imaging with US. *Radiology* 1988:167:179–182.

63. Koenig RW, Pedro MT, Heinen CPG, Schmidt T et al. High resolution ultrasonography in evaluating peripheral nerve entrapment and trauma. *Neurosurg Focus* 2009;26(2):E13.

64. Buchberger W, W, Schon G, Stresser K, Jungwith W. high resolution ultrasonography of the carpal tunnel. *J Ultrasound Med* 1991;10:531–537.

65. Bargfrede M, Schwennicke MC, Tumani H, Reimers CD. Quantitative ultrasonography in focal neuropathies as compared to clinical and EMG findings. *Eur J Ultrasound* 1999;10:21–29..

66. Martinolli C, Bianchi S, Gandolfo N et al. US of nerve entrapments in osteo-fibrous tunnels of the upper and lower limb. *Radiographics* 2000;20:199–217.

67. Stuart RM, Koh ESC, Brieidahl WH. Sonography of nerve pathology. *AJR Am J Roentgenol* 2004;182:123–129.

68. Reimers CD, Fleckenstein JL, Wittb TN et al. Muscular ultrasound in idiopathic inflammatory myopathies of adults. *J Neurol Sci* 1993, 116:82–92.

69. Adler RS, Garofalo G. Ultrasound in the evaluation of the inflammatory myopathies. *Curr Rheumatol Rep* 2009;11(4):302–308.

70. Jones A, Regan M, Ledingham J et al. Importance of placement of intra-articular steroid injections. *BMJ* 1993:307(6915):1329–1330.

71. Cunnington J, Marshall N, Hide G, et al. A randomized double blind, controlled, study of ultrasound guided corticosteroid injection in the joint of patients with inflammatory arthritis. *Arthritis Rheum* 2010;62(7):1862–1869.

72. Estrach C, Thompson RN. Why aren't we all doing ultrasound? *Rheumatology* (Oxford) 2009;48(9):1019–1020.

73. Bowen CJ, Dewbury K, Sampson M et al. Musculoskeletal ultrasound imaging of the plantar forefoot in patients with rheumatoid arthritis: inter-observer agreement between podiatrist and radiologist. *J Foot Ankle Res* 2008;1(1):5.

74. Kumar P, Bradley M, Swinkels A. With-day and day to day intra-rater reliability of ultrasonographic measurements of acromium-greater tuberosity distance. *Physiotherapy Theory Pract* 2010;26(5):347–351.

75. Naredo E, Bijlsma JW, Conaghan P et al. Recommendations for the content and conduct of EULAR musculoskeletal ultrasound courses. *Ann Rheum Dis* 2008;67(7):962–965.

76. Filippucci E, Meenagh G, Ciapetti A, et al. E-learning in ultrasonography; a web-based approach. *Ann Rheum Dis* 2007;66(7):962–965.

77. Naredo E, D'Agostino MA, Conaghan et al. Current state of musculoskeletal ultrasound training and implementation in Europe: results of a survery of experts and scientific societies. *Rheumatol* (Oxford) 2010;49(12):2438–2443.

78. Backhaus M, Burmester GR, Gerber T et al. Working group for musculo-skeletal ultrasound in the EULAR standing committee on International Clinical Studies including therapeutic trials. Guidelines for musculoskeletal ultrasound in rheumatology. *Ann Rheum Dis* 2001;60(7):641–649.

79. Filippucci E, Unlu Z, Farina A, Grassi W. Sonographic training in rheumatology: a self teaching approach. *Ann Rheum Dis* 2003;62(6):565–567.

80. Taggart AJ, Wright SA, Ball E, Kane D Wright G. The Belfast musculoskeletal ultrasound course. *Rheumatology* (Oxford) 2009;48(9): 1073–1076.

CHAPTER 68

Magnetic resonance imaging

S. Balamoody, Helena Marzo-Ortega,
and Philip J. O'Connor

Introduction

Magnetic resonance imaging (MRI) has established considerable utility in the assessment of musculoskeletal disorders over the last two decades. This is largely due to the unique capabilities of MRI to allow thorough visualization of soft tissues as well as bone. Providing reproducible three-dimensional (3D) imaging without ionizing radiation, excellent soft tissue contrast and well-defined anatomy makes MRI amenable to clinicians as a 'treatment road map' as well as for diagnosis. Despite its massive contribution towards the understanding of aetiopathogenesis in the commonest musculoskeletal disorders within the research field, the clinical utility of MRI in real practice is limited mainly by high running costs and long imaging times.

MRI has been instrumental in enabling further understanding into the pathogenesis and evolution of arthritis and remains a key diagnostic tool in many musculoskeletal disorders. Important advances include the identification of bone marrow oedema as a prognostic biomarker for erosion progression in rheumatoid arthritis (RA). MRI plays an important diagnostic role in axial spondyloarthritis (SpA), shortening the time to therapeutic intervention. The role of MRI in distinguishing pathologies in early undifferentiated arthritis and in osteoarthritis (OA), as well as its role as an outcome measure, continues to evolve. For now, MRI remains a sensitive imaging tool and provides unparalleled access to joint tissues.

Basic principles of MRI

The nuclear magnetic resonance phenomenon

MRI uses the property of charged nuclei in tissues to behave as a bar magnet. The hydrogen nucleus, often referred to as a 'spin', consists of a single positively charged proton constantly orbiting a single neutron, creating its own electromagnetic field. Placed within a strong external magnetic field, these align in one of two orientations, sometimes described as 'north' or 'south', which have different energy states. A slightly greater number will align in one direction.[1] The particles have energy and as such move within the constraints of their magnetic field. This movement is termed precession and occurs at a set frequency. Adding energy of the same frequency as this precession frequency produces a much greater tissue response,

the so-called 'nuclear magnetic resonance' (NMR) phenomenon. By varying the frequency of precession, an MR scanner can select which protons it adds energy to. Once these protons have been excited, the additional energy must be lost in order to return to their pre-excitation state. The energy is lost by two processes, T1 and T2 relaxation. An MR scanner can preferentially collect T1 and T2 relaxation information from tissues, giving images the differing tissue contrasts accordingly.

Standard image contrast

Contrast refers to the ability to distinguish different signal intensities, manifested as different shades of greyscale within an MR image. This allows differentiation between tissues and tissue qualities. In general, an MR scan will consist of several pulse sequences. These pulse sequences differ in their parameters in order to exploit properties of different tissues. In most cases, a single pulse sequence is inadequate to obtain all the information required and a combination of pulse sequences is required to interrogate the different tissues. T1, T2, and proton density refer to three basic types of contrast used (described as 'weighting'). These can be generated by altering pulse sequence parameters termed TR (repetition time) and TE (echo time). The commonest image sequences applied in the musculoskeletal setting are the T1 and T2 and proton density weighting (T1W, T2W, PDW).

T1 weighting sequences

T1-weighted (T1W) images are sensitive to fat (including fatty bone marrow) which gives a high signal whereas fluid will show as low signal. Highly proteinaceous fluids, certain blood degradation products, and melanin are high signal on T1W. There is good signal-to-noise ratio as T1 relaxation occurs relatively slowly; hence T1W images are considered good for anatomical definition. Cortical bone returns no signal and is shown better on T1W sequences, as a well-defined black stripe outlining bone marrow.

T2W/PDW weighting sequences

T2-weighted (T2W) images are fluid-sensitive and hence demonstrate fluid, oedema, and inflammation as high (or hyperintense) signal. Fat is also demonstrated as high signal on T2W imaging. Fluid-sensitive sequences are often combined with fat suppression techniques to enhance the visualization of fluid/inflammation within fatty tissues (e.g. bone marrow). T2 relaxation occurs relatively quickly and therefore these images can suffer reduced signal-to-noise ratios compared with T1W images. PDW images can be a good compromise, providing a balance between anatomical definition and pathology detection. When accompanied with fat suppression, proton density images are highly sensitive to pathology such as bone marrow oedema. T2-weighted images are less sensitive but more specific for pathology, hence both sequences are included in some imaging protocols

T2* (T2 star)—imaging of magnetic susceptibility

T2* relaxation is a component of T2 relaxation, occurring even faster than T2 relaxation. Paramagnetic or ferromagnetic structures are demonstrated as black, often with a characteristic 'blooming' artefact—a smudged outer margin. This sequence is useful in the detection of haemosiderin, making it useful for example in the diagnosis of pigmented villonodular synovitis (see 'Pigmented villonodular synovitis').

Fat suppression

Fat suppression is an essential technique for detection of bone marrow pathology, as well as for identifying the presence of fat within lesions. There are several methods of fat suppression, although the main two utilized in musculoskeletal imaging are short-tau inversion recovery (STIR) and (spectral) fat saturation. The STIR method produces global and homogeneous fat suppression and allows for quick imaging acquisition. The main disadvantage of STIR is being not completely lipid specific and hence other non-fat tissues may also have suppressed signal. The fat-saturation method, using a lipid-specific technique, is generally preferred for most musculoskeletal imaging. There are drawbacks to the fat-saturation method including sensitivity to magnetic field inhomogeneities resulting in artefact and substantially lengthened imaging times.[2] Fat saturation is essential with contrast-enhanced imaging to differentiate between high-signal gadolinium and high-signal fat on T1W images.

Further characterization of pathology—intravenous contrast agent

Gadolinium is a paramagnetic heavy metal with a valuable T1-relaxation shortening property. Intravenous (IV) injection of gadolinium accumulates in those tissues with increased vascularity, extracellular fluid volume, and capillary permeability. It is therefore good at demonstrating tumour and inflammatory pathology (Figure 68.1). Nephrogenic systemic fibrosis, a chronic debilitating condition, has been associated with IV gadolinium injection in subjects with chronic renal failure; this finding has led to restricted administration in individuals with pre-existing renal impairment.[3]

Contra-indications to MRI

Conventional MRI is safe for most people, but is contraindicated in people with any of the following: pacemaker, cochlear implants, metallic intraorbital foreign body, aneurysm clips, implanted devices (e.g. nerve stimulator). MRI is considered potentially unsafe in other scenarios and careful consideration is required to assess whether scanning can be permitted. Concerns for patient safety are generally related to the potential for the magnetic field to cause movement of metallic structures and/or the heating effect of the transmitted energy. Patients with internal metallic medical devices not uniformly contraindicated (e.g. shunts, stents) require these to be checked for MRI compatibility.

MRI assessment of arthritis

While much of the work in rheumatic conditions has involved imaging of small joints, MRI remains the preferred modality for imaging of deeper or larger joints such as hip joints and spine to demonstrate inflammatory or degenerative joint involvement or to exclude other pathologic processes such as avascular necrosis.

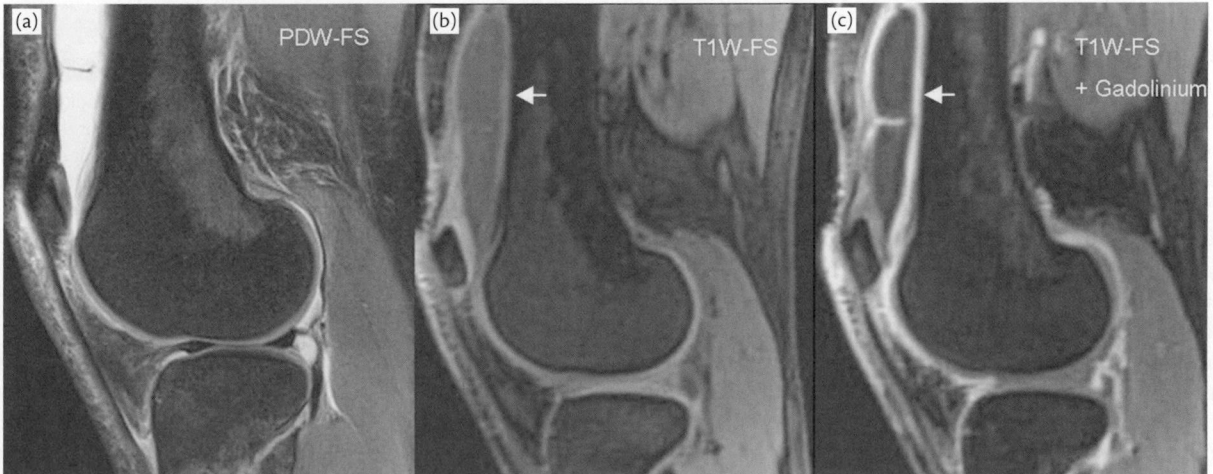

Fig. 68.1 Imaging of synovitis and the benefit of IV contrast: Sagittal knee images in the same patient of the suprapatellar pouch: (a) PDW fat-saturated (FS) image demonstrates high-signal distension of the suprapatellar pouch in keeping with an effusion. (b) T1W-FS image demonstrates intermediate signal of the synovium and low-signal fluid (thin arrow). (c) T1W post-IV contrast image clearly differentiates high signal of the enhancing synovium from the adjacent low-signal, non-enhancing fluid (thick arrow).
Courtesy of Claire Wenham Research Fellow at NIHR Leeds Musculoskeletal Biomedical Imaging Unit, Leeds, UK.

MRI features of acute inflammation

Synovitis

Active acute synovitis is considered a reversible feature of an inflammatory arthritis which may respond to therapy. Synovitis manifests as thickened synovium, sometimes causing distension of a joint or bursa, and demonstrating high signal on T2W/PDW images. Thickening of the synovial membrane may not always be readily identifiable in the presence of excess synovial fluid using fluid-sensitive sequences alone. T1W images are helpful as intermediate-signal synovium can be differentiated from low-signal fluid on careful inspection. Contrast-enhanced images are the gold standard, especially for detection of early changes,[4] but acquisition for routine detection of synovitis is not recommended as unenhanced MRI or ultrasound is generally adequate in most situations.

Pannus refers to focal areas of bulky fibrovascular tissue which occurs in the context of chronic synovitis and subsequent fibrotic change. Pannus therefore demonstrates low-grade inflammation histologically.[5] Pannus may also appear hypointense on MRI, reflecting a higher fibrous and lower cellular/vascular content.[6]

Tenosynovitis/tendonitis

The same signal characteristics seen in synovitis occur in inflammatory involvement of tendons and their tendon sheath. Tenosynovitis manifests as diffuse, smooth, high-signal swelling around the tendon due to thickening of the sheath (often containing excess fluid) surrounding the low-signal tendon. Ganglions of the tendon sheath can have a similar appearance but in general cause a more focal bulge, often to one side of the tendon.

Bone marrow oedema

In neonatal life bones are filled predominantly with 'red marrow' rich in haemopoietic cells. This is gradually replaced through childhood with fat or 'yellow marrow', a process which starts in the appendicular followed by the axial skeleton and from distal to proximal.[7] In adults, imaging of normal bones with fat-suppressed sequences in general displays marrow as homogeneously low signal. Some regions commonly retain red marrow in adulthood, such as the proximal femoral and humeral metaphyses, and consequently manifest as regions of intermediate signal on fat-suppressed (and T1W) imaging.

Consequently, bone marrow pathology is easily visualized as high signal within bone marrow on fat-suppressed fluid-sensitive sequences or contrast-enhanced images. Subchondral bone marrow oedema is typically represented as focal ill-defined high signal extending from the articular surface. Subchondral bone marrow oedema is a non-specific feature, with an extensive differential diagnosis (Box 68.1 and Figure 68.2). In some cases, there are other imaging features present/absent which help to narrow the differential diagnosis and, as always, clinical correlation is required. The histopathology of the bone marrow oedema lesion rarely represents simple interstitial oedema and the term 'bone marrow oedema' is considered an oversimplification. Depending on the aetiopathology, the same imaging appearance can represent variable degrees and combinations of interstitial oedema, increased vascular permeability/congestion, neoangiogenesis, inflammatory cellular infiltrate, necrosis, fibrosis, haemorrhage, and disorganized lipid content. For example, there is histological evidence that the high-signal 'oedema-like' lesions seen in the context of active sacroiliitis in ankylosing spondylitis or in RA peripheral joints do indeed

Box 68.1 Differential diagnosis of bone marrow oedema lesions

- Trauma, e.g. acute fracture, stress injuries
- Infection, e.g. septic arthritis
- Inflammatory arthropathy
- Other arthropathies, e.g. crystal arthropathy, osteoarthritis
- Vascular aetiologies, e.g. avascular necrosis, osteochondral lesions, complex regional pain syndrome
- Red marrow reconversion
- Paget's disease
- Bone marrow oedema syndrome
- Iatrogenic, e.g. radiotherapy
- Neoplasm, e.g. osteoid osteoma, leukaemia
- Reactive to adjacent soft tissue pathology

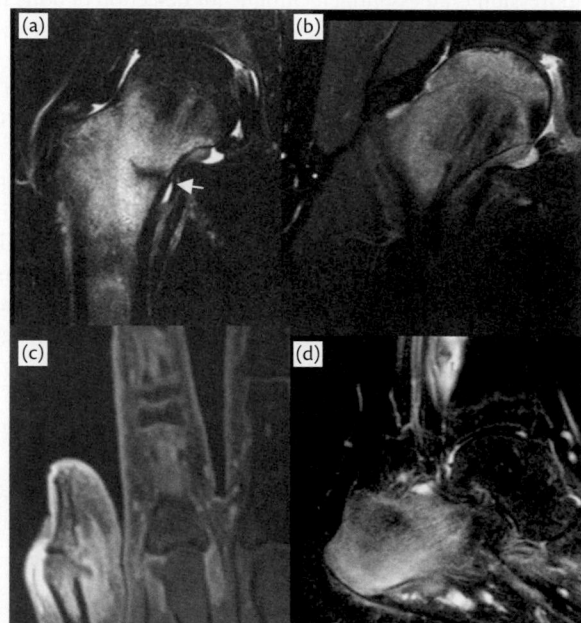

Fig. 68.2 Examples of bone marrow oedema in different conditions: (a) Diffuse bone marrow oedema in the femoral neck. Linear low signal at the medial cortex (white arrow) indicates the cause—stress fracture. (b) Transient osteoporosis of the hip: note subtle insufficiency fracture at the femoral articular margin. (c) Active rheumatoid arthritis; post-gadolinium image demonstrates bone marrow enhancement due to florid inflammation and synovial proliferation and enhancement at the thumb interphalangeal joint, and less severe changes in the index finger. (d) Calcaneal osteitis and plantar fasciitis in spondyloarthropathy.

represent an inflammatory process[8–11] or 'osteitis', a term frequently used to define the MRI appearance of bone marrow oedema. This more specific term technically should be used in reference to post-contrast images to indicate active inflammation. By contrast, in bone marrow oedema lesions of OA, predominant histological abnormalities include marrow necrosis, fibrosis, haemorrhage, and abnormal trabeculae. Bone marrow oedema severity on imaging is considered to have a relation to symptoms and prognosis for certain diseases such as RA[12] and avascular necrosis.[13]

Acute chondrolysis and subchondral destruction

Diffuse acute chondrolysis and subchondral destruction are characteristic features of acute joint infection. Cartilage destruction occurs rapidly, manifesting as intensely high signal on fluid-sensitive sequences. An irregular subchondral bone contour is an indication of a destructive process.

MRI features of joint structural damage

Plain radiography is the simplest and most efficient method of detecting established joint space loss and bone destruction. Although erosions can be visualized by MRI, CT remains the gold standard for cortical bone abnormalities and periarticular ossification, with the added value of being a 3D modality. The main drawback of CT is its significant ionizing radiation burden.

Erosions

Erosions characteristically represent focal bone loss at the joint interface, ranging from a few millemetres to several centimetres in size. Radiographic erosions are the hallmark of structural damage in inflammatory arthropathy. The erosion shape and specific location within the joint can give clues as to the aetiology e.g. psoriatic arthritis vs RA vs gout (Figure 68.3). Erosions seen on radiographs can also be seen on MRI. Because of its tomographic nature, MRI often detects more and smaller erosions than radiographs.

Joint space loss

Joint space loss is originally a radiographic term providing a surrogate estimate of cartilage loss. Loss of tissue in fibrocartilaginous structures such as menisci and labra which have become degenerate / torn can also contribute to reduction in joint space. In the case of meniscal tears in OA, the type of tear can give an indication as to whether this damage is primary or secondary to the process of joint degeneration. Meniscal extrusion outside the joint is often seen in OA, also contributing to joint space loss and abnormal distribution of force within the joint.[14]

Subchondral remodelling and osteophytes

The cumulative response of dynamic changes in subchondral bone architecture to abnormal joint biology and mechanics due to arthritis are also captured on MRI, particularly in slowly progressive diseases such as OA. Osteophytes are a pathognomonic feature of OA, occurring at the bone–cartilage junction. Subchondral sclerosis and attrition can be seen as diffuse low-signal areas on T1W imaging and flattening of the normal surface curvature. These features are less evident in diseases such as RA where bone destruction and inflammation are predominant. Subchondral cysts, a typical feature of OA, are well visualized as focal, well-defined hyperintense areas at the joint margin, often but not always in areas of bone marrow oedema. Subchondral cysts may be mistaken for erosions but can be differentiated from these by the intact overlying cortical bone.

Common arthritic diseases

Rheumatoid arthritis

The greatest advantage of MRI over ultrasound and radiography is its ability to clearly depict all the soft tissue structures involved in RA. In addition, MRI can depict subchondral bone pathology, in particular bone marrow oedema. Histological samples taken from joints undergoing surgery have confirmed that bone marrow oedema in RA has a prominent inflammatory component.[11,15]

Post-IV gadolinium MRI is considered the gold standard for imaging of synovitis. MRI correlation has been shown with other multiplanar modalities such as power Doppler ultrasound and in histopathological studies.[16,17]

MRI is more sensitive than radiography for the detection of erosions; identifying smaller and earlier changes,[18] with high sensitivity and specificity compared to the gold standard, CT.[19] There is, however, a lack of pathological correlation in the literature. Although cohort studies have demonstrated persistence and increased sites of MRI erosions in RA after 1–2 years, not all MRI erosions progress to radiographic erosions.[20] Precisely which factors determine progression remains controversial. Some studies show that a good level of correlation for detecting bone erosions between MRI and CT of metacarpophalangeal (MCP) and wrist joints is seen in RA patients, suggesting that MRI erosions represent a true destructive process.[19,21] Nevertheless plain radiography

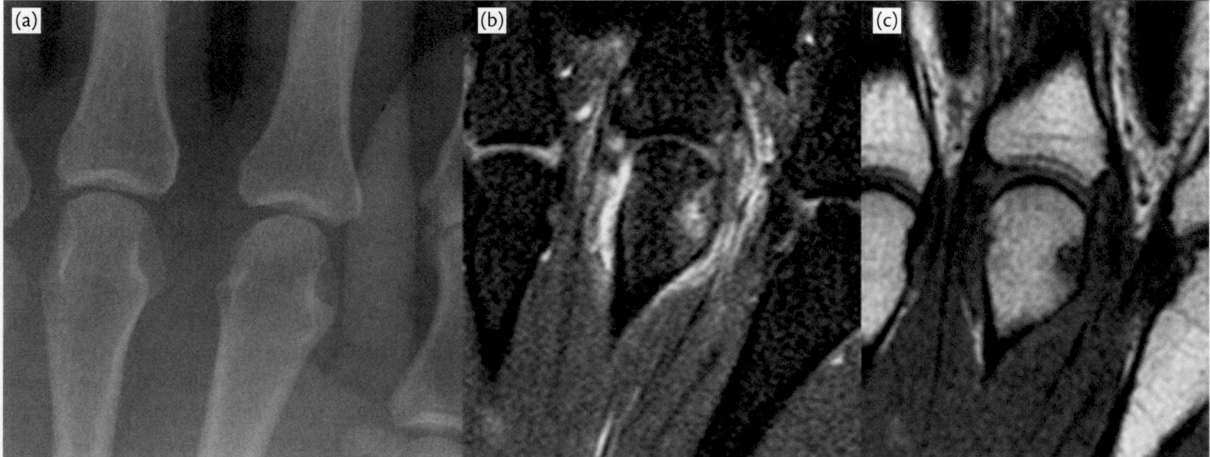

Fig. 68.3 Rheumatoid arthritis in the hand of a symptomatic patient: (a) Plain radiograph is unremarkable.(b) T2W fat-saturated image showing bone marrow, ill-defined high signal at the middle metacarpal head, and synovitis. (c) T1W image better demonstrates well-defined low-signal periarticular erosion in the middle metacarpal head and base of middle phalanx.

remains the gold standard for monitoring structural damage in RA, as the true prognostic significance of these MRI-determined erosions remain unclear.[22] Regression of MRI erosions has been observed with combination therapies.[23,24]

MRI and the pathogenesis of rheumatoid arthritis

MRI-detected erosions in RA can be seen early, within 6 weeks from symptom onset. Synovitis and bone marrow oedema are both considered markers of active inflammatory activity[22] and represent the forerunners of erosion formation in inflammatory arthritis. Progression of joint damage may also occur in part due to biomechanical factors.[25] In some studies bone marrow oedema has been shown to be a better predictor of increased joint destruction than single time-point measures of synovitis,[26-29] as bone marrow oedema probably represents a more direct inflammatory process effecting trabecular bone.

MRI in early diagnosis of rheumatoid arthritis

Early treatment of RA to delay and minimize irreversible joint destruction is now standard. Treat-to-target strategies have been implemented to ablate disease activity from symptom onset.[30] Early diagnosis requires having a low threshold of clinical suspicion supported by biochemical and imaging signs of joint inflammation, before overt erosive change occurs. Ultrasound and MRI are favoured for the purposes of early diagnosis, both modalities being more sensitive and specific than clinical examination and serum inflammatory markers.[31,32] The cost-effectiveness of widespread use of MRI in early diagnosis has yet to be shown. MRI has potential benefit as a prognostic tool, largely by the ability to depict bone marrow oedema which no other modality can detect.[27]

MRI outcomes in clinical trials

One of the main utilities of MRI in RA has been as an outcome measure in the clinical research setting to demonstrate the benefit of biologic therapies. Its success is due to its superior discriminatory ability and greater sensitivity to change in active joint inflammation as compared to conventional radiography, allowing for short observation periods and lower patient numbers when assessing for progression of structural damage.[33] The OMERACT RA-MRI score, involving semiquantitative assessment of synovitis, bone marrow oedema, erosions, and joint space narrowing,[34] is now widely used in clinical trials. MRI also allows for quantification of synovial inflammation by measuring early 'enhancement' or contrast augmentation after intravenous injections of gadolinium (see 'Compositional imaging of cartilage').[35]

Spondyloarthropathy

Traditionally, diagnostic imaging has been confined to the identification of radiographic sacroiliac joint (SIJ) abnormalities or sacroiliitis.[36] Although this approach is still widely applied in clinical practice, it is now well recognized that there may be several years' delay from the onset of clinical symptoms of back pain until the appearance of radiographic sacroiliitis.[36] MRI is highly sensitive to early and active SpA; sacroiliitis can be detected nearly a decade earlier.[37] This is of major relevance since individuals can experience levels of pain and disability at the early stages of disease comparable to those experienced by subjects with established or chronic disease.[38] Furthermore, individual response to biological therapies (the only treatments proven to be efficacious in these diseases) may be greater when initiated early in the disease process.[39,40]

MRI lesions in the sacroiliac joint in spondyloarthritis

A number of MRI lesions representative of active and chronic stages of disease have been described at the SIJ and spine in SpA. In the SIJ, active lesions include synovitis, ligamentous enthesitis, and subchondral bone marrow oedema. SIJ subchondral bone marrow oedema can be reliably detected as high signal in fat-suppressed or STIR sequences (Figure 68.4). These sequences have the same sensitivity as gadolinium-enhanced T1W images for the detection of bone marrow oedema.[41,42] Bone marrow oedema lesions can appear within a few weeks of onset of symptoms of inflammatory back pain.[43] although their natural history remains unclear. At the histopathological level, these 'oedematous' changes correspond to an inflammatory infiltrate with mononuclear cells found in biopsy samples.[8,10] Nevertheless, there is poor correlation between the amount of infiltrate found in the biopsies and MRI appearances of bone marrow oedema with MRI 'missing' more than half the lesions found at histology.

Chronic or structural lesions of the SIJ include fat infiltration, erosions, bone sclerosis, and ankylosis. These lesions are best characterized on T1W sequences. Fat infiltration is due to esterification of fatty acids and appears as bright signal both on T1W and T2W scans (except in fat-suppressed sequences where these lesions appear as low signal). Although thought to represent a postinflammatory process, this change can also be found in healthy individuals, where it is thought to represent normal ageing. Erosions are identified as full-thickness loss of the cortical bone in either side (iliac or sacral) of the SIJ. Erosions are easier to identify when multiple, as they can become confluent giving appearance to the so-called 'pseudowidening' of the sclerosis identified as low subchondral signal on all sequences.

MRI and classification criteria of axial spondyloarthritis

A major breakthrough in the clinical field in SpA occurred with the advent of the new classification criteria developed by the Assessment of SpondyloArthritis International Society (ASAS).[44] The notable change these criteria is the inclusion of MRI alongside radiography as imaging criterion, allowing for the early diagnosis of sacroiliitis in the absence of radiographic abnormalities.[45] In the clinical context it allows for early recognition of AS, as early as 3 months from symptom onset. To aid with implementation of these criteria, definition of a positive MRI of the SIJs in SpA has been proposed by an expert group based solely on the presence of subchondral bone marrow oedema,[46] and its utility is currently being reappraised.[47]

MRI lesions in the spine

The majority of functional burden experienced by patients with SpA is linked to disease affecting the spine rather than the SIJs. Direct association between inflammation in the early stages of disease and structural damage has been shown.[48] The thoracic spine is the most frequently affected area after the SIJ in AS, according to evidence from MRI studies.[49,50] Posterior element, costovertebral, and discovertebral change make up the bulk of spinal disease.

Active lesions are identified by high signal in fat-suppressed sequences with the corresponding low-intensity signal on T1W sequences at entheses, joints, and disc margins. Characteristic lesions include vertebral corner lesions, facet joint, and soft tissue or perifacetal lesions. Corner lesions can occur in the anterior or posterior corners, sometimes covering half and on occasions

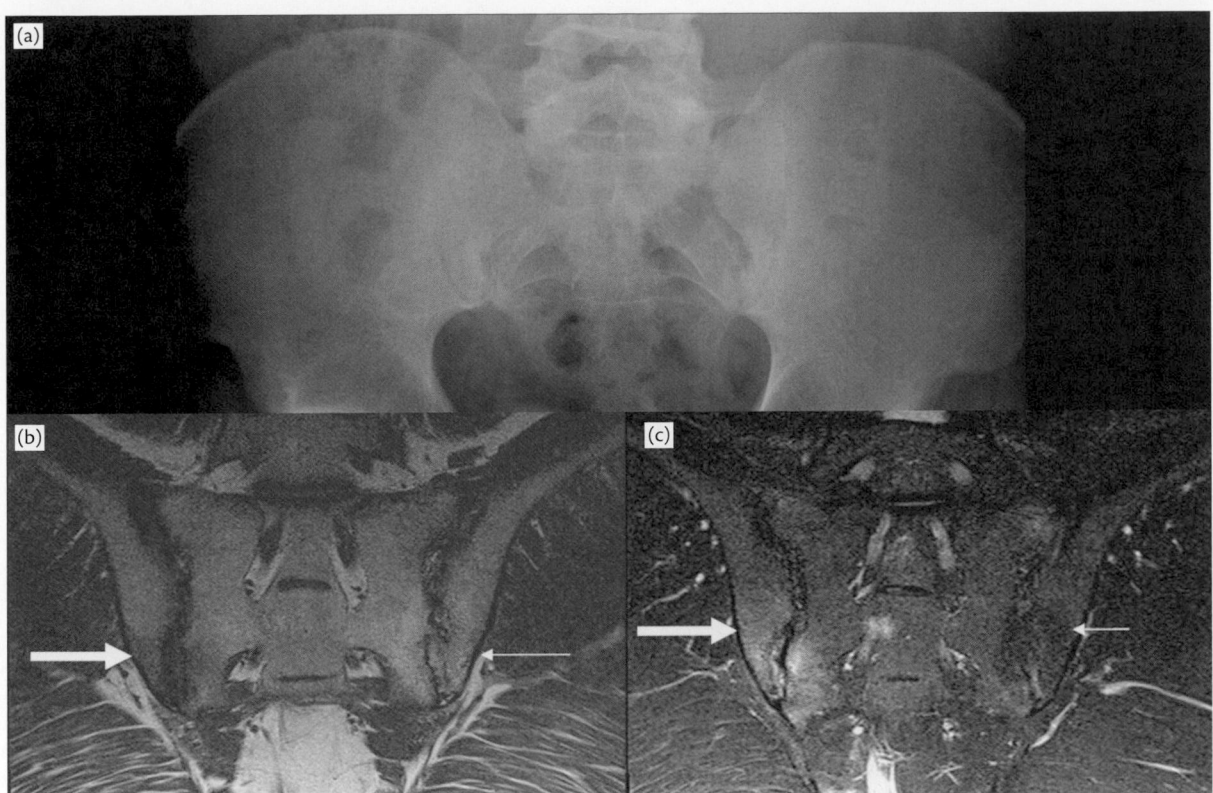

Fig. 68.4 Sacroiliitis in SpA: MRI will detect sacroiliitis years before conventional methods[56]: (a) Plain AP radiograph showing sclerosis and irregularity of the left sacroiliac joint (SIJ). (b) and (c) T1W and STIR and coronal oblique images of bilateral SIJs. *Active sacroiliitis*: right inferior SIJ demonstrates bone marrow oedema hyperintense STIR signal with corresponding low signal on T1W image (white thick arrows). *Chronic sacroiliitis*: left inferior SIJ shows joint space loss. Low STIR signal with corresponding high signal on T1W representing increased fat deposition—a postinflammatory feature (white thin arrows).

a whole vertebral body. Several studies have looked at the diagnostic utility of these lesions by assessing different disease groups such as degenerative spinal disease, spinal malignancy, and various other disorders, suggesting that a cut-off of at least three corner lesions is needed to diagnose SpA.[51] Posterior element lesions, although infrequent, appear to be highly specific of AS.[51,52] Costovertebral and costotransverse joints at the thoracic level can often be missed since routine scanning protocols of the spine may not include the lateral segments, hence missing highly specific lesions that may be crucial in the clinical context for diagnosis.[53,54] It is important for sagittal imaging to extend laterally to include the lateral aspect of the pedicles and costovertebral joints, and that these areas are carefully scrutinized. Although limited, there is mounting evidence that MRI-detected inflammatory spinal lesions may predict syndesmophyte formation[55,56] (see Figure 68.5). Spondylodiscitis (Andersson lesion) can masquerade as other causes of discitis.

In chronic disease, the main pathological feature is progressive axial ossification caused by bridging syndesmophytes along ligaments and annulus fibrosus which may eventually lead to the 'bamboo spine'. MRI, although sensitive to the inflammatory elements of SpA, is relatively insensitive to chronic syndesmophyte formation. Plain radiograph remains the gold standard for assessment of chronic SpA, although changes may take years to manifest. Fatty vertebral corner lesions detected on MRI are not a specific feature, but when present in high numbers these lesions are considered diagnostic of postinflammatory axial SpA.[57] Fatty corners are readily identifiable as high signal at vertebral corners on T1W

sequences, and mounting evidence suggests they may be predictive for syndesmophyte formation.[58] It remains to be demonstrated whether therapeutic strategies utilizing biologic therapies early would be able to delay or prevent the process of bone formation and spinal ossification using the new ASAS diagnostic criteria.

Osteoarthritis

MRI can directly assess hyaline cartilage, demonstrating a range of pathology from shallow defects to full-thickness loss; its tomographic nature demonstrates more frequent osteophytes than radiography. In established OA, MRI has also demonstrated frequent subchondral bone marrow lesions (with the appearance of bone marrow oedema) and synovitis. The is now mounting evidence for the use of MRI imaging as a more sensitive tool for detecting early OA.[59]

MRI has few indications in routine clinical management of OA, but can be useful in subjects with true knee joint locking (compared to the more common symptom of gelling), where identification of potentially remediable meniscal tears may be possible.[60,61] Anterior cruciate tears are considered a risk factor for accelerated OA, although recent reviews indicate that this may be due to the presence of meniscal tears.[62] High incidence of cartilage loss has also been noted in subjects post-meniscectomy.[63] Variable degrees of meniscal extrusion may accompany meniscal tears, leading to further abnormal mechanical load on the joint.

MRI predictors of progressive cartilage loss include the presence of meniscal extrusion, meniscal tears, and bone marrow lesions.[64]

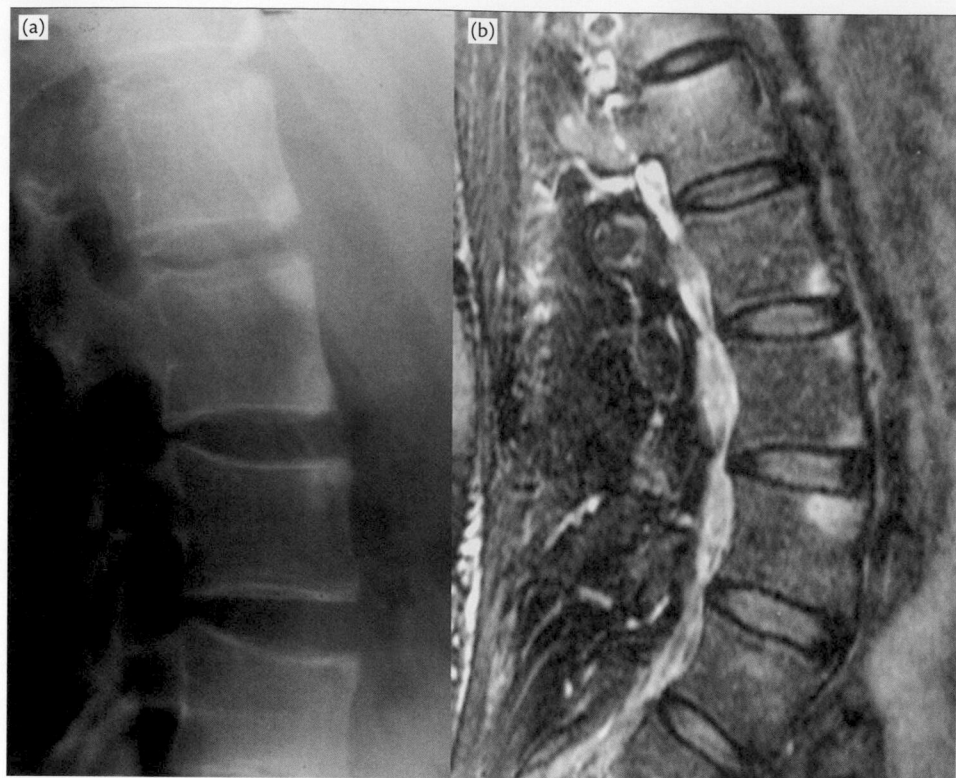

Fig. 68.5 (a) Lumbar spine MRI showing active inflammation in SpA at vertebral corners. (b) Sclerosis visible on radiograph in similar locations to change of active inflammation as in (a) (different patient).

Focal cartilage defects also predict subsequent increased rate of cartilage loss. Importantly, MRI has demonstrated certain OA pathological features to be associated with pain, including synovitis and bone marrow lesions.[62]

Undifferentiated arthritis

The role of MRI in early undifferentiated arthritis is yet to be established as there is a generalized lack of data on its potential diagnostic utility. Early MRI studies hinted at different patterns of joint involvement, with intra-articular synovial involvement found to be more common in RA and extrasynovial and capsular involvement found to be more common in seronegative or SpA type presentations.[65] However, these disease phenotypes are not always readily identifiable. Synovitis can have similar appearances in the various inflammatory arthropathies.[5] Features favouring psoriatic arthritis (PsA) rather than RA include the presence of dactylitis, periostiitis, and extracapsular/perientheseal soft tissue oedema. Tenosynovitis is considered to preferentially affect the extensor compartments in RA and the flexor compartments in PsA. Evaluation of disease distribution (proximal or distal) is essential, as with other modalities.

As a rule, MRI features should not be considered in isolation but in conjunction with radiographic findings which may indicate other features less apparent on MRI, e.g. subarticular osteoporosis or entheseal calcification. A recent systematic literature review concludes there is significant evidence for the combination of bone marrow oedema, synovitis, and erosion pattern as a prognostic indicator of future development of RA.[66] Bone marrow oedema has also been shown to be a predictor of future RA when found in metatarsophalangeal and wrist joints in early undifferentiated arthritis.[67] In this study by Duer-Jensen et al., the prediction model was stronger when bone marrow oedema was associated with other factors such as hand joint synovitis, morning stiffness and positive rheumatoid factor. The role of MRI may increase in the clinical setting with the advent of the new American College of Rheumatology (ACR) diagnostic criteria.[68]

Septic arthritis

Infection should always be considered and excluded in the case of an acute or subacute presentation of a monoarthritis. MRI has little ability to differentiate septic arthritis from other causes of acute inflammatory arthritis, so clinical and laboratory tests, including joint aspiration or biopsy, are often required for diagnosis. As with any inflammatory arthritis, bone marrow oedema, erosion, synovial thickening and enhancement, and effusions may be present. No imaging features alone or combined have been proven to differentiate between the septic and non-septic inflamed joint.[69] MRI can help to localize the presence of an effusion in deep joints which can then be targeted for aspiration. MRI is also useful for clarifying disease extent when surgical intervention is required. In the context of septic arthritis, the presence of high T2 oedema signal extending further than the subchondral bone rim, with corresponding T1 low signal, indicates osteomyelitis.

MRI can be particularly useful in certain clinical scenarios such as the diagnosis of spinal infection or in diabetics. A low threshold of suspicion is required for MRI in subjects presenting with insidious back pain and unusually high serum inflammatory markers to exclude a pyogenic discitis. Radiographic findings can be very subtle and, if undiagnosed, consequences can be severe. MRI features include high T2 signal within the intervertebral disc and adjacent oedema of the endplate and adjacent bone. Contiguous discs can be affected and there is often paraspinal soft tissue involvement. Another potential feature of spinal septic arthritis is epidural abscess formation—an indication for surgical intervention. Tuberculous infection of the spine should be considered in cases of subacute pain, and where suspected, whole spine imaging is indicated due to the high incidence of multifocal disease from subligamentous spread to non-contiguous vertebra and tracking of epidural and paravertebral infection.[70]

Gout

MRI is not often required in the imaging of suspected gout as radiographic findings are usually adequate, with typical features that differentiate from other arthritides. Atypical presentations of gout that may lead to the use of MRI include acute arthritis and chronic tophaceous gout. The disease is characterized by the presence of tophi, a focal accumulation of urate crystals, which often have a peri-articular or intra-articular location, but can also be located in the bone marrow or subcutaneous tissue. Tophi appear as intermediate signal on T1W imaging, a variable appearance on T2W imaging, usually low–intermediate signal, and variable post-gadolinium enhancement. In the advanced stages, erosions occur, often juxta-articular rather than periarticular and with a 'punched-out' or scooped appearance. Differential diagnosis includes other crystal arthropathies, pigmented villonodular synovitis, and amyloidosis (Figure 68.6).[71]

Miscellaneous

Benign proliferative disorders of the synovium

Large-joint monoarthritis refractory to conventional treatments can represent a considerable diagnostic challenge for the clinician. MRI can occasionally be helpful in this scenario. Three major subtypes of benign proliferative disorders of the synovium are readily identified by MRI: pigmented villonodular synovitis, lipoma arborescens, and synovial osteochondromatosis. For cases that do not show the typical imaging characteristics of these subtypes, diagnosis is more difficult. Despite the aid of various imaging modalities, histological assessment from synovial biopsy may be required to exclude a malignant synovial disease in some cases, especially where there is a single focus of synovial proliferation (i.e. nodular synovitis).

Pigmented villonodular synovitis

Pigmented villonodular synovitis (PVNS) typically presents as a non-inflammatory, occasionally erosive, monoarthropathy, most commonly affecting the knee or hip joints. MRI appearance is often characteristic, demonstrating nodular synovial proliferation with synovial haemosiderin deposition, typically evident as multiple low-signal foci on T1W and T2W sequences.[72] The low signal is further enhanced by the use of gradient echo sequences, which are even more susceptible to the ferromagnetic haemosiderin. Synovial masses can be substantial (Figure 68.7).

Lipoma arborescens

Lipoma arborescens is characterized as subsynovial villous fatty proliferation, most commonly occurring in the knee joint. Although the pattern of fat deposition within the synovium can be variable, MRI can easily characterize this condition[73] where joint effusions as well as periarticular erosions can be found. Onset of symptoms tends to be insidious over years, although the condition can eventually be quite debilitating, requiring synovectomy (Figure 68.8) Chronic oligoarthritis with low-grade synovial inflammation can give a similar appearance.

Synovial osteochondromatosis

Primary synovial osteochondromatosis is essentially a monoarthropathy due to chondroid metaplasia of the synovium, resulting in multiple synovial chondroid bodies which may eventually ossify. Large joints are most commonly affected. The condition is often more easily diagnosed radiographically due to the characteristic pattern of multiple intra-articular osseous bodies. The MRI appearance of these intra-articular bodies varies depending on the proportion of chondroid to osseous material.[74]

Bone marrow oedema syndrome

Bone marrow oedema syndrome (BMOS) has evolved over the last decade as an umbrella term for benign conditions previously known as transient osteoporosis, regional migratory osteoporosis,

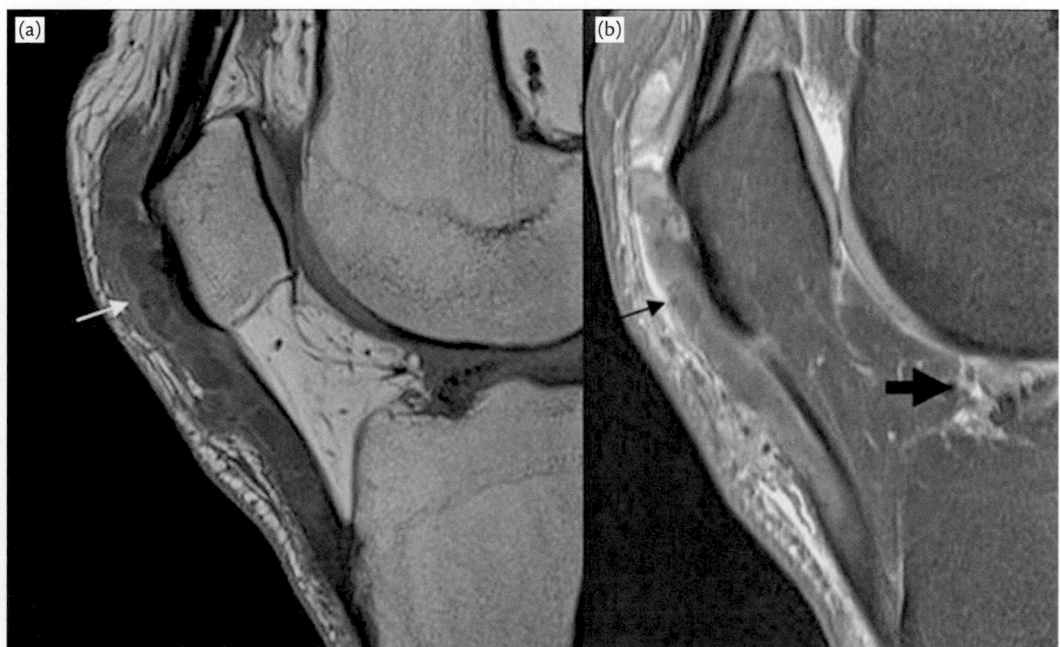

Fig. 68.6 Prepatellar tophi in gout. (a) Low signal on T1W (white arrow) and (b) intermediate–high signal on PDW/T2W (black arrow). Intra-articular tophus (thick black arrow).

or reflex sympathetic dystrophy (RSD). Differentiation between these conditions is usually by clinical presentation. The painful joint is characterized on MRI by rapidly spreading bone marrow oedema in a localized area of periarticular bone. The hip joint is most commonly affected, but the condition can present in the knee[75] and the foot.[76] The aetiopathology remains unclear; several theories have been proposed, but there is lack of evidence and concordance with the various manifestations. Clinical presentation with a painful limp of insidious onset typically occurs in young men, or in women in the third trimester of pregnancy. The condition may recur in other bone areas, hence the use of the previous term 'migratory'. Radiographs are insensitive in the first months.

MRI is very sensitive to bone marrow oedema, soft tissue and intra-articular synovial involvement and can also exclude diffuse articular surface damage, which is not a feature of BMOS. Focal regions of radiographic osteopenia may be evident later in the course of the condition. There are currently no useful laboratory diagnostic tests, except for exclusion of other diagnoses. In the majority of cases, transient osteoporosis will regress spontaneously after a period of 3–9 months.[77] RSD is a somewhat atypical manifestation as the pain may persist and result in chronic morbidity, and can be associated with skin changes and peripheral nervous symptoms.[78] BMOS is a diagnosis of exclusion and differentiation of other early presentations of conditions requiring prompt intervention such as

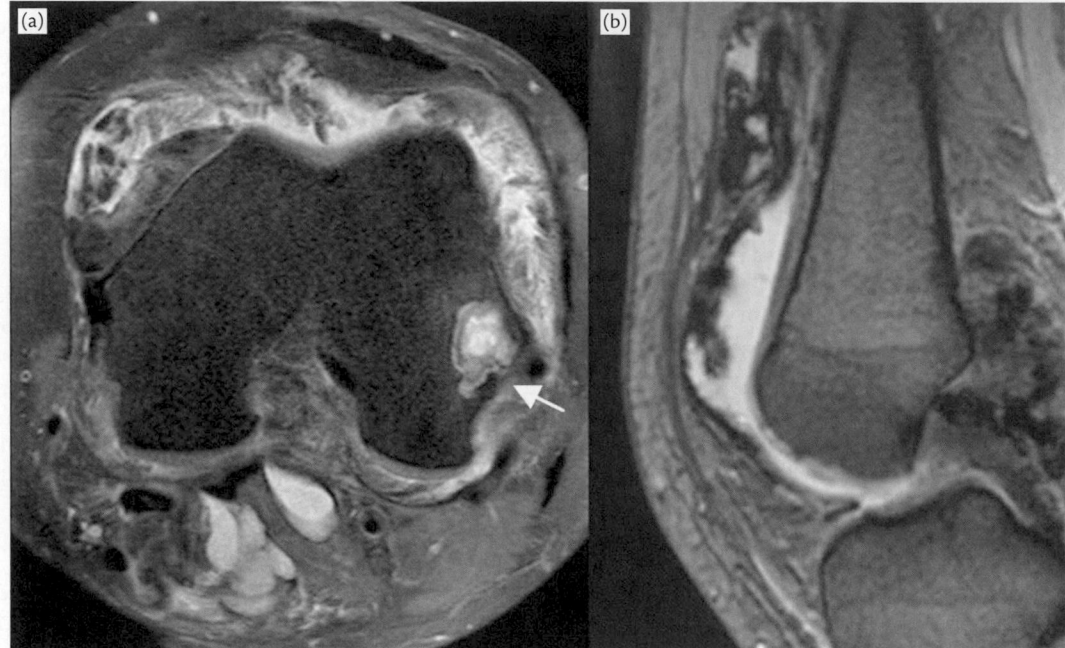

Fig. 68.7 Pigmented villonodular synovitis (PVNS): (a) Axial T2W image showing effusion and typical low-signal synovial thickening. Large erosion in the lateral femoral condyle (white arrow). (b) Gradient echo (T2* weighting). This sequence is useful in diagnosing PVNS, producing characteristic low-signal 'blooming artefact' from synovial haemosiderin deposition.

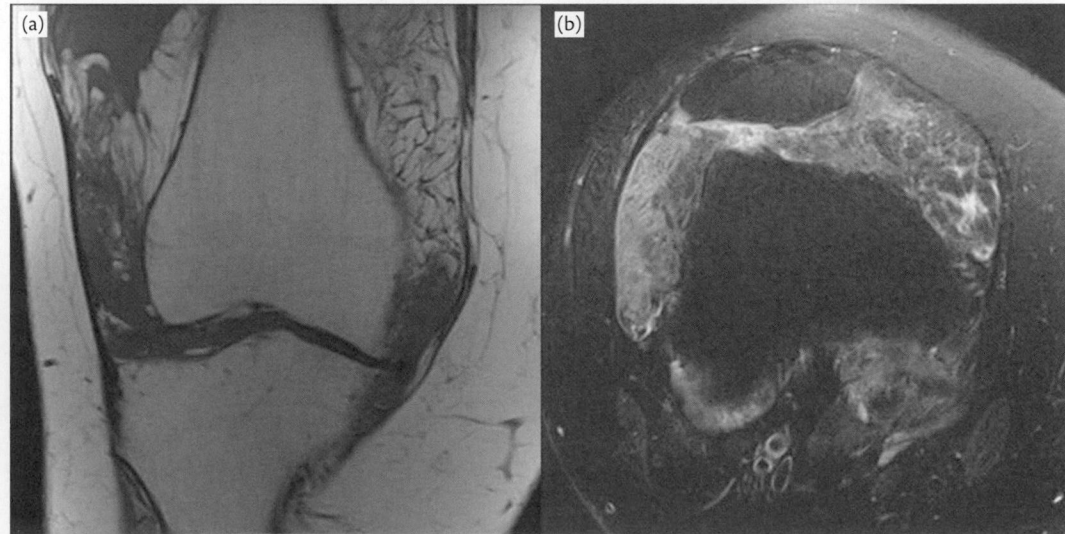

Fig. 68.8 T1W coronal and axial PDW fat-saturated (FS) images showing diffuse lobulated fatty proliferation of the knee synovium characteristic of lipoma arborhescens. PDW-FS images show increased signal laterally indicating superimposed oedema/inflammation.

avascular necrosis can be challenging. It has been suggested that BMOS and osteonecrosis are entities at different ends of the same spectrum. Sequential MRI is can be useful in these cases of diagnostic uncertainty (Figure 68.2b).[79]

Advanced MRI applications

Advanced imaging techniques

Ultrashort echo time imaging

Ultrashort echo time imaging (UTE) is a technique providing detailed visualization of short-T2 tissues. Tendons, entheses, ligaments, menisci, and cortical bone, which have T2 relaxation times of the order of 0.1–10 ms, are no longer 'invisible' and internal structure can be visualized.[80] Contrast enhancement can be

detected, showing neovascularity more extensively than power Doppler ultrasound.[81]

Whole-body MRI

Whole-body imaging (WB-MRI) has recently emerged as a screening technique applicable to several areas of musculoskeletal radiology. The main challenges to overcome are changes of patient positioning and manipulation of radiofrequency (RF) coils around the patient within a reasonable scan time and without compromising on spatial resolution. Multichannel MRI scanners, improved coil and sequence technology, and a continuously moving table within the bore have allowed advances in WB-MRI to occur with promising results so far. Scan techniques are different from tumour scanning techniques, with emphasis on peripheral assessment (see Figure 68.9). Weckbach et al. demonstrated that WB-MRI led to

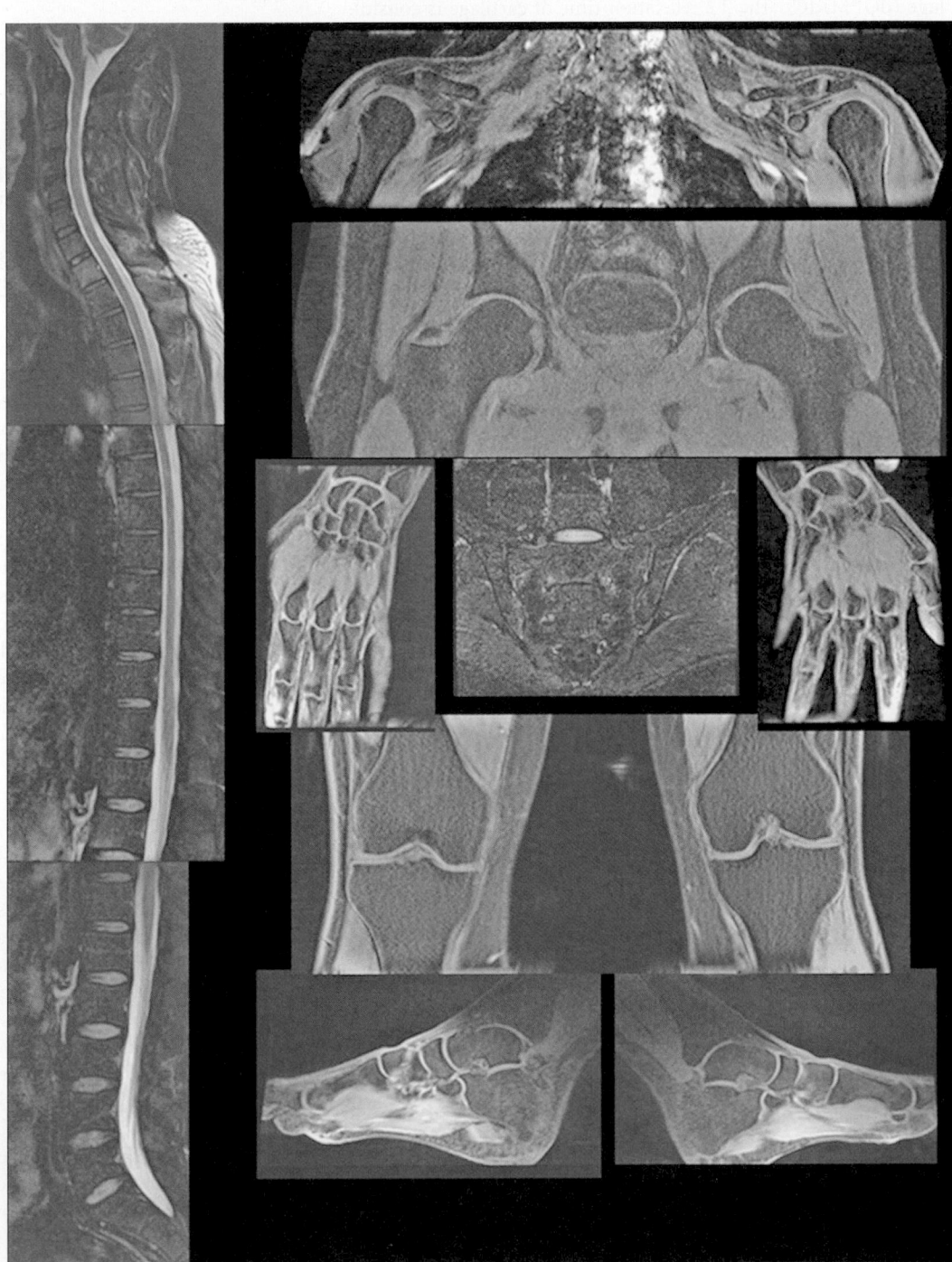

Fig. 68.9 Example of images acquired in whole-body imaging for undifferentiated arthritis. Scan time 40 minutes.
Courtesy of Dr R. Hodgson, NIHR Leeds Musculoskeletal Biomedical Research Unit, Leeds, UK.

upscaled therapy, particularly with anti-TNFα-blockade in 22 of 30 subjects with PsA.[82]

Compositional imaging of cartilage

Imaging tissue function rather than anatomical structure is a relatively new concept, with the potential to detect disease prior to structural damage has occurred. 'Mapping' image representation is often employed, whereby the value of a tissue parameter is calculated per voxel and represented as a colour-coded image. Some techniques have been employed investigating cartilage repair in clinical studies.[70] Further optimization of these techniques is required to demonstrate adequate robustness for large or multicentre clinical intervention trials. Proteoglycan depletion has been imaged by several techniques such as T1 rho mapping, sodium (Na) imaging, and delayed gadolinium enhancement MRI of cartilage (dGEMRIC). The T2 relaxation time of cartilage is considered to be a reflection of cartilage water content and the integrity of collagen fibril microstructure. In healthy cartilage, a characteristic variation in T2 from superficial to deep layers is depicted (Figure 68.10).

MRI as an outcome measure: applications in clinical trials

Imaging biomarker development

Recent growing interest in detection of OA in early or preclinical disease has been driven by the desire to identify potential therapeutic targets for early intervention. The National Institute of Health Osteoarthritis Initiative (NIH OAI) is a large study in the United States which has recruited almost 5000 subjects with the aim to identify biomarkers of early OA. Non-invasive methods of joint evaluation sensitive to early disease will require advanced MRI

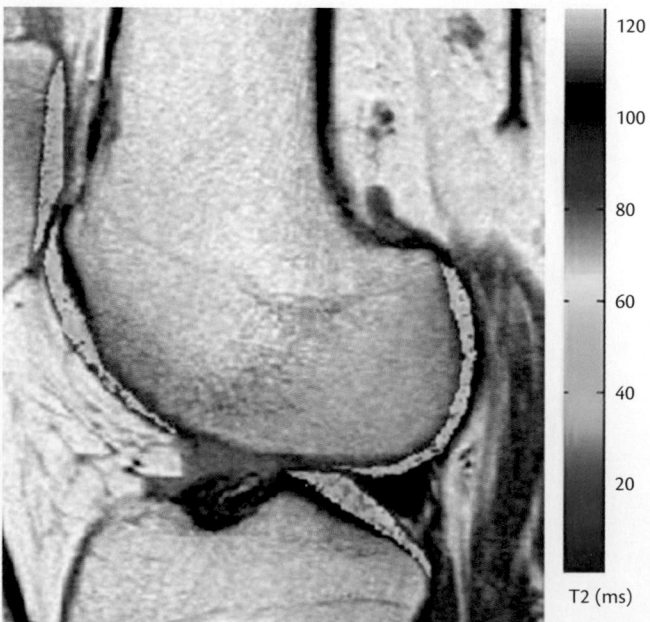

Fig. 68.10 T2 map of the knee overlaid on corresponding PDW MRI, showing per pixel variation in T2 relaxation reflecting collagen microstructure integrity. Courtesy of C.E. Hutchinson & T.G. Williams University of Manchester (UK), J.C. Waterton, AstraZeneca (Cheshire, UK) and M. Bowes, Imorphics (Manchester, UK). From work presented in ref. 94, partially funded by TSB and EPSRC.

techniques to investigate earlier changes of cartilage degradation, prior to the occurrence of cartilage loss.

Semiquantitative assessments

These systems are useful in giving a comprehensive overview of the joint, as opposed to quantitative imaging which assesses a single feature. Several scoring systems exist, e.g. for OA,[64,83] RA,[84,85] and SpA.[86,87]

Composite baseline semiquantitative scores encompassing synovitis, tenosynovitis, erosions and bone marrow oedema have been shown to exceed the ability of individual feature scores to predict future MRI erosions at 1 year in RA.[88] When the composite score is combined with clinical scores, long-term prediction of disease can be further enhanced, explaining 59% of the variation, as shown by McQueen et al.[89]

Quantitative assessments

The more precise measurement in quantitative analysis is considered to have better reproducibility, accuracy, and sensitivity than semiquantitative techniques. In general, the parameters measured fall into one of two categories: morphology (e.g. volume, thickness, surface area) or quality (e.g. signal intensity, enhancement rate, signal heterogeneity). These techniques have drawbacks, often requiring specialized software and trained operators, and are much more time consuming and costly than semiquantitative techniques.

Image analysis

Simple measurements of signal intensity can be made from a region of interest superimposed on the area of the feature to be analysed. Entire soft tissue structures or regions or pathology may be outlined in order to measure the volume of that structure. Various semi-automated techniques have been developed to assist segmentation, as the manual process is time consuming. Thresholding-related methods enable outlining of areas of a specified signal intensity range. Recent advances include the incorporation of statistical shape modelling into software which develops models which 'learn' the shape and appearance of particular structures of interest (e.g. cartilage, bone) from a pre-existing image dataset. The models can then be used to 'search' and automatically segment new images. These automated methods have yet to be widely validated, but will no doubt have an important role to play in future quantitative MRI research (Figure 68.11).

Dynamic contrast MRI

Dynamic contrast MRI (DCE-MRI) has been used in arthritis imaging, assessing enhancement rates of structures involved in active inflammation, e.g. synovitis, enthuses, and bone marrow. Multiple T1W acquisitions are obtained at intervals of several seconds, allowing a curve of signal intensity over time to be obtained. In active synovitis, curves characteristically demonstrate an initial rapid increase within the first 60 seconds then slow to eventually reach a plateau. Measures of synovial relative early enhancement rate (RER) measured within the first 60 seconds have been shown to correlate strongly with histological inflammation in several studies.[5,17] Higher RERs are considered to reflect increased synovial vascularity and capillary permeability, features of more aggressive active inflammation. Quantification of synovial vascular flow with power Doppler is possible; however, DCE-MRI enhancement

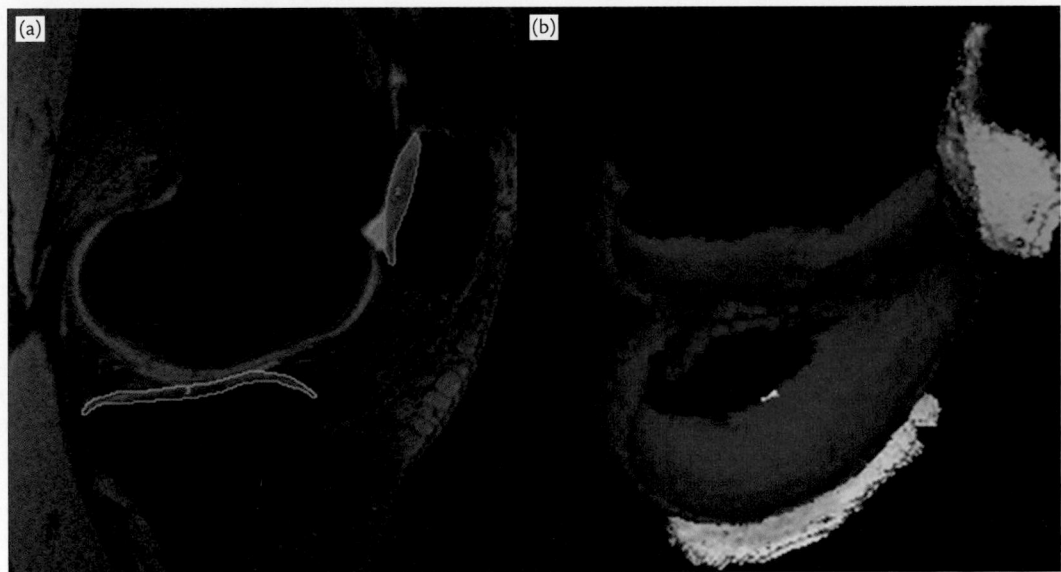

Fig. 68.11 Quantitative image analysis methods in cartilage quantitation: (a) Manual delineation (segmentation) of cartilage plates in the knee on single sagittal dual echo steady state (DESS) image. (b) Subsequent 3D rendered segmentation of total knee cartilage obtained from manual segmentation demonstrating patellar (green), femoral (red), medial tibial (yellow), and lateral tibial (blue) cartilage plates. Analysis performed using Analyze 10.0 (AnalyzeDirect, Overland Park, KS, USA). Courtesy of NIHR Leeds Musculoskeletal Biomedical Research Unit, Leeds, UK.

rates also reflect vascular permeability and allow for improved global synovial volume assessment.

DCE-MRI has been used both as a tool to probe further into the understanding of inflammatory arthritis and as an indicator of the 'aggressiveness' of disease activity. Synovial early enhancement rates correlate well with power Doppler ultrasound assessment of active synovial inflammation.[16] As a surrogate marker, DCE-MRI has proved useful in assessing response post-treatment to disease-modifying drugs and biological therapies in RA.[90,91] Baseline DCE-MRI measures have been found to predict RA progression in some studies.[92] One advantage of DCE-MRI is clear; being sensitive to small changes, it allows study cohorts to be small. The main drawback is that many methodological factors that can affect results, e.g. gadolinium injection dose/rate, or patient movement between series. Entire synovial assessment is preferable to single region of interest or single slice, due to substantial regional variation of synovitis within large joints in particular,[93] and this is increasingly being facilitated by advanced image analysis software applications.

Acknowledgements

The authors would like to acknowledge people who contributed to the images in this chapter. Dr Richard Hodgson, Head of MRI and Claire Wenham, Research Fellow at NIHR Leeds Musculoskeletal Biomedical Imaging Unit, Leeds, UK; T.G. Williams, University of Manchester, UK; J.C. Waterton, AstraZeneca (Cheshire, UK); and M. Bowes, Imorphics Ltd, Manchester, UK.

References

1. Hashemi RH, Bradley WG Jr. *MRI: the basics*. Williams & Wilkins, Baltimore, MD, 1997.

2. Delfaut EM, Beltran J, Johnson G et al. Fat suppression in MR imaging: techniques and pitfalls. *Radiographics*, 1999;19(2):373–382.

3. Leiner T, Kucharczyk W. NSF prevention in clinical practice: summary of recommendations and guidelines in the United States, Canada, and Europe. *J Magn Reson Imaging* 2009;30(6):1357–1363.

4. Tamai M, Kawakami A, Uetani M et al. Magnetic resonance imaging (MRI) detection of synovitis and bone lesions of the wrists and finger joints in early-stage rheumatoid arthritis: comparison of the accuracy of plain MRI-based findings and gadolinium-diethylenetriamine pentaacetic acid-enhanced MRI-based findings. *Mod Rheumatol* 2012;22(5):654–648.

5. McQueen FM. The MRI view of synovitis and tenosynovitis in inflammatory arthritis: implications for diagnosis and management. *Ann N Y Acad Sci* 2009;1154:21–34.

6. Konig H, Sieper J, Wolf KJ. Rheumatoid arthritis: evaluation of hypervascular and fibrous pannus with dynamic MR imaging enhanced with Gd-DTPA. *Radiology* 1990;176(2):473–477.

7. Kricun ME. Red-yellow marrow conversion: its effect on the location of some solitary bone lesions. *Skeletal Radiol* 1985;14(1):10–19.

8. Bollow M, Fischer T, Reisshauer H et al. Quantitative analyses of sacroiliac biopsies in spondyloarthropathies: T cells and macrophages predominate in early and active sacroiliitis- cellularity correlates with the degree of enhancement detected by magnetic resonance imaging. *Ann Rheum Dis* 2000;59(2):135–140.

9. François RJ, Neure L, Sieper J, Braun J. Immunohistological examination of open sacroiliac biopsies of patients with ankylosing spondylitis: detection of tumour necrosis factor alpha in two patients with early disease and transforming growth factor beta in three more advanced cases. *Ann Rheum Dis* 2006;65(6):713–720.

10. Marzo-Ortega H, O'Connor P, Emery P, McGonagle D. Sacroiliac joint biopsies in early sacroiliitis. *Rheumatology* (Oxford) 2007;46(7):1210–1211.

11. Jimenez-Boj E, Nöbauer-Huhmann I, Hanslik-Schnabel B et al. Bone erosions and bone marrow edema as defined by magnetic resonance imaging reflect true bone marrow inflammation in rheumatoid arthritis. *Arthritis Rheum* 2007;56(4):1118–1124.

12. Palosaari K, Vuotila J, Takalo R et al. Bone oedema predicts erosive progression on wrist MRI in early RA—a 2-yr observational MRI and NC scintigraphy study. *Rheumatology* (Oxford) 2006;45(12):1542–1548.

13. Ito H, Matsuno T, Minami A. Relationship between bone marrow edema and development of symptoms in patients with osteonecrosis of the femoral head. *AJR Am J Roentgenol* 2006;186(6):1761–1770.

14. Fukubayashi T, Kurosawa H. The contact area and pressure distribution pattern of the knee. A study of normal and osteoarthrotic knee joints. *Acta Orthop Scand* 1980;51(6):871–879.

15. Østergaard M, McQueen F, Bird P et al. The OMERACT Magnetic Resonance Imaging Inflammatory Arthritis Group—advances and priorities. *J Rheumatol* 2007;34(4):852–853.

16. Szkudlarek M, Court-Payen M, Strandberg C et al. Power Doppler ultrasonography for assessment of synovitis in the metacarpophalangeal joints of patients with rheumatoid arthritis: a comparison with dynamic magnetic resonance imaging. *Arthritis Rheum* 2001;44(9): 2018–2023.

17. Østergaard M, Stoltenberg M, Løvgreen-Nielsen P et al. Quantification of synovitis by MRI: correlation between dynamic and static gadolinium-enhanced magnetic resonance imaging and microscopic and macroscopic signs of synovial inflammation. *Magn Reson Imaging*, 1998;16(7): 743–754.

18. Farrant JM, Grainger AJ, O'Connor PJ. Advanced imaging in rheumatoid arthritis: part 2: erosions. *Skeletal Radiol* 2007;36(5):381–389.

19. Døhn UM, Ejbjerg BJ, Court-Payen M et al. Are bone erosions detected by magnetic resonance imaging and ultrasonography true erosions? A comparison with computed tomography in rheumatoid arthritis metacarpophalangeal joints. *Arthritis Res Ther* 2006;8(4):R110.

20. McQueen FM, Benton N, Crabbe J et al. What is the fate of erosions in early rheumatoid arthritis? Tracking individual lesions using x rays and magnetic resonance imaging over the first two years of disease. *Ann Rheum Dis* 2001;60(9):859–868.

21. Perry D, Stewart N, Benton N et al. Detection of erosions in the rheumatoid hand; a comparative study of multidetector computerized tomography versus magnetic resonance scanning. *J Rheumatol* 2005;32(2): 256–267.

22. McQueen F, Lassere M, Edmonds J et al. OMERACT rheumatoid arthritis magnetic resonance imaging studies. Summary of OMERACT 6 MR imaging module. *J Rheumatol* 2003;30(6):1387–1392.

23. Døhn UM, Ejbjerg B, Boonen A et al. No overall progression and occasional repair of erosions despite persistent inflammation in adalimumab-treated rheumatoid arthritis patients: results from a longitudinal comparative MRI, ultrasonography, CT and radiography study. *Ann Rheum Dis* 2011;70(2):252–258.

24. Østergaard M, Emery P, Conaghan PG et al. Significant improvement in synovitis, osteitis, and bone erosion following golimumab and methotrexate combination therapy as compared with methotrexate alone: a magnetic resonance imaging study of 318 methotrexate-naive rheumatoid arthritis patients. *Arthritis Rheum* 2011;63(12):3712–3722.

25. McGonagle D, Ash ZR, Hodgson RJ, Emery P, Radjenovic A. MRI for the assessment and monitoring of RA—what can it tell us? *Nat Rev Rheumatol* 2011;7(3):185–189.

26. Ashikyan O, Tehranzadeh J. The role of magnetic resonance imaging in the early diagnosis of rheumatoid arthritis. *Top Magn Reson Imaging* 2007;18(3):169–176.

27. Suter LG, Fraenkel L, Braithwaite RS. Role of magnetic resonance imaging in the diagnosis and prognosis of rheumatoid arthritis. *Arthritis Care Res* (Hoboken) 2011;63(5):675–688.

28. Conaghan PG, McQueen FM, Peterfy CG et al. The evidence for magnetic resonance imaging as an outcome measure in proof-of-concept rheumatoid arthritis studies. *J Rheumatol* 2005;32(12):2465–2469.

29. Hetland ML, Ejbjerg B, Hørslev-Petersen K et al. MRI bone oedema is the strongest predictor of subsequent radiographic progression in early rheumatoid arthritis. Results from a 2-year randomised controlled trial (CIMESTRA). *Ann Rheum Dis* 2009;68(3):384–390.

30. Smolen JS, Aletaha D, Bijlsma JW et al. Treating rheumatoid arthritis to target: recommendations of an international task force. *Ann Rheum Dis* 2010;69(4):631–637.

31. Goupille P, Roulot B, Akoka S et al. Magnetic resonance imaging: a valuable method for the detection of synovial inflammation in rheumatoid arthritis. *J Rheumatol* 2001;28(1):35–40.

32. Scirè CA, Montecucco C, Codullo V et al. Ultrasonographic evaluation of joint involvement in early rheumatoid arthritis in clinical remission: power Doppler signal predicts short-term relapse. *Rheumatology* (Oxford) 2009;48(9):1092–1097.

33. Quinn MA, Conaghan PG, O'Connor PJ et al. Very early treatment with infliximab in addition to methotrexate in early, poor-prognosis rheumatoid arthritis reduces magnetic resonance imaging evidence of synovitis and damage, with sustained benefit after infliximab withdrawal: results from a twelve-month randomized, double-blind, placebo-controlled trial. *Arthritis Rheum* 2005;52(1):27–35.

34. Østergaard M, Peterfy C, Conaghan P et al. OMERACT Rheumatoid Arthritis Magnetic Resonance Imaging Studies. Core set of MRI acquisitions, joint pathology definitions, and the OMERACT RA-MRI scoring system. *J Rheumatol* 2003;30(6):1385–1386.

35. Østergaard M, Conaghan PG, O'Connor P et al. Reducing invasiveness, duration, and cost of magnetic resonance imaging in rheumatoid arthritis by omitting intravenous contrast injection—Does it change the assessment of inflammatory and destructive joint changes by the OMERACT RAMRIS? *J Rheumatol* 2009;36(8):1806–1810.

36. Van der Linden S, Valkenburg HA, Cats A. Evaluation of diagnostic criteria for ankylosing spondylitis: a proposal for modification of the New York criteria. *Arthritis Rheum*, 1984;27:361–368.

37. Bennett AN, Marzo-Ortega H, Emery P, McGonagle D; Leeds Spondyloarthropathy Group. Diagnosing axial spondyloarthropathy. The new Assessment in SpondyloArthritis international Society criteria: MRI entering centre stage. *Ann Rheum Dis* 2009;68(6):765–767.

38. Rudwaleit M, Haibel H, Baraliakos X et al. The early disease stage in axial spondylarthritis: results from the German Spondyloarthritis Inception Cohort. *Arthritis Rheum* 2009;60(3):717–727.

39. Haibel H, Rudwaleit M, Listing J et al. Efficacy of adalimumab in the treatment of axial spondylarthritis without radiographically defined sacroiliitis: results of a twelve-week randomized, double-blind, placebo-controlled trial followed by an open-label extension up to week fifty-two. *Arthritis Rheum* 2008;58(7):1981–1991.

40. Barkham N, Keen HI, Coates LC et al. Clinical and imaging efficacy of infliximab in HLA-B27-Positive patients with magnetic resonance imaging-determined early sacroiliitis. *Arthritis Rheum* 2009;60(4): 946–954.

41. Madsen, KB, Egund N, Jurik AG. Grading of inflammatory disease activity in the sacroiliac joints with magnetic resonance imaging: comparison between short-tau inversion recovery and gadolinium contrast-enhanced sequences. *J Rheumatol* 2010;37(2):393–400.

42. Baraliakos X, Hermann KG, Landewé R et al. Assessment of acute spinal inflammation in patients with ankylosing spondylitis by magnetic resonance imaging: a comparison between contrast enhanced T1 and short tau inversion recovery (STIR) sequences. *Ann Rheum Dis* 2005;64(8):1141–1144.

43. Marzo-Ortega H, McGonagle D, O'Connor P et al. Baseline and 1-year magnetic resonance imaging of the sacroiliac joint and lumbar spine in very early inflammatory back pain. Relationship between symptoms, HLA-B27 and disease extent and persistence. *Ann Rheum Dis* 2009;68(11):1721–1727.

44. Rudwaleit M, van der Heijde D, Landewé R et al. The development of Assessment of SpondyloArthritis international Society classification criteria for axial spondyloarthritis (part II): validation and final selection. *Ann Rheum Dis* 2009;68(6):777–783.

45. Bennett AN, Marzo-Ortega H, Rehman A et al. The evidence for whole-spine MRI in the assessment of axial spondyloarthropathy. *Rheumatology* (Oxford) 2010;49(3):426–432.

46. Rudwaleit M, Jurik AG, Hermann KG et al. Defining active sacroiliitis on magnetic resonance imaging (MRI) for classification of axial spondyloarthritis: a consensual approach by the ASAS/OMERACT MRI group. *Ann Rheum Dis* 2009;68(10):1520–1527.

47. Aydin SZ, Maksymowych WP, Bennett AN et al. Validation of the ASAS criteria and definition of a positive MRI of the sacroiliac joint in an inception cohort of axial spondyloarthritis followed up for 8 years. *Ann Rheum Dis* 2012;71(1):56–60.

48. Machado P, Landewé R, Braun J et al. Both structural damage and inflammation of the spine contribute to impairment of spinal mobility in patients with ankylosing spondylitis. *Ann Rheum Dis* 2010;69(8):1465–1470.

49. Weber U, Hodler J, Jurik AG et al. Assessment of active spinal inflammatory changes in patients with axial spondyloarthritis: validation of whole body MRI against conventional MRI. *Ann Rheum Dis* 2010;69(4): 648–653.

50. Baraliakos X, Landewé R, Hermann KG et al. Inflammation in ankylosing spondylitis: a systematic description of the extent and frequency of acute spinal changes using magnetic resonance imaging. *Ann Rheum Dis* 2005;64(5):730–734.

51. Bennett AN, Rehman A, Hensor EM et al. Evaluation of the diagnostic utility of spinal magnetic resonance imaging in axial spondylarthritis. *Arthritis Rheum* 2009;60(5):1331–1341.

52. Maksymowych WP, Crowther SM, Dhillon SS, Conner-Spady B, Lambert RG. Systematic assessment of inflammation by magnetic resonance imaging in the posterior elements of the spine in ankylosing spondylitis. *Arthritis Care Res* (Hoboken) 2010;62(1):4–10.

53. Rennie WJ, Dhillon SS, Conner-Spady B, Maksymowych WP, Lambert RG. Magnetic resonance imaging assessment of spinal inflammation in ankylosing spondylitis: standard clinical protocols may omit inflammatory lesions in thoracic vertebrae. *Arthritis Rheum* 2009;61(9): 1187–1193.

54. Bochkova AG, Levshakova AV, Bunchuk NV, Braun J. Spinal inflammation lesions as detected by magnetic resonance imaging in patients with early ankylosing spondylitis are more often observed in posterior structures of the spine. *Rheumatology* (Oxford) 2010;49(4):749–755.

55. Baraliakos X, Listing J, Rudwaleit M, Sieper J, Braun J. The relationship between inflammation and new bone formation in patients with ankylosing spondylitis. *Arthritis Res Ther* 2008;10(5):R104.

56. Maksymowych WP, Chiowchanwisawakit P, Clare T et al. Inflammatory lesions of the spine on magnetic resonance imaging predict the development of new syndesmophytes in ankylosing spondylitis: evidence of a relationship between inflammation and new bone formation. *Arthritis Rheum* 2009;60(1):93–102.

57. Bennett AN, Rehman A, Hensor EM et al. The fatty Romanus lesion: a non-inflammatory spinal MRI lesion specific for axial spondyloarthropathy. *Ann Rheum Dis* 2010;69(5):891–894.

58. Chiowchanwisawakit P, Lambert RG, Conner-Spady B, Maksymowych WP. Focal fat lesions at vertebral corners on magnetic resonance imaging predict the development of new syndesmophytes in ankylosing spondylitis. *Arthritis Rheum* 2011;63(8):2215–2225.

59. Hunter DJ, Arden N, Conaghan PG et al. Definition of osteoarthritis on MRI: results of a Delphi exercise. *Osteoarthritis Cartilage* 2011;19(8):963–969.

60. Kääb MJ, Ito K, Clark JM, Nötzli HP. The acute structural changes of loaded articular cartilage following meniscectomy or ACL-transection. *Osteoarthritis Cartilage* 2000;8(6):464–473.

61. Englund M, Roos EM, Lohmander LS. Impact of type of meniscal tear on radiographic and symptomatic knee osteoarthritis: A sixteen-year follow-up of meniscectomy with matched controls. *Arthritis Rheum* 2003;48(8):2178–2187.

62. Hunter DJ, Zhang W, Conaghan PG et al. Systematic review of the concurrent and predictive validity of MRI biomarkers in OA. *Osteoarthritis Cartilage* 2011;19(5):557–588.

63. Cicuttini FM, Forbes A, Yuanyuan W, Rush G, Stuckey SL. Rate of knee cartilage loss after partial meniscectomy. *J Rheumatol* 2002;29(9):1954–1956.

64. Hunter DJ, Guermazi A, Lo GH et al. Evolution of semi-quantitative whole joint assessment of knee OA: MOAKS (MRI Osteoarthritis Knee Score). *Osteoarthritis Cartilage* 2011;19(8):990–1002.

65. McGonagle D, Gibbon W, O'Connor P et al. An anatomical explanation for good-prognosis rheumatoid arthritis. *Lancet* 1999;353(9147):123–124.

66. Machado PKR, Bombardier C, van der Heijde D. The value of magnetic resonance imaging and ultrasound in undifferentiated arthritis: a systematic review. *J Rheumatol* 2010;38(suppl 87):31–37.

67. Duer-Jensen A, Hørslev-Petersen K, Hetland ML et al. Bone edema on magnetic resonance imaging is an independent predictor of rheumatoid arthritis development in patients with early undifferentiated arthritis. *Arthritis Rheum* 2011;63(8):2192–2202.

68. Aletaha D, Neogi T, Silman AJ et al. 2010 rheumatoid arthritis classification criteria: an American College of Rheumatology/European League Against Rheumatism collaborative initiative. *Ann Rheum Dis* 2010;69(9):1580–1588.

69. Graif M, Schweitzer ME, Deely D, Matteucci T. The septic versus nonseptic inflamed joint: MRI characteristics. *Skeletal Radiol* 1999;28(11): 616–620.

70. Kaila R, Malhi AM, Mahmood B, Saifuddin A. The incidence of multiple level noncontiguous vertebral tuberculosis detected using whole spine MRI. *J Spinal Disord Tech* 2007;20(1):78–81.

71. Chen CK, Yeh LR, Pan HB et al. Intra-articular gouty tophi of the knee: CT and MR imaging in 12 patients. *Skeletal Radiol* 1999;28(2): 75–80.

72. Cheng XG, You YH, Liu W, Zhao T, Qu H. MRI features of pigmented villonodular synovitis (PVNS). *Clin Rheumatol* 2004;23(1):31–34.

73. Ryu KN, Jaovisidha S, Schweitzer M, Motta AO, Resnick D. MR imaging of lipoma arborescens of the knee joint. *AJR Am J Roentgenol* 1996;167(5):1229–1232.

74. Murphey MD, Vidal JA, Fanburg-Smith JC, Gajewski DA. Imaging of synovial chondromatosis with radiologic-pathologic correlation. *Radiographics* 2007;27(5):1465–1488.

75. Nikolaou VS, Pilichou A, Korres D, Efstathopoulos N. Transient osteoporosis of the knee. *Orthopedics* 2008;31(5):502.

76. Shariff SS, Baghla DP, Clark C, Dega RK. Transient osteoporosis of the foot. *Br J Hosp Med* 2009;70(7):402–405.

77. Starr AM, Wessely MA, Albastaki U, Pierre-Jerome C, Kettner NW. Bone marrow edema: pathophysiology, differential diagnosis, and imaging. *Acta Radiol* 2008;49(7):771–786.

78. Korompilias AV, Karantanas AH, Lykissas MG, Beris AE. Bone marrow edema syndrome. *Skeletal Radiol* 2009;38(5):425–436.

79. Steinbach LS, Suh KJ. Bone marrow edema pattern around the knee on magnetic resonance imaging excluding acute traumatic lesions. *Semin Musculoskelet Radiol* 2011;15(3):208–220.

80. Robson MD, Gatehouse PD, Bydder M, Bydder GM. Magnetic resonance: an introduction to ultrashort TE (UTE) imaging. *J Comput Assist Tomogr* 2003;27(6):825–846.

81. Hodgson R, Grainger AJ, O'Connor PJ et al. Imaging of the Achilles tendon in spondyloarthritis: a comparison of ultrasound and conventional, short and ultrashort echo time MRI with and without intravenous contrast. *Eur Radiol* 2011;21(6):1144–1152.

82. Weckbach S, Mendlik T, Horger W et al. Quantitative assessment of patellar cartilage volume and thickness at 3.0 tesla comparing a 3D-fast low angle shot versus a 3D-true fast imaging with steady-state precession sequence for reproducibility. *Invest Radiol* 2006;41(2):189–197.

83. Peterfy CG, Guermazi A, Zaim S et al. Whole-Organ Magnetic Resonance Imaging Score (WORMS) of the knee in osteoarthritis. *Osteoarthritis Cartilage* 2004;12(3):177–190.

84. Ejbjerg B, McQueen F, Lassere M et al. The EULAR-OMERACT rheumatoid arthritis MRI reference image atlas: the wrist joint. *Ann Rheum Dis* 2005;64 Suppl 1:i23–i47.

85. Conaghan P, Bird P, Ejbjerg B et al. The EULAR-OMERACT rheumatoid arthritis MRI reference image atlas: the metacarpophalangeal joints. *Ann Rheum Dis* 2005;64 Suppl 1:i11–i21.

86. Sieper J, Rudwaleit M, Baraliakos X et al. The Assessment of SpondyloArthritis international Society (ASAS) handbook: a guide to assess spondyloarthritis. *Ann Rheum Dis* 2009;68 Suppl 2:ii1–ii44.

87. Ostergaard M, McQueen F, Wiell C et al. The OMERACT psoriatic arthritis magnetic resonance imaging scoring system (PsAMRIS): definitions of key pathologies, suggested MRI sequences, and preliminary scoring system for PsA Hands. *J Rheumatol* 2009;36(8):1816–1824.

88. McQueen FM, Stewart N, Crabbe J et al. Magnetic resonance imaging of the wrist in early rheumatoid arthritis reveals progression of erosions despite clinical improvement. *Ann Rheum Dis* 1999;58(3):156–163.

89. McQueen FM, Benton N, Perry D et al. Bone edema scored on magnetic resonance imaging scans of the dominant carpus at presentation predicts radiographic joint damage of the hands and feet six years later in patients with rheumatoid arthritis. *Arthritis Rheum* 2003;48(7):1814–1827.

90. Hodgson RJ, Barnes T, Connolly S et al. Changes underlying the dynamic contrast-enhanced MRI response to treatment in rheumatoid arthritis. *Skeletal Radiol* 2008;37(3):201–207.

91. Reece RJ, Kraan MC, Radjenovic A et al. Comparative assessment of leflunomide and methotrexate for the treatment of rheumatoid arthritis, by dynamic enhanced magnetic resonance imaging. *Arthritis Rheum* 2002;46(2):366–372.

92. Hodgson RJ, O'Connor P, Moots R. MRI of rheumatoid arthritis image quantitation for the assessment of disease activity, progression and response to therapy. *Rheumatology* (Oxford) 2008;47(1):13–21.

93. Rhodes LA, Tan AL, Tanner SF et al. Regional variation and differential response to therapy for knee synovitis adjacent to the cartilage-pannus junction and suprapatellar pouch in inflammatory arthritis: implications for pathogenesis and treatment. *Arthritis Rheum* 2004;50(8):2428–2432.

94. Balamoody S, Hutchinson CE, Waterton JC et al. *Intra- and inter-scanner variability of knee cartilage T2 in human knees at 3.0T: a multi-vendor comparison study. Poster 1962. International Society of Magnetic Resonance in Medicine, Annual Meeting* 2009. Honolulu, Hawaii, USA.

CHAPTER 69

Computed tomography

Geoff Hide and Jennifer Humphries

Introduction

Computed tomography (CT) was developed by Godfrey Hounsfield in 1973[1] and rapidly acquired an essential role within diagnostic imaging. Images in CT are produced using a uniform X-ray beam produced in an X-ray tube which passes through the patient, is modified by interaction with the tissues it encounters, and is detected beyond the patient in a manner similar to the production of a conventional radiograph. However, CT differs from conventional radiography in that the X-ray source and the bank of detectors are mounted on opposite sides of a rotating circular gantry. Rotation of this gantry results in the beam passing through the patient's body from all sides during the course of a complete 360° rotation. The data obtained from the detectors can then be reconstructed by computer to produce an axial (horizontal) sectional image (or slice) of the area assessed.

In an older CT scanner, the table on which the patient was lying would then be advanced further through the gantry, typically by the same distance as the thickness of a slice, and another rotation would occur to produce the next image. The end result would be a series of images of the area scanned, much like the slices making up a loaf of bread. These images provided good anatomical detail within each slice but examinations were slow and the reconstruction of a series of slices to produce images in other planes (e.g. coronal or sagittal) yielded poor-quality results, even with the thinnest of slices. Modern CT scanners combine constant, synchronous gantry rotation and movement of the table to allow faster scanning and more importantly, permitting the entire area of interest to be scanned in a single, continuous X-ray exposure. This results in the X-ray beam effectively passing around the patient in a spiral fashion, and producing a single volume of data, rather than a series of individual slices. Such data can still be used to produce axial sectional images, but also permits high-quality reconstructions in other imaging planes as well as allowing volumetric and other three-dimensional images to be produced. Most recently, technological developments have allowed multiple banks of detectors to be placed adjacent to each other, with each bank obtaining its own dataset at the same time. These 'multislice' scanners can now be manufactured with several hundred detector banks, allowing exceptionally rapid scanning of large patient areas in polytrauma situations, or alternately, if the table remains stationary, imaging of the entire heart in a single contraction.

CT images

CT images are digital, consisting of multiple small squares or pixels (picture elements) arranged in a grid or matrix (Figure 69.1). Each pixel corresponds to a small volume of tissue (voxel) and is assigned a number which indicates the degree to which tissue in the voxel absorbs or deflects the X-ray beam. Such CT numbers (also known as Hounsfield units) range from 1000 (air) to +1000 (bone), with water assigned a value of zero. The CT number broadly reflects the average density of the tissue contained within that voxel. Although it is possible to display the entire range of CT numbers from 1000 to +1000 on a single image, it is difficult for an observer to perceive differences between some tissue types and usually the image

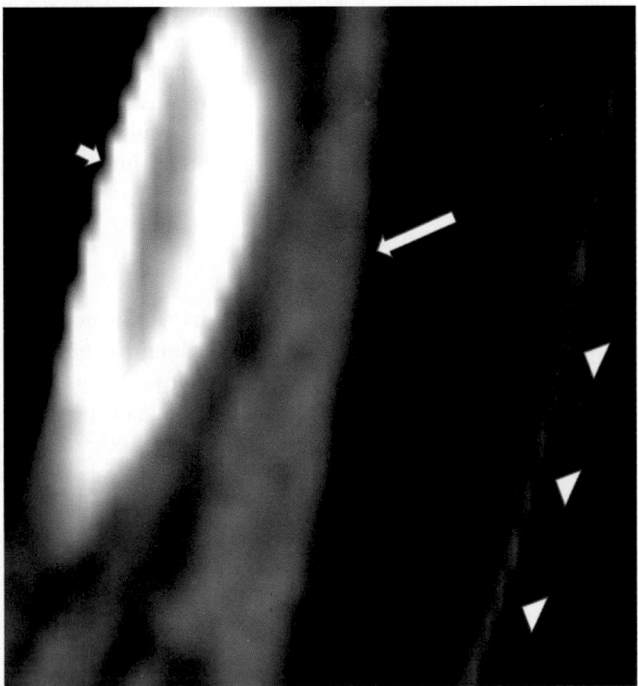

Fig. 69.1 CT image of the left chest wall which has been magnified to demonstrate the individual pixels making up the image. The black triangle top left is lung. Adjacent to this (from left to right) are rib (arrow), chest wall muscle (long arrow), subcutaneous fat and skin (arrowheads). Note how the edges of structures such as the rib demonstrate the square nature of the individual elements making up the image.

is shown in a manner which makes it easier to identify such differences (or contrast); this is termed 'windowing'. Here only a proportion of the possible CT number range is displayed, determined by the numerical width of the 'window' and its centre value. Window settings are used to highlight detail of soft tissue (where a typical width of 400 with a centre value of 40 is used), lung (width 1000/centre 700), or bone (width 2400/centre 200). In many situations, each CT image must be viewed on several different window settings in order to extract all of the available diagnostic information. For example, a CT examination of the chest must be viewed on soft tissue settings to identify lymph nodes at the hilum, at lung settings to detect small pulmonary metastases, and at bone settings to demonstrate destructive metastatic bone deposits. Window settings can be readily altered on most picture archiving and communication system (PACS) workstations. Similarly, CT numbers can be measured and give an indication of the prevalent tissue type in an area of interest. This can be useful to aid the detection of fat tissue, and is helpful in assessing certain bone and soft tissue tumours, and in detecting the presence of acute haemorrhage, which has a higher CT number than most other fluids because of its iron content.

The size of each individual pixel depends on the number of pixels making up the rows and columns within the image (termed the matrix size) and the extent of the anatomical tissue included within that matrix (termed the field of view). With a typical field of view of 25 cm × 25 cm and using a matrix size of 512 × 512, each pixel within the image would be approximately 0.5 mm in height and width. Previously in most CT systems, the pixel depth (which is equivalent to the thickness of each image slice) is considerably greater than this and consequently image detail (resolution) is higher in the original axial plane than when images are reconstructed in other planes. However, modern CT scanners with multislice technology are capable of producing such images with slice thicknesses also of 0.5 mm. In this situation, pixels are said to be 'isotropic', with height, width, and depth comparable, and hence essentially cubic in shape. As a consequence, reconstructed coronal or sagittal images have equivalent resolution to those in the axial plane, allowing high-quality reconstructions and volume images to be produced.

Radiation dose

Medical devices have contributed to an ever-increasing population radiation dose, and CT is now believed to contribute over 68% of the total dose from medical and dental examinations.[2] The use of CT has increased, with an estimated 3.4 million CT scans performed in the UK during 2008 compared to 1.4 million in 1997.[2] The dose received from a single CT scan of the pelvis is equivalent to the effective background radiation dose received by an individual over a period of 4.5 years or to 500 chest radiographs.[3] Health professionals consequently have a responsibility on to minimize dose received from CT examinations. First, and most importantly, any exposure to medical ionizing radiation must be justified and the use of other imaging modalities which do not use ionizing radiation should be considered before requesting a CT study. Referrers are required to understand the implications of their referrals for diagnostic imaging using ionizing radiation, including the responsibility to ensure the examination is not being repeated with excessive frequency, for example in the case of CT screening for recurrent malignant disease or pulmonary complications of drug therapy.

Where CT imaging is justifiable, several tactics can be implemented to ensure patient dose is 'as low as reasonably practicable' (ALARP) as set out in ICRP 2007,[4] such as scanning minimal anatomical area and using low-dose technique where this can maintain scans of adequate diagnostic quality.

A feature of modern CT scanners which has the potential to reduce radiation dose is the use of an automatic exposure control (AEC) system[5] which determines the required dose quantity by taking into account patient size and the variation in attenuation due to different anatomical structures within the scan field.[6] Use of AEC has to be monitored, however, as there are instances where image quality can be voluntarily reduced, for example when checking needle position during joint injections, and where the inadvertent use of AEC would result in an unnecessary attempt by the scanner to increase quality and consequently the patient dose.

Clinical applications

Trauma

Spinal and pelvic trauma

Rapid CT scanning, where necessary from 'head to heels', has become an integral component of the initial assessment of patients who have sustained major trauma. In such situations, time is critical and CT has contributed to a reduction in mortality and morbidity.[7] This imaging approach allows the acquisition of images of the head, chest, abdomen, pelvis, and extremities as necessary, which can all then be analysed for the presence of injuries while the patient is removed to a suitable area for further resuscitation and the scanner made ready for another casualty where required. The continuous dataset also allows the production of images of the spine, both axial sections and multiplanar reformats, the latter having been shown to be more accurate in the detection and characterization of spinal injuries than radiographs or axial CT images alone.[8]

Most traumatic fractures in the thoracic and lumbar spine occur at the most mobile region, the thoracolumbar junction (Figure 69.2). Injuries are rare below L2 and the thoracic cage acts as a splint, relatively protecting the thoracic spine between T1 and T10. Sagittal reconstructions in the thoracic region should include the sternum, as injuries in this area require high force and are often associated with other, non-contiguous spinal fractures or sternal fractures as well as spinal cord injury. Certain types of patient are at increased risk of spinal fracture with minor trauma, such as those suffering from ankylosing spondylitis or diffuse idiopathic skeletal hyperostosis, and MRI alone can be confusing. CT can readily clarify the nature of such injuries (Figure 69.3).

The complex nature of pelvic anatomy can make bony injuries difficult to identify and appreciate fully on plain radiographs, even when using supplementary views such as the Judet series. Axial CT images allow injuries to the bony pelvic ring or sacroiliac joint diastasis to be readily identified. Reconstructions in other planes allow more accurate assessment of the acetabular roof, and thick slab reformatted data can produce a 'CT equivalent' Judet series if required by surgeons less comfortable working directly with the CT images. Furthermore, since pelvic bone injuries are commonly associated with injuries to other pelvic structures, including major blood vessels, contrast enhancement may be used to detect arterial bleeding,[9] provided the modest additional time required is not considered to be detrimental to patient safety.

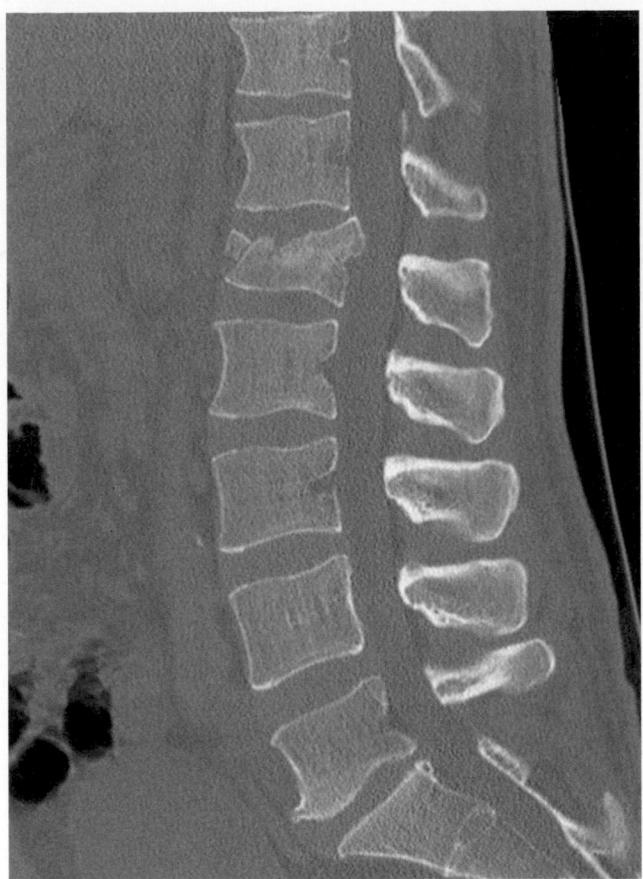

Fig. 69.2 Sagittal CT reconstruction of the lumbar spine showing a burst fracture of the L1 vertebral body. Note the buckling of the posterior vertebral body wall which can occur in such injuries.

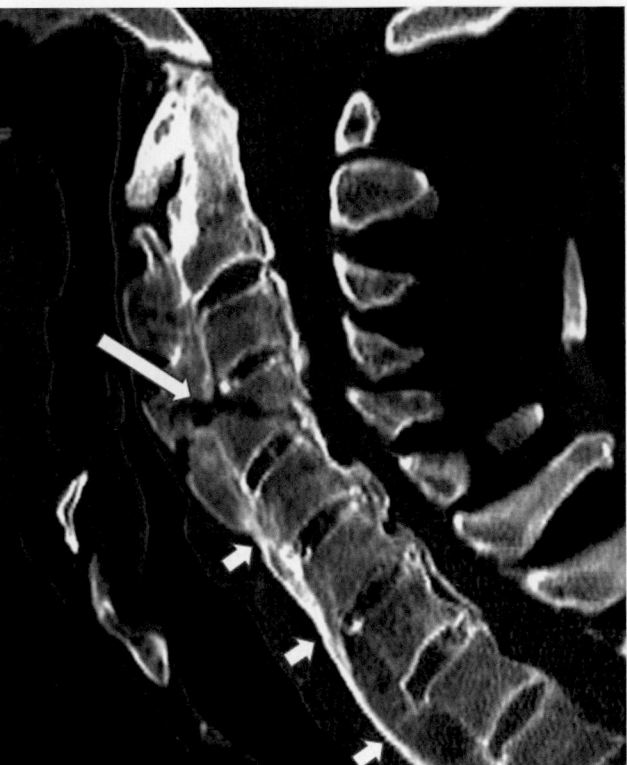

Fig. 69.3 Sagittal reconstruction CT image of the cervical spine in a patient with diffuse idiopathic skeletal hyperostosis who described neck pain following minor trauma. Note the extensive flowing ossification of the anterior longitudinal ligament (small arrows) and the oblique fracture line crossing the C4 vertebral body (long arrow). This continued through the posterior elements (not shown), indicating an unstable fracture.

Extremity trauma

CT plays a useful role in the management of patients with extremity fractures. The degree of comminution, position and size of fragments, integrity of articular surfaces, and some associated soft tissue injuries are frequently better shown on CT than on radiographs. Selection of patients for CT is usually determined in an orthopaedic trauma meeting, with radiography remaining the initial imaging modality—there are currently no centres in the United Kingdom using CT as a first line imaging investigation. There is consequently variation between (and frequently within) units as to which patients undergo CT, and the potential impact and cost of more extensive use is difficult to assess.

In the lower limb, complex injuries of the tibial plateau, ankle, and calcaneum may all benefit from the greater detail provided by CT (Figures 69.4 and 69.5). Management of tibial plateau fractures is determined by the pattern of injury, including depression of the articular surface. Such depression is better appreciated on CT than on radiographs, as is the morphology and position of fragments. CT modifies treatment in a significant proportion of patients with lower-extremity fractures.[10,11] CT similarly assists in planning management of complex ankle fractures, increasing the likelihood of satisfactory reconstruction of the articular surface in cases of displacement. CT is now pivotal in the diagnosis and management of intra-articular calcaneal fractures. The pattern of injury to the posterior facet of the subtalar joint, the degree of comminution of

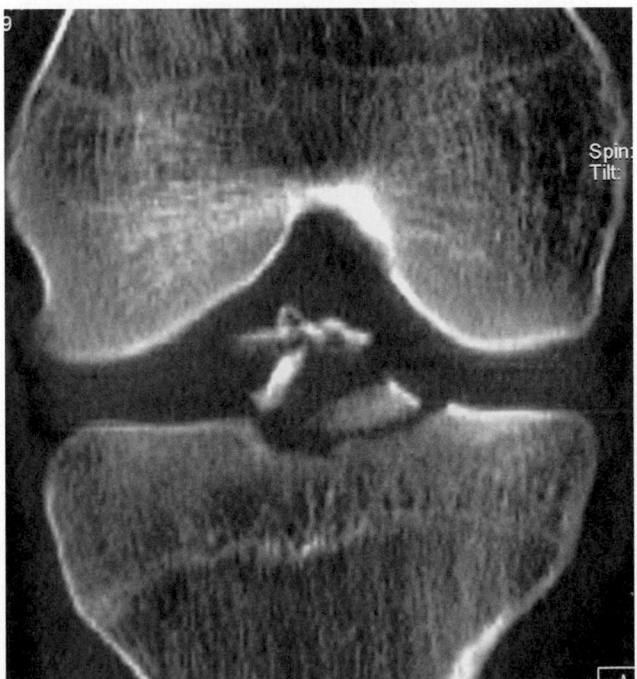

Fig. 69.4 Coronal reconstruction CT image of the right knee in a patient with a comminuted fracture of the tibial insertion of the anterior cruciate ligament. It was not possible to appreciate the degree of comminution on the corresponding MRI scan.

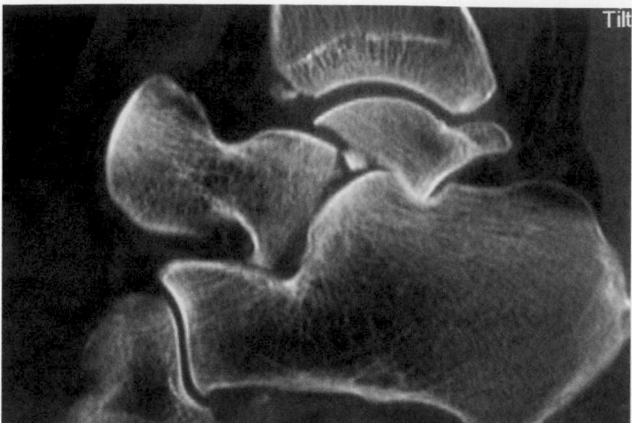

Fig. 69.5 Sagittal reconstruction CT image of the ankle in a patient with a displaced fracture of the body of the talus.

the lateral wall of the calcaneum and the sustentaculum tali, and the detection of involvement of the calcaneo-cuboid joint are all relevant features best shown on CT.[12] Associated soft tissue injuries may also be demonstrated such as dislocation or entrapment of tendons,[13] which may require surgical attention.

In the upper limb, experience of use of CT is greatest in injuries to the scaphoid (Figure 69.6), where it can identify fractures occult on radiographs.[14,15] Reconstructions aligned parallel to the long axis of the bone are particularly useful. These previously required precise patient positioning within the CT gantry, but modern CT systems are capable of obtaining volume data with isotropic voxels allowing rapid reconstruction in any desired imaging plane and from any original wrist position. CT may still have difficulty confirming an undisplaced fracture. Here, the ability of MRI to determine the presence of bone marrow oedema is advantageous.

CT provides useful information in suspected stress fracture (Figure 69.7) where the periosteal reaction and bone sclerosis observed on radiographs, occurring in a patient with a history of increasing pain and often no immediate link with trauma, raise understandable concerns about possible bone tumours. CT will frequently demonstrate the fracture line with the sclerotic region, as well as excluding other conditions such as osteoid osteoma.

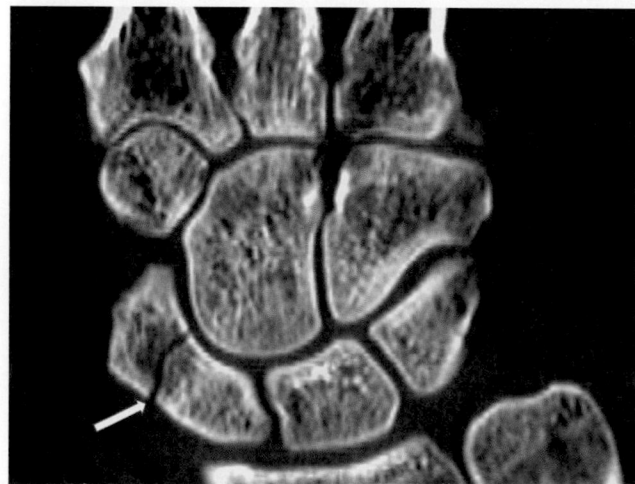

Fig. 69.6 Coronal reconstruction CT image of the wrist. Note the undisplaced fracture of the waist of the scaphoid (arrow).

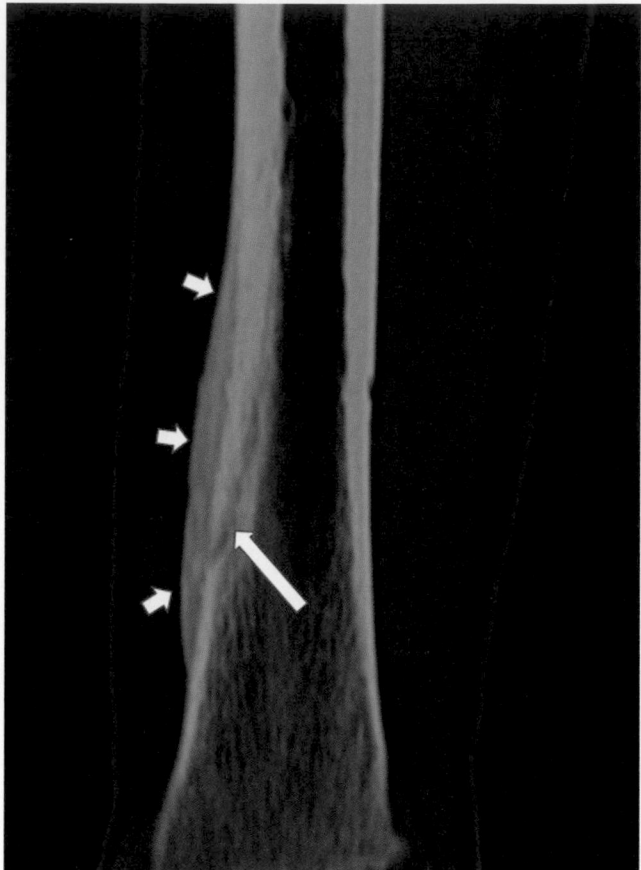

Fig. 69.7 Coronal reconstruction CT image of the tibia in a patient with a stress fracture. Note the periosteal reaction (small arrows) and the fracture line visualized within sclerosis affecting the medial cortex (long arrow).

Complications of trauma and its treatment

CT plays a useful role in the assessment of healing and the evaluation of complications related to surgical fixation.[16] The superior ability of CT to demonstrate cortical bone and medullary trabeculae makes it more useful than MRI in identifying fusion and callus bridging the fracture site. Following fracture healing, bone marrow appearances on MRI may remain abnormal for some time, leading to a false impression that fusion may not have occurred. Radiography can confirm bone healing, but overlapping of structures on the radiographs, even when two projections at 90° have been obtained, can lead to either under- or overestimation of the amount of fusion which has occurred.

Failure of bone healing to progress correctly following fracture can result in a range of complications. Malunion refers to fusion occurring with the final fracture positioning being abnormal and unsatisfactory. Non-union is classified as failure of fracture healing. There are several types of non-union: atrophic, hypertrophic, and infective. CT demonstrates differing appearances in each case.

Metalwork failure

Requests for evaluation of potential problems with orthopaedic hardware can be challenging to deal with satisfactorily, as the metalwork can interfere with all diagnostic imaging modalities. Radiographs remain the initial examination of choice and careful attention is required to identify subtle fractures of rods or screws which are sometimes diagnosed in hindsight. MR images

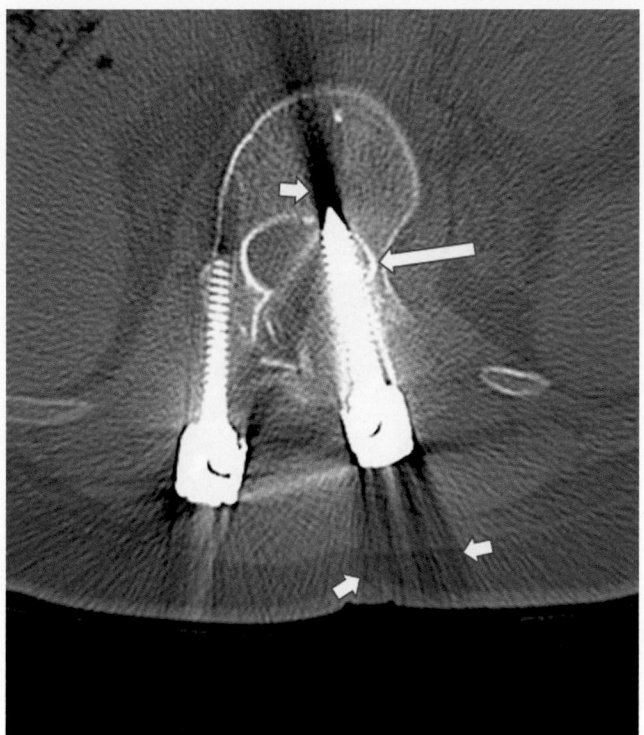

Fig. 69.8 Axial CT image of the lower thoracic spine in a patient with a scoliosis and fixation. Note the streak artefact from the metalwork (short arrows) and that the left-sided screw is malpositioned, crossing the spinal canal (long arrow).

are usually degraded by the distortion of the magnetic field such that they provide no useful information about the metalwork itself, although techniques now exist to allow assessment of soft tissues close to implants, particularly in patients with hip joint prostheses. CT is also affected by the presence of metal within the imaging field.[17] The density of the metal is significantly higher than that of bone and consequently considerably higher than the usual range of CT numbers. Attenuation of the CT beam due to interactions with the metal causes image deterioration and streak artefacts extending into surrounding tissues (Figure 69.8). Careful radiographic technique can reduce the effect of artefact observed. It is frequently possible to position the patient and/or the CT gantry in order to bring the long axis of metal screws into the imaging plane, concentrating the streak artefact into a minimum number of slices and improving the quality of the remainder of the examination. This manoeuvre is only applicable if the screw is known to be normal. Increasing image factors such as the tube voltage and current settings will improve image appearances, reducing noise and artefact but at the cost of increased dose and greater stress on the CT X-ray tube.

Producing images from the data using smooth reconstruction algorithms (similar to those used for soft tissue image reconstruction) rather than the harder algorithm more typically used for bone window images results in reduced artefact, and reconstructing image series with thicker slices may also improve quality by reduction of noise. Different sizes of implant and types of metal used in their construction can result in differing, not always predictable, degrees of artefact. It is frequently necessary to experiment with reconstructions in differing imaging planes and with various slice thicknesses before determining the optimum combination in any single case. Artefact is generally less conspicuous on images displayed on wide window settings.

Non-traumatic applications

Tarsal coalition

Tarsal coalition refers to the abnormal bridging of two or more tarsal bones by bony or fibrous tissue. Although congenital, the condition most commonly presents in late childhood or young adults, causing pain and stiffness in the foot. Secondary changes can occur in the ankle as a result of the restricted range of movement, resulting in a 'ball and socket' rather than hinge configuration. Other radiographic signs include the 'uninterrupted C' visible on lateral radiographs in bony talocalcaneal coalition (Figure 69.9). The condition is often difficult to assess adequately on radiographs and CT is helpful in further assessment, or in establishing the diagnosis in radiographically occult cases. Complete (osseous) coalitions are readily identifiable on CT due to the abnormal bony bridging of the affected structures. Incomplete coalitions (due to abnormal fibrous or cartilaginous bridging) are less obvious and best identified by observing the narrowed joint spaces and frequently associated secondary osteoarthritic changes. Talocalcaneal (Figure 69.10) and calcaneonavicular coalitions are the most commonly encountered, although other more unusual combinations also exist.

Spinal fusion/spondylolysis

CT provides better detail of cortical bone than does MRI and generally suffers less than MRI as a consequence of metal artefact. CT is therefore preferred for the assessment of bone fusion in the spinal column following surgery. In patients with scoliosis, MRI is used to identify underlying disorders of the spinal cord and craniocervical junction. MRI will demonstrate some bony segmentation or formation anomalies of the spinal column, but CT may be necessary to fully evaluate complex disorders (Figure 69.11). This is particularly

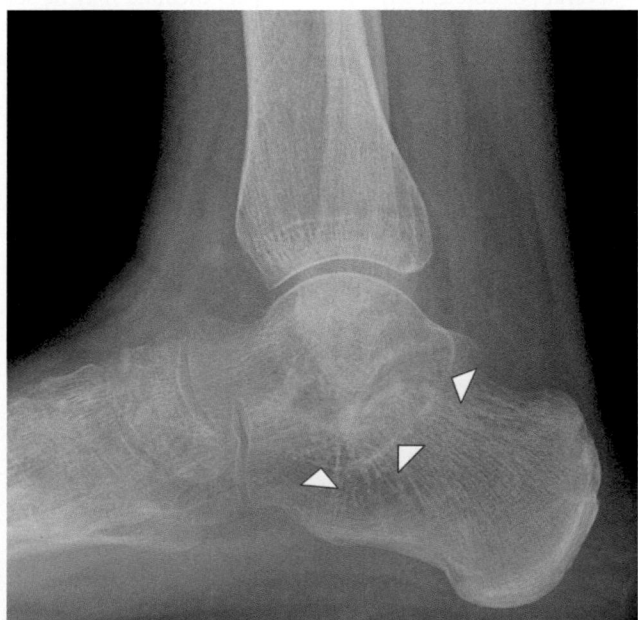

Fig. 69.9 Lateral radiograph of a patient with talocalcaneal coalition. Note the complete sclerotic line from the inferior aspect of the sustentaculum tali to the posterior aspect of the body of the talus (arrowheads). This line is normally interrupted.

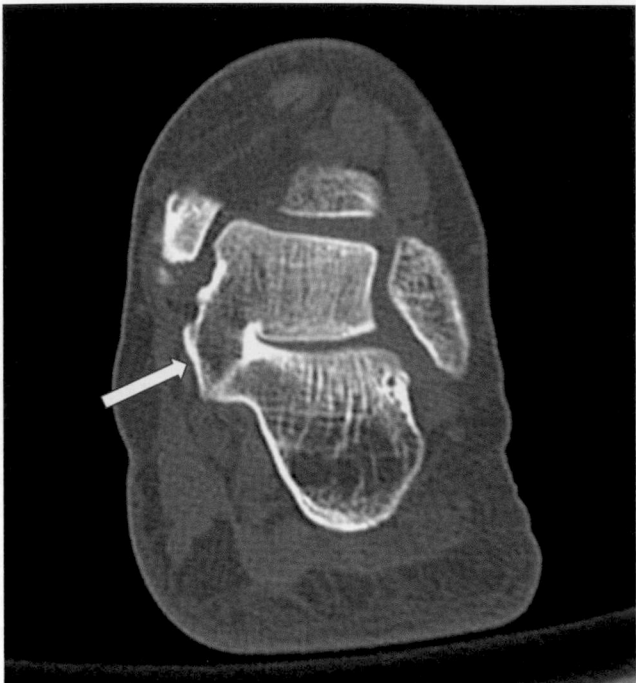

Fig. 69.10 Coronal CT image in the same patient as in Figure 69.9 demonstrates the talocalcaneal coalition (long arrow).

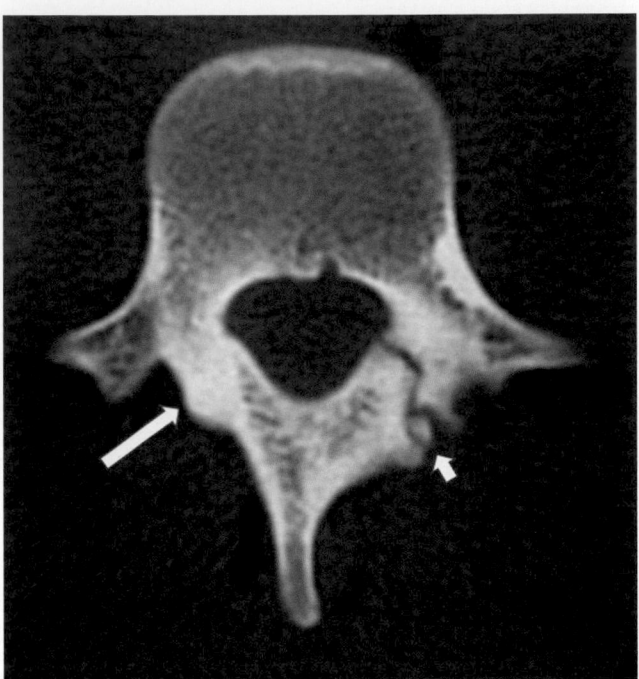

Fig. 69.12 Oblique axial CT image demonstrating a fractured left pars (arrow). Note the intact right pars (long arrow).

the case for the posterior elements where the small amount of medullary bone makes resolution of structures on MRI more difficult.

For similar reasons, CT provides additional information to MRI in cases of spondylosis (fracture of the pars interarticularis). On MRI, when continuous high T1 signal is seen through the pars, from the superior to the inferior articular facet, it can be considered normal as the examination has confirmed the presence of medullary fat. However, when continuous high T1 is not shown, there are several possible explanations. The pars medulla may be sclerotic, or simply too narrow in comparison to the thickness of the MRI slice, such that 'partial volume' artefact from the average of

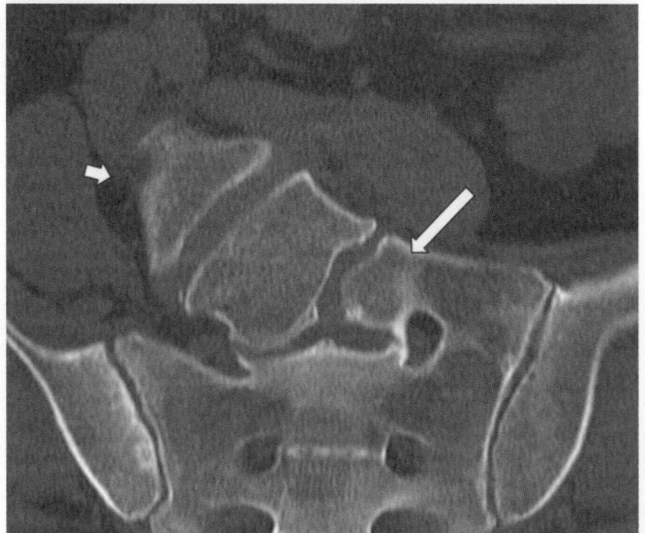

Fig. 69.11 Coronal CT image in a patient with a left-sided hemivertebra at the lumbosacral junction (long arrow) which is fused with the left sacral ala. Note the resulting right convex scoliosis (small arrow).

fat and cortical bone lowers the signal. Alternately, the pars may be fractured. CT can directly identify either intact or fractured cortex (Figure 69.12) and hence provide a more specific diagnosis, albeit at the cost of radiation exposure. Consequently, CT is often used in a second line 'targeted' manner when spondylolysis is considered a potential cause of low back pain.

Sequestrum/bone tumour characterization

Characterization of bone tumours remains most accurate on plain radiographs and this is unlikely to change. MRI is used for local tumour staging and is currently the optimal imaging modality to demonstrate the presence of fluid levels within a tumour and extension of tumour into joints. The role of CT in the local assessment of bone tumours is mainly in demonstrating and characterizing calcifications formed within and by the tumour, termed tumour matrix. The matrix produced by bone-forming (osseous) tumours is typically much more amorphous and cloud-like than that produced by cartilage-forming (chondroid) tumours, which is described as 'punctate' and commonly arranged in rings or arcs (Figure 69.13). CT provides greater detail of matrix than does either MRI or radiography, and hence can assist in identifying the likely cellular tumour type. CT also allows more accurate assessment of the degree of scalloping of endosteal cortex which can be seen in certain cartilage bone tumours. Enchondromas (benign) may scallop cortex, reducing its thickness by up to 66%,[18] but scalloping in excess of this is much more likely to indicate that a tumour is a malignant chondrosarcoma (Figure 69.14).

CT is the best imaging modality to demonstrate the nidus of an osteoid osteoma (Figure 69.15). within its surround shell of thickened, most typically cortical or periosteal, bone. Despite MRI being better for identifying bone marrow oedema, and the synovitis associated with those osteoid osteomas occurring within a joint, the nidus is frequently difficult to identify on MRI, with potential

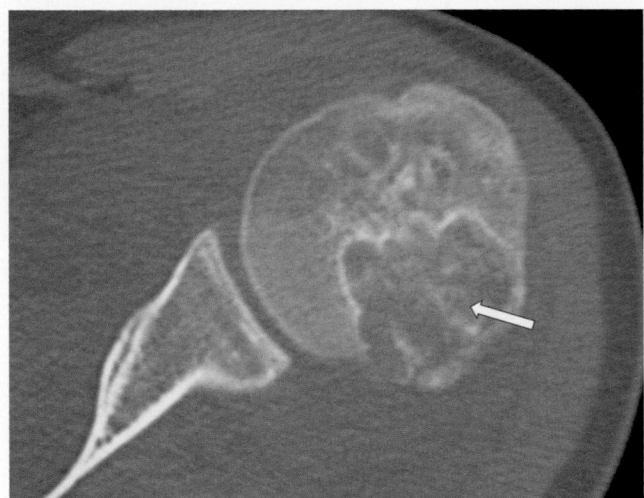

Fig. 69.13 Axial CT image of the left humeral head in a patient with a chondroblastoma. Note the 'rings and arcs' appearance of typical chondroid (cartilage) matrix within the lesion (long arrow).

for misdiagnosis as either a stress fracture or as an inflammatory arthropathy.

CT is a useful adjunct to MRI in the assessment of osteomyelitis. Although MRI is preferred for the demonstration of bone marrow oedema, bone and soft tissue fluid collections, it is less accurate at detecting the presence of a sequestrum, or sclerotic, avascularized bone fragment, which can act as a focus for recurrent infection following antibiotic therapy and frequently requires surgical removal. CT readily demonstrates such fragments (Figure 69.16) and is the better technique for confirming or excluding continuity of fragments with the remainder of the bone.

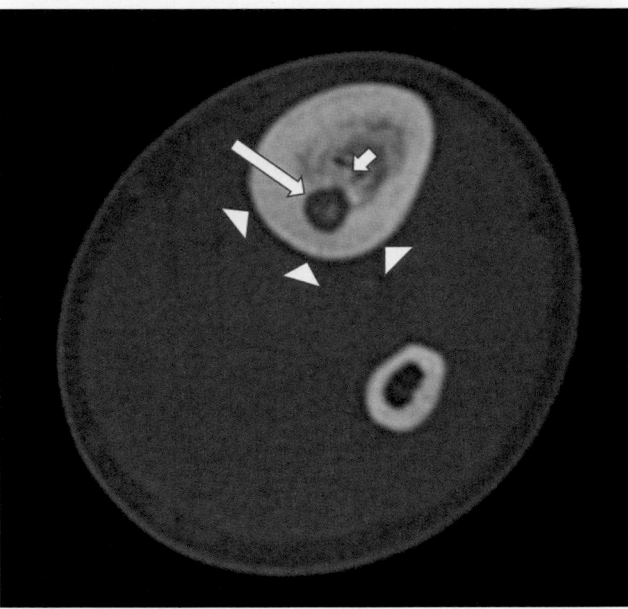

Fig. 69.15 Axial CT image in a patient with a tibial osteoid osteoma. Note the nidus (long arrow) and the surrounding reactive cortical thickening (arrowheads) and medullary sclerosis (small arrow).

Interventional CT

Arthrography

Conventional arthrography is now performed mainly to confirm accurate needle position prior to aspiration of joint fluid or more commonly, injection of anaesthetic and/or steroid. Diagnostic arthrography is more frequently combined with cross-sectional

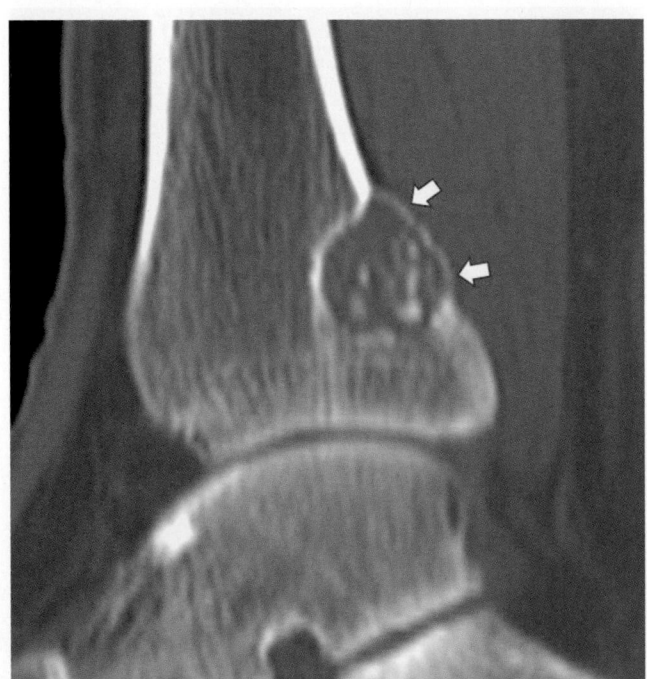

Fig. 69.14 Sagittal CT image of a cartilage tumour in the distal tibia. The lesion has caused significant scalloping and expansion of the posterior cortex (arrows), features much more typical of a malignant tumour than a benign enchondroma.

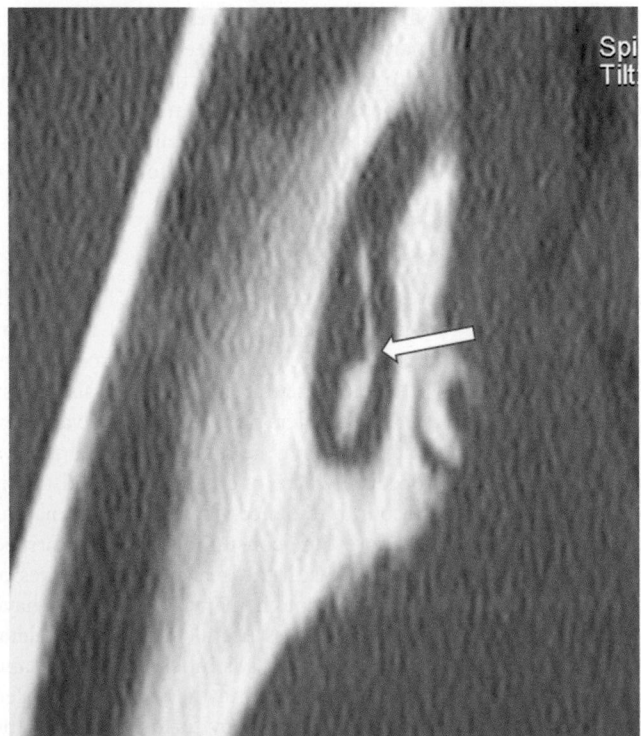

Fig. 69.16 Longitudinal CT reconstruction of a sequestrum with an area of osteomyelitis in the femur. Note the cavity within the area of cortical sclerosis containing the sequestrum (arrow).

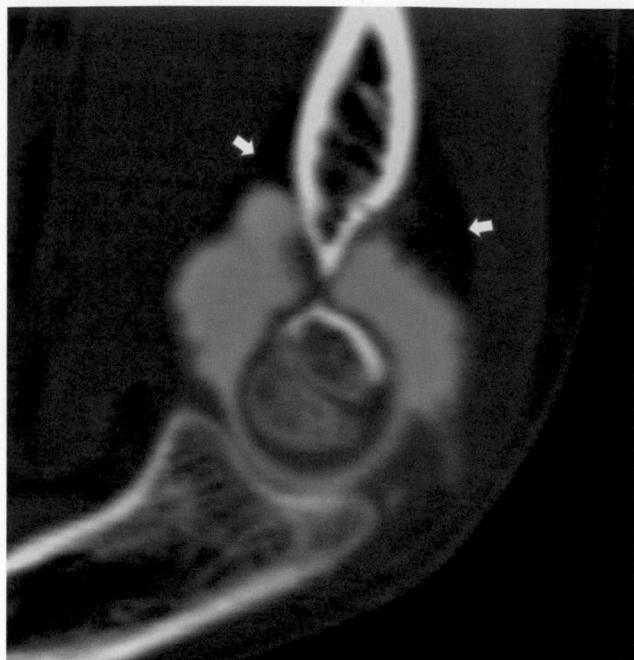

Fig. 69.17 Sagittal reconstruction image from a CT arthrogram of the elbow. Note how contrast displaces both the anterior and posterior fat pads from their normal locations (arrows)

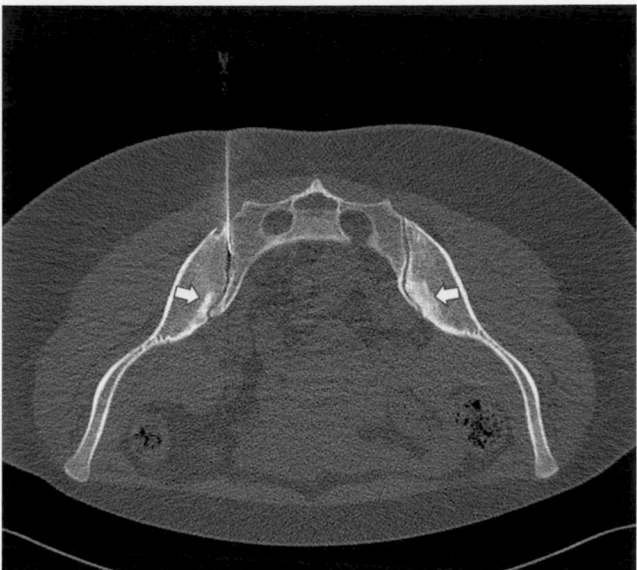

Fig. 69.18 Axial image from a CT-guided sacroiliac injection procedure. The image is relatively noisy due to the low-dose technique employed, but both needle and joint space can be easily identified. Note the subchondral sclerosis and erosions seen anteriorly, particularly on the iliac side of the joint, indicating sacroilitis (arrows). Such features are typically more extensive on the iliac side because of the protective effect of the thicker sacral articular cartilage.

imaging to take advantage of the latter's ability to produce detailed, sectional images through the joint of interest. MRI is the more common modality of choice, favoured partly because of its greater soft tissue and bone marrow imaging capability, and partly because of its lack of associated ionizing radiation. CT arthrography (Figure 69.17) may be used in patients in whom MRI is not possible, but also where the superior spatial resolution of CT is considered to be of paramount importance.[19] CT is also preferable when attempting to identify small calcified intra-articular loose bodies, which may be difficult to confirm on MRI. In such cases, CT is frequently performed both before and after contrast injection as small calcified bodies may become obscured within the pool of contrast.

CT-guided biopsy/injection

Interventional procedures may be performed in the CT suite itself. CT allows precise guidance of needles and is useful when performing injections into complex areas such as the sacroiliac joint (Figure 69.18). CT is also the most accurate modality to assist biopsy of bone lesions (Figure 69.19). It suffers from several disadvantages, however. Ionizing radiation dose may be higher than that from a similar fluoroscopic procedure where one is possible, and this is clearly significant if ultrasound guidance is a realistic alternative. Procedures are generally more time consuming when performed under CT guidance rather than with the 'real-time' modalities of fluoroscopy and ultrasound. Although many CT scanners have a 'CT fluoroscopy' option, this is less useful in musculoskeletal system interventions where bone access is inherently slower and requires the operator's hands to be within the scanner, exposed to the primary beam. Using CT fluoroscopy further increases the patient's cumulative skin radiation dose as well as that to the operator because the scanning plane is kept constant and continually exposes the same area of tissue.

Radiofrequency ablation of osteoid osteoma

Just as CT is the best modality to demonstrate an osteoid osteoma nidus, it also assists in percutaneous treatment. CT guidance allows positioning of a needle with a laser (or more commonly a radiofrequency tip) which can be used to ablate the nidus, avoiding the

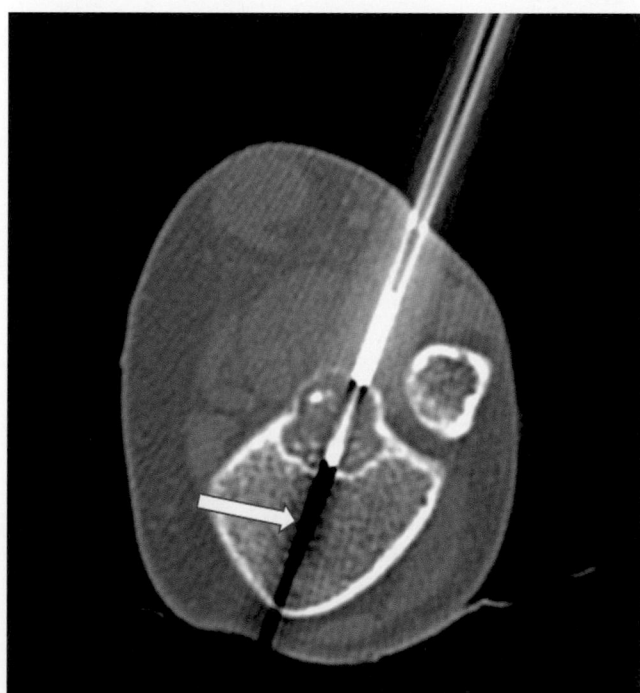

Fig. 69.19 Axial image from a CT-guided biopsy procedure performed for the patient with the lesion in Figure 69.14. The needle is well demonstrated. Note the streak artefact proceeding away from the needle tip (arrow). The biopsy confirmed the imaging suspicion of a chondrosarcoma.

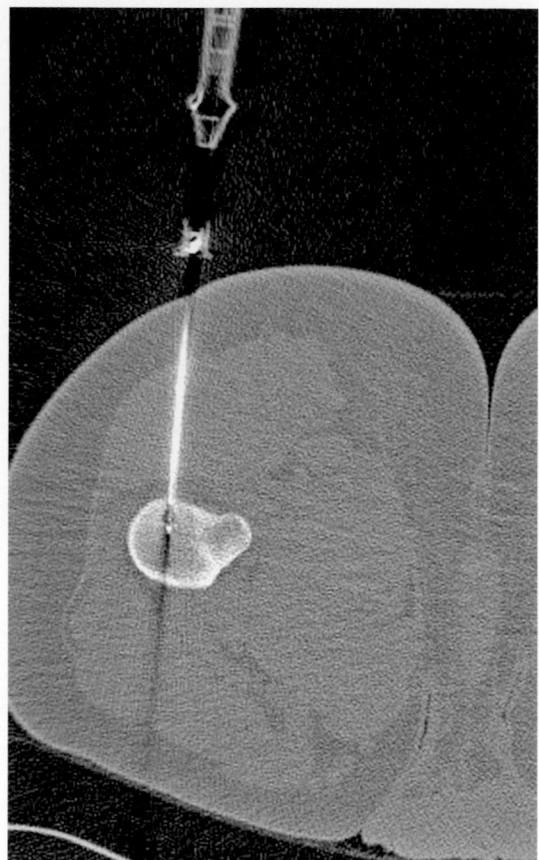

Fig. 69.20 Axial image from a CT-guided radiofrequency ablation procedure performed to treat a right femoral osteoid osteoma. Under CT guidance, such needles can be positioned with considerable accuracy.

need for a more extensive surgical resection with the associated risk of fracture (Figure 69.20). Radiofrequency ablation of osteoid osteoma has an extremely high therapeutic success rate of around 90%[20] from a single treatment and a minimal complication rate. Ablation has become the treatment of choice for osteoid osteoma except for the occasional lesion lying close to the spinal cord, typically in the pedicle or posterior vertebral body wall, where the potential risk of thermal injury to the cord in an anaesthetized patient makes a surgical procedure preferable.

New developments

Dual-energy CT is a recent development, not yet in widespread clinical use, which could offer potentially interesting features in several areas of musculoskeletal imaging. Dual-energy CT scanners produce images using two different X-ray sources of different energy levels (typically 80 kV and 140 kV) housed within the same gantry. The sources scan the patient simultaneously, resulting in two sets of spiral CT data. X-ray absorption within tissues is energy dependent and hence alters at different energy levels. Individual substances have their maximum X-ray absorption at different levels (e.g. iodine absorbs maximally at low energy levels and its absorption reduces significantly at higher levels) and this allows dual-energy CT to provide specific information about the chemical composition of individual tissues and areas within images. In rheumatology, the most obvious potential application is in the detection of monosodium urate tophi in gout,[21] allowing the diagnosis to be made without

recourse to joint aspiration and microscopy. Dual-energy CT also allows more refined assessment of ligament and tendon structures than has previously been possible with CT, but it is currently unclear whether this refinement will translate to a genuine clinical role for the modality in the assessment of soft tissue structures in the musculoskeletal system. MRI and ultrasound remain the modalities of choice, but dual-energy CT may be able to provide useful additional soft tissue information in patients undergoing CT for suspected fracture, for example after trauma to the knee. Dual-energy CT allows reduction in the artefact from metal implants and can consequently improve image quality and diagnostic value.[22]

References

1. Hounsfield GN. Computerized transverse axial scanning (tomography) I. Description of a system. *Br J Radiol* 1973;46:1016.
2. Hart D, Wall BF, Hillier MC, Shrimpton PC. *Frequency and collective dose for medical and dental X-ray examinations in the UK, 2008*. HPA-CRCE-012. Health Protection Agency, London, 2010.
3. European Commission. *Radiation protection 118: Referral guidelines for imaging*. Office for Official Publications of the European Communities, Luxembourg, 2001. Available at: http://ec.europa.eu/energy/nuclear/radioprotection/publication/doc/118_en.pdf.
4. ICRP. Recommendations of the International Commission on Radiological Protection (Users Edition). ICRP Publication 103 (Users Edition). *Ann ICRP* 2007;37(2–4).
5. McCollough CH, Bruesewitz MR, Kofler JM. CT dose reduction and dose management tools: Overview of available options. *Radiographics* 2006 26:503–512.
6. Coursey CA, Frush DP. CT and radiation: what radiologists should know. *Appl Radiol* 2008; 37: 22–29.
7. Ptak T, Rhea JT, Novelline RA. Experience with a continuous, single-pass whole-body multidetector CT protocol for trauma: the three-minute multiple trauma CT scan. *Emerg Radiol* 2001;8:250–256.
8. Jayashankar A, Udayasankar U, Sebastian S et al. MDCT of thoraco-abdominal trauma: an evaluation of the success and limitations of primary interpretation using multiplanar reformatted images vs axial images. *Emerg Radiol* 2008;15:29–34.
9. Stephen DJ, Kreder HJ, Day AC et al. Early detection of arterial bleeding in acute pelvic trauma. *J Trauma* 1999;47:638–642.
10. Wicky S, Blaser PF, Blanc CH et al. Comparison between standard radiography and spiral CT with 3D reconstruction in the evaluation, classification and management on tibial plateau fractures. *Eur Radiol* 2000;10:1227–1232.
11. Macarini L, Murrone M, Marini S et al. Tibial plateau fractures: evaluation with multidetector CT. *Radiol Med* 2004;108:503–514.
12. Bearcroft PWP. The use of spiral computed tomography n musculoskeletal radiology of the lower limb: the calcaneus as an example. *Eur J Radiol* 1998;28:30–38.
13. Ohashi K, Restrepo JM, El-Khoury GY et al. Peroneal tendon subluxation and dislocation: detection on volume-rendered images—initial experience. *Radiology* 2007;242:252–257.
14. Kiuru MJ, Haapamaki VV, Koivikko MP et al. Wrist injuries: diagnosis with multidetector CT. *Emerg Radiol* 2004;10:182–185.
15. Welling RD, Jacobson JA, Jamadar DA et al. MDCT and radiography of wrist fractures: radiographic sensitivity and fracture patterns. *Am J Roentgenol* 2008;190:10–16.
16. Krestan CR, Noske H, Vasilevska V et al. MDCT versus digital radiography in the evaluation of bone healing in orthopaedic patients. *Am J Roentgenol* 2006;186:1754–1760.
17. Barrett JF, Keat N. Artifacts in CT: recognition and avoidance. *Radiographics* 2004;24:1679–1691.
18. Murphey MD, Flemming DJ, Bovea SR et al. Enchondroma versus chondrosarcoma in the appendicular skeleton: differentiating features. *Radiographics* 1998;18:1213–1237.

19. Vande Berg BC, Lecouvet FE, Poilvache P et al. Anterior cruciate ligament tears and associated meniscal lesions: Assessment at dual-detector spiral CT arthrography. *Radiology* 2002;223:403–409.

20. Rosenthal DI, Hornicek FJ, Torriani M, Gebhardt MC, Mankin HJ. Osteoid osteoma: percutaneous treatment with radiofrequency energy. *Radiology* 2003;229:171–175.

21. Nicolaou S, Yong-Hing CJ, Galea-Soler S et al. Dual-energy CT as a potential new diagnostic tool in the management of gout in the acute setting. *AJR* 2010;194:1072–1078.

22. Bamberg F, Dierks A, Nikolaou K et al. Metal artefact reduction by dual energy computed tomography using monoenergetic extrapolation. *Eur Radiol* 2011;21:1424–1429.

CHAPTER 70

Nuclear medicine

Adil Al-Nahhas and Imene Zerizer

Introduction

The science of using radioactive tracers in the investigation and treatment of disease began in the early 20th century, and was soon followed by its introduction into clinical practice. The application was initially aimed at thyroid diseases, because early experiments used radioactive iodine, but the wide spectrum of diseases that could benefit from this novel technique was soon realized. Now nuclear medicine plays an important role in the management of cancer as well as diseases affecting cardiovascular, endocrine, renal, and musculoskeletal systems. This has been achieved through the introduction of hundreds of radiopharmaceuticals that target cellular and subcellular structures and functions, such as cell membrane receptors, glucose metabolism, hypoxia, and angiogenesis. These developments were paralleled by continuous innovation in imaging of these in-vivo events, through the introduction of high-resolution gamma cameras, positron emission tomography (PET) scanners, and more recently hybrid PET/CT cameras.

The principal of achieving a diagnostic or therapeutic effect using nuclear medicine techniques is the administration of a radioactive tracer in vivo (by IV injection, inhalation, or ingestion) that can target a physiological or pathological process. Once there, its distribution can be mapped by detecting its emitted gamma rays through special gamma cameras. However, radiotracers have no targeting potential and have to be 'made' to target disease process. This is achieved by binding the tracer with a chemical messenger (ligand) that is known to be attracted to a particular cellular or subcellular structure, or be part of a physiological process. This chemical bonding (labelling) is vital for the success of imaging or therapy. Examples in clinical practice include the labelling of technetium-99 m (^{99m}Tc) with methylene diphosphonate (^{99m}Tc-MDP) to visualize hydroxyapatite in bone scanning, or macraggregated albumin (^{99m}Tc-MAA), which is used in detecting pulmonary emboli. A novel method of detecting cancers is to detect their metabolic activity through increased glucose metabolism by labelling fluorine-18 (^{18}F) with a glucose precursor (^{18}F-FDG).

The real strength of nuclear medicine imaging is its ability to highlight the physiological nature and development of disease rather than its anatomy. A good example is the detection of bone metastases due to subtle changes in the hydroxyapatite structure caused by increased bony turnover, which will take up to 9 months to produce a sufficient shift in calcium mass to make it visible on traditional imaging. Likewise, small lymph nodes of 5–10 mm in diameter that are affected by lymphoma would be regarded as normal by CT criteria (lymph nodes need to be >1 cm to be regarded as malignant) while they can show intense metabolic activity on PET. In certain diseases, nuclear medicine is the only modality that can separate disease from normality, as in the use of postsynaptic imaging in Parkinson's disease.

Since the early 1950s, nuclear medicine procedures have been used in the investigation, treatment, and follow-up of major rheumatologic conditions. This chapter will focus on their use in imaging rheumatoid arthritis (RA), systemic lupus erythematosus (SLE), ankylosing spondylitis (AS), vasculitis, and myopathy as well as in treatment of inflamed joints (radiosynovectomy).

Rheumatoid arthritis

The pathophysiological processes involved in RA (activation of leucocytes, infiltration of the synovium, and neovascularization) have become the target of several nuclear medicine procedures—including bone scintigraphy, molecular targeting of inflammation, and glucose metabolism—that are used in the staging and follow-up of RA.

Bone scintigraphy

Since the 1970s there have been several reports that describe the utility of bone scintigraphy (BS) using ^{99m}Tc-labelled phosphonates in RA.[1] Ideally, a three-phase acquisition is performed to depict inflammatory changes. The perfusion phase (1 image per second for 60s) allows visualization of the increased vascularity that is commonly found in acute inflammatory processes. A blood-pool phase is then acquired to demonstrate equilibrium of arterial and venous flow, followed by a bone phase demonstrating the osteoblastic activity. Bone scans have been used to both confirm the diagnosis by identifying involved joints and in assessing response to treatment.

An acute inflammatory arthritis is characterized by increased vascularity and blood pooling in the affected joint and surrounding soft tissues as well as increased uptake in the periarticular bones on the bone phase (Figure 70.1). This is due to the synovitis and inflammation of the chondro-osseous zone which leads to oedema, blood vessel proliferation, and synovial hypertrophy.[2] Some authors have also described flushing of the fingers in the blood flow phase of the bone scan, due to vasodilatation secondary to microcirculatory disturbances that occur in RA.[3]

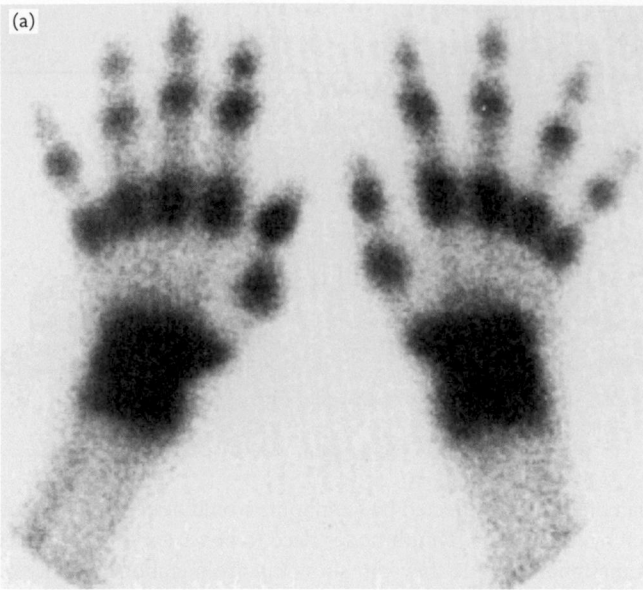

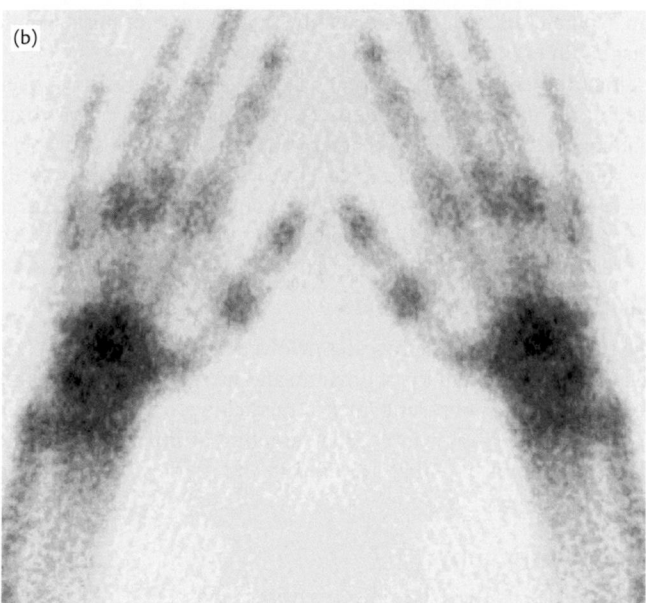

Fig. 70.1 Bone scan with $^{99\,m}$Tc HDP showing typical example of increased bone uptake in the small joints of both hands in acute rheumatoid arthritis (a) compared to uptake in a normal hand (b).

An early study by Mottenen et al. evaluated the role of BS in predicting the development of erosions in early RA in 13 patients.[4] The authors performed serial scintigraphy in patients diagnosed with RA at 0, 6, and 12 months. All except one of the joints that were to become eroded during the first 12 months were active on serial bone scans. Inactive joints on BS did not demonstrate erosions throughout the period of follow-up. The scintigraphic results also correlated with clinical activity and Larsen's index. The authors concluded that persistent activity on BS predates the onset of erosions and a negative BS excludes an active synovitis. This was supported by another retrospective study of 22 patients with RA which demonstrated that after a mean follow-up period of 3.6 years, none of the cohort with a negative BS had evidence of inflammatory joint disease.[5] Another study by Duncan et al. assessed the impact of BS

on patients' management.[6] A total of 136 bone scans were evaluated to confirm or exclude a clinical diagnosis and to localize the site of pain. BS was successful in excluding a diagnosis of RA in 87% and confirming a diagnosis in 80%. The patients' management altered based on the bone scan report in 43% of patients and the results prevented further investigations in 60% of cases. Despite these encouraging results, BS has several disadvantages, such as lack of specificity. This has led to the introduction of several other more specific agents to image inflammation.

Molecular targeted imaging

Radiolabelled white cells have been utilized to image inflammatory processes such as RA. Radiolabelling is carried out by separating leucocytes from the patient's own blood, which are incubated with radioactive tracers ($^{99\,m}$Tc-HMPAO or ^{111}In-oxine), washed, and suspended in plasma before being readministered intravenously to the patient. An early study has demonstrated that labelled white cells accumulated in clinically active knee joints and a 50–60% reduction in uptake was observed following treatment with local steroid injections.[7]

Antibodies against granulocyte-surface antigens, molecules within microorganisms, or antigens of such disease-related molecules have been radiolabelled to image inflammatory processes. Specific polyclonal IgG-type antibodies labelled with $^{99\,m}$Tc-HIG have been shown to accumulate in inflamed joints by binding with lymphocyte-surface antigens, which are found at sites of chronic inflammation. $^{99\,m}$Tc-HIG was shown to be more sensitive and accurate in diagnosing active, histologically proven synovitis,[8] and could predict the development of RA in patients with arthralgia, providing additional information to rheumatoid factor measurements.[9]

Immunoscintigraphy has also been utilized in monitoring disease and response to immunotherapy.[10] Recently, several antibodies, either chimeric or humanized, have been introduced into clinical practice to control the autoimmune inflammatory process that is the basis of RA. These can also be labelled, mainly with $^{99\,m}$Tc or ^{111}In, for imaging. Several monoclonal antibodies and their fragments such as anti-TNFα, anti-CD20, anti-CD3, anti-CD4, and anti-E-selectin antibody have been successfully used in imaging. These labelled antibodies not only offer the ability to stage the disease accurately and identify involved joints but can also offer a unique opportunity to identify patients who will benefit from treatment with therapeutic unlabelled antibodies.

Imaging with $^{99\,m}$Tc-labelled infliximab before and 3 months after intra-articular infliximab therapy has shown very specific uptake of $^{99\,m}$Tc-infliximab in inflamed joints, unlike normal joints that did not show any uptake,[11] with good correlation between pretherapy uptake and improvement in clinical symptoms post-treatment. Clinical improvement of symptoms and reduction of swelling were higher in patients with the higher uptake of $^{99\,m}$Tc-infliximab pretherapy and decrease of uptake after therapy.

Anti-E-selectin monoclonal antibody, overexpressed on the vasculature of inflamed tissue, has been labelled with ^{111}In or $^{99\,m}$Tc. A comparison between ^{111}In anti-E-selectin antibody and $^{99\,m}$Tc-HIG in 11 patients with active RA showed the former to have a higher sensitivity in the detection of active disease and correlated well with clinical scores of joint involvement.[12] Another study by the same authors demonstrated the feasibility and advantages of $^{99\,m}$Tc anti-E-selectin (1.2B6) antibody fragment over conventional $^{99\,m}$Tc HDP bone scanning and ^{111}In-anti-E-selectin.[13]

^{18}F-FDG PET/CT

^{18}F-FDG is a widely used PET radiopharmaceutical for tumour imaging. However, increased uptake of ^{18}F-FDG in inflamed joints has incidentally been noted in two oncology patients who were also suffering from RA.[14]

In addition, animal experiments have demonstrated that up to 29% of ^{18}F-FDG is not taken up by tumour cells alone but also by macrophages and surrounding granulation tissue.[15] Lin et al. demonstrated a correlation between TNFα, which enhances glucose entry into macrophages and metabolism in fibroblasts, and ^{18}F-FDG accumulation in experimental animal models.[16] These factors make ^{18}F-FDG PET a highly sensitive imaging modality for the detection and monitoring of inflammatory diseases and in particular synovitis. An early study comparing ^{18}F-FDG PET with gadolinium-enhanced MRI in 12 patients with RA demonstrated a correlation between enhancing pannus on MRI and ^{18}F-FDG accumulation.[17] The volume of enhancing pannus also showed a liner relationship with the total uptake value of the wrist and the regional uptake value.

Beckers et al. assessed ^{18}F-FDG uptake in 356 joints in 21 patients with active RA.[18] These authors found that ^{18}F-FDG uptake in the joints correlated well with clinical parameters (disease activity score, swelling, and tenderness), ultrasound findings of synovitis and synovial thickening, neovascularization as assessed on Doppler, and laboratory inflammatory markers (ESR and CRP). In addition, this study evaluated response to therapy. Sixteen knees in 16 patients with active RA were assessed using ^{18}F-FDG PET, dynamic MRI, and ultrsound pretreatment and at 4 weeks after anti-TNF treatment. The imaging studies were also correlated with CRP and matrix metalloproteinase-3 (MMP3) measurements. Changes in ^{18}F-FDG uptake after 4 weeks were observed in responding joints which correlated with reduced enhancement on MRI and serum CRP and MMP-3 levels. However, measurements of synovial thickening on ultrasound did not show a response, confirming the superior role of ^{18}F-FDG PET in depicting early metabolic changes following anti-TNF treatment. There is continued interest in the role of ^{18}F-FDG PET/CT in the assessment of RA, and a recent study has confirmed the correlation between CRP levels and ^{18}F-FDG uptake in large joints.[19]

All of the above studies emphasize the role of ^{18}F-FDG PET in the accurate staging of RA and assessment of joint activity following therapy with disease-modifying and anti-inflammatory drugs. However, despite its high sensitivity, ^{18}F-FDG PET lacks specificity since it accumulates in osteoarthritis. This has led to the introduction of novel PET tracers that can potentially be more accurate for RA diagnosis and treatment response.

Non-FDG PET/CT

Several experimental PET tracers have been investigated in an attempt to make an early diagnosis of RA by detecting subclinical synovitis. This is highly important to identify patients who are at risk of potentially serious RA complications, such as atlantoaxial subluxation, that require more intensive drug therapy and possible early intervention.

Imaging of macrophages was investigated using the PET tracer ^{11}C-(R)-PK11195, which binds to peripheral benzodiazepine receptors (PBRs) on macrophages. The study was performed in knee joints of 11 patients with RA and the findings were correlated with arthroscopy and immunohistochemistry staining of obtained samples.[20] The uptake of ^{11}C-(R)-PK11195 was significantly higher in severely inflamed joints than in joints with moderate or mild signs of inflammation. In addition, there was a significant correlation between tracer uptake and PBRs and CD68 staining of macrophages. There was significantly higher uptake in contralateral non-inflamed knee joints of RA patients than in the non-inflamed joints of control patients. This may indicate that ^{11}C-(R)-PK11195 can play a prognostic role since its uptake preceded clinically evident synovitis.

Van der Heijen et al. demonstrated that synovial tissue from RA patients expressed folate receptor beta on activated macrophages; this can be targeted for therapy using high-affinity-binding folate antagonists such as BCG 945.[21] A recent study investigated the use of ^{18}F-PEG-folate PET to image arthritis in a rat model and therefore facilitate the selection of patients for folate antagonist therapy.[22] Rats with induced arthritis showed a macrophage-rich inflammation in the synovial tissue of the affected joint, resembling synovitis in RA patients. ^{18}F-PEG-folate PET images in these rats clearly demonstrated the arthritic joints. Further studies are awaited to evaluate the role of ^{11}C-(R)-PK11195 in humans.

Systemic lupus erythematosus

Several clinical, laboratory, and imaging modalities are available for the diagnosis and assessment of response to treatment in SLE. Anatomic imaging modalities (CT/MRI) provide a high-quality assessment of structural changes relating to inflammation. However, these secondary changes take time to develop and therefore do not allow early detection of disease. Nuclear medicine studies offer the possibility of early disease detection before anatomical changes occur and follow-up of response to therapy.

Bone scintigraphy

The most important role of BS in SLE is in the detection of osteonecrosis, which occurs in 5–50% of SLE patients and mainly affects weight-bearing joints.[23] The femoral head is most commonly affected, followed by the humeral head, femoral condyle, and tibial plateau. ^{99m}Tc HDP depicts early osteonecrosis as a photopenic area in the affected bone due to necrosis of the bone with lack of osteoblastic reaction. This is followed by a hyperaemic stage with increased vascularity and tracer uptake at the margins of the infarction on a three-phase bone scan. Although a three-phase bone scan is highly sensitive in the detection of osteonecrosis, MRI has been found to be more sensitive in the early detection of osteonecrosis, depicting changes in bone marrow as a result of vascular insufficiency.[23]

Gallium-67 citrate scintigraphy

Gallium-67 (^{67}Ga) scintigraphy has been widely used in the assessment of suspected inflammation. Various mechanisms have been proposed for the accumulation of ^{67}Ga in inflammatory lesions, including binding to transferrin and lactoferrin, uptake by lysosomes in mononuclear phagocytes, and direct binding to the lymphocyte membrane.[24] Although its use in detecting inflammation has been reduced in favour of ^{18}F-FDG because of its unfavourable physical properties, it has been used in SLE is in the detection of nephritis and pulmonary complications among others.

Several studies have demonstrated that ^{67}Ga scintigraphy is an excellent screening test for the presence of acute interstitial nephritis.[25,26] Pagniez et al. demonstrated that significant renal ^{67}Ga uptake indicates active, potentially curable lesions.[25] Bakir et al. performed ^{67}Ga scans in 43 patients with SLE and reported that 89% of patients with active renal disease had positive ^{67}Ga scintigraphy whereas only 17% of patients with inactive renal disease had positive findings.[26] Lin et al. studied the role of ^{67}Ga scans in 47 patients with SLE in predicting a response to therapy.[27] They showed that patients with a positive ^{67}Ga renal scan (71.4% of the cohort) had a good response to treatment, while more than 88% of patients with a negative ^{67}Ga scan had a poor response.

Many patients with SLE will develop involvement of the lung, its vasculature, the pleura, and/or the diaphragm during the disease course. [67]Ga scintigraphy has been evaluated in the detection of alveolitis in SLE. Witt and colleagues found that significant ^{67}Ga accumulation was present in patients with alveolitis confirmed on brancheoalveolar lavage.[28] The severity of lung inflammation in 34 patients with SLE was also measured by quantitatively measuring the level of ^{67}Ga in the lungs (gallium uptake index, GUI) compared to 20 normal controls.[29] Higher values of GUI in SLE patients were detected compared to normal controls, and in patients with a flare-up or a negative chest radiograph compared to patients who have stable disease or a positive chest radiograph. This indicates that a positive chest radiograph finding may be a later manifestation of lung involvement in SLE. There are few publications describing the use of ^{67}Ga in myocarditis[30,31] and other vascular complications.[32,33]

Lung permeability studies

Measurements of the vascular permeability have been used for early detection of lung involvement in SLE. Dalcin et al. performed ^{99m}Tc-DTPA clearance in active and inactive SLE, compared with clinical data and disease activity, and showed pulmonary clearance to be faster in SLE patients with active disease compared to normal controls.[34] Lung uptake of ^{99m}Tc-HMPAO was compared in 20 SLE patients and 25 controls; uptake was higher in the patients with SLE, suggesting that this method may be useful in assessing pulmonary injury in SLE patients.[35]

^{18}F-FDG PET/CT

Lymph node involvement is a common early manifestation of active SLE, correlating well with constitutional symptoms. Patients with active SLE have been found to have activated T and B lymphocytes in their lymph nodes compared to those with inactive disease. Therefore, ^{18}F-FDG PET/CT has been utilized to visualize active lymphadenopathy in patients with SLE[36] as well as detecting early hepatosplenomegaly in SLE patients presenting with pyrexia of unknown origin.[37] ^{18}F-FDG PET/CT has also been shown to detect alteration in cerebral glucose uptake, oxygen consumption, and cerebral blood flow in SLE patients and was superior to MRI studies, which did not demonstrate any structural changes.[38]

A study that evaluated the role of ^{18}F-FDG PET/CT in 28 SLE patients with varying degrees of severity demonstrated reduced metabolic activity in at least one brain region in all patients with severe or mild central nervous system (CNS) symptoms (100%) as compared with patients without symptoms (40%).[39] In contrast, MRI images were abnormal in only 50% of patients with neuropsychiatric symptoms and in one of four patients (25%) without symptoms.

This suggests a correlation between metabolic changes on PET/CT and clinical symptoms that can be useful during follow-up.

In summary, 18F-FDG PET/CT is a useful imaging modality in the diagnosis of CNS involvement in SLE, particularly in the diagnosis of unclear cases, when other imaging modalities are negative and only minor neuropsychiatric symptoms are present. However, MRI scans are highly sensitive in detecting infarction and white matter lesions.

Ankylosing spondylitis

There is an estimated delay of approximately 8–10 years between the onset of symptoms and diagnosis of AS.[40] Early detection is therefore highly important to avoid delays in diagnosis and commence appropriate disease-modifying treatment. [99m]Tc HDP is commonly used in the diagnosis of sacroiliitis, which occurs early in the disease course. The most widely used method of assessment is the calculation the ratio of radiotracer uptake over the sacroiliac joint (SIJ) compared with the sacrum as a reference point (SIJ:S ratio). A study that assessed 137 patients with inflammatory back pain and 31 controls, found that ^{99m}Tc HDP had a sensitivity of 52.7% in the diagnosis of sacroilietis[41] in 112 of patients with AS (according to the modified New York criteria). A recent systemic review of published studies that evaluated the value of ^{99m}Tc HDP BS in the detection of sacroilieits has found an overall sensitivity of 50–55% and a specificity of 80%.[42] However, scintigraphy is usually negative in the fibrosclerotic stage compared to the persistence of radiological changes. Further studies have shown that MRI is more sensitive in early detection of sacroiliitis and, because of its lack of radiation burden, may be a preferred method for diagnosis particularly in young patients.[42]

Vasculitis

As in other rheumatologic conditions, the mechanism of uptake of radiopharmaceuticals in imaging vasculitis relies on its pathological features. Regardless of the different classifications, vasculitis is basically an inflammatory condition of blood vessels associated with leucocytic infiltration of the vessel wall with eventual destruction of the wall and surrounding tissues, resulting in serious consequences such as infarction. Conventional cross-sectional imaging can demonstrate the anatomical changes once the inflammatory process is well established but lack the ability to diagnose early inflammatory changes, which are potentially reversible and, if treatable, may have an impact on the long-term management of this condition.[43] Taking into account that the majority of patients present with non-specific symptoms, there is a need for a physiological imaging procedure that can show early disease for biopsy guidance.

[67]Ga-citrate has been used in the detection of inflammation in certain vasculitic conditions such as Wegner's granulomatosis and Kawasaki's disease since the early 1980s.[44,45] However, its mechanism of uptake (described earlier) and unfavourable physical criteria have reduced its use in clinical practice. Similarly, the use of labelled white cells[46] in this condition has been deemed inappropriate because of its complexity and low sensitivity.[47]

^{18}F-FDG PET

For reasons to do with the resolution of PET scanners (currently around 5 mm), the types of vasculitis most successfully evaluated with PET and PET/CT have been medium- and large-vessel vasculitis, particularly giant cell arteritis (GCA) and Takayasu's arteritis (TA).

Progress in this area has been aided by better understanding of the immunohistopathology underlying the inflammatory mechanism.[48] The 'respiratory burst' phenomenon occurs when resting cells are activated to phagocytes (i.e. neutrophils, eosinophils, and mononuclear phagocytes) and start metabolizing large quantities of glucose with increased rates (>50-fold) of oxygen uptake.[49] In addition, micro-autoradiography has shown high levels of ^{18}F-FDG accumulation in macrophages, activated lymphocytes, and granulation tissue,[50,51] mostly due to increased oxidative metabolism.[52]

In normal ^{18}F-FDG PET scans, the aorta and its main branches usually only demonstrate normal background uptake of activity due to the low numbers of metabolically active cells dispersed between the elastic layers of the arterial wall. This pattern becomes distinctly abnormal in large-vessel vasculitis. Individual case reports have documented a pattern of linear uptake along the walls of the involved vessels on ^{18}F-FDG PET scan in vasculitis associated with SLE,[53] TA,[54] and GCA.[55] Blockmans and colleagues studied 25 subjects with GCA or polymyalgia rheumatica (PR) with ^{18}F-FDG PET and compared them with 44 age-matched control subjects. Vascular uptake in the vessels of the thorax and legs was found in 76% of the affected group compared to 23% of normal controls (p < 0.0001) They reported a sensitivity of 56%, specificity of 98%, positive predictive value of 93%, and negative predictive value of 80%.[56] Another study by Meller et al. compared ^{18}F-FDG PET and MRI in 15 patients with GCA and TA. ^{18}F-FDG PET was shown to be better than MRI in identifying the extent of vasculitis, monitoring disease activity, and response to therapy; it correlated well with clinical and laboratory findings.[57] The study showed that early diagnosis is possible with ^{18}F-FDG PET in the absence of late complications such as stenosis or aneurysmal dilatation detected by angiography. This was also shown by our group in a smaller series of six newly diagnosed TA patients.[58] The high sensitivity of ^{18}F-FDG PET in detecting vasculitis was used as an argument to characterize PR as a type of vasculitis.[59] The value of ^{18}F-FDG in detecting brain abnormalities relating to TA has been shown in 4 out of 5 patients with TA.[60]

The hallmark of diagnosis is the linear increase in ^{18}F-FDG uptake along the vessel walls when compared to background (Figure 70.2). Quantitation of uptake using the standardized uptake value (SUV) does not necessarily reflect the disease severity and may be normal in highly active disease.[61] However, SUV is very useful in the follow-up of the same patient. A study by our group showed that ^{18}F-FDG PET was helpful in assessing response to therapy and reducing the need to perform arterial biopsies or repeat angiography. It involved 18 patients with TA who had ^{18}F-FDG PET, the results of which were compared with angiography and clinical scoring. The sensitivity, specificity, negative and positive predictive values for ^{18}F-FDG PET were 92%, 100%, 85%, and 100% respectively.[62]

Using an aorta-to-liver ratio in 23 patients with aortic involvement in GCA, Hautzel et al. recorded a sensitivity and specificity for ^{18}F-FDG PET of 89% and 95% respectively.[63] Using a similar technique, another recent study correlated ^{18}F-FDG uptake with clinical and laboratory parameters in 78 patients with vasculitis.[64] The authors concluded that FDG PET/CT could detect the extent and activity of large-vessel vasculitis in untreated patients with lower uptake in patients on steroids. This confirms the value of a baseline study before the initiation of therapy.

A recent systematic review of the literature on the diagnostic performances of ^{18}F-FDG PET for GCA found that linear or long-segmental pattern of ^{18}F-FDG uptake along the vessels is a

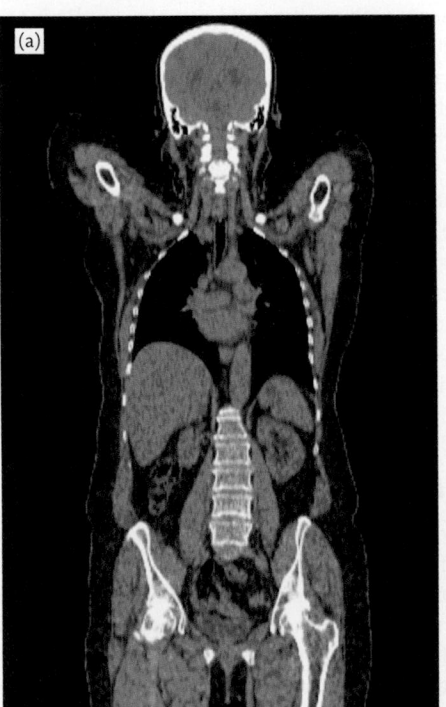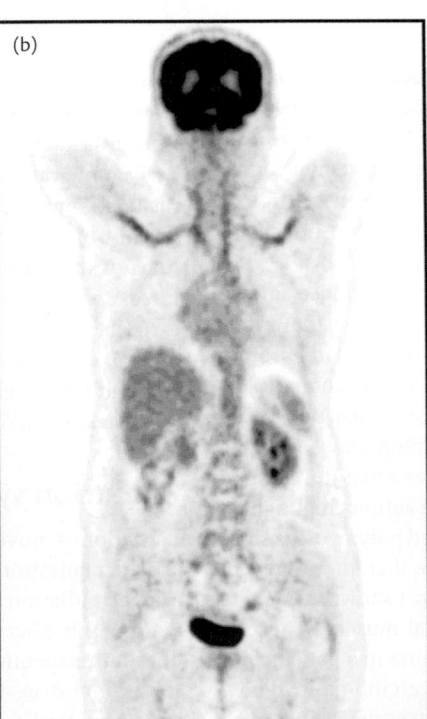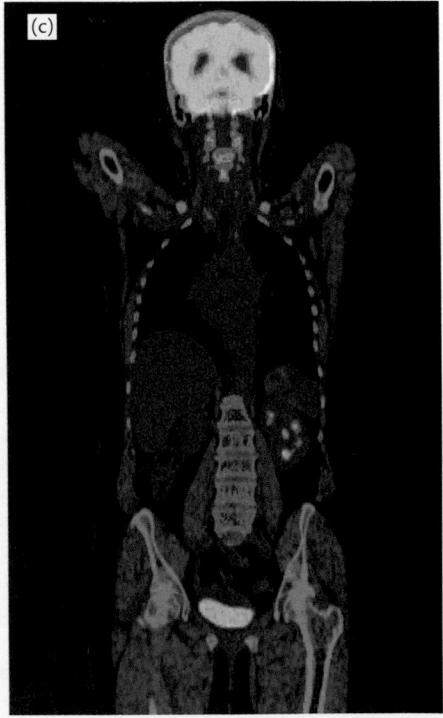

Fig. 70.2 Coronal images of CT (a), FDG PET (b), and fused PET/CT (c) of a 90 year old woman with bilateral axillary artery thrombosis, arthralgia and fatigue. Images (b) and (c) demonstrate increased FDG uptake in the carotid, subclavian, and axillary vessels, consistent with large-vessel vasculitis.

characteristic pattern of GCA, with meta-analysis of data showing sensitivity, specificity, positive and negative predictive values of 80%, 89%, 85%, and 88% respectively.[63]

Other rheumatologic conditions associated with vasculitis such as PR and GCA can benefit from PET imaging, although the literature is sparse and consists of small series or case reports.[65–68] In addition to increased ^{18}F-FDG uptake in involved large vessels, it was also documented that ^{18}F-FDG uptake was increased in involved joints.[66] Blockmans et al found uptake in large vessels to be a sensitive marker for GCA while uptake in the shoulders correlated significantly (p = 0.005) with the presence of PR.[67] More recently, Camellino and Cimmino conducted a literature search to look at the role of imaging in the management of PMR.[68] They found that MRI and PET were most promising in demonstrating interspinous bursitis, with PET frequently showing large-vessel vasculitis. They concluded that the full potential of these techniques is still unexplored.

Inflammatory myopathy

The aetiology of inflammatory myopathy is described elsewhere in this book. It is thought that the mechanisms leading to muscular damage include infiltration by T lymphocytes and macrophages, indirect effect of cytokines, and disturbance of the microcirculation. An increased risk of malignancy (lymphoma, lung, ovary, breast, and colon) at the time of diagnosis or later is associated with dermatomyositis (DM).

An accurate diagnosis of inflammatory myopathy requires a muscle biopsy, which may be difficult because of the heterogeneous nature of muscle involvement.[69] There is therefore a need for an imaging procedure that can depict the disease activity in involved muscle(s), identify a biopsy site, assess response to therapy, and aid in detecting associated malignancy.

^{18}F-FDG PET

There is no visible uptake in voluntary muscle during normal ^{18}F-FDG PET scan due to the low metabolic rate induced by strict prescan avoidance of almost all activities for 1 hour. If this restriction is ignored, variable muscle uptake is noticeable and may render the scan non-diagnostic.[70] Other than that, any muscle uptake would indicate abnormal metabolic activity such as that induced by inflammatory disease.

Early reports of the use of ^{18}F-FDG PET in assessing muscular disorders date back to the early 1990s. A report by Frey et al. described the metabolic activity of lumbar spine muscles involved in fibromyalgia using dynamic ^{18}F-FDG PET and found a significant backflow of glucose from affected muscles back into the vascular pool.[71] An interesting case report was published by Agriantonis et al. showing intense and diffuse muscle uptake in a patient as a manifestation of chronic graft versus host disease (GVHD). The authors highlighted the value of early detection of GVHD-associated polymyositis since it is readily treatable with immunosuppressive therapy to prevent devastating consequences.[72] Another case report showed the value of ^{18}F-FDG PET in revealing diffuse proximal muscle hypermetabolism in keeping with the inflammatory nature in a patient with DM. PET also showed the underlying adenocarcinoma involving the mediastinum.[73] We presented our limited experience in a small series of four patients who underwent ^{18}F-FDG PET for assessment of different types of inflammatory myopathy.[74] One of our cases

had a drug-induced myopathy in which ^{18}F-FDG PET showed significant uptake in upper and lower limb girdle muscles with resolution of uptake 4 months after stopping the offending drug. Our results suggested that ^{18}F-FDG PET is better suited to detect florid necrotizing/inflammatory myopathies and their response to therapy rather than low-grade disease, which needs further and larger studies.

A literature search for articles dealing with the role of PET in the diagnosis and assessment of response to therapy in inflammatory myopathy would, so far, reveal a small number of case reports and small series. This may reflect the fact that PET was, until recently, restricted to research purposes. Concern about using repetitive PET imaging in a benign conditions such as inflammatory myopathy is unjustifiable, because of the debilitating nature of the condition and the fact that PET can detect the associated malignancies, as discussed in the following section.

Use of PET in screening underlying malignancy

There are relatively more studies that show the role of ^{18}F-FDG PET and PET/CT in detecting malignancies associated with inflammatory myopathies. Current opinion suggests that polymyositis (PM) and dermatomyositis (DM) are potential paraneoplastic diseases that require cancer screening. Employing a multitude of conventional imaging techniques may not succeed in this task and a number of studies have demonstrated the value of ^{18}F-FDG PET in this respect.[73,75–77]

A recent study by Selva-O'Callaghan et al. assessed the cost-effectiveness of PET/CT in conventional cancer screening for patients with inflammatory myopathy.[75] They performed ^{18}F-FDG PET/CT in 55 patients with recent diagnosis of myositis and compared the results with those obtained using conventional screening including thoracolumbar CT, mammography, gynaecological examination, ultrasonography, and tumour marker analysis. Malignancies were detected in 9/55 patients with positive and negative predictive values for PET/CT of 85.7% and 93.8% compared to those obtained with conventional screening of 77.8% and 95.7%, respectively. The overall predictive value of both approaches was the same (92.7%). This indicated that the value of a single imaging procedure (PET) was comparable to that of broad conventional screening that included multiple tests.

Unfortunately, the role of PET is not well defined in the guidelines of the European Federation of Neurological Societies' task force report for screening in paraneoplastic syndromes.[78] However, a recent review recommends yearly PET/CT study for at least 3–5 years in patients with PM (moderate risk of associated cancer) and DM (high risk of associated cancer), especially those with positive anti-p155 autoantibodies.[75]

Radiation synovectomy

Radiation synovectomy/radiosynoviorthesis (RS) is the intra-articular injection of beta-emitting isotopes into joints to deliver a local radiation dose to the inflammatory process in the synovium. This direct irradiation of the synovial membrane can produce a therapeutic effect on persistent synovitis that is resistant to traditional drug treatment. The radiopharmaceuticals that have been used for RS are composed of small colloidal particles labelled to beta-emitting isotopes (yttrium-90, rhenium-186, erbium-169, samarium-153). Once injected into the joint these compounds are taken up by phagocytes, which are abundant in inflamed tissues, hence providing a localized radiation source within the joint. This allows these compounds to deliver a cytotoxic dose to the inflamed synovium.

The procedure is simple to carry out in the outpatient department, although it needs particular attention to radiation protection measures. Availability of the radioisotopes needs to be considered. The injected joints are immobilized for the first 24 hours and the patient may experience some increased pain for the first few days, which can be treated with simple analgesia. Most patients will experience a therapeutic effect within 3–4 weeks after treatment, and therapy can be repeated if clinically indicated.

RS has been successful in the treatment of early stage RA due to its effect on controlling the proliferation of the inflammatory process in the synovial membrane. However treatment may not be effective in advanced cases where there is significant secondary osteoarthritic damage[79]; significant osteoarthritis remains a contraindication for its use.

A meta-analysis of published data on the efficacy of RS has reported 51–100% success rates.[80] A placebo-controlled study evaluated RS in patients with mostly bilaterally affected joints.[81] Random selection of one knee to be treated with ^{90}Y colloid showed more than 50% of patients to benefit from RS 12 months after treatment. This was also found to be superior to other therapeutic procedures (except for surgical synovectomy) such as corticosteroid injections. Further studies have demonstrated the efficacy of RS in patients who became refractory to intra-articular injections of steroids. Jahangier et al. performed RS for RA knees in patients who had at least two failed injections of corticosteroids.[82] After 12 months, 78% of the knees in RA patients had been effectively treated with a sustained improvement in 57% of cases with resolution of joint effusion in 30% of patients. Another study has evaluated the role of ^{90}Y colloid injection alone compared to triamcinolone alone and combination treatment of triamcinolone and ^{90}Y colloid in the treatment of RA knees.[83] The authors found that ^{90}Y colloid alone was more effective in long-term control of symptoms than triamcinolone alone. However, short-term control of pain and joint effusion was similar using either ^{90}Y colloid alone or the combination of ^{90}Y colloid and triamcinolone.

In addition, RS has been used successfully in a wider spectrum of inflammatory arthritides ranging from spondyloathropathies such as AS to Paget's disease, hæmophiliac synovitis, and pigmented villonodular synovitis. Jahangier et al. observed good effects in psoriatic arthritis in 75% of cases and in AS in 76%.[84] Dawson et al., reported success rates of 50–90% in the control of pain in haemophilic arthritis.[85]

Conclusion

Nuclear medicine procedures are well suited to assist in the management of a variety of rheumatological conditions. Traditional tests such as bone, lung, gallium, and labelled white cell scans continue to be used in the diagnosis and follow-up of RA, SLE, and AS as well as in monitoring response to therapy. However, the recent introduction of PET/CT into clinical practice has provided an excellent imaging procedure that is capable of detecting molecular and submolecular changes with superb resolution and accurate localization. PET/CT has been used successfully in the detection of inflammatory changes in vasculitis, RA, and inflammatory

myopathy with the additional benefit of cancer screening in the latter. Newer PET radiopharmaceuticals that target activated macrophages such as ^{11}C-(R)-PK11195 and ^{18}F-PEG-folate are expected to improve the imaging of inflammation, which is the hallmark of most rheumatological conditions. In addition to imaging, nuclear medicine offers pain relief and improved joint performance through the intra-articular administration of beta emitters (radiosynovectomy), which has been found very useful in resistant synovitis.

References

1. Greyson ND. Radionuclide bone and joint imaging in rheumatology. *Bull Rheum Dis* 1979;30(7):1034–1038.
2. Stevens CR, Blake DR, Merry P, Revell PA, Levick JR. A comparative study by morphometry of the microvasculature in normal and rheumatoid synovium. *Arthritis Rheum* 1991;34(12):1508–1513.
3. Vaudo G, Marchesi S, Gerli R et al. Endothelial dysfunction in young patients with rheumatoid arthritis and low disease activity. *Ann Rheum Dis* 2004;63(1):31–35.
4. Mottonen TT, Hannonen P, Toivanen J, Rekonen A, Oka M. Value of joint scintigraphy in the prediction of erosiveness in early rheumatoid arthritis. *Ann Rheum Dis* 1988;47(3):183–189.
5. Shearman J, Esdaile J, Hawkins D, Rosenthall L. Predictive value of radionuclide joint scintigrams. *Arthritis Rheum* 1982;25(1):83–86.
6. Duncan I, Dorai-Raj A, Khoo K, Tymms K, Brook A. The utility of bone scans in rheumatology. *Clin Nucl Med* 1999;24(1):9–14.
7. Al Janabi MA, Jones AK, Solanki K et al. 99Tcm-labelled leucocyte imaging in active rheumatoid arthritis. *Nucl Med Commun* 1988;9(12):987–991.
8. de Bois MH, Tak PP, Arndt JW et al. Joint scintigraphy for quantification of synovitis with 99 mTc-labelled human immunoglobulin G compared to histological examination. *Clin Exp Rheumatol* 1995;13(2):155–159.
9. de Bois MH, Arndt JW, Speyer I, Pauwels EK, Breedveld FC. Technetium-99 m labelled human immunoglobulin scintigraphy predicts rheumatoid arthritis in patients with arthralgia. *Scand J Rheumatol* 1996;25(3):155–158.
10. Malviya G, Conti F, Chianelli M et al. Molecular imaging of rheumatoid arthritis by radiolabelled monoclonal antibodies: new imaging strategies to guide molecular therapies. *Eur J Nucl Med Mol Imaging* 2010;37(2):386–398.
11. Chianelli M, D'Alessandria C, Conti F et al. New radiopharmaceuticals for imaging rheumatoid arthritis. *Q J Nucl Med Mol Imaging* 2006;50(3):217–225.
12. Jamar F, Chapman PT, Manicourt DH et al. A comparison between 111In-anti-E-selectin mAb and 99Tcm-labelled human non-specific immunoglobulin in radionuclide imaging of rheumatoid arthritis. *Br J Radiol* 1997;70(833):473–481.
13. Jamar F, Houssiau FA, Devogelaer JP et al. Scintigraphy using a technetium 99 m-labelled anti-E-selectin Fab fragment in rheumatoid arthritis. *Rheumatology* (Oxford) 2002;41(1):53–61.
14. Scannell G. Leukocyte responses to hypoxic/ischemic conditions. *New Horiz* 1996;4(2):179–183.
15. Kaim AH, Weber B, Kurrer MO et al. Autoradiographic quantification of 18F-FDG uptake in experimental soft-tissue abscesses in rats. *Radiology* 2002;223(2):446–451.
16. Lin PW, Liu RS, Liou TH, Pan LC, Chen CH. Correlation between joint (F-18) FDG PET uptake and synovial TNF-alpha concentration: a study with two rabbit models of acute inflammatory arthritis. *Appl Radiat Isot* 2007;65(11):1221–1226.
17. Palmer WE, Rosenthal DI, Schoenberg OI et al. Quantification of inflammation in the wrist with gadolinium-enhanced MR imaging and PET with 2-(F-18)-fluoro-2-deoxy-D-glucose. *Radiology* 1995;196(3):647–655.
18. Beckers C, Jeukens X, Ribbens C et al. (18)F-FDG PET imaging of rheumatoid knee synovitis correlates with dynamic magnetic resonance and

sonographic assessments as well as with the serum level of metallopro-teinase-3. *Eur J Nucl Med Mol Imaging* 2006;33(3):275–280.

19. Kubota K, Ito K, Morooka M et al. Whole-body FDG-PET/CT on rheumatoid arthritis of large joints. *Ann Nucl Med* 2009;23(9):783–791.

20. van der Laken CJ, Elzinga EH, Kropholler MA et al. Noninvasive imaging of macrophages in rheumatoid synovitis using 11C-(R)-PK11195 and positron emission tomography. *Arthritis Rheum* 2008;58(11):3350–3355.

21. van der Heijden JW, Oerlemans R, Dijkmans BA et al. Folate receptor beta as a potential delivery route for novel folate antagonists to macrophages in the synovial tissue of rheumatoid arthritis patients. *Arthritis Rheum* 2009;60(1):12–21.

22. van der Laken CJ, de Greeuw I, Gent YJ et al;18FPEG-folate: a new potential macrophage PET tracer for imaging of arthritis. (abstract) *Arthritis Rheum* 2010;62 Suppl 10 :1613

23. Nagasawa K, Tsukamoto H, Tada Y et al. Imaging study on the mode of development and changes in avascular necrosis of the femoral head in systemic lupus erythematosus: long-term observations. *Br J Rheumatol* 1994;33(4):343–347.

24. Tsan MF. Mechanism of gallium-67 accumulation in inflammatory lesions. *J Nucl Med* 1985;26(1):88–92.

25. Pagniez DC, MacNamara E, Beuscart R et al. Gallium scan in the follow-up of sarcoid granulomatous nephritis. *Am J Nephrol* 1987;7(4):326–327.

26. Bakir AA, Lopez-Majano V, Hryhorczuk DO, Rhee HL, Dunea G. Appraisal of lupus nephritis by renal imaging with gallium-67. *Am J Med* 1985;79(2):175–182.

27. Lin WY, Lan JL, Wang SJ. Gallium-67 scintigraphy to predict response to therapy in active lupus nephritis. *J Nucl Med* 1998;39(12):2137–2141.

28. Witt C, Dorner T, Hiepe F et al. Diagnosis of alveolitis in interstitial lung manifestation in connective tissue diseases: importance of late inspiratory crackles, 67 gallium scan and bronchoalveolar lavage. *Lupus* 1996;5(6):606–612.

29. Kao CH, Lin HT, Yu SL, Wang SJ, Lan JL. Lung inflammation in patients with systemic lupus erythematosus detected by quantitative 67Ga-citrate lung scanning. *Nucl Med Commun* 1994;15(11):928–931.

30. Busteed S, Sparrow P, Molloy C, Molloy MG. Myocarditis as a prognostic indicator in systemic lupus erythematosus. *Postgrad Med J* 2004;80(944):366–367.

31. Jolles PR, Tatum JL. SLE myocarditis. Detection by Ga-67 citrate scintigraphy. *Clin Nucl Med* 1996;21(4):284–286.

32. Colamussi P, Trotta F, Ricci R et al. Brain perfusion SPET and proton magnetic resonance spectroscopy in the evaluation of two systemic lupus erythematosus patients with mild neuropsychiatric manifestations. *Nucl Med Commun* 1997;18(3):269–273.

33. Lin WY, Lan JL, Wang SJ. Lupus mesenteric vasculitis detected by Ga-67 scan. *Clin Nucl Med* 2001;26(8):726.

34. Dalcin PT, Barreto SS, Cunha RD et al. Lung clearance of 99 mTc-DTPA in systemic lupus erythematosus. *Braz J Med Biol Res* 2002;35(6):663–668.

35. Shih CM, Shiau YC, Wang JJ, Ho ST, Kao A. Increased lung uptake of technetium-99 m hexamethylpropylene amine oxime in systemic lupus erythematosus. *Respiration* 2002;69(2):143–147.

36. Rennen HJ, Boerman OC, Oyen WJ, Corstens FH. Imaging infection/inflammation in the new millennium. *Eur J Nucl Med* 2001;28(2):241–252.

37. Meller J, Sahlmann CO, Scheel AK. 18F-FDG PET and PET/CT in fever of unknown origin. *J Nucl Med* 2007;48(1):35–45.

38. Weiner SM, Otte A, Schumacher M et al. Alterations of cerebral glucose metabolism indicate progress to severe morphological brain lesions in neuropsychiatric systemic lupus erythematosus. *Lupus* 2000;9(5):386–389.

39. Weiner SM, Otte A, Schumacher M et al. Diagnosis and monitoring of central nervous system involvement in systemic lupus erythematosus: value of F-18 fluorodeoxyglucose PET. *Ann Rheum Dis* 2000;59(5):377–385.

40. Feldtkeller E, Khan MA, van der HD, van der LS, Braun J. Age at disease onset and diagnosis delay in HLA-B27 negative vs. positive patients with ankylosing spondylitis. *Rheumatol Int* 2003;23(2):61–66.

41. Goei The HS, Lemmens AJ, Goedhard G et al. Radiological and scintigraphic findings in patients with a clinical history of chronic inflammatory back pain. *Skeletal Radiol* 1985;14(4):243–248.

42. Song IH, Carrasco-Fernandez J, Rudwaleit M, Sieper J. The diagnostic value of scintigraphy in assessing sacroiliitis in ankylosing spondylitis: a systematic literature research. *Ann Rheum Dis* 2008;67(11):1535–1540.

43. Zerizer I, Tan K, Khan S et al. Role of FDG-PET and PET/CT in the diagnosis and management of vasculitis. *Eur J Radiol* 2010;73(3):504–509.

44. Sty JR, Chusid MJ, Dorrington A. Ga-67 imaging: Kawasaki disease. *Clin Nucl Med* 1981;6(3):112–113.

45. Alpert LI. Pulmonary uptake of gallium-67 in Wegener's granulomatosis. *Clin Nucl Med* 1980;5(2):53–54.

46. Williamson MR, Williamson SL, Seibert JJ. Indium-111 leukocyte scanning localization for detecting early myocarditis in Kawasaki disease. *AJR Am J Roentgenol* 1986;146(2):255–256.

47. Chen CC, Kerr GS, Carter CS et al. Lack of sensitivity of indium-111 mixed leukocyte scans for active disease in Takayasu's arteritis. *J Rheumatol* 1995;22(3):478–481.

48. Yamada S, Kubota K, Kubota R, Ido T, Tamahashi N. High accumulation of fluorine-18-fluorodeoxyglucose in turpentine-induced inflammatory tissue. *J Nucl Med* 1995;36(7):1301–1306.

49. Babior BM. The respiratory burst of phagocytes. *J Clin Invest* 1984;73(3):599–601.

50. Kubota R, Yamada S, Kubota K et al. Intratumoral distribution of fluorine-18-fluorodeoxyglucose in vivo: high accumulation in macrophages and granulation tissues studied by microautoradiography. *J Nucl Med* 1992;33(11):1972–1980.

51. Ishimori T, Saga T, Mamede M et al. Increased (18)F-FDG uptake in a model of inflammation: concanavalin A-mediated lymphocyte activation. *J Nucl Med* 2002;43(5):658–663.

52. Rudd JH, Warburton EA, Fryer TD et al. Imaging atherosclerotic plaque inflammation with (18F)-fluorodeoxyglucose positron emission tomography. *Circulation* 2002;105(23):2708–2711.

53. Hiraiwa M, Nonaka C, Abe T, Iio M. Positron emission tomography in systemic lupus erythematosus: relation of cerebral vasculitis to PET findings. *AJNR Am J Neuroradiol* 1983;4(3):541–543.

54. Hara M, Goodman PC, Leder RA. FDG-PET finding in early-phase Takayasu arteritis. *J Comput Assist Tomogr* 1999;23(1):16–18.

55. Turlakow A, Yeung HW, Pui J et al. Fludeoxyglucose positron emission tomography in the diagnosis of giant cell arteritis. *Arch Intern Med* 2001;161(7):1003–1007.

56. Blockmans D, Stroobants S, Maes A, Mortelmans L. Positron emission tomography in giant cell arteritis and polymyalgia rheumatica: evidence for inflammation of the aortic arch. *Am J Med* 2000;108(3):246–249.

57. Meller J, Strutz F, Siefker U et al. Early diagnosis and follow-up of aortitis with (18)FFDG PET and MRI. *Eur J Nucl Med Mol Imaging* 2003;30(5):730–736.

58. Andrews J, Al Nahhas A, Pennell DJ et al. Non-invasive imaging in the diagnosis and management of Takayasu's arteritis. *Ann Rheum Dis* 2004;63(8):995–1000.

59. Blockmans D, Maes A, Stroobants S et al. New arguments for a vasculitic nature of polymyalgia rheumatica using positron emission tomography. *Rheumatology* (Oxford) 1999;38(5):444–447.

60. Weiner SM, Vaith P, Walker UA, Brink I. Detection of alterations in brain glucose metabolism by positron emission tomography in Takayasu's arteritis. *Eur J Nucl Med Mol Imaging* 2004;31(2):300–302.

61. Kobayashi Y, Ishii K, Oda K et al. Aortic wall inflammation due to Takayasu arteritis imaged with 18F-FDG PET coregistered with enhanced CT. *J Nucl Med* 2005;46(6):917–922.

62. Webb M, Chambers A, Al Nahhas A et al. The role of 18F-FDG PET in characterising disease activity in Takayasu arteritis. *Eur J Nucl Med Mol Imaging* 2004;31(5):627–634.

63. Hautzel H, Sander O, Heinzel A, Schneider M, Muller HW. Assessment of large-vessel involvement in giant cell arteritis with 18F-FDG

PET: introducing an ROC-analysis-based cutoff ratio. *J Nucl Med* 2008;49(7):1107–1113.

64. Papathanasiou ND, Du Y, Menezes LJ et al. 18F-Fluorodeoxyglucose PET/CT in the evaluation of large-vessel vasculitis: diagnostic performance and correlation with clinical and laboratory parameters. *Br J Radiol* 2012;85(1014):e188–194.

65. Dos Anjos DA, Dos Anjos RF, de Paula WD, Sobrinho AB. F-18 FDG PET/CT in giant cell arteritis with polymyalgia rheumatica. *Clin Nucl Med* 2008;33(6):402–404.

66. Toriihara A, Seto Y, Yoshida K et al. F-18 FDG PET/CT of polymyalgia rheumatica. *Clin Nucl Med* 2009;34(5):305–306.

67. Blockmans D, de Ceuninck L, Vanderschueren S et al. Repetitive 18F-fluorodeoxyglucose positron emission tomography in giant cell arteritis: a prospective study of 35 patients. *Arthritis Rheum* 2006;55(1):131–137.

68. Camellino D, Cimmino MA. Imaging of polymyalgia rheumatica: indications on its pathogenesis, diagnosis and prognosis. *Rheumatology* (Oxford) 2012;51(1):77–86.

69. Walker UA. Imaging tools for the clinical assessment of idiopathic inflammatory myositis. *Curr Opin Rheumatol* 2008;20(6):656–661.

70. Yeung HW, Grewal RK, Gonen M, Schoder H, Larson SM. Patterns of (18)F-FDG uptake in adipose tissue and muscle: a potential source of false-positives for PET. *J Nucl Med* 2003;44(11):1789–1796.

71. Frey LD, Locher JT, Hrycaj P et al. (Determination of regional rate of glucose metabolism in lumbar muscles in patients with generalized tendomyopathy using dynamic 18F-FDG PET) *Z Rheumatol* 1992;51(5):238–242.

72. Agriantonis DJ, Perlman SB, Longo WL. F-18 FDG PET imaging of GVHD-associated polymyositis. *Clin Nucl Med* 2008;33(10):688–689.

73. Liau N, Ooi C, Reid C, Kirkwood ID, Bartholomeusz D. F-18 FDG PET/CT detection of mediastinal malignancy in a patient with dermatomyositis. *Clin Nucl Med* 2007;32(4):304–305.

74. Al-Nahhas A, Jawad A. PET/CT imaging in inflammatory myopathies. *Ann N Y Acad Sci.* 2011;1228:39–45.

75. Selva-O'Callaghan A, Grau JM, Gamez-Cenzano C et al. Conventional cancer screening versus PET/CT in dermatomyositis/polymyositis. *Am J Med* 2010;123(6):558–562.

76. Munoz MA, Conejo-Mir JS, Congregado-Loscertales M et al. The utility of positron emission tomography to find an occult neoplasm in a patient with dermatomyositis. *J Eur Acad Dermatol Venereol* 2007;21(10):1418–1419.

77. Berner U, Menzel C, Rinne D et al. Paraneoplastic syndromes: detection of malignant tumors using (18)FFDG-PET. *Q J Nucl Med* 2003;47(2):85–89.

78. Titulaer MJ, Soffietti R, Dalmau J et al. Screening for tumours in paraneoplastic syndromes: report of an EFNS task force. *Eur J Neurol* 2011;18(1):19–e3.

79. Franssen MJ, Boerbooms AM, Karthaus RP, Buijs WC, van de Putte LB. Treatment of pigmented villonodular synovitis of the knee with yttrium-90 silicate: prospective evaluations by arthroscopy, histology, and 99 mTc pertechnetate uptake measurements. *Ann Rheum Dis* 1989;48(12):1007–1013.

80. Kampen WU, Czech N. Methodologic issues in the assessment of the efficacy of radiation synovectomy for arthritis of the knee: comment on the article by Janangier et al. *Arthritis Rheum* 2007;56(1):385.

81. Bridgman JF, Bruckner F, Eisen V, Tucker A, Bleehen NM. Irradiation of the synovium in the treatment of rheumatoid arthritis. *Q J Med* 1973;42(166):357–367.

82. Jahangier ZN, Moolenburgh JD, Jacobs JW, Serdijn H, Bijlsma JW. The effect of radiation synovectomy in patients with persistent arthritis: a prospective study. *Clin Exp Rheumatol* 2001;19(4):417–424.

83. Urbanová Z, Gatterová J, Olejárová M, Pavelka K. Radiosynoviorthesis with 90Y—results of a clinical study. *Èes Revmatol* 1997;5:140–142.

84. Jahangier ZN, Jacobs JW, van Isselt JW, Bijlsma JW. Persistent synovitis treated with radiation synovectomy using yttrium-90: a retrospective evaluation of 83 procedures for 45 patients. *Br J Rheumatol* 1997;36(8):861–869.

85. Dawson TM, Ryan PF, Street AM et al. Yttrium synovectomy in haemophilic arthropathy. *Br J Rheumatol* 1994;33(4):351–356.

CHAPTER 71

Imaging in children

Karl Johnson

Introduction

In principle, the imaging of children with rheumatological disorders is no different from imaging adults; namely the most appropriate test done in a timely manner causing the least amount of distress or long-term complications. Any investigation needs to be clearly considered and affect clinical management. Successful imaging in children requires an understanding of the disease process, the anatomical variants that can occur in childhood, and the developmental needs of the child. As with all aspects of radiology, close collaboration and discussion between the requesting physician and radiologist will improve the quality of the service provided.

This chapter illustrates the specific demands of paediatric imaging. While reference will be made to the important radiological features of individual diseases, they are described in more detail in their appropriate sections.

Clinical indications

The imaging of children with rheumatological conditions is very patient specific with no absolute indications, or contra-indications, for any investigation at any point in the patient's clinical pathway. It is important that any investigation is used to influence management, be it to confirm a diagnosis, exclude potential other diagnoses, or alter management. It must be realized that attending a radiology department, regardless of how child-friendly, may be a daunting experience for a child, not to mention the potential resource implications on the parents/carers who have to accompany them, as well as the demand on the service provision and staffing of the radiology department. The exact choice of imaging will depend on the clinical question and the available resource.

Although radiographs are the commonest used investigation, in childhood arthropathies as well as other musculoskeletal conditions, the diagnosis of juvenile idiopathic arthritis (JIA) is a clinical one and does not depend upon the radiographic findings.[1] The routine screening of a child's bones with radiographs is not indicated. Also, in the early stages of JIA the radiographic features may be normal or relatively non-specific, such as periarticular osteopenia and soft tissue swelling. More importantly, radiographs are important in excluding other causes of joint symptomatology.[2]

Ultrasound is being increasingly used in the management of JIA, but the absolute indications for its use are more difficult to clearly define. The quality of the imaging is very much

operator dependent, whether the operator is a rheumatologist or a radiologist. Obviously, rheumatologists may have access immediately within the clinic setting to confirm or refute the presence of synovial thickening or effusion in the joint, whereas if an appointment needs to be made with the radiology department, this would be less amenable to immediate diagnosis. Ultrasound has the advantage of not involving ionizing radiation, but is relatively time-consuming.

The use of more complex investigations, such as CT and MRI, usually involves booked appointments and is less readily available. In some children, there may be requirement for sedation or general anaesthesia and their use should be more considered. MRI will often provide the most information about joint inflammation and underlying abnormalities.

The advantages and disadvantages of different methods are summarized in Table 71.1. With all investigations, discussion with a radiologist as to the most appropriate test which would answer the diagnostic question most easily and promptly is important. A strong working relationship between rheumatologists and radiologists is to be fully supported. The use of multidisciplinary team meetings can only aid this interaction.

Issues for paediatric imaging

The indications and appropriateness of any investigation which involves ionizing radiation (radiography, screening studies, CT and nuclear scintigraphy) needs to be fully justifiable as they all carry some long-term risk. The true long-term effects of diagnostic radiation exposure are not fully known, but any effects on young children are greater than that in adults.

To aid compliance, optimize image quality, and thus improve the diagnostic yield of an investigation, it is important that the child is pain-free, comfortable, and reassured.

The department should be 'child-friendly', but this is an euphemistic term and difficult to implement in practice: what might seem friendly and welcoming to a small child would be regarded as patronizing by a teenager. Regardless of the content, the decoration should extend down to the eye level of a child and try to appeal to all age groups. Bravery certificates and stickers are useful additions to help the compliance of younger children.

The child being pain-free is one of the best ways to achieve good compliance for any radiological investigation. It is important that adequate and timely pain relief is optimized to the time of the

Table 71.1 Advantages and disadvantages of different modalities in paediatric musculoskeletal imaging

Modality	Advantages	Disadvantages
Radiography	Low cost Good detail of bone injuries Readily available Relatively cheap High availability Good anatomical detail Helpful in differential diagnosis Reproducibility Validated assessment methods	Use of ionizing radiation Not sensitive in detecting inflamed and enhanced synovium, fibrocartilaginous structures, or bone marrow changes due to limited soft tissue contrast Limited and non-specific for diagnosis of early JIA changes at diagnosis Reveals late and often irreversible structural damage Projectional superimposition Unable to directly detect cartilage changes or damage 2D representation of a 3D body part
Ultrasound	Lack of ionizing radiation Non-invasive, well tolerated Relatively low cost Repeatability Possibility of examining several joint regions at one session Ability to visualize both inflammatory and destructive disease manifestations Potential for guiding interventions (e.g. intra-articular steroid injection) Portable Good anatomical detail Dynamic so can be used to assess function and useful for guided procedures such as biopsies and aspirations	Operator dependence Not all joints accessible, the whole joint space not assessed Reduced joint movement in case of joint tenderness and pain Small field of view Acoustic shadowing from overlying bones Difficult to standardize and centralize for clinical trials In small children, compliance may be difficult Relatively poor for air-filled and bony structures as these do not transmit sound. Deep structures can be difficult to visualize
MRI	Lack of ionizing radiation Marked soft tissue contrast Multiplanar tomographic imaging Early detection of erosive changes Soft tissue inflammation detection Direct visualization of cartilage Bone marrow oedema visualization	High cost Longer examination time Claustrophobia Relatively expensive Sedation or general anaesthesia required in the younger or uncooperative child Potential allergic contrast reaction Evaluation limited to one target joint Availability varies worldwide Cannot put pacing wires or patients with metallic fragments near the magnet
CT	High availability Multiplanar tomographic imaging Early detection of erosive changes Can be used for image guidance Relatively quick Good anatomical detail and bony detail	Use of ionizing radiation Not sensitive in detecting inflamed and enhanced synovium Reveals late and often irreversible structural damage Unable to directly detect cartilage changes or damage Sedation or general anaesthesia required in the younger or uncooperative child Potential allergic contrast reaction
Nuclear scintigraphy	Information about organ function Useful whole-body screening investigation Relative sensitive to bone turnover	Radiation dose Poor anatomical detail Use of ionizing radiation Sensitive but non-specific Need for sedation

examination and is age appropriate. Suitable explanation of the procedure and the reasons and consequences of the examination are important, and should be related to the child's age and development. Care must be taken not to exaggerate or elaborate, since one does not want to elicit fear in the child. Play specialists are useful in forming and developing a relationship of trust with the child and devising games and procedures which often help the child understand and cooperate with the radiology staff while being imaged. There is very little indication for the parents/carers of a child not to be present during the examination.

For longer examinations, particularly MRI and, to some extent, CT and nuclear scintigraphy, good compliance is needed. In the younger child, typically those under the age of 5 years, or those with developmental problems, cooperation for longer than a few minutes is often not possible and as a consequence, either sedation or general anaesthesia will be required. With a child under 1 month of age swaddling them after food allow them to fall asleep.

For most radiographic procedures, the required level of sedation is one which allows the child to remain stationary and asleep during the entire imaging acquisition time, but they should be relatively rousable if necessary.[3,4] General anaesthesia requires a suitably trained paediatric anaesthetist, as the child is in an unrousable state associated with loss of airway, control and respiratory depression. Full support staff, anaesthetic machinery, and monitoring equipment is needed and so may not be readily available in all institutions.

Imaging modalities

Radiography

Role of radiography in musculoskeletal practice

Radiographs have historically been the mainstay of imaging in paediatric joint disease. However, they involve a radiation burden to the patient and their sensitivity and specificity in detecting joint damage is less than that of ultrasound or MRI. In view of this, they should no longer be regarded as the routine monitor of disease progression in JIA (Figure 71.1).

The immature skeleton differs considerably from that of an adult, most notably due to the presence of cartilaginous elements and the presence of physes. Interpretation of imaging studies therefore requires an understanding of normal anatomy, normal development, and those variations in normality which could be confused with disease processes. There are exhaustive texts which provide

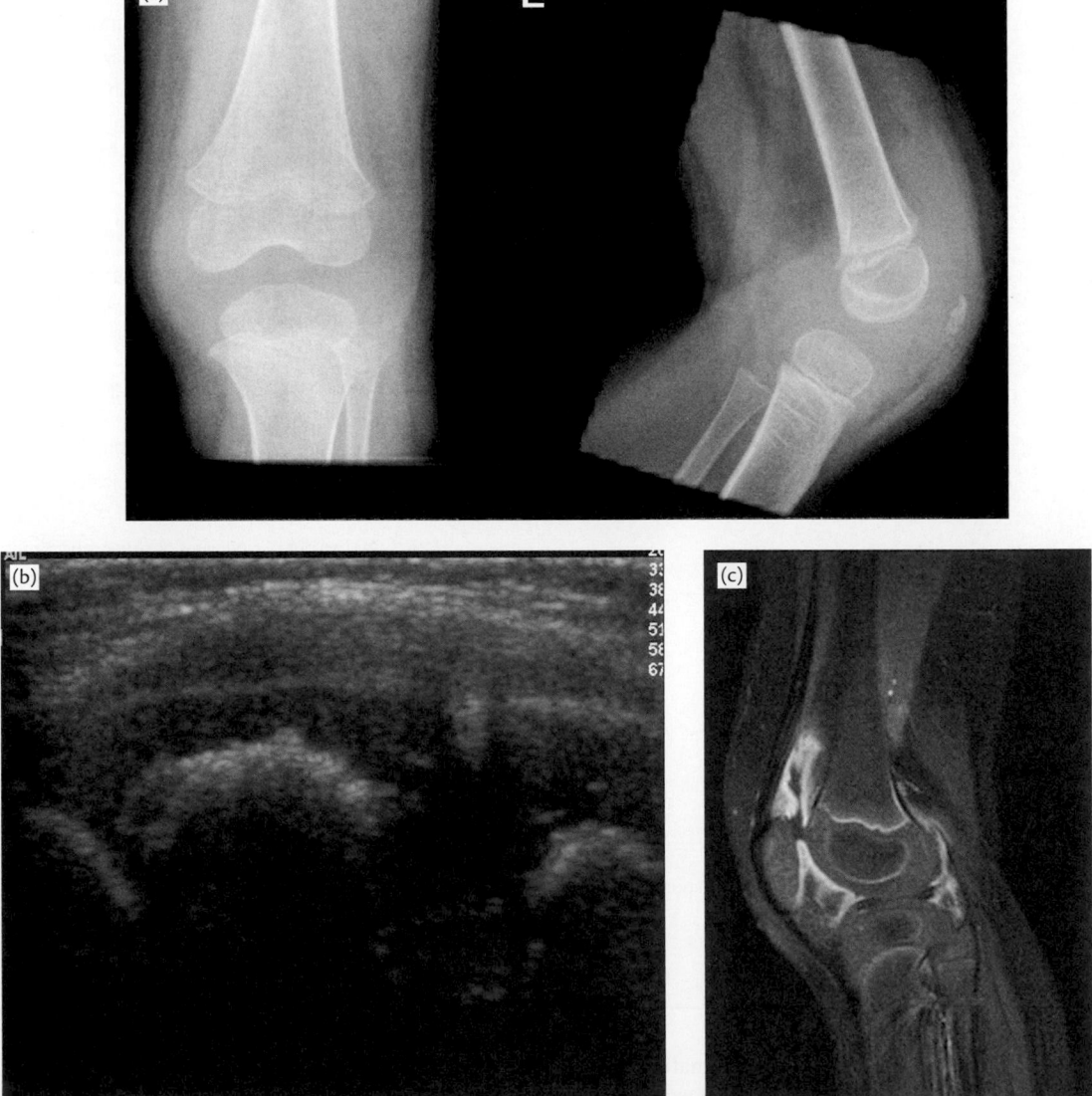

Fig. 71.1 Serial images in the same child showing the value of different imaging modalities: (a) Radiographs of the knee show extensive soft tissue swelling. No significant bony changes identified. (b) Ultrasound of the same patient shows a joint effusion and synovial thickening. (c) Postcontrast T1 fat-saturated MRI shows synovial thickening and a large joint effusion.

an extensive atlas of these normal variants.[5] In the growing skeleton, there are secondary cartilaginous growth centres around joints (epiphyses) and at the attachment of tendon ligaments to bone (apophyses) An epiphysis typically contributes to longitudinal growth of a bone while an apophysis does not, acting primarily as an insertion site. Both apophyses and epiphyses are separated from the adjacent bone by a physis. These cartilaginous structures are radiolucent on plain radiographs and CT scans and distinction from fractures and bone defects needs to be considered.[6] In the younger child, the epiphyses only become invisible after ossification, with the growth plate between the epiphysis and long bone being identifiable as a lucent line.

Differential diagnosis of joint disease

The differential diagnosis of arthritis in children is extensive and radiographs can be useful at diagnosis in either excluding or confirming the cause for the child's symptoms. An overview of the differential diagnosis of a childhood arthropathy is shown in Table 71.2 and the radiographic features of a number of conditions are shown in Figure 71.2.

Radiographs are most useful for traumatic and mechanical causes of damage. They are valuable in diagnosing avascular necrosis, at whatever site. Depending on the systemic disorder, they may either be diagnostic (such as skeletal dysplasias and storage disorders) or be essentially normal, such as in systemic lupus erythematosus (SLE). Typically, radiographs will diagnose focal malignant conditions (e.g. primary bone tumours), but are less sensitive for systemic malignancy (e.g. leukaemia). With infection, radiographs are often normal within the first few days or weeks and are of minimal value for septic arthritis. If septic arthritis is suspected, this should be regarded as a relative emergency and diagnosis made by aspiration culture of the joint fluid rather than from imaging.

Radiography in juvenile idiopathic arthritis

In JIA, there are a number of radiographic features which may or may not be present. These are not specific to JIA and need to be placed in the appropriate clinical context. The level of sensitivity for radiographs in detecting inflammatory arthritis, particularly in the acute phase, is very low. The timing and development of any radiographic features will depend on disease duration, severity, and the child's response to treatment.

In early disease, where there is often a hyperaemia associated with the joint inflammation, there may be visible soft tissue swelling and the development of periarticular osteopenia. The osteopenia may become more generalized if the child is treated with steroids or becomes generally immobile due to more widespread disease activity.[7-8]

Periostitis, often around the phalanges, metacarpals, and metatarsals, due to tendon and ligamental inflammation as well as joint disease, can occur relatively early. Classically, but not exclusively, this is seen in psoriatic arthropathy.[7,8,9]

Growth disturbance in the early stages of disease can result in advanced skeletal maturation and epiphyseal enlargement. This is a result of chronic hyperaemia and growth factor release. In more progressive disease, the accelerated maturation will result in early growth-plate fusion and eventually long-term limb shortening. Generalized skeletal remodelling is the result of abnormal muscle tractions, generalized growth disturbance, and limited mobility (Figure 71.3).[7-10]

Abnormal joint alignment, either subluxation, dislocation, or flexion extension deformities, can either result from synovial-based

Table 71.2 The differential diagnoses of childhood arthropathy

Inflammatory	Inflammatory disease: inflammatory bowel disease, sarcoid
	Malignancies: leukaemia, lymphoma, neuroblastoma
	Infection: septic arthritis, osteomyelitis, tuberculosis, lyme arthritis
	Systemic disease: systemic lupus erythematosus, vasculitis, juvenile dermatomyositis, systemic sclerosis
	Chronic recurrent multifocal osteomyelitis
	Transient joint effusion/synovitis
Mechanical	Trauma: accidental and non-accidental injury
	Osteochondroses
	Avascular necrosis and other degenerative disorders: Perthes', slipped upper femoral epiphysis, idiopathic chondrolysis
	Inherited: skeletal dysplasias, congenital dislocation of the hip
	Collagen disorders: e.g. Ehlers–Danlos, Marfan's, Stickler syndromes
	Tumours of cartilage, bone, or muscle:
	benign: osteoid osteoma, pigmented villonodular synovitis, haemangioma, lipoma arborescens
	malignant: synovial sarcoma, osteosarcoma, rhabdomyosarcoma
	Inherited metabolic disorders: hypophosphataemic rickets, hypo/hyperthyroidism, diabetes, purine metabolism
	Storage disorders e.g. mucopolysaccharidoses/lipidoses
	Haematological: haemophilia and haemoglobinopathy (sickle cell disease predominantly)
	Chronic infantile neurological cutaneous and arthritis syndrome (CINCA)
Idiopathic pain syndromes	Local: reflex sympathetic dystrophy
	Generalized: fibromyalgia

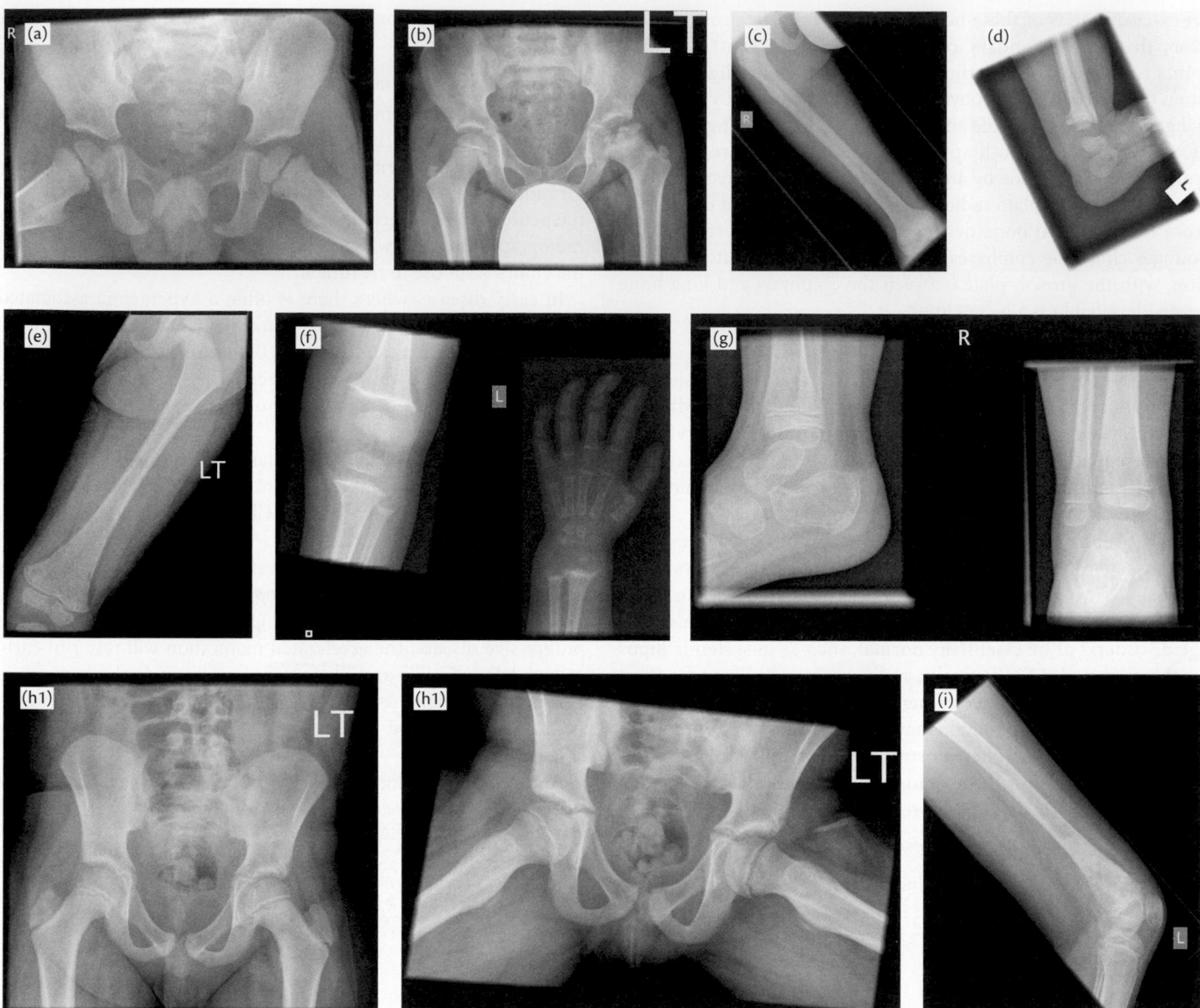

Fig. 71.2 Radiographic features of pathological process that can mimic juvenile idiopathic arthritis (JIA): (a) Early fragmentation and irregularity of the proximal left femoral epiphysis. Early Perthes' disease in a 4 year old. (b) AP radiograph in an 8 year old showing fragmentation and sclerosis of the left femoral epiphysis, a shallow left acetabulum, and some remodelling of the left femoral neck. These are the features of chronic Perthes' disease of the left hip. (c) Extensive sclerosis with some cortical expansion of the proximal right femoral metadiaphysis. Within the marked sclerosis, there is a small lucency. Features are of an osteoid osteoma. (d) An unexplained metaphyseal fracture of the distal left tibia in a 9 month old child. There is sclerosis and metaphyseal irregularity. Appearances are of a healing metaphyseal fracture of the distal left tibia. (e) Generalized osteopenia with some more focal lucency within the distal left femoral metadiaphysis and some very early periosteal new bone formation. There are corresponding changes within the femoral epiphysis. These are features of osteomyelitis of the distal left femur. (f) Extensive metaphyseal irregularity, metaphyseal widening, cupping and splaying with widening of the physeal growth plate around the knee joint and the wrist joint. Bones are osteopenic. Classic features of rickets. (g) Metaphyseal lucency of the distal left tibia in a child with leukaemia. (h) AP and frog lateral views of the pelvis in a 12 year old girl showing bilateral slipped upper femoral epiphyses. (i) Metaphyseal fracture (bucket-handle type) of the proximal left tibia. There is cortical destruction, soft tissue expansion, extensive spiculated periosteal reaction, and mixed sclerotic and lytic appearances in the distal left femoral metaphysis in a child with osteosarcoma.

disease or extra-articular damage and processes. In the more chronic treatment-resistant cases, synovial-based disease will lead to joint space narrowing, both cartilaginous and bony erosions, eventually leading to ankylosis (Figures 71.4 and 71.5).[7–10]

With the increasing use of disease-modifying and biological agents in the treatment of JIA, it is important that any assessment of response is reliable, objective, and safe. Consequently, because of the variations in growth and development which occur in the paediatric skeleton, the routine use of radiographs to assess disease, as is often used in adult practice, is questionable. Although a number of radiographic scoring systems have been proposed (Table 71.3) and a number of them validated, with the increasing use of ultrasound and MRI, their role is uncertain.[11–18] However, because of the easy availability and objectivity of scoring systems, their role cannot be completely dismissed.[19] Radiographs are limited in that they do not give any assessment of synovial thickness, size of effusions, or degree of inflammatory change.

Extra-articular rheumatologic disease

Radiographs have a significant role in detecting and monitoring extra-articular aspects of autoimmune and rheumatological conditions.

With the musculoskeletal system these may be complications of the primary disorder such as soft tissue calcification seen in juvenile dermatomyositis (JDMS; Figure 71.6) or iatrogenic, such as the extra-articular calcification seen after steroid joint injections in children with JIA. The differential diagnosis for soft tissue calcification in childhood is given in Table 71.4.

With autoimmune pulmonary disorders, radiographs may show progressive interstitial lung disease, which can be split into three groups based on the imaging findings: nodular, reticular (linear opacities), and reticular nodular (linear and nodular opacities).

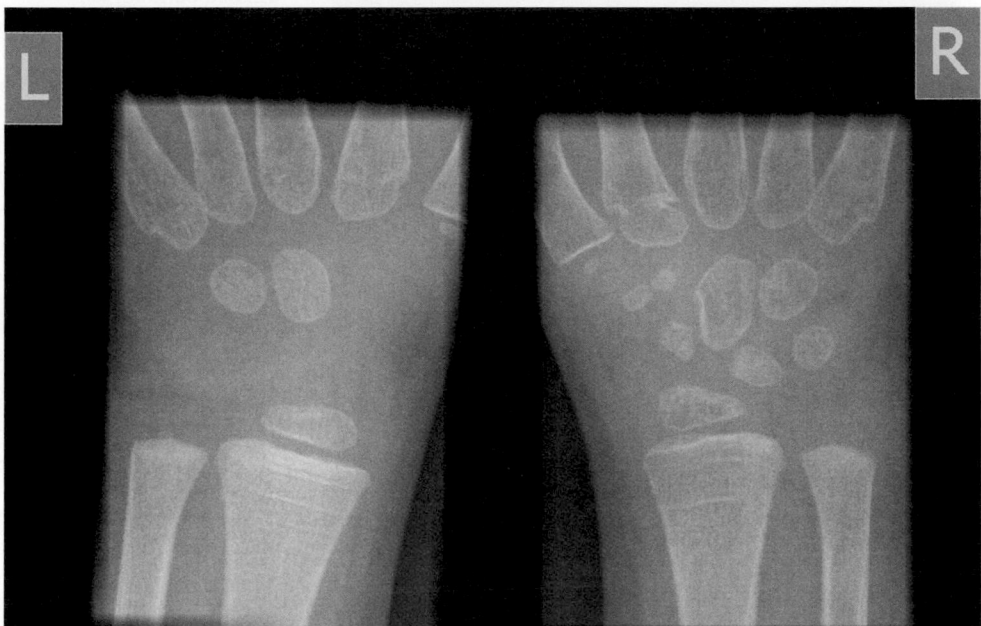

Fig. 71.3 Left and right AP radiographs of the wrist joint. The ossification of the right wrist joint is accelerated as a consequence of active disease within the joint. There is some generalized loss of joint space and cortical irregularity as a consequence of the disease process.

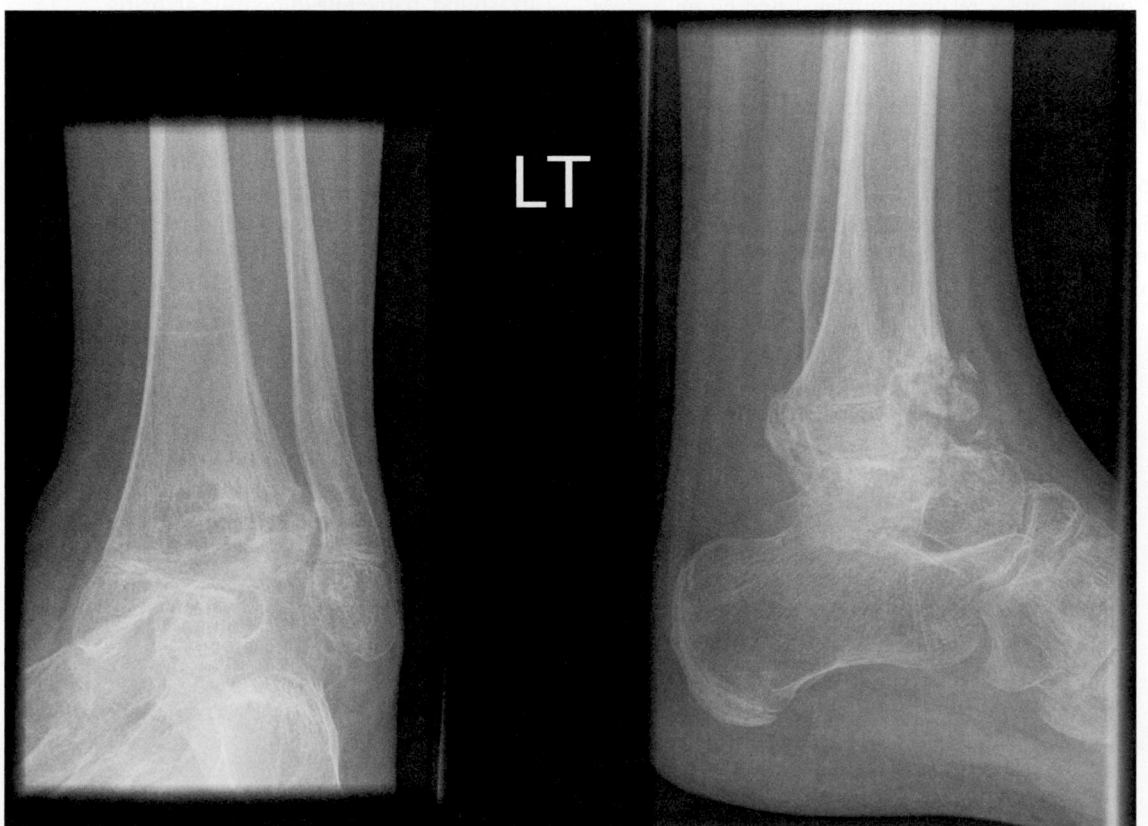

Fig. 71.4 AP and lateral radiographs of the left ankle showing severe joint destruction, extensive bony erosive changes, some early ankylosis, and fragmentation.

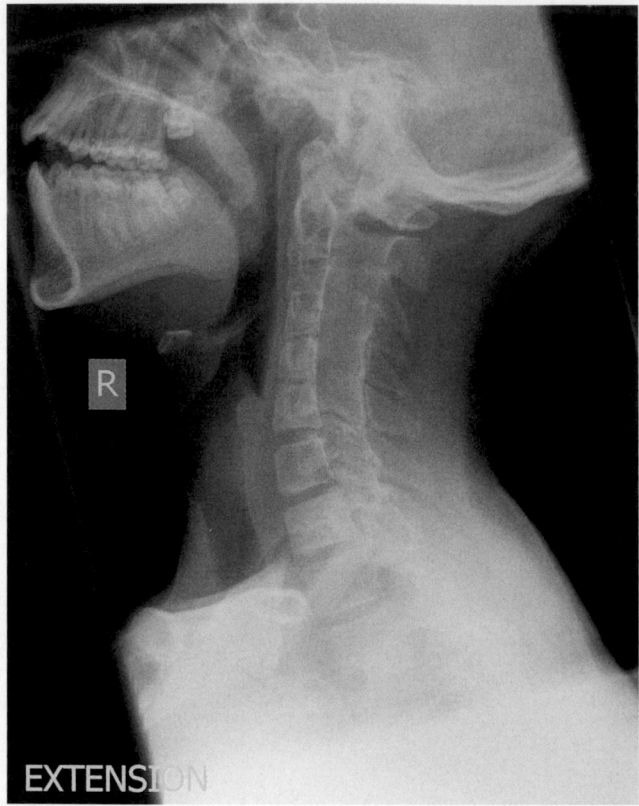

Fig. 71.5 Lateral cervical spine in a child with longstanding juvenile idiopathic arthritis shows extensive fusion of the facet joints and squaring of the vertebral bodies.

Pulmonary nodules are a relatively unusual finding on a chest radiograph in children. The clinical history is very important in determining the cause of lung nodules (Table 71.5). The use of high-resolution CT (HRCT) will improve the detection and determination of the lung changes.[20,21]

Ultrasonography

Ultrasound is increasingly being utilized in the management of paediatric musculoskeletal disorders. Apart from the fact that it does not involve ionizing radiation, it is relatively portable and can be used by a clinician within the consulting room, without the need for a referral to the radiology department. Ultrasound has the great advantage of being able to image joints, muscles, and tendons in real time motion. This allows the patient to reproduce signs and symptoms during the examination, and the stability and integrity of the joint can also be assessed. Any clinician using ultrasound must be aware of their own limitations and view the images within the appropriate clinical context, to avoid medico-legal consequences of missed pathology.

Role of ultrasound in musculoskeletal practice

Normal synovial membrane is too thin to be seen on ultrasound. Obviously with synovial hypertrophy, it becomes more visible. Synovium can be differentiated from joint effusion due to its vascularity and the fact it can be deformed with probe pressure (Figure 71.7). Increased blood flow on Doppler imaging is indicative of active synovitis, whereas it may be absent in chronic disease.

The joint capsule is a hypoechoic line separating the joint and para-articular soft tissues. Ligaments are also hypoechoic structures about the joint. Importantly, because of their fibrillar structure, they are anisotropic. When the ligament is perpendicular to the ultrasound beam it appears hyperechoic, and when visualized obliquely to the beam there is decreased reflection of sound, making it more hypoechoic.[22]

Tendons are also hyperechoic with a fibrillar echotexture and, like ligaments, demonstrate anisotropy. In children, the tendons often attach to hypoechoic cartilage that surrounds the ossification centre of the bone rather than the bone itself. A small amount of fluid around the tendon sheath is within normal limits.

Ultrasound in juvenile idiopathic arthritis

Within routine rheumatological practice, ultrasound is becoming of increasing clinical importance, and in a variety of anatomical areas it has been shown to be superior to clinical examination. There is increasing evidence that in children with JIA physical examination is neither highly sensitive or specific in identifying synovitis in a wide variety of joints. Ultrasonograhy has shown that subclinical synovitis is not uncommon. Some patients who meet the clinical criteria for remission may continue to show ongoing pathological features on joint ultrasound which may be suggestive of persisting

Table 71.3 Scoring systems

Scoring methods	Type of joints	Sample size	Authors	Reference number
Knee score	Knee	15	Pettersson et al.	18
Poznanski score	Wrist	94	Poznanski et al., Magni-Manzoni et al.	19, 20
Conventional and the modified Larsen's system	Wrists/hands	60	Doria et al.	21
Dijkstra composite score	Hand, foot and knee	66	Van Rossum et al.	22
Sharp and Larsen scoring systems	Wrist/hand	25	Rossi et al.	23
Adapted version of the Sharp/van der Heijde score	Wrist/hand	177	Ravelli et al.	24
Childhood arthritis radiographic score of the hip	Hip	148	Bertamino et al.	25

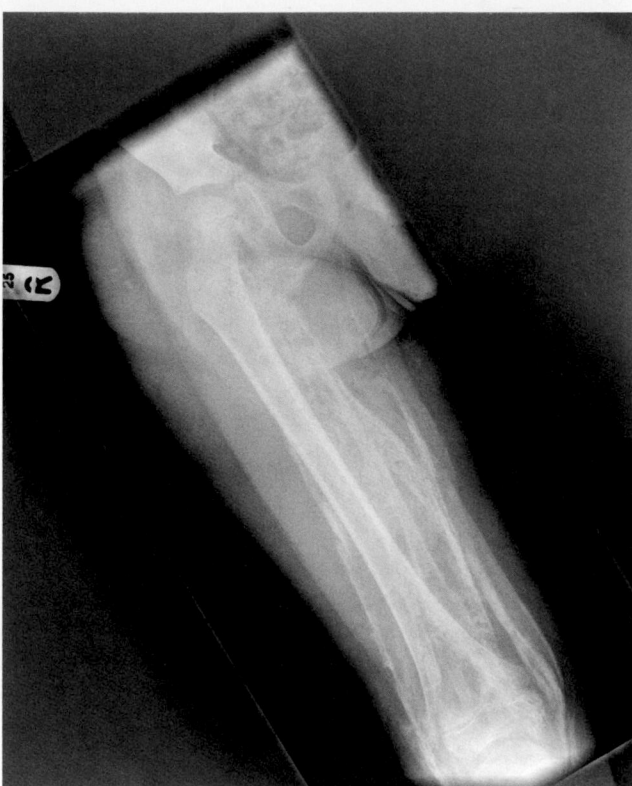

Fig. 71.6 Sheet calcification in the subcutaneous tissues of the right thigh in a child with juvenile dermatomyositis.

inflammation.[23–27] Within the ankle joint, ultrasound is more sensitive than clinical examination in determining tibiotalar joint effusions and for assessing tendonopathy.[28]

The implications for ultrasound screening in disease subclassification have yet to be fully evaluated, particularly with reference to subclinical synovitis which is detectable by ultrasound (and in some studies MRI as well). The current International League of Associations for Rheumatology (ILAR) classification determines if a child has oligoarthritis, extended oligoarthritis, or polyarthritis depending on the number of affected joints, based on clinical examination. Obviously, the addition of subclinical joint disease

Table 71.4 Causes of radiographic soft tissue calcification

Clumped/irregular calcification	Scleroderma
	Haemangioma
	Trauma (haematoma/burns/myositis ossificans)
	Synovial sarcoma
	Juvenile idiopathic arthritis (post joint injection)
	Tuberculosis.
	Parosteal osteosarcoma
	Parasitic infection
	Hyperparathyroidism
	Ehlers–Danlos syndrome
'Sheets' of calcification	Myositis ossificans progressiva
	Juvenile dermatomyositis

Table 71.5 Pulmonary nodules

Large pulmonary nodules	Metastatic lung disease, e.g. Wilm's tumour
	Single large nodule: consider round pneumonia
	Wegener's granulomatosis
	Aspergillosis
	Multiple haemangiomas
Small pulmonary nodules	Miliary TB
	Septic emboli (e.g. from central line infection)
	Fungal/candida disease in immunosuppressed patients
	Metastatic disease, e.g. rhabdomyosarcomas, osteosarcoma
	Past history of chickenpox pneumonia (calcified)
	Tuberous sclerosis and histiocytosis (usually cysts are also present)
	Sarcoid
Interstitial lung disease	Interstitial lung disease can be split into: nodular, reticular (linear opacities) and reticular nodular (linear and nodular opacities present)
Reticular	Heart failure causing interstitial oedema
	Idiopathic interstitial lung disease
	Alveolar proteinosis (ground-glass alveolar opacity also present)
	Radiation therapy
	Sarcoidosis (rare in children) nodules usually also present
	Lymphoma (rarely involves the lung parenchyma)
	Secondary to treatment, e.g. immunosuppressants such as tacrolimus
Reticular nodular	Histiocytosis (irregular cysts and nodules usually present)
	Sarcoidosis
	Tuberous sclerosis and neurofibromatosis

will alter a patient's classification, which may have important implications for inclusion in clinical trials or in the use of biological agents.[29,30]

The serial use of ultrasound is valuable in supplementing clinical assessment for disease monitoring and therapy. Ultrasound can be used to objectively assess the size of effusions and the degree of synovial proliferation. Response to steroid injections within the hips and knees has been documented. Colour Doppler provides an indication of the degree of vascularity of the synovial hypertrophy, and assessment of this vascularity may be useful in monitoring disease response.[31,32]

As well as detecting synovitis, ultrasound has been shown to have a role in the detection and evaluation of enthesitis in JIA. The detection of enthesitis is improved by the use of power Doppler and this has been shown to be superior to clinical examination. Particular areas which are useful for ultrasound evaluation are the Achilles, quadriceps insertion, gluteal insertion, and plantar fascia. Ultrasound can be used not only to visualize cartilage, but also assess its thickness.[33] However, ultrasound appears to be less

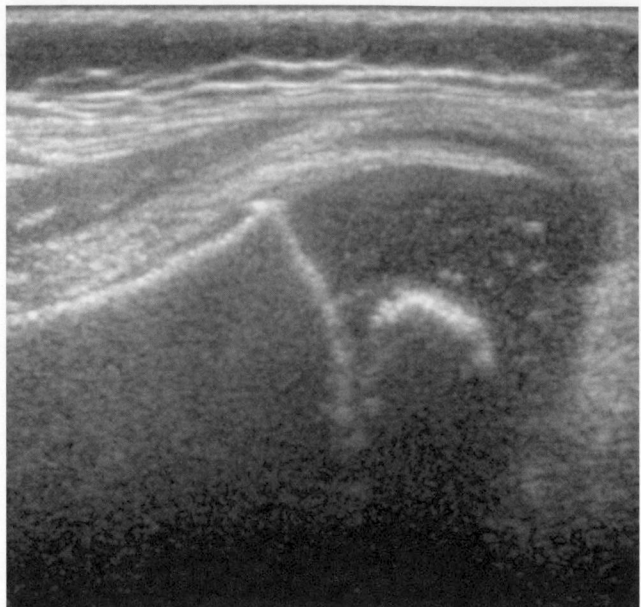

Fig. 71.7 Ultrasound of the distal femur show marked synovial thickening which is hypoechoic.

reliable in detecting bony erosions than MRI.[33–36] Tenosynovitis can often be detected by ultrasound and this is aided by the peripheral location of many structures. Distinguishing tenosynovitis from joint effusions is useful when subcategorizing JIA.[37,38]

Ultrasound contrast agents will improve detection and evaluation of the vascularity of synovium. This may prove useful in staging disease activity and monitoring disease response.[39,40]

Extra-articular rheumatological disease

The widespread use of ultrasound beyond the joint is well established and its use in rheumatological conditions will depend on the clinical situation. It is well recognized as a sensitive investigation of intra-abdominal pathology and for the assessment of vascular flow. Ultrasound can be used to determine the presence of pleural effusions within the chest and potentially as a guide to aspiration.

Ultrasound has been used to assess the signal intensity of muscle in children with JDMS. Inflamed muscle is relatively hyperechoic and the muscle fibres are typically slightly expanded in more active disease. However, in adult patients suspected of having dermatomyositis or polymyositis, contrast-enhanced ultrasound has been compared with MRI and biopsy findings and the sensitivity, specificity, and predictive values of ultrasound were found to be less than MRI.[41]

Magnetic resonance imaging

MRI does not use ionizing radiation, but utilizes the interaction of magnetic fields and radio waves to create an image. MRI scanners use very strong magnets, which can vary in strength from 0.25 to 3 T. (For comparison, the strength of the Earth's magnetic field is less than 60 μT.)

Positioning of the child within the magnet is important, so that they lie as close to the centre of the magnetic field as possible to improve signal homogeneity and reduce image artefacts. The use of a larger field of view (FOV) will improve the signal-to-noise ratio, but lead to reduction in spatial resolution. A smaller FOV

will increase spatial resolution, but will result in loss of signal, and there may need to be a compensatory increase in imaging time and the number of acquisitions.

Typical imaging systems are 1.5 T but there is an increasing availability of 3 T systems; the increased strength can be used to shorten examination times or improve image resolution. Tissue contrast on higher-level systems is not always reproducible, which may lead to interpretation problems if follow-up imaging is performed on different strength magnets, and consequently there may be a need to alter imaging sequences and parameters. With 3 T systems, there is potentially an increased risk from heating effect, noise, and bore size causing claustrophobia, which may cause some problems for some imaging of children.[42]

Depending on the send and receive parameters, the same tissue may appear bright or dark on the resultant image. In routine practice, the spin echo sequences are commonly used. These are termed either T1 weighted or T2 weighted, depending on the send and receive time of the radio waves used. A joint effusion is high signal on a T2-weighted sequence, and low signal on a T1-weighted dequence. Signal intensities of common structures on different sequences are listed in Table 71.6. In addition to these baseline echo sequences, vast numbers of other sequences and image protocols are available. Many of these are specific to certain manufacturers' own systems, but essentially they enable

Table 71.6 Common cause of high and low signal intensity appearances on T1- and T2-weighted spin echo sequences on 1.5 T MRI

T1-weighted image	
Low signal (dark)	Increased free water (oedema, tumour, infarction, inflammation, infection)
	Haemorrhage (hyperacute or chronic)
	Low density of protons (calcification, fibrous tissue, bone cortex)
	Flow void
High signal (bright)	Fat
	Subacute haemorrhage
	Melanin
	Protein-rich fluid
	Slow-flowing blood
	Paramagnetic substances: gadolinium, manganese, copper
	Calcification (rarely)
T2-weighted image	
Low signal (dark)	Low density of protons (calcification, fibrous tissue)
	Paramagnetic substances: deoxyhaemoglobin, methaemoglobin (intracellular), iron, ferritin, haemosiderin, melanin
	Protein-rich fluid
	Flow void
High signal (bright)	Increased water (oedema, CSF, tumour, infarction, inflammation, infection)
	Methaemoglobin (extracellular) in subacute haemorrhage
	Fat

the radiologist to tailor an MR examination to the exact clinical requirements.

Gadolinium is an intravenous contrast agent which is used with T1 weighted sequences; its uptake causes enhancement (increased signal) in areas of hypervascularity and disrupted cell membranes, hence inflamed synovium shows marked enhancement.

Role of MRI in musculoskeletal practice

The multiplanar ability, excellent image contrast, and tissue resolution of MRI is well recognized and its role in paediatric musculoskeletal disease is firmly established. In view of its relatively high cost, lengthy imaging time, and availability, MRI is not predominantly used as a first line investigation.

A water-sensitive sequences is needed for the detection of fluid, marrow oedema, and soft tissue inflammation. The most widely used are either short tau inversion recovery (STIR) or fat-suppressed T2-weighted spin echo sequences. On both these sequences, water is seen as high signal intensity. The signal intensity of muscle is typically higher on STIR sequences, so subtle change in muscle inflammation may be missed. Fat-suppressed T2 weighted sequences are more efficient, with more slices per given unit of time, but more susceptible to magnetic field in homogeneities and where the body part is outside the centre of the magnetic field.[42]

For general anatomy and assessment of the bone marrow, which is typically fatty from early childhood, a T1-weighted sequence is very useful. Proton density or intermediate weighted images have a relatively high signal-to-noise ratio and are helpful in depicting finer detail around joints. There are continuing developments in MR technology to create specific sequences for different anatomical areas within the joint. For instance, considerable research is being performed on imaging the cartilage and creating sequences which show the cartilage as high signal, and postprocessing techniques that allow measurements of the cartilage volume. Other sequences can demonstrate the level of hydration of the cartilage.[43–45]

Following gadolinium administration, normal enhancement occurs within the physis, the adjacent metaphyseal tissue, and the vascular channels supplying the epiphyseal ossification centre. Normal synovium, if not undetectable, may be seen as a thin, uniform rim around the articular surface. The addition of fat saturation techniques are valuable following gadolinium administration to suppress the high signal (T1 weighted) from adjacent fatty marrow, increasing the sensitivity of the imaging. STIR sequences should not be used in this regard as signal from gadolinium will also be suppressed.[5,42,43]

Contrast-enhanced MRI more reliably differentiates synovial inflammation, which shows increased contrast enhancement as it is of high signal on T1-weighted images, from non-enhancing joint effusions (Figure 71.8). Gadolinium will also discriminate between active hypervascular destructive pannus and inactive fibrous tissue. It is useful in evaluating infection, areas of avascular necrosis, and abscess formation.[46]

Clinical indications

MRI is sensitive and quite specific in detecting the site and severity of joint disease in children with arthritis, as well as assessing soft tissue and muscle involvement in other inflammatory conditions. It is the most sensitive imaging modality for the detection of ongoing synovial inflammation. MRI is superior to clinical examination and has been shown to detect persistent synovitis in subclinical patients as well as potentially predicting synovial disease in unaffected joints.[47] Its role is pivotal in selecting children for treatment options and monitoring treatment efficacy.[46,48]

It allows assessment of joints which are clinically difficult to image in other ways as well as being challenging to examine clinically, particularly the sacroiliac, temporomandibular, and subtalar joints (Figure 71.9).

Synovial inflammation

MRI is very sensitive in detecting synovial proliferation and assessing its extent and, in some cases, volume. The use of post gadolinium imaging is the most sensitive technique; this is either used with fat saturation techniques (where the signal intensity of fat is reduced) or with subtraction techniques (pre- and postcontrast images are subtracted from each other, just leaving the postcontrast changes). Gadolinium improves the contrast between enhancing hypervascular synovium and surrounding tissues. Post gadolinium images allow reliable differentiation from joint effusion and differentiation between destructive hypervascular synovium and more chronic inactive fibrotic tissue. It has been shown that the sensitivity of MRI is greater than that of clinical examination, and detection of subclinical synovium may predict disease extension.[46–49]

To assist in more objective measurement of disease, there has been an emphasis on measuring the degree and nature of inflammation with MRI. The measurement of synovial volume as a way of evaluating disease activity and response to treatment has been assessed within adult practice,[50] and the feasibility to do this in children is being researched.[51] It may be that synovial volume as a whole rather than maximum synovial thickness is the better marker for the degree of clinical synovitis. Certainly, reduction in synovial volume and a degree of enhancement correlates with improved clinical response.[52,53]

The other potentially objective measure of synovial activity is assessing the dynamics of contrast enhancement. Since the rate of contrast enhancement is increased by greater hypervascularity and capillary permeability, then the greater the inflammatory response within a tissue, the higher the rate of contrast enhancement. Dynamic contrast enhancement has been shown to be a sensitive and relatively accurate method of assessing synovitis and therapy response in adults.[54–55]

While both volume assessment and dynamic contrast enhancement are being increasingly utilized, they require a significant amount of postimaging processing, significant research resource, and appropriate computer software.

Bone marrow oedema

On MRI, the signal intensity of bone marrow will alter depending on the amount of haemopoietic and fatty marrow. Bone marrow oedema reflects the increased signal seen within the bone marrow on T2-weighted images, which in most cases reflects localized inflammation and increased water content (marrow oedema). Caution must be taken, as in certain individuals signal intensity changes may occur within the marrow which just reflects normal growth and maturation of the bone marrow.[55] This can cause confusion between normal physiological change and bone marrow oedema/early erosions. An understanding of normal physiological changes and the age of these changes is required. In particular, patchy signal change within the foot is well recognized and should not be confused with erosive disease.[56,57]

Localized bone marrow oedema has been shown to correlate with erosive damage in adults with rheumatoid arthritis.[58–60]

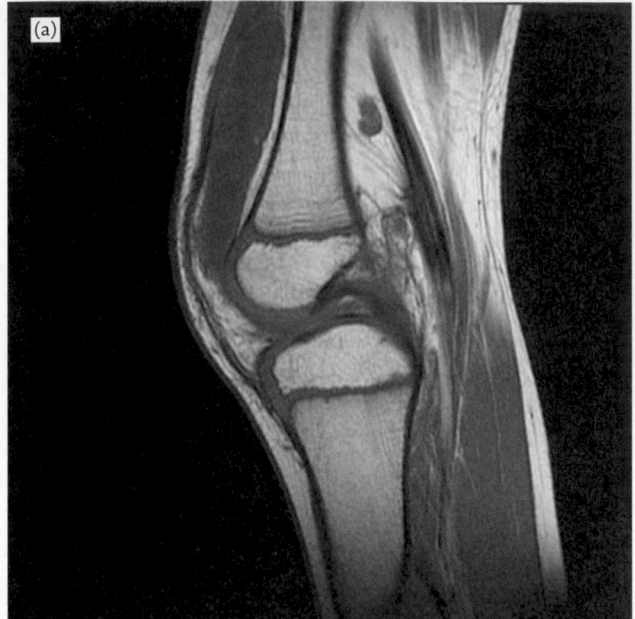
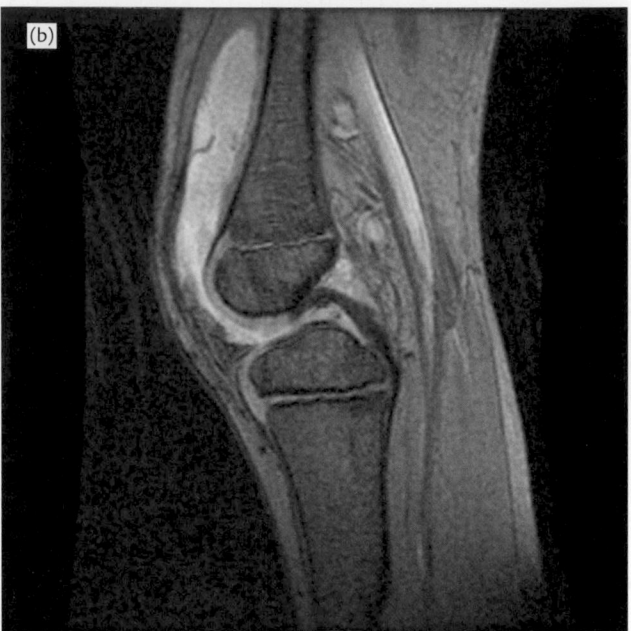
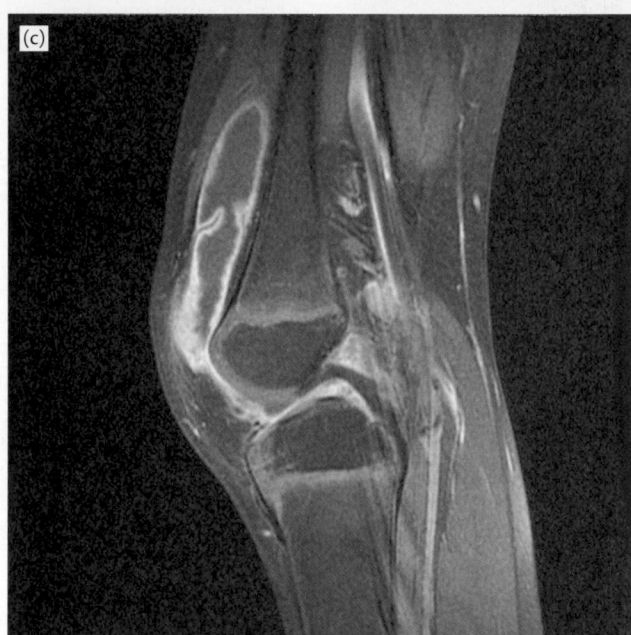

Fig. 71.8 Serial MRI demonstrating the use of gadolinium as a contrast agent: (a) T2-weighted sagittal image of the knee showing a large effusion and popliteal lymphadenopathy. (b) T1-weighted images in the same patient confirm the presence of the effusion and lymphadenopathy. (c) Postcontrast T1 fat-saturated image demonstrates the marked enhancement of the synovium (high signal intensity) surrounding the fluid (low signal intensity) within the suprapatellar bursa. The popliteal lymph nodes are also enhanced.

Histological studies in adults have shown that areas of bone marrow oedema on MRI contain inflammatory cellular infiltrates which may suggest a mechanism to explain the development of erosions.[61] The exact significance of bone marrow oedema and its prognostic evaluation in terms of erosive change in JIA is undefined. The presence of bone marrow oedema and its implication in terms of treatment in JIA is unknown.

Cartilage imaging

MRI is able to directly visualize both articular and growth (epiphyseal and physeal) cartilage. Consequently, a proper assessment of cartilage damage is possible. The assessment of cartilage has been

significantly improved in recent years by the use of dedicated MR sequences, allowing assessment of thinning, erosions and signal change.[42,43,45]

With ultra-short TE sequences, driven equilibrium Fourier, and steady-state free procession sequences, high-resolution volume acquisitions allow significant postprocessing manipulation to detect subtle surface irregularity and tiny focal defects of the articular cartilage.

Bone erosions

Bone erosions are typically well-defined subcortical lesions and may contain either fluid or synovial tissue. MRI is able to detect

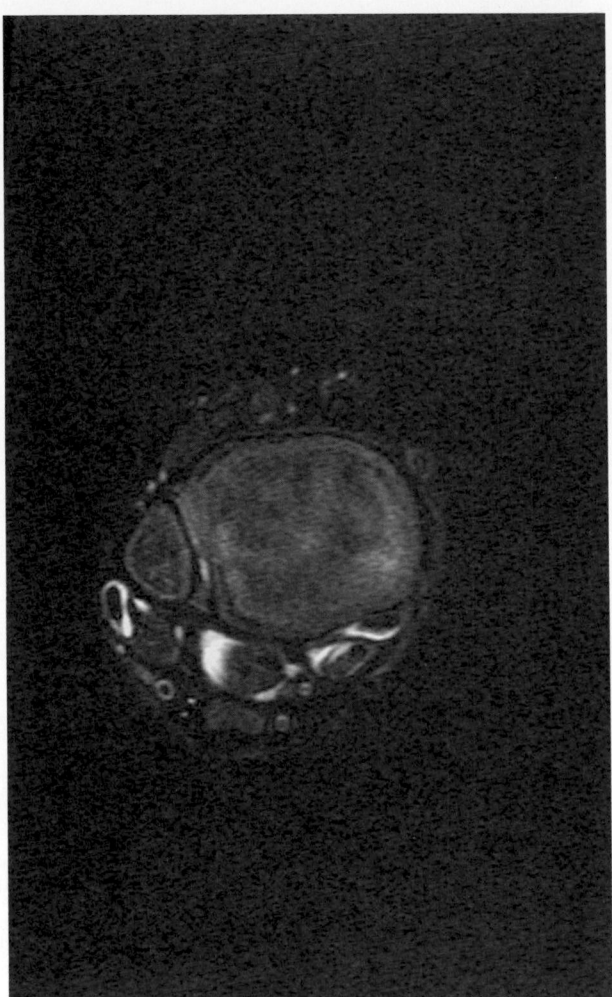

Fig. 71.9 Axial T2-weighted images through the ankle joint showing effusions around the extensor and peroneal tendons.

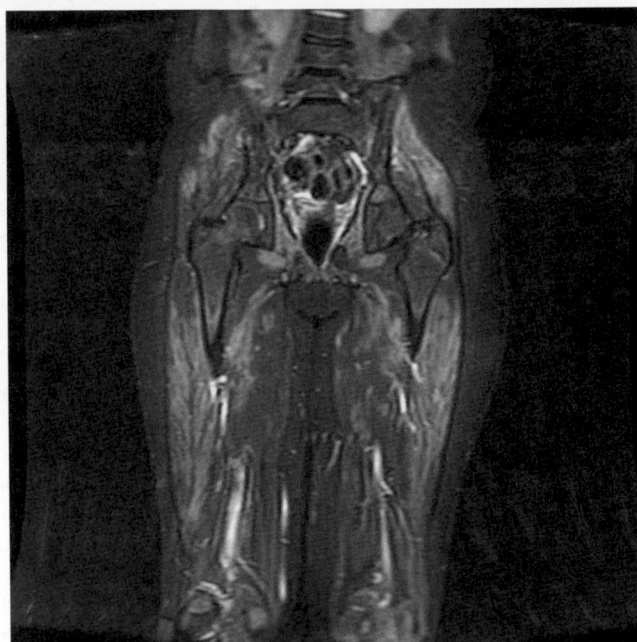

Fig. 71.10 Coronal STIR images in a child with juvenile dermatomyositis. There is bilateral symmetrical muscle oedema with a preponderance for proximal muscle involvement.

subchondral changes within the bone prior to any obvious radiographic changes. The significance and long-term outcome of the subchondral changes and whether or not they are true early erosions is a cause for debate. However, it is recognized that MRI is more sensitive in detecting erosions than either ultrasound or radiography.[33,34,58,61] Studies in adults demonstrate significant prognostic value of MR-detectable lesions with respect to long-term radiographic damage.[55,61,62,63] Erosions on MRI may be associated with cartilage loss. The bone defect may be fluid filled or filled with synovium; with the latter, there will be enhancement following gadolinium administration.

Muscle disease

MRI is the most sensitive investigation for evaluating myositis. Its specificity in classical JDMS is high. Abnormal increased signal intensity on T2-weighted images is seen in skeletal muscles in nearly all patients with acute symptoms of myositis; in JDMS, the distribution is typically proximal (Figure 71.10). The increased T2 signal is believed to represent an acute accumulation of extracellular water and recent-onset microinfarction. The use of whole-body MRI permits a global view of the muscle groups and is useful in clinical monitoring and follow-up. MRI can also facilitate biopsy.[64–67]

MRI techniques can be used to evaluate the degree of inflammatory activity within the muscle, which may provide an objective measure of disease activity. Techniques that have been employed include T2 mapping, which relies on relaxation times of the muscle.[68] Diffusion-weighted MRI can provide tissue fluid motion data to differentiate capillary blood flow from intra- and extracellular compartmental fluid.[67] Phosphorus spectroscopy has also been used to evaluate the constituents of inflammatory muscle.[69]

In more chronic disease, there is increased fat deposition within the muscle. Calcification deposition, which can occur in JDMS, may be related to signal change within the subcutaneous fat.[70]

Vascular imaging

Children who have a variety of autoimmune conditions may be at a significant risk of vascular and cerebral involvement. Magnetic resonance angiography (MRA) can provided detailed imaging of both peripheral and cerebral blood vessels and demonstrate stenoses or small aneurysms. HRCT is also very useful, but involves a radiation dose. In both CT and MRI the image quality is typically sufficient to avoid formal interventional angiography.

MRI is the modality of choice to assess for changes of cerebral vasculitis and SLE. In SLE, there may be focal infarcts and multiple areas of high signal on T2-weighted images, indicating microinfarcts. Multiple white-matter lesions are often associated with neuropsychiatric symptoms.

Computed tomography (CT)

CT utilizes X-radiation to produce an image. As opposed to conventional radiography where a single X-ray beam is passed through the body, with CT, multiple beams are passed through the patient and absorbed by a number of detectors. The current generation of dual-energy CT scanners have two X-ray beams of different voltage, allowing greater image manipulation, reduced radiation dose, and decreased scan times.

Role of CT in musculoskeletal practice

CT is very valuable in the assessment of skeletal injuries. It is the imaging modality of choice following major trauma, being both fast and sensitive in the detection of intracranial, thoracic, abdominal, and skeletal injures. It is essential in the acute management of the severely injured child.

CT is also useful in the assessment, treatment planning and follow-up of peripheral fractures. It is complementary to MRI in the evaluation of spinal pathology including spondylolysis.[71]

With regard to rheumatological conditions, the use of CT is relatively limited. It provides excellent resolution of bony detail, but it is not as sensitive as MRI in the assessment of soft tissues and intra-articular pathology. CT imaging involves a significant radiation dose and so there needs to be a clear indication for its use.

Within the chest, HRCT is the modality of choice for the assessment of lung parenchyma; it allows detection and characterization of the pattern of distribution of interstitial lung disease. CT angiography can be used to assess the vascular anatomy, including the detection of aneurysmal disease, stenosis, and thrombus.

Bone scintigraphy

Radionuclide imaging has a relatively limited role in the musculoskeletal system. It can be used to assess multiple foci, such as in multifocal osteomyelitis. It may be helpful in assessing for fractures or tumours. It has a limited role in the assessment of joint disease.

The procedures involve a relatively high radiation dose and while they are relatively sensitive, they are of low specificity. The most commonly used isotope is technetium-labelled methylene disphosphonate (^{99m}Tc-MDP). This isotope is taken up by osteoblasts and therefore reflects areas of increased bone turnover. ^{99m}Tc-MDP has a half-life of 6 hours, which means that half the radionuclide activity will have disappeared in 6 hours. The amount of activity to be injected will depend on the body weight and the age of the child. Less than 70% will be taken up by the bone and soft tissues, with the rest renally excreted. This will result in a relatively high affective dose to the body. Consequently, the use of bone scintigraphy should be reserved for specific cases.

The uptake of ^{99m}Tc-MDP in bone depends on the metabolism of phosphates which are absorbed by bone and absorbed into the matrix. The uptake is related to local blood supply, rate of bone turnover, the quantity of mineralized bone, local capillary permeability, and the fluid pressure within the bone. It is possible to image within an early vascular phase to assess the blood flow to a lesion followed by delayed static phases to assess bone turnover.

Single photon emission CT (SPECT) is a technique which increases spatial information, improving the sensitivity of the bone scan, particularly in those areas where there is overlapping bone, such as the spine.

The relative dose with radionuclide imaging is high and in most clinical situations an alternative, often non-ionizing investigation, can be employed. Whole-body MRI is being increasingly used instead of radionuclide studies to image the whole of the skeleton in order to assess for widespread skeletal lesions, such as metastases, and in Langerhans cell histiocytosis.

References

1. Petty RE, Southwood TR, Manners P et al. International League of Associations for Rheumatology. International League of Associations for Rheumatology classification of juvenile idiopathic arthritis: second revision, Edmonton, 2001. *J Rheumatol* 2004;31(2):390–392.

2. Johnson K. Imaging of juvenile idiopathic arthritis. *Pediatr Radiol* 2006;36(8):743–758.

3. Sury MR, Harker H, Begent J, Chong WK. The management of infants and children for painless imaging. *Clin Radiol* 2005;60(7):731–741.

4. Sury MR, Hatch DJ, Deeley T, Dicks-Mireaux C, Chong WK. Development of a nurse-led sedation service for paediatric magnetic resonance imaging. *Lancet* 1999;353(9165):1667–1671.

5. Keats TE, Anderson MW. *Atlas of normal roentgen variants that may simulate disease*, 7th edn. Mosby, St. Louis, MO, 2001.

6. Williams H. Normal anatomical variants and other mimics of skeletal trauma. In: Johnson KJ, Bache E (eds) *Imaging of pediatric skeletal trauma*. Springer, Berlin, 2008:91–118.

7 Breton S, Jousse-Joulin S, Finel E et al. Imaging approaches for evaluating peripheral joint abnormalities in juvenile idiopathic arthritis. *Semin Arthritis Rheum* 2012;41(5):698–711.

8 Johnson K. Imaging of juvenile idiopathic arthritis. *Pediatr Radiol* 2006;36(8):743–758.

9. Cohen PA, Job-Deslandre CH, Lalande G, Adamsbaum C. Overview of the radiology of juvenile idiopathic arthritis (JIA). *Eur J Radiol* 2000;33(2):94–101.

10. Anderson Gare B. Juvenile arthritis—who gets it, where and when? A review of current data on incidence and prevalence. *Clin Exp Rheumatol* 1999;17:367–374.

11. Pettersson H, Rydholm U. Radiologic classification of knee joint destruction in juvenile chronic arthritis. *Pediatr Radiol* 1984;14:419–421.

12. Poznanski AK, Hernandez RJ, Guire KE et al. Carpal length in children—a useful measurement in the diagnosis of rheumatoid arthritis and some congenital malformation syndromes. *Radiology* 1978;129:661–668.

13. Magni-Manzoni S, Rossi F, Pistorio A et al. Prognostic factors for radiographic progression, damage, and disability in juvenile idiopathic arthritis. *Arthritis Rheum* 2003;48(12):3509–3517.

14. Doria AS, de Castro CC, Kiss MH et al. Inter- and intrareader variability in the interpretation of two radiographic classification systems in juvenile rheumatoid arthritis. *Pediatr Radiol* 2003;33:673–681.

15. Van Rossum MA, Boers M, Zwinderman AH. Development of a standardized method of assessment of radiographs and radiographic changes in juvenile idiopathic arthritis: introduction of the Dijkstra composite score. *Arthritis Rheum* 2005;52:2865–2872.

16. Rossi F, Di Dia F, Galipo O et al. Use of the Sharp and Larsen scoring method in the assessment of radiographic progression in juvenile idiopathic arthritis. *Arthritis Rheum* 2006;55:717–723.

17. Ravelli A, Ioseliani M, Norambuena X et al. Adapted versions of the Sharp/van der Heijde score are reliable and valid for assessment of radiographic progression in JIA. *Arthritis Rheum* 2007;56:3087–3095.

18. Bertamino M, Rossi F, Pistorio A et al. Development and initial validation of a radiographic scoring system for the hip in juvenile idiopathic arthritis. *J Rheumatol* 2010;37:432–439.

19. Ravelli AJ. The time has come to include assessment of radiographic progression in juvenile idiopathic arthritis clinical trials. *Rheumatology* 2008;35(4):553–557.

20. van Zeggeren L, van de Ven AA, Terheggen-Lagro SW et al. High-resolution computed tomography and pulmonary function in children with common variable immunodeficiency. *Eur Respir J* 2011;38(6):1437–1443.

21. Kim EA, Lee KS, Johkoh T et al. Interstitial lung diseases associated with collagen vascular diseases: radiologic and histopathologic findings. *Radiographics* 2002;22 Spec No:S151–S165.

22. Fornage BD. The case for ultrasound of muscles and tendons. *Semin Musculoskelet Radiol* 2000;4(4):375–391.

23. Rebollo-Polo M, Koujok K, Weisser C et al. Ultrasound findings on patients with juvenile idiopathic arthritis in clinical remission. *Arthritis Care Res* (Hoboken) 2011;63(7):1013–1019.

24. Filippou G, Cantarini L, Bertoldi I et al. Ultrasonography vs. clinical examination in children with suspected arthritis. Does it make sense

to use poliarticular ultrasonographic screening? *Clin Exp Rheumatol* 2011;29(2):345–350.

25. Janow GL, Panghaal V, Trinh A et al. Detection of active disease in juvenile idiopathic arthritis: sensitivity and specificity of the physical examination vs ultrasound. *J Rheumatol* 2011;38(12):2671–2674.

26. Karmazyn B, Bowyer SL, Schmidt KM et al. US findings of metacarpophalangeal joints in children with idiopathic juvenile arthritis. *Pediatr Radiol* 2007;37(5):475–482.

27. Magni-Manzoni S, Epis O, Ravelli A et al. Comparison of clinical versus ultrasound-determined synovitis in juvenile idiopathic arthritis. *Arthritis Rheum* 2009;61(11):1497–1504.

28. Pascoli L, Wright S, McAllister C, Rooney M. Prospective evaluation of clinical and ultrasound findings in ankle disease in juvenile idiopathic arthritis: importance of ankle ultrasound. *JRheumatol* 2010;37(11): 2409–2414.

29. Haslam KE, McCann LJ, Wyatt S, Wakefield RJ. The detection of subclinical synovitis by ultrasound in oligoarticular juvenile idiopathic arthritis: a pilot study. *Rheumatology* (Oxford) 2010;49(1):123–127.

30. Wallace CA, Ruperto N, Giannini E. Preliminary criteria for clinical remission for select categories of juvenile idiopathic arthritis. Childhood Arthritis and Rheumatology Research Alliance; Pediatric Rheumatology International Trials Organization; Pediatric Rheumatology Collaborative Study Group. *J Rheumatol* 2004;31(11):2290–2294.

31. Strunk J, Strube K, Müller-Ladner U, Lange U. Three dimensional power Doppler ultrasonography confirms early reduction of synovial perfusion after intra-articular steroid injection. *Ann Rheum Dis* 2006;65(3):411–412.

32. Doria AS, Kiss MH, Lotito AP et al. Juvenile rheumatoid arthritis of the knee: evaluation with contrast-enhanced color Doppler ultrasound. *Pediatr Radiol* 2001;31(7):524–531.

33. Spannow AH, Pfeiffer-Jensen M, Andersen NT, Stenbøg E, Herlin T. Inter- and intraobserver variation of ultrasonographic cartilage thickness assessments in small and large joints in healthy children. *Pediatr Rheumatol Online J* 2009;7:12.

34. Malattia C, Damasio MB, Magnaguagno F et al. Magnetic resonance imaging, ultrasonography, and conventional radiography in the assessment of bone erosions in juvenile idiopathic arthritis. *Arthritis Rheum* 2008;59(12):1764–1772.

35. Wakefield RJ, Conaghan PG, Jarrett S, Emery P. Noninvasive techniques for assessing skeletal changes in inflammatory arthritis: imaging technique. *Curr Opin Rheumatol* 2004;16(4):435–442.

36. Malattia C, Damasio MB, Magnaguagno F et al. Magnetic resonance imaging, ultrasonography, and conventional radiography in the assessment of bone erosions in juvenile idiopathic arthritis. *Arthritis Rheum* 2008;59(12):1764–1772.

37. Rooney ME, McAllister C, Burns JF. Ankle disease in juvenile idiopathic arthritis: ultrasound findings in clinically swollen ankles. *J Rheumatol* 2009;36(8):1725–1729.

38. Hendry GJ, Gardner-Medwin J, Steultjens MP et al. Frequent discordance between clinical and musculoskeletal ultrasound examinations of foot disease in juvenile idiopathic arthritis. *Arthritis Care Res* (Hoboken) 2012;64(3):441–447.

39. De Zordo T, Mlekusch SP, Feuchtner GM et al. Value of contrast-enhanced ultrasound in rheumatoid arthritis. *Eur J Radiol* 2007;64(2):222–230.

40. Shahin AA, el-Mofty SA, el-Sheikh EA, Hafez HA, Ragab OM. Power Doppler sonography in the evaluation and follow-up of knee involvement in patients with juvenile idiopathic arthritis. *J Rheumatol* 2001; 60(3):148–155.

41. Weber MA, Jappe U, Essig M et al. Contrast-enhanced ultrasound in dermatomyositis- and polymyositis. *J Neurol* 2006; 253:1625–1632.

42. Jaramillo D, Laor T. Pediatric musculoskeletal MRI: basic principles to optimize success. *Pediatr Radiol* 2008;38(4):379–391.

43. Buchmann RF, Jaramillo D. Imaging of articular disorders in children. *Radiol Clin North Am* 2004;42(1):151–168, vii.

44. Kim HK, Laor T, Graham TB et al. T2 relaxation time changes in distal femoral articular cartilage in children with juvenile idiopathic arthritis: a 3-year longitudinal study. *AJR Am J Roentgenol* 2010;195(4):1021–1025.

45. Jazrawi LM, Alaia MJ, Chang G, Fitzgerald EF, Recht MP. Advances in magnetic resonance imaging of articular cartilage. *J Am Acad Orthop Surg* 2011;19(7):420–429.

46. Lamer S, Sebag GH. MRI and ultrasound in children with juvenile chronic arthritis. *Eur J Radiol* 2000;33(2):85–93.

47. Gardner-Medwin JM, Killeen OG, Ryder CA, Bradshaw K, Johnson K. Magnetic resonance imaging identifies features in clinically unaffected knees predicting extension of arthritis in children with monoarthritis. *J Rheumatol* 2006;33(11):2337–2343.

48. Küseler A, Pedersen TK, Gelineck J, Herlin T. A 2 year followup study of enhanced magnetic resonance imaging and clinical examination of the temporomandibular joint in children with juvenile idiopathic arthritis. *J Rheumatol* 2005;32(1):162–169.

49. Gylys-Morin VM, Graham TB, Blebea JS et al. Knee in early juvenile rheumatoid arthritis: MR imaging findings. *Radiology* 2001;220(3):696–706.

50. Cimmino MA, Bountis C, Silvestri E, Garlaschi G, Accardo S. An appraisal of magnetic resonance imaging of the wrist in rheumatoid arthritis. *Semin Arthritis Rheum* 2000;30(3):180–195.

51. Graham TB, Laor T, Dardzinski BJ. Quantitative magnetic resonance imaging of the hands and wrists of children with juvenile rheumatoid arthritis. *J Rheumatol* 2005;32(9):1811–1820.

52. Hodgson RJ, Barnes T, Connolly S et al. Changes underlying the dynamic contrast-enhanced MRI response to treatment in rheumatoid arthritis. *Skeletal Radiol* 2008;37(3):201–207.

53. Tan AL, Keen HI, Emery P, McGonagle D. Imaging inflamed synovial joints. *Methods Mol Med* 2007;135:3–26.

54. McQueen FM. The MRI view of synovitis and tenosynovitis in inflammatory arthritis: implications for diagnosis and management. *Ann N Y Acad Sci* 2009;1154:21–34.

55. Foster K, Chapman S, Johnson K. MRI of the marrow in the paediatric skeleton. *Clin Radiol* 2004;59(8):651–673.

56. Pal CR, Tasker AD, Ostlere SJ, Watson MS. Heterogeneous signal in bone marrow on MRI of children's feet: a normal finding? *Skeletal Radiol* 1999;28(5):274–278.

57. Zubler V, Mengiardi B, Pfirrmann CW et al. Bone marrow changes on STIR MR images of asymptomatic feet and ankles. *Eur Radiol* 2007;17(12):3066–3072.

58. McQueen FM, Benton N, Perry D et al. Bone edema scored on magnetic resonance imaging scans of the dominant carpus at presentation predicts radiographic joint damage of the hands and feet six years later in patients with rheumatoid arthritis. *Arthritis Rheum* 2003;48(7):1814–1827.

59. Gandjbakhch F, Conaghan PG, Ejbjerg B et al. Synovitis and osteitis are very frequent in rheumatoid arthritis clinical remission: results from an MRI study of 294 patients in clinical remission or low disease activity state. *J Rheumatol* 2011;38(9):2039–44.

60. Benton N, Stewart N, Crabbe J et al. MRI of the wrist in early rheumatoid arthritis can be used to predict functional outcome at 6 years. *Ann Rheum Dis* 2004;63(5):555–561.

61. Dalbeth N, Smith T, Gray S et al. Cellular characterisation of magnetic resonance imaging bone oedema in rheumatoid arthritis; implications for pathogenesis of erosive disease. *Ann Rheum Dis* 2009;68(2):279–282.

62. Haavardsholm EA, Bøyesen P, Østergaard M, Schildvold A, Kvien TK. Magnetic resonance imaging findings in 84 patients with early rheumatoid arthritis: bone marrow oedema predicts erosive progression. *Ann Rheum Dis* 2008;67(6):794–800.

63. McQueen FM, Dalbeth Predicting joint damage in rheumatoid arthritis using MRI scanning. *Arthritis Res Ther* 2009;11(5):124.

64. Tzaribachev N, Well C, Schedel J, Horger M. Whole-body MRI: a helpful diagnostic tool for juvenile dermatomyositis case report and review of the literature. *Rheumatol Int* 2009;29(12):1511–1514.

65. O'Connell MJ, Powell T, Brennan D et al. Whole-body MR imaging in the diagnosis of polymyositis. *AJR Am J Roentgenol* 2002;179(4):967–971.

66. Hernandez RJ, Keim DR, Sullivan DB, Chenevert TL, Martel WJ. Magnetic resonance imaging appearance of the muscles in childhood dermatomyositis. *Pediatrics* 1990;117(4):546–550.

67. Qi J, Olsen NJ, Price RR, Winston JA, Park JH. Diffusion-weighted imaging of inflammatory myopathies: polymyositis and dermatomyositis. *J Magn Reson Imaging* 2008;27(1):212–217.

68. Maillard SM, Jones R, Owens C etal. Quantitative assessment of MRI T2 relaxation time of thigh muscles in juvenile dermatomyositis. *Rheumatology* (Oxford) 2004;43(5):603–608.

69. Park JH, Niermann KJ, Ryder NM et al. Muscle abnormalities in juvenile dermatomyositis patients: P-31 magnetic resonance spectroscopy studies. *Arthritis Rheum* 2000;43(10):2359–2367.

70. Ladd PE, Emery KH, Salisbury SR et al. Juvenile ermatomyositis: correlation of MRI at presentation with clinical outcome. *AJR Am J Roentgenol* 2011;197(1):W153–W158.

71. Campbell RS, Grainger AJ, Hide IG, Papastefanou S, Greenough CG. Juvenile spondylolysis: a comparative analysis of CT, SPECT and MRI. *Skeletal Radiol* 2005;34(2):63–73.

CHAPTER 72

Assessment of synovial joint fluid

Engy Abdelattif and Anthony J. Freemont

Introduction

Normal synovial fluid

Normal synovial fluid (SF) enables joint lubrication[1] and cartilage nutrition.[2] It is formed from a transudate of plasma supplemented by other molecules (complex lipids, proteoglycans, and peptides), synthesized largely by fibroblast-derived type B synoviocytes.

There is no physical barrier between SF and the matrix of articular cartilage or synovium. This allows fluid flow through the tissues lining the joint, particularly during loading, and the development of a relatively uniform chemical environment.

Debris and particulate material are cleared from the joint by macrophage-derived type A synoviocytes. A lack of physical barriers allows inflammatory cells to migrate into the synovial fluid and chondrocytes to enter SF from the cartilage surface.

Thus normal SF is a viscous, hypocellular, fluid containing a mixture of synovium and cartilage-derived cells. Its chemical composition reflects that within the synovium and cartilage.

Synovial fluid in diseased joints

During disease, joints often swell by accumulation of SF. This reflects alterations in the permeability of the synovial vasculature.

The chemical and cellular composition of SF changes in disease with alterations of the environment in synovium and cartilage. Although some of the biochemical changes are predictable, others can only be explained on the basis of a degree of partitioning between synovium, SF, and cartilage, based on differences in their composition and the ease with which cells and molecules move within and between them. In addition, during disease, particulate material derived from, or formed within, the joint accumulates in SF.

The fact that the chemical, particulate, and cellular composition of synovial fluid changes with disease means that analysis of these components of SF can be used as the basis of diagnostic (and prognostic) tests. Particles and cells can be recognized by microscopy, and chemical biomarkers by assay.

Synovial fluid microscopy

SF microscopy has been carried out as a diagnostic test for years. Unfortunately it is not always done well, limiting its value to the rheumatologist.[3] As such, it does not have a high credibility. However, detailed microscopic analysis of SF by specialist histopathologists/cytopathologists can yield useful information about the nature of joint diseases and their prognosis.[4,5] For instance, in one published study[6] using algorithms based on microscopy alone (Figure 72.1) we examined 200 consecutive SF samples without knowledge of any clinical details, comparing blinded cytological and clinical diagnoses at the end of the study. Matching diagnoses were made in 35.5% and a short list of differential diagnoses (e.g. seronegative spondylarthropathy), was proffered, which included the clinical diagnosis, in a further 21.5%. Of the rest, 31.5% were correctly described as inflammatory or non-inflammatory and in 2.5% no diagnosis could be made. Only in 3.5% was a false-positive cytological diagnosis made.

Basic approach to synovial fluid microscopy

The following is a guide to show the diversity of cells and particles and how their identification can be used diagnostically.[7–9]

Specimen handling

As SF is 'fresh', it should be examined within 24 hours of aspiration. Examination should be undertaken in such a way as to minimize potential infection risks. Similarly, as inflammatory SF contains fibrin and tends to clot, it is essential that samples should reach the laboratory in anticoagulant. Crystalline anticoagulants should be avoided, for obvious reasons.[4]

Visual and microscopic examination of synovial fluid

The examination of SF is in four parts.

Visual analysis

The colour, turbidity, and presence of obvious particles are recorded. Colour gives important information (e.g. presence of haemorrhage or chromogen-producing organism) and turbidity gives data on the number of particles (cells, crystals, etc.) in the fluid.

Nucleated cell count

Manual counting using a haemocytometer chamber is the traditional way to count nucleated cells; nowadays automated computerized instruments are available.

For convenience of handling large numbers, the SF nucleated cell count is traditionally expressed as cells/mm^3. Normal SF contains

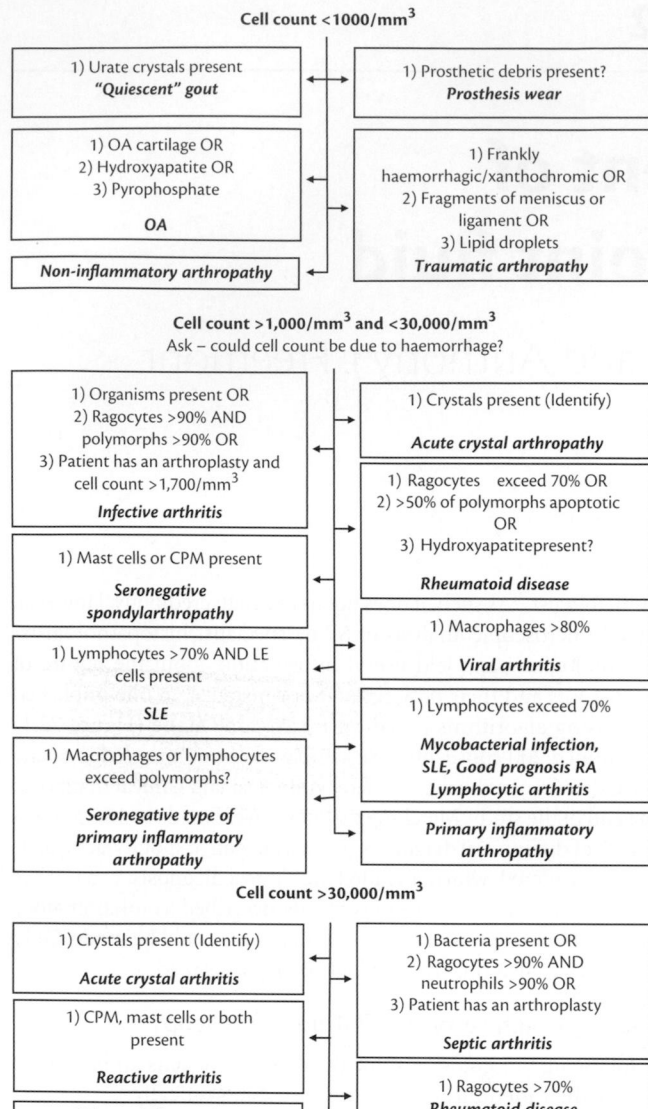

Cell count <1000/mm³

| 1) Urate crystals present
"Quiescent" gout | → | 1) Prosthetic debris present?
Prosthesis wear |

| 1) OA cartilage OR
2) Hydroxyapatite OR
3) Pyrophosphate

OA | → | 1) Frankly
haemorrhagic/xanthochromic OR
2) Fragments of meniscus or
ligament OR
3) Lipid droplets
Traumatic arthropathy |

| ***Non-inflammatory arthropathy*** |

Cell count >1,000/mm³ and <30,000/mm³
Ask – could cell count be due to haemorrhage?

| 1) Organisms present OR
2) Ragocytes >90% AND
polymorphs >90% OR
3) Patient has an arthroplasty and
cell count >1,700/mm³
Infective arthritis | → | 1) Crystals present (Identify)
Acute crystal arthropathy |

| 1) Mast cells or CPM present
***Seronegative
spondylarthropathy*** | → | 1) Ragocytes exceed 70% OR
2) >50% of polymorphs apoptotic
OR
3) Hydroxyapatite present?
Rheumatoid disease |

| 1) Lymphocytes >70% AND LE
cells present
SLE | → | 1) Macrophages >80%
Viral arthritis |

| 1) Macrophages or lymphocytes
exceed polymorphs?
***Seronegative type of
primary inflammatory
arthropathy*** | → | 1) Lymphocytes exceed 70%
***Mycobacterial infection,
SLE, Good prognosis RA
Lymphocytic arthritis*** |

| | | ***Primary inflammatory
arthropathy*** |

Cell count >30,000/mm³

| 1) Crystals present (Identify)
Acute crystal arthritis | → | 1) Bacteria present OR
2) Ragocytes >90% AND
neutrophils >90% OR
3) Patient has an arthroplasty
Septic arthritis |

| 1) CPM, mast cells or both
present
Reactive arthritis | → | 1) Ragocytes >70%
Rheumatoid disease |

| ***Primary inflammatory
arthropathy*** |

Fig. 72.1 Three diagnostic algorithms starting with the nucleated cell count, for the analysis of synovial fluid by microscopy.

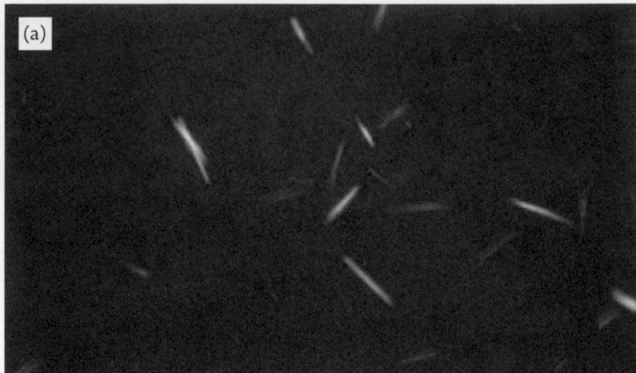

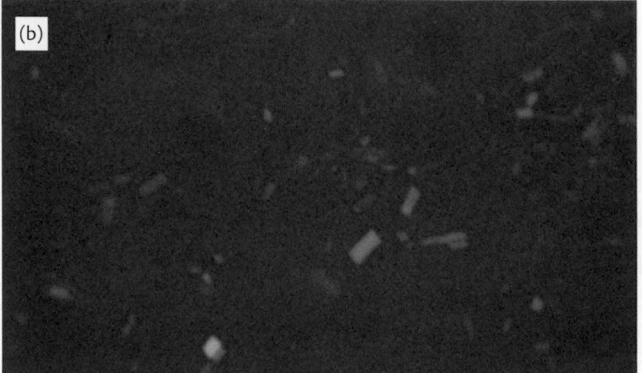

Fig. 72.2 Two different types of crystal (A, urate; B, pyrophosphate) viewed in polarized light with a quarter-wave interference plate. Note the difference in crystal shape and brightness, and the difference in colour of crystals with aligned long axes.

The sample is squeezed beneath a cover slip and examined for crystals, particles (synovial villi, fragments of meniscus/ligament, osteoarthritic cartilage), and one cell type, the ragocyte.

Crystals Crystals are a common finding in joints. The most frequently encountered are sodium urate, calcium pyrophosphate, lipid and hydroxyapatite. Detection is not as straightforward as is sometimes believed, but being able to obtain accurate, reproducible results has important clinical implications.[10,11] The easiest way to distinguish between crystal types is on the basis of shape, size, brightness in polarized light and how they interact with a phase-shifted polarized light path. In the latter it is customary to set up the microscope with a quarter-wave interference plate between the crossed polarizers. This creates a red background. Crystals placed between the quarter-wave plate and the analyser plate will shift the wavelength of the incident light and render the crystal coloured. Depending on the orientation of their long axes, crystals appear yellow or blue (Figure 72.2). The direction of the long axis of a crystal of a specific colour varies with the crystal type.

In very general terms the common crystals are:

♦ **Urate**: Crystals are 5–35 μm long, highly birefringent, needle-shaped, and soluble in water. Lipid crystals mimic urate but are insoluble in water and usually found in lipid droplets. Urate crystals are usually found on the background of acute inflammation, the most common presentation of gout. However, in some cases the interval between presentation and aspiration is such that the disease may be in a relatively quiescent phase and the fluid 'non-inflammatory' when aspiration occurs. In 1–2% of cases of acute gout there is a concomitant infection which may be masked by the acute crystal arthropathy.

fewer than 200 cells/mm³. In inflammatory joint disease the cell count is greater than 1000 cells/mm³ and in non-inflammatory arthropathies it is lower. Cell counts in excess of 30 000 cells/mm³ are restricted to a few clinical conditions: acute rheumatoid flares (including disease flares in patients previously stable on treatments with agents such as anti-tumour necrosis factor (TNF) drugs and septic, acute crystal. and reactive arthritis.

'Wet preparation' (WP)

This is shorthand for an unstained preparation viewed in a disorganized light path, formed by partially closing the condenser diaphragm on a conventional light microscope. The WP is also viewed in polarized light.

The WP is made by agitating the sample and aspirating a small amount using a conventional bulb pipette. Every effort should be made to include visible particles in the sample as they often sequester crystals.

◆ **Pyrophosphate**: Crystals are rhomboidal and appear less bright in polarized light than urate crystals. They accumulate in joints with increasing age and may cause no symptoms (chondrocalcinosis). In osteoarthritis (OA) crystals accumulate on the background of a non-inflammatory arthropathy.[12] Microscopy is particularly useful in distinguishing pseudogout from gout.

◆ **Hydroxyapatite**: Crystals indicate damage to calcified cartilage or underlying subarticular bone. This occurs most commonly in the non-inflammatory OA and inflammatory rheumatoid disease (RA), following joint replacement surgery, and in avascular bone necrosis. The crystals are small and granular, are not birefringent but can be rendered so by staining with Alizarin Red stain. 'Milwaukee shoulder' (and equivalents in other joints), is characterized by SF microspheroidal aggregates of hydroxyapatite crystals.[5]

◆ **Lipids** enter the joint through 'leaky' vessels in either long-standing inflammation or haemorrhage. They often appear as droplets with a Maltese cross pattern (liquid spherical crystal) when polarized or as urate-like needle-shaped crystals within a droplet of neutral fat. Occasionally lipids may themselves be phlogistic.[13] Intra-articular depot corticosteroid crystalloids may still be found up to 10 weeks after injection and may lead to the wrong diagnosis of pyrophosphate arthritis.

Other rarer crystals are also found in SF. For a full description see Freemont and Denton.[4]

Non-crystalline particles   These can consist of fragments from damaged intra-articular structures, fibrin, and material introduced accidently or therapeutically. The most common examples of the former are fragments of articular cartilage or, specifically in the knee, internal ligament and meniscus; the latter include, particles of metal, plastic polymer, and bone cement.

In OA, the most common disorder in which cartilage fragments appear in SF, tiny fragments of fibrillated cartilage, often containing chondrocyte clusters, can be identified (Figure 72.3) In knee trauma diagnostically useful fragments of meniscal fibrocartilage and intra-articular ligaments can be detected.

Wear of implant material can lead to foreign material within the joint. Modern plastic polymers used as articulating surfaces in joint prostheses (such as ultra-high-density polyethylene), bone cement, and composite (e.g. carbon fibre) fragments can be mistaken for crystals when they fragment. The presence of wear particles is not, in itself, evidence of loosening or failure, but wear particles are a feature of both actual and incipient loosening and are frequently present in patients with painful arthroplasties.

Ragocytes   Ragocytes are cells first described in RA.[14] They are not a cell type as such but rather a phenomenon in which any cell type (but most commonly polymorphs) accumulate large refractile granules within their cytoplasm. Despite their name ragocytes are not restricted to the SF in RA; however, finding that 70–90% of the nucleated cells in the WP are ragocytes is practically diagnostic of RA. Similarly, greater than 90% is a very strong independent biomarker of septic arthritis (specificity and sensitivity >90%).

Cytocentrifuge preparation

Adequate cytological analysis of SF requires a cytocentrifuge preparation. Optimal SF preparations involve diluting to 400 cells/mm³ and staining with Giemsa, except when septic arthritis is suspected, when the greatest likelihood of identifying organisms is afforded by diluting to 1200 cells/mm³ and staining with Gram stain.

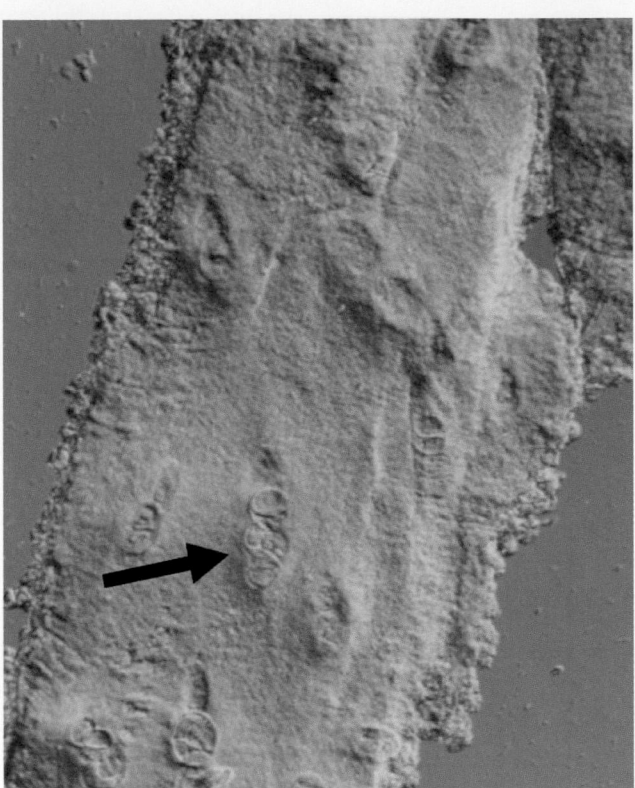

Fig. 72.3 Unstained osteoarthritic cartilage viewed in diffused light on a conventional light microscope. Note the chondrocyte clusters typical of osteoarthritis (arrowed).

Septic arthritis   Septic arthritis (SA) is an important but difficult diagnosis to make.[15] Careful microscopic examination of Gram-stained preparations is required (most SA is caused by Gram-positive organisms[16]).This approach detects microorganisms within 1–2 hours of the sample arriving in the laboratory (Figure 72.4). The greatest problems in diagnosing SA are failure to recognize Gram-negative organisms and distinguishing contaminating organisms from pathogens.

Immunosuppressed patients have an increasing incidence of non-suppurative infectious arthritis, particularly caused by mycobacteria and fungi.

In septic arthroplasty loosening SF cell counts as low as 1100 cells/mm³ plus neutrophil differentials in excess of 64% are described as sufficient evidence to diagnose infection in 98.6% of cases.[17]

Cell types and diagnosis   Many cell types are identifiable in Giemsa-stained cytocentrifuge preparations. The nature, and in some settings the proportion of cells (polymorphs, lymphocytes, macrophages, cytophagocytic mononuclear cells (CPM), and mast cells) are key diagnostic tools.

Neutrophils   Neutrophils predominate in the SF in most inflammatory arthropathies, and in haemarthroses. In the seronegative arthropathies, however, lymphocytes and macrophages may exceed polymorphs in number. Acute crystal and SA are the only disorders in which neutrophils regularly account for more than 95% of nucleated cells.

Lymphocytes   Finding a predominance of lymphocytes in a sample of SF from a patient with RA usually indicates a better long-term

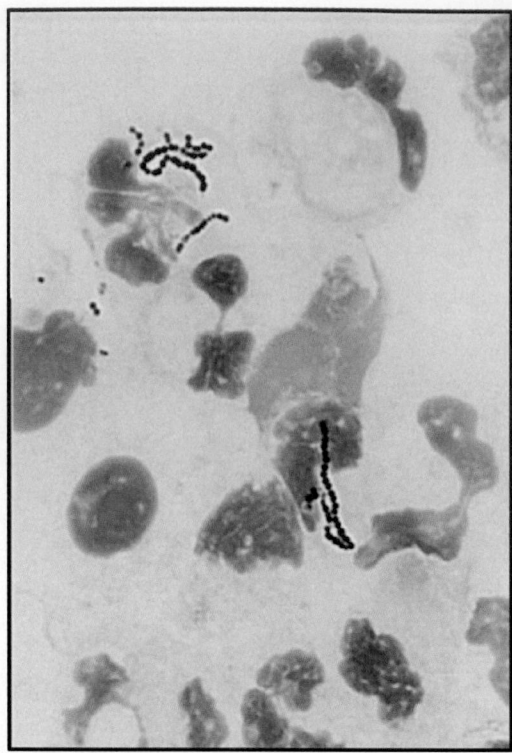

Fig. 72.4 Gram stain showing Gram-positive cocci in a sample of synovial fluid from a patient with septic arthritis.

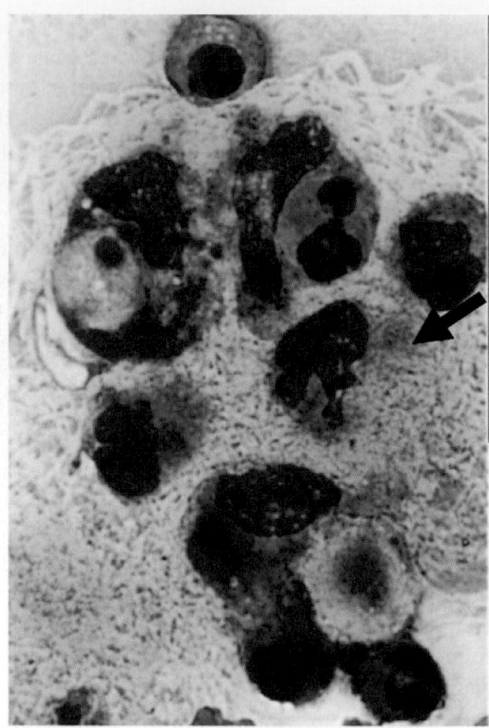

Fig. 72.5 Cytophagocytic mononuclear cells in a Giemsa-stained sample of synovial fluid from a patient with a seronegative spondylarthropathy. The arrow points to a polymorph apoptotic body in the cytoplasm of a macrophage.

prognosis for the joint. Lymphocytes also predominate in systemic lupus erythematosus (SLE).

Macrophages and CPM   Macrophages predominate in viral arthritis, Milwaukee shoulder and prosthetic-debris-induced arthropathy. CPM are macrophages that have phagocytosed apoptotic polymorphs (Figure 72.5). They are abundant in the seronegative spondyloarthropathies,[18] and if they are found a confident diagnosis can be made. In RA, apoptosis occurs in the absence of CPM formation.

Mast cells   Mast cells are seen most commonly in the seronegative spondyloarthropathies and in traumatic arthritis.[18]

The place of synovial fluid microscopy in diagnosis

Synovial biopsy is the investigation of choice in diseases where morphology is an imperative for diagnosis (e.g. granulomatous inflammation, villonodular synovitis); however, in almost every other clinical setting SF analysis is a more powerful diagnostic tool,[19] particularly in:

♦ differentiating between inflammatory and non-inflammatory arthropathies

♦ identifying specific disorders within these two groups

♦ diagnosing mono- and oligoarthropathies

♦ the rapid diagnosis of joint disease, in particular in suspected cases of SA where prognosis is inversely related to the delay in diagnosis.

Synovial fluid microbiology

Diagnosing infective arthritis is a major clinical problem and, as described, microscopic SF analysis has an important part to play.[20]

Culture is also important, but it is essential (and quick) to exclude crystal arthropathies by SF microscopy before sending specimens for culture. In addition to common bacterial joint pathogens (*Staphylococcus*, *Streptococcus*, etc.), *Neisseria*, *Salmonella*, *Mycobacterium tuberculosis*, fungi, and viruses requiring special culture methods should also be considered.

New techniques, particularly polymerase chain reaction (PCR) of SF looking for widely expressed nucleic acid sequences such as the 16S ribosomal component shared by many bacteria, may expand the future pool of diagnostic techniques.[21]

Serum procalcitonin (PCT) levels, used to diagnose systemic infection, are elevated in SA.[22] PCT levels are very variable in the SF in infective arthritis because of sequestration in fibrin (Figure 72.6) The role of PCT in infection is unknown but in the SF it binds to bacteria internalized in neutrophils (Figure 72.7), so it may have a role in opsonization.

Chemical changes in the synovial fluid in disease

Normal SF chemistry is extremely complex, as outlined in Table 72.1. As SF is in part a transudate, variations in disease may reflect alterations in either the blood or the joint. There is still a great deal to learn about the biochemical changes that occur in specific diseases, but the application of emerging 'omics' technology will make this possible.[23]

Most of the alterations in the biochemistry of SF relate to non-disease-specific processes, nevertheless they may be very useful in guiding therapy.

Levels of inflammatory mediators (cytokines,[24] proteases,[25] eicosanoids[26]) are elevated in the SF of 'non-inflammatory' and

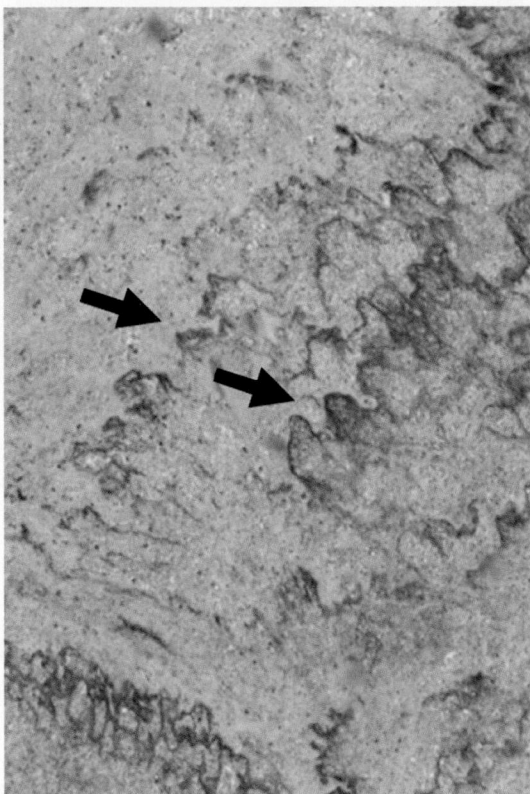

Fig. 72.6 Fibrin from the joint of a patient with septic arthritis stained by immunohistochemistry for procalcitonin (brown reaction product). Note the waves of deposition (arrowed).

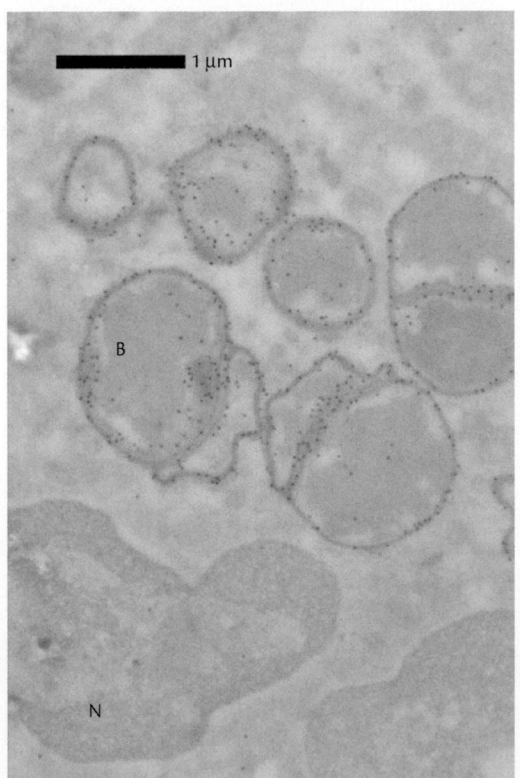

Fig. 72.7 Ultraimmunohistochemistry to localize procalcitonin in the cytoplasm of a polymorph from the synovial fluid of a patient with septic arthritis. The black circles are reaction product and are attached to bacterial (B) cell walls. The polymorph nucleus (N) can also be seen.

Table 72.1 Biochemical parameters of normal synovial fluid (indicative levels)

Osmolarity	300 mosmol/L
pH	7.44
PCO$_2$	6.0 kPa
PO$_2$	<4.0 kPa
Potassium	4.0 mmol/L
Sodium	135 mmol/L
Calcium	1.8 mmol/L
Urea	2.5 mmol/L
Uric acid	0.25 mmol/L
Glucose	100 mmol/L
Chondrotoin sulfate	40 mg/L
Hyaluronate	2.2 g/L
Total protein	25 g/L
Albumin	8 g/L
α_1-Antitrypsin	0.8 µg/L
Haptoglobin	90 mg/L
α_2-Macroglobin	0.3 g/L
IgG	2.6 g/L
IgA	0.9 g/L
IgM	0.2 g/L
IL-1b	20 pg/mL
IL-2	15 U/mL
TNFα	1.4 ng/mL
INFα	350 U/mL

Ig, immunoglobulin; IL, interleukin; INF, interferon; TNF, tumour necrosis factor.

'inflammatory' arthropathies. Antibodies (e.g. rheumatoid factor) have been described in SF, reflecting local production.

Changes in SF complement levels occur with local joint inflammation and, in RA, complement breakdown products correlate with the extent of synovitis. There is evidence that complement can be regulated by cartilage oligomeric matrix protein (COMP) in a disease-specific manner.[27]

Products of cartilage degradation assayed in SF change with tissue degradation in an enzyme-specific manner, exposing unique sites within the peptide chain. Similarly, synthesis of new proteoglycan molecules may result in expression of sugar motifs not usually found in adult cartilage. Assays of potential markers of synthesis and breakdown of collagens, proteoglycans, and a variety of noncollagenous proteins with connective tissue matrices are now being developed for research purposes and may gain use as diagnostic and prognostic tools.[28,29]

Conclusion

SF is: easy to aspirate, intimately associated with potentially diseased joint tissues, and increased in a broad spectrum of joint disorders. Despite this, it seems to have been an underexploited source of cellular and non-cellular biomarkers of diagnostic and prognostic value. An appraisal/reappraisal of new and old analytical technologies is required if the full potential of SF in patient diagnosis and management is to be realized.

References

1. Seror J, Merkher Y, Kampf N, et al. Articular cartilage proteoglycans as boundary lubricants: structure and frictional interaction of surface-attached hyaluronan and hyaluronan—aggrecan complexes. *Biomacromolecules* 2011;12(10):3432–3443.

2. Jackson A, Gu W. Transport properties of cartilaginous tissues. *Curr Rheumatol Rev* 2009;5(1):40.

3. Pal B, Nash J, Oppenheim B et al. Is routine synovial fluid analysis necessary? Lessons and recommendations from an audit. *Rheumatol Int* 1999;18(5–6):181–182.

4. Freemont AJ, Denton J. *Atlas of synovial fluid cytopathology.* Kluwer, Dordrecht, 1991.

5. Davis MJ, Denton J, Freemont AJ, Holt PJ. Comparison of serial synovial fluid cytology in rheumatoid arthritis: delineation of subgroups with prognostic implications. *Ann Rheum Dis* 1988;47(7):559–562.

6. Freemont AJ, Denton J, Chuck A, Holt PJ, Davies M. Diagnostic value of synovial fluid microscopy: a reassessment and rationalisation. *Ann Rheum Dis* 1991;50(2):101–107.

7. Swan A, Amer H, Dieppe P. The value of synovial fluid assays in the diagnosis of joint disease: a literature survey. *Ann Rheum Dis* 2002; 61(6):493–498.

8. Moreno MJ, Clayburne G, Schumacher HR Jr. Processing of noninflammatory synovial fluids with hyaluronidase for cytospin preparations improves the accuracy of differential counts. *Diagn Cytopathol* 2000;22(4):256–258.

9. McCarty DJ. Crystal identification in human synovial fluids. Methods and interpretation. *Rheum Dis Clin North Am* 1988;14(2):253–276.

10. Von Essen R, Holtta AM, Pikkarainen R. Quality control of synovial fluid crystal identification. *Ann Rheum Dis* 1998;57(2):107–109.

11. Pascual E, Sivera F, Andrés M. Synovial fluid analysis for crystals. *Curr Opin Rheumatol* 2011;23(2):161–169.

12. Rosenthal AK. Crystals, inflammation, and osteoarthritis. *Curr Opin Rheumatol* 2011;23(2):170–173.

13. Freemont AJ. What is the significance of synovial fluid lipid crystals in a patient with an isolated monoarthritis? *Br J Rheumatol* 1992;31(3):183–184.

14. Hollander JL, McCarty DJ Jr, Rawson AJ. The 'R.A. cell', 'ragocyte', or 'inclusion body cell'. *Bull Rheum Dis* 1965;16(1):382–383.

15. Mathews CJ, Coakley G. Septic arthritis: current diagnostic and therapeutic algorithm. *Curr Opin Rheumatol* 2008;20(4):457–462.

16. Ryan MJ, Kavanagh R, Wall PG, Hazleman BL. Bacterial joint infections in England and Wales: analysis of bacterial isolates over a four year period. *Br J Rheumatol* 1997;36(3):370–373.

17. Ghanem E, Parvizi J, Burnett RS, et al. Cell count and differential of aspirated fluid in the diagnosis of infection at the site of total knee arthroplasty. *J Bone Joint Surg Am* 2008;90(8):1637–1643.

18. Freemont AJ, Denton J. The disease distribution of synovial fluid mast cells and cytophagocytic mononuclear cells in inflammatory arthritis. *Ann Rheum Dis* 1985;44(5):312–315.

19. Johnson JS, Freemont AJ. A ten year retrospective comparison of the diagnostic usefulness of synovial fluid and synovial biopsy examination. *J Clin Pathol* 2001;54(8):605–607.

20. Mathews CJ, Weston VC, Jones A, Field M, Coakley G. Bacterial septic arthritis in adults. *Lancet* 2010;375(9717):846–855.

21. Bonilla H, Kepley R, Pawlak J et al. Rapid diagnosis of septic arthritis using 16S rDNA PCR: a comparison of 3 methods. *Diagn Microbiol Infect Dis* 2011;69(4):390–395.

22. Hügle T, Schuetz P, Mueller B et al. Serum procalcitonin for discrimination between septic and non-septic arthritis. *Clin Exp Rheumatol* 2008;26(3):453–456.

23. Williams A, Smith JR, Allaway D et al. Applications of proteomics in cartilage biology and osteoarthritis research. *Front Biosci* 2011;17,2622–2644.

24. Punzi L, Calò L, Plebani M. Clinical significance of cytokine determination in synovial fluid. *Crit Rev Clin Lab Sci* 2002;39(1):63–88.

25. Catterall JB, Cawston TE. Assays of matrix metalloproteinases (MMPs) and MMP inhibitors: bioassays and immunoassays applicable to cell culture medium, serum, and synovial fluid. *Methods Mol Biol* 2003;225:353–364.

26. Day RO, McLachlan AJ, Graham GG, Williams KM. Pharmacokinetics of nonsteroidal anti-inflammatory drugs in synovial fluid. *Clin Pharmacokinet* 1999;36(3):191–210.

27. Happonen KE, Saxne T, Aspberg A et al. Regulation of complement by cartilage oligomeric matrix protein allows for a novel molecular diagnostic principle in rheumatoid arthritis. *Arthritis Rheum* 2010;62(12):3574–3583.

28. Garvican ER, Vaughan-Thomas A, Innes JF, Clegg PD. Biomarkers of cartilage turnover. Part 1: Markers of collagen degradation and synthesis. *Vet J* 2010;185(1):36–42.

29. Garvican ER, Vaughan-Thomas A, Clegg PD, Innes JF. Biomarkers of cartilage turnover. Part 2: Non-collagenous markers. *Vet J* 2010; 185(1):43–49.

CHAPTER 73

Cardiopulmonary investigations

Benjamin E. Schreiber, Gregory J. Keir, and J. Gerry Coghlan

Introduction

Rheumatological conditions frequently involve the cardiac and respiratory systems. In this chapter we aim to survey appropriate investigations for common clinical indications and to review the strengths and weaknesses of the more commonly performed tests.

The need for cardiopulmonary investigations is driven by clinical concern. Cardiopulmonary investigations may be required as part of screening for disease in high-risk groups or to diagnose or guide treatment of disease.

There is a huge array of cardiac and pulmonary investigations available to the clinician. Obviously the clinical use of the tests cannot be encapsulated in one chapter. We present suggested investigation routes for particular clinical contexts, and then review individual investigations with their respective indications, strengths and weaknesses.

Indications

There is often considerable overlap in symptoms between diseases affecting the cardiac or respiratory symptoms in the setting of rheumatological disease. Shortness of breath, chest pain, and palpitations may be due to disease in either system and a detailed history and physical examination, coupled with an understanding of comorbidities common to individual rheumatological conditions, help to refine pretest probabilities. Furthermore, while virtually any component of the cardiac or respiratory system may be affected, 'typical' patterns of heart and lung involvement are recognized in individual rheumatologic diseases and this knowledge helps to further direct an appropriate investigation pathway.

Shortness of breath

Shortness of breath accompanied by symptoms of cough, wheeze, or sputum production suggests a primary respiratory process, and initial investigation with chest radiography, spirometry, and sputum analysis is appropriate. If cardiac involvement is suspected, electrocardiography, natriuretic peptides, and echocardiography may be useful.

At times, the cause for dyspnoea is not readily apparent following simple first-line investigations, and the diagnostic algorithm needs be broadened to include 'blind spots' which are more difficult to easily assess. Pulmonary vascular disease such as pulmonary hypertension, pulmonary thromboembolic disease and pulmonary vasculitis, interstitial lung involvement, and myocardial disease require a high index of suspicion to allow timely diagnosis.

Extrathoracic manifestations of rheumatological disease including musculoskeletal disease and deconditioning should also be considered when evaluating dyspnoea. Patients who are markedly short of breath without hypoxia may have non-cardiopulmonary causes of dyspnoea, and pulse oximetry with exercise, a simple, easily performed screening test, may provide vital information.

Cough

The British Thoracic Society distinguishes acute cough (<3 weeks) from chronic cough (>8 weeks).[1] Acute cough should be investigated with chest radiography if it is accompanied by haemoptysis, breathlessness, fever, chest pain, or weight loss. Patients with significant haemoptysis or any possibility of foreign body inhalation should be referred for urgent bronchoscopy. Patients with breathlessness and acute cough should be assessed for possible asthma or anaphylaxis. Patients with chronic cough should be investigated initially with chest radiography and spirometry with reversibility testing. If these show no obvious pulmonary pathology and there are no avoidable cough triggers, referral to a specialist clinic is recommended.

Chest pain

The current United Kingdom National Institute for Health and Clinical Excellence (NICE) guidelines (CG 95) group recommendations by the pretest probability of ischaemic heart disease. Patients with low probability (10–29%) are investigated with CT calcium scoring, those with intermediate probability (30–60%) are offered functional imaging, and those at high risk (61–90%) are offered coronary angiography.[2] Functional imaging modalities detect stress-induced wall motion abnormalities or hypoperfusion using nuclear medicine (MPS), echocardiography or MRI.

Syncope

European guidelines recommend initial investigation of patients with transient loss of consciousness with careful history, including assessing for a family history of premature coronary artery disease or sudden cardiac death, physical examination including orthostatic blood pressure measurements, and electrocardiogram (ECG). In patients with syncope even very subtle ECG abnormalities (such as T-wave inversion in septal leads) may be important. Additional investigations include carotid sinus massage in patients over the age of 40. Further investigations are guided by clinical suspicion: echocardiography in patients with known or suspected heart disease, ECG monitoring when there is suspicion of an arrhythmic cause, and orthostatic challenge when postural causes are suspected.[3]

Rheumatological considerations

The heart and lungs are affected in many ways in rheumatological disease, and the prevalence of differing complications is often difficult to accurately define. Many rheumatological diseases are relatively rare, with significant clinical heterogeneity in disease manifestations. Methodological differences in case ascertainment and differences in the definition of cardiac and pulmonary disease have further hampered accurate definition. Nonetheless, there are associations between certain rheumatological conditions and a predilection for particular cardiopulmonary complications. For instance, interstitial lung disease is seen as a complication of systemic sclerosis, rheumatoid arthritis, systemic lupus erythematosus, Sjögren's syndrome, polymyositis, dermatomyositis. and mixed connective tissue disease.[4] On the other hand, the aorta is commonly affected in temporal arteritis, long-standing ankylosing spondylitis, Cogan's syndrome, and relapsing polychondritis. Table 73.1 summarizes the more common cardiac and respiratory complications encountered in rheumatological disease, in addition to suggested investigations.

Cardiopulmonary tests

Chest radiography

Chest radiography is readily available, safe (with a radiation dose of 0.02 mSv per radiograph, equivalent to 3 days' background radiation in the United Kingdom[5]) and capable of detecting significant

Table 73.1 Common cardiac and respiratory complications, and suggested initial investigations, in various rheumatological diseases

Condition	Complications		Investigations to consider
	Cardiac	**Respiratory**	
Rheumatoid arthritis	Accelerated atherosclerosis	Pleural disease, interstitial lung disease, necrobiotic nodules, bronchiectasis, bronchiolotis	CXR, ECG
Gout	Increased risk of ischaemic heart disease		Address risk factors
Seronegative arthritides	Ischaemic heart disease. Aortic insufficiency	Apical lung fibrosis	Echo if suspicion
Systemic lupus erythematosus	Accelerated atherosclerosis, pericarditis, cardiomyopathy, myocarditis, endocarditis, conduction disorders	Pleural effusion, acute lupus pneumonitis/diffuse alveolar damage, interstitial lung disease, pulmonary haemorrhage, respiratory muscle weakness, pulmonary hypertension	CXR, ECG
Sjögren's syndrome	Interstitial lung disease. Lymphoma	Interstitial lung disease, bronchiectasis, lymphoproliferative disease	PFT, CXR, HRCT
Giant cell arteritis	Thoracic and abdominal aortic aneurysms	Pleural effusion (rare)	Regular CXR, abdominal ultrasound
Takayasu's arteritis	Large vessel vasculitis—stenoses, aneurysm	Pulmonary vasculitis, pulmonary haemorrhage	MRA, PET
Medium-vessel vasculitis (polyarteritis nodosa, Kawasaki's disease)	Coronary vasculitis	Pulmonary vasculitis, pulmonary haemorrhage	ECG, CXR, HRCT
Relapsing polychondritis	Valvular disease	Large-airway narrowing/collapse	Echo if suspicion
Behçet's disease	Coronary artery aneurysms, intracardiac thrombosis	Pulmonary artery aneurysms, pulmonary thromboembolic disease	V/Q, CTPA/MRA, pulmonary angiogram
Scleroderma	Chronic pericarditis, myocardial fibrosis	Interstitial lung disease, pulmonary hypertension	CXR, Echo, PFT, HRCT, RHC

CTPA, CT pulmonary angiography; CXR, chest radiography; ECG, electrocardiography; HRCT, high-resolution CT; MRA, MR angiography; PFT, pulmonary function testing; RHC, right heart catheterization; V/Q, ventilation–perfusion scanning.

pulmonary processes such as consolidation, effusion, pneumothorax and pulmonary oedema.

Diffuse pulmonary processes may be less reliably detected by chest radiography, and are more difficult to accurately characterize. About 10% of patients with significant diffuse interstitial diseases have normal chest radiographs.[6] Similarly, chest radiography has a high specificity but only a moderate sensitivity for diagnosing heart failure.[7–9] Importantly, it cannot reliably diagnose important causes of sudden shortness of breath as such aortic dissection, myocardial infarction, or cardiac arrhythmias.

Troponin

Troponin is released during myocardial ischaemia and is therefore important in the diagnosis of acute coronary syndromes. In patients with suspected myocarditis a raised troponin correlates strongly with presence of inflammation as detected by endomyocardial biopsy.[10]

A raised troponin is associated with higher mortality in several conditions, including heart failure,[11] acute pulmonary emboli,[12] severe exacerbations of chronic obstructive pulmonary disease (COPD),[13] and critical illness.[14]

However, raised troponins may also be seen in pericarditis, acute stroke, cardiac contusion, sepsis, and chronic kidney disease.

Brain natriuretic peptide

Brain natriuretic peptide (BNP) is released from the brain and from the heart. Cardiac secretion of BNP is seen in response to wall stress.[15] It may serve to counteract the vasoconstriction and sodium retention due to noradrenaline, endothelin, and angiotensin II in heart failure. It may also have a role in preventing cardiac collagen accumulation in heart failure.[16] It aids in diagnosis of heart failure in emergency settings.[17]

Raised BNP levels are associated with a worse prognosis in acute coronary syndromes,[18] stable angina,[19] chronic mitral regurgitation,[20] adult congenital heart disease,[21] pulmonary hypertension,[22] and non-cardiac surgery.[23]

Pulmonary function tests

Pulmonary function tests (PFTs) form a crucial part in diagnosis, staging of disease severity, and serial monitoring of many connective tissue disease (CTD)-associated lung diseases. Patterns of lung function impairment vary widely between rheumatological diseases, depending on the nature of the underlying pulmonary pathophysiological process as detailed in Table 73.2.[24]

Typical measurements made during pulmonary function testing include spirometric volumes, lung volumes performed with body plethysmography, and diffusing capacity of the lung. Spirometric volumes are the most readily available measures of lung function, and are highly reproducible when performed by trained personnel. Measurements consist of the forced expiratory volume in one second (FEV_1) and the total exhaled volume (vital capacity; VC) following a maximal inspiration. The forced expiratory ratio (FEV_1:FVC) is useful in differentiating obstructive (FEV_1:FVC <70) from restrictive (FEV_1:FVC >80) pulmonary processes, and flow–volume curves (which display inspiratory and expiratory flow rates for given lung volumes) provide similar information in a graphical form.[25] Examples of flow–volume curves in various diseases are provided in Figure 73.1.

Diffusing capacity of the lung (DL_{CO}) is a measure of the rate of diffusion of carbon monoxide (CO) across the blood–gas barrier into the pulmonary capillaries. DL_{CO} may be affected by a variety of pulmonary pathologic processes, including diseases of the lung parenchyma (e.g. emphysema), the interstitium, or the pulmonary vasculature, all leading to ventilation–perfusion mismatch. Of all lung function measures, DL_{CO} is most prone to measurement variation. The carbon monoxide transfer coefficient (K_{CO}) is derived by correcting the DL_{CO} for alveolar volume (DL_{CO}/V_A) and may be raised to supranormal levels (>100% predicted) in the presence of extrapulmonic restriction (respiratory muscle weakness, pleural disease).

The interpretation of PFT abnormalities can become considerably more complex where overlapping pathophysiological processes are present (e.g. concomitant pulmonary fibrosis and pulmonary hypertension in systemic sclerosis).

Bronchoscopy

Flexible bronchoscopy may aid substantially in clarifying the cause of respiratory symptoms in patients with rheumatological disease. It is a safe procedure (with an estimated mortality rate of up to 0.04%,

Table 73.2 Patterns of pulmonary function test abnormalities associated with rheumatological lung diseases.

	Restrictive lung disease	Obstructive lung disease	Pulmonary vascular disease	Extrapulmonary restriction
Total lung capacity	Reduced	Increased	Normal	Reduced
Spirometry	FEV_1 normal/↓ FVC ↓↓ FEV_1:FVC >80%	FEV_1 ↓↓ FVC normal/↑ FEV_1:FVC <70%	FEV_1 and FVC preserved	FEV_1 normal/↓ FVC ↓↓ FEV_1:FVC >80%
Diffusing capacity	Reduced	Reduced	Reduced	Normal/↓ K_{CO} ↑↑
Flow–volume curve	Preserved PEFR Tall, narrow expiratory curve	Reduced PEFR Upward concavity of expiratory curve	Normal	Normal or ↓ PEFR if muscle weakness is severe
Disease examples	Pulmonary fibrosis	Bronchiolitis, bronchiectasis Emphysema	Pulmonary hypertension	Pleural disease Respiratory muscle weakness

FEV_1, forced expiratory volume in 1 second; FVC, forced vital capacity; PEFR, peak expiratory flow rate; K_{CO}, carbon monoxide transfer coefficient: diffusing capacity corrected for alveolar volume (DL_{CO}/VA).

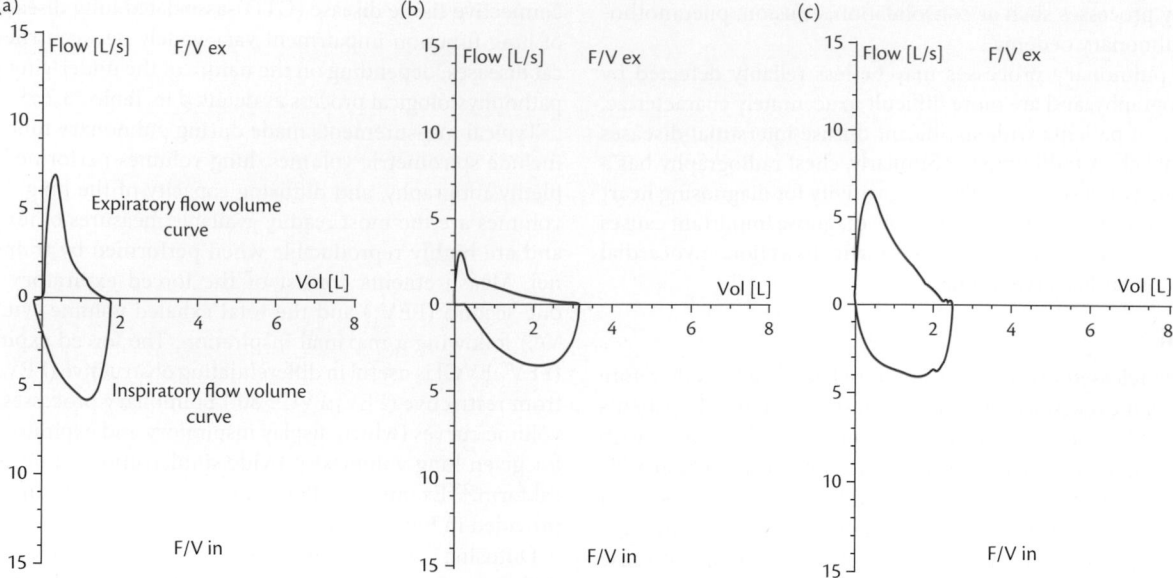

Fig. 73.1 (a) Flow–volume curves in a 58 year old woman with systemic sclerosis-associated non-specific interstitial pneumonia. The peak expiratory flow rate is preserved, but increased lung compliance results in rapid emptying of the lung and a tall, narrow expiratory flow–volume curve. (b) A 47 year old woman with rheumatoid arthritis associated obliterative bronchiolitis. The expiratory flow-volume curve demonstrates reduced peak expiratory flow rate and 'scooping out' of the curve, typical of small airways obstruction. (c) Normal flow–volume curves in a 37 year old woman with systemic sclerosis associated pulmonary hypertension. There was no significant interstitial lung disease or airways disease demonstrated on HRCT or at lung function.

and major complication rate of up to 0.12%),[26] and enables the direct visualization of airways to the level of the subsegmental bronchi, in addition to allowing various sampling manoeuvres to be performed.

Bronchoalveolar lavage (BAL) allows the sampling of cellular contents of the distal airways and alveolar space. When interpreted in conjunction with CT findings, BAL can be useful in distinguishing patterns of diffuse lung involvement, in identifying pulmonary haemorrhage, in the assessment of possible drug-induced pulmonary reactions, and in identifying pulmonary infections. The utility of BAL as a prognostic tool in CTD associated diffuse lung disease is unclear. One study has reported the presence of BAL eosinophilia to be associated with increased mortality in scleroderma associated non-specific interstitial pneumonia (NSIP), although similar data for other CTDs are lacking.[27]

In the setting of diffuse lung disease associated with rheumatological disease, transbronchial lung biopsy is often of limited diagnostic utility due to small biopsy size and sampling error due to the heterogeneous nature of lung involvement.[28] Furthermore, detailed clinical–pathological–radiological correlation of historical cohorts, and advances in CT imaging, have largely negated the need for surgical lung biopsy for diagnostic purposes in many rheumatologic diffuse lung diseases.

Electrocardiography

ECG provides information on cardiac rate and rhythm as well as indirect evidence of coronary artery disease, cardiomyopathy, pericardial effusion, pulmonary hypertension, and electrolyte abnormalities. It should therefore be performed in all patients with cardiac symptoms.

Echocardiography

Echocardiography has an established central role in the assessment of cardiac anatomy and function. In addition, it may detect

rheumatic complications such as aortic root dilatation, Liebman–Sacks endocarditis, amyloidosis, pulmonary hypertension, and pericardial effusion. Limitations of the technique should, however, be recognized. Detailed assessment of ventricular function is suboptimal with two-dimensional echocardiography, and echocardiography cannot exclude coronary artery disease.

Specialized techniques are available for specific indications. Echocardiography with pharmacological stress or exercise may reveal ischaemic myocardium. Transoesophageal echocardiography has improved detection of valvular function and vegetations. Bubble contrast echocardiography improves recognition of right-to-left shunts.

Experimental techniques include three-dimensional echocardiography to more accurately assess cardiac chamber size and function. There is much debate about optimal advanced imaging analysis techniques for cardiac function, with little consensus as to date.

Computed Tomography

The widespread utilization of computed tomography (CT) has greatly improved diagnostic accuracy for many rheumatological lung diseases. High-resolution CT (HRCT), utilizing thin-slice reconstructions, has become invaluable in identifying patients with suspected diffuse lung involvement and airways involvement.

CT evidence of pulmonary disease in rheumatological disease varies widely between series, and depends partly on the diligence with which it is sought. In one series of consecutive unselected patients with rheumatoid arthritis recruited from a general rheumatology clinic, the prevalence of interstitial abnormalities on HRCT was 19%.[29] The high sensitivity of CT in detecting pulmonary abnormalities poses challenges to the clinician in distinguishing trivial change from clinically significant disease. In addition to pulmonary manifestations of the underlying rheumatological disease, CT also plays an important role in identifying abnormalities associated with treatment (infection, drug-induced pulmonary reactions).

Figure 73.2 demonstrates common HRCT patterns of disease in various rheumatological diseases.

Cardiac catheterization

Left heart catheterization with percutaneous interventions (PCI) has an established role in patients with unstable angina and non-ST elevation myocardial infarction. It is associated with a reduction in myocardial infarction, refractory angina, and rehospitalization but not death. On the other hand, it is associated with periprocedural myocardial infarction and increased risk of bleeding.[30] Its role in patients with stable angina has been brought into question by the recent COURAGE and FAME trials. Major complications with PCI include a mortality rate of 0.4%, need for emergency CABG 0.2%, periprocedural myocardial infarction 0.8%.[31] The risk of stroke is 0.1–0.4%.[32]

Right heart catheterization is the gold standard investigation for the diagnosis of pulmonary hypertension. Pulmonary capillary wedge pressure or left ventricular end-diastolic pressure are measured to assess the contribution of the left heart to pulmonary pressures. Cardiac output is assessed by thermodilution or oxygen saturation (Fick method) to allow estimation of pulmonary vascular resistance. In some patients with pulmonary hypertension, a vasoreactivity test is performed to assess whether the patient may respond to calcium-channel antagonists.

Conventional pulmonary angiography may be performed at the same time, although nuclear medicine lung perfusion–ventilation scanning, CT pulmonary angiography, and MR pulmonary angiography are non-invasive alternatives.

Cardiac magnetic resonance imaging

Cardiac MR imaging (CMR) is a powerful non-invasive non-ionizing technique with the ability to depict cardiac anatomy, function, and tissue characterization. CMR can detect myocardial inflammation, perfusion defects, fibrosis, and coronary and great arteries aneurysms, making it a valuable tool for cardiovascular system assessment in selected patients with rheumatic diseases.

In the assessment of cardiac chamber volume and function, it has advantages over echocardiography in accuracy and reproducibility. The ability of CMR to assess myocardial inflammation is often useful in rheumatology. T2-weighted images detect tissue water content and cannot distinguish necrotic from inflamed tissue. Early and late gadolinium enhancement improves specificity for myocardial inflammation.[33] In addition, it can provide valuable information in autoimmune conditions affecting the cardiovascular system such as Takayasu's arteritis, Behçet's syndrome, and systemic sclerosis. The

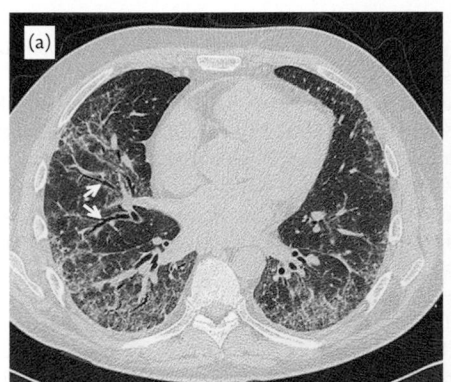
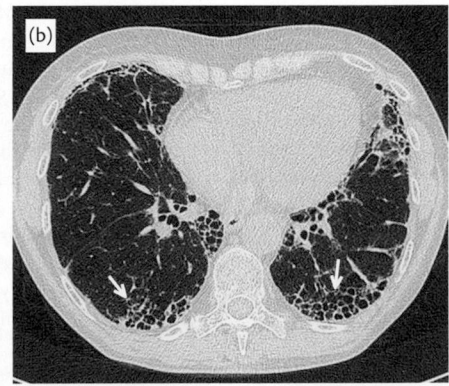
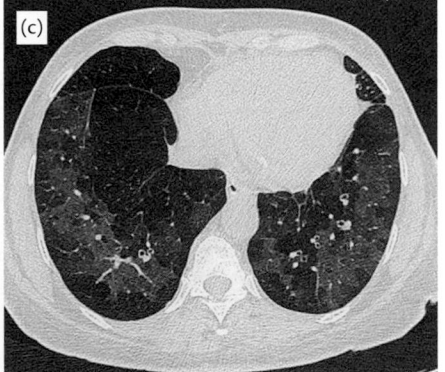
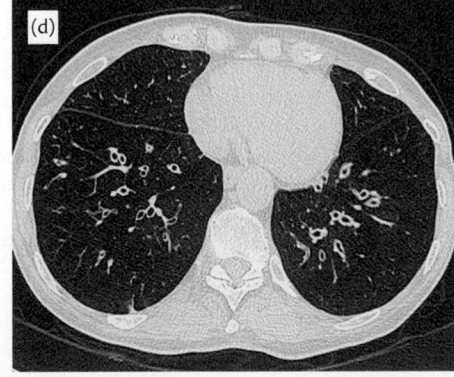
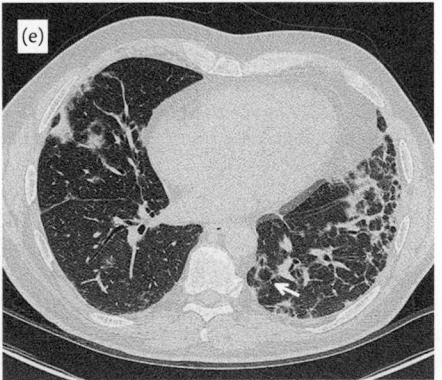

Fig. 73.2 (a) Systemic sclerosis associated non-specific interstitial pneumonia (NSIP). There is extensive reticular shadowing and ground-glass change, with evidence of traction bronchiectasis (arrows). NSIP is the most frequently observed radiological and histological pattern of diffuse lung disease in systemic sclerosis. (b) Rheumatoid arthritis associated usual interstitial pneumonia (UIP). There is a coarse subpleural reticular pattern, with evidence of honeycomb lung destruction (arrow). UIP is the most frequently observed pattern of diffuse lung disease in rheumatoid arthritis. (c) Obliterative bronchiolitis associated with rheumatoid arthritis. A mosaic attenuation pattern is present, with a mixture of low attenuation (blacker) and normal attenuation lung. In the blacker lung, there is a reduction in calibre and number of vessels (due to hypoxic vasoconstriction). Mild bronchial wall thickening is also present. (d) Sjögren's syndrome associated with bronchiectasis. The airways are thick walled and dilated. In normal lung, the airway is of the same calibre, or smaller, than its accompanying blood vessel. (e) Organizing pneumonia associated with polymyositis/dermatomyositis. There are bilateral areas of patchy consolidation, in some areas displaying a perilobular pattern (arrow), characteristic of organizing pneumonia.

role of CMR is not fully elucidated in rheumatic disease and only small case series have been published to date.[34]

CMR has several drawbacks. It is expensive and time consuming. Good images require the patient to be able to breath-hold for 5–10 seconds, and most implanted pacemakers and cardiac devices are not MRI compatible. Patients with claustrophobia often find the procedure very difficult. Highly irregular rhythms can affect the image quality. Finally, nephrogenic systemic fibrosis due to gadolinium has increasingly been described and MRI with gadolinium is relatively contraindicated in patients with eGFR below 30 mL/min.[35]

Conclusion

There is a huge and growing array of specialized cardiac and respiratory tests, many of which are beyond the scope of this chapter. These include cardiopulmonary exercise testing, tilt table testing, CT angiography and coronary calcium scoring, intracardiac and intravascular ultrasound, sleep studies, lung perfusion scanning, VATS procedures, and lung biopsy. However, these tests are for use by cardiac and pulmonary specialists. We have emphasized initial investigations which are appropriate for common cardiac and respiratory symptoms, and highlighted cardiac and respiratory complications associated with rheumatological conditions.

References

1. Morice AH, McGarvey L, Pavord I. British Thoracic Society Cough Guideline Group. Recommendations for the management of cough in adults. *Thorax* 2006;61 Suppl 1:i1–i24.
2. www.nice.org.uk/guidance/CG95
3. Moya A, Sutton R, Ammirati F et al.; Task Force for the Diagnosis and Management of Syncope; European Society of Cardiology (ESC); European Heart Rhythm Association (EHRA); Heart Failure Association (HFA); Heart Rhythm Society (HRS), Guidelines for the diagnosis and management of syncope (version 2009). *Eur Heart J* 2009;30(21):2631–2671.
4. Castelino FV, Varga J. Interstitial lung disease in connective tissue diseases: evolving concepts of pathogenesis and management. *Arthritis Res Ther* 2010;12(4):213.
5. Hart D, Wall BF. UK population dose from medical X-ray examinations. *Eur J Radiol* 2004;50(3):285–291.
6. Stark P. Evaluation of diffuse lung disease by plain chest radiography. In: Basow DS (ed.) *UpToDate*. UpToDate, Waltham, MA, 2011.
7. Kennedy S, Simon B, Alter HJ, Cheung P. Ability of physicians to diagnose congestive heart failure based on chest X-ray. *J Emerg Med* 2011;40(1):47–52.
8. Knudsen CW, Omland T, Clopton P et al. Diagnostic value of B-Type natriuretic peptide and chest radiographic findings in patients with acute dyspnea. *Am J Med* 2004;116(6):363–368.
9. Studler U, Kretzschmar M, Christ M et al. Accuracy of chest radiographs in the emergency diagnosis of heart failure. *Eur Radiol* 2008;18(8):1644–1652.
10. Lauer B, Niederau C, Kühl U et al. Cardiac troponin T in patients with clinically suspected myocarditis. *J Am Coll Cardiol* 1997;30(5):1354.
11. Horwich TB, Patel J, MacLellan WR, Fonarow GC. Cardiac troponin I is associated with impaired hemodynamics, progressive left ventricular dysfunction, and increased mortality rates in advanced heart failure. *Circulation* 2003;108(7):833.
12. Becattini C, Vedovati MC, Agnelli G. Prognostic value of troponins in acute pulmonary embolism: a meta-analysis. *Circulation* 2007;116(4):427.
13. Baillard C, Boussarsar M, Fosse JP et al. Cardiac troponin I in patients with severe exacerbation of chronic obstructive pulmonary disease. *Intensive Care Med* 2003;29(4):584.
14. Lim W, Qushmaq I, Devereaux PJ et al. Elevated cardiac troponin measurements in critically ill patients. *Arch Intern Med* 2006;166(22):2446.
15. Steiner J, Guglin M. BNP or NTproBNP? A clinician's perspective. *Int J Cardiol* 2008;129(1):5–14.
16. Tamura N, Ogawa Y, Chusho H et al. Cardiac fibrosis in mice lacking brain natriuretic peptide. *Proc Natl Acad Sci U S A* 2000;97(8):4239.
17. Maisel AS, Krishnaswamy P, Nowak RM et al. Breathing Not Properly Multinational Study Investigators. Rapid measurement of B-type natriuretic peptide in the emergency diagnosis of heart failure. *N Engl J Med* 2002;347(3):161.
18. de Lemos JA, Morrow DA, Bentley JH et al. The prognostic value of B-type natriuretic peptide in patients with acute coronary syndromes. *N Engl J Med* 2001;345(14):1014.
19. Schnabel R, Lubos E, Rupprecht HJ et al. B-type natriuretic peptide and the risk of cardiovascular events and death in patients with stable angina: results from the AtheroGene study. *J Am Coll Cardiol* 2006;47(3):552.
20. Pizarro R, Bazzino OO, Oberti PF et al. Prospective validation of the prognostic usefulness of brain natriuretic peptide in asymptomatic patients with chronic severe mitral regurgitation. *J Am Coll Cardiol* 2009;54(12):1099–1106.
21. Giannakoulas G, Dimopoulos K, Bolger AP et al. Usefulness of natriuretic Peptide levels to predict mortality in adults with congenital heart disease. *Am J Cardiol* 2010;105(6):869–873.
22. Nagaya N, Nishikimi T, Uematsu M et al. Plasma brain natriuretic peptide as a prognostic indicator in patients with primary pulmonary hypertension. *Circulation* 2000;102(8):865–870.
23. Ryding AD, Kumar S, Worthington AM, Burgess D. Prognostic value of brain natriuretic peptide in noncardiac surgery: a meta-analysis. *Anesthesiology* 2009;111(2):311–319.
24. Wells AU. Pulmonary function tests in connective tissue disease. *Semin Respir Crit Care Med* 2007;28(4):379–388.
25. West JB. *Pulmonary pathophysiology: the essentials*, 6th edn. Lippincott Williams & Wilkins, Philadelphia, PA, 2003.
26. British Thoracic Society Bronchoscopy Guideline Committee: a subCommittee of the Standards of Care Committee of the British Thoracic Society. British Thoracic Society guidelines on diagnostic flexible bronchoscopy. *Thorax* 2001 56: (Suppl I); i1–i21.
27. Bouros D, Wells AU, Nicholson AG et al. Histopathologic subsets of fibrosing alveolitis in patients with systemic sclerosis and their relationship to outcome. *Am J Respir Crit Care Med* 2002;165:1581–1586.
28. Bradley B, Branley HM, Egan JJ et al.; British Thoracic Society Interstitial Lung Disease Guideline Group, British Thoracic Society Standards of Care Committee; Thoracic Society of Australia; New Zealand Thoracic Society; Irish Thoracic Society. Interstitial lung disease guideline: the British Thoracic Society in collaboration with the Thoracic Society of Australia and New Zealand and the Irish Thoracic Society. *Thorax* 2008;63 Suppl 5:v1–v58.
29. Dawson JK, Fewins HE, Desmond J, Lynch MP, Graham DR. Fibrosing alveolitis in patients with rheumatoid arthritis as assessed by high resolution computed tomography, chest radiography, and pulmonary function tests. *Thorax* 2001;56:622–627.
30. Hoenig MR, Aroney CN, Scott IA. Early invasive versus conservative strategies for unstable angina and non-ST elevation myocardial infarction in the stent era. *Cochrane Database Syst Rev* 2010;3:CD004815.
31. Moschovitis A, Cook S, Meier B. Percutaneous coronary interventions in Europe in 2006. *EuroIntervention* 2010;6(2):189–194.
32. Hamon M, Baron JC, Viader F, Hamon M. Periprocedural stroke and cardiac catheterization. *Circulation* 2008;118(6):678–683.
33. Mavrogeni S, Vassilopoulos D. Is there a place for cardiovascular magnetic resonance imaging in the evaluation of cardiovascular involvement in rheumatic diseases? *Semin Arthritis Rheum* 2011;41(3):488–496.
34. Wassmuth R, Schulz-Menger J. Cardiovascular magnetic resonance imaging of myocardial inflammation. *Expert Rev Cardiovasc Ther* 2011; 9(9):1193–1201.
35. Dichstein K, Ørn S. Clinical utilities of cardiac MRI. *E-journal of Cardiology Practice* 2008;6(39). www.escardio.org/communities/councils/ccp/e-journal/volume6/Pages/vol6n39.aspx

CHAPTER 74

Electrophysiology

Julian Blake

Introduction

Clinical neurophysiology is a diagnostic discipline that uses the recording of bioelectrical signals from the central and peripheral nervous systems and from skeletal muscle in the examination of patients with neurological disease. It includes nerve conduction studies (NCS), needle electromyography (needle EMG), electroencephalography (EEG), and evoked cortical responses such as somatosensory and visual evoked potentials. Only those aspects related to the study of the peripheral nervous system and neuromuscular function are discussed in this chapter.

Neurophysiological consultation

A neurophysiological consultation includes taking an appropriate history and clinical examination as well as performing the neurophysiological assessment. Some patients may find the examination uncomfortable and they should be warned about this. However, it should not be over emphasized as anxiety prior to the examination undoubtedly increases the discomfort. Special care is needed with pacemakers and patients may need cardiac monitoring during the examination and a pacemaker check afterwards. The presence of implantable defibrillators is a significant contraindication. Pregnancy is not a contraindication to electrical stimulation. Needle EMG is often likened to acupuncture and is of similar discomfort to a venepuncture. Warfarin is a relative contraindication to needle examination and a recent INR of less than 2.5 is desirable. These aspects should be discussed with the neurophysiologist.

Methodology

Nerve conduction

Any sizeable nerve that is accessible can be studied. Action potentials are evoked by transcutaneous stimulation of a peripheral nerve with stimulus intensity more than sufficient to produce a maximum response. A supramaximal stimulus consists of a pulsed square wave current of 0–100 mA, usually of 0.1 ms duration. Where a nerve is deep or is hypoexcitable due to demyelination the duration may need to be increased up to 1 ms. The resultant evoked action potential is recorded with surface electrodes at a measured distance from the stimulating surface electrode. The amplitude of the evoked response is recorded and the conduction velocity calculated.

Needle electromyography

With a needle electrode placed in a muscle, action potentials can be recorded from individual muscle fibres or motor units (a group of muscle fibres supplied by one axon) in response to a voluntary contraction. Although there are objective quantitative techniques for this part of the examination, in routine clinical practice this assessment is most often performed subjectively by observation of the action potential representation on a display and listening through a loudspeaker. EMG is used to determine if a deficit of motor function is secondary to nerve dysfunction (neurogenic) or due to primary muscle disease (myopathic). It also allows one to work out the anatomy of a nerve lesion.

Spontaneous activity

The muscle being studied must be completely relaxed. A muscle should be nearly silent on insertion of the needle. If one is near the neuromuscular junction, a characteristic 'endplate noise' is heard. In acutely denervated muscle, myositis, and many myopathies, muscle fibres generate spontaneous, low-amplitude, very brief potentials called fibrillations which are a relatively non-specific feature of disturbed muscle physiology. Fibrillations may occur for months to years if a denervated muscle does not fully reinnervate.

Other spontaneous activity is also seen which may imply more specific diagnoses. Infrequent spontaneously firing motor units (fasciculations) are normal but, if plentiful, suggest chronic denervation as seen in motor neuron disease. Some types of spontaneous and rapidly firing motor units, complex repetitive discharges, and myokymic or neuromyotonic discharges may be seen in proximal compressive lesions, denervation and peripheral demyelination. Myotonic discharges are seen with clinical myotonia.

Motor unit

The shape, duration, firing rate, and amplitude of the individual motor unit action potentials are assessed.

Acute denervation results in a reduced number of motor units which fire at increased frequency. Their morphology remains normal for several weeks after axonal loss. Chronic denervation results in the reinnervation of previously denervated motor units by axonal regeneration and intramuscle collateral axonal sprouting, with consequent increase in amplitude and complexity resulting in polyphasia.

Primary muscle disease is characterized by the presence of many low-amplitude, brief, and polyphasic motor units which fire very easily and rapidly in response to voluntary activation at low levels of muscle contraction.

Interference pattern

At maximal voluntary contraction the number of motor units and fullness of the overall envelope of electrical activity is assessed, referred to as the interference pattern. Denervation from any cause results in the reduction of the number of motor units that can be activated and thereby also a reduction of the interference pattern. In myopathic processes there is a very full, low-amplitude interference pattern at low levels of contraction.

Definitions

Amplitude

The amplitude of an axon-generated action potential recorded with intracellular electrodes is fixed around 100 mV. It is due to the depolarization of the cell (axon or muscle) from its resting membrane potential of around -70 mV to the maximum depolarized state of +30 mV. In the case of an axon this rise is due to the rapid opening of voltage-gated sodium channels clustered at the node of Ranvier.

Compound action potential

The compound action potential (CAP) is recorded using surface electrodes in response to stimulating a peripheral nerve with a supramaximal stimulus. It is the result of the summation of all of the individual axon-generated action potentials.

The CAP amplitude is related to the number of axons stimulated. There are several reasons (beyond the scope of this discussion) why this is an oversimplification but, in general, it holds true. Loss of axons therefore results in a fall in amplitude and loss of function, either loss of sensation or weakness.

The amplitude of the CAP using standard surface electrodes is greatly influenced by the distance from the generator (muscle or axon) to the recording electrode. This results in a very large variability of amplitudes between different nerves, muscles, and subjects, making the provision of normative data nearly impossible. The amplitude is affected by skin thickness, sex, occupation, weight, and age.

Sensory action potential

The sensory action potential (SAP) is the recorded surface potential change in response to the stimulation of only sensory fibres. These are the large myelinated fibres that are relayed centrally via the dorsal columns of the spinal cord.

The isolation of the SAP requires the ability to stimulate a pure sensory nerve such that no motor fibres are included. There are many pure sensory nerves such as the median and ulnar digital and superficial radial nerves in the upper limb and the sural and superficial peroneal nerves in the lower limb. Stimulation of any one of these nerves with a supramaximal stimulus generates a near-synchronized volley of action potentials in the large myelinated sensory axons. The amplitude is measured in μV and the normal amplitude falls in the range of 5–100 μV depending on the nerve examined (Figure 74.1).

Compound muscle action potential

Unlike the sensory recordings, there are no pure motor nerves that can be easily recorded from. The isolation of motor axons requires

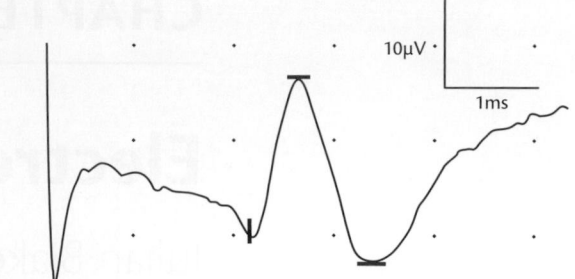

Fig. 74.1 Median sensory action potential. Conduction velocity of 54.5 m/s is measured to the first positive peak, shown by vertical bar latency marker of 2.2 ms over a distance of 12 cm. The action potential amplitude of 18 μV is measured between the two horizontal bars.

an indirect approach, recording from a muscle. The action potential generated in a muscle in response to stimulation of a nerve must be the result of stimulation of motor axons only.

A supramaximal stimulus of motor axons causes activation of the muscle at the neuromuscular junctions and a near-synchronized depolarization of all of the muscle fibres, resulting in a compound muscle action potential (CMAP). CMAPs are much bigger than SAPs and are measured in mV in the range of 2–20 mV depending on the muscle and nerve being studied.

Conduction velocity

Conduction velocity (CV) of axons is largely determined by their diameter and myelination. The larger the axon, and the greater the distance between nodes of Ranvier, the faster it will convey the action potential.

A peripheral nerve is made up of a mixture of fibre types. The majority of the nerve fibres in a peripheral nerve are small-diameter, slowly conducting, unmyelinated or thinly myelinated fibres that convey autonomic functions and information about pain and temperature. Unfortunately routine neurophysiology cannot examine these and their assessment requires esoteric techniques.

Only the large, fast-conducting, myelinated fibres generate electrical signals big enough to be recorded with surface electrodes. CV is calculated by dividing the distance between stimulation electrode and the recording point by the time taken for the generation of an action potential at the recording point in seconds, and is measured in m/s. The first electrical deflection from the baseline represent the time at which the action potential arrives at the recording site due to the fastest conducting fibres. As a general rule the normal recorded velocities are in the region of 50–60 m/s in the upper limb and 40–50 m/s in the lower limb. This is due to the fact that axons taper, being large at the cell body and thinner at their distal end. The main variable influencing CV in the non-diseased state is temperature. Cooling by 1 °C may reduce velocity by 2 m/s. Temperature is therefore controlled to 30–32 °C during the examination.

Disturbance of the myelin or loss of large, fast-conducting axons results in a fall in CV. Conduction slowing on its own does not lead to symptoms or clinical signs.

Measuring sensory CV is simple. A sensory nerve is stimulated at one point and recorded from either upstream (orthodromic) or downstream (antidromic). The distance between these two points divided by the time taken by the action potential to travel between them gives the velocity.

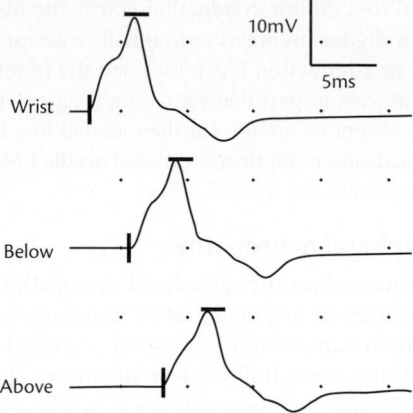

Fig. 74.2 Ulnar motor study recording from abductor digiti minimi. Vertical bars mark the onset latencies of motor responses stimulating at the wrist, below the elbow, and above the elbow. The distal motor latency (DML = 2.5 ms) to stimulation at the wrist is measured to the top vertical bar. The conduction velocities are 65 m/s in the forearm and 45 m/s around the elbow. Motor amplitudes are 13.6 mV at the wrist, 13.0 mV below the elbow, and 10.9 mV above the elbow.

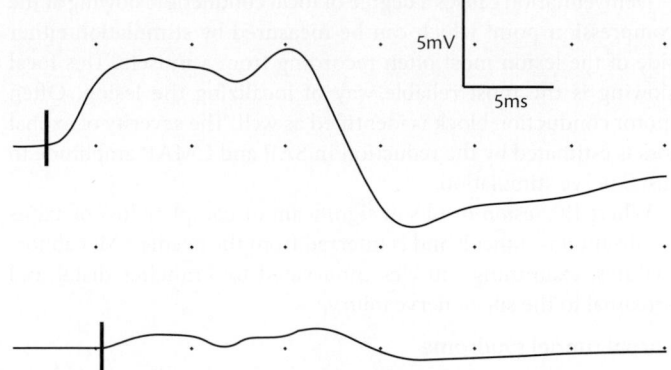

Fig. 74.3 Motor conduction block at the fibula head. Amplitude of compound muscle action potential from tibialis anterior stimulating below the fibula head is 4.8 mV and stimulating above the fibula head is 0.9 mV. The conduction velocity across the fibula head is 27 m/s (RR >40 m/s).

Motor CV is a little more complicated because of the indirect method of recording from motor fibres using the CMAP. It is not possible to calculate a velocity between the stimulation point of a motor nerve and the onset of the CMAP as there is an unknown delay in transmission across the neuromuscular junction and generation of an action potential in the muscle. Therefore motor fibres are stimulated at two separate points. The distance between these points is divided by the difference in onset of the CMAP generated by each stimulus. Motor CV is often measured in multiple segments along the nerve, stimulating at accessible points (Figure 74.2).

Distal motor latency

The distal motor latency (DML) is an important measure of the speed of motor conduction at the very distal end of the nerve. It is measured in milliseconds (ms). The DML is dependent on the distance from the stimulation point to the muscle and also on the CV of the motor axons. The recording distance is usually around 8 cm and results in a normal DML of 3–5 ms. This is variable between nerve–muscle arrangements being studied. There are a number of clinical situations where the distal motor nerve is more affected than more proximal parts.

Mixed nerve action potential

The mixed nerve action potential is the term used to identify the response to stimulation of a named nerve which includes both motor and sensory axons. Most of the amplitude is, however, due to stimulation of sensory fibres as these are usually more numerous than motor axons. It is measured in a similar way to sensory conduction, stimulating the nerve at one point and recording at another, either orthodromically or antidromically.

Conduction block and temporal dispersion

The concept of conduction block generates a lot of confusion. Most commonly it is seen in entrapment neuropathies and is the result of a segment of demyelination at a point of compression. An action potential cannot reliably travel along a demyelinated axon. The axon nevertheless remains viable and is also able to generate an action potential both proximal and distal to the segment that

has no myelin, but not through the segment. In the case of a motor nerve, stimulation distally elicits a motor response but not when the nerve is stimulated proximal to the demyelinated lesion. This usually affects only a proportion of axons in a nerve, so the result is a motor response that is smaller to proximal stimulation than it is to distal stimulation (Figure 74.3).

The amplitude of a motor response may be reduced not due to failure of conduction through a demyelinated segment but due to variable severity of demyelination resulting in an increased range of conduction velocities. This causes a prolongation of the CMAP or temporal dispersion. This is often wrongly described as conduction block.

Another situation where conduction block is seen is following trauma or peripheral nerve infarction where there is acute axonal damage An axon divided from its cell body may be able to generate an action potential for up to 10 days after injury. Thus in the early phase after injury, stimulation of the distal segment of the nerve elicits an action potential but stimulation of the proximal part of the nerve cannot. This is sometimes referred to as pseudo conduction block.

F wave and H reflex

Although in principle very proximal conduction velocities can be measured, the latency of the F wave is most often used as an indirect measure of proximal conduction. The F wave is a non-physiological reflex dependent on the retrograde stimulation of the motor nerve. A motor action potential can travel the wrong way along the axon to the anterior horn cell where it can generate a reflex action potential which then travels back down the motor axon in the normal physiological direction evoking a recordable motor response distally. Any delay in the time taken for this reflex (F latency) with normal distal conduction implies proximal slowing and demyelination. The Hoffman reflex (H reflex) is used in a similar way but is a physiological response dependent on the stretch reflex arc and stimulation of the 1A afferents from the muscle spindle. It is the neurophysiological counterpart of the tendon reflex.

Clinical application

Entrapment neuropathies

As already mentioned, entrapment of a nerve may cause a segment of demyelination but there is frequently axonal damage in varying amounts.

Demyelination causes a degree of focal conduction slowing at the compression point which can be measured by stimulation either side of the lesion most often recording from a muscle. This focal slowing is the most reliable way of localizing the lesion. Often motor conduction block is identified as well. The severity of axonal loss is estimated by the reduction in SAP and CMAP amplitude to distal nerve stimulation.

Where the lesion results in significant or complete loss of axons localization is difficult and is inferred from the needle EMG abnormalities, examining muscles innervated by branches distal and proximal to the site of nerve injury.

Carpal tunnel syndrome

The neurophysiological examination of patients with carpal tunnel syndrome (CTS) represents a paradigm of neurophysiology and of other entrapment neuropathies.

The aim is to confirm the focal nature of the neuropathy at the wrist and grade its severity. The median nerve SAP is normally recorded by stimulating a median-innervated digit and recording over the median nerve proximal to the carpal tunnel. This is compared to either the ulnar or radial SAP. In a mild or early neuropathy only slowing of conduction may be seen but as the condition progresses axonal degeneration occurs with a fall in SAP amplitude. The DML to abductor policis brevis is measured to determine the degree of distal motor slowing. As with sensory conduction, evidence of motor slowing and demyelination normally occur before loss of axons and CMAP amplitude reduction.

A variety of short-segment nerve studies are used to demonstrate focal carpal tunnel slowing such as a median palm to wrist sensory CV and a comparison of the DML to the second lumbrical (median innervated) to that of the second interosseous (ulnar innervated) muscles.

Endstage CTS results in the loss of recordable median motor and sensory responses, preventing confirmation of the focal nature of the original lesion. Neurophysiology for CTS is not usually required for diagnosis but is needed for planning treatment and predicting outcome. Patients with mild or severe neurophysiological abnormalities have been shown to respond less well to surgical decompression compared to those with moderate changes.

Other entrapment neuropathies

The principles used to study CTS apply to other entrapment neuropathies.

Focal slowing or conduction block in the radial nerve when compressed in the spiral grove is usually difficult to show but if a patient with a wrist drop has loss of radial sensation but a normal radial SAP it can be inferred that there is conduction block somewhere along the nerve. When accompanied by normal needle EMG of triceps and reduced motor unit recruitment in brachioradialis, the lesion would clearly localize to somewhere between the nerve branches to each of these muscles. One would also be able to say that the lesion is demyelinating and, as long as it was acute, it would be expected to recover within 8–12 weeks from onset (the time taken to remyelinate a nerve). Where the SAP is attenuated and the needle EMG demonstrates acute denervation a degree of axonal damage would be evident and the time to recovery would depend on axonal regeneration from the site of injury, traditionally said to occur at the rate of 1 mm/day.

Acute foot drop is assessed in the same way. The superficial peroneal SAP is measured in the foot; loss or attenuation of the response implies axonal loss. Motor conduction across the fibular head to either extensor digitorum brevis or to tibialis anterior is measured; focal slowing or conduction block localizes the lesion and would confirm it as at least in part demyelinating (Figure 74.3). If motor responses are absent or attenuated then axonal loss has occurred and further localization requires additional needle EMG of muscles both above and below the knee.

Axonal peripheral neuropathy

An axonal motor and sensory peripheral neuropathy is characterized by attenuation of SAP and CMAP amplitudes. In the early phase of a length-dependent pathological process this will affect distal fibres in the lower limbs before significant changes in the upper limbs. Conduction velocities are generally within normal limits but, in certain circumstances, the motor conduction velocities may be mildly slowed due to the preferential loss of the largest and fastest axons.

Pure sensory neuropathies are encountered where only attenuation of SAPs is demonstrated. This might be seen in some presentations of diabetic neuropathy and in hereditary sensory and autonomic neuropathies (HSAN). Diseases of sensory ganglia such as due to Sjögren's or paraneoplastic neuropathies will produce similar features but the neurophysiological abnormalities may be either patchy or uniform but not length dependent.

Pure motor neuropathies are also seen. These are usually distal hereditary motor neuropathies (dHMN). The diagnosis requires the demonstration of normal sensory conduction and attenuation of motor responses, along with denervation of distal limb muscles on needle EMG.

Demyelinating peripheral neuropathy

The cardinal feature of a demyelinating neuropathy is CV slowing. Uniform slowing of conduction is a feature of hereditary motor and sensory neuropathies (HMSN or Charcot–Marie–Tooth disease, CMT) and patchy, variable slowing suggestive of acquired neuropathies such as acute inflammatory demyelinating polyneuropathy (AIDP or Guillian–Barré syndrome) and chronic inflammatory demyelinating polyneuropathy (CIDP). It is increasingly recognized that this distinction is not absolute and the neurophysiologist's clinical experience and pattern recognition ability becomes important under these circumstances. A not infrequent cause of failure of CIDP to respond to treatment is a misdiagnosis of X-linked CMT (CMTX). The neurophysiological features of CIDP, CMTX, and classical diabetic neuropathy may be indistinguishable.

Radiculopathy

Neurophysiology does not have a significant role in the diagnosis of radiculopathy, which is investigated better with MRI. Consideration of the neurophysiology of radiculopathy, however, illustrates some important principles. When a nerve root is injured the lesion is usually proximal to the dorsal root ganglion and described as being preganglionic. Afferent sensory information to the spinal cord is interrupted and the patient will have sensory disturbance or numbness in the distribution of the nerve root but, because the peripheral sensory axons are still connected to the sensory cell body, the peripheral sensory conduction remains normal. Conversely the motor axons that are divided in the root lose their connection with the anterior horn cell body and degenerate, resulting in denervation of muscles in that root distribution. The combination of numbness and weakness with normal sensory conduction but denervation usually indicates a preganglionic root lesion.

Vasculitis

Peripheral nerve vasculitis causes a variety of neurophysiological patterns, the most classical of which results from mononeuritis multiplex. This typically results in loss of both SAP and CMAP when stimulating the affected nerve at any point along its course. Occasionally there are a few surviving axons through the infarcted area of nerve with recordable, albeit severely attenuated, responses. Needle EMG of supplied muscles shows acute denervation changes. A source of confusion results from the fact that, if the nerve is examined within 10 days of symptom onset, the distal axons can still generate action potentials, mimicking the neurophysiological features of conduction block. In practice this should not present a diagnostic problem, and this possibility should not delay the neurophysiological examination. The suspicion of peripheral nerve vasculitis is a rare instance where the clinical presentation requires urgent neurophysiological examination.

Some more indolent vasculitic conditions may result in the gradual accruing of motor and sensory deficits with progressive attenuation of SAP and CMAP amplitudes in a distal and symmetrical fashion, which can be neurophysiologically indistinguishable from a length-dependent peripheral neuropathy. A high index of suspicion is required and the diagnosis may need to be confirmed with a nerve biopsy.

Motor neuronopathy

The term motor neuronopathy refers to diseases of anterior horn cells. When the neurophysiology shows isolated motor axon loss the possibility of anterior horn cell disease must be considered. The neurophysiological clue to the diagnosis is the lack of length-dependence of motor axon loss with proximal muscles such as paraspinal muscles showing similar signs of denervation to distal limb muscles. A prerequisite for this diagnosis is the absence of both sensory symptoms and neurophysiological sensory abnormalities.

Neurophysiologically the features are those of a preganglionic lesion and similar to a root lesion.

Primary muscle disease

The examination of a patient with a primary muscle disease needs needle EMG. As already mentioned the myopathic EMG pattern is of low amplitude, rapidly recruiting and polyphasic motor units. The pattern is often non-specific and the main role of neurophysiology is to exclude a neurogenic cause, suggesting the need for a muscle biopsy.

Neuromuscular junction disorders

Neuromuscular junction disorders are characterized neurophysiologically by a progressive fall in CMAP amplitude in response to repetitive motor nerve stimulation at 3 Hz. This is referred to as a decrement. Postsynaptic conditions such as myasthenia gravis are distinguished from presynaptic ones such as Lambert–Eaton myasthenic syndrome (LEMS) by the response of the CMAP amplitude to 15 s of maximal voluntary contraction. The latter condition shows a post contraction increment greater than twice the CMAP amplitude at rest. This is due to a presynaptic influx of calcium and results in increased acetylcholine release. The quantitative technique of single-fibre EMG is also used to measure the increased variability of conduction velocity and decreased reliability of synaptic transmission which occurs in neuromuscular junction disorders.

Further reading and resources

American Association of Neuromuscular and Electrodiagnostic Medicine: www.aanem.org

Bland JD. Do nerve conduction studies predict the outcome of carpal tunnel decompression? *Muscle Nerve* 2001;24(7):935–940.

Preston DC, Shapiro BE. *Electromyography and neuromuscular disorders*, 2nd edition. Elsevier Butterworth Heinemann, Philadelphia, PA, 2005.

Michell A. Understanding EMG. Oxford University Press 2013

Neuromuscular Home Page, Neuromuscular Diseases Center, Washington University, St Louis, MO USA: http://neuromuscular.wustl.edu

SECTION 8

Management of rheumatic disease

CHAPTER 75

Patient education

David Walker and Ben Thompson

Introduction

Patient education is recognized as essential for the management of musculoskeletal disorders. National and international guidelines invariably state its importance,[1,2] while moral and practical arguments for its value are persuasive. Patients have a right to know about their health and treatment, while education enables patients to contribute to decisions about their health, access appropriate help, and behave in ways which could improve their future health.

While there may be consensus that patient education is a 'good thing', evidence-based guidance describing how health professionals should develop and provide educational resources is not available, nor are tools to decide if education is effective. Equally, there is no clear consensus about what constitutes 'effective' education—i.e. the precise changes we should be expecting education to have on patients. This chapter therefore goes beyond this acceptance of patient education as beneficial for patients, and examines topics including its scope and aims, the practical steps patients take to learn about their condition, and the challenges faced by those who develop, provide or evaluate educational resources for patients. It summarizes the current evidence and opinion around patient education, and suggests methods to improve education and learning for patients in the future.

Definition and aims

Patient education is a broad term which is difficult to define. The term adopts different meanings in different circumstances, relates to a variety of resources and interventions according to the situation and audience, and aims to achieve broad but ill-defined benefits. Its use overlaps and is used interchangeably with concepts such as health literacy,[3] patient participation,[4] and self-management.[5] Kate Lorig's definition of patient education is the most widely used in rheumatology, and was adopted by the Cochrane review of education for people with rheumatoid arthritis[6]:

> any set of planned, educational activities designed to improve patients' health behaviors and/or health status. ... The purpose is to maintain or improve health, or, in some cases, to slow deterioration.[7]

By suggesting that only *planned* activities meet her definition, Lorig excludes much of the learning that patients carry out independently, for example through searches for information on the internet, or during routine consultations with health professionals. These methods of education may be the most effective for patients,

or the most commonly used. Equally, while health professionals may view education as a way of '*improving* patients' health behaviours', this aim may not be shared by patients themselves. Instead, patients may view education as a way of obtaining new ideas about treatments, or evaluating the health care they are receiving. Thus, if an educational resource does not reflect the aims and needs of patients then they are unlikely to choose to use it, and it will be unsuccessful because of a lack of uptake. These differences between the aims of providers of education and patients themselves need to be considered, and should be reflected in the design and aims of such resources.

The World Health Organization (WHO) also offers a definition of 'Therapeutic Patient Education' which has influenced practice in Europe:

> Therapeutic Patient Education (TPE) helps patients acquire or maintain the skills they need to manage their life with a chronic disease in the best possible way. It covers organized activities, including psychosocial support, designed to make patients fully aware about their disease and to inform them about care, hospital organization and procedures, and health- and disease-related behaviours. It helps patients and their families understand and deal with the disease and its treatment together, in order to maintain or even improve quality of life.[8]

This definition does not limit patient education to processes separate from routine care and, in contrast to Lorig, focuses on *informing* patients about their behaviour rather than *improving* it. It also acknowledges the need for patients' families to be included in attempts to provide education for people with chronic illnesses.

The aims of patient education deduced from these definitions are therefore not only to increase patients' knowledge about their condition and treatment, but are also focused on changing their behaviour and, ultimately, improving their health. This perspective of education as a 'therapy' is supported by examining the outcome measures used in studies of educational interventions, which include a range of physical, psychological, behavioural, and health status measures. The potential of such interventions to achieve benefits for society by reducing economic costs through a decrease in participants' utilization of healthcare has also been recognized by both academics and policy-makers.[9]

However, there are wider functions of education which are not recognized by such definitions, or by the research studies designed to evaluate them. As well as broadly trying to help patients 'feel better' in terms of their physical, psychological health, and social participation, and the potential societal benefits of economic savings, it can also improve relationships between patients and their healthcare professionals, providing patients with sources of help they can return to if they encounter problems in the future. There are also benefits for health professionals themselves. These are rarely emphasized in the literature but are important when deciding whether to invest resources in patient education; it can reduce health professionals' workload, and may increase patients' willingness to participate in research studies.

As well as educating patients it is also important to educate the wider population—health education—for two principal reasons. First, so that society does not disadvantage people with musculoskeletal conditions, making adaptations in the case of physical disability and understanding the symptoms and challenges they may face. Secondly, in the case of inflammatory arthritis, to encourage early presentation to medical professionals, in turn leading to earlier treatment which has been shown to be more effective.[10] Most of the delay to diagnosis for rheumatoid arthritis (RA) is the delay in the patient presenting to the GP rather than the GP referring to the hospital.[11] Health beliefs such as 'It's only arthritis and there isn't much they can do about that' should be challenged and consigned to the past.

Historical overview

Many of the social, demographic, and medical changes during the last century have contributed to the growing interest in and need for high-quality patient education. A greater proportion of the population now live for considerable periods with one or more chronic illnesses, and health systems have shifted focus from the treatment of acute illness to long-term 'incurable' conditions such as arthritis. These changes have in turn prompted changes to how healthcare systems are envisaged, with self-care at the base of a healthcare pyramid in the United Kingdom.[9] Self-care is the care taken by individuals towards their own health and well-being, including those of their family and communities. It increases the scope for patients to participate in decisions about their health care, a role in which they require both information and the skills to appraise it. The traditional model of a paternalistic doctor and a compliant patient has to some extent been replaced with ideas of partnership and 'patient participation'.[4]

Simultaneously, the concept of 'patient consumerism' has become more prevalent—the refusal of patients to accept the 'medical dominance' of doctors, and a desire to 'shop around' for the best health care available.[12] Patients are therefore more inclined to seek out the information on which to base these types of decisions. At the same time, such information has become more accessible, in part because of the growth of the internet.

However, this demand for information from patients is not universal and a proportion of patients are content not to know about their condition,[13] or do not wish to participate in decisions about their care.[14] Similarly, the idea that education can lead to a fully informed, autonomous patient has been criticized, especially if the aim of the intervention is to increase compliance with medical care.[15] At the same time, some commentators have suggested that 'patient empowerment'—the expectation that patients will take control of their illness and treatment—is not necessarily in their interests.[16]

Patient education has changed alongside these developments, from interventions which focused on the transfer of knowledge

in the 1970s, to more sophisticated interventions which focus on patients' self-care and decision making, and are often based on psychological theory. Social learning theory,[17] and the related concept of self-efficacy, are fundamental to self-management programmes such as those developed by Kate Lorig. Social learning theory upholds the importance of demonstrating or 'modelling' appropriate health behaviours. Self-efficacy refers to an individual's confidence in their ability to perform a task or specific behaviour successfully.

Methods of delivering patient education

Learning can take place in many settings, and can occur independently of health care and health professionals. The first point of education may be at the time of diagnosis where information will be offered by the clinician, usually verbally and written. This will be against the background of a narrative that the patient has developed to explain their symptoms and current health state. The narrative is developed around their health beliefs on causation and treatment, which may not necessarily be credible to the clinician.[18] Further contact with professionals provides opportunities for question-and-answer learning as well as formal education about things such as drugs. Studies of where patients get information and how they value it suggest information from clinicians, particularly doctors, is rated most highly.[19] Good communication is at the heart of education and many communication models exist, of which the Cambridge Calgary model remains a current favourite.[20]

More formal education is often done in groups because they are thought to be efficient in terms of professional time. There has been speculation over whether a professional group leader is necessary and whether a lay leader may be equally or more effective.[21] This has led to initiatives around self-management and 'expert patients' and to the Expert Patient Programme in the United Kingdom.[22] It is proposed that the lay leader for such groups acts as a role model for attendees, making them more likely to change health behaviours. This has been both evaluated[23] and criticized.[24]

Research into such interventions for ankylosing spondylitis has shown that group self-management education could improve self-efficacy scores but not measures of the disease itself.[25] A study of physiotherapy-led education for exercises in anyklosing spondylitis (AS) showed better spinal mobility at 9 months.[26] Similarly, studies in RA and osteoarthritis (OA) have shown an effect of education on pain and self-management.[27]

Overall, studies have failed to show a clinically significant long-term benefit from group education, though in part this may reflect the challenges in designing appropriate trials and measuring any resulting changes. The benefits of groups include the ability of participants to share their experiences, and learn from each other. At the same time, they are less able to offer attendees specific advice and address their learning needs and queries. Equally, some patients are unwilling to attend groups because of the time commitment, or because they do not want to discuss their own health in a public setting.

One-to-one education by a health professional is more resource intensive, but commonly occurs as part of routine care. It has the advantage of offering information tailored to that individual, and has shown very good satisfaction with patients. Probably because the resource implications make it less attractive to healthcare providers, there is less published research on one-to-one education, but there is a similar lack of long-term benefit.[28] One-to-one is the usual format for educating patients prior to commencement of new drugs and a study has shown better adherence to the medication following this.[29]

Written information is also widely used, and Arthritis Research UK has produced information in leaflet and booklet form for more than 50 years. They produce written information on diseases and drugs as well as more generic information on topics such as pain; footwear; gardening, and sex. They produce more than 2 million leaflets and booklets, delivered free to patients and professionals.[30] These have been evaluated[31] and, in a substudy on RA, were shown to increase knowledge, improve pain and depression, but no effect was shown on overall health. Such booklets are valued highly by patients, principally because they offer a definitive information source which, if handed to them by their clinician, has been endorsed by their health professional.

The use of written information raises the issue of language and the decoding and understanding of it, i.e. literacy. In a study from Glasgow[32] 15% of participants were found to be functionally illiterate. There was association between this and social factors and use of health services. It is therefore unlikely in this group that the handing out of a densely worded leaflet will produce much useful education. One initiative to make information more accessible is the production of 'mind maps' of some booklets by Arthritis Research UK (see Figure 75.1). These are much more visual, using pictures spreading out from a central icon, and use fewer words. Patients are able to look at the pictures while the text is read to them. It was expected that they would have utility for people whose first language was not English and in those with specific learning difficulties. In an evaluation for RA[33] the 15% functional illiteracy was confirmed, but knowledge transfer was greater for the literate participants and if anything enhanced by the mind map in these people. The illiterate participants in this study were generally globally challenged rather than having a particular problem with written English. The mind map may have utility in people with dyslexia and people whose first language is not English.

On the same theme there are diseases such as osteomalacia that are more common in people from ethnic minorities. Arthritis Research UK has translated the osteomalacia booklet into five languages with matching audiotapes. These have been evaluated[34] and show the huge problems of producing such translations that are culturally as well as language sensitive. Similarly, the images used on the osteomalacia mind map have been redrawn with input from the populations involved.[35] One set of images was found to be suitable for all languages including English.

Beyond specifically produced and edited information as above there is the internet. There are huge resources of information out

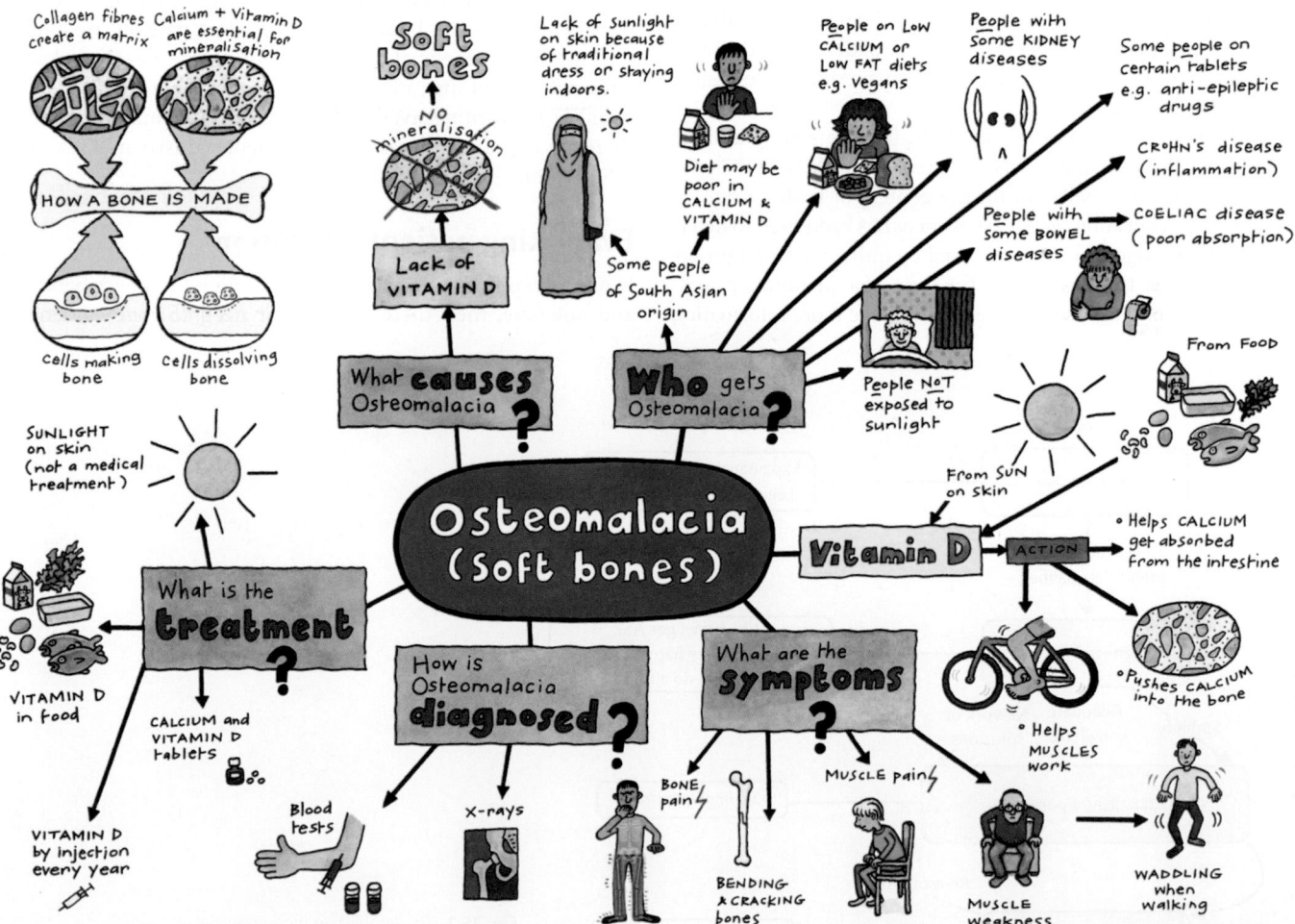

Fig. 75.1 An example mind map, in this instance referring to osteomalacia. Reproduced with kind permission from Arthritis Research UK.

there and many of them are very good. However, there is also information that is misleading or taken out of context, which may not be helpful. Patients using the internet as a source of information need to be aware of the lack of provenance of some sites and choose what to access. Exactly how they do this will undoubtedly be the subject of research and debate. The internet is a very convenient way to access information and educational resources and allows greater interactivity and timeliness. In a recent survey of professionals accessing internet resources, the provenance of the material was judged the most important feature, followed by speed and ease of access.[36] It is hoped that patients will learn to make similar discriminations.

Content and timing of patient education

As part of the process of education, patients should accumulate knowledge and skills to help them manage and cope with their musculoskeletal condition. Knowledge may include such diverse topics as an understanding of the pathophysiology of their condition, action to take in the event of developing new symptoms, and how to take medication safely. Relevant skills include managing pain, appraising new information, negotiating the healthcare system, and learning to cope with chronic illness. However, there is such variation between individuals' conditions and backgrounds that a universal and comprehensive curriculum is not practical. There is also a balance between what patients want to know, and what health professionals judge is useful for them to know—that is, knowledge or skills that are likely to improve patients' health. These two viewpoints must be reconciled when considering the content of any education programme.

Needs assessment within the wider healthcare setting aims to bring about changes in the provision of care which benefit the population as a whole, usually within the context of finite resources. Within patient education, needs assessment has been used to determine the knowledge and skills required by individuals or a group. In some instances this has been in the form of a quantitative questionnaire regarding topics the patient would like more information

about.[37] While these may offer healthcare providers some useful information about what patients want, they are unlikely to offer a comprehensive account of what they need, which relies on health professionals' assessment of their circumstances, and judgements about what they would find useful and potentially improve their condition.

Alongside debate about the content which should be provided for patients is a debate about when it should be provided. Issues related to timing have been considered in relation to patients' 'readiness to learn'.[38] and their 'stages of change'.[39] However, both these concepts view education as consistently and undoubtedly beneficial for patients, and view patients' judgements not to engage with education as inherently flawed.

Recent work focusing on the choices and practical steps patients with AS take to learn about their condition has proposed an alternative model with respect to the timing of education.[40] This work observed that patients' search for information was influenced by the stage of their condition (see Figure 75.2). When first diagnosed, patients began a rapid search for information, searching for the answers to three broad and challenging questions—'Why have I got AS?', 'What is going to happen to me and my family?', and 'What can I do about it?'. Later, when their health, their health care and their social lives are more stable, they become 'established'; their search for information slows, and is orientated towards solving or adapting to new problems as and when they arise.

It is therefore not possible to be prescriptive about the content of patient education, because the topics that patients are likely to find useful or beneficial are dependent on the health and social circumstances of the individual. The range of potential topics and quantity of learning available to patients are immense, and yet there are broad topic areas which patients consistently search for information.

Evaluating patient education

If one is expecting educational interventions to affect behaviour and outcome, then there is a similar need to have evidence of

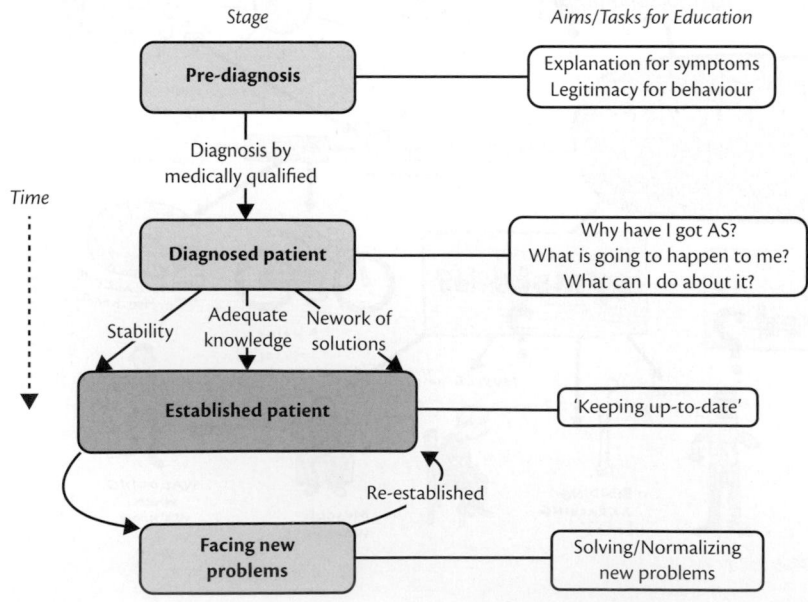

Fig. 75.2 The established patient model.

From Thompson B. Education and learning for people with ankylosing spondylitis. MD thesis, Newcastle University, 2011.

effectiveness and lack of harm as with any other intervention. It has always been necessary to show effectiveness and lack of harm for a drug to get a licence, yet education is something health professionals do every day with patients. The need to examine this interaction and any supporting material scientifically to measure and improve effects has been adopted more slowly.

This partially explains the relative lack of studies; however, the complexity of the methodology and outcome measures required for educational interventions is also a major factor. Educational intervention studies have been judged to be of poorer quality than those of the pharmacological industry.[41] However, this is principally for structural reasons, as discussed below. A typical study of educational needs will involve a qualitative phase to identify the issues, then a quantitative phase to explore these in a larger population. A study of the effectiveness of an educational intervention will usually show a change in knowledge or confidence, but showing a change of behaviour is much more difficult. Kirkpatrick's hierarchy[42] (see Figure 75.3) displays this in pyramid form with patient satisfaction at the bottom, going through knowledge and skill acquisition, then change of behaviour to a peak of better health outcomes for the patient and society at large. Change is progressively more difficult to show, and confounding factors are more likely to explain the differences between study groups the further up the pyramid you go.

Equally, for the results of such studies to be generalizable, the study population should be adequately described and be similar to the population to which the results are to be applied. In pharmacological studies, this can usually be achieved by detailing variables which could influence the effect of the drug, such as the age, gender, ethnicity, comorbidity, or even genotype of the participants. While these variables are also likely to be important in deciding whether educational interventions are applicable to a particular population, an additional range of variables may influence the outcome of educational interventions, and less is known about their potential effect. Therefore, consideration should also be given to variables which are less easy to describe, such as participants' level of education, previous experience of patient education, social circumstances, personality, educational needs, and expectations. Patients who are recruited for group educational studies are not representative of the wider population with arthritis, with more female, elderly, and well-educated patients volunteering.[43] The discrepancy is probably influenced by the significant time commitment required from participants, and thus the need to either sacrifice other activities or to have sufficient leisure time in order to attend. This does reduce our ability to generalize the results of such trials to those populations who may actually have more to gain from education—those who have lower levels of previous educational attainment, lower social class, and who have poorer outcomes with respect to their arthritis.

Improving patient education

Patient education can be improved by health professionals increasing the quality of education they offer patients, and through the production of high-quality research which will inform our future practice.

In the case of the former, patient education can influence the greatest number of patients if it is part of routine care—not just an optional extra to be chosen by those who are highly motivated but may have less to gain. This routine care involves offering verbal and written information, especially at the time of diagnosis and changes to health or treatment, allowing time for questions, and even prompting to find out what information they have already found through their own searches. It is important to appreciate the role health professionals play in recommending educational resources to patients, endorsing their use, and acknowledging their need for information about their condition. Health professionals need to be aware of the resources, including groups, that are available locally, and be prepared to offer them to patients. They should also be alert for areas of unmet need, either for groups of patients or for individuals, and seek to address these. Strategies to identify those patients who would benefit from additional support and education should be utilized. However, education also needs to be convenient, and increasingly, this means using the internet. As part of education, patients gain from learning about the experience of other patients, and this too can be accessed through different online resources such as social media, charities, and resources such as healthtalkonline.[44]

Research around this topic has focused on the evaluation of resources in the form of randomized trials, and 'measuring the measurable' is certainly useful when looking to compare interventions and learn more about their effects. However, as already discussed, this is challenging and may neglect important effects and benefits of education. At the same time, research which could be considered the 'basic science' of educational research can be enlightening and produce new ideas for methods of helping patients. Qualitative research has helped to describe and understand the questions and problems patients face as they learn to cope with their musculoskeletal condition, and the resources they choose to use, and how they use them. At the same time we can learn about groups of patients who may benefit from different approaches, such as those for whom English is not their first language, or have low previous educational attainment. There remains a great deal more to learn about the optimum methods to offer information to patients, and help them to learn the skills they need.

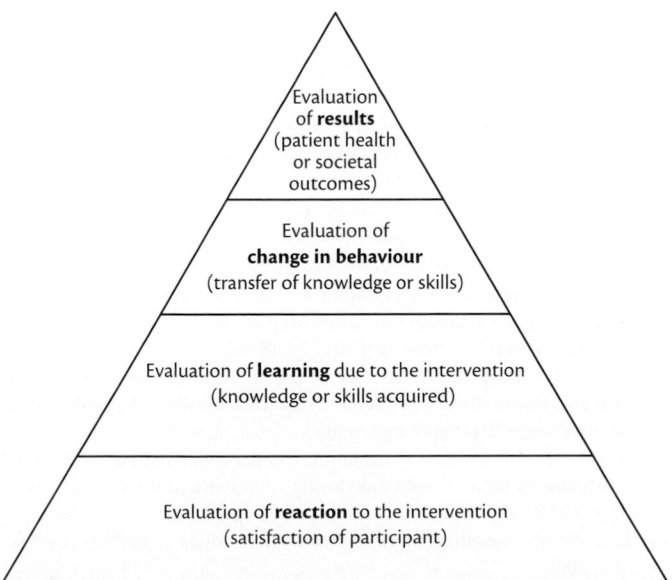

Fig. 75.3 Kirkpatrick's hierarchy—evaluating educational interventions. Adapted from Kirkpatrick DL, Kirkpatrick JD. Evaluating training programs, 3rd edn. Berrett-Koehler, San Francisco, CA, 2006.

Evaluation of **results** (patient health or societal outcomes)

Evaluation of **change in behaviour** (transfer of knowledge or skills)

Evaluation of **learning** due to the intervention (knowledge or skills acquired)

Evaluation of **reaction** to the intervention (satisfaction of participant)

Conclusion

We have presented an overview of patient education for people with musculoskeletal conditions, illustrating the range of resources available, evidence regarding their effect on patients, and the challenges for researchers and practitioners in this field. It has become an increasingly important topic as patients become more involved in decisions about their care, and shoulder increasing responsibility for their own health and health care. However, the time, money, and expertise required to provide education can be substantial, and solutions need to be found from limited resources. The use of technology, including social media and online resources, is likely to continue to change this field. Overall, though, it is important to remember that patients will continue to learn about their condition and the best ways to cope and adapt to it; our challenge as health professionals is to aid them in their learning as effectively as we can. Patient education is not a process imposed on passive patients; instead, it is about enabling patients to learn, and identifying patients who would benefit from additional help in this process.

References

1. National Institute for Health and Clinical Excellence. *The management of rheumatoid arthritis in adults CG79)*, 2009. Available at: www.nice.org.uk/nicemedia/pdf/CG79NICEGuideline.pdf. Accessed 08/04/2012.

2. National Institute for Health and Clinical Excellence. *The care and management of osteoarthritis in adults (CG59)*, 2009. Available at: www.nice.org.uk/nicemedia/live/11926/39557/39557.pdf. Accessed 08/04/2012.

3. Nutbeam D. Health literacy as a public health goal: a challenge for contemporary health education and communication strategies into the 21st century. *Health Promot Int* 2000;15(3):259–267.

4. Coulter A. Paternalism or partnership? Patients have grown up—and there's no going back. *BMJ* 1999;319(7212):719–720.

5. Newman S, Mulligan K, Steed L. What is meant by self-management and how can its efficacy be established?, *Rheumatology* 2001;40(1):1–4.

6. Riemsma RP, Kirwan JR, Taal E, Rasker JJ. Patient education for adults with rheumatoid arthritis, *Cochrane Database Syst Rev* 2003;2:CD003688.

7. Lorig K. *Patient education: a practical approach*, 2nd edn. Sage, London, 1996.

8. WHO (Europe). *Therapeutic patient education: continuing education programmes for health care providers in the field of prevention of chronic diseases: report of a WHO working group*. World Health Organization, Copenhagen, Denmark, 1998.

9. Department of Health (UK). Self care—a real choice: self-support a practical option, 2005. Available at: www.dh.gov.uk/en/Publicationsandstatistics/Publications/PublicationsPolicyAndGuidance/DH_4100717. Accessed: 8/4/2012.

10. van der Linden MPM, le Cessie S, Raza K et al. Long-term impact of delay in assessment of patients with early arthritis *Arthritis Rheum* 2010;62(12):3537–3546.

11. Kumar K, Daley E, Carruthers DM et al. Delay in presentation to primary care physicians is the main reason why patients with rheumatoid arthritis are seen late by rheumatologists. *Rheumatology* 2007;46:1438–1440.

12. Lupton D. Consumerism, reflexivity and the medical encounter. *Soc Sci Med* 1997;45(3):373–381.

13. Kjeken I, Dagfinrud H, Mowinckel P et al. Rheumatology care: Involvement in medical decisions, received information, satisfaction with care, and unmet health care needs in patients with rheumatoid arthritis and ankylosing spondylitis, *Arthritis Rheum* 2006;55(3):394–401.

14. May C. Patient autonomy and the politics of professional relationships. *J Adv Nurs* 1995;21(1):83–87.

15. Fahrenfort M. Patient emancipation by health education: an impossible goal? *Patient Educ Couns* 1987;10:25–37.

16. Salmon P, Hall G. Patient empowerment or the emperor's new clothes. *J Roy Soc Med* 2004;97:53–56.

17. Bandura A. *Social learning theory*. Prentice-Hall, Englewood Cliffs, NJ, 1977.

18. Donovan J. Patient education and the consultation: the importance of lay beliefs. *Ann Rheum Dis* 1991;50(Suppl 3):418–421.

19. Buckley LM, Vacek P, Cooper SM. Educational and psychosocial needs of patients with chronic disease. A survey of preferences of patients with rheumatoid arthritis. *Arthritis Care Res* 1990;3(1):5–10.

20. Silverman J, Kurtz S, Draper J. *Skills for communicating with patients*. Radcliffe Publishing, Oxford, 1998.

21. Lorig K, Feigenbaum P, Regan C et al. A comparison of lay-taught and professional-taught arthritis self-management courses. *J Rheumatol* 1986;13(4):763–767.

22 Expert Patients Programme. www.expertpatients.co.uk/. Accessed 08/04/12.

23. Kennedy A, Reeves D, Bower P et al. The effectiveness and cost effectiveness of a national lay-led self care support programme for patients with long-term conditions: a pragmatic randomised controlled trial. *J Epidemiol Community Health* 2007;61(3):254–261.

24. Taylor D, Bury B. Chronic illness, expert patients and care transition. *Sociol Health Illness* 2007;29(1):27–45.

25. Barlow J, Barefoot J. Group education for people with arthritis. *Patient Educ Couns* 1996;27(3):257–267.

26. Hidding A, van der Linden S, Boers M et al. Is group physical therapy superior to individualized therapy in ankylosing spondylitis? A randomized controlled trial. *Arthritis Care Res* 1993;6(3):117–125.

27. Hammond A, Bryan J, Hardy A. Effects of a modular behavioural arthritis education programme: a pragmatic parallel-group randomized controlled trial, *Rheumatology* 2008;47(11):1712–1718.

28. Branch VK, Lipsky K, Nieman T, Lipsky PE. Positive impact of an intervention by arthritis patient educators on knowledge and satisfaction of patients in a rheumatology practice. *Arthritis Care Res* 1999;12(6):370–375.

29. Hill J, Bird H, Johnson S. Effect of patient education on adherence to drug treatment for rheumatoid arthritis: a randomised controlled trial, *Ann Rheum Dis* 2001;60(9):869–875.

30. Arthritis Research UK. *Arthritis Research Campaign: annual review 2008–09*, 2010. Available at: www.arthritisresearchuk.org/.

31. Barlow J, Pennington D, Williams N, Hartley P, Bishop P. *An evaluation of the arthritis and rheumatism council patient literature materials*. Arthritis Research UK, London, 1995.

32. Gordon MM, Hampson R, Capell HA, Madhok R. Illiteracy in rheumatoid arthritis patients as determined by the Rapid Estimate of Adult Literacy in Medicine (REALM) score. *Rheumatology* 2002;41(7):750–754.

33. Walker D, Adebajo A, Heslop P et al. Patient education in rheumatoid arthritis: the effectiveness of the ARC booklet and the mind map. *Rheumatology* 2007;46(10):1593–1596.

34. Samanta A, Johnson MRD, Guo F, Adebajo A. Snails in bottles and language cuckoos: an evaluation of patient information resources for South Asians with osteomalacia. *Rheumatology* 2009;48:299–303.

35. Walker DJ, Robinson SM, Jagatsinh Y et al. A survey of the images used on the ARUK Osteomalacia Mind-Map in relation to cultural background. *J Visual Commun Med* 2011;34:58–62.

36. Walker DJ, Margham T. The use of the internet to search for education and information: the views of the musculoskeletal professionals. *Rheumatology* 2011;50 (Suppl 3):iii57.

37. Ndosi ME, Hill J, Hale C, Adebajo A. Gender differences of educational needs among patients with ankylosing spondylitis and psoriatic arthritis. *EULAR Conference, Barcelona, 2007*.

38. Bastable SB. *Essentials of patient education*. Jones & Bartlett, Boston, MA, 2006.

39. Prochaska JO, Diclemente C. Towards a comprehensive, transtheoretical model of change and addictive behaviors. In: Miller W, Heather N(eds) *Applied clinical psychology*. Plenum Press, New York, 1998:3–24.

40. Thompson B. *Education and learning for people with ankylosing spondylitis*. MD thesis, Newcastle University, 2011.

41. Boutron I, Tubach F, Giraudeau B, Ravaud P. Methodological differences in clinical trials evaluating nonpharmacological and pharmacological treatments of hip and knee osteoarthritis. *JAMA* 2003;290(8):1062–1070.

42. Kirkpatrick DL, Kirkpatrick JD. *Evaluating training programs*, 3rd edn. Berrett-Koehler, San Francisco, CA, 2006.

43. Hawley D. Psycho-educational interventions in the treatment of arthritis. *Baillieres Clin Rheumatol* 1995;9(4):803–823.

44. DipEX (2012). www.healthtalkonline.org. Accessed 08/04/2012.

CHAPTER 76

Multidisciplinary treatment

Sarah Ryan, Jo Adams, Anne O'Brien, and Anita Williams

Introduction

This chapter explores the evidence base for multidisciplinary treatment from four of the main disciplines involved in the care of people with a long-term musculoskeletal condition: nursing, physiotherapy, occupational therapy, and podiatry. Multidisciplinary treatments occur alongside medical and surgical treatment and involve working in partnership with the patient and with other members of the multidisciplinary team to optimize outcomes.

Nursing

Rheumatology nurse specialists (RNSs) are considered an essential member of the nursing team by both professional and patient organizations. The majority of RNSs are primarily involved in the care and management of people with rheumatoid arthritis (RA). The main role functions of a RNS[1] are shown in Box 76.1.

Three randomized controlled studies (RCTs)[2-4] have demonstrated the positive impact that the RNS can have on the patient's physical and psychological health, including improvements in pain, anxiety, function, and perceptions of self-control over the condition. Hill et al.[2] is a key reference, as this is the first RCT to evaluate the impact of a rheumatology nurse specialist.

Providing support following diagnosis

Following a diagnosis of RA the patient is often referred to the RNS to commence disease-modifying anti-rheumatic drug (DMARD)

Box 76.1 The role functions of the rheumatology nurse specialists

◆ Patient education

◆ Drug monitoring

◆ Psychological support: ongoing from the time of diagnosis

◆ Running telephone advice lines

◆ Running nurse-led clinics for patients with RA

◆ Coordinating care

◆ Assessment, administration and ongoing management of patients receiving biological therapy

---

therapy and receive ongoing psychological support, as the patient commences the process of adapting to living with a long-term condition. In the United Kingdom, in accordance with the National Institute for Health and Clinical Excellence (NICE) guidelines,[5] patients will often commence more than one DMARD. As DMARDs may take several months to provide maximal efficacy, the nurse will carry out a biopsychosocial assessment to identify the impact of the condition and to work with the patient to address those areas of the individual's life where the condition is having the greatest impact.

Many rheumatology nurses also provide one-to-one education or develop multidisciplinary education programmes. In addition they will ensure that the patient has access to the rheumatology telephone advice line, which has become an integral part of most rheumatology services.[6] The telephone advice line is commonly used by patients when they experience an increase in their inflammatory symptoms or notice a possible medication side effect.

Many RNSs run their own follow-up clinics for patients with RA. The main objectives of these clinics are to ensure that the RA is well controlled and the patient is achieving optimum physical, psychological and social function. Monitoring the safety and efficacy of disease-modifying anti-rheumatic drugs (DMARDs) and biological therapies is also a major component of the RNS role as detailed in Box 76.2.[7-8]

Physiotherapy

Physiotherapy (physical therapy) is a key component of multidisciplinary rheumatology management. Physiotherapists, often key patient motivators, have important assessment, treatment and educational roles with patients of all ages. Physiotherapists undertake detailed musculoskeletal (MSK) assessments identifying key functional problems which are likely to impact on treatment outcome, negotiate functional goals with patients, and identify practical approaches to maximizing activities of daily living (ADL). During consultation, physiotherapists are well positioned to identify self-efficacy issues as well as education needs. Some physiotherapists work in extended practitioner roles which include the ordering of investigations, injecting joints and supplementary prescribing.

Box 76.2 The nurse's role in drug monitoring

- Assessing safety in administration, e.g. ensuring that methotrexate is taken on a weekly basis

- Monitoring for any drug reactions that have occurred, e.g. gastrointestinal, skin, urinary abnormalities, and chest manifestations

- Requesting and interpreting appropriate haematological and biochemical investigations

- Assessing for evidence of increased disease activity and increasing the dose of or adding additional DMARD treatment where indicated; some RNS also administer intra-articular joint injections

- Providing the patient with the opportunity to discuss any problems or concerns, e.g. whether they can have a vaccination

- Accessing other care needs and referring where appropriate to other members of the multidisciplinary team

The aims of physiotherapy are to:

- reduce pain/ stiffness

- improve (or maintain) joint range and muscle strength

- maximize physical functioning to achieve optimal quality of life.

The evidence base supporting physiotherapy continues to evolve and therapists continue to provide empirical evidence to support their treatments.

Exercise prescription may often be simple—e.g. encouraging postsurgical mobility, improving transfers from sitting to standing, climbing stairs—but will be fundamental to successful mobility in daily life. In other cases specific rehabilitation of key muscle groups or joints will be the key to return to function.

Exercises in arthritis are often prescribed in conjunction with other modalities to address pain[9] and swelling (e.g. using ice or heat therapy) but they are also used to improve joint range, proprioception, and/or muscle strength, all of which may have a prophylactic effect, as in osteoarthritis,[10] and a positive treatment effect.

Anxiety relating to exacerbating inflamed joints with exercise has been proven to be unfounded and physiotherapists continue to promote the positive effects of aerobic and strengthening exercises in particular[11] (this paper by Vliet Vlieland and van den Ende is a key reference, offering, a contemporary review of the literature focusing on conservative and self-management interventions.) Targeting key muscle groups around weightbearing joints will also aim to improve joint stability and thus optimize not only joint mobility, but functioning. Other exercise prescriptions will focus on optimizing cardiopulmonary fitness and aerobic capacity.[12] There is some evidence for the benefits of t'ai chi exercises (frequently popular with patients) in terms of balance and proprioception.[13]

Limited evidence supports electrical stimulation in management of RA.[14] Transcutaneous electrical nerve stimulation (TENS) intends to relieve pain with some arthritis patients,[15] but dosage is relevant: only 'acupuncture-like TENS' appears to have an analgesic effect. Low-level laser therapy is used less often, but has few side effects and has been shown to provide short-term relief of pain and morning stiffness in RA patients.[16]

Heat therapies are well liked, versatile, and commonly used at home e.g. in the form of hot packs. Wax and hydrotherapy are also used for analgesic purposes. Heat reduces muscle spasm and provides short-term reduction in pain and disability. Heat also reduces acute and subacute low back pain, especially if exercise is added,[17] and short-term analgesic benefits are reported for superficial moist heat in RA. Short-term pain relief has been described with hydrotherapy in osteoarthritis (OA), and it is generally enjoyed and accepted by patients.[18] Cryotherapy (ice), another easy modality to use at home, has been shown to have a beneficial effect on knee range of movement, strength, and function as well as reducing swelling, although the effect on pain is not significant in the OA knee.[19]

Pain reduction and improvements in physical functioning have been demonstrated in a few limited studies using acupuncture for peripheral joint OA.[20] However, other studies in low back pain suggest that acupuncture may be an effective adjunct to other physiotherapy techniques.[21]

A growing evidence base supports the physiotherapist's role in reducing impairment, minimizing disability, and maximizing patient participation. Exercise and education remain fundamental components of their interventions.

Occupational therapy

Occupational therapists aim to improve people's ability to perform daily activities and valued life roles at work, in the home, at leisure, and socially,[22] utilizing a biopsychosocial model.[23-25] The role of the occupational therapist within the multidisciplinary team is to:

- improve a person's ability to perform daily tasks and valued life roles

- facilitate successful adaptation to disruptions in lifestyle

- prevent loss of function

- improve and maintain psychological status.[26]

Occupational therapists evaluate people's specific activities that may be affected by their illness and work closely with them to help

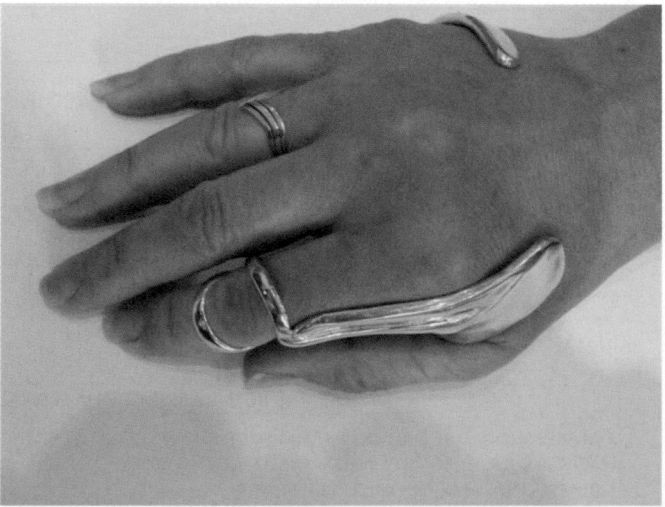

Fig. 76.1 A tailor-made palmar and metacarpal phalangeal splint support.
Reproduced with kind permission of Christina Macleod, Occupational Therapy Department, Royal Hampshire County Hospital, Winchester.

adapt their occupation or activity, the person, and/or the environment. Occupational therapists work within primary and secondary health care delivering effective components to rheumatology rehabilitation,[27] and many are also based in community social services. Here, occupational therapists are ideally positioned to actively assist people to manage and adapt home, work, and community environments using housing adaptations and equipment to facilitate optimum functional ability.[28]

Using a biomechanical model, occupational therapists with specialist skills in regional upper limb and hand rehabilitation work with the person to provide active exercise home programmes[29] and splint provision.[30] These interventions aim to support and protect inflamed, damaged joints and maintain intrinsic muscle strength and functional ability in valued life roles affected by disease processes. Figure 76.1 illustrates an example of a tailor-made splint to provide additional support to metacarpal, proximal phalangeal,

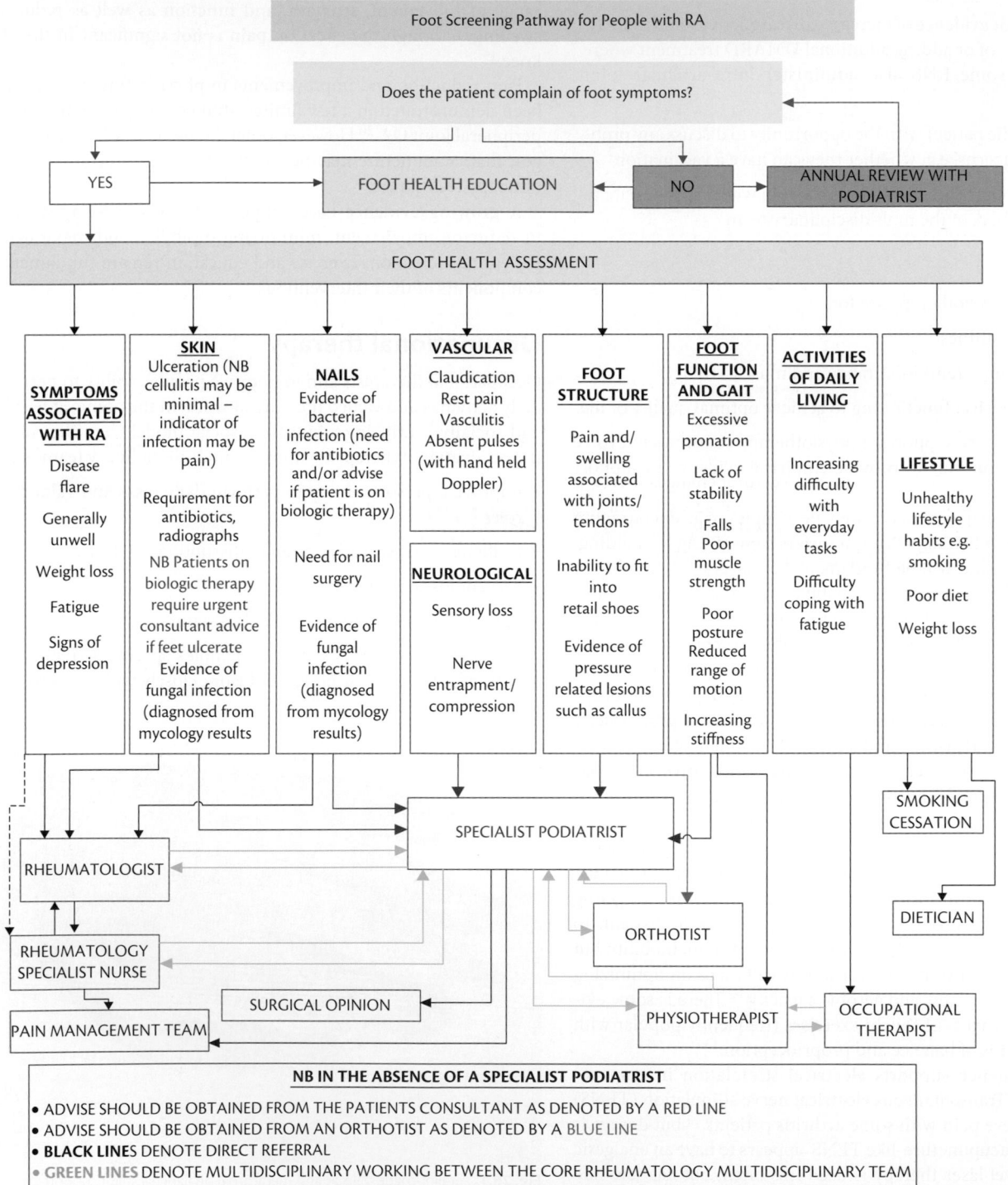

Fig. 76.2 Foot screening pathway for people with rheumatoid arthritis.

From Williams AE, Davies S, Graham A et al. Guidelines for the management of foot health problems associated with rheumatoid arthritis. Musculoskeletal Care 2011;**92**:86–92.

and palmar arches affected by RA in a competitive professional horse rider.

Rehabilitative/compensatory techniques are used to assess and advise regarding the provision of assistive equipment such as chair raises, tap turners, adapted computer keyboards, and wheelchairs and can be supported by an ergonomic assessment of peoples' work and leisure performance.

Home structural adaptations assessed and managed by the social service occupational therapy team may include provision of grab rails, stair lifts, ramps, and ground-floor adaptations. These cost-effective interventions can maintain a person's functional independence, delay performance loss, reduce home falls, and maintain healthy life styles.[31,32] Occupational therapists will also be placed with work rehabilitation and employability schemes to support and enable active living. Access to these services and specialized occupational therapists is recommended within a national clinical care guideline for people with arthritis.[24]

An educational behavioural approach is employed by occupational therapists to encourage and support people to be active partners in their health care and to adopt a range of self-management behaviours such as joint protection and fatigue management.[33]

Podiatry

Many rheumatic diseases have the potential to impact negatively on the feet.[34–35] However, in those with RA, life-limiting foot problems are prevalent[36–37] and persistent, even when the disease is in remission or well managed by systemic therapy.[37–42] Pain and changes in foot structure can severely affect gait and mobility,[40] thereby impacting on quality of life.[41] Structural changes increase both the duration and magnitude of plantar pressures[42] resulting in the formation of hyperkeratosis, and the development of foot ulcers[43] and infection.

Podiatrists are considered the experts in foot health and have a crucial role in the diagnosis, assessment, management, and periodic review of foot and ankle problems for people with rheumatic diseases[44–45] including RA.[46–47] The use of foot orthoses and specialist therapeutic footwear are recommended by both the Arthritis and Musculoskeletal Alliance (ARMA)[46] and NICE,[47] who also recommend that people with RA should have access to foot health assessment and management early in the disease process.

Good links can be established with podiatry services, supported with local screening (Figure 76.2) and referral guidelines that will ensure that foot health is managed in the most appropriate way,[48] especially for those patients on biological therapy who may be at risk of foot ulceration.

Specialist podiatrists assess, monitor, and manage some of the more demanding complications such as significant structural changes, peripheral arterial disease, vasculitis, neuropathy, bacterial and fungal infections of the skin and nails, and ulceration, and can carry out nail surgery for persistent nail deformity and infections. Those specialist podiatrists with extended skills use ultrasonography to both aid diagnosis and guide steroid injections which are effective for targeting localized, inflamed joints when the general disease is controlled. Additionally, all podiatrists who are registered with the Health Professions Council are now able to safely and competently access, supply and administer the range of prescription-only medicines and pharmacy-only medicines available on the approved list of medicines.

In early disease, where there is minimal joint damage and capability for self-management, the combination of medical and local foot health management minimizes the effects of joint and soft tissue involvement. This is achieved through offloading the forefoot and rearfoot control with rigid foot orthoses (Figure 76.3) that aim to control the abnormal alignment of joints and improve function, but this has to be done before the joint changes become irreversible.[49]

Instruction on self-care of the skin and nails can be given to the patient so that they can carry out simple foot hygiene tasks.

Where there are established foot problems (intermediate stage) the focus is on minimizing progressive changes and reduction of symptoms, with maintenance of independence and participation a priority. Orthotic intervention tends to be more accommodative or palliative though still improving control and support. Footwear advice becomes more relevant as the structural changes in the feet (toe deformity, increased width, pressure areas, and hyperkeratosis) mean that patients need guidance as to the styles of footwear that can accommodate both the foot and the orthoses. Judicious sharp debridement of hyperkeratosis may have some therapeutic effect from the patient's perspective, but is not recommended if pressure relief is not provided.[48]

In longstanding disease (late stage), progressive structural changes contribute to further mechanical stresses causing pes plano valgus foot position with significant forefoot deformity. Management focuses on maintenance of good tissue viability, and palliative orthoses designed to protect the plantar aspect of the foot, often requiring specialist therapeutic footwear.[53] If the non-surgical interventions fail to relieve symptoms then a referral for consultation about surgical options is recommended.[47]

Conclusion

This chapter has identified the roles and functions of four different professionals involved in the care of people with musculoskeletal conditions. Where research evidence is available this has been used to discuss the merits and limitations of multidisciplinary treatments delivered by nurses, physiotherapists, occupational therapists and podiatrists. It is additionally recognized that people with musculoskeletal conditions will have varying physical, psychological, and

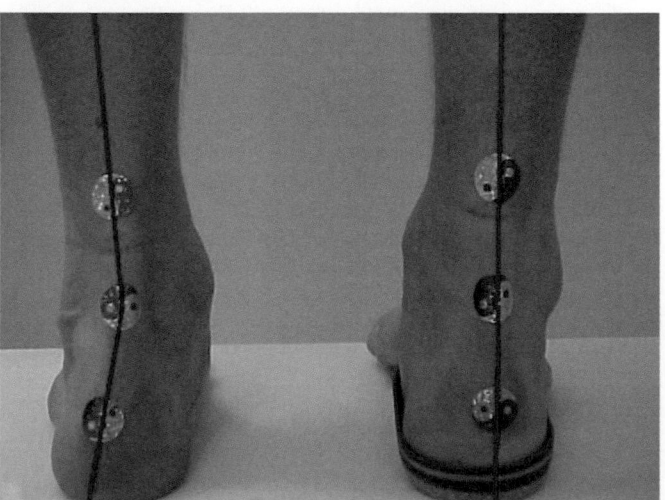

Fig. 76.3 Realignment of an everted rearfoot (left foot) with foot orthoses (right foot).

social needs that may require input from other health professionals including psychologists, dietitians, social workers, pharmacists, and orthotists.

References

1. RCN. *Rheumatology nursing: a survey exploring the performance and activity of rheumatology nurses.* Royal College of Nursing, London, 2009.

2. Hill J, Bird HA, Harmer R, Wright V, Lawton C. An evaluation of the effectiveness, safety and acceptability of a nurse practitioner in a rheumatology outpatient clinic. *Br J Rheumatol* 1994;33:283–288.

3. Tijhuis GT, Zwindermann AH, Hazes JMW et al. A randomised comparison of care provided by a clinical nurse specialist, an inpatient team and a day patient team in rheumatoid arthritis. *Arthritis Care Res* 2002;45:280–286.

4. Ryan S, Hassell AB, Lewis M, Farrell A. Impact of a rheumatology expert nurse on the wellbeing of patients attending a drug monitor clinic. *J Adv Nurs* 2006;53(3):277–286.

5. NICE. *Rheumatoid arthritis: national clinical guideline for management and treatment of adults (CG79).* National Institute of Health and Clinical Effectiveness, London, 2009.

6. Thwaites C. Rheumatology telephone advice lines. *Musculoskeletal Care* 2004;2(2):120–126.

7. Ryan S, Voyce MA. The role of the nurse in drug therapy. Chapter 3 in Ryan S (ed) *Drug therapy in rheumatology nursing.* Wiley, Chichester, 2007:171–172.

8. RCN. *Assessing, managing and monitoring biologic therapies for inflammatory arthritis.* Royal College of Nursing, London, 2009.

9. Fransen M, McConnell S, Hernandez-Molina G, Reichenbach S. Exercise for osteoarthritis of the hip. *Cochrane Database Syst Rev* 2009;3:CD007912.

10. Segal NA, Glass NA, Felson DT et al. Effect of quadriceps strength and proprioception on risk for knee osteoarthritis. *Med Sci Sports Exerc* 2010;42(11):2081–2088.

11. Vliet Vlieland TP, van den Ende CH. Nonpharmacological treatment of rheumatoid arthritis. *Curr Opin Rheumatol* 2011;23(3):259–264.

12. Breedland I, van Scheppingen C, Leijsma M, Verheij-Jansen NP, van Weert E. Effects of a group-based exercise and educational program on physical performance and disease self-management in rheumatoid arthritis: a randomized controlled study. *Phys Ther* 2011;91:879–893

13. Uhlig T, Fongen C, Steen E, Christie A, Ødegård S. Exploring Tai Chi in rheumatoid arthritis: a quantitative and qualitative study. *BMC Musculoskelet Disord* 2010;11:43.

14. Pelland L, Brosseau L, Casimiro L et al. Electrical stimulation for the treatment of rheumatoid arthritis. *Cochrane Database Syst Rev* 2002;2:CD003687.

15. Brosseau L, Yonge KA, Welch V et al. Transcutaneous electrical nerve stimulation (TENS) for the treatment of rheumatoid arthritis in the hand. *Cochrane Database Syst Rev* 2003;2:CD004377.

16. Casimiro L, Brosseau L, Welch V et al. Therapeutic ultrasound for the treatment of rheumatoid arthritis. *Cochrane Database Syst Rev* 2002;3:CD003787.

17. French SD, Cameron M, Walker BF, Reggars JW, Esterman AJ. Superficial heat or cold for low back pain. *Cochrane Database Syst Rev* 2006;1:CD004750.

18. Bartels EM, Lund H, Hagen KB et al. Aquatic exercise for the treatment of knee and hip osteoarthritis. *Cochrane Database Syst Rev* 2007;4:CD005523.

19. Brosseau L, Yonge KA, Welch V et al. Thermotherapy for treatment of osteoarthritis. *Cochrane Database Syst Rev* 2003;4:CD004522.

20. Manheimer E, Cheng K, Linde K et al. Acupuncture for peripheral joint osteoarthritis. *Cochrane Database Syst Rev* 2010;1:CD001977.

21. Furlan AD, van Tulder MW, Cherkin D et al. Acupuncture and dry-needling for low back pain. *Cochrane Database Syst Rev* 2005;1:CD001351.

22. Hammond A. What is the role of the occupational therapist? *Best Pract Res Clin Rheumatol* 2004;18(4):491–505.

23. National Collaborating Centre for Chronic Conditions. *Osteoarthritis: National clinical guideline for care and management in adults.* Royal College of Physicians, London, 2008.

24. NICE. *Rheumatoid arthritis. National clinical guideline for management and treatment in adults (CG79).* National Institute for Health and Clinical Excellence, London, 2009.

25. *Standards of care for people with inflammatory arthritis.* Arthritis and Musculoskeletal Alliance, London, 2004.

26. *Occupational therapy clinical guidelines for rheumatology.* College of Occupational Therapists, London, 2003.

27. Steultjens EM, Dekker J, Bouter LM et al. Occupational therapy for rheumatoid arthritis. *Cochrane Database Syst Rev* 2004;1:CD003114.

28. Heywood F, Turner L. *Better outcomes, lower costs: implications for health and social care budgets of investment in housing adaptations, improvements and equipment: a review of the evidence.* Stationary Office, London, 2007.

29. Hammond A, Young A, Kidao R. A randomised controlled trial of occupational therapy for young people with early rheumatoid arthritis. *Ann Rheum Dis* 2004;63:23–30.

30. Adams J. A research report on the effectiveness of silver ring splints in preventing interphalangeal joint hyperextension during functional activity. *J Rheumatol Occup Ther* 2008;23(1): 19–21.

31. DiMonaco M, Vallero F, De Toma E. A single home visit by an occupational therapist reduces the risk of falling after hip fracture in elderly women: a quasi-randomised controlled trial. *J Rehabil Med* 2008;40(6):446–450.

32. Gitlin L. Conducting research on home environments: lessons learned and new directions. *Gerontologist* 2003;43(5): 628–637.

33. Bodenheimer T, Lorig K, Holman H, Grumbach K. Patient self-management of chronic disease in primary care. *JAMA* 2002;288(19): 2469–2475.

34. Hyslop E, McInnes IB, Woodburn J, Turner DE. Foot problems in psoriatic arthritis: high burden and low care provision. *Ann Rheum Dis* 2010;69(5):928.

35. Sari-Kouzel H, Hutchinson CE, Middleton A et al. Foot problems in patients with systemic sclerosis. *Rheumatology (Oxford)* 2001;40(4):410–413.

36. Grondal L, Tengstrand B, Nordmark B, Wretenberg P, Stark A. The foot: still the most important reason for walking incapacity in rheumatoid arthritis: distribution of symptomatic joints in 1,000 RA patients. *Acta Orthop* 2008;79(2):257–261.

37. Otter SJ, Lucas K, Springett K et al. Foot pain in rheumatoid arthritis prevalence, risk factors and management: an epidemiological study. *Clin Rheumatol* 2010;29(3):255–271.

38. van der Leeden M, Steultjens MP, van Schaardenburg D, Dekker J. Forefoot disease activity in rheumatoid arthritis patients in remission: results of a cohort study. *Arthritis Res Ther* 2010;12:R3.

39. Otter SJ, Lucas K, Springett K et al. Comparison of foot pain and foot care among rheumatoid arthritis patients taking and not taking anti-TNFα therapy: an epidemiological study. *Rheumatol Int* 2011;31(11):1515–1519.

40. Turner DE, Helliwell PS, Siegel KL, Woodburn J. Biomechanics of the foot in rheumatoid arthritis: identifying abnormal function and the factors associated with localised disease 'impact'. *Clin Biomech* (Bristol, Avon) 2008;23:93–100.

41. Wickman AM, Pinzur MS, Kadanoff R, Juknelis D. Health-related quality of life for patients with rheumatoid arthritis foot involvement. *Foot Ankle Int* 2004;25:19–26.

42. Woodburn J, Helliwell PS. Relation between heel position and the distribution of forefoot plantar pressures and skin callosities in rheumatoid arthritis *Ann Rheum Dis* 1996;55:806–810.

43. Firth J, Hale C, Helliwell P, Hill J, Nelson EA. The prevalence of foot ulceration in patients with rheumatoid arthritis. *Arthritis Care Res* 2008;59:200–205.

44. Arthritis and Musculoskeletal Alliance. *Standards of care*, 2004. Available at: www.arma.uk.net/care.html

45. PRCA. *Standards of care for people with musculoskeletal foot health problems*, 2008. Available at: www.prcassoc.org.uk/standards-project.

46. ARMA. *Standards of care for people with inflammatory arthritis*. Arthritis and Musculoskeletal Alliance, London, 2004.

47. NICE. *Guidelines for the management for the adult with rheumatoid arthritis (CG79)*, 2009. Available at: http://guidance.nice.org.uk/CG79/Guidance/pdf/English. Consulted May 2011.

48. Williams AE, Davies S, Graham A et al. Guidelines for the management of foot health problems associated with rheumatoid arthritis *Musculoskeletal Care* 2011;9(2):86–92.

49. Woodburn J, Hennessy K, Steultjens MP, McInnes IB, Turner DE. Looking through the 'window of opportunity': is there a new paradigm of podiatry care on the horizon in early rheumatoid arthritis? *J Foot Ankle Res* 2010;3:8.

50. Farrow SJ, Kingsley GH, Scott DL. Interventions for foot disease in rheumatoid arthritis: a systematic review. *Arthritis Rheum* 2005;53(4):593–602.

Sources of patient information

Arthritis Care: www.arthritiscare.org.uk
Arthritis Research UK: www.arthritisresearchuk.org/
National Rheumatoid Arthritis Society: www.nras.org.uk

CHAPTER 77

Cyclooxygenase inhibitors

Burkhard Hinz and Kay Brune

Mode of action and side effects of cyclooxygenase inhibitors

Biochemical basis

In 1971, Vane showed that the anti-inflammatory action of non-steroidal anti-inflammatory drugs (NSAIDs) rests in their ability to inhibit the activity of the cyclooxygenase (COX) enzyme, which in turn results in a diminished synthesis of proinflammatory prostaglandins.[1] This action is considered a major factor of the mode of action of NSAIDs, although not the only one. The pathway leading to the generation of prostaglandins has been elucidated in detail. Within this process, the COX enzyme (also referred to as prostaglandin H synthase) catalyses the first step of the synthesis of prostanoids by converting arachidonic acid into prostaglandin H_2, which is the common substrate for specific prostaglandin synthases (Figure 77.1). The enzyme is bifunctional, with fatty-acid COX activity (catalysing the conversion of arachidonic acid to prostaglandin G_2) and prostaglandin hydroperoxidase activity (catalysing the conversion of prostaglandin G_2 to prostaglandin H_2). In the early 1990s, COX was demonstrated to exist as two distinct isoforms.[2,3] COX-1 is constitutively expressed as a 'housekeeping' enzyme in nearly all tissues, and mediates physiological responses (e.g. cytoprotection of the stomach, platelet aggregation). COX-2, expressed by cells that are involved in inflammation (e.g. macrophages, monocytes, synoviocytes), has emerged as the isoform that is primarily responsible for the synthesis of prostanoids involved in pathological processes, such as acute and chronic inflammatory states (Figure 77.1). The expression of COX-2 is regulated by a broad spectrum of other mediators involved in inflammation. Accordingly, glucocorticoids have been reported to inhibit the expression of the COX-2 isoenzyme.[2]

Side effects dependent on COX-1 inhibition

All conventional NSAIDs interfere with the enzymatic activity of both COX-1 and COX-2 at therapeutic doses.[4] In fact, many of the side effects of NSAIDs (e.g. gastrointestinal ulceration and bleeding, platelet dysfunctions) are due to a suppression of COX-1-derived prostanoids. Likewise, COX-1 inhibition confers hypersensitivity to aspirin and other chemically unrelated NSAIDs in 5–20% of patients with chronic asthma and in an unknown fraction of patients with chronic urticaria–angioedema. Here, inhibition of COX-1 leads to activation of the lipoxygenase pathway and production of cysteinyl leukotrienes that induce bronchospasm and nasal obstruction. Asthmatic patients who are intolerant to NSAIDs produce low levels of bronchodilatatory prostaglandin E_2 (probably because of a lack of COX-2), and have increased levels of leukotriene C4 synthase and reduced levels of metabolites (lipoxins) released through the transcellular metabolism of arachidonic acid.[5]

Analgesic action dependent on COX-2 inhibition

On the other hand, inhibition of COX-2-derived prostanoids facilitates the anti-inflammatory, analgesic, and antipyretic effects of NSAIDs. Inflammation causes an increased synthesis of COX-2-dependent prostaglandins, which sensitize peripheral nociceptor terminals and produce localized pain hypersensitivity. Prostaglandins regulate the sensitivity of so-called polymodal nociceptors that are present in nearly all tissues. A significant proportion of these nociceptors cannot be easily activated by physiological stimuli such as mild pressure or some increase of temperature.[6] However, following tissue trauma and subsequent release of prostaglandins, 'silent' polymodal nociceptors become excitable to pressure, temperature changes, and tissue acidosis.[7] This process results in a phenomenon called hyperalgesia—in some instances allodynia. Prostaglandin E_2 and other inflammatory mediators facilitate the activation of tetrodotoxin-resistant Na^+ channels in dorsal root ganglion neurons.[8–10] Another important target of protein kinase A-mediated phosphorylation is the capsaicin receptor (transient receptor potential vanilloid 1, TRPV1), a non-selective cation channel of sensory neurons involved in the sensation of temperature and inflammatory pain.[11–13] TRPV1 responds to temperature above 40 °C and to noxious stimuli including capsaicin, the pungent component of chili peppers, and extracellular acidification. On the basis of this mechanism, prostaglandins produced during inflammatory states may significantly increase the excitability of nociceptive nerve fibres, including reactivity to temperatures below 40 °C (i.e., body temperature), thereby contributing to the activation of 'sleeping' nociceptors and the development of burning pain. As such, it appears reasonable that at least a part of the peripheral antinociceptive action of COX inhibitors arises from prevention of this peripheral sensitization. Apart from sensitizing peripheral nociceptors, prostaglandins also act in the central nervous system to produce central hyperalgesia. Experimental data suggest that both acidic and non-acidic COX inhibitors antagonize central

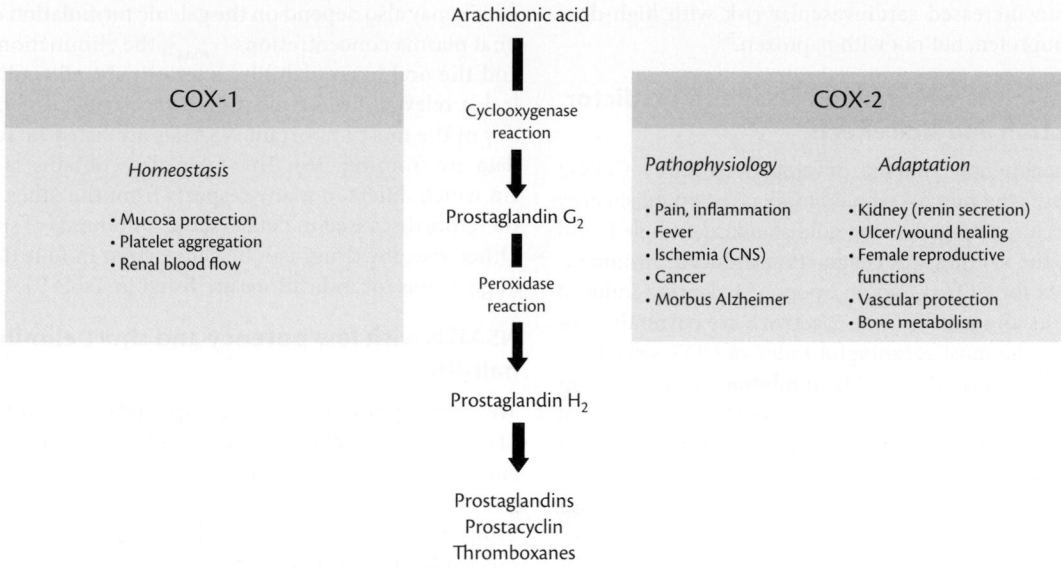

Arachidonic acid

COX-1		COX-2	
Homeostasis		*Pathophysiology*	*Adaptation*

Cyclooxygenase reaction

Prostaglandin G$_2$

Peroxidase reaction

Prostaglandin H$_2$

Prostaglandins
Prostacyclin
Thromboxanes

COX-1 — *Homeostasis*
- Mucosa protection
- Platelet aggregation
- Renal blood flow

COX-2 — *Pathophysiology*
- Pain, inflammation
- Fever
- Ischemia (CNS)
- Cancer
- Morbus Alzheimer

COX-2 — *Adaptation*
- Kidney (renin secretion)
- Ulcer/wound healing
- Female reproductive functions
- Vascular protection
- Bone metabolism

Fig. 77.1 Physiological and pathophysiological roles of COX-1 and COX-2.

hyperalgesia in the dorsal horn of the spinal cord by modulating the glutamatergic signal transfer from nociceptive C fibres to secondary neurons, which propagate the signals to the higher centres of the central nervous system. Some COX-2 is expressed constitutively in the dorsal horn of the spinal cord, and becomes upregulated briefly after a trauma, such as damage to a limb, in the corresponding sensory segments of the spinal cord.[14] The induction of spinal cord COX-2 expression may facilitate transmission of the nociceptive input. In line with a role of COX-2 in central pain perception, Smith et al.[15] reported that selective COX-2 inhibition suppressed inflammation-induced prostaglandin levels in cerebrospinal fluid, whereas selective inhibition of COX-1 was inactive in this regard. These observations were substantiated by findings showing a widespread induction of COX-2 expression in spinal cord neurons and in other regions of the central nervous system following peripheral inflammation.[16] Several mechanisms have been proposed to underlie the facilitatory action of prostaglandin E$_2$ on central pain sensation. Baba et al.[17] showed that prostaglandin E$_2$ at relatively high concentrations directly depolarizes wide dynamic range neurons in the deep dorsal horn. More convincingly, prostaglandin E$_2$ at significantly lower concentrations reduces the inhibitory tone of the neurotransmitter glycine on to neurons in the superficial layers of the dorsal horn[18] by phosphorylation of the specific glycine receptor subtype GlyRα3,[19] thereby causing a disinhibition of spinal nociceptive transmission. In another study, the same group has identified prostaglandin E$_2$ receptors of the EP$_2$ receptor subtype as key signalling elements in spinal inflammatory hyperalgesia,[20] thus opening new avenues for the development of new analgesics.

Side effects dependent on COX-2 inhibition

The hypothesis that selective inhibition of COX-2 might have therapeutic actions similar to those of NSAIDs, but without causing the unwanted side effects elicited by COX-1 inhibition, was the rationale for the development of selective COX-2 inhibitors. However, the simple concept of COX-2 being an exclusively proinflammatory and inducible enzyme cannot be sustained in the light of diverse experimental and clinical findings. Accordingly, COX-2

has also been shown to be expressed under basal conditions in organs including the ovary, uterus, brain, spinal cord, kidney, cartilage, bone, and even the gut, suggesting that this isozyme may play a more complex physiological role than previously recognized (for review see ref. 21).

In line with this view, a permanent blockade of COX-2-dependent prostaglandins, including prostacyclin, is the currently most plausible explanation for the cardiovascular hazard conferred by long-term use of selective and non-selective COX-2 inhibitors. In fact, prostacyclin, which is suppressed by over 60% by both NSAIDs and selective COX-2 inhibitors,[22] is not only a potent inhibitor of platelet aggregation, but also interferes with processes leading to hypertension, atherogenesis, and cardiac dysfunction. In this context changes in arterial blood pressure have been proposed to underlie the long-term cardiovascular side effects of both NSAIDs and COX-2 inhibitors. The involvement of COX-2 in human renal function is supported by numerous clinical studies that showed that COX-2 inhibitors, similar to NSAIDs, can cause peripheral oedema, hypertension, and exacerbation of pre-existing hypertension by inhibiting water and salt excretion by the kidneys.[23–25] These observations are of major importance given that relatively small changes in blood pressure could have a significant impact on cardiovascular events. In patients with osteoarthritis, increases in systolic blood pressure of 1–5 mmHg have been associated with 7100–35 700 additional ischaemic heart disease and stroke events over 1 year.[26]

It has been suggested that both degree and time-course of intravascular COX-2 inhibition might determine the differential profile of cardiovascular side effects associated with NSAIDs and COX-2 inhibitors.[27–29] Claims that NSAIDs inhibit COX-1 thereby conferring cardioprotection proved wrong since platelet COX-1 activity has to be suppressed by more than 95% to translate into inhibition of platelet aggregation.[30] Such a complete COX-1 inhibition over the whole dosing interval is only achieved by low-dose aspirin and in some individuals by high-dose naproxen (500 mg twice daily).[30,31] Other NSAIDs such as ibuprofen and diclofenac suppress COX-1 (>95%) only at peak plasma concentrations. This is consistent with an increased cardiovascular risk with high-dose diclofenac and ibuprofen, but not with naproxen.[32]

COX inhibition in the whole blood assay as a predictor of analgesic action and side effects

Among the experimental systems developed to study COX-2 selectivity of drugs, the human whole blood assay established by Patrono's group[33] has emerged as the gold standard. Whole blood assays, based on the synthesis of coagulation-induced thromboxane B_2 as an index for COX-1 and on lipopolysaccharide-induced prostaglandin E_2 as an index of COX-2 activity, are currently considered to provide the most meaningful index of COX selectivity. In these assays, the selectivity of COX inhibition is measured in a physiological milieu which takes into account the differential binding of drugs to plasma proteins. According to Huntjens et al.[34] ex-vivo COX-2 inhibition in the whole blood assay by approximately 80% is expected to result in analgesia due to the fact that the analgesic therapeutic plasma concentration of a COX inhibitor correlates with its inhibitory concentration $(IC)_{80}$ (the concentration that leads to 80% inhibition) on COX-2 in the human whole blood assay. By contrast, only in excess of 95% suppression of thromboxane B_2 formation translates into clinically relevant inhibition of platelet aggregation,[30] thus predicting whether a drug might cause cardioprotection (and bleeding) or not. In addition, ex-vivo COX-2 inhibition measurements from whole blood has been suggested as a potential surrogate to estimate cardiovascular risk.[27-29]

Non-steroidal anti-inflammatory drugs (acidic antipyretic analgesics)

Based on the finding that aspirin at high doses (>3 g/day) not only inhibits fever and pain but also interferes with inflammation, Winter developed an assay to search for drugs with a similar profile of anti-inflammatory activity.[35] Amazingly, all substances that survived the test of experimental pharmacology and clinical trials turned out to be acids with a high degree of lipophilic–hydrophilic polarity, similar pK_a values, and a high degree of plasma protein binding (for reviews see refs 36–38).

Later it turned out that high concentrations of these acidic compounds are reached in bloodstream, liver, spleen, and bone marrow (due to high protein binding and an open endothelial layer of the vasculature), but also in body compartments with acidic extracellular pH values.[39] The latter type of compartments includes the inflamed tissue, the wall of the upper gastrointestinal tract, and the collecting ducts of the kidneys. Concerning gastrointestinal toxicity, there are, in fact, at least two major components contributing to the ulcerogenic action of NSAIDs in the stomach: a topical irritant effect on the epithelium and the ability to suppress prostaglandin synthesis.[40-43] Topical irritant properties are confined to acidic NSAIDs which accumulate in gastric epithelial cells because of the phenomenon of 'ion trapping'.[44]

Apart from aspirin, all of these compounds differ in their potency, i.e., the single dose necessary to achieve a certain degree of effect ranges from a few milligrams (e.g. lornoxicam) to about 1 g (e.g. salicylic acid). They also differ in their pharmacokinetic characteristics, i.e. the speed of absorption (time to peak, t_{max};

which may also depend on the galenic formulation used), the maximal plasma concentrations (c_{max}), the elimination half-life ($t_{1/2}$), and the oral bioavailability. Interestingly, all traditional NSAIDs lack a relevant degree of COX-2 selectivity.[4] The key characteristics of the most important NSAIDs are listed in Table 77.1 (most data are from ref. 36). This table also contains the data on aspirin which differs in many respects from the other NSAIDs and is therefore discussed in detail (see 'Compounds of special interest'). Otherwise, the drugs can be categorized in four different groups. Suggestions for indications are listed in Table 77.2.

NSAIDs with low potency and short elimination half-life

The prototype of this type of compounds is ibuprofen. Other drugs of this group are salicylates and mefenamic acid. The latter does not appear to offer major advantages. By contrast, this and other fenamates are rather toxic at overdosage (central nervous system). The drugs of this group are particularly useful for blocking occasional mild inflammatory pain.

In the following the pharmacology of ibuprofen is addressed in more detail. Depending on its galenic formulation, fast or slow absorption of ibuprofen may be achieved. A fast absorption of ibuprofen was observed following administration of the respective lysine salt.[45] The bioavailability of ibuprofen is close to 100% and the elimination is always fast, even in patients suffering from mild or severe impairment of liver or kidney function.[36] Ibuprofen is used as single doses ranging from 200 mg to 1 g. A maximum dose of 3.2 g per day (United States) or 2.4 g (Europe) for rheumatoid arthritis is possible. At low doses ibuprofen appears particularly useful for the treatment of acute occasional inflammatory pain. High doses of ibuprofen may also be administered, although with less benefit, for the treatment of chronic rheumatic diseases. Remarkably, at high doses the otherwise harmless compound has been shown to result in an increased incidence of gastrointestinal side effects.[46] In some countries ibuprofen is also administered as the pure S-enantiomer, which comprises the active entity of the racemic mixture in terms of COX inhibition. On the other hand, a substantial conversion of the less potent COX inhibitor R-ibuprofen (comprises 50% of the usual racemic mixture) into the active S-enantiomer has been observed following administration of the racemic mixture.[47]

NSAIDs with high potency and short elimination half-life

These drugs are predominantly prescribed for the treatment of rheumatic (arthritic) pain. The most widely used compound of this group is diclofenac. Other drugs of this group are lornoxicam, flurbiprofen, and indomethacin (very potent), but also ketoprofen and fenoprofen (less active). All of the latter drugs show a high oral bioavailability and good effectiveness, but also a relatively high risk of unwanted drug effects.[48]

Diclofenac appears to be less active on COX-1 as compared to COX-2.[4,49] This is taken as a reason for the relatively low incidence of gastrointestinal side effects of diclofenac.[48] The limitations of diclofenac result from its usual formulation (monolithic acid-resistant coated dragée or tablet). In fact, retention of such formulations

Table 77.1 Physicochemical and pharmacological data of acidic antipyretic analgesics

Pharmacokinetic/chemical subclasses	pK$_a$	Binding to plasma proteins	Oral bioavailability	t_{max}[a]	$t_{1/2}$[b]	Single dose (maximal daily dose) for adults
Low potency/short elimination half-life						
Salicylates						
Aspirin	3.5	50%–70%	~50% dose-dependent	~15 min	~15 min	0.05–1 g[c] (~6 g)
Salicylic acid	3.0	80%–95% dose-dependent	80%–100%	0.5–2 h	2.5–4.5 h dose-dependent	0.5–1 g(~6 g)
2-Arylpropionic acids						
Ibuprofen	4.4	99%	100%	0.5–2 h	2 h	200–800 mg (2.4 g)
Anthranilic acids						
Mefenamic acid	4.2	90%	70%	2–4 h	1–2 h	250–500 mg (1.5 g)
High potency/short elimination half-life						
2-Arylpropionic acids						
Flurbiprofen	4.2	>99%	No data	1.5–3 h	2.5–4(–8) h	50–100 mg (200 mg)
Ketoprofen	5.3	99%	~90%	1–2 h	2–4 h	25–100 mg (200 mg)
Aryl-/heteroarylacetic acids						
Diclofenac	3.9	99.7%	~50% dose-dependent	1–12 h[e] very variable	1–2 h	25–75 mg (150 mg)
Indometacin	4.5	99%	~100%	0.5–2 h	2–3(–11) h[d] very variable	25–75 mg (200 mg)
Oxicams						
Lornoxicam	4.7	99%	~100%	0.5–2 h	4–10 h	4–12 mg (16 mg)
Intermediate potency/intermediate elimination half-life						
Salicylates						
Diflunisal	3.3	98%–99%	80%–100%	2–3 h	8–12 h dose-dependent	250–500 mg (1 g)
2-Arylpropionic acids						
Naproxen	4.2	99%	90%–100%	2–4 h	12–15 h[d]	250–500 mg (1.25 g)
Arylacetic acids						
6-Methoxy-2-naphthyl-acetic acid (active metabolite of nabumetone)	4.2	99%	20%–50%	3–6 h	20–24 h	0.5–1 g (1.5 g)
High potency/long elimination half-life						
Oxicams						
Piroxicam	5.9	99%	~100%	3–5 h	14–160 h[d]	20–40 mg; initial: 40 mg
Tenoxicam	5.3	99%	~100%	0.5–2 h	25–175 h[d]	20–40 mg; initial: 40 mg
Meloxicam	4.08	99.5%	89%	7–8 h	20 h[e]	7.5–15 mg

[a]Time to reach maximum plasma concentration after oral administration.

[b]Terminal half-life of elimination.

[c]Single dose for inhibition of thrombocyte aggregation, 50–100 mg; single analgesic dose, 0.5–1 g.

[d]Enterohepatic circulation.

[e]Monolithic acid-resistant tablet or similar galenic form.

Table 77.2 Indications for antipyretic analgesics

Acute and chronic pain, produced by inflammation of different etiology	High dose	Middle dose	Low dose
Acidic antipyretic analgesics (anti-inflammatory antipyretic analgesics, NSAIDs)[a]			
Arthritis: chronic polyarthritis (RA, AS (Morbus Bechterew), acute gout (gout attack)	Diclofenac, indometacin, ibuprofen, piroxicam (phenylbutazone)[b]	Diclofenac, indometacin, ibuprofen, piroxicam, (phenylbutazone)[b]	No
Cancer pain (e.g. bone metastasis)	(Indometacin)[c], diclofenac[c], ibuprofen[c], piroxicam[c]	(Indomethacin)[c], diclofenac[c], ibuprofen[c], piroxicam[c]	Aspirin[d], ibuprofen[c]
Active arthrosis (acute pain-inflammatory episodes)	No	Diclofenac, indometacin, ibuprofen, piroxicam	Ibuprofen, ketoprofen
Myofascial pain syndromes (antipyretic analgesics are often prescribed but of limited value)	No	Diclofenac, ibuprofen, piroxicam	Ibuprofen, ketoprofen
Posttraumatic pain, swelling	No	(Indometacin), diclofenac, ibuprofen	Aspirin[d], ibuprofen[c]
Postoperative pain, swelling	No	(Indometacin), diclofenac, ibuprofen	Ibuprofen
Non-acidic antipyretic analgesics			
Acute pain and fever	Pyrazolinones[g] (high dose)	Pyrazolinones[g] (low dose)	Paracetamol (high dose is toxic)
Spastic pain (colics)	Yes	Yes	No
Conditions associated with high fever	Yes	Yes	No
Cancer pain	Yes	Yes	Yes
Headache, migraine	No	Yes	Yes[f]
General disturbances associated with viral infections	No	Yes[e]	Yes

AS, ankylosing spondylitis; RA, rheumatoid arthritis.

[a]Dosage range of NSAIDs and example of monosubstances (but note dosage prescribed for each agent).

[b]Indicated only in gout attacks.

[c]Compare the World Health Organization sequence staged scheme for cancer pain.

[d]Blood coagulation and renal function must be normal.

[e]If other analgesics and antipyretics are contraindicated, e.g. gastroduodenal ulcer, blood coagulation disturbances, or asthma.

[f]In particular patients.

[g]Given the fact that pyrazolinone derivatives (phenazone, propyphenazone, dipyrone) are not available in the United Kingdom, the pharmacology of these drugs is not further addressed in this chapter.

in the stomach for hours or even days may cause retarded absorption of the active ingredient.[36] Moreover, diclofenac has a considerable first-pass metabolism that causes its limited (about 50%) oral bioavailability. Consequently, a lack of therapeutic effect may require adaptation of the dosage or change of the drug. New formulations (microencapsulations, salts, etc.) remedy some of these deficits.[50] The slightly higher incidence of liver toxicity associated with diclofenac may result from the high degree of first-pass metabolism, but other interpretations appear feasible. Previously, it has been demonstrated that pharmacologically relevant concentrations of diclofenac are generated through limited but sustained bioactivation following oral administration of aceclofenac.[49] As aceclofenac per se does not interfere with the COX enzymes, diclofenac seems to confer a major part of the pharmacological action of aceclofenac. Interestingly, metabolic generation of diclofenac after administration of a 100 mg dose of aceclofenac was associated with an apparently improved COX-2 selectivity as compared to a 75 mg dose of a sustained-release diclofenac formulation.[49]

NSAIDs with intermediate potency and intermediate elimination half-life

The third group is intermediate in potency and speed of elimination and comprises drugs such as naproxen and diflunisal. Because of its slow absorption, diflunisal is rarely used anymore.

The use of naproxen has been associated with a potential cardioprotective effect. Indeed, evidence suggests that continuous and regular administration of naproxen 500 mg administered twice daily can affect platelet COX-1 activity and subsequent platelet aggregation throughout the dosing interval in some, but not all, patients.[31] In line with this notion, a meta-analysis of 138 (published and unpublished) randomized trials[32] concluded that the incidence of serious vascular events is similar between a COX-2 inhibitor and any non-naproxen COX inhibitor and that the risk of naproxen is in the placebo range. On the other hand, ulcer bleeds are seen more frequently with naproxen than with ibuprofen, which does not cause lasting platelet inhibition.[51]

NSAIDs with high potency and long elimination half-life

The fourth group consists of the oxicams (meloxicam, piroxicam, and tenoxicam). These compounds are characterized by a high degree of enterohepatic circulation, slow metabolism, and slow elimination.[36] Because of their long half-life (days), oxicams are not drugs of first choice for the treatment of acute pain of short duration. The main indication of the oxicams is inflammatory pain that persists for days, i.e. pain resulting from cancer (bone metastases) or chronic polyarthritis. The high potency and long persistence in the body may be the reason for the somewhat higher incidence of serious adverse drug effects in the gastrointestinal tract and in the kidney observed in the presence of these drugs.[48]

Compounds of special interest

Aspirin, the prototype NSAID, deserves special discussion. This drug irreversibly inactivates both COX-1 (highly effective) and COX-2 (less effective) by acetylating an active-site serine. Consequently, this covalent modification interferes with the binding of arachidonic acid at the COX active site. Most cells compensate the enzyme loss due to acetylation by aspirin via de-novo synthesis of this enzyme. However, as platelets are unable to generate fresh enzyme, a single dose of aspirin may suppress platelet COX-1-dependent thromboxane synthesis for the whole lifetime of thrombocytes (8–11 days) until new platelets are formed.

Following oral administration, aspirin is substantially cleaved before, during, and shortly after absorption, to yield salicylic acid. Consequently, the oral bioavailability is low and the plasma half-life of aspirin is only about 15 min. Aspirin may be used as a solution (effervescent) or as a (lysine) salt, allowing very fast absorption, distribution, and pain relief. Aspirin may cause bleeding from existing ulcers due to its long-lasting anti-platelet effect and topical irritation of the gastrointestinal mucosa.[52] The inevitable irritation of the gastric mucosa may be acceptable in otherwise healthy patients. Aspirin should not be used in pregnant women (premature bleeding, closure of ductus arteriosus) or children before puberty (Reye's syndrome) in addition to the contraindications pertinent to all NSAIDs.

When low doses of aspirin (≤100 mg) are administered, aspirin acetylates the COX-1 isozyme of platelets presystemically in the portal circulation before aspirin is deacetylated to salicylate in the liver. By contrast, COX-2-dependent synthesis of vasodilatory and antithrombotic prostacyclin by vascular endothelial cells outside the gut is not altered by low-dose aspirin. The reason for this phenomenon lies in the rapid cleavage of aspirin leaving little if any unmetabolized aspirin after primary liver passage. Thus, low-dose aspirin has its only indication in the prevention of thrombotic and embolic events.

Another problem concerns the use of low-dose aspirin together with other COX-2-selective or non-selective NSAIDs. In this context, it has been shown that the combination of low-dose aspirin with COX-2-selective inhibitors may abrogate the gastrointestinal-sparing effects of the latter compounds.[46,53] Moreover, ibuprofen and naproxen (the latter at higher than over-the-counter doses) can interfere with the anti-platelet activity of low-dose aspirin when they are coadministered.[54,55] The underlying mechanism might be a competitive inhibition at the acetylation site of platelet COX-1. The clinical implication of this interaction is unclear. It is, however,

potentially important because the cardioprotective effect of aspirin, when used for secondary prevention of myocardial infarction, could be decreased or negated if NSAIDs are used too. In this context a small epidemiological study of survivors of myocardial infarction suggested that concurrent ibuprofen but not diclofenac undermined the efficacy of aspirin in preventing a second myocardial infarction.[56] Therefore, current recommendations by the United States Food and Drug Administration (FDA)[57] advise patients who use immediate-release aspirin and require concurrent ibuprofen to take a single dose of 400 mg ibuprofen at least 30 minutes or longer after aspirin ingestion, or more than 8 hours before aspirin ingestion.

Selective COX-2 inhibitors

Selective inhibitors of the COX-2 enzyme, also referred to as coxibs, have been developed as substances with therapeutic actions similar to those of NSAIDs, but without causing gastrointestinal side effects. By definition, a substance may be regarded as a selective COX-2 inhibitor if it causes no clinically meaningful COX-1 inhibition at maximal therapeutic doses. Selective COX-2 inhibitors currently used in rheumatology are the sulfonamide celecoxib and the methylsulfone etoricoxib. Of these, celecoxib is the only COX-2 inhibitor available in the United States. Differences in physicochemical characteristics are reflected in different pharmacokinetic behaviour (Table 77.3; for review see ref. 58). Due to its very poor solubility, the absorption of celecoxib is relatively slow and incomplete; this compound undergoes considerable first-pass metabolism (20%–60% oral bioavailability). Both factors limit celecoxib's utility for treatment of acute pain. In addition, its rate of elimination ($t_{1/2}$ ~6–12 h) appears to be highly variable.[27,59,60] Etoricoxib is eliminated from the body slowly ($t_{1/2}$ ~20–26 h) and is absorbed at a fast rate, which appears to cause its fast onset of action. In fact, peak plasma concentrations of etoricoxib are reached within 1 hour of administration in both healthy volunteers and patients who had undergone hip surgery.[61] In another study addressing the analgesic effect of single oral doses of etoricoxib in the treatment of pain after dental surgery, the median time to onset of analgesia was 24 minutes for etoricoxib 120 mg, 180 mg, and 240 mg, and 30 minutes for etoricoxib 60 mg.[62] Both COX-2 inhibitors undergo oxidative drug metabolism by cytochrome P450 (CYP) enzymes. Celecoxib has been shown to inhibit the metabolism of the CYP2D6 substrate metoprolol, a widely used β-blocker.[60]

The hypothesis that selective COX-2 inhibitors may provide an improved risk-benefit ratio in terms of gastrointestinal safety as compared with conventional NSAIDs was tested in three large phase 3 clinical trials on a total of 35 000 patients. In the Gastrointestinal Outcomes Research (VIGOR) study[63] and the Therapeutic Arthritis Research and Gastrointestinal Event Trial (TARGET)[55] rofecoxib and lumiracoxib (both drugs were subsequently withdrawn due to cardiovascular or hepatotoxic side effects) were found to decrease the risk of confirmed gastrointestinal events (including ulcerations, bleedings, and perforations) associated with traditional NSAIDs by more than 50%. In the Celecoxib Long-term Arthritis Safety Study (CLASS), however, a significant beneficial effect of celecoxib was only evident when the definition of upper gastrointestinal endpoints was expanded to include symptomatic ulcers.[47] Moreover, outcomes of the first 6 months were published instead of the complete 1-year data of this study.

Table 77.3 Physicochemical and pharmacological data of selective COX-2 inhibitors

	COX-1/COX-2 ratio[a]	Binding to plasma proteins	V_d[b]	Oral bioavailability	t_{max}[c]	$t_{1/2}$[d]	Primary metabolism[e] (cytochrome P450 enzymes)	Recommended daily dose for adults
Sulfonamides								
Celecoxib	30	~97%	455 l	20%–60%	2–4 h	6–12 h	Oxidation (CYP2C9, 3A4)[e]	200 mg (1 × 200 mg or 2 × 100 mg) for OA 200 mg (2 × 100 mg)–400 mg (2 × 200 mg) for RA
Methylsulfons								
Etoricoxib	344	~92%	120 l	100%	~1 h	20–26 h	Oxidation to 6-hydroxy-methyletoricoxib (major role, CYP3A4; ancillary role, CYP2C9, 2D6, 1A2)	30–60 mg for OA 90 mg for RA 120 mg for acute gouty arthritis

OA, osteoarthrosis; RA, rheumatoid arthritis.

[a]Ratio of IC_{50} values (IC_{50} COX-1/IC_{50} COX-2) in the human whole blood assay.

[b]Volume of distribution.

[c]Time to reach maximum plasma concentration after oral administration.

[d]Terminal half-life of elimination.

[e]Compounds may inhibit CYP2D6.

Indeed, the risk of peptic ulcers in high-risk patients taking a COX inhibitor can be significantly reduced by concomitant administration of proton-pump inhibitors.[64,65] This combination, however, does not provide protection against damage caused by COX inhibitors in the lower gastrointestinal tract. Accordingly, a double-blind, placebo-controlled trial using capsule endoscopy revealed celecoxib to be associated with considerably fewer small-bowel mucosal breaks than naproxen plus omeprazole.[66] These data are supported by the recently published CONDOR (Celecoxib versus omeprazole and diclofenac in patients with osteoarthritis and rheumatoid arthritis) trial that was performed on patients with osteoarthritis or rheumatoid arthritis at increased gastrointestinal risk receiving either celecoxib 200 mg twice a day or diclofenac slow release 75 mg twice a day plus omeprazole 20 mg once a day. This study has shown a lower risk of clinical outcomes throughout the gastrointestinal tract in patients treated with celecoxib than in those receiving diclofenac plus omeprazole.[67]

In accordance with a decisive role of COX-1 in aspirin-induced asthma, COX-2 inhibitors are well tolerated by aspirin-sensitive asthmatic patients in several re-exposure studies.[68–71] However, these findings are as yet not seen as proof and the product information of all COX-2 inhibitors still regards aspirin-induced asthma as a contraindication.

COX-2 inhibitors have been associated with an increased incidence of cardiovascular side effects. In fact, in placebo-controlled randomized clinical studies rofecoxib and celecoxib were shown to increase the incidence of myocardial infarctions and other cardiovascular reactions after a prolonged period of treatment.[72,73] With respect to the original purpose of these studies, i.e. adenomatous polyposis prevention study with rofecoxib (APPROVE) and adenoma prevention with celecoxib (APC), both trials demonstrated a significant reduction in new adenoma formation associated with the use of COX-2 inhibitors in patients with a previous history of colorectal carcinomas. Moreover, in high-risk patients short-term

treatment with valdecoxib or parecoxib was associated with an increased number of severe thromboembolic events.[74] These observations had various pharmaco-political consequences: rofecoxib (Vioxx) and valdecoxib (Bextra) were withdrawn from the market; and regulatory bodies were prompted to request changes in the labelling of both selective and non-selective COX inhibitors, including those available for over-the-counter use.[75] To minimize this risk, the respective substances should be taken at the lowest effective dose for the shortest possible duration of treatment.[76,77]

In contrast to COX-2 inhibitors, no placebo-controlled randomized trial was designed to define the cardiovascular risk of NSAIDs. However, a recently published meta-analysis of 138 randomized trials[32] concluded that the incidence of serious vascular events is similar between a COX-2 inhibitor and any non-naproxen NSAID, and that the risk of naproxen is in the placebo range. The summary rate ratio for vascular events, compared with placebo, was 0.92 for naproxen, 1.51 for ibuprofen, and 1.63 for diclofenac. Furthermore, population-based nested case-control studies have shown an increased risk of myocardial infarction associated with the current use of both COX-2 inhibitors and traditional NSAIDs.[78,79] Finally, comparable rates of thrombotic cardiovascular events have been reported for the highly selective COX-2 inhibitor etoricoxib and the traditional NSAID diclofenac in the MEDAL study programme,[80] which involved around 35 000 patients with osteoarthritis or rheumatoid arthritis, suggesting that there is presently no rationale for a further differentiation of COX-2 inhibitors and NSAIDs in terms of cardiovascular safety.

Paracetamol

Paracetamol (acetaminophen) possesses weak anti-inflammatory but efficient analgesic and antipyretic activity. It is one of the most widely used over-the-counter antipyretic and analgesic drugs worldwide and is recommended as first-line therapy for pain associated with osteoarthrosis.[81] Typical further indications of paracetamol are fever and pain occurring in the context of viral infections as well as headache. Paracetamol is also used in children, but despite its somewhat lower toxicity in juvenile patients, fatalities due to involuntary overdosage have been reported.

Despite its improved gastrointestinal safety profile as compared to NSAIDs, paracetamol is unique in causing a dose-dependent hepatotoxic effect: A small proportion of paracetamol is metabolized to the highly toxic nucleophilic N-acetyl-benzoquinoneimine that is usually inactivated by reaction with sulfhydryl groups in glutathione. However, following ingestion of large doses of paracetamol, hepatic glutathione is depleted, resulting in covalent binding of N-acetyl-benzoquinoneimine to DNA and structural proteins in parenchymal cells (e.g. in liver and kidney; for review see ref. 82). Under these circumstances, dose-dependent, potentially fatal hepatic necrosis may occur. When detected early, overdosage can be antagonized within the first 12 h after intake of paracetamol by administration of N-acetylcysteine that regenerates detoxifying mechanisms by replenishing hepatic glutathione stores. Accordingly, paracetamol should not be given to patients with seriously impaired liver function. As a matter of fact, excessive doses of paracetamol are the most common cause of acute liver failure.[83] Remarkably, nearly half of paracetamol-associated cases are caused by unintentional overdose due to taking multiple products containing this drug.[83] In addition, there is increasing evidence that paracetamol may still elicit transient liver enzyme elevations and possibly hepatotoxicity at maximum therapeutic doses (i.e. 4 g daily), particularly in patients with risk factors (e.g., chronic alcohol use, malnutrition, concurrent use of inducers of the cytochrome P450 enzyme).[84–87] Accordingly, too short or insufficient pain relief associated with paracetamol's fast elimination (Table 77.4) or limited potency should be considered as an additional factor leading to overdosages with this drug.

Although paracetamol was discovered over 100 years ago and has been extensively used for over 50 years, its mode of action is still a matter of debate. For more than three decades it was commonly stated that paracetamol acts centrally and is at best a weak inhibitor of prostaglandin synthesis by COX-1 and COX-2.[88] This concept is based on early work by Flower and Vane[89] who showed that prostaglandin production in brain is 10 times more sensitive to inhibition by paracetamol than that in spleen. Instead, several data published during the past few years suggest a tissue-dependent inhibitory effect of paracetamol on the activity of both central and peripheral COX enzymes. Whereas NSAIDs and COX-2 inhibitors inhibit COX by competing with arachidonic acid for entering the COX reaction,[90,91] paracetamol has been suggested to act as a reducing agent within the peroxidase site. In brief, paracetamol quenches a protoporphyrin radical cation. The latter generates the

tyrosine radical in the COX site which is responsible for catalysing oxygenation of arachidonic acid.[92,93] In view of the fact that hydroperoxides oxidize the porphyrin within the peroxidase site, COX inhibition by paracetamol is hampered by high peroxide levels. Therefore, high extracellular levels of peroxide in the inflamed tissue may also explain why paracetamol does not suppress inflammation associated with rheumatoid arthritis.[94,95] On the other hand it is noteworthy that paracetamol decreases tissue swelling following oral surgery in humans, with activity very similar to that of ibuprofen.[96,97] Thus, the notion that paracetamol has only weak anti-inflammatory properties rather than it causes no anti-inflammatory action at all appears to be more favourable.

In addition, a recent clinical investigation suggests a preferential COX-2 inhibition by paracetamol in human whole blood. Accordingly, oral administration of 1000 mg paracetamol to human volunteers was shown to inhibit blood monocyte COX-2 by more than 80%, i.e. to a comparable degree as NSAIDs and selective COX-2 inhibitors.[98] In this study paracetamol displayed approximately fourfold selectivity for inhibition of COX-2 both in vitro and in vivo.[98] By contrast, a COX-1 blockade relevant for inhibition of platelet function (>95%) was not achieved.[98] With respect to the above mentioned 'peroxide theory', further experiments revealed that paracetamol elicits the most pronounced COX-2 inhibition in human whole blood when compared to the recombinant enzyme or freshly prepared human monocytes,[98] thus confirming the dependence of its potency as COX-2 inhibitor on the oxidant/anti-oxidant status of the surrounding system. As a matter of fact, human plasma (containing various enzymatic and non-enzymatic anti-oxidant components) may provide favourable conditions in this respect. Collectively, preferential COX-2 inhibition may explain why short-term administration of paracetamol at recommended single doses elicits no measurable toxic effect on the gastrointestinal tract,[99] does not inhibit platelet function,[54,100] and provokes less bronchoconstriction in aspirin-sensitive asthmatics than NSAIDs.[101] On the other hand, these findings raise concerns in particular to the hitherto proposed cardiovascular safety of the drug and the poorly investigated gastrointestinal safety under conditions of long-term treatment.

In contrast to the inflamed tissue, endothelial cells possess low levels of peroxide, making an undisturbed COX-2 inhibition by paracetamol possible.[93] In line with this notion, paracetamol was found to inhibit COX activity in human endothelial cells[102] and to diminish the urinary excretion of a stable prostacyclin metabolite in humans.[102,103] In addition, epidemiological data found that regular consumption of paracetamol is associated with a significantly higher relative risk for development of hypertension compared with no use[104] and that a frequent consumption of paracetamol has nearly the same risk for major cardiovascular events as NSAIDs.[105]

Table 77.4 Physicochemical and pharmacological data of paracetamol

Chemical/pharmacological class	Binding to plasma proteins	Oral bioavailability	t_{max}[a]	$t_{1/2}$[b]	Single dose (maximal daily dose) for adults
Aniline derivatives					
Paracetamol (acetaminophen)	5–50%, dose-dependent	70–100%, dose-dependent	0.5–1.5 h	1.5–2.5 h	0.5–1 g (4 g)

[a]Time to reach maximum plasma concentration after oral administration.
[b]Terminal half-life of elimination.

These epidemiological data are supported by a recently published randomized, double-blind, placebo-controlled, crossover study demonstrating that paracetamol induces a significant increase in ambulatory blood pressure in patients with coronary artery disease.[106] Collectively, these data raise concerns on the hitherto presumed cardiovascular safety of paracetamol, making further randomized trials necessary.

The favourable gastrointestinal tolerability of paracetamol as compared to NSAIDs is often cited with regard to a 7-day randomized trial, where healthy volunteers receiving paracetamol 4 g/day showed no significant difference from the placebo group in terms of gastric mucosal injuries.[107] Unfortunately, no long-term endoscopy study has been performed with paracetamol so far. However, observational studies suggest that higher doses of paracetamol taken for a longer period of time may elicit a gastrointestinal risk. In a first of these studies, Garcia-Rodriguez' group analysed upper gastrointestinal complications in almost one million patients receiving paracetamol and/or NSAIDs during a five-year investigation period. The relative risks for paracetamol showed a clear dose-dependence with an adjusted relative risk (RR) for paracetamol of 3.6 at doses greater than 2 g.[99] In addition, combined administration of NSAID and paracetamol was associated with a synergistic increase of RR.[108] These results were supported by a retrospective cohort study showing an increased risk of hospitalization due to gastrointestinal events (ulcer, perforation, bleeding in upper or lower gastrointestinal tract) among elderly patients requiring analgesic treatment following the use of NSAIDs in combination with paracetamol as compared with use of NSAIDs alone.[109] The authors explained this finding by paracetamol's additional COX-1 inhibition which is plausible in view of data showing paracetamol to augment diclofenac's inhibitory action on platelet aggregation in a synergistic manner,[110] A combined use of NSAID and paracetamol was also addressed in a recently published randomized, active controlled trial on almost 900 participants with chronic knee pain, most of them fulfilling American College of Rheumatology (ACR) criteria for knee osteoarthritis.[111] On the basis of haemoglobin levels measured the authors state that paracetamol 3 g/day may cause similar degrees of blood loss as ibuprofen 1.2 mg/day, and that the combination of the two appears to be additive, or even synergistic in terms of the number of individuals with a greater than 2 g/dL decrease in haemoglobin.[111] Further investigations on paracetamol's long-term gastrointestinal impact are therefore strongly advised.

Future developments

The available traditional antipyretic analgesics and selective COX-2 inhibitors still leave space for additional compounds. In past years, inhibition of the microsomal prostaglandin E synthase I that is coexpressed with COX-2 under diverse inflammatory conditions has been suggested to represent a potential target for treatment of inflammatory pain.[112] From the pharmacological point of view an inhibition of this enzyme would open the opportunity to inhibit the production of COX-2-dependent proinflammatory prostaglandins without a concomitant blockade of COX-2-dependent prostacyclin, which confers various protective actions in the cardiovascular and renal system. Finally, targeting of individual prostaglandin receptor subtypes may permit a separation

of desired and unwanted effects of NSAIDs. Recently, blockade of the EP_2 receptor has attracted attention as a possible target for centrally acting anti-hyperalgesic agents.[20] Alternative strategies might interfere with targets beyond prostanoid synthases or prostanoid receptors, such as transient receptor potential channels, tetrodotoxin-resistant sodium channels and inhibitory glycine receptors (for review see ref. 113). Currently, however, therapy of arthritis and arthritic pain has to rely on COX inhibitors whose diverse pharmacokinetics and adverse reaction profiles should be considered in daily practice.

References

1. Vane JR. Inhibition of prostaglandin synthesis as a mechanism of action for aspirin-like drugs. *Nat New Biol* 1971;231(25):232–235.
2. Masferrer JL, Zweifel BS, Seibert K, Needleman P. Selective regulation of cellular cyclooxygenase by dexamethasone and endotoxin in mice. *J Clin Invest* 1990;86(4):1375–1379.
3. Xie WL, Chipman JG, Robertson DL, Erikson RL, Simmons DL. Expression of a mitogen-responsive gene encoding prostaglandin synthase is regulated by mRNA splicing. *Proc Natl Acad Sci U S A* 1991;88(7):2692–2696.
4. Patrignani P, Panara MR, Sciulli MG et al. Differential inhibition of human prostaglandin endoperoxide synthase-1 and -2 by nonsteroidal anti-inflammatory drugs. *J Physiol Pharmacol* 1997;48(4):623–631.
5. Picado C. Mechanisms of aspirin sensitivity. *Curr Allergy Asthma Rep* 2006;6(3):198–202.
6. Schaible HG, Schmidt RF. Time course of mechanosensitivity changes in articular afferents during a developing experimental arthritis. *J Neurophysiol* 1988;60(6):2180–2195.
7. Neugebauer V, Geisslinger G, Rümenapp P et al. Antinociceptive effects of R(-)- and S(+)-flurbiprofen on rat spinal dorsal horn neurons rendered hyperexcitable by an acute knee joint inflammation. *J Pharmacol Exp Ther* 1995;275(2):618–628.
8. Akopian AN, Sivilotti L, Wood JN. A tetrodotoxin-resistant voltage-gated sodium channel expressed by sensory neurons. *Nature* 1996;379(6562):257–262.
9. England S, Bevan S, Docherty RJ. PGE2 modulates the tetrodotoxin-resistant sodium current in neonatal rat dorsal root ganglion neurones via the cyclic AMP-protein kinase A cascade. *J Physiol* 1996;495(2):429–440.
10. Gold MS, Reichling DB, Shuster MJ, Levine JD. Hyperalgesic agents increase a tetrodotoxin-resistant Na+ current in nociceptors. *Proc Natl Acad Sci U S A* 1996;93(3):1108–1112.
11. Lopshire JC, Nicol GD. Activation and recovery of the PGE2-mediated sensitization of the capsaicin response in rat sensory neurons. *J Neurophysiol* 1997;78(6):3154–3164.
12. Caterina MJ, Leffler A, Malmberg AB et al. Impaired nociception and pain sensation in mice lacking the capsaicin receptor. *Science* 2000;288(5464):306–313.
13. Davis JB, Gray J, Gunthorpe MJ, et al. Vanilloid receptor-1 is essential for inflammatory thermal hyperalgesia. *Nature* 2000;405(6783):183–187.
14. Beiche F, Scheuerer S, Brune K, Geisslinger G, Goppelt-Struebe M. Up-regulation of cyclooxygenase-2 mRNA in the rat spinal cord following peripheral inflammation. *FEBS Lett* 1996;390(2):165–169.
15. Smith CJ, Zhang Y, Koboldt CM, et al. Pharmacological analysis of cyclooxygenase-1 in inflammation. *Proc Natl Acad Sci U S A* 1998;95(22):13313–13318.
16. Samad TA, Moore KA, Sapirstein A et al. Interleukin-1beta-mediated induction of Cox-2 in the CNS contributes to inflammatory pain hypersensitivity. *Nature* 2001;410(6827):471–475.
17. Baba H, Kohno T, Moore KA, Woolf CJ. Direct activation of rat spinal dorsal horn neurons by prostaglandin E2. *J Neurosci* 2001;21(5):1750–1756.

18. Ahmadi S, Lippross S, Neuhuber WL, Zeilhofer HU. PGE2 selectively blocks inhibitory glycinergic neurotransmission onto rat superficial dorsal horn neurons. *Nat Neurosci* 2002;5(1):34–40.

19. Harvey RJ, Depner UB, Wässle Het al. GlyR alpha3: an essential target for spinal PGE2-mediated inflammatory pain sensitization. *Science* 2004;304(5672):884–887.

20. Reinold H, Ahmadi S, Depner UB et al. Spinal inflammatory hyperalgesia is mediated by prostaglandin E receptors of the EP2 subtype. *J Clin Invest* 2005;115(3):673–679.

21. Hinz B, Brune K. Cyclooxygenase-2—10 years later. *J Pharmacol Exp Ther* 2002;300(2):367–375.

22. McAdam BF, Catella-Lawson F, Mardini IA et al. Systemic biosynthesis of prostacyclin by cyclooxygenase (COX)-2: the human pharmacology of a selective inhibitor of COX-2. *Proc Natl Acad Sci U S A* 1999;96(1):272–277.

23. Catella-Lawson F, McAdam B, Morrison BW et al. Effects of specific inhibition of cyclooxygenase-2 on sodium balance, hemodynamics, and vasoactive eicosanoids. *J Pharmacol Exp Ther* 1999;289(2): 735–741.

24. Whelton A, Maurath CJ, Verburg KM, Geis GS. Renal safety and tolerability of celecoxib, a novel cyclooxygenase-2 inhibitor. *Am J Ther* 2000;7(3):159–175.

25. Schwartz JI, Vandormael K, Malice MP et al. Comparison of rofecoxib, celecoxib, and naproxen on renal function in elderly subjects receiving a normal-salt diet. *Clin Pharmacol Ther* 2002;72(1):50–61.

26. Singh G, Miller JD, Huse DM et al. Consequences of increased systolic blood pressure in patients with osteoarthritis and rheumatoid arthritis. *J Rheumatol* 2003;30(4):714–719.

27. Hinz B, Dormann H, Brune K. More pronounced inhibition of cyclooxygenase 2, increase in blood pressure, and reduction of heart rate by treatment with diclofenac compared with celecoxib and rofecoxib. *Arthritis Rheum* 2006;54(1):282–291.

28. García Rodríguez LA, Tacconelli S, Patrignani P. Role of dose potency in the prediction of risk of myocardial infarction associated with non-steroidal anti-inflammatory drugs in the general population. *J Am Coll Cardiol* 2008;52(20):1628–1636.

29. Hinz B, Brune K. Can drug removals involving cyclooxygenase-2 inhibitors be avoided? A plea for human pharmacology. *Trends Pharmacol Sci* 2008;29(8):391–397.

30. Reilly IA, FitzGerald GA. Inhibition of thromboxane formation in vivo and ex vivo: implications for therapy with platelet inhibitory drugs. *Blood* 1987;69(1):180–186.

31. Capone ML, Tacconelli S, Sciulli MG et al. Clinical pharmacology of platelet, monocyte, and vascular cyclooxygenase inhibition by naproxen and low-dose aspirin in healthy subjects. *Circulation* 2004;109(12):1468–1471.

32. Kearney PM, Baigent C, Godwin J et al. Do selective cyclo-oxygenase-2 inhibitors and traditional non-steroidal anti-inflammatory drugs increase the risk of atherothrombosis? Meta-analysis of randomised trials. *BMJ* 2006;332(7553):1302–1308.

33. Patrignani P, Panara MR, Greco A et al. Biochemical and pharmacological characterization of the cyclooxygenase activity of human blood prostaglandin endoperoxide synthases. *J Pharmacol Exp Ther* 1994;271(3):1705–1712.

34. Huntjens DR, Danhof M, Della Pasqua OE. Pharmacokinetic-pharmacodynamic correlations and biomarkers in the development of COX-2 inhibitors. *Rheumatology (Oxford)* 2005;44(7):846–859.

35. Winter CA, Risley EA, Nuss GW. Carrageenin-induced edema in hind paw of the rat as an assay for anti-inflammatory drugs. *Proc Soc Exp Biol Med* 1962;111:544–552.

36. Brune K, Lanz R. Pharmacokinetics of non-steroidal anti-inflammatory drugs. In: Bray MA, Bonta IL, Parnham MJ (eds) *Handbook of inflammation. The pharmacology of inflammation*, Vol. 5. Elsevier Science, Amsterdam, 1985:413–449.

37. Hinz B, Dorn CP, Shen TY, Brune K. Anti-inflammatory–antirheumatic drugs. In McGuire JL (ed.) *Pharmaceuticals—classes, therapeutic agents, areas of application*, Vol. 4. Wiley-VCH, Weinheim, 2000:1671–1711.

38. Brune K, Renner B, Hinz B. Using pharmacokinetic principles to optimize pain therapy. *Nat Rev Rheumatol* 2010;6(10):589–598.

39. Brune K, Glatt M, Graf P. Mechanism of action of anti-inflammatory drugs. *Gen Pharmacol* 1976;7(1):27–33.

40. McCormack K, Brune K. Classical absorption theory and the development of gastric mucosal damage associated with the non-steroidal anti-inflammatory drugs. *Arch Toxicol* 1987;60(4):261–269.

41. Price AH, Fletcher M. Mechanisms of NSAID-induced gastroenteropathy. *Drugs* 1990;40(5):1–11.

42. Wallace JL. Nonsteroidal anti-inflammatory drugs and gastroenteropathy: the second hundred years. *Gastroenterology* 1997;112(3):1000–1016.

43. Somasundaram S, Rafi S, Hayllar J et al. Mitochondrial damage: a possible mechanism of the 'topical' phase of NSAID induced injury to the rat intestine. *Gut* 1997;41(3):344–353.

44. Brune K, Rainsford KD, Schweitzer A. Biodistribution of mild analgesics. *Br J Clin Pharmacol* 1980;10:279S–284S.

45. Geisslinger G, Menzel S, Wissel K, Brune K. Single dose pharmacokinetics of different formulations of ibuprofen and aspirin. *Drug Invest* 1993;5:238–242.

46. Silverstein FE, Faich G, Goldstein JL et al. Gastrointestinal toxicity with celecoxib vs nonsteroidal anti-inflammatory drugs for osteoarthritis and rheumatoid arthritis: the CLASS study: A randomized controlled trial. Celecoxib Long-term Arthritis Safety Study. *JAMA* 2000;284(10):1247–1255.

47. Rudy AC, Knight PM, Brater DC, Hall SD. Stereoselective metabolism of ibuprofen in humans: administration of R-, S- and racemic ibuprofen. *J Pharmacol Exp Ther* 1991;259(3):1133–1139.

48. Henry D, Lim LL, Garcia Rodriguez LA et al. Variability in risk of gastrointestinal complications with individual non-steroidal anti-inflammatory drugs: results of a collaborative meta-analysis. *BMJ* 1996;312(7046):1563–1566.

49. Hinz B, Rau T, Auge D et al. Aceclofenac spares cyclooxygenase 1 as a result of limited but sustained biotransformation to diclofenac. *Clin Pharmacol Ther* 2003;74(3):222–235.

50. Hinz B, Chevts J, Renner B et al. Bioavailability of diclofenac potassium at low doses. *Br J Clin Pharmacol* 2005;59(1):80–84.

51. Goldstein JL, Eisen GM, Agrawal N et al. Reduced incidence of upper gastrointestinal ulcer complications with the COX-2 selective inhibitor, valdecoxib. *Aliment Pharmacol Ther* 2004;20(5):527–538.

52. Kimmey MB. Cardioprotective effects and gastrointestinal risks of aspirin: maintaining the delicate balance. *Am J Med* 2004;117: 72S–78S.

53. Schnitzer TJ, Burmester GR, Mysler E, et al.; TARGET Study Group. Comparison of lumiracoxib with naproxen and ibuprofen in the Therapeutic Arthritis Research and Gastrointestinal Event Trial (TARGET):reduction in ulcer complications: randomised controlled trial. *Lancet* 2004;364(9435):665–674.

54. Catella-Lawson F, Reilly MP, Kapoor SC et al. Cyclooxygenase inhibitors and the antiplatelet effects of aspirin. *N Engl J Med* 2001;345(25):1809–1817.

55. Capone ML, Sciulli MG, Tacconelli S et al. Pharmacodynamic interaction of naproxen with low-dose aspirin in healthy subjects. *J Am Coll Cardiol* 2005;45(8):1295–1301.

56. MacDonald TM, Wei L. Effect of ibuprofen on cardioprotective effect of aspirin. *Lancet* 2003;361(9357):573–574.

57. U.S. Food and Drug Administration. FDA Science Paper: Concomitant use of ibuprofen and aspirin: potential for attenuation of the anti-platelet effect of aspirin. 9/8/2006 . Available at: www.fda.gov/cder/drug/infopage/ibuprofen/default.htm.

58. Brune K, Hinz B. Selective cyclooxygenase-2 inhibitors: similarities and differences. *Scand J Rheumatol* 2004;33(1):1–6.

59. Werner U, Werner D, Pahl A et al. Investigation of the pharmacokinetics of celecoxib by liquid chromatography-mass spectrometry. *Biomed Chromatogr* 2002;16(1):56–60.

60. Werner U, Werner D, Rau T et al. Celecoxib inhibits metabolism of cytochrome P450 2D6 substrate metoprolol in humans. *Clin Pharmacol Ther* 2003;74(2):130–137.

61. Renner B, Zacher J, Buvanendran A et al. Absorption and distribution of etoricoxib in plasma, CSF, and wound tissue in patients following hip surgery—a pilot study. *Naunyn Schmiedebergs Arch Pharmacol* 2010;381(2):127–136.

62. Malmstrom K, Sapre A, Couglin H et al. Etoricoxib in acute pain associated with dental surgery: a randomized, double-blind, placebo- and active comparator-controlled dose-ranging study. *Clin Ther* 2004;26(5):667-679.

63. Bombardier C, Laine L, Reicin A et al.; VIGOR Study Group. Comparison of upper gastrointestinal toxicity of rofecoxib and naproxen in patients with rheumatoid arthritis. VIGOR Study Group. *N Engl J Med* 2000;343(21):1520–1528.

64. Chan FK, Hung LC, Suen BY et al. Celecoxib versus diclofenac and omeprazole in reducing the risk of recurrent ulcer bleeding in patients with arthritis. *N Engl J Med* 2002;347(26):2104–2110.

65. Lai KC, Chu KM, Hui WM et al. Celecoxib compared with lansoprazole and naproxen to prevent gastrointestinal ulcer complications. *Am J Med* 2005;118(11):1271–1278.

66. Goldstein JL, Eisen GM, Lewis B et al.; Investigators. Video capsule endoscopy to prospectively assess small bowel injury with celecoxib, naproxen plus omeprazole, and placebo. *Clin Gastroenterol Hepatol* 2005;3(2):133–141.

67. Chan FK, Lanas A, Scheiman J et al. Celecoxib versus omeprazole and diclofenac in patients with osteoarthritis and rheumatoid arthritis (CONDOR): a randomised trial. *Lancet* 2010;376(9736):173–179.

68. Dahlén B, Szczeklik A, Murray JJ; Celecoxib in Aspirin-Intolerant Asthma Study Group. Celecoxib in patients with asthma and aspirin intolerance. The Celecoxib in Aspirin-Intolerant Asthma Study Group. *N Engl J Med* 2001;344(2):142.

69. Stevenson DD, Simon RA. Lack of cross-reactivity between rofecoxib and aspirin in aspirin-sensitive patients with asthma. *J Allergy Clin Immunol* 2001;108(1):47–51.

70. Szczeklik A, Nizankowska E, Bochenek G et al. Safety of a specific COX-2 inhibitor in aspirin-induced asthma. *Clin Exp Allergy* 2001;31(2):219–225.

71. Woessner KM, Simon RA, Stevenson DD. The safety of celecoxib in patients with aspirin-sensitive asthma. *Arthritis Rheum* 2002;46(8):2201–2206.

72. Bresalier RS, Sandler RS, Quan H, et al.; Adenomatous Polyp Prevention on Vioxx (APPROVe) Trial Investigators. Cardiovascular events associated with rofecoxib in a colorectal adenoma chemoprevention trial. *N Engl J Med* 2005;352(11):1092–1102.

73. Solomon SD, McMurray JJ, Pfeffer MA, et al.; Adenoma Prevention with Celecoxib (APC) Study Investigators. Cardiovascular risk associated with celecoxib in a clinical trial for colorectal adenoma prevention. *N Engl J Med* 2005;352(11):1071–1080.

74. Nussmeier NA, Whelton AA, Brown MT et al. Complications of the COX-2 inhibitors parecoxib and valdecoxib after cardiac surgery. *N Engl J Med* 2005;352(11):1081–1091.

75. U.S. Food and Drug Administration. FDA News: FDA announces series of changes to the class of marketed non-steroidal anti-inflammatory drugs (NSAIDs). Available at: www.fda.gov/bbs/topics/news/2005/NEW01171.html.

76. European Medicines Agency. *Public statement: European Medicines Agency concludes action on COX2 inhibitors*. London, 27 June 2005.

77. European Medicines Agency. *EMEA, Press release: European Medicines Agency update on non-selective NSAIDs*. London, 17 October 2005.

78. Hippisley-Cox J, Coupland C. Risk of myocardial infarction in patients taking cyclo-oxygenase-2 inhibitors or conventional non-steroidal anti-inflammatory drugs: population based nested case-control analysis. *BMJ* 2005;330(7504):1366.

79. Singh G, Mithal A, Triadafilopoulos G. Both selective COX2 inhibitors and non-selective NSAIDs increase the risk of acute myocardial infarction in patients with arthritis: selectivity is with the patient, not with the drug class. *Annual European Congress of Rheumatology, Vienna*, 8–11 June 2005, Abstract OP0091.

80. Cannon CP, Curtis SP, FitzGerald GA, et al.; MEDAL Steering Committee. Cardiovascular outcomes with etoricoxib and diclofenac in patients with osteoarthritis and rheumatoid arthritis in the Multinational Etoricoxib and Diclofenac Arthritis Long-term (MEDAL) programme: a randomised comparison. *Lancet* 2006;368(9549): 1771–1781.

81. Schnitzer TJ; American College of Rheumatology. Update of ACR guidelines for osteoarthritis: role of the coxibs. *J Pain Symptom Manage* 2002;23(4):S24–S30.

82. Seeff LB, Cuccherini BA, Zimmerman HJ, Adler E, Benjamin SB. Acetaminophen hepatotoxicity in alcoholics. A therapeutic misadventure. *Ann Intern Med* 1986;104(3):399–404.

83. Schilling A, Corey R, Leonard M, Eghtesad B. Acetaminophen: old drug, new warnings. *Cleve Clin J Med* 2010;77(1):19–27.

84. Watkins PB, Kaplowitz N, Slattery JT et al. Aminotransferase elevations in healthy adults receiving 4 grams of acetaminophen daily: a randomized controlled trial. *JAMA* 2006;296(1):87–93.

85. Krähenbuhl S, Brauchli Y, Kummer O et al. Acute liver failure in two patients with regular alcohol consumption ingesting paracetamol at therapeutic dosage. *Digestion* 2007;75(4):232–237.

86. Larson AM. Acetaminophen hepatotoxicity. *Clin Liver Dis* 2007;11(3):525–548.

87. Schwartz J, Stravitz T, Lee WM; American Association for the Study of Liver Disease Study Group. AASLD position on acetaminophen. www.aasld.org/about/publicpolicy/Documents/Public%2520Policy%2520Documents/AcetaminophenPosition.pdf.

88. Botting RM. Mechanism of action of acetaminophen: is there a cyclooxygenase 3? *Clin Infect Dis* 2000;31:S202–S210.

89. Flower RJ, Vane JR. Inhibition of prostaglandin synthetase in brain explains the anti-pyretic activity of paracetamol (4-acetamidophenol). *Nature* 1972;240(5381):410–411.

90. Loll PJ, Picot D, Ekabo O, Garavito RM. Synthesis and use of iodinated nonsteroidal antiinflammatory drug analogs as crystallographic probes of the prostaglandin H2 synthase cyclooxygenase active site. *Biochemistry* 1996;35(23):7330–7340.

91. Gierse JK, Koboldt CM, Walker MC, Seibert K, Isakson PC. Kinetic basis for selective inhibition of cyclo-oxygenases. *Biochem J* 1999;339(3):607–614.

92. Ouellet M, Percival MD. Mechanism of acetaminophen inhibition of cyclooxygenase isoforms. *Arch Biochem Biophys* 2001;387(2): 273–280.

93. Boutaud O, Aronoff DM, Richardson JH, Marnett LJ, Oates JA. Determinants of the cellular specificity of acetaminophen as an inhibitor of prostaglandin H(2)synthases. *Proc Natl Acad Sci U S A* 2002;99(10):7130–7135.

94. Boardman PL, Hart FD. Clinical measurement of the anti-inflammatory effects of salicylates in rheumatoid arthritis. *Br Med J* 1967;4(5574):264–268.

95. Ring EF, Collins AJ, Bacon PA, Cosh JA. Quantitation of thermography in arthritis using multi-isothermal analysis. II. Effect of nonsteroidal anti-inflammatory therapy on the thermographic index. *Ann Rheum Dis* 1974;33(4):353–356.

96. Skjelbred P, Løkken P. Paracetamol versus placebo: effects on post-operative course. *Eur J Clin Pharmacol* 1979;15(1):27–33.

97. Bjørnsson GA, Haanaes HR, Skoglund LA. A randomized, double-blind crossover trial of paracetamol 1000 mg four times daily vs ibuprofen 600 mg: effect on swelling and other postoperative events after third molar surgery. *Br J Clin Pharmacol* 2003;55(4):405–412.

98. Hinz B, Cheremina O, Brune K. Acetaminophen (paracetamol) is a selective cyclooxygenase-2 inhibitor in man. *FASEB J* 2008;22(2):383–390.

99. García Rodríguez LA, Hernández-Díaz S. Relative risk of upper gastrointestinal complications among users of acetaminophen and nonsteroidal anti-inflammatory drugs. *Epidemiology* 2001;12(5):570–576.

100. Mielke CH Jr. Comparative effects of aspirin and acetaminophen on hemostasis. *Arch Intern Med* 1981;141(3):305–310.

101. Jenkins C, Costello J, Hodge L. Systematic review of prevalence of aspirin induced asthma and its implications for clinical practice. *BMJ* 2004;328(7437):434.

102. O'Brien WF, Krammer J, O'Leary TD, Mastrogiannis DS. The effect of acetaminophen on prostacyclin production in pregnant women. *Am J Obstet Gynecol* 1993;168(4):1164–1169.

103. Grèen K, Drvota V, Vesterqvist O. Pronounced reduction of in vivo prostacyclin synthesis in humans by acetaminophen (paracetamol). *Prostaglandins* 1989;37(3):311–315.

104. Forman JP, Stampfer MJ, Curhan GC. Non-narcotic analgesic dose and risk of incident hypertension in US women. *Hypertension* 2005;46(3):500–507.

105. Chan AT, Manson JE, Albert CM et al. Nonsteroidal antiinflammatory drugs, acetaminophen, and the risk of cardiovascular events. *Circulation* 2006;113(12):1578–1587.

106. Sudano I, Flammer AJ, Périat D et al. Acetaminophen increases blood pressure in patients with coronary artery disease. *Circulation* 2010;122(18):1789–1796.

107. Lanza FL, Codispoti JR, Nelson EB. An endoscopic comparison of gastroduodenal injury with over-the-counter doses of ketoprofen and acetaminophen. *Am J Gastroenterol* 1998;93(7):1051–1054.

108. Garcia Rodríguez LA, Hernández-Díaz S. The risk of upper gastrointestinal complications associated with nonsteroidal anti-inflammatory drugs, glucocorticoids, acetaminophen, and combinations of these agents. *Arthritis Res* 2001;3(2):98–101.

109. Rahme E, Barkun A, Nedjar H, Gaugris S, Watson D. Hospitalizations for upper and lower GI events associated with traditional NSAIDs and acetaminophen among the elderly in Quebec, Canada. *Am J Gastroenterol* 2008;103(4):872–882.

110. Munsterhjelm E, Niemi TT, Ylikorkala O, Silvanto M, Rosenberg PH. Characterization of inhibition of platelet function by paracetamol and its interaction with diclofenac in vitro. *Acta Anaesthesiol Scand* 2005;49(6):840–846.

111. Doherty M, Hawkey C, Goulder M et al. A randomised controlled trial of ibuprofen, paracetamol or a combination tablet of ibuprofen/paracetamol in community-derived people with knee pain. *Ann Rheum Dis* 2011;70(9):1534–1541.

112. Jakobsson PJ, Thorén S, Morgenstern R, Samuelsson B. Identification of human prostaglandin E synthase: a microsomal, glutathione-dependent, inducible enzyme, constituting a potent novel drug target. *Proc Natl Acad Sci U S A* 1999;96(13):7220–7225.

113. Zeilhofer HU, Brune K. Analgesic strategies beyond the inhibition of cyclooxygenases. *Trends Pharmacol Sci* 2006;27(9):467–474.

CHAPTER 78

Analgesics

Joanne Foo, Benazir Saleem, and
Philip G. Conaghan

Introduction

Pain is personal and complex in its origins. Pain is the predominant presenting symptom of most musculoskeletal conditions and varies in intensity, character, and duration. Musculoskeletal pain can originate from peripheral sites such as the synovium, tendons, ligaments, enthuses, and muscle, and be modified by spinal cord interactions and the central nervous system (CNS). Inflammation leads to hypersensitivity termed peripheral sensitization, which acts through polymodal recruitment of nociceptors as well as the silent nociceptors for activation.[1] The discordance of perception to pain and actual evidence of damage or inflammation has led to the concept of central pain contributing to chronic pain.[2] The detailed physiology of pain is discussed elsewhere in this textbook (Chapter 59). This chapter provides an overview of current, commonly used analgesics, including paracetamol, opioids, and therapies for neuropathic pain. Non-steroidal anti-inflammatory drugs (NSAIDs) are reviewed in Chapter 77). Some novel therapies are also briefly mentioned.

General principles of pain management

The World Health Organization (WHO) Pain Ladder was developed as a conceptual model to guide the management of cancer pain and provided five simple recommendations for the correct use of analgesics[3]:

- *Oral administration of analgesics.* The oral form of medication should be used whenever possible.

- *Analgesics should be given at regular intervals.* To relieve pain adequately, it is necessary to respect the duration of the medication's efficacy and to prescribe the dosage to be taken at definite intervals in conjunction with the patient's level of pain.

- *Analgesics should be prescribed according to pain intensity as evaluated by a scale of intensity of pain.*

- *Dosing of pain medication should be adapted to the individual.* There is no standardized dosage in the treatment of pain. Every patient will respond differently. The correct dosage is one that will allow adequate relief of pain, without producing intolerable side effects.

- *Analgesics should be prescribed with a constant concern for detail.* For example, the regularity of analgesic administration is crucial for the adequate treatment of pain.

Over the years there have been modifications to the ladder so that it can be used for non-cancer pain, with four steps:

1. Non-opioid analgesics or NSAIDs

2. Weak opioids

3. Strong opioids (oral administration or transdermal patch)

4. Nerve block/epidurals/patient controlled analgesia pump/neurolytic block therapy/spinal stimulators.

Paracetamol

Paracetamol, also known as acetaminophen, is one of the most commonly used non-narcotic analgesics; it is also an anti-pyretic agent. Acetaminophen is *N*-acetylaminophenol, the active metabolite of phenacetin. The antipyretics commonly used in the 1800s consisted of preparations of natural compounds such as cinchona bark, from which quinine is derived, or galenicals based on willow bark, the earliest source of salicylate. Two alternatives were subsequently developed, acetanilide in 1886 and phenacetin in 1887, both of which possessed both antipyretic and analgesic properties. It was established that paracetamol was a major metabolite of both phenacetin and acetanilide and subsequently recommended as a safer option. In the 1950s its use became widespread after evidence of its effectiveness when compared to aspirin was reported.

Mechanism of action

Research indicates that paracetamol inhibits prostaglandin synthesis, in a similar way to aspirin (see Chapter 77). This is through central and peripheral inhibition of both cyclooxygenase (COX) enzymes 1 and 2.[4] Paracetamol is thought to favour COX-2 inhibition. This preferred mode of action is particularly important in the presence of peroxide which is present in higher levels in inflamed tissues. The inhibitory effect of paracetamol on COX-1 becomes paradoxically inhibited in such circumstances. Paracetamol's lack of effect in reducing inflammation in rheumatoid arthritis (RA) can be explained by the levels of arachidonic acid and peroxide in the

RA tissues. Although traditionally known as a pure analgesic, the comparative effects of paracetamol and ibuprofen demonstrated in reducing oral inflammation postoperatively[5] supports the possible anti-inflammatory effects of this drug.[4]

Pharmacokinetics

When taken orally, paracetamol is rapidly and almost completely absorbed, reaching peak levels in 30–60 minutes. The plasma half-life is approximately 2 hours and the duration of action is approximately 4 hours. The drug is widely distributed and is approximately 20–50% plasma bound. Paracetamol is present in breast milk but at low levels (10–15 μg/mL). As paracetamol is metabolized in the liver and eliminated by the renal pathway, the metabolites can be hepatotoxic and nephrotoxic. The therapeutic effects of paracetamol may be decreased when given concomitantly with barbiturates, carbamazepine, isoniazid, rifampicin, and sulfinpyrazone as a result of increased metabolism. Cholestyramine may decrease the absorption of paracetamol.

Side effects

Paracetamol is a common over-the-counter drug used alone and in combination for pain control. In the United Kingdom, an estimate of recent annual consumption was 3500 million 500 mg tablets.[6] Hepatotoxicity is a well-known though uncommon adverse event with paracetamol use, usually in the context of overdosage. This may be deliberate or attributed to the fast clearance of paracetamol leading to risk of overuse. Acute hepatotoxicity may occur when a single dose of 10–15 g or more is taken. Doses of 20–25 g or more can be fatal. The risk of hepatotoxicity when taking paracetamol is increased in the presence of alcohol and NSAIDs.

Paracetamol has recently been associated with a small risk of causing gastrointestinal bleeding at a dose of 2 g daily or higher.[7-9] Doherty et al.[9] performed a randomized controlled trial looking at the use of ibuprofen, paracetamol, and a combination of both in a community population. The use of ibuprofen and paracetamol together was shown to be more effective in pain relief. However decreased haemoglobin levels were observed in all treatment groups. The risk was higher in the elderly, with dosages of 2 g/day or more, and with combination therapy. In their population, paracetamol at 3 g/day caused a similar degree of blood loss as ibuprofen 1200 mg/day. Epidemiological data supports increased upper gastrointestinal complications with use of paracetamol at a dose of 2 g/day or more; doses below this level did not show an increased risk.[8] Rahme et al.[10] reviewed hospitalization of patients due to gastrointestinal events in patients who used paracetamol alone and in combination with NSAIDS over a 6 year period and showed increased risk with combination therapy. In terms of cardiovascular effects, epidemiological studies also showed regular use of paracetamol increased risk of hypertension and cardiovascular events similarly to traditional NSAIDS.[4] This is further supported by a randomized double-blind placebo controlled trial showing increased ambulatory blood pressure levels in patients with existing coronary artery disease taking paracetamol.[11] This study looked at patients receiving paracetamol 1 g three times a day for 2 weeks, which resulted in increased blood pressure readings.

Clinical indications

Paracetamol is a widely used antipyretic and analgesic. It is not recommended for the primary treatment of inflammatory rheumatic conditions but is commonly used to treat mechanical and degenerative pain. It is recommended as first line therapy by the United Kingdom's National Institute of Clinical Excellence (NICE) for the management of lower back pain[12] and osteoarthritis (OA),[13] and by European League Against Rheumatism (EULAR) for the management of knee, hip, and hand OA.[14-16] However there is concern over its efficacy: the most recent systematic review of OA therapies[17] demonstrated a very low effect size for paracetamol in OA trials. Emerging data on its safety (see above) suggest caution in dosing, especially in combination with NSAIDs.

Opioid analgesics

The opium poppy, *Papaver somniferum*, is the most prevalent source of opioid analgesics, which have been used medicinally since the beginning of recorded history. The most important therapeutically active compounds found in the opium poppy are the alkaloids codeine and morphine.

Mechanism of action

Opioids work by binding to specific receptors of the CNS (mu, kappa, and delta) mounting an inhibitory effect of neurotransmission through G proteins. These receptors are present throughout the nervous system from the brain to the spinal cord. Most of the analgesic effect appears to come from activation of mu receptors. Activation of mu receptors leads to inhibition of neurotransmitters (including noradrenaline, acetylcholine, and the neuropeptide substance P) that would usually activate the pain pathway. Opioids have a central effect on both presynaptic and postsynaptic receptors.[18] Full opioid agonists act by direct stimulation of opioid receptors as outlined above. Most common opioids are full agonists (morphine, diamorphine, pethidine, and fentanyl). Buprenorphine is a partial agonist that binds with very high affinity to receptors but with both agonistic and antagonistic properties; however, no ceiling effect on analgesia has been observed and studies have demonstrated that full analgesic effect occurs with less than 100% receptor occupancy.[19]

Pharmacokinetics

Opioid plasma half-life and duration of action vary between the individual opioid agents. Morphine is a commonly used opioid drug. It has low lipid solubility resulting in longer duration of action but a latent onset of action due to its slow penetration of the blood–brain barrier.[20] Morphine can be administered orally, subcutaneously, intramuscularly, intravenously, rectally, via epidural, and intrathecally. When morphine is taken orally, only approximately 40–50% reaches the CNS after 30 minutes for immediate release and 90 minutes for slow-release preparations.[21] Elimination half-time for morphine is roughly 120 minutes.[20]

Diamorphine is more lipophilic and has more analgesic effect compared to morphine with a rapid onset of action. It is metabolized initially to monoacetylmorphine which crosses the blood–brain barrier rapidly and is therefore more potent than morphine. However, it undergoes extensive hepatic first-pass metabolism leading to low bioavailability. Dosing of diamorphine to morphine is roughly 2 to 1 in ratio and can be given via the same routes. It has a half-life of 2–3 minutes.

Codeine has weak opioid binding affinity for mu receptors, with half the potency of morphine and a half-life of

3 hours. Codeine is usually prescribed orally (doses of 30–60 mg 6 hourly). Smaller doses are used in combination preparations with paracetamol or anti-inflammatories. Codeine has anti-tussive and anti-diarrhoeal properties. There is evidence to show that the analgesic response and anti-diarrhoeal effect of codeine are under the genetic control of CYP2D6 (isozyme).[22] Part of the analgesic effect of codeine is mediated by its O-demethylated metabolite, morphine. In poor metabolizers, codeine may not have the desired analgesic effect as they are unable to convert codeine to morphine.[22]

Dihydrocodeine is similar in structure to codeine: it is a semisynthetic opioid analgesic with mu-receptor binding properties and a half-life of 4 hours. Oxycodone is a semisynthetic derivative of thebaine and similar in chemical structure to natural opioids.[22] Oxycodone has binding capacity for multiple receptors including kappa receptors. When taken orally, it has high bioavailability with a half-life of 3 hours.

Sustained-release analgesics have the advantages in maintaining a stable plasma concentration for a prolonged period of time, with improved patient compliance and satisfaction. Many opioid preparations are available in such formulations, requiring dosing every 8–12 hours. More recently 24 hour sustained-release preparations have been developed,[23] such as a 24 hourly morphine preparation that has been shown to improve sleep quality in chronic pain related to OA.[24] Other preparations of slow-release analgesics are the widely used transdermal patches.

Fentanyl is administered transdermally, parentally, and is also available transbucally; it is a very strong opioid agonist, with highly lipophilic characteristics therefore binds strongly to plasma proteins. It binds mainly to mu receptors. The fentanyl patch has a latent time of 6–12 hours before the onset of action, lasting 3–6 days, and after removal clearance takes up to 24 hours. Fentanyl is metabolized mainly in the liver to an inactive component called norfentanyl and excreted renally. Transdermal fentanyl has a half-life of approximately 17 hours.

A buprenorphine transdermal patch is also available, at a range of strengths (e.g. 5–20 μg/hour) for weekly use. It has a long half-life of approximately 30 hours. As well as an analgesic effect, it also has an anti-hyperalgesic effect, possibly through antagonism of kappa receptors; it may therefore be suitable for neuropathic pain. In the elderly, transdermal buprenorphine is relatively easy to use and is unaffected by renal function, therefore useful in patients with renal impairment.[19]

Tramadol is part of the opioid family, oral preparations being absorbed quickly with reduced first-pass metabolism. Its maximum dose is 400 mg/day. Elimination half-life is 4–6 hours. Sustained-release tramadol given 12 hourly or 24 hourly may improve sleep pattern related to pain, and quality of physical function.[23] Tramadol is also available in combination with paracetamol and has been shown to be efficacious in management of both acute and chronic pain including lower back pain, OA, and fibromyalgia, improving pain, function, and quality of life. The effect is comparable to combination preparations of paracetamol and codeine with some evidence for less constipation.[25]

Some caution should be taken in interpreting equivalent analgesic opioid dosing (often in morphine equivalents, e.g. 200 mg of oral codeine or 150 mg tramadol are equivalent to 10 mg of parenteral morphine), as most of the reported equivalencies are based on acute dosing and not the chronic use as is employed for

many musculoskeletal problems. Also, renal impairment must be considered for those agents with metabolites excreted renally.

Side effects

Opioid analgesia, when used short term, can cause nausea through centrally acting chemoreceptors, constipation from delayed gastric emptying, histamine release leading to pruritus, sedation, and respiratory depression. The latter two toxicities are dose related and can lead to coma in high doses. Other effects include meiosis, muscle rigidity, bradycardia, and mood changes. When opioids are used long term, there is recognized tolerance and chemical dependence which can lead to unpleasant withdrawal symptoms. Transdermal opioids can also have local reactions such as erythema and pruritus.

Tolerance refers to reduced effect from a drug after prolonged exposure. Tolerance to opioids is widely recognized; when tolerance occurs, a larger dose may be required to achieve a given effect. Receptor desensitization is thought to play an important role by the functional uncoupling of opioid receptors from G proteins. Tolerance is usually associated with prolonged use of opioids; while some clinicians use opioid rotation to address this, there are no recommendations for best practice.

Dependence can occur after a short period of opioid use and is characterized by a withdrawal response when the drug is stopped. The *International Statistical Classification of Diseases and Related Health Problems* (ICD-10) defines opioid dependence as 'a cluster of behavioural, cognitive, and physiological phenomena that develop after repeated substance use and that typically include a strong desire to take the drug, difficulties in controlling its use, persisting in its use despite harmful consequences, a higher priority given to drug use than to other activities and obligations, increased tolerance, and sometimes a physical withdrawal state.'[26] Generally, problems of dependence are very uncommon in the use of opioids at standard recommended doses for pain management.

Opioid hyperalgesia refers to a paradoxical response to opioids, with an increased perception of pain.[27] It is proposed to occur with chronic opioid use and is characterized by pain persisting or increasing with increased opioid dose. It is difficult to determine clinically if a patient reporting increasing pain is experiencing a change in pathology, tolerance to their opioid, or opioid hyperalgesia. At present small study numbers with varying study designs makes this problem difficult to understand. Opioid-induced endocrinopathy (potentially following suppression of the hypothalamic–pituitary–adrenal axis) is also poorly understood, and while in-vitro and animal studies have suggested opioid-related immunosuppression, this has not been reported as a significant problem in human studies.

Clinical indications

The role of opioids in the management of acute pain, postsurgical pain, and chronic cancer pain is clearly established. However, the role of opioid therapy for chronic non-cancer pain remains an area of debate. There is some evidence that opioids may provide clinically significant pain relief in a proportion of individuals with chronic non-cancer pain.[28] A review from the Cochrane Collaboration in 2009 addressed the use of opioids to treat OA of the knee or hip[29]; the review examined 10 study trials that included transdermal fentanyl and oral morphine, oral codeine, oral oxycodone, and oral oxymorphone, but studies of tramadol were excluded. The review found that opioid drugs were more effective than control interventions for relieving pain and improving function, but there were no differences in effect according to type or potency of opioid or the duration of treatment. However, given adverse events observed were more frequent compared to controls, the review concluded that 'the small to moderate beneficial effects of non-tramadol opioids are outweighed by the large risks of adverse events.' Clearly this risk/benefit needs to be defined carefully for individual patients, many of whom have no other analgesic options. All modern evidence-based OA guidelines recommend the use of opioids, with the most recent Osteoarthritis Research Society International (OARSI) meta-analysis supporting the benefits of opioid therapy.[30]

Patients with RA perceive pain to be their predominant impairment and report pain management as their highest priority.[31] As the analgesic properties of opioids do not depend on the presence of active inflammation, they are potential analgesic options in RA patients with persistent pain despite the use of disease-modifying anti-rheumatic drugs (DMARDs). The presence of opioid receptors on peripheral afferent nerves within joints also suggests that opioids may have peripheral analgesic effects in addition to their effect on the CNS.[32] Also, intra-articular nociceptive nerve fibres may contribute to joint inflammation via the release of neuropeptides such as substance P and calcitonin gene-related peptide, which raises the possibility that opioids may also act to inhibit joint inflammation.[33,34] A Cochrane review of 11 studies examined the role of opioid therapy in the treatment of RA pain.[35] It was concluded that there was limited evidence that weak oral opioids may be effective analgesics, but adverse effects were common and may offset the benefits of this class of medications.

It has been recommended that patients with chronic musculoskeletal pain avoid the long-term use of opioids unless the benefits outweigh the risks, in which case use should be regularly monitored.[27] The American Colllege of Rheumatology (ACR) Pain Management Task Force advises:

> The prescription of opioids must be done thoughtfully, since patients who may receive the greatest benefit may also be the same as those who are likely to abuse these agents. Better understanding of the risks and benefits of opioids should be mandated for all rheumatologists so that these medications can be safely, albeit selectively, used in patients with certain chronic rheumatologic disorders.[36]

Treatment of neuropathic pain

Neuropathic pain has been defined as 'pain arising as direct consequence of a lesion or disease affecting the somatosensory system.'[37] Neuropathic pain is manifested through a dysfunction of the nervous system at central or peripheral levels characterized by often disabling, constant and diffuse discomfort including hypersensitivity, altered sensitivity and reduced sensitivity. Such pain is often poorly localized and common examples are diabetic neuropathy, trigeminal neuralgia, postherpetic pain, or phantom limb pain.

Antidepressants
Mode of action
Tricyclic antidepressants (TCAs, e.g. amitriptyline, nortriptyline), selective serotonin reuptake inhibitors (SSRIs, e.g. fluoxetine, paroxetine, sertraline), and serotonin noradrenaline reuptake inhibitors (SNRIs, e.g. duloxetine, milnacipran) work to maintain serotonin and noradrenaline levels in the CNS by blocking their reuptake into nerve endings.

Side effects
TCAs can cause anticholinergic side effects of dry mouth, urinary retention, blurring of vision, and constipation. Less common side effects include tremor, palpitations, and somnolence. They can also lower seizure threshold.[38] In elderly people these drugs may result in falls and fainting episodes from postural hypotension. Men may experience erectile dysfunction. In some patients, weight gain has been reported. Venlafaxine, an SNRI, on the other hand can cause hypertension and gastrointestinal side effects as well as adversely effecting sexual function.

Clinical indications
Antidepressants such as TCAs and serotonin uptake inhibitors may be used to treat neuropathic pain. A Cochrane review of 61 randomized control trials showed a minimum to moderate benefit in relief of neuropathic pain. Three studies examined venlafaxine, and a number needed to treat (NNT) of 3 was achieved using TCAs and venlafaxine for at least moderate pain relief.[39] Analgesia was seen to be achieved quicker and at a smaller dose in comparison to the antidepressant effects.

A systematic review of antidepressants in the management of neuropathic pain generally indicated that TCAs and SNRIs are effective in chronic painful states with the strongest evidence being for use in fibromyalgia.[40] In other rheumatic conditions associated with chronic pain, there may be benefit of using antidepressants for managing sleep and fatigue symptoms.

A systematic review of amitryptyline vs placebo use in fibromyalgia[41] showed consistent benefit in patients with fibromyalgia with the use of amitriptyline 25 mg daily (<8 weeks duration) compared to a dose of 50 mg daily or placebo. However, limitations of included studies did not allow definite conclusions to be made. Another systematic review looking at the use of antidepressants in fibromyalgia patients showed that amitriptyline (25–50 mg daily) improved pain, fatigue, depression symptoms, sleep, and overall quality of life. Some domains in fibromyalgia improved with SSRIs (paroxetine, fluoxetine and sertraline) as well as SNRIs (duloxetine and milnacipran).[42]

Neuroleptics
Anticonvulsants are used to treat epilepsy but evidence shows benefit for some of these drugs in treatment of pain, particularly from nerve damage such postherpetic neuralgia, diabetic neuropathy, and neuropathic pain. These agents have also been reported to be effective in fibromyalgia.[43–45]

Mode of action
Some anticonvulsants act by blocking sodium channels leading to membrane stabilization resulting in reduced pain sensitization. Gabapentin acts on an auxillary alpha-2-delta subunit of a calcium channel, inhibiting influx of calcium and neurotransmission.[46] Pregabalin acts similarly to gabapentin in calcium channels, but also affects other neurotransmitters (glutamate, noradrenaline, and substance P) to reduce neuroexcitability.[47]

Side effects
The use of anticonvulsants is largely limited by their side effects which include sedation, cognitive suppression, tremors, and

gastrointestinal side effects. In higher doses, they can also cause hepatotoxicity and haematological problems. Less common effects on metabolism can lead to increased body weight.[48] Commonly used anticonvulsant drugs and their side effects are presented in Table 78.1.

Clinical indications

Carbamazepine has been shown to be effective in trigeminal neuralgia.

A recent review[43] reported efficacy for the use of pregabalin in management of neuropathic pain and in fibromyalgia. A dose between 300 mg and 600 mg daily was found to be effective but a lower dose of 150 mg daily was found to be ineffective, except for pain control in postherpetic neuralgia. NNT for moderate to significant benefit at 600 mg daily doses was also better demonstrated for postherpetic neuralgia and painful diabetic neuropathy in comparison to fibromyalgia.

In 2011, Moore et al.[44] reviewed the use of gabapentin in treating neuropathic pain. Moderate effectiveness of gabapentin (1200 g or more daily) was shown for neuropathic pain from postherpetic neuralgia, painful complications of diabetes, nerve injury pain, phantom limb pain, fibromyalgia, and trigeminal neuralgia.

Novel therapies

In an attempt to reduce bowel dysfunction and constipation due to opioids, a combination preparation of slow-release oxycodone and naloxone (the latter metabolized in the liver and providing opioid antagonism in the gut but not in the CNS) has been developed and licensed in the European Union.[49]

Tapentadol is a novel analgesic now licensed for use in the United States for moderate to severe acute pain. It is a centrally acting drug with dual mechanism in a single molecule acting as an opioid mu-receptor agonist and noradrenaline reuptake inhibitor; the latter action increases transmission in spinal cord inhibitory pathways, resulting in reduced pain sensation. Tapentadol has demonstrated effectiveness in trials of chronic lower back pain, OA knee pain, and diabetic neuropathy. Extended-release formulations are available. Side effects of tapentadol during phase II and phase III trials include nausea, diarrhoea, anxiety, and dizziness.[50,51] Its role compared to traditional opioid analgesics remains to be clarified.

Nerve growth factor (NGF) is a neurotropin which has effects on the nervous system and other non-neuronal cells (mast cells, monocytes, basophils).[52] The release of mediators sensitizing pain nociceptors is triggered partly by tropomyosin-related kinase A (TrkA), which is activated by NGF. TrkA also contributes directly to pain sensation by activating a signalling pathway.[52] A number of antagonists to this neurotropin are in development. Tanezumab is a humanized monoclonal IgG2 antibody against NGF. Lane et al.[53] demonstrated improvement in pain (45–62% from baseline), stiffness, and physical function in patients with moderate to severe knee OA when treated with tanezumab injections given 8 weeks apart. Transient symptoms of abnormal peripheral sensation have been reported in patients receiving tanezumab. The further development of anti-NGF therapies has been complicated by increased rates of joint replacement in patients receiving these agents in clinical trials; work is ongoing to understand if this represents direct drug toxicity or is related to an analgesic effect on already damaged joints.

Conclusion

Most of the traditional analgesic options have been available for many years, with well-defined efficacy and significant toxicity profiles. New formulations or delivery systems may improve their applicability. However, with the growth of genomic and molecular data related to pain pathways and management, it is hoped that new classes of analgesics will soon be forthcoming.

Table 78.1 Common side effects of anticonvulsants

Drug	Adverse effects
Pregabalin	CNS—dizziness, poor concentration, drowsiness, visual disturbances (diplopia, blurred vision, visual field defect), disturbance in muscular function, memory, speech, parasthesias
	Gastrointestinal—dry mouth, nausea, vomiting, weight gain
	Haematological—thrombocytopaenia, neutropaenia, Stevens–Johnson syndrome (rare)
	Other—peripheral oedema, fatigue
Carbamazepine	CNS—headache, ataxia, drowsiness, nausea, vomiting, blurring of vision, dizziness, unsteadiness (dose related, more common in elderly patients)
	Haematological—idiosyncratic blood dyscrasias, aplastic anaemia and agranulocytosis
	Other—Stevens–Johnson syndrome/toxic epidermal necrolysis rare), hyponatraemia
	Close monitoring of liver dysfunction (induces hepatic enzymes) and blood required
Gabapentin	Gastrointestinal—nausea, vomiting, gingivitis, diarrhoea, abdominal pain, dyspepsia, constipation, dry mouth or throat, flatulence, weight gain, increased appetite, anorexia
	CNS—confusion, emotional lability, depression, vertigo, anxiety, nervousness, abnormal thoughts, drowsiness, dizziness, malaise, ataxia, convulsions, movement and speech disorder, amnesia, tremor, insomnia, headache, paraesthesia
	Haematological—neutropenia (rare)

References

1. Schaible HG, Ebersberger A, Natura G. Update on peripheral mechanisms of pain: beyond prostaglandins and cytokines. *Arthritis Res Ther* 2011;13:210–218.
2. Merskey H, Bogduk N. *Classification of chronic pain*, 2nd edn. IASP Press, Seattle, 1994.
3. WHO. *Cancer pain relief*. World Health Organization, Geneva, Switzerland, 1986.
4. Hinz B, Brune K. Paracetamol and cyclooxygenase inhibition: is there a cause for concern? *Ann Rheum Dis* 2012;71:20–25.
5. Bjørnsson GA, Haanaes HR, Skoglund LA A randomized, double-blind crossover trial of paracetamol 1000 mg four times daily vs ibuprofen 600 mg: effect on swelling and other postoperative events after third molar surgery. *Br J Clin Pharmacol* 2003;55:405–412.
6. Sheen CL, Dillon JF, Bateman DN, Simpson KJ, MacDonald TM. Paracetamol toxicity: epidemiology, prevention and costs to the healthcare system. *Q J Med* 2002;95(9):609–619.
7. González-Pérez A, Rodríguez LA. Upper gastrointestinal complications among users of paracetamol. *Basic Clin Pharmacol Toxicol* 2006;98(3):297–303.

8. García Rodríguez LA, Hernández-Díaz S. Relative risk of upper gastrointestinal complications among users of acetaminophen and nonsteroidal anti-inflammatory drugs. *Epidemiology* 2001;12(5):570–576.

9. Doherty M, Hawkey C, Goulder M. et al. A randomised controlled trial of ibuprofen, paracetamol or a combination tablet of ibuprofen/paracetamol in community-derived people with knee pain. *Ann Rheum Dis* 2011;70(9):1534–1541.

10. Rahme E, Barkun A, Nedjar H et al. Hospitalizations for upper and lower GI events associated with traditional NSAIDs and acetaminophen among the elderly in Quebec, Canada. *Am J Gastroenterol* 2008;103:872–882.

11. Sudano I, Flammer AJ, Periat D et al. Acetaminophen increases blood pressure in patients with coronary artery disease. *Circulation* 2010;122:1789–1796.

12. National Institute for Health and Clinical Excellence. *Early management of persistent non-specific low back pain NICE (CG88)*, 2009. Available at: www.nice.org.uk/nicemedia/pdf/CG88QuickRefGuide.pdf

13. National Institute for Health and Clinical Excellence. *The care and management of osteoarthritis in adults (CG 59)*, 2008. Available at: www.nice.org.uk/nicemedia/pdf/CG59NICEguideline.pdf

14. Pendleton A, Arden N, Dougados M et al. EULAR recommendations for the management of knee osteoarthritis: report of a task force of the Standing Committee for International Clinical Studies Including Therapeutic trials (ESCISIT). *Ann Rheum Dis* 2000;59:936–944.

15. Zhang W, Doherty M, Leeb BF et al. EULAR evidence based recommendations for the management of hand osteoarthritis: Report of a Task Force of the EULAR Standing Committee for International Clinical Studies Including Therapeutics (ESCISIT) *Ann Rheum Dis* 2007;66(3):377–388.

16. Zhang W, Doherty M, Arden N et al. EULAR evidence based recommendations for the management of hip osteoarthritis: report of a task force of the EULAR Standing Committee for International Clinical Studies Including Therapeutics (ESCISIT). *Ann Rheum Dis* 2005;64(5):669–681.

17. Zhang W, Nuki G, Moskowitz RW et al. OARSI recommendations for the management of hip and knee osteoarthritis: part III: Changes in evidence following systematic cumulative update of research published through January 2009. *Osteoarthritis Cartilage* 2010;18(4):476–499.

18. Chahl LA. Opioids—mechanisms of action. Experimental and clinical pharmacology. *Aust Prescr* 1996;19:63–65

19. Pergolizzi J, Aloisi AM, Dahan A et al. Review article: current knowledge of buprenorphine and its unique pharmacological profile. *Pain Practice* 2010;10(5):428–450.

20. Trescot AM, Datta S, Lee M, Hansen H. Opioid pharmacology. *Pain Physician* 2008;11(2 Suppl):S133–S153.

21. Stoelting RK. *Pharmacology, physiology & anesthetic practice*, 2nd edn. Lippincott Williams & Wilkins, Baltimore, MD, 1991.

22. Mikus G, Weiss J. Influence of CYP2D6 genetics on opioid kinetics, metabolism and response. *Curr Pharmacogenomics* 2005;3:43–52.

23. Snidvongs S, Mehta V. Recent advances in opioid prescription for chronic non-cancer pain. *Postgrad Med J* 2012;88:66–72.

24. Rosenthal M, Moore P, Groves E et al. Sleep improves when patients with chronic OA pain are managed with morning dosing of once a day extended-release morphine sulfate (AVINZA): findings from a pilot study. *J Opioid Manag* 2007;3:145–154.

25. Schug SA. Combination analgesia in 2005—a rational approach: focus on paracetamol-tramadol. *Clin Rheumatol* 2006;25(Suppl 1):S16–S21

26. WHO. Chapter V: Classification of mental and behavioural disorders. Clinical descriptions and diagnostic guidelines. In: *International statistical classification of diseases and related health problems, 10th revision (ICD-10)*. World Health Organization, Geneva, Switzerland, 2005.

27. Crofford L.J. Adverse effects of chronic opioid therapy for chronic musculoskeletal pain. *Nat Rev Rheumatol* 6;2010:191–197.

28. Noble M, Tregear SJ, Treadwell JR et al. Long-term opioid management for chronic noncancer pain (Review). *Cochrane Database Syst Rev* 2010;1:CD006605.

29. Nüesch E, Rutjes AWS, Husni E, Welch V, Jüni P. Oral or transdermal opioids for osteoarthritis of the knee or hip. *Cochrane Database Syst Rev* 2009;4:CD003115.

30. Zhang W, Nuki G, Moskowitz RW et al. OARSI recommendations for the management of hip and knee osteoarthritis: part III: Changes in evidence following systematic cumulative update of research published through January 2009. *Osteoarthritis Cartilage* 2010;18(4):476–499.

31. Heiberg T, Kvien TK. Preferences for improved health examined in 1,024 patients with rheumatoid arthritis: pain has highest priority. *Arthritis Rheum* 2002;47(4):391–397.

32. Lang LJ, Pierer M, Stein C, Baerwald C. Opioids in rheumatic diseases. *Ann N Y Acad Sci* 2010;1193(1):111–116.

33. Fields HL, Emson PC, Leigh BK, Gilbert RF, Iversen LL. Multiple opiate receptor sites on primary afferent fibres. *Nature* 1980;284(5754):351–353.

34. McDougall JJ. Arthritis and pain. Neurogenic origin of joint pain. *Arthritis Res Ther* 2006;8(6):220–230.

35. Whittle SL, Richards BL, Husni E, Buchbinder R. Opioid therapy for treating rheumatoid arthritis pain. *Cochrane Database Syst Rev* 2011;11:CD003113.

36. Borenstein D, Altman R, Bello A et al. Report of the American College of Rheumatology Pain Management Task Force. *Arthritis Care Res* 2010;62:590–599.

37. Haanpää M, Attal N, Backonja M. NeuPSIG guidelines on neuropathic pain assessment. *Pain* 2011;152(1):14–27.

38. Nelson JC. Tricyclic and tetracyclic drugs. In: Schatzberg AF, Nemeroff CB (eds) *The American Psychiatric Publishing textbook of psychopharmacology*, 4th edn. American Psychiatric Publishing, Washington, DC, 2006:263–263.

39. Saarto T, Wiffen PJ. Antidepressants for neuropathic pain. *Cochrane Database Syst Rev* 2007;4:CD005454.

40. Perrot S, Javier RM, Marty M, Le Jeunne C, Laroche F. Is there any evidence to support the use of anti-depressants in painful rheumatological conditions? Systematic review of pharmacological and clinical studies. *Rheumatology (Oxford)* 2008;47(8):1117–1123.

41. Nishishinya B, Urrútia G, Walitt B et al. Amitriptyline in the treatment of fibromyalgia: a systematic review of its efficacy. *Rheumatology* (Oxford) 2008;47(12):1741–1746.

42. Üçeyler N, Häuser, W. Sommer C. A systematic review on the effectiveness of treatment with antidepressants in fibromyalgia syndrome. *Arthritis Care Res* 2008;59:1279–1298.

43. Moore RA, Straube S, Wiffen PJ, Derry S, McQuay HJ. Pregabalin for acute and chronic pain in adults. *Cochrane Database Syst Rev* 2009;3:CD007076.

44. Moore RA, Wiffen PJ, Derry S, McQuay HJ. Gabapentin for chronic neuropathic pain and fibromyalgia in adults. *Cochrane Database Syst Rev* 2011;3:CD007938.

45. Arnold LM, Goldenberg DL, Stanford SB et al. Gabapentin in the treatment of fibromyalgia: a randomized, double-blind, placebo-controlled, multicenter trial. *Arthritis Rheum* 2007;56(4):1336–1344.

46. van Hooft JA, Dougherty JJ, Endeman D, Nichols RA, Wadman WJ. Gabapentin inhibits presynaptic Ca (2+) influx and synaptic transmission in rat hippocampus and neocortex. *Eur J Pharmacol* 2002;449(3):221–228.

47. Lauria-Horner BA, Pohl RB. Pregabalin: a new anxiolytic. *Expert Opin Investig Drugs* 2003;12(4):663–672.

48. Swann AC. Major system toxicities and side effects of anticonvulsants. *J Clin Psychiatry* 2001;62(Suppl 14):16–21.

49. Clemens KE, Mikus G. Combined oral prolonged-release oxycodone and naloxone in opioid-induced bowel dysfunction: review of efficacy and safety data in the treatment of patients experiencing chronic pain. *Expert Opin Pharmacother* 2010;11(2):297–310.

50. Vadivelu N, Timchenko A, Huang Y, Sinatra R. Tapentadol extended-release for treatment of chronic pain: a review. *J Pain Res* 2011;4: 211–218.

51. Afilalo M, Etropolski MS, Kuperwasser B et al. Efficacy and safety of tapentadol extended release compared with oxycodone controlled release for the management of moderate to severe chronic pain related to osteoarthritis of the knee: a randomized, double-blind, placebo- and active-controlled phase III study. *Clin Drug Investig* 2010;30(8):489–505.

52. Covaceuszach S, Marinelli S, Krastanova I et al. Single cycle structure-based humanization of an anti-nerve growth factor therapeutic antibody. *PLoS One* 2012;7(3):e32212.

53. Lane NE, Schnitzer TJ, Birbara CA et al. Tanezumab for the treatment of pain from osteoarthritis of the knee. *N Engl J Med* 2010;14; 363(16):1521–1531.

CHAPTER 79

Glucocorticoids

Johannes W. G. Jacobs, Cornelia M. Spies,
Johannes W. J. Bijlsma, and Frank Buttgereit

Introduction

Glucocorticoids are anchor drugs of therapeutic regimens in most inflammatory and autoimmune rheumatic conditions, because of their effectiveness, versatility and low cost (Box 79.1). Basic mechanisms and effects, indications, adverse advents and monitoring of glucocorticoid therapy in rheumatology and new developments are discussed here with emphasis on clinically relevant implications.

Characteristics of glucocorticoids

Structure and classification

Steroid hormones and cholesterol are characterized by a sterol skeleton; the term 'steroid' refers to this basic sterol nucleus. On the basis of their main functions, steroid hormones can be classified into sex hormones, mineralocorticoids, and glucocorticoids. Mineralocorticoids and glucocorticoids are synthesized in the adrenal cortex, hence the terms 'corticosteroid' and 'corticoid' for

---

Box 79.1 Reasons for the wide usage of glucocorticoids in rheumatology

- Low cost
- Applicable in many drug combinations, additive effect
- Wide spectrum of anti-inflammatory and immunosuppressive actions
- Clear dose–effect relationship, wide dosing range, many dose steps
- Various routes of administration available
- Short lag time of effect
- Predictable effect
- Relatively mild toxicity, when used cautiously
- Inhibitory effect on radiographic progression in early rheumatoid arthritis
- Long-term clinical experience
- High percentage of responders

---

these hormones. The main natural mineralocorticoid is aldosterone, and the main natural glucocorticoid is cortisol (hydrocortisone). Natural glucocorticoids also have mineralocorticoid effects, but synthetic glucocorticoid drugs have less mineralocorticoid and clearly more glucocorticoid potency (Table 79.1). It is more precise to use the term glucocorticoid than the term corticosteroid when referring to one of the glucocorticoid drugs.[1]

Absorption and protein binding

Most orally administered glucocorticoids are absorbed readily, probably within about 30 minutes. The bioavailability of prednisone and prednisolone is high. The affinity of the individual glucocorticoids to bind to plasma proteins (transcortin, also called corticosteroid-binding globulin, and albumin) varies (Table 79.1). Transcortin binds glucocorticoids more strongly than does albumin; only unbound glucocorticoids are pharmacologically active. Patients with low levels of plasma protein, such as albumin (e.g. because of liver diseases or chronic active inflammatory diseases), are more susceptible to effects and side effects of glucocorticoids. In liver disease, an additional argument for dose adjustment is reduced metabolic clearance of glucocorticoids; see next section.

Conversion into active hormones and vice versa; pharmacology

Glucocorticoids with an 11-keto instead of an 11-hydroxy group, such as cortisone and prednisone, are inactive prohormones, which have negligible glucocorticoid bioactivity because of their very low affinity for the glucocorticoid receptor. They must be reduced in the liver to their biologically active 11-hydroxy configurations, cortisol and prednisolone respectively. Prednisone and prednisolone preparations are considered approximately bioequivalent, but in patients with severe liver disease it is rational to prescribe prednisolone instead of prednisone. The intracellular enzyme 11β-hydroxysteroid dehydrogenase (11β-HSD) type 1 activates the glucocorticoid prohormones. Although this enzyme can also promote the reverse reaction by dehydrogenation, leading to inactivation of active glucocorticoids, its activating activity predominates. In contrast, the isoenzyme 11β-HSD type 2 has only dehydrogenase activity, so converting active glucocorticoids to their inactive forms.

Table 79.1 Pharmacodynamics of glucocorticoids used in rheumatology

	Equivalent glucocorticoid dose (mg)	Relative glucocorticoid activity	Relative mineralocorticoid activity[a]	Protein binding[b]	Half-life (h) in plasma	Biological half-life (h)
Short-acting						
Cortisone	25	0.8	0.8	–	0.5	8–12
Cortisol	20	1	1	++++	1.5–2	8–12
Intermediate-acting						
Methylprednisolone	4	5	0.5	–	>3.5	18–36
Prednisolone	5	4	0.6	++	2.1–3.5	18–36
Prednisone	5	4	0.6	+++	3.4–3.8	18–36
Triamcinolone	4	5	0	++	2–>5	18–36
Long-acting						
Dexamethasone	0.75	20–30	0	++	3–4.5	36–54
Betamethasone	0.6	20–30	0	++	3–5	36–54

[a]Clinical signs: sodium and water retention, leading to oedema and hypertension, and potassium depletion.
[b]–, none; ++, high; +++, high to very high; ++++, very high.

Glucocorticoids have biologic half-lives longer than their plasma half-lives (see Table 79.1); with its biological half-life, prednisolone can be dosed once daily for most diseases. Maximal effects of glucocorticoids lag behind peak serum concentrations. Serum half-life of prednisolone is increased by decreased rates of metabolism in patients with renal disease or liver cirrhosis, and in elderly patients, which means that a given dose may have a greater effect in these individuals. Several other pharmacological mechanisms could be involved in the variability of glucocorticoid sensitivity in patients.[2] Prednisolone can be removed by haemodialysis, but, overall, the amount removed does not require dose adjustment in patients on haemodialysis.

Drug interactions

Cytochrome P450 (CYP) is a family of isozymes responsible for the biotransformation of several drugs. Drug interactions can be based either on induction or on inhibition of these enzymes. An example of induction of CYP isozymes is rifampin-induced non-responsiveness to prednisone in inflammatory diseases, which is clinically relevant.[3] Inhibitors of CYP are, for example, ketoconazole and grapefruit juice; the effect of grapefruit juice intake is likely to be of limited clinical significance.[4] Ketoconazole also interferes with endogenous glucocorticoid synthesis and is therefore used to treat hypercortisolism.[5]

Basic mechanisms of actions

Glucocorticoids influence the transcription of about 1% of the entire genome, which is an exceptionally broad spectrum of effects for a single class of endogenous hormones and hormonal drugs.

Genomic mechanisms

Glucocorticoid receptors are present in almost all tissues; genomic mechanisms constitute most glucocorticoid actions. Genomic mechanisms require passing of glucocorticoid molecules through the cell membrane—glucocorticoids are lipophilic, have a low molecular mass and thus can pass easily—binding, to the cytosolic glucocorticoid receptor, formation of the receptor–glucocorticoid complex, and translocation of this complex into the nucleus and, finally, influencing gene expression via transactivation and transrepression (Figure 79.1).

In the post-transcriptional phase, by decreasing the stability of messenger RNA via induction of ribonucleases, glucocorticoid receptor–glucocorticoid complexes also may inhibit protein synthesis, e.g. of interleukin (IL)-1, IL-6, granulocyte-macrophage colony-stimulating factor (GM-CSF), and inducible cyclooxygenase (COX)-2.[6]

Non-genomic mechanisms

Compared to genomic effects, non-genomic effects are more rapid, occurring within seconds or minutes. Non-genomic effects can involve membrane-bound glucocorticoid receptors. Dexamethasone targets these receptors on T lymphocytes, which rapidly impairs T lymphocyte receptor signalling and immune response.[7] Non-genomic actions without involvement of glucocorticoid receptors occur via physicochemical interactions with biological membranes, altering cell function. For instance, the resulting inhibition of calcium and sodium cycling across the plasma membrane of immune cells contributes to rapid immunosuppression and reduced inflammation.[8] However, for most of the effects of glucocorticoids, the underlying genomic and non-genomic basic mechanisms cannot clinically be discriminated very well.

Pharmacological effects

The spectrum of glucocorticoid effects is summarized in Figure 79.2.

Immunosuppression and immunomodulation

Immune cells, adhesion molecules, and cytokines

Glucocorticoids reduce activation, proliferation, differentiation, and survival of a variety of inflammatory cells, summarized in

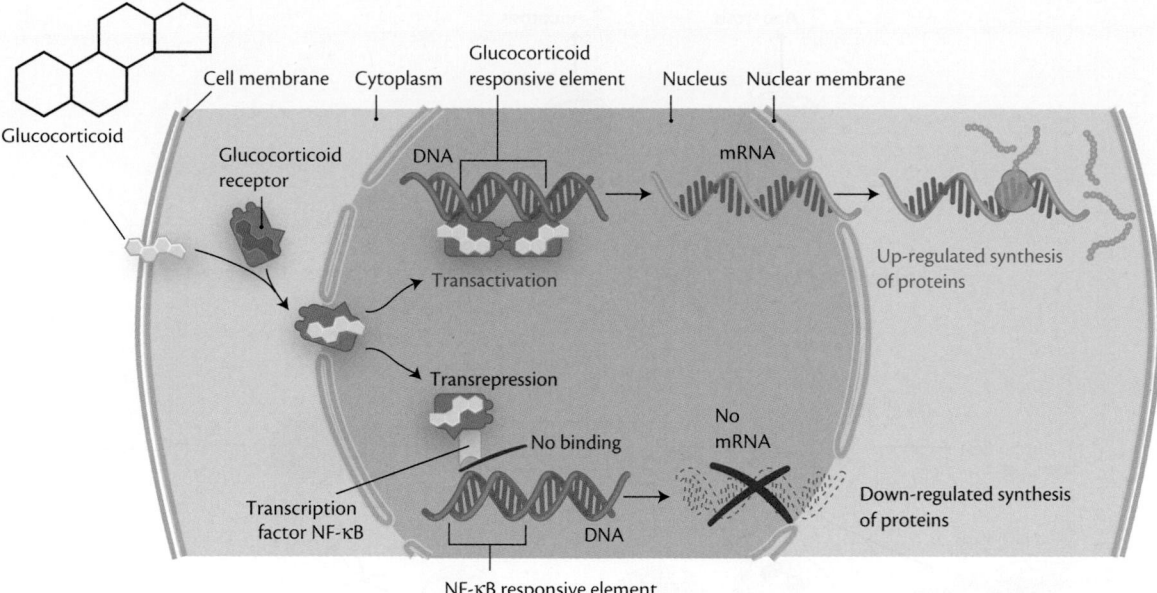

Fig. 79.1 Genomic action of glucocorticoids. Of the isoforms α and β of the glucocorticoid receptor, only the α isoform, common in all target tissues, binds to glucocorticoids. The glucocorticoid receptor–glucocorticoid complex rapidly migrates into the nucleus, where a dimer of the complex binds to specific consensus sites of the DNA, glucocorticoid-responsive elements, leading to an upregulated synthesis of certain regulatory proteins (**transactivation**), mainly responsible for unwanted metabolic effects of glucocorticoid therapy. The interaction of glucocorticoid receptor–glucocorticoid complex (as monomer) with transcriptional factors, such as NFκB, inhibits binding of these transcriptional factors to specific consensus sites in the DNA. This results in downregulation of (predominantly proinflammatory) protein synthesis (**transrepression**).[78] Selective glucocorticoid receptor agonists almost selectively exhibiting transrepression could result in less adverse effects than glucocorticoids.[77]
Adapted from Jacobs JWG, Bijlsma JWJ. Glucocorticoid therapy. In: Firestein CS, Budd RC, Harris ED et al. (eds) *Kelley's textbook of rheumatology*, 8th edn. Saunders Elsevier, Philadelphia, 2009:863–881.

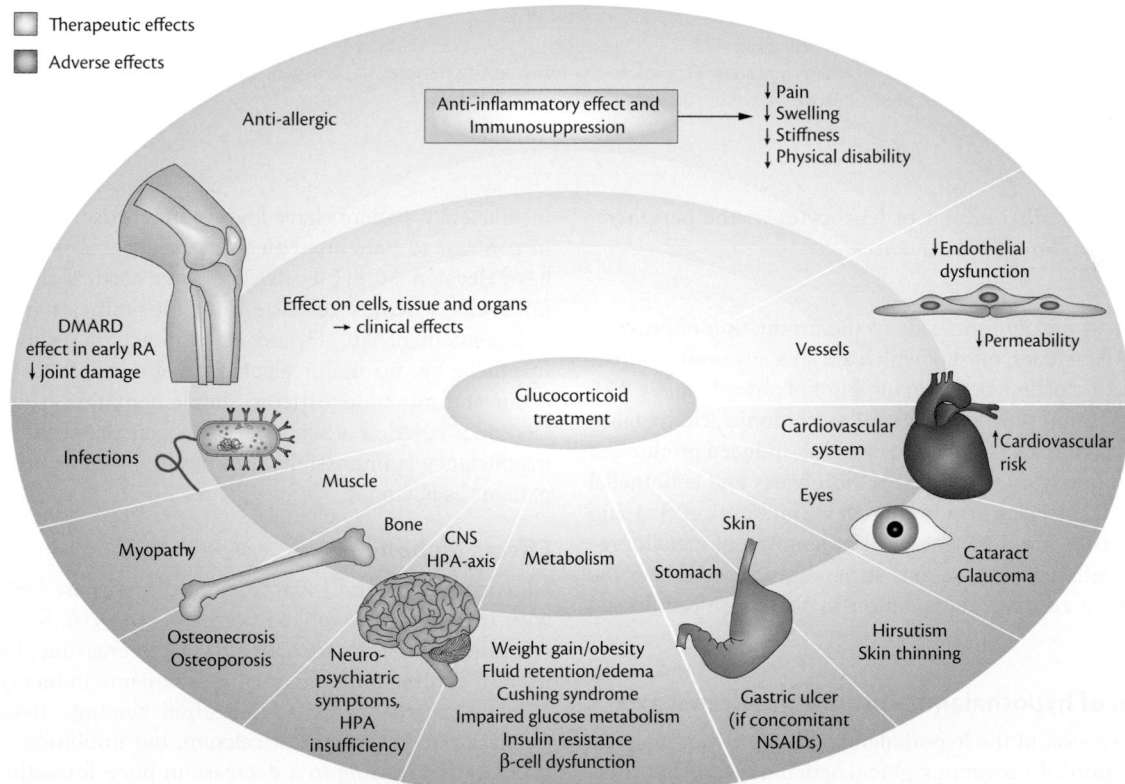

Fig. 79.2 Clinical effect spectrum of glucocorticoids. Upper part: wanted effects. Lower part: range of adverse effects, dependent on dose and duration of the glucocorticoid therapy. DMARD, disease-modifying anti-rheumatic drug; RA, rheumatoid arthritis; CNS, central nervous system; HPA, hypothalamic–pituitary–adrenal axis; NSAID, non-steroidal anti-inflammatory drug; CV, cardiovascular.
Adapted from Hoes JN, Jacobs JWG, Buttgereit F, Bijlsma JWJ. Current view of glucocorticoid co-therapy with DMARDs in rheumatoid arthritis. *Nat Rev Rheumatol* 2010;6:693–702, with permission.

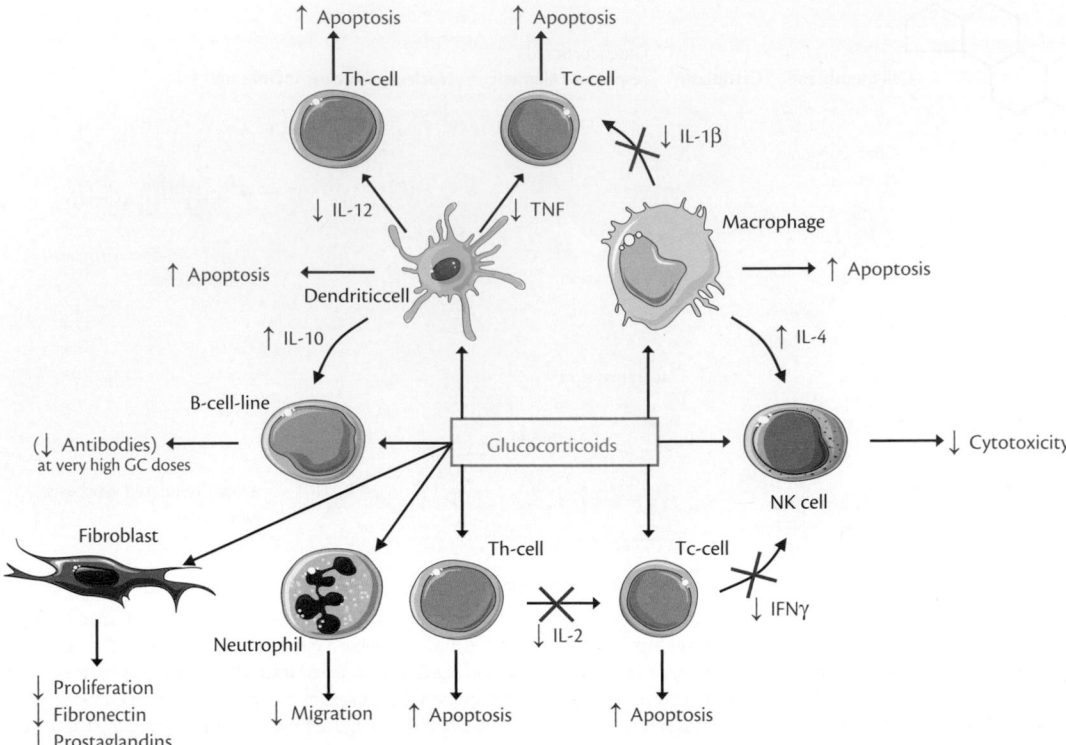

Fig. 79.3 Glucocorticoid effects (in red type) on the interplay of inflammatory cells and cytokines.[9] The production of proinflammatory cytokines, such as interleukin (IL)-1β and tumour necrosis factor (TNF) is inhibited and the production of anti-inflammatory cytokines, such as IL-10, by macrophages and dendritic cells is stimulated. Glucocorticoids promote apoptosis of macrophages, dendritic cells, and T cells. All these effects result in inhibition of immune responses. Downregulation of adhesion molecules decreases migration of neutrophils and increases the number of circulating neutrophils,[79] increasing the total leucocyte blood count, although there is decreased myelopoiesis and bone marrow release of other leucocyte subsets.

↓, decreased; ↑, increased; IFNγ, interferon-γ; NK cell, natural killer cell; Tc-cell, cytotoxic T lymphocyte; Th-cell, T-helper lymphocyte.

Adapted from Sternberg EM. Neural regulation of innate immunity: a coordinated nonspecific host response to pathogens. *Nat Rev Immunol* 2006;6:318–328, with permission. Figure was made using Servier Medical Art (www.servier.com).

Figure 79.3.[9] The redistribution of leucocytes in the peripheral blood has no clear clinical consequences.

Enzymes

Arachidonic acid metabolism leads to the production of prostaglandins and leukotrienes, most of which are strongly proinflammatory. Via induction of lipocortin (an inhibitor of phospholipase A2), glucocorticoids inhibit the formation of arachidonic acid metabolites. Glucocorticoids also inhibit the cytokine-induced production of COX-2 in monocytes/macrophages, fibroblasts and endothelial cells. In addition, glucocorticoids are potent inhibitors of IL-1 and tumour necrosis factor (TNF)-induced production of metalloproteinases, especially collagenase and stromelysin,[10] which are the main effectors of cartilage degradation in the chronic inflamed joint.

Suppression of hypothalamic–pituitary–adrenal axis

Chronic suppression of the hypothalamic–pituitary–adrenal axis by administration of exogenous glucocorticoids leads by negative feedback loops on corticotropin-releasing hormone (CRH) and adrenocorticotropic hormone (ACTH) to failure in pituitary ACTH release and thus to partial functional adrenal atrophy with loss of cortisol secretory capability: secondary adrenal insufficiency. Patients have low serum cortisol and ACTH levels, in contrast to patients with primary adrenal insufficiency, who have elevated ACTH levels. The outer cortical zone involved in mineralocorticoids (aldosterone) biosynthesis is functionally independent of ACTH and stays intact in secondary adrenal insufficiency; no major electrolyte abnormalities in the blood occur and mineralocorticoid supplementation is not necessary. Certain prediction of secondary, glucocorticoid-induced, adrenal insufficiency is impossible; if in doubt, it seems prudent to treat patients as having it.

Effects on bone

Glucocorticoids and inflammatory diseases are both associated with increased generalized bone loss and risk for osteoporotic fractures, while glucocorticoids by decreasing disease activity also inhibit inflammatory mechanisms inducing bone loss. Glucocorticoids decrease intestinal calcium absorption and increase renal excretion of calcium, but inhibition of osteoblast proliferation leading to a decrease in bone formation seems the most important cause of osteoporosis.[11] This topic is addressed in detail in Chapter 142.

In early rheumatoid arthritis (RA), glucocorticoids also have positive effects of on bone; the joint-sparing effect is probably based on the inhibition of proinflammatory cytokines such as IL-1 and TNF,[12] which stimulate osteoblasts and T lymphocytes to produce receptor activator of nuclear factor kappa B (RANK) ligand (RANKL). RANKL binding to its receptor RANK on osteoclast precursor cells leads to differentiation and activation of osteoclasts, and subsequently to bone resorption, periarticular osteopenia, and formation of bone erosions in patients with RA.[13]

Applications in rheumatology

In this chapter, systemic glucocorticoid therapy is discussed. Intralesional and intra-articular glucocorticoid injections are discussed in Chapter 87.

Often it is unclear what is exactly meant by semiquantitative terms used for doses, such as 'low' or 'high'. Based on pathophysiologic and pharmacokinetic data, standardization of terminology has been proposed:[1]

+ **low**: ≤7.5 mg

+ **medium**: >7.5 but ≤30 mg

+ **high**: >30 but ≤100 mg

+ **very high**: >100 mg prednisone equivalents per day

+ **pulse**: ≥250 mg prednisone equivalent per day for one or a few days.

Indications

The aims of glucocorticoid therapy differ for various rheumatic diseases; they range from symptomatic relief and disease-modifying effects to immunosuppressive and immunomodulatory actions. The specific indication determines route of administration, choice of drug (pharmacological properties), and dose. The dose and route of administration are related to clinical efficacy, speed of onset of action, and risk of adverse effects.

Table 79.2 gives an overview of general use of glucocorticoids in rheumatology. Some of the indications could at first glance be considered as questionable. For instance, in systemic sclerosis glucocorticoids, especially in high doses, are contraindicated because of the risk of scleroderma renal crisis, but they may be useful for myositis or interstitial lung disease complicating systemic sclerosis. The table shows that glucocorticoids form part of the primary therapeutic strategy in myositis, polymyalgia rheumatica, and systemic vasculitis. Moreover, they are frequently part of therapeutic

Table 79.2 General use of glucocorticoids in rheumatology

	Initial[a] oral dose			Intravenous, very high dose,[b] or pulse	Intra-articular injection
	Low[b]	Medium[b]	High[b]		
Arthritides					
Gouty arthritis, acute	–	2	2	–	2
Juvenile idiopathic arthritis	–	1	1	–	1
Osteoarthritis	–	–	–	–	1
Acute CPP crystal arthritis	–	–	–	–	2
Psoriatic arthritis	–	1	–	–	2
Reactive arthritis	–	–	–	–	1
Rheumatic fever	–	1	1	–	–
Rheumatoid arthritis	2	2	1	1	2
Collagen disorders					
Dermatomyositis, polymyositis	–	–	3	1	–
Mixed connective tissue disease	–	1	–	1	1
Polymyalgia rheumatica	–	3	–	1	–
Sjögren's syndrome, primary	–	–	1	–	–
Systemic lupus erythematosus	–	2	1	1	–
Systemic sclerosis	–	1	–	–	–
Systemic vasculitides in general					
	–	–	3	1	–

[a]Initial dose: dose at the start of therapy, will often be decreased in time depending on disease activity.

[b]Dose in prednisone equivalents a day: low, ≤ 7.5 mg; medium, >7.5 but ≤ 30 mg; high, >30 but ≤ 100 mg; very high, > 100 mg; pulse, ≥250 mg prednisone equivalent per day for one or a few days.[1]

–, rare use; 1, infrequent use, for therapy-resistant disease, complications, severe flare, major exacerbation, and for bridging the lag time of recently started therapy; 2, frequently added to/used as the basic therapeutic strategy; 3, basic part of the therapeutic strategy. Note: there may be considerable variation in uses between countries.

strategies for RA. For the other diseases, glucocorticoids are used as adjunctive therapy or not at all.

Doses and routes of administration

Aspects of systemic glucocorticoid use are discussed here; their use for specific rheumatological diseases is discussed in detail in the relevant chapters.

Oral low to high dose glucocorticoid therapy

Worldwide, glucocorticoids are used in 15–90% of RA patients,[14] given for their symptomatic effect and joint-sparing properties (i.e. disease-modifying effects), which have firmly been proven during the first 2 years of the disease,[15] most recently in the Computer Assisted Management of Early Rheumatoid Arthritis trial 2 (CAMERA-II study).[15a] Data on disease-modifying effects in long-standing RA are lacking, which is not to say these effects cannot be present. The benefit of glucocorticoid use during early disease remains detectable during the following years.[16,17]

Glucocorticoids are always combined with other disease-modifying drugs in early RA. In general, two dosing regimes can be discriminated: (1) starting 5–10 mg of prednisone equivalent per day during the first 2 years of the disease and (2) higher starting doses, e.g. 15–60 mg/day, followed by rapid tapering and continuation of a lower dose or stopping.

Next to RA, collagen disease and vasculitides, oral glucocorticoids are used to treat acute gout, especially in patients with contraindications to non-steroidal anti-inflammatory drugs (NSAIDs) and colchicine. For this use, typically 30–35 mg of prednisone equivalent during 5 days is prescribed.[18] A problem arises when the diagnosis is not proven, because septic arthritis may present similarly; furthermore, coincident septic and gouty arthritis have been described.[19] So this approach is only safe if the risk of septic arthritis is very low. Consequently it is probably safer and more effective to inject glucocorticoid intra-articularly following diagnostic aspiration.

Glucocorticoid pulse therapy

Pulse therapy is used in rheumatology primarily for remission induction, rapid disease suppression, and treatment of flares and severe complications (see Table 79.2). In active RA, pulse therapy is applied to bridge the lag time of recently initiated second-line anti-rheumatic treatment; although the duration of the effects varies, the beneficial effects—which are similar to effects of long-term methotrexate in patients with early RA[20]—generally last for about 6 weeks.[21] In systemic lupus erythematosus (SLE), osteonecrosis and psychosis seem to be more frequent side effects of pulse therapy compared to patients with RA, but these may also be complications of active SLE itself.

Alternate-day dosing

Alternate-day therapy uses a single dose administered every other morning, which is usually equivalent to, or higher than, twice the usual or pre-established daily dose. The rationale of this regimen is that the body, including the hypothalamic–pituitary–adrenal axis, is exposed to exogenous glucocorticoid only on alternate days. Alternate-day therapy is unsuccessful in most patients with a rheumatic disease; they often experience exacerbation of symptoms on the second day. This is in line with the clinical impression that a single dose of glucocorticoids daily is less effective in RA than half that dose given twice daily. In giant cell arteritis, alternate-day glucocorticoid therapy also is less effective than daily administration.[22] Alternate-day regimens are rarely used in rheumatology today except in patients with juvenile idiopathic arthritis, in whom this regimen results in less inhibition of body growth than does daily usage.[23]

Glucocorticoid-sparing drugs

For most inflammatory rheumatic diseases, other immunomodulatory drugs, including biologicals, are often added to therapy with glucocorticoids to improve efficacy. If this is done to decrease the glucocorticoid dose or the duration of this therapy, the added immunomodulatory drug is often referred to as a glucocorticoid-sparing agent. In polymyalgia rheumatica and giant cell arteritis, anti-malarials, ciclosporin, azathioprine, and more frequently methotrexate have been tried as glucocorticoid-sparing agents; half of the six randomized trials on methotrexate support its use in this situation.[24–26]

Stress regimes

Patients on long-term glucocorticoid medication should be instructed to double their daily glucocorticoid dose, or increase the dose to at least 15 mg prednisolone daily or equivalent, if they develop fever attributed to infection, and to seek medical help. In case of major surgery, given the unreliable prediction of adrenal suppression, many physicians recommend 'stress doses' of glucocorticoids, even for patients with a low risk of adrenal suppression. However, the scheme of 100 mg of hydrocortisone intravenously just before surgery, followed by an additional 100 mg every 6 hours for 3 days, is based on anecdotal information and is not always necessary.[27] Although conclusive evidence is scarce, other regimes with lower doses are used.[27,28] These include infusion continuously of 100 mg of hydrocortisone intravenously the first day of surgery, followed by 25–50 mg of hydrocortisone every 8 hours for 2 or 3 days. Another option is to administer the usual dose of oral glucocorticoid orally (or the equivalent) parenterally on the day of surgery, followed by 25–50 mg of hydrocortisone every 8 hours for 2 or 3 days. In cases of minor surgery, it is probably sufficient to double the oral dose or to increase the dose to 15 mg of prednisolone or equivalent daily for 1–3 days.

Tapering

Because of their potential adverse effects, glucocorticoids usually are tapered as soon as the disease being treated is under control. Tapering must be done carefully to avoid disease flares, and cortisol deficiency. Gradual tapering permits recovery of adrenal function. There is no standard scheme for tapering; it depends on the individual's disease, the disease activity, doses and duration of therapy, and clinical response. In general the lower the dose, the smaller the taper steps and the longer the period between steps. To taper high-dose prednisone, decrements of 10–5 mg every 1–2 weeks can be used to 30 mg; then 2.5 mg/day decrements every 2–4 weeks until 15 mg/day; thereafter, tapering steps of 1 mg each month or 2.5 mg every 7 weeks.

Glucocorticoids during pregnancy and lactation

The fetus is protected from exogenous (i.e. maternal) glucocorticoids via two mechanisms. First, glucocorticoids bound to transport proteins cannot pass the placenta. Second, the enzyme 11β-HSD in the placenta catalyses the conversion of active cortisol, corticosterone, and prednisolone into their inactive 11-dehydro-prohormones. As a result of these mechanisms, the maternal-to-fetal prednisolone blood concentration ratio is about 10:1. In contrast, dexamethasone has little or no affinity for transport proteins and is poorly metabolized by 11β-HSD in the placenta; its maternal-to-fetal blood concentration ratio is about 1:1. So if a pregnant woman has to be treated with glucocorticoids, prednisone, prednisolone, and methylprednisolone would be good choices to protect the unborn child. If the unborn child has to be treated, e.g. to induce lung maturation in a fetus at risk of preterm delivery or to treat congenital heart block associated with maternal Sjögren's syndrome, fluorinated glucocorticoids, such as betamethasone or dexamethasone, are indicated. The fear of physical and neurocognitive adverse effects has not been substantiated in children exposed to antenatal repeat doses of 12 mg betamethasone,[29] in contrast to adverse effects of early postnatal glucocorticoid exposure.[30] However, because of a small but increased risk of an oral cleft, it is advised to avoid high doses in the first trimester of pregnancy[31]; low to moderate doses of prednisone seem to be safe.[32]

Prednisolone and prednisone are excreted in small quantities in breast milk, but breastfeeding is generally considered safe for an infant whose mother on these drugs. Because curves of milk and serum concentrations for prednisolone are virtually parallel in time, the exposure of the infant seems minimized if breastfeeding is avoided during the first 4 hours after prednisolone dosing.[32]

Adverse effects and events

Often patents and physicians do not fully realize that the adverse effect spectrum of high-dose glucocorticoids differs from that of low-dose glucocorticoids.[33] This likely decreases adherence to treatment. In an investigation into patients' and physicians' perspectives on glucocorticoid therapy, osteoporosis, diabetes, and cardiovascular disease were ranked both by patients and rheumatologists within the top five of most worrisome adverse events; however, rheumatologists showed more concern about infections.[34]

There is lack of robust data on incidence of adverse effects of glucocorticoids; most data are derived from observational studies, which tend to overestimate adverse effects. First, in these studies there is bias by indication, i.e. that patients with the more severe disease are more frequently prescribed glucocorticoids. In these patients the risk of adverse effects is higher, based on their higher disease activity and their often more frequent comorbidities. Second, not all negative events are adverse effects of glucocorticoids; they could be manifestations of the disease,[35] and several negative effects on bone mass, lipids, endothelium, glucose metabolism, and infection risk are associated both with the disease treated and with glucocorticoids, especially at medium and high doses.[36–39] The adverse effects, at least of low-dose chronic glucocorticoid therapy, seem to be mild[33]; in fact glucocorticoid in lower doses, by inhibiting the inflammatory process, might counteract the negative effects of the disease mentioned above.

Infections

Epidemiological studies show that treatment with a daily dose of less than 10 mg of prednisone or equivalent leads to only a slightly increased risk of infection. An explanation might be that higher disease activity—adjusted for demographics, medications, and clinical factors—is associated with a higher risk of infections,[36] and that by lowering disease activity, the effect of the low-dose glucocorticoid on infection risk could be neutral. However, at doses of 20–40 mg daily, an increased infection risk is found (relative risk 1.3 to 3.6).[40] This risk increases with higher doses and longer duration of treatment.[41]

Glucocorticoid-treated patients with RA undergoing hand and wrist surgery while continuing this therapy appear to have no increased risk of wound infection or disturbed wound healing.[42]

Gastrointestinal adverse effects

Data from literature on the risk of peptic ulcer associated with oral glucocorticoids are inconclusive. The inhibition by glucocorticoids of the production of COX-2 without hampering the production of COX-1 is in line with studies that found no increased risk. In other studies, a relative risk of serious upper gastrointestinal peptic complications of about 2 was found.[43] When glucocorticoids are used in combination with NSAIDs, the relative risk of peptic ulcer disease and associated complications is estimated at about 4,[44] although this risk has been questioned.[45] Inflammatory disease and higher age are also risk factors for peptic ulcer disease.

Although glucocorticoids are usually listed as one of the many potential causes of pancreatitis, evidence for such an association is weak and difficult to separate from the underlying disease, such as vasculitis or SLE.[46] The risk of asymptomatic or symptomatic colonization of the upper gastrointestinal tract with *Candida albicans* is increased in patients treated with inhalation glucocorticoids and in those on systemic glucocorticoids, especially if combination immunosuppressive therapy is applied.[47]

Negative effects on bone
Osteoporosis

Fractures, especially of vertebral bodies, ribs, hips, and wrists, occur in 30–50% of patients on long-term glucocorticoid therapy. Many of the vertebral fractures are asymptomatic. Glucocorticoid-induced vertebral fractures occur at a higher bone mineral density (BMD) compared to postmenopausal vertebral fractures: BMD underestimates the risk of glucocorticoid-induced fractures. A negative effect of glucocorticoids also on bone structure seems important.[48] The topic of osteoporosis is comprehensively discussed in Chapter 142.

Osteonecrosis

Osteonecrosis has been attributed to fat emboli, microvascular obstruction of the blood vessels of the femoral head by marrow fat or oedema, and defective mending of stress fractures, depending on underlying diseases and risk factors. The mechanism of glucocorticoid-associated osteonecrosis may be osteocyte apoptosis as many apoptotic osteocytes were identified in femoral heads obtained at total hip replacement for glucocorticoid-associated osteonecrosis, which were absent in femoral heads with traumatic or sickle-cell osteonecrosis.[48]

Glucocorticoid-induced myopathy

Weakness in proximal muscles, especially of the lower extremities, may indicate glucocorticoid-induced myopathy. It is often suspected, but infrequently found; it occurs almost exclusively in patients treated with high doses (>30 mg/day prednisone or equivalent). Diagnosis is clinical and can be confirmed by a muscle biopsy specimen that reveals atrophy of type II fibres and lack of inflammation; there is no elevation of serum muscle enzymes. Treatment is withdrawal of the glucocorticoid if possible.

Metabolic and cardiovascular adverse effects and events

The risk of adverse cardiovascular events is twice as high in patients with RA as it is in the general population, similar to that in patients with type 2 diabetes mellitus.[49] This increased risk is probably caused by negative effects of chronic inflammation; by effects of treatment on conventional risk factors such as hypertension (secondary to use of NSAIDs, ciclosporin, and leflunomide), lipids, obesity, and glucose metabolism[50]; and by specific and unknown RA-related mechanisms. Consequently, guidelines published in 2010 recommend that a multiplication factor of 1.5 should be applied to cardiovascular risk scores for patients with severe or longstanding RA.[51] Increased cardiovascular risk has also been found in other inflammatory rheumatic diseases such as SLE and ankylosing spondylitis.[51] However, negative effects on conventional risk factors seem not to be adverse effects of low-dose glucocorticoids. Furthermore, atherosclerosis itself has been recognized as an inflammatory disease of arterial walls, for which glucocorticoids may be beneficial; glucocorticoids have been found to inhibit macrophage accumulation in injured arterial wall in vitro, possibly resulting in attenuation of the local inflammatory response.[52]

Glucose intolerance and type 2 diabetes mellitus

Glucocorticoids increase hepatic glucose production, induce insulin resistance, and probably also have a direct effect on the beta cells of the pancreas, resulting in enhanced insulin secretion. It may take only a few weeks before glucocorticoid-induced hyperglycaemia occurs on medium glucocorticoid doses, but in pulse therapy this effect is present within hours. In previously non-diabetic subjects, an odds ratio of 1.8 for the need to initiate antihyperglycaemic drugs during glucocorticoid therapy in doses of 10 mg or more of prednisone or equivalent per day was seen; the odds ratio was 3 for 10–20 mg, 5.8 for 20–30 mg, and 10.3 for 30 mg or more of prednisone or equivalent per day.[53] It is likely that the risk is higher in patients with other risk factors for diabetes mellitus, such as a family history of the disease, advanced age, obesity, and previous gestational diabetes. Controlling inflammation by disease-modifying anti-rheumatic drugs (DMARDs) including low-dose chronic glucocorticoid therapy may improve insulin sensitivity and subsequently reduce the risk of developing type 2 diabetes in RA patients.[37] Worsening of glucose control in patients with established diabetes mellitus is to be expected on medium to high glucocorticoid doses. Usually, glucocorticoid-induced diabetes is reversible when the drug is discontinued, unless there was pre-existing glucose intolerance.

Body fat and body weight

One of the most notable effects of long-term endogenous or exogenous glucocorticoid excess is the gain in total body and trunk fat.[54] Increased appetite occurs during glucocorticoid therapy leading to higher body weight; also, patients with active inflammatory diseases tend to lose weight, which is prevented with disease control by drugs, including glucocorticoids.[54a] A centripetal fat accumulation with thin extremities with atrophic skin and bruising is a characteristic feature of patients exposed to long-term high-dose glucocorticoids. Potential mechanisms include increased conversion of cortisone to cortisol in visceral adipocytes, hyperinsulinaemia, and a change in expression and activity of adipocyte-derived hormones and cytokines, such as leptin and TNF.[55] Protein loss resulting in muscle atrophy may also contribute to the change in body appearance, although protein loss or redistribution of fat is not always found.[54] Trials in patients with RA on low-dose glucocorticoids for a prolonged period showed only minor effects in fat distribution and body weight.[56,57]

Atherosclerosis and lipids

The effects on lipids and other cardiovascular risk factors of low-dose glucocorticoids in inflammatory diseases probably are different from those of medium and high doses,[50] or those of glucocorticoid therapy in non-inflammatory diseases. Low-dose glucocorticoids might improve dyslipidaemia associated with inflammatory disease[51,58]; in patients with RA using a glucocorticoid, a more favourable atherogenic index was found compared to that of patients without glucocorticoid therapy.[39] The interplay of disease activity, glucocorticoids, and adverse effects makes it difficult to judge the net adverse effects of glucocorticoids on cardiovascular risk and lipids.[59]

Hypertension and other mineralocorticoid effects

Cortisol in particular also has mineralocorticoid actions (Table 79.1), including reduced excretion of sodium and water and increased excretion of calcium and potassium, leading to hypokalaemia, especially when administered concomitantly with amphotericin B or potassium-depleting diuretics. Frequent clinical signs are oedema, weight gain, and increased blood pressure. However, low doses of synthetic glucocorticoids are not a cause of hypertension, in contrast to higher doses.[60] No formal studies addressing the effects of glucocorticoids in previously hypertensive patients have been performed. Glucocorticoids exerted no negative effects on myocarditis and idiopathic cardiomyopathy.[61,62]

Adverse effects on the eye

Cataract

Glucocorticoids stimulate the formation of especially posterior subcapsular cataract,[63] but the risk of cortical cataract is also increased, with an odds ratio of 2.6.[64] The likelihood and severity of this adverse effect depend on dose and duration of treatment. In patients treated with prednisone at a dose of 15 mg or more daily for at least 1 year, cataract is observed frequently, but cataract may also develop with long-term, low-dose therapy.[65] These cataracts are usually bilateral and progress slowly.

Glaucoma

Glucocorticoids may cause or aggravate glaucoma, especially in patients with a family history of open-angle glaucoma and patients receiving high doses; checks of intraocular pressure are then warranted. If intraocular pressure is found to be increased, patients need to be treated with medications that reduce pressure, often for a prolonged period after stopping the glucocorticoid.[66] Topical application of a glucocorticoid in the eye has a more pronounced effect on intraocular pressure than does systemic therapy.[67]

Adverse effects on skin and hair

Clinically relevant adverse effects of high-dose and long-term glucocorticoids on skin include cushingoid appearance, easy bruising, ecchymoses, skin atrophy, striae, disturbed wound healing, acne, perioral dermatitis, hyperpigmentation, facial redness, mild hirsutism, and thinning of scalp hair. The physician often considers these changes to be of minor clinical importance, but they may be disturbing to the patient.[68] No reliable data on the exact frequency of these adverse effects are available, but they are dependent on duration of therapy and dose.[65]

Psychological adverse effects

Glucocorticoid treatment is associated with a variety of behavioural symptoms.[69] Although most attention is drawn toward infrequent overt psychiatric disturbances, e.g. depression and mania, less florid psychological manifestations more frequently occur, which may cause distress to patients.[68] These include depressed or elated mood (euphoria), insomnia, irritability, emotional instability, anxiety, memory failure, and other cognition impairments; they may also occur on withdrawal of glucocorticoids. The exact incidence is unknown and probably dependent on dose. A history of psychiatric illness does not predict occurrence, nor do previous glucocorticoid-induced psychiatric disturbances or previous treatment(s) free of such disturbances.[69]

Prophylactic measures and monitoring

Some prophylactic measures during glucocorticoid therapy are evidence based. If comedication with an NSAID is needed, consider cotreatment with a proton pump inhibitor or misoprostol, and/or prescribe a COX-1 sparing NSAID,[33] dependent on the individual patient's risk of peptic ulcer and cardiovascular disease. Adequate use of calcium, vitamin D, and bisphosphonates according to national or international guidelines minimizes the risk of osteoporosis.

Recommendations have been formulated on the management of systemic glucocorticoid therapy in rheumatic diseases (Table 79.3),[70] as well on monitoring of patients receiving low-dose glucocorticoid therapy.[34] Overall, additions to standard monitoring of patients with an inflammatory disease should include screening for osteoporosis, and pretreatment assessments of fasting blood glucose levels, risk factors for glaucoma, and a check for ankle oedema.[34] For patients receiving medium or high doses of glucocorticoids monitoring should be intensified, but specific guidelines for use of these doses do not yet exist. In future clinical trials of glucocorticoid-based therapies for RA, comprehensive monitoring and reporting of treatment-related adverse effects is advised, to obtain more reliable data on the spectrum, incidence, and severity of adverse effects.[34]

New developments

Increased knowledge about modes of action of glucocorticoids and pathophysiological backgrounds of rheumatic diseases creates opportunities for new developments to optimize the effects

Table 79.3 The 10 EULAR recommendations on systemic glucocorticoid therapy in rheumatic diseases[70]

1a	The adverse effects of glucocorticoid therapy should be considered and discussed with the patient before glucocorticoid therapy is started
1b	This advice should be reinforced by giving information regarding glucocorticoid management
1c	If glucocorticoids are to be used for a more prolonged period of time, a 'glucocorticoid card' should be issued to every patient, with the date of commencement of treatment, the initial dosage, and the subsequent reductions and maintenance regimens
2a	Initial dose, dose reduction, and long-term dosing depend on the underlying rheumatic disease, disease activity, risk factors, and individual responsiveness of the patient
2b	Timing may be important, with respect to the circadian rhythm of both the disease and the natural secretion of glucocorticoids
3	When it is decided to start glucocorticoid treatment, comorbidities and risk factors for adverse effects should be evaluated and treated where indicated. These include hypertension, diabetes, peptic ulcer, recent fractures, presence of cataract or glaucoma, presence of (chronic) infections, dyslipidaemia, and comedication with NSAIDs
4	For prolonged treatment, the glucocorticoid dosage should be kept to a minimum and a glucocorticoid taper should be attempted in case of remission or low disease activity. The reasons to continue glucocorticoid therapy should be regularly checked
5	During treatment, patients should be monitored for body weight, blood pressure, peripheral oedema, cardiac insufficiency, serum lipids, blood and/or urine glucose and ocular pressure depending on individual patient's risk, glucocorticoid dose, and duration
6a	If a patient is started on prednisone >7.5 mg daily and continues on prednisone for more than 3 months, calcium and vitamin D supplementation should be prescribed
6b	Antiresorptive therapy with bisphosphonates to reduce the risk of glucocorticoid-induced osteoporosis should be based on risk factors, including BMD measurement
7	Patients treated with glucocorticoids and concomitant NSAIDs should be given appropriate gastroprotective medication, such as proton pump inhibitors or misoprostol, or alternatively could switch to a COX-2 selective inhibitor
8	All patients on glucocorticoid therapy for longer than 1 month, who will undergo surgery, need perioperative management with adequate glucocorticoid replacement to overcome potential adrenal insufficiency
9	Glucocorticoids during pregnancy have no additional risk for mother and child
10	Children receiving glucocorticoids should be checked regularly for linear growth and considered for growth hormone replacement in case of growth impairment

BMD, bone mineral density; COX, cyclooxygenase; NSAID, non-steroidal anti-inflammatory drug.

and to decrease adverse effects of these agents.[71] For instance, a modified-release prednisone tablet is now available. When taken in the evening, the delayed prednisone release mimics the natural circadian rhythm of cortisol and effectively targets the nocturnal release of proinflammatory cytokines, especially IL-6. This results in more reduction of morning stiffness in RA compared to taking prednisone early in the morning.[72] Further research is needed and is under way.[73] Combining glucocorticoids with agents that selectively amplify their anti-inflammatory activity, e.g. the platelet-activation blocking agent dipyridamole, could improve the risk–benefit ratio by reducing the effective dose.[74] Another such compound under development is nitric oxide.[75] Glucocorticoid-containing liposomes, which accumulate at sites of inflammation, enabling less-frequent dosing, are also being studied.[76] Selective glucocorticoid receptor agonists causing less DNA transactivation than conventional glucocorticoids could be associated with fewer metabolic and endocrine adverse effects.[77]

Conclusion

◆ Glucocorticoids are still the most effective, broadly applicable and cheapest immunosuppressive drugs.

◆ The risk of adverse effects of a glucocorticoid is patient, dose, and time dependent and is generally overestimated.

◆ Glucocorticoids have disease-modifying properties in early RA.

◆ For low-dose glucocorticoid therapy, monitoring as part of good clinical care in rheumatic patients in daily practice needs only to be extended with screening for osteoporosis, and pretreatment assessments of fasting blood glucose levels, risk factors for glaucoma, and a check for ankle oedema.

References

1. Buttgereit F, da Silva JA, Boers M et al. Standardised nomenclature for glucocorticoid dosages and glucocorticoid treatment regimens: current questions and tentative answers in rheumatology. *Ann Rheum Dis* 2002;61:718–722.
2. Barnes PJ, Adcock IM. Glucocorticoid resistance in inflammatory diseases. *Lancet* 2009;373:1905–1917.
3. Carrie F, Roblot P, Bouquet S et al. Rifampin-induced nonresponsiveness of giant cell arteritis to prednisone treatment. *Arch Intern Med* 1994;154:1521–1524.
4. Varis T, Kivisto KT, Neuvonen PJ. Grapefruit juice can increase the plasma concentrations of oral methylprednisolone. *Eur J Clin Pharmacol* 2000;56:489–493.
5. Bornstein SR. Predisposing factors for adrenal insufficiency. *N Engl J Med* 2009;360:2328–2339.
6. Ristimaki A, Narko K, Hla T. Down-regulation of cytokine-induced cyclo-oxygenase-2 transcript isoforms by dexamethasone: evidence for post-transcriptional regulation. *Biochem J* 1996;318 (Pt 1):325–331.
7. Harr MW, Rong Y, Bootman MD, Roderick HL, Distelhorst CW. Glucocorticoid-mediated inhibition of Lck modulates the pattern of T cell receptor-induced calcium signals by down-regulating inositol 1,4,5-trisphosphate receptors. *J Biol Chem* 2009;284:31860–31871.
8. Buttgereit F, Wehling M, Burmester GR. A new hypothesis of modular glucocorticoid actions: steroid treatment of rheumatic diseases revisited. *Arthritis Rheum* 1998;41:761–767.
9. Sternberg EM. Neural regulation of innate immunity: a coordinated nonspecific host response to pathogens. *Nat Rev Immunol* 2006;6:318–328.
10. DiBattista JA, Martel-Pelletier J, Wosu LO et al. Glucocorticoid receptor mediated inhibition of interleukin-1 stimulated neutral metallopro-

tease synthesis in normal human chondrocytes. *J Clin Endocrinol Metab* 1991;72:316–326.
11. De Nijs RN. Glucocorticoid-induced osteoporosis: a review on pathophysiology and treatment options. *Minerva Med* 2008;99:23–43.
12. Moreland LW, Curtis JR. Systemic nonarticular manifestations of rheumatoid arthritis: focus on inflammatory mechanisms. *Semin Arthritis Rheum* 2009;39:132–143.
13. Haugeberg G, Strand A, Kvien TK, Kirwan JR. Reduced loss of hand bone density with prednisolone in early rheumatoid arthritis: results from a randomized placebo-controlled trial. *Arch Intern Med* 2005;165:1293–1297.
14. Sokka T, Toloza S, Cutolo M et al. Women, men, and rheumatoid arthritis: analyses of disease activity, disease characteristics, and treatments in the QUEST-RA study. *Arthritis Res Ther* 2009;11:R7.
15. Kirwan JR, Bijlsma JW, Boers M, Shea BJ. Effects of glucocorticoids on radiological progression in rheumatoid arthritis. *Cochrane Database Syst Rev* 2007;CD006356.
15a. Bakker MF, Jacobs JW, Welsing PM et al. Low-dose prednisone inclusion in a methotrexate-based, tight control strategy for early rheumatoid arthritis. A randomized trial. *Ann Intern Med* 2012;156:329–339.
16. Landewé RB, Boers M, Verhoeven AC et al. COBRA combination therapy in patients with early rheumatoid arthritis: long-term structural benefits of a brief intervention. *Arthritis Rheum* 2002;46:347–356.
17. Jacobs JW, Van Everdingen AA, Verstappen SM, Bijlsma JW. Followup radiographic data on patients with rheumatoid arthritis who participated in a two-year trial of prednisone therapy or placebo. *Arthritis Rheum* 2006;54:1422–1428.
18. Janssens HJ, Janssen M, van de Lisdonk EH, van Riel PL, van WC. Use of oral prednisolone or naproxen for the treatment of gout arthritis: a double-blind, randomised equivalence trial. *Lancet* 2008;371:1854–1860.
19. Jarrett MP, Grayzel AI. Simultaneous gout, pseudogout, and septic arthritis. *Arthritis Rheum* 1980;23:128–129.
20. Jacobs JW, Geenen R, Evers AW et al. Short term effects of corticosteroid pulse treatment on disease activity and the wellbeing of patients with active rheumatoid arthritis. *Ann Rheum Dis* 2001;60:61–64.
21. Weusten BL, Jacobs JW, Bijlsma JW. Corticosteroid pulse therapy in active rheumatoid arthritis. *Semin Arthritis Rheum* 1993;23:183–192.
22. Hunder GG, Sheps SG, Allen GL, Joyce JW. Daily and alternate-day corticosteroid regimens in treatment of giant cell arteritis: comparison in a prospective study. *Ann Intern Med* 1975;82:613–618.
23. Avioli LV. Glucocorticoid effects on statural growth. *Br J Rheumatol* 1993;32 Suppl 2:27–30.
24. Ferraccioli G, Salaffi F, De Vita S, Casatta L, Bartoli E. Methotrexate in polymyalgia rheumatica: preliminary results of an open, randomized study. *J Rheumatol* 1996;23:624–628.
25. Jover JA, Hernandez-Garcia C, Morado IC et al. Combined treatment of giant-cell arteritis with methotrexate and prednisone. a randomized, double-blind, placebo-controlled trial. *Ann Intern Med* 2001;134:106–114.
26. Caporali R, Cimmino MA, Ferraccioli G et al. Prednisone plus methotrexate for polymyalgia rheumatica: a randomized, double-blind, placebo-controlled trial. *Ann Intern Med* 2004;141:493–500.
27. Marik PE, Varon J. Requirement of perioperative stress doses of corticosteroids: a systematic review of the literature. *Arch Surg* 2008;143:1222–1226.
28. Salem M, Tainsh RE, Jr., Bromberg J, Loriaux DL, Chernow B. Perioperative glucocorticoid coverage. A reassessment 42 years after emergence of a problem. *Ann Surg* 1994;219:416–425.
29. Wapner RJ, Sorokin Y, Mele L et al. Long-term outcomes after repeat doses of antenatal corticosteroids. *N Engl J Med* 2007;357:1190–1198.
30. Yeh TF, Lin YJ, Lin HC et al. Outcomes at school age after postnatal dexamethasone therapy for lung disease of prematurity. *N Engl J Med* 2004;350:1304–1313.

31. Park-Wyllie L, Mazzotta P, Pastuszak A et al. Birth defects after maternal exposure to corticosteroids: prospective cohort study and meta-analysis of epidemiological studies. *Teratology* 2000;62:385–392.

32. Temprano KK, Bandlamudi R, Moore TL. Antirheumatic drugs in pregnancy and lactation. *Semin Arthritis Rheum* 2005;35:112–121.

33. da Silva JAP, Jacobs JWG, Kirwan JR et al. Safety of low dose glucocorticoid treatment in rheumatoid arthritis: published evidence and prospective trial data. *Ann Rheum Dis* 2006;65:285–293.

34. van der Goes MC, Jacobs JWG, Boers M et al. Monitoring adverse events of low-dose glucocorticoids therapy: EULAR recommendations for clinical trials and daily practice. *Ann Rheum Dis* 2010;69:1913–1919.

35. Hoes JN, Jacobs JW, Verstappen SM, Bijlsma JW, van der Heijden GJ. Adverse events of low-to-medium-dose oral glucocorticoids in inflammatory diseases: a meta-analysis. *Ann Rheum Dis* 2009;68:1833–1838.

36. Au K, Reed G, Curtis JR et al. Extended report: high disease activity is associated with an increased risk of infection in patients with rheumatoid arthritis. *Ann Rheum Dis* 2011;70:785–791.

37. Wasko MC, Kay J, Hsia EC, Rahman MU. Diabetes mellitus and insulin resistance in patients with rheumatoid arthritis: risk reduction in a chronic inflammatory disease. *Arthritis Care Res (Hoboken)* 2011;63:512–521.

38. Klarenbeek NB, van der Kooij SM, Huizinga TJ et al. Blood pressure changes in patients with recent-onset rheumatoid arthritis treated with four different treatment strategies: a post hoc analysis from the BeSt trial. *Ann Rheum Dis* 2010;69:1342–1345.

39. Peters MJ, Vis M, van Halm VP et al. Changes in lipid profile during infliximab and corticosteroid treatment in rheumatoid arthritis. *Ann Rheum Dis* 2007;66:958–961.

40. Stuck AE, Minder CE, Frey FJ. Risk of infectious complications in patients taking glucocorticosteroids. *Rev Infect Dis* 1989;11:954–963.

41. Wolfe F, Caplan L, Michaud K. Treatment for rheumatoid arthritis and the risk of hospitalization for pneumonia: associations with prednisone, disease-modifying antirheumatic drugs, and anti-tumor necrosis factor therapy. *Arthritis Rheum* 2006;54:628–634.

42. Jain A, Witbreuk M, Ball C, Nanchahal J. Influence of steroids and methotrexate on wound complications after elective rheumatoid hand and wrist surgery. *J Hand Surg Am* 2002;27:449–455.

43. Garcia Rodriguez LA, Hernandez-Diaz S. The risk of upper gastrointestinal complications associated with nonsteroidal anti-inflammatory drugs, glucocorticoids, acetaminophen, and combinations of these agents. *Arthritis Res* 2001;3:98–101.

44. Piper JM, Ray WA, Daugherty JR, Griffin MR. Corticosteroid use and peptic ulcer disease: role of nonsteroidal anti-inflammatory drugs. *Ann Intern Med* 1991;114:735–740.

45. Filaretova L, Podvigina T, Bagaeva T, Bobryshev P, Takeuchi K. Gastroprotective role of glucocorticoid hormones. *J Pharmacol Sci* 2007;104:195–201.

46. Saab S, Corr MP, Weisman MH. Corticosteroids and systemic lupus erythematosus pancreatitis: a case series. *J Rheumatol* 1998;25:801–806.

47. Gupta KL, Ghosh AK, Kochhar R et al. Esophageal candidiasis after renal transplantation: comparative study in patients on different immunosuppressive protocols. *Am J Gastroenterol* 1994;89:1062–1065.

48. Weinstein RS. Glucocorticoids, osteocytes, and skeletal fragility: the role of bone vascularity. *Bone* 2010;46:564–570.

49. Peters MJ, van Halm VP, Voskuyl AE et al. Does rheumatoid arthritis equal diabetes mellitus as an independent risk factor for cardiovascular disease? A prospective study. *Arthritis Rheum* 2009;61:1571–1579.

50. Wei L, MacDonald TM, Walker BR. Taking glucocorticoids by prescription is associated with subsequent cardiovascular disease. *Ann Intern Med* 2004;141:764–770.

51. Peters MJ, Symmons DP, McCarey D et al. EULAR evidence-based recommendations for cardiovascular risk management in patients with rheumatoid arthritis and other forms of inflammatory arthritis. *Ann Rheum Dis* 2010;69:325–331.

52. Poon M, Gertz SD, Fallon JT et al. Dexamethasone inhibits macrophage accumulation after balloon arterial injury in cholesterol fed rabbits. *Atherosclerosis* 2001;155:371–380.

53. Gurwitz JH, Bohn RL, Glynn RJ et al. Glucocorticoids and the risk for initiation of hypoglycemic therapy. *Arch Intern Med* 1994;154:97–101.

54. Nordborg E, Schaufelberger C, Bosaeus I. The effect of glucocorticoids on fat and lean tissue masses in giant cell arteritis. *Scand J Rheumatol* 1998;27:106–111.

54a. Jurgens MS, Jacobs JWG, Geenen R et al. Increase of body mass index in a tight controlled methotrexate-based strategy with prednisone in early rheumatoid arthritis: side effect of the prednisone or better control of disease activity? *Arthritis Care Res* 2013; 65: 88–93.

55. Stewart PM, Tomlinson JW. Cortisol, 11 beta-hydroxysteroid dehydrogenase type 1 and central obesity. *Trends Endocrinol Metab* 2002;13:94–96.

56. Van Everdingen AA, Jacobs JW, Siewertsz Van Reesema DR, Bijlsma JW. Low-dose prednisone therapy for patients with early active rheumatoid arthritis: clinical efficacy, disease-modifying properties, and side effects: a randomized, double-blind, placebo-controlled clinical trial. *Ann Intern Med* 2002;136:1–12.

57. Wassenberg S, Rau R, Steinfeld P, Zeidler H. Very low-dose prednisolone in early rheumatoid arthritis retards radiographic progression over two years: A multicenter, double-blind, placebo-controlled trial. *Arthritis Rheum* 2005;52:3371–3380.

58. Garcia-Gomez C, Nolla JM, Valverde J et al. High HDL-cholesterol in women with rheumatoid arthritis on low-dose glucocorticoid therapy. *Eur J Clin Invest* 2008;38:686–692.

59. Davis JM, III, Maradit-Kremers H, Gabriel SE. Use of low-dose glucocorticoids and the risk of cardiovascular morbidity and mortality in rheumatoid arthritis: what is the true direction of effect? *J Rheumatol* 2005;32:1856–1862.

60. Panoulas VF, Douglas KM, Stavropoulos-Kalinoglou A et al. Long-term exposure to medium-dose glucocorticoid therapy associates with hypertension in patients with rheumatoid arthritis. *Rheumatology* (Oxford) 2008;47:72–75.

61. Mason JW, O'Connell JB, Herskowitz A et al. A clinical trial of immunosuppressive therapy for myocarditis. The Myocarditis Treatment Trial Investigators. *N Engl J Med* 1995;333:269–275.

62. Latham RD, Mulrow JP, Virmani R, Robinowitz M, Moody JM. Recently diagnosed idiopathic dilated cardiomyopathy: incidence of myocarditis and efficacy of prednisone therapy. *Am Heart J* 1989;117:876–882.

63. Carnahan MC, Goldstein DA. Ocular complications of topical, peri-ocular, and systemic corticosteroids. *Curr Opin Ophthalmol* 2000;11:478–483.

64. Klein BE, Klein R, Lee KE, Danforth LG. Drug use and five-year incidence of age-related cataracts: The Beaver Dam Eye Study. *Ophthalmology* 2001;108:1670–1674.

65. Huscher D, Thiele K, Gromnica-Ihle E et al. Dose-related patterns of glucocorticoid-induced side effects. *Ann Rheum Dis* 2009;68:1119–1124.

66. Garbe E, LeLorier J, Boivin JF, Suissa S. Risk of ocular hypertension or open-angle glaucoma in elderly patients on oral glucocorticoids. *Lancet* 1997;350:979–982.

67. Tripathi RC, Parapuram SK, Tripathi BJ, Zhong Y, Chalam KV. Corticosteroids and glaucoma risk. *Drugs Aging* 1999;15:439–450.

68. van der Goes MC, Jacobs JW, Boers M et al. Patient and rheumatologist perspectives on glucocorticoids: an exercise to improve the implementation of the European League Against Rheumatism (EULAR) recommendations on the management of systemic glucocorticoid therapy in rheumatic diseases. *Ann Rheum Dis* 2010;69:1015–1021.

69. Warrington TP, Bostwick JM. Psychiatric adverse effects of corticosteroids. *Mayo Clin Proc* 2006;81:1361–1367.

70. Hoes JN, Jacobs JW, Boers M et al. EULAR evidence-based recommendations on the management of systemic glucocorticoid therapy in rheumatic diseases. *Ann Rheum Dis* 2007;66:1560–1567.

71. Buttgereit F, Burmester GR, Straub RH, Seibel MJ, Zhou H. Exogenous and endogenous glucocorticoids in rheumatic diseases. *Arthritis Rheum* 2011;63:1–9.

72. Buttgereit F, Doering G, Schaeffler A et al. Efficacy of modified-release versus standard prednisone to reduce duration of morning stiffness of the joints in rheumatoid arthritis (CAPRA-1): a double-blind, randomised controlled trial. *Lancet* 2008;371:205–214.

73. Bijlsma JW, Jacobs JW. Glucocorticoid chronotherapy in rheumatoid arthritis. *Lancet* 2008;371:183–184.

74. Jacobs JW, Bijlsma JW. Innovative combination strategy to enhance effect and diminish adverse effects of glucocorticoids: another promise? *Arthritis Res Ther* 2009;11:105.

75. Baraldi PG, Romagnoli R, Del Carmen NM et al. Synthesis of nitro esters of prednisolone, new compounds combining pharmacological properties of both glucocorticoids and nitric oxide. *J Med Chem* 2004;47:711–719.

76. Hofkens W, Grevers LC, Walgreen B et al. Intravenously delivered glucocorticoid liposomes inhibit osteoclast activity and bone erosion in murine antigen-induced arthritis. *J Control Release* 2011;152:363–369.

77. Schacke H, Berger M, Rehwinkel H, Asadullah K. Selective glucocorticoid receptor agonists (SEGRAs): novel ligands with an improved therapeutic index. *Mol Cell Endocrinol* 2007;275:109–117.

78. Rhen T, Cidlowski JA. Antiinflammatory action of glucocorticoids—new mechanisms for old drugs. *N Engl J Med* 2005;353: 1711–1723.

79. Cronstein BN, Kimmel SC, Levin RI, Martiniuk F, Weissmann G. A mechanism for the antiinflammatory effects of corticosteroids: the glucocorticoid receptor regulates leukocyte adhesion to endothelial cells and expression of endothelial-leukocyte adhesion molecule 1 and intercellular adhesion molecule 1. *Proc Natl Acad Sci U S A* 1992;89:9991–9995.

CHAPTER 80

Immunosuppressants

Joanna Ledingham and Sarah Westlake

Methotrexate

Methotrexate (MTX) is used with therapeutic benefit, to treat a wide range of rheumatological disorders. In the United Kingdom its only rheumatic licence is for rheumatoid arthritis (RA).[1]

The use of MTX progressively rose during the 1980s and it is now considered the gold standard DMARD.[2] It also has efficacy in other inflammatory arthritides, connective tissue diseases (CTDs), and vasculitides.[2–4]

Pharmacology

MTX is a structural analogue of folic acid. Its exact mechanism of action is unknown. In high doses, used to treat malignancy, it inhibits DNA synthesis by inhibiting the reduction of dihydrofolate to tetrahydrofolate. In lower rheumatological doses it probably acts on multiple pathways including cytokine production, adenosine and arachidonic acid metabolism, and cell apoptosis.

For rheumatic diseases doses of 7.5–30 mg once weekly (licensed dose up to 25 mg) are used. MTX can be given orally, intramuscularly, or subcutaneously. At higher doses (>17.5 mg), parenteral absorption and bioavailability may be better than oral. The onset of action is usually 6–12 weeks.

Toxicity

MTX is contraindicated in pregnancy and breastfeeding. It should be stopped, in men and women, 3 months prior to conception. Effective contraception is essential for all couples with a woman of childbearing age.

MTX should not be started in patients with current sepsis or bone marrow failure.

Important MTX drug interactions are with other folate inhibitors, particularly trimethoprim and septrin; these should not be used with MTX. Theoretically, non-steroidal anti-inflammatory drugs (NSAIDs) may interact with MTX by impairing renal function, thereby reducing renal excretion and leading to haematological toxicity; in practice, with appropriate monitoring, this combination is safe and effective. MTX dose reduction should be considered in patients with renal impairment.

Rheumatological MTX doses are usually well tolerated. Most adverse effects are mild and do not require discontinuation. Some deaths have, however, been reported.

Nausea and oral ulceration are the most common adverse events(1–10%). These usually respond to symptomatic treatment. Coprescription of folic acid reduces their incidence. Parenteral administration may reduce gastrointestinal side effects.

Elevated liver function tests (LFTs) occur in approximately 10% of patients; most changes are mild, sporadic, and not linked to the rarer complication of cirrhosis. Risk factors for hepatotoxicity are as for non-MTX-linked liver disease (increasing age, obesity, heavy alcohol consumption, and diabetes) and should be minimized wherever possible. Persistently raised LFTs (>3× upper limit of normal) despite MTX dose reduction/discontinuation requires further investigation.

Cirrhotic complications are very rare (0.01%), more common with psoriatic arthritis (PsA) and can occur despite normal LFTs and hepatic imaging. Routine liver biopsy or serum procollagen III monitoring is not currently recommended in the United Kingdom.

Pulmonary complications are uncommon (0.1–1%) but potentially fatal pneumonitis, an idiosyncratic hypersensitivity reaction, is well recognized.[5] Symptoms (breathlessness and dry cough typically developing over several days) usually develop early in treatment (most within 1 year). Prompt recognition, discontinuation of MTX and investigation (high-resolution CT and possibly biopsy) is recommended. High-dose oral or intravenous steroids may hasten recovery and rechallenge is not recommended. Underlying lung disease has been linked with pneumonitis mortality so MTX should be used with caution in patients with established lung disease. Routine chest radiography (CXR) or pulmonary function test monitoring is not helpful.

Infections, including opportunistic infections such as disseminated herpes zoster, are common with MTX. Other factors (e.g. chronic disease, steroids, diabetes) contribute to this risk. Patients and clinicians should be vigilant for infection. MTX can be continued during minor infections but should be stopped with severe or opportunistic infections requiring antibiotics.

Leucopenia, thrombocytopenia, and anaemia are uncommon with MTX (0.1–1%). Most episodes respond to temporary dose reduction or MTX cessation. Severe pancytopenia is uncommon but is linked with renal impairment, hypoalbuminaemia, accidental overdose, and coprescription of other anti-folate drugs.[6] Fatal cases are reported. Severe leucopenia requires MTX cessation and may respond to folinic acid rescue.[7] Macrocytosis commonly occurs but does not require MTX withdrawal.

Rheumatoid nodules can develop or increase with MTX and regress with MTX dose reduction or cessation.[8]

There is no conclusive evidence for an increased risk of malignancy with MTX.[9,10]

Other information

MTX-treated patients should not receive live vaccines. Pneumovax and annual flu vaccination are recommended. Varicella zoster immune globulin (VZIG) can be considered for patients exposed to chickenpox or shingles.[7]

MTX may be associated with a decreased risk of cardiovascular disease in RA patients.[11]

Sulphasalazine

Sulphasalazine (SSP) has been used to treat RA since the 1940s.[12] Following 30 years of limited use, SSP was confirmed as an effective DMARD.[13] SSP is licensed for use in RA; it is unlicensed but commonly used for seronegative spondyloarthropathies (SPA).[1] It has no other rheumatic uses.

Pharmacology

SSP consists of sulphapyridine (SP) and 5-aminosalicylic acid (5-ASA). The majority of SSP is converted to SP and 5-ASA following enzymatic breakdown in the large intestine.[14] Studies suggest that SP has the main DMARD effect.[14] SP has immunomodulatory actions, to date not fully established, in addition to potential antibiotic effects. 5-ASA may have anti-inflammatory effects only.[14]

SSP is available as a tablet (500 mg) or syrup.[1] The dose is incrementally increased to a standard maintenance dose of 1 g twice daily (maximum 3 g daily or 40 mg/kg per day). Clinical effect should be achieved within 6–12 weeks.[7]

Toxicity

The main contraindication to SSP is sulphonamide allergy.[1,7]

SSP should be used with caution while breastfeeding.[7,15]

SSP has no cumulative toxicity. Most serious side effects occur early (within 3–6 months) and reverse promptly on SSP withdrawal.[9,16,17]

Nausea and rarely vomiting, are the most common side effects, causing estimated withdrawal rates of 10–15%. Nausea usually occurs early, generally eases with time and can be reduced by use of the enteric-coated tablet, taking SSP with food and increasing the dose more gradually.[9,16,17] Centrally acting anti-emetics can be beneficial, suggesting a central, not local, effect.[9]

Mucocutaneous reactions are common.[9,16,17] Dose reduction or temporary SSP withdrawal may allow milder symptoms to settle; severe rashes require SSP withdrawal and rechallenge is not advised.[9]

Diarrhoea and abdominal pain causes withdrawal in up to 5%; these do not result from structural change within the bowel, small-bowel bacterial overgrowth, or pseudomembranous colitis.[9]

Neuropsychiatric complications (headaches, irritability, anxiety) occur in up to 19% and may necessitate SSP withdrawal.[9,16,18]

Haematological complications occur in 1–3%.[9,16,17,19]

Mild neutropenia, lymphopenia, and thrombocytopenia may correct with no action or temporary dose reduction/drug holiday.

Severe neutropenia is reversible, can be life threatening, and necessitates SSP withdrawal; rechallenge is not recommended.[9] Very rarely aplastic anaemia is reported.[17,19,20]

Megaloblastic anaemia and significant haemolysis are rare but a rise in mean corpuscular volume is relatively common (70%) and the cause for this is not fully understood.[9,19] SSP, despite competitively antagonizing folic acid, does not directly affect folic acid levels.[21] Macrocytosis does not usually require SSP withdrawal.

Minor LFT abnormalities occur in up to 3%, do not require SSP withdrawal, and do not predict the rarer severe acute hepatic complications that do require SSP withdrawal.[9,22]

Pneumonitis is extremely rare (<0.1%), usually occurs early, and requires SSP withdrawal; eosinophilia and pulmonary infiltrates are often found in conjunction with rash and fever.[23]

Azoospermia occurs in some males but rapidly reverses on stopping treatment.[15,24]

Persistent reduced immunoglobulin levels occur in up to 10% but do not link with increased infection risk.[9]

Other information

SSP can cause orange discolouration of body fluids—this can stain soft contact lenses and discolour urine.

SSP can be continued if required during pregnancy provided adequate folic acid intake is ensured.[7,25]

Monitoring requirements

See Table 80.1.

Leflunomide

Leflunomide is the newest DMARD licensed for treatment of RA and PsA.[1] It is not commonly used for other rheumatic conditions.

Pharmacology

Leflunomide, N-(3-trifluromethylphenyl)-5-methylisoaazole-4-carboxamide, inhibits pyrimidine synthesis, resulting in blockage of T-cell proliferation. It is a prodrug that is rapidly converted to its active metabolite. It has a long half-life (1–4 weeks).[26] At a dose of 20 mg daily (licensed maintenance dose 10–20 mg) it reaches a steady state in 7 weeks. This period can be shortened by using a loading dose of 100 mg daily for 3 days. Time to onset of action is 3–12 weeks.[7]

Toxicity

Pregnancy is contraindicated with leflunomide. Couples with a woman of childbearing age must use reliable contraception. Women planning pregnancy should stop leflunomide 2 years before conception or undergo a washout (see 'Other information'). Men should use reliable contraception for 3 months after stopping leflunomide.[1,7]

Lefunomide should not be started in the presence of active sepsis, severely impaired bone marrow function, immunodeficiency, or liver disease.

Leflunomide interacts with warfarin.[1]

Leflunomide has a similar side-effect profile to MTX and SSP.[26] because of its long half-life side effects typically persist for longer. Minimal data are available on long-term toxicity.

Gastrointestinal side effects (nausea, dyspepsia, abdominal pain, and diarrhoea) are common (1–10%).[27] Diarrhoea is more

Table 80.1 Guidelines for monitoring DMARD therapy

Drug	Pretreatment	FBC	U&E, Creat 1	LFT	BP	Urine dipstick protein	Frequency/comment
Azathioprine	FBC, U&E, LFT, creatinine, **TPMT assay**	√	√	√	–	–	*FBC and LFT*—**weekly for 6 weeks**; then **2 weekly** until dose stable for **6 weeks**; then **monthly** After dose increase: FBC and LFTs after **2 weeks**, then **monthly** If dose and results stable for **6 months** consider reducing to **3 monthly** In **heterozygote** TPMT patients, **monthly** monitoring should continue *U&E, creatinine*—**6 monthly**
Ciclosporin	FBC, U&E, LFT, Creatinine: twice 2 weeks apart to obtain mean value creatinine clearance or equivalent Fasting lipids BP: <140/90 twice, 2 weeks apart	√	√	√	√	–	*U&E*—**every 2 weeks** until dose and results stable for **3 months**; then **monthly** *FBC and LFT*—**monthly** until dose and results stable for **3 months; thereafter 3 monthly** *BP*—at each attendance. BP >140/90 twice, 2 weeks apart—treat hypertension. If BP cannot be controlled, stop ciclosporin. Once BP controlled can restart ciclosporin *Fasting lipids*—check periodically
IM Gold	FBC, U & E, LFT & creatinine, urinalysis	√	–	–	–	√	Prior to each injection *FBC and urinalysis* *Enquire about skin rashes or mouth ulcers*
Hydroxychloroquine	FBC, U&E, LFT Identify visual impairment not corrected by glasses Record near visual acuity of each eye (with glasses if worn) using a test type or reading chart If abnormality, refer first to optometrist	–	–	–	–	–	*Annual review either by an optometrist or enquiring about visual symptoms, rechecking visual acuity and assessing for blurred vision using the reading chart.* *Discuss with ophthalmologist if on treatment for >5 years* **Patients should also be advised to report any visual disturbance**
Leflunomide	FBC, U&E, LFT, creatinine. BP twice, 2 weeks apart. If >140/90 treat before starting leflunomide Body weight	√	–	√	√	–	*FBC, LFT*—**every month** for 6 months; once if stable, **2 monthly thereafter** If other immunosuppressant or hepatotoxic agent are coprescribed **monthly tests long term** *BP*—at each visit *Weigh*—at each visit
Methotrexate (oral/IM or SC)	FBC, U&E, LFT CXR (within the last 6 months) Pulmonary function test in selected patients	√	√	√	–	–	*FBC, U&E, LFT* **every 2 weeks** until dose and monitoring **stable for 6 weeks**; thereafter **monthly**, until the dose and disease is stable for a year. Thereafter consider reducing monitoring **to every 2–3 months**

(Continued)

Table 80.1 (*Continued*)

Drug	Pretreatment	FBC	U&E, Creat 1	LFT	BP	Urine dipstick protein	Frequency/comment
Folic acid							*Dyspnoea or dry cough*—assess at each visit
Mycophenolate mofetil	FBC, U&E, LFT, CXR (within the last 6 months)	√	–	–	–	–	*FBC*—**weekly** until dose **stable for 4 weeks** then **fortnightly for 2 months; monthly thereafter**
D-Penicillamine	FBC, U&E, creatinine, urinary protein	√	–	–	–	√	*FBC and urinalysis*—**every 2 weeks** until dose and monitoring stable for **3 months; monthly thereafter**
Sulfasalazine	FBC, U&E, LFT, creatinine	√	–	√	–	–	*FBC, LFT*—**monthly for 3 months**. If dose and results **stable for 3 months**, then **3 monthly**. If dose increase, repeat **bloods after 1 month**; if stable revert to usual monitoring regime If **after first year** dose and results are stable, frequency of **6 monthly** tests for second year **After 2 years** of stable dose and results, no monitoring required

The BSR/BHPR guidelines on DMARD therapy provides further information on actions to take in the light of monitoring test results.[7] Note that in addition to absolute values a rapid fall or rise and a consistent upward or downward trend in any value should prompt caution and extra vigilance.

From the BSR guidelines for DMARD monitoring.[95]

common with use of the loading dose, typically occurs within the first 3 months, and often settles with symptomatic treatment or with dose reduction.[9] Significant weight loss has been reported.[28]

Raised LFTs occur in 10% and usually improve with dose reduction/treatment cessation.[9] Cirrhosis and fatal liver disease can occur and caution is recommended particularly with concomitant use of other hepatotoxic drugs (e.g. MTX and NSAIDs) and in patients with other risk factors for liver disease.[29] Alcohol intake should be limited.[7]

An increase in blood pressure (BP), usually mild, is commonly seen (1–10%). BP should be controlled prior to and during treatment. Severe, uncontrolled hypertension may require leflunomide withdrawal.[7]

Rashes and alopecia occur in 1–10%. Both respond to dose reduction or cessation if severe.[9]

Leucopoenia, anaemia, and thrombocytopenia are uncommon (0.1–1%) [9]; severe cases may require leflunomide cessation and washout (see 'Other information').

Rare cases of pneumonitis are reported.[30]

Cases of peripheral neuropathy have been reported, typically after 6 months of treatment.[31] Drug cessation is associated with the best outcome and most cases improve.

Other information

In the event of severe complications, or before conception, a washout procedure can be considered to expedite drug elimination. Leflunomide should be stopped and either cholestyramine or activated charcoal given for 11 days. Confirmation of active metabolite concentrations below 20 μg/litre is recommended before conception.[1,7]

Advice on immunization is as for MTX.

Monitoring

See Table 80.1.

Hydroxychloroquine and other anti-malarials

Anti-malarials have been used to treat rheumatic diseases since the 1950s.[32] Hydroxychloroquine (HCQ) is licensed to treat RA and CTDs.[1] Chloroquine is also licensed to treat inflammatory conditions but is rarely used.[1] Mepracrine and dapsone are sometimes used off license to treat discoid lupus and cutaneous vasculitides respectively.

Pharmacology

HCQ is administered orally.[7] Its DMARD actions are not well understood, but it is known to impair phago/lysosomal function and inhibit Toll-like receptors.[33] HCQ has a long half-life (approximately 40 days)[9], reaches a steady state concentration after about 6 months, and takes longer than other DMARDs to take effect (3–6 months).[9,34]

A typical dose of HCQ is 200–400 mg daily.[7] The dose should not exceed 6.5 mg/kg per day.[1]

Toxicity

Pre-existent maculopathy is a contra-indication.[7]

HCQ may reduce seizure thresholds and exacerbate psoriasis so should be used with caution in patients with epilepsy or psoriasis [7]

HCQ is relatively safe in pregnancy and can be continued if breast feeding.[15]

Anti-malarials generally have better toxicity profiles than other DMARDs. In particular, there is no significant increased risk of infection.

Gastrointestinal (nausea, vomiting, abdominal pain) and neurological (headache, dizziness and tinnitus) side effects are uncommon (0.1–1%) and usually respond to dose reduction.

Skin rashes are rare (0.01–0.1%); if severe, drug cessation is recommended.

Ocular toxicity is the major concern with HCQ. 'Bullseye' retinopathy can progress to blindness even with drug withdrawal but is rare with rheumatological doses (<6.5 mg/kg per day).[35] Blurring of vision is more common (0.1–1%) but resolves on stopping treatment.[9] The role of retinopathy screening is much debated.

Monitoring

See Table 80.1.

Gold (sodium aurothiomalate)

Gold therapy was first investigated for RA in the 1920s, having been used for tuberculosis in the preceding 30 years.[36] It became the most commonly prescribed DMARD before losing popularity to newer treatments with better efficacy:toxicity profiles.[9] Gold only has a licence for RA but has been used to treat seronegative arthritis; it has no well-established role in treating other rheumatic diseases.[1]

Pharmacology

Therapeutic gold is a water-soluble compound of sodium aurothiomalate (a sulphur moiety attached to gold). It localizes to synovium (larger amounts in inflamed synovium), in synovial fluid[37] and up to 60% can remain in the body for up to 25 years.[9,37] Gold is concentrated in the liver, bone marrow, lymph nodes, skin, and muscle as it binds highly to protein.[9,38]

Gold's mode of action is not fully understood. It has effects on B-cell and macrophage function, osteoclastic bone resorption, interleukin production, and signal transduction.[9] Interaction with thiol groups on cell membranes and proteins is postulated to be key in its actions.[39]

Gold is given as an intramuscular injection. A test dose (10 mg) precedes doses ranging from 20–50 mg weekly; once response is achieved (usually with a cumulative dose of 500 mg) injection frequency is reduced to monthly.[1] Clinical benefit should be seen within 3–6 months.[1,7]

Toxicity

The main contraindications to gold are pregnancy and breastfeeding.[1,7]

Gold should only be used with caution in patients with severe renal or hepatic impairment and in those with systemic lupus erythematosus (SLE), porphyria, previous exfoliative dermatitis, significant pulmonary fibrosis, necrotizing enterocolitis, or a history of blood dyscrasias.[1,7,37]

Tolerance is less good than many DMARDs, with 30% withdrawal rates over the first year of treatment.[9,40]

Mucocutaneous reactions account for up to 60% of adverse reactions.[41] Mild reactions may settle with topical treatments and/or reduced injection dose or frequency; more severe rashes require gold withdrawal.[41] Pruritus accompanies most rashes (85%), can occur alone, and may settle with anti-histamines. Rising eosinophilia can herald a rash.[38] Exfoliative dermatitis is rare but requires gold withdrawal with no rechallenge; rechallenge can be considered for other rashes.[41]

Renal toxicity (most commonly membranous glomerulonephritis) presents with proteinura in approximately 8% [9,40,42,43] Renal complications are immune mediated and generally reverse with gold withdrawal; reversal may take months or years.[43] Proteinuria with no glomerular abnormality can occur and will often reverse with dose reduction. Gold-induced nephrotic syndrome usually occurs within the first year (75%) and requires gold withdrawal.[43]

Acute facial flushing (nitritoid reaction) occurs in 5%; other symptoms include sweating, nausea, vomiting, dizziness, fainting, and rarely acute coronary and/or cerebral ischaemia.[9,44] Reactions generally reduce with ongoing treatment but are more common in those on angiotensin converting enzyme (ACE) inhibitors.[45] Patients should be observed for half an hour after their initial doses.

Haematological abnormalities develop in up to 3%. Thrombocytopenia occurs most commonly (up to 18 months after treatment has stopped) and slow-onset changes will often reverse on reducing dose or frequency.[9] All acute haematological changes, including aplastic anaemia and thrombocytopenia, require gold withdrawal with no rechallenge.[9] Eosinophilia can occur in up to 40%.[46] Hypogammaglobulinaemia that may reverse on stopping treatment is also reported.[47]

Gold-induced colitis is a rare (<1%) but serious complication.[48] It usually occurs within 3 months and after just small doses of gold but can also present late in treatment.[47,48] It is slow to settle with gold withdrawal and supportive treatment and has a high linked mortality (26%).[47,48]

Chrysiasis (blue discolouration) reflects gold deposition in the cornea and skin; it develops after long-term treatment and does not usually require gold withdrawal.[9,49]

Rarer complications include 'gold lung', hepatotoxicity, pancreatitis, and neurological complications (peripheral neuropathy, Guillain–Barré type syndrome, encephalopathy, cranial nerve palsies).[9,38,50,51]

Other information

Advice on immunization is as for MTX.

Monitoring requirements

See Table 80.1.

D-Penicillamine

D-Penicillamine (DPA) was originally used to treat Wilson's disease. It was used for RA when it was found to dissociate rheumatoid factor in the 1960s.[52] DPA has a licence for RA and has particularly been used to treat extra-articular features such as nodulosis.[1,53]

DPA has been used in scleroderma due to its inhibition of collagen cross-linking.[54,55] It has no significant role in the management of other rheumatic diseases and its use has progressively declined with the introduction of more effective, less toxic therapies.[56,57]

Pharmacology

DPA is an amino acid with a thiol side chain that can be formed synthetically or through acid hydrolysis of penicillin.[9,38,57] Its mode of action is not fully understood although the thiol side chain is thought to be important.[57] DPA has no effect on B-cell function but inhibits T helper-cell function (CD4).[57] It reduces rheumatoid factor titres and, by reducing proliferation of fibroblasts, may have an impact on RA pannus formation.[57,58]

DPA is given orally. The starting dose is 125 mg daily with monthly 125 mg increases in dose as required to 500 mg.[1] Beneficial effects take 12–24 weeks to achieve.[7]

DPA should be taken on an empty stomach. Absorption is reduced by iron, calcium, vitamin supplements. and indigestion medication.[9,57] Through unknown mechanisms, indomethacin and chloroquine have been linked with raised blood levels of DPA.[57]

Toxicity

DPA is contraindicated in SLE and should only be used with caution with pregnancy and lactation.[1,7,37,59]

DPA toxicity limits its use and is linked with higher doses, but there is no clear cumulative dose effect.[9]

Mucocutaneous reactions are common (10–20%) and can occur both early and late in treatment.[9,38] Milder reactions (mouth ulcers, stomatitis, pruritus) may respond to symptomatic treatments and/ or DPA dose reduction or temporary withdrawal. DPA-induced pemphigus requires urgent DPA withdrawal and pemphigus treatment.[9]

Hypogeusia or dysgeusia (altered or lost sense of taste) occur in 10–20%,[9] usually occur early (within 6 weeks) and settle after 2–3 months. Early-onset anorexia and nausea will also usually settle with time.

Renal and bone marrow toxicity are the major concerns with DPA, occurring in 10–15% and 5–10% respectively.[9] Isolated haematuria often reflects non-drug-related pathology but significant haematuria and proteinuria require further investigation for potential glomerulonephritis (usually membranous; rarely crescentic).[60–62]

DPA-associated pancytopenia, neutropenia, and thrombocytopenia usually respond to dose reductions or drug withdrawal.[9,38]

DPA can trigger several clinical conditions.[9,38] DPA-induced lupus differs from non-drug-induced lupus with the production of single-stranded (ss) DNA but not double-stranded (ds) DNA antibodies. DPA-induced myasthaenia gravis, polymyositis, and dermatomyositis all reverse with time on DPA withdrawal. Rarely a syndrome resembling Goodpasture's (without the anti-glomerular basement membranes antibodies) and an obliterative bronchiolitis can develop.

Mammary hyperplasia is also a rare side effect.[9,37,38]

Other information

Advice on immunization is as for MTX.

Monitoring requirements

See Table 80.1.

Azathioprine

Azathioprine was originally developed for transplant medicine. In the United Kingdom its only rheumatic disease license is for RA.[1] Its use in RA has declined. Off-licence efficacy has been shown for seronegative arthritides and CTDs.[63]

Pharmacology

Oral azathioprine is metabolized to 6-mercaptopurine and thereafter 6-thioquanine, the main active metabolite. Azathioprine reduces circulating B and T lymphocytes.[64] Thiopurine methyltransferase (TPMT) is the key inactivation enzyme. TPMT activity is autosomal dominantly inherited.[7,65]

Azathioprine is typically started at a dose of 1 mg/kg per day, increasing after 4–6 weeks up to 2–3 mg/kg.[1] The onset of action is 6–12 weeks.[7]

Toxicity

TPMT levels should be measured prior to treatment.[7] Low TPMT activity is linked with myelosuppression (up to 86%) and azathioprine is contraindicated in these patients.[64] With intermediate TPMT activity the risk of myelosuppression is increased (approximately fourfold); azathioprine can be prescribed with caution using lower initial doses if clinically indicated. Patients with high TPMT activity may require larger doses for clinical effects.[7]

Azathioprine is not recommended during pregnancy.[15] Effective contraception is recommended for all couples with a woman of childbearing age. For some women the potential risks of stopping treatment may outweigh those of continued treatment and, with informed consent, azathioprine may be continued during pregnancy.[7]

Breastfeeding is not recommended during treatment.[1]

Azathioprine has multiple drug interactions.[1] The most important are:

- allopurinol: reduce azathioprine dose to 25%
- ACE inhibitors: an alternative DMARD/anti-hypertensive should be considered due to risk of anaemia
- warfarin: higher warfarin doses may be required
- SSP and co-trimazole: avoid if possible as increased risk of bone marrow toxicity.

Nausea and vomiting are the commonest adverse events (10%).[7] They can be treated symptomatically, but often lead to drug withdrawal. Diarrhoea and oral ulceration are less common (<5%). Hepatitis is rare and usually responds to drug cessation. Pancreatitis is an uncommon (<1%) idiosyncratic reaction that requires azathioprine withdrawal without rechallenge.[9]

Rashes are relatively common (<5%), typically occur early and respond to drug cessation.[9]

Significant neutropenia requires azathioprine withdrawal and cautious reintroduction at a lower dose on resolution.[9]

Macrocytosis is common, occurs early[9] and does not require azathioprine withdrawal.[7]

Infection risk is probably increased with azathioprine (2%).[9] Therapy should be stopped during severe infections but can usually be restarted on resolution.

With rheumatological doses there is probably a small increased risk of lymphoproliferative and skin malignancies.[64] The situation is complicated by the increased risk associated with inflammatory disease.

Other information

Advice on immunization is as for MTX.

Effective sun protection is advised.[1]

Monitoring

See Table 80.1.

Mycophenolate mofetil

Mycophenolate mofetil (MMF) was first used in transplant medicine.[66] It has no rheumatic disease licenses but is increasingly used to treat CTDs and vasculitis.[1,7,67] MMF has no significant role in treating inflammatory arthropathies.[64]

Pharmacology

MMF is a prodrug that is activated to mycophenolic acid (MPA).[68] MPA suppresses T- and B-cell proliferation and affects cellular endothelial adhesion, reducing lymphocyte accumulation at sites of inflammation.[64]

For rheumatic diseases oral doses of 1–2 g daily are used. The daily dose is usually increased weekly from 500 mg to a tolerated maintenance dose. The onset of action is typically 6–12 weeks.[7]

Toxicity

MMF should not be started in the presence of sepsis or bone marrow failure.

MMF is not recommended during pregnancy or breastfeeding.[7]

Most MMF toxicity data comes from the higher doses (2–3g daily) used in transplant medicine; the toxicity profile of MMF is similar to azathioprine.[66]

Diarrhoea, nausea, vomiting and abdominal pain are the commonest side effects (20–36%).[66]

Leucopenia occurs in up to 35% and severe neutropenia in 0.5%. These usually occur in the first 6 months of treatment. Neutropenia often responds to temporary drug cessation.[7] Upon resolution MMF can be cautiously reintroduced at half the previous dose. Anaemia and thrombocytopenia are also common (8–13%).[7]

The incidence of viral infections is increased with MMF.[66]

The incidence of malignancies, particularly non-Hodgkin's lymphoma, is increased.[69]

Other information

Advice on immunization is as for MTX.

Monitoring

See Table 80.1.

Ciclosporin

Ciclosporin was initially used in transplant medicine.[70] It was first used to treat RA in the 1970s.[9] Its only rheumatic license is for RA[1] but it has efficacy in PsA and some CTDs.[71] Poor tolerability limits its use.[2]

Pharmacology

Ciclosporin targets calcineurin, inhibiting the production of interleukin (IL)-2 by T lymphocytes. It predominantly inhibits T helper cells and T-cell-dependent B-cell responses.[72]

Ciclosporin is orally administered and metabolized in the liver by the cytochrome P450 isoenzyme CYP 3A4. Drugs may alter ciclosporin levels by inducing or inhibiting this enzyme.[73]

For RA a starting dose of 2.5 mg/kg per day in two divided doses is given.[1,7] This can be increased gradually after 6 weeks to a maximum dose of 4 mg/kg per day. The lowest effective dose should be used as toxicity is dose dependent.[7] The time to response is typically 3 months.

Toxicity

Ciclosporin is contraindicated in pregnancy and breastfeeding.[74]

Ciclosporin should not be started in patients with renal or hepatic failure, uncontrolled hypertension, sepsis, or electrolyte imbalance.[7]

Ciclosporin has multiple drug interactions; use of a data sheet is recommended before initiating or adding other drugs.[1] The most notable interactions are:

- other nephrotoxic drugs, including NSAIDS
- colchicine
- potassium-sparing diuretics
- some calcium channel blockers
- grapefruit juice.

Adverse events with the low doses used rheumatologically are generally mild and reversible. However, toxicity causes drug withdrawal within the first year in up to 15%.[9]

A dose-related decrease in glomerular filtration rate (GFR) is common (1–10%),[75] is usually reversible, and responds to dose reduction or cessation.[75] The risk is greatest in elderly patients and with comcomitant use of nephrotoxic drugs.[9] Irreversible renal damage can occur with long-term use of more than 5 mg/kg per day.[9]

Increases in BP are common (up to 33%), dose related,[64] and should be treated (note drug interactions) before ciclosporin is reduced or stopped.[7]

Headaches, parasthesiae, and tremor are common (1–10%), dose related,[9] and typically respond to dose reduction or cessation.

The risk of viral infections (e.g. herpes simplex and zoster) is increased.[9] Ciclosporin can be continued with minor infections but should be suspended with more severe infections.

Hirsutism and hypertrichosis are common (1–10%).[9] In severe cases drug cessation should be considered.

Nausea, vomiting, and diarrhoea are common and often respond to symptomatic measures.[75]

Gum hyperplasia can be severe, necessitating drug cessation; resolution can take months.[9]

Leucopenia, anaemia, and thrombocytopenia are relatively rare (0.01–0.1%) compared to other DMARDs.[9] In severe cases dose reduction or cessation should be considered.

The risk of skin malignancies and lymphoma may be increased, particularly with long-term immunosuppression (data from transplant patients).[9,76] This is of particular importance for PUVA-treated PsA patients.[76]

Hepatotoxicity is very rare but is seen in overdose.[9] Raised transaminases should prompt investigation of other causes.[7] Dose reduction or cessation may be needed.

Other information

Advice on immunization is as for MTX.

Monitoring

See Table 80.1.

Cyclophosphamide

Cyclophosphamide (CP) was initially developed as a more selective cytotoxic agent for malignant cells.[77] Rheumatologically it is used to treat severe disease or major organ involvement with many inflammatory, vasculitic, and CTDs.[1,78,79] The availability of less toxic drugs limits its use in RA to severe disease and extra-articular features such as RA vasculitis.[1,79]

Pharmacology

CP is well absorbed orally (over 90% bioavailability) and is activated in the liver by cytochrome P450; phosphoramide mustard is the main active metabolite.[38,77,80] CP and its metabolites are renally excreted. Acrolein is one renally excreted metabolite that is linked with bladder toxicity.[9,81]

CP is an alkylating agent that prevents DNA replication and has an effect on both B- and T-cell function and the production of immunoglobulins.[77,82] Maximal effects are seen on rapidly dividing cells, but all cells are affected.[82]

CP can be given orally or intravenously.[1] Oral doses are usually 50–150 mg per day (maximum 2 mg/kg per day or 200 mg).[78] 'Pulsed' oral CP can also be prescribed.[83]

Intravenous (IV) doses usually range from 0.5–1 g (maximum 1500 mg) per infusion with infusions repeated at variable frequencies dependent on the clinical condition; most commonly every 2–4 weeks.[1,78] IV CP is ideally given in the morning to reduce bladder stasis overnight; IV fluids and high oral water intake during and after treatment encourage diuresis.[1,78] Mesna (2-mercaptothane sulphonate) and anti-emetics are recommended coprescriptions to reduce side effects.[78,83] Treatment duration should be minimized given the cumulative toxicity. CP usually takes effect over 2–3 weeks but oral CP can take up to 6–12 weeks.

Toxicity

Pregnancy and breastfeeding are contraindicated while on treatment and for 3 months and 36 hours after treatment respectively.[1]

Toxicity limits CP use and is generally dose dependent. Many side effects are reduced with IV CP regimes.[84]

Infection risk is increased and CP should be used with caution in those with high infection risk.[1,78] Infection risk is independent of haematological complications of CP and is more common with oral regimes.[84] Neutropenic sepsis can be fatal but most haematological changes are reversible; their peak incidence is at days 8–14 after IV CP.[38]

Prophylactic treatment against *Pneumocystis jirovecii* and consideration of anti-fungal and anti-staphylococcal treatment is recommended for many treatment regimes.[78] Pretreatment tuberculosis (TB) screening is recommended.[78]

Serious bladder toxicity is more common with oral regimes and links with cumulative dose and duration of treatment.[84] Dysuria can occur in up to 45%.[9] Haemorrhagic cystitis occurs in 10–43%, can range in severity and persist for up to 3 months.[9] CP rechallenge is not recommended after haemorrhagic cystitis due to the linked risks of bladder fibrosis and cancer.[9] Bladder malignancy is a dose-dependent complication and can occur up to 15 years after treatment has stopped; the risk is increased 31-fold compared to the general population.[85] Bladder complications can be reduced with mesna.[1]

Malignancies are more common with oral CP and are significant, dose-dependent, long-term complications.[85,86] Malignancy can develop many years after stopping CP and occurs more frequently in smokers.[86] No significant increase in mortality is reported and this probably reflects the high incidence of non-fatal bladder and skin malignancies.

Infertility is a major concern with CP—the risks are lower with pulsed IV CP and increase with increasing age, higher doses, and longer duration of treatment.[87]

Alopecia occurs in up to 63% of patients on oral CP; this again is dose dependent and usually reverses with CP dose reduction or withdrawal.[9]

Nausea and vomiting are also common (up to 64% with oral CP).[9]

Reversible reductions in immunoglobulins occur in up to 20% and patients have an impaired response to immunizations.[9]

Other information

As dialysis removes CP, administration should occur after dialysis in dialysed patients.[77]

As active metabolites are renally excreted, doses need to be reduced with renal impairment.[1,78]

Effective skin sun protection is advised

Advice on immunization is as for MTX.

Pretreatment sperm and oocyte cryopreservation should be considered.[78]

Monitoring requirements

For IV CP—pre- and 10 day post-treatment full blood count (FBC) and urea and electrolytes (U&E); urine dipstick prior to each treatment.[78]

For oral CP—FBC and U&E pretreatment, weekly for month 1, 2 weekly for months 2–3, then monthly. Regular urine dipstick.[78]

Vigilance for skin and other malignancies and annual cervical screening.

Minocycline and antibiotic regimes

Although not licensed for RA use, antibiotic regimes (tetracyclines, particularly minocycline used alone or in combination with other antibiotics) have been used to treat RA, having been found to have immunomodulatory effects. These treatments are tolerated well and a meta-analysis has shown benefit of tetracyclines with equivalent effects of minocycline to HCQ.[88,89]

Chlorambucil

Toxicity limits chlorambucil use in RA to the management of severe DMARD-resistant disease.[9,90,91] With proven reduction in mortality chlorambucil is mainly used to treat secondary AA amyloid. Given its cumulative dose toxicity, the smallest dose for the shortest duration is recommended.

Thalidomide

Thalidomide is a potent immunosuppressant[92] that can successfully (off-licence) treat resistant Behçet's syndrome or skin manifestations of SLE.[92,93] Teratogenicity and irreversible neuropathy limit its use.[93,94]

References

1. *British national formulary*, 62nd edn. Pharmaceutical Press, London, 2011.
2. Gaujoux-Viala C, Smolen JS, Landewe R et al. Current evidence for the management of rheumatoid arthritis with synthetic disease-modifying antirheumatic drugs: a systematic literature review informing the EULAR recommendations for the management of rheumatoid arthritis. *Ann Rheum Dis* 2010;69(6):1004–1009.
3. Jeurissen ME, Boerbooms AM, van de Putte LB. Methotrexate therapy in connective tissue diseases: a review of the literature. *Neth J Med* 1989;35(1–2):44–58.
4. Ash Z, Gaujoux-Viala C, Gossec L et al. A systematic literature review of drug therapies for the treatment of psoriatic arthritis: current evidence and meta-analysis informing the EULAR recommendations for the management of psoriatic arthritis. *Ann Rheum Dis* 2012;71(3):319–336.
5. Cannon GW. Methotrexate pulmonary toxicity. *Rheum Dis Clin North Am* 1997;23(4):917–937.
6. Gutierrez-Urena S, Molina JF, Garcia CO, Cuellar ML, Espinoza LR. Pancytopenia secondary to methotrexate therapy in rheumatoid arthritis. *Arthritis Rheum* 1996;39(2):272–276.
7. Chakravarty K, McDonald H, Pullar T et al. BSR/BHPR guideline for disease-modifying anti-rheumatic drug (DMARD) therapy in consultation with the British Association of Dermatologists. *Rheumatology (Oxford)* 2008;47(6):924–925.
8. Kerstens PJ, Boerbooms AM, Jeurissen ME et al. Accelerated nodulosis during low dose methotrexate therapy for rheumatoid arthritis. An analysis of ten cases. *J Rheumatol* 1992;19(6):867–871.
9. Capell H, Madhok R, McInnes IB. *Practical prescribing guidelines in rheumatoid arthritis*. Martin Dunitz, London, 2003.
10. Dawson TM, Starkebaum G, Wood BL, Willkens RF, Gown AM. Epstein-Barr virus, methotrexate, and lymphoma in patients with rheumatoid arthritis and primary Sjogren's syndrome: case series. *J Rheumatol* 2001;28(1):47–53.
11. Westlake SL, Colebatch AN, Baird J et al. The effect of methotrexate on cardiovascular disease in patients with rheumatoid arthritis: a systematic literature review. *Rheumatology (Oxford)* 2010;49(2):295–307.
12. Swartz N. The treatment of rheumatic polyarthritis with acid azo compounds. *Rheumatol* 1948;4:56–60.
13. McConkey B, Amos RS, Durham S et al. Sulphasalazine in rheumatoid arthritis *BMJ* 1980;280(6212):442–444.
14. Pullar T, Hunter JA, Capell HA. Which component of sulphasalazine is active in rheumatoid arthritis? *BMJ (Clin Res Ed)* 1985;290(6481):1535–1538.
15. Janssen NM, Genta MS. The effects of immunosuppressive and anti-inflammatory medications on fertility, pregnancy, and lactation *Arch Intern Med* 2000;160(5):610–619.
16. Amos RS, Pullar T, Bax DE, Situnayake D, Capell HA, McConkey B. Sulphasalazine for rheumatoid arthritis: toxicity in 774 patients monitored for one to 11 years. *BMJ (Clin Res Ed)* 1986; 293(6544):420–423.
17. Box SA, Pullar T. Sulphasalazine in the treatment of rheumatoid arthritis. *Br J Rheumatol* 1997;36(3):382–386.

18. Farr M, Scott DG, Bacon PA. Side effect profile of 200 patients with inflammatory arthritides treated with sulphasalazine. *Drugs* 1986;32 Suppl 1:49–53.

19. Farr M, Tunn EJ, Symmons DP, Scott DG, Bacon PA. Sulphasalazine in rheumatoid arthritis: haematological problems and changes in haematological indices associated with therapy *Br J Rheumatol* 1989;28(2):134–138.

20. Jick H, Myers MW, Dean AD. The risk of sulfasalazine- and mesalazine-associated blood disorders *Pharmacotherapy* 1995;15(2):176–181.

21. Grindulis KA, McConkey B. Does sulphasalazine cause folate deficiency in rheumatoid arthritis? *Scand J Rheumatol* 1985;14(3):265–270.

22. Aithal GP. Hepatotoxicity related to antirheumatic drugs. *Nat Rev Rheumatol* 2011;7(3):139–150.

23. Parry SD, Barbatzas C, Peel ET, Barton JR. Sulphasalazine and lung toxicity. *Eur Respir J* 2002;19(4):756–764.

24. Toovey S, Hudson E, Hendry WF, Levi AJ. Sulphasalazine and male infertility: reversibility and possible mechanism. *Gut* 1981;22(6):445–451.

25. van Leuven SI, Franssen R, Kastelein JJ, Levi M, Stroes ES, Tak PP. Systemic inflammation as a risk factor for atherothrombosis. *Rheumatology (Oxford)* 2008;47(1):3–7.

26. Keystone E, Haraoui B. *Disease-modifying antirheumatic drugs 4: leflunomide*. In: Hochberg MC et al. (eds) Rheumatology, 3rd edn. Elsevier Science, Amsterdam, 2003:431–438.

27. Van Riel PL, Smolen JS, Emery P et al. Leflunomide: a manageable safety profile. *J Rheumatol Suppl* 2004;71:21–24.

28. Coblyn JS, Shadick N, Helfgott S. Leflunomide-associated weight loss in rheumatoid arthritis. *Arthritis Rheum* 2001;44(5):1048–1051.

29. Weinblatt ME, Dixon JA, Falchuk KR. Serious liver disease in a patient receiving methotrexate and leflunomide. *Arthritis Rheum* 2000;43(11):2609–2611.

30. Inokuma S. Leflunomide-induced interstitial pneumonitis might be a representative of disease-modifying antirheumatic drug-induced lung injury. *Expert Opin Drug Saf* 2011;10(4):603–611.

31. Alcorn N, Saunders S, Madhok R. Benefit-risk assessment of leflunomide: an appraisal of leflunomide in rheumatoid arthritis 10 years after licensing. *Drug Saf* 2009;32(12):1123–1134.

32. Kersley GD, PALIN AG. Amodiaquine and hydroxychloroquine in rheumatoid arthritis. *Lancet* 21 Nov 1959;2(7108):886–888.

33. Katz SJ, Russell AS. Re-evaluation of antimalarials in treating rheumatic diseases: re-appreciation and insights into new mechanisms of action. *Curr Opin Rheumatol* 2011;23(3):278–281.

34. Tett SE. Clinical pharmacokinetics of slow-acting antirheumatic drugs. *Clin Pharmacokinet* 1993;25(5):392–407.

35. Finbloom DS, Silver K, Newsome DA, Gunkel R. Comparison of hydroxychloroquine and chloroquine use and the development of retinal toxicity. *J Rheumatol* 1985;12(4):692–694.

36. Forestier J. Rheumatoid Arthritis and its treatment by gold salts. *J Lab Clin Med* 1935;20:827.

37. *Medicines compendium*. Datapharm Communications, Leatherhead, 2007.

38. Firestein GS, Budd RC, Harris ED, Jr et al. (eds) *Kelley's textbook of rheumatology*, 8th edn. Saunders Elsevier, Philadelphia, PA, 2008.

39. Jeon KI, Jeong JY, Jue DM. Thiol-reactive metal compounds inhibit NF-kappa B activation by blocking I kappa B kinase. *J Immunol* 2000;164(11):5981–5989.

40. van Jaarsveld CH, Jahangier ZN, Jacobs JW et al. Toxicity of anti-rheumatic drugs in a randomized clinical trial of early rheumatoid arthritis *Rheumatology (Oxford)* 2000;39(12):1374–1382.

41. Taukumova LA, Mouravjoy Y, Gribakin SG. Mucocutaneous side effects and continuation of aurotherapy in patients with rheumatoid arthritis *Adv Exp Med Biol* 1999;455:367–373.

42. Ward JR, Williams HJ, Egger MJ et al. Comparison of auranofin, gold sodium thiomalate, and placebo in the treatment of rheumatoid arthritis. A controlled clinical trial. *Arthritis Rheum* 1983;26(11):1303–1315.

43. Hall CL, Fothergill NJ, Blackwell MM et al. The natural course of gold nephropathy: long term study of 21 patients. *BMJ (Clin Res Ed)* 1987;295(6601):745–748.

44. Arthur AB, Klinkhoff A, Teufel A. Nitritoid reactions: case reports, review, and recommendations for management *J Rheumatol* 2001 Oct;28(10):2209–2212.

45. Healey LA, Backes MB. Nitritoid reactions and angiotension-converting-enzyme inhibitors *N Engl J Med* 1989;321(11):763.

46. Davis P, Menard H, Thompson J, Harth M, Beaudet F. One-year comparative study of gold sodium thiomalate and auranofin in the treatment of rheumatoid arthritis. *J Rheumatol* 1985;12(1):60–67.

47. Stuckey BG, Hanrahan PS, Zilko PJ, Owen ET. Hypogammaglobulinemia and lung infiltrates after gold therapy *J Rheumatol* 1986;13(2):468–469.

48. Jackson CW, Haboubi NY, Whorwell PJ, Schofield PF. Gold induced enterocolitis. *Gut* 1986;27(4):452–456.

49. Leonard PA, Moatamed F, Ward JR, Piepkorn MW, Adams EJ, Knibbe WP. Chrysiasis: the role of sun exposure in dermal hyperpigmentation secondary to gold therapy. *J Rheumatol* 1986;13(1):58–64.

50. Scott DL, Bradby GV, Aitman TJ, Zaphiropoulos GC, Hawkins CF. Relationship of gold and penicillamine therapy to diffuse interstitial lung disease. *Ann Rheum Dis* 1981;40(2):136–141.

51. Edelman J, Donnelly R, Graham DN, Percy JS. Liver dysfunction associated with gold therapy for rheumatoid arthritis *J Rheumatol* 1983;10(3):510–511.

52. Jaffe IA. The effect of penicillamine on the laboratory parameters in rheumatoid arthritis. *Arthritis Rheum* 1965;8(6):1064–1079.

53. Dash S, Seibold JR, Tiku ML. Successful treatment of methotrexate induced nodulosis with D-penicillamine. *J Rheumatol* 1999;26(6):1396–1399.

54. Nimni ME, Bavetta LA. Collagen defect induced by penicillamine. *Science* 1965;150(698):905–907.

55. Clements PJ, Wong WK, Hurwitz EL et al. The Disability Index of the Health Assessment Questionnaire is a predictor and correlate of outcome in the high-dose versus low-dose penicillamine in systemic sclerosis trial. *Arthritis Rheum* 2001;44(3):653–661.

56. Fries JF, Williams CA, Ramey D, Bloch DA. The relative toxicity of disease-modifying antirheumatic drugs. *Arthritis Rheum* 1993; 36(3):297–306.

57. Munro R CH. Disease modifying drug series: penicillamine. *Br J Rheumatol* 1997;36:104–109.

58. Matsubara T, Hirohata K. Suppression of human fibroblast proliferation by D-penicillamine and copper sulfate in vitro. *Arthritis Rheum* 1988;31(8):964–972.

59. Bell CL, Graziano FM. The safety of administration of penicillamine to penicillin-sensitive individuals. *Arthritis Rheum* 1983;26(6):801–803.

60. Bacon PA, Tribe CR, Mackenzie JC et al. Penicillamine nephropathy in rheumatoid arthritis. A clinical, pathological and immunological study. *Q J Med* 1976;45(180):661–684.

61. Chakravarty EF, Sanchez-Yamamoto D, Bush TM. The use of disease modifying antirheumatic drugs in women with rheumatoid arthritis of childbearing age: a survey of practice patterns and pregnancy outcomes. *J Rheumatol* 2003;30(2):241–246.

62. Leonard PA, Bienz SR, Clegg DO, Ward JR. Hematuria in patients with rheumatoid arthritis receiving gold and D-penicillamine *J Rheumatol* 1987;14(1):55–59.

63. Luqmani RA, Palmer RG, Bacon PA. Azathioprine, cyclophosphamide and chlorambucil. *Baillieres Clin Rheumatol* 1990;4(3):595–619.

64. Furst DE CP. Immunosuppressives. In: Hochberg MC et al. (eds) Rheumatology, 3rd edn. Elsevier Science, Amsterdam, 2003:439–448.

65. Clunie GP, Lennard L. Relevance of thiopurine methyltransferase status in rheumatology patients receiving azathioprine *Rheumatology (Oxford)* 2004;43(1):13–18.

66. Hood KA, Zarembski DG. Mycophenolate mofetil: a unique immunosuppressive agent. *Am J Health Syst Pharm* 1997;54(3):285–294.

67. Hiemstra TF, Jones RB, Jayne DR. Treatment of primary systemic vasculitis with the inosine monophosphate dehydrogenase inhibitor mycophenolic acid. *Nephron Clin Pract* 2010;116(1):c1–c10.

68. Furst DE. Leflunomide, mycophenolic acid and matrix metalloproteinase inhibitors. *Rheumatology (Oxford)* 1999;38 Suppl 2:14–18.

69. Eugui EM, Allison AC. Immunosuppressive activity of mycophenolate mofetil. *Ann N Y Acad Sci* 1993;685:309–329.

70. Calne RY. Immunosuppression for organ grafting—observations on cyclosporin A. *Immunol Rev* 1979;46:113–124.

71. Gossec L, Smolen JS, Gaujoux-Viala C et al. European League Against Rheumatism recommendations for the management of psoriatic arthritis with pharmacological therapies. *Ann Rheum Dis* 2012;71(1):4–12.

72. Tsokos GC. Immunomodulatory treatment in patients with rheumatic diseases: mechanisms of action. *Semin Arthritis Rheum* 1987 Aug;17(1):24–38.

73. Ptachcinski RJ, Venkataramanan R, Burckart GJ. Clinical pharmacokinetics of cyclosporin. *Clin Pharmacokinet* 1986;11(2):107–132.

74. Dijkmans BA. Safety aspects of cyclosporin in rheumatoid arthritis. *Drugs* 1995;50 Suppl 1:41–47.

75. Tugwell P, Bombardier C, Gent M et al. Low-dose cyclosporin versus placebo in patients with rheumatoid arthritis. *Lancet* 1990;335(8697):1051–1055.

76. Muellenhoff MW, Koo JY. Cyclosporine and skin cancer: an international dermatologic perspective over 25 years of experience. A comprehensive review and pursuit to define safe use of cyclosporine in dermatology *J Dermatolog Treat* 2012;23(4):290–304.

77. Moore MJ. Clinical pharmacokinetics of cyclophosphamide. *Clin Pharmacokinet* 1991;20(3):194–208.

78. Lapraik C, Watts R, Bacon P, Carruthers D, Chakravarty K, D'Cruz D, et al. BSR and BHPR guidelines for the management of adults with ANCA associated vasculitis. *Rheumatology (Oxford)* 2007;46(10):1615–1616.

79. Suarez-Almazor ME, Belseck E, Shea B, Wells G, Tugwell P. Cyclophosphamide for treating rheumatoid arthritis *Cochrane Database Syst Rev* 2000;4:CD001157.

80. Grochow LB, Colvin M. Clinical pharmacokinetics of cyclophosphamide. *Clin Pharmacokinet* 1979;4(5):380–394.

81. Cox PJ. Cyclophosphamide cystitis—identification of acrolein as the causative agent. *Biochem Pharmacol* 1979;28(13):2045–2049.

82. Fauci AS, Wolff SM, Johnson JS. Effect of cyclophosphamide upon the immune response in Wegener's granulomatosis. *N Engl J Med* 1971;285(27):1493–1496.

83. Dawisha SM, Yarboro CH, Vaughan EM et al. Outpatient monthly oral bolus cyclophosphamide therapy in systemic lupus erythematosus *J Rheumatol* 1996;23(2):273–278.

84. Guillevin L, Cordier JF, Lhote F et al. A prospective, multicenter, randomized trial comparing steroids and pulse cyclophosphamide versus steroids and oral cyclophosphamide in the treatment of generalized Wegener's granulomatosis *Arthritis Rheum* 1997;40(12):2187–2198.

85. Radis CD, Kahl LE, Baker GL et al. Effects of cyclophosphamide on the development of malignancy and on long-term survival of patients with rheumatoid arthritis. A 20-year followup study. *Arthritis Rheum* 1995;38(8):1120–1127.

86. Baker GL, Kahl LE, Zee BC et al. Malignancy following treatment of rheumatoid arthritis with cyclophosphamide. Long-term case-control follow-up study. *Am J Med* 1987;83(1):1–9.

87. Mok CC, Lau CS, Wong RW. Risk factors for ovarian failure in patients with systemic lupus erythematosus receiving cyclophosphamide therapy. *Arthritis Rheum* 1998;41(5):831–837.

88. Stone M, Fortin PR, Pacheco-Tena C, Inman RD. Should tetracycline treatment be used more extensively for rheumatoid arthritis? Metaanalysis demonstrates clinical benefit with reduction in disease activity. *J Rheumatol* 2003;30(10):2112–2122.

89. O'Dell JR, Blakely KW, Mallek JA, Eckhoff PJ, Leff RD, Wees SJ, et al. Treatment of early seropositive rheumatoid arthritis: a two-year, double-blind comparison of minocycline and hydroxychloroquine *Arthritis Rheum* 2001;44(10):2235–2241.

90. Cannon GW, Jackson CG, Samuelson CO, Jr et al. Chlorambucil therapy in rheumatoid arthritis: clinical experience in 28 patients and literature review. *Semin Arthritis Rheum* 1985;15(2):106–118.

91. Jackson CG, Williams HJ. Disease-modifying antirheumatic drugs. Using their clinical pharmacological effects as a guide to their selection *Drugs* 1998;56(3):337–344.

92. Tseng S, Pak G, Washenik K, Pomeranz MK, Shupack JL. Rediscovering thalidomide: a review of its mechanism of action, side effects, and potential uses. *J Am Acad Dermatol* 1996;35(6):969–979.

93. Gardner-Medwin JM, Smith NJ, Powell RJ. Clinical experience with thalidomide in the management of severe oral and genital ulceration in conditions such as Behcet's disease: use of neurophysiological studies to detect thalidomide neuropathy *Ann Rheum Dis* 1994;53(12):828–832.

94. Parman T, Wiley MJ, Wells PG. Free radical-mediated oxidative DNA damage in the mechanism of thalidomide teratogenicity. *Nat Med* 1999;5(5):582–585.

95. British Society for Rheumatology. *Quick reference guideline for monitoring of disease-modifying anti-rheumatic drug (DMARD) therapy.* To accompany *Disease-modifying anti-rheumatic drug (DMARD) therapy guideline—April 2008.* Available at: www.rheumatology.org.uk/includes/documents/cm_docs/2009/d/dmard_grid_november_2009.pdf

CHAPTER 81

Signalling pathway inhibitors

Roy Fleischmann

Introduction

The treatment of rheumatoid arthritis (RA) has evolved significantly over the past 50 years with the realization that the disease is most likely to respond to early aggressive therapy with the lowest disease activity obtainable as the goal of therapy.[1] Methotrexate (MTX) has been the cornerstone of therapy for the last 25 years.[2,3] With the advent of biological agents having multiple mechanisms of action, including molecules that inhibit tumour necrosis factor alpha (TNFα) interleukin (IL)-1, IL-6, costimulation, or depletion of B cells, especially in combination with MTX, more patients are reaching lower disease activity with the hope that this will lead to less future disability. These biological agents, however, are all injectable and expensive; along with their safety profile, this limits the numbers of patients who have access to them. In addition, not all patients respond to these medications, and a number who do respond still have moderate or severe disease activity.

For years there has been an effort to develop orally administered small molecules targeting intracellular signalling pathways, which would be safe and efficacious in the treatment of RA. Among the first compounds investigated were ones that inhibit p38 MAP kinases (MAPK). These are intracellular enzymes in signalling pathways activated by inflammatory cytokines, pathogens, and growth factors. They ultimately regulate the transcriptional activation of several genes, including those encoding TNFα, IL-1, and IL-6. Activated p38 MAPK is found in the synovial lining and endothelium of vessels in RA synovium and studies have shown that inhibition of p38 MAPK suppresses production of inflammatory cytokines. Animal arthritis models have demonstrated reduction in paw swelling and joint damage with these compounds. A number of molecules (SCIO 469, Pamapimod, VX-702, BMS-582949, ARRY-797, and ARRY-162) have been evaluated in phase 1 and phase 2 trials but their development was discontinued as either clinical efficacy was not observed or dose-related toxicity was seen.[4,5]

Oral inhibitors that target the more upstream protein tyrosine kinases, such as spleen tyrosine kinase (SyK) and the JAK family of kinases have been investigated in phase 3 clinical studies; at least one JAK inhibitor, tofacitinib, has demonstrated efficacy in a variety of clinical situations in RA. The efficacy and safety profile of these small molecule drugs shares many similarities with that of the biological agents approved for use, with some differences from these agents and from each other. Because these compounds are oral small molecules but have clinical efficacy similar to approved biologics, they have the potential to be utilized after MTX, before a biologic, or, after failure of one or more biological agents.

SyK is a non-receptor protein tyrosine kinase; it is a modulator of immune signalling in cells bearing Fcγ-activating receptors including B cells, mast cells, macrophages, neutrophils, and synoviocytes. SyK binds to the cytoplasmic region of receptors that contain the immune-receptor tyrosine-based activation motif (ITAM) and receptor binding results in ITAM phosphorylation activating SyK. SyK activation activates downstream MAPKs, Pi3K, and phospholipase C with resultant increase in IL-6 and matrix metalloproteinase (MMP) production.[6] An oral agent that inhibits SyK, R788 (fostamatinib disodium), a prodrug of the active metabolite R406, was studied in phase 3 clinical trials.

Janus kinases (JAKs) bind the cytoplasmic region of transmembrane-cytokine receptors. After receptor–ligand interaction, various JAKs are activated, resulting in tyrosine phosphorylation of the receptor and subsequent activation of STATs (signal transducer and activators of transcription), which act as transcription factors.[7] JAKs consist of four types: JAK1, JAK2, JAK3, and tyrosine kinase (TyK). JAKs work in pairs as homo- or heterodimers. The combination of JAK3/1 is primarily expressed in haematopoietic cells and is critical for signal transduction from the common gamma chain of the receptors for IL-2, IL-4, IL-7, IL-9, IL-15, and IL-21 on the plasma membrane to the nuclei of immune cells while the combination of JAK1/2 is important for the signalling of interferon (IFN)γ, G-CSF, IL-6, and IL-23.[7–9] Baricitinib (INCB028050) is a selective orally bioavailable JAK1/JAK2 inhibitor in development in RA which is currently in phase 3 trials; the results of phase 2 studies in methotrexate (MTX) incomplete responders (IR) designed to show efficacy have been reported in abstract form only at the time of writing. Tofacitinib is an orally available JAK 3/1/2 antagonist that has now been approved by the FDA for the treatment of RA.

SyK inhibitor

Fostamatinib has been investigated in several phase 2 and phase 3 clinical trials. The proof-of-concept trial was a randomized, double-blind, placebo-controlled study in 189 patients who had active RA despite receiving MTX.[10] Patients were treated with fostamatinib 50, 100, or 150 mg or placebo twice a day The twice-daily 100 and 150 mg doses were statistically superior to placebo in achieving the primary endpoint of an American College of Rheumatology (ACR) 20 response at month 3 (65%, 72% vs 38%, p <0.01; the 100 and 150 mg twice-daily doses were also statistically superior to placebo for ACR 50 and 70 response rate. 26% of patients receiving 100 mg twice daily and 49% receiving 150 mg achieved a DAS28 score less than 2.6 compared to 8% in the placebo group, which was also statistically significant. Responses were seen as early as week 1. The most common adverse events are summarized in Table 81.1 and included abdominal complaints (diarrhoea, nausea, gastritis, dyspepsia, and abdominal pain), hypertension, neutropenia, oedema, and increased alanine transaminase (ALT).

The second phase 2 study[11] was a similar design in 457 RA patients who were also MTX incomplete responders (MTX IR). The primary endpoint was the ACR 20 response at month 6; fostamatinib 100 mg twice daily and 150 mg once daily were compared to placebo. Both doses were statistically superior to placebo in achieving an ACR 20 response at month 6 (ACR 20: 67%, 57%, 35% in the 100 mg twice daily, 150 mg four times daily, and placebo groups, respectively (p < 0.001)). Statistically significant differences were seen for both doses compared to placebo for an ACR

50 response but only for the 100 mg twice daily dose for an ACR 70 response. A DAS28 score of less than 2.6 was observed in 31% of the 100 mg twice daily and 21% of the 150 mg daily groups vs 7% in the placebo group (p = 0.003). Improvement in function, as measured by a change in Health Assessment Questionnaire—Disability Index (HAQ-DI) and Short Form 36 (SF-36) scores, was recently reported.[12] Diarrhoea was seen in 19%, 12% and 3% of patients in the 100 mg twice daily, 150 mg daily, and placebo groups, respectively; 7%, 5%, and 1% respectively developed neutropenia; hypertension was seen in 29% of combined fostamatinib treated patients vs 17% in the placebo group (mean 3 mm increase in systolic blood pressure by month 1 in the fostamatinib group vs a 2 mm decline in the placebo group); 23% of the patients taking fostamatinib required initiation or change of anti-hypertensive medication vs 7% in the placebo group. Fostamatinib was reduced to 100 mg daily in 5% of patients for gastrointestinal symptoms, in 4% for elevation of aminotransferase, and in 3% for hypertension (Table 81.1) [13]

Fostamatinib 100 mg twice daily vs placebo has been investigated in a 3 month study in 219 patients with active RA who had failed TNFα inhibitors.[14] Fostamatinib failed to achieve the primary endpoint of a statistically significant difference in the ACR 20 response at month 3 vs placebo (38% vs 37%). A secondary endpoint, decrease in synovitis score on MRI, was achieved. Based on the results of the phase 2 studies, fostamatinib advanced to phase 3 trials both in patients with an incomplete response to DMARDs, including MTX, and in those who have failed TNFα inhibitors. In these trials, fostamatinib 100 mg twice daily was being compared to fostamatinib 100 mg twice daily for 4 weeks followed by 150 mg daily vs placebo. However, a phase 2b study comparing fostamatinib monotherapy to placebo at week 6 and to adalimumab monotherapy at week 24 was reported at EULAR 2013 (OP0048), prior to the conclusion of phase 3 studies. Multiple doses of fostamatinib were superior to placebo in reduction of DAS28 (CRP) at week 6 but adalimumab monotherapy was more effective than all doses of fostamatinib at week 24. Furthermore the previously noted adverse events of diarrhea and hypertension were again evident and the development of fostamatinib in RA was subsequently halted. The failure of this compound may be compound- rather than target- specific and other inhibitors of Syk are currently in development.

JAK3/1/2 inhibitor

Tofacitinib is an orally administered inhibitor of JAK 3, 1, and 2. Three multinational phase 2 trials have been reported.[15–17] These trials demonstrated efficacy of tofacitinib, both as monotherapy and in combination with MTX, with respect to ACR responses, HAQ improvement,[18] and achievement of DAS28 score less than 2.6. With respect to safety, tofacitinib was associated with dose-dependent development of neutropenia and lipid elevation, and an increase in mean serum creatinine. A clinically significant increase in ALT or aspartate aminotransferase (AST) was not seen with tofacitinib monotherapy but was seen in combination with MTX. Serious infectious episodes (SIE) occurred more frequently in patients treated with tofacitinib than those treated with placebo.

Based on the results of the three phase 2 trials, a large phase 3 programme was initiated to investigate tofacitinib as

Table 81.1 Fostamatinib: important adverse events with incidence rate 2/100 per year or more[12]

Adverse events	All placebo PY 109 (n = 273)	All fostamatinib PY 1038 (n = 803)
	Incidence per 100 PY (%)	Incidence per 100 PY (%)
Neutropenia	0.9 (0.4%)	8.3 (10.7%)
Anaemia	4.6 (1.8%)	3.5 (4.5%)
Diarrhoea	14.6 (5.9%)	21.4 (27.6%)
Abdominal pain/discomfort	11.0 (4.4%)	9.0 (11.6%)
Nausea	10.1 (4.0%)	8.0 (10.3%)
Vomiting	2.7 (1.1%)	4.7 (6.1%)
Peripheral oedema	0.9 (0.4%)	2.2 (2.9%)
Upper RTIs	32.9 (13.2%)	19.5 (25.2%)
Urinary tract infection	11.0 (4.4%)	9.8 (12.7%)
Increased liver transaminases	5.5 (2.2%)	8.3 (10.7%)
Dyslipidaemia	6.4 (2.6%)	2.4 (3.1%)
Headache	13.7 (5.5%)	8.7 (11.2%)
Dizziness	3.7 (1.5%)	3.9 (5.0%)
Hypertension	12.8 (5.1%)	17.6 (22.8%)

IR/100 PY, incidence per 100 patient-years; PY, patient-years; RTIs: respiratory tract infections.

monotherapy[19]; in combination with DMARDs in patients who had an incomplete response to DMARDs[20]; in combination with MTX in patients who had an incomplete response to MTX (in which radiographic progression was assessed)[21]; compared to adalimumab in patients who had an incomplete response to MTX, who were TNF inhibitor (TNFI) naive and who were eligible for treatment with a TNFI[22]; in patients who had failed TNF inhibitors and were taking background MTX[23]; and compared to MTX in patients who were MTX naive.[24] Based on the results of the phase 2 studies, tofacitinib 5 and 10 mg twice daily were chosen as the optimal doses for the phase 3 trials, considering efficacy and safety.

Study design in the phase 3 studies

The study plans of the six reported phase 3 studies were similar (Figure 81.1). In five trials, patients with active disease who had failed one or more DMARDs were studied; in the sixth trial, patients who were naive to MTX were treated with tofacitinib 5 or 10 mg twice daily or MTX as monotherapy. In the comparator to adalimumab study, the patients could not have been treated with a TNF inhibitor (TNFI) previously; in the TNFI failure study, all patients had failed at least one TNFI. The MTX incomplete responder study required the patient to have been treated with MTX, with an incomplete response; the DMARD incomplete responder study included patients with an incomplete response to DMARDs, which included MTX; stable background non-steroidal anti-inflammatory drugs (NSAIDs) and prednisone up to 10 mg a day were allowed in all studies. Patients who were initially treated with placebo and who did not have a decrease in tender and swollen joints of 20% or more at month 3 were advanced to treatment with tofacitinib at a preassigned dose of 5 mg or 10 mg twice daily. At month 6, all patients in the placebo group were switched to tofacitinib, again at preassigned doses. In the TNFI failure study, although there was a similar rescue at month 3 for patients treated with placebo, the study ended at month 6. In all studies other than the TNFI failure study, approximately 75% of patients were not from the United States or western Europe.

Phase 3 monotherapy study in DMARD incomplete responders

This study was conducted in 610 RA patients with active disease who had failed one or more DMARDs, which could have been a biological agent.[19] They received either 5 or 10 mg of tofacitinib twice daily orally as monotherapy (no concomitant DMARD) or placebo. The coprimary endpoints at month 3 were ACR 20 response, change from baseline in HAQ-DI, and percentage of patients achieving disease activity score 28—erythrocyte sedimentation rate (DAS28-ESR) less than 2.6. Both doses of tofacitinib were statistically superior to placebo in achieving an ACR 20/50/70 response and improvement in HAQ-DI, with benefit maintained to month 6. Patients switching to tofacitinib at month 3 showed a response similar to patients originally treated with tofacitinib. There were no statistical differences among the placebo, tofacitinib 5 mg or 10 mg groups with respect to achieving DAS28-ESR less than 2.6 (Table 81.2).

In this study, the placebo group had a higher incidence of serious adverse events (SAE), 4.9% vs less than 1%, and the incidence of liver test abnormalities was similar between the monotherapy and placebo groups.

Phase 3 DMARD incomplete responders study

In a study in DMARD incomplete responders continuing DMARDs, 792 RA patients who had failed one or more DMARDs, which could have been a biologic agent, were treated with either 5 or 10 mg of tofacitinib twice daily or placebo orally in combination with a continued background DMARD.[20] The coprimary endpoints at month 3 were the HAQ-DI change from baseline and at month 6, the ACR 20, response and the percentage of patients achieving DAS28-ESR less than 2.6. All three primary endpoints were met (Table 81.2).

Phase 3 MTX incomplete responders with radiographic outcomes study

A study in 800 MTX incomplete responders also assessed radiographic outcomes.[20] The coprimary endpoints were the HAQ-DI change from baseline at month 3 and the ACR 20 response, the change in the van der Heijde modified Sharp score (vdHmTSS)

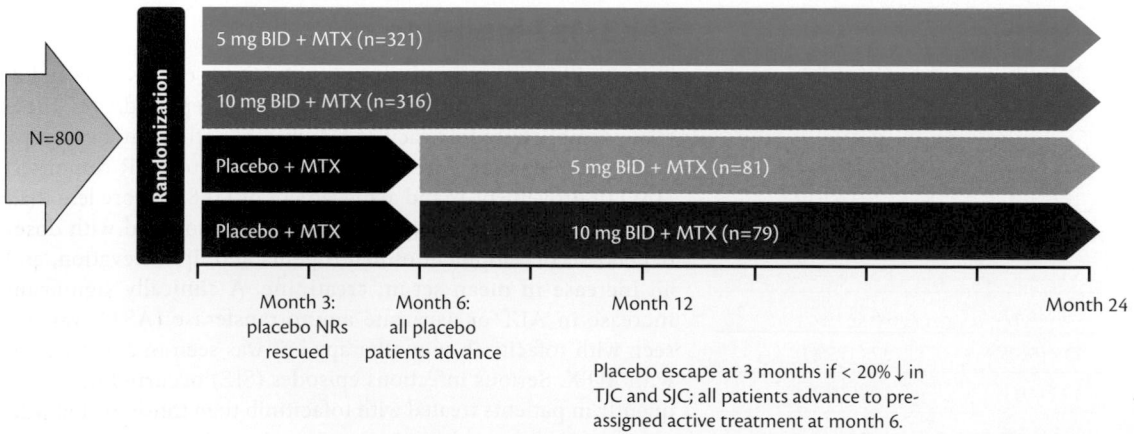

Fig. 81.1 Example of the plan for MTX IR assessing radiologic progression. Placebo patients were predetermined as to whether they would advance to 5 or 10 mg tofacitinib twice daily. Placebo patients were advanced to tofacitinib at month 3 if tender and swollen joints did not improve at least 20%; all placebo patients were advanced to tofacitinib at month 6. Patients on tofacitinib who did not improve by 20% or more at month 3 remained on their dose of tofacitinib.

Table 81.2 Clinical, functional, and radiographic results in tofacitinib phase 3 trials

	Mono N = 610			DMARD IR N = 792			MTX IR N = 800			Tofa/ADA vs Pbo N = 717				TNF IR N = 399			MTX naive N =952		
	P	5	10	P	5	10	P	5	10	P	5	10	ADA	P	5	10	MTX	5	10
ACR 20	27	60	68	31	53	58	25	52	62	28	52	53	47	24	42	48	51	69	72
ACR 50	13	31	37	10	28	35	25	35	50	12	37	35	28	8	27	28	34	50	56
ACR 70	6	15	20	2	10	10	10	15	25	2	20	22	9	2	14	11	15.	29	38
DAS↓	0.9	1.9.	2.0	NR	NR	NR	NR	NR	NR	1	2	2	1.9	0.9	1.9	2.1	2.2	2.8	3
DAS<2.6	4	6	10	2.7	11	15	2	7	18	1	7	13	6	2	7	11	13	20	23
HAQ-DI↓	.19	.50	.57	.21	.46	.56	.15	.40	.54	.24	.55	.61	.49	.18	.43	.48	.68	.86	.98
mTSS↑	ND	ND	ND	ND	ND	ND	.47	.12	.06	ND	ND	ND	ND	ND	ND	ND	.84	.18	.04

5, tofacitinib 5 mg po BID; 10, tofacitinib 10 mg po BID; ADA, adalimumab; DMARD IR, tofacitinib in DMARD incomplete responder study; Mono, tofacitinib monotherapy study; MTX, methotrexate; MTX IR, tofacitinib in MTX incomplete responders; ND, not done; NR, not reported; P, placebo; TNF IR, tofacitinib in TNFI incomplete responder study; Tofa/ADA vs Pbo, comparator trial of tofacitinib and adalimumab compared to placebo.

All studies 3 month endpoint, non-responder imputation, except Tofa/ADA vs Pbo = 6 months, DMARD IR DAS28 <2.6 and MTX IR = 6 months ACR50/70 without advancement penalty.

All statistically significant at p ≤ 0.05 except DAS < 2.6 in the monotherapy study; TSS progression in the 5 mg tofacitinib group (and thus p values not computed for change in HAQ-DI or DAS28 <2.6 per protocol).

from baseline, and the percentage of patients achieving DAS28-ESR less than 2.6 at month 6. Statistically significant improvements were seen in the ACR 20 response and in achievement of DAS28-ESR less than 2.6 versus placebo at month 6, and improvement of the HAQ-DI at month 3. At month 6, the change from baseline in the vdHmTSS, compared to placebo, was statistically significant for the 10 mg twice daily dose but not for the 5 mg twice daily dose (Table 81.2).

Phase 3 MTX incomplete responders comparing tofacitinib to adalimumab

A study of tofacitinib or adalimumab (as active comparator) in 717 patients on background MTX again used coprimary endpoints at month 3 of HAQ-DI change from baseline and at month 6, the ACR20 response, and the percentage of patients achieving DAS28-ESR less than 2.6.[22] Statistically significant changes were seen in both tofacitinib groups and adalimumab compared to placebo for each of these primary endpoints (Table 81.2).

Phase 3 TNFI incomplete responders study

A 6 month study was conducted in 399 RA patients with active disease despite concurrent MTX therapy who had failed one or more TNF inhibitor.[23] Subjects were treated with either 5 or 10 mg of tofacitinib twice daily or placebo in combination with background MTX. The majority of patients were from Europe and North America. The coprimary endpoints at month 3 were the HAQ-DI change from baseline, the ACR20 response, and the percentage of patients achieving DAS28-ESR less than 2.6; there was a statistically significant difference between both doses of tofacitinib and placebo for all three endpoints (Table 81.2).

Phase 3 monotherapy in patients naive to MTX study

A 24 month study was conducted in 952 RA patients with active disease who were naive to MTX.[24] Subjects were treated with either 5 or 10 mg of tofacitinib twice daily or MTX, titrated to 20 mg a week, as monotherapy. The coprimary endpoints at

Table 81.3 Important safety data from pooled phase 2, 3, and long-term extension studies of tofacitinib[26]

Event	% of patients
TEAE	66.2
Infections	39.7
Hb↓ ≥2 g or <8 g	2.5
AST/ALT >3 × ULN	1.1/1.7
ANC <1500	0.5
Creatinine↑ >33%	12.2

AST/ALT, aspartate/alanine aminotransferases; ANC, absolute neutrophil count; Hb, haemoglobin; TEAE, treatment-emergent adverse event; ULN, upper limit of normal.

Tofacitinib 5 or 10 mg po BID; 3227 patients; 3118 patient-years; mean treatment 349 days; 441 (13.7%) discontinued; 223 (6.9%) due to adverse event (AE); 42 (1.3%) due to lack of efficacy (LOE); serious adverse event (SAE): 337 patients (10.9%) incidence rate (IR): 11.34 (per 100 patient-years); serious infectious episode (SIE): 93 patients (2.9%) IR: 3.01 (per 100 patient-years)

month 6 were the change in the modified Sharp score and the ACR 70 response; there was a statistically significant difference between both doses of tofacitinib and MTX for both endpoints (Table 81.2).

JAK1/2 inhibitor

A 12 week phase 2A study was conducted in 302 patients who were MTX IR. Subjects continued MTX and were treated with placebo or baricitinib 1, 2, 4 or 8 mg orally once a day.[25] The primary endpoint was the combined ACR 20 response at week 12 of the combined 4 mg and 8 mg groups; there was a statistically significant difference between the combined groups (ACR 20 76% vs 41%, p <0.001) for the combined groups Both 4 mg and 8 mg once daily achieved statistically significant differences from placebo in ACR 20, ACR 50 and ACR 70 responses, DAS28 remission and improvement in HAQ and had an adverse event profile similar to

Table 81.4 Tofacitinib 5/10 mg BID: deaths and serious infections: phase 3 and long-term extension studies[27]

	Tofa (phase 3) n=3030	Pbo n=681	ADA n=204	Tofa (LTE) n=3227
Deaths n (%)	12 (0.4)	1 (0.15)	1 (0.49)	20 (0.62)
Events/100 pt-yrs	0.57	0.49	0.56	0.64
SIE n(%)	61(2)	3(0.44)	3(1.5)	93(2.9)
Events/100 pt-yrs	2.91	1.48	1.67	2.99

Deaths: 12 Phase 3: 5 infections, 3 other, 2 cardiovascular (CV), 1 trauma and 1 unknown; 20 long-term extension (LTE): 8 CV, 3 infection, 2 other, 1 cancer, 1 cardiac, and 5 unknown; infections: rate infectious episodes (IE) ≈ monotherapy or disease-modifying anti-rheumatic drugs (DMARDs); Rate serious infectious episodes (SIE) Tofacitinib 10 vs 5 ≈ in Phase 3; Rate of SIE in LTE: 10 > 5: (4.9 vs. 2.3) opportunistic infection (OI), uncommon. Herpes zoster >5% in LTE

tofacitinib.[25] The 4 mg dose was found to have significantly less adverse effects than 8 mg, and 4 mg is the dose being explored in phase 3 trials.

Safety

The safety profile of tofacitinib was similar in phase 2 and 3 trials and open-label extensions (Tables 81.3 and 81.4).[26,27]

Summary and clinical impact

The oral kinase inhibitors appear to be clinically effective. Fostamatinib was shown to be efficacious in MTX IR in two phase 2 studies but further development has been halted due to a combination of insufficient efficacy (as monotherapy compared to adalimumab) and adverse events. There is one report of baricitinib in MTX IR which showed that 4 mg and 8 mg orally once daily is clinically effective with a safety profile similar to tofacitinib; the 4 mg dose is the dose being explored in phase 3 trials, which should define it's clinical efficacy and safety.

Tofacitinib has been shown to be effective in multiple studies including use as monotherapy, in DMARD IR, in MTX IR, and in TNF inhibitor failures; it was comparable to adalimumab in patients with an IR to MTX. In MTX naive patients, both 5 mg and 10 mg orally twice daily were superior to MTX clinically, functionally and inhibiting radiographic progression. Both 5 mg and 10 mg twice daily are effective in improving patient-reported outcomes such as improvement in the HAQ-DI and SF-36.

Fostamatinib is associated with adverse effects of diarrhoea, hypertension, and liver test abnormalities. Tofacitinib is associated with neutropenia; elevation of lipids, liver tests, and creatinine; and anaemia in some patients. Similar adverse events were seen with baricitinib. With all three medications it appears that there is an increase in serious infections similar to the biological therapies currently approved; opportunistic infections have been described with tofacitinib as well, especially herpes zoster.

Clearly, regulatory authorities, as well as payers, will have a significant voice as to where these agents are used in the treatment paradigm; their decisions will be based on cost, cost-effectiveness, and safety. As the agents are oral, they should be more convenient, and one would hope cheaper, than biological agents. This could affect their uptake significantly.

Preliminary data have been reported with another molecule that inhibits JAK3[28]; this compound was found to be effective as monotherapy in a phase 2A study. Too few patients were studied to determine if this compound will have a distinct efficacy and safety profile to tofacitinib.

Rheumatologists are comfortable with biological agents, and know what to expect with respect to efficacy and safety. It will take time for them to become equally comfortable with these oral agents. Nonetheless, they should provide an attractive alternative for patients with active RA who cannot tolerate or do not respond to traditional oral DMARDs or biological agents.

Acknowledgements

No funding received for this manuscript. Consultant and study grants from Pfizer, Lilly, Vertex. Study grants from Astra-Zeneca.

References

1. Smolen JS, Aletaha D, Bijlsma JW et al. Treating rheumatoid arthritis to target: recommendations of an international task force. *Ann Rheum Dis* 2010;69:631–637.
2. Weinblatt ME, Coblyn JS, Fox DA et al. Efficacy of low-dose methotrexate in rheumatoid arthritis. *N Engl J Med* 1985;312:818–822.
3. Weinblatt ME, Kaplan H, Germain BF et al. Methotrexate in rheumatoid arthritis. A five-year prospective multicenter study. *Arthritis Rheum* 1994;37:1492–1498.
4. Cohen S, Fleischmann R. Kinase inhibitors: a new approach to rheumatoid arthritis treatment. *Curr Opin Rheumatol* 2010;22:330–335.
5. Fleischmann R. Novel small-molecular therapeutics for rheumatoid arthritis. *Curr Opin Rheumatol* 2012;24:335–341.
6. Bajpai M. Fostamatinib, a Syk inhibitor prodrug for the treatment of inflammatory diseases. *IDrugs*. 2009;12:174–185.
7. Ghoreschi K, Jesson MI, Li X et al. Modulation of innate and adaptive immune responses by tofacitinib (CP-690,550). *J Immunol* 2011;186:4234–4243.
8. Ghoreschi K, Laurence A, O'Shea JJ. Janus kinases in immune cell signaling. *Immunol Rev* 2009;228:273–287.
9. Fridman JS, Scherle PA, Collins R et al. Selective inhibition of JAK1 and JAK2 is efficacious in rodent models of arthritis: preclinical characterization of INCB028050. *J Immunol* 2010;184:5298–5307.
10. Weinblatt ME, Kavanaugh A, Burgos-Vargas R et al. Treatment of rheumatoid arthritis with a Syk kinase inhibitor: a twelve-week, randomized, placebo-controlled trial. *Arthritis Rheum* 2008;58:3309–3318.
11. Weinblatt ME, Kavanaugh A, Genovese MC et al. An oral spleen tyrosine kinase (Syk) inhibitor for rheumatoid arthritis. *N Engl J Med* 2010;363:1303–1312.
12. Weinblatt ME, Kavanaugh A, Genovese MC et al. Effects of fostamatinib (R788), an oral spleen tyrosine kinase inhibitor, on health-related quality of life in patients with active rheumatoid arthritis: analysis of patient-reported outcomes from a randomized, double-blind, placebo-controlled trial. *J Rheumatol* 2013;40:369–378.

13. Kavanaugh A, Weinblatt ME, Genovese MC et al. Longer-term safety of fostamatinib (R788) in patients with rheumatoid arthritis—analysis of clinical trial data from up to 2 years of exposure. *Arthritis Rheum* 2011;63:S1018.

14. Genovese MC, Kavanaugh A, Weinblatt ME et al. An oral Syk kinase inhibitor in the treatment of rheumatoid arthritis: a three-month randomized, placebo-controlled, phase II study in patients with active rheumatoid arthritis that did not respond to biologic agents. *Arthritis Rheum* 2011;63:337–345.

15. Kremer JM, Bloom BJ, Breedveld FC et al. The safety and efficacy of a JAK inhibitor in patients with active rheumatoid arthritis: Results of a double-blind, placebo-controlled phase IIa trial of three dosage levels of CP-690,550 versus placebo. *Arthritis Rheum* 2009;60:1895–1905.

16. Kremer JM, Cohen S, Wilkinson BE et al. A Phase 2B dose-ranging study of the oral JAK inhibitor tofacitinib (CP-690,550) versus placebo in combination with background methotrexate in patients with active rheumatoid arthritis and inadequate response to methotrexate alone. *Arthritis Rheum* 2012;64(4):970–981.

17. Fleischmann R, Cutolo M, Genovese MC et al. Phase 2B dose-ranging study of the oral JAK inhibitor tofacitinib (CP-690,550) or adalimumab monotherapy versus placebo in patients with active rheumatoid arthritis with an inadequate response to DMARDs. *Arthritis Rheum* 2012;64(3):617–629.

18. Coombs JH, Bloom BJ, Breedveld FC et al. Improved pain, physical functioning and health status in patients with rheumatoid arthritis treated with CP-690,550, an orally active Janus kinase (JAK) inhibitor: results from a randomised, double-blind, placebo-controlled trial. *Ann Rheum Dis* 2010;69:413–416.

19. Fleischmann R, Kremer J, Cush J et al. Placebo-controlled trial of tofacitinib monotherapy in rheumatoid arthritis. *N Engl J Med* 2012;367:495–507.

20. Kremer J, Li Z, Hall S et al. Tofacitinib (CP-690,550), an oral jak inhibitor, in combination with traditional DMARDs: phase 3 study in patients with active rheumatoid arthritis with inadequate response to DMARDs. *Ann Rheum Dis* 2011;70:611.

21. van der Heijde D, Tanaka Y, Fleischmann R et al. Tofacitinib (CP-690,550) in patients with rheumatoid arthritis on methotrexate: 12-month data from a 24-month phase 3 randomized radiographic study. *Arthritis Rheum* 2013;65:559–570.

22. van Vollenhoven RF, Fleischmann R, Cohen S et al. Tofacitinib or adalimumab versus placebo in rheumatoid arthritis. *N Engl J Med* 2012;367:508–519.

23. Burmester G, Blanco R, Charles-Schoeman C et al. Tofacitinib (CP-690,550) in combination with methotrexate in patients with active rheumatoid arthritis with an inadequate response to tumour necrosis factor inhibitors: a randomised phase 3 trial. *Lancet* 2013; 381(9865):451–460.

24. Lee E, Hall S, van Vollenhoven R et al. Radiographic, clinical and functional comparison of tofacitinib monotherapy versus methotrexate in methotrexate naive patients with rheumatoid arthritis. *Arthritis Rheum* 2012;64:S1049 (Abstract 2486).

25. Keystone E, Taylor P, Genovese M et al. Safety and efficacy of LY3009104 (JAK1/JAK2 inhibitor) in RA patients with inadequate response to MTX (Study I4V-MC-JADA). *Ann Rheum Dis* 2012;71(Suppl 3):LB0005.

26. Wollenhaupt J, Silverfield J, Lee EB et al. Tofacitinib (CP-690,550), an oral Janus kinase inhibitor in the treatment of rheumatoid arthritis: open-label, long term extension studies up to 36 months. *Arthritis Rheum* 2011;63:S152.

27. Cohen S, Radominski S, Asavantanabodee P et al. Tofacitinib (CP-690,550), an oral Janus kinase inhibitor: analysis of infections and all-cause mortality across phase 3 and long term extension studies in patients with rheumatoid arthritis. *Arthritis Rheum* 2011;63:S153.

28. Fleischmann R, Spencer-Green G, Fan F et al. Dose ranging study of VX-509, an oral selective JAK3 inhibitor, as monotherapy in patients with active rheumatoid arthritis (RA). *Arthritis Rheum* 2011; 63:LB3.

CHAPTER 82

Anti-cytokine biologics

Andrew J. K. Östör

Introduction

Produced in living systems, biologics comprise a group of recombinant proteins including antibodies and cytokine inhibitors. Following their introduction a seismic shift has occurred in the management of rheumatoid arthritis (RA) and a therapeutic landscape without them now seems inconceivable. The ascent of biologics occurred as a consequence of greater understanding of the proinflammatory mediators involved in the disease. At the vanguard has been tumour necrosis factor alpha (TNFα) antagonism and we now have five such agents at our disposal (infliximab, etanercept, adalimumab, certolizumab, golimumab)[1] as well as the interleukin (IL)-6 antagonist tocilizumab (Elliott et al.[1] is a key reference: the first randomized controlled trial (RCT) to show benefit of anti-TNF therapy in RA). These biologics are beneficial in a variety of clinical settings, including early and late disease, and have an acceptable safety profile. Not all anti-cytokine therapies have been successful, however, with the cost–benefit ratio of IL-1 antagonism with anakinra being deemed less favourable. A number of novel anti-cytokine biologics are in clinical trials which will increase the options to achieve individualized treatment and disease remission.

Aetiopathogenesis of rheumatoid arthritis

It is clear that cytokines are critical in the pathogenesis of RA, with the best-characterized being TNFα and IL-6. Their upregulation leads to the pathological manifestations of the condition including synovitis, and cartilage and bone destruction. Although the CD4+ T cell holds primacy as the orchestrator of the cell-mediated immune response in RA, it largely acts by stimulating other cells to produce cytokines including TNFα, IL-1, and IL-6.[2] Blocking cytokines therefore became a tantalizing prospect for treatment.

The pathogenesis of RA is discussed in detail in Chapter 109.

Properties of anti-cytokine biologics

A number of anti-TNF biologics exist, including monoclonal antibodies and a receptor fusion protein. Tocilizumab is an anti-IL-6 receptor monoclonal antibody and anakinra a recombinant IL-1 receptor antagonist. The agents currently available are listed in (Table 82.1).

Efficacy

Evidence base

Multiple RCTs using anti-cytokine biologics, usually in combination with methotrexate (MTX), have shown benefit, including signs and symptoms of disease, radiographic progression, function, and quality of life. In general these drugs work rapidly, with many patients experiencing improvement within weeks. Furthermore, a dramatic slowing of radiographic damage has resulted in an unprecedented alteration in the natural history of RA. Interestingly, an uncoupling of radiographic and clinical response was observed in some patients following TNF blockade, with slowing of bony damage even without a clear symptomatic response.[3] Tocilizumab has also been found to slow radiographic progression.[4]

Anti-cytokine biologics have led to significant benefits in patient-reported outcomes, with multiple trials showing improvement in function and quality of life indicators such as the Health Assessment Questionnaire (HAQ) and Sort Form 36 (SF-36). A systematic review of the efficacy of TNF antagonists calculated a number needed to treat of 5–6 for at least an acceptable response (ACR 20).[5] A recent Cochrane review found that the overall efficacy of biologic agents was similar, with the exception of anakinra which resulted in poorer responses.[6]

Anti-TNFα agents and productivity in rheumatoid arthritis

Several studies have shown that TNF inhibition increases the likelihood of remaining employed and reduces both presenteeism (reduced productivity) and absenteeism. This occurs in early and longstanding disease and in both 'real world' practice and clinical trials.[7–9] In the PROWD study, for example, job loss was significantly lower in patients receiving combination therapy with adalimumab than in those treated with MTX monotherapy.[10] Improvement in this area clearly has enormous health economic implications.

Window of opportunity

One of the most important lessons to emerge from research into RA treatment has been the need to treat patients as early in the disease process as possible and to adopt a tight control paradigm (see Chapter 112). Investigation continues to determine the optimal point to introduce anti-cytokine agents, but the benefits of targeting early disease have been clearly demonstrated.[9,11,12] (Goekoop-Ruiterman et al.[11] is a key reference, demonstrating

Table 82.1 Properties of anti-cytokine biological agents

Generic drug name	Chemical structure	Year of first approval	Brand name	Half-life	Dosage
Etanercept	Recombinant human soluble p75 TNFα receptor fusion protein	1998	Enbrel	70–132 h	25 mg twice weekly or 50 mg weekly SC
Infliximab	Recombinant chimeric monoclonal antibody to TNFα	1999	Remicade	9.5 days	3 mg/kg IV repeated 2 weeks and 6 weeks after the first infusion, then every 8 weeks
Adalimumab	Recombinant fully human monoclonal antibody to TNFα	2002	Humira	10–20 days	40 mg SC fortnightly
Golimumab	Recombinant fully human monoclonal antibody to TNFα	Apr 2009	Simponi	7–20 days	50 mg SC monthly
Certolizumab Pegol	Pegylated recombinant humanized anti-TNFα antibody Fab fragment	May 2009	Cimzia	14 days	400 mg SC at 0, 2 & 4 weeks then 200 mg fortnightly
Tocilizumab	Recombinant humanized monoclonal antibody to the IL-6 receptor	January 2009	Actemra (also RoActemra)	8–14 days	8 mg/kg IV monthly
Anakinra	Recombinant IL-1 receptor antagonist	November 2001	Kinaret	4–6 h	100 mg SC daily

that early intervention with combination therapy results in optimal outcomes.)

Further management issues

Anti-cytokine biologics are not always successful and failure of these drugs may occur due to:

- non-response (primary inefficacy)

- inefficacy following initial response (secondary inefficacy)

- incomplete response (patient remains in an unacceptably high disease state)

- toxicity

Failure of biologic agents has been most characterized for TNF antagonists, because they were first to market. Significant observational data has confirmed the benefit of switching to an alternative anti-TNF following loss of response with a first. However, only one RCT, using golimumab, has confirmed these observational data.[13] Other biologics found to be effective following failure of TNF antagonism include tocilizumab, rituximab, and abatacept.[14] A potentially important cause for a loss of response is immunogenicity, which can occur with any biologic.[15] Infliximab appears the most immunogenic of the anti-TNF drugs, with anti-infliximab antibodies also associated with infusion reactions.

Coprescription of MTX improves the efficacy of TNF blockade efficacy but many patients do not tolerate this disease-modifying anti-rheumatic drug (DMARD). Adalimumab, etanercept, and certolizumab are licensed for monotherapy when MTX is contraindicated or is not tolerated, as is tocilizumab. However tocilizumab is the only agent to show superiority to MTX when compared head-to-head as monotherapy and it appears that maximal response to tocilizumab is independent of background MTX.[16,17] (Jones et al.[16] is a key reference: the first study to show superiority of a biological agent when given as monotherapy when compared with MTX

monotherapy). Tocilizumab may also be used with non-MTX DMARDs with significant benefit.[18]

IL-1 antagonism

Despite positive evidence from animal models, blockade of IL-1 in humans has been less successful.[6] Apart from the reduced efficacy compared with other anti-cytokine biologics, the daily subcutaneous injections were less well tolerated by patients.

Safety of anti-cytokine biologics

As cytokines are critical for homeostasis, it may be anticipated that blockade of these molecules would result in a number of deleterious effects. In general, however, the major side-effect profile of anti-cytokine biologics has been favourable.[6] As more than 2 million patients worldwide have received infliximab, adalimumab, and/or etanercept for a variety of conditions, there is substantial real world experience. In addition, national biologic registries have been developed to monitor long-term safety (see Chapter 34). The British Society for Rheumatology Biologics Register (BSRBR) was formulated to detect an increased risk of lymphoma with TNF blockade, but a wealth of further safety data has been forthcoming.

No increased risk of lymphoma has been seen to date. However, the register has demonstrated that anti-TNF therapy is associated with an increased risk of serious infection. This occurs particularly in the first 3–6 months of the treatment where the risk almost doubled compared to controls taking non-biologic DMARDs.[19] A recent report has also confirmed an increased hospitalization rate for varicella infections compared with the general population, although the absolute risk remains low.[20]

Rarer side effects may be missed because of their short-term nature and the homogeneous group of patients used in clinical trials. A case in point was the reactivation of latent tuberculosis (TB) infection with anti-TNF agents observed in postmarketing surveillance. The risk appears less with etanercept, possibly due to its construct and mechanism of action.[21] Consequently, screening is now mandatory for latent TB infection prior to starting TNF antagonists. A substantial reduction in TB cases has been seen as a result. Other serious opportunistic infections reported following TNFα antagonism include reactivated histoplasmosis, listeriosis, pulmonary aspergillosis, and pneumocystis pneumonia, although these are all rare.

Other safety issues with TNF antagonism

Demyelination

One unexpected adverse event was demyelinating disease. Although the number of cases was no greater than would be expected in the general population, the results of two clinical trials found a worsening of multiple sclerosis in patients with known disease.[22,23] The precise role of anti-TNF agents in triggering demyelination is unclear, but they are contraindicated in patients with a known history, or family history, of such disorders.

Autoantibodies

Autoantibody production has been documented in patients receiving TNF antagonists, especially infliximab, with up to 60% of patients developing new anti-nuclear antibodies (ANA).[24] Lupus like syndromes have rarely been reported but the symptoms are usually mild and respond to stopping the medication. However, occasional patients have developed anti-dsDNA antibodies associated with renal or cerebral lupus.

Heart failure

As TNFα is upregulated in heart failure, trials were undertaken to determine whether blocking this cytokine would be beneficial. However, a worsening of heart failure was seen in these studies including some deaths.[25,26] Despite this observation a review of TNF antagonist use in RA found no worsening of heart failure relative to controls.[27] As RA increases cardiovascular risk per se, the true role that TNF antagonism plays in relation to cardiac disease remains unclear. Nonetheless, TNF antagonists remain contraindicated in patients with severe heart failure.

Malignancy

Given the immunosuppressive effects of the TNF antagonists, concerns exist regarding the development of malignancy, especially after prolonged use. For solid tumours, data from the United States National Cancer Institute and the Swedish register is reassuring, with no evident increased risk.[28,29] The data overall regarding the development of lymphoproliferative malignancies is reassuring. TNFα antagonists have been implicated in the development of bone marrow suppression although all reported cases were in patients with chronic RA receiving multiple medications.

Interstitial lung disease

Uncontrolled reports exist of a worsening of interstitial lung disease in patients treated with biologics, especially anti-TNF agents.[30] At the same time, observational data from the BSRBR are reassuring.[31] Vigilance must be employed, however, in any patient treated with biologics with pre-existing lung disease.

Tocilizumab

Like the anti-TNF agents, tocilizumab has been found to have an acceptable safety and tolerability profile. The experience is less than with anti-TNF agents as tocilizumab has only recently been licensed. The most common side effects in clinical trials were infections such as nasopharyngitis; however, a small but significant increase in serious infection was also seen, consistent with the rate with other biologic agents.[32]

Lower gastrointestinal complications have been described with tocilizumab, such as diverticular perforation, at a rate of 1.9 per 1000 patient years.[33] This is slightly higher than with traditional DMARDs and anti-TNF agents but less than with corticosteroids or NSAIDs.

A reduction in neutrophil count below 1×10^9/litre occurred in 3.4% of patients receiving tocilizumab 8 mg/kg plus DMARDs in controlled trials, approximately one-half of these occurring within 8 weeks of starting therapy. Despite this, no increase in infections was seen. Transient elevations in alanine/aspartate transaminases (ALT/AST) have also been observed particularly in patients who received tocilizumab plus DMARDs, especially MTX.

As the lipid profile represents a 'negative' acute-phase response, reduction of inflammation leads to an elevation in lipids. This has been seen with anti-TNF agents and tocilizumab. Approximately 24% of patients receiving tocilizumab experienced sustained elevations in total cholesterol to 6.2 mmol/litre or more, with 15% experiencing a sustained increase in low-density lipoprotein (LDL) to 4.1 mmol/litre or more. No increase in cardiovascular events was seen in patients with a rise in lipid parameters, although longer-term data are required. As inflammation itself leads to an increase in cardiovascular disease, attempts to block this should be beneficial with respect to cardiovascular risk.

Tocilizumab does not appear to reactivate TB or lead to the emergence of ANAs. There is also no evidence at present that tocilizumab increases the risk of malignancy.

Biological combination therapy

Trials using combinations of biological agents have not been successful, including etanercept with anakinra and abatacept with etanercept.[34,35] An increased risk of adverse events, including serious infections, was seen without an improvement in efficacy. Therefore combining biologics is not currently recommended.

Precautions and contraindications

Anti-TNF

Contraindications to use include active TB or other active infection as well as moderate to severe heart failure and demyelination. Their use is also cautioned in patients with a history of malignancy, blood dyscrasias, and chronic obstructive pulmonary disease as well as certain viral infections, including hepatitis B and C, and alcoholic hepatitis.

Anti-IL-6

Similar precautions exist as for anti-TNF agents. Inhibition of C-reactive protein (CRP), and neutropenia in some patients, requires vigilance as signs and symptoms of sepsis may be masked. Tocilizumab should also be used with particular caution in patients with a history of diverticulitis. Monitoring of lipids, hepatic enzymes, neutrophils, and platelets is required.

Use in pregnancy/breast feeding

The use of anti-cytokine drugs in pregnancy and breast feeding is currently contraindicated. This is in part because generally these agents are coprescribed with MTX. Data from spontaneous reports and registries has been encouraging, however, with reports of normal pregnancies in patients receiving anti-cytokine biologics.[36] Further data are required in this area, and with regard to their use during breastfeeding.

Monitoring

Prior to treatment routine screening should include full blood count (FBC), U&E, and liver function tests (LFT), as well as chest radiograph (CXR), followed by FBC and LFTs every 3 months (many patients will be receiving concurrent MTX therefore monitoring for this will suffice).

In relation to anti-IL-6 therapy lipids should be checked prior to treatment and then following 3 months of treatment. FBC and LFTs should be monitored monthly in the first 3 months of treatment then at 2–3 monthly intervals.

Vigilance for possible exacerbation of interstitial lung disease (ILD) is required, but serial CXRs are not recommended.

Guidelines and recommendations for anti-TNF agents

The licences for TNF antagonists and tocilizumab require the failure of at least one conventional DMARD prior to their prescription. In addition a number of guidelines have been developed for the use of anti-cytokine therapies in RA. The European League Against Rheumatism (EULAR) guidelines provide robust recommendations for the management of RA. They state that if the treatment target, such as disease remission, is not achieved following the first DMARD strategy in the presence of poor prognostic factors, or in patients responding insufficiently to DMARDs, then biological therapy should be considered. These individuals may be considered for combination DMARDs plus a biologic at the outset if poor prognostic features are present.[37] The ACR 2008 guidelines largely concur with the EULAR recommendations.

In the United Kingdom the role of the National Institute for Health and Clinical Excellence (NICE) is principally to determine the health economic implications of therapeutic interventions. The threshold for obtaining a biologic in the United Kingdom is currently high. However, due to the emerging evidence base the British Society for Rheumatology (BSR) has revised their guidelines regarding eligibility for biologic treatment.[38]

Pharmaco-economics

Although biologic therapy is expensive, in the region of £10 000 per patient per year, this should be set against the enormous societal impact of RA. Up to 50% of patients become work disabled within 10 years of disease onset and the total cost of RA in Europe has been estimated as €45.3 billion annually.[39] The cost of biologics will fall once patents expire, biosimilars arrive, and further agents are developed.

Future

Anti-cytokine therapy is well embedded in the management of moderate to severe RA but not all patients respond to the current agents. Research continues to identify biomarkers of response and prognostic factors to individualize treatment. A number of novel anti-cytokine therapies are being trialled, such as anti-IL-17 and anti-IL12/23. However, it remains to be seen whether these will have an advantage over the currently available drugs. In addition, the pre-eminence of anti-cytokine therapy for RA may be challenged if the promise of intracellular small molecule therapies (e.g. JAK/STAT inhibitors) is realized (see Chapter 81).

Over the next few years, treat-to-target strategies will ensure early review of patients with brisk escalation of treatment to switch off the aberrant immune-inflammatory process. The future is consequently bright for patients with RA, especially when biologics are used at the appropriate time in order to maximize the chance of remission.

Conclusion

Perhaps in no area of medicine have the recent therapeutic advances been as great as in RA. This has largely been due to biologic therapies, of which we have the greatest experience with anti-cytokine agents. TNFα antagonists currently rule supreme in the hierarchy of biologics due to their efficacy and safety in the long term; however, IL-6 receptor blockade is developing a solid track record. Thankfully for patients we now have the ability to profoundly alter the natural history of RA resulting in outcomes unimaginable even a decade ago.

Case history

A 63 year old woman with a 3 year history of seropositive, non-erosive RA presented with a flare of disease over 2 months. She had previously been well controlled on MTX 25 mg/week, folic acid 5 mg/week, and hydroxychloroquine 200 mg twice daily. Her erythrocyte sedimentation rate (ESR) was 47 mm/h and her DAS28 was 5.6. She was finding it increasing difficult to work and was considering early retirement although she loved her job as the manager of a care home for elderly people. It was decided to commence anti-TNF therapy and after 6 weeks she had responded well with a DAS28 of 3.1. After 6 months of the biologic her disease was in remission (DAS28 2.4), she was working, and playing golf in her spare time.

References

1. Elliott MJ, Maini RN, Feldmann M et al. Randomised double-blind comparison of chimeric monoclonal antibody to tumour necrosis factor α (cA2) versus placebo in rheumatoid arthritis. *Lancet* 1994;344: 1105–1110.
2. Choy EH, Panayi GS. Cytokine pathways and joint inflammation in rheumatoid arthritis. *N Engl J Med* 2001; 344:907–916.
3. Smolen JS, Han C, Bala M et al., ATTRACT Study Group. Evidence of radiographic benefit of treatment with infliximab plus MTX in rheumatoid arthritis patients who had no clinical improvement: a detailed subanalysis of data from the anti-tumor necrosis factor trial in rheumatoid arthritis with concomitant therapy study. *Arthritis Rheum* 2005; 52:1020–1030.
4. Kremer JM, Blanco R, Brzosko M, Burgos-Vargas R, Halland AM, Vernon E, Ambs P, Fleischmann R. et al. Tocilizumab inhibits structural joint damage in rheumatoid arthritis patients with inadequate responses to methotrexate: results from the double-blind treatment phase of a randomized placebo-controlled trial of tocilizumab safety and prevention of structural joint damage at one year. *Arthritis Rheum.* 2011;63:609–621.

5. Alberto Alonso-Ruiz A, Pijoan Jose Ignacio Pijoan, Ansuategui Eukene Ansuategui, Arantxa Urkaregi, Marcelo Calabozo, and Antonio Quintana et al. Tumor necrosis factor alpha drugs in rheumatoid arthritis: systematic review and metaanalysis of efficacy and safety *BMC Musculoskelet Disord.* 2008; 9:52.

6. Singh JA, Christensen R, Wells GA et al. Biologics for rheumatoid arthritis: an overview of Cochrane reviews. *Cochrane Database Syst Rev* 2009;(4):CD007848.

7. Kavanaugh A, Smolen JS, Emery P et al. Effect of certolizumab pegol with methotrexate on home and work place productivity and social activities in patients with active rheumatoid arthritis. *Arthritis Rheum* 2009; 61: 1592–1600.

8. Smolen JS, Han C, van der Heijde D et al. Infliximab treatment maintains employability in patients with early rheumatoid arthritis. *Arthritis Rheum* 2006; 54: 716–722.

9. Emery P, Breedveld FC, Hall S et al. Comparison of methotrexate monotherapy with a combination of methotrexate and etanercept in active, early, moderate to severe rheumatoid arthritis (COMET): a randomised, double-blind, parallel treatment trial. *Lancet* 2008; 372: 375–382.

10. Bejarano V, Quinn M, Conaghan PG et al. Effect of early use of the anti-tumor necrosis factor adalimumab on the prevention of job loss in patients with early rheumatoid arthritis. *Arthritis Rheum* 2008;59:1467–1474.

11. Goekoop-Ruiterman YPM, de Vries-Bouwstra JK, Allart CF et al. Clinical and radiographic outcomes of four different treatment strategies in patients with early rheumatoid arthritis (the BeSt study): A randomized, controlled trial. *Arthritis Rheum* 2005;52:3381–3390.

12. van der Heijde D, Breedveld FC, Kavanaugh A et al. Disease activity, physical function, and radiographic progression after longterm therapy with adalimumab plus methotrexate: 5-year results of PREMIER. *J Rheumatol* 2010;37:2237–2246.

13. Smolen JS, Kay J, Doyle MK et al.; GO-AFTER study investigators. Golimumab in patients with active rheumatoid arthritis after treatment with tumour necrosis factor alpha inhibitors (GO-AFTER study): a multicentre, randomised, double-blind, placebo-controlled, phase III trial. *Lancet* 2009;374:210–221.

14. Smolen JS, Aletaha D, Koeller M, Weisman MH, Emery P. New therapies for treatment of rheumatoid arthritis. *Lancet* 2007;370:1861–1874.

15. Bartelds GM, Krieckaert CL, Nurmohamed MT, et al. Development of antidrug antibodies against adalimumab and association with disease activity and treatment failure during long-term follow-up. *JAMA* 2011;305:1460–1468.

16. Jones G, Sebba A, Gu J et al. Comparison of tocilizumab monotherapy versus methotrexate monotherapy in patients with moderate to severe rheumatoid arthritis: The AMBITION study. *Ann Rheum Dis* 2010;69:88–96.

17. Dougados M, Kissel K, Sheeran T et al. Adding tocilizumab or switching to tocilizumab monotherapy in methotrexate inadequate responders: 24-week symptomatic and structural results of a 2-year randomised controlled strategy trial in rheumatoid arthritis (ACT-RAY). *Ann Rheum Dis* 2013;72(1):43–50.

18. Genovese MC, McKay JD, Nasonov EL et al. Interleukin-6 receptor inhibition with tocilizumab reduces disease activity in rheumatoid arthritis with inadequate response to disease-modifying antirheumatic drugs: The tocilizumab in combination with traditional disease-modifying antirheumatic drug therapy study. *Arthritis Rheum* 2008;58:2968–2980.

19. Galloway JB, Hyrich KL, Mercer LK et al.; BSRBR Control Centre Consortium; British Society for Rheumatology Biologics Register. Anti-TNF therapy is associated with an increased risk of serious infections in patients with rheumatoid arthritis especially in the first 6 months of treatment: updated results from the British Society for Rheumatology Biologics Register with special emphasis on risks in the elderly. *Rheumatology* 2011;50:124–131.

20. García-Doval I, Pérez Zafrilla B, Descalzo MA et al.; BIOBADASER 2.0 Study Group. Incidence and risk of hospitalisation due to shingles and chickenpox in patients with rheumatic diseases treated with TNF antagonists. *Ann Rheum Dis* 2010;69:1751–1755.

21. Gardam MA, Keystone EC, Menzies R et al. Anti-tumour necrosis factor agents and tuberculosis risk: mechanisms of action and clinical management. *Lancet Infect Dis* 2003;3:148–155.

22. Mohan N, Edwards ET, Cupps TR et al. Demyelination occurring during anti-tumor necrosis factor alpha therapy for inflammatory arthritides. *Arthritis Rheum* 2001;44:2862–2869.

23. The Lenercept Multiple Sclerosis Study Group and The University of British Columbia MS/MRI Analysis Group. TNF neutralization in MS: results of a randomized, placebo-controlled multicenter study. *Neurology* 1999;53:457–465.

24. Lipsky PE, van der Heijde DMFM, St Clair EW et al. Infliximab and methotrexate in the treatment of rheumatoid arthritis. *N Engl J Med* 2000;343:1594–1602.

25. Chung ES, Packer M, Lo KH, Fasanmade AA, Willerson JT; Anti-TNF Therapy Against Congestive Heart Failure Investigators. Randomized, double-blind, placebo-controlled, pilot trial of infliximab, a chimeric monoclonal antibody to tumor necrosis factor-alpha, in patients with moderate-to-severe heart failure: results of the anti-TNF Therapy Against Congestive Heart Failure (ATTACH) trial. *Circulation* 2003; 107:3133–3140.

26. Mann DL, McMurray JJ, Packer M et al. Targeted anticytokine therapy in patients with chronic heart failure: results of the Randomized Etanercept Worldwide Evaluation (RENEWAL). *Circulation* 2004;109: 1594–1602.

27. Wolfe F, Michaud MS. Congestive heart failure in rheumatoid arthritis: rates, predictors and the effect of anti-TNF therapy. *Am J Med* 2004;116:305–311.

28. Keystone CE. Safety of biologic therapies—an update. *J Rheumatol* 2005;32 Suppl 74:8–12.

29. Askling J, van Vollenhoven RF, Granath F et al. Cancer risk in patients with rheumatoid arthritis treated with anti-tumor necrosis factor alpha therapies: does the risk change with the time since start of treatment? *Arthritis Rheum* 2009;60(11):3180–3189.

30. Hadjinicolaou AV, Nisar MK, Bhagat S et al. Non-infectious pulmonary complications of newer biological agents for rheumatic diseases—a systematic literature review. *Rheumatology* 2011;50:2297–2305.

31. Dixon WG, Hyrich KL, Watson KD, Lunt M; BSRBR Control Centre Consortium, Symmons DP; British Society for Rheumatology Biologics Register. Influence of anti-TNF therapy on mortality in patients with rheumatoid arthritis-associated interstitial lung disease: results from the British Society for Rheumatology Biologics Register. *Ann Rheum Dis* 2010;69:1086–1091.

32. Campbell L, Chen C, Bhagat SS, Parker RA, Östör AJ. Risk of adverse events including serious infections in rheumatoid arthritis patients treated with tocilizumab: a systematic literature review and meta-analysis of randomized controlled trials. *Rheumatology* 2011;50:552–562.

33. Gout T, Ostör AJ, Nisar MK. Lower gastrointestinal perforation in rheumatoid arthritis patients treated with conventional DMARDs or tocilizumab: a systematic literature review. *Clin Rheumatol* 2011;30: 1471–1474.

34. Genovese MC, Cohen S, Moreland L, Lium D, Robbins S, et al. Combination therapy with etanercept and anakinra in the treatment of patients with rheumatoid arthritis who have been treated unsuccessfully with methotrexate. *Arthritis Rheum* 2004;50:1412–1419.

35. Weinblatt M, Schiff M, Goldman A et al. Selective costimulation modulation using abatacept in patients with active rheumatoid arthritis while receiving etanercept: a randomised clinical trial. *Ann Rheum Dis* 2007;66:228–234.

36. Verstappen SM, King Y, Watson KD, Symmons DP, Hyrich KL; BSRBR Control Centre Consortium, BSR Biologics Register. Anti-TNF therapies and pregnancy: outcome of 130 pregnancies in the British Society for Rheumatology Biologics Register. *Ann Rheum Dis* 2011;70:823–826.

37. Smolen JS, Landewé R, Breedveld FC et al. EULAR recommendations for the management of rheumatoid arthritis with synthetic and biological disease-modifying antirheumatic drugs. *Ann Rheum Dis* 2010;69:964–975.

38. Deighton C, Hyrich K, Ding T et al.; BSR Clinical Affairs Committee & Standards, Audit and Guidelines Working Group and the BHPR. BSR and BHPR rheumatoid arthritis guidelines on eligibility criteria for the first biological therapy. *Rheumatology (Oxford)* 2010;49(6):1197–1199.

39. Lundkvist J, Kastang F, Kobelt G. The burden of rheumatoid arthritis and access to treatment: health burden and costs. *Eur J Health Econ* 2008;8(Suppl 2):S49–S60.

Sources of patient information

American College of Rheumatology (ACR): www.rheumatology.org
Arthritis Care: www.arthritiscare.org.uk
Arthritis Research Campaign (ARC): www.arthritisresearchuk.org
British Society for Rheumatology (BSR): www.rheumatology.org.uk
DAS on line: www.das-score.nl
European League Against Rheumatism (EULAR): www.eular.org
National Institute for Health and Clinical Excellence (NICE): www.nice.org.uk
National Rheumatoid Arthritis Society (NRAS): www.nras.org.uk

CHAPTER 83

Rituximab and abatacept

John D. Isaacs and Philip M. Brown

Introduction

In contrast to cytokine blockade, which targets downstream mediators of joint inflammation, anti-cellular biologics target cells that are proposed to coordinate the immunopathology of rheumatoid arthritis (RA) (Figure 83.1). Currently available agents target two key players in RA pathogenesis: B cells and T cells. B cells are targeted and killed by rituximab, whereas T cells are modulated by abatacept, which interferes with their activation without killing them.

Rituximab

Rituximab is a chimeric human IgG1 monoclonal antibody (mAb) that targets the four-transmembrane phosphoprotein CD20. The function of CD20 is not fully elucidated, but involves calcium signalling and the formation of lipid rafts. Rituximab binds to CD20 and induces cell lysis by antibody-mediated cellular cytotoxicity, complement mediated cell lysis, and promotion of apoptosis. CD20 is expressed on pre-B cells and mature B cells, but not plasma cells or pluripotent B-cell precursors. Consequently, rituximab results in rapid B-cell depletion with subsequent recovery and minimal impairment of pre-existing humoral immunity. CD20 is also expressed on a minor proportion of mature T cells. These produce interleukin (IL)-1β and tumour necrosis factor alpha (TNFα) although the relevance of their depletion to rituximab efficacy is unclear.[1]

Efficacy

Six randomized controlled trials (RCTs) have investigated rituximab in RA (Table 83.1). In each study rituximab was administered as two infusions given 14 days apart. The first compared rituximab monotherapy, rituximab plus cyclophosphamide, and rituximab plus methotrexate (MTX) vs MTX monotherapy in MTX inadequate responders.[2] At 24 weeks, all active treatment groups demonstrated superiority over MTX monotherapy. By 48 weeks, however, only the combination groups retained superiority and responses were more robust with MTX cotherapy. The second phase 2 study (DANCER) compared 500 mg and 1000 mg infusions of rituximab.[3] Both were effective but 1000 mg led to more American College of Rheumatology70 (ACR70) and European League Against Rheumatism (EULAR) good responses. This trial also compared regimes for minimizing cytokine release reactions (see 'Adverse effects'). Earlier trials had combined premedication with intravenous methylprednisolone (days 1 and 15) with oral prednisolone on days 2–14 but DANCER concluded that the latter was unnecessary.

The phase 3 REFLEX study confirmed rituximab's efficacy, in combination with MTX, in patients who had failed at least one anti-TNF agent (current licensed indication).[4] The primary outcome (ACR 20 at 24 weeks) was achieved by 51% of rituximab recipients and only 18% in the placebo group, who continued MTX and received placebo infusions. ACR 50 and 70 responses were achieved in 27 and 12% (rituximab) vs 5 and 1% (placebo). EULAR moderate and good responses were seen in 50% and 15% respectively (rituximab), vs 20% and 2% (placebo). There were also improvements in fatigue, function, and quality of life outcomes. In addition, radiographic joint damage was reduced by active treatment at 52 and 104 weeks.[5] The benefits of rituximab have subsequently been confirmed in MTX inadequate responders, in the SERENE and MIRROR studies, as well as in MTX-naive patients in the IMAGE study, but neither of these is a licensed indication.[6–8] While rituximab's licence requires cotherapy with MTX, postmarketing data suggest that leflunomide may also provide effective background therapy.[9] Table 83.1 summarizes phase 2 and 3 trials with rituximab.

Although B-cell depletion occurs rapidly following rituximab infusions, the maximum therapeutic effect may not be seen for 12–16 weeks. The duration of benefit following a course of treatment is variable but is usually at least 6 months. There is some evidence that more robust responses are experienced by patients who are seropositive for rheumatoid factor (RF), anti-citrullinated peptide autoantibodies (ACPA), or both. Most clinical trials contain too few seronegative patients to robustly address this question, but pooled trial data and registry data support this observation.[10,11] Other response predictors are being actively sought, but none has been validated. However, emerging evidence suggests that response may relate to the depth of B-cell depletion.[12] Patients with higher circulating memory B-cell and plasmablast counts at baseline may also respond less well.[13–15] However, these observations require validation and currently have minimal utility in the clinic.

Mode of action

There are three potential mechanisms by which B-cell depletion could improve RA symptoms. The first is via an effect on circulating

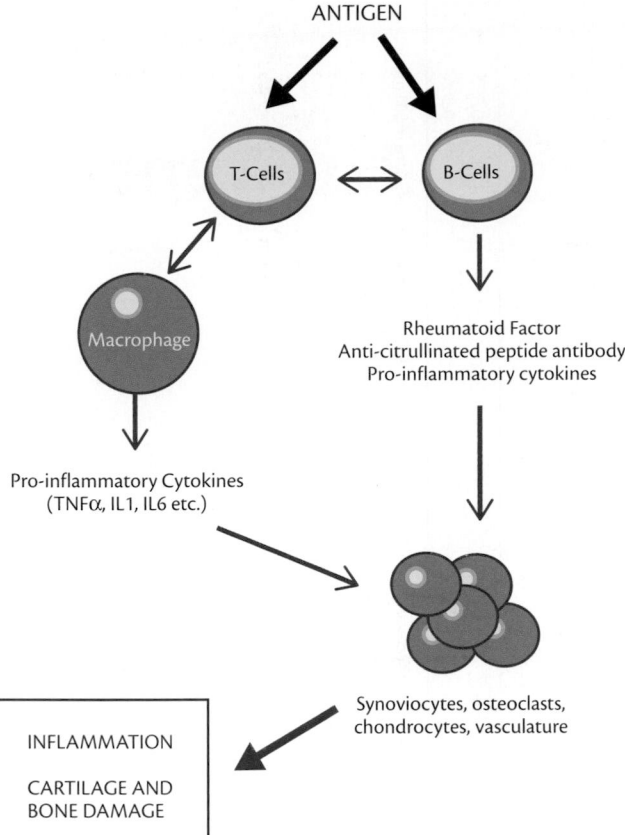

ANTIGEN

T-Cells ↔ B-Cells

Macrophage

Rheumatoid Factor
Anti-citrullinated peptide antibody
Pro-inflammatory cytokines

Pro-inflammatory Cytokines
(TNFα, IL1, IL6 etc.)

Synoviocytes, osteoclasts,
chondrocytes, vasculature

INFLAMMATION

CARTILAGE AND
BONE DAMAGE

Fig. 83.1 A simplifed model of RA pathogenesis. T and B cells respond to autoantigen by releasing proinflammatory cytokines and autoantibodies (B cells only). These two lymphocyte classes also interact with one another directly, as well as with other cell types such as macrophages. Ultimately, via soluble mediators and by direct interaction, they activate joint resident cells such as synoviocytes, osteoclasts. and chondrocytes and also generate an acute inflammatory reaction within the joint, ultimately leading to joint damage and destruction. By targeting B cells and T cells respectively, rituximab and abatacept act 'upstream' in RA pathogenesis compared to biologics that target proinflammatory cytokines.

autoantibody levels, although treatment leads to a variable reduction and rarely results in their complete disappearance from serum.[16] Furthermore, there is no clear evidence for a direct pathogenic role for either RF or ACPA in RA. A second possibility relates to loss of cytokine production by depleted B cells, but the relatively slow onset of action argues against this. Thirdly, B-cell presentation of antigen to autoreactive T cells could provide an explanation, consistent with rituximab's slow onset of action. Direct evidence in humans is lacking but there are supportive preclinical data.[17] Biomarker studies have not so far demonstrated a clear association between synovial B-cell depletion and rituximab efficacy, although a small, uncontrolled study suggested that synovial plasma cell depletion could be of importance.[18]

Safety

The safety of rituximab in RA has been investigated using a pooled analysis of 8 randomized trials and 2 long-term, open-label extensions, incorporating 3194 patients and 11 962 patient-years of experience.[19] Follow-up was from 1 to 9.5 years and number of rituximab courses between 1 and 17.

Infusion reactions

The commonest adverse reactions, affecting approximately one-third of patients receiving rituximab for the first time, are infusion reactions. These coincide with B-cell lysis and are generally mild in patients receiving premedication with methylprednisolone, an analgesic/anti-pyretic, and an anti-histamine. Common symptoms include headache, pruritus, throat irritation, flushing, rash, and pyrexia. Severe reactions occur in less than 1% of patients, and include chest and throat tightness, and hypotension; resuscitation facilities should therefore always be available during infusions. The incidence and severity of infusion reactions is lower with the second infusion of the first course and with subsequent courses.

Infections

The incidence of serious infections with rituximab is similar to other biologic therapies at 3.94 (confidence interval 3.60–4.31) per 100 patient-years in the aforementioned pooled analysis. The risk does not apparently increase with multiple courses. Commonest infections are bacterial affecting the respiratory tract, skin, urinary tract, and bowel. Unlike TNF blockade, opportunistic infections are rare and reactivation of tuberculosis (TB) has not been reported. Although most RA patients will have previously received TNF blockade and therefore been screened for TB, the incidence of reactivation is also low in patients receiving rituximab for non-Hodgkin's lymphoma. Rare cases of progressive multifocal leucoencephalopathy have been reported in RA patients receiving rituximab, although in almost all cases there was another potential contributing factor.[20] Nonetheless patients must receive a patient alert card with each infusion and be monitored for new neurological symptoms or signs. There are also rare reports of hepatitis B reactivation, occasionally resulting in fulminant hepatitis. Hepatitis B status should therefore be ascertained before therapy in relevant populations and local monitoring guidelines followed.[21]

Repeated courses of rituximab result in reduced levels of circulating IgM (incidence of 22% in the pooled analysis referred to above), although this is not associated with heightened infection risk. IgG levels below the normal range are less common, affecting 3.5% in the pooled analysis. Patients with a low IgG level have a higher serious infection risk than those who never develop a low IgG. The enhanced infection risk predates the fall in IgG levels, however, implying a common predisposing factor such as age or glucocorticoid use.[19] Other risk factors for serious infection include comorbidities such as diabetes, chronic lung or heart disease, and extra-articular disease.[22]

Vaccination

Live or attenuated vaccines are not recommended in patients receiving immunosuppressive drugs (see Chapter 94). Several studies report a reduced response to killed vaccines following rituximab.[23,24] RA patients should therefore receive necessary vaccines at least 4 weeks before a course of treatment.

Pregnancy and breastfeeding

Rituximab crosses the placenta and can deplete B cells in the fetus. It should not be administered during pregnancy and contraception is recommended for 12 months following treatment. Rituximab should also not be given to breastfeeding women.

Table 83.1 Rituximab clinical trials

Trial	Comparator	Intervention	Background Therapy	Follow-up	ACR 20 (%)	ACR 50 (%)	ACR 70 (%)	ΔDAS28	ΔGm-TSS	Ref
Edwards et al (Phase 2a)	MTX	RTX (2 × 1 g); RTX & CPM; RTX (2 × 1 g) & MTX	—	24 weeks	38	65* 76# 73#	13	33NS 41# 43#	5	15NS 15NS 23*	-1.3	-2.2# -2.6a -2.6a	—	—	2
				48 weeks	20	33NS 49# 65#	5	15NS 27# 35*	0	10NS 10NS 15*	—	—	—	—	
DANCER (Phase 2b)	Placebo	RTX (2 × 500 mg); RTX (2 × 1 g)	MTX	24 weeks	28	53a 54a	13	33a 34a	5	13* 20a	-0.67	-1.79a -2.05a	—	—	3
REFLEX (Phase 3)	Placebo	RTX (2 × 1 g)	MTX	24 weeks	18	51b	5	27b	1	12b	-0.4	-1.9b	—	—	4
				52 week	—	—	—	—	—	—	—	—	2.31	1.00#	
				104 weeks	—	—	—	—	—	—	—	—	2.81	1.14b	
SERENE (Phase 3)	Placebo	RTX (2 × 500 mg); RTX (2 × 1 g)	MTX	24 weeks	23.3	54.5b 50.6b	9.3	26.3b 25.9b	5.2	9.0NS 10.0NS	-0.75	-1.76b -1.69b	—	—	7
	RTX (2 × 500 mg)	RTX (2 × 1 g)		48 weeks	55.7	57.6NS	32.9	34.1NS	12.6	13.5NS	-1.96	-2.02NS	—	—	
MIRROR (Phase 3)	2 × RTX (2 × 500 mg)	RTX (2 × 500 mg) + (2 × 1 g); 2 × RTX (2 × 1 g)	MTX	48 weeks	64	64NS 72NS	39	39NS 48NS	20	19NS 23NS	-2.3	-2.4NS -2.6NS	—	—	6
IMAGE (Phase 3)	Placebo	2 × RTX (2 × 500 mg); 2 × RTX (2 × 1 g)	MTX	52 weeks	64	77* 80b	42	59b 65b	25	42b 47b	-2.06	-3.05b -3.21b	1.08	0.65NS 0.36a	8

ACR 20/50/70, percentage of patients achieving 20/50/70% reduction in American College of Rheumatology score; CPM, cyclophosphamide; MTX, methotrexate; NS, not statistically significant; RTX, rituximab (two infusions of 500 mg or 1000 mg 15 days apart); ΔDAS28, mean change in DAS28 score; ΔGm-TSS, mean change in Genant modified total Sharp score.
The MIRROR study investigated the effects of a second course of rituximab delivered after 24 weeks.

*p < 0.05; #p < 0.01; ap < 0.001; bp < 0.0001.

Malignancy

There has been no statistically significant increase in the rate of malignancies following the use of rituximab for RA.[19]

Place in therapeutic algorithm

Rituximab, with concomitant MTX, is licensed in the United Kingdom for the treatment of RA in patients who have failed to have an adequate response to other disease-modifying anti-rheumatic drugs (DMARDs), including at least one TNF inhibitor. NICE guidelines are broadly in line with the licence. In practice rituximab is sometimes used as first biologic therapy where there is a (relative) contraindication to TNF blockade, such as interstitial lung disease, prior history of malignancy, or demyelinating illness.

Treatment and retreatment with rituximab

In RA, rituximab is administered as two infusions of 1000 mg, given 15 days apart, in combination with MTX. Retreatment should be considered only if there is a significant response, measured at 12–16 weeks, and should not be offered any more frequently than every 6 months. Critically (and unfortunately), neither serial B-cell measurements nor any other blood biomarker predict symptomatic relapse, which therefore must be based on clinical measures. There is continued debate on the optimal retreatment regime: treatment on disease flare vs regular retreatment (e.g. every 6 months) vs treatment-to-target. However, current expert opinion suggests treatment-to-target provides the optimal strategy, combining better disease control while minimizing the risk of overtreatment.[21] Uncontrolled data suggest that the response to rituximab may improve with subsequent treatment courses.[25] Furthermore, occasional patients who fail to benefit from an initial course may respond to a second course.

Use in other diseases

Two RCTs have studied rituximab for the treatment of Sjögren's syndrome.[26,27] Although small, both found statistically significant improvements in disease symptom scores and objective measures of disease activity compared to placebo.

EXPLORER was a phase 2/3 study comparing rituximab with placebo in 257 patients with moderate to severely active extrarenal systemic lupus erythematosus (SLE).[28] Patients continued on background therapy and also received tapered prednisone. There was no difference in primary or secondary outcome measures between the groups over 52 weeks of observation. In the phase 3 LUNAR study, 144 patients with lupus nephritis were randomized to rituximab or placebo in addition to starting mycophenylate mofetil, pulsed methylprednisolone, and tapered prednisone.[29] Again, rituximab failed to show superiority over placebo at 52 weeks. SLE is a complex disease, rendering clinical trial design problematic. In both EXPLORER and LUNAR there were biomarker (dsDNA, complement) improvements with rituximab and clinical benefits could still be seen in future studies with distinct designs.

Rituximab was non-inferior to daily oral cyclophosphamide at achieving prednisone-free remission at 6 months in newly diagnosed or relapsing ANCA-associated vasculitis. In this double-blind randomized trial, the 197 participants also received pulsed methylprednisolone plus tapered prednisone.[30] In a small study (n = 44) in ANCA-associated renal vasculitis, sustained remission at 12 months was high in patients receiving either rituximab or pulsed intravenous cyclophosphamide as induction therapy, in addition to standard glucocorticoids. There was also no difference in adverse events.[31] Thus rituximab may provide an alternative to cyclophosphamide in ANCA-associated vasculitis. Confirmatory and longer-term studies are now required.

Abatacept

Abatacept (CTLA4-Ig) is a genetically engineered fusion protein, comprising the extracellular domain of cytotoxic T-lymphocyte-associated antigen-4 (CTLA-4) linked to a modified Fc segment of human IgG1. T cells require two key signals for activation to occur. The first is an antigen-specific signal, triggered when the T-cell receptor recognizes its cognate MHC/peptide combination on an antigen-presenting cell (APC). The second, costimulatory, signal is triggered when T-cell CD28 binds either CD80 or CD86 on the APC. Following activation, the T cell upregulates CTLA-4. This molecule outcompetes CD28 for binding to CD80 and CD86, providing negative feedback and switching off T-cell activation (Figure 83.2). Abatacept is a soluble form of CTL-4 and similarly competes with CD28, depriving T cells of costimulation. This prevents activation of naive, and potentially memory, T cells. The mutation in the abatacept Fc reduces binding to complement and Fc-γ receptors, minimizing cytotoxicity to APC.

Efficacy

Phase 3 trials studied abatacept in patients with an inadequate response to MTX (AIM) and in patients failing TNF blockade (ATTAIN).[32,33] In AIM, patients were randomized to abatacept (approximately 10 mg/kg monthly) or placebo. ACR 20/50/70 responses for abatacept and placebo groups were 67.9 vs 39.7%, 39.9 vs 16.8%, and 19.8 vs 6.5% respectively at 6 months and DAS28 remission was achieved in 14.8% and 2.8% respectively. Clinically significant improvements in HAQ-DI were achieved in 63.7 vs 39.9% of patients at 12 months. Mental and physical domains of the SF-36, as well as fatigue, improved with abatacept, and radiographic progression was also retarded.[32] In ATTAIN patients received abatacept or placebo, following a washout of anti-TNF for current users. Background DMARDs (mostly MTX) were continued. The primary endpoint was at 6 months, when response rates in abatacept and placebo groups were 54 and 19% (ACR 20), 20 and 4% (ACR 50), and 10 and 1% (ACR 70). A HAQ-DI improvement of 0.3 or more was achieved by 47.3 vs 23.3% of patients in each group, and DAS28 remission was achieved in 10.0 vs 0.8% of patients.

An indirect head-to-head trial randomized patients to abatacept, infliximab, or placebo.[34] The primary outcome compared abatacept and placebo for Disease Activity Score (DAS) reduction at 6 months but the study design allowed an indirect comparison between abatacept and infliximab. There was no difference at 6 months but at 12 months ACR 20 was achieved by 72.4 of patients receiving abatacept vs 55.8% receiving infliximab, ACR 50 by 45.5 vs 36.4%, and ACR 70 by 26.3 vs 20.6%. DAS low disease activity was achieved by 35.3 vs 22.4% and DAS remission by 18.7 vs 12.2%. Table 83.2 summarizes phase 2 and 3 trials with abatacept.

Abatacept has also been investigated in MTX-naive as well as in undifferentiated arthritis patients.[35,36] Although data from both trials were encouraging, neither group of patients is included in abatacept's licence.

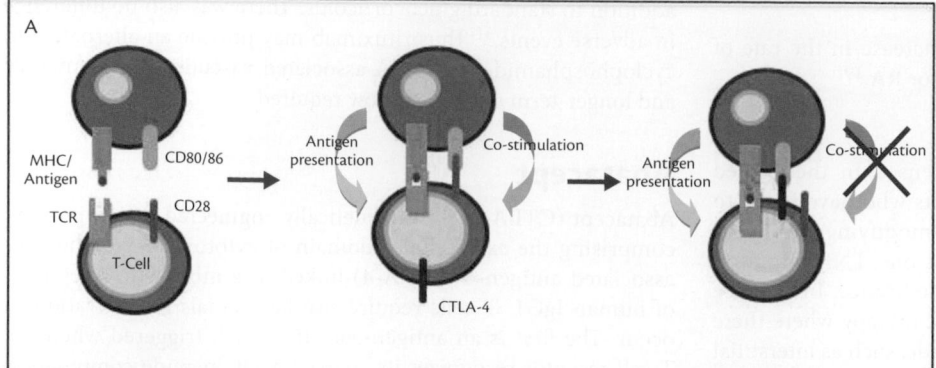
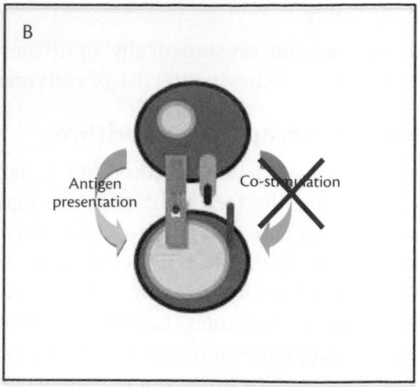

Fig. 83.2 T-lymphocyte activation and the effect of abatacept. (A) Activation of T lymphocytes (T cells) involves interaction of an MHC–antigen complex on an antigen-presenting cell (APC) with the T-cell receptor (TCR)—signal 1. This then allows interaction of CD80 or CD86 on the APC with CD28 on the T cell, providing costimulation—signal 2—and resulting in activation of the T cell. Subsequently there is upregulation of CTLA-4 on the T cell which competes with CD28 for CD80/86, antagonizing the costimulatory signal and simultaneously providing an inhibitory signal to the T cell. (B) Abatacept is a soluble form of CTLA-4 and therefore reduces T-cell costimulation by competing with CD80/86.

Mode of action

Abatacept deprives T cells of their key costimulatory signal. Immune dogma suggests that the dominant downstream effect is to inhibit activation of naive T cells. However, heterogeneity is increasingly recognized amongst memory T cells, with at least some requiring costimulation for their continued activity.[37] Furthermore, under some circumstances lack of costimulation can result in an anergic T cell, which cannot subsequently respond to antigen.[38] In this regard, the dynamics of the clinical response to abatacept are intriguing. Compared to cytokine blockade the onset of response to abatacept may be slower, although in both AIM and ATTAIN ACR 20 improvements were statistically superior to placebo by day 15. However, patient retention appears high with abatacept, with some evidence that the quality of response improves with time. Caution is required when interpreting 'as observed' data because only responders continue on therapy. However in a modified intention-to-treat analysis of ATTAIN, for example, DAS (CRP) low disease activity and remission were achieved by 18.3 (95% CI 13.0–23.5%) and 11.1 (6.8–15.3%) of patients at 6 months, increasing to 32 (24.6–39.4%) and 20.3 (13.9–26.6%) at 2 years.[39] Radiographic studies are also consistent with further slowing of joint damage with prolonged therapy. A possible interpretation of these data is that costimulation blockade leads to a gradual 'switching off' of T-cell responses, although direct evidence is lacking.

A small (n = 15) synovial biopsy study revealed minimal depletion of B cells (which express CD80 and CD86), and a reduction in levels of interferon (IFN)-γ, interleukin (IL)-1β, IL-6, matrix metalloprotein (MMP)-1 and MMP-3 in responders, suggesting a 'downstream' effect of costimulation blockade on other cell populations.[40] A preclinical study demonstrated an inhibition of T-cell activation with abatacept and secondary effects on B-cell function and antibody production, consistent with reductions in autoantibody titres documented in clinical trials.[41]

Safety

Infusion reactions were more common with abatacept than with placebo in AIM (9% vs 4%) and ATTAIN (5% vs 3%). Infections and serious infections were either numerically higher with abatacept (AIM) or similar to placebo (ATTAIN). Opportunistic infections were rarely reported and most serious infections were bacterial. A recent integrated safety review, incorporating more than 1000 patient-years of observation, reported slightly more serious infections with abatacept compared to placebo over 12 months of observation (3.47 vs 2.41 events/100 patient-years respectively) but no further increase in risk with long-term therapy.[42] Furthermore, a recent Cochrane review of biological therapies (not limited to RA) suggested that, using indirect comparisons, short-term abatacept use was associated with fewer serious adverse events and serious infections than other biological drugs.[43] During the first 12 months of the ATTEST study, serious adverse events (SAEs; 9.6 vs 18.2%) and serious infections (1.9 vs 8.5%) were fewer with abatacept than with infliximab, and all five reported opportunistic infections (herpes encephalitis, pseudomonas pneumonia, peritoneal TB, pneumocysitis pneumonia, and pulmonary TB) occurred with infliximab.[34] There was no signal relating to malignancy or autoimmune adverse events in the integrated safety review. Nonetheless when abatacept was combined with other biological drugs, an increase in both serious adverse events and serious infections was documented, without additional clinical benefit.[44,45]

Pregnancy and breastfeeding

Very limited information is available around the safety of abatacept during pregnancy or breastfeeding. Consequently, abatacept should not be administered during pregnancy and contraception is recommended for 14 weeks after the last dose.

Place in therapeutic algorithm

In the United Kingdom abatacept is licensed for use in combination with MTX, in patients who have failed treatment with one or more DMARDs. Unlike rituximab, its licence permits use before a TNF inhibitor. However, NICE guidelines restrict its use to third-line biological therapy when a patient develops side effects with rituximab, or second-line when rituximab is contraindicated. Abatacept is also licensed for the treatment of moderate to severe juvenile idiopathic

Table 83.2 Abatacept clinical trials

Trial	Comparator	Intervention	Background therapy	Follow-up	ACR 20 (%)	ACR 50 (%)	ACR 70 (%)	DAS28 < 2.6 (%)	ΔGm-TSS	Ref
AIM	Placebo	Abatacept	MTX	6 months	39.7 67.9[b]	16.8 39.9[b]	6.5 19.8[b]	2.8 14.8[b]	— —	32
				12 months	39.7 73.1[b]	18.2 48.3[b]	6.1 28.8[b]	1.9 23.8[b]	0.53 0.25*	
ATTAIN	Placebo	Abatacept	MTX	6 months	19.5 50.4[b]	3.8 20.3[b]	1.5 10.2[a]	0.8 10[b]	— —	33
ATTEST	Placebo	Abatacept; infliximab	MTX	6 months	41.8 66.7[b] 59.4[a]	20.0 40.4[b] 37.0[a]	9.1 20.5* 24.2[a]	2.9 11.3 12.8	— —	34
	Infliximab	Abatacept (indirect comparison)	MTX	12 months	72.4 55.8*	36.4 45.5[NS]	20.6 26.3[NS]	12.2 18.7[NS]	— —	
-	Placebo	Abatacept	MTX	12 months	— —	42.3 57.4[a]	27.3 42.6[a]	23.3 41.4[a]	0.63 1.06*	35

ACR 20/50/70, percentage of patients achieving 20/50/70% reduction in American College of Rheumatology score; DAS28 <2.6, percentage of patients meeting DAS28 criteria for disease remission (score <2.6); MTX, methotrexate; ΔGm-TSS, change in Genant modified total Sharp score (median in AIM, mean in 4th study).

Abatacept was administered at a concentration of 10 mg/kg as fortnightly infusions for 3 doses, then monthly.

*p < 0.05; # p < 0.01; [a]p < 0.001; [b]p < 0.0001.

arthritis (JIA) in patients who have failed at least one TNF inhibitor (patients aged ≥6; see Chapter 84). Abatacept is administered as infusions of approximately 10 mg/kg, fortnightly for the first three doses and then monthly. A subcutaneous formulation is currently in late-phase clinical development and is non-inferior to intravenous abatacept.[46]

Conclusion

Improved understanding of RA pathogenesis has allowed anti-cytokine biologics to be complemented by direct targeting of lymphocytes. Both rituximab and abatacept, targeting B and T cells respectively, are currently licensed for the treatment of RA. Their safety is broadly comparable to the anti-TNF biologics, and to one another, although the risk of TB reactivation is much less. Rituximab has very rarely been associated with the development of Progressive Multifocal Leucoencephalopathy, but may be safer than TNF blockade in patients with a history of malignancy. Between them, rituximab and abatacept provide additional options for patients in whom TNF blockade has failed or is contraindicated. Abatacept's licence permits its use as a first-line biologic but several guidelines, e.g. NICE, reserve its use for more refractory disease.

References

1. Wilk E, Witte T, Marquardt N et al. Depletion of functionally active CD20+ T cells by rituximab treatment. *Arthritis Rheum* 2009;60(12):3563–3571.

2. Edwards JC, Szczepanski L, Szechinski J et al. Efficacy of B-cell-targeted therapy with rituximab in patients with rheumatoid arthritis. *N Engl J Med* 2004;350(25):2572–2581.

3. Emery P, Fleischmann R, Filipowicz-Sosnowska A et al. The efficacy and safety of rituximab in patients with active rheumatoid arthritis despite methotrexate treatment: results of a phase IIB randomized, double-blind, placebo-controlled, dose-ranging trial. *Arthritis Rheum* 2006;54(5):1390–1400.

4. Cohen SB, Emery P, Greenwald MW et al. Rituximab for rheumatoid arthritis refractory to anti-tumor necrosis factor therapy: Results of a multicenter, randomized, double-blind, placebo-controlled, phase III trial evaluating primary efficacy and safety at twenty-four weeks. *Arthritis Rheum* 2006;54(9):2793–2806.

5. Keystone E, Emery P, Peterfy CG et al. Rituximab inhibits structural joint damage in patients with rheumatoid arthritis with an inadequate response to tumour necrosis factor inhibitor therapies. *Ann Rheum Dis* 2009;68(2):216–221.

6. Rubbert-Roth A, Tak PP, Zerbini C et al. Efficacy and safety of various repeat treatment dosing regimens of rituximab in patients with active rheumatoid arthritis: results of a Phase III randomized study (MIRROR). *Rheumatology* 2010;49(9):1683–1693.

7. Emery P, Deodhar A, Rigby WF et al. Efficacy and safety of different doses and retreatment of rituximab: a randomised, placebo-controlled trial in patients who are biological naive with active rheumatoid arthritis and an inadequate response to methotrexate (Study Evaluating Rituximab's Efficacy in MTX iNadequate rEsponders (SERENE)). *Ann Rheum Dis* 2010;69(9):1629–1635.

8. Tak PP, Rigby WF, Rubbert-Roth A et al. Inhibition of joint damage and improved clinical outcomes with rituximab plus methotrexate in early active rheumatoid arthritis: the IMAGE trial. *Ann Rheum Dis* 2011;70(1):39–46.

9. Chatzidionysiou K, Lie E, Nasonov E et al. Effectiveness of disease-modifying antirheumatic drug co-therapy with methotrexate and leflunomide in rituximab-treated rheumatoid arthritis patients: results of a 1-year follow-up study from the CERERRA collaboration. *Ann Rheum Dis* 2012;71(3):374–377.

10. Isaacs JD, Ferraccioli G. The need for personalised medicine for rheumatoid arthritis. *Ann Rheum Dis* 2011;70(1):4–7.

11. Chatzidionysiou K, Lie E, Nasonov E et al. Highest clinical effectiveness of rituximab in autoantibody-positive patients with rheumatoid arthritis and in those for whom no more than one previous TNF antagonist has failed: pooled data from 10 European registries. *Ann Rheum Dis* 2011;70(9):1575–1580.

12. Dass S, Rawstron AC, Vital EM et al. Highly sensitive B cell analysis predicts response to rituximab therapy in rheumatoid arthritis. *Arthritis Rheum* 2008;58(10):2993–2999.

13. Roll P, Dorner T, Tony HP. Anti-CD20 therapy in patients with rheumatoid arthritis: predictors of response and B cell subset regeneration after repeated treatment. *Arthritis Rheum* 2008;58(6):1566–1575.

14. Vital EM, Dass S, Rawstron AC et al. Management of nonresponse to rituximab in rheumatoid arthritis: predictors and outcome of re-treatment. *Arthritis Rheum* 2010;62(5):1273–1279.

15. Owczarczyk K, Lal P, Abbas AR et al. A plasmablast biomarker for non-response to antibody therapy to CD20 in rheumatoid arthritis. *Sci Transl Med* 2011;3(101):101ra92.

16. Teng Y, Hashemi M, Levarht N et al. Depleting effects of anti-CD20 monoclonal antibodies in blood, bone marrow and synovium of patients with refractory rheumatoid arthritis. *Ann Rheum Dis* 2007;66(Suppl II):439.

17. Takemura S, Klimiuk PA, Braun A, Goronzy JJ, Weyand CM. T cell activation in rheumatoid synovium is B cell dependent. *J Immunol* 2001;167(8):4710–4718.

18. Thurlings RM, Vos K, Wijbrandts CA et al. Synovial tissue response to rituximab: mechanism of action and identification of biomarkers of response. *Ann Rheum Dis* 2008;67(7):917–925.

19. van Vollenhoven RF, Emery P, Bingham CO, 3rd et al. Long-term safety of rituximab in rheumatoid arthritis: 9.5-year follow-up of the global clinical trial programme with a focus on adverse events of interest in RA patients. *Ann Rheum Dis* 2012 Nov 7 [Epub ahead of print]

20. Clifford DB, Ances B, Costello C et al. Rituximab-associated progressive multifocal leukoencephalopathy in rheumatoid arthritis. *Arch Neurol* 2011;68(9):1156–1164.

21. Buch MH, Smolen JS, Betteridge N et al. Updated consensus statement on the use of rituximab in patients with rheumatoid arthritis. *Ann Rheum Dis* 2011;70(6):909–920.

22. Gottenberg JE, Ravaud P, Bardin T et al. Risk factors for severe infections in patients with rheumatoid arthritis treated with rituximab in the autoimmunity and rituximab registry. *Arthritis Rheum* 2010;62(9):2625–2632.

23. Bingham CO, 3rd, Looney RJ, Deodhar A et al. Immunization responses in rheumatoid arthritis patients treated with rituximab: results from a controlled clinical trial. *Arthritis Rheum* 2010;62(1):64–74.

24. van Assen S, Holvast A, Benne CA et al. Humoral responses after influenza vaccination are severely reduced in patients with rheumatoid arthritis treated with rituximab. *Arthritis Rheum* 2010;62(1):75–81.

25. Keystone E, Fleischmann RM, Emery P et al. Repeated treatment courses of rituximab in rheumatoid arthritis: sustained efficacy in patients with an inadequate response to one or more TNF inhibitors. *Ann Rheum Dis* 2007;66(Suppl II):432.

26. Dass S, Bowman SJ, Vital EM et al. Reduction of fatigue in Sjögren syndrome with rituximab: results of a randomised, double-blind, placebo-controlled pilot study. *Ann Rheum Dis* 2008;67(11):1541–1544.

27. Meijer JM, Meiners PM, Vissink A et al. Effectiveness of rituximab treatment in primary Sjögren's syndrome: A randomized, double-blind, placebo-controlled trial. *Arthritis Rheum* 2010;62(4):960–968.

28. Merrill JT, Neuwelt CM, Wallace DJ et al. Efficacy and safety of rituximab in moderately-to-severely active systemic lupus erythematosus: the randomized, double-blind, phase II/III systemic lupus erythematosus evaluation of rituximab trial. *Arthritis Rheum* 2010;62(1):222–233.

29. Rovin BH, Furie R, Latinis K et al. Efficacy and safety of rituximab in patients with active proliferative lupus nephritis: The lupus

nephritis assessment with rituximab (LUNAR) study. *Arthritis Rheum* 2012;64(4):1215–1226.

30. Stone JH, Merkel PA, Spiera R et al. Rituximab versus cyclophosphamide for ANCA-associated vasculitis. *N Engl J Med* 2010;363(3): 221–232.

31. Jones RB, Tervaert JW, Hauser T et al. Rituximab versus cyclophosphamide in ANCA-associated renal vasculitis. *N Engl J Med* 2010;363(3):211–220.

32. Kremer JM, Genant HK, Moreland LW et al. Effects of abatacept in patients with methotrexate-resistant active rheumatoid arthritis: a randomized trial. *Ann Intern Med* 2006;144(12):865–876.

33. Genovese MC, Becker JC, Schiff M et al. Abatacept for rheumatoid arthritis refractory to tumor necrosis factor alpha inhibition. *N Engl J Med* 2005;353(11):1114–1123.

34. Schiff M, Keiserman M, Codding C et al. Efficacy and safety of abatacept or infliximab vs placebo in ATTEST: a phase III, multi-centre, randomised, double-blind, placebo-controlled study in patients with rheumatoid arthritis and an inadequate response to methotrexate. *Ann Rheum Dis* 2008;67(8):1096–1103.

35. Westhovens R, Robles M, Ximenes AC et al. Clinical efficacy and safety of abatacept in methotrexate-naive patients with early rheumatoid arthritis and poor prognostic factors. *Ann Rheum Dis* 2009;68(12): 1870–1877.

36. Emery P, Durez P, Dougados M et al. The impact of T-cell co-stimulation modulation in patients with undifferentiated inflammatory arthritis or very early rheumatoid arthritis: a clinical and imaging study of abatacept. *Ann Rheum Dis* 2010;69(3):510–516.

37. Floyd TL, Koehn BH, Kitchens WH et al. Limiting the amount and duration of antigen exposure during priming increases memory T cell requirement for costimulation during recall. *J Immunol* 2011;186(4):2033–2041.

38. Schwartz RH. A cell culture model for T lymphocyte clonal anergy. *Science* 1990;248(4961):1349–1356.

39. Genovese MC, Schiff M, Luggen M et al. Efficacy and safety of the selective co-stimulation modulator abatacept following 2 years of treatment in patients with rheumatoid arthritis and an inadequate response to anti-TNF therapy. *Ann Rheum Dis* 2008;67(4):547–554.

40. Buch MH, Boyle DL, Rosengren S et al. Mode of action of abatacept in rheumatoid arthritis patients having failed tumour necrosis factor blockade: a histological, gene expression and dynamic magnetic resonance imaging pilot study. *Ann Rheum Dis* 2009;68(7):1220–1227.

41. Platt AM, Gibson VB, Patakas A et al. Abatacept limits breach of self-tolerance in a murine model of arthritis via effects on the generation of T follicular helper cells. *J Immunol* 2010;185(3):1558–1567.

42. Schiff M. Abatacept treatment for rheumatoid arthritis. *Rheumatology (Oxford)* 2011;50(3):437–449.

43. Singh JA, Wells GA, Christensen R et al. *Adverse effects of biologics: a network meta-analysis and Cochrane overview.* John Wiley & Sons, Chichester, 2011.

44. Weinblatt M, Combe B, Covucci A et al. Safety of the selective costimulation modulator abatacept in rheumatoid arthritis patients receiving background biologic and nonbiologic disease-modifying antirheumatic drugs: A one-year randomized, placebo-controlled study. *Arthritis Rheum* 2006;54(9):2807–2816.

45. Weinblatt M, Schiff M, Goldman A et al. Selective costimulation modulation using abatacept in patients with active rheumatoid arthritis while receiving etanercept: a randomised clinical trial. *Ann Rheum Dis* 2007;66(2):228–234.

46. Weinblatt ME, Schiff M, Valente R, et al. Head-to-head comparison of subcutaneous abatacept versus adalimumab for rheumatoid arthritis: findings of a phase IIIb, multinational, prospective, randomized study. *Arthritis Rheum* 2013;65(1):28–38.

CHAPTER 84

Biologics in paediatric rheumatic diseases

Daniel J. Lovell, Nicolino Ruperto, Hermine I. Brunner, and Alberto Martini

Introduction

In the last 15 years the treatment approaches for children with rheumatic diseases have been dramatically changed as a result of the introduction of an ever-enlarging number of biological therapies. These biological therapies target a vast number of proteins and receptors central to the pathogenesis of the disease. In paediatric rheumatology, these biological therapies have been focused primarily on juvenile idiopathic arthritis (JIA) and to a lesser extent, on children with systemic lupus erythematosus (SLE). The treatment for JIA, including the expectations for treatment efficacy, has been revolutionized by the introduction of biologics. In this chapter the results of key efficacy and safety studies in JIA and SLE are described.

Biologics in juvenile idiopathic arthritis

Systemic juvenile idiopathic arthritis

Systemic JIA is characterized by prominent systemic features, such as fever, rash, and serositis. Anti-tumour necrosis factor (TNF) agents have been shown to be less effective in systemic JIA.[1] Findings from previous studies have suggested a major pathogenic role for interleukin (IL)-6[2-4] and for IL-1.[5] Indeed, a controlled withdrawal trial and several uncontrolled studies have shown the efficacy of tocilizumab[5] and anakinra.[6,7] In a double-blind controlled trial of tocilizumab against placebo in systemic JIA with or without systemic features, at the end of the 12 week double-blind phase 85% of those on tocilizumab and 24% of those on placebo (p <0.001) demonstrated an ACR Paediatric 30 level of response plus absence of fever. At week 52, 80% of those on tocilizumab were demonstrating an ACR Paediatric 70 level of response with no fever and 59% an ACR Paediatric 90 level of response without fever.[8] Two double-blind placebo-controlled trials of canakinumab (a new monoclonal antibody against IL-1) in children with systemic JIA with active systemic features have also been completed. In the first trial patients were randomly assigned to a single injection of canakinumab or placebo and assessed at day 15. Eighty-four per cent of those receiving canakinumab compared to only 10% of those receiving placebo demonstrated an ACR Paediatric 30 level of response and no fever (p <0.001). In the second trial, which used a randomized withdrawal design, at the end of the open-label phase of the study (median 113 days), 73% of the patients demonstrated at least an ACR Paediatric 50 level of response and no fever and 31% had inactive disease. In the randomized withdrawal phase the median time to flare was 236 days in the placebo group; the median was not observable in the canakinumab group, since less than 50% of the patients had a flare (p = 0.003 by the log-rank test).[9,10]It has been hypothesized that the early introduction of treatment with anakinra could be associated with a substantial prevention of refractory arthritis.[11] This hypothesis needs to be substantiated by prospective randomized trials. Another anti-IL-1 agent is rilonacept, for which very little information has been reported.[12]

According to the pattern of response to anti-IL-1 therapy, two subpopulations can be identified[13]: one with a pronounced, complete response to IL-1 blockade and another that is resistant to treatment or has an intermediate response. These two subpopulations do not differ in IL-1 in-vitro production or in serum cytokine concentrations, but only in the number of joints affected and in neutrophil counts. Patients with fewer joints affected or with a higher neutrophil count have an increased probability of responding to anti-IL-1 treatment. Thus, systemic JIA can be stratified into at least two subgroups on the basis of the response to IL-1 blocking agents and therefore on the possible pathogenic relevance of this cytokine.[14]

Polyarticular juvenile idiopathic arthritis

Currently JIA is classified, according to the International League Against Rheumatism (ILAR)[15,16] classification, criteria, into seven distinct clinical phenotypes, some of which appear to be rather definite disease entities, while others still appear to include heterogeneous conditions.[14,17] Since there are several JIA categories to be studied, most of the clinical trials described in the following paragraphs employed the concept of polyarticular-course JIA. This functional category groups patients with extended oligoarthritis, polyarthritis rheumatoid factor (RF) positive or negative, and systemic arthritis without active systemic features. Other than the studies in polyarticular forms of JIA, specific studies have been implemented so far only for systemic JIA while evidence for other JIA categories is scarce.[18] In the following sections the current evidence about the most widely used drugs, for children with polyarticular-course JIA, is summarized. In most of the trials a randomized withdrawal design has been used,[19] in which eligible children are treated in an open-label fashion with the experimental therapy for a few months, after which responders are randomized in a double-blind fashion either to continue the experimental therapy or to switch to placebo to look for disease flare.

Anti-tumour necrosis factor agents

TNF is a proinflammatory cytokine that plays a central role in the pathogenesis of JIA.[14] Three anti-TNF agents have so far been tested in randomized clinical trials (RCTs) in polyarticular-course JIA and have shown comparable efficacy and safety.

Etanercept

A controlled trial with a withdrawal design has shown the efficacy of etanercept, at a dose of 0.4 mg/kg subcutaneously twice a week (it can also be administered at 0.8 mg/kg once per week), in patients with JIA who were resistant or intolerant to methotrexate.[20] A total of 76 patients enrolled in the original trial have received the drug for at least 8 years with 28 of them reaching at least an American College of Rheumatology (ACR) 70 level of improvement,[21] at the last available observation. In the registry run by the Pediatric Rheumatology Collaborative Study Group (PRCSG) in North America of the 397 patients treated with etanercept alone or in combination with methotrexate for 3 years, a total of 218 (55%) discontinued, with the most frequent reasons being insufficient therapeutic effect, remission, or other[22]; patients treated with etanercept were generally with longer disease duration (40.7–58.1 months) when compared to the group newly treated with methotrexate (20.2 months). Etanercept was the first biological agent registered for use in JIA. Other studies have confirmed the remarkable and rapid efficacy of etanercept in JIA,[23–25] including restoration of normal growth in children with JIA,[22] and improved quality of life.[25]

Infliximab

A controlled trial with methotrexate (MTX) plus either infliximab or placebo failed to demonstrate a statistically significant difference in its primary outcome at 3 months.[26] However, by week 52, response to infliximab was similar to that observed with etanercept. Of note, although the two dosages used (3 and 6 mg/kg per infusion) were of comparable efficacy, patients receiving 3 mg/kg had a more frequent occurrences of serious adverse events, infusion reactions, antibodies to infliximab, and newly induced antinuclear and anti-double-stranded DNA antibodies. Therefore, 6 mg/kg is the dose recommended in paediatric rheumatology practice. Infliximab is not registered for use in JIA.

Adalimumab

A controlled trial with a withdrawal design has also shown the efficacy of adalimumab[27] for patients who were either methotrexate naive or methotrexate resistant or intolerant. Seventy-four per cent of patients not receiving methotrexate and 94% of those receiving methotrexate responded by week 16 with sustained response after 104 weeks of treatment. Overall, safety and efficacy were comparable to those observed with the other anti-TNF agents. Adalimumab is registered for JIA both in the United States (at a fixed dose of

20 mg every 2 weeks for children <30 kg and 40 mg/every 2 weeks for children ≥30 kg) and in Europe (24 mg/m²/every 2 weeks, maximum dose 40 mg).

Other anti-TNF agents

Other agents such as golimumab are undergoing phase 3 trials while for others, such as certolizumab, there is no public information available concerning future JIA trials.

Combined therapy

Although no specific studies exist in children, the results of the adalimumab trial as well as a retrospective analysis of the German registry[28] suggest that, in children, anti-TNF agents are more effective if combined with methotrexate. Similarly, no studies have been performed to assess the disease-modifying potential of biological agents on disease progression in JIA although a retrospective analysis has suggested that etanercept may reduce radiographic progression.[29] More recently, some evidence suggested early aggressive therapy with methotrexate and infliximab seems to be more effective than therapy with methotrexate alone or in combination with another disease-modifying anti-rheumatic drug (DMARD).[30]

Abatacept

Abatacept is a soluble, fully human fusion protein that consists of the extracellular domain of CTLA-4, linked to a modified Fc portion of human immunoglobin G1, which does not activate complement. Abatacept competitively binds to CD80 or CD86, where it selectively inhibits T-cell activation, and potentially affects many downstream cytokines and cell types involved in the immunopathogenesis of autoimmune disease. Its efficacy has been shown in a double-blind randomized controlled withdrawal trial in 190 patients with polyarticular-course JIA and inadequate response or intolerance to at least one DMARD, including anti-TNF drugs.[31] After 4 months of treatment an ACR Pediatric 50 was reached by 50% of the patients (and 25% of the patients who previously failed an anti-TNF). Durable efficacy was confirmed also in the long-term open-label extension phase also in patients who did not initially respond.[32] Treatment was also accompanied by a significant improvement in health-related quality of life.[33] Abatacept is registered for use in JIA in both the United States and Europe at a dose of 10 mg/kg of abatacept intravenously every 28 days in JIA patients at least 6 years old.

Tocilizumab

Tocilizumab was evaluated in polyarticular JIA patients using a double-blind, randomized, controlled withdrawal study design. After 16 weeks of open-label treatment with tocilizumab, ACR Pediatric 30, 50, 70, and 90 levels of response were seen in 89%, 83%, 62%, and 26%, respectively. In the withdrawal phase, 48% of those randomized to placebo flared compared to 26% of those continuing tocilizumab (p = 0.0035).[48]

Other JIA subtypes

The evidence for the treatment of other JIA subtypes such as enthesitis related arthritis (ERA) or psoriatic arthritis is scanty and comes mainly from retrospective case series. The largest body of evidence is from the Dutch registry,[18]where 22 JIA patients with ERA were treated with etanercept or adalimumab suggesting that treatment with anti-TNF seem effective also in this ILAR category. No information is available for the treatment with biologics of psoriatic arthritis patients.

Biologics in systemic lupus erythematosus

The pathogenesis of SLE involves a complex interplay between genetic and environmental factors and the adaptive and innate immune systems.[34] B-cell abnormalities leading to autoantibody production play a central role in SLE pathogenesis. Biological agents targeting specific pathways (i.e. T–B lymphocyte interaction, cytokines, and complement) have been proposed as new treatment tools for SLE.[35] B-cell targeted therapies, including anti-B lymphocyte stimulator (BLyS) and anti-CD20 monoclonal antibodies (mABs), are at the forefront of new SLE treatments.[36] Belimumab, a human mAb that binds to BLyS and thereby prevents it from activating various receptors and slows B-cell proliferation, was recently the first biological medication approved for the treatment of SLE in adults. Conversely, data on the safety and effectiveness of belimumab when used in children and adolescents with SLE are not available at present, but a paediatric trial is active at the time of writing.

Whereas belimumab only blocks soluble BLyS, the mAb LY2127399 also blocks membrane-bound BLyS and is in phase 3 trials in adults with SLE that are due to report results in 2013. The fusion protein atacicept combines immunoglobulin with a segment of the TNF receptor superfamily member TACI is also in phase 2/3 study. Because TACI binds both BLyS and the related TNF superfamily cytokine APRIL (a proliferation inducing ligand), it promises an advantage over belimumab.[37]

By lowering the number of circulating B cells and thereby decreasing autoantibody levels, anti-CD20 mABs like rituximab have been tested in SLE. Yet despite several clinical trials of the drug in SLE and regular off-label use, conclusive evidence of its efficacy has remained elusive. Compared to anti-CD20 blockage by 30%, the anti-CD22 mAB epratuzumab leads to a decrease in the number of B cells by 90% in early studies. There are at least 20 other biologic agents in clinical trials of SLE. Among others, there are phase 2/3 studies in adults with SLE that are testing biologic agents that block APRIL together with BLyS, T lymphocytes, T-lymphocyte activation antigens, interferon-α, or the interferon receptors. In phase 1 study are biologics blocking phosphdiesterase 4 and TNFα, IL-6, ICOSLG (inducible T-cell costimulator ligand), and JNK (Jun N-terminal kinase).

Targeted biological therapies show great promise in SLE treatment but additional studies are needed to define their role in SLE treatment.[34] Studies on the pathogenesis of SLE will open a new era of tailored patient-specific therapy.

Safety of biologics

With over a decade of international widespread use, the safety profile of the anti-TNF biologics is rather well characterized in children with JIA. To date, the safety signal with anti-TNF biological therapy in children with JIA is for the most part similar to that seen with use in adults with rheumatoid arthritis (RA). Safety data with the newer biological therapies in JIA are less extensive and limited primarily to the RCTs and open-label extension studies of the JIA patients in the trials. Safety data with biological agents in other rheumatic diseases are even more limited. Unique childhood safety issues are described below. An excellent review of safety of biological therapies in JIA patients was published in 2010.[38]

Anti-TNF agents

The safety of etanercept has been described in a randomized placebo-controlled trial,[20] up to 8 years of open-label follow-up of children in the randomized trial,[39] a drug-specific registry,[40] and as part of several national biologics registries.[23,24,28] In the controlled trial there were three cases of primary varicella infection that followed a complicated course. Those three cases had been treated as one would varicella infection in healthy children—observation only. Subsequently, there was an adoption in the remainder of that trial and other studies of anti-TNF therapies in JIA patients of the recommendation to evaluate and treat varicella infections in JIA patients on anti-TNF therapies as one would for infection in other moderately immunocompromised children and subsequently very few complicated varicella infections have been seen in JIA patients on anti-TNF agents.[23,24,28] In the drug-specific etanercept registry, the rates of adverse events (AEs), serious AEs (SAEs), medically important infections, and autoimmune events were similar in those treated with methotrexate alone, etanercept alone, and the combination of etanercept and methotrexate. No cases of demyelinating disease, tuberculosis, malignancy, or death were reported in the 594 patients in this registry, of whom 397 received etanercept therapy either alone or in combination with methotrexate.[40] However, the experience has not been so positive in other studies. There are several ongoing national registries of all JIA patients treated with etanercept in Germany, the Netherlands, and England. In the German registry, in 322 JIA patients treated with etanercept (592 patient-years of exposure), there were 12 SAEs; treatment was permanently stopped due to AE in 11 patients including 1 cancer (thyroid carcinoma) and 1 cerebral demyelination. There were no opportunistic infections or lupus-like syndromes.[23] In a recent publication from this same registry, there were 5 cases of malignancy out of 1260 JIA patients treated with etanercept.[41] In the Dutch registry, in 146 JIA patients (313 patient-years of exposure) there were nine SAEs; treatment was permanently stopped due to AE in six. Three new autoimmune diseases were noted: one case each of sarcoidosis, ulcerative colitis, and Crohn's disease and one case of tuberculosis (TB), but no cases of demyelinating disease, opportunistic infection, or cancer, and no patients died while on etanercept therapy.[24] In the British registry, in 483 JIA patients treated with etanercept (941 patient-years of exposure), 21 patients discontinued the etanercept due to toxicity: 5 discontinued due to infections, 10 due to non-infectious central nervous system (CNS) events (headaches 2, depression 1, anxiety attacks 1, hallucinations 1, optic neuritis 1, blurred vision 1 and uveitis flare 1) and 6 due to other events. One patient developed inflammatory bowel disease (IBD), there were no opportunistic infections, and no patient died while on etanercept therapy.[42]

The safety profile of adalimumab has been less well established. In a phase 3 trial of adalimumab in JIA patients, in 171 JIA patients treated with adalimumab for up to 104 weeks, 14 patients demonstrated a serious adverse event including 7 serious infections; 12 patients discontinued adalimumab due to toxicity. No malignancies, opportunistic infections, TB, demyelinating diseases, new autoimmune diseases and deaths were seen in this population.[27]

The safety profile of infliximab was studied in a phase III RCT in 122 children with JIA with up to 52 weeks of infliximab exposure. In this study, 60 patients were treated with infliximab 3 mg/kg per infusion, 60 patients received placebo infusions for 14 weeks and then 57 of these patients received infliximab 6 mg/kg per infusion for up to 38 weeks. Overall, there were 26 SAEs on infliximab including 6 serious infections including 1 case of pulmonary TB and 3 mild opportunistic infections (thrush 2, herpes zoster 1). Antibodies to infliximab were seen in 38% of those on 3 mg/kg and 12% of those on 6 mg/kg. Infusions reactions were seen 3–4 times more commonly in those with anti-infliximab antibodies. There were 31 of 117 patients on infliximab who developed an infusion reaction but in only 6 patients was it serious.[26]

The role of anti-TNF therapies in the development of cancer in JIA patients is not clearly understood at this time. In 2009, the United States Food and Drug Administration (FDA) reported on 48 malignancies in children and adolescents who had been treated with an anti-TNF agent. Arthritis was the reason for the anti-TNF treatment in 19 of the 48 cases (JIA 15, juvenile ankylosing spondylitis 3, juvenile psoriatic arthritis 1). There was a large variety of types of cancer. The FDA concluded there may be an increased risk of lymphoma and other cancers associated with the use of anti-TNF agents in children and required that black-box warning language be added to the labelling information for all anti-TNF biologics.[41] However, there are several problems with the FDA database. They have only numerator data in the reporting system and estimated the number of children on anti-TNF agents from external databases of prescribing information; the database combines several paediatric diseases in addition to JIA that are known to have differing rates and types of malignancies (e.g. IBD); and the comparisons are with healthy populations of children, not to children with the disease not treated with biologics. In the German JIA registry, 5 malignancies were reported out of 1260 patients on biological therapy. All had received other immunosuppressants prior to the biologic and several had received more than one biological therapy prior to developing the malignancy. They concluded from this data that the 'benefit/risk ratio has not changed even in light of the rare occurrences of malignancies' and supported the continued careful use of the biologics in those in whom there was an appropriate indication, use of other more traditional therapies first, and ongoing careful monitoring for any suggestion of a malignancy.[41] In a biologic-naive population of patients with JIA and matched healthy controls from the Swedish Patient Registry, those JIA patients with disease onset before 1987 were not at increased risk of cancer, whereas JIA identified in 1987–1999 was significantly associated with incident lymphoproliferative malignancies (relative risk 4.2, 95% confidence interval 1.7–10.7) and cancers overall (relative risk 2.3, 95% confidence interval 1.2–4.4) Sensitivity analysis failed to identify an associated factor with the increased rate.[43] This study suggests that there may be an increased rate of cancer in JIA patients independent of biological therapy and that any future studies of cancer risk with biological therapies needs to include biologic-naive JIA patients as the comparison group rather than healthy children.

Other biologics

The clinical experience with biologics other than the anti-TNF agents is significantly smaller. Abatacept is a T-cell costimulation inhibitor that has been approved for the treatment of JIA. In a phase III trial with 190 JIA patients, in the open-label lead-in phase in which all subjects received abatacept, there were six SAEs (three JIA flares, one each varicella, ovarian cyst, and acute lymphoblastic leukaemia). In the double-blind phase of the study, the rate of

AEs did not differ between the abatacept and placebo groups.[31] In a long-term open-label follow-up study of the participants in the trial (n = 153), there were six serious infections, no cases of TB, no opportunistic infections, and one case of multiple sclerosis.[32] An international registry to assess the safety of abatacept for up to 10 years of therapy began enrolment in 2013.

Anakinra is an IL-1 blocking biologic that has been studied in children. In 86 patients with polyarticular JIA, in an open-label lead-in, double-blind randomized withdrawal design treatment with anakinra 1 mg/kg per day for up to 19 months, there was only one serious adverse event thought to be due to anakinra (nephrosis). There were no cases of malignancy, TB, opportunistic infections, or deaths.[44] In a trial of anakinra in 44 patients with systemic JIA, one patient developed Crohn's disease and another hepatitis.[7]

In the phase 3 study of tocilizumab in 112 SJIA patients, there were 39 SAEs including 19 infections (4 varicella, 2 herpes zoster) and 3 MAS events. Opportunistic infection, TB, and cancer were not reported. Three deaths occurred during tocilizumab therapy (1 pneumothorax, 1 auto accident, and 1 streptococcal sepsis). Death also occurred in three patients who received tocilizumab and who had withdrawn from the study (pulmonary hypertension in 2, MAS in 1). Neutropenia developed in 17% and elevation of aminotransferase levels more than 2.5 times the upper limit of normal in 19% of the SJIA patients in the trial.[8]

In the trials of canakinumab in SJIA, there were 23 SAEs in those on canakinumab (13 infections and 3 episodes of MAS). No opportunistic infections, TB, or cancer were observed. Thrombocytopenia was seen in 6% and neutropenia in 6% of those on canakinumab. Two patients died in the trial (urosepsis and MAS in 1, pulmonary hypertension and MAS in 1).[10] In the trial of canakinumab in polyarticular forms of JIA, there were 12.5 SAEs per 100 patient-years of exposure and no deaths, opportunistic infections or malignancies were seen.[48]

Role of biologics in recent treatment recommendations for juvenile idiopathic arthritis

The ACR developed recommendations for the safest and most effective treatment of JIA, based on the available scientific evidence and consensus among stakeholders. Inherent to the guidelines is the necessity that the recommendations require frequent updates to adequately reflect the results from new studies and changes in treatment preferences of healthcare providers.[45] The recommendations are meant to function as a reference and do not serve as a substitute for individualized patient assessment and clinical decision-making, especially when conducted by specialist clinicians familiar with the treatment of JIA. Rather than the ILAR JIA classification, the ACR recommendations employ five so-called 'treatment groups'. They are (a) history of arthritis of four or fewer joints; (b) history of arthritis of five or more joints; (c) active sacroiliac arthritis; (d) systemic arthritis with active systemic features; and (e) systemic arthritis with active arthritis without active systemic features. Treatment recommendations also consider the presence of risk factors for poor outcome as well as the degree of JIA disease activity within each treatment group. It should be noted that the three disease activity levels (mild, moderate, severe) are subjective and not strictly evidence based. Patients with inactive disease were not considered. In a broad sense, the low disease activity level is meant to represent patients at the lowest disease activity level for

Table 84.1 American College of Rheumatology 2010 recommendations for juvenile idiopathic arthritis

Disease activity treatment group	Disease activity	Mainstay of treatment	Poor prognostic features	Treatment progression	Adjunct treatments
4 or fewer joints involved	Mild Moderate Severe	NSAIDs JI MTX, sulfasalazine, leflunomide TNF antagonists	Arthritis of hip or cervical spine Arthritis of ankle or wrist **plus** marked or prolonged inflammatory marker elevation Radiographic damage	Trial of NSAID monotherapy for up to 2 months[a] to achieve disease control For continuous moderate or high severe disease activity, treatment escalation or change after 3 months **with** and after 6 months **without** poor prognostic factors	NSAIDS prn JI prn
5 or more joints involved	Mild Moderate Severe	NSAIDS JI MTX, sulfasalazine, leflunomide TNF antagonists or abatacept	Arthritis of hip or cervical spine Positive RF or ACPA Radiographic damage		
Active sacroiliac arthritis	Mild Moderate Severe	NSAIDS JI MTX, sulfasalazine TNF antagonists	Radiographic damage of any joint		
Systemic arthritis with active systemic features (and without active arthritis);	Mild Moderate Severe	NSAIDs Glucocorticosteroids IL-1 inhibition	6-month duration of significant active systemic disease; requirement for treatment with systemic glucocorticoids	NSAID monotherapy no longer than 1 month for fever or arthritis Assessment of MTX failure after 3 months of therapy for continuous moderate or high severe disease activity	NSAIDs and glucocorticoids prn with IL-1 inhibition
Systemic arthritis with active arthritis (and without active systemic features)	Mild Moderate Severe	NSAIDs MTX TNF antagonists, IL-1 inhibition Abatacept	Arthritis of hip Radiographic damage		NSAIDS prn Joint injections prn

[a]2 weeks for active systemic features.

ACPA, anti-citrullinated peptide antibodies; IL, interleukin; JI, joint injections; MTX, methotrexate; NSAID, non-steroidal anti-inflammatory drug; prn, as the need arises; RF, rheumatoid factor; TNF, tumour necrosis factor.

which a majority of clinicians may consider altering the current medication regimen, and the high disease activity level is meant to represent patients with disease activity that is equivalent to or higher than the 'average' patient who may have been enrolled in a clinical trial of the medications under consideration. The ACR treatment guidelines for JIA are shown in Table 84.1.

Conclusion

In the last decade there have been dramatic advances in the treatment of JIA thanks to the availability of biological agents, the implementation of an adequate paediatric legislation [46,47] to require the performance of clinical testing of new agents in children and the existence of two large, not-for-profit paediatric rheumatology research networks, the Paediatric Rheumatology International Trials Organization (PRINTO) and the Pediatric Rheumatology Collaborative Study Group (PRCSG), covering most of the paediatric rheumatology centres worldwide. Despite progress, there are still problems to be solved including a better understanding of the long-term safety of the drugs as well as to provide more efficacious treatments for those patients that fail to adequately respond to current therapies.

References

1. Quartier P, Taupin P, Bourdeaut F et al. Efficacy of etanercept for the treatment of juvenile idiopathic arthritis according to the onset type. *Arthritis Rheum* 2003;48(4):1093–1101.
2. De Benedetti F, Martini A. Is systemic juvenile rheumatoid arthritis an interleukin 6 mediated disease? *J Rheumatol* 1998;25(2): 203–207.
3. De Benedetti F, Massa M, Pignatti P et al. Serum soluble interleukin 6 (IL-6) receptor and IL-6/soluble IL-6 receptor complex in systemic juvenile rheumatoid arthritis. *J Clin Invest* 1994;93:2114–2119.
4. De Benedetti F, Alonzi T, Moretta A et al. Interleukin 6 causes growth impairment in transgenic mice through a decrease in insulin-like growth factor-I—A model for stunted growth in children with chronic inflammation. *J Clin Invest* 1997;99(4):643–650.
5. Yokota S, Imagawa T, Mori M et al. Efficacy and safety of tocilizumab in patients with systemic-onset juvenile idiopathic arthritis: a randomised, double-blind, placebo-controlled, withdrawal phase III trial. *Lancet* 2008;371(9617):998–1006.
6. Pascual V, Allantaz F, Arce E, Punaro M, Banchereau J. Role of interleukin-1 (IL-1) in the pathogenesis of systemic onset juvenile idiopathic arthritis and clinical response to IL-1 blockade. *J Exp Med* 2005;201(9):1479–1486.
7. Quartier P, Allantaz F, Cimaz R et al. A multicentre, randomised, double-blind, placebo-controlled trial with the interleukin-1 receptor

antagonist anakinra in patients with systemic-onset juvenile idiopathic arthritis (ANAJIS trial). *Ann Rheum Dis* 2011;70(5):747–754.

8. De Benedetti F, Brunner H, Ruperto N et al. Randomized trial of tocilizumab in systemic juvenile idiopathic arthritis. *N Engl J Med* 2012;367(25):2385–2395.

9. Ruperto N, Quartier P, Wulffraat N et al. A phase II study to evaluate dosing and preliminary safety and efficacy of canakinumab in systemic juvenile idiopathic arthritis with active systemic features. *Arthritis Rheum* 2012;64(2):557–567.

10. Ruperto N, Brunner H, QuartierP et al. Two randomized trials of canakinumab in systemic juvenile idiopathic arthritis. *N Engl J Med* 2012;367(12):2396-2406.

11. Nigrovic PA, Mannion M, Prince FH et al. Anakinra as first-line disease-modifying therapy in systemic juvenile idiopathic arthritis: report of forty-six patients from an international multicenter series. *Arthritis Rheum* 2011;63(2):545–555.

12. Hayward K, Wallace CA. Recent developments in anti-rheumatic drugs in pediatrics: treatment of juvenile idiopathic arthritis. *Arthritis Res* 2009;11(1):216–227.

13. Gattorno M, Piccini A, Lasiglie D et al. The pattern of response to anti-interleukin-1 treatment distinguishes two subsets of patients with systemic-onset juvenile idiopathic arthritis. *Arthritis Rheum* 2008;58(5):1505–1515.

14. Prakken B, Albani S, Martini A. Juvenile idiopathic arthritis. *Lancet* 2011;377(9783):2138–2149.

15. Petty RE, Southwood TR, Baum J et al. Revision of the proposed classification criteria for juvenile idiopathic arthritides: Durban, 1997. *J Rheumatol* 1998;25(10):1991–1994.

16. Petty RE, Southwood TR, Manners P et al. International league of associations for rheumatology classification of juvenile idiopathic arthritis: Second revision, Edmonton, 2001. *J Rheumatol* 2004;31(2):390–392.

17. Martini A. Are the number of joints involved or the presence of psoriasis still useful tools to identify homogeneous disease entities in juvenile idiopathic arthritis? *J Rheumatol* 2003;30(9):1900–1903.

18. Otten MH, Prince FH, Twilt M et al. Tumor necrosis factor-blocking agents for children with enthesitis-related arthritis—data from the Dutch Arthritis and Biologicals in Children Register, 1999–2010. *J Rheumatol* 2011;38(10):2258–2263.

19. Giannini EH, Lovell DJ, Silverman ED et al. Intravenous immunoglobulin in the treatment of polyarticular juvenile rheumatoid arthritis: a phase I/II study. *J Rheumatol* 1996;23(5):919–924.

20. Lovell DJ, Giannini EH, Reiff A et al. Etanercept in children with polyarticular juvenile rheumatoid arthritis. *N Engl J Med* 2000;342(11): 763–769.

21. Giannini EH, Ruperto N, Ravelli A, Lovell DJ, Felson DT, Martini A. Preliminary definition of improvement in juvenile arthritis. *Arthritis Rheum* 1997;40(7):1202–1209.

22. Giannini EH, Ilowite NT, Lovell DJ et al. Effects of long-term etanercept treatment on growth in children with selected categories of juvenile idiopathic arthritis. *Arthritis Rheum* 2010;62(11):3259–3264.

23. Horneff G, Schmeling H, Biedermann T et al. The German etanercept registry for treatment of juvenile idiopathic arthritis. *Ann Rheum Dis* 2004;63(12):1638–1644.

24. Prince FH, Twilt M, ten Cate R et al. Long-term follow-up on effectiveness and safety of etanercept in juvenile idiopathic arthritis: the Dutch national register. *Ann Rheum Dis* 2009;68(5):635–641.

25. Prince FH, Geerdink LM, Borsboom GJ et al. Major improvements in health-related quality of life during the use of etanercept in patients with previously refractory juvenile idiopathic arthritis. *Ann Rheum Dis* 2010;69(1):138–142.

26. Ruperto N, Lovell DJ, Cuttica R et al. A randomized, placebo-controlled trial of infliximab plus methotrexate for the treatment of polyarticular-course juvenile rheumatoid arthritis. *Arthritis Rheum* 2007;56(9):3096–3106.

27. Lovell DJ, Ruperto N, Goodman S et al. Adalimumab with or without methotrexate in juvenile rheumatoid arthritis. *N Engl J Med* 2008;359(8):810–820.

28. Horneff G, De Bock F, Foeldvari I et al. Safety and efficacy of combination of etanercept and methotrexate compared to treatment with etanercept only in patients with juvenile idiopathic arthritis (JIA): preliminary data from the German JIA Registry. *Ann Rheum Dis* 2009;68(4):519–525.

29. Nielsen S, Ruperto N, Gerloni V et al. Preliminary evidence that etanercept may reduce radiographic progression in juvenile idiopathic arthritis. *Clin Exp Rheumatol* 2008;26(4):688–692.

30. Tynjala P, Vahasalo P, Tarkiainen M et al. Aggressive combination drug therapy in very early polyarticular juvenile idiopathic arthritis (ACUTE-JIA): a multicentre randomised open-label clinical trial. *Ann Rheum Dis* 2011;70(9):1605–1612.

31. Ruperto N, Lovell DJ, Quartier P et al. Abatacept in children with juvenile idiopathic arthritis: a randomised, double-blind, placebo-controlled withdrawal trial. *Lancet* 2008;372(9636):383–391.

32. Ruperto N, Lovell DJ, Quartier P et al. Long-term safety and efficacy of abatacept in children with juvenile idiopathic arthritis. *Arthritis Rheum* 2010;62(6):1792–1802.

33. Ruperto N, Lovell DJ, Li T et al. Abatacept improves health-related quality of life, pain, sleep quality and daily participation in subjects with juvenile idiopathic arthritis. *Arthritis Care Res* 2010;62(11):1542–1551.

34. Rahman A, Isenberg DA. Systemic lupus erythematosus. *N Engl J Med* 2008;358(9):929–939.

35. Murdaca G, Colombo BM, Puppo F. Emerging biological drugs: A new therapeutic approach for systemic lupus erythematosus. An update upon efficacy and adverse events. *Autoimmun Rev* 2011;11(1):56–60.

36. Editorial. Landmark lupus approval opens door for next wave of drugs. *Nat Rev Drug Discov* 2011;10(4):243–245.

37. Davidson A. Targeting BAFF in autoimmunity. *Curr Opin Immunol* 2010;22(6):732–739.

38. Hashkes PJ, Uziel Y, Laxer RM. The safety profile of biologic therapies for juvenile idiopathic arthritis. *Nat Rev Rheumatol* 2010;6(10): 561–571.

39. Lovell DJ, Reiff A, Ilowite NT et al. Safety and efficacy of up to eight years of continuous etanercept therapy in patients with juvenile rheumatoid arthritis. *Arthritis Rheum* 2008;58(5):1496–1504.

40. Giannini EH, Ilowite NT, Lovell DJ et al. Long-term safety and effectiveness of etanercept in children with selected categories of juvenile idiopathic arthritis. *Arthritis Rheum* 2009;60(9):2794–2804.

41. Horneff G, Foeldvari I, Minden K, Moebius D, Hospach T. Report on malignancies in the German juvenile idiopathic arthritis registry. *Rheumatology* (Oxford) 2011;50(1):230–236.

42. Southwood TR, Foster HE, Davidson JE et al. Duration of etanercept treatment and reasons for discontinuation in a cohort of juvenile idiopathic arthritis patients. *Rheumatology* (Oxford) 2011;50(1): 189–195.

43. Simard JF, Neovius M, Hagelberg S, Askling J. Juvenile idiopathic arthritis and risk of cancer: a nationwide cohort study. *Arthritis Rheum* 2010;62(12):3776–3782.

44. Ilowite N, Porras O, Reiff A et al. Anakinra in the treatment of polyarticular-course juvenile rheumatoid arthritis: safety and preliminary efficacy results of a randomized multicenter study. *Clin Rheumatol* 2009;28(2):129–137.

45. Beukelman T, Patkar NM, Saag KG et al. 2011 American College of Rheumatology recommendations for the treatment of juvenile idiopathic arthritis: initiation and safety monitoring of therapeutic agents

for the treatment of arthritis and systemic features. *Arthritis Care Res (Hoboken)* 2011;63(4):465–482.

46. Regulation (EC) no 1901/2006 of the European parliament and of the Council of 12 December 2006 on medicinal products for paediatric use and amending Regulation (EEC) No 1768/92, Directive 2001/20/EC, Directive 2001/83/EC and Regulation (EC) No 726/2004. *Official Journal of the European Union* 27 Dec 2006;L378:1–19.

47. Ruperto N, Martini A, for the Paediatric Rheumatology International Trials Organization (PRINTO). Use of unlabelled and off licence drugs in children. A European paediatric rule is needed to protect children. *BMJ* 2000;320(7243):1210–1211.

48. Brunner HI, Ruperto N, Zuber Z, et al. Efficacy and safety of tocilizumab in patients with polyarticular juvenile idiopathic arthritis: data from a phase 3 trial. *Arthritis Rheum* 2012: 60(10 Supplement):S682-3.

CHAPTER 85

Stem cell therapies

Alan Tyndall and Jacob M. van Laar

Introduction

Stem cells are cells capable both of self-replenishment and of providing progenitor cells for various tissues. There are different types, including **totipotent** (able to develop into a complete individual), **pluripotent** (able to develop into any tissue type), and **multipotent** (able to develop into various subgroups of a tissue type (Figure 85.1). Despite the enormous promise of using pluripotent embryonal stem cells (ESC) in regenerative medicine, problems regarding teratoma development and ethical aspects of ESC acquisition hamper progress. Recently it has been shown that insertion of certain developmental genes into adult differentiated somatic cells may 'reprogram' them back to an ESC-like phenotype; these are called induced pluripotent stem cells (iPSC) (Figure 85.1). Although this avoids the ethical issues of stem cell source, the teratoma development risk is still present. On the other hand, adult or 'postnatal' multipotent stem cells have none of these issues and are in clinical practice. Haematopoietic stem cells (HSC) have been used for decades to fully replenish a host's haematopoietic system after chemical and/or radiation ablation for malignant disorders. This was recently adopted to treat severe autoimmune disease.[1]

Definitions

- **Autologous haematopoietic stem cell transplantation (HSCT)** refers to the use of the patient's own HSC to rebuild an ablated haematopoietic system.

- **Allogeneic HSCT** is the use of another healthy donor's HSC. These need to be mobilized from the bone marrow, or directly harvested via bone marrow aspiration (which mostly needs a general anaesthetic).

- **Mobilization** is the process of driving the HSC from the bone marrow into the peripheral blood using growth factors such as granulocyte colony-stimulating factor (G-CSF) and/or cyclophosphamide (CYC). The HSC are then harvested via leukapheresis.

- **Graft manipulation or purging** is the process of purifying for wanted cells in the graft, e.g. CD34+ HSC using a column, or negatively selecting unwanted cells such as lymphocytes with antibodies.

- **Conditioning** is the protocol used to ablate the unwanted cells in the patient, e.g. leukaemia or solid tumour with chemicals and/radiation. Often antibodies to lymphocytes are also used to deplete the immune system. The haemato/immune system is mostly also ablated, hence the requirement for the HSCT to restore vital functions.

- **Myeloablative conditioning** occurs when the HSC are killed by the conditioning regimen, usually involving busulphan and/or radiation, and the ensuing severe cytopenia requires an HSCT—otherwise the patient would die from marrow failure.

- **Non-myeloablative** refers to a regimen which does not result in significant cytopenia, but due to immunosuppression, allows the donor graft to avoid being rejected by the host.

- **Reduced-intensity conditioning** occurs when the stem cells are not killed but require time to reconstitute the haematopoietic system. The HSCT is used to reduce the critical cytopenic period and hence toxicity.

- **Reconstitution** is the process of recovery following HSCT; haematopoietic reconstitution usually takes 11–14 days but immune reconstitution may take months (e.g. B cells) or several years (e.g. CD4 naive T cells) in adults due to thymic involution.

Haematopoietic stem cell transplantation in autoimmune disease

Over 1500 patients have received a HSCT, mostly autologous, as treatment for a severe autoimmune disease (AD) since the start of the international project in 1997.[1] A recent retrospective analysis of 900 patients from the European League Against Rheumatism (EULAR) combined database showed that the majority had multiple sclerosis (MS; n = 345) followed by systemic sclerosis (SSc; n = 175), systemic lupus erythematosus (SLE; n = 85, rheumatoid arthritis (RA; n = 89), juvenile idiopathic arthritis (JIA; n = 65), and idiopathic thrombocytopenic purpura (ITP; n = 37). An overall 85% 5-year survival and 43% progression-free survival was seen, with 100-day transplant-related mortality (TRM) ranging between 1% (RA) and 11% (SLE and JIA).[2] Around 30% of patients in all disease subgroups had a complete response, often durable despite full immune reconstitution. In many, e.g. SSc, morphological improvement such as reduction of skin collagen and normalization

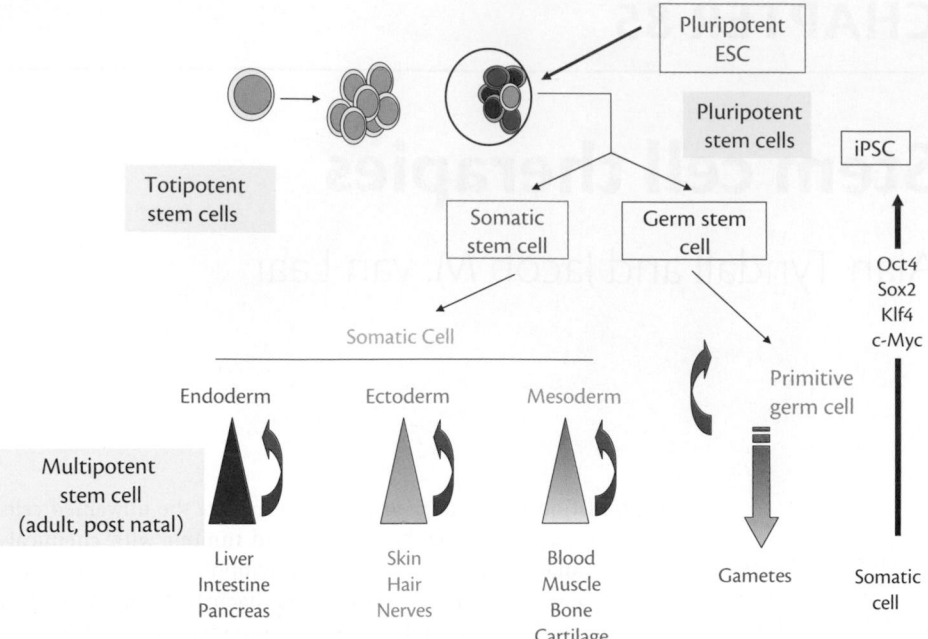

Fig. 85.1 Stem cell development.

of microvasculature was documented, beyond any predicted known effects of intense immunosuppression alone. It is hoped that the results of the three running large prospective randomized controlled trials (RCTs) will allow modification of the protocols to reduce the high TRM which relates to regimen intensity, age of patient, and comorbidity.

The concept of immune ablation, or at least severe reduction, and 'resetting' of autoimmunity arose from coincidental case reports (HSCT given for malignancy with coexisting AD improvement)[2] and was corroborated by animal model data.[3] The first patient published receiving an HSCT for an AD had SSc with pulmonary artery hypertension,[4] responded satisfactorily, and is still stable 15 years later.

From the outset, an international collaboration ensued which is committed to establishing the place, if any, of HSCT in the treatment of severe therapy-resistant AD in the context of prospective randomized clinical trials, coupled with mechanistic side studies[1]. Although many protocols were employed, they basically ranged from less aggressive, e.g. CYC 200 mg/kg plus anti-thymocyte globulin (ATG) to more intensive, e.g. total body irradiation (TBI) plus CYC/ATG and CD34 selection.

Up to one-third of patients in all groups experienced a significant clinical improvement, including full and drug-free sustained remissions.[5] In some of those studied (SLE, MS, and SSc patients), remission was sustained despite full immune reconstitution. In SLE, the authors demonstrated that humoral responses to recall antigens (tetanus, polio, measles, and mumps) were ablated following autologous HSCT, as would be expected, but in addition, eradication of autoantibodies such as anti-double stranded DNA was also achieved coincident with clinical remission in five cases.[6] Following immune reconstitution, a comparison between the patients' and normal subjects' T-cell receptor Vβ repertoires showed a fully normal pattern. Importantly, no patient had relapsed in the 8 year follow-up reported. Similar findings were described in seven MS patients who remained in remission up to 3 years post-transplant despite

regaining a normal T-cell repertoire.[7] These findings are particularly important, since at the onset of the project many considered autologous HSCT to be doomed to failure, given that the identical 'autoaggressive' immune system was being given back to the patient. However, the initial choice of autologous over allogeneic HSCT was mainly based on the lower toxicity of autologous HSCT, mainly due to absence of graft-vs-host disease (GvHD). It is now appreciated that in many patients who achieved clinical remission, the autoaggressive immune system was 'debulked' rather than fully ablated, allowing re-establishment of normal immune regulation, in part due to increased Treg numbers and activity.[8]

Several groups have described reduced collagen deposition in skin[9] (Figure 85.2) and normalization of microvasculature in SSc patients[10,11] (Figure 85.3) following autologous HSCT. None of these observations are readily explained by either sustained immunosuppression or direct effects on fibroblasts and endothelial cells, and suggest a more profound modulation of the inflammatory niche by mechanisms yet to be fully elucidated. Currently three large prospective randomized trials are running: ASTIS (Autologous Stem cell Transplantation International Scleroderma), SCOT (Scleroderma Cyclophosphamide Or Transplant), and ASTIC (Autologous Stem cell Transplantation International Crohn's). See Table 85.1; further details are available on the respective websites. ASTIS and SCOT are similar in patient selection, control arms, and endpoints, but the transplant protocols differ. SCOT employs a more intense regimen including TBI. Each has experienced its own toxicity issues, all previously known in HSCT medicine. Only time will tell which approach, if any, imparts a clinically useful and durable outcome; ASTIS has finished recruitment (156 patients). The primary endpoint is event-free survival, events being defined as death or end-organ (renal, cardiac or pulmonary) failure. SCOT finished recruitment in May 2011 and ASTIC is nearing its target of 40 patients.[12]

A smaller phase II randomized trial in SSc showed a positive outcome in the 10 transplanted patients compared with 9 control

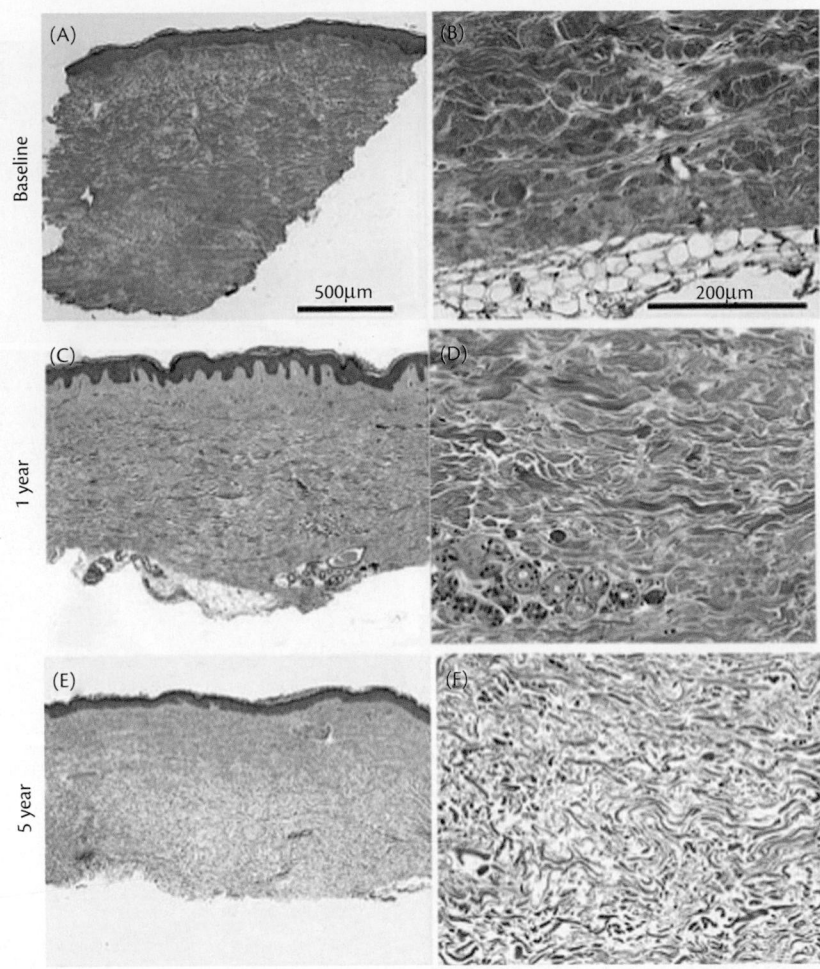

Fig. 85.2 Resolution of skin fibrosis after autologous haematopoietic stem cell transplant. Resolution of dermal fibrosis after high-dose immunosuppressive therapy (HDIT) and autologous haematopoietic cell transplant (HCT). Full-thickness skin biopsies from patient no. 11, collected at baseline and then at 1 and 5 years after HDIT, were histologically evaluated (H&E). The skin biopsies performed after HDIT were performed at a site adjacent to the baseline skin biopsy. The biopsies in the left column were taken at original magnification ×5, and those in the right column were taken at original magnification ×20. All sections were stained with H&E. (A) Skin biopsy was obtained before HDIT and autologous HCT. Pandermal sclerosis from the dermal–epidermal border to the hypodermis (subcutaneous fat) was observed. The epidermis is mildly acanthotic (thickened) with loss of rete ridges. The reticular dermis is replaced by dense compact collagen without normal fascicular bundles or dermal appendages. This pretransplantation skin biopsy was determined as grade 5 dermal fibrosis. The thickness of the dermis was measured at more than 2 mm. (B) In the higher-power magnification, the straightened dermal–subcutaneous border demonstrates the abnormal, densely packed, homogenized collagen. (C) The skin biopsy at 1 year after HDIT was determined to be a grade 2 dermal fibrosis and has less fibrosis than at baseline. The low-power magnification view shows crowded collagen fascicles with focal areas of residual thickened bundles. (D) A higher-power view of the 1 year skin biopsy from panel C shows thin and collagen bundles admixed with residual thick, straightened, hypereosinophilic collagen bundles without dense homogenization at baseline. The residual eccrine unit lacks any surrounding adipose tissue. (E) The skin biopsy at 5 years shows complete resolution of the dermal fibrosis (grade 0) with a reduction in the thickness of the dermis from baseline to 1 mm. The collagen bands in the dermis are thin with a relative increase in the intervening extracellular matrix (space between the collagen bands). The dermal–epidermal border remains straightened with loss of rete ridges. (F) A higher-power view of collagen in the lower reticular dermis demonstrates the change to thin wavy bundles separated by increased ground substance.
Reproduced from [Annals of the Rheumatic Diseases, Aschwanden M, Daikeler T, Jaeger KA, et al., 67, pp.1057–9 2008] with permission from BMJ Publishing Group Ltd.

patients who received CYC1 g/m^2 for 6 months.[13] The conditioning regimen was CYC 200 mg/kg plus five doses of rabbit ATG, each one accompanied by 1 g of intravenous methyl prednisolone. The primary endpoint at 12 months was based on a percentage improvement of the modified Rodnan skin score (mRSS) and/or pulmonary status. Although the low toxicity and positive outcome was gratifying, the low numbers of patients and short follow-up were not conclusive.[13]

Treatment-related mortality

A major issue for physicians dealing with AD was and is that patients rarely die immediately from their disease. However, a growing

literature had suggested that uncontrolled systemic inflammation leads to premature atherosclerosis and cardiovascular deaths,[14] as well as toxicity from chronic immunosuppression, especially glucocorticoids. Despite this, it is still a challenge for a rheumatologist, neurologist, or gastroenterologist to accept an immediate TRM of 5–10%, especially since long-term benefits have yet to be demonstrated. The hypothesis is that in a randomized prospective trial of HSCT vs conventional treatment, early toxicity from TRM would eventually be surpassed by later deaths and/or organ failure from disease progression in the control arm (Figure 85.4). This has yet to be proven.

Apart from the well-known acute toxicity of HSCT (infection and bleeding during the aplastic period and late infection during the

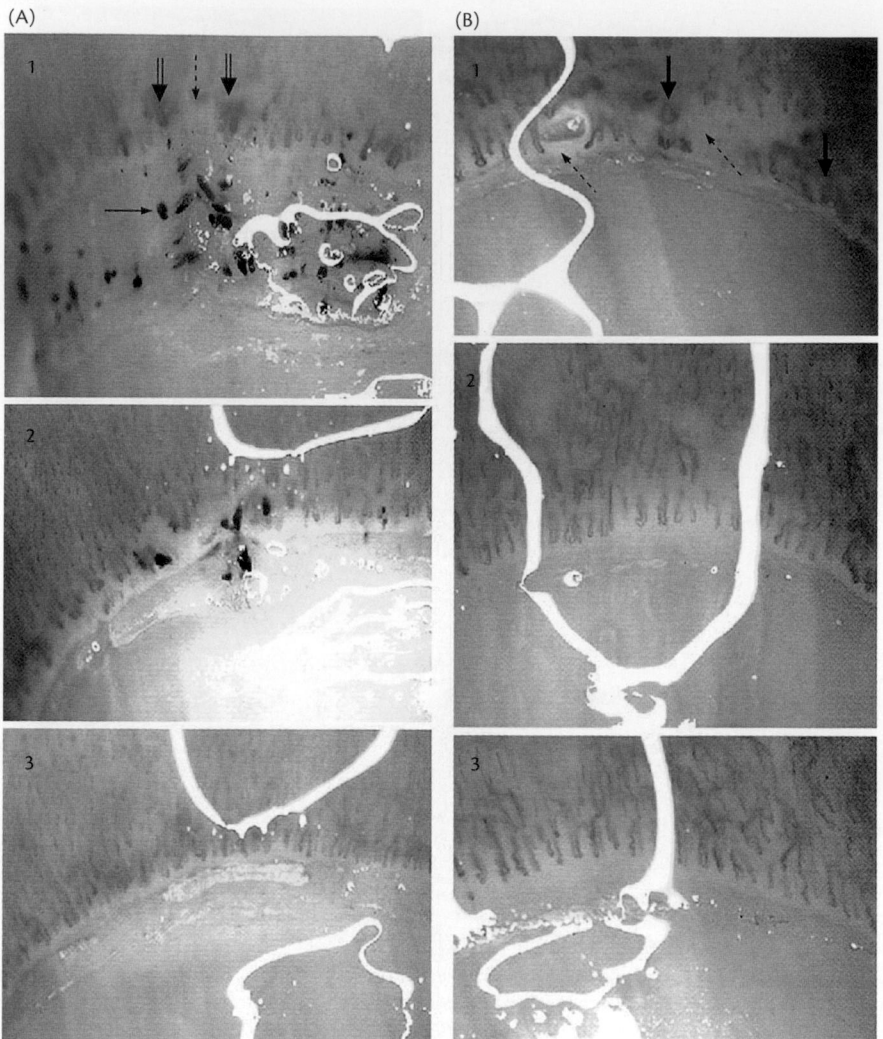

Fig. 85.3 Normalization of microcapillaries after haematopoietic stem cell transplantation (HSCT) in two patients with systemic sclerosis (SSc) (A) and mixed connective tissue disease (MCTD) (B). (A) Patient 1, fourth finger on the right hand. Panel 1: reduced translucency. Massive capillary bleedings (arrow), enlarged capillaries (arrow), and avascular regions (arrow, dotted line) before treatment. Panel 2: remarkable increase in capillary density and reduced bleedings but still some avascular regions after mobilization. Panel 3: normalized capillary number, size, and architecture with no bleedings 5 months after HSCT. (B) Patient 2, fourth finger on the left hand. Panel 1: severe disarrangement, multiple giant capillaries (arrow, double lined) and large avascular fields (arrow, dotted line) before mobilization. Panel 2: increase in capillary numbers and reduced avascular areas. Loss of giant capillaries after mobilization. Panel 3: further increase in capillary density with only hypovascularized regions. Normalization of the capillary architecture but still many capillaries with slightly pathological shapes. White stripes correspond to light reflections from the oily skin surface.

Reproduced with permission from Nash RA, Mcsweeney PA, Crofford U, et al. High-dose immunosuppressive therapy and autologous hematopoietiè cell transplantation for severe systemic sclerosis: long-term follow-up of the US multicenter pilot study. Blood 2007;110:138.

T-cell reconstitution phase), several other factors emerged during the programme. Some SSc patients experienced serious lung toxicity from TBI, while others suffered a scleroderma renal crisis during the conditioning phase, attributed to a combination of rapid fluid and electrolyte shifts and high-dose glucocorticoids given as prophylaxis for ATG-induced cytokine storm. In some children with JIA a fatal macrophage activation syndrome occurred, thought to be infection triggered and due to the profound immunosuppression resulting from TBI and CD34 purging.[15] These toxicity problems were mostly eliminated by lung shielding, concurrent angiotensin converting enzyme (ACE) inhibition, and reduced intensity of the regimen respectively. However, an inevitable TRM will always exist, which must be weighed against the potential long-term benefit, a calculation that requires efficacy data from the randomized trials.

Late complications include not just the well-known fungal and other opportunistic infections during the T-cell reconstitution phase (which may last up to 2 years or more) but also the emergence of second autoimmunity.[16] It is almost always antigen specific— e.g. platelet, erythrocyte, thyroid—and often, but not always, resolves as the Treg network is reconstituted. However some patients have succumbed from this, e.g. acquired haemophilia A antibodies after HSCT for MS.[17]

Non-response and relapse

Two-thirds of transplanted patients either did not respond or responded then relapsed. The factors determining this remain elusive, but some studies in RA suggested that clinical responders (n = 5) had a larger number of cells at baseline expressing CD3,

Table 85.1 Large randomized clinical trials of autologous haematopoietic stem cell transplantation in autoimmune disease

	ASTIS	SCOT	ASTIC
Principle investigator	J. van Laar, UK	K. Sullivan, USA	C. Hawkey, UK
Target	156 patients	70 patients	40 patients
Transplant regimen	CYC 200 mg/kgATG (rabbit)7.5 mg/kg CD34 selection	CYC 120 mg/kgATG (equine) 90 mg/kgTBI 800 cGy, CD34 selection	CYC 200 mg/kg ATG 7.5 mg/kg Unselected graft
Control arm	Monthly CYC 750 mg/m² IVI ×12	Monthly CYC 750 mg/m² IVI ×12	Mobilization then delayed transplant for 12 months
Primary endpoint	Alive at 2 years without endstage organ failure	Composite endpoint (death, end-organ failure) at 54 months	Proportion of patients in sustained remission at 1 year
Current status	Finalized: last patient randomized Oct 2009	Recruitment ends May 2011	37/40 patients randomized

ASTIC, Autologous Stem cell Transplantation International Crohn's Disease; ASTIS, Autologous Stem cell Transplantation International Scleroderma; ATG, anti-thymocyte globulin; CYC, cyclophosphamide; IVI, intravenous infusion; SCOT, Scleroderma Cyclophosphamide Or Transplant; TBI, total body irradiation.

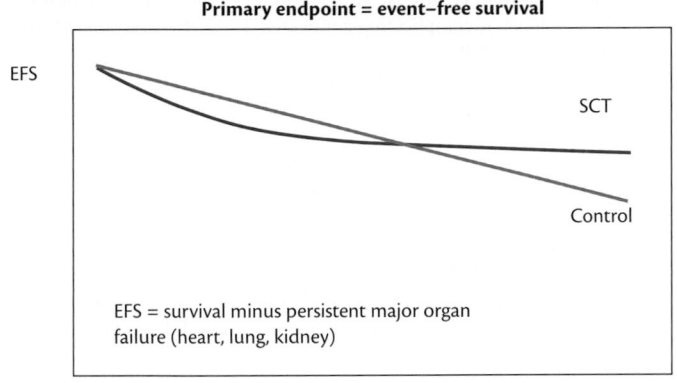

Primary endpoint = event–free survival

EFS

SCT

Control

EFS = survival minus persistent major organ
failure (heart, lung, kidney)

Sample size 150 patients based on 10-yr accrual, 11-yr follow-up;
Alpha = 0.05, power = 0.67, HR = 0.5; intention-to-treat

Fig. 85.4 Early vs late event-free survival power calculation for ASTIS.

CD4, CD27, CD45RA, CD45RB, and CD45RO in synovium (p <0.05), higher activity on HIg scans (p = 0.08), and a trend towards higher concentrations of C-reactive protein (CRP) in serum than non-responders (n = 2). Subsequent remissions and relapses in responders paralleled reduction and re-expression, respectively, of T-cell markers. A relatively increased expression of CD45RB and CD45RO on synovial CD3+ T cells was seen after HDC + ASCT. No correlations were found between Disability Activity Scale (DAS) and changes in B cells or macrophage infiltration or synoviocytes.[18]

Summary

Autologous HSCT for severe AD has demonstrated remarkable clinical, laboratory, and morphological improvement in many patients, but at a high price including a TRM up to 10% in some conditions. Retrospective analysis from established databases is inevitably incomplete, especially in those patients 'lost to follow-up' and assumed to be still alive. The advent of biologic agents has reduced the need for more radical therapies such as HSCT in RA and MS, but for SSc and severe forms of Crohn's disease it still remains an option. The results of the prospective RCTs will be critical in deciding the future of this treatment.

Allogeneic HSCT for AD has been performed and a summary of 35 patients so treated showed up to 50% remission induction in some AD subgroups.[19] However, the lack of a clear advantage over autologous HSCT and the risk of GvHD relegates this to a second-line strategy at the moment.

Mesenchymal stem cell transplantation for autoimmune disease

Mesenchymal stem cells (MSC) are stromally derived adult progenitor cells, more accurately called multipotent mesenchymal stromal cells, since their true 'stemness' has not been established. They may be derived from various tissues including bone marrow, placenta and umbilical cord, fat, and teeth. Although a heterogeneous group of progenitor cells, they have been defined by consensus as being plastic adherent, bearing certain stromal surface markers (CD76, CD90, CD105) and lacking hematopoietic cell markers such as CD11a, CD14, CD19, CD34, CD45, and MHC class II. In addition they should have at least adipogenic, osteogeneic, and chondrogenic differentiation potential.[20]

Since MSC were first applied in humans for HSC graft enhancement over 15 years ago,[21] there has since developed a major interest in their potential for immune modulating, anti-inflammatory, and tissue protective properties, including AD.[22] Originally considered as 'regenerative' due their ability to transdifferentiate into other tissues, it is now appreciated that the positive effects seen in vitro, in animal models, and in some clinical studies is most likely due to their capacity to initiate various paracrine events, resulting in tissue protection. Some of these effects are via soluble factors such as tissue growth factor (TGF)-β, 2,3-indoleamine dioxygenase, soluble HLA-G, and others via cell–cell contact and reprogramming of target cells.[23] In addition, MSC seem to display certain special properties such as immune privilege (survival in allogeneic environments) and active homing to distressed tissues via surface molecules such as CXCR4. They also preferentially home to tumour stroma,[24] potentially inhibiting tumour immune surveillance.

The role of the MSC in normal tissue homeostasis and repair is not fully clear, but it seems likely that they participate in the inflammatory niche, possibly as part of the resolution phase of injury. Their origin in adult animals is also not defined fully, but potential sources are from pericytes released from blood vessels during injury,[25] epidermal to mesenchymal transition, especially in lung and kidney,[26] and direct release from the bone marrow.

Clinical experience

Following many positive animal models of inflammation, organ transplant, autoimmunity, critical ischaemia, radiation damage, and tissue scarring, MSC entered clinical trials for inflammatory disorders, first in GvHD, then later MS, Crohn's disease (including fistula closure), SLE, and SSc (reviewed by Duijvestein et al.[22]). In addition, many trials relating to ischaemia in myocardium, central nervous system, kidney, and limbs have been performed.

Despite this activity, only 14 phase I/II clinical trials in AD have been published, all of less than 20 patients. Two large randomized prospective trials in Crohn's disease and GvHD were reported as failing to reach their primary endpoints, but as yet have not been published in the peer-reviewed literature.

There is a lack of standardization of cell product regarding heterogeneity, potency, impact of expansion media on phenotype, and suitability of source. Many expansion media employ growth factors such as fibroblast growth factor (FGF)-β, which has been shown to induce proliferation dependent MHC class II expression[27] and in one study, suspected karyotypic changes.[28] The clinical trials so far have used MSC derived from various sources including fat, bone marrow, placenta, and umbilical cord, the former two being either autologous or allogeneic. MSC from the bone marrow of AD patients have been shown to be defective regarding certain functions such as differentiation potential and hematopoietic support, but seem as equally potent as healthy allogeneic MSC in terms of in-vitro anti-proliferative potential.

The efficacy data so far available are difficult to interpret due to variable pre-MSC transplant treatment regimens, non-standardized outcome measures, and lack of long-term follow-up. So far no acute toxicity signals have emerged from the experience of around 1000 patients, though longer-term data are important regarding tumour surveillance.

Future directions

Clearly further small phase I/II trials will not shed further light on the long-term benefit of MSC and we now need larger, randomized double-blind clinical trials, including mechanistic side studies. There are major gaps in our knowledge such as duration of engraftment, impact on normal tissues and organs, and phenotypic changes occurring in the MSC when exposed to the inflammatory/ ischemic target tissue. At least interferon-γ and FGF-β will both cause expression of MSC class II on MSC, and in the latter case, this molecule is able to present antigen.[27] It would seem that costimulating molecules are never expressed by MSC, thus rendering the expression of MHC class II molecules potentially 'tolerogenic'. Several groups are planning such studies; the EULAR Stromal Cell Group is finalizing a prospective, double-blind comparative multicentre trial in lupus nephritis using allogeneic MSC, and an MS consortium a prospective comparative trial using autologous MSC.

It will require a determined effort from investigators, regulators, and industry to determine through adequately powered, prospective clinical trials the potential benefit of MSC transplantation in AD and other human disorders. As many of these are investigator-initiated, strategy-based studies, the bureaucratic burden may hamper development.

References

1. Tyndall A, Gratwohl A. Blood and marrow stem cell transplants in autoimmune disease: a consensus report written on behalf of the European League against Rheumatism (EULAR) and the European Group for Blood and Marrow Transplantation (EBMT). *Bone Marrow Transplant* 1997;19:643–645.

2. Jacobs P, Vincent MD, Martell RW. Prolonged remission of severe refractory rheumatoid arthritis following allogeneic bone marrow transplantation for drug-induced aplastic anaemia. *Bone Marrow Transplant* 1986;1:237–239.

3. Knaan-Shanzer S, Houben P, Kinwel-Bohre EP, van Bekkum DW. Remission induction of adjuvant arthritis in rats by total body irradiation and autologous bone marrow transplantation. *Bone Marrow Transplant* 1991;8:333–338.

4. Tamm M, Gratwohl A, Tichelli A, Perruchoud AP, Tyndall A. Autologous haemopoietic stem cell transplantation in a patient with severe pulmonary hypertension complicating connective tissue disease. *Ann Rheum Dis* 1996;55:779–780.

5. Gratwohl A, Passweg J, Bocelli-Tyndall C et al. Autologous hematopoietic stem cell transplantation for autoimmune diseases. *Bone Marrow Transplant* 2005;35:869–879.

6. Alexander T, Thiel A, Rosen O, et al. Depletion of autoreactive immunologic memory followed by autologous hematopoietic stem cell transplantation in patients with refractory SLE induces long-term remission through de novo generation of a juvenile and tolerant immune system. *Blood* 2009;113:214–223.

7. Muraro PA, Douek DC, Packer A et al. Thymic output generates a new and diverse TCR repertoire after autologous stem cell transplantation in multiple sclerosis patients. *J Exp Med* 2005;201:805–816.

8. van Wijk F, Roord ST, Vastert B et al. Regulatory T cells in autologous stem cell transplantation for autoimmune disease. *Autoimmunity* 2008;41:585–591.

9. Nash RA, McSweeney PA, Crofford LJ et al. High-dose immunosuppressive therapy and autologous hematopoietic cell transplantation for severe systemic sclerosis: long-term follow-up of the US multicenter pilot study. *Blood* 2007;110:1388–1396.

10. Fleming JN, Nash RA, McLeod DO et al. Capillary regeneration in scleroderma: stem cell therapy reverses phenotype? *PLoS One* 2008;3:e1452.

11. Aschwanden M, Daikeler T, Jaeger KA et al. Rapid improvement of nailfold capillaroscopy after intense immunosuppression for systemic sclerosis and mixed connective tissue disease. *Ann Rheum Dis* 2008;67:1057–1059.

12. Couzin-Frankel J. Immunology. Replacing an immune system gone haywire. *Science*;327:772–774.

13. Tyndall A. Stem cells: HSCT for systemic sclerosis—swallows and summers. *Nat Rev Rheumatol* 2011;7(11):624–626.

14. Bartoloni E, Shoenfeld Y, Gerli R. Inflammatory and autoimmune mechanisms in the induction of atherosclerotic damage in systemic rheumatic diseases: two faces of the same coin. *Arthritis Care Res* (Hoboken) 2011;63:178–183.

15. Mohyeddin Bonab M, Yazdanbakhsh S, Lotfi J et al. Does mesenchymal stem cell therapy help multiple sclerosis patients? Report of a pilot study. *Iran J Immunol* 2007;4:50–57.

16. Yamout B, Hourani R, Salti H et al. Bone marrow mesenchymal stem cell transplantation in patients with multiple sclerosis: a pilot study. *J Neuroimmunol* 2010;227:185–189.

17. Karussis D, Karageorgiou C, Vaknin-Dembinsky A et al. Safety and immunological effects of mesenchymal stem cell transplantation in patients with multiple sclerosis and amyotrophic lateral sclerosis. *Arch Neurol* 2010;67:1187–1194.

18. Riordan NH, Ichim TE, Min WP, et al. Non-expanded adipose stromal vascular fraction cell therapy for multiple sclerosis. *J Transl Med* 2009;7:29.

19. Liang J, Zhang H, Hua B et al. Allogeneic mesenchymal stem cells transplantation in treatment of multiple sclerosis. *Mult Scler* 2009;15:644–646.

20. Garcia-Olmo D, Herreros D, Pascual I et al. Expanded adipose-derived stem cells for the treatment of complex perianal fistula: a phase II clinical trial. *Dis Colon Rectum* 2009;52:79–86.

21. Ciccocioppo R, Bernardo ME, Sgarella A, et al. Autologous bone marrow-derived mesenchymal stromal cells in the treatment of fistulising Crohn's disease. *Gut* 2011;60:788–798.

22. Duijvestein M, Vos AC, Roelofs H et al. Autologous bone marrow-derived mesenchymal stromal cell treatment for refractory luminal Crohn's disease: results of a phase I study. *Gut* 2010;59:1662–1669.

23. Nevskaya T, Ananieva L, Bykovskaia S et al. Autologous progenitor cell implantation as a novel therapeutic intervention for ischaemic digits in systemic sclerosis. *Rheumatology* (Oxford) 2009;48:61–64.

24. Christopeit M, Schendel M, Foll J et al. Marked improvement of severe progressive systemic sclerosis after transplantation of mesenchymal stem cells from an allogeneic haploidentical-related donor mediated by ligation of CD137L. *Leukemia* 2008;22:1062–1064.

25. Liang J, Zhang H, Hua B et al. Allogenic mesenchymal stem cells transplantation in refractory systemic lupus erythematosus: a pilot clinical study. *Ann Rheum Dis* 2010;69:1423–1429.

26. Sun L, Wang D, Liang J et al. Umbilical cord mesenchymal stem cell transplantation in severe and refractory systemic lupus erythematosus. *Arthritis Rheum* 2010;62:2467–2475.

27. Carrion F, Nova E, Ruiz C et al. Autologous mesenchymal stem cell treatment increased T regulatory cells with no effect on disease activity in two systemic lupus erythematosus patients. *Lupus* 2010;19:317–322.

28. Liang J, Gu F, Wang H et al. Mesenchymal stem cell transplantation for diffuse alveolar hemorrhage in SLE. *Nat Rev Rheumatol* 2010;6:486–489.

CHAPTER 86

Tissue engineering

Andrew McCaskie, Paul Genever,
and Cosimo De Bari

Introduction

The field of tissue engineering has developed rapidly over the last few decades and is of great relevance to musculoskeletal therapy and intervention. Early definitions of tissue engineering emerged in the late 1980s[1] and early 1990s and described tissue engineering as an interdisciplinary science involving life sciences and engineering to bring about biological substitutes that restore, maintain, or improve tissue function.[2] At the time, loss or failure of an organ or tissue was already seen as a frequent, devastating, and costly problem in human health care and three tissue engineering strategies were proposed: (1) cell and cell substitutes; (2) tissue-inducing substances; and (3) cells placed within matrices.[2] Even at this early stage, Langer identified the need to develop treatments to create new cartilage and improve bone repair (mesodermal applications). The scope of tissue engineering is both ambitious and broadly based and includes many branches of biological and engineering disciplines. Over the years there have been developments in both science and technology and the understanding of how to apply them clinically and so new terms and definitions have been developed. Regenerative medicine has been defined as

> an emerging interdisciplinary field of research and clinical applications focused on the repair, replacement, or regeneration of cells, tissues, or organs to restore impaired function resulting from any cause, including congenital defects, disease, and trauma. It uses a combination of several technological approaches that moves it beyond traditional transplantation and replacement therapies. These approaches may include, but are not limited to, the use of stem cells, soluble molecules, genetic engineering, tissue engineering, and advanced cell therapy.[3]

More recently this has been shortened to a single explanatory sentence: regenerative medicine replaces or regenerates human cells, tissue, or organs, to restore or establish normal function.[4]

A further term to consider is cell therapy. This has recently been considered in the context of regenerative medicine and was defined as 'the therapeutic application of cells regardless of cell type or clinical application' and was considered a 'platform' technology, useful to a regenerative approach.[5]

Regenerative strategies—cells, scaffolds, and factors

We can now consider how the strategies defined above can be applied and used within musculoskeletal clinical applications. It is useful to consider the relevant anatomy, such as bone, cartilage, muscle, tendon, ligament, and meniscus. Each tissue can be considered in a simplified manner as a mixture of cells and extracellular matrix. The type of cell will influence the biology of the tissue, e.g. cartilage formation with chondrocytes or bone formation with osteoblasts and the matrix will provide a three-dimensional biological and structural environment. The interaction between a cell and its environment is complex but important as it can direct cell function. At the micro- and nanoscale, cell behaviour is influenced by factors such as cell signalling molecules and the properties of surfaces (chemistry and topography). Beyond the small-scale considerations, the fully assembled tissue must provide the intended function and in the case of the musculoskeletal system this can involve significant mechanical performance, e.g. load transmission across a joint.

Tissue engineering strategies are often considered in a simplified form in terms of cells, scaffolds, and additional factors, although it should be noted that successful translation of such a strategy is more complex (Figure 86.1). There are many variations of usage and combination and it is not necessary for all three to be provided by the proposed treatment. However, the regenerative approach must produce both the quantity and quality of target tissue at the level of the cell, matrix, and environment. Moreover, the regenerated tissue must interact with the host tissue with a seamless biological and functional interface.

Cells

The cell biology of musculoskeletal tissue is of great importance in a regenerative approach. Some orthopaedic applications such as bone graft incorporation, require osteogenesis (osteoblasts) whereas cartilage defects require chondrogenesis (chondrocytes). Some applications may utilize fully differentiated cell types, but recently research has looked to consider the role of stem cells. The multipotent stromal cell/mesenchymal stem cell (MSC) serves many

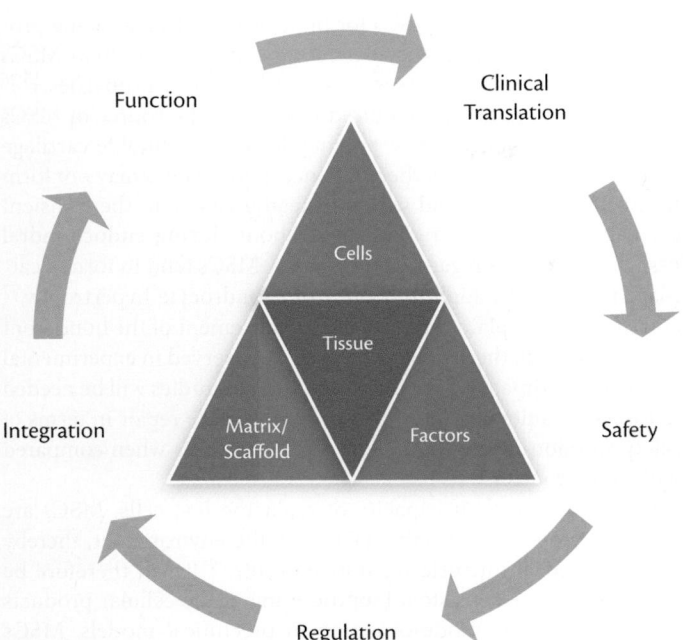

Fig. 86.1 Schematic representation of some key issues relating to tissue engineering and clinical translation.

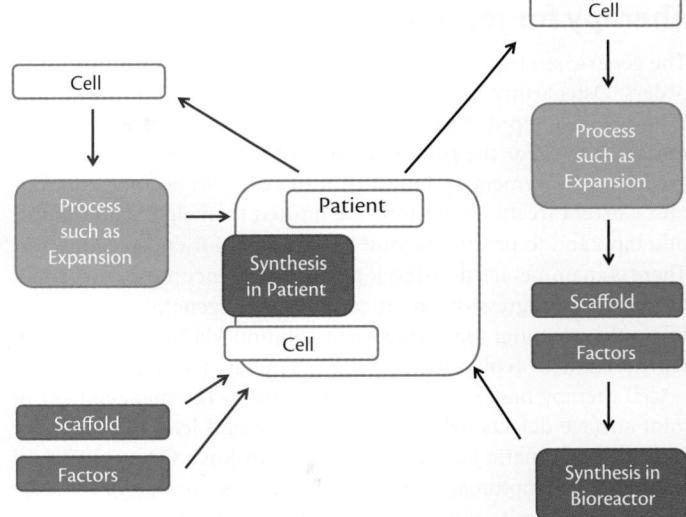

Fig. 86.2 Schematic representation of translational pathways in musculoskeletal regenerative medicine.

important functions within the body including repair and has the potential to differentiate into different cell phenotypes e.g. bone, cartilage, muscle, and tendon lineages. It has the advantage of being available within the adult and in many locations, such as bone marrow, fat, blood, and synovium.[6–9] In addition, relatively simple ex-vivo expansion and differentiation techniques have been developed for use in research and clinical applications. MSCs appear to have an immune-privileged or even an immunosuppressive function following transplantation. In trials of osteogenesis imperfecta, where allogeneic bone marrow-derived MSCs were given to patients after bone marrow transplantation, MSC engraftment was shown and a marked increase in patient recovery was detected.[10] Embryonic stem cells (ESCs) are pluripotent and clearly also have the ability to differentiate into relevant skeletal tissue groups, as well as cell and tissue types from all three embryonic germ layers. There are, however, ethical considerations associated with the use of ESCs in therapies and the need for defined protocols for osteo/chondrogenic differentiation.

Therapeutic adult stem cells, such as MSCs, could be used with or without culture expansion and with the target tissue synthesis taking place in the laboratory or in the human (Figure 86.2). In both approaches, these tissue progenitor cells are central to cell-based tissue engineering strategies that have been described[11,12]:

- local targeting of connective tissue progenitor cells
- homing connective tissue progenitor cells to new areas
- physically transplanting connective tissue progenitor cells
- transplantation of culture-expanded or modified connective tissue progenitor cells
- transplantation of fully formed tissue.

Scaffolds

The extracellular component of a therapy is often called a scaffold and must facilitate the cell repair processes (such as migration, proliferation, differentiation). In musculoskeletal applications it may also fulfil some biomechanical requirements such as load transmission. Several different types of support materials are available, ranging from natural and synthetic biomaterials and nano-textured scaffolds through to complex self-assembling peptide gels, with different compositional features, including polymers, ceramics, and metals. Increasingly sophisticated bioengineering approaches have been developed to allow precise control over the geometry and architecture of the desired scaffold.[13] When considering the design and selection of scaffolds the following features have been described[11]:

- preservation of tissue volume
- porosity that can allow mass transport of nutrients
- porosity that can allow tissue and vascular ingrowth
- a surface optimized for cell attachment migration proliferation and differentiation
- the degradation property that allows regeneration and does not cause local toxicity.

Factors

The interaction between a cell and the scaffold can be facilitated by various factors. This includes a range of secreted factors including hormones and locally released cytokines and growth factors.[14] For example, exposure of MSCs to bone morphogenic proteins (BMPs) can induce osteogenic differentiation. Furthermore, it may be important to consider the mechanical and chemical composition of the tissue from which the cells were initially derived. For example, MSCs are believed to exist in a specialized microenvironment, or niche, which can support the MSCs, protect from damaging stimuli and promote niche exit when appropriate differentiation stimuli are received, with growing evidence supporting a perivascular location.[15] A deeper knowledge of the in-vivo stem cell niche and its structure and organization in different tissue types will also contribute to new strategies for bioengineering scaffolds.

Therapy for joint disorders

The generic strategies described above can be applied to joint disorders. Osteoarthritis (OA) is the most common joint disease and is an increasing problem in our society as people age and wish to remain active. For the patient, quality of life is reduced because of the loss of movement and joint pain increases to become continuous. Current treatment options are limited to analgesia and physiotherapy, and to prosthetic joint replacement for endstage disease. There is an unmet need to develop new treatment options that could halt disease progression, at an early stage. Regenerative medicine offers the potential for a long-term solution via biological repair, regeneration, or replacement of the degenerate joint tissues.

Cell therapy has proved very promising in the management of joint surface defects, which if untreated could lead to secondary OA. Post-traumatic OA represents 13% of knee OA and 73% of ankle OA.[16] Symptomatic chronic full-thickness defects of the knee joint surface require surgical intervention for symptom relief and to prevent evolution towards OA. Current treatment options include microfracture and autologous chondrocyte implantation (ACI).[17,18] Microfracture involves creating a surgical communication between the joint space and the subchondral bone and marrow, which can be achieved by using a sharp awl. The theoretical basis for the cartilage regeneration is the release from the marrow space of adult stem cells. ACI involves two surgical procedures. In the first, cartilage is obtained from the patient's joint surface but from an area not required for joint function. From this cartilage, chondrocytes can be obtained and expanded in vitro. A second surgical procedure is carried out to place the expanded chondrocytes within the area of cartilage damage, either membrane bound or secured by a periosteal flap.

ACI was first described in 1994 by Brittberg and colleagues,[19] who reported treatment of symptomatic defects of the joint surface in humans by implantation of autologous, culture-expanded articular chondrocytes underneath a periosteal flap. Chondrocytes were obtained with a cartilage biopsy from an uninvolved and minor loadbearing area of the same joint surface. This study showed symptomatic relief in 14 out of 16 patients with lesions of the femoral condyle at 2 years follow-up. Currently, ACI represents the gold standard of cell therapy for cartilage repair with up to 20 years' follow-up showing ACI being an effective and durable solution for the treatment of large full-thickness cartilage lesions of the knee joint.[20]

Chondrocytes are difficult to grow in culture as they rapidly undergo dedifferentiation, resulting in the loss of their capacity to form cartilage in vivo.[21] MSCs are easy to isolate and culture expand, are chondrogenic, and therefore are attractive chondrocyte substitutes in an ACI-like procedure. For these reasons, the use of MSCs for joint surface repair is intensively sought and has been explored to reconstruct joint surface over eburnated condyles in patients with advanced OA.[22] MSCs could be implanted as undifferentiated cells, either in suspension or in combination with biomaterial scaffolds, while the addition of chondrogenic factors could enhance repair cartilage tissue formation.[23]

As discussed earlier, MSCs are known to be present in many connective tissues of the adult human body.[9] For example, MSCs can be derived from the adult human synovial membrane,[24] which is often exuberant in joint disorders and is therefore removed in diagnostic arthroscopic procedures. Excessive synovium could therefore

be a precious source of MSCs for biological joint-resurfacing protocols. However, there is evidence indicating that human MSCs from different tissues possess distinct biological properties,[25,26] and therefore studies are required to identify the source of MSCs with superior chondrogenic potency leading to durable cartilage repair tissue. In addition, there is concern that MSCs may not form hyaline-like cartilage and would instead give rise to the transient cartilage tissue that is replaced with bone during endochondral ossification. In this regard, bone marrow MSCs tend to form a cartilage tissue with a high frequency of chondrocyte hypertrophy,[27] and this could explain the excessive advancement of the bone front at the expense of the articular cartilage as observed in experimental animals.[28] Ultimately, preclinical and clinical studies will be needed to assess the suitability of MSCs for joint surface repair in terms of safety and non-inferiority in clinical effectiveness when compared with chondrocytes.

In addition to their capacity of replacing lost cells, MSCs are also likely to provide trophic factors to the environment, thereby enhancing local intrinsic reparative events.[29] It will therefore be crucial to ensure consistent bioprocessing of the cellular products while studying its mode of action in preclinical models. MSCs could also be implanted immediately after their purification in a one-step procedure, without culture expansion. Minimally manipulated cellular preparations would simplify the regulatory paths of autologous procedures but would equally require quality controls also including identity characterization and potency assessment.

The use of allogeneic MSCs would allow upscalable production of quality-controlled cell preparations, readily available for implantation. This would enhance consistency and abate costs, thus facilitating large-scale distribution for routine clinical application. MSCs appear suitable for allogeneic transplantation for their immune privilege and immunomodulatory properties, although these remain controversial due to conflicting results.[30] In addition, the differentiation into a mature phenotype of the implanted MSCs may result in the loss of the immunological privilege with consequent rejection.[31]

OA is often confined to one or a few large weightbearing joints and therefore intra-articular administration of allogeneic MSCs is being explored, supported by the promising data obtained in a preclinical goat model of OA induced by medial meniscectomy and resection of the anterior cruciate ligament.[32] In this model, intra-articular administration of bone marrow MSCs resulted in the regeneration of a meniscal-like tissue and retarded progression of OA.

In addition to the use of ex-vivo manipulated MSCs, another possible approach contemplates the activation of intrinsic regenerative mechanisms, e.g. by using medications that target the endogenous MSCs that are naturally present in the joint (see Figure 86.2). Several joint-associated tissues such as synovial membrane and fluid, fat pad, periosteum, bone marrow, and even the articular cartilage itself, have been reported to contain cells that, after isolation and culture expansion, display properties of MSCs, but their location and functional roles remain to be elucidated.

Recently, the use of a double nucleoside labelling scheme in a clinically relevant mouse model of joint surface injury[33] allowed the identification and characterization of endogenous resident MSC niches in the knee joint synovium in vivo.[34] An understanding of the molecular regulation of MSC niches in health and joint disorders will provide the scientific basis for the development of novel interventions that enhance intrinsic regenerative mechanisms in order to treat or even prevent OA. This could be achieved by local administration of drugs or via the controlled release of specific growth factors or morphogens using, for instance, bioactive scaffolds. Another key step will be the identification of the appropriate molecular signal(s) to be delivered. The evidence that the BMP and Wnt signalling pathways are activated in adult articular cartilage in response to mechanical injury[35] suggests that these signalling pathways could be part of a programme of remodelling or repair and therefore possible therapeutic targets to achieve joint tissue repair. Modulation of the Wnt and BMP signalling pathways within the joint environment is likely to affect stem cell fates and related tissue remodelling.

Conclusion

Tissue engineering, regenerative medicine, and cell therapies have developed significantly over the last few decades and are applicable to a wide range of musculoskeletal applications. Many strategies have been identified that would potentially benefit patients but the future will require successful translation from the laboratory into clinical practice. It is important to identify clinical targets where there is both clinical need and an informed view that the approach is likely to be successful. There are already examples of bone substitutes being used for bone loss and expanded chondrocytes being used to regenerate cartilage. The future will see more complex applications such as fracture healing and osteoarthritis. To deliver this, an interaction must be facilitated between many stakeholders such as scientific researchers, clinicians, healthcare providers, industry, regulatory organizations, and of course the patients themselves. The challenge is to provide treatments that are effective and safe but are also cost effective and available to all who require them. The original scope of tissue engineering was to improve upon end-stage treatments such as joint replacement, which utilize metal and plastic. As we move forward, we may see regenerative approaches that attempt to achieve repair and regeneration at an earlier stage, using advanced biomaterials and cell-based technologies.

References

1. Skalak R, Fox CF. Tissue engineering: proceedings of a workshop, held at Granlibakken, Lake Tahoe, California, February 26–29, 1988, Liss, New York, 1988.
2. Langer R, Vacanti JP. Tissue engineering. *Science* 1993;260(5110):920–926.
3. Greenwood HL, Singer PA, Downey GP et al. Regenerative medicine and the developing world. *PLoS Med* 2006;3(9):e381.
4. Mason C, Dunnill P. A brief definition of regenerative medicine. *Regen Med* 2008;3(1):1–5.
5. Mason C, Brindley DA, Culme-Seymour EJ, Davie NL. Cell therapy industry: billion dollar global business with unlimited potential. *Regen Med* 2011;6(3):265–272.
6. Friedenstein AJ, Chailakhjan RK, Lalykina KS. The development of fibroblast colonies in monolayer cultures of guinea-pig bone marrow and spleen cells . *Cell Tissue Kinet* 1970;3(4):393–403.
7. Friedenstein AJ, Piatetzky S, II, Petrakova KV. Osteogenesis in transplants of bone marrow cells. *J Embryol Exp Morphol* 1966;16(3):381–390.
8. Pittenger MF, Mackay AM, Beck SC et al. Multilineage potential of adult human mesenchymal stem cells. *Science* 1999;284(5411):143–147.
9. Augello A, Kurth TB, De Bari C. Mesenchymal stem cells: a perspective from in vitro cultures to in vivo migration and niches. *Eur Cell Mater* 2010;20:121–133.
10. Horwitz EM, Gordon PL, Koo WK et al. Isolated allogeneic bone marrow-derived mesenchymal cells engraft and stimulate growth in children with osteogenesis imperfecta: Implications for cell therapy of bone. *Proc Nat Acad Sci U S A* 2002;99(13):8932–8937.
11. Patterson TE, Kumagai K, Griffith L, Muschler GF. Cellular strategies for enhancement of fracture repair. *J Bone Joint Surg Am* 2008;90 Suppl 1:111–119.
12. Arthur A, Zannettino A, Gronthos S. The therapeutic applications of multipotential mesenchymal/stromal stem cells in skeletal tissue repair. *J Cell Physiol* 2009;218(2):237–245.
13. Hollister SJ. Porous scaffold design for tissue engineering. *Nat Mater* 2005;4(7):518–524.
14. Corsi KA, Schwarz EM, Mooney DJ, Huard J. Regenerative medicine in orthopaedic surgery. *J Orthop Res* 2007;25(10):1261–1268.
15. Crisan M, Yap S, Casteilla L et al. A perivascular origin for mesenchymal stem cells in multiple human organs. *Cell Stem Cell* 2008;3(3):301–313.
16. Buckwalter JA, Saltzman C, Brown T. The impact of osteoarthritis: implications for research. *Clin Orthop Relate Res* 2004;427(Suppl):S6–S15.
17. De Bari C, Pitzalis C, Dell'Accio F. Reparative medicine: from tissue engineering to joint surface regeneration. *Regen Med* 2006;1(1):59–69.
18. Roberts S, Genever P, McCaskie A, De Bari C. Prospects of stem cell therapy in osteoarthritis. *Regen Med* 2011;6(3):351–366.
19. Brittberg M, Lindahl A, Nilsson A et AL. Treatment of deep cartilage defects in the knee with autologous chondrocyte transplantation. *N Engl J Med* 1994;331(14):889–895.
20. Peterson L, Vasiliadis HS, Brittberg M, Lindahl A. Autologous chondrocyte implantation: a long-term follow-up. *Am J Sports Med* 2010;38(6):1117–1124.
21. Dell'Accio F, De Bari C, Luyten FP. Molecular markers predictive of the capacity of expanded human articular chondrocytes to form stable cartilage in vivo. *Arthritis Rheum* 2001;44(7):1608–1619.
22. Wakitani S, Imoto K, Yamamoto T et al. Human autologous culture expanded bone marrow mesenchymal cell transplantation for repair of cartilage defects in osteoarthritic knees. *Osteoarthritis Cartilage* 2002;10(3):199–206.
23. Gelse K, von der Mark K, Aigner T, Park J, Schneider H. Articular cartilage repair by gene therapy using growth factor-producing mesenchymal cells. *Arthritis Rheum* 2003;48(2):430–441.
24. De Bari C, Dell'Accio F, Tylzanowski P, Luyten FP. Multipotent mesenchymal stem cells from adult human synovial membrane. *Arthritis Rheum* 2001;44(8):1928–1942.
25. Sakaguchi Y, Sekiya I, Yagishita K, Muneta T. Comparison of human stem cells derived from various mesenchymal tissues: superiority of synovium as a cell source. *Arthritis Rheum* 2005;52(8):2521–2529.
26. De Bari C, Dell'Accio F, Karystinou A et al. A biomarker-based mathematical model to predict bone-forming potency of human synovial and periosteal mesenchymal stem cells. *Arthritis Rheum* 2008;58(1):240–250.
27. Scotti C, Tonnarelli B, Papadimitropoulos A et al. Recapitulation of endochondral bone formation using human adult mesenchymal stem cells as a paradigm for developmental engineering. *Proc Nat Acad Sci U S A* 2010;107(16):7251–7256.
28. Qiu YS, Shahgaldi BF, Revell WJ, Heatley FW. Observations of subchondral plate advancement during osteochondral repair: a histomorphometric and mechanical study in the rabbit femoral condyle. *Osteoarthritis Cartilage* 2003;11(11):810–820.
29. Munoz JR, Stoutenger BR, Robinson AP, Spees JL, Prockop DJ. Human stem/progenitor cells from bone marrow promote neurogenesis of endogenous neural stem cells in the hippocampus of mice. *Proc Nat Acad Sci U S A* 2005;102(50):18171–18176.
30. MacDonald GI, Augello A, De Bari C. Role of mesenchymal stem cells in reestablishing immunologic tolerance in autoimmune rheumatic diseases. *Arthritis Rheum* 2011;63(9):2547–2557.
31. Chen X, McClurg A, Zhou GQ, McCaigue M, Armstrong MA, Li G. Chondrogenic differentiation alters the immunosuppressive property of bone marrow-derived mesenchymal stem cells, and the effect is

partially due to the upregulated expression of B7 molecules. *Stem Cell* 2007;25(2):364–370.

32. Murphy JM, Fink DJ, Hunziker EB, Barry FP. Stem cell therapy in a caprine model of osteoarthritis. *Arthritis Rheum* 2003;48(12):3464–3474.

33. Eltawil NM, De Bari C, Achan P, Pitzalis C, Dell'accio F. A novel in vivo murine model of cartilage regeneration. Age and strain-dependent outcome after joint surface injury. *Osteoarthritis Cartilage* 2009;17(6):695–704.

34. Kurth TB, Dell'accio F, Crouch V et al. Functional mesenchymal stem cell niches in adult mouse knee joint synovium in vivo. *Arthritis Rheum* 2011;63(5):1289–1300.

35. Dell'Accio F, De Bari C, El Tawil NM et al. Activation of WNT and BMP signaling in adult human articular cartilage following mechanical injury. *Arthritis Res Ther* 2006;8(5):R139.

CHAPTER 87

Injection therapy

Philip Platt and Ismael Atchia

Introduction

Targeted injection for joint and soft tissues pathologies have been reported as far back as the 1930s though the outcomes with initial agents such as glycerin, formalin, and petroleum jelly were poor. Hydrocortisone was found to be more promising and Professor J.L. Hollander was a pioneer in the field with his publications in the 1950s of the results of tens of thousands of injections performed.[1,2] From early on, it was realized that the high solubility of hydrocortisone was perhaps one of the reasons for the short duration of action. Since then glucocorticoid esters with lower solubility have been preferred. Injection therapy has become a core treatment in musculoskeletal medicine.

Injection therapy is usually indicated in the treatment of inflammatory arthritis or soft tissue inflammation affecting structures such as tendons and bursae, but is also used in degenerative conditions. There is evidence of prolonged benefit from intra-articular steroid therapy in rheumatoid arthritis (RA). Joint injection has an important role as an adjunct to disease-modifying anti-rheumatic drug (DMARD) treatment, in achieving tight control in RA. The role of injections in the management of osteoarthritis (OA) has remained poorly defined and its use highly variable. Other intra-articular injections such as hyaluronic acid, silicone, glucosamine, non-steroidal anti-inflammatory drugs (NSAIDs), yttrium, and botulinum have been used,[3,4] as well as novel agents such as tropisetron (a 5 HT-3 receptor antagonist)[5] and interleukin(IL)-1 receptor antagonist.[6] The most widely used by far remain glucocorticoids followed by hyaluronic acid.[4] These agents are reviewed in this chapter with regard to their safety and efficacy.

Injection techniques

Clinically guided injection

Joint injection has usually been performed using anatomical landmarks to guide the needle into the joint. This technique is also referred as 'blind injection'. The ability to perform the procedure accurately depends on the experience and skill of the physician. It relies on clear understanding of static and functional anatomy of the target area and ability to palpate and identify joint contours. The method for identifying different joints and soft tissue areas are covered later in this chapter. Any clinician starting to perform injections will experience a learning curve, with increased accuracy over time. The advantage of the clinically guided technique is that, in experienced hands, this procedure can be easily and quickly performed within the clinic room setting. One of the potential drawbacks is the uncertain accuracy, unless there is a positive aspirate of synovial fluid. Surrogate criteria for accuracy such as low resistance on injecting can be misleading since periarticular structures such as fat pads around joints can be readily infiltrated.

A small number of studies have addressed the accuracy of injection and reported surprisingly low accuracy. Jones et al.,[7] using methylprednisolone mixed with contrast agent, demonstrated that the accuracy of blind joint injection was only 50% for injections performed at common sites such as the knee and shoulder. However more recent studies have revealed better results, indicating that accuracy probably remains physician dependent.[8]

Image-guided injection

A variety of imaging methods, including fluoroscopic screening, CT scanning, and more recently ultrasound and MRI, have been used to better localize needle placement.[9–13] Fluoroscopy screening improves accuracy but requires radiology staff and a suitably equipped environment, and involves exposure to radiation and injection of contrast material. CT scanning provides more detailed bony imaging and is the preferred option for sacroiliac joint injection but is also associated with radiation exposure. MRI, on the other hand, is safe and detailed imaging of structures is possible. However, like CT, it can (usually) only be performed in a radiology department and is relatively expensive.

Musculoskeletal ultrasound (MSUS)-guided injection does not involve radiation, allows dynamic images to be obtained, and in view of its portability makes it possible to perform procedures in the clinic setting. The use of ultrasound guidance is discussed further in this chapter; the other image-guided modalities tend to be practised by radiologists.

Ultrasound enables the visualization of soft tissue structures and can distinguish synovial fluid and synovial proliferation. Ultrasound can therefore confirm the indication for an injection and determine the most direct and safest route for needling, which avoids neurovascular structures or tendons. There are two techniques of ultrasound-guided injection, direct and indirect. For the indirect method, ultrasound is used to visualize the structures and determine the depth of the target area from the skin surface. The

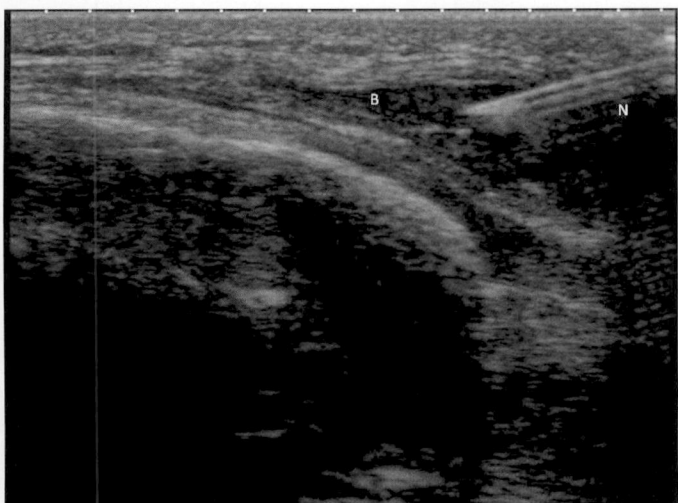

Fig. 87.1 Ultrasound-guided injection of the prepatellar bursa with real time visualization of the needle (N) and distension of the bursa (B) around the needle tip.

skin is then marked and the injection performed without further use of the ultrasound.

The direct method depends on direct visualization of the target structures and then real time visualization of the needle as shown in Figure 87.1. Injecting the target area can be confirmed from its distension and/or visualization of the material injected, which is hypoechoic for saline or lidocaine and hyperechoic for steroid or steroid/air mixture. Direct ultrasound-guided injections can be technically challenging as they rely on manual dexterity and coordination; usually the dominant hand is used for the syringe, with the probe being held by the non-dominant hand. There are situations when the needle will not be readily visualized, and the maintenance of asepsis during the procedure is clearly of paramount importance.

Glucocorticoid injections

Effects of steroids

The rationale for using steroids in inflammatory arthritis is their broad anti-inflammatory properties based on inhibition of prostaglandin, leukotriene, and proinflammatory cytokine production (see Chapter 79).[14,15] There are steroid receptors within the nucleus of all cells, including synoviocytes, which modulate transcription and expression of cellular proteins. A small study in RA has shown downregulation of a number of proinflammatory cytokines following a single intra-articular injection of triamcinalone,[16] but there are no similar human in-vivo data for OA. The first intra-articular steroids used, such as hydrocortisone acetate, were relatively water soluble, and therefore could permeate through the synovial membrane easily, with poor retention in the joint.[17] Since then less water-soluble forms, such as methylprednisolone acetate, triamcinolone acetonide, and triamcinolone hexacetonide, have been preferred. However, triamcinolone acetonide and trimacinolone hexacetonide are usually avoided for tendons and superficial structures because there is some evidence of increased tendon rupture and skin/fat atrophy.[18–20]

There is good evidence for prolonged benefit of intra-articular glucocorticoids in RA and juvenile idiopathic arthritis (JIA).[21,22]

On the other hand, meta-analyses of OA studies have failed to demonstrate benefit of more than 3 weeks. Recent studies in hip OA have demonstrated more prolonged benefit,[23–25] with evidence of synovitis being a predictor of prolonged response.[26]

There have been no clinical trials comparing both the long-term efficacy and safety between different steroid agents and preparations. One randomized controlled trial (RCT) revealed superior duration of benefit of triamcinolone hexacetonide and triamcinolone acetonide compared to hydrocortisone in the treatment of RA of the knee.[27] Other RCTs have demonstrated efficacy over placebo for OA of large joints and for conditions such as carpal tunnel syndrome. However, there is no consensus with regards to the dose, although there is some agreement that the dose should be proportionate to the size of the joint and perhaps to the degree of inflammation within a joint.

There are wider variations with regard to whether local anaesthetic is used and what volume. Surgeons tend to use higher volumes because they undertake more injections for diagnostic rather than therapeutic purposes. However, there is some debate whether immediate pain reduction from injection is solely due to adequate infiltration of the pathological structure with local anaesthetic as opposed to the possible placebo effect associated with injections.[28]

The overall evidence tends to indicate improved clinical outcomes for accurately delivered glucocorticoid injections.[7–9] However, for sacroiliac joint injections, a recent study revealed that periarticular deposition of glucocorticoid is as effective as accurate intra-articular injection.[29]

Risks/side effects of steroids

Intra-articular injection is a safe procedure but can nevertheless be associated with some adverse effects. These can be related to local trauma in and around the joint, and local or systemic adverse reactions to the injected agent. Postinjection flare is thought to be due to a reactive synovitis to the glucocorticoid crystals and usually should not last more than 24 hours. The most feared complication is septic arthritis, which is associated with significant morbidity and mortality.[30] The incidence of septic arthritis from joint injection is extremely low and usually quoted at around 1:10 000 to 1:20 000.[3,4,31,32] Hollander quoted 18 cases out of 250 000 injections performed and other more recent reviews suggest an even lower risk (4.6 per 100 000 based on a survey of 40 rheumatologists in the United Kingdom,[33] 2 in 100 000 by Gray et al.[34]). French data reported a septic arthritis rate as low as 1/162 000 when glucocorticoid packaged into a sterile syringe was used.[35] Of concern, however, are recent data from Iceland identifying a rate of 0.037%,[36] though this study did not document injection technique used or the clinicians performing the injections.

There is no clear indication whether full aseptic technique reduces the risk compared to the no-touch technique.[37] Overall, when the risk is so low, it is difficult to prove causality. Even if joint infection follows an injection, unless the timeframe precludes an alternative explanation it is important to remember that septic arthritis may also reflect underlying immune compromise secondary to disease factors (such as in RA) or the immunosuppressant effects of drugs.

Haemarthrosis is another potential complication of injection, but the risk is extremely low unless there is an underlying bleeding tendency. Salvati et al.[38] reported 2 cases of postprocedure haemarthrosis on their series of 15 patients on warfarin, but the INR of these 2 patients was between 3.8 and 5. In contrast, in the prospective study by Thumboo et al.,[39] of 32 soft tissue and joint injection/aspiration procedures the INR was less than 3 or well controlled in all patients and no cases of bleeding occurred. Thus as long as the INR is less than 3, warfarin therapy should not be a contraindication for intra-articular or soft tissue injection. Extra care should be taken to avoid vascular injuries particularly for the small joints, carpometacarpal (CMC), and ankle joint injections. There are reports not just of trauma to blood vessels, but also of cases of arterial emboli from the low-solubility steroids blocking arterioles.

Steroid injections have been linked to cartilage loss in some non-primate animal studies. Triamcinolone hexacetonide injections have been linked to increased progression of cartilage loss in the hands and the hip joint in juvenile arthritis,[40,41] although it is unclear from these observational data whether more aggressive disease in patients given this treatment option or the steroid injection itself was responsible for cartilage loss. In a large prospective RCT of patients receiving multiple intra-articular joint injections for knee OA followed over 2 years, there was no evidence of increased loss of cartilage in the injection group.[42] Our personal view is that this concern has been exaggerated and has resulted in unfounded restrictions in the frequency of intra-articular injections of steroids. This particularly is relevant for an inflamed joint, where untreated inflammation within the joint itself is almost certainly more likely to lead to cartilage loss than any injected glucocorticoid.

There can be systemic effects from local injections although studies have revealed that the effects, even for concurrent multiple joint injections, are minimal when compared with intramuscular steroid. There is no evidence to suggest long-term complications such as osteoporosis, hypertension, weight gain, and diabetes, which are associated with systemic glucocorticoids. Systemic effects are more pronounced in the first 24 hours and patients may experience facial flushing. Diabetic patients may experience higher than usual blood glucose levels, particularly in the first 24 hours following injection. There have been case reports of extremely rare side effects such as steroid psychosis after steroid injection.

Indications/contraindications

Glucocorticoid injections are administered for therapeutic benefits but, usually in combination with local anaesthetic, may also be administered for diagnostic purposes. The therapeutic benefits are reduction in pain by reduction of inflammation and preventing relapse of swelling/synovitis. In mono or oligo inflammatory arthritis, injection is often a better option than systemic steroid or immunosuppressant treatment.

In musculoskeletal presentations when the pathology is not clear (e.g. complex shoulder pain or lower limb/back pain), particularly when surgery is contemplated, a diagnostic injection may be indicated. In these situations a large volume of local anaesthetic is often used (usually in combination with steroid) and bupivacaine or another longer-acting local anaesthetic is preferred. If there is immediate benefit or significant benefit noted within a few hours of the injection, then the area infiltrated is probably the source of the patient's symptoms. However, in cases of intermittent pain, it may not be possible to ascertain the immediate response from the injection and then the potentially longer-acting steroid may clarify the diagnosis. However, the delayed response to an injection may not necessarily confirm the site of pain, since this may be due to the systemic action of the steroid. Finally, interpretation of a patient's response is further complicated by the strong placebo response to injections.

In summary, there is good rationale for performing joint/soft tissue steroid injections, but further evidence is required to ascertain whether medium/long-term outcomes depend on type of steroid, accuracy of injection, timing/frequency of injection, added benefit of local anaesthetic, and impact of other medical co morbidities, or psychological effects on perceived response.

Method

The techniques for clinically guided injections and also for ultrasound-guided injections of different structures are discussed below. There are common considerations for the different anatomical areas (summarized in Box 87.1). Either a no-touch technique or aseptic technique should be used. With the no-touch technique the target area is palpated to identify the joint contour or soft tissue structure. The overlying skin is then marked, preferably by indentation of the nail or with the tip of a pen. Pen marks, even with special skin marker pens, are best avoided as they may become indistinct with skin cleaning. Once the skin is marked, it is cleaned with an alcohol swab, ideally more than once, or with disinfectant such as chlorhexidine in alcohol, and then without touching the skin again, the injection is performed.

Aseptic technique will consist of sterilizing a wider skin area overlying the region of interest. The area is then usually isolated with sterile drapes. The clinician is gowned and will be using sterile gloves, and hence palpation of the area will not lead to loss of sterility.

When the injection is performed using direct visualization on ultrasound, the ultrasound probe needs to be cleaned with chlorhexidine spray/solution. The chlorhexidine in alcohol spray/solution absolves the requirement for gel, but otherwise sterile gel can be used. Some practitioners advocate the use of sterile sheaths

---

Box 87.1 General principles for joint injections

- Assess indications/contraindications
- Obtain written or verbal consent
- Glucocorticoid: higher dose for large joints
- Local anaesthetic: preinfiltrated or premixed steroid preparation; consideration for total volume
- Identification of anatomical landmarks
- Image guidance or assisted when appropriate/ultrasound to confirm effusion or synovitis
- Aseptic technique or no-touch technique
- Avoid injecting against significant resistance (except for entheses)
- Aspirate before injecting
- Reconsider/avoid injection if aspirate is bloody or potentially infected
- Provide postinjection advice about rest, postinjection flare, analgesia

and gel to cover the ultrasound probe as the preferred method to maintain sterility during the injection.

Injections can consist of just one syringe with one needle, e.g. injection of steroid or premixed steroid/lidocaine preparation. However, one needle and three syringes are usually required for joints needing aspiration and injection: once the area is infiltrated with local anaesthetic, usually all the way into the joint capsule, the syringe is disconnected from the needle, then another syringe is used for aspiration, and then finally a third syringe containing the steroid is connected. In these circumstances, the overall procedure takes longer, requiring handling of the needle end to change the syringe, and the no-touch technique is best avoided. Some practitioners do not infiltrate with local anaesthetic first, using just two syringes. In the paediatric setting the skin can be anesthesized with prior application (about 45 minutes before the procedure) of local anaesthetic cream, such as lidocaine/prilocaine (EMLA). Another option is refrigerant spray such as ethyl chloride, which is applied until the skin turns white, and then the procedure is carried out.

Patients should be always be made aware of the risk of septic arthritis and informed of the symptoms and signs to monitor. This should be distinguished from flare of pain during the first 24 hours, which can be the result of a transient synovitis to glucocorticoid crystals. Excessive weightbearing of the injected joint should usually be avoided for 24 hours following the injection.

Upper limbs

Glenohumeral joint

The joint capsule usually connects and communicates with the biceps tendon. The joint is usually accessed using the anterior or posterior approach; the lateral approach may cause damage to the rotator cuff tendons. Joint injection is indicated for suspected inflammation of the joint and/or if there is associated global restriction of movement.

Anterior approach

* Posture: patient either comfortably sitting up or lying supine.

* Anatomical landmarks: the coracoid process is identified below the distal part of the clavicle. The joint is just lateral and probably easier to access just inferior/lateral to the coracoid process (Figure 87.2).

* Needle: 23 or 21G.

* Approach: aim towards the acromion or fairly perpendicular; usually a 'give' is felt.

* Caution: risk of biceps tendon rupture. In obese patients it can be difficult to feel the bony landmarks. Longer needle may be required and care taken not to advance the needle medially to avoid lung injury.

Posterior approach

* Posture: patient sitting in an upright position and approach from behind.

* Anatomical landmarks: the acromion is palpated at its distal end and at the junction of the spine of the scapula. The area 1 cm under the acromion is marked.

* Needle: 23 or 21G.

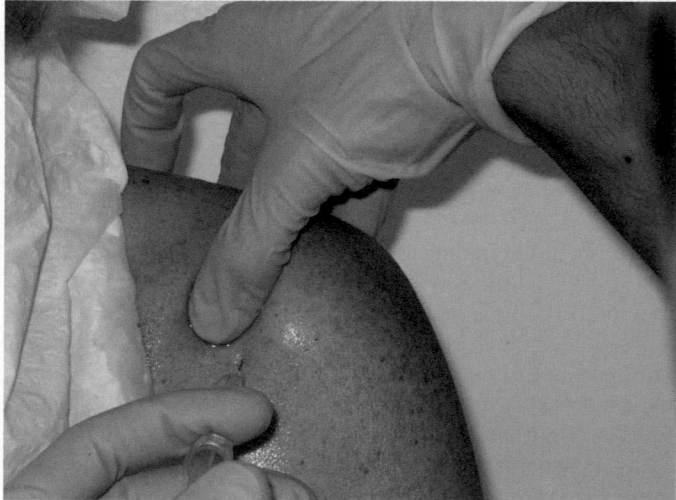

Fig. 87.2 Shoulder joint injection. Anterior approach with thumb of free hand positioned over the coracoid process and needle inserted just inferior and lateral.

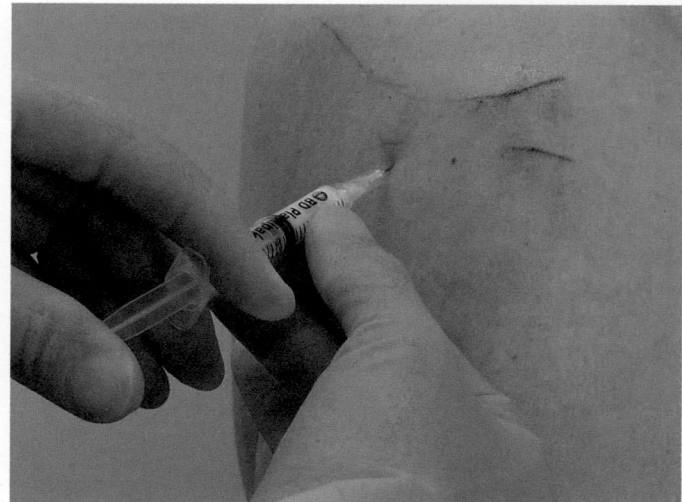

Fig. 87.3 Subacromial joint injection. The inferior margin of the acromium is outlined.

* Approach: needle is inserted and targeted towards the coracoid process, which can be palpated with the free hand. Aim as deep as possible or if bone contact withdraw slightly. Inject without resistance.

* Caution: the glenohumeral joint from this approach may be more than 3–4 cm deep even for average-sized patients.

Subacromial bursa

This is a large bursa between the deltoid and the rotator cuff tendons/muscles. Isolated bursitis is uncommon. Bursitis is usually associated with underlying rotator cuff pathology or impingement.

* Posture: patient sitting comfortably with the arm vertical and relaxed. The acromion is palpated and the gap between it and the humeral head felt. The skin is marked 1–1.5 cm below the inferior margin of the acromion (Figure 87.3).

* Needle: 23 or 21G.

* Approach: once the skin is punctured, aim the needle upwards under the acromion. Either infiltrate with local anaesthetic first then change syringe for the steroid or inject directly with steroid.

* Caution: the potential space can be obliterated in a full-thickness tear with superior migration of the humeral head.

Acromioclavicular joint

Indicated when there is localized tenderness over the joint. It is very superficial and a small joint, therefore only a small volume can be used. The gap is very difficult to feel and movement of the shoulder can make it easier to feel the joint line. Otherwise the joint can be easily visualized on ultrasound. When performed under clinical guidance, the joint is approached verticaly down but with ultrasound the approach can be modified and adapted to avoid any osteophytes.

Elbow joint

Lateral approach

* Posture: patient sitting with arm resting comfortably. The lateral epicondyle is palpated and the radial head palpated-supination/ pronation of the arm will facilitate. The entry point is just proximal to the radial head.

* Needle: 23G.

* Approach: once the skin is punctured, direct needle into the joint space. Target may be less than 1 cm deep.

* Caution: this is a difficult joint to inject in the absence of effusion.

Posterior approach

* Posture: patient sitting with palm down. The olecranon and lateral epicondyle are identified. The olecranon groove is just proximal to the olecranon.

* Needle: 23G.

* Approach: skin is marked over the olecranon groove and needled directed vertically. With ultrasound guidance, the needle is inserted more proximally and then aimed towards the olecranon at an angle of about 45°, with direct visualization of the needle (Figure 87.4).

Lateral epicondyle

Injection is indicated for epicondylitis (tennis elbow) with point tenderness over the area or discomfort on resisted wrist extension.

* Posture: elbow flexed at about 90°, arm resting. The lateral epicondyle is readily palpable and most tender spot identified.

* Needle: 23G.

* Approach: ideally the skin is marked 0.5 cm away from the point of maximum tenderness. Once skin is punctured, the needle is then 'tunnelled' to reach the musculotendinous insertion area (Figure 87.5). If point of entry is directly above the area, the steroid may be infiltrated subcutaneously and this can result in skin atrophy. This risk is minimized by using hydrocortisone.

* Caution: the insertion area is tough and resistance felt during this injection

Medial epicondyle

Injection indicated for golfer's elbow with tenderness over the medial epicondyle or with pain on resisted wrist flexion.

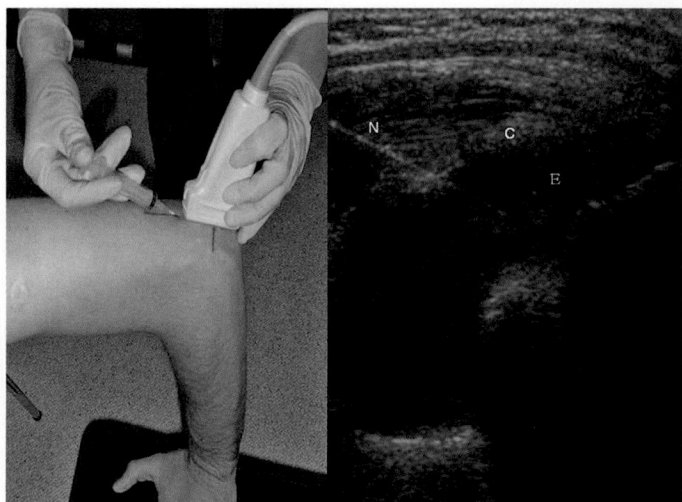

Fig. 87.4 Elbow joint injection. Posterior approach, under direct ultrasound visualization of the needle (N) going through the joint capsule (C) targeting the joint effusion (E).

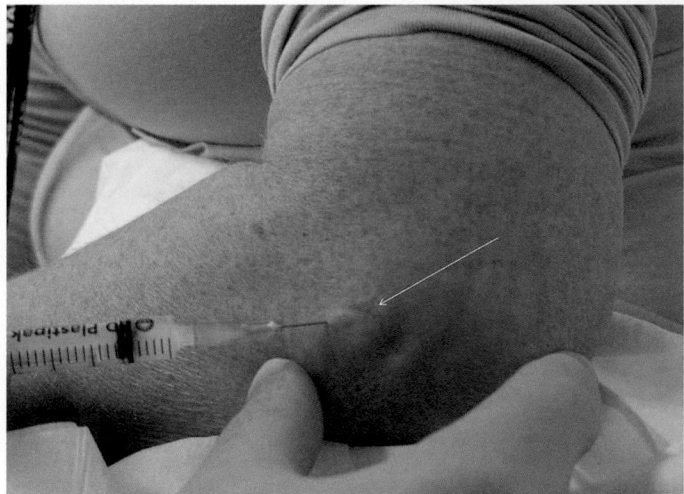

Fig. 87.5 Injection of lateral epicondyle. The point of maximum tenderness over the lateral epicondyle is marked (arrow) and needle inserted about 0.5 cm away and directed to the target area.

* Needle: 23G.

* Approach: skin marked 0.5 cm away. Avoid injection into the ulnar groove and check with patient about tingling/pins and needles which may indicate contact of needle with the ulnar nerve.

* Caution: ulnar nerve injury

Wrist

It is not possible to inject individual carpal joints under clinical guidance. Usually the gap between the distal radius and the scaphoid and lunate is palpated with the wrist in flexion. This is the target for injection.

* Posture: hand resting on a pillow with wrist flexed.

* Needle: 23 or 25G.

♦ Approach: Approach distally with needle at 60–90° angle (Figure 87.6).

♦ Caution: avoid the overlying extensor tendons

First carpometacarpal joint

OA of this joint is common and can be associated with localized tenderness on palpation and crepitus on movement. The thumb is gently flexed and extended and the joint line felt in the snuffbox between the extensor pollicus longus tendon and the combined tendon sheath of the extensor pollicus brevis and adductor pollicus longus. The radial artery should be palpated to ensure it does not lie along the joint line in the snuff box. If this is the case, then the joint should be approached just anterior to the combined tendon sheath of the extensor pollicus brevis and adductor pollicus longus.

♦ Needle: 23 or 25G.

♦ Approach: gentle flexion of the thumb. Approach distally with needle at 60–90° angle (Figure 87.7).

♦ Caution: avoid the radial artery.

Carpal tunnel

The median nerve runs just deep to the flexor retinaculum, with palmaris longus overlying the area. Palmaris longus tendon is identified by juxta opposing thumb and little finger. Skin marked just ulnar to the tendon on the distal palmar crease (Figure 87.8).

♦ Needle: 25G.

♦ Approach: needle at around 45°. Retract if patient feels increased tingling or pins and needles.

♦ Caution: avoid lidocaine.

Metacarpophalangeal joint

In the absence of effusion the target area is the joint line which is located distal to the knuckle crest and felt by passive movement of the finger and gentle pull/distraction. The extensor tendon overlying the joint is identified.

♦ Approach: distally at angle of 60°. Skin punctured lateral to extensor tendon and aiming under the tendon (Figure 87.9).

♦ Needle: 25G.

♦ Caution: risk of trauma to neurovascular structures.

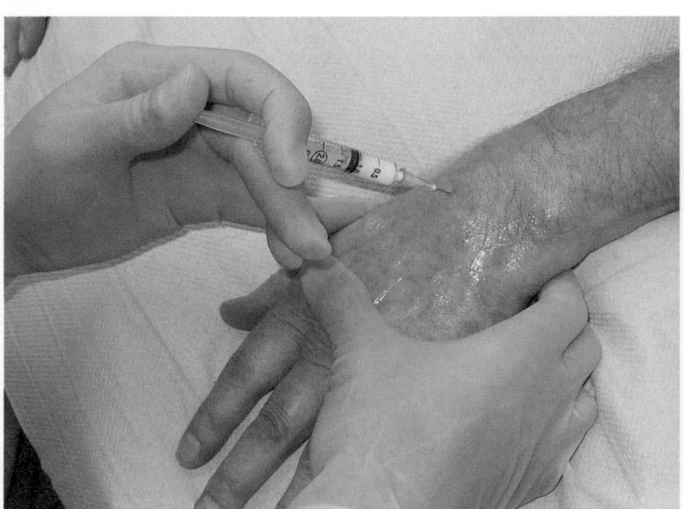

Fig. 87.6 Wrist joint injection.

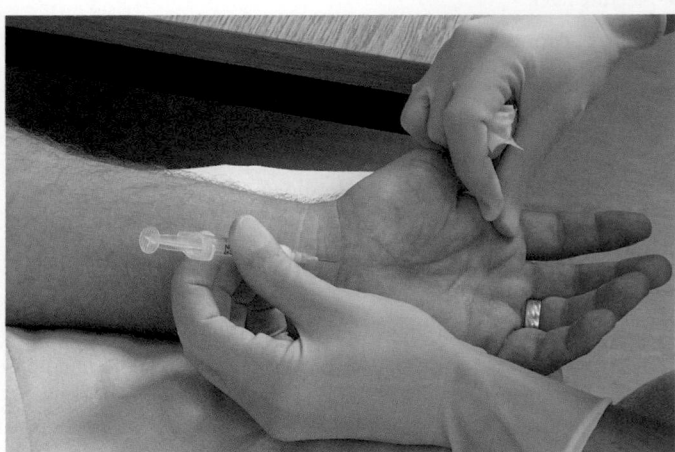

Fig. 87.8 Carpal tunnel injection.

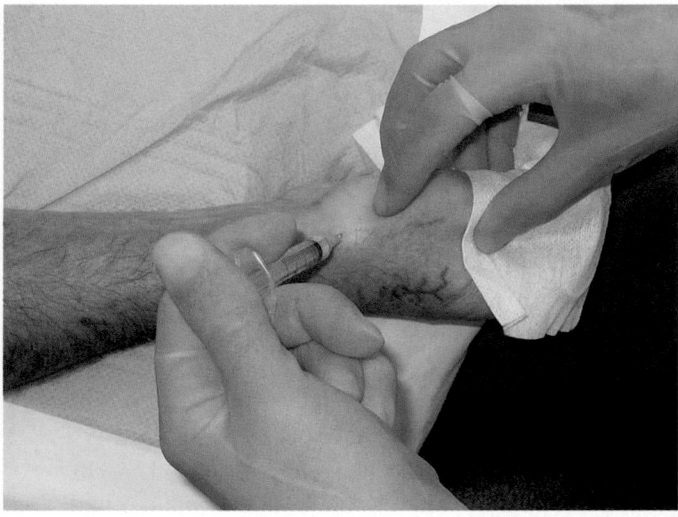

Fig. 87.7 Carpometacarpal joint injection. The thumb is flexed and gently pulled with the free hand to aid injection.

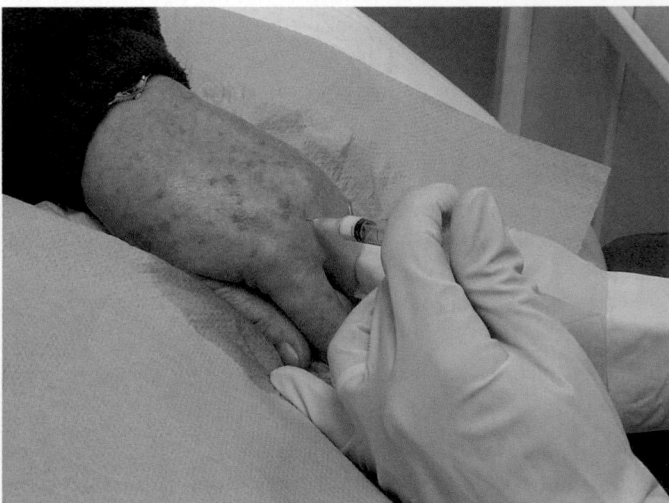

Fig. 87.9 Metacarpophalangeal joint injection. The joint line is marked just lateral to the extensor tendon. The finger is gently pulled with the free hand.

Interphalangeal joint

Joint line felt by passive movement of the joint.

◆ Approach: skin punctured just lateral to extensor tendon aiming under the tendon.

◆ Needle: 25G.

◆ Caution: risk of trauma to neurovascular structures.

De Quervain's tenosynovitis

Inflammation of the extensor pollicis brevis and/or the abductor pollicis longus. There can be associated swelling, crepitus or localized pain over the tendon.

◆ Approach: area of tenderness or swelling along the tendon usually in the snuff box area. Tangentially along the tendon.

◆ Needle: 23 or 25G.

◆ Caution: avoid injecting against resistance.

Flexor tenosynovitis

May be associated with history of triggering with triggering on examination, flexion of digit, or swelling of the tendon

◆ Approach: proximal approach tangentially to 30°, skin punctures around palmar crease and aiming distally (Figure 87.10).

◆ Needle: 25G.

Lower limbs

Hip joint

Injection of the hip joint is usually performed under image guidance only, though there are reports of clinically guided injection technique with reasonable accuracy rate.

Approach (ultrasound guided)

The hip joint can be accurately injected under ultrasound guidance using the direct approach. The patient lies flat and the hip joint and capsule are visualized as shown in Figure 87.11. The area on the skin is then marked and the injection prepared. Under direct visualization, local anaesthetic is infiltrated and distension of skin and then underlying fascia and muscles are seen. Resistance is usually felt just before puncture of the capsule. Once within the capsule,

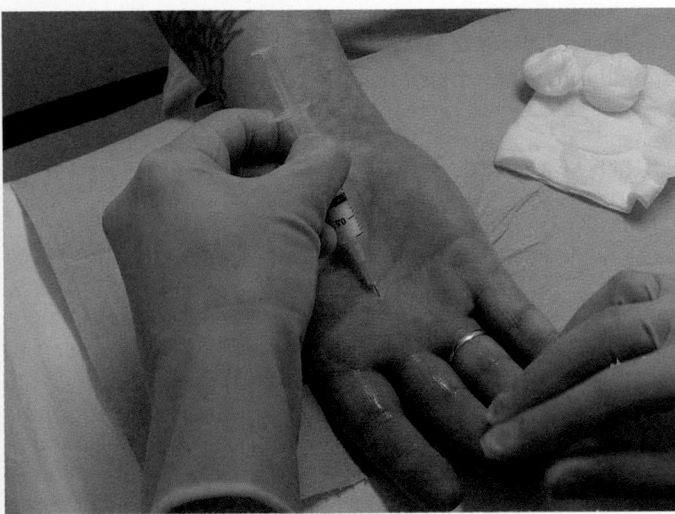

Fig. 87.10 Flexor tendon sheath injection.

accuracy can be further confirmed with visualization of distension of the capsule.

◆ Needle: spinal needle 21G.

Greater trochanteric bursa

Pain in this area is not always related to confirmed presence of bursitis. The most common bursitis is that underneath the gluteus maximus and is usually located on the posterolateral aspect of the greater trochanter. There are a large number of bursae in the area. Even in the absence of effusion, patients may benefit from injection of the painful area.

◆ Posture: usually patient lies on the contralateral side with the leg straight and the affected side leg flexed. Alternatively both hips can be in flexion, in fetal position, for this procedure.

◆ Approach: the tender area is marked and infiltrated. Perpendicular, aiming to touch bone and then retracting by a few millimetres, but response may improve by infiltrating a wider area (withdrawing and changing direction of the needle then infiltrating).

◆ Needle: 21G.

◆ Caution: even in thin people the bursa is deeper than the perceived depth on manual palpation and long needles are often required.

Knee

The joint can be approached medially, laterally, and via a suprapatellar approach. The infrapatellar approach is best avoided as the patellar tendon can easily be damaged.

◆ Posture: patient lies on the couch with the knee extended but not fully in order to ensure the patella is mobile and not locked in extension.

◆ Needle: 21G

Medial approach

Site of entry is just below the midline of the patella. Needle trajectory is horizontal and towards the suprapatellar area. Gentle pressure on the lateral patella may help to increase the gap, particularly in the presence of osteophytes in OA.

Lateral approach

Site of entry is just inferior to the margin of the upper and middle third of the patella (Figure 87.12). Pressure on the medial patellar may increase the gap underneath the patella.

Ankle joint

The talotibial joint is best accessed anteriorly by identifying a gap between the overlying tendons, usually just lateral to anterior tibialis (Figure 87.13). Dorsalis pedis artery should be palpated as anatomical variations exist and may be more medial than expected in some patients and occasionally the safest approach may be just medial to the anterior tibialis tendon.

◆ Posture: position the foot in neutral or plantarflexion, approaching from the distal end at an angle of about 45–90°.

◆ Needle: 23G.

◆ Caution: injury to overlying tendon and dorsalis pedis artery.

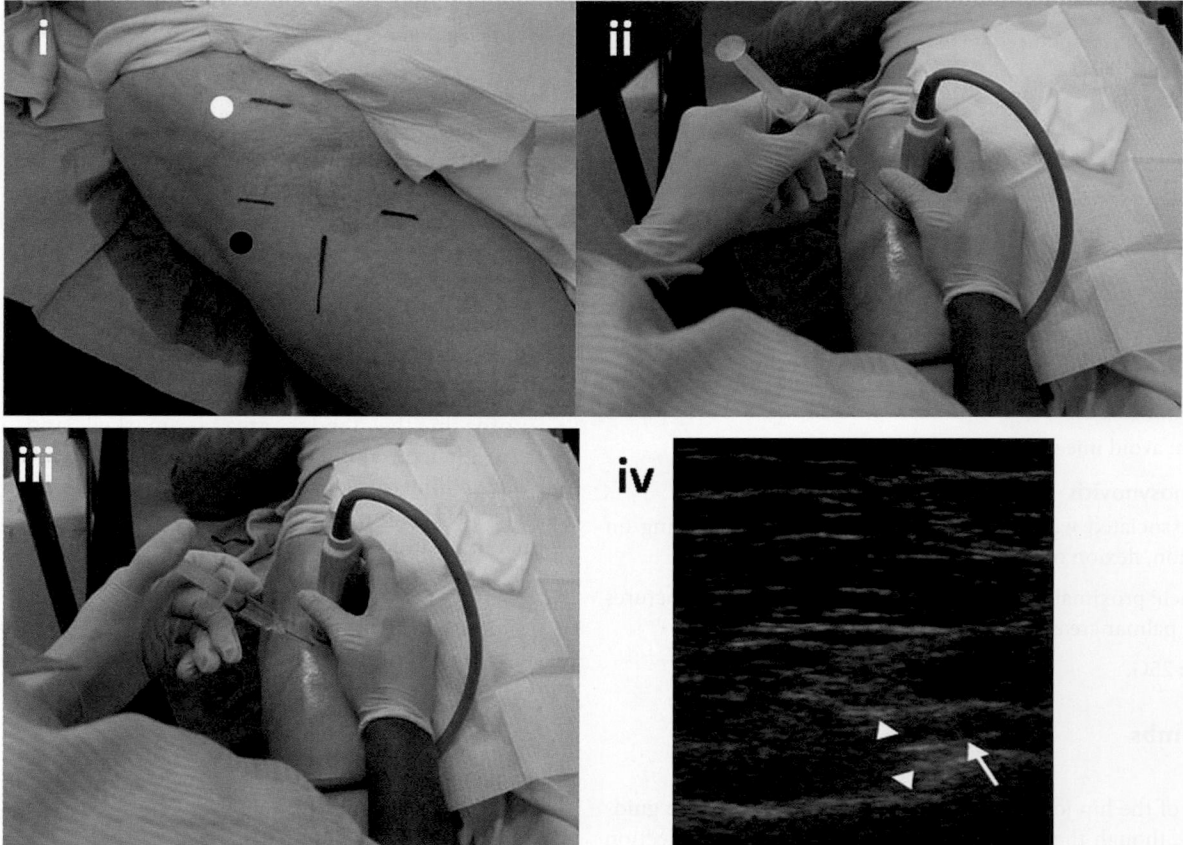

Fig. 87.11 Ultrasound-guided hip joint injection. The area is scanned and probe position marked (image i—white circle denoting level of anterior superior iliac spine and black circle at the level of greater trochanter) before thorough skin and probe cleaning. Using a spinal needle, the skin is punctured and infiltrated with local anaesthetic and then the needle advanced and deeper layers injected with local anaesthetic (images ii and iii). Once capsule is punctured (image iv) accuracy is ascertained with demonstration of capsular distension (arrowheads) and hyperechoic steroid infiltration (arrow).

Talonavicular joint

Patients not responding to ankle joint injection may have talonavicular involvement which can be missed clinically. Ultrasound can easily identify and differentiate between inflammation of the ankle joint and talonavicular joint and is also useful to guide injection.

- Approach: the probe is positioned so that that the talonavicular joint is in the midline. The needle is then inserted right next to the midline of the probe, aiming vertically to the joint capsule.
- Needle: 23 G

Subtalar joint

Pain around the ankle can be due to the subtalar joint. The subtalar joint is difficult to inject and usually 'blind' injection results in infiltration of the sinus tarsi rather than the joint. Because the joint is covered by the malleoli it is difficult to visualize, and hence, even with ultrasound it is difficult to inject accurately. The joint can be approached medially, but because of the overlying tendons and neurovascular structures on the medial side, the lateral approach is usually preferred.

- Approach: the joint line is felt just inferior and anterior to the lateral malleolus. Inversion/eversion of the foot may help to identify the joint line.
- Needle: 23G.

Metatarsophalangeal joint

The joint line is identified dorsally by movement of the toe. The gap/joint line may be more easily identified by gentle pulling of the toe. The extensor tendon is identified and point of entry of needle should be just medial or lateral to this structure.

- Needle: 25G
- Caution: injury to extensor tendon or neurovascular structures.

Tendons

Swelling around the ankle can be related to tendon swelling or subcutaneous oedema rather than joint pathology. Inflamed tendon sheaths can respond well to steroid injections. Posterior tibialis is located posterior to the medial malleolus, anterior tibialis anterolateral, and peroneal tendons posterior to the lateral malleolus. Achilles tendon is usually not injected as there is no tendon sheath and direct infiltration of steroid within the tendon substance may

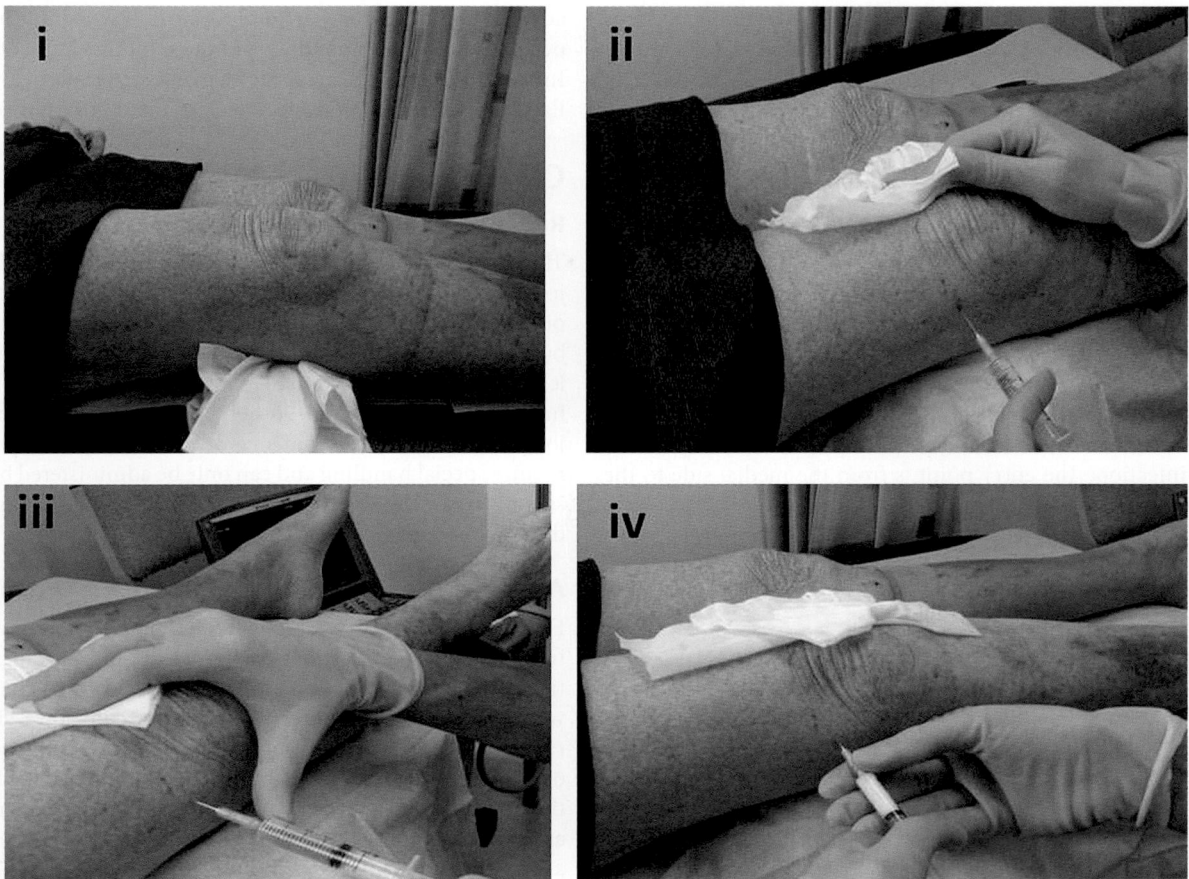

Fig. 87.12 Knee joint aspiration and injection. Knee joint is approached on the lateral aspect in slightly flexed position and skin marked inferior to the patella (image i, in this case close to the proximal border of the patella). Skin surface is cleaned and needle directed horizontally with free hand pressing on the medial side. Local anaesthetic is infiltrated (image ii) up to the joint which is then aspirated (image iii), syringe then changed and the knee then injected with corticosteroid (image iv).

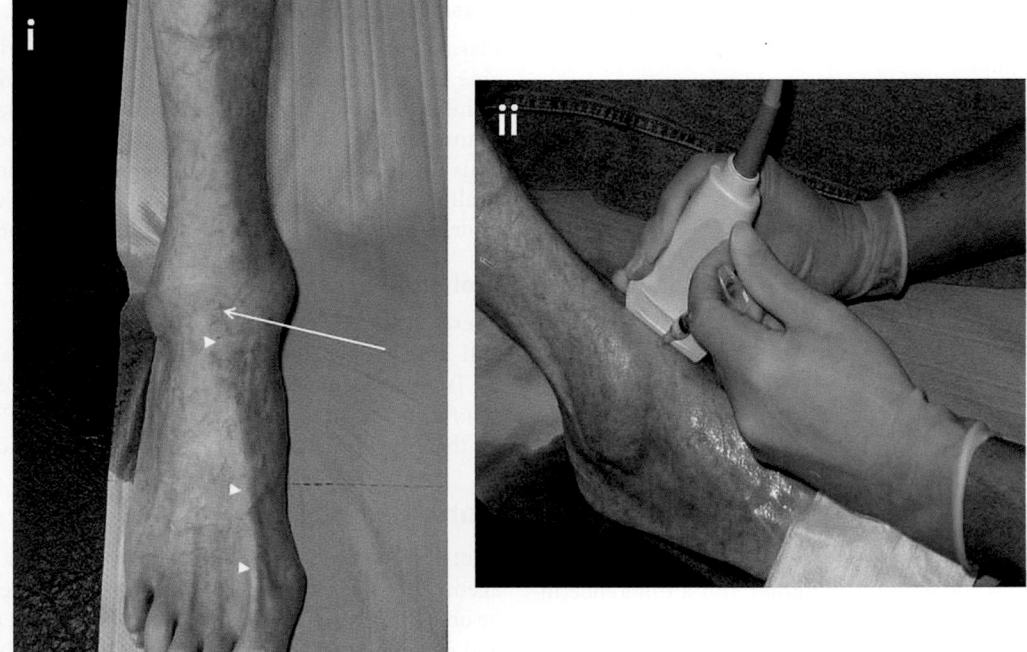

Fig. 87.13 Ankle joint injection. Here the gap (white arrow) between the anterior tibialis and extensor hallucis longus (outlined by the arrowheads) is marked. Ultrasound is helpful to ensure the location of dorsalis pedis and to visualize joint distension.

lead to rupture. Pain/tenderness around the insertion/calcaneus may be due to retrocalcaneal bursitis, which may respond to intrabursal injection.

- Needle: 23 or 25G.
- Caution: avoid injecting against resistance. Use ultrasound if available.

Plantar fasciitis

Heel pain can be due to plantar fasciitis relating to localized tenderness of the proximal fascia close to insertion to the calcaneus. Ultrasound enables measurement of the thickness and aids in the diagnosis of the condition.

- Approach: direct approach through the sole is usually avoided due to the thickness of the overlying skin and possible increased risk of infection. The entry point is from the medial side to the area of maximum tenderness.
- Needle: 23G.
- Caution: small risk of causing rupture.

Hyaluronic acid injections

Hyaluronic acid, also known as hyaluronan, is a high molecular weight glycosaminoglycan present in synovial fluid. It is thought to be critical for the homeostasis of the joint, in part because it provides the viscosity and elastic properties of the synovial fluid. These properties depend on both the concentration and molecular weight of the hyaluronan. In OA, the hyaluronan is lower both in molecular weight and in concentration. Hence the rationale for injecting hyaluronans into OA joints is to increase these properties towards normal—this is termed viscosupplementation. Hyaluronan acts not just as a viscous lubricant but also as a shock absorber during physical activities. Also, there are data suggesting that hyaluronans may act as immunomodulators, and as facilitators of solute exchange, as well as having other properties.[43] These may contribute to their clinical benefit which, in some studies, far outlasts their half-life within the synovial fluid.

Types of hyaluronic acid

There are different types of hyaluronic acids with variable molecular weights, high molecular weight forms usually staying longer in the joints.[44] Macromolecular derivates of hyaluronic acid, mainly of avian cartilage origin, or combinations of hyaluronans and more recently non-animal products, designed to avoid allergic reactions, are available for injections. Most of these products are licensed as devices rather than drugs and they are relatively expensive when compared with injectable glucocorticoid.

Efficacy/safety

There have been numerous studies demonstrating efficacy for the treatment of OA of different joints. These tend to demonstrate more prolonged benefit compared to glucocorticoid for mild to moderate OA.[45,46] However, review of the literature has highlighted some methodological issues for individual studies and a difference in outcomes for different preparations, with no direct studies comparing different hyaluronans. Subsequent RCTs directly comparing glucocorticoids with hyaluronic acid have failed to demonstrate increased duration of benefit with hyaluronic acid.[23,26,47] The local

adverse events are similar to glucocorticoid. Significant flare can occur and can last more than 24 hours, mimicking septic arthritis. In our experience, the presence of an effusion leads to higher risk of flares and any effusion needs to be aspirated prior to injection.

Other injections

Radiation/chemical synovectomy

This treatment can be considered for patients with inflammatory joint disease refractory to treatment including intra-articular steroid injections. Accuracy is extremely important not only for efficacy but also to minimize complications, as extra-articular injection can lead to significant soft tissue irritation. Different radio nucleotides have been used, yttrium-90 being commonly used for the knee joint, with significant evidence of efficacy.[48,49] These substances require special handling and can only be administered by clinicians suitably trained and meeting local requirements. They are contraindicated in pregnancy.

Arthroscopic washout with/without steroid injections

For knee OA, the KIVIS study revealed superior duration of benefit from arthroscopic washout compared to intra-articular glucocorticoid injection.[50] For inflammatory knee arthritis, arthroscopic washout followed by injection was found to have significantly reduced relapse rate when compared with either arthroscopy washout without injection or with intra-articular glucocorticoid injection.[51] However in these two studies the patients were not blinded and it has been previously demonstrated that sham arthroscopy has a strong placebo effect. In addition, arthroscopy is more invasive, with potentially increased risks of complications and is usually only performed by an orthopaedic surgeon in theatre. However there are some rheumatologists who have developed expertise in performing arthroscopies, which can be performed in a suitable non-theatre environment.

Plasma-rich products

Plasma-rich products have been used particularly in sports medicine for the treatment of ligament and tendon injuries such as Achilles tendinopathy. The underlying principle is to provide an injured area with natural growth factors isolated from an autologous blood sample, which is thought to be safe and to promote healing. There is some evidence supporting its use for soft tissue injuries but minimal evidence to support intra-articular use.[52,53]

Biologics

There have been case series reporting efficacy of intra-articular anti-TNF in the treatment of inflammatory knee arthritis. However, RCTs have not shown any benefit from either anakinra in knee OA[54] or of infliximab in inflammatory knee arthritis.[55] The evidence so far therefore does not justify the use of intra-articular biologics.

Conclusion

Joint and soft tissue injections remain a critical aspect of the management of musculoskeletal conditions. Informed consent should be obtained from the patient, taking into account the potential risks and side effects (Box 87.2). The indications for the procedure need to be carefully assessed and in expert hands, injection therapy is safe and effective, causing no or very little discomfort to patients.

| Box 87.2 | Joint injections: contraindications and risks |

Contraindications

Absolute

- Local infection
- Systemic infection
- Allergy to local anaesthetic or glucocorticoid preparation
- Arthroplasty

Relative

- Anticoagulation
- Bleeding diathesis
- Syncope after previous procedures
- Poorly controlled or unstable diabetes
- Imminent surgery to target joint
- Overlying skin psoriasis

Side effects and complications

Early (within 1–2 hours)

- Pain at injection site
- Bleeding/bruising
- Syncope
- Facial flushing
- Anaphylaxis
- Nerve trauma

Delayed

- Disturbed diabetic control
- Post injection flare
- Subcutaneous/skin atrophy and depigmentation
- Tendon rupture
- Septic arthritis
- Soft tissue calcification
- Avascular necrosis

References

1. Hollander JL, Brown EM, Jr., Jessar RA et al. Local anti-rheumatic effectiveness of higher esters and analogues of hydrocortisone. *Ann Rheum Dis* 1954;13(4):297–301.
2. Hollander JL, Moore R. Studies in osteo-arthritis using intra-articular temperature response to injection of hydrocortisone acetate and prednisone. *Ann Rheum Dis* 1956;15(4):320–326.
3. Ayral X. Injections in the treatment of osteoarthritis. *Best Pract Research Clin Rheumatol* 2001;15(4):609–626.
4. Uthman I, Raynauld JP, Haraoui B. Intra-articular therapy in osteoarthritis. *Postgrad Med J* 2003;79(934):449–453.
5. Samborski W, Stratz T, Mackiewicz S, Muller W. Intra-articular treatment of arthritides and activated osteoarthritis with the 5-HT3 receptor antagonist tropisetron. A double-blind study compared with methylprednisolone. *Scand J Rheumatol Suppl* 2004;119:51–54.
6. Chevalier X, Giraudeau B, Conrozier T et al. Safety study of intraarticular injection of interleukin 1 receptor antagonist in patients with painful knee osteoarthritis: a multicenter study. *J Rheumatol* 2005;32(7):1317–1323.
7. Jones A, Regan M, Ledingham J et al. Importance of placement of intraarticular steroid injections. *BMJ* 1993;307(6915):1329–1330.
8. Cunnington J, Marshall N, Hide G et al. A randomized, double-blind, controlled study of ultrasound-guided corticosteroid injection into the joint of patients with inflammatory arthritis. *Arthritis Rheum* 2010;62(7):1862–1869.
9. Eustace J, Brophy, DP, Gibney RP, Bresnihan B, Fitzgerald O. Comparison of the accuracy of steroid placement with clinical outcome in patients with shoulder symptoms. *Ann Rheum Dis* 1997;56:59–63.
10. Raza K, Lee C, Pilling D et al. Ultrasound guidance allows accurate needle placement and aspiration from small joints in patients with early inflammatory arthritis. *Rheumatology* (Oxford) 2003;42(8):976–979.
11. Weidner S, Kellner W, Kellner H. Interventional radiology and the musculoskeletal system. *Best Pract Research Clin Rheumatol* 2004;18(6):945–956.
12. Adler RS, Sofka CM. Percutaneous ultrasound-guided injections in the musculoskeletal system. *Ultrasound Q* 2003;19(1):3–12.
13. Karim Z, Brown AK, Quinn M et al. Ultrasound-guided steroid injections in the treatment of hip osteoarthritis: comment on the letter by Margules. *Arthritis Rheum* 2004;50(1):338–339; author reply 339–340.
14. Weiss MM, Weiss MM. Corticosteroids in rheumatoid arthritis. *Semin Arthritis Rheum* 1989;19(1):9–21.
15. Boers M, Boers M. The case for corticosteroids in the treatment of early rheumatoid arthritis.[see comment]. *Rheumatology* (Oxford) 1999;38(2):95–97.
16. Alex P, Szodoray P, Arthur E et al. Influence of intraarticular corticosteroid administration on serum cytokines in rheumatoid arthritis. *Clin Rheumatol* 2007;26(5):845–848.
17. Derendorf H, Mollmann H, Gruner A, Haack D, Gyselby G. Pharmacokinetics and pharmacodynamics of glucocorticoid suspensions after intra-articular administration. *Clin Pharmacol Ther* 1986;39(3):313–317.
18. Beardwell A. Subcutaneous atrophy after local corticosteroid injection. *Br Med J* 1967;3(5565):600.
19. Habib GS, Saliba W, Nashashibi M. Local effects of intra-articular corticosteroids. *Clin Rheumatol* 2010;29(4):347–356.
20. Price R, Sinclair H, Heinrich I, Gibson T. Local injection treatment of tennis elbow—hydrocortisone, triamcinolone and lignocaine compared. *Br J Rheumatol* 1991;30(1):39–44.
21. McCarty DJ. Treatment of rheumatoid joint inflammation with triamcinolone hexacetonide. *Arthritis Rheum* 1972;15(2):157–173.
22. McCarty DJ, Harman JG, Grassanovich JL, Qian C. Treatment of rheumatoid joint inflammation with intrasynovial triamcinolone hexacetonide. *J Rheumatol* 1995;22(9):1631–1635.
23. Qvistgaard E, Christensen R, Torp-Pedersen S, Bliddal H. Intra-articular treatment of hip osteoarthritis: a randomized trial of hyaluronic acid, corticosteroid, and isotonic saline. *Osteoarthritis Cartilage* 2006;14(2):163–170.
24. Kullenberg B, Runesson R, Tuvhag R, Olsson C, Resch S. Intraarticular corticosteroid injection: pain relief in osteoarthritis of the hip? *J Rheumatol* 2004;31(11):2265–2268.
25. Robinson P, Keenan AM, Conaghan PG. Clinical effectiveness and dose response of image-guided intra-articular corticosteroid injection for hip osteoarthritis. *Rheumatology.* 2007;46(2):285–291.
26. Atchia I, Kane D, Reed MR, Isaacs JD, Birrell F. Efficacy of a single ultrasound-guided injection for the treatment of hip osteoarthritis. *Ann Rheum Dis* 2011;70(1):110–116.
27. Blyth T, Hunter JA, Stirling A. Pain relief in the rheumatoid knee after steroid injection. A single-blind comparison of hydrocortisone succinate, and triamcinolone acetonide or hexacetonide. *Br J Rheumatol* 1994;33(5):461–463.

28. Zhang W, Robertson J, Jones AC, Dieppe PA, Doherty M. The placebo effect and its determinants in osteoarthritis: meta-analysis of randomised controlled trials. *Ann Rheum Dis* 2008;67(12):1716–1723.

29. Hartung W, Ross CJ, Straub R et al. Ultrasound-guided sacroiliac joint injection in patients with established sacroiliitis: precise IA injection verified by MRI scanning does not predict clinical outcome. *Rheumatology* 2010;49(8):1479–1482.

30. Matthews, C, Weston WC, Jones A, Field M, Coakley, G. Bacterial septic arthritis in adults. *Lancet* 2010; 375(9717): 846–855

31. Nallamshetty L, Buchowski Jacob M, Nazarian Levon A et al. Septic arthritis of the hip following cortisone injection: case report and review of the literature. *Clin Imaging* 2003;27(4):225–228.

32. Cole BJ, Schumacher HR, Jr. Injectable corticosteroids in modern practice. *Journal of the American Academy of Orthopaedic Surgeons.* 2005;13(1):37–46.

33. Pal B, Morris J. Perceived risks of joint infection following intra-articular corticosteroid injections: a survey of rheumatologists. *Clin Rheumatol* 1999;18(3):264–265.

34. Gray RG, Tenenbaum J, Gottlieb NL. Local corticosteroid injection treatment in rheumatic disorders. *Semin Arthritis Rheum* 1981;10(4):231–254.

35. Seror P, Pluvinage P, d'Andre FL, Benamou P, Attuil G. Frequency of sepsis after local corticosteroid injection (an inquiry on 1 160 000 injections in rheumatological private practice in France). *Rheumatology* 1999;38(12):1272–1274.

36. Geirsson AJ, Statkevicius S, Vikingsson A. Septic arthritis in Iceland 1990–2002: increasing incidence due to iatrogenic infections. *Ann Rheum Dis* 2008: 67(5): 638–643.

37. Charalambous CP, Tryfonidis M, Sadiq S, Hirst P, Paul A. Septic arthritis following intra-articular steroid injection of the knee—a survey of current practice regarding antiseptic technique used during intra-articular steroid injection of the knee. *Clin Rheumatol* 2003;22(6):386–390.

38. Salvati G, Punzi L, Pianon M et al. [Frequency of the bleeding risk in patients receiving warfarin submitted to arthrocentesis of the knee]. *Reumatismo* 2003;55(3):159–163.

39. Thumboo J, O. Duffy J D. A prospective study of the safety of joint and soft tissue aspirations and injections in patients taking warfarin sodium. *Arthritis and rheumatism* {Arthritis-Rheum}. 1998;41(4):736–739.

40. Alarcón Segovia D, Ward LE. Marked destructive changes occurring in osteoarthric finger joints after intra-articular injection of corticosteroids. *Arthritis Rheum* 1966;9(3):443–463.

41. Sparling M, Malleson P, Wood B, Petty R. Radiographic followup of joints injected with triamcinolone hexacetonide for the management of childhood arthritis. *Arthritis Rheum* 1990;33(6):821–826.

42. Raynauld JP, Buckland-Wright C, Ward R et al. Safety and efficacy of long-term intraarticular steroid injections in osteoarthritis of the knee: a randomized, double-blind, placebo-controlled trial.

[erratum appears in Arthritis Rheum 2003;48(11):3300]. *Arthritis Rheum* 2003;48(2):370–377.

43. Moreland LW. Intra-articular hyaluronan (hyaluronic acid) and hylans for the treatment of osteoarthritis: mechanisms of action. *Arthritis Res Ther* 2003;5(2):54–67.

44. Brandt KD, Smith GN, Jr., Simon LS. Intraarticular injection of hyaluronan as treatment for knee osteoarthritis: what is the evidence?[see comment]. *Arthritis Rheum* 2000;43(6):1192–1203.

45. Lo GH, LaValley M, McAlindon T, Felson DT. Intra-articular hyaluronic acid in treatment of knee osteoarthritis: a meta-analysis. *JAMA* 2003;290(23):3115–3121.

46. Bellamy N, Campbell J, Welch V et al. Viscosupplementation for the treatment of osteoarthritis of the knee. *Cochrane Database Syst Rev* 2006;2:CD005321.

47. Richette P, Ravaud P, Conrozier T et al. Effect of hyaluronic acid in symptomatic hip osteoarthritis: a multicenter, randomized, placebo-controlled trial. *Arthritis Rheum* 2009;60(3):824–830.

48. Sledge CB, Atcher RW, Shortkroff S et al. Intra-articular radiation synovectomy. *Clin Orthop* 1984;182:37–40.

49. van der Zant FM, Boer RO, Moolenburgh JD et al. Radiation synovectomy with (90)Yttrium, (186)Rhenium and (169)Erbium: a systematic literature review with meta-analyses. *Clin Exp Rheumatol* 2009;27(1):130–139.

50. Arden NK, Reading IC, Jordan KM, Thomas L, Platten H, Hassan A, et al. A randomised controlled trial of tidal irrigation vs corticosteroid injection in knee osteoarthritis: the KIVIS Study. *Osteoarthritis Cartilage* 2008;16(6):733–739.

51. van Oosterhout M, Sont JK, Bajema IM, Breedveld FC, van Laar JM. Comparison of efficacy of arthroscopic lavage plus administration of corticosteroids, arthroscopic lavage plus administration of placebo, and joint aspiration plus administration of corticosteroids in arthritis of the knee: A randomized controlled trial. *Arthritis Rheum* 2006;55(6):964–970.

52. de Jonge S, de Vos RJ, Weir A et al. One-year follow-up of platelet-rich plasma treatment in chronic Achilles tendinopathy: a double-blind randomized placebo-controlled trial. *Am J Sports Med* 2011;39(8):1623–1629.

53. Kon E, Filardo G, Di Martino A, Marcacci M. Platelet-rich plasma (PRP) to treat sports injuries: evidence to support its use. *Knee Surg Sports Traumatol Arthrosc* 2011;19(4):516–527.

54. Chevalier X, Goupille P, Beaulieu AD et al. Intraarticular injection of anakinra in osteoarthritis of the knee: a multicenter, randomized, double-blind, placebo-controlled study. *Arthritis Rheum* 2009;61(3):344–352.

55. van der Bijl AE, Teng YKO, van Oosterhout M et al. Efficacy of intraarticular infliximab in patients with chronic or recurrent gonarthritis: a clinical randomized trial. *Arthritis Rheum* 2009;61(7):974–978.

CHAPTER 88

Diet and obesity

Dorothy Pattison

Introduction

The role of diet in the management of rheumatic disease is being increasingly recognized. Dietary manipulation includes not only measures targeted at obesity but also the introduction or removal of specific nutritional substances.

Osteoarthritis

The primary dietary intervention in the management of osteoarthritis (OA) is the prevention and treatment of obesity. Weight reduction may be influential in slowing disease progression in these patients, particularly of knee OA,[1] and surgical intervention may be avoided. Weight reduction improves the outcome of joint replacement surgery in obese patients. This is an important issue given the increase in both the frequency of knee OA and of partial and total knee arthroplasty for primary OA especially in younger adults (<60 years of age) over recent decades.[2,3] Although no single reason has been identified to explain these findings, an increasingly older and obese population are likely contributing factors. In addition, weight reduction can be part of the management of and impact on related comorbidities.

Pharmacological treatments for OA remain generally palliative and symptomatic and there is little evidence that progression of disease is affected. Drugs can also cause unwanted side effects for some patients. Therefore, the possible use of alternative symptom-relieving treatments, including diet and dietary supplements, is of interest to both health professionals and patients.

Obesity

Obesity is a well-recognized risk factor for the development of OA.[4] A high body mass index (BMI) is also associated with more severe disease in terms of greater pain levels[5] and the need for joint replacement surgery.[6]

Every step taken increases the load on the hip or knee joint by around three to five times body weight, hence the physical stresses imposed on the joints by excessive body weight are considerable.[4] Each kilogram of weight loss will result in a fourfold reduction in the load exerted, for example on the knee, per step during daily activities. Despite this, the effect of obesity on the progression of OA, specifically joint space narrowing, has not been consistently shown. Some studies have shown a higher rate of joint space narrowing in obese subjects compared to non-obese, while others have found no association between obesity and disease progression in knee OA.[7,8] However, a longitudinal study of 3585 subjects aged at least 55 years, with radiographic data at baseline and follow-up, found that a high BMI was associated with loss of joint space in knee OA but not at the hip.[9] The disparity in these results could be due to several factors including study design, patient selection, loss to follow-up, and for knee OA, the degree of knee malalignment. The way in which these joint structures are built and maintained contributes to the development and progression of OA.

Increasing adiposity is also associated with an increased frequency of and worsening symptoms in OA of non-weightbearing joints: for example, primary nodal OA of the hand.[10] This affects mainly middle-aged women in sedentary roles, which cannot be attributed to the effect of increased physical load. This association is most likely related to the metabolic activity of adipose tissue, secreting various inflammatory mediators and hormones, such as cytokines, tumour necrosis factor (TNF), and leptin. The biological activity of adipose tissue may be integral in the aetiology and progression of OA. Thus, a reduction in adipose tissue rather than body weight alone may be responsible for improvement in symptoms.[4] It is most likely the aetiology of OA involves an interaction between mechanical and systemic factors.[3] A study of 22 obese patients with knee OA who completed a weight control programme for 6 weeks clearly demonstrated that reducing fat mass and increasing physical activity gave greater symptomatic relief that could be explained by the reduction in body weight alone.[11] Other clinical trials have also shown that body weight reduction in combination with increased physical activity can improve pain and stiffness symptoms, primarily in OA knee.[12] Patients who are overweight or obese should participate in weight loss programmes aimed at reducing fat mass, particularly abdominal fat mass.[11] Early intervention with dietary guidance and an exercise programme is effective to reduce symptoms of OA.[12]

Comorbidities

Factors consistent with the metabolic syndrome, such as hypertension, hypercholesterolaemia, and insulin resistance are prevalent in OA, in some cases independent of obesity, demonstrating the involvement of significant systemic and metabolic components in the aetiology of OA.[13] However, the efficacy of dietary therapy in cases where hyperlipidaemia and other factors of the metabolic syndrome are present in this population has yet to be demonstrated.[14]

Nutrition and orthopaedic surgery

Hip and knee replacement surgery is mainly performed for OA in late middle age and elderly patients, although recent data suggests an increase in surgery in younger age groups.[2,3] Lower levels of haemoglobin, ferritin, albumin, and protein intakes have been demonstrated in OA and RA patients 10 days after joint replacement surgery compared to preoperative levels, thus impeding postoperative recovery.[15] Poor nutritional status is particularly relevant in elderly and/or frail patients. Nutritional support administered as part of a rapid-recovery programme for lower extremity arthroplasty has demonstrated improved postoperative recovery in elderly patients (measured as decreased hospital length of stay) undergoing hip replacement.[16] Malnutrition remains a somewhat unrecognized, yet preventable, problem in hospital patients and highlights the need for ongoing education on clinical nutrition.

Dietary supplements

Glucosamine and chondroitin

Glucosamine is found naturally in the body. It plays an important role in the synthesis of glycosaminoglycans and glycoproteins which are the building blocks of many structures of the joints. Chondroitin also occurs naturally in the body and is a vital part of joint cartilage. The compound chondroitin sulphate is a complex sugar derived from the cartilage of cows, pigs, and sharks.

Results from randomized controlled trials (RCTs) examining the effectiveness of chondroitin and glucosamine are conflicting. Studies reporting sizeable effects on joint pain tend to be of poor quality and/or small sample size, whereas larger, methodologically robust trials generally found only small or no effects.[14] A meta-analysis of 20 studies of glucosamine in the management of OA of the knee and hip included 2570 patients. Pooled results from studies using a preparation of glucosamine sulphate (1500 mg/day) in patients with symptomatic OA failed to show benefit in pain and function.[17] A more recent meta-analysis of RCTs of glucosamine, chondroitin, or a combination of both included a pooled analysis of 3803 patients with hip or knee OA. No clinically relevant effect of either supplement or in combination was found on perceived joint pain or minimal joint space width.[18] Both meta-analyses reported that glucosamine/chondroitin is safe, compared with placebo.

Herbal and other dietary supplements

As pharmacological treatments for OA are ineffective in some patients and some, such as non-steroidal anti-inflammatory drugs (NSAIDs), can have serious side effects, many patients frequently turn to complementary/alternative medicines (see Chapter 89).

Many manufacturers of dietary supplements claim that their product will reduce symptoms or even alter the course of disease, but there is only weak scientific evidence to support the use of nutritional supplements in the management of OA. Most types of supplements promoted for the treatment of OA are unlikely to cause harm, but some plant-based remedies can be toxic.

A recent systematic review of herbal medicines and plant extracts (oral or topical) in OA included 12 RCTs and 2 systematic reviews. Moderately strong evidence (defined as 3 RCTs or more with significant clinically relevant benefits) was available for one preparation—a compound of plant extracts (Phytodolor), thought to inhibit prostaglandins and inflammatory mediators.[19] Devil's claw (*Harpagophytum procumbens*) and avocado soybean unsaponifiables (ASU) preparations have shown favourable outcomes in at least two RCTs, but for all other oral preparations included in the review there was only weak or no compelling evidence of efficacy.[20]

As yet there is no convincing evidence that fish oil supplementation provides clinical benefit in the clinical management of OA.

Gout

Gout is a common arthritis caused by the deposition of monosodium urate crystals within joints, and usually related to chronic hyperuricaemia. Large-scale studies have identified a number of associations between dietary factors and gout and a substantial burden from comorbidities. Patient education, appropriate lifestyle advice, and treatment of comorbidities are an important part of the management of patients with gout. Evidence supports gradual weight loss with exercise, limiting the consumption of purine-rich foods, sugary drinks, and alcohol, especially beer, not only to reduce the risk of gout but also that of hypertension, dyslipidaemia, and insulin resistance.[21]

Diet therapies in rheumatoid arthritis

RA is a chronic, inflammatory joint disorder that can last for decades, and although pharmacological intervention has been the mainstay of treatment, not all patients respond, and non-drug therapies have a definite place in disease management.[22] Poor eating patterns and nutritionally inadequate diets have consistently been found in people with RA.[23,24] There are various reasons for malnutrition in RA and these should be explored with the individual patient in the clinical setting.

- The pain and fatigue associated with RA can impair appetite considerably, particularly during an acute flare-up.

- The effects of RA on mobility, functional ability, and manual dexterity can make shopping, food preparation and cooking difficult, complex, and tiring.

- Medications for RA can cause nausea and anorexia or interact with nutrients. Examples of the former include NSAIDs and of the latter the effect of methotrexate on folate metabolism.

- So-called 'diets for arthritis' are popular with patients but lack scientific evidence and are very likely to compromise nutritional status

Dietitians and rheumatology occupational therapists (OT) work together to assess dietary intake, functional ability, and the living environment and advise patients how to improve circumstances and help to maintain a desirable nutritional status.

Dietary supplements

Antioxidants

Dietary antioxidant nutrients are associated with the risk of developing inflammatory arthritis.[25,26] A lower intake of vitamin C (lowest third compared to the highest) increased the risk of developing inflammatory polyarthritis more than threefold (adjusted odds ratio 3.3, 95% confidence interval 1.4–7.9).[25] Lower levels of serum antioxidants have been found in healthy individuals who went on to develop RA than those who did not develop the disease.[27] Because of the study design it is not possible to identify the reason for this: for example, whether it was a low consumption of dietary antioxidants, or antioxidant depletion due to increased activity of the endogenous immune system activity, or a combination of factors.

A recent systematic review concluded that there is no robust evidence that antioxidant supplements, vitamins A, C, E and selenium, provide any symptomatic benefit in patients with RA, OA or other inflammatory conditions.[28] However, individual patients may get some symptomatic improvement with these supplements and if taken in the recommended doses they do not cause harmful side effects.

Dietary fatty acids

The polyunsaturated fatty acids (PUFAs), omega-6 (n-6) and omega-3 (n-3) have several functions but of most importance in arthritis is their function as precursors of inflammatory mediators, including prostaglandins and leukotrienes. Conversion of the n-3 PUFA, α-linolenic acid (ALA) to long-chain n-3 PUFAs eicosapentaenoic acid (EPA) and docosahexaenoic acid (DHA) and of the n-6 PUFA linoleic acid (LA) to the long-chain n-6 PUFAs dihomo-γ-linolenic acid (DGLA) and arachidonic acid (AA) requires competition for the same enzyme systems. Exogenous sources of AA come primarily from the consumption of meat and meat products whereas oily fish provide the richest source of EPA and DHA. The inflammatory series 2 prostaglandins (PGE_2) and series-4 leukotrienes (LTB_4) originate from AA, whereas EPA is metabolized to the less inflammatory series 3 prostaglandins (PGE_3) and series-5 leukotrienes (LTB_5). EPA-derived PGEs can attenuate the proinflammatory effects of PGE_2 and LTB_4 and decrease the formation of proinflammatory n-6 eicosanoids, but only if the intake of EPA is sufficiently high compared to that of AA. n-3 PUFAs do this by decreasing the amount of AA in inflammatory cell membrane phospholipids and competitively inhibiting the production of AA-derived eicosanoids from cyclooxygenase (COX) and 5-LOX (Figure 88.1).[29,30] n-3 PUFAs can also decrease the production of proinflammatory cytokines (e.g. interleukin-1-beta and alpha (IL-1β, IL-1α) and TNF) and of reactive oxygen species.

Clinical trials of fish oil supplementation in RA have shown consistently favourable outcomes. Evidence from clinical trials of fish oil supplementation has shown that n-3 PUFA-rich supplements taken for a period of 3 months can significantly reduce the tender joint count (mean difference −2.9; p = 0.001) and duration of early morning stiffness (mean difference −25.9 min; p = 0.01) in patients with RA.[31] Furthermore, a meta-analysis of data from 17 RCTs of fish oil supplementation in RA found that n-3 PUFAs taken over 3–4 months significantly reduced patient-reported joint pain (p = 0.03); minutes of morning stiffness (p = 0.003); number of painful and/or tender joints (p = 0.003), and NSAID consumption (p = 0.01).[32] The potential for long-chain n-3-rich cod liver oil supplements to reduce the need for NSAIDs in RA patients has also been shown. In RA patients who consumed 10 g of fish oil, containing 2.2 g n-3 PUFA, daily for 9 months, 40% of patients in the treatment group were able to reduce NSAID consumption by 30% compared with only 10% in the placebo group.[33]

The possible use of n-3 PUFA supplementation as an adjunctive treatment for joint pain associated with RA, with a corresponding

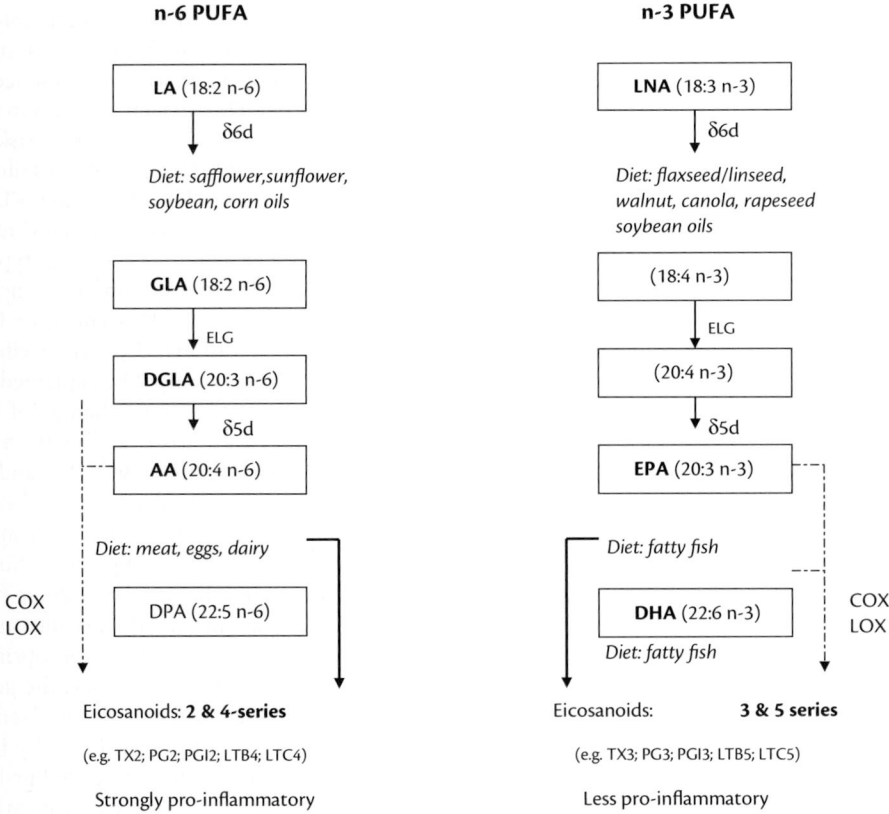

Fig. 88.1 Metabolism of n-6 and n-3 fatty acids. Key: LA: Linoleic acid; GLA: Gamma-linolenic acid; DGLA: Dihimo-gamma-linolenic acid; AA: Arachidonic acid; DPA: Docosapentaenoic acid; LNA: Linolenic acid; EPA: Eicosapentaenoic acid; DHA: Docosahexaenoic acid; COX: Cyclooxygenases; LOX: Lipoxygenases; ELG: Elongase; PG: Prostaglandin; LT: Leukotrienes; TX: Thromboxanes

reduction in NSAID use, thus attenuating the risk of gastrointestinal and/or cardiovascular side effects associated with these drugs, is not routinely considered in clinical practice.[33]

The benefits gained from increasing n-3 PUFA intake are thought to be enhanced by a simultaneous reduction in the consumption of n-6 PUFAs, thus increasing the n-3 PUFA to n-6 PUFA ratio.[34] It is of some note that over the past 100 years or so, the Western diet has become increasingly rich in n-6 PUFAs while the consumption of n-3 PUFAs has been decreasing.

Other supplements

As in many people with chronic diseases, the use of dietary therapies and complementary and alternative medicines (CAMs) are popular in patients with RA.

Common supplements include cod liver oil, evening primrose oil, iron, garlic, apple cider vinegar, vitamin C, selenium, B vitamins, calcium, general multivitamins and antioxidant supplements; extract of New Zealand green-lipped mussel; gamma-linolenic acid (GLA)-rich oils such as evening primrose oil, borage seed oil, or blackcurrant seed oil.[35,36] There is only weak or no evidence to support the use of these supplements in the management of RA symptoms. Gastrointestinal side effects were increased with GLA supplementation.[36]

Food intolerance and exclusion diets

Starvation greatly reduces symptoms in RA; for example, in the pre/postoperative state. It has been reported that the withdrawal of food in patients with RA results in a decreased production of the chemical mediators of inflammation but with the return of symptoms on the reintroduction of foodstuffs.[37]

Observational studies have reported food intolerance in RA patients, most commonly to milk, corn, wheat, and azo dyes, but there is no evidence that the prevalence of food intolerance is greater than in the general population or that the practice of food avoidance can be recommended to RA patients.[38] However, self-imposed food restrictions are popular with RA patients, most commonly citrus fruits, tomatoes, vinegars, pickles, dairy products, red meat, and alcohol. Clearly, the greater the number of foods avoided the greater the risk of malnutrition or nutrient deficiency.

Vegetarian and vegan diets

Vegetarian diets (preceded by fasting) for up to 4 months duration have resulted in symptomatic benefits in RA such as duration of morning stiffness, number of tender and swollen joints, and joint pain. However, there have been only a few studies, all with small sample size and at high risk of confounding.[39] Evidence is lacking for the routine use of vegan diets in the management of RA symptoms.

Although symptomatic improvements are experienced after fasting and/or elemental diet or vegetarian diet, the reasons for this are unclear. It is possible that the effect of excluding certain foods on symptoms of RA correlates with a reduction in antibodies to a food antigen,[40] or that inflammatory activity is attenuated by caloric restriction or reduction in gut involvement. However, these effects could also be a result of coincidental disease remission or weight loss, or due to a placebo effect.[37]

Mediterranean-type diet

Despite the folklore a 'diet for arthritis' has never been proven. However, there is evidence to support the role of n-3 fatty acids in the amelioration of inflammation and RA symptoms, with some epidemiological evidence for a role of antioxidants in reducing the risk of inflammatory arthritis.[25,26,41] Although conflicting results have been reported, high red meat consumption may have a role in increasing the risk of developing RA.[42,43] These studies have investigated foods individually, but collectively they form the basis of a Mediterranean-type diet which may provide symptomatic benefit in patients with RA. Studies of other foods and nutrients which have been investigated for a role in the aetiology of RA have been reviewed elsewhere.[44]

A modified Mediterranean diet followed for 3 months resulted in a significant reduction in disease activity (DAS28 score), functional ability (Health Assessment Questionnaire (HAQ) score), and improved vitality, compared to following a control diet.[45] Despite an increase in reported consumption of antioxidant-rich foods in the Mediterranean diet group, the levels of plasma antioxidants and urinary malondialdehyde (MDA), a marker of oxidative stress, did not change, although plasma levels of vitamin C, retinol, and uric acid were inversely correlated to variables related to RA disease activity.[46]

In a study which used a very different approach, women with established RA (n = 75) who came from socially deprived areas of Glasgow completed a 6 week educational programme with an emphasis on cooking and eating a 'Mediterranean-type' diet. Controls (n = 55) were given general healthy eating information only. Compared with controls, women in the intervention group reported a healthier dietary intake and showed significant improvement in patient global assessment at 6 months, pain score at 3 and 6 months, duration of early morning stiffness at 6 months, and HAQ score at 3 months.[47]

Comorbidities

Obesity is common in RA patients, partly due to a reduction in physical activity as a consequence of their symptoms of pain, stiffness, and poor mobility. Obesity is associated with the presence of traditional cardiovascular disease (CVD) risk factors as it is in the general population.[48] Patients with RA have an increased risk of CVD, especially ischaemic heart disease (IHD) and heart failure, and more than 50% of premature deaths in RA are due to CVD.[49] In fact, recent studies suggest that CVD mortality and morbidity in RA are of similar magnitude to that seen in people with type 2 diabetes mellitus.[50] The increase in risk of CVD observed in RA may be because traditional risk factors for CVD occur more frequently in RA, or that they have an additional deleterious effect. Alternatively, some of the excess CVD risk might be explained by the adverse impact of inflammation and immune changes of RA on blood vessel walls.[49] Abdominal fat is associated with insulin resistance and inflammatory load in patients with RA and in such patients is distributed differently between visceral and subcutaneous compartments, with visceral fat being more strongly associated with CVD risk than subcutaneous adiposity.[51] Since RA is an independent risk factor for IHD, cardiovascular risk assessment should be applied in all patients and dietary measures to treat obesity and CVD risk factors offered where appropriate. Although hyperlipidaemia is less frequent in RA than the general population, a meta-analysis confirmed that dyslipidaemia might affect up to half of all patients with RA, principally low levels of high-density lipoprotein (HDL) cholesterol.[52] Further studies are required to assess the value of dietary modification for dyslipidaemia and obesity in this population. However, until more is known the best strategy is to manage risk factors as for the general population, along with aggressive treatment of disease activity. Future research is needed to establish whether using lower targets for cholesterol and blood pressure management will be of benefit of CVD risk factors.

Anaemia in rheumatoid arthritis

Tiredness and fatigue are common in RA, caused in part by anaemia, a well-recognized complication of RA, even early on in disease.[53] The most common is a normochromic normocytic anaemia related to disease severity in the so-called 'anaemia of chronic disease' (ACD), in which iron and ferritin levels are not reduced, and responds to better disease control. Iron deficiency may be caused either by blood loss from chronic gastrointestinal ulceration and long-term NSAID or by a poor diet. Iron supplements are recommended for the former but not necessarily for the latter, where the deficiency can be corrected if foods rich in iron are eaten regularly (e.g. lean red meat especially offal, eggs, green leafy vegetables, pulses, dried fruits, and fortified breakfast cereals). The absorption of iron from food is enhanced if a source of vitamin C is eaten at the same time. A glass of orange juice at mealtimes is a good example. It should not be assumed that anaemia in RA is due to ACD, and all patients should be screened for other causes, especially vitamin deficiencies as these are so easily corrected, and further prevented with the correct nutritional and dietary advice.

Osteoporosis

Patients with RA and other forms of inflammatory arthritis are at an elevated risk of developing osteoporosis (see Chapter 142). RA is an independent risk factor for osteoporosis, thus risk assessments should be applied in all patients and dietary measures to maintain bone mass offered where appropriate. Dietary advice focuses on an appropriate calcium intake from the diet (e.g. from dairy products including low fat types; fruit and vegetables, especially green leafy vegetables; soya drinks with added calcium, and fish with edible bones). Calcium supplementation is usually only necessary when dietary intake is insufficient, combined with inadequate exposure to sunlight. Dietary sources of vitamin D are few: they include oily fish, eggs, fortified breakfast cereals, and margarines.

Other forms of arthritis and arthralgia

Systemic lupus erythematosus

Systemic lupus erythematosus (SLE) is an autoimmune disease that primarily affects young women, particularly of Afro-Caribbean and Asian origin. Evidence is lacking for any definite dietary triggers although anecdotal experience may be relevant to individual patients. Adults with SLE have an increased risk of cardiovascular mortality and morbidity, compared with the general population, with the risk increasing with disease duration, although this complication is apparent even in the early years of the disease.[49] As well as the standard and intensive treatment of active disease, the recommended management strategy for SLE should include screening for and management of traditional cardiovascular risk factors using at least the same targets as used for the general population. Future research is needed to establish if more aggressive management of obesity, cholesterol levels, and blood pressure, for example, will be of benefit.[49]

Vitamin D and joint pain

There has been increased interest in the role of vitamin D in musculoskeletal conditions in recent years since the measurement of vitamin D levels are now readily available.

The findings of a recent study in Ireland are of some relevance. Of 231 consecutive new patients to general rheumatology clinics 70% had vitamin D deficiency (defined as ≤53 nmol/litre) and 26% had severe deficiency (defined as ≤25 nmol/litre).[54] In patients diagnosed with OA and inflammatory joint disease 62% and 69% respectively were deficient in vitamin D.

Osteomalacia is a bone disease caused by chronic and severe calcium, vitamin D, or phosphate depletion of any cause. Bone pain, muscle weakness, tenderness, and difficulty walking are common manifestations of osteomalacia. In past years the most common causes of osteomalacia were malabsorption or prolonged lack of exposure to sunlight. However, nutritional deficiency, often in combination with UV light deficiency, is now a more common issue in the United Kingdom.

References

1. Richette P, Poitou C, Garnero P et al. Benefits of massive weight loss on symptoms, systemic inflammation and cartilage turnover in obese patients with knee osteoarthritis. *Ann Rheum Dis* 2011;70(1):139–144.

2. Leskinen J, Eskelinen A, Huhtala H, Paavolainen P, Remes V. The incidence of knee arthroplasty for primary osteoarthritis grows rapidly among baby-boomers—a population-based study. *Arthritis Rheum* 2012;64(2):423–428.

3. Sowers MR, Karvonen-Gutierrez CA. The evolving role of obesity in knee osteoarthritis. *Curr Opin Rheumatol* 2010;22(5):533–537.

4. Aspden RM. Obesity punches above its weight in osteoarthritis. *Nat Rev Rheumatol* 2011;7(1):65–68.

5. Marks R. Obesity profiles with knee osteoarthritis: correlates with pain, disability, disease progression. *Obesity* 2007;15(7):1867–1874.

6. Liu B, Balkwill A, Banks E et al. Relationship of height, weight and body mass index to the risk of hip and knee replacements in middle-aged women. *Rheumatology (Oxford)* 2007;46(5):861–867.

7. Niu J, Zhang, YQ, Torner J et al. Is obesity a risk factor for progressive radiographic knee osteoarthritis? *Arthritis Rheum* 2009;61(3):329–335.

8. Le Graverand MP, Brandt K, Mazzuca SA, Raunig D, Vignon E. Progressive increase in body mass index is not associated with a progressive increase in joint space narrowing in obese women with osteoarthritis of the knee. *Ann Rheum Dis* 2009;68(11):1734–1738.

9. Reijman M, Pols HA, Bergink AP et al. Body mass index associated with onset and progression of osteoarthritis of the knee but not of the hip: the Rotterdam Study. *Ann Rheum Dis* 2007;66(2):158–162.

10. Yusuf E, Nelissen RG, Ioan-Facsinay A et al. Association between weight or body mass index and hand osteoarthritis: a systematic review. *Ann Rheum Dis* 2010;69(4):761–765.

11. Toda Y, Toda T, Takemura S et al. Change in body fat, but not body weight or metabolic correlates of obesity, is related to symptomatic relief of obese patients with knee osteoarthritis after a weight control program. *J Rheumatol* 1998;25(11):2181–2186.

12. Messier SP, Loeser RF, Miller GD et al. Exercise and dietary weight loss in overweight and obese older adults with knee osteoarthritis: the Arthritis, Diet, and Activity Promotion Trial. *Arthritis Rheum* 2004;50(5):1501–1510.

13. Hart DJ, Doyle DV, Spector TD. Association between metabolic factors and knee osteoarthritis in women: the Chingford Study. *J Rheumatol* 1995;22(6):1118–1123.

14. National Collaborating Centre for Chronic Conditions. *Osteoarthritis: The care and management of osteoarthritis in adults. NICE clinical guideline 59.* Royal College of Physicians, London, 2008.

15. Haugen M, Homme KA, Reigstad A, Teigland J. Assessment of nutritional status in patients with rheumatoid arthritis and osteoarthritis undergoing joint replacement surgery. *Arthritis Care Res* 1999;12(1):26–32.

16. Berend KR, Lombardi AV, Mallory TH. Rapid recovery protocol for peri-operative care of total hip and total knee arthroplasty patients. *Surg Technol Int* 2004;13:239–247.

17. Towheed TE, Maxwell L, Anastassiades TP et al. Glucosamine therapy for treating osteoarthritis. *Cochrane Database Syst Rev* 2005;2:CD002946.

18. Wandel S, Jüni P, Tendal B et al. Effects of glucosamine, chondroitin, or placebo in patients with osteoarthritis of hip or knee: network meta-analysis. *BMJ* 2010;341:c4675.

19. Ernst E, Chrubasik S. Phyto-anti-inflammatories. A systematic review of randomized, placebo-controlled, double-blind trials. *Rheum Dis Clin North Am* 2000;26(1):13–27.

20. Long L, Soeken K, Ernst E. Herbal medicines for the treatment of osteoarthritis: a systematic review. *Rheumatology* (Oxford) 2001;40(7):779–793.

21. Choi HK. A prescription for lifestyle change in patients with hyperuricemia and gout. *Curr Opin Rheumatol* 2010;22(2):165–172.*

22. Vliet Vlieland TPM, Pattison D. Non-drug therapies in early rheumatoid arthritis. *Best Pract Res Clin Rheumatol* 2009;23(1):103–116.

23. Morgan SL, Anderson AM, Hood SM et al. Nutrient intake patterns, body mass index and vitamin levels in patients with rheumatoid arthritis. *Arthritis Care Res* 1997;10(1):9–17.

24. Stone J, Doube A, Dudson D, Wallace J. Inadequate calcium, folic acid, vitamin E, zinc and selenium intake in rheumatoid arthritis patients: results of a dietary survey. *Semin Arthritis Rheum* 1997;27(3):180–185.

25. Pattison DJ, Silman AJ, Goodson NJ et al. Vitamin C and the risk of developing inflammatory polyarthritis: prospective nested case-control study. *Ann Rheum Dis* 2004;63(7):843–847.

26. Pattison DJ, Symmons DPM, Lunt M et al. Dietary beta-cryptoxanthin and inflammatory polyarthritis: results from a population-based prospective study. *Am J Clin Nutr* 2005;82(2):451–455.

27. Heliövaara M, Knekt P, Aho K et al. Serum antioxidants and risk of rheumatoid arthritis. *Ann Rheum Dis* 1994;53(1):51–53.

28. Canter PH, Wider B, Ernst E. The antioxidant vitamins A, C, E and selenium in the treatment of arthritis: systematic review of randomised controlled trials. *Rheumatology* (Oxford) 2007;46(8):1223–1233.

29. Yaqoob P, Pala HS, Cortina-Borja M, Newsholme EA, Calder PC. Encapsulated fish oil enriched in alpha-tocopherol alters plasma phospholipid and mononuclear cell fatty acid compositions but not mononuclear cell functions. *Eur J Clin Invest* 2000;30(3):260–274.

30. Calder PC. n-3 Polyunsaturated fatty acids, inflammation, and inflammatory diseases. *Am J Clin Nutr* 2006;83(6 Suppl):1505S–1519S.*

31. Fortin PR, Lew RA, Liang MH et al. Validation of a meta-analysis: the effects of fish oil in rheumatoid arthritis. *J Clin Epidemiol* 1995;48(11):1379–1390.

32. Goldberg RJ, Katz J. A meta-analysis of the analgesic effects of omega-3 polyunsaturated fatty acid supplementation for inflammatory joint pain. *Pain* 2007;129(1–2):210–223.

33. Galarraga B, Ho M, Youssef HM et al. Cod liver oil (n-3 fatty acids) as an non-steroidal anti-inflammatory drug sparing agent in rheumatoid arthritis. *Rheumatology* (Oxford) 2008;47(5):665–669.

34. Adam O, Beringer C, Kless T et al. Anti-inflammatory effects of a low arachidonic acid diet and fish oil in patients with rheumatoid arthritis. *Rheumatol Int* 2003;23(1):27–36.

35. Cobb CS, Ernst E. Systematic review of marine nutriceutical supplement in clinical trials for arthritis: the effectiveness of the New Zealand green-lipped mussel Perna canaliculus. *Clin Rheumatol* 2006;25(3):275–284.

36. Cameron M, Gagnier JJ, Chrubasik S. Herbal therapy for treating rheumatoid arthritis. *Cochrane Database Syst Rev* 2011;2:CD002948.

37. Kavanaghi R, Workman E, Nash P et al. The effects of elemental diet and subsequent food reintroduction on rheumatoid arthritis. *Br J Rheumatol* 1995;34(3):270–273.

38. van de Laar MA, van der Korst JK. Food intolerance in rheumatoid arthritis. I. A double-blind, controlled trial of the clinical effects of the elimination of milk allergens and azo dyes. *Ann Rheum Dis* 1992;51(3):298–302.

39. Müller H, de Toledo FW, Resch KL. Fasting followed by vegetarian diet in patients with rheumatoid arthritis: a systematic review. *Scand J Rheumatol* 2001;30(1):1–10.

40. Hafström I, Ringertz B, Spångberg A et al. A vegan diet free of gluten improves the signs and symptoms of rheumatoid arthritis: the effects on arthritis correlate with a reduction in antibodies to food antigen. *Rheumatology* (Oxford) 2001;40(10):1175–1179.

41. Cerhan JR, Saag KG, Merlino LA, Mikuls TR, Criswell LA. Antioxidant micronutrients and risk of rheumatoid arthritis in a cohort of older women. *Am J Epidemiol* 2003;157(4):345–354.

42. Pattison DJ, Symmons DPM, Lunt M et al. Dietary risk factors for the development of inflammatory polyarthritis: evidence for a role of red meat consumption. *Arthritis Rheum* 2004;50(12):3804–3812.

43. Benito-Garcia E, Feskanich D, Hu FB, Mandl LA, Karlson EW. Protein, iron, and meat consumption and risk for rheumatoid arthritis: a prospective cohort study. *Arthritis Res Ther* 2007;9(1):R16.

44. Pattison DJ, Symmons DPM, Young A. Does diet have a role in the aetiology of rheumatoid arthritis? *Proc Nutr Soc* 2004;63(1):137–143.

45. Sköldstam L, Hagfors L, Johansson G. An experimental study of a Mediterranean diet intervention for patients with rheumatoid arthritis. *Ann Rheum Dis* 2003;62(3):208–214.

46. Hagfors L, Leanderson P, Sköldstam L, Andersson J, Johansson G. Antioxidant intake, plasma antioxidants and oxidative stress in a randomized, controlled, parallel, Mediterranean dietary intervention study on patients with rheumatoid arthritis. *Nutr J* 2003;2:5.

47. McKellar G, Morrison E, McEntegart A et al. A pilot study of a Mediterranean-type diet intervention in female patients with rheumatoid arthritis living in areas of social deprivation in Glasgow. *Ann Rheum Dis* 2007;66(9):1239–1243.

48. Stavropoulos-Kalinoglou A, Metsios GS, Panoulas VF et al. Associations of obesity with modifiable risk factors for the development of cardiovascular disease in patients with rheumatoid arthritis. *Ann Rheum Dis* 2009;68(2):242–245.

49. Symmons DPM, Gabriel SE. Epidemiology of CVD in rheumatic disease, with a focus on RA and SLE. *Nat Rev Rheumatol* 2011;7(7):399–408.

50. van Halm VP, Peters MJ, Voskuyl AE et al. Rheumatoid arthritis versus diabetes as a risk factor for cardiovascular disease: a cross-sectional study, the CARRE Investigation. *Ann Rheum Dis* 2009;68(9):1395–1400.

51. Giles JT, Allison M, Blumenthal RS et al. Abdominal adiposity in rheumatoid arthritis: Association with cardiometabolic risk factors and disease characteristics. *Arthritis Rheum* 2010;62(11):3173–3182.

52. Steiner G, Urowitz MB. Lipid profiles in patients with rheumatoid arthritis: mechanisms and the impact of treatment. *Semin Arthritis Rheum* 2009;38(5):372–381.

53. Young A, Koduri G. Extra-articular manifestations and complications of rheumatoid arthritis. *Best Pract Res Clin Rheumatol* 2007;21(5):907–927.

54. Haroon M, Bond U, Quillinan N, Phelan MJ, Regan MJ. The prevalence of vitamin D deficiency in consecutive new patients seen over a 6-month period in general rheumatology clinics. *Clin Rheumatol* 2011;30(6):789–794.

CHAPTER 89

Alternative therapies

Edzard Ernst

Introduction

This chapter is aimed at briefly summarizing the evidence regarding a range of alternative therapies for rheumatic conditions. As this is a very broad area, the focus is on areas where recent reliable evidence has become available.

Definitions

The terminology around alternative medicine is confusing. Ill-defined terms such as 'complementary', 'natural', 'holistic', or 'integrative' medicine are frequently used almost interchangeably. To avoid misunderstandings, this chapter merely discusses specific interventions and, as far as possible, avoids such umbrella terms. Short definitions of the alternative therapies covered in this chapter are provided in Table 89.1.[1]

Prevalence

The prevalence of the use of alternative therapies varies considerably from country to country. There is, however, general agreement that pain caused by rheumatic conditions is high on the list of reasons for patients to try alternative therapies. The lifetime prevalence of alternative therapy usage in the United Kingdom is 51% for pain and 38% for arthritis.[2]

Acupuncture

Acupuncture typically involves manual needling at specific points, but many variations of this theme exist. Numerous (around 1000) clinical trials have been published and are summarized repeatedly in systematic reviews. A recent overview included 57 systematic reviews of acupuncture for pain published since 2000.[3] Unanimously positive conclusions from more than one high-quality systematic review existed for only neck pain. The National Institute for Health and Clinical Excellence (NICE) recently recommended acupuncture as a treatment of persistent low back pain but not for osteoarthritis of the knee. For both indications, the evidence from systematic reviews is predominantly but not unanimously positive.[3]

Acupuncture is associated with sizeable placebo effects and only some trials adequately control for them. There is also evidence that the (non-verbal) interactions between the acupuncturist and the patient modify the clinical outcome.[4] As acupuncturists are never blinded to group allocation, this factor cannot easily be controlled for in clinical trials and may thus influence their results.

Several large prospective studies suggest that acupuncture is relatively safe; only about 10% of patients experience mild, transient adverse effects.[5] These studies have been conducted with relatively well-trained acupuncturists in the West, and their findings may thus not apply to other situations. Serious adverse effects, including death, continue to be associated with acupuncture.[3]

Chiropractic spinal manipulation

Chiropractors mostly but not exclusively treat back pain. NICE has recently recommended spinal manipulation or mobilization for persistent low back pain. Yet the evidence is not as straightforward as it may seem; a more recent Cochrane review included 26 randomized controlled trials (RCTs) and concluded that 'high quality evidence suggests that there is no clinically relevant difference between spinal manipulative therapy and other interventions for reducing pain and improving function in patients with chronic low back pain'.[6] Therefore other factors such as cost or safety (see below) should determine the choice of the optimal therapeutic approach.

For other rheumatic conditions, the evidence is even less convincing. Based on 33 RCTs, a Cochrane review demonstrated that, when combined with exercise, spinal manipulation treatments are beneficial for neck pain but, when done alone, they are not.[7] We concluded, in a systematic review of four RCTs which tested the effectiveness of chiropractic spinal manipulation for neck pain, that none of the studies 'convincingly demonstrated the superiority of chiropractic spinal manipulation over other interventions'.[8]

For other rheumatic conditions, including fibromyalgia and carpel tunnel syndrome, the evidence fails to suggest that chiropractic spinal manipulation is an effective treatment.[9] Reviews that arrive at more positive conclusions are misleading as they are not specifically of chiropractic manipulation but also include modalities such as exercise and other physical therapies (e.g. Schneider et al.[10]).

Chiropractic is associated with sizeable placebo effects which are difficult to control for in clinical trials.[11] Thus some of the outcomes seen in some of the RCTs might not rely on any specific effects of chiropractic spinal manipulation.

Chiropractic spinal manipulations are associated with an extraordinarily high rate of adverse effects. About one-half of all patients

Table 89.1 Definition of some relevant alternative therapies

Therapy	Definition
Acupuncture	Insertion of a needle into the skin and underlying tissues in special sites known as points for therapeutic or preventive purposes
Chiropractic	A health profession concerned with the diagnosis, treatment, and prevention of mechanical disorders of the musculoskeletal system, and the effects of these disorders on the function of the nervous system and general health. There is an emphasis on manual treatments including spinal manipulation or adjustment
Herbal medicine	The medical use of preparations that contain exclusively plant material
Homeopathy	A therapeutic method, often using highly diluted preparations of substances whose effects when administered to healthy subjects correspond to the manifestations of the disorder (symptoms, clinical signs and pathological states) in the unwell patient
Magnet therapy (static)	Application of static magnetic fields for therapeutic purposes
Massage therapy	A method of manipulating the soft tissue of body areas using pressure and traction (with primary focus on 'Swedish massage')
Osteopathy	Form of manual therapy (and diagnosis) involving the manipulation of soft tissues and the mobilization or manipulation of peripheral and spinal joints
Qigong	An Asian healing art that uses gentle, focused, exercises for mind and body to increase and restore the flow of qi (life energy) or to accumulate qi with the aim of encouraging and accelerating the healing process
T'ai chi	A system of movements and postures rooted in ancient Chinese philosophy and martial arts used to enhance mental and physical health

From Ernst et al.[1]

experience mild to moderate symptoms for one or two days.[12] In addition, several hundred cases of severe complications are on record. They are frequently caused by vertebral arterial dissections after neck manipulations (e.g. Di Fabio[13], Ernst[14]). Considering these risks, it is difficult to conclude that chiropractic is associated with a positive risk–benefit profile.

Herbal and other supplements

Two systematic reviews of herbal and other dietary supplements have been published by the charity Arthritis Research UK. One was based on seven RCTs and concluded that 'there is insufficient evidence on any complementary and alternative medicine, taken orally or applied topically, for fibromyalgia'.[15] The second review included 56 RCTs of supplements for the treatment of osteoarthritis (OA). It found

consistent evidence that capsaicin gel and S-adenosyl methionine were effective in the management of OA. There was also some consistency to the evidence that Indian Frankincense, methylsulphonylmethane and rose hip may be effective. For other substances with promising evidence, the evidence base was either insufficiently large

or the evidence base was inconsistent. Most of the CAM [complementary and alternative medicine] compounds studied were free of major adverse effects.[16]

A Cochrane review of herbal medicines for rheumatoid arthritis (RA) included 22 RCTs.[17] The authors found that:

there is moderate evidence that oils containing GLA [gamma-linolenic acid] ((evening primrose, borage, or blackcurrant seed oil) afford some benefit in relieving symptoms for RA, while evidence for Phytodolor® N is less convincing. *Tripterygium wilfordii* products may reduce some RA symptoms, however, oral use may be associated with several side effects.[17]

Specifically reviewing the RCT evidence for Ayurvedic herbal medicine for RA, we found seven such studies. The quality of these trials was disappointing and we concluded that they 'fail to show convincingly that such treatments are effective therapeutic options'.[18]

Even though many studies and systematic reviews have investigated the efficacy of chondroitin and glucosamine for osteoarthritis, the results continue to be contradictory. This is perhaps best summarized by quoting two recent and authoritative systematic reviews. Black et al. provided an overview of five systematic reviews and concluded that 'there was evidence that glucosamine sulphate shows some clinical effectiveness in the treatment of osteoarthritis of the knee'.[19] Yet a more recent meta-analysis arrived at far less optimistic conclusions: 'Compared with placebo, glucosamine, chondroitin, and their combination do not reduce joint pain or have an impact on narrowing of joint space'.[20]

The safety of supplements is a complex issue for which generalizations are problematic. Some seem to cause little more adverse effects than placebo, while others are outright toxic.[21] Other safety issues to consider are interactions with prescription drugs, contamination (e.g. with heavy metals), and adulteration with prescription drugs. Thus risk–benefit profiles have to be checked for each category and perhaps even for every preparation on offer.

Homeopathy

Homeopathy is perhaps the most implausible of all alternative treatments. Yet it is popular in many countries, particularly for the treatment of chronic conditions. Therefore it is relevant to know the evidence related to this subject.

A systematic review included four RCTs of homeopathy for osteoarthritis. Because of the low number and quality of the studies no firm conclusions regarding effectiveness were deemed possible.[22] Another systematic review included four RCTs of homeopathy for fibromyalgia. Because of the paucity of the trial data, no firm conclusions could be drawn about the effectiveness of homeopathic remedies.[23] A recent RCT was aimed at assessing whether the benefit many patients suffering from RA seem to experience after consulting a homeopath is due to specific effects of the homeopathic remedy or the non-specific effect of the consultation. The study used a factorial cross-over design and the conclusions could not have been clearer: 'homeopathic consultations but not homeopathic remedies are associated with clinically relevant benefits…'.[24]

Homeopathy is generally considered to be risk-free. This may apply to the homeopathic remedy but not necessarily to the homeopath. For instance, homeopaths frequently advise patients to forego effective treatments in favour of homeopathy.[25] On balance, therefore, the risk–benefit profile of homeopathy is not positive.

Magnet therapy

Many patients suffering from rheumatic conditions wear static magnets in the form of bracelets, belts, inlays, etc. in the hope of reducing pain effectively. Our systematic review of nine RCTs testing the effectiveness of this approach came to a sobering conclusion:

> The evidence does not support the use of static magnets for pain relief, and therefore magnets cannot be recommended as an effective treatment. For osteoarthritis, the evidence is insufficient to exclude a clinically important benefit, which creates an opportunity for further investigation.[26]

Direct adverse effects of static magnets are not to be expected. Yet, considering the often considerable costs of such devices, patients should be discouraged from using them.

Massage therapy

There are many variations of massage therapy—e.g. Shiatsu, Bowen technique, soft tissue massage, lymph drainage, Rolfing—of which 'Swedish' or classical muscle massage is the best-researched and most popular.

A Cochrane review included 13 RCTs of massage therapy for low back pain. Eight of these studies were of poor methodological quality. Even though most results suggested effectiveness, the authors drew cautious conclusions: 'Massage might be beneficial for patients with subacute and chronic non-specific low back pain…'.[27]

A systematic review of 19 RCTs of massage therapy for neck pain arrived at even more cautious conclusions. Most of the studies were of low quality and only six tested massage as a stand-alone therapy. The authors stated that 'the effectiveness of massage for neck pain remains uncertain'.[28]

A systematic review of massage for fibromyalgia symptoms included six RCTs. All of them suggested short-term benefits but all had serious methodological limitations. Therefore the author concluded that the RCT data provide 'modest support for the use of massage therapy in treating fibromyalgia'.[29] For other rheumatic conditions, the evidence related to massage therapy is too scarce to arrive at meaningful verdicts.

The risks of adequately administered massage therapy are very minor. The adverse effects that have been reported are rare and mostly due to inadequate technique or incompetent therapists.[30]

Osteopathy

Osteopathy is a manual treatment with many similarities to chiropractic (see above). In the United States, osteopaths are a fully recognized medical profession that today uses most conventional treatments alongside osteopathic techniques. In most other countries, osteopaths are considered alternative practitioners. Thus, in the United States, osteopaths would treat any condition, whereas elsewhere they would mostly treat musculoskeletal complaints.

A systematic review including six RCTs of osteopathic manipulations for low back pain concluded that this approach generates greater pain reductions than a range of active control interventions, placebo, or no treatment at all.[31] Our own systematic review of osteopathy for any type of musculoskeletal pain included 16 RCTs.[32] Their methodological quality was mostly poor. Only five of these studies suggested that osteopathy might cause more pain reduction than various control interventions. The evidence for other rheumatic conditions is scarce and unconvincing.[1,33]

Like other physical treatments, osteopathy might be associated with relatively large placebo effects. These are difficult to control for in RCTs. Thus some of the positive results might at least partly rely on non-specific results rather than specific effects of the treatment per se.

Osteopathy is, like chiropractic, associated with both frequent mild and infrequent serious adverse effects.[34] However, osteopathic techniques tend to be less forceful and less often include rotational thrusts of the cervical spine. Thus serious complications such as vertebral artery dissection seem to occur less frequently than with chiropractic.[34]

Qigong

Qigong is a traditional Chinese method; two different forms can be differentiated. External qigong is a form of 'energy healing' where a therapist channels healing 'energy' into a patient's body. This 'energy' allegedly stimulates the body's capacity to heal itself.

A systematic review of external qigong for reducing pain from any condition included five RCTs.[35] Some of these studies suggested positive effects; however, most were burdened with significant flaws. Thus firm conclusions about the effectiveness of this approach are not possible.

Internal qigong uses gentle, slow, meditative exercises. This allegedly increases the flow of energy through the body which, in turn, stimulates the body's healing capacity. A systematic review of this approach for reducing pain of any origin included four RCTs and three non-randomized studies.[36] Most of these studies included patients suffering from musculoskeletal problems. Again, most trials were of disappointing methodological quality. Even though these data included several encouraging results, the overall conclusion was that the totality of the evidence is less than convincing.

No serious risks have been associated with either form of qigong.

T'ai chi

T'ai chi is a meditative form of aerobic exercise involving slow movements, relaxation, and deep breathing techniques. It originates from China and has recently become popular in many Western countries.

Our systematic review included nine RCTs of t'ai chi for osteoarthritis most of which had significant methodological flaws.[37] A meta-analysis generated a positive effect on pain, physical function, and joint stiffness compared with a range of control interventions. Because of the relative small number of RCTs and their often weak designs, the conclusion had to be cautious.

For RA the evidence is less convincing. A systematic review found just two RCTs and three non-randomized studies.[38] Even though some positive results were reported in some trials for t'ai chi on disability, quality of life, and mood of patients with RA, the more rigorous RCTs failed to demonstrate any relevant clinical benefit.

T'ai chi is generally regarded as safe and no serious complications are to be expected.

Conclusion

This overview indicates that, in general, the evidence related to alternative therapies for rheumatic conditions is scarce. Few rigorous trials are available from which to draw firm conclusions about their efficacy in common rheumatic diseases. For less common rheumatic conditions, good evidence is almost entirely absent (e.g. Chou[39]). The safety of these approaches remains grossly under-researched. Thus it is impossible to be certain whether any alternative treatments generate more benefit than harm.

Even in areas where the evidence seems encouraging, important caveats persist. For instance, the quality of the research is often disappointing. Another concern is the clinical relevance of any documented effects. In most cases, they are small and thus questionable. In no case are they demonstrably superior to those of conventional therapeutic options.

Thus it seems that the popularity of alternative treatments is currently not supported by the findings from reliable scientific investigations.

References

1. Ernst E, Pittler MH, Wider B, Boddy K. *Complementary therapies for pain management. An evidence-based approach.* Elsevier, London, 2007.

2. Hunt KJ, Ernst E. Patient's use of CAM: results from the Health Survey for England 2005. *FACT* 2010;15(2):101–103.

3. Ernst E, Lee MS, Choi TY. Acupuncture: Does it alleviate pain and are there serious risks? A review of reviews. *Pain* 2011;152:755–764.

4. Suarez-Almazor ME, Looney C, Liu YF et al. A randomized controlled trial of acupuncture for osteoarthritis of the knee: effects of patient-provider communication. *Arthritis Care Res* 2010;62:1229–1236.

5. White A, Hayhoe S, Hart A, Ernst E. Adverse events following acupuncture: prospective survey of 32000 consultations with doctors and physiotherapists. *BMJ* 2001;323:485–486.

6. Rubinstein SM, van Middelkoop M, Assendelft WJ, de Boer MR, van Tulder MW. Spinal manipulative therapy for chronic low-back pain: an update of a Cochrane review. *Spine* 2011;36(13):E825–E846.

7. Gross AR, Hoving JL, Haines TA et al. A Cochrane review of manipulation and mobilization for mechanical neck disorders. *Spine* 2004;29:1541–1548.

8. Ernst E. Chiropractic spinal manipulation for neck pain—a systematic review. *J Pain* 2003;4:417–442.

9. Ernst E. Chiropractic manipulation for non-spinal pain—a systematic review. *N Z Med J* 2003;116:1–9.

10. Schneider M, Vernon H, Ko G, Lawson G, Perera J. Chiropractic management of fibromyalgia syndrome: a systematic review of the literature. *J Manip Physiol Ther* 2009;32:25–40.

11. Ernst E, Harkness EF. Spinal manipulation: a systematic review of sham-controlled, double-blind, randomized clinical trials. *J Pain Symptom Manage* 2001;24:879–889.

12. Senstad O, Leboeuf-Yde C, Borchgrevink C. Frequency and characteristics of side effects of spinal manipulative therapy. *Spine* 1997;22:435–441.

13. Di Fabio RP. Manipulation of the cervical spine: risks and benefits. *Physical Ther* 1999;79:50–65.

14. Ernst E. Manipulation of the cervical spine: a systematic review of case reports of serious adverse events, 1995–2001. *Med J Aust* 2002;176:376–380.

15. De Silva V, El-Metwally A, Ernst E, Lewith G, Macfarlane GJ. Evidence for the efficacy of complementary and alternative medicine in the management of fibromyalgia: a systematic review. *Rheumatology* 2010;49(6):1063–1068.

16. De Silva V, El-Metwally A, Ernst E, Lewith G, Macfarlane GJ. Evidence for the efficacy of complementary and alternative medicines in the management of osteoarthritis: a systematic review. *Rheumatology* 2011;50(5):911–920.

17. Cameron M, Gagnier JJ, Chrubasik S. Herbal therapy for treating rheumatoid arthritis. *Cochrane Database Syst Rev* 2011;16[2]:CD002948.

18. Park J, Ernst E. Ayurvedic medicine for rheumatoid arthritis: a systematic review. *Semin Arthritis Rheum* 2005;34:705–713.

19. Black C, Clar C, Henderson R, MacEachern C et al. The clinical effectiveness of glucosamine and chondroitin supplements in slowing or arresting progression of osteoarthritis of the knee: a systematic review and economic evaluation. *Health Technol Assess* 2009;13(52):1–148.

20. Wandel S, Jüni P, Tendel B et al. Effects of glucosamine, chondroitin, or placebo in patients with osteoarthritis of hip or knee: network meta-analysis. *BMJ* 2010;341:c4675.

21. Ernst E, Pittler MH, Wider B, Boddy K. *The desktop guide to complementary and alternative medicine*, 2nd edn. Elsevier Mosby, Edinburgh, 2006.

22. Long L, Ernst E. Homeopathic remedies for the treatment of osteoarthritis a systematic review. *Br Homeopathic J* 2001;90:37–43.

23. Terry R, Perry R, Ernst E. An overview of systematic reviews of complementary and alternative medicine for fibromyalgia. *Clin Rheumatol* 2012;31(1):55–66.

24. Brien S, Lachance L, Prescott P, McDermott C, Lewith G. Homeopathy has clinical benefits in rheumatoid arthritis patients which are attributable to the consultation process not the homeopathic remedy. A randomised controlled clinical trial. *Rheumatology* 2011;50(6):1070–1082.

25. Ernst E. Is homeopathy a clinically valuable approach? *Trends Pharmacol Sci* 2005;26(11):547–548.

26. Pittler MH, Brown EM, Ernst E. Static magnets for reducing pain: systematic review and meta-analysis of randomised trials. *CMAJ* 2007;177(7):736–742.

27. Furlan AD, Imamura M, Dryden T, Irvin E. Massage for low-back pain. *Cochrane Database Syst Rev* 2008;8(4):CD001929.

28. Ezzo J, Haralsson BG, Gross AR et al. Massage for mechanical neck disorders: a systematic review. *Spine* 2007;32(3):353–362.

29. Kalichman L. Massage therapy for fibromyalgia symptoms. *Rheumatol Int* 2010;30(9):1151–1157.

30. Ernst E. The safety of massage therapy. *Rheumatology* (Oxford) 2003;42:1101–1106.

31. Licciardone JC, Brimhall AK, King LN. Osteopathic manipulative treatment for low back pain: a systematic review and meta-analysis of randomized controlled trials. *BMC Musculoskelet Disord* 2005;6:43.

32. Posadzki P, Ernst E. Osteopathy for musculoskeletal pain patients: a systematic review of randomized controlled trials. *Clin Rheumatol* 2011;30(2):285–291.

33. Romano M, Negrini S. Manual therapy as a conservative treatment for adolescent idiopathic scoliosis: a systematic review. *Scoliosis* 2008;23:2.

34. Terrett AGJ. *Current concepts in verebrobasilar complications following spinal manipulation.* NCMIC, Clive, Iowa, 2001.

35. Lee MS, Pittler MH, Ernst E. External qigong for pain conditions: a systematic review of randomized clinical trials. *J Pain* 2007;8(11):827–831.

36. Lee MS, Pittler MH, Ernst E. Internal qigong for pain conditions: A systematic Review. *J Pain* 2009;10(11):1121–1127.

37. Kang JW, Lee MS, Posadzki P, Ernst E. T'ai chi for the treatment of osteoarthritis: a systematic review and meta-analysis. *BMJ Open* 2011;1(1):e000035.

38. Lee MS, Pittler MH, Ernst E. Tai chi for rheumatoid arthritis: systematic review. *Rheumatology* 2007;46(11):1648–1651.

39. Chou CT. Alternative therapies: what role do they have in the management of lupus? *Lupus* 2010;19(12):1425–1429.

CHAPTER 90

Principles of upper limb surgery

Ian McNab and Chris Little

Introduction

Inflammatory arthritis primarily involves synovial tissue. The associated immune response releases cytokines and degradative enzymes that lead to articular cartilage destruction, and the attenuation of joint-stabilizing ligaments and tendons. The mainstay of treatment of inflammatory joint disease is medical control of synovitis. However, if the symptoms persist despite optimal medical management and, in particular, once irreversible joint damage has occurred, reconstructive surgical treatment may be indicated. Wherever possible this should be undertaken before the patient becomes severely incapacitated; salvage options exist where irreversible damage has arisen, but prophylactic interventions are better.

Most patients referred for a surgical opinion on the management of a rheumatic disease have rheumatoid arthritis (RA), but the surgical principles of managing most inflammatory arthropathies are similar. This chapter therefore focuses primarily on the principles of managing RA, using this as an exemplar for similar conditions. Box 90.1 shows the investigations that may be required prior to surgery.

Operative treatment

Patient fitness should be optimized, ideally with good medical control of synovitis and no chest, urinary, or skin sepsis. Care must be taken perioperatively with renal function, hydration, and increased steroid requirements (see Chapter 93).

Surgical treatment forms only a part of the continuing management of the patient by the whole medical team. Active disease and the use of glucocorticoids are not contraindications to surgery, although the timing of surgery will need to consider cycles of biological or some immune-suppressive treatments.

Ultimately a successful outcome for patients (especially when undergoing upper limb surgery) is determined by matching the correct patient to the correct procedure, meticulous attention to surgical detail and technique, and especially by the motivation and hard work of the nurses, physiotherapists, occupational therapists, and patients themselves, during their postoperative rehabilitation (see Box 90.2).

Box 90.2 General perioperative considerations

+ Timing of surgery in relation to medical treatment/control of arthritis (optimized with DMARDs—usually continued)

+ Use of immunosuppressants and/or steroids increases the risk of infection

+ Past medical history, general health, treatment history

+ Cardiovascular and respiratory assessment, poor jaw mobility, micrognathia, reduced lung capacity, range of cervical spine movement (imaging to exclude subluxation), anticipate potential anaesthetic problems

+ Walking ability and use of suitable walking aids, presence of significant lower limb problems, thoracolumbar spine problems

+ Skin condition (including ulcers or thin skin)

+ Presence/treatment of vasculitis

+ Presence/treatment of osteoporosis

+ Anaemia of chronic disease

+ Polyarticular involvement with contractures—risk of pressure sores, requires careful positioning/padding

+ Home environment, and functional abilities/requirements

+ Optimization of occupational therapy, physiotherapy, splints, and aids

---

Box 90.1 Investigations prior to surgery

+ Plain radiograph (usually suffices)

+ Ultrasound scan (synovium, tendon, ligament)

+ MRI

+ Biopsy (confirm diagnosis, exclude infection)

The order of procedures should be tailored to the individual. Operations most likely to be successful are usually performed first, in order to build patient confidence. It is usually best to correct lower limb abnormalities before addressing upper limb problems because of the potential for damage to upper limb reconstructions with subsequent use of walking aids. In patients who require intubation, it is essential to check their clinical and radiographic cervical spine mobility and stability. Patients are susceptible to perioperative pressure sores and peripheral compression neuropathies.

Upper limb surgical management

Rapid improvements in medical treatment appear to be impacting on the course and pattern of RA presenting to upper limb surgeons. However, RA continues to cause pain and impaired function for patients, many of whom still require reconstructive surgery to their shoulders, elbows, hands, and wrists. The basic principles of this surgery are to preserve hand function and to maintain stable, comfortable proximal upper limb joints that will allow the patient to position their hand in space adequately, so that it can perform its essential functions.

Patient assessment and planning upper limb surgery

Initially, patients adapt their activities to accommodate their reduced upper limb function. However, if their function and pain continue to deteriorate despite maximal medical therapy, physiotherapy, occupational therapy, functional aids, and night splintage (to slow the progression of deformities), then they may require surgical intervention.

Patients with these complex and challenging upper limb, hand, and wrist problems require a highly integrated approach to their assessment and treatment. This is often best provided at a combined medical and surgical RA clinic. The extended multidisciplinary team includes rheumatologists, radiologists, nurses, physiotherapists, occupational therapists, surgeons, and anaesthetists (see Box 90.3 for a checklist prior to upper limb surgery).

The primary goals of any surgical treatment are to help alleviate pain and to maintain or improve function. A secondary consequence of correcting deformities may also be an improved appearance, particularly of the hand.

In addition to careful patient selection, and meticulous surgical planning and technique, extremely careful physiotherapy and hand therapy are also required to ensure success following all of the procedures listed below.

Indications and timing of surgery

The indications for and the timing of surgery are discussed in the sections relating to each anatomical region in the upper limb. However, these general principles must be carefully tailored to each individual patient's clinical presentation, general health, the current status of their RA, their optimal medications and the degree of disease control, the available physiotherapy and occupational therapy support, and their social and functional requirements and abilities (for home, work, and hobbies).

In patients who require multiple surgical interventions, careful planning is required as to which order to perform the procedures, and on which occasions. This initial plan may need to be adjusted as the programme of surgical treatment progresses.

Box 90.3 Surgical assessment checklist prior to hand and upper limb surgery

- Global upper limb examination: shoulder and elbow movements—positioning the hand in space for function (above the head, behind the back); adequate shoulder abduction and external rotation is required for regional anaesthetic and surgical positioning
- Test forearm rotation: supination and pronation requires free movement of both the proximal and distal radioulnar joints (elbow and wrist).
- Assess distal radioulnar joints and extensor tendons
- Assess carpal tunnel and flexor tendons
- Wrist movement should be approximately 50:50 radiocarpal and midcarpal joint function
- Check thumb CMC and MCP joints and look for swan-neck and boutonnière deformities
- Check fingers for MCP disease, ulnar drift or subluxation, abnormalities of PIPs and DIPs, and the presence of swan-neck and boutonnière deformities
- Test the intrinsic muscles which flex the MCP and extend the PIP joints and are placed under maximum tension when the MCP joints are passively extended and the PIP joints are passively flexed
- Intrinsic tightness test: compare PIP flexion with the MCP joint in extension vs flexion
- Assess skin and nails
- Neurovascular assessment—specifically check for nerve compression

CMC, carpometacarpal; DIP, distal interphalangeal; MCP, metacarpophalangeal; PIP, proximal interphalangeal.

Because lower limb generally requires the patient to mobilize with walking aids (so weightbearing through the upper limbs) postoperatively, these should usually be addressed prior to embarking on upper limb surgery.

If multiple-level surgery is required in the upper limb itself, it is generally best to correct problems sequentially working from proximal towards more distal joints, or to address the most symptomatic or severely affected region first.

The concept of performing a 'winner procedure' as the first operation is also important. These procedures should have both predictable and good results without undue rehabilitation requirements that will hopefully ensure the patient's first experience of surgery is a positive one. Therefore, replacement arthroplasty of the shoulder or elbow, or arthrodesis (or arthroplasty) of the wrist is often undertaken first.

Occasionally, urgent surgery is required to prevent sudden further deterioration. For example, following rupture of the extensor tendons to the little finger, urgent excision of the ulnar head and tenosynovectomy is required to prevent multiple extensor tendon ruptures.

Shoulder

Acromioclavicular joint

This is commonly affected by rheumatoid synovitis, often with radiographic changes, but because symptoms are similar to those from rotator cuff disease it is important to determine the source of pain. The typical features of acromioclavicular joint (ACJ) involvement in RA are:

- Pain usually well localized to the joint.
- Pain reproduced by high arc (>120°—end of range) elevation movements (abducting the outstretched arm above the patient's head) and by horizontal flexion (crossing the arm towards the opposite shoulder when elevated by 90°; the 'scarf test').
- The ACJ is tender.

Initial treatment is by intra-articular steroid. Since the orientation of the joint varies (lateral clavicle often over- or underrides the acromion), a plain radiograph shows the best angle for the needle. Surgery should be considered if this fails to improve the symptoms; excision arthroplasty (arthroscopically removing the lateral centimetre of the clavicle) improves symptoms in 80% of patients

Glenohumeral joint

The radiographic pattern of disease may be

- dry (with loss of joint space, bony sclerosis, and marked stiffness)
- wet (with marked synovitis, marginal humeral head erosions, and central glenoid erosion)
- resorptive (with marked bone loss, often with glenoid loss down to or beyond the coracoid process).

Intra-articular steroid injections can give good transient relief. The degree of bone loss, particularly from the glenoid, often makes total shoulder replacement inadvisable, due to problems with securely fixing a glenoid component in place, and hemiarthroplasty (humeral head replacement) is usually used, giving good pain control but limited improvement in function. Reverse geometry replacements (with a ball—glenosphere—placed in the glenoid, and a cup in the proximal humerus) carries potential advantages where the cuff is deficient, but glenoid bone loss will often render this inadvisable.

Rotator cuff

Impingement pain is felt in the region of the deltoid insertion with arm elevation. Rest and night pain occurring in a similar area suggests that a cuff tear is present (seen in up to 40%) with loss of movement due to pain or altered shoulder mechanics if the tear is large (which may give rise to a lag sign, with the patient unable to maintain the position of the passively placed arm, indicating a massive tear).

Initial non-operative treatment is indicated, with steroid injections into the subacromial bursa and physiotherapy to improve scapular positioning, because cuff repair is often technically difficult due to poor tissue quality, which would result in a high rate of repeat tears. Arthroscopic surgery to debride the bursa often helps those patients who respond transiently to non-operative treatments (even those with full-thickness cuff tears). Fistula formation from the arthroscopic port sites is more common than in non-rheumatoid patients.

Elbow

Ulnohumeral and radiocapitellar joints

This can present with:

- diffuse pain around the elbow
- stiffness, with loss of function; elbow flexion/extension and forearm rotation can be affected, causing difficulty with positioning the hand.
- instability due to bone erosion and soft tissue attenuation ('flail elbow').

Radiographic changes do not directly correlate with symptoms. Intra-articular steroid injections may help transiently with the pain from synovitis; optimizing systemic disease control is also required for longer-term improvement. Some patients, particularly those with lateral pain and restricted forearm rotation, are helped in the medium term by radial head excision coupled with a synovectomy; however, symptoms commonly recur.

Joint replacement components may be unlinked (surface replacement of the distal humerus and proximal ulna, with excision of the radial head), with stability dependent on soft tissue balance and reconstructions. Alternatively, linked components can be used (the humeral and ulnar components are connected, providing stability but potentially increasing mechanical loosening with time), particularly in flail elbows. 'Sloppy hinge' implants allow a little varus/valgus tilt between linked components to minimize mechanical loosening.

In the absence of complications, pain control is usually good and motion improved by around 20° of flexion/extension. The risk of infection or wound breakdown and nerve damage (ulnar nerve) is greater than with other commonly replaced large joints (hip/knee), and radiographic loosening is common (but may be asymptomatic, particularly given the polyarticular nature of the patient's disease). The 5 year implant survival rate (with revision surgery as the end-point) is 90%.

Ulnar nerve compression

Symptomatic ulnar nerve compression is surprisingly uncommon in rheumatoid patients, given that subclinical disease and neurophysiological changes are very common. Presentation is with:

- intermittent tingling in the little and ring fingers (with or without objective sensory changes)
- intrinsic wasting (especially of the first dorsal interosseous muscle)
- irritability of the ulnar nerve behind the medial epicondyle.

Failure to improve with simple avoidance of local pressure and prolonged flexion indicates the need for neurophysiological testing (to confirm nerve compression at the elbow) and a surgical review. Simple surgical decompression would not be recommended if it leaves the nerve in a 'hostile' bed; anterior transposition is preferred.

Posterior interosseous nerve palsy

This is usually due to local compression by cysts from the elbow joint, compression by local fibrous bands or vasculitis. Presentation is with wrist drop and the inability to dorsiflex fingers at the MCP. Remember that IP joint extension can be achieved by the hand intrinsic muscles, which are innervated by the ulnar and median nerves.

It is important to exclude extensor tendon attrition rupture (due to tenosynovitis and distal radioulnar joint synovitis at the wrist) and extensor mechanism subluxation at the MCPJ as the cause of the dropped fingers (see Box 90.4). Surgical exploration to decompress the nerve and to remove any local swelling is the treatment of choice.

Olecranon bursitis and rheumatoid nodules

In patients with RA, the olecranon bursa is a common site of pressure and friction. Pressure avoidance with or without aspiration of the bursa is the initial treatment of choice. Surgical excision is possible, but carries the potential for healing problems and prolonged drainage.

Hand and wrist

RA in the hand can affect multiple joints, but especially the wrist and distal radio ulnar joint (DRUJ), the metacarpophalangeal (MCP) and proximal interphalangeal (PIP) joints of the fingers and the carpometacarpal (CMC) and MCP joints of the thumb. In addition to the direct destruction of articulating joint surfaces, the synovitis associated with RA causes attenuation and

---

Box 90.4 Differential diagnosis of apparent finger extension lag

- Posterior interosseous nerve palsy caused by elbow synovitis (a tenodesis test will show intact extensor tendons producing finger extension during maximal passive wrist flexion)

- Extensor tendon rupture (loss of both active finger extension and passive extension on the tenodesis test)

- EDC tendon sagittal band rupture allowing subluxation of the extensor tendon into the valley between the metacarpal heads (if fingers are first placed in extension, allowing the extensor tendons to align centrally over the dorsum of the metacarpal heads, this position can be maintained actively; if fingers are first placed in flexion the subluxed extensor tendons cannot actively extend the MCP joints)

- Locked trigger finger (usually also has flexion of the PIP)

- Locked MCP joint (usually in osteoarthritis with active and passive extension except for the last 40° at MCP joint), or MCP joint subluxation

- Dupuytren's disease

EDC, extensor digitorum communis; MCP, metacarpophalangeal; PIP, proximal interphalangeal.

---

rupture of important joint-stabilizing ligaments and tendons, which leads to progressive joint subluxation and dislocation, and to the development of several characteristic zigzag collapse deformities in the hand. Fibrosis and contracture of the intrinsic muscles of the hand also contributes to the development of finger deformities.

Loss of finger extension is a common presentation; Box 90.4 outlines how to establish the cause, which will help management planning.

Distal radioulnar joint and extensor tendon surgery

Tenosynovitis (either flexor or extensor) that fails to respond to full medical treatment for 3–6 months (including steroid injection) may benefit from surgical tenosynovectomy, which may also reduce the rate of tendon rupture. Joint synovectomy may decrease symptoms but does not halt the progression of joint disease.

Caput ulna syndrome

Caput ulna syndrome is due to extensor tenosynovitis associated with DRUJ synovitis, leading to erosion and dorsal subluxation of the ulnar head through the dorsal joint capsule and consequent extensor tendon rupture. Extensor digiti minimi (EDM) and EDC to little finger usually rupture first, causing an extensor lag to the little finger. The other EDC tendons may then sequentially rupture from the ulnar side, creating a much more difficult reconstructive problem; rapid surgical intervention can prevent this. The surgical options are listed in Table 90.1.

Carpal tunnel and flexor tendon problems

Flexor tenosynovitis associated with carpal tunnel syndrome may occasionally be the first presenting feature of RA. If it fails to respond rapidly to steroid injections, it may require urgent carpal tunnel decompression (through an extended approach) with a flexor tenosynovectomy. Flexor tenosynovitis in the digits may cause triggering or result in the presence of a greater passive than active range of motion. If this persists despite medical management and steroid injections a tenosynovectomy may be performed (preserving the A1 pulley to prevent bowstringing and ulnar drift). Flexor pollicis longus (FPL) is the most common flexor tendon to rupture (Mannerfelt syndrome), due to palmar wrist synovitis and prominent bone spurs from the scaphoid and trapezium, along with flexor digitorum profundus (FDP) to the index finger. If the thumb interphalangeal (IP) joint is stiff or ankylosed, then function may be maintained without intervention. If not, the options for surgical reconstruction include arthrodesis of the thumb IP joint; repair or palmaris longus grafting of the FPL tendon; transfer of ring finger FDS tendon to FPL. Rupture of finger flexor tendons is less common but may require similar tendon repair, grafting, or transfers. Careful rehabilitation is required following all these procedures.

Wrist

Synovitis causes progressive attenuation and destruction of the intrinsic intercarpal ligaments and the extrinsic intracapsular ligaments of the wrist. The scapholunate ligament may rupture and the whole carpus tends to slide down the articular surface of

Table 90.1 Surgical options for caput ulna syndrome

Procedure	Comments
Ulnar head excision (Darrach procedure) plus soft tissue stabilization of the distal ulna	Most commonly perfomed for RA where there is often significant destruction of the ulnar head
Hemi-resection ulna head plus soft tissue interposition/stabilization (Bowers procedure)	A possibility in earlier disease, as it requires an intact/reconstructable TFCC
DRUJ arthrodesis plus pseudarthrosis proximal to the ulnar head (Sauve Kapandji procedure)	A proven alternative that has the theoretical advantage of maintaining some support to the ulnar carpus, so possibly reducing ulnar translation of the carpus. However, it can give unreliable results, and create almost unsalvageable problems from ulnar stump instability unless executed with precise techniques
Prosthetic ulnar head replacement (partial or total)	Established implants and techniques are now available, but as long-term results are not yet known, this is mainly performed by specialist hand surgeons and/or is reserved as a secondary salvage procedure
Extensor tenosynovectomy and tendon repairs, grafts, or transfers, plus retinaculum transposition (deep to the tendons)	Usually combined with one of the above procedures. Many reconstructive options are available and the exact combination of procedures is tailored to the findings at the time of surgery. Rupture of EDM and EDC to the little finger is commonly reconstructed by transferring the EIP tendon from the index finger. EDC to the ring finger can be transferred ('piggy-backed') onto the adjacent intact EDC tendon to the middle finger or combined with the EDM reconstruction. Multiple extensor tendon ruptures may require the transfer of additional motors, such as FDS from the ring finger.
Rehabilitation following tendon reconstruction	From 2 weeks after surgery gentle controlled range of motion exercises are commenced from a custom splint

DRUJ, distal radioulnar joint; EDC, extensor digitorum communis; EDM, extensor digiti minimi; EIP, extensor indicis proprius; FDS, flexor digitorum superficialis; RA, rheumatoid arthritis; TFCC, triangular fibrocartilage complex.

Table 90.2 Surgical options for wrist problems in rheumatoid arthritis

Procedure	Comments
Synovectomy of the wrist (open or arthroscopic)	May be useful in the early stage of the disease with joint preservation but significant synovitis that is resistant to medical therapy
ECRL to ECU transfer	Useful if the wrist joint surfaces are still healthy, to dynamically correct radial deviation of the carpus and metacarpals, prior to addressing finger MCP joint ulnar deviation
Radiolunate arthrodesis (or radioscapholunate arthrodesis)	Indicated with isolated radiocarpal joint involvement, early ulnar translation of the carpus, and preservation of >60° arc of motion. This will prevent further radiocarpal joint subluxation and preserves some midcarpal joint movement
Total wrist arthrodesis (using a dorsal wrist fusion plate, or intermedullary metacarporadial pins)	Indicated when both radiocarpal and midcarpal joints are involved, there is significant subluxation and pain, and <60°arc of motion is preserved
Total wrist arthroplasty	Historically, it has proved difficult to design and implant reliable total wrist prostheses. Until the long-term results of newer implants are known, this procedure should be performed in specialist hand surgery units. One approach has been to perform an arthroplasty on the dominant wrist, thus preserving some dexterity and flexion for performing tasks (such as personal hygiene), and to perform an arthrodesis on the non-dominant wrist, thus ensuring a stable wrist for power activities
Correction and stabilization of wrist subluxation and deformity	Restores a relatively normal carpal and metacarpal alignment, creating a stable base upon which the thumb and fingers can be reconstructed and can function

ECRL, extensor carpi radialis longus; ECU, extensor carpi ulnaris.

the radius into ulnar translation, palmar subluxation, and supination, with a secondary radial deviation of the metacarpals. The degree of surgical intervention required is matched to the level of the patient's pain and existing range of motion, the stage of the disease, and the pattern of joint destruction. Surgical options are listed in Table 90.2.

Thumb

Common problems are summarized in Table 90.3.

Metacarpophalangeal joints of the fingers

Common problems are summarized in Table 90.4.

Table 90.3 Common problems affecting the thumb

Problem/deformity	Comment
Synovitis	If it commences primarily in the thumb MCP joint, it causes a boutonnière deformity, but if it commences primarily in the CMC joint, it causes a swan-neck deformity
Boutonnière deformity	MCP joint synovitis leads to EPB tendon rupture, weakness of proximal phalanx extension, and progressive 'buttonholing' of the metacarpal head through the extensor apparatus. EPL subluxes anterior to the axis of MCP joint rotation, causing progressive flexion of the MCP joint and extension of the IP joint—a 'Z collapse' deformity
Early flexible boutonnière deformity	May be treated by transferring EPL on to the distal stump of EPB at the proximal phalanx base (some IP joint extension will be maintained by the intrinsic muscles)
Moderate late rigid boutonnière deformity (MCP flexion <45°)	May be pain free and functional, requiring only occasional splintage
Painful severe late rigid boutonnière deformity (MCP flexion >45°)	May be treated by MCP joint arthrodesis, plus lengthening of the EPL tendon, or IP joint arthrodesis, to reduce the disabling IP joint hyperextension
Boutonnière deformity with associated CMC involvement	Requires correction of the metacarpal position by performing a CMC joint excision arthroplasty, and an arthrodesis of the MCP joint etc. as above
Swan-neck deformity	CMC joint synovitis attenuates the anterior oblique ligament causing dorsal subluxation of the metacarpal base, and a 'thumb in the palm' deformity. Associated progressive MCP joint hyperextension and EPL subluxation palmar to the axis of rotation of the IP joint, and so IP joint hyperflexion, create the characteristic deformity
Symptomatic disabling swan-neck deformity	Requires correction of the metacarpal position by performing a CMC joint excision arthroplasty, and an arthrodesis of the MCP joint (or occasionally a MCP joint palmar plate advancement, if the joint remains healthy)
Thumb MCP joint ulnar collateral ligament insufficiency	Might be amenable to soft tissue reconstruction if the joint remains healthy, but often MCP joint arthrodesis is a more reliable procedure

CMC, carpometacarpal; EDC, extensor digitorum communis; EPB, extensor pollicis brevis; EPL, extensor pollicis longus; IP, interphalangeal; MCP, metacarpophalangeal.

Table 90.4 Common problems affecting finger MCP joints

Problem/deformity	Comment
MCP joint synovitis	Causes attenuation of the joint capsule and collateral ligaments, and progressive ulnar drift and palmar subluxation of the base of the proximal phalanx
Ulnar drift	Multifactorial: there is a natural 'push' towards MCP joint ulnar deviation caused by power gripping with the wrist in ulnar deviation; changes at the wrist described above cause the metacarpals to deform into radial deviation placing ulnar bias onto the EDC tendon's direction of pull; MCP joint synovitis also causes attenuation of the stabilizing sagittal bands and EDC tendon subluxation down the ulnar side of the metacarpal heads
Palmar subluxation	Driven by attenuation of the thin dorsal capsule, the powerful long flexor tendons to the fingers, and intrinsic muscle fibrosis and tightness
Early MCP joint ulnar drift	May be halted or corrected by the careful use of a resting night splint, and the modification of activities and walking aids etc. to minimize the ulnar deviation forces placed on the fingers
Splintage or surgical intervention to correct wrist deformities	This is also important when either preventing or correcting finger MCP joint ulnar deviation
MCP joint synovectomy and soft tissue rebalancing (± crossed intrinsic transfer)	Occasionally useful in the presence of well-preserved joint surfaces and synovitis resistant to medical intervention. Releasing the ulnar-sided tight intrinsic tendon will allow deformity correction; the tendon can be transferred to the radial side of the adjacent digit, so providing a corrective force to that ray as well as releasing a deforming force from its 'home' ray
MCP joint silicon arthroplasty and soft tissue rebalancing (± crossed intrinsic transfer)	When performed carefully (often simultaneously on multiple fingers) can produce excellent results with good pain relief and correction of deformity, the maintenance of about 45° of flexion, and around 90% implant survival at 5 years. When the silicon spacer eventually fractures, if no symptoms or deformity develop, then no intervention is required

EDC, extensor digitorum communis; MCP, metacarpophalangeal.

Proximal interphalangeal joints of the fingers

Common problems are summarized in Table 90.5.

Table 90.5 Common problems affecting finger PIP joints

Problem/deformity	Comment
PIP joint synovitis	Affecting predominantly either the dorsal or palmar structures, in combination with intrinsic muscle contracture, results in the characteristic Z-shaped RA finger deformities
Boutonnière deformity	This progressive deformity starts with the PIP joint synovitis causing attenuation of the central slip and weakness of PIP joint extension. The intrinsic muscles are employed increasingly in an attempt to extend the IP joints and the lateral bands sublux in a palmar direction, until they pass the axis of rotation and become flexors of the PIP joint. Intrinsic muscle action and contracture drives further PIP joint flexion and DIP joint extension
Early mild flexible boutonnière deformity (PIP joint contracture <30°)	May correct with a simple 'Fowler's' release of the central third of the extensor tendon (performed at the junction of the proximal and middle thirds of the middle phalanx)
Moderate flexible boutonnière deformity (PIP joint contracture >30°)	If passively correctable with a healthy joint, the deformity may respond to a careful procedure to shorten the central slip with release and dorsal relocation and suturing of the lateral bands (± Fowler's release, for residual DIP joint hyperextension)
Severe rigid boutonnière deformity (PIP joint contracture >60° and DIP joint contracture >20°)	If symptomatic, with such a poor range of PIP joint motion, the most reliable procedure is a PIP joint arthrodesis using K-wires and tension band (± Fowler's release, for residual DIP joint hyperextension)
Swan-neck deformity	PIP joint synovitis causes attenuation of the palmar plate and the transverse retinacular ligament, allowing PIP joint hyperextension and dorsal subluxation of the lateral bands. Intrinsic muscle tightness and shortening of the extensor apparatus drive the finger further into MCP joint flexion, PIP joint hyperextension, and DIP joint flexion
Early flexible swan-neck deformity	During active flexion (possibly with some passive assistance) the finger may suddenly snap from hyperextension into flexion, often with some pain. Treatment options include: ◆ Trialling the use of an extension block 'silver ring' splint ◆ Stabilizing the palmar aspect of the PIP joint with a tenodesis using one of the FDS tendon slips ◆ Reconstructing the oblique retinacular ligament with the ulnar lateral band (Litteler's procedure), or a tendon graft ◆ Rerouting one lateral band through the flexor tendon sheath at the level of the PIP joint (Zancolli procedure)
Late rigid swan-neck deformity	If symptomatic, with PIP joint damage, the most reliable procedure is a PIP joint arthrodesis in a better position for function (± shortening of the distal part of EDC to correct DIP flexion, or DIP arthrodesis)

DIP, distal interphalangeal; EDC, extensor digitorum communis; FDS, flexor digitorum superficialis; MCP, metacarpophalangeal; PIP, proximal interphalangeal, RA, rheumatoid arthritis.

CHAPTER 91

Principles of lower limb surgery

Peter Wall, Matthew Wyse, and Damian Griffin

Introduction

Surgical intervention for lower limb rheumatological disease can be broadly divided into five categories: injections, joint-preserving procedures, soft tissue procedures, arthrodesis, and arthroplasty. The art of surgery is in the effective use of these interventions in the course of a patient's disease. Modern practice usually involves a combined care approach between physicians and surgeons in order to manage diseases such as rheumatoid arthritis (RA) and expedite surgery at the most propitious moment. The focus of this chapter is not the details of surgery; rather, the timing, preoperative planning, and reducing the risk of surgery once a decision to operate has been made.

Planning surgery

Timing of surgical interventions

It is no longer acceptable for orthopaedic surgeons to work in isolation. For diseases such as RA it is regarded as good practice for patients to be managed by a multidisciplinary team including orthopaedic surgeons (see Case history 1). The timing of elective surgery should be made by the multidisciplinary team in order to address such issues as alterations to disease-modifying drugs (although this remains controversial; see Chapter 92) and prompt surgical input for cases of imminent or acute tendon rupture.[1,2]

Case history 1

Ankle fusion for rheumatoid arthritis

A 60 year old retired woman with RA was managed by a team including a rheumatologist and an orthopaedic surgeon. She had bilateral painful flat feet and a history of tibialis posterior tendon rupture bilaterally. Surgery involving a calcaneal osteotomy and spring ligament reconstruction was undertaken 5 years previously. The patient's symptoms were worsening in the left foot, and shoe orthotics no longer controlled her symptoms. Radiographs showed significant arthritis of subtalar and midfoot joints. A decision was made to undertake left triple joint arthrodesis (subtalar, talonavicular, and calcaneocuboid joints). At 6 month follow-up the patient was able to walk to the shops comfortably again.

Lower limb arthroplasty used to be reserved for patients with cases of severe symptomatic arthritis, but this philosophy is now changing. Although surgery should not be undertaken when the risks will outweigh the benefits, it should not be restricted to only those patients with the most severe symptoms. Evidence is building that the health benefit of arthroplasty surgery is less in those patients whose surgery is delayed.[3]

Preoperative assessment

It is now routine for patients scheduled for elective surgery in the United Kingdom to attend a preoperative assessment clinic. The purpose of these clinics is to improve the provision of patient information and care by careful preoperative evaluation of the patient with coexisting diseases.[4] An assessment of the patient's general health is made and further tests may be arranged depending on the patient's ASA grade (American Society of Anaesthesiologists grade—a simple scale which describes fitness to undergo an anaesthetic) and the level of surgery being undertaken. Tests that may be considered include blood tests (full blood count, renal function, random glucose, and clotting), electrocardiogram (ECG) and urine analysis (dipstick tests for pH, protein, glucose, ketones, blood/haemoglobin).[5]

Imaging

Imaging is essential for adequate preoperative planning and postoperative follow-up. Plain radiographs are used most frequently to make an assessment of lower limb joints. Two radiographic views are required as a minimum for any joint. Arthroplasty surgeons use these images to template a prosthesis before it is inserted (see Figure 91.1) so that they can anticipate any special implant sizes or designs that may be required. Weightbearing radiographs are usually preferred in order to appreciate the joint under normal load. Plain radiographs are also taken after surgery both in the early postoperative phase to check adequate alignment and placement of the prosthesis and in the longer term to check for any early signs of wear or loosening of the prosthesis.

Other imaging modalities include:

◆ CT: examples of application include accurately measuring the length of long bones and identifying exact bony anatomy and orientation prior to surgery.

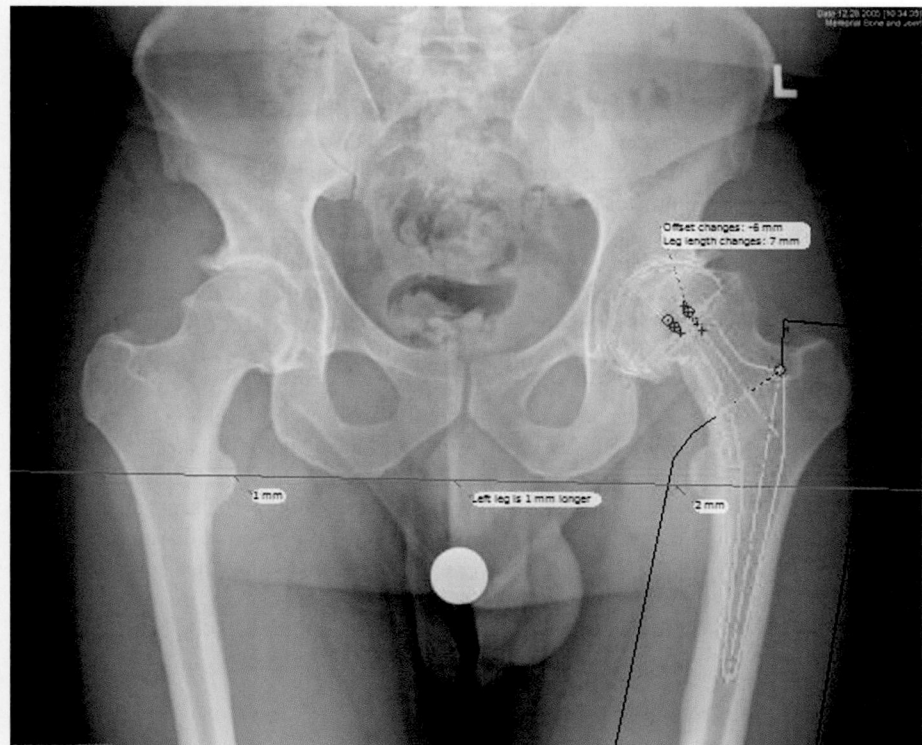

Fig. 91.1 Pelvis radiograph showing preoperative templating of a total hip arthroplasty.
Reproduced with kind permission from Voyant Health Support.

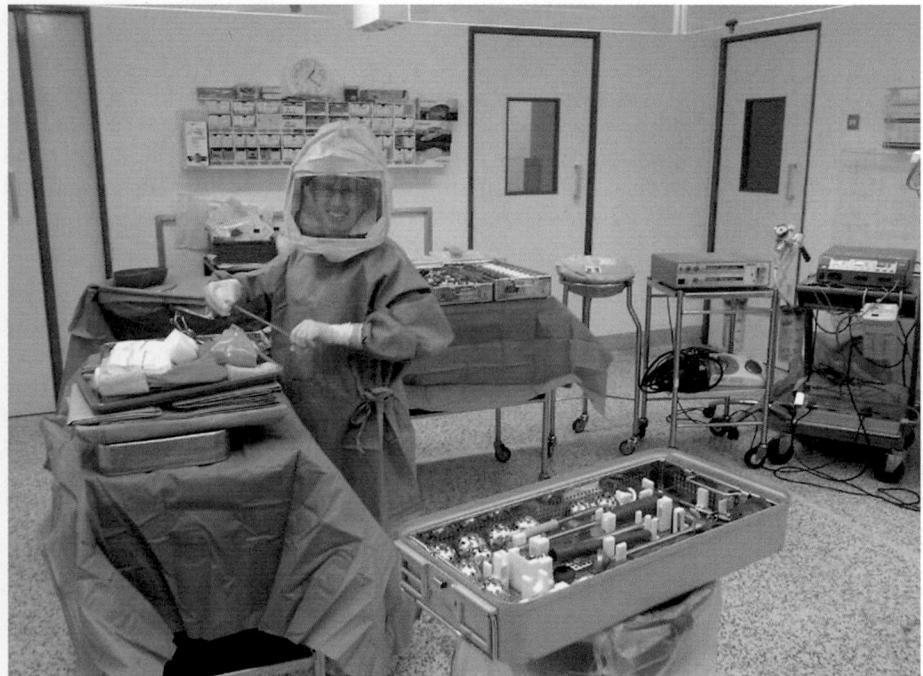

Fig. 91.2 Modern ultraclean theatre with laminar flow hood and staff member wearing hood and suit with exhaust system.

- MRI: examples of application include checking the integrity of soft tissues around a joint or determining the extent of articular cartilage damage within a joint prior to embarking on arthroscopic or arthroplasty surgery.

- Ultrasound can be used to guide intervention within soft tissues, particularly needle aspiration or injection.

General surgical principles

Theatre design and practice

In the United Kingdom it is regarded as good practice for procedures involving bony exposure to be undertaken in an operating theatre with laminar flow (ultraclean theatre) and for the operating surgeon and assistants to wear sterile suits and helmets with an exhaust system (see Figure 91.2). These principles are based on evidence that these measures significantly reduce the risk of sepsis.[6] Other important factors that reduce bacterial counts in theatre include staff covering their noses with masks, all body piercings being covered, and all scrub staff removing finger rings.[7–9]

Anaesthesia and analgesia

Anaesthesia for lower limb surgery can be divided into three broad categories; general anaesthesia, neuroaxial anaesthesia, and peripheral nerve blockade. The choice in an individual patient will be determined by patient preference, coexisting morbidity, and site of surgery. There is no evidence to support one technique over any other in respect of mortality or long-term outcomes. However, virtually all surgery in the lower limb can be performed with a neuroaxial technique such as a spinal anaesthetic unless there are absolute contraindications such as anticoagulation therapy or patient refusal. Neuroaxial techniques have advantages in providing better early analgesia and early mobilization and reduced morbidity such as nausea and vomiting. Peripheral nerve blocks may be used as a sole technique but most commonly are used to supplement general and spinal anaesthesia and to provide postoperative analgesia. Blocks may be single-shot techniques whereby a bolus of local anaesthetic is deposited around a nerve or plexus, or a catheter may be placed in proximity to the nerve for continuous infusion of local anaesthetic or repeated boluses. The duration of effect depends on the agent used and the site of the block: a single shot of long-acting local anaesthetic such as bupivacaine or ropivacaine may give up to 24 hours of analgesia although 12–18 hours is more typical (see Table 91.1).

Enhanced recovery programme (ERP) or fast-track surgery refers to a package of interventions designed to lead to early mobilization and discharge from hospital. Recent evidence also suggests that ERP may reduce postoperative mortality rates.[10] The ERP approach is widely employed for patients undergoing hip or knee arthroplasty. The key interventions are detailed preoperative assessment; optimizing comorbidities; providing patient information and reassurance so that patient expectations are managed; and minimizing preoperative starvation. The anaesthetic technique will avoid opiates and peripheral nerve blockade although short-acting neuroaxial blockade is often employed. The postoperative analgesia regime will be based around paracetamol, non-steroidal anti-inflammatory drugs (NSAIDs) and novel analgesics such as gabapentin commenced preoperatively and continued regularly postoperatively. If opiates are required the oral route will be used. In the postoperative phase oral intake will be encouraged, and the patient mobilized as rapidly as tolerated. Typically an ERP for arthroplasty will reduce the length of in-patient stay to 3 days or so.

Skin preparation and cleaning

Surgical sites with significant hair coverage require shaving, which should be undertaken just before surgery—the trauma of shaving induces proliferation of local skin bacteria which could increase the risk of infection if undertaken hours or days before surgery (the evidence supporting this is equivocal).[11] Surgical site skin antisepsis is achieved with either alcohol, chlorhexidine, or aqueous povidone-iodine based solution.

Controlling and managing blood loss

A surgeon can minimize the amount of blood lost during surgery by careful tissue handling and adequate haemostasis with sutures and diathermy during dissection. It is the role of both the surgeon and the anaesthetist to manage blood loss in a safe and controlled manner. Surgery should proceed with minimal disruption and the patient should recover without too many side effects from anaemia. Intraoperatively the surgeon, anaesthetist, and scrub nurse communicate in order to estimate the amount of blood being lost, using information from:

◆ blood at the surgical site

◆ soakage and increased weight of surgical swabs

◆ amount of blood in suction containers

◆ patient's physiology including pulse, blood pressure, and urine output.

Antifibrinolytic agents such as tranexamic acid are becoming increasingly popular in lower limb arthroplasty and revision surgery to help reduce the amount of blood lost during surgery and reduce postoperative transfusion requirements.[12] Tranexamic acid is a relatively cheap intervention and has a low side effect profile.

Tourniquets

Tourniquets are routinely used for knee, ankle, and foot procedures. Modern tourniquets are made from padded material and use a pneumatic pressure cuff to exert their limb-occlusive effects. They are regarded as safe devices under normal use and have small microcomputers to regulate cuff pressures to within 1% of the intended setting.[13] Complications from tourniquets increase with time.[13] The maximum safe duration of application is not known; however, most surgeons would regard a tourniquet time beyond 2 hours as excessive.

Table 91.1 Examples of peripheral nerve blocks for lower limb surgery

Surgical site anaesthesia	Peripheral nerve block	Duration of analgesia
Hip	Lumbar plexus	8–12 hours
Hip	Femoral nerve	12–18 hours
Knee	Femoral nerve (±sciatic nerve)	12–18 hours
Foot and ankle	Sciatic nerve or popliteal fossa (tibial nerve)	12–24 hours
Toes and forefoot	Ankle (posterior tibial nerve, saphenous, deep and superficial peroneal nerve ± sural nerve)	12–18 hours

Blood transfusions

Allogenic packed red cells are the most common type of transfusion in orthopaedics.[14] Blood transfusions increase a patient's oxygen-carrying capacity in the circulation. Blood should not be used to expand intravascular volume. The threshold for initiating allogenic blood transfusion is controversial. In a young, healthy patient blood losses of 30–40% can typically be controlled with crystalloids alone and, provided a patient is asymptomatic and has an adequate intravascular volume, haemoglobin levels of 7 g/dL or even lower are safe.[15,16] When surgeon and anaesthetist anticipate significant volumes of blood loss it is usual practice to cross-match sufficient blood to allow a surplus using a maximum blood- ordering schedule. This schedule is based on historical data either locally or nationally for the procedure being undertaken.[14] Autologous blood transfusions are becoming more popular in orthopaedic practice. Blood donated by the patient preoperatively or salvaged during/after the operation can be used, and this removes the risk of infectious disease transmission associated with allogenic blood transfusions. There is evidence that the use of autologous blood salvaged after lower limb joint arthroplasty reduces the need for allogenic blood transfusions.[17]

Surgical procedures

Joint injection

Joint injections can be used to diagnose lower limb pathology. Patients typically have numerous aches and pains, and attributing these to a specific disease or joint can be difficult from history and examination alone. Administration of local anaesthetic to a joint will temporarily reduce or abolish intra-articular pain and allow the surgeon to determine the likely success of proposed future surgery. Joint injections are also used therapeutically, particularly administration of steroids. There is also emerging evidence that administration of hyaluronic acid to a joint can provide relief of symptoms in the short to medium term (see Case history 2).[18,19]

Case history 2

Total knee arthroplasty for osteoarthritis

A 45 year old man with osteoarthritis of his knee and hypertension initially obtained relief from analgesia and hyaluronic acid injections. However, the pain deteriorated and he was unable to continue working as a schoolteacher. The decision was made to undertake total knee arthroplasty. The patient attended a preoperative assessment clinic, and 2 weeks later was admitted for surgery. Three months after the operation, the patient returned to fulltime work. He continues to be satisfied with the outcome 5 years postoperatively.

Arthroscopy

Arthroscopy can be used to aid diagnosis (actual visualization of the pathology or taking tissue biopsies). The hip, knee, and ankle are the joints typically examined. Hip and ankle arthroscopy require traction in order to distract the joint surfaces sufficiently to allow instrument access, which is via portals inserted through small incisions. Irrigation of the joint is required with normal saline under pressure, which has a tamponade effect on any small bleeding blood vessels and helps distend the synovial cavity. A rigid endoscope with a light source attached is inserted through one of the portals and via a series of lenses and a video camera an image is collected, magnified and projected on to a monitor. Probes, grabbers, shavers, and burrs can be inserted through other portals allowing therapeutic procedures to be undertaken. The therapeutic options of arthroscopy are expanding rapidly with advances in instrument technology: see Table 91.2 and Case history 3 for some examples.

Case history 3

Knee arthroscopy for meniscal tear

A 42 year old woman experienced intermittent 'locking' of her right knee, and the knee 'gave way' occasionally. These symptoms prevented her from continuing with recreational running. A course of physiotherapy provided no symptom relief. Investigation by her GP revealed a meniscal tear on MRI. Knee arthroscopy was undertaken as a day-case procedure. This confirmed a degenerative medial meniscal tear, which was debrided. Postoperative rehabilitation was supervised by a physiotherapist. The patient was able to return to running after 12 weeks.

The use of arthroscopic knee washouts as a treatment for osteoarthritis remains controversial and no clinical benefit has been shown in either the short or the long term.[20]

Arthrodesis

Arthrodesis (joint fusion) remains a reliable method of relieving the pain of arthritis where future stiffness is not going to be a significant problem. In order to achieve joint fusion articular cartilage needs to be removed from all surfaces, which are then held rigidly opposed to one another using either internal or external fixation. Fusion of the joint should be done in the most functional position and it should avoid significantly altering the normal mechanical axis of the lower limb. A specific risk of arthrodesis is non-union, which if painful will require further surgery. With the success of total joint arthroplasty, hip and knee

---

Table 91.2 Examples of interventions possible with lower limb arthroscopy

Joint	Treatable pathology	Typical length of in-patient stay
Hip	Correction of femoroacetabular impingement	1–2 days
Knee	Debridement of a degenerate meniscal tear	<24 hours
Knee	Synovectomy for rheumatoid arthritis	<24 hours
Ankle	Synovectomy for rheumatoid arthritis	<24 hours
Ankle	Cartilage debridement during arthroscopic assisted ankle fusion	1–2 days

fusion is now uncommon. Ankle fusion, however, remains a popular procedure for arthritis because ankle arthroplasty has not enjoyed the same success as hip and knee arthroplasty.

Joint-preserving procedures

Many techniques have been described over the years in order to delay the need for arthroplasty and slow the progression of arthritis. Osteotomies have been successfully used in the hip, knee, ankle, and foot in order to realign the joint and offload areas of symptomatic arthritis.

Corrective surgery for joint shape abnormalities is an area of interest in hip surgery at present. Femoroacetabular impingement (FAI), sometimes called hip impingement, describes a collection of subtle deformities of the hip which cause impingement between the femoral neck and anterior rim of the acetabulum.[21] Excess contact forces between the proximal femur and the acetabular rim during the terminal motion of the hip lead to lesions of the acetabular labrum and the adjacent acetabular cartilage.[21] FAI seems to be associated with progressive articular degeneration and probably accounts for a large proportion of idiopathic osteoarthritis.[22] Although many surgeons have been reporting favourable results (reduced pain and improved hip function) from shape-corrective surgery for FAI (see Case history 4), it is not yet clear if this surgery has any effect on the development of subsequent osteoarthritis.[23]

Case history 4

Shape-corrective surgery for femoroacetabular impingement

A 30 year old man, a farmer who played recreational cricket for a local village team, had right groin pain for 4–5 years. There was no evidence of groin hernias or hip osteoarthritis. Physiotherapy provided no relief and made his symptoms worse. Examination with right hip in flexion and internal rotation reproduced the pain. Imaging (radiographs and MRI) suggested femoroacetabular impingement with a labral tear. Arthroscopic femoral head–neck junction reshaping and labral tear debridement was undertaken. Postoperative rehabilitation was supervised by a physiotherapist. The patient resumed his farming work and playing cricket pain free after 16 weeks.

Soft tissue procedures

The aim of this group of procedures is to improve joint function and/or correct deformity. Some procedures may be undertaken in isolation, such as:

- tendon transfers of the foot and ankle for tendon rupture secondary to RA (see Case history 1)

- synovectomy for florid synovitis refractory to medical treatment.

Alternatively, soft tissue surgery may be used to augment a bony procedure and improve the overall effect; examples include:

- release of the collateral ligaments during total knee arthroplasty to improve alignment

- adductor longus release to correct adduction deformity after total hip arthroplasty

- tightening of medial collateral ligaments after osteotomy correction of hallux valgus.

Arthroplasty

Arthroplasty encompasses any refashioning of the joint and includes excision arthroplasty such as a girdlestone procedure for the hip. Total joint arthroplasty remains one of the most successful treatment options for arthritis of the hip and knee.[24,25] Sir John Charnley can be credited with the most significant advances in artoplasty surgery.[26] It was the success of his 'low friction arthroplasty' that also stimulated significant improvements in the design of total joint arthroplasty prostheses.[24] There are numerous designs of modern total hip and knee prostheses; the main differences/choices to be made are (1) the mode of fixation, e.g. uncemented or cemented designs and (2) the bearing surface, e.g. metal on polyethylene, metal-on-metal, ceramic-on-ceramic. Recently metal-on-metal bearing surfaces have been associated with higher than average failure rates.[27] The reasons for this are not completely clear but seem to relate to metal wear debris causing local soft tissue reactions.[28] For this reason many researchers and governing bodies, particularly in the United Kingdom, no longer advocate the use of metal-on-metal bearings.[27]

The lifespan of total hip replacements in the United Kingdom is expected to be greater than 90% at 10 years, with similar survival rates reported for contemporary total knee replacements.[29,30] As previously mentioned, total ankle arthroplasty has not enjoyed the same success as the hip and knee with survival rates of approximately 70% at 10 years.[31] The main risks of total joint arthroplasty are outlined in Table 91.3.

Risks

Infection

Surgical site infection (SSI) represents a significant risk when undertaking lower limb surgery. The effect on a patient can be profound (see Case history 5), with mortality rates doubled amongst those patients with a SSI.[32] It is estimated that SSI leads to an additional hospital stay of 6.5 days at a cost of £3246 per patient.[33] Early infection rates in patients undergoing total joint arthroplasty were historically 5–10%, but this has now reduced to approximately 1%, as a result of measures including prophylactic antibiotics and modern theatre design and clothing.[34] Ensuring that patients have clean healthy skin, no open wounds, good dental hygiene, and screening

Table 91.3 Details of the main risks of lower limb arthroplasty

Total joint arthroplasty	Main procedure-specific risks
Hip	Dislocation, leg length discrepancy, loosening, and infection
Knee	Difficulty kneeling, loosening, and infection
Ankle	Poor wound healing, early failure due to infection or loosening

for asymptomatic urinary tract infections and meticillin-resistant *Staphylococcus aureus* (MRSA) preoperatively are important factors in minimizing the potential for bacteraemia at the time of surgery, and subsequent SSI.

Case history 5
Infected total hip arthroplasty
A 75 year old retired man with type 2 diabetes mellitus underwent right-sided total hip replacement. Two months after the operation he had increased right hip pain and an erythematous wound. Joint aspiration and blood cultures were taken and evidence of *Staphylococcus aureus* infection was found. The hip replacement was removed and the patient left with a temporary girdlestone. After 3 months of intravenous antibiotics there was no evidence of ongoing infection. A further hip replacement was inserted at 4 months. At 1 year follow-up the patient was mobilizing and pain free.

Antibiotics

Prophylactic antibiotics are now routinely used when implants are inserted during lower limb arthroplasty, where their value in preventing SSI significantly outweighs the risks and cost of the antibiotic; the value in lower limb surgery not involving insertion of an implant remains equivocal.[33] The American Academy of Orthopaedic Surgeons has issued recommendations for prophylactic antibiotics in total joint arthroplasty:[35]

♦ The antibiotic used for prophylaxis should be carefully selected, consistent with current recommendations and or local guidelines, taking into account the issues of resistance and patient allergies.

♦ Timing and dosage of antibiotic administration should optimize the efficacy of the therapy.

♦ Duration of prophylactic antibiotic administration should not exceed the 24 hour postoperative period.

Venous thromboembolism

Lower limb surgery lasting more than 60 minutes represents a significant risk factor for venous thromboembolism and as a result many patients receive some form of chemical (typically low molecular weight heparin) and/or mechanical (intermittent pneumatic calf compression pumps) venous thromboprophylaxis intraoperatively and in the immediate postoperative period. The National Institute of Health and Clinical Excellence recommends continuing chemical prophylaxis in hip and knee arthroplasty cases for 28–35 days and 10–14 days respectively.[36]

There are a number of newer oral anticoagulants, either thrombin or factor Xa inhibitors, licensed for prevention of postoperative thromboembolism. These are typically oral preparations taken once or twice daily. The oral preparations have the advantage that they are easier to take than self-administering low molecular weight heparins at home.

It is essential to consider other simple measures in order to reduce a patient's risk of a thrombembolic event including:

♦ encouraging patients to stop smoking

♦ encouraging overweight patients to lose weight preoperatively

♦ adequate hydration perioperatively

♦ early mobilization of patients postoperatively.

Despite risk reduction venous thromboembolic events still occur, with an incidence of approximately 1%.[37] Patients suspected of having either a deep vein thrombosis or pulmonary embolism should be commenced on therapeutic doses of low molecular weight heparin pending confirmatory imaging. Imaging should be expedited to minimize the duration of antithrombotic agent use in those patients who have a subsequent negative result, in order to reduce the risk of iatrogenic bleeding at the site of surgery.

Effectiveness of surgery

Despite the risks, most patients who undergo lower limb orthopaedic surgery experience an improved health-related quality of life; however, there are significant variations between procedures.[38] Modern healthcare systems increasingly measure the cost-effectiveness of treatments in order to rationalize resources. Both hip and knee arthroplasty have a proven track record of providing a significant and prolonged effect on health-related quality of life and are considered procedures that provide a cost-effective solution for arthritis (see Case history 2).[38–40]

Conclusion

Lower limb surgery is now principally undertaken with the oversight of a multidisciplinary team from diagnosis and preoperative assessment, right through to postsurgery follow-up. Modern surgery focuses on risk reduction, particularly infection and venous thromboembolism, in order to maximize the potential benefits. The outcome of most lower limb procedures is favourable; however, total hip and knee arthroplasty remain two of the most effective procedures for achieving pain relief in patients with arthritis. A new understanding of the aetiology of primary hip osteoarthritis (FAI) has led to some exciting surgical advances in treatment, which are likely to be explored for effectiveness over the next decade.

References

1. National Institute for Health and Clinical Excellence. *Rheumatoid arthritis: The management of rheumatoid arthritis in adults (CG79)*, 2009. www.nice.org.uk/CG79

2. Jain A, Maini R, Nanchahal J. Disease modifying treatment and elective surgery in rheumatoid arthritis: the need for more data. *Ann Rheum Dis* 2004;63(5):602–603.

3. Hajat S, Fitzpatrick R, Morris R et al. Does waiting for total hip replacement matter? Prospective cohort study. *J Health Serv Res Policy* 2002;7(1):19–25.

4. AAGBI Safety Guideline. *Pre-operative assessment and patient preparation: the role of the anaesthetist.* www.aagbi.org/sites/default/files/preop2010.pdf

5. National Institute for Health and Clinical Excellence. *Preoperative tests: the use of routine preoperative tests for elective surgery (CG3)*, 2003. www.nice.org.uk/cg3

6. Lidwell OM. Air, antibiotics and sepsis in replacement joints. *J Hosp Infect* 1988, 11 Suppl C:18–40.

7. Woodhead K, Taylor EW, Bannister G et al. Behaviours and rituals in the operating theatre. A report from the Hospital Infection Society Working Party on Infection Control in Operating Theatres. *J Hosp Infect* 2002;51(4):241–255.

8. Bartlett GE, Pollard TC, Bowker KE, Bannister GC. Effect of jewellery on surface bacterial counts of operating theatres. *J Hosp Infect* 2002;52(1):68–70.

9. Kelsall NK, Griggs RK, Bowker KE, Bannister GC. Should finger rings be removed prior to scrubbing for theatre? *J Hosp Infect* 2006;62(4):450–452.

10. Malviya A, Martin K, Harper I, Muller SD, Emmerson KP, Partington PF, Reed MR: Enhanced recovery program for hip and knee replacement reduces death rate. *Acta Orthop* 2011;82(5):577–581.

11. Tanner J, Norrie P, Melen K. Preoperative hair removal to reduce surgical site infection. *Cochrane Database Syst Rev* 2011;11:CD004122.

12. Alshryda S, Sarda P, Sukeik M et al. Tranexamic acid in total knee replacement: a systematic review and meta-analysis. *J Bone Joint Surg Br* 2011;93(12):1577–1585.

13. Noordin S, McEwen JA, Kragh JF, Jr, Eisen A, Masri BA. Surgical tourniquets in orthopaedics. *J Bone Joint Surg Am* 2009;91(12):2958–2967.

14. Lemos MJ, Healy WL. Blood transfusion in orthopaedic operations. *J Bone Joint Surg Am* 1996;78(8):1260–1270.

15. Hebert PC, Wells G, Blajchman MA et al. A multicenter, randomized, controlled clinical trial of transfusion requirements in critical care. Transfusion Requirements in Critical Care Investigators, Canadian Critical Care Trials Group. *N Engl J Med* 1999;340(6):409–417.

16. Murphy MF, Wallington TB, Kelsey P et al. Guidelines for the clinical use of red cell transfusions. *Br J Haematol* 2001;113(1):24–31.

17. Gannon DM, Lombardi AV, Jr., Mallory TH et al. An evaluation of the efficacy of postoperative blood salvage after total joint arthroplasty. A prospective randomized trial. *J Arthroplasty* 1991;6(2):109–114.

18. Sun SF, Hsu CW, Sun HP et al. The effect of three weekly intra-articular injections of hyaluronate on pain, function, and balance in patients with unilateral ankle arthritis. *J Bone Joint Surg Am* 2011;93(18):1720–1726.

19. Wang CT, Lin J, Chang CJ, Lin YT, Hou SM. Therapeutic effects of hyaluronic acid on osteoarthritis of the knee. A meta-analysis of randomized controlled trials. *J Bone Joint Surg Am* 2004;86(3):538–545.

20. National Institute for Health and Clinical Excellence. *Arthroscopic knee washout, with or without debridement, for the treatment of osteoarthritis (IPG230)*, 2007. www.nice.org.uk/IPG230

21. Lavigne M, Parvizi J, Beck M et al. Anterior femoroacetabular impingement: part I. Techniques of joint preserving surgery. *Clin Orthop Relat Res* 2004;418:61–66.

22. Beck M, Kalhor M, Leunig M, Ganz R. Hip morphology influences the pattern of damage to the acetabular cartilage: femoroacetabular impingement as a cause of early osteoarthritis of the hip. *J Bone Joint Surg Br* 2005;87(7):1012–1018.

23. Clohisy JC, St John LC, Schutz AL. Surgical treatment of femoroacetabular impingement: a systematic review of the literature. *Clin Orthop Relat Res* 2010, 468(2):555–564.

24. Charnley J. The long-term results of low-friction arthroplasty of the hip performed as a primary intervention. *J Bone Joint Surg Br* 1972;54(1):61–76.

25. Culliford DJ, Maskell J, Beard DJ et al. Temporal trends in hip and knee replacement in the United Kingdom: 1991 to 2006. *J Bone Joint Surg Br* 2010;92(1):130–135.

26. Charnley J: Arthroplasty of the hip. A new operation. *Lancet* 1961;1(7187):1129–1132.

27. Smith AJ, Dieppe P, Vernon K, Porter M, Blom AW. Failure rates of stemmed metal-on-metal hip replacements: analysis of data from the National Joint Registry of England and Wales. *Lancet* 2012;380(9855):1759–1766.

28. Langton DJ, Jameson SS, Joyce TJ et al. Accelerating failure rate of the ASR total hip replacement. *J Bone Joint Surg Br* 2011;93(8):1011–1016.

29. National Institute for Health and Clinical Excellence. *Guidance on the selection of prostheses for primary total hip replacement (TA2)*. http://publications.nice.org.uk/guidance-on-the-selection-of-prostheses-for-primary-total-hip-replacement-ta2

30. Hossain F, Patel S, Haddad FS. Midterm assessment of causes and results of revision total knee arthroplasty. *Clin Orthop Relat Res* 2010;468(5):1221–1228.

31. Henricson A, Nilsson JA, Carlsson A: 10-year survival of total ankle arthroplasties: a report on 780 cases from the Swedish Ankle Register. *Acta Orthop* 2011;82(6):655–659.

32. Kirkland KB, Briggs JP, Trivette SL, Wilkinson WE, Sexton DJ. The impact of surgical-site infections in the 1990s: attributable mortality, excess length of hospitalization, and extra costs. *Infect Control Hosp Epidemiol* 1999;20(11):725–730.

33. Scottish Intercollegiate Guidelines Network. *Antibiotic prophylaxis in surgery: a national clinical guideline (SIGN 104)*, 2008. Available at: www.sign.ac.uk/pdf/sign104.pdf

34. Hamblen DL. Surgical management of the infected arthroplasty. *J Hosp Infect* 1988;11 Suppl C:48–56.

35. American Academy of Orthopaedic Surgeons. *Information statement: recommendations for the use of intravenous antibiotic prophylaxis in primary total joint arthroplasty*, 2004. www.aaos.org/about/papers/advistmt/1027.asp

36. National Institute for Health and Clinical Excellence. *NICE Pathways: Orthopaedic surgery; elective hip or knee replacement*, 2011. http://pathways.nice.org.uk/pathways/venous-thromboembolism/venous-thromboembolism-orthopaedic-surgery#content=view-node%3Anodes-elective-hip-or-knee-replacement

37. Januel JM, Chen G, Ruffieux C et al. Symptomatic in-hospital deep vein thrombosis and pulmonary embolism following hip and knee arthroplasty among patients receiving recommended prophylaxis: a systematic review. *JAMA* 2012;307(3):294–303.

38. Jansson KA, Granath F. Health-related quality of life (EQ-5D) before and after orthopedic surgery. *Acta Orthop* 2011;82(1):82–89.

39. Rasanen P, Paavolainen P, Sintonen H et al. Effectiveness of hip or knee replacement surgery in terms of quality-adjusted life years and costs. *Acta Orthop* 2007;78(1):108–115.

40. *Measuring effectiveness and cost effectiveness: the QALY*. www.nice.org.uk/newsroom/features/measuringeffectivenessandcosteffectivenesstheqaly.jsp

Sources of patient information

American Academy of Orthopaedic Surgeons. Informed patient learning modules. http://orthoinfo.aaos.org/informedPatient.cfm

Arthritis Research UK: www.arthritisresearchuk.org/arthritis-information.aspx

National Health Service: www.nhs.uk/Pages/HomePage.aspx

CHAPTER 92

Principles of spine surgery

Jeremy Fairbank and Nuno Batista

Introduction

This chapter considers the main ways that surgery can be applied to clinical problems affecting the spine (Box 92.1). In the last 20 years there have been dramatic advances in implant design, surgical techniques, and imaging. There have also been advances in clinical evidence for surgical techniques. How much this has translated into improved outcomes is hard to measure. Back pain remains a major clinical challenge. The application of surgery to treating back pain can be effective, but also has the capacity to make a bad situation worse. The spine is the critical supporting structure of the trunk and the head and protects the spinal cord and cauda equina. It is normally 'straight' in the coronal plane and with well-defined curves in the sagittal plane. It is also flexible in the cervical and lumbar regions. The orientation and 'balance' of the spine are critical to its proper function. Loss of sagittal balance is a cause of disability, contributed to not only by spinal deformity (almost always progressive kyphosis), but also by pelvic orientation and lower limb deformity (usually hip and knee arthritis).

Evidence of efficacy has lagged behind surgical capability, although important clinical trials are beginning to emerge, with improving methodology to cope with the complex issues that surround surgical interventions.

Epidemiology

The datasets on the Hospital Episode Statistics website (www. hesonline.nhs.uk) provide a summary of spinal surgical procedures carried out in England in 2010–2011.[1] The United Kingdom Department of Health has also reported on work done by working groups on the delivery of spinal surgery.[2] The Spinal Taskforce document can be found at www.ukssb.com/pages/News-and-Information.html

In many clinical areas it is well known that surgical rates tend to be higher in the United States than elsewhere. There are large variations within the country as well. The most striking difference between the United States and Europe is the rapidly rising rate (and costs) of spinal fusion for back pain, especially in older patients.[3] The reasons for this are complex, and include rapid development in implants with strong marketing, reimbursement strategies, and widespread use of expensive bone substitutes and bone morphogenic proteins to promote spinal fusion.[4]

Roles of surgery

Surgery for radicular pain and neurological compression

Surgery has a clear role in the management of acute spinal cord compression, whether by trauma, tumour, epidural haematoma, or spinal kyphosis.

Cauda equina compression

This is managed surgically. The main causes are disc prolapse, either massive with a wide spinal canal or less massive with a narrow spinal canal. Tumours and epidural haematomas can also present with cauda equina syndrome. This condition is important because the long-term consequences of urinary and faecal incontinence and sexual dysfunction are devastating. It is a major cause of litigation in the United Kingdom because of diagnostic or treatment delays. The common presentations are of severe back pain, unilateral or (more typically) bilateral leg pain, some relief with sitting, loss of perianal sensation (loss of feeling when wiping the bottom), and bladder retention or incontinence. It is a diagnosis that must always be considered. Diagnosis is clinical (especially loss of perineal sensation unilaterally or bilaterally) and by urgent MRI scan. The presentation may be seen in individuals with severe uncontrolled back pain. Treatment is surgical decompression as soon as feasible. More details can be found in Lavy et al.[5]

Nerve root compression

This is usually caused by disc herniation (prolapse). Other pathologies include tumour, infection, or neuritis. MRI scans of asymptomatic individuals detect disc herniation in up to 25%. Genetics

---

Box 92.1 Aims of spinal surgery

- Alter the balance and orientation of the spine
- Fix one or more segments of the spine to another with implants, secured in the long term by establishing a spinal fusion
- Decompress the spinal cord and emerging nerve roots
- Excise or palliate both malignant and benign tumours
- Contribute to the management of infection
- Insert implants to replace diseased parts and to restore mobility

explains 60% of the aetiology of new cases, with minimal contributions from environmental factors such as smoking and trauma.[6] True nerve root pain has a lifetime prevalence of less than 5%. Root pain caused by disc prolapse is usually preceded by back pain. The interval varies from a few minutes to years. Although back pain may coexist, the severity of the leg pain predominates. The majority of symptomatic disc herniation occurs at L4/5 or L5/S1, usually involving the L4, L5, or S1 nerve roots.

Lumbosacral nerve root pain radiates in the distribution of one or more dermatomes and may be associated with neurological deficits. Pain is exacerbated by coughing and sneezing, walking and standing. Night pain is common. Pain may be relieved by lying and flexing the spine. Root pain (sciatica) can be extremely severe, and associated with numbness and parasthesiae. Weakness may be experienced with poor push-off, flapping gait, and foot drop. The appearance of foot drop is sometimes associated with pain improvement. Perineal numbness, and associated bladder or bowel symptoms, are important indicators of cauda equina syndrome but the latter may be associated with pain severity and analgesic intake. Examination should include an assessment of sensation to both light touch and pinprick. Straight leg raising is restricted. We prefer to flex the hip and knee first, and then gradually and gently extend the knee. This allows assessment of hip pain, and is unfamiliar to experienced patients with illness behaviour. Weakness should be sought particularly in extension of the great toe and foot, foot eversion, and knee extension. Ankle and knee reflexes must be recorded.

Imaging is best done by MRI (CT and/or myelography may be used). Disc herniations are seen in up to 25% of normal scans, so it is essential to interpret the scan in the light of the clinical picture. Large discs tend to respond better to surgical treatment than small ones. Attention should be paid to the vertebral canal diameter. Small canals give more trouble than large ones. Look out for other contributing factors to nerve pain such as lateral recess and exit foraminal stenosis.

Nerve root pain

Nerve root pain caused by disc herniation usually gets better. Unfortunately the timescale is unpredictable. Clinical practice, observational data, and now some useful randomized controlled trials (RCTs) have given reasonably clear guidance on management. Evidence shows no benefit of non-operative treatments compared to natural history. However, explanation and analgesia, possibly combined with muscle relaxants, are important. Epidurals (either spinal or caudal) do not alter natural history, though the short-term relief of root pain may be convenient for some. Surgery may be indicated from 8 weeks from onset, unless there is evidence of cauda equina involvement or progressive neurological deficit, when surgery is indicated straight away. This strategy is informed by the trials of Weber,[7] the SPORT study,[8] and, most recently Peul et al.[9] who compared early with delayed surgical intervention. All of these favour early surgery over non-operative care in the short/medium term. The patient has to weigh up the risks of persisting pain, nerve damage, cauda equina damage (rare but devastating), dural tears, and recurrence against a 90% chance of relief of nerve root pain but not back pain. Earlier studies give a recurrence rate of 10% in 10 years, but Peul et al.[9] found 20% at 2 years.

Strong indications for surgical intervention are bladder and bowel involvement and progressive motor deficit. Relative indications for surgical intervention are failure of conservative treatment. Conservative treatment should last for at least 6 weeks and not more than 3–4 months, and result in improvement in the patient's symptoms and signs. Rarely, a patient will not respond to any form of pharmacological or physical pain control, in which case their severe incapacitating pain merits urgent surgical consideration. Recurrent episodic pain may also respond to surgery. Patients with significant motor deficit and diminished straight leg raising eventually recover just as well with non-surgical intervention.[7] However, often these patients are in extreme pain and will not wait for the benefits of conservative care. Occasionally, they present with a history of severe pain which has resolved while the neurologic deficit has increased. This rare patient is also a surgical candidate.

Disc herniation in young patients

The young patient with a disc herniation deserves special consideration because of the high proteoglycan content of the discal material (responsive to chymopapain) and the prevalence of disc protrusions rather than disc extrusions in this age group. The optimum treatment is chemonucleolysis rather than surgical intervention. Unfortunately chyomopapain is not currently available for commercial reasons, although there are hopes that it may return to the market. Surgery can be effective but the recurrence rate is significantly higher than with chymopapain.

Recurrence and scarring

The patient who has successful relief of sciatica after disc excision has a 5–20% chance of a recurrent disc rupture causing sciatica. Unfortunately, most recurrent disc herniations are at the same level and on the same side, and scar tissue from the previous surgery introduces a new element in diagnosis and treatment. Scarring 'tacks' down the dura to the back of the disc space so that a smaller amount of herniated nuclear material may produce significant pain and neurologic deficit in the relatively immobile nerve root. Because of the immobility of the scarred dura, transdural ruptures, although rare, can occur. Almost invariably the scar between the dura and the disc restricts migration of the recurrent disc fragments, i.e. on exploration they are routinely found opposite the disc space.

Health Technology Assessment has recently published a review of 'sciatica' which has conflated referred pain and root pain, and not addressed severity or failed treatment in its literature review.[10]

Spinal stenosis and neurogenic claudication

It is curious that neurogenic claudication, causing back and leg pain with walking, has taken such a long time to be recognized. Spinal stenosis was described in 1954 by Verbiest.[11] It causes a syndrome that is usually easy to recognize, including difficulty with walking (neurogenic claudication). Once considered rare, it is now clear that this syndrome occurs frequently with advancing years. Verbiest recognized two forms, developmental and acquired. Developmental stenosis may be localized to a single level or involve the whole spine. It is almost universally present in achondroplasia. People with narrow canals are probably more likely to run into trouble with back symptoms than those with wide canals, although the evidence for this statement is not robust. Acquired stenosis is associated with distortions of the spinal canal and exiting nerve root canals. This is secondary to disc degeneration causing narrowing of the disc space, disc bulges, and herniations. This in turn distorts facet joints, which degenerate and throw out osteophytes. The ligamentum flavum loses its elasticity and tends to crumple and thicken, occupying the vertebral canal and compressing the thecal sac and nerve roots. All of this is more marked when the lumbar spine is extended, particularly during standing and walking, and less marked when sitting or squatting. Many patients find they cannot lie on their back and have to sleep in a fetal position.

Neurogenic claudication refers to the symptoms experienced secondary to spinal stenosis. Typically patients present with a gradual onset of back, buttock, and/or leg pain which progressively limits their ability to walk or stand, but is relieved by sitting, bending or squatting. It may take 10 minutes or more to recover—much slower than vascular claudication. Many are helped with walking aids such as a supermarket trolley. Some are all right walking fast but cannot dawdle. Others just have trouble standing still. Severity frequently varies from day to day. Patients may also report lower limb fatigue, a feeling that the legs will give way, a sensation of heaviness, paraesthesia, cramp, or coldness; 12% report bladder disturbance. A few develop an acute drop foot, which can be painless. Objectively, those who are severely affected may have a simian stance or a wide-based gait. People with spinal stenosis can usually fully flex and have unrestricted straight leg raise. When sitting they are often bent forward and many are most comfortable standing when flexed or squatting.

Management of neurogenic claudication

Investigation is by imaging of the lumbar spine, usually with MRI (Figure 92.1). Where this is unavailable or contraindicated, CT or myelography are inferior substitutes. It is important to exclude other causes of claudication, such as peripheral vascular disease. MRI is best at demonstrating both bony and soft tissue stenosis, but there is a lack of correlation between severity of radiological and clinical findings. For example, 20% of asymptomatic people over the age of 65 have radiological spinal stenosis.

Non-operative treatment includes explanation, which can often be highly effective, simple analgesics such as paracetamol and sometimes non-steroidal anti-inflammatory drugs (NSAIDs). One trial has supported the use of gabapentin; epidural steroids may help; walking aids including portable seats and all-terrain rollators with a seat fitted; light rucksacks (many find carrying shopping in bags increases their symptoms).

Surgery involves decompressing the cauda equina, lateral recesses, and exit foramina, depending on the radiological anatomy, clinical symptoms, and signs. This can be achieved by a variety of techniques ranging from laminectomy to microdecompression. There is controversy concerning the use of fusion either with or without implants. Fusion is more commonly employed in the United States than elsewhere. It is more likely to be used if the patient has a degenerative spondylolisthesis. This condition most commonly occurs at L4/5, and is much more frequent in women than in men. There is a range of devices that can be inserted between the spinous processes to maintain the motion segment in flexion. The role of these devices and their duration of action remain controversial.

The outcome of surgery depends on comorbidity and age.[12] Patients over the age of 80 tend to have worse outcomes (but they also have more comorbidity). As a rule of thumb 70% of patients will have a good outcome.[13] The Swedish Spine Register data suggests that this figure may be optimistic (reporting good outcomes in only 55%). Even so, few will obtain the walking capacity of their fit contemporaries.[13,14] Complication rates vary, but for decision-making, we tell patients 5% will be worse off and may regret the decision to proceed with surgery. This may be due to root damage, cauda equina damage, impaired vascularity, infection, and recurrence. It is not always possible to tell why outcome is poor in a particular case, but it is important to ensure that the decompression was complete.

Surgery for back pain

Patients with chronic low back pain are frequently referred to orthopaedic surgeons. The majority of these patients do not require surgical treatment, and should be managed by non-operative means. A small proportion may benefit from surgical stabilization of the spine or disc replacement.

The surgeon and patient have to take a decision after weighing up the risks and benefits of the procedure (often hard to define) against the disability. Spinal fusion may be regarded as either an attempt

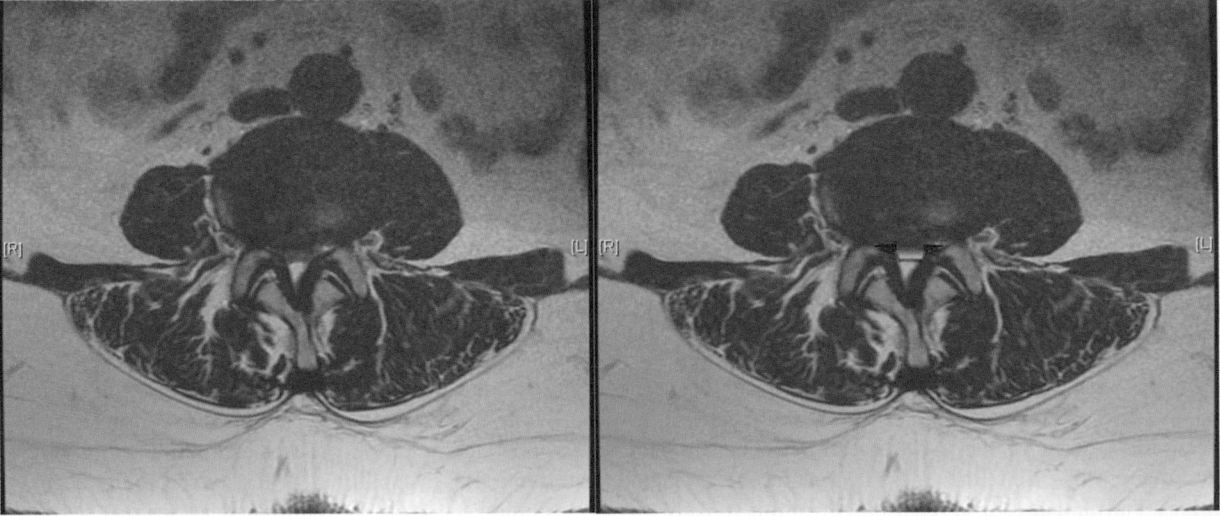

Fig. 92.1 Spinal stenosis (lumbar spine). The second image highlights the vertebral canal available for the cauda equina (blue). The areas for the transiting nerve roots (or lateral recesses) are coloured red. In a normal spine, both the blue and the red areas would be much larger, giving much more space for the neurological structures.

to speed up the natural progress of degenerative changes towards a functional ankylosis or a prevention of progressive deformity or instability. The aim is to reduce the severity of back pain and improve functional ability. Our understanding of spinal pain is developing rapidly. Peripheral pain generators are of two major types, nociceptive (tissue) and neuropathic (nerve). Distinguishing between them is important because the causes and treatments are different. Ideally, the causes of both types of pain will be identified and treated, resulting in pain relief. The experience of pain is modulated in the central nervous system (CNS) by the spinal cord and many parts of the brain. The surgeon has to be alert to these complexities, as surgery can usually only influence pain generated outside the CNS. Surgeons may be able to influence CNS pain in a variety of ways that are outside the scope of this chapter.[15] Surgery has great capacity to harm so surgeons, and others recommending surgery or referring to surgeons, need to be aware of the influence of what they say on patients' experience and attitude to pain.

The treatment of spine-related pain conditions may include active core stabilization exercises, body mechanics training, passive modalities, spinal injections, and surgery. Comprehensive management of acute and chronic spinal pain also includes a rational pharmacologic approach and may include the use of NSAIDs, oral steroids, opioids, antidepressants, neuropathic agents, and sleep agents. Nociceptive pain is generally responsive to NSAIDs and opioids. Conditions associated with inflammation, bone pain, and joint disease are particularly responsive to NSAIDs.

Neuropathic pain is relatively resistant to NSAIDs and opioids, although they may be helpful in certain cases. The major classes of medications useful for neuropathic pain include tricyclic antidepressants, anticonvulsants, and sodium channel blockers.

The evidence on which to base treatment decisions is developing.[16] A variety of less invasive interbody fusion techniques have emerged, but no well-designed clinical trials have yet been reported. Several randomized trials of spinal fusion have now been completed. In Sweden, Fritzell and others showed an outcome advantage of fusion over conventional physiotherapy, but could show no difference between 3 different surgical techniques.[17] Brox et al.[18] in Norway and Fairbank et al.[19] in the United Kingdom could show no advantage of surgery over intensive rehabilitation. These trials have caused controversy, especially in the United States, where there are high rates of surgery for back pain. Long-term follow-up of these patients suggest that these results are maintained.

'Soft' or flexible fusion, using a variety of posterior devices, has been practiced for 20 years, but no large trial has been completed. The rationale remains experimental, not least because of our poor understanding of intersegmental biomechanics in relation to pain. Many ingenious devices have been developed to alter these, but results are anecdotal.

Disc replacement has evolved in the last 30 years, with only cohort studies reported until two trials approved by the United States Food and Drug Aaministration. The Charite study was against a BAK anterior cage procedure (now abandoned) that showed non-inferiority.[20] The ProDisc study showed non-inferiority over 360§ fusion using an unvalidated version of the Oswestry Disability Index (www.mapi-trust.org/services/questionnairelicensing/catalog-questionnaires/266-odi.[21] Both these trials show a non-statistically significant advantage to disc replacement, and it is likely that they were underpowered. No study against rehabilitation has yet been reported. Surgeons should consider the difficulties of selecting

patients and the high risks of revision surgery before recommending this procedure. A Norwegian study group has reported an RCT of disc replacement vs intensive rehabilitation with a statistically better Oswestry Disability Index (ODI) improvement in the surgical group, although this did not meet their predefined criteria of clinically significant difference.[9,22] This study is the first RCT of disc replacement that was not commercially funded.[10]

Rationale

It is assumed that back pain may be generated from the low back by 'mechanical' means or through a source of 'inflammatory' agents (usually assumed to be the intervertebral disc) irritating neural tissues.

◆ **Mechanical back pain** is generated by movement, and may be controlled by rest or immobilization by external splintage (corsets, braces, plaster), or internal splintage (fusion, with or without internal fixation, or limitation of movement by special implants). In some cases there may be instability of the spine, actual or perceived, which can be controlled by spinal fusion.

◆ **Inflammatory pain** may be managed surgically by excision of a whole disc, or at least a substantial part of it, and replacement of it by allograft or autograft bone, cages made of various materials containing bone, or artificial disc prostheses designed to replace either the nucleus or whole disc.

◆ Both mechanical and inflammatory pain may be involved in patients with previous root decompression surgery.

Unfortunately, reality has not always followed expectation, and the results of treatment have varied considerably. Carragee used discography to identify 'best bet' patients for spinal fusion.[23] Only 27% met his strict criteria of success compared with 72% of a control-spondylolisthesis group.

Spinal instability

Spinal stability is a much abused term. There are at least four ways in which this can be conceived:

1. In **mechanical terms**, as summarized in White and Punjabi's[24] definition of stability for a functional spinal unit—i.e. two vertebrae and an intervening three joint complex (a disc and two facet joints).

2. In **temporal terms**, where symptoms wax and wane more or less predictably with time. Some patients report increasing frequency and duration of attacks of pain.

3. In **perceptual terms**, where the spine feels unstable although no abnormal motion or position can be detected by conventional radiography.

4. In **postural terms**, where the whole spine is unbalanced.

White and Punjabi[24] defined stability as 'a condition of the spine under normal physiological loading where there is neither abnormal strain nor excessive or abnormal motion in the functional spinal unit'. The functional spinal unit is a motion segment, consisting of bone, disc, and bone, as well as its supporting joints, ligaments, and muscles. Instability is the loss of the ability of the spine under physiological loads to maintain relationships between vertebrae in such a way that there is neither damage or subsequent irritation to the spinal cord or nerve roots and, in addition, there is no development of incapacitating deformity or pain from structural changes.

Perceived or functional instability is sometimes called 'instability syndrome'. The patient complains of giving way, getting stuck, a ratchety flexion in the spine, and, occasionally, a sensation of disconnection of the top of the body from the bottom. Panjabi's hypothesis is based on a concept that a single trauma or cumulative microtrauma causes subfailure injuries of the ligaments and embedded mechanoreceptors leading to disturbed muscle control.[25] Harris has suggested that mismatch between expected and actual proprioceptive information may be a potent source of 'distress' in the CNS, experienced as pain.[26] There is a strong body of evidence suggesting proprioceptive dysfunction in chronic back pain patients, but there is little evidence for mechanical instability as a cause of back pain.

Sagittal balance

Humans stand and walk best if they can keep their frame in balance. This means that, when standing, the head is over the hips, which are in turn over the heels. In other words the gravity line goes through the cervicothoracic junction and the lumbosacral joint. Deviations from this (usually forwards) overload the posterior lumbar musculature and require compensatory pelvic rotation, hip extension and knee flexion. In a standing lateral radiograph the sacrum is vertical, as the pelvis is maximally rotated backwards. All may be well at skeletal maturity, but loss of balance may follow kyphosis due to disc degeneration and fractures. Imbalance has become increasingly recognized as an important cause of back pain. Surgery can be used to correct imbalance by osteotomy or facetectomy during fusion, but milder cases may well respond to rehabilitation and exercise.

Assessment of instability

A good history is essential. The 'ideal' patient for spinal fusion may have some or all of the following characteristics: a nonsmoking 'normal citizen'; no litigation outstanding or other potential secondary gains from their pain; a clear history; and a crescendo of symptoms, but with pain-free or low-pain intervals. Some patients with recurrent attacks of pain report prodromal symptoms preceding an attack. Surgeons have tried many methods to identify good responders: for example, a trial period in external splintage, or a rational response to discography. External fixation has also been tried, but has not proved popular because of complications and poor predictive ability. Flexion–extension radiographs have been used for many years, but their value is very limited. Standing views may be of value if the gravity line or whole body can be included. This approach remains experimental.

Confounding factors

A technically correct operation achieving a solid fusion may not relieve pain, and indeed it can make it worse. Failures of the surgical approach can be attributed to two main areas: the patient and the surgical methodology.

The patient

1. Patient selection. Often significant psychosocial factors contribute to the extent of pain- related distress and disability. Even the most experienced surgeons can be caught out. Some surgeons make use of psychological questionnaires to aid in the selection of patients, but there is no good study to show that using these methods improves results. Ideally a pain psychologist should identify the degree of psychosocial involvement before the surgeon embarks upon surgical treatment. Pain-related distress should be treated first.

2. Poor recognition of sagittal imbalance.

3. The wrong levels may be selected for surgery.

4. Smoking cigarettes has been associated with a high pseudarthrosis rate in many studies.

5. Involvement in litigation or worker's compensation has long been recognized as being associated with poor clinical results.

Surgical methodology

The objective of most procedures is to obtain a solid bony fusion, avoiding damage to the surrounding soft tissues. A wide variety of methods are available, and comparisons between them are difficult. Posterolateral fusions tend to be easier to perform, but are probably less reliable in terms of both fusion rates and in immobilizing a segment (or functional spinal unit). Interbody fusions, either from the back or from the front, are more likely to fuse with instrumentation, but are technically more difficult to perform, and carry a higher risk of complication. Spinal instrumentation has evolved rapidly, increasing in complexity and expense. It has been difficult to demonstrate that its use has any advantage. Some studies, but not all, suggest that the use of instrumentation increases the fusion rate. Unfortunately this is not necessarily accompanied by an improvement in clinical results. The evidence base supports the use of uninstrumented posterolateral fusion as best option with lowest complication rate.

Discography

It is likely that a significant proportion of patients have discogenic or segmental pain. Proponents of this view use provocative discography to identify painful segments. Discography can identify segments where pain is reproduced by injection of saline into the disc and adjacent normal discs. It identifies patients with inappropriate responses (over-reaction to local anaesthetic or skin penetration by needle) and inappropriate or multilevel response to disc injection. The 'normal' disc is usually pain free when injected. There is a large literature on this, but many studies are flawed. Carragee's studies are a good starting point. He was able to demonstrate a predictive value for discography of only 50–60% in spinal fusion patients. In a cohort of 'normal' subjects who had discography, Carragee has found an increased incidence of disc degeneration, back pain, and back surgery.[27] This suggests discography should be used with extreme caution.

Other surgical indications

Spinal deformity

Spinal deformity (mainly scoliosis and kyphosis) affects children and adults. Surgery has an important part to play in management, depending on age (growth potential), aetiology, severity, and comorbidity. There is not space in this chapter to discuss this in detail, and the reader is referred to the *Oxford Textbook of Trauma and Orthopaedics*.[28] Adult deformity in both sagittal and coronal planes is an increasing issue as the population ages in better general health.

Tumours

Primary spinal tumours, both CNS and bony, are rare. They may present with pain, progressive neurological deficit, and spinal deformity. It can be challenging to diagnose the few cases in the generality of these common presenting symptoms. Continuous, atypical, and night pains should lower the threshold for obtaining an MRI scan to exclude such tumours. Surgical treatment is often required.

In contrast, metastases in the spine are extremely common, perhaps affecting 50% of cancer cases. Recent trials have supported the use of surgical management for uncontrolled pain and particularly for spinal cord compression. In the United Kingdom the National Institute for Health and Clinical Excellence (NICE) has issued guidance supporting the use of surgery combined with radiotherapy rather than radiotherapy alone.[29]

Trauma

The main indications for surgery of the injured spine are actual or potential instability of the spine likely to cause pain, deformity, and loss of function. There are also indications when neurological integrity is at risk. This is a complex area outside the scope of this book. The reader is referred to the *Oxford Textbook of Trauma and Orthopaedics*.[28]

Infection

Spinal tuberculosis was one of the first topics explored with high-quality clinical studies by the Medical Research Council in the United Kingdom after the Second World War. These and later studies confirmed the value of antimicrobial treatment with or without surgery. Surgery has a role when there is actual or potential spinal deformity (mainly kyphosis) that is threatening spinal cord function.

Non-specific infection of the spine can be very serious and even life threatening. Surgery may be needed for diagnosis and reconstruction of the spine. Details of this are beyond the scope of this textbook.

Cervical stenosis

Cervical stenosis may be congenital or acquired. Absolute (antero-posterior canal diameter <10 mm) or relative (10–13 mm diameter) stenosis predisposes the patient to development of radiculopathy, myelopathy, or both from relatively minor disc pathology or trauma. Minor trauma such as hyperextension may lead to a central cord syndrome even without overt skeletal manifestations. In relative stenosis, radicular symptoms usually predominate. Surgery may serve a prophylactic function but is usually reserved for patients who develop myelopathy or radiculopathy.

Cervical rheumatoid spondylitis

Cervical spine involvement is common in rheumatoid arthritis (RA) and is usually a result of pannus formation at the synovial joints between the dens and the ring of C1, resulting in destruction of the transverse ligament, the dens or both causing instability. Basilar invagination and subaxial subluxation may also occur but are less frequent. Neck pain, decreased range of movement, crepitation, and occipital headaches are the more common complaints. Neurological impairment in patients with RA usually occurs gradually and is often overlooked or attributed to other joint disease; it

is therefore essential to look for subtle neurological signs. Surgery may not reverse significant neurological deterioration but it can stabilize it. Indications for surgical stabilization include instability, pain, and neurologic deficit.

References

1. www.hesonline.nhs.uk/Ease/servlet/ContentServer?siteID=1937&categoryID=205.
2. *Organising quality and effective spinal services for patients: a report for local health communities by the Spinal Taskforce.* Department of Health, London. Available at: www.dh.gov.uk/en/Publicationsandstatistics/Publications/PublicationsPolicyAndGuidance/DH_114528.
3. Weinstein JN, Lurie JD, Olson PR, Bronner KK, Fisher ES. United States' trends and regional variations in lumbar spine surgery: 1992–2003. *Spine* 2006;31(23):2707–2714.
4. Deyo R. Trend, major medical complications, and charges associated with surgery for lumbar spinal stenosis in older adults. *JAMA* 2010;303(13):1259–1265.
5. Lavy C, James A, Wilson-MacDonald J, Fairbank J. Cauda equina syndrome. *BMJ* 2009;338:b936.
6. Battié M, Videman T, Kaprio J et al. The Twin Spine Study: contributions to a changing view of disc degeneration. *Spine J* 2009;9(1):47–59.
7. Weber H. Lumbar disc herniation: a controlled, prospective study with ten years of observation. *Spine* 1983;8:131–140.
8. Weinstein J, Lurie J, Tosteson T et al. Surgical versus nonoperative treatment for lumbar disc herniation four-year results for the Spine Patient Outcomes Research Trial (SPORT). *Spine* 2008;33(25):2789–2800.
9. Peul W, van Houwelingen H, van den Hout W et al. Surgery versus prolonged conservative treatment for sciatica. *N Engl J Med* 2007;356(22):2245–2256.
10. Lewis P, Williams N, Matar H et al. The clinical effectiveness and cost-effectiveness of management strategies for sciatica: systematic review and economic model. *Health Technol Assess* 2011;15(39):1–578.
11. Verbiest H. A radicular syndrome from developmental narrowing of the lumbar vertebral canal. *J Bone Jt Surg Br* 1954;36B:230–237.
12. Malmivaara A, Slatis P, Heliovaara M et al. Surgical or nonoperative treatment for lumbar spinal stenosis?: a randomized controlled trial. *Spine* 2007;32(1):1–8.
13. Jansson K-Å, Blomqvist P, Granath F, Németh G. Spinal stenosis surgery in Sweden 1987-1999. *Eur Spine J* 2003:535–541.
14. Pratt R, Fairbank J, Virr A. The reliability of the shuttle walking test, the Swiss spinal stenosis questionnaire, the Oxford spinal stenosis score, and the Oswestry disability index in the assessment of patients with lumbar spinal stenosis. *Spine* 2002;27:84–91.
15. Tracey I. Getting the pain you expect: mechanisms of placebo, nocebo and reappraisal effects in humans. *Nat Med* 2010;16(11):1277–1283.
16. Mirza S, Deyo R. A systematic review of randomized trials comparing lumbar fusion surgery to nonoperative care for treatment of chronic back pain. *Spine* 2007;32(7):816–823.
17. Fritzell P, Hägg P, Wessburg P, Nordwall A. 2001 Volvo award winner in clinical studies: lumbar fusion versus nonsurgical treatment for chronic low back pain. A multicenter randomized controlled trial from the Swedish lumbar spine group. *Spine* 2001;26:2521–2534.
18. Brox J, Sørensen R, Friis A et al. Randomized clinical trial of lumbar instrumented fusion and cognitive intervention and exercises in patients with chronic low back pain and disc degeneration. *Spine* 2003;28(17):1913–1921.
19. Fairbank J, Frost H, Wilson-MacDonald J et al. Randomised controlled trial to compare surgical stabilisation of the lumbar spine with an intensive rehabilitation programme for patients with chronic low back pain: the MRC spine stabilisation trial. *BMJ* 2005;330(7502):1233.
20. Fairbank J, Hashimoto R, Dailey A, Patel A, Dettori J. Does patient history and physical examination predict MRI proven cauda equina syndrome? *Evid Based Spine Care J* 2011;2(4):27–33.

21. Guyer RD, McAfee PC, Banco RJ et al. Prospective, randomized, multicenter Food and Drug Administration investigational device exemption study of lumbar total disc replacement with the CHARITE artificial disc versus lumbar fusion: five-year follow-up. *Spine J* 2009;9(5):374–386.

22. Zigler JE, Delamarter RB. Five-year results of the prospective, randomized, multicenter, Food and Drug Administration investigational device exemption study of the ProDisc-L total disc replacement versus circumferential arthrodesis for the treatment of single-level degenerative disc disease. *J Neurosurg Spine* 2012;17(6):493–501.

23. Carragee E, Tanner C, Kharana S et al. The rates of false-positive lumbar discography in select patients without low back symptoms. *Spine* 2000;25:1373–1381.

24. White A, Panjabi M. *Clinical biomechanics of the spine*, 2nd edn. Lippincott, Philadelphia, 1990.

25. Panjabi MM. A hypothesis of chronic back pain: ligament subfailure injuries lead to muscle control dysfunction. *Eur Spine J* 2006;15(5):668–676.

26. Harris A. Hypothesis: cortical origin of pathological pain. *Lancet* 1999;354:1464–1466.

27. Carragee EJ, Don AS, Hurwitz EL et al. 2009 ISSLS prize winner: does discography cause accelerated progression of degeneration changes in the lumbar disc: a ten-year matched cohort study. *Spine* 2009;34(21):2338–2345

28. Bulstrode C, Wilson-MacDonald J, Eastwood D et al. *Oxford textbook of trauma and orthopaedics*, 2nd edn. Oxford University Press, Oxford, 2011.

29. *Metastatic spinal cord compression: diagnosis and management of adults at risk of and with metastatic spinal cord compression (CG75).* NICE, London, 2008.

CHAPTER 93

Perioperative management of immunosuppression

Loreto Carmona and Maria Galindo

Introduction

Surgery is a common necessity for many rheumatic patients. Current therapeutic approaches have resulted in a lower frequency of reconstruction and replacement surgery, but some patients may still need surgery to regain function or control pain. Other non-orthopaedic interventions, both elective and emergency surgical procedures, may be also required at any given point. We, as rheumatologists, must recognize and communicate the risks of surgery in our patients, which are often higher than in non-rheumatic disease patients, and which are frequently under recognized by other specialists. Additionally, many patients are on immunosuppressive medications that must be managed appropriately at the time of elective surgery.

Surgical complications can range from minimal, such as wound dehiscence or numbness, to death, and include loss of function, excess blood loss, non-healing of the surgical wound, and infection.[1] Many risk factors for surgical complications have been recognized. These can be grouped into those related to (1) the patient's general health and specific rheumatic condition, (2) the ailment that lead to the operation, and (3) the procedure itself.[2] The patient's health and condition may determine the anaesthetic procedure to be used, and other arrangements, like the operating table, or the availability of extra blood. Sometimes it may determine the delay or indeterminate cancellation of surgery. It may also have an impact on the patient's recovery after surgery. The ailment requiring surgery may also influence the outcome and complications; cardiac surgery or neck surgery, for instance, increases the risk of perioperative mortality. The procedure itself may be revised in the light of added risk factors.

Aspects that should be acknowledged and corrected before surgery

Before elective surgery, some patient characteristics must be documented, and corrected if possible, in order to minimize the risk of surgery.[3] The anaesthetist and the physician in charge of the postoperative period must be aware of these, and a rheumatologist should be available at all times if not routinely involved in perioperative care. The following are a suggested list of aspects that should be considered and notified to the anaesthetist and surgeon:

◆ The **site of arthritic involvement** may itself be a source of risk. Cervical spine involvement may complicate anaesthesia by impeding cervical extension and endotracheal intubation, with the associated serious risk of spinal cord damage when there is instability. Other forms of anaesthesia should therefore be used in these patients, and the operating table adapted to the posture of the spine. Cord impingement may delay elective surgery until treated.

◆ **Airway involvement** may also complicate anaesthetic procedures. Crycoaritenoid arthritis, for instance, may interfere with intubation. This rare manifestation of rheumatoid arthritis (RA) should be fully treated before surgery, to avoid the potential need for tracheostomy.

◆ **Lung disease**, secondary either to the rheumatic condition or to its treatment, may increase the rate of pulmonary complications during anaesthesia. Preoperative recommendations are (in addition to a complete set of lung function tests, chest radiograph, and blood gases) avoidance of smoking or inhaling smoke for at least 4 weeks, bronchodilator therapy, or breathing exercises.

◆ **Anaemia** is frequent in patients with chronic inflammation, and orthopaedic surgery, especially that of large joints, may cause large loss of blood. All procedures aimed to reduce blood loss during surgery and to bring the patient to their optimum haemoglobin level before operation should be fully implemented.

◆ **Osteoporotic bones**, secondary to immobilization, glucocorticoids, age, and other causes, should be taken into account when mobilizing the patient, and when deciding the best prosthetic stem to use in a specific joint replacement.

◆ **Vasculitis** may underlie the lack of healing of a skin ulcer or a surgical wound. Surgery should consequently be delayed until the vasculitis is under control.

◆ **Heart involvement** should be fully checked before surgery and corrected if possible, as heart abnormalities are responsible for over one-third of intraoperative deaths.

◆ The **background risk of infection** should be taken into account. The risk of infection is increased in many rheumatic patients, especially those with lupus or RA, or with concomitant diabetes, and even more if they are immunosuppressed. The risk of infectious complications after surgery in a patient with RA, for instance, is nearly three times greater than that of osteoarthritis patients.[4] Antibiotic prophylaxis should therefore be considered for all surgery, independent of the apparent baseline risk of infection.

Perioperative use of immunosuppression

Any surgical operation is a stressful situation for an already stressed body; furthermore, patients on glucocorticoids may have a disrupted response to stress. Additionally, immunosuppressants may affect inflammation and local immune responses, which are necessary for proper wound healing, thereby potentially resulting in undesirable postoperative complications. The use of immunosuppression has been linked to the slow healing of surgical wounds and to an increased risk of infectious complications. On the other hand, stopping immunosuppressive medication may leave the patient at undesirable levels of disease activity, which itself may delay rehabilitation and require treatment escalation. Furthermore, in diseases such as RA, disease activity may reduce immune function. Factors such as blood count, drug type and dose, previous postoperative complications, type of surgery, and other factors should be taken into account when deciding how to manage perioperative immunosuppression. The timing of treatment discontinuation and reinstatement perioperatively also differs significantly among rheumatologists and even national guidelines vary. In a questionnaire sent to 200 randomly selected rheumatologists, Steuer et al.[5] reported the consensus on this issue: (1) 35% of respondents were concerned about disease-modifying antirheumatic drugs (DMARDs) increasing postoperative complications; (2) 14% 'always' advised stopping DMARDs perioperatively; (3) 48% advocated 'sometimes' stopping drugs perioperatively, depending on patient characteristics; (4) the timing of stopping treatment preoperatively and restarting after surgery also differed significantly among rheumatologists (from 1 week to more than 4 weeks). Even within in the same centre practice may vary.[4,6]

Unfortunately, only very limited data are available to support any decision and most available evidence comes from observational studies, only a few of which are of acceptable quality. While there is some information on the impact of non-steroidal anti-inflammatory drugs (NSAIDs), glucocorticoids and methotrexate (MTX), in the perioperative period,[7–10] we lack such data on DMARDs other than MTX, including biologics (e.g. TNF antagonists). In these cases, recommendations are rarely based on clinical trial evidence but more commonly on pharmacological considerations, experimental and animal models, and extrapolation from trials with the same drug in other diseases. Clearly, the implementation of randomized controlled trials in the perioperative period is complicated, as shown by Alarcon et al. in a clinical trial of three perioperative strategies that never reached the pre-planned sample size.[11] The main obstacle to participation was preconceived opinions on perioperative immune suppression, both from the rheumatologists and the orthopaedic surgeons. Curiously, physicians were equally divided between those who thought it unethical to suspend immunosuppressant therapy and those who thought that it was unethical to continue it.

Ultimately the objective is clearly to obtain a balance between maintaining disease control and avoiding an unfavourable impact on wound healing and postoperative complications.[9] To accomplish this, and prior to surgery, it is mandatory to document all medications that the patient is taking, including supplements and alternative medicines. All medications whose abrupt discontinuation may lead to increased morbidity should be maintained; it may even be necessary to substitute a parenteral form temporarily. All medications that may pose a surgical risk and are not essential for the patient's perioperative condition should be discontinued. A judgement should then be made on all other medications. For those drugs with limited or no data in this setting, the use of pharmacokinetic properties and biological effects of each drug may assist the judgement.[2]

Glucocorticoids

Glucocorticoids are clearly associated with skin fragility that may delay the healing process and also increase the risk of infection. It is generally believed that patients receiving long-term glucocorticoid therapy require supplemental perioperative (stress) doses owing to presumed suppression of the hypothalamic–pituitary–adrenal (HPA) axis (see Chapter 79). This hormonal system determines the body's response to stress, including surgical stress, which ranges from minimal to very high depending on the type of surgery. Failure to provide supplemental perioperative glucocorticoid therapy may result in adrenal crisis, although recent pooled evidence shows that this is not always the case if patients continue to receive their usual daily dose.[12] The anaesthetist, surgeon, and intensivist must be aware that the patient was receiving suppressive doses of glucocorticoids, necessitating close perioperative haemodynamic monitoring and the use of stress doses of hydrocortisone in patients with volume-refractory hypotension. As a rule, there is no risk of HPA axis suppression when the steroid treatment has been given for less than 3 weeks, the dose administered is lower than 5 mg/day of prednisone or equivalent, or if used on alternate days. The axis is more clearly suppressed when the dose is in excess of 20 mg/day of prednisone and it has been used for more than 3 weeks or when the patient has iatrogenic Cushing's syndrome. To avoid complications, such as refractory hypotension or haemorrhage, patients with a high suspicion of suppressed HPA axis should follow a regime of parenteral hydrocortisone perioperatively. No regime has demonstrated superiority over others,[2,3,10,13] but, as a rule, patients should receive 50 mg of hydrocortisone intraoperatively, then every 8 hours for 48–72 hours postoperatively in patients undergoing major surgery.[12]

Classical disease-modifying drugs in the perioperative period

Methotrexate

Since 1991, several studies have been published in which the use of perioperative MTX was analysed.[11,14–19] Most of these studies were observational and retrospective in nature. A randomized unblinded prospective 1 year follow-up study in 338 RA patients undergoing orthopaedic surgery reported less infections in patients who continued on MTX compared to those who stopped it (1% vs 25%; p<0.001) and did not present any RA flare, while 8% of those who stopped MTX flared.[16] A systematic review concluded that continuing MTX during the perioperative period is at least as safe as discontinuing it, but with better prognosis in terms of disease activity, in patients undergoing elective orthopaedic surgery.[20] There may be, however, two exceptions to this general recommendation: patients with renal failure and elderly patients, in whom haematological toxicity risk may be increased given the special conditions of surgery. In these cases, some authors recommend discontinuation of MTX a week before surgery and reintroduction 1–2 weeks after the intervention, depending on evolution.

Leflunomide

A randomized controlled trial showed that the risk of infectious complications associated with maintaining leflunomide was not different from that if the drug was discontinued.[21] This contradicted previous observational data suggesting increased infectious complications, compared to MTX, if the drug was continued perioperatively.[22] The strength of the evidence supports continuation of leflunomide perioperatively.

Sulfasalazine

Clinical data are lacking on the perioperative use of sulfasalazine. The half-life is 6–10 hours; elimination is primarily renal. There are no studies which provide definite answers as to whether and for how long the drug should be discontinued perioperatively. In a large study on postoperative infections with TNF antagonists, sulfasalazine use was shown to be a protective factor against infections, therefore providing indirect evidence for continuation.[23] Importantly, given that the glomerular filtration rate may be reduced after surgery in predisposed patients, withholding sulfasalazine at least on the day of surgery is reasonable.

Azathioprine

In a retrospective study of postoperative wound complications after orthopaedic surgery, azathioprine was not associated with delayed wound healing.[24] A retrospective study that evaluated the influence of immunosuppressive therapy on postoperative complications in patients with Crohn's disease undergoing abdominal surgery found that azathioprine was not associated with postoperative complications, including intraabdominal infections.[25] Given these findings, and the fact that azathioprine is administered early after kidney transplantation, this drug may be considered safe. Therefore, the drug needs to be withheld only on the day of surgery, when an empty stomach is required anyway.

Hydroxychloroquine

A study on risk factors for wound healing did not find any association between antimalarials and postoperative complications.[24] Bibbo et al. analysed the results of foot and ankle surgery in RA and did not find an increased risk of poor wound healing or postoperative infections associated with the use of hydroxychloroquine (for NSAIDs, steroids, MTX, or gold).[7] Hydroxychloroquine was used in the past to prevent postoperative venous thromboembolism after various orthopaedic surgical procedures, and despite some controversy about its benefit, the drug was considered to be well tolerated, and haemorrhagic complications or impaired wound healing were not increased.[26]

Based upon a long elimination half-life of approximately 40–50 days, and a toxicity profile generally classified as low, the continuation of hydroxychloroquine before and after surgery is deemed reasonable.

Biological agents in the perioperative period

TNF antagonists

Many studies have analysed perioperative exposure to anti-TNF agents,[23,27–35] most of which are neither adequately designed nor powered to answer whether the number and nature of complications is increased by discontinuation of the TNF antagonist during the perioperative period. In the British Society for Rheumatology Biologics Register (BSRBR), over 1500 surgeries, including patients with RA who had received anti-TNF treatment at any time prior to surgery, were studied with respect to exposure 28 days preceding surgery and serious infections occurring within 30 days of surgery.[28] The rate of infections in the exposed group was 7%, equal to the rate of the comparison control group on non-biologic DMARDs, and higher than the rate in the group in which the TNF antagonist was stopped (5%). Although the risk association does not reach statistical significance, and many unmeasured confounders may be at play, the authors recommend caution. This abstract did not comment on the risk of perioperative RA flares in patients discontinuing anti-TNF therapy.

Guidelines on the use of anti-TNF give specific recommendations on the perioperative management of these agents, which are based on expert opinion but a low level of evidence. The British[36] and the Spanish guidelines[37] recommend suspension of anti-TNF 2–4 weeks prior to elective surgery, depending on the drug half-lives.

Rituximab

The experience on the perioperative use of rituximab is driven mainly by the transplant literature. Rituximab is used in the prevention of transplant rejection and, as such, it is administered in the 4 months previous to surgery.[38] No distinct complications have been attributed to rituximab in this case. In fact, complete clearance of rituximab takes longer than 2 months, and this would require a prolonged interval between previous exposure and surgery. The transplant literature suggests that there is no need to discontinue rituximab prior to surgery, although it would be advisable to wait at least 2 weeks after last dosing to avoid delayed infusion reactions.

Abatacept, tocilizumab, and newer TNF antagonists

There is insufficient evidence to guide the perioperative use of newer biologics, and the manufacturers do not provide any specific guidance on the matter. Recommendations should probably align with those of TNF antagonists.

Other considerations

NSAIDs

NSAIDs may prolong the bleeding time, which may result in greater blood loss. Aspirin's effect on platelets may be long lasting, and it is recommended to suspend it 5–7 days prior to surgery and recommence it 72–96 hours after surgery. Other NSAIDs have shorter effects, with no requirement to suspend dosing for longer than 2–5 days prior to surgery, depending on half-lives of the individual

Table 93.1 Summary of recommendations on the perioperative use of immunosuppressive drugs

Drug	Before surgery	Day of surgery	After surgery
Glucocorticoids	Inform the anaesthetist, surgeon, and intensivist Haemodynamic monitoring	Haemodynamic monitoring Use stress doses of hydrocortisone if volume-refractory hypotension	Haemodynamic monitoring Use stress doses of hydrocortisone if volume-refractory hypotension
If <3 weeks + <5 mg/day of prednisone or equivalent (or on alternate days):	No action	No action—fasting	Reintroduce at same dosing
If >20 mg/day of prednisone + >3 weeks or iatrogenic Cushing's syndrome	No action	50 mg of hydrocortisone parenteral intraoperatively[12]	50 mg of hydrocortisone every 8 hours for 48–72 hours[12]
If intermediate situations:	No action	Hydrocortisone 25–50 mg or no action (fasting)	Hydrocortisone 25–50 mg every 8 hours for 48 hours or simply reintroduce steroids
Methotrexate	If >65 years old or renal failure discontinue 1 week before surgery. Other situations—no action[20]	No action—fasting	If >65 years old or renal failure wait 1–2 weeks All others, reintroduce as soon as oral medication can be provided
Leflunomide	No action[21]	No action—fasting	Reintroduce as soon as oral medication can be provided
Sulfasalazine	No action[23]	No action—fasting	Reintroduce as soon as oral medication can be provided
Azathioprine	No action[25]	No action—fasting	Reintroduce as soon as oral medication can be provided
Hydroxychloroquine	No action[7,24]	No action—fasting	Reintroduce as soon as oral medication can be provided
TNF antagonists	Suspend 2–4 weeks[a] prior to surgery[36]	No action	Reintroduce after 1 week
Rituximab	Wait 2 weeks after last dosing	No action	Reintroduce after 1 week
Abatacept	Wait 4 weeks after last dosing	No action	Reintroduce after 1 week

[a]Etanercept and adalimumab 2 weeks, infliximab 4 weeks.

drugs. They can be reintroduced from 48 hours after surgery if needed.

Risk factors for infectious complications

When deciding a perioperative strategy it is important to take into account other factors, especially those associated with an increased risk of infections, such as age, diabetes, renal failure, or comorbidities such as lung disease.[28,39,40] There is no clear association between disease activity in RA, for instance, and surgical complications. Hämäläinen et al. in a case-control study for risk factors of postoperative problems (136 cases; 1:2 controls), did not find any association with disease duration, Steinbrocker status, erythrocyte sedimentation rate (ESR), or rheumatoid factor.[39] However, surgical factors and factors related to the admission itself were associated, such as a prolonged admission,[39] the day of admission (apparently the risk seems higher on specific days),[39] the ischaemic time,[39] and the type of surgery (greater risk of major complications in knee replacement and hand and wrist synovectomy).[39,41,42] A final but very important factor would be a history of previous postoperative infections.[4,39]

Conclusion

The surgical risk must be carefully weighed against benefits in all rheumatic patients, especially in those using immunosuppressive medications and suffering multiple comorbid conditions. Where the benefits appear to outweigh the risks, a comprehensive health status and medication checklist should be used to uncover reversible risk factors that require attention, and to plan medication around surgery. Recommendations on the perioperative use of immunosuppressive drugs are summarized in Table 93.1. The support of the treating rheumatologist during the perioperative period is essential.

References

1. Shaw M, Mandell BF. Perioperative management of selected problems in patients with rheumatic diseases. *Rheum Dis Clin North Am* 1999;25(3):623–638, ix.
2. Ortiz García A. Management of problematic clinical situations in rheumatoid arthritis patients: Surgery. *Reumatol Clin* 2009;5(S1):61–65.
3. Haynie RL, Yakel J. Perioperative management of the rheumatoid patient. *J Foot Ankle Surg* 1996;35(2):94–100.

4. Bongartz T, Halligan CS, Osmon DR et al. Incidence and risk factors of prosthetic joint infection after total hip or knee replacement in patients with rheumatoid arthritis. *Arthritis Rheum* 2008;59(12):1713–1720.

5. Steuer A, Keat AC. Perioperative use of methotrexate—a survey of clinical practice in the UK. *Br J Rheumatol* 1997;36(9):1009–1011.

6. Halligan CR, Matteson EL, Osmon DR et al. Perioperative management of disease modifying antirheumatic agents and postoperative prosthesis infection in patients with rheumatoid arthritis undergoing total joint arthroplasty. *Arthritis Rheum* 2005;57(10 Suppl):S334.

7. Bibbo C, Anderson RB, Davis WH, Norton J. The influence of rheumatoid chemotherapy, age, and presence of rheumatoid nodules on postoperative complications in rheumatoid foot and ankle surgery: analysis of 725 procedures in 104 patients [corrected]. *Foot Ankle Int* 2003;24(1):40–44.

8. Busti AJ, Hooper JS, Amaya CJ, Kazi S. Effects of perioperative antiinflammatory and immunomodulating therapy on surgical wound healing. *Pharmacotherapy* 2005;25(11):1566–1591.

9. Pieringer H, Stuby U, Biesenbach G. Patients with rheumatoid arthritis undergoing surgery: how should we deal with antirheumatic treatment? *Semin Arthritis Rheum.* 2007 Apr;36(5):278–286.

10. Rosandich PA, Kelley JT, 3rd, Conn DL. Perioperative management of patients with rheumatoid arthritis in the era of biologic response modifiers. *Curr Opin Rheumatol* 2004;16(3):192–198.

11. Alarcon GS, Moreland LW, Jaffe K et al. The use of methotrexate perioperatively in patients with rheumatoid arthritis undergoing major joint replacement surgery: will we ever have consensus about its use? *J Clin Rheumatol* 1996;2(1):6–8.

12. Marik PE, Varon J. Requirement of perioperative stress doses of corticosteroids: a systematic review of the literature. *Arch Surg* 2008;143(12):1222–1226.

13. Cornia PB, Anawalt BD. Rational use of perioperative corticosteroid supplementation in patients at risk for acute adrenal insufficiency. *Hosp Physician* 2003;39(10):39–44, 8.

14. Bridges SL, Jr., Lopez-Mendez A, Han KH, Tracy IC, Alarcon GS. Should methotrexate be discontinued before elective orthopedic surgery in patients with rheumatoid arthritis? *J Rheumatol* 1991;18(7):984–988.

15. Carpenter MT, West SG, Vogelgesang SA, Casey Jones DE. Postoperative joint infections in rheumatoid arthritis patients on methotrexate therapy. *Orthopedics* 1996;19(3):207–210.

16. Grennan DM, Gray J, Loudon J, Fear S. Methotrexate and early postoperative complications in patients with rheumatoid arthritis undergoing elective orthopaedic surgery. *Ann Rheum Dis* 2001;60(3):214–217.

17. Murata K, Yasuda T, Ito H et al. Lack of increase in postoperative complications with low-dose methotrexate therapy in patients with rheumatoid arthritis undergoing elective orthopedic surgery. *Mod Rheumatol* 2006;16(1):14–19.

18. Sany J, Anaya JM, Canovas F et al. Influence of methotrexate on the frequency of postoperative infectious complications in patients with rheumatoid arthritis. *J Rheumatol* 1993;20(7):1129–1132.

19. Wluka A, Buchbinder R, Hall S, Littlejohn G. Methotrexate and postoperative complications. *Ann Rheum Dis* 2002;61(1):86–87.

20. Loza E, Martinez-Lopez JA, Carmona L. A systematic review on the optimum management of the use of methotrexate in rheumatoid arthritis patients in the perioperative period to minimize perioperative morbidity and maintain disease control. *Clin Exp Rheumatol* 2009;27(5):856–862.

21. Tanaka N, Sakahashi H, Sato E et al. Examination of the risk of continuous leflunomide treatment on the incidence of infectious complications after joint arthroplasty in patients with rheumatoid arthritis. *J Clin Rheumatol* 2003;9(2):115–118.

22. Fuerst M, Mohl H, Baumgartel K, Ruther W. Leflunomide increases the risk of early healing complications in patients with rheumatoid arthritis undergoing elective orthopedic surgery. *Rheumatol Int* 2006;26(12):1138–1142.

23. den Broeder AA, Creemers MC, Fransen J et al. Risk factors for surgical site infections and other complications in elective surgery in patients with rheumatoid arthritis with special attention for anti-tumor necrosis factor: a large retrospective study. *J Rheumatol* 2007;34(4):689–695.

24. Escalante A, Beardmore TD. Risk factors for early wound complications after orthopedic surgery for rheumatoid arthritis. *J Rheumatol* 1995;22(10):1844–1851.

25. Colombel JF, Loftus EV, Jr., Tremaine WJ et al. Early postoperative complications are not increased in patients with Crohn's disease treated perioperatively with infliximab or immunosuppressive therapy. *Am J Gastroenterol* 2004;99(5):878–883.

26. Loudon JR. Hydroxychloroquine and postoperative thromboembolism after total hip replacement. *Am J Med* 1988;85(4A):57–61.

27. Arkfeld DG, Kasraeian S, Metyas S, Itomura J. Use of anti-TNF agents in 15 rheumatoid arthritis patients undergoing total elbow arthroplasty. *Ann Rheum Dis* 2007;66(Suppl II):534.

28. Dixon W, Lunt M, Watson K, Hyrich KL, BSR Control Centre Consortium, Symmons DP. Anti-TNF therapy and the risk of serious post-operative infection: results from the BSR Biologics Register (BSRBR). *Ann Rheum Dis* 2007;66(Suppl II):118.

29. Hirano Y, Kojima T, Kanayama Y et al. Influences of anti-tumour necrosis factor agents on postoperative recovery in patients with rheumatoid arthritis. *Clin Rheumatol* 2010;29(5):495–500.

30. Kawakami K, Ikari K, Kawamura K et al. Complications and features after joint surgery in rheumatoid arthritis patients treated with tumour necrosis factor-alpha blockers: perioperative interruption of tumour necrosis factor-alpha blockers decreases complications? *Rheumatology* (Oxford) 2010;49(2):341–347.

31. Ruyssen-Witrand A, Gossec L, Salliot C et al. Complication rates of 127 surgical procedures performed in rheumatic patients receiving tumor necrosis factor alpha blockers. *Clin Exp Rheumatol* 2007;25(3):430–436.

32. Corrao S, Pistone G, Arnone S et al. Safety of etanercept therapy in rheumatoid patients undergoing surgery: preliminary report. *Clin Rheumatol* 2007;26(9):1513–1515.

33. Giles JT, Bartlett SJ, Gelber AC et al. Tumor necrosis factor inhibitor therapy and risk of serious postoperative orthopedic infection in rheumatoid arthritis. *Arthritis Rheum* 2006;55(2):333–337.

34. Kanazawa T, Nishida K, Hashizume K et al. Risk factors for surgical site infection and perioperative protocol in patients with rheumatoid arthritis receiving etanercept. *Ann Rheum Dis* 2011;70(Suppl 3):420.

35. Shergy WJ, Phillips RM, Hunt RE, Hernandez J. Infliximab and its impact on surgical outcomes in patients with rheumatoid arthritis. *Ann Rheum Dis* 2005;64(Suppl II):465–466.

36. Ledingham J, Deighton C. Update on the British Society for Rheumatology guidelines for prescribing TNFalpha blockers in adults with rheumatoid arthritis (update of previous guidelines of April 2001). *Rheumatology* (Oxford) 2005;44(2):157–163.

37. Tornero Molina J, Sanmarti Sala R, Rodriguez Valverde V et al. [Update of the Consensus Statement of the Spanish Society of Rheumatology on the management of biologic therapies in rheumatoid arthritis]. *Reumatol Clin* 2010;6(1):23–36.

38. Crocchiolo R, Castagna L, El-Cheikh J et al. Prior rituximab administration is associated with reduced rate of acute GVHD after in vivo T-cell depleted transplantation in lymphoma patients. *Exp Hematol* 2011;39(9):892–896.

39. Hamalainen M, Raunio P, Von Essen R. Postoperative wound infection in rheumatoid arthritis surgery. *Clin Rheumatol* 1984;3(3):329–335.

40. Dixon WG, Watson K, Lunt M et al. Rates of serious infection, including site-specific and bacterial intracellular infection, in rheumatoid arthritis patients receiving anti-tumor necrosis factor therapy: results from the British Society for Rheumatology Biologics Register. *Arthritis Rheum* 2006;54(8):2368–2376.

41. Harigane K, Mochida Y, Ishii K, et al. Short duration of antimicrobial prophylaxis is recommended for orthopaedic surgery in patients with rheumatoid arthritis. *Ann Rheum Dis* 2011;70(Suppl3):714.

42. Rosas I, Marcial-Barba D, Montejo J, Sánchez-Guerrero J. Incidence of major complications after primary total hip or total knee replacement in patients with rheumatoid arthritis. *Arthritis Rheum* 2006;58(10 Suppl):S197.

CHAPTER 94

Vaccination in immunocompromised adults

Sander van Assen and Marc Bijl

Introduction

The aim of vaccination is to prevent or mitigate diseases by artificially inducing immunity. **Active vaccination** triggers the immune system to provide (protective) humoral and cell-mediated immune responses against the vaccine-preventable disease, while **passive vaccination** refers to the administration of exogenously produced antibodies for protection.

Most vaccines confer protection by eliciting B-cell responses leading to the production of antibodies directed against infectious or toxic agents, but neutralizing immune effector responses can also be T-cell mediated. An adequately functioning immune system is required to respond with protective immunity following vaccination. Therefore, patients with a compromised immune system may not be able to elicit protective immune responses, although they are most in need of preventive measures against infections.

In patients with autoimmune inflammatory rheumatic diseases (AIIRD) an immunocompromised state can result from treatment with immunosuppressive agents, or from the AIIRD itself, e.g. functional asplenia, hypocomplementaemia, or the presence of damaged organs serving as a locus minoris resistentiae.

An important issue with regard to vaccination is safety, in particular in patients with autoimmune diseases. The antigenic stimulus of vaccination might trigger a broader non-specific response, potentially resulting in increased activity of the underlying autoimmune disease.

Epidemiology of vaccine-preventable infections in patients with AIIRD

Infection risk is increased in patients with AIIRD. Especially pulmonary infections occur more frequently, and the mortality and morbidity of these infections are increased. Vaccines are available against influenza, *Streptococcus pneumoniae*, and *Haemophilus influenzae* b (Hib), which cause the majority of pulmonary infections in the general population. Here we summarize the epidemiology of vaccine-preventable infections (VPI) in patients with AIIRD.

In patients with AIIRD the incidence of influenza is unknown; however, the risk of hospital admission for pneumonia or influenza has been demonstrated to be higher in older patients (≥65 years) with rheumatic diseases and vasculitis compared to the elderly population in general.[1] Comparisons of the incidence of *S. pneumoniae* infection between patients with AIIRD and the general population are lacking.[1] In an uncontrolled prospective cohort of 45 patients with systemic lupus erythematosus (SLE) treated with rituximab (RTX), cyclophosphamide, and methylprednisolone, one patient developed pneumococcal pneumonia and septicaemia.[1]

The incidence of herpes zoster (HZ) in rheumatoid arthritis (RA) ranges from 0.55 up to 11.1/1.000 patient-years (PY) in prospective cohort studies.[1] RA per se is a risk factor for HZ, as are the use of steroids (relative risk (RR) point estimates 1.41–2.52); anti-tumour necrosis factor alpha (TNFα), in particular infliximab and adalimumab (RR point estimates 1.38–2.44); and the combination of TNFα-blocking agents and steroids (RR estimate 2.44).[1] Non-biologic disease-modifying anti-rheumatic drugs (DMARDs), with or without steroids, also increase the risk (cyclophosphamide 4.2-fold, azathioprine 2.1-fold, leflunomide 1.4-fold, non-biologic DMARDs and steroids 2.39-fold).[1] However, combination therapy with etanercept and methotrexate (MTX) may not increase the risk for HZ.[1] In SLE, the risk of HZ is increased 5- to 16-fold compared to the general population. The incidence of HZ was 18.3/1.000 PY in SLE patients.[1] HZ risk correlates with the use of cyclophosphamide, azathioprine, and steroids in combination with other immunosuppressive drugs.[1] The risk may be lower for mycophenolic acid compared with cyclophosphamide (RR 0.36) A randomized controlled trial (RCT) showed that SLE patients treated with RTX, along with background immunosuppressives including steroids, developed HZ more often than the placebo groups.[1] No increase in incidence of HZ during flares of SLE has been demonstrated.[1] In granulomatosis with polyangiitis (GPA) patients treated with standard immunosuppressives with or without etanercept, the incidence of HZ was high compared with the general population

(45/1.000 PY vs 1.2–4.8/1.000 PY). A serum creatinine level of 1.5 mg/dL or more increased the risk of developing HZ by a factor of 6.3.[1] The incidence of HZ is also high in patients with polymyositis/dermatomyositis (PM/DM): 27.2/1.000 PY.[1]

Human papillomavirus (HPV) infection occurs more often in SLE patients compared with healthy controls (24.6% vs 10.4%), also with the high-risk subtype HPV-16 (4.7–53% vs 1.2–6.7%).[1] The cumulative prevalence rises from 13.1% at baseline (11.7% high-risk subtype) to 25.5% (21.4% high-risk subtype) after 3 years. The incidence of HPV infection was 17/1.000 patient-months. The most common newly acquired HPV subtype was HPV-16, followed by HPV-18, -56 and -58. Only 31.8% of all incident infections were cleared.[1] For SLE patients the risk factors for HPV infection are the same as those for the general population, in addition to anti-nuclear antibodies (ANA) in excess of 320.[1]

Efficacy of vaccination in patients with AIIRD

Since at least some VPI occur more often in patients with AIIRD, the efficacy of vaccination in these patients should be addressed. Preferably, studies evaluating the efficacy of vaccination should use clinical endpoints. Unfortunately, only one vaccination study meets this criterion. All other studies investigated vaccines by measuring the humoral and/or cell-mediated immune response as a surrogate, although correlate of protection is often lacking for these measures. For influenza a haemagglutination inhibition (HI) titre of 40 or more is considered protective; however, this has never been validated for AIIRD patients. For pneumococcal, HZ, and HPV vaccination a correlate of protection is unknown, therefore a rise in titre following vaccination is predominantly used to address the efficacy.

Influenza vaccine

A reduction in pneumonitis, acute bronchitis or viral infection was found in RA patients and SLE patients who received influenza vaccine compared to those who did not.[1] Other studies have shown similar efficacy of seasonal influenza vaccination in RA patients compared to healthy controls, based on a HI titre of 40 or more. In most studies neither DMARDs nor TNFα blocking treatment hampered the humoral response.[1] Two studies reported a modestly impaired response in anti-TNFα users, not resulting in a lower percentage of seroprotection.[1] In contrast to DMARDs and TNFα-blocking treatment, RTX severely hampers the immune response following influenza vaccination.[1] In the first 8–12 weeks after treatment with RTX no antibody response was induced; 6–10 months after RTX the antibody response was partially restored.[1]

A modestly reduced response to influenza vaccination in SLE patients but also comparable efficacy of subunit influenza vaccine have been found in SLE patients compared to healthy controls.[1] In most studies the use of immunosuppressive drugs did not affect the vaccination response[1]; however, a lower response to vaccination in SLE patients on azathioprine, steroids, and hydroxychloroquine[1] has also been observed. The vast majority of studies assessing the effect of disease activity on the humoral response following influenza vaccination in RA and SLE patients did not show a reduced response during active disease.[1] Also in patients with GPA and systemic sclerosis (SSc) similar responses

following influenza vaccination compared to healthy controls were found.[1]

Vaccination for the novel influenza A/H1N1v (A/California 7/2009) virus that emerged in Mexico in 2009 provided useful insight into vaccination responses in patients with AIIRD, because virtually no pre-existent immunity to the novel influenza strain was present. Seroprotection rates for patients with RA, SLE, AS, PsA, and DM were impaired compared to healthy controls following vaccination with a A/H1N1v-vaccine with and without adjuvants,[2–6] although one study in SLE patients did not show significant differences in response.[7] Biologics, B-cell depletion, DMARDs (except antimalarials and sulphasalazine) and lymphocytopenia negatively influenced the humoral response.[3–6] Interestingly, a second dose of vaccine 3–4 weeks after the first one could overcome the hampered response,[3,6] as has also been shown for seasonal influenza vaccination in SLE patients.[8]

Cellular immune responses following influenza vaccination have also been addressed in a limited number of studies. A small study on RA patients treated with RTX found no difference in interferon (IFN) γ production by CD4 cells following influenza vaccination compared to healthy controls.[9] Cell-mediated immune responses in patients with GPA are comparable to those in healthy controls.[10] However, in SLE patients cell-mediated responses to influenza vaccination are hampered, as demonstrated by IFNγ-ELISpot and intracellular cytokine staining.[11] This may have been caused by the concomitant use of immunosuppressive drugs. It should be emphasized that the exact contribution of cell-mediated immunity to protection against influenza following influenza vaccination remains unknown.

Pneumococcal vaccine

The efficacy of pneumococcal vaccination is difficult to determine, as no generally accepted response criteria have been defined. Moreover, different vaccines (polysaccharide and conjugate vaccine) are available containing antigens with different numbers of pneumococcal serotypes.

Unvaccinated RA patients treated with MTX have a RR of 9.7 for developing pneumonia compared to those vaccinated with 23-valent polysaccharide pneumococcal vaccine.[12] Compared to healthy controls, similar as well as lower humoral responses to pneumococcal vaccines have been demonstrated in RA patients.[1] MTX alone or combined with TNFα-blocking agents negatively influenced the response, whereas TNFα-blocking agents alone did not reduce efficacy of pneumococcal vaccination in most studies. This held true for 23-valent polysaccharide as well as 7-valent conjugate pneumococcal vaccine.[1,13,14] The same was found for psoriatic arthritis (PsA) and anklylosing spondylitis (AS) patients. However, the response to pneumococcal polysaccharide vaccine was markedly reduced in RA patients vaccinated 28 weeks after RTX administration.[1]

In SLE patients similar or reduced/low responses to pneumococcal vaccine have been found,[1] not influenced by the combined use of steroids and azathioprine or cyclophosphamide.[1] RA and SLE disease activity did not influence the efficacy of vaccination.[1]

Hepatitis B vaccine

A response to hepatitis B (HBV) vaccination could be demonstrated in the majority of patients with RA, SLE, AS, and Behçet's disease (BD), irrespective of the use of steroids or DMARDs.[1] In AS patients the use of TNFα-blocking agents severely hampered the response to

HBV vaccine.[1] Low patient numbers and the lack of appropriately controlled studies make firm conclusions impossible.

Tetanus toxoid vaccine

Tetanus toxoid vaccination seems to be efficacious in RA and SLE patients.[1] The use of steroids and DMARDs, but also RTX when administered 24 weeks before tetanus vaccination, did not reduce efficacy.[1] The efficacy of tetanus vaccination may be reduced during active disease in SLE patients, but not in RA patients.[1]

Haemophilus influenzae b (Hib) vaccine

Eighty-eight per cent of SLE patients developed a protective antibody titre against Hib, with a trend towards a lower response in those using immunosuppressive drugs.[1]

Box 94.1 EULAR recommendations for vaccination in adult patients with autoimmune inflammatory rheumatic diseases

1. The vaccination status should be assessed in the initial work-up of patients with AIIRD.

2. Vaccination in patients with AIIRD should ideally be administered during stable disease.

3. Live attenuated vaccines should be avoided whenever possible in immunosuppressed patients with AIIRD.

4. Vaccination in patients with AIIRD can be administered during the use of DMARDs and TNFα blocking agents, but should ideally be administered before starting B-cell-depleting biological therapy.

5. Influenza vaccination should be strongly considered for patients with AIIRD.

6. 23-valent polysaccharide pneumococcal vaccination should be strongly considered for patients with AIIRD.

7. Patients with AIIRD should receive tetanus toxoid vaccination in accordance to recommendations for the general population. In case of major and/or contaminated wounds in patients who received RTX within the last 24 weeks, passive immunization with tetanus Ig should be administered.

8. Herpes zoster vaccination may be considered in patients with AIIRD.

9. HPV vaccination should be considered in selected patients with AIIRD.

10. In hyposplenic/asplenic patients with AIIRD influenza, pneumococcal, *Haemophilus influenzae* b, and meningococcal C vaccinations are recommended.

11. Hepatitis A and/or B vaccination is only recommended in patients with AIIRD who are at risk.

12. AIIRD patients who plan to travel are recommended to receive their vaccinations according to general rules, except for live attenuated vaccines, which should be avoided whenever possible in immunosuppressed patients with AIIRD.

13. BCG vaccination is not recommended in patients with AIIRD.

Source: van Assen et al.[16]

Safety of vaccination in patients with AIIRD

In patients with AIIRD the antigenic stimulation applied by vaccination might theoretically lead to exacerbations of the underlying autoimmune disease. Few randomized trials have addressed the safety of vaccination in patients with AIIRD. However, several pre–post-vaccination studies are available that compare disease activity before and after vaccination, using every patient as their own control.

Influenza vaccine

Two controlled trials and several pre–post studies showed no increase in RA disease activity following influenza vaccination.[1] Similarly, SLE patients who are vaccinated against influenza do not develop more disease flares than unvaccinated patients in most studies, whereas a few uncontrolled studies reported mild flares (up to 35%) or renal flares with glomerulonephritis (1 of 29 SLE patients).[1] Also, in GPA patients receiving influenza vaccination a difference in the occurrence of disease flares was not found compared to GPA patients who did not receive influenza vaccination, and no flares were registered in SSc patients who received (virosomal) influenza vaccine.[1]

Vaccination of AIIRD patients with both the non-adjuvanted and adjuvanted 2009 pandemic influenza A/H1N1 vaccine also appeared safe. Flares of SLE occurred as often following vaccination as in a control population (11% vs 10.5%)[15] and no rise in disease activity scores following vaccination was found.[1,2,4,6,7] Moreover, the levels of autoantibodies remained unchanged.[1,15]

Pneumococcal vaccine

In pre–post vaccination studies in RA and SLE patients no increase in disease activity following pneumococcal vaccination was demonstrated.[1] Similarly, vaccination did not increase disease activity in PsA and Sjögren's syndrome (SjS).[1]

Hepatitis B vaccine

HBV vaccination did not lead to increased disease activity in 22 vaccinated RA patients compared to 22 unvaccinated patients,[1] and in 28 SLE patients no significant change was recorded in Systemic Lupus Erythematosus Disease Activity Index (SLEDAI) score after each vaccine dose.[1] In a study of 13 BD patients, three developed oral aphthae following HBV vaccination but otherwise no increase in disease activity was observed.[1]

Recommendations

A European League Against Rheumatism (EULAR) task force was set up in the spring of 2009 to develop evidence-based recommendations for vaccination of adult patients with AIIRD. Thirteen recommendations were formulated (Box 94.1). The basis for the recommendations are the increased incidence of certain VPI in patients with AIIRD and the efficacy of most vaccines in patients with AIIRD, even when treated with immunomodulating agents (rituximab being an exception). The aforementioned data, suggesting that vaccination is safe in patients with AIIRD, were considered to be of great importance when formulating the recommendations.[16]

References

1. van Assen S, Elkayam O, Agmon-Levin N et al. Vaccination in adult patients with auto-immune inflammatory rheumatic diseases: A

systematic literature review for the European League Against Rheumatism evidence-based recommendations for vaccination in adult patients with auto-immune inflammatory rheumatic diseases. *Autoimmun Rev* 2011;10(6):341–352.

2. Saad CG, Borba EF, Aikawa NE et al. Immunogenicity and safety of the 2009 non-adjuvanted influenza A/H1N1 vaccine in a large cohort of autoimmune rheumatic diseases. *Ann Rheum Dis* 2011;70(6):1068–1073.

3. Gabay C, Bel M, Combescure C et al. Impact of synthetic and biologic disease-modifying antirheumatic drugs on antibody responses to the AS03-adjuvanted pandemic influenza vaccine: a prospective, open-label, parallel-cohort, single-center study. *Arthritis Rheum* 2011;63(6):1486–1496.

4. Elkayam O, Amir S, Mendelson E et al. Efficacy and safety of vaccination against pandemic 2009 influenza A (H1N1) virus among patients with rheumatic diseases. *Arthritis Care Res* (Hoboken) 2011;63(7):1062–1067.

5. Iwamoto M, Homma S, Onishi S et al. Low level of seroconversion after a novel influenza A/H1N1/2009 vaccination in Japanese patients with rheumatoid arthritis in the 2009 season. *Rheumatol Int* 2012;32(11):3691–3694.

6. Mathian A, Devilliers H, Krivine A et al. Factors influencing the efficacy of two injections of a pandemic 2009 influenza A (H1N1) non-adjuvanted vaccine in systemic lupus erythematosus. *Arthritis Rheum* 2011;63(11):3502–3511.

7. Lu CC, Wang YC, Lai JH et al. A/H1N1 influenza vaccination in patients with systemic lupus erythematosus: safety and immunity. *Vaccine* 2011;29(3):444–450.

8. Holvast A, van Assen S, de Haan A et al. Effect of a second, booster, influenza vaccination on antibody responses in quiescent systemic lupus erythematosus: an open, prospective, controlled study. *Rheumatology* (Oxford) 2009;48(10):1294–1299.

9. Arad U, Tzadok S, Amir S et al. The cellular immune response to influenza vaccination is preserved in rheumatoid arthritis patients treated with rituximab. *Vaccine* 2011;29(8):1643–1648.

10. Holvast A, de Haan A, van Assen S, Stegeman CA et al. Cell-mediated immune responses to influenza vaccination in Wegener's granulomatosis. *Ann Rheum Dis* 2010;69(5):924–927.

11. Holvast A, van Assen S, de Haan A et al. Studies of cell-mediated immune responses to influenza vaccination in systemic lupus erythematosus. *Arthritis Rheum* 2009;60(8):2438–2447.

12. Coulson E, Saravanan V, Hamilton J et al. Pneumococcal antibody levels after pneumovax in patients with rheumatoid arthritis on methotrexate. *Ann Rheum Dis* 2011;70(7):1289–1291.

13. Kapetanovic MC, Roseman C, Jonsson G, Truedsson L. Heptavalent pneumococcal conjugate vaccine elicits similar antibody response as standard 23-valent polysaccharide vaccine in adult patients with RA treated with immunomodulating drugs. *Clin Rheumatol* 2011;30(12):1555–1561.

14. Kapetanovic MC, Roseman C, Jonsson G et al. Antibody response is reduced following vaccination with 7-valent conjugate pneumococcal vaccine in adult methotrexate-treated patients with established arthritis, but not those treated with tumor necrosis factor inhibitors. *Arthritis Rheum* 2011;63(12):3723–3732.

15. Urowitz MB, Anton A, Ibanez D, Gladman DD. Autoantibody response to adjuvant and nonadjuvant H1N1 vaccination in systemic lupus erythematosus. *Arthritis Care Res* (Hoboken) 2011;63(11):1517–1520.

16. van Assen S, Agmon-Levin N, Elkayam O et al. EULAR recommendations for vaccination in adult patients with autoimmune inflammatory rheumatic diseases. *Ann Rheum Dis* 2011;70(3):414–422.

CHAPTER 95

Vaccination in immunocompromised children

Marloes Heijstek, Mario Abinun, and Nico Wulffraat

Introduction

Recommendations from the European League Against Rheumatism (EULAR) exist for the immunization of children with rheumatic diseases (Table 95.1).[1] These are also applicable to patients with autoinflammatory diseases, because of similarities in clinical presentation and medication use.

Several issues need consideration when vaccinating immunocompromised hosts:

- Efficacy refers to the capacity of vaccinations to prevent infections.

  - Often, antibody responses are taken as surrogate endpoints for efficacy.

  - The immunogenicity can be reduced due to the immunosuppressed status.

- Safety depends on the disease, the vaccine, and the degree of treatment-induced immunosuppression.

  - Safety is determined by the rate of adverse events and the effect of vaccinations on the underlying disease.

- A clear distinction must be made between live-attenuated vaccines and non-live (killed) composite vaccines.

  - In immunosuppressed hosts, the risk of live-attenuated vaccines reverting to the virulent form, or inducing complications similar to those seen in the naturally occurring disease, must be weighed against the risks of natural infection.

Immunosuppression in patients with rheumatic or autoinflammatory diseases

All patients on high-dose glucocorticoids, high-dose disease-modifying antirheumatic drugs (DMARDs), and/or biologicals are considered immunocompromised. The doses are deemed fully immunosuppressive are listed in Table 95.2.

Live-attenuated vaccines in immunocompromised patients

It is recommended to adhere to national vaccination guidelines for the live-attenuated vaccines, unless patients are immunosuppressed due to high-dose DMARDs, high-dose glucocorticoids, or biologicals, when it is recommended to withhold these vaccines. However, booster live-attenuated vaccines can be considered when essential on a case-by-case basis, carefully weighing the risk of infections versus the hypothetical risks of vaccine adverse effects (Table 95.1). This is supported by studies showing that live-attenuated booster vaccines were safe in patients on standard doses of methotrexate (MTX) and low-dose glucocorticoids. Boosters are considered safer then primary live-attenuated vaccines, as patients have already built up (protective) immunity. Therefore, primary live-attenuated vaccines theoretically have higher risk of reverting to the virulent form of the pathogen, thereby inducing infection. Fortunately, primary vaccines are mostly administered prior to onset of the disease. However, when this is not the case, live-attenuated vaccines should be withheld in patients on high-dose immunosuppressive drugs and biologicals.

Bacillus Calmette–Guérin vaccine

The Bacillus Calmette–Guérin (BCG) vaccination against tuberculosis is included in national immunization programmes of countries where tuberculosis is endemic. In juvenile patients on anti-TNFα treatment, severe tuberculosis infections have been reported. In patients living in endemic areas, BCG vaccination should be administered prior to initiating immunosuppressive drugs. BCG vaccination is contraindicated in patients with cellular immunodeficiency syndromes and in severely immunosuppressed patients.[1] It is recommended to withhold BCG vaccination during active Kawasaki disease, because local inflammation at the BCG vaccination site can occur in up to 50% of these patients.[2] The efficacy of BCG vaccination in immunocompromised patients is unknown.

Table 95.1 Recommendations for vaccination of paediatric patients with rheumatic diseases

Recommendation	Grade[d] (A–D)
Live-attenuated vaccines	
Adhere to national vaccination guidelines[a] for live-attenuated vaccines unless patients are on high-dose DMARDs[b], high-dose glucocorticoids,[b] or biologicals	C
Withhold live-attenuated vaccines in patients on high-dose DMARDs,[b] high-dose glucocorticoids,[b] or biologicals. However, essential booster vaccinations can be considered on a case-by-case basis weighing the risk of infections vs the hypothetical risk of vaccine-induced adverse events	D
Booster vaccinations against VZV, MMR, and YFV can be considered in patients on methotrexate <15 mg/m^2 per week or low-dose glucocorticoids	C
Assess VZV infection and vaccination history, especially in patients anticipating high-dose immunosuppressive therapy[b] or biologicals. In case of a negative history, VZV vaccine should be considered, ideally before initiating immunosuppressive therapy[c]	D
Non-live vaccines	
When indicated according to national guidelines[a], non-live vaccines can be administered even when using glucocorticoids, DMARDs or anti-TNFα therapy	C
Adhere to national vaccination guidelines[a] for vaccination against HVA, tetanus, diphtheria, pertussis, Hib, pneumococci, and meningococci	B/C
Adhere to national vaccination guidelines[a] for vaccination against HVA, poliovirus, Japanese encephalitis, typhoid fever, rabies, cholera or tick-borne encephalitis	D
Consider annual influenza vaccination in all immunocompromised patients	D
When vaccinations against Hib, pneumococci and meningococci are not included in national vaccination programmes,[a] these vaccinations are recommended for patients with complement deficiency or functional asplenia. These vaccinations can be considered in patients on high-dose immunosuppressive drugs[b] or biologics prior to commencing therapy[c]	D
Adhere to national vaccination guidelines[a] for vaccination against HPV. Given the higher risk of HPV infection in female SLE patients, these patients should be advised to be vaccinated in the adolescence	D
Immunosuppressive drugs	
Measure pathogen-specific antibody concentrations after vaccination in patients on high dose glucocorticoids[b] or rituximab. This can also be considered in patients on anti-TNFα treatment	C
Measure pneumococcal strain-specific antibody concentrations after the pneumococcal polysaccharide vaccine in patients on methotrexate at time of vaccination	C
Vaccinate prior to commencing rituximab whenever possible	C
In patients with a contaminated wound, administer tetanus immunoglobulin if treated with rituximab in the past 6 months	D

DMARDs, disease-modifying anti-rheumatic drugs; Hib, *Haemophilus influenzae* type B; HVA, hepatitis A virus; HVB, hepatitis B virus; HPV, human papillomavirus; MMR, measles, mumps, rubella; SLE, systemic lupus erythematosus; TNF, tumour necrosis factor; VZV, varicella zoster virus; YFV, yellow fever virus

[a]National vaccination guidelines worldwide can be found via http://apps.who.int/immunization_monitoring/en/globalsummary/scheduleselect.cfm

[b]High-dose DMARDs are defined as intravenous pulse therapy, ciclosporin >2.5 mg/kg per day, sulphasalazine >40 mg/kg per day or 2 g/day, azathioprine >3 mg/kg, cyclophosphamide orally >2.0 mg/kg per day, leflunomide >0.5 mg/kg per day, or 6-mercaptopurine >1.5 mg/kg per day. High-dose glucocorticoids are dosages ≥2 mg/kg or ≥20 mg/day for ≥2 weeks.

[c]Generally 2–4 weeks is recommended before immunosuppressive therapy is commenced.

[d]The grade of recommendation is based on the level of evidence. Grade A recommendations are based on the highest level of evidence (meta-analysis of randomized controlled trials); grade D recommendations are based on consensus.

Adapted from Heijstek et al.[1]

Measles, mumps, rubella vaccine

The measles, mumps, rubella (MMR) vaccination is included in national immunization programmes worldwide. It is safe and efficacious when patients are not immunosuppressed by treatment. MMR booster vaccination does not aggravate JIA disease and has good immunogenicity, even in patients on standard dose MTX or low dose glucocorticoids.[3,4-4a] In these patients MMR booster vaccination can be considered.

Varicella zoster virus vaccine

Several countries have included varicella zoster virus (VZV) vaccination in their immunization programme. Case reports exist of severe disseminated primary VZV or zoster infections in patients on anti-TNFα therapy or MTX. Therefore, it is recommended to assess VZV infection and vaccination history, especially in patients anticipating high-dose immunosuppressive therapy or biologicals. In case of a negative history for VZV infection or vaccination,

Table 95.2 Immunosuppressive doses of anti-rheumatic drugs

Drug	Dose considered fully immunosuppressive
Glucocorticoids	>2 mg/kg or a total dose >20 mg/day during at least 2 weeks
Disease-modifying anti-rheumatic drugs (at a dose above the standard dosages)	
Methotrexate	15 mg/m^2 per week
Ciclosporin	2.5 mg/kg per day
Sulphasalazine	40 mg/kg per day up to 2 g/day
Azathioprine	1–3 mg/kg per day
Cyclophosphamide	0.5–2.0 mg/kg per day
Leflunomide	0.25–0.5 mg/kg per day
6-Mercaptopurine	1.5 mg/kg per day
Intravenous pulse therapy	
Methylprednisolone	Any
Cyclophosphamide	Any
Biologicals	Any

vaccination should be considered before initiation of immunosuppressive therapy.

The VZV vaccine is safe and efficacious when patients are not immunosuppressed by treatment.[1] Booster vaccinations against VZV can be considered in patients on MTX less than 15 mg/m^2 per week or low-dose glucocorticoids,[5] as the vaccine is at least relatively immunogenic.[5,6] A mild self-limiting varicella-like rash can occur, whereas severe adverse effects such as generalized varicella infection or disease flares are highly uncommon.

Yellow fever virus and oral poliovirus vaccine

It is recommended to follow national vaccination guidelines and to withhold the yellow fever virus (YFV) and oral poliovirus vaccine in patients on high-dose glucocorticoids, high-dose DMARDs, or biologicals. No information exists on these vaccines in juvenile patients. In adults with rheumatic diseases on various immunosuppressive drugs, including biologicals, YFV booster does not cause severe adverse events and has good immunogenicity.[1] Thus, booster vaccinations against yellow fever can be considered in patients on MTX less than 15 mg/m^2 per week or low-dose glucocorticoids.

Non-live composite vaccines in immunocompromised patients

Non-live composite vaccines administered through national vaccination programmes are safe and immunogenic in juvenile patients with rheumatic or autoinflammatory diseases even when using glucocorticoids, DMARDs, and/or anti-TNFα therapy (Table 95.1).[7–9]

Human papillomavirus vaccine

As patients with systemic lupus erythematosus (SLE) have higher risk of persistent human papillomavirus (HPV) infections,

premalignant lesions, and cervical cancer than healthy subjects, they should be vaccinated before they become sexually active.[10,10a] In all other patients, it is recommended to adhere to national vaccination guidelines.

Seasonal influenza virus vaccine

Seasonal influenza virus vaccination is recommended for children at high risk for influenza complications. Older patients with rheumatic diseases have an increased risk for influenza with a beneficial effect of vaccination, but it is unknown whether juvenile patients are at higher risk of (complicated) influenza infections.

Seasonal influenza vaccination is safe and immunogenic, even in patients on glucocorticoids or DMARDs.[11–14] Anti-TNFα treatment can suppress the antibody response, although this does not result in lower protection rates. Based on the potential increased risk of (complicated) influenza infections and the safety and immunogenicity of non-live influenza vaccines, annual influenza vaccination should be considered in immunocompromised patients.

Meningococcal, pneumococcal, and *Haemophilus influenzae* type b vaccine

Patients with SLE and JIA with functional asplenia or complement deficiencies (C3, C5–9) are at increased risk for infections with encapsulated bacteria such as meningococci, pneumococci, and *Haemophilus influenzae* type b (Hib). In countries where these vaccinations are not routinely administered, they are recommended for these patients. Immunocompromised patients travelling into countries where the meningococcal vaccine is not routinely administered are at increased risk of meningococcal infection. Additionally, patients receiving anti-TNFα agents and IL-1 receptor blocking agents may have increased susceptibility to pneumococcal infections.[15] These vaccines should be considered in patients prior to therapy with high-dose immunosuppressive drugs or biologicals. The monovalent meningococcal conjugate vaccine against serogroup C and the 7-valent pneumococcal conjugate vaccine are safe and immunogenic in JIA patients.[16,17-17a] The immunogenicity may be reduced in patients on high dose immunosuppressive drugs or biologicals.

Effects of immunosuppressive drugs on the efficacy of vaccinations

Glucocorticoids

It is recommended to measure vaccine responses through pathogen-specific antibody concentrations in patients on high-dose glucocorticoids.[14] Low-dose glucocorticosteroids do not reduce serologic responses. Hence, measuring antibody concentrations after immunization is not required in patients on low-dose glucocorticoids.[11]

Disease-modifying anti-rheumatic drugs

Patients on a standard MTX dose (15 mg/week) can be safely vaccinated with non-live and live-attenuated vaccines.[3–5] The standard MTX dose does not reduce the immunogenicity of vaccines,[8,11,14] except for the pneumococcal polysaccharide vaccine (PPV), and possibly other polysaccharide vaccines.[1,14] It is recommended to measure pneumococcal serotype-specific antibody concentrations after PPV in patients on MTX at time of vaccination. If responses are insufficient, conjugate vaccines should be considered, since these vaccines are more immunogenic in immunocompromised patients. Studies on other DMARDs are scarce and too diverse to draw conclusions.

Biologicals

Anti-TNFα treatment does not reduce the protection rate of non-live composite vaccines although it can lower the titre of vaccination-induced antibodies.[1,16] It is recommended to measure vaccine responses in patients on anti-TNFα treatment at time of vaccination.

Rituximab (anti-B cell monoclonal antibody) blunts the humoral immune response up to 6 months after treatment.[1,14] It is recommended to vaccinate prior to rituximab use or to measure vaccine responses in patients on rituximab at time of vaccination. Patients with a contaminated wound and treated with rituximab in the past 6 months should be given tetanus immunoglobulin.

As data on other biologicals are lacking, measuring established antibody concentrations after vaccination and withholding live-attenuated vaccines is prudent.

Conclusion

Patients with rheumatic or autoinflammatory diseases treated with high-dose glucocorticoids, high-dose DMARDs, or biologicals are immunocompromised. Vaccination is crucial in these patients, given their increased risks of infections.[1]

Generally, immunogenicity of vaccines is good with some exceptions:

- Responses are reduced in patients on high-dose glucocorticoids and rituximab.

- MTX reduces responses to (pneumococcal) polysaccharide vaccines.

- Anti-TNFα can lower vaccine-induced antibody concentrations.

Offering vaccination before immunosuppressive drugs and/or measuring antibodies after immunization is suggested.

Overall, vaccinations do not increase disease activity and do not cause severe adverse events. Non-live vaccines are safe, but it is recommended to withhold live-attenuated vaccines in patients on high-dose immunosuppressive drugs and biologicals. However, booster vaccinations can be considered when essential[18].

References

1. Heijstek MW, Ott de Bruin LM, Bijl M et al. EULAR recommendations for vaccination in paediatric patients with rheumatic diseases. *Ann Rheum Dis* 2011;70:1704–1712.

2. Uehara R, Igarashi H, Yashiro M et al. Kawasaki disease patients with redness or crust formation at the Bacille Calmette-Guerin inoculation site. *Pediatr Infect Dis J* 2010;29:430–433.

3. Borte S, Liebert UG, Borte M et al. Efficacy of measles, mumps and rubella revaccination in children with juvenile idiopathic arthritis treated with methotrexate and etanercept. *Rheumatology* (Oxford) 2009;48:144–148.

4. Heijstek MW, Pileggi GC, Zonneveld-Huijssoon E et al. Safety of measles, mumps and rubella vaccination in juvenile idiopathic arthritis. *Ann Rheum Dis* 2007;66:1384–1387.

4a. Heijstek MW, Kamphuis S, Armbrust W, Swart J, Gorter S, de Vries LD, Smits GP, van Gageldonk PG, Berbers GA, Wulffraat NM. Effects of the live attenuated measles-mumps-rubella booster vaccination on disease activity in patients with juvenile idiopathic arthritis: a randomized trial. JAMA. 2013 Jun 19;309(23):2449-56.

5. Pileggi GS, de Souza CB, Ferriani VP. Safety and immunogenicity of varicella vaccine in patients with juvenile rheumatic diseases receiving methotrexate and corticosteroids. *Arthritis Care Res* (Hoboken). 2010;62:1034–1039.

6. Lu Y, Bousvaros A. Varicella vaccination in children with inflammatory bowel disease receiving immunosuppressive therapy. *J Pediatr Gastroenterol Nutr* 2010;50:562–565.

7. Erguven M, Kaya B, Hamzah OY et al. Evaluation of immune response to hepatitis A vaccination and vaccine safety in juvenile idiopathic arthritis. *J Chin Med Assoc* 2011;74:205–208.

8. Kasapcopur O, Cullu F, Kamburoglu-Goksel A et al. Hepatitis B vaccination in children with juvenile idiopathic arthritis. *Ann Rheum Dis* 2004;63:1128–1130.

9. Kashef S, Ghazizadeh F, Derakhshan A et al. Antigen-specific antibody response in juvenile-onset SLE patients following routine immunization with tetanus toxoid. *Iran J Immunol* 2008;5:181–184.

10. Tam LS, Chan PK, Ho SC et al. Natural history of cervical papilloma virus infection in systemic lupus erythematosus—a prospective cohort study. *J Rheumatol* 2010;37:330–340.

10a. Heijstek MW, Scherpenisse M, Groot N, Tacke C, Schepp RM, Buisman AM, Berbers GA, van der Klis FR, Wulffraat NM. Immunogenicity and safety of the bivalent HPV vaccine in female patients with juvenile idiopathic arthritis: a prospective controlled observational cohort study. *Ann Rheum Dis*. 2013 May 30.

11. Kanakoudi-Tsakalidou F, Trachana M, Pratsidou-Gertsi P et al. Influenza vaccination in children with chronic rheumatic diseases and long-term immunosuppressive therapy. *Clin Exp Rheumatol* 2001;19:589–594.

12. Malleson PN, Tekano JL, Scheifele DW et al. Influenza immunization in children with chronic arthritis: a prospective study. *J Rheumatol* 1993;20:1769–1773.

13. Ogimi C, Tanaka R, Saitoh A et al. Immunogenicity of influenza vaccine in children with pediatric rheumatic diseases receiving immunosuppressive agents. *Pediatr Infect Dis J* 2010;30:208–211.

14. Van Assen S, Agmon-Levin N, Elkayam O et al. EULAR recommendations for vaccination in adult patients with autoimmune inflammatory rheumatic diseases. *Ann Rheum Dis* 2011;70:414–422.

15. Abinun M. An overview of infectious complications in children on new biologic response-modifying agents. *Pediatr Health* 2010;4:509–517.

16. Farmaki E, Kanakoudi-Tsakalidou F, Spoulou V et al. The effect of anti-TNF treatment on the immunogenicity and safety of the 7-valent conjugate pneumococcal vaccine in children with juvenile idiopathic arthritis. *Vaccine*. 2010;28:5109–5113.

17. Zonneveld-Huijssoon E, Ronaghy A, Van Rossum MA et al. Safety and efficacy of meningococcal c vaccination in juvenile idiopathic arthritis. *Arthritis Rheum* 2007;56:639–646.

17a. Stoof SP, Heijstek MW, Sijssens KM, van der Klis F, Sanders EA, Teunis PF, Wulffraat NM, Berbers GA. Kinetics of the long-term antibody response after meningococcal C vaccination in patients with juvenile idiopathic arthritis: a retrospective cohort study. *Ann Rheum Dis*. 2013 Mar 16.

18. Wraith DC, Goldman M, Lambert PH. Vaccination and autoimmune disease: what is the evidence? *Lancet* 2003;362:1659–1666.

CHAPTER 96

Principles of management of juvenile idiopathic arthritis

Nicolino Ruperto and Angelo Ravelli

Introduction

The management of juvenile idiopathic arthritis (JIA) is based on a combination of pharmacological interventions, physical and occupational therapy, and psychosocial support.[1,2] (Ravelli and Martini[2] is a key reference, providing a comprehensive review of the epidemiology, classification, clinical features, aetiopathogenesis, outcome, and management of JIA.) The goal of treatment should be to induce disease remission, to control pain, to facilitate normal nutrition and growth, to preserve physical and psychological well-being, and to prevent long-term damage related to the disease or its therapy. Although we still do not possess medications that are able to cure the disease, prognosis has greatly improved in the recent years owing to major progresses in therapy. These advances have increased the expectation for disease control.[3–6]

The optimal approach to the management of a child with JIA is based on a multidisciplinary team composed of a paediatric rheumatologist, specialist nurse, physical therapist, occupational therapist, and psychologist.[1] Patient and family education and integration of parents' and children's perception of the disease course and effectiveness of therapeutic interventions in the clinical assessment are important to facilitate adherence to the management programme and therapeutic benefit.[7]

Because JIA is not a single disease, treatment approaches must recognize the differences between subtypes.[8–10] However, a rational therapeutic strategy is hampered by the inability to identify early in the disease course which children will experience a benign and self-remitting course and which children will go on to have unremitting disease with substantial risk of joint destruction and serious functional impairment.

Results of therapeutic studies in adult patients with rheumatoid arthritis (RA) are not applicable to children with JIA not only because children cannot be considered as young adults, but also because childhood arthritis is different from adult-onset RA. Furthermore, the pharmacological issues and safety concerns relating to the use of medications in growing individual deserve special consideration.

Medical management of juvenile idiopathic arthritis

Non-steroidal anti-inflammatory drugs

Non-steroidal anti-inflammatory drugs (NSAIDs) have traditionally been the mainstay treatment for all forms of JIA. Their role remains important and most children are started on an NSAID. A 4–6 week trial of an individual NSAID is necessary to assess its efficacy. However, since NSAIDs are not disease modifying, they are used more to treat pain, stiffness, and the fever associated with systemic arthritis. Only a few NSAIDs are approved for use in children: the most commonly used are naproxen, ibuprofen, and indomethacin. They are usually well tolerated and side effects are less common than in adults. However, the parents and patients should be advised to take the medication with food to minimize the risk of gastric upset. The utility of antacids, histamine$_2$-receptor antagonists, misoprostol, and proton pump inhibitors for prophylaxis against serious NSAID-induced gastrointestinal complications in children with chronic arthritis is unclear. Experience with cyclooxygenase (COX)-2 inhibitors in the paediatric age range is scarce.[11,12] Meloxicam, an inhibitor of both COX-1 and COX-2, has proven to be effective and safe in children in a controlled trial.[11] The NSAIDs that are commonly used in JIA and their doses are presented in Table 96.1.

Corticosteroids

Intra-articular injections

Intra-articular corticosteroid (IAC) injections are widely used in the management of children with JIA to induce short-term relief of inflammation symptoms and functional improvement, and to obviate the need for regular systemic therapy.[13,14] Nowadays, it is thought that many paediatric rheumatologists are using IACs as their first approach in oligoarticular JIA. In children with this subtype, local IAC therapy has been shown to enable correction of joint contractures, prevention of leg-length discrepancy, discontinuation of oral medications, resolution of Baker's cysts, and improvement of tenosynovitis. However, the strategy of performing multiple

Table 96.1 Non-steroidal anti-inflammatory drugs commonly used in children with juvenile idiopathic arthritis

Chemical class/drug	Dose (mg/kg/day)	Maximum dose (mg/day)	Doses per day
Salicylate			
Aspirin	80–100 (<25 kg) 2500 mg/m² (>25 kg)	4900	2–4
Propionic acid derivatives			
Naproxen	10–20	1000	2
Ibuprofen	30–40	2400	3–4
Ketoprofen	2–4	300	3–4
Flurbiprofen	3–4	300	2–4
Oxaprozin	10–20	1200	1
Acetic acid derivatives			
Indomethacin	1.5–3	200	2–3
Tolmetin	20–30	1800	3–4
Sulindac	4–6	400	2
Diclofenac	2–3	150	3
Etodolac	10–20	1000	1
Oxicams			
Meloxicam	0.25	15	1
Piroxicam	0.2–0.3	20	1
Nabumetone	30	2000	1
Pyrazole derivative			
Celecoxib	>2 yr old, 10–25 kg: 100 >2 yr old, 25–50 kg: 200	200	2

IAC injections is used by some clinicians in children with polyarthritis to induce prompt remission of synovitis, while simultaneously initiating therapy with disease-modifying agents (DMARDs) and/or biological agents.[15,16] Multiple IAC injections are meant to have the potential advantage of avoiding many side effects of systemic corticosteroids and selectively targeting the inflamed joints. Triamcinolone hexacetonide, which is more effective and has a longer effect than other forms of injectable corticosteroids, is universally recognized among paediatric rheumatologists as the medication of choice for intra-articular administration in JIA. However, use of a more soluble agent for smaller or difficult-to-access joints has been advised to avoid local side effects related to extravasation of triamcinolone hexacetonide from the joint space.[13] The dosage regimen of corticosteroid preparations currently used at the authors' centre is reported in Table 96.2.

Systemic corticosteroids

Patients whose disease is not well controlled by a course of NSAIDs or IAC therapy and an appropriate programme of physical therapy are candidates to receive more aggressive interventions. Moderate or high-dose systemic corticosteroid therapy is usually reserved to the management of the extra-articular manifestations of systemic JIA.[17] These include high fever unresponsive to NSAIDs; severe anaemia, myocarditis, or pericarditis; and macrophage activation syndrome. Intravenous methylprednisolone (30 mg/kg per day to a maximum of 1 g/day on 1–3 consecutive days) is effective in controlling systemic and articular features of the disease, but its effect is often short-lived. In the other subtypes of JIA, corticosteroids should be used very selectively because their potential deleterious effects, especially on bone and growth, might outweigh any benefits to articular disease. A course of low-dose prednisone could be considered for reduction of pain and stiffness in patients with severe polyarthritis who are unresponsive to other therapies or who are awaiting the full therapeutic effect of a disease-modifying agent. There is no evidence that systemic corticosteroids are disease modifying in childhood arthritis.

Methotrexate

Methotrexate (MTX) has become the second-line agent of choice for children with persistently active arthritis because of its effectiveness and acceptable toxic effects.[18,19] Improvement in patients is usually seen after 6–12 weeks. The efficacy of this drug was established in a controlled trial in 1992 at a dose of 10 mg/m² per week given orally.[20] A subsequent randomized study has shown that MTX exerts its maximum therapeutic effect with parenteral administration of 15 mg/m² per week. There was no additional advantage in giving higher doses up to 30 mg/m² per week.[21] The greatest efficacy of MTX has been seen in patients with extended oligoarthritis, whereas the systemic-onset subtype may be the least responsive. The observation of a decrease in the rate of radiographic progression in two small uncontrolled studies has suggested that MTX may possess a disease-modifying effect.[22,23] It is not clear when a patient can stop taking MTX after the achievement of clinical remission because the disease will flare in up to 60% of patients after discontinuing the drug. Recently, a 12 month

Table 96.2 Type and dose of corticosteroid preparations used for intra-articular injections at the authors' centre

Joint	Corticosteroid	Dose
Shoulder	TH	1 mg/kg (max 40 mg)
Elbow	TH	0.75 mg/kg (max 30 mg)
Wrist	TH	0.25–0.5 mg/kg[a] (max 20 mg)
Hand (metacarpophalangeal and interphalangeal)	MP	5–10 mg[a]
Hip	TH	1 mg/kg (max 40 mg)
Knee	TH	1 mg/kg (max 40 mg)
Ankle	TH	0.75 mg/kg (max 30 mg)
Subtalar and intertarsal	MP	20–40 mg[a]
Foot (metatarsophalangeal and interphalangeal)	MP	5–20 mg[a]
Tendon sheaths	MP	20–40 mg%[a]

TH, triamcinolone hexacetonide; MP, methylprednisolone acetate.
[a]Depending on the child's size.

vs 6 month withdrawal of MTX was not found to reduce the relapse rate in JIA patients in remission.[24] Tests to monitor complete blood counts, liver enzymes, and renal function are recommended during MTX administration, although the optimal frequency of testing is unclear.[25] The supplementation of folic or folinic acid may help prevent the occurrence of liver enzyme abnormalities, oral ulcerations, and nausea. Leflunomide is an alternative option for patients unresponsive or intolerant to MTX.[26] However, experience with this drug in childhood arthritis is still scarce. Because leflunomide is teratogenic, young females of childbearing potential must have a negative pregnancy test before starting this medication and must practice appropriate contraception.

Sulfasalazine

Some studies have shown that sulfasalazine is able to improve arthritis in the late-onset oligoarticular group and in patients with juvenile spondyloarthropathies.[27,28] However, adverse reactions were frequently reported, especially rashes, gastrointestinal symptoms, and leucopenia, and led to discontinuation of the drug in a sizable proportion of patients. Administration of this medication in systemic arthritis is considered contraindicated, owing to the marked severity of side effects seen in patients with this JIA subset.

Ciclosporin

There are no controlled studies of ciclosporin in JIA. Small series have shown that this medication can be effective in patients refractory to MTX.[29] In systemic JIA, ciclosporin may be more beneficial for control of fever than for the treatment of arthritis and may enable corticosteroid dose reduction and may be distinctly efficacious in the management of macrophage activation syndrome.[30,31]

Combination therapies

Encouraging results have been reported in a small uncontrolled study of combination therapy with MTX and ciclosporin in patients refractory to MTX monotherapy.[32] A recent randomized trial has provided evidence that synthetic DMARDs in combination (MTX, sulfasalazine, and hydroxychloroquine) may be superior than MTX treatment alone in polyarticular JIA.[33]

Thalidomide

Thalidomide has been found to be effective in treatment-resistant systemic arthritis, both for systemic features and arthritis.[34] No significant adverse effects were noticed. However, use of this medication requires careful surveillance of the teratogenic effect and the development of peripheral neuropathy.

Autologous stem cell transplantation

Complete drug-free remission was achieved in around half of patients with long-standing and unresponsive systemic and polyarticular JIA who underwent autologous stem cell transplantation (ASCT).[35] However, since several issues remain open regarding the ASCT protocol, it should still be regarded as an experimental procedure for patients with very severe and unremitting disease. In the very rare patients who develop amyloidosis, alkylating agents such as chlorambucil may be beneficial.

Biologicals

The greatest advance in the treatment of JIA has been the introduction of biologic response modifiers, which offer a very effective therapeutic option for the treatment of patients who are resistant to conventional anti-rheumatic medications, namely MTX.[36] The development of these medications has been made possible by the advances in the understanding of the immune system, which have shed light on pathways involved in inflammation and self-tolerance and provided new targets for treatment of rheumatologic conditions. Biological agents have been designed to target key cytokines implicated in JIA, including tumour necrosis factor (TNF)α, interleukin (IL)-1, and IL-6 as well as signalling molecules involved in the regulation of B-cell and T-cell responses.

The efficacy of three anti-TNF agents (etanercept, infliximab, and adalimumab) and of the inhibitor of T-lymphocyte activation abatacept has been shown in the polyarticular form of the disease.[37–40] Anti-IL-1 (anakinra and canakinumab) and anti-IL-6 (tocilizumab) treatments have been found to be efficacious in systemic JIA, a disease that responds less well to anti-TNF drugs.[41–46] Biological medications are often used early in the course of JIA and are an effective treatment for arthritis, extra-articular manifestations of systemic disease, and uveitis. As seen for MTX, many patients experience a flare of symptoms after discontinuation of biological therapy.[47] Patients with JIA may, therefore, need to receive many years of biological therapy. Although the experience gained so far has shown that biological agents are overall safe in children with chronic arthritis, use of these medications in the paediatric population raises questions about risk of infections (particularly opportunistic infections and tuberculosis), response to vaccination, development of autoimmune phenomena, and long-term effects on immune surveillance and possible risk of malignancy.[48,49] Additional data concerning long-term safety of these drugs will be provided by the large-scale pharmacovigilance studies that are under way. The use of biologics in combination may be associated with increased infection risk and is not recommended. Details relating to biological therapies and the management of macrophage activation syndrome, a serious and potentially fatal complication seen most commonly in systemic JIA, are given in other chapters.

Treatment of problems associated with juvenile idiopathic arthritis

Iridocyclitis

In iridocyclitis, early diagnosis is fundamental for the success of therapy. The initial approach consists of glucocorticoid and mydriatic eye drops. In patients with disease resistant to topical therapy, systemic corticosteroid administration or subtenon injection of corticosteroids, or both, may be necessary. In disease not controlled by these interventions, several immunosuppressive medications have been considered effective, including MTX, ciclosporin, and alkylating agents. However, no controlled trials have been done. The efficacy of etanercept is controversial, whereas infliximab has been anecdotally reported to be of benefit.[50] A recent study has suggested that adalimumab is more efficacious than infliximab in maintaining remission of chronic childhood uveitis.[51] In a small case series, abatacept treatment was found to lead to sustained improvement in severe anti-TNFα-resistant JIA-related uveitis.[52]

Growth retardation and osteoporosis

Some studies have shown that human recombinant growth hormone could be beneficial in treatment of severe growth retardation in JIA.[53,54] The administration of oral alendronate has been associated with an increase in bone mineral density in paediatric patients with diffuse connective tissue diseases, including JIA, who had a low bone mass or fragility fractures.[55] However, the potential long-term toxic effects of bisphosphonates on the growing skeleton remains a matter of concern.[56] Oral calcium supplementation was found to have only a marginal effect on bone mineral density in children with JIA who were not receiving corticosteroids.[57]

Physical and occupational therapy

Physiotherapy and occupational therapy are important components of the therapeutic approach to any patients with JIA.[58] Physical therapy in children with arthritis should be performed by a therapist specifically knowledgeable in paediatrics and experienced in the treatment of JIA. The aim of physical therapy is to keep or restore joint function and alignment as much as possible and achieve a normal pattern of mobility. Orthotic devices can be very useful in selected patients. Children with persistent flexion contractures may require serial night splinting or even serial casting to help correction. Due to improvement in pharmacological management and earlier disease control, serious functional disability and joint deformities are becoming less frequent. There is, therefore, an increasing need for physiotherapists to focus on broader issues, such as fitness, stamina, and bone strength.

An important aim of the management is to foster the normal psychosocial and social development of the child and to tackle possible difficulties caused by the disease or its consequences on family life. Participation in peer-group activities and regular attendance to school (including, whenever possible, the physical education programme) should be strongly encouraged. Children should be left largely free to establish their own level of activity, including the choice of the sport they wish to practice. Swimming and cycling, which do not put substantial weight on joints, are suitable sport activities. Appropriate attention to psychosocial issues, with the possible help of a paediatric psychologist, can potentially have a positive impact on the well-being of the child. Overprotection of the ill child and neglect of siblings is a common parental reaction, but should be avoided by early intervention. Education and counselling of the child with chronic arthritis and the parents about the present state of knowledge regarding outcome and therapy should be provided by the physician at the time of the first visit and repeated, as needed, during the subsequent clinical course.

Role of nurses

Nurses may play an important role in educating patients and parents on several issues, including handling and administration of traditional anti-rheumatic drugs and the newer biologicals, adverse effects of medications and monitoring of toxicity, importance of compliance with physicians' prescriptions, cautions and risks related to immunization, harmful impact of alcohol and smoking on health, and need to avoid pregnancy while taking medications with teratogenic potential. The European League Against Rheumatism (EULAR) recommendations for vaccination in paediatric patients with rheumatic diseases have been published recently.[59]

Role of surgical treatment

In selected situations, surgical approaches to irreversible joint contractures, dislocations, or joint replacement may be indicated. However, nowadays the role of orthopaedic surgery in the management of JIA is much more limited than in the past. The long-term outcome of children with joint disease is not altered by prophylactic synovectomy. However, this surgical intervention may be useful to prolong the duration of remission of synovitis in a frequently relapsing joint. Care must be taken to prevent a postsurgical contracture. Arthroscopic surgery greatly reduces the morbidity associated with synovectomy.

Transition to adult care

The transition to adult care is a process that should start when a child reaches adolescence.[60] However, preparation of the child and family should be initiated as soon as the diagnosis is made and updated as the child matures. A successful transition requires an accurate planning and the coordinated participation of the patient, the family, and the paediatric and adult services. Adolescents should be encouraged gradually to take control of their disease management. Particular attention should be paid to fostering independent living skills and self-advocacy. Training in self-management, communication, and decision-making, conducted individually or in group sessions, may be helpful. Vocational evaluation and advice is welcome. The overall goal of transition is to help the adolescent or young adult to become more independent in managing healthcare needs and to assume adult roles such as a student, worker, parent, and partner.

American College of Rheumatology recommendations for the treatment of juvenile idiopathic arthritis

In 2011, the American College of Rheumatology (ACR) issued a set of recommendations aimed to assist physicians in selecting the safest and most effective treatment of JIA,[61] which were developed applying the Research and Development/University of California at Los Angeles (RAND/UCLA) Appropriateness Method and following the principles of the Appraisal of Guidelines for Research and Evaluation instrument (AGREE, at www.agreecollaboration. org). This process was based on a step-up approach, which mandates the subsequent administration of medications with greater potency once the previous treatment has failed. Instead of considering all International Leagues of Associations of Rheumatology (ILAR) categories of JIA individually, children with JIA were grouped into distinct 'treatment groups'. Recommendations were proposed for five treatment groups and were tailored according to the level of disease activity and the presence of features of poor prognosis specific for each treatment group. Three levels of disease activity were defined: low, moderate, and high. The state of inactive disease/clinical remission was not considered. Tapering or discontinuation of medications for patients with inactive disease was also not considered. In addition to the recommendations regarding treatment effectiveness, a guidance for the safety monitoring of the medications used in JIA is provided. A summary of the ACR recommendations for the treatment of JIA is presented in Box 96.1. Currently, the recommendations for systemic JIA are being revised to take into account the recently published trials on tocilizumab and canakinumab.[45,46]

Box 96.1 Summary of the American College of Rheumatology recommendations for the treatment of juvenile idiopathic arthritis

General recommendations that apply to all treatment groups

Intra-articular corticosteroids

- Recommended for active arthritis regardless of concurrent therapy or JIA treatment group
- Triamcinolone hexacetonide is the preferred injectable corticosteroid preparation
- A duration of clinical response to intra-articular corticosteroids of less than 4 months may imply a need for escalation of systemic therapy
- Intra-articular corticosteroid injection(s) that result in clinical improvement of arthritis for more than 4 months may be repeated, as needed

Methotrexate with TNFα inhibitors

- Continuing methotrexate when initiating etanercept or adalimumab is recommended for patients who had a partial previous clinical response to methotrexate
- Continuing methotrexate when initiating etanercept or adalimumab is uncertain for patients who had a poor previous clinical response to methotrexate
- It is assumed that methotrexate be continued when initiating infliximab

History of arthritis of four or fewer joints

NSAID monotherapy (without intra-articular corticosteroids)

- Patients with low disease activity, without joint contracture, and without poor prognostic features
- Continuation of NSAID monotherapy for more than 2 months is inappropriate for patients with active arthritis, irrespective of poor prognostic features

Intra-articular corticosteroids (with or without additional therapy)

- All patients with active arthritis

Methotrexate

- As initial treatment for patients with high disease activity and poor prognostic features
- Following initial intra-articular corticosteroid injection(s), patients with high disease activity without poor prognostic features and patients with moderate disease activity and poor prognostic features
- Following repeated intra-articular corticosteroid injection(s), patients with moderate disease activity without poor prognostic features, and patients with low disease activity and poor prognostic features

Sulfasalazine

- Following intra-articular corticosteroid injection(s) or an adequate trial of NSAIDs, patients with enthesitis-related arthritis

and moderate or high disease activity, irrespective of poor prognostic features

TNFα inhibitors

- Patients who have received intra-articular corticosteroid injection(s) and 3 months of methotrexate and have moderate or high disease activity and poor prognostic features
- Patients who have received intra-articular corticosteroid injection(s) and 6 months of methotrexate and have high disease activity without poor prognostic features
- Patients with enthesitis-related arthritis who have received intra-articular corticosteroid injection(s) and sulfasalazine and have moderate or high disease activity, irrespective of poor prognostic features

History of arthritis of five or more joints

NSAID monotherapy (without intra-articular corticosteroids)

- Uncertain as initial therapy
- Continuation of NSAID monotherapy for more than 2 months is inappropriate for patients with active arthritis, irrespective of poor prognostic features

Methotrexate

- As initial treatment for patients with high disease activity, irrespective of poor prognostic features, and patients with moderate disease activity and poor prognostic features
- Following approximately 1 month of NSAIDs, patients with low disease activity and poor prognostic features
- Following 1–2 months of NSAIDs, patients with moderate disease activity without poor prognostic features

Leflunomide

- Recommended as potential alternative to methotrexate

TNFα inhibitors

- Patients who have received 3 months of methotrexate or leflunomide and have moderate or high disease activity, irrespective of poor prognostic features
- Patients who have received 6 months of methotrexate or leflunomide and have low disease activity, irrespective of poor prognostic features

Switching from one TNFα inhibitor to another

- Patients who have received the current TNFα inhibitor for 4 months and have moderate or high disease activity, irrespective of poor prognostic features

Abatacept

- Patients who have received a TNFα inhibitor for 4 months and have high disease activity, irrespective of poor prognostic features, or moderate disease activity and poor prognostic features

- Patients who have received more than one TNFα inhibitor sequentially and have moderate or high disease activity, irrespective of poor prognostic features, or low disease activity and poor prognostic features

Switching from abatacept to a TNFα inhibitor

- Patients who have received abatacept for 3 months and have high disease activity and poor prognostic features
- Patients who have received abatacept for 6 months and have moderate or high disease activity, irrespective of poor prognostic features

Rituximab

- Patients (particularly if rheumatoid factor-positive) who have received a TNFα inhibitor and abatacept sequentially and have high disease activity, irrespective of poor prognostic features, or moderate disease activity and poor prognostic features

Active sacroiliac arthritis

TNFα inhibitors

- Patients who have received an adequate trial of NSAIDs and have high disease activity and poor prognostic features
- Patients who have received 3 months of methotrexate and have high disease activity, irrespective of poor prognostic features, or moderate disease activity and features of poor prognosis
- Patients who have received 6 months of methotrexate and have moderate disease activity without poor prognostic features
- Patients who have received 3 months of sulfasalazine and have moderate or high disease activity, irrespective of poor prognostic features
- Patients who have received 6 months of sulfasalazine and have low disease activity and poor prognostic features

Systemic arthritis with active systemic features (and without active arthritis)

NSAID monotherapy

- Appropriate during the clinical evaluation of possible systemic arthritis
- Uncertain as initial or continued therapy for patients with active fever
- Inappropriate for patients with active fever and physician global assessment ≥ 7 out of 10
- Inappropriate for a duration greater than 1 month in patients with active fever

Systemic corticosteroids (with or without additional therapy)

- Patients with active fever and physician global assessment ≥7 out of 10
- Following up to 2 weeks of NSAIDs, all patients with fever

Anakinra

- All patients with active fever and poor prognostic features, irrespective of current therapy

- All patients with sustained or newly-developed fever while receiving corticosteroids

Methotrexate

- Inappropriate

Systemic arthritis with active arthritis (and without active systemic features)

NSAID monotherapy (with or without intra-articular corticosteroids)

- Patients with low disease activity without poor prognostic features
- Continuation of NSAID monotherapy for more than 1 month uncertain for patients with any level of disease activity, irrespective of poor prognostic features

Methotrexate

- All patients with active arthritis following one month or less of NSAID monotherapy (with or without intra-articular corticosteroids), irrespective of poor prognostic features

Anakinra

- Patients who have received methotrexate and have moderate or high disease activity, irrespective of poor prognostic features
- Patients who have received methotrexate and a TNFα inhibitor or methotrexate and abatacept and have moderate or high disease activity, irrespective of poor prognostic features

TNFα inhibitors

- Patients who have received methotrexate for 3 months or anakinra and have moderate or high disease activity, irrespective of poor prognostic features

Abatacept

- Patients who have received methotrexate and a TNFα inhibitor and have high disease activity, irrespective of poor prognostic features, or moderate disease activity and poor prognostic features

Calcineurin inhibitors

- Inappropriate

See Beukelman et al.[59] for the definitions of treatment groups, levels of disease activity, and poor prognostic features.

Recommendations provided for patients with systemic JIA do not to apply in case of clinical and laboratory evidence of macrophage activation syndrome or other severe complications, such as serositis, that require specific changes in therapy.

Recommendations for systemic JIA do not incorporate recent data relating to use of the IL-6 inhibitor tocilizumab or the IL-1 inhibitors canakinumab or rilonacept, which were not available at the time when the recommendations were developed.

British Society for Paediatric and Adolescent Rheumatology Standards of Care for children and young people with juvenile idiopathic arthritis

The development of the standards of care by the British Society for Paediatric and Adolescent Rheumatology (BSPAR) was inspired by the belief that all children with JIA have the right to equitable access to the highest quality of care, regardless of their geographic location, and that their care should be based on current evidence and be delivered by experienced multidisciplinary teams. The aim of the standards is to help these teams to improve the service they provide by formulating a statement of the minimum set of standards of care for children, adolescents, and young adults with JIA.[62] Of the 27 standards that were promulgated, the following 4 were highlighted as fundamental:

◆ encouragement of patients with JIA and their families to participate in the management of their disease

◆ providing an adequate training to all professionals likely to come into contact with a patient with JIA

◆ pursuing a holistic approach with focus on functional and psychosocial issues in addition to control of disease activity

◆ development of clinical networks for paediatric rheumatology.

Another major area of concern was the delay in access to specialist care. The BSPAR standards recommend that all patients with suspected JIA be seen by a paediatric rheumatologist within 10 weeks of onset of symptoms and within 4 weeks of the referral. This advice is aimed to increase the awareness of JIA, facilitate its early recognition by physicians, and urge referral to specialist teams. Ensuring early diagnosis to all children with JIA is a challenging task, as in many parts of the world specialist teams are rare. However, even where they exist, delay in diagnosis or access is still common.[63]

Other important recommendations incorporated in the BSPAR standards are that children with incident or suspected JIA be managed by a paediatric rheumatology multidisciplinary team, that JIA patients have prompt access to the drugs required to control their disease, that monitoring of therapy be conducted according to established guidelines, that 'tight' disease control be implemented in patients with active disease, that ophthalmologic assessment be made according to current guidelines, and that all young people with JIA have a planned and coordinated transition from the paediatric to the adult service. Beside the standards of care, the BSPAR outlined the optimal structure of the paediatric rheumatology multidisciplinary team, which should include a 'core multidisciplinary team', composed of members required by every JIA patients (e.g. paediatric rheumatologist, paediatric rheumatology nurse specialist, ophthalmologist, paediatric physiotherapist), and an 'extended multidisciplinary team', composed of members required if clinically indicated (e.g. play therapist, orthodontist, orthopaedic surgeon). In an editorial and a letter commenting the standards, it was argued that the goal of achievement of inactive disease and remission was not clearly formulated. Considering that therapeutic approaches and medications are now available to make disease remission an attainable objective for many, if not most, patients with JIA, it has been suggested that the standards be revised to include as overriding goal the achievement of clinical remission or, at least, minimal disease activity.[64,65]

References

1. Petty RE, Cassidy JT. Chronic arthritis in childhood. In: Cassidy JT, Petty RE, Laxer RM, Lindsley CB (eds). *Textbook of pediatric rheumatology*, 6th edn. Elsevier Saunders, Philadelphia, PA,2011:211–235.
2. Ravelli A, Martini A. Juvenile idiopathic arthritis. *Lancet* 2007;369:767–778.
3. Martini A, Lovell DJ. Juvenile idiopathic arthritis: state of the art and future perspectives. *Ann Rheum Dis* 2010;69:1260–1263.
4. Ruperto N, Giannini EH, Pistorio A et al. Is it time to move to active comparator trials in juvenile idiopathic arthritis? A review of current study designs. *Arthritis Rheum* 2010;62:3131–3139.
5. Wallace CA, Giannini EH, Huang B, Itert L, Ruperto N. American College of Rheumatology provisional criteria for defining clinical inactive disease in select categories of juvenile idiopathic arthritis. *Arthritis Care Res* 2011;63:929–936.
6. Consolaro A, Bracciolini G, Ruperto N et al. Remission, minimal disease activity and acceptable symptom state in juvenile idiopathic arthritis. *Arthritis Rheum* 2012;64(7):2366–2374.
7. Filocamo G, Consolaro A, Schiappapietra B et al. Introducing a new approach into clinical care of children with juvenile idiopathic arthritis: the juvenile arthritis multidimensional assessment report. *J Rheumatol* 2011;38:938–953.
8. Hashkes PJ, Laxer RM. Medical treatment of juvenile idiopathic arthritis. *JAMA* 2005;294:1671–1684.
9. Hayward K, Wallace CA. Recent developments in anti-rheumatic drugs in pediatrics: treatment of juvenile idiopathic arthritis. *Arthritis Res Ther* 2009;11:216.
10. Ruperto N, Martini A. Current medical treatments for juvenile idiopathic arthritis. *Front Pharmacol* 2011;2:60.
11. Ruperto N, Nikishina I, Pachanov ED et al. A randomized, double-blind clinical trial of two doses of meloxicam compared with naproxen in children with juvenile idiopathic arthritis: short- and long-term efficacy and safety results. *Arthritis Rheum* 2005;52:563–572.
12. Reiff A, Lovell DJ, Adelsberg JV et al. Evaluation of the comparative efficacy and tolerability of rofecoxib and naproxen in children and adolescents with juvenile rheumatoid arthritis: a 12-week randomized controlled clinical trial with a 52-week open-label extension. *J Rheumatol* 2006;33:985–995.
13. Scott C, Meiorin S, Filocamo G et al. A reappraisal of intra-articular corticosteroid therapy in juvenile idiopathic arthritis. *Clin Exp Rheumatol* 2010;28:774–781.
14. Bloom BJ, Alario AJ, Miller LC. Intra-articular corticosteroid therapy for juvenile idiopathic arthritis: report of an experimental cohort and literature review. *Rheumatol Int* 2011;31:749–756.
15. Southwood TR. Report from a symposium on corticosteroid therapy in juvenile chronic arthritis. *Clin Exp Rheumatol*. 1993;11:91–94.
16. Lanni S, Bertamino M, Consolaro A et al. Outcome and predicting factors of single and multiple intra-articular corticosteroid injections in children with juvenile idiopathic arthritis. *Rheumatology* 2011;50:1627–1634.
17. Ravelli A, Lattanzi B, Consolaro A, Martini A. Glucocorticoids in paediatric rheumatology. *Clin Exp Rheumatol* 2011; 29(5 Suppl.68):S148-S152.
18. Ravelli A, Martini A. Methotrexate in juvenile idiopathic arthritis: answers and questions. *J Rheumatol* 2000; 27: 1830–1833.
19. Gutierrez-Suarez R, Burgos-Vargas R. The use of methotrexate in children with rheumatic diseases. *Clin Exp Rheumatol* 2010;28(Suppl.61):S122–S127.
20. Giannini EH, Brewer EJ, Kuzmina N et al. Methotrexate in resistant juvenile rheumatoid arthritis. Results of the U.S.A.-U.S.S.R. double-blind, placebo-controlled trial. The Pediatric Rheumatology Collaborative Study Group and The Cooperative Children's Study Group. *N Engl J Med* 1992;326:1043–1049.

21. Ruperto N, Murray KJ, Gerloni V et al. A randomized trial of parenteral methotrexate in intermediate versus higher doses in children with juvenile idiopathic arthritis who failed standard dose. *Arthritis Rheum* 2004;50:2191–2201.

22. Harel L, Wagner-Weiner L, Poznanski AK et al. Effects of methotrexate on radiologic progression in juvenile rheumatoid arthritis. *Arthritis Rheum* 1993;36:1370–1374.

23. Ravelli A, Viola S, Ramenghi B et al. Radiologic progression in juvenile chronic arthritis patients treated with methotrexate. *J. Pediatr* 1998;133:262–265.

24. Foell D, Wulffraat N, Wedderburn LR et al. Methotrexate withdrawal at 6 vs 12 months in juvenile idiopathic arthritis in remission: a randomized clinical trial. *JAMA* 2010;303:1266–1273.

25. Ortiz-Alvarez O, Morishita K, Avery G et al. Guidelines for blood test monitoring of methotrexate toxicity in juvenile idiopathic arthritis. *J Rheumatol* 2004;31:2501–2506.

26. Silverman E, Mouy R, Spiegel L et al. Leflunomide or methotrexate for juvenile rheumatoid arthritis. *N Engl J Med* 2005;352:1655–1666.

27. van Rossum MA, Fiselier TJ, Franssen MJ et al. Sulfasalazine in the treatment of juvenile chronic arthritis: a randomized, double-blind, placebo-controlled, multicenter study. Dutch Juvenile Chronic Arthritis Study Group. *Arthritis Rheum* 1998;41:808–816.

28. Burgos-Vargas R, Vazquez-Mellado J, Pacheco-Tena C et al. A 26 week randomised, double blind, placebo controlled exploratory study of sulfasalazine in juvenile onset spondyloarthropathies. *Ann Rheum Dis* 2002;61:941–942.

29. Reiff A, Rawlings DJ, Shaham B et al. Preliminary evidence for cyclosporin A as an alternative in the treatment of recalcitrant juvenile rheumatoid arthritis and juvenile dermatomyositis. *J Rheumatol* 1997;24:2436–2443.

30. Mouy R, Stephan JL, Pillet P et al. Efficacy of cyclosporine A in the treatment of macrophage activation syndrome in juvenile arthritis: report of five cases. *J Pediatr* 1996;129:750–754.

31. Ravelli A, De Benedetti F, Viola S, Martini A. Macrophage activation syndrome in systemic juvenile rheumatoid arthritis successfully treated with cyclosporine. *J Pediatr* 1996;128:275–278.

32. Ravelli A, Moretti C, Temporini F et al. Combination therapy with methotrexate and cyclosporine A in juvenile idiopathic arthritis. *Clin Exp Rheumatol* 2002;20:569–572.

33. Tynjälä P, Vähäsalo P, Tarkiainen M et al. Aggressive combination drug therapy in very early polyarticular juvenile idiopathic arthritis (ACUTE-JIA): a multicentre randomised open-label clinical trial. *Ann Rheum Dis* 2011;70:1605–1612.

34. Lehman TJ, Schechter SJ, Sundel RP et al. Thalidomide for severe systemic onset juvenile rheumatoid arthritis: A multicenter study. *J Pediatr* 2004; 145: 856–857.

35. Wulffraat NM, van Rooijen EM, Tewarie R et al. Current perspectives of autologous stem cell transplantation for severe juvenile idiopathic arthritis. *Autoimmunity* 2008;41:632–838.

36. Ruperto N, Martini A. Emerging drugs to treat juvenile idiopathic arthritis. *Expert Opin Emerg Drugs* 2011;16:493–505.

37. Lovell DJ, Giannini EH, Reiff A et al. Etanercept in children with polyarticular juvenile rheumatoid arthritis. *N Engl J Med* 2000; 342:763–769.

38. Ruperto N, Lovell DJ, Cuttica R et al. A randomized, placebo-controlled trial of infliximab plus methotrexate for the treatment of polyarticular-course juvenile rheumatoid arthritis. *Arthritis Rheum* 2007;56:3096–3106.

39. Ruperto N, Lovell DJ, Quartier P et al. Abatacept in children with juvenile idiopathic arthritis: a randomised, double-blind, placebo-controlled withdrawal trial. *Lancet* 2008;372:383–391.

40. Lovell DJ, Ruperto N, Goodman S, Reiff A, Jung L, Jarosova K, et al. Adalimumab with or without methotrexate in juvenile rheumatoid arthritis. *N Engl J Med* 2008;359:810–820.

41. Pascual V, Allantaz F, Arce E, Punaro M, Banchereau J. Role of interleukin-1 (IL-1) in the pathogenesis of systemic onset juvenile idiopathic arthritis and clinical response to IL-1 blockade. *J Exp Med* 2005;201:1479–1486.

42. Quartier P, Allantaz F, Cimaz R et al. A multicentre, randomised, double-blind, placebo-controlled trial with the interleukin-1 receptor antagonist anakinra in patients with systemic-onset juvenile idiopathic arthritis (ANAJIS trial). *Ann Rheum Dis* 2011;70:747–754.

43. Woo P, Wilkinson N, Prieur AM et al. Open label phase II trial of single, ascending doses of MRA in Caucasian children with severe systemic juvenile idiopathic arthritis: proof of principle of the efficacy of IL-6 receptor blockade in this type of arthritis and demonstration of prolonged clinical improvement. *Arthritis Res Ther* 2005;7:R1281–R1288.

44. Yokota S, Imagawa T, Mori M et al. Efficacy and safety of tocilizumab in patients with systemic-onset juvenile idiopathic arthritis: a randomised, double-blind, placebo-controlled, withdrawal phase III trial. *Lancet* 2008;371:998–1006.

45. Ruperto N, Brunner HI, Quartier P et al. Canakinumab in systemic juvenile idiopathic arthritis: 2 randomized trials. *N Engl J Med* 2012;367:2396–2406.

46. De Benedetti F, Brunner HI, Ruperto N et al. Randomized trial of tocilizumab in systemic juvenile idiopathic arthritis. *N Engl J Med* 2012;367:2385–2395.

47. Prince FH, Twilt M, Simon SC et al. When and how to stop etanercept after successful treatment of patients with juvenile idiopathic arthritis. *Ann Rheum Dis* 2009;68:1228–1229.

48. Hashkes PJ, Uziel Y, Laxer RM. The safety profile of biologic therapies for juvenile idiopathic arthritis. *Nat Rev Rheumatol* 2010;6:561–571.

49. Ruperto N, Martini A. Pediatric rheumatology: JIA, treatment and possible risk of malignancies. *Nat Rev Rheumatol* 2011;7:6–7.

50. Richards JC, Tay-Kearney ML, Murray K, Manners P. Infliximab for juvenile idiopathic arthritis-associated uveitis. *Clin Exp Ophthalmol* 2005;33:461–468.

51. Simonini G, Taddio A, Cattalini M et al. Prevention of flare recurrences in childhood-refractory chronic uveitis: an open-label comparative study of adalimumab versus infliximab. *Arthritis Care Res* 2011;63:612–618.

52. Zulian F, Balzarin M, Falcini F et al. Abatacept for severe anti-tumor necrosis factor alpha refractory juvenile idiopathic arthritis-related uveitis. *Arthritis Care Res* 2010;62:821–825.

53. Bechtold S, Ripperger P, Hafner R, Said E, Schwarz HP. Growth hormone improves height in patients with juvenile idiopathic arthritis: 4-year data of a controlled study. *J Pediatr* 2003;143:512–519.

54. Saha MT, Haapasaari J, Hannula S, Sarna S, Lenko HL. Growth hormone is effective in the treatment of severe growth retardation in children with juvenile chronic arthritis. Double blind placebo-controlled followup study. *J Rheumatol* 2004;31:1413–1417.

55. Bianchi ML, Cimaz R, Bardare M et al. Efficacy and safety of alendronate for the treatment of osteoporosis in diffuse connective tissue diseases in children: a prospective multicenter study. *Arthritis Rheum* 2000;43:1960–1966.

56. Marini JC. Do bisphosphonates make children's bones better or brittle? *N Engl J Med* 2003;349:423–426.

57. Lovell DJ, Glass D, Ranz J et al. A randomized controlled trial of calcium supplementation to increase bone mineral density in children with juvenile rheumatoid arthritis. *Arthritis Rheum* 2006;54:2235–2242.

58. Hafner R, Spamer M. Rehabilitation of children. In: Isenberg DA, Maddison PJ, Woo P, Glass D, Breedveld FC. *Oxford textbook of rheumatology*, 3rd edn. Oxford University Press, Oxford, 2004:269–279.

59. Heijstek MW, Ott de Bruin LM, Bijl M et al. EULAR recommendations for vaccination in paediatric patients with rheumatic diseases. *Ann Rheum Dis* 2011;70:1704–1712.

60. White PH. Transition: a future promise for children and adolescents with special health care needs and disabilities. *Rheum Dis Clin North Am* 2002;28:687–703, viii.

61. Beukelman T, Patkar NM, Saag KG et al. 2011 American College of Rheumatology recommendations for the treatment of juvenile idiopathic arthritis: Initiation and safety monitoring of therapeutic agents for the treatment of arthritis and systemic features. *Arthritis Care Res* 2011;63:465–482.

62. Davies K, Cleary G, Foster H, Hutchinson E, Baildam E. BSPAR Standards of Care for children and young people with juvenile idiopathic arthritis. *Rheumatology* 2010;49:1406–1408.

63. Foster H, Rapley T. Access to pediatric rheumatology care—A major challenge to improving outcome in juvenile idiopathic arthritis. *J Rheumatol* 2010; 37:2199–2202.

64. Wallace CA. Developing standards of care for patients with juvenile idiopathic arthritis. *Rheumatology* 2010;49:1213–1214.

65. Beresford MW, Cleary AG, Foster HE et al. Comment on: Developing standards of care for patients with juvenile idiopathic arthritis. *Rheumatology* 2010;49:2227–2229.

CHAPTER 97

Anti-rheumatic drugs in pregnancy and lactation

Tarnya Marshall and Rita Abdulkader

Introduction

Autoimmune diseases affect males and females at childbearing ages. With the introduction of new agents, early aggressive disease control is possible early, but the influence on fertility, safety during pregnancy, and lactation are not yet fully understood.

The assessment of safety of drugs in pregnancy and during lactation relies on a limited body of evidence, based mainly on observational studies and case reports. Although studies in animals help inform experience, some drug effects prove to be species specific and extrapolation of this data to humans may be inappropriate. Additionally, when interpreting the effect of a drug and reports of adverse effects, two factors should be remembered:

◆ When the outcome of pregnancy exposed to a particular drug is considered, there is no 'normal' control group for comparison, and congenital malformation and other pregnancy-related complications could occur in the' normal' population.

◆ The effect of the underlying disease and its severity on the outcome of pregnancy need to be appreciated. This is usually difficult to predict and at times is not well described.

Although many women with autoimmune diseases notice improvement in their symptoms during pregnancy, some experience no improvement at all and some will have disease flares requiring treatment which may influence pregnancy outcomes. In general, if the disease control is achieved prior to pregnancy, this continues throughout pregnancy in most women provided they are compliant with appropriate treatment.[1]

Postpartum, however, autoimmune diseases tend to flare: for example 90% of rheumatoid arthritis (RA) patients will suffer a flare of their disease within 3 months of delivery,[2] requiring treatment that might affect the nursing infant.

In light of these issues, discussion should be undertaken early so that conception is planned. Patients of childbearing age should be counselled at drug initiation of the potential effects of their treatment on fertility and on the outcome of pregnancy if inadvertent exposure occurs.

The physician and patient should ideally plan future pregnancies, so that remission of the disease has been achieved where possible, that treatments compatible with pregnancy have been initiated, and that others with known risks to the fetus have been discontinued.

The decision to continue or stop any drugs in these patients should be taken on a case by case basis, after balancing the benefits of controlling active disease in the mother and the outcome of the pregnancy against possible risks to the fetus posed by the exposure to any drug.

Clearly, there is always a risk of an unplanned pregnancy resulting in inadvertent exposure to drugs. When this occurs, there should be a new literature review to establish emerging data, and discussion involving an obstetrician and the patient about the risks to the pregnancy. Further information can be sought about teratogenicity risk from the UK Teratology Information Services when drug exposure has occurred. Termination of pregnancy is not always indicated; however, close monitoring with screening for deformities is advisable in cases where the teratogenic risk of the key drugs is not clearly established or where there is significant risk.[3]

Non-steroidal anti-inflammatory drugs

Pregnancy

Population-based cohort studies show that the use of non-steroidal anti-inflammatory drugs (NSAIDs) in early pregnancy does not increase the risk of congenital deformities,[3] despite some reports of increased risk of cardiac septal defects, gastroschisis, and oral cleft associated with their use.[1,3] Additionally, there have been reports of increased risk of miscarriages in women taking NSAIDs, especially when these were used around the time of conception.[4,5]

The experience in women taking selective inhibitors of cyclooxygenase-2, however, has not been reported[3,4] and avoidance during pregnancy is recommended.[6]

Other than low-dose aspirin(<100 mg daily), the use of NSAIDs in late pregnancy was found to cause significant adverse effects in the fetus.[5] Administration of these drugs at this stage could lead to constriction and premature closure of the ductus arteriosus with reports of resulting pulmonary hypertension in the infant. NSAIDs may also impair renal function in the fetus, leading to reduced urine output and oligohydroamnios. These effects are evident from week 20 of pregnancy.[3,5] Additionally, there are reports of increased susceptibility to bleeding in newborns exposed to some NSAIDs and high-dose aspirin late in pregnancy, including central nervous system haemorrhage.[5] Current advice, therefore, is to discontinue NSAIDs by week 32 of pregnancy. Before this their use is relatively safe, especially if agents with a short half-life are used and with the lowest effective doses.[3,5]

There are reports of epidural haematomas in mothers undergoing epidural anaesthesia while taking low-dose aspirin. Some experts advise cessation of treatment a week before a planned delivery, but the individual risks should be assessed and aspirin continued if the risks of stopping aspirin, such as in anti-phospholipid syndrome, outweigh the risks of bleeding complications.[5]

Lactation

Aspirin should be avoided in breastfeeding women because of the risk of Reye's syndrome;[6] however, if continuing treatment is considered essential, then caution should be exercised especially with doses above 100 mg.[5] Other NSAIDs are considered compatible with breastfeeding.[2]

When prescribing NSAIDs for nursing mothers, drugs with a long half-life should be avoided,[2] and mothers should be advised to take the drug at or shortly after breastfeeding to reduce the exposure of the infant to these drugs.[2,5] Ibuprofen in particular is preferred because of its short half-life and very low excretion in breast milk.[2,4]

Fertility

The effects of NSAIDs on fertility are uncertain. Their use has been implicated in reports of impaired fertility in women[4]; this is theoretically related to the role of cyclooxygenase enzymes in the rupture of the luteinized follicle.[3,4] However, the prevalence and significance of the luteinized unruptured follicle syndrome (LUFS) in women using NSAIDS remains to be established.[3]

Women attempting to conceive should preferably use NSAIDS intermittently and infrequently. Discontinuation of treatment should be considered in a woman who has had difficulty conceiving.[3,4]

Corticosteroids

Pregnancy

Placental transfer of corticosteroids varies according to their structure, leading to differences in fetal exposure to these drugs. Non-fluorinated corticosteroids such as prednisolone and methylprednisolone are subject to extensive metabolism by the placenta, resulting in only 10% of the maternal dose reaching the fetus.[5,7] On the other hand, fluorinated corticosteroids such as betamethasone and dexamethasone are less metabolized in the placenta, allowing significant effects on the fetus. When corticosteroids are used for maternal indications, non-fluorinated agents should be used to minimize unnecessary in-utero exposure.

In addition to those side effects encountered in non-pregnant patients, there are also pregnancy-related side effects, such as an increased risk of premature rupture of the membranes.[5,7] Although the use of corticosteroids does not cause an increased frequency of infections in newborn babies, prolonged high doses (>15 mg prednisolone) may lead to an increased risk of intrauterine infection.[3,5]

The use of corticosteroids in pregnancy is not associated with major teratogenic effect. Only rarely are cataract and adrenal suppression reported in infants exposed to high-dose corticosteroids.[5]

However, there has been concern about a small increase in the risk of cleft palate/cleft lip with corticosteroid use in the first trimester. This concern was raised by a meta-analysis which reported a 3.3-fold increase in the odds ratio of cleft lip and/or palate after first-trimester exposure to corticosteroids.[8] This was not supported by subsequent studies. At worst, therefore, the risk would increase the incidence from 1/1000 in the general population to 3/1000.[4]

There is conflicting evidence regarding the relationship between administration of corticosteroids during pregnancy and low birthweight. The difficulty arises from separating the complications of the underlying maternal disease requiring treatment, and the effects of the drugs.[3,5] A dose of 5–15 mg of prednisolone daily does not seem to increase the risk of intrauterine growth restriction.[3]

On balance, when steroids are needed, the lowest effective dose should be administered especially during early pregnancy. The mother should be monitored closely for side effects of treatment, and consideration should be given to adding calcium and vitamin D supplements if corticosteroid treatment throughout pregnancy is required.

Finally, a stress dose should be considered in cases of acute illness and in the peripartum period.[3]

Lactation

There is no evidence that the small amounts of corticosteroids excreted in breast milk have an adverse effect on the nursing infant. Therefore they are considered compatible with breastfeeding.[2,5]

In patients taking high doses of corticosteroids, a period of 4 hours between administration and breast feeding is recommended to minimize the infant's exposure to these drugs.[5,7]

As in pregnancy, consideration should be given to calcium and vitamin D supplements.

Fertility

There are no reports of corticosteroids having an adverse effect on fertility.[7]

Hydroxychloroquine

Hydroxychloroquine is an anti-malarial drug with mild disease-modifying actions in RA and causes a reduction in systemic lupus erythematosus (SLE) of fatigue, skin, arthralgia, and mucous membrane symptoms.

Pregnancy

Although hydroxychloroquine crosses the placenta, there is no evidence of toxicity in the fetus at the doses used in treating rheumatic diseases. Although the drug manufacturer advises against treatment with hydroxychloroquine during pregnancy in the summary of product characteristics (SPC), this is not borne out in clinical practice. In animal studies, ototoxicity and retinal pigmentation have been described but these have not been reported in human pregnancies when children were followed up to 26 months of age.[4,9]

Successful pregnancy outcome in SLE is dependent on tight disease control, and several studies have shown that discontinuing treatment in pregnant lupus patients is detrimental to disease control, with an increase in disease flares reported. In those patients who continue hydroxychloroquine, lower maintenance doses of prednisolone are required.[10]

Lactation

Although hydroxychloroquine is excreted in breast milk, levels are very low and are not thought to be sufficient to cause infant toxicity. Guidance from national bodies is conflicting, with the American Academy of Paediatrics[11] advocating continuing therapy, whereas British Society for Rheumatology (BSR) guidance advocates stopping treatment.[6,12]

Risk and benefits of treatment should be discussed with the patient, and if they wish to continue breastfeeding this should be done with caution, recognizing that autoimmune disease often flares postpartum.

Fertility

There are no reports of adverse effects on fertility.

Sulfasalazine

Most of the evidence available for sulfasalazine in pregnancy and lactation is derived from studies in patients with inflammatory bowel disease.

Pregnancy

Sulfasalazine is known to inhibit the absorption and metabolism of folic acid. Therefore, adequate folate supplements should be given to the expectant mother before and during pregnancy. Although sulfasalazine crosses the placental barrier, it seems to have little effect on the fetus.[13] It is advised, however, that the dose used does not exceed 2 g/day during pregnancy.[5]

There have been scattered case reports of congenital malformation in children of mothers taking sulfasalazine during pregnancy, but the direct association with sulfasalazine remains to be established.[13,14] Additionally, a case of fetal haemolytic anaemia has been described, in which intrauterine blood transfusion was required.[15] However, the majority of published data has found no association with congenital malformations, or increased risk of kernicterus in full-term newborn infants.[16–18]

Lactation

Sulfasalazine use is considered safe in nursing mothers,[1,11] despite its excretion at low levels in breast milk. There appears no link with kernicterus in full-term infants.[16] Caution is advised, however, in premature babies and those deficient in glucose-6-phosphate dehydrogenase (G6PD).[6] There is one case report of bloody diarrhoea in an infant breastfed by a mother prescribed sulfasalazine in whom no other cause could be found.[19]

Fertility

Sulfasalazine use results in reversible infertility in men due to oligospermia, reduced sperm motility, and increased abnormal sperm forms.

A drug-free period of 3 months is recommended prior to conception as it may take up to 2.5 months for normal spermatogenesis and therefore fertility to return.[20,21] Additionally, there may be an increased risk of congenital abnormalities in the offspring of these men during this period.[22]

Methotrexate

Pregnancy

The majority of data is from patients treated with high-dose methotrexate for malignancy; much less is known about pregnancy in women taking low doses. In high doses, methotrexate is known to be teratogenic and as a result, it is sensible to advise against pregnancy in patients on lower doses.

Studies in animals showed that methotrexate is embryotoxic. Exposure to methotrexate during the first trimester is associated with increased risk of fetal death, and a risk of major congenital anomalies, including craniofacial and limb defects; severe neurological anomalies such as anencephaly, hydrocephaly, and meningomyelocele; and growth retardation.[3,23]

Methotrexate is retained in tissue for months after administration and should therefore be discontinued at least 3 months before attempting conception.[6] The manufacturer takes a more cautious opinion and advises a 6 month interval. Women should continue folic acid supplements prior to and during pregnancy.

Lactation

Methotrexate should be avoided during breastfeeding. It is present in breast milk, and may accumulate in the infant tissues.[11]

Fertility

Methotrexate does not appear to affect female fertility. In men, a reversible effect on fertility has been described,[24] although this may have been due to the effect of other coprescribed medicines.[25] It remains to be established whether methotrexate in men is teratogenic, so current advice is to stop treatment for at least 3 months prior to conception.[6]

Leflunomide

Pregnancy

Leflunomide is contraindicated in pregnancy as animal studies have shown marked teratogenicity. In rats, skeletal and central nervous system deformities, in addition to low birthweight and increased death rate after birth, are reported in pregnancies with leflunomide exposure.[4] Data for safety in human pregnancies is restricted mostly to case reports. Although no fetal abnormalities have been described, the current recommendation on the basis of animal studies is to avoid treatment in pregnancy.

Leflunomide's active metabolite A77 1726 is slowly eliminated and levels can be detected in plasma for up to 2 years after the last dose.[1] Patients who wish to consider a pregnancy should be advised to stop leflunomide for at least 2 years before conception, although a washout procedure can be undertaken to accelerate elimination using agents such as colestyramine or activated charcoal. This requires 11 days of colestyramine, an unpalatable agent, in a dosage of 8 g three times a day, or charcoal at a dose of 50 g four times a day. With either procedure, the active metabolite concentration should be measured on two occasions 14 days apart, and its concentration should be less than 20 µg/litre before attempting conception by men or women.[6] The washout procedure is also advised in the event of unplanned pregnancy in women prescribed leflunomide. For women using oral contraception and requiring washout, it should be pointed out that the absorption of oestrogen and progesterone may also be affected, and that additional contraceptive methods are required.[26,27]

Lactation

The effects of leflunomide on the nursing infant are not known; it is therefore contraindicated during lactation.

Fertility

There are no known adverse effects of leflunomide on fertility in women; in men it may cause a reversible reduction in sperm count. Men taking leflunomide are advised that reliable contraception should be used, and that a washout procedure as outlined above should be performed 3 months before conception.

Azathioprine

Azathioprine is a prodrug. It is metabolized in the liver to 6-mercaptopurine, its active metabolite.

Pregnancy

Animal studies have shown potential teratogenicity, but there is no recurrent pattern of congenital anomalies reported in humans.[4] Most of the available data are derived from transplant patients and those with inflammatory bowel disease. Although an increased risk of intrauterine growth restriction and preterm delivery are reported, these could be related to disease severity rather than an effect of the drug.[4] Azathioprine and its metabolites are found in low concentrations in fetal blood after administration to the mother. The fetal liver is deficient in inosinate pyrophosphorylase, the enzyme required to convert azathioprine to its active metabolite; this may shield the fetus from harmful effects.[7,28] A decision to continue treatment during pregnancy should follow a careful assessment of risk vs benefit and a discussion with the patient.

In mothers continuing treatment, it is best to restrict the dose to 2 mg/kg or less to avoid haematopoietic suppression in the newborn.[3]

Lactation

Azathioprine is present in breast milk in low concentrations but it does not cause harm in the neonate and is therefore considered safe during lactation.[1] In one study there was no increased risk of infection in the breastfed offspring of mothers taking azathoprine and all children had mental and physical progress suitable for age in early childhood.[29]

Fertility

Azathioprine does not affect fertility in men or women. There is no convincing evidence of teratogenicity in men who father children during treatment.[30]

Mycophenolate mofetil

Mycophenolate mofetil is metabolized to mycophenolic acid. Most of the available data in pregnancy are derived from its use in organ transplant patients.

Pregnancy

Evidence from case reports and animal models suggests that mycophenolate mofetil is teratogenic, and it is therefore contraindicated in pregnancy and patients should stop treatment at least 6 weeks prior to conception.

Exposure to mycophenolate mofetil during pregnancy may result in low birthweight, premature birth, and an increased incidence of birth defects.[1] The most observed deformities involve the mouth (microtia, cleft lip and palate, micrognathia), ear (auditory canal atresia), fingers (short fingers and hypoplastic nails), and eyes (hypertelorism, ocular coloboma). There are also reports of renal, central nervous system, diaphragmatic, and cardiovascular malformations.

A distinctive phenotype has been described with in-utero exposure to mycophenolate mofetil: EMFO tetrada (ear, mouth, finger, ocular/organ malformations).[31]

Breastfeeding

Animal studies confirm that mycophenolate mofetil is excreted in breast milk. It should therefore be avoided in breastfeeding mothers.[6]

Fertility

Mycophenolate mofetil is not associated with reduced fertility in either men or women and does not adversely affect spermatogenesis. Drug company files (Roche Pharma, safety update) reported the outcome of 45 pregnancies where paternal mycophenolate mofetil exposure occurred. In this series, six cases of fetal malformations were described: foot, mouth, bladder, and chromosomal. Although the association with treatment is difficult to confirm, the incidence of abnormalities is high and the current advice for men is to stop mycophenolate mofetil for at least 3 months prior to conception.[5]

Ciclosporin

The data for the safety of ciclosporin in pregnancy and lactation are mainly derived from the transplant literature.

Ciclosporin passes the placental barrier, but its use has not been shown to increase the incidence of birth defects in exposed infants. This is supported by data from the United States National Transplantation Pregnancy Registry.[32] A meta-analysis reporting 410 pregnancies with history of exposure to ciclosporin also found no increase in risk of congenital malformations. The odds ratio for low birthweight and prematurity did not achieve statistical significance; however, they are reported at a rate of 56.3%. It is difficult to ascertain if this rate is related to the underlying disease or the influence of the drug.[5,33]

Ciclosporin could therefore be continued during pregnancy, preferably at the lowest effective dose, if the benefit of continuing the drug outweighs the risks. Maternal blood pressure and renal function should be even more closely monitored than usual during pregnancy. Where ciclosporin can be stopped, advice is to discontinue therapy at least 6 weeks prior to conception.[1]

Lactation

Ciclosporin is present in breast milk; there are reports of patients continuing treatment while nursing with no significant adverse effects.[2] However, there are insufficient safety data and the consensus is that breastfeeding should be avoided in women taking ciclosporin.[11]

Fertility

There are no reports of adverse effects on fertility in women.

Although ciclosporin has been shown to cause reversible impairment of testicular function and reduced fertility in rats,[34,35] this has not been observed in men.[36] However, unexplained infertility may warrant a break from therapy if clinically appropriate. There are no reports of male-mediated teratogenicity relating to the use of ciclosporin, and the decision to continue treatment while attempting conception should be tailored to the individual patient.

Cyclophosphamide

Cyclophosphamide is absolutely contraindicated in the first trimester of pregnancy; women should use a reliable contraceptive method during treatment and for 3 months afterwards.

Cyclophosphamide teratogenicity has been demonstrated in animal studies and observed in human pregnancies.[5] Although the administration of cyclophosphamide in the first trimester does not always result in fetal anomalies,[5] significant birth defects are observed with its use, including craniofacial, distal limb, ear, and visceral malformations, in addition to growth retardation.[5,7]

Cyclophosphamide use after the first trimester should only be considered if there is a significant risk to the life of the expectant mother from the underlying disease.[4,7] Although it is not associated with structural defects in the fetus, it may result in adverse effect on the infant's later neurological development, and may also cause growth delay and bone marrow suppression.[5] The outcome of these pregnancies is likely to be poor for the fetus, possibly reflecting the severity of the underlying maternal disease.[4]

Lactation

Cyclophosphamide is excreted in breast milk; therefore women receiving treatment should avoid breastfeeding during and for 36 hours after treatment.[6,11]

Fertility

There are isolated reports of birth defects in the babies born to fathers treated with cyclophosphamide. A causative relationship has not been proven, but men should be advised to avoid conception during treatment and for 3 months after.[1,5]

Cyclophosophamide has toxic effects on reproduction in men and women. These are present with both oral and intravenous administration. In women there is a risk of up to 40% of permanent amenorrhoea due to cyclophosphamide treatment. This risk is mainly related to cumulative dose and the age of the patient, being lowest below the age of 25, and highest above the age of 31.[5] In one study, permanent amenorrhoea was observed in 12% of women who were treated with 7 doses of cyclophosphamide (0.5–1.0 g/m^2 body surface area) increasing to 39% of women treated with 15 doses. There was also a significant increase in the incidence of amenorrhoea with age independent of the dose prescribed.[37] In men, on the other hand, the risk of infertility is unpredictable and can occur at any age, and at any dose.[5]

If time allows, men and women should be offered fertility preservation measures, such as cryopreservation and sperm banking. Additionally, the use of gonadotropin-releasing hormone agonists (GnRHa) in women may help protect the ovarian function; although the evidence for its use is still developing, it is unlikely to be associated with harm and, in our opinion, should be considered in patients below 40 years of age should a future pregnancy be desirable.[38,39]

Gold

Gold compounds should be avoided during pregnancy as they cross the placenta and have been detected in fetal tissues.[6,7] Gold is also excreted in breast milk and is absorbed by the nursing infant; it should be therefore avoided in breastfeeding mothers.[6]

Penicillamine

Penicillamine is teratogenic in animal studies. Serious connective tissue abnormalities are reported in babies exposed to penicillamine in utero. It should be avoided in pregnant and breastfeeding patients.[6,7]

Biological agents

The data regarding biological treatment in pregnancy and lactation are limited as these are relatively new agents. Placental transfer differs between agents and depends on the molecular structure of the drug. For example, monoclonal antibodies are transferred by the placenta increasingly in the second and third trimesters, whereas fusion proteins have much less placental transfer, which in turn is minimal for agents that do not contain the fragment crystallizable region (Fc) of the immunoglobulin.[40]

The safety of biologics in pregnancy is collected via national registries and case reports, and as tumour necrosis factor alpha (TNFα) inhibitors were developed ahead of newer agents, more data is available for their safety. The need for ongoing treatment with biologic agents during pregnancy should be assessed on an individual basis following discussion with the patient.

TNFα inhibitors

Experience with TNFα inhibitors in pregnancy is limited. The data come from case reports, small case series, some controlled studies, and drug registries.

The BSR guidelines advise precaution in pregnancy for both men and women.[41] Therapy should only be continued if the risk of stopping is perceived to be high. In those cases where treatment is continued, monoclonal antibodies should be stopped by week 30, due to significant transplacental transfer. The long-term effects of in-utero exposure remain to be established.[40]

There is some controversy around the association of TNFα inhibitor use with VACTER (vertebral, anal, cardiac, tracheal, oesophageal, renal) anomalies. This was reported by one study which found an increase in congenital VACTER spectrum in women treated with infliximab or etanercept in early pregnancy.[42] Due to flaws in methodology and design, most experts agree that no association could be deduced from this study between TNFα inhibitors and fetal abnormalities. The lack of association with birth defects is also borne out in the literature of TNFα inhibitors in patients with inflammatory bowel disease.[43,44]

Despite the lack of evidence for teratogenicity with the use of these treatments, there may be an increased risk of miscarriage and fetal loss. Whether this is the effect of TNFα inhibitors or the underlying disease process remains unclear. Some studies showed no difference in miscarriage in pregnancies with history of exposure to TNFα inhibitors comparing to non-exposed pregnancies.[3]

However, the British Society for Rheumatology Biologics Register (BSRBR) has reported the outcome of 130 pregnancies in patients exposed to TNFα inhibitor treatment before or at conception. An increased rate of spontaneous abortion was noted among patients who received TNFα treatment. These women have severe disease to be able to access biological therapy, as defined by NICE, but levels of disease activity have not to date been reported in this cohort of women and this may be a confounding factor.[45]

Fertility

TNFα inhibitors have not been shown so far to have any adverse effects on fertility or male-mediated teratogenicity.

Etanercept

Etanercept is recombinant human TNF receptor (p75) Fc fusion protein.

Manufacturer advice

The manufacturer advises discontinuing etanercept at least 3 weeks before conception, and to avoid breastfeeding during treatment.

Pregnancy

Etanercept is not teratogenic in animals. Very low levels of etanercept cross the placenta, possibly due to the low affinity of etanercept to neonatal IgG transporter (FcRn).[40]

As discussed earlier, the suggestion of an association with VACTER anomalies with etanercept has been given little weight so far.

Lactation

Etanercept is present in breast milk in low levels. It is unlikely to have significant effects on the nursing infant. However, the current advice from the manufacturer is to avoid breastfeeding while receiving treatment.[40,46]

Adalimumab

Manufacturer advice

The manufacturer advises avoiding treatment during pregnancy and lactation, and discontinuing treatment for up to 5 months before conception in women and before commencing breastfeeding.

Pregnancy

In animals, it does not seem that adalimumab results in birth defects. Cases of successful human pregnancies while exposed to adalimumab were reported with no harmful effects on the fetus.[28]

Breastfeeding

There is insufficient data about the safety of the administration of adalimumab while breastfeeding. It is not also known if adalimumab is absorbed by the nursing infant after ingestion. The manufacturer advises discontinuation of treatment for at least 5 months before commencing breastfeeding.

Fertility

No adverse effects were reported.

Infliximab

Infliximab is a chimeric IgG1 monoclonal antibody to TNFα.

Pregnancy

The current advice from the manufacturer is to stop treatment 6 months before conception. If continuing treatment is deemed necessary, ongoing treatment is not recommended beyond the latter part of the second trimester.

Infliximab does not appear to cause congenital malformation in the fetus. It does not actively cross the placenta during the first trimester, but it is transferred during late second and third trimester. It is detectable in newborn serum for a few months after delivery.[40]

The limited available data does not show an association with increased infection risk. However concern has been raised about live vaccinations in young children, which should be delayed at least 6 months after delivery, if treatment was continued during pregnancy.[47] There is one case report of fatal disseminated Bacille Calmette–Guérin (BCG) infection after BCG vaccination in a 4.5 month old baby exposed to infliximab in utero throughout pregnancy.[48]

Lactation

Infliximab is present in breast milk. Case reports of patients continuing treatment while on infliximab revealed no adverse effect, however. The manufacturer advises no breastfeeding for 6 months after discontinuation.

Certulizumab

Certulizumab is a Fab fragment of an anti-TNFα monoclonal antibody.

Pregnancy

The current advice from the manufacturer is not to use certulizumab during pregnancy, and to use contraception up to 5 months after the last dose.

Data about the use in pregnancy is limited to few case reports with favourable outcomes.[40] There is no evidence of teratogenic effect in animal studies. Additionally, no transfer across the placenta was noted in rats. Unlike whole IgG antibodies, certulizumb lacks the Fc region necessary for active transfer across the placenta. Theoretically, certulizumab may have advantages over other TNFα inhibitors because of this, although this is an area for further research.[28,40]

Lactation

It is not known if certulizumab is excreted in breast milk, and breastfeeding should therefore be avoided in women receiving treatment.

Fertility

The manufacturer reports a trend on reduced sperm count with effect on motility in rodents with no effect on fertility. The significance of this in humans is still to be established.

Golimumab

The manufacturer advises adequate contraception and avoiding breastfeeding for 6 months after the last dose.

Pregnancy

No harm has been demonstrated in animal studies. There is limited data in humans and use during pregnancy should be considered only if essential.[6]

Lactation

Golimumab is present in milk in animal studies, although this is yet to be established in women. The manufacturer advises avoiding breastfeeding for 6 months after the last dose.

Fertility

No data available.

Rituximab

Rituximab is a monoclonal B-cell-depleting antibody.

Pregnancy

The manufacturer advises avoiding pregnancy and breastfeeding for 12 months after treatment as rituximab crosses the placenta. Animal studies revealed no evidence of teratogenicity, but experience in human pregnancies is limited. The effects of exposure early in the pregnancy are not yet clear. Case reports have shown that exposure during the second and third trimester resulted in serum levels of rituximab similar to the mother's, and was associated with B-cell depletion in the newborn.[40] Spontaneous recovery of B-cell numbers was complete within 6 months.[3] The long-term effects of this early B-cell depletion are not known.

Rituximab should, therefore, be avoided during pregnancy unless benefit to the mother outweighs possible risks to the baby, otherwise contraception should be recommended up to 12 months after the last dose.[6]

Lactation

Rituximab is excreted in animal milk. Breastfeeding should be avoided for 12 months after treatment, as advised by the manufacturer.

Abatacept

Abatacept is a CTLA4 and human immunoglobulin fusion protein which acts as a selective costimulation modulator inhibiting the activation of T cells.

Pregnancy

There are insufficient data about the use of abatacept in human pregnancies. In animal studies there is no evidence of teratogenicity. Limited changes in the immune function were noted in rats at 11 times a human dose of 10 mg/kg.[49] Current advice is to avoid unless treatment is essential[6]; patients should be advised to use contraception up to 14 weeks after the last dose (manufacturer's advice).

Lactation

It is not clear if abatacept is excreted in human milk. The current advice from the manufacturer is to discontinue treatment 14 weeks before breastfeeding.

Fertility

No adverse effects on fertility are noted in animal studies; there are no available data in humans.

Anakinra

Anakinra is the recombinant form of the human interleukin-1 receptor (IL-1R) antagonist.

There are insufficient data about safety in human pregnancy, although there is no evidence of harm in animal studies. Current advice is to avoid treatment during pregnancy. Additionally, patients should be advised to use contraception during treatment.

Lactation

It is yet to be established if anakinra is excreted in human milk, and breastfeeding should be avoided during treatment.

Tocilizumab

Tocilizumab is an interlukin-6 receptor (IL-6R) monoclonal antibody.

Pregnancy

The manufacturer advises stopping treatment 3 months before conception. The *British National Formulary* (BNF), however, advises 6 months before conception.

Animal studies revealed increased risk of spontaneous abortions and fetal death at a high dose. There is some emerging data about the safety of tocilizumab in human pregnancy, but these are still insufficient to recommend its safety.

Lactation

It remains to be established if tocilizumab is excreted in breast milk and there are insufficient safety data in breastfed infants to date.

References

1. Watts R, Clunie G, Hall F, Marshall T (eds). *Oxford desk reference: Rheumatology*. Oxford University Press, New York, 2009.
2. Østensen M, Motta M. Therapy insight: the use of antirheumatic drugs during nursing. *Nat Clin Pract Rheumatol* 2007;3(7):400–406.
3. Østensen M, Förger F. Management of RA medications in pregnant patients. *Nat Rev Rheumatol* 2009;5(7):382–390.
4. Elliott AB, Chakravarty EF. Immunosuppressive medications during pregnancy and lactation in women with autoimmune diseases. *Womens Health* (Lond Engl) 2010;6(3):431–440.
5. Østensen M, Khamashta M, Lockshin M et al. Anti-inflammatory and immunosuppressive drugs and reproduction. *Arthritis Res Ther* 2006;8(3):209.
6. Joint Formulary Committee. *British national formulary*, 61st edn. British Medical Association and Royal Pharmaceutical Society, London, 2011.
7. Janssen NM, Genta MS. The effects of immunosuppressive and anti-inflammatory medications on fertility, pregnancy, and lactation. *Arch Intern Med* 2000;160(5):610–619.
8. Park-Wyllie L, Mazzotta P, Pastuszak A et al. Birth defects after maternal exposure to corticosteroids: prospective cohort study and meta-analysis of epidemiological studies. *Teratology* 2000;62(6):385–392.
9. Costedoat-Chalumeau N, Amoura Z et al. Safety of hydroxychloroquine in pregnant patients with connective tissue diseases: a study of one hundred thirty-three cases compared with a control group. *Arthritis Rheum* 2003;48(11):3207–3211.
10. Clowse ME, Magder L, Witter F, Petri M. Hydroxychloroquine in lupus pregnancy. *Arthritis Rheum* 2006;54(11):3640–3647.
11. American Academy of Pediatrics Committee on Drugs. Transfer of drugs and other chemicals into human milk. Pediatrics 2001;108(3):776–789.
12. Chakravarty K, McDonald H, Pullar T et al. BSR/BHPR guideline for disease-modifying anti-rheumatic drug (DMARD) therapy in consultation with the British Association of Dermatologists. *Rheumatology* (Oxford). 2008;47(6):924–925.
13. Brar H, Einarson A. Effects and treatment of inflammatory bowel disease during pregnancy. *Can Fam Physician* 2008;54(7):981–983.
14. Newman NM, Correy JF. Possible teratogenicity of sulphasalazine. *Med J Aust* 1983;1(11):528–529.
15. Bokström H, Holst RM, Hafström O et al. Fetal hemolytic anemia associated with maternal sulfasalazine therapy during pregnancy. *Acta Obstet Gynecol Scand* 2006;85(1):118–121.
16. Esbjörner E, Järnerot G, Wranne L. Sulphasalazine and sulphapyridine serum levels in children to mothers treated with sulphasalazine during pregnancy and lactation. *Acta Paediatr Scand* 1987;76(1):137–142.
17. Nørgård B, Czeizel AE, Rockenbauer M, Olsen J, Sørensen HT. Population-based case control study of the safety of sulfasalazine use during pregnancy. *Aliment Pharmacol Ther* 2001;15(4):483–486.

18. Willoughby CP, Truelove SC. Ulcerative colitis and pregnancy. *Gut* 1980;21(6):469–474.

19. Branski D, Kerem E, Gross-Kieselstein E et al. Bloody diarrhea—a possible complication of sulfasalazine transferred through human breast milk. *J Pediatr Gastroenterol Nutr* 1986;5(2):316–317.

20. O'Moráin C, Smethurst P, Doré CJ, Levi AJ. Reversible male infertility due to sulphasalazine: studies in man and rat. *Gut* 1984;25(10):1078–1084.

21. Toovey S, Hudson E, Hendry WF, Levi AJ. Sulphasalazine and male infertility: reversibility and possible mechanism. *Gut* 1981;22(6):445–451.

22. Moody GA, Probert C, Jayanthi V, Mayberry JF. The effects of chronic ill health and treatment with sulphasalazine on fertility amongst men and women with inflammatory bowel disease in Leicestershire. *Int J Colorectal Dis* 1997;12(4):220–224.

23. Corona-Rivera JR, Rea-Rosas A, Santana-Ramírez A et al. Holoprosencephaly and genitourinary anomalies in fetal methotrexate syndrome. *Am J Med Genet A* 2010;152A(7):1741–1746.

24. Heetun ZS, Byrnes C, Neary P, O'Morain C. Review article: Reproduction in the patient with inflammatory bowel disease. *Aliment Pharmacol Ther* 2007;26(4):513–533.

25. French AE, Koren G; Motherisk Team. Effect of methotrexate on male fertility. *Can Fam Physician* 2003;49:577–578.

26. Electronic Medicines Compendium (eMC). Summary of product characteristics for Arava 10, 20 and 100mg tablets. Datapharm Communications, Leatherhead. [updated 12/05/2011; cited 09/09/2011]. Available at: www.medicines.org.uk/EMC/medicine/7480/SPC/Arava+10%2c+20+and+100mg+Tablets/

27. Electronic Medicines Compendium (eMC). Summary of product characteristics for leflunomide film-coated tablets. Datapharm Communications, Leatherhead. [updated 14/07/2011;cited 09/09/2011]. Available at: www.medicines.org.uk/EMC/medicine/24155/SPC/Leflunomide+film-coated+tablets/

28. Gisbert JP. Safety of immunomodulators and biologics for the treatment of inflammatory bowel disease during pregnancy and breast-feeding. *Inflamm Bowel Dis* 2010;16(5):881–895.

29. Angelberger S, Reinisch W, Messerschmidt A et al. Long-term follow-up of babies exposed to azathioprine in utero and via breastfeeding. *J Crohns Colitis* 2011;5(2):95–100.

30. Heetun ZS, Byrnes C, Neary P, O'Morain C. Review article: Reproduction in the patient with inflammatory bowel disease. *Aliment Pharmacol Ther* 2007;26(4):513–533.

31. Merlob P, Stahl B, Klinger G. Tetrada of the possible mycophenolate mofetil embryopathy: a review. *Reprod Toxicol* 2009;28(1):105–108.

32. Armenti VT, Radomski JS, Moritz MJ et al. Report from the National Transplantation Pregnancy Registry (NTPR): outcomes of pregnancy after transplantation. *Clin Transpl* 2004:103–114.

33. Bar Oz B, Hackman R, Einarson T, Koren G. Pregnancy outcome after cyclosporine therapy during pregnancy: a meta-analysis. *Transplantation* 2001;71(8):1051–1055.

34. Hisatomi A, Fujihira S, Fujimoto Y et al. Effect of Prograf (FK506) on spermatogenesis in rats. *Toxicology* 1996;109(2–3):75–83

35. Seethalakshmi L, Flores C, Khauli RB, Diamond DA, Menon M. Evaluation of the effect of experimental cyclosporine toxicity on

male reproduction and renal function. Reversal by concomitant human chorionic gonadotropin administration. *Transplantation* 1990;49(1):17–19.

36. Xu L, Han S, Liu Y et al. The influence of immunosuppressants on the fertility of males who undergo renal transplantation and on the immune function of their offspring. *Transpl Immunol* 2009;22(1-2):28–31.

37. Boumpas DT, Austin HA 3rd, Vaughan EM et al. Risk for sustained amenorrhea in patients with systemic lupus erythematosus receiving intermittent pulse cyclophosphamide therapy. *Ann Intern Med* 1993;119(5):366–369.

38. von Wolff M, Montag M, Dittrich R et al. Fertility preservation in women—a practical guide to preservation techniques and therapeutic strategies in breast cancer, Hodgkin's lymphoma and borderline ovarian tumours by the fertility preservation network FertiPROTEKT. *Arch Gynecol Obstet* 2011;284(2):427–435.

39. Clowse ME, Behera MA, Anders CK et al. Ovarian preservation by GnRH agonists during chemotherapy: a meta-analysis. *J Womens Health (Larchmt)* 2009;18(3):311–319.

40. Ostensen M, Förger F. Treatment with biologics of pregnant patients with rheumatic diseases. *Curr Opin Rheumatol* 2011;23(3):293–298.

41. Ding T, Ledingham J, Luqmani R et al. Standards, Audit and Guidelines Working Group of BSR Clinical Affairs Committee; BHPR. BSR and BHPR rheumatoid arthritis guidelines on safety of anti-TNF therapies. *Rheumatology* (Oxford) 2010;49(11):2217–2219.

42. Carter JD, Ladhani A, Ricca LR, Valeriano J, Vasey FB. A safety assessment of tumor necrosis factor antagonists during pregnancy: a review of the Food and Drug Administration database. *J Rheumatol* 2009;36(3):635–641.

43. Schnitzler F, Fidder H, Ferrante M et al. Outcome of pregnancy in women with inflammatory bowel disease treated with antitumor necrosis factor therapy. *Inflamm Bowel Dis* 2011;17(9):1846–1854.

44. Zelinkova Z, de Haar C, de Ridder L et al. High intra-uterine exposure to infliximab following maternal anti-TNF treatment during pregnancy. *Aliment Pharmacol Ther* 2011;33(9):1053–1058.

45. Verstappen SM, King Y, Watson KD, Symmons DP, Hyrich KL; BSRBR Control Centre Consortium, BSR Biologics Register. Anti-TNF therapies and pregnancy: outcome of 130 pregnancies in the British Society for Rheumatology Biologics Register. *Ann Rheum Dis* 2011;70(5):823–826.

46. Keeling S, Wolbink GJ. Measuring multiple etanercept levels in the breast milk of a nursing mother with rheumatoid arthritis. *J Rheumatol* 2010;37(7):1551.

47. Djokanovic N, Klieger-Grossmann C, Pupco A, Koren G. Safety of infliximab use during pregnancy. *Reprod Toxicol* 2011;32(1):93–97.

48. Cheent K, Nolan J, Shariq S, Kiho L, Pal A, Arnold J. Case report: fatal case of disseminated BCG infection in an infant born to a mother taking infliximab for Crohn's disease. *J Crohns Colitis* 2010;4(5):603–605.

49. Electronic Medicines Compendium (eMC). Summary of product characteristics for ORENCIA 250 mg powder for concentrate for solution for infusion. Datapharm Communications, Leatherhead. [updated 06/07/2011; cited 09/09/2011].Available at: www.medicines.org.uk/EMC/medicine/19714/SPC/ORENCIA+250+mg+powder+for+concentrate+for+solution+for+infusion/

Infection in rheumatic disease

SECTION 9

Infection in
rheumatic disease

CHAPTER 98

Septic arthritis in adults

Laura McGregor, Monica N. Gupta, and Max Field

Infections in native joints

Epidemiology

The sudden onset of monoarthritis in a synovial joint can arise from a variety of causes (Table 98.1) but the most likely is trauma or inflammation. Acute joint pain and swelling should always be regarded as a significant clinical event because joint infection has a high morbidity[1] and 11% mortality.[2] The incidence of septic arthritis (SA) in Europe is estimated to be 4–10 per 100 000 patient years per year.[3] However, these figures may be an underestimate because many analyses fail to take account of patients with negative microbiology in whom SA is suspected. The recent rising incidence may be due to an ageing population, increased use of immunosuppressant therapy, and increased surgical intervention. Five-year survival is poor irrespective of whether bacteria are isolated from synovial fluid or not, with over 30% mortality in each group.[4]

Risk factors

Although children are susceptible, SA occurs at any age. Adult patients, especially those with underlying joint disease, including osteoarthritis (OA) and in particular rheumatoid arthritis (RA), are at greater risk. Social deprivation[2] and increasing age are also risk factors. Currently 17% of the United Kingdom population is over 65 years of age, a figure due to rise to 23% by 2035,[5] suggesting that SA incidence is likely to increase. Elderly patients are also more likely to have undergone joint replacement surgery, and by 2010 an estimated 6% of the United Kingdom population will have undergone arthroplasty.[6] The elderly population are also more likely to have comorbidities that predispose to SA, including diabetes mellitus, malignancy, and renal disease (especially haemodialysis patients). In addition, recurrent infections of respiratory or urinary tracts or in cutaneous ulceration all confer an increased risk, which might explain the increased predisposition in more impoverished populations. Intravenous drug users are also predisposed to SA, often in unusual sites of infection and with atypical organisms.[3] The increasingly widespread use of biological therapies for inflammatory rheumatic and bowel diseases has also led to an increased SA incidence. Patients with RA receiving anti-tumour necrosis factor (TNF) therapy for less than 1-year have a twofold increase in risk compared with patients treated with disease-modifying anti-rheumatic drugs (DMARDs) alone.[7] However, RA patients needing anti-TNF therapy typically have longer disease duration, more severe disease, and more joint replacements, and are therefore already in a high-risk group.

Pathopysiology

Mechanisms behind SA pathogenesis are unclear but clues can be found in patients and animal models. Native joint infections usually follow bacterial colonization in a primary source, spread via the bloodstream.[1] SA develops in up to 90% of mice after intravenous

Table 98.1 Differential diagnosis of acute pain in a single joint

Common	Acute monoarthritis of systemic disease
Septic arthritis	Systemic lupus erythematosus
Crystal arthropathies	Vasculitides (ANCA positive and negative)
Reactive arthritides	Henoch–Schönlein purpura
Lyme disease	Behçet's disease
Plant thorn synovitis	Bacterial endocarditis
Other infections (mycobacterial, viral)	Familial Mediterranean fever
Trauma	**Bone disease**
Loose bodies	Paget's disease
Stress fracture	Osteomyelitis
Ischaemic necrosis	Osteogenic/osteoid tumours
Haemarthrosis	Metastatic disease
Acute monoarthritis of polyarthritis	**Monoarthritis of non-inflammatory disease**
Psoriatic arthritis	Osteoarthritis
Rheumatoid arthritis	Charcot joint
Juvenile inflammatory arthritides	Storage diseases (haemochromatosis)

ANCA, anti-neutrophil cytoplasmic antibodies.

injection of staphylococci[8] or streptococci,[9] supporting this hypothesis, but these models are complicated by high mortality from infection. In humans, inflammatory cytokines are found in SA synovial fluids,[10] and metalloproteinases have also been found. This implies that cytokine production could activate intra-articular enzymes leading to joint damage after infection.

Pathogenesis of SA is probably multifactorial, depending on interactions between bacteria and their ability to bind to synovial tissues, evade the immune response and stimulate joint damage. *Staphylococcus aureus* has a variety of receptors (microbial surface components recognizing adhesive matrix molecules, MSCRAMMs) that mediate attachment to joint tissues or implanted devices.[11] Cell-surface alpha-haemolysin on staphylococci adheres to host cell-surface membranes and produces pores in them, leading to cell death.[12] Some proteins facilitate bacterial entry into osteoblasts, implying a potential role in osteomyelitis, and others could be implicated in apoptosis via a host caspase-dependant mechanism, thereby accelerating joint destruction.[13] Injection of bacteria genetically altered to be deficient in staphylococcal protein A (SPA) in the mouse model results in less severe SA than that following injection of wild-type bacteria.[11] The mechanism remains unclear but because SPA binds IgG, interferes with complement binding, and restricts bacterial opsonization and phagocytosis, altered clearance of bacteria deficient in SPA may explain the lesser degree of articular damage. Similarly, variations in sialic acid content in streptococcal cell-wall polysaccharides may explain different degrees of joint damage in mice after injection of different strains of streptococci. Bacterial cell-wall antigens in *Neisseria gonorrhoeae* can also inactivate complement, enable survival inside neutrophils[14] and adversely affect immune-mediated removal of Gram-negative bacteria. Neisseria also have endotoxin activity, which may be a 'virulence factor' activating mediators of joint destruction.

Host factors are also important in SA. MHC class II antigens bind to staphylococcal exotoxin TSST-1 and activate T cells by linking with the T-cell receptor beta chain. Injection of staphylococci producing TSST-1 induce synovitis with clonal T-cell expansion, expression of the interleukin (IL)-2 receptor, and production of gamma-interferon (IFNγ) in synovial T cells,[15] whereas injection of bacteria lacking TSST-1 causes synovial inflammation less frequently.[16] Other mechanisms behind bacterial interaction with host cells may involve Toll-like receptors (TLRs). Peptidoglycans in Gram-positive bacteria interact with macrophage TLR-2 increasing intracellular NFκB production, which increases IL-1 and TNFα synthesis,[17] which in turn can stimulate metalloproteinase production.

The roles of proinflammatory cytokines and those that control inflammation in SA are not clear from experiments in animal models. Administration of IFNγ, which upregulates macrophage activation, worsens arthritis in both mouse models,[18,19] confirming a role for T cells. Infected murine synovial tissue T cells contain messenger RNA for IL-4 and IL-10, which downregulate the immune response, but their role in human disease remains uncertain. Removal of IL-10 worsens the clinical and histological features of SA,[20,21] implying IL-10 may control inflammation after infection. The role for IL-4 is less clear. In the streptococcal model IL-4 deficiency worsens arthritis,[22] whereas in the staphylococcal model IL-4 gene deletion limits arthritis development.[23]

The role of macrophage-derived cytokines, particularly TNFα, is in augmenting a wide variety of cellular and humoral host responses

to infection. TNFα can also directly restrict growth of intracellular bacteria. Removal of TNFα leads to accelerated growth of *Listeria monocytogenes* in infected tissue following enteric infection.[24] In septic shock in animals, neutralization of TNFα before inoculation of bacteria led to reduced mortality. However, in human clinical trials in septic shock an increase in mortality was noted. The role for TNFα in the pathogenesis of RA is increasingly apparent. Patients with RA are susceptible to native joint SA, possibly because of increased vascular flow to synovial tissues, previous damage to the joint, or DMARD therapy to control arthritis. Since licensing of TNF blockade as an RA treatment, nearly 20% of patients on these treatments have suffered serious infections,[25] often without an apparent 'septic' response. In a recently published British Society of Rheumatology Biologics Registry retrospective analysis[7] of patients receiving anti-TNF, a twofold increase of RA patients developing SA was shown compared to DMARDs alone. The risk appears greatest within the first year of treatment and falls in later years, suggesting a possible differing role for TNFα in response to early and late infections, but this has yet to be characterized.

Currently, there is no consistent information from animal models to explain the role of TNFα and IL-1. Neutralizing TNFα and IL-1 in a rabbit *S. aureus* model of SA before inoculation prevented arthritis development; whereas inactivation 24 hours after inoculation treatment was ineffective.[26] This suggests that macrophage-derived cytokines may be implicated in microbial clearance, as well as synovitis in SA. However, in mice with TNFα and IL-1 receptor genes both deleted, staphylococcal inoculation led to more aggressive joint disease,[23,26] possibly by allowing more bacteria access to the joints. In the streptococcal model, TNFα was not implicated but limitation of IL-1β and IL-6 production 1 hour after bacterial inoculation reduced joint destruction,[27] and this effect could be overcome by injecting exogenous IL-1β and IL-6. This suggests that IL-1 and IL-6 overproduction by monocytes and macrophages is also implicated in the pathogenesis of early joint damage.

The reasons for conflicting results in different models remain unclear and there may be no unifying hypothesis. However, interactions between different bacteria and host blood vessels, mononuclear phagocytic system, and inflamed synovium are clearly important. Equally, cytokines from T cells and macrophages are probably implicated, but, as their roles can vary during different phases of infection, their effects in the in-vivo models will need more detailed study if mechanisms of inflammation in joint infection are to be accurately elucidated.

Clinical features

History

Patients usually complain of an acutely painful single swollen joint, but up to 20% of patients have identifiable polyarticular infection (Table 98.2) The history should include the patient's age and occupation, together with a social history to include use of illicit drugs. To further differentiate causes of acute joint pain a history of prescribed medications, as well as information concerning sexual and travel history, should be obtained. Pain and joint stiffness, its temporal pattern, aggravating and relieving factors should also be sought. A systemic enquiry can help to aid the diagnosis, and specific enquiries regarding purulent sputum, dysuria, penile/vaginal discharge, leg ulceration, or recent joint surgery should be made. History of fever occurs in 50–57%,[2,28] and sweats/rigors are reported in only 30%, and these are therefore not essential for

Table 98.2 Joints most frequently affected in septic arthritis

Site	USA[1,a]	France[47,a]	Scotland[2,b]	Saudi Arabia[48,b]
Knee	68%	33%	56%	50%
Hip	9%	22%	16%	25%
Polyarticular	19%	11%	15%	8%
Shoulder	15%	12%	4%	16%
Wrist	15%	NR	4%	NR
Ankle	7%	NR	2%	NR
Elbow	10%	NR	2%	NR
Sternoclavicular	NR	NR	2%	NR
Sacro-iliac	NR	11%	NR	NR

NR, not recorded.
[a]Retrospective study.
[b]Prospective study.

diagnosis. Immunosuppressive therapy for any disease may mask typical features of inflammation, so a high index of suspicion is required.

Examination

The Regional Examination of the Musculoskeletal System (REMS; see Chapter 6) may be used to identify articular abnormalities. Physicians should look, feel, and move the joint to assess function, comparing the affected joint and normal side for evidence of more widespread disease. Examination of the acutely swollen joint will show signs of inflammation (pain, erythema, swelling, heat, and disability). The presence of synovial swelling and/or effusion, joint instability, limited movement, and deformity necessitate investigation. Local periarticular tenderness without joint swelling could indicate enthesitis, tendinitis, or bursitis, or possibly primary bone disease. In those patients with an inflammatory polyarthritis, the affected septic joints are likely to have signs out of keeping with global underlying disease activity. Large joints are the most commonly affected (Table 98.2).

Untreated *Neisseria gonorrhoeae* infection can also lead to a destructive arthritis, but can be asymptomatic. It should be suspected in sexually active patients presenting with migratory arthralgias, tenosynovitis, and skin rashes with vesicles.

Investigations

Prompt aseptic synovial aspiration is of paramount importance in diagnosis and treatment of SA and should take place prior to antibiotic administration (Figure 98.1). Although individual hospital admission policies may differ, many uncomplicated patients with SA can be managed in a rheumatology setting without recourse to surgical intervention. However, a suspected infected prosthetic joint should be referred to the orthopaedic surgical team for aspiration in theatre.[29]

Synovial fluid is usually cloudy with a high white cell count (WCC). Immediate microscopy is recommended to identify cell types, Gram stain for bacteria, and polarized light microscopy for uric acid or calcium pyrophosphate dihydrate disease (CPPD) crystals.[29] Causative organisms are seen in up to 57% of synovial fluid.[3] The value of performing quantitative WCC in synovial fluid aspirated from native joints is debated as it lacks the sensitivity to differentiate between infection and inflammation.[30] Low synovial fluid glucose, high lactate,[31] and procalcitonin are reported in SA. Evidence that these can separate infectious from inflammatory arthritis is lacking, and so they are not performed in routine practice. Neisseria organisms are fastidious with low yields from culture, but polymerase chain reaction (PCR) can detect Neisseria-specific DNA. Arthroscopic synovial biopsy is rarely necessary, but in tuberculosis may be required for diagnosis. Bone biopsy may be needed to identify causative organisms in non-resolving osteomyelitis.

Blood cultures should be performed routinely, prior to antibiotic therapy. The commonest joint infections result from haematogenous spread, and in some cases blood cultures may identify bacteria when synovial fluid cultures do not. At presentation, erythrocyte sedimentation rate (ESR) and C-reactive protein (CRP) are almost invariably raised, with CRP being the more discriminatory.[32] The WCC is normal at presentation in 37% of SA patients, but in those with RA this figure rises to 50%. Impaired renal and liver function predicts a poorer outcome.[2] Evaluation of potential distant sites of infection should be determined by clinical presentation, including chest radiograph, urine cultures, and swabs from skin ulcers as well as oral, anal, and genital sites in patients with suspected Neisseria infection.

A range of imaging studies can assist in diagnosis of an acute monoarthritis but only a few are salient for SA. Plain radiographs show soft tissue swelling and previous joint damage from whatever cause, but often show no evidence of the joint destruction that may be apparent later. In anaerobic infections (the least common cause of SA), gas may be seen in the joint cavity. Nevertheless, radiographs can be helpful in providing evidence of an alternative diagnosis such as chondrocalcinosis. The quickest way to localize synovitis and to target aspiration is ultrasound, which can also discriminate between joint effusion, and more superficial cellulitis, bursitis or tenosynovitis. MRI (Figure 98.2a) can also assist in distinguishing between potential differential diagnoses and is helpful in demonstrating additional osteomyelitis (Figure 98.2c). Radionucleotide scans (Figure 98.2b) will not be able to differentiate between infection and inflammation, but labelled white call scans can identify areas of infection when the primary source of infection is uncertain.

Suspected SA

When there is a clinical suggestion of SA from the patients' history and examination, but routine investigations fail to isolate any bacteria, the other immediate investigations (as outlined above) are equally likely to be abnormal and outcomes (including mortality) are identical when compared patients with bacterial proven SA.[33] Long-term mortality outcomes are also similar between patients with bacteria-proven and suspected SA.[4] Hence, absence of systemic symptoms and normal microbiological investigations should never negate a strong clinical suspicion.

Organisms

The most commonly detected organisms in SA (Table 98.3) include staphylococci, streptococci, and Gram-negative bacteria.[2] Infection with multiple organisms is increasingly recognized.[2] *S. aureus* is the prominent organism in retrospective and prospective published series with prevalence in SA remaining unchanged for many years.[34] In addition to an increasing resistance to penicillin G noted in the 1970s, the prevalence of methicillin-resistant *S. aureus* (MRSA) detection is rising.[33] In the past, isolates of coagulase-negative

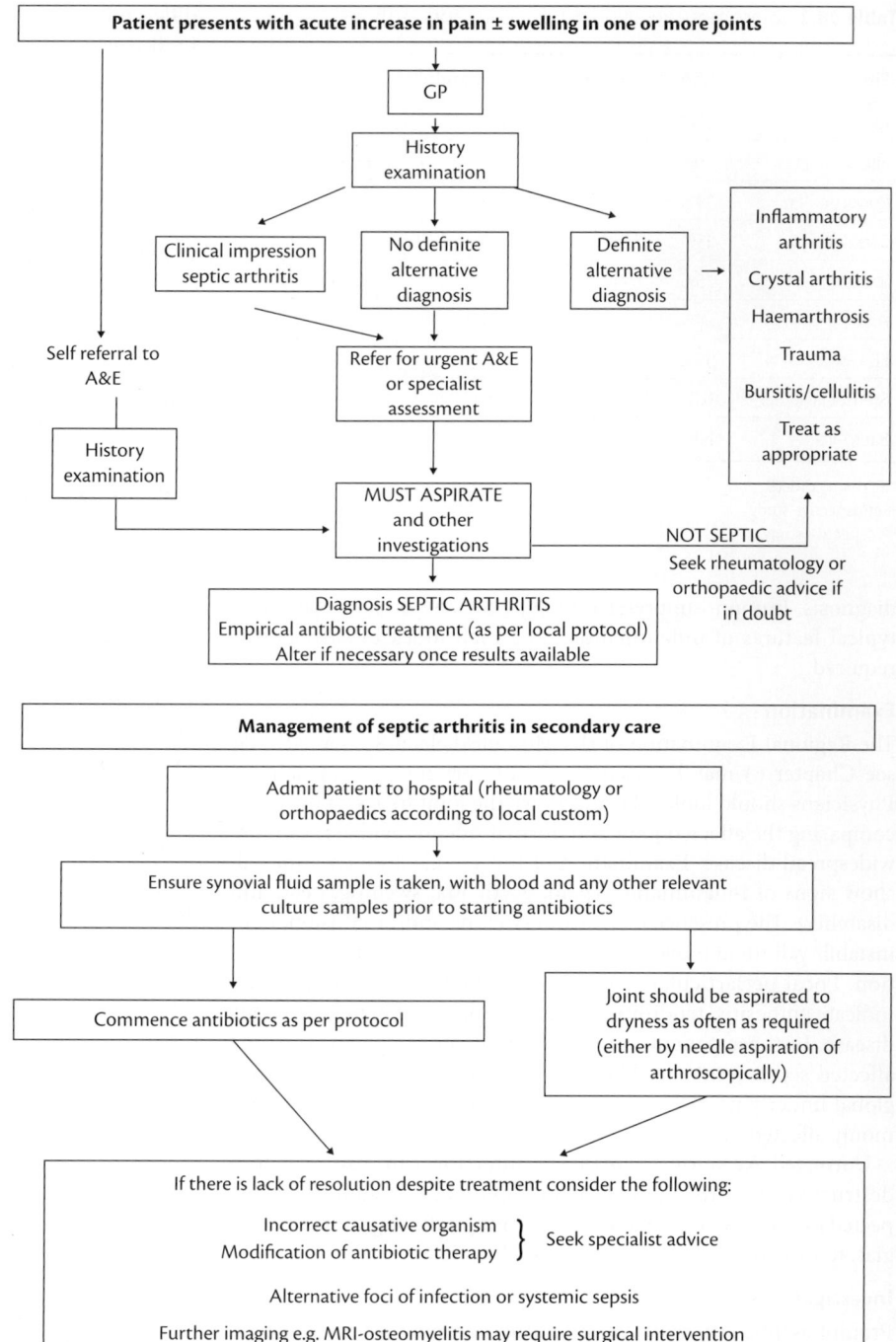

Fig. 98.1 British Society of Rheumatology (BSR) guidelines for management of the acutely hot swollen joint.

staphylococci, commonly *S. epidermidis*, were regarded as contaminants, but frequent detection in patients following recent joint surgery has raised awareness of this organism's significance.[33] Analysis of streptococci implicated in SA shows that group A (the most pathogenic) account for around 40%, group B for 30%, and group G for the remainder. Most patients with streptococcal SA were aged 50 years or older and often had comorbidities: autoimmune disease, chronic wounds, diabetes mellitus, and neoplasia. *S. pneumoniae* is alpha-haemolytic and is an important cause of pneumonia but is an uncommon pathogen in streptococcal SA.[34,35]

Gram-negative bacteria, especially those belonging to the family Enterobacteriaceae, are an increasing cause of bone and joint

infections.[35] Elderly patients and those with urinary tract infections and chronic illness (particularly diabetes mellitus, sickle cell anaemia, neoplasia, connective tissue disease, and after renal transplantation) were found to be most susceptible.

Anaerobes including bacteroides, *Propionibacterium acnes*, and some anaerobic Gram-positive cocci are isolated in less than 7% of cases of SA, often in combination with aerobes. Free gas in the joint on plain radiograph, or foul-smelling synovial fluid could suggest an anaerobic infection. Synovial fluid should be cultured for at least 2 weeks because of the slow growth of these organisms. Sensitivity testing is mandatory because many species are multidrug resistant.

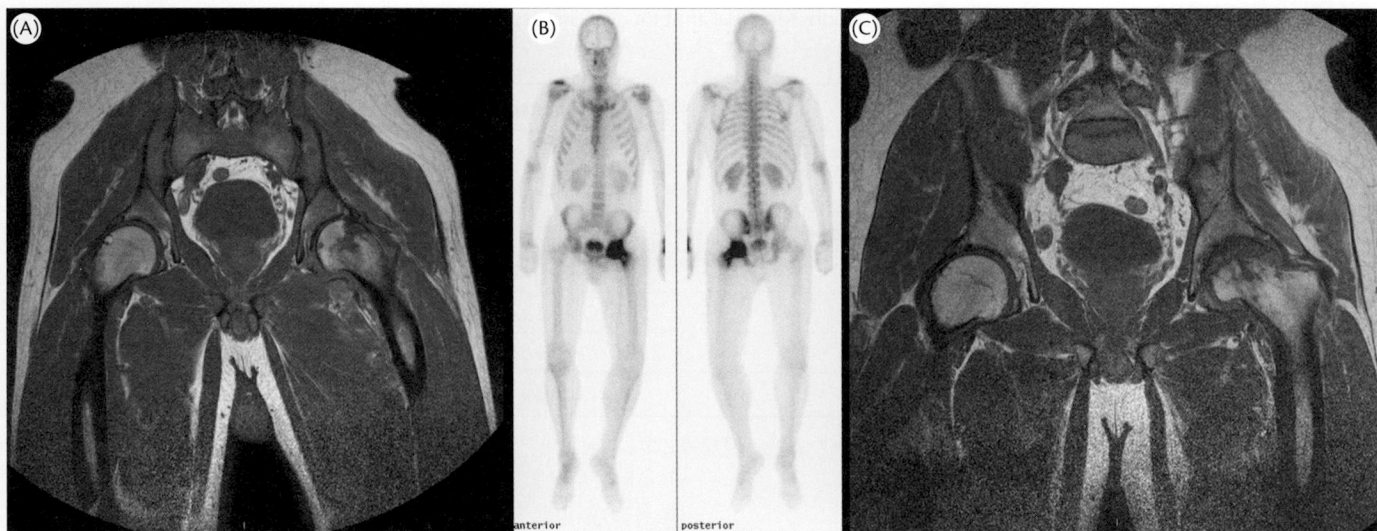

Fig. 98.2 Evolution of an infected left hip joint despite antibiotic therapy: (A) Initial MRI scan of an infected left hip at day 3 showing destruction of the femoral head. (B) Technetium isotope bone scan at day 3 showing uptake of radioactivity in the left hip joint. (C) MRI scan at week 8 showing further destruction of left femoral head and acetabulum.
Figures provided by Dr D. Colville, Department of Nuclear Medicine, Glasgow Royal Infirmary.

N. gonorrhoeae was isolated from the synovial fluid in 12% of SA cases seen in aboriginal Australians,[36] a much higher percentage than that reported recently in European studies (Table 98.3). Infection can be asymptomatic, but should be suspected in sexually active patients presenting with migratory arthralgias, tenosynovitis, and skin rashes with vesicles.

Mycobacteria and fungi rarely cause SA. Special microbiological techniques are required to enable confirmation and a high index of suspicion is necessary in potentially infected individuals.

Treatment

The BSR, British Health Professionals in Rheumatology (BHPR), and British Orthopaedic Association (BOA) guidelines published in 2006 (Figure 98.1) provide a framework on which to base treatment.[29] Prompt treatment is required to reduce the associated morbidity and mortality. Joints should be aspirated to dryness, with repeated aspirations necessary if effusions reaccumulates. Surgical intervention in uncomplicated cases does not appear to confer benefit compared with repeated aseptic joint aspiration. Antibiotic therapy should be guided by local prescribing protocols, and instituted before culture results are available, but preferably after joint aspiration. Individual patient risk factors and the likelihood of a causative organism should help to determine an appropriate antibiotic until culture and sensitivity results are known (Table 98.4). Although there is no evidence to support the route or treatment duration of antibiotics in patients with SA, the general consensus is that at least 2 weeks of parenteral therapy followed by 4 weeks of oral therapy is required. Monitoring for signs and symptoms of sepsis or shock should be undertaken and treated appropriately. Orthopaedic intervention with arthroscopy and wash out of the affected joint may be required if signs do not settle with conservative measures.[29] Physiotherapy in the recovery period is important in order to maintain function.

Table 98.3 Bacteria isolated (%) from patients with proven septic arthritis

Bacteria	The Netherlands[49,b]	England and Wales[50,a]	France[47,a]	Australia[36,a]	USA[1,a]	Scotland[2,b]
Staphylococcus aureus	44	40	56	37	34	60
Staphylococcus epidermidis	NR	NR	NR	NR	NR	9
Streptococci	21	28	10	21	28	28
Escherichia coli	6	6	9	1	10	9
Pseudomonas	3	2	4	1	2	0
Haemophilus	6	7	0	1	2	0
Neisseria gonorrhoea	0	1	3	12	0	0
Anaerobes	2	1	2	3	8	2

NR, not recorded.
[a]Retrospective study.
[b]Prospective study.

Table 98.4 Summary of United Kingdom recommendations for initial antibiotic use in suspected septic arthritis after obtaining bacterial culture (dependent on local protocols)

Clinical situation	Suggested antibiotic
No risk of atypical organisms	IV flucloxacillin. Local policy may add IV gentamycin or oral fusidic acid
No risk of atypical organisms but penicillin allergic	Clindamycin or 2nd/3rd generation cephalosporin
High risk of Gram-negative infection (elderly ±UTIs or recent bowel surgery)	2nd/3rd generation cephalosporin (flucloxacillin may be in local policy)
Discuss with microbiologist	MRSA risk (recent in-patient, nursing home resident, leg ulcers, etc.)
Vancomycin together with 2nd/3rd generation cephalosporin	Discuss with microbiologist
Possible gonococcus or meningococcus	Ceftriaxone or similar (depends on local policy)
Patient needing intensive care or high-risk IV drug users	Discuss with microbiologist

IV, intravenous; MRSA, methicillin-resistant Staphylococcus aureus; UTI, urinary tract infection.
Adapted from Matthews et al.[29]

Corticosteroids and bisphosphonates

Suppression of an excessive immune response with corticosteroids could be a more effective treatment regimen for *S. aureus* SA than use of antibiotics alone. Tarkowski and colleagues showed that, in mice treated with intraperitoneal cloxacillin together with intraperitoneal corticosteroid, the prevalence, severity, and mortality associated with SA induced by *S. aureus* inoculation was significantly reduced compared with mice treated with intraperitoneal cloxacillin alone.[37]

A randomized double-blind, placebo-controlled trial assessed dexamethasone treatment for SA in 123 children, given in parallel with standard antibiotic treatment, reduced duration of infection and subsequent joint damage when compared to antibiotics alone.[38] However, there are no studies in the adult population—a potential subject for further clinical trials.

The addition of bisphosphonates to an intraperitoneal treatment regimen of corticosteroids and antibiotics seems to add further clinical benefit in the staphylococcus animal model. This finding could be due to a decrease in osteoclast activity and a consequent reduction in skeletal destruction, and again may warrant further study in the human population.[39]

Infections in prosthetic joints

Prosthetic joints have brought relief to many millions of patients since the middle of the 20th century. Infection in primary joint replacements, is fortunately rare (1–3%), but in patients with RA and following an infected first replacement the frequency is higher. BSR/BOA guidelines suggest that suspected prosthetic joint infection should be referred to orthopaedic surgery for treatment.[29] Increased risks for prosthetic joint infection include infection at a distant site, the presence of a malignancy, a history of joint arthroplasty, other comorbid conditions (RA, diabetes mellitus), simultaneous bilateral joint replacement, and an operative time in excess of 2.5 hours.[40]

Contamination during implantation is considered to result in early (up to 3 months) or delayed up to 24 months) infections, but those after 24 months (late) probably result from joint infection via the blood stream as with native joint infection. Patients usually present with local pain at rest and on movement. Examination of infected joints may show a sinus, indicating a need for prosthesis removal. However, signs of inflammation may be found in early or delayed infections but are less likely in late infections.

ESR can be high for months and the CRP for up to 3 weeks following routine arthroplasty and so are of limited value during acute infections. Nevertheless, in delayed joint prosthesis infection, an elevated CRP and ESR have a high sensitivity (88% and 75% respectively) compared to 45% for high WCC. Low inflammatory markers at presentation have a good negative-predictive value.

Radiographs in infected prosthetic joints may show loosening (Figure 98.3a), subperiosteal bone growth, and rarely transcortical sinus tracts. Bone scans using technetium-99 m-labelled methylene diphosphonate can be positive for up to 12 months after replacement surgery[41] but are useful in patients with suspected delayed infection (Figure 98.3b). CT and MRI are of limited value because of the metal in the joints. However, indium-labelled white cell scans can be helpful (Figure 98.3c), especially when compared to the marrow-suppressed signal from the same scan which confirms the uptake in the femoral component (Figure 98.3d).

Joint aspiration may help differentiate infection from joint loosening. Gram-stained smear of synovial fluid has high specificity (>97%) but low sensitivity (<20%).[42] Synovial fluid WCC in excess of 1700/mm³ and neutrophils greater than 65% has a 97% sensitivity,[43] but these figures are reduced in patients with inflammatory arthritis. *S. aureus* accounts for most early and recurrent infections, but delayed infections often result from skin contaminants like coagulase-negative staphylococci. If surgery is required, best microbiological results are obtained if three samples of tissue from the joint capsule, synovial lining, bone–cement interface, and samples from purulent material or sequestra are taken.[40] Ideally, antimicrobial therapy should be stopped for at least 2 weeks before revision surgery, and perioperative antibiotics should be withheld until all tissue cultures have been obtained. If this approach is followed and at leaat one out of three specimens show bacterial growth then the probability of prosthetic joint infection is over 94%.[42]

A variety of factors affect interactions between hosts and joint implants. Fibronectin-binding proteins on staphylococci enhance bacterial adherence to joint prostheses, limiting efficient bacterial removal. *S. epidermidis* can degrade polysaccharides and form an exopolysaccharide glycocalyx on artificial surfaces which protect bacteria from phagocytosis.[44] The heat resulting from bone cement mixing around the shafts of prostheses can cause bone necrosis,

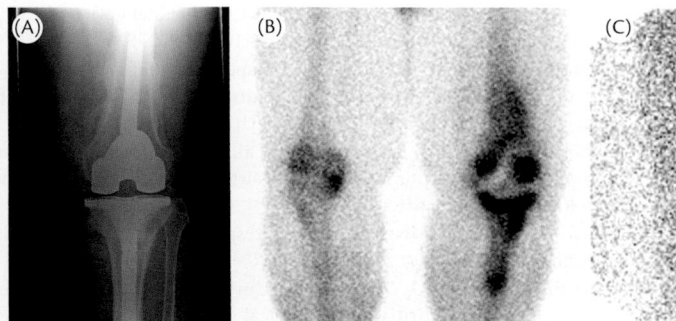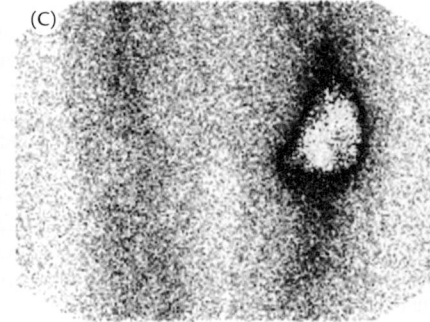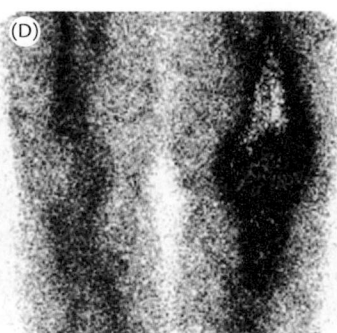

Fig. 98.3 Infected femoral component of a left knee prosthesis: (A) Routine radiograph showing area of loosening round the femoral and tibial components of the prosthesis. (B) Technetium isotope bone scan showing increased uptake in the femoral and tibial components. (C) Indium-labelled white cell scan showing increased uptake around the femoral component and in the local bone marrow. (D) Simultaneous technetium scan shows bone marrow uptake in both components confirming that a concentration of radioactivity in the white cell scan (C) is the result of the focus of infection in the femoral component.
Figures provided by Dr D. Colville, Department of Nuclear Medicine, Glasgow Royal Infirmary.

providing a nidus for infection, and bone cement itself can inhibit neutrophil and complement functions, as can the implant itself.

As in native joint infection, not all patients with infected prosthetic joints require joint removal. Patients with joint pain and swelling of less than 3 weeks with a stable prosthesis may not need surgery but may be candidates for antibiotics and implant retention, possibly with debridement.[45] Equally, long-term antibiotic treatment may be necessary for patients if risks of surgery are too great. However, late infections require most patients to undergo a two-stage process, removing infected prosthesis, debriding of infected bone, and stabilizing the joint with an antibiotic-impregnated spacer. After 6 weeks of intravenous antibiotics (according to local protocols) and reimplantation of a second implant the success rate can be as high as 90%.[46]

Prevention of prosthetic joint infections

Preoperative evaluation of a patient for occult infection, such as periodontal disease or bacteriuria, is warranted, and any infection should be successfully treated before proceeding to joint replacement. Perioperative antibiotic prophylaxis significantly reduces rates of early joint infection after initial replacement. The role of antibiotic prophylaxis to prevent late prosthetic joint infection during procedures that lead to transient bacteraemia is more controversial. The incidence of late infection in prosthetic joints because of procedure-related bacteraemia is 10–100 cases per 100 000 patients per year. The cost of providing antibiotic prophylaxis to all patients with prosthetic joints is not inconsiderable and its efficacy is unknown. Similarly, the effect of more intensive therapy in treating infected prosthetic joints in RA patients is also unknown and until long-term studies from the British Society for Rheumatology Rheumatoid Arthritis Register (BSRBR) of biological and routine DMARD treatments are available, patients should be counselled on risks and benefits of antibiotic prophylaxis.

Conclusion

In an acute monoarthritis with classical symptoms of acute inflammation, SA should be considered as the most likely diagnosis, and should be treated immediately after appropriate investigations, particularly culture of synovial fluid, blood, and any possible sites of infection. Treatment for native joint infection outlined in BSR and

BOA guidelines includes repeated aspiration to dryness and intravenous antibiotics to cover common organisms, but locally derived antibiotic guidelines should be used in each case. Lack of bacterial culture results in a patient with suspected SA should not delay treatment, as outcomes are no different from those in bacteria-proven SA. Treatment of infected prosthetic joint infection should always be referred to orthopaedic surgeons for investigation and treatment, which may include removal of the infected prosthesis as well as long-term intravenous antibiotic therapy.

References

1. Goldenberg DL, Cohen AS. Acute infectious arthritis. A review of patients with non gonococcal joint infections. *Am J Med* 1976;60:369–377.
2. Gupta MN, Sturrock RD, Field M. A prospective 2 year study of 75 patients with adult-onset septic arthritis. *Rheumatology* (Oxford) 2001;40:24–30.
3. Weston VC, Jones AC, Bradbury N, Fawthorpe F, Doherty M. Clinical features and outcome of septic arthritis in a single UK health district 1982–1991. *Ann Rheum Dis* 1999;58:214–219.
4. Gupta MN, Field M. Gupta MN, Field M. Long term outcome from septic arthritis on five year follow up. A prospective study. *Rheumatology* (Oxford) 2004; ii131 (Poster abstract No 336).
5. UK National Statistics 2011.
6. National Joint Registry, 8th Annual Report, 2011.
7. Galloway JB, Hyrich KL, Mercer UK et al. Risk of septic arthritis in patients with rheumatoid arthritis and the effect of anti-TNF therapy: results from the British Society for Rheumatology Biologics Register. *Ann Rheum Dis* 2011;70(10):1810–1804.
8. Bremell T, Abdelnour A, Tarkowski A. Histopathological and serological progression of experimental Staphylococcus aureus arthritis. *Infect Immun* 1992;60:2976–2985.
9. Puliti M, Bistoni F, von Hunolstein C, Orefeci G, Tissi L. Severity of group B streptococcal arthritis in selected strains of laboratory mice. *Infect Immun* 2001;69:551–555.
10. Osiri M, Ruxrungtham K, Nookhai S, Ohmoto Y, Deesomchok U. IL-1beta, IL-6 and TNF-alpha in synovial fluid of patients with non gonococcal arthritis. *Asian Pacific J Allergy Immunol* 1988;16:155–160.
11. Palmquist n, Foster T, Tarkowski A, Josefsson E. Protein A is a virulence factor in Staphylococcal aureus arthritis and septic death. *Microbial Pathol* 2002;33:239–249.
12. Bantel H, Sinha B, Domschke W et al. α-Toxin is a mediator of Staphylococcal aureus- induced cell death and activates caspases via the intrinsic death pathway independently of death receptor signalling. *J Cell Biol* 2001;155:637–648.

13. Bayles KW, Wesson CA, Lion LE et al. Intracellular Staphylococcus aureus escapes the endosome and induces apoptosis in epithelial cells. *Infect Immun* 1998;66:336–342.

14. Lorenzen DR, Gunther D, Pandit J et al. Neisseria gonorrhoeae porin modifies the oxidative burst of human professional phagocytes. *Infect Immun* 2000;68:6215–6222.

15. Abdelnour A, Bremmel T, Holmdahl R, Tarkowski A. Clonal expansion of T lymphocytes causes arthritis and mortality in mice infected with toxic shock syndrome toxin-1-producing staphylococci. *Eur J Immunol* 1994;24:1161–1166.

16. Bremmel T, Tarkowski A. Preferential induction of septic arthritis and mortality by super antigen-producing staphylococci. *Infec Immun* 1995;63:4185–4187.

17. Barnes PJ, Karin M. Nuclear Factor-kB—a pivotal transcription factor in chronic inflammatory diseases. *N Engl J Med* 1997;336:1066–1071.

18. Zhao YX, Tarkowski A. Role of Europhiles in experimental septicaemia and septic arthritis induced by Staphylococcus aureus. *Infec Immun* 1997;155:5736–5742.

19. Puliti M, von Hunolstein C, Bistoni F et al. Influence of interferon-gamma administration on the severity of experimental group B streptococcal arthritis. *Arthritis Rheum* 2000;43(12):2678–2686.

20. Gjertsson I, Hultgren OH, Tarkowski A. Interleukin-10 ameliorates the outcome of Staphylococcus aureus arthritis by promoting bacterial clearance. *Clin Exp Immunol* 2002;130:409–414.

21. Puliti M, von Hunolstein C, Verwaerde C et al. Regulatory role of interleukin 10 in experimental Group B Streptococcal arthritis. *Infect Immun* 2002;70(6):2862–2868.

22. Tissi l, Bistoni F, Puliti M. IL-4 deficiency decreases mortality but increases severity of arthritis in experimental Group B Streptococcus infection. *Mediators Inflamm* 2009;394021.

23. Hultgren OH, Eugster HP, Sedgwick JD, Korner H, Tarkowski A. TNF/Lymphotoxin-a double mutant mice resist septic arthritis but display increased mortality in response to Staphylococcus aureus. *J Immunol* 1998;161:5937–5942.

24. Beretich GR, Carter PB, Havell RA. Roles for tumour necrosis factor and gamma interferon in resistance to enteric listeriosis. *Infect Immun* 1998;66(5):2368–2373.

25. Kroesen S, Widmer AF, Tyndall A, Haster P. Serious bacterial infection in patients with rheumatoid arthritis under anti-TNF-alpha therapy. *Rheumatology* (Oxford) 2003;42(5):617–621.

26. Hultgren OH, Svensson L, Tarkowski A. Critical role of signalling through IL-1 receptor for development of arthritis and sepsis during Staphylococcal aureus infection. *J Immunol* 2002;168:5207–5212.

27. Tissi L, Puliti M, Barluzzi R et al. Role of tumour necrosis factor alpha, interleukin-1B and interleukin-6 in a mouse model of Group B Streptococcal arthritis. *Infect Immun* 1999;67:4545–4550.

28. Margaretten ME, Kohlewes J, Moore D, Bent S. Does this adult patient have septic arthritis? *JAMA* 2007;297(13):1478–1488.

29. Matthews C, Coakley G, Field M et al. BSR & BHPR, BOA, RCGP &BSAC Guideline for management of the hot swollen joint in adults. *Rheumatology* 2006;45:1039–1041.

30. McGillicuddy DC, Shah KH, Friedberg RP, Nathanson LA, Edlow JA. How sensitive is the synovial fluid white blood cell count in diagnosing septic arthritis? *Am J Emerg Med* 2007;25(7):749–752.

31. Matthews CM, Weston VC, Jones A et al. Bacterial septic arthritis in adults. *Lancet* 2009;374:1–10.

32. Ernst AA, Weiss SJ, Tracy LA, Weiss NR. Usefulness of CRP and ESR in predicting septic joints. *South Med J* 2010;103(6):522–526.

33. Gupta MN, Sturrock RD, Field M. Prospective comparative study of patients with culture proven and high suspicion of adult onset septic arthritis. *Ann Rheum Dis* 2003;62:327–331.

34. Dubost JJ, Soubrier M, De Champs C et al. No changes in the distribution of organisms responsible for septic arthritis over a 20 year period. *Ann Rheum Dis* 2002;61(3):267–269.

35. Bouza E, Munoz P. Micro-organisms responsible for osteo-articular infections. *Baillieres Best Pract Res Clin Rheumatol* 1999;13(1):21–35.

36. Morgan DS, Fisher D, Merianos A, Currie BJ. An 18 year clinical review of septic arthritis from tropical Australia. *Epidemiol Infect* 1996;117:423–428.

37. Sakiniene E, Bremell T, Tarkowski A. Addition of corticosteroids to antibiotic treatment ameliorates the course of experimental Staphylococcus aureus arthritis. *Arthritis Rheum* 1996;39(9):1596–1605.

38. Harel L, Prais D, Bar-On E et al. Dexamethasone therapy for septic arthritis in children: results of a randomised double-blind placebo-controlled study. *J Pediatr Orthop* 2011;31(2):211–215.

39. Verdrengh M, Carlsten H, Ohlsson C, Tarkowski A. Addition of bisphosphonate to antibiotic and anti-inflammatory treatment reduces bone resorption in experimental Staphylococcus aureus-induced arthritis. *J Orthop Res* 2007;25(3):304–310.

40. Del Pozo JL, Patel R. Infection associated with prosthetic joints. *N Engl J Med* 2009;361:787–794.

41. Smith SL, Wastie ML, Forster I. Radionucleotide bone scintigraphy in the detection of significant complications after total knee joint replacement. *Clin Radiol* 2001;56:221–224.

42. Atkins BL, Athanasou N, Deeks JJ et al. Prospective evaluation of criteria for microbiological diagnosis of prosthetic joint infection at revision athroplasty. The OSIRIS Collaborative Study Group. *J Clin Microbiol* 1998;36:2932–2939.

43. Trampuz A, Hassen AD, Osmon DR et al. Synovial fluid leucocyte count and differential for the diagnosis of prosthetic knee infection. *Am J Med* 2004;117:556–562.

44. Costerton JW, Irvin RT, Cheng KJ. The role of bacterial surface structures in pathogenesis. *Crit Rev Microbiol* 1981;8(4):303–338.

45. Byren I, Bejon P, Atkins BL et al. One hundred and twelve infected athroplasties treated with DAIR (debridement, antibiotics and implant retention): antibiotic duration and outcome. *J Antimicrob Chemother* 2009;63:1264–1271.

46. Brandt CM, Duffy MCT, Berbari EF et al. Staphylococcus aureus prosthetic joint infection treated with prosthesis removed and delayed reimplantation arthroplasty. *Mayo Clin Proc* 1999;74:553–558.

47. Le Dantec L, Maury F, Flipo RM et al. Peripheral pyogenic arthritis. A study of one hundred seventy-nine cases. *Rev Rheum Engl Ed* 1996;63(2):103–110.

48. Al Arfaj AS. A prospective study of the incidence and characteristics of septic arthritis in a teaching hospital in Riyadh, Saudi Arabia. *Clin Rheumatol* 2008;27(11):1403–1410.

49. Kaandrop CJE, van Schaardenburg D, Krijnen P, Habbema JDF, van de Laae MAFJ. Risk factors for septic arthritis in patients with joint disease: a prospective study. *Arthritis Rheum* 1995; 38:1819–1825.

50. Ryan MJ, Kavanagh R, Wall PG, Hazelman BL. Bacterial joint infections in England and Wales; analysis of bacterial isolates over a four year period. *Br J Rheumatol* 1997;36:370–373.

CHAPTER 99

Bone and joint infections in children

Priya Sukhtankar, Julia Clark, and Saul N. Faust

Introduction

This chapter describes the range of paediatric bone and joint infections, focusing on osteomyelitis (OM), both acute and chronic; septic arthritis (SA); and tuberculous osteomyelitis. In addition, special situations such as immunodeficiency, complications of surgery, children with sickle cell disease, and infections caused by multiresistant organisms and hospital-acquired infections are discussed.

Bone and joint infections are relatively uncommon in children, and may be challenging to diagnose and treat. While laboratory investigations and imaging aid diagnosis, clinical signs are vital in informing the diagnosis and management of children of different ages with bone and joint infections. This chapter discusses the features suggestive of OM/SA in children of different ages, and investigations to aid diagnosis.

The involvement of multidisciplinary medical and surgical teams is essential to provide optimal care. Bone biopsy of infected joints may be indicated to identify organisms, although it may not always be technically possible or feasible due to lack of resources.

Certain laboratory tests have more relevance than others, and normal values should be interpreted with caution. Conventional microscopy and culture of bone and joint samples or blood cultures from children with OM/SA has a diagnostic yield as low as 12% in many western European paediatric populations including the United Kingdom, but rates of up to 50% have been reported in selected case series. Newer specific molecular tests appear to be useful in achieving a microbiological diagnosis.

The use of imaging varies with the suspected site of infection, the age of the child, and the resources available locally. Importantly, radiological features of infection may not be present in early disease.

The clinical course and prognosis depends on the causative organism, the mode of infection, and risk factors of the patient. However, more favourable outcomes occur with early diagnosis and prompt treatment with appropriate antimicrobial therapy. Complications of OM and SA in children vary according to age and depend on the extent of disease.

Epidemiology

The incidence of osteomyelitis (OM) and SA in children in the United Kingdom was estimated to be 2.9 new cases per 100 000 in 2001,[1,2] but is currently the subject of a national clinical study. Unpublished data from Southampton, Newcastle, and South London show an admission rate of between 0.048 and 0.07 per 1000 child years in all children from 0 to 18 years. In high-risk groups and in tropical countries the incidence is significantly higher, particularly of chronic osteoarticular infection (OAI). In sub-Saharan Africa HIV-positive and malnourished children are at increased risk of SA and OM due to immunocompromise.[3] This region also has a high incidence of sickle cell disease, which increases the risk of OAI.

Half of children with acute OM are 0–5 years old. Boys are approximately twice as likely to be affected by OM or SA as girls, although there is no gender predilection in the first year of life.[4] There no longer appears to be a link with social deprivation in resource-rich countries.[1]

Bone and joint infections are the second most common infections children with sickle cell disease after pneumonia and pneumococcal septicaemia.[5] This is discussed further under aetiology and pathophysiology.

Tuberculous SA and osteomyelitis are increasing, especially in countries where HIV is highly endemic. In the United Kingdom this tends to be a disease of immigrant populations from countries where the prevalence of tuberculosis (TB) is high, for example the Indian subcontinent.[6] These infections represent 1–2% of all TB, and 10–20% of all extrapulmonary disease. Tuberculous bone and joint disease mainly affects adolescents. Only 50% of these will have concurrent pulmonary TB. TB typically involves synovial joints and spine; osteomyelitis of long bones is less common.[7,8] Tuberculous infection of the spine (Pott's disease) accounts for up to 50% of tuberculous OM/SA.

Definitions

Osteomyelitis is inflammation of bone, usually due to bacterial infection, but occasionally due to fungal infection. It can be broadly divided into three groups:

◆ **Acute or haematogenous osteomyelitis (AHOM)**: this is the most common form of osteomyelitis in infants and young children. Organisms are seeded to the bone or joint via the circulation during an episode of bacteraemia. Children with sickle cell disease and immunodeficiency such as chronic granulomatous disease are at increased risk.

- **Subacute or focal osteomyelitis**: this generally occurs in older children, often secondary to penetrating injury or surgical-site infection. Organisms are directly inoculated to the site of infection via puncture wound, or from adjacent infection.
- **Chronic osteomyelitis**: this occurs if osteomyelitis is left untreated or partially treated and can lead to abscess formation, pathological fracture, and sequestration. It is most common following focal osteomyelitis owing to its insidious course in resource-rich countries. In resource-poor countries, or where access to health care is not readily available, it follows AHOM and is more common.[9]

The clinical course of these types of infections depends on the age of the child, additional pathology and the causative organism.

- **SA** is infection within a joint, either due to haematogenous spread, extension of osteomyelitis into the adjacent joint, or direct inoculation of the joint itself.
- **Tuberculous osteomyelitis** is infection of a long bone, or spine with *Mycobacterium tuberculosis*. There is caseation and granuloma formation. This infection almost always involves the adjacent joint, causing tuberculous SA.
- **Osteoarticular infection (OAI)**: in this chapter the term refers to either OM and/or SA.
- **Discitis (diskitis)** is specifically infection and/or inflammation of an intervertebral disc.

Pathophysiology and aetiology

Acute (haematogenous) osteomyelitis

Organisms enter bone via the nutrient artery. There is some evidence based on clinical observation that infection of the bone is associated with microtrauma of the growth plate. This is supported by experiments using animal models.[10,11] A subclinical nidus of necrotic bone may form where infection can become established.

If osteomyelitis remains untreated inflammatory exudate spreads from infected region into haversian canals and canals of Volkmann towards the periosteum. This compresses blood supply further, resulting in bone necrosis, which goes on to form a sequestrum and/or sinus.

The metaphyseal region of long bones is most commonly affected as this has rich blood supply and bacteria are deposited in tight capillary loops where blood flow is slow. Once adhesion has occurred the bacteria proliferate into vascular tunnels. They can then invade metaphyseal cartilage. Metaphyseal capillaries also have very low numbers of phagocytic cells in the endothelium and therefore have limited protection against bacterial organisms.

In older children the growth plate acts as a barrier to extension of infection as blood vessels do not cross this layer of cartilage. Importantly, neonates have transphyseal vessels that traverse the growth plate into the epiphysis, which can lead to more extensive infection with more likely spread into the adjacent joint.[11] In adolescents, where the physis has ossified, the barrier also disappears, allowing extension and contiguous SA.

Subacute or focal osteomyelitis

Organisms usually enter the bone or joint directly from a puncture wound, such as an animal bite, or ingrowing toenail. These infections often present insidiously with localized inflammation, and are more likely to become chronic if unrecognized or misdiagnosed as soft tissue infection.

Surgical-site infection is caused by a similar range of organisms to acute haematogenous osteomyelitis. External fixation of fractures is a significant risk factor.[12,13] Resistant organisms are likely to be hospital-acquired, and can be persistent and difficult to treat where indwelling metalwork,[14] or devices such as bone-implanted hearing aids,[15] are present.

Chronic osteomyelitis

This occurs if the initial infection is left untreated (or is partially untreated), and was common in the preantibiotic era. If treatment is not initiated, abscess formation, and chronic suppuration with a leaking sinus can occur. This can lead to lifelong deformity, or may necessitate amputation.[16]

Septic arthritis

Infection of the joint can occur secondary to direct haematogenous seeding of bacteria to the joint, or as an extension of OM.[17] Notably SA occurs in up to 76% of neonates with bone infection.[18,19] If osteomyelitis extends into the adjacent joint it is likely to cause significant damage to the growth plate.

Organisms

Many organisms cause bone and joint infections (Table 99.1), in particular those mentioned in this section.

Staphylococcus aureus

The most common OAI-causing organism worldwide is *Staphylococcus aureus*, which has specific binding factors for fibronectin and laminin. Strains causing osteomyelitis have also been found to express adhesins for collagen and bind to bone and connective tissue.[20]

In the United Kingdom the majority of infections caused by *S. aureus* are meticillin-sensitive (MSSA). However, in other countries (such as the United States), community as well as hospital-acquired infections may be meticillin resistant (MRSA).[21] If there is a history of travel to countries where community-acquired MRSA (CA-MRSA) is common this should be considered and antibiotic therapy adapted accordingly. Patients with CA-MRSA OM/SA are also at increased risk of deep vein thrombosis (DVT).[21,22]

Panton–Valentine leucocidin (PVL) producing strains of *S. aureus* are relatively uncommon in OM/SA in the United Kingdom and also tend to be associated with acquisition of infection in other countries such as the United States. Around 60% of PVL *S. aureus* is MSSA.[23] However, if PVL is suspected it is important to request additional testing. Expression of PVL is associated with depletion of leucocytes, tissue necrosis, severe systemic illness, and destructive bone disease.[24]

Risk factors for PVL *S. aureus* include communities living in close contact, contact sports, and previous history of skin abscesses. MRSA and PVL-producing strains have been noted to cause higher fever and more significantly raised inflammatory markers than non-PVL-producing MSSA.[25]

Kingella kingae

Kingella kingae is a facultative anaerobic Gram-negative organism that has been recognized as an important pathogen in OM

Table 99.1 Microorganisms causing osteoarticular infections in children in the United Kingdom

Organism frequency

Common

Staphylococcus aureus (MSSA), 44–80%

Kingella kingae, 14–50% (increased <36 months)

Rare

Meticillin-resistant S aureus, (MRSA) 40–50% in USA, rare in UK

Panton Valentine Leucocidin (PVL) MSSA

Group A Streptococcus (GAS)

Group B Streptococcus (GBS), Escherichia coli (neonate)

Non-typeable Haemophilus spp. (incidence unknown), Haemophilus influenzae type b (non-immunized or immunodeficient)

Streptococcus pneumoniae, Coagulase-negative staphylococcus (CoNS) (subacute)

Very rare at any age (increased in immunodeficiency and where specific risk factors occur)

Pseudomonas aeruginosa (usually inoculation injuries and therefore >1 year old)

Neisseria gonorrhea, Neisseria menigitidis (neonate, adolescent)

Mycobacterium tuberculosis (older children as OAI develops 2 years from primary infection)

Salmonella spp. (sickle cell disease) Non-tuberculous mycobacteria (associated with defects of IFNg/IL12 pathway)

Klebsiella spp. Bartonella henselae, Fusobacterium spp. (often multifocal)

Aspergillus spp., Candida albicans (neonate, damaged bone, CGD)

Nocardia asteroides, Serratia spp. (CGD)

Age-specific organisms

Neonate:

GBS, MSSA E coli and other gram-negatives, Candida albicans

<2 years:

MSSA, K kingae, S pneumoniae, H influenzae type b Non-typeable Haemophilus spp., E coli, MSSA PVL

2–5 years:

MSSA, K kingae, GAS, S pneumoniae, H influenzae type b, Non-typeable Haemophilus spp., Pseudomonas spp., Coagulase negative staphylococcus (subacute) MSSA PVL>5 years

MSSA,MSSA PVL, MRSA

Adapted from Managing bone and joint infection in children, Faust et al, Archives of Disease in Childhood, 2012 Jun;97(6):545–53.

and SA in young children for the last two decades. One study has suggested that *K. kingae* is more likely to be detected if bone and joint aspirates are cultured in broth,[26] although this has not been replicated elsewhere and has not been the case in clinical practice in the United Kingdom. New molecular methods including specific targeted polymerase chain reaction (PCR) are more likely to demonstrate the organism.[27] Often carried in the nasopharynx, the major clinical manifestation in children is in bone and joint disease, although it also causes endocarditis and has been described as a causative agent in brain abscesses.

Streptococci

Streptococcus pneumoniae is a less common cause of OM/SA in children, despite being a relatively common cause of bacteraemia. When seen it is mainly in infants and in immunocompromised children.

Group A β-haemolytic streptococci more commonly cause bone and joint infections. This is a common cause of skin and soft tissue infections, particularly following chickenpox.

Haemophilus influenzae

Haemophilus influenzae was a major cause of OM and SA in children prior to the introduction of the *H. influenza* type B (Hib) vaccination in the late 1980s and early 1990s. It should be considered in unvaccinated and immunocompromised children.

Pseudomonas aeruginosa

This is an uncommon cause of osteomyelitis in general. However, it is an important cause of subacute focal osteomyelitis of the foot, and usually involves a puncture wound such as stubbed toe or blister. Puncture wounds through a shoe are a particular risk factor.[28–30] Cases of acute haematogenous spread of *P. aeruginosa* are also reported.

Mycobacterium tuberculosis

Mycobacterium tuberculosis is an increasingly important pathogen worldwide. Fifty percent of children with TB present with no active pulmonary focus. In children pulmonary TB may be 'silent' with no signs or symptoms.[31] Initial infection can be missed, and subsequent bone and joint infection may not become apparent until several years later. Fifty percent have spinal involvement and the remainder have infection of long bones and synovial joints.

Spread of *M. tuberculosis* to osteoarticular sites is usually haematogenous. Occasionally there is direct contamination of a joint, or spread from an adjacent lymph node. Tuberculous osteomyelitis is usually characterized by necrotizing (caseating) granulomatous inflammation. Weightbearing joints are most commonly involved. In the spine the lower thoracic and lumbar vertebrae usually involved and spread occurs into adjacent discs and vertebrae, although there may be 'skip' lesions.

The organism usually enters the spine via arterioles supplying the anterior end plate and then spreads posteriorly. Spread to the intervertebral disc occurs late in the disease.[32] Pott's disease is vertebral osteomyelitis with paravertebral abscess, frequently associated with extensive bone destruction. Spinal tuberculosis is most common in adolescents and can present with vertebral collapse. Gibbus deformity occurs when there are multiple levels of collapse late in the disease.[33] Tuberculous dactylitis is largely a disease of young children (<10 years) and may remain unrecognized for long periods of time. It usually affects the hands, but can also affect the feet.[34] Extrapulmonary TB is more common in children who are coinfected with HIV, and also shows some female preponderance.[35]

Anaerobes

Anaerobic OAI is uncommon. However, in cases where there has been preceding history of trauma or surgery disrupting blood supply to the affected area, or in the skull where there has been mastoiditis or chronic otitis media, this should be considered. Anaerobes usually enter the site by direct contamination rather than via the haematogenous route.

Propionibacterium acnes is an aerotolerant anaerobe that causes postoperative infection, particularly following spinal surgery with metalwork. *Fusobacterium necrophorum* is an obligate anaerobe causing complicated mastoiditis with osteomyelitis.[36]

There are several case reports of non-tuberculous mycobacterial osteomyelitis, in both immunocompetent and immunocompromised children.[37–39]

Fungi

OAI caused by fungal infection, including yeasts and moulds, is extremely rare in immunocompetent hosts, although cases are documented in adults.[40] It affects children with neutropenia, chronic granulomatous disease, and premature and low-birthweight neonates. Fungaemia occurs most commonly in the intensive care setting.[41]

Candida species are the most common yeasts to cause systemic fungal infection, of which *C. albicans* is most common. Non-albicans candida species include *C. glabrata*, *C. kruseii*, and *C. parapsilosis*. These may be more virulent organisms than *C. albicans* and have different antifungal susceptibilities and resistance.

Aspergillus is the most common moulds implicated. Pathogenic species in humans include *A. fumigatus*, *A. flavus*, and *A. niger*. The most common sites of aspergillus OM are the spine, ribs, small bones, and chest wall.[42]

Other filamentous fungi found to cause opportunistic infection in immunocompromised patients are mucor, rhizopus, and fusarium.

Cryptococcus is a yeast found in soil, and has been described in a number of cases of fungal OAI. This organism is a cause of fungal meningitis in patients with HIV infection, but is occasionally seen as a cause of OAI in immunocompetent individuals.[43]

Special groups

Neonates

Neonates are more likely to have multifocal OM and to develop SA as infection spreads via transphyseal vessels. This is usually caused by haematogenous spread. Group B streptococcus is the most common organism and MSSA is also common. Coagulase-negative staphylococcus can also cause bacteraemia and seed to neonatal bones and joints. This organism should always be considered when indwelling central catheters are present.

Neonates are also more likely to develop fungal OM and SA, most commonly secondary to disseminated candidiasis. Risk factors for neonatal systemic fungal infection and subsequent OAI are prematurity, indwelling catheters, prolonged antibiotic use, and immune deficiency. Some 1–2% of infants with disseminated candidiasis will develop OM/SA. Infants less than 6 months old account for 85% of all paediatric fungal arthritis, which is most commonly caused by *C. albicans* or *C. parapsilosis*. Use of prophylactic fluconazole in neonatal intensive care units is changing the patterns of infection and susceptibility.[41]

Sickle cell disease

Sickle cell disease (SCD) is a most common genetic disease in defined areas of Africa and in migrant populations, affecting approximately 12 000 people in the United Kingdom. In 1999 the number of babies born with SCD in the United Kingdom was estimated to be 0.28 in 1000 per year.[44] In parts of sub-Saharan Africa the incidence is estimated at 3% of live births.[45]

Children with SCD, and to a lesser extent other haemoglobinopathies, are at increased risk of bone and joint infection. This may be difficult to distinguish clinically from ischaemic disease such as necrosis of the femoral head due to the SCD itself, and from sickle cell crisis. The increased risk of bone and joint infection is due to bone ischaemia, and small areas of necrotic bone allow a nidus of infection to form.

In sub-Saharan Africa 90% of children with SCD die before diagnosis, and the most common cause of death is sepsis.[46] In the United Kingdom at-risk infants are screened for SCD and will start penicillin prophylaxis once a diagnosis is made. In addition, Hib and conjugate pneumococcal vaccination reduce the risk of sepsis.

Non-typhoid salmonella bacteraemia is much more common in the SCD population. This can be attributed to impaired liver and splenic function, areas of devitalization of the bowel allowing translocation, and impairment of opsonization and phagocytosis. However, the reasons for salmonella bacteraemia in SCD are not fully understood.[47,48]

OM and SA in these patients is more likely to be caused by salmonella as a result of the increased risk of bacteraemia,[49] although MSSA infection remains an important cause.[50,51] The most commonly affected sites are long bones, in particular the tibia and humerus. Children with SCD are at greater risk of recurrence of OM/SA and treatment may be more challenging.

Immunocompromise

In immunosuppressed children MSSA remains the most common organism. However, if there is poor response to conventional therapy it is important to consider fungal infections such as *C. albicans*, *Aspergillus* , and less common organisms such as non-tuberculous mycobacteria, *Nocardia asteroides*, and anaerobes. Infection in immunocompromised children is more likely to be disseminated. OAI may be the first presentation and immunocompromise should be considered if there are atypical organisms, fungi, or multifocal or disseminated disease.

Children with acute leukaemia frequently present with bone pain. Once these patients have started chemotherapy they are at risk of neutropenia and thus at risk of infection. Bone and joint pain may therefore indicate OAI, or relapse of malignancy.[52] Children presenting with febrile neutropenia are usually treated with empiric intravenous antibiotic therapy assuming bacterial infection, which is usually not found to be OAI, and a high index of clinical suspicion is often required to detect the source of infection if the febrile episode does not resolve as expected.

Chronic granulomatous disease (CGD) is a rare inherited deficiency of NADPH oxidase causing failure of phagocytic cells to produce oxidants. Children with this disease are therefore particularly susceptible to infection with catalase-positive organisms, non-tuberculous mycobacteria, *Nocardia asteroides*, serratia, aspergillus: 25% of children with CGD develop OAI.[53] Chest wall and vertebral spread may occur from contiguous pneumonia. Haematogenous spread also occurs to limb bones, and the osteomyelitis may be multifocal.

Clinical features

Classically the child with OAI presents with fever, pain at the affected site, and often bone or joint swelling. The child may be systemically unwell, especially in acute haematogenous OM.

Infants may present with a pseudoparalysis—refusal to move the affected limb. Where the lower limb is affected toddlers may refuse to walk. In SA the joint is held in a fixed position that maximizes the joint space and reduces pain. For example, the hip may be held flexed, abducted and externally rotated.

Pyrexia of unknown origin is a presenting feature. OAI should be considered in all children with persistent fever where no cause is found, even if there are no focal signs.

Focal osteomyelitis generally presents insidiously. There may be history of puncture wound, and localized tenderness and swelling in an otherwise well child. This may be difficult to distinguish from overlying soft tissue infection, but is more persistent.

Tuberculous OAI can be challenging to diagnose. These children may have a very long history of pain. In particular, spinal pain may have been present for months or years. Often there is faltering growth or weight loss.

Discitis often presents with an irritable child with no obvious cause. Babies and young children in nappies may become distressed during nappy changes as the spine is flexed.

See Table 99.2 for a summary of aetiology and clinical features.

Table 99.2 Summary of aetiology and clinical features

Age	Organisms	Clinical features
Neonates	GBS, *Escherichia coli*/Gram-negatives, MSSA, *Candida albicans*, coagulase-negative staphylococcus	Irritability, fever, widespread pain often difficult to localize on examination
		Pseudoparalysis, erythema, bone or limb swelling. Several sites may be involved
		Pseudoparalysis of arm, looking like a delayed-onset Erb's palsy, classic of late-onset GBS OM of humeral head
		Bone or joint infection should be considered if there is a positive blood culture
<2 years	MSSA, *Kingella kingae*, *Streptococcus pneumoniae*, *Haemophilus influenzae* type b, non-typeable haemophilus, *E. coli*, GAS (especially in children following chickenpox), MSSA PVL (uncommon in the UK), MRSA PVL (very rare in the UK)	**Acute haematogenous osteomyelitis:**
		Usually short history, with an ill child in pain
		Fever of unknown origin
		Fever and malaise are frequent with bacteraemia but may be absent
2–5 years	MSSA, *K. kingae*, GAS, *S. pneumoniae*, non-typeable haemophilus, MSSA PVL (uncommon in the UK), MRSA PVL (very rare in the UK)	Refusal to move the limb or to weightbear, limp, erythema, bone or limb swelling, local tenderness
		Septic arthritis:
>5 years	MSSA, MRSA PVL (uncommon in the UK), MRSA PVL (very rare in the UK), *K. kingae*, pseudomonas	Usually a unifocal hot, immobile, tender peripheral joint, with pain on passive joint movement
		May have no focal signs
		Fever of unknown origin
		Subacute or chronic osteomyelitis:
		Longer history, maybe weeks, with no systemic symptoms
		History of penetrating wound
		Often no fever
		Less acute local signs with limp, refusal to move the limb or weightbear
		Local bony swelling or tenderness
		If left untreated can form fistulas, have purulent discharge
Discitis	Usually no organism is isolated	**Insidious onset, with no systemic illness**
		Fever is uncommon
		Back pain, refusal to sit, stand, or walk
		Refusal to flex the spine, local tenderness, irritability on nappy changing in infants
		Constipation or abdominal pain

GAS, group A streptococcus; GBS, group B streptococcus; MRSA, meticillin-resistant *Staphylococcus aureus*; MSSA, meticillin-sensitive *Staphylococcus aureus*; PVL, Panton–Valentine leucocidin.

The differential diagnoses of OM/SA include:

+ Trauma including non-accidental injury
+ Soft tissue infections—cellulitis, fasciitis
+ Malignancy—osteosarcoma, leukaemia, neuroblastoma
+ Reactive arthritis—secondary to viral infection
+ Haemarthrosis
+ Henoch–Scho?nlein purpura
+ Juvenile idiopathic arthritis—the commonest cause of monoarthritis in children
+ Infarction/bone necrosis, especially in SCD
+ Erb's palsy in neonates

Investigations and diagnosis

The clinical course and outcome of OAI is dependent on early treatment before tissue destruction can occur.[17] If clinical features suggest OM or SA, imaging and laboratory tests can confirm diagnosis and the extent of disease. They can then be used to monitor disease progression and resolution.

Laboratory tests

Initial tests when the child presents should include C-reactive protein (CRP) and erythrocyte sedimentation rate (ESR). These are more reliably increased than white cell count but normal values do not absolutely exclude OM or SA.[54] Values of ESR greater than 20 mm/hour and CRP greater than 20 mg/litre are found in more than 90% of children with OM or SA. ESR tends to peak on day 3–5 of infection, whereas CRP increases more rapidly and peaks on day 2 of hospitalization. ESR lags behind resolution of disease, and takes 2–3 weeks of to return to normal, whereas CRP takes around 1 week.[55]

The Kocher criteria are used in the emergency setting to aid diagnosis of a septic hip in a child presenting with hip pain. The original study to develop these rules was based on SA of the hip specifically. Kocher's criteria use four independent predictive factors: history of fever above 38.3 °C, non-weightbearing, ESR 40 mm/hour or longer, and white blood cell count greater than 12×10^6/dL. If all four features are present the likelihood of SA of the hip is 93%.[56,57] If a CRP level above 20 mg/litre is included, the likelihood increases to 97%.[58]

More recently studies have shown that the severity of infection with MRSA is greater than with MSSA and that CRP and ESR are higher in MRSA infection than in MSSA infection.[59]

Blood culture should be performed in all children with suspected bone and joint infection, ideally before starting antibiotic therapy. Blood cultures have been reported to be positive in up to 60% of cases.[60] However, these are mostly selected case series and rates of positive blood culture in OM/SA in the United Kingdom and Europe are often much lower.[2]

Full blood count and film should also be performed, as the differential diagnosis of bone and joint pains will include leukaemia, particularly if the spine is involved.

Due to the non-specificity of symptoms in neonates and ability of bacteria to cause widespread infection, a full septic screen including urine microscopy and culture, chest radiograph, and lumbar puncture should be performed.

If TB is suspected a tuberculin skin test (TST) and interferon gamma release assay (IGRA) should be done. These have similar sensitivity in children.[61] Negative TST and/or IGRA do not rule out TB, but are useful tools to aid diagnosis where history is suggestive of exposure to *M. tuberculosis*.

Direct samples from the affected bone or joint are usually taken surgically if indicated (bone biopsy), or occasionally via interventional radiology. CT- or ultrasound-guided aspiration of joints allows for reliable samples of the affected area.

All samples should be sent for microscopy and culture, and histology. Culture of bone and joint aspirates is important, but sensitivity remains low, even when methods are optimized.

However, molecular techniques such as PCR are being increasingly used to identify organisms in culture-negative disease. DNA is extracted from tissue and incubated with primers for the constant regions of 16S RNA gene.[62] The bacterial specific sequences between these regions are then amplified and the bacteria can be identified by entering the sequence into a database.[60,63]

Real-time PCR has been particularly useful for identifying *K. kingae* infections, and is one of the reasons this organism has been more recently recognized as an important cause of OM/SA.[63] This method is also used to identify PVL-producing strains of *S. aureus* when clinically suspected, using a PCR target specific for these strains.[64]

Imaging

Plain radiographs may show periosteal elevation or lytic change if infection has been present for more than 10 days. This is not a sensitive test and it is particularly difficult to see changes in the pelvis, ribs, sternum, and spine. Plain radiographs of the affected joint are usually performed, for example, in the non-weightbearing toddler to exclude fracture.

MRI is the gold standard for imaging OM and SA due to its higher sensitivity and specificity, and also as it does not involve ionizing radiation.[65] T2-weighted images show increased bone marrow intensity corresponding with oedema. T1-weighted images show darker bone marrow. These changes are not specific, but can be interpreted in the context of suspected bone infection. If abscess is suspected this is best demonstrated with fat suppression on T1-weighted image with gadolinium enhancement.[66] However, MRI is not always be practical in the acute setting when younger children are likely to require a general anaesthetic for the procedure. MRI is particularly important in the diagnosis of skeletal TB, and in spinal and pelvic osteomyelitis and discitis. Sparing of the intervertebral disc on imaging early in the disease is suggestive of TB.[32,33]

CT shows soft tissue changes and necrotic bone, and may be easier to perform in young children where general anaesthetic is not available. CT is also useful for providing guidance to interventional radiologists and surgeons when taking aspirates from sites of bone or joint infection.

Ultrasound scan be useful in SA to assess deep effusion, subperiostial collection and abscess formation. Its main use is in neonates, and in guided aspiration of joints.[67]

Technetium radionuclide bone scan (^{99m}Tc) or bone scintigraphy has high sensitivity and specificity but is now used less often due to the radiation burden. This technique may also give false-negative results in infancy. Scintigraphy can be useful where multifocal infection is more common, such as in immunocompromised children or those with SCD.[68]

Management

There are no agreed national or international guidelines for the management of paediatric OAI, although recent pragmatic guidelines have been published in the United Kingdom.[2,69] Management is multidisciplinary including paediatricians, orthopaedic surgeons, radiologists, and microbiologists. There remains limited high-quality evidence to guide therapy, although large prospective trials are currently being considered. Until now established practice has been based on expert opinion and history.[70,71]

Key steps in the management involve an initial decision regarding whether surgical intervention for diagnosis and/or treatment is required or feasible, as well as the choice of empirical intravenous antibiotic agent. The choice of antimicrobial agent for ongoing care will be guided by microbiology results. Subsequently decisions must be made surrounding the overall length of therapy, and whether to switch from intravenous to oral antibiotic agents.

Surgery

There is little high-quality evidence on which to base surgical practice of OAI at present, and decisions are therefore based on expert orthopaedic opinion.

Where a soft tissue collection or bone abscess is apparent radiologically, surgical drainage is recommended.[72] Immobilization of any surgically treated limb is also advisable.[2]

If OM/SA is diagnosed early by MRI scan and medical treatment is initiated successfully, surgical intervention is usually not required. Treatment response can be assessed by monitoring CRP and ESR, and the clinical status of the child.[9] Surgical drainage in acute OM is indicated if there is poor response to antibiotics after 48–72 hours.[71]

If SA is suspected, guided aspiration prior to starting antibiotic therapy is advisable to identify the organism where logistically possible. Ideally this should be before antibiotic therapy is initiated, unless a delay of more than 4 hours is anticipated. Arthroscopic drainage or washout of the joint is also indicated to reduce destruction of the synovium and cartilage by inflammatory cells. In SA of the hip, the role of surgery is considered more definite. Capsulotomy to drain the joint, and where pus is not identified, drilling of the femoral head to decompress any osteomyelitis to prevent necrosis, are indicated.[20] If PVL MSSA or MRSA is suspected it, aspiration and washout are considered essential as these organisms can cause rapid tissue destruction.[16,17] Where the spine is involved, orthotic support may be indicated especially if there is evidence of collapse on imaging.

Antibiotic therapy

See Table 99.3 for summary.

Initial empirical therapy

Once the child is clinically stable, the important aspects of medical management are antibiotic therapy and analgesia. The majority of children with OM/SA do not present overtly septic or unwell, and do not usually require resuscitation outside the neonatal period. It takes time to identify causative organisms, therefore initial therapy will usually be empirical, and is always intravenous. This must be tailored to provide best cover for the most likely organisms. Treatment should be initiated as soon as a diagnosis of OAI is made, or immediately following surgery for diagnosis or treatment.

Table 99.3 Summary table of antibiotics by age group

Neonate (<3 months)	Benzyl penicillin and gentamicin
	Or cefotaxime
	Add amoxicillin if listeria suspected
	Oral switch to co-amoxiclav
3 months–5 years	Cefuroxime
	Oral switch to cefalexin or co-amoxiclav
>5 years	Flucloxacillin or clindamycin
	Consider ceftazidime or ciprofloxacin if pseudomonas suspected
	Oral switch to co-amoxiclav suspension or flucloxacillin or clindamycin tablets

In neonates (preterm or <3 months of age), initial empiric therapy is the same as for other neonatal sepsis, and practice varies between centres. For example, benzylpenicillin with gentamicin, or cefotaxime are often first line. These regimes cover group B streptococcus, MSSA, and Gram-negative organisms. Cefotaxime also has good penetration into the cerebrospinal fluid. Ampicillin or amoxicillin are added until *Listeria monocytogenes* meningitis is excluded. In view of the haematogenous aetiology of OM/SA in neonates and immature immune system, it is advisable to do a full septic screen including lumbar puncture in this group.

In children 3 months to 5 years old, initial therapy should have potent activity against MSSA although this age group is at most risk of *K. kingae* infection, probably secondary to pharyngeal colonization.[73] Cefuroxime provides good cover for this and for MSSA as well as for group A streptococcus, non-typeable haemophilus infections, and *H. influenzae* type B in any children incompletely immunized.

In children 6 years and older, MSSA is by far the most common organism and high-dose intravenous flucloxacillin is the usual antibiotic therapy of choice, or clindamycin if penicillin allergic. If there is poor response to treatment after 48–72 hours of treatment, or if MRSA or PVL is suspected, clindamycin or linezolid can be added as a second agent (but see below for treatment in confirmed PVL staphylococcal infections).[59,65,72]

In children with puncture wounds of the feet, such as a nail through a sports shoe, pseudomonas should also be covered. The wound should be irrigated and debrided if necessary to remove debris, and tetanus vaccination status checked.

Duration of intravenous therapy and oral switch

In recent years, many have advocated the reduction of risks associated with long-term intravenous therapy with early switch to oral therapy.[69,71,74] Small clinical studies have shown a similar cure rate between short courses of intravenous antibiotic therapy with oral continuation vs long-course intravenous therapy. In selected cases, acute SA has also been treated with a total course of 2 weeks of antibiotic therapy.[69,75]

Oral switch can be considered early after 48 hours if disease is uncomplicated osteomyelitis, and there is clinical improvement.[76] The child should be afebrile and able to take oral food and fluids.[74] CRP should also have fallen consistently.[9] Pragmatically this could be to one third of the original value or to less than 20 mg/mL. Conversely, if there is continued pyrexia and inflammatory markers are not falling, intravenous therapy should be reviewed, and further imaging and surgical intervention considered as above.[2]

The decision of which agent to use when to switch to switching to oral therapy is also dependent on palatability and frequency of administration of the drug. Flucloxacillin and clindamycin suspensions are unpalatable and poorly tolerated, and adherence to these medications is poor.[77] They are therefore not a good first choice in young children who cannot take tablets, despite their excellent oral bioavailability and tissue penetration.[71]

Co-amoxiclav and cefalexin suspensions are generally well tolerated and these are good alternatives for oral switch in any children unable to take tablets. In older children who can take tablets, flucloxacillin or clindamycin can be continued orally.[77]

The total duration of intravenous antibiotic therapy required to effect complete cure is unknown, but most clinical practice is based on consideration of reduction of old textbook regimes of up to 6 weeks intravenous therapy for both uncomplicated and complex disease. Historic observational studies suggested a risk of relapse with antibiotic therapy of less than 3 weeks.[78,79]

In complicated disease—defined as where there is evidence of multifocal disease, significant bone destruction, abscess or pathological fracture, or immunocompromise[20]—the total duration of antibiotic therapy may be longer. Intravenous therapy may also be prolonged if the child is systemically unwell or unable to tolerate oral antibiotics. This group includes neonates, in whom oral antibiotics are unreliably absorbed, and intravenous therapy should be continued for 14–21 days.[20] Complex disease with significant collection may require up to 6 weeks intravenous antibiotics.

Where pseudomonas infection is suspected, anti-pseudomonal therapy should be initiated. Agents include ciprofloxacin and ceftazidime. Ciprofloxacin is has good oral availability, and can be used for oral switch. The wound should be irrigated and debrided if necessary to remove debris, and tetanus vaccination status checked.[28,80]

If PVL disease is suspected the latest Health Protection Agency guidelines should be used in the United Kingdom, and the case discussed with a specialist in infectious disease. This is a notifiable disease in the United Kingdom and contacts should be traced. It should be treated with flucloxacillin, if MSSA. If MRSA is confirmed, vancomycin or clindamycin may be used. Clindamycin, linezolid, or rifampicin inhibits protein synthesis and theoretically reduces toxin production. Addition of rifampicin to vancomycin therapy in MRSA OAI may also be advised by local microbiologists.[72]

Tuberculous osteomyelitis once confirmed should be treated according to National Institute for Health and Clinical Excellence (NICE) guidelines for *M. tuberculosis* infection. This is initially standard regimen of 4 months rifampicin, isoniazid, pyrazinamide, and ethambutol followed by 2 months rifampicin and isoniazid only. *M. tuberculosis* infections require close monitoring and repeat imaging is advised.

In immunocompromised children prolonged intravenous antibiotic therapy is indicated. These should be discussed with microbiology and paediatric infectious disease consultants. Many of these children will have been treated with antibiotics previously and may be colonized with resistant organisms.

If fungal osteomyelitis is suspected antifungal treatment is initiated, for example with amphotericin, caspofungin, posaconazole, or voriconazole. This should be discussed with specialist microbiologists or infectious disease paediatricians. There is limited

evidence available regarding the treatment of these infections, which frequently require surgical debridement.[42] Fluconazole and amphotericin B remain commonly used both in neonates and in older children at risk of fungal infection. Liver and renal functions require monitoring with most antifungal therapy. Echinocandins such as caspofungin and micafungin are a newer class of antifungals that effectively treat yeast infections such as candida and are fungicidal for these. Voriconazole and pozaconazole are also being used in persistent fungal infections.

Children with SCD should be managed with adequate analgesia and hydration where necessary. Intravenous cephalosporin is usual as empirical therapy, although failure of ceftriaxone treatment for salmonella is reported. If salmonella infection is suspected, quinolones may be of use in susceptible organisms.

Children with discitis should be treated with empiric anti-staphylococcal antibiotic therapy as this reduces duration of symptoms.

Complications

Children who have had OM/SA should be followed carefully, as seemingly uncomplicated cases may have altered growth or occasionally develop deformity. Pathological fracture following chronic OM is a well-recognized complication.[81]

Necrosis of the affected epiphysis and limb-length discrepancy are also seen. This is more common where there is a delay in treatment, or in response to treatment and following MRSA infections.[82] Complication rates of treatment regimens themselves are unclear.

Spinal osteomyelitis, and in particular destructive tuberculous disease, can lead to neurological complications associated with vertebral collapse including hemiplegia. This is preventable with regular follow-up and orthotic and physiotherapy input.

Conclusion

OAI in children is an uncommon but important diagnosis. Clinical features may be non-specific and variable. Imaging techniques aid diagnosis, and MRI is the most effective of these. The causative organisms vary with age and risk factors.

Empirical antibiotic therapy should target the most likely causative organisms within these groups. Surgical input to obtain samples, or decompress or stabilize bones and joints is sometimes necessary, and orthopaedic opinion should be sought. Complications are rare when OAI is diagnosed and treated in the acute phase.

Case history 1: Osteomyelitis in a child over 6 years old.

A 6 year old boy presented with a one-day history of right knee pain. He had played football in the park the day before, and was otherwise usually fit and well with no significant past medical history. On arrival at the Emergency Department he had a temperature of 38.5 °C. Examination of his legs showed reduced flexion and rotation of the right hip, which was warm to touch.

Blood tests showed a white blood cell count of 12×10^9/dL and CRP of 52 g/dL. Ultrasound scan showed an effusion in the right hip. Blood cultures showed no growth at 48 hours. Arthroscopic washout of the hip was performed, obtaining turbid fluid. His unifocal SA was treated empirically with intravenous flucloxacillin for 1 week with resolution of pain and fever. He was discharged with a further 3 weeks of oral co-amoxiclav, ensuring good drug adherence by using an oral antibiotic with good taste and suitable dose frequency regime.

Learning Points:

- Reduced range of movement, pain and fever suggest OAI.

- Knee pain may be referred pain from the hip.

- MSSA is the most likely organism, flucloxacillin is a good choice of intravenous antibiotic in this age group if there are no comorbidities.

Case history 2: Osteomyelitis in a younger child

A 5 year old boy presented to hospital with a 2 week history of left ankle pain. His mother thought he might have twisted it while playing. On examination he was reluctant to weight bear and the ankle was swollen and warm to touch. White blood cell count was 10×10^9/dL, and CRP was 25 mg/L.

Following normal ultrasound and plain radiographs, MRI of the ankle was performed and showed OM of the distal fibula, the report suggesting inflammation of 2–3 weeks duration. Blood cultures were negative but multiplex PCR subsequently confirmed *Kingella kingae* infection. He was treated with intravenous cefuroxime for 5 days, and discharged to complete 4 weeks cefalexin. Clinical symptoms resolved.

Learning points:

- Minor trauma is commonly present in the history, and may be a 'red herring'.

- Ultrasound scan and radiograph may appear normal and MRI can confirm diagnosis.

- Multiplex PCR is useful for the identification of *K. kingae*— which should be considered in all children up to 5 years.

Case history 3: Neonatal osteoarticular infection—beware limb pseudoparalysis

A 3 week old baby presented with a 3 day history of not moving the right leg. He was mottled and pyrexial, 38.5 °C at presentation. Full septic screen was performed that showed white blood cell count of 4×10^9/dL with neutrophil count of 2×10^9/dL. CRP was 77 g/dL. Lumbar puncture showed cerebrospinal fluid white cell count of less than 5/dL with normal protein and glucose 70% of plasma level (normal).

Clinical diagnosis of SA of the hip was made and washout performed. He was treated empirically with intravenous cefotaxime for 2 weeks initial period. As blood culture grew a fully sensitive group B streptococcus, treatment was changed to intravenous benzylpenicillin to complete a 6 week course of therapy.

Learning points:

- Pseudoparalysis in a neonate suggests OAI.

- Full septic screen is indicated in view of likely bacteraemia.

- Surgical washout is indicated in SA of the hip.

Case history 4: Tuberculous osteoarticular infection

A 14 year old Nepalese boy presented with a painful, discharging sinus on the anterior aspect of his left shoulder with reduced range of movement. He had been taking non-steroidal anti-infalammatory drugs (NSAIDs) for 6 weeks for pain and swelling. He was noted to be of short stature, below the 0.4th centile, and reported that he had had night sweats for some months. He also described worsening back pain for the last 2 years. Examination showed marked scoliosis.

White cell count was 12.2×10^9/dL, neutrophils 7×10^9/dL, CRP 43 g/dL and ESR 23 mm/hour. TST showed induration of 15 mm, IGRA was indeterminate. Culture of pus from the sinus showed no growth and acid-fast bacilli were not seen.

Technetium bone scan showed a lesion in the T12/L1 region of the spine, and in the left shoulder. MRI also showed multifocal spinal disease with collapse of the T12 vertebra. CT-guided biopsy of the spine was performed and culture grew a fully sensitive *M. tuberculosis*. Quadruple therapy of rifampicin, isoniazid, pyrazinamide, and ethambutol was started following the biopsy. This teenager also required a spinal brace and physiotherapy input before return to school and mobile activities.

Learning points:

- Tuberculous OAI may be chronic.

- Diagnosis may be challenging due to false-negative or equivocal IGRA or TST, and difficulty culturing the organism.

- Treatment is for at least 6 months and regular follow-up is required.

References

1. Blyth MJ, Kincaid R, Craigen MA, Bennet GC. The changing epidemiology of acute and subacute haematogenous osteomyelitis in children. *J Bone Joint Surg Br* 2001;83(1):99–102.

2. Faust SN, Clark J, Pallett A, Clarke NM. Managing bone and joint infection in children. *Arch Dis Child* 2012;97(6):545–553.

3. Lavy CB. Septic arthritis in Western and sub-Saharan African children—a review. *Int Orthop* 2007;31(2):137–144.

4. Vazquez M. Osteomyelitis in children. *Curr Opin Pediatr* 2002;14(1):112–115.

5. Topley JM, Cupidore L, Vaidya S, Hayes RJ, Serjeant GR. Pneumococcal and other infections in children with sickle-cell hemoglobin C (SC) disease. *J Pediatr* 1982;101(2):176–179.

6. Talbot JC, Bismil Q, Saralaya D et al. Musculoskeletal tuberculosis in Bradford—a 6-year review. *Ann R Coll Surg Engl* 2007;89(4):405–409.

7. Holland TS, Sangster MJ, Paton RW, Ormerod LP. Bone and joint tuberculosis in children in the Blackburn area since 2006: a case series. *J Child Orthop* 2010;4(1):67–71.

8. Teo HE, Peh WC. Skeletal tuberculosis in children. *Pediatr Radiol* 2004;34(11):853–860.

9. Paakkonen M, Kallio MJ, Kallio PE, Peltola H. Sensitivity of erythrocyte sedimentation rate and C-reactive protein in childhood bone and joint infections. *Clin Orthop Relat Res* 2010;468(3):861–866.

10. Norden CW. Experimental osteomyelitis. I. A description of the model. *J Infect Dis* 1970;122(5):410–418.

11. Wiley AM, Trueta J. The vascular anatomy of the spine and its relationship to pyogenic vertebral osteomyelitis. *J Bone Joint Surg Br* 1959;41-B:796–809.

12. Ramseier LE, Janicki JA, Weir S, Narayanan UG. Femoral fractures in adolescents: a comparison of four methods of fixation. *J Bone Joint Surg Am* 2010;92(5):1122–1129.

13. Sohn AH, Schwartz JM, Yang KY et al. Risk factors and risk adjustment for surgical site infections in pediatric cardiothoracic surgery patients. *Am J Infect Control* 2010;38(9):706–710.

14. Bucher BT, Guth RM, Elward AM et al. Risk factors and outcomes of surgical site infection in children. *J Am Coll Surg* 2011;212(6):1033–1038 e1.

15. Kraai T, Brown C, Neeff M, Fisher K. Complications of bone-anchored hearing aids in pediatric patients. *Int J Pediatr Otorhinolaryngol* 2011;75(6):749–753.

16. Brand RA. 50 Years ago in CORR: Osteomyelitis since the advent of antibiotics; a study of infants and children: Gordon M. Cottington, MD, Jay M. Riden, MD, and Albert B. Ferguson, Jr, MD CORR 1959;14:97–101. *Clin Orthop Relat Res* 2011;469(11):3257–3258.

17. Hartwig NG. How to treat acute musculoskeletal infections in children. *Adv Exp Med Biol* 2006;582:191–200.

18. Lunseth PA, Heiple KG. Prognosis in septic arthritis of the hip in children. *Clin Orthop Relat Res* 1979;139:81–85.

19. Peltola H, Vahvanen V. A comparative study of osteomyelitis and purulent arthritis with special reference to aetiology and recovery. *Infection* 1984;12(2):75–79.

20. Ohbayashi T, Irie A, Murakami Y et al. Degradation of fibrinogen and collagen by staphopains, cysteine proteases released from Staphylococcus aureus. *Microbiology* 2011;157(Pt 3):786–792.

21. Vander Have KL, Karmazyn B, Verma M et al. Community-associated methicillin-resistant Staphylococcus aureus in acute musculoskeletal infection in children: a game changer. *J Pediatr Orthoped* 2009;29(8):927–931.

22. Bouchoucha S, Benghachame F, Trifa M et al. Deep venous thrombosis associated with acute hematogenous osteomyelitis in children. *Orthop Traumatol Surg Res* 2010;96(8):890–893.

23. Cunnington A, Brick T, Cooper M et al. Severe invasive Panton-Valentine leucocidin positive Staphylococcus aureus infections in children in London, UK. *J Infect* 2009;59(1):28–36.

24. Lina G, Piemont Y, Godail-Gamot F et al. Involvement of Panton-Valentine leukocidin-producing Staphylococcus aureus in primary skin infections and pneumonia. *Clin Infect Dis* 1999;29(5):1128–1132.

25. Ju KL, Zurakowski D, Kocher MS. Differentiating between methicillin-resistant and methicillin-sensitive Staphylococcus aureus osteomyelitis in children: an evidence-based clinical prediction algorithm. *J Bone Joint Surg Am* 2011;93(18):1693–1701.

26. Yagupsky P, Dagan R. Kingella kingae: an emerging cause of invasive infections in young children. *Clin Infect Dis* 1997;24(5):860–866.

27. Ceroni D, Cherkaoui A, Ferey S, Kaelin A, Schrenzel J. Kingella kingae osteoarticular infections in young children: clinical features and contribution of a new specific real-time PCR assay to the diagnosis. *J Pediatr Orthop* 2010;30(3):301–304.

28. Inaba AS, Zukin DD, Perro M. An update on the evaluation and management of plantar puncture wounds and Pseudomonas osteomyelitis. *Pediatr Emerg Care* 1992;8(1):38–44.

29. UK Health Protection Agency. Polymicrobial bacteraemias and fungaemias in England, Wales, and Northern Ireland: 2009. *Health Protection Report* 2011 5(3). Available at: http://www.hpa.org.uk/hpr/archives/2011/hpr0311.pdf.

30. Brand RA, Black H. Pseudomonas osteomyelitis following puncture wounds in children. *J Bone Joint Surg Am* 1974;56(8):1637–1642.

31. Nicol MP, Zar HJ. New specimens and laboratory diagnostics for childhood pulmonary TB: progress and prospects. *Paediatr Respir Rev* 2011;12(1):16–21.

32. De Vuyst D, Vanhoenacker F, Gielen J, Bernaerts A, De Schepper AM. Imaging features of musculoskeletal tuberculosis. *Eur Radiol* 2003;13(8):1809–1819.

33. Teo HE, Peh WC. Skeletal tuberculosis in children. *Pediatr Radiol* 2004;34(11):853–860.

34. Ritz N, Connell TG, Tebruegge M, Johnstone BR, Curtis N. Tuberculous dactylitis—an easily missed diagnosis. *Eur J Clin Microbiol Infect Dis* 2011;30(11):1303–1310.

35. Zhang X, Andersen AB, Lillebaek T et al. Effect of sex, age, and race on the clinical presentation of tuberculosis: a 15-year population-based study. *Am J Trop Med Hyg* 2011;85(2):285–290.

36. Haidar R, Najjar M, Der Boghossian A, Tabbarah Z. Propionibacterium acnes causing delayed postoperative spine infection: review. *Scand J Infect Dis* 2010;42(6–7):405–411.

37. Petitjean G, Fluckiger U, Scharen S, Laifer G. Vertebral osteomyelitis caused by non-tuberculous mycobacteria. *Clin Microbiol Infect* 2004;10(11):951–953.

38. Williams B, Neth O, Shingadia D et al. Mycobacterium kansasii causing septic arthritis and osteomyelitis in a child. *Pediatr Infect Dis J* 2010;29(1):88–89.

39. van Ingen J, Looijmans F, Mirck P, Dekhuijzen R, Boeree M, van Soolingen D. Otomastoiditis caused by Mycobacterium abscessus, The Netherlands. *Emerg Infect Dis* 2010;16(1):166–168.

40. Sethi S, Siraj F, Kalra K, Chopra P. Aspergillus vertebral osteomyelitis in immunocompetent patients. *Indian J Orthopaed* 2012;46(2):246–250.

41. Chapman RL. Prevention and treatment of Candida infections in neonates. *Semin Perinatol* 2007;31(1):39–46.

42. Dotis J, Roilides E. Osteomyelitis due to Aspergillus species in chronic granulomatous disease: an update of the literature. *Mycoses* 2011;54(6):e686–e696.

43. Raftopoulos I, Meller JL, Harris V, Reyes HM. Cryptococcal rib osteomyelitis in a pediatric patient. *J Pediatr Surg* 1998;33(5):771–773.

44. Hickman M, Modell B, Greengross P et al. Mapping the prevalence of sickle cell and beta thalassaemia in England: estimating and validating ethnic-specific rates. *Br J Haematol* 1999;104(4):860–867.

45. Grosse SD, Odame I, Atrash HK et al. Sickle cell disease in Africa: a neglected cause of early childhood mortality. *Am J Prevent Med* 2011;41(6 Suppl 4):S398–S405.

46. Sadarangani M, Makani J, Komba AN et al. An observational study of children with sickle cell disease in Kilifi, Kenya. *Br J Haematol* 2009;146(6):675–682.

47. Anand AJ, Glatt AE. Salmonella osteomyelitis and arthritis in sickle cell disease. *Semin Arthritis Rheum* 1994;24(3):211–221.

48. Brown M, Eykyn SJ. Non-typhoidal Salmonella bacteraemia without gastroenteritis: a marker of underlying immunosuppression. Review Of cases at St. Thomas' Hospital 1970–1999. *J Infect* 2000;41(3):256–259.

49. Richards LH, Howard J, Klein JL. Community-acquired Salmonella bacteraemia in patients with sickle-cell disease 1969–2008: a single centre study. *Scand J Infect Dis* 2011;43(2):89–94.

50. Epps CH, Jr., Bryant DD, 3rd, Coles MJ, Castro O. Osteomyelitis in patients who have sickle-cell disease. Diagnosis and management. *J Bone Joint Surg Am* 1991;73(9):1281–1294.

51. Burnett MW, Bass JW, Cook BA. Etiology of osteomyelitis complicating sickle cell disease. *Pediatrics* 1998;101(2):296–297.

52. van der Have N, Nath SV, Story C et al. Differential diagnosis of paediatric bone pain: acute lymphoblastic leukemia. *Leukemia Res* 2012;36(4):521–523.

53. Winkelstein JA, Marino MC, Johnston RB et al. Chronic granulomatous disease. Report on a national registry of 368 patients. *Medicine* (Baltimore) 2000;79(3):155–169.

54. Unkila-Kallio L, Kallio MJ, Eskola J, Peltola H. Serum C-reactive protein, erythrocyte sedimentation rate, and white blood cell count in acute hematogenous osteomyelitis of children. *Pediatrics* 1994;93(1):59–62.

55. Paakkonen M, Kallio MJ, Kallio PE, Peltola H. Sensitivity of erythrocyte sedimentation rate and C-reactive protein in childhood bone and joint infections. *Clinical Orthop Relat Res* 2010;468(3):861–866.

56. Kocher MS, Mandiga R, Zurakowski D, Barnewolt C, Kasser JR. Validation of a clinical prediction rule for the differentiation between septic arthritis and transient synovitis of the hip in children. *J Bone Joint Surg Am* 2004;86-A(8):1629–1635.

57. Kocher MS, Zurakowski D, Kasser JR. Differentiating between septic arthritis and transient synovitis of the hip in children: an evidence-based clinical prediction algorithm. *J Bone Joint Surg Am* 1999;81(12): 1662–1670.

58. Caird MS, Flynn JM, Leung YL et al. Factors distinguishing septic arthritis from transient synovitis of the hip in children. A prospective study. *J Bone Joint Surg Am* 2006;88(6):1251–1257.

59. Williams DJ, Deis JN, Tardy J, Creech CB. Culture-negative osteoarticular infections in the era of community-associated methicillin-resistant Staphylococcus aureus. *Pediatr Infect Dis J* 2011;30(6): 523–525.

60. Kaplan SL. Challenges in the evaluation and management of bone and joint infections and the role of new antibiotics for gram positive infections. *Adv Exp Med Biol* 2009;634:111–120.

61. Machingaidze S, Wiysonge CS, Gonzalez-Angulo Y et al. The utility of an interferon gamma release assay for diagnosis of latent tuberculosis infection and disease in children: a systematic review and meta-analysis. *Pediatr Infect Dis J* 2011;30(8):694–700.

62. Rosey AL, Abachin E, Quesnes G et al. Development of a broad-range 16S rDNA real-time PCR for the diagnosis of septic arthritis in children. *J Microbiol Methods* 2007;68(1):88–93.

63. Ceroni D, Cherkaoui A, Ferey S, Kaelin A, Schrenzel J. Kingella kingae osteoarticular infections in young children: clinical features and contribution of a new specific real-time PCR assay to the diagnosis. *J Pediatr Orthoped* 2010;30(3):301–304.

64. Shallcross LJ, Williams K, Hopkins S et al. Panton-Valentine leukocidin associated staphylococcal disease: a cross-sectional study at a London hospital, England. *Clin Microbiol Infect* 2010;16(11):1644–1648.

65. Thomsen I, Creech CB. Advances in the diagnosis and management of pediatric osteomyelitis. *Curr Infect Dis Rep* 2011;13(5):451–460.

66. Chung T. Magnetic resonance imaging in acute osteomyelitis in children. *Pediatr Infect Dis J* 2002;21(9):869–870.

67. Rubin LP, Wallach MT, Wood BP. Radiological case of the month. Neonatal osteomyelitis diagnosed by ultrasound. *Arch Pediatr Adolesc Med* 1996;150(2):217–218.

68. Steer AC, Carapetis JR. Acute hematogenous osteomyelitis in children: recognition and management. *Paediatr Drugs* 2004;6(6):333–346.

69. Paakkonen M, Peltola H. Management of a child with suspected acute septic arthritis. *Arch Dis Child* 2012;97(3):287–292.

70. Weichert S, Sharland M, Clarke NM, Faust SN. Acute haematogenous osteomyelitis in children: is there any evidence for how long we should treat? *Curr Opin Infect Dis* 2008;21(3):258–262.

71. Zaoutis T, Localio AR, Leckerman K et al. Prolonged intravenous therapy versus early transition to oral antimicrobial therapy for acute osteomyelitis in children. *Pediatrics* 2009;123(2):636–642.

72. Lambert M. IDSA guidelines on the treatment of MRSA infections in adults and children. *Am Fam Physician* 2011;84(4):455–463.

73. Slonim A, Walker ES, Mishori E et al. Person-to-person transmission of Kingella kingae among day care center attendees. *J Infect Dis* 1998;178(6):1843–1846.

74. Peltola H, Paakkonen M, Kallio P, Kallio MJ. Short- versus long-term antimicrobial treatment for acute hematogenous osteomyelitis of childhood: prospective, randomized trial on 131 culture-positive cases. *Pediatr Infect Dis J* 2010;29(12):1123–1128.

75. Le Saux N, Howard A, Barrowman NJ et al. Shorter courses of parenteral antibiotic therapy do not appear to influence response rates for children with acute hematogenous osteomyelitis: a systematic review. *BMC Infect Dis* 2002;2:16.

76. Peltola H, Paakkonen M, Kallio P, Kallio MJ. Short- versus long-term antimicrobial treatment for acute hematogenous osteomyelitis of childhood: prospective, randomized trial on 131 culture-positive cases. *Pediatr Infect Dis J* 2010;29(12):1123–1128.

77. Baguley D, Lim E, Bevan A, Pallet A, Faust SN. Prescribing for children—taste and palatability affect adherence to antibiotics: a review. *Arch Dis Child* 2012;97(3):293–297.

78. Ring D, Johnston CE, 2nd, Wenger DR. Pyogenic infectious spondylitis in children: the convergence of discitis and vertebral osteomyelitis. *J Pediatr Orthoped* 1995;15(5):652–660.

79. Dich VQ, Nelson JD, Haltalin KC. Osteomyelitis in infants and children. A review of 163 cases. *Am J Dis Child* 1975;129(11):1273–1278.

80. Raz R, Miron D. Oral ciprofloxacin for treatment of infection following nail puncture wounds of the foot. *Clin Infect Dis* 1995;21(1):194–195.

81. Belthur MV, Birchansky SB, Verdugo AA et al. Pathologic fractures in children with acute Staphylococcus aureus osteomyelitis. *J Bone Joint Surg Am* 2012;94(1):34–42.

82. Sukswai P, Kovitvanitcha D, Thumkunanon V et al. Acute hematogenous osteomyelitis and septic arthritis in children: clinical characteristics and outcomes study. *J Med Assoc Thai* 2011;94 Suppl 3:S209–S216.

CHAPTER 100

Osteomyelitis

Jeremy Field and Neil Upadhyay

Epidemiology

The heterogeneity of osteomyelitis makes the true incidence in the United Kingdom unknown. Osteomyelitis resulting from bacteria spread via the bloodstream to bone is reported at between 10 and 100 per 100 000 in adults[1] and approximately 3 per 100 000 in children[2]; incidences in decline with rising living standards.

Osteomyelitis in adults more typically follows direct or contiguous spread of organisms to bone. Individuals sustaining open fractures, those who have undergone orthopaedic surgery, and those with systemic diseases such as diabetes, peripheral vascular disease, and rheumatoid arthritis have a greater prevalence of osteomyelitis than age- and sex- matched persons without such risk factors.[3–5]

Classification

Several classifications of osteomyelitis exist with none universally accepted. In general osteomyelitis is categorized as acute or chronic; the distinction is based on histological appearance rather than duration of infection. Acute osteomyelitis is defined by presence of inflammatory response cells. Persistent infection causes periosteal stripping, local ischaemia, and microvascular thrombosis. The result is tissue death. The presence of necrotic bone signals the end of the acute phase, independent of time.

The most accepted classification for osteomyelitis in adults is that of Cierny and Mader[6] (Table 100.1). It considers four anatomical stages of disease and emphasizes patient factors which influence both a hosts' response to infection and would-be treatments. Stages are interchangeable, altered by successful therapy, patient comorbidity optimization, or adjuvant treatments. Knowing the stage and host characteristic helps direct surgical treatment and correlates with prognosis.

Aetiopathogenesis

Bacterial inoculation of bone follows (1) haematogenous dissemination, (2) direct inoculation (open fracture, penetrating injury, surgery), or (3) contiguous spread from an adjacent infection (cellulitis, ulcer, infected prosthesis). Rarely adult osteomyelitis follows reactivation of earlier bone infection. The causative organism and pathogenesis will vary with patient age, immunosuppression, and mechanism of inoculation. All aetiological classes of osteomyelitis may progress to a chronic process.

Haematogenous osteomyelitis

The pathogenesis of haematogenous dissemination of microorganisms to bone varies with age. This reflects the differences in microbial causes for bacteraemia as a function of age.

Haematogenous spread to metaphyseal bone is the most common pathogenesis for osteomyelitis in healthy children. Their highly vascular bone with non-anastamosing capillary loops, prone to haemorrhage and infarction from minor trauma, can create a favourable environment for bacterial embolic settling. The growing ends of bone, in particular the distal femur and proximal tibia, are affected. In infants, concurrent septic arthritis is common; infection spreads from the metaphysis via transphyseal blood vessels to the epiphysis and then to the joint. At the age of 1 year the physis becomes avascular, limiting spread to the joint in older age groups.

Infection seeding to bone via the bloodstream is uncommon in healthy adults and unusual without an element of bone injury prior to inoculation. Adult patients with haematogenous osteomyelitis often have an underlying medical condition (Table 100.2). Osteomyelitis from haematogenous spread again typically affects metaphyseal bone but the metaphysis of long bones does not have the same predisposition for infection as seen in children; vertebrae and sternoclavicular and sacroiliac joints are often affected. Metaphyseal bone remains susceptible to infection since blood vessels make sharp angles that slow blood flow; this is particularly seen in venous sinusoids. The venous sinusoids additionally have reduced phagocytic activity, making them venerable to bacterial adherence and multiplication.

Haematogenous osteomyelitis is usually caused by a single pathogen. *Staphylococcus aureus* is far the commonest causative organism in children, accounting for more than 80% of cases. Groups A, C, and G β-haemolytic streptococcus and *Streptococcus pneumoniae* are also encountered in infants and children. *Haemophilus influenzae* is now not usually seen in the United Kingdom following introduction of conjugate Hib vaccination in childhood immunizations.[7] Group B streptococcal infection and enteric Gram-negative bacilli such as *E. coli* are seen in neonates.

In adults *S. aureus* is the common causative organism[8]; however, those with other medical comorbidities may have less common organisms isolated (Table 100.3). Staphylococcus species have numerous mechanisms to adhere to and invade into bone, and to survive within osteoblasts, allowing the bacteria to avoid contact with host defences and several antibiotic agents.[9]

Table 100.1 Cierney–Mader staging system. Patients' staging may be altered by successful therapy, host alteration, or treatment

Anatomical classification		Physiological classification	
Type I	Intramedullary osteomyelitis; nidus is endosteal, confined to intramedullary surfaces of bone, e.g. haematogenous osteomyelitis, infected fracture union following intramedullary nail stabilization	Normal physiological, metabolic and immunologic capabilities. Normal response to infection/surgery	Class A
Type II	Cortical bone osteomyelitis; infection limited to exterior of bone, e.g. infected fracture union with soft issue deficit; contiguous spread from decubitus or vascular ulcers	At risk of treatment failure due to local and systemic deficiencies predisposing to infection/poor wound healing (Table 100.2). Host reversal/optimization of comorbidities will improve outcomes to more closely parallel Class A patients	Class B
Type III	Cortical bone and marrow osteomyelitis; localized full thickness. Bone axially stable, e.g. infected fracture union following internal fixation	Poor physiological reserve. Morbidity of treatment greater than risk of disease or exceeds expected benefit. Palliative or non-curative therapy	Class C
Type IV	Circumferential involvement osteomyelitis; diffuse; axially unstable either before or after debridement, e.g. periprosthetic infections, infected non-unions		

There is increasing awareness of meticillin-resistant *S. aureus* (MRSA) in adults and this should be considered the infecting organism in high-risk patients (Box 100.1).

Direct inoculation and contiguous spread osteomyelitis

Infections following osteosynthesis or arthroplasty are rising in line with numbers performed. Rheumatoid arthritis has a higher incidence of delayed infection than osteoarthritis and is a significant factor in the late development of sepsis in arthroplasties.[10] Osteomyelitis from contiguous spread (overlying soft tissue infection or ulceration) is more common with diabetes and peripheral vascular disease becoming more prevalent.

Table 100.2 Systemic and local patient factors that affect the host's immunological, metabolic, and vascular response to an infecting organism

Systemic factors	Local factors
Diabetes mellitus	Arterial and venous insufficiency
Sickle cell disease	Chronic lymphoedema
Malignancy	Previous surgery
Extremes of age	Prosthetic material
Renal or hepatic failure	Extensive tissue scarring
Malnutrition	Neuropathy
Immune-modulating agents	Obesity
HIV/AIDS	Post-radiation fibrosis
Alcohol/parenteral drug abuse	
Chronic granulomatous disease	
Chronic hypoxia	

Chronic osteomyelitis is a progressive infection resulting in inflammatory destruction and necrosis of bone. It can become persistent as a result of inadvertent innate host immune responses to contain the infection, and bacterial adaptation regardless of patient's immune status. In an attempt to contain the infection host phagocytes generate toxic oxygen free radicals and release proteolytic enzymes which lyse surrounding tissue. Cytokines such as interleukin(IL)-1, IL-6, and tumour necrosis factor (TNF), released as part of the immune response, are potent osteolytic factors. In conjunction, some released metabolites such as prostaglandin E2 have the effect of decreasing the amount of bacterial inoculum required for infection.[11]

Chronic osteomyelitis is a biofilm infection.[12] Several bacteria (*S. aureus*, coagulase-negative staphylococci, and pseudomonas species), once attached to the surface of dead bone or prosthetic implants, produce a polysaccharide extracellular matrix within which colonies of microorganisms develop and mature. This biofilm microbial growth protects against natural host defences and antibiotic therapy. Although some antibiotics can penetrate the biofilm, the most effective treatment is surgical debridement.

Direct or contiguous infections tend to be localized and involve multiple organisms. *S aureus* predominates, but coagulase-negative staphylococci, pseudomonas species and enteric Gram-negative bacilli are all common,[13] especially in implant-related infections. Anaerobes such as clostridia may be involved following contaminated open fractures. *Pseudomonas aeruginosa* is the commonest infective organism from puncture wounds to the foot, particularly in diabetics.

Clinical features

In early stages of disease diagnosis is primarily clinical and often difficult, thus a raised index of suspicion is required particularly in certain patient groups (Table 100.2). History should identify conditions which predispose to infection, affect host response, and

Table 100.3 Potential aetiopathogen based on location of disease and patient characteristics

Location	Age/susceptibility factors	Organism
Haematogenous	Neonates	S. aureus, Group B streptococcus, enteric Gram-negative bacilli
	Children	S. aureus, Streptococcus pneumoniae, Group A,C, G, β-haemolytic streptococcus
	Adults	S. aureus (predominates unless comorbidities/post traumatic/post surgery)
	Elderly	S. aureus, enteric Gram-negative bacilli
	Sickle cell disease	Salmonella, S. pneumoniae, Haemophilus influenzae
	Immunocompromised	S. aureus, fungi, Bartonella henselae, mycobacterium species
	IVDU	S. aureus, enteric Gram-negative bacilli, MRSA, PVL S. aureus
Post-traumatic	Open fractures	S. aureus, polymicrobial Gram-negative aerobic bacilli, anaerobes such as clostridia
Periprosthetic	Prosthesis	S. aureus, Staph. epidermidis, polymicrobial, streptococcus species, pseudomonas, enteric Gram-negative bacilli
Dependent areas	Decubitus ulcers	S. aureus, pseudomonas, streptococci, anaerobic bacteria
Vertebrae: 50% lumbar 35% thoracic 15% cervical	Elderly Urinary tract sepsis Immunocompromised IVDU	S. aureus (in all groups), enteric Gram-negative bacilli, pseudomonas, Mycobacterium tuberculosis (most common in thoracic spine), brucella (especially in S. America, Middle East, and Mediterranean), candida
Tarsal bones	Diabetes Peripheral vascular disease Puncture wound	S. aureus, Pseudomonas aeruginosa, streptococcus, enterococcus, coagulase-negative staphylococcus, enteric Gram-negative bacilli, anaerobes
Sternoclavicular joint	Indwelling devices	S. aureus
	IVDU	S. aureus, β-haemolytic streptococcus, enteric Gram-negative bacilli, P. aeruginosa, PVL S. aureus, MRSA
Anywhere	Human/animal bite	S. aureus, pasteurella, Eikenella corrodens
	HIV/AIDS	Aspergillus, Candida albicans, mycobacterium
Acute multifocal osteomyelitis	Skin disorders such as palmoplantar pustulosis	Negative bone cultures and spontaneous healing without specific treatment

IVDU, intravenous drug use; MRSA, methicillin-resistant Staphylococcus aureus; PVL, Panton-Valentine leukocidin Staphylococcus aureus.

Box 100.1 Factors associated with increased risk of MRSA infection

- History of hospitalization
- Surgery
- Dialysis
- Residence in long-term care facility
- Permanent indwelling catheter or percutaneous medical device
- Previous MRSA isolation from patient
- Intravenous drug user

ascertain the most likely aetiological organism based on presence or absence of certain risk factors (Box 100.1). Malignant and benign tumours, bone cysts, non-infected non-unions, and acute bone infarcts may present with similar symptoms to osteomyelitis.

Acute osteomyelitis, particularly in children, will present with systemic symptoms of bacteraemia as well as local tenderness, reluctance to use affected limb, increased swelling, temperature, and erythema surrounding the involved bone. Symptoms are a function of the host response to infection; thus in many adults with reduced immunity the response is variable and may, even in severe disease, be mild and difficult to localize.

Clinical manifestations of chronic osteomyelitis are often localized and, although they always involve surrounding soft tissues, can be subtle with minimal swelling, erythema, or raised temperature. Symptoms may follow an open injury, surgery, or skin ulcer. Infection could occur almost immediately, within days, or have a more insidious onset over weeks to months after injury, operation, or earlier infection. Patients may have indwelling prosthetic material and a history of preceding treatments to date. Longstanding poorly localized pain, deformity, axial instability, limb shortening, sinus tract, and chronic wounds overlying bone or surgical hardware may signify underlying infection. Bone may be seen or felt at the base of a deep ulcer or wound, a clinical finding highly predictive of underlying bone involvement.[14]

The arterial and venous system should be assessed and the limb examined for neuropathy.

Investigations

There are no specific blood tests to confirm osteomyelitis. In acute cases, acute-phase proteins such as white cell count, C-reactive protein (CRP) and erythrocyte sedimentation rate (ESR) will be raised but are often normal in chronic infection. If raised, monitoring CRP may help assess effectiveness of antibiotic therapy.[15] Doppler ultrasonography or angiography may be indicated if arterial or venous insufficiency is suspected.

Imaging

Anterior-posterior and lateral radiographs (including oblique views in the hand or foot) of the affected area should first be requested but may show no abnormality in early disease. It will take many days to weeks for radiographic findings such as periosteal reaction, periosteal lifting, cortical breaches, bone destruction, and involucrum to develop (Figures 100.1, Figure 100.2a). Initial radiographs will aid exclusion of differential diagnoses such as osteoporotic fracture or metastasis, identify implants, and complement later imaging tests. In chronic osteomyelitis osseous changes are apparent but some initial findings may also represent non-infective aetiologies such as bone healing following fracture or surgical sequelae; thus, further imaging may be required.

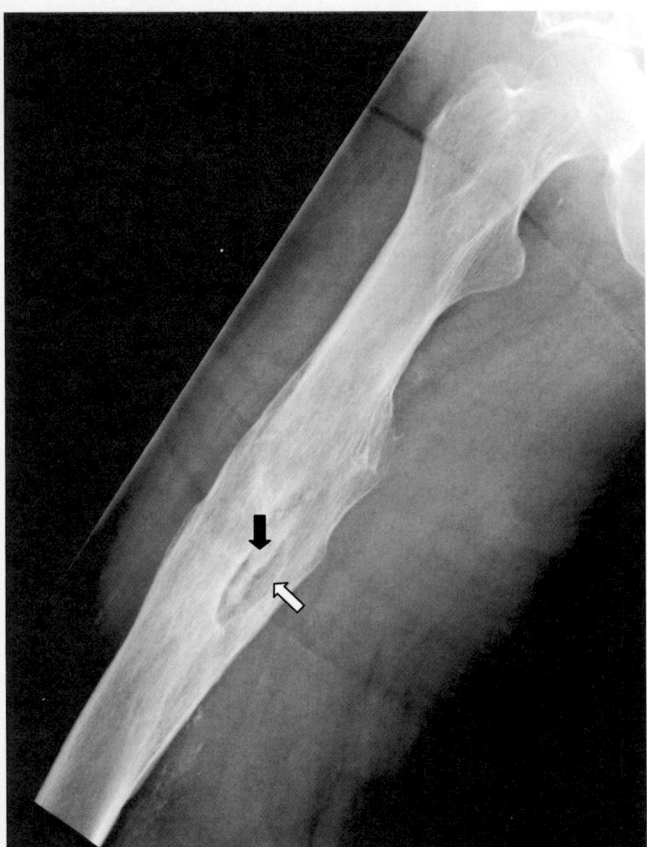

Fig. 100.1 Chronic osteomyelitis of femur. The inflammatory exudate (pus) spreads into the vascular channels raising the intraosseous pressure, slowing blood flow, and resulting in ischaemic necrosis of bone. The devascularized necrotic bone fragments may separate; these are known as sequestra (black arrow). New bone continues to form in response; the less dense area surrounding the sequestra (white arrow) is the involucrum.

CT is sensitive for bone destruction but again demonstrates little abnormality in early disease. CT is useful in chronic osteomyelitis prior to surgery for delineating bone disease.

MRI is highly sensitive and will detect early inflammatory changes of osteomyelitis within days of onset (Figure 100.2b).[16] Later in the disease it will demonstrate necrotic bone, abscess, sequestra and sinus formation, and define extent of tissue involvement. MRI has a low specificity differentiating osteomyelitis from other inflammatory conditions or normal postoperative changes, and may be limited from artefacts from metallic implants. It is therefore not helpful in assessing response to treatment.

Indium-111-labelled white cell scintigraphy can provide useful early information and is more specific than three-phase technetium-99m bone scan in identifying an area of infection. Isotope scanning is inferior to other forms of diagnostic imaging but may be useful in suspected prosthetic infections,[17] and can be used to evaluate response to treatment and confirm eradication of infection. Fluorodeoxyglucose positron emission tomography (FGD-PET) has been reported to have the highest diagnostic accuracy for confirming or excluding diagnosis of chronic osteomyelitis in the axial skeleton[18] but is not widely available.

Management of osteomyelitis

There are no set guidelines for antibiotic therapy. Each hospital has its own preferred regimes. Aetiological diagnosis is key since treatment success is directly related to knowledge of pathogen sensitivity.[19] Bacterial identification may come from multiple blood cultures, biopsy of affected area, or samples sent following surgical debridement. Cultured swabs or fluid from sinuses correlates poorly with underlying deep infective flora, and aspiration of deep fluid collections or percutaneous biopsies in chronic osteomyelitis may provide false-negative results since the organisms are distributed sparsely.[20] Most microbiological departments will only perform a standard microscopy, culture, and sensitivity (MC&S). If unusual pathogens are suspected from clinical history the microbiology department should be informed.

False-negative growth is common when empirical treatment is commenced prior to culture. In such situations histology will confirm the underlying infective process and exclude other pathological processes. The genome of many microorganisms is known and molecular detection methods such as polymerase chain reaction (PCR) can be used when standard methods do not confirm a causative organism. Mass spectrometry, pulsed field gel electrophoresis, and DNA pyrosequencing has improved pathogen detection and characterization and may well be the method of diagnosis in the future but is not universally accepted or available at present.[21,22]

Treatment of acute osteomyelitis

A combined focused antimicrobial and surgical approach should be considered in all cases of osteomyelitis; however, antimicrobial therapy alone may suffice for treatment of acute osteomyelitis in children and some adults diagnosed early. Patients with diabetic foot infections may require surgical debridement, but revascularization of the limb and appropriate antimicrobial therapy may be sufficient for healing to occur. Vertebral osteomyelitis without neurological symptoms is treated with antibiotic therapy alone. Empirical antibiotics can be commenced to cover clinically suspected pathogens after cultures are taken in acute cases (Table 100.4). Osteomyelitis

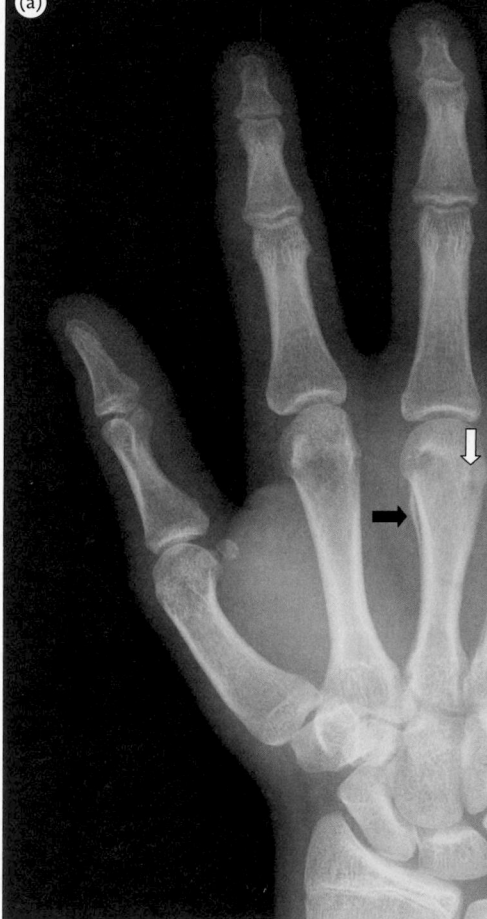

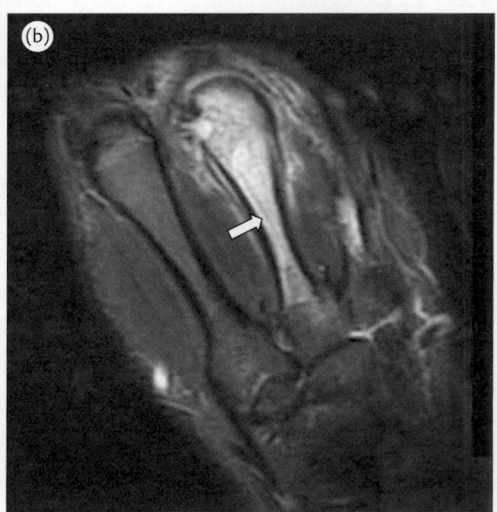

Fig. 100.2 This patient with type 1 diabetes presented with a 2 week history of swelling and erythema centred over third metacarpal of hand. He had sustained a penetrating injury several weeks prior that required no formal treatment. (a) Radiograph demonstrates periosteal reaction (black arrow) and lytic bone area (white arrow). (b) MRI (T2 fat-suppressed image) showing diffuse oedema within third metacarpal (white arrow) and swelling of surrounding tissue. A bone biopsy was taken which revealed *Staphylococcus aureus*. The patient was successfully treated with 14 days intravenous antibiotics followed by 28 days oral antibiotics.

Table 100.4 First-line intravenous/oral antibiotics for osteomyelitis in adults (comorbidities include diabetes, rheumatoid arthritis, immunocompromised, intravenous drug users)

Adults **without** comorbidities		Adults **with** comorbidities or vertebral osteomyelitis	
First-line IV/PO antibiotics	Penicillin allergy	First-line IV/PO antibiotics	Penicillin allergy or diabetic foot osteomyelitis
Samples to determine causative organism should be taken prior to commencement of antibiotics (multiple blood cultures/bone biopsy) In the absence of acute local or systemic upset there is no urgency to commence empiric antibiotic treatment		Multiple blood cultures should be taken prior to commencement of antibiotics	
Benzylpenicillin 2.4 g IV QDS *plus* Flucloxacillin 2 g IV QDS *plus* Sodium fusidate 500 mg[a] PO TDS *or* Rifampicin 600 mg[a] BD	Clindamycin 1.2 g IV QDS	Flucloxacillin 2 g IV QDS *plus* Sodium fusidate 500 mg[a] PO TDS *plus* Ciprofloxacin 750 mg PO BD	Clindamycin 1.2 g IV QDS[c] *plus* Ciprofloxacin 750 mg PO BD
If high risk for MRSA based on patient characteristics			
Teicoplanin 600 mg[b] IV OD after loading doses			
plus			
Fusidin 500 mg PO TDS *or* rifampacin 600 mg[a] BD			

BD, twice daily;IV, intravenous; PO, by mouth; QDS, four time a day; TDS, three times a day; MRSA, methicillin resistant *S. aureus*.
[a]Monitor liver function.
[b]Teicoplanin levels should be checked day 5: aim for serum levels 20–60 mg/litre.
[c]If concern about high levels of *Clostridium difficile* locally, consider teicoplanin.

arising from *Mycobacterium tuberculosis* is often successfully treated with multidrug antibiotic regimes but should be discussed with infectious disease or respiratory physicians (see Chapter 103) with surgery reserved for cases requiring bone stabilization or decompressive spinal surgery for neurological complications.

If appropriate, the limb should be elevated, splinted to rest the soft tissues, and comorbidities addressed. Targeted multidrug antibiotic therapy can be instituted once organisms and sensitivities are determined. There is no clarity on optimum duration of intravenous antibiotics. If the patient systemically improves, surrounding tissues settle and the causative organism identified with known sensitivities, antibiotic agents may be converted to oral. Two weeks of parenteral antibiotics followed by 4 weeks oral is often prescribed but this should be flexible depending on patient response to treatment. In some adults 72 hours of intravenous antibiotics may be appropriate, and often 24–48 hours is adequate in children, followed by the targeted oral agents.

Treatment of chronic osteomyelitis

Complex infections do not permit application of general algorithms and are best treated in dedicated centres. Treatment recommendations are based on expert opinion rather than randomized control trials. They broadly include limb salvage, amputation, and palliative treatment.

Patients require optimization of comorbidities. If indicated, vascular reconstruction prior to orthopaedic and plastic surgical intervention will prove beneficial in long-term results. If angioplasty or arterial bypass is performed surgical debridement should be delayed for up to 3 months to allow optimal reperfusion of tissues.

Limb salvage

Meticulous surgical debridement is required,[23] i.e. removal of the infected segment of bone, surrounding infected tissues or retained implants (such as plates, screws, and joint replacements). An oncologic approach—complete (i.e. wide) excision—is often adopted. Prosthetic material in situ should be considered colonized and a potential nidus for recurrence. That said, bones will heal in the presence of active infection provided stability is maintained. Well-fixed implants can be removed at a later stage.[24] Infected arthroplasties generally require immediate removal, commencement of treatments to eradicate infection, and staged revision. The exception is a stable implant and a known organism of lower virulence (such as coagulase-negative staphylococcus) in a patient with comorbidities that make further surgery high risk.

In patients with long-bone disease staged reconstruction may be required: In Cierny–Mader stage IV disease, and occasionally in stage III disease (Table 100.1), debridement results in a large bone and soft tissue defect. Appropriate management of this space is essential to prevent infection recurrence. Soft tissue and bone reconstruction should not be considered separate procedures, since complete and good-quality soft tissue cover is required to ensure survival of new callus formation.

Two methods widely used to bridge the bone defect are (1) insertion of a cancellous bone graft and (2) circular frame (Ilizarov/Taylor special frame) callus-distraction osteogenesis. The cancellous bone graft is a feasible method to bridge defects less than 6 cm in size, provided infection-free well-vascularized soft tissue cover is attainable and good contact between graft and living cancellous

bone is achieved.[25] This may be difficult to accomplish, thus the callus-distraction technique is the gold standard for bridging larger osseous defects provided there is sufficient bone to create a transport segment.[26] Bone is fractured at the proximal metaphysic (corticotomy) and the segment between the newly created metaphyseal fracture and defect is slowly transported through the defect left by debridement and later docked to the distal, disease-free bone. Growth of new bone (regenerated) follows the transported metaphyseal bone segment (Figure 100.3). The technique is labour intensive and requires extended periods of treatment (averaging 9 months). It can be combined with muscle flaps provided adequate preprocedure planning ensures that injury to the flap is avoided during bone transport.

In patients with comorbidities or those who will not tolerate prolonged reconstruction, acute shortening—i.e. removing osteomyelitis segment and immediately approximating the bone ends—is a reasonable option. The tibia can be shortened up to 4 cm, the femur 6 cm, and humerus 5 cm. An orthosis can later be prescribed to correct lower limb length discrepancy.

There is no consensus on optimum method of delivery or duration of antibiotics following surgery. Antibiotic-loaded spacers can be used on occasions to deliver high concentrations of antimicrobial therapy between reconstructive operations. Four to six weeks of parenteral therapy has become the standard.[27] The rationale behind this regime is recognition that bone takes 3–4 weeks to revascularize. Many centres will continue oral antibiotics for a further 6 weeks after parenteral therapy. In one-third of cases, no organisms are identified thus postoperative antibiotic regimes need to cover *S. aureus* and other probable pathogens based on patient characteristics (Table 100.3).

Amputation or palliative treatment

In a subgroup of patients with chronic infection and concomitant systemic disease, intervention will not alter prognosis. Persistent infection, pain, deformity, and even chronic suppuration are not absolute indications for treatment. These patients may benefit from amputation or disease-controlling measures such as limited debridements/evacuation of collections and long-term suppressive antibiotic therapy. Amputation does not guarantee eradication of infection.[28]

Prognosis

Prognosis depends on the number of risk factors, duration of infection before treatment, and the patient's overall health. The different aetiologies require differing medical and surgical strategies but early diagnosis and appropriate intervention in an otherwise well or fully optimized patient should lead to recovery.

Dedicated units treating complex chronic cases report 98% infection-free patients at 2 years, falling to 92% at 4 years and 90% at 8 years. Recurrence of disease may occur early (shortly after stopping antibiotics) or late. The tendency for infection to relapse sometimes years after apparently successful therapy suggests remission (or arrest) rather than cure of treated osteomyelitis. Outcome is related to host type. A review of 2207 patients treated over a 26 year period showed primary treatment to be successful in 96% of healthy patients (success defined as infection free at 2 year follow-up); this success rate fell to 73% in patients classed to have local and systemic comorbidities.

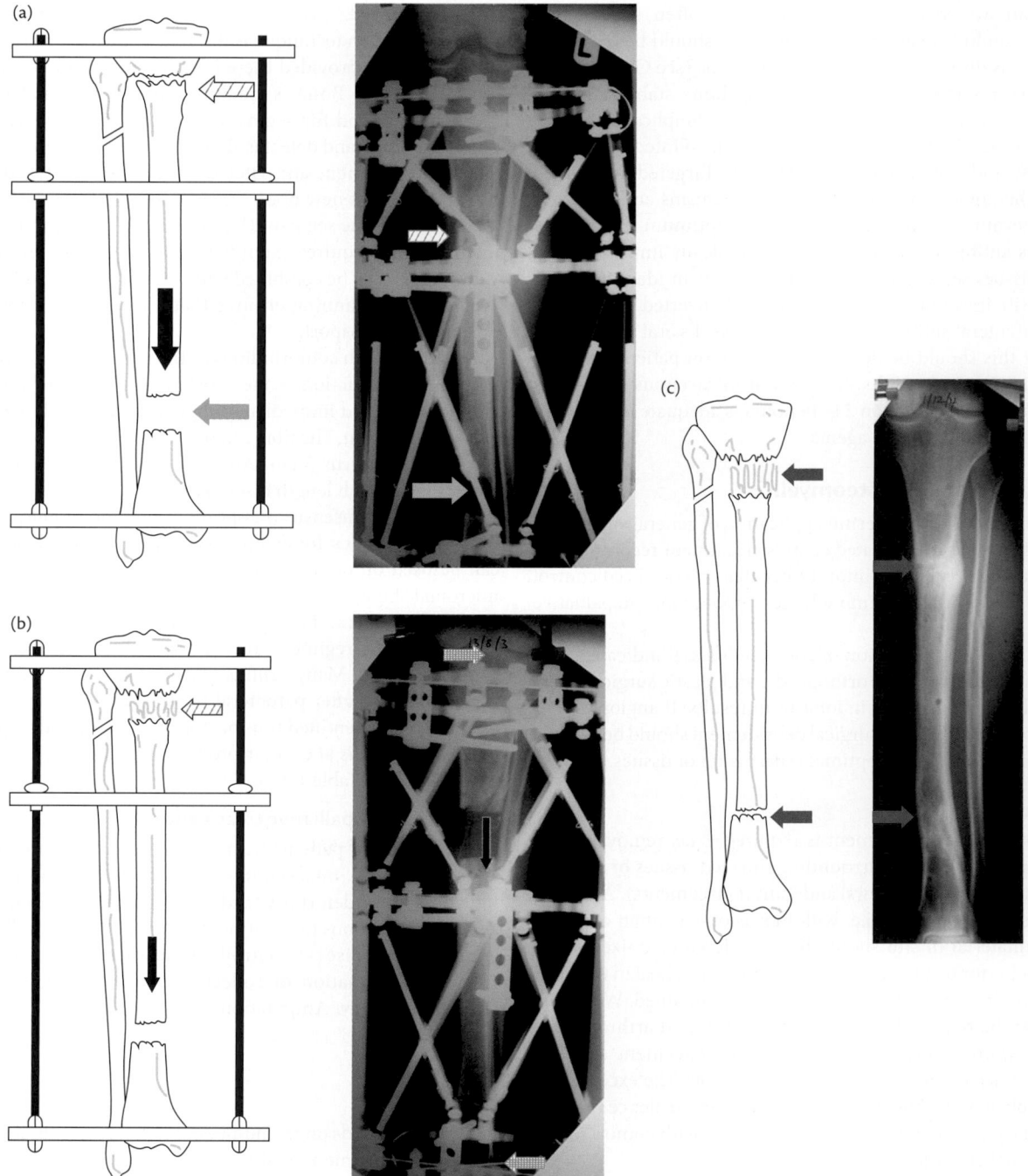

Fig. 100.3 The radiographs and illustration from left to right show the process of bone transport with use of a ring fixator to treat a bone defect following debridement of infected bone. (a) The 3 cm defect following debridement is seen (grey arrow). A corticotomy is made proximally at the metaphysis (grey striped arrow). (b) the segment between is transported down in the direction of black arrow to docking site of the distal tibia. The regenerate (grey crossed arrow) is what follows behind the corticotmy. (c) The same tibia following successful treatment (red arrows show remodelled segments).

Acknowledgements

We wish to acknowledge Dr Robert Jackson (consultant microbiologist) and Mr James Livingstone (consultant limb reconstruction surgeon).

References

1. Berendt AR, McNally M. Osteomyelitis. In: *Oxford textbook of medicine*, 4th edn, Oxford University Press, Oxford, 2003.
2. Blyth MJ, Kincaid R, Craigen MA, Bennet GC. The changing epidemiology of acute and subacute haematogenous osteomyelitis in children. *J Bone Joint Surg Br* 2001;83:99–102.
3. Lew DP, Waldvogel FA. Osteomyelitis. *Lancet* 2004;364:369–379.
4. Lavery LA, Armstrong DG, Wunderlich RP et al. Risk factors for foot infections in individuals with diabetes. *Diabetes Care* 2006;29:1288–1293.
5. Doran MF, Crowson CS, Pond GR, O'Fallon WM, Gabriel SE. Frequency of infection in patients with rheumatoid arthritis compared with controls: a population-based study. *Arthritis Rheum* 2002;46:2287–2293.
6. Cierny G III, Mader JT, Penninck JJ. A clinical staging system for adult osteomyelitis. *Clin Orthop Relat Res* 2003;414:7–24.
7. Howard AW, Viskontas D, Sabbagh C. Reduction in osteomyelitis and septic arthritis related to Haemophilus influenzae type B vaccination. *J Pediatr Orthop* 1999;19:705–709.
8. Lew DP, Waldvogel FA. Osteomyelitis. *N Engl J Med* 1997;336:999–1007.
9. Ciampolini J, Harding KG. Pathophysiology of chronic bacterial osteomyelitis. Why do antibiotics fail so often? *Postgrad Med J* 2000;76:479–483.
10. Bengtson S. Prosthetic osteomyelitis with special reference to the knee: risks, treatment and costs. *Ann Med* 1993;25:523–529.
11. Klosterhalfen B, Peters KM, Tons C et al. Local and systemic inflammatory mediator release in patients with acute and chronic posttraumatic osteomyelitis. *J Trauma* 1996;40:372–378.
12. Gristina AG, Costerton JW. Bacterial adherence to biomaterials and tissue. The significance of its role in clinical sepsis. *J Bone Joint Surg Am* 1985;67:264–273.
13. Mader JT, Landon GC, Calhoun J. Antimicrobial treatment of osteomyelitis. *Clin Orthop Relat Res* 1993;295:87–95.
14. Grayson ML, Gibbons GW, Balogh K, Levin E, Karchmer AW. Probing to bone in infected pedal ulcers. A clinical sign of underlying osteomyelitis in diabetic patients. *JAMA* 1995;273:721–723.
15. Ferard G, Gaudias J, Bourguignat A, Ingenbleek Y. C-reactive protein to transthyretin ratio for the early diagnosis and follow-up of postoperative infection. *Clin Chem Lab Med* 2002;40:1334–1338.
16. Kapoor A, Page S, Lavalley M, Gale DR, Felson DT. Magnetic resonance imaging for diagnosing foot osteomyelitis: a meta-analysis. *Arch Intern Med* 2007;167:125–132.
17. Del Pozo JL, Patel R. Clinical practice. Infection associated with prosthetic joints. *N Engl J Med* 2009;361:787–794.
18. Termaat MF, Raijmakers PGHM, Scholten HJ et al. The accuracy of diagnostic imaging for the assessment of chronic osteomyelitis: a systematic review and meta-analysis. *J Bone Joint Surg Am* 2005;87:2464–2471.
19. Conterno LO, da Silva Filho CR. Antibiotics for treating chronic osteomyelitis in adults. *Cochrane Database Syst Rev* 2009;8:CD004439.
20. Perry CR, Pearson RL, Miller GA. Accuracy of cultures of material from swabbing of the superficial aspect of the wound and needle biopsy in the preoperative assessment of osteomyelitis. *J Bone Joint Surg Am* 1994;73:745–749.
21. Fenollar F, Roux V, Stein A, Drancourt M, Raoult D. Analysis of 525 samples to determine the usefulness of PCR amplification and sequencing of the 16S rRNA gene for diagnosis of bone and joint infections. *J Clin Microbiol* 2006;44:1018–1028.
22. Sontakke S, Cadenas MB, Maggi RG, Diniz PP, Breitschwerdt EB. Use of broad range16S rDNA PCR in clinical microbiology. *J Microbiol Methods* 2009;76:217–225.
23. Simpson AH, Deakin M, Latham JM. Chronic osteomyelitis. The effect of the extent of surgical resection on infection-free survival. *J Bone Joint Surg Br* 2001;83:403–407.
24. Berkes M, Obremsky WT, Scannell B et al. Maintenance of hardware after early postoperative infection following fracture internal fixation. *J Bone Joint Surg Am* 2010;92:823–828.
25. Dinh P, Hutchinson BK, Zalavras C, Stevanovic MV. Reconstruction of osteomyelitis defects. *Semin Plast Surg* 2009;23:108–118.
26. Green SA. Osteomyelitis. The Ilizarov perspective. *Orthop Clin North Am* 1991;22:515–521.
27. Lazzarini L, De Lalla F, Mader JT. Long bone osteomyelitis. *Curr Infect Dis Rep* 2002;4:439–445.
28. Cierny G. Surgical treatment of osteomyelitis. *Plast Reconstr Surg* 2011;127 Suppl 1:190S–204S.

CHAPTER 101

Lyme borreliosis

Andreas Krause and Volker Fingerle

Definition

Lyme borreliosis (LB) is an infectious disease endemic in the northern hemisphere with a broad spectrum of clinical manifestations mainly affecting skin, joints and nervous system. The causative agent of LB, *Borrelia burgdorferi sensu lato*, is transmitted by hard ticks belonging to the *Ixodes ricinus/I. persulcatus* complex. Most cases heal completely, either spontaneously or after antibiotic therapy. Only rarely does the pathogen persist chronically or, by infection-triggered immunopathological mechanisms, does a chronic Lyme arthritis occur.

Epidemiology

LB occurs in a belt-like area between 40° and 60°N latitude around the world, corresponding to the abundance of vector-competent hard ticks, *I. persulcatus and I. scapularis* in North America, *I. ricinus* in Europe, and *I. persulcatus* in Asia. The highest incidences are reported from the north-eastern United States and central/eastern Europe (300 cases/100 000 or more). The rate appears to have increased significantly over the past 10–20 years, although this observation may be due mostly to increased awareness, advanced reporting, and improved diagnosis of the disease. Antibodies against *B. burgdorferi* can be detected in about 5–25% of healthy adults (rate of subsided infection or seroprevalence), depending among other things on age, region, and risk of exposure. The rate of infected ticks varies broadly but is usually 10–30%. The risk of being infected with *B. burgdorferi* by a tick bite varies considerably and is entirely dependent on the local tick infection rate and duration of the tick bite.[1,2]

Aetiology and pathogenesis

B. burgdorferi sensu lato refers to a heterogeneous group of highly mobile spirochaetes, of which at least five genospecies can cause LB in humans in Europe: *B. burgdorferi sensu stricto*, *B. garinii*, *B. afzelii*, *B. bavariensis*, and *B. spielmanii*. The pathogens differ, among other things, by their geographical distribution (in the United States, only *B. burgdorferi sensu stricto* has been found so far; Europe is dominated by *B. garinii* and *B. afzelii*), their adaptation to different hosts and, which is clinically significant, by the preferred affliction of different organ systems (organotropism). Although all five genospecies may be pathogens causing erythema migrans (EM),

B. burgdorferi sensu stricto preferably affects joints. Acrodermatitis chronica atrophicans (ACA) is, in the vast majority of cases, caused by *B. afzelii*, and *B. spielmanii* has been isolated only from skin so far. This organotropism of the pathogen is not absolute, but it at least partially explains the various clinical manifestations and different forms of disease.[3]

The pathogen is transmitted during the blood meal of infected ticks. In this, the tick and the borrelia both experience complex processes of adaptation until the pathogens may emigrate from the midgut of the ticks, invade the salivary glands, and finally infect the host via the saliva.[4] The best-studied example is the differential expression of the surface proteins (Osp) OspA and OspC of *B. burgdorferi*. OspA is the dominant surface protein in the tick that has not yet sucked, with which it anchors to the intestinal wall by a receptor that is primarily upregulated in the intestines of infected ticks. During the act of sucking, OspA is downregulated and OspC is upregulated, which allows borrelia to disseminate into the salivary glands. There, OspC binds the tick saliva protein Salp15 that, among other things, suppresses the antibody-mediated killing and the activation of CD4+ T cells in the host. Therefore, after the start of a tick bite it usually takes several hours until successful pathogen transmission can take place.[4,5]

In the skin, the spirochaetes spread locally at first, which is noticeable as the typical centrifugal expansion of the EM. Haematogenous and probably also lymphogenous spreading of the pathogens with colonization of various organs may occur even in the first days of the infection. Clinical manifestations of LB are thus the expression of a direct infection of the respective organ at first. The observation that on the one hand, infections can also be asymptomatic and that on the other hand, a few pathogens can cause a severe inflammatory reaction, demonstrates the importance of the host immune response and the pathogen–host interaction in the pathogenesis of the disease.

Relatively little is known about the natural course of borrelia infection in humans. In every phase of the infection or disease, spontaneous healing of the disease can occur even without antibiotic therapy. On the other hand, *B. burgdorferi* can persist in the host for many years despite an intense immune response. Among other things, the pathogen protects itself by escaping to immunologically privileged sites, complement resistance, and change in the antigen structure against the elimination by the immune system. It is possible that this pathogen persistence is not associated with symptoms in every case.[5]

B. burgdorferi has several mechanisms for spreading in the host after transmission and escaping attack by the immune system. These include the corkscrew-like motion (rotation around the longitudinal axis) by endoflagella; the expression of numerous proteins interacting with the extracellular matrix such as plasminogen-binding proteins, fibrinogen-binding protein BBK32, decorin-binding proteins A and B, integrin-binding protein p66, and the glycosaminoglycan-binding protein Bgp. Erp (OspE-related) and CRASP (complement regulator-acquiring surface proteins) that bind factor H and factor H-like protein I, inhibit complement activation depending on the species (*B. afzelii* is resistant to complement, *B. garinii* is sensitive to complement); and also the formation of the membrane attack complex as well as opsonization for complement-dependent phagocytosis and the mortification of the pathogens. The differential expression and true antigenic variation of surface proteins, especially of the *vlsE* gene products, impair an effective specific immune response.

The non-specific immune response is stimulated in particular by surface lipoproteins of *B. burgdorferi*. By binding to Toll-like receptors, especially TLR 2/1 and TLR 2/6 heterodimers, activation of macrophages and initiation of an inflammatory reaction with release of proinflammatory chemokines and interleukins including IL-17 occurs. At the same time, the specific humoral and cellular immune response is activated, which is characterized by a predominant Th1 response and a relatively slowly developing antibody formation.[5]

Adequate antibiotic therapy usually results in pathogen elimination and healing of the infection. Nevertheless, there are a few patients with Lyme arthritis who have lasting joint symptoms despite repeated antibiotic therapy. In the United States, this applies to an estimated 10% of patients; Europe does not have good epidemiological data for this. The immunopathogenesis of this so-called 'antibiotic-resistant' Lyme arthritis is still poorly understood. Available results argue against pathogen persistence as a cause, without being able to exclude it completely. Infection-triggered immunological mechanisms are suspected instead. The association of antibiotic-resistant cases with antibody formation against OspA and certain *HLA DRB1* alleles binding the $OspA_{163-175}$ peptide led to suspicions of an immunological cross-reaction, e.g. with homologous human LFA-1 structures as a cause. However, further studies could not confirm this autoimmune hypothesis and rather indicated that the prolonged immune response may be adequate and targeted against persistent antigens. Recent studies suggest that a Th17 response induced via NapA (neutrophil-activating protein A) could play a crucial role in the pathogenesis of Lyme arthritis. The question of which immunological mechanisms lead to chronic Lyme arthritis (which, ultimately, heals spontaneously within a few years) thus remains unclear.[5]

Clinical picture

The manifestations of the disease are individually variable and can heal spontaneously in every phase of the disease or can be brought to healing by appropriate antibiotic therapy.

Clinically proven is the division of LB into an early phase (early localized and early disseminated) and a late phase (persisting infection) with different clinical pictures and a varied response to antibiotic therapy (Table 101.1).[1,2,6,7]

The EM, by far the most common clinical manifestation of LB, starts with a latency of 2–30 (mean 7–14) days at the site of the tick bite as a reddish-livid, only rarely pruritic, painless erythema. The characteristic ring shape with a central papule (site of the tick bite) may develop over time by central healing. After dissemination of the pathogen, multiple EM or the borrelial lymphocytoma (lymphadenosis cutis benigna Bäfverstedt) may occur as further early skin manifestations. The late borreliosis of the skin, ACA, most frequently affects the extremities and starts as a bluish-livid inflammatory process of the skin with oedematous swelling. The atrophy of skin and subcutaneous fat tissue occurs only in the further course of the disease, which may last for many years. The ACA is often associated with arthropathies and polyneuropathies in the area of the affected skin.[2,67]

Early neuroborreliosis develops as the second most common manifestation of LB after an average incubation period of 3–6 weeks. The typical manifestation is the Garin–Bujadoux–Bannwarth meningoradiculoneuritis with nocturnally more pronounced pseudoradicular pain and cranial nerve pareses, most frequently affecting the facial nerve (one or both sides). Especially children show marked symptoms of meningitis. Late manifestations involving the central nervous system with myelitis, encephalitis, or encephalomyelitis are very rare but usually take a chronic course. Vasculitides in the area of the central nervous system are very rare.[1,2,8]

Lyme carditis is observed in less than 5% of patients and can lead to variable degrees of atrioventricular (AV) blocks with dizziness, palpitations, or syncopations. An involvement of other internal organs is possible but usually without clinical significance.[1,2,6]

Rheumatological symptoms may occur relatively early in the disease, i.e. within a few weeks after infection, as arthralgias, myalgias, or mild, transient arthritides of individual joints. However, the typical Lyme arthritis manifests itself in the late phase of the disease, i.e. several weeks to months after pathogen transmission.

The arthritis usually starts as a monoarthritis or oligoarthritis that is intermittent at first, later persistent. In 85% of these cases, at least one knee is affected. The ankle and elbow joints may be involved as well, while an affliction of the finger joints, especially in the form of a polyarthritis, is practically never observed. Also, an involvement of the sacroiliac joints or the spine does not occur in Lyme arthritis. Analysis of the synovia in acute arthritis shows significantly increased cell numbers of up to 50 000/μL with a predominance of neutrophils. Concomitant manifestations in the locomotor system are bursitides and tenosynovitides. Aside from the myalgias particularly observed in early phases, the late Lyme borreliosis can lead in rare cases to a manifest, proximally more pronounced myositis with muscle weakness and muscle atrophies.[1,2,6,7,9]

Diagnostics

The tentative diagnosis of LB is always made based on the clinical symptoms at first; laboratory diagnostics then serve to substantiate the diagnosis. Aside from the skin manifestations of LB, which can often be diagnosed clinically, the symptoms are often ambiguous and require the exclusion of differential diagnoses (Tables 101.2–101.4) For the diagnosis of neuroborreliosis, cerebrospinal fluid diagnostics with detection of pleocytosis and autochthonous antibody production should always be performed. Without direct pathogen detection in the joint, Lyme arthritis can be diagnosed with sufficient certainty only after appropriate differential diagnostics and under observation of the diagnostic criteria.

Table 101.1 Clinical manifestations in Lyme borreliosis

Organ system/stage of illness	Manifestations	Commentary
Non-specific symptoms		
Early stage	Malaise, headache, low fever, arthralgias, myalgias, swollen lymph nodes	May be severe, no respiratory or gastrointestinal symptoms
Late stage	See early stage	Mostly less pronounced
Skin		
Early stage	Erythema migrans	Expanding, not markedly elevated erythematous skin lesion (>5 cm largest diameter), with or without central clearing, distinct edge. 2–30 days after tick removal. Often seronegative. Multiple lesions (disseminated form) more often in the USA
	Borrelial lymphocytoma	Rare. Painless bluish-red node or plaque, predelection site: ear lobe or scrotum in children, on or near the nipple in adults
Late stage	ACA, not present in the USA	Mainly extensor site of extremities. After initial oedematous swelling, long standing red to bluish-red lesion, later on skin atrophy. Sometimes polyneuropathy, juxta-articular fibroid nodes and skin induration. Chronic course
Nervous system		
Early stage	Meningoradiculitis (Bannwarth syndrome; Europe), meningitis predominantly USA. Rare: CNS manifestations, vasculitis	Bannwarth: painful radiculitis that typically exacerbates at night, cranial nerve pareses (mostly facial nerve). Signs of meningitis
Late stage	Meningitis, myelitis, encephalitis, encephalomyelitis, peripheral neuropathy	Very rare, chronic course. Mostly encephalitis and/or myelitis with spastic syndrome, spastic-atactic gait disorder, micturition. Encephalopathy with cognitive disturbance or isolated PNP described in the USA. In Europe PNP only in association with ACA
Heart		
Early stage	Myopericarditis	Rare, typically atrioventricular block of varying degree, usually total recovery
Late stage	Chronic cardiomyopathy, ventricular extrasystolia	Questionable, single cases
Musculoskeletal		
Early stage	Arthralgia, myalgia	Sometimes transient arthritis
Late stage	Arthritis, myositis, bursitis, enthesitis	Initially intermittent, later on persistent arthritis of large joints, mostly affecting the knee, no axial involvement, myositis rare
Other		
Early stage	Conjunctivitis, uveitis anterior und posterior, papillitis, episcleritis	Rare, chorioiditis characteristic, may result in persisting visual loss
	Hepatomegaly, hepatitis, splenomegaly	Usually not clinically relevant
Late stage	Vasculitis	Rare, may result in ischemia

ACA, acrodermatitis chronica atrophicans; CNS, central nervous system; PNP, polyneuropathy.

Detection of pathogens by culture and polymerase chain reaction

Suitable materials are skin biopsies, cerebrospinal fluid, synovial fluid, and synovial membrane. The cultivation of *B. burgdorferi* is very time consuming (6 weeks or more) and is offered by only a few laboratories. Polymerase chain reaction (PCR) can quickly and sensitively detect borrelial DNA, but should be interpreted with caution. It is crucial that a positive result is verified regarding specificity (e.g. by sequencing or probes), which typically allows precise identification of the detected species. The diagnostic sensitivity of PCR and culture averages 50–70% in case of

skin biopsies (EM or ACA) and 10–30% in case of cerebrospinal fluid from patients with early neuroborreliosis. PCR can detect borrelia DNA in the joint fluid of 50–70% of patients with Lyme arthritis, while detection by culture extremely rarely succeeds here.[2,3,6,8,10]

Serology

Serological testing should be requested exclusively in case of sufficient clinical probability (≥20%), otherwise the positive predictive value of a positive test result is too small. If an examination is performed for a suspected late manifestation, however, the negative

Table 101.2 Diagnostic criteria for Lyme arthritis

Clinical criteria		Laboratory criteria	
Essential	**Supporting**	**Essential**	**Supporting**
Mono- or oligoarthritis of large joints (predominantly knee, also ankle, elbow, shoulder)	Other Lyme borreliosis manifestations or tick bite in patient´s history	Detection of *B. burgdorferi*-specific IgG antibodies (typically high titre)	Detection of *B. burgdorferi* from synovial fluid or tissue by PCR or cultur
Exclusion of differential diagnoses, no axial involvement		Synovial fluid (if obtainable) with neutrophilic pleocytosis	

predictive value is very good, especially if there are only unspecific symptoms.

For the detection of antibodies, a sensitive immunoassay (EIA) is used as a screening test. Positive results are confirmed by immunoblot to exclude unspecific reactions or cross-reactions. Especially in the early phase of LB, the serology can often still be negative. As a rule, specific IgM antibodies increase within 3 weeks after pathogen transmission, while IgG antibodies may be detected approximately 3 weeks later. In late manifestations, significantly elevated IgG antibody levels are usually found. An IgG-negative result therefore excludes a late manifestation of LB with high probability. IgM antibodies are in suspected late manifestations without diagnostic value.

With suspected neuroborreliosis, the diagnosis can be confirmed by demonstrating a lymphocytic pleocytosis, protein elevation, and intrathecal *B. burgdorferi*-specific antibody production in the cerebrospinal fluid.

As a rule, serological follow-up examinations after antibiotic therapy of an LB do not result in relevant findings. The success of the therapy can only be seen clinically. Neither the persistence of specific IgM antibodies nor IgG antibodies alone justify further therapeutic measures.[2,3,8,10]

Methods not to be recommended for diagnostics

Among the non-evaluated and therefore not recommended tests are antigen tests from bodily fluids, PCR from urine or ticks, the detection of a decreased CD57+/CD3– lymphocyte subpopulation, the lymphocyte transformation test (LTT), HLA-DR subtyping, the detection of so-called 'cystic forms', dark field microscopy, and the visual contrast sensitivity test (VCS).[2,38]

Therapy

Antibiotic treatment should be initiated as soon as possible after diagnosis, to shorten the course of the disease and to prevent the development of further manifestations or a chronic disease process. The treatment is stage-oriented and symptom-oriented. Doxycycline, amoxicillin, and ceftriaxone are the drugs of choice. Development of resistance to these antibiotics has not yet been proven, but *B. burgdorferi* shows primary resistance to numerous substances including gyrase inhibitors and sulfonamides. The therapy recommendations summarized in Table 101.5 are essentially the same as the recommendations or guidelines supported by numerous medical societies.[2,8,11,12]

Course and prognosis

In the early phase, one treatment cycle virtually always leads to healing of the disease. After antibiotic treatment of late manifestations, it is often only in the course of several weeks or months that a gradual remission is seen, so that it frequently takes several months until the therapeutic success can be assessed. It is important to note that new manifestations of the disease do not occur after antibiotic therapy.

Severe courses of LB and only partial recoveries have been described, especially involving the central nervous system and the

Table 101.3 Differential diagnosis in Lyme borreliosis (important examples)

Erythema migrans	Insect-bite reaction, erysipelas, tinea, erythema anulare centrifugum, initial morphea, granuloma anulare, parvovirus B19 infection in children
Lyme carditis	Other (mainly viral) infections, coronary disease, non-infectious systemic diseases
Neuroborreliosis	Viral infections (e.g. tick-borne encephalitis), herpes zoster (pre eruption), spinal disc herniation, periarthropathia humeroscapularis, cervicobrachialgia, neoplastic infiltration, Guillain–Barré syndrome, multiple sclerosis
Borrelial lymphocytoma	Insect-bite reaction, foreign body granuloma, gynaecomastia, lymphomas and pseudolymphomas
Acrodermatitis chronica atrophicans	Chronic venous insufficiency, morphea, scleroderma, cortisone side effect, frostbite, erythromelalgia, acrocyanosis, skin atrophy
Lyme arthritis	Gout, pseudogout, septic arthritis, Löfgren´s syndrome, viral arthritis, psoriatic arthritis, reactive arthritis, enteropathic arthritis, rheumatoid arthritis (atypically beginning)

Table 101.4 Recommendations for a diagnostic approach

Tentative diagnosis	Antibody detection (serology)	Sensitivity	Puncture or biopsy for PCR/culture	Sensitivity
Early manifestations				
Erythema migrans	Only in atypical cases: immediately and follow up[a]	20–50%	Only in atypical cases: skin biopsy	50–70%
Borrelial lymphocytoma	Essential. If unclear, follow up[a]	70–90%	Skin biopsy; also for histology	?
Early neuroborreliosis (Bannwarth, meningitis, etc.)	Essential. CSF/serum pair. Demonstration of intrathecal specific antibody synthesis and signs of CSF inflammation. If unclear, follow up[a]	70–90%	CSF	10–20%
Late manifestations				
Lyme arthritis	Essential. Detection of specific IgG antibodies and usually broad spectrum of bands in the IgG-immunoblot in serum	90–100%	PCR from synovia or synovialis, positive culture extremely rare; joint aspiration diagnostics incl. cell count and differentiation	50–70% (only PCR)
Acrodermatitis chronica atrophicans	Essential detection of specific IgG antibodies and broad spectrum of bands in the IgG-immunoblot in serum	90–100%	Skin biopsy; also for histology	50–70%
Late neuroborreliosis	Essential. CSF/serum pair. Demonstration of intrathecal specific IgG antibody synthesis and signs of chronic CSF inflammation	90–100%	PCR and culture from CSF typically negative	

CSF, cerebrospinal fluid; PCR, polymerase chain reaction.
[a]Question: Seroconversion, significant rise in titre.

Table 101.5 Recommended antimicrobial regimens for treatment of patients with Lyme borreliosis for adults

Manifestation	Drug	Dosage per day	Duration, days (range)	Strength of recommendation
Erythema migrans	Doxycycline	1 × 200 mg or 2 × 100 mg PO	10–21	A
	Amoxicillin	3–4 × 500–1000 mg PO	14–21	
	Cefuroxime	2 × 500 mg PO	14–21	
	Azithromycin[a]	500 mg PO	7–10	
		or 2 × 500 mg day 1, 500 mg days 2–5	5	
Neuroborreliosis[c]	Ceftriaxone	1 × 2 g IV	14–21	A
	Cefotaxime	3 × 2 g IV	14–21	
	Penicillin G	4 × 5 MU IV	14–21	
	Doxycycline[b]	200–300 mg PO	14–21	
Carditis[d]	Ceftriaxone	1 × 2 g IV	14	D
	Cefotaxime	3 × 2 g IV	14	
	Penicillin G	4 × 5 MU IV	14	
Arthritis, acrodermatitis chronica atrophicans	Doxycycline	1 × 200 mg or 2 × 100 mg PO	30	B
	Amoxicillin	3 × 500–1000 mg	30	NA
	Ceftriaxone	1 × 2 g IV	14–21	NA
	Cefotaxime	3 × 2 g IV	14–21	

IV, intravenous; PO, oral; MU, mega units; NA, not available..
[a]Only for patients intolerant to doxycycline, amoxicillin, and cefuroxime.
[b]Only in uncomplicated cases; possibly 300 mg/day needed.
[c]For late neuroborreliosis IV therapy for 14–28 days.
[d]In first-degree atrioventricular block and PR <30 ms oral therapy for 14–21 days.

locomotor system, but fortunately are rare. Thus, LB is a serious disease with potentially grave organ manifestations, but generally with a benign course especially if it is detected and treated early.

While a *B. burgdorferi* infection, on the one hand, frequently takes a self-limiting course, the pathogen, on the other hand, may in rare cases persist for many years and cause a prolonged disease course. This is particularly true for the chronic neuroborreliosis with involvement of the central nervous system, as well as the ACA. These diseases usually heal only after thorough antibiotic therapy and in part with irreversible organ defects. This may also be true for Lyme arthritis, which can take a course over many years if left untreated. Rarely, it may persist for years—chronically—despite repeated courses of antibiotic treatment. This so-called treatment-resistant Lyme arthritis is presumably caused by infection-triggered immunopathological mechanisms. However, also these chronic arthritides most often slowly regress, but sometimes only after several years.

Clearly to be distinguished from these well-defined clinical courses of LB are patients who fear they are suffering from chronic LB because of unspecific symptoms and positive (sometimes even despite of negative) serology. These are particularly the patients who report persisting symptoms after antibiotic therapy of a confirmed LB in the sense of a so-called 'post-Lyme syndrome'. Despite a clear improvement of objective clinical signs these patients frequently complain about fatigue, impaired concentration, headaches or arthralgias and myalgias.[2,6,13,14] These symptoms can usually be assigned to a prolonged convalescence after successful therapy. Therapy studies, including those from Europe, show that the regression of symptoms especially of late manifestations can take weeks to months and that the success of therapy can be fully evaluated only after several months. Residuals of the disease persisting over longer time periods or only partial recoveries after antibiotic treatment are possible but rare.

Many patients also tend to assign new symptoms to the past LB. As the serology in these patients remains positive and does not permit a statement on the success of therapy, and furthermore direct pathogen detection or exclusion of infection is not possible with certainty, many fear that the past therapy was not sufficient. Follow-up studies, however, show that most symptoms reported after treated LB do not occur more frequently than in control groups without a history of borreliosis, aside from mild neurological residuals such as facial nerve weakness after acute neuroborreliosis or arthralgias after Lyme arthritis. Moreover, it could be demonstrated that an intensive antibiotic therapy over 90 days remains without effect in this situation as well. There are many indications that these are unspecific symptoms unrelated to LB that are not an expression of pathogen persistence and thus do not respond to antibiotic therapy.[12,15]

Aside from this, there is a large group of patients seeking help who never had certain symptoms of LB but ultimately only a 'seroprevalence titre' as evidence of a previous infection. For various reasons, these often desperate patients are convinced that they suffer from chronic LB. The need to explain the symptoms (for patients and their doctors), lack of knowledge about the actual course of the disease, uncontrolled misinformation such as can be found on the internet,

and the behaviour of some self-appointed borreliosis specialists with in part dubious, self-developed, and unevaluated diagnostic and therapeutic regimens, are only a few reasons contributing to this development.[13] The response of some symptoms to antibiotics, though usually only short-term and incomplete, seems to further support the tentative diagnosis. However, this 'treatment response' is usually due to non-specific effects of the drugs and to placebo effects. Numerous scientific studies argue unequivocally against the hypothesis that these patients suffer from LB, especially since there is no evidence for pathogen persistence and since even the most intensive antibiotic therapies are unsuccessful in the long term.

References

1. Stanek G, Wormser GP, Gray J, Strle F. Lyme borreliosis. *Lancet* 2012;379(9814):461–473.
2. Wormser GP, Dattwyler RJ, Shapiro ED et al. The clinical assessment, treatment, and prevention of lyme Lyme disease, human granulocytic anaplasmosis, and babesiosis: clinical practice guidelines by the Infectious Diseases Society of America. *Clin Infect Dis* 2006;43(9):1089–1134.
3. Wilske B, Fingerle V, Schulte-Spechtel U. Microbiological and serological diagnosis of Lyme borreliosis. *FEMS Immunol Med Microbiol* 2007;49(1):13–21.
4. Hovius JW, van Dam AP, Fikrig E. Tick-host-pathogen interactions in Lyme borreliosis. *Trends Parasitol* 2007;23(9):434–438.
5. Samuels DS, Radolf JD (eds) *Borrelia: molecular biology, host interaction and pathogenesis*. Caister Academic Press, Caister, Norfolk, 2010:548.
6. EUCALB European Concerted Action on Lyme Borreliosis (EUCALB). www.eucalb.com
7. Stanek G, Fingerle V, Hunfeld KP et al. Lyme borreliosis: clinical case definitions for diagnosis and management in Europe. *Clin Microbiol Infect* 2011;17(1):69–79.
8. Mygland A, Ljostad U, Fingerle V et al. EFNS guidelines on the diagnosis and management of European Lyme neuroborreliosis. *Eur J Neurol* 2010;17(1):8–16
9. Schnarr S, Franz JK, Krause A, Zeidler H. Infection and musculoskeletal conditions: Lyme borreliosis. *Best Pract Res Clin Rheumatol* 2006;20(6):1099–1118.
10. Aguero-Rosenfeld ME, Wang G, Schwartz I, Wormser GP. Diagnosis of lyme borreliosis. *Clin Microbiol Rev* 2005;18(3):484–509.
11. Société de Pathologie Infectieuse de la Langue Française. [Lyme borreliosis: diagnostic, therapeutic and preventive approaches. 16th consensus conference on anti-infective therapy. Organized by SPILF with the participation of: Collège des Universitaires de Maladies Infectieuses et Tropicales, Société Française de Dermatologie, Société Française de Microbiologie, Société Française de Neurologie, Société Française de Rhumatologie, Société Nationale Française de Medicine Interne.]. *Med Mal Infect* 2007;37 Suppl 3:S153–S174.
12. Oksi J, Nikoskelainen J, Hiekkanen H et al. Duration of antibiotic treatment in disseminated Lyme borreliosis: a double-blind, randomized, placebo-controlled, multicenter clinical study. *Eur J Clin Microbiol Infect Dis* 2007; 26(8):571–581
13. Klempner MS, Hu LT, Evans J et al. Two controlled trials of antibiotic treatment in patients with persistent symptoms and a history of Lyme disease. *N Engl J Med* 2001;345(2):85–92.
14. Auwaerter PG, Bakken JS, Dattwyler RJ et al. Antiscience and ethical concerns associated with advocacy of Lyme disease. *Lancet Infect Dis* 2011;11(9):713–719.
15. Feder HM, Jr., Johnson BJ, O'Connell S et al. A critical appraisal of 'chronic Lyme disease'. *N Engl J Med* 2007;357(14):1422–1430.

CHAPTER 102

Viral arthritis

Stanley J. Naides

Introduction

Viruses may affect the joints by a number of mechanisms. The mechanisms employed vary with the infecting virus based on mode of tissue entry, tissue tropism, mechanisms of replication, direct viral effects on cellular functions, the ability to establish persistent infection, local immune response, expression of host-like antigens, ability to alter host antigens, host age and genetic makeup, and the infection history of the host. Several viruses directly infect the cells of the synovium. The mechanism of injury may be through lysis of target cells. The target cells may die by one of three mechanisms. First, viral infection may result in classic cell necrosis with karyorrhexis. Second, the virus may initiate the cellular machinery for programmed cell death, or apoptosis. Third, the virus may express virally encoded cell surface antigens that elicit an immune response, that in turn targets killing of virally-infected cells.

Direct infection may also result in non-lytic mechanisms of viral arthritis pathogenesis. Viruses may coopt normal cell functions in such a way as to alter normal cell function. Viral gene products may transactivate host cell genes. Immune activation may result from cell surface expression of normally sequestered autoantigens or viral antigens or virally encoded cytokines. The infected cell would become a target for immune attack or the focus of recruitment of cytokine responsive cells. Viral infection leading to expression of viral antigens on the cell surface may serve as a novel foreign antigen and elicit an immune response. Alternatively, molecular mimicry of host autoantigens may break immune tolerance, resulting in generation of autoimmune responses. Immune complex disease may result when the humoral response generates sufficient antibody to cause deposition of immune complexes either locally, at the site of viral infection, or systemically with deposition of circulating immune complex in synovium.

Parvovirus B19

Human parvovirus B19 is a member of the family *Parvoviridae*, genus *erythrovirus*, consisting of parvoviruses autonomously replicating in erythroid precursors. B19 is a non-enveloped, single-stranded DNA virus measuring approximately 23 nm in diameter. Although infection of other tissue types may occur, viral replication is usually not as efficient in cells other than erythroid progenitors.

Epidemiology

B19 infection is common and geographically widespread. Seroepidemiological studies of community outbreaks of B19 infection demonstrate that a large proportion of B19 infections remain asymptomatic or present as undiagnosed non-specific viral illnesses. Approximately 50% of the general adult population has serological evidence of past B19 infection. Outbreaks of B19 infection occur in late winter and spring, although epidemics have also been reported in summer and autumn. Within a community, B19 outbreaks tend to cycle every 3–5 years, representing the period of time for a fresh cohort of susceptible children to enter the school system. Since the seroprevalence of anti-B19 IgG antibodies is only approximately 50% in adults, these periodic outbreaks often involve susceptible adults as well. The risk of infection in susceptible adults with multiple exposures may be as high as 50%. Workers in occupations with increased exposure to children, such as schoolteachers, daycare workers, and hospital personnel, have increased risk of infection.[1] Sporadic cases occur between outbreaks. Transmission is via nasopharyngeal secretions.

The incubation period between infection and onset of symptoms is 7–18 days. In human volunteer studies, introduction of B19 nasally was followed in 7 days by a flu-like illness associated with viraemia, viral shedding in nasal secretions, and areticulocytosis. At approximately 11 days after infection, an incipient anti-B19 IgM antibody response was associated with clearing of viraemia, cessation of nasal shedding of virus, and a second phase of clinical illness characterized by rash, arthralgia, and arthritis. Onset of the anti-B19 IgG antibody response occurred almost concurrently with the IgM response.[2] In natural infections, the temporal separation between the two phases of clinical illness is often blurred.

Additional B19-like viruses have been isolated and represent genotypic variants of the original B19 isolates, now designated genotype 1 and found worldwide. Genotype 2 consists of A6, LaLi/K71, and Vx strains. Genotype 3 consists of the V9 virus and related isolates. Protein homology between genotypes is 96–97% and no antigenic differences have been identified. Genotypes have similar biological behaviour and clinical presentations.

Clinical features

B19 is the cause of transient aplastic crisis in the setting of chronic haemolytic anaemia.[3] B19 causes erythema infectiosum, or fifth disease, a common rash illness of children characterized by bright red

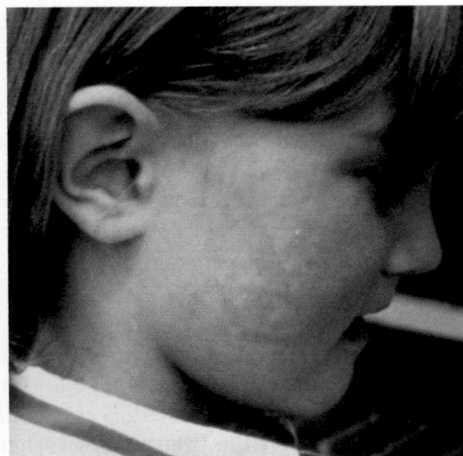

Fig. 102.1 Classic 'slapped cheeks' of a child with erythema infectiosum, or fifth disease, caused by parvovirus B19.

Reproduced with permission from Human parvovirus infection. *American Family Physician* 1989;39(1):165–169. Copyright © 1989 American Academy of Family Physicians. All Rights Reserved.

'slapped cheeks' and a macular, maculopapular, and occasionally vesicular or haemorrhagic eruption on the torso and extremities (Figure 102.1). While infection in children may be asymptomatic, when symptoms do occur they tend to be mild and include sore throat, headache, fever, cough, anorexia, vomiting, diarrhoea, and arthralgia. Erythema infectiosum may also be seen in adults not previously infected. In adults, the rash tends to be subtler and the bright red 'slapped cheeks' absent. A number of uncommon dermatologic manifestations of B19 infection have been reported including a vesiculopustular eruption, purpura with or without thrombocytopenia, Henoch–Schönlein purpura, and a 'gloves and socks' erythema.

B19 infection may be associated with paraesthesias in the fingers. Rarely, progressive arm weakness has occurred, as has numbness of the toes. In such instances, nerve conduction studies show mild slowing of nerve conduction velocities and decreased amplitudes of motor and sensory potentials.[3]

B19 may infect the fetus, causing hydrops fetalis on the basis of either B19-induced anaemia or viral cardiomyopathy. B19 has been reported to less commonly cause pancytopenia, isolated anaemia, thrombocytopenia, leucopenia, myocarditis, neuropathy, hepatitis, or vasculitis.[3,4] Patients with congenital or acquired immune deficiencies, including prior chemotherapy for lymphoproliferative disorders, immunosuppressive therapy, or AIDS may fail to clear B19 infection, causing chronic or recurrent anaemia, thrombocytopenia, or leucopenia. B19 infection is the leading cause of pure red cell aplasia in AIDS patients.

Among B19-infected immunocompetent children under 10 years of age, arthralgia may occur in about 5% and joint swelling in only approximately 3%. In adolescents, joint pain and swelling occurs in about 12% and 5%, respectively. However, joint pain occurs in about 77% and joint swelling in 60% of adults 20 years of age or older.[5] In adults, B19 infection may be associated with a severe flu-like illness in which polyarthralgia and joint swelling are prominent. The distribution of involved joints is rheumatoid-like with prominent symmetric involvement of the metacarpophalangeal, proximal interphalangeal, wrist, knee, and ankle joints. Patients usually experience sudden-onset polyarthralgia or polyarthritis.

Onset of joint symptoms may or may not be preceded by a viral prodrome consisting of fever, malaise, chills, and myalgias. Most adults present with acute, moderately severe, symmetric polyarthritis that usually starts in the hands or knees and within 24–48 hours spreads to include the wrists, ankles, feet, elbows, and shoulders. Spinal involvement is uncommon. Joint symptoms in adults are usually self-limited, but a minority of adults have prolonged symptoms. Of those with chronic symptoms, approximately two-thirds have continuous symptoms of morning stiffness and arthralgia with intermittent flares. The remaining one-third are symptom free between flares. Morning stiffness is prominent. Rheumatoid factor may be present in low to moderate titre during the acute phase of infection but usually resolves.[6] Anti-DNA, anti-lymphocyte, anti-nuclear antibodies, and anti-phospholipid antibodies may also be found acutely. Joint erosions and rheumatoid nodules have not been reported. Chronic B19 arthropathy may last for years. Several weeks after the initial infection, symptoms of acute synovitis tend to resolve. Joint pain and stiffness remain prominent features in patients who continue to have symptoms. Approximately 12% of patients presenting with 'early synovitis' have B19-induced rheumatoid-like arthropathy, the majority of whom are women.[3] Adults usually lack the classic slapped-cheek rash seen in children.

The distribution of joint involvement in B19 arthropathy and its symmetry may suggest a diagnosis of rheumatoid arthritis (RA). An initial report of a HLA DR4 association was not supported by further study. The absence of rheumatoid nodules or joint destruction aids in the differential diagnosis of B19 arthropathy from classic, erosive RA.[3]

Diagnosis

Diagnosis is based on laboratory confirmation in the appropriate clinical setting. While detection of B19 virions or DNA in serum during viraemia is confirmatory, these have usually resolved when the patient presents with joint symptoms. The diagnosis of a *recent* B19 infection is usually confirmed by detection of anti-B19 IgM antibody. Commercially available tests use recombinant empty capsids for antibody detection.[3]

The anti-B19 IgM antibody response is usually positive for at least 2 months following onset of joint symptoms, but may wane shortly thereafter. However, the IgM antibody may be detectable in occasional patients for 6 months or longer. Because of the high seroprevalence of anti-B19 IgG in the adult population, detection of anti-B19 IgG antibody shortly after presentation of acute-onset joint symptoms in a patient, in the absence of anti-B19 IgM, suggests past B19 infection and other diagnoses should be entertained. Failure to obtain B19 serological testing at presentation may leave the diagnostic IgM antibody response undetected, leading to failure to diagnosis B19 arthropathy in those patients in whom joint symptoms persist. Testing for B19 DNA at the time of arthropathy presentation is unlikely to be useful. Finding B19 DNA in synovium in chronic arthropathy is of questionable diagnostic value given that B19 DNA is found in synovium in half of healthy military recruits undergoing arthroscopy for injury using sensitive polymerase chain reaction (PCR) techniques.[3,6,7]

Pathogenesis

Anti-B19 IgM antibody and acute-phase IgG antibody (less than 1 week after inoculation) recognize determinants on the major capsid protein, VP2. In convalescent serum, anti-B19 IgG antibody recognizes determinants on the minor capsid protein VP1 structural protein.[8] Since B19 VP1 and VP2 are products of alternate transcription of the same open reading frame, VP1 contains an additional 227 N-terminal amino acids not present in VP2. VP1 therefore contains unique determinants not present in the truncated form represented by VP2; these determinants may be in the unique non-overlapping N-terminal region or, alternatively, represent conformational differences in the sequences shared between the two proteins. Western blot analysis of serum from individuals with congenital immune deficiency, prior chemotherapy, or AIDS, demonstrated the absence of convalescent anti-B19 IgG antibodies directed against VP1. These sera were unable to neutralize B19 virus in experimental bone marrow culture systems.[8] In the absence of neutralizing antibodies to B19, B19 persists in the bone marrow and may cause chronic or intermittent suppression of one or more haematopoietic lineages.

B19 NS1 is a member of the superfamily 3 of helicases found in DNA viruses. In non-erythroid cells, B19 fails to transcribe capsid mRNA, but does produce intact NS1[4] that induces apoptosis in the host cell[9–11] and damages host cell DNA by single strand nicking and bulky adduct formation (protein–DNA covalent bonding).[12] Presentation of self-DNA modified by covalent linkage to viral proteins may allow the immune system to break tolerance by activating anergic B lymphocytes though viral peptide recognition.[12] This mechanism may explain the detection of DNA antibodies in acute B19 infection and the prevalence of B19 antibodies in patients with systemic lupus erythematosus (SLE). It also suggests a role for B19 and other viruses with superfamily 3 helicases, e.g. EBNA in Epstein–Barr virus, in breaking tolerance to self-DNA in SLE.[12]

Management

There is no specific vaccine or treatment for B19 infection at this time. Neutralizing activity to B19 is found in commercially available pooled immunoglobulin because of the high seroprevalence of anti-B19 IgG antibodies in the adult population. Intravenous immunoglobulin has been successful in the treatment of bone marrow suppression and B19 persistence in immunocompromised patients. However, this may not be applicable to chronic arthropathy patients as viraemia is usually absent by onset of joint symptoms; treatment is symptomatic with non-steroidal anti-inflammatory agents (NSAIDs).

Rubella virus

Rubella virus is the sole member of the genus *rubivirus* in the *Togaviridae* family of enveloped RNA viruses. The spherical rubella virion measures 50–70 nm in diameter with a 30 nm dense core. An envelope is acquired by budding at vesicles or the cell surface. Spike-like projections on the envelope measuring 5–6 nm contain haemagglutinin activity detected by agglutination of erythrocytes from a variety of animal species.[13]

Epidemiology

Rubella host range is restricted to humans. Transmission is by nasopharyngeal secretions with peak incidence in late winter and spring. Widespread rubella vaccination altered the epidemiology of rubella infection which had previously occurred in 6–9 year cycles mostly in children. Now, the age profile has shifted toward young adults and infection rates are 10–20% of those in the pre-vaccine era. More recent rubella outbreaks in college students and in adults underscore the public health need for maintaining vaccination programmes.

Incubation time from infection to onset of rash is 14–21 days. Viraemia occurs 6–7 days before skin eruption, peaks immediately prior to eruption, and clears within 48 hours of rash. Virus shedding in nasopharyngeal secretions may be detected from 7 days before and until 14 days after skin eruption, but is maximal just before onset of rash until 5–6 days after eruption.[14]

Clinical features

The spectrum of clinical disease in children and adults ranges from asymptomatic infection to a classic syndrome of low-grade fever, rash, coryza, malaise, and prominent posterior cervical, postauricular, and occipital lymphadenopathy. Constitutional symptoms may precede the skin eruption by 5 days. The eruption may vary during a brief 2–3 day period, starting as a morbilliform facial eruption before spreading to the torso, and upper then lower extremities. The eruption may coalesce on the face and clear as the extremities become involved. Alternatively, the eruption may be limited to a transient blush.

Joint complaints are common in adult infection, especially in women. Joint symptoms may occur 1 week before or after onset of the rash. Joint involvement is usually symmetric and may be migratory, resolving over a few days to 2 weeks. Arthralgias are more common than frank arthritis. Stiffness is prominent. The metacarpophalangeal and proximal interphalangeal joints of the hands, the knees, wrists, ankles and elbows are most frequently involved. Periarthritis, tenosynovitis, and carpal tunnel syndrome may be seen. In some patients, symptoms may persist for several months or years.[15]

Current vaccination with live attenuated vaccine, RA27/3, has a complication rate of 15–25% characterized by arthralgia, myalgia, arthritis, and paraesthesias. The pattern of joint involvement is similar to natural infection. Arthritis usually occurs 2 weeks after inoculation and typically lasts less than a week. However, in some patients postvaccination rubella arthritis may persist for more than a year.[16]

In children, two syndromes of rheumatological interest may occur. In the 'arm syndrome,' a brachial radiculoneuropathy causes arm and hand pain, and dysaesthesias that are worse at night. The 'catcher's crouch' syndrome is a lumbar radiculoneuropathy characterized by popliteal fossa pain on arising in the morning. Those affected assume a 'catcher's crouch' position. The pain gradually decreases through the day. Both syndromes occur 1–2 months after vaccination. The initial episode may last up to 2 months, but recurrences are usually shorter in duration. Episodes may recur for up to 1 year, but there is no permanent damage.[17]

Diagnosis

Rubella is readily cultured from tissues and body fluids including throat swabs. Rubella RNA may be detected in tissue of body fluids by reverse transcription polymerase chain reaction (RT-PCR) amplification. Presence of anti-rubella IgM antibody or anti-IgG antibody seroconversion is diagnostic of rubella infection. Anti-rubella IgM and IgG are usually present at onset of joint symptoms. IgM antibody peaks 8–21 days after symptoms then decreases over the next 4–5 weeks to undetectable levels in most patients. Therefore, detection of anti-rubella IgM indicates recent infection, usually in the last 1–2 months. Since anti-rubella IgG rises rapidly over a period of 7–21 days after onset symptoms, a diagnosis of rubella infection based on IgG serology can only be made with paired acute and convalescent sera.[14]

Pathogenesis

Failure to mount an adequate immune response to specific epitopes may allow rubella virus to persist in patients with rubella arthritis. Virus may be detected in synovial fluid during arthritis flares and in lymphocytes years after symptom resolution. Onset of rash and arthritis is coincident with the appearance of antibodies, including neutralizing antibodies to whole virus, suggesting a role for antibody or immune complexes in the synovitis.[14]

Management

NSAIDs may be used for symptom control. Low to moderate doses of steroids have been used to control symptoms and viraemia.

Hepatitis B virus

Hepatitis B virus (HBV) is a member of the family *Hepadnaviridae*, genus *orthohepadnavirus*. HBV is an enveloped double-stranded DNA icosahedral virus measuring 42 nm in diameter, the 'Dane' particle.[18]

Epidemiology

HBV is transmitted by parenteral and sexual routes. HBV infection occurs worldwide, but prevalence of hepatitis B surface antigen (Australian antigen) is higher in Asia, the Middle East, and sub-Saharan Africa. The prevalence in China may be as high as 10% compared to 0.01% in the United States. There is no known seasonality to primary HBV infections. Most acute infections in endemic regions occur at an early age, with many acquired perinatally from infected mothers, and are usually asymptomatic; incidence of infection in children may be as high as 5% annually, with gradual decline of carriage rates and specific antibody with advanced age. In developed countries, most infections are acquired in adulthood during sexual or needle exposures. Adult infection is more often associated with acute hepatitis; of those with hepatitis, 5–10% develop persistent infection. In endemic regions, HBV is a common cause of chronic liver disease and a leading cause of hepatocellular carcinoma.[18]

Clinical features

The incubation period from infection to hepatitis is usually 45–120 days. A preicteric prodromal period lasting several days to a month may be associated with fever, myalgia, malaise, anorexia, nausea, and vomiting. Significant viraemia occurs early in infection; soluble immune complexes with circulating hepatitis B surface antigen (HBsAg) are formed as anti-hepatitis B surface antigen antibodies (HBsAb) are produced. Immune-complex-mediated severe arthritis often occurs abruptly, concurrent with urticaria. Joint involvement is usually symmetric with simultaneous involvement of several joints at onset, but arthritis may be migratory or additive. The joints of the hand and knee are most often affected, but wrists, ankles, elbows, shoulders, and other large joints may be involved as well. Fusiform swelling may be seen in the small joints of the hand. Morning stiffness is common. Arthritis and urticaria may precede jaundice by days to weeks and may persist several

weeks after jaundice, but usually subside soon after onset of jaundice. Patients who develop chronic active hepatitis or chronic HBV viraemia may have recurrent arthralgias or arthritis. Polyarteritis nodosa (PAN) is frequently associated with chronic hepatitis B viraemia.

Diagnosis

Urticaria in the presence of polyarthritis should raise the possibility of HBV infection. Acute hepatitis may be asymptomatic, but elevated bilirubin and transaminases are usually present when the arthritis appears. Joint fluid examination is not diagnostic. At the time of arthritis onset, peak levels of serum HBsAg are detectable. Virions, viral DNA, viral polymerase, and hepatitis B e antigen may be detectable in serum. Anti-hepatitis B core antigen IgM antibodies are present and indicate acute HBV infection, as opposed to past or chronic infection.[19]

Pathogenesis

HBV arthritis is thought to be mediated by immune complex deposition in synovium. Immune complexes containing HBsAg, antibody, and complement components may be detected.

Management

Management is limited to supportive measures including NSAIDs.

Hepatitis C virus

Hepatitis C virus (HCV) is a member of the family *Flaviviridae*, genus *hepacivirus*. It is an enveloped single-stranded RNA spherical virus measuring 38–50 nm in diameter.

Epidemiology

HCV is distributed worldwide. Seroprevalence is less than 1% in developed Western countries but is higher in Africa and Asia where it may cause one-quarter or more of acute and chronic hepatitides. HCV is transmitted by the parenteral route; sexual transmission is rare. HCV genotypic variants have been described and these differ in their pathogenicity including severity of disease and response to interferon-α. HCV has 6 major genotypes groups or clades and over 50 genotypic subtypes.[20] As with other positive-strand RNA viruses, the viral polymerase is error prone, generating variants at a high rate.

Clinical features

Acute HCV infection is usually benign. Up to 80% of post-transfusion infections are anicteric and asymptomatic, even though liver transaminases may be markedly elevated acutely. Subsequently and prior to cirrhosis, liver enzymes are usually minimally elevated to normal. HCV is strongly associated with HBV-negative hepatocellular carcinoma, especially in Africa and Japan.

Acute-onset polyarthritis in a rheumatoid distribution, including the small joints of the hand, wrists, shoulders, knees, and hips, may occur in acute HCV infection.[21] HCV is often associated with type II cryoglobulinaemia in established infection. It may present as essential mixed cryoglobulinaemia, a triad of arthritis, palpable purpura, and cryoglobulinaemia. Indeed, a majority of patients originally described as having essential mixed cryoglobulinaemia had HCV infection. HCV infection is also seen in non-essential secondary cryoglobulinaemia although less commonly. The presence of detectable anti-HCV antibodies in essential mixed cryoglobulinaemia is associated with more severe cutaneous involvement, e.g. Raynaud's phenomena, purpura, livedo, distal ulcers, and gangrene. HCV RNA may be found in 75% of cryoprecipitates from patients with essential mixed cryoglobulinaemia and anti-HCV antibodies.[22]

Diagnosis

Serological tests utilize an array of antigens in an enzyme immunoassay; a recombinant strip immunoblot assay (RIBA) is confirmatory. RT-PCR is used for diagnosis, identification of genotype, and detection of sequence variants associated with drug resistance.[23] A minority of patients may have HCV RNA detectable by PCR amplification methods in the absence of a positive serology. Transaminase levels may not reflect severity of viral load, hepatitis, or cryoglobulinaemia because hepatocytes die by apoptosis allowing hepatocyte content to be cleared by apoptotic mechanisms.[24]

Pathogenesis

Chronic HCV infection can lead to cirrhosis, endstage liver failure, and hepatocellular carcinoma but the mechanisms by which they occur are not known. HCV infection persists despite vigorous antibody response to an array of viral epitopes. The high rate of mutation in the envelope protein is responsible for emergence of neutralization escape mutants and quasispecies.[25] HCV is suspected to elicit cryoglobulins because HCV envelope glycoprotein has antibody Fc receptor properties that allow epitope spreading from HCV to bound immunoglobulin Fc.[26]

Management

Intravenous interferon-α has been shown to be efficacious in the treatment of chronic HCV hepatitis and HCV-associated cryoglobulinaemia. Ribavirin in combination with interferon-α2b, or higher doses of interferon-α2b alone when tolerated, improve response rates. Pegylation of interferon lengthens drug half-life. However, interferon therapy is often associated with undesirable side effects that discourage completion of the therapeutic course; relapse after completion of the initial course of therapy is common. Those with cryoglobulinaemic vasculitis failing interferon therapy may require immunosuppressive therapy. There is controversy whether interferon therapy precipitates autoimmune disease such as autoimmune thyroiditis. Inhibitors of the viral non-structural protein NS3/4A protease and NS5B polymerase, and other drugs, hold further therapeutic promise.[27] These agents will become available in 2014 and promise high rates of viral eradication after shorter courses of oral therapy. This promise has prompted recommendations for routine screening of at-risk populations.

Retroviruses

Human immunodeficiency virus (HIV)

Several musculoskeletal syndromes have been described in HIV-infected patients. Initial HIV infection may be associated with a transient flu-like illness with arthralgias. Later, three pain syndromes not associated with synovitis may be seen.[28] The concurrence of RA and HIV is thought to be very rare. An acute symmetric polyarthritis involving the small joints of the hands and the wrists has been described but it was associated with periosteal new bone formation about the involved joints, a feature not seen in RA.

Subacute oligoarticular arthritis primarily of the knees and ankles may cause severe arthralgia and disability but is transient, peaks in intensity within 1–6 weeks, and responds to NSAIDs. Synovial fluid is non-inflammatory. Mononuclear cell infiltrates may be seen in the synovium of the involved joints. In Brazil, a similar presentation has been described amongst heterosexual men with HIV and arthritis, with 83.5% polyarthritis, 16.5% oligoarthritis, and 97.5% symmetrical, almost always involving lower extremities and about a one-quarter with involvement of the great toe. Erythrocyte sedimentation rate (ESR) exceeded 100 mm/hour in more than one-half of cases. Rheumatoid factor was negative, synovial fluid sterile and non-inflammatory, and radiographs normal. Successive bouts resolved in 2–5 weeks with NSAIDs.[29]

As many as 10% of HIV-infected patients may experience 'painful articular syndrome' characterized by intermittent severe joint pain predominantly of the shoulders, elbows, and knees that lasts about a day. The pain may be incapacitating and require short-term narcotic analgesics. Fibromyalgia has been reported in HIV-infected patients with prevalence as high as 29% in one series. The role of HIV and other potential agents in these pain syndromes remains to be clarified. In addition to arthritis, disseminated interstitial lymphocytosis syndrome (DILS) may be seen in AIDS patients. In affected patients, a CD8-positive lymphocyte infiltrate of salivary glands causes parotid swelling. This entity needs to be differentiated from classic Sjögren's syndrome.[30]

Patients with reactive arthritis do not have sacroiliitis or anterior uveitis, nor do they present with the classic triad of arthritis, urethritis, and uveitis. The prevalence of HLA B27 positivity appears to be lower in the HIV-infected patients compared to non-HIV-associated reactive arthritis. In Africa where the route of HIV transmission is predominantly heterosexual, approximately 40% of HIV patients with joint symptoms in Zimbabwe have reactive arthritis, and another 40% have a pauciarticular presentation without extra-articular features characteristic of reactive arthritis.[31] In the United States, psoriatic arthritis limited to a pattern of asymmetric oligoarthritis may be seen in as many as one-third of HIV-infected patients with psoriasis, but the overall incidence of psoriasis does not appear to be significantly increased. Whether the different patterns of rheumatic disease expression are attributable to HIV infection itself or coinfection with other agents remains controversial.[32]

Human T lymphocyte leukaemia virus 1

Human T lymphocyte leukaemia virus (HTLV) is found in Japan, the Caribbean, South America, and sub-Saharan Africa where 1% of the population may be infected. HTLV-1 causes asymptomatic infection, leukaemia or lymphoma, myelopathy, or tropical spastic paraparesis, uveitis, or opportunistic infections. An association with inclusion body myositis has been reported. HTLV-1 is endemic in defined localities in Japan, historically associated with early European trade, where oligoarthritis and a nodular rash have been typical presentations. The patients have positive serology for anti-HTLV antibodies. Type C viral particles are seen in skin lesions. The presence of atypical synovial cells with lobulated nuclei and T cell synovial infiltrates suggests direct involvement of the synovial tissue by the leukemic process.[33] Patients with HTLV-1 infection may also have sicca symptoms. A number of reports associate HTLV-1 infection with Sjögren's syndrome, as well as autoimmune thyroid disease.[34]

Alphaviruses

Chikungunya virus

Chikungunya virus was originally isolated during an epidemic of febrile arthritis in Tanzania in 1952–1953. The local tribal word, chikungunya, 'that which twists or bends up', was applied to the virus and the disease. Retrospectively, it is likely that similar epidemics occurred in Indonesia, Africa, India, Asia, and possibly the southern United States from 1779 to 1828.[35]

Epidemiology

Chikungunya virus is transmitted from its reservoir hosts (baboons, monkeys, and, in Senegal, *Scotophilus* bat species) to humans by *Aedes* mosquitoes in south and west central Africa, Thailand, Vietnam, and India. *Mansonia africana* and mosquitoes from other genera may also act as vectors. In a 1964 epidemic in Bangkok, Thailand, an estimated 40 000 patients out of an urban area of 2 million were infected and 31% of the prospectively studied cohort seroconverted to chikungunya virus antibody positivity. Globalization may contribute to increasing risk of spread. An outbreak in Malaysia in 1998–1999 was attributed to migrant workers from endemic areas. A major outbreak occurred in the Emilia-Romagna region of north-eastern Italy in the summer of 2007.[36] The reinfestation of *Aedes aegypti* and the introduction of *Ae. albopictus* into the western hemisphere raises the spectre of an expanded geographic distribution.

Clinical features

Chikungunya fever has explosive onset associated with fever and severe arthralgia. The incubation period is usually 2–3 days but ranges over 1–12 days. Constitutional symptoms, rash and fever to 40 °C are accompanied by rigors. The acute illness may last 2–3 days with a range of 1–7 days. Suffusion of the conjunctiva is prominent. Sore throat, pharyngitis, headache, photophobia, retro-orbital pain, anorexia, nausea, vomiting, and abdominal pain may accompany the acute illness. Lymphadenopathy may be tender but is usually not massive. Following the acute illness, fever may resolve for 1–2 days before recrudescence. Polyarthralgia is migratory and predominantly affects the small joints of the hands, wrists, feet, and ankles with less prominent involvement of the large joints. Previously injured joints may be more severely affected. Stiffness and swelling may occur but large effusions are uncommon. In severe cases, symptoms may persist for months. Approximately 10% of patients have joint symptoms 1 year after infection. Generalized myalgia and back and shoulder pain are common. A destructive arthropathy may occur in a few adult patients with chronic symptoms. Low-titre rheumatoid factor may be found in those with longstanding symptoms.

Skin eruption is characterized by facial and neck flushing, followed by macular or maculopapular eruption beginning 1–10 days after illness onset. Typically, a rash occurs on day 2–5 and is associated with defervescence. The rash may last 1–5 days and may recur with fever. It is located on the torso, extremities, and occasionally the face, palms, and soles. It may be pruritic. In some patients, involved skin desquamates.[37] Isolated petechiae and mucosal bleeding may occur, usually without significant haemorrhage.

Symptoms in children tend to be milder. Nausea, vomiting, pharyngitis, and facial flushing are prominent features. Arthralgia, arthritis, and rash are uncommon, and milder and briefer in duration when present. Children may present with mild dengue-like haemorrhagic fever, headache, pharyngeal injection, vomiting, abdominal pain, constipation, diarrhoea, cough, or lymphadenopathy. Maternal–fetal transmission may result in severe neonatal infection.

Diagnosis

Chikungunya fever should be considered in any febrile patient resident in or returning from endemic areas. A history of epidemic occurrence should be sought. O'nyong-nyong virus, Mayaro virus, Ross River virus, rubella virus, parvovirus B19, dengue, and HBV infections may present similarly. Synovial fluid shows decreased viscosity with poor mucin clot, 2000–5000 white cells/mm³. Therefore, the definitive diagnosis depends on laboratory confirmation.

Virus may be isolated during days 2–4 after infection. Haemagglutination and complement fixation assays and neutralizing antibody assays have been replaced by RT-PCR methods.[38]

Pathogenesis

Following mosquito bite, intense viraemia occurs within 48 hours. Viraemia begins to wane around day 3. The appearance of hemagglutination inhibition activity in neutralizing antibodies clears the viraemia. Involved skin shows erythrocyte extravasation from superficial capillaries and perivascular cuffing. The virus absorbs to human platelets causing aggregation, suggesting a mechanism for bleeding. Synovitis in chikungunya fever probably results from direct viral infection of synovium.[35]

Management

Management for the patient is supportive. During the acute attack, range of motion exercises ameliorate stiffness. NSAIDs are useful. However, chloroquine phosphate (250 mg/day) has been used when NSAIDs failed.

O'nyong-nyong virus

O'nyong-nyong virus is closely related to chikungunya virus. It was first described in the Acholi province of north-western Uganda in February, 1959, where its name means 'joint breaker.' Within 2 years, it had spread through Uganda and the surrounding region, affecting 2 million people. Serologically determined attack rates ranged from 50% to 60% with up to 78% of infected individuals becoming symptomatic. Disease spread at a rate of 2–3 km daily. After the epidemic, the virus was not detected again until it was isolated from *Anopheles funestus* mosquitoes in Kenya in 1978. *A. gambiae* also serves as a vector. Serological surveys indicate that o'nyong-nyong virus is endogenous. The non-human vertebrate reservoir for the virus is not known. In 1996–1997, o'nyong-nyong virus again appeared during an outbreak in south central Uganda.[39]

Clinical features

O'nyong-nyong fever is clinically similar to chikungunya infections. The incubation period lasts at least 8 days and is followed by sudden-onset polyarthralgia/polyarthritis. Four days later, appearance of skin eruptions is typically associated with improvement in joint symptoms. The eruption is uniform in nature and lasts 4–7 days before fading. The fever is not prominent but postcervical lymphadenopathy may be marked. Knees and ankles are most commonly affected. Arthralgias last 2–21 days with 1–14 days of immobilization.[40] Although residual joint pain often persists, there appear to be no long-term sequelae.

Diagnosis

Differential diagnosis includes chikungunya fever, igbo ora virus infection, and measles. Viral isolation by intracerebral injection into suckling mice produces runting, rash, and alopecia. Haemagglutination inhibition or complement fixation tests identify the virus. The differential diagnosis is similar to that of chikungunya fever. Mouse anti-sera raised against chikungunya virus or o'nyong-nyong virus react equally well with o'nyong-nyong virus, but o'nyong-nyong anti-sera do not react well with chikungunya virus. The mechanisms of o'nyong-nyong virus pathogenesis are unknown.[35]

Management

Management is symptomatic. Patients typically recover without long-term sequelae.

Igbo ora virus

Igbo Ora virus is serologically similar to chikungunya and o'nyong-nyong viruses. Initially, a single patient with fever, sore throat, and arthritis was identified. In 1984, an epidemic of fever, myalgias, arthralgias, and skin eruption occurred in the Ivory Coast. The term 'igbo ora' was coined: it means 'the disease that breaks your wings'. The virus was isolated from *A. funestus* and *A. gambiae* mosquitoes, and from affected individuals. Domestic animals show a higher seroprevalance than humans, suggesting that humans are a secondary host. Growth in culture in VERO and MRC5 causes lysis while growth in MDCK and MA104 cells is less cytotoxic.[41]

Ross River virus (epidemic polyarthritis)

Epidemics of fever and rash have been observed in Australia since 1928. Isolation of Ross River virus from mosquitoes, its serological association with epidemic polyarthritis, and the isolation of the virus from epidemic polyarthritis patients in Australia confirmed Ross River virus as the etiologic agent of epidemic polyarthritis.[35] Antibodies to Ross River virus have been observed in the sera of endogenous populations in Papua New Guinea, West New Guinea, the Bismarck Archipelago, Rossel Island, and the Solomon Islands. From 1979 to 1980, a major epidemic of febrile polyarthritis occurred in Fiji, affecting over 40 000 individuals. Serological surveys suggested that a low level of Ross River virus infection was present throughout the Fijian islands before 1979 but that following the epidemic, up to 90% of the residents of some communities had antibody. A similar epidemic occurred in the Cook Islands early in 1980. Antibodies to Ross River virus are not found in the Asiatic zone west of Weber's line (a hypothetical line separating the Australian biogeographic zone from the Asiatic zone).

In Australia, both endemic cases and epidemics occur in temperate and tropical zones. Significant numbers of cases are reported in Queensland and New South Wales, although cases and outbreaks are described in other regions as well. Seroprevalence may reach only 6–15% in temperate coastal zones but is 27–39% in the plains of the Murray Valley river system.[42] High rainfall, which increases mosquito populations, usually precedes epidemic periods. Cases occur from the spring through the fall.

The major vectors are *Ae. vigilax* on the eastern coast of Australia and *Ae. camptorhynchus* in southern Australia, where the mosquito breeds in salt marshes. *Culex annulirostris* is a fresh-water breeding vector. Other Australian *Aedes* species and *Mansonia uniformus* may also serve as vectors. Several mammalian species may serve as intermediate hosts, including domestic animals, rodents, and marsupials. In the Pacific island outbreaks, *Ae. polynesiensis*, *Ae. aegypti*, *Ae. vigilax*, and *C. annulirostris* may have contributed as well.

In Queensland, annual rates of disease range from 31.5 to 288.3 per 100 000 person years.[43] During epidemics in Fiji and New South Wales, the majority of those infected were symptomatic. While male and female infection rates were similar, there was a predominance of women in presenting cases. Children have a case/infection ratio lower than adults.

Clinical features

Arthralgias occur abruptly after a 7–11 day incubation period.[35] A macular, popular, or maculopapular skin eruption, that may be pruritic, typically follows onset of arthralgia by 1–2 days; in some patients, rash may precede or follow joint symptoms by 11 days or 15 days, respectively. Occasionally, vesicles, papules, or petechiae are seen. The trunk and extremities are typically involved although involvement of the palms, soles, and face may occur. The rash resolves by fading to a brownish discoloration or by desquamation. Despite the name of the disease, one-half of patients have no fever, and in those who do, modest fevers may last only 1–3 days. Headache, nausea, and myalgia are common. Mild photophobia, respiratory symptoms, and lymphadenopathy may occur.

A majority of patients have severe, incapacitating arthralgia. Joint distribution is often asymmetric and migratory, commonly involving the metacarpophalangeal and finger interphalangeal joints, wrists, knees, and ankles. Shoulders, elbows, and toes may also be involved. Axial, hip, and temporomandibular involvement occasionally occurs. Arthralgias are worse in the morning and after periods of inactivity. Mild exercise tends to improve joint symptoms. One-third will have frank synovitis. Polyarticular swelling and tenosynovitis are common. As many as one-third have paraesthesias, or palm or sole pain. Some patients have classic carpal tunnel syndrome. Half of all patients are able to resume their activities of daily living within 4 weeks although residual polyarthralgia may be present. Joint symptoms recur but episodes of relapse gradually resolve. A few patients will continue to have joint symptoms for up to 3 years.[44]

Diagnosis

The diagnosis of Ross River virus infection should be considered in anyone with a febrile arthritis in the appropriate geographic setting. Acute rubella arthritis may present in a similar fashion, although the signs and symptoms of an upper respiratory infection are more prominent in rubella. Patients may present without a rash. The differential diagnosis then would include early seronegative RA, SLE, parvovirus B19 infection, HBV infection, HCV infection, other alphavirus infections, Henoch–Schönlein purpura, and drug hypersensitivities. In those individuals who develop vesicles, differential from varicella or the occasional parvovirus B19 infection would need to be considered.

Synovial fluid cell counts range from 1500 to 13 800 cells/mm^3. Monocytes and vacuolated macrophages dominate with few neutrophils. Virus has been isolated only from antibody-negative sera. In the Australian epidemics prior to 1979, patients were antibody positive at the time of presentation. However, in the Pacific island epidemics of 1979–80, patients remained viraemic and serologically negative for up to a week following onset of symptoms. Ross River virus antigen is detectable by fluorescent antibody staining of C6/36 cells inoculated with acute patient serum. Virus in serum is stable for up to a month at 0 to −10 °C.

Pathogenesis

Ross River viral antigen may be detected by specific immunofluorescence in monocytes and macrophages early, but intact virus is not identifiable by electron microscopy or cell culture.[35] The dermis shows mild perivascular mononuclear cell, mostly T lymphocytic, infiltrate in both erythematous and purpuric eruptions. The purpuric form of eruption also shows extravasation of erythrocytes. Synovium demonstrates synovial lining layer hypertrophy, vascular proliferation, and mononuclear cell infiltration. Viral RNA can be found by RT-PCR. Ross River virus antigen may be found in epithelial cells in the erythematous or purpuric skin lesions, and in the perivascular zone in the erythematous lesion.[45]

Management

Management of the acute infection is symptomatic. Aspirin or NSAIDs provide relief for joint pain. Corticosteroids may shorten time of recovery and do not appear to exacerbate symptoms.[46] Occasional patients may develop more persistent joint symptoms, but full recovery is usual.

Barmah forest virus

This circulates in the same geographic areas as does Ross River virus and presents in a similar fashion. A major outbreak occurred in summer and autumn of 2002 and 2003.[47]

Sindbis virus

Sindbis virus is the prototype alphavirus used for molecular virology studies. It was isolated from *Culex* mosquitoes in the Egyptian village of the same name in 1952.

Epidemiology

Sindbis virus infection occurs in Sweden, Finland, and the neighbouring Karelian isthmus of Russia where it is known locally as Okelbo disease, Pogosta disease, or Karelian fever, respectively.[35] *Aedes*, *Culex*, and *Culiseta* species transmit the virus to humans. Birds are an intermediate host. Cases are confined to predominantly forested areas where seroprevalence is approximately 5%. Individuals involved in outdoor activities or occupations are at risk. Sindbis virus infection has also been reported as sporadic cases and small outbreaks in Uganda, South Africa, Zimbabwe, Central Africa, and Australia.[35]

Clinical features

Skin eruption and arthralgia are the initial symptoms although one may precede the other by a few days. Fever may be present although it is not high. Constitutional symptoms including headache, fatigue, malaise, nausea, vomiting, pharyngitis, and paraesthesias may be present but are usually not severe. Macular skin eruptions typically begin on the torso, spreading to the arms and legs, palms, soles, and occasionally head. The macules may evolve to papules that have a tendency to vesiculate. Vesiculation is particularly prominent on pressure points, including the palms and soles. As the eruption fades, a brownish discoloration is left. Vesicles on the palms and soles may become haemorrhagic. The rash may recur during convalescence.

Arthralgia and arthritis involve the small joints of the hands and feet, wrists, elbows, ankles, and knees. Occasionally, the axial skeleton becomes involved. Tendonitis is common, often involving the extensor tendons of the hand and the Achilles tendon. Non-erosive chronic arthropathy is common in both Swedish and Finnish reports, with up to one-half of patients having symptoms 2.5 years after onset. A smaller number have symptoms as long as 5–6 years after infection.[48]

Diagnosis

Haemagglutination inhibition and complement fixation tests may establish the diagnosis. Antibodies appear during the first week of illness. A real time RT-PCR assay for detection of Sindbis viral RNA has been developed.

Pathogenesis

Little is known about the pathogenesis of Sindbis virus disease. Virus has been isolated from a skin vesicle in the absence of viraemia. Skin lesions show perivascular oedema, haemorrhage, lymphocytic infiltrates, and areas of necrosis. Sindbis virus is capable of replication in human macrophages which are activated to release proinflammatory cytokines including macrophage inhibitory factor, tumour necrosis factor α, interleukin (IL)-1β, and IL-6. Antiviral IgM may persist for years, raising the possibility that Sindbis virus arthritis is associated with viral persistence and direct viral effect on the synovium.

Management

Management is supportive.

Mayaro virus

This virus was first recognized in Trinidad in 1954 and has caused epidemics in Bolivia and Brazil. Mayaro virus is transmitted from monkey to man by *Haemogogus* mosquitoes in the South American tropical rain forest. Mayaro virus was responsible for an outbreak in Belterra, Brazil in 1988 with 800 out of 4000 exposed latex gatherers becoming infected. The clinical attack rate was 80%. Illness was characterized by sudden onset of fever, headache, dizziness, chills, and arthralgias in the wrists, fingers, ankles, and toes. About 20% had joint swelling. Unilateral inguinal lymphadenopathy was seen in some patients. Leucopenia was common. Viraemia was present during the first 1–2 days of illness. After 2–5 days, fever resolved but a maculopapular rash on the trunk and extremities appeared. The rash lasted about 3 days. Recovery was usually complete, although some patients had persistent arthralgias at 2 month follow-up.[49]

Cases were detected in 2007–2008 in Manaus, the urban capital of Amazonas state in western Brazil, suggesting that the infection is endemic in the area.[50] Imported cases have been identified in non-endemic areas of Brazil and in the United States and France after travel from the endemic area in the Brazil–Bolivia–Peru inter-border region, and in the Netherlands after travel from Surinam, an area not reported to have Mayaro virus. Of interest, Mayaro virus has been isolated from a bird in Louisiana, raising the spectre of emergence of Mayaro virus in North America.

Other viruses

Apart from specific viral infections noted above in which arthralgia and/or arthritis is typically a prominent feature, there are a host of commonly encountered viral infections in which joint involvement is occasionally seen. Children with varicella have been reported rarely to develop brief monoarticular or pauciatricular arthritis that is thought to be viral in origin; in both children and adults, knee arthritis has been reported. Adults who develop mumps occasionally develop small- or large-joint synovitis lasting up to several weeks. Arthritis may precede or follow parotitis by up to 4 weeks.

Infection with adenovirus and coxsackieviruses A9, B2, B3, B4, and B6 have been associated with recurrent episodes of polyarthritis, pleuritis, myalgia, rash, pharyngitis, myocarditis, and leucocytosis. Epstein–Barr virus associated mononucleosis is frequently accompanied by polyarthralgia, but occasional monoarticular knee arthritis occurs. Polyarthritis, fever, and myalgias due to echovirus 9 infection have been reported in a few cases. Arthritis associated with herpes simplex virus or cytomegalovirus infections are likewise rare. *Herpes hominis* occasionally causes arthritis of the knee known as herpes gladiatorum because it is seen in wrestlers. Vaccinia virus has been associated with non-bacterial postvaccination knee arthritis as a rare complication.

References

1. Gillespie SM, Cartter ML, Asch S et al. Occupational risk of human parvovirus B19 infection for school and day-care personnel during an outbreak of erythema infectiosum. *JAMA* 1990;263:2061–2065.

2. Anderson MJ, Higgins PG, Davis LR et al. Experimental parvoviral infection in humans. *J Infect Dis* 1985;152:257–265.

3. Naides SJ. Parvoviruses. In: Specter S, Hodinka RL, Young SA, Wiedbrauk DL (eds) *Clinical virology manual*, 4th edn. ASM Press, Washington DC, 2009:546–561.

4. Karetnyi YV, Beck PR, Langnas AN, Naides SJ. Human parvovirus B19 infection in acute fulminant liver failure. *Arch Virol* 1999;144:1713–1724.

5. Ager EA, Chin TDY, Poland JD. Epidemic erythema infectiosum. *N Engl J Med* 1966;275:1326–1331.

6. Naides SJ, Scharosch LL, Foto F, Howard EJ. Rheumatologic manifestations of human parvovirus B19 infection in adults. Initial two-year clinical experience. *Arthritis Rheum* 1990;33:1297–1309.

7. Soderlund-Venermo M, Hokynar K, Nieminen J, Rautakorpi H, Hedman K. Persistence of human parvovirus B19 in human tissues. *Pathol Biol (Paris)* 2002;50:307–316.

8. Kurtzman GJ, Cohen B J, Field AM et al. Immune response to B19 parvovirus and an antibody defect in persistent viral infection. *J Clin Invest* 1989;84:1114–1123.

9. Poole BD, Karetnyi YV Naides SJ. Parvovirus B19-induced apoptosis of hepatocytes. *J Virol* 2004;78:7775–7783.

10. Poole BD, Zhou J, Grote A, Schiffenbauer A, Naides SJ. Apoptosis of liver-derived cells induced by parvovirus B19 nonstructural protein. *J Virol* 2006;80:4114–4121.

11. Kivovich V, Gilber, L, Vuento M, Naides SJ. Parvovirus B19 genotype specific amino acid substitution in NS1 reduces the protein's cytotoxicity in culture. *Int J Med Sci* 2010;7:110–119.

12. Poole BD, Kivovich V, Gilbert L, Naides SJ. Parvovirus B19 Nonstructural protein-induced damage of cellular DNA and resultant apoptosis. *Int J Med Sci* 2011;8:88–96.

13. Frey TK. Molecular biology of rubella virus. *Adv Virus Res* 1994;44:69–160.

14. Hobman T C, Chantler JK. Rubella virus. In: Knipe DM, Howley PM, Griffin DE et al (eds) *Field's virology*, 5th edn. Lippincott Williams & Wilkins, Philadelphia, PA, 2007:1069–1100.

15. Ueno Y. Rubella arthritis. An outbreak in Kyoto. *J Rheum* 1994;21:874–876.

16. Geier DA, Geier MR. A one year followup of chronic arthritis following rubella and hepatitis B vaccination based upon analysis of the Vaccine Adverse Events Reporting System (VAERS) database. *Clin Exp Rheumatol* 2002;20:767–771.

17. Schaffner W, Fleet WF, Kilroy AW et al. Polyneuropathy following rubella immunization: a follow-up study and review of the problem. *Am J Dis Child* 1974;127:684–688.

18. Seeger C, Zoulim F, Mason WS. Hepatitis B virus. In: Knipe DM, Howley PM, Griffin DE et al (eds) *Field's virology*, 5th edn. Lippincott Williams & Wilkins, Philadelphia, PA, 2007:2977–3029.

19. Hoofnagle JH. Serologic markers of hepatitis B virus infection. *Annu Rev Med* 1981;32:1–11.

20. Bhandari BN, Wright TL. Hepatitis C: an overview. *Annu Rev Med* 1995;46:309–317.

21. Siegel LB, Cohn L, Nashel D. Rheumatic manifestations of hepatitis C infection. *Semin Arthritis Rheum* 1993;23:149–154.

22. Munoz-Fernandez S, Barbado FJ, Martin Mola E et al. Evidence of hepatitis C virus antibodies in the cryoprecipitate of patients with mixed cryoglobulinemia. *J Rheumatol* 1994;21:229–233.

23. Chevaliez S, Pawlotsky JM. Use of virologic assays in the diagnosis and management of hepatitis C virus infection. *Clin Liver Dis* 2005;9:371–382.

24. Calabrese F, Pontisso P, Pettenazzo E et al. Liver cell apoptosis in chronic hepatitis C correlates with histological but not biochemical activity or serum HCV-RNA levels. *Hepatology* 2000;31:1153–1159.

25. Shimizu YK, Hijikata M, Iwamoto A et al. Neutralizing antibodies against hepatitis C virus and the emergence of neutralization escape mutant viruses. *J Virol* 1994;68:1494–1500.

26. Wundschmann S, Medh J D, Klinzmann D, Schmidt WN, Stapleton JT. Characterization of hepatitis C virus (HCV) and HCV E2 interactions with CD81 and the low-density lipoprotein receptor. *J Virol* 2000;74:10055–10062.

27. Cheng KC, Gupta S, Wang H et al. Current drug discovery strategies for treatment of hepatitis C virus infection. *J Pharmacy Pharmacol* 2011;63:883–892.

28. Kaddu-Mukasa M, Ssekasanvu E, Ddumba E, Thomas D, Katabira ET. Rheumatic manifestations among HIV positive adults attending the Infectious Disease Clinic at Mulago Hospital. *African Health Sci* 2011;11:24–29.

29. Ntsiba H, Ngandeu-Singwé M, Makita-Bagamboula C, Yala F. [Human immunodeficiency virus associated arthritis in Congo Brazzaville]. *Med Mal Infect* 2007;37:758–761.

30. Reveille JD. The changing spectrum of rheumatic disease in human immunodeficiency virus infection. *Semin Arthritis Rheum* 2000;30:147–166.

31. Davis P, Stein M. Human immunodeficiency virus-related connective tissue diseases: a Zimbabwean perspective. *Rheum Dis Clin N Amer* 1991;17:89–97.

32. Cuellar M L, Espinoza L R Rheumatic manifestations of HIV-AIDS. *Bailliere's Best Prac Res Clin Rheum* 2000;14:579–593.

33. Nishioka K, Nakajima T, Hasunuma T, Sato K. Rheumatic manifestation of human leukemia virus infection. *Rheum Dis Clin N Amer* 1993;19:489–503.

34. Hida A, Imaizumi M, Sera N et al. Association of human T lymphotropic virus type I with Sjogren syndrome. *Ann Rheum Dis* 2010;69:2056–2057.

35. Griffin DE. Alphaviruses. In Knipe DM, Howley PM, Griffin DE et al. (eds) *Field's virology*, 5th edn. Lippincott Williams & Wilkins, Philadelphia, PA, 2007:1023–1067.

36. Moro ML, Gagliotti C, Silvi G et al. Chikungunya virus in North-Eastern Italy: a seroprevalence survey. *Am J Trop Med Hyg* 2010;82:508–511.

37. Halstead SB, Udomsakdi S, Singharaj P, Nisalak A. Dengue and chikungunya virus infection in man in Thailand:1962–1964. III. Clinical, epidemiologic, and virologic observations on disease in non-indigenous white persons. *Am J Trop Med Hyg* 1969;18:984–996.

38. Hasebe F, Parquet MC, Pandy BD et al. Combined detection and genotyping of Chikungunya virus by a specific reverse transcription-polymerase chain reaction. *J Med Virol* 2002;67:370–374.

39. Sanders EJ, Rwaguma EB, Kawamata J et al. O'nyong-nyong fever in south-central Uganda:1996–1997: description of the epidemic and results of a household-based seroprevalence survey. *J Infect Dis* 1999;180:1436–1443.

40. Kiwanuka N, Sanders EJ, Rwaguma EB et al. O'nyong-nyong fever in south-central Uganda:1996–1997: clinical features and validation of a clinical case definition for surveillance purposes. *Clin Infect Dis* 1999;29:1243–1250.

41. Olaleye OD, Omilabu SA, Baba SS Growth of Igbo-Ora virus in some tissue cultures. *Acta Virol* 1990;34:367–371.

42. Boughton CR, Hawkes RA, Naim HM, Wild J, Chapman B. Arbovirus infections in humans in New South Wales. Seroepidemiology of the alphavirus group of togaviruses. *Med J Aust* 1984;141:700–704.

43. Kelly-Hope LA, Kay BH, Purdies DM, Williams GM. The risk of Ross River and Barmah Forest virus disease in Queensland: implications for New Zealand. *Aust N Z J Public Health* 2002;26:69–77.

44. Fraser JR, Ratnamohan VM, Dowling JP, Becker GJ, Varigos GA. The exanthem of Ross River virus infection: histology, location of virus antigen and nature of inflammatory infiltrate. *J Clin Pathol* 1983;36:1256–1263.

45. Fraser JRE. Epidemic polyarthritis and Ross River virus disease. *Clin Rheum Dis* 1986;12:369–388.

46. Mylonas AD, Harley D, Purdie DM et al. Corticosteroid therapy in an alphaviral arthritis. *J Clin Rheumatol* 2004;10:326–330.

47. Quinn HE, Gatton ML, Hall G, Young M, Ryan PA. Analysis of Barmah Forest virus disease activity in Queensland, Australia:1993–2003: identification of a large, isolated outbreak of disease. *J Med Entomol* 2005;42:882–890.

48. Kurkela S, Helve T, Vaheri A, Vapalahti O. Arthritis and arthralgia three years after Sindbis virus infection: clinical follow-up of a cohort of 49 patients. *Scand J Infect Dis* 2008;40:167–173.

49. Pinheiro FP, Freitas RB, Travassos da Rosa JF et al. An outbreak of Mayaro virus disease in Belterra, Brazil. I. Clinical and virological findings. *Am J Trop Med Hyg* 1981;30:674–681..

50. Mourão MP, Bastos MD, de Figueiredo RP et al. Mayaro fever in the city of Manaus, Brazil: 2007–2008. *Vector Borne Zoonotic Dis* 2011;12:42–46.

CHAPTER 103

Mycobacterial diseases

Rita Abdulkader and Richard A. Watts

Introduction

Tuberculosis (TB) and leprosy are the main diseases caused by mycobacteria. Their manifestations result from chronic granulomatous infections caused by *M. tuberculosis* and *M. leprae*. These are obligate intracellular aerobic acid fast bacilli. Atypical mycobacteria such as *M. avium-intracellulare* and *M. marinum* are uncommon causes of musculoskeletal infection.

Tuberculosis

Epidemiology

The World Health Organization (WHO) reported 8.8 million new cases of tuberculosis in 2010.[1] Despite a fall in the number of reported cases, TB still poses a significant health challenge globally. Efforts to control the disease are hampered by the prevalence of HIV infection, and the emergence of multidrug resistant (MDR) and extremely drug resistant (XDR) TB.[2] Extrapulmonary TB including musculoskeletal infection is commoner in immunocompromised patients. These patients are also at a higher risk of developing MDR TB.[2] Musculoskeletal infection accounts for 1–3% of all TB infections; it can occur at any age, but it is rare in infancy.[3]

Transmission of the pathogen in the majority of cases is from a human host with active pulmonary disease via droplets. Host factors largely determine the course of the infection. The risk is increased in immunocompromised individuals, through HIV coinfection or medication. Malnutrition, substance abuse, and the presence of chronic disease are also associated with increased risk.[2] After reaching the pulmonary alveoli, the bacilli are phagocytosed by macrophages where they multiply. The resulting inflammatory response leads to the formation of granulomata typical of tuberculosis, consisting of a necrotic caseating centre, multinucleated giant cells, epitheloid cells, and peripheral lymphocytes. The primary infection is symptomatic in only one-third of patients.[2] Cell-mediated immune response is important in containing the infection, and this occurs in most cases. Afterwards, the bacilli remain dormant within the macrophages for many years. During this time the patient is completely asymptomatic and non-infectious. The tuberculin skin test is usually positive. This is recognised as latent TB. Reactivation of latent TB is responsible for 90% of active TB cases in adults. Active TB will develop in 10% of immunocompetent individuals with latent TB during their lifetime, most commonly within the first 2 years of the infection.[2]

Clinical manifestations

Early diagnosis and treatment of musculoskeletal TB is an important factor in reducing long-term damage and possible disability. However, this is usually challenging and a high index of suspicion is required to establish the diagnosis early. The infection usually develops after haematogenous dissemination of the bacilli; however, transmission via lymphatic vessels, local reactivation of latent microorganisms, or less commonly direct invasion from an adjacent site may also occur.[4,5] The course of the disease is usually indolent over weeks to months. Delay in diagnosis for several months is common. Systemic symptoms of fever, weight loss, malaise, and night sweats may point to the diagnosis, although they are frequently absent.[6] Active pulmonary disease is present in less than 50% of cases.[3]

The most common site of infection is the spine in about 50% of cases. Extraspinal TB usually manifests as monarthritis in a large weight bearing joint. Osteomyelitis and soft tissue infection including myositis, bursitis, and tenosynovitis are rarer. Poncet's disease, a reactive arthritis to *M. tuberculosis* infection, is occasionally reported, but its occurrence as an entity is debatable.

Spinal tuberculosis (Pott's disease)

The lower thoracic and upper lumbar spine is most commonly affected. The infection usually begins at the anterior aspect of the vertebra, adjacent to the superior or inferior endplates. It can directly spread across the subchondral plate to the adjacent disc or track beneath the longitudinal anterior and posterior ligaments sparing the disc.[7] With progression of the infection, the vertebral body collapses and anterior wedging occurs. Gibbus formation and vertebral instability may ensue. The slow progression of intervertebral disc involvement helps differentiate spinal tuberculosis from pyogenic infections in adults.[8] The posterior elements are affected in TB, and this distinguishes TB from other bacterial infections[5]; however, it raises the possibility of metastatic malignancy (Figure 103.1).[3] The typical appearance is of two adjacent vertebrae affected with disc destruction and paravertebral abscess. Single vertebral or skip lesions are less frequent (Figure 103.2).[4] After healing, vertebral ankylosis occurs.

The most common symptom is pain, which is usually worse at night, waking the patient up from sleep. Patients may present after vertebral collapse with kyphosis, or with neurological complications. A paravertebral collection can track along fascial planes and discharge in distant locations. In the lumbar spine, cold abscesses can involve the iliopsoas muscle, tracking along its sheath to the groin or thigh.[3] In the thoracic spine they can track along the ribs to the anterior chest wall. In the neck, a retropharyngeal abscess may develop and cause compressive symptoms with hoarseness,

dysphagia, and stridor. Neurological symptoms may result from local oedema and vascular congestion, from direct compression due to vertebral collapse, or from posterior extension of a cold abscess. Less commonly intramedullary tuberculoma have been implicated and very rarely spinal vascular thrombosis and infarction can occur.[9,10] Symptoms vary from difficulty in walking, or radicular pain, to a more severe picture of cauda equina syndrome, paraplegia, or quadriplegia. Tuberculosis can involve the atlanto-axial articulation, resulting in instability. Neurological involvement at this level can cause irreversible quadriplegia. Even after healing, neurological complications can occur as a result of spinal stenosis, gibbus formation, or peridural fibrosis.[9] A shorter duration of symptoms and slow progression indicate a better diagnosis when neurological symptoms occur. The presence of paraplegia, flaccid paralysis, myelomalacia, or a syrinx on MRI carries a worse prognosis.[9]

Tuberculous arthritis

Tuberculous arthritis occurs in 30% of cases of musculoskeletal TB.[8] It is most commonly monoarticular, affecting weightbearing joints. Sacroiliac, shoulder, elbow, and ankle joints may also be affected.[11] Multifocal disease is encountered in 10% of cases.[8]

Symptoms include pain, stiffness, effusion, and synovial thickening with minimal inflammation. Compared to pyogenic infections, cartilage loss occurs late in the disease.[11] Rice bodies may form with longstanding disease. Sinuses may be complicated by secondary infection. Eventually, joint deformity and fibrous ankylosis develop (Figure 103.3).

Tubercular osteomyelitis

This is a rare form of skeletal TB. The commonest sites affected include the tibia, femur and short bones in the hands and feet.[3] Multifocal disease may be encountered in immunocompromised

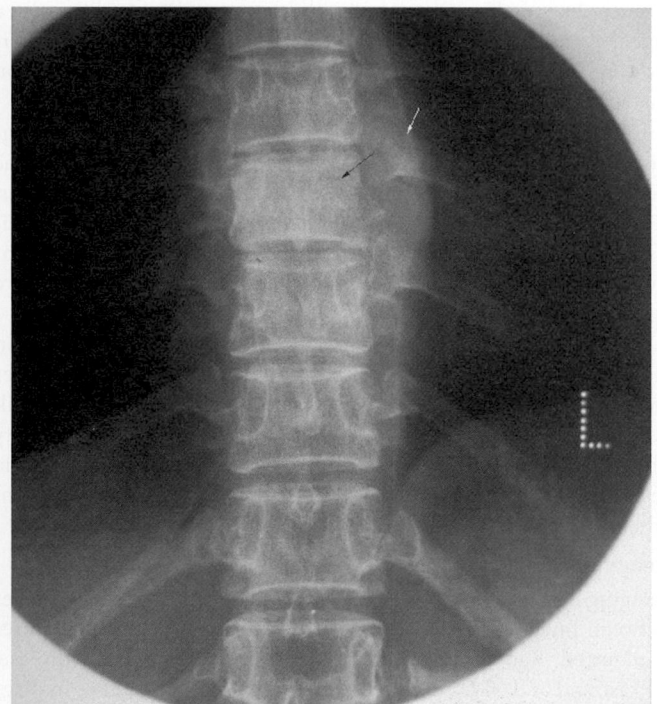

Fig. 103.1 Thoracic spine radiograph showing destruction of the left pedicle of T8 (black arrow) with associated paravertebral soft tissue mass (white arrow). Disc spaces are preserved. The differential diagnosis also includes malignancy.

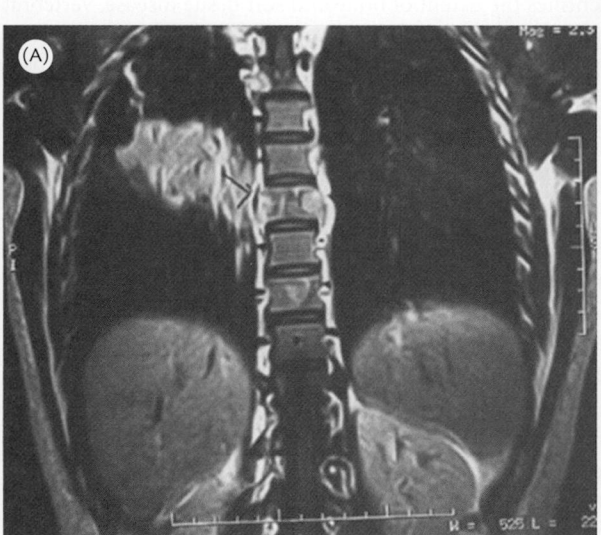

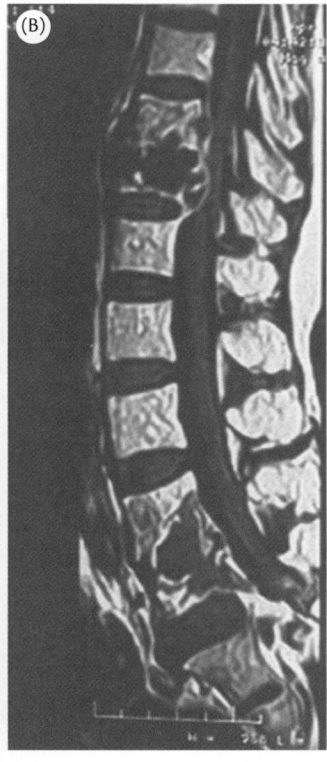

Fig. 103.2 MRI of an adolescent girl showing a tuberculous focus of infection at the mid-dorsal level together with a pulmonary lesion.

Fairbank, J. Oxford Textbook of Trauma and Orthopaedics

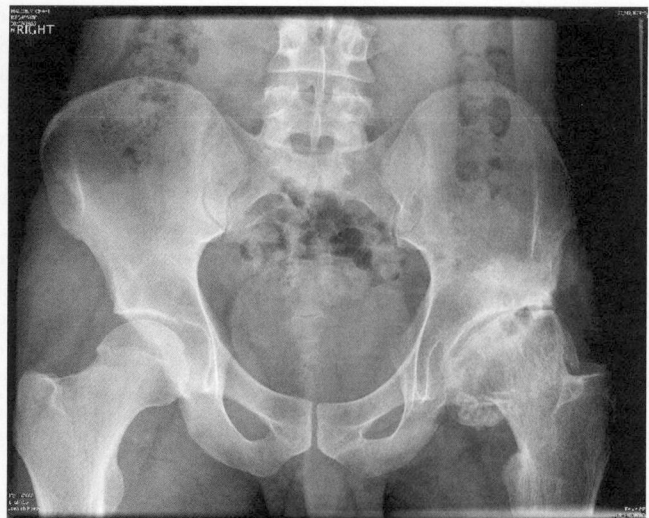

Fig. 103.3 Tuberculosis of the left hip with narrowing of the joint space, lateral erosive changes, and secondary marginal osteophytes. The femoral head is expanded and flattened.

patients.[11] The infection usually affects the metaphysis of the long bones, and may spread to the adjacent joint. In children, extension across the growth plate is characteristic of TB.[3,9] Clinical features include mild pain, tenderness, soft tissue swelling, and sinus formation. Pathological fractures may occur.

A less common type is cystic TB, which may be multifocal, and is most commonly encountered in the lower limbs in children. In adults it tends to affect the axial skeleton.[3]

Dactylitis is usually painless, affecting children under 6 years of age in 85% of cases. It can be difficult to differentiate from chronic osteomyelitis.[8]

Investigations and diagnosis

The diagnosis of musculoskeletal TB relies on a combination of clinical, radiological, histological, and microbiological features. No one test rules out the diagnosis. In areas where TB is endemic, treatment should be initiated if the clinical picture and radiological features are suggestive of the diagnosis.[9]

Laboratory tests

Inflammatory markers are usually raised, with evidence of anaemia and lymphocytosis. In 10% of patients both the white blood cell count (WBC) and erythrocyte sedimentation rate (ESR) are normal.[5] Testing for HIV should be considered.

The tuberculin skin test is positive in most cases. However, its usefulness is limited in endemic areas and it is not specific to *M. tuberculosis*; false-positive results are encountered with previous BCG vaccination. A negative test does not rule out *M. tuberculosis* especially in immunocompromised individuals.

Interferon-gamma release assays (IGRA) may support the diagnosis. They are performed on whole blood or mononuclear cells to detect the presence of T cells previously sensitized to *M. tuberculosis* through release of interferon-gamma. As they use proteins specific to *M. tuberculosis*, previous BCG vaccine does not affect the result of IGRAs. However, they are unable to differentiate active from latent TB. A negative test does not rule out active TB. Serological tests for antibodies to *M. tuberculosis* are

not recommended in routine practice due to discrepancies in their sensitivity and specificity.

Tissue or fluid samples for microbiological and histological confirmation can be obtained through open biopsy or using imaging guidance. Samples should be stained for acid-fast bacilli (AFB) using Ziehl–Neelsen or auramine fluorescent stain, which provide a quick diagnostic method, but with low sensitivity. Additionally, a smear does not differentiate atypical mycobacteria from *M. tuberculosis*. The identification of typical necrotizing granulomata on histopathological examination strongly suggests the diagnosis.

Culture from an aspirate or biopsy is the gold standard for diagnosis. It is important to avoid culturing fistula fluid because of the presence of secondary infections, which may confuse the diagnosis. Culture is time consuming but it allows assessment of drug sensitivity. Liquid-based media culture give quicker results than conventional solid-based media. With the use of automated liquid culture systems, positive results may be obtained within 2 weeks.[6,7]

Nucleic acid amplification using polymerase chain reaction (PCR) techniques is more sensitive than AFB staining, and quicker than cultures. Experience in using this method in skeletal TB is still accumulating. Reports suggest a sensitivity of 78% and specificity of 100%.[10] This technique detects the presence of the mycobacteria regardless of their activity, and this should be taken into account when interpreting the results.

Imaging studies

Imaging may aid the diagnosis. The sensitivity and specificity varies between imaging techniques and correlation with clinical pictures is required. Radiographs have low sensitivity early in the disease. Ultrasound and MRI scan are the main imaging modalities in diagnosis and assessment of bursitis, myositis, and tenosynovitis. Isotope bone scintigraphy can help in localizing the infection, but false-negative results were reported in 35% of cases of spinal disease.[3]

Spine

Plain radiographic changes require 3–5 months to develop with destruction of about 50% of trabecular bone occurring before changes are detected.[8] Disc space narrowing and demineralization of endplates occur. Erosions without reactive sclerosis are characteristic of TB infection. Scalloping of the vertebra results from the presence of a paraspinal abscess.[3] Asymmetry of the psoas shadow may be seen.[9] Later, wedge fracture develops.

CT identifies the extent of bone and soft tissue disease, vertebral fragmentation (exploded vertebra appearance),[8] and the presence of paraspinal abscesses. The presence of calcification within a paraspinal abscess is characteristic of TB infection.[5]

MRI is the modality of choice, with a sensitivity of 100% and specificity of 88%.[7] MRI detects early bone marrow oedema, disc involvement, and endplate changes. Relative preservation of the intervertebral disc (floating disc), disruption of the endplate, and the presence of paravertebral soft tissue are features with high sensitivity and specificity.[7] It is also useful in the assessment of soft tissue disease (cold abscesses, horseshoe appearance), and the cause and extent of neurological involvement.

Tuberculous arthritis

The features on plain radiography are usually non-specific. The Phemister triad is a combination of juxtaarticular osteopenia, peripheral osseous erosions, and gradual loss of joint space, and is suggestive of TB arthritis.[11] Osteolytic lesions and cartilage loose bodies occur as the disease progresses. Occasionally wedge-shaped areas of necrosis are present on both sides of the joint (kissing sequestra).[11] MRI is the modality of choice for early diagnosis. The synovial membrane typically is hypointense on T2-weighted images and enhanced with gadolinium.[8]

Osteomyelitis

Osteopenia and osteolytic lesions with little or no periosteal reaction are demonstrated on plain radiography.[3] Multiple oval lesions are observed in the cystic form.[11] In dactylitis, cystic expansion of the bone with coarse trabecular pattern and periosteal reaction occur, this appearance is termed spina ventosa.[8] MRI scan allows a detailed assessment including sinus tracts and abscesses.

Treatment

The mainstay of treatment is chemotherapy. Surgery plays a supportive role in selected cases. Anti-tuberculosis drugs have excellent tissue penetration in bone and joint, and chemotherapy is effective in 90% of cases. Compliance is important to avoid developing drug resistance.[9]

The first-line drugs used in treatment of TB are isoniazid, rifampicin, ethambutol, and pyrazinamide. Treatment regimens usually consist of two phases, an initial phase and a continuation phase. Treatment should include isoniazid and rifampicin throughout, in addition to ethambutol and pyrazinamide for the initial 2 months. Daily regimens are recommended.

Monitoring for side effects is important. Baseline full blood count, kidney function, and liver function should be obtained. Liver function should be monitored in the presence of pre-existing liver disease or significant risk factors. Visual acuity and green–red discrimination should be monitored with ethambutol.[12,13] The physician should be alert to possible interactions, especially between rifampicin and HIV treatment.[13] Treatment should be continued for 6–9 months in extraspinal TB.[2,12,13] The length of treatment in spinal disease is controversial. The Medical Research Council trials suggested that uncomplicated spinal TB can be treated successfully with multidrug regimens for 6 months. However, many argue that treatment should be at least for 9 months to reduce relapse rates. In complicated cases 12–18 months treatment may be required.[7,9] MDR TB (resistance to isoniazid and rifampicin) is suspected when improvement is delayed, with continuous bony destruction or the appearance of new lesions after 3–5 months of treatment.[7] Every effort should be then made to ascertain sensitivity. Treatment is with 4–6 drugs for at least 24 months in spinal disease.[7] Surgery may play a role in these patients.

Surgical treatment is usually reserved for resistant disease and complications. In spinal disease, intervention should be considered with the development or worsening of neurologic deficit. Other indications for surgery include panvertebral disease, spinal instability, or significant kyphosis.[7] In joint disease osteotomy, arthrodesis, and joint replacement may be indicated.[9]

Tumour necrosis factor inhibitors and tuberculosis

The introduction of tumour necrosis factor (TNF) inhibitors for the treatment of rheumatoid arthritis (RA) is associated with an increased rate of latent TB reactivation. The risk is three- to fourfold higher with infliximab and adalimumab compared to etanercept. There is an increased incidence of extrapulmonary and disseminated TB.[14,15]

Patients starting treatment with TNF inhibitors should be monitored closely for signs of TB reactivation, especially within the first year. Reactivation may occur after cessation of treatment, and monitoring should continue for at least 6 months afterwards.

All patients should be screened for the presence of latent TB before initiating TNF inhibitors. Identification of risk factors, history of previous exposure or infection, and a chest radiograph are mandatory. Tuberculin skin test is even less reliable in patients on immunosuppressive treatment, and false-negative rates are more frequent. IGRAs are more sensitive in these patients, and are recommended. If TNF inhibitors are indicated in cases of previous exposure, infection, or evidence of latent or active TB, they should be managed in close liaison with a TB specialist.

Atypical mycobacterial skeletal infection

Skeletal infections with atypical mycobacteria occur mainly through direct inoculation after trauma, surgical intervention, or intraarticular corticosteroid injections. Haematogenous dissemination with multifocal disease is encountered in immunocompromised patients.[4] Unlike *M. tuberculosis*, atypical mycobacteria are present in the soil and water and are not obligate parasites.[4] Synovitis and tenosynovitis are most commonly caused by *M. avium-intracellulare*, *M. haemophilum*, and *M. marinum*. Joint disease was also reported less commonly with *M. fortuitum*, *M. abscessus*, *M. chelonae*, and *M. kansasii*. Osteomyelitis has been reported particularly following surgical procedures. These microorganisms are usually resistant to conventional anti-tuberculosis drugs. Multidrug regimens containing azithromycin, clarithromycin, fluroquinolones, or aminoglycosides may be used depending on the sensitivity of the mycobacteria. Rifampicin is also used in *M. avium-intracellulare* and *M. haemophilum* infections. *M. kansasii* responds to treatment with isoniazid, ethambutol, and rifampicin. Prolonged durations of treatment in addition to surgical excision and debridement are usually required.[16]

Leprosy (Hansen's disease)

Epidemiology

In 2010, 228 474 new cases of leprosy were reported to WHO from 130 countries around the world.[17] The prevalence of leprosy has been falling over the last decade, but it is still the leading infectious cause of disability worldwide. At the time of diagnosis, nerve damage is already present in one-third of cases.[18] Leprosy can affect people of any age, but it is extremely rare in those younger than 1 year old. In adults lepromatous leprosy is commoner in males, with a male to female ratio of 2:1. In children tuberculoid leprosy is usual.[19] HIV infection does not increase the risk of infection and is not associated with more severe manifestations or treatment resistance.[20]

Pathogenesis

Leprosy is mainly caused by *M. leprae*. A newly identified mycobacterium, *M. lepromatosis*, may also cause lepromatous leprosy. Humans are the main reservoir of the pathogen. The mode of transmission is not well established, but is most likely through respiratory droplets from person to person. The possibility of transmission from animals was suggested with the identification of a strain of *M. leprae* in the southern United States, which infects both wild armadillos and humans.

Most individuals exposed to leprosy do not develop the infection. The risk increases in close household contacts, especially with increased bacterial load.[18] Genetic factors play a role in the susceptibility to the infection and the clinical expression of the disease.[19]

The interaction between *M. leprae* and the immune system of the host accounts for the variation in clinical manifestations of leprosy. In tuberculoid leprosy, evidence of specific cell-mediated response is present, with formation of organized granulomata with predominance of CD4+ T cells and a positive lepromin skin test. In lepromatous leprosy, there is evidence of a humoral but not cell-mediated response to *M. leprae*. Granulomata are absent in the lesions with preponderance of CD8+ T cells and the skin test is negative.[19,20]

Clinical features

M. leprae has a predilection for Schwann cells and macrophages. The incubation period varies from only few months to decades. The disease progresses slowly, mainly affecting the skin and peripheral nerves.

In tuberculoid leprosy, there are few asymmetrical macules with low numbers of bacilli. These macules are usually well defined, dry, and hypopigmented with reduced sensation. Neuropathy is asymmetrical with thickening of the involved nerve and early loss of sensory and motor function. The ulnar and common peroneal nerves are most commonly affected. In lepromatous leprosy, macules, nodules, papules or plaques may occur. They are numerous and symmetrical. High bacterial load exists in nasal secretions and skin lesions. Saddlenose deformity from septal perforation, keratitis, iridocyclitis, and testicular scarring and atrophy occur. Symmetrical peripheral neuropathy develops gradually, later in the disease. Intermediate forms of the disease exist in between these two polar types.

Leprosy reactions are episodes of acute inflammation, which interrupt the course of the chronic disease, possibly resulting in major nerve damage. Concurrent infection, pregnancy, and physical and emotional stress are some of the predisposing events. Reactions may occur after initiation or completion of treatment.[18] There are two types of leprosy reactions:

◆ **Type 1 reactions** are cell-mediated immune reactions. They occur in borderline forms of leprosy resulting in neuritis, formation of new skin lesions, and inflammation of existing ones. They may occur after treatment initiation (reversal reaction) or in the context of worsening immunity (downgrading).

◆ **Type 2 reactions** (erythema nodosum leprosum) are immune complex mediated. They occur in multibacillary disease, usually within 2 years after starting treatment, and present with systemic symptoms, fever, tender nodules, arthritis, eye symptoms, and neuritis.[18,19,21]

Skeletal involvement in leprosy occurs as a consequence of peripheral neuropathy. Neuropathic arthropathy results in joint destruction in weightbearing joints, hands, and feet. Ulcers and secondary infections complicate the picture. A 'licked candy stick' appearance on plain radiographs occurs from tapering osteolysis. Resorption of digits and toes may occur. Polyarticular inflammatory arthritis occurs during leprosy reactions. It is usually short lived, mainly affecting hands and feet. A chronic inflammatory arthritis mimicking rheumatoid arthritis, sacroiliitis, and tenosynovitis have also been reported.[21]

M. leprae osteomyelitis is rare; it usually results from direct extension of the infection from the overlying skin. Haematogenous spread is less common.

Classification of leprosy

The Ridley and Jopling classification identifies five forms according to the clinical and histopathological features: two polar forms, tuberculoid (TT) and lepromatous leprosy (LL), and three intermediate forms, borderline tuberculoid (BT), mid-borderline (BB), and borderline lepromatous (BL). Classification systems proposed by WHO rely either on skin smear results or the number of skin lesions. In paucibacillary disease, skin smears are negative at all sites. The presence of positive smears at any site indicates multibacillary leprosy. Classification according to the number of skin lesions is used to determine the treatment regimen:

◆ **paucibacillary leprosy**: five or fewer skin lesions

◆ **multibacillary leprosy**: six or more skin lesions.

Investigations

A clinical diagnosis of leprosy can be made in the presence of one of the following features:

◆ the presence of a skin lesion consistent with leprosy, with definite loss of sensation, with or without nerve thickening

◆ positive skin smears or tissue biopsy.

Identification of the pathogen on microscopy in slit-skin smears, usually taken from a peripheral site (earlobes), nasal smears, tissue biopsies, or synovial fluid is the gold standard for diagnosis but sensitivity is low in paucibacillary disease. Culture of *M. leprae* is not used in routine practice, as the organism can only be cultured in murine footpads and armadillos and not *in vitro*. Several months are required for positive results. The detection of antiphenolic glycolipid-1 antibodies (PG-1) may assist the diagnosis. They are positive in 90% of LL, and 40 to 50% of paucibacillary disease.[21] *M. leprae* identification using PCR is a sensitive tool but is not routinely used in clinical practice. The lepromin test is positive in tuberculoid leprosy, indicating the presence of cell-mediated immunity.

Treatment

Multidrug treatment should be used to avoid the emergence of drug resistance. Reconstructive surgery may improve the functional outcome and reduce residual disability.

The regimen recommended by WHO includes dapsone 100 mg/day and rifampicin 600 mg once a month for 6 months in paucibacillary disease. In multibacillary disease, clofazimine 300 mg once a month and 50 mg/day is added to this regimen; treatment should continue for a year. A single skin lesion is treated with one dose of rifampicin 600 mg with ofloxacin 400 mg, and minocycline 100 mg.

The treatment of leprosy reactions aims to control symptoms and reduce nerve damage. Symptomatic treatment may suffice in mild cases. Relapse occurs frequently and monitoring is required.[18] Type1 reaction is treated with high-dose oral steroids, reduced every 2–4 weeks for 4–6 months.[19] In severe or recurrent type 2 reactions, high-dose corticosteroid is usually needed for 3 months. Clofazimine is used if the response is unsatisfactory or there are significant side effects with corticosteroids. Pentoxifylline can also be used in these cases. Thalidomide is effective especially in reducing recurrence, however, it is not recommended by WHO because of the risk of malformations associated with its use in pregnancy.

Patient on anti-leprosy drugs should not stop their treatment during reactions.

References

1. WHO. *Global tuberculosis control 2011*. World Health Organization, Geneva. Available at: www.who.int/tb/publications/global_report/2011/gtbr11_full.pdf

2. Sia IG, Wieland ML. Current concepts in the management of tuberculosis. *Mayo Clin Proc* 2011;86(4):348–361.

3. Burrill J, Williams CJ, Bain G et al. Tuberculosis: a radiologic review. *Radiographics* 2007;27(5):1255–1273.

4. Gardam M, Lim S. Mycobacterial osteomyelitis and arthritis. *Infect Dis Clin North Am* 2005;19(4):819–830

5. De Backer AI, Mortelé KJ, Vanschoubroeck IJ et al. Tuberculosis of the spine: CT and MR imaging features. *JBR-BTR* 2005;88(2):92–97.

6. Agrawal V, Patgaonkar PR, Nagariya SP. Tuberculosis of spine. *J Craniovertebr Junction Spine* 2010;1(2):74–85.

7. Jain AK. Tuberculosis of the spine: a fresh look at an old disease. *J Bone Joint Surg Br* 2010;92(7):905–913.

8. Andronikou S, Bindapersad M, Govender N et al. Musculoskeletal tuberculosis—imaging using low-end and advanced modalities for developing and developed countries. *Acta Radiol* 2011;52(4):430–441.

9. Spiegel D, Singh G; Banskota A. Tuberculosis of the musculoskeletal system. *Techn Orthopaed* 2005;20(2):167–178.

10. Franco-Paredes C, Díaz-Borjon A, Senger MA, Barragan L, Leonard M. The ever-expanding association between rheumatologic diseases and tuberculosis. *Am J Med* 2006;119(6):470–477.

11. De Backer AI, Vanhoenacker FM, Sanghvi DA. Imaging features of extraaxial musculoskeletal tuberculosis. *Indian J Radiol Imaging* 2009;19(3):176–186.

12. Joint Tuberculosis Committee of the British Thoracic Society. Chemotherapy and management of tuberculosis in the United Kingdom: recommendations 1998. *Thorax* 1998;53(7):536–548.

13. Blumberg H, Burman W, Chaisson R et al. American Thoracic Society/Centers for Disease Control and Prevention/Infectious Diseases Society of America: treatment of tuberculosis. *Am J Respir Crit Care Med* 2003;167:603–662.

14. Ledingham J, Deighton C; the British Society for Rheumatology Standards, Guidelines and Audit Working Group (SGAWG). Update on the British Society for Rheumatology guidelines for prescribing TNFa blockers in adults with rheumatoid arthritis. *Rheumatology* 2005;44:157–163

15. Dixon W, Hyrich K, Watson K, Lunt M et al. BSR BR Control Centre Consortium, Drug-specific risk of tuberculosis in patients with rheumatoid arthritis treated with anti-TNF therapy: Results from the British Society for Rheumatology Biologics Register (BSRBR). *Ann Rheum Dis* 2010;69:522–528.

16. Griffith DE, Aksamit T, Brown-Elliott BA et al.; ATS Mycobacterial Diseases Subcommittee; American Thoracic Society; Infectious Disease Society of America. An official ATS/IDSA statement: diagnosis, treatment, and prevention of nontuberculous mycobacterial diseases. *Am J Respir Crit Care Med* 2007;175(4):367–416.

17. WHO. Leprosy update. *Wkly Epidemiol Rec* 2011;86(36):389–399. Available at: www.who.int/wer/2011/wer8636.pdf

18. Rodrigues LC, Lockwood DNJ. Leprosy now: epidemiology, progress, challenges, and research gaps. *Lancet Infect Dis* 2011;11(6):464–470.

19. Pinheiro RO, de Souza Salles J, Sarno EN, Sampaio EP. Mycobacterium leprae-host-cell interactions and genetic determinants in leprosy: an overview. *Future Microbiol* 2011;6(2):217–230.

20. Lockwood DN, Lambert SM. Human immunodeficiency virus and leprosy: an update. *Dermatol Clin* 2011;29(1):125–128

21. Chauhan S, Wakhlu A, Agarwal V. Arthritis in leprosy. *Rheumatology* 2010;49(12):2237–2242.

CHAPTER 104

Brucellar arthritis

Esperanza Merino and Eliseo Pascual

Introduction

Infection of the joints is the most frequent local complication of brucellosis, and a common cause of infectious arthritis in countries where the disease is endemic.

Epidemiology

Brucellosis is a worldwide zoonosis that has affected humans for at least 2000 years[1] and has managed to elude eradication even in most developed countries. Renewed scientific interest has been fuelled by its recent re-emergence and enhanced surveillance in many areas of the world.[2] More than 500 000 new cases occur annually, but it is estimated that the number of brucella-infected individuals may be up to 26 times higher, because brucellosis remains underdiagnosed and under-reported.[2]

The disease is prevalent in countries of the Mediterranean basin, the Near East, South America, and possibly sub-Saharan Africa. The epidemiology has now changed significantly because several areas traditionally considered to be endemic have achieved control of the disease.

In northern Europe the disease is considered to have been eradicated. In southern countries its incidence has reduced greatly, although small areas remains endemic in the south of Spain, Italy, and around Portugal. However, in many Asian republics of the former Soviet Union, the Balkan peninsula, and Turkey it remains a major public health problem. In the United States cases of brucellosis occur mostly in California and Texas due to ingestion of unpasteurized products or related to travel to endemic areas in Mexico. Most areas of Latin America have achieved control of the disease but in Mexico, Argentina, and Peru the disease remains endemic. Nowadays infection is acquired during foreign travel or from consumption of infected marketed dairy products, mainly in immigrant populations.

In endemic countries brucellosis is more prevalent in the 15–35 year age group,[3] but in Western countries the age-specific incidence was highest in persons 60–69 years of age, mainly first-generation immigrants who keep closer contact with their homelands.[4] Male predominance is observed only in the working age group and in countries where brucellosis is related to occupational exposure.

Brucellosis occurs naturally in domesticated animals, and its transmission to humans most often occurs through consumption of infected, unpasteurized dairy products (especially raw milk, soft cheese, butter, and ice cream), direct contact and care of infected animals (sheep, cattle, goats, pigs), or inhalation of their secretions.[5] Patients often recall possibly infected animals or their unpasteurized products, but this evidence may be missing. The disease can be accidentally acquired by laboratory personnel.[6] Rare human-to-human transmission has been reported.

General characteristics of the organism

Brucella species are small, non-motile facultative intracellular aerobic rods that can multiply within phagocytic cells with humans as end hosts. Gram staining demonstrates single, tiny, Gram-negative coccobacilli. Brucella species can survive up 2 days in milk at 8 °C, up to 3 weeks in frozen meat, and up to 3 months in goat cheese. They remain viable in animal excretions for more than 40 days, but are sensitive to heat, disinfectants, and pasteurization. Brucella are slow growing and require specific culture conditions, including prolonged incubation (as long as 30 days in some media).

There are six brucella species, four of which are recognized human zoonoses: *Brucella melitensis*, *B. abortus*, *B. suis*, and *B. canis*. The majority of human cases worldwide are attributed to *B. melitensis* and in general, *B. melitensis* and *B. suis* are more virulent for humans than *B. abortus* or B. *canis*.[5] The complete sequencing of the *B. melitensis*, *B. abortus*, and *B. suis* genomes was achieved in 2001–2.[7]

After infection, brucella are readily ingested by polymorphonuclear leucocytes and macrophages, reaching local lymph nodes; the organisms replicate intracellularly and bacteria from lysed cells can infect other cells or disseminate systemically. A majority of brucella are rapidly eliminated by phagolysosomal fusion, but 15–30% survive.[6,8,9] During the intracellular stage, brucella display a range of survival strategies to suppress host immune response: they can inactivate the innate immune system, withstand the direct action of complement and other bactericidal substances, and evade the action of polymorphonuclear cells and macrophages. Brucella can establish long-lasting infection within host cells, and they promote the chronicity of infection. Cell-mediated immunity appears to be the principal mechanism of recovery and partial resistance to subsequent reinfection. Interferon-gamma activates the bactericidal function in macrophages to hamper the intracellular survival of brucella, then cytotoxicity of CD8 and gamma-delta T cells destroys the infected macrophages and finally Th1-type antibodies opsonize the pathogen to facilitate phagocytosis.[10] Antibody response, although important for diagnostic purposes, appears to play a minor role in the immune response to the infection.

In humans, brucella infection results in the formation of non-caseating sarcoidosis-like granulomas, consisting of epithelioid cells, polymorphonuclear leucocytes, lymphocytes, and some giant cells. The granulomatous response is typical of *B. abortus*, the granulomas produced by *B. melitensis* are very small, and *B. suis* infection is accompanied by chronic abscess formation.[11]

General characteristics of the disease

Human brucellosis is a systemic infection that may present with a broad spectrum of clinical manifestations and its complications can affect almost all organs and systems. The manifestations of the disease are non-specific, and no combination of signs or symptoms can be considered as characteristic.[12] The bulk of human disease is caused by *B. melitensis* and *B. abortus* and their clinical presentation is similar, although comparative studies are few. The incubation period after contact is usually 1–4 weeks although it may be as long as several months; localized disease may present after an asymptomatic/paucisymptomatic undiagnosed acute phase.[6,13] Epidemiological data suggest that brucellosis occurs in 40–50% of contacts.[3] The term 'chronic brucellosis' was coined in the preantibiotic era, referring to patients with persistent symptoms of disease after treatment of brucellosis, but in the majority a bacteriologically proven relapse or localized disease can be diagnosed.

Insidious onset of fever is almost universal with night sweats (with a peculiar, mouldy odour) followed in 40–50% by arthralgias, myalgias, and low back pain or arthritis.[14] Constitutional symptoms—weight loss, weakness fatigue, malaise, and headache—occur in 20–40%. Hepatosplenomegaly is found about one-third of patients, and lymphadenopathy in about 10%. Other manifestations including neurobrucellosis, endocarditis, hepatitis, and epididimo-orchitis may occur. Childhood brucellosis generally exhibits a more benign course in terms of the rate and severity of complications.[15] Subclinical disease occurs, and may heal spontaneously, but patients may present with relapses following previous subclinical disease, or with late, localized complications, simulating a very long incubation period.

Relapse following treatment occurs in about 5–15%, generally within the first 6 months after treatment, and it has been related to inadequate choice of antibiotics, shortened treatment duration, poor compliance, or localized infection.[16]

Brucellar arthritis

General considerations

Arthralgia is more common in brucellosis than in other febrile illnesses. It has been recorded in 70% of patients with brucellosis, with similar frequency in children or adults[3]; its presence may be a clue to the disease.

Bone scinitigraphy in patients with brucellosis and musculoskeletal symptoms has been reported as being frequently abnormal, often in multiple sites; some of the minor musculoskeletal symptoms of these patients may result from localized infection. Since the treatment of brucellar arthritis and that of uncomplicated brucellosis is the same, once brucellosis is diagnosed, it is not worthwhile searching for arthritis to explain minor or unclear musculoskeletal symptoms.

The reported prevalence of ostearticular involvement ranges from 20% to 60%: 20% in Spain,[17] 28.5% in Iran,[18] 42% in Greece,[12] 47.7% in Saudi Arabia,[19] 59.2% in Macedonia,[20] 25.3% in Turkey,[3] and 25% in the United States.[21]

The bulk of musculoskeletal involvement is most often large joint, sacroiliitis, and spondylitis. The frequency varies according to the characteristics of the reported patients; in general sacroiliitis predominates in younger adults and as a result of *B. mellitensis* infection, while spondylitis is observed in older patients, and peripheral arthritis occurs in all ages, predominating in children and young adults. The discrepancies in the frequency and distribution of ostearticular brucellosis relate to the characteristics of the examined population, stages of the diseases, diversity of definition of the cases, nature of the causative agent, and diagnostic procedures undergone, as well as the prospective/retrospective nature of studies.

Arthritis of peripheral joints

Large peripheral joints are a common site of localized infection. In all age groups, the hip is the most common location, followed by the knee. Ankles, shoulders, elbows, wrists, and sternoclavicular joints contribute a small percentage of cases. Although brucellosis arthritis is generally monoarticular; oligoarticular and polyarticular arthritis have been reported in one-fifth to one-half of the patients with arthritis.[22–25] Involvement of the small joints of hands and feet is rare, although a 'rheumatoid like' distribution may occur.

Peripheral joint arthritis often, but not necessarily always, predominates over other disease manifestations. It usually occurs during the acute phase of the disease or during a relapse, and fever or other general symptoms of the disease frequently accompany the arthritis, which tends to be symptomatic from the start; so the patients tend to seek prompt medical attention. The joints are swollen and painful, and an effusion is generally seen. Joint inflammation is not as intense as it is in some septic arthritides due to pyogenic organisms, and there is seldom obvious redness or unusual warmth in the skin. Six cases of arthritis of in prosthetic joints have been reported.[26] Local complications, such as popliteal cyst rupture also occur.[24]

If diagnosis or treatment is delayed the joint is damaged, resulting in radiological abnormalities with joint space narrowing and damage to the joint surfaces, similar to other infectious arthritides. The interval between initiation of infection and the appearance of structural damage in the joint tends to be longer than in pyogenic arthritides, but probably shorter than in tuberculosis. The sequelae of infection depends on timing of treatment; when treatment is started early enough, no sequelae develop.

Bursitis and tenosynovitis due to *B. melitensis*, *B. abortus*, and *B. suis* may also occur.

Sacroiliitis

The sacroiliac joint is frequently involved. The incidence ranges from 30% to 75% in recent series[3,18,22]; in our own experience in Spain it is 36%. Sacroiliitis is uncommon in children and seems an unusual complication of *B. abortus* and *B. suis*.

Sacroiliitis tends to occur in the acute, febrile phase of the disease, is usually unilateral but can be bilateral, and is usually symptomatic from the start[27]; other joints can be simultaneously affected. In some patients the pain becomes so intense that for two or three days they can hardly move from the bed,[28] and many have severe pain when walking. Radiation of pain to the buttock, posterior thigh, and even below is not unusual. In these patients, any movement of the leg is very painful, and hip manoeuvres or straight leg elevation may seem positive: in this setting, clinical differentiation of sacroiliitis from hip disease or sciatica may be difficult. Gently tapping on the lower surface of the heel while the patient keeps the leg extended usually localizes the pain to the sacroiliac area. Other sacroiliac manoeuvres may result too painful and be difficult to interpret. Evaluation of patients with less intense symptoms is easier with standard manoeuvres.

Radiological exploration in the early stage of disease is normal, but within 2–3 weeks radiological abnormalities such as blurring of the subchondral osseous line, narrowing and widening of the interosseous line, and narrowing and widening of the interosseous space (changes which are similar to septic sacroiliac arthritis) are observed (Figure 104.1). Bone scintigraphy provides early evidence of sacroiliitis in most cases (Figure 104.2).[22] MRI may detect early bone marrow oedema and intra-articular synovial fluid.[29]

Symptoms ease rapidly after introduction of antimicrobial treatment, indicating its infectious nature, and no sequelae or later joint disease occurs. Though possibly very painful, brucellar sacroileitis is a mild disease associated with a good outcome similar to that observed for patients with uncomplicated brucellosis.

Spondylitis

Brucellar spondylitis is most often seen in adult and elderly patients, frequently men (probably due to a higher frequency of occupational disease in many countries and not a real sex difference). Reported percentages vary according to the characteristics of the series and are higher in series where bone scintigraphy has been used for diagnosis reaching 50% of the musculoskeletal focal disease.[22] The lumbar spine is most frequently affected, followed by dorsal and less frequently cervical spine.[30,31] In contrast to peripheral arthritis or sacroiliitis, spondylitis is often a later feature. In a prospectively collected series of 96 patients 91% were febrile and 88% had chills or rigor,[30] but patients may also present with only vague symptoms of a general infectious disorder, and be afebrile.

Systemic features tend to occur when spinal infection presents shortly after disease onset. Presentation of spinal disease is often insidious, and its hallmark is local pain of variable intensity, often moderate, which may allow the patient to maintain a fairly normal life. Pressure or percussion of the spinous processes of the affected

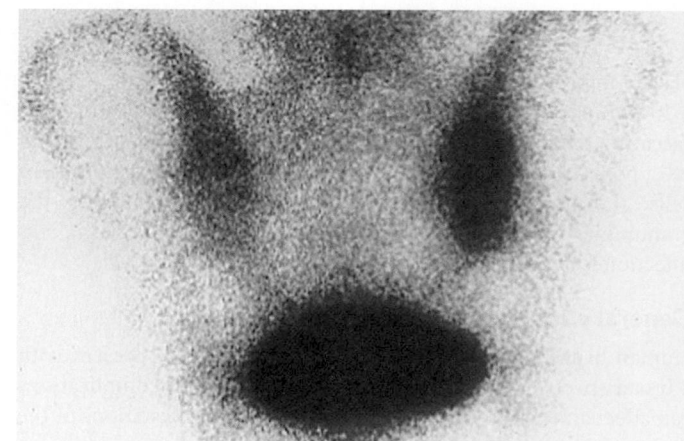

Fig. 104.2 Bone scan of the posterior pelvis of a patient with left brucellar sacroiliitis of short duration and normal radiograph.

vertebrae often reproduces the pain and paravertebral muscles may be tender. Cord or nerve root compression due to epidural abscesses (more frequent in cervical spondylitis) can occur. Small paravertebral abscesses or paravertebral masses are frequent and psoas abscesses occur.[30] These abscesses clear with medical treatment. The newer imaging techniques allows easy detection of lesions that were formerly overlooked. Material obtained from the abscesses is usually sterile. Some patients can develop epidural abscesses from the infected disc space. Compression of the medulla or nerve roots is found more frequently in cervical spondylitis, which should be considered a severe manifestation of the disease.

In the very early phase, radiography of the affected segments is normal. After 2 months, nearly all patients show radiographic alterations. The first sign is narrowing of the disc, without bone abnormalities. Later, two different changes are seen in the limiting vertebral endplates: a limited form with an erosion, generally in the anterosuperior vertebral angle, with sclerotic base, which is considered to be characteristic of brucellar spondylitis (Figure 104.3); and a diffuse form, in which the corresponding vertebral endplates show erosions, accompanied by narrowing of the disc space (Figure 104.3). Early signs of repair occur, with the appearance of osteophytes. Both pathological and radiological data suggest that the infection begins in the vertebra, and then spreads to the disc. In a series of 35 patients with brucellar spondylitis in whom MRI was carried out,[32] 32 of them had involvement in only a single spine region: 31 had diffuse disease of a disc space, two of them had focal disease at an anterior vertebral angle, and one had diffuse disease at a disc space and focal disease at another level. The two remaining patients had contiguous involvement of multiple levels (>2). Paraspinal masses were noted in 22/35, epidural masses in 27/35, and masses with root compression in 19/35. In this series one patient underwent laminectomy, but none developed neurological sequelae. Bone scintigraphy frequently shows increased uptake at the level of the affected disc space, even when radiologically normal.

Spondylitis heals with antimicrobial treatment (requiring a longer duration than in the other locations of arthritis) and residual pain may remain. Early diagnosis and treatment, and consequently less structural damage, are followed by a better recovery.

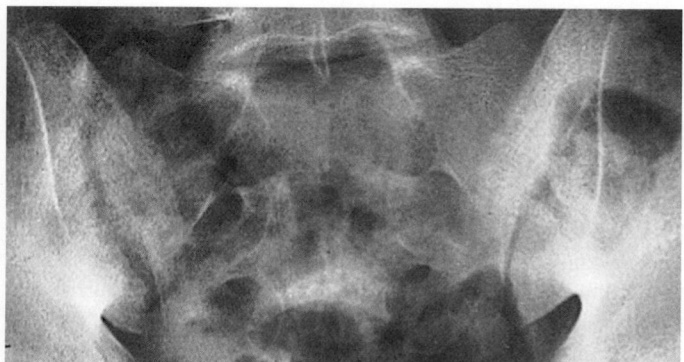

Fig. 104.1 Radiograph of the sacroiliac joints, showing widening and erosions of the right joint in a patient with long-standing brucellar sacroiliitis.

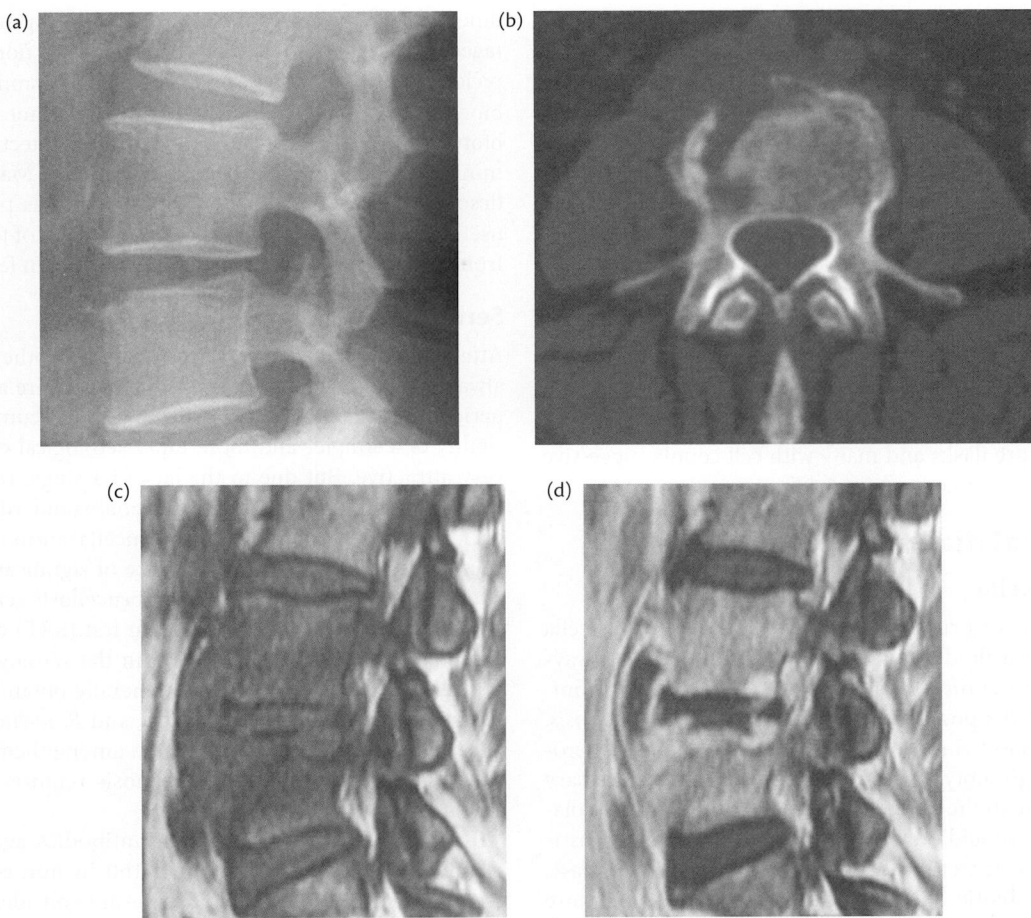

Fig. 104.3 Brucellar infection at the lumbar spine. (a) Lateral radiograph of lumbar vertebrae, showing an upper corner lesion, with sclerotic base in L4, considered characteristic of brucellar spondylitis. Reduction in the height of the disc space is also seen. (b) CT section across the upper vertebral plateau of L4 showing an anterior lytic lesion and adjacent soft tissue mass. (c) T1-weighted MRI showing a sagittal section: there is marked oedema in the bodies of the L3 and L4 vertebrae, narrowing of the disc space, and a mass bulging anteriorly; intravertebral lesions connected to the disc space are also seen. (d) Same sagittal cut, gadolinium enhanced. Areas of inflammation are now seen light, including the intravertebral lesions indicating that they are vascularized, and an anterior dark abscess is seen.
Figure kindly provided by Dr Jaime Fernández Campillo.

Diagnostic investigations

Clinical approach

The clinical features of brucellosis are non-specific. The manifestations of brucellar joint disease are similar to those of other infectious peripheral or axial arthritides, and may also resemble some inflammatory arthritides; presentation can be acute, but usually less than pyogenic infections. Nevertheless, in the following circumstances, appropriate testing for brucellosis should always be done:

- in all undiagnosed arthritides, with features fitting those of brucellosis, occurring in areas where the disease is endemic, or in patients with a history of possible exposure to the disease through travel to endemic areas, ingestion of possibly contaminated imported products, or in exposed laboratory workers

- in all cases of undiagnosed acute unilateral sacroiliitis

- in all cases of undiagnosed disc-space infection, especially those with radiological evidence of localized vertebral angle infection, or infection of multiple levels.

About 25% of patients do not recall exposure to possibly infected animals or unpasteurized dairy products.

Due to the lack of a single standardized laboratory test, diagnosis of human brucellosis remains difficult. Brucella cultures require special prolonged processing and have a low yield. Serology is more rapid and effective, although there is not an internationally standardized test since adequate cut-off points have to be defined for each test and for different populations (related to endemicity). In the near future, molecular techniques may revolutionize the laboratory diagnosis of human brucellosis.

General laboratory features

The laboratory features of brucellosis are non-specific. Although white blood cell counts are usually normal, leucocytosis is observed in about 9% of patients and if found, focal disease should be considered. Leucopenia and thrombocytopenia are seen with similar frequencies (10%) and anaemia in 25%.[33] Minor abnormalities in hepatic enzymes are common.

The erythrocyte sedimentation rate (ESR) and C-reactive protein (CRP) are usually elevated[18,20] and normal values are not unusual in late and localized forms such as spondylitis.

There were no significant laboratory differences between brucellosis with or without osteoarticular forms, except for a higher rate of anaemia in patients without osteoarticular involvement.[18]

Synovial fluid analysis

Published data of synovial fluid analysis in brucellar arthritis are scarce. Unlike bacterial arthritis caused by other microorganisms, in brucellar arthritis, the synovial fluid leucocyte count is frequently less than 50 000/mm^3, with a predominance of lymphomononuclear cells.[26,28,34,35] and 6000–18000/mm^3.

Glucose levels were within normal limits in the above series. Lactic acid levels have also been found to be normal. *B. melitensis* has been isolated from some of the above synovial fluids. Our own unpublished data from 18 prospectively studied patients showed different results. The cell counts were 3200–90000/mm^3; glucose was low in some of the fluids (0–100 mg/dL, (mean 47) and lactic acid was also high on a few occasions (13–138 mg/dL, (mean 74). *B. melitensis* was recovered from 73% of those fluids, many cultured in blood culture flasks and many with cell counts suggestive of non-infectious inflammatory synovial fluid.

Bacteriological diagnosis

Isolation of brucella

Definitive diagnosis of brucellosis requires isolation of brucella from blood, synovial fluid, or other sources, and should always be attempted when the disease is suspected. It provides a definitive diagnosis, and the possibility of differentiating *B. melitensis*, *B. abortus*, and *B. suis*, which is not possible with the usual serological tests, although subtyping of brucella species is not necessary for treatment.[36] Due to the specific requirements of brucella isolation, the laboratory should be warned when brucellosis is a possibility. Isolation rates are variable depending on the stage of disease, previous use of antibiotic, the clinical specimen, and the culture methods.[36] Bacteraemia is an early event in brucellosis, so isolation rates are much higher during first 2 weeks of symptoms (80–90% in acute forms, and 30–70% in more chronic cases), also depending on the technical approach.[37] The recovery rate of brucella is improved when blood samples are taken in the pyrexial phase and by collecting multiple blood samples or material from infection sites; bacterial isolation is also highly dependent on the total volume of the sample.[36] Bone marrow culture is considered the gold standard for the diagnosis of brucellosis, since it is more sensitive than blood cultures, the time to detection is shorter, and the sensitivity is not reduced by prior use of antibiotics.[36]

Brucella are slow-growing organisms, often requiring longer incubation. Although they will grow in the usual media the rate of recovery is low and different enriched media, prolonged culture times, and subcultures have been used. The classic biphasic (solid and liquid) Ruiz-Castañeda blood culture medium is still in use but growth is slow and may require up to 30 days; it is a simple medium that does not require special laboratory conditions. Semiautomated methods are more effective, considerably shortening the time to detection (<4 days).[38] Recovery of brucella from body fluids is higher using this blood culture system, and it has been recommended to inoculate synovial fluid in blood culture flasks and processed in automated blood culture systems.[26]

Despite the better performance of these culture systems, a prolonged incubation period and periodic subcultures for at least 4 weeks are still recommended to reliably exclude a brucella infection. The lysis-centrifugation technique provides rapid diagnoses (2–3 days) and has higher sensitivity independent of the stage of illness.[26,39,40] The newer continuous monitoring methods are advantageous because of their shorter time to detection.[36] Colonies suspicious for brucella can be confirmed with a commercially available biochemical test such as API 20 NE or semiautomated metabolic biotyping systems that facilitate the rapid detection from culture, minimizing the risk of laboratory infection.[36] Matrix-assisted laser desorption/ionization mass spectrometry has proved to be very useful in the direct identification of members of the genus brucella from culture plates and blood culture bottles in few minutes.[41]

Serological diagnosis

Attempts to isolate brucella from blood or other sources are not always successful; besides, culture may require a long incubation period and still show no growth. In these circumstances, the possibility of a simpler and more rapid serological diagnosis remains very attractive. But due to the lack of a single reliable laboratory test, the unavailability of international standardization, the high background prevalence of anti-brucella antibodies in endemic countries, and long-term persistence of significant antibody titres after successful treatment, human brucellosis remains difficult to diagnose.[36] The serum agglutination test (SAT) remains generally accepted as the reference method in the serological diagnosis of brucellosis. The antigen used is generally obtained from *B. abortus*, and it reacts against *B. abortus*, and *B. melitensis*, and *B. suis*, but does not allowing differentiation among them. The non-cross-reacting *B. canis* serological diagnosis requires specific antigen preparations.[42]

The SAT detects agglutination antibodies against brucella in serum; SAT titres greater than 1:160 in non-endemic areas or greater than 1:320 in endemic areas are considered as consistent with active brucellosis if accompanied by clinical symptoms. A four-fold or greater rise in brucella agglutination titre between acute and convalescent phase serum (>2 weeks apart) studied at the same laboratory may prove infection. Definitive cure correlates well with lower SAT titres, although 3–5% of clinically cured patients maintain significant SAT titres. False negative rates are high (1) in the early course of the disease (even bacteraemic patients may present with titre <1:160); (2) in the setting of immunosuppression; and (3) in the presence of blocking antibodies or the so-called 'prozone' phenomenon (inhibition of agglutination at low dilutions due to an excess of antibodies, detected by the brucellar Coombs test) that occurs in late or focal brucellosis or during relapses. These blocking antibodies increase over agglutinating antibodies along the course of infection and the Coombs test is routinely recommended as an extension of the SAT.

Enzyme-linked immunosorbent assay (ELISA) allows a better interpretation of the clinical situation; besides, the measurement of specific antibodies may detect occasional patients undiscovered by other serological tests.[36] ELISA is more sensitive than SAT in chronic and past brucellosis, but in acute cases SAT show the same results and is simpler and less expensive.[36]

The Rose Bengal test (RBT) is a rapid slide-type agglutination assay and because of its simplicity is used as screening test for human brucellosis. Although overall sensitivity and specificity reported by RBT varies widely in a recent review comparing 208 sera from patients with brucellosis, 20 contacts with no brucellosis and 1559 controls, a diagnostic titre greater than 4 in the RBT resulted in 87.4% sensitivity (infected patients) and 100% specificity.

The simplicity and affordability of the RBT make it close to the ideal test for screening, especially for small hospitals and laboratories.[43]

The classical serologic tests, such as the SAT and Coombs test, are labour-intensive and time-consuming. Brucellacapt (Vircell, Granada, Spain) is a simpler test showing better reproducibility that detects total anti-brucella antibodies. It has been shown to be superior to the SAT in all stages of disease including relapses and has a similar yield to the Coombs test; it is recommended for use in endemic countries.[44,23,45,46]

Treatment

There have been three important recommendations in recent times: WHO/FAO (WHO 2006),[47] the Ionnina recommendations for the treatment of human brucellosis,[48] and a *BMJ* review on the subject.[49] As first-line treatment for uncomplicated brucellosis all recommended combined regimens include doxycycline for 6 weeks (Table 104.1). WHO recommended adding rifampicin for 6 weeks, however, it has become apparent that aminoglycosides are a better choice than rifampicin and at Ionnina the recommended first choice added streptomycin (2–3 weeks) to doxycycline. Besides this, the doxycicline–rifampicin combination has been widely used because of the difficulties of administering streptomycin in less well-resourced areas. Because of the greater availability of gentamycin and its lesser ototoxicity the *BMJ* review recommends 2 weeks of gentamycin added to the 6 weeks of doxycycline based on extensive studies which support the combination.[50,51]

Interestingly, it has been shown that brucella isolated from relapsing patients shows similar sensitivities to those of the original isolate,[52] and the limited capacity to produce resistance has been confirmed in more recent reports,[53] although drug resistance has been reported. Relapses or late, localized disease may result from insufficient duration of treatment, poor compliance, or unrecognized focal disease in apparently uncomplicated brucellosis and too short treatment. In any case uncertainties about brucellosis treatment remain, and better treatment regimens are required for patients with difficult or severe disease. In this setting triple therapy with either co-trimoxazole or a quinolone is added to a regimen of doxycycline/rifampicin or doxycycline/gentamycin has been used with promising results.

Brucella spondylitis

Most brucellar complications respond well to standard regimens; however, brucellar spondylitis, neurobrucellosis, endocarditis, and localized suppurative lesions warrant special consideration. An 'impossible meta-analysis'—described as such by the authors because of the heterogeneity of the studies on which it is based—on the results of the treatment of brucellar spondylitis concluded that what matters for the outcome is the duration of treatment, rather than the drug regimen used.[54] Although this meta-analysis did not conclude that streptomycin-containing regimens might be superior, the slight superiority of doxycycline/streptomycin (or gentamycin) in uncomplicated brucellosis underlines the frequent statement that the outcome of spondylitis may potentially be improved when such regimens are used. Although the optimal duration of therapy remains undefined, the available data supports a duration of not less than 3 months[48,30] and probably 6 months,[49,55] with streptomycin or gentamicin during the first 3 weeks. Large paravertebral or abscesses have been drained percutaneously with CT guidance, but they may also respond well to antibiotic treatment. Surgery has been reserved for exceptional cases or epidural abscess and progressive signs of neurological deficit. Lack of controlled trials in these less usual situations requires careful evaluation of the individual cases. Brucellar spondylitis has a good prognosis, and under medical treatment patients recover in 1–3 months. Brucella antibody titres have been recommended to assess therapeutic efficacy and resolution of the disease.[36] In peripheral arthritis regular drainage of the affected joints appears unnecessary, as it is done in pyogenic arthritis to avoid joint damage.

In children up to 8 years of age, co-trimoxazole plus rifampin for 4–6 weeks and doxycycline plus rifampicin in older children are the recommended treatments for uncomplicated brucellosis. In those with osteoarticular disease a regimen containing an aminoglycoside is considered more effective: co-trimoxazole for 6 weeks plus a parenteral aminoglycoside (gentamicin or streptomycin) for the first 14 days of therapy is recommended for children under 8 years of age, and for children over 8 year of age co-trimoxazole should be changeable for an oral tetracycline.[56] The systematic review and meta-analysis of randomized controlled trials made by Skalky supports the use of co-trimoxazole monotherapy for a prolonged period of time (up to 6 months), and this may be useful in some circumstances.

Prevention

Brucellosis may be prevented by vaccination of domestic animals. When the occurrence of brucellosis is controlled in animal reservoirs the incidence in humans show a significant decline, but this requires a sustained vaccination programme over several years. Vaccination for the prevention of human brucellosis is not available.

Postexposure prophylaxis after laboratory exposure to brucella isolates should be offered as soon as brucella exposure has been identified.

Table 104.1 Recommendations for the treatment of uncomplicated brucellosis in non-pregnant adults

	WHO 2006	Ioannina 2007[48]	BMJ 2008[49]
First-line regimen	Doxycycline+rifampicin 6 weeks	Doxycycline 6 weeks+ Streptomycin 2–3 weeks	Doxycycline 6 weeks+gentamicin 2 weeks or Doxycycline +rifampicin 6 weeks+ +gentamicin 2 weeks
Alternative	Tetracycline 6 weeks+ Streptomycin 2–3 weeks	Doxycycline+rifampicin 6 weeks	Doxycycline 6 weeks+ Streptomycin 2 weeks

Modified from Skalsky et al.[49]

References

1. Capaso L. Bacteria in two-millennia—old cheese, and related epizoonoses in Roman populations. *J Infect* 2002;45:122–127.

2. Pappas G, Papadimitriou P, Akritidis N, Christou L, Tsianos EV. The new global map of human brucellosis. *Lancet Infect* 2006;6:91–99.

3. Buzgan T, Kasim, Karahocagil M et al. clinical manifestations and complications in 1208 cases of brucellosis: a retrospective evaluation and review of the literature. *Int J Infect Dis* 2010;14:e469–e478.

4. Al Dahourk S, Neubuer H, Hensel A et al. Changing epidemiology of human brucellosis, Germany 1962–2005. *Emerg Infect Dis* 2007;13(12): 1895–1890.

5. Pappas G, Akritidis N, Bosilkowski M,Tsianos E. Brucellosis. *N Engl J Med* 2005;352:2325.

6. Fiori PL, Mastandrea S, Rappelli P, Capuccinelli P. Brucella abortus infection acquired in microbioloby laboratorios. *J Clin Microbiol* 2000;38:2005.

7. Delvecchio VG, Kapatral V, Redkar RJ et al. The genome sequence of the facultative intracellular pathogen Brucella melitensis. *Proc Natl Acad Sci U S A* 2002;99:443–448.

8. Barquero-Calvo E, Chaves-Olarte E, Weiss DS et al. Brucella abortus uses a stealthy strategy to avoid activation of the innate immune system during the onset of infection *PLoS One* 2007;2:e631.

9. Gorvel JP, Moreno E. Brucella intracellular life: from invasion to intracellular replication. *Vet Microbiol* 2002;90:281–297.

10. Ko J, Splitter GA. Molecular host-pathogen interaction in brucellosis: current understanding and future approaches to vaccine development for mice and humans. *Clin Microbiol Rev* 2003;16:65.

11. Doganay M, Aygen B. Human brucellosis: an overview. *Int J Infect Dis* 2003;7:173.

12. Andriopoloulos P, Tsironi M, Defletereos S, Aessopos A, Assimakapoulos G. Acute brucellosis: presentation, diagnosis and treatment of 144 cases. *Int J Infect Dis* 2007;11:52–57.

13. Mantur BG, Amarnath SK, Shinde RS. Review of clinical and laboratory features of human brucellosis. *Indian J Med Microbiol* 2007;25:188.

14. Vassalos CM, Economou V, Vassalou E, Papadopoulou C. Brucellosis in humans: why is it so elusive? *Vet Med Mycol* 2009;20:63–73.

15. Logan LK, Jacobs NM, McAurely JB, Weinstein R, Anderson EJ. A multicenter retrospective study of childhood brucellosis in Chicago, Illinois from 1986 to 2008. *Int J Infect Dis* 2011;15:e812–e817.

16. Hasanjani Roushan MR, Mohrez M, Smailnejad Gangi SM, Solemani Amiri MJ Hajahmadi M. Epidemiological features and clinical manifestations in 469 patients with brucelosis in Babol, northern Iran. *Epidemiol Infect* 2004;132:1109.

17. Ruiz-Mesa JD, Rodríguez-Contreras PR, Gil B et al. Study of 1595 brucellosis cases in Almeria province (1972–86) based on epidemiological data from disease reporting. *Rev Clin Esp* 2002;202:577–582.

18. Hashemi SH, Keramat F, Ranjbar M et al. Ostearticular complications of brucellosis in Hamedan, an endemic area in the west of Iran. *Int J Infect Dis* 2007;11:486–500.

19. El-Desouki MI, Benjamin RS. Diagnostic value of quantitative sacroiliac joint scintigraphy in brucellosis. *Clin Nucl Med* 1999;24:10:756–758.

20. Bosilkovski M, Krteva L, Dimzova M, Kondva I. Brucellois in 418 patients from the Balkan Peninsula: exposure-related differences in clinical manifestations, laboratory test results and therapy outcome. *Int J Infect Dis* 2007;11:342–347.

21. Troy SB, Rickman LS, Davis CE. Brucellosis in San Diego: epidemiology and species-related differences in acute presentations. *Medicine* (Baltimore) 2005;84(3):174–187.

22. Heidari P, Heidari B. Rheumatologic manifestations of brucellosis. *Rheumatol Int* 2011;31(6):721–724.

23. Bosilkovski M, Katerian S, Zaklina S, Ivan V. The role of Brucellacapt tt for follow-up patients with brucellosis. *Comp Immunol Microbiol Infect Dis* 2010:33(5):435–442.

24. Geyik MF, Gür A, Nas K et al. Musculoskeletal involvement in brucellosis in different age groups: a study of 195 cases. *Swiss Med Wkly* 2002;132:98–105.

25. Batlle E, Pascual E, Salas E et al. Brucellar arthritis: an study of 86 prospectively collected patients. *Br J Rheumatol* 1989;28 (Suppl 2):25.

26. Cerit ET, Aydin M, Azap A. A case of brucellar monoarthritis and review of the literature. *Rheumatol Int* 2012;32(5):1465–1468.

27. Hizel, K, Guzel O, Dizbay M et al. Age and duration of disease as factors affecting clinical findings and sacroiliitis in brucellosis. *Infection* 2007;35(6):434–437.

28. Mousa AR, Elhag KM, Khogali M, Marafie AA. The nature of human brucellosis in Kuwait: study of 379 cases. *Rev Infect Dis* 2011;10:211–217.

29. Arkun R, Mete BD. Musucloskeletal brucellosis. *Sem Musculoskel Radiol* 2011;15(5): 470–479.

30. Colmenero JD, Ruiz-Mesa JD, Plata A et al. Clinical findings, therapeutic approach and outcome of brucellar vertebral osteomyelitis. *Clin Infect Dis* 2008;46:426–433.

31. Turgut M, Turgut AT, Kosar U. Spinal brucellosis: Turkish experience based on 452 published during the last century. *Acta Neurochir* 2006; 148: 1033–1044.

32. Solera J, Lozano E, Martínez-Alfaro E et al. Brucellar spondylitis: review of 35 cases an dlitature survey. *Clin Infect Dis* 1999;29:1440.

33. Franco MP, Mulder M, Gilman RH, Smits HL. Human brucellosis. *Lancet* 2007,7:775–786.

34. Gotuzzo E, Alarcón GS, Bocanegra TS et al. Articular involvement in human brucellosis: a retrospective analysis of 304 cases. *Semin Arthritis Rheum* 1982: 12,245–255..

35. Andononopoulos AP, Asmakopoulos G, Anastasiou E, Bassaris HP. Brucella arthritis. *Scand J Rheumatol* 1986;15(4):377–380.

36. Al Dahouk S, Nöckler K. Implications of laboratory diagnosis on brucellosis therapy. *Expert Rev Anti Infect Ther* 2011;9(7):833–845.

37. Espinosa BJ, Chacaltana J, Mulder M et al. Comparison of culture techniques at differents stages of brucellosis. *Am J Trop Med Hyg* 2009;80(4): 625–627.

38. Baysallar M, Aydogan H, Kilic A et al. Evaluation of the BacT/ALERT and BACTEC 9240 automated blood cultures systems for growth time of Brucella species in a Turkish tertiary hospital. *Med Sci Monit* 2006;12(7):235–238.

39. Mantur BG, Mangalgi S. Evaluation of conventional Castañeda and lysis centrifugation blood culture techniques for the diagnosis of human brucellosis. *J Clin Microbiol* 2004;42(5):4327.

40. Cetin ES, Kaya S, Bemici M, Aridogan BC. Comparison of the BACTEC blood culture system versus conventional methods for culture of normally sterile body fluids. *Adv Ther* 2007;24(6):1271–1277.

41. Ferreira L, Vega Casño S, Sánchez-Juanes et al. Identification of Brucella by MALDITOF mass spectrometry: fast and reliable identification from agar plates and blood cultures. *PLoS ONE* 2010;12:e4235.

42. Lucero NE, Escobar BI, Ayala SM, Jacob N. Diagnosis of human brucellosis caused by Brucella canis. *J Med Microbiol* 2005;54(5):457–461.

43. Díaz R, Casanova A, Ariza J, Moriyón I. The Rose Bengal test in human brucellosis: a neglected test for the diagnosis of a neglected disease. *PLoS One* 2011;5(4):1–7.

44. Casanova A, Ariza J, Rubio M, Masuet C, Diaz R. Brucellacapt versus classical test in the serological diagnosis and management of human brucellosis. *Clin Vaccine Immunol* 2009;16:844–851.

45. Mantur BG, Amarnath SK, Parande AM et al. Comparison of a novel immunocapture assay with standard serological methods in the diagnosis of brucellosis. *Clin Lab* 2011;57(5–6):333–341.

46. Özdemir M, Feyzioglu B, Kurtoglu MG et al. A comparison of immunocapture agglutination and ELISA methods in serological diagnosis of Brucellosis. *Int J Med Sci* 2011;8:428–432..

47. Corbel MJ. *Brucellosis in humans and animals.* WHO/CDS/EPR/2006.7. World Health Organization, Geneva, 2006.

48. Ariza J, Bosilkovsky M, Casacio A et al Perspectives for the treatment of brucellosis in the 21st century: The Ioannina Recommendations. *PLos Med* 2007;4(12):e317–317.

49. Skalsky K, Yahav D, Bishara J et al. Treatment of human brucellosis: systematic review and meta-analysis of randomised controlled trials. *BMJ* 2008;336:1–8.

50. Solera J, Espinosa A, Martínez-Alfaro E et al. Treatment of human brucellosis with doxycycline and gentamicin. *Antimicrob Agents Chemother* 1997;41:80–84.

51. Hasanjani Roushan MR, Mohraz M, Hajiahmadi M, Ramzani A, Valayati AA. Efficacy of gentamicin plus doxycycline versus streptomycin plus doxycycline in the treatment of brucellosis humans. *Clin Infect Dis* 2006;42:1075–1080.

52. Ariza J, Bosch J, Gudiol F, Liñares J, Viladrich PF, Martín R. Relevance of in vitro antimicrobial susceptibility of Brucella melitensis to

53. Turkmani A, Ionnidis A, Christidou A et al. In vitro susceptibilities of Brucella melitensis isolates to eleven antibiotics. *Ann Clin Microbiol Antimicrob* 2006;5:24.

54. Pappas G, Scitariadis S, Akritidis N, Tsianos E. Treatment of brucella spondylitis: lessons from an impossible meta-analysis and initial report of efficacy of a fluoroquinolones-containing regimen. *Int J Antimicrob Agents* 2004;24:502–507.

55. Bouaiz MC, Ladeb MF, Cahkroun M, Chaabane S. Spinal brucellosis: a review. *Skeletal Radiol* 2008;37:785–790.

56. American Academy of Pediatrics. Brucellosis. In: Pickering LD (ed) *Red Book: 2009 Report of the Committee on Infectious Diseases*, 28th edn. American Academy of Pediatrics, Elk Grove Village, IL, 2009:237.

relapse rate in human brucellosis. *Antimicrob Agents Chemother* 1986;30:958–960.

CHAPTER 105

Parasitic infection

Olabambo Ogunbambi and Yusuf I. Patel

Introduction

Parasitism defines the relationship between two organisms, where the host provides both habitat and nourishment to the parasite. In order to establish itself within the environment of the host, the parasite must develop the ability to evade or tolerate the immune response of the host.[1] Pathogenicity depends on a variety of factors including host fitness and parasitic virulence.[2]

Immunity to parasites

Host immune responses to parasites are geared to eliminate the foreign organism, and include both innate and specific immune responses. Innate responses involve complement-mediated lysis and macrophage/neutrophil phagocytosis and killing. Some parasites evade complement-mediated lysis by altering surface molecules that bind complement or by acquiring host proteins that inhibit complement pathways (e.g. CD55, decay accelerating factor). The tegument of helminths makes them resistant to neutrophil and macrophage cytocidal mechanisms.

Specific immune responses appear to segregate into two groups: cellular immunity against protozoa mediated through CD4-driven macrophage activation or CTL (cytotoxic T-lymphocyte) responses, and antibody (IgE) or eosinophil (major basic protein)-mediated defence against helminthic infections.

Immune responses against parasites may in fact produce some of the damage seen in the host. Examples include the fibrosis and granuloma formation in schistosomiasis, immune complex deposition in malaria and schistosomiasis, autoimmune myocarditis, and neuropathy in Chagas' disease caused by *Trypanosoma cruzi*.[3] Autoimmune disease in chronic parasitic infections may be associated with molecular mimicry.[4]

Parasites use a number of mechanisms to evade the host immune system (Box 105.1). These are crucial adaptations in ensuring the survival of the species from the point of view of the parasite, but equally may contribute significantly to the pathology seen in the host.

Epidemiology

Parasitic infections are a particular problem in developing countries. In developed countries, they usually occur in isolated outbreaks or in people who have been travelling to endemic areas. An increased incidence of parasitic disease is found throughout the

---

Box 105.1 Immune evasive mechanisms

Anatomic sequestration

- Intracellular replication (malaria, toxoplasma)
- Cyst formation (entamoeba)
- Residence within the intestinal lumen (helminths)

Antigen masking

- Parasite acquires surface coat of host proteins (schistosomiasis)

Antigenic variation

- Antigenic shift with stages of parasitaemia (malaria)
- Continuous variation of surface antigens (African trypanosomiasis)

Antigen shedding

- Loss of surface antigen spontaneously or after antibody binding (*E. histolytica*, trypanosomes, schistosome larvae)

Resistance to host immune effector mechanisms

- Development of tegument (resistant to antibodies, complement, or CTL attack)
- Inhibition of complement (various mechanisms)
- Resistance to phagocytosis (various mechanisms)
- Resistance to antibody (production of ectoenzymes)

---

world amongst patients infected with HIV.[5] Even in endemic areas, direct parasitic involvement of the musculoskeletal system is relatively rare. Systematic epidemiologic studies are lacking and therefore the true prevalence of rheumatic manifestations in parasitic infections remains unknown. No specific manifestations or rheumatic syndromes have been identified in association with parasitic infection. Diagnostic criteria for 'parasitic rheumatism' have been suggested, but because of its relatively low prevalence, together with other problems related to conducting epidemiological studies in developing countries, there has not been a rigorous study of 'parasitic rheumatism' and its diagnostic criteria. Where data is available, the musculoskeletal manifestations are varied and the outcome usually very good either with or without therapy.[6]

Differential diagnosis and investigations

Parasitic infection as a cause of rheumatic disease is not frequently considered in the primary differential diagnosis. Factors that must alert the clinician to a parasitic association include:

◆ patients from endemic areas

◆ patients who have travelled to endemic areas

◆ elevation of eosinophil count

◆ failure to respond to anti-inflammatory therapy

◆ coincidental identification of parasitic infection in index patient.

Initiation of relevant investigations for parasitic infection depends on the clinician having a heightened level of awareness for the association of parasitic infection and musculoskeletal disease. An appropriate search for parasites and/or their immune phenomena may assist in making a diagnosis. This includes a search in blood, urine, and faeces, and where appropriate, tissue for histological analysis.[7] Direct identification of parasitic material in muscle, synovium, and bone has highlighted the role of parasitic infections in causing musculoskeletal disease. However, it is rare to find parasites at the site of pathology and this depends on the type of parasite involved. Parasitic material has been identified at the site of musculoskeletal pathology in cases with cysticercosis, gnathostomiasis, filariasis, Guinea worm infestation, hydatid disease, malaria, schistosomiasis, strongyloidiasis, toxocariasis, toxoplasmosis, trichinella infections, and trypanosomiasis. With the advent of molecular methods of identification of parasites, including specific polymerase chain reaction (PCR) techniques, the percentage of cases with identifiable 'parasitic material' may increase in future.[8] Developments in imaging techniques may also aid diagnosis. Typical ultrasonographic and MRI features have been described for certain parasites, e.g. muscular cysticercosis.[9]

More often, rheumatic syndromes are associated as a remote manifestation accompanying a parasitic infection elsewhere in a given individual. In this case, parasitic material may be identified at a site remote from the musculoskeletal system, or immune phenomena may indicate the possibility of a parasitic infection. These include elevated blood eosinophils (usually with nematode infections), infiltration of eosinophils into tissue, specific anti-parasitic antibodies, deposition of immune complexes, and signs of immune damage such as granuloma formation or fibrosis.

Parasites are broadly classified into two groups, protozoa and helminths. A wide variety of parasites from both groups have been associated with rheumatic manifestations (Tables 105.1 and 105.2). These include oligoarthritis, polyarthritis resembling rheumatoid arthritis, enthesitis, myositis and myopathic syndromes, and vasculitis, either localized or systemic. However, no specific 'parasitic syndrome' has been identified, and the pathogenesis remains uncertain. Evidence exists for both direct parasitic involvement of musculoskeletal tissue as well as possible reactive arthritis or immune-mediated mechanisms causing the rheumatic manifestations.

Treatment

The optimal approach to therapy has not been firmly established for many of the parasitic musculoskeletal manifestations and therapy remains largely empirical. Some patients only require non-steroidal anti-inflammatory drugs (NSAIDs) to control symptoms while others need specific anti-parasitic therapy or direct removal of the parasite (Tables 105.1 and 105.2). Complete resolution of symptoms and signs has been reported with anti-parasitic therapy, particularly where strong evidence of infection has been found. No formal studies have been conducted to assess the need for anti-parasitic therapy in all patients. Several of the anti-parasitic agents are relatively toxic, so a trial of therapy should not be undertaken lightly. Where clinical suspicion is high, and particularly where evidence exists for parasitic infestation, a trial of therapy may be undertaken under close supervision. Typically, therapeutic responses to anti-parasitic therapy occurs where standard anti-inflammatory therapy and/or steroids have previously failed.

Infections due to amoebae and *Blastocystis* spp. can be treated with metronidazole[56] or tinidazole. *Blastocystis* spp. also respond to nitazoxanide.[57] Flagellates (e.g. *Giardia*) generally respond to metronidazole or tinidazole.[58] The benzimidazole albendazole is a useful alternative. Therapeutic choices for malaria are complicated by resistance to traditional therapies such as chloroquine, particularly for *Plasmodium falciparum*. Chloroquine usually followed by primaquine remains effective, however, for most forms of non-falciparum malaria. Falciparum malaria in areas of chloroquine resistance requires combination therapy based on artemesinin derivatives, atovaquone–proguanil, quinine, or mefloquine.

Intestinal nematodes are generally sensitive to benzimidazoles such as albendazole or mebendazole. However, the response to therapy is variable. Pyrantel pamoate is effective against *Ascaris* spp. and *Ancylostoma* spp. Ivermectin is also effective against several nematodes although not considered the drug of choice. The treatment of filarial worms has traditionally been based on the use of diethylcarbamazine or ivermectin, particularly for endemic disease. However, these agents are associated with significant side effects. An alternative initial agent for the individual patient is doxycycline, which targets endosymbiotic bacteria.[59]

Intestinal cestode infestations due to *Taenia solium* and *T. saginata* usually respond to praziquantel which remains the drug of choice. Niclosamide and albendazole may also be effective. Tissue cestodes (larval forms) may respond to a number of agents including benzimidazoles. However, the need for specific anthelmintic therapy is unclear in these cases. In addition, other measures such as steroid therapy and surgical removal of cysts are often required.[46] Schistosomes and many trematodes are sensitive to praziquantel. The drug of choice for the liver fluke *Fasciola hepatica* is triclabendazole. Newer anthelmintics include nitazoxanide, tribendimidine, and artemisinine derivatives; however, their role is yet to be determined in treatment of rheumatic manifestations of parasitic infections.

In addition to uncertainty related to outcome measures, there is the possibility of exacerbating musculoskeletal symptoms on initiation of anti-parasitic therapy. This is more of a problem when treating tissue-invasive parasites, and varies with type of parasite, parasite load, and the drug used.[60] A policy of 'start low and go slow' should help avoid most major complications of therapy but there may be a need for concomitant steroids, particularly in the Mazzotti reaction described in the treatment of filariasis with diethylcarbazine or ivermectin.[61,62]

Table 105.1 Protozoa have been associated with a variety of musculoskeletal manifestations. Therapeutic choices and references of case reports or case series are indicated

Protozoa	Musculoskeletal manifestations	Therapy	Reference	
Blastocystis spp	Asymmetric oligoarthritis Infectious arthritis	Metronidazole Iodoquinol	Tejera et al. (2012)	10
Cryptosporidium	Reactive arthritis	Nsaids Paromomycin	Hay et al. (1987)	11
Entamoeba histolytica	Reactive arthritis Infective arthritis Vasculitis cutaneous Intestinal	Metronidazole Metronidazole Metronidazole	Than-saw et al. (1993) Demircin et al. (1998)	12 13
Entamoeba hartmanni	Reactive arthritis	Metronidazole	Schirmer et al. (1998)	14
Giardia lamblia	Asymmetrical oligoarthritis Infectious arthritis Symmetrical polyarthritis Vasculitis	Metronidazole Tinidazole	Woo and Panayi (1984)	15
Isospora belli	Reactive arthritis Myositis Vasculitis	Trimethoprim-sulfamethoxazole	Gonzales-Domingues et al. (1994)	16
Microsporidia	Myositis	Albendazole	Coyle et al. (2004)	17
Plasmodium spp	Symmetrical polyarthritis Polymyositis Vasculitis	Chloroquine, quinine, pyrimethamine/ sulfadoxine	Swash and Scwartz (1993)	18
Sarcocystis spp	Myositis Vasculitis	Co trimoxazole	Van Den Enden et al. (1995)	19
Toxoplasma gondii	Arthritis (Still's like) Myositis Vasculitis	Pyrimethamine, sulfadiazine	Balleari et al. (1991) Carmeni et al. (1991)	20 21
Trypanosoma spp American— *cruzi* African—*rhododiense, gambiense*	Polymyositis Vasculitis	Suramin, eflornithine, nifurtimox Benzimidazole, nifurtimox pentamidine, melarsoprol	Damien et al. (1994) Ferreira at el. (1997)	22 23

Table 105.2 Helminth infections causing musculoskeletal manifestations are summarized, with therapeutic choices and selected references indicated

Helminth	Musculoskeletal Manifestations	Therapy	Reference	
Ancylostoma (A duodenale)	Arthritis	Mebendazole	Bissonnette and Beaudet (1983)	24
Ascaris (A. lumbricoides)	Arthritis Vasculitis	Mebendazole Mebendazole	Chaughan et al. (1990)	25
Dirofilaria (D. immitis, D. tenuis)	Arthritis (reactive) Vasculitis (pulmonary)	Self-limiting Surgical resection	Flieder and Moran (1999)	26
Dracunculus (D.medinensis)	Arthralgia Myalgia Arthritis	Metronidazole Niridazole Arthrotomy	Garf (1985) Kothari et al. (1968) Reddy and Sivaramappa (1968)	27 28 29

(Continued)

Table 105.2 (*Continued*)

Helminth	Musculosketal Manifestations	Therapy	Reference	
Echinococcus spp (Hydatid)	Arthralgia Arthritis Myalgia Vasculitis Bone lesions	Albendazole Surgical excision	Bakkaloglu et al. (1994)	30
Fasciola	Vasculitis	Triclabendazole	Llanos et al. (2006)	31
Gnathostoma	Soft tissue mass Nodular panniculitis	Surgical excision Albendazole	Thomas et al. (2009)	32
Loa Loa (filiaria)	Arthritis vasculitis	Aspirate NSAID	Bouvet et al. (1977)	33
Onchocerca (filarial)	Arthritis Myositis	Diethylcarbamazine Ivermectin	Carme et al. (1989)	34
Paragonimus spp	Myalgia, weakness	Praziquantel	Sohn et al. (2009)	35
Schistosoma spp	Arthralgia Polyarthritis Oligoarthritis Enthesopathy Infectious arthritis Sacroiliitis Vasculitis (cerebral)	Niridazole Niridazole Praziquantel Steroids	Clement et al. (1979) Atkin et al. (1986) Bassiouni and Kamel (1984)	36 37 38
Spirometra spp (Sparganosis)	Tissue mass	Surgical excision Thiabendazole	Lee et al. (2010)	39
Strongyloides (S stercoralis)	Arthralgia, Arthritis Infectious arthritis Reactive arthritis Sacroiliitis Polyarthritis	Thiabendazole Albendazole Ivermectin Albendazole	Bocanegra et al. (1981) Akoglu (1984) Richter et al. (2006) van Kuijk et al. (2003)	40 41 42 43
Taenia multiceps (Coeneurosis)	Nodules in subcutaneous tissue and muscle	Surgical excision	Templeton (1968)	44
Taenia saginata	Polyarthritis	Praziquantel	Bocanegra (1981)	40
Taenia solium (cysticercus)	Bone infection Myopathy Vasculitis Localized muscle cysticercosis Generalized muscular pseudohypertrophy	Albendazole Mebendazole Albendazole, Praziquantel Surgical excision Corticosteroids	Estanol et al. (1986) Nagaraj et al. (2007) Chopra et al. (1986)	45 46 47
Toxocara (T. canis, T. catis)	Arthalgia/arthritis Panniculitis Transient myositis Eosinophilic arthritis	Diethylcarbamazine Mebendazole Self-limiting Ivermectin	William and Roy (1981) Walsh et al. (1988) Rayes and Lambertucci (2000)	48 49 50
Trichinella (Trichinella spp)	Myalgia myositis Vasculitis	Pyrantel Pamoate Mebendazole Albendazole Thiabendazole	Durlin-Ortiz et al. (1992) Frayha (1981)	51 52
Trichuris (T. trichuria)	Arthritis	Mebendazole	Treusch et al. (1981)	53
Wuchereria (filiaria)	Arthralgi a/Arthritis Myositis vasculitis	Diethylcarbamazine Diethylcarbamazine	Chaturverdi et al. (1993) Narasimhan et al. (1992)	54 55

References

1. Zelmer DA. An evolutionary definition of parasitism. *Int J Parasitol* 1998;28:531–533.

2. Poulin R, Combes C. The concept of virulence: interpretations and implications. *Parasitol Today* 1999;15(12):474–475.

3. Abbas AK, Lichtman AH, Pober JS. *Cellular and molecular immunology*, 3rd edn. W.B. Saunders, Philadelphia PA,1997.

4. Abu-Shakra M, Buskila D, Shoenfeld Y. Molecular mimicry between host and pathogen: examples from parasites and implication. *Immunol Lett* 1999;67:147–152.

5. Mannheimer SB, Sloave R. Protozoal infections in patients with AIDS. Cryptosporidiosis, isosporiasis, cyclosporiasis, and microsporidiosis. *Infect Dis Clin North Am* 1994;8:483.

6. Ferraccioli GF, Mercadanti M, Salaffi F et al. Prospective rheumatological study of muscle and joint symptoms during *Trichinella nelsoni* infection. *Q J Med* 1988;69:973–984.

7. Garcia LS. Diagnosis of parasitic infections: collection, processing and examination of specimens. In: Murray PR et al. *Manual of clinical microbiology* 6th edn. ASM Press, Washington DC, 1995:1145–1158.

8. Weiss JB. DNA probes and PCR for diagnosis of parasitic infections. *Clin Microbiol Rev* 1995;8:113.

9. Tripathy SK, Sen RK, Akkina N et al. Role of ultrasonography and magnetic resonance imaging in the diagnosis of intramuscular cysticercosis. *Skeletal Radiol* 2012;41(9):1061–1066.

10. Tejera B, Grados D, Martinez-Morillo M et al. Artritis reactiva por Blastocystis hominis. *Reumatol Clin* 2012;8(1):50–51.

11. Hay EM, Windfield J, McKendrick MW. Reactive arthritis associated with cryptosporidium enteritis. *BMJ* 1987;295:248.

12. Than-Saw, Mar-Mar-Nyein, Oo MM et al. Isolation of *Entamoeba histolytica* from arthritic knee joint *Trop Geogr Med* 1992;44(4):355–358.

13. Demircin G, Oner A, Erdoğan O, Bülbül M, Memiş L. Henoch Schönlein purpura and amebiasis. *Acta Paediatr Jpn* 1998;40(5):489–491.

14. Schirmer M, Fischer M, Rossboth DW et al. Entamoeba hartmanni: a new causative agent in the pathogenesis of reactive arthritis? *Rheumatol Int* 1998;18(1):37–38.

15. Woo P, Panayi GS. Reactive arthritis due to infestation with Giardia lamblia. *J Rheumatol* 1984;11:719.

16. Gonzalez-Dominguez J, Roldan R, Villanueva JL et al. *Isospora belli* reactive arthritis in a patient with AIDS. *Ann Rheum Dis*1994;53:618–619.

17. Coyle CM, Weiss LM, Rhodes LV 3rd et al. Fatal myositis due to the microsporidian Brachiola algerae, a mosquito pathogen *N Engl J Med* 2004;351(1):42–47.

18. Swash M, Scwartz MS. Malaria myositis. *J Neurol Neurosurg Psychiatry* 1993;56:1238.

19. Van Den Enden E, Praet M, Joos R et al. Eosinophilic myositis resulting from sarcocystosis. *J Trop Med Hyg* 1995;98(4):273–276.

20. Balleari E, Cutolo M, Accardo S Adult-onset Still's disease associated with *Toxoplasma gondii* infection. *Clin Rheumatol* 1991;10:326–327.

21. Carmeni G, Toto A, Martusciello S et al. Vascular involvement and toxoplasma infection. *Br J Dermatol* 1991;124:14.

22. Damian MS, Dorndorf W, Burkhardt H et al. Polyneuritis and myositis in *Trypanosoma gambiense* infection. *Dtsch Med Wochenschr* 1994; 119/49:1690–1693.

23. Ferreira MS, Nishioka Sde A, Silvestre MT et al. Reactivation of Chagas disease in patients with AIDS. *Clin Infect Dis* 1997;25(6):1397–1400.

24. Bissonnette B, Beaudet F. Reactive arthritis with eosinophilic synovial infiltrations. *Ann Rheum Dis* 1983;42:466–468.

25. Chauhan A, Scott DGI, Neuberger J, Gaston JSH, Bacon PA. Churg-Strauss vasculitis and ascaris infection. *Ann Rheum Dis* 1990;49:320–322.

26. Flieder DB, Moran CA. Pulmonary dirofilariasis: a clinicopathologic study of 41 lesions in 39 patients. *Hum Pathol* 1999;30(3):251–256.

27. Garf AE. Parasitic rheumatism: rheumatic manifestations associated with calcified Guinea worm. *J Rheumatol* 1985;12:976–979.

28. Kothari ML, Pardnani DS, Mehta L, Anand MP. Guinea-worm arthritis of knee joint. *Br Med J* 1968;iii(5615):435–436.

29. Reddy CR, Sivaramappa M. Guinea-worm arthritis of knee joint. *Br Med J* 1968;i(5585):155–156.

30. Bakkaloglu A, Soylemezoglu O, Tinaztepe K et al. A possible relationship between polyarteritis nodosa and hydatid disease. *Eur J Paediatr* 1994;153:469.

31. Llanos C, Soto L, Sabugo F et al. Systemic vasculitis associated with *Fasciola hepatica* infection *Scand J Rheumatol* 2006;35(2):143–146.

32. Thomas B, Ciocan D, Jacobson M et al. Cutaneous gnathostomiasis in New York City. *J Cutan Pathol* 2009;36(1) (abstract).

33. Bouvet JP, Therizol M, Auquier L. Microfilarial polyarthritis in a massive Loa Loa infestation. *Acta Trop* 1977;34(3):281–284.

34. Carme B, Mamboueni JP, Copin N et al. Clinical and biological study of Loa-Loa filariasis in Congolese. *Am J Trop Med Hyg* 1989;41:331–337.

35. Sohn BS, Bae YJ, Cho YS, Moon HB, Kim TB. Three cases of paragonimiasis in a family. *Korean J Parasitol* 2009;47(3):281–285.

36. Clement A, Treves R, Pitrou E. Articular manifestations in Schistosoma mansoni and their regression under niridazole treatment *Rhumatologie* 1979;31(9):343–346.

37. Atkin SL, Kamel M, El-Hady AMA et al. Schistosomiasis and inflammatory polyarthritis: a clinical, radiological and laboratory study of 96 patients infected by *S. mansoni* with particular reference to the diarthrodial joint. *Q J Med* 1986;59:479–487.

38. Bassiouni M, Kamel M. Bilharzial arthropathy. *Ann Rheum Dis* 1984;43:806–809.

39. Lee KJ, Myung NH, Park HW. A case of sparganosis in the leg. *Korean J Parasitol* 2010;48(4):309–312.

40. Bocanegra TS, Espinoza LR, Bridgeford PH et al. Reactive arthritis induced by parasitic infestation. *Ann Intern Med* 1981;94:207–209.

41. Akoglu T, Tuncer I, Erken E et al. Parasitic arthritis induced by *Strongyloides stercoralis*. *Ann Rheum Dis* 1984;43:523–525.

42. Richter J, Müller-Stöver I, Strothmeyer H et al. Arthritis associated with *Strongyloides stercoralis* infection in HLA B-27-positive African. *Parasitol Res* 2006;99(6):706–707.

43. van Kuijk AWR, Kerstens PJSM, Perenboom RM et al. Early onset polyarthritis as presenting feature of intestinal infection with *Strongyloides stercoralis*. *Rheumatology* 2003;42(11):1419–1420.

44. Templeton AC. Human coeneurosis infection: a report of 14 cases from Uganda. *Trans Roy Soc Trop Med Hyg* 1968;62:251–255.

45. Estanol B, Corona T, Abad P. A prognostic classification of cerebral cysticercosis: therapeutic implications. *J Neurol Neurosurg Psychiatr* 1986;49:1131–1134.

46. Nagaraj C, Singh S, Joshi A, Trikha V. Cysticercosis of biceps brachii: a rare cause of posterior interosseous nerve syndrome. *Joint Bone Spine* 2008;75(2):219–221.

47. Chopra JS, Nand N, Jain K, Mittal R, Abrol L. Generalized muscular pseudohypertrophy in cysticercosis *Postgrad Med J* 1986;62(726): 299–300.

48. William D, Roy S. Arthritis and arthralgia associated with toxocaral infestation. *BMJ* 1981;283:192.

49. Walsh SS, Robson WJ, Hart CA Acute transient myositis due to *Toxocara*. *Arch Dis Child* 1988;63:1087–1088.

50. Rayes AA, Lambertucci JR. Human toxocariasis as a possible cause of eosinophilic arthritis. *Rheumatology* 2001;40:109.

51. Durán-Ortiz JS, Garcia de la Torre J, Orozco-Barocio I et al. Trichinosis with severe myopathic involvement mimicking polymyositis. Report of a family outbreak. *J Rheumatol* 1992;19, 310–312.

52. Frayha RA. Trichinosis related polyarteritis nodosa. *Am J Med* 1981;71:307–312.

53. Treusch PJ, Swatnam RE, Woelke BJ. Eosinophilic joint effusion and intestinal nematodiasis. *Ann Emerg Med* 1981;10:614–615.

54. Chaturvedi P, Gawdi AM, Parkhe K, Harinath BC, Dey SK. Arthritis in children: an occult manifestation of Bancroftian filariasis. *Indian J Pediatr* 1993; 60(6):803–807.

55. Narasimhan C, George TJ, Thomas George K et al. *W. bancrofti* as a causal agent of polymyositis. *J Assoc Physicians India* 1992;40(7): 471–472.

56. Nigro L, Larocca L, Massarelli L et al. A placebo-controlled treatment trial of *Blastocystis hominis* infection with metronidazole *J Travel Med* 2003;10(2):128.

57. Rossignol JF, Kabil SM, Said M, Samir H, Younis AM. Effect of nitazoxanide in persistent diarrhea and enteritis associated with *Blastocystis hominis*. *Clin Gastroenterol Hepatol* 2005;3(10):987.

58. Cañete R, Escobedo AA, González ME, Almirall P, Cantelar N. A randomized, controlled, open-label trial of a single day of mebendazole versus a single dose of tinidazole in the treatment of giardiasis in children *Curr Med Res Opin* 2006;22(11):2131.

59. Hoerauf A, Volkmann I, Hamelmann C et al. Endosymbiotic bacteria in worms as targets for a novel chemotherapy in filiriasis. *Lancet* 2000;355(9211):1242–1243.

60. Bocanegra TS. Parasitic involvement. In: Oxford textbook of rheumatology, 2nd edn. Oxford University Press, Oxford, 1998: 945–954.

61. Ottesen EA. Description of mechanisms and control of reactions to treatment in human filiriases. *Ciba Found Symp* 1987;127:265–283.

62. Kumaraswami V, Ottesen EA, Vijeyasekaran V et al. Ivermectin for the treatment of *Wuchereria bancrofti* filariasis: efficacy and adverse reactions. *JAMA* 1988;259:3150–3153.

CHAPTER 106

Fungal arthritis

Carol A. Kemper and Stanley C. Deresinski

Introduction

Fungal infection of joints is an uncommon but challenging clinical problem whose recognition and management is often belated. A high degree of suspicion for fungal infection must be maintained in the face of persistent monoarticular or, less commonly, asymmetric polyarticular, arthritis, especially in an immunosuppressed host. Fungal joint infection most often results from the haematogenous dissemination of the pathogen from a primary portal of infection (usually pulmonary) directly to the synovial tissue, or occurs as the result of infection of para-articular bone with subsequent rupture into a joint space. Less commonly, such infection occurs as the result of direct inoculation of the organism into the joint space or synovial tissue. An inflammatory, aseptic arthritis may also occur in association with certain fungal infections (e.g. coccidioidomycos is,histoplasmosis) as a consequence of the immune response to the organism, rather than a result of infection of the joint space itself.

Epidemiology

Only a handful of fungi, perhaps five or six species at most, are responsible for most human mycotic musculoskeletal infections (Table 106.1),[1,2] but virtually all of the approximately 100 fungi pathogenic in humans have been reported to cause infection of bones and/or joints. The frequency with which fungal arthritis occurs, its clinical presentation, and its outcome varies depending on the specific pathogen as well as upon host variables. For example, fungal arthritis due to the endemic dimorphic fungi, such as *Histoplasmosis capsulatum*, *Blastomycosis dermatiditis*, and *Coccidioides immitis*, is often seen in patients without overt immunodeficiency. In contrast, infection due to candida species is usually found in association with intravascular infection in individuals with readily apparent host factors, such as indwelling central venous catheters (often in association with the administration of long-term antibiotic therapy and/or parenteral nutrition), haemodialysis, or intravenous drug use. Defects in cellular immunity are critical to the dissemination of certain fungi from their initial portal of infection and the secondary infection of joint spaces. Patients with haematological malignancy, haematopoietic and organ transplant recipients, and those receiving long-term corticosteroids and immunosuppressive therapy (including biological agents for rheumatoid arthritis) are especially at risk for fungal arthritis due to candida. Rarely, joint infection occurs secondary to direct inoculation of the organism

into the joint during aspiration or injection, trauma, or surgical intervention. Unlike the other fungi, infection with *C. albicans* and related yeasts is ordinarily the consequence of host invasion by endogenous colonizing organisms. In contrast, exposure to *B. dermatiditis*, *C. immitis*, *H. capsulatum*, or *Paracoccidioides brasiliensis* primarily occurs because of exposure within an endemic area (see Table 106.1). Two of the more common fungi found in joint space infections, *C. neoformans* and *Sporothrix schenckii*, have a worldwide distribution.

Clinical picture

The clinical presentation of joint infection is generally indolent, although the onset of some infections, such as those due to *B. dermatiditis*, candida species, and occasionally other fungi, may be acute, with hot, erythematous, tender joints and accompanying fever. The presentation may thus resemble an acute bacterial septic arthritis. Most cases, however, present with the usual findings of monoarticular (or occasionally asymmetric polyarticular) arthritis with decreased range of motion, tenderness, and swelling. There is often evidence of joint effusion; but in some cases of chronic infection due to *C. immitis*, joint swelling may be due to synovial proliferation rather than the accumulation of fluid. The initial list of differential diagnoses may therefore be quite broad, and includes septic arthritis, rheumatoid arthritis, mycobacterial infection, brucellosis, and pigmented villonodular synovitis. While fungal arthritis may present in the setting of widespread fungal infection, in many instances there is little clinical evidence of extra-articular infection. Large weightbearing joints, particularly the knee, are the usual targets. Radiographic findings that may be seen with varied frequency, depending include erosion of juxta-articular cortex, osteoporosis, and associated para-articular osteomyelitis. Clinically important information about joint integrity and the presence of otherwise unapparent para-articular osteomyelitis may be provided by MRI, which has greater sensitivity and resolution than other conventional techniques (see Chapter 68). Synovial fluid examination reveals an elevated white blood cell count. Although candidal and blastomycotic joint infections typically present with frankly purulent synovial fluid with a predominance of polymorphonuclear leucocytes, the other fungi often cause lesser degrees of inflammation with lower cell counts and variable predominance of either polymorphonuclear leucocytes or lymphocytes. The protein concentration is usually in excess of 3.0 g/dL while the glucose concentration is

Table 106.1 Risk factors for infection and the clinical setting of fungal joint infection

Organism	Endemicity	Host risk factors	Mode of infection	Joint involvement
Candida spp.	Normal human commensal	Haematological malignancy, immunodeficiency, neonates, indwelling catheters, central catheters, long-term antibioticuse, exogenous steroids	Haematogenous, rarely direct inoculation from trauma or injections	Monoarticular; predominately large joints (knee 70%)
Coccidioides immitis	Arizona, New Mexico, California	Usually immunocompetent host	Haematogenous	Monoarticular (90%); predominately knee and ankle
Blastomyces dermatitidis	Ohio, Missouri, Mississippi river valley, south-eastern USA, Africa, Middle East	Usually immunocompetent host (>90%)	Haematogenous rarely direct inoculation	Monoarticular (90%); knee ankle, elbow, and wrist
Sporothrix schenkii	Worldwide	Alcoholic, diabetic, rarely severely immunocompromised	Haematogenous, may be direct inoculation	Monoarticular (50%), polyarticular (50%); knee, ankle, wrist, small joints of the hand
Histoplasma capsulatum	Ohio, Missouri, Mississippi river valleys, Central and South America	Both normal and immuno- deficient hosts (e.g. AIDS)	Haematogenous	Monoarticular; knee, wrist, small joints of the hand
Cryptococcus neoformans	Worldwide	Organ transplant, AIDS, haematological, malignancy, diabetes, exogenous steroids	Haematogenous	Monoarticular (65%), polyarticular (35%); knee(60%), ankle, wrist, sterno/acromio-clavicular
Paracoccidioides brasiliensis	Central and South America	Immunocompetent host	Haematogenous	

low to normal. Routine direct examination (e.g. Gram stain) usually does not reveal the organism, but cytological preparations are useful in the diagnosis of blastomycosis, cryptococcus, and, to a lesser degree, coccidioidomycosis. Culture of synovial fluid or synovial tissue usually yields the organism. Synovial tissue histopathology is variable and often non-specific, as in infection due to *S. schenckii* in which the organisms are few and difficult to visualize. A granulomatous reaction is most commonly observed. The use of additional diagnostic procedures, such as blood cultures, bone marrow examination and culture, antibody tests, or tests for the detection of fungal antigen in serum or other body fluids, depends upon the clinical setting and the suspected aetiology. Tests of delayed dermal hypersensitivity to fungal antigens are generally not useful for diagnostic purposes. Some infections may cause tenosynovitis in the absence of osteomyelitis or arthritis. Tenosynovitis may occur as the result of haematogenous dissemination or direct inoculation, and is most often associated with *S. schenkii* infection, and less frequently, with infections due to *C. immitis* and *C. neoformans*. During the primary pulmonary infection with *C. immitis*, an acute self-limiting arthritis or periarthritis, commonly referred to as 'desert rheumatism', may be seen in association with erythema nodosum, erythema multiforme, and occasionally hilar adenopathy. Thus, the clinical picture may resemble sarcoidosis.

Management

Amphotericin B remains the initial therapeutic agent of choice for many serious fungal infections, especially for those who are severely immunosuppressed, have life-threatening or central nervous system disease, or who have failed azole therapy. Lipid-associated or -complexed formulations of amphotericin allow the administration of higher dosages of drug with less toxicity than the conventional

formulation, but are substantially more expensive. The triazoles, fluconazole and itraconazole, especially in the outpatient setting, have similar efficacy but reduced toxicity and morbidity compared to amphotericin B. Newer azoles, voriconazole and posaconazole, are available. The echinocandins caspofungin, anidulafungin, and micafungin may prove to have a role in the treatment of selected infections. 5-fluoroctosine (5-FC) is used much less frequently.

Individual mycoses

Aspergillus

Aspergillus rarely results in joint space infection. Severely immunosuppressed hosts, such as those with haematopoetic and organ transplants, haematological malignancy and intra-articular steroid injection, are at greatest risk for aspergillus infection.[3] Clinically apparent pulmonary infection is present in two-thirds of patients with disseminated aspergillus. Haematogenous dissemination of the organism is implicated in most cases, although introduction of the organism into the joint space has occurred during surgical or arthroscopic procedures, or as a result of trauma.

Voriconazole is the treatment of choice for life-threatening invasive aspergillus infection, but amphotericin B, caspofungin, posaconazole, and micafungin are alternatives.

Blastomycosis

Blastomycosis is an uncommonly encountered mycotic infection endemic in parts of the United States (Table 106.1). *B. dermatiditis* is a thermal dimorph whose mycelial phase is thought to reside in soil. Primary pulmonary infection maybe acute, subacute, or subclinical, but is usually self-limited; chronic infections are unusual. Haematogenous dissemination is relatively frequent during the initial phase of the disease, leading to infection at almost any body site. Skin and bones are the most frequent sites of dissemination (25–60%), and only 2.5–8% of patients develop joint infection.[4] Patients with particularly severe pulmonary disease or miliary involvement, or those who are immunocompromised, are at the greatest risk for dissemination.[5] Myalgias and arthralgias are common during the acute pulmonary phase of the disease, but erythema nodosum is not. The arthritis is monoarticular in more than 95% of cases with the knee most commonly involved (see Table 106.2). Joint pain is often acute in onset and patients usually appear toxic. In contrast to coccidioidal arthritis, active pulmonary disease is present in more than 90% of patients with joint involvement, and more than 70% have evidence of additional dissemination. Synovial fluid findings are similar to those seen in candida arthritis. Definitive diagnosis requires growth of the organism. A presumptive diagnosis may be made by visualization of the yeast in synovial biopsy specimens.

Itraconazole is the drug of choice for most forms of the disease; amphotericin B is reserved for the more severe forms. Newer azoles such as voriconazole and posaconazole have a limited role in the treatment of pulmonary blastomycosis.[6]

Candida species

C. albicans is a normal commensal of humans, and endogenous colonization is the source of most infections by candida species. Deep tissue infection generally occurs after amplification of colonization during an intervening immunodeficient state or during administration of broad-spectrum antibacterial therapy coupled with breaches in integumentary and mucosal barriers. Candida infection of joints is typically the consequence of haematogenous dissemination (often from indwelling intravenous catheters in predisposed immunodeficient hosts or in intravenous drug users).[7] Joints previously afflicted by rheumatoid arthritis appear to be at increased risk of infection with candidal organisms (Table 106.1).

Candida joint infection is acute in approximately two-thirds of cases. The large joints are most commonly affected. Synovial fluid examination demonstrates a markedly elevated white blood cell count with a predominance of polymorphonuclear leucocytes (Table 106.2). Candida can be observed on Gram stain. Histological examination of synovium reveals mononuclear cell infiltration but usually an absence of granulomata. Synovial fluid or tissue consistently yield the organism in culture. Recovery of the organism from blood cultures may provide an important clue to the aetiology of the joint process.

Intravenously administered amphotericin B, with or without 5-FC, remains the standard of treatment for immediately life-threatening infection.[8] Fungal susceptibility studies, performed by a reliable laboratory, may help to guide therapy in more complicated cases. Caspofungin may also prove efficacious. Repeated joint aspiration is usually indicated. Surgical debridement, both to confirm the diagnosis and to remove infected tissues, is often necessary (in addition to antifungal chemotherapy), particularly in cases of hip joint infection.

Prosthetic joint infection

Fungal infection of total joint arthroplasties is rare.[9] Infection is a consequence of implantation of skin microflora during surgery. The infections are clinically low-grade, and indolent. Pain, decreased range of motion, and peri-articular swelling are common. Sinus tracts may be seen. Radiographs show evidence of loosening and adjacent areas of osteolysis indicative of osteomyelitis.

Technetium pyrophosphate and gallium nitrate scans are not useful, since they are often positive in the presence of a loosened prosthesis, regardless of the presence of infection. Consistent with a more subacute presentation, synovial fluid white blood cell counts are less inflammatory than that typically seen in native joint infections (4000–15 000/mm^3).

Table 106.2 Clinical and laboratory data helpful in the diagnosis of fungal joint infection

Organism	Serology	Synovial fluid white cell count	Synovial glucose	Synovial fluid examination	Culture
Candida spp.	Not useful	Frankly purulent, <100 000/mm^3	Variable, low to normal	20% positive	Blood and/or synovial fluid, >95% positive
Coccidioides immitis	Complement fixation, immunodiffusion diagnostic	<50 000/mm^3, mononuclear cells	Low	Rarely positive	Synovial fluid, >95% positive
Blastomyces dermatitidis	Low sensitivity, low specificity	Frankly purulent, <100 000/mm^3 polymorphonuclear	Variable, low to normal	By cytological preparation, 90% positive	Synovial fluid, 50% positive
Sporothrix schenkii	Not available	2000–60 000/mm^3 lymphocytes and polymorphonuclear	Variable, low to normal	Rarely positive	Synovial tissue more often positive than synovial fluid
Histoplasma capsulatum	Complement fixation, immunodiffusion diagnostic			Not helpful	Blood and/or synovial fluid, 20–25% positive
Cryptococcus neoformans	Cryptococcal antigen diagnostic	200–5000/mm^3	Variable, usually normal	Indian ink very helpful	Blood and/or synovial fluid, 80% positive
Paracoccidioides brasiliensis	Serum antibody			Not helpful	Usually positive, slow growth (>4 weeks)

Amphotericin B, with or without fluconazole,[9] in combination with removal of the prosthesis and other foreign material, and debridement of affected tissue is the initial treatment of choice.

Coccidioidomycosis

Coccidioides immitis is endemic to soils, with most cases resulting from exposure to airborne arthroconidia (Table 106.1). Risk factors include ethnicity (especially African and Pacific Island ancestry), male gender, and immunosuppression (Table 106.1). Upon reaching the alveoli of the infected host, the organism, a tissue dimorph, converts to the spherule–endospore phase. Approximately one-half of infected patients become symptomatic and, in the vast majority of these, the infection is self-limiting with influenza-like symptoms. Transient arthralgias or aseptic inflammatory arthritis, which probably represents an immunologically mediated inflammatory process similar to erythema nodosum, occur in 3–5% of patients with primary pulmonary coccidioidomycosis. Treatment consists of the administration of non-steroidal anti-inflammatory agents.

Clinically important extrapulmonary dissemination occurs in fewer than 0.5% of cases. Most cases that occur outside an endemic area are the result of travel to an endemic area by someone with no pre-existing immunity.

Skeletal infection occurs in up to 10–50% of patients with disseminated disease, and is frequently multicentric with axial involvement.[10,11] Monoarticular arthritis occurs in more than 90% of cases, with large weightbearing joints, particularly the knee and ankle, being most frequently affected. Although the larger joints are more commonly involved in adults, the small joints of the hand appear to be more commonly affected in children. At the time of presentation with joint disease, occult sites of dissemination are present in up to 25% of cases. Extrapulmonary sites of infection, including meningeal, bone, and joint infection, should, therefore, be avidly sought for in any patient with disseminated coccidioidomycosis. Some patients may initially present with an acutely inflamed joint, but most infections are indolent with progressive effusion and synovial thickening. The diagnosis of joint infection is often delayed, and chronic infection frequently results in significant articular and bony destruction with resultant loss of joint function (see Figure 106.1a). Occasionally, chronic arthrocutaneous fistulas develop with drainage of synovial fluid (Figure 106.1b). Radiographic examination may be unremarkable during the initial phase of infection; effusion, and erosion of articular cortex and adjacent osteoporosis are commonly seen as the infection progresses. MRI in adults with coccidioidal arthritis frequently reveals synovitis, subarticular bone loss, and loss of cartilage, but less frequent marrow involvement.[11]

Synovial fluid is inflammatory with total white blood cell counts as high as 50 000/mm³ (Table 106.2). Culture of synovial fluid yields the organism in approximately 50% of cases, usually within 3–6 days. Greater yield is seen with culture and histological examination of synovial tissue. The affected proliferative synovium, which often invades cartilage and articular surfaces, exhibits granulomatous villonodular inflammatory changes with the characteristic endosporulating spherules visible on microscopic examination. Most importantly, if coccidioidomycosis infection is suspected, the microbiology laboratory must be notified because of the significant biohazard represented by this organism in culture. Several serological techniques are available for establishing the diagnosis.

Among the endemic fungal infections, coccidioidomycosis is the most recalcitrant to therapy. Patient prognosis depends upon the extent of dissemination to other sites, particularly the central nervous system. Treatment consists of systemic administration of antifungal agents. Amphotericin B remains the treatment of choice in many cases, especially for those with life-threatening disease, central nervous system involvement, and immunosuppression, as well as those who have failed appropriate azole therapy. Patients with disseminated disease often receive a total of 1.0–2.5 g of amphotericin B.[12] Patients with skeletal infection may do better in response to itraconazole rather than fluconazole.[13] Continued therapy is indicated until remission has been achieved, as defined by objective clinical measures, and improvement in serological and radiographic data. Lifelong therapy for disseminated infection is often necessary. The need for synovectomy and debridement of infected bone and tissue remain controversial. Despite appropriate medical and surgical intervention, the joint infection often remains progressive and disabling.

Cryptococcosis

Cryptococcus neoformans is worldwide in distribution. Skin test surveys suggest that subclinical infection is quite common in normal

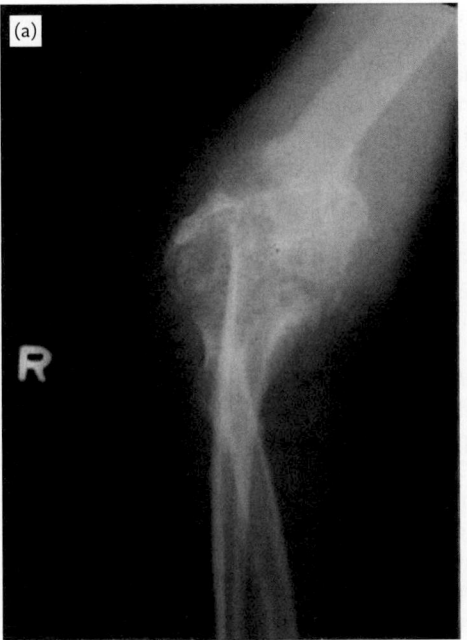

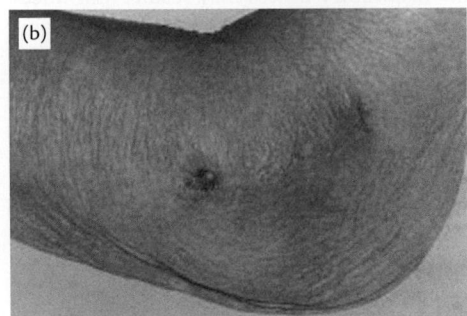

Fig. 106.1 (a) Radiograph of the right elbow demonstrating destruction of the articular cortex and osteomyelitis of contiguous bone, and (b) sinus formation in an elderly woman with chronic coccidioidal arthritis of many years' duration despite multiple courses of antifungal therapy.
Courtesy of Jesse Hofflin.

hosts. Clinical disease occurs predominantly, but not exclusively, in individuals with defects in cellular immunity (Table 106.1). Patients with renal failure and HIV infection are especially vulnerable to infection with this encapsulated yeast. The primary portal of entry for the organism is believed to be the respiratory tract, although clinical recognizable pulmonary infection is infrequent. Haematogenous dissemination leads to varying organ involvement, although the organism has a particular predilection for the brain and meninges.

Cryptococcal arthritis, frequently associated with areas of contiguous osteomyelitis and osteomyelitis, occurs in up to 10% of patients with systemic disease.[14] Although soft tissue swelling, inflammation, and frank cellulitis have been reported in cases of cryptococcal joint infection, most cases are indolent in presentation. The knee is involved in approximately 60% of reported cases, followed by an equal number of cases in the sternoclavicular and acromioclavicular joints, elbow, wrist, and ankle (Table 106.2). Approximately one-third of the cases are polyarticular. Radiographs demonstrate an erosive arthritis and juxta-articular osteomyelitis. CT scans often show evidence of surrounding soft tissue inflammation. *C. neoformans* can be visualized using Indian ink. Examination of the synovial fluid reveals a white blood cell count of 200–20 000/mm^3, with a predominance of mononuclear cells. The peripheral white blood cell count and erythrocyte sedimentation rate are often normal.

Amphotericin B may be administered as initial therapy in most cases of life-threatening, disseminated infection. Many experts advocate the concomitant administration of 5-FC for approximately 4 weeks for more severe infection. Once the systemic disease is under control and the joint disease is improving, consideration can be given to completing treatment with fluconazole. Debridement may be useful, especially in cases with significant synovial thickening and peri-articular extension of infection.

Histoplasmosis

Histoplasmosis capsulatum is endemic to many areas within the temperate zones of the world, but is most heavily concentrated in the Ohio, Mississippi, and Missouri River valleys of the United States (Table 106.1). The organism is a thermal dimorph with the mycelial phase existing in soil, generally in association with bird and bat guano. Large outbreaks occur in urban endemic areas. Speleologists throughout the world may be at risk. Upon inhalation by the human or animal host, microconidia reach the alveoli where they convert to the yeast phase. While more than 95% of infections are subclinical, a flu-like respiratory illness may result from infection. Haematogenous dissemination is rare and occurs most commonly in patients with impaired cellular immunity. People with HIV infection who travel to or have previously lived in an endemic area are at risk for reactivation disease.

Immunologically mediated arthralgias and aseptic inflammatory arthritis, similar to that reported for coccidioidomycosis, are common in primary histoplasmosis.[15] Erythema nodosum and erythema multiforme may also occur. During a single outbreak of acute histoplasmosis in 381 symptomatic patients, 16 (4.1%) developed arthralgias and 6 (1.6%) developed aseptic arthritis.[15] The knees, ankles, wrists, and small joints of the hands were the most common sites of involvement; approximately 50% of the cases were polyarticular. The synovial fluid is inflammatory. This clinical problem is self-limited and is treated with non-steroidal anti-inflammatory agents. In contrast to candidiasis and

coccidioidomycosis, infection of the synovium or joint space by *H. capsulatum* is exceedingly rare.[16] Juxta-articular osteomyelitis is often present. Joint involvement is usually monoarticular and has been reported in both apparently immunologically normal and compromised hosts.

The diagnosis of histoplasmosis can be made by culture of both blood and infected sites, including synovial fluid, and histologic demonstration of the infecting organism. The organism is readily cultivated on a variety of media. Detection of histoplasma antigen in serum or urine is useful in the diagnosis of disseminated histoplasmosis. Although both false-positive and false-negative results occur, antibody tests may be useful.

Amphotericin B remains the initial treatment of choice for severe, life-threatening forms of histoplasmosis. Itraconazole, is effective for mild to moderately severe infection.[17]

Paracoccidioidomycosis

Paracoccidioidomycosis is endemic only to areas of Central and South America where it is the most commonly encountered respiratory mycotic infection. *Paracoccidioides brasiliensis* is thermally dimorphic, and as is true for the other dimorphic fungi, conidia released by the mycelial phase of the fungus are inhaled and convert to the yeast phase in the alveoli. Acute, self-limited pulmonary infection may occur, although most patients present with chronic pulmonary disease and evidence of chronic haematogenous dissemination, including painful granulomata of the skin, lymphadenopathy, and ulceration of mucous membranes. Osteoarticular infection is typically multifocal with osteomyelitis of long bones; lesions are ostelytic without sclerosis or periosteal reaction.[18] Articular involvement occurs in one-third, but primary arthritis is rare. Infection is most common in children and adolescents. The diagnosis is usually made on the basis of visualization of the organisms in synovial fluid or tissues, or by culture. Serological tests have been utilized with varying success.

Although the disease is rarely encountered outside endemic areas, the diagnosis should be suspected in any individual at epidemiological risk. Paracoccidioidomycosis primarily occurs in individuals without evidence of immune dysfunction,

Amphotericin B is effective in the treatment of disseminated paracoccidioidomycosis, although itraconazole (and ketoconazole) appear as effective in the treatment of less severe cases.[19] Relapses after treatment are common, and chronic suppressive therapy with one of the azoles or a sulfonamide is therefore recommended.

Sporotrichosis

Sporothrix schenckii, a tissue dimorph, is commonly found on decaying vegetation and in soil in many areas of the world. Infections are both sporadic and epidemic. In contrast to the other soil fungi, cutaneous disease occurs secondary to the inoculation of the organism as a result of trauma to the skin. The lymphocutaneous form, with the development of an ulcer at the site of cutaneous inoculation and proximal nodules in the area of lymphatic drainage, is the most common manifestation of infection.[20] People at particular risk for this infection include rose cultivators and those who handle soil and sphagnum moss.

While arthralgias occur in approximately 2% of those with acute cutaneous or lymphocutaneous disease, infection of the joint space with *S. schenkii* is rare, having occurred in only 1 of 3300 patients (0.03%) in a large outbreak of sporotrichosis.[21] Arthritis may occur in the presence of widespread dissemination to other sites, but is much more common as an isolated finding.[22] Bayer and colleagues described 44 cases of sporotrichal joint infection, 20% of which were associated with systemic and pulmonary disease.[22] Most cases of sporotrichal arthritis are, therefore, believed to be due to haematogenous dissemination of the organism, although some cases may be the result of articular extension of infection from an adjacent site of osteomyelitis or skin infection or, occasionally, from direct inoculation of the organism into the joint. The majority of patients with systemic infection have predisposing underlying disease, including myeloproliferative disorders, malignancy, chronic corticosteroid use, and alcoholism.

Sporotrichal arthritis is an indolent and slowly progressive infectious process that predominantly affects the knee and other large weightbearing joints, although the small joints of the hand and wrist are also commonly affected. Calhoun and colleagues described 11 cases of systemic sporotrichosis; 8 involved the skeletal system with a total of 12 joints being affected, including the wrist (63%), knee (%), ankle (25%), and elbow and phalanx (13% each).[23] Monoarticular and polyarticular involvement occurs with equal frequency. Most cases present as a slowly progressive synovitis or tenosynovitis with pain, warmth, swelling, and restricted range of motion.[22,24]

Radiographic abnormalities are seen in more than 90% of cases, possibly reflecting the chronicity of infection prior to diagnosis. Osteoporosis of contiguous bone is the most common radiographic finding, followed by soft tissue swelling with effusion, punched-out osteolytic lesions, articular cartilage erosion, and joint space narrowing (Figure 106.2b,c).[22,25]

Synovial fluid white blood cell count is reported to range from 2800 to 60 000/mm^3 (Table 106.2). The diagnosis may be delayed because of the isolated nature of the infection, the rarity of visualizing the organism on smears of synovial fluid, the often non-specific nature of synovial histopathology (which may resemble that of rheumatoid or tuberculous arthritis), and the paucity of organisms in tissue (see Figure 106.2d). Asteroid bodies, often said to be pathognomonic of sporotrichosis, may, in fact, be seen in other infections. Isolation of the organism in culture is the cornerstone of diagnosis. Synovial tissue is more likely to yield the organism (usually within 5 days) than is synovial fluid.

Itraconazole is recommended for osteoarticular sporotrichosis, with amphotericin B as a second-line agent. Surgical debridement may also be necessary on occasion, but should be reserved for persistent culture positivity and in cases of tenosynovitis.

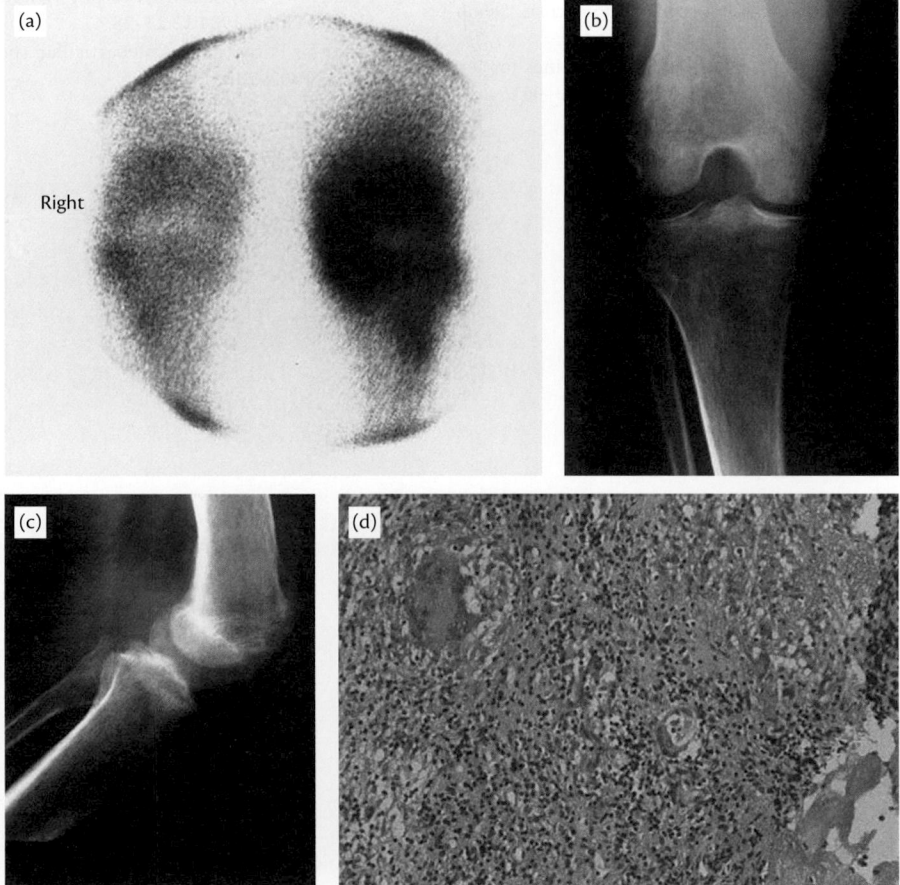

Fig. 106.2 (a) Bone scintigraphy, using technetium-99m, demonstrating intense uptake of the radionuclide in the left knee of a patient with synovitis due to Sporothrix schenckii. (b and c) Radiographs of the left knee from a patient with Sporothrix schenckii, demonstrating only patchy osteopenia of the distal femur and proximal tibia. (d) Granulomatous reaction with typical giant cells of synovium obtained from the same patient. Organisms were not visualized with this stain or with Gomori–methamine silver or periodic acid–Schiff (PAS) stains and the diagnosis was made by recovery of the organism in culture from the synovial tissue. Haematoxylin and eosin, original magnification ×200.
Courtesy of Jesse Hofflin.

References

1. Cuellar ML, Silveira LH, Espinoza LR. Fungal arthritis. *Ann Rheum Dis* 1992;51:690–697.
2. Cuellar ML, Silveira LH, Citera G, Cabrera GE, Valle R. Other fungal arthritides. *Rheum Dis Clin N Am* 1993;19:439–455..
3. Golmia R, Bello I, Marra A et al. Aspergillus fumigatus joint infection: a review. *Semin Arthritis Rheum* 2011;40:580–584.
4. McDonald PB, Black GB, MacKenzie R. Orthopaedic manifestations of blastomycosis. *J Bone Joint Surg* 1990;72A:860–864.
5. Davies SF, Sarosi GA. Clinical manifestations and management of blastomycosis in the compromised patient. In: Warnock DW, Richardson MD (eds) *Fungal infection in the compromised patient*, 2nd edn. Wiley, Chichester, 1991:215–229.
6. Bariola JR, Vyas KS. Pulmonary blastomycosis. *Semin Respir Crit Care Med* 2011;32(6):745–753.
7. Marina N, Flynn P, Rivera G, Hughes W. *Candida tropicalis* and *Candida albicans* fungemia in children with leukemia. *Cancer* 1991;68:594–599.
8. Mills EJ, Perri D, Cooper C et al. Antifungal treatment for invasive Candida infections: a mixed treatment comparison meta-analysis. *Ann Clin Microbiol Antimicrob* 2009;8:23.
9. Dutronc H, Dauchy FA, Cazanave C et al. Candida prosthetic infection: case series and literature review. *Scand J Infect Dis* 2010;42:890–895.
10. Deresinski SC. Coccidioidomycosis of the musculoskeletal system. In: Stevens D (ed.) *Coccidioidomycosis*. Plenum Press, New York, 1980:195–212.
11. Taljanovic MS, Adam RD Musculoskeletal coccidioidomycosis. *Semin Musculoskelet Radiol* 2011;15:511–526.
12. Galgiani J, Ampel NH, Catanzaro A et al. Practice guidelines for the treatment of coccidioidomycosis. *Clin Infect Dis* 2000;30:658–661.
13. Galgiani JN, Catanzaro A, Cloud GA et al. Comparison of oral fluconazole and itraconazole for progressive, nonmeningeal coccidiodomycosis: a randomized, double-blind trial. *Ann Intern Med* 2000;133:676–686.
14. Stead KJ, Klugman KP, Painter ML, Koornhof HJ. Septic arthritis due to Cryptococcus neoformans. *J Infect* 1988;17;139–145.
15. Rosenthal J, Brandt KD, Wheat JL, Slama TG. Rheumatologic manifestations of histoplasmosis in the recent Indianapolis epidemic. *Arthritis Rheum* 1983;26:1065–1070.
16. Weinberg, JM, Ali R, Badve S, Pelker RR. Musculoskeletal histoplasmosis. A case report and review of the literature. *J Bone Joint Surg* 2001;83A:1718–1722.
17. McKinsey Ds, McKinsey JP. Pulmonary histoplasmosis. *Semin Respir Crit Care Med* 2011;32:735–744.
18. Monsignore LM, Martinez R, Simao MN et al. Radiologic findings of osteoarticular infection in paracoccidioidomycosis. *Skeletal Radiol* 2012;41:203–208.
19. Kwon-Chung, KJ, Bennett JE. Paracoccidioidomycosis. In: Kwon-Chung KJ, Bennett JE (eds) Medical mycology. Lea & Febiger, Philadelphia, PA, 1992:594–619.
20. Belknap BS. Sporotrichosis. *Dermatol Clin* 1989;7:193–202.
21. Lurie HI. Five unusual cases of sporotrichosis from South Africa showing lesions in muscles, bones, and viscera. *Br J Surg* 1963;50:585–591.
22. Bayer AS, Scott VJ, Guze LB. Fungal arthritis. III. Sporothrichal arthritis. *Semin Arthritis Rheum* 1979;9:66–74.
23. Calhoun, DL, Waskin H, White MP et al. Treatment of systemic sporotrichosis with ketoconazole. *J Infect Dis* 1991;13:47–51.
24. Chang, AC, Destouet JM, Murphy WA. Musculoskeletal sporotrichosis. *Skeletal Radiol* 1984;12:23–28.
25. Jones N. Photo quiz. Osteoarticular sporothrichosis. *Clin Infect Dis* 1999;29:202–203.

CHAPTER 107

Opportunistic infection

Saraswathi Murthy and Susan Hopkins

Introduction

Approximately 400 000 adults (>600 per 100 000) living in the United Kingdom are affected by rheumatological diseases.[1] Infections in patients with rheumatological disease are common and contribute to morbidity and mortality in this group. This is largely due to an intrinsic immunomodulatory effect of the disease itself and end-organ damage; or due to the use of corticosteroids, disease-modifying anti-rheumatic drugs (DMARDs), and now more commonly biological agents.

Progression of rheumatoid arthritis (RA) disease has been associated with a greater likelihood of developing infection[2,3]; greater than twice the risk of the general population with risk of respiratory and skin and soft tissue infections most likely.[4] A recent European study looking at a cohort of 1000 systemic lupus erythematosus (SLE) patients found that 25% of patient deaths were due to infection alone.[5] Among patients with systemic sclerosis a recent study found that one-third of deaths not directly related to the disease itself were due to infection.[6]

The potential to acquire any infection relates to alterations in the host immune system, damage to epithelial barriers, and organ dysfunction related to the disease process. Low complement levels, impaired lymphocyte response and activation, as well as defective apoptosis and phagocytosis play a role in the immunodeficient state related to rheumatological disease. Skin damage from vasculitic disease or systemic sclerosis creates an impaired barrier in the normal defence innate defence system allowing for skin and soft tissue infection. Lung fibrosis related to RA, vasculitides, or systemic sclerosis (SSc) may alter the immunological milieu and increase the likelihood of pulmonary infection.

The use of biological agents continues to increase and although they have proven effective in controlling these disease processes they are unfortunately associated with an increase in bacterial, fungal, and viral infections including tuberculosis (TB) and non-tuberculous mycobacteria. The frequent use of corticosteroids in rheumatological disease has been consistently shown to increase the rate of bacterial, fungal, and viral infections. There appears to be a dose-related and cumulative dose relationship to this which needs to be taken into account with each patient.

There is therefore an increasing need for guidance in managing the patient with rheumatological disease who develops infection and, moreover, guidance on the prevention of developing infection is of paramount importance. This may be in the form of screening tests at the time of diagnosis, line care, vaccination, or secondary prophylaxis. This chapter provides an overview of the factors that potentiate infection risk within rheumatological diseases and with pharmacological therapies, the common infections encountered, their initial management, and preventable measures that should be undertaken.

Role of underlying disease in infection

RA has been shown to be an independent risk factor for hospitalization with a serious infection.[4] All infections are more common in RA patients than in the general population.[2–4] RA almost doubles the risk of developing community-acquired pneumonia, the likelihood of which correlates directly with disease activity.[7] Atrophic skin over affected joints allows microbial penetration of the skin and soft tissue. Rheumatoid vasculitis can result in ulceration of the skin, distal ischaemia of the digits, and ultimately gangrenous changes with resultant infection.

Neutropenia and splenomegaly, such as occurs in Felty's syndrome, results in splenic sequestration of immune complexes and neutrophils and renders the patients susceptible to encapsulated bacterial organisms (*Streptococcus pneumoniae*, *Haemophilus influenzae*, *Neisseria meningitidis*).

Other forms of arthritic disease such as psoriatic arthritis, ankylosing spondylitis, and enteropathic arthritis have a lower intrinsic risk of infection.[8]

SLE is associated with a significant risk of developing infection, and 50% of hospitalizations are related to infection.[9] One-quarter of deaths in lupus patients are caused by infection,[5] and infection is the second most common cause of death in the first 5 years after disease diagnosis.[10] Infection occurs predominantly in the respiratory, urinary, and skin systems and to organisms that take advantage of the gaps in the innate immune system posed by lupus itself.[5,9–13] A greater risk of developing infections in SLE has been shown with a SLE disease activity index (SLEDAI) score over 12, longer disease duration, renal involvement, and serological markers such as positive anti-dsDNA antibody levels.[9,11,14–17] Hypocomplementaemia and hyposplenism especially associated with lupus render the active lupus patient susceptible to infections with encapsulated organisms and non-typhoidal salmonella.[10] Mannose-binding lectin (MBL) polymorphism in SLE has been shown to increase the infection risk.[10,18] The active lupus patient is therefore more susceptible to viruses, mycobacterial disease, and fungal and protozoal infections.[9,18–20] Diagnosis of infection in the lupus patient may prove difficult as both infection and lupus flares cause a systemic inflammatory response and clinicians must be vigilant to intervene early in sepsis to improve outcome.

A recent large, multicentre prospective study[6] demonstrated that 33% of non-systemic sclerosis-related deaths were from infection or, put another way, in the overall cohort more than 1 in 8 deaths were infection related. Polymyositis and dermatomyositis are not commonly studied with regard to risk of infection but recent studies show that infection is also one of the leading causes of death in this patient group, representing approximately 30% of all patient deaths.[12,21]

Luqmani et al.[22] showed that the mortality within the first year of diagnosing Wegener's granulomatosis is nine times greater than in the general population and the most common cause of death is infection(32%) followed by active vasculitis and renal disease. In another study[23] looking at the long-term survival in 535 ANCA-positive vasculitis patients (Wegener's granulomatosis and microscopic polyangiitis) most deaths occurred within the first year and almost one-half of these deaths were infection related. It is important to note that all of the patients were on a combination of immunosuppressants.

Role of immunosuppressant treatment in infection

Glucocorticoids have a vital role in the management of patients with rheumatological disease,[1] to various degrees at different points in the disease history. They inhibit synthesis of the majority of cytokines including interleukin(IL)-1, interferon-gamma (INFγ) and tumour necrosis factor alpha (TNFα) while also reducing the production and impairing the function of macrophages. Although neutrophilia is a common feature of steroid use, this apparent increase in blood is related to the inability of these cells are to migrate to tissues where they are required. Leucocyte function is also impaired and is thought to be related to inhibition of endothelial adhesion. As a result, patients treated with glucocorticoids are at significant risk of developing infection with bacterial fungal or viral pathogens.[24,25] In a large cohort study, glucocorticoids use increased the relative risk of serious infection (requiring intravenous antibiotics or hospitalization) almost threefold.[26] The risk of opportunistic infections with doses equivalent to more than 10 mg of prednisolone daily or intravenous boluses of corticosteroids is clearly demonstrated.[25,27] Developing active TB infection on a DMARD is almost twice as likely if it is in combination with steroid rather than DMARD monotherapy.[28] Low-dose corticosteroids (<5–10 mg prednisolone) appear to have little or no significant infection risk whereas high daily doses (>20–30 mg) are associated with significant risk.[24,29–31] Few studies have looked at what the cut-off for the 'safe' dose of steroid would be and this would invariably depend on multiple factors related to the individual and disease.

The DMARDs have varying effects on the immune system and as a consequence some are much more strongly associated with different infections than others. Methotrexate is particularly associated with infections. Greenberg et al.[27] demonstrated an infection rate of 30.9 per 100 person-years in methotrexate users compared to other DMARDs (24.4 per 100 person-years). A recent systematic review[31] looking at methotrexate monotherapy for RA showed the greatest risk of infection is within the first 2 years of use.

Cyclophosphamide causes bone marrow suppression, reduced lymphocyte proliferation, and hypogammaglobulinaemia. In one study, it increased the risk of infection even more than glucocorticoids (relative risk of 3.3 compared to 2.6 for steroids).[26] Azathioprine and lefluonamide are also associated with infection.[26,32] Other DMARDs including gold, antimalarials, D-penicillamine, and sulfasalazine generally cause a state of hypogammaglobulinaemia and have not been linked to significant risks for developing infection in comparison to glucocorticords.[26,32,33]

The use of biological agents is a rapidly evolving area targeting specific parts of the immune system, which has changed management of autoimmune and rheumatological disease profoundly. Consequently the effects that this has on the rate and types of infections that can be acquired or reactivated are still being determined, especially as new agents are being licensed for use continuously.

Monoclonal antibodies against TNFα, such as infliximab, adalimumab and golimumab, and the soluble TNFα receptor fusion protein etanercept have been associated with a high risk of infection.[25,27,28,34–40] Higher incidences of intracellular pathogen-related infections occur with anti-TNF.[25,37] Both new infections and reactivations of TB are strongly associated with anti-TNF drugs (RR 1.6–25.1).[34] Infliximab is currently the most associated with serious infections,[25,31,37] although the 2011 Cochrane review[41] demonstrated that certolizumab was also associated with a high risk of serious infections. Infliximab confers twice the risk of TB reactivation compared to etanercept[34] and has been shown to cause a much faster presentation with a median interval from commencing treatment of only 12 weeks.[36,42] Non-tuberculous mycobacterial infection, most commonly *Mycobacterium avium*, has also been strongly associated with anti-TNF use.[43]

Rituximab results in a state of hypogammaglobulinaemia.[44] There does not appear to be a significant risk of opportunistic infection and no association has been shown relating to TB infection.[39,45,46] Some association has been made with rituximab and cytomegalovirus (CMV) and JC virus, leading to progressive multifocal leucoencephelopathy (PML).[47]

Tocilizumab, a monoclonal IL-6 antibody, has shown greater rates of bacterial, not opportunistic, infection during its use than rituximab or anti-TNF agents at 5.3 per 100 patient-years, though this may be related to comorbidities or previous DMARD history.[48] The effect of abatacept and anakinra on the incidence of infection remains unclear.[46]

Changing biological agents has appears to confer a greater rate of developing infections requiring hospitalization,[39] although patients switching regimens tend to have a larger number of comorbidities. Infections occur more often at the start of treatment and the risk of developing serious infection reduces with time.[35,43] Particular care should be taken around the time of therapy switches and commencement of new therapies, especially as the effects of infection may mimic the adverse effects of the drugs.

Diagnosis and treatment of infections

When managing patients with chronic multisystem disease, and especially while using immunomodulatory therapies, the clinician must be ever vigilant for early signs of infection. These individuals may not present with conventional symptoms and signs: inflammatory response will be suppressed; blood inflammatory markers and cerebrospinal fluid (CSF) white cell counts may be low or normal. A thorough knowledge of the travel, occupational, and medical history is essential to develop an accurate differential diagnosis.

When an acute infective process occurs on immunosuppressants, where possible these should be stopped immediately and recommenced after the infection is treated. Corticosteroids should of course not be stopped suddenly and may even need to be increased during serious infections to compensate for adrenal suppression despite infection risk.

Infection empiric guidelines for specific organisms and syndromes are outlined in Tables 107.1 and 107.2. However, where a patient is slow to respond, or has a rapidly evolving clinical picture, consultation with the local infection expert is recommended.

The infections that are common in the community and hospitals are even more frequent in this population. These common infections are outlined in this section and summarized in Table 107.2.

Pneumonia

The most common causes of lower respiratory tract infections in patients with rheumatological illness are similar in aetiology to the general population. Aspiration pneumonia is included in the differential for many rheumatological patients with altered dysmotility syndromes, which most commonly becomes secondarily infected with anaerobic and Gram-negative species. Opportunistic infection is uncommon but must be considered when managing these patients: the most frequent opportunistic pathogens are *Pneumocystic jirovecii*, cryptococci, mycobacteria, and CMV. These should be considered if there is a poor clinical response to antibacaterials.

Appropriate clinical specimens should be taken prior to commencing antimicrobial therapy including: sputum samples, urinary antigens (pneumococcal and legionella), and acute and convalescent serology. When present, pleural effusions should be aspirated and sent for microbiological culture. Where individuals do not improve with empiric anti-bacterial treatment, further diagnostic samples such as bronchoalveolar lavage (BAL) should be performed especially to determine the presence of a fungal or viral pathogens. Empirical antibiotics according to the appropriate local and national guidelines are appropriate relating to the severity of infections—commonly amoxicillin or co-amoxiclav.[49] If clinical evidence of severe pneumonia is present then the addition of atypical cover with a macrolide is recommended (e.g. clarithromycin).

Skin, soft tissue, bone and joint infection

Cellulitis is most commonly caused by *Staphylococcus aureus* or streptococci (group A, C, or G). Initial therapy should treat these organisms: flucloxacillin with or without penicillin. Recent healthcare interactions, preceding trauma, animal bites or scratches, and fresh or salt water exposure are important historical aspects to consider in determining whether additional empirical antimicrobial treatments are required for Gram-negative pathogens or multidrug-resistant organisms. Blood cultures and/or samples from tissue and pus can assist in the microbiological diagnosis.

Osteomyelitis can either occur from haematogenous spread or, more commonly, is due to contiguous lesions that are infected. This occur commonly in individuals with chronic peripheral ulceration. MRI is the recommended imaging modality as it has excellent sensitivity of 81–100% and reasonable specificity (67–96%), allowing changes to be seen as early as 3–7 days from onset of infection.[50,51] Nuclear imaging modalities such as the three-phase bone scan, although sensitive (73–100%) can be poorly specific and often ambiguous when other inflammatory causes are present (presenting as false-positive results) or when vascular supply is poor (false-negative results).

Meningitis

CSF findings for the common types of meningitis are outlined in Table 107.3. In the immunocompromised, *Listeria monocytogenes* is an important additional pathogen. Encapsulated organisms are important pathogens in those with splenic dysfunction.

Table 107.1 Common infection syndromes and their management

Infection type	Management
Vascular access device	Send blood cultures, line site swab
	Remove VAD if SIRS
	Send catheter tip for culture
	Start empiric antimicrobials (e.g. vancomycin and gentamicin)
Lower respiratory tract	Obtain sputum for culture
	Consider nasopharyngeal swab for respiratory viruses
	Consider acute and convalescent serology
	Start empirical therapy according to local guidelines (e.g. amoxicillin and clarithromycin)
	Further investigations if not improving at day 3–4
Skin and soft tissue	MRSA screen
	Isolate suspected streptococcal infection for initial 24 h of treatment
	Obtain tissue samples for culture if exposed ulcer/bone
	Aspirate joint prior to antibiotics
	Empiric treatment according to local guidelines. Tailor treatment with culture results
	Consider radiograph of affected limb ±MRI scan for deep collections/osteomyelitis
Urinary tract	Send urine culture prior to therapy
	Review previous cultures if available to tailor treatment (especially where multidrug-resistant organisms may be present)
	Initial treatment according to local empirical guidelines
Infective endocarditis	Await blood culture results
	Echo—determine effect and suitability for emergency valve replacement
	Chase MRSA screen
Meningitis	CT scan and lumbar puncture pre-antibiotics if this can happen within 2–4 h
	Send CSF for bacteria, viral, fungal, and TB culture
	Indian ink/cryptococcal antigen
	Aciclovir only if evidence of encephalitis
Disseminated infections (e.g. TB, viruses, fungi, tropical)	Discussion with specialist infection unit

CSF, cerebrospinal fluid; MRSA, methicillin-resistant *S. aureus*; SIRS, systemic inflammatory response syndrome; TB, tuberculosis.

Table 107.2 Common infection aetiologies in immunocompetent and suppressed hosts

Gram stain	Grouping	Important species	Infections	Focused treatments
Gram-positive cocci	Staphylococci	*Staphylococcus aureus* (MRSA and MSSA)	Skin and soft tissue infections, bacteraemia, endocarditis, osteomyelitis and septic arthritis	MSSA: Flucloxacillin MRSA: Glycopeptide
		CNS, e.g. *S. epidermidis, S. lugdenensis*	Device-associated infections: CVC, prosthetic joints	
	Streptococci and related organisms	Haemolytic streptococci	Skin and soft tissue infections, bacteraemia, endocarditis, osteomyelitis and septic arthritis, pharyngitis ('strep throat')	Penicillin
		Pneumococci	Pneumonia, meningitis, sinusitis	Penicillin, 3rd-generation cephalosporin
		Enterococci	Urinary tract and abdominal/biliary sepsis	Amoxicillin or glycopeptide
Gram-positive bacilli	Anaerobic bacteria	*Clostridium* spp. (e.g. *C. tetani, C. difficile*) *Actinomyces israelii*	Tetanus, *C. difficile* associated diarrhoea/pseudomembranous colitis Actinomycosis—GI, dental, respiratory	
	Other important	*Listeria monocytogenes*	Bacteraemia, meningitis	Amoxicillin
Gram-negative bacilli	Enterobacteriaciae	**GI commensals** *Escherichia coli, Klebsiella* spp., *Proteus* spp., *Enterobacter* spp., *Citrobacter* spp.		According to sensitivities Co-amoxiclav, Ciprofloxacin, Cephalosproins, Carbopenems
		GI pathogens *Salmonella typhi & paratyphi* Non-typhoidal salmonella	Gastrointestinal disease, bacteraemia, biliary tract disease and recurrent infection	3rd generation cephalosporins, quinolones
		Shigella spp., *Campylobacter* spp.	Acute gastorenterintis	Ciprofloxacin, clarithromycin
	Non-enterobacteriacaie	*Pseudomonas aeriginosa* And other environmental organisms less frequently *Acinetobacter* spp *Stenotophomonas* spp	Healthcare-associated pneumonia (including ventilator), cellulitis (esp. in those with ulcers or underlying immunosuppressive condition) Device-associated UTI and bacteraemia	
Gram-negative cocci		*Neisseria meningitis*	Bacteraemia, meninigitis	
Fungal	Candida spp	*Candida albicans*	Mucositis, vaginitis Bacteraemia, device related infection, endocarditis	Fluconazole
		Non-albicans species: *Candida glabrata, krusii* etc		Caspofungin, amphotericin

CNS, coagulase-negative staphylococci; CVC, central venous catheter; GI, gastrointestinal; MRSA, methicillin-resistant *S. aureus*, MSSA. methicillin-sensitive *S. aureus*; UTI, urinary tract infection.

Table 107.3 Common cerebrospinal fluid findings

	Protein (g/L)	CSF glucose: serum glucose ratio	White cells (per µL)	White cell differential	Appearance	Added tests to CSF
Normal	0.18–0.45	0.6	<5	Mononuclear	clear	–
Viral	Raised (usually <1)	normal	Raised (usually <1000)	Mononuclear	clear	Viral NAAT (liaise with virology lab)
Bacterial	Raised (usually >1)	Low (<0.6)	Raised (often >1000)	neutrophils	turbid	Gram stain and culture
Tuberculosis	Raised	Low	Raised	Lymphocytes	Turbid/clear	Acid-fast bacilli smear TB culture NAAT (liaise with microbiologist)
Listeria	Raised	Normal/low	Raised	lymphocytes	Turbid/clear	Gram stain Culture
Cryptococcus	Raised/normal	Normal/low	Normal/raised	monocytes	clear	Indian ink Cryptococcal antigen

CSF, cerebrospinal fluid; NAAT, nucleic acid amplification techniques; TB, tuberculosis.

Cell-mediated immunodeficiency, often iatrogenic in rheumatology patients, weakens the response to other organisms, such as nocardia, mycobacteria, and cryptococci—which, although rare, may cause central nervous system (CNS) infection.

Immunocompromised individuals may not be able to mount the usual response to infection and often the CSF white cell count is not raised. Therefore clinicians must be prudent when diagnosing meningitis but also when managing these cases as low CSF white cell count is a poor prognostic factor in bacterial meningitis.[52]

Other multiorgan infections

Non-typhoidal salmonella

Non-typhoidal salmonella—facultative anaerobic Gram-negative rods—belong to the *Enterobacteriaceae* group and are spread via the faeco-oral route in contaminated water or food. Salmonella is the most common cause of bacteraemia in lupus patients.[17] Approximately one-third of infected individuals die from overwhelming sepsis.[14] The organism can easily be grown from blood cultures and once bacteraemia is confirmed metastatic infection should be considered, especially determining whether there is intra-abdominal or bone and joint infection. Treatment of disseminated diseases is guided by antimicrobial susceptibility testing but is usually with a fluoroquinolone or third-generation cephalosporin.

Tuberculosis

In 2010, TB accounted for 1.1 million deaths (in non-HIV-infected individuals) and there were 8.8 million new cases of TB.[53] The bacilli replicate relatively slowly and eventually the host mounts a significant cell-mediated response which destroys cells and surrounding tissues. In untreated or uncontained infection the bacilli spread by eruption of the caseating granulomas in which they are held into the airways of surrounding parenchyma. Haematogenous spread allows for disseminated infection and can involve any organ. TNFα plays an important role in the control of tuberculous disease as macrophages form granulomas where the mycobacteria are contained. Diagnosis of active TB involves radiological and microbiological evidence.

The organism is microbiologically confirmed through specific stains (Ziehl–Nielsen and Auramine) and nucleic acid amplification tests (NAATs). IFNγ release assays and tuberculin skin tests are not useful in the diagnosis of active infection, as a negative result does not rule out the diagnosis.[54]

Treatment for pulmonary TB involves 6 months of antimicrobials and is longer in disseminated (miliary) disease and drug-resistant cases. Latent TB diagnosis and treatment is discussed in the 'Prevention of infection' section.

Non-tuberculous mycobacteria

Atypical or non-tuberculous mycobacteria (NTM) include over 50 species of environmental organisms that can be found in water and soil. In immunocompromised individuals these traditionally non-virulent organisms can cause largely cavitatory pulmonary infections in addition to skin and soft tissue infection, bone and joint infection, and lymphadenitis. Disseminated infection has been reported in individuals on anti-TNF agents.[43,54] Standard mycobacteriological cultures from tissue or pus will facilitate growth of organisms. Treatment and duration of treatment is dependent on the mycobacterium species, the site of infection, and other underlying conditions. Specialist input from infectious disease or respiratory physicians should be sought.

Nocardia

Nocardia, a Gram-positive bacillus, causes granulomatous pulmonary infections mainly in immunocompromised hosts.[55] It is abundant in soil and water and inhaled into the lungs where it can cause a variety of presentations including nodularity, cavitations, or lung abscess. Disseminated disease is more likely in immunodeficient individuals through haematogenous spread leading to granulomas and abscesses in multiple organs.[56] These are slow-growing organisms that can take 4–6 weeks to grow, in specialized media. Nocardia requires treatment over many months (4–12 months) that often includes co-trimoxazole (see Table 107.2). Antibiotic susceptibility varies according to species[57] and in cases of disseminated or severe infections more than one agent should be used according to susceptibility patterns.

Herpesviridae

Herpes simplex

The complete range of clinical syndromes associated with herpes simplex virus (HSV) types 1 and 2 may be seen in rheumatological patients. Antivirals—aciclovir or valaciclovir—are used to treat infection in immunocompromised patients with disseminated infections. With continued immunosuppression after infection or recurrent disabling attacks, secondary prophylactic antivirals may be considered for both HSV-1 and HSV-2.

Varicella zoster

Immunocompromised patients are more prone to reactivation of varicella zoster (VZV), severe disease with a prolonged recovery period, and complications including pneumonitis, hepatitis, encephalitis, and secondary bacterial infection over lesions.[58] Immunocompromised hosts should receive early antiviral treatment (aciclovir and valaciclovir) and intravenous treatment in disseminated disease. In continued states of immunosuppression after infection, secondary prophylaxis may be considered.

Cytomegalovirus

Higher rates of disseminated CMV disease have been reported with azathioprine, cyclophosphamide, and anti-TNF agents.[25] Antivirals such as ganciclovir, foscarnet, and cidofovir can be used to treat disease in immunocompromised patients. In continued states of immunosuppression after infection, secondary prophylactic antivirals may be considered.

Epstein–Barr virus

A close relationship appears to exist between SLE and Epstein–Barr virus (EBV) where disease activity of lupus has been followed by reactivation of EBV; studies suggest that a particular CD8 T-cell defect specific to EBV has been shown in lupus patients.[59] Chronic infection is rare but can cause an ongoing clinical picture of fever, lymphadenopathy, cytopenias, and hepatosplenomegaly; the patient has a persistently high-level viraemia which cannot be controlled into a latent state and can rarely lead to fulminant disease and death. Other complications include cancers such as Hodgkin's lymphoma, Burkitt's lymphoma, and nasopharyngeal carcinoma.

JC virus

JC virus is a dsDNA human polyomavirus mainly described in HIV-positive individuals causing PML. With the recent development of more immunosuppressive treatments for various conditions including autoimmune diseases, case reports have been published of non-HIV patients infected with JCV.[60-62] The virus commonly causes an infection within brain cells that forms white matter demyelinating plaques visible on MRI. Cognitive impairment ensues, with varying degrees of motor dysfunction and in some cases speech and language impairment, visual disturbances, and seizure activity. The disease is ultimately fatal. These cases are rare but clinicians should be aware and include this disease in the differential in the context of neurological changes in autoimmune disease. Virus can be detected in urine and CSF but confirmatory methods use brain tissue samples for histological examination and electron microscopy. In those with autoimmune disease a relationship between rituximab use and PML is documented; isolated cases have occurred in association with infliximab.[48,63] Unfortunately there are no curative therapies and management is largely symptomatic.

Hepatitis B virus

Hepatitis B virus (HBV) reactivation or flares in the disease have also been widely associated with rituximab use and is also documented with other immunosuppressants.[64-66] Reactivation of chronic hepatitis B with anti-TNF agents is approximately 40%.[67] It is thought to be related to the profound circulating B-cell suppression which is essential in controlling the virus. Those who are HBsAg positive should be commenced on a nucleoside or nucleotide analogue antiviral prior to immunosuppression.[66-68] This is generally commenced at least 1 week prior to immunosuppressants and continued for 6–12 months from cessation.

Baseline serology should be done before commencing immunsuppressants in individuals with autoimmune disease. Those individuals with positive serology should be reviewed by a viral hepatitis specialist.[9,64,66,69] If a flare of HBV occurs during immunosuppressant therapy, immunosupressants should be stopped and prompt antiviral treatment should be commenced. Sudden flares in hepatitis and fulminant hepatitis have also been reported after stopping methotrexate.[70,71]

Fungal infections

Candida

Candida, a yeast, is often found in the environment and is a normal body commensal of the skin and genitourinary tract. Immunosuppression is a major risk factor for developing invasive candida infection as both the humoral and cell-mediated immune systems fight invasion of the organism.[72] Invasive disease most often occurs from an infected vascular access device (VAD)[72] and can cause bloodstream infection leading to endocarditis, osteomyelitis, and prosthetic joint infections. All cases of candida bloodstream infection should have a formal ophthalmological assessment to search for endophthalmitis and an echocardiogram for endocarditis. Uncontrolled disseminated disease can occur in heavy immunosuppression where multiple microabscesses can occur in multiple organs.

Candida can be cultured using standard microbiological techniques and culture media. A prolonged course of therapy is required and often involves amphotericin B or fluconazole if susceptible.

Aspergillus

Aspergillus, a mould, occurs in patients with chronic lung disease and those with immune deficiencies including active disease states and iatrogenic deficiency.[25,73,74] It may affect many organs, including eyes with keratitis, sinuses with chronic infection, and brain with ring-enhancing lesions found on CT scanning. The diagnosis is confirmed with classical radiological findings and serum galactomannan antigen, an antigen generated by the aspergillus. Parenteral amphotericin B, voriconazole, or caspofungin are the antifungals of choice (see Table 107.2). Some patients with a poor response to antifungals require surgical resection to debulk the disease.

Pneumocystis jiroveci

Pneumocystis jiroveci (formerly known as Pneumocystis carinii) has also been reported in those on immunosuppressive medication.[75] It is an environmental fungus that individuals encounter on multiple occasions but does not usually cause disease unless host defences are impaired. It is thought to spread via aerosolized particles and is most likely to result in lower respiratory tract infection which presents with a dry cough and reduced exercise tolerance. The best diagnostic method is by BAL with cytological examination using silver staining and microscopy. First-line treatment is with high-dose co-trimoxazole although there are alternatives, such as clindamycin and primaquine if co-trimoxazole is not tolerated. Individuals with pneumocystis infection are at risk of spontaneous pneumothorax.[76] Empirical prophylaxis is not considered appropriate but may be considered after treated pneumocystis infection in those remaining on immunosuppressants.

Cryptococci

Cryptococcus neoformans is a ubiquitous, yeast-like organism that causes systemic infections in the immunocompromised host. It can be cultured from trees, soil, or fruit contaminated with bird droppings. It is thought to enter the system via aerosolized particles and eventual haematogenous spread to other organs, mainly the brain, but can cause disseminated and pulmonary disease.[77] Cryptococcal meningitis causes varying symptoms of raised intracranial pressure, although sometimes a persistent headache is the only manifestation. Serum and CSF cryptococcal antigen tests can assist in the diagnosis and serial tests are useful in determining a therapeutic response. Treatment usually involves amphotericin and flucytosine. Secondary prophylactic antifungals are recommended while individuals remain immunosuppressed.

Histoplasma

Histoplasmosis is a granulomatous infection caused by *Histoplasma capsulatum*, a dimorphic fungus, the mycelial form of which is found in soil and in bird or bat droppings. It is endemic in temperate climates such as the mid-west and south-east United States, Africa, Asia, and parts of Australia. Inhalation of particles is the usual method of entry. Severity of disease is dependent on comorbidities, immunodeficiency affecting T cells, increasing age and inoculum size. TNF and IFNγ play a vital role in the immune response to *H. capsulatum* and hence the use of immunosuppressants when individuals are living or visiting endemic regions at risk. It is important that laboratory staff are aware of the differential diagnosis, to ensure that specimens are appropriately examined in specialist conditions. Urine and serum antigen testing are also used. Treatment involves itraconazole or amphotericin B and length of treatment is dependent on the extent of infection.

Other unusual infections

Other unusual infections may occur such as cryptosporidiosis (causing a chronic diarrhoea and sclerosing cholangitis), strongyloides, leishmaniasis, toxoplasmosis, and endemic fungal diseases such as coccidiomycosis and blastomycosis. All of these syndromes require a detailed travel history and specialist diagnostic tests. Infectious disease consultation should be considered in those with travel history to endemic areas for these diseases, and is essential to the management of these conditions.

Prevention of infection

The prevention of infection is an intrinsic part of the ongoing care and management of individuals with autoimmune disease. This is particularly important before starting immunosuppressant treatment, especially with agents that modify particular parts of the immune system and increase the risk to certain infections.

Vascular access devices

Many rheumatology patients require a VAD, often centrally placed and in place for prolonged periods. These devices are associated with a higher risk of catheter-related bloodstream infections (CRBSIs).[78,79] Infection prevention measures using the National Institute for Health and Clinical Excellence (NICE) guidelines, *Saving lives* tools and Centers for Disease Control (CDC) guidelines can dramatically improve rates of CRBSIs and must be implemented for all patients with venous access.[78,80–82] This includes choosing the appropriate VAD, following aseptic protocols for placement and subsequent use, and prompt removal when alternative measures are available. A study by Pronovost et al.[78] implemented 5 steps in 103 intensive care unit patients (hand-washing, full barrier care during insertion, cleaning skin surfaces with chlorhexidine, avoiding femoral VAD, and removing unnecessary VAD) to prevent CRBSI and managed to reduce the overall median rate of infection from 2.7 at baseline to 0 at up to 18 months after. Local guidelines should be in place for VAD insertion and continuing care.

Vaccinations and immunization against infection

Vaccines attempt to provide immunity to a person by using altered organisms or their components to induce an immune response, which is reactivated when the organism is encountered. Live attenuated vaccines use laboratory-grown organisms with weakened virulence. Inactivated vaccines use grown components of an organism that are then 'killed' prior to use and do not induce as long-lasting a response as live vaccines, often requiring booster injections periodically. When using vaccines it is important to consider that the patient may not produce antibodies readily, especially where deficiencies or alterations in the standard cell-mediated response exist. Therefore some cases may require repeat vaccination and all cases require other measures to be taken to prevent infection.

Live vaccines are contraindicated in those who are pregnant or immunosuppressed—which according to United Kingdom, European, and American guidelines include those on DMARDs, biological agents, and high-dose steroids.[83–85] (The United Kingdom Department of Health 'Green Book' defines 'high-dose' steroids as ≥40 mg prednisolone daily use for more than 1 week compared to the CDC guidelines of prednisolone 20 mg or more daily for >14 days.) It is generally accepted that this state of immunosuppression remains for at least 1 month for corticosteroid use and 6 months for DMARD use.[83,84] Low-dose steroid, methotrexate (<0.4 mg/kg per week) and azathioprine (<3 mg/kg per day) may be safe for some live vaccines such as the herpes zoster vaccine.[84,86] Before starting immunosuppressants all patients should be considered for vaccination as appropriate and the course should be completed at least 2 weeks before the immunosuppressants commence.

Active immunization

The recommended vaccinations for patients with chronic disease and immunosuppression are outlined in Table 107.4. The important characteristics of some vaccines are considered here.

The 23-serotype polysaccharide pneumococcal vaccine (PPV) is an inactivated polysaccharide vaccine which covers 23 serotypes of pneumococcus, accounting for 88% of all pneumococcal infection.[86] It is recommended for use in asplenic or hyposplenic patients, those over 65 years of age, and patients with chronic

Table 107.4 Prevention of infection

Infection-associated risk	Method of prevention	Approach
Vascular access device	VAD insertion and care protocols Patient education	Staff education, competency assessment and audits of practice
Influenza	Vaccination Postexposure prophylaxis	Annual vaccine recommended
Pneumococcal disease	Vaccination	23 serotype PPV Vaccine every 5 years recommended
Hyposplenism	Vaccination	Meningococcal ACW135Y, HiB, Pneumococcal vaccine recommended
VZV	Screening and active vaccination Passive vaccination	Consider pre-immunosuppression active vaccine Postexposure VZIg
Hepatitis B	Screening and vaccination	If negative, consider vaccination prior to immunosuppression If positive, pre-treatment or early antiviral treatment; refer to specialist.
CMV	Screening and monitor	If previous symptomatic infection, monitor CMV viral load Consider prophylaxis if previous invasive infection
Fungal	No current recommendations	Consider prophylaxis if previous invasive infection
PCP	No current recommendations	Consider prophylaxis if previous infection
TB	Screening and treatment	IGRA prior to immunosuppressants Treatment if IGRA positive
Tropical diseases	Appropriate vaccination, prophylaxis and education	Refer to travel clinic prior to travel abroad

CMV, cytomegalovirus; IGRA, interferon-gamma releasing assay; PCP, pneumocystis pneumonia; TB, tuberculosis; VAD, vascular access device; VZV, varicella zoster virus.

disease. Individuals on immunosuppressant therapy (methotrexate and anti-TNF) have a reduced response to this vaccine with reduced antibody titres 1 month and 1 year after vaccination.[86,87] Concerns about disease flare after vaccination have also been raised but this has not been demonstrated.[88] It is recommended that this vaccine is administered every 5 years to those with autoimmune disease, with or without immunosuppressant therapy.

Influenza vaccines are inactivated vaccines that are required annually as the composition of these vaccines changes yearly, based on expert group consensus of circulating strains. The vaccine response may be reduced in these patients and some suggest considering repeat vaccination after 3 weeks.[83,89] There is a reduced response to the vaccine with rituximab use, azathioprine, and moderate to high-dose steroids (>10 mg prednisolone daily) but a reasonable response with anti-TNF use has been observed.[86] Household contacts and carers should also be vaccinated to ensure adequate protection, especially in those who show poor seroconversion.[83]

VZV vaccine is a live attenuated vaccine that has been contraindicated for use in patients who are immunosuppressed but may be given to those with autoimmune diseases prior to immunosupressants.[43,90] In those with autoimmune disease it has been shown to reduce infection risk by 51% and postherpetic neuralgia by 66% 3 years after vaccination.[53]

Passive immunization

Intravenous immunoglobulin delivers passive immunity against certain infections. Varicella zoster immunoglobulin (VZIg) should be considered in immunosuppressed patients who are exposed to cases of zoster infection—both chickenpox and shingles—from 48 hours prior to rash developing until crusting of vesicles. VZIg use does not preclude infection and therefore if these patients develop early signs of infection they should be given empirical antivirals. Immunoglobulin use alters the normal immune response to vaccine and therefore use of vaccines should be delayed until 3 months after immunoglobulin administration.[83]

Prophylactic antimicrobials

Medical prophylaxis is generally not recommended in those on immunosuppressive drugs for autoimmune disease unless the patient is asplenic or has a history of invasive infection. Where invasive bacterial, viral, or fungal disease has occurred, the case should be discussed with a microbiologist or infectious diseases physician to consider use of prophylactic antimicrobials, as previously discussed for individual infections. Routine prophylactic antibiotics to prevent infective endocarditis in patients with autoimmune disease and those undergoing immunosuppressive treatment are not recommended.[91,92] Certain individuals should be given prophylaxis prior to certain procedures only (see Table 107.4).

Latent tuberculosis infection

Up to 10% of patients with latent TB infection (LTBI) develop reactivation of the disease. The use of immunomodulatory drugs in rheumatological or autoimmune diseases allow reactivation of LTBI to occur, through dysregulation of the granulomatous process.

According to published guidelines, prior to starting immuno-suppressive therapy including long-term glucocorticoid therapy (prednisolone >15 mg/day for >2–4 weeks), DMARDs, or bio-logical agents, individuals should be assessed for active and latent TB.[9,34,93-95] An accurate history of previous TB exposure, diagno-sis, or treatment should be taken and a clinical examination done to look for signs of active TB, particularly lymphadenopathy. A chest radiograph should be taken to determine whether there are radio-logical appearances of active or old TB. If there are signs of active TB, referral to a TB specialist physician is recommended. If there is a confirmed diagnosis of active TB, treatment with anti-TNF agents should ideally be deferred until at least 2 months of appropriate TB therapy has been taken.[94]

For those with no TB history and no active TB on chest radio-graph, further tests should be performed.[42,94,96]

The current United Kingdom guidelines recommend the use of blood INFγ release assays and IGRA to diagnose LTBI in immu-nocompromised patients, as they are appear to be more sensitive in this population.[42,93,94,97] IGRAs are in-vitro blood tests using antigens that detect a T-cell response to TB antigens by releasing measured INFγ. Positive IGRA tests require prompt treatment for LTBI in those due to undergo immunosuppressive treatment if the risk of treatment (mainly hepatotoxicity) is less than the risk of reactivation. Those deemed at high risk of hepatotoxicity should be monitored 3–4 monthly and warned of TB symptoms. Standard LTBI therapy is 3 months of combination rifampicin and isoniazid or alternatively 6 months of isoniazid monotherapy.[93]

Vaccination against TB uses a live attenuated vaccine derived from *Mycobacterium bovis* that confers up to 70–80% protection depending on individual response.[83] It is generally not recom-mended over the age of 16 years and as it is a live vaccine is also contraindicated in individuals on immunosuppressive therapy.

Conclusion

Rheumatic and autoimmune disease creates a state of immune dys-function and dysregulation that must be taken into account when dealing with infections in these patients. Furthermore, the disease process can lead to end-organ damage that creates an environment for microorganisms to invade or proliferate. The therapies used to treat rheumatic and autoimmune disease target various points in this already altered immune system, making this set of patients more vulnerable to infective agents. Thus those patients diagnosed with these rheumatic diseases should be screened and vaccinated appro-priately for those common infections during their routine medical visits. Before commencing any immunosuppressant therapy they should be screened for underlying chronic infections such as TB. Clinicians must remain highly vigilant in identifying the early signs of infection, being aware of the likely standard and opportunistic infections that may occur.

References

1. National Collaborating Centre for Chronic Conditions. *Rheumatoid arthritis: national clinical guideline for management and treatment in adults*. Royal College of Physicians, London, 2009.
2. Au K, Reed G, Curtis JR et al. High disease activity is associated with an increased rate of infection in patients with rheumatoid arthritis. *Ann Rheum Dis* 2011;70:785–791.
3. Thomas E, Symmons DP, Brewster DH, Black RJ, Macfarlane GJ. National study of cause specific mortality in rheumatoid arthritis, juve-nile chronic arthritis and other rheumatic conditions: a 20 year follow up. *J Rheumatol* 2003;30:958–965.
4. Franklin J, Lunt M, Bunn D, Symmons D, Silman A. Risk and predictors of infection leading to hospitalisation in a large primary-care-derived cohort of patients with inflammatory polyarthritis. *Ann Rheum Dis* 2007;66:308–312.
5. Cervera R, Khamashta MA, Font J et al. Morbidity and mortality in systemic lupus erythematosus during a 10-year period: a comparison of early and late manifestations in a cohort of 1,000 patients. *Medicine* (Baltimore) 2003;82(5):299–308.
6. Tyndall AJ, Bannert B, Vonk M et al. Causes and risk factors for death in systemic sclerosis: A study from the EULAR scleroderma trialsand research (EUSTAR) database. *Ann Rheum Dis* 2010;69:1089–1815.
7. Vinogradova Y, Hippisley-Cox J, Coupland C. Identification of new risk factors for pneumonia: population-based case-control study. *Br J Gen Pract* 2009;59(567):329–338.
8. Foque-Aubert A, Jette-Paulin L, Combescure C et al. Serious infections in patients with ankylosing spondylitis with and without TNF block-ers: a systematic review and meta-analysis of randomised and placebo-controlled trials. *Ann Rheum Dis* 2010;69:1756–1761.
9. Barber C, Gold WL, Fortin PR. Infections in the lupus patient: perspec-tives on prevention. *Curr Opin Rheumatol* 2011;23(4):358–365.
10. Doria A, Canova M, Tonon M et al. Infections as triggers and compli-cations of systemic lupus erythematosus. *Autoimmun Rev* 2008;8(1):24–28.
11. Falagas ME, Manta KG, Betsi GI, Pappas G. Infection-related morbidity and mortality in patients with connective tissue diseases: a systematic review. *Clin Rheumatol* 2007;26(5):663–670.
12. Chen IJ, Tsai WP, Wu YJ et al. Infections in polymyositis and dermato-myositis: analysis of 192 cases. *Rheumatology* (Oxford) 2010;49(12):2429–2437.
13. Pego-Reigosa JM, Medeiros DA, Isenberg DA. Respiratory manifesta-tions of systemic lupus erythematosus: old and new concepts. *Best Pract Res Clin Rheumatol* 2009;23(4):469–480.
14. Tsao CH, Chen CY, Ou LS, Huang JL. Risk factors of mortality for salmonella infection in systemic lupus erythematosus. *J Rheumatol* 2002;29(6):1214–1218.
15. Cho YN, Kee SJ, Lee SJ et al. Numerical and functional deficiencies of natu-ral killer T cells in systemic lupus erythematosus: their deficiency related to disease activity. *Rheumatology* (Oxford) 2011;50(6):1054–1063.
16. Jeong SJ, Choi H, Lee HS et al. Incidence and risk factors of infection in a single cohort of 110 adults with systemic lupus erythematosus. *Scand J Infect Dis* 2009;41(4):268–274.
17. Lim E, Koh WH, Loh SF, Lam MS, Howe HS. Non-typhoidal salmo-nellosis in patients with systemic lupus erythematosus. A study of fifty patients and a review of the literature. *Lupus* 2001;10(2):87–92.
18. Navarra SV, Leynes MS. Infections in systemic lupus erythematosus. *Lupus* 2010;19(12):1419–1424.
19. Fessler BJ. Infectious diseases in systemic lupus erythematosus: risk factors, management and prophylaxis. *Best Pract Res Clin Rheumatol* 2002;16(2):281–291.

20. Morton M, Edmonds S, Doherty AM et al. Factors associated with major infections in patients with granulomatosis with polyangiitis and systemic lupus erythematosus treated for deep organ involvement. *Rheumatol Int* 2012;32(11):3373–3382.

21. Marie I, Hachulla E, Cherin P et al. Opportunistic infections in polymyositis and dermatomyositis. *Arthritis Rheum* 2005;53(2):155–165.

22. Luqmani R, Suppiah R, Edwards CJ et al. Mortality in Wegener's granulomatosis: a bimodal pattern. *Rheumatology* (Oxford) 2011;50(4):697–702.

23. Flossmann O, Berden A, de Groot K et al. Long-term patient survival in ANCA-associated vasculitis. *Ann Rheum Dis* 2011;70(3):488–494.

24. Dixon WG, Kezouh A, Bernatsky S, Suissa S. The influence of systemic glucocorticoid therapy upon the risk of non-serious infection in older patients with rheumatoid arthritis: a nested case-control study. *Ann Rheum Dis* 2011;70(6):956–960.

25. Salmon-Ceron D, Tubach F et al. Drug-specific risk of non-tuberculosis opportunistic infections in patients receiving anti-TNF therapy reported to the 3-year prospective French RATIO registry. *Ann Rheum Dis* 2011;70(4):616–623.

26. Bernatsky S, Hudson M, Suissa S. Anti-rheumatic drug use and risk of serious infections in rheumatoid arthritis. *Rheumatology* (Oxford) 2007;46(7):1157–1160.

27. Greenberg JD, Reed G, Kremer JM et al. Association of methotrexate and tumour necrosis factor antagonists with risk of infectious outcomes including opportunistic infections in the CORRONA registry. *Ann Rheum Dis* 2010;69(2):380–386.

28. Brassard P, Kezouh A, Suissa S. Antirheumatic drugs and the risk of tuberculosis. *Clin Infect Dis* 2006;43(6):717–722.

29. Hoes JN, Jacobs JW, Verstappen SM, Bijlsma JW, Van der Heijden GJ. Adverse events of low- to medium-dose oral glucocorticoids in inflammatory diseases: a meta-analysis. *Ann Rheum Dis* 2009;68(12):1833–1838.

30. Ruyssen-Witrand A, Fautrel B, Saraux A, Le-Loet X, Pham T. Infections induced by low-dose corticosteroids in rheumatoid arthritis: a systematic literature review. *Joint Bone Spine* 2010;77(3):246–251.

31. Salliot C, van der Heijde D. Long-term safety of methotrexate monotherapy in patients with rheumatoid arthritis: a systematic literature research. *Ann Rheum Dis* 2009;68(7):1100–1104.

32. Jenks KA, Stamp LK, O'Donnell JL, Savage RL, Chapman PT. Leflunomide-associated infections in rheumatoid arthritis. *J Rheumatol* 2007;34(11):2201–2203.

33. Caporali R, Caprioli M, Bobbio-Pallavicini F, Montecucco C. DMARDS and infections in rheumatoid arthritis. *Autoimmun Rev* 2008;8(2):139–143.

34. Solovic I, Sester M, Gomez-Reino JJ et al. The risk of tuberculosis related to tumour necrosis factor antagonist therapies: a TBNET consensus statement. *Eur Respir J* 2010;36(5):1185–1206.

35. Leombruno JP, Einarson TR, Keystone EC. The safety of anti-tumour necrosis factor treatments in rheumatoid arthritis: meta and exposure-adjusted pooled analyses of serious adverse events. *Ann Rheum Dis* 2009;68(7):1136–1145.

36. Keane J, Gershon S, Wise RP et al. Tuberculosis associated with infliximab, a tumor necrosis factor alpha-neutralizing agent. *N Engl J Med* 2001;345(15):1098–1104.

37. Nam JL, Winthrop KL, van Vollenhoven RF et al. Current evidence for the management of rheumatoid arthritis with biological disease-modifying antirheumatic drugs: a systematic literature review informing the EULAR recommendations for the management of RA. *Ann Rheum Dis* 2010;69(6):976–986.

38. Tubach F, Salmon D, Ravaud P et al. Risk of tuberculosis is higher with anti-tumor necrosis factor monoclonal antibody therapy than with soluble tumor necrosis factor receptor therapy: The three-year prospective French Research Axed on Tolerance of Biotherapies registry. *Arthritis Rheum* 2009;60(7):1884–1894.

39. Curtis JR, Xie F, Chen L, Baddley JW, Beukelman T, Saag KG, et al. The comparative risk of serious infections among rheumatoid arthritis patients starting or switching biological agents. *Ann Rheum Dis* 2011;70(8):1401–1406.

40. Bernatsky S, Habel Y, Rahme E. Observational studies of infections in rheumatoid arthritis: a metaanalysis of tumor necrosis factor antagonists. *J Rheumatol* 2010;37(5):928–931.

41. Singh JA, Wells GA, Christensen R et al. Adverse effects of biologics: a network meta-analysis and Cochrane overview. *Cochrane Database Syst Rev* 2011;2:CD008794.

42. Wallis RS, Ehlers S. Tumor necrosis factor and granuloma biology: explaining the differential infection risk of etanercept and infliximab. *Semin Arthritis Rheum* 2005;34(5 Suppl 1):34–38.

43. Winthrop KL, Chang E, Yamashita S, Iademarco MF, LoBue PA. Nontuberculous mycobacteria infections and anti-tumor necrosis factor-alpha therapy. *Emerg Infect Dis*2009;15(10):1556–1561.

44. Cambridge G, Leandro MJ, Edwards JC et al. Serologic changes following B lymphocyte depletion therapy for rheumatoid arthritis. *Arthritis Rheum* 2003;48(8):2146–2154.

45. Kelesidis T, Daikos G, Boumpas D, Tsiodras S. Does rituximab increase the incidence of infectious complications? A narrative review. *Int J Infect Dis* 2011;15(1):e2–e16.

46. Salliot C, Dougados M, Gossec L. Risk of serious infections during rituximab, abatacept and anakinra treatments for rheumatoid arthritis: meta-analyses of randomised placebo-controlled trials. *Ann Rheum Dis* 2009;68(1):25–32.

47. Riminton DS, Hartung HP, Reddel SW. Managing the risks of immunosuppression. *Curr Opin Neurol* 2011;24(3):217–223.

48. Nishimoto N, Miyasaka N, Yamamoto K et al. Long-term safety and efficacy of tocilizumab, an anti-IL-6 receptor monoclonal antibody, in monotherapy, in patients with rheumatoid arthritis (the STREAM study): evidence of safety and efficacy in a 5-year extension study. *Ann Rheum Dis* 2009;68(10):1580–1584.

49. Lim WS, Baudouin SV, George RC et al. BTS guidelines for the management of community acquired pneumonia in adults: update 2009. *Thorax* 2009;64 Suppl 3:iii1–55.

50. Dinh MT, Abad CL, Safdar N. Diagnostic accuracy of the physical examination and imaging tests for osteomyelitis underlying diabetic foot ulcers: meta-analysis. *Clin Infect Dis* 2008;47(4):519–527.

51. Hankin D, Bowling FL, Metcalfe SA, Whitehouse RA, Boulton AJ. Critically evaluating the role of diagnostic imaging in osteomyelitis. *Foot Ankle Spec* 2011;4(2):100–105.

52. Vibha D, Bhatia R, Prasad K et al. Clinical features and independent prognostic factors for acute bacterial meningitis in adults. *Neurocrit Care* 2010;13(2):199–204.

53. WHO Report. *Global tuberculosis control 2011*. World Health Organization, Geneva, 2011.

54. van Ingen J, Boeree MJ, Dekhuijzen PN, van Soolingen D. Mycobacterial disease in patients with rheumatic disease. *Nat Clin Pract Rheumatol* 2008;4(12):649–656.

55. Yildiz O, Doganay M. Actinomycoses and Nocardia pulmonary infections. *Curr Opin Pulm Med* 2006;12(3):228–234.

56. Hara H, Wakui F, Ochiai T. Disseminated Nocardia farcinica infection in a patient with systemic lupus erythematosus. *J Med Microbiol* 2011;60(Pt 6):847–850.

57. Munoz J, Mirelis B, Aragon LM et al. Clinical and microbiological features of nocardiosis 1997–2003. *J Med Microbiol* 2007;56(Pt 4):545–550.

58. Sayeeda A, Al Arfaj H, Khalil N, Al Arfaj AS. Herpes zoster infections in SLE in a university hospital in Saudi Arabia: risk factors and outcomes. *Autoimmune Dis* 2011;2011:174891.

59. Larsen M, Sauce D, Deback C et al. Exhausted cytotoxic control of Epstein-Barr virus in human lupus. *PLoS Pathog* 2011;7(10):e1002328.

60. Pavlovic AM, Bonaci-Nikolic B, Kozic D et al. Progressive multifocal leukoencephalopathy associated with mycophenolate mofetil treatment in a woman with lupus and CD4+ T-lymphocyte deficiency. *Lupus* 2012;21(1):100–102.

61. Viallard JF, Ellie E, Lazaro E, Lafon ME, Pellegrin JL. JC virus meningitis in a patient with systemic lupus erythematosus. *Lupus* 2005;14(12): 964–966.

62. Boren EJ, Cheema GS, Naguwa SM, Ansari AA, Gershwin ME. The emergence of progressive multifocal leukoencephalopathy (PML) in rheumatic diseases. *J Autoimmun* 2008;30(1–2):90–98.

63. Major EO. Progressive multifocal leukoencephalopathy in patients on immunomodulatory therapies. *Annu Rev Med* 2010;61:35–47.

64. Gentile G, Foa R. Viral infections associated with the clinical use of monoclonal antibodies. *Clin Microbiol Infect* 2011;17(12): 1769–1775.

65. Furst DE, Keystone EC, Fleischmann R et al. Updated consensus statement on biological agents for the treatment of rheumatic diseases, 2009. *Ann Rheum Dis* 2010;69 Suppl 1:i2–29.

66. Ferri C, Govoni M, Calabrese L. The A, B, Cs of viral hepatitis in the biologic era. *Curr Opin Rheumatol* 2010;22(4):443–450.

67. Vassilopoulos D. Should we routinely treat patients with autoimmune/rheumatic diseases and chronic hepatitis B virus infection starting biologic therapies with antiviral agents? Yes. *Eur J Intern Med* 2011;22(6):572–575.

68. European Association for the Study of the Liver. EASL Clinical practice guidelines: management of chronic hepatitis B virus infection. *J Hepatol* 2012;57(1):167–185.

69. Mastroianni CM, Lichtner M, Citton R et al. Current trends in management of hepatitis B virus reactivation in the biologic therapy era. *World J Gastroenterol* 2011;17(34):3881–3887.

70. Ito S, Nakazono K, Murasawa A et al. Development of fulminant hepatitis B (precore variant mutant type) after the discontinuation of low-dose methotrexate therapy in a rheumatoid arthritis patient. *Arthritis Rheum* 2001;44(2):339–342.

71. Hagiyama H, Kubota T, Komano Y et al. Fulminant hepatitis in an asymptomatic chronic carrier of hepatitis B virus mutant after withdrawal of low-dose methotrexate therapy for rheumatoid arthritis. *Clin Exp Rheumatol* 2004;22(3):375–376.

72. Ruhnke M, Rickerts V, Cornely OA et al. Diagnosis and therapy of Candida infections: joint recommendations of the German Speaking Mycological Society and the Paul-Ehrlich-Society for Chemotherapy. *Mycoses* 2011;54(4):279–310.

73. Ben-Ami R, Lewis RE, Kontoyiannis DP. Enemy of the (immunosuppressed) state: an update on the pathogenesis of Aspergillus fumigatus infection. *Br J Haematol* 2010;150(4):406–417.

74. Chen HS, Tsai WP, Leu HS, Ho HH, Liou LB. Invasive fungal infection in systemic lupus erythematosus: an analysis of 15 cases and a literature review. *Rheumatology* (Oxford) 2007;46(3):539–544.

75. Yoshida Y, Takahashi Y, Minemura N et al. Prognosis of pneumocystis pneumonia complicated in patients with rheumatoid arthritis (RA) and non-RA rheumatic diseases. *Mod Rheumatol* 2012;22(4):509–514.

76. Festic E, Gajic O, Limper AH, Aksamit TR. Acute respiratory failure due to pneumocystis pneumonia in patients without human immunodeficiency virus infection: outcome and associated features. *Chest* 2005;128(2):573–579.

77. Li SS, Mody CH. Cryptococcus. *Proc Am Thorac Soc* 2010;7(3):186–196.

78. Pronovost P, Needham D, Berenholtz S et al. An intervention to decrease catheter-related bloodstream infections in the ICU. *N Engl J Med* 2006;355(26):2725–2732.

79. Weeks KR, Goeschel CA, Cosgrove SE, Romig M, Berenholtz SM. Prevention of central line-associated bloodstream infections: a journey toward eliminating preventable harm. *Curr Infect Dis Rep* 2011;13(4): 343–349.

80. Gold JA, Simmons K. The 100,000 lives campaign: saving lives in Wisconsin and the nation. *WMJ* 2006;105(8):89–90.

81. O'Grady NP, Alexander M, Burns LA et al. Guidelines for the prevention of intravascular catheter-related infections. *Am J Infect Control* 2011;39(4 Suppl 1):S1–34.

82. NICE. *Infection: prevention and control of healthcare-associated infections in primary and community care (CG 139)*. NICE, London, 2012.

83. Department of Health. *Immunisation against infectious disease—'The Green Book'*. Available at: http://immunisation.dh.gov.uk/category/the-green-book/

84. National Center for Immunization and Respiratory Diseases. General Recommendations on Immunization Recommendations of the Advisory Committee on Immunization Practices (ACIP). *MMWR Recomm Rep* 2011; 60(2):1–64.

85. van Assen S, Agmon-Levin N, Elkayam O et al. EULAR recommendations for vaccination in adult patients with autoimmune inflammatory rheumatic diseases. *Ann Rheum Dis* 2011;70(3):414–422.

86. Gluck T, Muller-Ladner U. Vaccination in patients with chronic rheumatic or autoimmune diseases. *Clin Infect Dis* 2008;46(9):1459–1465.

87. Elkayam O, Ablin J, Caspi D. Safety and efficacy of vaccination against streptococcus pneumonia in patients with rheumatic diseases. *Autoimmun Rev* 2007;6(5):312–314.

88. Conti F, Rezai S, Valesini G. Vaccination and autoimmune rheumatic diseases. *Autoimmun Rev* 2008;8(2):124–128.

89. Saad CG, Borba EF, Aikawa NE et al. Immunogenicity and safety of the 2009 non-adjuvanted influenza A/H1N1 vaccine in a large cohort of autoimmune rheumatic diseases. *Ann Rheum Dis* 2011;70(6): 1068–1073.

90. Garcia-Doval I, Perez-Zafrilla B, Descalzo MA et al. Incidence and risk of hospitalisation due to shingles and chickenpox in patients with rheumatic diseases treated with TNF antagonists. *Ann Rheum Dis* 2010;69(10):1751–1755.

91. Habib G, Hoen B, Tornos P et al. Guidelines on the prevention, diagnosis, and treatment of infective endocarditis (new version 2009): the Task Force on the Prevention, Diagnosis, and Treatment of Infective Endocarditis of the European Society of Cardiology (ESC). Endorsed by the European Society of Clinical Microbiology and Infectious Diseases (ESCMID) and the International Society of Chemotherapy (ISC) for Infection and Cancer. *Eur Heart J* 2009;30(19):2369–2413.

92. Wilson W, Taubert KA, Gewitz M et al. Prevention of infective endocarditis: guidelines from the American Heart Association: a guideline from the American Heart Association Rheumatic Fever, Endocarditis, and Kawasaki Disease Committee, Council on Cardiovascular Disease in the Young, and the Council on Clinical Cardiology, Council on Cardiovascular Surgery and Anesthesia, and the Quality of Care and Outcomes Research Interdisciplinary Working Group. *Circulation* 2007;116(15):1736–1754.

93. BTS recommendations for assessing risk and for managing Mycobacterium tuberculosis infection and disease in patients due to start anti-TNF-alpha treatment. *Thorax* 2005;60(10):800–805.

94. National Collaborating Centre for Chronic Conditions. *Tuberculosis: Clinical diagnosis and management of tuberculosis, and measures for its prevention and control*. Royal College of Physicians (UK), National Institute for Health and Clinical Excellence, London, 2006.

95. Saag KG, Teng GG, Patkar NM et al. American College of Rheumatology 2008 recommendations for the use of nonbiologic and biologic disease-modifying antirheumatic drugs in rheumatoid arthritis. *Arthritis Rheum* 2008;59(6):762–784.

96. Pinto LM, Grenier J, Schumacher SG et al. Immunodiagnosis of tuberculosis: state of the art. *Med Princ Pract* 2012;21(1):4–13.

97. Vassilopoulos D, Tsikrika S, Hatzara C et al. Comparison of two gamma interferon release assays and tuberculin skin testing for tuberculosis screening in a cohort of patients with rheumatic diseases starting anti-tumor necrosis factor therapy. *Clin Vaccine Immunol* 2011;18(12): 2102–2108.

CHAPTER 108

Rheumatic fever

Andrew Steer

Introduction

Acute rheumatic fever is an autoimmune disease that follows infection with a bacterium, the beta-haemolytic Lancefield group A streptococcus (*Streptococcus pyogenes*). It affects multiple systems including the heart, the joints, the brain, and the skin. Only the effects on the heart can lead to permanent illness; the chronic changes to the valves of the heart are called rheumatic heart disease. Acute rheumatic fever can be primary (a first episode in a patient without a prior episode of rheumatic fever and without evidence of established rheumatic heart disease) or recurrent. Recurrent episodes of rheumatic fever lead to cumulative damage to the cardiac valvular tissues and worsening rheumatic heart disease.

Epidemiology

Acute rheumatic fever was common in industrialized nations including the United Kingdom in the 1800s and early 1900s until its frequency decreased over the course of the first half of the 20th century (Figure 108.1).[1] Much of the reduction in the rate of rheumatic fever occurred before the introduction of antibiotics and therefore this decrease was thought to be mostly due to improvements in living conditions and hygiene with an associated interruption in the transmission of group A streptococci.[1] Cases of rheumatic fever still occur in industrialized countries, however, and outbreaks of rheumatic fever have been reported as recently as the 1980s.[2-4] Overall the incidence of acute rheumatic fever in countries such as the United Kingdom is low (<1 per 100 000), and in the United States acute rheumatic fever is an uncommon hospital admission representing 14.8 cases per 100 000 paediatric hospital admissions.[5]

By contrast, high rates of acute rheumatic fever and rheumatic heart disease are found in developing countries and in populations of indigenous peoples living in industrialized countries.[6,7] There are over 330 000 new cases of acute rheumatic fever each year in children aged 5–14 years worldwide. The highest rates of acute rheumatic fever have been documented in Aboriginal children aged 5–14 in the Northern Territory of Australia (>500 cases per 100 000). More than 2.4 million children aged 5–14 years have rheumatic heart disease worldwide and 94% of these are in developing countries.[6]

Primary episodes of acute rheumatic fever occur mainly in children aged 5–15 years, and are rare in people aged over 30 years. Recurrent episodes remain relatively common in adolescents and young adults up until the age of around 35 years.[8] There is no clear gender predilection for acute rheumatic fever. Most epidemiologic surveys of rheumatic fever and rheumatic heart disease have observed an association with low socio-economic status, most probably related to levels of crowding.[9] There is no definitive evidence for a racial predisposition to rheumatic fever, but there appear to groups at particularly high risk, including Pacific Island populations and Aboriginal Australians.[5,9–11]

Between 3 and 6% of any population may be susceptible to acute rheumatic fever and this susceptibility appears to be inherited.[8,12] Familial clustering of cases of acute rheumatic fever have been found, and there is weak concordance in monozygotic twins.[13,14] Particular HLA class II alleles appear to be associated with rheumatic fever susceptibility including *HLA DRB1*0701* and *DQA1*0201* alleles and *DRB1*0701-DQA1*0201* and *DRB1*13-DQA1*0501-3-DQB1*0301* haplotypes.[15] The D8/17 antigen is expressed on B cells and may act as a binding site for the group A streptococcus on these cells,[16] and there is a strong association in a number of populations between the expression of D8/17 antigen and rheumatic

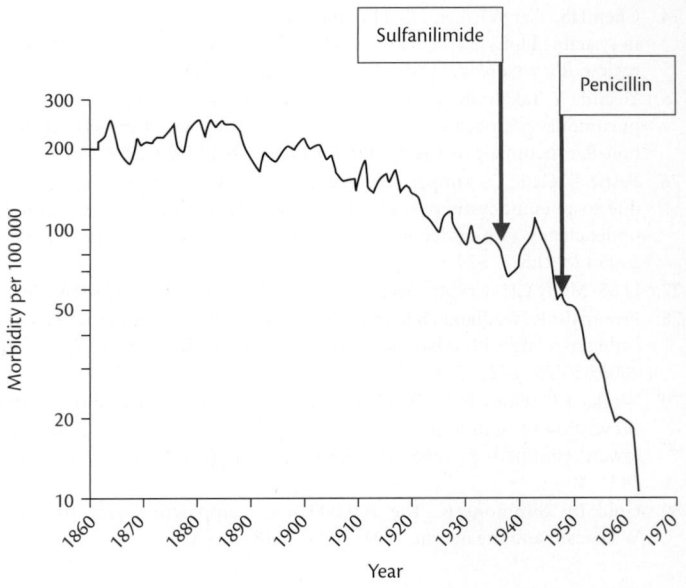

Fig. 108.1 The falling incidence of rheumatic fever in Denmark 1860–1970.[77]
Lennon D. Acute rheumatic fever in children—recognition and treatment. Pediatric Drugs. 2004;6(6):363–73.

including in the United States, Australia, Israel, Russia, Mexico, and Chile,[17–19] although this association is not universal.[20,21]

Aetiopathogenesis

Acute rheumatic fever is the result of an interaction between a group A streptococcal strain with certain undefined features that confer an ability to cause acute rheumatic fever, and a host with an inherited susceptibility. This interaction leads to an autoimmune response directed against cardiac, synovial, subcutaneous, epidermal, and neuronal tissues. Traditional teaching states that rheumatic fever follows pharyngitis but not pyoderma, although this has been questioned.[22]

The exact nature of the pathogenesis of rheumatic fever is still to be determined, but it is believed that both cross-reactive antibodies and cross-reactive T cells play a role in the disease, and that molecular mimicry between group A streptococcal antigens and human host tissue is the basis of this cross-reactivity (Figure 108.2).[23] With a severe initial attack and with repeated attacks, rheumatic granulomatous inflammation manifests in the myocardium as Aschoff bodies leading to chronic rheumatic heart disease.[24]

Diagnostic criteria

The diagnosis of rheumatic fever is a clinical one. The Jones criteria were established in 1944 to aid clinicians in making the diagnosis of acute rheumatic fever.[25] These criteria divide the clinical features of rheumatic fever into major and minor manifestations. The criteria were modified in 1956,[26] revised in 1965,[27] revised again in 1984,[28] and updated in 1992.[29] The 1992 update is the most widely used version today (Table 108.1), but the criteria are currently under revision again.

It should be noted that the Jones criteria are intended as guidelines only, designed to aid clinicians in the exercise of their clinical judgment, not replace it. The Jones criteria are often applied in a different manner in high-risk populations as recommended by some international and national health authorities, including the World Health Organization (Table 108.1).[8,30] It may be appropriate, therefore, to consider immigrants from rheumatic fever endemic developing countries as high risk, particularly if they are newly arrived.

Clinical features

The diagnosis of rheumatic fever can be complex and requires attention to all of the manifestations of acute rheumatic fever, while considering other, often more likely, diagnoses for each manifestation. Each clinical manifestation is considered below.

Major manifestations of acute rheumatic fever

Arthritis

Polyarthritis, along with fever, is one of the most common presenting symptoms of rheumatic fever. Joint involvement occurs in more than 75% of first attacks of rheumatic fever, and may be a major manifestation (polyarthritis) or a minor manifestation (polyarthralgia or aseptic monoarthritis). However, because of the broad differential diagnosis of arthritis, including viral and reactive arthropathies, septic arthritis, and systemic lupus erythematosus (SLE), it is the most challenging diagnostic feature of rheumatic fever. The classic history of joint involvement in acute rheumatic fever is one of asymmetrical, large joint (especially knees, ankles,

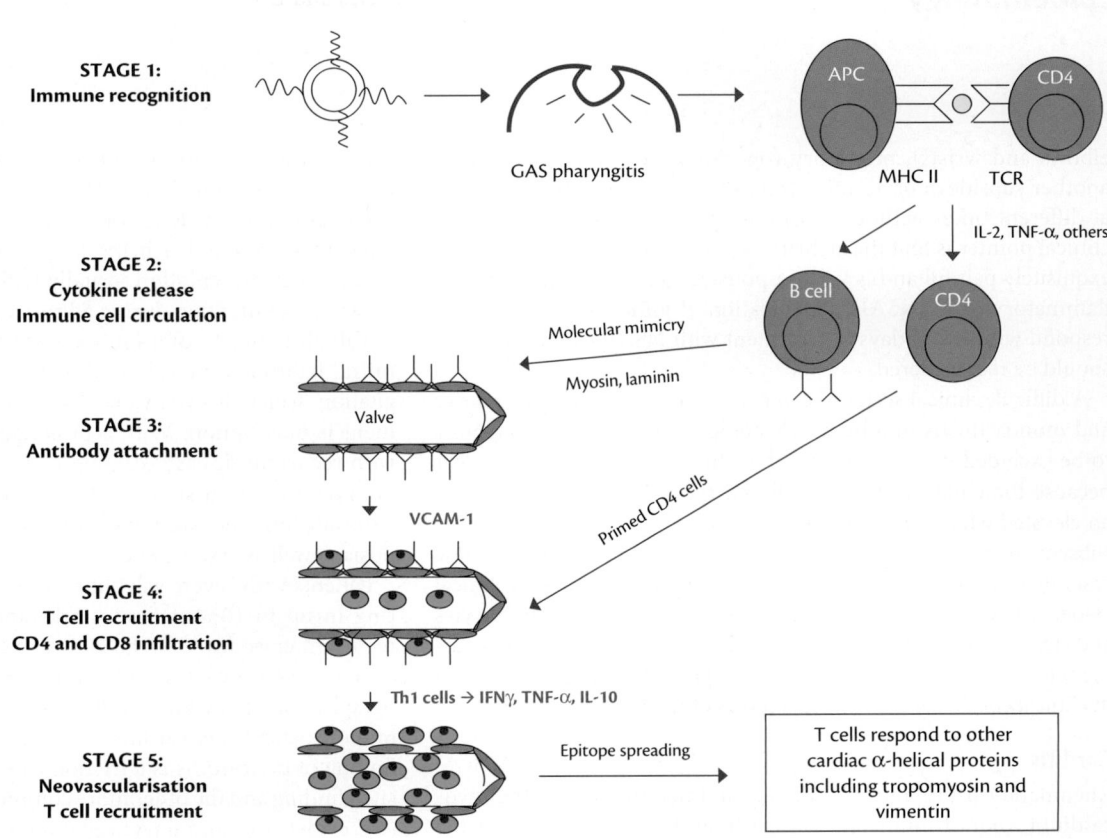

Fig. 108.2 A proposed model of the pathogenesis of acute rheumatic fever.

Table 108.1 The Jones criteria for the diagnosis of acute rheumatic fever[29]

Major manifestations	Carditis	
	Polyarthritis	
	Chorea	
	Erythema marginatum	
	Subcutaneous nodules	
Minor manifestations	Clinical:	Polyarthralgia or aseptic monoarthritis
		Fever
	Laboratory:	Elevated acute-phase reactants (CRP or ESR)
		Prolonged P-R interval on electrocardiogram
Evidence of antecedent group A streptococcal infection		Elevated or rising streptococcal antibody titres (ASOT, ASD B)
		Positive throat culture or rapid streptococcal antigen test
		Major/minor criteria
Initial episode of rheumatic fever		Two major, or
		One major and two minor manifestations
Recurrent rheumatic fever in a patient with known past rheumatic fever or established rheumatic heart disease		Two major, or
		One major and two minor manifestations

Notes: All of the above clinical manifestations assume that other more likely diagnoses have been excluded. There are a couple of important caveats to remember when applying the Jones criteria:
♦ In a patient in whom arthritis is considered as a major manifestation, arthralgia cannot be considered as a minor manifestation.
♦ In a patient in whom carditis is considered as a major manifestation, prolonged P-R interval cannot be considered as a minor manifestation.
♦ Chorea does not require evidence of a preceding group A streptococcal infection.

In populations at high risk of acute rheumatic fever and rheumatic heart disease (high-risk populations have been defined as a population where the incidence of rheumatic fever is >30 per 100 000 and/or the prevalence of rheumatic heart disease is >2 per 1000),[74] some authorities suggest modifications to the Jones criteria:
♦ Echocardiographic evidence of valvulitis without clinical findings (so-called subclinical carditis) may be considered as a major manifestation.[30]
♦ Monoarthritis or polyarthralgia may be considered as a major manifestation.[30]
♦ A recurrence in a patient with evidence of established rheumatic heart disease may be diagnosed by the presence of at least two minor manifestations plus evidence of a recent group A streptococcal infection provided that other diagnoses have been excluded.[8]

elbows and wrists), migratory (one joint becoming inflamed as another subsides), or additive (multiple joints becoming inflamed at different times without subsiding) polyarthritis. An important clinical pointer is that the arthritis of acute rheumatic fever is often exquisitely painful and is very responsive to non-steroidal anti-inflammatory drug (NSAID) medication; if joint symptoms do not respond within 2–3 days of treatment with NSAIDs, the diagnosis should be reconsidered.

A difficult clinical scenario can be the child presenting with fever and monoarthritis in a high-risk population.[31] The first diagnosis to be excluded is septic arthritis but this diagnosis is usually clear because the child appears unwell and the joint aspirate will show an elevated white cell count that is predominantly neutrophils with subsequent positive bacterial culture. However, a proportion of these cases may be rheumatic fever, particularly if there are there is clinical evidence of carditis and the joint fluid is predominantly lymphocytes and sterile.[32] In this scenario it is prudent to withhold NSAID treatment to observe for the development of polyarthritis, thereby aiding in clinical confirmation of the diagnosis of rheumatic fever.

Carditis

Rheumatic carditis refers to the active inflammation of the myocardium, endocardium, and pericardium that occurs in rheumatic fever. Carditis occurs in 50–80% of first episodes of rheumatic fever, predominantly as a valvulitis.[2,33,34] In many patients with rheumatic fever evidence of carditis can be found at presentation along with fever and arthritis, but in some patients signs of carditis appear after presentation, usually within the first 2–6 weeks, and repeated examination during admission is therefore important.[35]

Valvulitis most commonly affects the mitral valve leading to mitral regurgitation, followed by the aortic valve as aortic regurgitation. Isolated aortic valve disease without mitral valve involvement is uncommon. With a prolonged and severe first attack or with recurrent disease scarring may lead to stenotic lesions, predominantly mitral stenosis. Diagnosis of valvulitis can be made clinically but echocardiography has assumed a central role in diagnosis as well as assessment of severity (see 'Investigations' below).

Patients with severe valvulitis can develop cardiac failure, occurring in up to 10% of first attacks and then more commonly in recurrent episodes.[36,37] The clinical signs of cardiac failure should be augmented by chest radiograph (Figure 108.3) and echocardiography. Patients with carditis rarely present with chest pain, and in these patients pericarditis should be suspected. The main clinical finding of pericarditis is a friction rub. Pericarditis is rarely an isolated finding and the other more common clinical features of carditis (e.g. evidence of mitral regurgitation) should be carefully sought.

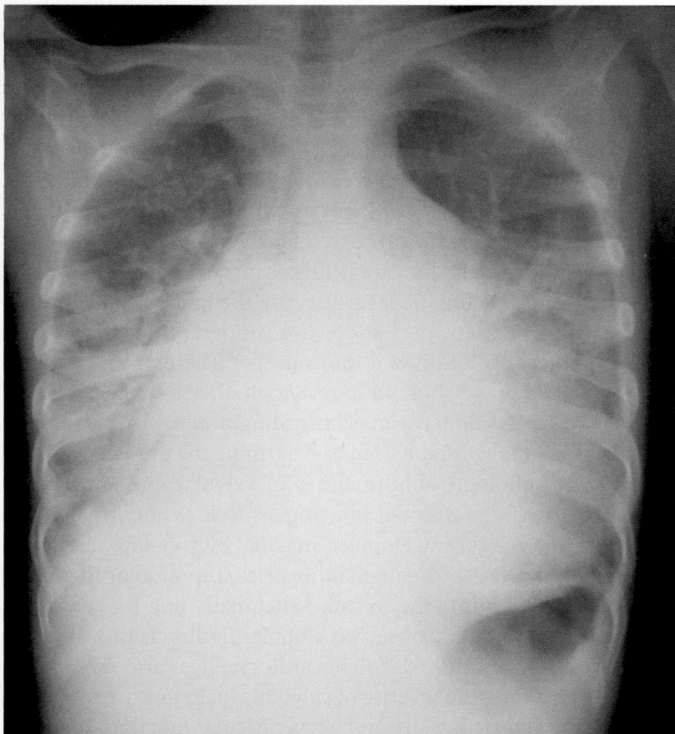

Fig. 108.3 Chest radiograph of biventricular failure secondary to rheumatic fever.[78] Steer AC, Kado J, Colquhoun S, Noonan S, Babitu T. Awareness of rheumatic heart disease. Lancet. 2006;367:2118.

Chorea

Sydenham's chorea, also known as St Vitus' dance, was first described in the 1600s.[38] Chorea can present alongside the other manifestations of rheumatic fever (where it occurs in approximately 10% of first episodes), and also as an isolated presentation without fever or other features of rheumatic fever when it is called 'pure chorea'.[39–41]

Chorea consists of purposeless, involuntary, uncoordinated, rapid movements of the body, especially involving the hands, feet, face, and tongue.[38] Chorea particularly affects adolescent females.[38] There history may initially be subtle, with the child becoming fidgety at school and home, with subsequent clumsiness noted before more florid, uncoordinated, and erratic movements appear. There is often an associated history of emotional lability and other personality changes.[42] An extremely useful point on history and examination is that chorea always disappears with sleep, and is made more pronounced by purposeful movements. The head is often involved with erratic movements of the face that resemble grimaces, grins, and frowns. Severe cases may put patients at risk of self-injury or impair their ability to feed themselves. Choreiform movements can affect the whole body, or just half the body (hemichorea). Recurrence of rheumatic chorea can occur, often associated with pregnancy or the oral contraceptive pill.[43]

The diagnosis of rheumatic chorea is a clinical one, but there are a number of useful clinical signs on examination. Examination of the tongue is important; the patient with chorea will be unable to maintain protrusion of the tongue, and the tongue itself can be involved, often described as a 'bag of worms'. When the patient is asked to grasps the examiner's hands, there is a rhythmic, uncontrollable squeezing, so-called 'milkmaid's grip' sign. When the patients hands are extended, there is flexion of the wrists and

extension of the fingers, so-called 'spooning' sign. When the hands are held above the head, there is turning outwards of the arms and palms, so-called 'pronator' sign. The differential diagnosis of chorea includes SLE, drug intoxication, Wilson's disease, tic disorders, Huntington's chorea, and intracranial tumours.

Because pure chorea may occur up to 6 months after the inciting group A streptococcal infection, evidence of recent group A streptococcal infection may be absent and is not required for diagnosis.[44] Patients with chorea often have a mildly elevated erythrocyte sedimentation rate (ESR). All patients with chorea should have an echocardiogram because of the high likelihood of cardiac involvement.[45]

Erythema marginatum

Erythema marginatum is a distinctive clinical sign of rheumatic fever; however, it is an uncommon manifestation occurring in less than 5% of cases and is rarely found in the absence of carditis and/or arthritis. The rash is a non-pruritic, non-painful blanching evanescent pink rash with a rounded or serpiginous edge that is well-defined (Figure 108.4). Individual lesions begin as a macule and expand with central clearing. The lesions can vary greatly in size and appear mostly on the trunk and proximal limbs but never on the face. The lesions may appear and then disappear before the examiner's eyes, and have been described as 'smoke rings'.

Subcutaneous nodules

Subcutaneous nodules are an uncommon finding in rheumatic fever, occurring in less than 5% of cases. They are firm, mobile, and painless lumps, 0.5–2 cm in diameter; they may occur in crops and are found mainly over the extensor surfaces or bony protuberances particularly on the hands, feet, occiput, and back. They usually appear after the onset of acute rheumatic fever and last from days to 3 weeks. They are strongly associated with carditis.

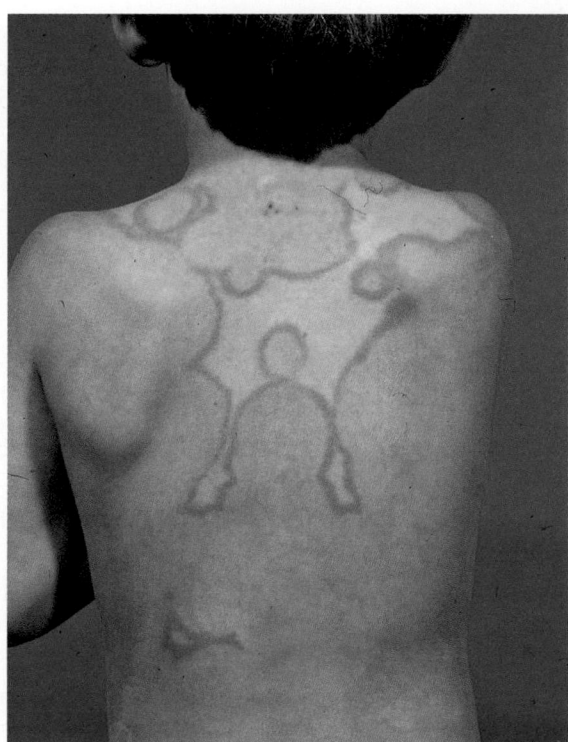

Fig. 108.4 Erythema marginatum.

Minor manifestations of acute rheumatic fever

Minor manifestations are used to support the diagnosis of rheumatic fever when only a single major manifestation is present; the diagnosis of a first episode of rheumatic fever should not be made on the basis of minor manifestations alone.

Clinical findings

Fever is a common finding, occurring in nearly all cases at the onset of the illness. Most patients will have fever in excess of 39 °C, but fever in of 38 °C measured orally, rectally, or tympanically is considered significant.

Arthralgia refers to pain in one or more joints without objective evidence of inflammation. In rheumatic fever arthralgia often has similar features to the polyarthritis described above; that is, it is migratory, asymmetric, and affects large joints.

Laboratory findings

There are two key laboratory findings that are considered minor manifestations of acute rheumatic fever: elevated acute-phase reactants (ESR and C-reactive protein (CRP)) and prolonged P-R interval on electrocardiogram (see 'Investigations').

Investigations

The diagnosis of rheumatic fever requires a series of investigations (Box 108.1).[30] Investigations are required for: (1) confirming/excluding the presence of carditis (chest radiograph and echocardiography); (2) determining the severity of carditis if present (chest radiograph and echocardiography); (3) determining the presence of minor manifestations (elevated acute-phase reactants, prolonged P-R interval on electrocardiogram); (4) establishing evidence of preceding group A streptococcal infection (throat swab, rapid group A streptococcal antigen test, streptococcal serology); and (5) exclusion of differential diagnoses.

Chest radiograph

A chest radiograph should be performed in all cases in whom carditis is suspected.[46] In patients with carditis the radiograph may demonstrate chamber enlargement and frank congestive cardiac failure secondary to valvulitis and valvular dysfunction (Figure 108.3).

Box 108.1 Minimum investigations for the diagnosis of acute rheumatic fever

- Erythrocyte sedimentation rate (ESR)
- C-reactive protein (CRP)
- Electrocardiogram (ECG)
- Chest radiograph if clinical or echocardiographic evidence of carditis
- Echocardiogram (consider repeating after 1 month if negative)
- Throat swab (preferably before giving antibiotics)—culture for group A streptococci and/or rapid antigen test for group A streptococci
- Anti-streptococcal serology (anti-streptolysin O and anti-DNase B titres, repeat 10–14 days later if first test not confirmatory)

Echocardiography

The 1992 update of the Jones criteria does not allow inclusion of echocardiography findings alone as a criterion for carditis. However, it is clear that echocardiography allows at least accurate confirmation of clinical findings and objective measurement of severity of valvular lesions.[34,47] With increasing experience it appears that echocardiographic evidence alone (so-called subclinical carditis) is sufficient to determine the presence of valvulitis, especially in high-risk populations.[48] Subclinical carditis occurs in approximately 15% of cases of acute rheumatic fever because the first episode of rheumatic carditis is often mild and echocardiographic findings may precede clinical evolution of a murmur.[35,49] Therefore, all patients with suspected acute rheumatic fever, whether they have clinical carditis or not, should have an echocardiogram.

Echocardiography can be used to determine the presence of characteristic morphologic abnormalities of valvular and subvalvular tissue using two-dimensional imaging, as well as abnormalities of flow across the valve using Doppler imaging. Morphological changes include mitral valve thickening and restricted motion of the mitral valve leaflet that leads to the so-called rheumatic 'dog-leg deformity', and the most commonly observed Doppler finding is that of mitral regurgitation (Figure 108.5).[50] Echocardiography is also very important in determining the severity of valvulitis including assessment of left atrial and ventricular size and left ventricular function, and these findings inform clinical decision-making regarding management.

Electrocardiogram

Conduction abnormalities occur in up to 33% of first episodes of rheumatic fever.[2] Prolonged P-R interval is a non-specific finding, occurring in some healthy people. However, a prolonged P-R interval that resolves over the course of an episode of rheumatic fever is a useful diagnostic feature. Second-degree, and even complete heart block, are less common but can occur (Figure 108.6).[51]

Inflammatory markers

The most reliably elevated acute-phase reactants in rheumatic fever are the ESR (≥30 mm/h) and the CRP (≥30 mg/L). The peripheral

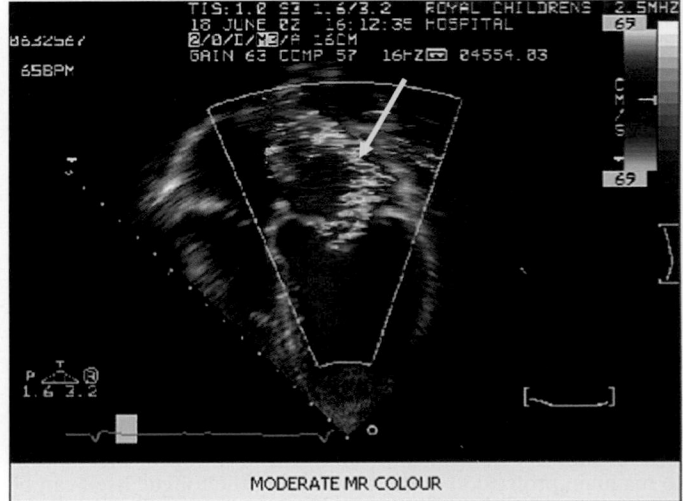

Fig. 108.5 Mitral regurgitation on echocardiogram (arrow indicates the mitral regurgitant jet into the left atrium).

Reproduced from Carapetis, J Rheumatic Heart Disease in Developing Countries, N Engl Jnl Med 357;5 (2007) pp. 439–441 with permission from Massachusetts Medical Society.

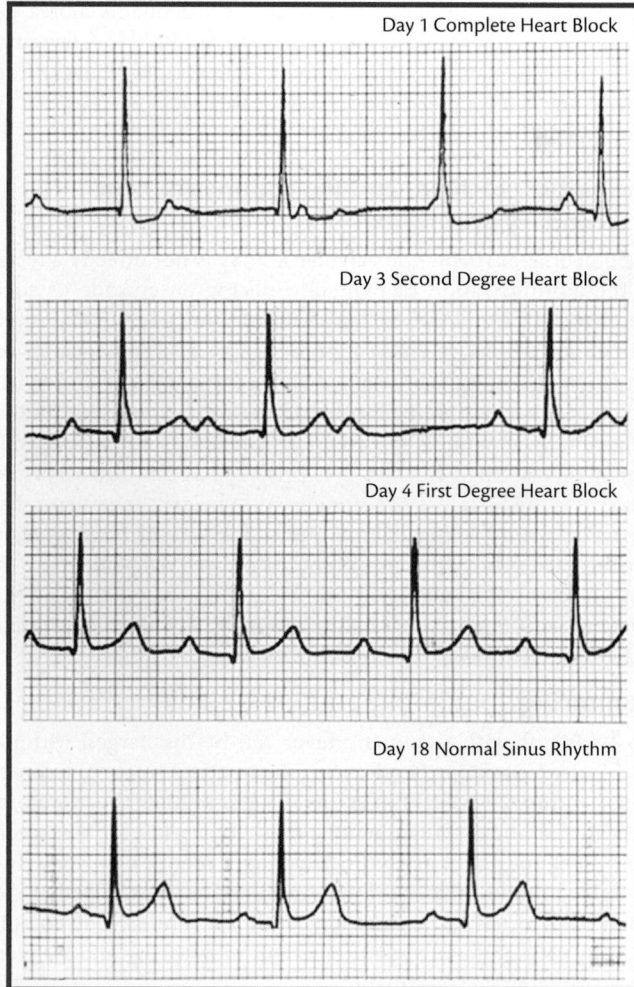

Fig. 108.6 Electrocardiogram showing heart block in acute rheumatic fever.[79] Bishop W, Currie B, Carapetis J, Kilburn C. A subtle presentation of acute rheumatic fever in remote northern Australia. Aust N Z J Med. 1996 Apr;26:241–2.

white cell count is less reliably elevated and is not included in the 1992 Jones criteria update.[29]

Supporting evidence of preceding streptococcal infection

Evidence of a preceding group A streptococcal infection should be sought in all cases of suspected rheumatic fever. Absence of a serologic response to streptococcal antigens and/or absence of microbiologic evidence of group A streptococcal pharyngitis makes the diagnosis of rheumatic fever highly unlikely, except in the case of pure chorea.

A throat swab for bacterial culture on blood agar and/or rapid antigen test should be taken, although less than 10% of throat swabs are positive for group A streptococcus,[52] reflecting the postinfectious nature of the disease—i.e. the group A streptococcus is eradicated before onset of the disease. As a result, streptococcal antibody titres are key in confirming the diagnosis of rheumatic fever. The most commonly used tests are the anti-streptolysin O (ASO) titre and the anti-deoxyribonuclease B (ADB) titre. It is generally recommended that paired titres be taken, i.e. an acute titre and a convalescent titre (usually taken 14–28 days after the initial titre). A positive result is defined as a rise in titre of twofold or more.[53] However, a titre greater than

Table 108.2 Recommended upper limits of normal for anti-streptolysin O and anti-DNase B titres[54,75,76]

Age group (years)	Upper limit of normal	
	ASO titre (IU/mL)	Anti-DNase B titre (IU/mL)
2–4	160	240
5–9	240	320–640
10–12	320	480–640
>12	400	200

the upper limit of normal at the initial testing is also considered positive (Table 108.2).[54]

Management

While treatment can shorten the acute inflammation of rheumatic fever, all of the various manifestations will resolve of their own accord, except for carditis. Carditis can lead to chronic rheumatic heart disease, but none of the treatments used in the acute phase of rheumatic fever can alter the course of progression to rheumatic heart disease.[55] However, good compliance with secondary prophylaxis over time can positively alter the progression of rheumatic heart disease. The aims of the management of acute rheumatic fever are summarized in Box 108.2.

Confirmation of the diagnosis of rheumatic fever

All patients with acute rheumatic fever should be admitted so that the diagnosis can be confirmed and so that the clinical features and severity of the attack can be assessed. Some patients in whom the diagnosis has already been confirmed and who have a mild attack may be able to be managed as an outpatient after an initial period of stabilization.

Management of arthritis and arthralgia

The first-line treatment is salicylate therapy, based on extensive experience with aspirin in acute rheumatic fever, although there

---

Box 108.2 Aims of the management of acute rheumatic fever

1 Confirm the diagnosis of acute rheumatic fever

2 Provide symptomatic treatment and to shorten the acute inflammatory phase, particularly for joint involvement which can be very painful

3 Determine the presence and severity of carditis, and manage cardiac failure if present

4 Manage chorea if present

5 Commence secondary prophylaxis in all patients

6 Monitoring in hospital

7 Provide education for the patient and the patient's family about rheumatic fever and rheumatic heart disease, and emphasize the importance of compliance to secondary prophylaxis

8 Ensure that follow-up is arranged

is increasing experience with NSAIDs such as ibuprofen and naproxren.[56-58] Naproxen has been used successfully including in one small randomized controlled trial,[59] and some experts recommend it because of its twice-daily dosing and more favourable side-effect profile. Aspirin can have a dramatic effect on the both arthritis and fever in patients with rheumatic fever, and if there is little or no response after 2–3 days of therapy then the diagnosis should be reconsidered. A particularly important group of patients are those with suspected acute rheumatic fever that have monoarthritis. These patients should be admitted and observed for the appearance of another affected joint and it may be necessary to withhold anti-inflammatory therapy and use paracetamol or codeine to manage the pain of arthritis until the diagnosis can be confirmed.

The duration of anti-inflammatory treatment is dictated by the clinical response and improvement in inflammatory markers (ESR, CRP). Many patients need anti-inflammatory therapy for only 1–2 weeks when there is a good clinical response with resolution of pain and when inflammatory markers normalize. In some patients joint symptoms may recur following cessation of treatment (so-called 'rebound phenomenon')—this does not indicate recurrence, and can be treated with another course of anti-inflammatory therapy.[60] Some patients who still have symptoms or elevated inflammatory markers at 2 weeks may require anti-inflammatory therapy for up to 6 weeks. A very small subset of patients (<5%) require 6 months or more of anti-inflammatory therapy.

Management of carditis

Most patients with mild or moderate carditis without cardiac failure do not require any specific therapy. In general, salicylates, NSAIDs, intravenous immunoglobulin (IVIG), and glucocorticoid therapy are not recommended in the treatment of carditis because their use has not been directly associated with a reduction in residual rheumatic heart disease.[55,61]

All patients with cardiac failure require an urgent echocardiogram and review by a cardiologist. Patients require bed rest with gradual ambulation as tolerated. Diuretic therapy results in improvement in most cases, and the addition of other therapy such as an angiotensin converting enzyme (ACE) inhibitor or digoxin should be undertaken in consultation with a cardiologist. Rarely, more severe cardiac failure is present and it is in this situation that some clinicians prescribe glucocorticoid therapy; anecdotal experience suggests that glucocorticoids can more rapidly improve severe cardiac failure.[61] Acute surgery is rarely attempted unless there is valve leaflet or chordal rupture with associated torrential and life-threatening regurgitation.

Management of chorea

Most patients with chorea do not require treatment as it is benign and self-limiting.[62] Reassurance and a quiet and calm environment often suffice. However, occasionally patients have chorea that is so severe that it may interrupt activities of daily living including eating, may become very distressing to family members, and may even place the patient at risk of serious injury. In these circumstances treatment with valproic acid or carbamazepine is appropriate. Valproic acid may be more effective than carbamazepine,[63] but carbamazepine is preferred as first line because of the potential for liver toxicity with valproic acid.[30] Haloperidol should be avoided, as should combinations of agents. Aspirin has no effect on rheumatic chorea. Anecdotal reports suggest that prednisolone can reduce

symptom severity and shorten the course of Sydenham's chorea, but randomized studies have found conflicting results.[64,65] A few small studies of IVIG have appeared to show a more rapid recovery from chorea, but IVIG should be reserved for treatment of cases that are refractory to first-line treatments.[49,65,66]

Antibiotic treatment and the commencement of secondary prophylaxis

The outcome of rheumatic valvular lesions is not directly affected by the administration of penicillin during an episode of acute rheumatic fever.[67] However, the administration of penicillin is recommended to ensure eradication of group A streptococci in the throat whether there has been a positive throat culture or not. The choice is either oral penicillin for 10 days or a single injection of benzathine penicillin G. Intravenous penicillin is not necessary. In general benzathine penicillin G is preferred as this also serves the purpose as the first dose of secondary prophylaxis. In patients with bona-fide allergy to penicillin, a macrolide such as erythromycin, clarithromycin, or azithromycin should be used. As penicillin is the first-line choice for secondary prophylaxis it is recommended that a patient with reported penicillin allergy be investigated carefully and it may be necessary to consult with an allergist.

Monitoring

Most patients with rheumatic fever can be discharged within 2 weeks of presentation, and anti-inflammatory treatment can be ceased within 6 weeks if not earlier. Progress should be monitored clinically, although inflammatory markers weekly for 4–6 weeks can be helpful, particularly in detecting a rebound episode. It is advisable to repeat the echocardiogram at 4–6 weeks whether carditis was detected or not. Patients with a severe episode complicated by cardiac failure require careful monitoring and frequent echocardiographic assessment.

Education

Education is a key component of the management of all patients with rheumatic fever because of the necessity of ongoing long-term preventive measures. The disease, and its implications, should be explained to the patient and family with the aid of printed educational materials. Patients should be aware that in the long term they are at risk of repeated episodes of acute rheumatic fever and of developing chronic rheumatic heart disease; 30–50% of all patients with rheumatic fever will develop rheumatic heart disease and this risk increases to more than 70% if the initial attack is severe or if there has been at least one recurrence.[68]. Therefore, secondary prophylaxis to prevent recurrent attacks is very important, particularly as 75% of recurrences occur within 2 years of the first attack and more than 90% occur within the first 5 years.[31]

Adequate follow-up and adherence to secondary prophylaxis

The management of a patient with rheumatic fever does not end at discharge because of the implications of the diagnosis for the development of rheumatic heart disease. The main priority of long-term management is to ensure adherence to secondary prophylaxis. Secondary prophylaxis involves regular administration of penicillin (usually intramuscular benzathine penicillin G) to patients with a history of acute rheumatic fever or with established rheumatic heart disease for many years. Intramuscular benzathine penicillin

Table 108.3 Duration of secondary prophylaxis following rheumatic fever

Category	Duration
Rheumatic fever without carditis	5 years or until age 21 years (whichever is longer)
Rheumatic fever with carditis that has resolved	10 years or until age 21 years (whichever is longer)
Rheumatic fever with carditis that has led to residual rheumatic heart disease	10 years or until age 40 years (whichever is longer); Sometimes lifelong if very severe disease

Adapted from the American Heart Association and the American Academy of Pediatrics.[72]

reduces streptococcal pharyngitis by 71–91% and reduces recurrent rheumatic fever by 87–96%.[69] Secondary prophylaxis can also reduce the severity of rheumatic heart disease, can reduce mortality from rheumatic heart disease and can lead to regression of mild rheumatic heart disease in 50–70% of patients who are fully adherent over a decade.[70,71]

Recommendations on the frequency of intramuscular injections and the duration of secondary prophylaxis varies between authorities.[8,30,72] Most patients can be started on 4-weekly injections and if there is a 'breakthrough' episode of rheumatic fever can be switched to a 3-weekly regimen.[73] The duration of secondary prophylaxis is determined by a number of factors including age, time since last episode of rheumatic fever, and severity of disease (Table 108.3).[8]

Conclusion

Rheumatic fever is a multisystem, autoimmune, inflammatory condition that follows infection with group A streptococci. Rheumatic fever is now uncommon in industrialized countries, but remains a major public health concern in many tropical developing countries. Patients typically present with fever and arthritis, but may also present with carditis, chorea, and/or characteristic skin and soft tissue findings. Of greatest long-term concern is the presence of carditis, manifesting as a valvulitis that can progress to chronic rheumatic valvular disease, a condition associated with considerable morbidity and premature mortality. The first priority in management is to make an accurate clinical diagnosis of rheumatic fever as there is a broad differential diagnosis for a number of the clinical features of rheumatic fever. Once the diagnosis is made, the aim of management is to treat the inflammation of rheumatic fever and to can adequately assess and manage any cardiac involvement. Secondary prophylaxis is the mainstay of long-term management and patients require antibiotic prophylaxis for at least 5 years and often much longer.

References

1. Quinn RW. Comprehensive review of morbidity and mortality trends for rheumatic fever, streptococcal disease, and scarlet fever: the decline of rheumatic fever. *Rev Infect Dis* 1989;11:928–953.
2. Veasy LG, Tani LY, Hill HR. Persistence of acute rheumatic fever in the intermountain area of the United States. *J Pediatr* 1994;124:9–16.
3. Veasy LG, Wiedmeier SE, Orsmond GS et al. Resurgence of acute rheumatic fever in the intermountain area of the United States. *N Engl J Med* 1987;316:421–427.
4. Johnson DR, Stevens DL, Kaplan EL. Epidemiologic analysis of group A streptococcal serotypes associated with severe systemic infections, rheumatic fever, or uncomplicated pharyngitis. *J Infect Dis* 1992;166:374–382.
5. Miyake CY, Gauvreau K, Tani LY, Sundel RP, Newburger JW. Characteristics of children discharged from hospitals in the United States in 2000 with the diagnosis of acute rheumatic fever. *Pediatrics* 2007;120:503–508.
6. Carapetis JR, Steer AC, Mulholland EK, Weber M. The global burden of group A streptococcal diseases. *Lancet Infect Dis* 2005;5(11):685–694.
7. Steer AC, Carapetis JR. Prevention and treatment of rheumatic heart disease in the developing world. *Nat Rev Cardiol* 2009;6:689–698.
8. *Rheumatic fever and rheumatic heart disease: report of a WHO Expert Consultation.* World Health Organization, Geneva, 2004.
9. Steer AC, Carapetis JR, Nolan TM, Shann F. Systematic review of rheumatic heart disease prevalence in children in developing countries: the role of environmental factors. *J Paediatr Child Health* 2002;38:229–234.
10. Chun LT, Reddy DV, Yamamoto LG. Rheumatic fever in children and adolescents in Hawaii. *Pediatrics* 1987 Apr;79:549–552.
11. Chun LT, Reddy V, Rhoads GG. Occurrence and prevention of rheumatic fever among ethnic groups of Hawaii. *Am J Dis Child* 1984;138:476–478.
12. Carapetis JR, Currie BJ, Mathews JD. Cumulative incidence of rheumatic fever in an endemic region: a guide to the susceptibility of the population? *Epidemiol Infect* 2000;124:239–244.
13. Wilson MG, Schweitzer MD, Lubschez R. The familail epidemiology of rheumatic fever: genetic and epidemiologic studies. *J Pediatr* 1943;22:468–492.
14. Taranta A, Torodsag S, Metrakos J, Jeiger W, Uchida I. Rheumatic fever in monozygotic and dizygotic twins. *Circulation* 1959;20:778.
15. Guedez Y, Kotby A, El-Demellawy M et al. HLA class II associations with rheumatic heart disease are more evident and consistent among clinically homogeneous patients. *Circulation* 1999;99:2784–2790.
16. Kemeny E, Husby GW, Williams RC Jr, Zabriskie JB. Tissue distribution of antigen(s) defined by monoclonal antibody D8/17 reacting with B lymphocytes of patients with rheumatic heart disease. *Clin Immunol Immunopathol* 1994;72(35–43).
17. Harel L, Zeharia A, Kodman Y et al. Presence of the d8/17 B-cell marker in children with rheumatic fever in Israel. *Clin Genet* 2002;61(4):293–298.
18. Harrington Z, Visvanathan K, Skinner NA et al. B-cell antigen D8/17 is a marker of rheumatic fever susceptibility in Aboriginal Australians and can be tested in remote settings. *Med J Aust* 2006;184:507–510.
19. Khanna AK, Buskirk DR, Williams RC, Jr et al. Presence of a non-HLA B cell antigen in rheumatic fever patients and their families as defined by a monoclonal antibody. *J Clin Invest* 1989;83:1710–1716.
20. Weisz JL, McMahon WM, Moore JC et al. D8/17 and CD19 Expression on lymphocytes of patients with acute rheumatic fever and Tourette's disorder. *Clin Diagn Lab Immunol* 2004;11(2):330–336.
21. Kaur S, Kumar D, Grover A et al. Ethnic differences in expression of susceptibility marker(s) in rheumatic fever/rheumatic heart disease patients. *Int J Cardiol* 1998;64:9–14.
22. McDonald M, Currie BJ, Carapetis JR. Acute rheumatic fever: a chink in the chain that links the heart to the throat? *Lancet Infect Dis* 2004;4:240–245.
23. Guilherme L, Kalil J, Cunningham MW. Molecular mimicry in the autoimmune pathogenesis of rheumatic heart disease. *Autoimmunity* 2006;39(1):31–39.
24. Kumar V, Fausto N, Abbas A. *Robbins & Cotran pathologic basis of disease*, 7th edn. W.B. Saunders, Philadelphia, 2004.
25. Jones TD. The diagnosis of rheumatic fever. *J Am Med Assoc* 1944;126:481–484.
26. Rutstein DD. Report of the committee on standards and criteria for programs of care of the council of rheumatic fever and congenital heart disease of the American Heart Association: Jones criteria (modified) for guidance in the diagnosis of rheumatic fever. *Circulation* 1956;13:617–620.

27. Stollerman GH, Markowitz M, Taranta A, Wannamaker LW, Whittemore R. Committee report: Jones criteria (revised) for guidance in the diagnosis of rheumatic fever. *Circulation* 1965;32:664–668.

28. Committee of rheumatic fever and bacterial endocarditis of the American Heart Association: Jones Criteria (revised) for guidance in the diagnosis of rheumatic fever. *Circulation* 1984;69:204A–208A.

29. Steer AC, Carapetis JR. Acute rheumatic fever and rheumatic heart disease in indigenous populations. *Pediatr Clin North Am* 2009;56:6.

30. National Heart Foundation of Australia and Cardiac Society of Australia and New Zealand. *Diagnosis and management of acute rheumatic fever and rheumatic heart disease in Australia: an evidence-based review.* NHFA, Melbourne, 2006.

31. Carapetis JR, Currie BJ. Rheumatic fever in a high incidence population: the importance of monoarthritis and low grade fever. *Arch Dis Child* 2001;85:223–227.

32. Mataika R, Carapetis JR, Kado J, Steer AC. Acute rheumatic fever: an important differential diagnosis of septic arthritis. *J Trop Paediatr* 2008;54(3):205–207.

33. Steer AC, Kado J, Jenney AW et al. Acute rheumatic fever and rheumatic heart disease in Fiji: prospective surveillance, 2005–2007. *Med J Aust* 2009;190(3):133–135.

34. Vasan RS, Shrivastava S, Vijayakumar M et al. Echocardiographic evaluation of patients with acute rheumatic fever and rheumatic carditis. *Circulation* 1996;94:73–82.

35. Abernethy M, Bass N, Sharpe N et al. Doppler echocardiography and the early diagnosis of carditis in acute rheumatic fever. *Aust N Z J Med* 1994;24:530–535.

36. Meira ZMA, Goulart EMA, Colosimo EA, Mota CC. Long term follow up of rheumatic fever and predictors of severe rheumatic valvar disease in Brazilian children and adolescents. *Heart* 2005;91:1019–1022.

37. Kamblock J, Nguyen L, Pagis B et al. Acute severe mitral regurgitation during first attacks of rheumatic fever: clinical spectrum, mechanisms and prognostic factors. *J Heart Valve Dis* 2005;14:440–446.

38. Colony HS, Malamud N. Sydenham's chorea; a clinicopathologic study. *Neurology* 1956;6:672–676.

39. Sanyal SK, Thapar MK, Ahmed SH, Hooja V, Tewari P. The initial attack of acute rheumatic fever during childhood in North India; a prospective study of the clinical profile. *Circulation* 1974;49:7–12.

40. Jamal M, Abbas KA. Clinical profile of acute rheumatic fever in children. *J Trop Pediatr* 1989;35:10–13.

41. Carapetis JR, Currie BJ. Rheumatic chorea in northern Australia: a clinical and epidemiological study. *Arch Dis Child* 1999;80:353–358.

42. Swedo SE, Leonard HL, Schapiro MB et al. Sydenham's chorea: physical and psychological symptoms of St Vitus dance. *Pediatrics* 1993;91:706–713.

43. Leys D, Destee A, Petit H, Warot P. Chorea associated with oral contraception. *J Neurol* 1987;235:46–48.

44. Taranta A, Stollerman GH. The relationship of Sydenham's chorea to infection with group A streptococci. *Am J Med* 1956;20:170–175.

45. Elevli M, Celebi A, Tombul T, Gokalp AS. Cardiac involvement in Sydenham's chorea: clinical and Doppler echocardiographic findings. *Acta Paediatr* 1999;88:1074–1077.

46. Gentles TL, Colan SD, Wilson NJ, Biosa R, Neutze JM. Left ventricular mechanics during and after acute rheumatic fever: contractile dysfunction is closely related to valve regurgitation. *J Am Coll Cardiol* 2001;37:201–207.

47. Jaffe WM, Roche AH, Coverdale HA et al. Clinical evaluation versus Doppler echocardiography in the quantitative assessment of valvular heart disease. *Circulation* 1988;78(2):267–275.

48. Tubridy-Clark M, Carapetis JR. Subclinical carditis in rheumatic fever: A systematic review. *Int J Cardiol* 2007;119(1):54–58.

49. Voss LM, Wilson NJ, Neutze JM et al. Intravenous immunoglobulin in acute rheumatic fever: a randomized controlled trial. *Circulation* 2001;103:401–406.

50. Remenyi B, Wilson N, Steer A et al. World Heart Federation criteria for echocardiographic diagnosis of rheumatic heart disease—an evidence-based guideline. *Nat Rev Cardiol* 2012;9(5):297–309.

51. Reeves BM. Complete heart block complicating acute rheumatic fever. *J Paediatr Child Health* 2011;47:844–845.

52. Martin DR, Voss LM, Walker SJ, Lennon D. Acute rheumatic fever in Auckland, New Zealand: spectrum of associated group A streptococci different from expected. *Pediatr Infect Dis J* 1994;13:264–269.

53. Wannamaker LW, Ayoub EM. Antibody titers in acute rheumatic fever. *Circulation* 1960;21:598–614.

54. Kaplan EL, Rothermel CD, Johnson DR. Antistreptolysin O and anti-deoxyribonuclease B titers: normal values for children ages 2 to 12 in the United States. *Pediatrics* 1998;101:86–88.

55. Albert DA, Harel L, Karrison T. The treatment of rheumatic carditis: a review and meta-analysis. *Medicine* (Baltimore) 1995;74:1–12.

56. Illingworth RS, Lorber J, Holt KS. Acute rheumatic fever in children: a comparison of six forms of treatment in 200 cases. *Lancet* 1957;273:653–659.

57. Dorfman A, Gross JI, Lorincz AE. The treatment of acute rheumatic fever. *Pediatrics* 1961;27:692–706.

58. Bywaters EGL, Thomas GT. Bed rest, salicylates and steroid in rheumatic fever. *Br Med J* 1961;1:1628–1634.

59. Hashkes PJ, Tauber T, Somekh E et al. Naproxen as an alternative to aspirin for the treatment of arthritis of rheumatic fever: a randomized trial. *J Pediatr* 2003;143:399–401.

60. Feinstein AR, Spagnuolo M, Gill FA. The rebound phenomenon in acute rheumatic fever. I. Incidence and significance. *Yale J Biol Med* 1961;33:259–278.

61. Cilliers AM, Manyemba J, Saloojee H. Anti-inflammatory treatment for carditis in acute rheumatic fever. *Cochrane Database Syst Rev* 2003:CD003176.

62. Lessof MH, Bywaters EG. The duration of chorea. *Br Med J* 1956(4982):1520–1523.

63. Pena J, Mora E, Cardozo J, Molina O, Montiel C. Comparison of the efficacy of carbamazepine, haloperidol and valproic acid in the treatment of children with Sydenham's chorea: clinical follow-up of 18 patients. *Arq Neuropsiquiatr* 2002;60:374–377.

64. Paz JA, Silva CAA, Marques-Dias MJ. Ranomized double-blind study with prednisone in Sydenham's chorea. *Pediatr Neurol* 2006;34:264–269.

65. Garvey MA, Snider LA, Leitman SF, Werden R, Swedo SE. Treatment of Sydenham's chorea with intravenous immunoglobulin, plasma exchange, or prednisone. *J Child Neurol* 2005;20:424–429.

66. Swedo SE. Sydenham's chorea. A model for childhood autoimmune neuropsychiatric disorders. *JAMA* 1994;272:1788–1791.

67. Mortimer EA, Jr., Vaisman S, Vigneau A. The effect of penicillin on acute rheumatic fever and valvular heart disease. *N Engl J Med* 1959;260:101–112.

68. Stollerman GH. *Rheumatic fever and streptococcal infection.* Grune & Stratton, New York, 1975.

69. Manyemba J, Mayosi BM. Penicillin for secondary prevention of rheumatic fever. *Cochrane Database Syst Rev* 2002:CD002227.

70. Sanyal SK, Berry AM, Duggal S, Hooja V, Ghosh S. Sequelae of the initial attack of acute rheumatic fever in children from north India. A prospective 5-year follow-up study. *Circulation* 1982;65:375–379.

71. Feinstein AR, Stern EK, Spagnuolo M. The prognosis of acute rheumatic fever. *Am Heart J* 1964;68:817–834.

72. Gerber MA, Baltimore RS, Eaton CB et al. Prevention of Rheumatic Fever and Diagnosis and Treatment of Acute Streptococcal Pharyngitis: A Scientific Statement From the American Heart Association Rheumatic Fever, Endocarditis, and Kawasaki Disease Committee of the Council on Cardiovascular Disease in the Young, the Interdisciplinary Council on Functional Genomics and Translational Biology, and the Interdisciplinary Council on Quality of Care and Outcomes Research: Endorsed by the American Academy of Pediatrics. *Circulation* 2009;119(11):1541–1551.

73. Lue HC, Wu MH, Hsieh KH et al. Rheumatic fever recurrences: controlled study of 3-week versus 4-week benzathine penicillin prevention programs. *J Pediatr* 1986;108:299–304.

74. Steer AC, Carapetis JR. Acute rheumatic fever and rheumatic heart disease in indigenous populations. *Pediatr Clin North Am* 2009;56:1401–1409.

75. Gray GC, Struewing JP, Hyams KC et al. Interpreting a single antistreptolysin O test: a comparison of the 'upper limit of normal' and likelihood ratio methods. *J Clin Epidemiol* 1993;46:1181–1185.

76. Karmarkar MG, Venugopal V, Joshi L, Kamboj R. Evaluation & revaluation of upper limits of normal values of anti-streptolysin O and ant-deoxyribonuclease B in Mumbai. *Indian J Med Res* 2004;119 (suppl):26–28.

77. Lennon D. Acute rheumatic fever in children—recognition and treatment. *Pediatr Drugs* 2004;6(6):363–373.

78. Steer AC, Kado J, Colquhoun S, Noonan S, Babitu T. Awareness of rheumatic heart disease. *Lancet* 2006;367:2118.

79. Bishop W, Currie B, Carapetis J, Kilburn C. A subtle presentation of acute rheumatic fever in remote northern Australia. *Aust N Z J Med* 1996;26:241–242.

SECTION 10

Rheumatoid arthritis

CHAPTER 109

Pathogenesis of rheumatoid arthritis

Ranjeny Thomas and Andrew P. Cope

Introduction

Rheumatoid arthritis (RA) is an autoimmune disease in which chronic inflammation predominates. Inflammation is systemic, targeting articular tissues, and predisposing to cardiovascular comorbidity and increased susceptibility to infectious pathogens, combining to reduce life expectancy by up to 10 years in severe cases. The clinically described syndrome we recognize as RA encompasses a spectrum of clinical entities underpinned by distinct genetic, molecular, and cellular signatures. Heterogeneity translates to variable and unpredictable outcomes, in spite of widely adopted treatment programmes focused on early, intensive therapy. Accordingly, defining these phenotypes in the laboratory has become a priority, with the long-term goal of stratification of disease subtypes, and adopting the most appropriate therapy at an individual patient level. Here, we describe genetic associations, immune and inflammatory responses, and the effector pathways characteristic of RA, and how this knowledge has advanced our understanding of disease pathogenesis.

The inflamed rheumatoid synovium

The rheumatoid synovium is a prototypic inflammatory effector site that has taught us much about autoimmune, inflammatory, and destructive mechanisms.[1] From these studies therapeutic targets have been elucidated and used successfully to suppress disease in clinical rheumatology practice. Synovial tissue from normal joints consists of a lining layer of macrophages and fibroblasts from one to three cells thick, associated with a loose, vascularized, connective tissue sublining layer. The lining layer of macrophages and fibroblasts in inflamed RA synovial tissue is hyperplastic, and the sublining is infiltrated by inflammatory cells. In inflammation, vascular endothelial cells are activated, and angiogenesis and high endothelial venule development are evident. Foci of activated dendritic cells (DC), T cells, and inflammatory macrophages are recruited adjacent to vessels. B cells infiltrate RA synovial tissue and, in a subset of patients, form distinct germinal centres associated with follicular DC. Although neutrophils are infrequent in the tissue, they are abundant in inflamed synovial fluid.

RA is driven by autoimmune processes involving antigen presentation by DC to autoreactive T cells and production of autoantibodies by autoreactive B cells. However, the pathological consequences of these processes on joints are not driven directly by T cells or autoantibodies themselves, but by inflammatory products of macrophage and synovial fibroblast effector cells,[2] and by the destructive consequences of proliferative, tissue-invasive pannus derived from 'transformed' synovial fibroblasts,[3] as well as the bone-destructive effects of osteoclasts derived from tissue monocyte precursors.[4] Therapeutic interventions targeting immuno-inflammatory pathways are highly effective. These include inhibition of T-cell costimulation by antigen-presenting cells (APC) through targeting of B7–CD28 interactions (CTLA4-Ig; known as abatacept), inhibition of B-cell function through depletion of B-cell subsets with anti-CD20 monoclonal antibody (rituximab), and inhibition of inflammatory cytokines through tumour necrosis factor (TNF), interleukin (IL)-6 or Janus kinase (JAK) inhibitors. This directly reflects the role of these pathways as critical (and, very likely, multifunctional) control points in disease progression.

Leucocyte migration in response to inflammatory conditions increases the cellularity of the synovial tissue. It is orchestrated by secretion of chemokines and the upregulation of adhesion molecules expressed by endothelial cells which in turn promote cell rolling, adhesion, and transmigration. Increased tissue cellularity provokes hypoxia, stimulating angiogenic and cellular stress pathways and resulting in tissue damage, manifest as necrosis and apoptosis.[1] Post-translational modifications of protein antigens, such as citrullination and carbamylation, occur under conditions of stress and damage. Such modified self-antigens may be presented to the immune system both by DC and other APC such as B cells locally and by migratory DC in joint-draining lymph nodes.

Cell populations recruited to RA synovium through inflamed endothelium are enriched for T and B lymphocytes, monocytes, conventional and plasmacytoid DC, and other innate immune cells such as NK and NKT cells, mast cells, and neutrophils.

T cells in the synovium express a memory phenotype characterized by CD45RO, and activation or differentiation markers such as CD40-ligand, LFA-1, NKG-2D, ICOS, CCR5, and CX3CR1. Synovial fluid and synovial tissue are enriched in terminally differentiated or ageing CD45RO[neg] memory cells which have re-expressed CD45RA, and which are deficient in the expression of CD27 and CD28.[5] Although poorly proliferative, these T cells produce cytokines (including IFNγ, IL-6, TNF, and IL-10), may be cytotoxic, and may express low levels of T-cell receptor zeta (TCRζ, reducing the capacity for TCR-mediated signalling.[6] RA synovial T cells therefore resemble normal T cells activated by IL-2, IL-6, and TNF more closely than T cells activated through the TCR. These cytokine-activated bystander T cells may chronically stimulate effector responses through cell-to-cell interactions with synovial fibroblasts or macrophages.[7] CD4+IFNγ+IL-17+ T cells are also found in synovial fluid and tissue. as are FoxP3+ regulatory T cells. In RA peripheral blood (PB), enrichment of CD16+ inflammatory monocytes correlates with disease activity.[8]

Subtypes of RA synovium include highly inflammatory tissue containing ectopic lymphoid tissue and germinal centres, tissue containing granulomas, tissue infiltrated by scattered lymphocyte infiltrates, and fibrotic tissue lacking significant infiltrates. These subphenotypes are associated to some extent with clinical features, and with specific gene expression profiles. A gene expression-profiling study of RA synovial tissue demonstrated at least two distinct profiles. One was highly inflammatory, involving genes associated with immunoglobulins (Ig) and innate and adaptive immunity, including STAT-1 and IFNγ-mediated gene activation. Upon immunohistochemical staining, the tissues with this subphenotype contained germinal centres, and organized lymphoid tissue, with expression of CCL19 and CXCR4 and CXCR5. IL-7 was expressed by fibroblast-like synoviocytes, macrophages, and endothelial cells close to T cells, likely supporting ectopic lymphoid development and T-cell survival in the synovium. Patients with this synovial subphenotype on average had higher clinical disease activity.[9] In contrast, the less inflammatory synovial subphenotype showed greater expression of genes associated with tissue remodelling and repair, including members of the Wnt signalling pathway, and matrix metalloproteinase (MMP) activity.

The 'at-risk' subject

The European League Against Rheumatism (EULAR) Study Group for Risk Factors for RA has published guidelines focusing on the preclinical and very earliest clinically apparent stages of disease.[10] Specific phases of RA are proposed, and terminology suggested for describing each stage of disease (Figure 109.1). This provides a framework to define the temporal relationship between genetic, environmental, and immuno-inflammatory factors that confer risk for RA, and will underpin the development of risk stratification and prediction models in the future. Genetic and environmental risk factors are important components of risk stratification.

Genetic factors

Disease concordance rates for twins are 15–30% (monozygotic) and 5% (dizygotic), with heritability estimates of up to 60%.[11] The major histocompatibility complex (MHC), which is highly polymorphic, contributes about one-third of this genetic susceptibility. Specific *HLA-DRB* gene variants mapping to amino acids 70–74 of DRβ-chains are strongly associated with RA (Figure 109.2).[12] This region encodes a conserved amino acid sequence (the 'shared epitope' or SE) in the HLA-DR antigen-binding groove, common to multiple RA-associated DR alleles. Specific polymorphisms at amino acid positions 11, 71, and 74 of the DRβ chain associate with the highest risk for seropositive RA. Amino acids 71 and 74 form part of the positively charged fourth anchoring pocket (P4), which would preferentially bind non-polar amino acids, such as citrulline, but not arginine. Tightly bound modified peptide antigens are then available for presentation to the T-cell antigenic receptor. Accordingly, RA-specific anti-citrullinated protein autoantibodies (ACPA), which reflect autoimmunity towards a group of citrulline-modified autoantigens, are much more likely to occur in SE+ patients.[13]

The majority of other susceptibility variants, identified through genome-wide association studies (GWAS), confer low to moderate risk with low penetrance (<50% increased risk per variant).[14] These include *PADI4, CD28, CTLA4, CD2-CD58, PTPRC,* and *CD40* (molecular determinants of lymphocyte activation), *CD3Z, PTPN22, PRKCQ, IL2-IL-21, IL2RA, IL2RB, RBPJ, PIP4K2C,* and *REL* (transducer modules of TCR signalling and regulators of IL-2 gene expression and IL-2R signalling), *STAT4,* and *TNFRSF14* (inducers of lineage-specific cytokine gene expression and persistence of memory T cells). Thus, genetic risk for ACPA+ RA is not only linked with genes modifying peptide antigen presentation, but also with variation in genes involved in T-cell activation, differentiation and effector function. Other genetic variants, such as *AFF3, TRAF1-C5, TRAF6, TNFAIP3, CCL21, CCR6, IRF5, BLK, TAGAP, FCGR2A, PXK, SPRED2, PRDM1,* and *IL6ST* may perturb cell

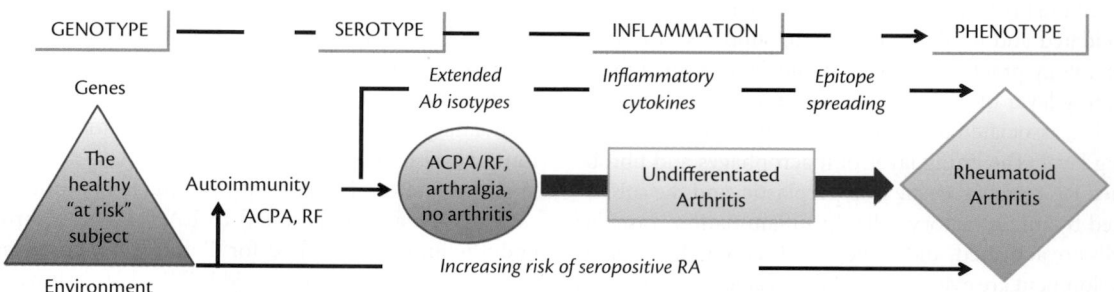

Fig. 109.1 The natural history of rheumatoid arthritis—from at-risk subject to expression of disease. An at-risk subject is likely to progress through multiple phases before disease onset. Inheritance of genetic variants associated with disease susceptibility and exposure over time to environmental factors (the 'exposome') initiates autoimmunity. This is manifest through detection of autoantibodies in serum which may be detectable for many years before the onset of symptoms (such as arthralgia). Autoantibody-positive arthralgia subjects may then progress to a phase of undifferentiated arthritis (clinically apparent swollen joints), before fulfilling disease classification criteria for rheumatoid arthritis. Not all at-risk subjects will pass through these phases in the same way; the timing and order of these stages may vary, and some subjects may reach multiple checkpoints over a short period of time.

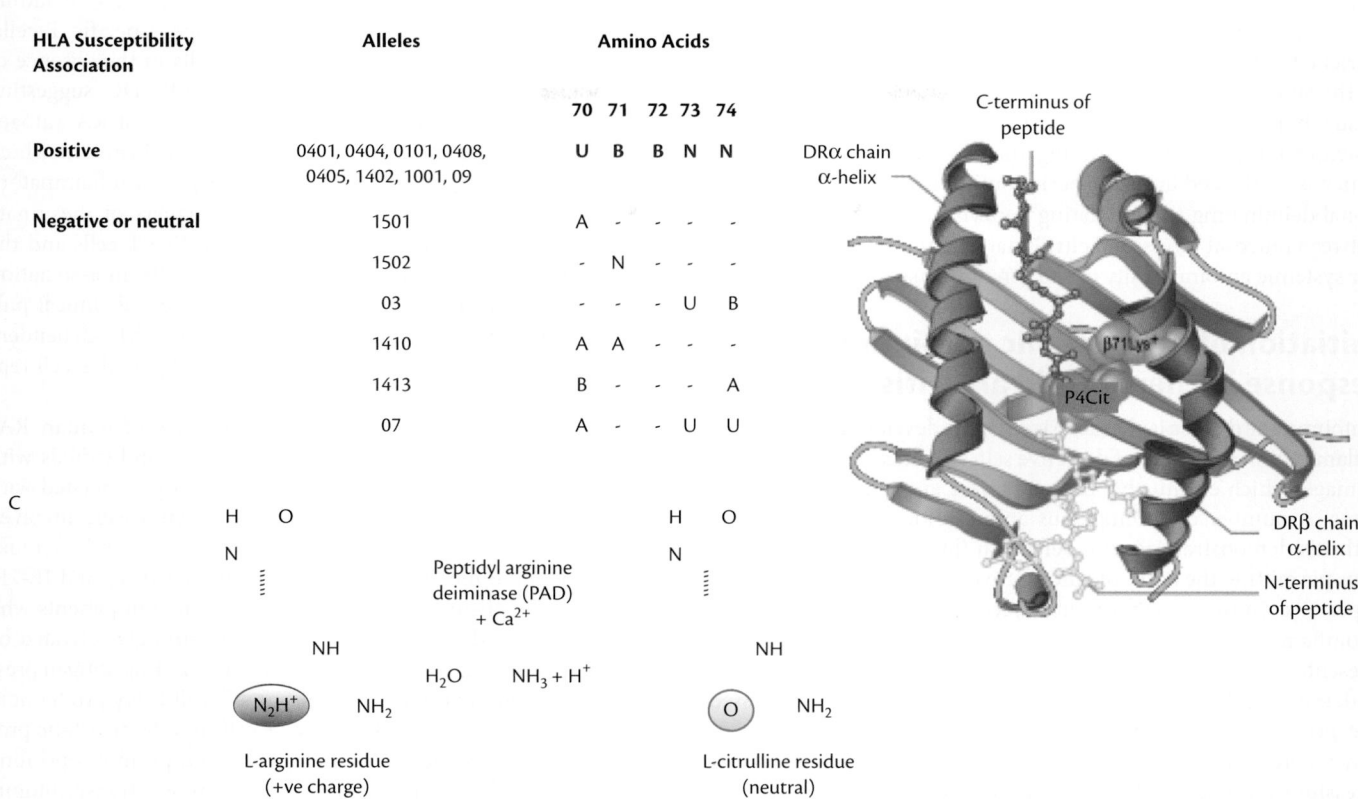

A

HLA Susceptibility Association	Alleles	Amino Acids				
		70	71	72	73	74
Positive	0401, 0404, 0101, 0408, 0405, 1402, 1001, 09	U	B	B	N	N
Negative or neutral	1501	A	-	-	-	-
	1502	-	N	-	-	-
	03	-	-	-	U	B
	1410	A	A	-	-	-
	1413	B	-	-	-	A
	07	A	-	-	U	U

Fig. 109.2 Basis for the association between anti-citrullinated protein autoantibodies (ACPA) and HLA susceptibility in rheumatoid arthritis (RA). Specific *HLA-DR* gene variants mapping to amino acids 70–74 of DRβ-chains are strongly associated with RA. (A) This region encodes a conserved amino acid sequence (the 'shared epitope' or SE) in the HLA-DR antigen-binding groove, found in multiple RA-associated DR alleles. Polymorphisms at amino acid positions 11, 71, and 74 of the DRβ chain have highest risk for seropositive RA. A, negatively charged amino acid; B, positively charged amino acid; U, polar uncharged amino acid; N, hydrophobic amino acid. (B) Amino acids 71 (green) and 74 form part of the positively charged fourth anchoring pocket (P4), which preferentially binds non-polar amino acids, such as citrulline (orange), but not the positively charged amino acid arginine. (C) Citrullination occurs in antigen-presenting cells under stress and is associated with conversion of a positive to a neutral charge. Tightly bound modified peptide antigens are then available for presentation to the T-cell antigenic receptor. Thus, RA-specific ACPA, which reflect autoimmunity towards a group of citrulline-modified autoantigens, are much more likely to occur in SE+ patients.

differentiation and innate inflammatory pathways but their functional significance has yet to be determined.

Specific genotypes, including *DRB1*04*, cosegregate with distinct clinical features including ACPA^pos, erosive disease. Genetic associations for ACPA^neg disease are distinct from ACPA^pos disease, with major differences in the MHC region, including *HLA-DRB1*03*, as well as *IRF5* and mannose-binding lectin. However, certain *HLA-DRB1* alleles (*DRB1*0103*, *0402*, *1102*, *1103*, *1301*, *1302*, and *1304*) confer lower disease risk, and reduced radiographic progression in RA even in the presence of one copy of a susceptibility *HLA-DRB1* allele, suggesting that specific subsets of MHC class II genes may confer an independent protective role.[15]

Environmental factors

Low concordance rates for twins with RA point to non-inherited disease risk factors.[16] The 'exposome' is proposed as the total environmental exposures of an individual over his or her lifetime, and is comparable in molecular complexity to the genome and proteome. It includes infectious and non-infectious agents which stimulate host cells or damage mucosal sites. Attention has focused on the gastrointestinal and respiratory tracts as principle

sites of exposure. Smoking contributes approximately 25% of the population-attributable risk of RA. Smoking interacts with all SE alleles to increase RA risk—particularly ACPA^+ RA—although this ACPA-specificity is not observed in all populations.[17] Citrullination of proteins is more likely during cellular inflammation, stress, and autophagy. Whereas bronchoalveolar lavage (BAL) cells from healthy smokers contained citrullinated proteins, cells from non-smokers did not.[18] Such proteins are also found in inflamed RA joints. Thus stress-inducing environmental agents, such as smoking, obesity, and exposure to toxins such as silica and mineral oils, may promote expression of post-translationally modified neoantigens. On the other hand, factors such as red wine and statins, which reduce oxidative stress, and pregnancy, which promotes immune tolerance, reduce RA risk.[16]

The symbiont microbial communities that colonize mammals (the 'microbiota') constitute attractive environmental risk factors since they are acquired from around the time of birth and, although modified by diet or physiology, are remarkably stable. Preclinical mouse models have defined links between segmented filamentous bacterial species in small intestine, lamina propria, or large intestine and the rapid emergence of IL-17-expressing effector T cells in the context of autoimmunity, including inflammatory arthritis.[19] A recent study in patients with RA has highlighted *Prevotella* species, a Gram-negative anaerobe of the *Bacteroides* genus, as being enriched in the gut of patients with early but not established RA.[20]

The similarities between RA and periodontal disease—inflamed tissue, bone erosion, associations with tobacco smoke, and MHC polymorphism—and the finding that *Porphyromonas gingivalis*. which is implicated in severe periodontitis, expresses its own functional deiminating ('citrullinating') enzyme, provide a second link between mucosal 'stress' and citrullinated antigens, which may trigger systemic autoimmunity in the genetically susceptible host.[21]

Initiation of the systemic autoimmune response in rheumatoid arthritis

Autoimmune disease is characterized by the development of chronic inflammation as a result of defective self-tolerance, leading to tissue damage, which eventually becomes severe enough to cause symptoms. A number of spontaneous animal models of autoimmune arthritis demonstrate genetic defects in thymic negative selection, thus permitting the entry of autoreactive T cells into the peripheral repertoire. In the periphery, subsequent genetic or environmental proinflammatory pressure on the innate immune control of antigen presentation may more readily trigger the activation of these T cells and, thus, the development of autoimmune disease.[22] As discussed, the priming of autoantigen-specific responses in patients with genetic predisposition to RA very likely follows an inflammatory or stressful trigger sensed by DC. Bone-marrow-derived professional APC specialize in antigen presentation to T cells. Although multiple subsets of DC with specialized functions have been described in different tissues, they can be simply classified as conventional myeloid-derived DC and plasmacytoid DC. Conventional DC in the resting or steady state are termed 'immature', and in this state they very efficiently take up and process antigen from their local environment.

In response to pathogen- or danger-associated molecular patterns (PAMPs and DAMPs), or to signals derived from T-cell crosstalk, DC undergo phenotypic and functional changes referred to as 'maturation', which influence their antigen-presenting function. Immature DC take up antigen, while receiving and recognizing environmental signals. Ligation of receptors, including Fc receptors, integrins, C-type lectins, Toll-like receptors (TLR), nucleotide-binding oligomerization domain (NOD) proteins, and RIG-I like receptors signal to DC during this process. As a result, maturing DC secrete cytokines, and express chemokine receptors including CCR7, enabling migration to the T-cell rich areas of lymph nodes. Mature DC also express high levels of MHC and T-cell costimulatory molecules, including CD80 and CD86, which enhance their capacity to present captured antigen to T cells in lymphoid organs.[23] DC express CD40 which, when engaged by CD40-ligand expressed by activated CD4+ T cells, promotes NFκB activation. This enhances MHC molecule expression and the production of IL-12p70 among other cytokines, and promotes DC survival.[24] Chemokines secreted by DC, such as CCL5, CCL3, and CXCL-10, recruit T cells, monocytes, NK cells, and other DC into the local environment, further amplifying the inflammatory response.

Autoantigen-specific T cells can be identified in RA patients and at-risk subjects using tetramers—fluorescent reagents that bind TCRs specific for particular HLA-DR–self-peptide complexes[25]—or by stimulation of T cells with autoantigens in vitro. Synovial and PB DC have been shown to present RA self-antigens, including HC-gp39 and citrullinated peptides, to antigen-specific T cells. Synovial fluid DC stimulate autologous T cells in the absence of exogenous antigen much more effectively than PB DC, suggesting that their MHC molecules are loaded with relevant RA autoantigens.[26] In murine models of inflammatory arthritis, in which autoreactive T cells are enriched in the periphery, inflammatory (usually microbial, including microbiota) triggers of the innate immune system provoke priming of autoreactive T cells and the generation of antigen-specific autoreactive B cells, in association with follicular-helper T cells (Tfh). For example, subclinical pulmonary fungal infection promotes spontaneous Th17-dependent inflammatory arthritis in SKG mice, whose peripheral T-cell repertoire is enriched in autoreactive T cells.[22]

How do these models relate to pathogenesis of human RA? PB gene profiling studies in seropositive at-risk individuals with arthralgia have identified signatures significantly associated with imminent RA development. Overexpressed genes were involved in type I IFN-mediated immunity, haematopoiesis, and chemokine and cytokine-mediated immunity, including IFNγ and IL-7R. In contrast, B-cell-related genes were upregulated in patients who did not go on to develop arthritis.[27] DC are strongly activated by type I IFN, inducing IL-12 production and promoting antigen presentation to CD4+ and CD8+ T cells, and T-cell IFNγ production. IL-7 triggers low-affinity self-reactive T cells into homeostatic proliferation and conversion to memory cells, and promotes priming of efficient T-cell responses by DC.[28] Interestingly, transcriptomic profiling data parallel genetic associations in RA with the pathways of DC activation, NFκB activity, and T-cell activation and effector function predominating.[29] Taken together, the animal and human data suggest that low-affinity autoreactive T cells in at-risk subjects differentiate into effector cells, with the capacity for synovial migration and activation of other innate inflammatory cells, once a signalling threshold for DC activation and IL-7 secretion has been overcome. The development of chronic inflammation also implies that normal mechanisms of effector T-cell regulation are dampened or defective, in part a consequence of exposure to proinflammatory cytokines TNF and IL-1.[30]

A variety of self-antigens is implicated in the development and progression of RA, including joint-derived proteins, such as type II collagen and human cartilage derived glycoprotein HC gp39, and ubiquitous antigens, such as the endoplasmic reticulum stress protein BiP and other stress proteins. Post-translationally modified proteins, including citrullinated and carbamylated self-antigens, and glycosylated IgG Fc, are major RA autoantigens. Autoantigenic citrullinated self-proteins include vimentin, fibrinogen, type II collagen, and α-enolase. Not only do HLA-DR SE alleles provide a receptive peptide binding groove for citrullinated epitopes, but they also disturb T-cell homeostasis. CD4+ T cells in both SE+ RA patients and HLA-DR4+ healthy controls show features consistent with reduced thymic T-cell output to the peripheral repertoire, an increased proliferative drive for naive T cells towards self-antigens, increased immune senescence, and restricted diversity of the TCR repertoire.[31] In such a relatively lymphopenic setting, homeostatic proliferation—associated with IL-7—lowers the threshold for T-cell activation in response to antigen.

What happens in the synovium before and after the disease starts? Recent studies examined immune cell infiltration in synovial biopsies taken from healthy controls, autoantibody (ACPA or RF) positive non-RA patients, and patients with undifferentiated arthritis. In some subjects, a diagnosis of RA was made within 2 years, and in others, arthritis remitted. Somewhat surprisingly, synovial tissues of autoantibody-positive non-RA subjects and healthy controls appeared similar. In contrast, synovial biopsies from patients with undifferentiated arthritis contained inflammatory cell infiltrates, and these were not significantly different from patients with early RA.[32] These studies suggest that systemic autoimmunity precedes clinical and histological evidence of inflammatory arthritis, and that specific events associated with inflammatory cell migration to synovial tissue associate with clinical onset.

There is evidence of ongoing immuno-inflammatory activity in PB prior to the clinical diagnosis of RA. For example, established RA is associated with an acute phase response, manifested by elevations of hepatic proteins including C-reactive protein (CRP), IL-6, and fibrinogen, and associated with procoagulant activity in the blood. These systemic manifestations provoke high-density cholesterol reductions, fatigue, raised erythrocyte sedimentation rate (ESR), and reduced insulin sensitivity. A study of preclinical sera stored prior to RA onset demonstrated that autoantibodies were associated with elevated cytokines in serum, including IL-1, IL-6, IL-12p70, and CRP, predicting development of seropositive RA (Figure 109.1).[33] Elevated expression of increasing numbers of cytokines were predictive of shorter duration to disease onset. Together these studies suggest that autoreactivity and systemic inflammation precede RA, but that the initiating inflammatory process might derive from tissue(s) other than the synovium, such as sites of microbial colonization.

The synovial stromal response

The synovial stroma—made up of fibroblast-like synoviocytes (FLS) and resident macrophages—expresses a wide range of pattern recognition receptors (PRR) that equip these cells to sense 'danger' in their environment, such as components of bacterial cell wall and viral nucleic acids, fibrinogen fragments, HMGB-1, hyaluronan, and other fragments derived from host tissues following damage or stress. Synovial tissue stromal cells, which are rather heterogeneous at the cellular level and expressing markers similar to bone marrow stroma, respond to such stimuli in a variety of ways. Firstly they undergo semi-autonomous hyperplasia, over time becoming anchorage-independent and expanding in situ as a result of reduced contact inhibition and active attenuation of apoptosis. Cell-to-cell adhesion is regulated by integrins and cadherins; the synovial lining of cadherin-11-deficient mice is hypoplastic, with impaired invasiveness and inflammatory responses.[34] Activated FLS are an abundant source of cytokines, chemoattractants, and enzymes that target the matrix of articular cartilage, such as MMPs and A disintegrin-like and metalloproteinase with thrombospondin (ADAMTS) 4 and 5, which have potent aggrecanase activity.[3] Epigenetic modifications, and microRNA expression profiles, may promote cytokine-independent activation of inflammatory and destructive pathways in FLS.[35] These characteristics equip FLS with invasive properties reminiscent of transformed cells, associated with reduced apoptosis, upregulated proto-oncogenes and defective tumour suppressor genes.[3] RANK ligand+ FLS also support the differentiation of osteoclasts from monocyte-derived precursors. This allows FLS to breach cortical bone and to enter the bone marrow, promoting inflammatory reactions such as osteitis (bone marrow oedema) early in the evolution of the disease.

Synovial stromal cells provide a niche that supports the survival of infiltrating leucocytes, through cell contact and the production of soluble factors such as type I interferons. FLS are also proangiogenic, in response to hypoxic conditions and endoplasmic reticulum stress in inflamed synovium, supporting the formation in some patients of tertiary lymphoid structures. Serial synovial biopsies from RA patients demonstrate dissolution of these lymphoid structures after B-cell depletion (anti-CD20)[36] and, in murine models of arthritis, enhanced lymphatic drainage and egress of resident leucocytes following TNF inhibition.[37]

Cellular mediators of the effector response in situ

Both Th1 cells secreting IFNγ, and Th17 cells secreting IL-17, are found in RA synovium. Th1 cells activate macrophages to produce proinflammatory cytokines, and induce immunoglobulin class switching by B cells, to complement-fixing antibodies. IFNγ also has important regulatory effects through induction of nitric oxide and indoleamine 2,3-dioxygenase (IDO). IL-17 stimulates FLS and osteoclastogenesis, and also provokes cartilage and extracellular matrix destruction in vitro, independent of TNF and IL-1. Synovial DC are involved in antigen presentation, local inflammation, joint destruction, and immune regulation. Their production of IL-12 and IL-23 maintains and promotes differentiation of Th1 and Th17 cells respectively. Differentiation of Th17 requires TGF-β, IL-6, and IL-1β and low signal strength T-cell activation associated with low levels of IL-2 or increased numbers of Treg—all features of RA synovium.[38] TGF-β has both proinflammatory and anti-inflammatory effects, including the promotion of regulatory T-cell differentiation and the maintenance of DC in an immature state. These DC tend to be located close to the synovial lining layer. FoxP3+ Treg cells suppress both effector T cells and innate immune cells, to regulate inflammation.[39] Treg cells are enriched in synovial fluid and tissue of patients with RA, juvenile inflammatory arthritis (JIA), and other inflammatory arthritic conditions, and in some studies also RA PB[39]. In JIA, Treg suppressor function is associated with reduced disease activity, and suppression appears more effective in the joint than in PB.[40] In RA PB, reduced in-vitro suppression of TNF and IFNγ production was demonstrated in active disease, and this improved with TNF inhibitors.[41] In murine models, inflammatory arthritis can be suppressed by induction of functional Treg cells, and more severe disease, or a more extended repertoire of joint involvement, is exacerbated by depletion of Treg or deficiency of Foxp3.[42,43]

Mature conventional, and plasmacytoid DC accumulate perivascularly in inflamed synovium, associated with T- and B-cell follicles.[44] They display evidence of in-vivo activation, with upregulation of MHC molecules, CD86 and RelB, and production of proinflammatory cytokines in response to stimulation with immune complexes or TLR agonists, HMGB-1, or heat shock proteins. Mature conventional DC are associated with synovial cells expressing CCL19 and CCL21.[44,45] CCL19 expression can trigger formation of tertiary lymphoid structures similar to those in RA synovial tissue. In RA synovium, such germinal centre-like structures support autoantibody production, since they express activation-induced cytidine deaminase (AID) and are surrounded by ACPA-producing plasma cells.[46]

T follicular helper (FH) cells have not been studied in RA in any depth, but murine models demonstrate their importance in the induction of autoantibody-secreting B cells. These CD4+ cells differentiate upon T-cell activation and costimulation in draining lymph nodes; indeed, the higher the affinity of antigen activation, the more T cells are recruited into the Tfh lineage.[47] Tfh express ICOS and CXCR5, secrete large amounts of IL-21, and provide help to B cells for long-lived antibody responses. In a murine model of arthritis, the costimulation blocker abatacept suppressed the development of antigen-specific Tfh and thus B-cell autoreactivity in antigen-induced arthritis.[48] In another model, recipients of cotransferred Tfh and Th17 T-cell subsets developed autoantibodies and inflammatory arthritis.[49] Given that Th17 development is promoted by low-affinity antigen presentation, these data support the contention that optimal development of inflammatory arthritis may be promoted by a mix of T-cell responses to antigens presented by APC with both low and high affinity. These effector mechanisms may require multiple regulatory mechanisms, including Tregs and lytic NK cells.[49]

B cells also play multiple roles in RA—as antibody-producing cells, as APC, and as regulatory cells. B cells have been shown to be activated by immune complexes containing chromatin through the B-cell receptor and TLR9, to produce rheumatoid factor.[50] The pathogenic role of B cells is demonstrated by the lack of development of arthritic models in the absence of B cells, suppression of disease by anti-CD20 mAb, and transfer of disease using anti-collagen II or anti-GPI autoantibodies in mice. In RA patients, it is not clear whether the efficacy of anti-CD20 is due to depletion of pathogenic autoantibodies or the reduction of antigen-presenting B cells. Antibodies may activate Fc receptors expressed by monocytes, DC, neutrophils, mast cells, or platelets and, by activating the alternate pathway of complement, result in the proinflammatory effects of C5a. Nonetheless, B cells represent a large APC compartment, predominantly involved in perpetuation of antigen presentation, after priming by DC has occurred at disease initiation. The regulatory B-cell subset represents an attractive approach for immune modulation in RA. Regulatory B cells secrete IL-10 and this was shown to be induced after CD40 ligation in a murine model[51].

Macrophages and fibroblasts are critical mediators of inflammation and joint destruction in RA. They are the major producers of proinflammatory cytokines, including TNF, GM-CSF, IL-1β, IL-6, IL-10, and chemokines such as IL-8 and MCP-1, as well as MMPs. Blockade of TNF and IL-6 are highly effective therapies in RA. Monocytes and macrophages are APC, and monocytes can differentiate under inflammatory conditions into DC or osteoclasts. They engage in T- and NK-cell cross-talk to promote proinflammatory cytokine production. Monocytes also have beneficial roles in RA, including clearance of apoptotic bodies and immune complexes, secretion of regulatory molecules including tissue inhibitors of MMPs, and wound healing. The balance between inflammatory and healing activities of monocytes and macrophages depends on local stimuli, including TLR ligands, cytokines, and damage-associated molecules. Macrophages and FLS are highly enriched in RA synovial tissue, particularly at the cartilage–pannus junction.[3,52]

Pathways to cartilage destruction

Articular cartilage matrix is composed of a network of type II, IX, and XI collagens responsible for tensile strength.[53] The other major component is the large proteoglycan aggrecan providing compressive resistance; biglycan, decorin, fibromodulin, the matrilins, and cartilage oligomeric matrix protein (COMP) contribute to the extracellular matrix (Figure 109.3). Chondrocytes, whose proliferative capacity is limited, maintain a stable equilibrium between the synthesis and the degradation of these matrix components, with a half-life of more than 100 years for type II collagen and a half-life for aggrecan core protein up to 24 years.[53] They adapt to low oxygen tensions by upregulating hypoxia-inducible factor (HIF)-1α, which can stimulate the expression of glucose transporter proteins (GLUT) and angiogenic factors as well as genes associated with cartilage anabolism and chondrocyte differentiation, including Sox9 and type II collagen. In spite of this, the regenerative potential of cartilage is poor.

In RA, cartilage destruction arises as a consequence of several distinct but temporally and spatially related events. Cartilage integrity is lost early, through exposure to the inflammatory milieu. Synovial IL-1 and TNF (as well as adipokines alone or in synergy with other cytokines), induce nitric oxide (NO) production through inducible nitric oxide synthetase and prostaglandins such as PGE2, in both FLS and chondrocytes. IL-1 also induces the production of proteinases involved in cartilage destruction including MMP-1, MMP-3, MMP-8, and MMP-13. This, together with loss of protective factors such as lubricin, perturbs the protein-binding characteristics of articular cartilage and permits the attachment of FLS to cartilage matrix through syndecan-4 and integrin-dependent pathways. Human chondrocytes also express TLR-1, TLR-2, and TLR-4. Activation of TLR-2 by IL-1, TNF, peptidoglycans, or fibronectin fragments further increases production of MMPs, NO, PGE, and proangiogenic factors such as VEGF. Inflammation also reduces collagen II mRNA synthesis in cartilage. Anti-inflammatory cytokines such as IL-4, IL-10, and IL-13, as well as PPAR-α agonists, may exert anabolic effects, retarding cartilage damage, in part through stimulation of IL-1 receptor antagonist expression.

The MMPs collagenase (MMP-1, MMP-8, and MMP-13), gelatinase (MMP-2 and MMP-9), stromelysin (MMP-3), and membrane type I MMPs (MT1-MMP; MMP-14) target native collagens and proteoglycans, and are expressed by inflamed RA synovium.[54] Indeed, MMP-1 is produced largely by chondrocytes at the cartilage–pannus junction while MMP14 is expressed at the surface of FLS and is important for cartilage invasion. However, ADAMTS-4 and ADAMTS-5 are considered to be the dominant effectors of proteoglycan destruction.[55] Cathepsin K also degrades matrix through its capacity to hydrolyse collagen I and II at multiple sites within the triple helical region. Counter-regulatory networks are evident in articular cartilage and inflamed synovium, including TIMPs, induced by such cartilage protective factors as TGFβ. TIMP-3 is a particularly potent inhibitor of ADAMTS-4 and -5.[56]

Cartilage degradation to cartilage matrix fragments can be used to monitor disease progression and to predict long-term outcomes; serum levels of COMP, YKL-40/HCgp-39, and MMP correlate with joint destruction. Monoclonal antibodies (mAb) recognizing specific N- or C-terminal sequences of the cleaved protein also detect cartilage degradation. The best-characterized are the C2C

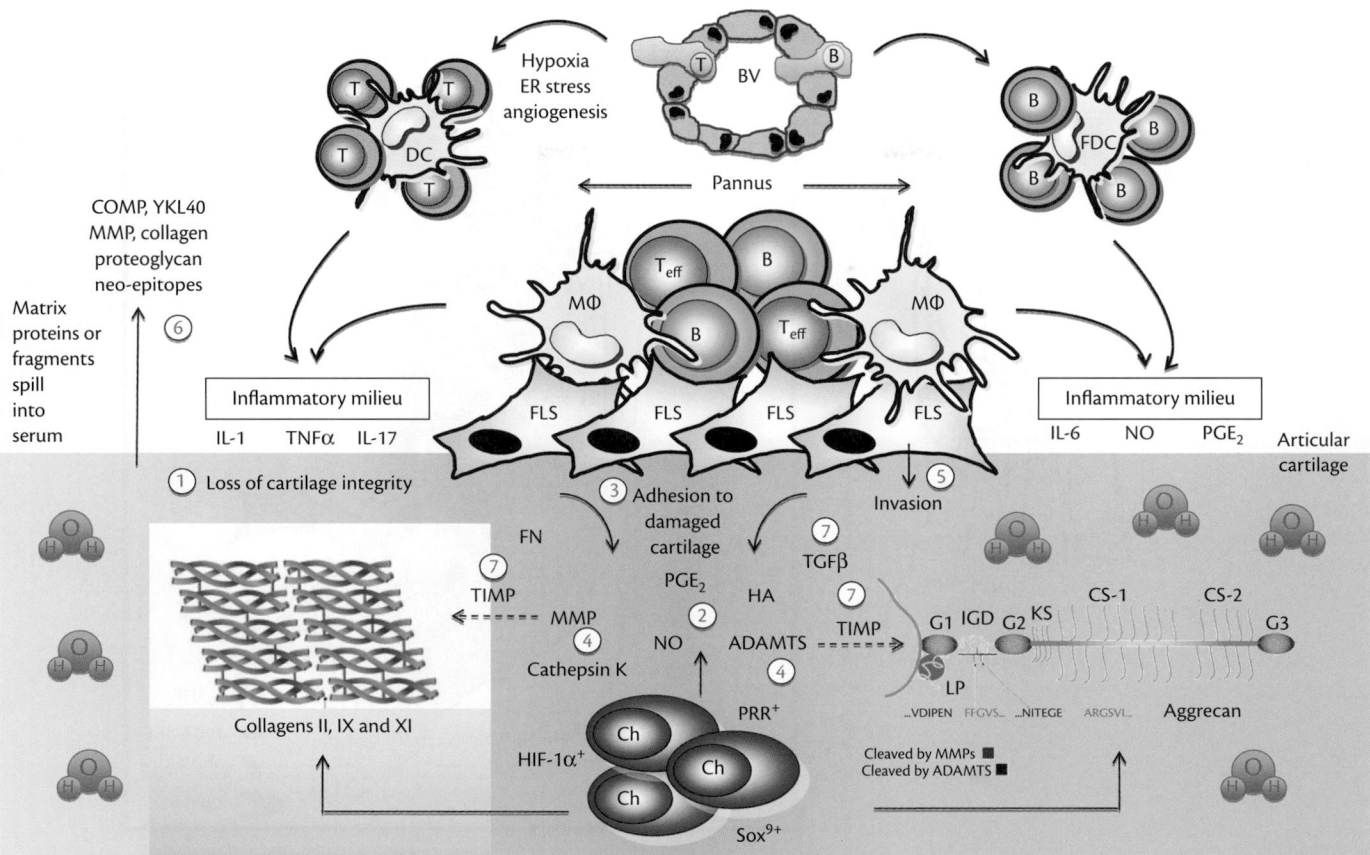

Fig. 109.3 Pathways to destruction of articular cartilage. The major components of articular cartilage are triple helical collagen fibrils (II, IX, and XI), proteoglycans (aggrecan, biglycan, decorin, fibromodullin) and water (H-O-H). (1) An early event in cartilage destruction is loss of cartilage integrity following exposure of cartilage to the inflammatory milieu. (2) Synovial pannus and chondrocytes are a rich local source of inflammatory mediators. (3) Fibroblast-like synoviocytes (FLS) adhere to damaged cartilage. (4) Proteinases of the matrix metalloproteinase (MMP) and A disintegrin-like and metalloproteinase with thrombospondin (ADAMTS) family cleave matrix proteins (see cleavage sites in the IGD for MMP and ADAMTS), further destroying cartilage integrity, (5) promoting invasion of FLS and (6) releasing matrix proteins and their fragments into the synovial joint, spilling over into serum. (7) Counter-regulatory networks exist which serve to inhibit the catabolic process, including anti-inflammatory cytokines such as TGFβ and IL-10, and tissue inhibitors of metalloproteinases (TIMPS). B, B lymphocyte; Ch, chondrocytes; CS, chondroitin sulfate; FN, fibronectin fragments; HA, hyaluronan; IGD, interglobular domain on aggrecan KS, keratan sulfate glycosaminoglycan side chains; Mφ, macrophages; NO, nitric oxide; PRR, pattern recognition receptor; T, T lymphocytesulfsulf.

antibodies, which detect cleavage of triple helical collagen II, and a panel of mAb to neoepitopes of chondroitin and keratan sulfate as well as the specific aggrecanase (VIDIPEN) and MMP (NITEGE) cleaveage sites within the interglobular G1 domain of aggrecan.[56] Once refined and validated, these biomarkers could become valuable surrogates of cartilage destruction, especially when monitoring early responses to therapy. The radiographic outcomes of cartilage damage measure more advanced changes, including joint space narrowing and erosion of cartilage and bone.

Mechanisms of bone resorption

Bone destruction and joint deformity are closely associated with poor joint function. Periarticular bone erosion is initiated at mechanically vulnerable periosteal surfaces adjacent to articular cartilage, such as the second and third metacarpals and fifth metatarsal, and is thought to precede focal articular bone loss.[57] Histological analysis of these erosion-prone sites suggests that microdamage arises adjacent to collateral ligament insertions, especially on the radial side. The resulting 'bare area' is invaded by

fibrovascular synovial tissue, evolving into inflammatory synovium in direct contact with bone at what is termed the cartilage–pannus junction. Synovitis exacerbates the damage, breaching cortical bone and allowing access of the synovial pannus into the bone marrow cavity. Lymphocyte aggregates gradually replace marrow fat. This manifests as bone marrow oedema, or osteitis, one of the earliest signs of joint inflammation using MRI (Figure 109.4).

During pathogenic bone erosion, physiological bone remodelling by osteoclasts (the bone-resorbing cell) and ostoeblasts (the bone-forming cell) is uncoupled.[4] Osteoclasts are specialized multinucleate, calcitonin-receptor-expressing cells equipped with molecular and enzymatic machinery (cathepsin K and tartrate-resistant acid phosphatase) to attach to bone and cartilage matrix proteins and to digest mineralized tissues. The resulting resorption pits are replaced by inflamed synovial tissue, providing an abundant source of osteoclast precursors and additional proteinases, further exacerbating bone destruction. Osteoclast differentiation is regulated by M-CSF, which amplifies monocyte differentiation to osteoclasts, RANKL, and inflammatory cytokines including TNF which itself promotes M-CSF action, and IL-1, which decreases osteoclast apoptosis.[58]

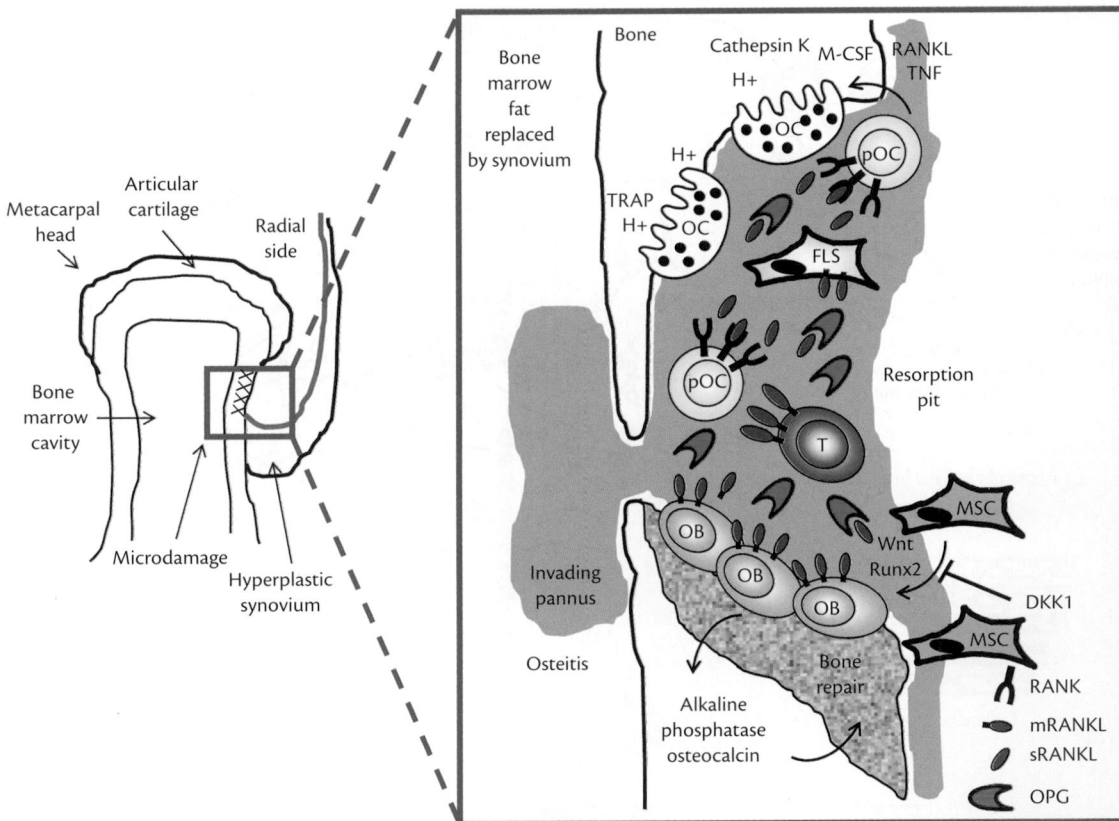

Fig. 109.4 Pathways to the erosion of bone. Microdamage to cortical bone occurs at vulnerable sites. This allows adhesion and activation of osteoclasts, which carry the machinery to digest mineralized tissues, breaching the bone marrow cavity and allowing access to invading pannus. Osteoclasts are derived from monocyte precursors and require M-CSF, RANKL, and TNFα signals for differentiation. Osteoblasts are derived from mesenchymal stromal cells in which Runx2 and Wnt provide key lineage signals. Levels of RANKL and OPG determine osteoclast differentiation and activation status, while factors such as DKK-1 influence osteoblast differentiation by inhibiting Wnt signalling. DKK-1, Dickkopf-1; FLS, fibroblast-like synoviocytes; mRANKL/sRANKL, membrane/soluble RANK ligand; M-CSF, macrophage colony stimulating factor; MSC, mesenchymal stromal cell; OB, osteoblast; OC, osteoclast; OPG, osteoprotegerin; pOC, precursor osteoclast; RANK, receptor activator of NFκB;T, T cell; TRAP, tartrate-resistant acid phosphatase.

RANKL is normally produced by osteoblasts, and in RA synovium by FLS and activated T cells.

Bone-forming osteoblasts are derived from mesenchymal stromal cells.[4] Lineage differentiation is induced by the Wnt family of glycoproteins. As osteoblasts mature, they produce and mineralize bone matrix, at the same time downregulating expression of RANKL, and upregulating production of osteoproteregin (OPG), a soluble RANKL decoy receptor. In RA, serum RANKL/OPG levels may be a surrogate biomarker of osteoclast activity in vivo.

Proinflammatory cytokines in inflamed joints impair the capacity of osteoblasts to produce bone and to repair bone erosions through reduction of Runx2 (a transcription factor controlling osteoblast differentiation), alkaline phosphatase, and osteocalcin expression. They may induce RANKL and RANK expression, while reducing OPG, and uncouple Wnt signalling, to inhibit the differentiation of osteoblasts and chondroblasts. Agents which suppress osteoclast differentiation and activation, including TNF inhibitors, OPG:Fc, the anti-RANKL monoclonal antibody denosumab, IL-1Ra, or bisphosphonates, fail to adequately repair bone lesions. This demonstrates the impact of factors inhibiting bone formation, and why healing remains a relatively rare event, even in patients in clinical remission.

Persistence vs resolution of inflammation

The capacity to keep innate immune inflammatory responses in check despite exposure of mucosal surfaces to the universe of organisms is in large part due to innate regulatory and anti-inflammatory factors. The devastating pathology arising in mice and humans as a consequence of deficiencies of such elements attests to this.[59]

Pathways that promote immune and tissue homeostasis are overexpressed in inflamed RA joints, in spite of the ongoing inflammatory process. These include the anti-inflammatory cytokines IL-10 and TGFβ and specific cytokine inhibitors including soluble cytokine receptors such as sTNF-R, receptor antagonists like IL-1Ra, receptor 'sheddases' such as ADAM17 and TIMPs, which cleave receptors from the cell surface, and suppressors of cytokine signal transduction (e.g. A20/TNFAIP3—an intracellular inhibitor of NFκB signalling) and SOCS (a family of suppressors of cytokine signalling). Other factors limit the stability of inflammatory cytokine mRNAs (e.g. tristetraprolin), or shorten the activity of signalling intermediates (e.g. IκBα which inhibits NFκB and mitogen-activated protein kinase (MAPK) phosphatases, which inactivates MAPK and annexin 1, all of which are induced by corticosteroids). Indoleamine 2,3-dioxygenase (IDO), expressed by DC, suppresses effector functions by consuming the essential amino acid tryptophan, producing kynurenine catabolites. Pro-resolving mediators derived from polyunsaturated fatty acids, such as resolvin E2, stimulates host protection throughout the innate inflammatory response, by reducing neutrophil chemotaxis, promoting phagocytosis and anti-inflammatory cytokine production, and downregulating integrin expression. Persistent disease activity implies that intrinsic regulatory or inhibitory mechanisms are insufficient to suppress chronic inflammation; supplementation of endogenous TNF inhibitors with pharmacological neutralization of TNF suggests that homeostasis can be restored.

Immune regulatory cells, besides Tregs, are also enriched in inflamed RA synovium. Mesenchymal stromal cells exert potent anti-proliferative and anti-inflammatory effects and contribute to the tissue repair response as precursors of osteoblasts and chondrocytes. These cells likely contribute to the tissue remodelling and repair signature that predominates in a subgroup of patients.

Conclusion

Research over the last decade has contributed to important advances in our understanding of the factors that put individuals at high risk of developing RA. Pathways of innate immunity and the cells contributing to the earliest events are now better appreciated. The distinctive features and aberrations of adaptive immune responses in RA patients are being uncovered, and many of the end-organ effector pathways that lead to cartilage destruction and bone erosion have now been identified. Major challenges for the future will be to apply targeted therapies that induce rapid and sustained remission without compromising host defence (e.g. through antigen-specific therapy), coupled to well-tolerated regimens for drug tapering and withdrawal. As insights into methods of risk stratification evolve, primary prevention will become the next major goal. This will best be realized through:

- an understanding of disease pathogenesis at a molecular and cellular level such that the full spectrum of disease subtypes is appreciated, and can be used more efficiently to predict outcomes and the best therapies for both individual patients and those at highest risk of developing disease

- insights into the inherited and acquired perturbations of immunity and inflammation and their impact on the disease over time

- detailed knowledge of the clinical and biological remission state (immunological tolerance) and how to measure it.

References

1. Firestein GS. Evolving concepts of rheumatoid arthritis. *Nature* 2003;423(6937):356–361.
2. McInnes IB, Schett G. Cytokines in the pathogenesis of rheumatoid arthritis. *Nat Rev Immunol* 2007;7(6):429–442.
3. Muller-Ladner U, Ospelt C, Gay S, Distler O, Pap T. Cells of the synovium in rheumatoid arthritis. Synovial fibroblasts. *Arthritis Res Ther* 2007;9(6):223.
4. Walsh NC, Crotti TN, Goldring SR, Gravallese EM. Rheumatic diseases: the effects of inflammation on bone. *Immunol Rev* 2005;208:228–251.
5. Weng NP, Akbar AN, Goronzy J. CD28(-) T cells: their role in the age-associated decline of immune function. *Trends Immunol* 2009;30(7):306–312.
6. Zhang Z, Gorman CL, Vermi AC et al. TCRzetadim lymphocytes define populations of circulating effector cells that migrate to inflamed tissues. *Blood* 2007;109(10):4328–4335.
7. Brennan F, Foey A. Cytokine regulation in RA synovial tissue: role of T cell/macrophage contact-dependent interactions. *Arthritis Res* 2002;4 Suppl 3:S177–S182.
8. Rossol M, Kraus S, Pierer M, Baerwald C, Wagner U. The CD14(bright) CD16+ monocyte subset is expanded in rheumatoid arthritis and promotes expansion of the Th17 cell population. *Arthritis Rheum.* 2012; 64(3):671–677.
9. van Baarsen LG, Wijbrandts CA, Timmer TC et al. Synovial tissue heterogeneity in rheumatoid arthritis in relation to disease activity and biomarkers in peripheral blood. *Arthritis Rheum* 2010;62(6):1602–1607.
10. Gerlag DM, Raza K, van Baarsen LG et al. EULAR recommendations for terminology and research in individuals at risk of rheumatoid arthritis: report from the Study Group for Risk Factors for Rheumatoid Arthritis. *Ann Rheum Dis.* 2012;71(5):638–641.
11. MacGregor AJ, Snieder H, Rigby AS et al. Characterizing the quantitative genetic contribution to rheumatoid arthritis using data from twins. *Arthritis Rheum.* 2000;43(1):30–37.
12. Gregersen PK, Silver J, Winchester RJ. The shared epitope hypothesis. An approach to understanding the molecular genetics of susceptibility to rheumatoid arthritis. *Arthritis Rheum* 1987;30(11):1205–1213.
13. Huizinga TW, Amos CI, van der Helm-van Mil AH et al. Refining the complex rheumatoid arthritis phenotype based on specificity of the HLA-DRB1 shared epitope for antibodies to citrullinated proteins. *Arthritis Rheum* 2005;52(11):3433–3438.
14. Gregersen PK, Olsson LM. Recent advances in the genetics of autoimmune disease. *Annu Rev Immunol* 2009;27:363–391.
15. van der Helm-van Mil AH, Huizinga TW, Schreuder GM et al. An independent role of protective HLA class II alleles in rheumatoid arthritis severity and susceptibility. *Arthritis Rheum* 2005;52(9):2637–2644.
16. Scott IC, Steer S, Lewis CM, Cope AP. Precipitating and perpetuating factors of rheumatoid arthritis immunopathology: linking the triad of genetic predisposition, environmental risk factors and autoimmunity to disease pathogenesis. *Best Pract Res Clin Rheumatol* 2011;25(4): 447–468.
17. Padyukov L, Silva C, Stolt P, Alfredsson L, Klareskog L. A gene-environment interaction between smoking and shared epitope genes in HLA-DR provides a high risk of seropositive rheumatoid arthritis. *Arthritis Rheum* 2004;50(10):3085–3092.
18. Makrygiannakis D, Hermansson M, Ulfgren AK et al. Smoking increases peptidylarginine deiminase 2 enzyme expression in human lungs and increases citrullination in BAL cells. *Ann Rheum Dis* 2008;67(10): 1488–1492.
19. Wu HJ, Ivanov, II, Darce J et al. Gut-residing segmented filamentous bacteria drive autoimmune arthritis via T helper 17 cells. *Immunity* 2010;32(6):815–827.
20. Scher JU, Abramson SB. The microbiome and rheumatoid arthritis. *Nat Rev Rheumatol.* 2011;7(10):569–578.
21. Lundberg K, Wegner N, Yucel-Lindberg T, Venables PJ. Periodontitis in RA—the citrullinated enolase connection. *Nat Rev Rheumatol* 2010; 6(12):727–730.
22. Yoshitomi H, Sakaguchi N, Kobayashi K et al. A role for fungal {beta}-glucans and their receptor Dectin-1 in the induction of autoimmune arthritis in genetically susceptible mice. *J Exp Med* 2005;201(6): 949–960.
23. Lutzky V, Hannawi S, Thomas R. Cells of the synovium in rheumatoid arthritis. Dendritic cells. *Arthritis Res Ther* 2007;9(4):219.
24. O'sullivan B, Thomas R. CD40 and dendritic cell function. *Crit Rev Immunol* 2003;23(1–2):83–107.
25. Snir O, Rieck M, Gebe JA et al. Identification and functional characterization of T cells reactive to citrullinated vimentin in HLA-DRB1*0401-positive humanized mice and rheumatoid arthritis patients. *Arthritis Rheum* 2011;63(10):2873–2883.
26. Thomas R, Davis LS, Lipsky PE. Rheumatoid synovium is enriched in mature antigen-presenting dendritic cells. *J Immunol* 1994;152(5):2613–2623.

27. van Baarsen LG, Bos WH, Rustenburg F et al. Gene expression profiling in autoantibody-positive patients with arthralgia predicts development of arthritis. *Arthritis Rheum* 2010;62(3):694–704.

28. Saini M, Pearson C, Seddon B. Regulation of T cell-dendritic cell interactions by IL-7 governs T-cell activation and homeostasis. *Blood* 2009;113(23):5793–5800.

29. Gregersen PK, Amos CI, Lee AT et al. REL, encoding a member of the NF-kappaB family of transcription factors, is a newly defined risk locus for rheumatoid arthritis. *Nat Genet* 2009;41(7):820–823.

30. Ehrenstein MR, Evans JG, Singh A et al. Compromised function of regulatory T cells in rheumatoid arthritis and reversal by anti-TNFalpha therapy. *J Exp Med* 2004;200(3):277–285.

31. Schonland SO, Lopez C, Widmann T et al. Premature telomeric loss in rheumatoid arthritis is genetically determined and involves both myeloid and lymphoid cell lineages. *Proc Natl Acad Sci U S A* 2003;100(23):13471–13476.

32. van de Sande MG, de Hair MJ, van der Leij C et al. Different stages of rheumatoid arthritis: features of the synovium in the preclinical phase. *Ann Rheum Dis* 2011;70(5):772–777.

33. Deane KD, O'Donnell CI, Hueber W et al. The number of elevated cytokines and chemokines in preclinical seropositive rheumatoid arthritis predicts time to diagnosis in an age-dependent manner. *Arthritis Rheum* 2010;62(11):3161–3172.

34. Lee DM, Kiener HP, Agarwal SK, et al. Cadherin-11 in synovial lining formation and pathology in arthritis. *Science* 2007;315(5814):1006–1010.

35. Ospelt C, Reedquist KA, Gay S, Tak PP. Inflammatory memories: is epigenetics the missing link to persistent stromal cell activation in rheumatoid arthritis? *Autoimmunity Rev* 2011;10(9):519–524.

36. Thurlings RM, Vos K, Wijbrandts CA et al. Synovial tissue response to rituximab: mechanism of action and identification of biomarkers of response. *Ann Rheum Dis* 2008;67(7):917–925.

37. Polzer K, Baeten D, Soleiman A et al. Tumour necrosis factor blockade increases lymphangiogenesis in murine and human arthritic joints. *Ann Rheum Dis* 2008;67(11):1610–1616.

38. Purvis HA, Stoop JN, Mann J et al. Low-strength T-cell activation promotes Th17 responses. *Blood* 2010;116(23):4829–4837.

39. Oh S, Rankin AL, Caton AJ. CD4+CD25+ regulatory T cells in autoimmune arthritis. *Immunol Rev* 2010;233(1):97–111.

40. Ruprecht CR, Gattorno M, Ferlito F et al. Coexpression of CD25 and CD27 identifies FoxP3+ regulatory T cells in inflamed synovia. *J Exp Med*. 2005;201(11):1793–1803.

41. Nadkarni S, Mauri C, Ehrenstein MR. Anti-TNF-alpha therapy induces a distinct regulatory T cell population in patients with rheumatoid arthritis via TGF-beta. *J Exp Med* 2007;204(1):33–39.

42. Capini C, Jaturanpinyo M, Chang HI et al. Antigen-specific suppression of inflammatory arthritis using liposomes. *J Immunol* 2009;182(6):3556–3565.

43. Morgan ME, Sutmuller RP, Witteveen HJ et al. CD25+ cell depletion hastens the onset of severe disease in collagen-induced arthritis. *Arthritis Rheum* 2003;48(5):1452–1460.

44. Pettit AR, MacDonald KP, O'sullivan B, Thomas R. Differentiated dendritic cells expressing nuclear RelB are predominantly located in rheumatoid synovial tissue perivascular mononuclear cell aggregates. *Arthritis Rheum* 2000;43(4):791–800.

45. Page G, Lebecque S, Miossec P. Anatomic localization of immature and mature dendritic cells in an ectopic lymphoid organ: correlation with selective chemokine expression in rheumatoid synovium. *J Immunol* 2002;168(10):5333–5341.

46. Humby F, Bombardieri M, Manzo A et al. Ectopic lymphoid structures support ongoing production of class-switched autoantibodies in rheumatoid synovium. *PLoS Med* 2009;6(1):e1.

47. Fazilleau N, McHeyzer-Williams LJ, Rosen H, McHeyzer-Williams MG. The function of follicular helper T cells is regulated by the strength of T cell antigen receptor binding. *Nat Immunol* 2009;10(4):375–384.

48. Platt AM, Gibson VB, Patakas A et al. Abatacept limits breach of self-tolerance in a murine model of arthritis via effects on the generation of T follicular helper cells. *J Immunol* 2010;185(3):1558–1567.

49. Leavenworth JW, Wang X, Wenander CS, Spee P, Cantor H. Mobilization of natural killer cells inhibits development of collagen-induced arthritis. *Proc Natl Acad Sci U S A*. 2011;108(35):14584–14589.

50. Leadbetter EA, Rifkin IR, Hohlbaum AM et al. Chromatin-IgG complexes activate B cells by dual engagement of IgM and Toll-like receptors. *Nature* 2002;416(6881):603–607.

51. Mauri C, Gray D, Mushtaq N, Londei M. Prevention of arthritis by interleukin 10-producing B cells. *J Exp Med* 2003;197(4):489–501.

52. Kinne RW, Stuhlmuller B, Burmester GR. Cells of the synovium in rheumatoid arthritis. Macrophages. *Arthritis Res Ther* 2007;9(6):224.

53. Otero M, Goldring MB. Cells of the synovium in rheumatoid arthritis. Chondrocytes. *Arthritis Res Ther* 2007;9(5):220.

54. Hembry RM, Bagga MR, Reynolds JJ, Hamblen DL. Immunolocalisation studies on six matrix metalloproteinases and their inhibitors, TIMP-1 and TIMP-2, in synovia from patients with osteo- and rheumatoid arthritis. *Ann Rheum Dis* 1995;54(1):25–32.

55. Arner EC. Aggrecanase-mediated cartilage degradation. *Curr Opin Pharmacol* 2002;2(3):322–329.

56. Nagase H, Kashiwagi M. Aggrecanases and cartilage matrix degradation. *Arthritis Res Ther* 2003;5(2):94–103.

57. McGonagle D, Tan AL, Moller Dohn U, Ostergaard M, Benjamin M. Microanatomic studies to define predictive factors for the topography of periarticular erosion formation in inflammatory arthritis. *Arthritis Rheum* 2009;60(4):1042–1051.

58. Theill LE, Boyle WJ, Penninger JM. RANK-L and RANK: T cells, bone loss, and mammalian evolution. *Ann Rev Immunol* 2002;20:795–823.

59. Nguyen LT, Jacobs J, Mathis D, Benoist C. Where FoxP3-dependent regulatory T cells impinge on the development of inflammatory arthritis. *Arthritis Rheum* 2007;56(2):509–520.

CHAPTER 110

Rheumatoid arthritis—diagnosis

Daniel Aletaha and Helga Radner

Introduction

Rheumatoid arthritis (RA) affects approximately 1% of the adult population.[1] Currently RA is considered to be a chronic disease for which there is no cure, but remission, as a state where no active disease is present, has become an achievable goal with optimal treatment. At the same time, for the function and quality of life of patients with RA, it is crucial to recognize RA early and treat it effectively from the beginning. Both disability and the enormous costs of the disease are a function of disease activity over time. The ultimate goals are therefore to treat RA early and persistently until remission is present.

The challenge of treatment of early RA is not the lack of effective medicines, but rather ethical and economic considerations related to risk-benefit and cost-benefit. Overtreating patients with potentially self-limiting or non-destructive disease by using disease-modifying anti-rheumatic drugs (DMARDs) is still often feared. The flipside of the coin is the potential undertreatment of patients with true RA, which—particularly in its early phases—can have accelerated structural consequences. This damage cannot be reversed even by optimal delayed treatment.[2,3] At the same time, prolonged use of non-steroidal anti-inflammatory drugs (NSAIDs) in patients with undifferentiated arthritis also carries significant risk of adverse events.[4] In fact, some of the DMARDs could possibly be considered safer than some of the NSAIDs, particularly if the latter are employed over longer periods of time.[5,6] With these thoughts on the table one can draw a hypothetical risk (i.e. overtreatment or undertreatment)/benefit ratio for patients presenting with undifferentiated arthritis or arthritis that is not yet worked up. This leads to a necessary note regarding the terminology and semantics that are used: the term 'early' arthritis is used to indicate the duration of the symptom 'arthritis'; 'undifferentiated' on the other hand, although also early in terms of symptom duration, is used to indicate that no specific diagnosis has yet been made. This is a challenging concept, as the lack of a specific diagnosis is related to the amount of effort that has been put into the work-up. Usually some basic work-up is deemed to be present, if the term 'undifferentiated' is used, e.g. typical lupus arthritis could otherwise be called undifferentiated just because the doctor has not examined the patients and not noted the typical rash, the Raynaud's, and has not ordered the immunological tests that would have shown high antinuclear antibodies and complement activation. In theory, however, there might also be the case of chronic undifferentiated arthritis following the above logic.

Figure 110.1 depicts the scenarios of late, delayed, and early diagnosis of RA in regard to the respective risk/benefit of subsequent treatment or lack of treatment, respectively. Scenarios are split for two principal therapeutic options: immediate DMARD treatment in every patient with early arthritis, or DMARD treatment only upon an established diagnosis of RA. The sequence from panel A to panel C indicates that the risk/benefit ratio for either therapeutic approach improves with an earlier timing of the definite diagnosis. Patients diagnosed earlier (panels B and C of Figure 110.1) would benefit from an earlier 'correction' of the therapeutic approach (DMARDs or symptomatic) preventing overtreatment in patients without RA, and undertreatment in those with RA, and thus improving the overall risk/benefit ratio of the respective therapeutic strategy.

It can be deduced from the above that the question of whether RA should be treated before or only after establishing the definite diagnosis is secondary, but that the timing of the diagnosis in relation to the duration of symptoms is key in both approaches. DMARD institution before diagnosis may, however, be difficult for legal reasons in many countries or settings.

A few thoughts need to be considered in this context: first, the true risk of overtreatment with DMARDs in patients with undifferentiated arthritis is not yet completely clear, particularly when a diagnosis will be established within a reasonable time frame anyway; neither is the risk of prolonged symptomatic treatment, e.g. with NSAIDs, which may also be considerable. Second, early aggressive intervention in undifferentiated arthritis often leads to the challenging situation in which some patients with true RA may be prevented from eventually being diagnosed due to resolution of their symptoms, or, vice versa, some patients with self-limiting arthritis might be misdiagnosed as RA in clinical remission. Only withdrawal of therapy may reveal the underlying chronic condition, which is a diagnostic dilemma in clinical practice. Finally, in Figure 110.1 it is assumed that the diagnostic properties of criteria

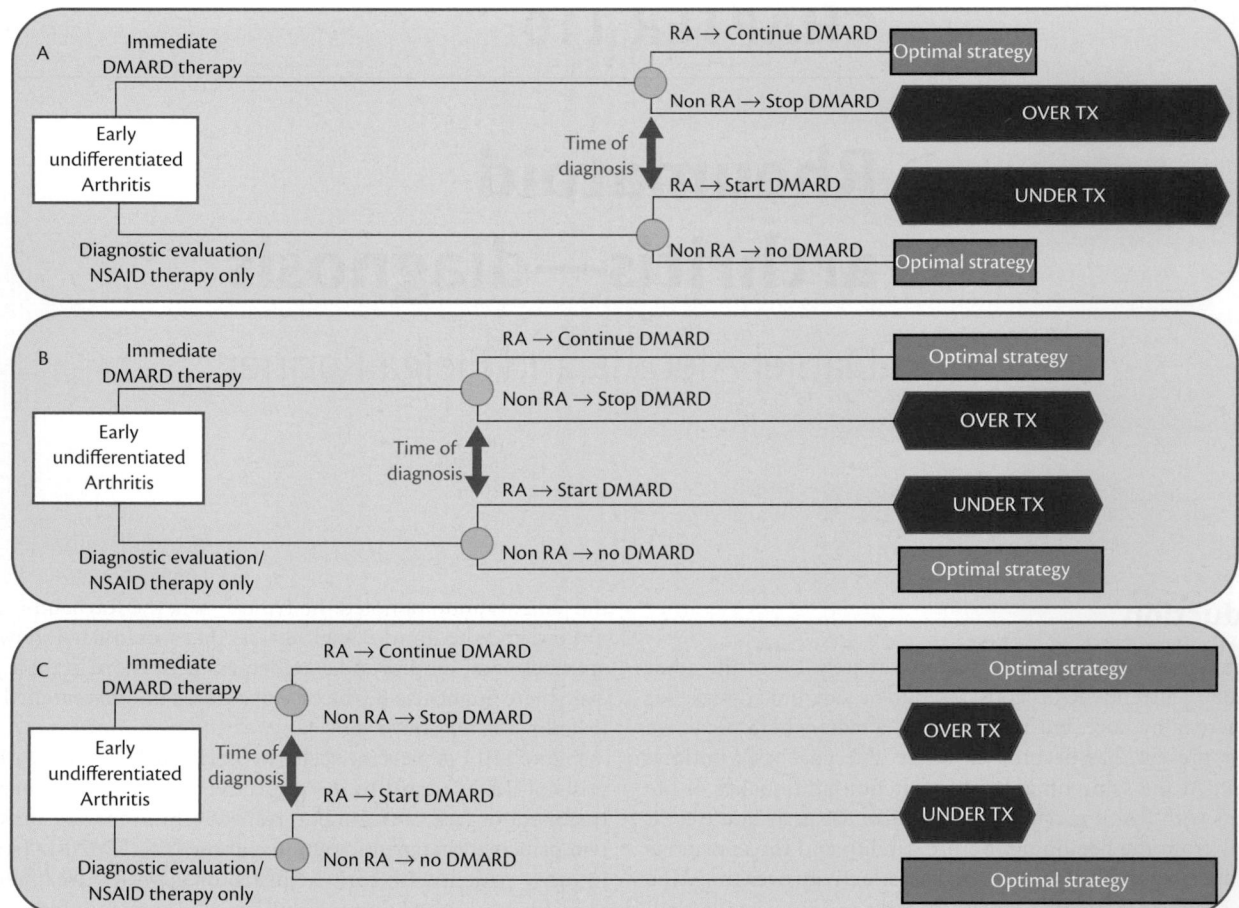

Fig. 110.1 Consequences of delayed diagnosis. Three scenarios of risk/benefit are depicted for (A) late, (B) delayed, and (C) early diagnosis of definite rheumatoid arthritis (RA). Physicians face two principal therapeutic options: immediate disease-modifying anti-rheumatic drug (DMARD) treatment in every patient with early arthritis (top option in each panel), or DMARD treatment only upon an established diagnosis of RA (bottom option in each panel). The sequence from panel A to panel C indicates that the risk/benefit ratio for both options improves with an earlier timing of the definite diagnosis of RA.

will be similar at all stages of the disease, while in reality any diagnostic approach will likely be more accurate when more time has elapsed since the onset of symptoms.

All these considerations come into play when one aims to diagnose (and treat) RA early, but in fact currently no diagnostic criteria exist. In the following, we discuss the principal approach to patients presenting with arthritis, looking at the potential differential diagnoses of RA, as well as algorithms and criteria that may be helpful in eventually establishing an accurate diagnosis of RA.

Initial evaluation of patients presenting with new-onset arthritis

The terminology for patients with recent onset of their arthritis is often confusing. While 'early arthritis' may not mean more than a mere description of a temporal notion, many see a difference from 'undifferentiated arthritis'. The term 'undifferentiated' implies that some efforts have already been taken to determine the type of disease underlying the symptom 'arthritis'. This leads to the question of which steps reasonably need to be taken in order to be able to label early arthritis as 'undifferentiated'. For that purpose, an algorithm has recently been proposed to delineate the evaluative steps in the work-up of patients with new-onset inflammatory arthritis

(Figure 110.2), which can either lead to a specific diagnosis or to the classification as 'undifferentiated'.[7] This includes evaluation for a history of trauma, as well as evaluating the clinical presentation of the affected joint. The major initial distinction would be between acutely inflamed ('red hot') arthritis and other forms of arthritis. The former should arouse the suspicion of crystal-induced arthritis or septic arthritis, and although demographic and contextual factors may help to differentiate these two (e.g. age, gender, history, and lifestyle), arthrocentesis is necessary to make the specific diagnosis, as the therapeutic consequences are very different.

Synovial fluid analysis is of greatest use to distinguish between inflammatory and non-inflammatory arthropathy, usually affecting one or a few joints. Among the former are those types of inflammatory arthritis that need immediate care, particularly septic arthritis (see Chapter 98), in which the prognosis rapidly worsens with time to effective diagnosis and treatment. In fact, if the synovial fluid analysis is typical, then a confident diagnosis can be made already at this stage. This includes the presence of a high leucocyte count, positive Gram staining, or the presence of crystals (Figure 110.3). In clinical reality, the synovial fluid analysis will often enough not be diagnostic.

In general, after exclusion of crystal- or infection-related arthritis, a relatively large set of differential diagnoses is to be considered, which is different in patients with mono-, oligo-, and polyarthritis

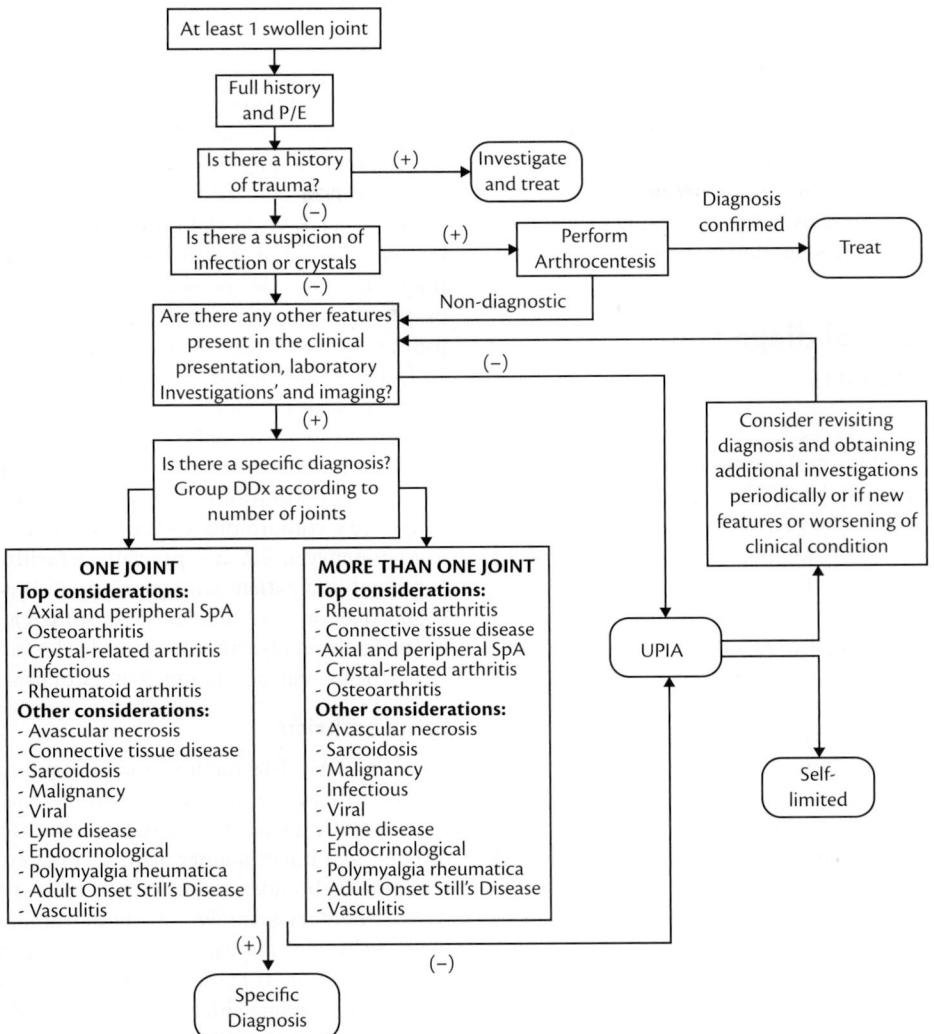

Fig. 110.2 Flowchart to establishing a specific diagnosis (Dx) in new onset arthritis in at least a single swollen joint. The starting point is a full history and physical examination (P/E). After exclusion of trauma, and acute inflammatory events such as gout and septic arthritis, a specific diagnosis may be established in the presence of suggestive clinical, laboratory, or imaging features, where the differential diagnoses (DDx) differ according to the number of swollen joints involved. If no specific diagnosis can be established, the presentation may be labelled as 'undifferentiated arthritis' (in the algorithm shown as 'UPIA' for undifferentiated peripheral inflammatory arthritis). This status needs to be re-evaluated periodically, as undifferentiated arthritis may evolve into specific diagnosis over time.

Reproduced with permission from Hazlewood G, Aletaha D, Carmona L et al. Algorithm for identification of undifferentiated peripheral inflammatory arthritis: a multinational collaboration through the 3e initiative. J Rheumatol Suppl 2011;87:54–58.

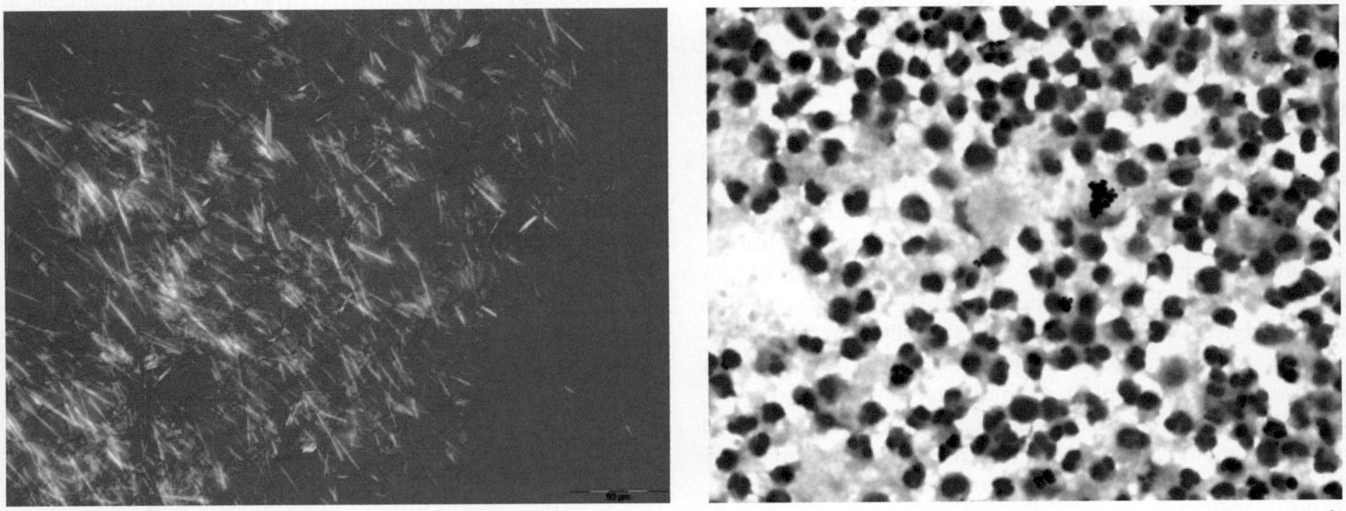

Fig. 110.3 Microscopic synovial fluid analysis: (A) crystal arthritis: evidence of intracellular needle shaped crystals; (B) septic arthritis showing positive Gram stain of cocci in typical formation; *Staphylococcus aureus*

Courtesy of Prof. Stefan Winkler, Division of Infectious Diseases, Medical University Vienna, Austria.

(Figure 110.2).[7] The most important of these are discussed in the following section.

If no specific diagnosis can be established, the presentation can be labelled as undifferentiated arthritis. As the state of 'undifferentiated' in fact is a lack of definitive diagnosis, and hence is provisional, this state needs to be revisited periodically, for evolving diagnostic hints, although the presentation may turn out to be self-limiting disease (Figure 110.2).

Important differential diagnoses of rheumatoid arthritis

Viral polyarthritis

Several types of viral infections can mimic RA by leading to the typical polyarthritis of the small joints. This differs from RA in that viral polyarthritis can last from days to weeks, but is less frequently seen over the course of months, although some patients can develop a chronic arthropathy lasting for 6 months or longer.[8] A variety of viruses can lead to arthralgia, fewer even to arthritis, the most important among the latter being the hepatitis viruses (particularly hepatitis B and C virus, HBV and HCV), as well as parvovirus B19 and rubella.

Parvovirus B19 is the cause of erythema infectiosum (also called 'fifth disease'). It is typically a benign self-limiting disease of childhood that goes along with rash, fever, and commonly also arthritis. Less frequently, it may cause aplastic anaemia, which is a life-threatening disease. Joint involvement can impressively mimic RA by a symmetrical involvement of the small finger joints.

Patients with infectious origin of their polyarthritis may not be seronegative for rheumatoid factor, as many viral agents induce transient seropositivity.[8] Therefore determination of anti-cyclic citrullinated peptides (CCP) antibodies may be of more help in these circumstances, as they are less likely to be positive in diseases other than RA.[9,10] Virus-specific serological testing may be helpful to identify patients with recently acquired parvovirus infection, or to identify patients with HBV- or HCV-associated arthritis in the differential diagnosis. The treatment remains symptomatic—NSAIDs in most cases. If arthritis persists after clearance of the infection, then one might not speak of viral arthritis any more, but the viral infection may be considered the trigger of an autoimmune disease, such as RA, in which case DMARDs may be used. Both symptomatic (NSAIDs) and disease-modifying agents are often problematic in the context of viral hepatitis.

Peripheral spondylarthropathy

Several forms of spondylarthropathies (SpA) are known, many of which can cause peripheral arthritis. Recently, classification criteria for peripheral SpA have been put forward,[11] which imply arthritis, enthesitis, or dactylitis ('sausage digit') as an important feature. In combination with other typical SpA features diagnosis of SpA can be established as follows. If one of the three starting symptoms mentioned above is present, then one of the following characteristics is sufficient for a classification: psoriasis, uveitis, inflammatory bowel disease, preceding infection (indicative of reactive arthritis), positive HLA-B27, and evidence of sacroiliitis on MRI. If two of the starting symptoms are present, then a history of inflammatory bowel disease or family history of sacroiliitis is already sufficient. If all three of the symptoms are present, the patient is directly classifiable.

Over and above the classification of peripheral SpA, joint distribution of the different peripheral SpA may help in the diagnostic process, such as the fact that reactive arthritis typically affects the larger joints of the lower extremity in an asymmetric fashion.[12] Although psoriatic arthritis and RA can in most cases be well distinguished based on the criteria of the classification system, the fact that RA often is also seronegative, and that joint manifestations may precede the skin manifestations in psoriatic arthritis by years,[13] may complicate the diagnostic process: a diagnosis of psoriatic arthritis can be made in patients who also have psoriasis and who are seronegative for rheumatoid factor (RF) and antibodies directed to citrullinated peptides (ACPA); on the other hand, a diagnosis of RA may be established in psoriasis patients with a symmetric polyarthritis who are positive for rheumatoid factors or ACPA, since skin psoriasis is very common, and therefore can also simply be a comorbidity to RA. One may occasionally speak of an overlap between RA and psoriatic arthritis, if seropositive disease is present in a patient with psoriasis and radiographic changes are supportive for either diagnosis. In some patients with a symmetric inflammatory polyarthritis, the only clue to the diagnosis of psoriatic arthritis may be a family history of psoriasis.

Lyme arthritis

Lyme arthritis, a late manifestation of Lyme disease (see Chapter 101), occurs primarily in individuals who live in or travel to Lyme disease endemic areas. Lyme arthritis is characterized by intermittent or persistent inflammatory arthritis in a few large joints, especially the knee,[14] shoulder, ankle, elbow, temporomandibular joint, and wrist. Migratory arthralgias without frank arthritis may occur during early localized or early disseminated Lyme disease.

The diagnosis of Lyme arthritis may be supported by serologic testing for borrelia, which should only be done in patients presenting with undiagnosed inflammatory arthritis in endemic areas. In several respects, Lyme arthritis is different from RA as, for example, involvement of the small joints of the hands and feet is uncommon. Aside from serological testing, a positive history of erythema migrans or a tick bite may be suggestive of Lyme disease.

Sarcoid arthritis

Arthritis seen with sarcoidosis most commonly affects the ankles and knees, and less frequently, the wrist, metacarpophalangeal, and proximal interphalangeal joints. It may thus be a relevant differential diagnosis to RA in some cases. In contrast to RA, sarcoidosis can present with a variety of skin and ocular manifestations, such as erythema nodosum or uveitis, with bilateral hilar lymphadenopathy, and elevated serum concentrations of angiotensin converting enzyme (ACE). In some cases sarcoidosis presents with the typical triad of erythema nodosum, hilar lymphadenopathy, and bilateral ankle arthritis (Löfgren's syndrome). Treatment of mild forms of sarcoid arthritis includes NSAIDs whereas more severe cases, particularly those with pulmonary involvement, require the use of glucocorticoids. A high proportion of patient with sarcoidosis have non-progressive, spontaneous remitting disease: only a small proportion require immunosuppressive agents.

Other systemic rheumatic diseases

Early RA may be difficult to distinguish from the arthritis of systemic lupus erythematosus (SLE), Sjögren's syndrome, dermatomyositis, or overlap syndromes, such as mixed connective tissue disease. In contrast with RA, these disorders are generally characterized by the presence of other systemic features such as rashes, Raynaud's syndrome, dry mouth or dry eyes, myalgia or myositis, renal or haematological abnormalities, and by various autoantibodies not seen in RA. Additionally, in connective tissue disease, particularly SLE, the values and responses of the erythrocyte sedimentation rate (ESR) and C-reactive protein (CRP) may be less well correlated with each other than in RA. Whereas both are commonly raised in RA, the CRP is often normal or only minimally elevated in patients with active SLE even when the ESR is elevated.

Polymyalgia rheumatica

Polymyalgia rheumatica (PMR) and osteoarthritis (OA, see below) are common differential diagnoses of RA in the elderly population. PMR is an inflammatory rheumatic disease that is typically associated with marked myalgias of the shoulder girdle and the hips, and affects individuals over the age of 50.[15] It can sometimes be mistaken for RA if the presentation includes arthritis of the small joints of the hands.[16] PMR arthritis may be distinguished from RA by the fact that it tends to be milder, more limited, often asymmetric, with rapid response of symptoms to moderate doses of glucocorticoids, the often unduly high ESR, and the seronegativity for RF and ACPA. However, some cases ultimately diagnosed as RA may start with polymyalgia-like symptoms.[16]

Osteoarthritis of the hand

Osteoarthritis (OA) can be confused with RA in the middle-aged or older patient when the small joints of the hands are involved. However, arthritis in OA is different from RA with respect to the distribution of joint involvement, the clinical type of arthritis, and the structural and serological findings.

OA of the fingers typically affects the distal interphalangeal joints causing the so-called Heberden's nodes in this area, as well as the carpometacarpal joint of the thumb—both joint areas are not usually involved in RA, and in fact, are therefore explicitly excluded from the current classification criteria for RA (see further below). Joint swelling is hard and bony in OA, while it is soft in RA. Morning stiffness is typical in both OA and RA, but it is usually transient or lasts no more than a few minutes in OA, while it typically lasts more than 30–60 minutes in RA.

Structural investigations by conventional radiographs in OA are characterized by joint space narrowing that is asymmetric and accompanied by periarticular osteophytes, while the typical erosions of RA are not seen. OA is classically associated with the absence of RFs and ACPAs, and normal levels of acute-phase reactants. However, RFs may be present, usually in low titre, consistent with the generally old age of this patient population.

Critical diagnostic features of rheumatoid arthritis

Joint pattern

Arthritis in RA usually is a polyarthritis of insidious onset,[17] affecting primarily the proximal interphalangeal (PIP), metacarpophalangeal (MCP), and wrist joints, as well as the ankles and the metatarsophalangeal (MTP) joints. All other joints can also be affected by RA, with the exception of the distal interphalangeal (DIP) joints. A monoarthritic onset of RA is less common, affecting larger joints, and usually evolves to typical polyarthritis that includes the small joints over time. Occasionally, RA may start as palindromic rheumatism, characterized by episodes of joint inflammation affecting one to several joint areas for hours to days, with intermittent periods without symptoms that may last from days to months.[18] Palindromic rheumatism may also develop into other systemic disorders, such as SLE, or resolve over time. Particularly in elderly patients, RA may evolve from an initial polymyalgia-like presentation.[16] Typically, arthritis in RA is accompanied by morning stiffness of at least 30–60 minutes until maximum improvement.

Serology

RFs occur in 70–80% of patients with RA. Their diagnostic utility is limited by their relatively poor specificity since they are found in 5–10% of healthy individuals, 20–30% of those with SLE, virtually all patients with mixed cryoglobulinaemia (usually caused by hepatitis C virus infections), and many other inflammatory conditions. Higher titres of RF have greater specificity for RA.[19] The prevalence of RF positivity in healthy individuals rises with age. Antibodies to citrullinated peptides/proteins (ACPA) are usually measured by enzyme-linked immunosorbent assays (ELISA) using CCP as antigen. Anti-CCP antibodies have a similar sensitivity and specificity to (particularly high levels of) RF for RA, although some argue that they may be more specific,[9,10] which is still a matter of debate. The specificity is greater in patients with higher levels of anti-CCP antibodies.

Acute-phase reactants

Elevations of the ESR and/or CRP level are typically seen in inflammatory conditions such as RA. The degree of elevation of these acute-phase reactants correlates with the severity of inflammation and the structural damage that will occur over time.[20] Although increased levels of acute-phase reactants are not specific for RA, they are often useful for distinguishing inflammatory from non-inflammatory musculoskeletal conditions, such as OA. Therefore elevation of acute-phase reactants was also included in the 2010 classification criteria (see below). On the other hand, occasionally normal acute-phase reactants may also occur in untreated patients with RA.

The 2010 classification criteria for rheumatoid arthritis

The major problem for most inflammatory rheumatic diseases is that there are no diagnostic criteria. All criteria available are classification criteria, and the major difference here is that classification criteria are developed to minimize errors at the group level (e.g. for the purpose of including most homogeneous patient populations in clinical trials of a given disease), while they inherently accept the possibility of misclassification in the individual. On the other hand, the goal of diagnostic criteria is to be correct in the individual most of the time, as often the diagnosis is linked with more or less harmful therapies, as also discussed at the beginning of this chapter. The value of a diagnostic test also depends on the a priori suspicion of disease ('pretest probability'). From this, it becomes clear why diagnostic criteria are scarce.

Until 2010, the classification criteria for RA in use were those by the American College of Rheumatology (ACR) dating from 1987.[21] These criteria have been increasingly debated in the recent past, because of their lack of sensitivity in early disease, given that they were derived using mostly patients with long-standing, established RA.[22] The best example is the inclusion of erosions in these criteria as a feature for diagnosis, which over time contradicted clinical practice, which emphasized the importance of preventing structural damage instead of waiting for irreversible stigmata of RA to occur. Before the introduction of the new criteria, many rheumatologists indicated that their treatment decision was independent of fulfilment of the ACR 1987 classification criteria.[23] Rheumatoid nodules are likewise rarely seen in early disease, and therefore even more weight is put on the remaining six variables, including erosions. In addition, new diagnostic tools, such as testing for ACPA, have emerged in recent years which tends to be at least as sensitive and specific as RF for diagnosis of RA.[10]

A joint working group of the ACR and the European League Against Rheumatism (EULAR) aimed to develop new classification criteria for RA that would replace the 1987 criteria. The work was performed between 2007 and 2010 and included a three-step approach including a data analysis phase using early arthritis cohorts, a consensus science phase, and a refinement phase. These final criteria and the detailed methodology were published in the two journals associated with the ACR and EULAR.[24–27]

As shown in Table 110.1, the 2010 criteria are made up of four domains, including the number and type of the affected joints, serology (RF and ACPA), acute-phase reactants (CRP and ESR), and the duration of symptoms. For evaluation of a patient's classification, the highest category within each domain is taken, and the four scores are added together. The maximum possible score is 10, and a score of 6 or more indicates the presence of definitely classifiable RA. The details of how the various categories and domains are defined are given in the footnotes to Table 110.1. Another way to classify RA, based on the same rules, is by the tree algorithm depicted in Figure 110.4.

Inherent to classification criteria is the fact that they do not work in all individuals who can theoretically be tested. It is very important to understand the target population of the new classification criteria, that is, who they were developed to be applied to. As can be seen in the top part of Table 110.1, the target population for the criteria is well defined: the 2010 criteria may be applied to any patient who presents with at least one clinically swollen joint, for which another disease is not the most likely cause. These limitations were introduced to increase the specificity of the new criteria, and to prevent patients with e.g. gout or obvious SLE being tested with the criteria.

With imaging techniques such as MRI or ultrasonography rapidly developing, it is frequently discussed how these methods can be integrated into the new classification criteria . In this regard, it is important to make two distinctions: for the definition of the target population it is essential to have at least one clinically swollen joint. At this stage, the presence of imaging synovitis without clinical synovitis does not render a patient eligible for application of the criteria. In contrast, once clinical synovitis is confirmed, any imaging method may be used to further explore the extent of arthritis, which may increase the points achieved in the 'joint distribution' category.

The other important issue in imaging is the question about the relevance of erosions, and when to perform standard radiographic investigations. In this respect, a major objective of the new criteria was to not bias against the diagnosis of RA in individuals who are not yet erosive. Structural joint damage is now a major (bad) outcome of RA but not a feature required for classification. Therefore, the scoring system does not give any weight to erosions,

Table 110.1 2010 ACR/EULAR classification criteria for rheumatoid arthritis

Target population (Who should be tested?)

(1) Patient with *at least one joint* with definite clinical synovitis (swelling)

Exception: patients with erosive disease typical for RA, or those with a history compatible with prior fulfilment of the 2010 criteria, or those who have previously fulfilled the 2010 criteria, should be directly classified as RA. A detailed algorithm for the use of radiographic evidence of erosions is presented in Figure 110.6.

(2) Synovitis is *not better explained* by another disease

In case of any doubt or uncertainty about the presence of an alternative diagnosis, the requirement of this rule is fulfilled.

Classification criteria for RA (Score-based algorithm: add score of categories A–D)

A score of **≥6/10** is needed for a definite classification of a patient with RA. Although patients with a score <6/10 are not classifiable as RA, their status can be reassessed and the criteria might be fulfilled cumulatively over time.

(A) Joint involvement[a]	
1 large[b] joint	0
2–10 large joints	1
1–3 small[c] joints (with or without involvement of large joints)	2
4–10 small joints (with or without involvement of large joints)	3
>10 joints[d] (at least one small joint)	5
(B) Serology[e] (at least one test result is needed for classification)	
Negative RF *AND* negative ACPA	0
Low positive RF *OR* low positive ACPA	2
High positive RF *OR* high positive ACPA	3
(C) Acute-phase reactants[f] (at least one test result is needed for classification)	
Normal CRP *AND* normal ESR	0
Abnormal CRP *OR* abnormal ESR	1
(D) Duration of symptoms[g]	
<6 weeks	0
≥6 weeks	1

ACPA, anti-citrullinated protein/peptide antibodies; CRP, C-reactive protein; ESR, erythrocyte sedimentation rate; RF, rheumatoid factor; ULN, upper limit of normal.
[a]Joint involvement refers to any *swollen* or *tender* joint on examination, which may be confirmed by imaging evidence of synovitis. Distal interphalangeal joints (DIPs), 1st carpometacarpal (CMC) joint, and 1st metatarso-phalangeal (MTP) joint are *excluded from assessment*. Categories of joint distribution are classified according to the location and number of the involved joints, with placement into the highest category possible based on the pattern of joint involvement.
[b]Large joints refer to shoulders, elbows, hips, knees, and ankles.
[c]Small joints refer to the metacarpophalangeal (MCP) joints, proximal interphalangeal (PIP) joints, metatarsophalangeal (MTP) joints 2–5, thumb interphalangeal (IP) joints, and wrists.
[d]In this category, at least one of the involved joints must be a small joint; the other joints can include any combination of large and additional small joints, as well as other joints not specifically listed elsewhere (e.g. temporomandibular, acromioclavicular, sternoclavicular, etc.)
[e]Negative refers to international unit (IU) values that are ≤upper limit of normal (ULN) for the lab and assay; low positive refers to IU values that are >ULN but ≤3× ULN for the lab and assay; high positive refers to IU values that are >3× ULN for the lab and assay. Where RF is only available as positive or negative, a positive result should be scored as 'low positive' for RF.
[f]Normal/abnormal is determined by local laboratory standards.
[g]Duration of symptoms refers to patient self-report of the duration of signs or symptoms of synovitis (e.g. pain, swelling, tenderness) of joints that are clinically involved at the time of assessment, regardless of treatment status.
Adapted from Aletaha et al.[24,25]

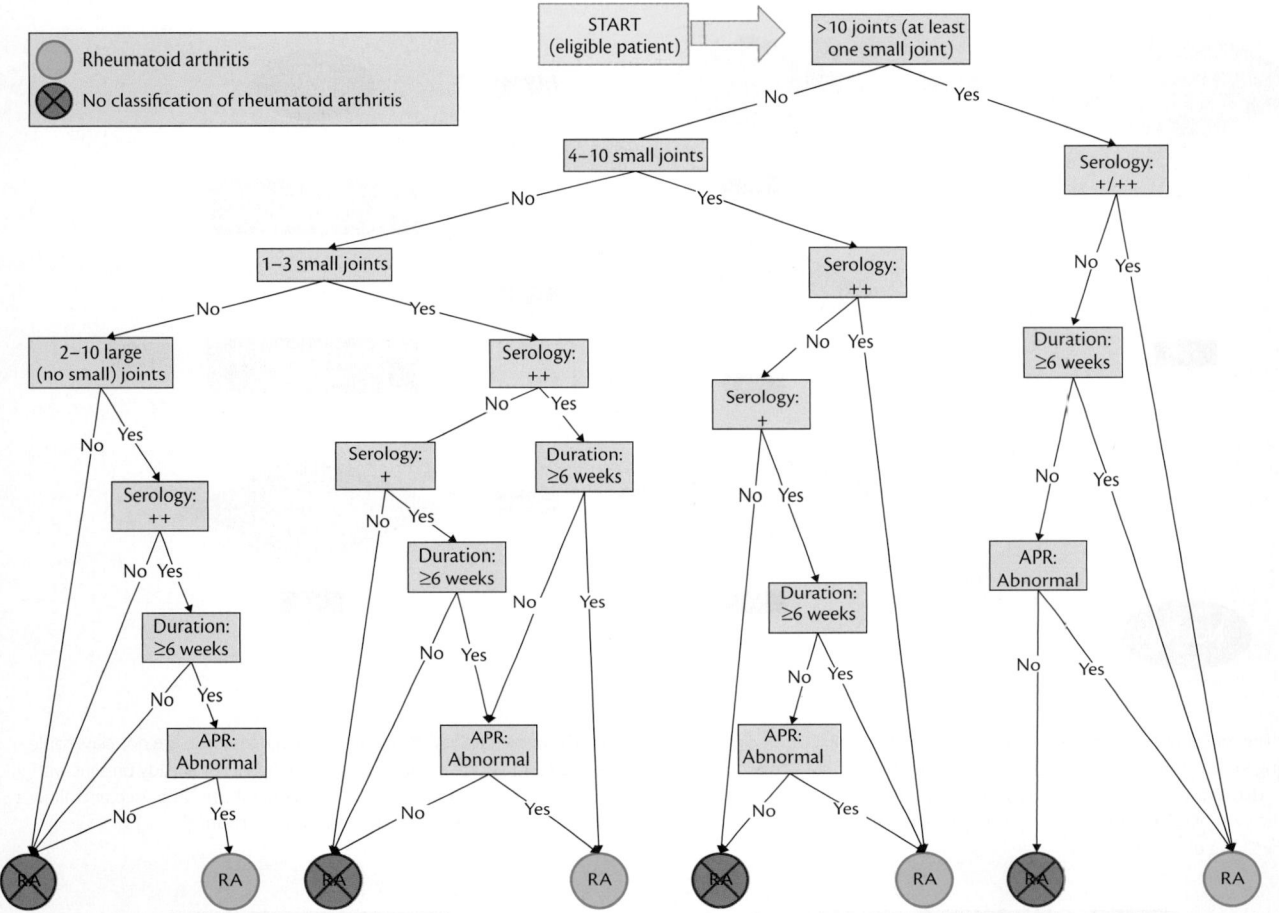

Fig. 110.4 Tree algorithm to classify definite rheumatoid arthritis (green circles) or to exclude its current presence (red circles) among those who are eligible to be assessed by the new criteria. For definitions of categories (e.g. serology: +, ++, or joint regions), see footnotes to Table 110.1.

Taken from the original publication: 2010 rheumatoid arthritis classificationcriteria: an American College of Rheumatology/European League Against Rheumatismcollaborative initiative. Aletaha D, Neogi T, Silman AJ, Funovits J, Felson DT, Bingham CO 3rd et al Ann Rheum Dis. 2010 Sep;69(9):1580–8.

and thus does not penalize individuals without structural damage. At the same time there remains the—currently more theoretical—situation of patients with long-standing disease, who have not yet been classified, but may have become less active over time ('burnt-out' disease). For these patients, an option has been introduced, which allows immediate classification by presence of typical radiographic evidence of RA. Typical erosiveness of RA has recently been defined as erosions in more than three joints.[28] This is shown in Figure 110.5.

Therefore, comparing the 2010 classification criteria to those developed in 1987, many aspects have remained while several have changed. The radiographic changes are not weighted into the new scoring system, while patients with long-standing unclassified disease, who do not fit the criteria, can be classified on the basis of their typical joint destruction alone. Rheumatoid nodules have completely disappeared in the new classification system, mainly due to their low prevalence, and thus low diagnostic value, in early disease. The joint distribution remains similar to the 1987 scoring system, as the weight remains on polyarthritis (which at some level inherently includes symmetric disease) and on small joints. Serological changes were expanded from the mere use of RF to also include ACPA, and to a consideration of the antibody level (negative vs low positive vs high positive). Duration was introduced as a separate item in the new system, while it was integrated in the

joint activity items of the 1987 criteria, and elevated acute-phase response was newly introduced.

Classification vs diagnosis of rheumatoid arthritis

The distinction between classification and diagnosis is crucial: classification criteria aim to define a homogenous disease group for clinical and epidemiological studies. To this end, they aim at differentiating a specified rheumatic disease from other diseases (or healthy individuals). Classification criteria thus aim for a good group categorization (usually characterized by sensitivity, specificity, positive and negative predictive values, and likelihood ratios). In contrast, the clinical diagnosis aims at the correct individual categorization, to minimize misdiagnosis at the individual level.

Inherent in these concepts is the fact that classification and diagnostic criteria will not always categorize individuals into the same group (Figure 110.6). This leads to the issue of false-positive and false-negative classification when compared to clinical diagnosis, which is not a deficiency of any classification system, but rather a matter of fact. Since classification criteria will inevitably be applied by clinicians, for diagnostic purposes, it is important to emphasize that a clinician can at any time overrule the classification result using clinical judgement. In other words, clinicians may establish a diagnosis in unclassified patients, as well as decide not to treat classified patients for the lack of a clinical diagnosis (Figure 110.6).

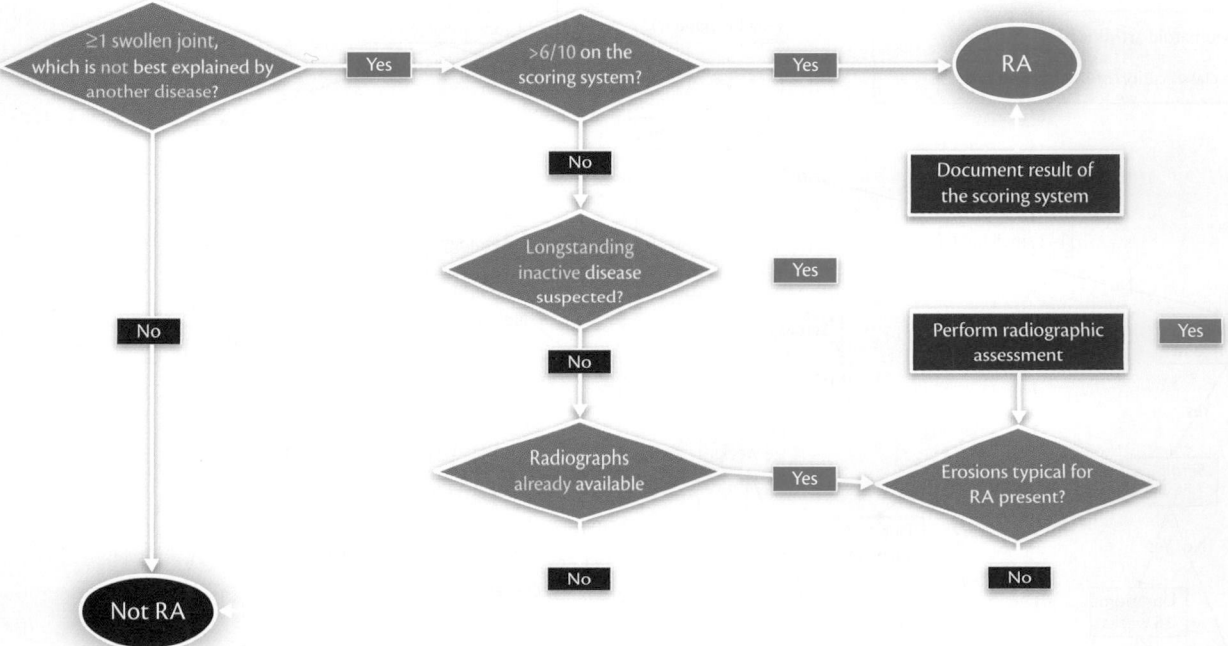

Fig. 110.5 The role of radiographic examination in the 2010 ACR/EULAR classification criteria. The figure depicts an algorithm for patients who are not classifiable by the scoring system, but who are either suspected to have long-standing (unclassified) disease (decision node in the middle of the figure) or already present with radiographic damage, which may then not be ignored (decision node at the bottom). In these two instances, information from radiographs may be used and allow a direct classification of RA in case of presence of typical RA erosions. The definition of 'erosiveness typical for RA' has recently been put forward.[28]
Taken from the Slidekit of EULAR and ACR.

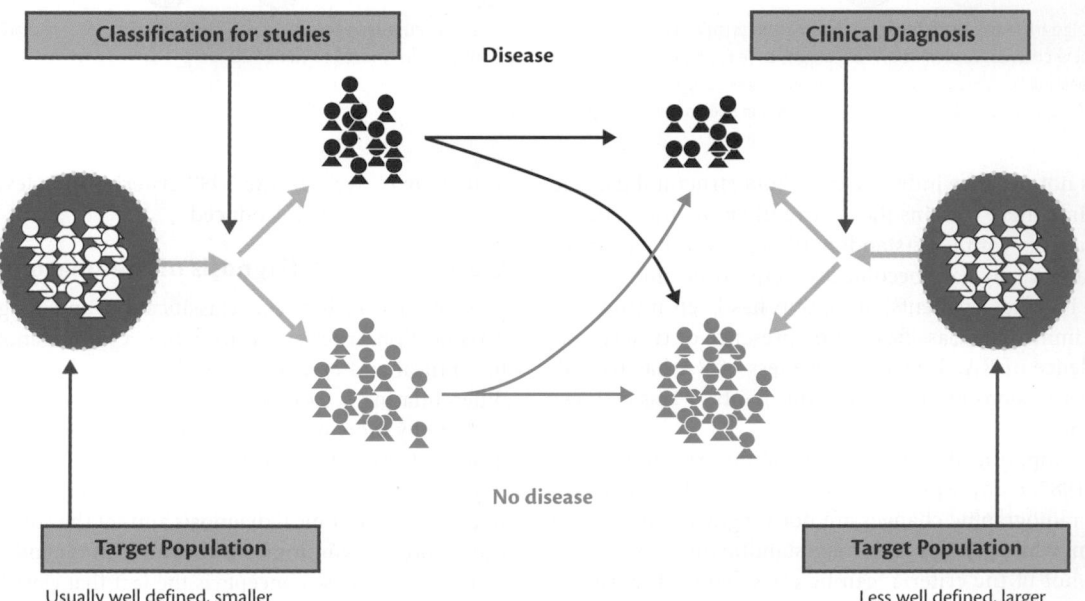

Fig. 110.6 Classification vs diagnosis. The target population for classification is usually smaller and better defined than that for diagnosis, as classification is used for study purposes. Both, classification criteria and diagnostic criteria categorize individuals as diseased or not diseased. The figure implies that there might be considerable overlap between these groups. From a clinical perspective a diagnosis can be established and treatment may be initiated, even if the classification result is negative.
Reproduced from the Slidekit of EULAR and ACR.

A typical scenario for a false-positive classification by the 2010 classification criteria is a patient with osteoarthritis of the hand with one swollen PIP joint. Such a patient would score highly on the joint distribution domain (also tenderness is counted as 'joint activity') and would likely present with a symptom duration of 6 weeks or more, and hence be classified as having RA. Vice versa, patients seronegative for RF and ACPA are prone to false-negative classification: once zero points are achieved in the serology domain, and given the fact that only one point each may be acquired from the acute-phase response and the symptom duration domain, this means that patients need to show a joint distribution in the top category. In other words, this means that seronegative patients need at least 10 active joints for their disease to be classified as RA. Inherent to the label of a 'diagnosis' is the fact that some sort of therapeutic intervention usually ensues.

It is important to mention in this context that the fulfilment of the new criteria can also be achieved cumulatively, that is, through repeated assessments over time, and in case of adequate previous documentation, also retrospectively.

Conclusion

In summary, the correct diagnosis of RA still remains a challenge, and it remains the task of the rheumatologist. Because of the large number of potential differential diagnoses, and the ability of RA to present in a very heterogeneous way, no criteria can replace the judgement and experience of the rheumatologist in this respect. Nevertheless, classification criteria may help to guide the rheumatologist in this difficult task of establishing a diagnosis, the importance of which still lies in the therapeutic implication for the patient. It is inherent to the concept of classification that it will differ from a clinical diagnosis in a potentially significant portion of individuals. As most current treatment algorithms indicate that treatment should be initiated immediately after the diagnosis of RA,[29] the rheumatologist is charged to lead and accelerate the diagnostic process by using algorithms, criteria, and other tools so as to avoid the most dangerous mistake in treatment of RA: delay.

References

1. Kvien TK. Epidemiology and burden of illness of rheumatoid arthritis. *Pharmacoeconomics* 2004;22(2 Suppl):1–12.
2. Nell VP, Machold KP, Eberl G, Stamm TA, Uffmann M, Smolen JS. Benefit of very early referral and very early therapy with disease-modifying anti-rheumatic drugs in patients with early rheumatoid arthritis. *Rheumatology* (Oxford) 2004;43(7):906–914.
3. Landewe RB, Boers M, Verhoeven AC et al. COBRA combination therapy in patients with early rheumatoid arthritis: long-term structural benefits of a brief intervention. *Arthritis Rheum* 2002;46(2):347–356.
4. Bijlsma JW. Patient benefit-risk in arthritis—a rheumatologist's perspective. *Rheumatology* (Oxford) 2010;49 Suppl 2:ii11–ii17.
5. Fries JF, Williams CA, Bloch DA. The relative toxicity of nonsteroidal antiinflammatory drugs. *Arthritis Rheum* 1991;34(11):1353–1360.
6. Fries JF, Williams CA, Ramey D, Bloch DA. The relative toxicity of disease-modifying antirheumatic drugs. *Arthritis Rheum* 1993;36(3): 297–306.
7. Hazlewood G, Aletaha D, Carmona L et al. Algorithm for identification of undifferentiated peripheral inflammatory arthritis: a multinational collaboration through the 3e initiative. *J Rheumatol Suppl* 2011;87:54–58.
8. Moore TL. Parvovirus-associated arthritis. *Curr Opin Rheumatol* 2000;12(4):289–294.
9. Avouac J, Gossec L, Dougados M. Diagnostic and predictive value of anti-cyclic citrullinated protein antibodies in rheumatoid arthritis: a systematic literature review. *Ann Rheum Dis* 2006;65(7):845–851.
10. Nishimura K, Sugiyama D, Kogata Y et al. Meta-analysis: diagnostic accuracy of anti-cyclic citrullinated peptide antibody and rheumatoid factor for rheumatoid arthritis. *Ann Intern Med* 2007;146(11): 797–808.
11. Rudwaleit M, van der HD, Landewe R et al. The Assessment of SpondyloArthritis International Society classification criteria for peripheral spondyloarthritis and for spondyloarthritis in general. *Ann Rheum Dis* 2011;70(1):25–31.
12. Dougados M, van der Linden S, Juhlin R et al. The European Spondylarthropathy Study Group preliminary criteria for the classification of spondylarthropathy. *Arthritis Rheum* 1991;34(10):1218–1227.
13. Gladman DD, Shuckett R, Russell ML, Thorne JC, Schachter RK. Psoriatic arthritis (PSA)—an analysis of 220 patients. *Q J Med* 1987;62(238):127–141.
14. Steere AC, Schoen RT, Taylor E. The clinical evolution of Lyme arthritis. *Ann Intern Med* 1987;107(5):725–731.
15. Dasgupta B, Cimmino MA, Maradit-Kremers H et al. 2012 provisional classification criteria for polymyalgia rheumatica: a European League Against Rheumatism/American College of Rheumatology collaborative initiative. *Ann Rheum Dis* 2012;71(4):484–492.
16. Healey LA. Polymyalgia rheumatica and seronegative rheumatoid arthritis may be the same entity. *J Rheumatol* 1992;19(2):270–272.
17. Fleming A, Crown JM, Corbett M. Early rheumatoid disease. I. Onset. *Ann Rheum Dis* 1976;35(4):357–360.
18. Maksymowych WP, Suarez-Almazor ME, Buenviaje H et al. HLA and cytokine gene polymorphisms in relation to occurrence of palindromic rheumatism and its progression to rheumatoid arthritis. *J Rheumatol* 2002;29(11):2319–2326.
19. Nell VPK, Machold KP, Eberl G et al. The diagnostic and prognostic significance of autoantibodies in patients with early arthritis. *Ann Rheum Dis* 2003;62(Suppl 1):OP0015.
20. van Leeuwen MA, van Rijswijk MH, van der Heijde DM et al. The acute-phase response in relation to radiographic progression in early rheumatoid arthritis: a prospective study during the first three years of the disease. *Br J Rheumatol* 1993;32 Suppl 3:9–13.
21. Arnett FC, Edworthy SM, Bloch DA et al. The American Rheumatism Association 1987 revised criteria for the classification of rheumatoid arthritis. *Arthritis Rheum* 1988;31(3):315–324.
22. Silman AJ, Symmons DP. Selection of study population in the development of rheumatic disease criteria: comment on the article by the American College of Rheumatology Diagnostic and Therapeutic Criteria Committee. *Arthritis Rheum* 1995;38(5):722–723.
23. Aletaha D, Eberl G, Nell VP, Machold KP, Smolen JS. Attitudes to early rheumatoid arthritis: changing patterns. Results of a survey. *Ann Rheum Dis* 2004;63(10):1269–1275.
24. Aletaha D, Neogi T, Silman AJ et al. 2010 Rheumatoid arthritis classification criteria: an American College of Rheumatology/European League Against Rheumatism collaborative initiative. *Arthritis Rheum* 2010;62(9):2569–2581.
25. Aletaha D, Neogi T, Silman AJ et al. 2010 rheumatoid arthritis classification criteria: an American College of Rheumatology/European League Against Rheumatism collaborative initiative. *Ann Rheum Dis* 2010;69(9):1580–1588.
26. Funovits J, Aletaha D, Bykerk V et al. The 2010 American College of Rheumatology/European League Against Rheumatism classification criteria for rheumatoid arthritis: methodological report phase I. *Ann Rheum Dis* 2010;69(9):1589–1595.
27. Neogi T, Aletaha D, Silman AJ et al. The 2010 American College of Rheumatology/European League Against Rheumatism classification criteria for rheumatoid arthritis: Phase 2 methodological report. *Arthritis Rheum* 2010;62(9):2582–2591.
28. van der Heijde D, van der Helm-van Mil AH, Aletaha D et al. EULAR definition of erosive disease in light of the 2010 ACR/EULAR rheumatoid arthritis classification criteria. *Ann Rheum Dis* 2013;72(4):479–481.
29. Smolen JS, Landewe R, Breedveld FC et al. EULAR recommendations for the management of rheumatoid arthritis with synthetic and biological disease-modifying antirheumatic drugs. *Ann Rheum Dis* 2010;69(6):964–975.

CHAPTER 111

Rheumatoid arthritis— clinical features

Eugen Feist and Gerd-R. Burmester

Early rheumatoid arthritis

Introduction and epidemiology

Rheumatoid arthritis (RA) is the most frequent chronic systemic autoimmune disease with joint involvement. It affects approximately 0.5% of the adult population of Europe and North America. Females are two- to fourfold more frequently affected and predisposed to develop a more severe disease manifestation. The incidence of disease increases with age and plateaus around 60 years.

Different genetic and environmental factors are involved in the pathogenesis of disease, and have an influence on the risk for developing RA. The incidence rates show a considerable variation even within Europe from south to north, from 16.5 to 29 cases per million people.[1] The risk for first-degree relatives of affected persons to develop RA is increased.[2] In genetically predisposed cohorts, such as some tribes of Native Americans, the prevalence of RA can reach up to 5%, whereas in less prone populations such as in China the prevalence is about 2.8 to 3.5 cases in 10 000 individuals.[1]

Disease onset and diagnosis

The onset of articular symptoms is usually insidious as mono-, oligo- or polyarthritis with pain, soft tissue swelling, and sometimes warmth as a correlate of acute synovitis (Figure 111.1). The predominantly affected joints include small finger joints (the metacarpophalangeal (MCP) and proximal interphalangeal (PIP) joints), wrists and forefeet, especially the metatarsophalangeal joints (MTP). For unknown reasons, the distal interphalangeal (DIP) joints are not affected. In addition to articular manifestations with pannus formation, joint effusion, bursitis, and risk of cartilage as well as bone destruction, periarticular symptoms can include tendinitis, tenosynovitis, epicondylitis, carpal tunnel syndrome, and myalgias. Involvement of shoulder and hip joints is relatively rare in early RA but common in patients with established and late-onset disease. In relation to the severity of the local and systemic inflammatory response, the disease process can be accompanied by nonspecific symptoms such as long-lasting morning stiffness affecting the joints, generalized weakness with loss of energy, fatigue, weight loss, fever, and early functional joint impairment.[3,4] In this context, depression and fatigue in close relation to the inflammatory process of RA can cause psychological stress and a significant reduction of

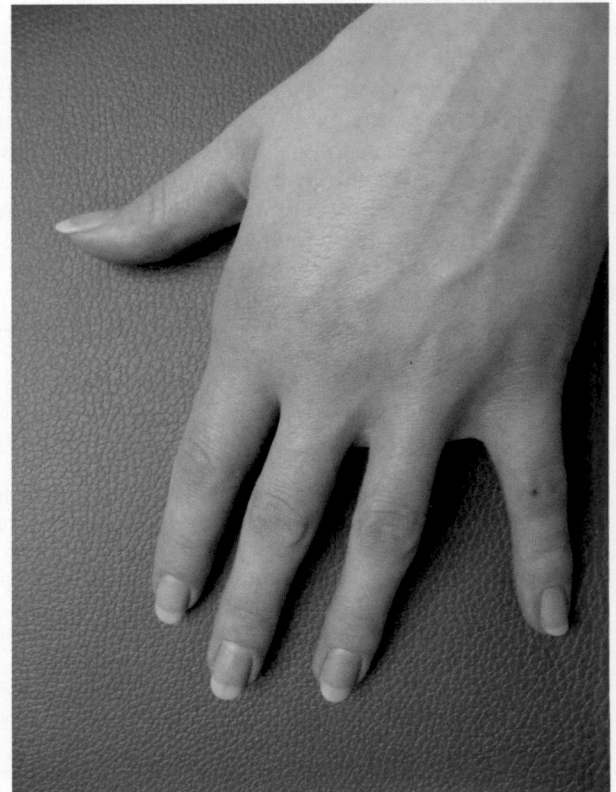

Fig. 111.1 Patient with early rheumatoid arthritis presenting with swelling and pain of the first and second metacarpophalangeal (MCP) joints of the left hand.

quality of life. High levels of disability have a negative impact on social participation and psychological functioning of patients.

The pattern of joint involvement is of particular importance for the differential diagnosis and separation from e.g. psoriatic arthritis or osteoarthritis, where the DIP joints are typically affected (Table 111.1, see also Chapter 110). If the disease presents with mono- or oligoarthritic symptoms, follow-up examinations are usually required to exclude peripheral spondylarthritides such as reactive arthritis. In patients with systemic onset and presentation with fever, vasculitic skin lesions, and internal organ

Table 111.1 Frequent differential diagnoses for rheumatoid arthritis (see Chapter 110)

Differential diagnosis	Frequent clinical findings for differentiation	Typical laboratory findings	Typical imaging findings
Psoriatic arthritis	Psoriatic skin lesions, different involvement patterns, asymmetric arthritis, irregular deformities, involvement of DIP joints, arthritis mutilans, enthesopathy, fasciitis, dactylitis with 'sausage digit', spinal involvement	Seronegative for RF and ACPA, association with HLA-B27	Ultrasound and MRI with detection of bursitis–tenosynovitis and joint synovitis. Radiographs may show erosive arthritis, missing periarticular osteoporosis, ossifying periostitis, acroosteolysis with resorption of the distal phlangeal tufts, arthritis mutilans with massive periarticular bone resorption, 'pencil in cup' deformity, spinal syndesmophytes and sacroilitis
Polymyalgia rheumatica	Proximal musculoskeletal symptoms with bursitis–tenosynovitis and synovitis	Seronegative for ACPA, strongly elevated ESR	Ultrasound and MRI with detection of bursitis–tenosynovitis of subdeltoid and subacromial bursae, trochanteric bursae and long head of the biceps, interspinous bursae in the neck and back, shoulder and hip joint synovitis
Reactive arthritis	Asymmetric mono- or oligoarthritis, other manifestations (conjunctivitis, urethritis, colitis, enthesitis)	Seronegative for RF and ACPA, positive serology or detection of infectious agent	Ultrasound and MRI with detection of bursitis–tenosynovitis and joint synovitis, non-erosive arthritis
Lyme arthritis	Asymmetric mono- or oligoarthritis, other manifestations (meningitis, encephalitis, carditis, enthesitis)	Seronegative for RF and ACPA, positive serology (IgM and/or IgG) and/or PCR result for *Borrelia burgdorferi*	Ultrasound and MRI with detection of bursitis–tenosynovitis and joint synovitis, non-erosive arthritis
Gout	Attacks of asymmetric mono- or oligoarthritis, gouty tophi	Seronegative for RF and ACPA, elevated serum uric acid (may be normal/low during acute attack), detection of urate crystals by polarized light microscopy	Intra- and para-articular erosions and intraosseous calcifications due to deposits of urate crystals, secondary osteoarthritic changes, dual-energy CT with detection of tophi and urate deposits
Haemochromatosis	Arthropathy with frequent symmetrical involvement of MCP II and III joints, pronounced degenerative changes, accumulation of iron in other organs especially liver with altered function	Seronegative for RF and ACPA, increased serum ferritin and transferrin saturation test, mutations of the *HFE* gene	Prominent degenerative changes with subchondral cyst formation, sclerosis, thinning of cartilage, and osteophytes
Osteoarthritis	Degenerative changes with involvement of DIP and PIP joints (Heberden's and Bouchard's nodes)	Seronegative for RF and ACPA, normal inflammatory markers	Degenerative changes with asymmetric joint space narrowing, subchondral cyst formation, sclerosis, thinning of cartilage, and osteophytes

ACPA, anti-citrullinated peptide antibodies; DIP distal interphalangeal; ESR, erythrocyte sedimentation rate; MCP, metacarpophalangeal; PIP, proximal interphalageal; PCR, polymerase chain reaction; RF, rheumatoid factor.

involvement, e.g. serositis or vasculitis, further differential diagnoses include systemic lupus erythematosus (SLE) or systemic vasculitis. Polymyalgia rheumatic (PMR) is another common inflammatory disorder that has to be considered as a differential diagnosis, especially in elderly patients. In addition to the typical proximal musculoskeletal symptoms of PMR affecting shoulder–neck as well as pelvic regions, an overlap with RA can be frequently seen in patients with peripheral joint involvement (PMR/late-onset RA or LORA overlap). Another distinct arthritic disease is characterized by remitting, seronegative, symmetric synovitis with pitting oedema of hands and forefeet (known as RS3PE syndrome). Further differential diagnoses of arthritic manifestations include acute and chronic sarcoidosis, other connective tissue diseases, Lyme disease, and gouty arthritis. Haemochromatosis with joint involvement is characterized by predominant degenerative changes affecting typically the second and third MCP joints, but can also cause soft tissue swelling and arthritic symptoms. An obscure disorder termed 'palindromic rheumatism' presents with variable episodes of arthritis flares affecting one or more joints. Typically, these attacks resolve without any sequelae after hours or days. However, in approximately one-third of affected patients the disease can progress into classical RA.

Laboratory markers play an important role for diagnosis, follow-up, evaluation and prognosis of patients. At disease onset the presence of rheumatoid factor (RF) and of antibodies against citrullinated protein/peptide antigens (ACPA) are important diagnostic markers and allow differentiation from other distinct forms of arthritides.[5] In approximately one-half of ACPA positive patients with undifferentiated arthritis, the diagnosis of RA was confirmed within the first year of follow-up.[6] So far the assays for ACPA are not internationally standardized; the most widely used and established antigen is a synthetic peptide (cyclic citrullinated peptide, CCP). Another licensed and commercially available assay with comparable diagnostic performance employs citrullinated and mutated vimentin (MCV) as antigen.[7] In Table 111.2, typical laboratory findings in patients with RA are summarized. Interestingly, as the first preclinical sign of disturbances in the immune system with formation of an auto-inflammatory response, RF, and ACPA as well as slowly rising levels of C-reactive protein (CRP) can be detected even years before the onset of articular disease manifestation in some patients.[8,9]

Conventional radiographic examinations (including wrists, hands, and forefeet as well as other affected joints) are still the gold standard for the documentation of the erosive nature and progress of RA, but provide relatively low sensitivity for detection of early soft tissue and erosive bone changes. Therefore, as useful imaging techniques for documentation of the inflammatory soft tissue process in early RA, ultrasound including power Doppler examination (US with PD: visualization of effusion, synovitis, hyperaemia, bursitis, tenosynovitis, and eventually erosions) and MRI (more sensitive than US for early detection of erosions, and additional visualization of bone oedema) should be used.[10] Bone scintigraphy can differentiate inflammatory from degenerative joint processes, but—besides irradiation exposure—provides a rather low diagnostic specificity and also low image resolution. In case of active disease, radiographic examinations can be recommended every 6–12 months to assess joint damage and adapt therapy appropriately. In contrast, MRI and especially US can be useful tools to frequently assess disease activity.

Classification criteria

Novel classification criteria for RA were recently introduced by an American College of Rheumatology/European League Against Rheumatism (ACR/EULAR) initiative.[11,12] The goal of these classification criteria was to improve early differentiation of patients with RA from other causes of arthritis. The main purpose was to facilitate the early initiation of disease modifying anti-rheumatic drug (DMARD) therapy and to support the performance of clinical studies in the field of early RA (see Chapter 110). Patients with a score of at least 6 points are classified as having RA. Scoring should only be done if information from at least one serological test (RF or ACPA) is available. In this context, high-level positive autoantibodies were defined as a result of at least three times the upper limit of normal. In fact, the introduction and weighting of ACPA and inflammatory markers would allow classification as RA of a patient with involvement of only one small joint or two large joints in case of symptom duration of at least 6 weeks. However, it should be pointed out that these criteria are not meant for the *diagnosis* of early RA and that before applying them other inflammatory joint disorders have to be excluded. In addition, patients with typical radiologic changes would per se classify as RA in the absence of other explanations.

Table 111.2 Laboratory findings in patients with rheumatoid arthritis with relevance for disease activity, diagnosis and prognosis

Laboratory parameter	Finding	Relevance
CRP	Slight to moderate increase	Inflammatory marker (acute-phase reaction) Prognostic marker for erosive disease
ESR	Slight to moderate increase	Inflammatory marker (chronic process)
Erythrocytes and haemoglobin levels	Reduced, slight to moderate anaemia	Active inflammatory disease, anaemia due to overexpression of IL-6 with induction of hepcidin causing disturbances in iron metabolism
Thrombocytes	Increased, slight to moderate thrombocytosis	Active inflammatory disease
Leucocytes	Increased, slight to moderate leucocytosis	Inflammatory process
Immunoglobulin levels	Slight to moderate increase	Inflammatory marker (chronic process)
Iron metabolism	Iron levels reduced and ferritin increased	Disturbances in iron metabolism due to induction of hepcidin and increase of ferritin as inflammatory marker (acute-phase reaction)
Lipid levels	Decrease of total cholesterol and LDL	Inflammatory marker (chronic process)
Rheumatoid factor (RF, measurement of IgM and IgA subtypes)	Positive titres in international units (>20 IU)	Diagnostic marker with moderate sensitivity, specificity and positive predictive value. Prognostic marker for erosive and systemic disease, Autoantibodies against Fc part of human IgG
ACPA, measurement of IgG subtypes)	Positive titres (no international standardization)	Diagnostic marker with moderate sensitivity, but high specificity and positive predictive value. Prognostic marker for erosive and systemic disease. Autoantibodies against citrullinated epitopes of different antigens (such as fibrinogen, vimentin, α-enolase, collagen type II and as artificial antigen, CCP)

ACPA, anti-citrullinated peptide antibodies; CCP, cyclic citrullinated peptide; CRP, C-reactive protein; ESR, erythrocyte sedimentation rate; RF, rheumatoid factor.

The earlier revised ACR classification criteria dating from 1987 provided good specificity for established RA.[13] The main limitations of these criteria are reflected by the incorporation of signs and symptoms that are more present in advanced disease such as symmetric polyarthritis, rheumatoid nodules, and radiological changes. Furthermore, ACPAs, as the most specific biomarkers for diagnosis of RA nowadays, were not routinely available when these criteria were introduced. Therefore, these criteria are not very useful for differentiation of patients with early arthritis.

Established and advanced rheumatoid arthritis

Symptoms and diagnosis

Involvement of musculoskeletal apparatus

Small joints

The inflammatory process of RA predominantly affects small joints, leading to synovitis with pannus formation and clinically evident signs and symptoms of arthritis. In the joint region, the influence on bone metabolism and the destructive nature of disease manifest as periarticular bone demineralization, and irreversible destruction of cartilage as well as articular bone. First erosions are frequently found at the insertion region of the joint capsule, where pannus tissue starts to invade into the naked bone structures not covered by cartilage.

As signs of advanced disease in the upper limb, the involvement of carpal bones and MCP joints causes ulnar drift, often in combination with radial deviation of the wrist and flexion deformities (Figure 111.2). Typical wrist deformities include volar subluxation of the hand with a visible sliding at the radiocarpal joint and radial deviation of the carpal bones (Figure 111.3). Involvement of the radioulnar joint can lead to instability and dorsal subluxation of the ulnar head with a 'piano key' phenomenon on downward pressure. The resulting instability and mechanical tension of the ulnar head can eventually cause rupture of carpal extensor tendons.

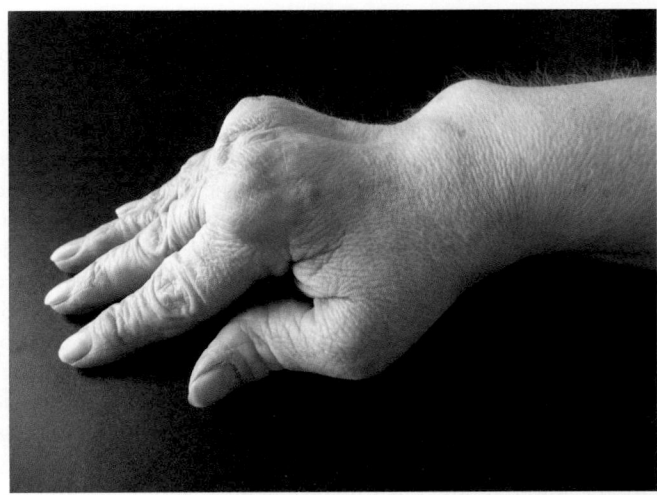

Fig. 111.3 Patient with rheumatoid arthritis presenting with volar subluxation of the right hand with a visible sliding at the radiocarpal joint and Z-deformity (or 90–90 thumb) with flexion of the first metacarpophalangeal joint and hyperextension of the interphalangeal joint.

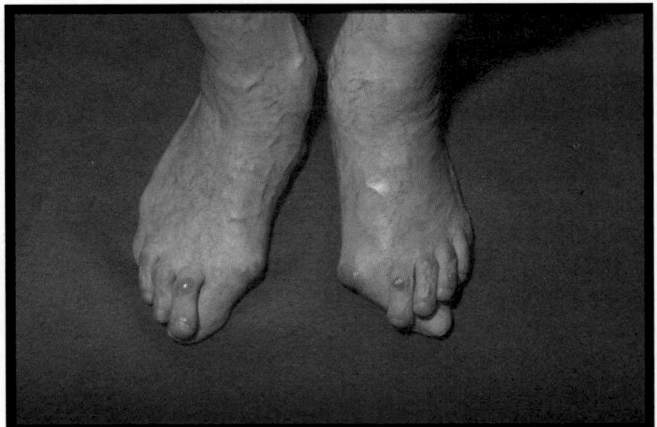

Fig. 111.4 Typical forefoot deformities in a patient with rheumatoid arthritis with clawing of the toes and dislocation of the metatarsophalangeal (MTP) joints.

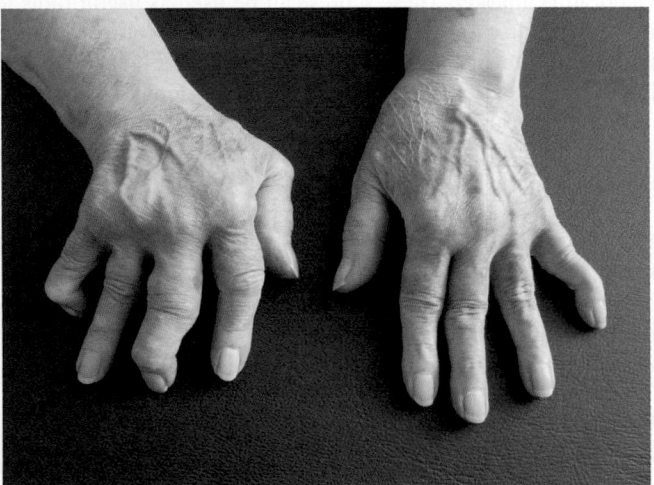

Fig. 111.2 Patient with rheumatoid arthritis presenting with a radial deviation (right wrist), swan-neck deformity with hyperextension of the proximal interphalangeal (PIP) and flexion of distal interphalangeal (DIP) joints (digits 3 right and 5 on both sides) and boutonnière deformity with flexion of the PIP and hyperextension of DIP joints (digits 2–4 left).

Involvement of MCP and PIP joints is typically symmetric and can lead to articular destruction, subluxation, or dislocation and finally, as an endstage change, to an ankylosis of joints. Tenosynovitis of tendon sheaths can cause typical finger deformities such as Z-deformity of the thumb, swan-neck deformity, and boutonnière deformity (Figures 111.2 and 111.3). Furthermore, tenosynovitis of the carpal flexor tendons can lead to compression of the median nerve causing carpal tunnel syndrome with altered/lost sensation of the thumb, index, and middle fingers predominantly, in association with a characteristic pattern of weakness. Another typical sign of established RA is atrophy of interosseous muscles of the hand mainly due to reduced use as a consequence of joint pain and stiffness. As in early RA, the DIP joints are typically not involved even in advanced stages of disease.

As signs of advanced disease in the lower limbs, involvement of the metatarsophalangeal (MTP) joint is very common, frequently leading to forefoot deformities (Figure 111.4). Synovitis with erosive bone changes as well as tenosynovitis especially of the flexor tendons can cause clawing of the toes and dorsal dislocation of the MTP joints.

Another occasional but relevant manifestation of RA can affect the temporomandibular joints, with resulting painful limitation of mouth opening.

Large and medium-sized joints

At the upper limbs, involvement of the elbow is often accompanied by considerable synovitis with effusion in the olecranon fossa and bursitis, leading to a reduction of extension, flexion, and supination (Figure 111.5). Shoulder involvement often starts with bursitis and tenosynovitis of the biceps tendon. In patients with advanced disease, synovitis can cause erosions and destruction of the glenohumeral joint. Furthermore, rupture of tendons including parts of the rotator cuff are frequently observed in patients with shoulder involvement. Taken together, all these manifestations can cause significant functional loss in such basic daily activities as eating, washing, and dressing.

At the lower limbs, knee involvement is very common and presents with synovitis, bursitis with effusion especially in the supra patellar recess, and erosive lesions. Popliteal bursitis (Baker's cyst) is associated with risk of popliteal vein compression, which can lead to thrombosis and subsequently, life-threatening pulmonary embolism. Rupture of a Baker's cyst can cause acute pain and inflammatory swelling of the soft tissue compartment of the lower leg and also thrombotic complications. At the knee joint, functional loss is associated with a reduction of extension and instability as a result of laxity in the collateral and cruciate ligaments. Subsequently, progressive valgus deformity can occur, especially in women with a physiological valgus position. Due to involvement of the tibiotalar and subtalar joints, a progressive flattening of the longitudinal foot arch can further increase valgus deformity of the legs (Figure 111.4). Furthermore, involvement of the ankle joints can cause considerable functional deficits interfering with walking ability. In long-standing and poorly controlled RA, prosthetic joint replacement is frequently required for knee and hip joints.

Axial joints

The most critical involvement of the axial joints in RA affects the cervical spine. Particularly, inflammatory changes of the atlantoaxial joint (C1–C2) with destabilization and atlantoaxial dislocation represents a potentially life-threatening complication. This process is typically driven by synovitis, most commonly in the space between the transverse ligament of the atlas and the posterior part of the dens. Ventral atlantal dislocation has to be considered if the space between the anterior dens border and atlas arch increases to 5 mm or more. Vertical dislocation of the dens can occur in conjunction with a ventral atlantal dislocation but also in isolation, leading to a rising of the dens position sometimes even passing the foramen magnum line. Erosive changes of the dens are particularly associated with the risk of dens fracture causing compression of the cervical cord and basilar invagination. This severe complication can lead to paraplegia potentially accompanied by fatal respiratory paralysis. Therefore, functional cervical radiographs and/or MRI are strongly recommended in patients with suspected cervical involvement (pain in the neck, headache, pain with projection to shoulder and upper extremities, paraesthesiae or numbness of upper extremities). Instability in the atlantoaxial joint must be excluded especially before procedures leading to hyperflexion of the cervical spine such as during physiotherapy, dental care, and intubation. In case of proven instability, wearing a stiff collar and surgical stabilization are appropriate measures.

Disease assessment in daily practice

Several composite scores are useful and established in daily practice for assessment of disease activity in patients with RA (Table 111.3).[13,14] These scores include the number of tender and swollen joints (usually out of 28 defined joints), patient's and physician's global assessment of disease activity on a visual analogue scale (VAS) as well as levels of acute-phase reactants (erythrocyte sedimentation rate (ESR) or CRP). The Disease Activity Score using 28 joint counts (DAS28) is a frequently used measure for disease activity in RA.[15] The score is calculated by a complex mathematical formula providing a good sensitivity to change of disease activity. However, it is important to note that a limitation of the DAS28 includes a rather high false-positive rate for remission. The main advantage of the Simplified Disease Activity Index (SDAI) and Clinical Disease Activity Index (CDAI) is the ability to evaluate disease activity without using a calculator.[16] The CDAI even allows immediate scoring without the need for a laboratory marker. These scores can be used as useful tools for monitoring disease activity and tight disease control and can guide treatment decisions. For assessment of joint damage and disease progression in stable RA, conventional radiographic examinations can be recommended once a year. In active, early or resistant disease, radiologic re-evaluation at shorter intervals (e.g. 6 months) can be recommended.

The Stanford or Modified Health Assessment Questionnaires (HAQ) are frequently used to assess functional disability in daily practice.[17,18] Functional disability as such is influenced by age, female sex, disease duration, disease activity reflected by the number of affected joints (particularly in early disease), and radiological joint damage (particularly in established disease).

Prognostic markers, course of disease, and outcome

RA is a severe systemic autoimmune disease with increased morbidity and mortality compared to the general population of the same age and gender. Furthermore, the disease is characterized by disability, reduced quality of life, and high levels of work instability. Pain, joint destruction, progressive loss of mobility, and reduced ability to care for oneself are closely related features of RA.

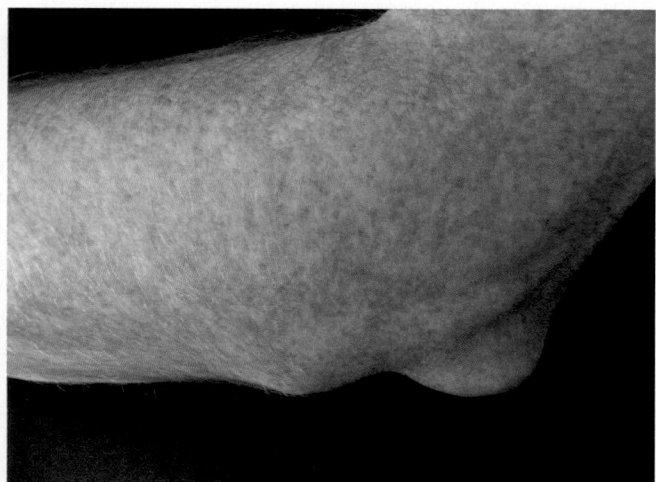

Fig. 111.5 Patient with rheumatoid arthritis presenting with involvement of the elbow accompanied by effusion in the olecranon fossa and bursitis, plus a rheumatoid nodule distal to olecranon bursitis.

Table 111.3 Composite scores for disease activity in rheumatoid arthritis[13,14,16]

Tool	Calculation	Cut-off for remission
DAS28 (ESR)	$(0.56 \times TJC1/2) + (0.28 \times SJC1/2) + (0.7 \times \ln[ESR]) + (0.014 \times PtGA)$	<2.6
CDAI	SJC + TJC + PhGA + PtGA	≤2.8
SDAI	SJC+ TJC + PhGA + PtGA + CRP (mg/dl)	≤3.3
New ACR/EULAR remission criteria 2011		
For clinical trials		
Boolean criteria or	SJC, TJC, PtGA, CRP	all ≤1
Index-based criteria	SDAI SJC+ TJC + PhGA + PtGA + CRP (mg/dl)	≤3.3
For clinical practice		
Boolean criteria or	SJC, TJC, PtGA	all ≤1
Index-based criteria	CDAI SJC + TJC + PhGA + PtGA	≤2.8

APR, acute-phase reactant; CDAI, Clinical Disease Activity Index; CRP, C-reactive protein; ESR, erythrocyte sedimentation rate; PhGA, physician global activity; PtGA, patient global activity; SDAI, Simplified Disease Activity Index; SJC, swollen joint count; TJC, tender joint count.

Since RA is a heterogeneous disease with a highly variable course and outcome, it is important to predict the course of disease and adjust treatment options individually. The spectrum includes patients with remitting flares, patients with mild disease manifestations without erosive arthritis, and also severe, progressively destructive disease and even refractory cases. The differentiation of clinically distinct subgroups is also reflected by distinct serological and genetic characteristics (see Chapter 109). In this context, the prognosis and outcome of joint involvement is influenced by several independent factors. The following predictors for severe and erosive disease have been identified so far: female gender, early detection of erosive changes, elevated acute-phase reactants (ESR and/or CRP) as well as seropositivity for RF and/or ACPA.[19] High autoantibody titres for RF and ACPA are also indicative for more severe and systemic disease.

The outcome of patients with RA with respect to joint involvement has been significantly improved over recent decades due to major advances in diagnostics, treatment strategies, and the development of novel drugs. Under optimal treatment conditions, even patients with long-standing disease can present without joint damage or disability. In this context, it is particularly important to start effective treatment within the so-called 'window of opportunity' before such changes occur. It remains to be determined whether the outcome with respect to extra-articular disease manifestations (e.g. systemic manifestations and amyloidosis) as well as comorbidities (e.g. cardiovascular events and lymphoma) will also be influenced by more recent treatment approaches.

Extra-articular manifestations in rheumatoid arthritis

Extra-articular disease manifestations reflect the systemic nature of RA and play a significant role in prognosis and treatment decisions.[20] Since involvement of internal organs is frequent, detailed organ examination and, if required, interdisciplinary management of complications is necessary.

Rheumatoid nodules

Subcutaneous rheumatoid nodules belong to the frequent extra-articular disease manifestations primarily in seropositive patients with severe and active disease. However, with increasingly effective use of conventional and biological DMARDs the occurrence of subcutaneous nodules has decreased and is now rare. They present predominantly at the extensor surfaces of the upper limb, along the forearm (Figure 111.5) and fingers, but can occasionally be found at other periarticular regions such as the Achilles tendon and in internal organs, e.g. in the lung parenchyma and myocardium.[21] In some patients, the occurrence of subcutaneous nodules is paradoxically pronounced during treatment with methotrexate (MTX). Since the clinical manifestation of rheumatoid nodules is very typical, histological examination is usually not necessary. However, with atypical presentations or in cases of symptomatic nodules (e.g. due to pressure effects), biopsy or removal of the tissue reveals a granulomatous lesion with focal central fibrinoid necrosis surrounded by fibroblasts.

Eye involvement

Eye involvement includes the frequent occurrence of secondary Sjögren's syndrome as well as the rarer and mild complication of episcleritis and the potentially severe manifestation of scleritis and keratitis.[22] Secondary Sjögren's syndrome occurs in about one-quarter of patients and is characterized by typical sicca symptoms of eyes and mouth. Treatment should be symptomatic with substitution of saliva and tears. The incidence of episcleritis in patients with RA is less than 1%. The clinical manifestations are usually mild to asymptomatic with separation of diffuse and nodular episcleral types of inflammation. The prevalence of scleritis is lower with clinical symptoms of pain, vascular injection, photophobia and visual disturbance (Figure 111.6). Clinically, scleritis can be classified as anterior (approximately 90% of cases) vs posterior localization, and by the inflammatory process in non-necrotizing (diffuse or nodular) and necrotizing (often painless, affecting approximately 10% of cases) forms. Importantly, scleritis has to be considered as an emergency situation, since it can progress to eye perforation with resulting blindness. Often in conjunction with scleritis, the most severe eye involvement includes peripheral ulcerative keratitis (PUK, corneal 'melt'). This typically painless manifestation occurs primarily in patients with long-lasting RA, which may be clinically inactive, and is associated with a high risk of ocular perforation and subsequent blindness. Therapy of inflammatory and severe eye

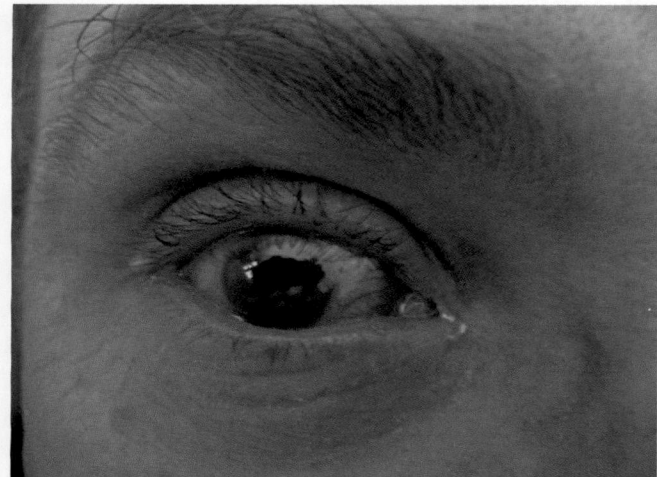

Fig. 111.6 Patient with rheumatoid arthritis presenting with acute scleritis with pain, vascular injection, photophobia, and visual disturbance.

involvement in RA includes topical and systemic administration of anti-inflammatory and potentially highly potent immunosuppressive drugs in close interdisciplinary cooperation.

Haematological and systemic manifestations

Blood cell count disturbances in association with disease activity in RA are presented in Table 111.2. Benign lymphadenopathy is another common finding in active and chronic RA and must be differentiated from non-Hodgkin's lymphoma in suspicious cases. As a systemic form of RA, Felty's syndrome is characterized by chronic neutropenia, splenomegaly, destructive joint involvement, high positive results for autoantibodies (RF and ACPA), and rheumatoid nodules. Felty's syndrome affects about 1% of cases and usually requires an intensive immunosuppressive treatment strategy.

Vasculitis

Vasculitis is now rare and associated with disease severity and activity in RA. The most frequent manifestation is cutaneous vasculitis of small to medium-sized vessels leading to necrosis and ulceration, predominantly of the lower legs. Furthermore, vasculitis may cause peripheral neuropathy either symmetrical 'glove and stocking' or mononeuritis multiplex with loss of sensory and motor conduction. Organ-specific vasculitis may lead to infarction including myocardial infarction or stroke, or damage of other internal organs by affecting e.g. mesenteric arteries with abdominal pain, digestive symptoms, and bowel ischaemia. Laboratory results usually reveal a strong inflammatory response (elevated CRP and ESR levels) as well as signs of an immune-complex-mediated vasculitis (e.g. high titres of RF, positive results for cryoglobulins, and low levels of complement). Treatment of vasculitic manifestations includes optimal anti-rheumatic treatment with immunosuppressive drugs, including glucocorticoids, but also optimal management of traditional cardiovascular risk factors.

Lung and cardiac involvement

Lung involvement in RA is frequent and under-recognized.[20,23] Pleuritis might occur at onset of disease and can cause progressive respiratory distress due to accumulating pleural fluid. However, in some asymptomatic patients with minor effusion, pleuritis is detected only incidentally by routine imaging. Furthermore, interstitial lung disease usually of mild to moderate severity is quite common. Approximately 6% of patients will develop clinical symptoms due to pulmonary fibrosis and pulmonary hypertension, especially in long-standing disease. It is important to keep in mind that interstitial lung disease is also a rare but important adverse effect of MTX therapy. However, this toxicity often occurs within weeks of MTX initiation and has a subacute to acute onset with rapidly progressive respiratory symptoms. Interstitial lung disease can also present as nodular lung disease in association with rheumatoid nodules.

In the context of serositis, pleuritis may be associated with exudative pericarditis. Pericarditis with acute chest pain, dyspnoea, and pericardial effusion represents the most frequent heart manifestation in RA. Since this condition can lead to pericardial tamponade, close monitoring by echocardiographic examination is required. Chronic constrictive pericarditis can lead to right-sided heart failure. Involvement of the myocardium and endocardium can also occur as well as conduction defects and coronary arteritis due to vasculitis. In cases of active inflammatory heart or lung involvement, especially in patients with acute serositis, immunosuppressive treatment is indicated and usually includes glucocorticoids.

Amyloidosis

Secondary amyloidosis due to chronic persistent inflammation is a severe and potentially underdiagnosed condition. Deposition of amyloid A interferes especially with renal function and may lead to terminal renal failure requiring dialysis. Mortality in affected patients is strongly increased and, therefore, early recognition and effective anti-inflammatory regimes with suppression of the inflammatory cascade are the treatment goals. With the introduction of effective therapeutic approaches, amyloidosis is increasingly rare in daily practice.

Comorbidity in rheumatoid arthritis

Mortality and disability in RA is significantly influenced by comorbidities such as cardiovascular disease (myocardial infarction and stroke), infections, osteoporosis, overlapping autoimmune diseases, and lymphoma. Therefore, management of comorbidities is of major relevance for treatment decisions and individual prognosis.

Infection

The incidence of infections including severe infections is significantly increased in patients with RA, due to effects on the immune system of the autoimmune disease itself as well as the prescription of immunosuppressive drugs. The risk profile includes infections of soft tissue and skin, respiratory and urinary tracts, as well as joints and bones. Early diagnosis and treatment are essential. For example, in every suspected case of septic arthritis, an immediate aspiration of synovial fluid must be performed for microscopic and cultural diagnostics.

It is important to note that concomitant medication, especially the use of glucocorticoids, is a well-known risk factor for recurrent infections. Furthermore, increased risk for infections is also a relevant safety issue for all biologics.[24] However, there are certain differences between the compounds. It has been shown in clinical trials and registries that blocking of the cytokine tumour necrosis factor alpha (TNFα) is associated with an increased risk of opportunistic infections, including reactivation of latent tuberculosis. In contrast, up to now there is no evidence for the same risk under the B- and T-cell directed drugs rituximab and abatacept.[25,26] For all biologics except rituximab, screening for latent tuberculosis is a standard procedure before starting therapy. Furthermore, prophylactic vaccination using killed or inactivated vaccines is nowadays strongly recommended for patients with RA prior to initiation of immunosuppressive therapy especially biologics (including but not limited to vaccinations against tetanus, hepatitis B, influenza, and pneumococcal vaccines; see Chapter 94).[27] In contrast, immunization with live or attenuated vaccines is not recommended in immunocompromised patients with RA. In some patients, especially those undergoing treatment with immunosuppressive drugs, signs and symptoms of infections can be hidden or atypical. For example, under treatment with biologics such as tocilizumab, the inflammatory response against infectious agents might be suppressed with lack of increase in CRP levels.

Cardiovascular risk

The risk for cardiovascular events is strongly increased in RA from the beginning of the disease process and is comparable to that for patients with diabetes mellitus.[28] RA should therefore be considered as an independent risk factor for cardiovascular disease, with myocardial infarction, congestive heart failure and stroke representing the main complications for mortality.[29] The vascular changes can be best described by a premature atherosclerosis, which is associated with prolonged increased inflammatory parameters such as ESR and CRP, extra-articular features of RA, and the use of glucocorticoids. In addition, increasing evidence suggests that particularly seropositive patients and patients with extra-articular disease manifestations have the highest risk of developing cardiovascular complications.[30] Since the process of premature atherosclerosis appears to associate with disease activity, effective anti-inflammatory treatment is the appropriate preventive approach. In this context, a reduced risk for cardiovascular events is emerging from registries, due to use of traditional DMARDs as well as biologics such as TNF blockers. In the prevention and management of cardiovascular disease, traditional risk factors such as smoking, hypertension, diabetes, and hypercholesterolaemia must be considered appropriately. It should be noted that in active RA the measurable lipid levels are suppressed due to the inflammatory response. Therefore, higher levels of cholesterol appear frequently after the initiation of an effective therapy. Under such circumstances, the use of statins should be considered, especially since they may beneficially influence both vascular risk as well as disease activity.

Osteoporosis

The association of RA with an increased risk of generalized bone loss and osteoporosis is well documented. It has been shown that the risk of osteoporosis in patients with RA is increased approximately twofold in males and females. As a consequence, the risk for vertebral as well as non-vertebral fractures (especially hip, pelvis, humerus, tibia, and fibula) is also increased. Development of osteoporosis is driven by several factors including release of proinflammatory cytokines such as IL6 with impact on bone metabolism but also simply immobilization due to pain and functional impairment. Long-standing, particularly active, disease and low body mass index (BMI), which may be a manifestation of disease activity, are predictive factors. Therefore, osteoporosis can also be addressed as an extra-articular manifestation of RA. In addition, prolonged exposure to glucocorticoids is a risk factor for the development of secondary osteoporosis. Therefore, early initiation of preventive measures (e.g. calcium, if not sufficient in the diet, vitamin D supplementation, bisphosphonates) and consequent treatment of manifest osteoporosis are part of the standard care of RA.

Malignancies

The risk for development of certain malignancies is slightly increased in patients with RA. Amongst them, the incidence of non-Hodgkin's lymphoma (most frequent subtype large-cell B-cell lymphoma) is increased approximately two- to fourfold compared to the healthy population.[31] With a clear association to active and severe disease, development of non-Hodgkin's lymphoma can be considered as a long-term risk in uncontrolled and refractory patients.[32] Furthermore, data from meta-analyses showed an increased risk for lung cancer and potentially decreased risk for colorectal and breast cancer compared with the general population.[33] So far the available data for patients under biologics, especially TNF blockers, showed an overall unchanged risk for the development of non-Hodgkin's lymphoma.[24] On the other hand, the anti-CD20 antibody rituximab represents a preferable biological option for patients with coexistent or previous B-cell lymphoma.

Overlapping autoimmune diseases

RA is frequently accompanied by or overlaps with other systemic and non-systemic autoimmune diseases. Under certain circumstances the manifestations are inseparable, such as in patients with polymyalgia rheumatica in association with late-onset RA as well as in patients with mixed connective tissue diseases, secondary Sjögren's syndrome or SLE; in the latter, seropositive patients can present with an erosive arthritis ('rhupus'). Furthermore, potentially due to a common genetic predisposition, the incidence of multiple sclerosis, myasthenia gravis, and autoimmune thyroiditis as well as autoimmune liver diseases are increased in patients with RA. If repeatedly positive anti-phospholipid antibodies are detectable in patients with RA and vascular thrombosis or characteristic pregnancy morbidity, secondary anti-phospholipid syndrome must be considered.

Conclusion

RA is a heterogeneous disease with involvement of the musculoskeletal system but potentially also other organs. Risk factors for aggressive disease include the inflammatory response, the formation of autoantibodies, and internal organ involvement. RA is closely associated with different comorbidities including cardiovascular disease and malignancies. Active and uncontrolled disease leads to loss of function, early invalidity and an overall increased mortality rate. Therefore, early diagnosis, application of novel classification criteria, stratification of patients according to prognostic markers, and appropriate treatment are crucial for the best outcome.

References

1. Alamanos Y, Voulgari PV, Drosos AA. Incidence and prevalence of rheumatoid arthritis, based on the 1987 American College of Rheumatology criteria: a systematic review. *Semin Arthritis Rheum* 2006;36(3):182–188.
2. Grant SF, Thorleifsson G, Frigge ML et al. The inheritance of rheumatoid arthritis in Iceland. *Arthritis Rheum* 2001;44(10):2247–2254.

3. Suurmeijer TP, Waltz M, Moum T et al. Quality of life profiles in the first years of rheumatoid arthritis: results from the EURIDISS longitudinal study. *Arthritis Rheum* 2001;45(2):111–121.

4. Hakkinen A, Arkela-Kautiainen M, Sokka T, Hannonen P, Kautiainen H. Self-report functioning according to the ICF model in elderly patients with rheumatoid arthritis and in population controls using the multidimensional health assessment questionnaire. *J Rheumatol* 2009;36(2):246–253.

5. van Venrooij WJ, Zendman AJ, Pruijn GJ. Autoantibodies to citrullinated antigens in (early) rheumatoid arthritis. *Autoimmun Rev* 2006;6(1):37–41.

6. Avouac J, Gossec L, Dougados M. Diagnostic and predictive value of anti-cyclic citrullinated protein antibodies in rheumatoid arthritis: a systematic literature review. *Ann Rheum Dis* 2006;65(7):845–851.

7. Bang H, Egerer K, Gauliard A et al. Mutation and citrullination modifies vimentin to a novel autoantigen for rheumatoid arthritis. *Arthritis Rheum* 2007;56(8):2503–2511.

8. Nielen MM, van Schaardenburg D, Reesink HW et al. Increased levels of C-reactive protein in serum from blood donors before the onset of rheumatoid arthritis. *Arthritis Rheum* 2004;50(8):2423–2427.

9. Nielen MM, van Schaardenburg D, Reesink HW et al. Specific autoantibodies precede the symptoms of rheumatoid arthritis: a study of serial measurements in blood donors. *Arthritis Rheum* 2004;50(2):380–386.

10. Tan YK, Conaghan PG. Imaging in rheumatoid arthritis. *Best Pract Res Clin Rheumatol*;25(4):569–584.

11. Aletaha D, Neogi T, Silman AJ et al. Rheumatoid arthritis classification criteria: an American College of Rheumatology/European League Against Rheumatism collaborative initiative. *Arthritis Rheum* 2010;62(9):2569–2581.

12. Aletaha D, Neogi T, Silman AJ et al. rheumatoid arthritis classification criteria: an American College of Rheumatology/European League Against Rheumatism collaborative initiative. *Ann Rheum Dis* 2010;69(9): 1580–1588.

13. Felson DT, Smolen JS, Wells G et al. American College of Rheumatology/European League Against Rheumatism provisional definition of remission in rheumatoid arthritis for clinical trials. *Arthritis Rheum* 63(3):573–586.

14. Felson DT, Smolen JS, Wells G et al. American College of Rheumatology/European League against Rheumatism provisional definition of remission in rheumatoid arthritis for clinical trials. *Ann Rheum Dis* 70(3): 404–413.

15. Prevoo ML, van 't Hof MA, Kuper HH et al. Modified disease activity scores that include twenty-eight-joint counts. Development and validation in a prospective longitudinal study of patients with rheumatoid arthritis. *Arthritis Rheum* 1995;38(1):44–48.

16. Aletaha D, Smolen J. The Simplified Disease Activity Index (SDAI) and the Clinical Disease Activity Index (CDAI): a review of their usefulness and validity in rheumatoid arthritis. *Clin Exp Rheumatol* 2005;23(5 Suppl 39):S100–S108.

17. Bruce B, Fries JF. The Stanford Health Assessment Questionnaire: dimensions and practical applications. *Health Qual Life Outcomes* 2003;1:20.

18. Bruce B, Fries JF. The Stanford Health Assessment Questionnaire: a review of its history, issues, progress, and documentation. *J Rheumatol* 2003;30(1):167–178.

19. Visser K, Goekoop-Ruiterman YP, de Vries-Bouwstra JK et al. A matrix risk model for the prediction of rapid radiographic progression in patients with rheumatoid arthritis receiving different dynamic treatment strategies: post hoc analyses from the BeSt study. *Ann Rheum Dis*; 69(7):1333–1337.

20. Turesson C, O'Fallon WM, Crowson CS, Gabriel SE, Matteson EL. Extra-articular disease manifestations in rheumatoid arthritis: incidence trends and risk factors over 46 years. *Ann Rheum Dis* 2003;62(8):722–727.

21. Raven RW, Weber FP, Price LW. The necrobiotic nodules of rheumatoid arthritis; case in which the scalp, abdominal wall, involving striped muscle, larynx, pericardium, involving myocardium, pleurae, involving lungs, and peritoneum were affected. *Ann Rheum Dis* 1948;7(2):63–75.

22. McGavin DD, Williamson J, Forrester JV et al. Episcleritis and scleritis. A study of their clinical manifestations and association with rheumatoid arthritis. *Br J Ophthalmol* 1976;60(3):192–226.

23. Saag KG, Kolluri S, Koehnke RK et al. Rheumatoid arthritis lung disease. Determinants of radiographic and physiologic abnormalities. *Arthritis Rheum* 1996;39(10):1711–1719.

24. Nam JL, Winthrop KL, van Vollenhoven RF et al. Current evidence for the management of rheumatoid arthritis with biological disease-modifying antirheumatic drugs: a systematic literature review informing the EULAR recommendations for the management of RA. *Ann Rheum Dis*; 69(6):976–986.

25. Campbell L, Chen C, Bhagat SS, Parker RA, Ostor AJ. Risk of adverse events including serious infections in rheumatoid arthritis patients treated with tocilizumab: a systematic literature review and meta-analysis of randomized controlled trials. *Rheumatology (Oxford)*; 50(3):552–562.

26. Buch MH, Smolen JS, Betteridge N et al. Updated consensus statement on the use of rituximab in patients with rheumatoid arthritis. *Ann Rheum Dis*; 70(6):909–920.

27. Singh JA, Furst DE, Bharat A et al. 2012 update of the 2008 American College of Rheumatology recommendations for the use of disease-modifying antirheumatic drugs and biologic agents in the treatment of rheumatoid arthritis. *Arthritis Care Res* (Hoboken) 2012;64(5):625–639.

28. Lindhardsen J, Ahlehoff O, Gislason GH et al. The risk of myocardial infarction in rheumatoid arthritis and diabetes mellitus: a Danish nationwide cohort study. *Ann Rheum Dis*; 70(6):929–934.

29. Maradit-Kremers H, Nicola PJ, Crowson CS, Ballman KV, Gabriel SE. Cardiovascular death in rheumatoid arthritis: a population-based study. *Arthritis Rheum* 2005;52(3):722–732.

30. Turesson C, McClelland RL, Christianson TJ, Matteson EL. Severe extra-articular disease manifestations are associated with an increased risk of first ever cardiovascular events in patients with rheumatoid arthritis. *Ann Rheum Dis* 2007;66(1):70–75.

31. Zintzaras E, Voulgarelis M, Moutsopoulos HM. The risk of lymphoma development in autoimmune diseases: a meta-analysis. *Arch Intern Med* 2005;165(20):2337–2344.

32. Baecklund E, Iliadou A, Askling J, Ekbom A, Backlin C, Granath F, et al. Association of chronic inflammation, not its treatment, with increased lymphoma risk in rheumatoid arthritis. *Arthritis Rheum* 2006;54(3): 692–701.

33. Smitten AL, Simon TA, Hochberg MC, Suissa S. A meta-analysis of the incidence of malignancy in adult patients with rheumatoid arthritis. *Arthritis Res Ther* 2008;10(2):R45.

CHAPTER 112

Rheumatoid arthritis—management

Chris Deighton

Introduction

Rheumatoid arthritis (RA) management has been revolutionized in the past 20 years.[1,2] Where remission was once an aspiration, it is now common to see patients with no or minimal disease activity, no progressive damage on joint imaging, and consequently no disability.[1-3] This has resulted in improved mortality, ability to work, and reductions in joint replacements.[4-6]

Influential international and national RA management guidelines have been published (see Box 112.1).[1,7-11] Guidelines are helpful for several reasons:

- RA is common, affecting up to 1% of the population.

- Low incidence means that primary care physicians (PCPs) may see only new RA patients less than once per year.[12,13] Guidelines promote awareness of symptoms and signs of new disease, and clues that synovitis will persist.

- RA is very expensive for national economies. In the United Kingdom direct care costs to the National Health Service are £560 million per year, with additional costs to the economy of sick leave and work-related disability at £1.8 billion a year.[13] Implementation of national guidelines, particularly in treating early and intensively, would save money in the national economy,[13] with similar conclusions in international studies.[14]

- The provision and quality of care for RA shows marked variation which guidelines can decrease, and set benchmarks for high-quality care.[13]

- The advent of biological therapies has given rheumatology the ability to consume large amounts of healthcare resources, but the responsibility to spend this appropriately. Treating disease early and intensively may decrease, or at least delay, the need for biologics.[15,16]

Some examples of key international and national guidelines are listed in Box 112.1. The following is a summary of key recommendations that are common to these guidelines:

- There is a need for early diagnosis and rapid referral to specialist care (see Chapter 110). Any persistent joint inflammation, irrespective of the distribution of joints affected, should be referred

> **Box 112.1** Key national and international rheumatoid arthritis management guidelines
>
> - EULAR recommendations for the management of rheumatoid arthritis with synthetic and biological disease-modifying anti-rheumatic drugs[1]
> - American College of Rheumatology 2008 recommendations for the use of nonbiologic and biologic disease-modifying anti-rheumatic drugs in rheumatoid arthritis[8]
> - National Institute of Health and Clinical Excellence clinical guideline 79. Rheumatoid arthritis: national guideline for management and treatment in adults[7]
> - Scottish Intercollegiate Guidelines Network. Management of early rheumatoid arthritis. a national clinical guideline, 2011[9]
> - British Society for Rheumatology and British Health Professionals in Rheumatology guideline for the management of rheumatoid arthritis (the first 2 years)[10]
> - British Society for Rheumatology and British Health Professionals in Rheumatology guideline for the management of rheumatoid arthritis (after the first 2 years)[11]

for a specialist opinion. Inflammatory arthritis is a clinical diagnosis, based on signs and symptoms of inflammation in joints. Although PCPs may perform blood tests, waiting for the results should not lead to a delay in specialist referral. Even more importantly, if test results are available, normal inflammatory markers and negative serology should not put PCPs off referring promptly. This is particularly the case if poor prognostic clinical signs are evident, such as small-joint disease of the hands and feet. The more joints that are affected, the worse the outcome. In most countries the main component of the delay between patients developing initial symptoms and starting disease-modifying anti-rheumatic drugs (DMARDs) is the delay in seeing PCPs in the first place.[12] Public health campaigns need to emphasize the signs and symptoms of inflammatory arthritis, so that patients do not delay seeing their PCPs (see Figure 112.1).

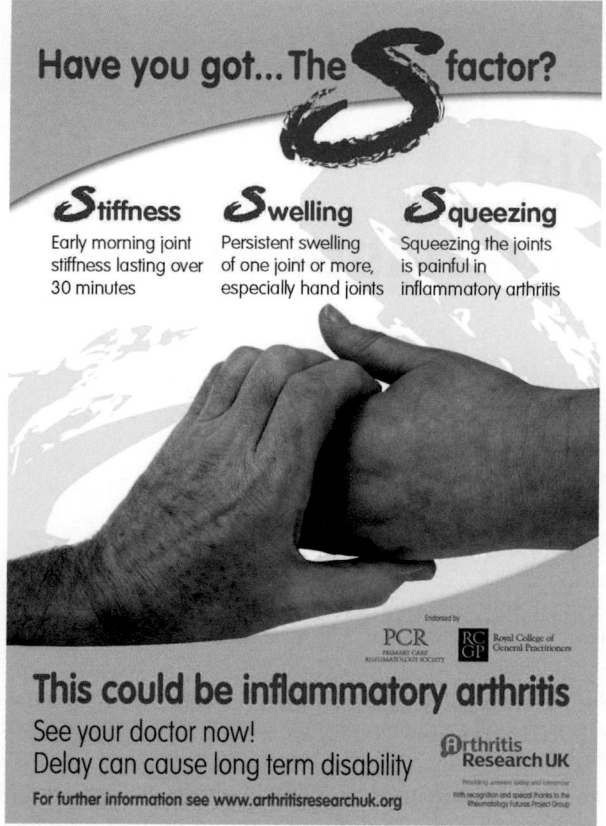

Fig. 112.1 The S Factor Campaign in the United Kingdom to highlight awareness of early inflammatory arthritis.
Reproduced with permission of Arthritis Research UK.

◆ Early intensive treatment of active RA is needed. If treatment is not initiated within the 'window of opportunity', the chances of influencing long-term outcomes is profoundly diminished.[17]

◆ Early disease should be followed up closely and documented objectively, to ensure adequate disease activity suppression.

◆ For early and established disease there should be availability of education on self-management and the need for medication, and ongoing access to the MDT. Prompt access should be available for any flare-ups of the disease, with flexible follow-up based more on the need of the patient rather than the convenience of the clinic.

◆ For established and stable disease, annual review should be available (see below).

There are controversies in the management of RA due to either different interpretations of or lack of evidence, or because the label of RA covers a broad diversity of disease expression. These include:

◆ the need for the same intensive interventions in all patients, irrespective of disease activity or prognostic markers, and whether DMARD monotherapy or combination therapy is appropriate

◆ the role of steroids

◆ the appropriate introduction of biological therapies.

The next section expands on these issues.

Early intervention

Remission is easier to achieve and maintain by prompt treatment.[1,2] Immunopathological changes in the first 3 months of RA lead to self-perpetuation of the disease, and become increasingly difficult to influence.[17] Sustained remission translates into less radiological damage and less disability. In the early stages of disease the disability index Health Assessment Questionnaire (HAQ) is determined largely by inflammation which is amenable to intervention, but as time goes by the HAQ is more governed by increasing joint damage which is less responsive to medical therapy. Aletaha and colleagues pooled six trials looking at remission, and demonstrated that the ability to influence HAQ decreased progressively with delays in treatment.[18] The Finnish RA Combination Therapy (FIN-RACo) study showed that early suppression of disease activity resulted in a greater likelihood of maintaining work capacity at 5 years, and was maintained for up to 11 years.[19] The Norfolk Arthritis Register demonstrates that sustained remission is less likely to show deterioration of function over 5 years.[20]

However there are still frustrating delays in patients initiating DMARDs. In the United Kingdom the Early Rheumatoid Arthritis Network demonstrated median delays of 8 months.[21] The National Audit Office Report found that people with RA visit a GP on average four times before being referred to a specialist for diagnosis.[13]

In early intervention a balance should be struck between overtreating self-limiting inflammatory arthritis, and undertreating poor-prognosis aggressive RA. Trials have attempted to address this with interventions in early undifferentiated synovitis. In the PROMPT trial treatment with weekly methotrexate reduced and delayed the number of patients transforming from undifferentiated arthritis to RA at 1 year (mainly anti-citrullinated protein antibodies (ACPA) positive patients), with radiological progression diminished also, but no improvement in remission rates.[22] The STIVEA trial gave three intramuscular injections of 80 mg of methylprednisolone or placebo at weekly intervals to patients with early inflammatory polyarthritis (4–10 weeks' duration); methylprednisolone resulted in a modest but significant decrease in the percentage of patients who needed DMARDs at 6 months (61% vs 76%, p = 0.015) and an increase in resolution of arthritis at 1 year (19.8% vs 9.9%, p = 0.05).[23] By contrast, a single dose of methylprednisolone in the SAVE trial did not change disease progression.[24] In arthralgia patients positive for rheumatoid factor (RF) or ACPA two injections of 100 mg of dexamethasone reduced antibody titres at 6 months compared with placebo, but did not prevent progression to arthritis.[25] The ADJUST trial compared 6 months of abatacept (a T-cell costimulation inhibitor biological drug) against placebo in undifferentiated arthritis.[26] At a year there was a decrease in the proportion of patients who developed RA in the abatacept group, though this did not reach significance (46% vs 67%). In a small study infliximab (10 patients) was used against placebo (7 patients) in undifferentiated arthritis of less than 1 year's duration which had relapsed after a steroid injection.[27] The use of infliximab showed modest short-term relief but did not prevent the development of RA.

Biomarkers to predict who will transform from arthralgias or undifferentiated arthritis into RA do not currently exist to warrant widespread use of steroids, DMARDs, or biologics. Methotrexate, and steroid injections, could be considered in patients with early persistent synovitis who are ACPA positive. ACPA and/or RF status should be assessed in all early persistent synovitis patients because of the diagnostic specificity,[28–30] prognostic assistance,[28,30] and potential to influence therapy decisions.[22] However, in any patient in whom RA is suspected irrespective of serology, a low threshold for starting DMARDs should operate, because the diagnosis is not always easy, and the consequences of delaying DMARDs can be serious.[1]

The current label of RA covers a heterogeneous spectrum of disease. It would be useful to be able to stratify patients according to risk of progression, with patients with poor prognoses being treated very aggressively from the start with combinations of DMARDs and steroids, whereas patients with good prognoses might receive more cautious DMARD monotherapy. A validated prediction rule has been developed using information regularly collected in clinic: patient age and gender, number and types of joints involved, duration of morning stiffness, C-reactive protein (CRP) level, RF and ACPA levels.[31] Such indices can help management decisions, as advocated by guidelines.[1,8]

Multidisciplinary support for patients from the start, and throughout the course of the disease, is vital.[7,9,10] All patients must be informed about our understanding of the disease and the need for interventions, and receive the opportunity for early education on how to best manage their own disease.[7] Specialist nurses often provide follow-up monitoring of DMARDs and disease activity. Access to physiotherapy and occupational therapy is also important from disease onset. The impact of RA on patients, particularly their social roles, can be devastating, as well as affecting carers.

Treating to target

The concept

Treatment should aim for remission preferably, or low disease activity where this cannot be achieved, and this should be sustained to avoid disease progression and disability. The American College of Rheumatology (ACR) and the European League Against Rheumatism (EULAR) have agreed criteria on remission which are a tender joint count, swollen joint count, CRP (in mg/dL), and patient global assessment (0–10 scale) all being less than or equal to 1, or when the Simplified Disease Activity Index (SDAI) is 3.3 or less.[32] Although designed for clinical trials, this is bound to influence clinical practice. Four key approaches are needed for early RA:

- Patients should be seen regularly to ensure that inflammation is suppressed quickly and permanently. The National Institute for Health and Clinical Excellence (NICE) guidelines advocate monthly clinic visits for early active RA, based on studies such as TICORA,[7,33] where frequent visits with action taken for active disease were associated with excellent outcomes. EULAR guidelines suggest every 1–3 months [1]

- Patients should have a formal assessment of their disease activity. Validated measures include the Disease Activity Score (DAS), the 28 joint Disease Activity Score (DAS28—see Figure 112.2), the SDAI, and the Clinical Disease Activity Index (CDAI).[34] Although there are criticisms of scores such as the DAS28,[2,16] they are better than a 'physician's global assessment', and record a figure in the patient record, without which there is no target to aim for.[2]

- Inflammation must be suppressed quickly. Disease activity at 3 months is a good predictor of long-term outcomes.[2] Combinations of DMARDs may extend the window of opportunity for influencing long-term outcomes,[35] but there is no room for complacency.

- Each follow-up occasion on which the target DAS is not achieved needs treatment intervention.[1,2,7] Individual inflamed joints can be injected with steroids, or for more widespread disease activity, an intramuscular injection or course of oral steroids might be used. Steroids alone should not be relied upon in the long term, and DMARDs also need to be adjusted or changed to aim for prolonged disease suppression. This may mean increasing the dosage of established DMARDs, adding others in, or using alternative drugs if they are not working or causing side effects.[1,7]

Methotrexate as the anchor drug

For patients with early active RA methotrexate should be included in the DMARD regimen, because:

- It is as good as any other conventional DMARD, and in head-to-head studies in early RA compares favourably with anti-TNF. In the BeSt trial monotherapy arm, 44% of methotrexate patients were in remission at 6 months, and 32% at 2 years follow-up.[36] An observational cohort comparing methotrexate with sulfasalazine found similar outcomes, but greater erosion suppression with methotrexate.[37]

- There is considerable experience of methotrexate in combination regimens with other DMARDs and biological therapies.[1,7]

- The dose is highly adjustable, with higher doses (20–30 mg once weekly) more efficacious than lower (7.5–15 mg).[1]

- Patients are more likely to stay on methotrexate longer, due to sustained efficacy, and good long-term tolerability.[38]

- It is available orally and subcutaneously. With intolerance of tablets, or limited efficacy, switching to subcutaneous injections improves bioavailability, increases efficacy, and decreases toxicity.[39]

- Methotrexate is cheaper than most other DMARDs, and considerably cheaper than biologics.

Not all new patients need to go onto methotrexate. In some there may be an absolute contraindication. The evidence for using methotrexate either alone or in combination has largely been generated in trials on 'active' RA (defined in different trials in different ways). Evidence is lacking in patients with milder or palindromic RA, where other monotherapies may be just as appropriate.[1,9]

Monotherapy or combination therapy?

There are disagreements between guidelines on whether methotrexate should be used as mono- or combination therapy in early RA. EULAR guidelines argue for initial monotherapy usually,[1] and NICE for combination therapy in early active disease[7] The arguments against combination therapies are:

- Methotrexate can work very effectively as a monotherapy.[1]

- Combination therapies have a higher rate of toxicity.[40] If drugs with similar side-effect profiles are administered concomitantly it is difficult to judge which drug might be responsible for a certain side effect (e.g. elevated alanine transaminase in a patient

Which joints are <u>tender</u>? (please tick)   Which joints are <u>swollen</u>? (please tick)

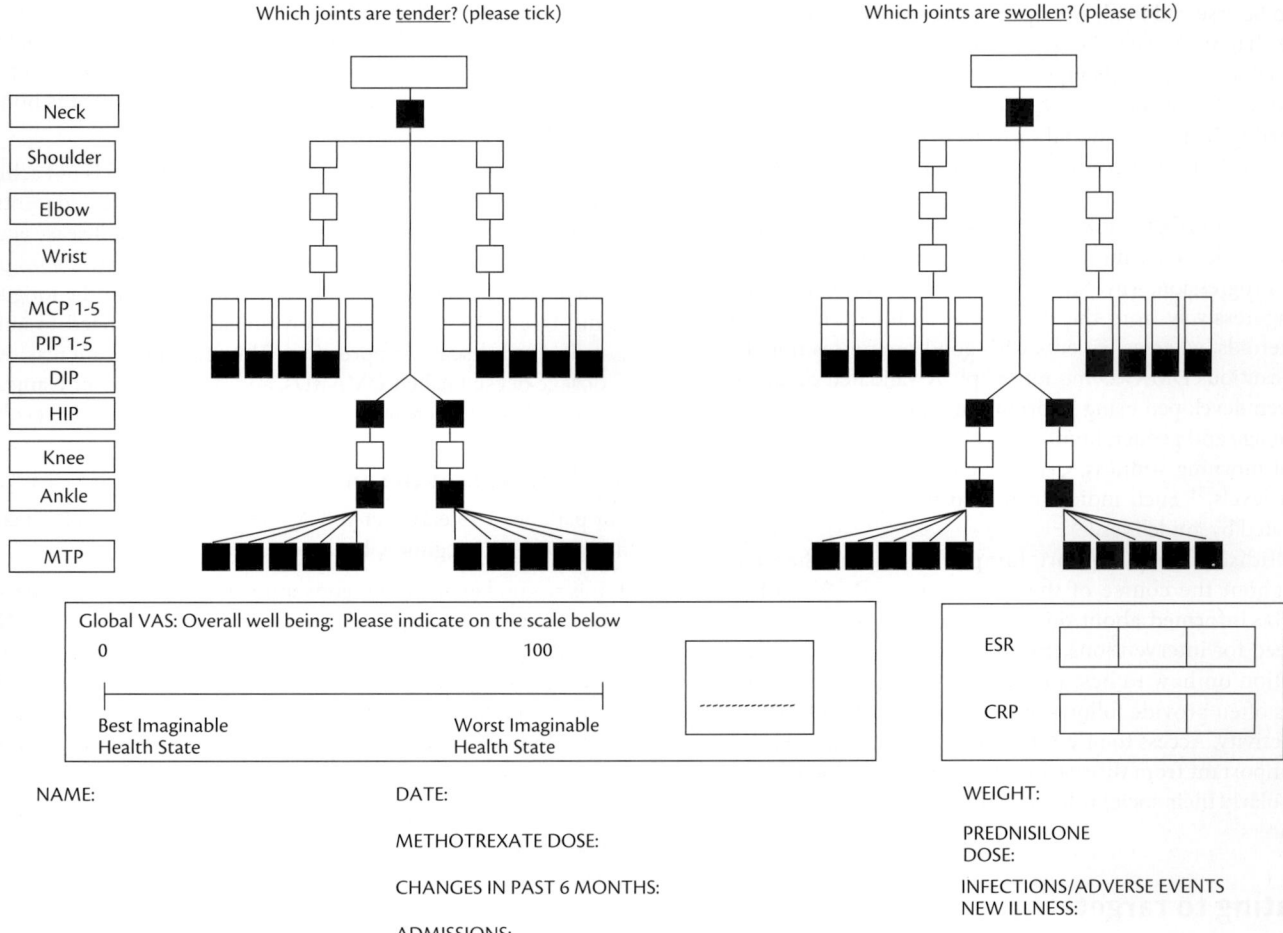

Fig. 112.2 The joints included in the DAS28 and the form used for recording disease activity at the Royal Derby Hospital (United Kingdom). This consists of a tender joint count, swollen joint count, measure of inflammation (usually ESR, though a CRP version is available) and a visual analogue score of global health (1–100). The calculation is complex, but calculators are readily available (e.g. www.4s-dawn.com/DAS28/DAS28.html)

recently starting methotrexate and sulfasalazine). If combination therapy is effective it is difficult to know whether this is due to just one or more of the agents.

- Combination therapies are more expensive than monotherapies and may require more monitoring tests.

- A recent trial of step-up therapy starting with sulfasalazine compared with combination therapy from the start showed no significant differences in outcomes.[33]

Arguments for combination therapies include:

- They are more efficacious than monotherapies. A meta-analysis supported this.[40] The combination of methotrexate with biological therapies is more efficacious than the single drugs.[41] However, in many trials, steroids were included in the combination arm which might account for improved and more rapid outcomes.[1] Comparisons of combination therapies with monotherapies without steroids have sometimes not shown significant differences in efficacy.[1]

- They may extend the window of opportunity for influencing long-term outcomes, and should be used when there have been DMARD delays.[35]

- Combination therapies are more cost-effective than monotherapies, due to a greater ability to postpone the need for expensive biological therapies.[42] Four-year follow-up data from the BeSt study showed that 39% of sequential monotherapy patients needed to start infliximab and methotrexate at some stage during the follow-up period. However, in the sequential step-up combination therapy, only 11% went on to anti-TNF, and 20% of the combination therapy with tapered steroids,[43] suggesting that combination therapies are superior to monotherapies in decreasing the need for biologics.

- Some trials suggest sustained benefits for patients on combination therapy compared with monotherapies,[44,45] whereas others have shown a convergence of long-term outcomes irrespective of the initial treatment strategy.[46]

In deciding for each individual patient which is the appropriate treatment strategy, the most important principle is to suppress inflammation quickly and sustain this. All is well if this can be achieved with monotherapy.

Alternatives to methotrexate include sulfasalazine, leflunomide, and intramuscular gold injections.[1] In the EULAR guidelines these drugs were given priority over other DMARDs because systematic reviews found no evidence that these drugs are inferior to methotrexate.[1] Hydroxychloroquine was deemed to be a weaker DMARD in isolation, and having a place in milder disease, or in combination therapy regimens, but showing inferiority to sulfasazine in inhibiting structural damage.[1] The ACR guidelines on DMARD therapy give a useful overview on DMARD combinations.[8] The best evidence is for methotrexate with hydroxychloroquine, leflunomide, or sulfasalazine, and triple therapy combining methotrexate with sulfasalazine and hydroxychloquine.[8]

The role of steroids

Steroids are the best way of getting active RA under rapid control, with greater potency than non-steroidal anti-inflammatory drugs (NSAIDs), because they act on numerous inflammatory pathways, not just antagonizing cyclooxygenase.[47] A meta-analysis has shown they are disease modifying, unlike NSAIDs.[48] They are often safe where there are contra-indications to NSAIDs (e.g. ischaemic heart disease, asthma, renal disease).

There are several ways of employing steroids.

- Inject inflamed joints as and when they occur, though the role of this approach is limited in active polyarthritis.

- Give regular intramuscular injections in the early phases of the disease, e.g. TICORA where active disease was treated with monthly injections up to a total of 120 mg of methylprednisolone either into inflamed joints or intramuscularly.[33]

- Give a tapered oral regimen, starting on a high dose and tailing this down as the disease is controlled, e.g. COBRA where patients start on 60 mg of prednisolone with methotrexate and sulfasalazine, and the steroids are gradually tapered subsequently.[45]

- Use longer-term low-dose steroids. There are no trials comparing high-dose tapered steroids against longer-term low-dose regimens.[1] Although steroids are invaluable in rapidly dampening active inflammation while waiting for other DMARDs to become effective, their long-term use should be avoided wherever possible. They are also useful in managing disease flare-ups, either in the early stages of attempting to induce remission, or in established disease. However, difficulties in weaning patients off steroids, or the need to use recurrent steroids for repeated flares of disease, should result in adjustments to other DMARDs.[7] The safety of glucocorticoids is an important aspect of the EULAR guidelines on the management of steroid treatment.[49]

In treating to target, all aspects of the patients and their disease need to be taken into account. Some patients may get a useful drop in DAS, yet still have ongoing grumbling synovitis that can damage joints. MRI evidence shows that patients 'in remission' can still erode joints due to clinically silent synovitis.[50] Early inflammatory arthritis EULAR guidelines advocate radiography of affected joints every 6–12 months to assess progression of joint damage.[51] DMARDs should be adjusted accordingly when there is ongoing structural damage, even if the disease activity appears to be well controlled. Likewise, in patients appearing to be in remission, any DMARD decreases should be performed slowly and cautiously, with ongoing documentation of both disease activity and structural damage on imaging.[52]

Biological agents

The introduction of biologics to RA and other inflammatory arthropathies has had a huge impact on improving the control of poor-prognosis and refractory disease. In RA, biologics have the following advantages over DMARDs:

- Most conventional DMARDs were discovered by serendipity, and there is ongoing debate on how they specifically work. Biologics were designed with an increasing understanding of the pathogenesis of RA to specifically block cytokines, cells, or interactions between cells that are critical in RA pathogenesis.

- Unlike conventional DMARDs where benefits are delayed, anti-TNF and other biologics can work quickly with symptom-relieving benefits, as well as profound disease-modifying capabilities in preventing disease progression.

- They can have dramatic benefits where conventional therapies have failed.

The disadvantages of biological therapies are:

- They are very expensive compared with conventional DMARDs.

- As monotherapies in early RA, they are no more efficacious than methotrexate, which makes it challenging to suggest that they are cost-effective.[53] They are better at slowing radiological progression than single conventional DMARDs, though a meta-analysis of anti-TNF vs conventional combination therapies suggests no significant differences.[54]

- They cannot be administered orally, which adds to costs for intravenous therapies, and inconvenience for subcutaneous drugs compared with tablets.

- They increase the risk of infections. For anti-TNF therapies this is particularly in the first 6 months of treatment,[55] but vigilance is required for emerging infections while patients continue on biologics. Specific infections such as tuberculosis (TB) need to be screened for at baseline as this decreases the risk.[56]

- There is concern over long-term administration of cytokine and cell blockers, particularly with regard to malignancies, and immunosuppression-associated rare infections (e.g. progressive multifocal leucoencephalopathy reports with rituximab[57]). Because anti-TNF therapies have the longest track record, considerable data have accumulated from national registers that are largely reassuring for the predisposition to solid malignancies and lymphomas, though concerns around increased risks of skin cancers remain, and patients need to be counselled about this.[58,59]

Anti-TNF therapies currently take precedence as they were the first RA biologics, and unlike some other biologics, are licensed for patients who fail on DMARDs. The best time to introduce anti-TNFs is debatable. EULAR and ACR guidelines suggest a place for first-line use in patients with poor-prognosis RA.[1,8] However, there is a lack of biomarkers to accurately predict the course of RA, and some of these patients can do very well on standard DMARDs. Health economic modelling has largely failed to demonstrate that widespread use of first-line anti-TNF therapy is good use of limited healthcare resources.[53] Most health economies restrict anti-TNF use to patients who fail on conventional DMARDs (usually at least methotrexate), and have ongoing active disease (set differently across nations).[60] Other biologics are currently largely used in patients who have failed anti-TNF, because of licensing restrictions, or national guidelines. Health economic models could potentially lead to advocating first-line anti-TNF use with accurate predictions of which patients would do badly on conventional therapies (with poor efficacy or high toxicity), and who would do well on anti-TNF. This would be even more cost-effective if anti-TNFs could induce remission and then be withdrawn and replaced by cheaper drugs. Infliximab could be used in this way, such as in the BeSt study, where 50% of patients were able to stop anti-TNF and be maintained on conventional DMARDs,[46] and sustained benefits over 8 years from a smaller study using 1 year of initial infliximab with methotrexate maintenance thereafter.[61] More research on biomarkers to predict disease course and response to therapies, and on the health economics of targeted early anti-TNF therapy, is needed, before health economies would advocate widespread use of early biologics. Alternatively, the price of biologics needs to drop considerably, with maintained evidence of long-term safety.

If widespread first-line anti-TNF therapy is currently unlikely, then should anti-TNF be introduced after the failure of one, or several DMARDs? The SWEFOT trial is informative. The addition of infliximab for patients who failed to reach low levels of disease activity after 3 months of methotrexate monotherapy resulted in better outcomes than the addition of sulfasalazine and hydroxychloroquine.[62] Furthermore, in the BeSt trial, patients in any arm who failed on methotrexate had only approximately a 12% chance of responding to other conventional therapies.[43] Consequently, patients failing on early DMARDs, particularly methotrexate, should have access to anti-TNF, instead of inappropriate faith in trials of more conventional DMARDs.

There are discrepancies in national guidelines on eligibility criteria for anti-TNF.[60] Most nations define active disease worthy of biologics as a DAS28 score greater than 3.2, whereas others, including the United Kingdom, pitch this cut-off at 5.1.[16,60] The latter level is inappropriately high, and should be reduced because:

* A sustained DAS28 between 3.2 and 5.1 is not benign disease, with radiological progression, functional decline, and loss of work not much less than patients with higher disease activity. If a patient on combination conventional therapy has a DAS28 greater than 3.2, they are not being controlled satisfactorily.[16,21,63]

* Patients with a DAS28 of less than 5.1 starting anti-TNF therapy do just as well as, if not better than, patients with higher DAS28, with decreased disease activity, and improved functional ability.[16,64,65]

If a patient fails on their first anti-TNF, either through toxicity, or no response (primary non-responders), or because of gradual loss of response (secondary non-responders), there is emerging evidence on the next-best strategy. For secondary non-responders, there may be a greater chance of responding to a second anti-TNF than for primary non-responders.[66] If patients have had adverse reactions to a first anti-TNF, there is a greater chance that they will have toxicity with a second.[67] Irrespective of why the first anti-TNF was stopped, patients may do better on rituximab as the second biologic compared to a second anti-TNF.[68] This appeals to healthcare funders because rituximab is significantly cheaper than anti-TNF if administered less frequently than 6 monthly.[69] Patients who are seropositive for RF and/or ACPA respond better to rituximab, though a health economic model from NICE still suggested it was more cost-effective to use rituximab in seronegative disease than a second anti-TNF.[69,70] For other biologics, rheumatologists are spoilt for choice. There are now five anti-TNFs (etanercept, infliximab,

adalimumab, golimimumab, certolizumab), a B cell depleter (rituximab), an IL-6 inhibitor (tocilizumab), a T-cell costimulatory molecule inhibitor (abatacept), and an IL-1 inhibitor (anakinra—though this is of lesser efficacy than other biologics, and consequently restricted access in some health economies). There are extremely limited head-to-head comparisons between these drugs, but indirect comparisons suggest similar efficacy in biologic-naive patients, and in patients failing on a first anti-TNF.[1,71] There are some differences in toxicity profiles that might lead a clinician to choose one drug over another,[72] but there is a need for further research to elucidate biomarkers that might guide clinicians on the best biologic for each patient, perhaps based on cytokine profiles, or cellular infiltrates in synovial biopsies,[73] or pharmacogenetics.[74] Currently the choice of biologics is governed by national guidelines and intuitive guess work.

Established disease: annual review

The NICE and British Society for Rheumatology (BSR) guidelines recommend that all patients with established disease have at least an annual review with the MDT in order to check for progression of articular disease, manifestations of extra-articular disease, emergence of comorbidities (particularly the increased risk of cardiovascular morbidity[75]), and the need for referrals to members of the MDT, such as physiotherapy, occupational therapy, podiatry, and orthopaedic surgery.[7,11] An overview of what this might include is in Table 112.1. Annual review also gives an opportunity to review medication to ensure ongoing efficacy with preferably remission, or at least a level of disease control that the patient finds satisfactory with minimal interference with their lives. For patients in remission, it should be considered whether they could be as well controlled with less DMARDs, either by stopping drugs if they are on combination therapy, or decreasing doses. The first priority should be to decrease steroids, or at least reduce the dose, in the minority of patients who have to stay on them long term. Any reduction should be performed cautiously and slowly. There may be opportunities to decrease biological agents also, tapering them down whenever possible, but with close monitoring to ensure ongoing excellent control, and restoring previous drug regimens if synovitis is returning.[1]

Complications of articular disease in which inflammation has been inadequately controlled include deformity of joints, pain due to mechanical damage, rupture of tendons (particularly finger extensors), and compression of nerves through synovial hypertrophy and deformity (e.g. carpal tunnel syndrome). Where pain and nerve compression cannot be controlled by conservative approaches, orthopaedic surgeons should be involved quickly to optimize surgical management plans. Where joint function is compromised by deformity or tendon rupture, the opinions of orthopaedic surgeons, physiotherapists, and occupational therapists, should be sought promptly.[7]

Conclusion

Influential guidelines on RA management agree on most key recommendations. Early diagnosis of persistent synovitis, and identification of poor prognostic markers, is essential. Rapid intervention is vital with drugs that suppress inflammation, slow down damaging disease components, and prevent disability.

Table 112.1 The components of an annual review

Assessment	Methods of assessment and references
Disease activity and drug assessment for efficacy and toxicity ♦ If in remission or low levels of disease activity, consider cautious reduction of DMARDs or biologics (including steroids if appropriate) ♦ If ongoing active disease, adjust or change DMARDs or biologics	DAS28 or similar validated measure of disease activity (see Figure 112.2[34])
Functional ability and damage to joints and soft tissues. Consider involving the MDT and Orthopaedics where appropriate. Cervical spine disease needs assessment[76]	Examination, radiographs, ultrasound, HAQ-DI[77]
Comorbidities such as hypertension, ischaemic heart disease, osteoporosis, depression	EULAR cardiovascular risk management guidelines[75] Osteoporosis guidelines (e.g.[78,79]) Depression screening (e.g. Beck Depression Inventory)[80]
Check for extra-articular complications,[81] particularly: ♦ Anaemia of chronic disease, Felty's syndrome, drug-induced abnormalities, non-Hodgkin's lymphoma ♦ Pulmonary involvement; pleural disease, interstitial disease, cricoarytenoid joint involvement ♦ Cardiac involvement; pericarditis, myocardial disease ♦ Ocular involvement; keratoconjunctivitis sicca (Sjögren's syndrome), episcleritis, scleritis, ulcerative keratitis ('corneal melt') ♦ Neurological involvement; entrapment neuropathies, cervical myelopathy, peripheral neuropathy ♦ Hepatic and renal abnormalities, amyloidosis ♦ Vasculitis (e.g. skin and nailfold infarcts, ulcers, sensory neuropathy)	Full medical history and examination with urinalysis, blood screen, and other investigations as appropriate
Assess the effect the disease is having on the quality of the person's life, and their understanding of the disease and management	For example, quality of life measures (generic such as EQ-5D,[82] or disease-specific such as RAQoL[83]), ability to work, enjoy hobbies, participate fully in social roles, ability to manage their own condition, need for educational updates

DAS, Disease Activity Score; DMARD, disease-modifying anti-rheumatic drug; EQ-5D, EuroQol; HAQ-DI, Health Assessment Questionnaire Disability Index; MDT, multidisciplinary team.

The label of RA covers a broad spectrum of disease severity, and there is controversy on

♦ whether the same interventions are needed for all patients
♦ whether monotherapy or combination treatment is appropriate
♦ the role of steroids in RA
♦ the appropriate introduction of biological therapies.

Treating to specified targets is optimal evidence-based practice, where patients are reviewed regularly for disease activity assessments, and inadequate control rectified. Aiming for remission is the ultimate goal, though for some patients minimal disease activity may be appropriate. Patient education addressing self-management is important, and the MDT needs to be involved from the start to minimize the impact on quality of life of the patient.

For established disease, rapid access is important for flares, and to consider whether disease management could be improved. An intermittent overview of established disease is important with access to the MDT, and assessments for comorbidities and complications of the disease itself. An informed patient needs to be central to all decision making.

References

1. Smolen JS, Landewé R, Breedveld FC et al. EULAR recommendations for the management of rheumatoid arthritis with synthetic and biological disease-modifying anti-rheumatic drugs. *Ann Rheum Dis* 2010;69(6):964–975;
2. Smolen JS, Aletaha D, Bijlsma JWJ et al. Treating rheumatoid arthritis to target: recommendations of an international task force. *Ann Rheum Dis* 2010;69(4):631–637;
3. Felson DT, Smolen JS, Wells G et al. American College of Rheumatology/European League Against Rheumatism provisional definition of remission in rheumatoid arthritis for clinical trials. *Ann Rheum Dis* 2011;70(3):404–413.
4. van Nies JA, de Zong Z, van-der Helm-van Mil AH et al. Improved treatment strategies reduce the increased mortality risk in early RA patients. *Rheumatology* 2010;49(11):2210–2216.
5. Ziegler S, Huscher D, Karberg K et al. Trend in treatment and outcomes of rheumatoid arthritis in Germany 1997-2007: results from the National Database of the German Collaborative Arthritis Centres. *Ann Rheum Dis* 2010;69(10):1803–1808.
6. Louie GH, Ward MM. Changes in the rates of joint surgery among patients with rheumatoid arthritis in California, 1983-2007. *Ann Rheum Dis* 2010;69(5):868–871.
7. National Institute of Health and Clinical Excellence. *Clinical Guideline 79. Rheumatoid Arthritis. National Guideline for management and treatment in adults.* National Collaborating Centre for Chronic Conditions, Royal College of Physicians, London, 2009. Available at: http://guidance.nice.org.uk/CG79/Guidance/pdf/English (accessed 28 October 2011);
8. Saag KG, Teng GG, Nivedita MP et al. American College of Rheumatology 2008 Recommendations for the Use of Nonbiologic and Biologic Disease-Modifying Antirheumatic Drugs in Rheumatoid Arthritis. *Arthritis Rheum*, 2008;59(6):762–784;

9. Scottish Intercollegiate Guidelines Network. *Management of early rheumatoid arthritis: A national clinical guideline.* Available at: www.sign.ac.uk/guidelines/fulltext/123/index.html (accessed 28 October 2011).

10. Luqmani R Hennell S Estrach C et al. British Society for Rheumatology and British Health Professionals in Rheumatology Guideline for the Management of Rheumatoid Arthritis (the first 2 years). *Rheumatology* 2006;45(9):1167–1169.

11. Luqmani R, Hennell S, Estrach C et al. British Society for Rheumatology and British Health Professionals in Rheumatology Guideline for the Management of Rheumatoid Arthritis (after the first two years). *Rheumatology (Oxford)* 2009;48(4):436–439.

12. Raza K, Stack R, Kumar K et al. Delays in assessment of patients with rheumatoid arthritis: variations across Europe. *Ann Rheum Dis* 2011;70(10):1822–1825.

13. National Audit Office. *Services for people with rheumatoid arthritis.* The Stationery Office, London, 2009. Available at: www.nao.org.uk/publications/0809/services_for_people_with_rheum.aspx (accessed 28 October 2011).

14. Schoels M, Wong J, Scott DL et al. Economic aspects of treatment options in rheumatoid arthritis: a systematic literature review informing the EULAR recommendations for the management of rheumatoid arthritis. *Ann Rheum Dis* 2010;69(6):995–1003.

15. The King's Fund and the Rheumatology Futures Group. *Perceptions of patients and professionals on rheumatoid arthritis care.* Kings Fund, London, 2009. Available at www.rheumatology.org.uk/../rheumatology_futures_group_project.pdf (accessed 28 October 2011).

16. Deighton C, Hyrich K, Ding T et al. BSR and BHPR rheumatoid arthritis guidelines on eligibility criteria for the first biological therapy. *Rheumatology (Oxford)* 2010;49(6):197–199.

17. Hyrich KL. Patients with suspected rheumatoid arthritis should be referred early to rheumatology. *BMJ* 2008;336(7637):215–216.

18. Aletaha D, Smolen J, Ward MM. Measuring function in rheumatoid arthritis: identifying reversible and irreversible components. *Arthritis Rheum* 2006;54(9):2784–2792.

19. Rantalaiho V, Korpela M, Hannonen P et al. The good initial response to therapy with a combination of traditional disease-modifying antirheumatic drugs is sustained over time: the eleven-year results of the Finnish rheumatoid arthritis combination therapy trial. *Arthritis Rheum* 2007;60(5):1222–1231.

20. Scire CA, Verstappen SMM, Mirjafari H et al. Reduction of long-term disability in inflammatory polyarthritis by early and persistent suppression of joint inflammation: Results from the Norfolk Arthritis Register. *Arthritis Care Res* 2011;63(7):945–952.

21. Kiely P, Williams R, Walsh D, Young A; Early Rheumatoid Arthritis Network. Contemporary patterns of care and disease activity outcome in early rheumatoid arthritis. *Rheumatology (Oxford)* 2009;48(1):57–60.

22. van Dongen H, van Aken J, Lard LR et al. Efficacy of methotrexate treatment in patients with probable rheumatoid arthritis: a double-blind, randomised, placebo-controlled trial. *Arthritis Rheum* 2007;56(5):1424–1432.

23. Verstappen SMM, McCoy MJ, Roberts C et al. Beneficial effects of 3-week course of intramuscular glucocorticoid injections in patients with very early inflammatory polyarthritis.: results of the STIVEA trial. *Ann Rheum Dis* 2010;69(3):503–509.

24. Machold KP, Landewé R, Smolen JS et al. The Stop Arthritis Very Early (SAVE) trial, an international multicentre, randmised, double-blind, placebo-controlled trial on glucocorticoids in very early arthritis. *Ann Rheum Dis* 2010;69(3):495–502.

25. Bos WH, Dijkmans BA, Boers M, van der Stadt RJ, van Schaardenburg D. Effect of dexamethasone on autoantibody levels and arthritis development in pateitns with arthralgia: a randomised trial. *Ann Rheum Dis* 2010;69(3):571–574.

26. Emery P, Durez P, Dougados M et al. Impact of T-cell costimualtion modulation in patients with undifferentiated inflammatory arthritis or very early rheumatoid arthritis: a clinical and imaging study of abatacept (the ADJUST trial). *Ann Rheum Dis* 2010;69(3):510–516.

27. Saleem B, Mackie S, Quinn M et al. Does the use of tumour necrosis factor antagonist therapy in poor prognosis, undifferentiated arthritis prevent progression to rheumatoid arthritis? *Ann Rheum Dis* 2008;67(8):1178–1180.

28. Machado P, Castrejon I, Katchamart W et al. Multinational evidence-based recommendations on how to investigate and follow-up undifferentiated peripheral inflammatory arthritis: integrating systematic literature research and expert opinion of a broad international panel of rheumatologists in the 3E Initiative. *Ann Rheum Dis* 2011;70(1):15–24.

29. Whiting PF, Smidt N, Sterne JAC et al. Systematic review: accuracy of anti–citrullinated peptide antibodies for diagnosing rheumatoid arthritis. *Ann Intern Med* 2010;152(7):456–464.

30. Farragher TM, Lunt M, Plant D et al. Benefit of early treatment in inflammatory polyarthritis patients with anti-cyclic citrullinated peptide antibodies versus those without antibodies. *Arthritis Care Res* 2010;62(5):664–675.

31. van-der Helm-van Mil AH, le Cassie S, van Dongen H et al. A prediction rule for disease outcome in patients with recent-onset undifferentiated arthritis: how to guide individual treatment decisions. *Arthritis Rheum* 2007;52(1):36–41.

32. Felson DT, Smolen JS, Wells G et al. American College of Rheumatology/European League Against Rheumatism Provisional Definition of remission in rheumatoid arthritis clinical trials. *Ann Rheum Dis* 2011;70(3):404–413.

33. Saunders SA, Capell HA Stirling A et al. Triple therapy in early active rheumatoid arthritis: A randomized, single-blind, controlled trial comparing step-up and parallel treatment strategies. *Arthritis Rheum* 2008;58(5):1310–1317.

34. Aletaha D, Smolen JS. The definition and measurement of disease modification in inflammatory rheumatic diseases. *Rheum Dis Clin North Am* 2006;32(vii):9–44.

35. Möttönen T, Hannonen P, Korpela M et al. Delay to institution of therapy and induction of remission using single-drug or combination disease modifying anti-rheumatic drug therapy in early rheumatoid arthritis. *Arthritis Rheum* 2002;46(4):894–898.

36. van der Kooij SM, de Vries-Boerstra JK, Goekoop-Ruiterman, YPM et al. Limited efficacy of conventional DMARDs after initial methotrexate failure in patients with recent onset rheumatoid arthritis treated according to the disease activity score. *Ann Rheum Dis* 2007;66(10):1356–1362.

37. Hider SL, Silman A, Bunn D et al. Comparing the long-term clinical outcome of treatment with methotrexate or sulfasalzine prescribed as the first disease-modifying drug in patients with inflammatory polyarthritis. *Ann Rheum Dis* 2006;65(11):1449–1455.

38. Salliott C, van der Heijde D. Long-term safety of methotrexate monotherapy in patients with rheumatoid arthritis: a systematic literature research. *Ann Rheum Dis* 2009;68(7):1100–1104.

39. Braun J, Kästner P, Flaxenberg P et al. Comparison of the clinical efficacy and safety of subcutaneous versus oral administration of methotrexate in patients with active rheumatoid arthritis: results of a six-month, multicenter, randomized, double-blind, controlled, phase IV trial. *Arthritis Rheum* 2008;58(1):73–81.

40. Choy EH, Smith C, Dore CJ et al. A meta-analysis of the efficacy and toxicity of combining disease modifying drugs in rheumatoid arthritis based on patient withdrawal. *Rheumatology (Oxford)* 2005;44(11):1414–1421.

41. Nixon R, Bansback N, Brennan A. The efficacy of inhibiting tumour necrosis factor alpha and interleukin 1 in patients with rheumatoid arthritis: a meta-analysis and adjusted indirect comparisons. *Rheumatology* (Oxford) 2007;46(7):1140–1147.

42. Tosh JC, Wailoo AJ, Scott DL, Deighton CM. Cost-effectiveness of combination on biologic disease-modifying antirheumatic drug

strategies in patients with early rheumatoid arthritis. *J Rheumatol* 2011;38(8):1593–1600.

43. van der Kooij SM, Goekoop-Ruiterman YP, de Vries-Bouwstra JK et al. Drug-free remission, functioning and radiographic damage after 4 years of response-driven treatment in patients with recent-onset rheumatoid arthritis. *Ann Rheum Dis* 2009;68(6):914–921.

44. Rantalaiho V, Korpela M, Laasonen L et al. Early combination disease-modifying antirheumatic drug therapy and tight disease control improve long-term radiologic outcome in patients with early rheumatoid arthritis: the 11-year results of the Finnish Rheumatoid Arthritis Combination Therapy trial. *Arthritis Res Ther* 2010;12(3), R122.

45. van Tuyl LH, Boers M, Lems WF et al. Survival, comorbidities and joint damage 11 years after the COBRA combination therapy trial in early rheumatoid arthritis. *Ann Rheum Dis* 2010;69(5):807–812.

46. Klarenbeek NB, Güler-Yüksel M, van der Kooij SM et al. The impact of four dynamic, goal-steered treatment strategies on the 5-year outcomes of rheumatoid arthritis patients in the BeSt study. *Ann Rheum Dis* 2011;70(6):1039–1046.

47. Spies CM, Bijlsma JW, Burmester GR, Buttgereit F. Pharmacology of glucocorticoids in rheumatoid arthritis. *Curr Opin Pharmacol* 2010;10(3):302–307.

48. Kirwan JR, Bijlsma JWJ, Boers M, Shea B. Effects of glucocorticoids on radiological progression in rheumatoid arthritis. *Cochrane Database Syst Rev* 2007;1:CD006356.

49. Hoes JN, Jacobs JW, Boers M et al. EULAR evidence-based recommendations on the management of systemic glucocorticoid therapy in rheumatic diseases. *Ann Rheum Dis* 2007;68(12):1560–1567.

50. Brown AK, Quinn MA, Karim Z et al. Presence of significant synovitis in rheumatoid arthritis patients with disease-modifying antirheumatic drug-induced clinical remission. *Arthritis Rheum* 2006;54(12):3761–3773.

51. Combe B, Landewe R, Lukas C et al. EULAR recommendations for the management of early arthritis: report of a task force of the European Standing Committee for International Clinical Studies Including Therapeutics (ESCISIT). *Ann Rheum Dis* 2007;66(1):34–45.

52. O'Mahony R, Richards A, Deighton C, Scott D. Withdrawal of disease-modifying antirheumatic drugs in patients with rheumatoid arthritis: a systematic review and meta-analysis. *Ann Rheum Dis* 2010;69(10):1823–1826.

53. van der Velde G, Pham B, Machado M *et al.* Cost-effectiveness of biologic response modifiers compared to disease-modifying antirheumatic drugs for rheumatoid arthritis: a systematic review. *Arthritis Care Res* (Hoboken) 2011;63(1):65–78.

54. Ma MH, Kingsley GH, Scott DL. A systematic comparison of combination DMARD therapy and tumour necrosis inhibitor therapy with methotrexate in patients with early rheumatoid arthritis. *Rheumatology* (Oxford) 2010;49(1):91–98.

55. Galloway JB, Hyrich KL, Mercer LK et al. Anti-TNF therapy is associated with an increased risk of serious infections in patients with rheumatoid arthritis especially in the first 6 months of treatment: updated results from the British Society for Rheumatology Biologics Register with special emphasis on risks in the elderly. *Rheumatology* (Oxford) 2011;50(1):124–131.

56. Gómez-Reino JJ, Carmona L, Angel Descalzo M; Biobadaser Group. Risk of tuberculosis in patients treated with tumor necrosis factor antagonists due to incomplete prevention of reactivation of latent infection. *Arthritis Rheum* 2007;57(5):756–761.

57. Clifford DB, Ances B, Costello C et al. Rituximab-associated progressive multifocal leukoencephalopathy in rheumatoid arthritis. *Arch Neurol* 2011;68(9):1156–1164.

58. Askling J, Fahrbach K, Nordstrom B et al. Cancer risk with tumor necrosis factor alpha (TNF) inhibitors: meta-analysis of randomized controlled trials of adalimumab, etanercept, and infliximab using patient level data. *Pharmacoepidemiol Drug Saf* 2011;20(2):119–130.

59. Mariette X, Matucci-Cerenic M, Pavelka K et al. Malignancies associated with tumour necrosis factor inhibitors in registries and prospective observational studies: a systematic review and meta-analysis. *Ann Rheum Dis* 2011;70(11):1895–1904.

60. Emery P. Rheumatoid arthritis: International disparities in access to anti-TNF therapy. *Nat Rev Rheumatol* 2011;7(4),197–198.

61. Bejarano V, Conaghan PG, Quinn MA, Saleem B, Emery P. Benefits 8 years after a remission induction regime with an infliximab and methotrexate combination in early rheumatoid arthritis. *Rheumatology* (Oxford) 2010;49(10):1971–1974.

62. van Vollenhoven RF, Ernestam S, Geborek P et al. Addition of infliximab compared with addition of sulfasalazine and hydroxychloroquine to methotrexate in patients with early rheumatoid arthritis (Swefot trial: 1-year results of a randomised trial. *Lancet* 2009;374(9688):459–466.

63. Conaghan PG, Hensor EM, Keenan AM, Morgan AW, Emery P; YEAR Consortium. Persistently moderate DAS-28 is not benign: loss of function occurs in early RA despite step-up DMARD therapy. *Rheumatology* (Oxford) 2010;49(10):1894–1899.

64. Hyrich KL, Deighton C, Watson K, Symmons DPM, Lunt M. Benefit of anti-TNF therapy in rheumatoid arthritis patients with moderate disease activity. *Rheumatology* 2009;48(10):1323–1327.

65. Keystone E, Freundlich B, Schiff M, Li J, Hooper M. Patients with moderate rheumatoid arthritis (RA) achieve better disease activity states with etanercept treatment than patients with severe RA. *J Rheumatol* 2009;36(3):522–531.

66. Deighton C. Therapy: what should we do after the failure of a first anti-TNF? *Nat Rev Rheumatol* 2009;5(11):596–597.

67. Hyrich KL, Lunt M, Watson KD, Symmons DP, Silman AJ; British Society for Rheumatology Biologics Register. Outcomes after switching from one anti-tumor necrosis factor alpha agent to a second anti-tumor necrosis factor alpha agent in patients with rheumatoid arthritis: results from a large UK national cohort study. *Arthritis Rheum* 2007;56(1):13–20.

68. Finckh A, Ciurea A, Brulhart L et al. B cell depletion may be more effective than switching to an alternative anti-tumor necrosis factor agent in rheumatoid arthritis patients with inadequate response to anti-tumor necrosis factor agents. *Arthritis Rheum* 2007;56(5):1417–1423.

69. National Institute for Health and Clinical Excellence. *Technology appraisal 195 (2010). Rheumatoid arthritis—drugs for treatment after failure of a TNF inhibitor*. Available at: http://guidance.nice.org.uk/TA195 (accessed 31 October 2011)

70. Chatzidionysiou K, Lie E, Nasonov E *et al* , Highest clinical effectiveness of rituximab in autoantibody-positive patients with rheumatoid arthritis and in those for whom no more than one previous TNF antagonist has failed: pooled data from 10 European registries. *Ann Rheum Dis* 2011;70(9):1575–1580.

71. van Vollenhoven RF. Unresolved issues in biologic therapy for rheumatoid arthritis. *Nat Rev Rheumatol* 20117(4):205–215;

72. Kiely PDW, Deighton C, Dixey J, Östör AJK. Biologic agents for rheumatoid arthritis—negotiating the NICE technology appraisals. *Rheumatology* (Oxford) 2012;51(1):24–31.

73. de Hair MJ Harty LC, Gerlag DM et al. Synovial tissue analysis for the discovery of diagnostic and prognostic biomarkers in patients with early arthritis. *J Rheumatol* 2011;38(9):2068–2072.

74. Davila L, Ranganathan P. Pharmacogenetics: implications for therapy in rheumatic diseases. *Nat Rev Rheumatol* 2011;7(9):537–550.

75. Peters MJL, Symmons DPM, McCarey D et al. EULAR evidence-based recommendations for cardiovascular risk management in patients with rheumatoid arthritis and other forms of inflammatory arthritis. *Ann Rheum Dis* 2010;69(2):325–331.

76. Neva MH, Häkkinen A, Mäkinen H et al. High prevalence of asymptomatic cervical spine subluxation in patients with rheumatoid arthritis waiting for orthopaedic surgery. *Ann Rheum Dis* 2006;65(7):884–888.

77. Aramis: HAQ. http://aramis.stanford.edu/HAQ.html (accessed 28 October 2011)

78. National Osteoporosis Guideline Development Group (2009). Available at www.shef.ac.uk/NOGG/index.html (accessed 28 October 2011)

79. Broy SB, Tanner SB; FRAX(*) Position Development Conference Members. Official Positions for FRAX® clinical regarding rheumatoid arthritis from Joint Official Positions Development Conference of the International Society for Clinical Densitometry and International Osteoporosis Foundation on FRAX®. *Clin Densitom* 2011;14(3):184–189.

80. Pincus T, Hassett AL, Callahan LF. Criterion contamination of depression scales in patients with rheumatoid arthritis: the need for interpretation of patient questionnaires (as all clinical measures) in the context of all information about the patient. *Rheum Dis Clin North Am* 2009;35(4):861–864, xi–xii.

81. Young A, Koduri G. Extra-articular manifestations and complications of rheumatoid arthritis. *Best Pract Res Clin Rheumatol* 2007;21(5):907–927.

82. EuroQol. A standardised instrument for use as a measure of health outcome. Available at: www.euroqol.org/eq-5d/what-is-eq-5d.html (accessed 28 October 2011).

83. de Jong Z, van der Heijde D, McKenna SP, Whalley D. The reliability and construct validity of the RAQoL: a rheumatoid arthritis-specific quality of life instrument. *Br J Rheumatol* 1997;36(8):878–883.

Spondyloarthropathies

SECTION 11

Spondyloarthropathies

CHAPTER 113

Ankylosing spondylitis

Joachim Sieper

Introduction and definition

The hallmarks of ankylosing spondylitis (AS) are inflammation of the sacroiliac joints (SIJ) and spine associated with clinical symptoms such as pain and stiffness in the back, followed in a significant proportion of patients by new bone formation.[1] The name dates from around 1900 when a diagnosis could only be made clinically when a patient had already advanced ankylosis of the spine. With the increased use of radiography it became clear in the 1930s that the disease normally starts in the SIJ and that the SIJs are involved in at least 95% of patients.[2] On this basis radiographic sacroiliitis has become an important part for diagnosis and is an essential criterion in the 1984 modified New York classification criteria for AS (Figure 113.1).[3] But already by this time the term 'ankylosing spondylitis' was no longer really adequate because patients fulfilled these criteria just based on radiographic sacroiliitis, with or without ankylosis of the spine.

However, radiographs detect only structural damage as a consequence of inflammation and not inflammation itself. As a consequence the European Spondylarthropathy Study Group (ESSG) criteria[4] and the Amor criteria[5] for spondyloarthropathies already covered around 1990 patients with back symptoms but normal radiographs. The increasing use of MRI from the 1990s on made it quite clear that chronic changes visible on radiographs (structural damage) is preceded by inflammation,[6] often by several years. Finally, in 2009 the Assessment in Spondylo-Arthritis international Society (ASAS) published new classification criteria for axial SpA which cover both patients with and without radiographic sacroiliitis and for which active sacroiliitis as shown on MRI is an important finding (Figure 113.2).[7] Therefore, instead of AS the term axial spondyloarthritis (SpA) should rather be used in future, with AS being just one part of a continuous spectrum.[7,8]

The term SpA compromises traditionally different diseases such as AS, psoriatic arthritis, reactive arthritis, arthritis/spondylitis associated with inflammatory bowel disease (IBD), and undifferentiated SpA. These diseases have in common that patients present with a similar clinical picture, either predominantly axial or predominantly peripheral or as an overlap between these two patterns, and with a varying association with HLA B27.[9] Recently, ASAS developed and published, in addition to the already mentioned criteria for axial SpA, new classification criteria for predominantly peripheral SpA.[10] For such an approach the pattern of clinical presentation—either predominantly axial or peripheral—is more relevant and the absence or presence of predisposing or associated diseases such as IBD, psoriasis, or a preceding infection is just recorded. In the current chapter only axial SpA is discussed, and peripheral manifestations only if associated with axial disease.

Epidemiology

Axial SpA is a disease which starts normally in the third decade of life, rarely (<5%) at an age older than 45 years, but in 10–20% of patients even between the ages of 10 and 20 years.[11] Thus, mostly young people are affected early in the course of the disease. Interestingly, HLA B27-positive patients have the first symptoms about 10 years earlier in comparison to HLA B27-negative patients.[12]

The male/female ratio is estimated to be 2:1, in early cases without radiographic visible chronic changes approaching even 1:1, indicating that women—for unclear reasons—seem to develop chronic changes later and less often.[1]

The prevalence of axial SpA correlates directly with the prevalence of HLA B27[13,14] in a given population and has been estimated to be between 0.1% and 1.4% in different parts of the world.[9] Recent investigations from France,[15] the United States,[16] and Lithuania[17] showed that the overall prevalence of SpA (including axial and peripheral SpA) is similar to that for rheumatoid arthritis (RA).

No clear data are yet available about the relative prevalence of patients with non-radiographic (nr) axial SpA in comparison to those with radiographic axial SpA (fulfilling the modified New York criteria for AS) among the axial SpA group. Several projects have recently screened for axial SpA patients in primary care. If these patients were then referred to the rheumatologist the proportion of axial nr SpA was reported to be 25–60%, confirming that this a relevant subgroup.[18–20] The progression from non-radiographic to radiographic sacroiliitis has recently been estimated to be around 12% over a follow-up period of 2 years.[21] There is still a gap of 5–10 years between the onset of symptoms and a diagnosis of AS in these patients,[11] probably because diagnosis relied in the past mostly on the presence of structural damage as seen on radiographs.

1. Clinical criteria:

a. Low back pain and stiffness for more than 3 months which improves with exercise, but is not relieved by rest.

b. Limitation of motion of the lumbar spine in both the sagittal and frontal planes.

c. Limitation of chest expansion relative to normal values correlated for age and sex.

2. Radiological criterion:

Sacroiliitis grade ≥ 2 bilaterally or grade 3-4 unilaterally

Definite ankylosing spondylitis if the radiological criterion is associated with at least 1 clinical criterion.

Fig. 113.1 Modified New York criteria for ankylosing spondylitis.
Reproduced with permission of John Wiley & Sons, Inc.

In patients with ≥ 3 months back pain and age at onset <45 years

Sacroiliitis on imaging* plus ≥ 1 SpA feature#	OR	HLA-B27 plus ≥ 2 other SpA features#

#SpA features
- inflammatory back pain
- arthritis
- enthesitis (heel)
- uveitis
- dactylitis
- psoriasis
- Crohn's/colitis
- good response to NSAIDs
- family history for SpA
- HLA-B27
- elevated CRP

*Sacroiliitis on imaging
- active (acute) inflammation on MRI highly suggestive of sacroiliitis associated with SpA
- definite radiographic sacroiliitis according to mod NY criteria

n=649 patients with back pain;
Sensitivity: 82.9%, Specificity: 84.4%
Imaging alone: Sensitivity: 66.2%, Specificity: 97.3%

Fig. 113.2 ASAS classification criteria for axial spondyloarthritis.
Reproduced with permission from British Medical Journal and with permission from ASAS.

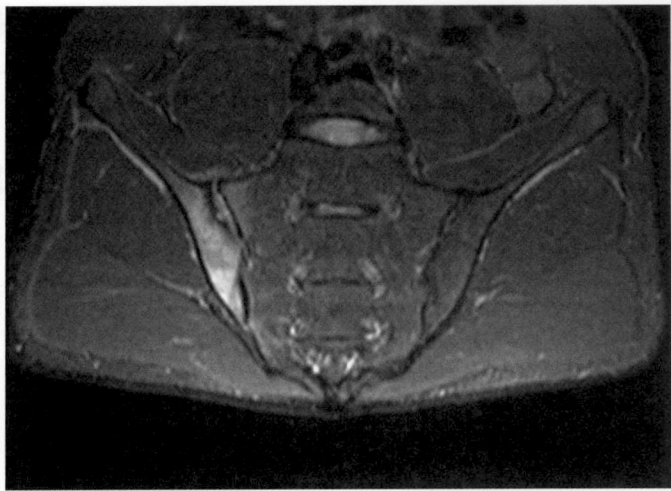

Fig. 113.3 MRI of sacroiliac joints (SIJ): active sacroiliitis (hyperintense signal) shown on a short tau inversion recovery (STIR) MRI sequence in the ileum and in the upper part of the sacrum of the right SIJ.

Classification criteria and diagnosis

For classification and partly also for diagnosis of AS, the 1984 modified New York criteria for AS have been used in the past.[3] The presence of radiographic sacroiliitis (at least either grade 2 bilaterally or grade 3 unilaterally) is essential for the fulfilment of these criteria, plus one clinical criterion: either morning stiffness with improvement by exercise but not by rest or restriction of spinal mobility (Figure 113.1). However, both radiographic sacroiliitis and restriction of spinal mobility occur relatively late in the course of the disease and therefore these criteria are not suitable for classification/diagnosis of early cases. These are included in the recently developed ASAS criteria for axial SpA which cover patients with and without radiographic changes in the SIJ (Figure 113.2).[7] These criteria should be applied in the presence of chronic back pain (> 3 months) starting at an age younger than 45 years. Sacroiliitis on imaging remains important, not only if visible on radiographs but also when subchondral bone marrow oedema as evidence of active bony inflammation can be seen on MRI (Figure 113.3).[22]

Although the imaging arm has good specificity (97.3%) the sensitivity is not optimal (only 66.2%). Therefore a clinical arm was added which is fulfilled if a positive HLA B27 is present plus two other SpA-typical features, always in the presence of chronic back

pain starting at an age less than 45 years. With both arms these new criteria reach a specificity of 84.4% and a sensitivity of 82.9%.

There are differences between classification criteria and a diagnosis of a certain disease. Classification criteria always give a clear yes/no answer (fulfilled or not), with the aim of getting a relatively homogenous population for inclusion into a clinical trial, for example. A diagnostic approach has to be more flexible, resulting in certain probabilities that a diagnosis can be made, dependent on the number and nature of the parameters being positive (positive likelihood ratio). Furthermore, for diagnosis negative findings should also be taken into account, which is not the case for classification criteria. Finally, the pretest probability of a disease needs to be known if parameters are used for diagnosis, while the pretest probability does not matter for classification criteria because the diagnosis should already have been made before inclusion into a trial.[8] Two overlapping possible diagnostic approaches have been proposed. For the first one, presence or absence of all for axial SpA-relevant parameters are looked for and weighted according to the likelihood ratio (calculated from the sensitivity and specificity of this patameter) and the post-test probability can be estimated based on an assumed pretest probability of 5% for axial SpA among patients presenting with chronic back pain.[8] In Figure 113.4 a more structured diagnostic approach is presented with the evaluation of clinical parameters coming first, together with radiographs of the SIJ, followed by laboratory parameters such as HLA B27 and C-reactive protein (CRP) and, finally, by MRI.[23]

Both for classification and diagnosis MRI has become an important new tool for axial SpA, especially for active inflammatory lesions (subchondral bone marrow oedema). To make this visible one of the following MRI sequences must be used: short tau inversion recovery (STIR), T2-weighted sequence with fat suppression, or T1 sequence with application of a contrast agent (such as gadolinium) with fat suppression. In many centres the STIR sequence is preferred and is normally sufficient. A positive MRI of the SIJ (active inflammation) has been defined as the presence of subchondral bone marrow oedema at at least two sites or

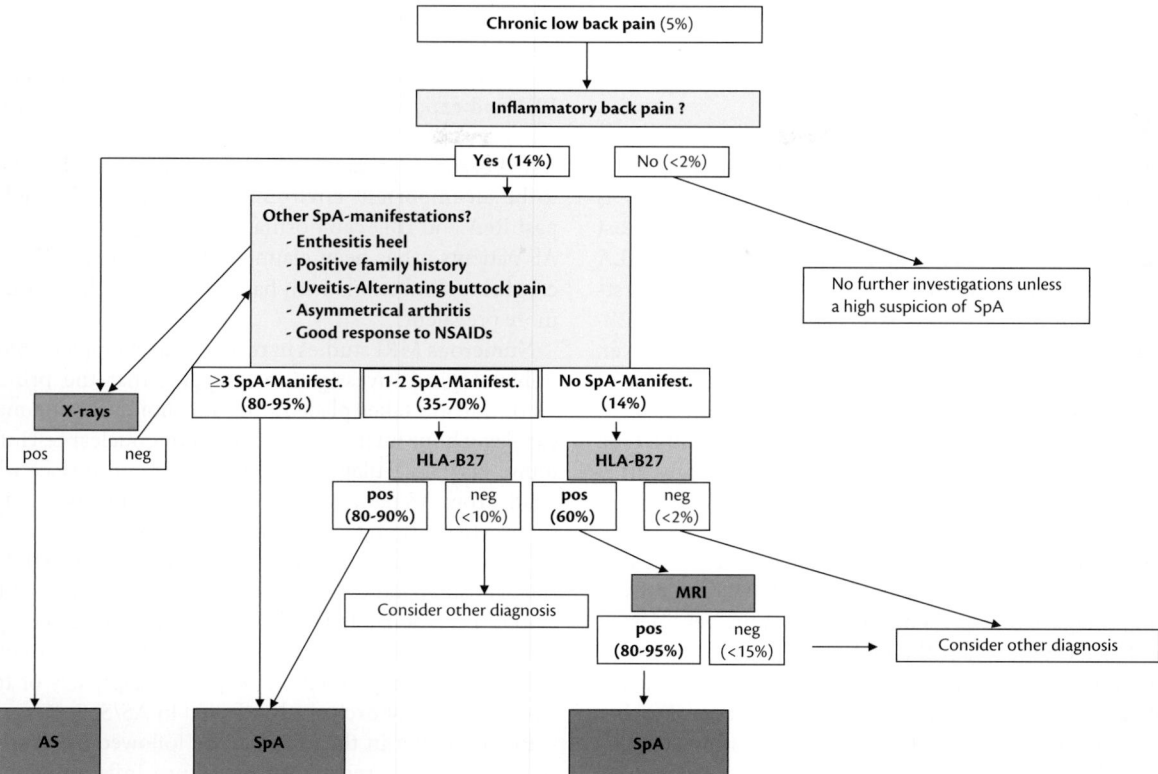

Fig. 113.4 Diagnostic algorithm in axial spondyloarthritis.
With permission from British Medical Journal and with permission from ASAS.

one site visible on at least two subsequent slices.[22] An example of a clearly positive MRI is show in Figure 113.3. Obviously, differential diagnosis of diseases which can also cause subchondral bone marrow oedema, such as mechanical burden, infection, and/or tumour, has to be taken into account and should be excluded. More recently, more attention has also been paid to T1 sequences which can show early chronic changes such as replacement of bone marrow by fatty lesions and/or erosions.[24] However, at the moment the exact value of T1 findings in a diagnostic approach has not yet agreed on.

Normally the spine is affected later in the course of the disease, so classification criteria focus on the SIJ. In the spine, as in the SIJ, the disease starts with inflammation, such as spondylitis anterior, spondylitis posterior, spondylodiscitis or involvement of the facet joints.[25] Figure 113.5 shows a typical example of a patient with advanced disease with multiple syndesmophytes.

An **elevated CRP** (or erythrocyte sedimentation ratio, ESR) is found in only about 60% of AS patients who are clinically active, although CRP-positive patients seem to have a worse prognosis regarding radiographic progression on the one hand,[21] but respond better to TNF blocker treatment on the other hand[26] (see also below).

Recently **referral parameters** have been proposed and have been tested in primary care in patients presenting with chronic back pain. If symptoms start at an age lower than 45 years and if the patient complains about inflammatory back pain and/or if the patient has been tested positive for HLA B27, a diagnosis of

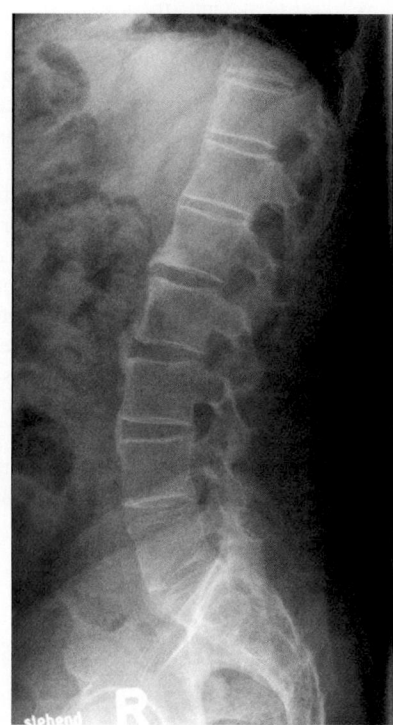

Fig. 113.5 Radiographs of the spine: lateral radiograph view of the lumbar and lower thoracic spine with widespread syndesmophyte formation in a patient with ankylosing spondylitis.

axial SpA was made in 25–60% of these patients after referral to a rheumatologist.[18–20,27]

Aetiopathogenesis

It has been estimated that about 90% of the pathogenesis of AS is genetically determined and that the contribution of HLA B27 is about 50% of the genetic risk, making HLA B27 by far the most important risk factor.[28] The chance of developing AS/SpA in HLA B27-positive individuals is about 5%, in HLA B27-positive first-degree relatives from AS patients it is 12–20%, but in HLA B27-negative relatives from AS patients it is less than 1%.[29] However, despite intensive research, the role of HLA B27 in the pathogenesis of AS/SpA has not yet been clarified.[9,30,31] More than 30 HLA B27 subtypes have been described and HLA B2705, B2702, and B2704 are the ones most often be associated with AS. Interestingly, HLA B2709—present in Sardinia—and HLA B2706—present in Asia—are not associated, although they differ by only one or two amino acids in the peptide-binding groove of the molecule from the disease-associated subtypes HLA B2705 or B2704, respectively. These findings suggest that presentation of certain peptides by HLA B27 to T cells can explain the pathogenesis, although such peptides have not yet been identified. However, HLA B27 subtyping does not have any relevance for daily clinical practice. Further hypotheses are based on the fact that HLA B27 can behave differently from other HLA molecules. The 'HLA B27 misfolding' hypothesis claims that misfolding of the HLA B27 heavy chain in the cytoplasm induces a rather non-specific inflammatory reaction, and the 'B27 homodimer' hypothesis suggests that the B27 heavy chains can form homodimers on the cell surface which can then also present peptides to T cells, but in this case to CD4+ T cells.

ARTS-1 (endoplasmatic reticulum amino peptidase), a peptide relevant for processing peptides in the cytoplasm of cells, and IL-23 receptor (R) genetic polymorphisms have also been associated with AS.[30] The relative contribution of the genes to the susceptibility to AS can be estimated by using the population-attributable risk fraction analysis, which is 90% for HLA B27, 26% for ARTS-1, and 9% for IL-23.[32] Most recently it was found that the ARTS-1 polymorphism is only relevant in HLA B27-positive but not HLA B27-negative patients, indicating that the interaction between peptide processing and peptide presentation might play a relevant role in the pathogenesis of AS.[33] Associations of other genes with AS have also been described,[9] but they are less strong than the ones discussed here.

AS/SpA can be found worldwide and its occurrence is predominantly dependent on the frequency of HLA B27 in a given population. Therefore, the environmental factors contributing to the pathogenesis are probably rather non-specific. Because AS can occur after a preceding reactive arthritis (ReA) or in the context of IBD and exposure to bacteria (bacterial infection of the urogenital or gastroenteral tract in case of ReA, or exposure to gut bacteria because of a damaged mucosa in case of IBD) bacteria seem to be an important environmental factor.[1] Although present or past ReA and IBD can normally only be found in less than 10% of AS patients it has been claimed that sublinical IBD[34] or subclinical chronic infections with bacteria such as chlamydia[35] are much more prevalent.

Numerous MRI studies in recent years,[6] supplemented by immunohistological investigations, suggest that the primary inflammation in AS takes place in the subchondral bone marrow at the cartilage–bone interface.[36] Indeed, mononuclear cell infiltrates were found only if cartilage was left on the bone surface when femoral heads from AS patients were investigated histologically, indicating that cartilage (antigens) might be a primary target of the immune process.[37] However, it is currently not clear how HLA B27, bacterial exposure, and cartilage interact and which part of the immune system is responsible for the link between these components. An additional necessary and possibly initiating factor might be microtrauma of cartilage/bone at weightbearing parts of the skeleton, which are almost exclusively affected in AS/SpA.[38]

Inflammation in the bone can be followed by new bone formation as part of a repair process. Once inflammation has caused damage of the bone, the process of new bone formation can probably no longer be influenced and/or prevented by anti-inflammatory drugs such as TNF blockers.[39] The molecular basis of the interaction between inflammation and new bone formation is currently not clear but is under intensive investigation.[40]

Clinical features

Spinal symptoms—pain and stiffness

The symptoms are dominated by pain and stiffness in the spine, focusing on the lower back, reflecting inflammation in the SIJ and/or lumbar spine. Mostly later in the course of the disease the thoracic and cervical spine can also be affected.[1] Typical is the so called 'inflammatory back pain' (IBP) which is characterized by morning stiffness (normally >30 minutes) which improves with exercise but not with rest, and/or by awakening in the second half of the night because of back pain. This kind of pain starts normally at an age less than 45 years. Several sets of clinical criteria for the characterization of IBP have been developed (Figure 113.6),[41–43] with comparable sensitivity and specificity. However, these do not go beyond about 80% each, clearly indicating that the presence of IBP alone is

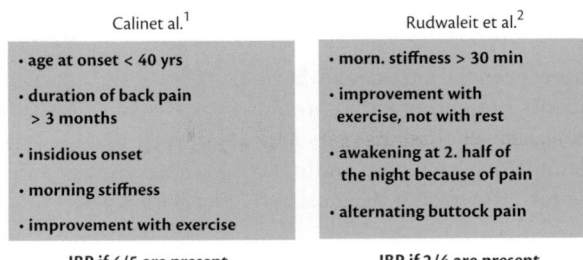

Fig. 113.6 Different sets of criteria for inflammatory back pain.
With permission from ASAS.

not sufficient for the diagnosis of SpA and that absence of IBP does not exclude a diagnosis of axial SpA.

Disease activity is normally measured by using the Bath Ankylosing Spondylitis Activity Index (BASDAI) which is a composite index from 0 (= no symptoms) to 10 (= maximal symptoms) on a numeric scale.[44] The BASDAI is a patient-based questionnaire including questions about fatigue, pain in the spine, pain at peripheral joints and entheses, and morning stiffness (Figure 113.7). Function is measured, again by using a patient-based questionnaire, using the Bath Ankylosing Spondylitis Functional Index (BASFI) on a similar numeric rating scale between 0 and 10.[45] Recently, ASAS has developed and proposed a new Ankylosing Spondylitis Disease Activity Score(ASDAS) which includes the CRP value as well as patients' reported outcome measures (Figure 113.8).[46,47]

Restriction of spinal mobility

Restriction of spinal mobility and function is caused early in the course of the disease by inflammation in the axial skeleton, but later on by new bone formation in the spine.[48] Most typically, syndesmophytes develop from the corner of the vertebral bodies, potentially resulting in an ankylosis of the spine. But ossification of the facet joints, for example, can also contribute to restriction of spinal mobility. However, it must be emphasized that only a small proportion of patients with axial SpA develop an advanced ankylosis. Spinal mobility should be measured using the established Bath Metrology Ankylosing Spondylitis Index (BASMI), which quantifies forward motion of the lumbar spine (modified Schober test), lateral flexion of the lumbar spine, tragus to wall (or occiput to wall) distance, cervical rotation and intermalleolar distance (measuring mobility of the hip joint). A BASMI score between 0 (no restriction) and 10 (maximal restriction) is preferred[49] over a score between 0 and 2 because the former is more sensitive to change. In addition, chest expansion (difference between inspiration and expiration) can be measured in the fourth intercostal level anteriorly.[25]

Long-term outcome is closely related to formation of syndesmophytes in the spine, potentially resulting in ankylosis. The strongest predictor for syndesmophyte progression on follow-up is the presence of syndesmophytes at baseline.[50,51] Interestingly, an elevated CRP has most recently also been be associated with radiographic progression both of the spine[51] and the SIJ.[21]

In more advanced disease osteoporosis of the spine, can occur with the potential consequence of osteoporotic fractures.

1. How would you describe the overall level of fatigue/tiredness you have experienced?

none 0 – 1 – 2 – 3 – 4 – 5 – 6 – 7 – 8 – 9 – 10 very severe

2. How would you describe the overall level of AS neck, back or hip pain you have had?

none 0 – 1 – 2 – 3 – 4 – 5 – 6 – 7 – 8 – 9 – 10 very severe

3. How would you describe the overall level of pain/swelling in joints other than neck, back hips you have had?

none 0 – 1 – 2 – 3 – 4 – 5 – 6 – 7 – 8 – 9 – 10 very severe

4. How would you describe the level of discomfort you have had from an area tender to touch or pressure?

none 0 – 1 – 2 – 3 – 4 – 5 – 6 – 7 – 8 – 9 – 10 very severe

5. How would you describe the level of morning stiffness you have had from the time you wake up?

none 0 – 1 – 2 – 3 – 4 – 5 – 6 – 7 – 8 – 9 – 10 very severe

6. How long does your morning stiffness last from the time you wake up?

0 – 1 – 2 – 3 – 4 – 5 – 6 – 7 – 8 – 9 – 10

0 hour 1 hour 2 or more hours

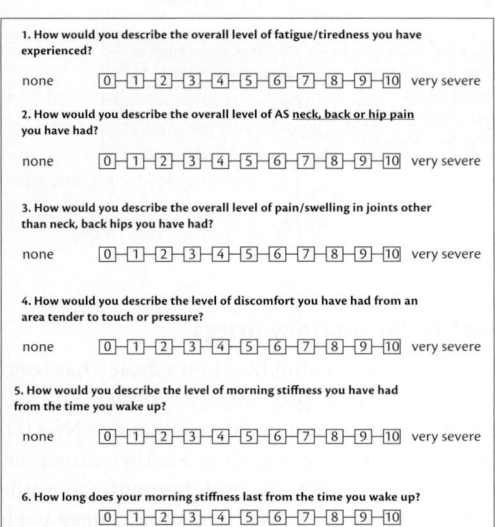

Calculation of BASDAI:

- Compute the mean of questions 5 and 6.
- Calculate the sum of the values of question 1-4 and add the result to the mean of questions 5 and 6.
- Divide the result by 5.

Alternatively, a VAS between 0 and 10 cm or 0 and 100 mm can be used. ASAS prefers to use a NRS.

Fig. 113.7 The Bath Ankylosing Spondylitis Disease Activity Index (BASDAI).
With permission from ASAS.

Calculation of the ASDAS

$ASDAS_{CRP}$

0.12 ×Total Back Pain	+	0.06 × Duration of Morning Stiffness	+	0.11 × Patient Global	+	0.07 × Peripheral pain/Swelling	+	0.58 × Ln(CRP+1)

$ASDAS_{ESR}$

0.08 ×Total Back Pain	+	0.07 × Duration of Morning Stiffness	+	0.11 × Patient Global	+	0.09 × Peripheral pain/Swelling	+	0.29 × √ESR

$ASDAS_{CRP}$ is the preferred ASDAS but the $ASDAS_{ESR}$ can be used in case CRP is not available.

CRP in mg/l; all patient assessments on a 10 cm scale.

Fig. 113.8 Calculation of the Ankylosing Spondylitis Activity Score (ASDAS).
With permission from ASAS.

Extraspinal rheumatic manifestations

Peripheral arthritis—often transient—is reported by about 30% patients with axial SpA. Typically, the arthritis is asymmetrical and affects predominantly the lower limbs. Mono- or oligoarthritis is most frequent, but polyarthritis is possible. Structural bone damage such as erosions or ankylosis is rare in peripheral joints.[1,52]

Enthesitis

Inflammation at the insertion sites of tendons or ligaments at bone is called enthesitis and is a typical manifestation in any SpA, including axial SpA patients. Enthesitis is reported in 30–50% of patients with axial SpA/AS. Similarly to arthritis, it occurs predominantly at the lower limbs, such as the insertion site of the Achilles tendon or the plantar fascia at the calcaneus or in the pelvis, but it can also occur in the upper limbs, such as the elbows or at the insertion of the supraspinatus tendon at the greater tuberosity of the humerus.[10,52] Enthesitis is normally quite painful and can be accompanied by a considerable restriction of function, especially if occurring in a lower limb. Swelling is normally only observed if the adjacent soft tissue, such as the bursae, is also affected. Currently there is no general agreement on which imaging method can or should be used for the investigation of enthesitis. MRI seems to be superior for the detection of subchondral bone marrow oedema, while ultrasound seems to be better for the investigation of soft tissue inflammation.

Extra-articular manifestations

Current or history of uveitis anterior can be found in 30–40% of AS patients. Flares of uveitis are reported in 15–20% of AS patients per year. Uveitis is typically anterior, sudden in onset (painful red eye), acute, self-limiting, and unilateral but alternating from one eye to the other.[53]

A concomitant diagnosis of psoriasis is found in about 10% and of IBD in about 5% of AS patients. Psoriasis and IBD most often, but not always, precedes the diagnosis of AS.

Other organs can be involved such as kidney, lung, or heart, but these are rare manifestations.[1] Whether these manifestations are related to the level of clinical disease activity and inflammation is not known, but seems to be likely. Amyloidosis can occur in patients who are highly active over a long time.

Management

Recently, an updated version of the ASAS/EULAR recommendations for the management of AS[54] (Figure 113.9) and of the more specific ASAS recommendation for the treatment of axial SpA with TNF blockers[55] have been published (Figure 113.10).

Physiotherapy

This is still an important part of the treatment strategy. It helps to improve spinal mobility and to reduce pain and stiffness in the spine. Patients should be educated by a physiotherapist about an exercise programme and should carry this out daily, long term. Exercises concentrate on extension and rotation of the spine to prevent fixed flexion of the spine.

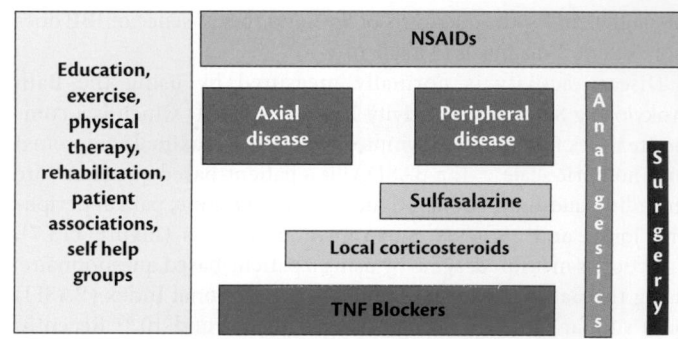

Fig. 113.9 ASAS/EULAR recommendations for the management of ankylosing spondylitis.
With permission from the Journal of Rheumatology and with permission from ASAS.

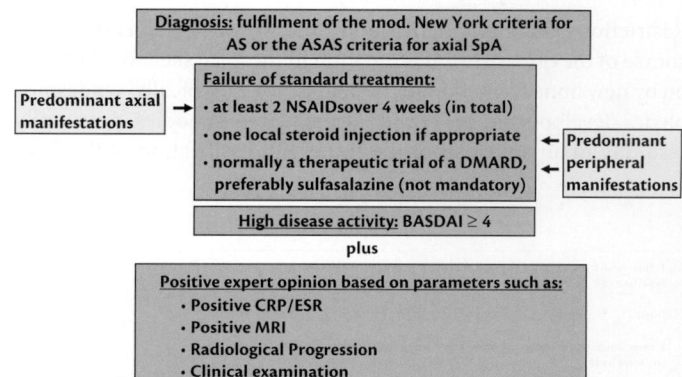

Fig. 113.10 ASAS recommendations for the treatment of ankylosing spondylitis with TNF blockers.
With permission from the Journal of Rheumatology and with permission from ASAS.

Non-steroidal anti-inflammatory drugs

NSAIDs form the basis of drug treatment. Their efficacy has been proven in many trials and is most probably due to their anti-inflammatory properties.[56,57] There is no evidence that one NSAID, including the COX-2 selectives, is better than another. However, for unknown reasons patients might respond differently to available NSAIDs and treatment with at least two should have been tried before a patient is regarded as being NSAID-refractory. As long as patients are symptomatic and the NSAID is well tolerated, patients should be treated with a full dose on a daily basis. Upper dose limits of NSAIDs normally used for the treatment of AS have recently been published.[58] A small reduction of the CRP serum level in AS patients treated with NSAIDs has been reported.[59]

There is also evidence from one prospective randomized clinical trial (RCT) that patients treated with continuous (daily) NSAIDs show less radiographic progression in the spine over a 2 year follow-up period compared to patients treated only on demand.[60] However, further confirmation of this interesting finding is needed before definite conclusions can be drawn. Thus, currently the aim in the treatment of axial SpA patients with NSAIDs is to get the patient free of symptoms.

There is less data about the efficacy of NSAIDs for the treatment of peripheral SpA manifestations such as peripheral arthritis or enthesitis, but they are nonetheless used as first-line treatment here also.

Glucocorticoids

Steroids do not play a major role in the treatment of axial SpA. Normally a dose of 20–30 mg prednisolone per day, a treatment quite effective in RA, for example, shows only a small or no effect on spinal symptoms. Glucocorticoid treatment might be tried for peripheral arthritis, while its effect in enthesitis is less clear. Short-term effects of high-dose glucocorticoid pulse therapy has been reported but its long-term effect is not clear and has not been studied in a controlled trial. Local glucocorticoid injection in the SIJ, peripheral joints, or entheses can be effective and should be considered especially when just one site is affected.[54]

Disease-modifying anti-rheumatic drugs

Similarly to steroids, conventional disease-modifying anti-rheumatic drugs (DMARDs) such as methotrexate, sulfasalazine, or leflunomide have shown no efficacy in the treatment of patients with AS or axial SpA.[54]

TNF blockers

Treatment with a biological TNF blocker is quite effective in patients with active AS who fail conventional therapy such as NSAIDs. In addition to the already mentioned BASDAI, BASFI, and ASDAS the ASAS improvement criteria are used for the evaluation of a treatment effect in clinical trials. For this, four domains—patient global, pain, function, and inflammation (the mean value for questions 5 and 6 on morning stiffness in the BASDAI)—are used. ASAS 20 (%), ASAS 40 (%), and ASAS partial remission are the normal improvement criteria.[61,62] An ASAS 40 or a BASDAI 50 (%) improvement is seen in 40–50% of patients treated with any of the approved TNF blocking agents: infliximab (5 mg/kg body weight intravenously every 6–8 weeks),[63] etanercept (50 mg subcutaneously once a week),[64] adalimumab (40 mg subcutaneously every other week),[65] or golimumab (50 mg subcutaneously once a month).[66] An improvement of clinical symptoms can often be observed after a few days, and a plateau of the clinical response rate is normally reached after 3–6 months of treatment. Follow-up data from the first clinical TNF blocker trials are now available for up to 8 years without new or specific safety signals over time. Between 10 and 20% of patients per year stop TNF blocker treatment in the clinical trial follow-ups and in the registries. The reasons for stopping are side effects, inefficacy, and others, but no specific reason is obvious. For those who stay on the drug a further small improvement of signs and symptoms can even be observed over the years. Small clinical trials and clinical experience indicate that in a proportion of patients the interval between the injections can be prolonged. This should be considered after about 6 months if patients are in remission. The interval should be adjusted to the patient's symptoms. Normally patients can tell quite accurately when symptoms come back. However, it is not clear at the moment in how many of the patients an interval prolongation (or a dose reduction) is possible. About 80–90% of patients relapse if TNF blockers are withdrawn completely.

Objective signs of inflammation such as CRP or active bone inflammation on MRI also improve considerably, although the reduction of the MRI-visible inflammation is reached only by 70–80% of patients and only a minority of AS patients become free of inflammation on MRI when treated with a TNF blocker.[67,68]

There have been reports in AS that immunogenic antibodies can develop against TNF blockers, especially against the monoclonal antibodies,[69] which can reduce efficacy and might increase the likelihood of a hyperergic reaction to the drug. It has therefore been discussed, based on data from combination therapies in RA and Crohn's disease, that combining TNF blocker treatment with a DMARD might increase efficacy. However, two trials comparing infliximab treatment alone vs infliximab plus methotrexate did not show superiority for the combination therapy.[70,71] Thus, currently TNF blockers should be given only as monotherapy in AS.

Although the development of immunogenic anti-drug antibodies might be overcome by increase of the drug dose in some cases, this has not been formally tested and the role of dose increase in case of inefficacy or loss of efficacy has not been well investigated. However, if treatment is switched from one TNF blocker to another an ASAS 40 response rate can still be expected in 38% of patients (compared to 59% in case of no prior TNF blocker exposure) in one investigation.[72] Patients respond better if response is lost over time compared to patients who show no response at the start of treatment. In another report a decrease of the BASDAI by 2 points was still observed in patients who switched to a second and third TNF blocker in comparison to a decrease of 3 BASDAI points in patients on their first TNF blocker.[71]

Some of the other biologics which are effective in RA have also been tested in AS. Anakinra,[73] rituximab,[74] abatacept,[75] and monoclonal antibodies against the IL-6 receptor are not effective in AS. Trials with other biologics directed against IL-17 or against the p40 chain of IL-12 and IL-23, for example, are currently ongoing.

More recently, TNF blocker trials have also been performed in patients, or including patients, with non-radiographic axial SpA. The clinical response rate was even higher in these trials compared to AS patients (with radiographic sacroiliitis) with a clinical remission rate of up to 50%.[76–78] A good response on MRI inflammation in the SIJ and/or spine was also found. Currently several phase 3 clinical trials with the TNF blocking agents that are approved for AS are under way in patients with non-radiographic axial SpA according to the ASAS classification criteria with the aim to get an extension of the AS label. In 2012, adalimumab became the first TNF blocker to be approved by the European Medicine Agency (EMA), based on the results of a phase 3 trial,[79] for the treatment of adults with severe axial SpA without radiographic evidence of AS but with objective signs of inflammation by elevated CRP and/or MRI, who have had an inadequate response to, or are intolerant to, NSAIDs.

TNF blocker treatment did not retard formation of syndesmophytes if AS patients were treated over 2 years.[80] Whether this is the case when patients are treated earlier before the occurrence of early structural damage or whether TNF blockers have to be combined with other treatments to avoid new bone formation has yet to be seen.

Prediction of response to TNF blockers

In the analysis of several AS trials and one study in patients with non-radiographic axial SpA, short symptom duration (overlapping with young age at time of treatment) and elevated CRP performed very consistently best as predictors for a good clinical response.[80] Better function was also predictive, probably indicating reversible changes.[26] Active bone inflammation on MRI and positivity for HLA B27 were less predictive, and less consistent in the different analyses. Furthermore, in two trials in patients with axial SpA (including patients with nr axial SpA) using active MRI inflammation and short symptom duration as an essential inclusion criterion, clinical remission was reached in 50%, confirming that short symptom duration and objective signs of inflammation (such as positive CRP and/or inflammation on MRI) are the most important predictors.[77,78] It has also been proposed that these prediction parameters can be combined in a kind of matrix to predict response even better.[81]

Effect of TNF blocker treatment on peripheral and extra-articular manifestations

Manifestations of peripheral SpA such as arthritis, enthesitis, or dactylitis were not primary outcome parameters in any of the AS trials. However, an improvement was reported in most of the studies, although this was mostly non-significant, probably because of the small number of patients in these subgroups.

Infliximab, etanercept, and adalimumab have also been approved for the treatment of psoriasis; infliximab and adalimumab are licensed for the treatment of Crohn's disease and ulcerative colitis. Thus, it can expected that these associated manifestations, if present, also improve when patients are treated with a TNF blocker licensed for this indication. No controlled trials are available for the treatment of active uveitis anterior; however, the flare rates are reduced if AS patients are treated with a TNF blocker.[82-84]

Recommendations for the treatment of AS/axial SpA with TNF blockers

ASAS has recently updated the international recommendations for the treatment of active AS.[55] Failure of conventional treatment includes only NSAIDs; no previous DMARD therapy is asked for the axial manifestations. Importantly, the correct diagnosis now includes, in addition to AS according to the modified New York criteria, also patients who fulfil the new ASAS criteria for axial SpA (Figure 113.3), based on the published results on the good efficacy of TNF blockers in this indication. The judgement on disease activity is based on an elevated BASDAI (≥4), but should be supplemented by a positive expert opinion, normally based on other (objective) signs of inflammation such as CRP, MRI-visible inflammation, or other clinical manifestations. The expert is normally the treating rheumatologist with experience in spondyloarthritis and in TNF blocker treatment. Response should be assessed after at least 12 weeks of treatment, which should be continued if there is an improvement in the BASDAI of at least 50% or an improvement of at least 2 points on the 0–10 BASDAI scale.

National recommendations e.g. in the United Kingdom,[85] Canada,[86] and the United States (www.spondylitis.org/physician_resources/guidelines.aspx) have normally followed these ASAS recommendations, partly with small modifications, but have not yet extended the indication to patients with axial SpA according to the ASAS criteria. The British National Institute for Health and Clinical Excellence (NICE) (www.nice.org.uk/143) recommends only adalimumab or etanercept for the treatment of severe active AS if all of the following criteria are fulfilled: (1) diagnosis of AS according to the modified New York criteria; (2) sustained active spinal disease demonstrated by a BASDAI score of at least 4 and at least 4 cm on the 0–10 pain visual analogue scale; (2) these should be demonstrated on two occasions at least 12 weeks apart; (4) conventional treatment with two or more NSAIDs taken sequentially at maximum tolerated or recommended dosage over 4 weeks has failed to control symptoms.

Conclusion

The new term 'axial spondyloarthritis' comprises both patients with early inflammation in the SIJ and patients with radiographic evidence of sacroiliitis. New diagnostic approaches and new classification criteria have been developed to cover the whole group and to allow an early diagnosis. Active inflammation of subchondral bone marrow as shown on MRI plays an important role for early diagnosis. HLA B27 is the strongest known pathogenetic factor. Symptoms are present predominantly in the pelvis and the spine, but extraspinal manifestations are frequent. Besides regular physiotherapy there are only two types of drugs which have been proven to be effective: NSAIDs and TNF blockers. Recommendations for the treatment of ankylosing spondylitis and axial SpA with TNF blockers have been developed.

References

1. Braun J, Sieper J. Ankylosing spondylitis. *Lancet* 2007;369(9570): 1379–1390.
2. Sieper J, Braun J, Rudwaleit M, Boonen A, Zink A. Ankylosing spondylitis: an overview. *Ann Rheum Dis* 2002;61 Suppl 3:iii8–iii18.
3. van der Linden S, Valkenburg HA, Cats A. Evaluation of diagnostic criteria for ankylosing spondylitis. A proposal for modification of the New York criteria. *Arthritis Rheum* 1984;27(4):361–368.
4. Dougados M, van der Linden S et al. The European Spondylarthropathy Study Group preliminary criteria for the classification of spondylarthropathy. *Arthritis Rheum* 1991;34(10):1218–1227.
5. Amor B, Dougados M, Mijiyawa M. Criteria of the classification of spondylarthropathies. *Rev Rhum Mal Osteoartic* 1990;57(2):85–89. Criteres de classification des spondylarthropathies.
6. Braun J, Bollow M, Eggens U et al. Use of dynamic magnetic resonance imaging with fast imaging in the detection of early and advanced sacroiliitis in spondylarthropathy patients. *Arthritis Rheum* 1994;37(7):1039–1045.
7. Rudwaleit M, van der Heijde D, Landewe R et al. The development of Assessment of SpondyloArthritis international Society classification criteria for axial spondyloarthritis (part II): validation and final selection. *Ann Rheum Dis* 2009;68(6):777–783.
8. Rudwaleit M, Khan MA, Sieper J. The challenge of diagnosis and classification in early ankylosing spondylitis: do we need new criteria? *Arthritis Rheum* 2005;52(4):1000–1008.
9. Dougados M, Baeten D. Spondyloarthritis. *Lancet* 2011;377 (9783):2127–2137.

10. Rudwaleit M, van der Heijde D, Landewe R et al. The Assessment of SpondyloArthritis International Society classification criteria for peripheral spondyloarthritis and for spondyloarthritis in general. *Ann Rheum Dis* 2011;70(1):25–31.

11. Feldtkeller E, Khan MA, van der Heijde D, van der Linden S, Braun J. Age at disease onset and diagnosis delay in HLA B27 negative vs. positive patients with ankylosing spondylitis. *Rheumatol Int* 2003;23(2):61–66.

12. Rudwaleit M, Haibel H, Baraliakos X et al. The early disease stage in axial spondylarthritis: Results from the German spondyloarthritis inception cohort. *Arthritis Rheum* 2009;60(3):717–727.

13. Khan MA. HLA B27 and its subtypes in world populations. *Curr Opin Rheumatol* 1995;7(4):263–269.

14. Reveille JD, Hirsch R, Dillon CF, Carroll MD, Weisman MH. The prevalence of HLA B27 in the United States: Data from the U.S. National Health and Nutrition Examination Survey, 2009. *Arthritis Rheum* 2011.

15. Saraux A, Guillemin F, Guggenbuhl P et al. Prevalence of spondyloarthropathies in France: 2001. *Ann Rheum Dis* 2005;64(10):1431–1435.

16. Helmick CG, Felson DT, Lawrence RC et al. Estimates of the prevalence of arthritis and other rheumatic conditions in the United States. Part I. *Arthritis Rheum* 2008;58(1):15–25.

17. Adomaviciute D, Pileckyte M, Baranauskaite A et al. Prevalence survey of rheumatoid arthritis and spondyloarthropathy in Lithuania. *Scand J Rheumatol* 2008;37(2):113–119.

18. Brandt HC, Spiller I, Song IH et al. Performance of referral recommendations in patients with chronic back pain and suspected axial spondyloarthritis. *Ann Rheum Dis* 2007;66(11):1479–1484.

19. Poddubnyy D, Vahldiek J, Spiller I et al. Evaluation of 2 screening strategies for early identification of patients with axial spondyloarthritis in primary care. *J Rheumatol* 2011;38(11):2452–2460.

20. Braun A, Saracbasi E, Grifka J, Schnitker J, Braun J. Identifying patients with axial spondyloarthritis in primary care: how useful are items indicative of inflammatory back pain? *Ann Rheum Dis* 2011;70(10):1782–1787.

21. Poddubnyy D, Rudwaleit M, Haibel H et al. Rates and predictors of radiographic sacroiliitis progression over 2 years in patients with axial spondyloarthritis. *Ann Rheum Dis* 2011;70(8):1369–1374.

22. Rudwaleit M, Jurik AG, Hermann KG et al. Defining active sacroiliitis on magnetic resonance imaging (MRI) for classification of axial spondyloarthritis: a consensual approach by the ASAS/OMERACT MRI group. *Ann Rheum Dis* 2009;68(10):1520–1527.

23. van den Berg R, de Hooge M, Rudwaleit M et al. ASAS modification of the Berlin algorithm for diagnosing axial spondyloarthritis: results from the SPondyloArthritis Caught Early (SPACE)-cohort and from the Assessment of SpondyloArthritis international Society (ASAS)-cohort. *Ann Rheum Dis* 2012 Nov 8. [Epub ahead of print]

24. Weber U, Lambert RG, Pedersen SJ et al. Assessment of structural lesions in sacroiliac joints enhances diagnostic utility of magnetic resonance imaging in early spondylarthritis. *Arthritis Care Res* (Hoboken) 2010;62(12):1763–1771.

25. Sieper J, Rudwaleit M, Baraliakos X et al. The Assessment of SpondyloArthritis international Society (ASAS) handbook: a guide to assess spondyloarthritis. *Ann Rheum Dis* 2009;68 Suppl 2:ii1–ii44.

26. Rudwaleit M, Listing J, Brandt J, Braun J, Sieper J. Prediction of a major clinical response (BASDAI 50) to tumour necrosis factor alpha blockers in ankylosing spondylitis. *Ann Rheum Dis* 2004;63(6):665–670.

27. Hermann J, Giessauf H, Schaffler G, Ofner P, Graninger W. Early spondyloarthritis: usefulness of clinical screening. *Rheumatology* (Oxford) 2009;48(7):812–816.

28. Brown MA, Kennedy LG, MacGregor AJ et al. Susceptibility to ankylosing spondylitis in twins: the role of genes, HLA, and the environment. *Arthritis Rheum* 1997;40(10):1823–1828.

29. Brown MA, Laval SH, Brophy S, Calin A. Recurrence risk modelling of the genetic susceptibility to ankylosing spondylitis. *Ann Rheum Dis* 2000;59(11):883–886.

30. Thomas GP, Brown MA. Genetics and genomics of ankylosing spondylitis. *Immunol Rev* 2010;233(1):162–180.

31. Tam LS, Gu J, Yu D. Pathogenesis of ankylosing spondylitis. *Nat Rev Rheumatol* 2010;6(7):399–405.

32. Burton PR, Clayton DG, Cardon LR et al. Association scan of 14,500 nonsynonymous SNPs in four diseases identifies autoimmunity variants. *Nat Genet* 2007;39(11):1329–1337.

33. Evans DM, Spencer CC, Pointon JJ et al. Interaction between ERAP1 and HLA B27 in ankylosing spondylitis implicates peptide handling in the mechanism for HLA B27 in disease susceptibility. *Nat Genet* 2011;43(8):761–767.

34. Mielants H, Veys EM, Cuvelier C et al. The evolution of spondyloarthropathies in relation to gut histology. III. Relation between gut and joint. *J Rheumatol* 1995;22(12):2279–2284.

35. Carter JD, Gerard HC, Espinoza LR et al. Chlamydiae as etiologic agents in chronic undifferentiated spondylarthritis. *Arthritis Rheum* 2009;60(5):1311–1316.

36. Maksymowych WP. Ankylosing spondylitis—at the interface of bone and cartilage. *J Rheumatol* 2000;27(10):2295–2301.

37. Appel H, Kuhne M, Spiekermann S et al. Immunohistochemical analysis of hip arthritis in ankylosing spondylitis: evaluation of the bone-cartilage interface and subchondral bone marrow. *Arthritis Rheum* 2006;54(6):1805–1813.

38. McGonagle D, Emery P. Enthesitis, osteitis, microbes, biomechanics, and immune reactivity in ankylosing spondylitis. *J Rheumatol* 2000;27(10):2302–2304.

39. Sieper J, Appel H, Braun J, Rudwaleit M. Critical appraisal of assessment of structural damage in ankylosing spondylitis: implications for treatment outcomes. *Arthritis Rheum* 2008;58(3):649–656.

40. Schett G, Coates LC, Ash ZR, Finzel S, Conaghan PG. Structural damage in rheumatoid arthritis, psoriatic arthritis, and ankylosing spondylitis: traditional views, novel insights gained from TNF blockade, and concepts for the future. *Arthritis Res Ther* 2011;13 Suppl 1:S4.

41. Calin A, Porta J, Fries JF, Schurman DJ. Clinical history as a screening test for ankylosing spondylitis. *Jama* 1977;237(24):2613–2614.

42. Rudwaleit M, Metter A, Listing J, Sieper J, Braun J. Inflammatory back pain in ankylosing spondylitis: a reassessment of the clinical history for application as classification and diagnostic criteria. *Arthritis Rheum* 2006;54(2):569–578.

43. Sieper J, van der Heijde D, Landewe R et al. New criteria for inflammatory back pain in patients with chronic back pain: a real patient exercise by experts from the Assessment of SpondyloArthritis international Society (ASAS). *Ann Rheum Dis* 2009;68(6):784–788.

44. Garrett S, Jenkinson T, Kennedy LG et al. A new approach to defining disease status in ankylosing spondylitis: the Bath Ankylosing Spondylitis Disease Activity Index. *J Rheumatol* 1994;21(12):2286–2291.

45. Calin A, Garrett S, Whitelock H et al. A new approach to defining functional ability in ankylosing spondylitis: the development of the Bath Ankylosing Spondylitis Functional Index. *J Rheumatol* 1994;21(12):2281–2285.

46. Lukas C, Landewe R, Sieper J et al. Development of an ASAS-endorsed disease activity score (ASDAS) in patients with ankylosing spondylitis. *Ann Rheum Dis* 2009;68(1):18–24.

47. Machado P, Landewe R, Lie E, et al. Ankylosing Spondylitis Disease Activity Score (ASDAS): defining cut-off values for disease activity states and improvement scores. *Ann Rheum Dis* 2010;70(1):47–53.

48. Landewe R, Dougados M, Mielants H, van der Tempel H, van der Heijde D. Physical function in ankylosing spondylitis is independently determined by both disease activity and radiographic damage of the spine. *Ann Rheum Dis* 2009;68(6):863–867.

49. Jones SD, Porter J, Garrett SL et al. A new scoring system for the Bath Ankylosing Spondylitis Metrology Index (BASMI). *J Rheumatol* 1995;22(8):1609.

50. Baraliakos X, Listing J, Rudwaleit M et al. Progression of radiographic damage in patients with ankylosing spondylitis: defining the central role of syndesmophytes. *Ann Rheum Dis* 2007;66(7):910–915.

51. Poddubnyy D, Haibel H, Listing J et al. Baseline radiographic damage, elevated acute phase reactants and cigarette smoking status predict radiographic progression in the spine in early axial spondyloarthritis. *Arthritis Rheum* 2012;64(5):1388–1398.

52. Rudwaleit M, Feldtkeller E, Sieper J. Easy assessment of axial spondyloarthritis (early ankylosing spondylitis) at the bedside. *Ann Rheum Dis* 2006;65(9):1251–1252.

53. Zeboulon N, Dougados M, Gossec L. Prevalence and characteristics of uveitis in the spondyloarthropathies: a systematic literature review. *Ann Rheum Dis* 2008;67(7):955–959.

54. Braun J, van den Berg R, Baraliakos X et al. 2010 update of the ASAS/EULAR recommendations for the management of ankylosing spondylitis. *Ann Rheum Dis* 2011;70(6):896–904.

55. van der Heijde D, Sieper J, Maksymowych WP et al. 2010 Update of the international ASAS recommendations for the use of anti-TNF agents in patients with axial spondyloarthritis. *Ann Rheum Dis* 2011;70(6):905–908.

56. Sieper J, Klopsch T, Richter M et al. Comparison of two different dosages of celecoxib with diclofenac for the treatment of active ankylosing spondylitis: results of a 12-week randomised, double-blind, controlled study. *Ann Rheum Dis* 2008;67(3):323–329.

57. van der Heijde D, Baraf HS, Ramos-Remus C et al. Evaluation of the efficacy of etoricoxib in ankylosing spondylitis: results of a fifty-two-week, randomized, controlled study. *Arthritis Rheum* 2005;52(4):1205–1215.

58. Song IH, Poddubnyy DA, Rudwaleit M, Sieper J. Benefits and risks of ankylosing spondylitis treatment with nonsteroidal antiinflammatory drugs. *Arthritis Rheum* 2008;58(4):929–938.

59. Barkhuizen A, Steinfeld S, Robbins J et al. Celecoxib is efficacious and well tolerated in treating signs and symptoms of ankylosing spondylitis. *J Rheumatol* 2006;33(9):1805–1812.

60. Wanders A, Heijde D, Landewe R et al. Nonsteroidal antiinflammatory drugs reduce radiographic progression in patients with ankylosing spondylitis: a randomized clinical trial. *Arthritis Rheum* 2005;52(6):1756–1765.

61. Anderson JJ, Baron G, van der Heijde D, Felson DT, Dougados M. Ankylosing spondylitis assessment group preliminary definition of short-term improvement in ankylosing spondylitis. *Arthritis Rheum* 2001;44(8):1876–1886.

62. Brandt J, Listing J, Sieper J et al. Development and preselection of criteria for short term improvement after anti-TNF alpha treatment in ankylosing spondylitis. *Ann Rheum Dis* 2004;63(11):1438–1444.

63. van der Heijde D, Dijkmans B, Geusens P et al. Efficacy and safety of infliximab in patients with ankylosing spondylitis: results of a randomized, placebo-controlled trial (ASSERT). *Arthritis Rheum* 2005;52(2):582–591.

64. Davis JC, van der Heijde DM, Braun J et al. Sustained durability and tolerability of etanercept in ankylosing spondylitis for 96 weeks. *Ann Rheum Dis* 2005;64(11):1557–1562.

65. van der Heijde D, Kivitz A, Schiff MH et al. Efficacy and safety of adalimumab in patients with ankylosing spondylitis: results of a multicenter, randomized, double-blind, placebo-controlled trial. *Arthritis Rheum* 2006;54(7):2136–2146.

66. Inman RD, Davis JC, Jr., Heijde D et al. Efficacy and safety of golimumab in patients with ankylosing spondylitis: results of a randomized, double-blind, placebo-controlled, phase III trial. *Arthritis Rheum* 2008;58(11):3402–3412.

67. Braun J, Landewe R, Hermann KG et al. Major reduction in spinal inflammation in patients with ankylosing spondylitis after treatment with infliximab: results of a multicenter, randomized, double-blind, placebo-controlled magnetic resonance imaging study. *Arthritis Rheum* 2006;54(5):1646–1652.

68. Sieper J, Baraliakos X, Listing J et al. Persistent reduction of spinal inflammation as assessed by magnetic resonance imaging in patients with ankylosing spondylitis after 2 yrs of treatment with the anti-tumour necrosis factor agent infliximab. *Rheumatology* (Oxford) 2005;44(12):1525–1530.

69. de Vries MK, Wolbink GJ, Stapel SO et al. Decreased clinical response to infliximab in ankylosing spondylitis is correlated with anti-infliximab formation. *Ann Rheum Dis* 2007;66(9):1252–1254.

70. Breban M, Ravaud P, Claudepierre P et al. Maintenance of infliximab treatment in ankylosing spondylitis: results of a one-year randomized controlled trial comparing systematic versus on-demand treatment. *Arthritis Rheum* 2008;58(1):88–97.

71. Lie E, van der Heijde D, Uhlig T et al. Effectiveness of switching between TNF inhibitors in ankylosing spondylitis: data from the NOR-DMARD register. *Ann Rheum Dis* 2011;70(1):157–163.

72. Rudwaleit M, Van den Bosch F, Kron M, Kary S, Kupper H. Effectiveness and safety of adalimumab in patients with ankylosing spondylitis or psoriatic arthritis and history of anti-tumor necrosis factor therapy. *Arthritis Res Ther* 2010;12(3):R117.

73. Haibel H, Rudwaleit M, Listing J, Sieper J. Open label trial of anakinra in active ankylosing spondylitis over 24 weeks. *Ann Rheum Dis* 2005;64(2):296–298.

74. Song IH, Heldmann F, Rudwaleit M et al. Different response to rituximab in tumor necrosis factor blocker-naive patients with active ankylosing spondylitis and in patients in whom tumor necrosis factor blockers have failed: a twenty-four-week clinical trial. *Arthritis Rheum* 2010;62(5):1290–1297.

75. Song IH, Heldmann F, Rudwaleit M et al. Treatment of active ankylosing spondylitis with abatacept: an open-label, 24-week pilot study. *Ann Rheum Dis* 2011;70(6):1108–1110.

76. Haibel H, Rudwaleit M, Listing J et al. Efficacy of adalimumab in the treatment of axial spondylarthritis without radiographically defined sacroiliitis: results of a twelve-week randomized, double-blind, placebo-controlled trial followed by an open-label extension up to week fifty-two. *Arthritis Rheum* 2008;58(7):1981–1991.

77. Barkham N, Keen HI, Coates LC et al. Clinical and imaging efficacy of infliximab in HLA B27-Positive patients with magnetic resonance imaging-determined early sacroiliitis. *Arthritis Rheum* 2009;60(4):946–954.

78. Song IH, Hermann K, Haibel H et al. Effects of etanercept versus sulfasalazine in early axial spondyloarthritis on active inflammatory lesions as detected by whole-body MRI (ESTHER): a 48-week randomised controlled trial. *Ann Rheum Dis* 2011;70(4):590–596.

79. Sieper J, van der Heijde D, Landewe R et al. Efficacy and safety of adalimumab in patients with non-radiographic axial spondyloarthritis: results of a randomised placebo-controlled trial (ABILITY-1). *Ann Rheum Dis* 2012 Jul 7 [Epub ahead of print].

80. van der Heijde D, Landewe R, Baraliakos X et al. Radiographic findings following two years of infliximab therapy in patients with ankylosing spondylitis. *Arthritis Rheum* 2008;58(10):3063–3070.

81. Vastesaeger N, van der Heijde D, Inman RD et al. Predicting the outcome of ankylosing spondylitis therapy. *Ann Rheum Dis* 2011;70(6):973–981.

82. Braun J, Baraliakos X, Listing J. et al. Differences in the incidence of flares or new onset of inflammatory bowel diseases in patients with ankylosing spondylitis exposed to therapy with anti-tumor necrosis factor alpha agents. *Arthritis Rheum* 2007;57(4):639–634.

83. Rudwaleit M, Rodevand E, Holck P et al. Adalimumab effectively reduces the rate of anterior uveitis flares in patients with active ankylosing spondylitis: results of a prospective open-label study. *Ann Rheum Dis* 2009;68(5):696–701.

84. Sieper J, Koenig A, Baumgartner S et al. Analysis of uveitis rates across all etanercept ankylosing spondylitis clinical trials. *Ann Rheum Dis* 2010;69(1):226–229.

85. Keat A, Barkham N, Bhalla A et al. BSR guidelines for prescribing TNF-alpha blockers in adults with ankylosing spondylitis. Report of a working party of the British Society for Rheumatology. *Rheumatology* (Oxford) 2005;44(7):939–947.

86. Maksymowych WP, Gladman D, Rahman P et al. The Canadian Rheumatology Association/Spondyloarthritis Research Consortium of Canada treatment recommendations for the management of spondyloarthritis: a national multidisciplinary stakeholder project. *J Rheumatol* 2007;34(11):2273–2284.

CHAPTER 114

Psoriatic arthritis

Laura C. Coates and Philip S. Helliwell

Introduction

Although inflammatory arthritis associated with psoriasis has been recognized for many years, there was controversy about whether it represented a separate disease entity, or simply the co-existence of rheumatoid arthritis (RA) and psoriasis. Psoriatic arthritis (PsA) was recognized as a separate disease by the American Rheumatism Association (now the American College of Rheumatology) in 1964, and is now classified as a member of the spondyloarthropathy spectrum.[1,2] PsA was initially defined by Moll and Wright as 'an inflammatory arthritis in the presence of psoriasis with a usual absence of rheumatoid factor',[3] but more robust classification criteria have now been developed.[4] Although it was thought initially to be a relatively benign disorder, more recent work has demonstrated the destructive and progressive nature of the disease with increased mortality and significant cardiovascular comorbidity. At the same time advances in treatment, and in particular with biological drugs, have provided effective tools with which to control the disease.

Epidemiology

Although there is a relative paucity of research in this area, it has been suggested by multiple studies that the prevalence of arthritis in patients with psoriasis, particularly those with peripheral inflammatory arthritis, is higher than population controls.[5] In the Norfolk Arthritis Register (NOAR) cohort, the prevalence of psoriasis was 9.5% in patients with new-onset arthritis, higher than in the general population.[6]

A number of studies have attempted to estimate the incidence and prevalence of PsA but results have varied. A systematic review of papers revealed a median incidence rate of 6 per 100 000 population (range 0.1–23) and a median prevalence of 180 per 100 000 population (range 1–420).[7] However, there is an increase in the incidence and prevalence of PsA,[7,8] possibly as a result of increased recognition.

Among patients with psoriasis, the prevalence of PsA has been reported as varying between 6% and 42%,[9] highlighting the variable definitions used in these studies. However, the development of the CASPAR criteria has provided a more robust tool for classifying disease and a recent study showed a prevalence of approximately 14% when using these criteria among patients with psoriasis in a community setting.[10]

Recently, significant research effort has been invested into the development of screening tools to identify PsA among populations of psoriasis patients.[11] These instruments are self-completed questionnaires which, when scored, provide cut-offs for detecting PsA: they are used to identify patients who should be referred to rheumatologists. The use of such tools should increase the identification of PsA as it is known that cases of PsA exist undiagnosed in dermatology clinics.[12] This work has been given further impetus by the finding of asymptomatic ultrsonographic enthesitis in psoriasis patients.[13]

The majority of patients develop psoriasis prior to the onset of arthritis, even though it may not have been diagnosed by a physician previously. However, up to 20% of patients develop arthritis first, which may cause misdiagnosis and confusion until the psoriasis becomes apparent.[14] A longitudinal cohort over a 30 year period found the following clinical features were associated with the development of PsA: psoriatic nail changes, scalp psoriasis, and intergluteal/perianal psoriasis.[15] No specific association with subtype of psoriasis was found. Also of interest is the usual lack of association between disease activity in the skin and joints, although clinical anecdote suggests that this may occur in those cases which have simultaneous appearance of skin and joint disease.

Classification

The concept of the spondyloarthropathies (SpA) was first introduced by Moll and Wright in the 1970s.[16] Anklyosing spondylitis (AS) is considered as the 'prototype' SpA with typical features such as sacroiliitis, a high prevalence of HLA B27, and only minimal clinical variation. However, PsA shows significant clinical heterogeneity, which provides additional challenges for classification. New classification criteria are either 'standalone' such as the CASPAR criteria (see below) or the inclusive axial and peripheral spondyloarthropathy criteria which subsume PsA.[17]

The CASPAR criteria (Table 114.1) include characteristic dermatological, clinical and radiological features and have both high sensitivity and very high specificity.[4] Reassuringly, the Moll and Wright criteria are nested within the CASPAR criteria. Despite the wide acceptance of the CASPAR criteria a number of areas require further clarification. First, there have been doubts on the suitability of the criteria for early disease,[18] but a recent study found good sensitivity/specificity for these criteria in people presenting with less than 2 years of disease.[19] Secondly, the criteria have inevitably been used as diagnostic criteria and, although they were not designed for this purpose, there is some evidence that they work

Table 114.1 The CASPAR criteria

Inflammatory articular disease (joint, spine, or entheseal), with three or more points from the following:		
1. Evidence of psoriasis (one of a, b, c)	(a) Current psoriasis[a]	Psoriatic skin or scalp disease present today as judged by a rheumatologist or dermatologist
	(b) Personal history of psoriasis	A history of psoriasis that may be obtained from patient, family doctor, dermatologist, rheumatologist, or other qualified healthcare provider
	(c) Family history of psoriasis	A history of psoriasis in a first- or second-degree relative according to patient report
2. Psoriatic nail dystrophy		Typical psoriatic nail dystrophy including onycholysis, pitting and hyperkeratosis observed on current physical examination
3. A negative test for rheumatoid factor		By any method except latex but preferably by ELISA or nephelometry, according to the local laboratory reference range
4. Dactylitis (one of a, b)	(a) Current	Swelling of an entire digit
	(b) History	A history of dactylitis recorded by a rheumatologist
5. Radiological evidence of juxta-articular new bone formation		Ill-defined ossification near joint margins (but excluding osteophyte formation) on plain radiographs of hand or foot

Specificity 0.987, sensitivity 0.914.
[a]Current psoriasis scores 2 whereas all other items score 1.

well in this context.[20] Thirdly, the criteria are only applicable to people with inflammatory musculoskeletal disease: defining what is meant by this requires further work.

Clinical spectrum

PsA is a heterogenous disease and there have been a number of attempts to subgroup patients according to their clinical presentation. Moll and Wright described the five classic subgroups (monoarthritis/oligoarthritis, distal interphalangeal (DIP)-predominant disease, RA-like polyarticular disease, pure axial involvement, and arthritis mutilans) (Figure 114.1).[3] More recently it has become clear that these groups are not robust and can change with time and treatment.[21] It is also clear that assessing joints with other modalities, such as imaging, can alter the subgroup to which patients belong, ultrasound being more sensitive than clinical examination.[22] A more simple grouping of patients into axial and peripheral, with the latter divided into oligo- and polyarthritis, has the advantage of simplicity and may provide a better basis to take forward as there is evidence that a polyarticular onset is associated with a worse outcome.[23]

Certain clinical features suggest PsA. Common presentations are oligoarticular disease, with perhaps just one or two very swollen joints, nail disease, and enthesis. The presence of dactylitis is very suggestive, although other causes of dactylitis (such as gout, sarcoid, and tuberculosis) should be considered in the differential diagnosis.[24] DIP involvement can be misleading as inflammatory osteoarthritis (OA) in this joint can look identical: sometimes the age of the patient and the lack of family history of OA indicate the significance of involvement at this joint. Symmetrical polyarthritis is probably the most frequent subtype of PsA and overlap with RA can lead to misidentification and problems with nosology. It is of paramount importance to take a good family history and to inspect both nails and 'hidden' areas for psoriasis, particularly the natal cleft (Figure 114.2). Despite typical clinical presentations,

rheumatologists in practice still overlook some of the vital clinical signs.[25]

The foot is commonly involved in PsA and first presentation may be to a podiatrist. PsA may present with dactylitis (more common than in the hands), enthesitis (at the calcaneum but also at the insertion of tibialis posterior and peroneus brevis), arthritis (in metatarsophalangeal and midtarsal joints), and skin and nail changes, although the latter are easily confused with fungal infection. Foot problems are often overlooked in rheumatology and may result in unnecessary disability and pain.[26]

Dactylitis

Dactylitis (Figure 114.3A) is one of the hallmark clinical features of PsA, occurring in up to half of all cases.[27,28] Dactylitis is seen more often in the foot, and more often in the fourth toe.[29] Of interest is the fact that most tissues of the digit are affected by inflammation in active, tender dactylitis.[30] Dactylitis is a marker of severity in the ipsilateral digit and may be a marker of severity overall.[29] Chronic, non-tender, diffuse dactylitic swelling occurs in PsA and is regarded as less of an indicator of active disease although MRI abnormalities differ in quantitative terms only.[30] Rarely unilateral limb oedema is seen in PsA and this may be an extreme example of 'limb dactylitis'.

Enthesitis

Entheses, the point of attachment of ligaments and tendons to bone, are widely distributed in the body. The major entheses of the lower limb around the calcaneum provide the hallmark features of enthesitis (Figure 114.3B) in PsA and other spondyloarthropathies.[1] However, enthesitis may underlie most of the changes found in the spine and it has even been suggested that enthesitis is the primary pathological lesion in the peripheral joints in PsA.[31] Reliable clinical assessment of enthesitis has remained elusive, with poor correlation between ultrasonographic enthesitis and tenderness, with higher sensitivity of ultrasonography.[32]

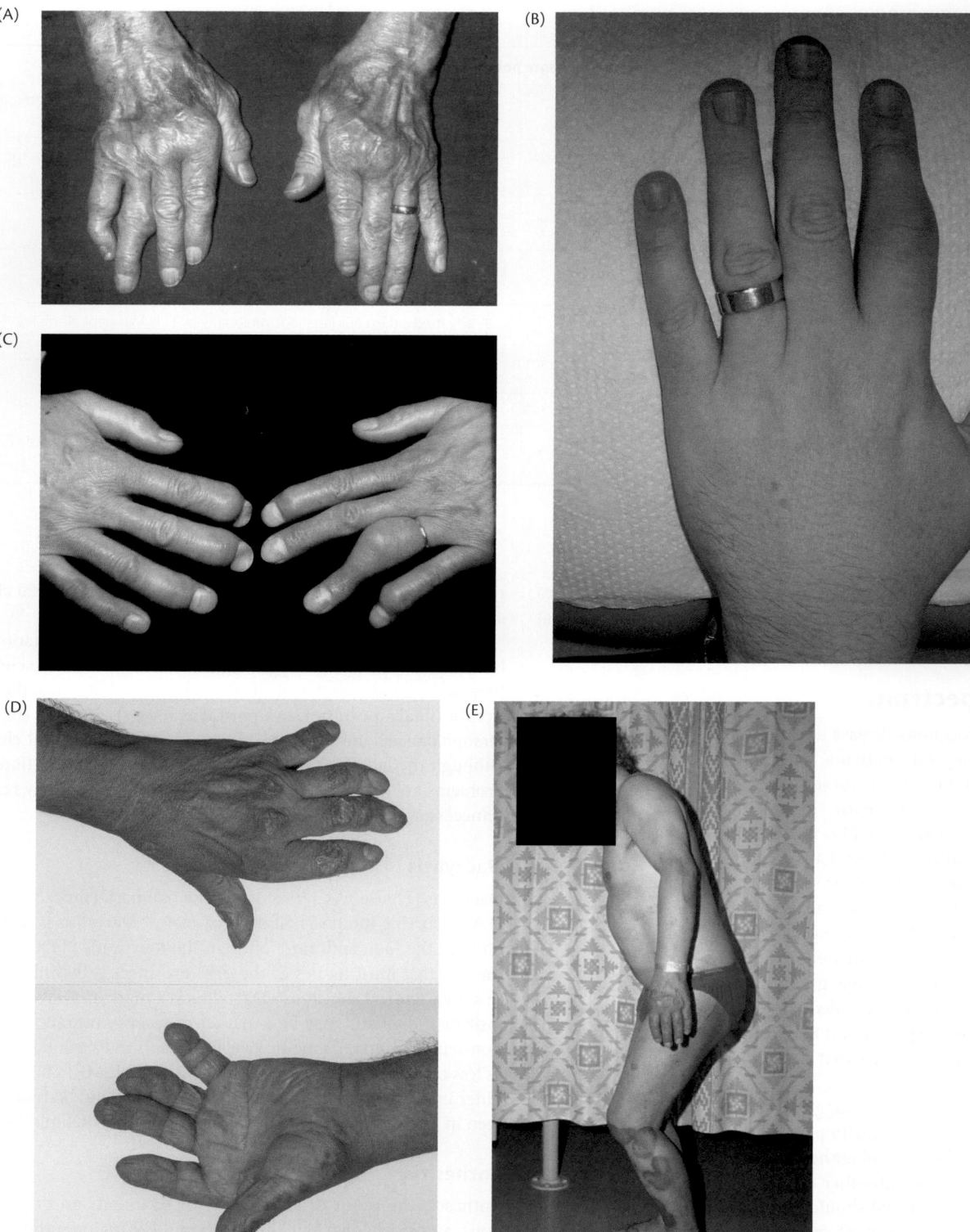

Fig. 114.1 The five clinical subgroups described by Moll and Wright [3]: (A) symmetrical polyarthritis resembling rheumatoid arthritis; (B) oligoarthritis; (C) distal interphalangeal joint predominant; (D) arthritis mutilans; (E) predominant axial involvement.

Reproduced with kind permission from Springer Science+Business Media from Atlas of Psoriatic Arthritis, Mease, Philip J.; Helliwell, Philip S. (Eds.) 1st Edition., 2008.

Axial involvement

It is to be expected that axial disease similar to AS is found in PsA, but notable differences in radiological phenotype have been described.[33,34] The differences can be summarized as both quantitative (less of sacroiliitis and new bone formation) and qualitative (paravertebral ossification and morphologically different syndesmophytes in PsA). In PsA it is also likely that syndesmophytes occur in the absence of sacroiliitis, something of an anathema in AS where sacroiliitis is assumed to precede syndesmophytes.[35] It is also noteworthy that axial involvement defined radiologically is more prevalent than clinical axial involvement, perhaps reflecting the lower pain thresholds observed in PsA.[36]

Juvenile psoriatic arthritis

The classification criteria for juvenile arthritis continue to be the subject of much debate. Juvenile arthritis is uncommon, and juvenile PsA uncommon within this group. The Edmonton (ILAR) criteria provided a clear division for PsA within children but at the expense of excluding those who have enthesitis or inflammatory back pain and those who are rheumatoid factor (RF) positive.[37] It is clear that juvenile PsA is biphasic in onset with peaks at less than 5 years, where the skin disease may present with guttate psoriasis, and over 10 years. The older children tend to have an equal sex ratio and present with peripheral and axial symptoms with enthesitis. Younger children are female predominant, have more wrist and small joint involvement in hands and feet, and may be anti-nuclear antibody (ANA) positive, but are distinguishable from oligoarticular juvelile idiopathic arthritis (JIA) by the pattern of joint involvement and the association with psoriasis.[38]

Prognosis and mortality in psoriatic arthritis

Early studies suggested that PsA was a relatively mild arthropathy and, by implication, that there was little morbidity and no increase in mortality in this condition.[39] However, even these early studies reported a high prevalence of deaths due to cardiovascular disease. This is now increasingly recognized as an important comorbidity of psoriasis and PsA and has been amply demonstrated in a number of studies.[40–42] The mechanisms behind this risk continue to be investigated but a higher prevalence of the metabolic syndrome and therefore traditional risk factors for cardiovascular disease (hypertension, obesity, diabetes) are likely to be significant factors.[43,44]

Laboratory features

C-reactive protein (CRP) is elevated in only about one-half of cases with PsA and the search for a reliable biomarker for outcome in PsA continues.[45] Although PsA is typically considered to be seronegative for RF, RF positivity does occur in PsA and has been recorded in up to 13% of cases.[28] In the 588 patients with PsA recruited to develop the CASPAR criteria, approximately 5% of patients had a positive RF compared to 76% in the RA control group. The estimates for prevalence of anti-CCP antibodies in PsA vary from 6% to 16% in

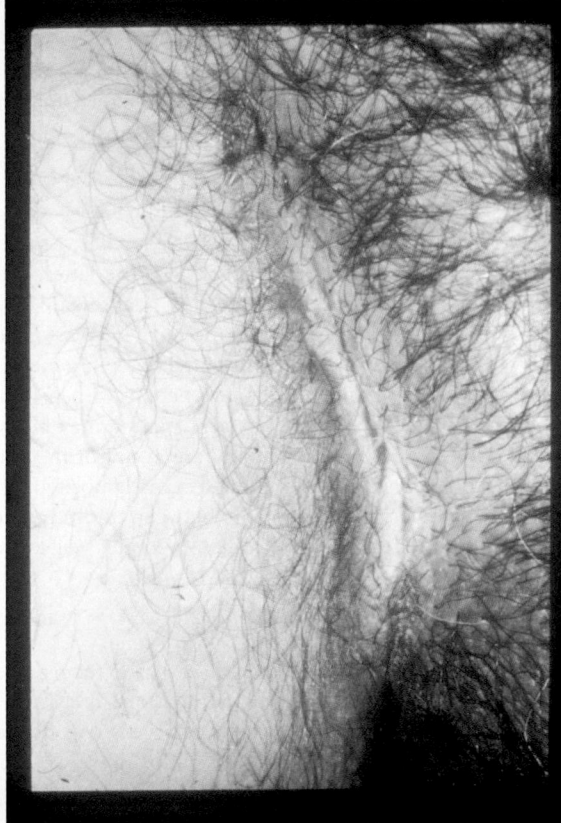

Fig. 114.2 'Hidden' psoriasis in the natal cleft. This may be the only skin manifestation, and the patient may be unaware of it.

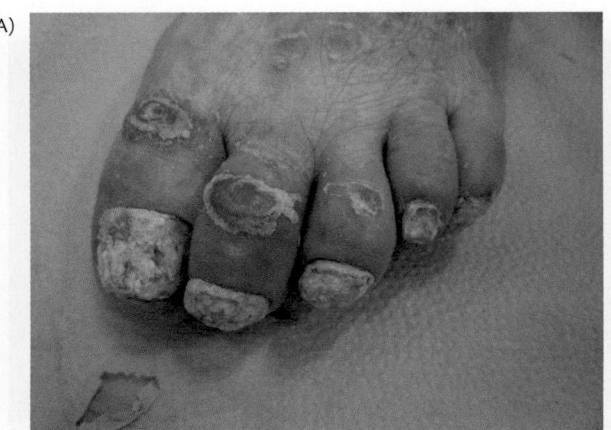
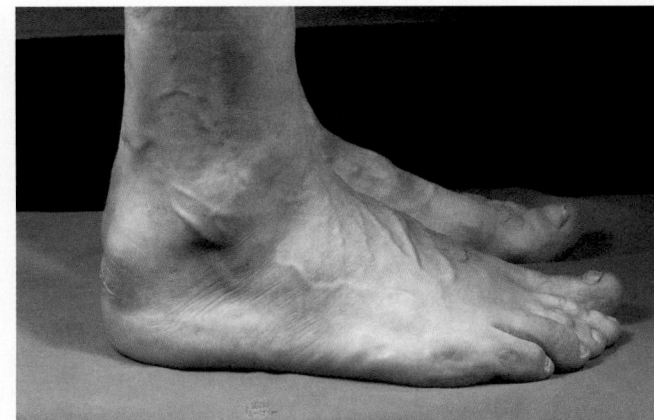

(A)　　　　(B)

Fig. 114.3 Dactylitis and enthesitis: (A) dactylitis of toes; (B) enthesitis of Achilles tendon insertion

different cross-sectional studies.[46–49] Interestingly, patients with polyarticular PsA are no more likely to be RF positive than those with oligoarthritis but nearly all studies have shown a significant association between polyarthritis and CCP. CCP positivity in PsA seems to be associated with a greater risk of aggressive, erosive disease and higher joint counts and may be a marker for developing arthritis mutilans.[46]

Imaging features

Plain radiography

In PsA radiographic damage is not as severe as that seen in RA matched for disease duration,[50] but even early on in the course of disease around 27% have evidence of erosions on radiographs and this increases to 47% at 2 years despite conventional treatment with disease-modifying anti-rheumatic drugs (DMARDs).[51]

Key radiographic features of PsA have been defined as joint erosions, joint space narrowing (JSN), bony proliferation, osteolysis (including pencil-in-cup deformity), ankylosis, and new bone formation at entheses, both central and peripheral.[52] Erosive changes are marginal (similar to RA) but become irregular with disease progression because of new bone formation adjacent to the erosions.[53] Severe erosions lead to the pencil-in-cup deformity due to new bone formation in conjunction with osteolysis (Figure 114.4A).[54] Whiskery juxta-articular new bone formation was the only radiographic feature that separated PsA from other inflammatory arthritides in the CASPAR study (Figure 114.4B).[4]

However, some of these findings have been challenged. For example, in the CASPAR study, comparing RA with PsA (where radiographs were read blind to diagnosis) found a limited number of unique features.[4] For example, osteolysis at a peripheral joint was not found to discriminate between RA and PsA. Osteolysis was characteristic of PsA only if it occurred at the DIP joint—osteolysis at proximal interphalangeal (PIP) joints and metacarpophalangeal joints (MCP) was seen equally in RA. Further, the only distinguishing plain radiographic features of PsA were irregular new bone formation adjacent to small joints of the hand and foot and irregular new bone in the pelvis, particularly at sites of attachment of inguinal ligament, Sartorius, and rectus femoris muscles.[55] Axial changes (discussed above) did not appear as distinctive radiological features of PsA because there were a significant number of cases of AS in the matched controls.

MRI

Although synovitis in PsA and RA is indistinguishable on MRI scanning,[56] features of enthesitis, dactylitis, and spondylitis are in accordance with the appearances of the SpA group of disorders and can be used to differentiate the two conditions.[57] Jevtic and coworkers[58] first described the extensive extracapsular inflammation seen in PsA. Bone oedema, widely accepted to be a surrogate for inflammation, is commonly described as an MRI feature of PsA and can be found extensively at juxta-articular sites.[57]

Ultrasonography

Ultrasound (US) has emerged as an extremely useful non-invasive means of imaging soft tissues and, in particular, entheses.[59] Entheseal imaging with US provides a bedside assessment of the morphological and vascular changes and is more sensitive than clinical examination. Indeed, there may be a role for US examination of cases of psoriasis as a means of early diagnosis of PsA.[13]

Pathogenesis

It seems likely that PsA results from an interplay between genetic susceptibility and environmental triggers. Of the latter, the two most recorded are infection and trauma. The relationship between guttate psoriasis, streptococcal infection, and PsA was discussed in the early 1980s,[60] and more recently infections in general have been associated with the onset of PsA in people with psoriasis.[61] Studies have suggested that acute physical trauma may be associated with the onset of PsA,[62] and many are aware of the concept of PsA as a deep Koebner phenomenon, originally posited by Moll and Wright.[16] However, the relationship between trauma and onset of arthritis is not unique to PsA: this phenomenon is well known in OA and has also been reported in RA.[63]

Genetic factors

PsA is known to be a highly heritable disease: the recurrence risk (ΛS; risk to siblings/risk in general population) of PsA is estimated at 27,[64] which is higher than for psoriasis (ΛS between 4 and 11).[65] An Icelandic study found risk ratios of 39, 12, 3.6, 2.3, and 1.2 respectively in first- to fifth-degree relatives.[66] Thirty per cent of the genetic susceptibility to psoriasis is found in the major histocompatability complex (MHC) class I region on chromosome 6p21.3 (psoriasis susceptibility 1, PSORS1) where HLA Cw*0602 is

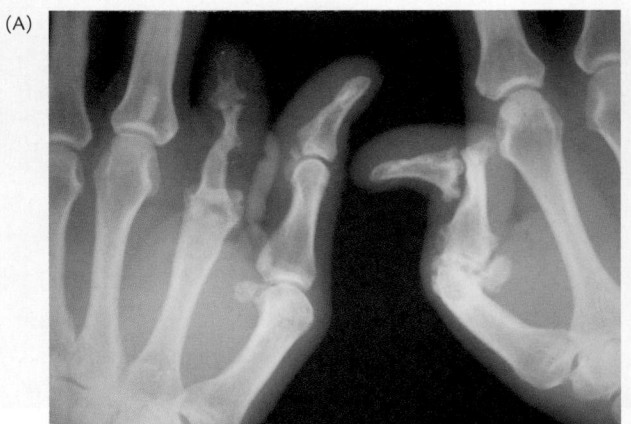

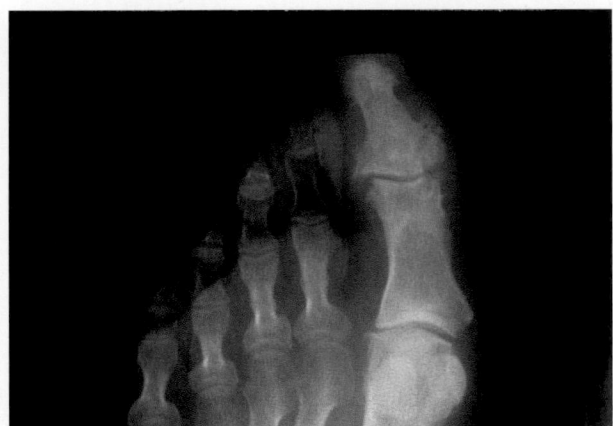

Fig. 114.4 Plain radiographic findings: (A) osteolysis in toes; (B) whiskery new bone formation in toes (arrow).

the susceptibility allele.[67] The frequency of *HLA Cw*0602* is also increased in PsA but only for patients with type I psoriasis and not those with type II psoriasis,[68] suggesting that its major influence is on the age of onset of psoriasis, not susceptibility to PsA.

HLA B27, typically associated with AS, is also found to be associated with psoriatic spondylitis although the frequency of B27 positivity is much lower overall in PsA patients.[69] HLA B38 and HLA B39 have been shown to be associated with peripheral PsA and, additionally, the shared epitope (HLA DRB1) in association with erosive polyarticular disease.[70]

Genome-wide association studies (GWAS) have also shown associations including alleles of the interleukin (IL)-12B and IL-23 receptor gene in both psoriasis[67] and PsA.[71,72] Later GWAS have confirmed the above associations and discovered new loci in signalling pathways in both skin barrier dysfunction (for psoriasis) and innate (NFκB and INF) and adaptive (CD8 and Th17) immune systems.[73]

Pathways for inflammation and new bone formation

Since PsA is such an heterogeneous disease it is not surprising that there is wide heterogeneity in the cells and cytokines found in this disorder. As a marker of the end result of these processes bone morphology provides an insight into the mechanisms involved. As mentioned above, both bone destruction and bone formation can be observed: separately these processes are seen exclusively in RA and AS respectively, thus emphasizing the mixed manifestations of this disease. In AS there is evidence that inflammation and new bone formation occur independently,[74] and this may be a clue to the different manifestations of PsA. In a mouse model of inflammation and ankylosing enthesitis, inhibition of tumour necrosis factor (TNF) has no impact on ankylosis,[75] whereas targeting bone morphogenetic protein is effective.[76] In addition to the TGFβ superfamily of growth factors and cytokines, other morphogenetic signalling pathways may also have relevance in spondyloarthropathy and in PsA. For example, blocking Dickkopf-1, a Wnt receptor antagonist, causes fusion of both sacroiliac and peripheral joints in an animal model.[77]

Immunological mechanisms

The acquired immune system may be less important in PsA than in RA. Material taken from synovial biopsies may be helpful in determining the key cells and cytokines. Beaten et al.[78,79] found significant differences between RA and PsA synovium. In the RA group were highly specific intracellular citrullinated peptides and monoclonal antibody 12A (in 44% and 46% respectively) and increased lining layer thickness, whereas the SpA group showed greater vascularity, increased CD163 and ICAM-1, and a higher number of polymorphonuclear cells. The mononuclear cell may provide the link between the articular and extra-articular manifestations of this disease.[80] The mononuclear cell can differentiate into macrophages, dendritic cells, and osteoclasts. Elevated osteoclast precursors have been found in PsA,[81] and monocytes may have a role in the development of atherosclerotic plaques.[82] Mention has already been made of the IL-23 gene in psoriasis and PsA. IL-23, released by dendritic cells and keratinocytes in psoriatic skin, leads to proliferation of Th17 lymphocytes which in turn produce IL-17, an important cytokine in inflammatory arthritis and psoriasis. This may explain

in part the relative efficacy of anti-T-cell therapies in psoriasis and RA and, to a lesser extent, PsA. TNF is a key proinflammatory cytokine, and blockade of TNF in vitro causes a downregulation of multiple proinflammatory cytokines. Research in PsA found high levels of TNF both in psoriatic plaques in the skin and in synovial fluid taken from active arthritic joints,[83] providing a rationale for treatment of PsA with this class of drugs.

Disease assessment

PsA is a heterogeneous disorder affecting peripheral and axial joints as well as having other features such as dactylitis, enthesitis, and skin and nail disease. Although not all these clinical features may occur together at any one time, it is important to be able to capture them all in order to assess their impact on the patient and the response, which may not be consistent across features, to treatment. This may be carried out in each individual domain or as a composite measure. A composite measure is one way of assessing all relevant clinical outcomes in one single instrument. In PsA the science of outcome measurement has lagged behind other diseases, such that many current measures are 'adopted' from RA. These include the American College of Rheumatology (ACR) responder index,[84] a simplified version adapted for PsA (Psoriatic Arthritis Response Criteria, PsARC)[85] and the Disease Activity Score for 28 joints (DAS28)[86] although the latter does not assess the joints of the foot and ankle which are commonly involved in PsA.

A number of additional composite measures for assessing disease activity in PsA have been proposed. A composite measure for defining 'minimal disease activity' (MDA) has been validated and includes assessments of joints, skin, entheses, and physical function.[87] The MDA criteria define a low disease state and can be used as a responder index in addition to a target for treatment interventions. Three other disease-specific measures have been suggested. First, an adaptation of the Disease Activity index for Reactive Arthritis (DAREA) has been renamed the Disease Activity index for PSoriatic Arthritis (DAPSA).[88] Second, a weighted articular responder index, the Psoriatic Arthritis Joint Activity Index (PsAJAI), has been developed from pooled data from RCTs of biologic agents in PsA.[89] In both of these instruments, the analytic method used in their development led to factoring out skin disease, which was therefore recommended to be measured separately from the musculoskeletal components, as has been the case with the ACR and DAS scoring systems. Third, a domain-based approach has been proposed with the development of a composite measure known as the Composite Psoriatic Disease Activity Index (CPDAI) which assesses disease severity separately in joints, skin, entheses, dactylitis, and spine and sums the individual scores.[90] In addition, two new disease activity scores have been developed; the first uses similar methodology to the DAS and is called the PASDAS, and the second uses an approach using predefined cut-offs for acceptable disease states, the so-called desirability function.[90a]

Treatment

As indicated in the previous section, PsA is a complex and heterogeneous disease and the key to optimal treatment is to consider all aspects of the disease. The more complex patients with PsA will require treatment input from both a rheumatologist and a dermatologist to allow optimal management of their condition. Good communication between these specialties and with primary care is important for managing treatment.

Little research has been done on different treatment regimes and protocols for PsA, particularly in comparison to RA. Given the complexities of presentation it seems likely that different algorithms will be required for different subgroups, particularly since a polyarticular onset is likely to indicate the group with the worst prognosis. The most commonly used regime in PsA is a step-up model where treatment is escalated gradually in the case of non-response. Treatment guidelines were published by the GRAPPA group in 2006 based on a full literature review and expert consensus.[91] They outline the different treatments that are considered efficacious for the five main domains of PsA (see Figure 114.5). More recently the European League Against Rheumatism (EULAR) has published evidence-based recommendations with a detailed algorithm independent of clinical subgroup.[92] Evidence for individual drugs and approaches, with the exception of topical treatments is summarized below.

The use of intra-articular steroids

Despite widespread use, there is little data to support the use of intra-articular (IA) steroids in PsA. Expert opinion is that IA glucocorticoid injections may be used in persistent mono- or oligoarthritis with good clinical results.[93] There is observational evidence of benefit in a longitudinal database with 41% of joints improved at 3 months, although one-third of these relapsed within 12 months.[94]

Non-steroidal anti-inflammatory drugs

The use of NSAIDs to treat PsA has been recommended for many years, and in mild cases, they are often recommended as the only therapy.[95] However there is a lack of randomized trials to support their use. Only one randomized controlled trial (RCT) has compared a standard NSAID to placebo,[96] with four RCTs comparing different NSAIDs.[97,98] In addition to the standard concerns about gastrointestinal (GI) toxicity caused by NSAIDs and their risks in renal impairment, there is a concern about NSAIDs worsening skin psoriasis. The potential for this flare of skin lesions was highlighted by dermatologists in case reports.[99] However, in the five RCTs discussed above, there was no evidence of an effect on psoriasis.[93]

Disease-modifying drugs

Small molecules

Standard DMARDs are routinely used in PsA despite a paucity of evidence for their use in this condition. There is no evidence

to support the use of gold salts in PsA,[93] although anti-malarials may have weak benefit. The use of these two drugs has been discouraged because of an anecdotal risk of deterioration in skin, although the evidence for the latter with the use of anti-malarials seems fallacious.[100] Interest in methotrexate (MTX) for the treatment of PsA evolved following its use in RA for arthritis and studies showing efficacy in psoriasis. Historically the evidence is poor,[101–103] and a Cochrane review calculated only a moderate effect size of 0.65 based on both patients' and physicians' global assessments, but the confidence intervals included zero.[104] An analysis of the Norwegian DMARD (NOR-DMARD) register identified 526 cases treated with MTX (n = 380) or anti-TNF ± MTX (n = 146). Those patients in the MTX group showed a similar improvement in both tender and swollen joint counts to those treated with TNF. The drug adherence rates at 6 months were similar in both groups, with adverse event being the commonest reason for withdrawal in both groups.[105] The only fully powered RCT of oral MTX found no significant difference from placebo in the primary outcome but doses of MTX were only 15 mg weekly in the majority of patients.[106]

The evidence for the use of sulfasalazine is supported by multiple RCTs, reported in a Cochrane review,[104] although effect sizes were small. Only one small study has attempted to assess the impact of sulfasalazine on radiographic damage, with no evidence that sulfasalazine slows or stops the progression of radiographic joint damage.[107]

The benefit of leflunomide for both skin and joints has been demonstrated in an RCT[108] and a further 24 week open-label study confirmed the efficacy and safety of leflunomide in daily clinical practice.[109] Radiographic outcomes were not assessed.

Ciclosporin is more often used for the skin than the joints but may be of use where both skin and joints are problematic and therapy with MTX is suboptimal. The latter strategy is supported by an RCT using ciclosporin added to MTX partial responders which found both PASI score and US-detected synovitis showed a greater improvement with combination treatment.[110]

Biological agents

A summary of the results from the key trials of TNF blockers is shown in Table 114.2. In the United Kingdom, National Institute of Clinical Excellence (NICE) guidance on the use of TNF inhibitors in PsA advises that the patient must have active disease (three

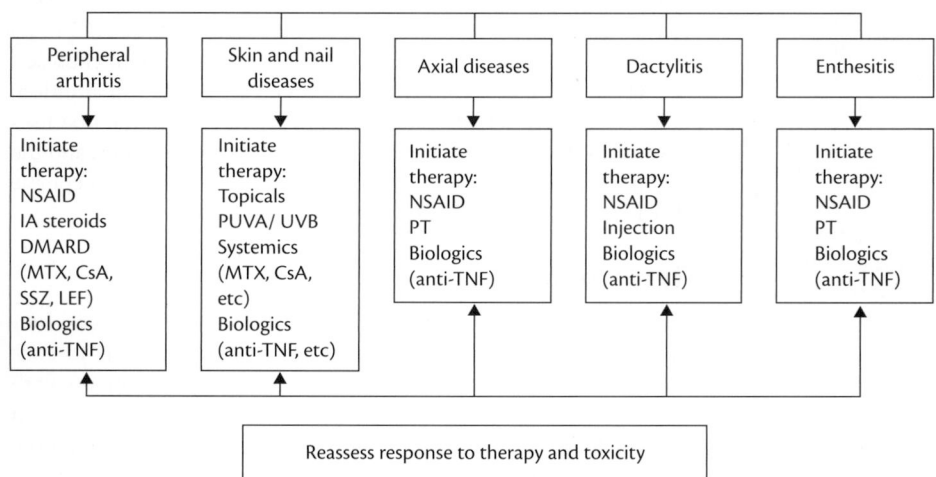

Fig. 114.5 The GRAPPA treatment guidelines.[127] Reproduced from Annals of the Rheumatic Diseases, Ritchlin CT, Kavanaugh A, Gladman DD, Mease PJ, Helliwell P, Boehncke WH et al. Treatment recommendations for psoriatic arthritis. 68(9):1387–1394. With permission from *BMJ* Publishing Group Ltd.

Table 114.2 Summary of trials of TNF inhibitors in psoriatic arthritis

Drug	N	Inclusion	Baseline TJC	Baseline SJC	PsARC	ACR20	ACR50	ACR70
Adalimumab 40 mg eow[128]	100	≥3 TJC and ≥3 SJC	25.3	18.2	51	39	25	14
Adalimumab 40 mg eow[117]	313	≥3 TJC and ≥3 SJC	23.9	14.3	62	52	36	20
Etanercept 25 mg biw[111]	60	≥3 TJC and ≥3 SJC	20 (median)	14 (median)	87	73	50	13
Etanercept 25 mg biw[129]	205	≥3 TJC and ≥3 SJC	20.4	15.9	72	59	38	11
Golimumab 50/100 mg monthly[118]	405	≥3 TJC and ≥3 SJC	22.5	12	73/72	51/45	30/28	12/17
Infliximab 5 mg/kg 8 weekly[113]	104	≥5 TJC and ≥5 SJC	23.7	14.6	75	65	46	29
Infliximab 5 mg/kg 8 weekly[115]	200	≥5 TJC and ≥5 SJC	24.6	13.9	77	58	36	15

biw, twice a week; eow, every other week; SJC swollen joint count; TJC, tender joint count.

swollen and tender joints) and have failed two or more conventional DMARDs (http://guidance.nice.org.uk/TA199).

Etanercept was the first anti-TNF therapy to be tested in a randomized trial in patients with PsA, demonstrating an impressive response to treatment with 87% of etanercept-treated patients achieving a PsARC response compared with 23% of placebo-treated patients.[111] A larger phase 3 study, demonstrated retardation of radiographic disease progression at 12 months.[112]

Following on from successful trials of infliximab in the treatment of psoriasis, a phase 2 RCT of infliximab in PsA (Infliximab Multinational Psoriatic Arthritis Controlled Trial or IMPACT) showed a significant benefit in terms of arthritis, skin disease, enthesitis, and dactylitis.[113] Further analysis on this trial showed a halt in radiographic progression with infliximab therapy over the 12 month treatment time.[114] A larger phase 3 study (IMPACT 2) followed, confirming the efficacy of infliximab in terms of improving disease activity and reducing progression in radiographic damage compared to placebo.[115,116] This larger group also allowed a more thorough assessment of safety. Further studies of other anti-TNF drugs have included adalimumab[117] and golimumab.[118] The safety profile of anti-TNF drugs within the studies seems acceptable, with infection and elevation of liver transaminases the most worrisome.

New drugs and other biologicals

Many biologics used in RA have shown relatively disappointing results in PsA, including abatacept[119] and rituximab.[120] Results of trials with tociluzimab (an IL-6 blocker), and secukinumab (anti-IL-17) are awaited. Apremilast, an orally active inhibitor of phosphodiesterase-4, shows efficacy in psoriasis and PsA equivalent to methotrexate but less than monoclonal antibody inhibitors of tumour necrosis factor (TNFi).[121-123]

Ustekinumab is a human monoclonal antibody that binds to the p40 subunit present on both human IL-12 and IL-23. It therefore prevents binding of these interleukins to the IL-12Rβ1 receptor, blocking this signalling pathway. Studies in skin psoriasis have shown a significant response to ustekinumab,[124] and a phase II trial has shown benefit in PsA.[125]

Surgical options

Surgery may be required for 'endstage' large joints such as the hip and knee. Unless routine antibiotic cover is used there is evidence to suggest a higher rate of superficial and deep infection in PsA.[126]

Patients may also develop psoriasis in the operation scar as part of the Koebner phenomenon.

References

1. Helliwell PS, Wright V. Psoriatic arthritis: clinical features. In: Klippel JH, Dieppe PA (eds) *Rheumatology*. Mosby, London,1998:6.21.1–6.21.8.
2. Helliwell P, Wright V. Seronegative spondarthritides. In: Anderson JAD(ed) *Clinical rheumatology international practice and research: epidemiological, sociological and environmental aspects of rheumatology*. Balliere Tindall, London 1987:491–524.
3. Moll JMH, Wright V. Psoriatic arthritis. *Semin Arthrits Rheum* 1973;3: 51–78.
4. Taylor WJ, Gladman DD, Helliwell PS, Marchesoni A, Mease PJ, Mielants H. Classification criteria for psoriatic arthritis. *Arthritis & Rheumatism* 2006;54(8):2665–2673.
5. FitzGerald O, Dougados M. Psoriatic arthritis: one or more diseases? *Best Pract Res Clin Rheumatol* 2006;20(3):435–450.
6. Harrison BJ, Silman AJ, Barrett EM, Scott DG, Symmons DP. Presence of psoriasis does not influence the presentation or short-term outcome of patients with early inflammatory polyarthritis. *J Rheumatol* 1997;24(9): 1744–1749.
7. Alamanos Y, Voulgari PV, Drosos AA. Incidence and prevalence of psoriatic arthritis: a systematic review. *J Rheumatol* 2008;35(7):1354–1358.
8. Wilson FC, Icen M, Crowson CS, McEvoy MT, Gabriel SE, Kremers HM. Time trends in epidemiology and characteristics of psoriatic arthritis over 3 decades: a population-based study. *J Rheumatol* 2009;36(2):361–367.
9. O'Neill T, Silman AJ. Psoriatic arthritis. Historical background and epidemiology. *Baillieres Clin Rheumatol* 1994;8(2):245–261.
10. Ibrahim G, Waxman R, Helliwell PS. The prevalence of psoriatic arthritis in people with psoriasis. *Arthritis Care Res* 2009;61(10):1373–1378.
11. Qureshi A, Dominguez P, Duffin K et al. Psoriatic arthritis screening tools. *J Rheum* 2008;35:1423–1425.
12. Reich K, Kruger K, Mossner R, Augustin M. Epidemiology and clinical pattern of psoriatic arthritis in Germany: a prospective interdisciplinary epidemiological study of 1511 patients with plaque-type psoriasis. *Br J Dermatol* 2009;160(5):1040–1047.
13. Gisondi P, Tinazzi I, El Dalati G et al. Lower limb enthesopathy in patients with psoriasis without clinical signs of arthropathy: a hospital-based case control study. *Ann Rheum Dis* 2008;67(1):26–30.
14. Kane D, Pathare S. Early psoriatic arthritis. *Rheumatic Dis Clin North Am* 2005;31(4):641–657.
15. Wilson FC, Icen M, Crowson CS et al. Incidence and clinical predictors of psoriatic arthritis in patients with psoriasis: A population-based study. *Arthritis Rheum* 2009;61(2):233–239.
16. Wright V, Moll JMH. *Seronegative polyarthritis*. North Holland, Amsterdam, 1976.

17. Rudwaleit M, van der HD, Landewe R et al. The Assessment of SpondyloArthritis International Society classification criteria for peripheral spondyloarthritis and for spondyloarthritis in general. *Ann Rheum Dis* 2011;70(1):25–31.

18. Di Angelo S, Mennillo G, Cutro M et al. Sensitivity of the classification of psoriatic arthritis criteria in early psoriatic arthritis. *J Rheumatol* 2009;36(2):368–370.

19. Coates L, Conaghan P, Emery P et al. Sensitivity and specificity of the classification of psoriatic arthritis criteria in early psoriatic arthritis. *Arthritis Rheum* 2012;64(10):3150–3155.

20. Chandran V, Schentag CT, Gladman DD. Sensitivity and specificity of the CASPAR criteria for psoriatic arthritis in a family medicine clinic setting. *J Rheumatol* 2010;35(10):2069–2070.

21. Jones SM, Armas JB, Cohen MG et al. Psoriatic arthritis: outcome of disease subsets and relationship of joint disease to nail and skin disease. *Br J Rheumatol* 1994;33(9):834–839.

22. Wakefield RJ, Green MJ, Marzo-Ortega H et al. Should oligoarthritis be reclassified? Ultrasound reveals a high prevalence of subclinical disease. [see comment]. *Ann Rheum Dis* 2004;63(4):382–385.

23. Gladman DD, Farewell VT, Nadeau C. Clinical indicators of progression in psoriatic arthritis: multivariate relative risk model. *J Rheumatol* 22(4):675–679, 1995.

24. Rothschild BM, Pingitore C, Eaton M. Dactylitis: implications for clinical practice. *Semin Arthritis Rheum* 1998;28(1):41–47.

25. Gorter S, van der Heijde DMFM, vander Linden S et al. Psoriatic arthritis: performance of rheumatologists in daily practice. *Ann Rheum Dis* 2002;61:219–224.

26. Hyslop E, McInnes IM, Woodburn J, Turner D. Foot problems in psoriatic arthritis: high burden and low care provision. *Ann Rheum Dis* 2010;69(5):928.

27. Helliwell P, Marchesoni A, Peters M, Barker M, Wright V. A re-evaluation of the osteoarticular manifestations of psoriasis [see comments]. *Br J Rheumatol* 1991;30(5):339–345.

28. Gladman DD, Shuckett R, Russell ML, Thorne JC, Schachter RK. Psoriatic arthritis (PSA)—an analysis of 220 patients. *Q J Med* 1987;238:127–141.

29. Brockbank JE, Stein M, Schentag CT, Gladman DD. Dactylitis in psoriatic arthritis: a marker for disease severity? *Ann Rheum Dis* 64(2):188–190, 2005.

30. Healy PJ, Groves C, Chandramohan M, Helliwell PS. MRI changes in psoriatic dactylitis extent of pathology, relationship to tenderness and correlation with clinical indices. *Rheumatology* 2008;47(1):92–95.

31. McGonagle D, Conaghan P, Emery P. Psoriatic arthritis: a unified concept 20 years on. *Arthritis Rheum* 1999;42(6):1080–1086.

32. Balint PV, Kane D, Wilson H, McInnes IB, Sturrock RD. Ultrasonography of entheseal insertions in the lower limb in spondyloarthropathy. *Ann Rheum Dis* 2002;61(10):905–910.

33. Helliwell PS, Hickling P, Wright V. Do the radiological changes of classic ankylosing spondylitis differ from the changes found in the spondylitis associated with inflammatory bowel disease, psoriasis, and reactive arthritis? *Ann Rheum Dis* 1998;57(3):135–140.

34. McEwen C, Di Tata D, Lingg C et al. A comparative study of ankylosing spondylitis and spondylitis accompanying ulcerative colitis, regional enteritis, psoriasis and Reiter's disease. *Arthritis Rheum* 1971;14:291–318.

35. Taylor WJ, Zmierczak HG, Helliwell PS. Problems with the definition of axial and peripheral disease patterns in psoriatic arthritis. *J Rheumatol* 32(6):974–977, 2005.

36. Buskila D, Langevitz P, Gladman DD, Urowitz S, Smythe H. Patients with rheumatoid arthritis are more tender than those with psoriatic arthritis. *J Rheumatol* 1992;19:1115–1119.

37. Petty RE, Southwood TR, Manners P et al. International League of Associations for Rheumatology classification of juvenile idiopathic arthritis: second revision, Edmonton, 2001. *J Rheumatology* 2004;31:390–392.

38. Stoll M, Nigrovic P, Gotte A, Punaro M. Clinical comparison of early onset psoriatic and non-psoriatic oligoarticular juvenile idiopathic arthritis. *Clin Exp Rheumatol* 2011;29(582):588.

39. Roberts MET, Wright V, Hill AGS, Mehra AC. Psoriatic arthritis: follow-up study. *Ann Rheum Dis* 1976;35:206–212.

40. Wong K, Gladman DD, Husted J, Long JA, Farewell VT. Mortality studies in psoriatic arthritis: results from a single outpatient clinic. I. Causes and risk of death.[see comment]. *Arthritis Rheum* 1997;40(10):1868–1872.

41. Gelfand JM, Troxel AB, Lewis JD et al. The risk of mortality in patients with psoriasis: results from a population-based study. *Arch Dermatol* 2007;143(12):1493–1499.

42. Peters MJ, van der Horst-Bruinsma IE, Dijkmans BA, Nurmohamed MT. Cardiovascular risk profile of patients with spondylarthropathies, particularly ankylosing spondylitis and psoriatic arthritis. *Semin Arthritis Rheum* 2004;34(3):585–592.

43. Husted JA, Thavaneswaran A, Chandran V et al. Cardiovascular and other co-morbidities in patients with psoriatic arthritis: a comparison with patients with psoriasis. *Arthr Care Res* 2011;63(12):1729–1735.

44. Gisondi P, Tessari G, Conti A et al. Prevalence of metabolic syndrome in patients with psoriasis: a hospital-based case/control study. *Br J Dermatol* 2007;157(1):68–73.

45. Ritchlin CT, Qureshi AA, De Vlam K et al. Biomarkers in psoriasis and psoriatic arthritis: GRAPPA 2008. *J Rheumatol* 2010;37(2):462–467.

46. Bogliolo L, Alpini C, Caporali R et al. Antibodies to cyclic citrullinated peptides in psoriatic arthritis. *J Rheumatol* 2005;32(3):511–515.

47. Korendowych E, Owen P, Ravindran J, Carmichael C, McHugh N. The clinical and genetic associations of anti-cyclic citrullinated peptide antibodies in psoriatic arthritis. *Rheumatology* (Oxford) 2005;44(8):1056–1060.

48. Alenius GM, Berglin E, Rantapaa Dahlqvist S. Antibodies against cyclic citrullinated peptide (CCP) in psoriatic patients with or without joint inflammation. *Ann Rheum Dis* 2006;65(3):398–400.

49. Shibata S, Tada Y, Komine M et al. Anti-cyclic citrullinated peptide antibodies and IL-23p19 in psoriatic arthritis. *J Dermatol Sci* 2009;53(1):34–39.

50. Sokoll KB, Helliwell PS. Comparison of disability and quality of life in rheumatoid and psoriatic arthritis. *J Rheumatol* 2001;28(8):1842–1846.

51. Kane D, Stafford L, Bresnihan B, Fitzgerald O. A prospective, clinical and radiological study of early psoriatic arthritis: an early synovitis clinic experience. *Rheumatology* 2003;42:1460–1468.

52. van der HD, Sharp J, Wassenberg S, Gladman DD. Psoriatic arthritis imaging: a review of scoring methods. *Ann Rheum Dis* 2005;64 Suppl 2:ii61–ii64.

53. Ory PA, Gladman DD, Mease PJ. Psoriatic arthritis and imaging. *Ann Rheum Dis* 2005;64 Suppl 2:ii55–ii57.

54. Taylor WJ, Porter GG, Helliwell PS. Operational definitions and observer reliability of the plain radiographic features of psoriatic arthritis. *J Rheumatology* 2003;30(12):2645–2658.

55. Helliwell PS, Porter G, CASPAR study group. Sensitivity and specificity of plain radiographic features of peripheral enthesopathy at major sites in psoriatic arthritis. *Skeletal Radiol* 2007;36(11):1061–1066.

56. Cimmino MA, Parodi M, Innocenti S et al. Dynamic magnetic resonance of the wrist in psoriatic arthritis reveals imaging patterns similar to those of rheumatoid arthritis. *Arthritis Res Ther* 2005;7(4):R725–R731.

57. McQueen F, Lassere M, Ostergaard M. Magnetic resonance imaging in psoriatic arthritis: a review of the literature. *Arthritis Res Ther* 2006;8(2):207.

58. Jevtic V, Watt I, Rozman B et al. Distinctive radiological features of small hand joints in rheumatoid arthritis and seronegative spondyloarthritis demonstrated by contrast-enhanced (Gd-DTPA) magnetic resonance imaging. *Skeletal Radiol* 1995;24(5):351–355.

59. D'Agostino MA. Ultrasound imaging in spondyloarthropathies. *Best Pract Res Clin Rheumatol* 2010;24:693–700.

60. Vasey FB, Deitz C, Fenske NA, Germain BF, Espinoza LR. Possible involvement of Group A streptococci in the pathogenesis of psoriatic arthritis. *J Rheumatol* 1982;9:719–722.

61. Eder L, Law T, Chandran V et al. Association between environmental factors and onset of psoriatic arthritis in patients with psoriasis. *Arthritis Care Res* 2011;63(8):1091–1097.

62. Scarpa R, Del Puente A, di Girolamo C et al. Interplay between environmental factors, articular involvement, and HLA-B27 in patients with psoriatic arthritis. *Ann Rheum Dis* 1992;51:78–79.

63. Julkunen H, Rajanen JA, Kataja J. Severe trauma as an aetiological factor in rheumatoid arthritis. *Scand J Rheum* 1974;3:97–102.

64. Gladman DD, Farewell VT, Pellett F, Schentag C, Rahman P. HLA is a candidate region for psoriatic arthritis. evidence for excessive HLA sharing in sibling pairs. *Hum Immunol* 2003;64(9):887–889.

65. Bhalerao J, Bowcock AM. The genetics of psoriasis: a complex disorder of the skin and immune system. *Hum Mol Genet* 1998;7(10):1537–1545.

66. Karason A, Love TJ, Gudbjornsson B. A strong heritability of psoriatic arthritis over four generations—the Reykjavik Psoriatic Arthritis Study. *Rheumatology* (Oxford) 2009;48(11):1424–1428.

67. Nograles KE, Brasington RD, Bowcock AM. New insights into the pathogenesis and genetics of psoriatic arthritis. [*Nat Clin Pract Rheumatol* 2009;5(2):83–91.

68. Ho PY, Barton A, Worthington J et al. Investigating the role of the HLA-Cw*06 and HLA-DRB1 genes in susceptibility to psoriatic arthritis: comparison with psoriasis and undifferentiated inflammatory arthritis. *Ann Rheum Dis* 2008;67(5):677–682.

69. Queiro-Silva R, Torre-Alonso JC, Tinture-Eguren T, Lopez-Lagunas I. The effect of HLA-DR antigens on the susceptibility to, and clinical expression of psoriatic arthritis. *Scand J Rheumatol* 2004;33(5):318–322.

70. Korendowych E, Dixey J, Cox B, Jones S, McHugh N. The influence of the HLA-DRB1 rheumatoid arthritis shared epitope on the clinical characteristics and radiological outcome of psoriatic arthritis. *J Rheumatol* 2003;30(1):96–101.

71. Liu Y, Helms C, Liao W et al. A genome-wide association study of psoriasis and psoriatic arthritis identifies new disease loci. *PLoS Genet* 2008;4(3):e1000041.

72. Huffmeier U, Lascorz J, Bohm B et al. Genetic variants of the IL-23R pathway: association with psoriatic arthritis and psoriasis vulgaris, but no specific risk factor for arthritis. *J Invest Dermatol* 2009;129(2):355–358.

73. Huffmeier U, Uebe S, Ekici AB et al. Common variants at TRAF3IP2 are associated with susceptibility to psoriatic arthritis and psoriasis. *Nat Genet* 2010;42(11):996–999.

74. van der HD, Landewe R, Einstein S et al. Radiographic progression of ankylosing spondylitis after up to two years of treatment with etanercept. *Arthritis Rheum* 2008;58(5):1324–1331.

75. Lories RJ, Derese I, De Bari C, Luyten FP. Evidence for uncoupling of inflammation and joint remodelling in a mouse model of spondylarthritis. *Arthritis Rheum* 2007;56(2):489–497.

76. Lories RJ, Derese I, Luyten FP. Modulation of bone morphogenetic protein signalling inhibits the onset and progression of ankylosing enthesitis. *J Clin Invest* 2005;115(6):1571–1579.

77. Lories RJ, Luyten FP. Osteoimmunology: Wnt antagonists: for better or worse? *Nat Rev Rheumatol* 2009;5(8):420–421.

78. Bennett PH, Wood PHN. Population studies of the rheumatic diseases. Proceedings of the 3rd International Symposium, New York, 1966. Excerpta Medica, Amsterdam, 1968.

79. Kruithof E, Baeten D, De Rycke L et al. Synovial histopathology of psoriatic arthritis, both oligo- and polyarticular, resembles spondyloarthropathy more than it does rheumatoid arthritis. *Arthritis Res Ther* 2005;7(3):R569–R580.

80. Ritchlin CT, Proulx S, Schwartz E. Translational perspectives on psoriatic arthritis. *J Rheumatol* 2009;36(Suppl 83):30–34.

81. Ritchlin CT, Haas Smith S, Li P, Hicks D, Schwartz E. Mechanisms of TNF alpha and RANKL mediated osteoclastogenesis and bone resorption in psoriatic arthritis. *J Clin Invest* 2003;111:821–831.

82. Ritchlin C. Psoriatic disease—from skin to bone.[*Nat Clin Pract Rheumatol* 2007;3(12):698–706.

83. Partsch G, Steiner G, Leeb BF et al. Highly increased levels of tumor necrosis factor-alpha and other proinflammatory cytokines in psoriatic arthritis synovial fluid. *J Rheumatol* 1997;24(3):518–523.

84. Felson DT, Anderson JJ, Boers M et al. American College of Rheumatology. Preliminary definition of improvement in rheumatoid arthritis.[see comment]. *Arthritis Rheum* 1995;38(6):727–735.

85. Clegg DO, Reda DJ, Mejias E et al. Comparison of Sulfasalazine and Placebo in the Treatment of Psoriatic Arthritis: A Department of Veterans Affairs Cooperative Study. [Article]. *Arthritis Rheum* 1996;39(12):2013–2020.

86. Prevoo M, van Gestel A, van t'Hof VA et al. Remission in a proposed study of patients with rheumatoid arthritis. American Rheumatism Association preliminary criteria in relation to the disease activity score. *Br J Rheumatol* 1996;35(11):1101–1105.

87. Coates LC, Fransen J, Helliwell PS. Defining minimal disease activity in psoriatic arthritis: a proposed objective target for treatment. *Ann Rheum Dis* 2010;69(1):48–53.

88. Nell-Duxneuner VP, Stamm TA, Machold KP et al. Evaluation of the appropriateness of composite disease activity measures for assessment of psoriatic arthritis. *Ann Rheum Dis* 2010;69(3):546–549.

89. Gladman DD, Tom BDM, Mease PJ, Farewell VT. Informing response criteria for psoriatic arthritis (PsA). II: Further considerations and a proposal—the PsA joint activity index. *J Rheumatology* 2010;37(12):2559–2565.

90. Mumtaz A, Gallagher P, Kirby B et al. Development of a preliminary composite disease activity index in psoriatic arthritis. *Ann Rheum Dis* 2011;70:272–277.

90a. Helliwell PS, FitzGerald O, Fransen J et al. The development of candidate composite disease activity and responder indices for psoriatic arthritis (GRACE project). *Ann Rheum Dis* 2012 Jul 13 [Epub ahead of print].

91. Ritchlin CT, Kavanaugh A, Gladman DD et al. Treatment recommendations for psoriatic arthritis. *Ann Rheum Dis* 2009;68(9):1387–1394.

92. Gossec L, Smolen JS, Gaujoux-Viala C et al. European League Against Rheumatism recommendations for the management of psoriatic arthritis with pharmacological therapies. *Ann Rheum Dis* 2012;71(1):4–12.

93. Soriano ER, McHugh NJ. Therapies for peripheral joint disease in psoriatic arthritis. A systematic review. *J Rheumatol* 2006;33(7):1422–1430.

94. Eder L, Chandran V, Schentag CT et al. Time and predictors of response to tumour necrosis factor-α blockers in psoriatic arthritis: an analysis of a longitudinal observational cohort. *Rheumatology* 2010;49(7):1361–1366.

95. Cuellar ML, Citera G, Espinoza LR. Treatment of psoriatic arthritis. *Baillieres Clin Rheumatol* 1994;8(2):483–498.

96. Sarzi-Puttini P, Santandrea S, Boccassini L, Panni B, Caruso I. The role of NSAIDs in psoriatic arthritis: evidence from a controlled study with nimesulide. *Clin Exp Rheumatol* 2001;19(1 Suppl 22):S17–S20.

97. Lassus A. A comparative pilot study of azapropazone and indomethacin in the treatment of psoriatic arthritis and Reiter's disease. *Curr Medical Res Opin* 1976;4(1):65–69.

98. Lonauer G, Wirth W. [Controlled double blind study on the effectiveness and adverse effects of acemetacin and indomethacin in the treatment of psoriatic arthritis]. *Arzneimittelforschung* 1980;30(8A):1440–1444.

99. Griffiths CE. Therapy for psoriatic arthritis: sometimes a conflict for psoriasis. *Br J Rheumatol* 1997;36(4):409–410.

100. Gladman DD, Blake R, Brubacher B, Farewell VT. Chloroquine therapy in psoriatic arthritis. *J Rheumatol* 1992;19(11):1724–1726.

101. Black RL, O'Brien WM, Vanscott EJ et al. Methotrexate therapy in psoriatic arthritis;double-blind study on 21 patients. *J Am Med Assoc* 1964;189:743–747.

102. Willkens RF, Williams HJ, Ward JR et al. Randomized, double-blind, placebo controlled trial of low-dose pulse methotrexate in psoriatic arthritis. *Arthr Rheum* 1984;27:376–381.

103. Espinoza LR, Zakraoui L, Espinoza CG et al. Psoriatic arthritis: clinical response and side effects to methotrexate therapy. *J Rheumatol* 1992;19:872–877.

104. Jones G, Crotty M, Brooks P. Interventions for psoriatic arthritis. *Cochrane Database Syst Rev* 2000;3:CD000212.

105. Heiberg MS, Kaufmann C, Rodevand E et al. The comparative effectiveness of anti-TNF therapy and methotrexate in patients with psoriatic arthritis: 6 month results from a longitudinal, observational, multicentre study. *Ann Rheum Dis* 2007;66(8):1038–1042.

106. Kingsley G, Kowalczyk A, Taylor H et al. Methotrexate is not disease modifying in psoriatic arthritis: the MIPA trial. *Arthritis Rheum* 2010;62(Suppl 10):664.

107. Rahman P, Gladman DD, Cook RJ, Zhou Y, Young G. The use of sulfasalazine in psoriatic arthritis: a clinic experience. *J Rheumatol* 1998;25(10):1957–1961.

108. Kaltwasser JP, Nash P, Gladman D et al. Efficacy and safety of leflunomide in the treatment of psoriatic arthritis and psoriasis: a multinational, double-blind, randomized, placebo-controlled clinical trial. *Arthritis Rheum* 2004;50(6):1939–1950.

109. Behrens F, Meier L, Thaci D, Burkhardt H. Efficacy of leflunomide in psoriatic joint and skin disease: results from a large German prospective observational study of psoriatic arthritis treated with leflunomide (OSPAL). *Ann Rheum Dis* 66 (SII), 99. 2007.

110. Fraser AD, van Kuijk AW, Westhovens R et al. A randomised, double blind, placebo controlled, multicentre trial of combination therapy with methotrexate plus ciclosporin in patients with active psoriatic arthritis. *Ann Rheum Dis* 2005;64(6):859–864.

111. Mease PJ, Goffe BS, Metz J et al. Etanercept in the treatment of psoriatic arthritis and psoriasis: a randomised trial. [see comment]. *Lancet* 2000;356(9227):385–390.

112. Mease PJ, Kivitz AJ, Burch FX et al. Etanercept treatment of psoriatic arthritis: safety, efficacy, and effect on disease progression. *Arthritis Rheum* 2004;50(7):2264–2272.

113. Antoni CE, Kavanaugh A, Kirkham B et al. Sustained benefits of infliximab therapy for dermatologic and articular manifestations of psoriatic arthritis: results from the infliximab multinational psoriatic arthritis controlled trial (IMPACT).[erratum appears in *Arthritis Rheum*. 2005;52(9):2951]. *Arthritis Rheum* 2005;52(4):1227–1236.

114. Kavanaugh A, Antoni CE, Gladman D et al. The Infliximab Multinational Psoriatic Arthritis Controlled Trial (IMPACT): results of radiographic analyses after 1 year. *Ann Rheum Dis* 2006;65(8):1038–1043.

115. Antoni C, Krueger GG, de Vlam K et al. Infliximab improves signs and symptoms of psoriatic arthritis: results of the IMPACT 2 trial. *Ann Rheum Dis* 2005;64(8):1150–1157.

116. van der Heijde D, Kavanaugh A, Gladman DD et al. Infliximab inhibits progression of radiographic damage in patients with active psoriatic arthritis through one year of treatment: Results from the induction and maintenance psoriatic arthritis clinical trial 2. *Arthritis Rheum* 2007;56(8):2698–2707.

117. Mease PJ, Gladman DD, Ritchlin CT et al. Adalimumab for the treatment of patients with moderately to severely active psoriatic arthritis: results of a double-blind, randomized, placebo-controlled trial. *Arthritis Rheum* 2005;52(10):3279–3289.

118. Kavanaugh A, McInnes I, Mease P et al. Golimumab, a new human tumor necrosis factor alpha antibody, administered every four weeks as a subcutaneous injection in psoriatic arthritis: Twenty-four-week efficacy and safety results of a randomized, placebo-controlled study. *Arthritis Rheum* 2009;2009/04/01(4):976–986.

119. Mease P, Genovese M, Ritchlin C et al. Abatacept in the treatment of patients with psoriatic arthritis: results of a six-month, multicenter, randomized, double-blind, placebo-controlled, phase II trial. *Arthritis Rheum* 2009;63(4):939–948.

120. Mease PJ, Genovese MC, Ritchlin CT et al. Rituximab in psoriatic arthritis: results of an open label trial. *Ann Rheum Dis* 2010;69(Suppl3):116 2010.

121. Schett G, Wollenhaupt J, Papp K et al. Apremilast is active in the treatment of psoriatic arthritis (PsA). *Arthritis Rheum* 60(10), S1258. 2009.

122. Papp K, Cather JC, Rosoph L et al. Efficacy of apremilast in the treatment of moderate to severe psoriasis: a randomised controlled trial. *Lancet* 2012;380(9843):738–746.

123. Kavanaugh A, Mease P, Gomez-Reino J et al. Apremilast, an oral phosphodiasterase 4 inhibitor, in patients with psoriatic arthritis: results of a phase 3, randomised, controlled trial. *Arthritis Rheum* 2012;64(S10):L13 (abstract).

124. Papp KA, Langley RG, Lebwohl M et al. Efficacy and safety of ustekinumab, a human interleukin-12/23 monoclonal antibody, in patients with psoriasis: 52-week results from a randomised, double-blind, placebo-controlled trial (PHOENIX 2). *Lancet* 2008;371(9625):1675–1684.

125. Gottlieb AB, Menter A, Mendelsohn A et al. Ustekinumab, a human interleukin 12/23 monoclonal antibody, for psoriatic arthritis: randomised, double-blind, placebo-controlled, crossover trial. *Lancet* 2009;373:633–640.

126. Menon T, Wroblewski BM. Charnley low friction arthroplasty in patients with psoriasis. *Clin Orthop* 1983;248:108–111.

127. Ritchlin CT, Kavanaugh A, Gladman DD et al. Treatment recommendations for psoriatic arthritis. *Ann Rheum Dis* 2009;68(9):1387–1394.

128. Genovese MC, Mease PJ, Thomson GT et al. Safety and efficacy of adalimumab in treatment of patients with psoriatic arthritis who had failed disease modifying antirheumatic drug therapy. *J Rheumatol* 2007;34(5):1040–1050.

129. Mease PJ, Kivitz AJ, Burch FX et al. Etanercept treatment of psoriatic arthritis: safety, efficacy, and effect on disease progression. *Arthritis Rheum* 2004;50(7):2264–2272.

CHAPTER 115

Reactive arthritis and enteropathic arthropathy

J. S. Hill Gaston

Definitions

The term 'reactive arthritis' is often used loosely to cover any form of arthritis which can be linked to preceding infection. This produces a large group of diseases with little in common as far as their clinical features or pathogenesis are concerned, for example, postviral arthritis, poststreptococcal arthritis, and Lyme disease. It is preferable to reserve the term 'reactive arthritis' (ReA) for the clearly identified clinical syndrome which falls naturally within the spondyloarthropathies on clinical, immunogenetic, and pathogenetic grounds. This syndrome is usually triggered by infection with a relatively small number of organisms and forms an important part of the differential diagnosis of acute oligo- and mono arthritis (Table 115.1). Other forms of arthritis seen in relation to infection are best termed 'postinfectious'.

There are several examples of disorders linking the gastrointestinal tract and arthritis, ReA following gastroenteritis being an obvious example, along with the arthritis associated with Crohn's disease or ulcerative colitis. Both the latter are classified within the spondyloarthropathies, but other forms of arthritis are sometimes included in the 'enteropathic' grouping such as Whipple's disease, arthritis associated with coeliac disease, and other syndromes. This chapter is divided into two sections, the first dealing with ReA, and the second with other forms of enteropathic arthritis.

Reactive arthritis

Historical perspective

An association between urethritis and arthritis has been known for nearly 500 years. Many authors attribute the first description of ReA to van Forest in the 1500s, and a description in Spanish literature by Lopez de Hinojosos in Mexico City in 1578 has been recognized. By the beginning of the 19th century the syndrome was clearly recognized, but inevitably in a prebacteriological era 'venereal arthritis' encompassed both postgonococcal arthritis and true ReA, mainly due to *Chlamydia trachomatis*. Nevertheless, some of the case descriptions, particularly those which mention prominent eye involvement, very likely represent ReA. Brodie described six cases in 1818 and a survey of early case records in London

Table 115.1 Infections that trigger arthritis

Reactive arthritis	Postinfectious arthritis
Common triggering infections	Postviral arthritis
Salmonella	Parvovirus
Campylobacter	Rubella
Yersinia	Mumps
Shigella	HIV
Chlamydia trachomatis	Hepatitis B and C
Occasional triggering infections	Arboviruses
Chlamydia pneumoniae	Other case reports (e.g. herpesviruses)
Clostridium difficile	Bacterial infections
M. bovis BCG (intravesical)	Streptococci
Mycoplasma (e.g. *U. urealyticum*)	Rheumatic fever
Rare triggering infections	Poststreptococcal arthritis
Many case reports of infection, particularly of the intestine, including:	Neisseria
	Gonococcal arthritis
Giardia	Meningococcal arthritis
Cryptosporidium	Lyme disease (Borrelia)
Chlamydia psittaci	Brucella
Hafnia alvei	Whipple's disease (*Tropheryma whippeli*)
Vibrio parahaemolyticus	
and many other single case reports	

hospitals shows that the condition was commonly recognized from 1820 onwards, accounting for a significant proportion of hospital admissions.[1]

A link between gastrointestinal infection and reactive arthritis was noted in the early years of the 20th century and outbreaks of dysentery in the trenches of the First World War led to classical descriptions by Fiessinger and Leroy in 1916, and also by Hans Reiter. Although the term 'Leroy–Fiessinger–Reiter syndrome' is sometimes encountered, it is the name of Reiter which has come to be associated with ReA, and the terms 'Reiter's syndrome' and 'reactive arthritis' have often been used interchangeably. There are several cogent reasons for bringing this practice to an end and abandoning the term 'Reiter's syndrome'. First, Reiter was clearly not the first to describe ReA; disease associated with dysentery was first reported by Vossius in 1904. Secondly, Reiter did not shed any useful light on its pathogenesis, erroneously attributing it to spirochaetal infection. Thirdly, and more practically, the triad of arthritis, conjunctivitis, and urethritis/cervicitis has often been taken to imply that Reiter's syndrome is the form of ReA secondary to genitourinary infection, missing the point that the urethritis in his original description was also 'reactive', following bacillary dysentery. There are no prognostic implications associated with the classical triad and therefore no clinical value in singling out Reiter's triad as a subsection of reactive arthritis. Lastly, several authors have felt the eponym inappropriate in view of Reiter's later enthusiasm for the Nazi party.

Case definition

Classification criteria for reactive arthritis present difficulties. Since ReA is one of the spondyloarthropathies, criteria such as those devised by Amor[2] or the European Spondyloarthropathy Study Group (ESSG)[3] can be applied. More recently the international ankylosing spondylitis assessment group (ASAS) has put forward criteria for both axial and peripheral spondyloarthritis.[4,5] The success of these criteria is variable; on the one hand many cases of ReA do not have sufficient features to satisfy the Amor criteria. On the other hand, most cases would meet the ESSG criteria, or either of the ASAS criteria, but these criteria are very wide-ranging and do not allow ReA to be distinguished from undifferentiated spondyloarthropathy. Unfortunately all current criteria fail to deal adequately with cases with no preceding *symptomatic* gastrointestinal or genitourinary infection. In these cases, a link to preceding infection depends on adequate laboratory investigation (see below). While diagnostic and classification criteria continue to be debated, a suggested working definition is presented in Box 115.1. This groups:

1. patients with classical clinical features (oligoarthritis, predominantly of the lower limbs, and/or inflammatory back pain, with extra-articular signs, including enthesitis) **plus** proven preceding infection with one of the organisms known to trigger reactive arthritis, irrespective of preceding symptoms

2. patients with proven preceding infection **plus** arthritis with no diagnostic features

3. patients with classical clinical features **without** proven preceding infection.

This definition avoids separating patients with identical clinical manifestations on the basis of the skills of the microbiological laboratory, or failing to include patients with new inflammatory disease of joints or entheses after proven, but asymptomatic, infection with reactive arthritis-associated organisms. The latter are often seen in follow-up of cohorts of patients from outbreaks of food poisoning. Indeed, in a recent series, the proportion of patients with

> **Box 115.1** Working definition of reactive arthritis
>
> - Classical clinical features:
>   - asymmetric oligoarthritis, lower limbs predominate
>   - enthesitis
>   - extra-articular signs and proven infection by salmonella, campylobacter, yersinia, shigella, or chlamydia (whether symptomatic or not)
> - Classical clinical features and proven infection by other organisms (e.g. *Clostridium difficile*, *Mycobacterium bovis*, BCG)
> - Any acute inflammatory arthritis (including monoarthritis) and proven infection by ReA-associated bacteria
> - Classical clinical features and preceding diarrhoea or urethritis/cervicitis, infection not proven

a clinical diagnosis of ReA in whom a triggering infection could be identified after appropriate investigations was very similar in patients with a preceding symptomatic infection and those with no such history. Practically, it is worth considering the diagnosis of ReA in any patient presenting for the first time with acute oligo- or monoarticular synovitis, in whom no other diagnosis (sepsis, crystal arthropathies, etc.) can be made. This allows adequate history, physical examination, and diagnostic tests to be performed, so that a definite diagnosis of ReA can be made.

Epidemiology

Given the difficulties in case definition, accurate epidemiological studies on incidence and prevalence present problems. There are two possible approaches. In the first, the proportion of patients with ReA can be measured in clinics designed to examine all cases of early synovitis. One such study in Oslo measured an incidence of 9.6 per 100 000, equally divided between cases due to *Chlamydia trachomatis* and enteric infection.[6] Previous estimates of chlamydia-induced arthritis of 5 per 100 000 have also been recorded.[7] The difficulty with this approach is that it cannot take account of mild cases not referred to early synovitis clinics, cases where arthritis is short lived, or cases with inflammatory back pain or enthesitis in the absence of synovitis. The alternative approach has been to take advantage of food poisoning outbreaks, when an entire population infected with an organism at a particular time can be followed up prospectively. Patients are sent questionnaires on the occurrence of arthritic symptoms subsequent to their exposure to the infection, and those reporting symptoms are examined by a rheumatologist. Although the incidence of ReA in food poisoning outbreaks varies substantially, several series report incidences ranging from 5% to 25%, with an additional percentage of patients developing arthritic symptoms but not meeting criteria for ReA. These figures are interesting in relation to a comprehensive United Kingdom study on the community incidence of enteric infections in a population of 460 000. This showed a combined incidence of campylobacter, salmonella, and yersinia infection confirmed by stool culture of 17.7 per 1000. Interestingly, particularly for yersinia, the number of cases identified in the community survey was substantially higher than those in the same population who presented to their family physician. This means that many of the cases of yersinia infection were too mild to require medical attention. Combining these results would give an estimate of ReA in the community of 100–200 per 100 000, not including cases induced by chlamydia. Although a large proportion of these cases may have mild self-limiting disease, the figures suggest that the incidence calculated on the basis of patients seen at early synovitis clinics is a serious underestimate.

The incidence of ReA may be declining; this decline seems particularly marked for chlamydia-associated arthritis. This is not due to any decline in the overall incidence of chlamydia infection in Western countries—quite the opposite, with the incidence in the United Kingdom doubling through the 1990s to 50 000 cases per year, with a further doubling over the next decade to 123 000 in 2008. This suggests that other factors must be affecting the incidence of chlamydia-induced arthritis. This could include differences in the organism—whole-genome sequencing of chlamydiae is now able to identify different 'subspecies' which do not necessarily correspond to the serovar classification, so that 'arthritogenic' chlamydiae might be identified. Other changes may involve the host; chlamydia infection is now commonly acquired in early teenage years. At this age few subjects will have been previously infected with related organisms, such as *Chlamydia pneumoniae,* an infection whose overall incidence has declined with improved socioeconomic conditions. In the 20th century many subjects acquiring *C. trachomatis* in their third decade would previously have experienced *C. pneumoniae* infection in childhood or adolescence. It has been shown that such infection has the potential to prime the immune system for more vigorous responses to *C. trachomatis,*[8] which would be relevant to the occurrence of arthritis.

Infections with salmonella and with campylobacter increased substantially in the 1990s in the United Kingdom, without a notable increase in the incidence of ReA, and then have declined in recent years as public health measures have been implemented. Again the lack of a relationship between incidence of infection and ReA is striking, and suggests that changes in immunological memory in those who now become infected has somehow altered their susceptibility to arthritis

Pathogenesis

Since ReA is a member of the spondyloarthropathy group, pathogenesis of these conditions can be considered together, and is discussed in detail elsewhere (see Chapters 113 and 114). However, its clear association with infection by known bacteria, and its usual acute presentation, means that ReA lends itself to investigation, and much work has been done in the last 20 years. From this three factors have emerged as critical to pathogenesis: the infecting organism; the immune response elicited by infection, particularly that mounted by T lymphocytes; and genetic influences, principally HLA B27. Interestingly, all of these are important in rat HLA B27 transgenic models of spondyloarthropathy [9]; in this model arthritis requires infection (gut flora rather than specific pathogens), T lymphocytes (especially CD4+ T cells), and an appropriate genetic background in addition to transgenic B27, since disease incidence varies in different inbred rats.

The list of bacteria which commonly cause ReA is quite short (Table 115.1). Another set of organisms has been implicated in ReA on multiple occasions, but their contribution to ReA incidence is relatively small. Lastly, there are many single case reports implicating particular infections. In these cases, there is always uncertainty about whether the organism provoked true ReA or simply a

postinfectious arthritis, but where classical extra-articular features are noted (as distinct from only positivity for HLA B27), the reports are convincing. Very similar organisms, e.g. *Shigella flexnerii* and *Shigella sonnei,* have previously been associated with very different rates of ReA, with *S. sonnei* infection rarely being reported as a cause of ReA in series from the United States; but, interestingly, a recent survey of shigella-infected patients in Finland found a majority of the arthritis cases to be triggered by *S. sonnei.*[10] Thus differences in the ability of an organism to trigger ReA may not be consistent in all populations, and investigations focused on the differences between such organisms to identify arthritogenic factors may not be informative.

Contrary to previous expectations, there is now substantial evidence that bacteria or their antigens reach the affected joints in ReA. Bacterial antigens were first demonstrated in phagocytic cells within the joint using immunofluorescence and immunoblotting techniques.[11,12] This has been shown for salmonella, yersinia, and shigella, and since phagocytic cells in peripheral blood were also shown to contain antigen,[13] it seems likely that there is traffic from the site of infection to the affected joint. Most studies to demonstrate nucleic acids of enteric bacteria in ReA joints have been negative,[14] but by using the more sensitive technique of reverse transcription polymerase chain reaction (RT-PCR), ribosomal RNA from *Yersinia pseudotuberculosis* was unequivocally demonstrated in a ReA joint.[15] The demonstration of bacterial RNA is particularly important since, unlike DNA, this has a relatively short half-life and its presence implies that transcriptionally active organisms can reach the joint, although ribosomal RNA has a longer half-life than that of messenger RNA. Evidence that intact *C. trachomatis* reaches the joint is much stronger, with detection by both PCR and RT-PCR[16,17] and the demonstration of organisms (albeit with atypical morphology) by electron microscopy or immunofluorescence.[18] Interestingly, in all these studies evidence for organisms or their antigens in the joint has been obtained long after the initial infection, strongly suggesting that these organisms can persist at low levels, perhaps in sites such as lymphoid tissue associated with the gut or genital tract. This persistence may relate to their ability to survive intracellularly. Such persistence has been demonstrated, even after 'curative' antibiotics, but dormant intracellular organisms that divide infrequently may be insensitive to conventional antibiotics—this reasoning has led to new attempts to treat chlamydia-associated ReA with novel combinations of antibiotics (see below).

Affected joints in ReA have a substantial infiltrating T-cell population, including both CD4+ and CD8+ T cells. Some of these T cells may have trafficked from the gut or genitourinary tract because the synovium shares 'addressins' (molecules which determine which T cells are recruited) with the mucosal-associated lymphoid tissue (MALT).[19] This may apply to the inflamed synovium since it is unlikely that there is normal traffic of lymphocytes through the normal paucicellular synovial membrane. The preference for weight-bearing joints in ReA might reflect pre-existing microtrauma and hence increased monocyte and lymphocyte traffic to such joints, delivering both antigen and antigen-specific T cells. Prominent responses to arthritis-triggering bacteria have been demonstrated in both CD4+ and CD8+ populations, most work having been done on the experimentally more tractable CD4+ T cells.[20,21] Organism-specific clones have been obtained and their specificities identified (e.g. Goodall et al.,[22] Mertz et al.[23]). In several studies bacterial hsp60 has emerged as a major target antigen,[24–26] although this is a common feature of T-cell-mediated responses to intracellular bacteria. Hsp60 is a good candidate for 'molecular mimicry', since there are large numbers of conserved peptides in human and bacterial hsp60, so that T cells stimulated by bacterial hsp60 might conceivably cross-react with human hsp60 and generate autoimmunity. This was not found when analysed with T-cell clones,[27] though the possibility was raised in a non-clonal analysis.[26] Generally evidence for molecular mimicry is lacking and the significance of CD4+ T-cell responses to bacterial hsp60 for ReA pathogenesis is not known. Likewise the attractive idea that bacteria-specific CD8+ T cells restricted by HLA B27 would make an autoreactive response to a joint-specific antigen has not received experimental support, although yersinia- and chlamydia-reactive, B27-restricted T-cell clones have been isolated from ReA joints.[28,29] Analysis of T-cell-receptor expression has shown expansions of multiple clones in both CD4+ and CD8+ subsets of blood and joint,[30] with CD8+ expansions commonest in the joint. It may be that both subsets are involved in disease. In the ReA which frequently occurs in HIV-infected individuals in sub-Saharan Africa, the arthritis is associated with modest diminution in CD4+ T-cell counts rather than profound levels of CD4+ T-cell depletion,[31] suggesting that CD4+ T cells are required for arthritis—an observation in agreement with the B27 transgenic model.[32] The cytokines produced by synovial bacteria-specific T cells are generally proinflammatory, particularly interferon-gamma (IFNγ) and/or interleukin (IL)-17 produced by the Th1 or Th17 subsets of CD4+ T cells[33–35]; increased quantities of IL-17 have also been noted in ReA synovial fluid.[36]

HLA B27 is associated with the occurrence of ReA,[37,38] but strikingly with severe disease.[39] Patients with prolonged course, recurrent attacks, or evolution to chronic arthropathy are very likely to be B27+.[40] The B27+ patients also have activated neutrophils and enhanced monocyte production of tumour necrosis factor alpha (TNFα).[41,42] However, B27 is not necessary for ReA to develop, and ascertaining B27 status is not useful diagnostically, although it may help predict prognosis. How B27 acts remains frustratingly unclear. It is assumed, but not proven, that the role of HLA B27 is identical in all spondyloarthropathies. There are currently three main theories proposed for the role of HLA B27 in spondyloarthritis[43]: first, that it involves its classical function in presenting antigenic peptides to T cells, and that there is an 'arthritogenic' peptide which binds to B27: secondly, that HLA B27 is able to form heavy chain dimers which are surface expressed, interact with receptors (KIR and LILR) on lymphocytes and antigen-presenting cells, altering their function[44]; thirdly, that inefficient B27 heavy chain folding in the endoplasmic reticulum generates cellular stress which alters cytokine production, favouring proinflammatory responses, particularly those involving IL-23 and differentiation of IL-17-producing cells.[45,46] Recent genome-wide association studies (GWAS) have revealed a large number of genes associated with anklosing spondylitis (AS).[47] Several involve responses to IL-23 (especially the IL-23 receptor) and genes expressed by Th17 cells. In addition, ERAP-1 is an enzyme whose function is to trim antigenic peptides to the correct length for fitting into the groove of class I MHC molecules such as HLA B27. Importantly, an association between *ERAP1* polymorphisms and AS is confined to HLA B27+ patients.[48] Whether there is an association between ERAP-1 and ReA remains to be determined. Its association with AS points to the importance of the antigenic peptides which are both presented by HLA B27 and form an important part of its molecular structure. A hypomorphic allele of *ERAP1* is protective[49]; this would fit with either the 'arthritogenic' peptide hypothesis—fewer arthritogenic peptides would be generated—or with models which require efficient surface expression of HLA B27, e.g. for the generation of B27 heavy chain dimers.

Bacterial products are initially detected by the innate immune system, particularly the Toll-like receptors (TLR) expressed on phagocytic cells, and a polymorphism in TLR2 (*R753Q*) has been reported to be associated with acute salmonella-induced ReA, with 6/48 patients having this rare variant as compared to 0/27 patients infected by salmonella without developing arthritis and 2/91 healthy controls.[50] This finding needs confirmation in larger studies, but in principle polymorphisms in TLRs, or other receptors for bacteria products, which could alter cytokine production in response to peptidoglycan, lipopolysaccharide (LPS), or bacterial nucleic acids could play an important role in susceptibility to ReA.

Clinical features

Preceding illness

A history of urethritis (dysuria or discharge) or diarrhoea must be specifically sought for several reasons. The interval between these symptoms and the development of arthritis means that patients may not connect these apparently unrelated events. Moreover, preceding infection may be virtually asymptomatic—chlamydia infection in women is notoriously silent, and in men these symptoms or a sexual history are often not volunteered spontaneously. Of gastrointestinal infections, salmonella and shigella are likely to produce symptoms in those who develop ReA, whereas in yersinia-related arthritis many patients have subclinical or mild gastrointestinal symptoms.

Arthritis

ReA is usually an asymmetric oligoarthritis, generally involving fewer than six joints, with a tendency to affect the lower limbs preferentially. Some patients may have arthralgias at sites in addition to those affected by synovitis. Community surveys of patients infected by ReA-associated organisms also reveal patients with polyarticular arthralgia, but these tend not to present to rheumatologists since the symptoms are mild and resolve spontaneously. In rheumatology practice any joint can be affected, and a proportion of patients have monarthritis. Affected joints generally become rapidly hot and swollen, and large effusions can develop especially in the knee. The evolution of joint involvement is such as to make septic arthritis or crystal-induced arthritis likely differential diagnoses. There is a real possibility of patients being treated for a culture-negative septic arthritis if a full history is not obtained from the patient or careful examination made for extra-articular signs of ReA. The arthritis can have features seen in other forms of spondyloarthropathy. Dactylitis, resembling that seen in psoriatic arthritis, occurs in ReA, and many patients experience low back or buttock pain due to acute sacroiliitis. The arthritis is generally most severe in the first few weeks following its onset, followed by substantial improvement over the next few weeks. However, mild but significant symptoms often persist 6–12 months before full resolution. Patients need reassurance during this phase that complete resolution is still probable. In addition, not all patients experience a 'monophasic' disease and both exacerbations and involvement of new joints can occur, even in those in whom the disease eventually settles completely.

Extra-articular disease

One of the characteristic features of spondyloarthropathies is the presence of **enthesitis** (inflammation of ligamentous and tendinous insertions) and it has been argued that synovitis in spondyloarthropathies is secondary to enthesitis.[51] Whether or not this is so, the presence of enthesitis is often helpful in making a diagnosis of ReA, with the Achilles tendon insertion and plantar fascia the commonest sites of involvement. Enthesitis may be mild, particularly in relation to active synovitis at other sites, and so the patient may not report symptoms, particularly if not weightbearing. Other ligamentous insertions involving the pelvis and chest wall may be symptomatic, and some low back symptoms may represent enthesitis.

Conjunctivitis is a classical feature of ReA but is usually painless and often transitory. It may not be evident when the patient presents with arthritis, and a history should be sought from the patient (or relatives who may have noticed red eyes). Persistent eye inflammation and painful eyes raise the question of acute anterior uveitis, but this is much less common in ReA. It requires full ophthalmological assessment.

Skin and mucous membranes can be involved. Keratoderma blennorhagica is histologically identical to psoriasis, and most commonly seen on the soles of the feet, although it can also involve the hands and trunk. Its site, and the fact that it is painless, means that again it needs to be sought directly, since patients may not have noticed it. **Balanitis** is also asymptomatic and may not be readily apparent, particularly in the uncircumcised. The occurrence of balanitis, like urethritis, does not imply a genitourinary aetiology for the ReA. Ulcerative lesions in the mouth and soft palate are also seen but are usually asymptomatic. Lastly, erythema nodosum has been noted in ReA associated with yersinia.

In general, extra-articular disease is associated with severity of arthritis, a less favourable prognosis, and HLA B27 positivity. The most severe extra-articular manifestations are aortitis and cardiac conduction disorders but fortunately these are rare. Table 115.2 shows the frequency of joint and extra-articular involvement in a number of series of ReA patients.[52]

Differential diagnoses

Differential diagnoses are listed in Box 115.2. In patients who present with an acute arthritis, the principal differential diagnoses are septic arthritis and crystal arthropathies. Other forms of postinfectious arthritis enter the differential, particularly postgonococcal

Table 115.2 Frequency (%) of extra-articular signs in reactive arthritis[a]

Lesion	Enteric infection	Sexually acquired infection
Keratoderma and psoriaform lesions	1–2	10–30
Circinate balanitis	5–25; higher in shigella	40–70
Conjunctivitis	6–20; higher in shigella	25–40
Oral ulcers	2–5	10–30
Erythema nodosum	7 (mainly yersinia)	0
Reactive urethritis	10–30	N/A

[a]Data from Angulo and Espinoza[52] combined with other published series.

Box 115.2 Differential diagnosis of reactive arthritis

- Septic arthritis
- Postinfectious arthritis
  - Lyme disease
  - poststreptococcal or neisseria infection
  - viral arthritis
- Crystal arthropathies
- Other spondyloarthopathies
- Early rheumatoid arthritis
- Behçet's disease
- Sarcoidosis
- Trauma, sports injury

or postmeningococcal arthritis, along with arthritis due to streptococci and Lyme disease. Although streptococcal infection rarely gives rise to rheumatic fever, except under conditions of social deprivation, an inflammatory oligoarthritis strongly resembling ReA is seen,[53] but classical extra-articular features are not present. In subacute disease, it is sometimes difficult to distinguish ReA from other forms of spondyloarthropathy, particularly if there is no history of preceding infection and no laboratory evidence to implicate specific infections. The term 'undifferentiated spondyloarthropathy' is rightly applied to these cases, with the possibility that psoriasis or inflammatory bowel disease (IBD) will declare themselves as time goes on.

Laboratory investigations

Investigations are directed towards excluding the major differential diagnoses, and thereafter to establishing the organism responsible for triggering the disease.

General investigations

In acute ReA severe enough to present to hospital, there is usually a major acute-phase response (ESR >100, CRP 100–200 mg/litre) and neutrophilia. Other biochemical investigations are not generally helpful, although serum urate should be checked. Classical autoantibodies such as rheumatoid factor (RF) and anti-nuclear antibodies (ANA) are absent, and although positive anti-neutrophil cytoplasmic antibodies have been described, they are not diagnostically useful. The antibodies are not directed against proteinase-3 or myeloperoxidase, unlike those seen in granulomatosis with polyangiitis (Wegener's) and microscopic polyangiitis.

Microbiology

Tests to exclude septic arthritis or other forms of postinfectious arthritis

Microscopy, Gram stain, and culture of synovial fluid is the single most important investigation to diagnose septic arthritis, together with blood cultures and culture of any other possible site of infection, including throat swab for streptococci. Application of PCR techniques may establish the triggering agent in ReA (see below), but may also be helpful in the diagnosis of mycobacterial infection, borreliosis, and Whipple's disease. Antibody responses to strepto-coccal antigens, including both anti-streptolysin and anti-DNaseB, should be sought, along with antibodies to borrelia in patients who have been in endemic areas. Viral antibodies may also be checked, particularly IgM antibodies to parvovirus, Epstein–Barr virus (EBV), and cytomegalovirus (CMV). Note that IgG antibodies will very often be present since infection with these viruses is endemic, and so only IgM antibodies are diagnostically useful. In appropriate geographic regions antibodies to Ross river virus or chikungunya can also be measured.

Identification of ReA-associated organisms

An excellent account of microbiological tests useful in the diagnosis of ReA is available.[54] By definition, ReA and associated bacteria are not cultured from affected joints, but the organisms may be identi-fied by stool cultures in enteric arthritis, and cultures of swabs from the genitourinary tract or urine in chlamydia infection. Nucleic acid amplification techniques are now favoured for diagnosing *C. trachomatis* infection and avoid invasive swabs while maintain-ing high sensitivity. Their use should allow a higher proportion of patients with chlamydia-induced ReA to be positively diagnosed. *C. pneumoniae* can also be diagnosed by PCR on sputum. There has been interest in using PCR diagnostically in chlamydia-induced ReA to identify organisms in infected joints, but thus far reliable techniques have not emerged. Although some laboratories have reported that a high proportion of chlamydia-induced ReA cases are positive for the organism by PCR, the test can never establish 100% specificity. This is because, in populations in whom chlamy-dia infection is frequent, chlamydiae may well traffic to joints of those affected by e.g. rheumatoid disease in the same way that they do in ReA.

Serological techniques can also be used to establish preceding infection. Current chlamydia serology is unsatisfactory since there are difficulties in distinguishing antibodies to *C. trachomatis* and *C. pneumoniae*, and the incidence of antibodies to the latter can be very high in the general population. Specialized techniques meas-uring antibody bound to purified organisms, and comparing the titre of antibodies to *C. trachomatis* and *C. pneumoniae*, can estab-lish specificity, but are not used routinely. New techniques using recombinant chlamydial antigens may allow more specific and sen-sitive serological tests for chlamydial infection, but these are not yet in use.

There are also problems with the serology of enteric infections, mainly because certain populations have previously encountered salmonella and campylobacter in foods such as chicken and eggs, and developed antibodies. In acute disease, measurement of sal-monella-specific IgM (the Widal test), or IgM responses to other enteric organisms, can be useful but has low sensitivity. Since high titres of IgG antibodies to organisms such as salmonella or campy-lobacter are not uncommon in the general population, it is prefer-able to demonstrate a rising titre of IgG antibodies or high levels of persistent IgA antibodies to the organism of interest. IgA has a shorter half-life than IgG, so persistence of high titres of specific IgA antibodies is often taken to indicate persistent infection.

ReA-triggering organisms also elicit prominent T-cell-mediated responses and the possibility of these being useful diagnostically has been considered. The responses are most easily detectable in syno-vial fluid, but because they only demonstrate T-cell memory for the organism, they cannot provide more than supporting evidence that

a particular episode of arthritis is due to the organism recognized by synovial fluid T cells. They may have some negative diagnostic value—for instance, it would be very unusual for a patient to have chlamydia-triggered ReA without a T-cell response to chlamydia being detectable in the joint. However, as noted in discussion of PCR tests, patients with rheumatoid arthritis (RA) can incidentally become infected with ReA-associated organisms and will then have organism-specific T cells detectable in their affected joints.

In summary, for routine investigation of ReA, stool should be cultured, chlamydia sought by PCR, and antibodies to yersinia and camplyobacter measured. Other tests require further study for their validation.

Tissue typing

HLA B27 testing has no diagnostic value since ReA often occurs in B27-negative patients. However, it is still worth doing to help establish prognosis, since this is less favourable in B27+ patients. HLA B27+ patients may warrant earlier treatment with disease-modifying drugs (see below) or closer follow-up to detect relapse or chronic spondyloarthropathy.

Radiology

Radiological examination of acutely affected joints is not helpful in the diagnosis of ReA, but may aid in establishing differential diag-noses, for example, by showing chondrocalcinosis. Chest radio-graph may reveal hilar adenopathy in sarcoidosis, or occasionally in yersinia infection which can cause a sarcoid-like illness. Although sacroiliac joint involvement is common acutely in ReA, radio-graphic abnormality is not. MRI is a more sensitive indicator of enthesitis and/or synovitis in the sacroiliac joint. Ultrasonography can also demonstrate enthesitis and distinguish oedema of tendon and ligament insertions from bursitis. Bone isotope scintigraphy may also be useful to demonstrate joint inflammation, especially in the sacroiliac joints, and also enthesopathy, but has mainly been superseded by MRI. In patients in whom disease persists, radio-logical changes can develop, with erosion of affected joints, includ-ing the sacroiliac joints, and the formation of new bone, which can be seen as either periostitis in the hands and feet or spur formation at entheses such as the plantar ligament insertion. Erosions may also be present at these same sites. In chronic ReA, paravertebral ossification may be seen in the lumbar spine; unlike ankylosing spondylitis this is often asymmetric. Atlantoaxial subluxation has also been described in chronic ReA.

Treatment

Symptomatic treatment

Patients require conventional measures to treat acutely inflamed joints, including non-steroidal anti-inflammatory drugs (NSAIDs), joint aspiration with injection of depot steroid preparations (when septic arthritis has been excluded), together with analgesia and phys-iotherapy to maintain range of motion and regain the muscle power and bulk which is lost during acute inflammation. In severe disease, systemic corticosteroids may be used but injection of affected joints is preferable. Extra-articular disease does not call for specific treat-ment, with the exception of uveitis which requires topical steroids. Of the triggering infections, only chlamydia infection generally requires specific treatment in its own right, with conventional short-term antibiotic regimes using tetracyclines or azithromycin.

Specific treatment

Current opinion on the pathogenesis of ReA would suggest two specific treatment strategies. If disease is maintained by persistent infection and trafficking of triggering organisms to affected joints and entheses, long-term antibiotics should hasten resolution of the disease. On the other hand, if disease is mainly maintained by an aberrant immune response, triggered by infection but later directed against components of the joint, immunosuppressive treatment would be indicated. Unfortunately, evidence from therapeutic trials does not yet allow us to distinguish definitively between these hypotheses.

There have been several trials of prolonged doses of antibiotics in ReA. When tetracycline was used to treat episodes of non-gono-coccal urethritis very promptly, there was a decrease in the number of episodes of ReA, but in this instance treatment was administered prior to the onset of arthritis.[55] The first trial to treat established ReA using lymecycline did not show efficacy overall, but a subgroup of patients with chlamydia-induced arthritis had a decreased disease duration.[56] Patients with chronic yersinia infection, diagnosed by showing organisms in intestinal mucosa or gut lymphoid tissue, and with wider symptomatology than ReA, were reported to respond to ciprofloxacin in an uncontrolled trial. These findings prompted controlled trials but those in enteric ReA have shown no therapeutic advantage of 3 months' treatment with ciprofloxacin,[57–59] nor did a similar trial of azithromycin, which has activity against both enteric organisms and chlamydia, show benefit.[60] Likewise 4 months' doxycycline was no more effective than 10 days' in chlamydia-induced disease.[61] This does not necessarily imply that disease is not maintained by persistent infection, since organisms may be relatively resistant to ciprofloxacin or azithromycin when not actively dividing. This argument led to a recent trial aiming to target both bacterial gene transcription and protein synthesis using combinations of antibiotics—rifampicin and azithromycin/doxycycline for 6 months. The patients chosen had longstanding disease (>10 years) and had RT-PCR evidence of persistent chlamydia infection (*C. trachomatis* or *C. pneumoniae*). In a double blind placebo-controlled trial impressive improvements were noted at 6 months.[62] This intriguing result in a relatively small trial requires confirmation.

Disease-modifying agents used in rheumatoid disease have also been tested in ReA, although in many trials ReA patients have been included along with patients with other forms of spondyloarthropathy.[63] One difficulty in these trials is that the rate of spontaneous remission in ReA is high, so that large numbers of patients would need to be tested to have adequate power to show a therapeutic effect. If extrapolation from other forms of spondyloarthropathy is justified, both sulfasalazine and methotrexate should be useful, but the effect of sulfasalazine is relatively modest.[64] It is reasonable to withhold disease-modifying drugs for the first 3 months in ReA and reserve their use for those whose disease is not settling (particularly if they are B27+), or who have involvement of new joints. Therapies directed against TNFα, having proved useful in both AS and psoriatic arthritis, have been shown to be effective in patients with intractable chronic ReA,[65] with no evidence of recrudescence of infection by 'latent' triggering organisms. An antibody to IL-6 receptor has also recently been reported to be useful in such cases.[66]

Prognosis

Many patients with ReA are young, otherwise healthy, and used to an active lifestyle. To these individuals ReA, even when self-limiting, is a major life event, particularly since cases seen in hospital practice commonly take months to resolve. Patients therefore need considerable reassurance that there is an 80% chance of complete resolution of their symptoms within the first year, with a further 10% settling in the following year. Prognosis is less favourable in those who have disease severe enough to require hospitalization and who are B27+. Progression to chronic disease in 16% was recorded in one series, with recurrent attacks of reactive disease in a further 22%,[67] and some eventually have disease which resembles AS.[68] The tendency to trivialize the disease because its prognosis is generally so much better than that of RA needs to be resisted. Although many ReA patients may have future episodes of gastroenteritis or urethritis without recurrence of arthritis, it is advisable for patients to minimize their risk of recurrent infection, particularly younger patients who may need advice on foreign travel and barrier contraception.

Enteropathic arthropathy

Although ReA due to enteric infection falls within the definition of enteropathic arthritis, this section discusses forms of arthritis other than ReA which are associated with gut inflammation. These include others within the spondyloarthropathy group, along with the arthritis associated with coeliac disease, and Whipple's disease.

Spondyloarthropathies associated with gut inflammation

Crohn's disease and ulcerative colitis

The association between IBD and arthropathy has long been recognized.[69] Although estimates of the incidence of arthritis vary, several large series from different geographical areas suggest approximately 10% of IBD patients have peripheral arthritis, with a somewhat higher incidence in Crohn's disease as compared to ulcerative colitis. An additional proportion of patients (~5%) have axial disease indistinguishable from AS, while asymptomatic sacroiliitis is even commoner (15–20%). Arthritis in IBD is associated with other extragastrointestinal features, and is present in 30–60% of patients with uveitis or skin lesions such as erythema nodosum and pyoderma gangrenosum. Arthritis is also commonly accompanied by enthesopathy, as in other spondyloarthropathies. The idea of linkage between spondyloarthopathies and IBD is given greater credence by ileocolonoscopy studies which have shown that up to 60% of patients with ankylosing spondylitis or undifferentiated spondyloarthopathy have subclinical inflammatory lesions in the gut[70,71]; a proportion of these patients progress to overt clinical IBD. The situation has been further clarified by subclassification of the peripheral arthritis of IBD into patients with fewer than five involved joints (type I) and those with five or more involved joints (type II).[72] Type I patients mainly have asymmetric involvement of predominantly lower limb joints (often a monoarthritis, particularly at onset), whereas type II patients have symmetric polyarticular small joint involvement in a rheumatoid-like distribution. Further analysis suggests that only type I patients can be regarded as falling within the spondyloarthopathy group. Like ReA, 80% with type I arthritis have self-limiting disease and active arthritis is associated with relapse of IBD in 80%. In contrast, 80% of type II patients have persistent disease and a much less marked association between active arthritis and IBD relapse. These clinical observations are underpinned by the associations with the relatively rare MHC class II allele, *HLA DRB*0103*, seen in both type I arthritis (relative risk 12) and ReA due to enteric infection. The same allele has also been found to be increased in IBD patients with AS, or with IBD and uveitis. An association with B27 was also described, but this was weaker for type I disease than for ReA. In contrast, type II disease showed no association with either B27 or DRB*0103, but instead a weak association with HLA B44. The pathogenesis of the peripheral arthritis in IBD likely has many features in common with ReA. Whereas specific pathogens are required to provoke the gastrointestinal inflammation which produces ReA in the presence of susceptibility genes (HLA B27 and others), the same genes predispose to arthritis in response to the gastrointestinal inflammation of IBD. IBD is considered to be an aberrant response to normal gut bacteria—loss of tolerance of the host microbiome.[73] As in ReA, further genetic influences, again including B27, may lead to chronicity with established sacroiliitis and axial disease, rather than self-limiting peripheral arthritis. Unlike classical AS, HLA B27 is only found in 50% of the IBD patients with spondylitis, suggesting that other genetic factors can substitute for B27. In a different genetic background, other patterns of arthritis are seen, including the rheumatoid-like type II arthritis.

Treatment is directed at the underlying IBD, and for type I peripheral arthritis effective control of IBD allows resolution of arthritis. This is not the case for type II arthritis or for spondylitis, and these require treatment in their own right. NSAIDs and methotrexate, which are generally appropriate in the management of inflammatory arthritis, can both exacerbate IBD, although methotrexate is also sometimes used to treat IBD, and COX-2 selective NSAIDs are suggested not to have the same risks as non-selective drugs. In contrast, sulfasalazine, and more recently, anti-TNFα antibodies, have been found to be effective for both IBD and its associated arthritis.

Pouchitis

Patients treated by proctocolectomy for ulcerative colitis commonly have a pouch fashioned by ileo-anal anastomosis to avoid ileostomy. The pouch develops inflammation in 20–40% of patients, possibly due to bacterial overgrowth, and this 'pouchitis' responds to antibiotics, particularly metronidazole. A proportion of patients with pouchitis also develop an arthritis which has features of spondyloarthopathy including lower limb involvement, enthesitis, and sacroiliitis.[74,75] Other extra-articular features such as iritis and erythema nodosum have been described. The development of pouchitis and associated arthritis is much commoner in patients operated on for ulcerative colitis than in those requiring colectomy for familial polyposis, perhaps indicating a genetic predisposition to make inflammatory responses to gut flora. Some authors have described a close relationship between the severity of pouchitis and arthritis (similar to type I arthritis in IBD) with recovery following pouch removal in some cases. Clinically significant arthritis associated with pouchitis is relatively uncommon, but a larger proportion (30%) of patients complain of arthralgia involving hands and knees; in these cases a relationship with pouch inflammation is not evident.[76]

Coeliac disease

Inflammatory arthritis complicating coeliac disease has been recognized for two decades,[77] but is relatively rare. The disease is generally an oligo- or monoarthritis, with preferential involvement of lower limb joints. Lumbar spine and sacroiliac joint involvement have also been described, but there is no clear association with HLA B27.

In fact the genes which increase susceptibility to coeliac disease are those involved in other autoimmune disorders such as RA, type I diabetes, and autoimmune thyroid disease rather than those associated with spondyloarthritis.[78] The best evidence that the arthritis is causally related to coeliac disease, and not an incidental finding, is the observation that both gut and joint disease respond to a gluten-free diet. Joint symptoms can precede gastrointestinal symptoms; indeed, coeliac disease can be silent in one-third of cases with arthritis, so investigation of unexplained seronegative arthritis by measuring anti-endomysial antibodies is appropriate, followed by endoscopy and biopsy in antibody-positive patients. This approach is justified since untreated coeliac disease carries an increased risk of lymphoma. Note that measuring antibodies to gliadin is much less satisfactory since such antibodies are sometimes present in patients with polyclonal increases in immunoglobulins, such as those with RA. In keeping with genetic predisposition to various forms of autoimmunity, an increased incidence of coeliac disease (~6%) among patients with juvenile idiopathic arthritis (JIA) has been reported.[79]

Whipple's disease

Understanding of this disease was advanced enormously by the discovery of the causative organism, using the molecular approach of amplifying bacterial ribosomal RNA (rRNA) genes which have sequences which are conserved in all bacteria.[80] This allows the use of 'universal' primers which amplify rRNA from all bacteria. Sequencing the product allows particular bacteria to be identified since rRNA genes also possess species-specific sequences. In the case of the Whipple's bacillus, a previously undescribed unique sequence was identified in the rRNA PCR product, and consistently found in jejunal biopsies from Whipple's disease patients. The organism, named *Tropheryma whippelii*, is related to actinomycetes, and has now been cultured, though it grows very slowly. It is not uncommon in the environment, and can be found in normal individuals' saliva or duodenal secretions (but not normal jejunal biopsies). It does not usually establish infection, suggesting that Whipple's patients have some impairment of their immune response. Although bacteria have long been implicated in Whipple's disease, identification of a specific organism has allowed more accurate diagnosis and indicates that there are patients, including some with arthropathy, who do not have the histological changes in the gut previously required for diagnosis. PCR has shown the presence of the organism in the joints,[81] and culture from synovial fluid has also been achieved.[82]

Whipple's disease is a rare (incidence $1:10^6$) systemic disorder, and the commonest triad of symptoms is weight loss, diarrhoea, and arthralgia or arthritis.[83] Oligo- or polyarthritis are seen, often with involvement of large joints. Spondyloarthropathy features are generally absent, although a high frequency of HLA B27 has been observed in some series, and uveitis is seen. The arthritis can precede other features by up to 8 years, and PCR diagnosis may allow cases to be identified and treated before they develop systemic symptoms. Diagnosis can also be made by immunohistology using organism-specific antibodies. The diagnosis should be considered in patients with persistent seronegative oligoarthritis. The infection can also involve the central nervous system, heart valves, and lungs; treatment is with long courses of trimethoprim/sulphamethoxazole. Its efficacy can be monitored by determining whether patients remain PCR positive. These have persistent infection which may require a change in antibiotics. Given that some cases of Whipple's disease will not be recognized, especially in the absence of gut symptoms, such patients may be classified as seronegative RA and eventually receive TNFα-blocking drugs when they fail to respond to disease-modifying anti-rheumatic drugs (DMARDs). Since the disease is driven by an intracellular bacterium, inhibition of TNFα is potentially disastrous, and dissemination of the organism with severe endocarditis has been reported in these circumstances.[84]

References

1. Storey GO, Scott DL. Arthritis associated with venereal disease in nineteenth century London. *Clin Rheumatol* 1998;17(6):500–504.

2. Amor B, Dougados M, Mijiyawa M. Critères de classification des spondylarthropathies. *Rev Rhum Mal Ostéoartic* 1990;57:85–89.

3. Dougados M, van der Linden S, Juhlin R et al. The European Spondylarthropathy Study Group preliminary criteria for the classification of spondylarthropathy. *Arthritis Rheum* 1991;34(10):1218–1227.

4. Sieper J, Rudwaleit M, Baraliakos X et al. The Assessment of SpondyloArthritis international Society (ASAS) handbook: a guide to assess spondyloarthritis. *Ann Rheum Dis* 2009;68 Suppl 2:ii1–ii44.

5. Rudwaleit M, van der Heijde D, Landewe R et al. The Assessment of SpondyloArthritis international Society classification criteria for peripheral spondyloarthritis and for spondyloarthritis in general. *Ann Rheum Dis* 2011;70(1):25–31.

6. Kvien TK, Glennas A, Melby Kn et al. Reactive arthritis: incidence, triggering agents and clinical presentation. *J Rheumatol* 1994;21(1):115–122.

7. Kvien T, Glennas A, Melby K, Husby G. The natural history of reactive arthritis. *Rheumatology in Europe* 1995;24:15–19.

8. Telyatnikova N, Gaston JSH. Prior exposure to infection with Chlamydia pneumoniae can influence the T-cell-mediated response to Chlamydia trachomatis. *FEMS Immunol Med Microbiol* 2006;47(2):190–198.

9. Tran TM, Dorris ML, Satumtira N, Richardson JA, Taurog JD. Additional human beta-2 microglobulin curbs HLA-B27 heavy chain misfolding and promotes arthritis and spondylitisbut not colitis in male B27 transgenic rats. *Arthritis Rheum* 2005;52:S447.

10. Hannu T, Mattila L, Siitonen A, Leirisalo-Repo M. Reactive arthritis attributable to Shigella infection: a clinical and epidemiological nationwide study. *Ann Rheum Dis* 2005;64(4):594–598.

11. Granfors K, Jalkanen S, von Essen R et al. Yersinia antigens in synovial fluid cells from patients with reactive arthritis. *N Engl J Med* 1989;320:216–221.

12. Granfors K, Jalkanen S, Lindberg A et al. Salmonella lipopolysaccharide in synovial cells from patients with reactive arthritis. *Lancet* 1990;335:685–688.

13. Granfors K. Host-microbe interaction in reactive arthritis: Does HLA-B27 have a direct effect? *J Rheumatol* 1998;25(9):1659–1661.

14. Nikkari S, Rantakokko K, Ekman P et al. Salmonella-triggered reactive arthritis: use of polymerase chain reaction, immunocytochemical staining, and gas chromatography-mass spectrometry in the detection of bacterial components from synovial fluid. *Arthritis Rheum* 1999;42(1):84–89.

15. Gaston JSH, Cox C, Granfors K. Clinical and experimental evidence for persistent Yersinia infection in reactive arthritis. *Arthritis Rheum* 1999;42(10):2239–2242.

16. Taylor-Robinson D, Gilroy C, Thomas B, Keat A. Detection of *Chlamydia trachomatis* DNA in joints of reactive arthritis patients by polymerase chain reaction. *Lancet* 1992;340:81–82.

17. Schumacher H, Arayssi T, Branigan P et al. PCR study for bacterial DNA in normal synovium. *Arthritis Rheum* 1997;40:S269.

18. Nanagara R, Li F, Beutler A, Hudson A, Schumacher HR, Jr. Alteration of Chlamydia trachomatis biologic behavior in synovial membranes. Suppression of surface antigen production in reactive arthritis and Reiter's syndrome. *Arthritis Rheum* 1995 Oct;38(10):1410–1417.

19. Salmi M, Jalkanen S. Human leukocyte subpopulations from inflamed gut bind to joint vasculature using distinct sets of adhesion molecules. *J Immunol* 2001;166(7):4650–4657.

20. Gaston JSH, Life PF, Merilahti Palo R et al. Synovial T lymphocyte recognition of organisms that trigger reactive arthritis. *Clin Exp Immunol* 1989;76:348–353.

21. Sieper J, Braun J, Wu P, Kingsley G. T-cells are responsible for the enhanced synovial cellular immune response to triggering antigen in reactive arthritis. *Clin Exp Immunol* 1993;91(1):96–102.

22. Goodall JC, Yeo G, Huang M, Raggiaschi R, Gaston JSH. Identification of Chlamydia trachomatis antigens recognized by human CD4+ T lymphocytes by screening an expression library. *Eur J Immunol* 2001;31:1513–1522.

23. Mertz AK, Wu P, Sturniolo T et al. Multispecific CD4+ T cell response to a single 12-mer epitope of the immunodominant heat-shock protein 60 of Yersinia enterocolitica in Yersinia-triggered reactive arthritis: overlap with the B27-restricted CD8 epitope, functional properties, and epitope presentation by multiple DR alleles. *J Immunol* 2000;164(3):1529–1537.

24. Gaston J, Life P, Bailey L, Bacon P. *In vitro* responses to a 65kD mycobacterial protein by synovial T cells from inflammatory arthritis patients. *J Immunol* 1989;143:2594–2600.

25. Hermann E, Lohse AW, van der Zee R et al. Synovial fluid derived Yersinia reactive T cells responding to human 65 kDa heat shock protein and heat stressed antigen presenting cells. *Eur J Immunol* 1991;21(9):2139–2143.

26. Thiel A, Wu P, Lanowska M et al. Identification of immunodominant CD4+ T cell epitopes in patients with Yersinia-induced reactive arthritis by cytometric cytokine secretion assay. *Arthritis Rheum* 2006;54(11):3583–3590.

27. Deane KH, Jecock RM, Pearce JH, Gaston JS. Identification and characterization of a DR4-restricted T cell epitope within chlamydia heat shock protein 60. *Clin Exp Immunol* 1997;109(3):439–445.

28. Appel H, Kuon W, Kuhne M et al. Use of HLA-B27 tetramers to identify low-frequency antigen-specific T cells in Chlamydia-triggered reactive arthritis. *Arthritis Res Ther* 2004;6(6):R521–R534.

29. Matyszak MK, Gaston JS. Chlamydia trachomatis-specific human CD8+ T cells show two patterns of antigen recognition. *Infect Immun* 2004;72(8):4357–4367.

30. Allen RL, Gillespie GMA, Hall F et al. Multiple T cell expansions are found in the blood and synovial fluid of patients with reactive arthritis. *J Rheumatol* 1997;24(9):1750–1757.

31. Njobvu P, McGill P. Human immunodeficiency virus related reactive arthritis in Zambia. *J Rheumatol* 2005;32(7):1299–1304.

32. Taurog JD, Dorris ML, Satumtira N et al. Spondylarthritis in HLA-B27/human beta2-microglobulin-transgenic rats is not prevented by lack of CD8. *Arthritis Rheum* 2009;60(7):1977–1984.

33. Schlaak J, Hermann E, Ringhoffer M et al. Predominance of Th1 type T cells in synovial fluid of patients with Yersinia induced reactive arthritis. *Eur J Immunol* 1992;22:2771–2776.

34. Thiel A, Wu PH, Lauster R, Braun J, Radbruch A, Sieper J. Analysis of the antigen-specific T cell response in reactive arthritis by flow cytometry. *Arthritis Rheum* 2000;43(12):2834–2842.

35. Shen H, Goodall JC, Gaston JSH. Frequency and phenotype of T helper 17 cells in peripheral blood and synovial fluid of patients with reactive arthritis. *J Rheumatol* 2010;37(10):2096–2099.

36. Singh AK, Misra R, Aggarwal A. Th-17 associated cytokines in patients with reactive arthritis/undifferentiated spondyloarthropathy. *Clin Rheumatol* 2011;30(6):771–776.

37. Aho K, Ahvonen P, Lassus A, Sievers K, Tiilikainen A. HL-A antigen 27 and reactive arthritis. *Lancet* 1973;ii:157–159.

38. Brewerton DA, Caffrey M, Nicholls A et al. Reiter's disease and HL-A 27. *Lancet* 1973;2(7836):996–998.

39. Ekman P, Kirveskari J, Granfors K. Modification of disease outcome in Salmonella-infected patients by HLA-B27. *Arthritis Rheum* 2000;43(7):1527–1534.

40. Leirisalo-Repo M, Helenius P, Hannu T et al. Long-term prognosis of reactive salmonella arthritis. *Ann Rheum Dis* 1997 Sep;56(9):516–520.

41. Anttonen K, Orpana A, Leirisalo-Repo M, Repo H. Aberrant TNF secretion by whole blood in healthy subjects with a history of reactive

arthritis: time course in adherent and non-adherent cultures. *Ann Rheum Dis* 2006;65(3):372–378.

42. Kuuliala K, Orpana A, Leirisalo-Repo M, Repo H. Neutrophils of healthy subjects with a history of reactive arthritis show enhanced responsiveness, as defined by CD11b expression in adherent and non-adherent whole blood cultures. *Rheumatology* (Oxford) 2007;46(6):934–937.

43. Gaston JSH. Mechanisms of disease: the immunopathogenesis of spondyloarthropathies. *Nat Clin Pract Rheumatol* 2006;2(7):383–392.

44. Kollnberger S, Bowness P. The role of B27 heavy chain dimer immune receptor interactions in spondyloarthritis. *Adv Exp Med Biol* 2009;649: 277–285.

45. DeLay ML, Turner MJ, Klenk EI et al. HLA-B27 misfolding and the unfolded protein response augment interleukin-23 production and are associated with Th17 activation in transgenic rats. *Arthritis Rheum* 2009;60(9):2633–2643.

46. Goodall JC, Wu C, Zhang Y et al. Endoplasmic reticulum stress-induced transcription factor, CHOP, is crucial for dendritic cell IL-23 expression. *Proc Natl Acad Sci U S A* 2010;107:17698–17703.

47. Reveille JD, Sims AM, Danoy P et al. Genome-wide association study of ankylosing spondylitis identifies non-MHC susceptibility loci. *Nat Genet* 2010;42(2):123–127.

48. Evans DM, Spencer CC, Pointon JJ et al. Interaction between ERAP1 and HLA-B27 in ankylosing spondylitis implicates peptide handling in the mechanism for HLA -B27 in disease susceptibility. *Nat Genet* 2011;43(8):761–767.

49. Kochan G, Krojer T, Harvey D et al. Crystal structures of the endoplasmic reticulum aminopeptidase-1 (ERAP1) reveal the molecular basis for N-terminal peptide trimming. *Proc Natl Acad Sci U S A* 2011;108(19): 7745–7750.

50. Tsui FW, Xi N, Rohekar S et al. Toll-like receptor 2 variants are associated with acute reactive arthritis. *Arthritis Rheum* 2008;58(11):3436–3438.

51. McGonagle D, Lories RJU, Tan AL, Benjamin M. The concept of a 'synovio-enthesal complex' and its implications for understanding joint inflammation and damage in psoriatic arthritis and beyond. *Arthritis Rheum* 2007;56(8):2482–2491.

52. Angulo J, Espinoza L. The spectrum of skin, mucosa and other extra-articular manifestations. *Bailliere's Clin Rheumatol* 1998;12(4):649–664.

53. Deighton C. beta-Haemolytic Streptococci and Reactive Arthritis in Adults. *Ann Rheum Dis* 1993;52(6):475–482.

54. Wollenhaupt J, Schnarr S, Kuijpers JG. Bacterial antigens in reactive arthritis and spondarthritis. Rational use of laboratory testing in diagnosis and follow-up. *Bailliere's Clin Rheumatol* 1998;12(4):627–647.

55. Bardin T, Enel C, Cornelis F et al. Antibiotic treatment of venereal disease and Reiter's syndrome in a Greenland population. *Arthritis Rheum* 1992;35:190–194.

56. Lauhio A, Leirisalo Repo M, Lahdevirta J, Sikku P, Repo H. Double-blind, placebo-controlled study of three-month treatment with lymecycline in reactive arthritis with special reference to chlamydia arthritis. *Arthritis Rheum* 1991;34:6–14.

57. Sieper J, Fendler C, Laitko S et al. No benefit of long-term ciprofloxacin treatment in patients with reactive arthritis and undifferentiated oligoarthritis—A three-month, multicenter, double-blind, randomized, placebo-controlled study. *Arthritis Rheum* 1999;42(7):1386–1396.

58. Wakefield D, McCluskey P, Verma M et al. Ciprofloxacin treatment does not influence course or relapse rate of reactive arthritis and anterior uveitis. *Arthritis Rheum* 1999;42(9):1894–1897.

59. YliKerttula T, Luukkainen R, YliKerttula U et al. Effect of a three month course of ciprofloxacin on the outcome of reactive arthritis. *Ann Rheum Dis* 2000;59(7):565–570.

60. Kvien TK, Gaston JS, Bardin T et al. Three month treatment of reactive arthritis with azithromycin: a EULAR double blind, placebo controlled study. *Ann Rheum Dis* 2004;63(9):1113–1119.

61. Putschky N, Pott HG, Kuipers JG et al. Comparing 10-day and 4-month doxycycline courses for treatment of Chlamydia trachomatis-reactive arthritis: a prospective, double-blind trial. *Ann Rheum Dis* 2006;65(11):1521–1524.

62. Carter JD, Espinoza LR, Inman RD et al. Combination antibiotics as a treatment for chronic Chlamydia-induced reactive arthritis: a double-blind, placebo-controlled, prospective trial. *Arthritis Rheum* 2010;62(5):1298–1307.

63. Dougados M, Vanderlinden S, Leirisalorepo M et al. Sulfasalazine in the treatment of spondylarthropathy: A randomized, multicenter, double-blind, placebo-controlled study. *Arthritis Rheum* 1995;38(5): 618–627.

64. Egsmose C, Hansen TM, Andersen LS et al. Limited effect of sulphasalazine treatment in reactive arthritis. A randomised double blind placebo controlled trial. *Ann Rheum Dis* 1997;56(1):32–36.

65. Meyer A, Chatelus E, Wendling D et al. Safety and efficacy of anti-tumor necrosis factor alpha therapy in ten patients with recent-onset refractory reactive arthritis. *Arthritis Rheum* 2011;63(5):1274–1280.

66. Tanaka T, Kuwahara Y, Shima Y et al. Successful treatment of reactive arthritis with a humanized anti-interleukin-6 receptor antibody, tocilizumab. *Arthritis Rheum.* 2009;61(12):1762–1764.

67. Leirisalo-Repo M. Prognosis, course of disease, and treatment of the spondyloarthropathies. *Rheum Dis Clin North Am* 1998;24(4): 737–751, viii.

68. Kaarela K, Jantti JK, Kotaniemi KM. Similarity between chronic reactive arthritis and ankylosing spondylitis.A 32-35-year follow-up study. *Clin Exp Rheumatol* 2009;27(2):325–328.

69. Haslock I, Wright V. The musculoskeletal complications of Crohn's disease. *Medicine* 1973;52:217–225.

70. Leirisalorepo M, Turunen U, Stenman S, Helenius P, Seppala K. High frequency of silent inflammatory bowel disease in spondylarthropathy. *Arthritis Rheum* 1994;37(1):23–31.

71. Mielants H, Veys E, Cuvelier C, De Vos M. Course of gut inflammation in spondylarthropathies and therapeutic consequences. *Baillieres Clin Rheumatol* 1996;10:147–164.

72. Orchard T, Wordsworth B, Jewell D. Peripheral arhropathies in inflammatory bowel disease: their articular distribution and natural history. *Gut* 1998;42:387–391.

73. Kaser A, Zeissig S, Blumberg RS. Inflammatory bowel disease. *Annu Rev Immunol* 2010;28:573–621.

74. Abi Karam G, Awada H, Nasr F, Uthman I. Ileal pouchitis and arthritis. *Semin Arthritis Rheum* 2003;33(3):215.

75. Balbir-Gurman A, Schapira D, Nahir M. Arthritis related to ileal pouchitis following total proctocolectomy for ulcerative colitis. *Semin Arthritis Rheum* 2001;30(4):242–428.

76. Thomas PD, Keat AC, Forbes A, Ciclitira PJ, Nicholls RJ. Extraintestinal manifestations of ulcerative colitis following restorative proctocolectomy. *Eur J Gastroenterol Hepatol* 1999;11(9):1001–1005.

77. Bourne J, Kumar P, Huskisson E et al. Arthritis and coeliac disease. *Ann Rheum Dis* 1992;44:592–598.

78. Lettre G, Rioux JD. Autoimmune diseases: insights from genome-wide association studies. *Hum Mol Genet.* 2008;17(R2):R116–R121.

79. Stagi S, Giani T, Simonini G, Falcini F. Thyroid function, autoimmune thyroiditis and coeliac disease in juvenile idiopathic arthritis. *Rheumatology* (Oxford) 2005;44(4):517–520.

80. Relman DA, Schmidt TM, MacDermott RP, Falkow S. Identification of the uncultured bacillus of Whipple's disease. *New Engl J Med* 1992;327:293–301.

81. O'Duffy JD, Griffing WL, Li CY, Abdelmalek MF, Persing DH. Whipple's arthritis—Direct detection of Tropheryma whippelii in synovial fluid and tissue. *Arthritis Rheum* 1999;42(4):812–817.

82. Puechal X, Fenollar F, Raoult D. Cultivation of Tropheryma whipplei from the synovial fluid in Whipple's arthritis. *Arthritis Rheum* 2007;56(5):1713–1718.

83. Schneider T, Moos V, Loddenkemper C et al. Whipple's disease: new aspects of pathogenesis and treatment. *Lancet Infect Dis* 2008;8(3): 179–190.

84. Ansemant T, Celard M, Tavernier C et al. Whipple's disease endocarditis following anti-TNF therapy for atypical rheumatoid arthritis. *Joint Bone Spine* 2010;77(6):622–623.

Arthropathies primarily occurring in childhood

CHAPTER 116

Juvenile idiopathic arthritis

Eileen Baildam

Introduction

Juvenile idiopathic arthritis (JIA) is the current terminology for chronic arthritis in childhood that is not related to another multisystem disorder.[1] JIA is the most common chronic arthritis in childhood with an annual incidence of 1/10 000 in the United Kingdom, with reports from elsewhere varying from 2 to 20 per 100 000 and published prevalences of 16 to 150/100 000.[1-5] JIA is currently defined as arthritis of unknown aetiology beginning before the child's 17th birthday and persisting for at least six 6 weeks and where known causes have been excluded. The term JIA encompasses a heterogeneous group of conditions with variable clinical features and prognosis. The term JIA is also used for patients who reach adulthood and aims to emphasize the difference from adult-onset rheumatoid arthritis (RA).[1-5] It is known that many patients have ongoing problems into adulthood and although lasting disease remission may occur in some patients, as many as 50% of children will go into adult life with ongoing, active disease.[6] A recent multicentre study by Wallace 2005 illustrated the relapsing and remitting nature of the disease.[7] In this study 196 of 437 JIA patients followed for 7 years achieved a 1 year period without any active disease features were taking medication. However, less than 20% had two consecutive years without disease related symptoms and only 4% had a 5 year disease-free period.[7]

JIA affects more girls than boys, although the gender distribution varies with different subgroups; e.g. in the oligoarticular, polyarticular and psoriatic subtypes the gender ratio is 2:1 females to males although it is more equal in systemic JIA and there are more boys affected in the enthesitis-related arthritis (ERA) group.[3] Notably, in patients with associated uveitis, females are more affected.[8] The management of JIA requires specialist multidisciplinary expertise and increasingly the approach is early and aggressive intervention with potent immunosuppressive treatments. Details about management, treatment, outcomes and outcome measures are given elsewhere in this textbook.

Differential diagnosis of juvenile idiopathic arthritis

The differential diagnosis of JIA is broad (Box 116.1). The diagnosis is one of exclusion requiring careful clinical assessment, knowledge of normal development, and judicious use and interpretation of investigations. Serious and potentially life-threatening conditions

---

Box 116.1 The differential diagnosis of pain in childhood

Life-threatening conditions
- Malignancy (leukaemia, lymphoma, bone tumour)
- Sepsis (septic arthritis, osteomyelitis)
- Non-accidental injury

Joint pain with no swelling
- Hypermobility syndromes
- Idiopathic pain syndromes (reflex sympathetic dystrophy, fibromyalgia)
- Orthopaedic syndromes (e.g. Osgood–Schlatter disease, Perthes' disease)
- Metabolic (e.g. hypothyroidism, lysosomal storage diseases)

Joint pain with swelling
- Trauma
- Infection
- Septic arthritis and osteomyelitis (viral, bacterial, mycobacterial)
  - Reactive arthritis (post-enteric, sexually acquired)
  - Infection related (rheumatic fever, post-vaccination)
- Juvenile idiopathic arthritis
- Arthritis-related inflammatory bowel disease
- Connective tissue diseases (systemic lupus erythematosus, scleroderma, dermatomyositis, vasculitis)
- Sarcoidosis
- Metabolic (e.g. osteomalacia, cystic fibrosis, lysosomal disorders)
- Haematological (e.g. haemophilia, haemoglobinopathy)
- Tumour (benign and malignant)
- Chromosomal (e.g. Down's related arthritis)
- Autoinflammatory syndromes (e.g. periodic syndromes, chronic recurrent multifocal osteomyelitis)
- Developmental/congenital (e.g. spondyloepiphyseal dysplasia)

need to be considered (including infection, malignancy, and non-accidental injury); infections must be considered in the context of the immunocompromised and geographical areas where certain infections are endemic (e.g. Lyme disease and rheumatic fever). The reader is directed to other chapters in the textbook (Chapters 1, 5, 12–14, 99) for further information. Misunderstandings about the nature of pain in JIA, the misplaced expectation that children present with pain, and that normal investigations exclude the diagnosis are a cause of many missed or delayed diagnoses.[9] Conversely, many children with chronic musculoskeletal pain are misdiagnosed as having arthritis. In childhood, infective disease is much more frequent, and genetic disorders, immune deficiency states, and metabolic disorders are more commonly diagnosed than in adults. Comorbidity can associate with arthritis, e.g. children with chromosomal disorders (such as Down's syndrome, Turner's syndrome, velocardiofacial syndrome) and inflammatory bowel disease (IBD) have an increased risk of inflammatory arthritis.[10–14]

Early diagnosis of JIA rests on suspicion and awareness that young children and especially preverbal children, may present without apparent pain. Presentations may be vague and based on observations from parents or carers (such as limp) or a change in behaviour, mood, or avoidance of activities. Joint swelling can be difficult to detect especially if the changes are symmetrical. Examination often reveals joint involvement that is seemingly asymptomatic. Investigations including acute-phase reactants are often normal and radiographs are usually normal in early disease. Increasingly ultrasound is used, albeit there is a lack of standardized assessment and interpretation of normal and abnormal changes in the growing joint. Autoantibodies are not diagnostic; anti-nuclear antibodies (ANA) may be detected in many children with transient illness and also normal healthy children. Rheumatoid factor (RF) is invariably negative in JIA and again is not diagnostic. However, in the presence of JIA, autoantibodies are useful regarding prognosis; ANA increase the risk of uveitis and RF associates with a guarded prognosis. The absence of definite joint swelling should not discount a potential diagnosis of JIA; referral for specialist opinion from paediatric rheumatology is advised, and especially before contemplating invasive procedures (such as arthroscopy, synovial biopsy, or MRI), which are invariably not necessary to confirm the diagnosis. If MRI is required, then gadolinium should be given as enhancement is helpful to detect synovitis.

Definitions, classification criteria, and diagnostic criteria

Box 116.2 and Table 116.1[1,15] summarize the International League of Associations for Rheumatology (ILAR) classification of JIA, clinical features, definitions, and exclusion criteria for each subtype.[16–18] The subtypes are largely based on clinical features and in clinical practice some children are unclassifiable; for example, a patient with both systemic-onset JIA and psoriasis. The ILAR criteria have replaced previous criteria and are used internationally but have not been validated prospectively.

Oligoarticular juvenile idiopathic arthritis

This is the most common presentation of JIA and further subdivided into persistent and extended oligoarticular disease by the course (Box 116.2 and Box 116.3). Oligoarticular JIA affects up

---

Box 116.2 ILAR classification of juvenile idiopathic arthritis subtypes

Oligoarthritis—arthritis of 4 or fewer joints within the first 6 months

i Persistent—affecting not more than 4 joints throughout the disease process

ii Extended—extending to affect more than 4 joints after the first 6 months

Polyarthritis—arthritis of 5 or more joints within the first 6 months

Subdivided according to presence of rheumatoid factor (RF)

i RF-positive

ii RF-negative

Systemic arthritis—arthritis with or preceded by quotidian (daily) fever for at least 3 days, accompanied by one or more of:

1 Evanescent erythematous rash

2 Lymphadenopathy

3 Hepatomegaly and/or splenomegaly conditions

4 Serositis

(Mandatory exclusion of infective and malignant; arthritis may not be present early in course)

Psoriatic arthritis—arthritis and psoriasis or arthritis with at least 2 of:

1 Dactylitis

2 Nail pitting or onycholysis

3 Psoriasis in first-degree relative

Enthesitis-related arthritis—arthritis and enthesitis or arthritis or enthesitis with 2 of:

1 Sacroiliac joint tenderness of inflammatory lumbosacral pain

2 HLA B27 antigen

3 Onset after age 6 years in a male

4 Acute (symptomatic) anterior uveitis

5 History of HLA B27-associated disease in a first-degree relative

Undifferentiated arthritis—arthritis that fulfils criteria in no or more than two of the above categories

Adapted from Petty et al.[1]

---

to 50–60% of JIA cases[1,19–20]; the majority are girls (80%) with a peak age of onset in early childhood (1–3 years of age). The onset may be insidious and asymptomatic and blood tests may be normal, leading to a delay in diagnosis. However, the joint may be stiff especially in the morning and after rest, and this may lead to limping in lower limb joints or reluctance to push up on an arm in upper limb joints. The joint may feel slightly warm and may be swollen with a reduced range of movements, but these findings may be subtle and difficult to detect (especially in toddlers). Knees and ankles (Figure 116.1) are the most commonly affected joints and

Table 116.1 Summary of clinical features of juvenile idiopathic arthritis (JIA) subtypes

JIA subtype	Clinical features	%	Onset	Gender ratio (female:male)	Uveitis risk
Systemic-onset JIA	Fever, rash, and arthritis. Arthritis may be absent at presentation	4–17	Throughout childhood and in adults	1:1	Very low
Oligoarticular JIA	≤4 joints affected. Monoarthritis most frequent	27–60	Early childhood peak 2–4 years	5:1	High
Persistent oligo JIA	Disease remains oligoarticular at 6 months from onset and throughout its course	(40)			High
Extended oligo JIA	Oligoarticular at 6 months from onset and then subsequent polyarticular extension	(20)			The highest
Polyarticular JIA	Affecting ≥5 joints within the first 6 months from onset				Significant
RF-positive polyarticular JIA	Polyarticular arthritis and most like adult-onset RA	2–7	Late childhood or early adolescence into adulthood	3:1	Low
RF-negative polyarticular JIA	RF polyarticular disease	11–30	Early peak 2–4 years and late peak 6–12 years	3:1	Significant
Psoriatic arthritis	Can be diagnosed without signs of psoriasis, with arthritis and at least 2 of dactylitis, nail pitting or oncholysis, psoriasis in a first-degree relative	2–11		1:1	Significant
ERA	Arthritis and enthesitis or arthritis or enthesitis with at least 2 of: sacroiliac joint tenderness or inflammatory lumbosacral pain (or both), HLA B27-positive, onset in boy over 6 years, acute anterior uveitis, HLA B27-associated disease[a] in a first-degree relative. Spondylitis rare in childhood. Terminology ankylosing spondylitis in adulthood	1–11		1:7	Usually acute anterior uveitis but may be mixed
Unclassified		11–21			Moderate

ERA, enthesitis-related arthritis; JIA, juvenile idiopathic arthritis; RA, rheumatoid arthritis. RF, rheumatoid factor.
[a]Ankylosing spondylitis, enthesitis-related arthritis, sacroileitis with inflammatory bowel disease, Reiter's syndrome, or acute anterior uveitis.
Adapted from the 2001 Edmonton Revision of Durban Criteria.[1]

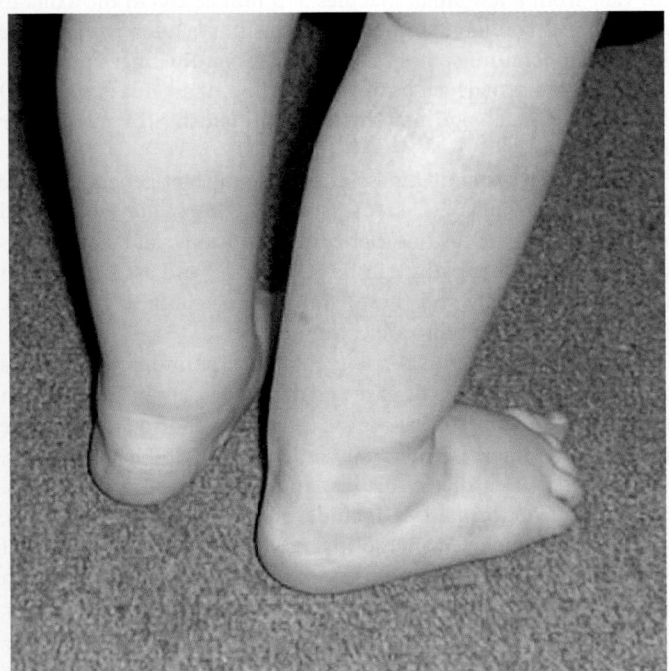

Fig. 116.1 Swollen ankles in oligo juvenile idiopathic arthritis.

50% present with a monoarthritis.[21–23] However most joints can be involved, including the temporomandibular joint (TMJ). The disease can be relatively mild and self-resolving or remitting permanently after a single intra-articular steroid injection. Repeated injections may be required and there is a low threshold for use of methotrexate and biologics, especially with extended disease. In approximately 50% of cases there will be an evolution to extended oligoarticular disease where after 6 months from onset 5 or more joints become involved.[21,22]

Many cases have a positive anti-nuclear factor (up to 85%) and many will develop uveitis. Although uveitis may occur in most types of JIA, numerically the majority of cases will be in the oligoarticular subtype and the risk is highest in the young girls with a positive anti-nuclear factor. Sequelae of long-standing inflammation of joints in oligo JIA include overgrowth and subsequent premature fusion of the epiphyses. Involvement of the knee, for example, may result in unequal leg lengths leading to secondary scoliosis, and prominent bony enlargement with genu valgum. At other sites uncontrolled inflammation can result in inequality of digit length, micrognathia, and flexion contractures. Joint damage and functional limitation are much less common with modern approaches to treatment but are still seen and usually reflect delay in access to specialist care.

Juvenile idiopathic arthritis involving multiple joints

Many types of arthritis in childhood involve multiple joints (defined as ≥5 joints). This can be seen in both types of polyarticular JIA (RF positive or negative). In systemic-onset JIA with a polyarticular course there is sometimes resolution of the systemic features after the first illness flare, such that the disease course is otherwise very like a RF-negative JIA. Extended oligoarticular JIA involves five or more joints but only after the first 6 months of initial illness where up to four joints have been involved. There is a high risk of associated uveitis in many of the polyarticular types of JIA as well as in oligoarticular disease. Polyarticular involvement is also seen in psoriatic arthritis and in ERA. Constitutional symptoms of fatigue, morning stiffness, poor appetite, anaemia, and raised inflammatory markers do occur. If gastrointestinal features are prominent it is important to exclude coeliac disease and IBD, both of which can have associated arthritis which may precede the bowel symptoms. There is, conversely, an increased risk of coeliac disease in association with JIA also. If fever is a major feature then systemic JIA must be considered.

Polyarticular JIA is subdivided into RF-positive (with positive results on two tests measured at least 6 weeks apart) or RF-negative polyarticular JIA. These subtypes affect 25–40% of JIA cases.[1,19,20] All joints can be involved in polyarticular JIA and in many cases most joints are simultaneously affected. Cervical spine and TMJ disease often coexist. Joints may be swollen (Figures 116.2 and 116.3) or simply painful and tender with reduction in function (this is so-called 'dry synovitis'). RF-positive polyarticular JIA accounts for only 5–10% of JIA and resembles adult-onset RA with a guarded prognosis and propensity for nodule formation. Disease onset is typically in children older than 8 years but more common in adolescence, with 90% being girls. The exact role of anti-citrullinated protein/peptide antibodies (ACPA) in polyarticular JIA is unclear in contrast to adult RA. RF-negative polyarticular JIA may be anti-nuclear factor positive and in either case there is an increased risk of uveitis.

Systemic-onset juvenile idiopathic arthritis

Systemic-onset juvenile idiopathic arthritis (SJIA) is increasingly perceived as an autoinflammatory disorder,[23,24] accounts for

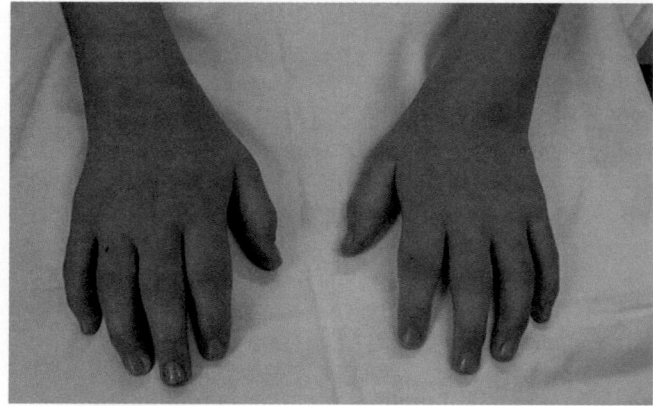

Fig. 116.3 Swollen fingers and wrists in polyarticular juvenile idiopathic arthritis.

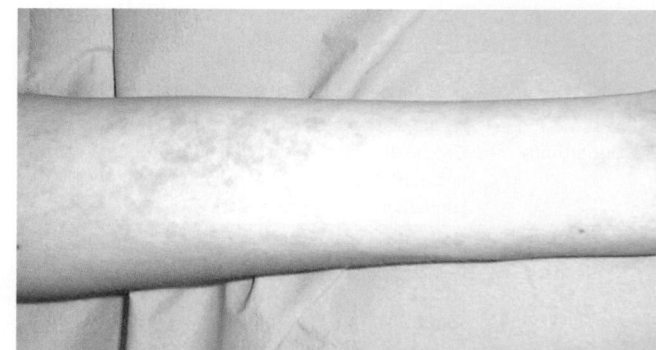

Fig. 116.4 Rash in systemic juvenile idiopathic arthritis.

approximately 10% of JIA,[25] and is characterized by a fever with a daily pattern of one or more regular fever spikes with a subnormal or hypothermic dip after spikes.

There is a characteristic systemic rash (Figure 116.4) which comes and goes, is maculopapular, salmon pink, often pruritic, and can vary from a few small macules 3–5 mm across in the axilla to a widespread confluent and urticarial rash. It is often worse at the time of temperature spikes or in the evening. Koebner's phenomenon (where a rash develops in a scratch line, or an area of pressure) is a useful clinical sign may help to distinguish SJIA from other febrile illnesses.

Features of a systemic illness include significant general malaise with arthralgia, myalgia, serositis causing chest and abdominal pain from pleural effusions, pericardial effusions, and sterile peritonitis. Lymphadenopathy can be generalized and associated with hepatosplenomegaly and these lymph nodes can also be painful. Headaches and irritability are common.

Although pleural effusions are common, pulmonary disease is rare, but interstitial lung disease and deranged pulmonary function tests have been reported.[26] Rare radiographic abnormalities include transient pneumonitis, interstitial reticular and nodular infiltrates, pleural and pericardial effusions, and patchy pleural infiltrates. Pathological abnormalities include pulmonary haemosiderosis, lymphoid follicular bronchiolitis, and lymphocytic interstitial pneumonitis. Arthritis of the cricoarytenoid joints can present with hoarseness or stridor (as can occur in polyarticular disease). Severe chest pain may be caused by pericarditis and may lead to tamponade. Chronic and constricting pericarditis is rare.[27,28] Clinically apparent myocarditis is rare (but potentially fatal without urgent

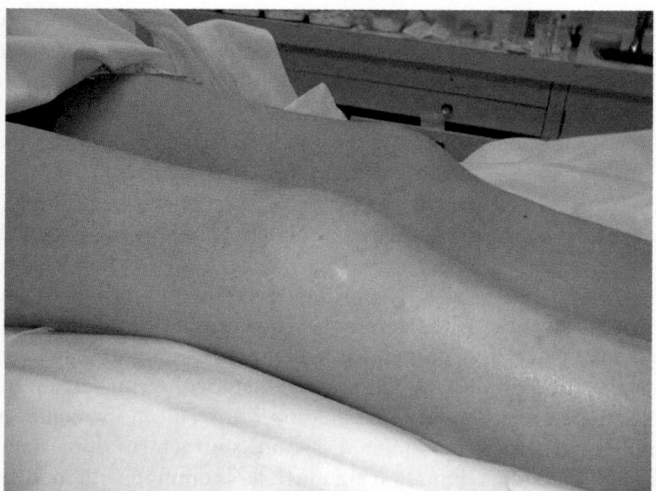

Fig. 116.2 Swollen knees in polyarticular juvenile idiopathic arthritis, with quadriceps wasting.

treatment with steroids), but subclinical myocarditis may occur in up to 10–12%.[27] Some cases with mild coronary dilatation have been observed although no cases of coronary artery aneurysms have been reported.[27,28]

Asymptomatic anterior uveitis is distinctly uncommon, although steroid-induced cataracts can occur, necessitating eye screening. Arthritis can be absent in the early weeks of disease onset and, in an unwell child with fever and rash, the differential diagnosis remains broad and infection and malignancy must be excluded. Neurological features are rare and if present raise the possibility of systemic vasculitis or macrophage activation syndrome (MAS),[29] which is a serious life-threatening complication.

Laboratory findings

Laboratory findings in SJIA include a marked inflammatory response with raised erythrocyte sedimentation rate (ESR) and C-reactive protein (CRP), leucocytosis, neutrophilia, anaemia, thrombocytosis, hypoalbuminaemia, and hypergammaglobulinaemia. A markedly raised serum ferritin is helpful, albeit not diagnostic of SJIA with or without MAS. Other suggestive features of MAS include cytopenias, low fibrinogen, unexpectedly normal or low ESR for the level of the CRP, liver derangement, raised triglycerides, and raised D-dimer levels in the serum.

Course of disease

Arthritis usually develops within the first few weeks or months of presentation and can be in an oligoarticular pattern or more commonly polyarticular and severe, resulting in joint damage. Tenosynovitis is common and can be associated with exuberant synovial thickening and bursal formation around the shoulder, wrists, knees, and ankles as well as around the flexor tendons of the hands and toes. This swelling and any associated joint effusions can come and go rapidly in association with temperature spikes and can be very painful. In the long term bony ankylosis is a characteristic feature in SJIA and especially in the cervical spine, wrist, and tarsus. Damage to the growth plates can occur rapidly and can lead to micrognathia or brachdactyly.[30] Chronic destructive arthritis is reported in up to 50% of patients although with modern drug treatment regimes it is anticipated that the prognosis is better.[31]

SJIA is a heterogeneous subtype and can follow a monocyclic, polycyclic, or persistent course. It can be severe, with potential for mortality and severe morbidity; management approaches focus on potent immunosuppression, usually with high-dose corticosteroids initially, parenteral methotrexate, and biologics especially with IL-6 and IL-1RA blockade as detailed in Chapter 96.

Psoriatic arthritis

Initially juvenile onset psoriatic arthritis was diagnosed when a child with arthritis went on to develop frank psoriasis, but it is now generally accepted that the term can be applied to children with arthritis who also have dactylitis, nail changes, and/or a history of psoriasis in a first-degree relative. This subtype is diagnosed in about 5–7% of cases of JIA.[32] There appear to be two peaks in age at onset, one at the age of 2 years and another in late childhood. Younger patients are more likely to exhibit dactylitis and small-joint involvement and to be female, and are more likely to progress to polyarticular disease. Older patients are more likely

to have enthesitis, axial joint disease, and to remain oligoarticular. Psoriatic JIA can be erosive and severely damaging to joints, is usually asymmetrical (Figure 116.5), and can cause significant local bony overgrowth and deformity. Uveitis occurs in around 8–10% of patients with psoriatic disease and it is vital that they are referred for uveitis screening.[33]

Enthesitis-related arthritis

ERA is an HLA B27-associated subtype of JIA characterized by inflammation of the entheses and/or the axial spine as well as peripheral joint disease. It affects 11–16% of children and young people with JIA.[34,35] In the past this type of JIA was called juvenile ankylosing spondylitis, seronegative enthesopathy and arthropathy (SEA) syndrome, or undifferentiated juvenile spondylarthropathy. Enthesitis is defined as discretely localized inflammation at the point of insertion of tendons, ligaments, joint capsules, or fascia to bone.

In a recent cohort study of 32 newly diagnosed ERA patients with a median age of 12.5 years, the median number of tender entheses at presentation was 2 (IQR 0–5); 21 subjects (66%) had at least 1 tender enthesis. The most frequently affected entheses were the patellar ligament insertion at the inferior pole of the patella, the plantar fascial insertion at the calcaneus, the Achilles tendon insertion at the calcaneus, and the plantar fascial insertion at the metatarsal heads. Enthesitis was usually symmetrical. The median number of active joints was 2 (IQR 0–4) and arthritis most commonly affected the sacroiliac (SI) joints, knees, and ankle joints.[34]

Diagnosing sacroiliitis in children and young people is based on reported pain and pain on SI stretch tests in combination with the gold standard of changes on MRI scan. Signs on MRI include synovial fluid in the SI joint, bone marrow oedema, subchondral sclerosis, bone erosions or irregularities, periarticular fat deposition, and SI anklyosis.[35] Sacroiliitis is often over-diagnosed on the plain radiograph with the growing epiphyses mimicking ostieitis to a non-paediatric specialist radiologist.[36]

Symptomatic acute anterior uveitis is present in up to 40% of adult patients[37] and in around 9.8% of children with spondyloarthritis, and chronic uveitis can also occur.[35]

In children the development of sacroiliitis and frank ankylosing spondylitis may take 5–10 years to develop. Juvenile onset ankylosing spondylitis appears to be a progressive disease, associated

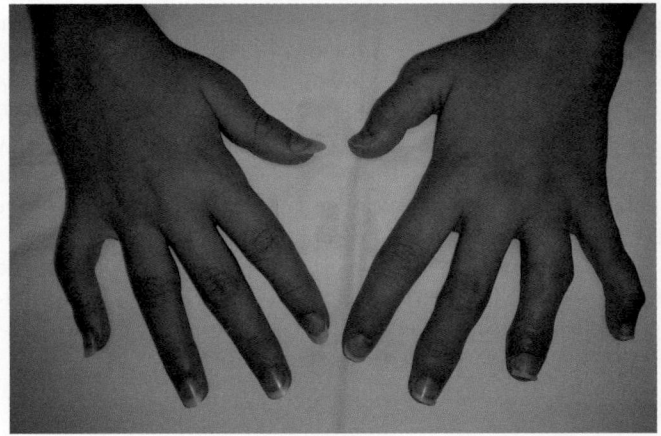

Fig. 116.5 Asymmetrical small-joint involvement in psoriatic juvenile idiopathic arthritis.

with a significant delay in diagnosis and with a worse functional outcome.[38]

Extra-articular associated disorders—uveitis

JIA-associated uveitis is one of the leading causes of blindness worldwide and the importance of ongoing screening may not be fully appreciated by families and clinical teams alike. Uveitis can present with symptoms such as blurred vision, reduced visual acuity, photophobia, occasionally with pain and redness around the iris, an irregular pupil, a change in colour of the iris, and sometimes with a visible hypopyon. However, small children adapt so quickly that they do not notice an impairment in their own vision. Parents may only suspect problems when the child becomes clumsy. By this stage there is likely to be severe inflammation and secondary complications such as glaucoma, cataracts, fibrosis, and scarring within the eye, which may be irreversible. For this reason it is vital that all children are referred as soon as possible after diagnosis of JIA for screening to the local ophthalmology department. This needs to be done with regular slit-lamp examinations and usually requires dilation of the pupil at least for the first examination. The frequency and duration of eye screening is dependent on the JIA subtype and the presence of uveitis.

In older published series rates of uveitis in JIA vary from 4% to 24.4%.[39] More recent studies have suggested rates of 13.1% of 1081 patients with JIA in a study by Saurenmann,[40] and 12% of 3271 JIA patients in a large German cohort study.[41] The most frequent incidence was in the extended oligoarticular group where 25% had uveitis and the persistent olioarticular group where 16% were affected. Predictors of uveitis were younger age at onset of arthritis, ANA positivity, and JIA subtype. Uveitis is very unusual in SJIA but rarely can occur, as can steroid-induced cataracts. Uveitis is often acute with a painful red eye in enthesitis-related JIA, but this is not always the case and chronic uveitis can also occur in this group of patients. In all other types of JIA, including psoriatic disease, uveitis can occur. The median onset of uveitis after diagnosis of arthritis was 5.5 months, with uveitismanifesting between 2–5 years in 16% and after 5 years in 7%. In 70% of cases uveitis is bilateral and this increases to 77% of the oligo JIA cases. Approximately 77% developed uveitis before their 7th birthday. Anterior uveitis is the most common anatomical type of arthritis (83%), intermediate uveitis 9%, posterior uveitis 1%, and panuveitis in 7%.[42] In 45% of patients complications of uveitis are already seen at the initial screen, emphasizing the asymptomatic nature of this uveitis and the need for rapid diagnosis of JIA so that the eye screening can be started as soon as possible. Ocular complications are seen in up to 65–86% of patients with uveitis 3–5 years after initial diagnosis and many patients are unfortunately legally blind at first presentation to the ophthalmologist. Long-term follow-up studies after 20 years have revealed surprisingly poor outcomes.[41,43]

The management of JIA-associated uveitis can be complex and requires close collaboration with ophthalmologists and rheumatologists to ensure rapid access to screening, facilitate systemic therapies to be started early and optimize visual outcomes.

References

1. Petty RE, Southwood TR, Manners P et al. International League of Associations for Rheumatology classification of juvenile idiopathic arthritis; second revision. Edmonton, 2001. *J Rheumatol* 2004:31:390–392.

2. Ravelli A, Martini A. Juvenile idiopathic arthritis. *Lancet* 2007;369:767–778.

3. Symmons DP, Jones M, Osborne J et al. Pediatric rheumatology in the United Kingdom: data from the British Pediatric Rheumatology Group National Diagnostic Register. *J Rheumatol* 1996;23:1975–1980.

4. Gortmaker SL, Sappenfield W. Chronic childhood disorders: prevalence and impact. *Pediatr Clin North Am* 1984;34(31):390–392.

5. Prakken, B, Albani S, Martini A. Juvenile idiopathic arthritis. *Lancet* 2011;377:2138–2149/

6. Minden K, Kiessling U, Listing J et al. Prognosis of patients with juvenile chronic arthritis and juvenile spondyloarthropathy. *J Rheumatol* 2000;27:2256–2263.

7. Wallace CA, Huang B, Bandeira M, Ravelli A, Giannini EH: Patterns of clinical remission in select categories of juvenile idiopathic arthritis. *Arthritis Rheum* 2005;52:3554–3562.

8. Cassidy JT, Petty RF. Juvenile rheumatoid arthritis. In Cassidy JT, Petty RE (eds) *Textbook of paediatric rheumatology*, 4th edn. W.B. Saunders, Philadelphia, 2001:218–322.

9. Foster HE, Rapley T. Access to pediatric rheumatology care—a major challenge to improving outcome in juvenile idiopathic arthritis. *J Rheumatol* 2010;37(11):2199–2202.

10. Padmakumar B, Evans Jones LG, Sills JA Is arthritis more common in children with Down syndrome? *Rheumatology* 2002;41(10):1191–1193.

11. Juj H, Emery H. The arthropathy of Down syndrome: an underdiagnosed and under-recognized condition. *J Pediatr* 2009;154(2):234–238.

12. Accorinti M, La Cava M, Speranza S, Pivetti-Pezzi P. Uveitis in Turner's syndrome. *Graefes Arch Clin Exp Ophthalmol* 2002;240(7):529–532.

13. Verloes A, Curry C, Jamar M et al. Juvenile rheumatoid arthritis and del(22q11) syndrome: a non-random association. *J Med Genet* 1998;35(11):943–947.

14. Gottlieb C, Li Z, Uzel G, Nussenblatt RB, Sen HN. Uveitis in DiGeorge syndrome: a case of autoimmune ocular inflammation in a patient with deletion 22q11.2. *Ophthalmic Genet* 2010;31(1):24–29.

15. Petty RE, Southwood TR, Manners P et al. International League of Associations for Rheumatology classification of juvenile idiopathic arthritis: second revision, Edmonton, 2001. International League of Associations for Rheumatology. *J Rheumatol* 2004;31(2):390–392.

16. Beresford MW. Juvenile idiopathic arthritis, new insights into classification, measures of outcome, and pharmacology. *Pediatric Drugs* 2011;13(3):161–173.

17. Prince FHM, Otten MH, van Suijlekom-Smit LW. Diagnosis and management of juvenile idiopathic arthritis. *BMJ* 2011;342:95–102.

18. Berntson L, Fasth A, Andersson-Gäre B et al.; Nordic Study Group. Construct validity of ILAR and EULAR criteria in juvenile idiopathic arthritis: a population based incidence study from the Nordic countries. International League of Associations for Rheumatology. European League Against Rheumatism. *J Rheumatol* 2001;28(12):2737–2743.

19. Thomson W, Barrett JH, Donn R et al. Juvenile idiopathic arthritis classified by the ILAR criteria: HLA associations in UK patients. *Rheumatology* (Oxford) 2002;41(10):1183–1189.

20. Berntson L, Andersson Gäre B et al.; Nordic Study Group. Incidence of juvenile idiopathic arthritis in the Nordic countries. A population based study with special reference to the validity of the ILAR and EULAR criteria. *J Rheumatol* 2003;30(10):2275–2282.

21. Weiss JE, Ilowite NT. Juvenile idiopathic arthritis. *Rheum Dis Clin North Am* 2007;33(3):441–470, vi.

22. Minden K, Niewerth M, Listing J et al. Long-term outcome in patients with juvenile idiopathic arthritis. *Arthritis Rheum* 2002;46(9):2392–2401.

23. Ramanan AV, Grom AA. Does systemic-onset juvenile idiopathic arthritis belong under juvenile idiopathic arthritis? *Rheum* 2005;44:1350–1353.

24. Sikora KA, Grom AA. Update on the pathogenesis and treatment of systemic arthritis. *Current Opin Pediatr* 2011;23:640–646.

25. Scheider R, Laxer RM. Systemic onset juvenile rheumatoid arthritis. *Ballieres Clin Rheumatol* 1998;12(2):245–269.

26. Wagener JS, Taussig LM, DeBenedetti C, Lemen RJ, Loughlin GM. Pulmonary function in juvenile rheumatoid arthritis. *J Pediatr* 1981;99(1):108–110.

27. Goldenberg J, Ferraz MB, Pessoa AP et al. Symptomatic cardiac involvement in juvenile rheumatoid arthritis. *Int J Cardiol* 1992;34:57–62.

28. Binstadt BA, Levine JC, Nigrovic PA et al. Coronary artery dilation among patients presenting with systemic-onset juvenile idiopathic arthritis. *Pediatrics* 2005;116(1):e89–93.

29. Gupta S, Weitzman S. Primary and secondary hemophagocytic lymphohistiocytosis: clinical features, pathogenesis and therapy. *Expert Rev Clin Immunol* 2010;6(1):137–154.

30. MacRae VE, Farquharson C, Ahmed SF. The pathophysiology of the growth plate in juvenile idiopathic arthritis. *Rheumatology* 2006;45:11–19.

31. Calabro JJ, Holgerson WB, Sonpal GM, Khoury MI. Juvenile rheumatoid arthritis: a general survey of 100 patients observed for 15 years. *Semin Arthritis Rheum* 1976;5:257–298.

32. Krumrey-Langkammerer M, Hafner R. Evaluation of the ILAR criteria for juvenile idiopathic arthritis. *J Rheumatol* 2001;28:2544–2547.

33. Stoll ML, Zurakowski D, Nigrovic LE et al. Patient with juvenile psoriatic arthritis comprise two distinct populations. *Arthritis Rheum* 2006;54(11):3564–3572.

34. Weiss PF, Andrew J, Behrens EM et al. Enthesitis in an inception cohort of enthesitis-related arthritis. *Arthritis Care Res* 2011;63(9):1307–1312.

35. Stoll ML, Bhore R, Dempsey-Robertson M, Punaro M. Spondyloarthritis in a pediatric population: risk factors for sacroiliitis. *J Rheumatol* 2010;37(11):2402–2408.

36. Bollow M, Beidermann T, Kannenberg J et al. Use of dynamic magnetic resonance imaging to detect sacroiliitis in HLA-B27 positive and negative children with juvenile arthritides. *J Rheumatol* 1998;25:556–564.

37. Muñoz-Fernández S, de Miguel E, Cobo-Ibáñez T et al. Enthesis inflammation in recurrent acute anterior uveitis without spondylarthritis. *Arthritis Rheum* 2009;60(7):1985–1990.

38. Stone M, Warren RW, Bruckel J et al. Juvenile onset ankylosing spondylitis is associated with worse functional outcomes than adult onset ankylosing spondylitis. *Arthritis Care Res* 2005;53(3):445–451.

39. Kotaniemi K, Kautiainen H, Karma A, Aho K. Occurrence of uveitis in recently diagnosed juvenile chronic arthritis. A prospective study. *Ophthalmology* 2001;108:2071–2075.

40. Saurenmann RK, Levin AV, Feldman BM et al. Prevalence, risk factors, and outcome of uveitis in juvenile idiopathic arthritis, a long-term follow-up study. *Arthritis Rheum* 2007;56(2):647–657.

41. Heiligenhaus A, Niewerth M, Ganser G, Heinz C, Minder K; German Uveitis in Childhood Study Group. Prevalence and complications of uveitis in juvenile idiopathic arthritis in a population based nation-wide study in Germany: suggested modification of the current screening guidelines. *Rheumatology* 2007;46(6):1015–1019.

42. Ying Q, Acharya NR. Juvenile idiopathic arthritis associated uveitis. *Curr Opin Ophthalmol* 2010;21(6):468–472.

43. Anesi SD, Foster CS. Importance of recognizing and preventing blindness from juvenile idiopathic arthritis-associated uveitis. *Arthritis Care Res* (Hoboken) 2012;64(5):653–657.

SECTION 13

Systemic lupus erythematosus

CHAPTER 117

Systemic lupus erythematosus—clinical features and aetiopathogenesis

Caroline Gordon

Epidemiology of systemic lupus erythematosus

Systemic lupus erythematosus (SLE) is associated with multiple genetic and environmental risk factors that have been discussed in Chapter 42. The importance of environmental factors acting on the genetic background is manifest by the observation that only 24% of identical twin pairs are concordant for lupus, and for dizygotic twins the risk is 1 in 50 (2%) for both developing the disease.[1]

Prevalence of lupus

The prevalence of lupus around the world is summarized in Table 117.1.[2,3] In the United Kingdom, carefully conducted studies to assess the prevalence of lupus were undertaken in the early 1990s. The largest study from Birmingham using multiple methods of case ascertainment and clinical assessment of all suspected cases referred by hospital doctors or general practitioners confirmed that the point prevalence of lupus in adults in 1992 was 27.7 per 100 000, suggesting that about 1 in 3500 people have lupus.[4] Lupus was 14 times more common in women than men with a prevalence in adult women of 49.6/100 000 and 3.6/100 000 in adult men. Lupus may be underdiagnosed in men, as the gender ratio has been 14 females to each male for over 20 years in the Birmingham study. The prevalence was highest in patients of Afro-Caribbean origin, irrespective of place of birth. Lupus was found to affect 206.0/100 000 Afro-Caribbean adult women compared with 90.6/100 000 South Asian women from India or Pakistan, and 36.2/100 000 women of white European background. Patients of Afro-Caribbean origin aged 30–39 had the highest prevalence (405/100 000), were the youngest at disease onset, and were most likely to have renal disease.

Studies over the last 20 years in the United States have yielded higher prevalence, with rates between 32 and 150/100 000,[5] than either the United Kingdom studies or previous United States studies undertaken between 1965 and 1995, which suggested a mean prevalence of about 24/100 000. Recent studies in Michigan and Georgia (USA) using multiple methods of case ascertainment in

Table 117.1 Worldwide prevalence of systemic lupus erythematosus

Region	Place	Population	Rate/100,000
Europe	Sweden	C	68
	Norway	C	45
	Iceland	C	36
	Finland	C	28
	Ireland	C	25
	Denmark	C	22
	Spain	C, Af	34
	Greece	C	38
	UK (Leicester)	C, A	26
	UK (Nottingham)	C, AC	25
	UK (Birmingham)	C, AC, A	28
	Saudi Arabia	Ar	19
America	USA (Ward)	C, AA	241
	USA (Hochberg)	C, AA	124
	USA (Rochester)	C	122
	USA (California)	AA, H, A, P, C	108
	USA (Pennsylvania)	AA, H, A, P, C	150
	USA (Arizona)	H	103
	Alaskan Indians	N	112
	Canada	N, C	22
Oceania	Australia	C, Aau	45

A, Asian; AA, African-American; A Au, Aboriginal Australian; AC, Afro-Caribbean; Af, African; Ar, Arabic; C, Caucasian (white European); H, Hispanic; N, North American Indian; P, Pacific Islander.

areas with about 50% black population have found a mean annual prevalence rate of lupus of 73/100 000.[6–8] The rates in women were about 10 times higher than the rates in males. Black women not only had the highest prevalence (at about 190/100 000) in both Michigan and Georgia, but also presented younger than white women, were more likely to have renal disease, and to develop end-stage renal disease.

Many studies from around the world have confirmed that lupus is rare before puberty and is most common in women in the reproductive age group, when the gender ratio is about 10 females to each male, whereas there is less female predominance in children and in older age groups (>50 years). Further studies are ongoing in the United States to confirm the prevalence in other racial/ethnic groups such as Hispanics, Chinese and American Indians. The LUMINA study has shown that Hispanics and African-Americans are at increased risk of developing lupus nephritis compared to populations of white European descent.[9] Several studies have shown that populations of Chinese origin have an increased risk of lupus and lupus nephritis.[10]

Incidence of lupus

The incidence of lupus around the world is summarized in Table 117.2.[2,3] Studies undertaken in the United Kingdom in the early 1990s suggested that the incidence of lupus was about 4 per 100 000 in Birmingham and Nottingham, and similar results were obtained from Sweden.[4,11,12] A more recent UK GP Research Database based study suggested than the mean incidence in the United Kingdom in participating general practices was 7.9/100 000 per year between 1990 and 1999.[13] However, the criteria for classification of cases

Table 117.2 Worldwide incidence of systemic lupus erythematosus

Region	Place	Population	Rate/100,000
Europe	Sweden	C	4.8
	Norway	C	2.6
	Iceland	C	3.3
	Denmark	C	2.5
	Spain	C	2.2
	Greece	C	1.9
	UK (Nottingham)	C, AC	4.0
	UK (Birmingham)	C, AC, A	3.8
	UK (GP)	C, AC, A	4.7
North America	Rochester	C	5.6
	Pennsylvania	C, AA	2.8
	Wisconsin	C	5.1
	Georgia	C, AA	5.6
	Michigan	C, AA	6.0
South America	Curacao	AC	4.6
	Brazil (Natal)	H	8.7

A, Asian; AA, African-American; AC, Afro-Caribbean; Af, African; Ar, Arabic; A Au, Aboriginal Australian; C, Caucasian (white European); GP, UK General Practice Database; H, Hispanic; N, North American Indian.

was not standardized, whereas most other studies required at least 4 out of 11 American College of Rheumatology (ACR) classification criteria for SLE. The rate varied widely between geographical regions and was highest in Northern Ireland, although studies on prevalence in Northern Ireland in 1993 had shown similar prevalence to Birmingham, at 25.4/100 000. In this GP database study the West Midlands incidence was 3.6/100 000, comparable to that found in Birmingham previously. The recent United States studies found incidence to be higher at about 5.5/100 000 per year in Michigan and Georgia, and to be highest in black females (about 13/100 000 per year).[6–8]

Pathology of systemic lupus erythematosus

Multiple immune abnormalities involving B and T cells, dendritic cells, and mononuclear phagocytes contribute to the development of lupus. Although cell-mediated mechanisms are involved in the pathology of lupus, it is the formation of immune complexes involving nucleic acids and autoantibodies that is the hallmark of the disease.[14] The mechanisms involved in the activation of B and T cells and the generation of autoantibodies are discussed further below. Tissue damage results from mechanisms resulting from direct binding of autoantibodies and from the activation of complement by immune complexes formed in the circulation or in the tissues. Levels of certain autoantibodies (anti-dsDNA, anti-C1q) and complement consumption can be used to assess disease activity. Lupus can affect all organs of the body and specific histological features may be seen, as for example with lupus nephritis. In general, there is infiltration of the tissues with mononuclear cells together with evidence of fibrinoid necrosis, formation of haematoxylin bodies containing chromatin and immunoglobulin, vascular inflammation and injury, deposition of immunoglobulin and complement, and in the skin disruption of the dermal–epidermal junction.

There is increasing evidence that the processing of immune complexes and of apoptotic cells is suboptimal and that this contributes to the development of lupus and flares at times of physical stress, such as after infection and UV light exposure, when increased production of apoptotic cells and immune complexes occurs. Genetic or acquired deficiency of the early components of complement (C1q, C2, or C4) and polymorphisms of the Fc gamma receptors are important risk factors for lupus because of the resulting deficits in handling apoptotic material and immune complexes.[15–19]

Not only is the adaptive immune response important in the development of lupus but there is increasing evidence for a role for the innate immune activation and production of type 1 interferons which may promote autoantibody formation. Genetic risk factors predisposing to lupus include a single-nucleotide polymorphisms in two interferon-related genes, those encoding tyrosine kinase 2 and interferon regulatory factor 5 (IRF5).[20–23] Even premature atherosclerosis, which is a common complication of lupus, is probably initiated and accelerated by immune mechanisms.[24]

Lupus is most common in women during the reproductive years, suggesting a role for sex hormones. Oestrogens in hormone replacement therapy and contraceptive pills can increase the risk of mild/moderate flares even in patients without severe disease activity.[25–27] Pregnancy, which is associated with much higher hormone levels, can cause the disease to flare severely, especially if lupus presents for the first time in pregnancy or established disease is not well controlled before pregnancy. The molecular mechanisms whereby oestrogens influence immune cell function and cytokine formation are not well understood but there is evidence that many cells of the immune system bear oestrogen receptors. Furthermore, lupus patients have recently been reported to develop antibodies to oestrogen receptor alpha that are associated with active disease and that on binding can cause activation and subsequent apoptosis of resting lymphocytes or induce proliferation of stimulated T cells.[28,29]

Autoantibodies in lupus

The presence of autoantibodies in the serum, particularly IgG antibodies to nuclear material, is the hallmark of lupus disease. However, autoantibodies directed against a large number of self-antigens (>40) in the cytoplasm and cell membranes as well as the nucleus are found in lupus patients, only a few of which are tested for in the clinic.[30] IgM autoantibodies can occur in healthy people, particularly after infections including glandular fever due to Epstein–Barr virus (EBV), but class switching to IgG antibodies is not usually seen. The anti-nuclear antibody (ANA) test is very sensitive, being positive in over 95% of lupus patients, but is not very specific as it is also positive in other diseases such as dermatomyositis and systemic sclerosis. Studies have shown that IgG autoantibodies can be found in the serum up to 9 years before the development of clinical features of lupus.[31] Deposition of autoantibodies and complement has been observed in the kidneys and skin. Although immunoglobulins that bind to a number of non-DNA antigens, including Ro (a ribonucleoprotein complex), La (an RNA-binding protein), C1q (a subunit of the C1 complement component), and Sm (nuclear particles consisting of several different polypeptides) can be observed in the serum and the kidney, it is the presence of antibodies that bind double stranded (ds)DNA in the kidney and in the serum that is considered one of the most typical features of lupus. Anti-dsDNA antibodies are highly specific for lupus and are present in 40–70% of patients with lupus but in less than 0.5% of healthy people or patients with other autoimmune diseases.[14] The levels of anti-dsDNA antibodies in serum usually reflect disease activity, with rises before flares though sometimes falls at the time of flare due to deposition of the antibodies in the tissues. Indeed, some of the autoantibodies observed in the kidney may be deposited in the tissue only after inflammatory processes expose nuclear antigens during apoptosis (programmed cell death). Nucleosomes are fragments of DNA and histone generated during apoptosis.[30] There is increasing evidence that anti-nucleosome antibodies are formed even before anti-dsDNA antibodies in response to dysfunctional clearance of apoptotic cells at times of stress,[18] and that antibodies to dsDNA, nucleosomes, and α-actinin are important in the pathogenesis of lupus nephritis.[32] Anti-nucleosome antibodies have been observed also in some skin biopsies from patients with lupus nephritis, but without rash.[33]

Photosensitive rashes are associated with anti-Ro antibodies. During pregnancy Ro antigens are exposed on the surface of fetal cardiac myocytes during remodelling of the heart. From about 16 weeks of gestation onwards, maternal anti-Ro or anti-La antibodies can cross the placenta and may interact with exposed Ro or La antigens, resulting in atrioventricular conduction defects. This can cause congenital complete heart block which may present at any time from week 16 to the neonatal period, but usually between weeks 16 and 32 of gestation. Fortunately this only occurs in 1–2% of babies born to mothers with anti-Ro antibodies or anti-La antibodies, though 5–10% of babies may develop UV-induced subacute lupus rash after birth, usually during the first 3 months of life due to placental transmission of these antibodies.[34,35]

Anti-NMDA-receptor antibodies have been found in the brain tissue of patients with cerebral lupus and animal studies have suggested that antibodies against the N-methyl-D-aspartate (NMDA) receptor may be important in the development of central nervous system lupus. NMDA is an excitatory amino acid released by neurons. Intravenous administration of serum from lupus patients containing antibodies against DNA and NMDA receptors induced cognitive impairment and hippocampal damage.[36]

Other autoantibodies are important in autoimmune haemolytic anaemia and thrombocytopenia. In these cases the autoantibody can bind to cell surface antigens, leading to immune-mediated destruction of red cells and platelets. Anti-phospholipid antibodies may also bind to platelets and are associated with thrombosis in lupus patients, as occurs in anti-phospholipid syndrome.[37]

Tissue damage by autoantibodies

There are two main theories of how tissue damage occurs in the kidney in patients with lupus nephritis, and similar mechanisms are thought to explain other lupus manifestations. Berden and colleagues have proposed that pathogenic, high-affinity, anti-dsDNA or anti-nucleosome autoantibodies bind to nucleosomes in the blood of patients with lupus and form antibody–nucleosome complexes that deposit in the renal glomerular basement membrane.[38] These complexes activate complement which initiates the development of glomerulonephritis. IgG antibodies have been shown to colocalize with extracellular chromatin in lupus nephritis in humans and mouse models of lupus.

The alternative model proposes that high-affinity anti-dsDNA and/or anti-nucleosome antibodies cross-react with proteins such as α-actinin in the kidney and have a direct pathogenic effect on renal cells. Renal podocytes are part of the glomerular filtration process and their function is dependent on α-actinin. Mouse monoclonal anti-DNA antibodies that cross-reacted with α-actinin were pathogenic and induced lupus nephritis after transfer into recipient mice, in contrast to monoclonal anti-DNA antibodies that did not cross-react with α-actinin, which were non-pathogenic in two studies. Anti-α-actinin antibodies are not specific for lupus but may act as a marker of renal involvement when found in the serum of lupus patients; however, anti-α-actinin antibodies have not been reported in renal biopsies from patients with lupus nephritis.[14]

Role of T cells

Interaction of a T-cell receptor (TCR) with antigen bound to a major histocompatibility complex (MHC) peptide on the surface of an antigen-presenting cell (APC)—which may be a dendritic cell, macrophage, or B cell—triggers a T-cell response. MHC gene haplotypes such as HLA A1, B8, DR3 are associated with an increased risk of immune responses to self-antigens, resulting in autoimmune diseases such as lupus. IgG antibodies with high-affinity binding to dsDNA are more strongly associated with tissue damage than IgM or lower-affinity IgG antibodies in mouse models of lupus and in humans. Production of high-affinity IgG antibodies requires a process known as T-cell help and is important in the pathogenesis of lupus.[14]

The generation of high-affinity antibodies is a multistep process that starts with the binding of antigen to a specific immunoglobulin on the surface of B lymphocytes (B cells). This stimulates the B lymphocytes to proliferate, migrate within germinal centres, and differentiate in the presence of signals from T lymphocytes, specifically from T helper (Th) cells.[30] Each T cell carries a surface-receptor molecule that binds to a particular antigen presented to the TCR in a complex with an MHC molecule on the surface of an APC. Presentation of the antigen–MHC complex and interaction with the TCR generates an activation signal but this alone is not sufficient to stimulate the T cell to produce all the signals required to induce B-cell differentiation. A second molecular interaction between the APC and the T cell is required, a process known as costimulation. There are several different pairs of costimulatory molecules, including the CD40–CD40 ligand and CD28–B7, which can generate the second signal required for T-cell activation and the subsequent generation of signals that induce B-cell proliferation and differentiation into the plasma cells that produce antibodies. Furthermore, the interaction of B and T cells and the stimulation of each other generates T-cell cytokines that promote B-cell proliferation and the switching of antibody production from IgM to IgG, and induces a change in the molecular structure of the secreted antibody so that it has higher affinity and binds more strongly to the target antigen. Agents that block costimulation can inhibit immune responses that depend on T-cell help. This includes cytotoxic T-lymphocyte–associated protein 4 (CTLA-4) on T cells that competes with CD28 to bind to B7 and can downregulate B-cell responses. CTLA-4 bound to an IgG1 molecule has been developed as a treatment for inflammatory immune-mediated diseases including rheumatoid arthritis and more recently lupus on this basis.[39]

Nucleosomes consist of a protein core of histones around which DNA winds. Histone-derived peptides H2B10-33, H416-39, H471-94, H391-105, H2A34-48, and H449-63 stimulate T cells from patients with lupus to produce cytokines.[14] Similar peptides stimulate T cells from lupus-prone mice but these peptides do not stimulate T cells from healthy people or non-lupus-prone mouse strains. It has been proposed that stimulation of these peptide-specific T cells would allow them to help B cells that respond specifically to antigenic epitopes derived from nucleosomes resulting in the production of high-affinity pathogenic autoantibodies. Nucleosomes contain B and T cell epitopes, and anti-nucleosome antibodies are present early and play a pathogenic role in the development of lupus. Anti-dsDNA antibodies are thought to be generated by similar process involving nucleosomes with T cells recognizing the histone-derived epitopes and B cells recognizing DNA (as T cells can only respond to protein-based epitopes).[30] This is reminiscent of hapten-carrier induction of antibodies in vaccine development and is likely to apply to the generation of anti-phospholipid antibodies as well, as only B-cell expressed Ig receptors can bind to phospholipids, while T cells react to protein antigens derived from membrane proteins.

The autoantigen-specific B and T cells that interact to produce pathogenic autoantibodies are not found in healthy people. Several mechanisms may be responsible for the absence of these cells, a phenomenon known as tolerance. These mechanisms include removal (deletion) of the autoreactive T and B cells, inactivation of the cells so that they are anergic, or a change in the light chain of the antibody expressed by an autoreactive B lymphocyte (so-called receptor editing) such that the antibody loses the ability to bind autoantigen. Furthermore the activation of Th cells and B cells can be suppressed by regulatory T cells (Tregs). Both the number and

function of regulatory T cells have been reported to be reduced in patients with lupus.[40] There is also an increased number of double negative (CD3+CD4−CD8−) T cells and of interleukin (IL)-17-producing T cells, and various early and late signalling abnormalities that contribute to the autoimmune process and provide novel targets for therapeutic intervention.[41]

Cytokines and lupus

Cytokines are protein messenger molecules that are produced by immune cells and play a key role in the development of innate and adaptive immune responses.[42,43] Cytokines may have stimulatory or suppressive effects depending on the ligand that they interact with and the activation state of the cell. Their production and effects are carefully regulated in a complex interacting network and anything that disturbs the cytokine environment (homeostasis) in one direction can have a variety of downstream effects, which may include effects that are the opposite of what is expected.

B lymphocyte stimulator

B lymphocyte stimulator (BLyS; also known as B-cell activating factor, BAFF) and APRIL (a proliferation-inducing ligand) are expressed by T cells, dendritic cells, monocytes, and macrophages but not by B cells. They are membrane proteins that can be released by proteolytic cleavage that are important for B-cell survival, differentiation, and function. In particular BLyS controls the final differentiation of mature, preimmune B cells and plays an important role in maintaining B-cell tolerance.[44] BLyS binds to three receptors: BCMA, TACI, and BR3 (also known as BAFFR). Pre-plasmablast mature B cells depend on BLyS as they express mostly BR3 and only a little TACI. Plasma cells express BCMA and TACI that bind BLyS and APRIL. Memory B cells are independent of BLyS and APRIL. T cells express BR3, though the role of BLyS in T-cell signalling is uncertain. Dendritic cells also express BLyS receptors and respond to BLyS by upregulating costimulatory molecules, chemokines, and IL-1 and IL-6 production.[42]

Aberrant BLyS expression is observed on many cell types and circulating BLyS levels are increased in some lupus patients. B cells and plasma cells can express high levels of BLyS and APRIL mRNA that correlate with anti-dsDNA antibodies and lupus disease activity. BLyS antagonists being developed for the treatment of lupus include belimumab (a monoclonal antibody that inactivates soluble BLyS)[45,46] and atacicept[47,48] (a fusion protein combining TACI and the Fc portion of IgG to bind BLyS and APRIL).

Interferons

Type I interferons (IFN-α and IFN-β) have important anti-viral, anti-proliferative, and immune modulatory functions.[42,43] Plasmacytoid dendritic cells are the major producers of IFN-α, but most cells can make this cytokine. The stimuli that induce it include viral and bacterial infections, self-nucleic acids, and nucleic-acid-containing immune complexes which engage with Toll-like receptors (TLRs). ssRNA-containing complexes engage TLR7 and TLR8 and dsDNA-containing complexes engage TLR9. IFN-α levels are increased in many lupus patients, especially with active disease, and type I interferon therapy has been found to induce a lupus-like syndrome. Raised IFN-α levels have been observed in healthy relatives of patients with lupus, confirming that other factors are required for disease manifestations to develop in susceptible people. IFN-α promotes B-cell activation, proliferation, antibody production, and class switching and can potentially promote survival of autoreactive B cells, since it can prevent B-cell apoptosis. Furthermore, IFN-α produced by APCs modulates Treg function, reducing Treg suppression of inflammation and T-cell proliferation.

It has been shown that IFN-α contributes to the initiation and persistence of lupus and is linked to the activation of specific genes involved in the development of lupus (e.g. *IRF5, IRF7*).[23] Upregulated expression of IFN-inducible genes has been observed using genome-wide expression profiling and this characteristic gene expression pattern is known as the IFN signature. However, this is not restricted to lupus as it has been found in patients with Sjögren's syndrome and systemic sclerosis as well. There have been two phase 1 trials of anti-IFN-α monoclonal antibodies (sifalimumab and rontalizumab) in which dose-dependent reduction in the interferon signature was observed in association with reduced disease activity,[49,50] and the results of phase 2 trials are awaited.

Interleukins

Interleukin-1 (IL-1) and the IL-1 receptor antagonist (IL-1RA) are produced by activated mononuclear phagocytes. Specific polymorphisms of the IL-1a and IL-1b genes are associated with increased risk for SLE and specific alleles of the IL-1RA gene are associated with increased severity of the disease.[43]

IL-2 levels are low in lupus patients and this may contribute to the reduced number of regulatory Tregs observed in SLE. IL-17 levels are increased in many lupus patients, probably due to increased numbers of double negative T cells and Th17 cells which produce IL-17 and a reduction in Treg cells that control Th17 cells.[41,43] Development of Th17 cells is promoted by increased levels of IL-6, IL-21, and IL-23 which have been observed in patients with lupus, especially with active disease. IL-17 promotes monocyte and neutrophil recruitment and together with BAFF/BLyS, provides help to B cells resulting in B-cell activation, proliferation, and differentiation promoting antibody production and class switching.

IL-4, IL-5, IL-10, and IL-13 are produced by Th2 cells and are involved in proliferation, activation and isotype switching of B cells.[43] Increased amounts of IL-4 and IL-4-producing cells have been reported in SLE patients. IL-10 has anti-inflammatory effects through its effects on Tregs and proinflammatory effects through its effects on B cells. In SLE patients, monocytes and B cells are the main producers of IL-10. Polymorphisms of the IL-10 and the IL-10 promoter gene and increased IL-10 levels in serum have been observed. A monoclonal antibody against IL-10 was tested for 21 days in 6 patients with lupus.[51] There was a beneficial effect on skin and joint manifestations and a steroid-sparing effect at 6 months, but all of the patients developed an immune response to the administered monoclonal antibody which prevented further trials of this agent. IL-13 levels are raised in lupus, which may be associated with a polymorphism of the IL-13 promoter gene.

There is considerable evidence that serum levels of IL-6 are elevated and correlate with lupus activity and anti-dsDNA antibody levels, and an increased frequency of IL-6-producing mononuclear cells that correlates with disease activity and response to treatment in SLE patients.[42,43] Autoreactive T-cell clones have been observed that produce large amounts of IL-6 which promotes B-cell activation and autoantibody formation in lupus patients. Elevated cerebrospinal fluid (CSF) levels of IL-6 have been found in patients with psychosis. Mesangial IL-6 has been observed in kidney samples,

and raised urinary levels of IL-6 have been observed in some active patients to associate with anti-dsDNA antibody levels and to fall after treatment. Tocilizumab is a humanized IgG1 monoclonal antibody against the α-chain of the IL-6 receptor that inhibits binding of IL-6 to membrane-bound and soluble IL-6 receptor.[52] An open-label phase I dose escalation study suggested that tocilizumab may be able to control SLE disease activity but there were concerns about the risk of neutropenia and infections that may limit the development of this therapeutic strategy.

IL-12 stimulates the differentiation of TH1 cells which produce IL-2 and IFN-γ.[43] In mouse models of lupus IFN-γ is pathogenic. The role of IFN-γ and of the IFN-γ receptor in human lupus is less clear. IL-27 synergizes with IL-12 to increase IFN-γ production and has both proinflammatory and anti-inflammatory properties but its role in SLE is not certain.[43,53] In mice, IL-27 can induce T cells to produce IL-21, and IL-27 has been shown to be important for the function of follicular Th cells in germinal centres that are essential for maturation and selection of high-affinity B-cell clones. There is increasing evidence that IL-27 has useful anti-inflammatory effects in several autoimmune models of diabetes and lupus. Deficiency of IL-27 receptor α-chain in a pristine induced mouse model of lupus resulted in a reduction in autoantibodies and glomerulonephritis. In a mouse model of SLE-like skin inflammation IL-27/IL-27 receptor α-subunit signalling appeared to be protective. Finally, there are reports suggesting that levels of IL-27 are reduced in patients with lupus nephritis[54] and that expression of urinary IL-27 mRNA increased significantly in patients with complete response but not in those with no response or partial response after 6 months of immunosuppressive therapy, supporting the concept that IL-27 may be associated with anti-inflammatory effects.[55]

IL-15 and IL-21 are part of the IL-2 superfamily.[43] The receptors of all three cytokines share the same γ-chain, and IL-15 and IL-21 share the IL-2β receptor as well. IL-15 is increased in lupus patients and like IL-2 can induce T cell and NK cell proliferation, but importantly for lupus, also promotes isotype switching in B cells. IL-21, in contrast to IL-15 and IL-2, is involved in B-cell activation and plasma cell differentiation. Certain polymorphisms of the IL-21 and IL-21recepor genes have been reported in SLE patients and decreased IL-21 receptor expression on peripheral B cells is associated with high levels of autoantibodies and nephritis in SLE patients, making IL-21 a therapeutic target.[56,57] However caution is required, as in the BXSB-Yaa mouse model of lupus, IL-21 can regulate immune responses and can have immunosuppressive effects mediated in part by induction of IL-10.

Tumour necrosis factor alpha

The role of Tumour necrosis factor alpha (TNFα) in lupus remains controversial. It is an important mediator of inflammation but may also help to control autoimmunity.[42,58] Patients with a variety of diseases treated with anti-TNFα monoclonal antibodies or soluble receptors may develop anti-nuclear antibodies and occasionally transient lupus-like syndromes. There is some evidence from the New Zealand Black/White (NZB/W) mouse models of lupus that have genetically determined low levels of TNFα that administration of exogenous TNFα is beneficial. However, these and other mouse models of lupus have evidence of TNFα in the kidney, and in humans, elevated levels of TNFα have been observed in serum, kidney, and skin samples of patients with active lupus. Administration of infliximab and rarely other TNF blockers in single cases and open-label studies involving at least 50 lupus patients have suggested that short-term induction therapy may be relatively safe but that long-term TNF blockade is associated with more risk.[59] Although long-term remission in patients with lupus nephritis, haemophagocytic syndrome, and interstitial lung disease have been reported, lupus arthritis tends to recur after cessation of therapy. Lupus flares do not occur even when there are transient increases in antibodies to dsDNA but increases in anti-phospholipid antibodies have been associated with vascular adverse events and there have been reports of bacterial infections, pneumonia, and urinary tract infections.

Presentation of systemic lupus

Lupus may present as a rapidly progressive condition with several systems involved over a few weeks or months, or as a slowly progressive condition with an increasing number of systems involved initially relatively mildly over several years. There are a wide variety of clinical and laboratory manifestations that may develop over time which are discussed below but each patient usually only demonstrates a few manifestations in a small number of systems at the same time.[60]

When assessing lupus patients it is important to distinguish reversible active inflammatory disease from thrombotic complications of anti-phospholipid syndrome, and to distinguish active lupus from chronic damage due to the accumulated effects of the disease and its therapy: for example lung fibrosis, myocardial infarction, or cataracts.[61] The possibility of infection and other comorbidity should be considered, especially as infection is a common trigger for lupus. Flares of active disease may also be triggered by UV light exposure, hormonal changes (oestrogens), and stress (e.g. major life events).

Constitutional features

The most common complaint of lupus patients is fatigue. It is important to be sure that fatigue is not due to a comorbid condition such as hypothyroidism, iron deficiency anaemia, depression, fibromyalgia, or chronic postviral or isolated chronic fatigue syndrome. Fatigue often contributes to the poor quality of life experienced by lupus patients.[62]

Fever with temperatures above 37.5 °C can occur due to lupus itself. It can also be due to comorbid conditions that need excluding including infection, lymphoma, and occasionally other malignant conditions. It is particularly important to bear in mind that lupus patients are more susceptible than healthy people to atypical infections, including tuberculosis (TB), pneumocystis, and cytomegalovirus (CMV) infection. Occasionally patients develop fungal infection secondary to cytotoxic therapy, or other infections which are more often associated with HIV infection. This is no coincidence, since both HIV infection and SLE are associated with low CD4 Th cell numbers, as lupus patients make antibodies to CD4+ T cells.

Lupus patients may develop reactive lymphadenopathy. This is most often seen in the early years of the disease course. A small number of patients present with Kikuchi–Fujimoto syndrome.[63,64] This is a necrotizing lymphadenitis that is known to predispose to autoimmune diseases including SLE and autoimmune hypothyroidism. Lymphadenopathy can also be due to infection, lymphoma[65] or other malignancy and needs to be investigated if the lymph nodes steadily enlarge. Fluctuating lymphadenopathy is more typical of lupus, particularly when there are other features of active lupus disease.

Anorexia and weight loss occur in some patients with active disease, particularly those with other constitutional features, and have the same differential diagnosis as fever and lympadenopathy. Anorexia and weight loss can also be due to depression or drug side effects. In addition, some patients who reduce their steroid dose or come off steroids altogether report quite marked weight loss, particularly if they put weight on while on higher doses of oral corticosteroids. For patients who have discontinued steroids completely there is always the risk that the original disease will return, but weight loss is rarely the first presenting feature of a lupus flare.

Mucocutaneous manifestations

Photosensitivity occurs in 50–60% of lupus patients, particularly those of white European origin, but is less common in those of African origin. Patients present most often with photosensitive maculopapular, subacute lupus, or discoid rashes. These rashes can also occur in the absence of photosensitivity. Subacute lupus rash may present as non-indurated psoriasiform and/or annular polycyclic lesions that resolve without scarring, but sometimes show postinflammatory dyspigmentation or telangiectasia. Rarer types of lupus rash are recognized.[66,67] The discoid lesions cause the most distress as they can be associated with scarring and may heal with either hypopigmentation or hyperpigmentation. Vasculitic rashes may also leave scarring with or without pigment changes, but subacute lupus and maculopapular lesions, including the generalized butterfly rash, usually resolve without any scarring or pigment change.

Reflex vasoconstriction of the blood vessels known as Raynaud's phenomenon is common in both the hands and feet. The characteristic three-colour change is white to blue with vasoconstriction, then red on rewarming, but two colour change is sometimes seen. It may also effect the other extremities, including the ear and the nose. Raynaud's and severe digital ischaemia can occur in patients exposed to drops in temperature of only 5–10 °C without going down to freezing and can result in significant digital infarction and gangrene. It is important to monitor the skin very carefully in these patients because of the risk of infection which can be difficult to treat due to the poor blood supply. These patients often require intravenous antibiotics and prolonged antibiotic courses to eradicate infection in the ischaemic extremities.

Vasculitic lesions can also progress to infarction and sometimes ulceration with a risk of secondary infection. Vasculitic lesions occur most commonly on the hands and feet, but can occur on all parts of the body and are typically associated with non-blanching purpuric rashes or subcutaneous erythema/nodules such as Janeway lesions as seen in subacute bacterial endocarditis, which is also due to immune complex deposition. Blistering lesions due to lupus are uncommon. The important differential diagnosis for localized areas of blisters in a dermatone distribution is herpes zoster (shingles) which is more common in patients on immunosuppressants. Rarely disseminated herpes zoster can occur with devastating consequences in patients without pre-existing immunity to this virus.[68]

Diffuse alopecia is more common than patchy alopecia. Diffuse alopecia often starts around the hairline and may be associated with irregular short hairs on the hairline in the frontal region known as lupus frizz, particularly in patients of African origin. Diffuse alopecia may persist longer than other features of active lupus disease after treatment is initiated. Patients may need reassurance that their hair will gradually stop falling out and will regrow. In some cases it may remain thinner than it used to be and it may change consistency and even colour. Patchy hair loss can resolve completely with treatment over time, but if there is an associated discoid rash that heals with scarring, the patch of alopecia is likely to persist.

Nasal and oral ulcers are quite common in lupus patients. They may be painful or painless The oral ulcers are indistinguishable from normal apthous ulcers and those that occur in Behçet's syndrome and Crohn's disease. They tend to occur in crops within the oral cavity including the pharynx, and they may persist longer than in people without lupus. Some patients get mucosal ulceration in other regions including the vagina but this is less common than nasal and oral ulceration. It is important to exclude herpes simplex infection when genital ulcers occur, particularly in immunosuppressed patients.

Oral and ocular dryness due to immune destruction of mucosal glands occurs with increasing age. It is known as secondary Sjögren's syndrome and is more common with patients with anti-Ro and anti-La antibodies. Primary Sjögren's syndrome can be distinguished by salivary and lacrimal gland enlargement at the beginning of the disease associated with early-onset oral and ocular dryness (keratoconjunctivitis sicca). In lupus, other manifestations of lupus precede the ocular and oral dryness. Damage to other mucosal tissues may occur, for example causing dry cough and dry vagina.

Musculoskeletal manifestations

Over 90% of lupus patients suffer from inflammatory synovitis and the remainder usually suffer from arthralgia with early morning stiffness and gelling after a period of rest. Inflammatory arthritis in lupus is usually a symmetrical polyarthritis affecting small joints but it may present as a monoarthritis or oligoarthritis affecting medium and occasionally large joints. It is non-erosive and is associated with joint tenderness and stiffness but more limited amounts of swelling than is seen in other forms of inflammatory arthritis such as rheumatoid and psoriatic arthritis. Nevertheless, effusions of the knees, ankles, wrists, and even the small joints of the hand may be seen. Patients with such severe inflammatory arthritis are prone to develop ligamentous laxity leading to the deformities known as Jaccoud's arthropathy.[69] This looks similar to the deformities of rheumatoid arthritis but is not associated with erosions. During the assessment of joints it is important not to attribute to lupus pain that is due to comorbid conditions such as osteoarthritis. Some patients will develop bony swellings at the distal and proximal interphalangeal joints due to Heberden's nodes or Bouchard's nodes as they get older.

Mild diffuse muscle pain (myalgia) associated with inflammatory arthralgia with a lot of early morning stiffness is likely to be due to lupus. However some patients have persistent diffuse tenderness around the joints and muscles due to fibromyalgia. Studies, particularly in North America, have shown that up to one-third of lupus patients can develop fibromyalgia, which is distinguished by the presence of multiple tender points typical of fibromyalgia. Thus it is important to do a full assessment when patients complain of joint and muscle pain to determine the underlying cause appropriately.

Inflammatory myositis tends to affect the proximal muscles of the arms and legs, and is the least common cause of myalgia. This is characterized by the development of proximal weakness in association with muscle tenderness, stiffness, and raised muscle enzymes. Patients who are anti-RNP antibody positive with features of an overlap syndrome or mixed connective tissue disease[70] consisting of lupus and systemic sclerosis are the most likely to develop inflammatory myositis. Important differential diagnoses to consider in patients with muscle weakness are steroid-induced myopathy and statin-induced myopathy.

Lupus patients are at increased risk of avascular necrosis which may affect the hip, shoulder, knee, wrist, or ankle. It is usually unilateral and presents in a single joint but it may affect more than one joint and become symmetrical over time. Although some studies have suggested that this is directly due to steroids, other studies have suggested that it is more likely to occur after periods of high disease activity[71] and it is probably the result of localized inflammatory vascular damage or thrombosis in certain bones, since it is not a generalized condition like steroid-induced osteoporosis. MRI scan is much better than plain radiographs at detecting early avascular necrosis. Avascular necrosis needs to be distinguished from other causes of acute single joint pain that present in the absence of a generalized disease flare, such as septic arthritis and osteoarthritis.

Respiratory features

Pleurisy is common in SLE and occurs in about 60% of patients. It can be difficult to distinguish left anterior chest pain due to pleurisy and pericarditis clinically, although pericardial pain is typically worse lying down and better sitting forward. It is important to distinguish both of these from musculoskeletal chest wall pain with localized tenderness. Pleuritic chest pain due to inflammation of the pleura is not necessarily associated with a pleural rub or effusion that can be detected clinically but small effusions may be picked up on radiographs (blunting of costophrenic angle), ultrasound, or CT scan. Large pleural effusions are rare and should be aspirated to exclude infection, including TB, and malignancy. Pleural thickening, like respiratory muscle weakness or shrinking lung syndrome which can occur in lupus, is associated with small-volume lungs with a restrictive defect on lung function tests and preserved diffusion factor.

Pulmonary embolism usually presents with pleuritic chest pain and is commonest in patients with anti-phospholipid antibodies. Pulmonary emboli may occur in patients with a prothrombolic tendency for other reasons, with or without a preceding history of deep vein thrombosis (DVT) in the leg. Recurrent small pulmonary emboli may present with shortness of breath on exertion without chest pain. Patients should be investigated with V/Q scan or CT pulmonary angiography (CTPA).

Interstitial lung disease is less common but more serious than pleurisy. It usually presents with increasing shortness of breath on exertion and dry cough. There is an acute form of alveolitis or pneumonitis that can deteriorate rapidly. This needs to be distinguished from pneumonia, heart failure, and adult respiratory distress syndrome (ARDS). Broad-spectrum antibiotics covering atypical infections may need to be started together with immunosuppression while awaiting the results of investigations, as respiratory failure can develop in a few days in up to 50% of patients. The subacute form of alveolitis is more common and progresses more slowly over several weeks or months. Both can result in permanent lung fibrosis if not treated promptly with intense immunosuppression. Patients should be investigated with lung function tests (restrictive deflect with impaired diffusion) and high-resolution CT (HRCT) scan initially which is much more sensitive than plain radiographs.[72] Lung function tests can be used to monitor for progression and response to therapy.

Cardiac features

Pericarditis occurs in about 60% of patients and presents with chest pain on inspiration that is worse lying down and better sitting forward, without chest wall tenderness. A pericardial rub and ECG abnormalities are not required for a clinical diagnosis of pericarditis. Echocardiography is the best way to assess whether or not there is a pericardial effusion. Rarely pericardial effusions can enlarge sufficiently to cause cardiac tamponade. As with large pleural effusions, large pericardial effusions should be investigated to exclude coexistent infection or malignancy.

Myocarditis due to lupus is rare and presents with heart failure or arrhythmias. Bradycardia or tachycardia may occur and may cause syncope which needs to be distinguished from epileptic seizures or drop attacks due to cerebral ischaemic events. Patients may require 24 hour ECG monitoring to confirm the arrhythmia. Myocarditis is usually biventricular and may be associated with pericarditis. Diagnosis usually requires cardiac enzymes, ECG, echocardiography, and a perfusion scan, cardiac MRI or angiography. Other causes of myocardial dysfunction include systemic or pulmonary hypertension, or myocardial ischaemia. Ischaemic heart disease secondary to atherosclerosis is more common than coronary vasculitis or thrombosis of coronary vessels in patients with anti-phospholipid syndrome (APS) and is an increasingly important cause of death in lupus patients.[24,73,74]

Endocardial disease is most often found as a coincidental finding as the time of echocardiography. Mitral and aortic valve lesions are more common than tricuspid and pulmonary valve lesions. Patients with pulmonary hypertension may present with tricuspid regurgitation and right ventricular failure. Less than 10% of patients deteriorate to the point that they need valve repair or replacement surgery. Some studies suggest that endocarditis is more common in patients with APS. Libman–Sachs endocarditis is the name given to the aseptic vegetations on heart valves in lupus patients. There is a risk that these will become infected during septicaemia, particularly in patients on immunosuppressants. These patients should be considered for antibiotic prophylaxis during surgical procedures, including complex dental procedures, and great care is needed with insertion of central lines.

Pulmonary hypertension is rare (<5%) but most common in patients with lupus anti-coagulant,[75] with or without a history of thromboembolism, and in patients with pulmonary fibrosis. Pulmonary hypertension, irrespective of the underlying cause, is associated with about 50% mortality in pregnancy, so echocardiography should be arranged in patients at high risk of this complication at the time of pre-pregnancy counselling before conception.[75] Prognosis has improved with the advent of therapy such as sildenafil and bosantan.[76]

Gastrointestinal manifestations

Gastrointestinal manifestations of lupus are often overlooked as they may be confused with drug side effects and comorbid conditions.[77]

Anorexia and nausea are the most common manifestations, but are more often due to drug side effects. Abdominal pain due to serositis with localized tenderness and even rebound and guarding can occur. Investigations including ultrasound and CT scan may be needed to look for comorbid conditions, particularly abscess and localized bowel disease. Ascites due to peritonitis from lupus occurs in some cases, but is uncommon. Aspirating the acidic fluid is usually required to exclude infection including TB and malignant cells. Acute abdominal pain with vomiting and constipation raises the possibility of subacute bowel obstruction which has been reported in SLE due to inflammation in the bowel wall. Diarrhoea can occur with protein-losing enteropathy and occasionally gut vasculitis but is usually drug related.

Right hypochrondrial pain with tenderness and thickening of the gallbladder in the absence of gallstones can occur due to vasculitis of the gallbladder wall. The diagnosis is confirmed by histology at cholecystectomy. Patients may develop lupus hepatitis which needs to be differentiated from viral-induced hepatitis and hepatitis due to drugs. Sclerosing cholangitis is less common in lupus than in systemic sclerosis. Acute pancreatitis due to vasculitis can occur in lupus. This is often attributed to steroids or azathioprine but is more often due to active disease that has not been controlled by immunosuppressive therapy.

Renal manifestations

Renal involvement is more prevalent and associated with higher risk of renal failure in patients of African or Chinese origin than in those of white European origin. Proliferative glomerulonephritis is most common in patients who are anti-dsDNA antibody positive, especially by crithidia or radioimmunoassay. Anti-C1q antibodies are associated with class 3 and class 4 proliferative glomerulonephritis as well. The World Health Organization (WHO) classification of lupus nephritis was revised in 2003 and Table 117.3 shows a simplified version of the International Society of Nephrology/Renal Pathology Society classification of lupus nephritis (LN).[78] More recently a European consensus statement has been developed that covers the classification of patients with LN, how classification affects the selection of treatment options and definitions of response, flare, induction, and maintenance.[79] Usually patients with class 1, 2, and 5 disease present with isolated proteinuria, whereas those with class 3 and class 4 disease present with a positive urinary sediment consisting of red cells, white cells and/or casts, and a lesser degree of proteinuria. However, nephrotic range proteinuria may develop in patients with class 3, 4, or 5 disease and the only way to establish the nature of the renal disease and the amount of activity and damage is by biopsy. It is important to arrange renal biopsy promptly in patients who develop reproducible proteinuria of more than 0.5 g in 24 hours or equivalent by polymerase chain reaction (PCR) (~50 mg/mmol on early morning spot urine), if there are casts, red cells, or white cells which are not attributable to other conditions such as menstrual blood loss or infection. In patients with isolated proteinuria it is acceptable not to biopsy unless the proteinuria rises above 2 g in 24 hours (~200 mg/mmol) unless the patient is developing renal impairment. Patients with anti-phospholipid antibodies, particularly those with APS, are at increased risk of developing APS-related nephropathy which is associated with a worse prognosis. Patients may progress to endstage renal disease requiring dialysis or transplantation with class 3, 4, or 5 disease if not diagnosed early and treated optimally, but class 5 disease is usually more slowly

Table 117.3 Simplified version of the International Society of Nephrology/Renal Pathology Society classification of Lupus Nephritis[78]

Class	Name	Features
I	Minimal mesangial lupus nephritis	Normal at light microscopy Mesangial deposits on immunofluorescence
II	Mesangial proliferative lupus nephritis	Mesangial hypercellularity or expansion with mesangial immune deposits Some subepithelial or subendothelial deposits on immunofluorescence by electron microscopy
III	Focal lupus nephritis	Involves <50% glomeruli. Active or inactive lesions typically with subendothelial deposits
IV	Diffuse lupus nephritis	Involves >50% glomeruli. Active or inactive diffuse, segmental or global endo-or extracapillary glomerulomephritis. Typically with subendothelial deposits. Divided into diffuse segmental when >50% of involved glomeruli have segmental lesions and diffuse global when >50% of involved glomeruli have global lesions
V	Membranous lupus nephritis	Global or segmental subepithelial immune deposits by light microscopy and immunofluorescence or electron microscopy, with or without mesangial changes Class V lupus nephritis may occur in combination with class III or class IV disease in which case both are diagnosed Class V disease may show advanced sclerosis
VI	Advanced sclerosis lupus nephritis	>90% of glomeruli globally sclerosed without residual activity

Table 117.4 The 19 American College of Rheumatology neuropsychiatric lupus syndromes

Central	Peripheral
Acute confusional state	Acute inflammatory demyelinating polyradiculoneuropathy (Guillain–Barré syndrome)
Aseptic meningitis	Autonomic disorder
Anxiety disorder	Mononeuropathy (single or multiplex)
Cerebrovascular disease	Myasthenia gravis
Cognitive dysfunction	Neuropathy, cranial
Demyelinating syndrome	Plexopathy
Headache (including migraine and benign intracranial hypertension)	Polyneuropathy
Mood disorder	
Movement disorders (including chorea)	
Myelopathy	
Psychosis	
Seizure disorders	

progressive unless it is associated with class 3 or 4 disease. Patients who fail to improve with therapy should be rebiopsied to determine whether there has been transformation to another class, increasing damage or other changes.

Neuropsychiatric features

In 1999 the ACR nomenclature and case definitions for neuropsychiatric lupus syndromes were reported.[80] These covered 19 clinical syndromes affecting the central and peripheral nervous systems (Table 117.4). Potential non-lupus causes and associations were described as well as the case definitions and investigations necessary for their reporting in patients with lupus. The aim of this work was to standardize the terminology used, so that these often uncommon syndromes reported by different investigators could be better compared. Sixteen of the syndromes are associated with neuronal damage and are more common in lupus patients than controls.[81] The EULAR SLE Task Force reported more recently on the investigations and treatment of neuropsychiatric manifestations of lupus.[82] Their systematic literature search highlighted that the diagnostic work-up of such patients should be the same as for other patients presenting with the same symptoms and signs, and should focus on excluding non-lupus causes. It can be difficult to attribute neuropsychiatric manifestations to lupus in the absence of other features of active lupus disease, although neuropsychiatric lupus may occur occasionally in the absence of other manifestations of

lupus and without typical lupus serology other than anti-nuclear antibodies.

The most common central nervous system (CNS) manifestations are headache, mood disorders, cognitive dysfunction, cerebrovascular accidents, seizures, psychosis, and acute confusional state. Less common manifestations are aseptic meningitis, movement disorders such as chorea, myelopathy (transverse or longitudinal), and a demyelinating syndrome that is often confused with multiple sclerosis.[83] Oligoclonal bands in the CSF, that are distinct from those in serum reflecting intrathecal immunoglobulin production, occur both in lupus patients with neuropsychiatric lupus disease and in multiple sclerosis. Thus the diagnosis of lupus demyelinating syndrome depends on MRI features being atypical for multiple sclerosis and the clinical situation (active lupus disease elsewhere).

Most headaches in lupus patients are due to migraine and tension headaches and these are not more common than they are in the normal population. Aseptic meningitis is a cause of severe headache where attribution to lupus can be made on the basis of the CSF findings (raised protein and lymphocytes) after exclusion of infection (viral, bacterial, fungal, and protozoal). Rarely lupus patients present with very severe, intractable headache that persists for at least 3 days and does not respond to opiate analgesia but does improve after administration of high-dose corticosteroids. This is what is meant by the term 'lupus headache', and, as with aseptic meningitis, the diagnosis should only be made after investigations to exclude other causes of such severe headache including CT or MRI brain scan and CSF examination. Other causes of such severe headaches in lupus patients that need to be excluded include malignant hypertension, cerebral or subarachnoid haemorrhage, cerebral abscess, uraemia, and other metabolic or drug-related disorders. Occasionally patients present with severe headache and papilloedema due to benign intracranial hypertension which may be due to lupus, obesity, or with a cerebral venous sinus thrombosis. The latter usually occurs in patients with APS. It is important to obtain CT or MR venography in patients in whom this is a possibility.

Anti-phospholipid antibodies can be associated with cerebrovascular accidents due to arterial thrombosis, seizures, myelopathy, demyelinating syndrome, and chorea. However, the commonest cause of a stroke is atherosclerosis, though occasionally there may be emboli from Libman–Sachs endocarditis or from carotid plaques. Cerebral vasculitis is rare. Seizures are commonest early in the disease course and are often self-limiting when the active disease is controlled, especially if the MRI brain scan is normal. However, if recurrent epileptic seizures occur, especially in the presence of an abnormal MRI scan, long-term anticonvulsant therapy is usually required. Myelopathy usually presents as a rapidly progressive transverse myelitis, but may affect multiple levels, often with early bladder involvement. It can be difficult to establish if the lesions are inflammatory or thrombotic and treatment for both may be needed while awaiting investigation results. It should be noted that the spinal MRI can be normal in the early stages and this should not prevent patients with classic clinical features being treated.

Mood disorders such as depression and anxiety, like headaches, are more often due to non-lupus causes including psychosocial issues than due to lupus. Psychosis may be due to lupus or to corticosteroids but is rare with prednisolone doses equivalent to 30 mg prednisolone daily or less. When in doubt, give patients more, not less, steroid, particularly if there is active lupus in other systems, together with an anti-psychotic agent.

Lupus patients may develop a relatively benign sensory neuropathy or more serious mixed sensory and motor cranial or peripheral mononeuropathy, or polyneuropathies (glove and stocking distribution or mononeuritis multiplex) due to vasculitis of the vasa nervorum. Rare peripheral conditions include acute inflammatory demyelinating polyradiculoneuropathy (presenting like Guillain–Barré syndrome), autonomic neuropathy, brachial or lumbar plexopathy, and myasthenia gravis. Nerve conduction studies are important in confirming and monitoring these peripheral conditions.

Ophthalmic manifestations

All layers of the eye can be affected by lupus.[84] The most common condition is inflammatory destruction of the conjunctival epithelium resulting in chronic irritation of the eyes with reduced tear production, known as keratoconjunctivitis sicca (dry eyes). This usually occurs in patients who are anti-Ro or anti-La antibody positive. In contrast to primary Sjögren's syndrome in which patients develop dry eyes and dry mouth due to mucosal glandular involvement early in the disease course, secondary Sjögren's syndrome tends to occur late in the course of lupus patients.

Patients with lupus may develop a benign, localized, and painless red eye condition due to episcleritis. Less common but more serious is inflammation of the choroid causing anterior uveitis and/or posterior uveitis. Anterior uveitis is distinguished from episcleritis by the more generalized redness and the presence of pain in the eye with photophobia in anterior uveitis. Posterior uveitis or chorioretinitis is more serious as the retina may be involved and this condition causes blurring and loss of vision and needs urgent management by an ophthalmologist. The formation of a hypopyon, as seen in Behçet's syndrome, is rare in lupus.

Scleritis and kerititis can occur in lupus but infectious causes of keratitis need to be sought. Scleritis can occur due to vasculitis in the sclera and occasionally is associated with thinning of the sclera as is seen in rheumatoid arthritis. Retinal vasculitis and optic neuritis are uncommon but devastating conditions that can lead to visual loss. Patients with anti-phospholipid antibodies are at risk of vaso-occlusive disease affecting retinal and choroidal vessels that may lead to anterior ischaemic optic neuropathy. Rarely diplopia and/or proptosis may occur due to orbital inflammation with myositis of the eye muscles. Prompt assessment by an ophthamologist is required to determine the diagnosis and to determine if treatment should be with immunosuppressives, anti-platelet drugs, and/or anticoagulation. Sometimes it is difficult to be sure whether the underlying pathology is inflammatory, thrombotic, or both and it is often important to exclude infection. Significant hydroxychloroquine toxicity causing visual loss is very uncommon.[85] Patients at greatest risk are those that have renal or liver impairment and/or have been treated with high dose (>6.5 mg/kg per day) and/or prolonged therapy (>10 years). In such cases macular degeneration due to hydroxychloroquine toxicity has to be distinguished from age-related macular degeneration.

Haematological manifestations

Leucopenia can be an important clue to the diagnosis of lupus, as it may be observed on a full blood count being done as part of the investigation of a patient not yet known to have lupus. It may also occur as a side effect of cytotoxic therapy in patients on therapy for established disease. The most typical feature due to lupus, found in over 90% of patients, is antibody-induced lymphopenia. This affects CD4 T cells most and leads to a low CD4:CD8 ratio as seen in HIV infection. Antibody-mediated neutropenia is much more uncommon, though it is found most often in patients of African descent. Antibody-mediated leucopenia is rarely associated with infection unless the total white count is less than 1×10^9/litre, but when there is such a severe leucopenia or lymphopenia ($<0.4 \times 10^9$/litre) there is an increased risk of opportunistic infections.

The most significant but least common haematological manifestation is antibody-mediated thrombocytopenia, which can cause significant bleeding with platelet counts below 50×10^9/litre. Idiopathic thrombocytotenic purpura may present before other features of lupus. Patients with APS often have platelet counts about $70–90 \times 10^9$/litre and this is paradoxically associated with an increased risk of thrombosis that may be venous and/or arterial, and with or without pregnancy complications.[37] In patients who are known to have APS it is important to not discontinue anti-platelet or anti-coagulant drugs unless the platelet count is less 30×10^9/litre because of the risk that they can develop a clinical thrombosis once the platelet count rises above 30×10^9/litre.

Anaemia of chronic disease is more common than autoimmune haemolytic anaemia. Haemolysis can be diagnosed if there is a positive Coombs' test and low haptoglobins, increased reticulocyte count, and/or raised non-conjugated bilirubin. Anaemia due to chronic inflammation that impairs utilization of iron needs to be distinguished from iron deficiency anaemia due to dietary deficiency and/or blood loss from the gut due to drugs or occasionally bowel involvement by the disease.

Obstetric issues

In the past, patients with lupus were recommended not to become pregnant. It is now recognized that most women can have a successful pregnancy as long as they do not have active lupus disease in the 6 months preceding conception, significant renal impairment, pulmonary hypertension, or other serious heart, lung, or neurological disease.[86] Infertility due to anti-ovarian antibodies is rare in lupus patients and when infertility occurs it is usually due to cyclophosphamide therapy, especially in those over 30 years of age.[87] It should be noted that low doses and short courses with less than 7 g cumulative dose in patients under 30 years of age is associated with a low risk of infertility. However, in those over 35 years of age cyclophosphamide usually induces the menopause. Lupus patients with anti-phospholipid antibodies may suffer recurrent pregnancy losses, particularly in the second or third trimester. APS also predisposes to pre-eclampsia and thrombosis in the mother during pregnancy.[37,86] The baby should be monitored for intrauterine growth restriction (IUGR) due to placental insufficiency during pregnancy so that the mother can be offered early delivery if necessary to avoid the risk of stillbirth. IUGR is most commonly due to APS but can occur in patients with active lupus, pre-eclampsia, and renal impairment. Fetal heart rate monitoring should start at 16 weeks' gestation in mothers with anti-Ro and anti-La antibodies because of the risk of congenital heart block.[34] This only occurs in about 1% of babies born to mothers with these antibodies though the risk is about 20% if the mother has had a previous baby with this condition. The risk of neonatal lupus syndrome presenting with a photosensitive rash due to anti-Ro and anti-La antibodies is about 10%.

Diagnosis and classification of lupus

The diagnosis of lupus is most reliably made by identifying typical clinical features of lupus associated with evidence of an immune complex mediated disease involving the production of autoantibodies. The ACR (formerly the American Rheumatological Association) classification criteria for SLE are often used as diagnostic criteria (Table 117.5). However, they were designed to provide criteria for patients going in to clinical research and not for diagnosis.[66,88,89] Patients are required to have at least 4 of the 11 criteria listed in Table 117.5 at any point in time to fulfil these criteria. More recently the Systemic Lupus International Collaborating Clinics (SLICC) group have proposed revised criteria for lupus as the ACR criteria do not include many features of lupus and allow patients to be classified even if they have not had autoantibodies or other serological abnormalities documented.[90] These new SLICC criteria allow a patient to be classified as having lupus if they have a classical renal biopsy, e.g. class IV glomerulonephritis and positive ANA or anti-dsDNA antibodies, but otherwise require at least four criteria from an expanded list of which at least one must be clinical and at least one a serological criterion (Table 117.6).[90]

Monitoring disease activity and distinguishing damage

Patients with lupus should be monitored at intervals depending on their disease manifestations, blood results, and therapy.[91,92] Patients with very active disease including renal involvement are usually seen 2–4 weekly and may require blood tests 1–2 weekly for monitoring their disease-modifying therapy, bearing in mind the risk of cytopenias due to the disease and the drugs. For patients with LN assessment is usually at least 3 monthly, even when they appear to be in remission, especially if immunosuppressive therapy is being reduced or has been discontinued, as flare may be asymptomatic. Rising titres of anti-dsDNA antibodies and/or falling complement

Table 117.5 The 11 revised criteria of the American College of Rheumatology for the classification of systemic lupus erythematosus

Malar rash	Fixed erythema, flat or raised, over the malar eminences tending to spare the nasolabial folds
Discoid rash	Erythematosus raised patches with adherent keratotic scaling and follicular plugging; atrophic scarring may occur in older lesions
Photosensitivity	Skin rash as a result of unusual reaction to sunlight, by patient history or physician observation
Oral ulcers	Oral or nasopharyngeal ulceration, usually painless, observed by a physician
Arthritis	Non-erosive arthritis involving two or more peripheral joints, characterized by tenderness, swelling, or effusion
Serositis	(a) Pleuritis—convincing history of pleuritic pain or rub heard by a physician or evidence of pleural effusion or (b) Pericarditis—documented by ECG or rub or evidence of pericardial effusion
Renal disorder	(a) Persistent proteinuria >0.5 g/day or >3+ if quantification not performed or (b) Cellular casts—may be red cell, haemoglobin, granular, tubular, or mixed
Neurological disorder	(a) Seizures—in the absence of offending drugs or known metabolic derangements; e.g. uraemia, ketoacidosis, or electrolyte imbalance; or (b) Psychosis—in the absence of offending drugs or known metabolic derangements; e.g. uraemia, ketoacidosis, or electrolyte imbalance
Haematological disorder	(a) Haemolytic anaemia—with reticulocytosis or (b) Leucopenia < 4.0×10^9/l on two or more occasions (c) Lymphopenia <1.5×10^9/l on two or more occasions (d) Thrombocytopenia <150×10^9/l
Immunological disorder	(a) Anti-dsDNA: antibody to asDNA in abnormal titre, or (b) Anti-Sm: presence of antibody to Sm nuclear antigen, orPositive finding of anti-phospholipid antibodies based on: (1) abnormal serum level of IgG or IgM anti-cardiolipin antibodies; (2) positive test for lupus anti-coagulant using a standard method, or (3) false-positive test for at least 6 months and confirmed by *Treponema pallidum* immobilization or fluorescent antibody absorption test
Positive ANA	Abnormal titre of ANA by immunofluorescence or an equivalent assay at any point in time in the absence of drugs

ANA, anti-nuclear antibody.

levels suggest that a lupus flare may occur though it is hard to predict when, so patients may need to be seen more frequently. For patients with stable low level activity or remission, with no renal involvement and no serological changes, lupus assessment may be 3–6 monthly. Assessment of patients requires a review of all systems including blood pressure, urinalysis, and measures of renal function, as well as full blood count and measurement of anti-dsDNA antibodies, C3 and C4.[61] If proteinuria is present, quantification should occur using measurement of 12 or 24 hour urine protein, protein:creatinine ratio, or albumin:creatinine ratio, and urine microscopy to identify red and white cells and casts. A urine sample should be sent for culture to exclude infection and other causes of

Table 117.6 Clinical and immunological criteria used in the SLICC classification criteria for systemic lupus erythematosus (see text)

Type of criterion	No.	Criterion	Description of components
Clinical	1	Acute cutaneous lupus	Lupus malar rash (do not count if malar discoid)
			Bullous lupus
			Toxic epidermal necrolysis variant of SLE
			Maculopapular lupus rash
			Photosensitive lupus rash
			Subacute cutaneous lupus
	2	Chronic cutaneous lupus	Classical discoid rash: localized (above the neck) generalized (above and below the neck)
			Hypertrophic (verrucous) lupus
			Lupus panniculitis (profundus)
			Mucosal lupus
			Lupus erythematosus tumidus
			Chillblains lupus
			Discoid lupus/lichen planus overlap
	3	Mucosal ulcers	Oral ulcers: palate, buccal, tongue
			Nasal ulcers
	4	Non-scarring alopecia	Diffuse thinning or hair fragility with visible broken hairs
	5	Synovitis involving two or more joints	Characterized by swelling or effusion, *or*
			Tenderness in two or more joints *and*
			≥30 minutes of morning stiffness
	6	Serositis	Typical pleurisy for >1 day *and/or* pleural effusions *and/or* pleural rub
			Typical pericardial pain (pain with recumbency improved by sitting forward) for >1 day *and/or* pericardial effusion *and/or* pericardial rub *and/or* pericarditis by ECG
	7	Renal	Urine protein/creatinine (or 24 h urine protein) representing 500 mg of protein/24 h, *and/or*
			Red blood cell casts
	8	Neurological	Seizures
			Psychosis
			Mononeuritis multiplex
			Myelitis
			Peripheral or cranial neuropathy
			Acute confusional state (*in the absence of other causes*)
	9	Haemolytic anaemia	
	10	Leucopenia, *or* Lymphopenia	White cell count <4000/mm³ at least once (*not due to drugs*), *or* Lymphocyte count <1000/mm³ at least once (*not due to drugs*)
	11	Thrombocytopenia	Platelet count <100 000/mm³ at least once
Immunological	1	ANA	Above laboratory reference range
	2	Anti-dsDNA antibodies	Above laboratory reference range, except ELISA: Twice above laboratory reference range
	3	Anti-Sm antibodies	Above laboratory reference range
	4	Anti-phospholipid antibodies	Lupus anti-coagulant
			False-positive RPR
			Medium or high titre anticardiolipin (IgA, IgG, or IgM)
			Anti-β₂ glycoprotein I (IgA, IgG, or IgM)
	5	Low complement	Low C3
			Low C4
			Low CH50
	6	Direct Coombs' test	*In the absence of haemolytic anaemia*

red and white cells in the urine should be considered (stone, contamination by menses or vaginal infection). Validated disease activity measures are recommended for use in clinical practice as well as clinical trials and outcome studies.[61,91,92] The most widely used are the BILAG-2004 index and the SLEDAI-2K, though other versions of SLEDAI are in use such as the SELENA-SLEDAI.[93] The patients' perspective should be captured using a generic health survey such as the SF-36 and/or a lupus-specific quality of life instrument such as the LupusQoL, as patients often have poor quality of life.[62,93]

Irreversible damage (scarring) due to the disease or its treatment should be distinguished from disease activity, as this will not respond to immunosuppressive therapy.[61] It is also important to identify comorbid conditions such as infection, malignancy, and drug side effects. Malignancy is slightly more common in lupus patients that expected, especially lymphoma, and lung cancer in smokers. However some cancers such as breast, ovary, endometrial, and prostate are less common than expected.[94] The SLICC/ACR Damage Index can be used to record damage in routine clinical practice and for research studies.[61,91] Damage items are recorded if a feature appears after the onset of lupus and persists at least 6 months or is associated with a classical scar such as myocardial infarction in which case it can be recorded immediately.

Outcome and causes of death

The survival in SLE patients has improved over the last 50 years from about 50% survival at 5 years after diagnosis in the 1950s to survival figures of up to 98% at 5 years and 95% survival at 10 years.[3] Prognosis for patients with renal involvement, African or Chinese descent, Hispanic ethnicity, and poor socio-economic background has been less good than for patients without these factors. The main causes of death are increasingly infection and cardiovascular disease (especially premature atherosclerosis secondary to lupus) rather than acute lupus disease. However, if access to good health care is limited by availability or cost there are still significant numbers of deaths due to lupus activity and renal failure in certain populations. In the multisite international SLE cohort (23 centres, 9547 patients) studied by the SLICC, the standardized mortality ratio (95% CI) was 2.4 (2.3–2.5).[73] The commonest causes of death in SLE patients (expressed as a standardized mortality ratio) were infections (9.0), renal disease (7.9), non-Hodgkin's lymphoma (2.8), lung cancer (2.3), and circulatory diseases (1.7). Increased risk of death was associated with female gender, younger age, shorter SLE duration, and black/African-American race. To improve outcomes, it is important that patients have access to high-quality care with prompt investigations and treatment of lupus and complications such as infection, hypertension, and atherosclerosis. Monitoring vaccination and smoking status, and ensuring that screening for comorbidities such as hypertension, hypercholesterolaemia, diabetes mellitus, metabolic syndrome, osteoporosis, cancer, and cervical dysplasia due to human papillomavirus (HPV) infection are important in addition to monitoring lupus if outcomes are to be improved.

References

1. Deapen D, Escalante A, Weinrib L et al. A revised estimate of twin concordance in systemic lupus erythematosus. *Arthritis Rheum* 1992;35(3):311–318.

2. Kumar K, Chambers S, Gordon C. Challenges of ethnicity in SLE. *Best Pract Res Clin Rheumatol* 2009;23(4):549–561.

3. Pons-Estel GJ, Alarcon GS, Scofield L, Reinlib L, Cooper GS. Understanding the epidemiology and progression of systemic lupus erythematosus. *Semin Arthritis Rheum* 2010;39(4):257–268.

4. Johnson AE, Gordon C, Palmer RG, Bacon PA. The prevalence and incidence of systemic lupus erythematosus in Birmingham, England. Relationship to ethnicity and country of birth. *Arthritis Rheum* 1995;38(4):551–558.

5. Cooper GS, Bynum ML, Somers EC. Recent insights in the epidemiology of autoimmune diseases: improved prevalence estimates and understanding of clustering of diseases. *J Autoimmun* 2009;33(3–4):197–207.

6. Lim SS, Drenkard C, McCune WJ et al. Population-based lupus registries: advancing our epidemiologic understanding. *Arthritis Rheum* 2009;61(10):1462–1466.

7. Drenkard CM, Bao G, Helmick CG et al. The Georgia Lupus Registry: differences in age-specific incidence rates between black and white females with SLE. *Arthritis Rheum* 2011;64(10 suppl):1847.

8. Somers EC, Marder W, Cagnoli PC et al. Population-based incidence estimates for systemic lupus erythematosus in the USA, 2002–2005: results from the Michigan Lupus Epidemiology and Surveillance (MILES) Program. *Arthritis Rheum* 2011;64(10 suppl):1849.

9. Burgos PI, McGwin G Jr, Pons-Estel GJ et al. US patients of Hispanic and African ancestry develop lupus nephritis early in the disease course: data from LUMINA, a multiethnic US cohort (LUMINA LXXIV). *Ann Rheum Dis* 2011;70(2):393–394.

10. Jakes RW, Bae SC, Louthrenoo W, Mok CC, Navarra SV, Kwon N. Systematic review of the epidemiology of systemic lupus erythematosus in the Asia-Pacific region: prevalence, incidence, clinical features, and mortality. *Arthritis Care Res* (Hoboken) 2012;64(2):159–168.

11. Hopkinson ND, Doherty M, Powell RJ. The prevalence and incidence of systemic lupus erythematosus in Nottingham, UK, 1989–1990. *Br J Rheumatol* 1993;32(2):110–115.

12. Stahl-Hallengren C, Jonsen A, Nived O, Sturfelt G. Incidence studies of systemic lupus erythematosus in Southern Sweden: increasing age, decreasing frequency of renal manifestations and good prognosis. *J Rheumatol* 2000;27(3):685–691.

13. Somers EC, Thomas SL, Smeeth L, Schoonen WM, Hall AJ. Incidence of systemic lupus erythematosus in the United Kingdom, 1990–1999. *Arthritis Rheum* 2007;57(4):612–618.

14. Rahman A, Isenberg DA. Systemic lupus erythematosus. *N Engl J Med* 2008;358(9):929–939.

15. Botto M, Walport MJ. C1q, autoimmunity and apoptosis. *Immunobiology* 2002;205(4–5):395–406.

16. Norsworthy P, Theodoridis E, Botto M et al. Overrepresentation of the Fc gamma receptor type IIA R131/R131 genotype in caucasoid systemic lupus erythematosus patients with autoantibodies to C1q and glomerulonephritis. *Arthritis Rheum* 1999;42(9):1828–1832.

17. Shao WH, Cohen PL. Disturbances of apoptotic cell clearance in systemic lupus erythematosus. *Arthritis Res Ther* 2011;13(1):202.

18. Munoz LE, Janko C, Schulze C et al. Autoimmunity and chronic inflammation—two clearance-related steps in the etiopathogenesis of SLE. *Autoimmun Rev* 2010;10(1):38–42.

19. Niederer HA, Clatworthy MR, Willcocks LC, Smith KG. FcgammaRIIB, FcgammaRIIIB, and systemic lupus erythematosus. *Ann N Y Acad Sci* 2010;1183:69–88.

20. Rhodes B, Vyse TJ. The genetics of SLE: an update in the light of genome-wide association studies. *Rheumatology* (Oxford) 2008;47(11):1603–1611.

21. Fairhurst AM, Wandstrat AE, Wakeland EK. Systemic lupus erythematosus: multiple immunological phenotypes in a complex genetic disease. *Adv Immunol* 2006;92:1–69.

22. Salloum R, Niewold TB. Interferon regulatory factors in human lupus pathogenesis. *Transl Res* 2011;157(6):326–331.

23. Niewold TB, Kelly JA, Kariuki SN et al. IRF5 haplotypes demonstrate diverse serological associations which predict serum interferon alpha activity and explain the majority of the genetic association with systemic lupus erythematosus. *Ann Rheum Dis* 2012;71(3):463–468.

24. Skaggs BJ, Hahn BH, McMahon M. Accelerated atherosclerosis in patients with SLE-mechanisms and management. *Nat Rev Rheumatol* 2012;8(4):214–223.

25. Buyon JP, Petri MA, Kim MY et al. The effect of combined estrogen and progesterone hormone replacement therapy on disease activity in systemic lupus erythematosus: a randomized trial. *Ann Intern Med* 2005;142(12 Pt 1):953–962.

26. Petri M, Kim MY, Kalunian KC et al. Combined oral contraceptives in women with systemic lupus erythematosus. *N Engl J Med* 2005; 353(24):2550–2558.

27. Sanchez-Guerrero J, Uribe AG, Jimenez-Santana L et al. A trial of contraceptive methods in women with systemic lupus erythematosus. *N Engl J Med* 2005;353(24):2539–2549.

28. Colasanti T, Maselli A, Conti F et al. Autoantibodies to estrogen receptor alpha interfere with T lymphocyte homeostasis and are associated with disease activity in systemic lupus erythematosus. *Arthritis Rheum* 2012;64(3):778–787.

29. Kassi E, Moutsatsou P. Estrogen receptor signaling and its relationship to cytokines in systemic lupus erythematosus. *J Biomed Biotechnol* 2010;2010:317452.

30. Gordon C, Salmon M. Update on systemic lupus erythematosus: autoantibodies and apoptosis. *Clin Med* 2001;1(1):10–14.

31. Arbuckle MR, McClain MT, Rubertone MV et al. Development of autoantibodies before the clinical onset of systemic lupus erythematosus. *N Engl J Med* 2003;349(16):1526–1533.

32. Manson JJ, Ma A, Rogers P et al. Relationship between anti-dsDNA, anti-nucleosome and anti-alpha-actinin antibodies and markers of renal disease in patients with lupus nephritis: a prospective longitudinal study. *Arthritis Res Ther* 2009;11(5):R154.

33. Grootscholten C, van Bruggen MC, van der Pijl JW et al. Deposition of nucleosomal antigens (histones and DNA) in the epidermal

basement membrane in human lupus nephritis. *Arthritis Rheum* 2003; 48(5):1355–1362.

34. Brucato A, Cimaz R, Caporali R, Ramoni V, Buyon J. Pregnancy outcomes in patients with autoimmune diseases and anti-Ro/SSA antibodies. *Clin Rev Allergy Immunol* 2011;40(1):27–41.

35. Izmirly PM, Llanos C, Lee LA, Askanase A, Kim MY, Buyon JP. Cutaneous manifestations of neonatal lupus and risk of subsequent congenital heart block. *Arthritis Rheum* 2010;62(4):1153–1157.

36. Faust TW, Chang EH, Kowal C et al. Neurotoxic lupus autoantibodies alter brain function through two distinct mechanisms. *Proc Natl Acad Sci* U S A 2010;107(43):18569–18574.

37. Ruiz-Irastorza G, Crowther M, Branch W, Khamashta MA. Antiphospholipid syndrome. *Lancet* 2010;376(9751):1498–1509.

38. van der Vlag J, Berden JH. Lupus nephritis: role of antinucleosome autoantibodies. *Semin Nephrol* 2011;31(4):376–389.

39. Merrill JT, Burgos-Vargas R, Westhovens R et al. The efficacy and safety of abatacept in patients with non-life-threatening manifestations of systemic lupus erythematosus: results of a twelve-month, multicenter, exploratory, phase IIb, randomized, double-blind, placebo-controlled trial. *Arthritis Rheum* 2010;62(10):3077–3087.

40. Chavele KM, Ehrenstein MR. Regulatory T-cells in systemic lupus erythematosus and rheumatoid arthritis. *FEBS Lett* 2011;585(23): 3603–3610.

41. Crispin JC, Kyttaris VC, Terhorst C, Tsokos GC. T cells as therapeutic targets in SLE. *Nat Rev Rheumatol* 2010;6(6):317–325.

42. Jacob N, Stohl W. Cytokine disturbances in systemic lupus erythematosus. *Arthritis Res Ther* 2011;13(4):228.

43. Poole BD, Niewold TB, Tsokos GC. Cytokines in systemic lupus erythematosus 2011. *J Biomed Biotechnol* 2012;2012:427824.

44. Cancro MP, D'Cruz DP, Khamashta MA. The role of B lymphocyte stimulator (BLyS) in systemic lupus erythematosus. *J Clin Invest* 2009; 119(5):1066–1073.

45. Navarra SV, Guzman RM, Gallacher AE et al. Efficacy and safety of belimumab in patients with active systemic lupus erythematosus: a randomised, placebo-controlled, phase 3 trial. *Lancet* 2011;377(9767):721–731.

46. Furie R, Petri M, Zamani O et al. A phase III, randomized, placebo-controlled study of belimumab, a monoclonal antibody that inhibits B lymphocyte stimulator, in patients with systemic lupus erythematosus. *Arthritis Rheum* 2011;63(12):3918–3930.

47. Dall'Era M, Chakravarty E, Wallace D et al. Reduced B lymphocyte and immunoglobulin levels after atacicept treatment in patients with systemic lupus erythematosus: results of a multicenter, phase Ib, double-blind, placebo-controlled, dose-escalating trial. *Arthritis Rheum* 2007;56(12):4142–4150.

48. Ginzler EM, Wax S, Rajeswaran A et al. Atacicept in combination with MMF and corticosteroids in lupus nephritis: results of a prematurely terminated trial. *Arthritis Res Ther* 2012;14(1):R33.

49. Yao Y, Richman L, Higgs BW et al. Neutralization of interferon-alpha/beta-inducible genes and downstream effect in a phase I trial of an anti-interferon-alpha monoclonal antibody in systemic lupus erythematosus. *Arthritis Rheum* 2009;60(6):1785–1796.

50. Merrill JT, Wallace DJ, Petri M et al. Safety profile and clinical activity of sifalimumab, a fully human anti-interferon alpha monoclonal antibody, in systemic lupus erythematosus: a phase I, multicentre, double-blind randomised study. *Ann Rheum Dis* 2011;70(11):1905–1913.

51. Llorente L, Richaud-Patin Y, Garcia-Padilla C et al. Clinical and biologic effects of anti-interleukin-10 monoclonal antibody administration in systemic lupus erythematosus. *Arthritis Rheum* 2000;43(8):1790–1800.

52. Kaly L, Rosner I. Tocilizumab—a novel therapy for non-organ-specific autoimmune diseases. *Best Pract Res Clin Rheumatol* 2012;26(1):157–165.

53. Pan HF, Tao JH, Ye DQ. Therapeutic potential of IL-27 in systemic lupus erythematosus. *Expert Opin Ther Targets* 2010;14(5):479–484.

54. Li TT, Zhang T, Chen GM et al. Low level of serum interleukin 27 in patients with systemic lupus erythematosus. *J Investig Med* 2010;58(5):737–739.

55. Kwan BC, Tam LS, Lai KB et al. The gene expression of type 17 T-helper cell-related cytokines in the urinary sediment of patients with systemic lupus erythematosus. *Rheumatology* (Oxford) 2009;48(12):1491–1497.

56. Li J, Pan HF, Cen H et al. Interleukin-21 as a potential therapeutic target for systemic lupus erythematosus. *Mol Biol Rep* 2011;38(6):4077–4081.

57. Dolff S, Abdulahad WH, Westra J et al. Increase in IL-21 producing T-cells in patients with systemic lupus erythematosus. *Arthritis Res Ther* 2011;13(5):R157.

58. Aringer M, Smolen JS. Therapeutic blockade of TNF in patients with SLE-promising or crazy? *Autoimmun Rev* 2012;11(5):321–325.

59. Aringer M, Houssiau F, Gordon C et al. Adverse events and efficacy of TNF-alpha blockade with infliximab in patients with systemic lupus erythematosus: long-term follow-up of 13 patients. *Rheumatology* (Oxford) 2009;48(11):1451–1454.

60. Smith PP, Gordon C. Systemic lupus erythematosus: clinical presentations. *Autoimmun Rev* 2010;10(1):43–45.

61. Griffiths B, Mosca M, Gordon C. Assessment of patients with systemic lupus erythematosus and the use of lupus disease activity indices. *Best Pract Res Clin Rheumatol* 2005;19(5):685–708.

62. McElhone K, Castelino M, Abbott J et al. The LupusQoL and associations with demographics and clinical measurements in patients with systemic lupus erythematosus. *J Rheumatol* 2010;37(11):2273–2279.

63. Hutchinson CB, Wang E. Kikuchi-Fujimoto disease. *Arch Pathol Lab Med* 2010;134(2):289–293.

64. Prignano F, D'Erme AM, Zanieri F, Bonciani D, Lotti T. Why is Kikuchi-Fujimoto disease misleading? *Int J Dermatol* 2012;51(5):564–567.

65. Bernatsky S, Ramsey-Goldman R, Rajan R et al. Non-Hodgkin's lymphoma in systemic lupus erythematosus. *Ann Rheum Dis* 2005;64(10):1507–1509.

66. Petri M. Review of classification criteria for systemic lupus erythematosus. *Rheum Dis Clin North Am* 2005;31(2):245–254, vi.

67. Klein RS, Morganroth PA, Werth VP. Cutaneous lupus and the Cutaneous Lupus Erythematosus Disease Area and Severity Index instrument. *Rheum Dis Clin North Am* 2010;36(1):33–51, vii.

68. Douglas KM, Gordon C, Osman H et al. Lupus and zoster. *Lancet* 2003;362(9384):616.

69. Santiago MB, Galvao V. Jaccoud arthropathy in systemic lupus erythematosus: analysis of clinical characteristics and review of the literature. *Medicine* (Baltimore) 2008;87(1):37–44.

70. Cappelli S, Bellando RS, Martinovic D et al. 'To be or not to be,' ten years after: evidence for mixed connective tissue disease as a distinct entity. *Semin Arthritis Rheum* 2012;41(4):589–598.

71. Fialho SC, Bonfa E, Vitule LF et al. Disease activity as a major risk factor for osteonecrosis in early systemic lupus erythematosus. *Lupus* 2007;16(4):239–244.

72. Devaraj A, Wells AU, Hansell DM. Computed tomographic imaging in connective tissue diseases. *Semin Respir Crit Care Med* 2007;28(4):389–397.

73. Bernatsky S, Boivin JF, Joseph L et al. Mortality in systemic lupus erythematosus. *Arthritis Rheum* 2006;54(8):2550–2557.

74. Gustafsson J, Simard JF, Gunnarsson I et al. Risk factors for cardiovascular mortality in patients with systemic lupus erythematosus, a prospective cohort study. *Arthritis Res Ther* 2012;14(2):R46.

75. Prabu A, Patel K, Yee CS et al. Prevalence and risk factors for pulmonary arterial hypertension in patients with lupus. *Rheumatology* (Oxford) 2009;48(12):1506–1511.

76. Johnson SR, Granton JT. Pulmonary hypertension in systemic sclerosis and systemic lupus erythematosus. *Eur Respir Rev* 2011;20(122): 277–286.

77. Sultan SM, Ioannou Y, Isenberg DA. A review of gastrointestinal manifestations of systemic lupus erythematosus. *Rheumatology* (Oxford) 1999;38(10):917–932.

78. Weening JJ, D'Agati VD, Schwartz MM et al. The classification of glomerulonephritis in systemic lupus erythematosus revisited. *J Am Soc Nephrol* 2004;15(2):241–250.

79. Gordon C, Jayne D, Pusey C et al. European consensus statement on the terminology used in the management of lupus glomerulonephritis. *Lupus* 2009;18(3):257–263.

80. The American College of Rheumatology nomenclature and case definitions for neuropsychiatric lupus syndromes. *Arthritis Rheum* 1999;42(4):599–608.

81. Ainiala H, Hietaharju A, Loukkola J et al. Validity of the new American College of Rheumatology criteria for neuropsychiatric lupus syndromes: a population-based evaluation. *Arthritis Rheum* 2001;45(5):419–423.

82. Bertsias GK, Ioannidis JP, Aringer M et al. EULAR recommendations for the management of systemic lupus erythematosus with neuropsychiatric manifestations: report of a task force of the EULAR standing committee for clinical affairs. *Ann Rheum Dis* 2010;69(12):2074–2082.

83. Bertsias GK, Boumpas DT. Pathogenesis, diagnosis and management of neuropsychiatric SLE manifestations. *Nat Rev Rheumatol* 2010;6(6):358–367.

84. Sivaraj RR, Durrani OM, Denniston AK, Murray PI, Gordon C. Ocular manifestations of systemic lupus erythematosus. *Rheumatology*(Oxford) 2007;46(12):1757–1762.

85. Ruiz-Irastorza G, Ramos-Casals M, Brito-Zeron P, Khamashta MA. Clinical efficacy and side effects of antimalarials in systemic lupus erythematosus: a systematic review. *Ann Rheum Dis* 2010;69(1):20–28.

86. Jain V, Gordon C. Managing pregnancy in inflammatory rheumatological diseases. *Arthritis Res Ther* 2011;13(1):206.

87. Hickman RA, Gordon C. Causes and management of infertility in systemic lupus erythematosus. *Rheumatology* (Oxford) 2011;50(9):1551–1558.

88. Tan EM, Cohen AS, Fries JF et al. The 1982 revised criteria for the classification of systemic lupus erythematosus. *Arthritis Rheum* 1982;25(11): 1271–1277.

89. Hochberg MC. Updating the American College of Rheumatology revised criteria for the classification of systemic lupus erythematosus. *Arthritis Rheum* 1997;40(9):1725.

90. Petri M, Orbai AM, Alarcon GS, Gordon C, Merrill JT, Fortin PR, et al. Derivation and validation of systemic lupus international collaborating clinics classification criteria for systemic lupus erythematosus. *Arthritis Rheum* 2012;64(8):2677–2686.

91. Mosca M, Tani C, Aringer M et al. European League Against Rheumatism recommendations for monitoring patients with systemic lupus erythematosus in clinical practice and in observational studies. *Ann Rheum Dis* 2010;69(7):1269–1274.

92. Mosca M, Tani C, Aringer M et al. Development of quality indicators to evaluate the monitoring of SLE patients in routine clinical practice. *Autoimmun Rev* 2011;10(7):383–388.

93. Yee CS, McElhone K, Teh LS, Gordon C. Assessment of disease activity and quality of life in systemic lupus erythematosus—new aspects. *Best Pract Res Clin Rheumatol* 2009;23(4):457–467.

94. Bernatsky S, Kale M, Ramsey-Goldman R, Gordon C, Clarke AE. Systemic lupus and malignancies. *Curr Opin Rheumatol* 2012;24(2):177–181.

CHAPTER 118

Systemic lupus erythematosus— management

Ida Dzifa Dey and David Isenberg

The challenge of managing systemic lupus erythematosus

Systemic lupus erythematosus (SLE) is a disease whose manifestations often fluctuate markedly. The most severe manifestations are not necessarily the most symptomatic. The goals of therapy are to control the patient's symptoms, suppress the underlying disease adequately, and prevent secondary organ damage. The correct regimen of drugs is that which achieves these aims, and balances the need to treat aggressively on occasions, mindful of the possible long-term side effects of the agents used.

Patients tend to be young and female. Since the disease is suppressed but not cured by treatment, patients may be faced with the prospect of taking potent drugs for years. The social and psychological effects of both the chronic disease and the necessity for continuing treatment must be recognized and addressed by physicians and patients. Potential effects of the drugs upon fertility or pregnancy are particularly important.

Non-pharmacological management

General measures include avoidance of UV radiation, especially in fair-skinned people since this may cause not only photosensitive rash, but also a more general flare of symptoms. Rest as appropriate, stress avoidance, prevention of infections, a diet low in saturated fats and high in fish oils, not smoking, and avoidance of oestrogen-containing contraceptive pills are also advised.

Recent studies suggest vitamin D deficiency may have a role in the aetiology of SLE and its supplementation may have possible benefits in the treatment of patients.

Vaccinations apart from 'live' vaccines in patients on greater than 10 mg prednisolone and/or immunosuppressives are safe. In patients on immunosuppressive therapy, there may be a reduction in vaccine efficacy but there is satisfactory humoral response to hepatitis A and B, influenza, and pneumococcal vaccine. It is important to update vaccinations before immunosuppressive or biological treatment. The use of hormone replacement in patients past the menopause is still controversial. The risk of disease flares when starting oestrogens after the menopause is small, but can occur.

Pharmacological management

Patients with SLE are treated with four main groups of drugs, often in combination. These are non-steroidal anti-inflammatory drugs (NSAIDs), anti-malarials, corticosteroids, and cytotoxic drugs. However, new biological therapies have been introduced, directed at particular cells or molecules implicated in the pathogenesis of the disease.

Recommendations about precisely when to commence therapy, the initial dose of a given drug, the likely response of a given symptom, and the duration of treatment vary widely. In Table 118.1, the broad indications for use of these four types of drugs are shown. In Table 118.2, suggestions are provided as to the initial doses and duration of treatment with the anti-malarials, corticosteroids, and cytotoxic drugs. These are intended purely as guidelines and there will be patients who require larger doses for longer periods of time. Tables 118.1 and 118.2 both make the point that different regimens of drugs are suitable for different manifestations of the disease.

Non-steroidal anti-inflammatory drugs

NSAIDs have no immune-modulating actions and lupus patients are at no lesser risk of gastrointestinal, cardiovascular, and renal complications of NSAIDs than other patients, and thus careful monitoring is required.

Several long-term studies have shown that both selective and non-selective cycloxygenase (COX) inhibitors, except naproxen, are associated with increased risk of cardiac infarction.

Hydroxychloroquine

Hydroxychloroquine (Plaquenil) is the anti-malarial drug of choice, with a better safety profile and tolerability than other anti-malarials such as chloroquine and quinacrine. The mechanism of action of anti-malarials is not fully understood but it is thought to work by

Table 118.1 Drug therapy in systemic lupus erythematosus

	NSAIDs	Anti-malarials	Corticosteroids	Cytotoxic agents
Malaise	+	+	+	–
Fever	+	–	+	–
Serositis	+	–	+	–
Arthralgia	+	+	+	–
Arthritis	+	+	+	+
Myalgia	+	+	+	–
Myositis	–	–	+	+
Malar/discoid rash	–	+	+	–
Pneumonitis	–	–	+	+
Carditis	–	–	+	+
Vasculitis	–	–	+	+
CNS disease	–	–	+[a]	? +
Renal	–	+	+	+
Haemolytic anaemia	–	–	+	+
Thrombocytopaenia	–	–	+	+
Raynaud's	–	–	?	?
Alopecia	–	–	?	?

+, usually beneficial; –, not beneficial; ?+, possible benefit; ?, dubious.
[a]Widely prescribed, but doubts remain that steroids are beneficial in many cases.

increasing the pH within the intracellular vacuoles thus interfering with antigen presenting in macrophages and other antigen-presenting cells (APCs) and inhibiting the activation of Toll like receptors.

Anti-malarials, in addition to their immunomodulatory and anti-inflammatory properties, are anti-hyperglycaemic, anti-thrombotic, and anti-hyperlipidemic even in those taking corticosteroids, thereby possibly having an influence on the development of atherosclerosis which is increased in SLE.

Hydroxychloroquine (HCQ) is commonly used in patients in whom the main symptoms are fatigue, rash, and arthralgia, without evidence of major organ involvement. It is, however, now thought to be beneficial to most patients with SLE because of this broad spectrum of beneficial effects. This claim is supported by a small randomized controlled trial (RCT)[1] and supported by findings from other studies of an increased relative risk of severe SLE flares in patients on HCQ who discontinued it compared to those who did not, a negative association in the development of renal flares, hypertension, thrombosis, and infection.

The Lupus in the Minorities and Nature versus nurture (LUMINA) cohort[2] showed a reduced risk of irreversible damage with HCQ use and other beneficial effects including increase survival, reduction in disease activity, thrombotic effects, and low lipid levels, supporting the notion that SLE patients who can tolerate it should be maintained on this treatment.

Anti-malarials occasionally cause mild gastrointestinal and cutaneous effects. The most troublesome but extremely rare side effect has been the effect of long-term use on the eye; this is more common with chloroquine which crosses the blood–retinal barrier more easily. Retinal toxicity sufficient to cause reduced visual acuity occurs in about 1 in 1800 cases. Recommendations for preventing retinal toxicity include not exceeding a maximum dose of 6.5 mg/kg lean body weight (i.e. 200–400 mg), reviewing baseline renal and hepatic tests and visual assessments. Patients should be referred to the ophthalmologist if they have visual impairment or age-related eye disease at baseline and if they develop reduction in peripheral vision, patchy central vision, or distorted central vision while on treatment.[3] Some units choose to carry out such monitoring every 6–12 months, though this is probably unnecessary as severe visual disturbances is very rare.

Many patients with cutaneous SLE respond well to HCQ, but a minority may require treatment with a combination of HCQ and quinacrine or with more potent agents such as dapsone, steroids, or rarely thalidomide.

Treatment with corticosteroids

Corticosteroids remain a mainstay of the treatment of SLE. These drugs (usually in moderate doses orally up to 30 mg/day) are used in severe arthritis, pleuritis, or pericarditis. Corticosteroids are used at higher dosages where SLE causes more severe effects, which may in some cases be life threatening, such as autoimmune haemolytic anaemia, thrombocytopenia, nephritis, and a wide range of neuropsychiatric problems.

Corticosteroids are usually prescribed orally but may also be given intramuscular or intravenously. Intravenous pulse therapy has been widely used. If given over a 15–20 min period there is a danger of reactive arthropathy, and in our experience intravenous pulses are best given slowly over a 3–4 h period. We use pulse therapy: for

Table 118.2 Recommendations for use of conventional immunosuppressive drugs in lupus

Symptom	Drugs to try	Dose and duration
Arthralgia Myalgia Lethargy	NSAIDs Hydroxychloroquine	Avoid in renal failure Start 400 mg/day for 3–4 months then reduce to 200 mg/day for 3–4 months, then to 200 mg five times week for 3–4 months; repeat courses may be necessary and annual retinal checks are probably unnecessary until patient has been on the drug for 5 years
Rash	Hydroxychloroquine Topical steroids or tacrolimus	
Arthritis	Prednisolone Hydroxychloroquine Methotrexate in refractory cases	Prednisolone: 20–40 mg per day initially for 2–4 weeks, reducing in 5–10 mg increments per week, if patient is responding; treatment is likely to be required for several months
Pleuritis and pericarditis	NSAIDs Anti-malarials, low-dose corticosteroids Refractory cases—azathioprine, MMF or cyclophosphamide	20–30 mg prednisolone per day then tapering doses, along the lines of arthritic treatment (above)
Autoimmune haemolytic anaemia/thrombocytopaenia	Corticosteroids often accompanied by azathioprine or cyclophosphamide ?Rituximab	60–80 mg prednisolone for 1–2 weeks reducing in 10 mg increments in response to the blood test results; aim for 2–2.5 mg/kg azathioprine; treatment will last for several months
Renal	Prednisolone plus cyclophosphamide or MMF Azathioprine or MMF for maintenance Rituximab for refractory cases	Induction: cyclophosphamide can be given by intravenous boluses—the Euro-Lupus nephritis regimen six fortnightly pulses of IV cyclophosphamide 500 mg. The older (NIH) regime using IV Cyclophosphamide of 750 mg–1g monthly for 6 months followed by 3 monthly infusions for 2 years is regarded as far too toxic Mycophenolate 1–3g/day may be required for several months to years; the ALMS trial showed this to be equivalent to cyclophosphamide use for getting patients into remission Maintenance: MMF 1–3 g/day is better than azathioprine at 2–3 mg/kg; treatment is likely to be required for several years
Central nervous system	Corticosteroids plus an appropriate drug, e.g. an anti-depressant, anti-convulsant, etc. ?Cyclophosphamide ?Rituximab	Controversial—but 20–60 mg prednisolone have been prescribed or IV pulse methylprednisolone (sometimes accompanied by azathioprine or IV cyclophosphamide pulses); treatment is likely to be required for months

IV, intravenous; MMF, mycophenolate mofetil; NSAIDs, non-steroidal anti-inflammatory drugs.

example, 500 mg–1 g methylprednisolone on three successive days for patients with severe disease not responding to oral corticosteroids. However, smaller pulse doses (100 mg) may be as efficacious and associated with fewer side effects.

Mild to moderate flares may be managed by increase of the normal steroid dose then rapid tapering down or by administration of an intramuscular steroid, e.g. depomedrone or triamcinolone.

The major side effects of corticosteroids include increased risk of infection, osteoporosis, diabetes, and hypertension. Chronic corticosteroid use has also been linked to the development of premature atherosclerosis. They are thus no panacea. It is important to take these side effects into account in planning a course of high-dose corticosteroids. The risk of osteoporosis must be considered in all patients who are going to take 7.5 mg prednisolone/day or more for a period of several months. Patients are advised to take calcium and vitamin D supplements to reduce the risk of corticosteroid-induced osteoporosis. Bisphosphonates, such as alendronate or residronate, which have a greater protective effect on bone may be used, but also have more side effects. Bone mineral density (DEXA) scanning offers a simple and effective way of monitoring bone loss, and should be repeated every 18–24 months in those on regular oral steroids.

Cytotoxic drugs

Cyclophosphamide

Cyclophosphamide (CYC) is an alkylating agent which is used in severe organ involvement in SLE; adequate evidence is lacking for its use in other organs except lupus nephritis.

The group from the National Institutes of Health (NIH) at Bethesda proposed that intravenous boluses of cyclophosphamide monthly for 6 months and subsequently every 3 months for 2 years compared to steroids alone, was the treatment of choice in patients with severe renal involvement and this was subsequently confirmed to be superior to pulse methylprednisolone alone in the long-term treatment of lupus nephritis.[4]

The problems of side effects with this drug in the long term—infertility or ovarian toxicity and increased risk of neoplasia—have made others more wary about its routine use, especially daily oral regimens. A shorter treatment protocol of six pulses of 500 mg cyclophosphamide fortnightly was compared to the standard NIH regime by the Euro-Lupus Nephritis Trial with a long-term follow-up of 10 years. Data from the trial suggest it may be as effective and safer than NIH regimen in controlling lupus nephritis though there is a high relapse rate, hence the need for maintenance therapy.[5]

In neuropsychiatric SLE there have been no adequate controlled trials of CYC though some believe it may be more effective than pulse corticosteroids especially in patients with seizures, optic neuritis, brainstem disease, and peripheral neuropathy.

Gonadotropin-releasing hormone analogue (GNRH-a) may help preserve ovarian function and is recommended especially in at-risk patients who are more than 30 years of age and receiving an average cumulative dose of more than 8 g.

Azathioprine

Azathioprine is a purine analogue; it is a prodrug that is metabolized into the active purine synthesis inhibitor 6-mercaptopurine, which affects T and B lymphocyte proliferation. Azathioprine is used in mucocutaneous, serositis and haematological manifestations of SLE for inducing disease remission. It may also be used as a steroid-sparing agent in cases where it proves difficult to reduce the dose of oral prednisolone without causing a flare. It is used widely as maintenance therapy after cyclophosphamide in lupus nephritis and other severe disease manifestations.

Thiopurines S-methyltransferase (TPMT) deactivates 6-mercaptopuirne into inactive metabolites; hence genetic polymorphisms of TPMT that reduce its activity can lead to excessive drug levels and toxicity. TPMT assays can be used to predict potential side effects which include reversible bone marrow suppression, hepatic toxicity and increase risk of infections.

Azathioprine should be used with caution in conjunction with other purine analogues such as allupurinol, if its use is inevitable, azathioprine dose should be reduced by 50–75%.

Methotrexate

There have been surprisingly few RCTs of methotrexate (MTX) in the treatment of SLE. Most have been retrospective, studying relatively few patients. There are some data to suggest that MTX may be useful for cutaneous lupus and be can used to treat anti-malarial resistant lupus arthritis and as a 'steroid sparer'.[6]

Some published small series report efficacy and improved prognosis in all neuropsychiatric SLE patients treated with intrathecal MTX and intrathecal dexamethasone refractory to conventional pulse methylprednisolone (MP).[7]

Mycophenolate mofetil

Mycophenolate mofetil (MMF) is a prodrug that is metabolized to mycophenolic acid which inhibits inosine-5-monophosphate dehydrogenase, inhibiting the de-novo pathway of purine synthesis and therefore B- and T-lymphocyte proliferation.

MMF is commonly used in cases of moderate to severe SLE that have proved resistant to other cytotoxic agents and there are case reports of its success in the treatment of patients with autoimmune haemolytic anaemia, thrombocytopenia, and anti-phospholipid syndrome. There is inadequate evidence for its use in refractory haematological and dermatological manifestations of SLE and its effectiveness in neuropsychiatric SLE is unproven.[8]

Experience in its use in solid organ transplantation suggested a better safety profile and tolerability than CYC, which had hitherto been the standard of care in the treatment of lupus nephritis. CYC has been dogged by concerns regarding its adverse effects, slow response, and failure to control lupus nephritis fully. A few clinical trials have suggested that MMF may be at least as effective or even superior to CYC in induction therapy and possibly safer. Results from the Aspreva Lupus Management Trial (ALMS), a large two-part RCT of 370 class III–V lupus nephritis patients designed to evaluate the superiority of MMF compared to CYC in a 24 month induction and subsequent maintenance therapy, however, failed to meet its primary endpoint of showing superiority of MMF to intravenous (IV) CYC as induction therapy. It had similar efficacy as CYC in short-term induction therapy in combination with corticosteroids with 56.2% response in the MMF group compared to 53.0% in I.V.CYC group. Secondary endpoints and adverse events were similar in both groups.[9] Intriguingly, the trial has shown statistically significant difference in response by different ethnic and racial groups to MMF vs CYC. Hispanic and black patients responded better to MMF compared to CYC, supporting findings from some earlier studies that in patients of African or Hispanic descent, IV CYC may be less effective for disease control. MMF was, however, effective in treating a wide variety of non-renal aspects of lupus in all racial and ethnic groups.[10]

The subsequent follow-up study has shown MMF to be better than azathioprine at maintaining patients in renal remission.[11] But invariably the question of the lower cost of azathioprine, and the relatively good response obtained from it, suggest it will continue to be used in patients with nephritis.

Beneficial results were obtained in the treatment of membranous glomerulonephritis (MGN) using moderate doses of MMF in combination with renoprotective and antiproteinuric therapy.

MMF may therefore be the treatment of choice in black and Hispanic populations, in patients who prefer the convenience of twice daily dosing vs monthly cyclophosphamide, and in women of childbearing age where there will be concerns about gonadal toxicity caused by IV CYC. Whatever immunosuppressive regime is chosen, a key element in managing renal lupus is controlling the blood pressure. Very often, in severe cases, a combination of antihypertensives (e.g. a diuretic, an angiotensin converting enzyme inhibitor, and a beta blocker) is required for adequate control.

For those patients in whom renal failure develops in spite of immunosuppressive therapy, dialysis and/or renal transplantation is required. There is equivalent patient and graft survival in SLE patients who receive renal transplantation compared to the general population, but recurrence of lupus nephritis appears to be frequent though not always tied with loss of the allograft and may present without clinical and serological confirmation of active disease.

Flow diagrams of the way we use drugs to treat the various aspects of lupus are shown in Figures 118.1 and 118.2.

Other 'standard' treatments

Leflunomide

Leflunomide is a synthetic isoxazol derivative known to inhibit the pyrimidine synthesis pathway, thus blocking RNA and DNA synthesis in T and B cells and inhibiting proliferation of these cells. It is well established in the treatment of rheumatoid and psoriatic arthritis and case reports suggest some level of efficacy in SLE arthropathy. Short-term studies of this drug in the treatment of SLE appeared to show it to be safe and reasonably efficacious in with significant reduction in Systemic Lupus Erythematosus Disease Activity Index (SLEDAI) scores in mild to moderate SLE. There are also suggestions of its possible role in the treatment of lupus nephritis. However, large long-term RCTs are needed to prove its efficacy.

Plasma exchange

The effectiveness of plasma exchange is not supported by the few small, non-controlled, randomized and retrospective studies. The concept was that the removal of circulating, presumptively pathogenic, immune complexes offered a therapeutic advantage. In practice, it became evident that in some patients a 'rebound' phenomenon occurred in which patients' symptoms and signs dramatically improved but returned within a few days or weeks. It is mainly used in severe therapy-resistant or life threatening disease such as refractory renal disease, neuropsychiatric manifestations, thrombotic thrombocytopenic purpura, or catastrophic anti-phospholipid syndrome, though its efficacy is not supported in clinical trials. This form of treatment requires good venous access and much patience on the part of both physician and patient, and is extremely expensive. As reviewed elsewhere,[12] controlled studies failed to provide convincing evidence of real benefit. Even combining plasma exchange with subsequent pulse cyclophosphamide

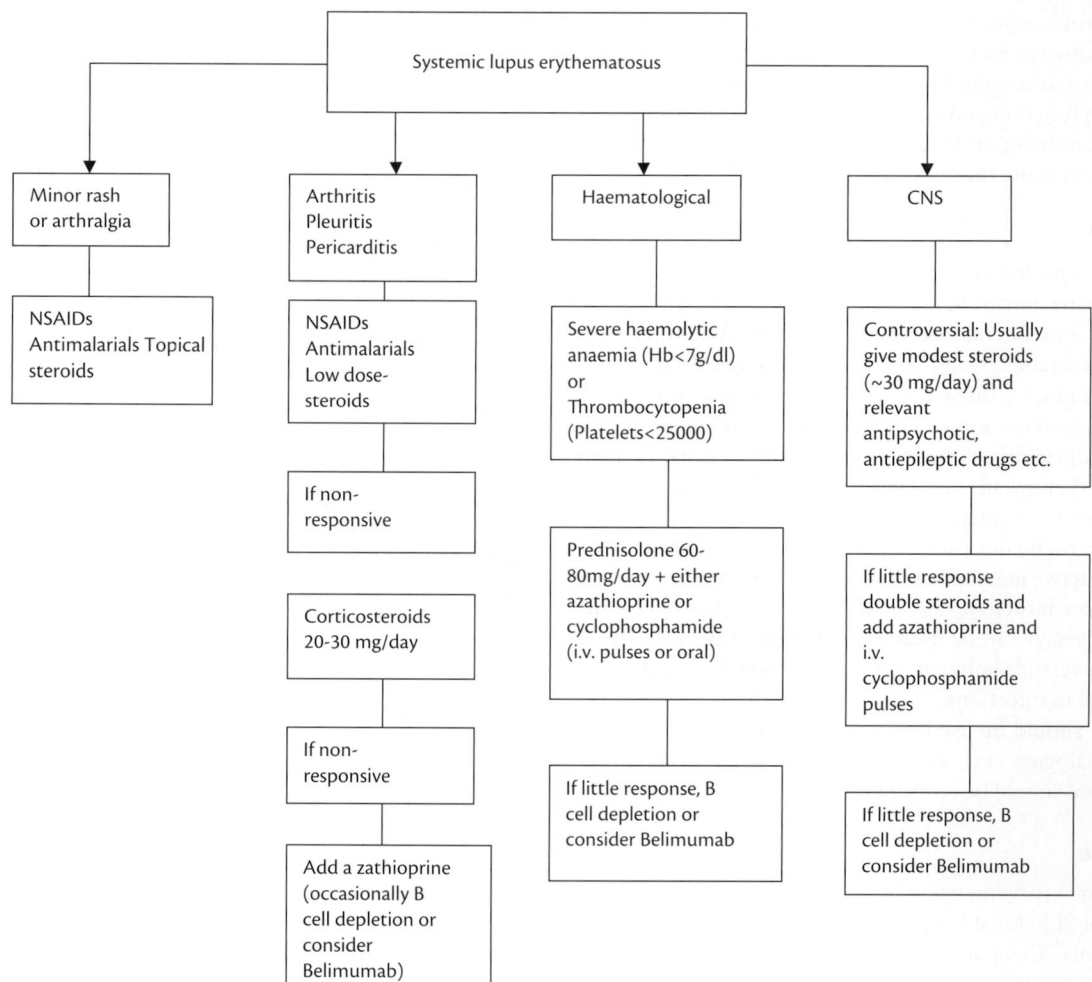

Fig. 118.1 Flow diagram of the management of non-renal systemic lupus erythematosus that forms the basis of our practice.

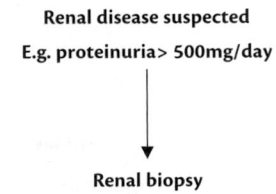

Renal disease suspected

E.g. proteinuria> 500mg/day

Renal biopsy

ISN/RPS Classification system

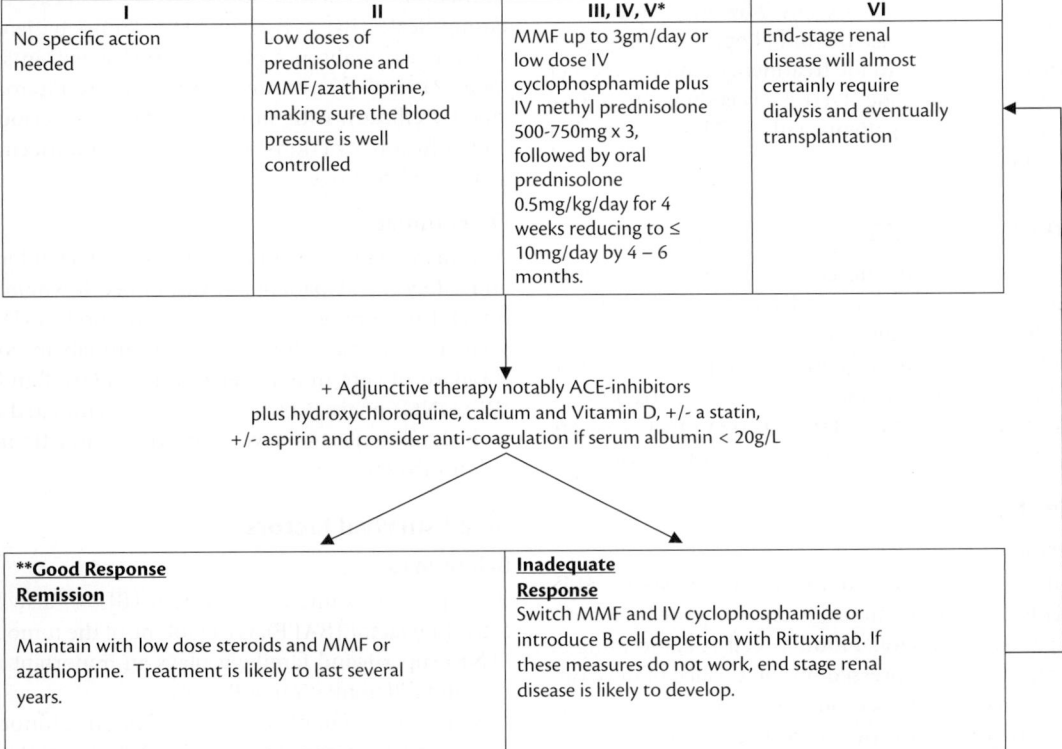

I	II	III, IV, V*	VI
No specific action needed	Low doses of prednisolone and MMF/azathioprine, making sure the blood pressure is well controlled	MMF up to 3gm/day or low dose IV cyclophosphamide plus IV methyl prednisolone 500-750mg x 3, followed by oral prednisolone 0.5mg/kg/day for 4 weeks reducing to ≤ 10mg/day by 4 – 6 months.	End-stage renal disease will almost certainly require dialysis and eventually transplantation

+ Adjunctive therapy notably ACE-inhibitors
plus hydroxychloroquine, calcium and Vitamin D, +/- a statin,
+/- aspirin and consider anti-coagulation if serum albumin < 20g/L

Good Response Remission	Inadequate Response
Maintain with low dose steroids and MMF or azathioprine. Treatment is likely to last several years.	Switch MMF and IV cyclophosphamide or introduce B cell depletion with Rituximab. If these measures do not work, end stage renal disease is likely to develop.

**= 50% reduction in proteinuria and stability on improvement in GFR in 6 – 12 months.

Fig. 118.2 Flow diagram of the management of renal systemic lupus erythematosus based on our own practice.

did not provide additional clinical benefit compared to pulse cyclophosphamide alone.

Diet therapy

Supplementation of the diet by fish oils has been shown to be beneficial in a double-blind cross-over study in which all the lupus patients were put on to low-fat diets; those who were concurrently taking 10 g/day of fish oil were shown to have done significantly better over a 6 month period.[13] With the concomitant use of steroids and the association of the metabolic syndrome with SLE patients, general advice on modifiable risk factors such as reduced salt, reduced saturated fat, increased fruits and vegetables, and regular exercise is beneficial. It has become more important to monitor lipid levels over time. Anti-malarials have been shown to lower these levels, but if this is unsatisfactory statins may be needed.

Intravenous high-dose gammaglobulin

Intravenous high-dose gammaglobulin (IVIG) is not a first-line treatment in SLE, but may have a role in cases resistant to other treatment modalities, IVIG is a blood product prepared from plasma composing of plasma proteins secreted by plasma cells. Most of the evidence for its use in SLE is anecdotal or obtained from small clinical trials, case series, and case reports. It may be effective in the treatment of immune thrombocytopenic purpura, immune neutropenia, myositis, serositis, and recurrent pregnancy losses in SLE. Monthly IVIG may be a useful alternative to intravenous cyclophosphamide in the treatment of lupus nephritis.[14] However, in most cases rituximab is now used in preference to IVIG. Good-quality research is needed to inform for its effective and appropriate use in SLE.

Ciclosporin A/neoral therapy

Following the failure of original attempts to use ciclosporin (because the dose was too high and caused nephrotoxicity),[15] there was something of a moratorium on its use in patients with SLE. Recently, several investigators have shown that a dose of 2.5–5 mg/kg provides reasonable disease control and enables steroid reduction over long-term follow-up. However, hypertrichosis develops in the majority of patients; it is best avoided in the presence of significant renal disease with close monitoring of blood pressure.

Some controlled trials seem to suggest it may be used in the maintenance treatment of membranous lupus nephritis and it may be as effective as azathioprine for maintenance therapy for diffuse proliferative lupus nephritis.[16]

Sex hormone therapy

Given the marked predilection of lupus for females, it is not surprising that attempts have been made to treat the condition by manipulating the level of sex hormones. One drug, danazol, an androgen with reduced virilizing capacity, has been used by several groups; as is so often the case with new drugs, the initial optimism has given way to the view that it adds little to the treatment of lupus. Another androgen, dehydroepiandrosterone (DHEA), was shown to reduce the requirement for steroids in patients with SLE but had modest effects at best in mild SLE.

Newer forms of therapy

The management of rheumatologic conditions is moving from 'serendipity to (immunological) sense'. Advances in knowledge of immunological reactions including T-cell activation, T cell–B cell collaboration, anti-dsDNA antibody production, deposition of anti-dsDNA antibody complexes, and complement activation are leading to the development of more targeted treatments that are showing promise in the management of this complex disease.

B-cell-targeted therapies

Anti-CD20 (rituximab)

B-cell dysregulation is involved in the pathogenesis of SLE. Rituximab (RTX) is a chimeric mouse/human monoclonal antibody directed against peripheral blood B-cell-specific antigen anti-CD20, a surface marker expressed on the surface of developing B cells and minimally expressed on the plasma cells. Initially introduced for the treatment of low grade B-cell follicular non-Hodgkin's lymphoma (NHL), it has shown promise in the treatment of chronic immune thrombocytopenic purpura (ITP), rheumatoid arthritis (RA), Sjögren's syndrome, vasculitis, and dermatomyositis.

Currently it has found use as an alternative to conventional immunosuppressive agents in SLE patients with active or severe disease resistant to other forms of treatment. Many studies report its effectiveness in inducing complete remission in lupus patients with a wide variety of clinical features including refractory lupus nephritis. It has been used with steroids alone (to minimize allergic reactions) or in combination with cyclophosphamide with improvements clinically, histopathologically, and in serological parameters.[17] Studies also show a positive long-term safety profile, but long-term monitoring is necessary.[18]

Successful reports from studies of the use of rituximab in central nervous system (CNS) involvement refractory to standard therapy showed rapid improvement in manifestations such as acute confusional state, cognitive dysfunction, psychosis, seizures, transverse myelitis, and vasculitis of the CNS.[19]

Despite this favourable response from multiple non-randomized studies, rituximab failed to reach its primary endpoints in the EXPLORER (non-renal lupus) and LUNAR (renal lupus) studies, a result that has been attributed to poor trial design with inadequate power to detect a realistic effect, heterogeneous selection of SLE patients, and the concomitant use of high doses of other immunosuppressive therapies. Ideally, further controlled studies with improved designs are necessary to characterize the place of RTX in the management of SLE.

Anti-CD22

Epratuzumab is a fully humanized recombinant monoclonal antibody against CD22 expressed on the surface of maturing B cells but not plasma cells.

Phase 2b studies in 90 patients with moderate to severe lupus showed significant improvements to British Isles Lupus Assessment Group Scale (BILAG) C or better, most patients had symptom reduction and absence of active disease within specific body systems. Particularly prominent was cardiorespiratory and neuropsychiatric efficacy, with similar incidence of serious adverse events and infusion reactions as placebo. A multicentre phase 3 trial started in late 2010.

Ocrelizumab

A humanized monoclonal antibody to CD20 has shown efficacy and safety in RA patients. It was hoped it would avoid the development of human anti-chimaeric antibodies (HACA) responses seen in rituximab; however, ocrelizumab in combination with standard of care in extrarenal SLE (BEGIN) and lupus nephritis (BELONG) phase 3 trials have been terminated due to problems with development of severe and opportunistic infections in East Asian subjects.

B-cell survival factors

Belimumab

B-lymphocyte stimulation protein (BLyS), also known as B-cell activating factor (BAFF), is a cytokine of the tumour necrosis factor (TNF) superligand family. It plays an important role in proliferation and differentiation of B cells.

Belimumab (Benlysta) is a human monoclonal antibody developed to recognize and inhibit the biological activity of BLyS. It has been approved for the treatment of SLE, becoming the first specifically targeted biological therapy for SLE to have been developed in 50 years. Phase 2 and 3 trials confirmed its biological activity and tolerability. Serologically active patients responded better to belimumab plus standard of care than standard of care alone, with response of 57.6% and 43.2% for 10 mg/kg compared to 43.6% and 33.85 for placebo in the BLISS-52 and BLISS-76 studies.[20,21]

Questions remain to be answered about the optimal patient population for its use, however. As belimumab has not been used in renal or CNS lupus it is not known whether it would be effective in these groups of patients, the duration of treatment, long-term adverse effects, and its place in the standard treatment protocols.

Atacicept, a chimeric molecule formed by a receptor for BAFF and a proliferation-inducing ligand (APRIL) with immunoglobulin (Ig) is also undergoing a major clinical trial in SLE.

B-cell tolerization

LJP 394 (abetimus sodium)

LJP 394 is a drug that was developed specifically to inactivate B cells which produce anti-dsDNA antibodies. The drug consists of four oligonucleotides, each 20 bases in length, which are attached to an inert scaffold. When these nucleotides bind surface Ig anti-dsDNA molecules on B cells, they can cross-link those molecules.

This leads to anergy or deletion of the B cells rather than activation, because the drug molecule does not carry any T-cell epitopes and cannot recruit T-cell help.

Although some early studies showed promise (appearing to reduce the rate of renal flares), a large trial failed to show any benefit and this approach is no longer being used.

Anti-cytokine agents

Interleukin (IL)-10 levels are consistently elevated in the blood of patients with SLE, and monoclonal anti-IL-10 antibodies have been used to treat six patients with SLE for 21 days each.[22] These patients reported improvements of the skin and joints, which persisted for up to 6 months in the majority of cases. Surprisingly, this approach has not been further pursued.

Increased TNF concentrations are found in the sera of SLE patients with increased deposits in skin and renal tissues. Anti-TNFα drugs used in RA have been associated with the production of anti-dsDNA antibodies and, rarely, the development of a lupus-like syndrome.[23]

An open-label study suggests that TNF blockade in combination with azathioprine may be effective in SLE patients with arthritis and skin disease. Lupus nephritis patients showed reduction in proteinuria and, despite the induction of lupus-specific autoantibodies, it was not associated with disease flares; further controlled studies are warranted.[24]

Inhibition of costimulatory molecules

Anti-CD40 ligand antibody

The interaction between CD40, which is present on APCs, and CD40 ligand (L) expressed on T cells provides an important costimulus to the activation of T cells. This interaction also has significant effects on B cells, for example augmenting B-cell responses to cytokines and causing antibody isotype switching.[25]

In a double-blind placebo-controlled trial, a humanized monoclonal antibody against CD40L (IDEC-131) showed no statistically significant differences in SLEDAI and adverse events with placebo. Blockade of the CD40L pathway was successful but not safe with another antibody, BG9588, and there are fears about this approach causing major vascular events.[26]

CTLA4-Ig

CTLA4-Ig (abatacept) has been effective in the treatment of psoriatic arthritis and RA. In murine lupus models it has been found to be effective in combination with cyclophosphamide in treating lupus nephritis; however, a clinical trial involving over 150 patients did not meet its endpoints.

Autologous haematopoietic stem cell transplantation

In SLE some promising results of non-myeloablative and mesenchymal stem cell transplantation in reducing disease activity, improving serological markers, and stabilization of renal function has been shown.[27] [28] However, this treatment is very demanding of the patients and must only be undertaken at centres where the technique is performed regularly.

Questions plaguing future, clearly needed, studies include deciding which patient groups would do well or badly, and clinical, serological, and organ system involvement to use as markers for patient selection. Long-term outcomes remain unknown, as well as the selection of optimal remission and maintenance regimes.

Management in special situations

Pregnancy

Since most patients with SLE are women in their childbearing years, the question of managing pregnancy is a significant issue for many. It is important to recognize that around 25% of lupus patient pregnancies do not go to full term (i.e. well in excess of the figure of approximately 10% of pregnancies in healthy women). Those patients with anti-phospholipid antibodies are especially likely to suffer recurrent miscarriages. Those with anti-Ro or anti-La antibodies have a small (1:20) chance of having a child with the neonatal lupus syndrome or congenital heart block. Those patients with renal disease have to be watched very closely during pregnancy and on occasion it may be hard to distinguish a renal flare from pre-eclamptic toxaemia. We strongly recommend comanaging SLE patients with an interested obstetrician.

Contraindications to pregnancy include severe pulmonary hypertension (symptomatic or systolic pulmonary artery pressure>50 mmHg), chronic renal failure (Cr >2.8 g/dl), heart failure, restrictive lung disease, previous severe preeclampsia despite aspirin or heparin, stroke, or a severe lupus flare within the past 6 months.

Drugs safe to take in pregnancy include NSAIDs (avoid after week 32 to prevent premature closure of ductus arterosius), anti-malarials, corticosteroids, ciclosporin, azathioprine, heparin, and low-dose aspirin. Try to keep prednisolone dose to 7.5 mg/day or less to prevent maternal adverse effects. NSAIDs, anti-malarials, corticosteroids, warfarin, heparin, and aspirin are safe for breast-feeding. Other immunosuppressive and biological drugs are contraindicated.[29]

In-vitro fertilization seems to be safe and successful, though there are reports of high maternal and complications in well-selected patients with SLE and anti-phospholipid syndrome (APS) though the evidence is mainly from case reports and small case series.

An overall guide to management is shown in Figure 118.3.

Coincident anti-phospholipid antibody syndrome

Perhaps 10% of patients with SLE also have APS and even more (around 25–35%) have anti-phospholipid antibodies. The 'balance of disease' may go in either direction and on occasion we have seen a patient deemed to have primary APS develop SLE over time. Mainly, however, in our experience SLE is diagnosed first.

Managing the APS component of those with both conditions is little different from patients who have primary APS. Problems may arise in particular when an overlap patient of this type presents with hypertension and mild proteinuria. Invariably a renal biopsy will be needed to ascertain to what extent the kidneys have been affected by multiple small thrombi and/or 'lupus' glomerulonephritis. In some patients, therapy with both immunosuppressive and long-term anticoagulants is needed.

Prognosis and survival

Studies on duration of disease and overall survival rates have frequently been confounded by the numbers of patients lost to follow-up and inadequate attention paid to the ethnic group, age of onset, and socio-economic status of individual patients. With these possible confounding factors in mind, and the division of lupus

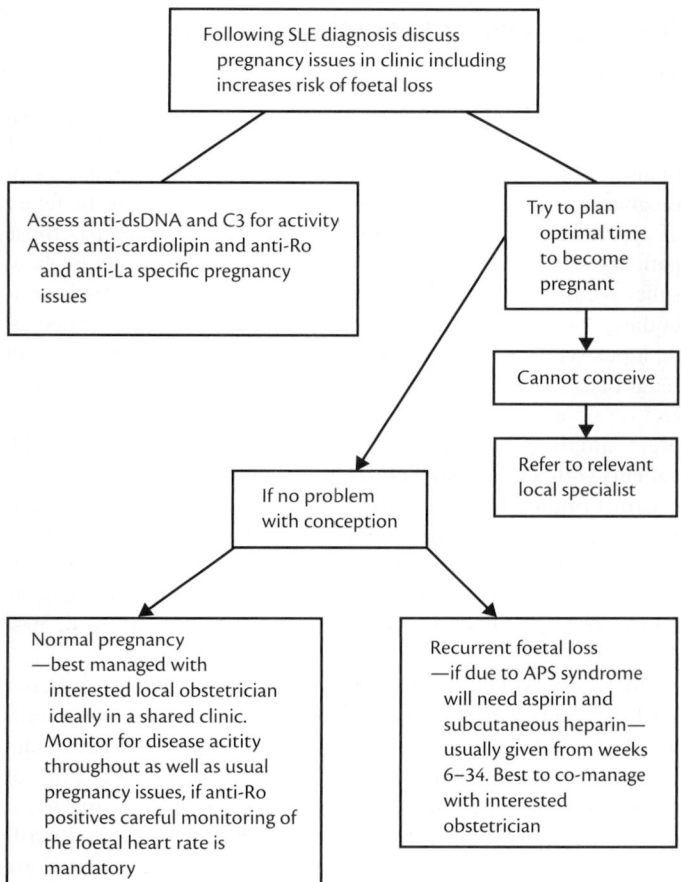

Fig. 118.3 Flow diagram of the management of systemic lupus erythematosus in pregnancy.

patients into those with overt nephritis and those without, it is reasonable to state that the 5 year survival in lupus is presently 90% or greater, but at 15 years only 60% of those with nephritis will still be alive compared to around 85% of those without nephritis. In the United States, it has been claimed that black lupus patients, males, those from poorer socio-economic groups and possibly children, have poorer survival, especially if nephritis is present. It has also been suggested that there exists a bimodal mortality curve. Patients who die within 5 years usually have very active disease, with a requirement for substantial doses of steroids and other immunosuppressives. Those patients dying much later tend to do so from cardiovascular disease and possibly infection. Overall, most lupus patients die from sepsis, malignancy, cardiovascular disease, and active generalized disease.

One of the most important steps for monitoring progress has been the development of reliable activity tools like the BILAG, SLEDAI and the Systemic Lupus Erythematosus International Collaborating Clinics (SLICC) damage index.

SLE is a multisystem disease and the involvement of different medical subspecialties in management of patients is strongly encouraged to ensure the best outcome for patients.

References

1. Canadian Hydroxychloroquine Study Group. A randomized study of the effect of withdrawing hydroxychloroquine sulphate in systemic lupus erythematosus. *N Engl J Med* 1991;324:150–154.

2. Alarcón GS, McGwin G, Bertoli AM et al., for the LUMINA Study Group. Effects of hydroxychloroquine on survival of patients with SLE:data from LUMINA, a multiethnic US Cohort (LUMINA). *Ann Rheum Dis* 2007;66:1168–1172.

3. Royal College of Ophthalmology. *Hydroxychloroquine and ocular toxicity recommendations on screening*, 2009. Available at: www.rcophth. ac.uk/page.asp?section=451&sectionTitle=Clinical+Guidelines

4. Boumpas DT, Austin HA, Balow JE et al. Controlled trial of pulse methylprednisolone versus two regimens of pulse cyclophosphamide in severe lupus nephritis. *Lancet* 1992;340(8822):741–745.

5. Houssiau FA, Vasconcelos C, D'Cruz D et al. The 10-year follow-up data of the Euro-Lupus Nephritis Trial comparing low-dose and high-dose intravenous cyclophosphamide. *Ann Rheum Dis* 2010;69(1):61–64.

6. Sato EL. Methotrexate therapy in systemic lupus erythematosus. *Lupus* 2001;10(3):162–164.

7. Zhou H, Zhang F, Tian X et al. Clinical features and outcome of neuropsychiatric lupus in Chinese: analysis of 240 hospitalized patients. *Lupus* 2008;17(2):93–99.

8. Mok CC. Mycophenolate mofetil for non-renal manifestations of systemic lupus erythematosus: a systematic review. *Scandinavian Journal of Rheumatology*. 2007;36(5):329–337.

9. Appel GB, Contreras G, Dooley MA et al. Mycophenolate mofetil versus cyclophosphamide for induction treatment of lupus nephritis. *J Am Soc Nephrol* 2009;20:1103–1112.

10. Isenberg D, Appel GB, Contreras G et al. Influence of race/ethnicity on response to lupus nephritis treatment: the ALMS study. *Rheumatology* 2010;49(1):128–140.

11. Dooley MA, Jayne D, Ginzler EM et al. Mycophenolate versus azathioprine as maintenance therapy for lupus nephritis. *N Engl J Med* 2011;365(20):1886–1895.

12. McClure CE, Isenberg DA. Does plasma exchange have any part to play in the management of systemic lupus erythematosus? In: Isenberg DA, Tucker LB (eds) *Controversies in rheumatology*. Martin Dunitz, London, 1997:75–86.

13. Walton AJ, Snaith ML, Locniskar M et al. Dietary fish oil and the severity of symptoms in patients with systemic lupus erythematosus. *Ann Rheum Dis* 1991;50(7):463–466.

14. Boletis JN, Ioannidis JP, Boki KA, Moutsoupoulos HM. Intravenous immunoglobulin compared with cyclophosphamide for proliferative lupus nephritis. *Lancet* 1999;354:569–570.

15. Isenberg DA, Snaith ML, Morrow WJ et al. Cyclosporin a for the treatment of systemic lupus erythematosus. *Int J Immunopharmacol* 1981;3(2):163–169.

16. Griffiths B, Emery P, Ryan V et al. The BILAG multi-centre open randomized controlled trial comparing ciclosporin vs azathioprine in patients with severe SLE. *Rheumatology* 2010;49(4):723–732.

17. Terrier B, Amoura Z, Ravaud P et al. Safety and efficacy of rituximab in systemic lupus erythematosus: Results from 136 patients from the French autoimmunity and rituximab registry. *Arthritis Rheum* 2010;62(8):2458–2466.

18. Lu TY, Ng KP, Cambridge G et al. A retrospective seven-year analysis of the use of B cell depletion therapy in systemic lupus erythematosus at university college london hospital: The first fifty patients. *Arthritis Care Res* 2009;61(4):482–487.

19. Tokunaga M, Saito K, Kawabata D et al. Efficacy of rituximab (anti-CD20) for refractory systemic lupus erythematosus involving the central nervous system. *Ann Rheum Dis* 2007;66(4):470–475.

20. Navarra SV, Guzmán RM, Gallacher AE et al. Efficacy and safety of belimumab in patients with active systemic lupus erythematosus: a randomised, placebo-controlled, phase 3 trial. *Lancet* 2011;377(9767):721–731.

21. Jacobi AM, Huang W, Wang T et al. Effect of long-term belimumab treatment on B cells in systemic lupus erythematosus: Extension of a phase II, double-blind, placebo-controlled, dose-ranging study. *Arthritis Rheum* 2010;62(1):201–210.

22. Llorente L, Richaud-Patin Y, García-Padilla C et al. Clinical and biologic effects of anti–interleukin-10 monoclonal antibody administration in systemic lupus erythematosus. *Arthritis Rheum* 2000;43(8):1790–1800.

23. Ioannou Y, Isenberg DA. Current evidence for the induction of autoimmune rheumatic manifestations by cytokine therapy. *Arthritis Rheum* 2000;43(7):1431–1442.

24. Aringer M, Houssiau F, Gordon C et al. Adverse events and efficacy of TNF-α blockade with infliximab in patients with systemic lupus erythematosus: long-term follow-up of 13 patients. *Rheumatology* 2009;48(11):1451–1454.

25. Kalunian KC, Davis JC, Merrill JT, Totoritis MC, Wofsy D; for the I-LSG. Treatment of systemic lupus erythematosus by inhibition of T cell costimulation with anti-CD154: A randomized, double-blind, placebo-controlled trial. *Arthritis Rheum* 2002;46(12):3251–3258.

26. Boumpas DT, Furie R, Manzi S et al. A short course of BG9588 (anti-CD40 ligand antibody) improves serologic activity and decreases hematuria in patients with proliferative lupus glomerulonephritis. *Arthritis Rheum* 2003;48(3):719–727.

27. Burt RK, Traynor A, Statkute L et al. Nonmyeloablative hematopoietic stem cell transplantation for systemic lupus erythematosus. *JAMA* 2006;295(5):527–535.

28. Liang J, Zhang H, Hua B et al. Allogenic mesenchymal stem cells transplantation in refractory systemic lupus erythematosus: a pilot clinical study. *Ann Rheum Dis* 2010;69(8):1423–1429.

29. Ruiz-Irastorza G, Khamashta M. Lupus and pregnancy: ten questions and some answers. *Lupus* 2008;17(5):416–420.

CHAPTER 119

Paediatric-onset systemic lupus erythematosus

Louise Watson and Michael W. Beresford

Introduction and epidemiology

Systemic lupus erythematous (SLE) is a rare, autoimmune, multisystem disorder. It is of unknown aetiology but it is characterized by the production of autoantibodies directed against nuclear antigens, including antinuclear antibodies (ANA), anti-extractable nuclear antibodies (ENA), and anti-double-stranded DNA antibodies (dsDNA).

SLE is rare in children, although around 20% of all cases of SLE will have an onset before adulthood.[1] The incidence of juvenile-onset SLE (JSLE) is reported to be 0.36–0.9 per 100 000 children per year.[2–7] In a similar manner to adult-onset disease, the incidence varies significantly according to racial background, with a higher incidence in patients of black African or Asian descent. Ethnicity may also influence disease phenotype, with an earlier disease onset and more nephritis seen in patients of black African or Asian origin.[8] Like most autoimmune conditions, SLE is more prevalent in females. However, the sex difference is less striking in JSLE than in adult-onset disease. In JSLE, the female to male ratio is around 5:1 in contrast to the 9:1 ratio seen in adult-onset SLE.[9]

Hormonal, environmental, and genetic factors play a contributory role in the development of JSLE. Hormonal influences, particularly oestrogen, contribute to disease activity, as illustrated in patients taking oral contraceptive medication or during pregnancy, both of which can trigger a flare of the disease. Men with Kleinfelter's syndrome (46XXY) are reported to have an increased risk of developing SLE.[10,11] Environmental factors including certain medications, UV exposure, and infectious stimuli such as the Epstein–Barr virus, all play a role.[12] Individuals with SLE have a genetic susceptibility to developing the disease, as the risk of autoimmunity in a first-degree relative is significantly higher than that of the general population.[13] Genetic contribution in JSLE may be more significant than that seen in adult-onset disease as the sex distribution is less striking, disease presents earlier and conditions, such as Aicardi–Goutiers syndrome with known genetic mutations present with a lupus phenotype in childhood.[14] Although genetic contribution is clearly very important in JSLE, it cannot be the entire cause as the concordance rate between monozygotic twins is only around 25%.[15]

JSLE also occurs in the context of rare inherited complement deficiencies, the most common of which is C1q deficiency. These deficiencies predispose patients to a high (>90%) chance of developing SLE over their lifetime and while C1q deficiency is phenotypically variable, children with C1q deficiency and SLE are often younger at disease onset, have a more severe disease course, and more cutaneous manifestations than patients with JSLE.[16]

Lupus-like disorders

Lupus-like features can present in children in a secondary form, either following the administration of certain drugs, so called 'drug-induced' lupus, or secondary to maternal lupus causing neonatal lupus in the newborn period. The medications with the highest risk of producing lupus-like features include the anti-hypertensive medication hydralazine, with features occurring in 5% of patients taking the medication, the anti-arrhythmic drug procainamide, and newer biologics including anti-TNFα therapy.[17] Drug-induced SLE is usually associated with transient autoantibodies and cutaneous manifestations, with occasional systemic features described mainly in neonatal lupus syndrome.[18] In infants of mothers with anti-Ro and/or anti-La antibodies congenital heart block can be seen and may lead to fetal death or in-utero cardiac failure. Once the infant is delivered they frequently require artificial cardiac pacing.[19] In both cases, symptoms typically resolve either with cessation of the offending medication or gradually over time.

Disease pathogenesis

An exaggerated immune response, characterized by an immune reaction directed against the nuclear components of one's own cells (thus autoantibody formation against nuclear material) underpins the pathophysiology of JSLE.

Adaptive immune system

Commonly observed nucleic autoantibodies include ANA, anti-ENA, and anti-dsDNA. Anti-ENAs include anti-Sm, -RNP, -Ro and -La antibodies. This response involves hyperactive immune cells and uncontrolled immune pathways with a reduced clearance of immune complexes and reduced tolerance to antigenic stimuli.

Increased and dysregulated apoptosis (programmed cell death) occurs in JSLE,[20] and defective clearance of the subsequent apoptotic material is characteristic of mouse-models of lupus[21] and SLE.[22] Autoantigens typical of lupus cluster in surface blebs of apoptotic cells, increasing their immune exposure.[23] Saturation of the normal physiological processes to safely remove this apoptotic debris leads to amplification of autoantigen exposure and the immune cascade.[24] Autoantibodies produced as a result of plasma B-cell activity are a component of the adaptive immune system response, and form immune complexes. These immune complexes activate complement cascades and can deposit in tissues, resulting in specific features of SLE including cutaneous lupus and lupus nephritis.[25]

Although the adaptive immune system mounts a very specific antibody response to self-nucleic components, failure of its regulation, and its working relationship with the innate immune system, has more recently been recognized.

Innate immune system

Monocytes and macrophages secrete chemokines, cytokines, and growth factors, causing inflammation and damage to both healthy and target tissues. Interferon alpha (INF-α) is one of the most frequently found cytokines in SLE.[26,27] Recent research has identified Toll-like receptors (TLRs), present within certain cells including lymphocytes, having a specific early role in SLE.[28] TLRs, normally able to discriminate between self and foreign material, identify host nucleic acids as foreign invaders activating the innate immune system. Increased expression of TLRs capable of recognizing SLE-associated autoantigens, including TLR9, occurs in JSLE.[29] Apoptotic neutrophils trigger TLR activation through their presentation of autoantigens and trigger activation of the type 1 INF-α pathway.[29,30]

TLR activation produces a surge of inflammatory cytokines, interacting with signalling pathways, and influencing the release of downstream proinflammatory cytokines including tumour necrosis factor alpha (TNFα) and interleukins (IL). Other important cytokines seen in JSLE include B-cell activating factor (BAFF)/B lymphocyte stimulator (BlyS), IL-10, and monocyte chemo attractant protein 1 (MCP-1).[31] Inadequate production of the regulatory T and B cells occurs which results from abnormally low levels of IL-2 and transforming growth factor beta (TGFβ), from T and natural killer (NK) cells.

Other important antibodies

The presence of certain autoantibodies related to the coagulation system, such as lupus anticoagulant (LA), anti-phospholipid antibodies (APAs), and anti-cardiolipin antibodies (ACAs), are also seen. Over recent years, disease registries have demonstrated an increased association with childhood anti-phospholipid syndrome and autoimmune disease than in adults.[32–34]

Diagnosis and monitoring

Diagnosis

A combination of clinical features and laboratory markers are used to diagnose SLE. Classification criteria developed by the American College of Rheumatology (ACR) are generally used in forming the diagnosis (see Table 119.1). Four out of the 11 stated criteria are highly suggestive of SLE.[35–37]

The multisystemic nature of the condition means that JSLE may present to any one of a multitude of different specialists, including

Table 119.1 American College of Rheumatology classification criteria

Criterion	Definition
1. Malar rash	Fixed erythema, flat or raised, over the malar eminences, tending to spare the nasolabial folds
2. Discoid rash	Erythematous raised patches with adherent keratotic scaling and follicular plugging; atrophic scarring may occur in older lesions
3. Photosensitivity	Skin rash as a result of unusual reaction to sunlight, by patient history or physician observation
4. Oral ulcers	Oral or nasopharyngeal ulceration, usually painless, observed by physician
5. Non-erosive arthritis	Involving two or more peripheral joints, characterized by tenderness, swelling, or effusion
6. Pleuritis or pericarditis	(1) Pleuritis—convincing history of pleuritic pain or rubbing heard by a physician or evidence of pleural effusion, *or* (2) Pericarditis—documented by ECG or rub or evidence of pericardial effusion
7. Renal disorder	(1) Persistent proteinuria >0.5 g/day or > 3+ if quantitation not performed, *or* (2) Cellular casts—may be red cell, haemoglobin, granular, tubular, or mixed
8. Neurological disorder	(1) Seizures—in the absence of offending drugs or known metabolic derangements e.g. uraemia, ketoacidosis, or electrolyte imbalance, *or* (2) Psychosis—in the absence of offending drugs or known metabolic derangements, e.g. uraemia, ketoacidosis, or electrolyte imbalance
9. Haematological disorder	(1) Haemolytic anaemia—with reticulocytosis, *or* (2) Leukopenia—<4000/mm³ on ≥2 occasions, *or* (3) Lymphopenia—<1500/mm³ on ≥2 occasions, *or* (4) Thrombocytopenia—<100 000/mm³ in the absence of offending drugs
10. Immunological disorder	(1) Anti-DNA—antibody to native DNA in abnormal titre, *or* (2) Anti-Sm—presence of antibody to Sm nuclear antigen, *or* (3) Positive finding of APA on: (a) an abnormal serum level of IgG or IgM anticardiolipin antibodies, (b) a positive test result for lupus anticoagulant using a standard method, or (c) a false-positive test result for at least 6 months confirmed by *Treponema pallidum* immobilization or fluorescent treponemal antibody absorption test
11. Positive ANA	An abnormal titre of ANA by immunofluorescence or an equivalent assay at any point in time and in the absence of drugs

ANA, antinuclear antibody; APA, anti-phosphlipid antibodies.

psychiatrists, haematologists, or nephrologists. This may contribute to a delay in the initial diagnosis if they are unfamiliar with childhood lupus. Some children may have lupus or evolving lupus without formally meeting the ACR criteria. The opinion of an experienced paediatric rheumatologist with experience of paediatric connective tissue disorders should be sought.

Typically patients with JSLE present with non-specific constitutional symptoms, such as fever, lymphadenopathy, lethargy, and weight loss, which can make the diagnosis difficult. These may or may not accompany end-organ disease. Musculoskeletal, cutaneous, haematological, and renal system involvement are common features of JSLE at presentation and can occur in varying severity. Less frequent but important manifestations are neurological symptoms and signs, which occur in up to 10% of JSLE patients and can present with headaches, altered consciousness, seizures, and even psychosis. Liver, ophthalmic, and especially cardiac and pulmonary involvement are all rare manifestations in the paediatric form of SLE.

General points to ask in history taking are outlined in Box 119.1. Clinical signs of lupus can also be defined by system/organ involvement as shown in Box 119.2.

The main differential diagnoses of JSLE include other systemic autoimmune conditions, for example juvenile dermatomyositis or systemic juvenile idiopathic arthritis, bacterial or viral infections, immunodeficiency, or malignancy. Thorough evaluation, investigation, and experience of these conditions are required to distinguish JSLE from these differential diagnoses.

Disease monitoring

In view of the characteristic multisystem nature of SLE and the complexity of the clinical features of JSLE, a number of disease activity assessment tools have been developed. These endeavour to assess and summarize overall disease activity, especially at time of disease flare. In JSLE two main disease activity tools have been used. Both of these were originally designed for adult-onset SLE and have been modified for use in childhood disease; initial versions of these tools have subsequently been validated for use in JSLE.[38,39] The SLE Disease Activity Index (SLEDAI) scoring system[40] evaluates the presence of multiple features of SLE at the time of completion or in the previous 10 days. This tool has been demonstrated to differentiate mild and moderate from severe disease activity and generates an overall disease activity score. Another commonly used tool is the British Isles Lupus Assessment Group (BILAG) disease activity score.[41] Often used for clinical trials, it is able to separate disease activity into different organ systems and score accordingly. It takes into account the disease features experienced by a patient in the past 4 weeks and is designed to reflect a clinician's intention to alter treatment.

Disease flares are defined as a measurable increase in disease activity in one or more organ systems involving new or worse clinical signs and symptoms and/or laboratory measurements. It must be considered clinically significant by the assessor and usually there would be at least consideration of a change or an increase in treatment.[42]

Investigations

Investigations assist clinicians in forming a diagnosis of JSLE, monitoring activity and assessing organ damage. Children with lupus often present with haematological involvement affecting any of the blood cell lines together with evidence of autoantibodies. Lymphopenia is almost universally seen, with neutropenia, thrombocytopenia, and haemolytic anaemia common. Over 90% will be ANA positive; however, the presence, or precise levels, of particular antibodies are poor indicators of disease activity and, as

with adults, may occur as an isolated finding in healthy individuals. Useful laboratory tests and the common findings in JSLE are shown in Table 119.2.

To formulate a diagnosis and discover the extent of systemic involvement, a detailed multisystem work-up of patients is critical. Exclusion of other potential differential diagnoses, which include malignancy and infectious diseases, is important. Repeated

---

Box 119.1 Signs and symptoms in the diagnosis of juvenile-onset systemic lupus erythematosus

Constitutional symptoms
- Pyrexia
- Weight loss
- Lymphadenopathy
- Fatigue/lethargy
- Anorexia

Mucocutaneous
- Malar erythema
- Discoid lesions
- Mucosal ulceration
- Alopecia
- Photosensitive skin

Neurological
- Headache
- Cognitive dysfunction
- Seizures
- Hallucinations

Cardiovascular and respiratory
- Dyspnoea
- Chest pain

Vasculitis
- Thromboembolism
- Cutaneous changes ± ulceration
- Raynaud's

Renal
- Oedema
- Haematuria

Gastrointestinal
- Colitis
- Pancreatitis
- Cholecystitis

Ophthalmic
- Proptosis

Box 119.2 System/organ involvement in juvenile-onset systemic lupus erythematosus

General assessment

- Weight, height centiles
- Systolic and diastolic blood pressure and centiles
- Lymphadenopathy
- Hepatosplenomegaly

Mucocutaneous

- Skin rashes (discoid lesions, malar erythema)
- Alopecia
- Periungal erythema
- Mucosal ulceration

Neurological

- Altered consciousness
- Acute delirium or psychosis
- Meningitis
- Demyelitis
- Peripheral or cranial neuropathy

Cardiovascular and respiratory

- Cardiac failure
- Pericardial or pleural effusion

Musculoskeletal

- Myositis
- Arthritis (poly or mono)
- Tendonitis

Vasculitis

- Cutaneous ulceration/phlebitis
- Raynaud's phenomenon
- Livido reticularis
- Thromboembolism

Renal

- Oedema (nephritic syndrome)

Gastrointestinal

- Ascites
- Jaundice
- Abdominal pain

Ophthalmic

- Uveitis, keratitis, episcleritis
- Optic neuritis

Table 119.2 Laboratory investigations and common findings in juvenile-onset systemic lupus erythematosus

Investigation	Features with JSLE
FBC, blood film	Anaemia, leucopenia (especially lymphopenia), thrombocytopenia
Direct Coombs' test	Haemolytic anaemia
U&E	Abnormal renal function
LFTs, bone profile	Hypoalbuminaemia (nephritic syndrome); elevated transaminases (hepatitis)
Creatinine kinase	May be elevated (myositis)
LDH	May be elevated (myositis)
CRP	Often low or normal, unless concurrent infection
ESR	Usually elevated
Complement (C3, C4)	Often reduced, particularly in renal lupus
Coagulation, INR, lupus anticoagulant	May be deranged, lupus anticoagulant positive
Ferritin	Often elevated due to inflammation
Immunoglobulins G,A,M	May get hypogammaglobulinaemia
ANA	Positive
Anti-dsDNA	Often positive, may reflect renal lupus
Anti- ENA (includes anti-Sm, -RNP, -Ro, -La)	May be present
Anticardiolipin antibodies IgG, IgM	May be present
Complement C1q levels and anti-C1q antibodies	May be C1q deficient or have C1q antibodies, especially seen in renal lupus
ANCA	Often normal (useful for differential diagnosis)
TFTs	
Urinalysis	
Urine albumin:creatinine ratio	

ANA, antinuclear antibodies; ANCA, anti?neutrophil cytoplasmic antibody; CRP, C-reactive protein; dsDNA, double-stranded DNA; ENA, extractable nuclear antibodies; ESR, erythrocyte sedimentation rate; FBC, full blood count; INR, international normalization ratio; LADH, lactate dehydrogenase; LFTs, liver function tests; TFTs, thyroid function tests; U&E, urea and electrolytes.

evaluation is crucial at times of disease flare to assess the extent of disease involvement, and over time to assess disease related damage.

Appropriate investigations need to be considered carefully and tailored to the individual patient, balancing the invasiveness of each procedure with the ability to establish a diagnosis and determine the extent of the disease process. Where appropriate, investigations may include: electrocardiograph, chest radiograph, echocardiography, bone marrow aspiration, lumbar puncture, MRI, angiography, tissue histology (skin, lymph nodes) and renal biopsy (if significant proteinuria, haematuria, altered renal function, or hypertension). Many of these procedures will require sedation, even the use of general anaesthesia, to perform the procedure safely and protect the young patient from painful experiences.

Management

The management of JSLE requires comprehensive and holistic multidisciplinary team (MDT) input to achieve optimal disease control and quality of life for children and young people with lupus. Key challenges include preventing disease progression, controlling symptoms, and minimizing adverse consequences of treatment while supporting the patient and their families through the enormous impact the diagnosis of JSLE may have upon them.

The multidisciplinary team

Because of the complexity of the disease, the care of a patient with JSLE requires involvement of multiple specialists preferably coordinated by a paediatric rheumatologist with experience of JSLE.[43] Nurse specialists have an essential role in liaison with the patient/ family and can be useful in educating the patient about the disease and medication and liaising with schools. Paediatric specialists such as dermatologists, nephrologists, and haematologists may assist with the initial diagnosis, management of disease flares, and long-term disease monitoring. Physiotherapists, occupational therapists, and play specialists can assist the patient with adapting and coping with the disease and have a role in rehabilitation following disease activity flares.

JSLE can have significant and debilitating neuropsychiatric manifestations, and significant psychosocial consequences can occur secondary to chronic disease in childhood. The MDT should therefore include paediatric psychologists who can assist the patients through such difficulties. The family general practitioner should be kept informed about medication regimens and any monitoring required in the primary care setting including the special circumstances surrounding vaccination (see Chapter 95 and section 'Vaccination schedule'). Clinical medical teams working closely with clinical research teams will have a positive impact on the patient and facilitate recruitment to studies to further our understanding of this condition.

Medical management

JSLE is generally more aggressive than the adult-onset form and frequently requires higher doses of corticosteroid treatment as well as more intensive immunosuppressive treatment. Optimum disease control requires repeated and regular review to optimize management. Undertreatment can be associated with increased symptoms, worsening growth, and poor educational abilities, and can hasten disease progression and tissue damage. On the other hand, overtreatment poses more drug toxicity and potentially more frequent, severe opportunistic infections.

The overall aim of treatment is to achieve symptomatic resolution, disease control, and improved quality of life by reducing disease progression and preventing further tissue damage. This is balanced against the potential side effects of immunosuppressive therapy, which bring an increased risk of infection and a long-term risk of malignancy.

In JSLE, corticosteroids still have a crucial role in disease control. Immunosuppressive treatment regimens usually consist of a period of intensive induction of remission therapy over 6–12 months to achieve disease quiescence followed by a period of long-term maintenance therapy to control disease and prevent disease flares. Disease flares are proactively screened for and aggressively treated.

Induction therapies

Induction treatment options include intravenous corticosteroids (e.g. intravenous methylprednisolone 30 mg/kg per day for 3 days, up to maximum 1 g/day) and long-term high-dose oral corticosteroids (e.g. 1–2 mg/kg per day, followed by gradual weaning regime) combined with a disease-modifying agent. Traditionally, intravenous cyclophosphamide has been used for major organ involvement in JSLE,[44] with azathioprine or methotrexate used for milder or moderate disease. More recently, mycophenolate mofetil (MMF) has offered an alternative therapeutic option, depending on the type of organ manifestation. For example, in cases of severe lupus nephritis, identified by the International Society of Nephrology/Renal Pathology Society (ISN/RPS)[45] as class III (focal) and IV (diffuse), cyclophosphamide and MMF have been shown to be equally effective in adult-onset SLE [46] and may be more effective in those of black African ethnicity.[47] However, in cases of other major organ involvement, or where there is concurrent severe systemic vasculitis, intravenous cyclophosphamide along with corticosteroids remains the preferred induction therapy. In circumstances of rapidly progressive life-threatening disease (typically involving the neurological or renal systems) plasma exchange and intravenous immunoglobulin can be effective short-term treatment options while awaiting response to cytotoxic and corticosteroid treatment.

Maintenance therapies

All patients should receive hydroxychloroquine (HCQ), unless contraindicated, as in cases of glucose-6-phospate dehydrogenase (G6PD) deficiency. Adult studies indicate that HCQ[48,49] has a disease-modifying role, reduces long-term risk of flares, and has a steroid-sparing and lipid-lowering effect. It can be particularly useful for skin and joint disease; indeed, occasionally some patients with mild disease can be managed with HCQ alone or with addition of low-dose corticosteroids only.

Maintenance therapy of JSLE usually involves the use of either azathioprine (AZA) or MMF as immunosuppressive therapy, with reports suggesting that MMF is equally efficacious, if not slightly superior to AZA.[50,51] These disease-modifying drugs are steroid sparing and usually initially administered in combination with oral prednisolone, which is gradually withdrawn as the disease permits. Maintenance therapy should be continued for several years to achieve ongoing disease remission, particularly during critical stages of childhood development and educational milestones. For disease manifesting predominantly in the musculoskeletal system, methotrexate can achieve a good clinical response.

Second-line treatments

Second-line therapies include some of the newer biological therapies including monoclonal B-cell antibodies (rituximab), which may be used in unresponsive disease.[52] Other therapies that can be used for recalcitrant, complex disease, not controlled by the above options, include ciclosporin and monoclonal antibodies against TNFα or newer biologic therapies outlined below. Thalidomide has been used effectively in patients with severe unremitting skin involvement, but clinicians have a duty to counsel patients appropriately about its teratogenic consequences and ensure adequate contraception in sexually active patients. The medications frequently prescribed, along with the most common side effects seen in children, are summarized in Table 119.3.

Treatment of relapses

Disease relapses require thorough investigation followed by treatment according to the severity of organ involvement. Disease activity tools can categorize flares into mild, moderate, and severe.[53] Milder flares may respond to a dose increase of their maintenance therapy or a short-term increase in oral corticosteroids. Moderate to severe disease flares are likely to need intravenous corticosteroid therapy to achieve remission and may need further cytotoxic treatment. Prompt recognition, intervention, and appropriate treatment of disease flares are important as disease damage can occur during periods of poor control. During each disease exacerbation and at each annual review a meticulous calculation of the cumulative cyclophosphamide dose exposure is essential.

New drug therapies

Newer biological therapies are usually derived from drug trials in adult SLE patients, which then become adapted for use in an unlicensed manner in children with SLE. The exact side effects likely to be experienced by children on these medications is therefore not known, and specific parental consent and education regarding the risks and benefits of new therapies is required.

Biological therapies currently under investigation primarily target B-cell function, although targets to several other parts of the immune system are beginning to emerge.

◆ **Belimumab** is a new drug that has shown promising results in adult SLE trials (e.g. BLISS-52 and BLISS-76[54]). Belimumab is a human monoclonal antibody that inhibits the survival and differentiation of B cells and immunoglobulin class switching by inhibiting BLyS/BAFF.

◆ **Epratuzumab** is a CD22 monoclonal antibody that inhibits B cells and is currently undergoing clinical trials in adult-onset SLE (http://clinicaltrials.gov/ct2/home).

◆ **Atacicept** has reached phase 2 trials and is a receptor analogue, inhibiting BAFF as well as APRIL, both of which are members of the TNF family; they reduce B-cell activity and immunoglobulin formation.

◆ **Tocilizumab**, a human monoclonal antibody, acts against IL-6 and has been tested in phase 1 studies of SLE with promising reduction in laboratory markers and a good safety profile.[55]

◆ **Ocrelizumab**, like rituximab, targets CD20+ B cells but is fully humanized and avoids the problem associated with chimeric products of human antibodies directed against the treatment.

◆ **Abatacept**, used in rheumatoid arthritis, tested in a double-blind randomized controlled trial (RCT) for adult SLE failed to show a significant reduction in new flares.[56] Abatacept modulates CD80/CD86:CD28, which is a costimulatory molecule that acts as an interface between regulatory and target T cells, resulting in the production of inhibitory factors such as IL-10.

Table 119.3 Frequently prescribed medications and common side effects seen in children

Medication	Indications	Common side effects
Corticosteroids	Induction and maintenance therapy	Adrenal suppression
	All moderate to severe cases; may be required for mild unremitting disease	Striae
		Obesity
		Mood alterations
		Growth failure
		Osteoporosis
Cyclophosphamide	Induction therapy, usually intravenous	Infertility
	Moderate to severe disease with organ involvement	Hair loss
		Increased risk of infection
		Nausea and vomiting
		Long-term increased risk of malignancy
Mycophenolate mofetil	Induction and maintenance therapy	Abdominal discomfort
	Moderate to severe cases	Diarrhoea
		Liver inflammation
		Increased risk of infection
		Teratogenic in pregnancy
Azathioprine	Maintenance treatment	Increased risk of infection
	Mild, moderate, or severe disease	Bone marrow suppression
Methotrexate	Maintenance treatment	Bone marrow suppression
		Musculoskeletal symptoms
		Liver inflammation
Hydroxychloroquine	All patients	Haemolytic anaemia in patients with G6PD
Rituximab	Second-line induction therapy in moderate to severe disease	Infusion reactions
		Increased risk of infection
		Potential malignancy risk
		Long-term data in children not available

◆ **Abetimus** is a synthetic immunomodulator, shown in phase 3 trials to reduce anti-dsDNA levels after inducing tolerance in B cells.[57]

◆ **Rigeromid** is a newer agent requiring long-term testing and acts via recognition by CD4+ T cells. Clinical trials in TLR inhibition are also under way (http://clinicaltrials.gov/ct2/home).

Growth and development

Patients with JSLE require particular consideration to their growth and development, with measurements and comparison to growth centile charts recommended every 3 months. Body mass index and pubertal assessment is also important during monitoring. Faltering growth and pubertal delay may be seen due to chronic disease or may occur secondary to treatment side effects.

Psychosocial well-being

Health consideration in terms of physical well-being is essential, but equally important is the acknowledgment of the patient's educational, emotional, and psychosocial needs.

Long-term consequences

The patients and their families need to be aware of the long-term consequences of JSLE secondary to both disease and treatment, including reduced fertility, long-term cardiovascular complications and the risk of future malignancy, particularly in cases requiring toxic immunosuppressant treatment or newer biologic therapies. The long-term consequences of the disease are very important in childhood disease as these patients have a lifetime of disease and treatment burden.

Research in JSLE

There is a great need to find more effective treatments in JSLE with fewer, more tolerable side effects. Achieving this in children requires international collaboration to produce large multicentre treatment trials. All patients with JSLE should be provided with an opportunity to take part in research to further the care and understanding of their condition. Paediatric-specific drug trials would allow a more accurate awareness of the childhood specific risks associated with new treatments and would assess the acceptability of administrating such medications to a childhood population.

The Paediatric Rheumatology International Trials Organization (PRINTO) is currently attempting to standardize definitions and management for SLE and have worked to define core sets of outcome measures for disease activity and disease damage assessment and definitions of improvement, to be used in clinical trials and outcome assessment studies in children with JSLE.[58] The overall goal of the PRINTO project is to have a standardized approach for the outcome evaluation of children with JSLE, allowing international trials.

Other management options

Bone marrow or stem cell transplant is considered in the rare cases of poorly controlled JSLE. It is reserved for severe cases and requires consensus from external expert reviewers, as it is associated with a significant mortality.

In cases of severe end-organ involvement other interventions may be required, for example renal transplant for advanced glomerulonephritis. These will not affect the systemic disease course and inflammation can reoccur in the transplanted organ, although surprisingly this is rare, perhaps because systemic immunosuppression is required to prevent organ rejection.

Topical immunosuppressive treatments can be used for isolated skin manifestations and laser therapy has been used to treat striae associated with corticosteroid use.

Compliance to treatment

As with many lifelong chronic conditions, poor compliance in JSLE can be an important factor contributing to worsening or poorly controlled disease. At every opportunity concordance with management should be explored in a sensitive way and may influence treatment options to suit the individual patient. A supportive partnership with the patient, family members and the MDT may assist with resolving compliance issues, which are frequently seen during adolescent years.

Vaccination schedule

Serological evaluation of viral status in relation to differential diagnosis is important, as well as determining immunity in relation to varicella and measles, as vaccination prior to immunosuppressive treatment is recommended where clinically possible.

All vaccines are strongly recommended except for live vaccines such as the measles, mumps, and rubella (MMR) vaccine, which are contraindicated while the patient is on immunosuppressive agents including corticosteroids. Live vaccines can only be given once the patient has been off treatment for greater than 3 months. In addition to scheduled vaccinations, which include the human papillomavirus (HPV) vaccine, the annual flu vaccine and pneumococcal vaccination are recommended. Patients who are not immune to measles and who come into contact with the condition should receive intravenous immunoglobulin. In response to contact with varicella, a non-immune patient should receive varicella zoster immunoglobulin and if symptoms develop intravenous aciclovir should be administered.

Prognosis

Long-term morbidity of JSLE is significant, related to both disease damage and treatment toxicity. The 10-year mortality rate remains around 10%, with the greatest improvement in mortality seen during the introduction and routine use of immunosuppressive medication and corticosteroid treatment. Children with SLE have a lower life expectancy than the general population, mainly due to an increased cardiovascular morbidity, with evidence of premature atherosclerosis when begins forming in childhood.[59,60]

More severe and active disease is associated with a worse life expectancy and JSLE has a higher risk of death than adult-onset SLE. Disease damage in JSLE should be monitored annually using the damage index Systemic Lupus International Collaborating Clinics/American College of Rheumatology (SLICC/ACR) Damage Index.[61] Designed and validated for use in adults, it provides a useful comparative tool for assessing the frequency and distribution of end-organ damage although a paediatric-specific damage index is required.

Conclusion

JSLE is a complex multisystemic disease requiring specialist assessment and careful monitoring. The disease shares many similarities to adult-onset SLE but an awareness of the differences is crucial. An experienced paediatric rheumatologist, working closely with a dedicated MDT, should lead the management of these patients. Children with this lifelong condition may have disease- and treatment-associated morbidity and a reduced life expectancy. Research into the pathophysiology of JSLE will provide important insight into childhood disease, which may be translational to adults and is crucial for developing more effective treatments to improve outcomes. Clinical trials in JSLE are urgently required to establish the optimum treatment regimens.

References

1. Tucker LB, Uribe AG, Fernandez M et al. Adolescent onset of lupus results in more aggressive disease and worse outcomes: results of a nested matched case-control study within LUMINA, a multiethnic US cohort (LUMINA LVII). *Lupus* 2008:17(4):314–322.

2. Huang JL, Yao TC, See LC. Prevalence of pediatric systemic lupus erythematosus and juvenile chronic arthritis in a Chinese population: a nation-wide prospective population-based study in Taiwan. *Clin Exp Rheumatol* 2004:22(6):776–780.

3. Huemer C, Huemer M, Dorner T et al. Incidence of pediatric rheumatic diseases in a regional population in Austria. *J Rheumatol* 2001:28(9):2116–2119.

4. Bowyer SL. Demography of a regional pediatric rheumatology patient population. *J Rheumatol* 1995:22(4):790–791.

5. Kaipiainen-Seppanen O, Savolainen A. Incidence of chronic juvenile rheumatic diseases in Finland during 1980–1990. *Clin Exp Rheumatol* 1996:14(4):441–444.

6. Houghton KM, Page J, Cabral DA, Petty RE, Tucker LB. Systemic lupus erythematosus in the pediatric North American Native population of British Columbia. *J Rheumatol* 2006:33(1):161–163.

7. Malleson PN, Fung MY, Rosenberg AM. The incidence of pediatric rheumatic diseases: results from the Canadian Pediatric Rheumatology Association Disease Registry. *J Rheumatol* 1996:23(11):1981–1987.

8. Hiraki LT, Benseler SM, Tyrrell PN et al. Ethnic differences in pediatric systemic lupus erythematosus. *J Rheumatol* 2009:36(11):2539–2546.

9. Brunner HI, Gladman DD, Ibanez D, Urowitz MD, Silverman ED. Difference in disease features between childhood-onset and adult-onset systemic lupus erythematosus. *Arthritis Rheum* 2008:58(2):556–562.

10. Sasaki N, Yamauchi K, Sato R et al. Klinefelter's syndrome associated with systemic lupus erythematosus and autoimmune hepatitis. *Mod Rheumatol* 2006:16(5):305–308.

11. Shiari R, Farivar S. Juvenile systemic lupus erythematosus associated with Klinefelter's syndrome: A case report. *Reumatol Clin* 2010:6(4):212–213.

12. Cooper GS, Wither J, Bernatsky S et al. Occupational and environmental exposures and risk of systemic lupus erythematosus: silica, sunlight, solvents. *Rheumatology* (Oxford) 2010:49(11):2172–2180.

13. Priori R, Medda E, Conti F et al. Familial autoimmunity as a risk factor for systemic lupus erythematosus and vice versa: a case-control study. *Lupus* 2003:12(10):735–740.

14. Ramantani G, Kohlhase J, Hertzberg C et al. Expanding the phenotypic spectrum of lupus erythematosus in Aicardi-Goutieres syndrome. *Arthritis Rheum* 2010:62(5):1469–1477.

15. Rahman A, Isenberg DA. Systemic lupus erythematosus. *N Engl J Med* 2008:358(9):929–939.

16. Al-Mayouf SM, Abanomi H, Eldali A. Impact of C1q deficiency on the severity and outcome of childhood systemic lupus erythematosus. *Int J Rheum Dis* 2011:14(1):81–85.

17. Chang C, Gershwin ME. Drug-induced lupus erythematosus: incidence, management and prevention. *Drug Saf* 2011:34(5):357–374.

18. Pain C, Beresford MW. Neonatal lupus syndrome. *Paediatr Child Health* 2007:17(6):223–227.

19. Jaeggi E, Laskin C, Hamilton R, Kingdom J, Silverman E. The importance of the level of maternal anti-Ro/SSA antibodies as a prognostic marker of the development of cardiac neonatal lupus erythematosus a prospective study of 186 antibody-exposed fetuses and infants. *J Am Coll Cardiol* 2010:55(24):2778–2784.

20. Midgley A, McLaren Z, Moots RJ, Edwards SW, Beresford MW. The role of neutrophil apoptosis in juvenile-onset systemic lupus erythematosus. *Arthritis Rheum* 2009:60(8):2390–2401.

21. Perry D, Sang A, Yin Y, Zheng YY, Morel L. Murine models of systemic lupus erythematosus. *J Biomed Biotechnol* 2011:2011:271694.

22. Midgley A, Mayer K, Edwards SW, Beresford MW. Differential expression of factors involved in the intrinsic and extrinsic apoptotic pathways in juvenile systemic lupus erythematosus. *Lupus* 2011:20(1):71–79.

23. Midgley A, Beresford MW. Cellular localization of nuclear antigen during neutrophil apoptosis: mechanism for autoantigen exposure? *Lupus* 2011:20(6):641–646.

24. Gaipl US, Munoz LE, Grossmayer G et al. Clearance deficiency and systemic lupus erythematosus (SLE). *J Autoimmun* 2007:28(2–3):114–121.

25. Toong C, Adelstein S, Phan TG. Clearing the complexity: immune complexes and their treatment in lupus nephritis. *Int J Nephrol Renovasc Dis* 2011:4:17–28.

26. Weckerle CE, Franek BS, Kelly JA et al. Network analysis of associations between serum interferon-alpha activity, autoantibodies, and clinical features in systemic lupus erythematosus. *Arthritis Rheum* 2011:63(4):1044–1053.

27. Crow MK, Kirou KA, Wohlgemuth J. Microarray analysis of interferon-regulated genes in SLE. *Autoimmunity* 2003:36(8):481–490.

28. Hackl D, Loschko J, Sparwasser T, Reindl W, Krug AB. Activation of dendritic cells via TLR7 reduces Foxp3 expression and suppressive function in induced Tregs. *Eur J Immunol* 2011:41(5):1334–1343.

29. Midgley AM, Thorbinson C, Beresford MW. Toll like receptor expression and their detection of nuclear self-antigen leading to immune activation in JSLE. *Rheumatology* (Oxford) 2012:51(5):824–832.

30. Guiducci C, Gong M, Xu Z et al. TLR recognition of self nucleic acids hampers glucocorticoid activity in lupus. *Nature* 2010:465(7300):937–941.

31. Jacob N, Stohl W. Cytokine disturbances in systemic lupus erythematosus. *Arthritis Res Ther* 2011:13(4):228.

32. Avcin T, Cimaz R, Rozman B. The Ped-APS Registry: the antiphospholipid syndrome in childhood. *Lupus* 2009:18(10):894–899.

33. Cervera R, Boffa MC, Khamashta MA, Hughes GR. The Euro-Phospholipid project: epidemiology of the antiphospholipid syndrome in Europe. *Lupus* 2009:18(10):889–893.

34. Avcin T, Cimaz R, Silverman ED et al. Pediatric antiphospholipid syndrome: clinical and immunologic features of 121 patients in an international registry. *Pediatrics* 2008:122(5):e1100–e1107.

35. Tan EM, Cohen AS, Fries JF et al. The 1982 revised criteria for the classification of systemic lupus erythematosus. *Arthritis Rheum* 1982:25(11):1271–1277.

36. Hochberg MC. Updating the American College of Rheumatology revised criteria for the classification of systemic lupus erythematosus. *Arthritis Rheum* 1997:40(9):1725.

37. Ferraz MB, Goldenberg J, Hilario MO et al. Evaluation of the 1982 ARA lupus criteria data set in pediatric patients. Committees of Pediatric Rheumatology of the Brazilian Society of Pediatrics and the Brazilian Society of Rheumatology. *Clin Exp Rheumatol* 1994:12(1):83–87.

38. Marks SD, Pilkington C, Woo P, Dillon MJ. The use of the British Isles Lupus Assessment Group (BILAG) index as a valid tool in assessing disease activity in childhood-onset systemic lupus erythematosus. *Rheumatology* (Oxford) 2004:43(9):1186–1189.

39. Brunner HI, Feldman BM, Bombardier C, Silverman ED. Sensitivity of the Systemic Lupus Erythematosus Disease Activity Index, British Isles Lupus Assessment Group Index, and Systemic Lupus Activity Measure in the evaluation of clinical change in childhood-onset systemic lupus erythematosus. *Arthritis Rheum* 1999:42(7):1354–1360.

40. Bombardier C, Gladman DD, Urowitz MB, Caron D, Chang CH. Derivation of the SLEDAI. A disease activity index for lupus patients. The Committee on Prognosis Studies in SLE. *Arthritis Rheum* 1992:35(6):630–640.

41. Isenberg DA, Rahman A, Allen E et al. BILAG 2004. Development and initial validation of an updated version of the British Isles Lupus Assessment Group's disease activity index for patients with systemic lupus erythematosus. *Rheumatology* (Oxford) 2005:44(7):902–906.

42. Ruperto N, Hanrahan LM, Alarcon GS et al. International consensus for a definition of disease flare in lupus. *Lupus* 2011:20(5):453–462.

43. Beresford MW, Davidson JE. Adolescent development and SLE. *Best Pract Res Clin Rheumatol* 2006:20(2):353–368.

44. Ardoin SP, Schanberg LE. The management of pediatric systemic lupus erythematosus. *Nat Clin Pract Rheumatol* 2005:1(2):82–92.

45. Weening JJ, D'Agati VD, Schwartz MM et al. The classification of glomerulonephritis in systemic lupus erythematosus revisited. *J Am Soc Nephrol* 2004:15(2):241–250.

46. Touma Z, Gladman DD, Urowitz MB et al. Mycophenolate mofetil for induction treatment of lupus nephritis: a systematic review and metaanalysis. *J Rheumatol* 2011:38(1):69–78.

47. Isenberg D, Appel GB, Contreras G et al. Influence of race/ethnicity on response to lupus nephritis treatment: the ALMS study. *Rheumatology* (Oxford) 2010:49(1):128–140.

48. Costedoat-Chalumeau N, Amoura Z, Hulot JS, Lechat P, Piette JC. Hydroxychloroquine in systemic lupus erythematosus. *Lancet* 2007:369(9569):1257–1258.

49. Fessler BJ, Alarcon GS, McGwin G Jr et al. Systemic lupus erythematosus in three ethnic groups: XVI. Association of hydroxychloroquine use with reduced risk of damage accrual. *Arthritis Rheum* 2005:52(5):1473–1480.

50. Dall'era M. Mycophenolate mofetil in the treatment of systemic lupus erythematosus. *Curr Opin Rheumatol* 2011:23(5):454–458.

51. Houssiau FA, Vasconcelos C, D'Cruz D et al. The 10-year follow-up data of the Euro-Lupus Nephritis Trial comparing low-dose and high-dose intravenous cyclophosphamide. *Ann Rheum Dis* 2010:69(1):61–64.

52. Podolskaya A, Stadermann M, Pilkington C, Marks SD, Tullus K. B cell depletion therapy for 19 patients with refractory systemic lupus erythematosus. *Arch Dis Child* 2008:93(5):401–406.

53. Brunner HI, Mina R, Pilkington C et al. Preliminary criteria for global flares in childhood-onset systemic lupus erythematosus. *Arthritis Care Res* (Hoboken) 2011:63(9):1213–1223.

54. Navarra SV, Guzman RM, Gallacher AE et al. Efficacy and safety of belimumab in patients with active systemic lupus erythematosus: a randomised, placebo-controlled, phase 3 trial. *Lancet* 2011:377(9767):721–731.

55. Illei GG, Shirota Y, Yarboro CH et al. Tocilizumab in systemic lupus erythematosus: data on safety, preliminary efficacy, and impact on circulating plasma cells from an open-label phase I dosage-escalation study. *Arthritis Rheum* 2010:62(2):542–552.

56. Merrill JT, Burgos-Vargas R, Westhovens R et al. The efficacy and safety of abatacept in patients with non-life-threatening manifestations of systemic lupus erythematosus: results of a twelve-month, multicenter, exploratory, phase IIb, randomized, double-blind, placebo-controlled trial. *Arthritis Rheum* 2010:62(10):3077–3087.

57. Cardiel MH, Tumlin JA, Furie RA et al. Abetimus sodium for renal flare in systemic lupus erythematosus: results of a randomized, controlled phase III trial. *Arthritis Rheum* 2008:58(8):2470–2480.

58. Ruperto N, Ravelli A, Murray KJ et al. Preliminary core sets of measures for disease activity and damage assessment in juvenile systemic lupus erythematosus and juvenile dermatomyositis. *Rheumatology* (Oxford) 2003:42(12):1452–1459.

59. Kamphuis S, Silverman ED. Prevalence and burden of pediatric-onset systemic lupus erythematosus. *Nat Rev Rheumatol* 2010:6(9):538–546.

60. Gonzalez B, Hernandez P, Olguin H et al. Changes in the survival of patients with systemic lupus erythematosus in childhood: 30 years experience in Chile. *Lupus* 2005:14(11):918–923.

61. Stoll T, Sutcliffe N, Mach J, Klaghofer R, Isenberg DA. Analysis of the relationship between disease activity and damage in patients with systemic lupus erythematosus—a 5-yr prospective study. *Rheumatology* (Oxford) 2004:43(8):1039–1044.

Further reading

Ardoin SP, Schanbery LE. Systemic lupus erythematosus. Chapter 152 in: Kliegman RM, Stanton B, Geme JS, Schor N, Behroman RE (eds) *Nelson textbook of pediatrics*, 19th edn. Saunders Elsevier, Philadelphia, PA, 2011.

Cassidy JT, Petter RE, Laxer R, Lindsley C. *Textbook of pediatric rheumatology*, 6th edn. Saunders Elsevier, Philadelphia, PA, 2011.

Sources of patient information

Lupus UK: www.lupusuk.co.uk

National Health Service patient information website: www.nhs.uk/Conditions/Lupus/Pages/Introduction.aspx

CHAPTER 120

Anti-phospholipid antibody syndrome

Munther A. Khamashta, Graham R. V. Hughes, and Guillermo Ruiz-Irastorza

Introduction

In 1983, few rheumatologists would have predicted the interest that the introduction of the anti-cardiolipin test would generate.[1] New autoantibodies turn up frequently in patients with systemic lupus erythematosus (SLE) and there may have seemed little reason why anti-cardiolipin antibodies should have merited any more than passing interest. However, their association with an unusual combination of clinical complications that included venous and arterial thrombosis, pregnancy loss, and thrombocytopenia attracted the attention of investigators from a variety of disciplines.[2] A chronology of the major developments in the unfolding of the anti-phospholipid syndrome (APS) story is listed in Box 120.1.

During the last three decades, considerable progress has been made in understanding anti-phospholipid antibodies (APA) and the disorder with which they are associated, but many questions remain unanswered, particularly those of pathogenesis and optimal treatment.[3]

Epidemiology

Efforts are being made in clinics throughout the world to assess the importance of APA in recurrent abortion, stroke, myocardial infarction, and epilepsy, among others. Prospective studies have shown an association between APA and the first episode of venous thrombosis,[4] the first myocardial infarction,[5] and the first ischaemic stroke.[6] A critical issue, therefore, is the identification of patients with APA who are at increased risk for a thrombotic event.

Many patients have laboratory evidence of APA without clinical consequence. APA, using standardized techniques, are detected in less than 1% of apparently normal individuals and in up to 3% of the elderly population without clinical manifestations of the APS. Among patients with SLE, the prevalence of APA is much higher, 30–40%.[7] For otherwise healthy control subjects, there are insufficient data to determine what percentage of those with APA will eventually have a thrombotic event or a complication of pregnancy consistent with the APS. In contrast, the APS may develop in

Box 120.1 Anti-phospholipid antibodies and the anti-phospholipid syndrome—history	
1906	Wasserman reaction (reagin)
1941	Reagin binds cardiolipin
1952	False-positive test for syphillis
1952	Lupus anti-coagulant
1960s	Lupus anti-coagulant: association with thrombosis
1970s	Lupus anti-coagulant is due to immunoglobulin
1975	Lupus anti-coagulant: association with recurrent miscarriages
1983	Anti-cardiolipin antibodies
1983–1985	Detailed clinical description of the anti-phospholipid syndrome (APS)
1985	APS—separate entity from lupus
1989	Lupus anti-coagulant and anti-cardiolipin: separate antibody subgroups
1990	Phospholipid-binding proteins (β2-glycoprotein I)
1990s	Animal models for APS
1999	Classification criteria for APS
2006	Classification criteria updated

50–70% of patients with both SLE and APA after 10–20 years of follow-up.[8]

The specificities of APA probably differ in various disorders. Large retrospective studies of patients with thrombotic complications suggest that those with lupus anti-coagulant and/or high concentrations of IgG anti-cardiolipin antibodies appear to be at greatest risk for thrombosis, whereas the risk of clotting appears to be much lower in patients with infection-related or drug-induced APA.

Genetic analyses and modelling studies strongly support a genetic basis for disease in families with the APS and suggest an autosomal dominant model of inheritance.[9] HLA studies have suggested associations with DR7, DR4, DRw53, DQw7, and C4 null alleles.

Detection of anti-phospholipid antibodies

APA are detected by a variety of laboratory tests, the most useful for identifying patients with the APS being the lupus anti-coagulant and the anti-cardiolipin antibody tests. These antibodies are distinct and separable immunoglobulins present alone or in combination.[10]

The autoantibodies sometimes bind phospholipids utilized in the Venereal Disease Research Laboratories (VDRL) test; hence, some patients may have a false-positive test for syphilis. However, the VDRL test is not positive frequently enough to make it valuable in diagnosing the APS.

The lupus anti-coagulant is a functional assay measuring the ability of APA to prolong clotting via their inhibition of the conversion of prothrombin to thrombin or the activation of factor X (both reactions are catalysed by phospholipids). Tests for the lupus anti-coagulant have been difficult to standardize, and no single test appears to be adequate. The test begins with an attempt to demonstrate an abnormal coagulation screening test, such as a prolonged activated partial thromboplastin time (APTT) , dilute Russell viper venom time, or kaolin clotting time. If any of these is positive, the test is repeated, using a sample in which the patient's plasma has been mixed with normal plasma. If the patient's disorder is a clotting deficiency, the test should become normal. If, on the other hand, lupus anti-coagulant or some other clotting inhibitor is present, the clotting time will remain prolonged. The presence of lupus anti-coagulant is confirmed by the return to normal of the clotting test after addition of freeze-thawed platelets or excess phospholipids, either of which bind the antibodies. The lupus anti-coagulant test must be performed on platelet-poor plasma.[10]

The anti-cardiolipin antibody test was introduced in 1983 and extensively improved since that time.[11] This test uses enzyme-linked immunosorbent assay (ELISA) to determine antibody binding to solid plates coated with either cardiolipin or other phospholipids. Serum or plasma samples may be used for the anti-cardiolipin assay. The availability of reference sera which are isotype specific (IgG and IgM) has greatly improved interlaboratory testing and quantification of anti-cardiolipin antibodies. IgA anti-cardiolipin reference sera are also now available. Many laboratories currently measure all three isotypes and sensitive kits are commercially available.

In general, positive lupus anti-coagulant tests are more specific for the APS, whereas anti-cardiolipin antibodies are more sensitive. The specificity of anti-cardiolipin antibodies for APS increases with the titre and is higher for the IgG than for the IgM isotype. However, some patients may have only a positive IgM test, and a few are only IgA positive.[10]

The observation that many anti-cardiolipin antibodies are directed at an epitope on β2-glycoprotein I led to the development of anti-β2-glycoprotein I antibody immunoassays.[12] Their presence has been included in the 2006 updated criteria for the classification of the APS.[13] The main clinical utility of anti-β2-glycoprotein I antibodies is when they appear in combination with other APA, since those patients triple positive for lupus anti-coagulant, anti-cardiolipin, and anti-β2-glycoprotein I antibodies are at the highest risk of thrombosis.[14] However, in some patients with clinical features of APS, anti-β2-glycoprotein I antibodies are rarely the sole antibodies detected.[15] Thus, multiple APA tests should be used in seeking the diagnosis of APS.

The clinical utility of APA assays for autoantibodies to phospholipids other than cardiolipin and to phospholipid-binding proteins other than β2-glycoprotein I, such as prothrombin, remains unclear.[10] However, new refined tests are expected in the near future that could improve the correct identification of patients with APS.

Pathogenesis

There is now good evidence, mainly from animal models, that APA can be pathogenic rather than a simple serological marker for APS. Passive transfer and active immunization of BALB/c mice with human or mouse anti-cardiolipin monoclonal antibodies induced features of the APS.[16,17] Also, atherosclerosis in a susceptible mouse model (the LDL-receptor knockout mouse) was accelerated by immunization with human anti-cardiolipin antibodies from an APS patient, providing additional evidence for a causal pathogenic effect.[18]

Mechanisms of thrombosis

APA alone are apparently unable to induce thrombotic manifestations per se. In this regard, a two-hit hypothesis has been suggested: APA (first hit) increases the risk of thrombotic events that occur in the presence of another thrombophilic condition (second hit).[19]

Precisely how APA relate to thrombosis is unknown. Several mechanisms have been proposed to explain the prothrombotic nature of the APS. The range of possible mechanisms includes effects of APA on platelet membranes, on endothelial cells, and on clotting components such as antithrombin, protein C, and protein S (Box 120.2).[20]

Box 120.2 Proposed mechanisms of thrombosis mediated by anti-phospholipid antibody

- Increase of tissue factor expression on monocytes and on endothelial cells
- Increase of platelet activation and aggregation
- Decrease of prostacyclin production and/or release by endothelial cells
- Complement activation
- Decrease of function of annexin A5
- Decrease of protein C activation
- Decrease of free protein S levels
- Decrease of antithrombin activation
- Interference with thrombomodulin function on endothelial cells
- Interference with the function of plasma β2-glycoprotein I
- Inhibition of tissue factor pathway inhibitor
- Direct injury to endothelium
- Induction of apoptosis on vascular cells
- Vascular activation and release of von Willebrand factor multimer
- Increase of endothelin-1
- Increase of plasminogen activator inhibitor-1
- Cross-reactivity to oxidized LDL
- Inhibition of factor XII/prekallikrein-mediated fibrinolytic activity

It is now accepted that APA can react with endothelial cells, monocytes, and platelets, mainly through the binding to β2-glycoprotein I expressed on cell membranes. Exogenous β2-glycoprotein I can bind to endothelial cells at the putative phospholipid binding site located in the fifth domain of the molecule. Binding of APA induces activation of endothelial cells, monocytes, and platelets. Adhesion molecules such as intercellular cell adhesion molecule-1 (ICAM-1), vascular cell adhesion molecule-1 (VCAM-1), and E-selectin are expressed by activated endothelial cells. Both endothelial cells and monocytes upregulate the production of tissue factor (TF).[21] Activated platelets increase the expression of glycoprotein IIb–IIIa and the synthesis of thromboxane A2 (TXA2). Many of these processes are mediated by nuclear factor-κB (NFκB) and p-38 mitogen-activated protein kinase (p-38 MAPK).[22] Recent studies in mice also suggest an important role of complement activation in aPL-induced thrombosis.[23]

The activation of endothelial cells, monocytes, and platelets induces a procoagulant state that is mainly mediated by the increased synthesis of TF and TXA2. Activation of the complement cascade, in combination with a 'second hit', results in clinical thrombosis. Traditional cardiovascular risk factors, which are present in more than 50% of patients with the APS, frequently play an important role.[2] Additionally, interaction of APA with proteins implicated in clotting regulation, such as prothrombin, factor X, protein C, and plasmin, may interfere with the inactivation of procoagulant factors and fibrinolysis.

Mechanisms of pregnancy loss

The mechanism of pregnancy loss associated with APA remains uncertain. Progressive thrombosis of the microvasculature of the placenta and subsequent infarction resulting in placental insufficiency, fetal growth restriction, and, ultimately, fetal loss, is a plausible explanation. The disruption of the annexin A5 shield seems to play an important additional role in the pathogenesis of the obstetric manifestations of the APS. Annexin A5 is a potent vascular and placental anti-coagulant protein with high affinity for negatively charged phospholipids. It is highly expressed at the interface between the fetus and the placenta, with its anti-coagulant effect resulting from the capacity to crystallize over phospholipid bilayers, which blocks their availability for coagulation reactions. APA interfere with annexin A5 function.[24]

Not all placentas examined, however, have shown areas of thrombosis or infarction and other mechanisms may be operative in these patients. Recently, in-vitro studies showed that APA may impair trophoblastic invasion and hormone production, thereby promoting not only early miscarriages but also fetal loss and uteroplacental insufficiency.[25] These findings provide strong evidence for a defective placentation mediated directly by APA that is not necessarily associated with thrombotic phenomena.[26] Complement activation can also have a major role in APS-related pregnancy loss.[27]

Clinical features

The APS is a non-inflammatory autoimmune disease. The most critical pathologic process is thrombosis, which results in most of the clinical features suffered by these patients. Any organ can be affected in this disorder; thus, the range of clinical features is extremely wide (Box 120.3).

Box 120.3 Clinical features of the anti-phospholipid syndrome

Major features

- Venous thrombosis: deep venous thrombosis,
- Budd–Chiari syndrome, and pulmonary thromboembolism
- Arterial thrombosis: strokes, transient ischaemic attacks, multi-infarct dementia, and myocardial infarction
- Pregnancy complications: recurrent pregnancy loss, intrauterine growth restriction, pre-eclampsia, and abruption

Associated clinical features

- Thrombocytopenia
- Leg ulcers, livedo reticularis, thrombophlebitis, and Sneddon's syndrome
- Heart valve lesions
- Transverse myelitis, chorea, and epilepsy
- Haemolytic anaemia, Coombs' positivity, and Evans' syndrome
- Pulmonary hypertension
- Cognitive impairment
- Chronic headache

Others (less common)

- Splinter haemorrhages
- Labile hypertension and accelerated atherosclerosis
- Ischaemic necrosis of bone
- Bone marrow necrosis
- Addison's disease
- Guillain–Barré syndrome and pseudo-multiple sclerosis
- Aumaurosis fugax
- Sensorineural hearing loss
- Renal artery and vein thrombosis and microangiopathy
- Retinal artery and vein thrombosis
- Digital gangrene

Thrombosis

Arterial and venous thromboses are among the main features of the APS. In contrast, thromboses associated with congenital thrombophilias, such as protein C, protein S, or antithrombin deficiency, factor V Leiden and factor II 20210A mutations, are almost all only venous. Vessels of all sizes may be affected, and the vascular pathological appearance has consistently been of bland occlusion without inflammatory infiltrates.[28]

In the venous circulation, thrombosis of the deep veins of the lower extremities has been reported most frequently.[29] They are often recurrent and may be accompanied by pulmonary embolism. It has been estimated that up to 19% of patients with deep-vein thrombosis and/or pulmonary thromboembolism have APS.

Recurrent pulmonary emboli or pulmonary veno-occlusive disease may be cause of pulmonary hypertension. Other reported venous sites of thrombosis include the axillary, ocular, renal, hepatic and sagittal veins, and the inferior vena cava. The APS is now considered one of the most frequent causes of the Budd–Chiari syndrome.[30] APA have been implicated in the development of adrenal vein thrombosis leading to adrenal insufficiency. Venous events usually occur at single sites and they can recur at the same or different sites, months or years apart.

Arterial thromboses are a major feature of the APS. As with venous thrombosis, arterial events usually occur at single sites and can recur months or years later. Occlusion of the intracranial arteries has been reported most frequently, with the majority of patients presenting with stroke or transient ischaemic attacks. However, cerebral infarctions may be silent. MRI scans may show changes that vary from single lesions to multiple, widely scattered infarcts (Figure 120.1). In some patients, untreated recurrent cerebral thrombosis can lead to multi-infarct dementia and cognitive impairment has been prominent in the presentation of some patients with the APS.[31] APA are now recognized as an important aetiological factor and may be present in 7% of all patients who have suffered a stroke. They should be sought especially in young patients with strokes, where they may account for up to 18%. Since emboli from heart valve vegetations may be responsible for cerebral infarction, it is advisable to perform echocardiograms on patients with APS who present with transient ischaemic attacks or brain infarction. Other arterial thromboses are less frequent, involving the retina, coronary, mesenteric, and peripheral arteries.[29] The clinical presentation depends on the anatomic site occluded.

Renal involvement in APS was first described in 1992.[32] Glomerular thrombotic microangiopathy is the most characteristic finding in APS nephropathy, albeit not exclusive of this syndrome, usually presenting with the triad of hypertension, proteinuria, and renal failure. Other histological lesions include fibrous intimal hyperplasia, focal cortical atrophy, and arterial occlusions have also been described.[33] Refractory hypertension secondary to renal artery stenosis can be also found.[34]

Pregnancy complications

Recurrent spontaneous pregnancy losses are one of the most consistent complications of the APS. Losses can occur at any stage of pregnancy, although miscarriages associated with APA are strikingly frequent during the second and third trimester (about 50% of cases). This differs from the pattern of pregnancy loss in the normal population, which usually occurs during the first trimester and is most often due to non-immunological factors: that is, morphological or chromosomal abnormalities. The rate of miscarriage in patients positive for APA is still uncertain, although testing for this antibody is becoming a routine investigation in women with recurrent miscarriages. Fewer than 2% of apparently normal pregnant women have either anti-cardiolipin antibody or lupus anti-coagulant in any titre, and less than 0.2% have high titre antibody. Hence, screening normal pregnant women has little value. Previous pregnancy history is of importance in determining the significance of a positive laboratory test for APA. It has been estimated that if a patient with lupus has a positive lupus anti-coagulant or at least moderate levels of IgG anti-cardiolipin antibodies, the risk of spontaneous miscarriage during the first pregnancy is 30% and if she has a history of at least two spontaneous miscarriages, the risk is 70% during the following pregnancy.

The risk of fetal loss is directly related to the antibody type and titres. A recent meta-analysis including 25 studies showed that lupus anti-coagulant has the strongest association with recurrent fetal losses before 24 weeks of gestation—odds ratio (OR) 7.79, 95% confidence interval (CI) 2.30–26.45—although it was not possible to analyse its association with miscarriages before 13 weeks.[35] IgG anti-cardiolipin antibodies (aCL) were associated with both early (OR 3.56, 95% CI 1.48–8.59) and late recurrent fetal losses (OR 3.57, 95% CI 2.26–5.65), women with moderate to high titres showing increased risk (OR 4.68, 95% CI 2.96–7.40). IgM aCL were also associated with late recurrent fetal losses (OR 5.61, 95% CI 1.26–25.03). On the other hand, no relationship was found between anti-β2GP1 and recurrent miscarriages (OR 2.12, 95% CI 0.69–6.53).

Despite the clear relation between APA and obstetric morbidity, it is not possible to predict which women will develop complications in pregnancy. However, an adverse previous obstetric outcome, a history of thrombosis, and triple positivity for lupus anti-coagulant, anti-cardiolipin and anti-β2-glycoprotein I antibodies have been identified as high-risk predictors.[36,37] In pregnancies that do not end in miscarriage or fetal loss, there is still a high incidence of intrauterine growth restriction, placental abruption, and premature delivery.

Other manifestations

Thrombocytopenia is common in patients with APA, though rarely severe enough to cause haemorrhage. The platelet count often

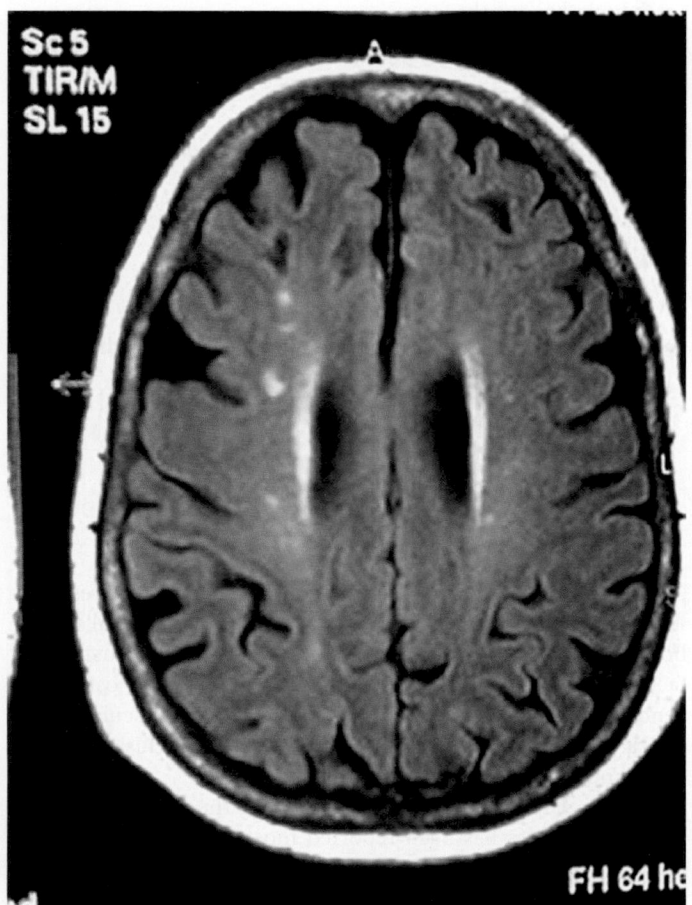

Fig. 120.1 MRI scan showing cerebral infarctions.

remains stable for many years; then, for reasons that are often obscure, the count drops, sometimes catastrophically. Occasionally, patients with APS may present only with severe thrombocytopenia and later develop pregnancy loss or thrombosis. This form of presentation was observed in a very small number of our patients with the syndrome.[38] Some patients with APA and thrombocytopenia also develop haemolytic anaemia with positive direct Coombs' test, a combination known as Evans' syndrome.

Epilepsy and chorea are less frequent manifestations of the APS and have, intriguingly, been seen to improve in some patients treated with anti-coagulants. Transverse myelopathy, though rare, has been strongly associated with the presence of APA.[39] However, more recent studies put such association into question.[40] Occasionally, in some patients with bizarre, transient/recurrent neurological signs and cerebral lesions resembling multiple sclerosis, APA have been detected in the absence of other immunological abnormalities. Its recognition is important as anti-coagulation therapy may be effective in these patients.[41]

Migraine is a common finding in patients with the APS, and often predates the diagnosis by many years. However, several prospective studies have not demonstrated a significant statistical association between migraine headaches and the presence of APA.[38]

Heart valve disease is strikingly associated with APA.[42] In some cases, this is due to a combination of valvular thrombosis and degeneration. The mitral valve is the most frequently affected, followed by the aortic valve. Insufficiency is more common than stenosis. Most patients with heart valve disease associated with APA are asymptomatic, though severe valvular dysfunction requiring surgical valve replacement has been reported. Emboli from sterile valvular vegetations can cause multiple cerebral lesions.[43] Large intracardiac thrombosis associated with APA can mimic atrial myxoma.

One of the most striking physical signs in patients positive for APA is livedo reticularis (Figure 120.2), sometimes widespread, sometimes subtle, for example, confined to a small area on the back of the wrist. Many cases of Sneddon's syndrome, defined as the clinical triad of stroke, livedo reticularis, and hypertension, may represent undiagnosed APS. More dramatic skin manifestations associated with vascular thrombosis include widespread skin ulceration, notably in the lower extremities (Figure 120.3). Clinically, some patients with APA may develop nail splinter haemorrhages and clubbing,

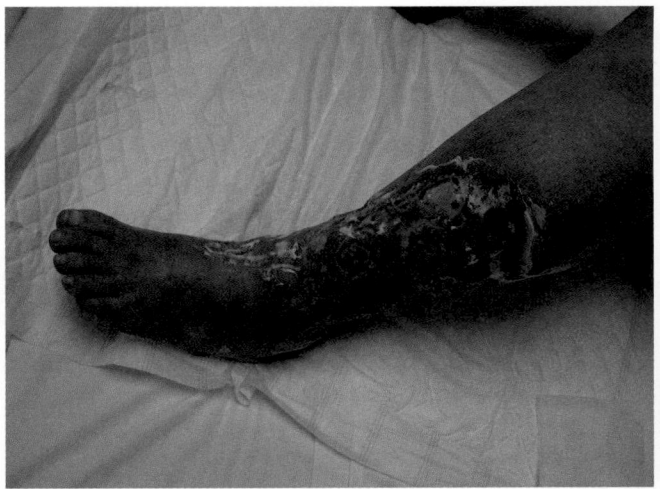
Fig. 120.3 Skin ulceration associated with vascular thrombosis.

posing major diagnostic difficulties, in those with heart valve disease, in differentiating from bacterial endocarditis.

Avascular necrosis of bone is an uncommon complication in lupus patients and clearly associated with high steroid dosage. We have noted an increased risk of avascular necrosis in individuals positive for APA, possibly as a result of small arterial occlusions, notably of the head of the femur.

Many patients with APS seem to develop widespread arteriopathy. The systemic narrowing of major arteries is similar in many respects to the widespread endarterial disease seen in some patients after heart–lung transplantation. Thus, APA might be associated with accelerated vascular disease, including atherosclerosis.[18]

Definition and classification criteria

An international consensus statement on classification criteria for definite APS was first published after a workshop in Sapporo, Japan, in 1998.[44] These criteria have recently been updated.[13] At least one clinical manifestation such as vascular thrombosis or pregnancy morbidity, together with positive laboratory tests, including lupus anti-coagulant, anti-cardiolipin and anti-β2-glycoprotein I antibodies, detected at least twice 12 weeks apart, are necessary to fulfil the classification criteria (Box 120.4). Other features of APS such as thrombocytopenia, haemolytic anaemia, transient cerebral ischaemia, transverse myelopathy or myelitis, livedo reticularis, cardiac valve disease, multiple sclerosis-like syndrome, chorea, and migraine were felt by the workshop to not have as strong an association and were excluded as classification criteria. This should not deter the clinicians from making the diagnosis or administering therapy if other causes of such features have been excluded.

Many of the patients reported to have the syndrome have lupus and can be regarded as having secondary APS. Some patients do not have any underlying systemic disease. These patients may be regarded as having primary APS. For research and classification purposes, the term 'primary' is useful, although there appear to be few differences in complications related to APA or in antibody specificity in the presence or absence of SLE.[29] Although some patients with primary APS progress to SLE, most do not show such progression.

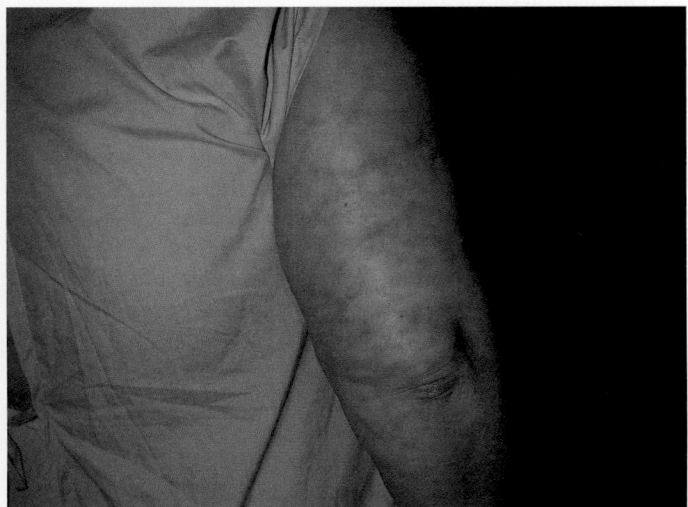
Fig. 120.2 Livedo reticularis.

Box 120.4 Criteria for the classification of definite anti-phospholipid syndrome

Clinical criteria

1. Vascular thrombosis

   One or more clinical episodes of arterial, venous, or small-vessel thrombosis, in any tissue or organ.
   Thrombosis must be confirmed by objective validated criteria (i.e. unequivocal findings of appropriate imaging studies or histopathology). For histopathological confirmation, thrombosis should be present without significant evidence of inflammation in the vessel wall.

2. Pregnancy morbidity

   (a) One or more unexplained deaths of a morphologically normal fetus at or beyond the 10th week of gestation, with normal fetal morphology documented by ultrasound or by direct examination of the fetus, *or*

   (b) One or more premature births of a morphologically normal neonate before the 34th week of gestation because of: (i) eclampsia or severe pre-eclampsia defined according to standard definitions or (ii) recognized features of placental failure, *or*

   (c) Three or more unexplained consecutive spontaneous abortions before the 10th week of gestation, with maternal anatomic or hormonal abnormalities and paternal and maternal chromosomal causes excluded.

   In studies of populations of patients who have more than one type of pregnancy morbidity, investigators are strongly encouraged to stratify groups of subjects according to (a), (b), or (c) above

Laboratory criteria

1. Lupus anti-coagulant present in plasma, on 2 or more occasions at least 12 weeks apart, detected according to the guidelines of the International Society on Thrombosis and Hemostasis (Scientific Subcommittee on LA/phospholipid-dependent antibodies).

2. Anti-cardiolipin antibody of IgG and/or IgM isotype in serum or plasma, present in medium or high titres (i.e. >40 GPL or MPL, or greater than the 99th percentile), on 2 or more occasions, at least 12 weeks apart, measured by a standardized ELISA.

3. Anti-β2 glycoprotein I antibody of IgG and/or IgM isotype in serum or plasma (in titres greater than the 99th percentile), present on 2 or more occasions, at least 12 weeks apart, measured by a standardized ELISA, according to recommended procedures.

Note: Definite anti-phospholipid syndrome may be diagnosed if at least one of the clinical criteria and at least one of the laboratory criteria are met. Modified from Miyakis et al.[13]

A minority of patients with the APS present with an acute and devastating syndrome characterized by multiple simultaneous vascular occlusions throughout the body, often resulting in death. This syndrome, termed 'catastrophic APS', is defined by the clinical involvement of at least three different organ systems over a period of days or weeks with histopathological evidence of multiple occlusions of large or small vessels.[45] Although the same clinical manifestations seen with primary and secondary APS occur as part of catastrophic APS, there are important differences in prevalence and in the calibre of the vessels predominantly affected.

Ischaemia of the kidneys, bowels, lungs, heart and/or brain are most frequent, but rarely adrenal, testicular, splenic, pancreatic, or skin involvement have been described. Occlusion of small vessels (thrombotic microangiopathy) is characteristic, resulting in symptoms related to dysfunction of the affected organs. Depending on the organs involved, patients may present with hypertension and renal impairment, acute respiratory distress syndrome (ARDS), alveolar haemorrhage and capillaritis, confusion and disorientation, or abdominal pain and distension secondary to bowel infarction. Precipitating factors of catastrophic APS include infections, surgical procedures, withdrawal of anti-coagulant therapy, and the use of drugs such as oral contraceptives.

Differential diagnosis

Careful family and personal history and physical examination of patients with unexplained thromboses are of the utmost importance as thrombotic events and, notably, venous thromboses often have explanations other than APS. The occurrence of other features of APS, such as livedo reticularis or obstetric complications, should alert the clinician. Vascular risk factors are frequent in patients with APS and thrombosis, thus its presence should not be a reason for not pursuing the diagnosis.

One of the most striking features of APS is the frequent observation of life-threatening thrombosis in the setting of thrombocytopenia. A number of other conditions can result in thrombocytopenia and thrombosis, including heparin-induced thrombocytopenia and thrombotic thrombocytopenic purpura.

Heparin-induced thrombocytopenia develops in 1–5% of patients receiving standard heparin and less frequently in those who receive low-molecular-weight preparations. This is due to the presence of an antibody which binds to platelet factor 4 and heparin. Approximately 10–20% of patients with substantial heparin-induced thrombocytopenia have venous or arterial thrombosis, including pulmonary, cardiac, and cerebral thrombosis. Thrombocytopenia typically develops approximately a week after exposure in persons not previously treated with heparin and sooner in those with previous exposure.

Thrombotic thrombocytopenic purpura is associated with neurological syndromes, but it is chiefly a microvascular disorder and confusion, seizures, or changes in the level of consciousness are more frequent than isolated, cerebral, large-vessel thrombosis. Microangiopathic haemolysis with evidence of schistocytes in peripheral blood is usually a prominent finding. Elevation in the serum level of lactate dehydrogenase is found in nearly all cases and is a sensitive marker of the severity of the disorder.

APS has been identified as a cause of first, second, and third trimester pregnancy losses as well as intrauterine growth restriction and pre-eclampsia. One of the major advances in the field of thrombophilia in the last few years has been the recognition that other thrombophilic states, such as factor V Leiden mutation and prothrombin 20210A mutation, also predispose to second and third trimester losses, as well as intrauterine growth restriction and pre-eclampsia.[46] It is important when considering the late pregnancy morbidity associated with APA to check that the history concurs with that of placental insufficiency. We have a number of women referred to our clinic with the diagnosis of APS on the basis of pregnancy loss where APA were an incidental finding. These women have proved to have pregnancy loss due to other causes such as premature labour secondary to an incompetent cervix.[26] Thus, history-taking and obtaining the post-mortem findings in previous pregnancy losses are very important.

Treatment

Given the diversity of clinical presentations and medical specialties involved, it is not surprising that treatment of APS has long been subject of intense debate. Fortunately, a consensus document has recently been agreed.[47] Some of these recommendations are supported by weak evidence and in others the consensus was not complete; however, these guidelines are a valuable tool for clinicians in order to decide therapy for individual patients with APS. A summary of recommendations is shown in Box 120.5.

Box 120.5 Recommendations for primary and secondary thromboprophylaxis in individuals with anti-phospholipid antibodies

General measures for anti-phospholipid antibody carriers

♦ A strict control of cardiovascular risk factors should be accomplished in all individuals with a high-risk antiphospholipid antibody profile,[a] irrespective of the presence of previous thrombosis, concomitant SLE or additional APS features

♦ All APA carriers should receive thromboprophylaxis with usual doses of LMWH in high-risk situations, such as surgery, prolonged immobilization, and puerperium

Primary thromboprophylaxis in SLE patients with anti-phospholipid antibodies

♦ In patients with SLE and positive lupus anti-coagulant or isolated persistent anti-cardiolipin antibodies at medium–high titres, primary thromboprophylaxis with hydroxychloroquine ± low-dose aspirin is recommended

Primary thromboprophylaxis in APA-positive individuals without SLE

♦ In non-SLE individuals with APA and no previous thrombosis, long-term primary thromboprophylaxis with low-dose aspirin is recommended in those with a high-risk APA profile, especially in the presence of other thrombotic risk factors

Secondary thromboprophylaxis

♦ Patients with either arterial or venous thrombosis and APA who do not fulfil criteria for APS should be managed in the same manner as APA-negative patients with similar thrombotic events

♦ Patients with definite APS and a first venous event should receive oral anti-coagulant therapy to a target INR 2.0–3.0

♦ Patients with definite APS and arterial thrombosis should be treated with warfarin at an INR >3.0 or combined anti-aggregant–anti-coagulant therapy (INR 2.0–3.0)

♦ The patient's bleeding risk should be estimated before prescribing high-intensity anti-coagulant or combined anti-aggregant–anti-coagulant therapy

♦ Non-SLE patients with a first non-cardioembolic cerebral arterial event, with a low-risk APA profile[b] and the presence of reversible trigger factors could individually be considered candidates for treatment with antiplatelet agents.

Duration of treatment

♦ Indefinite antithrombotic therapy is recommended in patients with definite APS and thrombosis

♦ In cases of first venous event, low-risk APA profile[b] and a known transient precipitating factor, anti-coagulation could be limited to 3–6 months.

Refractory and difficult cases

♦ In patients with difficult management due to recurrent thrombosis, fluctuating INR levels, major bleeding or at a high risk for major bleeding, alternative therapies could include long-term LMWH, hydroxychloroquine, or statins.

APA, anti-phospholipid antibody; APS, anti-phospholipid syndrome; INR, international normalized ratio; LMWH, low-molecular-weight heparin; SLE, systemic lupus erythematosus.
[a]High-risk APA profile: lupus anti-coagulant positivity, triple positivity (lupus anti-coagulant + anti-cardiolipin + anti-β2-glycoprotein I antibodies), isolated persistently positive anti-cardiolipin antibodies at medium–high titres.
[b]Low-risk APA profile: isolated, intermittently positive anti-cardiolipin or anti-β2-glycoprotein I at low–medium titres.
Modified from Ruiz-Irastorza et al.[47]

Primary thromboprophylaxis

Whether prophylactic treatment is indicated in patients with APA who have no history of thrombosis reminds an open question. No study has clearly demonstrated the benefit or harm of active therapy against placebo. General measures to control cardiovascular risk factors are recommended for all patients with APA. In fact, the most important prophylactic therapy may be the avoidance or reduction of smoking, obesity, high blood pressure, hypercholesterolaemia, and oestrogen-containing oral contraceptive pills or oestrogen replacement therapy.

SLE is considered by itself a risk factor for thrombosis. Thus, all patients with lupus and positive lupus anti-coagulant (alone or in combination with other APA) or with isolated persistent anti-cardiolipin antibodies at medium–high titres should be given primary thromboprophylaxis.[47] Hydroxychloroquine has shown protection against thrombosis in lupus patients, including those with APA.[48] Aspirin may also be effective in this setting.[49] However, no study has investigated whether combination therapy offers additional protection. Thus, given the general recommendation of hydroxychloroquine therapy in lupus patients, the addition of low-dose aspirin should be decided on an individual basis.

In asymptomatic carriers of APA without lupus, the decision regarding thromboprophylaxis should be best based on the APA profile. Aspirin thromboprophylaxis is suggested for those with a high-risk profile (lupus anti-coagulant, particularly triple-positive individuals), although the efficacy of this regime has not been demonstrated.[14,50] The presence of concomitant vascular risk factors should count in favour of starting low-dose aspirin. On the contrary, previous obstetric manifestations are not definitely associated with a higher thrombotic risk.[47]

The addition of low intensity oral anti-coagulation (international normalized ratio, INR~1.5) to low-dose aspirin has been tested in a recent randomized controlled trial (RCT).[51] This regime has not been more effective and, on the contrary, is poorly tolerated by the patients.

Prevention of recurrent thrombosis

There is good evidence that APS patients with thrombosis will be subject to recurrences, and these can be prevented by long-term antithrombotic therapy.[52,53] However, two important questions arise in this setting: (1) Should patients with APS receive the same therapy as the general population with similar manifestations? and (2) Should arterial and venous events be treated differently?

Two RCTs have compared high (target INR 3.0–4.0) with standard (target INR 2.0–3.0) intensity of anti-coagulation for the secondary thromboprophylaxis in patients with APS.[54,55] None of them found significant differences in efficacy or side effects between both regimes. However, given the overrepresentation of patients with first venous thromboembolism in both trials, the recommendation of warfarin therapy to a target INR 2.0–3.0 can only be extended to that subgroup.

Regarding arterial events, recommendations are more disputed. The APA and Stroke Study (APASS) supported the view that patients with stroke and APA not fulfilling classification criteria should be best treated as the general population.[56] On the other hand, patients with definite APS having arterial and/or recurrent events are at a higher risk for recurrences, even when treated with oral anti-coagulation to a target INR 2.0–3.0. As a whole, recurrences are very infrequent among patients effectively receiving oral anti-coagulation to an INR 3.0–4.0.[57] A small Japanese RCT has shown that combined therapy warfarin (target INR 2.0–3.0) plus low-dose aspirin is more effective and as safe as warfarin in monotherapy.[58] The current consensus recommends that patients with APS and arterial disease be treated with warfarin to a target INR of more than 3.0 or combined anti-coagulant–anti-aggregant therapy.[57]

Concerns exist over the validity of the INR in the control of oral anti-coagulant dosing if lupus anti-coagulant is present. The inhibitor occasionally increases the prothrombin time (PT) and, in turn, the INR, which may thus not reflect the true degree of anti-coagulation. This phenomenon seems to be more likely when certain recombinant thromboplastin reagents are used and can usually be circumvented by careful selection of the thromboplastin to be used for the PT test.[59]

High-intensity oral anti-coagulation therapy carries an inevitable risk of serious haemorrhage. In APS, serious bleeding complications may occur, but their risk is not higher than that observed in other thrombotic conditions warranting oral anti-coagulation.[60]

The role of steroids and immunosuppressive drugs in treatment of patients with APA and thrombosis is uncertain. Such drugs have severe side effects when given for prolonged periods and APA are not always suppressed by these agents. The use of these drugs is probably justified only in patients with repeated episodes of thrombosis despite adequate anti-coagulant therapy, that is, catastrophic APS. In this rare but life-threatening condition, combination therapy with heparin, steroids, and immunoglobulins, or plasmapheresis is recommended.[45]

The use of intra-arterial fibrinolysis has been described to be of benefit in patients with acute myocardial infarction associated with APA. Prostacyclin analogues (Iloprost) were also successfully used in patients with severe ischaemic necrotic toes associated with APS. Elective pulmonary thromboendarterectomy can be very effective and life-saving in selected patients with chronic thromboembolic pulmonary hypertension.

Prevention of pregnancy loss

The management of pregnancy in women known to have APS is also the subject of much debate and, as yet, there have been few RCTs. Antithrombotic therapy is the preferred treatment. Glucocorticoids and immunoglobulins have not demonstrated additional benefit compared with aspirin/heparin. Moreover, glucocorticoids may cause serious pregnancy complications, such as prematurity and hypertension.[36]

For therapeutic purposes during pregnancy, women with APS may be categorized into one of three groups: (1) those with recurrent early miscarriage (pre-embryonic or embryonic); (2) those with one or more prior fetal deaths (>10 weeks' gestation) or prior early delivery (<34 weeks' gestation) due to severe pre-eclampsia or placental insufficiency; and (3) those with previous thrombosis. Proposed recommendations for each of these groups are shown in Box 120.6.

Three RCTs[61–63] and one trial with consecutive treatment assignment[64] have compared low-dose aspirin alone vs combination therapy with heparin in women with APS, many of them with predominantly recurrent early miscarriage. In two studies the proportion of successful pregnancies significantly improved on adding unfractionated heparin to low-dose aspirin,[61,64] while the two other randomized trials, both using low-molecular-weight heparin (LMWH), found no differences.[62,63] It is noteworthy that the heterogeneity in the results is attributable to outcomes in women receiving aspirin only, who did strikingly worse in the two former studies. Remarkably, several observational studies have reported 79–100% pregnancy success rates with low-dose aspirin alone in this subgroup of women.[36] Despite the general recommendation of combined therapy with aspirin and heparin for all women with

---

Box 120.6 Recommended treatment of anti-phospholipid syndrome in pregnancy

APS with poor obstetric outcomes

Recurrent early (pre-embryonic or embryonic) miscarriage

- Low-dose aspirin *alone, or plus*:
- LMWH at thromboprophylactic doses

Fetal death (>10 weeks' gestation) or prior early delivery (<34 weeks' gestation) due to severe pre-eclampsia or placental insufficiency

- Low-dose aspirin, *plus*:
- LMWH at thromboprophylactic doses

APS with thrombosis

- Low-dose aspirin, *plus*:
- LMWH

APS, anti-phospholipid syndrome; LMWH, low-molecular-weight heparin.

obstetric APS, we believe that the option of monotherapy with aspirin cannot be discarded beforehand in the subgroup of women with recurrent early miscarriages. The selection of therapy should be decided on an individual basis, with pros and cons being discussed with the patient in the preconceptional counselling visit.

Women with APS and fetal losses have been studied much less extensively. However, fetal loss being a more severe and specific manifestation of the APS, combination therapy with aspirin and heparin is recommended by most authors.[36] When used for obstetric purposes, aspirin is best started before conception. No differences have been found between unfractionated heparin and LMWH combined with aspirin, thus any of them can be given, starting once pregnancy has been confirmed. Many centres are now using LMWH, since it has increased bioavailability and a longer half-life and can therefore conveniently be given once daily.

Patients with APS who have suffered a previous thrombosis need a different approach. In this group, low-dose aspirin and therapeutic dose heparin or LMWH at anti-coagulant doses are recommended.[36] The change from warfarin to heparin should be achieved prior to 6 weeks gestation to avoid warfarin embryopathy. Heparin does not cross the placenta and is not known to cause any adverse fetal effects. However, long-term use of heparin in pregnancy has been associated with osteoporosis in the mother. LMWH seems safer in this setting.[65] Heparin should be continued intrapartum and postpartum until women are rewarfarinized. Both warfarin and subcutaneous heparin are compatible with breastfeeding.

Antithrombotic coverage of the postpartum period is recommended also in women with APA and no previous thrombosis. The current recommendation is for prophylactic-dose heparin or LMWH, although the extension is variable from 1 to 6 weeks depending on the presence of additional risk factors.[66]

Most authorities agree that one of the main reasons for the improving outcome of APS pregnancies is closer obstetric surveillance. Viable anti-phospholipid pregnancies have a high incidence of obstetric and fetal complications, including intrauterine growth restriction, prematurity, and pre-eclampsia; hence, close monitoring and timely delivery may improve fetal outcome in these women. Preconception counselling is essential in order to estimate the chance of both fetal and maternal problems and to provide the patient with reliable information regarding her specific risk for complications and the expected management plan. Despite the good prognosis achieved with correct management, patients must also know that there is an increased risk of serious complications (miscarriage, thrombosis, fetal death, prematurity, pre-eclampsia). A complete set of APA and autoantibodies should be available before planning pregnancy. Women who have recently had thrombotic events, particularly stroke, should be advised to delay pregnancy.

All women with APS should be managed in a combined high-risk medical–obstetric clinic throughout the whole pregnancy. The general schedule includes more frequent visits as pregnancy progresses. Regular monitoring of blood pressure and urine analysis and timely Doppler studies of the uteroplacental circulation are essential part of the optimal care of these women.

Management of other manifestations of anti-phospholipid syndrome

Mild thrombocytopenia with platelet counts between 100 000 and 150 000/mm^3 are common in patients with APA and usually does not require intervention. In a minority of cases it can be severe. In these cases, corticosteroid therapy should be the treatment of choice. Several drugs have been used successfully to treat steroid-resistant thrombocytopenia in APS patients, including aspirin, intravenous gammaglobulin infusion, danazol, chloroquine, and dapsone. Splenectomy has been safely and successfully performed in some patients.[67]

Transverse myelitis and multiple sclerosis-like illnesses have been described in APS. Anecdotally, most clinicians dealing with APS or lupus with APS have seen patients initially labelled as 'probable multiple sclerosis'. Certainly the ischaemic changes produced by the APS in white matter may be indistinguishable on MRI from those of multiple sclerosis. Therefore, in some of these patients with multiple sclerosis-like illness, the importance of a treatable differential diagnosis—APS—cannot be underestimated.

There is a high prevalence of heart valve lesions in patients with APA. In some cases, valvular damage may result in significant haemodynamic compromise requiring surgery. Both biological and mechanical valves have been implanted with favourable results, although both bleeding and thrombotic complications have been reported in about one-half of the patients.[68]

It is important to distinguish the thrombotic microangiopathy found in some patients with APS from inflammatory forms of renal involvement. The physician will face this problem mainly in patients with SLE, and management with oral anti-coagulation or steroids will depend on the histological findings. The outcome of kidney transplantation in patients with SLEs and endstage renal failure appears to be similar to that of patients with renal failure from other causes. However, the presence of APA seems to be associated with a poorer prognosis. Post-transplant thromboembolic phenomena, recurrence of thrombotic microangiopathy in the graft despite anti-coagulation, and thrombosis of the graft's renal vein have all been reported.[69]

Prognosis

The long-term prognosis in patients with APS is primarily influenced by the risk of recurrent thrombosis. Although there are a number of studies of prognostic factors in SLE, only a few have addressed the possible role of APA. Lupus patients with APS are reported to accrue more damage and have higher mortality rates. Two studies have found that the prognosis of patients with primary APS is poor.[70,71] One-third of patients had organ damage and one-fifth were unable to perform everyday activities. A recent cohort study of 135 patients with APS, with concurrent systemic lupus in one-third of them, has shown that 29% of patients accrued damage and 5 died after a mean follow-up of 7.5 years. Arterial thrombosis and the presence of lupus were associated with an adverse prognosis.[72]

Anti-phospholipid syndrome in childhood

There have been relatively few reports of clinical associations of APA in children and the spectrum of clinical findings remains at present unknown. APA in childhood-onset SLE (see Chapter 119) have been described in several small clinical reports, occurring in one-third of the patients. The clinical manifestations are similar to those encountered in adults, particularly recurrent deep-vein thrombosis, strokes, and chorea. Devastating thrombotic complications of the APS in children have been reported, including digital ischaemia and myocardial infarction. The risk of maternal transmission of APA to infants during pregnancy is unknown, though there have been several case reports of thrombotic events in neonates of mothers with the APS.[73]

There is general agreement that long-term anti-coagulation is needed in children who experienced an anti-phospholipid-related thrombosis to prevent recurrences, but there is no consensus about the duration and intensity of this therapy. Given that the risk of recurrence might be lower in anti-phospholipid-positive children compared with adults, and considering the higher risk of haemorrhage during play and sports, it was suggested that intermediate-intensity anti-coagulation therapy targeted at an INR of 2.0–2.5 be performed in paediatric patients who have experienced an anti-phospholipid-related thrombosis.[74]

References

1. Harris EN, Gharavi AE, Boey ML et al. Anticardiolipin antibodies: detection by radioimmunoassay and association with thrombosis in systemic lupus erythematosus. *Lancet* 1983;2:1211–1214.

2. Hughes GRV. Thrombosis, abortion, cerebral disease and lupus anticoagulant. *BMJ* 1983;287:1088–1089.

3. Ruiz-Irastorza G, Crowther MA, Branch W, Khamashta MA. Antiphospholipid syndrome. *Lancet* 2010;376:1498–1509.

4. Ginsburg KS, Liang MH, Newcomer L et al. Anticardiolipin antibodies and the risk for ischemic stroke and venous thrombosis. *Ann Intern Med* 1992;117:997–1002.

5. Vaarala O, Mänttäri M, Manninen V. et al. Anti-cardiolipin antibodies and risk of myocardial infarction in a prospective cohort of middle-aged men. *Circulation* 1995;91:23–27.

6. Brey RL, Abbott RD, Curb JD et al. β2-glycoprotein I-dependent anticardiolipin antibodies and the risk of ischemic stroke and myocardial infarction: the Honolulu Heart Program. *Stroke* 2001;32:1701–1706.

7. Cervera R, Khamashta MA, Font J et al. Morbidity and mortality in systemic lupus erythematosus during a 5 year period: a multi-centre prospective study of 1000 patients. *Medicine* (Baltimore) 1999;78:167–175.

8. Petri M. Epidemiology of the antiphospholipid antibody syndrome. *J Autoimmun* 2000;15:145–151.

9. Goel N, Ortel TL, Bali D et al. Familial antiphospholipid antibody syndrome. *Arthritis Rheum* 1999;42:318–327.

10. Giannakopoulos B, Passam F, Ioannou Y, Krilis SA. How we diagnose the antiphospholipid syndrome. *Blood* 2009;113:985–994.

11. Tincani A, Balestrieri G, Allegri F et al. Overview on anticardiolipin ELISA standardization. *J Autoimmun* 2000;15:195–197.

12. Matsuura E, Igarashi Y, Yasuda T, Triplett DA, Koike T. Anticardiolipin antibodies recognize β2-glycoprotein I structure altered by interacting with an oxygen modified solid phase surface. *J Exp Med* 1994;179:457–462.

13. Miyakis S, Lockshin MD, Atsumi T et al. International consensus statement on an update of the classification criteria for definite antiphospholipid syndrome (APS). *J Thromb Haemost* 2006;4:295–306.

14. Pengo V, Ruffatti A, Legnani C et al. Incidence of a first thromboembolic event in asymptomatic carriers of high-risk antiphospholipid antibody profile: a multicenter prospective study. *Blood* 2011;118:4714–4718.

15. Cabral AR, Amigo MC, Cabiedes J, Alarcon-Segovia D. The antiphospholipid/cofactor syndromes: a primary variant with antibodies to β2-glycoprotein I but no antibodies detectable in standard antiphospholipid assays. *Am J Med* 1996;101:472–481.

16. Pierangeli SS, Gharavi AE, Harris EN. Experimental thrombosis and antiphospholipid antibodies: new insights. *J Autoimmun* 2000;15:241–247.

17. Sherer Y, Shoenfeld Y. Antiphospholipid syndrome: insight from animal models. *Curr Opin Hematol* 2000;7:321–324.

18. George J, Haratz D, Shoenfeld Y. Accelerated atheroma, antiphospholipid antibodies, and the antiphospholipid syndrome. *Rheum Dis Clin North Am* 2001;27:603–610.

19. Meroni PL, Riboldi P. Pathogenic mechanisms mediating antiphospholipid syndrome. *Curr Opin Rheumatol* 2001;13:377–382.

20. Rand JH. Molecular pathogenesis of the antiphospholipid syndrome. *Circ Res* 2002;90:29–37.

21. Pierangeli SS, Chen PP, Raschi E et al. Antiphospholipid antibodies and the antiphospholipid syndrome: pathogenic mechanisms. *Semin Thromb Hemost* 2008;34:236–250.

22. López-Pedrera C, Cuadrado MJ, Herández V et al. Proteomic analysis in monocytes of antiphospholipid syndrome patients: Deregulation of proteins related to the development of thrombosis. *Arthritis Rheum* 2008;58:2835–2844.

23. Pierangeli SS, Girardi G, Vega-Ostertag M et al. Requirement of activation of complement C3 and C5 for antiphospholipid antibody-mediated thrombophilia. *Arthritis Rheum* 2005;52:2120–2124.

24. Rand JH, Wu X-X, Quinn AS, Taatjes DJ. The annexin A5-mediated pathogenic mechanism in the antiphospholipid syndrome: role in pregnancy losses and thrombosis. *Lupus.* 2010;19:460–469.

25. Di Simone N, Raschi E, Testoni C et al. Pathogenic role of anti-beta 2-glycoprotein I antibodies in antiphospholipid associated fetal loss: characterisation of beta 2-glycoprotein I binding to trophoblast cells and functional effects of anti-beta 2-glycoprotein I antibodies in vitro. *Ann Rheum Dis* 2005;64:462–467.

26. Stone S, Khamashta MA, Poston L. Placentation, antiphospholipid syndrome and pregnancy outcome. *Lupus* 2001;10:67–74.

27. Girardi G, Redecha P, Salmon JE. Heparin prevents antiphospholipid antibody-induced fetal loss by inhibiting complement activation. *Nature Med* 2004;10:1222–1226.

28. Lie JT. Vasculitis in the antiphospholipid syndrome: culprit or consort? *J Rheumatol* 1994;21:397–399.

29. Cervera R, Piette JC, Font J et al. Antiphospholipid syndrome: clinical and immunologic manifestations and patterns of disease expression in a cohort of 1,000 patients. *Arthritis Rheum* 2002;46:1019–1027.

30. Espinosa G, Font J, Garcia-Pagan JC et al. Budd–Chiari syndrome secondary to antiphospholipid syndrome. Clinical and immunologic characteristics of 43 patients. *Medicine* (Baltimore) 2001;80:345–354.

31. Tektonidou MG, Varsou N, Kotoulas G, Antoniou A, Moutsopoulos HM. Cognitive deficits in patients with antiphospholipid syndrome: association with clinical, laboratory, and brain magnetic resonance imaging findings. *Arch Intern Med* 2006;166:2278–2284.

32. Amigo MC, Garcia-Torres R, Robles M, Bochicchio T, Reyes PA. Renal involvement in primary antiphospholipid syndrome. *J Rheumatol* 1992;19:1181–1185.

33. Tektonidou MG, Sotsiou F, Nakopoulou L, Vlachoyiannopoulos PG, Moutsopoulos HM. Antiphospholipid syndrome nephropathy in patients with systemic lupus erythematosus and antiphospholipid antibodies: prevalence, clinical associations, and long-term outcome. *Arthritis Rheum* 2004;50:2569–2579.

34. Paul SN, Sangle SR, Bennett AN et al. Vasculitis, antiphospholipid antibodies, and renal artery stenosis. *Ann Rheum Dis* 2005;64:1800–1802.

35. Opatrny L, David M, Kahn SR, Shrier I, Rey E. Association between antiphospholipid antibodies and recurrent fetal loss in women without autoimmune disease: a metaanalysis. *J Rheumatol* 2006;33:2214–2221.

36. Danza A, Ruiz-Irastorza G, Khamashta M. Antihospohlipid syndrome in obstetrics. *Best Pract Res Clin Obstet Gynaecol* 2012;26:65–76.

37. Ruffatti A, Calligaro A, Hoxha A et al. Laboratory and clinical features of pregnant women with antiphospholipid syndrome and neonatal outcome. *Arthritis Care Res* 2010;62:302–307.

38. Cuadrado MJ, Hughes GRV. Hughes (antiphospholipid) syndrome: clinical features. *Rheum Dis Clin North Am* 2001;27:507–524.

39. Alarcón-Segovia D, Delezé M, Oria CV et al. Antiphospholipid antibodies and the antiphospholipid syndrome in systemic lupus erythematosus: a

prospective analysis of 500 consecutive patients. *Medicine* (Baltimore) 1989;68:353–365.

40. Katsiari CG, Giavri I, Mitsikostas DD, Yiannopoulou KG, Sfikakis PP. Acute transverse myelitis and antiphospholipid antibodies in lupus. No evidence for anticoagulation. *Eur J Neurol* 2011;18:556–563.

41. Cuadrado MJ, Khamashta MA, Ballesteros A et al. Can neurologic manifestations of Hughes (antiphospholipid) syndrome be distinguished from multiple sclerosis? *Medicine* (Baltimore) 2000;79:57–68.

42. Zuily S, Regnault V, Selton-Suty C et al. Increased risk for heart valve disease associated with antiphospholipid antibodies in patients with systemic lupus erythematosus: Meta-Analysis of echocardiographic studies. *Circulation* 2011;124:215–224.

43. Roldan CA, Gelgand EA, Qualls CR, Sibbitt WL. Valvular heart disease as a cause of cerebrovascular disease in patients with systemic lupus erythematosus. *Am J Cardiol* 2005;95:1441–1447.

44. Wilson WA, Gharavi AE, Koike T et al. International consensus statement on preliminary classification criteria for definite antiphospholipid syndrome: report of an international workshop. *Arthritis Rheum* 1999;42:1309–1311.

45. Cervera R, Tektonidou M, Espinosa G et al. Task Force on Catastrophic Antiphospholipid Syndrome (APS) and non-criteria APS manifestations (II): thrombocytopenia and skin manifestations. *Lupus* 2011;20:174–181.

46. Kupferminc MJ, Eldor A, Steinman N et al. Increased frequency of genetic thrombophilia in women with complications of pregnancy. *N Engl J Med* 1999;340:9–13.

47. Ruiz-Irastorza G, Cuadrado M, Ruiz-Arruza I et al. Evidence-based recommendations for the prevention and long-term management of thrombosis in antiphospholipid antibody-positive patients: Report of a Task Force at the 13th International Congress on Antiphospholipid Antibodies. *Lupus* 2011;20:206–218.

48. Tektonidou MG, Laskari K, Panagiotakos DB, Moutsopoulos HM. Risk factors for thrombosis and primary thrombosis prevention in patients with systemic lupus erythematosus with or without antiphospholipid antibodies. *Arthritis Rheum* 2009;61:29–36.

49. Wahl DG, Bounameaux H, de Moerloose P, Sarasin FP. Prophylactic antithrombotic therapy for patients with systemic lupus erythematosus with or without antiphospholipid antibodies: do the benefits outweigh the risks? A decision analysis. *Arch Intern Med* 2000;160:2042–2048.

50. Erkan D, Harrison MJ, Levy R et al. Aspirin for primary thrombosis prevention in the antiphospholipid syndrome: a randomized, double-blind, placebo-controlled trial in asymptomatic antiphospholipid antibody-positive individuals. *Arthritis Rheum* 2007;56:2382–2391.

51. Cuadrado MJ, Bertolaccini ML, Seed PT et al. Low dose aspirin versus low dose aspirin plus low-intensity warfarin in the primary prevention of thrombosis: a prospective, multi-center, randomized, open, controlled trial, in patients positive for antiphospholipid antibodies (ALIWAPAS). *Rheumatology* (in press)

52. Khamashta MA, Cuadrado M-J, Mujic F et al. The management of thrombosis in the antiphospholipid-antibody syndrome. *N Engl J Med* 1995;332:993–997.

53. Brunner HI, Chan WS, Ginsberg JS, Feldman BM. Long-term anticoagulation is preferable for patients with antiphospholipid antibody syndrome. Result of a decision analysis. *J Rheumatol* 2002;29:490–501.

54. Crowther MA, Ginsberg JS, Julian J et al. A comparison of two intensities of warfarin for the prevention of recurrent thrombosis in patients with the antiphospholipid syndrome. *N Engl J Med* 2003, 349:1133–1138.

55. Finazzi G, Marchioli R, Brancaccio V et al. A randomized clinical trial of high-intensity warfarin vs. conventional antithrombotic therapy for the prevention of recurrent thrombosis in patients with the antiphospholipid syndrome (WAPS). *J Thromb Haemost* 2005;3:848–853.

56. Levine SR, Brey RL, Tilley BC et al; APASS Investigators. Antiphospholipid antibodies and subsequent thrombo-occlusive events in patients with ischemic stroke. *JAMA* 2004;291:576–584.

57. Ruiz-Irastorza G, Hunt BJ, Khamashta MA. A systematic review of secondary thromboprophylaxis in patients with antiphospholipid antibodies. *Arthritis Rheum* 2007;57:1487–1495.

58. Okuma H, Kitagawa Y, Yasuda T, Tokuoka K, Takagi S. Comparison between single antiplatelet therapy and combination of antiplatelet and anticoagulation therapy for secondary prevention in ischemic stroke patients with antiphospholipid syndrome. *Int J Med Sci* 2009;7:15–18.

59. Lawrie AS, Purdy G, Mackie IJ, Machin SJ. Monitoring of oral anticoagulant therapy in lupus anticoagulant positive patients with the antiphospholipid syndrome. *Br J Haematol* 1997;98:887–892.

60. Ruiz-Irastorza G, Khamashta MA, Hunt BJ et al. Bleeding and recurrent thrombosis in definite antiphospholipid syndrome: analysis of a series of 66 patients treated with oral anticoagulation to a target international normalized ratio of 3.5. *Arch Intern Med* 2002;162:1164–1169.

61. Rai R, Cohen H, Dave M, Regan L. Randomised controlled trial of aspirin and aspirin plus heparin in pregnant women with recurrent miscarriage associated with phospholipid antibodies (or antiphospholipid antibodies). *BMJ* 1997;314:253–257.

62. Farquharson RG, Quenby S, Greaves M. Antiphospholipid syndrome in pregnancy: a randomized, controlled trial of treatment. *Obstet Gynecol* 2002;100:408–413.

63. Laskin CA, Spitzer K, Clark C et al. Low molecular weight heparin and aspirin for recurrent pregnancy loss: results from the randomized, controlled HepASA trial. *J Rheumatol* 2009;36:279–287.

64. Kutteh WH. Antiphospholipid antibody-associated recurrent pregnancy loss: treatment with heparin and low-dose aspirin is superior to low-dose aspirin alone. *Am J Obstet Gynecol* 1996;174:1584–1589.

65. Sanson BJ, Lensing AW, Prins MH. et al. Safety of low-molecular weight heparin in pregnancy: a systematic review. *Thromb Haemost* 1999;81:668–672.

66. Royal College of Obstetricians and Gynaecologists. *Reducing the risk of thrombosis and embolism during pregnancy and the puerperium.* Green Top Guideline 37, 2009.

67. Galindo, M, Khamashta MA, Hughes GRV. Splenectomy for refractory thrombocytopenia in the antiphospholipid syndrome. *Rheumatology* 1999;38:848–853.

68. Erdozain JG, Ruiz-Irastorza G, Segura MI et al. Cardiac valve replacement in patients with antiphospholipid syndrome. *Arthritis Care Res* (Hoboken) 2012;641256–1260.

69. McIntyre JA, Wagenknecht DR. Antiphospholipid antibodies. Risk assessment for solid organ, bone marrow, and tissue transplantation. *Rheum Dis Clin North Am* 2001;27:611–631.

70. Ruiz-Irastorza G, Egurbide M-V, Ugalde J, Aguirre C. High impact of antiphospholipid syndrome on irreversible organ damage and survival of patients with systemic lupus erythematosus. *Arch Intern Med* 2004;164:77–82.

71. Erkan D, Yazici Y, Sobel R, Lockshin MD. Primary antiphospholipid syndrome: functional outcome after 10 years. *J Rheumatol* 2000;27:2817–2821.

72. Grika EP, Ziakas PD, Zintzaras E, Moutsopoulos HM, Vlachoyiannopoulos PG. Morbidity, mortality and organ damage in patients with antiphospholipid syndrome. *J Rheumatol* 2012;39:516–523.

73. Avcin T, Cimaz R, Meroni PL. Recent advances in antiphospholipid antibodies and antiphospholipid syndromes in pediatric populations. *Lupus* 2002;11:4–10.

74. Tucker LG. Antiphospholipid antibodies and antiphospholipid syndrome in children. In: Khamashta MA (ed.) *Hughes syndrome—antiphospholipid syndrome.* Springer, London, 2000:155–166.

Scleroderma

CHAPTER 121

Systemic sclerosis

Christopher P. Denton and Pia Moinzadeh

Introduction

'Scleroderma', a word meaning hard skin, is a part of many syndromes including localized and systemic scleroderma. Most of these disorders can occur at any stage of life, although the pattern of scleroderma occurring in childhood is different from that in the adult (see below). Scleroderma or systemic sclerosis has been confused with other diseases that have cutaneous features resembling it, for example scleromyxoedema, scleroedema, and primary amyloidosis (see Box 121.1). In this chapter we focus on systemic sclerosis (SSc) and localized scleroderma.

Systemic sclerosis

Systemic sclerosis (SSc) is a heterogeneous and rare, multisystem connective tissue disease, based on autoimmunological processes, vascular endothelial cell damage and an extensive activation of fibroblasts, causing a massive production and accumulation of extracellular matrix proteins and collagen. It is characterized by a large individual variability in the extent of skin and organ involvement, as well as in disease progression and prognosis.

Epidemiology

Systemic sclerosis (SSc; scleroderma) is an uncommon disorder and virtually all of the descriptive epidemiology is derived from retrospective or prospective reviews of patients attending hospitals or institutions serving a defined denominator population. Variations in incidence and prevalence rates of SSc patients seem to appear due to differences in disease definition/characterization, geographic differences, and methods of individual case ascertainment. Also the fact that patients are nowadays identified earlier due to better interdisciplinary medical care, increased awareness by physicians, and also due to improved survival rates because of growing treatment options, has changed incidence and prevalence rates in SSc patients. A summary of salient epidemiological data is given in Table 121.1.

Published data about incidence rates reported variations from 0.1 to 4.3 patients per 100 000 inhabitants, which is also true for the prevalence rates, which have risen from 1.5 to 34 patients per

---

Box 121.1 Spectrum of scleroderma and scleroderma-like syndromes

- Systemic sclerosis
- Localized scleroderma (morphoea)
- Eosinophilic fasciitis
- Sclerodermatous genodermatoses (e.g. progeria, acrogeria, Werner's disease)
- Acrodermatitis chronic atrophicans
- Eosinophilia-myalgia syndrome
- Scleredoema adultorum Buschke
- Scleredoema diabeticorum
- Scleromyxeodema
- Sclerodoema amyloidosis
- Nephrogenic systemic fibrosis
- Porphyria cutanea tarda
- Sclerodermatous chronic graft-vs-host disease
- Scleroderma-like lesions in malignancies (paraneoplastic scleroderma)
- Lichen sclerosus et atrophicans

Table 121.1 Variations in prevalence and incidence rates depending on study and country

Study	Incidence (patients per 100 000 per year)	Prevalence (patients per 100 000)
North-west Greece 1981–2002[4]	0.11	1.54
Pennsylvania 1978–1982[10]	0.18	No data
Tokyo 1988[2]	No data	2.1–5.3
South Australia 1993–2002[7]	0.15	2.14
Britain 1985–1986[8–9]	0.37	3.08
North-east England 2000[81]	No data	8.80
Detroit, USA 1989–1991[1]	1.9	27.6
North-west Spain 1988–2006[5]	2.3	27.7
North Italy 1999–2007[6]	4.3	34.0

100 000 inhabitants per year.[1-10] SSc seem to occur more frequently in the United States than in Europe (north–south gradient with lower rates in northern Europe), the United Kingdom, and Japan.[11] Currently the best estimate for United Kingdom prevalence overall is approximately 120 per million of the population. The formation of these geographical clusters may be due to genetic and/or environmental exposures, necessary for disease susceptibility, which occurs infrequently in the population. For example, clustering has been described close to two major international airports in the United Kingdom,[12] for a variety of autoimmune rheumatic diseases in the Republic of Georgia,[13] and there is a clearer cluster of systemic sclerosis in a region of Italy close to Rome.[14] In North America the highest prevalence has been observed among a population of Choctaw native Americans in Oklahoma.[15] The prevalence in these full-blooded Choctaws was 469 cases/100 000 (based on 14 cases) with a majority suffering from diffuse SSc and anti-topoisomerase antibodies.[15] There is growing evidence for a genetic basis for this high prevalence and ongoing studies are defining this in detail.[16] Scleroderma has a female excess (4F:1M overall, and in the childbearing years 15F:1M). Interestingly the peak of the female:male ratio in the major autoimmune connective tissue diseases, including SSc, is between the late teens and forties and some reports hypothesized that this is the time with the greatest changes in hormone levels.[17] Finally, again in contrast to other autoimmune rheumatic diseases, a growing number of environmental agents have been implicated in SSc.

Aetiopathogenesis

SSc is almost certainly multifactorial, involving genetic and environmental factors, and it is clear that a combination of genetic or environmental factors is responsible for the susceptibility to develop the disease.[18] SSc occurs mostly in females and gender may be one of the strongest genetic markers. There are several lines of evidence indicating familial or genetic predisposition to SSc. Besides gender, racial variations are also reported with a higher and also a more severe form of this disease in the black population. Furthermore, 50% of black women with scleroderma have the diffuse form, compared to only 25% of white women with SSc.[19]

Genetic factors

Studies of families with a member suffering from SSc have shown that another SSc case occur more frequently in these SSc-positive families (1.6%) in comparison to the general population (0.026%)[20] with a 13–14-fold increased relative risk for a first-degree relative.[20-21] Some authors have hypothesized that the clustering of SSc within families may also be associated with shared environmental factors, shared genes, or interactions between them (Table 121.2).[22]

Many centres worldwide have observed abnormal frequencies of the major histocompatibility complex (MHC) antigens associated with SSc. As one of the primary roles of MHC class II molecules is the presentation of processed antigen to the T-cell receptor (TCTR) on helper T lymphocytes resulting in an antigen-specific immune response, autoantibody subsets in scleroderma might be expected to show correlations with class II MHC polymorphism and indeed they do, although again they appear to be complex. Haplotypes of *DRB1*11-DQB1*0301* seem to be associated with

anti-topoisomerase antibodies in white Europeans.[23-24] Anti-centromere antibody was reported to be associated with *HLA DRB1*01, DQB1*0501*, and *DQB1 26 epi*,[22,25] while anti-RNA polymerase antibodies has been reported to be associated with *DRB1*0404, DRB1*11*, and *DQB1*03*.[23] Several studies suggest an association of *HLA DRB1*1302, DQB1*0604/0605* haplotypes with anti-fibrillarin positive patients,[26] while *HLA SRB1*0301* occurs in patients with anti-Pm-Scl antibodies.[27]

Studies coping with the whole-genome microarray expression studies of skin biopsies and circulating blood cells support the involvement of multiple and complex pathways in the development of SSc.[21]

These studies identified several genes involved in immune function, such as *IRF5* (interferon regulatory factor 5),[28] *CTGF*,[29] *BANK1*,[30] and *STAT4* (signal transducer and activator of transcription 4), *CD247*, *PTPN22* (protein tyrosine phosphatase non-receptor type 22), which are all associated with an increased susceptibility to SSc (see Table 121.3).[31-33] Candidate gene studies have confirmed these findings by identifying single nucleotide polymorphisms (SNPs), again associated with susceptibility to SSc.

Increasingly, gene expression profiling in SSc plays a major role in detecting and confirming genetic alterations, analysing skin biopsies as well as peripheral blood of SSc patients in comparison to healthy controls. After clustering the gene expression signatures depending on their expression pattern, Milano et al. found distinct subgroups of signatures which arranged patients into four different groups with a more inflammatory pattern, with a fibroproliferative signature for limited and diffuse forms, and a group of healthy controls and some SSc patients classified with a normal-like signature.[34]

Environmental factors

SSc and scleroderma-like syndromes have been reported in association with numerous different environmental toxins and drugs, including solvents (vinyl chloride, benzene, toluene, epoxy resins), drugs (bleomycin, cardiopa, pentazocine, cocaine, docetaxel, metaphenylenediamine), and other miscellaneous substances.[35] Furthermore, scleroderma was reported to occur especially in men who worked underground as coal and gold miners. In male patients with silicosis who are older than 40 years of age, the likelihood of developing SSc is approximately 190 times greater than in males who were never exposed to silica, and 50 times higher than in males without silicosis but exposed to silica dust.[36] Whether silicone gel implants and other silicone products may play a role in the development of scleroderma has also been discussed, but a recent meta-analysis showed no evidence that they trigger SSc.[37] However, most epidemiological studies have failed to show a significant association. There is still a lack of large epidemiological studies that might reveal a significant role for toxins and drugs in the development of scleroderma.

Immune events

An increasing number of immune abnormalities are being reported in SSc and the designation of SSc as an autoimmune disease now has widespread support. Some of the clinical features of scleroderma bear similarities to other autoimmune disorders such as systemic lupus erythematosus (SLE), dermatomyositis, and rheumatoid arthritis (RA), and there are also patients who have overlap syndromes or who have sequential development of more

Table 121.2 Autoantibodies and clinical associations

Autoantibodies	Characteristics
Anti-centromere antibodies	◆ ACA antibodies together with Raynaud phenomenon has been reported to be predictive for the development of SSc ◆ Associated with the limited form of SSc, vasculopathy, and calcinosis cutis ◆ In later stages patients have a higher risk of developing an isolated pulmonary arterial hypertension ◆ In 20–30% overall, very specific for scleroderma, frequency varies depending on ethnic background ◆ In IIF pattern on HEp-2 cells show punctuate spots (speckled pattern) in the nucleolus ◆ Solid-phase ELISA used for routine diagnostics in the clinic
Anti-topoisomerase antibodies	◆ Associated with the diffuse form of SSc, as well as a higher risk for lung fibrosis, renal crisis, severe heart involvement and digital ulcers ◆ In approximately 40% in overall, frequency varies depending on ethnic background (28–70%) ◆ <10% of patients with lSSc carry this kind of autoantibody ◆ In IIF it shows a homogenous and nucleolar pattern ◆ Solid-phase ELISA used for routine diagnostics in the clinic
Anti-RNA polymerase antibodies	◆ Highly specific for SSc ◆ Anti-RNAP I and III coexist, while anti-RNAP II is very rare ◆ Associated with the diffuse form of SSc, as well as a higher risk for renal crisis ◆ Survival rates are better than in those patients with anti-topoisomerase antibodies ◆ Fine speckled and nucleolar pattern in IIF ◆ Solid-phase ELISA used for routine diagnostics in the clinic
Anti-PmScl antibodies	◆ In approximately 4–11% overall, frequency varies depending on ethnic background ◆ In approximately 25% of SSc patients with myositis overlap, but just in 2% with SSc alone ◆ Associated with the limited form of SSc, usually with no severe internal organ manifestations ◆ In IIF) it shows a homogenous and nucleolar pattern
Anti-fibrillarin antibodies	◆ In approximately 4–10% patients with SSc ◆ More frequently found in African-American patients ◆ These patients usually have a diffuse form of SSc with peripheral vasculopathy, pulmonary hypertension, and myositis ◆ Nucleolar pattern (clumpy) in IIF

ELISA, enzyme-linked immunosorbent assay; IIF indirect immunofluorescence; SSc, system sclerosis.
Reviewed by Hamaguchi.[82]

than one autoimmune rheumatic disease. There is considerable evidence that abnormalities in both humoral and cell-mediated immunity occur in SSc, although the precise importance of these immunological events in the pathogenesis remains uncertain. The lack of a generalized immune dysfunction in SSc suggests that the derangement of immune-cell dysfunction may be specific to certain antigens or cells.[38–39] The association of SSc with particular major HLA antigens and the close association of certain HLA alleles with scleroderma-specific antibodies is indirect evidence for T-cell involvement in SSc. There is considerable evidence for T-cell activation in SSc, including an increased ratio of circulating CD4+:CD8+ cells,[40–41] reflecting an increased number of CD4+ and/or a reduced number of CD8+ lymphocytes. Consequently increased serum levels of T-cell derived cytokines, i.e. interleukins IL-2, IL-4, IL-10, IL-13, and IL-17, have been observed in scleroderma patients.[42–43] It is known that T cells provide major stimuli for collagen synthesis in fibroblasts but depending on the type of

T cells they have distinct roles in their influence on collagen production. The Th1 cells produce cytokines which are associated with the cellular immune response, including interferon-gamma (IFNγ), tumour necrosis factor alpha (TNFα), IL-1, IL-2, and IL-12, while the Th2 lymphocytes synthesize cytokines which are involved in the inflammatory processes of SSc, such as IL-4, IL-13, IL-5, IL-6, and IL-10. Another group of lymphocytes, namely the Th17 cells, produce cytokines (IL-17, IL-21, IL-22) which are involved in the inflammation but also regulation of processes[44–45] that are more frequently found in early stages of SSc, enhancing the production and deposition of extracellular matrix (ECM); see Table 121.4. Especially in SSc patients a predominance of Th2-polarized T cells have been found. Besides T cells, B cells are also found in involved skin. Several studies suggest that B cells are able to induce ECM production through secretion of IL-6 and tissue growth factor beta (TGFβ) and are involved in the production of autoantibodies (Figure 121.1, Table 121.4).

Table 121.3 Major non-HLA-associated systemic sclerosis susceptibility genes

Genes	Chromosome variant	Function
Innate immunity		
IRF5 (*Interferon regulatory factor 5*)	**7q32** rs2004640 rs2280714	◆ Central mediator of innate immunity ◆ Already found in several autoimmune diseases, such as SLE, Sjögren's syndrome, pernicious anaemia, RA as well as SSc ◆ Transcription factor with important role in the TLR signalling pathway ◆ Important in the activation of type I IFN genes ◆ Identified as potential risk factor for SSc; preferentially found in SSc patients suffering from the diffuse form with ATA positivity
T-cell differentiation and activation		
PTPN 22 (*Protein tyrosine phosphatase non-receptor type 22*)	**1p13.2** rs2476601	◆ Expressed in hematopoietic cells ◆ Acts as inhibitor of TCR signal transduction ◆ Reported to be associated with type I diabetes[83] as well as with RA, JIA, SLE, myasthenia gravis, generalized vitiligo, alopecia areata, and SSc (reviewed in[22]) ◆ Patients carrying the 620W allele showed a significant correlation with ATA positive
STAT4 (*Signal transducer and activator of transcription 4*)	**2q32.3** rs7574865	◆ Relevant for directing Th cells to the proinflammatory Th1 and Th17 lineages, induced by IL-12, IL-23, and type 1 IFN, leading to production of IFN-γ and IL-17[84] ◆ rs7574865 T allele seem to be a risk factor for SSc susceptibility, especially for patients with ACA positivity
Immune signalling		
BANK1 (*B-cell scaffold protein with ankryn repeats*)	**4q24** rs3733197 rs10516487	◆ *BANK1* gene encodes a B-cell-specific scaffold protein with ankyrin repeats ◆ Acts as a substrate for LYN tyrosine kinase[85] ◆ Both SNPs (rs3733197 and rs10516487) were found to be connected with the diffuse form of SSc[32]
BLK/C8orf13 (*B lymphocyte kinase*)	**8p23–22** rs13277113	◆ B-cell specific gene ◆ Close association to ACA positivity
CD247	**1q22–23** rs2056626	◆ Encodes the TCRζ subunit (component of the TCR-CD3 complex) involved in receptor signalling ◆ Associations found for SSc and SLE[85] (new susceptibility locus for SSc)[33]

ACA, anti-centromere antibodies; ATA, anti-topoisomerase-1; IFN, interferon; JIA, juvenile idiopathic arthritis; RA, rheumatoid arthritis; SLE systemic lupus erythematosus; SNP, single-nucleotide polymorphism; SSc, systemic sclerosis; TCR, T-cell receptor; TLR, Toll-like receptor.
Reviewed by Dieude et al.[22]

An increased number of lymphokine-activated killer and natural killer (NK) cells[46] have been reported in blood samples from patients with SSc.

Humoral abnormalities in SSc are most clearly reflected by the presence of autoantibodies with well-defined target epitopes; mapping of the precise binding sites for some of these is currently being undertaken in several centres.[47] About 97% of SSc patients have detectable anti-nuclear antibodies when HEp-2 lines are used as the detection tissue. Characteristic staining patterns for anti-nuclear antibodies within the nuclear and subnuclear structures are relatively specific,[48] and can be confirmed by more sophisticated tests.

The pathogenesis of SSc is still uncertain; it is likely that the development of both the fibrous and the vascular lesion is complicated and a the result of a number of key events.

Fibrosis

Fibrosis is a hallmark of a number of diseases including scleroderma, pulmonary fibrosis, atherosclerosis, liver cirrhosis, and keloids. Excess deposition of collagen and ECM protein in the skin and internal organs of patients with SSc was first demonstrated histopathologically many years ago, and this was confirmed by physical and biochemical means. Subsequently, techniques for culturing fibroblasts have provided valuable insight into the mechanisms involved in the synthesis of ECM components.

The observation that skin fibroblasts from scleroderma, or at least a subset of them, synthesize increased quantities of fibronectin, fibrillins, proteoglycan core proteins, and particularly collagens types I and III and to a lesser degree IV and VI was inferred from ex-vivo studies of skin biopsies, but the intriguing finding that this phenotype of matrix overproduction persists in tissue culture and could be passed on at cell division has provided a paradigm for the mechanisms underlying the development of fibrosis secondary to vascular and immunological perturbation.[49] Overproduction of type I collagen is a reflection of increased transcriptional activation of the two pro(I)collagen genes and of increased transcript stability. Transcriptional regulation of collagen genes has itself been a major area of biological study and a number of important cis-acting regulatory regions and factors interacting with these regions have been

Table 121.4 T cells and cytokines involved in pathogenesis of systemic sclerosis[44]

Cytokines	Function
Th1 lymphocytes	
IFN-γ	◆ Produced by Th1 cells, memory T CD8+ cells, dendritic and NK cells
	◆ Responsible for Th1 differentiation, the activation of B cells to produce immunoglobulins as well as the Th2 cytokine inhibition via IL-4 and IL-10 repression
TNFα	◆ Mainly produced by macrophages, APC, skin mast cells and keratinocytes
	◆ Important for neutrophil/lymphocyte recruitment
	◆ Proinflammatory and proapoptotic
IL-1	◆ Produced by Th1 cells, monocytes, macrophages, dendritic and endothelial cells
	◆ Important role for Th1 (together with IL-1β, IL-23) and Th17 (together with IL-1β, IL-6, and IL-23) differentiation
	◆ Proinflammatory
IL-2	◆ Produced by T lymphocytes
	◆ Stimulates NK and T CD8+ cells
	◆ Important for lymphocyte proliferation and differentiation to Th1 cells in the presence of IL-12 and IFN-ν as well as Th2 cells together with IL-4
	◆ Important for anti-inflammatory response associated with Th17 inhibition and Treg activation
IL-12	◆ Produced by monocytes, macrophages, dendritic cells as well as B lymphocytes
	◆ Important for Th1 differentiation, while inhibiting Th17 differentiation
	◆ Proinflammatory
Th2 lymphocytes	
IL-4	◆ Produced by Th2 cells, macrophages, mast cells and NK cells
	◆ Important for Th2 differentiation, Th1 cytokine inhibition as well as Treg differentiation
IL-5	◆ Produced by Th2 cells, as well as by mast cells and eosinophils
	◆ Important for B-cell differentaition
IL-6	◆ Produced by Th2 cells, macrophages, B lymphocytes as well as epithelial cells and fibroblasts
	◆ Important for Th2 differentiation, Th17 differentiation (together with TGFβ and IL-21), stimulation of inflammation due to inhibition of Treg differentiation and triggering of fibrosis due to stimulation of collagen production and inhibition of collagenase production
IL-13	◆ Produced by Th2, NK, and mast cells
	◆ Important for B-cell proliferation and differentiation as well as anti-inflammatory response and fibrosis
Th17 lymphocytes	
IL-17	◆ Produced by Th17 cells and NK cells
	◆ Proinflammatory and profibrotic
IL-21	◆ Produced by Th17 cells and NK cells
	◆ Important for Th17 response expansion
IL-22	◆ Produced by mature Th17 cells and Th2 cells and NK cells
	◆ Proinflammatory

APC, antigen-presenting cells; IFN, interferon; IL, interleukin; TGF, tissue growth factor; Th, T helper cell; TNF, tumour necrosis factor; Treg, regulatory T cell.
Adapted from Baraut et al.[44]

identified. More recent studies have implicated several ubiquitous transcription factors in collagen gene activation in SSc fibroblasts including the heterotrimeric factor CBF, the GC-sequence binding protein Sp1, and most recently Smad proteins and their coactivators. It seems likely that upstream regulators of these factors are disturbed in SSc and that this leads to greater levels or more active phosphorylated forms of the transcription factors. Another possibility is that genetic differences in these factors or their regulation contribute to severity or susceptibility to scleroderma, as part of the polygenic background to this disease.

Profibrotic cytokines and chemokines, such as TGFβ, CTGF, PDGF, endothelin-1, interleukins, and monocyte chemoattractant proteins (MCP-1 and -3), are involved in the initiation of fibrosis in scleroderma, and constitutive alterations in the production of some growth factors or responsiveness to their actions has been observed in scleroderma fibroblasts. One of the most potent of these is connective tissue growth factor and there is a body of evidence now suggesting that this could be an important autocrine factor in the maintenance of the scleroderma fibroblast phenotype. Several studies have shown that a lot of serum markers in SSc patients correlate positively with the extent of skin fibrosis in SSc patients (reviewed by Moinzadeh et al.[50]).

Vasculopathy

The most prevalent clinical manifestation of vascular abnormality is Raynaud's phenomenon, which is present in over 95% of SSc

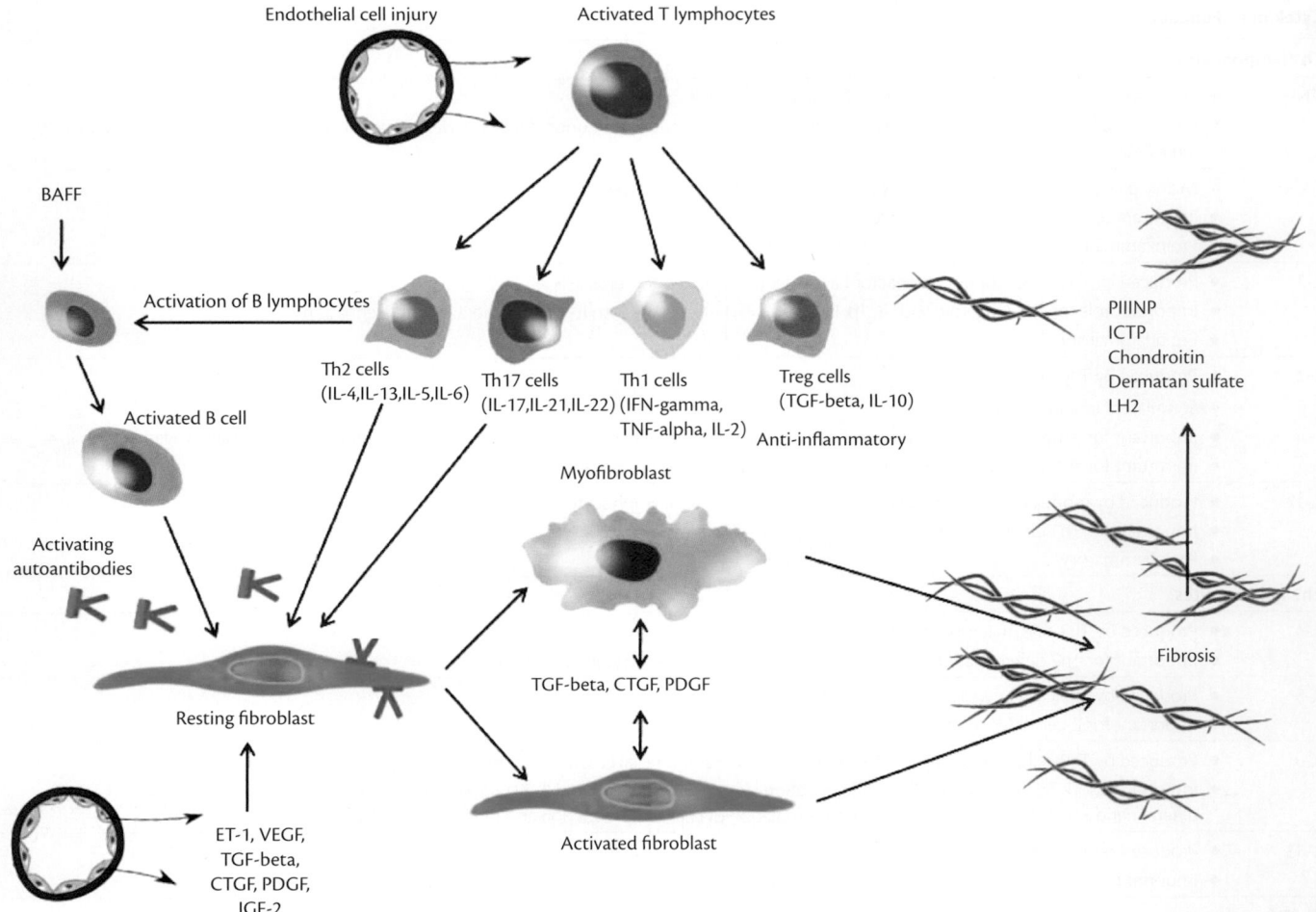

Fig. 121.1 Immunological mechanisms resulting in fibrosis.

patients. In addition, nailfold capillaroscopy is generally altered in SSc at the time of diagnosis. Indeed, the combination of Raynaud's phenomenon and characteristic nailfold capillary dilatation or drop-out offers one of the earliest opportunities to diagnose patients as they develop SSc and it has been proposed that these patients, especially when they also carry a hallmark autoantibody reactivity such as anti-centromere or anti-topoisomerase-1 reactivity, comprise a specific pre-scleroderma clinical subset of the disease.[51] It has also prompted reclassification of some of these cases as limited SSc.[52]

The pathological features of vascular damage, immune-cell activation, and fibrosis are believed to be closely linked in scleroderma.[53] In both localized and generalized disease many histological features are often shared, but the remainder of this discussion focuses on SSc. Detailed studies suggest that in both the skin and internal organs one of the earliest features is endothelial cell injury, initially at the ultrastructural level,[54] and that this is temporally and spatially associated with activation of perivascular fibroblasts and subsequent deposition of increased amounts of structurally normal ECM components. Inflammation is associated with early lesions leading to tissue oedema and leucocytic infiltration. Mononuclear cells predominate, with monocytes/macrophages amongst the

earliest cells within lesional tissue[55] followed later by lymphocytes, mainly carrying phenotypic markers of activated T lymphocytes and including a significant proportion of Ro+ 'memory' cells.

The precise role of vascular pathology in the pathogenesis of SSc remains uncertain. There is considerable evidence that endothelial cell activation and damage are early events in lesional and prelesional tissues but their importance in initiating or sustaining abnormalities in other cell types remains uncertain.

Data suggest that angiogenesis might be altered in scleroderma. The classical telangiectatic lesions of limited cutaneous disease, which are also common especially at later stages of diffuse cutaneous SSc, are consistent with local distruption of angiogenesis. The established fibrotic skin of scleroderma is relatively avascular and it is an attractive hypothesis that perhaps angiogenesis in scleroderma may be inadequate and perturbed. Elevated circulating levels of inhibitors of angiogenesis have been reported although tissue expression of angiogenic factors has not been shown to be consistently altered.

Clinical features

As discussed earlier, SSs is a very heterogeneous condition occurring at any age and including skin and internal organ manifestations.

Within each subtype the rate of progression and extent of damage varies.

Classification of different SSc subsets

The heterogeneity of SSc is caused by the range of disease manifestations that vary in extent and severity of organ involvement between each individual patient. However, Raynaud's phenomenon and skin sclerosis are almost always present. The extent of skin thickening helps to define patients into the two major SSc subsets, i.e. the limited and diffuse forms.

In 1980 the American College of Rheumatology (ACR) reported preliminary SSc classification criteria, for patients with definite disease.[56] The criteria are satisfied, and therefore the diagnosis is established, if either one major criterion (scleroderma proximal to the metacarpophalangeal or metatarsophalangeal joints) or at least two or more minor criteria (sclerodactyly, digital ulcerations and/or pitting digital scars and bibasilary pulmonary fibrosis) are found.

In 1988 LeRoy published a descriptive subclassification of limited vs diffuse SSc,[57] primarily just according to the extent of cutaneous involvement, but later, in 2001, LeRoy and Medsger[29] published amendments, which included the additional presence of autoantibodies and nailfold capillaroscopic alterations to identify also patients with early onset of SSc and just minimal skin sclerosis. To fulfil these criteria, it is essential that patients with early (limited) SSc have evidence of Raynaud's phenomenon plus scleroderma-specific autoantibodies and/or nailfold capillaroscopic manifestations.[58–59]

Patients with the diffuse form of SSc are defined by an early onset of Raynaud's phenomenon, usually within 1 year of onset of skin thickening. This subset is characterized by a very progressive course with skin involvement of trunk, face, upper arms, and thighs, within 1 year. These patients very frequently show anti-Scl 70 (anti-topoisomerase-I) or anti-RNAPIII antibodies,[57] with a higher risk of developing pulmonary fibrosis, cardiac involvement, and scleroderma renal crisis.

Limited cutaneous SSc is characterized by a long pre-existing history of Raynaud's phenomenon, usually several years before the appearance of the first skin changes in the extremities distal to the knee and elbow joints, and including facial skin.[57] This variant of SSc subset often (50–70%) shows anti-centromere antibodies (ACA) and is frequently associated with an isolated pulmonary arterial hypertension. The traditional acronym CREST (defining patients with calcinosis, Raynaud's phenomenon, oesophageal dysmotility, sclerodactyly, and teleangiectasias) is no longer used and all patients with these symptoms are assigned to the limited form of SSc.

Patients are said to have an overlap syndrome if they have the clinical features of SSc (according to the ACR criteria) or main symptoms of SSc simultaneously with those of other connective tissue diseases or other autoimmune diseases such as dermatomyositis, Sjögren's syndrome, SLE, vasculitis, or polyarthritis. These patients mostly have high titres of anti-U1-RNP, anti-nRNP, anti-fibrillarin, or anti-PM Scl antibodies.[60]

Patients classified as having early SSc, also known as undifferentiated SSc, show a positive Raynaud's phenomenon and at least one further aspect of SSc (positive nailfold capillary alterations, puffy fingers, pulmonary hypertension) and/or detectable scleroderma-associated autoantibodies without fulfilling the ACR criteria.[61]

Patients suffering from SSc without scleroderma are very rare and present with virtually no skin thickening, but with Raynaud's phenomenon, pulmonary hypertension, or other scleroderma features as well as ACA or other scleroderma-associated autoantibodies.[62]

Organ manifestation

Vasculopathy

Raynaud's phenomenon was first described by Maurice Raynaud in 1862 as episodic digital ischaemia provoked by cold and emotion, and appears in more than 90% of scleroderma patients. It is classically manifest by episodic pallor of the digits followed by cyanosis, suffusion, and/or pain and tingling (Figure 121.2). The blanching reflects digital arterial vasospasm, the cyanosis the deoxygenation of static venous blood, and the redness reactive hyperaemia following the return of blood flow (triphasic Raynaud's). Diagnostic procedures and therapeutic strategies are summarized in Table 121.5.

Important clues to secondary Raynaud's phenomenon on clinical evaluation are: the development of Raynaud's phenomenon either in very young children or after the age of 45 years; severe symptoms occurring all year round; digital ulcerations, which rarely, if ever occur in primary Raynaud's phenomenon; asymmetry of symptoms; and the recurrence of chilblains in an adult. Two simple, inexpensive, non-invasive procedures have high predictive power for detecting patients in the Raynaud's group who will have SSc in the future, namely patients with positive serum autoantibodies and alterations seen in the nailfold capillaroscopy. Nailfold capillaroscopy is a non-invasive and very useful tool to distinguish between patients with primary and secondary Raynaud's phenomenon and to visualize changes which are typical for early, active and late stages of SSc (Figure 121.3). In addition, laser Doppler perfusion imaging (LDPI), a non-invasive microvascular imaging technique, provides maps of the cutaneous blood flow.[63]

Some SSc patients are troubled by digital ulcerations which are associated with vasculopathy. This is the major external feature of structural vessel disease, probably due to thickened intima and luminal occlusions of vessels. Tender and painful pitting scars are observable and may progress to very painful ulcers, which have a major impact on quality of life with regard to activities of daily living—dressing, eating, etc. These ulcers occur on the tips of the fingers or toes, but may also be found over the extensor surfaces of the joints due to microtrauma or in association with calcinosis cutis. Further possible complications are critical digital ischaemia, paronychia, infections, gangrene, osteomyelitis, and finger pulp loss or amputation.

Cutaneous involvement

The changes in the skin usually proceed through three phases: early, established, and late. The early stage can be difficult to diagnose and a high level of suspicion is needed in the oedematous phase when the only feature may be puffiness of the hands and feet, most marked in the mornings. Oedema may be dependent and can lead to symptoms of neural compression including carpal tunnel syndrome. The face may feel slightly taut at this stage and Raynaud's phenomenon may be present. On examination there is a non-pitting oedema with intact epidermal and dermal appendages. The subsequent, often sudden, development of firm, taut, hidebound skin proximal to the metacarpophalangeal joints, adherent to deeper structures such as tendons and joints, causing limitation of their movement and subsequent contractures,

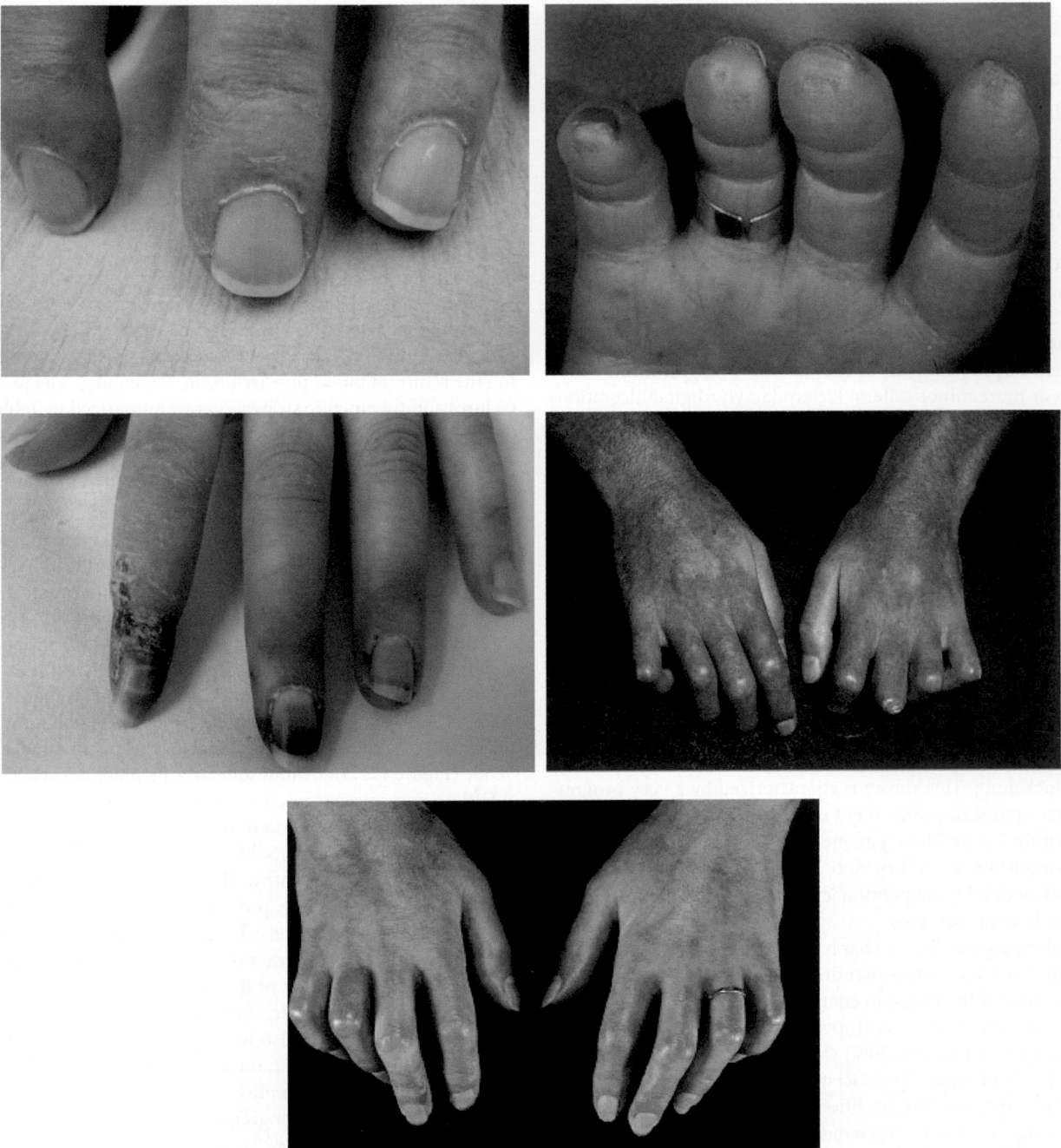

Fig. 121.2 Typical clinical features in the hands of patients with systemic sclerosis.

permits a definitive diagnosis in over 90% of patients. The epidermis thins, hair growth ceases, sweating is impaired, hypo- and hyperpigmentations (salt and pepper phenomenon) appear, and skin creases disappear.

Sclerotic changes limited to the fingers alone (sclerodactyly) do not have the same implications. The classical changes, once fully developed, can remain static for many years. Depending on the region of skin sclerosis, restricted mobility of joints with contractures and/or restricted chest excursion may appear. Typical facial features include teleangiectasiases, a beak-shaped nose as well as

reduced mouth aperture (microstomy) with a typical physiognomy of SSc patients (radial furrowing around the mouth, an expressionless stiff and mask-like facial appearance, and sclerosis of the frenulum). Besides cosmetic/aesthetic problems, in some cases skin sclerosis may also cause difficulties for eating and oral hygiene. The cutaneous or subcutaneous deposition of calcium (calcinosis cutis) usually occurs over pressure points (acral, joints) and is known as Thieberge–Weissenbach syndrome, if it appears extended next to joints. Diagnostic procedures and therapeutic strategies are summarized in Table 121.6.

Table 121.5 Diagnostic procedures and therapeutic strategies, including disease-modifying treatment options for the vascular system

Clinical feature	Diagnostic procedure	Therapeutic strategies
Vascular system		
RP	◆ RP provocation ◆ Nailfold capillaroscopy ◆ Serology	◆ General recommendations: avoid coldness, keep body warm, paraffin bath, heatable soles and gloves ◆ Vitamins and supplements: fish oil capsules, antioxidant vitamins, ginko biloba **Oral treatments** ◆ Calcium channel blockers: nifedipin (10–20 mg, three times daily); amlodipin or felodipin (10 mg once daily) ◆ Angiotensin-II-receptor 1 blocker: losartan (25–50 mg once daily) ◆ Serotonin reuptake inhibitors: luoxetin (20 mg once daily) ◆ Phosphodiesterase type 5 inhibitor: sildenafil (not licensed, trial in severe cases) **Topical treatment** ◆ GTN patches (1/2 of the patch located at the wrist, next to the vessels for 12 hours) **Intravenous treatment** ◆ Prostacyclin infusion: iloprost (0.5–2 ng/kg per minute over 6 h on 5 consecutive days) **Surgical treatment** ◆ Lumbar sympathectomy ◆ Radical microaretriolysis
Digital ulceration	◆ Clinical assessment for infection, necrosis, etc. ◆ Radiograph or MRI to exclude osteomyelitis	**Intravenous treatment** ◆ Prostacyclin infusion: iloprost (0.5–2 ng/kg per minute over 6 h on 5 consecutive days) **Oral treatments** ◆ Phosphodiesterase type 5 inhibitor: sildenafil (not licensed, trial in severe cases) ◆ Dual ET receptor antagonist: bosentan (reduce the frequency of new DUs in the future) ◆ Pain reliever ◆ Antibiotic treatment in case of infection **Topical treatment** ◆ Hydrocolloid wound dressing ◆ Hydrofibre dressing ◆ Vitamin E gel **Surgical treatment** ◆ Lumbar sympathectomy ◆ Radical microaretriolysis ◆ Amputation, debridement

RP, Raynaud's phenomenon.

Careful mapping of the degree and extent of skin involvement is the single best clinical technique for detecting the patient at risk for life-threatening involvement of internal organs. A number of scoring systems to quantify skin sclerosis have been developed. The most widely used is a modification of that proposed by Rodnan, consisting of a 0 to 3 grading at 17 skin sites (maximum score 51). The sites assessed in the modified skin score are summarized in Figure 121.4. The interobserver variability in the use of the modified Rodnan skin score in studies from the United Kingdom and United States is similar.[64]

Furthermore, new techniques for skin thickening scoring have been evaluated, such as 20 MHz ultrasound,[65] durometry,[66] cutometry,[67] elastometry,[68] and plicometry.[69] The evaluation of collagen bundles and inflammatory infiltrates is still only possible by taking skin biopsies with histological evaluation of the dermal skin thickness (see Table 121.6).

The natural history of skin involvement in SSc emphasizes that after 2–3 years plateauing of skin score and/or improvement even without effective treatment is often observable. Also, its use as a surrogate for outcome is supported by secondary analyses confirming that skin score at presentation reflects disease outcome at later time points.

Systemic features of disease

The patient with SSc must cope with a complex set of symptoms that range from features common to chronic diseases through to complaints attributable to specific visceral involvement. Fatigue and lethargy are common throughout the illness, although usually more pronounced in its early phases. Weight loss is almost universal in the diffuse cutaneous form but less common in the limited variety.

Gastrointestinal tract

The gastrointestinal tract is probably the most commonly involved internal organ system in SSc. More than 90% of patients with limited cutaneous and diffuse cutaneous SSc have oesophageal hypomotility and serious gastrointestinal disease has been estimated to occur in 50% of patients with limited cutaneous SSc.

(A)

(C)

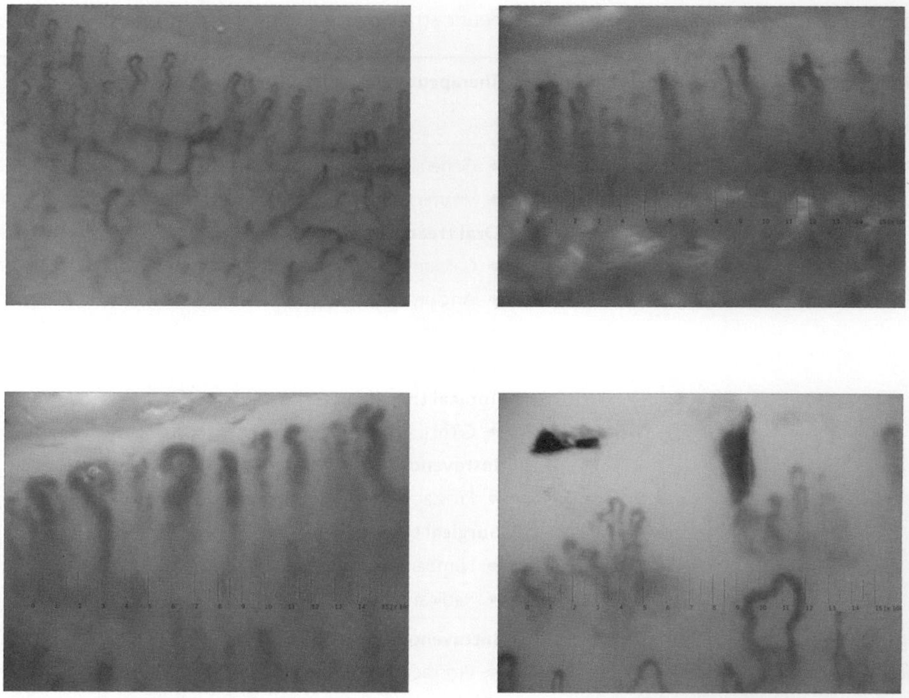

Fig. 121.3 Nailfold capillaroscopy with early, active, and late patterns of systemic sclerosis:[86]
(a) Normal capillaries (9–11 capillaries/mm with a regular order of capillary loops).
(b) Earlysystemic sclerosis pattern (few enlarged/ecstatic capillaries and a few haemorrhages, but normal density of capillaries). (c) Active pattern (multiple giant and enlarged/ecstatic capillaries with haemorrhages and also disordered capillaries due to development of capillary loss).
(d) Late pattern (completely disturbed architecture with multiple losses of capillaries and bushy capillaries (neovascularization); giant capillaries, and haemorrhages just occasionally visible).
Courtesy of Dr Kevin Howell, RFH Microvascular Laboratory.

Table 121.6 Diagnostic procedures and therapeutic strategies, including disease-modifying treatment options for the skin

Clinical feature	Diagnostic procedure	Therapeutic strategies
Skin thickening	◆ Clinical assessment ◆ mRSS ◆ Durometer ◆ 20 Mhz ultrasound ◆ Biopsy	General recommendations: skin care with moisturizing cream or ointments **Physical treatments** ◆ Lymphatic drainage/physiotherapy: for skin fibrosis, sclerodactyly, microstomia, dermatogenous contractures, puffy fingers ◆ Phototherapy: skin hardening, itchiness **Topical treatment** ◆ Steroids or calcineurin inhibitors: early stage of skin hardening with inflammation and itchiness **Systemic treatments** ◆ Steroids (just short dated due to side effects and risk of renal crisis) ◆ Ciclosporin (small studies showed improvement of skin score[87] ◆ Methotrexate (improvement in skin score reported)[88–90] ◆ Cyclophosphamide (trials have shown significant improvement in mRSS)[91–92]
Calcinosis cutis	◆ Clinical assessment ◆ Imaging (X-ray, MRI, CT)	**Caution: side effects have to be balanced** ◆ General recommendations: improve blood flow and keep hands warm ◆ Local corticosteroid injections ◆ Laser therapy ◆ Surgery ◆ Minocycline ◆ Bisphosphonate (oral)
Teleangiectases	◆ Clinical assessment	◆ Laser therapy ◆ Camouflage

mRSS, Modified Rodnan skin score.

Site	Maximum score		
Face	3		
Anterior chest	3		
Abdomen	3		
Subtotal	**9**		
		Right	Left
Upper arm		3	3
Forearm		3	3
Hand		3	3
Fingers		3	3
Thigh		3	3
Leg		3	3
Foot		3	3
		21	21
Maximum	**51**		

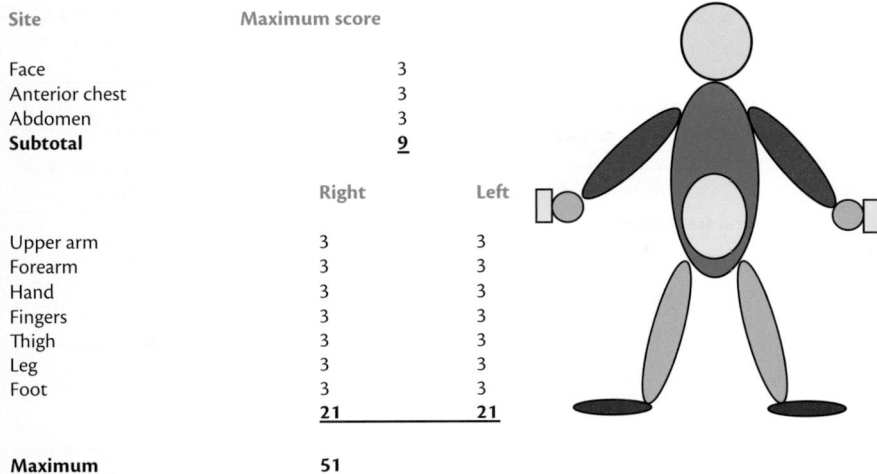

Scoring of each skin region determined by skin thickness and tethering:

0 = normal

1 = possible thickening

2 = definite thickening but mobile

3 = skin more thickened and fixed to deeper tissues "hide-bound"

Scoring system assessing 17 sites (omitting neck and back) with maximum of 54 is also widely used to avoid these sites which are often hard to accurately score.

Fig. 121.4 Standardized assessment of skin involvement in systemic sclerosis using a modified Rodnan skin score.

The earliest clinical symptoms may be quite subtle. Patients may experience difficulties in swallowing (dysphagia), retrosternal discomfort or even overt pain, which can be nocturnal, due to reflux and oesophagitis. Measurement of lower oesophageal pressure is frequently unacceptable to the patient and therefore in clinical practice the oesophageal transit time (quantitative oesophageal scintigraphy) is usually the preferred screening test. In those who have an abnormal scan and those who have severe dysphagia and/or heartburn, direct oesophago-/gastroscopy may be required to identify structural divisions such as hiatus hernia and oesophageal strictures as well as to identify Barrett's metaplasia at an early stage. Proton pump inhibitors are the drugs of first choice. Diagnostic procedures and therapeutic strategies are summarized in Table 121.7.

Small-bowel disease with hypomotility is a major problem in scleroderma and can lead to weight loss, cachexia, and malabsorption. The classical symptoms are of a change in bowel pattern, with loose, frequent, floating, foul-smelling stools, and abdominal distension. Once the disease is established, bacterial overgrowth with its associated malabsorption is a recurring problem, often punctuated by abrupt episodes of distension and adynamic ileus (pseudo-obstruction). Management of such patients is difficult and includes the rotational use of antibiotics, attempts to stimulate the bowel directly with prokinetics including erythomycin or domperidone, and on occasion total parenteral nutrition. Atony and hypomotility of the rectum and sigmoid colon is frequent and occurs early. Constipation is usually manageable with the use of dietary manipulation and stool volume expanders.

Surgery to the large bowel or any other part of the gastrointestinal tract must be viewed with great caution because it is not without risk and not always successful. As the gastrointestinal manifestations of SSc are frequent, and debilitating if not life-threatening, the goal in this area must be early detection, support, and control, thus permitting as active a life as possible.

Cardiopulmonary involvement

It is likely that cardiac involvement from scleroderma, although important and potentially life-threatening, is underdiagnosed. The cardiopulmonary system may be affected different ways, most often by fibrosis and pulmonary arterial hypertension (PAH). PAH is defined as a mean pulmonary pressure (mPAP) of at least 25 mmHg at rest combined with a pulmonary capillary wedge pressure of less than 15 mmHg, determined by right heart catheterization.[70]

Due to similar, overlapping clinical features, such as dyspnoea, non-productive cough, disturbed diffusion capacity, and cyanoses, it can sometimes be a challenge to distinguish between cardiac and pulmonary factors. PAH is the most common cause of disease-related death in SSc, replacing scleroderma renal crisis. PAH occurs in patients with limited and diffuse SSc, although the most typical cases are those of lSSc associated with isolated PAH, but there are also some patients with late-stage extensive interstitial lung fibrosis in SSc who develop a secondary PAH. In addition the heart can also be affected due to diffuse interstitial myocardial fibrosis, which leads to diastolic dysfunctions as well as restricted contractibility of the myocardium. These patients typically present symptoms such as cardiac arrhythmia, paroxysmal tachycardia, incomplete or complete right-heart blocks, and heart insufficiency.

All patients with SSc should be followed up at least annually with lung function tests and echocardiography. Further investigation such as the 6 minute walk test or high-resolution CT (HRCT) may

Table 121.7 Diagnostic procedures and therapeutic strategies, including disease-modifying treatment options for the gastrointestinal system and the kidneys

Clinical feature	Diagnostic procedure	Therapeutic strategies
Gastrointestinal involvement		
Reflux	◆ Gastro-oesophageal endcoscopy	◆ General recommendations: bed head elevated during the night, small meals **Oral treatments** ◆ Proton pump inhibitors: lansoprazole, omeprazole, etc. ◆ Procinetics: domperidone ◆ H_2 receptor antagonists: ranitidine
Dysphagia	◆ Oesophageal szintigraphy	◆ General recommendations: change of eating habits, small meals **Oral treatments** ◆ Prokinetics: domperidone, metoclopramide
GAVE	◆ Endoscopy	◆ Argon plasma coagulation
Diarrhoea Constipation	◆ Coloscopy	◆ General recommendations: change of eating habits **Oral treatments** ◆ Prokinetics: domperidone ◆ Antibiotics ◆ Laxative
Faecal incontinence	◆ Coloscopy ◆ Rectal manometry	◆ Solidifying liquid stools ◆ Biofeedback therapy ◆ Sacral nerve stimulation
Rectal prolapse	◆ Clinical assessment	◆ Surgery

help to determine possible cardiopulmonary involvement. Lung function testing is useful to give early signs for both lung fibrosis and PAH, in the form of impaired diffusion capacity (DL_{CO} ≤75%). To determine the presence of interstitial lung involvement, HRCT and/or chest radiograph should be used and these tests are generally performed at diagnosis, especially if there is any breathlessness or impaired lung function. Regular follow-up looking for cardiac involvement should also include transthoracic Doppler echocardiography, which can indicate a hypertrophy with or without enlargement of the right ventricle, paradoxical motion of the interventricular septum, tricuspid valve insufficiency, and pericardial effusion. In case of suspected PAH, right heart catheterization is still the gold standard, but it is an invasive diagnostic procedure.

Fibrotic changes in the myocardium in scleroderma have been demonstrated in biopsy specimens and at necropsy. Non-invasive imaging techniques such as MRI or spiral CT scanning may allow this to be determined more precisely. Indirect clues to cardiac involvement may be deduced from ECG or echocardiographic studies. Conduction defects are the most frequently observed disturbances. Typical features include QTc prolongation on 12-lead ECG. Later, conduction tissue fibrosis may lead to varying degrees of heart block including first- or second-degree block or complete heart block necessitating pacemaker implantation. Also the use of N-terminal brain natriuretic peptide (NTproBNP) in the patient's serum is helpful to detect right ventricular impairment.

The treatment of the cardiac manifestations of SSc is primarily supportive, empirical, and of moderate value. Diagnostic procedures and therapeutic strategies are summarized in Table 121.8.

Kidney involvement

This remains one of the most important complications of scleroderma and is amenable to treatment, although the prognosis is much better if appropriate management is instituted early. As with PAH, renal scleroderma is mainly a vascular disease. Both post- and antemortem studies suggest that epithelial and endothelial renal lesions occur before there is clinical evidence of renal disease in SSc,[71] and certainly precede any histological evidence of fibrosis. This supports the view that epithelial, and particularly endothelial, damage are important early events in the pathogenesis of scleroderma.[72] The best-characterized pattern of renal involvement in SSc is an acute or subacute renal hypertensive crisis. This generally occurs in patients with diffuse SSc within 5 years of disease onset. The overall incidence of scleroderma renal crisis is uncertain, with differences in the reported frequency even in series from the same unit. This variation probably reflects differences in incidence in the various subsets of SSc. Traub et al. proposed the following criteria to diagnose scleroderma renal crisis: abrupt onset of arterial hypertension greater than 160/90 mmHg, hypertensive retinopathy of at least grade III severity, rapid deterioration of renal function, and elevated plasma renin activity.[73] Other typical features include the presence of a microangiopathic haemolytic blood film and hypertensive encephalopathy, often complicated by generalized

Table 121.8 Diagnostic procedures and therapeutic strategies, including disease-modifying treatment options for the cardiopulmonary system

Clinical feature	Diagnostic procedure	Therapeutic strategies
Respiratory system		
Lung fibrosis	◆ Lung function test ◆ Imaging (X-ray/HRCT) ◆ Bronchioalveolar lavage	**Systemic treatments** ◆ Cyclophosphamide orally or IV ◆ Glucocorticosteroids (short dated) ◆ Azathioprine orally ◆ Mycophenolate mofetil orally vOxygen (if needed)
Cardiac system		
PAH	◆ Lung function test ◆ Electrocardiography ◆ Echocardiography ◆ 24 h blood pressure control ◆ Right heart catheterization	**Systemic treatments** ◆ Bosentan orally ◆ Sildenafil orally ◆ Epoprostenol orally ◆ Oxygen (if needed)
Cardiac myopathy	◆ Electrocardiography ◆ Echocardiography ◆ 24 h blood pressure control ◆ MRI	**Systemic treatments** ◆ Cyclophosphamide orally or intravenous ◆ Glucocorticosteroids (short dated) ◆ Azathioprine orally ◆ Mycophenolate mofetil orally ◆ Pacemaker (if needed)
Renal system		
Scleroderma renal crisis	◆ Regular blood pressure controls ◆ Ultrasound ◆ Serological renal profile ◆ Proteinuria analysis	**Systemic treatments** ◆ ACE inhibitors (high-dose) under blood pressure monitoring ◆ Iloprost intravenous

convulsions. It is generally considered important to perform a renal biopsy, once hypertension has been adequately controlled, especially if renal replacement therapy is being contemplated. This allows histological confirmation of the diagnosis and the exclusion of other causes for renal failure of abrupt onset, such as glomerulonephritis or the haemolytic uraemic syndrome.

Musculoskeletal system

Skeletal muscle is often involved in scleroderma. In many instances the weakness, pain, and atrophy results from disuse secondary to joint contractures or chronic disease. However, about 20% of patients have a chronic myopathy, characterized by mild weakness and atrophy of muscles, minimal elevation of creatine phosphokinase, few or no changes on electromyography, and subtle histological features showing focal replacement of myofibrils with collagen and perimysial and epimysial fibrosis without inflammatory change. A minority of patients exhibit an inflammatory myositis, usually categorized as an SSc–polymyositis overlap syndrome, sometimes indistinguishable from polymyositis; caution is required if this occurs in the context of early diffuse disease, when treatment with high-dose steroids might precipitate renal failure, and an alternative treatment should be considered.

A symmetrical polyarthritis, usually seronegative, anodular and non-erosive, is the presenting feature in a small number of patients destined ultimately to develop SSc. By 2 years, frequently much

earlier, the synovitis has subsided and classic cutaneous SSc is present, often developing abruptly over 1–3 months.

Management of systemic sclerosis

There have been major advances in treating many of the organ-specific complications of SSc. Critical ischaemia and severe Raynaud's phenomenon are improved by parenteral prostacyclin analogues; the management and outcome of scleroderma renal crisis has been transformed by use of angiotensin converting enzyme (ACE) inhibitors, and the morbidity from oesophagitis has been drastically cut by use of proton pump inhibitors. Added to this are the exciting developments in treating PAH and several encouraging retrospective studies suggesting that immunosuppression using cyclophosphamide may be effective in slowing the progression of SSc-associated fibrosing alveolitis (all symptomatic and disease-modifying treatments for SSc are listed in Tables 121.5–121.8). In addition to these developments, there is now a much clearer understanding of the heterogeneity and natural history of the major subsets of SSc and an appreciation of risk stratification, the use of serological markers, and proactive regular screening of patients for early signs of complications. Together, these factors make SSc a much more manageable disease.

The choice and evaluation of any treatment regimen are not easy because the disease is complex and the pathogenesis poorly understood; the disorder is heterogeneous and its extent, severity, and rate of progression are highly variable. Therapy must therefore be closely tailored to the individual patient involved. There is a tendency towards spontaneous stabilization and/or regression after a few years, particularly within the more benign and numerically larger subset of limited cutaneous SSc; and there is a paucity of both clinical and laboratory features for ascertaining improvement (or deterioration) in the disease, especially with respect to visceral change. Ultimately it is hoped that a better understanding of the pathogenesis of SSc, especially in its aggressive diffuse form, will identify key factors, pathways, or processes that can be targeted therapeutically. It is possible that targets will be stage- or subset-specific. There are already examples of pilot studies of anti-cytokine therapies using neutralizing antibodies or soluble receptors. Ultimately, small molecules that inhibit key pathways are likely to be the most successful form of treatment but these are presently a long way off.

It is generally considered that immunosuppressive strategies are most likely to be effective in the early stages of SSc when inflammatory features are prominent. A large number of agents have been tried but none has been shown in clinical trials to be definitely effective.

Localized scleroderma

This is distinguished from SSc not only by the absence of vasospasm, structural vascular damage, and involvement of internal organs, but also by the distribution of the dermal lesions, which may, depending on the subtype, follow a dermatomal pattern. It can appear in children and adults and depending on the subtype of localized scleroderma; children more frequently develop the linear form of SSc, while adults suffer commonly from the limited localized scleroderma form. The incidence varies between 0.4 and 2.7 per 100 000 inhabitants and it is also predominantly a female condition.[8,74–75] The pathogenesis of this disease is also still not fully understood, but some authors have reported that trauma, autoimmunity, drugs, radiation, and also infections might be triggers for this kind of disease.

Classification

The varied clinical features have led to the separation of four main varieties of localized scleroderma: limited and generalized forms of morphoea, and linear and frontal ('en coup de sabre') forms of localized scleroderma (see Figure 121.5 and Table 121.9).[76]

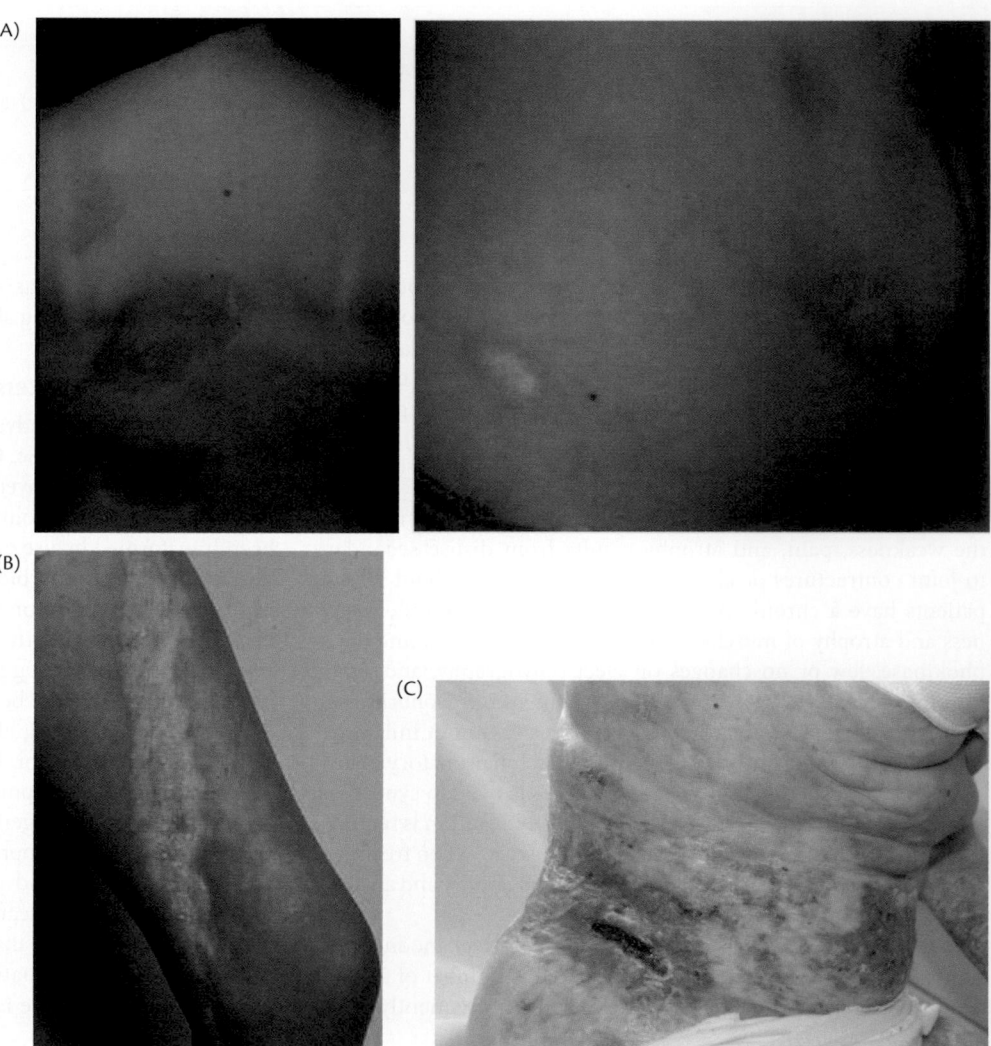

Fig. 121.5 Variants of localized scleroderma: (a) limited forms of morphoea (plaque type); (b) linear forms of morphoea (linear type, en coup de sabre, Parry–Romberg syndrome); (c) generalized forms of morphoea (generalized disabling form of morphoea).

Table 121.9 Classification of localized scleroderma[76]

Localized scleroderma	Subtypes	Clinical characteristics
Limited type	Morphoea (plaque type)	At least one lesion (>1cm), in one or two anatomic regions, such as back, abdomen, limbs, buttock, and/or neck. The lesions are usually initially erythematous, afterwards changing into indurated and central thickened plaques. The typical lilac ring can be used as an activity sign
	Guttata morphoea	Characterized by at least one lesion (<1cm), which are commonly visible at the trunk
	Atrophoderma of Pasini and Pierini	Hyperpigmented/erythematous atrophic patches, which are commonly located at the trunk. Interestingly, these lesions show no sclerotic process
Generalized type	Generalized localized scleroderma	The plaques of this form show a tendency to confluence at more than two anatomic areas into huge plaques
	Disabling pansclerotic morphoea	Generalized, diffuse sclerosis, involving the whole body of the patients and usually sparing only the extremities of the patients. It can be complicated by very painful and resistant ulcerations
	Eosinophilic fasciitis	Severe fibrosis of the deep fascia, characterized by symmetric skin sclerosis, oedema, and eosinophilia around the lower extremities
Linear type	Linear localized scleroderma	This type shows band-like lesions of sclerotic skin with possibly deep atrophy of the soft tissue. Patients develop this condition usually in the first or second decade of their life
	'en coup de sabre' type	Linear skin sclerosis and atrophy of subcutaneous tissue localized at the forehead. Typically children develop this form of linear scleroderma
	Progressive facial hemiatrophy@ (Parry–Romberg syndrome)	This is the more severe form of the linear variant with an involvement of one-half of the face defined by atrophy of subcutaneous tissue
Deep type	Deep morphoea	This form primarily involves the panniculus or fascia and therefore forms deep and bound down skin lesions

Morphoea

The **limited form** of morphoea includes plaque-type morphoea, guttata morphoea, and the atrophoderma of Pasini and Pierini. This form is characterized by changes that often begin with small, violaceous or erythematous skin lesions, which enlarge and progress to firm 'hidebound' skin with variable degrees of hypo- or hyperpigmentation. These lesions eventually settle into a waxy, white appearance with subsequent atrophy. Pruritus is often a problem with the early lesion. Lesions vary in diameter between 1 and 10 cm. The condition generally resolves within 3–5 years, although sometimes a patch may persist for more than 25 years.

The **generalized form** of morphoea includes generalized localized scleroderma and the disabling pansclerotic morphoea as well as eosinophilic fasciitis. These forms are characterized by the development of many patches covering a large surface area. The acral parts are usually spared, but the trunk and legs are often involved. Generalized morphea can be disfiguring and may continue to extend, resulting in contractures, disability, and troublesome ulceration that may occasionally become malignant. In guttate morphea there are multiple small, hypopigmented and pigmented papules 2–10 mm in diameter, with minimal sclerosis, and the lesions closely resemble those of lichen sclerosus et atrophicus. These lesions usually localize to the neck, shoulders, and anterior chest wall.

Linear form of localized scleroderma

The linear form of localized scleroderma includes the normal linear morphoea, en coup de sabre, and the Parry–Romberg syndrome. These patients are defined by sclerotic areas occurring in a linear, band-like pattern, often in a dermatome distribution. These areas often cross joint lines, and are associated with atrophy of the soft tissue, muscle, periosteum, bone, and occasionally synovium; they can lead to extensive growth defects in a limb or a part thereof, which can be extremely disfiguring. Fixed valgus or various deformities also occur, and scoliotic changes in the spine can develop as a result of inequalities in limb length. If the toes or fingers are involved, 'hammer toes' or 'claw hand' may develop. All of these changes are much more noticeable in a growing child and most cases of linear SSc tend to occur in childhood, as do most cases of en coup de sabre, a specialized form of linear disease. Lesions generally predominate on one side of the body although some degree of contralateral involvement is often present at later stages, suggesting that there may be a systemic process operating.

Frontal linear scleroderma ('en coup de sabre')

This gets its name because the lesion was originally considered to be reminiscent of the scar from a sabre wound so it was termed 'en coup de sabre'. It is a form of linear scleroderma occurring on the face or scalp; the linear lesion may assume a depressed, ivory appearance and is often associated with hemiatrophy of the face on the same side. It may also be associated with vascular abnormalities of the brain and also with morphoea lesions elsewhere. There is clinical overlap between this form of linear scleroderma and specific localized growth defects such as idiopathic hemifacial atrophy (Parry–Romberg syndrome). In the latter the overlying skin may be texturally normal or there may be skin changes resembling those of scleroderma. It is not uncommon for patients to present with morphea and then later develop linear lesions. This evolution should be anticipated extremely carefully, as the linear lesions tend to have much greater morbidity than the circumscribed patches of morphoea. The linear lesions may be quietly progressive for a long period, and lengthy follow-up is important.

Other forms

In addition, a small group of children has been described with morphoea and/or linear lesions who also have a synovitis, which can be demonstrated by infrared thermography. These patients have a raised erythrocyte sedimentation rate (ESR), rheumatoid factor (RF), and circulating autoantibodies. Such cases are unusual, but they have an accelerated course with rapid development of contractures. At the time of presentation, there may only be a small area of localized or linear scleroderma, distant from the joint symptoms. The ESR and RF are usually normal, but autoantibodies are often present. There is both a clinical and a biochemical association, the nature of which is unclear, between localized scleroderma and eosinophilic fasciitis, in which large sclerotic patches may also occur.

Evaluation

Evaluation of all forms of scleroderma is difficult. In the localized forms, charting of the involved areas is often cumbersome and imprecise. However, the size of the lesion can be recorded, leg length, limb circumferences, and posture can be monitored, and muscle function and neurological status assessed. Charting of new lesions is also essential. In addition, thermography can be used to assess the activity of localized disease,[77] and high-frequency ultrasound or MRI have also been used to determine the depth of localized scleroderma lesions. CT scans and MRI investigations are also useful to identify extracutaneous manifestations, such as subcortical calcifications, brain atrophy, and muscular, bone, and subcutaneous tissue involvement.

Different variants of skin scoring techniques are now used in patients with morphoea to assess the development over years and to see whether there are still signs for activity and progression. The Localized Scleroderma Clinical and Ultrasound group (LOCUS)[78] has validated a morphoea-specific skin scoring system which is used at 18 different body areas, classifying skin erythema, skin hardening, and new lesions. Laser Doppler flowmetry,[79] durometry,[80] elastometry, and cutometry[68] have also been used in clinical practice as well as in clinical trials to evaluate the progression of the skin hardening, as in patients with SSc.

Different therapy strategies can be used in morphoea patients depending on the type and the severity/extension, as listed in Table 121.10.

In addition to localized scleroderma and the more severe SSc, there are many other scleroderma-mimicking diseases, which have to be excluded and also considered as differential diagnoses. These disorders are briefly summarized in Box 121.1.

Table 121.10 Morphoea: treatment recommendations

Treatment	Comments
Topical treatments	
Topical steroids	Can be helpful in active stages of superficial morphoea subtypes
Topical calcipotriol	Can be beneficial for plaque-type superficial types of morphoea
Topical tacrolimus	Can improve skin lesions, especially in the erythematous, active stage of superficial morphoea types
Phototherapy	Initial UV dosage has to be adjusted after determining the individual MED for UVA1 and MPD for bath PUVA
UVA$_1$ phototherapy	◆ Phototherapy is known to have an anti-inflammatory and also an anti-fibrotic effect on sclerotic skin lesions ◆ **Caution**: especially in light-skinned patients, long-term consequences should be discussed in detail
Bath PUVA	◆ Phototherapy is known to have an anti-inflammatory and also an anti-fibrotic effect on sclerotic skin lesions ◆ Bath PUVA can be effective in early inflammatory stages of morphoea ◆ **Caution**: especially in light-skinned patients, long-term consequences should be discussed in detail
Systemic treatments	
Oral steroids	◆ Helpful in early acute stage of severe morphoea types and eosinophilic fasciitis ◆ **Caution**: side effects should be considered
Methotrexate	◆ Used in patients with generalized types of morphoea and active linear morphoea ◆ Can be used orally or subcutaneously, once per week
Physical treatments	
Physiotherapy	It is important to combine all systemic or topical treatments with physiotherapy, especially in patients with linear localized morphoea, to reduce skin contractures and defective positions of extremities **Caution**: physiotherapy should not be used in inflammatory active stages
Lymphatic drainage	Again the combination of physical and medicinal treatments is important in patients with linear localized morphoea **Caution**: lymphatic drainage should not be used in inflammatory active stages

MED, minimal erythema dose; MPD, minimal phototoxic dose; PUVA, psoralen ultraviolet A.

References

1. Mayes MD. Scleroderma epidemiology. *Rheum Dis Clin North Am* 2003;29(2):239–254.

2. Tamaki T, Mori S, Takehara K. Epidemiological study of patients with systemic sclerosis in Tokyo. *Arch Dermatol Res* 1991;283(6):366–371.

3. Medsger TA, Jr. Epidemiology of systemic sclerosis. *Clin Dermatol* 1994;12(2):207–216.

4. Alamanos Y, Tsifetaki N, Voulgari PV et al. Epidemiology of systemic sclerosis in northwest Greece 1981 to 2002. *Semin Arthritis Rheum* 2005;34(5):714–720.

5. Arias-Nunez MC, Llorca J, Vazquez-Rodriguez TR et al. Systemic sclerosis in northwestern Spain: a 19-year epidemiologic study. *Medicine* (Baltimore) 2008;87(5):272–280.

6. Lo Monaco A, Bruschi M, La Corte R, Volpinari S, Trotta F. Epidemiology of systemic sclerosis in a district of northern Italy. *Clin Exp Rheumatol* 2011;29(2 Suppl 65):S10–S14.

7. Roberts-Thomson PJ, Walker JG et al. Scleroderma in South Australia: further epidemiological observations supporting a stochastic explanation. *Intern Med J* 2006;36(8):489–497.

8. Silman A, Jannini S, Symmons D, Bacon P. An epidemiological study of scleroderma in the West Midlands. *Br J Rheumatol* 1988;27(4):286–290.

9. Silman AJ. Epidemiology of scleroderma. *Ann Rheum Dis* 1991;50 Suppl 4:846–853.

10. Steen VD, Medsger TA, Jr. Epidemiology and natural history of systemic sclerosis. *Rheum Dis Clin North Am* 1990;16(1):1–10.

11. Walker UA, Tyndall A, Czirjak L et al. Geographical variation of disease manifestations in systemic sclerosis: a report from the EULAR Scleroderma Trials and Research (EUSTAR) group database. *Ann Rheum Dis* 2009;68(6):856–862.

12. Silman AJ, Howard Y, Hicklin AJ, Black C. Geographical clustering of scleroderma in south and west London. *Br J Rheumatol* 1990;29(2):93–96.

13. Freni-Titulaer LW, Kelley DB, Grow AG et al. Connective tissue disease in southeastern Georgia: a case-control study of etiologic factors. *Am J Epidemiol* 1989;130(2):404–409.

14. Valesini G, Litta A, Bonavita MS et al. Geographical clustering of scleroderma in a rural area in the province of Rome. *Clin Exp Rheumatol* 1993;11(1):41–47.

15. Arnett FC, Howard RF, Tan F et al. Increased prevalence of systemic sclerosis in a Native American tribe in Oklahoma. Association with an Amerindian HLA haplotype. *Arthritis Rheum* 1996;39(8):1362–1370.

16. Tan FK, Arnett FC. Genetic factors in the etiology of systemic sclerosis and Raynaud phenomenon. *Curr Opin Rheumatol* 2000;12(6):511–519.

17. Oliver JE, Silman AJ. Why are women predisposed to autoimmune rheumatic diseases? *Arthritis Res Ther* 2009;11(5):252.

18. Nikpour M, Stevens WM, Herrick AL, Proudman SM. Epidemiology of systemic sclerosis. *Best Pract Res Clin Rheumatol* 2010;24(6):857–869.

19. Laing TJ, Gillespie BW, Toth MB et al. Racial differences in scleroderma among women in Michigan. *Arthritis Rheum* 1997;40(4):734–742.

20. Arnett FC, Cho M, Chatterjee S et al. Familial occurrence frequencies and relative risks for systemic sclerosis (scleroderma) in three United States cohorts. *Arthritis Rheum* 2001;44(6):1359–1362.

21. Agarwal SK, Tan FK, Arnett FC. Genetics and genomic studies in scleroderma (systemic sclerosis). *Rheum Dis Clin North Am* 2008;34(1):17–40; v.

22. Dieude P, Boileau C, Allanore Y. Immunogenetics of systemic sclerosis. *Autoimmun Rev* 2011;10(5):282–290.

23. Arnett FC, Gourh P, Shete S et al. Major histocompatibility complex (MHC) class II alleles, haplotypes and epitopes which confer susceptibility or protection in systemic sclerosis: analyses in 1300 Caucasian, African-American and Hispanic cases and 1000 controls. *Ann Rheum Dis* 2010;69(5):822–827.

24. Gladman DD, Kung TN, Siannis F et al. HLA markers for susceptibility and expression in scleroderma. *J Rheumatol* 2005;32(8):1481–1487.

25. Reveille JD, Owerbach D, Goldstein R et al. Association of polar amino acids at position 26 of the HLA-DQB1 first domain with the anticentromere autoantibody response in systemic sclerosis (scleroderma). *J Clin Invest* 1992;89(4):1208–1213.

26. Arnett FC, Reveille JD, Goldstein R et al. Autoantibodies to fibrillarin in systemic sclerosis (scleroderma). An immunogenetic, serologic, and clinical analysis. *Arthritis Rheum* 1996;39(7):1151–1160.

27. Marguerie C, Bunn CC, Copier J et al. The clinical and immunogenetic features of patients with autoantibodies to the nucleolar antigen PM-Scl. *Medicine* (Baltimore) 1992;71(6):327–336.

28. Dieude P, Guedj M, Wipff J et al. Association between the IRF5 rs2004640 functional polymorphism and systemic sclerosis: a new perspective for pulmonary fibrosis. *Arthritis Rheum* 2009;60(1):225–233.

29. Fonseca C, Lindahl GE, Ponticos M et al. A polymorphism in the CTGF promoter region associated with systemic sclerosis. *N Engl J Med* 2007;357(12):1210–1220.

30. Rueda B, Gourh P, Broen J et al. BANK1 functional variants are associated with susceptibility to diffuse systemic sclerosis in Caucasians. *Ann Rheum Dis* 2010;69(4):700–705.

31. Rueda B, Broen J, Simeon C et al. The STAT4 gene influences the genetic predisposition to systemic sclerosis phenotype. *Hum Mol Genet* 2009;18(11):2071–2077.

32. Dieude P, Guedj M, Wipff J et al. STAT4 is a genetic risk factor for systemic sclerosis having additive effects with IRF5 on disease susceptibility and related pulmonary fibrosis. *Arthritis Rheum* 2009;60(8):2472–2479.

33. Radstake TR, Gorlova O, Rueda B et al. Genome-wide association study of systemic sclerosis identifies CD247 as a new susceptibility locus. *Nat Genet* 2010;42(5):426–429.

34. Milano A, Pendergrass SA, Sargent JL et al. Molecular subsets in the gene expression signatures of scleroderma skin. *PLoS One* 2008;3(7):e2696.

35. Nietert PJ, Silver RM. Systemic sclerosis: environmental and occupational risk factors. *Curr Opin Rheumatol* 2000;12(6):520–526.

36. Mayes MD. Epidemiologic studies of environmental agents and systemic autoimmune diseases. *Environ Health Perspect* 1999;107 Suppl 5:743–748.

37. Janowsky EC, Kupper LL, Hulka BS. Meta-analyses of the relation between silicone breast implants and the risk of connective-tissue diseases. *N Engl J Med* 2000;342(11):781–790.

38. Lupoli S, Amlot P, Black C. Normal immune responses in systemic sclerosis. *J Rheumatol* 1990;17(3):323–327.

39. Padula SJ, Clark RB, Korn JH. Cell-mediated immunity in rheumatic disease. *Hum Pathol* 1986;17(3):254–263.

40. White B. Immune abnormalities in systemic sclerosis. *Clin Dermatol* 1994;12(3):349–359.

41. Degiannis D, Seibold JR, Czarnecki M, Raskova J, Raska K, Jr. Soluble and cellular markers of immune activation in patients with systemic sclerosis. *Clin Immunol Immunopathol* 1990;56(2):259–270.

42. Hasegawa M, Fujimoto M, Kikuchi K, Takehara K. Elevated serum levels of interleukin 4 (IL-4), IL-10, and IL-13 in patients with systemic sclerosis. *J Rheumatol* 1997;24(2):328–332.

43. Kurasawa K, Hirose K, Sano H et al. Increased interleukin-17 production in patients with systemic sclerosis. *Arthritis Rheum* 2000;43(11):2455–2463.

44. Baraut J, Michel L, Verrecchia F, Farge D. Relationship between cytokine profiles and clinical outcomes in patients with systemic sclerosis. *Autoimmun Rev* 2010;10(2):65–73.

45. Chizzolini C, Brembilla NC, Montanari E, Truchetet ME. Fibrosis and immune dysregulation in systemic sclerosis. *Autoimmun Rev* 2011;10(5):276–281.

46. Kantor TV, Whiteside TL, Friberg D, Buckingham RB, Medsger TA, Jr. Lymphokine-activated killer cell and natural killer cell activities in patients with systemic sclerosis. *Arthritis Rheum* 1992;35(6):694–699.

47. Bona C, Rothfield N. Autoantibodies in scleroderma and tightskin mice. *Curr Opin Immunol* 1994;6(6):931–937.

48. Tan EM. Antinuclear antibodies: diagnostic markers for autoimmune diseases and probes for cell biology. *Adv Immunol* 1989;44:93–151.

49. LeRoy EC. Increased collagen synthesis by scleroderma skin fibroblasts in vitro: a possible defect in the regulation or activation of the scleroderma fibroblast. *J Clin Invest*. 1974;54(4):880–889.

50. Moinzadeh P, Denton CP, Abraham D et al. Biomarkers for skin involvement and fibrotic activity in scleroderma. *J Eur Acad Dermatol Venereol* 2012;26(3):267–276.

51. Ihata A, Shirai A, Okubo T et al. Severity of seropositive isolated Raynaud's phenomenon is associated with serological profile. *J Rheumatol* 2000;27(7):1686–1692.

52. LeRoy EC, Medsger TA, Jr. Criteria for the classification of early systemic sclerosis. *J Rheumatol* 2001;28(7):1573–1576.

53. Denton CP, Xu S, Welsh KI, Pearson JD, Black CM. Scleroderma fibroblast phenotype is modulated by endothelial cell co-culture. *J Rheumatol* 1996;23(4):633–638.

54. Freemont AJ, Hoyland J, Fielding P, Hodson N, Jayson MI. Studies of the microvascular endothelium in uninvolved skin of patients with systemic sclerosis: direct evidence for a generalized microangiopathy. *Br J Dermatol* 1992;126(6):561–568.

55. Kraling BM, Maul GG, Jimenez SA. Mononuclear cellular infiltrates in clinically involved skin from patients with systemic sclerosis of recent onset predominantly consist of monocytes/macrophages. *Pathobiology* 1995;63(1):48–56.

56. Subcommittee for scleroderma criteria of the American Rheumatism Association Diagnostic and Therapeutic Criteria Committee. Preliminary criteria for the classification of systemic sclerosis (scleroderma). *Arthritis Rheum* 1980;23(5):581–590.

57. LeRoy EC, Black C, Fleischmajer R et al. Scleroderma (systemic sclerosis): classification, subsets and pathogenesis. *J Rheumatol* 1988;15(2):202–205.

58. Walker JG, Pope J, Baron M et al. The development of systemic sclerosis classification criteria. *Clin Rheumatol* 2007;26(9):1401–1409.

59. Nadashkevich O, Davis P, Fritzler MJ. Revising the classification criteria for systemic sclerosis. *Arthritis Rheum* 2006;55(6):992–993.

60. Bennett RM. Scleroderma overlap syndromes. *Rheum Dis Clin North Am* 1990;16(1):185–198.

61. LeRoy EC, Maricq HR, Kahaleh MB. Undifferentiated connective tissue syndromes. *Arthritis Rheum* 1980;23(3):341–343.

62. Poormoghim H, Lucas M, Fertig N, Medsger TA, Jr. Systemic sclerosis sine scleroderma: demographic, clinical, and serologic features and survival in forty-eight patients. *Arthritis Rheum* 2000;43(2):444–451.

63. Rosato E, Borghese F, Pisarri S, Salsano F. Laser Doppler perfusion imaging is useful in the study of Raynaud's phenomenon and improves the capillaroscopic diagnosis. *J Rheumatol* 2009;36(10):2257–2263.

64. Clements PJ, Lachenbruch PA, Ng SC et al. Skin score. A semiquantitative measure of cutaneous involvement that improves prediction of prognosis in systemic sclerosis. *Arthritis Rheum* 1990;33(8):1256–1263.

65. Moore TL, Lunt M, McManus B, Anderson ME, Herrick AL. Seventeen-point dermal ultrasound scoring system—a reliable measure of skin thickness in patients with systemic sclerosis. *Rheumatology* (Oxford) 2003;42(12):1559–1563.

66. Kissin EY, Schiller AM, Gelbard RB et al. Durometry for the assessment of skin disease in systemic sclerosis. *Arthritis Rheum* 2006;55(4):603–609.

67. Balbir-Gurman A, Denton CP, Nichols B et al. Non-invasive measurement of biomechanical skin properties in systemic sclerosis. *Ann Rheum Dis* 2002;61(3):237–241.

68. Enomoto DN, Mekkes JR, Bossuyt PM, Hoekzema R, Bos JD. Quantification of cutaneous sclerosis with a skin elasticity meter in patients with generalized scleroderma. *J Am Acad Dermatol* 1996;35(3 Pt 1):381–387.

69. NivesParodi M, Castagneto C, Filaci G et al. Plicometer skin test: a new technique for the evaluation of cutaneous involvement in systemic sclerosis. *Br J Rheumatol* 1997;36(2):244–250.

70. Wells AU, Steen V, Valentini G. Pulmonary complications: one of the most challenging complications of systemic sclerosis. *Rheumatology* (Oxford) 2009;48 Suppl 3:iii40–iii44.

71. Kovalchik MT, Guggenheim SJ, Silverman MH, Robertson JS, Steigerwald JC. The kidney in progressive systemic sclerosis: a prospective study. *Ann Intern Med* 1978;89(6):881–887.

72. Prescott RJ, Freemont AJ, Jones CJ, Hoyland J, Fielding P. Sequential dermal microvascular and perivascular changes in the development of scleroderma. *J Pathol* 1992;166(3):255–263.

73. Traub YM, Shapiro AP, Rodnan GP et al. Hypertension and renal failure (scleroderma renal crisis) in progressive systemic sclerosis. Review of a 25-year experience with 68 cases. *Medicine* (Baltimore) 1983;62(6):335–352.

74. Peterson LS, Nelson AM, Su WP et al. The epidemiology of morphea (localized scleroderma) in Olmsted County 1960–1993. *J Rheumatol* 1997;24(1):73–80.

75. Murray KJ, Laxer RM. Scleroderma in children and adolescents. *Rheum Dis Clin North Am* 2002;28(3):603–624.

76. Kreuter A, Krieg T, Worm M et al. [AWMF Guideline no. 013/066. Diagnosis and therapy of circumscribed scleroderma]. *J Dtsch Dermatol Ges* 2009;7 Suppl 6:S1–S14.

77. Birdi N, Shore A, Rush P et al. Childhood linear scleroderma: a possible role of thermography for evaluation. *J Rheumatol* 1992;19(6):968–973.

78. Arkachaisri T, Vilaiyuk S, Li S et al. The localized scleroderma skin severity index and physician global assessment of disease activity: a work in progress toward development of localized scleroderma outcome measures. *J Rheumatol* 2009;36(12):2819–2829.

79. Weibel L, Howell KJ, Visentin MT et al. Laser Doppler flowmetry for assessing localized scleroderma in children. *Arthritis Rheum* 2007;56(10):3489–3495.

80. Seyger MM, van den Hoogen FH, de Boo T, de Jong EM. Reliability of two methods to assess morphea: skin scoring and the use of a durometer. *J Am Acad Dermatol* 1997;37(5 Pt 1):793–796.

81. Allcock RJ, Forrest I, Corris PA, Crook PR, Griffiths ID. A study of the prevalence of systemic sclerosis in northeast England. *Rheumatology* (Oxford) 2004;43(5):596–602.

82. Hamaguchi Y. Autoantibody profiles in systemic sclerosis: predictive value for clinical evaluation and prognosis. *J Dermatol* 2010;37(1):42–53.

83. Bottini N, Musumeci L, Alonso A et al. A functional variant of lymphoid tyrosine phosphatase is associated with type I diabetes. *Nat Genet*. 2004;36(4):337–338.

84. Watford WT, Hissong BD, Bream JH et al. Signaling by IL-12 and IL-23 and the immunoregulatory roles of STAT4. *Immunol Rev*. 2004;202:139–156.

85. Allanore Y, Dieude P, Boileau C. Updating the genetics of systemic sclerosis. *Curr Opin Rheumatol* 2010;22(6):665–670.

86. Cutolo M, Pizzorni C, Secchi ME, Sulli A. Capillaroscopy. *Best Pract Res Clin Rheumatol* 2008;22(6):1093–1108.

87. Filaci G, Cutolo M, Scudeletti M et al. Cyclosporin A and iloprost treatment of systemic sclerosis: clinical results and interleukin-6 serum changes after 12 months of therapy. *Rheumatology* (Oxford) 1999;38(10):992–996.

88. van den Hoogen FH, Boerbooms AM, Swaak AJ et al. Comparison of methotrexate with placebo in the treatment of systemic sclerosis: a 24 week randomized double-blind trial, followed by a 24 week observational trial. *Br J Rheumatol* 1996;35(4):364–372.

89. Pope JE, Bellamy N, Seibold JR et al. A randomized, controlled trial of methotrexate versus placebo in early diffuse scleroderma. *Arthritis Rheum* 2001;44(6):1351–1358.

90. Das SN, Alam MR, Islam N et al. Placebo controlled trial of methotrexate in systemic sclerosis. *Mymensingh Med J* 2005;14(1):71–74.

91. Tashkin DP, Elashoff R, Clements PJ et al. Cyclophosphamide versus placebo in scleroderma lung disease. *N Engl J Med* 2006;354(25):2655–2666.

92. Nadashkevich O, Davis P, Fritzler M, Kovalenko W. A randomized unblinded trial of cyclophosphamide versus azathioprine in the treatment of systemic sclerosis. *Clin Rheumatol* 2006;25(2):205–212.

CHAPTER 122

Paediatric scleroderma and related disorders

Francesco Zulian

Juvenile systemic sclerosis

Introduction

Juvenile systemic sclerosis (JSSc) is a chronic, multisystem connective tissue disease characterized by sclerodermatous skin changes and widespread abnormalities of the viscera.

According to 1980 classification criteria of the American College of Rheumatology (ACR),[1] definite SSc requires the presence either of the major criterion (fibrosis/induration involving areas proximal to the metacarpophalangeal (MCP) or metatarsophalangeal (MTP) joints) or of two minor criteria (sclerodactyly, digital pitting scars, bibasilar pulmonary fibrosis). Subsequently, the widespread use of nailfold capillary microscopy, the discovery of SSc-specific autoantibodies and the early detection of Raynaud's phenomenon in patients who, years later, developed SSc, have raised the need for a more comprehensive classification.

Recently, an ad-hoc International Committee on Classification Criteria for Juvenile Systemic Sclerosis, following an evidence-dased and consensus-based methodology, developed new classification criteria for this rare paediatric disease.[2] According to these criteria, a patient aged less than 16 years, is classified as having JSSc if the one major (presence of skin sclerosis/induration proximal to MCP or MTP joint) and at least two of the 20 minor criteria listed in Box 122.1 are present.

Epidemiology

Onset of SSc in childhood is uncommon. A recent study from the United Kingdom reported an annual incidence rate of 0.27 per million children under the age of 16 years.[3] It has been estimated that approximately 3% of all patients had onset in childhood, and patients aged 10–20 years account for only 1.2–9% of all cases.[4]

JSSc occurs with equal frequency in boys and girls younger than 8 years old, whereas girls outnumber boys 3 to 1 when disease onset occurs in children who are older than 8 years.[5]

Aetiology and pathogenesis

The cause of diffuse SSc is unknown, despite significant advances in understanding of potential pathogenetic mechanisms. The disease can be represented as a tripartite process in which dysfunction of the immune system, endothelium, and fibroblasts gives rise to a heterogeneous phenotype that is characterized prominently by fibrosis. Since both aetiology and pathogenesis are similar to the more common adult disease the reader is referred to Chapter 121 for a detailed description.

Genetic background

The familial occurrence of JSSc is very rare, as confirmed by few case reports in which first-degree relatives of the same family were affected.[6] Just one report described JSSc monozygotic twins.[7]

Microchimerism, defined as the presence within one individual of cells derived from a different individual, was postulated as a possible cause of scleroderma. Microchimerism occurs in women who had previous pregnancies, individuals who have had blood transfusions, and children with cells from the mother or a twin. Maternal cells can persist in an immunocompetent offspring even in adult life, and fetus-derived haemopoietic cells may persist in the maternal circulation for many years postpartum. In scleroderma, circulating chimeric cells are increased in number[8] and have been described also in sclerodermatous skin.[9] These findings support the hypothesis that fetal anti-maternal graft-vs-host reactions might be involved in the pathogenesis of SSc,[10] but cannot explain the occurrence of scleroderma in men or in women who have never had children.

Clinical manifestations

Early signs and symptoms

Onset of the disease is usually insidious and the course prolonged. Generally, in children SSc may have two possible evolutions: a few children have a rapid development of internal organ failure leading to severe disability and eventually to death, whereas other patients experience a slow, insidious course of the disease with lower mortality.[11] The onset is often characterized by the development of isolated Raynaud's phenomenon which is usually associated with positive antinuclear antigens (ANA) and capillariscopy changes. Months or years later, tightening of the skin, especially of fingers and face, appearance of cutaneous telangiectases and symptoms related to internal organs involvement gradually develop.[5] Because of the subtle nature of this presentation, there is often a diagnostic delay of years.

The main signs and symptoms of JSSc are summarized in Table 122.1.

Box 122.1 PRES/ACR/EULAR provisional classification criteria for juvenile systemic sclerosis

Major criterion

Proximal sclerosis/induration of the skin

Minor criteria

Skin

◆ Sclerodactyly

Vascular

◆ Raynaud's phenomenon

◆ Nailfold capillary abnormalities

◆ Digital tip ulcers

Gastrointestinal

◆ Dysphagia

◆ Gastro-oesophageal reflux

Renal

● Renal crisis

◆ New-onset arterial hypertension

Cardiac

◆ Arrhythmias

◆ Heart failure

Respiratory

◆ Pulmonary fibrosis (HRCT/chest radiograph)

◆ DL_{CO}

◆ Pulmonary hypertension

Muskuloskeletal

◆ Tendon friction rubs

◆ Arthritis

◆ Myositis

Neurological

◆ Neuropathy

◆ Carpal tunnel syndrome

Serology

◆ Anti-nuclear antibodies

◆ SSc selective autoantibodies (anti-centromere, anti-topoisomerase I, anti-fibrillarin, anti-PM-Scl, anti-fibrillin. or anti-RNA polymerase I or III)

A patient aged less than 16 years is classified as having juvenile systemic sclerosis if the one major and at least two of the 20 minor criteria are present. This set of classification criteria has a sensitivity of 90%, a specificity of 96%, and a kappa statistic value of 0.86.

Adapted from Zulian et al.[2]

Table 122.1 Clinical features of juvenile systemic sclerosis at the time of diagnosis and during the overall course of the disease

	At diagnosis (%)	Overall course (%)
Skin		
Sclerodactily	45.8	66.0
Skin induration	73.9	82.4
Calcinosis	9.3	18.5
Peripheral vascular system		
Raynaud's phenomenon	74.7	84.2
Digital infarcts	18.8	28.9
Digital pitting	28.0	38.0
Abnormal capillaroscopy	24.7	51.7
Respiratory system		
Dyspnoea	9.9	17.9
Abnormal chest radiograph	12.1	28.9
Abnormal chest HRCT	4.7	23.0
Reduced DL_{CO}	8.0	26.7
Cardiac involvement		
Pericardial effusion	5.2	9.8
Heart failure	2.0	7.3
Pulmonary hypertension	1.3	7.2
Musculoskeletal system		
Muscle weakness	12.0	24.3
Arthritis	17.3	27.0
Arthralgia	26.4	36.0
Tendon friction rubs	5.6	11.3
Gastrointestinal system		
Dysphagia	9.9	23.7
Gastro-oesophageal reflux	8.0	30.0
Diarrhoea	1.3	9.9
Weight loss	18.0	27.2
Renal system		
Raised creatinine/proteinuria	3.3	5.2
Renal crisis	0.0	0.7
Hypertension	1.3	2.6
Nervous system		
Peripheral neuropathy	0.6	0.6
Abnormal brain MRI	1.9	2.6

Adapted from Martini et al.[5]

Skin disease

Cutaneous changes characteristically evolve in a sequence beginning with oedema, followed by induration resulting in marked tightening and contractures, and eventually atrophy.

During the sclerotic phase, the skin develops a waxy texture and becomes tight and bound to subcutaneous structures. This is particularly noticeable in skin of the dorsal surface of the digits, so-called sclerodactyly (Figure 122.1), and face; the characteristic expressionless, unwrinkled appearance of the skin may be the first clue to the diagnosis (Figure 122.2). These superficial abnormalities result in a shiny appearance of the skin accompanied by areas of hypo- or hyperpigmentation.

Telangiectases of the periungual nailfold is often the early location, and examination with an ophthalmoscope demonstrates capillary dropout, tortuous dilated loops, and occasionally distorted capillary architecture. Digital pitting, sometimes with ulceration and gangrene, occurs in the pulp of the fingertips as a result of ischaemia (Figure 122.3). Subcutaneous calcification, especially over the elbows, MCP joints, and knees, may occur, sometimes with ulceration of surrounding skin.

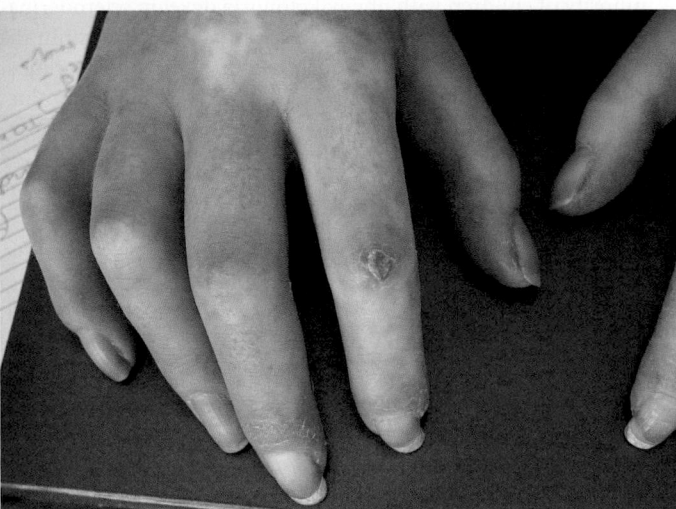

Fig. 122.1 Sclerodactyly in juvenile scleroderma.

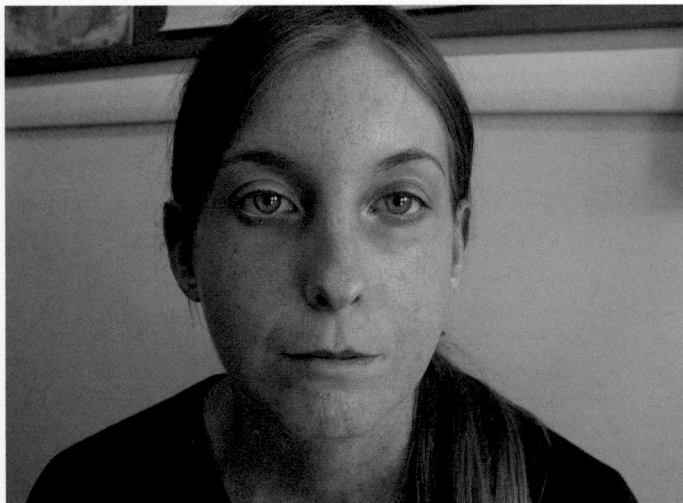

Fig. 122.2 Unwrinkled facial skin in early juvenile scleroderma.

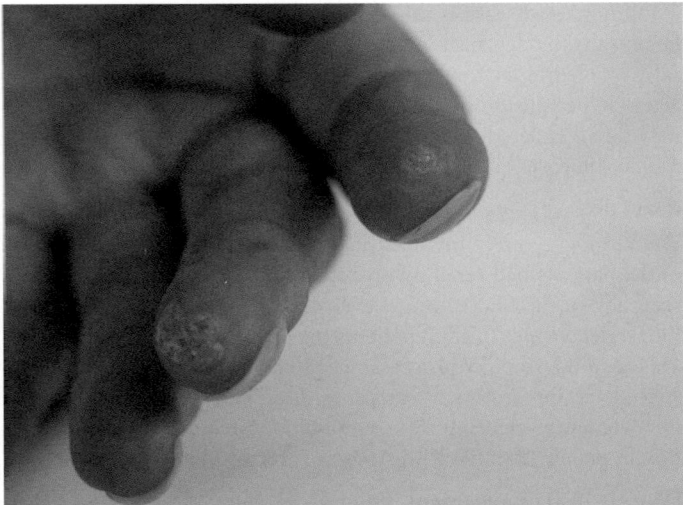

Fig. 122.3 Typical digital pits indicating ischaemia in scleroderma.

As already stated, Raynaud's phenomenon represents the first manifestation of the disease in 70% of children with JSSc preceding other manifestations, in some instances, by years.[12] During the overall course of the disease, Raynaud's phenomenon is also the most frequently reported symptom being present in 90% of children. In 10% it is complicated by digital infarcts.[5,12]

Musculoskeletal disease

Musculoskeletal symptoms characteristically occur at or near onset of the disease in one-third of children with JSS.[5] Morning stiffness, arthralgias, and arthritis are often the initial manifestations of the disease.

Joint contractures of insidious onset and limitation of motion are most common at the proximal interphalangeal (PIP) joints and elbows, but other joints can be affected. Muscle inflammation characterized by pain and tenderness occurs in up to one-fifth of children.

Gastrointestinal disease

Symptomatic gastrointestinal involvement affects around one-third of the patients but is much more frequent if the diagnosis is made instrumentally (barium swallow, scintigraphy, etc.).[5,12] Lesions of the mouth include mucosal telangiectases, reduced maxima mouth opening caused by skin thickening and tightness and, rarely, parotitis as part of the sicca syndrome. Although the oesophagus is involved, often quite early in the disease, many patients are asymptomatic and rarely present as heartburn with postural aggravation or dysphagia. Small-bowel involvement usually develops in association with oesophageal or colonic disease. Malabsorptive diarrhoea and delayed colonic transit, when present, reflect long-standing disease. Large-bowel disease is also often asymptomatic but may sometimes cause severe constipation, bloating, or diarrhoea.

Cardiopulmonary disease

The involvement of the cardiopulmonary system is the leading cause of morbidity and mortality.[11,13] Pericardial effusions are usually small and asymptomatic, although fever and retrosternal pain may accompany acute disease. Severe cardiomyopathy is rare, although it can be one of the causes of early death and require prompt and aggressive immunosuppressive treatment.[13]

Cardiac ischaemia may result from the equivalent of Raynaud's phenomenon of the coronary arteries and is a potential precursor of myocardial fibrosis.

Pulmonary disease is initially asymptomatic but later on it may be revealed by dry, hacking cough or dyspnoea on exertion and by rales or pleural friction rubs on physical examination. Pulmonary artery hypertension occurs in 7% of JSSc patients and, as in adults, may be an isolated vascular complication or consequence of pulmonary fibrosis.[5,12]

Renal disease

The kidney is rarely involved in JSSc. In the Padua database, 5% of the patients had renal involvement as increased urinary protein secretion or raised creatinine level, and only one patient developed renal crisis.[5] Since in adult patients the presence of anti-topoisomerase I antibody, rapidly progressing skin involvement, and high-dose steroids are predictors of early and often severe renal and cardiac involvement,[14] close monitoring of blood pressure and renal function in patients treated with steroids is recommended.

Neurological involvement

The rare neurological involvement consists of cranial neuropathy, especially of the sensory branch of the trigeminal nerve, or peripheral neuropathies.[5,15] Involvement of the central nervous system (CNS), as hypertensive encephalopathy, is usually a reflection of renal or pulmonary disease.

Differences from adult disease

As compared with adults, at diagnosis, children show a significantly less frequent involvement of all organs, except for the prevalence of arthritis which is equally frequent.[5,12,16] Differences from adults become less evident during follow-up with the exception of interstitial lung involvement, gastroesophageal dysmotility, and renal involvement which are significantly much more common in adults. Arthritis and muscle inflammation are slightly more common in children.[7] The limited cutaneous form, which is by far the most frequent in adults, is rare in children. It is possible that this subset may be underdiagnosed because young children with just isolated Raynaud's phenomenon and capillaroscopy changes are diagnosed during adolescence or early adulthood when the other typical features appear.

Differential diagnosis

Because JSSc usually involves internal organs, muscles, and skin, the differential diagnosis includes many disorders such as juvenile dermatomyositis mixed connective tissue disease, and other undifferentiated connective tissue diseases. In the following section the most common non-rheumatological conditions which enter into the differential diagnosis with JSSc are described.

Chronic graft-vs-host disease

Chronic graft-vs-host disease (GVHD) is a complication of allogeneic bone marrow transplantation for the treatment of marrow aplasia, leukaemia, or malignant diseases. GVHD results from the interaction between immunocompetent T lymphocytes from the donor and host cells bearing histocompatibility antigens that are recognized as foreign. The resulting scleroderma-like disease may follow acute GVHD or occur de novo up to 100 days after transplantation. It is characterized by dermatitis, usually beginning with erythema of the face, palms, soles and followed by hyper- or hypopigmentation. A hidebound skin and extreme tightening of the tendons and periarticular structures may severely limit motion. The histology in GVHD and SSc is similar but not identical.[17] Recent modifications of the chemotherapeutic preparation of the graft recipient have reduced the incidence of this complication.

Chemically induced scleroderma-like disease

Several chemicals have been implicated in the induction of scleroderma.[18] Bleomycin, an antineoplastic agent, causes skin changes resembling scleroderma and pulmonary fibrosis. This syndrome is not accompanied by Raynaud's phenomenon and may improve on cessation of the drug. Pentazocine, a non-narcotic analgesic drug, has been reported to cause cutaneous sclerosis with or without ulceration.[18]

The toxic oil syndrome, caused by ingestion of rapeseed cooking oil that contained unidentified contaminants, occurred in epidemic proportions in Spain in the early 1980s, and indications are that complications have been less severe in children.[19] The onset of the disease was characterized by fever, eosinophilia, dyspnoea caused by pulmonary oedema, a pruritic rash, and malaise. Scleroderma-like changes, involving both skin and internal organs, evolved over a period of months.

Phenylketonuria

A minority of children with phenylketonuria develop sclerodermatous skin lesions.[20] These lesions, which usually appear within the first year of life, are symmetric, poorly demarcated, and occur most frequently on the lower extremities and trunk. After the introduction of newborn metabolic screening in many countries, this complication has almost completely disappeared.

Syndromes of premature ageing

Two rare autosomal recessive disorders accompanied by dwarfing, premature ageing, and early death from atherosclerotic heart disease are associated with sclerodermatous skin changes. In **progeria**, the cutaneous changes usually develop before 1 year of age and are characterized by thickened, bound-down skin on the abdomen, flanks, proximal thighs, and upper buttocks (Figure 122.4).[21] During the second year of life, the skin becomes thinner, subcutaneous vascularization is more evident, and alopecia and nail dystrophy develop. **Werner's syndrome** most often presents in adolescence with generalized atrophy of muscle and subcutaneous tissue, greying of the hair, baldness, and scleroderma-like skin changes and ulcers involving the extremities.[22]

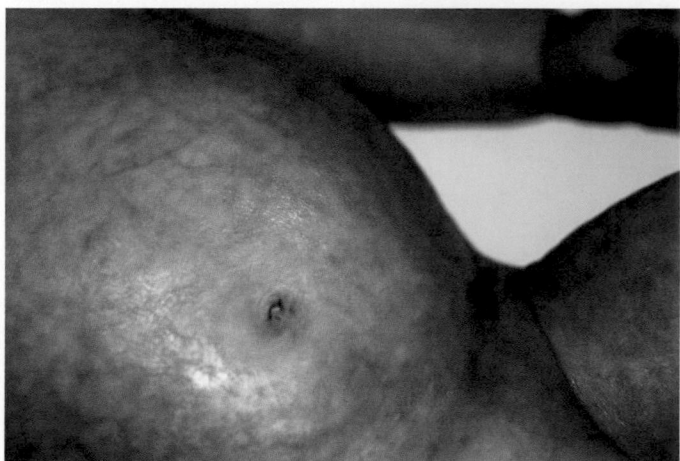

Fig. 122.4 Generalized trunkal sceroderma.

Scleroedema

Scleroedema is characterized by edematous induration of the face, neck, shoulders, thorax, and proximal extremities, but not the hands.[23] It usually follows β-haemolytic streptococcal infection with insidious onset and spontaneous resolution after 6–12 months. Dysphagia may be present, but Raynaud's phenomenon and telangiectases are not. Histologically, the dermis is thickened; there are multiple fenestrations between swollen collagen bundles, a scant perivascular lymphocytic infiltrate, and minimal deposits of acid mucopolysaccharides.

Autoantibodies

High-titre ANA are frequently present from the disease onset. The predominant patterns on HEp-2 cell substrate are speckled and nucleolar. ANA seropositivity in two large paediatric series was 81–97%, which is slightly lower than that reported in adults.[5,12] Anti-topoisomerase I (anti-Scl-70) autoantibodies are present in 28–34% of patients, while the prevalence of anti-centromere antibodies is lower in children than in adults (7% vs 23%).[5,16]

Anti-PM-Scl and anti-U1RNP antibodies correlate with scleroderma in overlap syndromes with muskuloskeletal involvement. Anti-RNA-polymerase III antibody is very unusual, in parallel with the rarity of renal involvement in JSSc.[12]

The frequency of rheumatoid factor (RF) and anti-cardiolipin antibodies (aCL) is similar in adults and children with SSc (RF17% vs 23%; aCL14.8% vs 10%).[5,16]

Clinical assessment and monitoring

Assessment of disease activity and severity in JSSc is difficult. For organ-based complications such as cardiac abnormalities, pulmonary fibrosis, pulmonary hypertension, or renal involvement, objective assessment is possible.

Electrocardiographic abnormalities include first-degree heart block, right and left bundle branch block, premature atrial and ventricular contractions, and non-specific T-wave changes. The most frequent cardiac arrhythmias in children are supraventricular, whereas ventricular arrhythmias do not occur very often.[24] Echocardiographic abnormalities in addition to pericardial effusions include thickening of the left ventricular wall and decreased left ventricular compliance. The two-dimensional echocardiogram is important in confirming early pulmonary hypertension by documentation of a dilated right ventricle with thickening of the ventricular wall and straightening of the septum. Right heart catheterization provides definitive confirmation but is often unnecessary.

Characteristic findings of respiratory tract involvement include a decrease in timed vital capacity (FVC) and forced expiratory flow (FEV), and decrease in CO diffusion (DL_{CO}).[25] Radiographic changes on chest radiograph correlate poorly with pulmonary function. High-resolution CT (HRCT) may confirm pulmonary disease despite a normal chest radiograph. In children, the most frequent HRCT findings are ground-glass opacification, subpleural micronodules, linear opacities, and honeycombing.[26]

Gastrointestinal involvement can be assessed by cine-oesophagogram that may document decreased or absent peristalsis in the lower part of the oesophagus with distal dilatation and, frequently, stricture and shortening of the oesophagus. Oesophageal motility studies by manometry and pH probe monitoring of the distal oesophagus for 12–24 hours provide more sensitive indicators of diminished lower sphincter tone and the presence of reflux.[27]

Skin involvement can be quantified by the modified Rodnan skin score (MRSS). The role of capillaroscopy in children is similar to that of adults and is discussed further elsewhere (Chapter 121).

A multidimensional severity score, named "J4S", an acronym which stays for Juvenile Systemic Sclerosis Severity Score, including growth parameters, skin and internal organs involvement has been recently reported[28] This is a simple instrument to assess disease severity in JSSc which includes nine clinical categories, scored from 0 to 8, weighting various organ involvements on the basis of their clinical importance. J4S may have several applications for the pediatric age group since it can be used, in daily clinical practice, to guide decision-making, to compare study populations and to identify potentially reversible aspects of the disease.

Treatment

The pharmacological management of patients with JSSc is challenging since no drug has been shown to be of unequivocal benefit in either children or adults with systemic sclerosis (Figure 122.5). Recently, an European League Against Rheumatism (EULAR) task force, including paediatric rheumatologists, has proposed some recommendations for the management of SSc.[29] As first-line therapy for Raynaud's phenomenon, calcium channel blockers, such as nifedipine or nicardipine, should be considered. For severe Raynaud's phenomenon with ischaemic digits or digital ulcers, iloprost, or other available intravenously delivered prostanoids, should be used.[30,31] Cyclophosphamide represents the drug of choice for the treatment of interstitial lung disease and, according to the experience in juvenile systemic lupus erythematosus (SLE), it should be administered as intravenous pulse therapy at a dosage of 0.5–1 g/m² every 4 weeks for at least 6 months.[32] To prevent cystitis, adequate hydration and frequent voiding must be emphasized.

Glucocorticoids, preferably prednisone at a dosage of 0.3–0.5 mg/kg per day, should be reserved for the treatment of myositis, arthritis, and tenosynovitis. Since several studies suggest that steroids are associated with a higher risk of scleroderma renal crisis, blood pressure and renal function should be carefully monitored. Methotrexate has been shown to improves skin score in early diffuse SSc in adults.[33] Accordingly, methotrexate should be the treatment of choice for the skin manifestations also for JSSc, especially in the early phase. With the same indication, mycophenolate mofetil may be a good alternative to methotrexate, especially in refractory disease or in case of intolerance[34].

Symptomatic treatments are essentially based on the principle of good clinical practice and include the use of proton pump inhibitors, such as omeprazole and lansoprazole, for prevention of gastroesophageal reflux disease and oesophageal ulcers; the use of prokinetic drugs, such as domperidone, for the management of symptomatic motility disturbances; and rotating antibiotics, such as metronidazole, ciprofloxacin, and doxycycline, to treat malabsorption due to bacterial overgrowth. Angiotensin converting enzyme (ACE) inhibitors (e.g. captopril, losartan) are effective for the long-term control of blood pressure and stabilization of renal function of scleroderma renal crisis.[35] With regard to new experimental drugs, such as bosentan and sildenafil for pulmonary arterial hypertension and digital ulcers, the paediatric experience is encouraging although still anecdotal.[36,37]

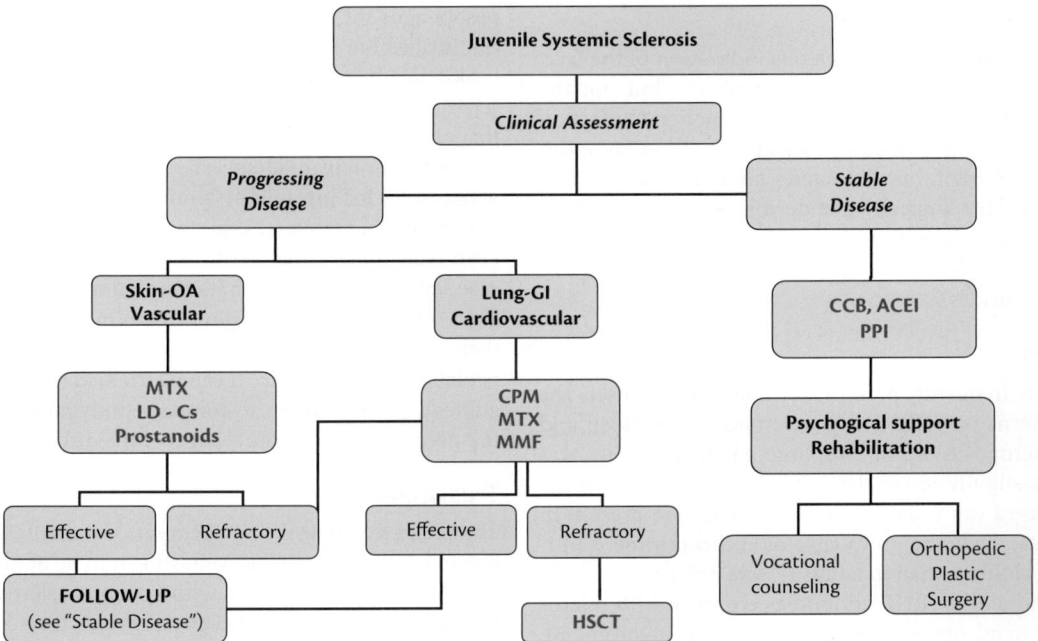

Fig. 122.5 Proposed flowchart for the management of juvenile systemic sclerosis.

One of the most innovative although aggressive approaches to therapy is immunoablation followed by reconstitution with autologous haemopoietic stem cell transplantation (HSCT). The rationale for this therapy is the ablation of self-reactive lymphocyte clones to block the autoimmune process. Recent studies reported that HSCT improved the skin score for 69% of patients, did not affect lung function, but halted pulmonary hypertension.[38] However, disease progression occurred in 19%, and 17% died of complications related to the procedure.[38] Because of this high mortality rate, HSCT should be carefully considered for paediatric patients, and it may only be a rational therapy early in the disease course before irreversible damage has resulted.

Course of the disease and prognosis

The ultimate prognosis of the child with JSSc depends primarily on the extent of visceral involvement. Skin tightness and joint contractures inevitably lead to severe disability. Cardiac arrhythmias may result from myocardial fibrosis and congestive heart failure is often a terminal event. Pulmonary interstitial disease and vascular lesions are probably universal, even if not clinically evident. Renal failure or acute hypertensive encephalopathy supervenes as a potentially fatal outcome in a few children. Nevertheless, the overall prognosis of SSc in children appears better than in adults. The survival of childhood-onset SSc at 5, 10, 15 and 20 years after diagnosis is 89%, 80–87.4%, 74–87.4%, and 69–82.5%, respectively—significantly higher than in adult-onset disease.[11,39] Death in JSSc is usually related to the involvement of cardiac, renal, and pulmonary systems.[11] Cardiomyopathy early in the disease course is rare and usually associated with diffuse cutaneous disease and features of polymyositis. An aggressive immunosuppressive treatment has been shown to be effective on muscle, skin, and lung involvement but hardly impairs progression of myocardial dysfunction.[11,13]

Localized sclerodermas

Localized sclerodermas are a group of disorders whose manifestations are confined to the skin and subdermal tissues and, with some exceptions, do not affect internal organs. There is no accepted uniform terminology; dermatologists typically use the term 'morphoea' and rheumatologists tend to use the term 'localized scleroderma' to refer to the same group of conditions.

Definition and classification

Localized scleroderma (LS) includes a number of conditions that are often grouped together. The classification used most widely currently includes five subtypes: circumscribed morphoea, linear scleroderma, generalized morphoea, pansclerotic morphoea, and the new mixed subtype where a combination of two or more of the previous subtypes is present (Table 122.2).[40]

- **Circumscribed morphoea** (CM) is characterized by oval or round circumscribed areas of induration with a central waxy, ivory colour surrounded by a violaceous halo (Figure 122.6). The superficial variety is usually confined to the dermis. Very rarely lesions are small, less than 1 cm in diameter (guttate). In the deep variety the entire skin feels thickened, taut, and bound down, and the primary site of involvement is the panniculus or subcutaneous tissue. CM lesions occur most frequently on the trunk and less often on the extremities or face.

- **Generalized morphoea**: This term is used when four or more individual plaques larger than 3 cm become confluent, involving at least two out of seven anatomical sites (head–neck, right upper extremity, left upper extremity, right lower extremity, left lower extremity, anterior trunk, posterior trunk) (Figure 122.7).

- **Linear scleroderma** is the most common subtype in children and adolescents.[41] It is characterized by one or more linear

Table 122.2 Preliminary classification of juvenile localized scleroderma

Type	Subtype	Features
1. Circumscribed morphea	(a) Superficial	Oval or round circumscribed areas of induration limited to epidermis and dermis, often with altered pigmentation and violaceous, erythematous halo (lilac ring). The lesions can be single or multiple
	(b) Deep	Oval or round circumscribed deep induration of the skin involving subcutaneous tissue extending to fascia and underlying muscle. The lesions can be single or multiple
		Sometimes the primary site of involvement is in the subcutaneous tissue without involvement of the skin
2. Linear scleroderma	(a) Trunk/limbs	Linear induration involving dermis, subcutaneous tissue and, sometimes, muscle and underlying bone and affecting the limbs and/or the trunk
	(b) Head	*En coup de sabre (ECDS)*—linear induration of the skin that affects the face and/or the scalp and sometimes involves muscle and underlying bone
		Parry–Romberg or progressive hemifacial athrophy—loss of tissue on one side of the face that may involve dermis, subcutaneous tissue, muscle. and bone. The skin is unaffected and mobile
3. Generalized morphoea		Induration of the skin starting as individual plaques (4 or more, >3 cm) that become confluent and involve at least two anatomical sites
4. Pansclerotic morphoea		Circumferential involvement of limb(s) affecting the skin, subcutaneous tissue, muscle and bone. The lesion may also involve other areas of the body without internal organ involvement
5. Mixed morphoea		Combination of two or more of the previous subtypes. The order of the concomitant subtypes, specified in brackets, follows their predominant representation in the individual patient, e.g. 'mixed (linear-circumscribed)'

Adapted from Laxer and Zulian.[40]

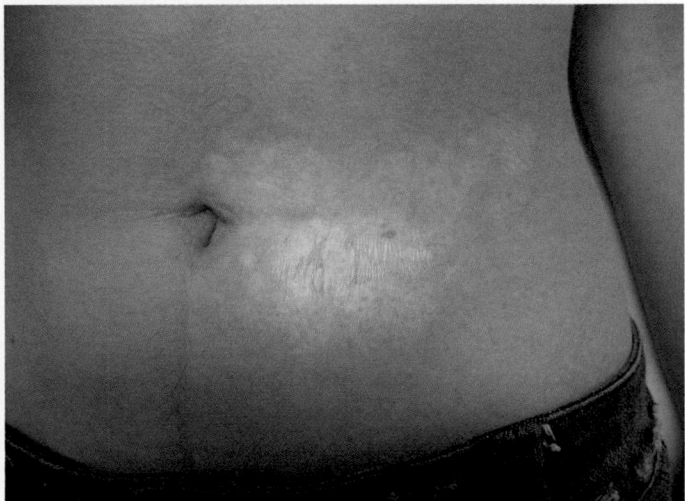
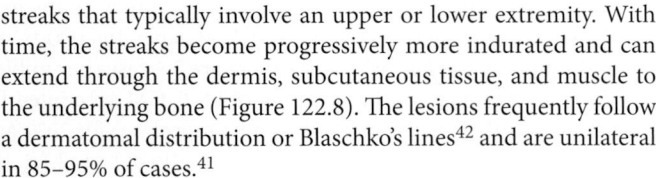

Fig. 122.6 Circumscribed morphoea.

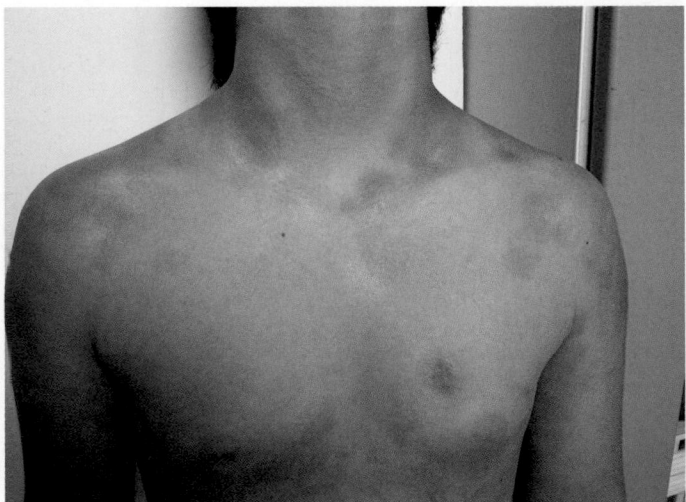

Fig. 122.7 Generalized morphoea.

streaks that typically involve an upper or lower extremity. With time, the streaks become progressively more indurated and can extend through the dermis, subcutaneous tissue, and muscle to the underlying bone (Figure 122.8). The lesions frequently follow a dermatomal distribution or Blaschko's lines[42] and are unilateral in 85–95% of cases.[41]

– The face or scalp may also be involved, as in the **en coup de sabre** (ECDS) variety. This term was applied historically because the lesion was reminiscent of the depression caused by a sword wound (Figure 122.9).

– The **Parry–Romberg syndrome** (PRS), characterized by a progressive hemifacial atrophy of the skin and tissue below the forehead, with mild or absent involvement of the superficial skin, is considered the severe end of the spectrum of ECDS

and for this reason included in the linear head subtype.[40,43] Evidence for this close relationship is the presence of associated disorders, including seizures and dental and ocular abnormalities, reported with similar prevalence in both conditions.[43]

In both circumscribed and linear morphoea subtypes, deep variants where the entire skin feels thickened, taut, and bound down can be present.[40]

◆ **Pansclerotic morphoea** is an extremely rare but severe disorder characterized by generalized full-thickness involvement of the skin of the trunk, extremities, face, and scalp with the sparing of the fingertips and toes (Figure 122.10).[44] The involvement of the entire body without internal organ involvement helps differentiate this from SSc. Recent reports have raised awareness of the possible evolution of chronic ulcers, frequently complicating

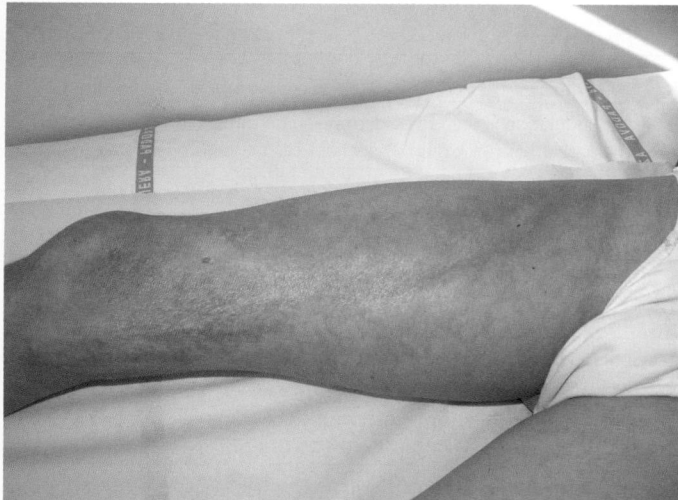

Fig. 122.8 Linear scleroderma.

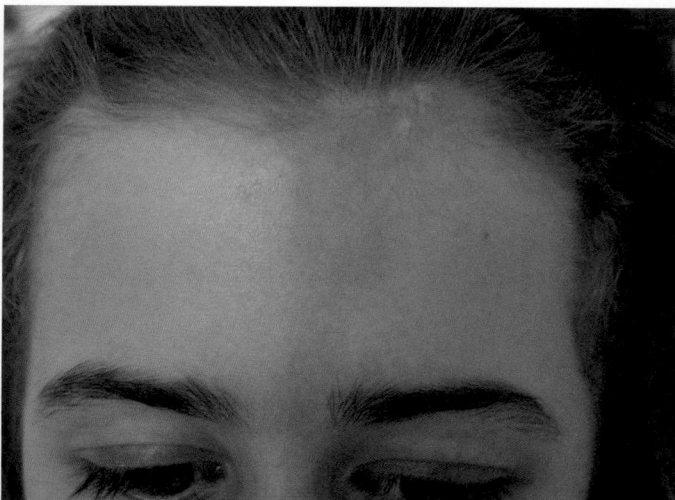

Fig. 122.9 Linear scleroderma 'en coup de sabre'.

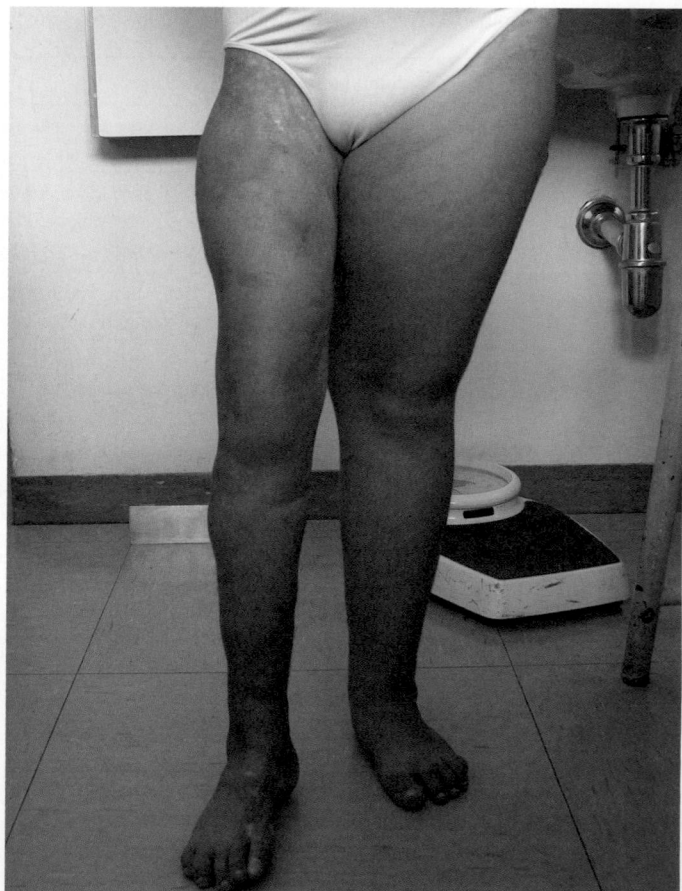

Fig. 122.10 Pansclerotic morphoea.

pansclerotic morphoea, to squamous cell carcinoma, a threatening complication already reported in SSc.[45,46]

◆ The **mixed subtype** results from a combination of two or more of the previous subtypes. The order of the concomitant subtypes, specified in brackets, follows their predominant representation in the individual patient, e.g. 'mixed (linear-circumscribed)'.[40]

Associated conditions

Other disorders not included in the more recent classification of LS can precede, follow, or be concomitant with LS.

◆ **Lichen sclerosus et atrophicus** is characterized by shiny white plaques often preceded by violaceous discoloration with some predilection for the anogenital area, wrists, and ankles. The superficial layers of the skin are usually involved.

◆ **Atrophoderma of Pasini and Pierini** is characterized by asymptomatic hyperpigmented atrophic patches usually on the trunk with well-demarcated borders. These lesions usually represent the end stage of LS.

◆ **Bullous morphoea** is a very rare subtype characterized by bullous lesions possibly resulting from a localized trauma or related to lymphatic obstruction from the sclerodermatous process.[47]

◆ In **eosinophilic fasciitis** the fascia is the predominant site of involvement.[48] The lesions typically involve the extremities, spare the hands and feet, and have an appearance that is described as 'peau d'orange'. Hypergammaglobulinemia and eosinophilia are often present.

Epidemiology

LS is more frequent than SSc but still a rare condition. In the general population the incidence of LS is 2.7 cases per 100 000,[49] and in children under the age of 16 years there are 3.4 cases per million per year.[3] In a population-based study of LS,[49] CM accounted for 56%, generalized morphoea for 13%, linear morphoea for 20%, and deep morphoea for 11%. The female-to-male ratio of LS is 2.4:1, the mean age at onset is approximately 7.3 years,[4] and there are no differences in the various LS subtypes.[41] The disease can start as early as at birth.[50] It can be misdiagnosed as skin infection, naevus, or salmon patch and this may lead to a consistent delay in diagnosis.

Aetiology and pathogenesis

The cause and pathogenesis of LS are unknown. Abnormalities of the immune system, regulation of fibroblasts, and production of collagen represent the most important points investigated by experimental studies. Multiple studies have demonstrated increased levels of cytokines and other molecules that influence fibroblasts and collagen synthesis.[51] Autoimmunity, environmental factors, infection, and trauma have all been associated with localized disease. It seems certain that autoimmunity plays an important role because of the multiplicity of abnormal serum antibodies that occurs in patients with LS and because of the association of similar cutaneous abnormalities in patients with chronic GVHD.[52]

The clinical and histopathological similarities of LS to chronic GVHD have suggested that non-self cells or chimerism may be involved in the pathogenesis of the disease.[53] A large number of chimeric infiltrating cells, mainly epithelial or dendritic cells, have been found in biopsies of LS patients.

Some drugs and environmental toxins have resulted in scleroderma-like reactions, including bleomycin, ergot, bromocriptine, pentazocine, carbidopa, and vitamin K_1.[54]

A few studies have examined a putative association of LS and *Borrelia burgdorferi*, the spirochete that causes Lyme disease. Many studies have documented evidence of infection with *B. burgdorferi* in patients with morphoea who live in areas endemic for Lyme disease, or have a history of tick bites.[55] This was not confirmed in patients with morphoea who do not live in endemic areas.[56] Trauma has been implicated in the initiation of lesions and particularly with the onset of eosinophilic fasciitis.[41,57]

Extracutaneous manifestations

One-fifth of patients with LS present extracutaneous manifestations and 4% of them may have multiple features.[58] Extracutaneous findings are more frequent in patients with linear scleroderma and consist essentially of arthritis (19%), neurological findings (4%), or other autoimmune conditions (3%). In these patients, organ impairment is milder and not life-threatening compared to SSc.

Articular involvement is the most frequent extracutaneous feature, and is more common in patients with linear scleroderma. The joint involved may be completely unrelated to the site of the skin lesion. Children with LS who develop arthritis often have a positive RF,[41] and sometimes an elevated erythrocyte sedimentation rate (ESR).

The most frequent neurological conditions are seizures and headaches, although behavioural changes and learning disabilities also have been described.[58,59] Abnormalities seen on MRI, such as calcifications, white matter changes, vascular malformations, and changes consistent with CNS vasculitis, also have been reported.[60] Gastro-oesophageal reflux is the only gastrointestinal complication reported so far.[61] In a cohort of 14 consecutive patients, oesophageal involvement was found in 8 (57%), 7 had pathological pH test findings, and in 4 of them, concomitant oesophageal dysmotility was also present.[61]

Ocular involvement has been reported in 3.2% of patients affected by LS.[62] As expected, two-thirds of patients with ocular manifestations have the ECDS subtype but, interestingly, the other third have no facial skin lesion. The most frequent lesions (42%) are on eyelids and eyelashes; one-third consists of anterior segment inflammation, such as anterior uveitis or episcleritis, the remaining are mainly CNS-related abnormalities. Although extracutaneous manifestations should be considered on every patient with LS, routine screening for internal organ manifestations (other than uveitis in linear scleroderma of the face) is generally not recommended.

Differential diagnosis

LS should be differentiated from systemic disease. In the most common form, linear scleroderma, the lesions are discrete, limited to a single extremity, and easily differentiated from SSc. The more difficult diagnostic challenge is to differentiate SSc from the diffuse and deep forms, such as pansclerotic morphoea. These patients, in contrast to those with SSc, rarely have Raynaud's phenomenon and do not develop symptomatic evidence of internal organ involvement. Occasionally, the deep forms of LS may be confused with juvenile idiopathic arthritis in that they can manifest with contractures of the hands, arthralgias, and sometimes synovitis and may have a positive RF test result. In cases such as these, further testing may document the presence of anti-histone antibodies, hypergammaglobulinaemia, and eosinophilia typical of the deep varieties of LS.

Laboratory findings

The diagnosis of LS is established on clinical grounds; no laboratory abnormality is diagnostic. Routine laboratory tests such as a complete blood cell count, blood chemistries, and urinalysis are normal. The acute-phase reactants, ESR and C-reactive protein (CRP), are usually within the normal ranges with the exception of the deep subtypes in which eosinophilia and hypergammaglobulinaemia may be found.[41,63]

RF is present in 25–40% of patients[41,58] and is often related to the presence of articular involvement.[4]

Autoantibodies are found in many patients with LS. ANA can be present in any subtype, with a frequency ranging from 23% to 73%.[41,63] Anti-histone antibodies (AHA) have been detected in 47% of patients with LS with a different prevalence in the various subtypes—higher in generalized morphoea, lower in CM.[64]

Anti-topoisomerase I antibodies (anti-Scl 70), a marker of SSc in adults, were found to be positive in 2–3% of children with LS but not in adults with LS.[41,64] Conversely, anti-centromere antibodies (ACA) were found in 12% of adults with LS but only in 1.7% of children.[41,65] Anti-DNA topoisomerase IIα antibodies (anti-topo IIα) were detected in 76% of patients with LS and in 85% of those with generalized morphoea.[66] Immunoblotting showed no cross-reactivity of anti-topo IIα with anti-topo I autoantibodies, which are almost exclusively detected in SSc. Anti-topo IIα, however, is not completely specific for LS, being present also in patients with SSc (14%), in those with SLE (8%), and even in dermatomyositis (10%). Anti-cardiolipin antibodies (aCL) have been found in 46% of the patients with LS and lupus anticoagulant (LAC) in 24% while β2-glycoproteinI (β2GPI) antibodies were absent.[67] In children aCL were found in 12.6% of patients.[41]

Serum concentrations of soluble interleukin(IL)-2 receptor have been increased in cases of LS and may differentiate active from inactive disease,[68] although this finding is not supported by all studies.[57]

Disease monitoring

Various methods for the clinical monitoring of LS have been developed but none has been validated in large cohort of patients.

A semiquantitative scoring method, the Localized Scleroderma Severity Index (LoSSI), is based on the evaluation of three parameters: lesion extension, intensity of inflammation, and new lesion development or existing lesion extension.[69] The extension score is based on the evaluation of 14 cutaneous anatomic sites, each divided into 3 segments; the intensity score is related to the degree of erythema of the lesion's edge and/or skin thickness by palpation. The last parameter is calculated on the basis of the appearance of new lesions or enlargement of the existing ones. The overall composite score ranges between 0 and 168. The limitation of this method is that it is quite subjective and does not evaluate the real size of the lesions.

A computerized skin score (CSS) method for the measurement of circumscribed lesions allows a more precise evaluation of the extension of each lesion.[70] It involves demarcating the indurate borders of the scleroderma lesions on an adhesive transparent film, transferring them to a card, scanning, and recording the data in a computer. Calculation of the affected area, performed by computer software, takes into account the child's growth and in this way allows the longitudinal monitoring of the lesions.

Infrared thermography (IT) has been shown to be of value in the detection of active LS lesions in children with high sensitivity (92%) but low specificity (68%).[71] The false-positive results are related to the fact that old lesions lead to a marked atrophy of skin, subcutaneous fat, and muscle, with increased heat conduction from deeper tissues. Laser doppler flowmetry (LDF) is another non-invasive method for the measurement of cutaneous microcirculation for the evaluation of scleroderma lesions.[72] LDF can detect the increase of blood flow in clinically active lesions. It represents a complementary tools in evaluating LS in the sense that while IT can quantitate thermographic changes of visible lesions and may reveal hidden active lesions, LDF can confirm the presence of active lesion and exclude activity in atrophic lesions. High-frequency ultrasound can detect several abnormalities of LS lesions such as increased blood flow, increased echogenicity due to fibrosis. and loss of subcutaneous fat[73]. The main limits of this tool are its operator dependency and the lack of standardization.

The use of MRI is indicated when CNS or orbital involvement are suspected,[74] and to demonstrate the depth of soft tissue lesions in the deep subtypes of LS.[75]

Treatment

Over the years, many treatments have tried for LS.[76] Management decisions must be based on the particular subtype of disease and the fact that these disorders may spontaneously enter remission after 3–5 years (Figure 122.6).

CM is generally of cosmetic concern only, and treatments with potentially significant toxicity are not justified., Treatment should therefore be directed towards topical therapies such as moisturizing agents, topical glucocorticoids, or calcipotriene.[76]

Phototherapy with ultraviolet (UV) represents another possible therapeutic choice for LS.[77] The use of UV light therapy, with or without chemical agents such as psoralen, has been reported to be beneficial for localized or superficial lesions in a number of studies. Limitations for the use of UV phototherapy in children are the need for prolonged maintenance therapy, leading to a high cumulative dosage of irradiation, and the increased risk for potential long-term effects such as skin ageing and carcinogenesis.[78]

The use of vitamin D or its analogues (topically and systemically) has been reported in several case series,[76] but in the only controlled trial, results did not show efficacy higher than placebo.[79]

When there is a significant risk for disability, such as in progressive linear scleroderma crossing joint lines and generalized or pansclerotic morphoea, systemic treatment, particularly with methotrexate, should be considered.[76] A weekly regimen of methotrexate of 10–15 mg/m^2 as a single oral or subcutaneous dose per week is recommended. During the first 3 months of therapy, a course of glucocorticoids should be used as adjunctive 'bridge therapy'. Recently, a randomized trial comparing a 12 month course of oral methotrexate (15 mg/m^2) for 12 months with a 3 month course of oral prednisone (1 mg/kg per day, maximum dose 50 mg) showed that methotrexate was effective and well tolerated in more than two-thirds of patients with JLS.[80] New lesions appeared in only 6.5% of methotrexate-treated patients compared with 16.7% of the prednisone group. Patients who do not respond to this treatment may be treated with mycophenolate mofetil at a dose of 500–1000 mg/m^2.[81] There are, to date, no published trials of biologics or combination treatments. Surgical reconstruction may be required if the disease has not been adequately controlled. Surgery should only be performed after the active phase of the disease has abated and when the child's growth is complete. Facial recontouring is a surgical treatment option that may improve quality of life in adolescents with facial asymmetry due to scleroderma ECDS.[82]

Course of the disease and prognosis

Unlike SSc, the prognosis with regard to survival for LS is usually benign. The course is characterized by an early inflammatory phase, with progression to multiple or extensive lesions, then stabilization, and finally improvement with softening of the skin and increased pigmentation around the lesions. In a population-based study of LS,[49] 50% of patients had documented skin softening of 50% or more or had disease resolution by 3.8 years after the diagnosis. A small number of patients had active disease for more than 20 years. One-fourth of patients with linear scleroderma and 44% of those with deep morphoea developed significant disability. Progression to systemic sclerosis occurs rarely in children.[83]

References

1. Preliminary criteria for the classification of systemic sclerosis (scleroderma). Subcommittee for scleroderma criteria of the American Rheumatism Association Diagnostic and Therapeutic Criteria Committee. *Arthritis Rheum* 1980;23:581–590.
2. Zulian F, Woo P, Athreya BH et al. The PRES/ACR/EULAR Provisional Classification Criteria for Juvenile Systemic Sclerosis. *Arthritis Rheum* 2007;57:203–212.
3. Herrick AL, Ennis H, Bhushan M, Silman AJ, Baildam EM. Incidence of childhood scleroderma in the UK and Ireland. *Arthritis Care Res* (Hoboken) 2010;62:213–218.
4. Mayes MD, Lacey JV Jr, Beebe-Dimmer J et al. Prevalence, incidence, survival, and disease characteristics of systemic sclerosis in a large US population. *Arthritis Rheum* 2003;48:2246–2255.
5. Martini G, Foeldvari I, Russo R et al. Systemic sclerosis in childhood: clinical and immunological features of 153 patients in an international database. *Arthritis Rheum* 2006;54:3971–3978.
6. Gray RG, Altman RD: Progressive systemic sclerosis in a family: case report of a mother and son and review of the literature. *Arthritis Rheum* 1977;20:35–41.
7. De Keyser F, Peene I, Joos R et al. Occurrence of scleroderma in monozygotic twins. *J Rheumatol* 2000;27:2267–2269.
8. Nelson JL, Furst DE, Maloney S et al. Microchimerism and HLA-compatible relationships of pregnancy in scleroderma. *Lancet* 1998;351:559–562.
9. Ohtsuka T, Miyamoto Y, Yamakage A et al. Quantitative analysis of microchimerism in systemic sclerosis skin tissue. *Arch Dermatol Res* 2001;293:387–391.

10. Artlett CM, Smith JB, Jimenez SA. Identification of fetal DNA and cells in skin lesions from women with systemic sclerosis. *N Engl J Med* 1998;338:1186–1191.

11. Martini G, Vittadello F, Kasapçopur Ö et al. Factors affecting survival in juvenile systemic sclerosis. *Rheumatology (Oxford)* 2009;48:119–222.

12. Scalapino K, Arkachaisri T, Lucas M et al. Childhood onset systemic sclerosis: classification, clinical and serologic features, and survival in comparison with adult onset disease. *J Rheumatol* 2006;33:1004–1013.

13. Quartier P, Bonnet D, Fournet JC et al. Severe cardiac involvement in children with systemic sclerosis and myositis. *J Rheumatol* 2002;29:1767–1773.

14. Perera A, Fertig N, Lucas M et al. Clinical subsets, skin thickness progression rate, and serum antibody levels in systemic sclerosis patients with anti-topoisomerase I antibody. *Arthritis Rheum* 2007;56:2740–2746.

15. Teasdall RD, Frayha RA, Shulman LE. Cranial nerve involvement in systemic sclerosis (scleroderma): a report of 10 cases. *Medicine (Baltimore)* 1980;59:149–159.

16. Della Rossa A, Valentini G, Bombardieri S et al. European multicentre study to define disease activity criteria for systemic sclerosis. I. Clinical and epidemiological features of 290 patients from 19 centres. *Ann Rheum Dis* 2001;60:585–591.

17. Penas PF, Jones-Caballero M, Aragues M et al. Sclerodermatous graft-vs-host disease: clinical and pathological study of 17 patients. *Arch Dermatol* 2002;138:924–934.

18. Owens GR, Medsger TA: Systemic sclerosis secondary to occupational exposure. *Am J Med* 1988;85:114–116.

19. Izquierdo M, Mateo I, Rodrigo M et al. Chronic juvenile toxic epidemic syndrome. *Ann Rheum Dis* 1985;44:98–103.

20. Lasser AE, Schultz BC, Beaff D et al. Phenylketonuria and scleroderma. *Arch Dermatol* 1978;114:1215–1217.

21. Jansen T, Romiti R: Progeria infantum (Hutchinson-Gilford syndrome) associated with scleroderma-like lesions and acroosteolysis: a case report and brief review of the literature. *Pediatr Dermatol* 2000;17:282–285.

22. Epstein CJ, Martin GM, Schultz AL et al. Werner's syndrome a review of its symptomatology, natural history, pathologic features, genetics and relationship to the natural aging process, *Medicine (Baltimore)* 1966;45:177–221.

23. Venencie PY, Powell FC, Su WP et al. Scleredema: a review of thirty-three cases. *J Am Acad Dermatol* 1984;11:128–134.

24. Wozniak J, Dabrowski R, Luczak D et al. Evaluation of heart rhythm variability and arrhythmia in children with systemic and localized scleroderma, *J Rheumatol* 2009;36:191–196.

25. Garty BZ, Athreya BH, Wilmott R et al. Pulmonary functions in children with progressive systemic sclerosis. *Pediatrics* 1991;88:1161–1167.

26. Koh DM, Hansell DM: Computed tomography of diffuse interstitial lung disease in children. *Clin Radiol* 2000;55:659–667.

27. Weber P, Ganser G, Frosch M et al. Twenty-four hour intraesophageal pH monitoring in children and adolescents with scleroderma and mixed connective tissue disease. *J Rheumatol* 2000;27:2692–2695.

28. La Torre F, Martini G, Russo R et al. A preliminary disease severity score for Juvenile Systemic Sclerosis. *Arthritis Rheum.* 2012;64(12):4143-50

29. Kowal-Bielecka O, Landewé R, Avouac J, et al. EULAR recommendations for the treatment of systemic sclerosis: a report from the EULAR Scleroderma Trials and Research group (EUSTAR). *Ann Rheum Dis* 2009;68(5):620–628.

30. Pope J, Fenlon D, Thompson A et al. Iloprost and cisaprost for Raynaud's phenomenon in progressive systemic sclerosis. *Cochrane Database Syst Rev* 2007;2:CD000953.

31. Zulian F, Corona F, Gerloni V et al. Safety and efficacy of iloprost for the treatment of ischaemic digits in paediatric connective tissue diseases. *Rheumatology (Oxford)* 2004;43(2):229–233.

32. Tashkin DP, Elashoff R, Clements PJ et al. Cyclophosphamide versus placebo in scleroderma lung disease. *N Engl J Med* 2006;354:2655–2666.

33. Pope JE, Bellamy N, Seibold JR et al. A randomized, controlled trial of methotrexate versus placebo in early diffuse scleroderma. *Arthritis Rheum* 2001;44:1351–1358.

34. Liossis SNC, Bounas A, Andonopulos AP Mycophenolate mofetil as first-line treatment improves clinically evident early scleroderma lung disease. *Rheumatology* (Oxford) 2006;45:1005–1008.

35. Steen VD, Costantino JP, Shapiro AP et al. Outcome of renal crisis in systemic sclerosis: relation to availability of angiotensin converting enzyme (ACE) inhibitors. *Ann Intern Med* 1990;113:352–357,.

36. García de la Peña-Lefebvre P, Rodríguez Rubio S, Valero Expósito M et al. Long-term experience of bosentan for treating ulcers and healed ulcers in systemic sclerosis patients *Rheumatology* (Oxford) 2008;47(4):464–466.

37. Lin HK, Wang JD, Fu LS. Juvenile diffuse systemic sclerosis/systemic lupus erythematosus overlap syndrome—a case report. *Rheumatol Int* 2012;32(6):1809–1811.

38. Van Laar JM, Farge D, Tyndall A. Stem cell transplantation: a treatment option for severe systemic sclerosis? *Ann Rheum Dis* 2008;67(suppl 3):35–38.

39. Foeldvari I, Zhavania M, Birdi N et al. Favourable outcome in 135 children with juvenile systemic sclerosis: results of a multinational survey. *Rheumatology (Oxford)* 2000;39:556–559.

40. Laxer RM, Zulian F. Localized scleroderma. *Curr Opin Rheumatol* 2006;18(6):606–613.

41. Zulian F, Athreya BH, Laxer RM et al. Juvenile localized scleroderma: clinical and epidemiological features in 750 children. An international study. *Rheumatology* (Oxford) 2006;45:614–620.

49. Peterson LS, Nelson AM, Su WPD et al. The epidemiology of morphea (localized scleroderma) in Olmsted County 1960–1993. *J Rheumatol* 1997;24:73–80.

42. Weibel L, Harper JI. Linear morphoea follows Blaschko's lines. *Br J Dermatol* 2008;159:175–181.

43. Jablonska S, Blaszczyk M, et al. Long-lasting follow-up favours a close relationship between progressive facial hemiatrophy and scleroderma en coup de sabre. *J Eur Acad Dermatol Venereol* 2005;19:403–404.

44. Diaz-Perez JL, Connolly SM, Winkelmann RK, et al. Disabling pansclerotic morphea in children. *Arch Dermatol* 1980;116:169–173.

45. Wollina U, Buslau M, Weyers W, et al. Squamous cell carcinoma in pansclerotic morphea of childhood. *Pediatr Dermatol* 2002;19:151–154.

46. Parodi PC, Riberti C, Draganic Stinco D et al. Squamous cell carcinoma arising in a patient with long standing pansclerotic morphea. *Br J Dermatol* 2001;144:417–419.

47. Daoud MS, Su WP, Leiferman KM, et al. Bullous morphea: clinical, pathologic, and immunopathologic evaluation of thirteen cases. *J Am Acad Dermatol* 1994;30:937–943.

48. Shulman LE. Diffuse fasciitis with hypergammaglobulinemia and eosinophilia: a new syndrome? *J Rheumatol* 1974;1 (Suppl 1):46.

50. Zulian F, Vallongo C, de Oliveira SKF, et al. Congenital localized scleroderma. *J Pediatr* 2006;149(2):248–251.

51. Liu B, Connolly MK. The pathogenesis of cutaneous fibrosis. *Semin Cutan Med Surg* 1998;17:3–11.

52. Aractingi S, Socie G, Devergie A et al. Localized scleroderma-like lesions on the legs in bone marrow transplant recipients: association with polyneuropathy in the same distribution. *Br J Dermatol* 1993;129:201–203.

53. McNallan KT, Aponte C, el-Azhary R et al. Immunophenotyping of chimeric cells in localized scleroderma. *Rheumatology* (Oxford) 2007;46:398–402.

54. Haustein UF, Haupt B. Drug-induced scleroderma and sclerodermiform conditions. *Clin Dermatol* 1998;16:353–366.

55. Aberer E, Stanek G, Ertl M et al. Evidence for spirochetal origin of circumscribed scleroderma (morphea). *Acta Derm Venereol* 1987;67:225–231.

56. Weide B, Schittek B, Klyscz T et al. Morphoea is neither associated with features of Borrelia burgdorferi infection, nor is this agent detectable in lesional skin by polymerase chain reaction. *Br J Dermatol* 2000;143:780–785.

57. Vancheeswaran R, Black CM, David J et al. Childhood-onset scleroderma: is it different from adult-onset disease? *Arthritis Rheum* 1996;39:1041–1049.

58. Zulian F, Vallongo C, Woo P et al. Localized scleroderma in childhood is not just a skin disease. *Arthritis Rheum* 2005;52:2873–2881.

59. Blaszczyk M, Krolicki L, Krasu M et al. Progressive facial hemiatrophy: central nervous system involvement and relationship with scleroderma en coup de sabre. *J Rheumatol* 2003;30:1997–2004.

60. Flores-Alvarado DE, Esquivel-Valerio JA, Garza-Elizondo M et al. Linear scleroderma en coup de sabre and brain calcification: is there a pathogenic relationship? *J Rheumatol* 2003;30: 193–195.

61. Guariso G, Conte S, Galeazzi F et al. Esophageal involvement in juvenile localized scleroderma: a pilot study. *Clin Exp Rheumatol* 2007;25:786–789.

62. Zannin ME, Martini G, Athreya BH et al. Ocular involvement in children with localized scleroderma: a multicenter study *Br J Ophthalmol* 2007;91(10): 1311–1314.

63. Falanga V, Medsger TA Jr, Reichlin M et al. Linear scleroderma: clinical spectrum, prognosis, and laboratory abnormalities. *Ann Intern Med* 1986;104: 849–857.

64. Sato S, Fujimoto M, Ihn H et al. Clinical characteristics associated with antihistone antibodies in patients with localized scleroderma. *J Am Acad Dermatol* 1994;31:567–571.

65. Ruffatti A, Peserico A, Glorioso S et al. Anticentromere antibody in localized scleroderma. *J Am Acad Dermatol* 1986;15:637–642.

66. Hayakawa I, Hasegawa M, Takehara K et al. Anti-DNA topoisomerase IIα autoantibodies in localised scleroderma. *Arthritis Rheum* 2004;50:227–232.

67. Sato S, Fujimoto M, Hasegawa M et al. Antiphospholipid antibody in localised scleroderma. *Ann Rheum Dis* 2003;62:771–774.

68. Ihn H, Sato S, Fujimoto M et al. Clinical significance of serum levels of soluble interleukin-2 receptor in patients with localized scleroderma. *Br J Dermatol* 1996;134:843–847.

69. Arkachaisri T, Pino S. Localized Scleroderma Severity Index and global assessments: a pilot study of outcome instruments. *J Rheumatol* 2008;35:650–657.

70. Zulian F, Meneghesso D, Grisan E et al. A new computerized method for the assessment of skin lesions in localized scleroderma. *Rheumatology* (Oxford) 2007;46:856–860.

71. Martini G, Murray KJ, Howell KJ et al. Juvenile-onset localized scleroderma activity detection by infrared thermography. *Rheumatology* 2002;41:1178–1182.

72. Weibel L, Howell KJ, Visentin MT et al. Laser Doppler flowmetry for assessing localized scleroderma in children. *Arthritis Rheum* 2007;56: 3489–3495.

73. Li SC, Liebling MS, Haines KA, et al. Ultrasonography is a sensitive tool for monitoring localized scleroderma. *Rheumatology* (Oxford) 2007;46(8):1316–1319.

74. Ramboer K, Dermaerel P, Baert AL, et al. Linear scleroderma with orbital involvement: follow up and magnetic resonance imaging [letter]. *Br J Ophthalmol* 81: 90–93, 1997.

75. Horger M, Fierlbeck G, Kuemmerle-Deschner J et al. MRI findings in deep and generalized morphea. *Am J Roentgenol* 2008;190: 32–39.

76. Zulian F. New developments in Localized scleroderma. *Curr Opin Rheumatol* 2008;20:601–607.

77. De Rie MA, Bos JD. Photochemotherapy for systemic and localized scleroderma. *J Am Acad Dermatol* 2000;43:725–726.

78. Staberg B, Wulf HC, Klemp P et al. The carcinogenic effect of UVA irradiation. *J Invest Dermatol* 1983;81:517–519.

79. Hulshof MM, Bouwes Bavinck JN, Bergman W et al. Double-blind, placebo-controlled study of oral calcitriol for the treatment of localized and systemic scleroderma. *J Am Acad Dermatol* 2000;43:1017.

80. Zulian F, Martini G, Vallongo C et al. Methotrexate in juvenile localized scleroderma: A randomised, double-blind, placebo-controlled trial. *Arthritis Rheum* 2011;63:1998–2006.

81. Martini G, Ramanan AV, Falcini F et al. Successful treatment of severe or methotrexate-resistant juvenile localized scleroderma with mycophenolate mofetil. *Rheumatology* (Oxford) 2009;48: 1410–1413.

82. Palmero ML, Uziel Y, Laxer RM et al. En coup de sabre scleroderma and parry-romberg syndrome in adolescents: surgical options and patient-related outcomes. *J Rheumatol* 2010;37:2174–2179.

83. Birdi N, Laxer RM, Thorner P, Fritzler MJ, Silverman ED. Localized scleroderma progressing to systemic disease. Case report and review of the literature. *Arthritis Rheum* 1993;36:410–415.

CHAPTER 123

Nephrogenic systemic fibrosis

Cate H. Orteu

Introduction

The first cases of nephrogenic systemic fibrosis (NSF) were identified in 1997 and published by Cowper in 2000.[1] He described a scleromyxoedema-like cutaneous fibrotic disease in patients with renal impairment. The common features of renal insufficiency and cutaneous fibrosis initially prompted the name nephrogenic fibrosing dermopathy (NFD).[2] When autopsy studies later showed evidence of systemic organ involvement the name was changed to NSF.[3]

Gadolinum-based contrast agents (GBCAs) are intravenous drugs used in diagnostic MRI procedures to enhance the image quality. In 2006 a temporal relationship between the use of GBCAs and the onset of symptoms of NSF was identified.[4,5] Subsequently, gadolinium (Gd) deposits were identified in affected skin,[6,7] and a significant association between GBCA exposure and NSF (odds ratio 26.7, 95% confidence interval 3.7–69.4) was confirmed.[8] Previous gadolinium exposure is documented in 89% of biopsy-proven published cases.[9] Its precise role and mode of action in triggering fibrosis in NSF is still the subject of investigation.

Epidemiology

In December 2011, there were 580 unconfounded cases of NSF in which a single type of GBCA was implicated cited on the European Medicines Agency (EMA) website,[10] 613 on the United States Food and Drug Administration (FDA) Medwatch website,[11] and over 360 cases being followed at the Yale international NSF disease registry.[12] NSF affects males and females equally and has been found in all ethnic groups. The mean age of onset is 52 years, with an age range of 8–87 years. The documented prevalence of NSF, based on clinical examination and skin biopsy, is 0.77% and 0.64% in cohorts of haemodialysis patients from Scotland and the United States respectively.[13,14] The prevalence of NSF in renal failure patients exposed to GBCA varies from 0–18%.[9] This variability reflects the type of GBCA used, the dose, the time interval in between doses, and the severity of underlying renal insufficiency. In commercially available contrast agents, Gd is bound to a ligand or chelate, to render it less toxic. Ionic and non-ionic, linear and cyclical preparations are available (Table 123.1). The stability of the Gd–chelate complex is dependent on its configuration and charge. In vitro, linear chelates are the least stable, and ionic macrocyclic chelates the most stable (by a factor of 10^5).[15] The greatest number of NSF cases are documented following exposure to the linear forms gadodiamide, gadoversetamide, and gadopentate dimeglumine,[10] which are more likely to release Gd into the tissues. Until 2008 these three products accounted for a majority of GBCA use worldwide. There are very few unconfounded cases reported after the use of macrocyclic GBCAs. Three cases have been attributed to gadobutrol, one of whom had had gadodiamide 7 years previously,[16,17] one case following multiple doses of gadoteridol,[18] and one after gadoterate, although this patient received another unknown GBCA 9 years earlier.[19] High cumulative GBCA exposure and administration of higher dosages (0.3 vs 0.1 mmol/kg) at shorter intervals have also been implicated.[20,21] High-dose GBCA was given in 87.5% of cases.[9,22] In one study, prevalence after exposure to two gadodiamide injections was 36% in patients with chronic kidney disease (CKD) stage 5.[23]

The incidence of new cases has reduced dramatically since 2007–2008 when screening of renal function was introduced and high-risk linear GBCAs became contraindicated in patients with glomerular filtration rate (GFR) less than 30 mL/min/1.73 m^2. The EMA now also recommends the avoidance of repeated GBCA exposures during the same imaging session and within 1 week of exposure, the avoidance of use in patients over 65 years and under 4 weeks of age, and in the peritransplant period for patients receiving liver transplants. A blood screen for renal function is recommended for all patients and mandatory for those given high-risk products. Additional recommendations include limiting the GBCA dose to 0.1 mmol/kg per scan, dialysing dialysis patients promptly after GBCA exposure, and delaying GBCA administration in patients with acute renal failure until renal function has recovered or dialysis has been initiated.[10,24]

Aetiopathogenesis

Risk factors for developing NSF have been identified. Renal impairment is present in 100% of cases and the highest risk is seen in patients with CKD 4 and 5 (GFR <30 mL/min).[19,21–23] In 79–85% of published cases, patients were on dialysis.[9,22] More rarely, NSF

Table 123.1 Types of gadolinium contrast agent and numbers of associated cases of nephrogenic systemic fibrosis

Gadolinium			NSF cases reported	
			Unconfounded	Confounded
Linear	Non-ionic	Gadodiamide, Omniscan*	438	90
		Gadoversetamide, OptiMARK *	7	11
	Ionic	Gadopentetate dimeglumine, Magnevist *	135	276
		Gadobenate dimeglumine, MultiHance **	0	8
		Gadoxetic acid disodium salt, Primovist **	0	0
		Gadofosveset trisodium, Vasovist **	0	0
Cyclic	Non-ionic	Gadoteridol, ProHance ***	1	13
		Gadobutrol, Gadovist ***	1	5
	Ionic	Gadoterate, Dotarem ***	1a	11

Product viewed as *high risk,** medium risk, *** low risk by EMA.
dPatient also exposed to another unknown GBCA 9 years prior to Dotarem.
Adapted from European Medicines Agency: www.ema.europa.eu

has been described in patients with CKD 3 (GFR 30–60 mL/min). In some of these cases, the eGFR may have been overestimated because of acutely deteriorating renal function. A recent meta-analysis suggests that patients with liver disease in the peritransplant period are at increased risk as a result of their susceptibility to acute renal impairment, rather than as a result of their liver disease per se.[25]

Several different lines of investigation support Gd as the main trigger for NSF. NSF usually develops 2–10 weeks (median 5 weeks) after Gd exposure.[22] Some cases have presented over a year later, and the role of Gd in these cases is controversial. One possible explanation for a delayed presentation may be that Gd, deposited in bone in individuals with normal renal function,[26] is later released from bone if renal function deteriorates. In patients with renal failure, the elimination half-life of GBCA is increased substantially from 1.3 to 120 hours, dramatically increasing the exposure time of tissues to Gd.[15,26]

Since not all renal failure patients exposed to GBCA develop NSF, other cofactors are likely.[20,21] Proinflammatory events such as recent vascular surgery, recent renal transplant failure, hypercoagulability, and thrombotic events often precede the onset of NSF.[20] Many such events may be associated with acute kidney injury (AKI) and/or be investigated using MR angiography or venography requiring high-dose Gd. In one study, concurrent infection resulted in a 25-fold increased risk of developing NSF.[27] The use of high-dose erythropoietin, universal in patients with endstage renal failure, may also contribute, since combinations of iron and erythropoietin enhance the cutaneous changes triggered by Omniscan in rats.[28]

Gd release from its chelate is influenced by the presence of ligands with high affinity for Gd, such as phosphate and carbonate, and/or the presence of metals that have high affinity for the Gd-binding ligand, such as Zn^{2+}, Cu^{2+}, or Fe^{3+}.[15] These metals compete with Gd and displace it from its ligand by a process known as transmetallation. Gd is then 'free' to be deposited in the tissues as insoluble Gd phosphate. Scanning electron microscopy together with energy-dispersive spectroscopy has confirmed the presence of such deposits in NSF lesional skin.[6,7] Frenzel et al. showed that the

dissociation of Omniscan occurs from day 1 in human serum and the release of free Gd^{3+} increases to over 20% over a 2 week period.[28] At low pH and in the presence of hyperphosphataemia, both often present in patients developing NSF,[21] the rate of Gd release is increased.[28] The Klotho protein signalling pathway and fibroblast growth factor-23 (FGF-23) may provide a link between renal impairment, hyperphosphataemia, and NSF.[17] FGF-23 is a phosphate-lowering factor. Klotho protein is responsible for converting FGF I (IIIc) receptor to a specific receptor for FGF-23. In renal failure, circulating FGF-23 levels increase, but the ability of the kidney to produce Klotho protein falls. As a result, phosphate levels may go unchecked, and excess FGF-23, unable to act on its own receptor, might cause fibrocyte activation via non-specific stimulation of other FGF receptors.

Further supportive evidence of a role for Gd comes from animal models.[26,28] In rats Gd has been identified in organs including skin, liver, and femur after injection of linear but not macrocyclic GBCAs. Repeated intravenous administration of linear, but not macrocyclic, GBCA can induce erythematous, ulcerated, crusted skin lesions with cellular infiltration and thickened collagen consistent with human NSF lesions. Upregulated production of proinflammatory and profibrotic cytokines including TIMP-1, tumour necrosis factor alpha (TNFα, and osteopotin have been observed in serum in this model.[29,30] Osteopontin regulates macrophage activity in response to calcification and cell–matrix interaction, and is a chemoattractant for dendritic cells and T lymphocytes, whereads TIMP-1-inhibits extracellular matrix (ECM) degradation. In humans, Gd compounds can upregulate expression of profibrotic cytokines and growth factors from peripheral blood mononuclear cells, and stimulate normal human fibroblasts in culture to proliferate and secrete increased amounts of ECM, hyaluronic acid, and collagen.[31] This effect can also be produced with the more stable macrocyclic GBCAs, but requires 10^5-fold higher doses.[32] These studies suggest that multiple repeat injections of low-stability GBCAs, even in the absence of renal impairment, could lead to gradual accumulation of Gd^{3+} in tissues until it reaches a level that triggers the fibrotic process.

Definitions and diagnostic criteria

The diagnosis of NSF is based on the presence of characteristic clinical features in the setting of CKD, and substantiated by skin histology on a deep biopsy extending at least into subcutaneous fat. Visualization and quantitation of Gd cannot be performed in most laboratories and is not essential to the diagnosis. A recent clinico-pathological scoring system to aid in diagnosis has been published by Cowper's group.[33]

Clinical features

In the early stages, erythema and oedema may predominate, often associated with burning pain or itch. Thickened erythematous to brawny plaques, papules, and nodules develop, producing a peau d'orange, cobblestone, or woody indurated appearance (Figure 123.1).

The pattern of cutaneous involvement is generally symmetrical, most commonly involving the extremities, especially the lower limbs (Figure 123.2).[34] In some series it was worse over fistula sites.[34] The trunk may be involved, but in contrast to scleroderma and scleromyxoedema, the face is spared. Rarely, diffuse involvement of the limbs, more closely resembling scleroderma, is seen. The cutaneous changes generally evolve over weeks, but in 5% a fulminant course is described.[12] Around 60% of patients develop joint contractures and reduced mobility. Other changes include yellow scleral plaques resembling pingueculae present in 20/408 published cases.[9] Autopsy studies have confirmed that NSF is associated with

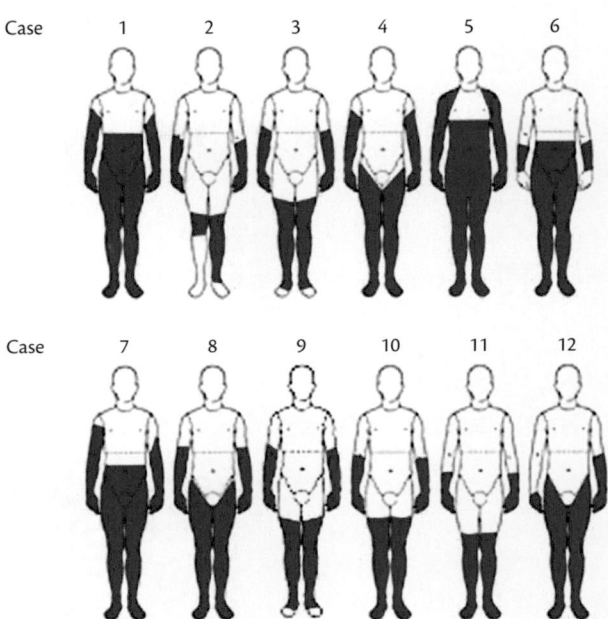

Fig. 123.2 Pattern of cutaneous involvement in 12 patients with nephrogenic systemic fibrosis.

Reprinted from Semin Arthritis Rheum, Vol 35 (4), Mendoza FA, et al., Description of 12 Cases of Nephrogenic Fibrosing Dermopathy and Review of the Literature, pp.238–249 (2006), with permission from Elsevier.

fibrotic damage to internal viscera including the heart, lungs, liver, oesophagus, skeletal muscle, dura, kidneys, and rete testes.[3,34] Calcification may also be present. Internal organ involvement was documented in 16/408 biopsy-confirmed published cases of NSF.[9]

Increased dermal cellularity with spindle and/or epithelioid cells is a key histopathological feature.[33] There is typically a massive infiltration of the dermis with CD34+ spindle-shaped and dendritic fibrocytes (Figure 123.3).[2,33,34]. These cells are thought to derive from the circulation and resemble cells which normally infiltrate injured tissue and are involved in wound healing. They exhibit dual staining with procollagen I. CD34+ cells may be less numerous during the later stages of the disease.[2,33] Elastic fibres are generally preserved and tram-tracking of CD34+ cell processes around a central elastic fibre is another key feature.[33] Small spicules of bone developing around elastic fibres are an uncommon but specific feature.[33] Mono- and multinucleate cells, dual staining for CD68 and factor XIIIa, may be present.[34] There are increased numbers of haphazardly arranged thick and thin collagen bundles throughout the dermis, surrounded by clefts. The process involves the entire dermis and extends deep, causing a widening of the septae of the subcutaneous fat, and sometimes extending into muscle. A variable increase in dermal mucin is seen.

Scleromyxoedema, scleredema, scleroderma, and eosinophilic fasciitis are the most important differential diagnoses (Table 123.2). Lipodermatosclerosis, porphyria cutanea tarda (sclerodermoid variant), and in the acute stages calciphylaxis, cellulitis, and panniculitis, should also be considered.

The prognosis is difficult to predict. A recent review by Zou identified 55/248 published cases in whom the disease improved, 63/248 in whom it remained stable, 25/248 in whom it progressed. 71 patients died. Although only 3 deaths were directly attributed to NSF, it may have contributed to death through reduced mobility, thrombotic complications, and malnutrition in others.[9]

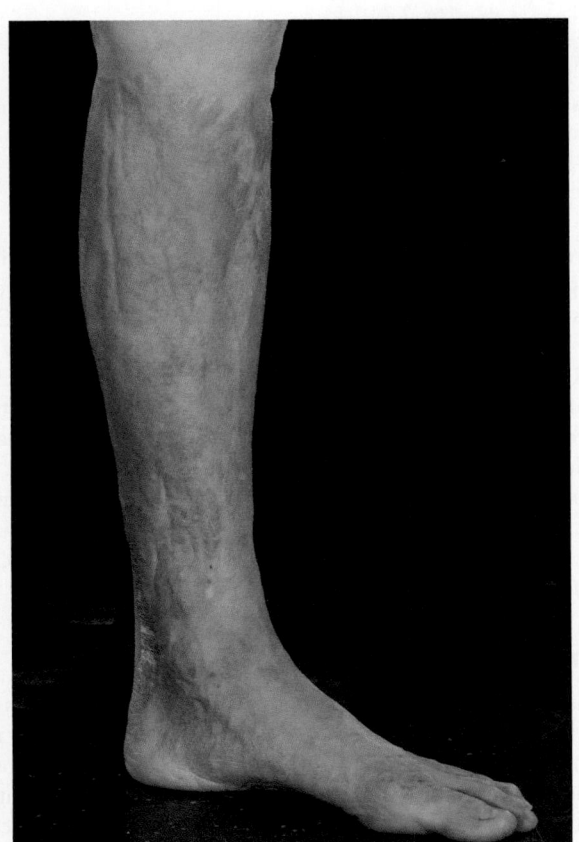

Fig. 123.1 Well-defined erythematous to brawny indurated plaques on the leg in a 34 year old woman with nephrogenic systemic fibrosis.

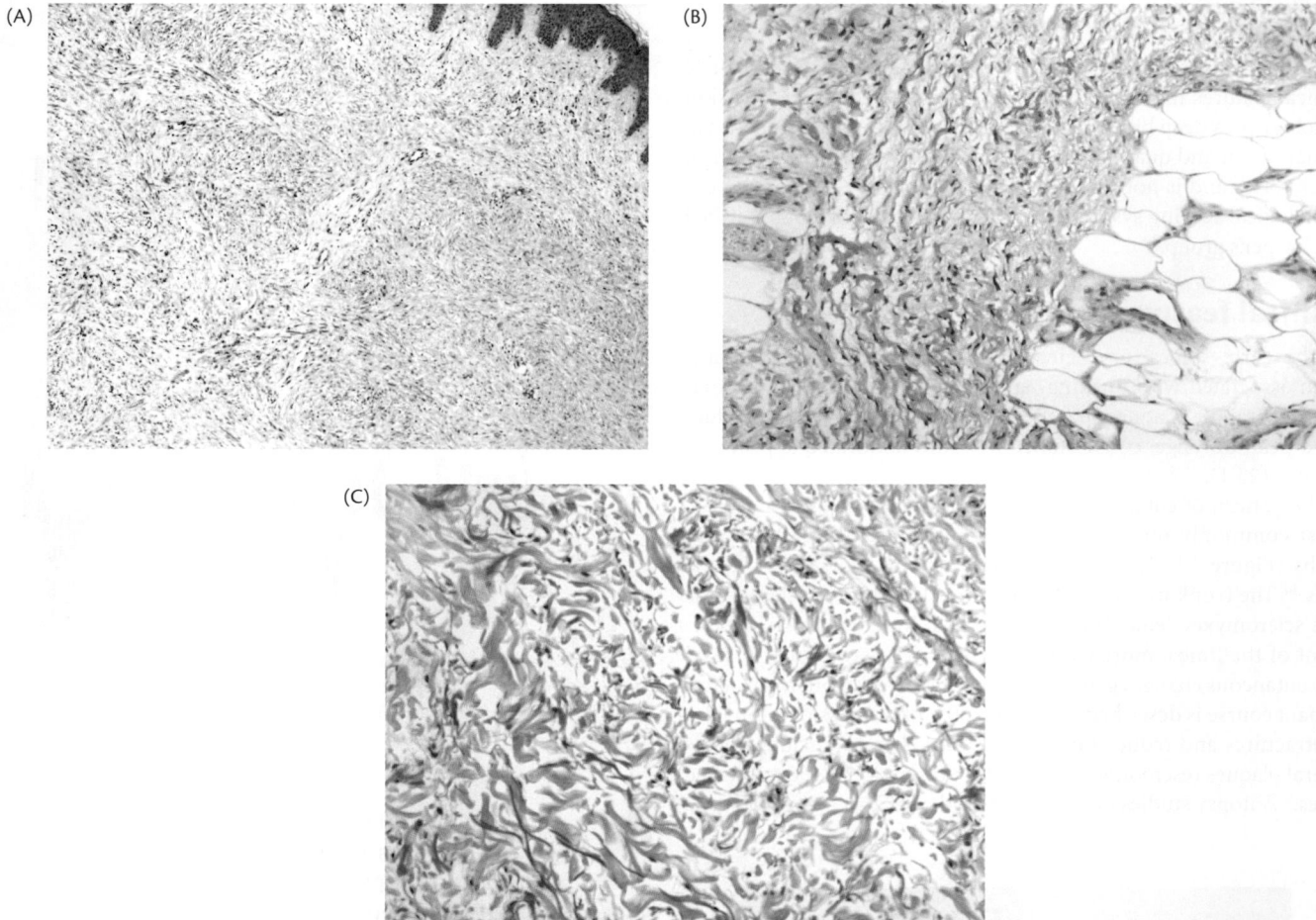

Fig. 123.3 Histopathological features in nephrogenic systemic fibrosis: (A) Low-power view, H&E stain ×40 mag, showing a markedly increased cellularity in the expanded dermis. Spindle and dendritic cells stain positively with CD34 (×40 mag). CD68+ epithelioid and dendritic cells are identified (×200 mag). Alcian blue stain reveals an excess of interstitial mucin (×100 mag). Elastic Van Giesen stain confirms preservation of the elastic network (×100 mag). (B) High-power view, H&E stain (×100 mag), showing increased numbers of spindle-shaped cells extending deep into the subcutis, in between the fat lobules. (C) High-power view, H&E stain (×100 mag), showing increased numbers of haphazardly arranged thick and thin collagen bundles separated by mucin-filled clefts (as seen on alcian blue stain).

Management

Improvement in renal function and renal transplantation have been associated with improvement or resolution of disease in some patients; up to 40% of cases in some reports.[9] Pain control and physical therapies to maintain mobility are essential. Most treatments are reported in anecdotal cases and small case series.[35] High-dose corticosteroids, thalidomide, methotrexate, pentoxifylline, cyclophosphamide, plasmapheresis, and intravenous immunoglobulins have all been tried but with generally disappointing results. More promising responses have been documented following prolonged extracorporeal photopheresis, ultraviolet UVA1 phototherapy, intravenous sodium thiosulphate, rapamycin, and more recently imatinib. Imatinib is an inhibitor of Abelson kinase (c-Abl) and platelet-derived growth factor (PDGF). c-Abl kinase is a target of transforming growth factor beta 1 (TGF-β1) signalling. This cytokine stimulates fibrocytes and its expression is upregulated in the tissues of patients with NSF.[30] Several reports have suggested that imatinib is effective in preventing and reversing fibrosis in some patients with NSF.[36]

Prevention is key. Current recommendations are that GBCA should be avoided, unless essential, and particularly in acute renal failure until after renal function returns or dialysis is initiated. Dosage should be maintained at 0.1 mmol/kg or below, and repeated exposures avoided, particularly within a week of each other. Cyclic ionic compounds should be used as first line in all patients with eGFR less than 30 mL/min, especially when there are associated proinflammatory conditions. All patients should have blood taken to screen for renal dysfunction.[10] Patients already on haemodialysis should be dialysed within 24 hours of receiving gadolinium. This approach seems to be effective. Perez Rodriguez showed a dramatic effect of risk factor screening on the incidence of NSF, reducing it from 36.5 cases/100 000 Gd-enhanced MRI in 2003–2006, to 4 cases/100 000 in 2007–2008.[37]

Conclusion

NSF is a systemic fibrosing condition which occurs in patients with renal impairment following the use of GBCA. The type (linear non-ionic), dose (>0.3 mmol/kg) and overall amount of Gd exposure, and degree of renal impairment (CKD5>CKD3) are important risk factors. Other cofactors include the presence of a metabolic acidosis and hyperphosphataemia which both increase the likelihood of Gd dissociation from its chelate and deposition in the tissues.

Table 123.2 Differential diagnosis of nephrogenic systemic fibrosis: comparative features of related skin diseases

	Nephrogenic systemic fibrosis	Eosinophilic fascitis	Scleromyxedema	Scleredema	Scleroderma
Collagen	Increased thick and thin collagen collagen, haphazard orientation	Thickened increased collagen	Thickened increased collagen, clefting	Swollen collagen bundles look fenestrated	Enlarged eosinophilic collagen bundles orientated parallel to skin surface Loss of adnexal structures
CD34+ fibrocytes	yes	No	Yes	No	No
Mucin (mainly hyaluronic acid)	+++++	No	++++	++	+
Depth of skin involvement	Into panniculus, (thickened septae)	Fat and deep fascia	To mid reticular dermis	Into subcutis (fat replaced by collagen)	Into subcutis fascia and muscle
Inflammation	No/less obvious	Yes, ± eosinophils	Perivascular upper cermis	No	Perivascular prominent
Typical site	Extremities, trunk	Extremities	Face hands forearms	Back, sides, neck, face. May involve tongue	Generalized
ANA	No	ANA± eosinophilia	± ANA	No	ANA++ ENA++
Other associations	Renal failure, gadolinium exposure	Polyclonal hypergammaglobulinaemia, morphoea, immune cytopenias, haematological malignancy	Paraprotein IgGλ	Diabetes, infection (especially streptococcal), paraprotein IgGκ, IgA, myeloma	

ANA, anti-nuclear antibodies; ENA.

Patients develop thickening of the skin on the limbs and trunk, often complicated by joint contractures and sometimes by fibrosis of internal organs. The disease improves in 22%, stabilizes in 25%, and progresses in the remainder. In 5% it has a fulminant course. Diagnosis is based on the typical clinical history and findings and a deep skin biopsy. Treatment is largely unsatisfactory and prevention by reducing exposure of patients to GBCA is essential.

References

1. Cowper SE, Robin HS, Steinberg SM et al. Scleromyxoedema-like cutaneous diseases in renal-dialysis patients. *Lancet* 2000;356(9234):1000–1001.

2. Cowper SE, Su LD, Bhawan J, Robin HS, LeBoit PE. Nephrogenic fibrosing dermopathy. *Am J Dermatopathol* 2001;23(5):383–393.

3. Ting WW, Stone MS, Madison KC, Kurtz K. Nephrogenic fibrosing dermopathy with systemic involvement. *Arch Dermatol* 2003;139(7):903–906.

4. Grobner T. Gadolinium—a specific trigger for the development of nephrogenic fibrosing dermopathy and nephrogenic systemic fibrosis? *Nephrol Dial Transplant* 2006;21(4):1104–1108.

5. Marckmann P, Skov L, Rossen K et al. Nephrogenic systemic fibrosis: suspected causative role of gadodiamide used for contrast-enhanced magnetic resonance imaging. *J Am Soc Nephrol* 2006;17(9):2359–2362.

6. Boyd AS, Zic JA, Abraham JL. Gadolinium deposition in nephrogenic fibrosing dermopathy. *J Am Acad Dermatol* 2007;56(1):27–30.

7. High WA, Ayers RA, Chandler J, Zito G, Cowper SE. Gadolinium is detectable within the tissue of patients with nephrogenic systemic fibrosis. *J Am Acad Dermatol* 2007;56(1):21–26.

8. Agarwal R, Brunelli SM, Williams K et al. Gadolinium-based contrast agents and nephrogenic systemic fibrosis: a systematic review and meta-analysis. *Nephrol Dial Transplant* 2009;24(3):856–863.

9. Zou Z, Ma L. Nephrogenic systemic fibrosis: review of 408 biopsy-confirmed cases. *Indian J Dermatol* 2011;56(1):65–73.

10. European Medicines Agency. *Assessment report for gadolinium-containing contrast agents.* Available at: www.ema.europa.eu/docs/en_GB/document_library/Referrals_document/gadolinium_31/WC500099538.pdf (accessed 20/01/2012).

11. U.S. Food and Drug Administration. *FDA Drug Safety Communication: New warnings for using gadolinium-based contrast agents in patients with kidney dysfunction.* Available at : www.fda.gov/Drugs/DrugSafety/ucm223966.htm. (accessed 20.01.2012).

12. Cowper SE. *Nephrogenic systemic fibrosis*, 2001–2011. International Center for Nephrogenic Systemic Fibrosis Research. Available at: www.icnsfr.org (accessed 20/12/2011).

13. Collidge TA, Thomson PC, Mark PBet al. Gadolinium-enhanced MR imaging and nephrogenic systemic fibrosis: retrospective study of a renal replacement therapy cohort. *Radiology* 2007;245(1):168–175.

14. Deo A, Fogel M, Cowper SE. Nephrogenic systemic fibrosis: a population study examining the relationship of disease development to gadolinium exposure. *Clin J Am Soc Nephrol* 2007;2(2):264–267.

15. Idee JM, Port M, Robic C et al. Role of thermodynamic and kinetic parameters in gadolinium chelate stability. *J Magn Reson Imaging* 2009;30(6):1249–1258.

16. Elmholdt TR, Jorgensen B, Ramsing M, Pedersen M, Olesen AB. Two cases of nephrogenic systemic fibrosis after exposure to the macrocyclic compound gadobutrol. *Nephrol Dial Transplant* 2010;3:285–287.

17. Wollanka H, Weidenmaier W, Giersig C. NSF after Gadovist exposure: a case report and hypothesis of NSF development. *Nephrol Dial Transplant* 2009;24 (12):3882–3884.

18. Reilly RF. Risk for nephrogenic systemic fibrosis with gadoteridol (ProHance) in patients who are on long-term hemodialysis. *Clin J Am Soc Nephrol* 2008;3(3):747–751.

19. Elmholdt TR, Pedersen M, Jorgensen B et al. Nephrogenic systemic fibrosis is found only among gadolinium-exposed patients with renal

insufficiency: a case-control study from Denmark. *Br J Dermatol* 2011; 165(4):828–836.

20. Prince MR, Zhang H, Morris M et al. Incidence of nephrogenic systemic fibrosis at two large medical centers. *Radiology* 2008;248(3):807–816.

21. Marckmann P, Skov L, Rossen K, Heaf JG, Thomsen HS. Case-control study of gadodiamide-related nephrogenic systemic fibrosis. *Nephrol Dial Transplant* 2007;22(11):3174–3178.

22. Braverman IM, Cowper S. Nephrogenic systemic fibrosis. *F1000 Med Rep* 2010;2:84.

23. Rydahl C, Thomsen HS, Marckmann P. High prevalence of nephrogenic systemic fibrosis in chronic renal failure patients exposed to gadodiamide, a gadolinium-containing magnetic resonance contrast agent. *Investig Radiol* 2008;43(2):141–144.

24. Leiner T, Kucharczyk W. NSF prevention in clinical practice: Summary of recommendations and guidelines in the United States, Canada, and Europe. *J Magn Reson Imaging* 2009;30:1357–1360.

25. Chow DS, Bahrami S, Raman SS et al. Risk of nephrogenic systemic fibrosis in liver transplantation patients. *AJR Am J Roentgenol* 2011; 197(3):658–662.

26. Morcos SK, Haylor J. Pathophysiology of nephrogenic systemic fibrosis: A review of experimental data. *World J Radiol* 2010;2(11):427–433.

27. Golding LP, Provenzale JM. Nephrogenic systemic fibrosis: possible association with a predisposing infection. *AJR Am J Roentgenol* 2008; 190(4):1069–1075.

28. Morcos SK. Experimental studies investigating the pathophysiology of nephrogenic systemic fibrosis; what did we learn so far? *Eur Radiol* 2011; 21(3):496–500.

29. Steger-Hartmann T, Raschke M, Riefke B et al. The involvement of pro-inflammatory cytokines in nephrogenic systemic fibrosis—a mechanistic hypothesis based on preclinical results from a rat model treated with gadodiamide. Exp Toxicol Pathol 2009;61(6):537–552.

30. Gupta A, Shamseddin MK, Khaira A. Pathomechanisms of nephrogenic systemic fibrosis: new insights. *Clin Exp Dermatol* 2011;36(7):763–768.

31. Edward M, Quinn JA, Burden AD, Newton BB, Jardine AG. Effect of different classes of gadolinium-based contrast agents on control and nephrogenic systemic fibrosis-derived fibroblast proliferation. *Radiology* 2010;256(3):735–743.

32. Varani J, DaSilva M, Warner RL et al. Effects of gadolinium-based magnetic resonance imaging contrast agents on human skin in organ culture and human skin fibroblasts. *Investig Radiol* 2009;44(2):74–81.

33. Girardi M, Kay J, Elston DM et al. Nephrogenic systemic fibrosis: clinicopathological definition and workup recommendations. *J Am Acad Dermatol* 2011;65(6):1095–1106 e7.

34. Mendoza FA, Artlett CM, Sandorfi N et al. Description of 12 cases of nephrogenic fibrosing dermopathy and review of the literature. *Semin Arthritis Rheum* 2006;35(4):238–249.

35. Hellman RN. Gadolinium-induced nephrogenic systemic fibrosis. *Semin Nephrol* 2011;31(3):310–316.

36. Elmholdt TR, Buus NH, Ramsing M, Olesen AB. Antifibrotic effect after low-dose imatinib mesylate treatment in patients with nephrogenic systemic fibrosis: an open-label non-randomized, uncontrolled clinical trial. *J Eur Acad Dermatol Venereol* 2013 Jun;27(6):779-84. doi: 10.1111/j.1468–3083. 2011.04398.x.

37. Perez Rodriguez J, Lai S, Ehst BD, Fine DM, Bluemke DA. Nephrogenic systemic fibrosis: incidence, associations, and effect of risk factor assessment—report of 33 cases. *Radiology* 2009;250(2):371–377.

Sources of patient information

European Medicines Agency. Questions and answers on the review of gadolinium-containing contrast agents, 2010. Available at: www.ema.europa.eu/docs/en_GB/document_library/Referrals_document/gadolinium_31/WC500099538.pdf

Food and Drug Administration. FDA requests boxed warning for contrast agents used to improve MRI images, 2007. Available at:www.fda.gov/NewsEvents/Newsroom/PressAnnouncements/2007/ucm108919.htm- Food and Drug Administration. Safety label changes for contrast agents, 2010. Available at:www.fda.gov/Safety/MedWatch/SafetyInformation/ucm235838.htm

Global Fibrosis Foundation. A not-for-profit organization whose mission is to help educate patients, families, and the medical community about NSF and other organ-specific fibrosing processes; to support research into prevention and treatment; and to advocate on behalf of patients. www.globalfibrosis.org/International Center for Nephrogenic Systemic Fibrosis Research (ICNSFR). www.icnsfr.org

Nephrogenic Systemic Fibrosis support group. http://health.groups.yahoo.com/group/nfd_support/

Myositis

CHAPTER 124

Polymyositis and dermatomyositis

Hector Chinoy and Robert G. Cooper

Introduction

The idiopathic inflammatory myopathies (IIM) are rare and heterogenous autoimmune diseases characterized by inflammation of skeletal muscle and other organ systems. The aetiopathology of IIM remains unknown, but genetic and environmental factors probably interact to produce disease.[1] Morbidity outcomes relate to skeletal muscle damage and to well-known complications such as cancer-associated myositis and interstitial lung disease (ILD). Adult-onset IIM can be broadly classified into polymyositis (PM), dermatomyositis (DM), and inclusion body myositis (IBM).

Epidemiology

Annual incidence rates for IIM vary from 2.18 to 8.7×10^{-6}.[2] Increased incidence rates have been observed over time and with age. The female to male incidence rate ratio in PM/DM varies between 1.5 and 2.4,[3] although in IBM prevalence rates are higher in men compared to women.[4] A higher incidence of PM/DM has been observed in black compared to white patients. The peak incidence of PM in adults is 40–60 years. The incidence of DM has two peaks, at 5–15 years and 45–65 years.[2]

Clinical and diagnostic criteria

Bohan and Peter introduced diagnostic criteria for myositis which remain the preferred criteria in clinical studies and trials worldwide (Table 124.1).[5,6] Further revised classification criteria have been proposed to take modern day diagnostics into account.[7] A further classification scheme has been developed following observations that specific HLA genotypes are associated with antibodies, which in turn predict clinical phenoypes.[8]

DM may be further subdivided. **DM *sine* dermatitis** describes patients where the rash is transient, subtle or absent, and/or where the histology pattern is in keeping with DM.[9] **Amyopathic DM** describes a subset whereby the rash is present in the absence of muscle weakness[10]; these patients may still be at risk of lung disease or malignancy. Patients without weakness, but who have slight creatine kinase (CK) elevation or disease activity on MRI/muscle biopsy, are described as having **hypomyopathic DM**.

There is a group of patients who have IBM clinically, but who do not meet the stringent histological requirements of the Griggs criteria.[11] In order to accommodate such patients, modified diagnostic criteria have been proposed by the MRC Centre for Neuromuscular Diseases (Table 124.2).[12]

Table 124.1 Bohan and Peter diagnostic criteria for polymyositis/dermatomyositis

Item	Description		
1	Symmetrical weakness of limb-girdle muscles and anterior neck flexors		
2	Muscle biopsy evidence typical of myositis		
3	Elevation of serum skeletal muscle enzymes, particularly CK		
4	Typical EMG features of myositis		
5	Typical DM rash, including heliotrope and Gottron's papules		
For the diagnosis of PM:		**For the diagnosis of DM:**	
Definite	All of items 1–4	Definite	Item 5 plus 3 of items 1–4
Probable	3 of items 1–4	Probable	Item 5 plus 2 of items 1–4
Possible	2 of items 1–4	Possible	Item 5 plus 1 of items 1–4

CK, creatine kinase; DM, dermatomyositis; EMG, electromyography; PM, polymyositis.
Exclusion criteria include congenital muscular dystrophies, central or peripheral neurological disease, infectious myositis, metabolic/endocrine myopathies, and myasthenia gravis.
Adapted from Bohan and Peter.[5,6]

Table 124.2 Proposed modified diagnostic criteria for inclusion body myositis

Pathologically defined IBM	
Conforming to the Griggs criteria[11]—invasion of non-necrotic fibres by mononuclear cells, and rimmed vacuoles, and either intracellular amyloid deposits or 15–18 nm filaments	
Clinically defined IBM	
Clinical features	Duration weakness >12 months
	Age >35 years
	Weakness of finger flexion > shoulder abduction AND of knee extension > hip flexion
Pathological features	Invasion of non-necrotic fibres by mononuclear cells or rimmed vacuoles or increased MHC-I, but no intracellular amyloid deposits or 15–18 nm filaments
Possible IBM	
Clinical criteria	Duration weakness >12 months
	Age >35 years
	Weakness of finger flexion > shoulder abduction OR of knee extension > hip flexion
Pathological criteria	Invasion of non-necrotic fibres by mononuclear cells or rimmed vacuoles or increased MHC-I, but no intracellular amyloid deposits or 15–18 nm filaments

From Hilton-Jones et al.[12]

Environmental risk factors

Infectious agents

Acute myopathies can ensue due to infection, with or without evidence of active muscle infection. Presentations include pyomyositis, rhabdomyolysis, or the self-limiting benign acute myositis.[13,14] Infectious agents such as cocksackie, cytomegalovirus, and toxoplasma and have been implicated in IIM, but studies have been largely unsuccessful in identifying evidence for specific infectious agents.[15,16]

Non-infectious agents

A number of drugs, foods, dietary supplements, and vaccinations have also been anecdotally associated with the onset of myositis (Table 121.3).

Genetic risk factors

Because of the scarcity of affected sibling pairs and twins, early evidence to suggest a genetic basis for IIM came from anecdotal familial aggregation and candidate gene studies.[17] Candidate gene studies provide the best evidence for a genetic basis in IIM. The strongest associations arise from the MHC region, as seen in other autoimmune diseases. Alleles forming part of the white European MHC common ancestral haplotype (HLA-A1-B8-Cw7-DRB1*0301-DQA1*0501-C4A*Q0) occur in strong linkage disequilibrium within white populations in northern and western Europe, and are associated with a large number of immunopathological diseases.[18] Thus, HLA-DRB1*0301 and HLA-DQA1*0501 are confirmed risk factors for white IIM.[17] The risk conferred by the common ancestral haplotype is further increased in patients who possess antisynthetase or anti-PM-Scl antibodies.[19]

A recent genome-wide association study in DM has suggested that many of the 'panautoimmunity' genes found in other autoimmune diseases are also important in DM susceptibility.[20]

Pathogenesis

Pathophysiology

As part of the adaptive immune response, both humoral and cell-mediated mechanisms are important in the pathogenesis of IIM. Evidence for a **humoral response** is as follows: (1) about 80% of patients with PM/DM possess autoantibodies; (2) B cells and plasma cell infiltrates are present in muscle tissue; (3) immunoglobulin transcripts are well represented in muscle tissue. The two differing patterns of distribution, location, and type of lymphocyte subsets in muscle biopsy tissue described below are suggestive of two differing **cell-mediated immune** pathways, which may overlap.[21]

Innate immune mechanisms require the presence of ancillary molecules, e.g. cytokines, chemokines, and their receptors. Proinflammatory cytokines such as interleukin (IL)-1α, IL-1β, tumour necrosis factor alpha (TNFα), type I interferons (INF-α and -β), and high-mobility group box 1 (HMGB1) are evident in PM/DM muscle tissue. IL-1α and HMGB1 may be present in muscle fibres in the absence of inflammatory infiltrates, suggesting a role in persisting weakness. A type I interferon gene signature is observed in muscle tissue and peripheral blood in PM/DM.[21] MHC class I expression in muscle fibres may link immune and non-immune mechanisms such as the endoplasmic reticulum stress response.

Muscle biopsy findings

Findings on muscle biopsy tissue may help to differentiate PM, DM, and IBM from each other. A pictorial representation of the muscle fibre is provided to aid interpretation (Figure 124.1).

DM

Early microvascular injury of muscle capillaries occurs through activation of the complement pathway and C5b-9 membranolytic attack complex deposition. Subsequent lysis of endothelial cells leads to necrosis of capillaries and perivascular inflammation. Ensuing focal capillary depletion, reduced capillary density, and muscle ischaemia on the periphery of the muscle fasciculus leads to perifascicular atrophy. T/B lymphocytes, macrophages, and plasma cells are the main inflammatory cells found, where B cells and CD4+ T helper (Th) cells predominate in a perimysial and perivascular distribution. MHC class I expression is limited to damaged fibres in the perifascicular region (Figure 124.2).[22]

Table 124.3 Non-infectious environmental agents linked with myositis

Agent	Exposure
Drugs, foods, and dietary supplements	D-Penicillamine
	Lipid-lowering drugs
	Fibrates
	HMG-CoA reductase inhibitors
	Leuprolide acetate
	Hydroxyurea
	Adulterated rapeseed oil (toxic oil syndrome)
	L-Tryptophan (eosinophilia myalgia syndrome)
	Ciguatera toxin
Biological agents	DTP, MMR, BCG, influenza, hepatitis A/B
Vaccines	INF-α
Cytokines	IL-2
Hormones	
	Growth hormone
Occupational exposures	Silica, cyanoacrylate glue
Other exposures	UV light, chimerism, graft vs host disease

Adapted from Reed and Ytterberg.[16]

PM

In PM and IBM, inflammatory infiltrates are endomysial, immunopathology is of an antigen-driven CD8+ T-cell cytotoxicity, and macrophages are involved in phagocytosis of necrotic cells. Inflammatory cell infiltrates surround and partially invade nonnecrotic muscle fibres which demonstrate strong expression of MHC class I antigen. MHC class I is upregulated on virtually all muscle fibres, regardless of the presence of inflammation,[23] but this not specific to IIM (Figure 124.2).[24]

IBM

As well as the changes described above, amyloid deposition, vacuolation, and inclusion bodies, if present, will help discriminate PM from IBM. B lymphocytes tend to be almost absent from the endomysium.[22] Rimmed vacuoles are round or polygonal small basophilic granules within vacuolar walls. The name IBM derives from clusters of cytoplasmic inclusions containing phosphorylated tau protein. Abnormal deposits accumulate in muscle fibres, including tiny amyloid deposits which immunoreact to Congo Red and other similar proteins.[25] Other characteristic findings in IBM include hypertrophic fibres, fibre-type grouping, ragged red fibres, fatty replacement, and loss of cyclooxygenase staining (Figure 124.2).

Necrotizing myopathy

Muscle biopsy findings from anti-signal recognition particle (SRP) positive cases demonstrate degenerating (necrosis) and regenerating fibres often invaded by macrophage-like cells, and C5b9 in capillaries of endomysial regions. MHC class I upregulation or mononuclear inflammatory cells are not evident.[26] In statin-induced myopathy, muscle biopsy findings again show myonecrosis, macrophagic infiltration and a paucity of B/T cell infiltrates.[27]

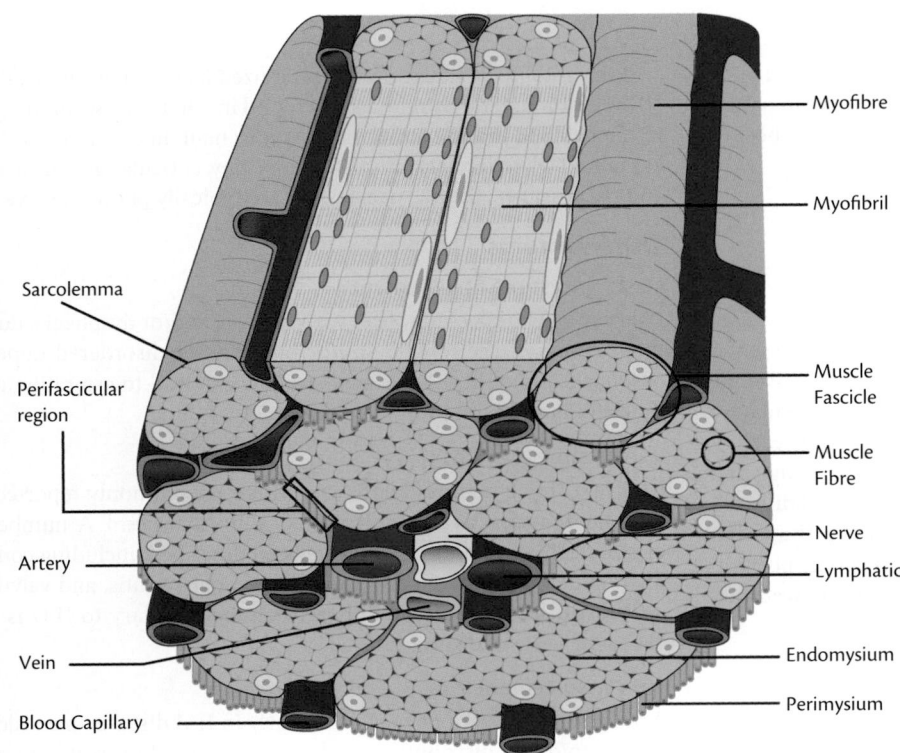

Labels: Sarcolemma, Perifascicular region, Artery, Vein, Blood Capillary, Myofibre, Myofibril, Muscle Fascicle, Muscle Fibre, Nerve, Lymphatic, Endomysium, Perimysium

Fig. 124.1 Pictorial representation of structures within skeletal muscle.

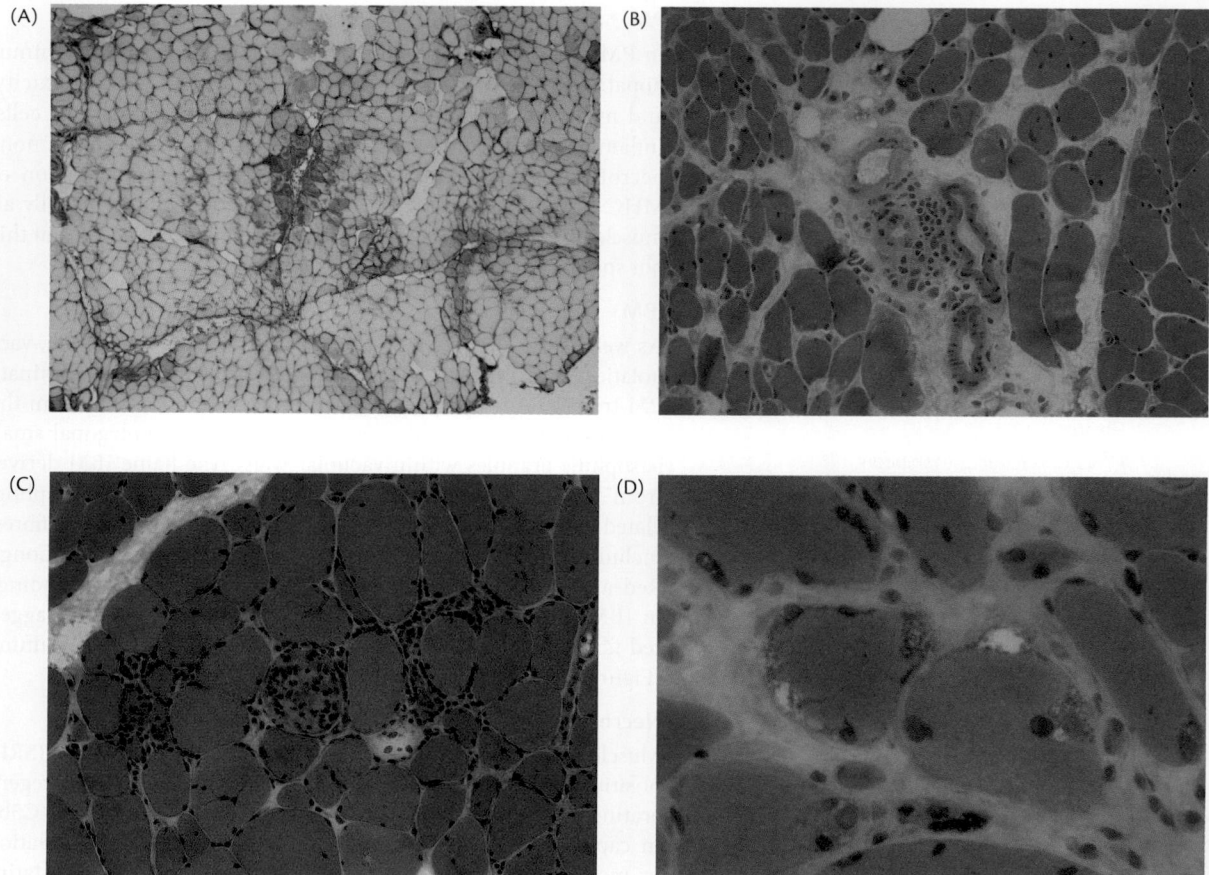

Fig. 124.2 Histopathological changes in idiopathic inflammatory myopathy: (A) Low-power view (×4) of perifascicular accentuation of HLA-1 expression and perifascicular atrophy in DM. (B) Perivascular inflammation in DM (H&E ×20). (C) Endomysial inflammation in PM attacking non-necrotic fibres. Also present are two necrotic fibres (H&E ×20). (D) Inclusion body myositis. Two vacuolated fibres with basophilic rimming; one of them also features an amphophilic inclusion body (H&E ×60).
Slides courtesy of Dr D. DuPlessis and Dr P. Pal, Salford Royal NHS Foundation Trust.

In paraneoplastic myopathy, perimysial staining for alkaline phosphatase, a paucity of inflammation, and a more widespread pattern of necrotic C5b-9 positive muscle fibres compared to SRP-positive myopathy, are observed.[28]

Clinical features

Muscle weakness

In IIM, the pattern of weakness is usually proximal, bilateral, and symmetrical over a period of weeks or months. Myalgia is present in only 25% of cases, typically early on in the disease course. Patients may report difficulty with tasks using the proximal musculature. Upper limb symptoms include difficulty combing hair or reaching up for objects above head height. Lower limb weakness is suggested by difficulty rising to a standing position from sitting and difficulty climbing steps or pavement curbs. Weakness in the abdominal musculature may cause difficulty sitting up from a supine position, and neck weakness may lead to problems keeping the head held upright. The facial musculature is generally spared.[29]

Rash

DM is defined according to classification criteria by the presence of characteristic rashes (Figure 124.3).

Skin vasculitis is an especially recognized feature of juvenile DM (JDM), although rarely may also be found in adult disease. Findings in the nail bed include abnormal tortuous nailfold capillaries, seen as nailfold telangiectasia or on capillaroscopy, cuticular overgrowth, and periungal erythema. Skin lesions are typically photosensitive.

Other systems

Gastrointestinal involvement

Pharyngeal weakness may lead to dysphonia and/or dysphagia, due to weakness of the tongue and/or pharynx, or disordered upper oesophageal motility.[29] A loss of swallow can lead to aspiration of food/fluids and aspiration pneumonia.

Cardiac involvement

Clinical cardiac manifestations in IIM are uncommonly reported, but may manifest as subclinical ECG abnormalities.[30] A number of other cardiac abnormalities have been described, including conduction defects, congestive cardiac failure, pericarditis, and valvular heart disease. Right-sided heart failure secondary to ILD is a common cause of death in IIM.[31]

Joint involvement

Articular manifestations may occur early in IIM disease, in a mild, rheumatoid-like distribution, and usually respond to treatment of

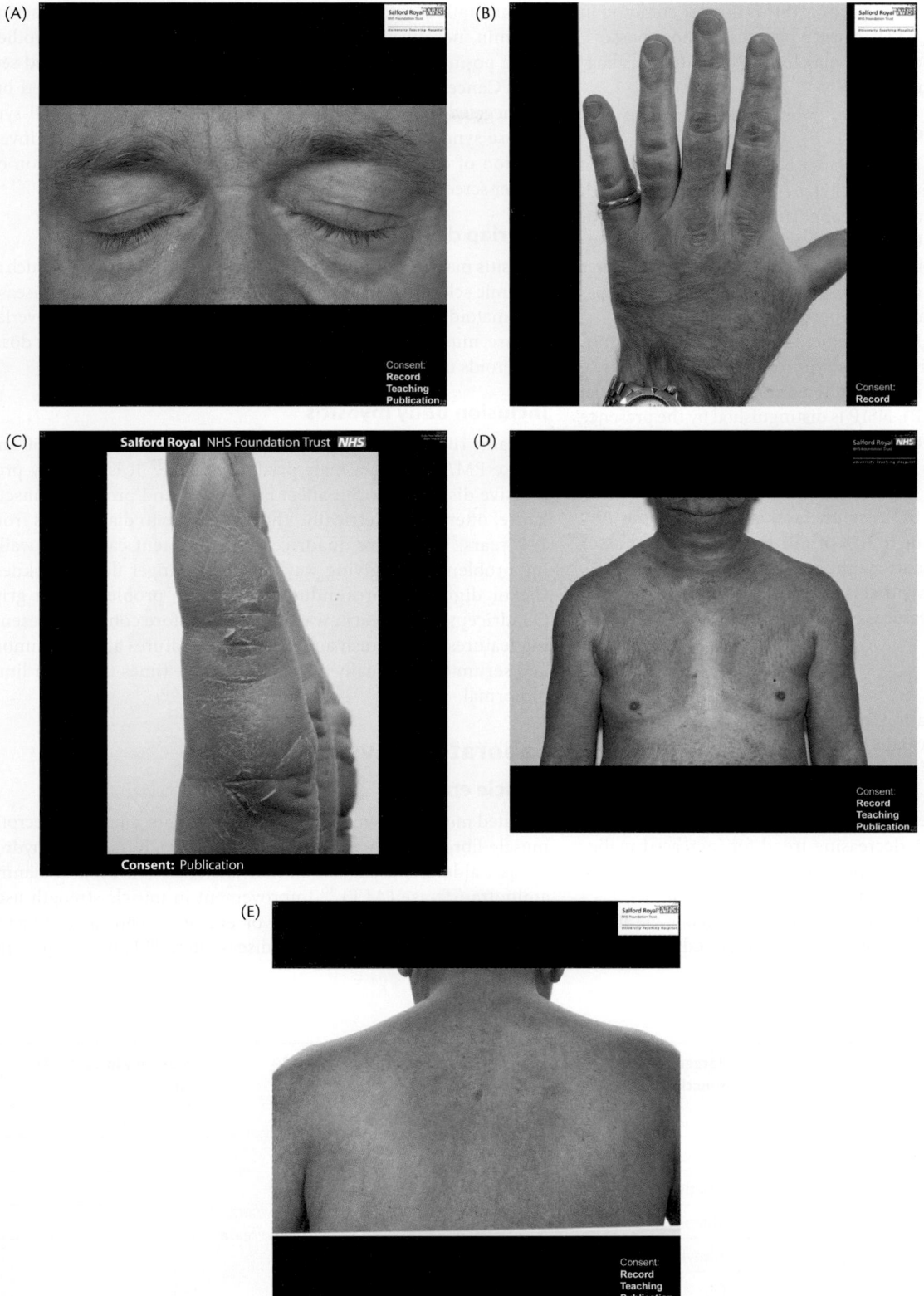

Fig. 124.3 Skin manifestations in idiopathic inflammatory myopathy: (A) Heliotrope rash, a violaceous discolouration affecting the upper eyelids often associated with periorbital oedema. (B) Gottron's papules, symmetrical, palpable erythematous rashes most commonly present on the extensor surface of the metacarpophalangeal or interphalangeal joints. (C) Mechanics' hands, hyperkeratosis, scaling and often painful fissuring of the skin in the tips and sides of the fingers, often mistaken for contact dermatitis, usually seen in the context of the anti-synthetase syndrome. (D) V sign, discrete and confluent macular erythema over the lower anterior neck and upper anterior chest. (E) Shawl sign, discrete and confluent macular erythema in a shawl distribution.

Image C courtesy of Dr Herman Mann.

the underlying disease.[32] Arthralgia or arthritis is more common in connective tissue disease (CTD)/overlap patients or those possessing anti-synthetase antibodies, and may lead to an initial misdiagnosis of inflammatory arthritis.

Respiratory involvement

ILD in the context of IIM (IIM-ILD) may be present in up to 65% of cases at diagnosis.[33] The severity of ILD presentation may vary, with some presenting subclinically, with abnormal chest radiographs or pulmonary function tests (PFTs) in the absence of cough or dyspnoea. Respiratory symptoms in IIM may be attributable to either intrinsic or extrinsic (e.g. aspiration pneumonia, respiratory muscle weakness, pulmonary arterial hypertension) lung disease.[34]

Clinical signs due to ILD involvement may range from asymptomatic to acute respiratory distress syndrome. The main forms of IIM-ILD are non-specific interstitial pneumonia (NSIP) and usual interstitial pneumonia (UIP). NSIP is distinguished by the presence of an inflammatory component, which is considered amenable to immunosuppression, and thus associated with a more favourable prognosis.[34]

Anti-Jo-1 (anti-histidyl-tRNA synthetase) is found in about 20% of PM/DM patients,[19] and up to 70% of anti-Jo-1 patients have associated ILD, as part of the anti-synthetase syndrome (Table 124.4). Patients possessing anti-synthetases, especially other than anti-Jo-1, may never develop features of myositis, or may only do so on subsequent follow-up.

Malignancy

A well-described association exists between malignancy and IIM, mainly based on population-based cohort studies, where the reported frequency of cancer in IIM ranges from 7% to 30%, and the risk is increased compared to population-matched control groups.[35] These studies clearly suggest that malignancy risk is greater in DM than PM. A decreasing trend for increased malignancy risk is observed over time post-IIM diagnosis, although risk may still be increased 5 years after the myositis diagnosis.[36]

Risk factors for malignancy include male gender, older age at disease onset, more severe skin or muscle disease, elevated erythrocyte sedimentation rate(ESR)/C-reactive protein (CRP), low serum albumin, negative result for routinely tested myositis antibodies, and a positive 155/140 antibody (TIF-1γ, see Table 124.4 and section 'Cancer screening'). The risk of malignancy is reduced but not negated in patients with other defined CTDs and the anti-synthetase syndrome. Further discussion about screening and investigation of cancer-associated myositis is found in the section on cancer screening.

Overlap disease

Myositis may also be found in association with other CTDs, such as systemic sclerosis, systemic lupus erythematosus, Sjögren's disease, rheumatoid arthritis, and as part of mixed CTD. In CTD/overlap disease, muscle involvement is usually less severe, and higher doses of steroids may not be required.

Inclusion body myositis

Sporadic IBM typically presents in patients over the age of 50 and unlike PM/DM, has a male predominance.[37] It is a slowly progressive disease that can affect both distal and proximal musculature, often asymmetrically. The mean time to diagnosis is from 1–9 years.[38] Selective quadriceps involvement can cause walking problems, legs giving way, and falls. Finger flexor weakness (flexor digitorum profundus) can lead to problems with grip. Quadriceps and forearm wasting are therefore common presenting features. A DM rash and other CTD features are uncommon, and serum CK is usually no more than five times the upper limit of normal.

Laboratory investigations

Muscle enzymes

Elevated muscle enzymes reflect the presence of injured or necrotic muscle fibres. Serum enzymes used include CK, lactate dehydrogenase, aldolase, aspartate aminotransferase (AST), and alanine aminotransferase (ALT).[39] Improvement in muscle strength usually lags behind normalization of enzymes, and an enzymatic rise may predict an impending disease flare.[40] However, patients

Table 124.4 Autoantibodies associated with myositis

Autoantibodies		Target autoantigen and function	Clinical phenotype	Frequency in adult IIM (%)
Myositis-specific antibodies				
Anti-aminoacyl-tRNA synthetases—associated with anti-synthetase syndrome				
	Anti-Jo-1	Histidyl	Myositis, mechanics' hands, Gottron's papules, arthritis, Raynaud's phenomenon, interstitial lung disease	11–20
	Anti-PL-7	Threonyl		2
	Anti-PL-12	Alanyl		1
	Anti-EJ	Glycyl		1–3
	Anti-OJ	Isoleucyl		1
	Anti-KS	Asparaginyl		<1
	Anti-Ha	Tyrosyl		<1
	Anti-Zo	Phenylalanyl		<1

(Continued)

Table 124.4 (*Continued*)

Autoantibodies		Target autoantigen and function	Clinical phenotype	Frequency in adult IIM (%)
Antibodies associated with acute necrotizing myopathy				
	Anti-SRP	Ribonucleoprotein complex comprising 6 polypeptides and 7SL RNA (intracytoplasmic protein translocation)	Acute necrotizing myopathy, high CK (up to 25 000), severe weakness, may be refractory to treatment. Usually respond well to steroids, but may flare on tapering thus requiring long-term immunosuppression	5
	Anti-200/100	HMG CoA reductase	Acute necrotizing myopathy, associated with statin use. Proximal weakness despite statin cessation. CK 2–35 000	unknown
Antibodies associated with adult dermatomyositis				
	Anti-Mi-2	Nucleosome remodelling histone deacetylase complex (nuclear transcription)	Cutaneous disease, milder muscle disease, acute onset, good response to treatment, lower mortality rates	5–10 (10–20% adult DM)
	Anti-155/140	TIF1-γ (nuclear transcription and cellular differentiation)	Severe cutaneous disease, cancer-associated myositis	5–10 (13–21% adult DM)
	Anti-NXP-2	Nuclear matrix protein 2 (p140) (nuclear transcription and RNA metabolism)	Cutaneous disease, systemic features, ILD (calcinosis more common in juveniles)	3
Antibodies associated with amyopathic dermatomyositis				
	Anti-SAE	Small ubiquitin-like modifier activating enzyme (post-translational modification)	Cutaneous disease precedes muscle disease	5
	Anti-MDA5	Melanoma-differentiation associated gene 5 (innate immune responses against viral infections)	Amyopathic dermatomyositis, rapidly progressive interstitial lung disease	Unknown
Myositis-associated antibodies				
	Anti-PM-Scl	Nucleolar protein complex (human exosome)	SSc overlap, Raynaud's phenomenon, interstitial lung disease	8–10 (50% myositis-scleroderma overlap syndrome)
	Anti-U1 RNP	U1 small nuclear RNP	Mixed CTD	10
	Anti-Ku	DNA-PK regulatory subunit	SSc overlap, interstitial lung disease	20–30
	Anti-Ro	Y1-Y5 RNP	Sjögren's overlap, frequently associated with Jo-1	10–20
	Anti-La	RNA polymerase III termination factor	Sjögren's overlap	5

Adapted from Hengstman et al.[44] and Hirakata.[45] Additional data from Casciola-Rosen et al.[46] and Gunawardena et al.[47]

may present with new active myosis or flare with normal muscle enzymes.[41] Other causes of raised muscle enzymes may be present (Box 124.1).

Muscle enzymes should thus not be used in isolation to monitor disease activity. In active disease, a CK increase can typically be tenfold. Increases above about 6000 may be seen but should prompt a search for other causes. A higher upper limit of normal may be seen in Afro-Caribbean patients. Cardiac troponin T may be raised in inflammatory myositis, in the absence of cardiac disease; cardiac troponin I does not correlate with skeletal muscle injury and is thus more accurate in assessing cardiac injury. Transaminases (ALT, AST) can be raised in IIM, which may lead to misdiagnosis of liver dysfunction during drug monitoring.

Other laboratory markers

The presence of urinary myoglobin may lead to the false-positive detection of blood on urinalysis testing—an absence of red blood cells is found on urine microscopy. ESR may be slightly raised and

Box 124.1 Causes of elevated creatine kinase other than inflammatory myositis

Muscle trauma

- Direct muscle injury
- Needle stick
- EMG
- Surgery
- Convulsions, delirium tremens

Diseases affecting muscle

- Myocardial infarction
- Rhabdomyolysis
- Metabolic or mitochondrial myopathies
- Muscular dystrophies
- Infectious myositis
- Amyotrophic lateral sclerosis (motor neuron disease)

Drug/toxin-induced myopathy

- Lipid-lowering agents, especially HMG CoA reductase inhibitors
- Alcoholic myopathy
- Drugs of abuse, e.g. cocaine, amphetamines, phencyclidine
- Malignant hyperthermia, neuroleptic malignant syndrome
- Other medications, e.g. zidovudine, colchicine, chloroquine, ipecac

Drug-induced myositis

- D-Penicillamine
- Interferon
- HMG-CoA-reductase inhibitors

Drug-induced CK elevation

- Inhibition of excretion, e.g. barbiturates, morphine, diazepam

Endocrine and metabolic abnormalities

- Hypothyroidism
- Hypokalaemia
- Hyperosmolar state or ketoacidosis
- Diabetic nephrotic syndrome with oedema
- Renal failure

Elevation of brain-type creatine kinase

- Central nervous system disease
- Tumours (e.g. gastrointestinal, bronchial)

Elevation without disease

- Strenuous, prolonged, and/or unaccustomed exercise
- Ethnic group (black > white)
- Increased muscle mass

Adapted from Targoff.[39]

CRP is not typically raised in acute inflammatory myositis; raised levels of inflammatory markers may suggest concurrent infection. Low serum creatinine may correlate with a general loss of muscle mass and atrophy.

Biomarkers including mucin-like glycoprotein KL-6, serum B-cell activating factor, and serum ferritin, have been described in IIM-ILD. The level of serum ferritin is higher in IIM-ILD, and may exceed 8000 ng/mL.[42]

Myositis-specific and associated autoantibodies

Great advances have been made over the last few years in our understanding of the relevance of myositis-specific and associated autoantibodies (MSA/MAA), in particular that an individual patient's antibody is predictable for their disease phenotype. Autoantibodies against nuclear or cytoplasmic antigens can be detected in 80–90% of IIM cases.[43] MSA are specific for inflammatory myositis, while MAA may also be detected in other rheumatic disorders without signs of inflammatory muscle disease; thus they are not specific to myositis (Table 124.4).

Clinical assessment

It is important to clinically differentiate disease activity from disease-induced tissue damage, to avoid immunosuppressing a patient with muscle weakness and no active inflammation, while treating disease activity in others, e.g. a patient who has ongoing inflammatory disease, but without CK elevation. The International Myositis Assessment and Clinical Studies (IMACS) Group have agreed core-set measures to assess myositis disease activity, including assessment of: (1) physician/patient global activity assessment by visual analogue scale; (2) muscle strength by manual muscle testing; (3) physical function; (4) muscle enzymes; (5) extraskeletal muscle disease.[41]

Muscle strength can be evaluated through isokinetic or isometric testing. Manual muscle testing (MMT) is widely used in clinical practice and a 0–10 point scale is used widely by the international myositis community (https://dir-apps.niehs.nih.gov/imacs/).[48] An abbreviated group of 8 proximal, distal, and axial muscles performs similarly to examination of 24 muscle groups.

Physical impairment may affect the function of patients, and can be measured with the Stanford Health Assessment Questionnaire (HAQ) which has been used as a measure of improvement in adult IIM trials.[41]

Muscle tissue is the primary organ affected in myositis, but other organs may also be involved.[49] The measures developed to assess disease activity include the Myositis Intention to Treat Index (MITAX) and the Myositis Activity Assessment by Visual Analogue Scales (MYOACT).[50] The Myositis Damage Index (MDI) assesses extent and severity of damage.[51]

Investigations

Muscle biopsy

Muscle biopsies can positively identify non-inflammatory myopathies, and differentiate between IIM subtypes. Open biopsy provides a large sample, thus reducing sampling error,[52] but is inconvenient, costly, and results in larger scars. The percutaneous conchotome method[53] is less invasive, and allows for repeat biopsies when monitoring disease activity or treatment response. Needle-based biopsy techniques, although yielding small samples, can produce adequate samples for diagnostics.

Vastus lateralis is usually selected for biopsy in IIM, although electromyography (EMG) (contralateral side to avoid contamination) and MRI can guide the choice of muscle group. Where extensive fatty replacement is present, the deltoid may provide better yield. Despite being more distal, tibialis anterior may also show characteristic changes and is technically an easier muscle to sample.

Neurophysiology

Neurophysiology provides an extension of the clinical examination in IIM and is important for the exclusion of non-inflammatory myopathies and neurogenic disorders. Classical (EMG) findings in IIM consist of: (1) early recruitment of low amplitude, short duration and polyphasic motor unit action potentials; (2) spontaneous fibrillations, positive sharp waves, and increased insertional activity; and (3) high-frequency complex repetitive discharges, which all correlate inversely with muscle strength in IIM patients. These changes are not specific for IIM and may also be seen in dystrophies and metabolic myopathy.[54] EMG has approximately 90% sensitivity for picking up inflammatory myopathy but this partly depends on the skill of the neurophysiologist.

Muscle imaging

MRI is a very sensitive non-invasive technique for localizing muscle oedema in inflammatory myositis. MRI allows sequential examination of large volumes of muscle and identification of focal myositis, and can also be used to target areas for muscle biopsy. However, mitochondrial/metabolic myopathies, dystrophies, or even motor neuron disease, may also manifest secondary inflammatory changes on MRI, thus the technique lacks specificity for IIM.

Muscle oedema is demonstrated as a multifocal or diffuse pattern of high signal intensity on T2-weighted sequences. Clearer images can be obtained with fat-suppressed (short tau inversion recovery, STIR) sequences (Figure 124.4).[55] Muscle atrophy is found on T1-weighted images as increased signal intensity, which correlates with disease-related damage.

Other investigations

If dysphagia is present, patients should be appropriately investigated with speech and language therapy assessment, barium swallow, and/or videofluoroscopy as appropriate.

Diagnosis of interstitial lung disease

PFTs may help detect subclinical ILD, and are useful for monitoring progression of disease or therapeutic response. ILD is suggested by a normal/raised FEV_1/FVC ratio, FVC or total lung capacity less than 80% predicted, and/or a decrease in diffusing capacity for carbon monoxide (DL_{CO}). Patients with respiratory muscle weakness may also present with a restrictive pattern and decreased DL_{CO}. A decreased DL_{CO} may also be seen in pulmonary hypertension. A number of biomarkers may be useful in the assessment of IIM-ILD (see Other laboratory markers).

Chest radiographs are also useful for screening and detection of ILD complications, e.g. pneumothoraces. High-resolution CT (HRCT) is sensitive and can also distinguish between fibrotic disease and active inflammation.[56] Irregular linear opacities with areas of consolidation and ground-glass attenuation suggest active inflammation. Honeycombing is suggestive of endstage lung disease with established fibrosis. Bronchoscopy and bronchoalveolar lavage may be useful to exclude opportunistic infections. The use of surgical biopsy in IIM-ILD is not routine in CTD-ILD patients unless diagnostic uncertainty remains.

Cancer screening

In addition to careful history-taking and examination, laboratory evaluation should include the following: full blood count, ESR, routine biochemistry, tumour markers, chest radiography, urinary cytology, and chest/abdomen/pelvis CT scans. Mammography and gynaecological examination is justified in female patients, as is testicular examination in males. Faecal occult blood testing and gastroscopy/colonoscopy should be carried out in all patients over 50 years of age. These investigations are of special importance in DM, and should be repeated yearly for at least 3 years following IIM

(A) 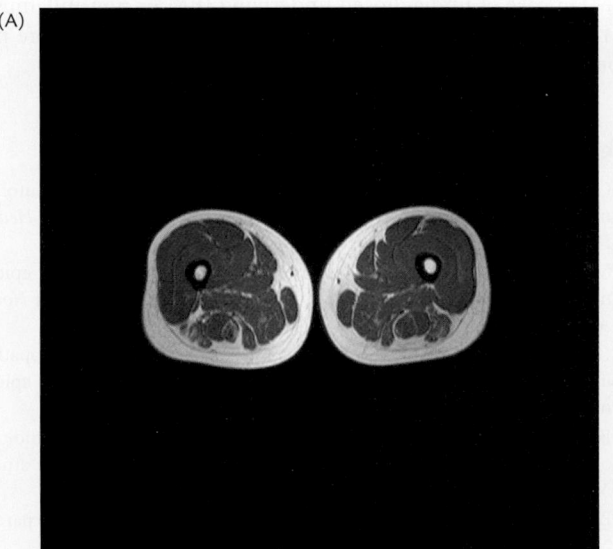 (B)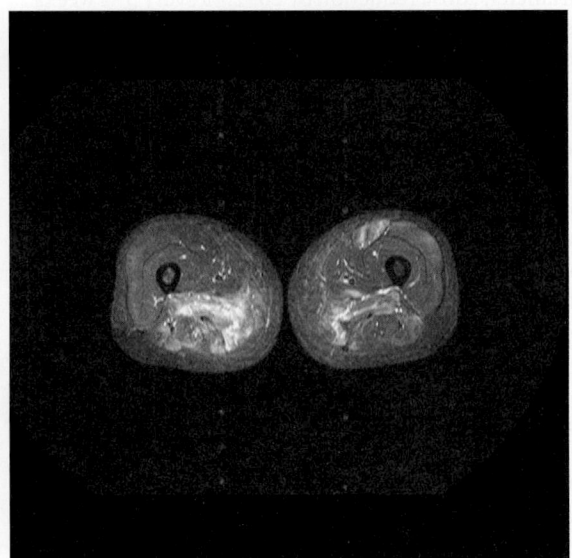

Fig. 124.4 MR changes in idiopathic inflammatory myopathy: (A) T1 and (B) axial STIR thigh sequence of a 34 year old patient with anti-SRP-positive dermatomyositis, CK>3000, proximal weakness. Muscle oedema (in white) is predominantly affecting the hamstrings.

diagnosis. The use of FDG-PET scanning appears to be comparable to conventional screening methods for detecting occult malignancy in the setting of myositis.[57]

A subtype of paraneoplastic necrotizing myopathy has been described in association with a wide spectrum of different solid tumour types. CK levels can vary from 8 to 100 times the normal range.[28]

Anti-TIF1-γ (p155/140) antibodies are found in about one-fifth of patients with adult and juvenile DM (Table 124.4). In adults, this antibody is 78% sensitive and 89% specific for the detection of cancer-associated myositis,[58,59] and generally not found in association with other MSA. Anti-TIF1-γ (p155/140) detection should prompt intensive cancer screening in DM patients for 3–5 years after myositis onset.

Differential diagnosis in myositis

There are many differential diagnoses when encountering an adult patient with muscle weakness where accurate clinical assessment is vital. For example, dystrophies tend to present at an earlier age, are slowly progressive, and do not respond to immunosuppression. Muscle weakness in myasthenia gravis or Eaton–Lambert syndrome may affect extraocular or bulbar musculature, and worsens with repetitive or prolonged use. Prominent muscle wasting, fasciculations, and brisk reflexes should alert to possible motor neuron disease which can also present with a raised CK. These conditions should be differentiated from IIM on EMG testing. Raised inflammatory markers and proximal stiffness may point towards polymyalgia rheumatica.

Mitochondrial disease, metabolic myopathies, and dystrophies may also mimic the presentation of IIM; a comprehensive discussion of these non-inflammatory myopathies is provided in Chapter 126.

Management and treatment of myositis

Initial treatment of choice in inflammatory myositis is with corticosteroids. The typical initial dose is 0.75–1 mg/kg (e.g. 60–80 mg prednisolone) per day for 3–4 weeks, and after normalization of CK and clinical parameters, dose reduction by 20–25% every 3–4 weeks until the lowest dose to control the disease is reached.[40] Treatment with intravenous methylprednisolone 1 g daily for 3 days may be necessary in aggressive disease.

Other treatments may be initiated for further control of disease and as steroid-sparing agents, e.g. methotrexate, azathioprine, ciclosporin, tacrolimus, cyclophosphamide, and mycophenolate mofetil (various trials reviewed by Oddis[40]). Intravenous immunoglobulin use has also been studied; a study in refractory DM showed improvement of muscle strength after 3 months.[60]

Plasma exchange has shown limited results in the treatment of myositis.[61] Anti-TNFα therapy is not recommended in IIM, where only variable improvements have been noted in serum muscle enzyme levels and muscle strength. The largest randomized placebo-controlled trial in IIM to date investigated rituximab with crossover at 8 weeks.[62] No significant difference in improvement was noted between the two arms at 12 months, but 83% of patients achieved the definition of improvements and a significant glucocorticoid-sparing effect was noted.

Exercise and rehabilitation programmes are safe and of benefit in stable treated myositis patients, improving function, aerobic fitness, and muscle strength. Creatine supplementation in addition to a home exercise programme is of benefit in clinically stable but weak PM/DM.[63] The issues of muscle weakness, loss of joint motion, and fatigue in myositis should be addressed in physiotherapy-led programmes.

Inclusion body myositis

IBM unfortunately does not respond to currently available pharmacological treatment. Due to inflammatory infiltrates observed in muscle biopsy tissue, steroids have been used to suppress inflammation, which may reduce the serum CK, but with no discernible improvement in muscle strength or attenuation of disease progression. Trials of a number of therapies, including intravenous immunoglobulin, anti-T-lymphocyte globulin, alemtuzumab, etanercept, IFNβ1-a, have all yielded mixed results, therefore none can currently be recommended for treatment.[38]

Lack of response

Patients may not respond to conventional treatment for a number of reasons[64]:

- Inadequate dose and/or length of treatment with glucocorticoids.

- Steroid-induced myopathy, manifesting usually as a deterioration of muscle strength without elevated CK levels after initial improvement.

- In patients with muscle atrophy, evidenced by MRI or muscle biopsy, immunosuppressive treatment will not be of help.

- Improvements in serum CK are not always associated with concurrent improvements in muscle strength, where there is often a delay.

- The presence of occult malignancy should always be considered, and comprehensive screening is recommended. Cancer-associated myositis should improve with treatment of the underlying neoplasia, but will depend on the type, stage, and grade of the tumour.

- Repeat biopsy should be considered in cases of disease-resistant IIM, in case of undiagnosed underlying IBM or non-inflammatory myopathy, especially if the initial biopsy findings were not specific for PM/DM.

References

1. Cooper GS, Miller FW, Pandey JP. The role of genetic factors in autoimmune disease: implications for environmental research. *Environ Health Perspect* 1999;107 Suppl 5:693–700.
2. Mastaglia FL, Phillips BA. Idiopathic inflammatory myopathies: epidemiology, classification, and diagnostic criteria. *Rheum Dis Clin North Am* 2002;28:723–741.
3. Cox S, Limaye V, Hill C, Blumbergs P, Roberts-Thomson P. Idiopathic inflammatory myopathies: diagnostic criteria, classification and epidemiological features. *Int J Rheum Dis* 2010;13:117–124.
4. Badrising UA, Maat-Schieman M, van Duinen SG et al. Epidemiology of inclusion body myositis in the Netherlands: A nationwide study. *Neurology* 2000;55:1385–1388.
5. Bohan A, Peter JB. Polymyositis and dermatomyositis (first of two parts). *N Engl J Med* 1975;292:344–347.
6. Bohan A, Peter JB. Polymyositis and dermatomyositis (second of two parts). *N Engl J Med* 1975;292:403–407.

7. Sultan SM, Isenberg DA. Re-classifying myositis. *Rheumatology* 2010;49:831–833.

8. Love LA, Leff RL, Fraser DD et al. A new approach to the classification of idiopathic inflammatory myopathy: myositis-specific autoantibodies define useful homogeneous patient groups. *Medicine* (Baltimore) 1991;70:360–374.

9. Dalakas MC, Hohlfeld R. Polymyositis and dermatomyositis. *Lancet* 2003;362:971–982.

10. Euwer RL, Sontheimer RD. Amyopathic dermatomyositis (dermatomyositis sine myositis). Presentation of six new cases and review of the literature. *J Am Acad Dermatol* 1991;24:959–966.

11. Griggs RC, Askanas V, DiMauro S et al. Inclusion body myositis and myopathies. *Ann Neurol* 1995;38:705–713.

12. Hilton-Jones D, Miller A, Parton M et al. Inclusion body myositis: MRC Centre for Neuromuscular Diseases, IBM workshop, London, 13 June 2008. *Neuromuscul Disord* 2010;20:142–147.

13. Ytterberg SR. Infectious agents associated with myopathies. *Curr Opin Rheumatol* 1996;8:507–513.

14. Mackay MT, Kornberg AJ, Shield LK, Dennett X. Benign acute childhood myositis: Laboratory and clinical features. *Neurology* 1999;53:2127.

15. Plotz PH, Rider LG, Targoff IN et al. NIH conference. Myositis: immunologic contributions to understanding cause, pathogenesis, and therapy. *Ann Intern Med* 1995;122:715–724.

16. Reed AM, Ytterberg SR. Genetic and environmental risk factors for idiopathic inflammatory myopathies. *Rheum Dis Clin North Am* 2002;28:891–916.

17. Chinoy H, Lamb JA, Ollier WE, Cooper RG. Recent advances in the immunogenetics of idiopathic inflammatory myopathy. *Arthritis Res Ther* 2011;13:216.

18. Price P, Witt C, Allcock R et al. The genetic basis for the association of the 8.1 ancestral haplotype (A1, B8, DR3) with multiple immunopathological diseases. *Immunol Rev* 1999;167:257–274.

19. Chinoy H, Salway F, Fertig N et al. In adult onset myositis, the presence of interstitial lung disease and myositis specific/associated antibodies are governed by HLA class II haplotype, rather than by myositis subtype. *Arthritis Res Ther* 2006;8:R13.

20. Miller FW, Cooper RG, Vencovsky J et al. Genome-wide association study of dermatomyositis reveals shared genetic risk factors with other autoimmune diseases [abstract]. *Arthritis Rheum* 2011;63:1678.

21. Nagaraju K, Lundberg IE. Polymyositis and dermatomyositis: pathophysiology. *Rheum Dis Clin North Am* 2011;37:159–171, v.

22. Dalakas MC. Muscle biopsy findings in inflammatory myopathies. *Rheum Dis Clin North Am* 2002;28:779–798, vi.

23. Nyberg P, Wikman AL, Nennesmo I, Lundberg I. Increased expression of interleukin 1alpha and MHC class I in muscle tissue of patients with chronic, inactive polymyositis and dermatomyositis. *J Rheumatol* 2000;27:940–948.

24. Karpati G, Pouliot Y, Carpenter S. Expression of immunoreactive major histocompatibility complex products in human skeletal muscles. *Ann Neurol* 1988;23:64–72.

25. Askanas V, Engel WK. Sporadic inclusion-body myositis and its similarities to Alzheimer disease brain. Recent approaches to diagnosis and pathogenesis, and relation to aging. *Scand J Rheumatol* 1998;27:389–405.

26. Miller T, Al-Lozi MT, Lopate G, Pestronk A. Myopathy with antibodies to the signal recognition particle: clinical and pathological features. *J Neurol Neurosurg Psychiatry* 2002;73:420–428.

27. Mammen AL, Chung T, Christopher-Stine L et al. Autoantibodies against 3-hydroxy-3-methylglutaryl-coenzyme A reductase in patients with statin-associated autoimmune myopathy. *Arthritis Rheum* 2011;63:713–721.

28. Levin MI, Mozaffar T, Al-Lozi MT, Pestronk A. Paraneoplastic necrotizing myopathy: clinical and pathological features. *Neurology* 1998;50:764–767.

29. Yazici Y, Kagen LJ. Clinical presentation of the idiopathic inflammatory myopathies. *Rheum Dis Clin North Am* 2002;28:823–832.

30. Lundberg IE. Cardiac involvement in autoimmune myositis and mixed connective tissue disease. *Lupus* 2005;14:708–712.

31. Danko K, Ponyi A, Constantin T, Borgulya G, Szegedi G. Long-term survival of patients with idiopathic inflammatory myopathies according to clinical features: a longitudinal study of 162 cases. *Medicine* (Baltimore) 2004;83:35–42.

32. Oddis CV. Inflammatory muscle disease: clinical features. In: Hochberg MC, Silman AJ, Smolen JS, Weinblatt ME, Weisman MH (eds) *Rheumatology*. Mosby, St Louis, 2003: 1537–1554.

33. Fathi M, Dastmalchi M, Rasmussen E, Lundberg IE, Tornling G. Interstitial lung disease, a common manifestation of newly diagnosed polymyositis and dermatomyositis. *Ann Rheum Dis* 2004;63:297–301.

34. Schnabel A, Hellmich B, Gross WL. Interstitial lung disease in polymyositis and dermatomyositis. *Curr Rheumatol Rep* 2005;7:99–105.

35. Madan V, Chinoy H, Griffiths CE, Cooper RG. Defining cancer risk in dermatomyositis. Part I. *Clin Exp Dermatol* 2009;34:451–455.

36. Buchbinder R, Forbes A, Hall S, Dennett X, Giles G. Incidence of malignant disease in biopsy-proven inflammatory myopathy. A population-based cohort study. *Ann Intern Med* 2001;134:1087–1095.

37. Engel WK, Askanas V. Inclusion-body myositis: Clinical, diagnostic, and pathologic aspects. *Neurology* 2006;66:S20–S29.

38. Solorzano GE, Phillips LH. Inclusion body myositis: diagnosis, pathogenesis, and treatment options. *Rheum Dis Clin North Am* 2011;37:173–183, v.

39. Targoff IN. Laboratory testing in the diagnosis and management of idiopathic inflammatory myopathies. *Rheum Dis Clin North Am* 2002;28:859–890, viii.

40. Oddis CV. Idiopathic inflammatory myopathy: management and prognosis. *Rheum Dis Clin North Am* 2002;28:979–1001.

41. Rider LG, Giannini EH, Harris-Love M et al. Defining clinical improvement in adult and juvenile myositis. *J Rheumatol* 2003;30:603–617.

42. Gono T, Kawaguchi Y, Hara M et al. Increased ferritin predicts development and severity of acute interstitial lung disease as a complication of dermatomyositis. *Rheumatology* (Oxford) 2010;49:1354–1360.

43. Targoff IN. Idiopathic inflammatory myopathy: autoantibody update. *Curr Rheumatol Rep* 2002;4:434–441.

44) Hengstman GJ, van Engelen BG, Vree Egberts WT, van Venrooij WJ. Myositis-specific autoantibodies: overview and recent developments. *Curr Opin Rheumatol* 2001;13:476–482.

45. Hirakata M. Humoral aspects of polymyositis/dermatomyositis. *Mod Rheumatol* 2000;10:199–206.

46. Casciola-Rosen LA, Pluta AF, Plotz PH et al. The DNA mismatch repair enzyme PMS1 is a myositis-specific autoantigen. *Arthritis Rheum* 2001;44:389–396.

47. Gunawardena H, Betteridge ZE, McHugh NJ. Myositis-specific autoantibodies: their clinical and pathogenic significance in disease expression. *Rheumatology* (Oxford) 2009;48:607–612.

48. Kendall FP, McCreary EK, Provance PG. *Muscles: testing and function*, 4th edn. Lippincott Williams and Wilkins, Baltimore:, MD, 1993.

49. Miller FW, Rider LG, Chung YL et al. Proposed preliminary core set measures for disease outcome assessment in adult and juvenile idiopathic inflammatory myopathies. *Rheumatology* (Oxford) 2001;40:1262–1273.

50. Sultan SM, Allen E, Oddis CV et al. Reliability and validity of the myositis disease activity assessment tool. *Arthritis Rheum* 2008;58:3593–3599.

51. Sultan SM, Allen E, Cooper RG et al. Interrater reliability and aspects of validity of the myositis damage index. *Ann Rheum Dis* 2011;70:1272–1276.

52. Mastaglia FL, Garlepp MJ, Phillips BA, Zilko PJ. Inflammatory myopathies: clinical, diagnostic and therapeutic aspects. *Muscle Nerve* 2003;27:407–425.

53. Dorph C, Nennesmo I, Lundberg IE. Percutaneous conchotome muscle biopsy. A useful diagnostic and assessment tool. *J Rheumatol* 2001;28:1591–1599.

54. Lynch MC, Cohen JA. A primer on electrophysiologic studies in myopathy. *Rheum Dis Clin North Am* 2011;37:253–268, vii.

55. Park JH, Olsen NJ. Utility of magnetic resonance imaging in the evaluation of patients with inflammatory myopathies. *Curr Rheumatol Rep* 2001;3:334–345.

56. Fathi M, Lundberg IE. Interstitial lung disease in polymyositis and dermatomyositis. *Curr Opin Rheumatol* 2005;17:701–706.

57. Selva-O'Callaghan A, Grau JM, Gamez-Cenzano C et al. Conventional cancer screening versus PET/CT in dermatomyositis/polymyositis. *Am J Med* 2010;123:558–562.

58. Chinoy H, Fertig N, Oddis CV, Ollier WE, Cooper RG. The diagnostic utility of myositis autoantibody testing for predicting the risk of cancer-associated myositis. *Ann Rheum Dis* 2007;66:1345–1349.

59. Trallero-Araguas E, Rodrigo-Pendas JA, Selva-O'Callaghan A et al. Usefulness of anti-p155 autoantibody for diagnosing cancer-associated dermatomyositis: A systematic review and meta-analysis. *Arthritis Rheum* 20112012;64(2):523–532.

60. Dalakas MC, Illa I, Dambrosia JM et al. A controlled trial of high-dose intravenous immune globulin infusions as treatment for dermatomyositis. *N Engl J Med* 1993;329:1993–2000.

61. Miller FW, Leitman SF, Cronin ME et al. Controlled trial of plasma exchange and leukapheresis in polymyositis and dermatomyositis. *N Engl J Med* 1992;326:1380–1384.

62. Oddis CV, Reed AM, Aggarwal R et al. Rituximab in the treatment of refractory adult and juvenile dermatomyositis (DM) and adult polymyositis (PM) the RIM study [abstract]. *Arthritis Rheum* 2010;62:3844.

63. Chung YL, Alexanderson H, Pipitone N et al. Creatine supplements in patients with idiopathic inflammatory myopathies who are clinically weak after conventional pharmacologic treatment: Six-month, double-blind, randomized, placebo-controlled trial. *Arthritis Rheum* 2007;57:694–702.

64. Mann HF, Vencovsky J, Lundberg IE. Treatment-resistant inflammatory myopathy. *Best Pract Res Clin Rheumatol* 2010;24:427–440.

Sources of patient information

Arthritis Research UK. www.arthritisresearchuk.org/arthritis_information/arthritis_types__symptoms/polymyositis_and_dermatomyosit.aspx

Fenton J. *Living with myositis—facts, feelings and future*, 2nd edn. Thoughtful Publications, London, 2006. www.livingwithmyositis.com/

Myositis Association (USA). www.myositis.org/template/page.cfm?id=3

Myositis support group UK. www.myositis.org.uk/guide_to_myositis.htm

Muscular Dystrophy Association (USA). www.mdausa.org/publications/fa-myosi.html

Muscular Dystrophy Campaign (UK). www.muscular-dystrophy.org/how_we_help_you/publications

CHAPTER 125

Paediatric polymyositis and dermatomyositis

Clarissa Pilkington and Liza McCann

Introduction

Juvenile dermatomyositis (JDM) is the commonest idiopathic inflammatory myopathy (IIM) in childhood with juvenile polymyositis (JPM) being extremely rare. Skeletal muscle inflammation leads to progressive weakness, which can be confused with tiredness in young children and needs to be distinguished from infectious myositis or neuromuscular disorders such as muscular dystrophy. JDM affects the skin with a typical rash, as well many other organs. JPM does not affect the skin and has little published literature. This chapter will focus predominantly on JDM.

Epidemiology

JDM has an annual incidence of 2–3 per million children per year. A UK British Paediatric Surveillance Unit survey (1992–3) found an incidence of 1.9 (sex ratio 5:1 girls to boys).[1] This was felt to be unusually low and under-representative of the true incidence. In 2000, the Juvenile Dermatomyositis National (UK and Ireland) Cohort and Biomarker Study and Repository for Idiopathic Inflammatory Myopathies was established. In the first 10 years of this study, 275 IIM patients were recruited from a UK-wide network using standardized data collection forms,[2] with 182 girls and 76 boys, giving a sex ratio of 2.39:1. This is closer to the ratio from the National Institute of Arthritis and Musculoskeletal and Skin Disease (NIAMS) registry in the United States, which collected 395 cases with a sex ratio of 2.3:1.[3] In the UK cohort, ethnic differences mainly reflected ethnicity of the United Kingdom population; 80% were white European. This was also true of the NIAMS registry, with 79% classed as white non-Hispanic or Hispanic. In the UK cohort, median age of onset was 6.3 years, but 37% of patients presented under the age of 4. The incidence of JPM is unknown, but the UK cohort included 7 cases of JPM (4 definite, 3 probable) out of a total of 275 IIM cases. Seasonal variations in the incidence of IIM have been suggested, with clustering of cases in one study of 55% with onset between February and April.[4] The UK 1992–3 survey saw variable clusters between years, with the largest between April and May 1992. It is thought that environmental triggers including viruses, photosensitivity, and noxious substances may interact in genetically predisposed individuals (see below), but no one viral trigger has been identified.

Diagnostic criteria for juvenile dermatomyositis

The most widely accepted diagnostic criteria are those suggested by Bohan and Peter in 1975 (Table 125.1).[5] JDM/JPM are usually defined with onset before the age of 16 (Europe) or 18 (America). Definite dermatomyositis requires a characteristic rash (heliotrope rash over eyelids with periorbital oedema, Gottron's papules) plus three of the four muscle features documented in Table 125.1. Definite polymyositis requires all four muscle criteria (excluding rash). Polymyositis is more common in adults than in children, and has different muscle biopsy features (inflammatory infiltrates often widespread, particularly CD8+ T cells). These diagnostic criteria were based on clinical observations and have not been tested for sensitivity or specificity against all appropriate disease confounders. Other diagnostic criteria have been proposed as more advanced investigative techniques (MRI, autoantibodies) have become available, but they suffer from the same drawbacks.

Recent international collaboration led to an American College of Rheumatology/European League Against Rheumatism (ACR/EULAR) funded classification criteria study for adult and paediatric IIM. The International Myositis Classification Criteria Project (IMCCP) working group included rheumatologists, neurologists, and dermatologists (adult and paediatric). Expertise was pooled to devise a questionnaire capturing major symptoms, physical findings, investigational results, and treatment responses for patients with inflammatory myopathies and confounding diseases. Data were collected on 262 DM, 240 PM, 200 JDM, 172 inclusion body myositis (IBM), and 601 comparator cases. These data will allow more robust classification criteria to be devised, enhance understanding of differential diagnoses, and enable clinical trials to recruit suitable patients.

Aetiopathogenesis

The aetiopathogenesis of JDM is poorly understood, but is likely to include a combination of environmental triggers in genetically susceptible individuals, causing immune dysregulation resulting in tissue inflammation. There is speculation as to the primary target of the inflammatory response; whether it is endothelium or muscle cells. Evidence supports both hypotheses. Autoimmune diseases

Table 125.1 Bohan and Peter diagnostic criteria[5]

	Feature	Details
1	Symmetrical weakness	Usually progressive, of the limb-girdle muscles.
2	Muscle biopsy evidence of myositis	Necrosis of type I and type II muscle fibres. Phagocytosis. Degeneration and regeneration of myofibres with variation in myofibre size with perifascicular atrophy. Endomysial, perimysial, perivascular or interstitial mononuclear inflammatory cells
3	Elevation of serum levels of muscle-associated enzymes	CK, LDH, aldolase,[a] transaminases (ALT/SGPT and AST/SGOT)
4	Electromyographic (EMG) triad of myopathy	Short, small, low-amplitude polyphasic motor unit potentials, fibrillation potentials, even at rest, bizarre high-frequency repetitive discharges
Definite JDM/JPM = presence of 3 out of 4 features (plus rash for JDM)		
Probable JDM/JPM = presence of 2 out of 4 features (plus rash for JDM)		
Possible JDM/JPM depends on the presence of one feature (plus rash for JDM)		

CK, creatine kinase; JDM, juvenile dermatomyositis; JPM, juvenile polymyositis; LDH, lactate dehydrogenase.
[a]Not routinely available in UK.

often run in families, suggesting a complex polygenic influence; variations at many genetic loci contributing to an autoimmune phenotype. Genetic studies require large case numbers to have sufficient power to reveal genetic effects. This is particularly difficult for rare diseases such as JDM. Recent collaboration has led to an international genetics consortium in myositis (MYOGEN) collecting a large number of DNA samples from adult and paediatric cases. Results are likely to confirm the importance of the human leucocyte region (HLA), but may lead to the discovery of previously unknown risk and protective alleles. Previous studies demonstrated alleles found in greater numbers in cases than controls (i.e. alleles conferring risk), as well those found in fewer cases than controls (protective alleles), some of which may be involved in regulation of autoreactive T cells. In white Europeans, known loci conferring risk are *HLAB*08*, *DRB1*0301*, *DQA1*0501*, whereas protective alleles are *DQA1*0201*, *DQA1*0101*, and *DQA*0102*.[6] Other loci involving proinflammatory cytokines are known to be risk factors for JDM (such as TNFα variant TNF308A, IL-1α, and IL-1β) and some are associated with more severe disease (calcinosis, ulceration). In the future, these may help clinicians tailor patient treatments according to genetic risk.

Autoantibodies in IIM can be divided into two categories. Myositis-specific antibodies (MSA) are more specific to myositis patients. Myositis-associated antibodies (MAA) are seen with different myositis subtypes and overlap syndromes (such as anti-PM-Scl in scleroderma overlap) and are also found in other autoimmune conditions. Although traditionally thought to occur more frequently in DM than JDM, recent studies have shown approximately 70% of JDM patients have detectable MSA or MAA.[7] Novel MSAs have been identified including anti-TIF1-gamma (anti-p155/140) and anti-NXP2 (anti-p140). In JDM, anti-TIF1-gamma (found in 23–29% of cases) was associated with worse skin disease and lipodystrophy, whereas in adult patients it was associated with malignancy. Anti-NXP2 in JDM cases was associated with increased risk of calcinosis.[8] In a study of 114 JDM patients, many cases were ANA positive with no identifiable MSA or MAA, suggesting that JDM patients may have autoantibodies not yet identified that differ from those found in adult DM, or may confer different risks than in DM.[7]

The perivascular infiltrates characteristic of JDM are made up of T cells, B cells, and macrophages. Activation of plasmacytoid dendritic cells (antigen-presenting cells that initiate immunity through the activation of naive T cells) may play a role in pathogenesis. Mature plasmacytoid dendritic cells are found in inflammatory lesions from JDM muscle biopsies, compared to scattered immature plasmacytoid dendritic cells seen in normal muscle tissue. These may induce T-cell-mediated responses leading to muscle damage, though it is not known what initiates initial maturation and collection of the cells.[9] Increased plasmacytoid dendritic cells have also been found in skin from JDM cases. An increase in mast cell numbers (compared to normal controls) was found in skin, both in areas affected by rash, and in unaffected areas, though not in muscle. This suggestion that a different mechanism may be present in skin inflammation is paralleled by clinical observation that skin and muscle inflammation do not mirror each other.

Cytokines are likely to play an important role in pathogenesis, particularly type 1 interferon, which is produced by activated plasmacytoid dendritic cells, and upregulates MHC class I proteins on muscle cells. Upregulation of MHC class I can be seen in muscle biopsies from JDM patients, even when there are few other changes, but this is not specific to JDM and can be seen in Duchenne's muscular dystrophy.

Microchimerism describes the presence of maternally derived cells (acquired in utero during fetal stages or neonatally around time of birth) in children and adults. These cells, found in the blood and inflammatory infiltrates of JDM patients more frequently than their healthy siblings or healthy controls, may cause a graft-vs-host response leading to the autoimmune process.

Clinical features: disease onset

Presenting symptoms of JDM can be variable (Table 125.2).[10–14] Skeletal proximal muscle weakness may be mild and manifest as fatigue and difficulty doing tasks. Many children adapt, so symptoms may not become apparent to parents for some time. Myalgia is often a predominant feature. Weakness is progressive and can become profound, starting with difficulty climbing stairs, combing hair, or lifting objects above the head (proximal weakness) and

Table 125.2 Features present (percentages) at presentation of juvenile dermatomyositis

Feature	Percentage with feature present at presentation of juvenile dermatomyositis				
	UK cohort (n = 151) 2006[10]	Toronto cohort (n = 105) 2002[11]	USA cohort (n = 79) 1998[12]	Danish cohort (n = 57) 2010[13]	European/Latin American cohort (n = 490) 2011[14]
Proximal muscle weakness	82	95	100	93	84.9
Gottron's (JDM rash)	88[a]	91	100	74	72.9
Arthritis	36	6	35	26	35.7
Dysphagia	29	24[b]	44	23	17.8
Skin ulceration	23	6	NA	16	6.3
Calcinosis	6	3	23	5	3.7
Fever (systemic features)	81[c]	16	65	30	30.8

NA, not available.
[a]Grouped as characteristic rash or Gottron's in UK cohort.
[b]Grouped as dysphagia or dysphonia in Toronto cohort.
[c]Grouped as fever or any other systemic symptom in UK cohort (including fatigue, alopecia, weight loss, headache, irritability, chest pain, abdominal pain, diarrhoea, melaena, haematuria).

progressing to an inability to roll over in bed. The truncal muscles most commonly affected are the neck flexors and abdominals. Children will be unable to lift their head off the pillow, but will use compensatory manoeuvres. Symmetrical proximal muscle weakness is typical, but as weakness progresses, distal muscles can become involved, resulting in poor grip strength. If palatal muscles are affected, there can be swallowing difficulties and change in voice (sometimes misdiagnosed as bulbar palsy). The commonest manifestation of swallowing difficulty is coughing during eating or drinking, which may not be noticed by parents until asked repeatedly. A recent study demonstrated high incidence of self-reported dysphagia in 18 adult patients with IIM and found symptoms follow a characteristic pattern.[15] In JDM, silent aspiration has been recognized in asymptomatic children, with swallow dysfunction or aspiration not restricted to those who were severely weak.[16]

Gowers' sign is an excellent screening test for pelvic girdle or lower extremity muscle weakness. Patients are asked to rise from lying supine or sitting on the floor. With muscle weakness, a typical pattern emerges (Gowers' positive):

◆ The child rolls prone, extending arms and legs far apart (reduces forces required for knee extension).

◆ With most weight on extended arms, they push the body backwards (shifts weight of trunk over extended legs). Early changes of muscle weakness include exaggerated torso flexion, wide base, and equinus posturing.

◆ To extend the hip, the child places hands onto their knees and 'walks' arms up the thighs until upright. Note: this is only seen when muscle weakness becomes more pronounced (children with mild disease are able to bend at the hips once knees extended).

The salient feature of Gowers' sign is turning prone to rise from a supine position. This is a normal developmental phase in toddlers, but is rarely seen in healthy children over the age of 3 years. Healthy toddlers or obese children may use a hand to push off the thigh or the floor, giving a false-positive Gowers'. It is therefore important to repeat the test if positive and may be helpful to ask children to get up from a kneeling position with arms folded across their chest. Although first described in Duchenne muscular dystrophy, Gowers' sign will be positive in many other conditions, including other types of muscular dystrophy, inflammatory myopathies, proximal pseudomyopathic disorders, spinal muscular atrophy, sarcoglycanopathy, and discitis. Children with juvenile idiopathic arthritis can have a positive Gowers' sign, particularly when they have active arthritis of the hips.[17]

Parents may not notice a rash (Figure 125.1), as it can be transient and precede the muscle weakness. The facial heliotrope rash over eyelids can be mistaken for sunburn, even when associated with periorbital oedema. Gottron's papules (erythematous plaques) can be mistaken for psoriasis, especially when affecting skin overlying the distal/proximal interphalangeal joints as well as the better known metacarpophalangeal joints. The rash can affect other areas of the body such as the back (shawl sign) and trunk. Generalized erythema or livedo-type rash can be seen. Skin ulceration can occur in severe cases over the flexor surfaces, trunk, or medial canthus of the upper eyelid (usually heals leaving a scar similar to a chickenpox lesion). Nail beds are often erythematous and swollen, with abnormal capillary dilatation. This is more easily seen magnified by KY jelly and an auroscope/ophthalmoscope, or with a capillaroscope.

Polyarticular arthritis occurs in one-third of patients, and can cause the myositis to be overlooked. Systemic features such as tiredness, weight loss, fevers, and irritability are common. Headaches, diarrhoea, alopecia, and mouth ulcers are less common. Lipoatrophy, although infrequent, can be associated with insulin resistance, and is often difficult to reverse. Interstitial lung disease and gut vasculitis (which can lead to perforation) are uncommon, but are associated with severe disease that can be fatal.

Calcinosis can be present at onset, or can develop later if disease is not controlled. Calcium can be deposited as nodules, usually in the subcutaneous layers or in the fascia around muscles. It can form sheets or liquefy to form pools of 'milk of calcium', which may be extensive enough to cause compartment syndrome. Calcium nodules can extrude from the skin and can cause tendons to shorten, especially the Achilles tendon.

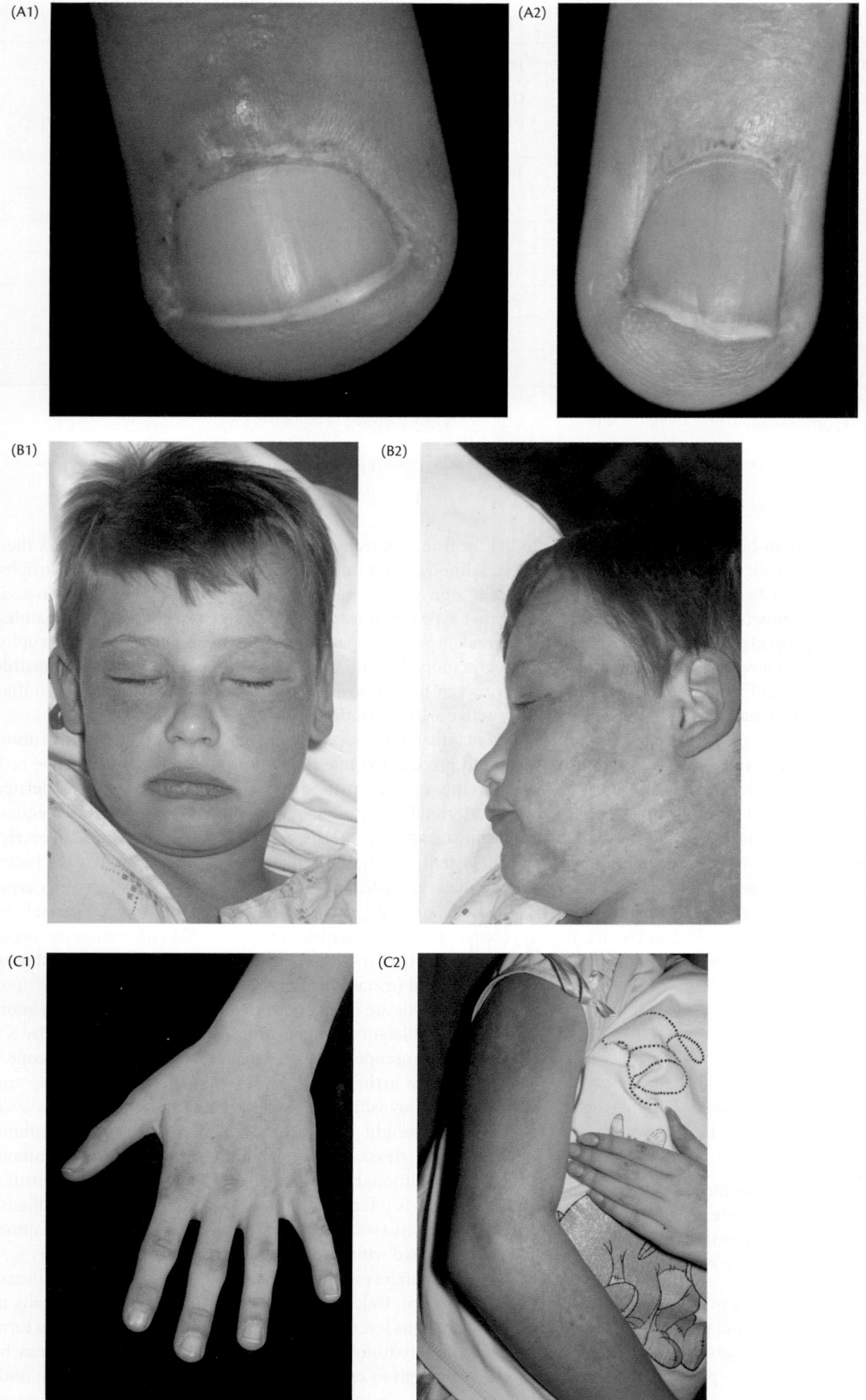

Fig. 125.1 Clinical signs of juvenile dermatomyositis: (A) nailfold capillary changes; (B) heliotrope and malar erythema; (C) rash on arm and Gottron's on hands.

Diagnosis

In typical cases, diagnosis of JDM is made clinically by the presence of classical rash and symmetrical proximal muscle weakness, supported by investigative results. However, no one investigation—muscle enzymes, MRI, electromyography (EMG), or muscle biopsy—is abnormal in all cases of JDM and therefore a high index of suspicion is required. The gold standard is still a tissue biopsy, but muscle inflammation in JDM affects muscle groups in a patchy manner, as well as being patchy within individual muscles. A biopsy can therefore look normal due to 'sampling' error or may look normal histologically, even when newer immunohistochemical stains (such as for MHC class I) pick up abnormalities. In atypical cases, it is crucial to undertake a biopsy to exclude muscular dystrophies and mitochondrial cytopathies.

In the absence of rash, diagnosis may be challenging and other causes of weakness including neuromuscular aetiologies need to be considered. It may be helpful to evaluate:

- onset of weakness: neonatal (hereditary causes)/infancy/childhood
- pattern of weakness: asymmetrical/symmetrical; proximal/distal/bulbar/cranial muscle (ptosis, facial weakness, dysphagia or dysarthria)
- time course: acute/subacute/chronic; episodic/persistent; progressive/non-progressive
- muscle features: pain/cramps/wasting
- presence of fatigue and its relationship to exercise
- associated features: sensory changes, abnormal reflexes; systemic/organ involvement; myotonia/hypertrophy, fever
- history of exposure to drugs or toxins
- family history: genetic causes/autoimmune disease.

The presence of myotonia (delayed relaxation of skeletal muscle following voluntary contraction; improves with repeated exercise), paramyotonia (gets worse with repeated exercise), or muscle hypertrophy may suggest neuromuscular causes. When primary pathology is in the nerve (cell body, axon or myelin), weakness is often more distal and associated with sensory loss. Disorders of the neuromuscular junction tend to cause patchy or diffuse weakness. Cranial weaknesses occur early. In contrast, muscle pathology tends to result in symmetrical, proximal, persistent weakness with less wasting, no sensory changes and normal reflexes (decreased only in areas of prominent weakness).[18]

Differential causes of systemic myopathy should be excluded before diagnosing inflammatory myopathy (Table 125.3).[19] Infections may be the cause of an acute myopathy or may trigger onset of JDM/JPM in susceptible individuals.[19] Fatigue, rather than weakness, is characteristic of endocrine myopathy. Constant weakness can be seen in myopathy due to systemic disease, whereas metabolic myopathy is classically associated with exercise-induced myalgia, exercise intolerance, and muscle cramps. Fatigue is a non-specific complaint but abnormal fatigability after exercise can be due to metabolic or mitochondrial myopathy or disorders of the neuromuscular junction.[19] Myalgia may be seen in infectious, inflammatory, drug-induced, or endocrine myopathy, but tends to be persistent in inflammatory muscle disorders and episodic in metabolic disease. Muscle cramps are usually benign but can be seen

in dehydration, hyponatraemia, and myxoedema. Muscle hypertrophy can be seen in hypothyroid myopathy, amyloidosis, sarcoidosis, neoplastic, or inflammatory processes.[20] Organ involvement should be considered (cardiac disease in particular is an important cause of mortality). The presence of optic atrophy or pigmented retinopathy suggests non-systemic causes. In adults, DM is associated with malignancy in approximately 24% of cases; this is thought to be due to an immune reaction to the tumour that cross-reacts with antigens in skin and muscle, leading to DM.[21] Although malignancy is reported in childhood myositis, it is so infrequent that routine assessment for occult malignancy is not warranted.

Inflammatory myopathy may be associated with other autoimmune diseases in 3–10% of cases.[22] The most common JDM overlap is with scleroderma, but any autoimmune disease may be seen including arthritis, lupus, or Sjögren's. A small minority of children have RNP+ve mixed connective tissue disease.[23] Vasculitis in the context of JDM should also be considered.

Muscle strength should be assessed at diagnosis and serially during follow-up. This can be achieved using the Childhood Myositis Assessment Scale (CMAS), a 14-item observational, performance-based instrument developed to evaluate muscle strength, physical function, and endurance in children with IIM. It addresses activities important in clinical assessment, such as timed neck flexion duration, ability to go from standing to seated position, and ability to perform sit-ups. The CMAS exhibits good reliability, construct validity, and responsiveness. A full description is provided on the ACR website (www.rheumatology.org). There is an important discrepancy between the CMAS scoring sheet found here and the original published by Lovell et al.,[24] due to typographical errors in the original article regarding scoring of certain variables (acknowledged by the authors, who agree the descriptions on the ACR website are correct). Normal scores for head lift manoeuvre and sit-ups are age and sex dependent and should be interpreted with caution, particularly in children less than 4 years of age.[25] Despite limitations, the CMAS is a valuable tool when used within its primary purpose to objectively and quantitatively compare a given patient's current performance with past performances. Although initially designed for research, it has been widely adopted as a reliable clinical tool for muscle strength assessment in units around the United Kingdom.[23]

Traditionally, muscle strength has been tested by five-point manual muscle testing (MMT), including the Medical Research Council Scale. However, recently, an expanded 0–10-point MMT scale has been used in therapeutic trials, postulated to be more sensitive in delineating weakness. The Kendal MMT-8 (Table 125.4) is now recommended, along with CMAS, as an outcome measure in JDM trials and is also a useful tool in clinical practice. The inclusion of a uniform set of muscle groups (including proximal, distal, and axial muscles with more emphasis on proximal and lower extremity muscle groups) with standardized scoring, should provide clinicians and researchers with more reliable MMT data in patients with juvenile PM/DM.[26]

Investigations should be carried out to exclude systemic causes of myopathy, confirm diagnosis of inflammatory myopathy (JDM/JPM), and determine extent of organ involvement. In light of this, blood tests should include inflammatory markers (erythrocyte sedimentation rate, C-reactive protein), renal function, liver function, muscle enzymes (creatine kinase, lactate dehydrogenase, aspartate aminotransferase, alanine aminotransferase, aldolase),

Table 125.3 Differential diagnosis of systemic myopathies[19]

Subgroup	Causes	Characteristics
Infectious	Viral: influenza, coxsackie B, HIV. Less common: adenovirus, parainfluenza	Acute weakness associated with prominent myalgia and painful muscle cramps affecting distal and proximal muscles. HIV myopathy is indistinguishable from idiopathic polymyositis clinically and histiologically
	Bacterial: *Staphylococcus aureus*, yersinia, streptococcus, anaerobic bacteria (e.g. clostridia). Less common: *Borrelia burgdorferi, Legionella pneumophila*	Suppurative myositis/pyomyositis. Rare in the West, but is seen in occasionally in AIDS patients
	Parasitic: protozoa, cestodes, nematodes	Focal or diffuse inflammatory myopathy ± neuropathy. May be associated with fever, myalgia, periorbital/facial oedema, or encephalopathy depending on cause
	Fungal: sporotripchosis, histomplasmosis, mucormycosis, cryptococcus, candidiasis	Uncommon but can be seen in immune-compromised patients. Can involve a single muscle group or may be diffuse. Mucormycosis can spread to the orbit causing ophthalmoplegia, proptosis or eyelid oedema
Endocrine	Hypothyroidism (proximal muscle weakness seen in one-third of patients)	Muscle complaints (pain, cramps, stiffness) frequent with proximal muscle weakness in one-third. Serum CK often elevated up to 10 times normal. Reflexes slow relaxing
	Hyperthyroidism	Often asymptomatic despite muscle weakness and atrophy on examination. Occasional bulbar muscle involvement with dysphagia, dysphonia, aspiration. Serum CK normal
	Hypoparathyroidism	Neuromuscular symptoms usually related to localized or generalized tetany, and if sustained, may cause elevation in CK
	Hyperparathyroidism	Proximal muscle weakness, muscle wasting, brisk reflexes. CK usually normal or slightly elevated
	Cushing's	Glucocorticoid excess (endogenous/exogenous) causes proximal weakness associated with cushingoid appearance. Muscle wasting may be striking
	Adrenal insufficiency (e.g. Conn's)	Muscle fatigue. Weakness typically mild. Serum CK may be elevated
	Agromegaly	Mild proximal muscle weakness without muscle atrophy
Metabolic myopathy associated with other systemic diseases	Vitamin D deficiency	Proximal muscle weakness and ataxic neuropathy. Pain due to osteomalacia. Progressive external ophthalmoplegia
	Hypokalaemia	Proximal or generalized weakness. Painless
	Hyperkalaemia	Weakness of cardiac and skeletal muscle likely secondary to effect on nerves
	Hypernatraemia	Proximal muscle weakness (rare). CK elevated
	Hypercalcaemia	Weakness with hyperreflexia
	Hypocalcaemia	Tetany more than weakness
	Hypophosphataemia	Acute severe areflexic weakness with rhabdomyolysis
	Chronic renal failure	Proximal limb weakness and bone pain. Painful myopathy may occur
	Hypomagnesaemia	Tetany with weakness
	Organ failure (cardiac, respiratory, hepatic failure)	Severe muscle wasting and complaints of weakness and fatigue
Drug- or toxin-induced myopathies	Glucocorticoid related	Proximal weakness and cushingoid features. CK usually normal
	Lipid lowering agents	Myalgia, malaise and muscle tenderness. Pain may be related to exercise. Proximal muscle weakness may be seen. CK elevated
	Alcohol and illicit drugs	Acute muscle weakness or painful chronic myopathy
	Other drugs, e.g. D-penicillamine, procainamide, L-tryptophan, amiodarone, chloroquine	Largely proximal muscle weakness, often painless
Paraneoplastic myopathy	Associated with numerous malignancies; most commonly ovary, lung, or gastrointestinal tract in Western nations (more common in adults but has been reported in children)	Myalgia and rapid progression of weakness involving proximal and distal muscles, pharyngeal and respiratory muscles. Tendency for more severe skin disease, less extramuscular or overlap features. CK normal or slightly elevated. MSA and MAA usually negative. Amyopathic DM also linked to malignancy
Critical illness myopathy	Thick filament myopathy, Acute necrotizing myopathy, cachetic myopathy	Major criteria include critical illness, difficulty with ventilator weaning and possible limb weakness. Myalgia less common. CK usually elevated

Table 125.4 Kendal MMT-8[26]

Muscle group (test right side only)	Starting position	Details
Neck flexion	Lying on back (completely flat bed)	Lift neck to 40° and place resistance on forehead
Shoulder abduction	From sitting	Shoulder abducted to 90°, arm straight at elbow, resistance placed at elbow
Elbow flexion	From sitting	Elbow flexed at 45°, supported with one hand, resistance at wrist
Wrist extension	Sitting	Forearm supported, hand pronated and wrist extended 60°, resistance on back of hand
Hip extension	Lying prone	Knee flexed to 90°, lift leg up, resistance on back of leg near knee
Hip abduction	Lying on side	Top leg slightly extended backwards, pelvis slightly rolled forward, abduct top leg, support pelvis. Resistance below knee, above ankle
Knee extension	Sitting over edge of bed	Knee extended but not locked, resistance placed above ankle. Modified if hamstrings tight (lean back onto elbows)
Ankle dorsiflexion	Lying on back	Dorsiflex the foot, resistance on top of foot
Score	**(maximum score = 80)**	
0	No movement	
1	Moves through partial range of movement in horizontal plane	
2	Moves through complete range of movement in horizontal plane	
3	Moves to completion of range of movement against resistance or moves to completion of range and holds against pressure or moves through partial range of movement in an anti-gravity position	
4	Gradual release from test position in an anti-gravity position	
5	Holds against test position (no added pressure)	
6	Holds test position against slight pressure	
7	Holds test position under slight to moderate pressure	
8	Holds test position under moderate pressure	
9	Holds test position under moderate to strong pressure	
10	Holds test position against strong pressure	

autoantibodies, thyroid function (plus other endocrine tests if relevant), virology/infection screen, bone profile (including parathyroid hormone and vitamin D). Other tests should be considered to look for other autoimmune disorders such as coeliac disease. Toxicology screen should be considered. Urine for albumin:creatinine ratio and microscopy should be taken, particularly if lupus overlap is suspected.

More than 20% of patients have normal creatine kinase (CK) at presentation,[10,13] and muscle enzymes may be normal despite ongoing active disease or disease flare. Likewise, inflammatory markers may be normal. Serum CK may help differentiate IIM from other causes of myopathy; if extremely high, Duchenne muscular dystrophy, muscle damage (rhabdomyolysis, trauma, injection), hypothyroidism, or immune polymyopathies should be considered. IIM tends to be associated with a moderately raised CK. This is also true of endocrine myopathy (hypothyroid, hypoparathyroid), asymptomatic dystrophy, metabolic or hereditary causes, exercise or trauma induced myopathy, drug toxicity, idiopathic hyperCKaemia, and certain races/genders (typically African American men).[18]

Antibody tests should be taken, including ANA and anti-ENA. Other antibody tests should be considered if overlap features are present and may include rheumatoid factor (RF), anti-dsDNA, anti-C1q antibody, and anti-thyroid antibodies. Tests for MSA and MAA (see above) are reliable, but currently not routinely available.

Traditional diagnostic criteria of JDM/JPM include EMG. This remains important if neuropathy is suspected, but an international survey of 118 clinicians from 92 centres (32 countries) caring for children with JDM found routine use of EMG was as low as 56%.[27] In contrast, MRI is increasingly used to help diagnose JDM/JPM and appears to be a valid indicator of disease activity. T2 weighted STIR images (fat suppressed) detect muscle inflammation and oedema in the subcutaneous tissue, myofascia, and skin. T1-weighted images may detect muscle atrophy and fatty infiltration. An MRI scoring system has been developed that objectively defines acute inflammatory change in JDM into four muscle groups and surrounding soft tissues.[28] Retrospective analysis of MRI scans by two paediatric radiologists showed fair to moderate agreement for all muscle groups and good intra-observer agreement between two readings. Further studies are needed. An evaluation of MRI in 45 children (36 with sufficient clinical data to assess duration of symptoms at time of MRI) with biopsy-proven JDM showed MRI appearance of muscle or fascia at diagnosis could not be used to predict clinical outcome, but abnormal increased signal intensity in subcutaneous fat had a high specificity (91%) for predicting ultimate progression to chronic or chronic ulcerative disease, independent of duration of symptoms at presentation.[29] Young children need sedation or general anaesthetic for MRI imaging. Musculoskeletal ultrasound may provide a safe, inexpensive, non-invasive means of supporting the clinical diagnosis of JDM and monitoring disease progression, without sedation. Ultrasound findings appear to correlate well with other markers of disease activity.[27]

Analysis of muscle biopsy tissue will often lead to confirmation of the diagnosis of JDM/JPM (Table 125.2). In order to determine the severity of JDM, an internationally agreed scoring system for muscle biopsies has been developed by consensus.[30] Muscle biopsies are scored using four domains: (1) inflammatory, (2) vascular/endothelial changes, (3) muscle fibre abnormalities (including staining for MHC class I overexpression), and (4) connective tissue changes. Prospective testing of this tool is underway. Greater understanding of muscle biopsy changes, including early abnormalities detected by advancing techniques, may allow prediction of disease course and prognosis.

The presence or extent of calcinosis should be determined by radiography (Figure 125.2) if clinically indicated. Investigations should also look for organ involvement including interstitial lung disease (chest radiograph, lung function tests, HRCT chest), cardiac involvement (ECG, echocardiogram), or abdominal pathology (ultrasound). A speech and language assessment may be needed with videofluoroscopy if there is dysphagia, dysphonia, or symptoms of aspiration. Nailfold capillaroscopy is helpful for distinguishing JDM from muscular dystrophies or other myopathies. It is a valuable marker of muscle and skin activity in JDM and has been found to be associated with other clinical measures of disease activity when analysed in 92 patients.[31] Within this cohort, 28 children had nailfold capillaroscopy at diagnosis; nailfold capillary density was reduced at onset but improved as the disease improved.

Disease course

Severity of disease can be difficult to judge at onset. Milder disease is usually monocyclic; a single episode, often recovering within a few years. Polycyclic disease course occurs with remissions and relapses, with the most severe disease being classed as 'chronic persistent': the disease may persist with no remission, for 15 years or more. Prior to the steroid era, one-third of JDM cases recovered, one-third were left with sequelae that caused severe disability, and one-third died.[32] Since the introduction of immunosuppressant medication, mortality has reduced significantly. In the first 10 years of the United Kingdom JDM Cohort and Registry Study, 285 patients were recruited (175 within 12 months of diagnosis), of which 3 died, giving an approximate mortality of 1%. This study has not recruited all British cases of JDM, and will not capture patients with severe disease who die prior to, or around time of diagnosis. In an international (European and South American) long-term follow-up study of 490 patients, mortality was 3.1%.[33] A prolonged course was predictive of poorer outcome, with persistently active disease at mean follow-up of 7.7 years in 40–60% of patients. In JDM, disease activity in the muscles often differs from that in the skin. Patients with prolonged disease course often have persistent skin activity even when myositis has come under control. One of the most difficult aspects of JDM to control once it has occurred is calcinosis. It is thought that increasing calcinosis is due to active disease and it can regress on treatment (unlike adult disease), but no one medication has been successful in halting progression of calcinosis. Cardiovascular mortality is significant in adult IIM. Subclinical cardiovascular changes are suggested in JDM and a recent study in a small number of adult patients with a history of definite or probable JDM (n = 8) found increased atherosclerotic burden compared to healthy controls.[34] Further studies are needed to assess long-term cardiovascular risk.

Disease activity and damage assessment tools

Disease severity at onset, as well as disease course, needs to guide aggressiveness of medical treatment. The multisystem aspect of disease makes assessments complex. Disease activity needs to be separated from disease damage. This can be difficult in paediatric

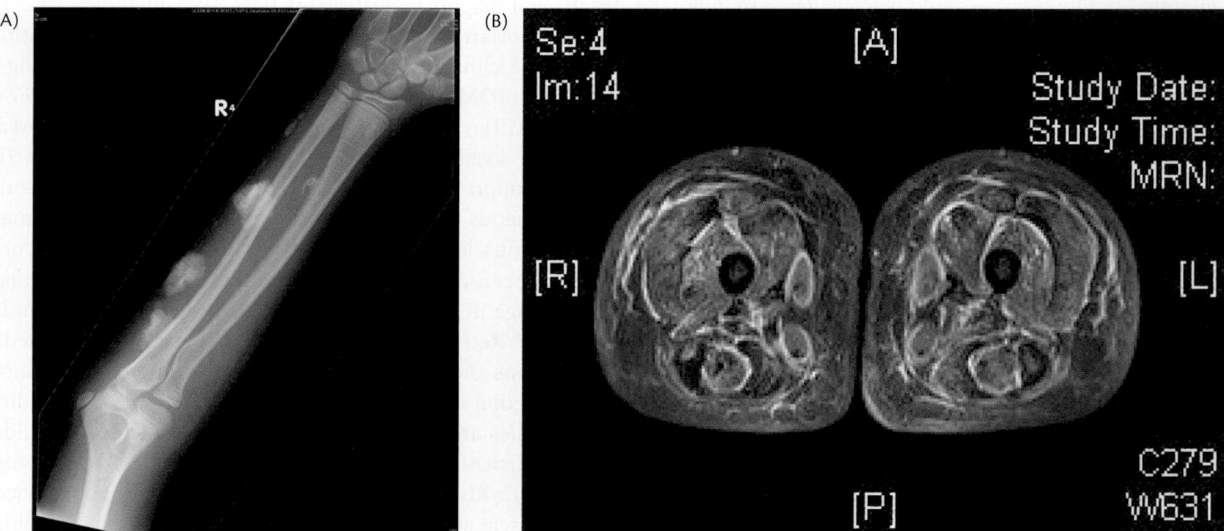

Fig. 125.2 Radiological signs of juvenile dermatomyositis: (A) radiograph of calcinosis; (B) MRI scan of thigh (axial STIR sequences) showing increased signal intensity (brightness) consistent with severe inflammation (myositis). Changes seen include soft tissue oedema, perifascicular oedema, and muscle oedema.

cases, where the power to repair is different from adults; during childhood, eroded bones can remodel, and calcinosis can regress and disappear. In order to study patients, disease activity assessment tools have been developed. The Disease Activity Score (DAS) rates muscle and skin disease.[35] A more comprehensive disease activity tool (MDAA) has been developed and standardized by an international group for use in adult and paediatric trials, but needs time and standardized training to be reliable. Two core set measures for clinical studies and criteria for response to treatment have been proposed for use in clinical trials. A separate disease damage tool (the Myositis Damage Index) has also been developed.[36]

Management

There are few published randomized controlled trials (RCTs) for myositis; most of the evidence base comes from case series and expert consensus. The first-line treatment for patients with JDM is corticosteroids. Evidence for use of steroids comes from the mortality rate of the presteroid era (one-third of patients),[32] compared to 10% in the early poststeroid era.[37] Route of administration has little evidence base, and varies depending on local healthcare systems and historical practice, but oral steroids are often started at 2 mg/kg, and maybe divided into two to four doses a day. The intravenous (IV) route may bypass absorption problems secondary to gut inflammation,[38] giving faster symptom control but with little effect on long-term outcome. In the United Kingdom, many centres start with IV followed by oral steroids.[23]

Drug treatment: disease-modifying drugs

Many centres use methotrexate (MTX) as the disease-modifying anti-rheumatic drug (DMARD) of choice, irrespective of disease severity. Over 90% of patients in the UK cohort study were given steroids and MTX.[23] There is evidence that early introduction of these drugs reduces incidence of calcinosis.[39] Previously, ciclosporin was used, based on a case series of 14 patients,[40] but it has been less frequently used since 2000,[14] when MTX became more widely utilized.[41] A randomized study to compare steroids (monotherapy) as first-line therapy vs steroids and MTX vs steroids and ciclosporin has been undertaken by PRINTO (the Paediatric Rheumatology International Trial Organization). Preliminary results show better response with MTX or ciclosporin compared to steroid alone. More side effects were seen with ciclosporin than MTX, supporting the usual UK practice of prednisolone and MTX as first-line treatment.

Intravenous immunoglobulin (IVIG) is widely used. An RCT in adult DM demonstrated effectiveness in 15 patients resistant to treatment.[42] In a Children's Arthritis and Rheumatology Research Alliance (CARRA) survey, physicians used IVIG for severe or refractory disease, and for significant skin disease.[43] In the United Kingdom, the Department of Health National Demand Programme for IVIG has approved IVIG for long-term use in JDM when alternative therapies have been used where appropriate (www.ivig.nhs.uk/clinicianinfo.html).

Other DMARDs used include azathioprine (often in combination with MTX), hydroxychloroquine, and mycophenolate mofetil (MMF). A retrospective case series of 12 patients showed improvement in myositis and skin rash with MMF including regression of calcinosis in one case.[44] Another retrospective case series showed improvement in muscle strength and skin rash at 6 months in 50 patients, with a further improvement in skin rash by 1 year.[45] Severe disease (such as skin ulceration, interstitial lung disease, and gastrointestinal perforation) is treated with IV cyclophosphamide; demonstrated to improve outcome in a retrospective case series of 12 patients with severe disease refractory to a combination of DMARDS.[46] Due to the side-effect profile of IV cyclophosphamide, it is reserved for patients with severe disease.

Anti-TNF (tumour necrosis factor) monoclonal antibodies have been used to treat IIM. An adult RCT of 16 patients refractory to treatment demonstrated improvement in muscle strength at 6 months in 9 of 11 patients on etanercept.[47] A retrospective case series of five JDM patients on infliximab showed improvements in all five,[48] and an updated case series from the UK cohort with 30 patients showed improvement in muscle strength, skin rash, and calcinosis.[49] The first international RCT in adult and juvenile DM has taken place using the anti-CD20 monoclonal antibody rituximab. Previous case series showed promising results in refractory patients. Although the trial failed to meet primary and secondary endpoints, the overall response rate, steroid-sparing effect, and retreatment response in a refractory group of patients suggest rituximab does have an effect.[50]

Anecdotal reports of treatments that have helped to treat calcinosis include diltiazem, infliximab, and bisphosphonates. Diclofenac is a useful non-steroidal anti-inflammatory drug (NSAID) to help inflammation around calcinotic deposits, and flucloxacillin can help secondary infection that may prolong or worsen calcinosis. In JDM, increasing calcinosis should be treated with more intense DMARD use, as widespread calcinosis causes severe morbidity and disability.

As JDM is rare, it will be difficult and expensive to undertake international RCTs. Many in the paediatric rheumatology community have advocated a system of using treatment plans to enrol all children with JDM. This system would parallel the system for childhood malignancies (which have allowed protocols to be evaluated and refined, leading to improved survival). To this end, CARRA have undertaken a survey of treatment practices in JDM,[43] followed by consensus conference to produce three consensus treatment plans for moderate severe cases of JDM.[51] Physicians can choose the treatment plan most akin to their practice and most suitable for their patient. Patient data are collected, and using statistics (taking into account intention to treat differences), plans can be compared and evaluated. The three consensus treatment plans are summarized in Table 125.5.

Non-drug treatment

The role of allied health professionals in the treatment of JDM is crucial: physiotherapists, clinical nurse specialists, occupational therapists, and psychologists provide important therapeutic input. It is important to prevent contractures as these can cause severe disability even when muscle strength has returned. Historically, active physiotherapy in the early stages of disease was discouraged, due to concerns that it would worsen inflammation and cause calcinosis. There is little evidence to support this; in a small study of JDM patients and normal controls, no increase was seen in muscle enzymes or MRI signal after undertaking a short exercise programme.[52] Patients with JDM have been shown to have impaired maximal aerobic exercise capacity when using a treadmill.[53] They can be helped to improve muscle strength and regain stamina through a targeted exercise programme.

Table 125.5 CARRA consensus treatment plans for moderately severe juvenile dermatomyositis[51]

Consensus treatment plan A	Consensus treatment plan B	Consensus treatment plan C
IV methylprednisolone 30 mg/kg/day (max 1g) × 3; may continue 1×/week (optional). Followed by: **Oral prednisone** 2 mg/kg/day (max 60 mg) once daily for 4 weeks, then decrease by 20% (as dictated by the treating physician)	**IV methylprednisolone** 30 mg/kg/day (max 1 g) × 3; may continue 1×/week (optional). Followed by: **Oral prednisone** 2 mg/kg/day (max 60 mg) once daily for 4 weeks, then decrease by 20% (as dictated by the treating physician)	**Oral prednisone** 2 mg/kg/day (max 60 mg) divided into twice daily doses for 4 weeks, then consolidate to once daily (as dictated by the treating physician)
Methotrexate (SC unless only oral possible); either 15 mg/m² or 1 mg/kg (maximum 40 mg) once weekly	**Methotrexate** (SC unless only oral possible), either 15 mg/m² or 1 mg/kg (maximum 40 mg) once weekly **IVIG** 2g/kg (max 70g), fortnightly for 3 doses, then monthly **Optional IV methylprednisolone** × 1 with each IVIG	**Methotrexate** (SC unless only oral possible). Lesser of 15 mg/m² or 1 mg/kg (maximum 40 mg) once weekly

A recent study of sleep and fatigue in patients with childhood rheumatic diseases, including 33 patients with JDM, found sleep was disturbed in approximately one-half of the patients, correlated with increased pain and decreased quality of life.[54] Children may need to return to school on a part-time basis initially, building up to full-time as they regain stamina. Liaison with schools is often beneficial. For families, coping with JDM and its impact on daily lives can be very difficult and support from experienced nurses, play specialists, and psychologists can be invaluable.

Case histories

Case history 1

6 year old girl: 2-year history of knee pain. Weakness implied by history of not being able to pull herself out of a swimming pool (twin sister had no difficulty). Frequent abdominal pain and poor growth compared to twin. Serum CK raised (2018 iu/litre), inflammatory markers (ESR, CRP) normal, ANA positive (>1:160), anti-ENA negative. O/E: Skin changes over MCP and PIPs suggestive of old Gottron's patches. Nailfold capillary changes seen using KY jelly and ophthalmoscope. Mild synovitis of wrists, decreased end range movement. Neck flexors and abdominal muscles weak, but normal muscle strength in limbs. MRI scan of thighs normal but muscle biopsy demonstrated changes consistent with JDM. Treatment started (steroid and methotrexate) with good response.

Learning points: Diagnosis of JDM was delayed in this child for the following reasons:

1. JDM considered unlikely because of normal inflammatory markers.

2. Skin features not recognized as old Gottron's.

3. Muscle weakness was subtle and required careful examination of neck flexor and abdominal muscles.

4. Muscle biopsy was needed to confirm diagnosis (MRI normal). MRI more likely to show abnormalities in acute phase (more oedema and inflammation).

Case history 2

12 year old boy: presented with rash, aching feet, shortness of breath, difficulty swallowing and nasal regurgitation. O/E: Rash typical of JDM (heliotrope changes, malar erythema with nasolabial involvement, Gottron's patches, nailfold capillary changes). CK and LDH elevated (2021 iu/litre and 1178 iu/litre respectively). ANA positive (1:160). EMG showed myopathic potential. MRI (T2 weighted) showed inflammatory changes consistent with JDM. Treated with intravenous methylprednisolone, followed by weaning course of oral steroid; good response. Two years later, complained of muscle weakness and tenderness. O/E: Active nailfold capillaries and Gottron's patches, weakness (CMAS score 15/53), mild restriction of elbows, knees, wrists and hips. Serum CK and LDH normal (61 iu/litre and 500iu/litre respectively). Treated with steroid (IV methylprednisolone followed by oral prednisolone) and methotrexate. Weakness improved, but skin remained active. Developed skin ulceration (armpits and elbow). Cyclophosphamide added with good effect.

Learning points:

1. Muscle enzymes may be normal in disease flares or later in disease.

2. Disease should be treated early and aggressively to obtain remission. Steroid monotherapy was inadequate and DMARD should have been added at presentation.

3. Stepwise approach needed; increase in immune-suppressive therapy if inadequate response. Cyclophosphamide indicated for severe ulcerative skin disease or major organ involvement.

Case history 3

4 year old boy: 2–3 months of tiredness, leg pain, not wanting to walk far; asking to go in buggy. Following holiday in Florida, developed sore throat, maculo-papular rash, particularly over axilla, violaceous skin rash over periorbital area, puffy eyes, erythema of nail beds and fingers. Two weeks later, developed generalized swelling of limbs and abdomen. Became extremely tired

with loss of appetite and activity. O/E: Lethargic, unwell with generalized oedema, violaceous macular rash over periorbital area, face, chin, neck, nail beds, knees and elbows. Macular-papular rash over both axillae, mild oral ulceration and gum swelling. Hepatomegaly (2–3cm), proximal muscle power of 3/10, distal power of 5/10, nasal speech. Muscle enzymes raised: CK 6926 iu/litre (5–120), LDH 3062 iu/litre (470–900). MRI showed significant increase in T2 signal bilaterally in the quadriceps and the thigh abductors consistent with myositis. Management: Treated with IV methyl prednisolone (high-dose, then maintenance) and subcutaneous methotrexate but developed skin ulceration in axillae: IV cyclophosphamide added for 6 doses. Muscle enzymes started to fall after the first week, but unable to tolerate oral steroids (abdominal pain and distension) for 3 months, requiring IV steroids (maintenance) daily via Hickman line. Remained on steroids for 18 months; stopped all treatment after 3.5 years. Muscle enzymes normalized by 4 months, but mild residual muscle weakness remained at 12 months. Currently well with no sequelae 4 years after stopping treatment.

Learning points:

1. In young children, parents may think their child is being lazy rather than weak.

2. Muscle enzymes recover faster than muscle strength.

Case history 4

4 year old Afro-Caribbean girl: presented to neurologist with difficulty climbing stairs, frequent falls, fatigue and joint pain. O/E: Facial rash around eyes and on neck. CK elevated (5000 iu/litre). Muscle biopsy consistent with JDM. Treated with oral prednisolone. Azathioprine added eight months later for recurrence of symptoms. Failed to improve – treated with IV steroids and ciclosporin. Eight months later she was osteoporotic and developed calcinosis in her right cheek. Transferred to rheumatology. O/E: Active capillary loop dilatations of nail beds, calcinosis in her left cheek, muscle strength of 3 to 7/10, patchy myositis on MRI thigh. CK normal, insignificantly raised LDH of 925 iu/litre (470–900). Treated with subcutaneous methotrexate, but soon flared and developed calcinosis on anterior chest wall. Infliximab added; calcinosis slowly regressed, with none in the chest 3 years later. Calcinosis of the cheek successfully removed by plastic surgeons.

Learning points:

1. Use DMARD early to control disease and prevent calcinosis. Add additional DMARD if calcinosis occurs (prolonged use often required for regression of calcinosis).

2. Surgical removal of calcinosis only if absolutely necessary; ensure disease controlled before surgery to prevent recurrence or discharging fistulae.

References

1. Symmons DP, Sills JA, Davis SM. The incidence of juvenile dermatomyositis: results from a nation-wide study. *Br J Rheumatol* 1995;34(8):732–736.

2. Martin N, Krol P, Smith S et al. A national registry for juvenile dermatomyositis and other paediatric idiopathic inflammatory myopathies: 10 years' experience; the Juvenile Dermatomyositis National (UK and Ireland) Cohort Biomarker Study and Repository for Idiopathic Inflammatory Myopathies. *Rheumatology* 2011;50(1):137–145.

3. Mendez EP, Lipton R, Ramsey-Goldman R et al. US incidence of juvenile dermatomyositis, 1995–1998: results from the National Institute of Arthritis and Musculoskeletal and Skin Diseases Registry. *Arthritis Rheum* 2003;49(3):300–305.

4. Medsger TA, Jr., Dawson WN Jr, Masi AT The epidemiology of polymyositis. *Am J Med* 1970;48(6):715–723.

5. Bohan A, Peter JB. Polymyositis and dermatomyositis (first of two parts). N Engl J Med 1975;292(7):344–347; second of two parts. N Engl J Med 1975;292(8):403–407.

6. Wedderburn LR, Rider LG Juvenile dermatomyositis: new developments in pathogenesis, assessment and treatment. *Best Pract Res Clin Rheumatol* 2009;23(5):665–678.

7. Wedderburn LR, McHugh NJ, Chinoy H et al. HLA class II haplotype and autoantibody associations in children with juvenile dermatomyositis and juvenile dermatomyositis-scleroderma overlap. *Rheumatology* (Oxford) 2007;46(12):1786–1791.

8. Gunawardena H, Wedderburn LR, Chinoy H et al. Autoantibodies to a 140-kd protein in juvenile dermatomyositis are associated with calcinosis. *Arthritis Rheum* 2009;60:1807–1814.

9. Lopez de Padilla CM, Vallejo AN, McNallan KT et al. Plasmacytoid dendritic cells in inflamed muscle of patients with juvenile dermatomyositis. *Arthritis Rheum* 2007;56:1658–1668.

10. McCann LJ, Juggins AD, Maillard SM et al. The Juvenile Dermatomyositis National Registry & Repository (UK & Ireland): Clinical characteristics of children recruited within the first 5 years. *Rheumatology* (Oxford) 2006;45(10):1255–1260.

11. Ramanan AV, Feldman BM. Clinical features and outcomes of juvenile dermatomyositis and other childhood onset myositis syndromes. *Rheum Dis Clin North Am* 2002;28(4):833–857.

12. Pachman LM, Hayford JR et al. Juvenile dermatomyositis at diagnosis: clinical characteristics of 79 children. *J Rheumatol* 1998;25(6):1198–1204.

13. Mathiesen PR, Zak M, Herlin T, Nielsen SM. Clinical features and outcome in a Danish cohort of juvenile dermatomyositis patients. *Clin Exp Rheumatol* 2010;28(5):782–789.

14. Guseinova D, Consolaro A, Trail L et al. Comparison of clinical features and drug therapies among European and Latin American patients with juvenile dermatomyositis. *Clin Exp Rheumatol* 2011;29(1):117–124.

15. Mulcahy KP, Langdon PC, Mastaglia F. Dysphagia in inflammatory myopathy: self-report, incidence, and prevalence. *Dysphagia* 2012;27(1):64–69.

16. McCann LJ, Garay SM, Ryan MM et al. Oropharyngeal dysphagia in juvenile dermatomyositis (JDM): an evaluation of videofluoroscopy swallow study (VFSS) changes in relation to clinical symptoms and objective muscle scores. *Rheumatology* 2007;46:1363–1366.

17. Chang RF, Mubarak SJ. Pathomechanics of Gowers' sign: a video analysis of a spectrum of Gowers' maneuvers. *Clin Orthop Relat Res* 2012;470(7):1987–1991.

18. Washington Neuromuscular Disease Centre. http://neuromuscular.wustl.edu.

19. Chawla J. Stepwise approach to myopathy in systemic disease. *Front Neurol* 2011;2:49.

20. Pachman L, Lipton R, Ramsey-Goldman et al. History of infection before the onset of juvenile dermatomyositis: results from the National Institute of Arthritis and Musculoskeletal and Skin Diseases Research Registry. *Arthritis Rheum* 2005;53(2):166–172.

21. Zahr ZA, Baer AN. Malignancy in myositis. *Curr Rheumatol Rep* 2011;13:208–215.

22. Feldman BM, Rider LG, Reed AM, Pachman LM. Juvenile dermatomyositis and other idiopathic inflammatory myopathies of childhood. *Lancet* 2008;371:2201–2212.

23. Martin N, Wedderburn LR, Pilkington CA, Davidson JE A survey of current practice in the management of Juvenile Dermatomyositis in the UK and Ireland. Abstract from the 17th Paediatric Rheumatology European Society Congress. *Clin Exp Rheumatol* 2011;29(Suppl):372.

24. Lovell DJ, Lindsley CB, Rennebohm RM et al. Development of validated disease activity and damage indices for the juvenile idiopathic inflammatory myopathies. II. The Childhood Myositis Assessment Scale (CMAS): a quantitative tool for the evaluation of muscle function. *Arthritis Rheum* 1999;42:2213–2219.

25. Rennebohm RM, Jones K, Huber AM et al. Normal scores for nine maneuvers of the Childhood Myositis Assessment Scale. *Arthritis Rheum* 2004;51(3):365–370.

26. Rider LG, Koziol D, Giannini EH et al. Validation of manual muscle testing and a subset of eight muscles for adult and juvenile idiopathic inflammatory myopathies. *Arthritis Care Res* (Hoboken) 2010;62(4):465–472.

27. Brown VE, Pilkington CA, Feldman BM, Davidson JE; Network for Juvenile Dermatomyositis, Paediatric Rheumatology European Society (PReS). An international consensus survey of the diagnostic criteria for juvenile dermatomyositis (JDM). *Rheumatology* (Oxford) 2006;45(8):990–993.

28. Davis WR, Halls JE, Offiah AC et al. Assessment of active inflammation in juvenile dermatomyositis: a novel magnetic resonance imaging-based scoring system. *Rheumatology* (Oxford) 2011;50(12):2237–2244.

29. Ladd PE, Emery KH, Salisbury SR et al. Juvenile dermatomyositis: correlation of MRI at presentation with clinical outcome. *AJR Am J Roentgenol* 2011;197(1):W153–W158.

30. Wedderburn LR, Varsani H, Li CK et al. International consensus on a proposed score system for muscle biopsy evaluation in patients with juvenile dermatomyositis: a tool for potential use in clinical trials. *Arthritis Rheum* 2007;57(7):1192–1201

31. Schmeling H, Stephens S, Goia C et al. Nailfold capillary density is importantly associated over time with muscle and skin disease activity in juvenile dermatomyositis. *Rheumatology* (Oxford) 2011;50(5):885–893.

32. Bitnum S, Daeschner CW Jr, Travis LB, Dodge WF, Hopps HC. Dermatomyositis. *J Pediatr* 1964;64:101–131.

33. Ravelli A, Trail L, Ferrari C et al. Long-term outcome and prognostic factors of juvenile dermatomyositis: a multinational, multicenter study of 490 patients, *Arthritis Care Res* 2010;62:63–72.

34. Eimer MJ, Brickman WJ, Seshadri R et al. Clinical status and cardiovascular risk profile of adults with a history of juvenile dermatomyositis. *J Pediatr* 2011;159:795–801.

35. Bode RK, Klein-Gitelman MS, Miller ML, Lechman TS, Pachman LM. Disease activity score for children with juvenile dermatomyositis: reliability and validity evidence. *Arthritis Rheum* 2003;49(1):7–15.

36. Lowry CA, Pilkington CA. Juvenile dermatomyositis: extramuscular manifestations and their management. *Curr Opin Rheumatol* 2009;21:575–580.

37. Spencer CH, Hanson V, Singsen BH et al. Course of treated juvenile dermatomyositis. *J Pediatr* 1984;105(3):399–408.

38. Rouster-Stevens KA, Gursahaney A, Ngai K-L, Daru JA, Pachman LM. Pharmacokinetic study of oral prednisolone compared with intravenous methyl-prednisolone in patients with juvenile dermatomyositis. *Arthritis Rheum* 2008;58:222–226.

39. Fisler RE, Liang MG, Fuhlbrigge RC, Yalcindag A, Sundel RP. Aggressive management of juvenile dermatomyositis results in improved outcome and decreased incidence of calcinosis. *J Am Acad Dermatol* 2002;47(4):505–511.

40. Heckmatt J, Saunders C, Peters AM et al. Cyclosporin in juvenile dermatomyositis. *Lancet* 1989;333:1063–1066.

41. Ramanan AV, Campbell-Webster N, Ota S et al. The effectiveness of treating juvenile dermatomyositis with methotrexate and aggressively tapered corticosteroids, *Arthritis Rheum* 2005;52:3570–3578.

42. Dalakas MC, Illa I, Dambrosia JM et al. A controlled trial of high-dose intravenous immune globulin infusions as treatment for dermatomyositis. *N Engl J Med* 1993;329(27):1993–2000.

43. Stringer E, Ota S, Bohnsack J et al. Treatment approaches to juvenile dermatomyositis across North America: The Childhood Arthritis and Rheumatology Research Alliance (CARRA) JDM treatment survey. *Rheumatology* 2010;37(9):1953–1961.

44. Dagher R, Desjonquères M, Duquesne A et al. Mycophenolate mofetil in juvenile dermatomyositis: a case series. *Rheumatol Int* 2012;32(3):711–716.

45. Rouster-Stevens KA, Morgan GA, Wang D, Pachman LM. Mycophenolate mofetil: a possible therapeutic agent for children with juvenile dermatomyositis. *Arthritis Care Res* (Hoboken) 2010;62(10):1446–1451.

46. Riley P, Maillard SM, Wedderburn LR et al. Intravenous cyclophosphamide pulse therapy in juvenile dermatomyositis. A review of efficacy and safety. *Rheumatology* (Oxford) 2004;43:491–496.

47. Muscle Study Group. A randomized, pilot trial of etanercept in dermatomyositis. *Ann Neurol* 2011;70(3):427–436.

48. Riley P, McCann LJ, Maillard SM et al. Effectiveness of infliximab in the treatment of refractory juvenile dermatomyositis with calcinosis. *Rheumatology* (Oxford) 2008;47(6):877–880.

49. Boulter EL, Beard L, Ryder C, Pilkington C. Effectiveness of anti-tumour necrosis factor-agents in the treatment of refractory juvenile dermatomyositis. *Arthritis Rheum* 2011;63(S),795.

50. Oddis CV, Reed AM, Aggarwal R et al. Rituximab in the treatment of refractory adult and juvenile dermatomyositis and adult polymyositis: A randomised, placebo-phase trial. *Arthritis Rheum* 2013;65(2):314–324.

51. Huber AM, Giannini EH, Bowyer SL et al. Protocols for the initial treatment of moderately severe juvenile dermatomyositis: results of a Children's Arthritis and Rheumatology Research Alliance Consensus Conference. *Arthritis Care Res* (Hoboken) 2010;62(2):219–225.

52. Maillard SM, Jones R, Owens C et al. Quantitative assessment of MRI T2 relaxation time of thigh muscles in juvenile dermatomyositis. *Rheumatology* (Oxford) 2004;43:603–608.

53. Takken T, Spermon N, Helders PJ, Prakken AB, Van Der Net J. Aerobic exercise capacity in patients with juvenile dermatomyositis. *J Rheumatol* 2003;30(5):1075–1080.

54. Aviel YB, Stremler R, Bensler SM et al. Sleep and fatigue and the relationship to pain, disease activity and quality of life in juvenile idiopathic arthritis and juvenile dermatomyositis. *Rheumatology* 2011;50:2051–2060.

Sources of patient/parent information

Robinson A, Reed A. Clinical features, pathogenesis and treatment of juvenile and adult dermatomyositis. *Nat Rev Rheumatol* 2011;7:664–675.

Juvenile Dermatomyositis Research Group: www.juveniledermatomyositis.org.uk

Myositis Association: www.myositis.org

Myositis Support Group: www.myositis.org.uk

Paediatric Rheumatology International Trials Organization: www.printo.it

CHAPTER 126

Non-inflammatory myopathies

Mark Roberts

Introduction

Non-inflammatory myopathies (NIM) are a diverse group of genetic disorders characterized by neuromuscular weakness, fatigue, muscle wasting, and pain due to inherited defects in proteins critical in the structural integrity and function of muscle fibre or in enzymes involved in energy production in this most metabolic tissue. The shared clinical and laboratory features (including elevated muscle enzyme levels, myopathic change on electromyography, and even inflammatory changes on muscle biopsy) of myositis and NIM frequently cause diagnostic confusion. Failure to distinguish these disorders will result in unnecessary immunosuppression, lack of screening for cardiorespiratory and other associations of NIM, and a missed opportunity for genetic counselling and potential future treatments. A strong index of suspicion is required in all patients presenting with neuromuscular syndromes if a long diagnostic odyssey is to be avoided. A clinically focused multidisciplinary approach, with a working knowledge of subtypes of NIM (as summarized in Box 126.1) is outlined in this chapter.

Clinical assessment: history

Weakness

Neuromuscular disorders commonly present with weakness, and focused enquiry into this symptom often accelerates a diagnosis of NIM. An accurate history documents the onset, nature and pattern, and progression of weakness, and is crucial in differentiating subtypes of NIM.

Reduced fetal movements and difficulties at delivery may suggest a congenital myopathy, metabolic, or myotonic disorder. Initially normal and then delayed motor milestones may suggest a muscular dystrophy such as Duchenne muscular dystrophy (DMD). It is common for weakness to be falsely attributed by doctor and patient alike to laziness, growing pains, or asthma in childhood, or to normal ageing or painful conditions in later life. A directive questioning style is required with questions such as 'when did you first use a stick?' Inquiries into sporting abilities, occupational history, and military service will often also help time the onset of symptoms, as will consultations with both patients and their relatives.

The nature and pattern of weakness is again often suggested by the history. Proximal weakness is seen in most NIM, and in the upper limbs causes practical difficulties reaching up to a shelf or combing

---

Box 126.1 Categories of non-inflammatory myopathies

Congenital myopathies

Myotonic disorders

- Myotonic dystrophy/dystrophica myotonica type 1 (DM1)
- Myotonic dystrophy type 2/proximal myotonic myopathy
- Myotonia congenita (Becker and Thomsen)

Dystrophinopathies

- Duchenne muscular dystrophy (DMD)
- Becker muscular dystrophy (BMD)
- Fascioscapular humeral muscular dystrophy (FSHD)
- Limb girdle muscular dystrophies (LGMD1 dominant, 2 recessive)

Metabolic myopathies

- Glycogen synthesis and glycogenolytic disorders
- Fatty acid oxidation defects

Other inherited myopathies

- Distal myopathies
- Myofibrillary myopathies
- Hereditary inclusion body myopathies
- Collagen disorders, e.g. Ulrich's, Bethlem

---

hair. Weakness in the legs presents with difficulty in rising from a low chair, climbing stairs, and stepping up on to a train or bus. Many patients with NIM either never run, or do so in an idiosyncratic fashion. Patients with distal weakness, for example in myotonic dystrophy (DM1), develop altered walking patterns (including high-stepping gaits) to prevent tripping, or may have problems turning a key or opening a jar. An inability to whistle, or to smile in family photographs, often indicates weakness of facial muscles (fascioscapular humeral muscular dystrophy (FSHD), or DM1). Speech and swallowing problems, and unexplained recurrent pneumonia may suggest weakness of bulbar musculature (DM1, and other dystrophies). Weakness of the cervical muscles will often lead to a complaint of the head falling forward ('head ptosis'), and is common in NIM including DMD and DM1. Shortness of breath on exertion, swimming in a front crawl, and lying flat all indicate involvement of respiratory musculature and are common in NIM.

The majority of NIM slowly progress as charted by a decline in motor function such as first use of a walking aid, furniture walking, and wheelchair use. Wheelchair dependence should always prompt consideration of NIM in patients with apparent steroid-resistant myositis and when correction of metabolic deficiencies such as hypocalcaemia, hypothyroidism, and vitamin D deficiency fails to improve clinical status.

Pain

Myalgia—muscle pain—is a common and relatively non-specific feature in both acquired (myositis) and genetic NIM, especially muscular dystrophies including FSHD and Becker muscular dystrophy (BMD), as well as less defined conditions such as fibromyalgia. Temperature-dependant exacerbation of myalgia may well indicate myotonia—delayed muscle relaxation. Specific enquiry into exercise-induced pain is useful in helping to identify metabolic myopathies, with glycogenolytic and fatty acid oxidation disorders associating with early and delayed pain respectively. A question such as 'Have you ever had Coca-Cola-coloured urine?' is useful in patients with muscle pain; it suggests myoglobinuria, and again suggests a metabolic disorder, particularly if a recurrent feature. Many NIM patients suffer with hip knee and lumbar spinal pain, whose presentation may predate the neuromuscular diagnosis.

Systemic enquiry

In patients with known NIM enquiry about cardiorespiratory symptoms is mandatory given common associations such as cardiomyopathy, cardiac arrhythmia, and respiratory failure. Equally, uncovering unexpected symptoms in patients suspected to have myositis such as palpitations (arrhythmias), blurring of vision (cataracts), deafness, and diabetes may suggest a multisystem disorder such as DM1 or a mitochondrial cytopathy.

Family history

Probing into a family history of neuromuscular disease/symptoms, facets of multisystem diseases, together with a gentle enquiry into cosanguinity together with causes of (including premature) death will often indicate the nature and pattern of inheritance of NIM. Examination of affected relatives, where permitted and practical, may also yield valuable insights into both diagnosis and prognosis, and is particularly useful when novel mutations in candidate genes of uncertain pathogenic significance are detected.

Clinical assessment: examination

Examination of the neuromuscular system seeks to confirm the distribution of muscular involvement suggested by the history, and to assess its severity using the MRC scale or (timed) functional tests e.g. the Gower s' manoeuvre. Weakness and wasting of proximal limb muscles are common to many muscle disorders, and only detailed examination will reveal physical signs suggestive of NIM:

Gait

Inspection of gait may reveal expected features such as a 'waddling' pattern, and additional signs such as an excessive lumbar lordosis (a very

common sign in NIM patients), foot drop (indicating distal weakness) and genu recurvatum in patients with severe quadriceps involvement.

Craniobulbar muscles

Cranial nerve signs are common in NIM. Weakness of facial muscles with reduced eye or lip closure is found in several NIM such as FSHD (Figure 126.1). Ptosis is a prominent feature in several muscular dystrophies, e.g. DM1 and oculopharngeal muscular dystrophy, and mitochondrial disease, and may be associated with compensatory overactivity in frontalis muscles. Involvement of extraocular muscles with strabismus and diplopia is found in several NIM, including mitochondrial disease and congenital myopathies. Bulbar palsies with a nasal dysarthria and a risk of aspiration are common in NIM, especially DM1. Neck extension weakness results in head drop and is common in DM1, and seen later in the clinical course of FSHD and acid maltase deficiency (Pompe's disease).

Limb muscles

Although most myopathies tend to cause symmetric proximal weakness, examination of the patient undressed can be justified as unanticipated muscular involvement may prove crucial in making a NIM diagnosis. A number of clinical algorithms are available to narrow the diagnosis.[2] Though not exhaustive, the following examples illustrate the utility of this approach:

- A generalized global reduction in muscle bulk is likely to indicate a congenital myopathy.

- Generalized muscle hypertrophy is seen in some congenital myotonic syndromes, producing the so-called Herculean appearance. Pseudohypertrophy, with fatty infiltration of weak muscles best seen in the calves, is seen in a number of dystrophies including

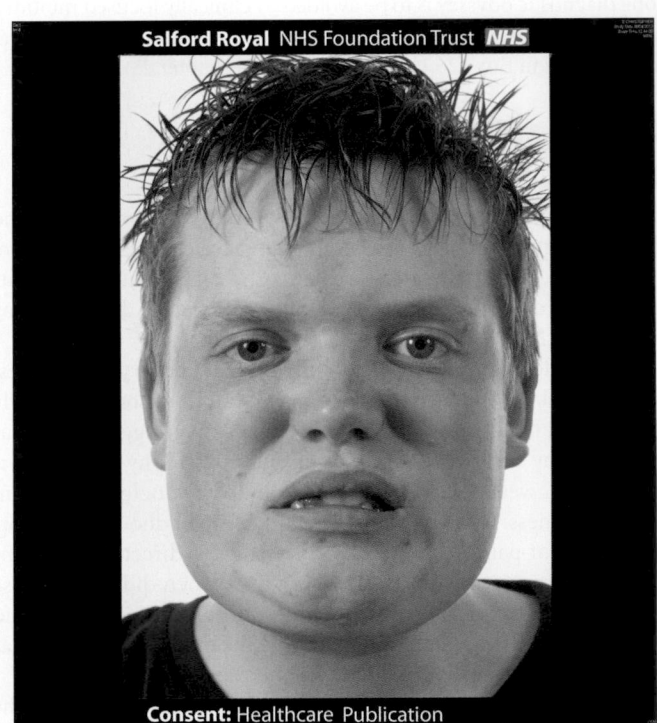

Consent: Healthcare Publication

Fig. 126.1 Fascioscapular humeral muscular dystrophy weakness of facial muscles with reduced smile, and widening of palpebral fissures.

BMD (Figure 126.2) and several LGMDs. Amyloid and glycogen deposition, e.g. Pompe's disease, may also lead to muscular hypertrophy including the tongue.

◆ Predominant proximal weakness of the lower limbs with an elevated creatine kinase (CK), in the absence of extraocular and facial weakness, and having considered DMD/BMD, may suggest a limb girdle muscular dystrophy (LGMD).

◆ Scapular winging is rare in myositis and is seen in a number of muscular dystrophies (including FSHD where it often asymmetric (Figure 126.3), and a number of LGMDs), metabolic syndromes such as Pompe's disease, and hereditary inclusion body myopathy with Paget's disease and dementia.

◆ Distal upper and lower limb involvement occurs in DM1, and a number of rare conditions including young-onset (e.g. Nonaka and Myoshi myopathies) and older-onset disorders (e.g. Welander's, tibial myopathy of Udd).[3]

◆ Myotonia, delayed relaxation of skeletal muscle following voluntary contraction, is seen prominently in myotonic dystrophies such as DM1 and ion-channel disorders such as myotonia congenital (but can occur in a subclinical form detectable on electromyography (EMG) in DM2 and Pompe's disease)

◆ Contractures are rare in acquired myopathic syndromes such as myositis but common in long-standing NIM with Achilles tendon shortening often resulting in toe walking in childhood with DMD and frequently requiring surgery or splinting. Finger and elbow contractures are uncommon even in NIM and are likely to indicate a disorder of collagen expression such as Bethlem myopathy, Emery–Dreifuss muscular dystrophy, and are also seen in some forms of LGMD.

◆ In DM1 deep tendon reflexes are reduced or absent; in other NIM reflexes are normal, except in disorders with associated neuropathy.

Spine

Involvement of paraspinal muscles is common in NIM including congenital myopathies, DMD, LGMD and metabolic myopathies such as Pompe's disease. Muscular weakness resulting in various combinations of undue prominence of the spinous processes, scoliosis, kyphosis, lordosis, or with contractures a rigid spine with limited forward flexion. Secondary disorders such as accelerated lumbar spondylosis, and hip dysfunction are common with an antalgic component to gait.

General examination

Cardiac and respiratory examination is prudent as these systems are often affected in NIM. Screening for cataracts and deafness is recommended if a multisystem disorder is suspected.

Neuromuscular investigations

Muscle enzymes

CK is expressed in a variety of tissues including heart, skeletal muscle, and liver. CK is elevated modestly in neurogenic disorders, and can be normal or significantly elevated in patients with both myositis and NIM. CK values greater than five times normal always indicate muscle disease. Persistently high CK levels (>10 times normal) are often found in patients with muscular dystrophies, including DMD and LGMD, and during episodes of rhabdomyolysis in

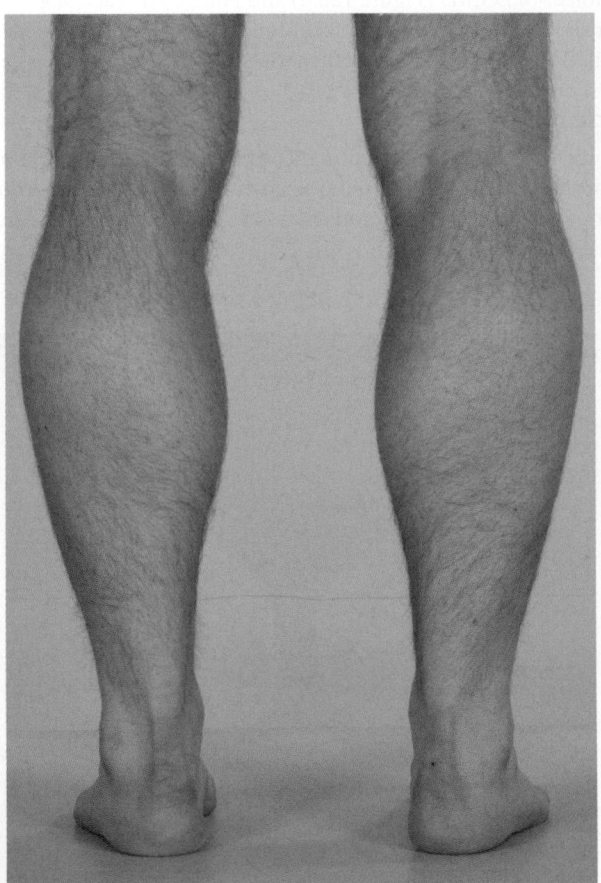

Fig. 126.3 Fascioscapular humeral muscular dystrophy striking asymmetric scapular winging, and excessive lumbar lordosis (same patient as shown in Figure 126.1).

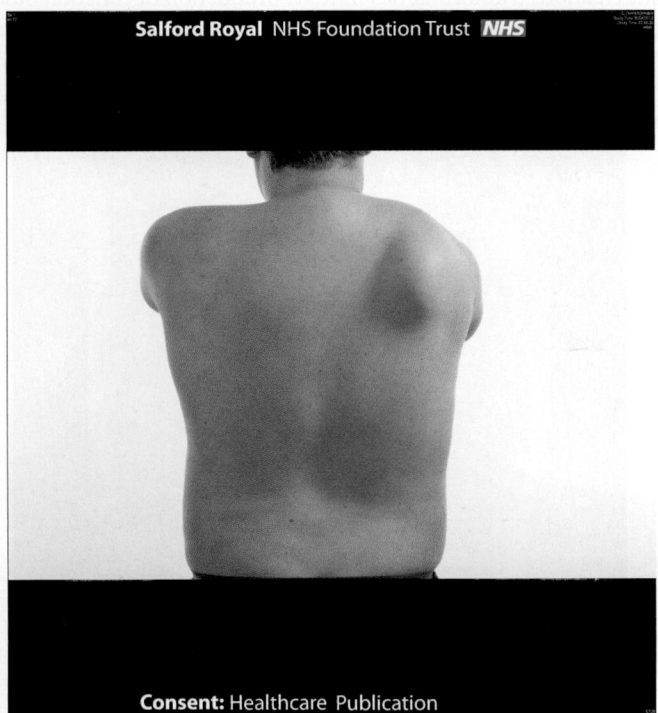

Consent: Healthcare Publication

Fig. 126.2 Becker muscular dystrophy pseudohypertrophy of calves.

patients with metabolic myopathies such as McArdle's disease. High variable CK levels may indicate myositis but also occur in NIM such as metabolic and myotonic myopathies.

Neurophysiology

Concentric needle electromyography (EMG) has a high sensitivity in distinguishing neurogenic and myopathic disorders. Muscle is normally electrically silent at rest. In neurogenic disorders positive sharp wave and fibrillation potentials are seen at rest in EMG studies, and on activation a reduced interference pattern is seen, reflecting the loss of motor neuron units. In chronic myopathy patients EMG reveals small-amplitude, short-duration motor unit potentials on activation and cannot reliably distinguish individual myopathic disorders, though spiky, unstable, and myotonic changes favour myositis and NIM respectively.

Muscle imaging

Ultrasound and CT can be useful in guiding muscle biopsies increasing their diagnostic yield. MRI scans of muscle can resolve selective muscle involvement more precisely, indicate pathological change (oedema and fatty change), and have been used for many years in the work-up of patients with suspected myositis. More recently MRI scans have been used in NIM, including congenital myopathies where the imaging phenotypes are providing diagnostic 'signatures' which may focus genetic tests and so reduce the diagnostic odyssey. MRI phenotypes are also being defined for some forms of LGMD (Figure 126.4) and Pompe's disease, speeding diagnosis, and with volumetric techniques may provide adjuncts to clinical measures in drug and other trials.

Muscle biopsy

Currently surgical open or percutaneous needle/conchotome muscle biopsies remain an essential diagnostic tool. Common features of myopathies include variation in muscle fibre size and increased internal nuclei.

Split and regenerating fibres with increased endomysial connective tissue are the hallmarks of musucular dystrophy. Immunological stains to define specific scarolemmal protein depletion in frozen sections and western blotting techniques help to distinguish subtypes of LGMD (Figures 126.5 and 126.6), confirmed by subsequent DNA analysis. Considerable care is required to not overinterpret inflammatory changes in dystrophic biopsies as these are relatively common, particularly in early stages of these diseases.

In metabolic myopathies accumulation of substrates such as glycogen and lipids may be apparent, though often such stains are normal and formal quantitation of enzyme in muscle, cultured skin fibroblast, or lymphocytes is often required in suspected cases.

Changes in oxidative enzymes such as cytochrome oxidase may suggest a mitochondrial disorder, with muscle providing a useful source of mitochondrial DNA for further analysis (Figure 126.7).

Inclusion bodies and other degenerative features may suggest a dystrophy or a still rarer myofibrillary diosorder

Descriptions of the pathologies seen in the more common NIM are now given in their order of frequency.

Myotonic disorders

DM1 or Stienhert's disease is the most common adult-onset inherited neuromuscular disorder with progressive wasting of the face, masticatory, neck, and distal limb muscles. The myotonia can be troublesome, and lessens as wasting advances. Associations of this multisystem condition are well known and include cardiac arrhythmias, cardiomyopathy, respiratory failure, cognitive dysfunction, somnolence, cataracts diabetes, hyopgonadism, and gastrointestinal dysfunction. DM1 is an autosomal dominant disorder with variable penetrance due to a trinucleotide (CTG) expansion in the untranslated *DMPK* gene on chromosome 19. This expansion is unstable, get larger in successive generations, and correlates with earlier, including congenital onset and worsening clinical phenotype—anticipation.[4] Abnormalities in RNA production or function other proteins coded for by neighbouring genes account for the diverse

(A)

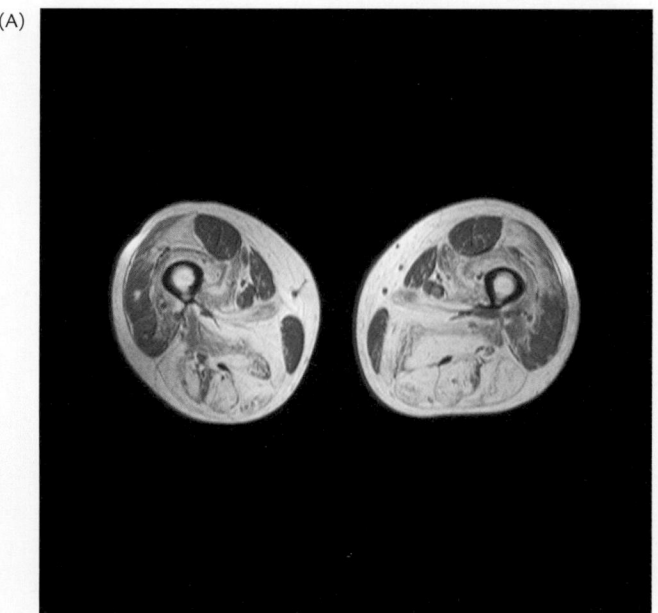

(B)

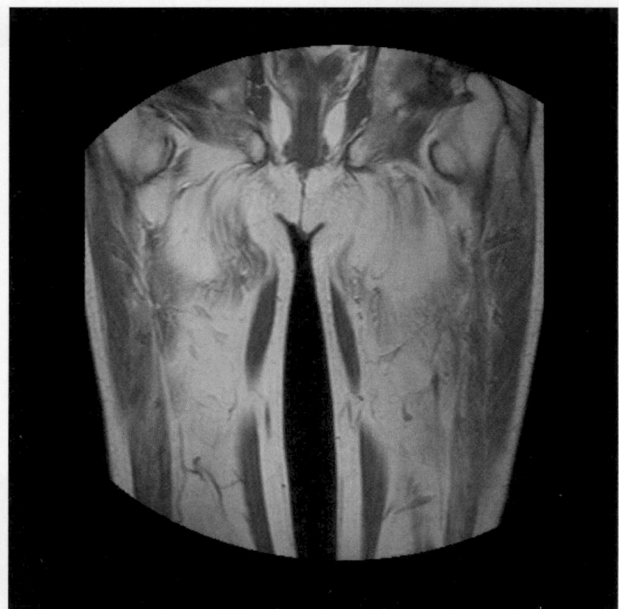

Fig. 126.4 Limb girdle muscular dystrophy 2I (common *FKRP* mutation). MRI scan: striking atrophy of hamstring muscles on axial (A) and sagittal (B) images.

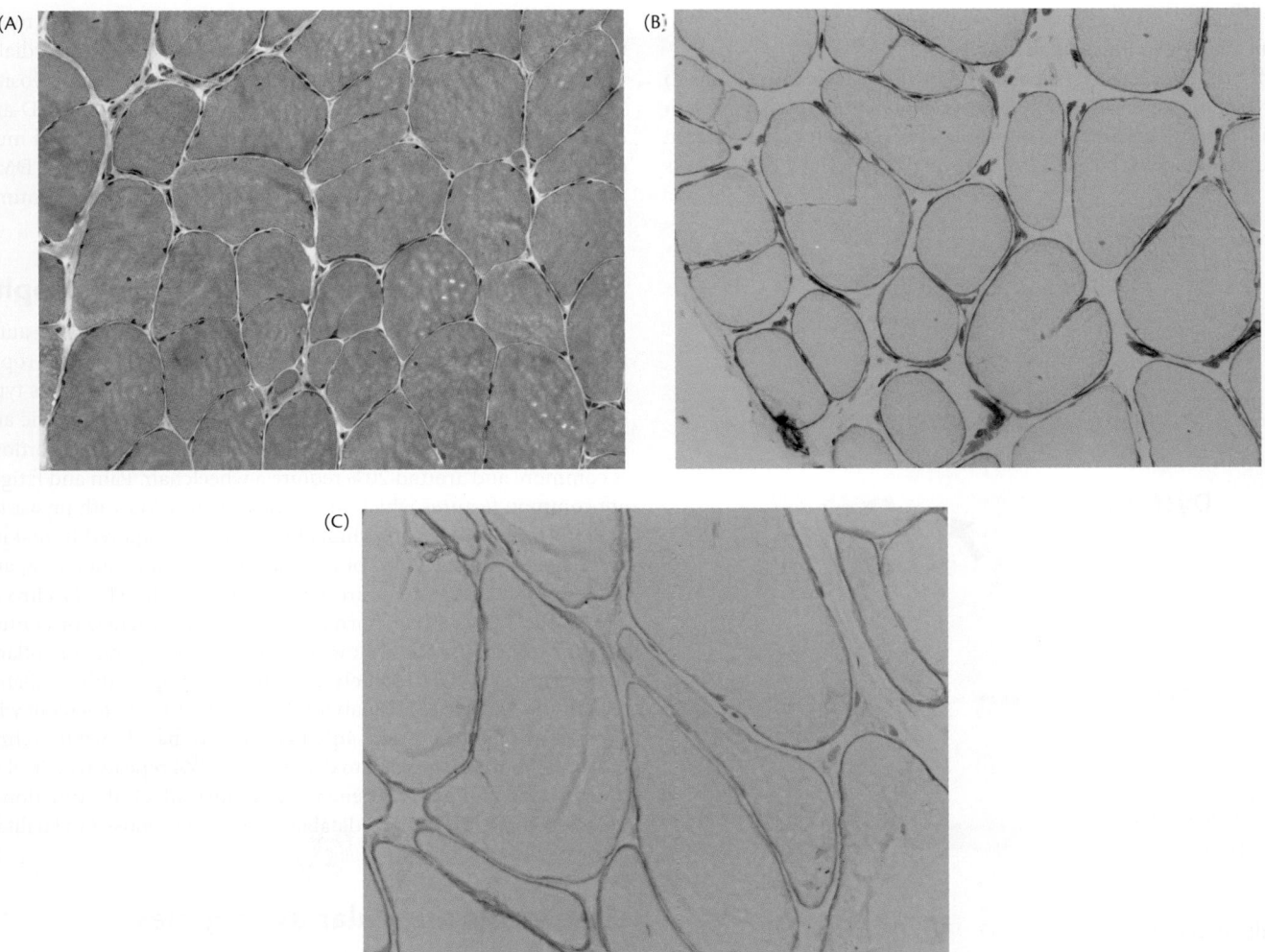

Fig. 126.5 Becker muscular dystrophy: (A) haematoxylin and eosin slide showing marked variation in muscle fibre size; (B) upregulation of dystrophin related protein/utrophin (brown sarcolemmal staining); (C) reduced staining with anti-dystrophin antibodies (DYS1).

features of the condition. DNA-based diagnosis is straightforward, can promote genetic counselling, and, with the availability of pre-implantation genetic diagnosis now possible, potentially reduce the impact and frequency of this life-shortening condition.[5]

DM2 or proximal myotonic myopathy is a less common, and generally milder, multisystem disorder due to a tetranucleotide (CCTG) expansion in the *ZNF9* gene on chromosome 3. Weakness is proximal and only in late stages distal. Muscle pain is a prominent feature, myotonia may only be detectable on EMG and rheumatologists may well be referred such patients. Paroxysmal atrial fibrillation is a common feature and a clue to the diagnosis, which is sometimes unmasked by the development of hypothyroidism.[6]

Myotonia congenita is a non-dystrophic condition with troublesome and occasionally painful myotonia, due to mutations in sarcolemmal chloride ion channels which can be inherited in a dominant (Thomsen) or recessive (Becker) fashion. The condition may mimic fibromyalgia but, of note, myotonia is aggravated by cold temperature, and improves with exercise. Muscle hypertrophy is common. Mexilitene may help myotonia and is currently undergoing clinical trials.

Dystrophinopathies, Duchenne and Becker muscular dystrophy

DMD and BMD are X-linked dominant allelic disorders due to mutations in the dystrophin gene, the largest gene in the body.

DMD is a severe disorder occurring in around 1/3000 live male births and associated with mutations (around one-third of which are spontaneous) which disrupt the open reading frame, resulting in stop codons, and little or no dystrophin production in muscle biopsies confirmed with western blotting. CK is often very high and may be detected in newborn screening programmes. Initial development is often normal, but by 2–3 years of age delayed motor milestones are apparent, and historically by 11 most boys are in a wheelchair, and die of cardiorespiratory failure in their late teens or early 20s. Patients have typical proximal neuromuscular phenotype with additional scoliosis (calf) pseudohypertophy and joint contractures. Mental retardation is frequent; skin ulceration and gastrointestinal problems including volvulus are less common. Early use of steroids defers both loss of ambulation and respiratory failure. Non-invasive ventilation and cardiac support (ACE inhibitors and atypical beta-blockers) prolong life by 10 years or more.[7]

Gene therapy shows promise and may alter the natural history with patients having a clinical course akin to BMD.[8]

BMD is less severe and is associated with in-frame mutations in the dytrophin gene with some protein product. BMD may present in mid childhood and even adulthood, and is likely to be referred to rheumatologists, particularly as myalgia (especially calf pain) is a common feature. CK is often elevated to 5000 iu/mL or more. Calf pseudohypertrophy, ECG changes with tall right precordial R waves, and family history enquiry distinguish BMD from myositis. Dilated cardiomyopathy can be a prominent feature of BMD and can be disproportionately severe when compared to skeletal muscle weakness. Particular care is needed in considering BMD/DMD manifesting carrier status in females where again it might mimic myositis.

Fascioscapular humeral muscular dystrophy

FSHD, or Landouzy–Dejerine syndrome, is a progressive autosomal dominant disorder with descending weakness and atrophy of facial, shoulder, and humeral muscles. Scapular winging is typically asymmetric and worse on the side of handedness. Pelvic and distal leg weakness also develops in most patients, lumbar lordosis is common, and around 20% require a wheelchair. Pain and fatigue are common features which might cause confusion with myosistis, or fibromyalgia. A strong clinical suspicion is required in making the diagnosis as one-third of patients are a de-novo mutation, and laboratory investigations are either non-specific (EMG chronic myopathic, CK is either normal or modestly elevated) or confusing (muscle biopsy may show dystrophic, neurogenic, or inflammatory features). Fortunately genetic testing is readily available, and around 95% of FSHD patients have a DNA rearrangement with shortening of chromosome 4q3. Recent work has shown this chromosomal shortening is due to deletion of D4Z4 repeats which allow derepression of the *DUX4* gene which in turn affects the function of nearby genes.[9] A European database has been proposed to facilitate clinical trials.[10]

Limb girdle muscular dystrophies

The term LGMD refers to significant numbers of both male and female patients with a high CK and predominately proximal lower limb weakness in the absence of phenotype suggestive of DMD/BMD or FSHD. This concept, first suggested by the Rare Muscles Diseases group in Newcastle, was initially controversial but with increasing linkage and DNA-based studies is now widely accepted. An alphabetical classification delineates rare

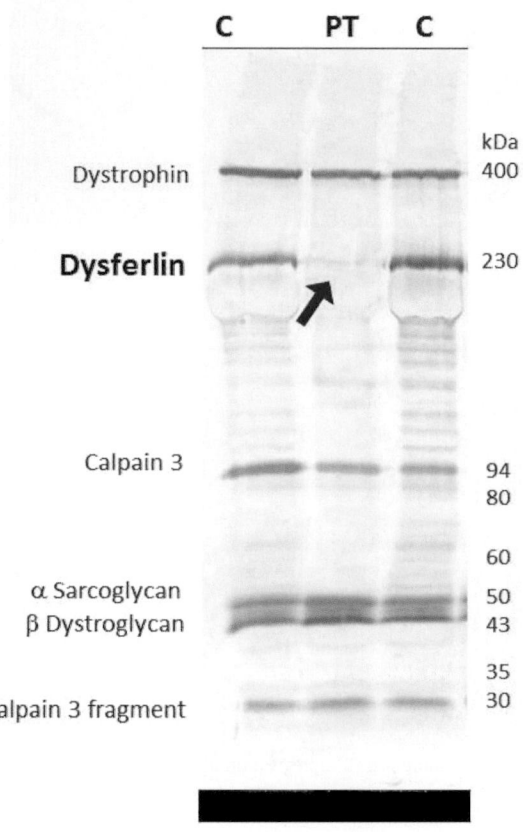

Fig. 126.6 Limb girdle muscular dystrophy 2B (complex heterozygote dysferlin mutation): western blot of leg muscle showing reduction in dysferlin band in patient (PT) compared to control (C).

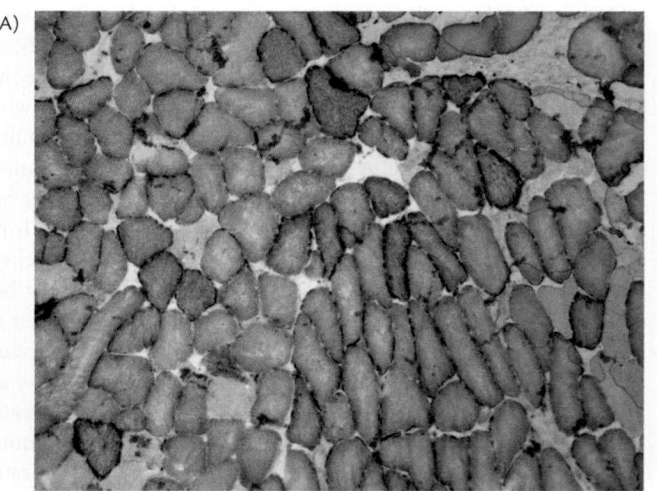

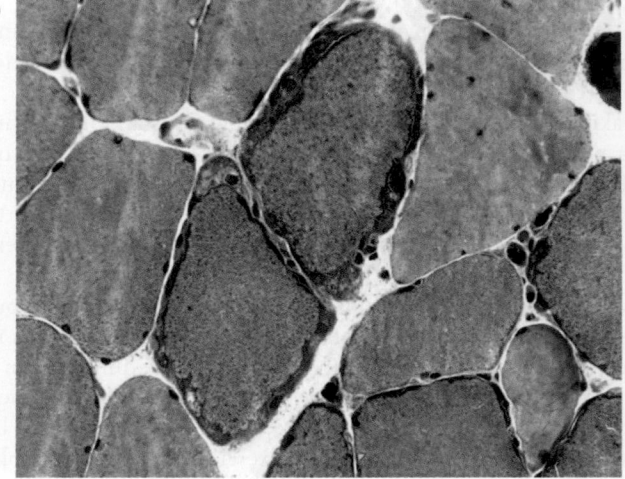

Fig. 126.7 Mitochondrial disorder (patient with POLG1 mutation) showing (A) muscle fibres deficient in cytochrome oxidase staining blue on COX/SDH preparation and (B) subsarcolemmal aggregates of mitochondria staining red ('ragged red') on Gomori trichome preparation.

autosomal dominant (LGMD1A–E) and more common recessive (LGMD2A–N) variants.

The frequent absence of a family history may readily cause diagnostic confusion with myositis, particularly as muscle biopsies in some forms of LGMD can show inflammatory features (e.g. LGMD2B),[11] as discussed in detail on www.jain-foundation.org.

Additional clinical features such as age of onset, pseudohypertophy (1C, 2D, 2E, 2I), scapular winging (2A,2I, 2N), selective quadriceps involvement without iliopsoas weakness (1B, 2B), rippling muscles (muscle movements with electrical silence on EMG, 1A) may suggest a particular variant though typically diagnosis depends on immunohistochemical and western blot analysis followed by a candidate gene approach.[12] Knowledge of the most prevalent LGMD in the local neuromuscular patient population, e.g. LGMD2I in the north-east of England, may facilitate DNA-based diagnosis and avoid muscle biopsy.[13]

Metabolic myopathies

Muscle pain, cramps, and fluctuating weakness are frequently seen in the rheumatology clinic. Occasionally these symptoms reflect metabolic myopathies—rare autosomal recessive conditions of muscle energy metabolism.[14] Metabolic disorders typically present with exercise-induced myalgia and rhabdomyolysis, or progressive myopathy.

McArdle's disease (glycogen storage disorder type V) is the most common glycogenolytic disorder and due to a deficiency of myophosphorylase; it is associated with muscle fatigue and pain within minutes of initiating activity, second wind phenomenon, painful contracture often lasting for days, rhabdomyolysis which can be complicated by renal failure, and in a minority with muscle weakness. Ischaemic lactate test and absent phoshorylase staining in muscle biopsies (Figure 126.8) support the diagnosis, with confirmatory DNA analysis now available. However, in a recent study of 59 patients non-exercise related chronic pain/fatigue was found in 42%.[15] and this and technical issues in muscle biopsy interpretation may delay diagnosis, prevent advice on diet such as sucrose and exercise,[16] and potentially contribute to a greater risk of renal failure.

Disorders of fatty acid oxidation are a group of inherited metabolic disorders of mitochondrial energy production. Most will present to paediatricians at an early age with multisystem problems such as hepatic failure.[17] Some milder phenotypes such as carnitine plamitoyl transferase 2 (CPTII) deficiency can remain asymptomatic until adulthood. Sporting stoics may have disregarded exercise-induced myalgia and present with postexercise rhabdomyolysis and uraemia. There is limited evidence that bezafibrate may help this disorder.[18]

Pompe's disease (glycogen storage disorder type II, acid maltase deficiency) is a rare, progressive, autosomal recessive disorder caused by deficiency of the lysosomal enzyme acid α-glucosidase (GAA) with glycogen accumulation in many tissues, especially muscle. There is a wide spectrum of disease. In infants with less than 1% of enzyme levels the condition is rapidly fatal with cardiorespiratory failure. In adult-onset cases, with higher enzyme levels, there is a wide range of phenotypes including fatigue, myalgia, limb girdle weakness, diaphragm involvement, and scoliosis, which could readily be confused with other NIM and myositis.[19,20] Standard laboratory investigations can be suggestive (myotonic discharges on paraspinal EMG, glycogen accumulation, and vacuoles on muscle biopsy) but crucially can be normal, particularly in milder late-onset cases. A high index of suspicion is required, as enzyme replacement therapy is now available which prolongs life in infants and stabilizes adult patients.[18,21,22] Fortunately dried blood spot analysis is now readily available and is a simple and reliable screen for Pompe's disease.

Mitochondrial diseases

Mutations in mitochondrial or nuclear DNA-encoded subunits of the mitochondrial respiratory chain cause fundamental defects in energy production within all cells. The energy requirements of muscle, with a high number of mitochondria per cell, ensure that myopathy is a common feature in mitochondrial disorders (MtD), which could result in confusion with both myositis and other NIM.

The clinical features of these MtD are typically diverse, variable, and multisystem, and a high index of suspicion is required in patients

(A)

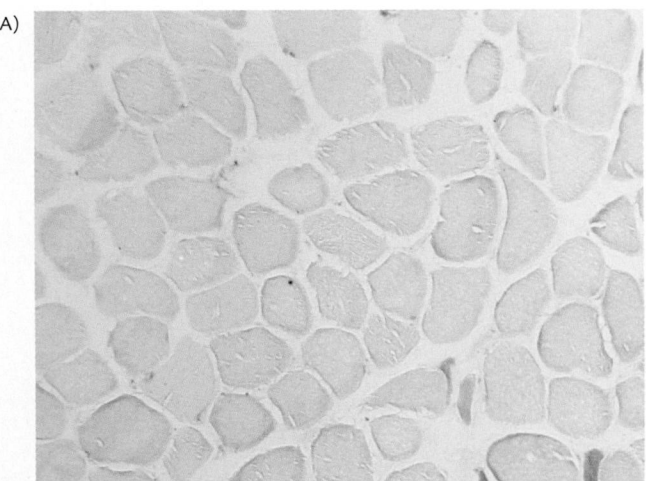

(B)

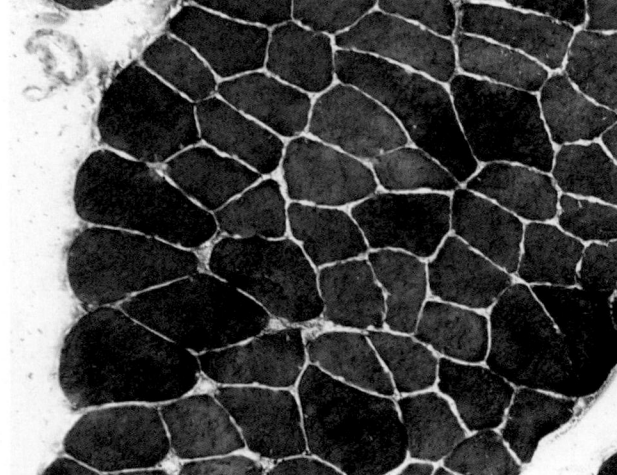

Fig. 126.8 McArdle's disease (glycogen storage disease type V) muscle biopsy showing absent phosphorylase staining (A) compared to control (B).

with myopathy who have additional features on clinical assessment such as exercise intolerance, deafness, diabetes, short stature, cognitive problems, epilepsy, peripheral neuropathy, cardiac arrhythmia, ptosis, and ophthamoplegia.[23] Regular cardiorespiratory and endocrine assessments are recommended in these patients.

Recognition of MtD syndromes, such as mitochondrial encephalomyopathy, lactic acidosis, and stroke-like episodes (MELAS), may prompt DNA-based diagnosis. Often other investigations such as a muscle biopsy are required to confirm the diagnosis, revealing defects such as cytochrome oxidase negativity, with disrupted mitochondrial structure and ragged red fibres.

Conclusion

Recognition of NIM in patients presenting with myopathy depends on an integrated clinical and laboratory assessment with a high index of suspicion if misdiagnosis of myositis is to be avoided. Novel markers of disease and in particular MRI scanning of muscles, together with other biomarkers, as well traditional techniques such as CK, EMG, and muscle biopsy will enable accurate diagnosis of NIM in most patients.

References

1. Sewry CA, Jimenez-Mallebrera C, Muntoni F. Congenital myopathies. *Curr Opin Neurol* 2008;21(5):569–575.
2. Pestronk A. *Neuromuscular diseases home page*, 2012 (cited 2012) Available at: http://neuromuscular.wustl.edu/.
3. Udd B. 165th ENMC International Workshop: distal myopathies 6–8th February 2009 Naarden, The Netherlands. *Neuromusc Disord* 2009;19(6):429–438.
4. Turner C, Hilton-Jones D. The myotonic dystrophies: diagnosis and management. *J Neurol Neurosurg Psychiatry* 2010;81(4):358–367.
5. Kakourou G, Dhanjal S, Mamas T et al. Preimplantation genetic diagnosis for myotonic dystrophy type 1 in the UK. *Neuromusc Disord* 2008;18(2):131–136.
6. Udd B, Meola G, Krahe R et al. Myotonic dystrophy type 2 (DM2) and related disorders report of the 180th ENMC workshop including guidelines on diagnostics and management 3–5 December 2010, Naarden, The Netherlands. *Neuromusc Disord* 2011;21(6):443–450.
7. Bushby K, Finkel R, Birnkrant DJ et al. Diagnosis and management of Duchenne muscular dystrophy, part 1: diagnosis, and pharmacological and psychosocial management. *Lancet Neurol* 2010;9(1):77–93.
8. Cirak S, Arechavala-Gomeza V, Guglieri M et al. Exon skipping and dystrophin restoration in patients with Duchenne muscular dystrophy after systemic phosphorodiamidate morpholino oligomer treatment: an open-label, phase 2, dose-escalation study. *Lancet* 2011;378(9791):595–605.
9. Lemmers RJLF, van der Vliet PJ, Klooster R et al. A unifying genetic model for facioscapulohumeral muscular dystrophy. *Science* 2010;329(5999):1650–1653.
10. Statland JM, Tawil R. Facioscapulohumeral muscular dystrophy: molecular pathological advances and future directions. *Curr Opin Neurol* 2011;24(5):423–428.
11. Bushby K, Norwood F, Straub V. The limb-girdle muscular dystrophies—diagnostic strategies. *Biochim Biophys Acta* 2007;1772(2):238–242.
12. Nagaraju K, Rawat R, Veszelovszky E et al. Dysferlin deficiency enhances monocyte phagocytosis—A model for the inflammatory onset of limb-girdle muscular dystrophy 2B. *Am J Pathol* 2008;172(3):774–785.
13. Norwood FLM, Harling C, Chinnery PF et al. Prevalence of genetic muscle disease in Northern England: in-depth analysis of a muscle clinic population. *Brain* 2009;132:3175–3186.
14. Smith EC, El-Gharbawy A, Koeberl DD. Metabolic myopathies: clinical features and diagnostic approach. *Rheum Dis Clin North Am* 2011;37(2):201–217.
15. Quinlivan R, Buckley J, James M et al. McArdle disease: a clinical review. *J Neurol Neurosurg Psychiatry* 2010;81(11):1182–1188.
16. Quinlivan R, Martinuzzi A, Schoser B. Pharmacological and nutritional treatment for McArdle disease (glycogen storage disease type V). *Cochrane Database Syst Rev* 2010;(12):CD003458.
17. Olpin SE. Fatty acid oxidation defects as a cause of neuromyopathic disease in infants and adults. *Clin Lab* 2005;51(5–6):289–306.
18. Angelini C, Semplicini C. Metabolic myopathies: the challenge of new treatments. *Curr Opin Pharmacol* 2010;10(3):338–345.
19. van den Berg LE, de Vries JM, Verdijk RM et al. A case of adult Pompe disease presenting with severe fatigue and selective involvement of type 1 muscle fibers. *Neuromusc Disord* 2011;21(3):232–234.
20. Desnuelle C, Salviati L. Challenges in diagnosis and treatment of late-onset Pompe disease. *Curr Opin Neurol* 2011;24(5):443–448.
21. Müller-Felber W, Horvath R, Gempel K et al. Late onset Pompe disease: clinical and neurophysiological spectrum of 38 patients including long-term follow-up in 18 patients. *Neuromusc Disord* 2007;17(9–10):698–706.
22. van der Ploeg AT, Clemens PR, Corzo D et al. A randomized study of alglucosidase alfa in late-onset Pompe's disease. *N Engl J Med* 2010;362(15):1396–1406.
23. McFarland R, Taylor RW, Turnbull DM. A neurological perspective on mitochondrial disease. *Lancet Neurol* 2010;9(8):829–840.

SECTION 16

Sjögren's syndrome

CHAPTER 127

Sjögren's syndrome— clinical features

Simon Bowman, John Hamburger,
Elizabeth Price, and Saaeha Rauz

Introduction

Sjögren's syndrome (SS) is named after Henrik Sjögren, a Swedish ophthalmologist, who published a doctoral thesis describing the condition in 1933.[1] He used the term 'keratoconjunctivitis sicca' to specifically distinguish the ocular surface features from those seen in vitamin-A deficiency (xerophthalmia) although the latter term is often used incorrectly to describe ocular dryness in SS ('xerostomia' is, however, legitimately used to describe oral dryness). Henri Gougerot, a French dermatologist had previously described three patients with sicca syndrome and salivary gland atrophy in 1925.[2] Jan Mikulicz-Radecki, an Austro-Polish surgeon, described the histological features in 1892 in a patient with parotid gland swelling.[3] As well as dryness of eyes and mouth, dryness of the trachea, skin, nose, vagina, and bowel are also common.

The distinction between primary SS (pSS) and secondary SS was set out in the 1960s.[4] The link with mucosa-associated lymphoid tissue (MALT) B-cell lymphoma was also reported,[5] and Chisholm and Mason described their scoring system for the histological features of salivary gland biopsies in pSS.[6] The anti-Ro (SS-A) and anti-La (SS-B) antibodies were first identified[7] in 1969 and subsequently shown to be associated with pSS, HLA DR3 and other human lymphocyte antigen (HLA) haplotypes[8] and the neonatal lupus syndrome.[9]

The glandular features and management of pSS and secondary SS are generally regarded as being similar although fibrosis, for example, is a more typical feature in scleroderma-related secondary SS. Unless otherwise stated, this chapter focuses on pSS.

Epidemiology

SS is a worldwide disease with a strong female bias—traditionally reported as 9:1 but possibly as high as 13:1.[10] Typically pSS presents in the fifth or sixth decade but can present at any age including, rarely, in childhood.

Classification criteria

In clinical practice it is up to the clinician to use their judgement in making a diagnosis of pSS. In research it is essential to have agreed classification criteria so that there is confidence that participants in a study have the specified condition. During the 1980s a number of classification criteria were proposed, with a major debate as to the advantages and disadvantages of each of these criteria.[11]

In 1988 a working group of 29 experts from 12 European countries initiated a study to develop consensus criteria and published their initial findings in 1993. The preliminary European criteria[12] included six components: symptoms of oral dryness identified through the presence of at least one out of three specified dry mouth questions and similarly for dry eyes, objective eye dryness, objective oral dryness, a positive labial salivary gland biopsy (>1 focus score/4 mm^2) and positive anti-Ro/La antibodies. Four out of the six components were required to make a diagnosis of pSS. Exclusion criteria were also proposed (head and neck radiotherapy, hepatitis C infection, AIDS, pre-existing lymphoma, sarcoidosis, graft-vs-host disease, use of anti-cholinergic drugs). These criteria were subsequently modified to require the presence of either positive anti-Ro/La antibodies or positive labial salivary gland biopsy to form the American–European Consensus Group (AECG) criteria,[13] thus requiring evidence of an immunological basis for the dryness. The diagnosis of pSS is also fulfilled if three of the four objective criteria are present. The criteria also propose that secondary SS is present if at least one oral or ocular symptom is present and two objective criteria (other than anti-Ro/La antibodies, as these are not associated with secondary SS in rheumatoid arthritis (RA) or scleroderma).

The AECG criteria are the most widely used 'gold standard' criteria for the classification of pSS in research studies. Criteria are never fixed in perpetuity, however, and as new technology such as ultrasound becomes more widely used or new data becomes available[14] further revision is likely. For example, one of the differences between the various criteria is whether to score a focus score of ≥1 or >1 as positive, and recent data suggests that the former is more closely linked with the clinical phenotype of pSS.[15]

Differential diagnosis of salivary gland enlargement and the IgG4 syndrome

Systemic diseases such as sarcoidosis can cause salivary gland enlargement. Metabolic or nutritional disorders such as diabetes, bulimia, and chronic alcohol excess can also cause generalized swelling of the glands (sialosis). HIV infection can cause the diffuse infiltrative lymphocytosis syndrome (DILS) (see below) and this together with other conditions will be discussed further in the section 'Oral features of Sjögren's syndrome' below. IgG4-related disease has recently been described.[16] Characteristic features include raised serum IgG4, IgG4-positive plasma cells infiltrating tissues, particularly the pancreas, causing autoimmune pancreatitis, and the salivary glands, resulting in swelling and/or dryness. There is no female bias, no association with anti-Ro/La antibodies, and generally a good response to corticosteroid therapy.

Prevalence

Initial research into the prevalence of pSS came up with estimates of up to 3% of the adult female population,[17] much higher than in subsequent reports. One explanation for this was the use of different, more permissive, classification criteria in the earlier studies.

More recent studies using the AECG criteria have estimated the prevalence in women in the United Kingdom at 0.1–0.4%.[18] Other studies using the AECG criteria have estimated the prevalence at around 0.2%[19] in the community and 0.05% in the hospital setting.[20]

Diagnostic autoantibodies

The best-described autoantibodies in pSS are the anti-Ro and anti-La antibodies, which are routinely identified as part of the ENA (extractable nuclear antigen) laboratory screen. The Ro autoantigen was originally identified as a 60 kDa ribonucleoprotein. A structurally distinct 52 kDa protein called Ro52 also colocalizes with Ro60 to surface membrane blebs on cells undergoing apoptosis where they may become targets of an autoimmune response. The 47 kDa La antigen is thought to be a transcription termination factor for RNA polymerase.

Approximately two-thirds of patients with pSS have anti-Ro antibodies and one-third have anti-La antibodies.[21] These figures, however, depend on the classification criteria used, referral bias, and access to labial salivary gland biopsy. Few patients have anti-La antibodies in the absence of anti-Ro antibodies and one suggestion is that the initial autoantibody response is directed against the Ro antigen and then 'spreads' to involve the La antigen as a secondary process.[22] Anti-Ro/La antibodies are also classically seen in patients with systemic lupus erythematosus (SLE), albeit at a lower frequency than in pSS. ANA and rheumatoid factor positivity are very commonly seen in pSS but are not sensitive or specific for the condition and hence are not included in the AECG classification criteria.

Other autoantibodies potentially related to pathogenesis

Other autoantibodies that have generated significant interest at times include anti-fodrin antibodies,[23] anti-muscarinic M3 receptor antibodies,[24] and anti-carbonic anhydrase antibodies,[25] as well as anti-ICA69 antibodies[26] and anti-aquaporin antibodies,[27] although this is not an exhaustive list.

Anti-muscarinic M3 receptor antibodies are of particular interest because the M3 receptor is found in exocrine cells and interference by anti-M3R autoantibodies with signalling through these receptors could explain reduced secretory function in pSS. Again, the

initial studies were promising, but more recent reports show conflicting results.[28]

Genetics, genomics, and proteomics

There have been no large-scale twin studies in pSS. Based on case reports and small studies, the estimated concordance rate for SS is low and the sibling prevalence likewise, suggesting that the heritability of SS is low and environmental factors play a greater role.[29]

pSS has been closely linked to the presence of particular genes of the human major histocompatibility complex (MHC) that encodes HLA proteins.[21,22] These links are principally between the HLA types and the anti-Ro/La autoantibodies rather than with the disease per se. Patients with high levels of both anti-Ro and anti-La antibodies have a very high (~90%) likelihood of being HLA DR3 DQ2 positive (typically associated with the *DRB1*03-DQB1*02-DQA1*0501* extended haplotype), whereas pSS patients who have high levels of anti-Ro antibody only and are negative for anti-La antibodies have an increased frequency of DR2(15) and DQ6 (typically associated with the *DRB1*1501-DQA1*0102-DQB1*0602* extended haplotype). Conversely, secondary SS in patients with RA is associated with HLA DR4,[30] emphasizing that the clinical and histopathological similarities between pSS and secondary SS do not extend into identical genetic backgrounds.

Other potential genetic markers include cytokine genes—e.g. for interleukins IL-10, IL-1 family, IL-6, and tumour necrosis factor (TNF)—MHC-related genes such as *TAP* and *TNF*, and the Ro/La autoantigens themselves.[31]

Gene expression profiling using microarray technology can be used to identify genes that are over- or underexpressed in particular circumstances, which may be relevant to disease pathogenesis. In pSS (and SLE and some other autoimmune disorders), one current theme, across a range of studies, is of overexpression of interferon (IFN)-inducible genes including Toll-like receptors, *STAT4*, *IRF5*, *BAFF*, and *MECP2*.[32] IFN is typically upregulated by viruses and this may provide a link between the 'disease trigger' in these disorders and subsequent pathogenic processes.

Microarray technology can also be extended to genotype large numbers of single nucleotide polymorphisms whose frequency can be compared in thousands of cases and controls to identify novel associations between genes and disease for further study. Such studies are now under way in pSS.

Another area of genetics that is currently of interest is that of epigenetics, i.e. the effects of processes such as DNA methylation or histone acetylation on gene expression, and some data is emerging in pSS in this field.[33]

Proteomics—the study of disease-associated variation in protein and peptide levels in biological samples—is another promising area of interest in pSS.[34]

Potential triggers

A number of viruses have been associated with a SS-like disease. Perhaps the best characterized is the hepatitis C virus (HCV).[35] HIV has been linked with a phenotype of swollen salivary and other glands infiltrated with CD8 cells (DILS).[36] Other potential viral associations that have been suggested include human herpesvirus 6, human T-lymphotropic virus type 1, cytomegalovirus, and Epstein–Barr virus. At present, however, there is no clear evidence to suggest that an infectious agent triggers pSS.

Mouse models

There are a number of mouse models for SS.[37] The best-known is the non-obese diabetic (NOD) mouse which develops diabetes mellitus at 2–3 months of age and an SS-like syndrome of salivary gland lymphocytic infiltration, anti-Ro/La and anti-muscarinic M3R antibodies and sicca features at 4 months. Another interesting model, particularly to explore the potential role of apoptosis and lymphoproliferation, is the MRL/lpr mouse. This has a genetic mutation of the lymphoproliferation (*lpr*) gene on chromosome 19, which encodes the structural gene for the Fas antigen involved in apoptosis and is typically a model for SLE. The mice also develop some features of RA and some SS-like features. There are a number of cytokine-transgenic mice including those for IL-6, IL-10, IL-12, IL-14, and BAFF, which develop some SS-like features. Antigen immunization graftvs host, gene knockout, and virus infection models also exist. Each of these models can be used to identify or investigate specific environmental or genetic components of the condition that might be difficult to isolate among the heterogeneity of human disease.

Immunopathology

The concept of 'autoimmune epitheliitis'[38] starts with the idea that individuals with a particular genetic background (e.g. HLA DR3 DQ2) and/or a permissive IFN gene profile (see above) (and predominantly women) are more likely to react to a triggering factor or factors (e.g. a virus?) with some form of initial tissue damage. This initial tissue insult could cause, for example, epithelial cell death (apoptosis) and hence the exposure of Ro and La in apoptotic blebs to the immune system and the generation of the anti-Ro/La autoantibodies.[39] It could explain the upregulation of 'non-specific' (innate) immunity e.g. of Toll-like receptors, interferons, and molecules involved in tissue breakdown such as metalloproteinases, the expression of HLA class II molecules on epithelial and endothelial cells primed to present antigens, and the upregulation of adhesion molecules on blood vessel walls that allows immune cells to enter the tissue and of a range of cytokines such as IL-6, IL-10, TNFα, IL-17, IL-23, and BAFF to mention but some.[40] BAFF/BlyS (B-cell activating factor/B-lymphocyte stimulator) has been of particular interest given the evidence for B-cell activation in pSS.[41,42] The assumption is that, once triggered, the process develops a momentum of its own with the tissue expressing homing molecules such as chemokines and their receptors drawing immune cells into the glands and stimulating their formation into organized self-perpetuating lymphoid structures that contribute to gland dysfunction, autoantibody formation, and lymphomatous transformation.[43–45]

Another aspect of the pathogenesis of pSS is the detailed mechanisms underpinning reduced glandular function. One component of this may be reduced hypothalamic–pituitary axis function and reduced sex-steroid levels having a direct downregulatory effect on glandular secretory function.[46] As described above, anti-muscarinic receptor antibody formation could interfere with normal acetylcholine signalling through the M3 receptors on the gland cells. Glandular cytokines themselves may increase cholinesterase activity, thus inhibiting normal stimulation of secretory mechanisms.[47] Abnormalities of water-specific membrane-channel proteins such as the aquaporins and other glandular proteins such as mucin proteins may also be contributory to this process.[48]

Oral features of Sjögren's syndrome

Symptoms

The major oral symptom of SS is that of dryness of the mouth (xerostomia). In younger individuals in particular, e.g. below 40 years of age, swelling of the parotid and/or submandibular salivary glands, often painless, is commonly the presenting feature.

Xerostomia is a common oral symptom[49] and most individuals with a complaint of oral dryness do not have a diagnosis of SS. The differential diagnosis of dry mouth can be classified according to whether there is salivary gland disease per se, resulting in glandular hypofunction, or whether the xerostomia is occasioned by other aetiological factors.

Other symptoms of oral dryness include reduced taste perception, difficulty in swallowing and speech, poor denture retention, bad breath, increased rate of dental decay, and possibly more marked periodontal disease (although this is a matter of debate), generalized oral discomfort with oral mucosal surfaces sticking together and to the teeth, and salivary gland swelling.

Xerostomia and its associated symptomatology have a significant impact on the quality of life, in terms of specific aspects of oral function as well as socially.[50,51]

Differential diagnosis of xerostomia

Xerostomia can result from the ingestion of various drugs, particularly but not exclusively those with anticholinergic activity (e.g. psychotropics including anti-depressants, anxiolytics and anti-psychotics), muscarinic antagonists (e.g. tamsolusin hydrochloride, ipratropium hydrochloride), anti-histamines, opiates, anti-hypertensives (e.g. beta-blockers; ACE inhibitors), proton pump inhibitors (e.g. omeprazole), head and neck radiotherapy, dehydration (e.g. poorly controlled diabetes), renal failure, acute anxiety, mouth breathing and rarely central lesions. Xerostomia can be a feature of oral dysasthaesias with no objective reduction in salivary flow rate. Such patients may complain of a constellation of oral symptoms, including burning sensations and unusual taste as well as oral dryness and their symptomatology is not uncommonly associated with anxiety states and occasionally, clinical depression. There may also be a history of low back pain, fibromyalgia, and irritable bowel syndrome.[52]

Primary salivary gland pathology, other than SS, that can cause salivary gland hypofunction includes sarcoidosis, HIV-associated salivary gland disease, graft-vs-host disease which produces an analogous condition to SS,[53] hepatitis C, sicca syndrome (dryness where there is no known obvious case for the salivary gland hypofunction) and very rarely salivary gland aplasia and ductal atresia which may be related to FGF10 missense mutations.[54]

A syndrome comprising histological evidence of sialadenitis, nodular osteoarthritis, and xerostomia ('SNOX') has also been described,[55] but in view of the frequency of the individual clinical features, clustering could also be expected to occur on a simple statistical basis.

Ageing per se is not a cause of xerostomia. Although there is a broadly linear reduction in the amount of functional acinar tissue within the salivary glands over time, this does not lead to clinically significant salivary gland hypofunction.[56] Xerostomia in the ageing population is more a function of intercurrent disease and medication rather than that of loss of acinar apparatus.[57]

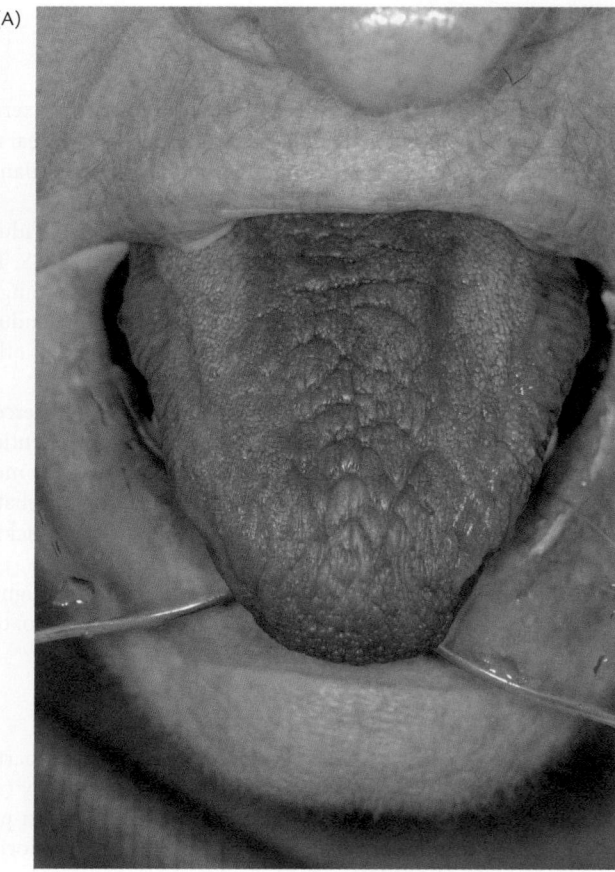

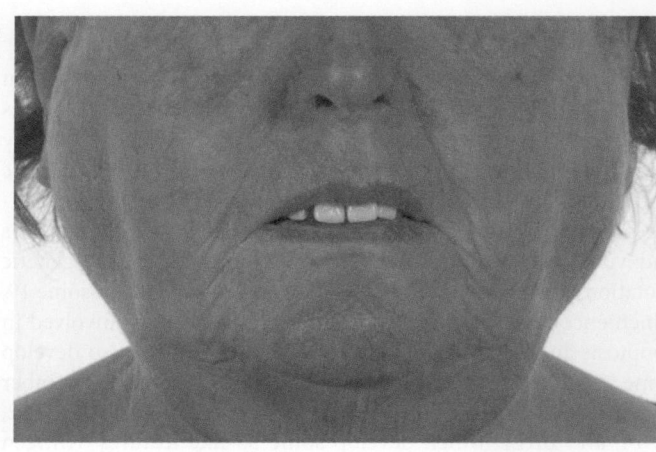

Fig. 127.1 (A) Dry, lobulated dorsum of tongue in a patient with long-standing Sjögren's syndrome. (B) Marked diffuse bilateral parotid swelling in a patient with primary Sjögren's syndrome.

Clinical signs of xerostomia

External signs of xerostomia may include angular cheilitis, dry flaky lips, and salivary gland swelling, involving any or all of the major salivary glands. However, these signs are not specific for dry mouth, and they may be indicative of a variety of other conditions (Figure 127.1).

Salivary gland swelling merits careful examination. Assessment should be made as to whether the swelling is diffuse or nodular, its texture, particularly if indurated, the presence of inflammation of the overlying skin, and associated VII nerve motor weakness or palsy in the case of parotid swellings, which frequently involve the lower pole of these glands.

Intraorally, milking the salivary glands may reveal thick mucoid saliva, sometimes containing blood or pus, which is suggestive of ascending infection, particularly when the swelling is painful. A history of pain associated with meal times suggests an obstructive aetiology of the swelling, which may be due to intraglandular ductal stenosis in SS, but other obstructive aetiologies including tumours must be excluded. Although bilateral salivary gland swelling due to tumours is uncommon it does occur and therefore bilateral salivary gland swelling should not necessarily be regarded as a reassuring sign (e.g. Warthin's tumour which may occur bilaterally at a frequency of 5–10%[58]).

Intraoral signs of xerostomia include those of a dry, sticky mucosa, with the gloved fingers sticking to the poorly lubricated mucosa; there is absence of a pool of saliva in the floor of the mouth and there may be difficulty in expressing saliva from the major duct openings. Oral clearance times are prolonged, leading to persistence of food debris around the mouth.[59] As a longer-term consequence of xerostomia, smooth-surface dental caries develops, particularly around the cervical margins of the dentition. Mucosal atrophy with fissuring especially of the dorsum of the tongue may present, sometimes with oral mucosal ulceration and superinfection with candida species.

Clinical assessment of the oral component of Sjögren's syndrome

Salivary gland involvement can be assessed objectively by measuring salivary flow rates, salivary gland biopsy, usually of the minor glands within the lower lip, and various imaging techniques. These modalities are described in detail in Chapter 128.

Ocular features of Sjögren's syndrome

The tear film and its dysfunction in pSS, including meibomian gland dysfunction

Dry eye is a critical component of pSS. Dry eye is defined as a multifactorial disease of the tears and ocular surface that results in symptoms of discomfort, visual disturbance, and tear film instability with potential damage to the ocular surface.[60] It is accompanied by increased tear film osmolarity and ocular surface inflammation. Dry eye occurs principally as a result of abnormalities of the lacrimal functional unit, which represents an integrated system consisting of the lacrimal glands, the ocular surface (cornea, conjunctiva), eyelids and meibomian glands (MG) together with the sensorimotor nerves that connect them.[61] The aetiopathogeneis of dry eye is broadly divided into aqueous deficient and evaporative forms, with the aqueous deficient component comprising of either SS dry eye (SSDE) or non-Sjögren's dry eye (NSDE).

Tear film pathology

The ocular surface is coated with a tear film, which is vital for lubrication, nutrition, and immunological defence of the eye. The tear film has a highly intricate structure, illustrated in Figure 127.2.[62] It consists of a negatively charged, hydrophilic mucinous glycocalyx synthesized by conjunctival goblet cells that limits adhesion of foreign debris or pathogens to the surface of the eye, and a more superficial aqueous phase secreted predominantly by the lacrimal gland that supports epithelial cell proliferation, maturation, and movement over the ocular surface.[63] The mucoaqueous gradient is critical for delivering essential nutrients and oxygen to the ocular surface and avascular cornea. The most superficial layer is a predominantly lipid layer secreted by the MG, which lie within the eyelids with their orifices behind the lash roots. Secreted lipids interact with aqueous proteins in a complex arrangement consisting of (1) proteins (lipocalin, lysozyme, surfactant proteins) intercalated with an outer non-polar lipid layer mediating tear film physical properties including surface tension and (2) long chain (O-acyl)-hydroxy fatty acids that form an intermediate surfactant polar lipid sublayer adjacent to the aqueous phase of the underlying mucoaqueous gradient. This lipoprotein construction not only confers tear film stability by minimizing evaporation and maintaining tear film integrity, it also forms an effective barrier protecting the eye from bacterial agents and organic matter.

SSDE is a principal cause of aqueous tear-deficient dry eye that results from lacrimal infiltration and/or destruction due to an immune-mediated process that releases inflammatory mediators into the tear film and ocular surface. The aqueous component evaporates at normal rates from a reduced pool of tears, resulting in both tear film and ocular surface epithelial cell hyperosmolarity.[64] This stimulates a cascade of signalling pathways involving MAP kinases and NFκB and the production of inflammatory cytokines perpetuating the autoimmune response.[65] An evaporative dry eye component secondary to loss of lipid layer due to MG obstruction, stagnation, dysfunction (MGD—Figure 127.3) and eventual destruction (with or without associated staphylococcal colonization and/or hypersensitivity) compounds ocular surface inflammation.

The basis for the dry eye symptoms is not fully understood, but activation of sensory nerves subserving nociception at the ocular surface is implicated.[66] This, together with a combination of tear film hyperosmolarity, rapid tear film break-up (TFBUT) in the interblink period, increased shear-stresses between the lids and globe due to reduced aqueous tear volume, reduced expression of mucins and lipids, the presence of inflammatory mediators, together with a hypersensitivity of the nociceptive sensory nerves, are likely candidates for neural activation and symptomatology.

Symptoms and signs

Patients typically complain of ocular discomfort described as dry, gritty, or burning of varying degrees of severity, ranging from mild and/or episodic discomfort frequently triggered by environmental stress, to severe, constant discomfort with visual disturbance, which in the severest cases may be constant and debilitating. The 'tear film dysfunction syndrome' describes a spectrum of conjunctival inflammation, staining of the ocular surface with vital dyes (fluorescein, lissamine green), reduced Schirmer's 1 test and TFBUT, increased debris and mucus clumping with or without filamentary keratitis, and MGD (Figure 127.3).[67] The symptoms and clinical features together formulate levels of dry eye disease severity, which provide a gauge for therapeutic strategies, although in some patients symptoms exceed clinical signs, presumably due to nociceptive sensory receptor hypersensitivity.[68] Photophobia is common and may be attributed to uveitis which is a rare complication of usually seropositive pSS, but should be recognized, as treatment with topical or systemic corticosteroid, or long-term maintenance with immunosuppression, may be required.

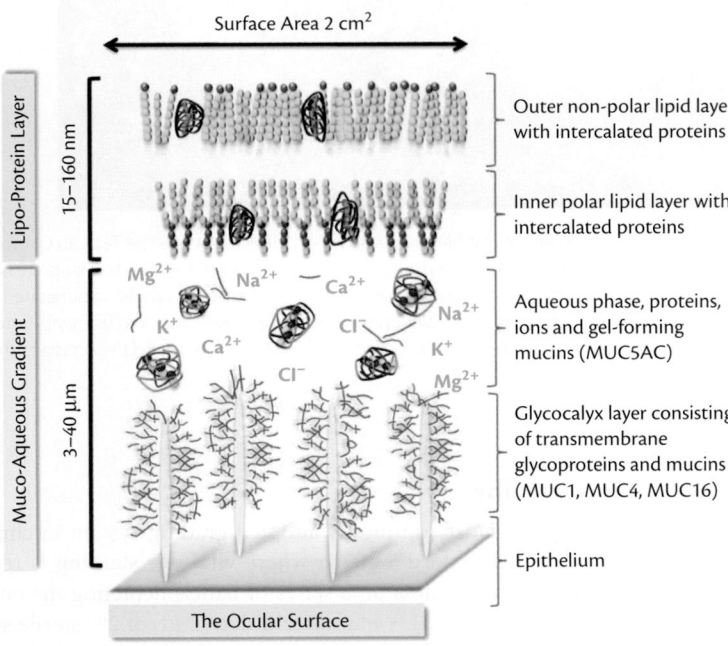

Surface Area 2 cm^2

Lipo-Protein Layer

15–160 nm

Outer non-polar lipid layer with intercalated proteins

Inner polar lipid layer with intercalated proteins

Muco-Aqueous Gradient

3–40 μm

Mg^{2+} Na^{2+} Ca^{2+}
K$^+$ Ca^{2+} Na^{2+}
            Cl$^-$ K$^+$
            Cl$^-$ Mg^{2+}

Aqueous phase, proteins, ions and gel-forming mucins (MUC5AC)

Glycocalyx layer consisting of transmembrane glycoproteins and mucins (MUC1, MUC4, MUC16)

Epithelium

The Ocular Surface

Fig. 127.2 Schematic representation of the tear film architecture (based on a novel model proposed by the International Meibomian Gland Dysfunction Workshop 2011). An outer lipoprotein layer confers architecture stability and reduces evaporation. The polar and non-polar lipids are secreted predominantly from the eyelid meibomian glands. The negatively charged glycocalyx, derived from the conjunctival goblet cells, reduces surface tension forces increasing the wettability of the ocular surface and forms a gradient with the largely lacrimal gland derived aqueous phase. The mucoaqueous component delivers essential nutrients (carbohydrates, proteins, enzymes, vitamins, hormones) to the ocular surface and the avascular structures of the external eye.

Based upon a novel model proposed by the International Meibomian Gland Dysfunction Workshop 2011. Reproduced with permission. © Rightsholder: Investigative Ophthalmology & Visual science.

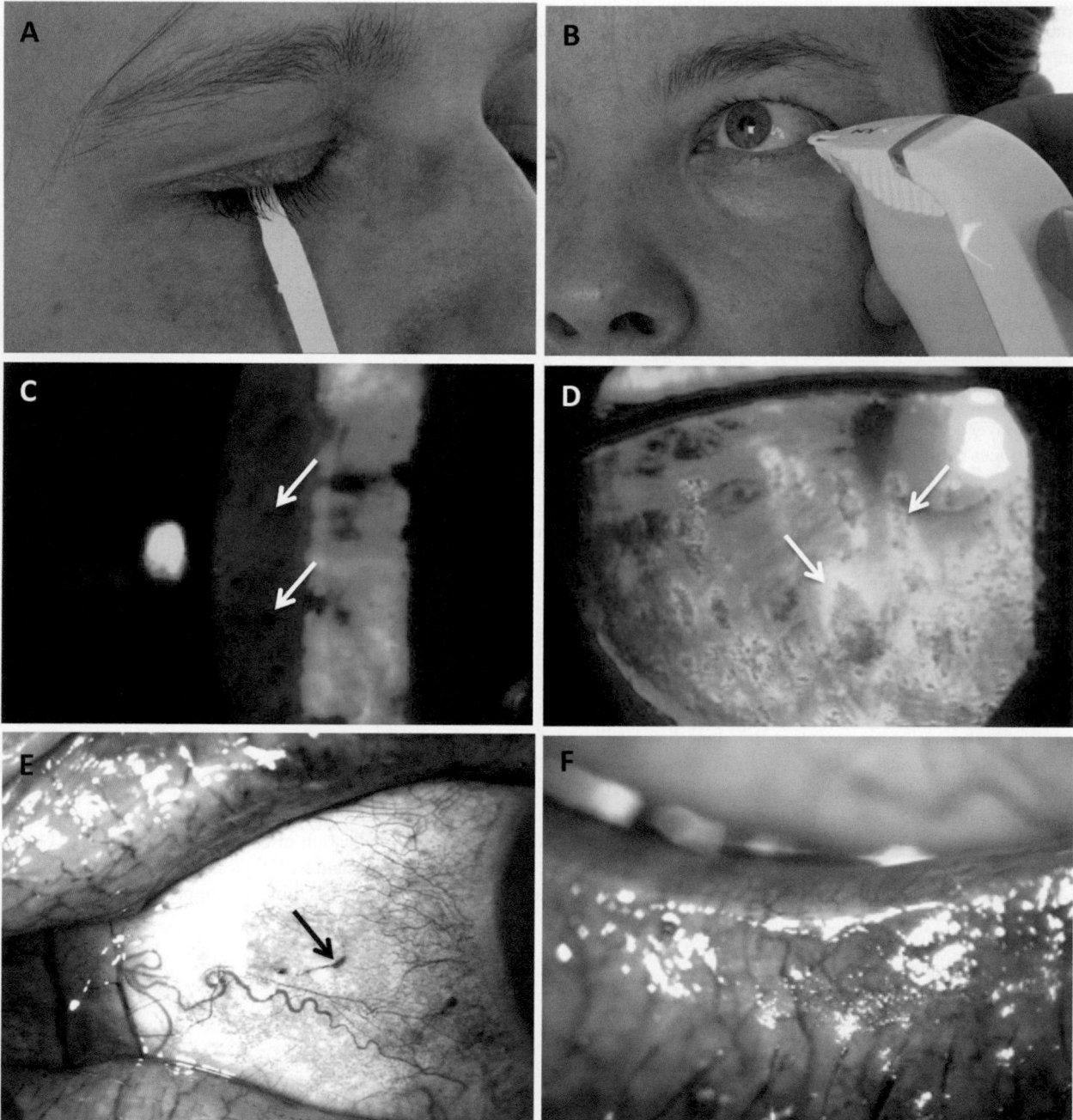

Fig. 127.3 Dry eye is traditionally diagnosed by (A) performing a Schirmer's I test, but measurement of tear film osmolarity using devices such as the TearLab Osmolarity System (B) has gained popularity as it provides an objective biomarker of dry eye severity. Tear film break-up time grades tear film stability (C)—note 'break-up' areas (arrows) in the fluorescein stained tear film—image taken 2 seconds after blink). Evaluating vital dye staining patterns with either (D) fluorescein showing punctate epithelial erosions on the corneal surface (arrows), or (E) lissamine green showing wedge-shaped staining of devitalized conjunctival epithelial cells and filaments (arrows) remain a key part of ocular examination. Meibomian gland dysfunction is more prevalent in pSS—(E) upper and lower lids, (F) lower lid. Note the telangiectasia at the eyelid margin (E, F)and inflammation at the mucocutaneous junction (F).

Objective assessment of dry eye

There is a wide range of clinical tests that may potentially be utilized in the assessment of SSDE.[69] These are frequently abridged to a practical sequence of taking a clinical history, grading the disease according to a symptom severity questionnaire, fluorescein TFBUT, ocular surface vital staining, and assessment of MGD.

Vital staining

Probably the most commonly adopted grading system in clinical practice is the Oxford Schema where vital dye staining is represented by punctate dots on a series of panels depicting the ocular surface (Figure 127.3).[70] Fluorescein dye (2 μL of 2% sterile solution) stains epithelial defects but has the disadvantage of a blurred staining pattern if slit-lamp reading with excitation and barrier filters is delayed. By contrast, staining with lissamine green is dose dependent, but maps devitalized epithelial cells that are present on the intact ocular surface.

Tear film break-up time

The TFBUT is a measure of tear film stability defined as the interval between the last complete blink and the first appearance of a dry spot or disruption in the tear film. It is performed by instilling 5 μL of 2% sodium fluorescein onto the bulbar conjunctiva; the patient instructed to blink naturally several times to distribute the fluorescein. Within 10–30 seconds of the fluorescein instillation, the patient is asked to stare straight ahead without blinking, and using a standard slit-lamp magnification (×10) and constant-intensity background illumination, the duration of the tear film integrity over the cornea is observed. A TFBUT of 10 seconds or more is considered to be normal, and a time of 5 seconds or less is reduced.

Schirmer's test

The Schirmer's 1 test without anaesthetic is considered the gold standard screening tool for dry eye.[71] The Schirmer's test I estimates unstimulated tear flow by inserting filter paper strips into the conjunctival sac over the lower lid margin, midway between the middle and outer third, with the eye closed in an anaesthetized eye (Figure 127.3). The strips are read at 5 minutes with a cut-off of 5 mm or less defining the probability of misclassification of patients with dry eye as 15% and of controls as 17%. In contrast, Schirmer's I with anaesthetic delivers an estimate of basal secretion, and Schirmer's II involves induction of 'reflex' secretion by irritating the nasal mucosa.

Tear film osmolarity

Because of its simplicity, increasing availability and affordability, osmolarity readings are becoming integral to dry eye assessment in the clinical setting for both ophthalmologists and rheumatologists. Osmolarity has the advantage of functioning as a non-invasive, easily performed, objective, continuously variable, clinical biomarker for dry eye severity.[72] Tear analysis is determined by a direct nanolitre specimen collection tool utilizing lab-on-a-chip technology. The test card for devices such as the TearLab Osmolarity System (Figure 127.3) is a single-use, polycarbonate lab-on-a-chip containing a sigmoidal nanofluidic channel collecting 50 nL of tear fluid sample by passive capillary action onto gold electrodes embedded in the card. Osmolarity values greater than 308 mOsm/L are generally indicative of dry eye disease (mild ⊠ 308 mOsm/L; moderate ⊠ 320 mOsm/L; severe >355 mOsm/L).

Impression cytology

Emerging objective assessment tools for quantifying disease include tear film proteomic analyses, ocular surface in-vivo confocal microscopy, and impression cytology of the conjunctiva coupled with flow cytometry to phenotype ocular surface damage and markers. The technique of impression cytology of the conjunctival epithelium provides a non-invasive histological evaluation of conjunctival epithelial morphology by using nitrocellulose filters to sample superficial epithelial cells followed by conventional histological stains for squamous metaplasia, keratinization, and inflammatory cells in situ.[73] Combined with flow cytometry of recovered sampled cells from a hydrophilic polyethersulfone filter, it provides a highly sensitive and specific tool that uses monoclonal antibodies for analysing expression of almost any cell marker allowing identification of conjunctival epithelial cells, inflammatory, cells and goblet cells.[72] Importantly, HLA-DR, which is minimally expressed in the healthy eye, is strongly overexpressed in cases of ocular surface inflammation and its measurement provides a biomarker of inflammatory dry eye disease activity.

Systemic features of Sjögren's syndrome

Fatigue

Seventy-five per cent of patients with pSS report mental and physical fatigue with levels of fatigue higher than healthy controls and similar to those affecting patients with other rheumatic diseases.[75] Fatigue is often the most disabling symptom,[76] and may correlate with night-time musculoskeletal pain causing sleep disturbance and anxiety. High levels of psychological distress are found in pSS patients and certain personality features (negativity, preoccupation with detail, perfectionism, and anxiety) prevalent in pSS[77] may contribute to fatigue.

Lymphoma

The prevalence of lymphoma increases from 3.4% in the first 5 years to 9.8% at 15 years.[78] The majority of lymphomas are of the MALT B-cell type and the risk is increased in Ro/La-positive patients. Presentation is usually with a firm, palpable swelling within the parotid gland or occasionally elsewhere. Open biopsy is usually essential (although fine-needle aspiration cytology may be useful initially in some cases) and CT scanning is helpful for staging. Treatment is generally with chemotherapy regimes that include rituximab. Occasionally, surgical excision and/or radiotherapy may be indicated. The prognosis is good, with a complete response to initial treatment in more than 90% of cases and 5 year disease-free survival of more than 75%. The median age of onset is in the mid-50s and the diagnosis of Sjögren's generally predates the lymphoma by a mean of 7 years. Predictive factors for later development of lymphoma include neutropenia, lymphadenopathy, and low C4 levels.[79]

Musculoskeletal

Arthralgia or arthritis are a presenting feature in one-third of cases and occur during the course of the disease in over one-half of cases.[80] The arthritis is generally peripheral, symmetrical, polyarticular, and intermittent. It is usually non-deforming and non-erosive, affects the metacarpophalangeal (MCP) and proximal interphalangeal (PIP) joints and wrists, and synovitis is generally mild.

Cutaneous

Dry skin affects at least 50% of cases and can cause pruritus. Treatment is with simple moisturizers and avoidance of perfumed products. Hypergammaglobulinaemic purpura affects about 9% of pSS patients[81] and causes a non-palpable purpura usually on the lower legs. It is associated with high immunoglobulin levels and histological examination demonstrates immune complex deposition. Subacute cutaneous lupus is a photosensitive, non-scarring rash, usually on the face, arms, and front of the chest. Treatment includes sun avoidance, the use of a high factor sunscreen, hydroxychloroquine, and occasionally additional immunosuppressive drugs.

Raynaud's phenomenon

Raynaud's phenomenon affects up to 80% of patients with pSS and may precede the sicca symptoms.[82] Precipitants such as smoking and beta-blockers should be avoided. Treatments include the calcium antagonists and ACE inhibitors.

Pulmonary

A chronic cough related to drying of the mucous membranes is common. Significant lung disease is rare. One study found plain radiograph abnormalities in 14% (most commonly fine reticular changes affecting the lower lobes) and abnormalities on high-resolution CT scanning in 34% (most commonly parenchymal linear opacities and bronchiolar abnormalities) but only 26% had symptoms; the majority of these were mild with poor correlation between symptoms, clinical signs, and radiological findings.[83]

Occasionally patients present acutely with lymphocytic interstitial pneumonitis (LIP). Clinical manifestations include fever, cough, and dyspnoea, with bibasilar pulmonary infiltrates consisting of dense interstitial accumulations of lymphocytes and plasma cells. LIP usually responds well to treatment with corticosteroids and the main differential diagnosis is infection.[84]

Neurological complications

A diffuse sensorimotor neuropathy may affect up to 25% of patients with pSS.[85] It usually presents insidiously and is probably not improved by treatment with steroids or cyclophosphamide,[86] but progress may be slowed with hydroxychloroquine.

Trigeminal neuropathy/neuralgia has been described in up to 5% of patients with pSS. It does not usually respond to treatment with corticosteroids and should be treated as for idiopathic trigeminal neuralgia. Mononeuritis multiplex is seen in less than 3% of pSS patients over their lifetime. It commonly affects the lateral popliteal nerve and may result in foot drop. It is associated with vasculitis and may respond to treatment with corticosteroids and cyclophosphamide.[84]

Autonomic neuropathy can cause a multitude of symptoms including postural hypotension, nocturnal diarrhoea, urinary retention, sweating, and dizziness, and may be under-recognized in SS. There is conflicting data on prevalence—it was not seen at all in one study,[88] affected 3% in a neurological case series [89] and 70% in a series focusing on gastrointestinal and urological features.[90] It is usually mild and may not require any specific treatment.

SS myelopathy can mimic multiple sclerosis (MS) and, although rare, distinction from MS is important as it may respond to immunosuppression.[91] Patients may present with paraplegia, sensory changes, and bladder dysfunction. Diagnosis requires MRI scanning, which shows white matter lesions and lumbar puncture, which demonstrates mild elevation of cerebrospinal fluid (CSF) protein and matched oligoclonal bands in CSF and serum.

Renal involvement

Significant renal disease is rare. One study found mild proteinuria (1.5–0.42 g/24 h) in 44% and distal renal tubular acidosis (RTA) in 33%.[92] The RTA patients tended to have a longer disease duration and were more likely to have proteinuria, hypertension, and raised creatinine than those without. The RTA was generally mild and often required no treatment or simple measures such as bicarbonate to restore the urine pH.

Symptoms of urinary dysfunction are common and Haarala and colleagues [90] found mild urinary symptoms in 61% of patients with SS compared with 27% of women without. Severe symptoms were seen in 14% and 7% respectively. Overall 27% of SS patients report urinary frequency and 36% complain of suprapubic pain. The frequency of urinary tract infection (UTI) in patients with pSS is not known but the frequency of recurrent UTI is increased from 6% in those with RA to 30% in those with coexistent SS.[94]

Interstitial cystitis is often seen in association with connective tissue diseases; 90% of sufferers are female. There is no good data on the prevalence in SS although one study suggests that SS is present in 23% of all patients with interstitial cystitis.[95]

Haematological

A mild normochromic anaemia is seen in approximately 20% of patients, leucopenia in 15%, and thrombocytopenia in 11%. Autoimmune haemolytic anaemia (AIHA) and neutropenia are occasionally reported.[96]

Thyroid disease

Thyroid disease, most commonly hypothyroidism, accompanies SS in up to 20% of cases.[97] Another interesting observation is that 37% of patients with autoimmune thyroid disease have an objectively dry mouth and 23% have objectively dry eyes.[98]

Gastrointestinal and liver involvement

Antibodies to tissue transglutaminase (TTG) are found in up to 5% of cases and confirmed coeliac disease in 4.5%,[99] a prevalence of approximately 10 times greater than expected.

Mild abnormalities of liver enzymes are found in 7% of cases,[100] with primary biliary cirrhosis (PBC)-associated autoantibodies in 6% of patients with SS and confirmed PBC in the majority of these.

Studies have shown mild elevation of pancreatic enzymes in about 35% of patients with SS[101] but more serious problems occur in no more than 1% of patients.

Biological

Hypocomplementaemia is seen in a subgroup of patients and is associated with a higher frequency of vasculitis, lymphoma, leucopenia, and cryoglobulinaemia.[11] It is an independent risk factor for the development of lymphoma. Hypergammaglobulinaemia is found in the majority of the Ro/La-positive patient group and is strongly associated with the presence of extraglandular manifestations.[102] A low positive dsDNA antibody has been described in a small proportion (<5%) of the Ro/La-positive patients.

Obstetric and gynaecological features of Sjögren's syndrome

Fertility and pregnancy

Fertility is normal in patients with SS, with a possible increased risk of recurrent miscarriage in the Ro/La-positive patients.[103] Neonatal lupus rash occurs in about 5% of live births in Ro/La positive women usually appearing at 6 weeks of age and lasting about 17 weeks before fading and clearing completely, although a few children have persistent depigmentation or telangiectasia. Congenital heart block (CHB) occurs in less than 2% of pregnancies in women with anti-Ro or -La antibodies[104] and may be detected by ultrasound scanning from about 16 weeks' gestation. Following an affected pregnancy the risk goes up to 17%[105] for subsequent pregnancies.

Seventy per cent of affected children survive but nearly all require pacemakers in the first few months of life.[106] Up to one-half of mothers are asymptomatic at the time of the birth although many go on to develop autoimmune disease later.[107]

Vaginal dryness and dyspareunia

Vaginal dryness affects 76% of women with SS compared to 5% of those without[108] and dyspareunia is a problem in 40%. Treatment includes the use of lubricating gels to aid intercourse and longer-acting vaginal moisturizers to improve moisture levels.

Prognosis and outcome

In general pSS is not associated with increased mortality, with the exception of patients who develop lymphoma.[106,110] There are, however, very major effects on patients and their quality of life, which in turn has health economic consequences, and these aspects are addressed in detail in the Chapter 128.

Acknowledgements

We would like to thank Dr Francesca Barone, Dr Wan-fai Ng, and Dr Arjan Vissink for critical reading of the manuscript.

Conflicts of interest

In the past few years Dr Simon Bowman has consulted for Merck-Sorrono and Takeda Pharmaceuticals and is in receipt of an Arthritis Research UK grant to which Roche Pharmaceuticals is contributing rituximab without charge.

References

1. Sjögren H. Zur kenntnis der keratoconjunctivitis sicca. *Acta Ophthalmol* 1933;11 (suppl II):1–151.
2. Gougerot H. Insuffisance progressive et atrophie des glandes salivarires et mugueuses de la bouche, des conjunctives (et parfois de muqueuses, nasale, laryngée, vulvaire) sécheresse de la bouche, des conjonctives. *Bull Med* (Paris) 1926;40:360–365.
3. Mikulicz J. Uber eine eigenartige symmetrische Erkrankung der Tranen- und Mundspeicheldrusen. In: Billroth GT (ed.) *Beitr. Chir. Fortschr.*, Stuttgart, 1892:610–630.
4. Bloch KJ, Buchanan WW, Wohl MJ, Bunim JJ. Sjögren's syndrome: a clinical, pathological, and serological study of sixty-two cases. *Medicine* 44:187–231, 1965.
5. Talal N, Bunim JJ. The development of malignant lymphoma in the course of Sjögren's syndrome. *Am J Med* 1964;36:529–540.
6. Chisholm DM, Mason DK. Labial salivary gland biopsy in Sjögren's syndrome. *J Clin Pathol* 1968;21:656–660.
7. Clark G, Reichlin M, Tomasi TB. Characterization of a soluble cytoplasmic antigen reactive with sera from patients with systemic lupus erythematosus. *J. Immunol* 1969;102:117–122.
8. Harley JB, Alexander EL, Bias WB et al. Anti-Ro(SSA) and anti-La(SSB) in patients with Sjogren's syndrome. *Arthritis Rheum* 1986;29:196–206.
9. Kephart DC, Hood AF, Provost TT. Neonatal lupus erythematosus: new serologic findings. *J Invest Dermatol* 1981;77:331–333.
10. Ramos-Casals M, Solans R, Rosas J et al.; GEMESS Study Group. Primary Sjögren syndrome in Spain: clinical and immunologic expression in 1010 patients. *Medicine* (Baltimore) 2008;87:210–219.
11. Manthorpe R, Anderson V, Jensen OA et al. Editorial comments to the four sets of criteria for Sjögren's syndrome. *Scand J Rheumatol* 1986;suppl 61:31–35.
12. Vitali C, Bombardieri S, Moutsopoulos HM et al. Preliminary criteria for the classification of Sjögren's syndrome. Results of a prospective concerted action supported by the European Community. *Arthritis Rheum* 1993;36(3):340–347.
13. Vitali C, Bombardieri S, Jonsson R et al. Classification criteria for Sjögren's syndrome: a revised version of the European criteria proposed by the American European Consensus Group. *Ann Rheum Dis* 2002;61:554–558.
14. Whitcher JP, Shiboski CH, Shiboski SC et al. ; Sjögren's International Collaborative Clinical Alliance Research Groups. A simplified quantitative method for assessing keratoconjunctivits sicca from the Sjögren's Syndrome International Registry. *Am J Ophthalmol* 2010;149:405–415.
15. Daniels TE, Cox D, Shiboski CH et al.; Sjögren's International Collaborative Clinical Alliance (SICCA) Research Groups. Associations between salivary gland histopathologic diagnoses and phenotypic features of Sjögren's syndrome (SS) among 1726 registry participants. *Arthritis Rheum* 2011;63(7):2021–2030.
16. Takahashi H, Yamamoto M, Suzuki C et al. The birthday of a new syndrome: IgG4-related diseases constitute a clinical entity. *Autoimmun Rev* 2010;9:591–594.
17. Thomas E, Hay EM, Hajeer A, Silman AJ. Sjögren's syndrome: A community-based study of prevalence and impact. *Br J Rheumatol* 1998;37:1069–1076.
18. Bowman SJ, Ibrahim GH, Holmes G, Hamburger J, Ainsworth JR. Estimating the prevalence among Caucasian women of primary Sjögren's syndrome in two general practices in Birmingham, UK. *Scand J Rheumatol* 2004;33:39–43.
19. Anagnostopoulos I, Zinzaras E, Alexiou I et al. The prevalence of rheumatic diseases in central Greece: a population survey. *BMC Musculoskelet Disord* 2010;26:11–98.
20. Goransson LG, Haldorsen K, Brun JG et al. The point prevalence of clinically relevant primary Sjögren's syndrome in two Norwegian counties. *Scand J Rheumatol* 2011;40:221–224.
21. Davies ML, Taylor EJ, Gordon C et al. Candidate T cell epitopes of the human La/SSB autoantigen. *Arthritis Rheum* 2002;46:209–214.
22. Rischmueller M, Lester S, Chen Z et al. HLA class II phenotype controls diversification of the autoantibody response in primary Sjögren's syndrome (pSS). *Clin Exp Immunol* 111;1998:365–371.
23. Haneji N, Nakamura T, Takio K et al. Identification of alpha-fodrin as a candidate autoantigen in primary Sjögren's syndrome. *Science* 1997;276:604–607.
24. Bacman S, Sterin-Borda L, Camusso JJ et al. Circulating antibodies against rat parotid gland M3 muscarinic receptors in primary Sjögren's syndrome. *Clin Exp Immunol* 1996;104:454–459.
25. Jonsson R, Haga H-J, Gordon TP. Current concepts on diagnosis, autoantibodies and therapy in Sjögren's syndrome. *Scand J Rheumatol* 2000;29:341–348.
26. Winer S, Astsaturov I, Cheung R et al. Primary Sjögren's syndrome and deficiency of ICA69. *Lancet.* 2002;360:1063–1069.
27. Steinfeld S, Cogan E, King LS et al. Abnormal distribution of aquaporin-5 water channel protein in salivary glands from Sjögren's syndrome patients. *Lab Invest* 2001;81:143–148.
28. Dawson LJ, Allison HE, Stanbury J, Fitzgerald D, Smith PM. Putative anti-muscarinic antibodies cannot be detected in patients with primary Sjogren's syndrome using conventional immunological approaches. *Rheumatology* 2004;43:1488–1495.
29. Anaya JM, Tobon GJ, Pineda-Tamayo R, Castiblanco J. Autoimmune disease aggregation in families of patients with primary Sjögren's syndrome. *J Rheumatol* 2006;33:2227–2234.
30. Mann DL, Moutsopoulos HM. HLA DR alloantigens in different subsets of patients with Sjögren's syndrome and in family members. *Ann Rheum Dis.* 1983 Oct;42(5):533–536.
31. Anaya J-M, Delgado-Vega AM, Castiblanco J. Genetic basis of Sjögren's syndrome. How strong is the evidence? *Clin Dev Immunol* 2006;13:209–222.

32. Emamian ES, Leon JM, Lessard CJ et al. Peripheral blood gene expression profiling in Sjögren's syndrome. *Genes Immunol* 2009;10:285–296.

33. González S, Aguilera S, Urzúa U et al. Mechanotransduction and epigenetic control in autoimmune diseases. *Autoimmun Rev.* 2011;10:175–179.

34. Hu S, Wang J, Meijer J et al. Salivary proteomic and genomic biomarkers for primary Sjögren's syndrome. *Arthritis Rheum* 2007;56:3588–3600.

35. Ramos-Casals M, Muñoz S, Medina F et al.; HISPAMEC Study Group. Systemic autoimmune diseases in patients with hepatitis C virus infection: characterization of 1020 cases (The HISPAMEC Registry). *J Rheumatol* 2009;36:1442–1448.

36. Itescu S, Winchester R. Diffuse infiltrative lymphocytosis syndrome: a disorder occurring in human immunodeficiency virus-1 infection that may present as a sicca syndrome. *Rheum Dis Clin North Am* 1992;18:683–697.

37. Lavoie TN, Lee BH, Nguyen CQ. Current concepts: mouse models of Sjögren's syndrome. *J Biomed Biotechnol* 2011:549107.

38. Skopouli FN, Moutsopoulos HM. Autoimmune epitheliitis: Sjögren's syndrome. *Clin Exp Rheumatol* 1994;12(suppl 11):S9–S11.

39. Bolstad AI, Eiken HG, Rosenlund B, Alarcon-Riquelme ME, Jonsson R. Increased salivary gland tissue expression of Fas, Fas ligand, cytotoxic T lymphocyte-associated antigen 4, and programmed cell death 1 in primary Sjögren's syndrome. *Arthritis Rheum* 2003;48:174–185.

40. Roescher N, Tak PP, Illei GG. Cytokines in Sjogren's syndrome: potential therapeutic targets. *Ann Rheum Dis* 2010;69:945–948.

41. Varin MM, Le Pottier L, Youinou P et al. B-cell tolerance breakdown in Sjögren's syndrome: focus on BAFF. *Autoimmun Rev* 2010;9:604–608.

42. Ittah M, Miceli-Richard C, Lebon P et al. Induction of B cell-activating factor by viral infection is a general phenomenon, but the types of viruses and mechanisms depend on cell type. *J Innate Immun* 2011;3:200–207.

43. Barone F, Bombardieri M, Rosado MM, Morgan PR, Challacombe SJ, De Vita S, Carsetti R, Spencer J, Valesini G, Pitzalis C. CXCL13, CCL21, and CXCL12 expression in salivary glands of patients with Sjogren's syndrome and MALT lymphoma: association with reactive and malignant areas of lymphoid organization. *J Immunol.* 2008;180:5130–5140.

44. Amft N, Curnow SJ, Scheel-Toellner D et al. Ectopic expression of the B cell-attracting chemokine BCA-1 (CXCL13) on endothelial cells and within lymphoid follicles contributes to the establishment of germinal center-like structures in Sjögren's syndrome. *Arthritis Rheum* 2001;44:2633–2641.

45. Xanthou G, Polihronis M, Tzioufas AG et al. 'Lymphoid' chemokine messenger RNA expression by epithelial cells in the chronic inflammatory lesion of the salivary glands of Sjögren's syndrome patients: possible participation in lymphoid structure formation. *Arthritis Rheum* 2001;44:408–418.

46. Johnson EO, Kostandi M, Moutsopoulos HM. Hypothalamic-pituitary-adrenal axis function in Sjögren's syndrome: mechanisms of neuroendocrine and immune system homeostasis. *Ann N Y Acad Sci* 2006;1088:41–51.

47. Dawson LJ, Christmas SE, Smith PM. An investigation of interactions between the immune system and stimulus-secretion coupling in mouse submandibular acinar cells: a possible mechanism to account for reduced salivary flow rates associated with the onset of Sjogren's syndrome. *Rheumatology* (Oxford) 2000;39:1226–1233.

48. Caffery B, Heynen ML, Joyce E et al. MUC1 expression in Sjogren's syndrome, KCS, and control subjects. *Mol Vis.* 2010;16:1720–1727.

49. Orellana MF, Lagravere MO, Boychuk DG, Major PW, Flores-Mir C. Prevalence of xerostomia in population-based samples: a systematic review. *J Public Health Dent* 2006;66(2):152–158.

50. Fox PC, Bowman SJ, Segal S et al. Oral involvement in primary Sjogren syndrome. *J Am Dent Assoc* 2008; 139:1592–1601.

51. Kamel UF, Maddison P, Whitaker R. Impact of primary Sjogren's syndrome on smell and taste: effect on quality of life. *Rheumatology* 2009; 48:1512–1514.

52. Mignogna MD, Pollio A, Fortuna G, et al. Unexplained somatic comorbidities in patients with burning mouth syndrome: a controlled clinical study. *J Orofacial Pain* 2011;25(2):131–140.

53. Imanguli MM, Atkinson JC, Mitchell SA. Salivary gland involvement in chronic graft versus host disease: prevalence, clinical significance and recommendations for evaluation. *Biol Blood Marrow Transplant* 2010;16(10):1362–1369.

54. Entesarian M, Dahlqvist J, Shashi V et al. FGF10 missense mutations in aplasia of lacrimal and salivary glands. *Eur J Hum Genet* 2007;15:379–382.

55. Kassimos DG, Shirlaw PJ, Choy EHS et al. Chronic sialadenitis in patients with nodal osteoarthritis. *Br J Rheumatol* 1997;36:1312–1217.

56. Ghezzi EM, Ship JA, Ageing and secretory reserve capacity of major salivary glands. *J Dent Res* 2003;82(10):844–848

57. Ghezzi EM, Wagner-Lange LA, Schork MA et al. Longitudinal influence of age, menopause, hormone replacement and other medications in on parotid flow rates in healthy women. *J Gerontol A Biol Sci Med Sci* 2000;55:M34–M42

58. Maiorano E, Lo Muzio L, Favia G, Piattelli A. Warthin's tumour: a study of 78 cases with emphasis on bilaterality, multifocality and association with other malignancies. *Oral Oncol* 2002;38(1):35–40

59. Yurtseven N, Gokalp S. Oral sugar clearance and other caries-related factors of stimulated whole saliva in patients with secondary Sjögren syndrome. *Quintessence Int* 2007; 38(3):e151–e157.

60. The definition and classification of dry eye disease: report of the Definition and Classification Subcommittee of the International Dry Eye Workshop (2007). *Ocular Surface* 2007;5(2):75–93.

61. Stern ME, Beuerman RW, Fox RI, et al. The pathology of dry eye: the interaction between the ocular surface and lacrimal glands. *Cornea* 1998;17(6):584.

62. Green-Church KB, Butovich I, Willcox M, et al. The International Workshop on Meibomian Gland Dysfunction: Report of the subcommittee on tear film lipids and lipid–protein interactions in health and disease. *Invest Ophthalmol Vis Sci* 2011;52(4):1979–1993.

63. Nichols KK, Foulks GN, Bron AJ, et al. The International Workshop on Meibomian Gland Dysfunction: executive summary. *Invest Ophthalmol Vis Sci* 2011;52(4):1922–1929.

64. Liu H, Begley C, Chen M et al. A link between tear instability and hyperosmolarity in dry eye. *Invest Ophthalmol Vis Sci* 2009;50(8):3671–3679.

65. De Paiva CS, Corrales RM, Villarreal AL, et al. Corticosteroid and doxycycline suppress MMP-9 and inflammatory cytokine expression, MAPK activation in the corneal epithelium in experimental dry eye. *Exp Eye Res* 2006;83(3):526–535.

66. Tuisku IS, Konttinen YT, Konttinen LM, Tervo TM. Alterations in corneal sensitivity and nerve morphology in patients with primary Sjögren's syndrome. *Exp Eye Res* 2008;86(6):879–885.

67. Behrens A, Doyle JJ, Stern L, et al. Dysfunctional tear syndrome: a Delphi approach to treatment recommendations. *Cornea* 2006;25(8):900–907.

68. Rosenthal P, Inna B, Jacobs D. Corneal pain without stain: Is it real? *Ocular Surface* 2009;7(1):28–40.

69. Foulks GN, Bron AJ. Meibomian gland dysfunction: a clinical scheme for description, diagnosis, classification, and grading. *Ocular Surface* 2003;1(3):107–126.

70. Bron AJ, Evans VE, Smith JA. Grading of corneal and conjunctival staining in the context of other dry eye tests. *Cornea* 2003;22(7):640–650.

71. van Bijsterveld OP. Diagnostic tests in the sicca syndrome. *Arch Ophthalmol* 1969;82(1):10–14.

72. Lemp MA, Bron AJ, Baudouin C, et al. Tear osmolarity in the diagnosis and management of dry eye disease. *Am J Ophthalmol* 2011;151(5):792–798.e1.

73. Pflugfelder SC, Huang AJ, Feuer W, et al. Conjunctival cytologic features of primary Sjogren's syndrome. *Ophthalmology* 1990;97(8):985–991.

74. Baudouin C, Brignole F, Becquet F et al. Flow cytometry in impression cytology specimens. A new method for evaluation of conjunctival inflammation. *Invest Ophthalmol Vis Sci* 1997;38(7):1458–1464.

75. Bowman SJ, Booth DA, Platts RG and UK Sjogren's Interest Group. Measurement of fatigue and discomfort in primary Sjogren's syndrome using a new questionnaire tool. *Rheumatology* 2004;43:758–764.

76. Theander L, Strombeck B, Mandl T, Theander E. Sleepiness or fatigue? Can we detect treatable causes of tiredness in primary Sjogren's syndrome? *Rheumatology* 2010;49(6):1177–1183.

77. Kariskos D, Mavragani CP, Sinno MH et al. Psychopathological and personality features in primary Sjogren's syndrome—association with autoantibodies to neuropeptides. *Rheumatology* 2010;49(9):1762–1769.

78. Solans-Laqué R, López-Hernandez A, Angel Bosch-Gil J et al. Risk, predictors and clinical characteristics of lymphoma development in primary Sjögren's syndrome. *Semin Arth Rheum* 2011;41(3):415–423.

79. Theander E, Henriksson G, Ljungberg O et al. Lymphoma and other malignancies in primary Sjögren's syndrome: a cohort study on cancer incidence and lymphoma predictors. *Ann Rheum Dis* 2006;65(6):796–803.

80. Fauchais AL, Ouattara B, Gondram G et al. Articular manifestations in primary Sjogren's syndrome: clinical significance and prognosis of 188 patients. *Rheumatology* 2010;49:1164–1172.

81. Ramos-Casals M, Anaya JM, Garcia-Carrasco M et al. Cutaneous vasculitis in primary Sjogren's syndrome: classification and clinical significance of 52 patients. *Medicine* 2004;83(2):96–106.

82. Davidson BK, Kelly CA, Griffiths ID. Primary Sjögren's syndrome in the North East of England: a long-term follow-up study. *Rheumatology* (Oxford) 1999; Mar;38(3):245–253.

83. Franquet T, Gimenez A, Monill JM, Diaz C, Geli C. Primary Sjogren's syndrome and associated lung disease: CT findings in 50 patients. *AJR* 1997;169:655–658.

84. Dalvi V, Gonzalez EB, Lovett L. Lymphocytic interstitial pneumonitis (LIP) in Sjögren's syndrome: a case report and a review of the literature. *Clin Rheum* 2007;26(8):1339–1343.

85. Sène D, Jallouli M, Lefaucheur JP et al. Peripheral neuropathies associated with primary Sjogren's syndrome: immunologic profiles of nonataxic sensory neuropathy and sensorimotor neuropathy. *Medicine* 2011;90(2):133–138.

86. Font J, Ramos-Casalas M, de la Red G et al. Pure sensory neuropathy in primary Sjögren's syndrome. Long-term prospective follow-up and review of the literature. *J Rheumatol* 2003;30:1552–1557.

87. Andonopoulos AP, Lagos G, Drosos AA, Moutsopoulos HM. The spectrum of neurological involvement in Sjogren's syndrome. *Br J Rheumatol* 1990;29(1):21–23.

88. Niemela RK, Hakala M, Huikuri HV, Airaksinen KE. Comprehensive study of autonomic dysfunction in a population with primary Sjogren's syndrome. No evidence of autonomic involvement. *J Rheumatol* 2003;30(1):74–79.

89. Mori K, Iijima M, Koike H et al. The wide spectrum of clinical manifestations in Sjogren's syndrome-associated neuropathy. *Brain* 2005;128(11):2518–2534.

90. Kovacs L, Papos M, Takacs R et al. Autonomic nervous system dysfunction involving the gastrointestinal and the urinary tracts in primary Sjogren's syndrome. *Clin Exp Rheumatol* 2003, 21;6:697–703.

91. Delalande S, de Seze J, Fauchais AL et al. Neurologic manifestations in primary Sjogren syndrome: a study of 82 patients. *Medicine* 2004;83(5):280–291.

92. Pertovaara M, Korpela M, Kouri T, Pasternack A. The occurence of renal involvement in primary Sjogren's syndreom: a study of 78 patients. *Rheumatology* 1999;38:1113–1120.

93. Haarala M, Alanen A, Hietarinta M, Kiilholma P. Lower urinary tract symptoms in patients with Sjogren's syndrome and systemic lupus erythematosus. *Int Urogynecol J Pelvic Floor Dysfunct* 2000;11(2):84–86.

94. Tischler M, Caspi D, Almog Y, Segal R, Yaron M. Increased incidence of urinary tract infection in patients with rheumatoid arthritis and secondary Sjogren's syndrome. *Ann Rheum Dis* 1992;51(5):604–606.

95. Van der Merwe K, Joop P, Yamada T, Sakamoto Y. Systemic aspects of interstitial cystitis, immunology and linkage with autoimmune disorders. *Int J Urol* 2003;10(s1):s35–s38.

96. Manganelli P, Fietta P, Quaini F. Haematologic manifestations of primary Sjogren's syndrome. *Clin Exp Rheumatol* 2006;24(4):438–448.

97. Kang JH, Lin HC. Comorbidities in patients with Primary Sjogren's syndrome: A registry based case control study. *J Rheumatology* 2010;37(6):1188–1194.

98. Coll J, Anglada J, Tomas S et al. High prevalence of subclinical Sjogren's syndrome features in patients with autoimmune thyroid disease. *J Rheumatol* 1997;24(9):1719–1724.

99. Luft LM, Barr SG, Martin LO, Chan EKL, Fritzler MJ. Autoantibodies to tissue transglutaminase in Sjogren's syndrome and related rheumatic diseases. *J Rheumatol* 2003;30(12):2613–2619.

100. Skopouli FN, Barbatis C, Moutsopoulos HM. Liver involvement in primary Sjogren's syndrome. *Br J Rheumatol* 1994:33;745–748.

101. Ostuni PA, Gazzetto G, Chieco-Bianchi F et al. Pancreatic exocrine involvement in primary Sjogren's syndrome. *Scand J Rheumatol* 1996;25(1):47–51.

102. ter Borg, EJ, Risselada AP, Kelder JC. Relation of systemic autoantibodies to the number of extraglandular manifestations in primary Sjogren's syndrome: a retrospective analysis of 65 patients in the Netherlands. *Semin Arthritis Rheum* 2011;40(6):547–551.

103. Mavragani CP, Ioannidis JP, Tzioufas AG, Hantoumi IE, Moutsopoulos HM. Recurrent pregnancy loss and autoantibody profile in autoimmune disease. *Rheumatology*1999;38(12):1228–1233.

104. Brucato A, Frassi M, Franceschini F et al. Risk of congenital complete heart block in newborns of mothers with anti-R/SSA antibodies detected by counterimmunoelectrophoresis: a prospective study of 100 women. *Arthritis Rheum* 2001;44(8):1832–1835.

105. Priori R. Pregnancy in Sjogren's syndrome and neonatal lupus. *Rheumatology* 2011;50(s3):iii12–iii13.

106. Waltuck J, Buyon JP. Autantibody associated congenital heart block: outcome in mothers and children. *Ann Intern Med* 1994;20(7):544–551.

107. Neiman, AR, Lee LA, Weston WL, Buyon JP. Cutaneous manifestations of neonatal lupus without heart block: characteristics of mothers and children enrolled in a national registry. *J Pediatr* 2000;137(5):674–680.

108. Lehrer S, Bogursky E, Yemini M, Kase NG, Birkenfield A. Gynaecologic manifestations of Sjogren's syndrome. *Am J Obstet Gynecol* 1994;170(3):835–837.

109. Voulgarelis M, Tzioufas AG, Moutsopoulos HM. Mortality in Sjögren's syndrome. *Clin Exp Rheumatol.* 2008;26(5 Suppl 51):S66–S71.

110. Theander E, Manthorpe R, Jacobsson LT. Mortality and causes of death in primary Sjogren's syndrome: a prospective cohort study. *Arthritis Rheum.* 2004;50:1262–1269.

CHAPTER 128

Sjögren's syndrome— management

Wan-Fai Ng, Arjan Vissink, Elke Theander, and Francisco Figueiredo

Introduction

To date, few therapeutic strategies for Sjögren's syndrome (SS) have been formally evaluated and treatment guidelines for SS have not been developed. The management approaches recommended are based on the collective experience of three large European tertiary referral centres for SS and relevant published data when available.

The most widely accepted classification criteria for SS are the American European Consensus Group (AECG) criteria. Diagnostic criteria are not available, but the AECG criteria may guide assessment of patients with suspected SS. In clinical practice, however, other investigations are usually necessary to exclude other conditions that mimic SS (Table 128.1) and to fully assess these patients (Table 128.2). The common diagnostic pitfalls in SS are listed in Box 128.1.

Disease assessment

Oral manifestations

Loss of salivary gland (SG) function is already prominent in the early stages of SS. The submandibular and sublingual glands, the most active glands at rest, are being affected first, whereas the parotid glands, which become active gland upon stimulation, appear to be affected last.[1] Thus, in early SS, xerostomia is often predominantly present at rest and at night. As the disease progresses and affects all SG, oral dryness is also present during the day with difficulties in chewing and swallowing food. Hyposalivation may also lead to difficulties in speaking, burning sensations in the mouth, a diminished ability to taste foods, and sensitivity to spicy or coarse foods.

Patients with advanced SG hypofunction have overt signs of mucosal dryness: cracked, peeling, and atrophic lips; pale and corrugated buccal mucosa; a smooth, reddened tongue with loss of the dorsal papillae or a fissured appearance. Dental erosion and caries are common and can be progressive despite vigilant oral hygiene. Greater accumulations of food debris at the smooth surfaces and cervical regions of the teeth also occur. SS patients are prone to oral infections, particularly candidiasis and fungal lesions of the mouth corners (angular cheilitis).

Chronic or episodic enlargement of the SG, especially the parotid and submandibular glands, is common. This is generally due to the underlying autoimmune inflammatory process. In the parotid glands this inflammatory process can occur unilaterally, but most often bilaterally. Glandular enlargement, especially the parotid glands, may also be due to lymphoma. Since the incidence of lymphomas is 15–20 times increased in SS patients, physicians should maintain a high index of suspicion on painless nodular glandular masses.[2]

Ocular manifestations

The grading scheme agreed at the 2007 International Dry Eye Workshop is the most widely used system for assessing the severity of dry eye.[3] It is based on the frequency and degree of severity of a combination of factors including discomfort, visual symptoms, conjunctival injection, conjunctival/corneal staining, corneal/tear signs (corneal filaments and tear debris), presence of meibomian gland diseases, tear break-up time, and Schirmer's score.[4]

Ocular symptoms questionnaires/patient-reported outcomes

Dry eye symptoms correlate poorly with objective assessments.[5] An accurate assessment of symptoms is essential, as often it is symptoms that dictate requests for treatment by patients. As a minimum, we recommend the use of the European League Against Rheumatism (EULAR) Sjögren's Syndrome Patient-Reported Index (ESSPRI).[6] In this instrument, ocular dryness, like oral dryness, is measured using a single Likert (0–10) scale. Additionally, a composite EULAR-sicca score defined as $[(2 \times \text{oral dryness} + \text{ocular dryness})/3]$ can be calculated.

The Ocular Surface Disease Index is a reliable and validated 12-item instrument for measuring dry eye-related ocular surface disability.[7] It is frequently used in specialized dry eye clinics and clinical trials.

Systemic assessment

Although oral and ocular dryness are the cardinal features of SS, dryness also occurs at the skin and other mucosal surfaces such as the respiratory tract, vagina, and vulva, which can cause symptoms mimicking other conditions. Therefore, clinicians should consider

Table 128.1 Differential diagnosis of Sjögren's syndrome and non-Sjögren's syndrome causes of sicca syndrome and salivary gland enlargement

	Differential diagnosis of SS	Non-SS causes of sicca syndrome	Non-SS causes of salivary gland enlargement
Infections	Viral infections: HIV, EBV, Hep A, B, C, HTLV-1, mumps	Viral infections	Viral or bacterial infections, mumps, HIV, EBV, CMV
Inflammatory	Sarcoidosis, amyloidosis	Sarcoidosis	Sarcoidosis
Endocrine/ metabolic	Lipoproteinaemia (types II, IV, V), diabetes	Endocrine: diabetes	Endocrine: diabetes, acromegaly Metabolic: alcohol excess, cirrhosis, lipoproteinaemia, chronic pancreatitis, bulimia, anorexia nervosa, endurance athletes
Malignancy	Lymphoma		Malignancy, irradiation
Iatrogenic		Irradiation	
Others	Fibromyalgia, chronic fatigue syndrome	Medications, psychogenic, age-related lacrimal gland disease, ocular hypoesthesia	Sialolithiasis, sialoadenitis, medications (e.g. isoproterenol)

CMV, cytomegalovirus; EBV, Epstein–Barr virus; GVHD, graft vs host disease; Hep, hepatitis; HTLV, human T-lymphotropic virus.

Table 128.2 Useful investigations for the diagnosis and assessment of Sjögren's syndrome

Systemic	Oral	Ocular
Essential		
Blood tests: FBC, electrolytes, Ur, Cr, liver enzymes, CK, TSH, ESR, CRP, G, Ig & EPS, C3, C4, ANA, RF, SSA/SSB, dsDNA *Urine:* Dipstick analysis *Imaging:* Chest radiograph	UWS Salivary gland biopsy	Schirmer's I test Tear film break-up time Ocular surface staining (e.g. Lissamin green, fluorescein or Rose Bengal staining)
If indicative		
Serology for hepatitis A, B, C, EBV & HIV; sACE, ENA, ACPA, AMA, cryoglobulins, amylase, HbA1c, haemolytic screen	Sialography	
Optional		
	SWS Selective sialometry Sialochemistry Ultrasound salivary glands MRI salivary glands Scintigraphy	Tear function index Impression cytology of the conjunctiva Tear osmolality Ocular surface disease index

ACPA, anti-citrullinated peptide antibodies; AMA, anti-mitochondrial antibodies; ANA, anti-nuclear antibodies; CK, creatinine kinase; Cr, creatinine; CRP, C-reactive protein; dsDNA, anti-ds DNA antibodies; ENA, extractable nuclear antigen; ESR erythrocyte sedimentation rate; FBC, full blood count; G, glucose; Ig & EPS, immunoglobulins and electrophoresis; RF, rheumatoid factor; sACE serum angiotensin converting enzyme; SWS, stimulated whole sialometry; TSH, thyroid stimulating hormone; Ur, urea; UWS, unstimulated whole sialometry.

dryness of these organs being a contributing factor to their presenting symptoms.

Furthermore, all SS patients should be assessed for systemic manifestations. For patients with secondary SS, this should also include the assessment of the disease activity and damage of the associated autoimmune rheumatic disease. To facilitate standardized evaluation of SS disease activity, the EULAR SS study group has developed a scoring system, the EULAR Sjögren's Syndrome Disease Activity Index (ESSDAI).[8,9] The ESSDAI also provides a useful framework for structured assessment of SS patients in clinics (Table 128.3). The ESSDAI consists of 12 domains: constitutional, lymphadenopathy, glandular, articular, cutaneous, pulmonary, renal, muscular, peripheral nervous system, central nervous system, haematological, and biological. These domains were selected on the basis of clinical experience, literature review, and a panel of

SS experts. Each domain is given a score of 0 (no activity), 1 (low activity), 2 (moderate activity), or 3 (high activity) with the exception of the constitutional, glandular, and biological domains which are scored between 0 and 2, and the central nervous system domain which is scored 0, 2, or 3. Each domain score is weighted according to its relative contribution to the overall disease activity. The total score is the sum of the weighted domain scores.

Patient-reported outcomes, functional capacity, quality of life

Dryness, fatigue and bodily discomfort are the most prominent clinical features of primary SS (pSS). In order to measure the impact of pSS on subjective well-being in clinical trials and clinical practice, the EULAR SS study group has developed the ESSPRI which give a composite total score defined as the mean of the Likert scores

(0–10) of dryness, fatigue, and pain.[6] Both ESSDAI and ESSPRI are sensitive to change in response to therapeutic intervention.[10]

Fatigue is an important and distressing symptom of pSS[11] and is a key predictor of reduced social activities and work productivity.[12,13] The best approach to assess fatigue has not been defined. A visual analogue scale (VAS) is often used, but numerous more complex instruments have also been applied.[14–16] The Profile of Fatigue (ProF) was developed specifically for pSS.[17–19] ESSPRI contains two Likert scales (0–10) on fatigue (physical and mental) and may also be used.[6]

Patients with established pSS have significantly impaired health-related quality of life (HRQL).[12,20,21] pSS patients may also have reduced functional capacities due to their symptoms of fatigue, dryness, and pain. There is currently no disease-specific instrument for measuring HRQL or functional capacity in SS. Therefore, generic tools such as EQ-5D (www.euroqol.org),[22] Short form (SF) health survey (www.sf-36.org),[23] Health Assessment Questionnaire (HAQ),[24] or appropriate instruments from the Patient-Reported Outcome Measurement System (PROMIS) (http://aramis.stanford.edu/HAQ.html) may be used.

Management

Oral manifestations

Management strategies are summarized in Box 128.2.

Preventive measures

Regular dental visits (3–4 monthly) and working closely with dentist and dental hygienist to maintain optimal dental health is important. Meticulous oral hygiene is essential for reducing the risk of developing new and recurrent carious lesions. Proper oral hygiene includes tooth brushing, flossing, the use of interproximal plaque removing agents, and mouth rinses. Regular use of topical fluorides is critical to control dental caries. Cariogenic foods (especially fermentable carbohydrates) and beverages should be minimized if possible. Chronic use of alcohol and caffeine can worsen oral dryness. Non-fermentable dietary sweeteners are recommended.

Salivary gland stimulation

Dry mucosal surfaces, difficulty in wearing dentures, accumulation of dental plaque and debris on surfaces normally cleansed by the mechanical washing action of saliva, difficulty in speaking, tasting, and swallowing may all benefit from strategies that stimulate salivary secretions. These strategies, however, will only be effective if there are residual functional SG cells. In long-standing SS, the atrophic

---

Box 128.1 Common diagnostic pitfalls in Sjögren's syndrome

- Symptoms such as fatigue and dryness may not always be reported by patients unless specifically sought by clinicians

- Objective tests can be positive despite the lack of symptoms (Note: SS can be diagnosed with 3 of the 4 objective AECG criteria met)

- Patients with dry eyes may notice 'intolerance of smoky environment', 'eye strain', 'intolerant of contact lens' rather than 'dryness'

- Dry eyes in contact lens users not further investigated for other underlying causes

- Patients with dry mouth may not report difficulty in swallowing *dry* food unless specifically asked

- Biopsy not performed in patients with negative anti-SSA/SSB

- Full history of medication (prescribed and non-prescribed) use and its relationship to the onset of sicca symptoms not obtained

- Lack of appreciation that there is no 'gold standard' test to diagnose dry eyes

---

Table 128.3 Suggested structured assessment of systemic disease activity of pSS

Organ systems	Symptoms	Signs
Constitutional and lymphatic	Fatigue, fever, night sweat, weight loss (unintentional)	Fever, lymphadenopathy, splenomegaly
Glandular	Glandular pain and swelling	Glandular tenderness and/or enlargement
Articular	Arthralgia, early morning stiffness	Synovitis
Cutaneous	Rash, pain, itch, skin ulceration or necrosis, cold extremities ± colour changes	Dry skin, rash (e.g. erythema multiforme, cutaneous vasculitis, urticaria, purpura, subacute cutaneous lupus), ulcer, Raynald's phenomenon
Pulmonary	Husky voice, breathlessness, persistent non-productive dry cough, chest pain	Pleural rub, crepitations, reduced breath sound, percussion dullness
Renal	Muscle weakness, bone pain, fatigue, renal colic	(Inappropriately) alkaline urine, hypercalciuria, urinary stone, proteinuria, haematuria
Muscular	Myalgia, weakness	Weakness
Peripheral nervous system	Paraesthesia, sensory deficit, weakness, ataxia, multiple sclerosis-like syndrome	Sensory changes, motor deficit, ataxia, mononeuritis multiplex
Central nervous system	Multiple sclerosis-like syndrome, cognitive impairment, seizures, headache	Optic neuritis, transverse myelitis, cranial neuropathy, meningism
Haematological and biological	Fatigue, easy bruising	Anaemia, bruises

Box 128.2 Management strategies for oral manifestations of Sjögren's syndrome

Preventive measures

◆ Regular dental visits (every 3–4 months, alternate between dentists and hygienists)

◆ Optimal oral hygiene (guidance from oral health professionals)

◆ Topical fluorides and remineralizing solutions

- Fluoride mouth rinse (0.1%, weekly)

- Neutral sodium fluoride gel (depending on the level of oral hygiene and residual level of salivary flow: from weekly to every second day; the gel is preferably applied with a custom-made tray)

  ◆ Avoid professional or over-the-counter fluoride gels as many of them are acidified which reduces patients' compliance (sore oral mucosa) and may damage the teeth (no saliva present to remineralize teeth)

◆ Diet modifications

- Avoid cariogenic food and beverages

- Minimize chronic use of alcohol and caffeine

- Use non-fermentable sweeteners (xylitol, sorbitol, aspartame, or saccharine) whenever possible

◆ If possible, avoid drugs that may worsen sicca symptoms (e.g. anti-depressants, anti-histamines, anti-cholinergics, anti-hypertensives, neuroleptics)

◆ Optimize treatment of other medical conditions that result in xerostomia (e.g. endocrine disorders, metabolic diseases, viral infections)

◆ Avoid other exacerbating factors

- Low-humidity atmospheres (e.g. air-conditioned buildings, windy locations)

- Irritants such as dust and cigarette smoke

Salivary gland stimulation

◆ Masticatory stimulation (e.g. sugar-free gums, lozenges, or pastilles)

◆ Combined gustatory and masticatory stimulatory

- Lozenges, mints, candies

- Water, with or without a slice of lemon

◆ Parasympathomimetic secretogogues

- Pilocarpine (5–7.5 mg, 3–4 times/day)

- Cevimeline (30 mg, 3 times/day)

Saliva replacement and other symptomatic treatments

◆ Relief of oral dryness (non-responders to systemic salivary stimulation)

- Increase humidification (e.g. air moisturizers, humidifiers)

- Frequent sips of water

- Oral rinses, gels, and mouthwashes

- Saliva substitutes

Treatment of complications

Oral candidiasis

◆ Topical anti-fungal drugs:

- Nystatin oral suspension (100,000U/1 ml, 4 times/day)

- Clotrimazole cream (1%, 2 times/day)

- Ketoconazole cream (2%, 1–2 times/day)

- Amphotericin B lozenge (10 mg, 4 times/day) or 100 mg/ml, 4 times/day)

- Systemic anti-fungal drugs:

- Fluconazole tablets (50–200 mg/day for 7–14 days)

- Itraconazole tablets (100–200 mg/day for 1–2 weeks)

◆ Dentures should be soaked in chlorhexine mouth rinse (0.2%) or a proprietary hypochlorite-containing denture soak at night

Angular cheilitis

◆ Usually a mixed infection with candidosis and *Staphylococcus aureus*. Therefore miconazole oral gel (24 mg/mL, 4 times/day for 7 days and continue for at least 2 days after clinical resolution of the lesions)

◆ Daktacort hydrocortisone cream (miconazole plus hydrocortisone; 1–2 times/day)

---

acinar fluid-producing cells are replaced by non-fluid-producing connective tissue cells which do not respond to stimulation.

◆ Masticatory and gustatory stimulation is the easiest to implement with few side effects. The combination of chewing and taste (e.g. sugar-free gums, mints, lozenges, candies) can be very effective in relieving symptoms. Special gum bases are available if regular chewing gums frequently sticking to the dry oral mucosa. If an acid is added, malic acid is preferred as it is less harmful to tooth substance and oral mucosa.

◆ Pilocarpine and cevimeline are muscarinic agonists which induce a transient increase in salivary output. Frequent but rarely severe or serious side effects include sweating, flushing, urinary urgency, and gastrointestinal discomfort. Parasympathomimetics are contraindicated in patients with uncontrolled asthma, narrow-angle glaucoma, or acute iritis and should be used with caution in patients with significant cardiovascular disease, Parkinson's disease, asthma, or chronic obstructive pulmonary disease. The recommended doses for pilocarpine are 5–7.5 mg 3–4 times daily but should be titrated for individuals to achieve the right balance between therapeutic benefits and adverse effects. The duration of action is 2–3 hours. Cevimeline (30 mg three times daily) has a longer duration of secretogogue activity (3–4 hours) but the onset of action is slower. Cevimeline is available in the United States, Canada, and Japan but not yet licensed in Europe.

Symptomatic treatment

Water, although less effective than natural saliva, is the most important fluid supplement for dry-mouth individuals. Sipping water and swishing it around the mouth throughout the day will help to moisten the oral cavity, hydrate the mucosa, and clear debris from the mouth. Careful water-drinking with meals will enhance taste perception, ease the formation of food bolus, and improve mastication and swallowing. It will also help prevent choking and aspiration.

However, aqueous solutions produce only transient relief from oral dryness, because the mucous membrane of xerostomic patients is inadequately coated by a protective glycoprotein layer and therefore its moisture is not retained.

Many oral rinses, mouthwashes, and gels are available for dry-mouth patients. Products containing alcohol, sugar, or strong flavourings which may irritate the sensitive, dry oral mucosa should be avoided. Saliva replacements are not well tolerated long-term, particularly when not instructed properly. To choose the best substitute for a SS patient, we recommend the following approaches:

- **Mild hyposalivation**: saliva substitutes are unlikely to be beneficial. Try gustatory or pharmacological stimulation.

- **Moderate hyposalivation**: if gustatory or pharmacological stimulation is ineffective, use saliva substitutes with low viscoelasticity, such as those containing carboxymethylcellulose, hydroxypropylmethylcellulose, mucin (porcine gastric mucin), or low concentrations of xanthan gum as base. During the night or other periods of severe oral dryness, oral gel can be helpful.

- **Severe hyposalivation**: a saliva substitute with gel-like properties should be used during the night and when daily activities are at a low level. During the day, use saliva substitutes with properties resembling the viscoelasticity of natural saliva, such as substitutes which have xanthan gum and mucin (particularly bovine submandibular mucin) as base.

Secondary infection of the oral mucosa with *Candida albicans* is common. A high index of suspicion for fungal disease should be maintained, and appropriate anti-fungal therapies instituted as necessary. Prolonged treatment may be needed to eradicate oral fungal infections. Avoid wearing dentures overnight and soak dentures in 0.2% chlorhexidine solution to prevent reinfections of the oral cavity by candida species living in the denture material.

Ocular manifestations

Most SS patients experience ocular surface irritation without long-term effects, although if it is left untreated, ocular surface damage and even visual impairment may ensue.

Overall, treatments aim at increasing ocular surface lubrication, stimulating secretion of or conserving tears, and targeting the associated ocular surface inflammation.[24] Treatments should be tailored to address the individual patient's needs and the severity of dry eye. Most treatments are palliative and do not treat the underlying condition. Management strategies are summarized in Box 128.3.

Preventive measures

If possible, patients should avoid dry, windy, or dusty environments which can exacerbate dry-eye symptoms. Similarly, the use of hair-dryers, central heating, air conditioning, or fans should be minimized, especially when these devices are directed towards the eyes.

Box 128.3 Management strategies for ocular manifestations of Sjögren's syndrome

Preventive measures

- Avoidance of exacerbating factors:
  - Avoid/restrict low humidity, dusty or windy environment
  - Avoid irritants such as dust and cigarette smoke
  - Avoid restrict and take regular breaks during activities that reduce blinking or provoke tear film instability (e.g. prolonged reading or computer use)
- Avoidance of drugs that may worsen sicca symptoms (e.g. anti-depressants, anti-histamines, anti-cholinergics, anti-hypertensives, neuroleptics)
- Optimized treatment of other conditions (e.g. ectropion, meibomian gland disease, lagophthalmos) that result in/aggravate dry eyes.
- Use of air moisturizers or moisture glasses

Improved ocular surface lubrication

- Tear substitution therapy (preservative-free preparations if frequent use is needed)
  - Low-viscosity eye-drops (e.g. cellulose derivatives) as frequently as needed
  - Medium- to high-viscosity eye-drops (e.g. carbomer gel 940) 3-4 times/day in more severe cases
  - Ophthalmic gels and ointments (at night)
- Mucolytic agents for sticky eyes or mucous threads/corneal filaments on eye examination
  - N-acetylcysteine 5% eye-drops (preservative-free, 2–3 times daily)
- Autologous serum eye-drops
- Systemic parasympathomimetic secretogogues
  - Pilocarpine (5–7.5 mg, 3–4 times/day) or cevimeline (30 mg, 3 times/day)
- Tear retention measures
  - Lacrimal punctum plugs/occlusion (moderate to severe dry eyes)

Reduction of ocular surface inflammation

- Topical immunomodulatory agents
  - Pulsed topical non-preserved corticosteroids (e.g. dexamethasone 0.1% eye-drops, 4 times daily twice daily for up to 8 weeks, taper dose or discontinue drops based on clinical findings and eye pressure)
  - Ciclosporin eye-drops
  - Dietary supplements: essential fatty acids (omega-3 and linoleic acid)

Other measures

- Treatment of blepharitis
  - Daily eyelid rubs with warm water and diluted baby shampoo, eyelid cleaning solutions, or wipes
  - Warm water compresses 2 times/day for 5 min
  - Topical antibiotics for anterior blepharitis if indicated (e.g. chloramphenicol ointment)

Spectacles, protective goggles, or glasses with lateral protection should be worn when aggravating environmental factors cannot be avoided. Humidifiers and house-plants can add moisture to the environment. Goggles should be used when swimming as chlorinated water and seawater can irritate the eyes.

Prolonged visual tasks with consequent reduced blink rate also aggravate dry eyes. Purposefully blinking, especially during computer use, and frequent resting of tired eyes with additional tear-drops can reduce discomfort.[25] Directing gaze downwards—by lowering computer screens, for example—may be helpful. Avoid rubbing the eyes as it can irritate them further.

Improving ocular surface lubrication
Topical tear supplementation
A key part of managing dry eye symptoms in SS patients is choosing the appropriate form of topical treatments. Most artificial tear substitutes fall into five main categories according to their active ingredients:

+ cellulose derivatives: carboxymethylcellulose, hydroxyethylcellulose, methylcellulose, ethylcellulose

+ polyvinyl derivatives: polyvinyl alcohol, polyvinylpyrolidone

+ viscosity agents: carbomer 940, hydroxypropyl-guar, chondroitin sulphate, sodium hyaluronate

+ paraffin ointments: white/yellow paraffin

+ osmoprotection agents.

Hypromellose eye-drops are inexpensive, well-tolerated, first-line treatments which should be used as frequently as necessary to alleviate symptoms. Persistent use of artificial tear-drops can produce a long-lasting improvement in tear stability.

Preservatives in many eye-drop preparations can exacerbate symptoms through direct toxicity to the ocular epithelium or via hypersensitivity. Therefore, preservative-free tear substitutes are recommended for patients who use these drops more than 4–5 times daily. When treatment is initiated patients should be given clear instructions on maintaining a high standard of hygiene and specific instructions regarding early disposal of preservative-free eye-drops, to reduce the risk of eye infections. Preservative-free eye-drops come from different sources which may involve special manufacturing procedures; they are therefore expensive and there can be supply problems at times.

Lubricant gels, with greater viscosity and longer retention time, may be used to supplement artificial tears. Paraffin ointments used before bedtime can help to reduce symptoms of waking up with uncomfortable eyes and minimize any blurring of vision associated with their use. The ointment should be warmed up before use to facilitate its instillation.

Topical mucolytics and autologous serum eye-drops
If mucous threads and/or corneal filaments are present, or if the patient complains of sticky eyes, particularly when waking, mucolytic agents such as acetylcysteine may be useful.

SS patients with severe dry eyes may benefit from autologous serum eye-drops. The therapeutic benefits are likely due to the growth factors and vitamins in the serum. A randomized controlled crossover trial comparing autologous serum eye-drops with conventional therapy demonstrated a significant improvement in conjunctival impression cytology and symptoms at months 3 and 6,

although Rose Bengal staining, Schirmer's test and fluorescein clearance test were not improved.[26]

Stimulating tear production
Secretagogues (pilocarpine, cevimeline) may improve dry-eye symptoms in patients with residual lacrimal gland function.[24] See section 'Salivary gland stimulation' for a detailed description of their use.

Tear retention/conservation
Temporary or permanent punctal occlusion is a useful adjunct treatment in patients with moderate to severe dry eyes by facilitating the retention of residual and artificial tears in the eyes.

Reduction of ocular inflammation
Ocular inflammation is a key pathogenetic factor in dry eyes.[4] Therefore, topical anti-inflammatory agents such as corticosteroids can result in complete symptom relief. Because of the potential risk of glaucoma and cataract, topical corticosteroids should be used only in the short term or as pulsed therapy. In the United States (not in Europe unless produced by local compounding pharmacies), ciclosporin eye-drops have been licensed as a treatment for dry eyes. Topical ciclosporin can ameliorate ocular surface inflammation, improve tear production, and alleviate dry-eye symptoms.[27]

Systemic immunosuppression therapies
These agents are usually reserved for SS patients with extraglandular manifestations and rarely used for ocular manifestations alone. Rituximab may improve ocular symptoms and signs.[28]

Other therapies
Two recent randomized, placebo-controlled clinical trials have shown that oral supplementation of omega-3 and -6 fatty acids improved ocular dryness, Schirmer's test results, and markers of ocular inflammation in patients with dry eye syndrome (some have SS),[29,30] but large-scale studies are needed to confirm these findings.

Meibomian gland dysfunction
Meibomian gland dysfunction (MGD) is defined as a chronic, diffuse abnormality of the meibomian gland, characterized by terminal duct obstruction and/or qualitative and quantitative changes in the glandular secretion, resulting in a defective tear-film lipid layer. Typical symptoms include eye irritation, stinging, and burning with clinically apparent chronic inflammation and ocular surface disease. Furthermore, MGD aggravates dry-eye symptoms through excessive evaporation and exacerbating inflammation. Treatments depend on the severity of MGD which include modulating diet, lid margin hygiene, warm glandular expression, topical emollient lubrication, systemic tetracyclines, and topical anti-inflammatory therapy.

Systemic manifestations
Current therapeutic strategies for the management of systemic manifestations of pSS are largely empirical based on experience from managing other autoimmune rheumatic conditions. They are summarized in Table 128.4.

Constitutional
pSS patients may experience constitutional symptoms such as fatigue, anorexia, pyrexia, and unintended weight loss. If severe, clinicians should consider investigations for underlying malignancy

Table 128.4 Management strategies for extraglandular manifestations of SS

Clinical feature		Management
Constitutional symptoms (severe fatigue, anorexia, weight loss, fever)		Consider investigations for malignancies
		NSAIDs
		Hydroxychloroquine (400 mg/day starting dose, titrate to lowest effective dose thereafter)
Arthralgia or myalgia		NSAIDs
		Consider hydroxychloroquine (200–400 mg/day)
Inflammatory arthritis		NSAIDs
		Hydroxychloroquine (400 mg/day starting dose, individual titration to lowest effective dose thereafter)
		Methotrexate (15 mg/week; max 25 mg)
		Sulphasalazine (2–3 g/day)
		Prednisolone (7.5–10 mg/day; max 15 mg)
Inflammatory myositis		Prednisolone (40–60 mg/day initially)
		Pulsed methylprednisolone or cyclophosamide if severe
		Methotrexate or azathioprine as maintenance
Skin involvement	Mild vasculitis	Analgesics
		Pressure stockings
	Moderate/recurrent vasculitis	Hydroxychloroquine (200–400 mg/day)
		Dapsone (50–100 mg/day)
		Colchicine (100 µg/day)
		Prednisolone (7.5–10 mg/day; max 15 mg)
	Polymorphic erythema	Hydroxychloroquine (400–800 mg/day)
		Prednisolone (7.5–10 mg/day; max 15 mg)
	Xerosis	Moisturizers, emollient
		Avoid alcohol-based or heavy perfumed skin products
Severe vasculitis or cryoglobulinaemia		Pulsed methylprednisolone
		Rituximab
		Intravenous immunoglobulin
Cardio-pulmonary involvement	Pleuritis/pericarditis	NSAIDs
		Prednisolone (15–20 mg/day; max 30 mg)
		Colchicine (100 µg/day)
	Interstitial pneumonitis	Prednisolone (60 mg/day)
		Rituximab
		Cyclophosphamide in resistant cases
Gastrointestinal	Oesophageal reflux	Proton pump inhibitors
	Primary biliary cirrhosis	Ursodeoxycholic acid
Neurological involvement	Pure sensory or 'small-fibre' neuropathy	Gabapentin
		Pregabalin
		Carbemazepam
		Citalopram
		Amitriptylline (beware of exacerbation of dryness)
	Severe PNS	Prednisolone (60 mg/day) or pulsed methylprednisolone
		Cyclophosphamide IV (750 mg/m^2/monthly; 6–12 times)
		Intravenous immunoglobulin
	CNS	Prednisolone (60 mg/day) with or without cyclophosphamide IV (750 mg/m^2/monthly; 6–12 times)
Renal involvement	Interstitial nephritis/renal tubular acidosis	Bicarbonate (personalized dose) ± potassium citrate (personalized dose)
		Prednisolone (15–60 mg/day, depending on severity of proteinuria or renal impairment)
	Nephrocalcinosis	Adequate hydration
		Potassium citrate
	Glomerulonephritis	Prednisolone (60 mg/day) with or without cyclophosphamide

CNS, central nervous system; PNS, peripheral nervous system.

in particularly lymphoma. Constitutional symptoms may respond to corticosteroid or hydroxychloroquine. High-dose or long-term use of corticosteroid should be avoided.

Articular

Analgesics or hydroxychloroquine can be considered for the treatment of musculoskeletal pain. Inflammatory arthritis can be treated with local or oral corticosteroid if transient and disease-modifying therapies such as hydroxychloroquine, methotrexate, or sulphasalazine if persistent.

Cutaneous

Xerosis (dry skin) should be managed symptomatically and photosensitivity dermatitis by avoidance of strong 'midday' sun and effective sun-screen. Mild cutaneous vasculitis is often self-limiting, therefore supportive treatment such as analgesics (e.g. non-steroidal anti-inflammatory drugs, NSAIDs) for pain and anti-histamines for pruritus usually suffice. For more severe or recurrent/persistent vasculitis and subacute cutaneous lupus erythematosus, hydroxychloroquine, dapsone, or colchicine can be used. Low/moderate dose of oral prednisolone and topical tacrolimus may also be considered. For more extensive vasculitis or with skin ulceration or necrosis, high-dose corticosteroid and other immunosuppressants such as cyclophosphamide, methotrexate, azathioprine, or mycophenolate are needed. For patients with resistant cutaneous vasculitis, plasmapheresis and intravenous immunoglobulins may be effective. Rituximab is an alternative, particularly for cryoglobulinaemia.

Pulmonary

Severe pulmonary manifestations such as interstitial pneumonitis require corticosteroid with or without immunosuppressive agents such as cyclophosphamide.

Genitourinary

For renal tubular acidosis, correction of acid–base imbalance with alkalis such as sodium bicarbonate or potassium citrate is usually sufficient to correct other metabolic aberrations such as hypokalaemia, hypercalciuria, and hypocalcaemia. Corticosteroid and other immunosuppressive therapy are needed for more severe cases or for glomerulonephritis or cryoglobulinaemia. Patients presenting with renal stones or nephrocalcinosis should be investigated for underlying renal acidosis. These patients should be advised to maintain adequate hydration. Potassium citrate is particularly effective as the potassium increases solubility of urinary calcium and citrate decreases urinary excretion of calcium. Subclinical renal manifestations such as mild proteinuria or metabolic disturbances can be managed conservatively. Symptoms of 'cystitis' such as dysuria or urinary frequency are not uncommon and may be due to a combination of vaginal dryness and/or vaginal thrush in women, urinary tract infections, autonomic dysfunction, or frequent fluid intake (to relieve oral dryness). Oestrogen cream may alleviate vaginal dryness and vaginal thrush or urinary tract infections should be treated with appropriate anti-microbial agents.

Muscular

Myalgia without myositis is managed conservatively. A slight rise in creatinine kinase without other evidence of overt myositis can be monitored. Prednisolone and methotrexate or azathioprine should be used if myositis is confirmed on electrophysiological studies or muscle biopsy or when associated with objective muscle weakness.

Neurological

Treatment of peripheral neuropathy depends on the underlying causes. Pure sensory neuropathy or small-fibre neuropathy are managed with analgesics or pain-modifying agents such as gabapentin, pregabalin, carbamazepam, or amitriptyline (patients should be warned of potential exacerbation of sicca symptoms). Mononeuritis multiplex is treated with corticosteroid and cyclophosphamide or other immunosuppressive therapies. Recovery can be slow and incomplete, however. Some forms of peripheral neuropathy especially those associated with vasculitis and cryoglobulinaemia, respond well to rituximab.[31] Central nervous system manifestations are extremely rare and usually treated with corticosteroid and cyclophosphamide. Intravenous immunoglobulin or rituximab can be considered in resistant cases.

Haematological or other biological abnormalities

Many isolated laboratory abnormalities that are commonly found in pSS patients, such as hypergammaglobulinaemia, mild lymphopaenia, thrombocytopaenia, or hypocomplementaemia, can be monitored and do not require specific treatment. Hypergammaglobulinaemia may improve with hydroxychloroquine. The presence of new onset or rising levels of paraproteinaemia or development of hypogammaglobulinaemia should prompt further investigations for the development of myeloma or lymphoma. The appropriate initial investigations depend on local practice and should be carried out in liaison with haematology specialists, but may include checking for urine Bence Jones proteins, serum lactate dehydrogenase, skeletal survey, and bone marrow biopsy. Stable levels of paraproteinaemia without evidence of malignant transformation can be monitored and do not normally require treatment.

Gastrointestinal

Proton pump inhibitors can be used for gastro-oesophageal reflux and ursodeoxycholic acid for patients with coexisting primary biliary cirrhosis.

Miscellaneous

Serositis such as pleuritis, pleural effusion, and pericarditis can be treated with anti-inflammatories. Corticosteroid may be used in more severe cases and in acute settings. Colchicine and hydroxychloroquine may be considered in persistent or recurrent disease.

Management of fatigue

In managing SS patients with disabling fatigue, it is pivotal that all potentially treatable factors that may contribute to the symptoms of fatigue (Box 128.4) are investigated, recognized, and appropriately managed. Sleep disturbance is common among pSS patients,[32–34] and the presence of sleep-disturbing sicca symptoms or pain should be adequately treated. Frequent awakening due to interstitial cystitis and overactive bladder can be alleviated by solifenacin, which is usually well-tolerated despite its anticholinergic effects. Sleep apnoea, if present, must be treated adequately. Depression and anxiety are not uncommon in pSS, and can cause tiredness and poor sleep.[12,34,35] Treatment with appropriate anti-depressive or anxiolytic drugs with low anticholinergic potential is indicated. Peripheral neuropathy and restless leg syndrome are common in pSS. Anaemia, thyroid dysfunction, and coeliac disease are other treatable causes associated with pSS, which may contribute to the

Box 128.4 Potential contributory factors to fatigue in primary Sjögren's syndrome

- Systemic inflammation and immune dysregulation
- Disturbed sleep (due to dryness, pain, irritable bladder, depression, anxiety, restless legs, nocturia from overhydration during the day)
- Anxiety and depression
- Secondary fibromyalgia
- Hypothyroidism
- Anaemia
- Coeliac disease
- Vitamin deficiencies (B_{12}, D)
- Pulmonary and renal dysfunction (rare!)
- Reduced physical capacity due to inactivity/sedentary lifestyle/kinesiophobia

symptom of fatigue. Reduced pulmonary and kidney function are less common, but should also be considered.

Some SS patients may experience the typical disabling feeling of exhaustion despite having all the above-mentioned treatable causes been either excluded or treated. Some may also suffer from secondary fibromyalgia-like symptoms with widespread musculoskeletal pain. For such patients, behavioural and psychological factors, such as a sedentary lifestyle with physical inactivity and low physical capacity, often accompanied by kinesiophobia and an exaggerated focus on bodily symptoms, should be explored and discussed. Coaching, behavioural therapy, regular physical activity, and learning of coping strategies may be useful in such cases.[36]

For patients with evidence of inflammation, considerable immune system activation and concomitant systemic disease activity from other organ systems, treatment with rituximab to reduce fatigue may be justified.[37,38]

Pregnancy in pSS

The main issue with regard to pregnancy in pSS patients is the risk of neonatal lupus syndrome with intrauterine fetal atrial ventricular (AV) heart block being the most severe complication. Women with antibodies to SSA (mainly antibodies to Ro-52) or SSB are at an increased risk with 2% of the pregnancies affected,[39,40] and up to 15–20% in patients who had a baby with neonatal lupus syndrome. pSS mothers may give birth to babies with lower birth weight and may have more frequent complications during deliveries compared to women in the general population.[41]

Pregnant pSS women with antibodies to SSA/SSB should be closely monitored by obstetricians with weekly assessment of the fetal heart rate between 14–30 weeks of gestation during which fetal heart blocks most commonly occur. Reduction or irregularity of the fetal heart rate may suggest intrauterine AV block and should be fully investigated promptly. First-degree AV block may resolve spontaneously, while second- and third-degree AV blocks usually persist or worsen. No evidence-based treatment is available, but high-dose dexamethasone or betamethasone (which cross the placenta, unlike prednisolone) has been used successfully and

without serious harm to the baby.[42,43] Babies with intrauterine AV block should be delivered at units where a cardiac pacemaker can be implanted immediately postpartum.

Management of lymphoma

Approximately 5–10% of pSS patients will develop lymphoma.[44–46] It is difficult to predict who will be affected and when and where the lymphoma will develop. Several risk factors have been identified, namely hypocomplementemia, cryoglobulinemia, cutaneous vasculitis, peripheral neuropathy, monoclonality in serum electrophoresis, and recurrent or persistent SG swelling.[45–47] More recently, cytopenias, especially CD4+ T-lymphocytopenia,[46,48] and the presence of germinal centre-like structures in the SG biopsies[48] have been linked with increased risk for lymphoma in pSS. Clinicians should give SS patients information on the risk and symptoms and signs that may be associated with malignancy, and advise them to seek prompt medical attention if these symptoms or signs occur. In addition, regular physical examinations of accessible structures such as lymph nodes and SGs should be performed and appropriate investigations arranged if signs and symptoms indicative of possible lymphoma are present. Despite improved awareness and clinical vigilance, lymphomas are frequently detected by chance. Effective screening programmes have not been developed.

Mucosa-associated lymphoid tissue (MALT) lymphomas, marginal zone lymphomas, and diffuse large B-cell (DLBC) lymphomas are the main types of lymphomas in pSS.[49] DLBC lymphoma, an aggressive high-grade malignancy, is associated with premature mortality in pSS.[50] Lymphoma can develop at any time between diagnosis and up to 30 years afterwards; MALT lymphomas usually develop earlier than the more aggressive types.[49]

Management of lymphoma is usually provided by haematologists or oncologists, and is tailored to individual patients depending on the site, grade, stage, and extent of the lymphoma. Some low-grade MALT lymphomas can be monitored without treatment. Localized MALT lymphomas may be excised surgically with or without radiotherapy. More aggressive or extensive lymphomas require treatment with chemotherapy, often in combination with rituximab (Figure 128.1).

Emerging therapies

Improved understanding of pSS pathogenesis and the development of biological therapies have led to potential new therapeutic strategies.[52–55] Neither infliximab nor etanercept is an effective treatment for pSS. Several case series and small randomized placebo-controlled clinical trials have demonstrated the efficacy of rituximab in the treatment of fatigue as well as other systemic manifestations of pSS. Rituximab can also improve oral and ocular dryness both subjectively and objectively especially in early pSS, and appears to be effective as a treatment for pSS-associated lymphomas. Nevertheless, large phase 3 clinical trials are needed to confirm these findings. Controlled trials with other B-cell targeted therapies such as epratuzumab, atacicept, and belimumab are underway.

Biological therapies targeting other immune pathways that have been implicated in pSS may also represent useful therapeutic strategies. For instance, blockade of interferon-α, interleukin (IL)-1 or IL-6 may be an attractive approach given their link with pSS pathogenesis and fatigue.

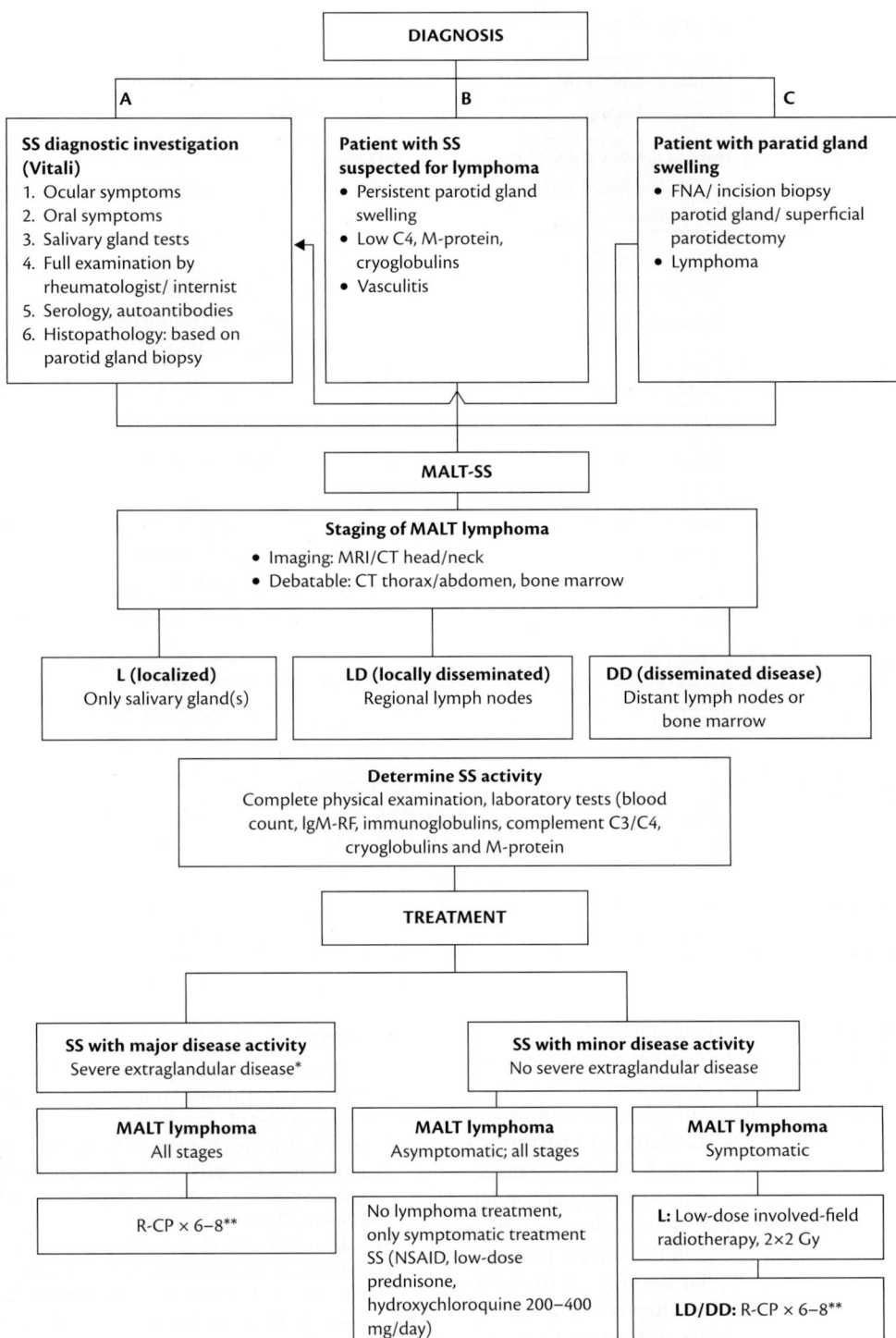

Fig. 128.1 Management of mucosa-associated lymphoid tissue-type lymphoma of parotid gland and associated Sjögren's syndrome (MALT-SS). FNA, fine needle aspiration; R-CP, rituximab with cyclophosphamide and prednisone; NSAID, non-steroidal anti-inflammatory drugs. *Extraglandular disease: polyarthritis/myositis, glomerulonephritis, nervous system involvement, cryoglobulinemic vasculitis, other severe organ involvement, serological abnormalities.
Reproduced from Pollard R P E et al Treatment of mucosa-associated lymphoid tissue- Lymphoma in sjogren's syndrome a retrospective clinical study J Rheumatol 2011; 38(10) 2198–2208 with permission.

Challenges

Effective management of SS remains a formidable challenge with several key obstacles yet to be overcome (Table 128.5). Success in improving the care for SS patients can only be achieved with a collaborative effort between clinicians, researchers, healthcare policymakers, and the pharmaceutical industry.

Conclusion

SS is a multisystem disease of unknown aetiology. Dryness, fatigue, and bodily pain are prominent symptoms which although not life-threatening are debilitating and associate with poor quality of life and substantial health economic cost. The AECG classification criteria are the current gold standard for SS; whether the recently

Table 128.5 Challenges in management of Sjögren's syndrome

Challenges	Underlying obstacle	Possible solutions
Diagnosis		
Avoid diagnostic delay	Lack of simple, reliable test for detecting early disease	Biomarker discovery (e.g. saliva proteomics?)
	Poor awareness of SS from the public and healthcare professionals	Increase public and healthcare professionals' awareness of SS
Disease assessment		
Predicting outcome	Heterogeneity of long-term outcome	Biomarker discovery
	Inadequate knowledge on the natural history of SS	Establish patient cohort or registry
		Epidemiological studies
Disease staging (e.g. disease reversibility)	Inadequate understanding of SS pathogenesis	Further basic science and clinical research
Treatment		
Improve the quality of saliva and tear substitutes	Saliva/tears are complex substances containing many different molecules which serves different functions	Further pharmaceutical research
Better treatment for fatigue	Poor understanding of the mechanistic basis of this symptom	Further basic science and clinical research
		Establish multidisciplinary clinic dedicated to fatigue management
Monitor progression of disease (e.g. lymphoma)	Inadequate understanding of SS pathogenesis	Further basic science and clinical research
Effective communication between different healthcare providers	Diversity of health problems of SS requiring different specialist care	Combined clinics
		Multidisciplinary meetings
		Develop local databases
Service provision and drug development		
Improve service provision in primary and secondary care	Poor awareness from healthcare professionals and policy-makers of the health economic impact of SS	Improve education of healthcare professionals including dentists and opticians
		Active engagement between policy-makers and clinicians
Encourage new drug development and clinical trials	SS is perceived to be a condition with high risk but low return by pharmaceutical industry	Active engagement between pharmaceutical industry, research funding bodies, researchers, and clinicians

introduced provisional American College of Rheumatology (ACR) classification criteria will replace the AECG criteria in research and in clinical practice is unclear at present. Assessment of SS patients should include glandular and extraglandular manifestations and lymphoma risk evaluation. The use of standardized instruments such as ESSDAI and ESSPRI is recommended. Optimal management of SS requires a multidisciplinary team consisting of specialists in oral medicine, ophthalmology, and rheumatology as well as other healthcare professionals depending on the clinical presentation. Both pharmacological and non-pharmacological interventions have a role in the management of SS. Replacement therapy and preventative measures are the mainstay of treatment for sicca symptoms but are only partially effective. The use of muscarinic receptor agonists is limited by side effects and poor efficacy in patients with severe glandular damage. Tear duct blockade and ciclosporin eye-drops may improve symptoms of ocular dryness and discomfort. Disease-modifying therapy for SS remains elusive but emerging biological therapies such as rituximab hold promise, especially for those with early disease.

Effective management of SS requires a better understanding of SS pathogenesis, development of more effective therapy as well as an increase in awareness of SS and its health economic impact among healthcare professionals, policy-makers, research funding bodies, the pharmaceutical industry, and the general public.

References

1. Pijpe J, Kalk WW, Bootsma H et al. Progression of salivary gland dysfunction in patients with Sjögren's syndrome. *Ann Rheum Dis* 2007;66(1):107–112.
2. Baimpa E, Dahabreh IJ, Voulgarelis M, Moutsopoulos HM. Hematologic manifestations and predictors of lymphoma development in primary Sjögren syndrome: clinical and pathophysiologic aspects. *Medicine* (Baltimore) 2009;88(5):284–293.
3. The definition and classification of dry eye disease: report of the Definition and Classification Subcommittee of the International Dry Eye Workshop (2007). *Ocular Surface* 2007;5(2):75–92.
4. Behrens A, Doyle JJ, Stern L et al. Dysfunctional tear syndrome: a Delphi approach to treatment recommendations. *Cornea* 2006;25(8):900–907.
5. Begley CG, Chalmers RL, Abetz L et al. The relationship between habitual patient-reported symptoms and clinical signs among patients with dry eye of varying severity. *Invest Ophthalmol Vis Sci* 2003;44(11):4753–4761.
6. Seror R, Ravaud P, Mariette X et al. EULAR Sjögren's Syndrome Patient Reported Index (ESSPRI): development of a consensus patient index for primary Sjögren's syndrome. *Ann Rheum Dis* 2011;70(6):968–972.
7. Schiffman RM, Christianson MD, Jacobsen G, Hirsch JD, Reis BL. Reliability and validity of the Ocular Surface Disease Index. *Arch Ophthalmol* 2000;118(5):615–621.
8. Seror R, Mariette X, Bowman S et al. Accurate detection of changes in disease activity in primary Sjögren's syndrome by the European League

Against Rheumatism Sjögren's Syndrome Disease Activity Index. *Arthritis Care Res* (Hoboken) 2010;62(4):551–558.

9. Seror R, Ravaud P, Bowman SJ et al. EULAR Sjögren's syndrome disease activity index: development of a consensus systemic disease activity index for primary Sjögren's syndrome. *Ann Rheum Dis* 2010;69(6):1103–1109.

10. Meiners PM, Arends S, Brouwer E et al. Responsiveness of disease activity indices ESSPRI and ESSDAI in patients with primary Sjögren's syndrome treated with rituximab. *Ann Rheum Dis* 2012;71(8):1297–1302.

11. Ng WF, Bowman SJ. Primary Sjögren's syndrome: too dry and too tired. *Rheumatology* (Oxford) 2010;49(5):844–853.

12. Meijer JM, Meiners PM, Huddleston Slater JJ et al. Health-related quality of life, employment and disability in patients with Sjögren's syndrome. *Rheumatology* (Oxford) 2009;48(9):1077–1082.

13. Westhoff G, Dorner T, Zink A. Fatigue and depression predict physician visits and work disability in women with primary Sjögren's syndrome: results from a cohort study. *Rheumatology* (Oxford) 2012;51(2):262–269.

14. Goodchild CE, Treharne GJ, Booth DA, Kitas GD, Bowman SJ. Measuring fatigue among women with Sjögren's syndrome or rheumatoid arthritis: a comparison of the Profile of Fatigue (ProF) and the Multidimensional Fatigue Inventory (MFI). *Musculoskelet Care* 2008;6(1):31–48.

15. Segal B, Thomas W, Rogers T et al. Prevalence, severity, and predictors of fatigue in subjects with primary Sjögren's syndrome. *Arthritis Rheum* 2008;59(12):1780–1787.

16. Cella D, Lai JS, Chang CH, Peterman A, Slavin M. Fatigue in cancer patients compared with fatigue in the general United States population. *Cancer* 2002;94(2):528–538.

17. Lwin CT, Bishay M, Platts RG, Booth DA, Bowman SJ. The assessment of fatigue in primary Sjögren's syndrome. *Scand J Rheumatol* 2003;32:33–37.

18. Goodchild CE, Treharne GJ, Booth DA, Kitas GD, Bowman SJ. Measuring fatigue among women with Sjögren's syndrome or rheumatoid arthritis: A comparison of the Profile of Fatigue (ProF) and the Multidimensional Fatigue Inventory (MFI). *Musculoskeletal Care* 2008;6(1):31–48.

19. Bowman SJ, Booth DA, Platts RG. Measurement of fatigue and discomfort in primary Sjögren's syndrome using a new questionnaire tool. *Rheumatology* 2004;43(6):758–764.

20. Strömbeck B, Ekdahl C, Manthorpe R, Wikström I, Jacobsson LT. Health-related quality of life in primary Sjögren's syndrome, rheumatoid arthritis and fibromyalgia compared to normal population data using SF-36. *Scand J Rheumatol.* 2000;29:20–28.

21. Champey J, Corruble E, Gottenberg JE et al. Quality of life and psychological status in patients with primary Sjögren's syndrome and sicca symptoms without autoimmune features. *Arthritis Rheum* 2006;55(3):451–457.

22. Bruce B, Fries JF. The Health Assessment Questionnaire (HAQ). *Clin Exp Rheumatol* 2005;23(5 Suppl 39):S14–S18.

23. Meiners PM, Meijer JM, Vissink A, Bootsma H. Management of Sjögren's syndrome. In: Weisman MH, Weinblatt ME, Louie JS, Van Vollenhove R (eds). *Targeted treatment of rheumatic diseases.* W.B. Saunders, Philadelphia, 2010:133–155.

24. Akpek EK, Lindsley KB, Adyanthaya RS et al. Treatment of Sjögren's syndrome-associated dry eye an evidence-based review. *Ophthalmology* 2011;118(7):1242–1252.

25. Lemp MA. Management of dry eye disease. *Am J Manag Care* 2008;14(3 Suppl):S88–S101.

26. Noble BA, Loh RS, MacLennan S et al. Comparison of autologous serum eye drops with conventional therapy in a randomised controlled crossover trial for ocular surface disease. *Br J Ophthalmol* 2004;88(5):647–652.

27. Sall K, Stevenson OD, Mundorf TK, Reis BL. Two multicenter, randomized studies of the efficacy and safety of cyclosporine ophthalmic emulsion in moderate to severe dry eye disease. CsA Phase 3 Study Group. *Ophthalmology* 2000;107(4):631–639.

28. Meijer JM, Meiners PM, Vissink A et al. Effectiveness of rituximab treatment in primary Sjögren's syndrome: a randomized, double-blind, placebo-controlled trial. *Arthritis Rheum* 2010;62(4):960–968.

29. Brignole-Baudouin F, Baudouin C, Aragona P et al. A multicentre, double-masked, randomized, controlled trial assessing the effect of oral supplementation of omega-3 and omega-6 fatty acids on a conjunctival inflammatory marker in dry eye patients. *Acta Ophthalmol* 2011;89(7):e591–597.

30. Wojtowicz JC, Butovich I, Uchiyama E et al. Pilot, prospective, randomized, double-masked, placebo-controlled clinical trial of an omega-3 supplement for dry eye. *Cornea* 2011;30(3):308–314.

31. Mekinian A, Ravaud P, Hatron PY et al. Efficacy of rituximab in primary Sjögren's syndrome with peripheral nervous system involvement: results from the AIR registry. *Ann Rheum Dis* 2012;71(1):84–87.

32. Gudbjörnsson B, Hetta J. Sleep disturbances in patients with systemic lupus erythematosus: A questionnaire-based study. *Clin Exp Rheum* 2001;19:509–514.

33. Walker J, Gordon T, Lester S et al. Increased severity of lower urinary tract symptoms and daytime somnolence in primary Sjögren's syndrome. *J Rheumatol* 2003;30(11):2406–2412.

34. Theander L, Strombeck B, Mandl T, Theander E. Sleepiness or fatigue? Can we detect treatable causes of tiredness in primary Sjögren's syndrome? *Rheumatology* (Oxford) 2010;49(6):1177–1183.

35. Valtysdóttir ST, Gudbjörnsson B, Lindquist U, Hällgren R, Hetta J. Anxiety and depression in patients with primary Sjögren's syndrome. *J Rheumatol* 2000;27:165–169.

36. Strombeck BE, Theander E, Jacobsson LT. Effects of exercise on aerobic capacity and fatigue in women with primary Sjögren's syndrome. *Rheumatology* (Oxford) 2007;46(5):567–571.

37. Dass S, Bowman SJ, Vital EM et al. Reduction of fatigue in Sjögren's syndrome with rituximab: results of a randomised, double-blind, placebo controlled pilot study. *Ann Rheum Dis* 2008;67(11):1541–1544.

38. Meijer J, Meiners P, Vissink A et al. Effective rituximab treatment in primary Sjögren's syndrome: A randomised, double-blind, placebo-controlled trial. *Arthritis Rheum* 2010;62(4):960–968.

39. Brucato A, Frassi M, Franceschini F et al. Risk of congenital complete heart block in newborns of mothers with anti-Ro/SSA antibodies detected by counterelectrophoresis. *Arthritis Rheum* 2001;44:1832–1835.

40. Salomonsson S, Dorner T, Theander E et al. A serologic marker for fetal risk of congenital heart block. *Arthritis Rheum* 2002;46(5):1233–1241.

41. Hussein SZ, Jacobsson LT, Lindquist PG, Theander E. Pregnancy and fetal outcome in women with primary Sjögren's syndrome compared with women in the general population: a nested case-control study. *Rheumatology* (Oxford) 2011;50(9):1612–1617.

42. Saleeb S, Copel J, Friedman D, Buyon JP. Comparison of treatment with fluorinated glucocorticoids to the natural history of autoantibody-associated congenital heart block. *Arthritis Rheum* 1999;42:2335–2345.

43. Theander E, Brucato A, Gudmundsson S et al. Primary Sjögren's syndrome—treatment of fetal incomplete atrioventricular block with dexamethasone. *J Rheumatol.* 2001;28(2):373–376.

44. Zintzaras E, Voulgarelis M, Moutsopoulos HM. The risk of lymphoma development in autoimmune diseases: a meta-analysis. *Arch Intern Med* 2005;165(20):2337–2344.

45. Ioannidis JP, Vassiliou VA, Moutsopoulos HM. Long-term risk of mortality and lymphoproliferative disease and predictive classification of primary Sjögren's syndrome. *Arthritis Rheum* 2002;46(3):741–747.

46. Theander E, Henriksson G, Ljungberg O et al. Lymphoma and other malignancies in primary Sjögren's syndrome: a cohort study on cancer incidence and lymphoma predictors. *Ann Rheum Dis* 2006;65(6):796–803.

47. Ramos-Casals M, Brito-Zeron P, Yague J et al. Hypocomplementaemia as an immunological marker of morbidity and mortality in patients with primary Sjögren's syndrome. *Rheumatology* (Oxford) 2005;44(1):89–94.

48. Theander E, Vasaitis L, Baecklund E et al. Lymphoid organisation in labial salivary gland biopsies is a possible predictor for the development of malignant lymphoma in primary Sjögren's syndrome. *Ann Rheum Dis* 2011;70(8):1363–1368.

49. Voulgarelis M, Ziakas PD, Papageorgiou A et al. Prognosis and outcome of non-Hodgkin lymphoma in primary Sjögren syndrome. *Medicine* (Baltimore) 2012;91(1):1–9.

50. Theander E, Manthorpe R, Jacobsson LTH. Mortality and causes of death in primary Sjögren's syndrome. *Arthritis Rheum* 2004;50(4):1262–1269.

51. Pollard RP, Pijpe J, Bootsma H et al. Treatment of mucosa-associated lymphoid tissue lymphoma in Sjögren's syndrome: a retrospective clinical study. *J Rheumatol* 2011;38(10):2198–2208.

52. Ramos-Casals M, Tzioufas AG, Stone JH, Siso A, Bosch X. Treatment of primary Sjögren syndrome: a systematic review. *JAMA* 2010;304(4):452–460.

53. Ng WF, Bowman SJ. Biological therapies in primary Sjögren's syndrome. *Expert Opin Biol Ther* 2011;11(7):921–936.

54. Kallenberg CG, Vissink A, Kroese FG, Abdulahad WH, Bootsma H. What have we learned from clinical trials in primary Sjögren's syndrome about pathogenesis? *Arthritis Res Ther* 2011;13(1):205.

55. Meiners PM, Vissink A, Kallenberg CG, Kroese FG, Bootsma H. Treatment of primary Sjögren's syndrome with anti-CD20 therapy (rituximab). A feasible approach or just a starting point? *Expert Opin Biol Ther* 2011;11(10):1381–1394.

Source of patient information

American Academy of Ophthalmology: (www.aao.org)

Arthritis Research UK: (www.arthritisresearchuk.org)

British Sjögren's Syndrome Association: (www.bssa.uk.net)

Nationale Vereniging Sjögren patiënten: (www.nvsp.nl)

NHS Choice: (www.nhs.uk/Conditions/Sjogrens-syndrome/Pages/Introduction.aspx)

Sjögren's Syndrome Foundation: (www.Sjogrens.org)

Tear Film & Ocular Surface Society: (www.tearfilm.org)

The Dry Eye Review: (www.thedryeyereview.com)

UK primary Sjögren's syndrome registry: (www.sjogrensregistry.org)

SECTION 17

Overlap/ undifferentiated syndromes

CHAPTER 129

Overlap/undifferentiated syndromes

Ariane Herrick

Introduction

'Undifferentiated connective tissue disease' (UCTD) and 'overlap syndromes' are difficult to define. Their existence in a separate chapter is justified by the clinical reality that many patients do not fit into the neat boxes of defined connective tissue diseases. First, we introduce the two terms.

Undifferentiated connective tissue disease

UCTD describes the situation when a patient has clinical and/or serological features which point to an underlying connective tissue disease, but there is insufficient evidence to make the diagnosis of any one specific connective tissue disease. If the patient is observed over time, then a defined connective tissue disease may evolve and if so, then this is usually within the first 5 years of disease, although it can be much later.

A complicating factor is that classification criteria for defined connective tissue diseases may change. For example, it is well recognized that the American College of Rheumatology (ACR) criteria for systemic sclerosis (SSc)[1] are insensitive to (especially early) limited cutaneous disease, and other criteria have therefore been proposed.[2,3] Until new classification criteria are validated and accepted, inevitably some clinicians will define disease on the basis of the proposed criteria, whereas others will not. The result is that one clinician's early SSc (using the proposed criteria) will be another's UCTD. This situation is analogous to the new classification criteria for rheumatoid arthritis (RA), which should lead to fewer diagnoses of 'undifferentiated arthritis'.[4,5]

Overlap syndromes

The term 'overlap syndrome' describes situations when a patient has features of more than one defined connective tissue disease. While many connective tissue diseases may overlap, the commonest to do so are systemic lupus erythematosus (SLE), SSc, inflammatory muscle disease (for the purposes of this review termed 'myositis') and Sjögren's syndrome (Figure 129.1). Each of these may also overlap with RA, and less frequently with other illnesses with an autoimmune component, for example vasculitis, and primary biliary cirrhosis.

If, despite overlapping clinical and/or serological features, the phenotype of one particular connective tissue disease predominates (or evolves over time), then a patient is often categorized (or recategorized)

as having that disease rather than an overlap syndrome. A problem is that there is no recognized hierarchy in which a defined connective tissue disease 'supersedes' the diagnosis of an overlap syndrome, or vice versa. For this reason (for example) one clinician's SSc with myositis is another clinician's SSc/myositis overlap.

Mixed connective tissue disease

Adding to the complexity of overlap syndromes is the diagnosis of 'mixed connective tissue disease' (MCTD). On the one hand this is sometimes considered the 'prototype' overlap syndrome, on the other hand some rheumatologists have debated whether it is a separate entity.[6] Most clinicians agree that a patient can only be assigned this diagnosis when positive for anti-U1 ribonucleoprotein (RNP) antibodies. However, U1 RNP antibody can also be positive in patients with SLE, SSc, and polymyositis, although most patients with high titres of U1 RNP antibodies have some 'overlap' connective tissue features. A further element of complexity is the suggestion that the term 'MCTD' should be dropped and 'undifferentiated autoimmune rheumatic disease' substituted.[7] The reality is that some patients diagnosed as having MCTD fulfil the criteria of one (or more) defined connective tissue disease but others do not.

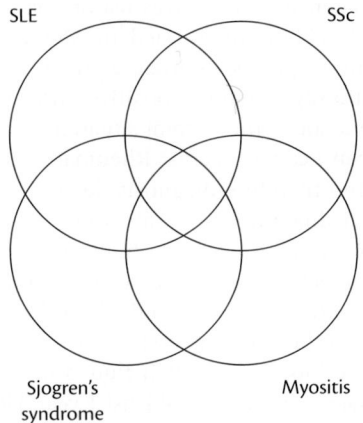

Fig. 129.1 Diagrammatic representation of overlap syndromes between systemic lupus erythematosus (SLE), systemic sclerosis (SSc), myositis, and Sjögren's syndrome. As shown, patients may overlap between two, three, or four defined diseases. The diagram does not illustrate how patients can overlap between SSc and Sjögren's syndrome alone, or between SLE and myositis alone.

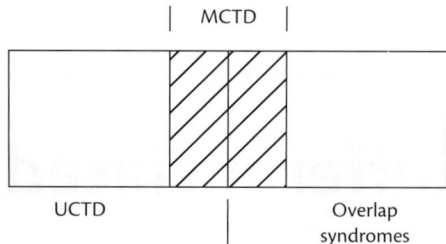

Fig. 129.2 The interrelationships between mixed connective tissue disease (MCTD), undifferentiated connective tissue disease (UCTD) and overlap syndromes.

If overlap syndromes are defined on the basis that the criteria for at least one defined connective tissue disease are met, then it could be argued that some patients with MCTD are 'undifferentiated' and some are 'overlaps' (Figure 129.2).

In this chapter, UCTD and overlap syndromes are considered separately, although it must be recognized that this is a somewhat false separation: both form part of the spectrum of multisystem connective tissue disease.

Undifferentiated connective tissue disease

Epidemiology

The incidence and prevalence of UCTD have not been studied, most likely reflecting the problems with definition (see next section). In the larger case series reported, the majority of patients are female (at least 90%) with a mean age of onset in the fourth to fifth decades.[8–11]

Definitions, classification criteria, and diagnostic criteria

LeRoy et al.[12] in 1980 first proposed the term 'undifferentiated connective syndromes' for those patients in the early stages of connective tissue disease, and who often presented with Raynaud's phenomenon and puffy fingers. These authors suggested that while many patients evolved into a defined connective tissue disease it was possible that some might remain 'undifferentiated', or remit.[12] As discussed below, it is now well recognized that many patients remain undifferentiated.

Thirty years later, different investigators have used different definitions for UCTD (summarized in Mosca et al.[13,14]). For example, some investigators require the presence of a non-organ-specific autoantibody, usually a positive anti-nuclear antibody (ANA),[8,11] others not.[15] The current situation is that there are no ACR or European League Against Rheumatism (EULAR) criteria for UCTD and therefore diagnosis depends largely on clinical judgement. A dilemma is that all connective tissue diseases 'have to start somewhere' and so a high proportion of patients with defined connective tissue disease at the time of first evaluation at a rheumatology clinic might have been diagnosed as having UCTD had they been assessed at an earlier stage of their disease. Therefore Mosca et al.[8,16] included in their cohort only patients with disease duration of at least 1 year. However, even in the cohort of patients with early connective tissue disease (disease less than 12 months' duration) described by Alarcon et al.[15] the majority of patients with undifferentiated disease remained undifferentiated or remitted.[17,18]

Mosca et al.[13,19] suggested the following preliminary classification criteria for stable UCTD:

- Signs and symptoms suggestive of a connective tissue disease, but not fulfilling criteria for defined connective tissue diseases
- Positive ANA
- Disease duration of at least 3 years (although patients with a shorter follow-up could be diagnosed as 'early UCTD').

Some investigators consider undifferentiated polyarthritis within the definition of UCTD. Although Williams et al.[17,18] and Bodoley et al.[10] included in their series patients with undifferentiated arthritis and with 'isolated' Raynaud's phenomenon, they conducted subanalyses of patients with other 'true' UCTD. For the purposes of this chapter, undifferentiated types of inflammatory arthritis are not included.

Aetiopathogenesis

As for the defined connective tissue diseases, this is unknown and has been less studied. While it is likely that there is a genetic component, this is an area requiring to be researched.

Clinical features

Essentially these are the clinical features of any of the connective tissue diseases, so long as the combination of clinical and serological features does not suffice to make a diagnosis of any one (or more) defined disease. Table 129.1 summarizes the clinical and laboratory features included in the classification criteria for SLE,[20,21] SSc,[1] myositis,[22] and Sjögren's syndrome.[23] It is very possible for a patient to present with one or more (sometimes several) of the features listed in the different classification criteria for these four diseases but remain 'undifferentiated' on the basis that no single set of classification criteria[1,20–23] is fulfilled. For example, a patient with arthralgia, tiredness, Raynaud's phenomenon, pulmonary fibrosis, leucopenia, and a positive ANA (titre 1/1000) does not fulfil any one set of criteria and so is 'undifferentiated'. Patients falling within the definition of UCTD may also have features of inflammatory arthritis (as long as they do not fulfil the criteria for RA) or of a connective tissue diseases other than SLE, SSc, myositis, or Sjögren's syndrome (again, as long as criteria of this are not fulfilled).

Raynaud's phenomenon is a very common presentation of UCTD, as originally described by LeRoy et al.[12] However, because UCTD may present with almost any clinical feature, some non-specific (e.g. fatigue) others organ based (e.g. pulmonary fibrosis, trigeminal neuralgia), patients may present to a number of different specialties. Some key clinical features/presentations (this is not a comprehensive list) include:

- **Raynaud's phenomenon**, with or without puffy fingers. This is a common presentation, reviewed by Mosca et al.[19] and reported in 33–56% of patients. Some clinicians seldom make the diagnosis of UCTD in the absence of Raynaud's phenomenon.

- **Fatigue**. Although this symptom is very common and non-specific, in the presence of a positive ANA (especially in high titre) it may indicate an underlying connective tissue disease (often undifferentiated).

- **Arthralgia (sometimes arthritis) and myalgia**. Again, these are non-specific, but especially if these occur with Raynaud's phenomenon and a positive ANA, may indicate UCTD.

Table 129.1 Clinical, haematological, and immunological features included in the classification criteria for systemic lupus erythematosus (SLE), systemic sclerosis (SSc), myositis, and Sjögren's syndrome (SS)

	SLE	SSc	Myositis	SS
Clinical features				
Mucocutaneous	Malar rash Discoid rash Photosensitivity Oral ulcers	Sclerodactyly (with or without more proximal skin thickening) Digital pitting	Rash of dermatomyositis	Dry eyes Dry mouth (criteria include a number of diagnostic tests for these[23])
Musculoskeletal	Arthritis		Proximal muscle weakness	
Other	Serositis—pleuritis or pericarditis Renal disorder—proteinuria or casts Neurologic disorder—seizures or psychosis Haematologic disorder—haemolytic anaemia, leucopenia, lymphopenia, thrombocytopenia	Pulmonary fibrosis	Raised muscle enzymes Abnormalities on electromyography Characteristic abnormalities on muscle biopsy	
Serological features				
	Anti-DNA Anti-Sm Antiphospholipid antibodies Abnormal titre of ANA			Anti-Ro Anti-La

- **Dry eyes and/or mouth**. These are common complaints in undifferentiated as well as other connective tissue diseases.

- **Interstitial lung disease**. This diagnosis should always prompt a search for an underlying connective tissue disease, which may be undifferentiated. Large series and review articles have reported low prevalences of pulmonary fibrosis in patients with UCTD.[9–11,19,24] Conversely, a substantial proportion of patients with interstitial pneumonia may have underlying autoimmune/connective tissue disease and the term 'lung-dominant connective tissue disease (CTD)' has been proposed.[25] Whether or not a patient with interstitial lung disease has an associated UCTD is clinically relevant because if so, then prognosis is improved.[26]

- **Leucopenia**. This is common, reported in 11% of the cohort of 213 patients with early disease reported by Alarcon et al.[15]

- **Serology**. Most patients with a diagnosis of UCTD have a positive ANA. In the cohort of patients described by Clegg[27] seen within 12 months of disease onset, 59% were ANA positive and as stated earlier, the presence of a non-organ specific antibody (usually ANA) has been required by some authors for diagnosis. A proportion of patients have other non-organ specific antibodies, for example anti-Ro, anti-La, or anti-U1 RNP.[27] Anti-thyroid antibodies may also be present (13% of 64 patients with 'stable' UCTD in the cohort of Mosca et al.[16] had autoimmune thyroid disease). In practice, often it is the finding of a positive ANA which alerts the clinician to the possibility of connective tissue disease, which may be undifferentiated.

Outcome

As first suggested by LeRoy et al.,[12] there are three possible outcomes of UCTD (Figure 129.3):

- evolution to a definite connective tissue disease

- persisting features of UCTD

- resolution.

Several case series have described these clinical outcomes in patients with UCTD. Table 129.2 summarizes some of the larger studies. A key point is that the majority of patients, especially those with disease duration of more than 1 year, never progress to a defined connective tissue disease but remain undifferentiated. Of these patients who remain undifferentiated, most have mild disease but some (e.g. those with lung fibrosis) may have severe even life-threatening disease.

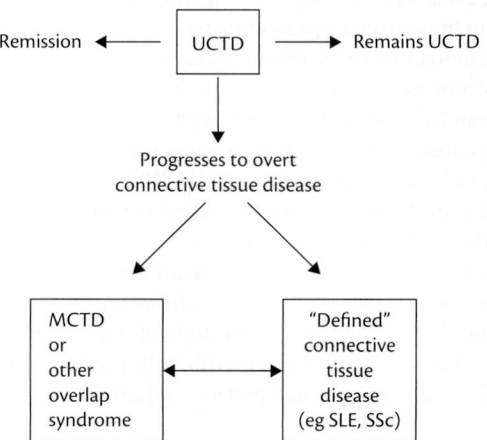

Fig. 129.3 Possible outcomes of undifferentiated connective tissue disease. The figure also illustrates how overlap syndromes and defined connective tissue diseases may transition from one to another.

Table 129.2 Clinical outcomes in undifferentiated connective tissue disease—summary table of some of the larger studies

Country	Number of patients	Duration of follow-up	Number (%) evolving into 'defined' connective tissue disease	Number (%) remaining undifferentiated	Number (%) of those remaining undifferentiated who remitted/became symptomatic
USA[a] [18]	115 (47 available for 10 year visit)[2]	10 years (5 year data is reported in [17])	20 (17%): 11 SLE 3 SSc 6 RA	66 (57%) at 1 year of whom 41 remained UCTD at 3 years, 29 at 5 years and 13 at 10 years[3]	10 of those not evolving to a connective tissue disease [c]
Italy[9]	165	5 years	10 (6%): 5 SLE (1 with SS, 1 with APS) 3 other SS, 1 myositis 1 MCTD	155 (94%)	19 (12% of 155)
Italy[16]	83	5 years (1 year data, describing 91 patients, reported in [8])	19 (23%): 18 SLE 1 SS	64 (77%)	0
Hungary[10]	665[b]	5 years	230 (35%): 87 RA 45 SS 28 SLE 26 MCTD 22 systemic vasculitis 19 SSc 3 myositis	435 (65%)	82 (19% of the 435)

APS, anti-phospholipid syndrome; MCTD, mixed connective tissue disease; RA, rheumatoid arthritis; SLE, systemic lupus erythematosus; SS, Sjögren's syndrome; SSc, systemic sclerosis; UTCD, undifferentiated connective tissue disease.
[a]Patients were only included if they had early disease (within 12 months of onset).
[b]Excluding patients with isolated Raynaud's phenomenon or unexplained polyarthritis.
[c]Percentages difficult to gauge because of numbers of withdrawals. Numbers do not include patients evolving to isolated Raynaud's phenomenon or to unexplained polyarthritis.

Evolution to a defined connective tissue disease may occur at any point but usually occurs early, within the first 2–5 years.[10,16] In some reported series, SLE was the connective tissue disease most likely to develop (Table 129.2). However, in the series of Bodoley et al.,[10] most 'evolvers' were to RA. The presenting clinical features may predict the pattern of evolution. For example, SSc may be more likely to develop than SLE in those patients presenting with severe Raynaud's phenomenon. The autoantibody profile may also help predict the most likely pattern of disease evolution: patients with anti-Sm patients, anti-double stranded (ds)DNA or ANA with a homogenous pattern are likely to progress to SLE,[28] patients with anti-Ro and anti-La antibodies to Sjögren's syndrome, those with U1 RNP antibodies to MTCD, and those with ANA with an anti-nucleolar pattern to SSc.[10] There is a substantial literature (not discussed in detail here) describing predictors of evolution to a SSc-spectrum disorder in patients with Raynaud's phenomenon[29,30]: abnormalities on nailfold capillaroscopy (Figure 129.4) and SSc-specific autoantibodies are independent predictors of progression (patients with both predictors are 60 times more likely to develop SSc than patients without either predictor).[29]

Management

There is no specific disease-modifying therapy for UCTD. Currently, treatment for any one individual is dictated by their clinical features.

For example, interstitial lung disease and pulmonary hypertension are generally treated similarly as in those with idiopathic disease. Raynaud's phenomenon may be severe, and should be treated as for Raynaud's secondary to SSc-spectrum disorders. Anti-malarials are often prescribed, especially in patients with arthralgia/arthritis, and findings from a retrospective study[31] suggested that anti-malarial therapy in patients with UCTD might delay progression to overt SLE. Although large case series described frequent use of (low-dose) steroids,[10,11] these should only be prescribed when there is clear evidence of an inflammatory component to the illness. Management is multidisciplinary and should have a strong emphasis on patient education: for example, patients with Raynaud's phenomenon should be told to report any persistent discolouration (suggesting a risk of critical ischaemia) or digital ulceration.

A key challenge is whether, in the future, early identification of underlying UCTD will allow early intervention to prevent disease progression, or at least to allow inclusion into clinical trials aimed at testing effectiveness of possible disease-modifying agents. For example, in the patient with Raynaud's phenomenon, early identification of nailfold capillaroscopic abnormality and/or disease-specific autoantibodies (predictive of an underlying SSc-spectrum disorder[29]) might in the future allow early commencement of vascular remodelling therapies. Early identification of interstitial

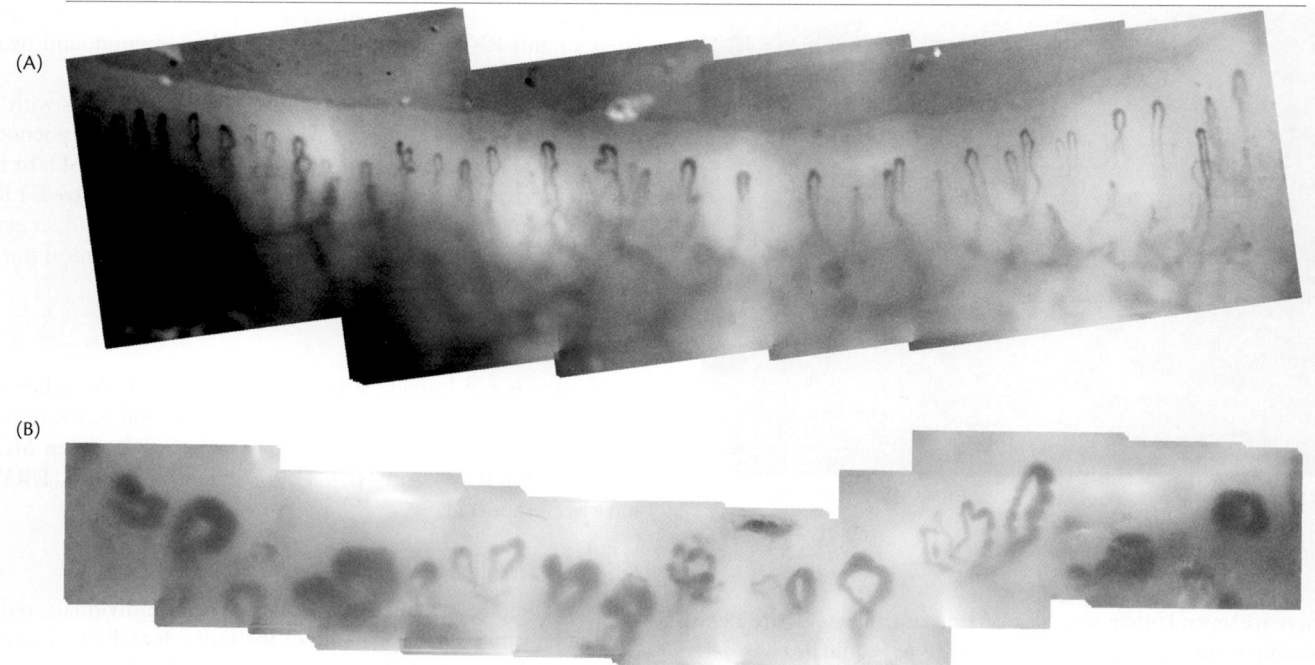

Fig. 129.4 (A) Normal nailfold capillaries in a healthy control subject compared to (B) abnormal capillaries in a patient with SSc, showing capillary enlargement, areas of avascularity, and loss of the normal nailfold architecture.

pneumonitis might similarly allow early intervention. However, first we need to identify effective disease-modifying agents.

Summary statement on UCTD

UCTD is difficult to define. A proportion of patients evolve to a defined connective tissue disease, and it will never be possible in all patients to separate completely the early stages of a defined connective tissue disease from UCTD. The key point for clinicians is to be especially vigilant in the first 3–5 years of disease onset, because evolution into a defined connective tissue disease is usually within this time frame. Therefore clinical stability after 3–5 years is reassuring. Treatment is based on symptoms and which (if any) internal organs are involved.

Overlap syndromes

Epidemiology

Most likely reflecting problems of definition (discussed below), the epidemiology of overlap syndromes has been little studied, similarly to the situation with UCTD. Of all the overlap syndromes, MCTD (a term first proposed in the early 1970s[32]) has been most researched, accepting that, as already mentioned, there has been considerable debate and controversy as to whether MCTD should be considered a separate disease entity.[6,7,33] For the purposes of this chapter, the term 'MCTD' is retained, given that much of the literature on overlap syndromes focuses on this, but MCTD should perhaps be viewed as an ill-defined entity within a broader group of overlap syndromes, with further overlap with UCTD (Figure 129.2). An epidemiological study of MCTD from Norway reported a mean age of adult-onset disease of 38 years, a female to male ratio of 3.3, a point prevalence of 3.8 per 100 000 adults, and an incidence of 2.1 per million adults per year.[34] These prevalence and incidence rates are lower than for SLE, SSc, and myositis.

Definitions, classification criteria, and diagnostic criteria

Definitions

The definition of overlap syndromes is likely to remain contentious. At one end of the spectrum is the viewpoint that most connective tissue diseases are overlaps, at the other end that 'overlaps' are not a useful concept but that most connective tissue diseases are highly heterogeneous, defined on the basis of their most prominent clinical features.

Nonetheless, the pragmatic approach is to state that overlap syndromes are diseases characterized by having features of more than one defined connective tissue disease. Some specific examples are defined as follows:

- **Mixed connective tissue disease**. As already mentioned, U1 RNP antibody (Figure 129.5) is generally considered a necessary prerequisite for diagnosis. The 'typical' patient with MCTD has overlapping features of SLE, SSc, and myositis.

- **SSc/polymyositis**. Patients with this overlap syndrome have features of both SSc and inflammatory muscle disease. Because myositis is common in SSc, many physicians would not define this as an overlap, but all part of the SSc-spectrum. A proportion of patients with this overlap have antibodies to PM-Scl.[35] However, this is a minority (in the order of 25%).[36] There are two antigens, PM-Scl-75 and PM-Scl-100. In a cohort of 280 patients with SSc, anti-PM-Scl-75/100 was associated not only with muscle involvement but also with lung disease and digital ulcers.[37]

- **SLE/RA**. Patients have features of both SLE and RA. For example, they might have erosive polyarthritis, low white blood and platelet counts, positive rheumatoid factor, positive ANA, and high levels of circulating dsDNA antibodies.

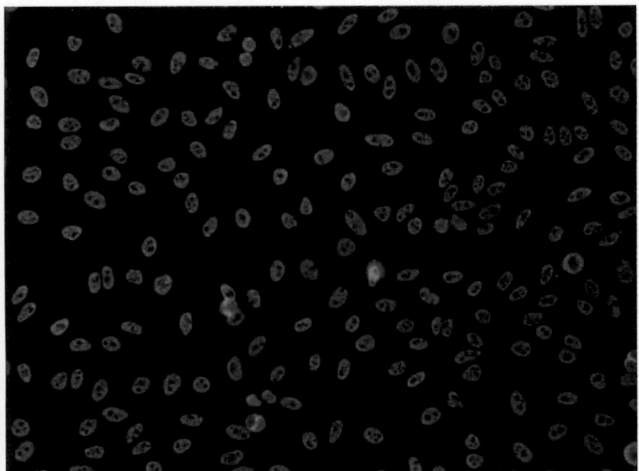

Fig. 129.5 Indirect immunofluorescent stain ng for ANA (U1 RNP antibodies) on HEP-2 cell line slides at 1 in 100 dilution.
Courtesy of Dr Hana Alachkar.

There are several other possible overlap syndromes (Figure 129.6). For example, the anti-synthetase syndrome[38,39] could be considered an overlap syndrome. This chapter confines itself to broad principles rather than describing details of individual syndromes.

Classification and diagnostic criteria

There are no ACR or EULAR criteria for overlap syndromes. Diagnostic criteria for MCTD have been suggested by different investigators.[40] Alarson-Segovia and Villareal[41] suggested that for a diagnosis of MCTD, a patient had to have (in addition to an anti-RNP antibody) three or more of: swollen hands, synovitis, myositis, Raynaud's phenomenon, and acrocyanosis (including one or both of synovitis and myositis). Kahn et al.'s criteria were similar,[42]

although insisting on Raynaud's phenomenon: these criteria stipulated an anti-RNP antibody, Raynaud's phenomenon, and two of: swollen fingers, synovitis, and myositis.

A key point is that a patient with U1 RNP antibodies with features typical of MCTD may evolve over the years into a phenotype more typical of another connective tissue disease (e.g. SLE or SSc) and that conversely a patient with SLE or SSc with positive U1 RNP antibodies may go on develop overlapping features and so evolve into a 'definite' MCTD (Figure 129.3). Neither the clinical nor the serological boundaries are clear-cut.

Aetiopathogenesis

While this is not known, it is likely that (as with the other connective tissue diseases) there are both genetic and environmental components to overlap syndromes. Associations between MCTD (and anti-U1 RNP) and HLA DR4[43–46] and also HLA DR2[45,46] have been reported.

Clinical and laboratory features

These are highly variable between and within individuals, reflecting the enormous heterogeneity of the individual defined connective tissue diseases, a heterogeneity which is further compounded when these occur in overlap. While all the possible 'combinations' constituting overlap syndromes will not be discussed here, the key features of MCTD deserve mention.

Features of mixed connective tissue disease

Common representing features include tiredness, Raynaud's phenomenon, arthralgias, and myalgias. The tiredness can be profound. Although swollen, puffy fingers (Figure 129.7) are said to be characteristic, these occur also in early inflammatory arthritis and in SSc. There is a large number of other possible presenting

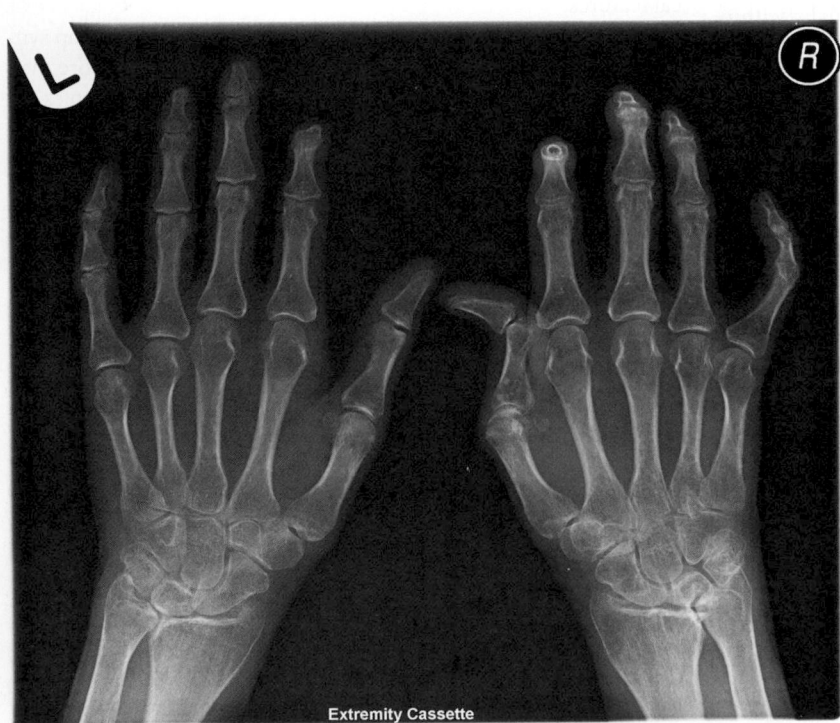

Fig. 129.6 Overlap syndrome of SSc and inflammatory arthritis. Hand radiograph showing acro-osteolysis of several of the distal phalanges, consistent with the diagnosis of SSc, and a Z-thumb deformity, consistent with the patient's inflammatory arthritis.

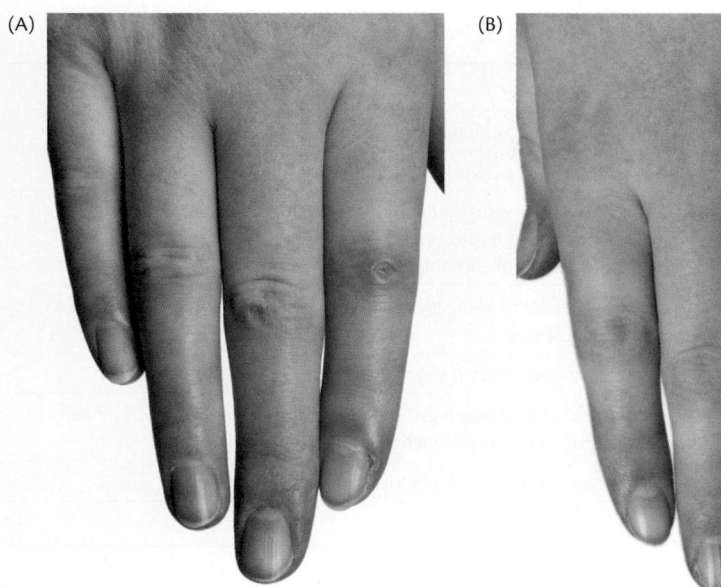

(A)   (B)

Fig. 129.7 (A) Right and (B) left hands showing puffy fingers (best shown on the left hand) and an ulcer over the right index proximal interphalangeal joint. Copyright Salford Royal NHS Foundation Trust.

features, including rashes and features reflecting the internal organ involvement of the disease. These possibilities include pulmonary arterial hypertension, interstitial lung disease (which can be fulminating),[47] trigeminal neuralgia, and aseptic meningitis. Renal involvement has generally been considered to be rare in patients who are anti-U1 RNP positive, but can occur.[46,48] Any of these clinical features may occur at any point in the time course of the disease, and it may be only after two or more of these features develop, and the U1 RNP antibody is tested, that the diagnosis is made.

Serology

As already stated, a positive RNP antibody (anti-U1 RNP) is a prerequisite for the diagnosis of MCTD, although RNP positivity is not specific for MCTD and, as stated earlier, can occur in patients with a defined connective tissue disease such as SLE and SSc. Anti-U1 RNP should be tested for if there is any clinical suspicion of connective tissue disease, especially in the presence of a high-titre ANA in a speckled pattern. Antibodies to Sm, Ro, and La also produce a speckled ANA pattern although these speckled patterns can be differentiated. It is now recognized that U1 RNP consists of RNA plus three different proteins (A, C, and a 68–70 kDa protein).[49] Most laboratories check for native U1 RNP which contains proteins 70P, A, and C.

Patients with MCTD may have other autoantibodies, including anti-dsDNA, anti-Ro, anti-La, and anti-cardiolipin antibodies.[46] The presence of these antibodies may be associated with specific features—for example, patients with anti-Ro and anti-La antibodies are likely to have features of Sjögren's syndrome. Other common laboratory features are hypergammaglobulinaemia and leucopenia (reported in 80% and 52% respectively of the original description of patients[32]).

Outcome

Outcome of overlap syndromes is highly variable, depending on the phenotype of the individual and whether this is predominantly (for example) of SLE or SSc. As stated earlier, patients with MCTD often evolve to SSc or SLE.[50] It has been suggested that whether MCTD evolves into SLE or SSc, or remains 'MCTD', is influenced by MHC antigens.[43]

Although it was originally thought that MCTD had a relatively benign course with a low prevalence of renal, cerebral, and pulmonary involvement,[32] this opinion has been revised and it is now recognized that patients with MCTD may have severe disease and that there is a significant mortality.[6,43,46,51] This reflects how a proportion of patients develop pulmonary arterial hypertension and other major organ involvement.[46,51,52] In the cohort of 47 patients described by Burdt et al.,[46] 23% developed pulmonary hypertension as diagnosed at right heart catheterization or at autopsy.

Management

At present there is no drug known to modify the underlying disease process in overlap syndromes in general or in MCTD in particular. This is unsurprising, given the definition issues.

Treatment is guided by experience from SLE, SSc, and myositis. The clinician has to assess which clinical features require specific treatment. Examples of commonly used treatments for some of the musculoskeletal, vascular, and internal organ involvements of overlap syndromes are given in Table 129.3.

Certain general points can be made:

◆ Patients should be kept under regular review, in order to identify any change in disease status which might require further assessment and management. For example, at the outpatient clinic patients should be asked about the development of any cardiorespiratory symptoms, examined for the presence of a loud pulmonary component to the second heart sound and for basal crackles, and investigations arranged as appropriate (ECG, echocardiogram, pulmonary function tests). A dipstick test of urine should be performed at each visit, looking for protein or blood. The blood count, biochemical profile, and acute-phase response should be monitored, and serological tests requested if appropriate (e.g. dsDNA antibodies and complement levels in the patient with an SLE overlap).

Table 129.3 Examples of treatments for some of the different features of overlap syndromes. This is not a comprehensive list

Clinical feature	Specific examples
Myositis	Steroids ± immunosuppression
Arthritis	Analgesics, NSAIDs, DMARDs including anti-malarials and methotrexate
Raynaud's phenomenon/digital ischaemia and ulceration	Conservative (non-drug) measures, vasodilators (e.g. calcium channel blockers), intravenous prostanoids for refractory ulceration or digital ischaemia (usually in combination with antibiotics)
Pulmonary arterial hypertension	Endothelin receptor antagonist, phosphodiesterase inhibitor, intravenous prostanoid therapy
Pulmonary fibrosis	Steroids ± immunosuppression
Renal disease	Steroids and immunosuppressants, depending on histology, ACE inhibitor (for proteinuria or for scleroderma renal crisis)
Gastro-intestinal disease	Proton pump inhibitors, antibiotics for bacterial overgrowth
Haematological involvement—haemolytic anaemia, thrombocytopenia	Steroids

ACE, angiotensin converting enzyme; DMARDs, disease-modifying anti-rheumatic drugs; NSAIDs, non-steroidal anti-inflammatory drugs.

◆ As with all connective tissue diseases, management is multidisciplinary, often involving different medical specialties as well as physiotherapy, occupational therapy, and podiatry. Patient education is a key aspect of management.

◆ A key point is to determine the inflammatory 'burden' in any one particular patient. This will be high when there is a strong SLE/myositis component, but may be low when most of the features are those of SSc. Steroids are commonly used for many of the inflammatory manifestations of MCTD and of other overlap syndromes.

◆ Pulmonary arterial hypertension is generally treated as in 'idiopathic' or SSc-related disease. However, if there is thought to be a significant inflammatory component to the overlap syndrome then steroids and/or immunosuppressants should also be considered.

◆ Pulmonary fibrosis should be treated as in other connective tissue diseases, usually with steroids and/or immunosuppressants accepting that the evidence base is weak, except for SSc-related pulmonary fibrosis when cyclophosphamide has been shown to confer modest benefit.[53,54]

◆ Caution needs to be exercised when steroids are prescribed for inflammatory features in patients with overlap syndromes which include SSc, especially if the SSc is of the diffuse cutaneous subtype. This is because steroids are a risk factor for scleroderma renal crisis.[55]

Summary statement on overlap syndromes

Patients with overlap syndromes fulfil the criteria of a defined connective tissue disease but in addition have clinical features of at least one other (and may fulfil the criteria for another). MCTD is characterized by overlapping features of SLE, SSc, and/or myositis with antibodies to U1 RNP. Management of overlap syndromes depends on the specific clinical manifestations. For example, a patient with a predominantly SLE phenotype, but with some features of SSc, will be managed mainly along 'SLE lines', but addressing also the SSc components (for example treatment of oesophageal dysmotility and/or of severe Raynaud's phenomenon).

Overall summary

UCTD and overlap syndromes form part of the broad spectrum of connective tissue disease. They are difficult to define, reflecting the heterogeneity of these diseases between and within individuals. Within any one individual the disease may evolve over time: different features of that disease may predominate at different times over the years.

UCTD and overlap syndromes are, at least in most patients, chronic conditions which range from the very mild (in some patients with UCTD) to the life-threatening. The key point for the clinician is early recognition of clinical features which require specific treatment. A major challenge over the next 10 years is to better understand the natural history of UCTD, in order to establish whether we can predict those patients who progress to severe disease and whether early immunosuppression and/or vascular remodelling agents might favourably influence prognosis.

Acknowledgement

I am grateful to Dr Hana Alachkar for her helpful comments on the text.

References

1. Masi AT, Rodnan GP, Medsger TA et al. Preliminary criteria for the classification of systemic sclerosis (scleroderma). *Arthritis Rheum* 1980;23(5):581–590.

2. LeRoy EC, Medsger TA. Criteria for the classification of early systemic sclerosis. *J Rheumatol* 2001;28:1573–1576.

3. Matucci-Cerinic M, Allanore Y, Czirják L et al. The challenge of early systemic sclerosis for the EULAR Scleroderma Trial and Research Group (EUSTAR) community. It is time to cut the Gordian knot and develop a prevention or rescue strategy. *Ann Rheum Dis* 2009;68:1377–1380.

4. Aletaha D, Neogi T, Silman AJ et al. 2010 rheumatoid arthritis classification criteria: an American College of Rheumatology/European League Against Rheumatism collaborative initiative. *Ann Rheum Dis* 2010;69:1580–1588.

5. Aletaha D, Neogi T, Silman AJ et al. 2010 rheumatoid arthritis classification criteria. An American College of Rheumatology/European League Against Rheumatism collaborative initiative. *Arthritis Rheum* 2010;62 (9):2569–2581.

6. Black C, Isenberg DA Mixed connective tissue disease—goodbye to all that. *Br J Rheumatol* 1992;31:695–700.

7. Swanton J, Isenberg D Mixed connective tissue disease: still crazy after all these years. *Rheum Dis Clin N Am* 2005;31:421–436.

8. Mosca M, Tavoni A, Neri R, Bencivelli W, Bombardieri S. Undifferentiated connective tissue diseases: the clinical and serological profiles of 91 patients followed for at least 1 year. *Lupus* 1998;7:95–100.

9. Danieli MG, Fraticelli P, Franceschini F et al. Five year follow up of 165 Italian patients with undifferentiated connective tissue diseases. *Clin Exp Rheumatol* 1999;17:585–591.

10. Bodolay E, Csiki Z, Szekanecz Z et al. Five year follow-up of 665 Hungarian patients with undifferentiated connective tissue disease (UCTD). *Clin Exp Rheumatol* 2003;21:313–320.

11. Vaz CC, Couto M, Medeiros D et al. Undifferentated connective tissue: a seven-center cross-sectional study of 184 patients. *Clin Rheumatol* 2009;28:915–921.

12. LeRoy EC, Maricq HR, Kahaleh MB. Undifferentiated connective tissue syndromes. *Arthritis Rheum* 1980;23:341–343.

13. Mosca M, Neri R, Bombardieri S. Undifferentiated connective tissue diseases (UCTD): a review of the literature and a proposal for preliminary classification criteria. *Clin Exp Rheumatol* 1999;17:615–620.

14. Mosca M, Tani C, Bombardieri S. Undifferentiated connective tissue diseases (UCTD): a new frontier for rheumatology. *Best Practice Res Clin Rheumatol* 2007;21(6):1011–1023.

15. Alarcon CS, Williams GV, Singer JZ et al. Early undifferentiated connective tissue disease. I. Early clinical manifestation in a large cohort of patients with undifferentiated connective tissues diseases compared with cohorts of well established connective tissue disease. *J Rheumatol* 1991;18:1332–1339.

16. Mosca M, Neri R, Bencivelli W, Tavoni A, Bombardiari S. Undifferentiated connective tissue disease: analysis of 83 patients with a minimum follow up of 5 years. *J Rheumatol* 2002;29:2345–2349.

17. Williams HJ, Alarcon GS, Neuner R et al. Early undifferentiated tissue disease. V. An inception cohort 5 years later: disease remissions and changes in diagnoses in well established and undifferentiated connective tissue diseases. *J Rheumatol* 1998;25:261–268.

18. Williams HJ, Alarcon GS, Joks R et al. Early undifferentiated connective tissue disease. VI. An inception cohort after 10 years: disease remissions and changes in diagnoses in well established and undifferentiated CTD. *J Rheumatol* 1999;26:816–825.

19. Mosca M, Tani C, Talarico R, Bombarieri S. Undifferentiated connective tissue diseases (UCTD): simplified systemic autoimmune diseases. *Autoimmunity Reviews* 2011;10:256–258.

20. Tan EM, Cohen AS, Fries JF et al. The 1982 revised criteria for the classification of systemic lupus erythematosus. *Arthritis Rheum* 1982;25(11):1271–1277.

21. Hochberg MC. Updating the American College of Rheumatology revised criteria for the classification of systemic lupus erythematosus. *Arthritis Rheum* 1997;40 (9),1725.

22. Bohan A, Peter JB. Polymyositis and dermatomyositis (second of two parts). *N Engl J Med* 1975;292:403–407.

23. Vitali C, Bombardieri S, Jonsson R et al. Classification criteria for Sjögren's syndrome: a revised version of the European criteria proposed by the American-European Consensus Group. *Ann Rheum Dis* 2002;61: 554–558.

24. Danieli MG, Fraticelli P, Salvi A, Gabrielli A, Danieli G. Undifferentiated connective tissue disease: natural history and evolution into definite CTD assessed in 84 patients initially diagnosed as early UCTD. *Clin Rheumatol* 1998;17:195–201.

25. Fischer A, West SG, Swigris JL, Brown KK, Du Bois RM. Connective tissue disease-associated interstitial lung disease: a call for clarification. *Chest* 2010;138:251–256.

26. Kinder BW, Shariat C, Collard HR et al. Undifferentiated connective tissue disease-associated interstitial lung disease: changes in lung function. *Lung* 2010;188:143–149.

27. Clegg DO, Williams HJ, Singer JZ. Early undifferentiated connective tissue disease. II. The frequency of circulating antinuclear antibodies in patients with early rheumatic diseases. *J Rheumatol* 1991;18:1340–1343.

28. Calvo-Alen J, Alarcon GA, Burgard SL et al. Systemic lupus erythematosus: predictors of its occurrence among a cohort of patients with early undifferentiated connective tissue disease: multivariate analyses and identification of risk factors. *J Rheumatol* 1996;23:469–475.

29. Koenig M, Joyal F, Fritzler MJ et al. Autoantibodies and microvascular damage are independent predictive factors for the progression of Raynaud's phenomenon to systemic sclerosis: a twenty-year prospective study of 586 patients, with validation of proposed criteria for early systemic sclerosis. *Arthritis Rheum* 2008;58:3902–3912.

30. Herrick AL, Cutolo M. Clinical implications from capillaroscopic analysis in patients with Raynaud's phenomenon and systemic sclerosis-spectrum disorders. *Arthritis Rheum* 2010;62:2595–2604.

31. James JA, Kim-Howard XR, Bruner BF et al. Hydroxychloroquine sulphate treatment is associated with later onset of systemic lupus erythematosus. *Lupus* 2007;16:401–409.

32. Sharp GC, Irvin WS, Tan EM, Gould RG, Holman HR. Mixed connective tissue disease—an apparently distinct rheumatic disease syndrome associated with a specific antibody to an extractable nuclear antigen (ENA). *Am J Med* 1972;52:148–159.

33. Smolen JS, Steiner G. Mixed connective tissue disease. To be or not to be? *Arthritis Rheum* 1998;41:768–777.

34. Gunnarsson R, Molberg O, Gilboe I-M, Gran JT. The prevalence and incidence of mixed connective tissue disease: a national multicentre survey of Norwegian patients. *Ann Rheum Dis* 2011;70:1047–1051.

35. Marguerie C, Bunn CC, Copier J et al. The clinical and immunogenetic features of patients with autoantibodies to the nucleolar antigen PM-Scl. *Medicine* 1992;71(6):327–336.

36. Oddis CV, Okano Y, Rudert WA et al. Serum autoantibody to the nucleolar antigen PM-Scl. *Arthritis Rheum* 1992;35(10):1211–1217.

37. Hanke K, Bruckner CS, Dahnrich C et al. Antibodies against PM/Scl-75 and PM/Scl-100 are independent markers for different subsets of systemic sclerosis patients. *Arthritis Res Ther* 2009;11(1):R22.

38. Marguerie C, Bunn CC, Beynon HL et al. Polymyositis, pulmonary fibrosis and autoantibodies to aminoacyl-tRNA synthetase enzymes. *Q J Med* 1990;77:1019–1038.

39. Betteridge Z, Gunawardena H, North J, Slinn J, McHugh N. Antisynthetase syndrome: a new autoantibody to phenylalanyl transfer RNA synthetase (anti-Zo) associated with polymyositis and interstitial pneumonia. *Rheumatology* 2007;46:1005–1008.

40. Alarcon-Segovia D, Cardiel MH. Comparison between 3 diagnostic criteria for mixed connective tissue disease. Study of 593 patients. *J Rheumatol* 1989;16:328–334.

41. Alarcon-Segovia D, Villareal M. Classification and diagnostic criteria for mixed connective tissue disease. In Kasukawa R, Sharp GC (eds) *Mixed connective tissue diseases and antinuclear antibodies*. Elsevier, Amsterdam, 1987:33–40.

42. Khan MF, Appelboom MT. Syndrome de Sharp. In: Khan MF, Peltier AP, Meyer O, Piette JC (eds) *Les maladies systemiques*, 3rd edn. Flammarion, Paris, 1991:545–556.

43. Gendi NST, Welsh KI, van Venrooij WJ et al. HLA type as a predictor of mixed connective tissue disease differentiation: ten-year clinical and immunogenetic follow up of 46 patients. *Arthritis Rheum* 1995;38: 259–266.

44. Genth E, Zarnowski H, Mierau R, Wohltmann D, Hartl PW. HLA-DR4 and Gm (1,3;5,21) are associated with U1-nRNP antibody positive connective tissue disease. *Ann Rheum Dis* 1987;46:189–196.

45. Hoffman RW, Rettenmaier LJ, Takeda Y et al. Human autoantibodies against the 70-kd polypeptide of U1 small nuclear RNP are associated with HLA-DR4 among connective tissue disease patients. *Arthritis Rheum* 1990;33(5):666–673.

46. Burdt MA, Hoffman RW, Deutscher SL et al. Long-term outcome in mixed connective tissue disease. *Arthritis Rheum* 1999;42:899–909.

47. Fernandes C, Bungay P, O'Driscoll BR, Herrick AL. Mixed connective tissue disease presenting with pneumonitis and pneumatosis intestinalis ('Radiological Vignette'). *Arthritis Rheum* 2000;43(3):704–707.

48. Reichlin M, Mattioli M. Correlation of a precipitin reaction to an RNA protein antigen and a low prevalence of nephritis in patients with systemic lupus erythematosus. *N Engl J Med* 1972;286:908–911.

49. Takeda Y, Wang GS, Wang RJ et al. Enzyme-linked immunosorbent assay using isolated (U) small nuclear ribonucleoprotein polypeptides as antigens to investigate the clinical significance of autoantibodies to these polypeptides. *Clin Immunol Immunopathol* 1989;50:213–230.

50. Van den Hoogen FHJ, Spronk PE, Boerbooms AMT et al. Long-term follow-up of 46 patients with anti-(U1)snRNP antibodies. *Br J Rheumatol* 1994;33:1117–1120.

51. Sullivan WD, Hurst DJ, Harmon CR et al. A prospective evaluation emphasising pulmonary invovlement in patients with mixed connective tissue disease. *Medicine* (Baltimore) 1984;63:92–107.

52. Prakesh UBS. Respiratory complications in mixed connective tissue disease. *Clin Chest Med* 1998;19:733–746.

53. Tashkin DP, Elashoff R, Clements PJ et al. Cyclophosphamide versus placebo in scleroderma lung disease. *N Engl J Med* 2006;354: 2655–2666.

54. Hoyles RK, Ellis RW, Wellsbury J et al. A multicenter, prospective, randomized, double-blind, placebo-controlled trial of corticosteroids and intravenous cyclophosphamide followed by oral azathioprine for the treatment of pulmonary fibrosis in scleroderma. *Arthritis Rheum* 2006;54:3962–3970.

55. Steen VD, Medsger TA. Case-control study of corticosteroids and other drugs that either precipitate or protect from the development of scleorderma renal crisis. *Arthritis Rheum* 1998;41:1613–1619.

Sources of patient information

Arthritis Research UK publishes a booklet on Raynaud's phenomenon. The Raynaud's and Scleroderma Association publishes leaflets on Raynaud's phenomenon and on MCTD.

SECTION 18

Vasculitis

CHAPTER 130

Vasculitis—classification and diagnosis

Richard A. Watts and David G. I. Scott

Introduction

The word vasculitis means inflammation of blood vessels; the blood vessel is the primary site of inflammation. The pathological consequence of such inflammation is destruction of the vessel wall, seen histologically as fibrinoid necrosis; hence the term 'necrotizing vasculitis'. Vasculitis may be localized to a single organ or vascular bed and be clinically insignificant, but more commonly it is generalized. Muscular arteries may develop focal or segmental lesions and these may be life threatening. Focal lesions, affecting part of the vessel wall, may lead to aneurysm formation and possible vessel rupture; segmental lesions (affecting the whole circumference) are more common and lead to stenosis or occlusion with distal infarction. The classification of vasculitis has been an area of controversy for many years, with specific classification criteria only relatively recently introduced. The early diagnosis of vasculitis is particularly important because of the significant morbidity and mortality of untreated disease. Appropriate use of immunological tests including anti-neutrophil cytoplasmic antibodies (ANCA) has proved to be most helpful in the assessment and diagnosis of small-vessel systemic vasculitides.

Classification of vasculitis

Kussmaul and Maier[1] are generally accepted as providing the first description of 'periarteritis nodosa' when they described a patient with a systemic illness characterized by numerous nodules along the course of small muscular arteries. Earlier descriptions suggest that the formal recording of this condition is at least 200 years old (reviewed by Matteson[2]).

Zeek[3] reviewed the literature relating to vasculitis and periarteritis nodosa and used the generic term 'necrotizing angiitis' to indicate the specific damage to the blood vessel wall rather than the presence of inflammation alone; she classified these into five distinct entities: (1) hypersensitivity angiitis, (2) allergic granulomatous angiitis, (3) rheumatic arteritis, (4) periarteritis nodosa, and (5) temporal arteritis. Most modern classifications are based on Zeek's work, which essentially combined histological changes and clinical features. Notable omissions from Zeek's classification were Wegener's granulomatosis (WG), microscopic polyangiitis (MPA), and Takayasu's arteritis (TA). Microscopic polyangiitis (originally

called microscopic polyarteritis) had been described by Davson[4] in 1948, but was not generally recognized until the 1990s following the description of its association with ANCA. WG, now renamed granulomatosis with polyangiitis (GPA),[5] and TA were not fully recognized in the English literature until after 1953.

The most widely accepted classification systems are still based on Zeek's original groupings, which reflect dominant vessel size but also an association with ANCA. There is considerable overlap in the size of vessels involved so it is important to define exactly what is meant by large-vessel, medium-vessel, and small-vessel vasculitis. This is reflected by the legend of Figure 130.1 which stresses 'more often' for large-vessel vasculitis and 'predominantly' for medium- and small-vessel vasculitis definitions. The most current classification system (Table 130.1 and Figure 130.2) recognizes that the small-vessel vasculitides can be differentiated by immunological testing into a group of ANCA-associated and a group of immune-complex-associated diseases. This classification also broadly reflects the therapeutic approaches that are applied to the different groups (Table 130.2). The small-vessel group associated with ANCA respond well to immunosuppression with cyclophosphamide and corticosteroids (and more recently to rituximab), whereas the large-vessel group require moderate to high-dose steroids and the small-vessel group associated with immune complexes usually require low-dose corticosteroids. Also, the ANCA-associated small-vessel group are those most likely to develop glomerulonephritis and renal failure. The medium-sized vessel group are not associated with ANCA and may respond to anti-viral therapy and plasma exchange (hepatitis B PAN) or intravenous immunoglobulin with or without corticosteroids (Kawaski). Biological drugs are being used with increasing frequency in these diseases and B-cell depletion using rituximab may be particularly helpful for early treatment of the ANCA-associated (replacing cyclophosphamide)[6] and some immune-complex-associated small-vessel diseases.

American College of Rheumatology (1990) criteria

In 1990 the American College of Rheumatology (ACR) proposed criteria for the classification of seven different vasculitides—giant cell arteritis (GCA), TA, granulomatosis with polyangiitis (Wegener's granulomatosis; GPA), eosinophilic granulomatosis with polyangiitis (Churg–Strauss syndrome; EGPA), polyarteritis

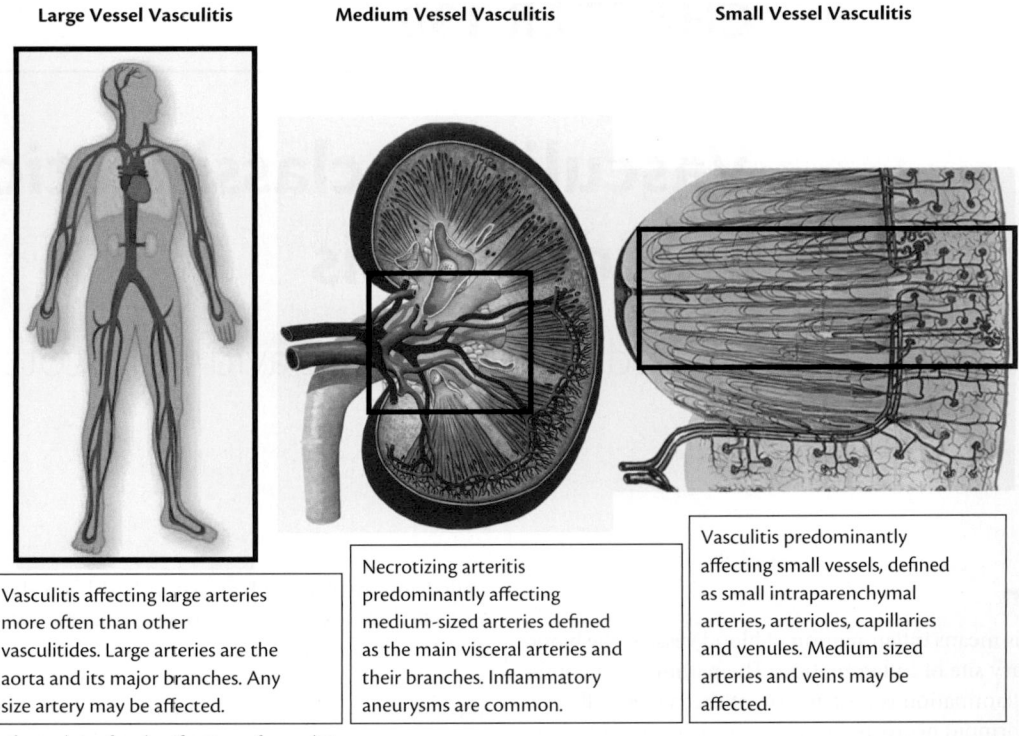

Large Vessel Vasculitis   **Medium Vessel Vasculitis**   **Small Vessel Vasculitis**

Vasculitis affecting large arteries more often than other vasculitides. Large arteries are the aorta and its major branches. Any size artery may be affected.

Necrotizing arteritis predominantly affecting medium-sized arteries defined as the main visceral arteries and their branches. Inflammatory aneurysms are common.

Vasculitis predominantly affecting small vessels, defined as small intraparenchymal arteries, arterioles, capillaries and venules. Medium sized arteries and veins may be affected.

Fig. 130.1 Definitions of vessel size for classification of vasculitis.
Reproduced with permission from Jennette JC et al. 2012 Revised International Chapel Hill Consensus Conference Nomenclature of Vasculitides. Arthritis and Rheumatism.
Copyright © 2012, John Wiley and Sons.

Table 130.1 Classification of the vasculitides by vessel size

Dominant vessel	Idiopathic (primary)	Probable aetiology (secondary)
Large	Takayasu	Syphilis
	Giant cell arteritis	Tuberculosis
		Aortitis—RA, AS
Medium	Polyarteritis nodosa (classical)	HBV associated polyarteritis nodosa
	Kawasaki's disease	
Small		
ANCA	Microscopic polyangiitis	Drugs (propylthiouracil, hydralazine)[a]
	Granulomatosis with polyangiitis	
	Eosinophilic granulomatosis with polyangiitis	
Immune complex	Anti-GBM disease	Cryoglobulinaemic (HCV)
	Cryoglobuinaemic vasculitis (non-HCV)	RA, SLE, Sjögren's syndrome
	IgA vasculitis	Serum sickness
	Hypocomplementaemic vasculitis	Drug induced[b]
Variable	Behçet's	
	Cogan's	

AS, ankylosing spondylitis; HBV, hepatitis B virus; HCV, hepatitis C virus; RA, rheumatoid arthritis; SLE, systemic lupus erythematosus.
[a]Most commonly induce MPO-ANCA.
[b]E.g. sulfonamides, penicillins, thiazide diuretics and many others.

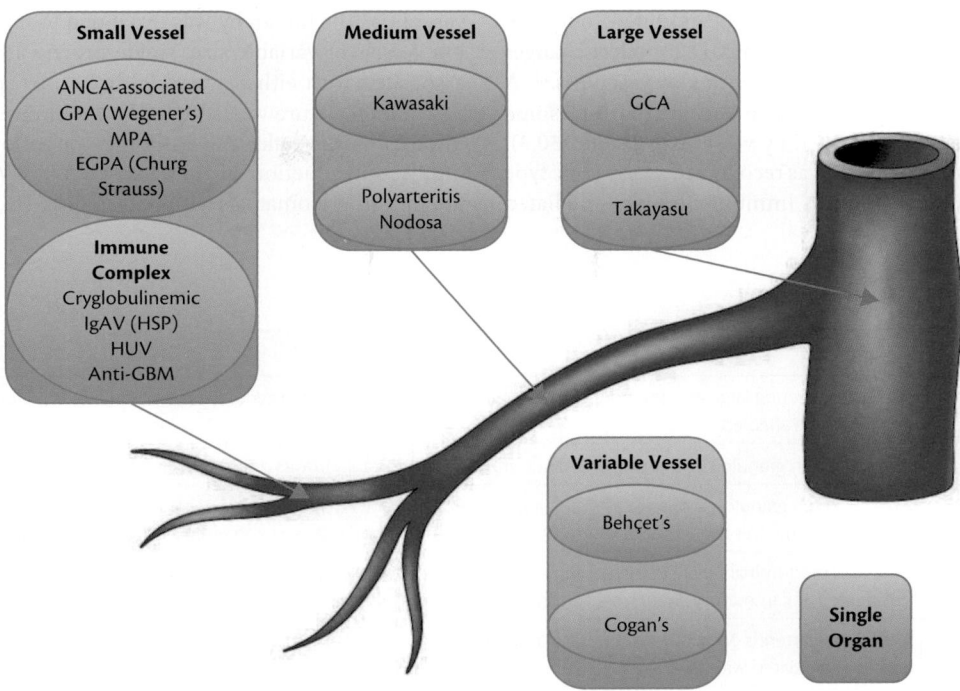

Fig. 130.2 Classification of vasculitis by vessel size.

Table 130.2 Relationship between vessel size and response to induction treatment

Dominant vessel	Corticosteroids alone	Cyclophosphamide and corticosteroids	Rituximab	Other treatments
Large arteries	+++	–	–	+
Medium arteries	+	++	–	++[a]
Small vessel (ANCA-associated)	+	+++	+++	+
Small vessel (immune complex)	++	+/–	+	++[a]

[a]Includes plasmapheresis, anti-viral therapy for hepatitis B-associated PAN and HCV-associated cryoglobulinaemia, and IVIg for Kawasaki disease.

nodosa (PAN), IgA vasculitis (Henoch–Schönlein purpura; IgAV), hypersensitivity vasculitis (HSV)—with sensitivities varying from 71.0% to 95.3% and specificities of 78.7–99.7%.[7–16] The most sensitive and specific criteria were found in EGPA, GCA, and TA; hypersensitivity (leucocytoclastic) vasculitis was the least well-defined condition. This development was important because it allowed epidemiological and clinical studies to be performed using established criteria. The ACR criteria have a number of drawbacks. The criteria were developed before the widespread introduction of ANCA testing, which now plays a key role in the diagnosis of many patients with GPA, MPA, EGPA (and also in PAN, because of its absence). In some circumstances ANCA may be used in place of tissue biopsy. The criteria also do not include MPA, which was not a term in common use during the 1980s. The criteria were established by comparing the clinical features of patients with established vasculitis, and identifying those features that contrasted between the different types of vasculitis. They were not established in an unselected group prior to the diagnosis of vasculitis or with other systemic diseases such as systemic lupus erythematosus (SLE) or other connective tissue diseases. The reliability of these criteria when used in patients in whom vasculitis is suspected but not yet diagnosed is poor.[17,18] However, it is important to stress that they were designed as classification criteria and not diagnostic criteria.

Chapel Hill Consensus definitions

In 1994, the Chapel Hill Consensus Conference (CHCC) produced definitions for vasculitis.[19] These included MPA, but they were not intended as either classification or diagnostic criteria. They recognized that histological data would not be available for all patients, especially when the clinical condition of the patient might preclude obtaining appropriate biopsies or the sample might not be representative and miss salient histological features. The concept of surrogate markers of vasculitis was therefore introduced. In addition, the importance of ANCA in diagnosis was recognized. However, neither surrogate markers nor ANCA were included in the definitions.

The CHCC definitions have recently been modified following an international consensus meeting held in 2011 to reflect changes in our understanding of the aetiopathogenesis of vasculitis.[20] A new tree hierarchy was developed which recognized that some conditions cannot be simply classified by vessel size (Table 130.3). ANCA-associated vasculitis (AAV) was recognized as a specific type of small-vessel vasculitis along with immune-complex-mediated vasculitis. The hierarchy was expanded to include vasculitis affecting vessels of variable size, single-organ vasculitis, and vasculitis associated with either systemic disease or specific aetiologies. A new nomenclature was adopted, with a move away from eponyms towards names reflecting pathology or aetiopathogenesis following the introduction of the term GPA for WG. The name 'eosinophilic granulomatosis with polyangiitis' (EGPA) was adopted for

Table 130.3 Revised Chapel Hill definitions

Name	Definition
Large-vessel vasculitis	Vasculitis affecting large arteries more often than other vasculitides. Large arteries are the aorta and its major branches. Any size artery may be affected
Takayasu's arteritis	Arteritis, often granulomatous, predominantly affecting the aorta and/or its major branches. Onset usually in patients <50 years
Giant cell arteritis	Arteritis, often granulomatous, usually affecting the aorta and/or its major branches, with a predilection for the branches of the carotid artery. Often involves the temporal artery. Onset usually in patients >50 years and often associated with polymyalgia rheumatica
Medium-vessel vasculitis	Vasculitis predominantly affecting medium-sized arteries defined as the main visceral arteries and their branches. Any size artery may be affected. Inflammatory aneurysms and stenoses are common
Polyarteritis nodosa	Necrotizing arteritis of medium-sized or small arteries without glomerulonephritis or vasculitis in arterioles, capillaries, or venules; and not associated with ANCA
Kawasaki's disease	Arteritis associated with the mucocutaneous lymph node syndrome and predominantly affecting medium-sized and small arteries. Coronary arteries are often involved. Aorta and large arteries may be involved. Usually occurs in infants and young children
Small-vessel vasculitis	Vasculitis predominantly affecting small vessels, defined as small intraparenchymal arteries, arterioles, capillaries and venules. Medium-sized arteries and veins may be affected
ANCA-associated vasculitis	Necrotizing vasculitis, with few or no immune deposits, predominantly affecting small vessels (i.e. capillaries, venules, arterioles and small arteries), associated with MPO-ANCA or PR3-ANCA. Not all patients have ANCA. Add a prefix indicating ANCA reactivity, e.g. PR3-ANCA, MPO-ANCA, ANCA-negative
Microscopic polyangiitis	Necrotizing vasculitis, with few or no immune deposits, predominantly affecting small vessels (i.e. capillaries, venules, or arterioles). Necrotizing arteritis involving small and medium-sized arteries may be present. Necrotizing glomerulonephritis is very common. Pulmonary capillaritis often occurs. Granulomatous inflammation is absent
Granulomatosis with polyangiitis (Wegener's)	Necrotizing granulomatous inflammation usually involving the upper and lower respiratory tract, and necrotizing vasculitis affecting predominantly small to medium-sized vessels (e.g., capillaries, venules, arterioles, arteries and veins). Necrotizing glomerulonephritis is common
Eosinophilic granulomatosis with polyangiitis (Churg–Strauss)	Eosinophil-rich and necrotizing granulomatous inflammation often involving the respiratory tract, and necrotizing vasculitis predominantly affecting small to medium-sized vessels, and associated with asthma and eosinophilia. ANCA is most frequent when glomerulonephritis is present
Immune complex small-vessel vasculitis	Vasculitis with moderate to marked vessel wall deposits of immunoglobulin and/or complement components predominantly affecting small vessels (i.e. capillaries, venules, arterioles and small arteries). Glomerulonephritis is frequent
Anti-GBM disease	Vasculitis affecting glomerular capillaries, pulmonary capillaries, or both, with basement membrane deposition of anti-basement membrane autoantibodies. Lung involvement causes pulmonary haemorrhage, and renal involvement causes glomerulonephritis with necrosis and crescents
Cryoglobulinaemic vasculitis	Vasculitis with cryoglobulin immune deposits affecting small vessels (predominantly capillaries, venules, or arterioles) and associated with cryoglobulins in serum. Skin and glomeruli are often involved
IgA vasculitis (Henoch–Schönlein)	Vasculitis, with IgA1-dominant immune deposits, affecting small vessels (predominantly capillaries, venules, or arterioles). Often involves skin and gut, and frequently causes arthritis. Glomerulonephritis indistinguishable from IgA nephropathy may occur
Hypocomplementaemic urticarial vasculitis (anti-C1q vasculitis)	Vasculitis accompanied by urticaria and hypocomplementemia affecting small vessels (i.e. capillaries, venules, or arterioles), and associated with anti-C1q antibodies. Glomerulonephritis, arthritis, obstructive pulmonary disease, and ocular inflammation are common.
Variable-vessel vasculitis	Vasculitis with no predominant type of vessel involved that can affect vessels of any size (small, medium, and large) and type (arteries, veins, and capillaries)
Behçet's disease	Vasculitis occurring in patients with Behçet's disease that can affect arteries or veins. Behçet's disease is characterized by recurrent oral and/or genital aphthous ulcers accompanied by cutaneous, ocular, articular, gastrointestinal, and/or central nervous system inflammatory lesions. Small-vessel vasculitis, thromboangiitis, thrombosis, arteritis and arterial aneurysms may occur

(Continued)

Table 130.3 (Continued)

Name	Definition
Cogan's syndrome	Vasculitis occurring in patients with Cogan's syndrome. Cogan's syndrome is characterized by ocular inflammatory lesions, including interstitial keratitis, uveitis, and episcleritis, and inner ear disease, including sensorineural hearing loss and vestibular dysfunction. Vasculitic manifestations may include arteritis (affecting small, medium or large arteries), aortitis, aortic aneurysms, and aortic and mitral valvulitis
Single-organ vasculitis	Vasculitis in arteries or veins of any size in a single organ that has no features that indicate that it is a limited expression of a systemic vasculitis. The involved organ and vessel type should be included in the name (e.g. cutaneous SVV, testicular arteritis, central nervous system vasculitis). Vasculitis distribution may be unifocal or multifocal (diffuse) within an organ. Some patients originally diagnosed with SOV will develop additional disease manifestations that warrant re-defining the case as one of the systemic vasculitides (e.g. cutaneous arteritis later becoming systemic polyarteritis nodosa, etc.)
Vasculitis associated with systemic disease	Vasculitis that is associated with and may be secondary to (caused by) a systemic disease. The name (diagnosis) should have a prefix term specifying the systemic disease (e.g. rheumatoid vasculitis, lupus vasculitis, etc.)
Vasculitis associated with probable aetiology	Vasculitis that is associated with a probable specific aetiology. The name (diagnosis) should have a prefix term specifying the association (e.g. hydralazine-associated microscopic polyangiitis, hepatitis B virus-associated vasculitis, hepatitis C virus-associated cryoglobulinemic vasculitis, etc.)

From Jennette et al.,[20] with permission.

Churg–Strauss syndrome and 'IgA vasculitis' (IgAV) for Henoch–Schönlein purpura. Definitions were developed for new categories of conditions including single-organ vasculitis, vasculitis associated with specific aetiologies including systemic disease (RA, SLE) and aetiologies such as infection (cryoglobulinaemia, hepatitis B and C), or drugs (e.g. propylthiouracil) (Table 130.3).

EMEA algorithm for classification of ANCA-associated vasculitis

In order to address the issues of lack of compatibility between the ACR (1990) criteria and the 1994 CHCC definitions for AAV and PAN; a consensus method of applying the two systems to facilitate epidemiology studies has been developed.[21] An algorithm was developed incorporating the key features of both systems. It is important to recognize that the algorithm was developed and validated for epidemiological studies rather than for clinical trials,[22] and its use in the latter setting requires validation. It also requires reassessment in light of the changes to the CHCC definitions made in 2011.

Polyarteritis nodosa and microscopic polyangiitis

One of the main problems with the ACR criteria is that they do not include MPA and consequently the ability to distinguish between PAN and MPA is poor. Henegar and colleagues recently conducted a detailed study of 949 patients with systemic vasculitis in the French Vasculitis Study Group database with the aim of developing better criteria for PAN.[23] They introduced the concept of negative predictive parameters in addition to positive ones. Of the original 10 ACR criteria they retained only 3 (hepatitis B virus antigen, arteriographic abnormalities, and polyneuropathy). They introduced 5 negative criteria including negative indirect immunofluorescence detection of ANCA. These criteria had 70.6% sensitivity against all vasculitis controls with 92.3% specificity. When compared against MPA there was 89.7% sensitivity and 83.1% specificity. The discriminant ability of this set of items performs better than the ACR (1990) criteria in all settings. These criteria remain to be validated as diagnostic criteria.

EULAR/PReS criteria for childhood vasculitis

A EULAR/PReS working group has recently developed classification criteria for childhood vasculitis (see Chapter 136) using a Delphi technique.[24] There was agreement to classify childhood vasculitis according to vessel size, with small-vessel diseases subdivided into granulomatous and non-granulomatous. Classification criteria were developed for IgAV (Henoch–Schönlein purpura), Kawasaki's disease (KD), childhood PAN, GPA, and TA. These criteria have not yet been validated.

In conclusion, the classification of vasculitis both for studies and for diagnostic purposes remains a considerable challenge. The new CHCC definitions are a useful step forward, but the development of validated criteria for both classification and diagnosis is urgently needed.[25]

Diagnosis of vasculitis

The diagnosis of vasculitis is often difficult, especially in early disease because of the heterogeneity of presentation and organ involvement. There are no diagnostic criteria, but classification criteria designed to differentiate one vasculitis from another rather than making the diagnosis. Vasculitis is an important diagnosis because of the potential consequences of untreated disease. The spectrum ranges from a minor rash to life-threatening systemic disease and vasculitis needs to be considered within the differential diagnosis of any multisystem disorder. Particularly severe consequences of vasculitis which must be avoided where possible include blindness or stroke in patients with GCA; renal failure leading to dialysis and possible death, especially in AAV; heart disease with coronary aneurysm formation in patients with KD prior to effective treatment. Granulomatosis with polyangiitis (Wegener's) historically had a very poor prognosis with a life expectancy of only 5 months from diagnosis in patients with renal involvement.[26] This was prior to the introduction of immunosuppressive treatment with cyclophosphamide and corticosteroids which have dramatically improved the outlook to a mortality of 11% at 1 year.[27] Early diagnosis and early treatment are therefore essential.

Vasculitis can affect the whole age spectrum from infancy (KD) through to the very elderly (age >90 years). Age has a very clear influence on the clinical phenotype. KD is entirely a disease of infancy occurring chiefly in children aged less than 2 years and very rarely after 5 years of age. IgAV (Henoch–Schönlein purpura) is mainly a disease of childhood and adolescence, but occurs infrequently in adults. At the other end of the spectrum GCA is uncommon before the age of 60 years but there is a rapid increase in age specific incidence peaking in those aged over 80 years. The AAV can occur at all ages but are most common in those aged 65–75 years.[28]

Increased diagnostic awareness over the past two decades especially has been associated with increased recognition of most vasculitides. This is particularly true for the AAV where introduction of ANCA testing in the 1980s greatly increased the recognition of the disease and decreased the diagnostic delay from 17 to 4 months.[29] Diagnostic delay is still a major problem, however, particularly for the rarer conditions. In GCA widespread recognition of the importance of quick introduction of glucocorticoid therapy in patients presenting with new-onset headache has reduced the risk of visual loss.[30]

A number of other diseases can mimic systemic vasculitis (Table 130.4). These mimics usually present with multiorgan illness or evidence of vascular damage or a combination of both. Simple blood tests such as the acute-phase response—erythrocyte sedimentation rate (ESR), C-reactive protein (CRP)—can be misleading as they may be elevated as a consequence of tissue damage rather than an underlying inflammatory process; tissue biopsy is still essential to identify non-inflammatory vascular changes such as embolism or thrombosis. Angiography shows aneurysms typically in PAN, but they have also been described in patients with atrial myxoma and subacute bacterial endocarditis.

A careful drug history is important, as many drugs have been associated with vasculitis. Most of these drugs have been described as causing a small-vessel vasculitis in the skin. Propylthiouracil and hydrallazine are associated with development of a systemic small vasculitis and the presence of MPO-ANCA. It is likely in these cases that the drugs act as a trigger for the vasculitis and withdrawal of the drugs may be sufficient to suppress the disease.[31] These patients may also require conventional immunosuppressive treatment, especially if there is significant organ- or life-threatening disease.

There are six essential components for making a diagnosis of vasculitis:

1. recognition that the patient might have vasculitis

2. a compatible clinical phenotype

3. consistent serology (e.g. ANCA) or radiology (e.g. angiography)

4. confirmation by histology

5. exclusion of mimics and secondary causes of vasculitis (see Table 130.4)

6. the increased certainty of diagnosis with time.

Presenting symptoms and signs

Presentation is often non-specific with features including low-grade fever, weight loss, and malaise which may last several months. Where the prodromal phase is short, reactive vasculitis such as IgAV (Henoch–Schönlein purpura) or a secondary vasculitis is more likely. Constitutional symptoms vary in intensity and may

Table 130.4 Vasculitis mimics

Systemic multisystem disease	
Infection	Infective endocarditis (neisseria, rikettsia)
Malignancy Paraneoplastic syndromes	Metastatic carcinoma
Occlusive vasculopathy	
Embolic	Cholesterol crystals
	Atrial myxoma
	Infection
Thrombotic	APS
	Procoagulant states
	Calciphylaxis
Others	Ergot
	Radiation
	Kohlmeier–Degos
	Severe Raynaud's
	Acute digital loss
	Exposure to cold
Angiographic mimics	
Aneurysmal	Congenital abnormalities
	Fibromuscular dysplasia
	Neurofibromatosis
	Marfan's
	Loyes–Dietz syndrome
	Ehlers–Danlos type IV
Occlusion	Amyloidosis
	Coarctation
Others	
	Scurvy
	Sweet syndrome
	Cocaine abuse
	Moyamoya disease

not be present in patients with organ-limited disease (e.g. cutaneous PAN). Kidney involvement can also present with relatively few systemic symptoms or signs, stressing the importance in all patients of repeated urinalysis for protein and blood.

Because of the widespread and different organ involvement in the various diseases, the clue to diagnosis is often the combination of involvement of one or more organs together with compatible blood tests. For example, the combination of proteinuria/haematuria with arthralgia and weight loss will make vasculitis particularly likely if accompanied by any one of the following: skin lesions such as purpura; chronic or persistent ENT symptoms such as nose bleeds/crusting; eye inflammation, particularly iritis/scleritis; neuropathy, particularly an acute motor neuropathy.

The range of organ involvement and the range of symptoms and signs is variable. Suggestive involvement of the skin includes palpable purpura, deep cutaneous ulcers in unusual sites, and skin infarction; ENT symptoms include epistaxis, crusting, sinusitis, and acute deafness; respiratory symptoms include non-productive cough, haemoptysis, shortness of breath, and wheezing; neurological symptoms range from mild sensory to widespread motor neuropathy, but the acuteness of onset is more indicative of an underlying vasculitis; gastrointestinal symptoms are often non-specific but include mouth ulcers, bloody diarrhoea, and non-specific abdominal pain. Although cardiac involvement is not uncommon, symptoms are usually non-specific such as chest pain and palpitations associated with arrhythmia. An acutely painful red eye suggesting iritis or scleritis associated with a multiorgan disease is also an important combination often indicating vasculitis. In patients with suspected larger-vessel vasculitis (TA or GCA) pulses should be assessed in four limbs together with blood pressure. Absence of pulses or differential blood pressure between limbs is suggestive of vasculitis.

An assessment tool developed for clinical trials in vasculitis is the Birmingham Vasculitis Score (BVAS). This is a useful aide mémoire for assessing patients with vasculitis and the detailed different organ involvement provide a useful reminder of the widespread nature of vasculitis and the more likely symptoms and signs associated with it. For large-vessel vasculitis, jaw claudication, visual disturbance, and temporal artery tenderness are particularly important features of GCA whereas for TA the absence of peripheral pulses or bruits over large arteries and tenderness over large arteries, particularly the carotid artery, are useful clinical findings.

Laboratory investigations

These may be divided into screening investigations of non-specific nature indicating inflammation, tests to identify specific organ involvement, and diagnostic investigations including serology (Box 130.1).

A patient with suspected systemic vasculitis should be assessed urgently, as the prognosis may be adversely affected by diagnostic delay. Renal involvement should be assessed with urinalysis as the presence of blood and protein with casts is indicative of glomerulonephritis. A poor long-term prognosis is associated with a raised serum creatinine at diagnosis.[27]

The non-specific investigations can sometimes provide useful clues to diagnosis. A full blood count will often reveal anaemia and in some cases this can be severe due to blood loss. If the white cell count reveals significant eosinophilia, the most likely diagnosis is EGPA (Churg–Strauss syndrome) or a drug reaction. A mild eosinophilia can be a feature of GPA (Wegener's). Leucopenia is unusual in systemic vasculitis and more likely to represent either severe sepsis or autoimmune diseases such as SLE, but has recently been described in vasculitis induced by levamisole-contaminated cocaine.[32] The acute-phase response (ESR and CRP) is almost always high in all types of vasculitis. Serum creatinine/eGFR are important screening tests but it is important to remember that significant renal impairment has to occur before there is a major change in these. Severe abnormalities of liver function is seen particularly in patients with hepatitis B or C associated disease but mild changes in the alkaline phosphatase or gamma-glutamyl transferase frequently just indicate low-grade inflammation. A thrombophilia screen is important to look for mimics such as a thrombotic tendency and plasma protein electrophoresis for systemic diseases such as myeloproliferative disorders.

Serology

ANCA testing is a vital part of vasculitis assessment, being associated particularly with a group of small-vessel vasculitides—GPA,

---

Box 130.1 Investigation of suspected vasculitis

General

- FBC anaemia, leucocytosis, eosinophils (eosinophilia suggestive of EGPA)
- Acute-phase response (ESR and CRP)
- Liver function

Assessment of organ involvement in all patients

- Urinalysis (proteinuria, haematuria, red cell casts), should be performed urgently in all patients in whom systemic vasculitis is suspected
- Renal function (creatinine clearance, quantification of protein leak if present using either 24 hour protein excretion or urine protein/creatinine ratio).
- CXR may show infiltrates, haemorrhage, granuloma (especially GPA, EGPA, MPA).
- Liver function.

Where appropriate

- Nervous system (nerve conduction studies in all four limbs, biopsy)
- Cardiac function (ECG, echocardiography)
- Gut (coeliac axis angiography)
- Biopsy of an affected organ should be obtained where possible to confirm diagnosis prior to treatment

Serological investigations

- ANCA: A cANCA pattern on indirect immunofluorescence and PR3 by ELISA are together strongly associated with GPA(>90%). pANCA and MPO is suggestive of MPA or EGPA. Both indirect immunofluorescence and ELISA for PR3/MPO should be performed in all patients
- ANA: ENA profile if positive ANA
- RF (may be positive in cryoglobulinaemic vasculitis or systemic rheumatoid vasculitis)
- Anti-cardiolipin antibodies (usually negative, but if positive consider anti-phospholipid syndrome and B2GPI antibodies).
- Complement (C3, C4 low in cryoglobulinaemic vasculitis)
- Cryoglobulins (suggestive of cryoglobulinaemic vasculitis)

Differential diagnosis

This is from vasculitis mimics (e.g. malignancy, cholesterol embolism, atrial myxoma, calciphylaxis—see Table 130.4) or infection (especially subacute bacterial endocarditis).

- Blood cultures
- Viral serology (HBV, HCV, HIV, CMV)
- Echocardiography (two-dimensional and/or transoesophageal)

ANA, anti-nuclear antibodies; ANCA, anti-neutrophil cytoplasmic antibodies; CMV, cytomegalovirus; CRP, C-reactive protein; CXR, chest radiograph; EGPA, eosinophilic granulomatosis with polyangiitis; ENA, extractable nuclear antigens; ESR, erythrocyte sedimentation rate; GPA, granulomatosis with polyangiitis; HBV, hepatitis B virus; HCV, hepatitis C virus; MPA, microscopic polyangiitis; RF, rheumatoid factor.

MPA, and EGPA. A negative ANCA is an important feature of classical PAN. ANCA testing needs to be undertaken carefully as non-specific ANCA staining on immunofluorescence can be associated with a range of systemic illnesses including infection and inflammatory bowel disease. Screening is frequently undertaken by immunofluorescence; with cytoplasmic staining being associated with proteinase-3 (PR3) specificity and GPA, and perinuclear staining with myeloperoxidase specificity and MPA and EGPA. However, reliance on indirect immunofluorescence (IIF) pattern alone is insufficient for diagnosis as this is less specific and ELISA testing for PR3 and myeloperoxidase (MPO) specificity is essential in all cases.[33] The combination of cANCA and PR3 is has a specificity of 90% for GPA and pANCA-MPO 75% for MPA.[34] ANCA titres may be influenced by treatment and ANCA can be negative in early mild or limited disease, particularly GPA. Other autoantibodies are also important for diagnosis. The presence of anti-nuclear antibodies (ANA) and DNA antibodies are highly suggestive of SLE, and specific ENA antibodies such as anti-Ro and -La are associated with Sjögren's syndrome as well as SLE. Rheumatoid factor is frequently present in low titre but anti-CCP antibodies are more specific for RA and likely to indicate the vasculitis being associated with RA. Complement levels (C3 and C4) are usually elevated in patients with systemic vasculitis as part of an acute inflammatory response: low levels usually indicate immune complex vasculitides (Table 130.1) such as SLE, hypocomplementaemic urticarial vasculitis, and cryoglobulinaemic vasculitis. Anti-cardiolipin antibodies are associated with the anti-phospholipid antibody syndrome—a mimic of systemic vasculitis causing skin or digital infarction as a consequence of thrombosis. Cryoglobulins are most frequently seen in cryoglobulinaemic vasculitis (often associated with hepatitis C infection) but low levels of cryoglobulins are not uncommon in other systemic vasculitides.

Organ-specific investigations

Assessment of kidney function such as eGFR, urinalysis, and urine protein excretion are important to identify that the kidney is involved and the function of the kidney. However, the most useful tissue for diagnostic assessment and prognosis is renal biopsy, particularly in the AAV. The characteristic change in AAV is a focal segmental necrotizing glomerulonephritis but the presence of crescents indicates more severe disease and the present of significant scarring reflects more chronic disease associated with a worse prognosis. Any significant organ involvement should trigger a specialist review which itself is an important part of investigation. Chest radiography may reveal a wide range of features; for example, nodules/fixed infiltrates in GPA, flitting shadowing in EGPA, and widespread changes indicating pulmonary haemorrhage in MPA. CT, bronchoscopy, and lung biopsy may be considered in some cases, again alongside specialist review. Orbital assessment is now highly specialized and investigations include orbital CT and MRI scanning. Subtle nerve involvement may only be detected by nerve conduction studies; nerve biopsy (sural and radial) are useful diagnostic tests if other tissue is not available for biopsy. The widespread nature of neurological involvement may require cerebrospinal fluid (CSF) examination, cerebral MRI and angiography (especially for isolated central nervous system vasculitis). Cardiac assessment includes ECG, echocardiography, and in some cases specialist cardiac MRI scanning and coronary angiography.

Investigations are also essential to exclude vasculitis mimics and secondary vasculitis. These include blood culture, viral screen, and echocardiography (to exclude rarities such as atrial myxoma and bacterial endocarditis as well as assessing possible cardiac involvement).

Coeliac axis and mesenteric angiography may be needed to diagnose PAN. The extent of large-vessel involvement in TA and GCA should be assessed using MR angiography; this enables assessment of inflammation as well the anatomical extent. Patients presenting with multisystem illness with no histological evidence in whom malignancy is suspected may be investigated by [18]FDG-PET scan. This is useful for demonstrating inflammation of large vessels in GCA and TA. Temporal artery biopsy is still the most useful diagnostic test for GCA; however, this must be performed within 10 days of the introduction of high-dose glucocorticoids, beyond this time the rate of positive biopsies decreases.

Conclusion

The diagnosis of systemic vasculitis depends on the presence of a pattern of supportive clinical features, supported by specific investigations (serology, radiology, etc.) and almost always confirmed by biopsy. It is also important to exclude other causes, particularly mimics of vasculitis and 'secondary' causes for vasculitis. Investigations can be inconclusive and vasculitis may be suspected and under these circumstances observation over time with repeat investigations and possibly a therapeutic trial of immunosuppressive drugs including corticosteroids. There are no current diagnostic (as opposed to classification) criteria. The development of diagnostic criteria is eagerly awaited and the evolution of Chapel Hill 1994 to Chapel Hill 2012 with updated definitions and descriptions of vasculitis have helped improve our understanding and classification of the different vasculitic diseases.

References

1. Kussmaul A, Maier R. Uber eine nicht bisher beschriebene eigenthumliche Arterienerkrankung (Periarteritis nodosa), die mit Morbus Brightii und rapid fortschreitender allgemeiner Muskelahmung einhergeht. *Deutsche Archiv Klin Med* 1866;1:484–518.

2. Matteson EL. A history of early investigation in polyarteritis nodosa. *Arthritis Care Res* 1999;12:294–302.

3. Zeek PM. Periarteritis nodosa; a critical review. *Am J Clin Pathol* 1952;22:777–790.

4. Davson J BJ, Platt R. The kidney in periarteritis nodosa. *Q J Med* 1948;17:175–202.

5. Falk RJ, Gross WL, Guillevin L et al. Granulomatosis with polyangiitis (Wegener's)': an alternative name for 'Wegener's granulomatosis'. A joint proposal of the American College of Rheumatology, the American Society of Nephrology, and the European League Against Rheumatism. *Arthritis Rheum* 2011; 863–864.

6. Ntatsaki E, Mooney J, Watts RA. Time to change the treatment paradigm of ANCA vasculitis.? Not yet. *Rheumatology* 2011; 1019–1024.

7. Fries JF, Hunder GG, Bloch DA et al. The American College of Rheumatology 1990 criteria for the classification of vasculitis. Summary. *Arthritis Rheum* 1990;33(8):1135–1136.

8. Arend WP, Michel BA, Bloch DA et al. The American College of Rheumatology 1990 criteria for the classification of Takayasu arteritis. *Arthritis Rheum* 1990;33(8):1129–1134.

9. Bloch DA, Michel BA, Hunder GG et al. The American College of Rheumatology 1990 criteria for the classification of vasculitis. Patients and methods. *Arthritis Rheum* 1990;33(8):1068–1073.

10. Calabrese LH, Michel BA, Bloch DA et al. The American College of Rheumatology 1990 criteria for the classification of hypersensitivity vasculitis. *Arthritis Rheum* 1990;33(8):1108–1113.

11. Hunder GG, Arend WP, Bloch DA et al. The American College of Rheumatology 1990 criteria for the classification of vasculitis. Introduction. *Arthritis Rheum* 1990;33(8):1065–1067.

12. Hunder GG, Bloch DA, Michel BA et al. The American College of Rheumatology 1990 criteria for the classification of giant cell arteritis. *Arthritis Rheum* 1990;33(8):1122–1128.

13. Leavitt RY, Fauci AS, Bloch DA et al. The American College of Rheumatology 1990 criteria for the classification of Wegener's granulomatosis. *Arthritis Rheum* 1990;33(8):1101–1107.

14. Lightfoot RW, Jr., Michel BA, Bloch DAet al. The American College of Rheumatology 1990 criteria for the classification of polyarteritis nodosa. *Arthritis Rheum* 1990;33(8):1088–1093.

15. Masi AT, Hunder GG, Lie JT et al. The American College of Rheumatology 1990 criteria for the classification of Churg-Strauss syndrome (allergic granulomatosis and angiitis). *Arthritis Rheum* 1990;33(8):1094–1100.

16. Mills JA, Michel BA, Bloch DA et al. The American College of Rheumatology 1990 criteria for the classification of Henoch-Schonlein purpura. *Arthritis Rheum* 1990;33(8):1114–1121.

17. Rao JK, Allen NB, Pincus T. Limitations of the 1990 American College of Rheumatology classification criteria in the diagnosis of vasculitis. *Ann Intern Med* 1998;129(5):345–352.

18. Watts RA, Suppiah R, Merkel PA, Luqmani RA. Systemic Vasculitis—is it time to reclassify. *Rheumatology* 2011; 50; 643–545.

19. Jennette JC, Falk RJ, Andrassy K et al. Nomenclature of systemic vasculitides. Proposal of an international consensus conference. *Arthritis Rheum* 1994;37(2):187–192.

20. Jennette JC, Falk RJ, Bacon PA et al. Revised International Chapel Hill Consensus Conference Nomenclature of the Vasculitides. *Arthritis Rheum* 2013;65(1):1–11.

21. Watts R, Lane S, Hanslik T et al. Development and validation of a consensus methodology for the classification of the ANCA-associated vasculitides and polyarteritis nodosa for epidemiological studies. *Ann Rheum Dis* 2007;66:222–227.

22. Liu LJ, Chen M, Yu F, Zhao MH, Wang HY. Evaluation of a new algorithm in classification of systemic vasculitis. *Rheumatology* (Oxford) 2008;47:708–712.

23. Henegar C, Pagnoux C, Puechal X et al. A paradigm of diagnostic criteria for polyarteritis nodosa: analysis of a series of 949 patients with vasculitides. *Arthritis Rheum* 2008;58:1528–1538.

24. Ozen S, Ruperto N, Dillon MJ et al. EULAR/PReS endorsed consensus criteria for the classification of childhood vasculitides. *Ann Rheumatic Dis* 2006;65:936–941.

25. Luqmani RA, Suppiah R, Grayson P, Merkel P, Watts RA. Nomenclature and classification of vasculitis—update on the ACR/EULAR diagosis and classification study (DCVAS). *Clin Exp Immunol* 2011;164 (suppl 1): 11–13.

26. Walton EW: Giant-cell granuloma of the respiratory tract (Wegener's granulomatosis). *Br Med J* 1958; 2:265–269.

27. Little MA, Nightingale P, Verburgh CA et al. Early mortality in systemic vasculitis: relative contribution of adverse events and active vasculitis. *Ann Rheum Dis* 2010;69:1036–1043.

28. Watts RA, Ntatsaki E. Epidemiology of systemic vasculitis. *Rheum Dis Clin North Am.* 2010;36:447–461.

29. Takala JH, Kautiainen H, Malmberg H, Leirisalo-Repo M. Incidence of Wegener's granulomatosis in Finland 1981–2000. *Clin Exp Rheumatol* 2008;26:S81–S85.

30. Gonzalez-Gay MA, Miranda-Filloy JA, Lopez-Diaz MJ et al. Giant cell arteritis in North Western Spain: a 25 year epidemiological study. *Medicine* (Baltimore) 2007;86:61–68.

31. Gao Y, Chen M, Yu F, Guo XH, Zhao MH. Long-term outcomes of patients with propylthiouracil induced anti-neutrophil cytoplasmic auto-antibody associated vascultiis. *Rheumatology* 2008;47:1515–1520.

32. Graf J, Lynch K, Yeh C-L et al. Purpura, cutaneous necrosis, and antineutrophil cytoplasmic antibodies associated with levamisole-adulterated cocaine. *Arthritis Rheum* 2011;63:3998–4001.

33. Savige J, Gillis D, Benson E et al. International consensus statement on testing and reporting of anti-neutrophil cytoplasmic antibodies (ANCA). *Am J Clin Pathol* 1999;111:507–513.

34. Hagen EC, Daha MR, Hermans J et al. Diagnostic value of standardised assays for anti-neutrophil cytoplasmic antibodies in idiopathic systemic vasculitis. EC/BCR project for ANCA assay standardisation. *Kidney Int* 1998;53:743–753.

CHAPTER 131

Clinical features of ANCA-associated vasculitis

Wolfgang L. Gross and Julia U. Holle

Definitions, classification criteria, disease stages, and epidemiology

The vasculitides are categorized according to the 1990 classification criteria of the American College of Rheumatology (ACR) and the 1994 Chapel Hill Consensus Definition (CCHD), which have recently (2012) been revised (Table 131.1).[1–4] The common feature of all ANCA-associated vasculitides (AAV) is small- to medium-size vessel vasculitis. Granulomatosis with polyangiitis (GPA, Wegener's) and eosinophilic granulomatosis with polyangiitis (EGPA, Churg–Strauss syndrome) are characterized by additional clinical and histological findings such as granulomatous lesions of the upper and/or lower respiratory tract in GPA and asthma, hypereosinophilia, and eosinophilic organ infiltration in EGPA. Recently, a four-step algorithm has been developed to distinguish between the vasculitides on the basis of the ACR criteria, the Chapel Hill Consensus Conference Criteria (CHCC) definitions, and the Lanham criteria for EGPA/CSS (Figure 131.1).[5] Importantly, these classification criteria and consensus definitions do not represent diagnostic criteria although they are often used as such in clinical practice. Yet, classification criteria and disease definitions should only be applied if the diagnosis of vasculitis is already established, to distinguish between the distinct forms. Diagnostic criteria in vasculitides are currently being developed.

The overall incidence of AAV is estimated at 10–20 million per year and the peak onset is from 65 to 74 years.[6] Most of the studies report stable incidence rates for the AAV over the past two decades (e.g. in the United Kingdom and Germany).[6] Incidence rates of 2.95–12 per million per year have been reported for GPA in Europe with lower rates in southern Europe (e.g. 2.95 per million per year in Spain[6]) compared to central and northern Europe (United Kingdom, Germany, and Norway[6]). In contrast, incidence rates of MPA are higher in Spain (11.6 per million per year) compared to other European countries (2.6–5.8 per million per year in Germany, Norway, and the United Kingdom).[6] Interestingly, a similar overall incidence rate was reported for GPA/MPA in Japan and the United Kingdom, but in Japan MPA was the predominant entity (83%) whereas GPA is more frequent in the United Kingdom (66%).[6] These findings suggest that GPA and MPA are genetically different diseases and linked to different ethnic backgrounds. EGPA

is generally rarer than the other AAV with an incidence of 1.0–3.0 per million per year.[6]

The AAV, particularly GPA, follow a stagewise course which has been formally defined by the European Vasculitis Study Group (EUVAS) in order to facilitate clinical studies and develop evidence-based treatment regimens for the different disease stages(Table 131.2).[7] Disease manifestations are restricted to the upper and lower respiratory tract in the localized disease stage. Importantly, there are no clinical signs of vasculitis and no constitutional symptoms in this stage. Typical initial nasal manifestations are bloody nasal discharge and crusting. Localized disease in GPA may be complicated by granulomatous inflammation and mass formation in sinuses, orbit and lungs (see below) which can lead to destruction of cartilage and bony structures.[8] Early systemic disease is defined as non-organ-threatening or life-threatening vasculitis and is characterized by manifestations such as episcleritis or purpura; the generalized stage corresponds to full-blown disease with organ-threatening vasculitis manifestations (e.g. crescentic necrotizing glomerulonephritis, pulmonary capillaritis). Acute organ failure is consistent with the severe disease stage (e.g. creatinine >500 µmol/litre).[7]

Organ manifestations of the AAV can be categorized according to disease extent index (DEI),[9] which is widely used in clinical practice to give an overview of organs involved. Disease activity and chronic organ damage induced by vasculitis or its treatment can be determined by validated scoring instruments such as the Birmingham Vasculitis Activity Score (BVAS) and the Vasculitis Damage index (VDI), respectively.[10–12]

Pathogenesis

Environmental and genetic risk factors

Occupational exposures such as to silica from specific farming tasks related to harvesting have been suggested to be associated with AAV in case-control studies,[13] but the data is controversial.[14] Furthermore, drugs have been implicated in the induction of ANCA and AAV (see below).

Anti-asthmatic medications such as leukotriene receptor antagonists, inhaled glucocorticoids such as fluticasone, inhaled β_2-mimetics such as salmeterole and omalizumab and other drugs such

a longer course of 12 cyclophosphamide pulses more effective than 6 in achievement of stable remission. Over one-third of EGPA patients suffer persisting steroid-dependent asthma after control of their vasculitis.

Induction treatment in children and the elderly

The approach to therapy and responsiveness to medication is the same in the young and the old as in other age groups, but drug selection and dosing may differ. In view of the fertility and malignancy risks of cyclophosphamide, alternative use of mycophenolate mofetil or rituximab has been suggested. Higher glucocorticoid doses, up to 2 mg/kg per day, are used in children, due to increased rates of elimination. Elderly patients are more likely to present with renal impairment and have a high risk of infective complications. It is important to reduce cyclophosphamide accordingly (Table 132.5). Lower cyclophosphamide dosing, fixed at 500 mg IV pulses, and reduced glucocorticoid exposure with more rapid tapering have been proposed. Glucocorticoid withdrawal in the remission period is desirable to reduce the risk of osteoporosis.

Remission maintenance therapy

Disease relapse occurs in 75% of GPA and 30% of MPA and EGPA cases by 5 years.[39] The goals of maintenance therapy are to prevent disease relapse while minimizing drug toxicity. Cyclophosphamide is withdrawn after 3–6 months and substituted by azathioprine 2 mg/kg per day, or methotrexate, up to 25 mg/week. They were equally effective for remission maintenance with similar safety risks in the WEGENT trial.[40] Methotrexate is excreted by the kidneys and should be avoided in the presence of renal impairment (GFR <50 mL/min). Although rare, concerns over methotrexate pneumonitis complicate its use in the presence of pulmonary vasculitis. Leflunomide, 20 mg/day, was superior to methotrexate for the prevention of relapse in a small GPA study but mycophenolate mofetil was less effective than azathioprine for relapse prevention after cyclophosphamide induction therapy.[41,42]

Prednisolone is either continued in conjunction with an immunosuppressive at doses of 5–10 mg/day or is withdrawn at the end of the induction phase. There is an increased relapse risk following steroid withdrawal which has to be balanced against the toxicity of long-term administration.[43]

There is no clear guidance as to how long remission maintenance treatment should be continued. The IMPROVE trial withdraw therapy 42 months after diagnosis, but withdrawal after 24 months has also been suggested. The various factors that influence relapse risk should be considered (Table 132.2) along with the likely consequences of relapse for the individual patient.[18,19] Most relapses are minor and do not increased the risk of death or organ failure, but delayed relapse diagnosis is a real concern and renal relapse increases the risk of ESRD. The most frequent factors that would support prolonged treatment are PR3-ANCA at diagnosis, ENT involvement, and persisting ANCA positivity.[44] There should be consideration for prolonged low-dose immunosuppression in these cases.

Management of relapse

The symptoms and signs of relapse in an individual patient reflect those present prior to the original diagnosis. The diagnosis of relapse needs to be differentiated from infection or other potential causes, including malignancy. Infection may precede and precipitate relapse and this is a particular issue with bacterial infections in respiratory tract relapse in GPA. Relapse is categorized as minor (non-severe), or major (severe) when vasculitic activity threatens vital organ function. Renal relapse is initially manifested by a return or increase in haematuria with proteinuria with subsequent deterioration in renal function and is usually, but not always, associated with ANCA positivity and rises in erythrocyte sedimentation rate (ESR) and CRP. Repeat renal biopsy is indicated if there is uncertainty as to whether or not renal relapse is occurring.

Minor relapse is treated by optimization of the background immunosuppressive, such as azathioprine or methotrexate, and increase in prednisolone to 0.5–1.0 mg/kg per day with a reducing regimen back to 5–10 mg/day. When the immunosuppressive dose is limited by adverse events, or if minor relapses recur, an alternative immunosuppressive or switch to rituximab should be considered. Major relapse is treated by introduction of cyclophosphamide or rituximab and a similar increase in prednisolone.[20] Data from the RAVE trial showed a higher rate of response to rituximab than to cyclophosphamide in this subgroup.[12]

Refractory disease

Progression of vasculitis despite induction therapy, failure to attain disease remission, and disease relapse while receiving maintenance therapy are defined as refractory disease (Table 132.3).[22] Before therapy is enhanced, causes for refractory disease—including infection, malignancy, and drugs—should be considered, as well as non-concordance with the prescribed regimen. Drug intolerance, especially to glucocorticoids or cyclophosphamide, and reductions in dosing due to intercurrent infection may also lead to primary treatment failure. This situation is associated with a high mortality due to the presence of organ failure and the risks of prolonged therapy.[45]

Progressive or non-responsive disease occurs in 5–10% and is treated with an increase in glucocorticoid, typically IV pulsed methylprednisolone 1000–3000 mg. Relative cyclophosphamide under dosing is indicated by a failure to induce lymphopenia and is more common with IV pulsed administration. A switch to daily oral cyclophosphamide or an increase in IV dosing has been suggested. Changing from cyclophosphamide to rituximab is now more attractive because rituximab is less likely to increase the infective risk. Failure to induce B-cell depletion indicates that rituximab will be ineffective. Where the response to rituximab appears slow, pulse cyclophosphamide can be added until response is seen, but cyclophosphamide is not routinely required with rituximab.

For resistant renal vasculitis or alveolar haemorrhage plasma exchange is used. Intravenous immunoglobulin reduces disease activity in refractory AAV but the effect lasts less than 3 months.[46] This option can be considered if conventional therapy is contraindicated, for example by infection or in pregnancy. A potential mechanism of immunoglobulin, as proposed in Kawasaki disease, is the neutralization of microbial toxins. Blockade of tumour necrosis factor alpha (TNFα) with infliximab or etanercept has led to remission when used also as an additional agent but prolonged use appears ineffective and it may increase the risks of infection.[24,47] Concerns over malignancy risk with anti-TNF therapy in vasculitis have not been supported by longer-term studies.[48]

Patients failing to achieve remission by 6 months, or possibly before, should have their non-glucocorticoid treatment reassessed as for progressive disease. Deoxyspergualin (Gusperimus) is an immunosuppressive with a range of activity on the innate and cognate immune systems that has demonstrated high response levels in refractory GPA.[49] Leucopenia is common but rapidly reversible and not accompanied by increased infection frequency. There does not appear to be a sustained effect after deoxyspergualin withdrawal when relapses are common. Lymphocyte, eosinophil, and macrophage depletion with the anti-CD52 therapeutic antibody alemtuzumab has led to sustained treatment-free remissions.[50] The profound, transient lymphopenia induced by alemtuzumab is poorly tolerated in those over 60 or with impaired renal function.

Those relapsing are treated as described above with multiple minor relapses or at least one major relapse requiring a change of immunosuppressive. Changing the non-cyclophosphamide immunosuppressive, for example from azathioprine to methotrexate, or vice versa, or switching to mycophenolic acid preparations or leflunomide, can be considered.[51,52] After a major relapse or after a failure of at least one alternative immunosuppressive for minor relapses, rituximab is indicated.

EGPA can pursue a primary progressive course requiring repeated courses of IV steroid; intravenous immunoglobulin and plasma exchange have also been used.[53] However, a more common problem in EGPA is relapse as glucocorticoids are reduced. Such patients are at risk of high glucocorticoid exposure and alternative strategies should be pursued to permit glucocorticoid reduction to conventional maintenance levels. A change in immunosuppressive may be effective in non-severe disease. Rituximab, alemtuzumab, interferon-α and mepolizumab, an anti-interleukin (IL)-5 monoclonal antibody, have been used in this setting.[54]

Management of damage

Ear, nose, and throat disease in GPA has a high risk of causing irreversible damage and chronic symptomatology. Collapse of the bridge of the nose can be corrected by bone or cartilage grafts and restorative procedures should be performed when the disease is thoroughly controlled and glucocorticoid doses at remission maintenance levels. Damage to the nasal mucosa results in nasal crusting, which provides a focus for infection as well as causing nasal obstruction. Regular nasal douching to remove the crusts and use of a topical aseptic cream, such as mupirocin, reduces associated symptoms and risk of infection.[55] Hearing loss is usually caused by eustachian tube obstruction and recurrent otitis media but may also result from damage to the eighth cranial nerve. Although some recovery may occur, chronic hearing loss is frequent. Subglottic, tracheal, or bronchial stenoses can be fibrotic in origin, reflecting previous episodes of vasculitic damage to the airways. They can progress to cause respiratory obstruction or, if at bronchial level, cause segmental or lobar obstruction, infection, and collapse. Physical dilatation by bougie or balloon can restore the lumen and antibiotics are usually required to control secondary infection. Multiple procedures may be required as well as subsequent intermittent surveillance by nasendoscopy or bronchoscopy.

The long-term outcome of alveolar haemorrhage is usually good with stable lung function, but a minority of patients present with overlapping features of ANCA vasculitis and pulmonary fibrosis.[56,57] The lung fibrosis can precede or follow vasculitis and be progressive, leading to respiratory failure despite control of vasculitis. This pattern is more commonly associated with the MPO-ANCA subtype.

Chronic kidney disease resulting from renal vasculitis is managed in a similar way to other causes of renal disease. Proteinuria rises during the recovery phase of renal vasculitis reflecting glomerular damage. Angiotensin converting enzyme (ACE) inhibition has been recommended to improve long-term renal outcomes without direct supporting evidence. Patients with reduced renal function are at high risk of ESRD if they have a further episode of renal vasculitis and need to be monitored with this in mind. Those developing ESRD can be supported by dialysis and their immunosuppressive treatment withdrawn in the absence of extrarenal disease. Peritoneal dialysis carries an increased risk of peritonitis and need for ongoing immunosuppression is a relative contraindication. Patients who develop ESRD should be considered for transplantation, which is a safe and effective option.[58] Adjusted outcomes for graft loss, death, or functional graft loss are at least as good in those patients with GPA compared to other causes of ESRD and vasculitic relapse is uncommon following transplantation. Patients who are transplanted survive better than those remaining on dialysis, when relapse is more frequent and often hard to control. Outcome in those patients who remain on dialysis is similar to other causes of ESRD. It has been conventional to wait at least 6 months after an episode of active vasculitis before transplanting. ANCA positivity at the time of transplantation does not appear to affect graft or patient survival, although an increase in graft vasculopathy was noted in one series.[59]

Adverse events

Improvement in survival has resulted from improved treatment strategies; however, adverse events associated with these treatments are now an important cause of death and morbidity. In the EUVAS studies mortality at 1 year was 11%. The cause of death was related to an adverse event of treatment in 59%, with infection being the most common factor (Figure 132.1).[26] Active vasculitis accounted for only 14% of deaths. This study highlights the burden of using non-selective immunosuppressant agents. Infection is also a common cause of morbidity, with 25% of patients developing infection in the first year, with respiratory tract infections and generalized septicaemia being the most common infections. Glucocorticoid and cytotoxic therapy both contribute to the increased risks of infection. An older study of 158 patients over a median of 8 years, which used prolonged oral cyclophosphamide, found that 50% of serious bacterial, fungal, and opportunistic infections occurred during periods of daily glucocorticoid therapy, with only 21% occurring on alternate-day glucocorticoids, 16% on single-agent cytotoxic therapy, and 12% while therapy-free.[6]

Infections

Those at risk of infection should be identified and interventions undertaken to reduce risk. Factors predictive of infection include age, severity of renal dysfunction, leucopenia, and intensity and duration of immunosuppression. *Pneumocystis jiroveci* infection occurs in AAV with an incidence of 0.85–12% usually within the first few months after diagnosis, when immunosuppressive therapy is most intense. Presentation is more acute than that commonly seen in HIV patients, with 41% having symptom duration of 3 days or less and high fevers with rapid onset of respiratory failure being common. Mortality rates of 47–62.5% are reported. Pneumocystis infection is associated with lymphopenia, oral cyclophosphamide,

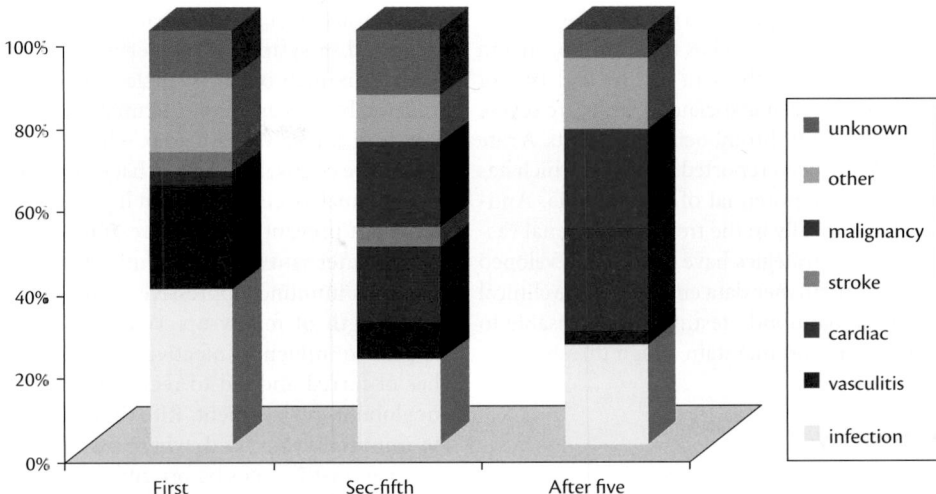

Fig. 132.1 Causes of death in 535 patients enrolled at diagnosis into prospective EUVAS trials in the first year, the second to fifth year and after five years.[14]
Reproduced from Annals of the Rheumatic Diseases, Flossmann O, Berden A, de Groot K, et al. 2011;70:488–494 with permission from the BMJ Publishing Group Ltd.

and steroid use. Prophylaxis against *P. jiroveci* with low-dose sulfamethoxaole/trimethoprim is recommended in patients receiving cyclophosphamide.[20] Herpes zoster varicella (HZV, shingles), occurs in AAV with a frequency of 4.5 episodes per 100 patient-years. While viral reactivation is linked to the intensity of immunosuppression, infections also occur following the switch to maintenance therapy.

Leucopenia is common, especially in those receiving oral cyclophosphamide, and is directly associated with infection and death.[39] It should be avoided with close monitoring. Leucopenic patients can safely be treated with granulocyte colony-stimulating factor (G-CSF). Influenza and pneumococcal immunization was safe and effective in 230 GPA patients and is recommended for AAV patients.[60] Live vaccines should be avoided in all patients taking immunosuppressives or prednisolone doses above 5 mg/day. In those AAV patients on standard maintenance therapy, maintenance of protective levels of antibody to other vaccines such as diphtheria, tetanus, and polio may be shorter than in immunocompetent patients and may require more frequent booster vaccinations.[61]

Malignancy

The incidence of cancer in treated AAV patients is 1.6–2.4 times higher than that in the general population. Immunosuppressive drugs contribute to this risk, especially a 4.8–33-fold risk of urothelial cancer and a 4.2–11-fold risk of leukaemia or lymphoma, attributed to cyclophosphamide, but proportionally higher rates of lymphoma and non-melanoma skin also occur.[6] Data collected from the EUVAS studies on patients recruited between 1995 and 2003 found an increased risk of all cancers of 1.7, largely driven by non-melanoma skin cancer.[52] The previously observed increased risk of bladder cancer and leukaemia was not seen, reflecting the reduced cyclophosphamide exposure in the EUVAS protocols. The degree of relative risk and bladder cancer frequency may have been a feature of relatively short follow-up; a French cohort study found a fivefold increase in risk for bladder cancer in AAV patients who had received cyclophosphamide. A Danish single-centre cohort study of 293 GPA patients recruited from 1973 to 1999 found an overall increased risk of 2.1, rising to 3.6 for bladder cancer and leukaemia, with no increased risk for these cancers in those receiving

a cyclophosphamide exposure below 36 g.[63] It appears probable that the bladder cancer risk is associated with cyclophosphamide exposure and length of follow-up, and strategies, such as IV pulse administration with hydration and mesna will minimize this risk. However, patients who have received cyclophosphamide require lifelong follow-up with prompt investigation by cystoscopy and urine cytology for the new onset or persistence of haematuria. Azathioprine increases the risk of skin malignancy and may contribute to lymphoma risk. Increased risks are detectable with more than 3 years' exposure in inflammatory bowel disease but have not been quantified in vasculitis. Patients receiving azathioprine should receive appropriate advice to minimize sun exposure and should be counselled and reviewed with these risks in mind.

Cardiovascular disease

Myocardial infarction rates were increased with a hazard ratio of 3.6 in a retrospective review of GPA patients enrolled in the Danish National Hospital Register. In addition, a retrospective study showed that patients with GPA and MPA, when matched for renal function and other traditional risk factors, had double the rate of cardiovascular events. Of 535 GPA and MPA patients enrolled in the EUVAS trials, 74 (14%) had had a cardiovascular event by 5 years, an increased risk of 3.7.[64] Those who were MPO-ANCA positive had higher risk than those with PR3-ANCA. Theories for the increased event rates in AAV include systemic inflammation and endothelial dysfunction, factors associated with increased cardiovascular risk in other inflammatory diseases. AAV patients in remission have impaired endothelial function and increased stiffness of large arteries, which has been reversed by TNFα blockade.[65] Renal dysfunction is an independent predictor of cardiovascular disease. Patients with AAV may also have an increased prevalence of traditional risk factors for atherosclerotic disease due to glucocorticoid treatment, which causes hypertension, dyslipidaemia, diabetes, and weight gain.

Thromboembolic disease

Although microthrombosis is a component of vasculitic pathology, the frequency of deep venous thrombosis and pulmonary embolism is also increased, being highest during periods of disease activity. A rate of 15% was reported in a prospective trial and in retrospective surveys rates of 1.8%/year for all AAV patients rising to 6.7–9%/year for those with active disease.[66] Autoantibodies to plasminogen and tissue plasminogen activator occur in the sera of 25% and 14% of AAV patients. Their presence has been associated with more severe renal outcomes and increased risk for thromboembolic events. A rate of thromboembolism of 8.1% has been reported in EGPA, which has been related to the thrombogenic potential of eosinophilia. Anti-coagulants have been used historically in the treatment of renal vasculitis but thromboprophylactic strategies have not been developed for AAV in the current era. Until further data emerges of the clinical utility of anti-plasminogen autoantibody testing, it is advisable to address conventional risk factors and maintain a high threshold for suspicion of thromboembolism.

Other drug-specific toxicity

Glucocorticoids

Glucocorticoids have a broad adverse event profile, including steroid-associated diabetes, avascular necrosis, and ocular cataract formation. Prophylaxis against osteoporosis and peptic ulceration has become routine, especially in those receiving high-dose glucocorticoids. Reduced bone mineral density is common in patients with AAV; in one study of 99 patients with AAV 57% had osteopenia and 21% had osteoporosis in at least one site; 7 out of 99 patients sustained fractures. Other studies also report high rates of fractures in AAV patients of 2.5–15%. Bisphosphonates are contraindicated in those with a GFR less than 30 mL/min.

Cyclophosphamide

The adverse events specific to cyclophosphamide, other than infection and bone marrow suppression, include hair loss, haemorrhagic cystitis, and infertility. Haemorrhagic cystitis occurs with a frequency of 0.5/100 patient-years and is associated with oral cyclophosphamide use and total exposure. Prevention of haemorrhagic cystitis is important, as an episode increases the risk of bladder cancer 5–7 times. The risk of haemorrhagic cystitis can be reduced by increased hydration and by concomitant treatment with mesna, which binds to the cyclophosphamide toxic metabolite acrolein. Fertility risks are discussed below.

Azathioprine

Myelosuppression is common with azathioprine and can occur early or later during its administration. Mutant polymorphisms in the thiopurine *S*-methyltransferase (*TPMT*) gene are associated with rapid and profound myelosuppression. Patients can be screened for common *TPMT* polymorphisms or for the biochemical activity of TPMT before commencing azathioprine. The significance of heterozygous states and borderline low activity levels is less clear, as many such patients tolerate azathioprine well. Azathioprine allergy or intolerance occurs in 5–10% and hypersensitivity reactions can be difficult to distinguish from infection or vasculitic relapse, but their onset within 2–3 weeks of commencing azathioprine is an indicator. Reactions are manifested by fevers, chills and rash, and interstitial nephritis can occur. Hepatotoxicity and cirrhosis are less common.

Rituximab

The use of rituximab is increasing in patients with AAV. No change in infection rates was observed when rituximab was substituted for cyclophosphamide in two induction trials.[11,12] Whether this reflects an infection risk with rituximab similar to cyclophosphamide or the role of concomitant high-dose steroid is unclear. Progressive multifocal leucoencephalopathy (PML), caused by the JC virus, has occurred in systemic lupus erythematosus (SLE) patients treated with rituximab but it is unclear whether the prevalence of PML is actually increased by rituximab in SLE. There has not been evidence of increased PML risk with rituximab in AAV but patients should be counselled that such a risk might exist. Infusion reactions to rituximab occur in 20% but have been mild without sequelae and have not prevented repeat treatment. Hypogammaglobulinaemia occurs after rituximab in a minority and is related to the use of previous immunosuppressives, cumulative exposure to rituximab, and length of follow-up. While mild reductions of IgG do not appear to influence infective risk, severe deficiency (to <3 g/litre) has occurred and led to recurrent infection and need for immunoglobulin replacement. Rituximab impairs the humoral response to immunizations, and, where possible, these should be administered at least 2 weeks before rituximab, or 4 months after it.

Fertility and pregnancy

Vasculitis activity and its therapy are threats to the fertility of patients with vasculitis. Loss of fertility is an important consequence of the disease, but the risks of this occurring can be considerably reduced with newer forms of treatment. As a chronic disease, vasculitis also causes psychosexual and relationship problems due to effects on self-esteem and mental well-being. Chronic kidney disease is a common consequence of renal vasculitis and depressed kidney function itself affects fertility in both women and men.

The major threat to fertility is cyclophosphamide exposure, which can result in primary ovarian failure. This is related to the total amount of cyclophosphamide administered and the age of the patient. Data from lupus nephritis suggests that a total cyclophosphamide exposure of 14–20 g results in infertility in over 50% of women aged over 32 years. The risk of infertility in those under 32 years is lower, around 10% in one series. Even if infertility is not induced, less severe ovarian damage leads to early menopause. Drugs that temporarily suppress ovarian function, such as goserelin, are used to reduce the risk of cyclophosphamide toxicity. Rituximab has been shown to be as effective as cyclophosphamide and can be used when cyclophosphamide avoidance is desirable. There have been concerns that cyclophosphamide may result in an increase in birth defects through damage to DNA in the unfertilized egg, but this has not proved to be the case. However, it is advisable to wait at least 6 months between stopping cyclophosphamide and attempting to conceive.

Cyclophosphamide directly affects sperm production in men. There is more potential for recovery by the generation of new sperm-forming cells when cyclophosphamide is withdrawn, although prepubertal boys are at greater risk of infertility than girls, with a threshold of 200 mg/kg deduced from nephritis trials. Sperm production does not usually recover to pretreatment levels and healthy sperm counts can remain depressed. It is likely that, in combination with non-specific effects of chronic illness, cyclophosphamide reduces male fertility. An alternative immunosuppressive used in vasculitis, methotrexate, also reduces sperm formation but has a lower risk of sustained effects after withdrawal. Egg preservation in women can be difficult because of the urgency in starting therapy, but semen preservation is quite feasible in men and can be considered before cyclophosphamide is commenced.

Methotrexate and mycophenolate mofetil, damage the fetus and must not be used in pregnant women or those attempting to conceive. Anti-inflammatory drugs and high-dose steroids also reduce fertility. The infective risks of the intrauterine coil are increased in those receiving immune suppression. Sexually transmitted diseases can be more problematic in immune suppressed patients and *Chlamydia trachomatis* infection results in infertility in women. Drug effects, especially high-dose steroids, vasculitic activity, and chronic illness reduce testosterone levels that can lead to reduced libido and erectile failure. Testosterone levels in the blood are readily measured and testosterone supplementation can correct the problem.

GPA has been diagnosed during pregnancy but this is rare and there is no evidence of an increased relapse risk during pregnancy or the postpuerperal period. The risks of pre-existing damage to the pregnancy, in particular to the kidneys, lungs, or heart, need to be considered before conception, and appropriate changes to medication made. Transmission of ANCA and a self-limiting vasculitis syndrome have been reported in the neonate, but this is probably a rare occurrence. The largest review of 22 pregnancies in AAV reported good fetal outcomes, the adverse events being pre-eclampsia in two pregnancies and one newborn with hypothyroidism and one with a cleft palate.

Future directions

Reducing diagnostic delay will have a major impact on outcomes but requires understanding of where patients present and subsequent referral pathways. Improved education of referring medical specialties and wider use of ANCA testing and urine analysis will facilitate earlier referral. Management in a subspecialist vasculitis clinic with rapid access to associated specialities including ENT and respiratory medicine allows a coordinated approach to patient care and optimal assessment of disease extent and treatment response. Careful supervision of therapy, especially cyclophosphamide and high-dose glucocorticoids, has led to major reductions in severe adverse events over the last 20 years and late treatment-related toxicity. This is likely to be further improved by the availability of rituximab as an alternative to cyclophosphamide.

Glucocorticoids, delayed treatment response, and a high relapse rate are important components of the unmet need of current vasculitis therapies. Potential alternatives to glucocorticoids, such as intravenous immunoglobulin or TNFα blockade have proved impractical or ineffective. Therapies targeted at other cytokine, complement, or immune components may provide an opportunity to reduce glucocorticoids, such as the use of mepolizumab in EGPA. Rituximab has not led to a lower relapse rate than cyclophosphamide and there is uncertainty as to how to prevent relapse after rituximab induction. Other B-cell targeted therapies may be more effective, or B-cell therapies may need to be continued during the remission phase.

The causes of impaired quality of life despite vasculitis remission are not understood, although subclinical disease activity is likely in some patients. Other factors include ongoing treatment toxicity, irreversible damage, and physical deconditioning. Newer therapies may impact on quality of life, but there is currently no evidence for rituximab doing so.

References

1. Walton EW. Giant-cell granuloma of the respiratory tract (Wegener's granulomatosis). *Br Med J* 1958;2:265–270.
2. Treatment of polyarteritis nodosa with cortisone: results after one year; report to the Medical Research Council by the collagen diseases and hypersensitivity panel. *Br Med J* 1957;1:608–611.
3. Leib ES, Restivo C, Paulus HE. Immunosuppressive and corticosteroid therapy of polyarteritis nodosa. *Am J Med* 1979;67:941–947.
4. Novack SN, Pearson CM. Cyclophosphamide therapy in Wegener's granulomatosis. *N Engl J Med* 1971;284:938–942.
5. Fauci AS, Wolff SM, Johnson JS. Effect of cyclophosphamide upon the immune response in Wegener's granulomatosis. *N Engl J Med* 1971;285:1493–1496.
6. Hoffman GS, Kerr GS, Leavitt RY et al. Wegener granulomatosis: an analysis of 158 patients. *Ann Intern Med* 1992;116:488–498.
7. van der Woude FJ, Rasmussen N, Lobatto S et al. Autoantibodies against neutrophils and monocytes: tool for diagnosis and marker of disease activity in Wegener's granulomatosis. *Lancet* 1985;1:425–429.
8. Savage CO, Winearls CG, Jones S, Marshall PD, Lockwood CM. Prospective study of radioimmunoassay for antibodies against neutrophil cytoplasm in diagnosis of systemic vasculitis. *Lancet* 1987;1:1389–1393.
9. Rasmussen N, Jayne D, Abramovicz D et al. European therapeutic trials in ANCA-associated systemic vasculitis: disease scoring, consensus regimens and proposed clinical trials. *Clin Exp Immunol.* 1995;101(Suppl 1):29–34.
10. Mathieson PW, Cobbold SP, Hale G et al. Monoclonal-antibody therapy in systemic vasculitis. *N Engl J Med* 1990;323:250–254.
11. Jones RB, Cohen Tervaert JW, Hauser T et al. Rituximab versus cyclophosphamide in ANCA-associated renal vasculitis. *N Engl J Med* 2010;363:211–220.
12. Stone JH, Merkel PA, Spiera R et al. Rituximab versus cyclophosphamide for ANCA-associated vasculitis. *N Engl J Med* 2010;363:221–232.
13. Bacon PA, Moots RJ, Exley A, Luqmani R, Rasmussen N. VITAL (Vasculitis Integrated Assessment Log) assessment of vasculitis. *Clin Exp Rheumatol* 1995;13:275–278.
14. Flossmann O, Berden A, de Groot K et al. Long-term patient survival in ANCA-associated vasculitis. *Ann Rheum Dis* 2011;70:488–494.
14a. Koike K, Fukami K, Yonemoto K et al. A new vasculitis activity score for predicting death in myeloperoxidase-antineutrophil cytoplasmic antibody-associated vasculitis patients. *Am J Nephrol* 2012;35:1–6.
15. Martinez Del Pero M, Walsh M, Luqmani R et al. Long-term damage to the ENT system in Wegener's granulomatosis. *Eur Arch Otorhinolaryngol* 2011;268:733–739.
16. Berden AE, Ferrario F, Hagen EC et al. Histopathologic classification of ANCA-associated glomerulonephritis. *J Am Soc Nephrol* 2010;21:1628–1636.
17. de Lind van Wijngaarden RA, Hauer HA, Wolterbeek R et al. Chances of renal recovery for dialysis-dependent ANCA-associated glomerulonephritis. *J Am Soc Nephrol* 2007;18:2189–2197.
18. Walsh M, Flossmann O, Berden A et al. Risk factors for relapse of antineutrophil cytoplasmic antibody-associated vasculitis. *Arthritis Rheum* 2012;64(2):542–548.
19. Pierrot-Deseilligny Despujol C, Pouchot J, Pagnoux C, Coste J, Guillevin L. Predictors at diagnosis of a first Wegener's granulomatosis relapse after obtaining complete remission. *Rheumatology* (Oxford) 2010;49(11):2181–2190.
20. Mukhtyar C, Guillevin L, Cid MC et al. EULAR Recommendations for the management of primary small and medium vessel vasculitis. *Ann Rheum Dis* 2008;68:310–317.
21. McKinney EF, Lyons PA, Carr EJ et al. A CD8(+) T cell transcription signature predicts prognosis in autoimmune disease. *Nat Med* 2010;16(5):586–591.
22. Hellmich B, Flossmann O, Gross WL et al. EULAR recommendations for conducting clinical studies and/or clinical trials in systemic vasculitis: focus on anti-neutrophil cytoplasm antibody-associated vasculitis. *Ann Rheum Dis* 2007;66:605–617.
23. Carrington CB, Liebow A. Limited forms of angiitis and granulomatosis of Wegener's type. *Am J Med* 1966;41:497–527.
24. Etanercept plus standard therapy for Wegener's granulomatosis. *N Engl J Med* 2005;352:351–361.
25. de Groot K, Harper L, Jayne DR et al. Pulse versus daily oral cyclophosphamide for induction of remission in antineutrophil cytoplasmic antibody-associated vasculitis: a randomized trial. *Ann Intern Med* 2009;150:670–680.

26. Little MA, Nightingale P, Verburgh CA et al. Early mortality in systemic vasculitis: relative contribution of adverse events and active vasculitis. *Ann Rheum Dis* 2010;69(6):1036–1043.

27. Jayne D, Rasmussen N, Andrassy K et al. A randomized trial of maintenance therapy for vasculitis associated with antineutrophil cytoplasmic autoantibodies. *N Engl J Med* 2003;349:36–44.

28. Jayne DR, Gaskin G, Rasmussen N et al. Randomized trial of plasma exchange or high-dosage methylprednisolone as adjunctive therapy for severe renal vasculitis. *J Am Soc Nephrol* 2007;18:2180–2188.

29. Walsh M, Catapano F, Szpirt W et al. Plasma exchange for renal vasculitis and idiopathic rapidly progressive glomerulonephritis: a meta-analysis. *Am J Kidney Dis* 2010;57:557–564.

30. De Groot K, Rasmussen N, Bacon PA et al. Randomized trial of cyclophosphamide versus methotrexate for induction of remission in early systemic antineutrophil cytoplasmic antibody-associated vasculitis. *Arthritis Rheum* 2005;52:2461–2469.

31. Silva F, Specks U, Kalra S et al. Mycophenolate mofetil for induction and maintenance of remission in microscopic polyangiitis with mild to moderate renal involvement—a prospective, open-label pilot trial. *Clin J Am Soc Nephrol* 2010;5(3):445–453.

32. Hu W, Liu C, Xie H et al. Mycophenolate mofetil versus cyclophosphamide for inducing remission of ANCA vasculitis with moderate renal involvement. *Nephrol Dial Transplant* 2008;23:1307–1312.

33. Guerry MJ, Brogan P, Bruce IN et al. Recommendations for the use of rituximab in anti-neutrophil cytoplasm antibody-associated vasculitis. *Rheumatology* (Oxford) 2012;51(4):634–643.

34. Jones RB, Ferraro AJ, Chaudhry AN et al. A multicenter survey of rituximab therapy for refractory antineutrophil cytoplasmic antibody-associated vasculitis. *Arthritis Rheum* 2009;60:2156–2168.

35. Berden AE, Jones RB, Erasmus DD et al. Tubular lesions predict renal outcome in antineutrophil cytoplasmic antibody-associated glomerulonephritis after rituximab therapy. *J Am Soc Nephrol* 2012;23(2):313–321.

36. Bakoush O, Segelmark M, Torffvit O, Ohlsson S, Tencer J. Urine IgM excretion predicts outcome in ANCA-associated renal vasculitis. *Nephrol Dial Transplant* 2006;21:1263–1269.

37. Cohen P, Pagnoux C, Mahr A et al. Churg-Strauss syndrome with poor-prognosis factors: A prospective multicenter trial comparing glucocorticoids and six or twelve cyclophosphamide pulses in forty-eight patients. *Arthritis Rheum* 2007;57:686–693.

38. Ribi C, Cohen P, Pagnoux C et al. Treatment of Churg-Strauss syndrome without poor-prognosis factors: a multicenter, prospective, randomized, open-label study of seventy-two patients. *Arthritis Rheum* 2008;58:586–594.

39. Booth AD, Almond MK, Burns A et al. Outcome of ANCA-associated renal vasculitis: a 5-year retrospective study. *Am J Kidney Dis* 2003;41:776–784.

40. Pagnoux C, Mahr A, Hamidou MA et al. Azathioprine or methotrexate maintenance for ANCA-associated vasculitis. *N Engl J Med* 2008;359:2790–2803.

41. Metzler C, Miehle N, Manger K et al. Elevated relapse rate under oral methotrexate versus leflunomide for maintenance of remission in Wegener's granulomatosis. *Rheumatology* (Oxford) 2007;46:1087–1091.

42. Hiemstra TF, Walsh M, Mahr A et al. Mycophenolate mofetil vs azathioprine for remission maintenance in antineutrophil cytoplasmic antibody-associated vasculitis: a randomized controlled trial. *JAMA* 2010;304(21):2381–2388.

43. Walsh M, Merkel PA, Mahr A, Jayne D. The effects of duration of glucocorticoid therapy on relapse rate in anti-neutrophil cytoplasm antibody associated vasculitis: A meta-analysis. *Arthritis Care Res* (Hoboken) 2010;62:1166–1173.

44. Sanders JS, Huitma MG, Kallenberg CG, Stegeman CA. Prediction of relapses in PR3-ANCA-associated vasculitis by assessing responses of ANCA titres to treatment. *Rheumatology* (Oxford) 2006;45:724–729.

45. Seror R, Pagnoux C, Ruivard M et al. Treatment strategies and outcome of induction-refractory Wegener's granulomatosis or microscopic polyangiitis: analysis of 32 patients with first-line induction-refractory disease in the WEGENT trial. *Ann Rheum Dis* 2010;69:2125–2130.

46. Jayne DR, Chapel H, Adu D et al. Intravenous immunoglobulin for ANCA-associated systemic vasculitis with persistent disease activity. *Q J Med* 2000;93:433–439.

47. Booth A, Harper L, Hammad T et al. Prospective study of TNFalpha blockade with infliximab in anti-neutrophil cytoplasmic antibody-associated systemic vasculitis. *J Am Soc Nephrol* 2004;15:717–721.

48. Silva F, Seo P, Schroeder DR et al. Solid malignancies among etanercept-treated patients with granulomatosis with polyangiitis (Wegener's): long-term followup of a multicenter longitudinal cohort. *Arthritis Rheum* 2011;63:2495–2503.

49. Flossmann O, Baslund B, Bruchfeld A et al. Deoxyspergualin in relapsing and refractory Wegener's granulomatosis. *Ann Rheum Dis* 2008

50. Walsh M, Chaudhry A, Jayne D. Long-term follow-up of relapsing/refractory anti-neutrophil cytoplasm antibody associated vasculitis treated with the lymphocyte depleting antibody alemtuzumab (CAMPATH-1H). *Ann Rheum Dis* 2008;67:1322–1327.

51. Koukoulaki M, Jayne DR. Mycophenolate mofetil in anti-neutrophil cytoplasm antibodies-associated systemic vasculitis. *Nephron Clin Pract* 2006;102:c100–c107.

52. Stassen PM, Tervaert JW, Stegeman CA. Induction of remission in active anti-neutrophil cytoplasmic antibody-associated vasculitis with mycophenolate mofetil in patients who cannot be treated with cyclophosphamide. *Ann Rheum Dis* 2007;66:798–802.

53. Nakamura M, Yabe I, Yaguchi H et al. Clinical characterization and successful treatment of 6 patients with Churg-Strauss syndrome-associated neuropathy. *Clin Neurol Neurosurg* 2009;111:683–687.

54. Kim S, Marigowda G, Oren E, Israel E, Wechsler ME. Mepolizumab as a steroid-sparing treatment option in patients with Churg-Strauss syndrome. *J Allergy Clin Immunol* 2010;125:1336–1343.

55. Laudien M, Lamprecht P, Hedderich J, Holle J, Ambrosch P. Olfactory dysfunction in Wegener's granulomatosis. *Rhinology* 2009;47:254–259.

56. Arulkumaran N, Periselneris N, Gaskin G et al. Interstitial lung disease and ANCA-associated vasculitis: a retrospective observational cohort study. *Rheumatology* (Oxford) 2011;50:2035–2043.

57. Hervier B, Pagnoux C, Agard C et al. Pulmonary fibrosis associated with ANCA-positive vasculitides. Retrospective study of 12 cases and review of the literature. *Ann Rheum Dis* 2009;68:404–407.

58. Geetha D, Eirin A, True K et al. Renal transplantation in antineutrophil cytoplasmic antibody-associated vasculitis: a multicenter experience. *Transplantation* 2011;91:1370–1375.

59. Little MA, Hassan B, Jacques S et al. Renal transplantation in systemic vasculitis: when is it safe? *Nephrol Dial Transplant* 2009;24:3219–3225.

60. Stassen PM, Sanders JS, Kallenberg CG, Stegeman CA. Influenza vaccination does not result in an increase in relapses in patients with ANCA-associated vasculitis. *Nephrol Dial Transplant* 2008;23:654–658.

61. van Assen S, Agmon-Levin N, Elkayam O et al. EULAR recommendations for vaccination in adult patients with autoimmune inflammatory rheumatic diseases. *Ann Rheum Dis* 2011;70:414–422.

62. Heijl C, Harper L, Flossmann O et al. Incidence of malignancy in patients treated for antineutrophil cytoplasm antibody-associated vasculitis: follow-up data from European Vasculitis Study Group clinical trials. *Ann Rheum Dis* 2011;70:1415–1421.

63. Faurschou M, Sorensen IJ, Mellemkjaer L et al. Malignancies in Wegener's granulomatosis: incidence and relation to cyclophosphamide therapy in a cohort of 293 patients. *J Rheumatol* 2008;35:100–105.

64. Suppiah R, Judge A, Batra R et al. A model to predict cardiovascular events in patients with newly diagnosed Wegener's granulomatosis and microscopic polyangiitis. *Arthritis Care Res* (Hoboken) 2011;63:588–596.

65. Booth AD, Jayne DR, Kharbanda RK et al. Infliximab improves endothelial dysfunction in systemic vasculitis: a model of vascular inflammation. *Circulation* 2004;109:1718–1723.

66. Merkel PA, Lo GH, Holbrook JT et al. Brief communication: high incidence of venous thrombotic events among patients with Wegener granulomatosis: the Wegener's Clinical Occurrence of Thrombosis (WeCLOT) Study. *Ann Intern Med* 2005;142:620–626.

CHAPTER 133

Large-vessel vasculitis

Nicolò Pipitone, Annibale Versari,
and Carlo Salvarani

Introduction

Giant cell arteritis (GCA) and Takayasu's arteritis (TAK) are primary systemic vasculitides mainly involving the aorta and its main branches. GCA was first described by Hutchinson in 1890, but the histological alterations of GCA were reported only in 1932 by Horton et al. TAK was first described by Morgagni in 1761, but is named after the Japanese ophthalmologist Takayasu, who reported a case with ocular involvement in 1908.[1,2]

Epidemiology

GCA affects almost exclusively subjects aged over 50 years at the time of diagnosis.[1,2] The incidence of GCA increases with advancing age, and peaks in the 70–79 years age group.[3] Females are affected two to three times more often than males.[3] GCA occurs predominantly in white people, and it is very rare in blacks and Asians. The highest incidence rates of GCA (>17/100 000 for individuals aged >50 years) have been reported in Scandinavian countries and North American populations of Scandinavian descent.[3] In contrast, the incidence of GCA is lower than 12/100 000 for those aged over 50 years in southern European countries.[3] The incidence of GCA has increased over the past decades, presumably as a consequence of heightened physician awareness.[3] A cyclic pattern in incidence rates of GCA has been observed.[4]

GCA and polymyalgia rheumatica (PMR) occur together more frequently than expected by chance alone. Around 16–21% of patients with PMR have clinical manifestations of GCA, while 40–60% of patients with GCA suffer from PMR.[4] PMR can develop before, simultaneously with, or after the onset of the clinical manifestations of GCA.[1] Furthermore, about 4% of patients with pure PMR (i.e. without clinical features of GCA) have temporal artery biopsy (TAB) lesions consistent with GCA,[5] while nearly one-third of patients with pure PMR have subclinical arteritis on imaging.[6] However, patients with PMR and clinically silent GCA are not at risk for ischaemic complications.

Mortality rates of patients with GCA are comparable to those of the general population.[7] An exception is the subset of GCA patients with thoracic aorta aneurysms, in which mortality is increased mainly due to thoracic aorta dissection.[8]

There is scanty data on the epidemiology of TAK. A population-based study of Olmsted County, Minnesota (USA) found an incidence rate of 2.6 cases/1 000 000 per year,[9] while a United Kingdom population study found an incidence rate of 0.8 cases/1 000 000 per year with a prevalence of 4.7/1 000 000.[10] Studies from East Asia on Asian subjects have reported higher incidence rates than in whites, but estimates are often biased by hospital-based study designs and imprecision in sampling. In Japan, an incidence rate of 1.5 cases/1 000 000/year[11] has been reported.[12] The female:male ratio is approximately 9:1 in Europe and Japan,[13,14] but close to 1.5:1 in India.[15] The typical age of onset is 20–30 years, but onset can also occur at paediatric ages.[13] The 5 year survival rates are in the range of 90–95%.[9] Mortality is increased in patients with severe vascular complications, including aneurysmal rupture, myocardial infarction, heart failure, and cerebrovascular accidents.[9]

Classification criteria

Criteria for the classification of GCA and TAK were published by the American College of Rheumatology (ACR) in 1990 (Tables 133.1 and 133.2).[16] These criteria were developed to distinguish a specific type of vasculitis among patients with various vasculitides, but not to differentiate patients with vasculitis from those without. Therefore, while they are helpful to recruit patients into clinical trials, it is not appropriate to use them to make a diagnosis of GCA or TAK, respectively, in individual patients.

There is also a set of criteria that classifies patients with TAK into five subtypes depending on the vessels involved on angiography (Table 133.3).[14] Typically, in white patients the branches of the aortic arch are most commonly (38–98%) involved, but the renal arteries and the abdominal aorta are also affected in approximately one-third of cases.[13] Involvement of other arteries is less frequent but by no means exceptional. Stenoses are by far the most common lesions, followed by occlusions, but dilatations and frank aneurysms are also recognized complications of TAK.[13]

Aetiology and pathogenesis

Genetics

The *HLA-DRB1*04* allele is associated with susceptibility to GCA.[2,18] Because MHC alleles function as antigen-presenting

Table 133.1 American College of Rheumatology 1990 classification criteria for giant cell arteritis[16]

Criterion	Definition
Age at disease onset ≥50 years	Development of symptoms or findings beginning at age ≥50
New headache	New onset of or new type of localized pain in the head
Temporal artery abnormality	Temporal artery tenderness to palpation or decreased pulsation, unrelated to arteriosclerosis of cervical arteries
Elevated ESR	ESR ≥50 mm/1st hour by the Westergren method
Abnormal artery biopsy	Biopsy specimen with artery showing vasculitis characterized by a predominance of mononuclear cell infiltration or granulomatous inflammation, usually with multinucleated giant cells

ESR, erythrocyte sedimentation rate.

For purposes of classification, a patient with vasculitis is said to have giant cell arteritis if at least three of these five criteria are present. The presence of any three or more criteria yields a sensitivity of 93.5% and a specificity of 91.2%.

From Hunder et al.[16]

Table 133.2 American College of Rheumatology classification criteria for Takayasu's arteritis[17]

Criteria	Definition
Age at disease onset	Development of symptoms or findings related to Takayasu's arteritis at age <40 years
Claudication of extremities	Development and worsening of fatigue and discomfort in muscles of one or more extremity while in use, especially the upper extremities
Decreased brachial artery pulse	Decreased pulsation of one or both brachial arteries
BP difference >10 mmHg	Difference of >10 mmHg in systolic blood pressure between arms
Bruit over subclavian arteries or aorta	Bruit audible on auscultation over one or both subclavian arteries or abdominal aorta
Arteriogram abnormality	Arteriographic narrowing or occlusion of the entire aorta, its primary branches, or large arteries in the proximal upper or lower extremities, not due arteriosclerosis, fibromuscular dysplasia, or similar causes: changes usually focal or segmental

BP, blood pressure.

For purposes of classification, a patient is said to have Takayasu's arteritis if at least three of the six criteria are present. The presence of any three or more criteria yields a sensitivity of 90.5% and a specificity of 97.8%.

From Arend et al.[17]

Table 133.3 Classification of Takayasu's arteritis based on the vessels involved on angiography

Type	Vessels involved
I	Branches from the aortic arch
IIa	Ascending aorta, aortic arch, and branches of the aortic arch
IIb	Ascending aorta, aortic arch and its branches, and thoracic descending aorta
III	Thoracic descending aorta, abdominal aorta, and/or renal arteries
IV	Abdominal aorta and/or renal arteries
V	Combined features of types IIb and IV

From Moriwaki et al.[14]

molecules, the association with the *HLA-DRB1*04* allele suggests that this allele may be implicated in presenting yet unidentified pathogenic antigens. In addition, this allele may be a marker of disease severity.[18] GCA is also associated with the *MHC B*15* allele as well as with the MHC class I chain-related gene A (*MICA*) *A5* allele independently of linkage disequilibrium with *HLA-B*15* and of the association with *HLA-DRB1*04*.[19] Functional polymorphisms of TNFα,[20] but not interleukins IL-6 or IL-12 have been linked to increased susceptibility to developing GCA.

Genetic factors may also play a role in determining susceptibility to TAK. The *HLA B52* and *B39* alleles are found with increased frequency in Japanese patients with TAK, although associations with *HLA* genes in different populations have proved inconsistent.[21] There are also reports of TAK cases in families and monozygotic twins.[21] Furthermore, different patterns of vascular involvement have been described in different ethnic groups.[21]

Aetiology

The aetiology of GCA remains unclear. Its higher incidence in Scandinavian countries and in populations of Scandinavian descent in North America suggest that both genetic and environmental risk factors may be involved. The infectious aetiology would also be consistent with observed cyclic patterns of incidence rates of GCA.[4] However, studies that have searched for evidence of infectious agents in the sera and in temporal artery specimens have provided conflicting results.[22] Such discrepancies do not necessarily rule out a pathogenic role for infection triggers and may be explained by a 'hit and run' mechanism of disease induction, i.e. triggering of the immune response by a microorganism followed by clearance of the offending agent. It is also conceivable that different agents may lead to the development of the same vasculitis in different individuals by activating similar immune pathways.

Traditional cardiovascular risk factors also modulate susceptibility to GCA. In particular, case-control studies have linked susceptibility to GCA to smoking and atherosclerosis.[23,24]

The aetiology of TAK is unknown. A number of infectious agents including *Mycobacterium tuberculosis* have been implicated as triggers, but none has conclusively been proven responsible.[21]

Pathology

Histologically, GCA is characterized by intimal hyperplasia and by a transmural inflammatory infiltrate mainly consisting of CD4+ lymphocytes and macrophages with a variable admixture of neutrophils and eosinophils. In addition, in approximately 50% of cases giant cells can be detected at the intima–media junction (Figure 133.1).[2] The affected arteries typically show 'skip' inflammatory changes most pronounced in the inner portion of the media adjacent to the internal elastic lamina, which appears disrupted.[25,26] However, in some cases the inflammation may be restricted to the vasa vasorum, to the periadventitial small vessels, or both (Figure 133.1).[27] These histological patterns have distinctive clinical correlations. More specifically, patients with inflammation confined to the vasa vasorum have clinical features similar to those of patients with transmural inflammation, whereas patients with periadventitial inflammation have lower inflammatory markers at diagnosis as well as less frequent constitutional and cranial manifestations including headache, scalp tenderness, and abnormalities of the temporal arteries.[27] In contrast, visual loss is equally represented in all patients with GCA regardless of their histological pattern.[27]

It is important to appreciate that marked fibrinoid necrosis is not part of the pathological abnormalities found in GCA. If a biopsy shows extensive fibrinoid necrosis, alternative diagnoses such as anti-neutrophil cytoplasmic antibodies (ANCA)-associated vasculitis (see Chapter 132) should be considered.

The histological alterations found in TAK are similar to, and often indistinguishable from, those observed in GCA.[28] The inflammatory infiltrate is mainly localized around the vasa vasorum in the adventitial layer and comprises B lymphocytes, αβ and γδ T lymphocytes, NK cells, dendritic cells, macrophages, and sometimes giant cells.[28]

Pathogenesis

A variety of cell types are involved in inducing and maintaining inflammation in GCA. Normally, large- and medium-sized arteries harbour dendritic cells located at the adventitia–media junction.[29] These dendritic cells express Toll-like receptors, which are able to stimulate the dendritic cells via their binding to specific ligands, including mediators synthesized or induced by infectious agents.[1] Dendritic cells in the temporal arteries from GCA patients have an activated phenotype, although the mechanisms leading to their activation are still in dispute. Activated dendritic cells release chemokines that recruit CD4+ lymphocytes and macrophages through the vasa vasorum into the vessel wall. In addition, they also

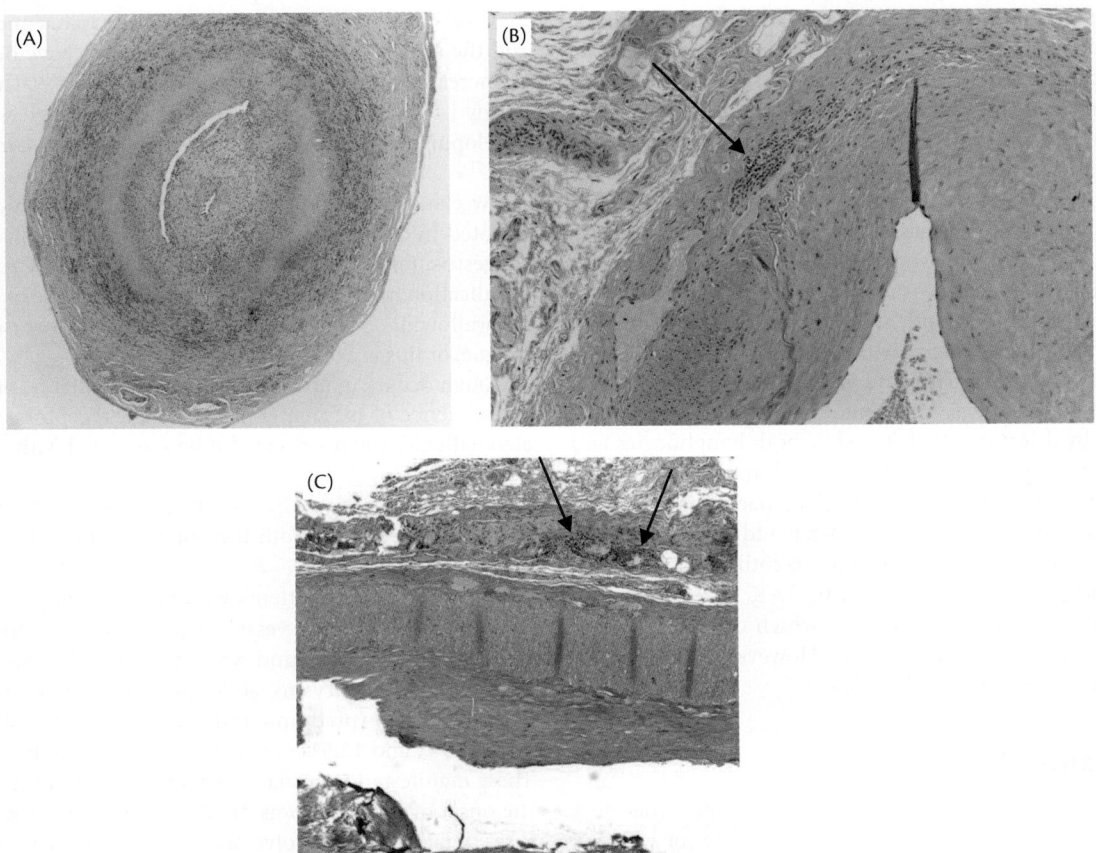

Fig. 133.1 Histological patterns of temporal arteries in giant cell arteritis: (A) Classical histological transmural inflammatory infiltrate with reduction in vessel lumen (H&E, 40×). (B) Vasa vasorum vasculitis (arrow). Note the preserved media and the lymphocytic infiltration around a small adventitial vessel (H&E, 100×). (C) Periadventitial inflammation characterized by small lymphocytic cuffs around periadventitial vessels (arrows). Note the preserved media (H&E, 20×).
Dr Alberto Cavazza, Pathology Department, Reggio Emilia Hospital.

provide costimulatory signals required for lymphocyte activation.[30] CD4+ lymphocytes are stimulated both by unknown antigens and by dendritic cells and, once activated, secrete the proinflammatory cytokines IL-1β, IL-2, IL-6, and interferon-γ.[30] In particular, interferon-γ is produced almost exclusively by a subset of CD4+ lymphocytes found in the adventitia.[30] Interferon-γ is found in most samples from patients with GCA but not in those from patients with PMR, and its expression correlates with the risk of developing GCA-related ischaemic complications.[30] These findings suggest that interferon-γ is critically involved in the pathogenesis of arteritis and of its ischaemic complications.[31] Interferon-γ acts, at least in part, by stimulating macrophages and, more specifically, by inducing the synthesis of platelet-derived growth factor (PDGF) by macrophages at the media–intima junction.[30] In turn, PDGF leads to intimal hyperplasia and thus to luminal narrowing or occlusion, which clinically translates into an increased risk of vascular ischaemic events.[32] Following stimulation by lymphocytes, macrophages (as well as circulating monocytes) also produce other inflammatory molecules, including TNFα, IL-1β, and IL-6.[33] Systemic release of inflammatory cytokines by monocytes plays a role in causing constitutional manifestations in both PMR and GCA.[33] However, IL-6 has not only a proinflammatory action, but also a protective effect against ischaemic events in GCA, since its expression in the temporal arteries and its circulating concentrations are significantly lower in patients with ischaemic complications.[34]

While adventitial macrophages specialize in producing proinflammatory cytokines, macrophages in the media primarily cause damage to the vessel wall and fragmentation of the internal elastic lamina by synthetizing matrix metalloproteinases and oxygen-derived free radicals.[1,33] These destructive processes are counterbalanced by tissue repair mechanisms including neoangiogenesis.[35] Mediators such as PDGF, IL-6, and vascular endothelial growth factor (VEGF) are mainly responsible for inducing tissue repair.[35]

An immune-mediated response also appears to be involved in the pathogenesis of TAK.[28] Because dendritic cells colocalize with lymphocytes, they may be involved in their activation. T-cell receptor (TCR) αβ and γδ gene usage is restricted, which suggests that T cells may target specific, yet unidentified, antigens. A possible target is a 65 kD heat shock protein, which is highly expressed in the media and vasa vasorum in TAK and is known to induce a strong response by γδ lymphocytes.[36] Lymphocytes and NK cells cause vascular injury by direct cytotoxicity, while both lymphocytes and macrophages release proinflammatory chemokines and cytokines, including TNFα, IL-1, and IL-6.[28] In addition, macrophages secrete matrix metalloproteinases and free oxygen radicals, leading to arterial wall damage, and PDGF, leading to intimal hyperplasia. A significant proportion of patients with TAK have circulating anti-endothelial cell antibodies (AECA), which can cause vascular complement-dependent cytotoxicity.[37] However, AECA are not consistently found in patients with TAK.[37]

Clinical manifestations

The onset of GCA is gradual, but can also be abrupt.[2] The most frequent symptom of GCA is new onset of headache (or worsening of pre-existing headache), which affects two-thirds of patients. The headache is predominantly localized to the temporal area, but may also be felt over other sites such as the occipital area.[2] The pain is often unrelenting and responds poorly to common painkillers. One-half of patients with GCA also report dysaesthesia of the scalp worsened by combing the hair, mostly associated with headache.

About one-half of patients have constitutional manifestations including fever, malaise, depression, anorexia, and weight loss.[1] The fever is usually low-grade, but it can reach 39–40 °C in about 15% of cases.[2] In a minority of patients, systemic manifestations can be the only features of GCA.

Partial or complete loss of vision in one or both eyes occurs in up to 20% of patients, most often at disease onset. Visual loss is typically related to anterior ischaemic optic neuropathy (AION) caused by occlusive arteritis of posterior ciliary artery and, less commonly, by retinal artery occlusion. Unilateral visual loss can be followed by visual loss in the other eye within a couple of weeks if the patient is not promptly treated with glucocorticoids. Rarely, posterior ischaemic optic neuropathy (PION) or cortical ischaemia is responsible for visual loss. Amaurosis fugax (transient visual loss) occurs in 10–15% of patients.[1] In nearly one-half of patients, amaurosis fugax heralds permanent visual loss if treatment with glucocorticoids is not started immediately.

Cerebrovascular ischaemic events, including transient ischaemic attacks and stroke, are a rare but recognized complication of GCA. These events are usually precocious and mostly due to vasculitis of the carotid or of the vertebrobasilar arteries. Intracranial vasculitis has been reported in patients with GCA, but only in extremely rare cases.[38] A moderately but not very high erythrocyte sedimentation rate (ESR) and C-reactive protein (CRP) at diagnosis, older age at diagnosis, hypertension, a past history of ischaemic heart disease, and the absence of systemic manifestations have been mapped to an increased risk of cranial ischaemic events.[39–41] The development of any ischaemic complication is also associated with the risk of developing subsequent ischaemic manifestations, including visual loss.[41]

Jaw claudication due to ischaemia of the masticatory muscles is noted in about one-half of patients. Jaw claudication is highly suggestive (although not pathognomonic) of GCA. Occasionally, claudication may affect the muscles of the tongue or those involved in swallowing. Severe ischaemia leading to necrosis of the scalp, tongue, or lips is exceedingly rare.[2,42]

Cough occurs in around 10% of GCA patients, presumably as a consequence of ischaemia of the cough receptors. Cough associated with GCA may or may not be associated with sore throat and hoarse voice.[2]

Peripheral neuropathy complicates GCA in approximately one-sixth of patients. Both the upper and the lower limbs may be affected.[1,2]

About 10–27% of patients with GCA develop clinical manifestations related to large-vessel involvement including arm claudication, arterial bruits, and heart murmurs.[2,43] More specifically, thoracic aorta aneurysms, abdominal aorta aneurysms, and large-vessel stenoses (predominantly of the upper limbs) develop in 9.3%, 6.5%, and 13.5% of unselected GCA patients, respectively.[44] These manifestations usually become apparent only 3–4 years after the onset of the symptoms of GCA. However, although overt features of large-vessel involvement are relatively late events in GCA, evidence of large-vessel involvement can be demonstrated early on in the disease course. A sensitive technique such as ^{18}F-fluorodeoxyglucose positron emission tomography (FDG-PET) is able to reveal large-vessel vasculitis in as many as 83% of patients with early GCA.[45] Other investigations such as colour Doppler sonography (CDS) and MRI are also able to document early large-vessel vasculitis.[46]

Compared to unselected patients with GCA, those with large-vessel vasculitis have less frequently cranial symptoms and a positive TAB,[8,43] while they have an increased risk of developing aortic aneurysms.[44] There also is a slightly increased risk of mortality due to thoracic aorta dissection. Yearly chest radiographs are recommended to screen for thoracic aorta aneurysms, while vascular imaging techniques are useful to study and monitor large-vessel disease.

PMR is the most frequent musculoskeletal manifestation of GCA, occurring in around 40% of patients.[1] Other musculoskeletal manifestations affect approximately 25% of patients and include carpal tunnel syndrome, non-erosive asymmetric peripheral arthritis (predominantly affecting the knees and wrists), and distal swelling with pitting oedema (also known as remitting symmetric seronegative synovitis with pitting edema, RS3PE).[1]

Other infrequent clinical manifestations of GCA include facial swelling, odontogenic pain, chin numbness, glossitis, submandibular swelling, audiovestibular dysfunction, diplopia, Charles Bonnet syndrome (visual hallucinations probably due to ischaemia of the visual pathways), pericardial and pleural effusions, myocardial infarction, female genital tract and breast involvement, syndrome of inappropriate antidiuretic secretion, dysarthria, and noises in the head (e.g. sounding like turbine engines and tree frogs).[1,2,47] These manifestations can usually be reversed by glucocorticoids.

Physical examination in GCA may reveal tenderness, thickening, nodules, and occasionally erythema of the superficial temporal arteries.[2] Temporal artery pulses may be decreased or absent. In patients with large-vessel involvement bruits may be heard, particularly over the epiaortic vessels.

TAK is traditionally considered a triphasic disease, although overlap between stages may occur.[48] Phase 1, or 'pre-pulseless' disease, is characterized by constitutional and musculoskeletal manifestations such as fatigue, fever, weight loss, myalgia, and joint pain. Arthritis proper is uncommon.[49] Vascular abnormalities are absent at this stage. Phase 2 involves manifestations related to vascular inflammation ('pulseless disease'). These include carotidodynia and clinical features due to insufficient vascular supply to limbs and organs, such as Raynaud's phenomenon, limb claudication, dizziness, and hypertension. Finally, phase 3 refers to the final or 'burnt out' stage, when inflammation has abated, but symptoms and signs of vascular insufficiency persist. Table 133.4 summarizes the frequency of the most common clinical manifestations in different countries.

Most patients develop manifestations of vascular insufficiency in the upper limbs, ranging from a feeling of numbness or coldness to claudication, Raynaud's phenomenon or, rarely, distal gangrene.[13,51] The lower limbs are less frequently affected.[51] Physical examination reveals decreased or absent arterial pulses, and arterial bruits consistent with stenosing vasculitis. Bruits are mainly heard over the carotid, subclavian, and abdominal arteries.[13,49] Differences exceeding 10 mmHg in blood pressure readings in the arms are noted in most patients.[13]

Neurological manifestations are reported by approximately one-third of patients and are related to involvement of the carotid or vertebral arteries.[13,51] Neurological features include headache, dizziness, lightheadedness, and less commonly ischaemic events, syncope, or seizures.[13,48]

Ocular disease in TAK can be due to hypoperfusion (typically in the presence of severe carotid stenosis), but can also to unrecognized, untreated hypertension or to glucocorticoid treatment. Blurred vision, often dependent on posture, is described by up to one-third of patients, but fully-fledged ischaemic retinopathy is rare.[49] Signs of ischaemic retinopathy resemble those seen in diabetes mellitus and include microaneurysms and venous beading.[49] Rarely, in advanced disease retinal haemorrhages, arteriovenous anastomoses, optic disk atrophy, and retinal detachment may occur.[49]

Hypertension is associated with renal artery stenosis and is observed in approximately one-half of patients.[13] This complication is more common in Chinese and Indian patients than in whites. Renal artery occlusion leading to renal failure ('Schrumpfniere') can cause refractory hypertension requiring nephrectomy of the

Table 133.4 Frequencies of main clinical manifestations of Takayasu's arteritis in different countries

Clinical manifestations	Country and number (n) of patients studied			
	Japan[50] (n = 52)	USA[51] (n = 60)	India[52] (n = 45)	Italy[13] (n = 104)
Constitutional manifestations	27%	43%	16%	ns
Musculoskeletal manifestations	ns	53%	31%	ns
Claudication	13%	70%	20%	62%
Vascular bruits	ns	80%	71%	94%
Reduced or absent arterial pulses	62%	60%	ns	92%
Asymmetric blood pressure readings	ns	47%	ns	83%
Hypertension	33%	33%	76%	58%
Dizziness	40%	35%	44%	30%
Carotidodynia	21%	32%	4%	ns

ns, not specified.

affected kidney. Blood pressure readings may be unreliable in the presence of vascular stenosis, and should be obtained in all four limbs to minimize the risk of spuriously low values. In patients with diffuse stenoses of all limbs, central blood pressure measurement may be required. There are also scattered reports of renal amyloidosis, glomerulonephritis, and mesangial disease associated with TAK.[49]

Heart involvement occurs in 8–40% of patients and can be multifactorial in origin.[49,51] Coronary artery involvement can cause angina, myocardial infarction, heart failure, and sudden death. Myocarditis has been documented histologically in some patients, while in others arteritis may cause aortic or, less commonly, mitral regurgitation.[48,49]

Pulmonary artery involvement is found in one-half of patients, although it remains subclinical in many of those affected.[48,49] Interstitial lung disease has also been occasionally noted.[49]

Intestinal involvement in TAK is seen in approximately 10% of patients.[53] It is often due to an associated Crohn's disease, but ulcerative colitis has also been reported.[53]

A variety of skin changes have been described in TAK, including erythema nodosum, pyoderma gangrenosum, panniculitis, facial lupus, and erythema multiforme.[49,53] Some of these changes may reflect an underlying inflammatory bowel disease.

There are no established criteria to assess disease activity in TAK. The National Institute of Health (NIH) criteria consider the disease active if a patient has new onset or worsening of at least two out of the following items: raised ESR, systemic features, manifestations of vascular ischaemia, and typical lesions on angiography.[51] However, the sensitivity of these criteria is only 39%.[51]

A newer tool is the Indian Takayasu Activity Score (ITAS), which assesses disease activity in six domains (one for systemic manifestations and five for organ involvement). Physician global opinion and inflammatory markers are also recorded. TAK is considered active if there is evidence of disease activity in at least one domain. However, false-negative results have been obtained using the ITAS in 31% of patients with active TAK.[54]

Investigations

Laboratory tests

Inflammatory markers, in particular the ESR and CRP, are usually raised at diagnosis before the onset of glucocorticoid treatment in GCA patients. Normochromic normocytic anaemia, thrombocytosis, hypoalbuminaemia, and raised α_2-globulin may also be present as part of the systemic inflammatory process. In a minority of cases the ESR and, less frequently, CRP may be normal at diagnosis.[2,55] Elevated inflammatory markers are useful to assess disease activity. The CRP is more specific than the ESR in measuring inflammation, and is thus better suited to assess disease activity and guide therapeutic decisions.[1,2] Flares and relapses are often heralded by an increase in inflammatory markers, but an increase in ESR or CRP does not necessarily portend worsening of disease activity.[1,2] Therefore, treatment decisions should not be based solely on the behaviour of markers of inflammation. A possible exception is ocular GCA (GCA affecting the eye only), where monitoring of inflammatory markers is the only way to assess disease activity, since by definition patients with ocular GCA have no symptoms or signs of GCA except for ocular involvement.

Approximately one-quarter of GCA patients with active disease have a raised alkaline phosphatase, which normalizes following the onset of glucocorticoid treatment.[56] Patients with active GCA also test positive for anti-cardiolipin antibodies more often than age- and gender-matched controls, but the presence of anti-cardiolipin antibodies is not associated with an increased risk of thrombosis.[57] Anti-cardiolipin antibody levels normalize after treatment onset, but may rise again during flares or relapses.

Occasionally, thyroid function tests may be abnormal.

About 70–80% of patients with active TAK have elevated inflammatory markers such as ESR and CRP.[9,51] Normocytic anaemia as well as moderate leucocytosis and thrombocytosis can also occur.[9] However, inflammatory markers have only limited sensitivity and specificity for active disease. In a study from the NIH, the ESR was raised in only 72% of patients with active disease and normal in only 56% of those in remission.[51] IL-6 may be a better indicator of disease activity, but is not routinely measured.[58] Hypergammaglobulinaemia is found in up to one-third of patients, while anti-nuclear antibodies and rheumatoid factor are usually negative.[9] AECA are neither sensitive nor specific and have no role in the diagnostic work-up or in assessing disease activity.

Temporal artery biopsy

TAB is considered the gold standard for the diagnosis of GCA. However, TAB is negative in at least 10% of patients with clinical GCA even when performed accurately 'by the book'.[59] There are a number of reasons why TAB may be negative in patients with GCA. First, inflammatory changes affect the temporal arteries in a segmental fashion, so that a 'sampling error' may occur if the particular vessel segment sampled is not inflamed. Second, in some patients with GCA the temporal arteries may be truly spared by the inflammatory process. Particularly patients with large-vessel involvement have negative TAB findings in a quite high proportion (42%) of cases.[43] Third, inadequate sampling, such as excision of small (<2 cm) vessel segments, may significantly contribute in clinical practice to obtaining false-negative biopsy findings. Finally, glucocorticoids therapy may decrease the rate of positive TAB findings. In newly diagnosed GCA patients treated with high-dose glucocorticoids, TAB is positive in 78% of patients treated for less than 2 weeks, in 65% of those treated for 2–4 weeks, but only in 40% of those treated for longer than 4 weeks.[60] Therefore, while glucocorticoid therapy should be promptly commenced if GCA is strongly suspected, it is preferable to perform TAB within 1 week or so of onset of glucocorticoid therapy.

Fundoscopy

All patients with suspected GCA and visual loss should undergo an ophthalmologic examination including fundoscopy. In most cases, acute visual loss in GCA is due to AION. A chalky white optic disc oedema on fundoscopy is typical of AION, representing infarction of the optic nerve head caused by vasculitis, while fluorescein angiography usually demonstrates extensive choroidal hypoperfusion.[61] Central retinal artery and cilioretinal artery occlusion are less common causes of visual loss[61] that can also been appreciated on ophthalmoscopy, although fluorescein angiography may be required to buttress the diagnosis.

PION is an infrequent cause of ischaemic visual loss in GCA.[61] It differs from AION, in that the optic disc has a normal appearance on fundoscopy in the acute phase, although optic disk pallor usually ensues 4–6 weeks later.[62] Finally, in extremely rare cases blindness in GCA can be the result of cortical ischaemia, which obviously leaves the optic disc intact.

Imaging techniques

CDS, magnetic resonance angiography (MRA), and contrast-enhanced CT angiography (CTA) can visualize both the vessel wall and the lumen of the aorta and its major branches.[46] All these techniques can aid in diagnosing early large-vessel vasculitis by demonstrating inflammation of the arterial wall before vascular complications develop. Early inflammatory signs are vessel wall thickening as well as the 'halo' sign on CDS (a hypoechoic rim surrounding the lumen of an inflamed artery), vessel wall oedema (on MRA) and contrast enhancement (on MRA and CTA).[46] These techniques are also useful to monitor luminal changes over time and may replace digital subtraction angiography (DSA) in this regard.[46] On a note of caution, it should be pointed out that vessels that appear unaffected on CDS, CT, and MRI may develop vessel lumen alterations later.[63] It should also be appreciated that inflammatory changes depicted by CDS, CT, and MRI may persist for a while despite clinical remission, particularly in the large vessels.[63] PET may be more specific for active vascular inflammation in this regard.[46] Finally, luminal changes need not always be due to active vasculitis. For instance, vessel stenosis may also be to postinflammatory scarring, while aneurysms may grow in size due to intraluminal pressure even after inflammation has abated.[46]

DSA can reveal stenoses or aneurysms of the large vessels, but cannot visualize the vessel wall. PET is very sensitive in revealing inflammation of large vessels, but does not provide anatomical details of the vessels involved. The choice of the particular technique to be used in the individual patient thus critically depends on the vessels to be examined and on the type of information that one wishes to obtain.[46]

All vascular imaging techniques are to some degree operator-dependent and should be performed and interpreted by physicians with an expertise in vasculitis.

MRI and CT

MRI is able to show increased vessel wall thickness and oedema of inflamed large vessels.[46] MRI performed with contrast medium can also show enhancing vascular lesions in inflamed arteries.[46] Because vessel wall thickening and oedema precede the development of stenoses or aneurysms, MRI can aid in diagnosing early large-vessel vasculitis at a stage when conventional angiography (which only depicts the vessel lumen) is still negative. MRI (and CT) are particularly useful in evaluating deep, large vessels such as the thoracic and the abdominal aorta, which are frequently involved in GCA and TAK (Figure 133.2). Both MRI and CT can be combined with angiography to document alterations of the vessel lumen. MRI and CT are overall equally sensitive and specific in assessing large-vessel alterations. Compared with CT, MRI has the advantage of not exposing patients to radiation, although it may spuriously accentuate the appearance of stenoses.[46]

Preliminary data suggests that high-field (1.5–3 T) MRI may be very sensitive and specific in showing temporal artery inflammation.[64] In contrast, lower-field (1 T) MRI of the temporal arteries has poor sensitivity (27.2%) although good specificity (88.9%) for diagnosing GCA defined according to the ACR criteria.[65]

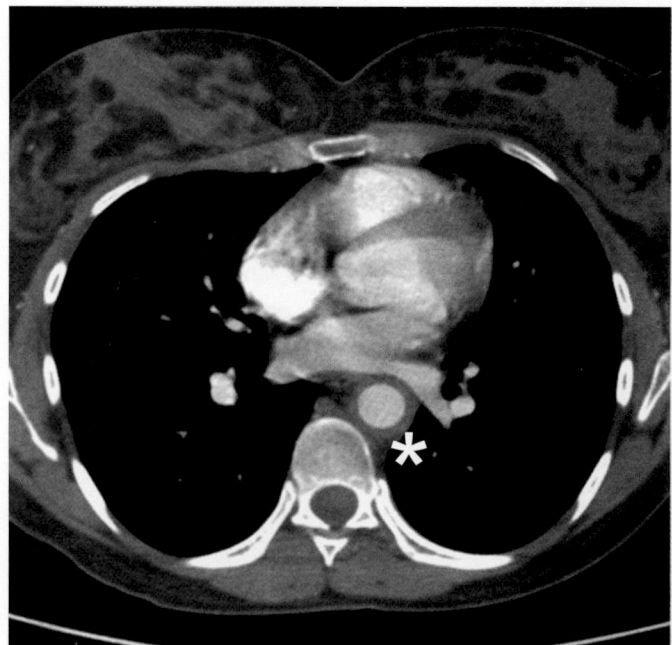

Fig. 133.2 Enhanced CT of a patient with giant cell arteritis involving the descending thoracic aorta (axial section). Note the thickened wall of the thoracic aorta (*).

Colour Doppler sonography

CDS combines imaging of the vessel wall with flow-velocity determination, and can thus assess both vessel anatomy and the lumen. The most specific and sensitive sign for the diagnosis of large-vessel vasculitis is a concentric hypoechogenic mural thickening ('halo' sign), reflecting vessel wall oedema.[66] This sign can be observed early on both in the temporal arteries and in the large vessels affected, and precedes the appearance of alterations of the vessel lumen such as stenoses or aneurysms (Figure 133.3). A recent meta-analysis which used a positive TAB as gold standard for the diagnosis of GCA demonstrated a sensitivity of 75% and a specificity of 83% for the halo sign in the temporal arteries.[67] The halo sign disappears within a few days to weeks from the temporal arteries following the onset of glucocorticoid treatment, whereas it may persist for longer periods of time in the large vessels involved.[46,66]

CDS has a 10-fold greater resolution than MRI or CT. Other advantages of CDS include its limited cost, the relatively short time required for the examination, and the absence of radiation. However, CDS is more operator-dependent than other imaging techniques. In addition, CDS cannot visualize some arteries covered by bones, such as the thoracic aorta, and may not image the abdominal aorta well when bowel gases and excessive fat tissue are interposed between the probe and the aorta.[46]

FDG-PET

PET (18F-Fluorodeoxyglucose positron emission tomography) is a nuclear medicine technique that is very sensitive in detecting increased uptake of a fluorine-labelled glucose analogue (FDG) by metabolically active cells, including inflammatory cells. PET is very useful in diagnosing large-vessel involvement because of its capacity to reveal inflammatory cell infiltration of the vessel wall, which

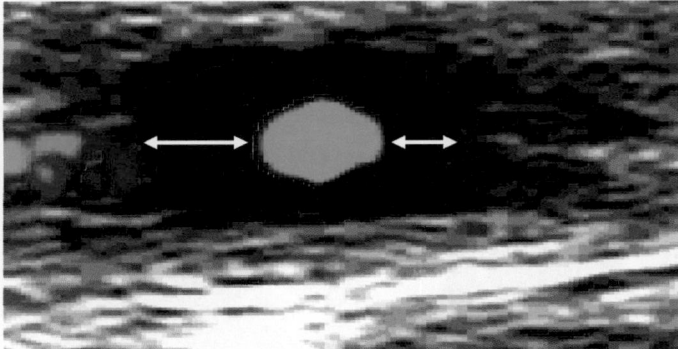

Fig. 133.3 Colour Doppler sonography of an inflamed temporal artery from a patient with giant cell arteritis (transverse section). The image shows the classical 'halo' sign, a hypoechoic rim (double arrows) around an inflamed temporal artery. Image courtesy of Dr Giuseppe Germanò, Department of Rheumatology, Reggio Emilia Hospital.

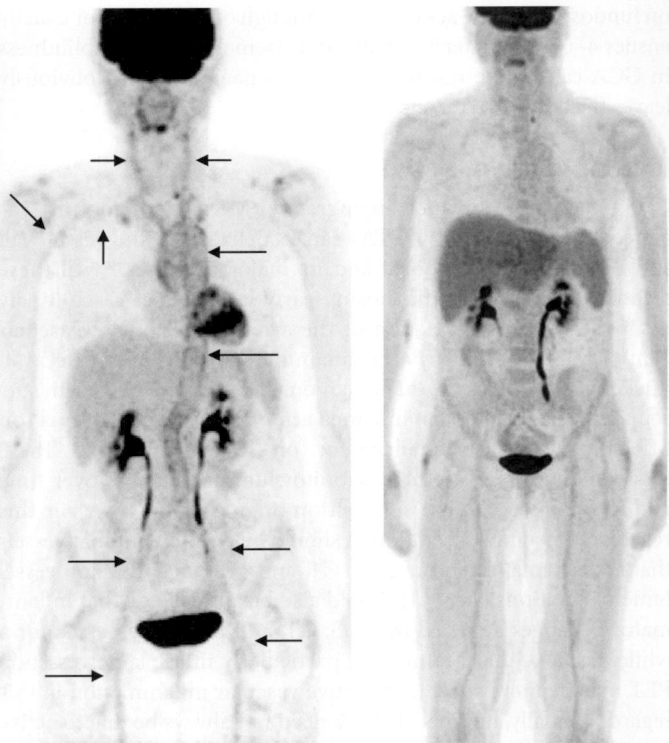

Fig. 133.4 ^{18}F-Fluorodeoxyglucose positron emission tomography of a patient with large-vessel giant cell arteritis before (A) and 6 months after onset of glucocorticoid therapy (B) (coronal sections). (A) Intense tracer uptake in the thoracic and abdominal aorta, and in the iliac, femoral, common carotid arteries bilaterally as well as in the right subclavian and axillary artery (arrows). (B) Resolution of the vascular uptake. (Images courtesy of Dr Annibale Versari, Department of Nuclear Medicine, Reggio Emilia Hospital.)

is one of the earliest events occurring in vasculitis (Figure 133.4).[46] In a study on 35 patients with new-onset, untreated GCA increased vascular uptake was observed in 83% of patients, mainly in the subclavian arteries (74%), in the aorta (>50%), and in the femoral arteries (37%).[45] A distinctive advantage of PET is its capacity to reveal both the grade and the extent of inflammation. Furthermore, because of its high sensitivity in revealing inflammation, PET may be a valuable tool in assessing disease activity over time, including response to therapy.[46] Compared with MRI, PET appears to be more sensitive in detecting vascular inflammation in the early stages of large-vessel vasculitis, and may also be superior in monitoring disease activity during immunosuppressive therapy.[46] However, the absence of validated criteria of disease activity hamper a proper assessment of the performance of PET.[68]

PET findings of vascular changes are not invariably due to vasculitis, and in fact may be secondary to atherosclerosis. Differentiating vasculitis from atherosclerosis is not always straightforward, but there are some clues that preferentially point to a diagnosis over the other (Box 133.1).[46] First, vasculitic lesions are usually characterized by more intense vascular uptake of FDG. Second, they have a smooth appearance that extends over long vascular segments, whereas atherosclerotic plaques are more irregular, with areas of high uptake close to others of lesser uptake. Finally, atherosclerosis and vasculitis tend to involve at least in part different types of vessel. Therefore, the pattern of vessels affected may provide some clues to the underlying disorder. Needless to say, vasculitis and atherosclerosis may also coexist in the same patient.

PET is minimally invasive and involves a very small dose of radiation. However, despite its merits, PET has some limitations. An important limitation is the lack of visualization of the temporal arteries, which is due both to the high background signal of the neighbouring brain and to the small diameter of the temporal arteries, which is below the resolution threshold of the PET scanners currently available.[46] Other limitations of PET are the high costs of the procedure, its long duration, and its limited availability.

Digital subtraction angiography

DSA is an excellent technique to document alterations of the vessel lumen such as stenoses or aneurysms in large-vessel vasculitis. Typical

---

Box 133.1 Differential diagnosis of established Takayasu's arteritis

Non-inflammatory vascular diseases

◆ Fibromuscular dysplasia
◆ Ehlers–Danlos syndrome
◆ Marfan syndrome
◆ Coarctation of the aorta
◆ Ergotism
◆ Neurofibromatosis

Diseases associated with large-vessel alterations

◆ Tuberculosis
◆ Syphilis
◆ Mycosis
◆ Spondyloarthropathies

Vasculitides involving large vessels

◆ Adamantiades–Behçet disease
◆ Cogan's syndrome
◆ Kawasaki's disease

angiographic findings are long, smooth vessel stenoses and, less frequently, occlusions and aneurysms.[46] However, none of these lesions occur early on. On the other hand, vessel wall thickening and mural oedema, which represent early vasculitic lesions, cannot be appreciated on angiography. Therefore, angiography is not useful in diagnosing early large-vessel vasculitis.[46] DSA also involves exposure to radiation and carries a risk of ischaemic complications due to the contrast medium.[46] Despite these limitations, angiography remains a helpful technique for guiding interventional procedures, and may also be used to monitor established lesions by means of serial angiograms.[46]

Management

Glucocorticoids

Glucocorticoids remain the cornerstone of treatment of GCA and TAK. In GCA, an initial dose of 40–60 mg daily of prednisone or its equivalent is adequate in most cases, while patients at high risk of developing ischaemic complications require higher dosages (in the range of 1 mg/kg per day). Pulse glucocorticoid therapy has been advocated for GCA patients with visual loss.[69] However, there is no evidence that pulse therapy is superior to oral glucocorticoids in preventing ischaemic complications including visual loss.[70] Regardless of the route of administration (oral or intravenous), glucocorticoids are very effective in rapidly preventing ischaemic complications, although they usually cannot reverse them.[71] Patients with active large-vessel vasculitis should receive glucocorticoids at appropriate dosages even in the absence of cranial vessel involvement to prevent vascular complications such as stenoses or aneurysms.

Alternate-day administration of glucocorticoids has been proposed to limit the occurrence of glucocorticoid-related adverse events. However, this regimen is associated with a much higher risk of relapses compared with daily treatment (70% vs 20%) and thus cannot be recommended.[72] Treatment with glucocorticoids at lower doses (10–40 mg/day) has also been proposed,[73] but there is insufficient evidence to support this regimen. Currently, the British Society for Rheumatology (BSR) recommends that the initial glucocorticoid dose be given for 3–4 weeks until clinical manifestations and laboratory alterations normalize. Subsequently, the glucocorticoid dose can be reduced by 10 mg every 2 weeks to 20 mg, then by 2.5 mg every 2–4 weeks to 10 mg, and then by 1 mg every 1–2 months provided there is no relapse.[74] Prophylaxis for osteoporosis should be implemented in all patients according to current guidelines.[74] Gradual tapering of glucocorticoids minimizes the risk of disease flares, although flares may still develop in some patients despite cautious tapering.[1,2] Flares are usually milder than clinical manifestations at onset, and can often be easily managed by increasing the glucocorticoid dosage.[75]

The majority of patients with GCA are able to discontinue glucocorticoids within 6 months to 2 years from the onset of treatment.[2] However, patients with PMR and GCA[76] and those with highly elevated inflammatory indices require longer glucocorticoid treatment.[40] A minority (up to one-third) of patients may require low-dose glucocorticoid treatment indefinitely.[77]

Glucocorticoids are also the mainstay of treatment of TAK. Although never formally tested in controlled trials, the NIH experience has shown their efficacy in improving clinical and laboratory parameters and preventing vascular complications.[9] The European League Against Rheumatism (EULAR) recommends that prednisone 1 mg/kg per day (maximum 60 mg/day) be used as induction therapy and slowly tapered after 1 month to a maintenance dose.[78] The vast majority (>90%) of TAK patients respond to glucocorticoids, but over two-thirds of them relapse upon tapering or discontinuation of glucocorticoid therapy.[79]

Immunosuppressive agents

Despite their remarkable efficacy, the use of glucocorticoids is fraught with many potential adverse events. Therefore, in patients with long-standing disease and in those at risk for glucocorticoid-related adverse events, the use of steroid-sparing agents should be considered.

Azathioprine

Azathioprine at a dose of 2 mg/kg per day has modest steroid-sparing properties in GCA. However, the effect of azathioprine becomes apparent only after over a year of continuous treatment.[80]

Azathioprine (2 mg/kg per day) is one of the steroid-sparing agents recommended by EULAR for use in patients with refractory TAK.[78] Azathioprine provides symptomatic benefit and prevents vascular complications.[81]

Cyclophosphamide

Cyclophosphamide can be efficacious in TAK,[78] but concerns about its toxicity limit its use in clinical practice.[52]

Methotrexate

Three randomized controlled trials have assessed the efficacy of methotrexate in recent-onset GCA with conflicting results. A meta-analysis based on the results of these studies has shown that methotrexate used as adjunctive treatment in GCA at a mean dosage of 11.1 mg/week reduced the risk of a first and a second relapse by 35% and 51%, respectively.[82] However, despite a lower cumulative glucocorticoid dose in the group of patients that received methotrexate, the incidence of glucocorticoid-related adverse events was similar in both groups. In addition, the effect of methotrexate was noticeable only after 24–36 weeks. It is unclear whether methotrexate used at a higher dosages could prove more effective and act more rapidly in curbing disease activity in GCA.

Methotrexate (20–25 mg/week) is recommended by EULAR as a steroid-sparing agent in patients with refractory TAK.[78] Methotrexate can improve clinical manifestations and halt progression of vascular complications.[83]

Mycophenolate mofetil

Mycophenolate mofetil ameliorates clinical manifestations and reduces serum levels of inflammatory markers in active TAK.[84]

Rituximab

A single report has described successful treatment of recalcitrant GCA with the monoclonal anti-CD20 (anti-B cell) antibody rituximab combined with cyclophosphamide.[85]

Rituximab also seems to be a useful option for refractory TA. Three patients with disease refractory to previous agents, including TNF blockers, were treated successfully with rituximab.[86]

TNFα-inhibitors

A randomized controlled trial (RCT) has shown that adding infliximab to prednisone provides no significant benefit over and above that provided by prednisone alone in patients with newly diagnosed GCA.[87] Therefore, TNFα inhibitors have no indication for the treatment of new-onset GCA.

In contrast, TNFα blocking agents might have some efficacy in patients with relapsing GCA. An RCT demonstrated that treatment with etanercept 25 mg twice weekly resulted in a lower cumulative prednisone dose after 12 months in patients who were unable to taper the prednisone dose below 10 mg/day.[88] Similarly, a small RCT and uncontrolled observations have shown that TNFα blockade with infliximab or etanercept was effective in reducing glucocorticoid requirements in patients with long-standing, relapsing GCA.[88,89]

The TNFα inhibitors etanercept (50 mg/week) and infliximab (3–5 mg/kg every 6–8 weeks) also induced remission in 60% of patients with TAK refractory to standard treatment.[15]

Tocilizumab

The IL-6 receptor antagonist monoclonal antibody tocilizumab has been used at a dose of 8 mg/kg per month in seven patients with GCA characterized by large-vessel involvement.[90,91] Three patients were treatment-naive and four had refractory GCA. All patients achieved a rapid and complete clinical response and normalization of the inflammatory markers, while the prednisone dosage could be tapered down within 12 weeks. However, it is unclear whether tocilizumab can effectively prevent GCA-related cranial ischaemic events; even more so, as IL-6 may arguably have a protective role against GCA-related ischaemic events.

Tocilizumab has proved effective in four patients with TAK, one of whom was treatment-naive, one resistant to glucocorticoids, and two resistant to multiple drugs.[91,92]

Aspirin

Two retrospective studies have suggested that low-dose aspirin might prevent ischaemic complications related to GCA. In one study, only 8% of the aspirin-treated patients presented with cranial ischaemic complications, compared with 29% of the non-aspirin-treated patients. In patients treated with glucocorticoids, addition of aspirin to glucocorticoids led to lower rates of cranial ischaemic complications (3%) compared to those observed in patients treated with glucocorticoids alone (13%).[93] In another study, only 16% patients on anti-platelet or anti-coagulant therapy suffered a GCA-related ischaemic event, compared with 48% of those not receiving such therapy.[94] However, these putative beneficial effects of aspirin have not been confirmed by other studies.[39,95] A prospective, controlled study is needed to formally assess the efficacy of aspirin for GCA patients, particularly those that are at risk of developing ischaemic complications.

Revascularization procedures

Revascularization procedures are indicated in patients with severe vascular stenoses. Both angioplasty and stenting have high (~90%) success rates, although restenosis may occur.[96,97] Bypass grafts provide the longest-lasting patency rates. Percutaneous balloon angioplasty provides good results for limited lesions. Timing surgery to remission reduces the risk of restenosis from 40–50% to 10%.[96,97] Nephrectomy is indicated if a kidney is non-functional owing to renal artery occlusion.

Differential diagnosis

Visual loss, usually due to AION, is a precocious manifestation, often heralding GCA. In patients with visual loss, diagnosing GCA is easy in the presence of the other typical clinical manifestations. However, some patients can present, at least initially, with isolated visual loss. In these cases, the diagnosis of GCA rests on the demonstration of elevated inflammatory markers and of a positive TAB. AION should be differentiated from non-arteritic AION (NAION). NAION is much more common than AION, affects almost exclusively elderly white patients, and is characterized by unilateral sudden visual loss in the absence of cranial of systemic manifestations suggestive of GCA. Contralateral eye involvement in NAION can occur, but less is less frequent than in AION. Fundoscopy usually shows hyperaemic (less often pale) oedema of the optic disk with a small cup to disc ratio.[62]

Approximately 15% of elderly patients with fever of unknown origin (FUO) are eventually diagnosed as having GCA.[98] In these patients, the diagnosis of GCA can be secured by TAB or, in some cases, by demonstrating large-vessel vasculitis using imaging procedures.

Temporal artery involvement is mostly due to GCA, but in the odd case may also be related to granulomatosis with polyangiitis (Wegener's) or primary systemic amyloidosis. In such cases histological findings point to the correct diagnosis.

A new onset of headache is also the most frequent main presenting symptom of primary central nervous system vasculitis; however, cerebral vasculitis is very rarely observed in GCA.[38]

Early, 'pre-pulseless' TAK should be differentiated from infections, FUO, malignancies, and early arthritis. A high index of suspicion and the use of imaging techniques are required to arrive at a correct diagnosis. Established TAK should be differentiated from other vasculopathies and diseases associated with large-vessel alterations (Box 133.1).[99]

In most cases, a diagnosis can be made by considering the features associated with the diseases and by the appropriate laboratory tests. Non-inflammatory vascular diseases can be distinguished from TAK by imaging. In older subjects, TAK should be differentiated from GCA. Age older than 40–50 years, shoulder stiffness, scalp tenderness and a lower frequency of vascular insufficiency of the upper limbs point away from TAK and towards GCA.[100] However, a subset of GCA patients may have only large-vessel vasculitis virtually indistinguishable from TAK.[99]

References

1. Salvarani C, Cantini F, Hunder GG. Polymyalgia rheumatica and giant-cell arteritis. *Lancet* 2008;372:234–245.
2. Salvarani C, Cantini F, Boiardi L, Hunder GG. Polymyalgia rheumatica and giant-cell arteritis. *N Engl J Med* 2002;347:261–271.
3. Gonzalez-Gay MA, Vazquez-Rodriguez TR, Lopez-Diaz MJ et al. Epidemiology of giant cell arteritis and polymyalgia rheumatica. *Arthritis Rheum* 2009;61:1454–1461.
4. Salvarani C, Gabriel SE, O'Fallon WM, Hunder GG. The incidence of giant cell arteritis in Olmsted County, Minnesota: apparent fluctuations in a cyclic pattern. *Ann Intern Med* 1995;123:192–194.
5. Gonzalez-Gay MA, Garcia-Porrua C, Amor-Dorado JC, Llorca J. Giant cell arteritis without clinically evident vascular involvement in a defined population. *Arthritis Rheum* 2004;51:274–277.
6. Blockmans D, De Ceuninck L, Vanderschueren S et al. Repetitive 18-fluorodeoxyglucose positron emission tomography in isolated polymyalgia rheumatica: a prospective study in 35 patients. *Rheumatology* (Oxford) 2007;46:672–677.
7. Pipitone N, Boiardi L, Bajocchi G, Salvarani C. Long-term outcome of giant cell arteritis. *Clin Exp Rheumatol* 2006;24:S65–S70.
8. Nuenninghoff DM, Hunder GG, Christianson TJ, McClelland RL, Matteson EL. Mortality of large-artery complication (aortic aneurysm, aortic dissection, and/or large-artery stenosis) in patients with giant

cell arteritis: a population-based study over 50 years. *Arthritis Rheum* 2003;48:3532–3537.

9. Hall S, Barr W, Lie JT et al. Takayasu arteritis. A study of 32 North American patients. *Medicine* (Baltimore) 1985;64:89–99.

10. Watts R, Al-Taiar A, Mooney J, Scott D, Macgregor A. The epidemiology of Takayasu arteritis in the UK. *Rheumatology* (Oxford) 2009;48:1008–1011.

11. Koide K. Takayasu arteritis in Japan. *Heart Vessels* Suppl 1992;7:48–54.

12. Toshihiko N. Current status of large and small vessel vasculitis in Japan. *Int J Cardiol* 1996;54 Suppl:S91–S98.

13. Vanoli M, Daina E, Salvarani C et al. Takayasu's arteritis: A study of 104 Italian patients. *Arthritis Rheum* 2005;53:100–107.

14. Moriwaki R, Noda M, Yajima M, Sharma BK, Numano F. Clinical manifestations of Takayasu arteritis in India and Japan—new classification of angiographic findings. *Angiology* 1997;48:369–379.

15. Jain S, Kumari S, Ganguly NK, Sharma BK. Current status of Takayasu arteritis in India. *Int J Cardiol* 1996;54 Suppl:S111–S116.

16. Hunder GG, Bloch DA, Michel BA et al. The American College of Rheumatology 1990 criteria for the classification of giant cell arteritis. *Arthritis Rheum* 1990;33:1122–1128.

17. Arend WP, Michel BA, Bloch DA et al. The American College of Rheumatology 1990 criteria for the classification of Takayasu arteritis. *Arthritis Rheum* 1990;33:1129–1134.

18. Gonzalez-Gay MA, Garcia-Porrua C, Ollier WE. Polymyalgia rheumatica and biopsy-proven giant cell arteritis exhibit different HLA-DRB1* associations. *J Rheumatol* 2003;30:2729.

19. Gonzalez-Gay MA, Rueda B, Vilchez JR et al. Contribution of MHC class I region to genetic susceptibility for giant cell arteritis. *Rheumatology* (Oxford) 2007;46:431–434.

20. Mattey DL, Hajeer AH, Dababneh A et al. Association of giant cell arteritis and polymyalgia rheumatica with different tumor necrosis factor microsatellite polymorphisms. *Arthritis Rheum* 2000;43:1749–1755.

21. Numano F. Differences in clinical presentation and outcome in different countries for Takayasu's arteritis. *Curr Opin Rheumatol* 1997;9:12–15.

22. Pipitone N, Salvarani C. The role of infectious agents in the pathogenesis of vasculitis. *Best Pract Res Clin Rheumatol* 2008;22:897–911.

23. Machado EB, Gabriel SE, Beard CM et al. A population-based case-control study of temporal arteritis: evidence for an association between temporal arteritis and degenerative vascular disease? *Int J Epidemiol* 1989;18:836–841.

24. Gonzalez-Gay MA, Pineiro A, Gomez-Gigirey A et al. Influence of traditional risk factors of atherosclerosis in the development of severe ischemic complications in giant cell arteritis. *Medicine* (Baltimore) 2004;83:342–347.

25. Lie JT. Illustrated histopathologic classification criteria for selected vasculitis syndromes. American College of Rheumatology Subcommittee on Classification of Vasculitis. *Arthritis Rheum* 1990;33:1074–1087.

26. Klein RG, Campbell RJ, Hunder GG, Carney JA. Skip lesions in temporal arteritis. *Mayo Clin Proc* 1976;51:504–510.

27. Restuccia G, Cavazza A, Boiardi L et al. Small-vessel vasculitis surrounding an uninflamed temporal artery and isolated vasa vasorum vasculitis of the temporal artery: two subsets of giant cell arteritis. *Arthritis Rheum* 2012;64:549–556.

28. Noris M. Pathogenesis of Takayasu's arteritis. *J Nephrol* 2001;14:506–513.

29. Han JW, Shimada K, Ma-Krupa W et al. Vessel wall-embedded dendritic cells induce T-cell autoreactivity and initiate vascular inflammation. *Circ Res* 2008;102:546–553.

30. Weyand CM, Goronzy JJ. Arterial wall injury in giant cell arteritis. *Arthritis Rheum* 1999;42:844–853.

31. Weyand CM, Hicok KC, Hunder GG, Goronzy JJ. Tissue cytokine patterns in patients with polymyalgia rheumatica and giant cell arteritis. *Ann Intern Med* 1994;121:484–491.

32. Kaiser M, Weyand CM, Bjornsson J, Goronzy JJ. Platelet-derived growth factor, intimal hyperplasia, and ischemic complications in giant cell arteritis. *Arthritis Rheum* 1998;41:623–633.

33. Wagner AD, Goronzy JJ, Weyand CM. Functional profile of tissue-infiltrating and circulating CD68+ cells in giant cell arteritis. Evidence for two components of the disease. *J Clin Invest* 1994;94:1134–1140.

34. Hernandez-Rodriguez J, Segarra M, Vilardell C et al. Elevated production of interleukin-6 is associated with a lower incidence of disease-related ischemic events in patients with giant-cell arteritis: angiogenic activity of interleukin-6 as a potential protective mechanism. *Circulation* 2003;107:2428–2434.

35. Weyand CM, Goronzy JJ. Pathogenic mechanisms in giant cell arteritis. *Cleve Clin J Med* 2002;69 Suppl 2:SII28–SII32.

36. Seko Y, Minota S, Kawasaki A et al. Perforin-secreting killer cell infiltration and expression of a 65-kD heat-shock protein in aortic tissue of patients with Takayasu's arteritis. *J Clin Invest* 1994;93:750–758.

37. Tripathy NK, Upadhyaya S, Sinha N, Nityanand S. Complement and cell mediated cytotoxicity by antiendothelial cell antibodies in Takayasu's arteritis. *J Rheumatol* 2001;28:805–808.

38. Salvarani C, Giannini C, Miller DV, Hunder G Giant cell arteritis: Involvement of intracranial arteries. *Arthritis Rheum* 2006;55:985–989.

39. Salvarani C, Della BC, Cimino L et al. Risk factors for severe cranial ischaemic events in an Italian population-based cohort of patients with giant cell arteritis. *Rheumatology* (Oxford) 2009;48:250–253.

40. Hernandez-Rodriguez J, Garcia-Martinez A, Casademont J et al. A strong initial systemic inflammatory response is associated with higher corticosteroid requirements and longer duration of therapy in patients with giant-cell arteritis. *Arthritis Rheum* 2002;47:29–35.

41. Salvarani C, Cimino L, Macchioni P et al. Risk factors for visual loss in an Italian population-based cohort of patients with giant cell arteritis. *Arthritis Rheum* 2005;53:293–297.

42. Paraskevas KI, Boumpas DT, Vrentzos GE, Mikhailidis DP. Oral and ocular/orbital manifestations of temporal arteritis: a disease with deceptive clinical symptoms and devastating consequences. *Clin Rheumatol* 2007;26:1044–1048.

43. Brack A, Martinez-Taboada V, Stanson A, Goronzy JJ, Weyand CM. Disease pattern in cranial and large-vessel giant cell arteritis. *Arthritis Rheum* 1999;42:311–317.

44. Bongartz T, Matteson EL. Large-vessel involvement in giant cell arteritis. *Curr Opin Rheumatol* 2006;18:10–17.

45. Blockmans D, De Ceuninck L, Vanderschueren S et al. Repetitive 18F-fluorodeoxyglucose positron emission tomography in giant cell arteritis: a prospective study of 35 patients. *Arthritis Rheum* 2006;55:131–137.

46. Pipitone N, Versari A, Salvarani C. Role of imaging studies in the diagnosis and follow-up of large-vessel vasculitis: an update. *Rheumatology* (Oxford) 2008;47:403–408.

47. Stone JH. Vasculitis: a collection of pearls and myths. *Rheum Dis Clin North Am* 2007;33:691–739, v.

48. Kerr GS. Takayasu's arteritis. *Rheum Dis Clin North Am* 1995;21:1041–1058.

49. Hall S, Buchbinder R. Takayasu's arteritis. *Rheum Dis Clin North Am* 1990;16:411–422.

50. Ueda H, Morooka S, Ito I, Yamaguchi H, Takeda T. Clinical observation of 52 cases of aortitis syndrome. *Jpn Heart J* 1969;10:277–288.

51. Kerr GS, Hallahan CW, Giordano J et al. Takayasu arteritis. *Ann Intern Med* 1994;120:919–929.

52. Samantray SK. Takayasu's arteritis: a study of 45 cases. *Aust N Z J Med* 1978;8:68.

53. Sharma BK, Jain S, Sagar S. Systemic manifestations of Takayasu arteritis: the expanding spectrum. *Int J Cardiol* 1996;54 Suppl:S149–S154.

54. Direskeneli H, Aydin SZ, Merkel PA. Assessment of disease activity and progression in Takayasu's arteritis. *Clin Exp Rheumatol* 2011;29:S86–S91.

55. Kyle V, Cawston TE, Hazleman BL. Erythrocyte sedimentation rate and C reactive protein in the assessment of polymyalgia rheumatica/giant cell arteritis on presentation and during follow up. *Ann Rheum Dis* 1989;48:667–671.

56. Kyle V, Wraight EP, Hazleman BL. Liver scan abnormalities in polymyalgia rheumatica/giant cell arteritis. *Clin Rheumatol* 1991;10:294–297.

57. Duhaut P, Berruyer M, Pinede L et al. Anticardiolipin antibodies and giant cell arteritis: a prospective, multicenter case-control study. Groupe de Recherche sur l'Arterite a Cellules Géantes. *Arthritis Rheum* 1998;41:701–709.

58. Noris M, Daina E, Gamba S, Bonazzola S, Remuzzi G. Interleukin-6 and RANTES in Takayasu arteritis: a guide for therapeutic decisions? *Circulation* 1999;100:55–60.

59. Salvarani C, Hunder GG. Giant cell arteritis with low erythrocyte sedimentation rate: frequency of occurence in a population-based study. *Arthritis Rheum* 2001;45:140–145.

60. Narvaez J, Bernad B, Roig-Vilaseca D et al. Influence of previous corticosteroid therapy on temporal artery biopsy yield in giant cell arteritis. *Semin Arthritis Rheum* 2007;37:13–19.

61. Hayreh SS, Podhajsky PA, Zimmerman B. Ocular manifestations of giant cell arteritis. *Am J Ophthalmol* 1998;125:509–520.

62. Rucker JC, Biousse V, Newman NJ. Ischemic optic neuropathies. *Curr Opin Neurol* 2004;17:27–35.

63. Tso E, Flamm SD, White RD et al. Takayasu arteritis: utility and limitations of magnetic resonance imaging in diagnosis and treatment. *Arthritis Rheum* 2002;46:1634–1642.

64. Bley TA, Wieben O, Uhl M et al. High-resolution MRI in giant cell arteritis: imaging of the wall of the superficial temporal artery. *AJR Am J Roentgenol* 2005;184:283–287.

65. Ghinoi A, Zuccoli G, Nicolini A et al. 1T magnetic resonance imaging in the diagnosis of giant cell arteritis: comparison with ultrasonography and physical examination of temporal arteries. *Clin Exp Rheumatol* 2008;26:S76–S80.

66. Schmidt WA, Kraft HE, Vorpahl K, Volker L, Gromnica-Ihle EJ. Color duplex ultrasonography in the diagnosis of temporal arteritis. *N Engl J Med* 1997;337:1336–1342.

67. Ball EL, Walsh SR, Tang TY, Gohil R, Clarke JM. Role of ultrasonography in the diagnosis of temporal arteritis. *Br J Surg* 2010;97:1765–1771.

68. Wenger M, Calamia KT, Salvarani C, Moncayo R, Schirmer M. Do we need 18F-FDG-positron emission tomography as a functional imaging technique for diagnosing large vessel arteritis? *Clin Exp Rheumatol* 2003;21:S1–S2.

69. Sailler L, Carreiro M, Ollier S et al. [Non-complicated Horton's disease: initial treatment with methylprednisolone 500 mg/day bolus for three days followed by 20 mg/day prednisone-equivalent. Evaluation of 15 patients.] *Rev Med Interne* 2001;22:1032–1038.

70. Chevalet P, Barrier JH, Pottier P et al. A randomized, multicenter, controlled trial using intravenous pulses of methylprednisolone in the initial treatment of simple forms of giant cell arteritis: a one year follow-up study of 164 patients. *J Rheumatol* 2000;27:1484–1491.

71. Pipitone N, Salvarani C. Improving therapeutic options for patients with giant cell arteritis. *Curr Opin Rheumatol* 2008;20:17–22.

72. Hunder GG, Sheps SG, Allen GL, Joyce JW. Daily and alternate-day corticosteroid regimens in treatment of giant cell arteritis: comparison in a prospective study. *Ann Intern Med* 1975;82:613–618.

73. Delecoeuillerie G, Joly P, Cohen dL, Paolaggi JB. Polymyalgia rheumatica and temporal arteritis: a retrospective analysis of prognostic features and different corticosteroid regimens (11 year survey of 210 patients). *Ann Rheum Dis* 1988;47:733–739.

74. Dasgupta B, Borg FA, Hassan N et al. BSR and BHPR guidelines for the management of giant cell arteritis. *Rheumatology* (Oxford) 2010;49:1594–1597.

75. Hachulla E, Boivin V, Pasturel-Michon U et al. Prognostic factors and long-term evolution in a cohort of 133 patients with giant cell arteritis. *Clin Exp Rheumatol* 2001;19:171–176.

76. Lundberg I, Hedfors E. Restricted dose and duration of corticosteroid treatment in patients with polymyalgia rheumatica and temporal arteritis. *J Rheumatol* 1990;17:1340–1345.

77. Graham E, Holland A, Avery A, Russell RW. Prognosis in giant-cell arteritis. *Br Med J Clin Res Ed* 1981;282:269–271.

78. Mukhtyar C, Guillevin L, Cid MC et al. EULAR recommendations for the management of large vessel vasculitis. *Ann Rheum Dis* 2009;68:318–323.

79. Maksimowicz-McKinnon K, Clark TM, Hoffman GS. Limitations of therapy and a guarded prognosis in an American cohort of Takayasu arteritis patients. *Arthritis Rheum* 2007;56:1000–1009.

80. De Silva M, Hazleman BL. Azathioprine in giant cell arteritis/polymyalgia rheumatica: a double-blind study. *Ann Rheum Dis* 1986;45:136–138.

81. Valsakumar AK, Valappil UC, Jorapur V et al. Role of immunosuppressive therapy on clinical, immunological, and angiographic outcome in active Takayasu's arteritis. *J Rheumatol* 2003;30:1793–1798.

82. Mahr AD, Jover JA, Spiera RF et al. Adjunctive methotrexate to treat giant cell arteritis: an individual patient data meta-analysis. *Arthritis Rheum* 2007;56:2789–2797.

83. Hoffman GS, Leavitt RY, Kerr GS et al. Treatment of glucocorticoid-resistant or relapsing Takayasu arteritis with methotrexate. *Arthritis Rheum* 1994;37:578–582.

84. Shinjo SK, Pereira RM, Tizziani VA, Radu AS, Levy-Neto M. Mycophenolate mofetil reduces disease activity and steroid dosage in Takayasu arteritis. *Clin Rheumatol* 2007;26:1871–1875.

85. Bhatia A, Ell PJ, Edwards JC. Anti-CD20 monoclonal antibody (rituximab) as an adjunct in the treatment of giant cell arteritis. *Ann Rheum Dis* 2005;64:1099–1100.

86. Hoyer BF, Mumtaz IM, Loddenkemper K et al. Takayasu arteritis is characterized by disturbances of B cell homeostasis and responds to B cell depletion therapy with rituximab. *Ann Rheum Dis* 2012;71:75–79.

87. Hoffman GS, Cid MC, Rendt-Zagar KE et al. Infliximab for maintenance of glucocorticosteroid-induced remission of giant cell arteritis: a randomized trial. *Ann Intern Med* 2007;146:621–630.

88. Martinez-Taboada VM, Rodriguez-Valverde V, Carreno L et al. A double-blind placebo controlled trial of etanercept in patients with giant cell arteritis and corticosteroid side effects. *Ann Rheum Dis* 2008;67:625–630.

89. Cantini F, Niccoli L, Salvarani C, Padula A, Olivieri I. Treatment of longstanding active giant cell arteritis with infliximab: report of four cases. *Arthritis Rheum* 2001;44:2933–2935.

90. Seitz M, Reichenbach S, Bonel HM et al. Rapid induction of remission in large vessel vasculitis by IL-6 blockade. A case series. *Swiss Med Wkly* 2011;141:w13156.

91. Salvarani C, Magnani L, Catanoso M et al. Tocilizumab: a novel therapy for patients with large-vessel vasculitis. *Rheumatology* (Oxford) 2012;51:151–156.

92. Salvarani C, Pipitone N. Treatment of large-vessel vasculitis: where do we stand? *Clin Exp Rheumatol* 2011;29:S3–S5.

93. Nesher G, Berkun Y, Mates M et al. Low-dose aspirin and prevention of cranial ischemic complications in giant cell arteritis. *Arthritis Rheum* 2004;50:1332–1337.

94. Lee MS, Smith SD, Galor A, Hoffman GS. Antiplatelet and anticoagulant therapy in patients with giant cell arteritis. *Arthritis Rheum* 2006;54:3306–3309.

95. Narvaez J, Bernad B, Gomez-Vaquero C et al. Impact of antiplatelet therapy in the development of severe ischemic complications and in the outcome of patients with giant cell arteritis. *Clin Exp Rheumatol* 2008;26:S57–S62.

96. Borg FA, Dasgupta B. Treatment and outcomes of large vessel arteritis. *Best Pract Res Clin Rheumatol* 2009;23:325–337.

97. Liang P, Hoffman GS. Advances in the medical and surgical treatment of Takayasu arteritis. *Curr Opin Rheumatol* 2005;17:16–24.

98. Calamia KT, Hunder GG. Giant cell arteritis (temporal arteritis) presenting as fever of undetermined origin. *Arthritis Rheum* 1981;24:1414–1418.

99. Wilke WS. Large vessel vasculitis (giant cell arteritis, Takayasu arteritis). *Baillieres Clin Rheumatol* 1997;11:285–313.

100. Michel BA, Arend WP, Hunder GG. Clinical differentiation between giant cell (temporal) arteritis and Takayasu's arteritis. *J Rheumatol* 1996;23:106–111.

CHAPTER 134

Polymyalgia rheumatica

Bhaskar Dasgupta

Introduction

Polymyalgia rheumatica (PMR), a common inflammatory condition of older people, is characterized by bilateral proximal pain and morning stiffness, an acute-phase response involving elevated erythrocyte sedimentation rate (ESR) and/or C-reactive protein (CRP), and a rapid response to corticosteroids. This widely prevalent condition is subject to variations of practice in primary and secondary care[1] and is a common indication for long-term steroid use in the community.[2] Patients are therefore vulnerable to the manifold adverse events associated with prolonged corticosteroid therapy.

Accurate assessment of patient-based outcomes, disease activity, and course of disease are critical to balance the benefits of corticosteroids against the increased risk of adverse outcomes such as diabetic complications and fractures. There is also considerable uncertainty regarding diagnosis and outcomes in PMR.[3] Initial features may be variable, e.g. PMR without an elevated ESR is reported in up to 22% of patients and common mimicking conditions can present with the polymyalgic syndrome. There is no gold standard test and several diagnostic criteria have been used. This may explain the lack of agreement in PMR diagnoses between primary care physicians and rheumatologists and revision of diagnoses in 5–23% of patients on long-term follow-up.

An international initiative to address this diagnostic conundrum has led to classification criteria for the polymyalgic syndrome.[4] Most clinicians consider a rapid resolution of symptoms with corticosteroid therapy a diagnostic hallmark of PMR, though some studies report slower responses in many patients and lack of response may indicate an incorrect diagnosis. However, there is little evidence on what constitutes a typical response and how it relates to longer-term outcomes or revisions of the initial diagnosis.

It is accepted that around one-half of patients have one or more relapses and median duration of corticosteroid treatment around 2–3 years. PMR appears to be a heterogeneous condition. The prognostic factors at presentation that affect this heterogeneity of disease course, clinical outcomes, and duration of treatment are ill understood. This chapter discusses (1) the epidemiology of PMR; (2) the burden of disease, including the economic burden; and (3) the impact of PMR, particularly the initial response to corticosteroid therapy, on clinical and patient-based outcomes (early and long term), and examines the relationship between laboratory measures and clinical outcomes, functional status, and changes in quality of life (QoL),[4] potential medical errors in the diagnosis and management of PMR, occurrence of preventable complications,[5] and guidelines and audit standards for diagnosis and management.

Epidemiology

The epidemiology and population burden of PMR is documented in a limited number of studies.[5] The incidence of PMR varies markedly according to geographical region, with much higher rates in countries in the northern latitudes. In northern United States, the average annual age- and sex-adjusted incidence of PMR per 100 000 population 50 years of age or over is estimated at 58.7.(95% CI 52.8–64.7) with a significantly higher incidence in females (69.8; 95% CI 61.2–78.4) than in males (44.8; 95% CI 37.0–52.6). The incidence in the northern United States is similar to the incidence estimates from Denmark (68.3 per 100 000) and Norway (112 per 100 000), but is substantially higher than the figures reported in Göteborg, Sweden (28.6 per 100 000), Reggio Emilia, Italy (12.7 per 100 000) and Lugo, Spain (18.7 per 100 000).

A recent large primary care database study from the United Kingdom reported an incidence of 84 per 100 000 with a female:male ratio of 2.0.[6] This is the only study that also reported a marked increase in the incidence of PMR throughout the 1990s, from 69 per 100 000 person-years in 1990 to 93 per 100 000 person-years in 2001. A similar temporal increase in incidence was not observed in other studies. It is unclear whether there is a true increase in incidence of PMR, or overdiagnosis or increased recognition of PMR over time.

The prevalence of PMR among individuals over 50 years of age in the year 2000 is estimated at 739 per 100 000, with a higher prevalence in females than in males.[7] The prevalence increases dramatically with age: from 21 per 100 000 for ages 50–54 years to 4213 per 100 000 for ages 90–95 years. With these prevalence estimates, 711 000 Americans are estimated to have PMR. Survival was also examined in various studies and they all indicate that survival in PMR patients is similar to that in the general population. This has been in part attributed to increased medical surveillance during the disease course.

Classification criteria

Difficulties in diagnosing and classifying patients with PMR unrelated to lack of training and expertise are inherent to accepted definitions of PMR. The proximal pain and stiffness syndrome, the commonly accepted phenotype of PMR, can occur at presentation in many other rheumatological and inflammatory illnesses, especially in older people. About one-half of patients diagnosed with PMR may have distal musculoskeletal manifestations such as peripheral arthritis, distal hand swelling with pitting oedema, and carpal tunnel syndrome. On the other hand, polymyalgic presentation is common, if not the rule, in late-onset rheumatoid arthritis and spondyloarthritis. Polymyalgia is also associated with giant cell arteritis (GCA) in 10–30% of cases. Heterogeneity in the clinical disease course, uncertainty regarding best disease assessment parameters, and the evolution of alternate diagnoses on follow-up complicate understanding and treatment of PMR. For all these reasons, recent guidelines on PMR opt for a safe and specific approach, preferring a relative underdiagnosis to an overdiagnosis of PMR.

A uniform responsiveness to low doses of corticosteroids has been assumed to be a cardinal feature of PMR. It is included in several popular diagnostic criteria and is commonly used by clinicians in both primary and secondary care to make a PMR diagnosis. However, there is little hard evidence to substantiate this assertion and a previous prospective inception cohort study of PMR showed that at 3 weeks after starting prednisolone 15 mg/day more than 55% failed a complete response to therapy as defined by greater than 70% improvement in pain, morning stiffness less than half an hour, and normal inflammatory markers.[10] This also emphasizes that clinical trials of disease-modifying anti-rheumatic drugs (DMARDs) and novel agents are needed to improve treatment efficacy in PMR.

In an international initiative sponsored by the European League Against Rheumatism (EULAR) and the ACR, candidate classification criteria for PMR were defined through systematic literature review, a three-phase consensus process, and a wider survey.[6] These criteria were then evaluated in a 6 month prospective cohort study of 125 patients with new-onset PMR and 169 non-PMR comparison subjects with conditions mimicking PMR. Potential criteria were assessed for their ability to discriminate PMR from other conditions and a scoring algorithm was developed.

New-onset bilateral shoulder pain in subjects aged 50 years or older and elevation of CRP and/or ESR are regarded as essential items for classification as PMR. The clinical scoring algorithm is based on morning stiffness in excess of 45 minutes (2 points), hip pain/limited range of motion (1 point), normal rheumatoid factor (RF) and/or anti-citrullinated protein antibody (ACPA) (2 points), and absence of peripheral joint pain (1 point). A score of 4 or more has 68% sensitivity and 78% specificity for discriminating all comparison subjects from PMR. The specificity is higher (88%) for discriminating shoulder conditions from PMR and lower (65%) for discriminating RA from PMR. The c-statistic for the scoring algorithm is 81%. The positive predictive value was 69% and the negative predictive value was 77%.

Ultrasound was performed in 120 PMR subjects, 154 comparison subjects (46 with RA and 47 with shoulder conditions), and 21 additional controls (not included in our study cohorts) who did not have shoulder conditions. Patients with PMR were more likely to have abnormal ultrasound findings in the shoulder (particularly subdeltoid bursitis and biceps tenosynovitis), and somewhat more likely to have abnormal findings in the hips than comparison subjects as a group (Table 134.1). PMR could not be distinguished from RA on the basis of ultrasound, but could be distinguished

Table 134.1 Polymyalgia rheumatica classification criteria: scoring algorithm. Required criteria: age≥50 years, bilateral shoulder aching, and abnormal CRP and/or ESR[a]

	Points without US 0–6	Points with US[b] 0–8
Morning stiffness >45 minutes	2	2
Hip pain or limited range of motion	1	1
Normal RF or ACPA	2	2
Absence of other joint involvement	1	1
At least 1 shoulder with subdeltoid bursitis and/or biceps tenosynovitis and/or glenohumeral synovitis (either posterior or axillary) AND at least 1 hip with synovitis and/or trochanteric bursitis	Not applicable	1
Both shoulders with subdeltoid bursitis, biceps tenosynovitis or glenohumeral synovitis	Not applicable	1

ACPA, anti-citrullinated protein antibody; CI, confidence interval; CRP, C-reactive protein; ESR, erythrocyte sedimentation rate; RF, rheumatoid factor; US, ultrasound.
[a]A score of 4 or more is categorized as PMR in the algorithm without US and a score of 5 or more is categorized as PMR in the algorithm with US.
[b]Optional ultrasound criteria.

from non-RA shoulder conditions and subjects without shoulder conditions. Adding ultrasound criteria of either both shoulders and/or a shoulder and hip showing typical abnormalities, an algorithm score of 5 or more has 66% sensitivity and 81% specificity for discriminating all comparison subjects from PMR. Ultrasound abnormalities at presentation were predictive of a good steroid response.

Pathogenesis

The pathogenesis of PMR is unclear, but one concept is that GCA and PMR are the opposite ends of the same spectrum with the absence of vascular involvement in pure PMR. Synovitis, bursitis, and tenosynovitis around the joints are all seen in PMR. Inflammation is initiated inside the tissue (synovium or bursa) with recognition of putative antigen by dendritic cells (DCs) or macrophages (Figure 134.1).[8] Activated DCs or macrophages secrete inflammatory mediators, including IL-1, IL-6, and tumour necrosis factor alpha (TNFα), which are responsible for the systemic features of the disease. They may then move to the central lymphoid organs, such as the lymph node and spleen, where they present antigen to the T cells. These T cells then migrate back to the synovium, enhance the adaptive immune response, and secrete further cytokines promoting local inflammation. A recent study has shown that vasoactive intestinal polypeptide, a neuropeptide, is locally produced inside the synovium. Vasoactive intestinal polypeptide (VIP) can induce a change in CD4+ T-cell phenotype from Th1 to Th2. Th2-type cells do not secrete interferon (IFN)-γ, which is a key cytokine in GCA pathogenesis. This may explain why most patients with PMR do not develop GCA. Two different T-cell subsets, Th17 (steroid-sensitive acute lesions) and Th1 (steroid-insensitive chronic lesions) may relate to the persistence of disease in GCA.[9] A similar mechanism for disease persistence may be relevant to PMR.

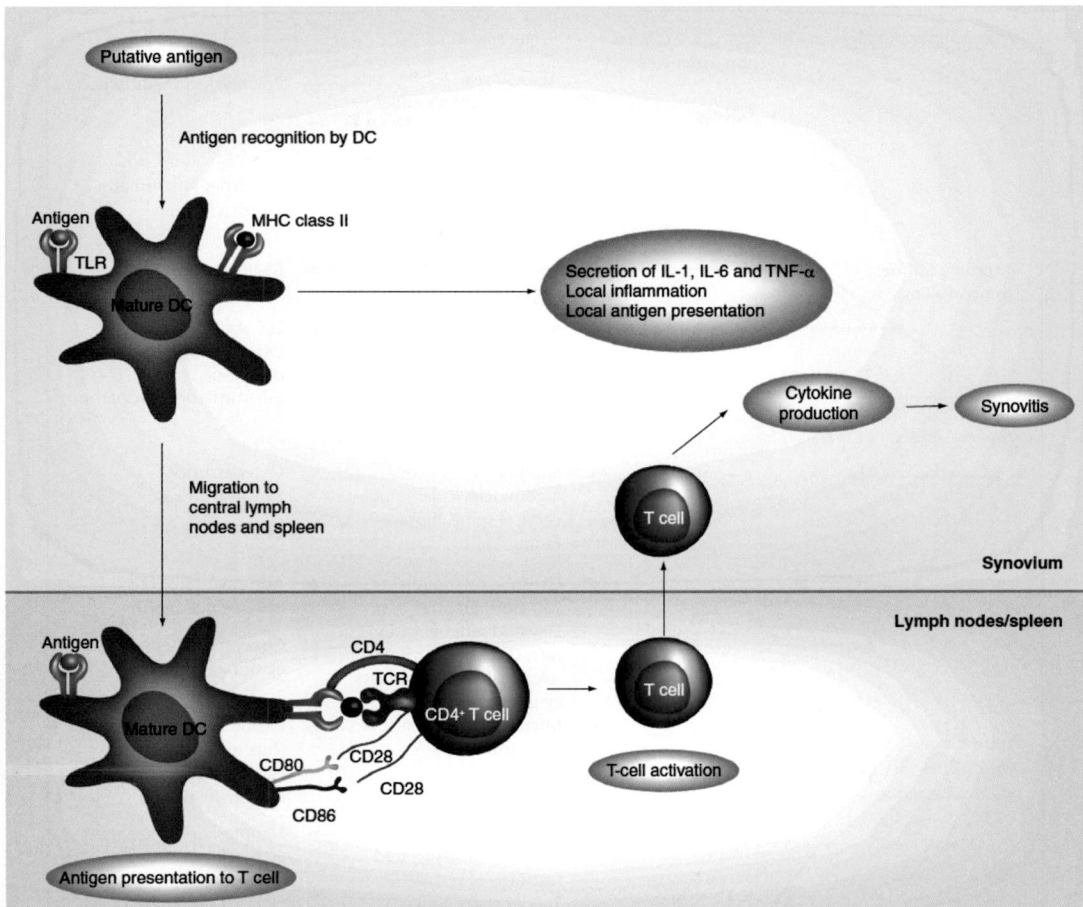

Fig. 134.1 Pathogenesis of polymyalgia rheumatica.
From Ghosh et al Expert Rev. Clin. Immunol. 6(6), 913–928 (2010).

Cytokines in polymyalgia rheumatica

Cytokines are the ultimate products fuelling the pathogenesis of PMR and GCA and are responsible for the systemic inflammatory response seen in these conditions. Therefore, modulating cytokine levels should lead to the amelioration of the disease process. Most studies regarding circulating cytokines focus on IL-6.[10] These studies show high levels of IL-6 in both PMR and GCA. The data on other cytokines (IL-1,IL-2, TNFα, IFN-γ, IL-10, and so on) are too scant to allow us to draw any definitive conclusions. Most studies in PMR have shown that levels of circulating IL-6 decrease significantly with the remission of clinical symptoms. IL-6 blockade could be a potential target for therapy, especially in PMR patients.

Evaluation of the patient with suspected polymyalgia rheumatica and pitfalls in diagnosis

Proximal pain and stiffness, hallmarks of the polymyalgic syndrome, can be features of several systemic inflammatory diseases. The disease usually starts abruptly with pain and stiffness in the shoulder, pelvic girdles, and neck. There may also be systemic features including fever, malaise, and weight loss. Patients may also present with distal features, especially hand arthritis, tenosynovitis, and carpal tunnel syndrome. PMR is present in approximately 50% of GCA patients and approximately 10% of PMR patients develop GCA.

The following are the key steps required:

1. **Establish the diagnosis** by ruling out mimics, considering clues to a non-PMR diagnosis and assessing any overlap with inflammatory arthritis or large-vessel vasculitis. A thorough history-taking, examination, and review of blood results is essential prior to prescription of steroids (see Figures 134.2 and 134.3). A pain diagram indicating the site of pain may be useful in improving accuracy of PMR diagnosis in primary care.

   Clues to a non-PMR diagnoses are: younger age of onset, chronic onset, peripheral arthritis, spinal involvement, pronounced systemic symptoms, neurological signs, very high CRP/ESR, lack of response to 15–20 mg prednisolone.

2. **Assess the severity** of the condition (based on intensity of pain, stiffness, disability, inflammatory markers).

3. **Imaging** with ultrasonography of shoulders, hips, peripheral joints, and temporal arteries may be helpful in establishing the diagnosis and excluding peripheral arthritis and GCA.

4. **Assess comorbidities** which may be relevant to choice of steroid dose.

5. **Make an individualized choice of steroid dose** and other therapy based on the above assessments and patient's preferences.

6. **Provide education** on the condition, its treatment, and potential complications, precautions, and monitoring requirements.

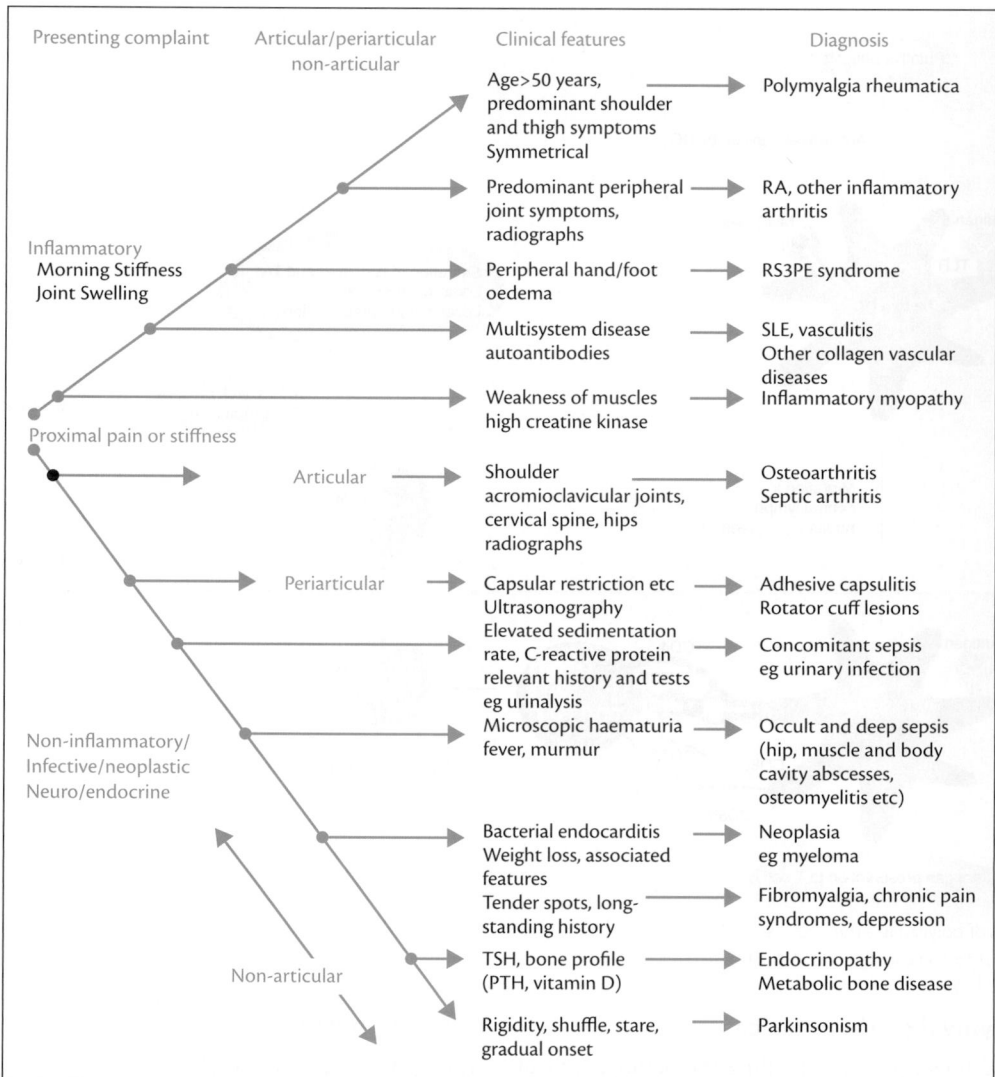

Fig. 134.2 A referral pathway for polymyalgia rheumatica (PMR) compatible with these guidelines is suggested in the Map of Medicine. CRP, C-reactive protein; CTD, connective tissue disease; ESR, erythrocyte sedimentation rate; FBC, full blood count; GCA, giant cell arteritis; IM, intramuscular; RA, rheumatoid arthritis; SLE, systemic lupus erythematosus; U&E, urea and electrolytes.

Reproduced from: Dasgupta B. Diagnosis and management of polymyalgia rheumatic. Clin Med 2010;10:270–4. Copyright © 2010 Royal College of Physicians. Reproduced with permission.

7. **Provide advice on range of motion exercises** for the shoulder and pelvic girdle muscles (with referral for physiotherapy if necessary).

Fallacies related to glucocorticoid use in polymyalgia rheumatica

An empirical trial of steroids should in no circumstances be used as an alternative to careful clinical evaluation of PMR. Recent reports show that 3–4 weeks after starting prednisolone 15 mg daily only 55% showed a complete response to therapy. Treatment with a moderate dose of prednisone, 15–20 mg daily as a single AM dose is indicated in PMR.[13,14] Under no circumstances should patients be given a larger dose of prednisone. Higher doses are unnecessary and only contribute to delays in diagnosis of another condition and lead to more corticosteroid morbidity. A 70% patient-reported global improvement with normalization of the ESR and CRP within

3–4 weeks indicates a complete response. If the initial response to treatment is not dramatic, do not continue treatment without considering other possible diagnoses. The corticosteroid dose should not be increased in an attempt to lower persistent elevation of acute-phase reactants without consideration of alternative diagnoses. High doses (often >40 mg/day) often employed as initial treatment for PMR are a source of diagnostic confusion as well as a rocky disease course.[13,14] They may serve to obscure systemic manifestations of potentially life-threatening diseases. Suppression of fever, malaise and weight loss in patients treated with high doses of corticosteroid can delay the diagnosis for example of malignancies or subacute bacterial endocarditis, with potentially life-threatening or life-limiting consequences.

The presence of swelling and early morning or inactivity stiffness of the peripheral joints should point the clinician towards an inflammatory arthritis such as RA or psoriatic arthritis.

A personal or family history of psoriasis or inflammatory bowel disease together with prominent inflammatory hip, back, or buttock

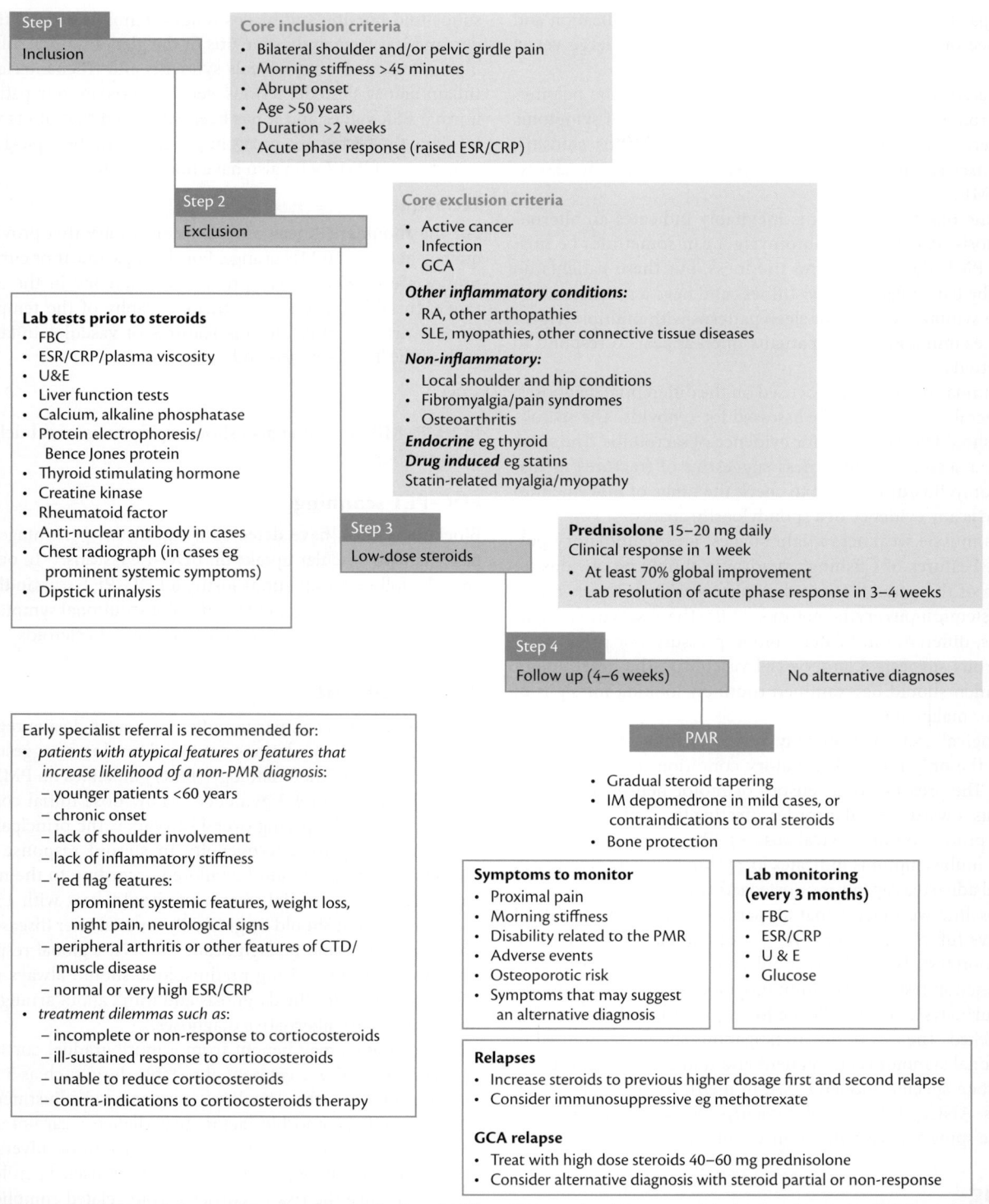

Fig. 134.3 Recommended approach for the evaluation of proximal pain and stiffness. PTH, parathyroid hormone; RA, rheumatoid arthritis; RS3PE, remitting, seronegative symmetrical synovitis with pitting oedema; SLE, systemic lupus erythematosus; TSH, thyroid stimulating hormone.
Reproduced from: Dasgupta B. Diagnosis and management of polymyalgia rheumatic. Clin Med 2010;10:270–4. Copyright © 2010 Royal College of Physicians. Reproduced with permission.

symptoms should make the clinician consider a late-onset seronegative spondyloarthropathy with sacroiliitis.

Severe back pain **without stiffness** might suggest vertebral metastases or myeloma. This is especially the case if red flag signs such as nocturnal pain, night sweats, anorexia, and significant weight loss are present. Although weight loss is common in PMR, loss of more than 14 lb (6 kg) is unusual and malignancies should be searched for.

High fevers can be caused by PMR, but should be investigated for other sources of infection, both common sources including urine and chest, and deep-seated infections, such as osteomyelitis, septic discitis and endocarditis, particularly if other systemic symptoms are prominent.

The presence of headache, visual symptoms, and jaw claudication should be recognized as GCA (40% of GCA patients have polymyalgia at onset). The presence of arm or leg claudication and prominence of systemic symptoms would suggest a large-vessel vasculitis.

ANCA-associated vasculitis can also present with the polymyalgic syndrome, and the clinician should enquire about symptoms of mesenteric ischaemia, nasal polyps, crusting, epistaxis, sinusitis, and late-onset asthma. Dipstick urinalysis is essential in the assessment of PMR.

A chronic onset of symptoms inevitably indicates an alternative diagnosis. Patients with fibromyalgia can sometimes be mistaken for PMR due to pain and tiredness, but these patients do not describe true inflammatory stiffness and have a prominence of depressive symptoms and poor sleep patterns with multiple trigger points on examination. Such patients often appear to respond to trial of steroids.

The examination should be focused on the differential diagnoses. All peripheral joints need to be assessed for synovitis. The sacroiliac joints should be examined for evidence of sacroiliitis. The spine should be assessed for tenderness suggestive of fractures/metastases/osteomyelitis/discitis and to check the range of movement to see if there is any evidence of a spondyloarthropathy.

Painless muscle weakness might suggest an inflammatory polymyositis. Features of Cushing's syndrome should be obvious on inspection of the patient. Discoid or photosensitive rashes might suggest systemic lupus erythematosus (SLE). The absence of peripheral pulses, difference in bilateral blood pressures, or presence of arterial bruits suggests a large-vessel vasculitis. The heart, lungs, and abdomen should be examined routinely looking for signs of infection or malignancy.

Neurological examination may reveal Parkinsonian features (which is the only non-inflammatory condition to produce true stiffness). The presence of a sensory or motor neuropathy in the arms points towards a local disorder affecting the neck, such as cervical disc protrusion or cervical abscess. The absence of systemic and lower limb symptoms indicates local shoulder pathology, such as bilateral adhesive capsulitis or osteoarthritis.

As a baseline we suggest that all patients with suspected PMR should have full blood count (FBC), urea and electrolytes (U&E), liver function tests (LFT), bone profile, CRP, creatine kinase (CK), thyroid function tests (TFTs), immunoglobulins and electrophoresis, basic urinalysis, urinary Bence Jones protein, and chest radiograph checked. The rest of the investigations should be tailored to the individual symptoms and patient and may include serum cortisol, prostate-specific antigen (PSA, in men), ANA, RF, anti-CCP antibodies, ANCA, CT chest/abdomen/pelvis, spinal radiographs, MRI of the spine and sacroiliac joints, and echocardiogram.

Imaging

It is recommended that ultrasound should be performed at first presentation. PMR is a heterogeneous disease with heterogeneous outcomes in disease course on follow-up. Patients may show features which are a mix of bursitis, tenosynovitis, synovitis, and large-vessel vasculitis on imaging.

Ultrasound

Ultrasound depicts characteristic pathologic findings of shoulders and hips that can aid in distinguishing PMR from other diseases that may mimic it.[11] Typical findings on ultrasound include subdeltoid bursitis and biceps tendon tenosynovitis at the shoulder, and less frequently synovitis of the glenohumoral joint. In the hips, ultrasound often reveals synovitis and trochanteric bursitis. Inflammatory shoulder lesions were observed even in patients with normal ESR values and it has been suggested that ultrasound may facilitate the correct diagnosis in patients with the typical proximal symptoms of PMR who also have normal ESR.

Technique

For the shoulders, linear probes are necessary that provide a frequency in the 6–10 MHz range. For the hips, linear or curved array probes are necessary that provide a frequency in the 5–8 MHz range. In addition, duplex ultrasonography of the temporal and axillary arteries often detects features of vascular inflammation such as the 'halo', stenosis and occlusions.

MRI

In PMR, MRI scanning also shows up features of subdeltoid/subacromial bursitis.

FDG-PET scanning

Blockmans et al. have detected a significant percentage of PMR patients with vascular uptake on FDG-PET scans.[12] In our experience the following situations justify a FDG-PET scan in the setting of either PMR or GCA: unexplained constitutional symptoms, limb claudication, persistent incomplete response to steroids.

Management

There are no trials comparing different steroid dosing regimens in PMR. The recommendations are based on doses suggested in the British Society of Rheumatology (BSR) guidelines on PMR and are mostly based on level 3 evidence.[13] Low-dose initial corticosteroids with gradual tapering over 1–2 years is the principal therapy. However, owing to heterogeneity in steroid response between patients, treatment should be tailored according to the needs of a particular patient. Initial treatment should start with 15 mg/day prednisolone and should be gradually tapered after disease control. The response should be significant (i.e. >70% global response). A lack of response to 15 mg prednisolone should always make the clinician reconsider the diagnosis and think about arranging other investigations for alternative diagnoses.

Some patients may benefit from a more gradual corticosteroid taper, or a period of treatment at a stable dose, such as 5 mg prednisolone for 3 months. The dose may also need adjustment, due to disease severity, comorbid factors (e.g. diabetes, cardiorespiratory, or renal disease), fracture risk, patient wishes, or adverse events. Intramuscular methylprednisolone may be used in milder cases and may reduce the risk of corticosteroid-related complications.[14] The initial dose is 120 mg intramuscularly repeated at 3–4-week intervals. The dose is then reduced by 20 mg every 2–3 months and given monthly. It is better to avoid non-steroidal anti-inflammatory drugs (NSAIDs), especially in very elderly patients and in those with renal impairment. Bone protection is advised for all patients.

Treatment of relapsing polymyalgia rheumatica

Relapse is defined as recurrence of symptoms of PMR or onset of GCA symptoms, such as headaches, jaw claudication, and visual symptoms, usually with a rise in ESR/CRP. Approximately 50% of patients relapse.[15] Clinical features of PMR may be mimicked by rotator cuff disease or shoulder osteoarthritis. An isolated rise of ESR or CRP, if not associated with clinical features of relapse, does not require an increase of immunosuppression. Speed of corticosteroid tapering and genetic factors have been postulated to influence the development of relapses in PMR. Initial relapses may be treated with a return to the previous higher dose. GCA relapse requires a high dose (40–60 mg) of prednisolone. Beyond two relapses, steroid-sparing agents such as methotrexate or azathioprine are usually used, but leflunomide has shown promise.[16] Current experience with randomized controlled trials of biological agents, such as infliximab or etanercept, is not generally encouraging.[10] An inability to wean off steroids or the development of new symptoms should make the clinician reassess the diagnosis.

Monitoring

Patients should be monitored for evidence of relapse, for disease-related complications, for steroid-related complications, and for symptoms that may suggest an alternative diagnosis. The best measures of disease activity and treatment response in PMR appear to be patient-reported global pain, hip pain, morning stiffness, physical function (MHAQ), mental function, and an inflammatory marker.[18] Ultrasound may have utility as an outcome measure. There is a need for specific biomarkers of disease activity in PMR. Poorly responsive PMR, persistent raised inflammatory markers, and constitutional symptoms may indicate large-vessel disease. Such patients may need echocardiography, PET, axillary artery ultrasound, and MRI to look for aortitis and large-vessel disease. Bone mineral density measurement may be required.

Conclusion

PMR may be an uncertain diagnosis and needs a stepwise assessment which includes inclusion and exclusion criteria and use of low-dose steroids. Subdeltoid bursitis or tenosynovitis visible on ultrasound appear to be key features. Meticulous monitoring for complications related to treatment and disease are required. The new EULAR/ACR classification criteria will facilitate uniform entry into clinical trials of novel therapies which are so urgently required for the condition. There appears to be an overlap with both GCA and large-vessel vasculitis as well as inflammatory arthritis.

References

1. Chakravarty K, Elgabani SHS, Scott DGI, Merry P. A district audit on the management of polymyalgia rheumatica and giant cell arteritis *Br J Rheumatol* 1994; 33:152–156.
2. Walsh LJ, Wong CA, Pringle M, Tattersfield AE. Use of oral corticosteroids in the community and the prevention of secondary osteoporosis: a cross sectional study. *BMJ* 1996;313:344–346.
3. Hutchings A, Hollywood J, Lamping D et al. Clinical outcomes, quality of life and diagnostic uncertainty in the first twelve months in polymyalgia rheumatica. *Arthritis Rheum* 2007;57(5):803–809.
4. Dasgupta B, Cimmino MA, Maradit-Kremers H et al. 2012 provisional classification criteria for polymyalgia rheumatica: a European League Against Rheumatism/American College of Rheumatology collaborative initiative *Ann Rheum Dis* 2012;71:484–492.
5. Doran MF, Crowson CS, O'Fallon WM, Hunder GG, Gabriel SE. Trends in the incidence of polymyalgia rheumatica over a 30 year period in Olmsted County, Minnesota USA *J Rheumatol* 2002;29:1694–1697.
6. Smeeth L, Cook C, Hall AJ. Incidence of diagnosed polymyalgia rheumatica and temporal arteritis in the United Kingdom 1990-2001 *Ann Rheum Dis* 2006;65:1093–1098.
7. Lawrence RC, Felson DT, Helmick CG, et al. Estimates of the prevalence of arthritis and other rheumatic conditions in the United States Part 2 *Arthritis Rheum* 2008;58(1):26–35.
8. Ma-Krupa W, Jeon MS, Spoerl S et al. Activation of arterial wall dendritic cells and breakdown of self-tolerance in giant cell arteritis. *J Exp Med* 2004;199:173–183.
9. Deng J, Younge BR, Olshen RA, Goronzy JJ, Weyand CM. Th17 and Th1 T-cell responses in giant cell arteritis *Circulation* 2010;121(7): 906–915.
10. Ghosh P, Borg FA, Dasgupta B. Current understanding and management of giant cell arteritis and polymyalgia rheumatic *Expert Rev. Clin Immunol* 2010;6(6):913–928.
11. Lange U, Piegsa M, Teichmann J, Neeck G. Ultrasonography of the glenohumeral joints – a helpful instrument in differentiation in elderly onset rheumatoid arthritis and polymyalgia rheumatica. *Rheumatol Int* 2000;19:185–189.
12. Blockmans D, De Ceuninck L, Vanderschueren S et al. Repetitive 18-fluorodeoxyglucose positron emission tomography in isolated polymyalgia rheumatica: a prospective study in 35 patients. *Rheumatology (Oxford)* 2007;46:672–677.
13. Dasgupta B, Borg FA, Hassan N et al. BSR and BHPR guidelines for the management of polymyalgia rheumatica. *Rheumatology (Oxford)* 2010;49:186–190.
14. Dasgupta B, Dolan AL, Fernandes L, Panayi G. An initially double-blind controlled 96 week trial of depot methylprednisolone against oral prednisolone in the treatment of polymyalgia rheumatica. *Br J Rheumatol* 1998;37:189–195.
15. Dejaco C, Duftner C, Cimmino MA et al. Definition of remission and relapse in polymyalgia rheumatica: Data from a literature search compared with a Delphi-based expert consensus. *Ann Rheum Dis* 2011;70:447–453.
16. Caporali R, Cimmino MA, Ferraccioli G et al. Prednisone plus methotrexate for polymyalgia rheumatica: a randomized, double-blind, placebo-controlled trial. *Ann.Intern. Med* 2004;141:493–500.
17. Matteson EL, Maradit-Kremers H, Cimmino MA et al. Patient-reported outcomes in polymyalgia rheumatica *J Rheum* 2012;39:4.

Sources of patient information

Polymyalgia Rheumatica & Giant Cell Arteritis UK (PMRGCAUK): www.pmrgcauk.com

CHAPTER 135

Behçet's syndrome

Sebahattin Yurdakul, Emire Seyahi, and Hasan Yazici

Introduction

Behçet's syndrome is a systemic vasculitis of unknown aetiology with a peculiar geographic distribution. Most cases are clustered around the countries of the Mediterranean basin, the Middle East, and the Far East. Its most dreaded complication, eye disease, is one of the leading causes of blindness in these regions.

In 1937, Behçet described in detail three patients with oral and genital ulceration, erythema nodosum, and hypopyon uveitis and proposed that this was a distinct entity. Subsequently, it was realized that many other clinical manifestations were part of this syndrome.[1] Table 135.1 lists the more important of these manifestations.

Epidemiology

The usual onset of the syndrome is in the third or fourth decade. The onset is rare in children and after the age of 45.

The male/female ratio is approximately equal but the syndrome has a more severe course in men and in young people. Worldwide, Turkey has the highest frequency with prevalence rates ranging from 2 to 42/10 000 based on five field surveys among the adult population.[2] Based on case registries, the prevalence is about 1/300 000 in northern Europe and 1/10 000 in Japan. The disease prevalence also shows ethnic variation in the same region: for example, ethnic Armenians living in Istanbul (Turkey) have a lower frequency of Behçet's syndrome (11/10 000) compared to that found in the general population (42/10 000).[3] Similarly, in a recent cross-sectional study disease frequency was significantly higher in North Africans (3.5/10 000) and Asians (1.8/10 000) compared to the native Europeans (0.2/10 000) living in a suburb of Paris (France). The study also showed that the overall frequency of Behçet's (0.7/10 000) was as frequent as those of other vasculitides (0.9/10 000) including polyarteritis nodosa, microscopic polyangiitis, granulomatosis with polyangiitis (Wegener's), and eosinophilic granulomatosis with polyangiitis (Churg–Straus).[4]

Clinical features

Skin and mucosal involvement

Oral aphthae

Behçet's syndrome only rarely occurs without oral ulceration, frequently also the first and most recurrent manifestation of the

Table 135.1 Clinical findings in Behçet's syndrome

Lesion	Frequency (%)
Aphthous ulcerations	97–100
Genital lesions	80–90
Skin lesions	80
Eye lesions	50
Arthritis	40–50
Thrombophlebitis	30
Neurological involvement	1–15
Gastrointestinal involvement	0–25

syndrome. It may precede the diagnosis by a mean of 8 (± 10) years.[5] Mostly oral ulcers in Behçet's syndrome are indistinguishable from what is seen in recurrent oral ulceration, but tend to be multiple and occur more frequently (Figure 135.1a). Large (major) ulcers are less frequent and herpetiform ulcers are rare. Major ulcers, however, can be very troublesome because they heal with scarring, which can even occlude the oropharynx. The minor ulcers do not as a rule leave scars. The histology reveals non-specific ulceration with necrotic material.

Genital ulceration

In male patients, 90% of genital ulcers occur on the scrotum and rarely on the penile shaft or on the glans penis. Urethritis is not observed, in contrast to reactive arthritis and sexually transmitted diseases. In the female, the labia (major and minor) are commonly affected (Figure 135.1b). As genital ulcers are usually deep and painful they affect the quality of life. Healing time is usually 2–4 weeks. Major ulcers (≥1 cm in diameter) almost always leave scars which are very specific for Behçet's syndrome.[6] Histologically, they are indistinguishable from what is seen in oral aphthae.

Skin lesions

The skin lesions of Behçet's syndrome can be divided into three main types:

- **Nodular lesions** resembling erythema nodosum: these are similar to idiopathic erythema nodosum and those due to other conditions (e.g. sarcoidosis). However, it has been shown that more elements of vasculitis are observed on histological sections of these lesions than in idiopathic erythema nodosum or to erythema nodosum due to other causes.[7,8] Sometimes superficial thrombophlebitis can be clinically indistinguishable from erythema nodosum.

- **Papulopustular lesions** also called acneiform lesions or simply acne: most papulopustular lesions are histologically very similar to ordinary acne. However, they differ from the latter in their propensity to occur also in the extremities in addition to the face and the trunk. Pustules associated with Behçet's syndrome are usually considered as non-infectious inflammatory lesions. However, a study showed that they were not sterile.[9] The predominant bacteria in pustules of Behçet patients were *Staphylococcus aureus* and *Prevotella* spp., whereas coagulase-negative staphylococci were more common in pustules from ordinary acne patients.

- Others lesions are leucocytoclastic vasculitis, necrotizing arteritis of the small and medium arteries, superficial thrombophlebitis, unclassifiable papules and pustules, and Sweet syndrome.[10]

The pathergy reaction (Figure 135.1c), a curious hyperreactivity of the skin to a needle prick, is peculiar to this syndrome. The only other condition in which it is known to be positive with any consistency is pyoderma gangrenosum. After a skin puncture with a needle, a papule or a pustule forms in 24–48 hours. Pathergy is seldom observed among patients in northern Europe or the United States. In patients from Japan and Turkey the reaction is positive in around 60–70% when tested repeatedly.

The mechanism of the pathergy reaction is still obscure. Surgical cleaning of the skin considerably dampens this reaction, which suggests that more than disrupting the integrity of the epidermis and dermis is operational. Immunophenotypic analysis of skin biopsy specimens of positive pathergy reactions suggest that the reaction consists of a delayed hypersensitivity reaction independent of a specific antigen. Skin biopsy specimens obtained at 48 hours after a needle prick showed marked cellular influxes into the injury site, leading to an exaggerated lymphoid Th1-type response.[11]

The propensity for inflammation in Behçet's syndrome can also be observed in the response to intradermal injections of monosodium urate crystals.[12]

Eye involvement

Eye involvement is one of the most serious manifestations of Behçet's syndrome (Figure 135.1d). Its overall rate is about 50%. Males and those with younger age of onset have an increased frequency. Females are less severely affected. Disease is bilateral in 90% of patients with ocular involvement.[13,14] The onset of eye disease is usually within 2–3 years of the development of the syndrome.[14]

Eye disease in Behçet's syndrome consists of a chronic relapsing posterior and anterior uveitis. Isolated anterior uveitis is found in only 10% of those with ocular involvement.[13] Hypopyon uveitis (Figure 135.1d) is very typical, although occasionally it can be

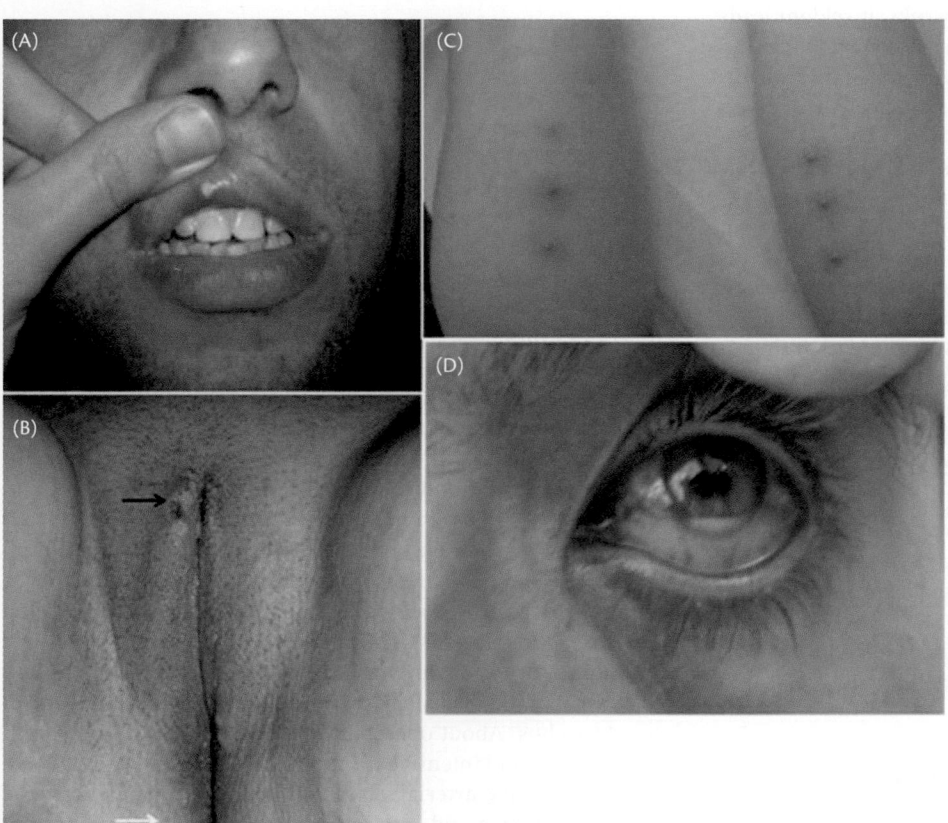

Fig. 135.1 Skin-mucosa and eye lesions in Behçet's syndrome. (A) Multiple oral ulcers on the mucosal side of the lips. (B) Multiple ulcers on the labia major (black arrow). A large scar on the perineum (white arrow). (C) Pathergy reaction. (D) Hypopyon.

observed in reactive arthritis. It is an accumulation of white cells and debris in the anterior chamber that precipitates to form a layer due to gravity. Hypopyon is seen in 10–20% of patients with eye disease and is almost always associated with severe retinal disease.

The basic retinal lesion is a vasculitis, which can lead to exudates, haemorrhages, venous thrombosis, papilloedema, and macular disease that frequently results in a hole. The pars plana is also involved. During an acute flare there is a marked influx of fibrin, inflammatory cells, and cellular debris into the vitreous. Recurrent inflammatory activity results in late complications such as anterior and posterior synechia, cataract, secondary glaucoma, macular degeneration, and finally phthysis bulbi.[13]

Male gender, posterior involvement, frequent attacks, strong vitreous opacity, and exudates alongside the retinal vascular arcade are poor prognostic factors.[15] The prognosis of the eye disease has been reported to be extremely poor in the past. Nearly three-quarters of patients with eye disease would eventually lose their vision more than 20 years ago, but loss of useful vision ensues in less than one-fifth of patients with Behçet's syndrome and eye involvement under treatment since 1990.[13,16] Severely impaired vision does not always mean an eventual loss of useful vision, and male patients with late-onset eye disease, and female patients overall have an improved visual prognosis.[13–16]

Musculoskeletal system

Involvement of the joints is seen in about one-half of the patients in the form of arthritis or arthralgia. There is usually a mono- or oligoarticular involvement but symmetrical disease of the wrist or elbow, which can be confused with rheumatoid arthritis, may occasionally be seen. Usually lasting a few weeks, it seldom leads to chronic synovitis and deformity. Erythema of the overlying skin is not seen. Erosions are uncommon. The synovial fluid is inflammatory with a good mucin clot and the histological changes are non-specific.

Knees are the most commonly affected joints, followed in frequency by ankles, wrists, and elbows. Back pain is quite rare in Behçet's syndrome and an increased prevalence of sacroiliac joint involvement has not been found in controlled studies. On the other hand, patients with Behçet's syndrome who had arthritis also had more acne lesions compared to controls, suggesting a link with the reactive arthritides.[17] Furthermore, the frequency of enthesopathy was found to be significantly increased among Behçet's syndrome patients with acne–arthritis compared with that among patients without arthritis.[18] These recent studies support the hypothesis that patients with Behçet's syndrome with arthritis and acne form a distinct cluster. Interestingly, this cluster shows also familial clustering.[19]

Local or generalized myositis is occasionally found in Behçet's syndrome. The muscle enzymes are not raised in the local forms and the histological features are indistinguishable from those seen in polymyositis.

Another musculoskeletal manifestation associated with Behçet's syndrome is aseptic necrosis of the bone. This is possibly related to vasculitis and not necessarily to steroid use.

Cardiovascular and pulmonary involvement

Cardiac involvement

Endocarditis, myocarditis, and pericarditis can all occur but are rare. Cases with intracardiac thrombosis, endomyocardial fibrosis, coronary vasculitis and ventricular aneurysms have also been reported. Intracardiac thrombosis is usually located in the right side of the heart and closely associated with pulmonary artery involvement.

Vascular involvement

Vascular disease develops in up to 40% of patients and has a definite male preponderance. Both veins and arteries are affected. However, venous involvement is more common than arterial disease (75% vs 25%). About 30% of the vascular events develop simultaneously at disease onset or before fulfilling the criteria.[20] Lower extremity vein thrombosis, pulmonary artery aneurysms, Budd–Chiari syndrome, and dural sinus thrombosis are reported to occur early. However, both vena cava thrombosis and non-pulmonary artery aneurysms are late findings developing in a median of 5 and 7 years.[5,20]

Venous lesions

Superficial and deep veins of the lower extremity are the most common sites of venous thrombosis, which constitute 60–80% of vascular lesions. The affected veins in descending order of frequency are femoral, popliteal, saphenous, and crural veins. Furthermore, chronic relapsing vein thromboses in the legs tend to precede other sites of major vessel involvement.

Chronic occlusion of the superior and the inferior venae cavae leads to the appearance of prominent venous collaterals on the thoracic and abdominal walls. Thrombotic involvement may extend from hepatic veins to femoral/iliac veins or vice versa. Hepatic vein thrombosis may cause Budd–Chiari syndrome which may lead to liver failure and death. On the other hand, superior vena cava thrombosis has a better outcome, despite its alarming presentation.

Arterial lesions

The frequency of arterial disease in Behçet's syndrome is relatively rare (2.5%).[20]

Pulmonary artery involvement is mainly manifested as aneurysms (Figure 135.2a,b) and, less often, as solo in-situ pulmonary artery thrombosis (Figure 135.2c). Often, both pathologies can be seen together.[21] In-situ pulmonary artery thrombosis has a clinical and prognostic picture similar to pulmonary artery aneurysms. Patients present with fever, chest pain, coughing, dyspnea, and hemoptysis and a high acute-phase response. They may also have mild pulmonary artery hypertension.[22] The involvement is usually bilateral and confined mostly to inferior lobes. In two-thirds of cases aneurysms may disappear with only medical treatment. Both aneurysms and thrombosis may heal without any arterial sequelae or by leaving occlusions or stenosis. Thoracic CT scans of these patients may also show parenchymal nodules (Figure 135.2d), consolidations, and cavities (Figure 135.2b) mimicking opportunistic infections.

Despite the high prevalence of venous thrombosis in Behçet's syndrome, pulmonary thromboembolism is extremely rare since thrombosis develops usually as a complication to the underlying extensive vasculitis and is tightly adherent to the vascular wall.

Pulmonary artery involvement causes significant morbidity and mortality.[21,23] This is usually due to the rupture of an aneurysm into a bronchus. About one-quarter of patients still die even with early diagnosis and intensive treatment.

Non-pulmonary arterial disease is manifested mostly in the form of aneurysms and located in the abdominal aorta, carotid (Figure 135.3), femoral, and popliteal arteries. Occlusions are seldom seen and have a better prognosis than that of the aneurysms.[24]

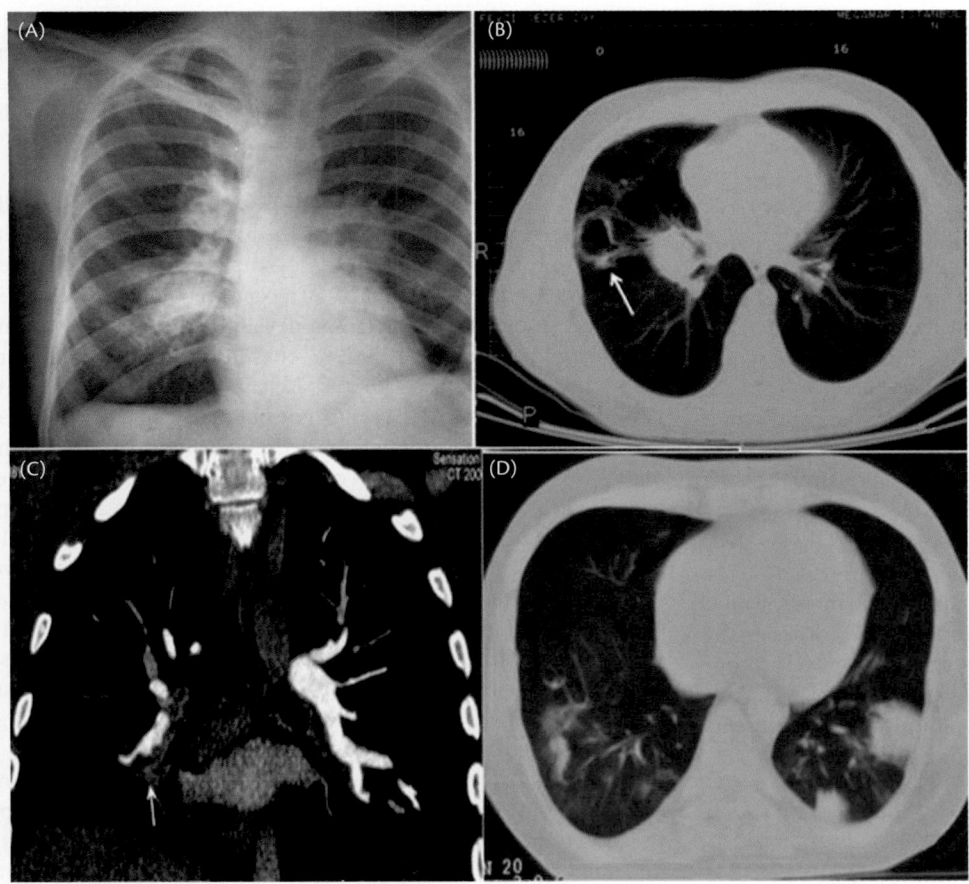

Fig. 135.2 Several pulmonary lesions in Behçet's syndrome. (A) Bilateral hilar opacities on the chest radiograph. (B) CT scan showing pulmonary artery aneurysm (red arrow) and a cavity (white arrow) in the right middle lobe. (C) Pulmonary artery thrombosis (arrow) in the right descending artery. (D) Nodular lesions in the lung.

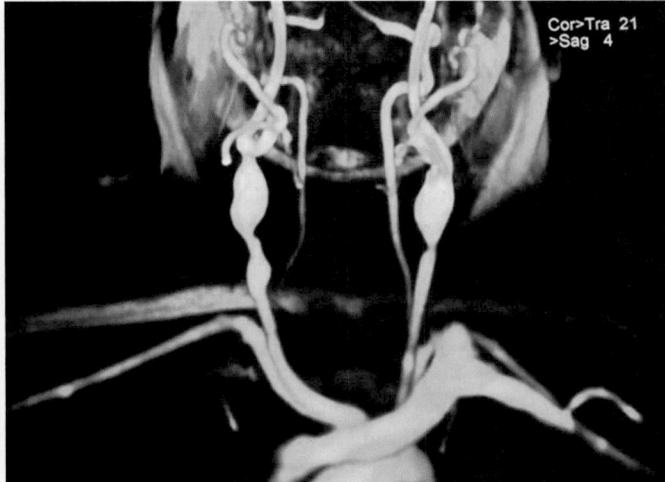

Fig. 135.3 Bilateral carotid artery aneurysms.

Atherosclerosis

Endothelial dysfunction and arterial stiffness have been well documented in Behçet's syndrome,[25] but clinical cardiovascular disease or its associated mortality seem not to be increased. The prevalence of angina and history of ischaemic heart disease was found to be similar between patients and non-diseased controls.[26] Evidence for subclinical atherosclerosis is also weak.[27]

Neurological involvement

The frequency of neurological involvement is around 5%. There are mainly two types, parenchymal disease (75–80%) and dural sinus thrombosis (10–20%).[28–30] The two types are rarely observed simultaneously in the same patient. Parenchymal disease is usually a late manifestation, developing after 5–10 years of disease onset. Male patients have more severe disease. It usually affects the brainstem, but hemispheric, meningeal, and spinal cord lesions are also seen.[31] The lesions are best demonstrated by MRI. In contrast to the other vasculitides, peripheral nerve disease is quite unusual.[28] Pyramidal signs, hemiparesis, behavioural–cognitive changes, and sphincter disturbances and impotence are the main clinical manifestations. Character disorders, impairment of memory and dementia, and other psychiatric symptoms may also occur.

Cerebrospinal fluid (CSF) findings are usually non-specific. An inflammatory CSF indicates a severe prognosis.

The lesions may progress to produce bulbar paralysis and this may often lead to disability and death.[28,29]

Dural sinus thrombosis is usually associated with other types of venous disease[32] and has a significantly better outcome.[28,29] It occurs earlier in the disease course. Severe headache, papilloedema, and motor ocular nerve palsies may be seen. Bilateral swollen optic disc is the most frequent sign. Persistent intracranial pressure may cause optic atrophy and blindness despite treatment.[33]

Headache is the most common neurological symptom in Behçet's syndrome.[34] It can be due to various causes such as parenchymal central nervous system (CNS) disease, dural sinus thrombosis, ocular inflammation, acute attacks of Behçet's syndrome itself, and coexisting primary headaches like migraine.

Gastrointestinal involvement

Gastrointestinal involvement is seen in about one-third of patients from Japan, but it is rare among patients in Turkey.[35,36] The basic pathology is that of mucosal ulceration. This is most commonly seen in the ileum, followed by the caecum and other parts of the colon. Enteroclysis findings are usually mild when compared with those seen in Crohn's disease.[37] Histologically, the ulcers are indistinguishable from those found in ulcerative colitis. The usual symptoms are abdominal pain and melena. A mass is often palpable in the abdomen. Ileocaecal ulcers have the worst prognosis, with a distinct tendency to perforate.

It must be emphasized that the differential diagnosis from Crohn's disease can be very difficult.[36]

Other clinical features

Renal involvement is seen much less frequently than one would expect in a systemic vasculitis. Glomerulonephritis is occasionally reported. Epididymitis and voiding dysfunction are well-recognized symptoms.

Amyloidosis of the AA type is seen sporadically, usually presents with nephrotic syndrome, and carries a grave prognosis.

Diagnosis

The full-blown Behçet's syndrome is easy to identify; the so-called incomplete forms sometimes cause problems. The main conditions that should be considered in the differential diagnosis are shown in Table 135.2.[38]

Using the presence of recurrent oral ulceration as mandatory, and with proper exclusions, the International Study Group criteria[39] require involvement of two other organ systems specified in the criteria for a diagnosis, or more correctly classification, of Behçet's syndrome (Table 135.3). In this scheme a positive pathergy test can replace involvement of an organ system.

Laboratory investigations

There are no laboratory findings specific for Behçet's syndrome. A moderate anaemia of chronic disease and leucocytosis are seen in 15% of patients. The erythrocyte sedimentation rate (ESR) is only mildly elevated, as is the C-reactive protein (CRP). Neither correlates well with disease activity.

The synovial fluid is usually inflammatory. The cell count is between 5000 and 50 000/mm^3 with neutrophils predominating. Despite this high cell count the mucin clot is usually good.

Serum immunoglobulins are sometimes elevated, while autoantibodies are absent. Complement levels may be high. Despite the pauci-immune nature of the basic disease process, anti-neutrophilic antibodies are not a feature of Behçet's syndrome.

Genetics and pathogenesis

Behçet's syndrome is an inflammatory vasculitis. The precise mechanisms that initiate and sustain the increased inflammatory state that characterizes the syndrome remain unknown.

Most cases are sporadic and do not show a mendelian inheritance pattern. On the other hand, familial cases exist and a sibling recurrence risk ratio (λ_s) of 11.4–52.5 has been reported.[40] In a recent study among a limited number of monozygotic twins the concordance for Behçet's syndrome was found to be 2/6 (95% CI −0.21–0.88).[41]

HLA B51 has been associated with Behçet's syndrome especially in areas where the syndrome shows the highest prevalence, but the strength of this association decreases in patients from the United Kingdom and the United States. A recent meta-analysis indicated that the risk of *HLA B51* carriers developing Behçet's syndrome is increased by a factor of 5.90.[42] Genes in linkage disequilibrium with *HLA B51* such as MHC class I chain related gene A (*MICA*) have also been linked to the syndrome but recent analyses in different ethnic groups have shown that *HLA B51* itself still confers the highest susceptibility. This was recently confirmed in two genome-wide studies.[43,44] Moreover, these studies also showed associations with non-HLA, *IL10*, and *IL23R-IL12RB2* loci. Interleukin (IL)-10 is an anti-inflammatory cytokine and a deficiency of this cytokine due to a mutation is certainly in line with the increased inflammation paramount in Behçet's syndrome. Non-HLA loci such as IL-10 variant and a variant between IL-23 and IL-12 receptors may also be operative. The exact direct role of HLA B51 in the pathogenesis is not known. Cross-reaction with self-peptides[45] and HLA B51 has been implicated as a potential mechanism.[46]

An infectious aetiology has been implicated in the pathogenesis since the original description. Herpes simplex virus type I[47] and streptococci (*S. oralis*) have been held responsible but a direct link has not been shown. The cellular and humoral immune response to mycobacterial heat shock proteins (HSP65) and to their human homologues—coupled with the production of uveitis in Lewis rats with some of these proteins—have also been proposed as a unifying mechanism that bridges the role of different microorganisms.[48]

Behçet's syndrome does not have the features of a classical autoimmune disorder such as female predominance, hypergammaglobulinaemia, a coexistent Sjögren's syndrome, autoantibodies, and a heightened T-cell response. Neutrophil hyperreactivity in the form of increased superoxide production, endothelial adhesion, chemotaxis, and phagocytosis have been reported and an animal model has linked increased superoxide production to the presence of HLA B51.[49]

Both the adaptive and innate immune systems are activated. While a Th1 predominant cytokine profile, a Th1 type tissue infiltration in cutaneous[11] and intestinal tissues, and elevated IL-17 levels are examples in favour of the adaptive system, the primed state of neutrophils, circulating polyclonal γδ T cells in the serum, and the decreased mannose binding leptin levels are in favour of the action of the innate immune system.[46,50]

A non-specific hyperreactivity as exemplified by the pathergy phenomenon constitutes an important feature of Behçet's syndrome. The spontaneous or induced overproduction of proinflammatory cytokines from mononuclear cells in Behçet's syndrome may also constitute an aspect of this non-specific hyperreactivity.[51]

No consistent coagulation abnormality has been found.[52] Increased factor V Leiden and prothrombin gene *G20210A* mutations have been observed mainly in patients with venous thrombosis but their exact roles in the pathogenesis have been inconclusive. Anti-endothelial cell antibodies, anti-phospholipid antibodies, and various endothelial cell activation markers have also been reported.

Table 135.2 Highlights of the clinical manifestations of Behçet's syndrome and differential diagnosis[38]

Manifestation	Comment	Differential diagnosis
Mouth ulcers	Similar in appearance to common aphthous ulcers, more frequent and frequently multiple	Reactive arthritis—painless ulceration
Genital ulcers	Most commonly scrotal or vulval, painful, recurrent, and usually with scarring. Urethral discharge and penile lesions very rare	Reactive arthritis
Skin	Acneiform lesions as common acne in appearance and histology but also at uncommon sites such as the extremities. Erythema nodosum-like lesions leaving pigmentation. Not psoriasis	Seronegative arthropathies; inflammatory bowel disease; sarcoidosis
Eyes	Panuveitis and retinal vasculitis, usually bilateral occurring within about 2 years of the onset of the disease. Conjunctivitis and sicca syndrome most unusual	Seronegative arthropathies
Joints	Monoarthritis in 50%, otherwise oligoarticular or polyarticular, involving relatively few joints; may be symmetrical; knees most frequently; intermittent resolving in 2–4 weeks or chronic and continuous; not involving sacroiliac joints or spine; deformity and erosions rare. Inflammatory synovial fluid with a good mucin clot	Inflammatory arthropathies
Peripheral arterial and venous disease	Subclinical peripheral large vein disease uncommon, usually involves large segments with skip areas without embolization; arteritis with occlusion and/or pseudoaneurysms; microaneurysms of the polyarteritic type very uncommon	Other vasculitides
Neurological involvement	Peripheral neuropathy with isolated cerebellar involvement very unusual, headaches with dural sinus thrombosis; vascular CNS lesions including transverse myelitis-type manifestation. Multiple sclerosis with aphthous ulcers a problem but no plaques on MRI	Multiple sclerosis
Pulmonary involvement	Haemoptysis associated with pulmonary artery aneurysm; pulmonary artery occlusion; pleural involvement uncommon; interstitial involvement very rare	Pulmonary embolism; any cause of haemoptysis
Gastrointestinal involvement	Severe abdominal pain; ulcerative lesions at any level but mainly in the ileocaecal region; mild gastrointestinal symptoms should not be associated with Behçet's syndrome	Inflammatory bowel disease
Cardiac disease	Pericarditis, valve lesions, and coronary artery involvement uncommon; rarely intracardiac thrombi	Valve lesions in seronegative arthropathies

From Barnes and Yazici.[38]

There is some debate whether Behçet's syndrome belongs to the group of autoinflammatory diseases; a group characterized by the episodic inflammatory attacks, specific mutations (e.g. pyrin, CARD, NOD), and the absence of specific autoantibodies. Most of these entities begin in infancy whereas paediatric Behçet's syndrome is not frequent. Paroxysmal attacks that last from a couple of hours to a couple of weeks with frequent serosal involvement and fever characterize autoinflammatory diseases, while they are not at all common in Behçet's syndrome. On the other hand the extensive vasculitis, the hypercoagulability, and the more severe disease among males are features of Behçet's syndrome that are not characteristic of the autoinflammatory conditions.

Finally, the presence of disease clusters, especially with the acne–arthritis clustering in families,[19] the differences in organ response to the same agent (see below), and differences in disease expression between different geographies suggest that what we call Behçet's syndrome today might be due to more than one pathophysiological pathway, or more simply, more than one disease.

Management

There are several important features of Behçet's syndrome that have to be taken into consideration when planning management:

- The usual course of the syndrome in any organ system is that of exacerbations and remissions with the overall activity generally

Table 135.3 International Study Group criteria for the diagnosis of Behçet's syndrome

Criterion	Definition
Recurrent oral ulceration	Aphthous or herpetiform lesions; recurring at least 3 times a year
Recurrent genital ulceration	Aphthous ulceration or scarring
Eye lesions	Anterior or posterior uveitis or cells in the vitreus body on slit-lamp examination or retinal vasculitis
Skin lesions	Erythema nodosum, pseudofolliculitis, papulopustular lesions or acneiform nodules, not related to glucocorticoids treatment or adolescence
Positive pathergy test	Papule or pustule formation at 48 h

Source: International Study Group for Behçet's Disease.[39]

abating with the passage of time; thus, the principal aim is to prevent irreversible structural damage, which is the outcome of the early stormy course.

- Being young and male are separate and additive negative prognostic factors.

- Eye disease usually has its onset, if at all, either initially or within the first few years.

◆ The syndrome can be fatal, especially in a young male patient.

◆ There are many patients with Behçet's syndrome who do not need any treatment other than reassurance.

Immunosuppressive drugs are the main line of treatment for eye involvement. Although corticosteroids have been used for a long time, there is no formal evidence that they are effective. Their short-term use over a few months, however, may shorten the duration of an attack.

Azathioprine at 2.5 mg/kg per day is useful in maintaining visual acuity and, perhaps more importantly, in preventing the emergence of new eye disease. Its early use in the disease course leads to a better long-term outcome. It is important that treatment is begun well before structural changes appear in the eye. The drug has also beneficial effects on oral and genital ulcerations, arthritis, and possibly thrombophlebitis. Because of its slow onset of action, it requires more than 3 months for efficacy at the recommended dosage. Ciclosporin is an effective and rapidly acting drug in sight-threatening and progressive uveitis, especially with retinal vasculitis of Behçet's syndrome. Problems with ciclosporin are its potential nephrotoxicity, especially at doses greater than 5 mg/kg per day, and the very frequent relapses after cessation of therapy. The high cost is another problem. Eye disease in remission for 2 years or more usually needs no further treatment. Young males, in general, need to be treated more vigorously. Once initiated, the usual course for cytotoxic or cyclosporin therapy is a minimum of 2 years, after which attempts at discontinuation are made. There is the concern that this medication not only tends to accelerate the development of CNS symptoms but also can cause CNS symptoms that can be confused with those in Behçet's syndrome itself.[53] Thus, its use is not recommended in patients with neurological involvement. In some patients, after a course for 6–8 months of combined azathioprine and ciclosporin, treatment is continued with azathioprine only. In more resistant cases azathioprine is used in combination with ciclosporin (both at conventional doses) for extended periods of time. Our uncontrolled experience with this mode of therapy in severe eye disease is quite favourable.

Data on biological agents such as interferon-α2a (IFN-α) and anti-tumour necrosis factor (TNFα) antagonists have been promising. IFN-α, subcutaneously, 3–6 MU/day, three times a week decreases the mucocutaneous lesions and is beneficial in posterior uveitis refractory to conventional medications.[54] Long-lasting remissions have been reported after stopping the drug.[55] Side effects include flu-like symptoms, liver enzyme elevations, cytopenias, and severe mood changes. Its drawbacks are high cost and frequent side effects. TNFα agents such as infliximab, etanercept, and adalimumab have been effective for various lesions of the disease, including eye, mucocutaneous, gastrointestinal, and neurological disease, and even pulmonary artery aneurysms. Among them infliximab has been the most commonly used anti-TNFα agent.[56,57] Infliximab is recommended as a first agent at a dosage of 5 mg/kg for sight-threatening uveitis as an add-on immunosuppressive therapy for patients who are refractory or intolerant to traditional immunosuppressives.[57] The initial response is generally seen within 24 hours, but relapses are frequent after withdrawal; therefore, continuous treatment are needed. The only placebo-controlled study with etanercept showed the drug significantly decreased the mucocutanous lesions in patients with mainly mucocutaneous lesions. Interestingly, however, it did not suppress the pathergy or the urate crystal skin response.[58] Its high cost, and side effects such

as an increased risk of tuberculosis and other infections, are still concerns.

The European League against Rheumatism (EULAR) has published recommendations for the therapy of Behçet's syndrome.[59,60] In ocular disease they suggest:

> If the patient has severe eye disease defined as >2 lines drop of visual acuity on a 10/10 scale, and/or retinal disease (retinal vasculitis or macular involvement), it is recommended that either ciclosporin or infliximab be used in combination with azathioprine and corticosteroids; alternatively, INF-α with or without corticosteroids could be used instead.

Concomitant use of other immunosuppressive agents together with the TNFα blocker has been suggested to prevent the development of antibody formation. IFN should not be used alongside an immunosuppressant because of the possibility of bone marrow suppression.

Structural eye damage can be managed surgically (i.e. vitrectomy) at specialized centres. However, results are not uniformly satisfactory. There is always the problem of new attacks of inflammation in surgically handled tissue in Behçet's syndrome. Also, already established disease in the retina cannot be helped by surgery. Local mydriatics should be used in the acute stage to prevent synechiae.

The oral and genital ulcers are usually well controlled by immunosuppressives and steroids. However, these should be reserved for more severe cases. Often, a local steroid preparation that adheres to fresh ulceration (such as triamcinolone acetonide oral paste) is all that is required.

A 2 year controlled trial has shown that colchicine is more effective than placebo in the treatment of mucocutaneous and joint symptoms and that this effect is especially prominent among females. Most notably, colchicine did not have any effect on the genital ulcerations in male patients.

Thalidomide at a dose of 100 mg/day can induce dramatic relief from oral and genital ulcers. Relapses are a rule after stopping treatment. Teratogenesis and polyneuropathy are the drawbacks of chronic thalidomide use.

Cyclophosphamide, either 2–2.5 mg/kg per day orally or 500–1500 mg weekly or monthly intravenous boluses, is required to treat those patients with severe cutaneous, arterial, or pulmonary vasculitis, or those with arterial aneurysms or vena caval involvement. There is no formal experience with any therapy for CNS disease; however, steroids, immunosuppressives, and biological agents are again used.

Gastrointestinal involvement is initially managed by sulfasalazine at a dosage of 2–6 g/day. Sometimes surgery is required, with resection of large segments of bowel. Usually, a good portion of uninvolved area should also be removed to prevent recurrences. Surgery is usually successful in aneurysms of peripheral vessels.

There is debate whether to use heparin or oral anticoagulants for the thrombophlebitis of Behçet's syndrome. Pulmonary embolism is seldom observed, as explained above. Further evidence that pulmonary emboli are rare comes from our recent observation that those lesions reported as pulmonary emboli in perfusion lung scans continue to persist after several months in Behçet's syndrome while, as a rule, they disappear in ordinary pulmonary emboli.[21] The role of anti-coagulation in deep vein thrombosis has not been evaluated in a controlled study. However, studies showed that anti-coagulant treatment is ineffective in preventing venous thrombosis.[61,62] In this setting, anti-platelet drugs (i.e. aspirin) are probably sufficient. We also use azathioprine in thrombophlebitis of Behçet's syndrome to suppress the disease activity in general.

Combination of these drugs with steroids or the combination of azathioprine and ciclosporin can be tried in cases resistant to a single agent.

In the absence of any hard data it is customary to stop treatment in a patient in remission after 2–4 years.

Prognosis

The disease intensity usually abates with the passage of time. On the other hand, it may cause several serious morbidities and a fatal outcome. A follow-up study of 20 years found an overall mortality rate of 10% among an inception cohort of 423 patients.[14] Standardized mortality ratios were specifically increased among young males while older males and females had a normal lifespan. Furthermore, the mortality rate was highest during the first 7 years of disease onset and had a tendency to decrease with time. Major causes of death were large-vessel (especially pulmonary artery) aneurysms and parenchymal CNS involvement. A more recent study reported a mortality rate of 5% among 817 patients followed for a median of 8 years.[63] Similarly, the mortality rate was increased among young patients and males.

References

1. Yazici H, Fresko I, Yurdakul S. Behçet's syndrome: disease manifestations, management, and advances in treatment. *Nat Clin Pract Rheumatol* 2007;3(3):148–155.

2. Yurdakul S, Yazici Y. Epidemiology of Behçet's syndrome and regional differences in disease expression. In Yazici Y, Yazici H (eds) *Behçet's syndrome*, 11th edn. Springer, New York, 2010:35–52.

3. Seyahi E, Tahir Turanli E, Mangan MS et al. The prevalence of Behçet's syndrome, familial Mediterranean fever, HLA-B51 and MEFV gene mutations among ethnic Armenians living in Istanbul, Turkey. *Clin Exp Rheumatol* 2010;28(4 Suppl 60):S67–S75.

4. Mahr A, Belarbi L, Wechsler B et al. Population-based prevalence study of Behçet's disease: differences by ethnic origin and low variation by age at immigration. *Arthritis Rheum* 2008;58 (12):3951–3959.

5. Ideguchi H, Suda A, Takeno M et al. Behçet disease:evolution of clinical manifestations. *Medicine* (Baltimore) 2011;90(2):125–132.

6. Mat MC, Goksugur N, Engin B, Yurdakul S, Yazici H. The frequency of scarring after genital ulcers in Behçet's syndrome: a prospective study. *Int J Dermatol* 2006;45(5):554–556.

7. Demirkesen C, Tüzüner N, Mat C et al. Clinicopathologic evaluation of nodular cutaneous lesions of Behçet syndrome. *Am J Clin Pathol* 2001;116 (3):341–346.

8. Kim B, LeBoit PE. Histopathologic features of erythema nodosum-like lesions in Behçet disease: a comparison with erythema nodosum focusing on the role of vasculitis. *Am J Dermatopathol* 2000;22(5):379–390.

9. Hatemi G, Bahar H, Uysal S et al. The pustular skin lesions in Behçet's syndrome are not sterile. *Ann Rheum Dis* 2004;63(11):1450–1452.

10. Jorizzo JL, Abernethy JL, White WL et al. Mucocutaneous criteria for the diagnosis of Behçet's disease: an analysis of clinicopathologic data from multiple international centers. *J Am Acad Dermatol* 1995;32(6): 968–976.

11. Melikoglu M, Uysal S, Krueger JG et al. Characterization of the divergent wound-healing responses occurring in the pathergy reaction and normal healthy volunteers. *J Immunol* 2006;177(9):6415–6421.

12. Cakir N, Yazici H, Chamberlain MA et al. Response to intradermal injection of monosodium urate crystals in Behçet's syndrome. *Ann Rheum Dis* 1991;50(9):634–636.

13. Tugal-Tutkun I, Onal S, Altan-Yaycioglu R, Huseyin Altunbas H, Urgancioglu M. Uveitis in Behçet disease: an analysis of 880 patients. *Am J Ophthalmol* 2004;138(3):373–380.

14. Kural-Seyahi E, Fresko I, Seyahi N et al. The long-term mortality and morbidity of Behçet syndrome: a 2-decade outcome survey of 387 patients followed at a dedicated center. *Medicine* (Baltimore) 2003; 82 (1):60–76.

15. Takeuchi M, Hokama H, Tsukahara R et al. Risk and prognostic factors of poor visual outcome in Behçet's disease with ocular involvement. *Graefes Arch Clin Exp Ophthalmol* 2005;243(11):1147–1152.

16. Taylor SR, Singh J, Menezo V et al. Behçet disease: Visual prognosis and factors influencing the development of visual loss. *Am J Ophthalmol* 2011;152(6):1059–1066.

17. Diri E, Mat C, Hamuryudan V et al. Papulopustular skin lesions are seen more frequently in patients with Behçet's syndrome who have arthritis: a controlled and masked study. *Ann Rheum Dis* 2001;60(11): 1074–1076.

18. Hatemi G, Fresko I, Tascilar K, Yazici H. Increased enthesopathy among Behçet's syndrome patients with acne and arthritis: an ultrasonography study. *Arthritis Rheum* 2008;58(5):1539–1545.

19. Karaca M, Hatemi G, Sut N, Yazici H. The papulopustular lesion/arthritis cluster of Behçet's syndrome also clusters in families. *Rheumatology* (Oxford) 2012;51(6):1053–1060.

20. Melikoglu M, Ugurlu S, Tascilar K et al. Large vessel involvement in Behçet's syndrome: A retrospective survey. *Ann Rheum Dis* 2008;67(Suppl II):67.

21. Seyahi E, Melikoglu M, Akman C et al. Pulmonary artery involvement and associated lung disease in Behçet syndrome: a series of 47 patients. *Medicine* 2012;91(1):35–48.

22. Seyahi E, Baskurt M, Melikoglu M et al. The estimated pulmonary artery pressure can be elevated in Behçet's syndrome. *Respir Med* 2011;105(11):1739–1747.

23. Hamuryudan V, Er T, Seyahi E et al. Pulmonary artery aneurysms in Behçet syndrome. *Am J Med* 2004;117(11):867–870.

24. Tuzun H, Seyahi E, Arslan C et al. Management and prognosis of non-pulmonary large arterial disease in 25 patients with Behçet disease from a single center. *J Vasc Surg* 2012;55(1):157–163.

25. Seyahi E, Yazici H. Atherosclerosis in Behçet's syndrome. *Clin Exp Rheumatol* 2007;25(4 Suppl 45):S1–S5.

26. Ugurlu S, Seyahi E, Yazici H. Prevalence of angina, myocardial infarction and intermittent claudication assessed by Rose Questionnaire among patients with Behçet's syndrome. *Rheumatology* (Oxford) 2008;47(4): 472–475.

27. Seyahi E, Ugurlu S, Cumali R et al. Atherosclerosis in Behçet's syndrome. *Semin Arthritis Rheum* 2008;38(1):1–12.

28. Akman-Demir G, Serdaroglu P, Tasçi B. Clinical patterns of neurological involvement in Behçet's disease: evaluation of 200 patients. The Neuro-Behçet Study Group. *Brain* 1999;122(Pt 11):2171–2182.

29. Siva A, Kantarci OH, Saip S et al. Behçet's disease: diagnostic and prognostic aspects of neurological involvement. *J Neurol* 2001;248(2):95–103.

30. Al-Araji A, Kidd DP. Neuro-Behçet's disease: epidemiology, clinical characteristics, and management. *Lancet Neurol* 2009;8(2):192–204.

31. Yesilot N, Mutlu M, Gungor O et al. Clinical characteristics and course of spinal cord involvement in Behçet's disease. *Eur J Neurol* 2007;14(7): 729–737.

32. Tunc R, Saip S, Siva A, Yazici H. Cerebral venous thrombosis is associated with major vessel disease in Behçet's syndrome. *Ann Rheum Dis* 2004;63(12):1693–1694.

33. Saadoun D, Wechsler B, Resche-Rigon M et al. Cerebral venous thrombosis in Behçet's disease. *Arthritis Rheum* 2009;61(4):518–526.

34. Saip S, Siva A, Altintas A et al. Headache in Behçet's syndrome. *Headache* 2005;45(7):911–919.

35. Yurdakul S, Tüzüner N, Yurdakul I, Hamuryudan V, Yazici H. Gastrointestinal involvement in Behçet's syndrome: a controlled study. *Ann Rheum Dis* 1996;55(3):208–210.

36. Cheon JH, Celik AF, Kim WH. Behçet's disease: gastrointestinal involvement. In: Yazici Y, Yazici H (eds) *Behçet's syndrome*, 11th edn. Springer, New York, 2010:165–188.

37. Korman U, Cantasdemir M, Kurugoglu S et al. Enteroclysis findings of intestinal Behcet disease: a comparative study with Crohn disease. *Abdom Imaging* 2003;28(3):308–312.

38. Barnes CG, Yazici H. Behçet's syndrome. *Rheumatology* (Oxford) 1999;38(12);1171–1174.

39. International Study Group for Behçet's Disease. Criteria for diagnosis of Behçet's disease. *Lancet* 1990;335(8697):1078–1080.

40. Gül A, Inanç M, Ocal L, Aral O, Koniçe M. Familial aggregation of Behçet's disease in Turkey. *Ann Rheum Dis* 2000;59(8):622–625.

41. Masatlioglu S, Seyahi E, Tahir Turanli E et al. A twin study in Behçet's syndrome. *Clin Exp Rheumatol* 2010;28(4 Suppl 60):S62–S66.

42. de Menthon M, Lavalley MP, Maldini C, Guillevin L, Mahr A. HLA-B51/B5 and the risk of Behçet's disease: a systematic review and meta-analysis of case-control genetic association studies. *Arthritis Rheum* 2009;61(10):1287–1296.

43. Remmers EF, Cosan F, Kirino Y et al. Genome-wide association study identifies variants in the MHC class I, IL10, and IL23R-IL12RB2 regions associated with Behçet's disease. *Nat Genet* 2010;42(8):698–702.

44. Mizuki N, Meguro A, Ota M et al. Genome-wide association studies identify IL23R-IL12RB2 and IL10 as Behçet's disease susceptibility loci. *Nat Genet* 2010;42(8):703–706.

45. Kurhan-Yavuz S, Direskeneli H, Bozkurt N et al. Anti-MHC autoimmunity in Behçet's disease: T cell responses to an HLA-B-derived peptide cross-reactive with retinal-S antigen in patients with uveitis. *Clin Exp Immunol* 2000;120(1):162–166.

46. Direskeneli H. Behçet's disease: infectious aetiology, new autoantigens, and HLA-B51. *Ann Rheum Dis* 2001;60(11):996–1002.

47. Sakane T, Takeno M, Suzuki N, Inaba G. Behçet's disease. *N Engl J Med* 1999;341(17):1284–1291.

48. Stanford MR, Kasp E, Whiston R et al. Heat shock protein peptides reactive in patients with Behçet's disease are uveitogenic in Lewis rats. *Clin Exp Immunol* 1994;97(2):226–231.

49. Takeno M, Kariyone A, Yamashita N et al. Excessive function of peripheral blood neutrophils from patients with Behçet's disease and from HLA-B51 transgenic mice. *Arthritis Rheum* 1995;38(3):426–433.

50. Inanc N, Mumcu G, Birtas E et al. Serum mannose-binding lectin levels are decreased in Behcet's disease and associated with disease severity. *J Rheumatol* 2005;32 (2):287–291.

51. Mege JL, Dilsen N, Sanguedolce V et al. Overproduction of monocyte derived tumor necrosis factor alpha, interleukin (IL) 6, IL-8 and increased neutrophil superoxide generation in Behçet's disease. A comparative study with familial Mediterranean fever and healthy subjects. *J Rheumatol* 1993;20(9):1544–1549.

52. Leiba M, Seligsohn U, Sidi Y et al.. Thrombophilic factors are not the leading cause of thrombosis in Behçet's disease. *Ann Rheum Dis* 2004;63(11):1445–1449.

53. Akman-Demir G, Ayranci O, Kurtuncu M et al. Cyclosporine for Behçet's uveitis: is it associated with an increased risk of neurological involvement? *Clin Exp Rheumatol* 2008;26(4 Suppl 50):S84–S90.

54. Kötter I, Vonthein R, Zierhut M et al. Differential efficacy of human recombinant interferon-alpha2a on ocular and extraocular manifestations of Behçet disease: results of an open 4-center trial. *Semin Arthritis Rheum* 2004;33(5):311–319.

55. Deuter CM, Zierhut M, Möhle A et al. Long-term remission after cessation of interferon-α treatment in patients with severe uveitis due to Behçet's disease. *Arthritis Rheum* 2010;62 (9):2796–2805.

56. Tugal-Tutkun I, Mudun A, Urgancioglu M et al. Efficacy of infliximab in the treatment of uveitis that is resistant to treatment with the combination of azathioprine, cyclosporine, and corticosteroids in Behçet's disease: an open-label trial. *Arthritis Rheum* 2005;52(8):2478–2484.

57. Sfikakis PP, Markomichelakis N, Alpsoy E et al. Anti-TNF therapy in the management of Behçet's disease-review and basis for recommendations. *Rheumatology* (Oxford) 2007;46(5):736–741.

58. Melikoglu M, Fresko I, Mat C et al. Short-term trial of etanercept in Behçet's disease: a double blind, placebo controlled study. *J Rheumatol* 2005;32 (1):98–105.

59. Hatemi G, Silman A, Bang D et al. Management of Behçet disease: a systematic literature review for the European League Against Rheumatism evidence-based recommendations for the management of Behçet disease. *Ann Rheum Dis* 2009;68(10):1528–1534.

60. Hatemi G, Silman A, Bang D et al. EULAR Expert Committee. EULAR recommendations for the management of Behçet disease. *Ann Rheum Dis* 2008;67(12):1656–1662.

61. Ahn JK, Lee YS, Jeon CH, Koh EM, Cha HS. Treatment of venous thrombosis associated with Behçet's disease: immunosuppressive therapy alone versus immunosuppressive therapy plus anticoagulation. *Clin Rheumatol* 2008;27(2):201–205.

62. Kahraman O, Celebi-Onder S, Kamali S et al. Long-term course of deep venous thrombosis in patients with Behçet's disease. *Arthritis Rheum* 2003;48(Suppl 9):S385.

63. Saadoun D, Wechsler B, Desseaux K et al. Mortality in Behçet's disease. *Arthritis Rheum* 2010;62(9):2806–2812.

CHAPTER 136

Paediatric vasculitis

Despina Eleftheriou and Paul A. Brogan

Introduction

Apart from relatively common vasculitides such as Henoch–Schönlein purpura (HSP) and Kawasaki's disease (KD), most of the primary vasculitic syndromes are rare in childhood, but when present are associated with significant morbidity and mortality.[1,2] Until recently clasifications in childhood vasculitis have been based on modifications of those used in adult populations. In 2005 the vasculitis working group of the Paediatric Rheumatology European Society (PRES) proposed preliminary classification criteria for some of the most common childhood vasculitides namely HSP, childhood polyarteritis nodosa (PAN), Wegener's granulomatosis (WG, now referred to as granulomatosis with polyangiitis (GPA) in adult classification systems), and Takayasu's arteritis (TA).[3] Subsequently, with support from the European League Against Rheumatism (EULAR), the Paediatric Rheumatology International Trials Organization (PRINTO) and PRES established a formal statistical validation process with a large-scale data collection that culminated in the final 2008 Ankara Consensus Conference.[4] Only paediatric diseases were considered, so giant cell arteritis was omitted.[3,4] Also a group of other vasculitides, including vasculitic disorders that did not fit into any category or fitted more than one, was defined. KD was not included since the clinical phenotype was already well described; nor are definitions for microscopic polyangiitis (too few cases included in dataset).[4] The general scheme for the classification of paediatric vasculitides is summarized in Box 136.1. This chapter summarizes the epidemiology, aetiopathogenesis, presenting clinical features, and current management strategies for paediatric vasculitides.

Predominantly small-vessel vasculitis

Henoch–Schönlein purpura

Epidemiology

HSP is the most common childhood primary systemic vasculitis.[1] Gardner-Medwin et al. reported a large population-based survey of 1.1 million children (aged <17 years old) from a multiethnic region of the United Kingdom.[1] The annual incidence was estimated to be 20.4 per 100 000 children in the United Kingdom, with greater incidence in children from the Indian subcontinent (24 per 100 000) compared

---

Box 136.1 Classification of childhood vasculitides[3–4]

Predominantly small-vessel vasculitis

Granulomatous

- Granulomatosis with polyangiitis (GPA, Wegener's)
- Churg–Strauss syndrome (CSS)

Non-granulomatous

- Microscopic polyangiitis
- Henoch–Schönlein purpura (HSP)
- Isolated cutaneous leukocytoclastic vasculitis
- Hypocomplementemic urticarial vasculitis

Predominantly medium-sized vessel vasculitis

- Childhood polyarteritis nodosa (PAN)
- Cutaneous polyarteritis
- Kawasaki disease (KD)

Predominantly large-vessel vasculitis

- Takayasu's arteritis (TA)

Other vasculitides

- Behçet's disease
- Vasculitis secondary to infection (including hepatitis B associated PAN), malignancies, and drugs, including hypersensitivity vasculitis
- Vasculitis associated with other connective tissue diseases
- Isolated vasculitis of the central nervous system (childhood primary angiitis of the CNS, cPACNS)
- Cogan's syndrome
- Unclassified

From Ozen et al.[3,4]

with white Europeans (17.8 per 100,000) and black (predominantly Afro-Caribbean) children (6.2 per 100 000).[1] Yang et al. reported an annual incidence of 12.9 per 100 000 children in Taiwan.[5]

Classification criteria

According to the new EULAR/PRINTO/PRES definition a patient is classified as having HSP in the presence of purpura or petechiae with lower limb predominance (mandatory criterion; Figure 136.1), plus one of the following four criteria[4]:

◆ abdominal pain

◆ histopathology showing typical leucocytoclastic vasculitis with predominant IgA deposit; or proliferative glomerulonephritis with predominant IgA deposit

◆ arthritis or arthralgia

◆ renal involvement (proteinuria or haematuria or presence of red blood cell casts).

In cases with purpura with atypical distribution a demonstration of IgA is required as a mandatory criterion, although in routine clinical practice skin biopsy with immunofluorescence is rarely performed. Another caveat regarding this point is that if the skin biopsy is taken in the centre of the necrotic lesion, IgA deposition may be falsely negative due to the presence of proteolytic enzymes. Despite some of the controversies surrounding inclusion of skin biopsy in the HSP classification criteria, the new definition provides sensitivity and specificity for classification of HSP (using other forms of vasculitis as controls) of 100% and 87% respectively.[4] It should be noted, however, that vasculitis classification criteria are not the same as diagnostic criteria, since they are designed to differentiate

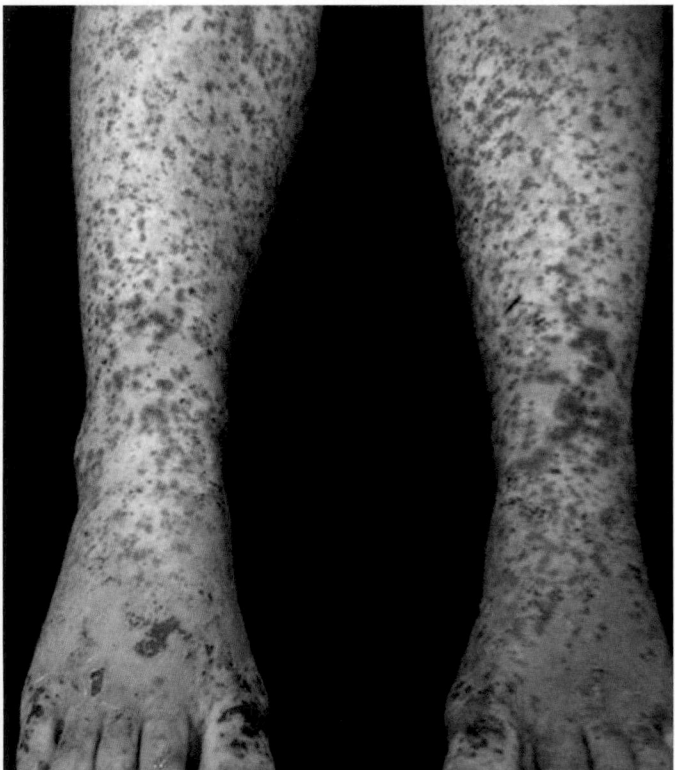

Fig. 136.1 Typical (severe) palpable purpura of Henoch–Schönlein purpura in a 13 year old female without renal involvement.

one form of vasculitis from another, rather than diagnose vasculitis in the first instance.

Aetiopathogenesis

As many as 50% of occurrences in paediatric patients are preceded by an upper respiratory tract infection.[6,7] HSP occurrence following occurring vaccination has also been described,[8] although this remains a contentious issue. Several infectious agents have been implicated, including group A streptococci, varicella, hepatitis B, Epstein–Barr virus, parvovirus B19, mycoplasma, campylobacter, and yersinia.[6]

It is suggested that IgA has a pivotal role in the pathogenesis of the disease, a hypothesis supported by the almost universal deposition of IgA in lesional vascular tissue.[9] Skin or renal biopsies demonstrate the deposition of IgA (mainly IgA1) in the wall of dermal capillaries and postcapillary venules and mesangium.[9] In addition, serum IgA levels have been reported to be increased during the acute phase of the disease, and a proportion of patients have circulating IgA-containing immune complexes and cryoglobulins.[10] Some studies have found IgA anti-neutrophil cytoplasmic antibodies (IgA-ANCA) in a proportion of patients with HSP, while others have shown an increase in IgA-rheumatoid factor, or IgA-anti-cardiolipin antibodies.[9] Recently, galactose deficiency of O-linked glycans in the hinge region of IgA1 has been reported in adults with IgA nephropathy and children with HSP.[11] Additionally, Hiasano et al. showed complement activation in the glomerulus through both the alternative and lectin pathways in patients with HSP nephritis.[12] IgA immune complexes and activation of complement lead to the formation of chemotactic factors (such as C5a), which in turn recruit polymorphonuclear leucocytes to the site of deposition,[13,14] resulting in further inflammation and necrosis of vessel walls, with concomitant thrombosis[9] and extravasation of erythrocytes from haemorrhage. The histological endpoint is that of a typical leukocytoclastic vasculitis.[9] The term 'leukocytoclasis' refers to the breakdown of neutrophils in lesional tissue, resulting in the characteristic nuclear debris or 'nuclear dust' observed, and is not specific for HSP.

Several genetic polymorphisms have been linked to HSP in various population cohorts.[15,16] On the whole, however, studies of this nature have been hampered by relatively small patient numbers and lack of power to be definitive or necessarily applicable to all racial groups.[16]

Clinical features

Skin involvement is typically with purpura which is generally symmetrical, affecting the lower limbs and buttocks in the majority of cases, the upper extremities being involved less frequently.[17,18] The abdomen, chest, and face are generally unaffected by purpura, although the face can be affected by angioedema. New crops of purpura may develop for several months after the disease onset, though generally fade with time.[17,18] Lesions can be induced by mild trauma. Angioedema and urticaria can also occur.[17,18] Around two-thirds of children have joint manifestations at presentation, with the knees and ankles most frequently involved.[17,18] Symptoms, which take the form of pain, swelling, and decreased range of movement, tend to be fleeting and resolve without the development of permanent articular damage.[7,17,18] Three-quarters of children develop abdominal symptoms ranging from mild colic to severe pain with ileus and vomiting.[7,17,18] Haematemesis and melaena are sometimes observed, due to mesenteric vasculitis.[17] Other serious complications include intestinal perforation and intussusception.[17] The latter may be difficult to distinguish from abdominal colic, and the incidence of intussusception is significant enough to warrant exclusion by ultrasound where suspected.[17] Acute pancreatitis is also described, although is a rare complication.[17]

Other organs less frequently involved include the central nervous system (cerebral vasculitis), gonads (orchitis may be confused with torsion of the testis), and lungs (pulmonary haemorrhage).[17] Ureteric obstruction has been reported.[17] Many cases follow an upper respiratory tract infection and the onset of the disorder may be accompanied by systemic symptoms including malaise and mild pyrexia.[17] Multiple organ involvement may be present from the outset of the disease, or alternatively an evolving pattern may develop, with different organs becoming involved at different time points over the course of several days to several weeks.[17] Recurrence of symptoms occurs in around one-third of cases, generally within 4 months of resolution of the original symptoms. Recurrences are more frequent in those with renal involvement.[17]

Reports of HSP nephritis indicate that between 20–61% of cases are affected with this complication. Renal involvement is normally manifest between a few days and a few weeks after first clinical presentation, but can occur up to 2 months or (rarely) more from presentation. There appears to be an increased risk of renal disease in those with bloody stools.[19] Renal involvement can present with varying degrees of severity. This includes isolated microscopic haematuria, proteinuria with microscopic or macroscopic haematuria, acute nephritic syndrome (haematuria with at least two of hypertension, raised plasma creatinine and oliguria), nephrotic syndrome (usually with microscopic haematuria), or a mixed nephritic–nephrotic picture.[17]

Most children do not require a tissue (renal and/or skin) biopsy diagnosis, with the exception of children with atypical skin findings, or suspected severe renal involvement. The skin lesion of HSP is that of a leucocytoclastic vasculitis with perivascular accumulation of neutrophils and mononuclear cells.[17] Immunofluorescence studies reveal vascular deposition of IgA and C3 in affected skin, though similar changes may be observed in skin unaffected by the rash.[17]

The renal lesion of HSP nephritis is characteristically a focal and segmental proliferative glomerulonephritis with IgA deposition (Figure 136.2). Severe cases with rapidly progressive glomerulonephritis can demonstrate crescentic glomerular changes on renal biopsy (Figure 136.2). Indications for diagnostic renal biopsy in children with HSP are[17,20]:

- nephritic/nephrotic presentation (urgent)

- raised creatinine, hypertension or oliguria (urgent)

- heavy proteinuria (Ua:Ucr persistently >100 mg/mmol) on an early morning urine sample at 4 weeks; serum albumin not necessarily in the nephrotic range

- persistent proteinuria (not declining) after 4 weeks

- impaired renal function (GFR <80 mL/min/1.73m²).

Management

The large majority of cases of HSP require symptomatic treatment only. Arthropathy is managed with rest and analgesia. Controversies concerning the use of corticosteroids in the treatment of HSP exist with regard to whether or not they can[1] reduce severity or duration

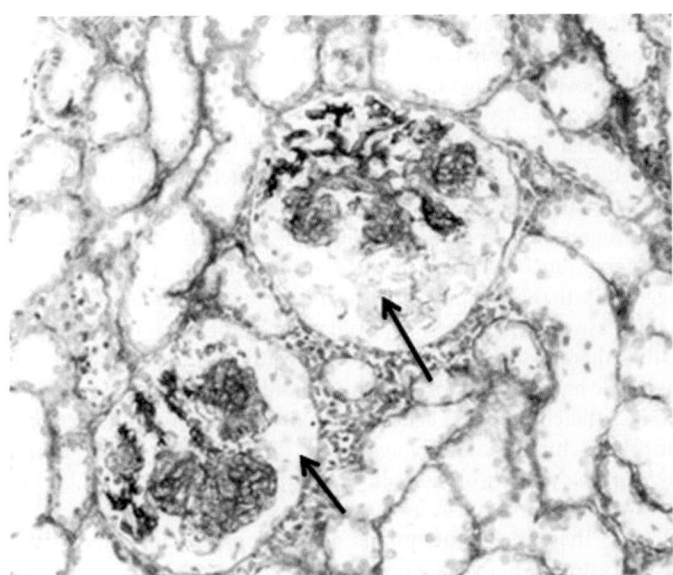

Fig. 136.2 Immunohistochemistry of renal histology from a 16-year-old male with Henoch–Schönlein purpura and heavy proteinuria. Diffuse mesangial matrix expansion and thickening of capillary walls. Strong diffuse granular mesangial and capillary wall IgA deposition. Fibrocellular crescentic change is also present in both the glomeruli (arrowed).

of disease,[2] decrease the risk of glomerulonephritis, and[3] prevent relapses of the disease.[21,22] Zaffanello and Fanos reviewed the treatment of HSP nephritis, concluding that currently prescribed treatments for HSP nephritis are not adequately guided by evidence obtained in robust randomized placebo-controlled trials with outcome markers related to the progression to end stage renal disease.[23] Current evidence is summarized in more detail below.

Treatment to prevent renal disease

Various treatment strategies and strategies aiming to prevent disease complications such as renal disease have been reported with variable effect. The efficacy of corticosteroids to prevent complications such as abdominal pain is still debated.[21,22] Chartapisak et al. recently systematically reviewed all published randomized controlled trials (RCTs) for the prevention or treatment of renal involvement in HSP.[24] Meta-analyses of four RCTs which evaluated prednisone therapy at presentation of HSP showed that there was no significant difference in the risk of development or persistence of renal involvement at 1, 3, 6, and 12 months with prednisone compared with placebo or no specific treatment. Thus it is becoming clearer that prophylactic corticosteroid does not prevent the onset of HSP nephritis. That said, there could still be a role for early use of corticosteroids in patients with severe extrarenal symptoms and in those with renal involvement, as suggested by the findings of a study performed by Ronkainen et al.[21] Prednisone (1 mg/kg per day for 2 weeks, with weaning over the subsequent 2 weeks) was effective in reducing the intensity of abdominal pain and joint pain. Prednisone did not prevent the development of renal symptoms but was effective in treating them if present; renal symptoms resolved in 61% of the prednisone patients after treatment, compared with 34% of the placebo patients.[21]

Treatment of rapidly progressive glomerulonephritis

There are good data indicating that crescents in >50% of glomeruli and nephrotic range proteinuria carry an unfavourable prognosis, thus highlighting the need for an effective intervention. Unfortunately, to date, there is only one RCT evaluating the benefit of treatment, which shows no difference in outcome using cyclophosphamide vs supportive therapy alone.[25] A major limitation of the study, however, is that it did not examine combined therapy, i.e. cyclophosphamide and corticosteroidsteroid, a regimen used in most other severe small-vessel vasculitides (see below). For patients with rapidly progressive glomerulonephritis (RPGN) with crescentic change on biopsy, uncontrolled data suggest that treatment may comprise aggressive therapy with corticosteroid, cyclophosphamide, and possibly plasma exchange,[26] as for other causes of crescentic nephritis. Other therapies such as ciclosporin, azathioprine, and cyclophosphamide have been reported by some authors to be effective.[17,26] As HSP is the commonest cause of rapidly progressive glomerulonephritis in childhood, more aggressive therapeutic approaches have been employed in some cases. Shenoy et al. reported 14 children with severe HSP nephritis treated successfully with plasma exchange alone.[26] These treatment options, although potentially important in select cases, are not yet supported by RCTs.

Treatment of HSP nephritis which is not rapidly progressive

Such patients may exhibit the following features: less than 50% crescents on renal biopsy, suboptimal glomerular filtration rate (GFR), heavy proteinuria which is not necessarily in the nephrotic range.[20] There are no robust clinical trials to guide therapy of this type of presentation. Many would advocate corticosteroids. Others advocate the addition of cyclophosphamide to corticosteroids in HSP nephritis with biopsy showing diffuse proliferative lesions or sclerosis, but with less than 50% crescentic change in patients who have ongoing heavy proteinuria. A typical regimen would comprise 8 weeks of oral cyclophosphamide (2 mg/kg per day) with daily prednisolone, converting to alternate-day prednisolone and azathioprine for a total of 12 months.[20] Published evidence for the efficacy of this approach is lacking, but this may be a reasonable option bearing in mind the adverse prognosis of children with HSP who have a nephritic–nephrotic phenotype. In patients with greater than 6 months duration of proteinuria an angiotensin converting enzyme (ACE) inhibitor may be indicated to limit secondary glomerular injury, although again the evidence to support this therapy is lacking.[23] Mycophenolate mofetil (MMF) has been reported in small case series as an effective treatment of recurrent skin, articular, and gastrointestinal symptoms as well as nephrotic-range proteinuria in children who failed to respond to systemic steroid therapy.[27,28]

Outcome

The majority of children with HSP make a full and uneventful recovery with no evidence of ongoing significant renal disease. Renal involvement is the most serious long-term complication of HSP. A study of long-term outcome of 78 subjects who had HSP nephritis during childhood (mean of 23.4 years after onset) demonstrated overall that initial findings on renal biopsy correlated well with outcome, but had poor predictive value in individual patients.[29] Forty-four per centof patients who had nephritic, nephrotic, or nephritic–nephrotic syndromes at onset had hypertension or impaired renal function, whereas 82% of those who presented with haematuria (with or without proteinuria) were normal.[29] Seven patients deteriorated clinically years after apparent complete clinical recovery. Sixteen of 44 full-term pregnancies were complicated by proteinuria and/or hypertension, even in the absence of active renal disease.[29]

Furthermore, Narchi systematically reviewed all published literature with regard to long-term renal impairment in children with HSP.[30] Twelve studies with 1133 children were reviewed. Renal involvement occurred in 34% of children; 80% had isolated haematuria and/or proteinuria while 20% had acute nephritis or nephrotic syndrome.[30] Renal complications, if they did occur, developed early—by 4 weeks in 85% and by 6 months in nearly all children.[30] Persistent renal involvement (hypertension, reduced renal function, nephrotic or nephritic syndrome) occurred in 1.8% of children overall but the incidence varied with the severity of the kidney disease at presentation, occurring in 5% of children with isolated haematuria and/or proteinuria but in 20% who had acute nephritis and/or nephrotic syndrome in the acute phase.[30] Children with significant renal impairment at presentation, and/or persistent proteinuria should undergo regular assessment of their GFR, e.g. at 1, 3, and 5 years after the acute episode of HSP.[20] Some instances of hypertension have been reported many years after normalization of renal function and urinalysis.[31] An increased incidence of pre-eclampsia has also been reported.[32]). Interestingly, in children who underwent repeat renal biopsies the majority of children with HSP still had IgA years later,[33] which could explain in part the late renal morbidity sometimes described. Thus it is clear that robust clinical trials for the treatment of moderate and severe HSP nephritis are urgently required. Lastly, it is recognized that HSP can occur in renal allografts.[34]

Acute haemorrhagic oedema of infancy

Acute haemorrhagic oedema of infancy (AHEI; Finkelstein–Seidlmayer syndrome) is often described as a variant of HSP that can affect young infants and toddlers under the age of 2 years.[35] More than 100 cases of this variant have been published in medical literature worldwide. Although initially considered a variant of HSP, it is now considered a separate entity, mainly because it predominantly affects the skin without the organ involvement described for typical HSP described above.[35] AHEI is characterized by the triad of fever; oedema (swelling of the skin); and rosette-, annular-, or targetoid-shaped purpura primarily over the face, ears, and extremities.[35] The cutaneous findings are dramatic both in appearance and in rapidity of onset, and are easily recognized once seen. The prognosis is usually excellent with resolution of the skin lesions within a few weeks without treatment, although attacks may recur.[35] Histopathology is typical of a leucocytoclastic vasculitis with occasional demonstration of perivascular IgA deposition.[35]

ANCA-associated vasculitides

Definitions, epidemiology, and classification

The ANCA-associated vasculitides (AAV) are considered in detail in Chapters 131 and 132. Although rare, AAV do occur in childhood and are associated with significant morbidity and mortality.[17]

The recently modified classification definition for GPA (formerly known as Wegener's granulomatosis) requires the presence of three out of the following criteria[4]:

- renal involvement (proteinuria or haematuria or red blood cell casts)
- positive histopathology (granulomatous inflammation within the wall of an artery or in the perivascular or extravascular area)
- upper airway involvement (nasal discharge or septum perforation, sinus inflammation)

- laryngo-tracheo-bronchial involvement (subglottic, tracheal, or bronchial stenosis)
- pulmonary involvement (chest radiograph or CT)
- ANCA positivity (by immunofluorescence, or by ELISA PR3 ANCA or MPO ANCA).

Sensitivity and specificity of the new EULAR/PRINTO/PRES criteria are 93% and 99% respectively for the classification of GPA from other forms of vasculitis in the young.[4]

Clinical features of granulomatosis with polyangiitis

From a clinical perspective in children it may be useful to think of GPA as having two forms: a predominantly granulomatous form with mainly localized disease with chronic course; and a florid, acute small-vessel vasculitic form characterized by severe pulmonary haemorrhage and/or rapidly progressive vasculitis or other severe vasculitic manifestation. These two broad presentations may coexist or present sequentially in individual patients.

In one case series of 17 children with GPA the frequency of different system involvement was: respiratory 87%, kidneys 53%, sinuses 35%, joints 53%, eyes 53%, nervous system 12%, skin 53%.[36] Another paediatric series of GPA reported even higher frequency of renal involvement with 22/25 cases having glomerulonephritis at first presentation, and only 1/11 patients who had renal impairment in that series recovered renal function with therapy.[37] In the most recent paediatric series of 65 children classified as having GPA, renal involvement was reported up to 75.4% of cases.[38] Dialysis was necessary in 7 patients (10.8%), and endstage renal disease was present in a single patient of that series.[38] Of note, renal involvement in GPA is recruited with increasing age which could account in part for the variation in reported renal involvement in paediatric GPA.

In a recent review of 33 cases of childhood Churg–Strauss syndrome (CSS), all patients had significant eosinophilia and asthma.[39] Furthermore histological evidence of eosinophilia and/or vasculitis was present in virtually all patients.[39] ANCA were found in only 25% of children with CSS.[39] There is considerable clinical overlap between CSS and primary hypereosinophilic syndromes in the young, and the differentiation of these two entities is challenging and beyond the scope of this chapter; the reader is referred to Kahn et al.[40]

Treatment of AAV

Treatment for paediatric AAV is broadly similar to the approach in adults, with corticosteroids, cyclophosphamide (usually 6–10 intravenous doses at 500–1000 mg/m^2 (maxiumm 1.2 g) per dose given 3–4 weekly; alternatively given orally at 2 mg/kg per day for 2–3 months), and in select patients plasma exchange (particularly for pulmonary capillaritis and/or rapidly progressive glomerulonephritis—'pulmonary–renal syndrome') routinely employed to induce remission.[2,41] Anti-platelet doses of aspirin (1–5 mg/kg per day, typically 37.5–75 mg/day) are empirically employed on the basis of the increased risk of thrombosis associated with the disease process.[42] Methotrexate may have a role for induction of remission in patients with limited GPA,[43] but is less commonly used as an induction agent in children with AAV. Recommendations regarding duration of maintenance therapy are based on adult trial data, with no clinical trials in children performed.

Biological therapy is also increasingly used to treat children with small-vessel vasculitis, including AAV and ANCA-negative vasculitides.[44] Agents used include rituximab, and anti-TNFα (etanercept, infliximab, and adalimumab).[44] These therapies are mainly reserved for children who have failed standard treatment, or in those patients where cumulative cyclophosphamide and/or corticosteroid toxicity is of particular concern.[44]

Outcome of AAV

The mortality for paediatric GPA from one recent paediatric series was 12% over a 17 year period of study inclusion.[36] Another paediatric series of GPA reported 40% of cases with chronic renal impairment at 33 months follow-up,[37] despite therapy.

For microscopic polyangiitis (MPA) in children, mortality during paediatric follow-up is reportedly 0–14%.[32,45] For CSS in children, the most recent series quotes a related mortality of 18%, all attributed to disease rather than therapy.[39]

Predominantly medium-vessel vasculitis

Polyarteritis nodosa

Definitions, epidemiology, and classification criteria

Polyarteritis nodosa (PAN) is a necrotizing vasculitis associated with aneurysmal nodules along the walls of medium-sized muscular arteries and is the condition classically described by Kussmaul and Maier in 1866.[46] Although comparatively rare in childhood it is the most common form of systemic vasculitis after HSP and KD.[46]

The new EULAR/PRINTO/PRES classification criteria for PAN[4] are:

- histopathological evidence of necrotizing vasculitis in medium-sized or small arteries or angiographic abnormality (aneurysm, stenosis, or occlusion) as a mandatory criterion, plus one of the following five:
  - skin involvement
  - myalgia or muscle tenderness
  - hypertension
  - peripheral neuropathy
  - renal involvement.

Sensitivity and specificity for these criteria were 73% and 100% respectively.[4]

Aetiopathogenesis

The immunopathogenesis leading to vascular injury in PAN is probably heterogeneous.[46] The mechanism of vascular inflammation most often implicated is mediated by immune complex deposition.[46] Infections including hepatitis B, parvovirus B19, cytomegalovirus, and HIV[46] have been implicated. PAN-like illnesses have additionally been reported in association with cancers and haematological malignancies.[32,46] However, these associations are rare in childhood. Streptococcal infection may be an important trigger, and indirect evidence suggests that bacterial superantigens may play a role in some cases.[47]

Genetic predisposing factors may make individuals vulnerable to develop PAN. Yalcinkaya et al. have recently reported on the prevalence of familial Mediterranean fever (FMF) mutations in 29 children with PAN showing that 38% of the patients were carriers of MEFV mutations.[48]

Clinical features

The main clinical features of systemic PAN are malaise, fever, weight loss, skin rash, myalgia, abdominal pain, and arthropathy.[49] In addition, there may be ischaemic heart and testicular pain, renal manifestations such as haematuria, proteinuria, and hypertension,[50,51] and neurological features such as focal defects, hemiplegia, visual loss, mononeuritis multiplex, and organic psychosis.[52,53] Skin lesions are variable and may masquerade as those of HSP or multiform erythema but can also be necrotic and associated with peripheral gangrene.[46] Livido reticularis is also a characteristic feature and occasionally subcutaneous nodules overlying affected arteries are present.[46] Systemic involvement is variable but the skin, the musculoskeletal system, the kidneys, and the gastrointestinal tract are most prominently affected, with cardiac, neurological, and respiratory manifestations occurring less frequently.[50,54] In some patients rupture of arterial aneurysms can cause retroperitoneal and peritoneal bleeding, with perirenal haematomata being a recognized manifestation of this phenomenon. This feature has been noted a number of times in Turkey where it has occurred in patients with the well-recognized association of PAN and FMF.[55]

The characteristic histopathological changes of PAN are fibrinoid necrosis of the walls of medium or small arteries with a marked inflammatory response within or surrounding the vessel wall.[46] Indirect evidence of the presence of medium-sizes artery vasculitis affecting the renal arteries may be obtained by demonstrating patchy areas of decreased isotope uptake within the renal parenchyma on technetium-99 m dimercaptosuccinic acid (DMSA) scanning of the kidneys.[46,56] However, the most valuable investigative procedure is selective visceral catheter digital subtraction arteriography (DSA).[56] Occasionally there is a requirement to undertake cerebral arteriography at the same examination (if there is suspicion of cerebral vasculitis), and in that setting the dose of contrast agent administered requires careful consideration, particularly in small children. Findings on catheter arteriography include aneurysms, segmental narrowing, and variations in the calibre of arteries together with pruning of the peripheral vascular tree.[56]

Magnetic resonance angiography (MRA) usually fails to detect small or microaneurysms although can demonstrate large intra- and extrarenal aneurysms and stenoses/occlusions of the renal arteries or their branches, and areas of ischemia and infarction.[57] Of note, MRA may overestimate vascular stenotic lesions,[46] and this is a particular caveat of this test in small children. CT angiography (CTA) may also be able to reveal larger aneurysms and occlusive lesions and demonstrate areas of renal cortical ischemia and infarction, but concerns regarding the significant radiation exposure and its lack of sensitivity for the detection of vasculitic changes affecting smaller arteries in comparison to catheter arteriography limit its use.[46]

Cutaneous polyarteritis nodosa is a form of vasculitis affecting small and medium-sized vessels limited (essentially) to the skin.[58] It is characterized by the presence of fever, subcutaneous nodular, painful, non-purpuric lesions with or without livedo reticularis occurring predominantly in the lower extremities, with no systemic involvement (except for myalgia, arthralgia and non-erosive arthritis).[46] The disease is well recognized in childhood and there are a number of reports in the literature.[46] In a recent international survey of childhood vasculitis approximately one-third of children identified as having PAN were categorized as cutaneous PAN

without systemic involvement.[32] The clinical course is characterized by periodic exacerbations and remissions that may persist for many years throughout childhood. The condition usually remains localized to the skin although a proportion of cases appear to evolve into full-blown systemic PAN in time, and clinicians need to be mindful of this possibility.[46]

Management

As in other forms of systemic necrotizing vasculitis, induction and remission phases of treatment are required.[46] Early diagnosis and treatment are key to successful outcomes.[46] The treatment of PAN involves the administration of high-dose corticosteroid with an additional cytotoxic agent such as cyclophosphamide to induce remission, typically for the first 3–6 months.[46,59] Empirically, aspirin has also been given as an anti-platelet agent by some clinicians.[46] Once remission is achieved maintenance therapy with daily or alternate-day prednisolone and oral azathioprine is frequently utilized for an additional 18 months. Adjunctive plasma exchange can be used during the induction phase of treatment in life- or organ-threatening situations.[46] Use of biological agents including anti-TNFα and rituximab is also described for children with systemic PAN, particularly those not responding to standard therapy or because of concern regarding cumulative cyclophosphamide toxicity.[44]

Treatment of cutaneous PAN is typically much less aggressive. Agents commonly utilized include low-dose prednisolone, anti-platelet agents (aspirin or dipyridamole), colchicine, hydroxychloroquine, or azathioprine.[46] However, in a few cases cutaneous PAN may progress over time to the systemic form of the disease and therefore require more aggressive therapy.[60] Cutaneous PAN may respond to non-steroidal anti-inflammatory drugs,[61] but can require oral corticosteroids in moderate dose to achieve remission.[46] When streptococcal infection is implicated penicillin may be effective.[62] Some clinicians recommend continuing prophylactic penicillin throughout childhood since relapses are common and occur in up to 25% of cases in association with further streptococcal infections.[62] In circumstances where there has been lack of response to standard treatment or concerns about possible steroid toxicity, intravenous immunoglobulin (IVIG) has been successfully utilized.[63] Some success has also been reported with the use of methotrexate, colchicine, dapsone, cyclophosphamide, pentoxyfylline, and chloroquine,[46] or (more commonly in the authors' opinion) hydroxychloroquine.

Outcome

PAN, unlike some other vasculitides such as GPA, appears to be a condition where permanent remission can be achieved. However, if treatment is delayed or inadequate, life-threatening complications can occur due to the vasculitic process. After treatment has commenced severe complications, especially infective, can arise as a sequel to the immunosuppressive drugs used. In comparison to the almost 100% mortality seen in the presteroid era, mortality rates are presently remarkably low—1.1% in a recent retrospective multicentre analysis.[32] However, this may not be truly reflective of mortality in circumstances of severe disease since in that series 30% of patients were considered to have cutaneous PAN.[32] A mortality rate of 10% was recently recorded from a major tertiary referral centre seeing predominantly children with aggressive advanced disease.[64] The impact of newer biological therapies on these outcomes is not yet clear-cut.

Kawasaki's disease

Definitions, epidemiology, classification

KD is an acute self-limiting systemic vasculitis predominantly affecting young children. It is of worldwide distribution with a male preponderance, an ethnic bias towards East Asian children, some seasonality, and occasional epidemics.[65,66] It is the second commonest vasculitic illness of childhood (the commonest being HSP) and the commonest cause of acquired heart disease in children in the United Kingdom and the United States.[67] The incidence in Japan is 138/100 000 in children younger than 5 years,[68] whereas in the United States[69] it is 17.1 and in the United Kingdom[70] 8.1 per 100 000 children less than 5 years old.

Aetiopathogenesis

The aetiology of KD remains unknown, but currently it is felt that some ubiquitous infectious agent produces an abnormal immunological response in a genetically susceptible subject that results in the characteristic clinical picture.[46,71] Pronounced seasonality and clustering of KD cases have led to the hunt for infectious agents as a cause. However, so far no single agent has been identified, a fact most recently highlighted by the negative results that emerged from studies examining the potential link between coronavirus infection and KD in Taiwan.[47,71] One debate regarding the cause of KD has centred around the mechanism of immune activation: conventional antigen vs superantigen (SAg).[72] A superantigen is also responsible for induction of coronary artery disease in a murine model of KD. Experimental mice develop coronary arteritis in response to intra-peritoneal injections of *Lactobacillus casei* wall extract (LCWE), providing a murine model of KD.[73] The peripheral immune activation within hours of LCWE injection is followed by local infiltration into cardiac tissue at day 3 with the inflammatory infiltrate consisting mainly of T cells.[73] This inflammatory response peaks at day 28 post injection and is accompanied by elastin breakdown with disruption of the intima and media, as well as aneurysm formation at day 42.[74] Rowley et al. reported three fatal cases of KD and observed IgA plasma cell infiltration into the vascular wall during the acute phase of the illness.[75] They observed that the IgA response was oligoclonal, more suggestive of a conventional antigenic process than a superantigenic-driven one.[75]

Although the clinical syndrome and occurrence of epidemics suggest an infectious cause for KD, a genetic contribution to risk is suggested by the much higher prevalence of the disease in Japan and Korea than elsewhere, and by increased prevalence within families with an increased relative risk to siblings compared to the general population.[6,16] Recently, a number of polymorphisms have been identified that appear to be linked to disease susceptibility in KD or the risk of coronary artery aneurysms.[16]

Clinical manifestations

The principal clinical features are fever persisting for 5 days or more, peripheral extremity changes (reddening of the palms and soles, indurative oedema and subsequent desquamation), a polymorphous exanthema (Figure 136.3), bilateral conjunctival injection/congestion, lips and oral cavity changes (reddening/cracking of lips as shown in Figure 136.3, strawberry tongue, oral and pharyngeal injection) and cervical lymphadenopathy (acute non-purulent).[46] For the diagnosis to be established according to the Diagnostic Guidelines of the Japan Kawasaki Disease Research Committee, five of six criteria should be present.[76] The North American recommendations for

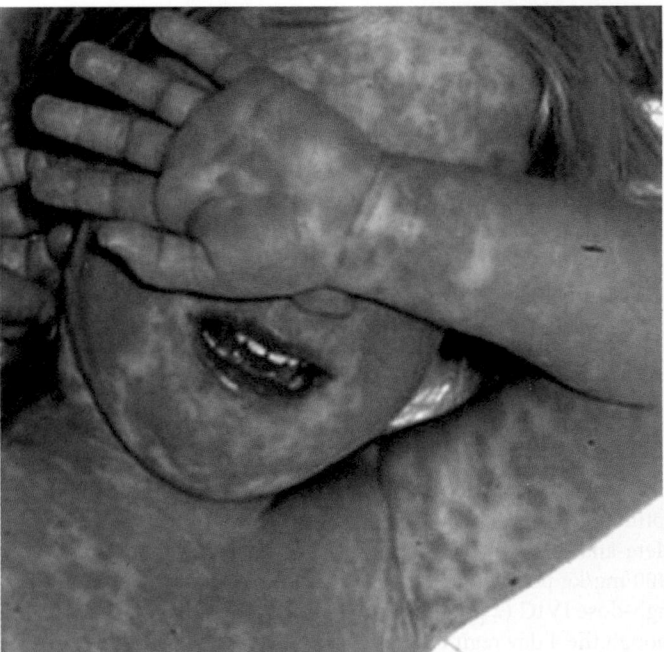

Fig. 136.3 Characteristic polymorphous exanthema and reddening of the lips in a 4 year old child with Kawasaki disease.
Courtesy of Prof N Klein "Training in Paediatrics" Edited by Mark Gardiner, Sarah Eisen, and Catherine Murphy, Oxford University Press.

the diagnosis are similar except that fever is a mandatory criterion and four of the remaining five criteria are required to establish the diagnosis.[66] If coronary artery aneurysms are present, fewer features are required for diagnostic purposes.[46,66] The cardiovascular features are the most important manifestations of the condition with widespread vasculitis affecting predominantly medium-sized muscular arteries, especially the coronary arteries. Coronary artery involvement occurs in 15–25% of untreated cases with additional cardiac features in a significant proportion of these including pericardial effusion, electrocardiographic abnormalities, pericarditis, myocarditis, valvular incompetence, cardiac failure, and myocardial infarction.[66] If looked for, damage to other medium-sized arteries including the major limb arteries, renal and other visceral arteries, and, at times, the aorta can be demonstrated.[46]

Other systemic involvement can occur including the gastrointestinal tract; the hepatobiliary tract, with hydrops of the gallbladder being well recognized; the respiratory tract (pneumonitis); and the central nervous system with aseptic meningitis and seizures, deafness, and arthropathy.[46] Renal manifestations include pyuria, proteinuria, tubulointerstitial nephritis, and renal failure.[46] The mechanism of the renal impairment is unclear although IVIG used in treatment may play a role.[46]

Another clinical sign that maybe relatively specific to KD is the development of erythema and induration at sites of BCG inoculations.[46] The mechanism of this sign is thought to be cross-reactivity of T cells in KD patients between specific epitopes of mycobacterial and human heat shock proteins.[77]

Routinely, two-dimensional echocardiography is the means of identifying coronary artery involvement acutely, and monitoring changes in the longer term.[65] Coronary catheter arteriography may have a role, particularly for monitoring the course of giant coronary artery aneurysms (>8 mm internal diameter), since in the longer term these can be associated with stenotic lesions at the inlet and/or outlet of the giant aneurysm, or in other circumstances where stenotic arterial lesions are suspected. This investigation provides little information about the microvasculature, however.[66] In addition, caution is advised regarding the timing of the timing of the timing of catheter coronary arteriography, since since this may be associated with significant risk of myocardial infarction if performed when the coronary vasculitis is still active. Dobutamine stress echocardiography has a role in follow-up evaluation of those with coronary artery aneurysms.[46] Spiral CTA and MRA have been advocated but the former is associated with significant radiation and the latter has limited resolution.[46]

Management

The management of KD is summarized in Figure 136.4. Early recognition and treatment of KD with aspirin and IVIG has been shown unequivocally by meta-analysis to reduce the occurrence of coronary artery aneurysms (CAA).[66,78] The prevalence of CAA is inversely related to the total dose of IVIG, 2 g/kg of IVIG being the optimal dose usually given as a single infusion over 12 hours.[66,78] Meta-analysis of RCTs comparing divided lower doses of IVIG (400 mg/kg per day for 4 consecutive days) vs a single infusion of high-dose IVIG (2 g/kg over 10 hours) has clearly shown that even though the 4 day regimen has some benefit, a single dose of 2 g/kg has a greater therapeutic effect in the prevention of CAA.[79]

IVIG resistance occurs in up to 20% of cases.[66] In those cases most advocate a second dose of IVIG based on the rationale that if there was an initial but temporary response, a second dose may adequately switch off the partially treated vasculitic process. Increasingly, however, many will consider the use of corticosteroids prior/or in addition to a second dose of IVIG.[80,81]

Regarding corticosteroid use in IVIG resistant to KD, there are apparently conflicting data from clinical trials. Inoue et al. reported on an RCT of 178 KD patients who were assigned to receive IVIG (2 g/kg) given over 2 consecutive days, or IVIG plus prednisolone sodium succinate (2 mg/kg per day) 3 times daily given by intravenous (IV) injection until the fever resolved, and then orally until the C-reactive protein (CRP) level normalized.[80] Patients in both groups received aspirin (30 mg/kg) and dipyridamole (2 mg/kg per day).[80] The addition of corticosteroid was associated with reduced CAA compared with IVIG alone: in those receiving IVIG and anti-platelet therapy, 11.4% had CAA at 1 month, compared with 2.2% in those receiving IVIG plus corticosteroids.[80] The duration of fever was shorter, and the CRP decreased more rapidly in the group of patients receiving corticosteroids.[80] In contrast Newburger et al. in a randomized, double-blind, placebo-controlled trial examined the effect of the addition of a single dose of intravenous methylprednisolone to standard therapy.[81] They found that this corticosteroid regimen did not improve the CAA outcome in these children.[81] Interestingly, a meta-analysis by Zhu et al. looked at all studies investigating the efficacy of corticosteroid therapy in KD by comparing it with standard IVIG and aspirin therapy. This analysis revealed a significant reduction in the rates of initial treatment failure among patients who received corticosteroid therapy in combination with IVIG compared to IVIG alone.[82] Furthermore, the use of corticosteroids reduced the duration of fever and the time required for CRP to return to normal.[82] Importantly, there was no increase in the frequency of coronary artery lesions in the patients receiving corticosteroids.[82] This meta-analysis therefore suggests that corticosteroids do have an important therapeutic role for the prevention of CAA, particularly in those resistant to a single IVIG dose, but that the dose and duration of corticosteroids is critical when considering this as adjunctive therapy in KD.

Infliximab, a chimeric monoclonal antibody against TNFα, has been reported to be effective for the treatment of IVIG-resistant KD.[83] In 13 of 16 patients with failed response to a single dose of IVIG who received infliximab, there was cessation of fever followed by reduction in CRP.[83] More recently, Burns et al reported on a multicentre, randomized, prospective trial of second IVIG infusion (2 g/kg) vs infliximab (5 mg/kg) in 24 children with acute KD and fever after initial failed treatment with IVIG.[84] There was resolution of fever within 24 hours in 11 of 12 subjects treated with infliximab, and in 8 of 12 subjects retreated with IVIG.[84] No significant differences were observed between treatment groups in the change from baseline for laboratory variables, fever, or echocardiographic assessment of coronary arteries.[84] These reports are encouraging, but further RCTs to establish the optimal management of KD, and in particular IVIG-resistant KD, are needed. Lastly, plasma exchange has been employed in refractory cases.[46]

In the convalescent phase of the condition, if aneurysms persist, anti-platelet therapy in the form of low-dose aspirin should be continued long term until the aneurysms resolve.[66] In the presence of giant aneurysms (>8 mm) warfarin is recommended in addition to aspirin.[85] Some patients may require coronary angioplasty or other revascularization procedure should ischaemic symptoms arise.[66]

Outcome

The outlook for KD patients is generally good. The standardized acute mortality ratio in Japan is 1.14.[86] Angiographic resolution 1–2 years after onset of disease has been observed in 50–70% of vessels with coronary aneurysms.[87] About 20% of patients who develop CAA during the acute disease will develop coronary artery stenoses and the risk is greater with giant (>8 mm) aneurysms.[87] However, there are data suggesting that in spite of seeming recovery, there could be long-term cardiovascular sequelae that persist into adult life.[46] In a study exploring the long-term outcomes of a cohort of 6576 patients with KD enrolled between 1982 and 2004 the mortality rate for patients without cardiac sequelae in the acute phase of the disease and for female patients with sequelae did not differ from the normal population.[86] The mortality rate of males with cardiac sequelae was, however, 2.4 times higher than the normal population.[86] Epidemiological studies from Japan have also demonstrated that late sequelae, especially in patients with large aneurysms, include myocardial ischaemia with a frequency of 3% within 4 years after the onset of the disease.[78] The study of late vasculopathy years after KD is therefore an important ongoing area of research to try to identify those patients who may in the future require interventions for the primary prevention of late cardiovascular complications.

Predominantly large-vessel vasculitis

Takayasu's arteritis

Definitions, epidemiology and classification

The onset of TA is most common during the third decade of life but has been well reported in young children.[88] The EULAR/PRES/PRINTO classification criteria for childhood TA are:

- angiographic abnormalities of the aorta or its main branches (also pulmonary arteries) showing aneurysm/dilatation (mandatory criterion), *plus* one of the five following criteria[4]:

  - pulse deficit or claudication

  - four-limb blood pressure discrepancy

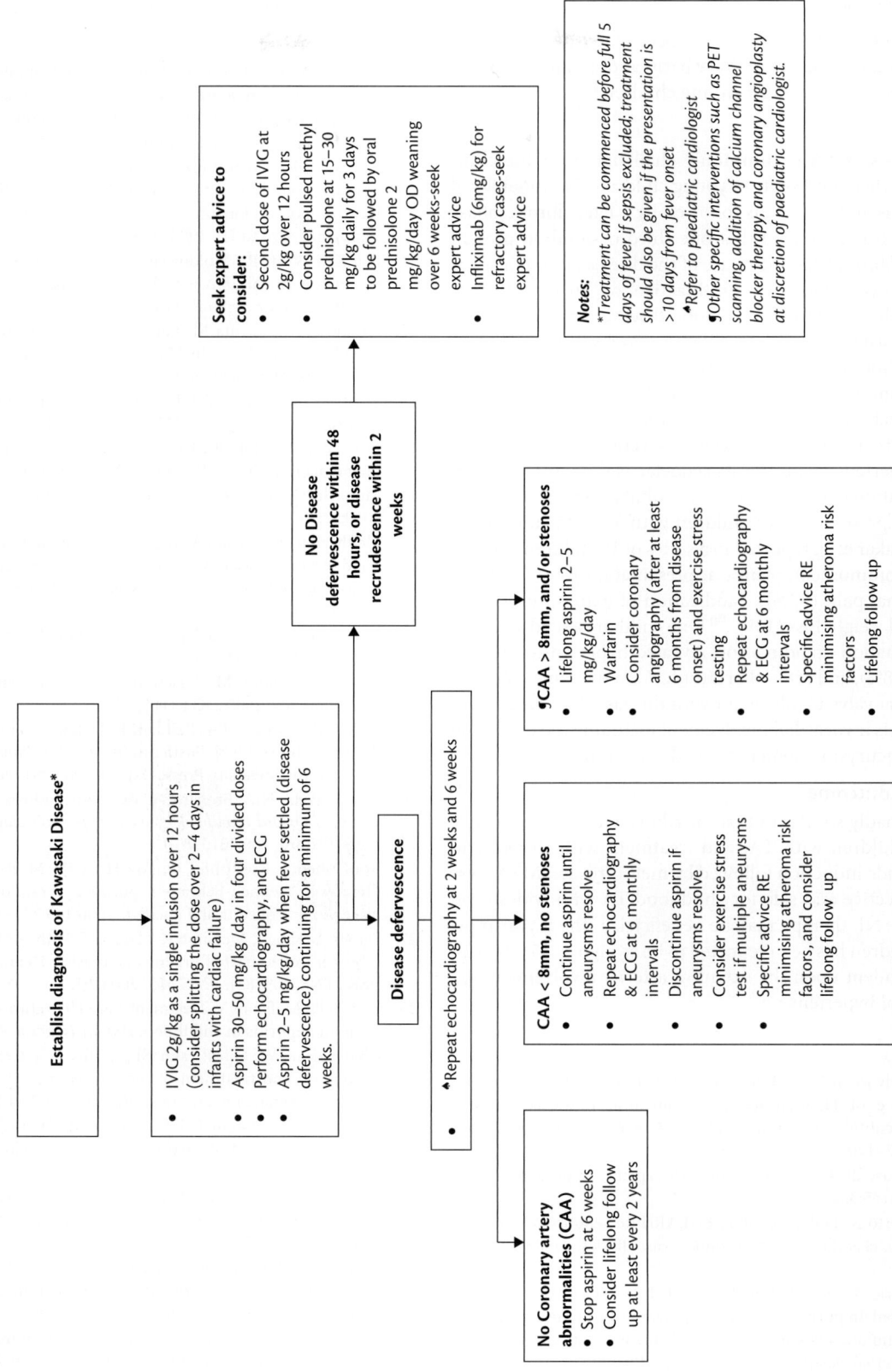

Establish diagnosis of Kawasaki Disease*

- IVIG 2g/kg as a single infusion over 12 hours (consider splitting the dose over 2–4 days in infants with cardiac failure)
- Aspirin 30–50 mg/kg /day in four divided doses
- Perform echocardiography, and ECG
- Aspirin 2–5 mg/kg/day when fever settled (disease defervescence) continuing for a minimum of 6 weeks.

Disease defervescence

△Repeat echocardiography at 2 weeks and 6 weeks

No Disease defervescence within 48 hours, or disease recrudescence within 2 weeks

Seek expert advice to consider:

- Second dose of IVIG at 2g/kg over 12 hours
- Consider pulsed methyl prednisolone at 15–30 mg/kg daily for 3 days to be followed by oral prednisolone 2 mg/kg/day OD weaning over 6 weeks-seek expert advice
- Infliximab (6mg/kg) for refractory cases-seek expert advice

No Coronary artery abnormalities (CAA)

- Stop aspirin at 6 weeks
- Consider lifelong follow up at least every 2 years

CAA < 8mm, no stenoses

- Continue aspirin until aneurysms resolve
- Repeat echocardiography & ECG at 6 monthly intervals
- Discontinue aspirin if aneurysms resolve
- Consider exercise stress test if multiple aneurysms
- Specific advice RE minimising atheroma risk factors, and consider lifelong follow up

¶CAA > 8mm, and/or stenoses

- Lifelong aspirin 2–5 mg/kg/day
- Warfarin
- Consider coronary angiography (after at least 6 months from disease onset) and exercise stress testing
- Repeat echocardiography & ECG at 6 monthly intervals
- Specific advice RE minimising atheroma risk factors
- Lifelong follow up

Notes:

*Treatment can be commenced before full 5 days of fever if sepsis excluded; treatment should also be given if the presentation is >10 days from fever onset

△Refer to paediatric cardiologist

¶Other specific interventions such as PET scanning, addition of calcium channel blocker therapy, and coronary angioplasty at discretion of paediatric cardiologist.

Fig. 136.4 Management of Kawasaki disease.

Reproduced from Oxford Specialist Handbook of Paediatric Rheumatology, ed Helen Foster and Paul Brogan. © Oxford University Press, 2012.

- bruits
- hypertension
- acute-phase response.

Familial occurrence of the disease has been extensively reported, leading to a hypothesis for a hereditary basis, and should be considered when the disease presents in young children.[89]

Clinical features

Clinical diagnosis of TA is commonly challenging for the clinician, especially when it presents in young children. An initial florid inflammatory vasculitic phase is followed by a later fibrotic phase of the illness.[88] It is estimated that one-third of children present within this late fibrotic/stenotic phase of the disease. It is a misconception that this is in some way an 'inactive', or 'burnt-out' stage of the disease, since progressive stenotic disease may be the consequence of persistent but low-level large-vessel vasculitic disease activity, but without evidence of conventional laboratory markers of systemic inflammation such as elevated CRP or increased erythrocyte sedimentation rate (ESR).[88] The time from onset of symptoms to diagnosis are variable, but can be several years.[4]

Although hypertension and/or its sequelae is the most common form of presentation in both children and adults,[90] the overall clinical spectrum at presentation of children with TA may differ from that in adults. Cakar et al. reported in a series of 19 children with TA that the most common complaints at presentation were headache (84%), abdominal pain (37%), claudication of extremities (32%), fever (26%), and weight loss (10%).[90] One child presented with visual loss. Examination on admission revealed hypertension (89%), absent pulses (58%), and arterial bruits (42%) in the same cohort.[90] Aortic and mitral valve involvement with the vasculitic process are recognized,[88] as is myocardial involvement including the formation of ventricular aneurysms, sometimes with calcification.[88]

Treatment and outcome

Treatment is broadly similar to that for adults with TA. Ozen et al. described six children with TA, and treatment with steroid and cyclophosphamide induction followed by methotrexate (MTX) was suggested as effective and safe for childhood TA with widespread disease.[88] Anti-TNF therapy may be beneficial.[91] The 5 year mortality rate in children has been reported to be as high as 35%,[88] with prognosis dependent upon the extent of arterial involvement and on the severity of hypertension.[88,90]

References

1. Gardner-Medwin JMM, Dolezalova P, Cummins C, Southwood TR. Incidence of Henoch-Schonlein purpura, Kawasaki disease, and rare vasculitides in children of different ethnic origins. *Lancet* 2002;360:1197–1202.
2. Dillon MJ. Vasculitis treatment—new therapeutic approaches. *Eur J Pediatri* 2006;165:351–357.
3. Ozen S, Ruperto N, Dillon MJ et al. EULAR/PReS endorsed consensus criteria for the classification of childhood vasculitides. *Ann Rheum Dis* 2006;65:936.
4. Ozen S, Pistorio A, Iusan SM et al. EULAR/PRINTO/PRES criteria for Henoch–Schönlein purpura, childhood polyarteritis nodosa, childhood Wegener granulomatosis and childhood Takayasu arteritis: Ankara 2008. Part II: Final classification criteria. *Ann Rheum Dis* 2010;69:798.
5. Yang YH, Hung CF, Hsu CR et al. A nationwide survey on epidemiological characteristics of childhood Henoch–Schönlein purpura in Taiwan. *Rheumatology* 2005;44:618.
6. Brogan PA. What's new in the aetiopathogenesis of vasculitis? *Pediatr Nephrol* 2007;22:1083–1094.
7. Trapani S, Micheli A, Grisolia F et al. Henoch Schonlein purpura in childhood: epidemiological and clinical analysis of 150 cases over a 5-year period and review of literature. *Semin Arthritis Rheum* 2005;35:143–153.
8. Chave T, Neal C, Camp R. Henoch–Schönlein purpura following hepatitis B vaccination. *Journal Dermatological Treat* 2003;14:179–181.
9. Yang YH, Chuang YH, Wang LC et al. The immunobiology of Henoch-Schönlein purpura. *Autoimmun Rev* 2008;7:179–184.
10. Coppo R, Basolo B, Mazzucco G et al. IgA1 and IgA2 in circulating immune complexes and in renal deposits of Berger's and Schönlein-Henoch glomerulonephritis. *Proceedings of the European Dialysis and Transplant Association* 1983;19:648.
11. Lau KK, Wyatt RJ, Moldoveanu Z et al. Serum levels of galactose-deficient IgA in children with IgA nephropathy and Henoch-Schönlein purpura. *Pediatr Nephrol* 2007;22:2067–2072.
12. Hisano S, Matsushita M, Fujita T, Iwasaki H. Activation of the lectin complement pathway in Henoch-Schönlein purpura nephritis. *Am J Kidney Dis* 2005;45:295–302.
13. Wyatt RJ, Kanayama Y, Julian BA et al. Complement activation in IgA nephropathy. *Kidney Int* 1987;31:1019–1023.
14. Motoyama O, Iitaka K. Henoch Schonlein purpura with hypocomplementemia in children. *Pediatr Int* 2005;47:39–42.
15. Monach PA, Merkel PA. Genetics of vasculitis. *Curr Opin Rheumatol* 2010;22:157.
16. Eleftheriou D, Brogan PA. The molecular biology and treatment of childhood systemic vasculitis in children. In: Hoimeister J, Willis D (eds) *Molecular and translational vascular medicine.* Elsevier, Amsterdam, 2012:35–70.
17. Brogan P, Eleftheriou D, Dillon M. Small vessel vasculitis. *Pediatr Nephrol* 2010;25:1025–1035.
18. Brogan PA, Dillon MJ. Vasculitis from the pediatric perspective. *Curr Rheumatol Rep* 2000;2:411–416.
19. Webb NJA, Brogan PA, Baildam EM. Renal manifestations of systemic disorders. In: Webb N, Postlethwaite R (eds) *Clinical paediatric nephrology.* Oxford University Press, Oxford, 2003:381–403.
20. Rees L, Webb NJA, Brogan PA. Vasculitis. In Rees L, Webb NJA, Brogan PA (eds) *Oxford handbook of paediatric nephrology.* Oxford University Press, Oxford, 2007:310–313.
21. Ronkainen J, Koskimies O, Ala-Houhala M et al. Early prednisone therapy in Henoch-Schönlein purpura: a randomized, double-blind, placebo-controlled trial. *J Paediatr* 2006;149:241–247.
22. Huber A, King J, McLaine P, Klassen T, Pothos M. A randomized, placebo-controlled trial of prednisone in early Henoch Schönlein Purpura [ISRCTN85109383]. *BMC Med* 2004;2:7.
23. Zaffanello M, Fanos V. Treatment-based literature of Henoch–Schönlein purpura nephritis in childhood. *Pediatr Nephrol* 2009;24:1901–1911.
24. Chartapisak W, Opastiraku SL, Willis NS, Craig JC, Hodson EM. Prevention and treatment of renal disease in Henoch-Schönlein purpura: a systematic review. *Arch Dis Child* 2009;94:132.
25. Tarshish P, Bernstein J, Edelmann CM. Henoch-Schonlein purpura nephritis: course of disease and efficacy of cyclophosphamide. *Pediatr Nephrol* 2004;19:51–56.
26. Shenoy M, Ognjanovic MV, Coulthard MG. Treating severe Henoch-Schönlein and IgA nephritis with plasmapheresis alone. *Pediatr Nephrol* 2007;22:1167–1171.
27. Nikibakhsh AA, Mahmoodzadeh H, Karamyyar M et al. Treatment of complicated Henoch-Schonlein purpura with mycophenolate mofetil: a retrospective case series report. *Int J Rheumatol* 2010;2010:254316.
28. Du Y, Hou L, Zhao C, Han M, Wu Y. Treatment of children with Henoch-Schonlein purpura nephritis with mycophenolate mofetil. *Pediatr Nephrol* 2011;27:1–7.
29. Goldstein AR, White RHR, Akuse R, Chantler C. Long-term follow-up of childhood Henoch-Schönlein nephritis. *Lancet* 1992;339:280–282.

30. Narchi H. Risk of long term renal impairment and duration of follow up recommended for Henoch-Schonlein purpura with normal or minimal urinary findings: a systematic review. *Arch Dis Child* 2005;90:916.

31. Ronkainen J, Nuutinen M, Koskimies O. The adult kidney 24 years after childhood Henoch-Schönlein purpura: a retrospective cohort study. *Lancet* 2002;360:666–670.

32. Ozen S, Anton J, Arisoy N et al. Juvenile polyarteritis: results of a multicenter survey of 110 children. *J Paediatr* 2004;145:517–522.

33. Algoet C, Proesmans W. Renal biopsy 2–9 years after Henoch Schönlein purpura. *Pediatr Nephrol* 2003;18:471–473.

34. Meulders Q, Pirson Y, Cosyns JP, Squifflet JP, van Ypersele SC. Course of Henoch-Schonlein nephritis after renal transplantation. Report on ten patients and review of the literature. *Transplantation* 1994;58:1179.

35. Caksen H, Odaba Odabaş D, Kösem M et al. Report of eight infants with acute infantile hemorrhagic edema and review of the literature. *J Dermatol* 2002;29:290.

36. Belostotsky VM, Shah V, Dillon MJ. Clinical features in 17 paediatric patients with Wegener granulomatosis. *Pediatr Nephrol* 2002;17:754–761.

37. Akikusa JD, Schneider R, Harvey EA et al. Clinical features and outcome of pediatric Wegener's granulomatosis. *Arthritis Care Res* 2007;57:837–844.

38. Cabral DA, Uribe AG, Benseler S et al. Classification, presentation, and initial treatment of Wegener's granulomatosis in childhood. *Arthritis Rheum* 2009;60:3413–3424.

39. Zwerina J, Eger G, Englbrecht M, Manger B, Schett G. Churg-Strauss syndrome in childhood: a systematic literature review and clinical comparison with adult patients. *Semin Arthritis Rheum* 2009;39: 108–115.

40. Kahn JE, Blétry O, Guillevin. Hypereosinophilic syndromes. *Best Pract Res Clin Rheumatol* 2008;22:863–882.

41. Brogan PA, Dillon MJ. The use of immunosuppressive and cytotoxic drugs in non-malignant disease. *Arch Dis Child* 2000;83:259.

42. Merkel PA, Lo GH, Holbrook JT et al. Brief communication: high incidence of venous thrombotic events among patients with Wegener granulomatosis: the Wegener's Clinical Occurrence of Thrombosis (WeCLOT) Study. *Ann Intern Med* 2005;142:620.

43. de Groot K, Rasmussen N, Bacon PA et al. Randomized trial of cyclophosphamide versus methotrexate for induction of remission in early systemic antineutrophil cytoplasmic antibodyûassociated vasculitis. *Arthritis Rheum* 2005;52:2461–2469.

44. Eleftheriou D, Melo M, Marks SD et al. Biologic therapy in primary systemic vasculitis of the young. *Rheumatology* 2009;48:978.

45. Hattori M, Kurayama H, Koitabashi Y. Antineutrophil cytoplasmic autoantibody-associated glomerulonephritis in children. *J Am Soc Nephrol* 2001;12:1493–1500.

46. Dillon MJ, Eleftheriou D, Brogan PA. Medium-size-vessel vasculitis. *Pediatr Nephrol* 2009;1:12.

47. Brogan PA, Shah V, Klein N, Dillon MJ. V restricted T cell adherence to endothelial cells: A mechanism for superantigen dependent vascular injury. *Arthritis Rheum* 2004;50:589–597.

48. YaInkaya Fûzakar Z, Kasapopur et al. Prevalence of the MEFV gene mutations in childhood polyarteritis nodosa. *J Paediatr* 2007;151:675–678.

49. Ozen S, Besbas N, Saatci U, Bakkaloglu A. Diagnostic criteria for polyarteritis nodosa in childhood. *J Pediatr* 1992;120:206–209.

50. Maeda M, Kobayashi M, Okamoto S et al. Clinical observation of 14 cases of childhood polyarteritis nodosa in Japan. *Acta Paediatr Jpn* 1997;39:277–279.

51. Cakar N, Ozcakar ZB, Soy D et al. Renal involvement in childhood vasculitis. *Nephron Clin Pract* 2008;108,c202–c206.

52. Engel DG, Gospe SM, Jr, Tracy KA, Ellis WG, Lie JT. Fatal infantile polyarteritis nodosa with predominant central nervous system involvement. *Stroke* 1995;26:699–701.

53. Tizard EJ, Dillon MJ. Wegener's granulomatosis, polyarteritis nodosa, Behcet's disease and relapsing polychondritis. In: Harper J, Oranje A,

Prose N (eds) *Textbook of pediatric dermatology*, 2nd edn. Blackwell, Oxford, 2006:1937–1952.

54. Ettlinger RE, Nelson AM, Burke EC, Lie JT. Polyarteritis nodosa in childhood a clinical pathologic study. *Arthritis Rheum* 1979;22:820–825.

55. Ozen S, Ben-Chetrit E, Bakkaloglu A et al. Polyarteritis nodosa in patients with familial Mediterranean fever (FMF): A concomitant disease or a feature of FMF? *Semin Arthritis Rheum* 2001;30:281–287.

56. Brogan PA, Davies R, Gordon I, Dillon MJ. Renal angiography in children with polyarteritis nodosa. *Pediatr Nephrol* 2002;17:277–283.

57. Schmidt WA. Use of imaging studies in the diagnosis of vasculitis. *Curr Rheumatol Rep* 2004;6:203–211.

58. Daoud MS, Hutton KP, Gibson LE. Cutaneous periarteritis nodosa: a clinicopathological study of 79 cases. *Br J Dermatol* 1997;136:706–713.

59. Jayne D. Current attitudes to the therapy of vasculitis. *Kidney Blood Press Res* 2003;26:231–239.

60. Siberry GK, Cohen BA, Johnson B. Cutaneous polyarteritis nodosa. Reports of two cases in children and review of the literature. *Arch Dermatol* 1994;130:884–889.

61. David J, Ansell BM, Woo P. Polyarteritis nodosa associated with streptococcus. *Arch Dis Child* 1993;69:685–688.

62. Fink CW. The role of the streptococcus in poststreptococcal reactive arthritis and childhood polyarteritis nodosa. *J Rheumatol Suppl* 1991;29:14.

63. Uziel Y, Silverman ED. Intravenous immunoglobulin therapy in a child with cutaneous polyarteritis nodosa. *Clin Exp Rheumatol* 1998;16:187.

64. Brogan PA, Shah V, Dillon MJ. Polyarteritis nodosa in childhood. Abstract, 10th International Vasculitis and ANCA Workshop, Cleveland, 2002.

65. Brogan PA, Bose A, Burgner D et al. Kawasaki disease: an evidence based approach to diagnosis, treatment, and proposals for future research. *Arch Dis Child* 2002;86:286.

66. Newburger JW, Takahashi M, Gerber MA et al. Diagnosis, treatment, and long-term management of Kawasaki disease: a statement for health professionals from the Committee on Rheumatic Fever, Endocarditis and Kawasaki Disease, Council on Cardiovascular Disease in the Young, American Heart Association. *Circulation* 2004;110:2747.

67. Shulman ST, De Inocencio J, Hirsch R. Kawasaki disease. *Pediatr Clin North Am* 1995;42:1205.

68. Yanagawa H, Nakamura Y, Yashiro M et al. Incidence survey of Kawasaki disease in 1997 and 1998 in Japan. *Pediatrics* 2001;107:e33.

69. Holman RC, Curns AT, Belay ED, Steiner CA, Schonberger LB. Kawasaki syndrome hospitalizations in the United States;1997 and 2000. *Pediatrics* 2003;112:495.

70. Harnden A, Alves B, Sheikh A. Rising incidence of Kawasaki disease in England: analysis of hospital admission data. *BMJ* 2002;324:1424.

71. Yeung RSM. Kawasaki disease: update on pathogenesis. *Curr Opin Rheumatol* 2010;22:551.

72. Herman A, Kappler JW, Marrack P, Pullen AM. Superantigens: mechanism of T-cell stimulation and role in immune responses. *Annu Rev Immunol* 1991;9:745–772.

73. Lehman TJA, Walker SM, Mahnovski V, McCurdy D. Coronary arthritis in mice following the systemic injection of group b Lactobacillus casei cell walls in aqueous suspension. *Arthritis Rheum* 1985;28:652–659.

74. Duong TT, Silverman ED, Bissessar MV, Yeung RSM. Superantigenic activity is responsible for induction of coronary arteritis in mice: an animal model of Kawasaki disease. *Int Immunol* 2003;15:79.

75. Rowley AH, Baker SC, Shulman ST et al. Detection of antigen in bronchial epithelium and macrophages in acute Kawasaki disease by use of synthetic antibody. *J Infect Dis* 2004;190:856.

76. *Diagnostic guidelines for Kawasaki disease*, 5th edn. Japan Kawasaki Disease Research Committee Tokyo, 2002.

77. Sireci G, Dieli F, Salerno A. T cells recognize an immunodominant epitope of heat shock protein 65 in Kawasaki disease. *Mol Med* 2000;6:581–590.

78. Durongpisitkul K, Gururaj VJ, Park JM, Martin CF. The prevention of coronary artery aneurysm in Kawasaki disease: a meta-analysis on the efficacy of aspirin and immunoglobulin treatment. *Pediatrics*1995;96:1057.

79. Newburger JW, Takahashi M, Beiser AS et al. A single intravenous infusion of gamma globulin as compared with four infusions in the treatment of acute Kawasaki syndrome. *N Engl J Med* 1991;324:1633–1639.

80. Inoue Y, Okada Y, Shinohara M et al. A multicenter prospective randomized trial of corticosteroids in primary therapy for Kawasaki disease: clinical course and coronary artery outcome. *J Paediatr* 2006;149:336.

81. Newburger JW, Sleeper LA, McCrindle BW et al. Randomized trial of pulsed corticosteroid therapy for primary treatment of Kawasaki disease. *N Engl J Med* 2007;356:663–675.

82. Zhu B, Lv H, Sun L, Zhang J et al. A meta-analysis on the effect of corticosteroid therapy in Kawasaki disease. *Eur J Pediatri* 2012;171:571–578.

83. Burns JC, Mason WH, Hauger SB et al. Infliximab treatment for refractory Kawasaki syndrome. *J Paediatr* 2005;146:662–667.

84. Burns JC, Best BM, Mejias A et al. Infliximab treatment of intravenous immunoglobulin-resistant Kawasaki disease. *J Paediatr* 2008;153:833–838.

85. Sugahara Y, Ishii M, Muta H et al. Warfarin therapy for giant aneurysm prevents myocardial infarction in Kawasaki disease. *Pediatr Cardiol* 2008;29:398–401.

86. Nakamura Y, Aso E, Yashiro M et al. Mortality among persons with a history of kawasaki disease in Japan: mortality among males with cardiac sequelae is significantly higher than that of the general population. *Circ J* 2008;72:134.

87. Kato H, Sugimura T, Akagi T et al. Long-term consequences of Kawasaki disease: a 10-to 21-year follow-up study of 594 patients. *Circulation* 1996;94:1379.

88. Gulati A, Bagga A. Large vessel vasculitis. *Pediatr Nephrol* 2010;25:1037–1048.

89. Morishita KA, Rosendahl K, Brogan PA. Familial Takayasu arteritis—a pediatric case and a review of the literature. *Pediatr Rheumatol Online J* 2011;9:6.

90. Cakar N, Yalcinkaya F, Duzova A et al. Takayasu arteritis in children. *J Rheumatol* 2008;35:913.

91. Hoffman GS, Merkel PA, Brasington RD, Lenschow DJ, Liang P. Anti-tumor necrosis factor therapy in patients with difficult to treat Takayasu arteritis. *Arthritis Rheum* 2004;50:2296–2304.

CHAPTER 137

Miscellaneous vasculitides

Richard A. Watts and Eleana Ntatsaki

Introduction

This chapter covers a wide range of individual conditions, which come under the umbrella of the term vasculitis. Where appropriate we have followed the Chapel Hill Classification and Nomenclature system.[1]

Immune complex small-vessel vasculitis

Hypocomplementaemic urticarial vasculitis

Hypocomplementaemic urticarial vasculitis (HUV) is defined as a vasculitis accompanied by urticaria and hypocomplementaemia affecting small vessels (i.e. capillaries, venules, or arterioles), and associated with anti-C1q antibodies. Common clinical features include glomerulonephritis, arthritis, and ocular inflammation (uveitis, scleritis, and episcleritis). The urticarial wheals may be accompanied by central purpura, are more painful, and tend to persist for longer (24–72 hours) compared to those of chronic urticaria (<24 hours). Laboratory findings include low complement levels of classical pathway, namely C1q, C2, C3, and C4, together with an acute-phase response. Antibodies against C1Q are invariably present in HUV, and this 100% sensitivity suggests a pathogenic role.[2] Systemic glucocorticoids can control the attack and prevent relapses. The urticarial lesions respond poorly to antihistamines. Patients may have significant morbidity and mortality, most commonly caused by chronic obstructive pulmonary disease and acute laryngeal oedema.

IgA vasculitis (Henoch–Schönlein purpura)

This is a vasculitis with IgA1–dominant immune deposits affecting small vessels. It typically involves the skin, gut, and glomeruli and is associated with arthralgia and arthritis.[3] It is predominately a childhood disease (see Chapter 136) but occurs rarely in adults, in whom it may be a more severe disease. The typical rash is erythematous papules followed by non-thrombocytopaenic purpura and is characteristically the presenting feature (Figure 137.1). A small proportion of patients (8%) with renal involvement and a mixed nephrotic/nephritic picture develop chronic renal failure. Most cases are self-limiting, but patients with severe skin or renal disease may need immunosuppressive therapy.

Cryoglobulinaemic vasculitis

Cryoglobulinaemic vasculitis is a rare small-vessel vasculitis that is often associated with hepatitis C virus (HCV) infection. Cryoglobulinaemia is the presence in the serum of immunoglobulins that precipitate in vitro at temperatures below 37 °C. Cryoglobulins are classified according to the clonality and type of the immunoglobulins[4]:

- type I consists of monoclonal immunoglobulin, either IgM or IgG
- type II are a mixture of monoclonal IgM and polyclonal IgG
- type III are a mixture of polyclonal IgM and IgG.

Types II and III are also known as mixed cryoglobulins as they have both IgG and IgM components.

A strong association is recognized between HCV infection and predominately type II cryoglobulinaemia. Hepatitis B (HBV) infection can also be associated with mixed cryoglobulinaemia. Cryoglobulinaemic vasculitis is more common in areas endemic for HCV and has a predilection for women (3:1).[5]

The clinical features of cryoglobulinaemic vasculitis were first described by Meltzer and colleagues in 1966.[6] The triad of purpura, arthralgia, and weakness, accompanied by organ dysfunction constitute the typical presentation in less than 40% of patients with cryoglobulinaemia.[7] The most frequently affected internal organs are peripheral nerves (polyneuropathy, mononeuritis multiplex of acute onset, or peripheral neuropathy of subacute gradual onset), kidneys (nephritic syndrome or nephritic urinary sediment due to mesangial proliferative glomerulonephritis in 40%) and joints

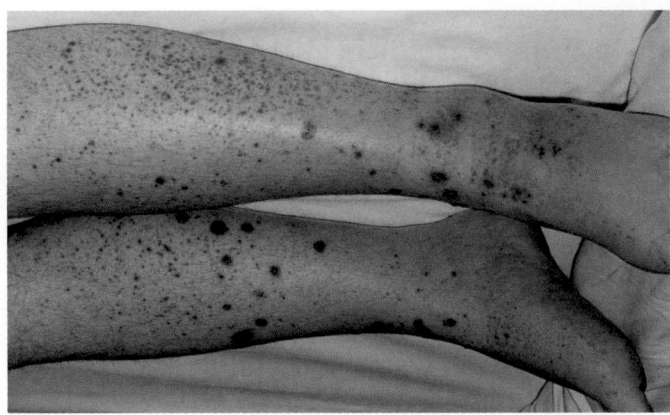

Fig. 137.1 Typical purpuric rash on a patient with IgA vasculitis.

(arthralgia or non-erosive arthritis in 10%). Systemic symptoms such as fever, weight loss, and myalgia are common. Purpura is the most typical cutaneous manifestation; however, urticaria, livedo, exanthema, acral necrosis, and leg ulcers may also occur. Raynaud's phenomenon is seen in 20% of cases.[8]

There are no standardized or validated diagnostic or classification criteria for cryoglobulinaemic vasculitis. Diagnosis is based on clinical presentation and the presence of circulating cryoglobulins. Viral serology together with appropriate tissue biopsy differentiates the diagnosis from the other systemic vasculitides.

High titres of rheumatoid factor (RF) are present in 70% of patients. Anti-neutrophil cytoplasmic antibodies (ANCA), antinuclear antibodies (ANA) and anti-cardiolipin antibodies are usually absent and complement levels are low in 90% of cases. Sample collection and handling is crucial when testing for cryoglobulins. The blood should be collected in pre-warmed syringes, transported, clotted, and centrifuged at 37–40 °C. The serum is thereafter stored at 4 °C for 7 days. Type I cryoglobulins precipitate within hours whereas mixed cryoglobulins can take days to precipitate.[9]

More than 90% of cases of cryoglobulinaemia have a recognized underlying cause. Therapy is focused on treating the cause of the disorder rather than simple symptomatic management. A combination of pegylated interferon-α and ribavarin is the therapeutic cornerstone for HCV-related cryoglobulinaemic vasculitis. Current consensus suggests that severe or life-threatening disease should be treated with steroids and cyclophosphamide together possibly with plasma exchange.[10] B-cell depleting therapies, although promising, should currently be reserved for severe refractory cases while the results of randomized trials are awaited.[4]

Anti-glomerular basement membrane disease

Anti-glomerular basement membrane (GBM) disease (Goodpasture's syndrome) is a vasculitis affecting glomerular capillaries, pulmonary capillaries, or both, with basement membrane deposition of anti-basement membrane autoantibodies. Lung involvement causes pulmonary haemorrhage, and renal involvement causes glomerulonephritis with necrosis and crescents.

Anti-GBM disease is an autoimmune disorder that mostly presents as rapidly progressive glomerulonephritis and pulmonary haemorrhage together with raised titres of antibodies against the GBM. The target autoantigens are the non-collagenous (NC1) regions of the α3 and to a lesser extent the α5 chains of type IV collagen. Treatment is generally immunosuppression combined with plasma exchange.[11]

Single-organ vasculitis

Single-organ vasculitis is a condition where the inflammatory process affecting the vessel walls appears to be localized to a single organ and there is no evidence to suggest local expression of a systemic process. Vasculitis may be unifocal or diffuse within the affected organ. Typical examples of diffuse forms of single-organ vasculitis include primary angiitis of the central nervous system (CNS), and cutaneous leucocytoclastic vasculitis.

Cutaneous vasculitis

Cutaneous vasculitis is one of the most frequent expressions of vasculitis; the appearances can be quite varied and a number of different types have been described.

Leucocytoclastic vasculitis

Leucocytoclastic vasculitis is one of the most common types of skin vasculitis in adults and it usually affects the lower legs. Lesions range from palpable purpura to urticarial plaques and haemorrhagic bullae. Leucocytoclasis is the destruction of cell nuclei with accumulation of nuclear dust. Chronic disease may result in ulceration. Precipitants include drugs (e.g. sulphonamides and penicillins), infection, or foreign protein (serum sickness) and therefore the condition is sometimes referred to as a hypersensitivity vasculitis. The prognosis is generally good with spontaneous resolution of lesions following withdrawal of the trigger. Development of systemic features such as arthralgia, abdominal pain, or haematuria should prompt assessment for systemic vasculitis and is indicative of a worse prognosis.

Cutaneous polyarteritis nodosa

Cutaneous polyarteritis nodosa is a chronic relapsing arteritis of subcutaneous and deep dermal small and medium-sized vessels. By definition, visceral organs are spared. Progression to systemic disease is rare. The cutaneous lesions are painful nodules which may ulcerate and occur most frequently on the lower legs (Figure 137.2). There may be marked livedo reticularis. There are no diagnostic markers and the diagnosis is made on the typical lesions and histology. Treatment usually requires glucocorticoids in moderate doses. Other agents that have been used include sulphapyridine, dapsone, and stanazolol. The role of other immunosuppressants is uncertain.[12]

Erythema elevatum diutinum and granuloma faciale

These represent rare but distinctive forms of localized chronic cutaneous leucocytoclastic vasculitis with no systemic involvement

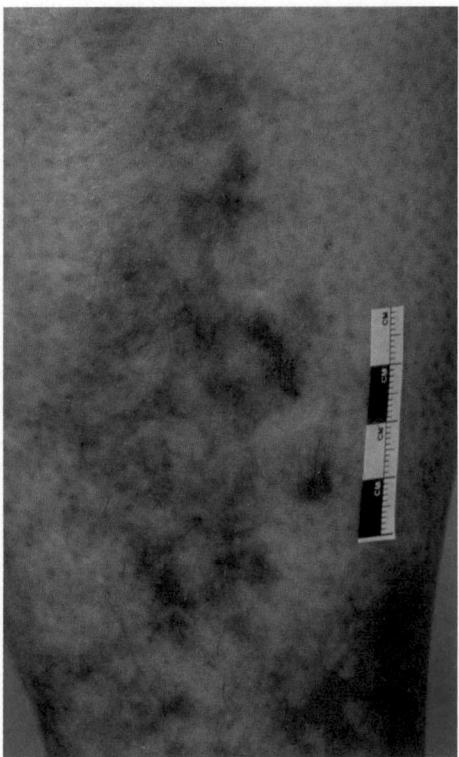

Fig. 137.2 Typical cutaneous lesions and livedo reticularis on a patient with cutaneous polyarteritis nodosa.

and unknown aetiology. Erythema elevatum diutinum presents with oedematous purplish-brown plaques over the back of hands, elbows, or knees which slowly enlarge and heal over months or years with fibrosis. Granuloma faciale is a persistent well-defined smooth papule and plaque on the face consisting of one or more pink-brown lesions.[13,14]

Isolated central nervous system angiitis (primary angiitis of the CNS)

CNS vasculitis is one of the rarest forms of vasculitis, with a large differential diagnosis. Due to a lack of validated diagnostic criteria it often poses a difficult challenge for the clinician. Primary angiitis of the central nervous system (pACNS) refers to disease confined to the brain, spinal cord, and overlying leptomeninges. Secondary CNS vasculitis occurs in the context of vascular inflammation caused either by systemic vasculitis, lymphoproliferative disease, infection (herpes zoster, syphilis, brucellosis, HIV), sarcoid, or amyloidosis.[15]

Typical presentation of pACNS is with headaches and behavioural/mental changes lasting a few weeks. Intermittent confusion and focal neurological changes such as aphasia, hemiparesis, seizures, transient ischaemic attacks, and strokes may also occur. Vision is commonly affected with visual defects in 1 in 5 patients and decreased acuity in 1 in 10 patients.

The diagnosis of CNS angiitis is usually based on a combination of MRI, cerebrospinal fluid (CSF), and biopsy findings.[16] Routine laboratory investigations are important in excluding secondary CNS vasculitis. However, inflammatory markers are not a reliable guide for monitoring disease activity or response to treatment. CSF abnormalities are found in 88% of patients and consist of elevated white cells and protein. Cerebral imaging is abnormal in 97% of patients and may reveal cerebral infarction in 50% of the patients. Intracranial haemorrhage is not as common (~10%). MRI has been shown to have a high positive predictive value in children.[17] Gadolinium enhancing of the leptomeninges may be useful in guiding a biopsy.

Biopsy of the leptomeninges, although only 75–80% sensitive, is necessary for a definitive diagnosis. Histological features of granulomatous vasculitis with or without acute necrosis or lymphocytic pattern support a diagnosis of primary CNS vasculitis. A biopsy can also prove useful in excluding other forms of vascular inflammation, malignancy and infection.

Treatment remains empirical. Induction therapy is with high-dose corticosteroids (1 mg/kg, maximum 60 mg and then tapered to 10 mg at 6 months; or intravenous methylprednisolone in severe cases) combined with intravenous cyclophosphamide in patients with poor prognosis. Maintenance therapy with oral corticosteroid is rarely required beyond 18 months. Refractory disease may respond to immunosuppression with mycophenolate mofetil or biologic therapy, although there is little evidence to support this. Relapse is not uncommon occurring in up to one-quarter of patients followed for 13 months in adults, whereas in children relapse rates are lower.[18]

Other organs

Several case series and individual reports have described patients with isolated vasculitis of the abdominal, gastrointestinal,[19] or genitourinary system,[20] breast, ascending aorta,[21] and skeletal muscle.[22]

Depending on the organ affected, clinical, serological, and histopathological features are helpful in diagnosing the severity of the inflammatory process. There are no features in the history, examination, laboratory testing, radiological, or angiographic investigations that are specific for the diagnosis of single-organ vasculitis. Histology is crucial for definitive diagnosis but may be indistinguishable from systemic syndromes.

In contrast to the systemic vasculitides the prognosis of single focal-organ vasculitis is very good as excision of the affected organ can be curative.[20,21] However, the prognosis is worse where ischaemic or haemorrhagic complications of the visceral organs or dissection/rupture of the aortic arch develop. Even forms of single-organ vasculitis may require treatment with systemic immunosuppressants if diffuse and severe disease is present depending on the organ involved.

It is very important to exclude systemic illness at the time of diagnosis and throughout the period of treatment and follow-up, as well as infection, malignancy, and other systemic autoimmune diseases. Progression to systemic disease is unusual even without immunosuppression. However, as many of the systemic vasculitides present initially as a localized process, it is important to remain vigilant and look out for features that are associated with progression to systemic disease.[23]

Infection and vasculitis

The notion of infection acting as a trigger for autoimmunity is not new. Infection may induce de-novo expression and relapse of vasculitis.[24] This may occur via direct microbial toxicity affecting the endothelium, either by invasion or the effect of microbial toxins. Humoral or cellular immune responses can lead to vasculitis via immune complex pathways (such as in HCV and cryoglobulinaemia) and also through mechanisms of molecular mimicry and superantigens.[25,26]

An increasing number of organisms are implicated in triggering vasculitis (Table 137.1). Identifying an infectious origin of vasculitis is of paramount importance as treatment strategies will need to include effective antimicrobial drugs.[27] Infection can also be a consequence of intensive immunosuppressive treatment for vasculitis.

Bacterial infections

Direct invasion of blood vessels by pyogenic organisms (e.g. staphylococcus and streptococcus) is a well-described cause of vasculitis, as is septic haematogenous embolization. Vessels previously damaged due to atheroma and surgery are more susceptible and conditions such as diabetes mellitus are predisposing. Bacterial infections with meningococcus or gonococcus can affect small vessels, causing necrotizing vasculitis or thrombosis. This can lead to maculopapular or purpuric lesions which when aspirated can isolate the organisms. In 50% of cases the microorganism can be isolated from blood cultures and prompt targeted antimicrobial therapy to eliminate the infective cause of the secondary vasculitis.[27]

A wide variety of bacteria including streptococcus, staphylococcus, klebsiella, pseudomonas, and more unusual microorganisms such as haemophilus and brucella have been reported to cause large-vessel arteritis. Although rare, it usually presents with the formation of mycotic aneurysms. Salmonella aortitis usually affects the abdominal aorta presenting with fever and abdominal and back pain. Predisposing conditions such as diabetes, intravenous drug

Table 137.1 Infection and vasculitis

	Infection	Vessel involved	Typical clinical associations
Bacterial	*Staphylococcus*	LA, MA, SVMA,SVLC	Mycotic aneurysm
	Salmonella	LA, MA, SVMA,SVLC	Abdominal aortitis
	Mycobacteria	LA, MA, SVMA,SVLC	Erythema nodosum
	Streptococcus	LA, MA, SVMA,SVLC	Mycotic aneurysms
	Klebsiella	LA	Mycotic aneurysms (rare)
	Pseudomonas	LA	Mycotic aneurysms (rare)
	Hemophilus, Brucella	LA	Mycotic aneurysms (very rare)
	Yersinia	SVLC	Digital vasculitis
	Neisseriae	SVLC	Necrotizing vasculitis and thrombosis
	Pseudomonas	SVMA	Ecthyma gangrenosum
	Nocardia	SVMA	Ecthyma like lesions
	Rickettsiae	SVLC	Macular papular rash
	Borrelia burgdorferi	SVMA	CNS vasculitis
Viral	HBV	MA, SVMA, SVLC	PAN
	HCV	MA, SVMA, SVLC	Cryoglobulinaemic vasculitis, PAN
	HIV	MA, SVMA, SVLC	PAN large/medium/small-vessel vasculitis cerebral vasculitis
	parvovirus B19	MA, SVLC	PAN, purpuric rash
	CMV	SVMA, SVLC	Retinitis, Colitis, PAN
	Herpes/Varicella zoster	SVLC	Retinitis meningo-encephalomyelitis
	HTLV-1	SVMA	Necrotizing retinitis, cerebral vasculitis
Spirochaetal	*Treponema pallidum*	LA	Syphilitic aortitis
Fungal	*Coccidiomycosis*	LA	Basilar granulomatous meningitis

CMV cytomegalovirus; CNS central nervous system; HBV hepatitis B virus; HCV hepatitis C virus; HIV human immunodeficiency virus; HTLV-1 human T-cell lymphotropic virus type 1; LA, large arteries; MA, medium arteries; PAN, polyarteritis nodosa; SVLC, small-vessel leucocytoclastic vasculitis; SVMA, small vessels and medium arteries.

abuse, hypertension, malignancy, and immunodeficiency also play a role. Treatment is with intravenous antibiotics and surgery but mortality remains high.

Infections can also affect the course of primary vasculitides. *Staphylococcus aureus* nasal carriage has been linked with higher risk of relapse in patients with GPA and the relative risk is modulated by the type of staphylococcus and is greater in the presence of toxic-shock-syndrome toxin-1.[28]

Mycobacterial infections

Mycobacterial infections can affect all vessels types but in *Mycobacterium tuberculosis* infection veins are more vulnerable than arteries.[25] Tuberculous vasculitis presents clinically with erythema nodosum and histopathology confirms granulomatous panarteritis or thrombophlebitis. Acid-fast bacilli can also be isolated in or adjacent to the vessel wall.

M. leprae infection causes focal vascular lesions of arteries and veins with equal frequency. Erythema nodosum leprosum (painful cutaneous nodules evolving towards ulceration) of the small vessels and vasa vasorum vasculitis of large vessels are the most common presenting features.[27]

Viral infections

The link between hepatitis B infection (HBV) and polyarteritis nodosa (PAN) has been known for 40 years.[29,30] In France, falling HBV infection rates and the development of vaccines against HBV have been correlated with a decrease in HBV-associated PAN.[29,31] Despite that, 400 million people are infected worldwide and 20% of those may develop extrahepatic manifestations.[32] A recent systematic retrospective study of 348 PAN patients registered over 42 years compared patient characteristics and outcome according to HBV status. Patients with HBV-related PAN had more frequent peripheral neuropathy, abdominal pain, cardiomyopathy, orchitis, and hypertension compared with patients with non-HBV-related PAN. HBV-related PAN had significantly better relapse rates and mortality.[33] Treatment is with anti-viral therapy in addition to conventional immunosuppression in combination with plasma exchange.[29,34]

In HCV-associated autoimmune diseases, type 2 cryoglobulinaemia is present in 52% of cases.[34] HCV infection has also been associated with a PAN-type vasculitis with involvement of medium-sized arteries and a necrotizing vasculitis.[35] Anti-viral treatment (pegylated interferon-α and ribavarin) should be considered for all HCV-positive patients with underlying vasculitis.[4,34] Sustained elimination of HCV RNA is required for long-term suppression of vasculitis, and maintenance of anti-viral therapy is therefore required. Severe or life-threatening disease should be treated with steroids, cyclophosphamide, and possibly plasma exchange.[36] B-cell depletion is a future promising approach.[4]

HIV infection may cause vasculitis either directly or as a consequence of secondary opportunistic infection, particularly with cytomegalovirus or tuberculosis.[37,38] A number of patterns of vasculitis have been described including polyarteritis nodosa-like, hypersensitivity vasculitis, large-vessel disease, and cerebral vasculitis.[27] Vasculitis usually occurs in late HIV infection and treatment is difficult, combining anti-viral therapy, plasmapheresis, and short courses of corticosteroids.

Parvovirus B19, cytomegalovirus (CMV), and herpes zoster are the other major viruses that have been implicated in the pathogenesis of vasculitis.[25] Parvovirus has been associated with PAN and IgA vasculitis. Herpes zoster is associated with meningoencephalitis and retinitis while CMV is associated with colitis, PAN, and retinitis.[27]

Vasculitis and malignancy

Acute vasculitis may be the presenting feature of an undiagnosed malignancy. Vasculitis has been associated with a variety of malignancies, mainly haematological and more rarely solid malignancies (Table 137.2). Possible pathogenic mechanisms include immune complex formation, tumour antigens acting as a sensitizing antigen, malignant cell products stimulating vascular inflammation, and direct invasion. Malignancy may also occur as a result of toxic immunosuppressive treatments.

Malignancy developing in patients with a diagnosis of vasculitis

Hejil et al.[39] reviewed the incidence of malignancy in patients treated for ANCA-associated vasculitis (AAV) using follow-up data from European Vasculitis Study Group clinical trials. This analysis concerned 535 patients with newly diagnosed AAV from 15 European countries. During the 2650 person-years observation period, 50 cancers were diagnosed in 46 patients. The standardized incidence ratios (SIR) and their 95% confidence intervals were 1.58 (1.17–2.08) for cancers at all sites, 1.30 (0.90–1.80) for cancers at all sites excluding non-melanoma skin cancer (NMSC), 2.41 (0.66–6.17) for bladder cancer, 3.23 (0.39–11.65) for leukaemia, 1.11 (0.03–6.19) for lymphoma and 2.78 (1.56–4.59) for NMSC. Cancer rates for AAV patients treated with conventional immunosuppressive therapy were found to be higher than those expected for the general population. This difference was attributed to the increased incidence of NMSC.

A population-based cohort study from the Mayo clinic that compared 204 giant cell arteritis (GCA) patients with 407 age- and sex-matched subjects suggested that such patients are not at increased risk of cancer following disease diagnosis. The hazard ratio for developing cancer was 1.26 (95% CI 0.87–1.83) and there was no difference in overall mortality between the two groups.[40]

Malignancy associated with subsequent development of vasculitis

A review of 2800 patients with vasculitis and 69 000 patients with cancer identified 69 patients with both diagnoses. In 12 of those vasculitis occurred within 12 months of the malignancy.[41] Half of those patients had solid tumours and the rest had haematological malignancies including lymphoma, myeloma, and leukaemia. The most common type of vasculitis seen was cutaneous leucocytoclastic vasculitis.

Malignancy related to toxicity from vasculitis therapy

Knights et al. looked at the risk of developing bladder cancer in relation to cyclophosphamide treatment in patients with GPA and reported that the risk doubled for every 10 g increment of cyclophosphamide used.[42] Treatment duration of more than 1 year was associated with an eightfold increased risk of bladder cancer and the absolute risk reached 10% 16 years after diagnosis of GPA. A more recent review concluded that daily oral cyclophosphamide is associated with an increased risk of both haemorrhagic cystitis and bladder cancer, in a dose-dependent and/or duration-dependent

Table 137.2 Malignancy and vasculitis

Malignancy developing in patients with a diagnosis of primary systemic vasculitis	Malignancy associated with subsequent development of vasculitis	Malignancy related to toxicity from vasculitis therapy	Vasculitis associated with malignancy	Vasculitis mimicking malignancy
Bladder cancer	Myelodysplasia	Bladder cancer	GPA	GPA and Lymphoma
Lymphoma	Lymphoma	Lymphoma	PAN	Primary CNS vasculitis and brain neoplasms
Leukaemia	Hairy cell leukaemia	Leukaemia	IgAV	PAN and testicular cancer
Non-melanoma skin cancer	Myeloma	Squamous cell skin cancer	Cutaneous Leucocytoclastic Vasculitis	Paraneoplastic syndromes
Renal cell carcinoma	Solid tumours	Renal cell carcinoma	MPA	
Colon adenocarcinoma		Colonic cancer		
		Cholangiocarcinoma Breast cancer		

CNS, central nervous system; GPA, granulomatosis with polyangiitis; IgAV IgA vasculitis; MPA, microscopic polyangiitis; PAN, polyarteritis nodosa.

manner with an increased risk of bladder cancer years later.[43] Intravenous cyclophosphamide therapy, as prescribed for rheumatic diseases, was reported to carry a low risk of cystitis and probably also of bladder cancer.

In the Wegener's Granulomatosis Etanercept Trial (WGET study) there was an increased frequency of solid tumours in the etanercept group, including colonic cancer, cholangiocarcinoma, breast cancer, and renal cell carcinoma. The long-term follow-up data of the WGET cohort (43 months) showed that the incidence of solid malignancy remained increased, although it is uncertain if this represents the association between GPA and malignancy or whether it was a result of the treatment. Nevertheless, anti-TNF therapy with etanercept appeared to further increase the risk of malignancy observed in patients with GPA treated with cytotoxic agents and should be avoided in these patients.[44]

Other immunosuppressive drugs such as azathioprine have also been associated with malignancies such as lymphoma, squamous cell skin cancer, and leukaemia.

Vasculitis mimicking malignancy

Finally, vasculitis may also mimic malignancy. A large mass of inflammatory tissue associated with constitutional symptoms can easily be misdiagnosed as a malignancy. Differentiating between lymphoma and GPA of the upper airways can be very challenging. There are several case reports of localized vasculitis mimicking neoplasms. Examples include testicular PAN mimicking testicular neoplasms,[45] or primary angiitis of the CNS mimicking tumour-like brain lesions.[46,47] Paraneoplastic syndromes often present as cutaneous vasculitis and skin manifestations may represent the very first diagnostic sign of a neoplastic disease in about 1% of patients.[48]

Drugs and vasculitis

The commonest clinical feature of drug-induced vasculitis is leucocytoclastic vasculitis (see 'Leucocytoclastic vasculitis'). It usually presents with a purpuric rash affecting symmetrically the lower extremities. The rash disappears within several weeks of drug withdrawal but may scar or leave haemosiderosis. Laboratory findings may include leucocytosis, hypocomplementaemia, and raised acute-phase response, although these are non-specific. An eosinophilia can be suggestive of drug aetiology but is also a typical feature of eosinophilic granulomatosis with polyangiitis (EGPA, Churg–Strauss syndrome). MPO-ANCA may be present and sometimes reflects systemic involvement. The most frequent precipitants are hydralazine and propylthiouracil. Although the condition is usually self-limiting on withdrawal of the trigger drug, it may relapse. Treatment options depend on the underlying cause and mainly consist of removal of the precipitating factor. Non-steroidal anti-inflammatory drugs (NSAIDs) have been used with encouraging response in cases with coexisting arthralgia. Immunosuppressive therapy is recommended only in patients with vital organ involvement without requiring maintenance therapy.[49]

The development of EGPA has been associated with use of leukotriene inhibitors and the anti-IgE monoclonal antibody omalizumab, which may due to unmasking previous undiagnosed disease with reduction in glucocorticoid use.[50,51]

A number of recreational drugs such as heroin, cocaine, and methamphetamine have also been reported as vasculitis triggers and are mainly associated with cerebral vasculitis. Cocaine-induced midline destructive lesions may mimic the midfacial destructive change of GPA. Cocaine-levamisole induced vasculopathy is associated with cutaneous vasculitis, leucopenia, and ANCA positivity.[52,53]

Inflammatory rheumatic disease

Systemic rheumatoid vasculitis

Rheumatoid vasculitis is a destructive inflammatory process affecting the blood vessels of patients with long-standing severe rheumatoid arthritis (RA). It is an uncommon but potentially serious systemic disease manifestation that can affect all vessel sizes from aorta to capillaries in patients with seropositive disease.

During the 1990s and 2000s there have been significant changes in the treatment of RA with a focus on aggressive control of inflammation. These might have contributed to the significant incidence decrease reported by recent studies, both in the United Kingdom and the United States, estimating the current incidence of systemic rheumatoid vasculitis (SRV) at less than 4 per million.[54,55] The effects of genetic factors such as *HLA DRB1* shared epitope genotypes,[56] and environmental factors such as change in smoking status are also considered important.[57]

Rheumatoid vasculitis presents in a wide spectrum of organs and systems. Cutaneous changes, nailfold infarcts, peripheral nerve involvement, and systemic symptoms are the most common manifestations. Pulmonary, renal, and cardiovascular involvement (pericarditis) and more rarely ophthalmic involvement (corneal melt, scleritis) are also seen. The typical patient is male with nodular erosive seropositive disease with a severe disease course and extra-articular manifestations such as nodules and pulmonary fibrosis.

There are no validated diagnostic criteria for the definition of SRV. The classification criteria proposed by Scott and Bacon (Box 137.1)[58] are most commonly used.

Leg ulcers are multifactorial but common in RA patients. True vasculitic ulcers are painful, deep, punched-out lesions of acute onset in sites not typically associated with venous stasis ulceration.

The three main patterns of rheumatoid vasculitis are (1) isolated nailfold vasculitis (Figure 137.3) due to digital endarteritis with intimal proliferation, (2) venulitis and small-vessel arteritis characterized by rash, skin eruptions or purpura, and (3) necrotizing

---

Box 137.1 Proposed classification criteria (Scott and Bacon 1984) for systemic rheumatoid vasculitis

◆ Presence of one or more of the following criteria in a patient with RA:

- Mononeuritis multiplex or acute peripheral neuropathy

- Peripheral gangrene

- Biopsy evidence of acute necrotizing arteritis plus systemic illness (e.g. fever or weight loss)

- Deep cutaneous ulcers or active extra-articular disease (e.g. pleurisy, pericarditis, scleritis) if associated with typical digital infarcts or biopsy evidence of vasculitis

◆ Other causes of such lesions, such as diabetes and atherosclerosis should be excluded and nailfold or digital infarcts alone do not suffice for a diagnosis of SRV to be made

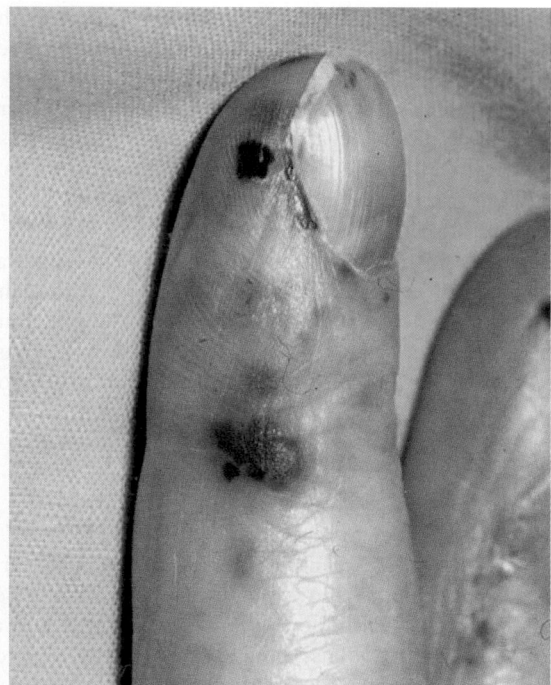

Fig. 137.3 Typical nailfold lesions on a patient with systemic rheumatoid vasculitis.

arteritis of small and medium-sized arteries with involvement of internal organs and peripheral nerves. Patients presenting with isolated nailfold vasculitis have a low risk of progressing from localized to systemic disease.[59] Peripheral nerve involvement occurs due to necrotizing vasculitis of the vasa nervosum. Acute mononeuritis multiplex is very specific to systemic vasculitis. A distal symmetric sensory or sensorimotor pattern of peripheral neuropathy is more commonly described.

There are no current evidence-based therapeutic guidelines for SRV. Treatment with cyclophosphamide and corticosteroids follows similar protocols to those used for AAV and is recommended for SRV with visceral involvement or active disease. Mild cases can be treated with disease-modifying anti-rheumatic drugs (DMARDs) such as methotrexate or azathioprine in combination with oral prednisolone. Isolated nailfold vasculitis may be treated symptomatically. Use of anti-TNF treatment is controversial. There is some supportive evidence for its use,[55] but also some case series reports propose a causal association between biologics and SRV.[60] Rituximab has also been successfully used.[61–63] Aggressive treatment of traditional risk factors for atherosclerotic disease and smoking cessation should also be pursued alongside mainstream treatment.

SRV has significant mortality and morbidity and should be recognized and treated promptly and aggressively. Its increasing rarity may prevent larger controlled trials from providing strong evidence-based management guidelines; therefore empirical treatment with cyclophosphamide and steroids is likely to remain the dominant therapeutic paradigm.

Seronegative spondyloarthopathies

The commonest form of vascular involvement in ankylosing spondylitis is an aortitis affecting predominately the aortic root and ascending aorta. Distal aortitis is less frequent. Aortic incompetence may present as a result of aortic root inflammation. Aortic incompetence occurs in up to 5% of cases of ankylosing spondylitis, 2.5% of cases of

reactive arthritis, and probably less frequently in the other seronegative spondyloarthropathies.[64] The duration of disease is associated with an increased risk of developing aortitis and is estimated at 10% for a patient diagnosed with ankylosing spondylitis for 30 years.

Echocardiography shows thickened aortic leaflets and histology reveals lymphocytic infiltration possibly with fibrosis in the aortic wall and aortic root. Obliterative endarteritis and fibrosis can be caused by vasculitis affecting the small arteries of the cardiac and aortic tissues.[65] Other types of large-vessel vasculitis such as Takayasu's arteritis have been described in patients with seronegative spondyloarthropathies.[66]

There is no evidence-based treatment for aortitis secondary to spondyloarthropathies, but anecdotal reports suggest the use of immunosuppressive drugs in cases of active inflammation. Surgery is particularly risky in the context of uncontrolled inflammation.

Systemic lupus erythematosus

The most common organ affected by vasculitis in systemic lupus erythematosus (SLE) is the skin.[65] Punch biopsy of cutaneous SLE lesions most commonly show findings of fibrinoid changes in the vessel walls composed of immunoglobulin and complement compatible with leucocytoclastic vasculitis.[67] Vasculitic skin lesions are usually found at the fingertips or toes, or on the extensor surface of the forearm. Vasculitis causing neurological, renal, or cardiac involvement is rare but may present as mononeuritis multiplex, progressive glomerulonephritis, and pericarditis respectively. Treatment of SLE-associated vasculitis is similar to that of ANCA-associated vasculitides. In most cases where vasculitis occurs in the course of SLE, it is unlikely to be AAV.

Sjögren's syndrome

Cutaneous vasculitis has been reported in 9–23% of patients with Sjögren's syndrome,[68] and is associated particularly with patients seropositive for Ro and La antibodies. Renal involvement presents with segmental necrotizing glomerulonephritis and treatment is the same as for AAV.

Anti-phospholipid antibody syndrome

In anti-phosphlipid syndrome (APS) the primary vascular pathology is thrombosis without evidence of vessel wall abnormality. It may present with recurrent arterial and venous thrombosis, peripheral gangrene, and organ infarction.[69] All these manifestations may mimic vasculitis. The presence of anti-cardiolipin antibodies combined with a typical clinical context establishes the diagnosis. Anticoagulation is the main treatment for APS.

Scleroderma

Despite the systemic vasculopathy associated with scleroderma, true vasculitis is considered rare.[65] Vasculitis occurs in the limited cutaneous form of scleroderma (SSc). Histologically it is typically leucocytoclastic and cutaneous. Treatment with immunosuppressives and corticosteroids is dependent on the severity of disease. AAV occurring with SSc has been reported in 37 patients with clinical features including include rapidly progressive glomerulonephritis, alveolar haemorrhage, limb ischaemia, and vasculitic skin rash. ANCA-associated glomerulonephritis in SSc patients occurs later, after several years of illness. Almost all cases of AAV in SSc were positive for MPO-ANCA. Differential diagnosis from scleroderma renal crisis is crucial as the treatment approach is significantly different. High doses of corticosteroids and immune suppression are recommended for severe AAV. In refractory cases, rituximab treatment may be considered.[70]

Variable vessel vasculitis

Relapsing polychondritis

Relapsing polychondritis (RP) is a rare immune-mediated condition characterized by inflammation and destruction of cartilage throughout the body. Males and females are equally affected with a peak age of onset at 50 years. There is an association with *HLA DR4*. Around 30% of cases are associated with other diseases, especially systemic vasculitis.

RP may present with non-specific symptoms like fever, weight loss, and fatigue. Clinical features include cartilage inflammation, with auricular inflammation being present in approximately 85% of patients. Characteristically, the cartilaginous part of the pinna is involved, sparing the non-cartilaginous lobe (Figure 137.4). Nasal chondritis occurs in about 50% of cases and may lead to saddle-nose deformity. Pulmonary involvement is the most serious complication of RP and affects half of the patients. Dyspnoea with stridor suggests tracheal involvement. Arthralgia is common, involving large and small joints and the axial skeleton. Ophthalmic manifestations include scleritis or episcleritis. Purpura is the most common skin involvement.

Laboratory features include raised inflammatory markers and immunology is typically negative. The diagnosis is made based on typical clinical features (Box 137.2).[71] Conditions such as GPA, lethal midline granuloma leading to nasal destruction, and infective perichondritis should be excluded.

Treatment is with NSAIDs for mild cases. Laryngotracheal involvement requires corticosteroids at high doses. Although there are no randomized controlled trials, immunosuppression with methotrexate, azathioprine, leflunomide, and ciclosporin has been reported to be effective. Anti-TNF and rituximab have also been used successfully in isolated case reports.[72,73]

MAGIC syndrome: mouth and genital ulcers with inflamed cartilage

First described in 1985 by Firestein,[74] the term 'MAGIC' as an acronym for 'mouth and genital ulcers with inflamed cartilage' was proposed to describe an overlap syndrome of RP and Behçet's disease. An immunological abnormality involving elastin as the possible target antigen was suspected to be common in both conditions. Clinical features include chondritis and oral aphthous ulcers, as well as ocular inflammation (mainly anterior uveitis or scleritis/episcleritis). Most patients also presented with genital ulcers and arthritis. Aneurysms seem to be a common complication of MAGIC syndrome (21.1%), even under immunosuppressants, and can require emergency surgery.[75] Anti-TNF may be used in order to control vascular inflammation and endovascular stent-grafting may be an alternative to surgery. Mainstay treatment is with azathioptine, methotrexate, or cyclophosphamide.

Cogan's syndrome

Cogan's syndrome (CS) is a rare inflammatory disease of unknown aetiology characterized by involvement of the eye and inner ear. It occurs mainly in young adults with a peak incidence in the 20s.

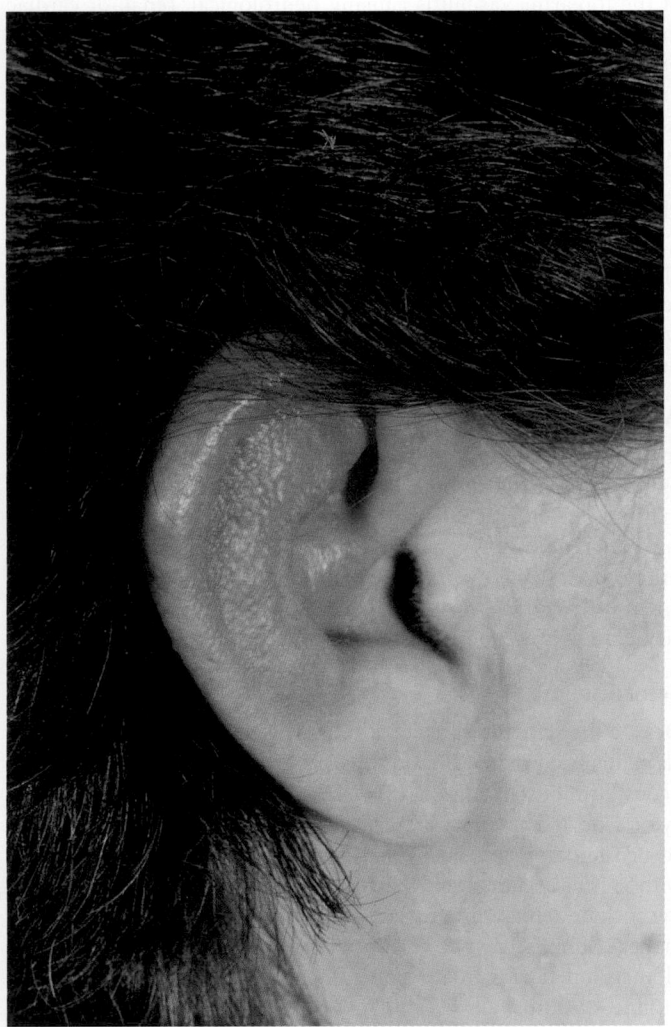

Fig. 137.4 Auricular cartilage inflammation on a patient with relapsing polychondritis.

Box 137.2 Proposed diagnostic criteria (McAdams 1976) for relapsing polychondritis

1. Recurrent chondritis of both auricles

2. Non-erosive seronegative inflammatory polyarthritis

3. Nasal chondritis

4. Inflammation of the ocular structures (conjunctivitis, keratitis, scleritis, episcleritis, uveitis)

5. Chondritis of the respiratory tract involving laryngeal and or tracheal cartilage

6. Cochlear and/or vestibular damage causing sensorineural hearing, tinnitus and/or vertigo

To establish diagnosis, a patient must fulfil one of the following:

◆ at least three of the above six criteria, *or*

◆ one or more of the criteria in conjunction with cartilage biopsy confirmation, *or*

◆ chondritis or two or more separate anatomical locations with response to steroids and/or dapsone

Although the true aetiology is unknown it is believed to result from an environmental trigger interacting with a genetically predisposed host. Infection may act as a precipitator: 25–33% of patients with CS have an antecedent flu-like illness.[76] However, antibiotic treatment is not effective.[77]

There are no validated diagnostic criteria for CS and therefore the diagnosis is based on demonstration of characteristic involvement of both the eye and the inner ear in a young adult. The predominant ocular feature is interstitial keratitis typically presenting with painful red eye, photophobia, and blurred vision. Diplopia, tearing, visual filed defect, and sensation of foreign body in the eye also occur frequently. Vestibular and auditory features include sudden onset vertigo, nausea, vomiting, tinnitus and hearing loss are also seen; symptoms that mimic attacks caused by Menière's disease. Systemic symptoms are often seen such as fever, weight loss, and fatigue, particularly at the initial stages. CS-related vasculitis may affect vessels of any size, but most commonly causes large-vessel vasculitis resembling TA. Neurological involvement is uncommon but may present with meningitis, encephalitis, psychosis, and seizures.

Laboratory tests may show an acute-phase response but immunological tests are usually negative. Corneal biopsies may show a plasma cell infiltrate and lymphocytes in the deeper layers of the cornea with scarring and neovascularization. The histology of vessels resembles GCA findings.

Treatment is with corticosteroids for acute flares and recurrences of ocular or auditory inflammation. Topical glucocorticoids are used for keratitis and anterior uveitis, whereas oral steroids are necessary for posterior scleritis and retinitis. Audiovestibular disease requires high-dose steroids (1–2 mg/kg per day). Additional immunosuppressive therapy with methotrexate, azathioprine; ciclosporin; tacrolimus, and cyclophosphamide maybe required for resistant disease. There are no controlled trials of therapy in CS and therefore the role of biologic agents remains undetermined.

Prognosis depends on disease activity. Although ocular outcomes are good, deafness remains the most common long-term sequel. If CS is complicated by large-vessel vasculitis this is generally associated with a poor prognosis.

References

1. Jennette JC, Falk RJ, Bacon PA et al. Revised International Chapel Hill Consensus Conference Nomenclature of the Vasculitides. *Arthritis Rheum* 2013;65(1):1–11.
2. Kallenberg CG. Anti-C1q autoantibodies. *Autoimmun Rev* 2008; 7(8):612–615.
3. Ozen S, Pistorio A, Iusan SM et al. EULAR/PRINTO/PRES criteria for Henoch-Schonlein purpura, childhood polyarteritis nodosa, childhood Wegener granulomatosis and childhood Takayasu arteritis: Ankara 2008. Part II: Final classification criteria. *Ann Rheum Dis* 2010; 69(5):798–806.
4. Ramos-Casals M, Stone JH, Cid MC, Bosch X. The cryoglobulinaemias. *Lancet* 2012;379(9813):348–360.
5. Sansonno D, Carbone A, De Re V, Dammacco F. Hepatitis C virus infection, cryoglobulinaemia, and beyond. *Rheumatology* (Oxford)2007;46(4):572–578.
6. Meltzer M, Franklin EC, Elias K, McCluskey RT, Cooper N. Cryoglobulinemia—a clinical and laboratory study. II. Cryoglobulins with rheumatoid factor activity. *Am J Med*1966;40(6):837–856.
7. Galli M, Invernizzi F, Monti G. In: Ball GV, Bridges L (eds) *Cryoglobulinaemic vasculitis*, 2nd edn. Oxford University Press, Oxford, 2008.
8. Watts RA, Scott DGI. Cryoglobulinaemic vasculitis. In: Watts RA, Scott DGI (eds) *Vasculitis in clinical practice*. Springer-Verlag, London, 2010:137–142.
9. Vermeersch P, Gijbels K, Marien G et al. A critical appraisal of current practice in the detection, analysis, and reporting of cryoglobulins. *Clin Chem* 2008;54(1):39–43.
10. Mukhtyar C, Guillevin L, Cid MC et al. EULAR recommendations for the management of primary small and medium vessel vasculitis. *Ann Rheum Dis* 2009;68(3):310–317.
11. Sanders JS, Rutgers A, Stegeman CA, Kallenberg CG. Pulmonary: renal syndrome with a focus on anti-GBM disease. *Semin Respir Crit Care Med* 2011;32(3):328–334.
12. Bastian L. Cutaneous polyarteritis. In: Ball G, Bridges S (eds) *Vasculitis*. Oxford University Press, Oxford, 2008:365–372.
13. Ziemer M, Koehler MJ, Weyers W. Erythema elevatum diutinum—a chronic leukocytoclastic vasculitis microscopically indistinguishable from granuloma faciale? *J Cutan Pathol* 2011;38(11):876–883.
14. Marcoval J, Moreno A, Peyr J. Granuloma faciale: a clinicopathological study of 11 cases. *J Am Acad Dermatol* 2004;51(2):269–273.
15. Calbrese LH, Duna GF. Vasculitis of the central nervous system. In: Ball GV, Bridges SL (eds) *Vasculitis*. Oxford University Press, Oxford, 2008:485–496.
16. Salvarani C, Brown RD, Jr, Calamia KT et al. Primary central nervous system vasculitis: analysis of 101 patients. *Ann Neurol* 2007;62(5):442–451.
17. Benseler SM, Silverman E, Aviv RI et al. Primary central nervous system vasculitis in children. *Arthritis Rheum* 2006;54(4):1291–1297.
18. Watts RA, Scott DG. Primary angiitis of the CNS. In: Watts RA, Scott DGI (eds) *Vasculitis in clinical practice*. Springer-Verlag, London, 2010.
19. Gonzalez-Gay MA, Vazquez-Rodriguez TR, Miranda-Filloy JA, Pazos-Ferro A, Garcia-Rodeja E. Localized vasculitis of the gastrointestinal tract: a case report and literature review. *Clin Exp Rheumatol* 2008;26(3 Suppl 49):S101–S104.
20. Hoppe E, de Ybarlucea LR, Collet J et al. Isolated vasculitis of the female genital tract: a case series and review of literature. *Virchows Arch* 2007;451(6):1083–1089.
21. Hernandez-Rodriguez J, Tan CD, Molloy ES et al. Vasculitis involving the breast: a clinical and histopathologic analysis of 34 patients. *Medicine* (Baltimore) 2008;87(2):61–69.
22. Prayson RA. Skeletal muscle vasculitis exclusive of inflammatory myopathic conditions: a clinicopathologic study of 40 patients. *Hum Pathol* 2002;33(10):989–995.
23. Burke AP, Virmani R. Localized vasculitis. *Semin Diagn Pathol* 2001; 18(1):59–66.
24. Kallenberg CG, Tadema H. Vasculitis and infections: contribution to the issue of autoimmunity reviews devoted to 'autoimmunity and infection'. *Autoimmun Rev* 2008;8(1):29–32.
25. Somer T, Finegold SM. Vasculitides associated with infections, immunization, and antimicrobial drugs. *Clin Infect Dis* 1995;20(4):1010–1036.
26. Lidar M, Lipschitz N, Langevitz P, Shoenfeld Y. The infectious etiology of vasculitis. *Autoimmunity* 2009;42(5):432–438.
27. Pagnoux C, Cohen P, Guillevin L. Vasculitides secondary to infections. *Clin Exp Rheumatol* 2006;24(2 Suppl 41):S71–S81.
28. Popa ER, Stegeman CA, Abdulahad WH et al. Staphylococcal toxic-shock-syndrome-toxin-1 as a risk factor for disease relapse in Wegener's granulomatosis. *Rheumatology* (Oxford)2007;46(6):1029–1033.
29. Guillevin L. Virus-induced systemic vasculitides: new therapeutic approaches. *Clin Dev Immunol* 2004;11(3–4):227–231.
30. Matteson EL. A history of early investigation in polyarteritis nodosa. *Arthritis Care Res* 1999;12(4):294–302.
31. Guillevin L. Virus-associated vasculitides. *Rheumatology* (Oxford)1999;38(7):588–590.
32. Cacoub P, Terrier B. Hepatitis B-related autoimmune manifestations. *Rheum Dis Clin North Am* 2009;35(1):125–137.
33. Pagnoux C, Seror R, Henegar C et al. Clinical features and outcomes in 348 patients with polyarteritis nodosa: a systematic retrospective study of

patients diagnosed between 1963 and 2005 and entered into the French Vasculitis Study Group Database. *Arthritis Rheum* 2010;62(2):616–626.

34. Kallenberg CG. What is the evidence for prophylactic antibiotic treatment in patients with systemic vasculitides? *Curr Opin Rheumatol* 2011;23(3):311–316.

35. Cacoub P, Maisonobe T, Thibault V et al. Systemic vasculitis in patients with hepatitis C. *J Rheumatol* 2001;28(1):109–118.

36. Lamprecht P, Gause A, Gross WL. Cryoglobulinemic vasculitis. *Arthritis Rheum* 1999;42(12):2507–2516.

37. Patel N, Khan T, Espinoza LR. HIV infection and clinical spectrum of associated vasculitides. *Curr Rheumatol Rep* 2011;13(6):506–512.

38. Chetty R. Vasculitides associated with HIV infection. *J Clin Pathol* 2001;54(4):275–278.

39. Heijl C, Harper L, Flossmann O et al. Incidence of malignancy in patients treated for antineutrophil cytoplasm antibody-associated vasculitis: follow-up data from European Vasculitis Study Group clinical trials. *Ann Rheum Dis* 2011;70(8):1415–1421.

40. Kermani TA, Schafer VS, Crowson CS et al. Malignancy risk in patients with giant cell arteritis: a population-based cohort study. *Arthritis Care Res* (Hoboken) 2010;62(2):149–154.

41. Hutson TE, Hoffman GS. Temporal concurrence of vasculitis and cancer: a report of 12 cases. *Arthritis Care Res* 2000;13(6):417–423.

42. Knight A, Askling J, Granath F, Sparen P, Ekbom A. Urinary bladder cancer in Wegener's granulomatosis: risks and relation to cyclophosphamide. *Ann Rheum Dis* 2004;63(10):1307–1311.

43. Monach PA, Arnold LM, Merkel PA. Incidence and prevention of bladder toxicity from cyclophosphamide in the treatment of rheumatic diseases: a data-driven review. *Arthritis Rheum* 2010;62(1):9–21.

44. Silva F, Seo P, Schroeder DR et al. Solid malignancies among etanercept-treated patients with granulomatosis with polyangiitis (Wegener's): long-term followup of a multicenter longitudinal cohort. *Arthritis Rheum* 2011;63(8):2495–2503.

45. Atis G, Memis OF, Gungor HS et al. Testicular polyarteritis nodosa mimicking testicular neoplasm. *Sci World J* 2010;10:1915–1918.

46. Tanei T, Nakahara N, Takebayashi S et al. Primary angiitis of the central nervous system mimicking tumor-like lesion—case report. *Neurol Med Chir* (Tokyo) 2011;51(1):56–59.

47. Qu SB, Khan S, Liu H. Primary central nervous system vasculitis mimicking brain tumour: case report and literature review. *Rheumatol Int* 2009;30(1):127–134.

48. Buggiani G, Krysenka A, Grazzini M et al. Paraneoplastic vasculitis and paraneoplastic vascular syndromes. *Dermatol Ther* 2010;23(6):597–605.

49. Gao Y, Chen M, Ye H et al. Long-term outcomes of patients with propylthiouracil-induced anti-neutrophil cytoplasmic auto-antibody-associated vasculitis. *Rheumatology* (Oxford) 2008;47(10):1515–1520.

50. Wechsler ME, Finn D, Gunawardena D et al. Churg-Strauss syndrome in patients receiving montelukast as treatment for asthma. *Chest* 2000;117(3):708–713.

51. Wechsler ME, Wong DA, Miller MK, Lawrence-Miyasaki L. Churg-Strauss syndrome in patients treated with omalizumab. *Chest* 2009; 136(2):507–518.

52. Poon SH, Baliog CR, Jr., Sams RN et al. Syndrome of cocaine-levamisole-induced cutaneous vasculitis and immune-mediated leukopenia. *Semin Arthritis Rheum* 2011;41(3):434–444.

53. Jacob RS, Silva CY, Powers JG et al. Levamisole-induced vasculopathy: a report of 2 cases and a novel histopathologic finding. *Am J Dermatopathol* 2012;34(2):208–213.

54. Ntatsaki E, Mooney J, Scott DGI, Watts RA. Systemic rheumatoid vasculitis in the biologic era. *Rheumatology* (Oxford) 2012;51(suppl 3):iii41.

55. Bartels CM, Bell CL, Shinki K, Rosenthal A, Bridges AJ. Changing trends in serious extra-articular manifestations of rheumatoid arthritis among United State veterans over 20 years. *Rheumatology* (Oxford) 2010;49(9):1670–1675.

56. Gorman JD, David-Vaudey E, Pai M, Lum RF, Criswell LA. Particular HLA-DRB1 shared epitope genotypes are strongly associated with rheumatoid vasculitis. *Arthritis Rheum* 2004;50(11):3476–3484.

57. Turesson C, Matteson EL. Vasculitis in rheumatoid arthritis. *Curr Opin Rheumatol* 2009;21(1):35–40.

58. Scott DG, Bacon PA. Intravenous cyclophosphamide plus methylprednisolone in treatment of systemic rheumatoid vasculitis. *Am J Med* 1984;76(3):377–384.

59. Watts RA, Carruthers DM, Scott DG. Isolated nail fold vasculitis in rheumatoid arthritis. *Ann Rheum Dis* 1995;54(11):927–929.

60. Ramos-Casals M, Brito-Zeron P, Munoz S et al. Autoimmune diseases induced by TNF-targeted therapies: analysis of 233 cases. *Medicine* (Baltimore) 2007;86(4):242–251.

61. Bartels CM, Bridges AJ. Rheumatoid vasculitis: vanishing menace or target for new treatments? *Curr Rheumatol Rep* 2010;12(6):414–419.

62. Hellmann M, Jung N, Owczarczyk K, Hallek M, Rubbert A. Successful treatment of rheumatoid vasculitis-associated cutaneous ulcers using rituximab in two patients with rheumatoid arthritis. *Rheumatology* (Oxford) 2008;47(6):929–930.

63. Maher LV, Wilson JG. Successful treatment of rheumatoid vasculitis-associated foot drop with rituximab. *Rheumatology* (Oxford)2006; 45(11):1450–1451.

64. Townend JN, Emery P, Davies MK, Littler WA. Acute aortitis and aortic incompetence due to systemic rheumatological disorders. *Int J Cardiol* 1991;33(2):253–258.

65. Hughes LB. Vasculitis in primary connective tissue diseases. In: Ball GV, Bridges SL (eds) *Vasculitis*, 2nd edn. Oxford University Press, Oxford, 2008:439–460.

66. Taharboucht S, Lanasri N, Laroche JP. Ankylosing spondylarthritis associated with Takayasu disease: a new case. *J Mal Vasc* 2010;35(4): 259–262.

67. Calamia KT, Balabanova M. Vasculitis in systemic lupus erythematosis. *Clin Dermatol* 2004;22(2):148–156.

68. Garcia-Carrasco M, Ramos-Casals M et al. Primary Sjogren syndrome: clinical and immunologic disease patterns in a cohort of 400 patients. *Medicine* (Baltimore) 2002;81(4):270–280.

69. Lie JT. Vasculitis in the antiphospholipid syndrome: culprit or consort? *J Rheumatol* 1994;21(3):397–399.

70. Arad U, Balbir-Gurman A, Doenyas-Barak K et al. Anti-neutrophil antibody associated vasculitis in systemic sclerosis. *Semin Arthritis Rheum* 2011;41(2):223–229.

71. McAdam LP, O'Hanlan MA, Bluestone R, Pearson CM. Relapsing polychondritis: prospective study of 23 patients and a review of the literature. *Medicine* (Baltimore) 1976;55(3):193–215.

72. Lahmer T, Treiber M, von Werder A et al. Relapsing polychondritis: An autoimmune disease with many faces. *Autoimmun Rev* 2010;9(8):540–546.

73. Leroux G, Costedoat-Chalumeau N, Brihaye B et al. Treatment of relapsing polychondritis with rituximab: a retrospective study of nine patients. *Arthritis Rheum* 2009;61(5):577–582.

74. Firestein GS, Gruber HE, Weisman MH et al. Mouth and genital ulcers with inflamed cartilage: MAGIC syndrome. Five patients with features of relapsing polychondritis and Behcet's disease. *Am J Med* 1985;79(1):65–72.

75. Mekinian A, Lambert M, Beregi JP et al. Aortic aneurysm in MAGIC syndrome successfully managed with combined anti-TNF-alpha and stent grafting. *Rheumatology* (Oxford) 2009;48(9):1169–1170.

76. Gluth MB, Baratz KH, Matteson EL, Driscoll CL. Cogan syndrome: a retrospective review of 60 patients throughout a half century. *Mayo Clin Proc* 2006;81(4):483–488.

77. Grasland A, Pouchot J, Hachulla E et al. Typical and atypical Cogan's syndrome: 32 cases and review of the literature. *Rheumatology* (Oxford) 2004;43(8):1007–1015.

SECTION 19

Osteoarthritis

CHAPTER 138

Pathogenesis of osteoarthritis

Tonia L. Vincent and Linda Troeberg

Structure and function of articular cartilage

Healthy articular cartilage provides a low-friction surface that facilitates smooth articulation of opposing bones (Figure 138.1). Chondrocytes are the only cell type present in cartilage, and they synthesize and are surrounded by a large volume of extracellular matrix (ECM), which gives the tissue its mechanical properties and hence enable its articulating function. The two most abundant components of the cartilage ECM are the protein collagen and the proteoglycan aggrecan.

Collagen provides cartilage with mechanical strength. The main type of collagen found in articular cartilage is type II collagen, a triple-helical collagen that forms strong, rope-like molecules which are cross-linked to form fibrils.[1] These are arranged tangentially near the articulating surface, and radially deeper within the tissue, to dissipate mechanical forces acting on the tissue.

Aggrecan is a proteoglycan, composed of a protein to which are attached many glycosaminoglycan (GAG) side chains (Figure 138.2). The protein 'core' is folded into three globular domains (called G1, G2, and G3) separated by interglobular regions. The GAGs (chondroitin sulfate and keratan sulfate) are attached in the extended region between G2 and G3. These aggrecan monomers aggregate into large extended complexes through interaction with link protein and hyaluronan. The GAGs are highly negatively charged, which draw water into the matrix and causes hydrostatic swelling of the matrix, providing resistance to compression.

The ECM is organized into different structural and functional regions. These can broadly be divided into the pericellular matrix (PCM), which surrounds individual chondrocytes, and the further removed matrix (comprised of the territorial and interterritorial matrices). Type II collagen and aggrecan are distributed in the further removed matrix and are largely absent from the PCM. The PCM is enriched for growth and regulatory factors that modulate the behaviour of the chondrocyte. For example, the PCM contains fibroblast growth factor 2 (FGF-2) that is released in response to mechanical loading and acts on chondrocytes through cell-surface FGF receptors.[2] Thus the extracellular matrix has two principal functions: (1) to withstand mechanical load and (2) to sense and respond to changes in the mechanical environment in order to maintain tissue homeostasis.

Changes to cartilage in osteoarthritis

OA is characterized by a number of changes within the cartilage. Most importantly, the cartilage ECM is progressively degraded, leading to loss of tissue and impairment of mechanical function. This degradation is not a passive wear-and-tear process, but is an active response of the tissue to an altered mechanical or biochemical environment. Chondrocytes alter their gene expression profile to take on a catabolic phenotype, synthesizing increased levels of proteolytic enzymes that degrade the cartilage ECM. In particular, chondrocytes synthesize collagenases that degrade collagen, and aggrecanases that degrade aggrecan. Degradation of these components leads to weakening of the cartilage ECM, causing surface roughening of the tissue and subsequent deep fibrillation of the matrix.

Some OA chondrocytes appear to have increased synthetic activity, suggesting that they attempt to repair the damage to the tissue. Safranin O staining of histological sections of OA cartilage shows increased proteoglycan around some chondrocytes (red staining in Figure 138.1).

Chondrocytes both proliferate, by a process of clonal expansion, and die in OA. Chondrocyte death occurs via various mechanisms, including apoptosis and necrosis and is often seen as empty lacunae on histological sections. Causes of chondrocyte death are postulated to involve mechanical injury and reactive oxygen species derived from dysfunctional mitochondria.[3]

Changes to other joint tissues in osteoarthritis

Early tissue responses in OA have mainly been studied at the level of the articular cartilage, indicating the early nature of these changes, and the largely chondrocentric view of those in the field. Other tissues of the joint are strongly altered in OA, especially the bone, capsule, and synovium. Bone changes in OA are early and pathognomonic and include thickening or sclerosis of the subchondral bone followed by reactive remodelling changes that lead to the formation of osteophytes, bone cysts, and epiphyseal expansion. These changes are diagnostic on plain radiographs and may represent mechano-adaptation to the altered mechanical environment.

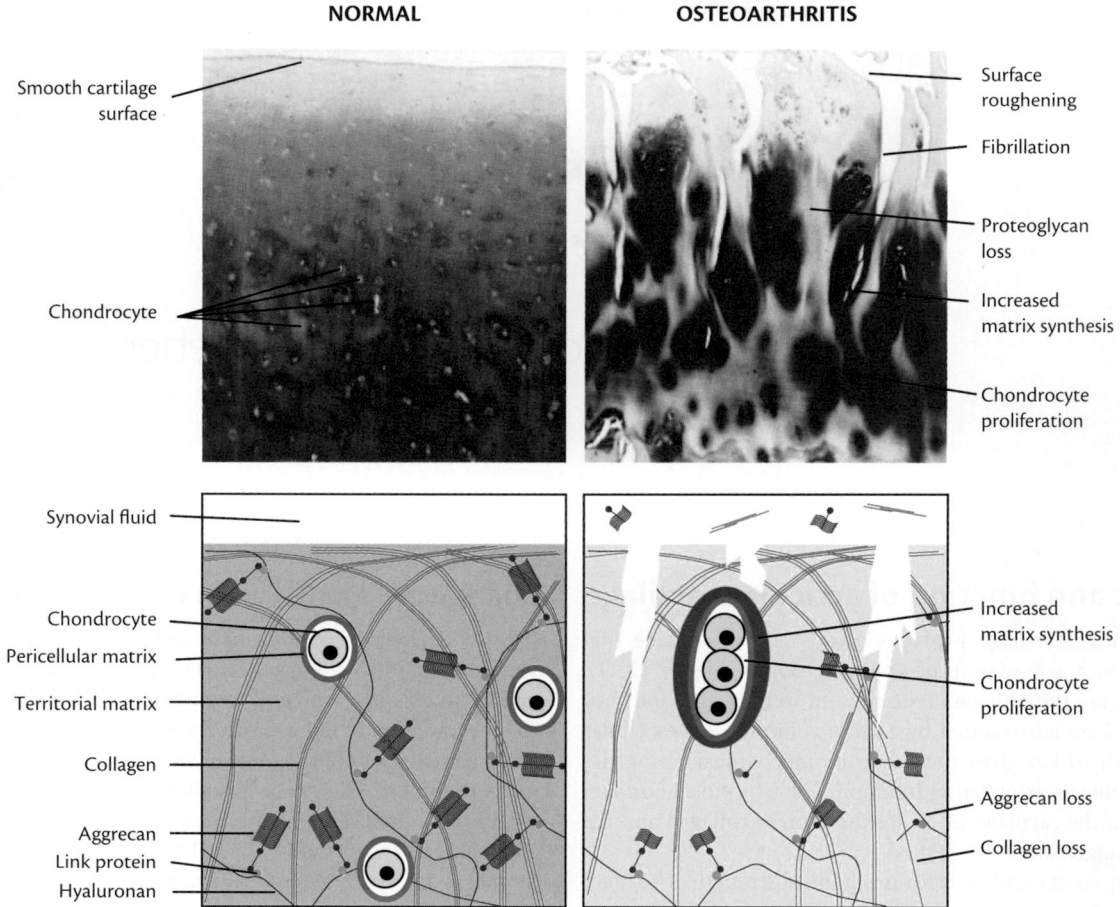

Fig. 138.1 Structure of normal and osteoarthritic cartilage. Histological sections (top panels) and diagrammatic representations (lower panels) of normal and osteoarthritic cartilage stained with the proteoglycan-reactive dye Safranin O. Aggrecan and other minor proteoglycans are uniformly distributed in normal cartilage, giving a uniform staining pattern. In osteoarthritis increased Safranin O staining is seen around some chondrocytes, indicative of anabolic attempts by the chondrocytes to repair the damage.

To what extent these changes are due to disease in the articular cartilage is unknown; whether subchondral bone changes predispose to cartilage loss (by altering the compliance of the tissue at the base of the cartilage) or whether bone remodels as a results of loss of integrity of the cartilage that protects it, is an argument that has raged for several decades. Some also regard these changes as an overzealous tissue repair response. It is of some interest that osteophytes form principally from the region of the joint where the synovium, periosteum, growth plate, and articular cartilage meet. Osteophytes form by a process of endochondral ossification (as is seen in long bone development) and typically have new cartilaginous caps that are indistinguishable from articular cartilage (Figure 138.2).[4]

Changes occurring in other tissues of the joint are less well studied. It is well accepted that the synovium is often thickened and may be moderately inflamed, especially at late stages of disease. Fibrotic change, laying down of a disorganized type I collagenous matrix, within the joint is common and affects tissues such as the capsule and menisci.

Early views of osteoarthritis pathogenesis

The concept that mechanical factors contribute to the development of OA cannot be overstated. Epidemiological data are compelling; OA is both a disease of joint overuse—seen in specific occupational settings such as cotton pickers (hand disease) and coal miners (back disease)—and is increased by joint injury. Both direct joint injury, e.g. through intra-articular fracture, and indirect injury, where the stabilizing structures of the joint (e.g. menisci and cruciate ligaments) are damaged, are associated with a substantially increased risk of developing OA.[5] Perhaps as many as 50% of individuals with meniscal injury will go on to develop OA within 5–10 years.[6] Moreover, a high percentage of individuals with age-related disease appear to have meniscal failure (in the absence of a history of injury), suggesting that this is an important consequence during ageing.[7] Individuals with deformities that change the loading patterns within a given joint are also at increased risk of disease, and these can be modified by osteotomy or joint distraction (where mechanical forces are absorbed by a temporary metal cage attached on either side of the joint).[8]

In a healthy joint there are a number of levels at which mechanical protection is enabled: within the joint itself, the ligaments, menisci and capsule provide stability, preventing excessive antero-posterior movement as well as rotational stress. The articular cartilage as well as the meniscus is uniquely adapted to withstand mechanical load. The orientation of collagen fibres and distribution of negatively charged proteoglycans protect the chondrocytes from compressive and shear forces generated by joint movement and fluid flow through the matrix. Outside the joint, engagement of muscles to

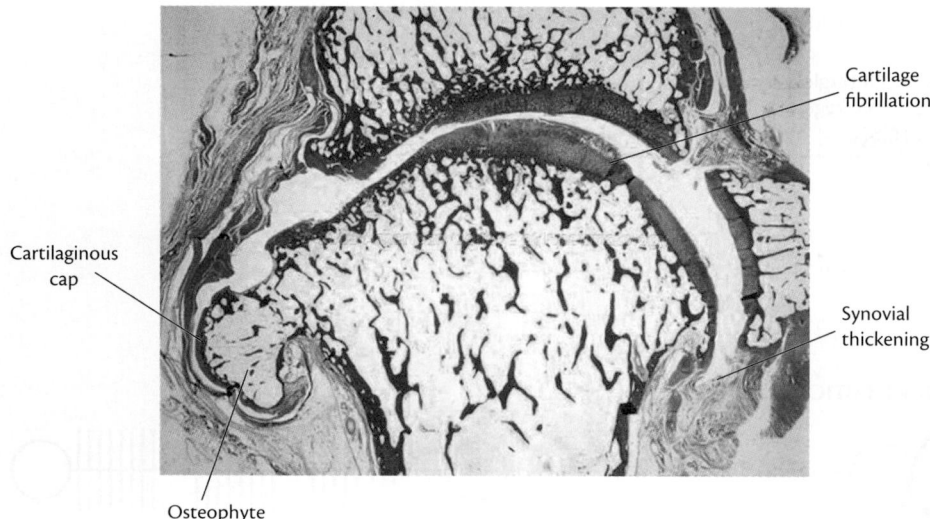

Cartilage fibrillation

Cartilaginous cap

Synovial thickening

Osteophyte

Fig. 138.2 Histological appearance of osteoarthritis in a metatarsal joint. Note uneven loss of articular cartilage (stained blue in this image) and dorsal osteophyte with cartilaginous cap. Other features include synovial and capsular thickening.

splint the joint during activity, as well as reflex actions that lead to deceleration of movement upon heel strike during the normal gait cycle are also likely to provide significant protection. Some of these responses are blunted with age.[5]

For many years these mechanical associations with disease were largely explained by passive attrition of joint tissues, so-called 'wear and tear'. It was thought that loss of lubrication of the joint surface may contribute to premature disease; the rationale for studies on intra-articular hyaluronan and lubricin, molecules that reduce frictional forces at the articular surface.[9] It was later in the 1950s when Maroudas[10] described a likely breakdown of the collagen fibres in the tissue and subsequently the discovery of proteases that specifically degraded components of the extracellular matrix, so-called matrix metalloproteinases (MMPs), that an active, enzymatically driven process of matrix destruction was proposed. One pivotal discovery in the early 1990s was finding fragments of aggrecan in the synovial fluid of patients with OA which had been cleaved at specific regions of the molecule. As none of the known MMPs at the time were predicted to cleave at this site it was proposed that this indicated a new disease-related enzyme activity that was termed 'aggrecanase'[11,12] (discussed further below).

Until this time, OA research was significantly limited by a number of factors. First, pathogenic mechanisms of disease tend to come from observations made in early human disease, and early OA was often subclinical or difficult to diagnose because the tools for making the diagnosis (plain radiographs) were too crude. Moreover, even when early disease could be identified, it was not possible, except in rare circumstances, to acquire joint tissues. Studies performed on late-stage cartilage (taken from joint replacement) have documented pathways activated in late disease, but do not provide insights into early molecular events. Analyses were also limited by the tissues themselves; cartilage is a paucicellular tissue and its highly negatively charged matrix posed many problems in the early days of molecular biology.

Using small-animal models to study osteoarthritis pathogenesis

Significant breakthroughs in pathogenic mechanism subsequently arose from rapid advances in accessible molecular tools, and in the widespread use of mechanically induced models of OA in mice,

which could be combined with genetic modification to interrogate the role of specific molecules in the disease process.[13] Joint instability-induced models of OA have been favoured in many studies as they recapitulate many of the features of human disease: insidious cartilage degradation, subchondral bone sclerosis, osteophyte formation, and pain that arises relatively late in the disease process (when significant cartilage has been lost).[14] There is little in the way of synovitis except in the immediate postoperative period and this differentiates them from some historical models such as those induced by intra-articular collagenase or monosodium iodoacetate injection. Surgical models are regarded as being good models of injury-induced OA, for which there is a good clinical corollary. Pathways that are identified in these models may or may not be relevant to age-related disease.[15]

The mouse has proved a tractable system in which it is possible, not only to investigate specific molecules in the course of OA, but to study all the tissues of the joint. Although the cartilage has been the focus of most studies thus far (the OA Research Society International (OARSI) guidelines for scoring these models are validated only for cartilage measurements),[16] an increasing number of studies are beginning to look at changes in bone, menisci, and synovium. Genetic modification is also becoming increasingly sophisticated with the creation of conditional and inducible knockout and overexpressing mice in which the gene of interest can be deleted/overexpressed in a tissue-specific manner and at specified times.

Molecular basis for osteoarthritis

Aggrecan degradation by aggrecanases

Degradation of aggrecan is a key early event in the pathogenesis of OA. Some studies suggest that aggrecan protects collagen from proteolytic degradation and that collagen degradation only occurs when aggrecan is lost from the tissue. Additionally, aggrecan degradation is thought to be reversible, while collagen loss is irreversible.[17] There has thus been considerable interest in identifying the enzyme(s) responsible for aggrecan degradation in OA, with numerous candidate enzymes proposed since the 1960s.[18]

In a landmark study, Sandy and colleagues analysed the synovial fluid of patients with early and late OA and patients who had experienced a recent knee injury.[11] They found that in all cases the synovial fluid contained aggrecan fragments with the N-terminal

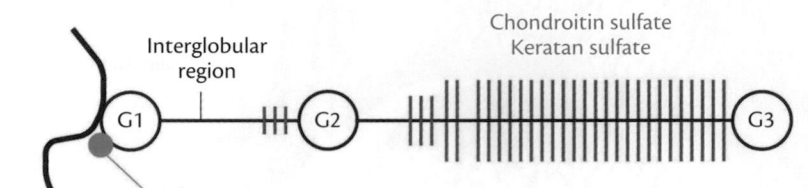

NORMAL AGGRECAN

Fig. 138.3 Structure of aggrecan in normal and osteoarthritic cartilage. Aggrecan consists of a core protein (blue) attached to chondroitin sulfate and keratan sulfate glycosaminoglycan chains (orange) that retain water in the cartilage matrix and hence enable resistance of the tissue to compression. In normal cartilage, aggrecan is immobilized in the cartilage matrix through interaction with link protein and hyaluronan. In osteoarthritic cartilage, ADAMTSs cleave aggrecan at the NITEGE[373]~[374]ARGSV bond in the interglobular domain between the G1 and G2 domains, releasing the majority of the molecule from the tissue. ADAMTSs and other enzymes can also cleave aggrecan at other sites, releasing smaller fragments from the tissue.

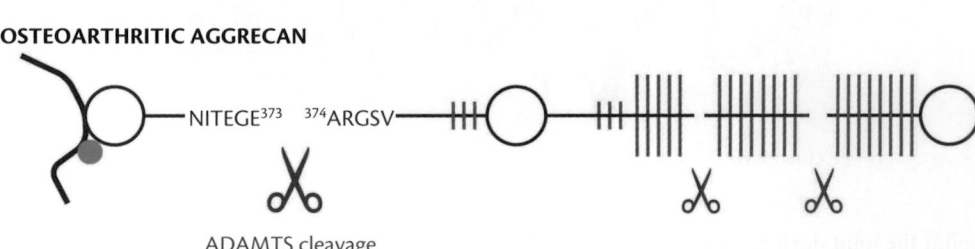

OSTEOARTHRITIC AGGRECAN

sequence [374]ARGSV. Cleavage at this site releases the water-bearing GAG-rich region of the molecule from the cartilage ECM, abrogating the function of the molecule (Figure 138.2). The MMPs, a family of zinc-dependent proteolytic enzymes, had been suggested to degrade aggrecan in OA cartilage, but these enzymes cleave aggrecan at the nearby DIPEN[341]~[342]FFGV site and are not active against the aggrecanase NITEGE[373]~[374]ARGSV site. This indicated that an unknown enzyme was responsible for pathological aggrecan cleavage in OA (see Figure 138.3).

Cleavage at the NITEGE[373]~[374]ARGSV bond was observed in vitro when cartilage explants were stimulated with inflammatory cytokines, enabling researchers to purify the aggrecanase enzyme from conditioned medium of bovine cartilage stimulated with interleukin-1 (IL-1).[19] Sequencing analysis revealed that the aggrecanase was a metalloproteinase, and that its active site is homologous to those of MMPs. The aggrecanases also contain additional domains not found in MMPs, such as disintegrin and thrombospondin domains, which determine substrate specificity and localization within the ECM. This family of proteinases are thus named as a disintegrin and metalloproteinase with thrombospondin domains (ADAMTS). Following discovery of aggrecanase 1 (designated ADAMTS-4), aggrecanase 2 (now designated ADAMTS-5, initially called ADAMTS-11) was later characterized.[20]

The importance of this family of proteases in vivo was then demonstrated by showing that mice lacking the gene for *Adamts5* had reduced disease following surgical joint destabilization compared to wild-type mice.[21] This experiment was a turning point in how OA was perceived, not only because it had identified the first realizable target for OA, but also it proved that disease was not a passive process of attrition, as the cartilage was preserved despite the joint being destabilized. Mice lacking genes for *Adamts4* were not protected, indicating that ADAMTS-5 was the primary aggrecanase in mice. Since then several other pathways have been shown to influence Adamts5 expression and activity in vivo.[15,22]

The relative importance of ADAMTS-4 and ADAMTS-5 in human OA is still under debate.[23] A limited number of studies have examined the effect of silencing specific proteases in human OA tissue (by molecular interference) and these suggest that, in humans, both ADAMTS-4 and ADAMTS-5 are important in driving aggrecan degradation. Several research groups are developing ADAMTS inhibitors as possible disease-modifying osteoarthritis drugs (DMOADs).[24] These are still in the early stages of development, but are reported to show some efficacy in animal OA models.

Collagen degradation by collagenases

In addition to aggrecan degradation, breakdown of collagen is a hallmark of osteoarthritic cartilage damage. Increased levels of collagen breakdown products are detectable in the cartilage ECM by immunohistochemistry,[25] and collagen fragments are found in the synovial fluid after joint injury and in patients with OA.[26]

Collagen is a very stable cross-linked protein and is resistant to cleavage by most proteinases, with only 6 of more than 500 proteinases in the human genome being capable of digesting triple-helical collagen. Five of these collagenases are members of the MMP family: MMP-1 (collagenase 1), MMP-8 (collagenase 2), MMP-13 (collagenase 3), MMP-2 (gelatinase A), and MT1-MMP (membrane-type MMP 1). The collagenases cleave collagen at a specific site, causing the triple helix to unravel and rendering it susceptible to further cleavage by non-collagenolytic proteinases (Figure 138.4).

MMP-13 is thought to be the primary cartilage collagenase in vivo. Expression of MMP-13 expression is increased in human OA cartilage, and mice overexpressing MMP-13 develop OA-like lesions.[22] Mice lacking the MMP-13 gene develop less severe cartilage damage in a surgical model of OA.[27] Several MMP-13 inhibitors are in the early stages of development, and some have been shown to reduce collagen breakdown and cartilage loss in animal models of OA.[24]

Global changes in chondrocyte gene expression

Global analyses of OA tissues have been performed at the mRNA and protein levels. Most of the studies published thus far have focused

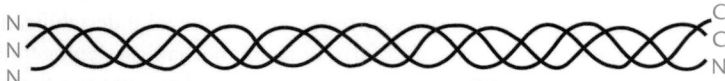

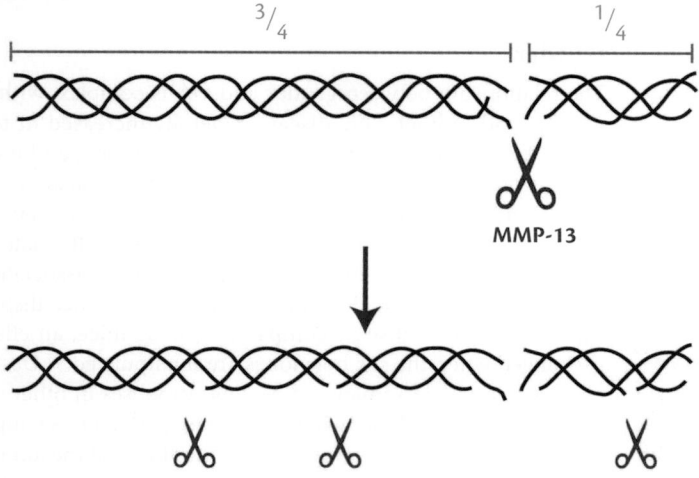

Fig. 138.4 Collagen degradation by collagenases. The main collagen found in cartilage is type II collagen, which is a triple helix composed of three α_1 (II) chains. These collagen molecules aggregate to form cross-linked fibrils. In osteoarthritic cartilage, collagenases such as MMP-13 initiate collagen degradation by unwinding the triple helix and cleaving the α_1 (II) chains at a specific site three-quarters of the length between the N-terminus (designated N) and the C-terminus (designated C) of the molecule. This destabilizes the helix, allowing collagenases or other non-collagenolytic proteases to cleave further, generating smaller fragments.

on the articular cartilage and have included proteomic (for proteins) and microarray (for mRNA) methodologies. Validation studies have tended to use quantitative RT-PCR (for RNA) and immunohistochemistry (for protein). In-situ hybridization (demonstration of the mRNAs within sections of mature joint tissue) remains challenging. Studies have been performed both in human tissue, acquired from individuals with established late disease, and preclinical models where early disease processes have generally been examined. For human studies, acquiring age-matched control samples is an ongoing difficulty.

The overall conclusion from these studies is that the chondrocytes in OA are highly active and express and secrete large numbers of proteins that promote catabolic processes within the joint as well as driving apparent repair/remodelling responses. Some of the genes identified by microarray are reminiscent of those activated during embryonic bone and cartilage development, such as type X collagen, Runx2, and the Wnt pathways, leading to the suggestion that OA to some extent recapitulates developmental processes.[28,29] They also reveal altered expression of many genes whose function in the joint is not yet known. Some consistent changes are seen, for instance chondrocytes from patients with late-stage OA express increased levels of collagen type II and VI at mRNA and protein levels,[30,31] but protease regulation in human studies has been inconsistent.[32–34] Interpretation of human studies is limited by large interpatient variability.

Gene expression profiling has been performed in rodent models of OA and is surprisingly consistent even when comparing rat with mouse, and across different models. For example, increased expression of *Mmp13* and *Adamts5* is seen in rats and mice following surgical injury to either the cruciate ligament or the meniscus.[35,36]

Growth factors in osteoarthritis

Chondrocyte proliferation and matrix synthesis in OA may be mediated by local production of growth factors. Many of these stimulate synthetic responses in chondrocytes in vitro and are upregulated in disease.[34] Some growth factors such as FGF-2 and osteogenic protein-1 (OP-1, also known as BMP-7) are thought to reside within the matrix and are released in a rapid and controlled fashion, albeit through mechanisms that are currently unclear.[2,37] Insulin-like growth factor (IGF)-1 also promotes matrix synthesis in vitro,[38] and may be tethered within the matrix attached to its binding protein.[39]

The transforming growth factors (TGFs) α and β are pleotropic molecules that have mixed functions in the joint, both promoting disease and likely protecting from it. In vitro, TGFβ promotes matrix synthesis and is regarded as an important anabolic factor in cartilage. It also has anti-catabolic actions including the ability to suppress cytokine-induced protease gene expression.[40] Loss of TGFβ signalling leads to development of OA in transgenic mice. Conversely, TGFβ has also been used to promote the development of OA in experimental models and probably plays roles in osteophyte formation and synovial hyperplasia.[40,41]

The role of growth factors in OA is complex and is not only dependent upon expression and bioavailability of the factor. Some growth factors, such as FGF-2 and TGF, may have unpredictable effects in vivo, which are dependent upon differential receptor expression and variable intracellular signalling responses.[42]

Inflammation in osteoarthritis

OA is not considered to be a classical inflammatory disease as the synovial fluid rarely contains high levels of neutrophils, and there is an absence of systemic inflammation. On the other hand, chemokines, cytokines, cytokine receptors, and other inflammatory mediators are expressed by connective tissue cells of the joint and could have a role in driving disease processes. Some of these have been investigated in knockout mice and have failed to demonstrate a pathogenic role. For instance, the IL-1α/β double knockout and TNFα knockout mice are not protected from development of OA following surgical joint destabilization.[43] The presence of synovitis in disease, and its relevance to OA progression is also controversial.[44] Synovitis is commonly found transiently in individuals following acute knee injury and also present in most patients (by MRI assessment) with late-stage painful disease,[45] but whether this contributes to cartilage degradation is unclear.

The presence of calcium pyrophosphate and other crystals within the joint may also contribute to inflammatory episodes in OA. Crystals are powerful activators of 'inflammasones' which drive caspase 1 activation and allow processing and secretion of cytokines including IL-1 and IL-18.[46] Uric acid levels correlate with disease and synovial levels of IL-1 and IL-18 in patients with OA.[47]

Perhaps the most compelling argument that OA is inflammatory is that it depends on the expression and activation of 'inflammatory response genes' such as *Adamts5* and *Mmp13*. These genes are normally induced by inflammatory cytokines through a network of intracellular inflammatory signalling pathways. These pathways and the induction of inflammatory response genes can also be induced by crude cartilage injury (cutting with a scalpel),[48] suggesting either that mechanical injury can induce inflammatory cytokines, or that the innate response to tissue injury can drive inflammatory response genes in the absence of cytokine release. The importance of this in vivo has been demonstrated by showing that early induction of proteases in the articular cartilage of mice after joint destabilization is prevented if the joint is paralysed.[36] Taken together these data present an attractive link between mechanical factors as strong aetiological agents in OA and the key role of proteases in disease. In essence it is necessary to define what is meant by inflammation and to distinguish between inflammation mediated by cells of the immune system (classical inflammation) and inflammation that is defined by the activation of inflammatory signalling pathways and by the induction of inflammatory response genes in cells that are not of immune origin—chondrocytes, fibroblasts etc. The fact that mechanical injury alone is able to activate these inflammatory pathways in non-immune cells has led to the use of the term 'mechanical cytokine'.

Epidemiological factors that influence the molecular pathogenesis of osteoarthritis

Ageing

Ageing is arguably the most important risk factor for the development of disease. In recent years a number of biological sequelae that are consequent upon ageing have been described in other systems/diseases, with the emerging paradigm that ageing is not simply a process of tissue wear over time, but is at least in part dependent upon the failure of various cellular pathways/mechanisms involved in growth, nutrition, and injury responses. The mitochondrion is increasingly seen as a principal offending organelle; it is responsible for the production of reactive oxygen species and for the manufacture of anti-oxidant genes such as superoxide dismutase.[49] Such genes are strongly regulated by inflammatory cytokine stimulation in articular cartilage. Failing mitochondria are removed by autophagy, a process that becomes defective in aged cartilage.[50] The molecular response to acute joint destabilization in the mouse (viewed as a form of acute mechanical derangement) is altered in aged vs young mice, suggesting that pathways that detect and respond to injurious pathways change with age also.[51] This may in part be due to the changes that occur in tissues over time such as glycosylation of matrix proteins and accumulation of turnover products within tissues.[52,53]

Gender

The relationship between gender and OA is complex, with symptomatic and radiographic disease generally increased in females. Most of these cases are in postmenopausal women, and increased disease in females is lost when one isolates those that are premenopausal. Indeed epidemiological studies point to a protective effect of oestrogen status, with the oral contraceptive pill, a late menopause, and hormone replacement therapy being associated with a degree of protection.[54] Premenopausal female mice display significantly reduced disease compared to male mice, an effect that is changed when the sex hormones are manipulated.[55] Oestrogens are important determinants of healing responses in other systems such as the skin and following brain injury,[56,57] so it is tempting to speculate that in OA, oestrogen alters the ability of the joint tissues to repair following injury.

Obesity

Obesity is a strong risk factor for OA. While this is in part due to increased mechanical loading of joints, adipokines synthesized in adipose tissue are also thought to contribute to OA pathogenesis by increasing joint inflammation.[58]

Genetics

Heritability of OA is in the region of 60% across all joints. Given this large heritability it is perhaps surprising that linkage studies have only identified a relatively small number of gene polymorphisms associated with disease (see Chapter 44), and these have frequently been of small effect size and not replicated in other cohorts. A recent genome-wide association study (GWAS) for OA has recently been published.[58a] Consistent with the linkage studies, only a handful of new genes were identified as being linked with the risk of OA (patients were identified on the basis of their needing a joint replacement) and the effect sizes were once again very small. Some further potential gene candidates were identified if patients were stratified according to joint site. Genes that we know are important in OA pathogenesis, e.g. *Adamts5* and *Mmp13*, have not come up in linkage or GWAS investigations. This is most likely explained either by the fact that these genes do not have polymorphic variants, or more likely that the principal level of regulation is post-translational (these proteases require extracellular processing to their active form), and transcriptional control of gene expression correlates poorly with tissue enzyme activity.

Another level at which genes are controlled (beyond their coding sequences) is epigenetically. Selective modification to either the DNA itself or to histone proteins, for instance by acetylation, is increasingly recognized as an important controller of how, where, and why certain genes are transcribed.[59] There are now many new epigenetic modifiers being identified, and the use of highly selective inhibitors of these is likely to reveal important levels of gene

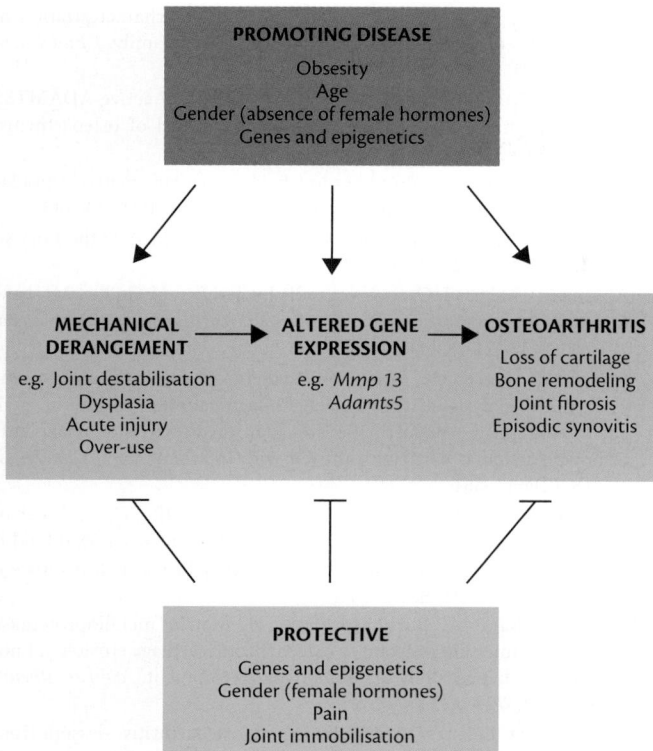

PROMOTING DISEASE
Obesity
Age
Gender (absence of female hormones)
Genes and epigenetics

MECHANICAL DERANGEMENT
e.g. Joint destabilisation
Dysplasia
Acute injury
Over-use

ALTERED GENE EXPRESSION
e.g. *Mmp 13*
Adamts5

OSTEOARTHRITIS
Loss of cartilage
Bone remodeling
Joint fibrosis
Episodic synovitis

PROTECTIVE
Genes and epigenetics
Gender (female hormones)
Pain
Joint immobilisation

Fig. 138.5 A summary of processes driving the pathogenesis of osteoarthritis.

expression in coming years. A summary of how these factors contribute to disease pathogenesis is shown in Figure 138.5.

Pathogenesis of pain in osteoarthritis

Most of the studies described thus far have focused on the structural features of the disease with pathogenic studies mainly geared towards finding structure-modifying targets. The correlation between structural damage and patient symptoms is not strong, and determining the processes that drive symptomatic disease is important. This is surprisingly difficult to do in human disease and in the main is reliant on careful correlative studies of pain with radiographic features (mainly MRI-based). Such studies have suggested likely candidates for pain in late OA. These include the presence of synovitis, which is invariably present (by gadolinium-enhanced MRI) in patients with late-stage painful OA.[60] Pain also likely arises from the bone where there is some correlation with the presence of subchondral bone oedema and osteophytes.[61] Cells lining vascular channels at the osteochondral junction are seen to express pain-sensitizing molecules such as nerve growth factor (NGF).[62] Clinical trials of anti-NGF in late-stage OA have demonstrated that this approach is efficacious in treating pain, although unfortunately a subgroup of patients developed accelerated disease in the index as well as non-index joints and this forced the United States Food and Drug Administration (FDA) to halt trials temporarily, although they have now been reinstated.[63,64] NGF was also demonstrated as an effective analgesic target in mice with OA.[65]

One very important feature of long-standing pain in OA is the development of central sensitization. This can be visualized in patients through functional and structural MRI studies of the brain.[66] Changes in the central nervous system (CNS) may identify those individuals for whom centrally acting drugs would improve their pain. They may also be able to predict which patients will do well with standard analgesia and following joint replacement.[67]

Future perspectives and limitations for osteoarthritis therapies

Most patients and practitioners would prioritize identifying new targets for pain and improving joint function over preservation of joint structure. However, the results from anti-NGF trials highlight the potential pitfalls of effective pain targeting and support the concept (which is not novel), that pain is a protective response in the joint, and mechanically offloading the joint because of pain is a way of limiting matrix breakdown. These results suggest that effective analgesia needs to be combined with disease-modifying drugs for optimal long-term patient benefit.

Another issue that is still unclear is which tissues should be targeted. Is OA a disease of cartilage, synovium, or bone? Targeting bone in OA is not a new concept, but has recently made headline news with the finding that strontium ranelate can act as a disease-modifying drug.[68] Although there is little mechanistic insight for its success, the trial nonetheless demonstrates a significant reduction in joint space narrowing over 3 years and a late reduction in pain compared to placebo. Whether these treatments are likely to become integrated into existing treatment guidelines will depend upon their reproducibility and cost-effectiveness, most probably linked to a demonstrable reduction in numbers of individuals needing joint replacement surgery.

Targeting cartilage is attractive if one believes that cartilage damage precedes bone change, but many patients present after significant damage has already taken place. Although a number of aggrecanase and collagenase inhibitors have been developed by industry, we still know little about how important these enzymes are once disease is established and whether inhibiting these pathways once significant cartilage is lost will be able to halt disease.

One new and exciting realization is that spontaneous intrinsic repair of articular cartilage may occur in certain individuals given the correct joint environment. For instance focal cartilage lesions, identified on arthroscopy, appear to heal well in approximately 30% of individuals. They are more likely to progress to OA if there is coexistent joint inflammation.[69] The mechanical environment is also critical and there are now a number of case studies and small series of individuals with established OA who appear to recover their joint space after a period (usually 3 months) of joint distraction.[8]

The most significant limitation that we face in trying to put novel targets into clinical trial is the lack of sensitive biomarkers of disease, either circulating or radiographic. These are essential for detecting early disease, predicting which patients will go on to develop severe disabling disease (and should therefore be treatment priorities), and assessing an individual's response to treatment. This is compounded by the insidious nature of the disease, the often late presentation (when significant joint damage has already occurred), and the broad pathogenic heterogeneity that is seen in late (and presumably also early) disease. Successful translation is most likely to come from selecting individuals with high risk of disease, e.g. following acute joint injury or strong family history, in which disease biomarkers can be studied and utilized in a more controlled setting. These are also likely to be the individuals for whom treatment is likely to be deemed most 'cost-effective' given that these individuals will develop OA at a young age, which will impact on their working lives. Tackling disability due to OA in the very old is likely to remain a huge challenge.

References

1. Gautieri A, Vesentini S, Redaelli A, Buehler MJ. Hierarchical structure and nanomechanics of collagen microfibrils from the atomistic scale up. *Nano Lett* 2011;11(2):757–766.

2. Vincent TL, McLean CJ, Full LE, Peston D, Saklatvala J. FGF-2 is bound to perlecan in the pericellular matrix of articular cartilage, where it acts as a chondrocyte mechanotransducer. *Osteoarthritis Cartilage* 2007;15(7): 752–763.

3. Kühn K. Cell death in cartilage. *Osteoarthritis Cartilage* 2004;12(1): 1–16.

4. Gelse K, Söder S, Eger W, Diemtar T, Aigner T. Osteophyte development—molecular characterization of differentiation stages. *Osteoarthritis Cartilage* 2003;11(2):141–148.

5. Brandt KD, Dieppe P, Radin EL. Commentary: is it useful to subset 'primary' osteoarthritis? A critique based on evidence regarding the etiopathogenesis of osteoarthritis. *Semin Arthritis Rheum* 2009;39(2):81–95.

6. Lohmander LS, Englund PM, Dahl LL, Roos EM. The long-term consequence of anterior cruciate ligament and meniscus injuries: osteoarthritis. *Am J Sports Med* 2007;35(10):1756–1769.

7. Englund M, Guermazi A, Roemer FW et al. Meniscal tear in knees without surgery and the development of radiographic osteoarthritis among middle-aged and elderly persons: The Multicenter Osteoarthritis Study. *Arthritis Rheum* 2009;60(3):831–839.

8. Intema F, Van Roermund PM, Marijnissen ACA et al. Tissue structure modification in knee osteoarthritis by use of joint distraction: an open 1-year pilot study. *Ann Rheum Dis* 2011;70(8):1441–1446.

9. Jones ARC, Chen S, Chai DH, Stevens AL, Gleghorn JP, Bonassar LJ, et al. Modulation of lubricin biosynthesis and tissue surface properties following cartilage mechanical injury. *Arthritis Rheum* 2009;60(1):133–142.

10. Maroudas AI. Balance between swelling pressure and collagen tension in normal and degenerate cartilage. *Nature* 1976;260(5554):808–809.

11. Sandy JD, Flannery CR, Neame PJ, Lohmander LS. The structure of aggrecan fragments in human synovial fluid. Evidence for the involvement in osteoarthritis of a novel proteinase which cleaves the Glu 373-Ala 374 bond of the interglobular domain. *J. Clin. Invest* 1992;89(5):1512–1516.

12. Lark MW, Bayne EK, Flanagan J et al. Aggrecan degradation in human cartilage. Evidence for both matrix metalloproteinase and aggrecanase activity in normal, osteoarthritic, and rheumatoid joints. *J Clin Invest* 1997;100(1):93–106.

13. Kamekura S, Hoshi K, Shimoaka T et al. Osteoarthritis development in novel experimental mouse models induced by knee joint instability. *Osteoarthritis Cartilage* 2005;13(7):632–641.

14. Inglis JJ, McNamee KE, Chia S-L et al. Regulation of pain sensitivity in experimental osteoarthritis by the endogenous peripheral opioid system. *Arthritis Rheum* 2008;58(10):3110–3119.

15. Vincent T, Williams R, Maciewicz R, Silman A, Garside P. Mapping pathogenesis of arthritis through small animal models. *Rheumatology* 2012;51(11):1931–1941.

16. Gerwin N, Bendele AM, Glasson S, Carlson CS. The OARSI histopathology initiative—recommendations for histological assessments of osteoarthritis in the rat. *Osteoarthritis Cartilage* 2010;18 Suppl 3:S24–S34.

17. Pratta MA Aggrecan protects cartilage collagen from proteolytic cleavage. *J Biol Chem* 2003;278(46):45539–45545.

18. Troeberg L, Nagase H. Proteases involved in cartilage matrix degradation in osteoarthritis. *Biochim Biophys Acta* 2012;1824(1):133–145.

19. Tortorella MD, Burn TC, Pratta MA et al. Purification and cloning of aggrecanase-1: a member of the ADAMTS family of proteins. *Science* 1999;284(5420):1664–1666.

20. Abbaszade I, Liu RQ, Yang F et al. Cloning and characterization of ADAMTS11, an aggrecanase from the ADAMTS family. *J Biol Chem* 1999;274(33):23443–23450.

21. Glasson SS, Askew R, Sheppard B et al. Deletion of active ADAMTS5 prevents cartilage degradation in a murine model of osteoarthritis. *Nature* 2005;434(7033):644–648.

22. Troeberg L, Nagase H. Proteases involved in cartilage matrix degradation in osteoarthritis. *Biochim Biophys Acta* 2012;1824(1):133–145.

23. Fosang AJ, Rogerson FM, East CJ, Stanton H. ADAMTS-5: the story so far. *Eur Cell Mater* 2008;15:11–26.

24. Alcaraz MJ, Megias J, Garcia-Arnandis I, Clerigues V, Guillen MI. New molecular targets for the treatment of osteoarthritis. *Biochem Pharmacol* 2010;80(1):13–21.

25. Dodge GR, Poole AR. Immunohistochemical detection and immunochemical analysis of type II collagen degradation in human normal, rheumatoid, and osteoarthritic articular cartilages and in explants of bovine articular cartilage cultured with interleukin 1. *J Clin Invest* 1989;83(2):647–661.

26. Lohmander LS, Atley LM, Pietka TA, Eyre DR. The release of crosslinked peptides from type II collagen into human synovial fluid is increased soon after joint injury and in osteoarthritis. *Arthritis Rheum* 2003;48(11):3130–3139.

27. Little CB, Barai A, Burkhardt D et al. Matrix metalloproteinase 13-deficient mice are resistant to osteoarthritic cartilage erosion but not chondrocyte hypertrophy or osteophyte development. *Arthritis Rheum* 2009;60(12):3723–3733.

28. Pitsillides AA, Beier F. Cartilage biology in osteoarthritis—lessons from developmental biology. *Nat Rev Rheumatol* 2011;7(11):654–663.

29. Corr M. Wnt-beta-catenin signaling in the pathogenesis of osteoarthritis. *Nat Clin Pract Rheumatol* 2008;4(10):550–556.

30. Hermansson M, Sawaji Y, Bolton M et al. Proteomic analysis of articular cartilage shows increased type II collagen synthesis in osteoarthritis and expression of inhibin betaA (activin A), a regulatory molecule for chondrocytes. *J Biol Chem* 2004;279(42):43514–43521.

31. Aigner T, Zhu Y, Chansky HH et al. Reexpression of type IIA procollagen by adult articular chondrocytes in osteoarthritic cartilage. *Arthritis Rheum* 1999;42(7):1443–1450.

32. Aigner T, Zien A, Gehrsitz A, Gebhard PM, McKenna L. Anabolic and catabolic gene expression pattern analysis in normal versus osteoarthritic cartilage using complementary DNA-array technology. *Arthritis Rheum* 2001;44(12):2777–2789.

33. Sato T, Konomi K, Yamasaki S et al. Comparative analysis of gene expression profiles in intact and damaged regions of human osteoarthritic cartilage. *Arthritis Rheum* 2006;54(3):808–817.

34. Karlsson C, Dehne T, Lindahl A et al. Genome-wide expression profiling reveals new candidate genes associated with osteoarthritis. *Osteoarthritis Cartilage* 2010;18(4):581–592.

35. Appleton CTG, Pitelka V, Henry J, Beier F. Global analyses of gene expression in early experimental osteoarthritis. *Arthritis Rheum* 2007;56(6): 1854–1868.

36. Burleigh A, Chanalaris A, Gardiner M et al. Joint immobilisation prevents murine osteoarthritis, and reveals the highly mechanosensitive nature of protease expression in vivo. *Arthritis Rheum* 2012;64(7):2278–2288.

37. Chubinskaya S, Kuettner KE. Regulation of osteogenic proteins by chondrocytes. *Int J Biochem Cell Biol* 2003;35(9):1323–1340.

38. Salmon WD, Daughaday WH. A hormonally controlled serum factor which stimulates sulfate incorporation by cartilage in vitro. *J Lab Clin Med* 1957;49(6):825–836.

39. Beattie J, Phillips K, Shand JH et al. Molecular recognition characteristics in the insulin-like growth factor (IGF)-insulin-like growth factor binding protein -3/5 (IGFBP-3/5) heparin axis. *J Mol Endocrinol* 2005;34(1):163–175.

40. Blaney Davidson EN, van der Kraan PM, van den Berg WB. TGF-β and osteoarthritis. *Osteoarthritis Cartilage* 2007;15(6):597–604.

41. Goldring MB. Update on the biology of the chondrocyte and new approaches to treating cartilage diseases. *Best Pract Res Clin Rheumatol* 2006;20(5):1003–1025.

42. Vincent TL. Fibroblast growth factor 2: good or bad guy in the joint? *Arthritis Res Ther*;13(5):127.

43. Fukai A, Kamekura S, Chikazu D et al. Lack of a chondroprotective effect of cyclooxygenase 2 inhibition in a surgically induced model of osteoarthritis in mice. *Arthritis Rheum* 2012;64(1):198–203.

44. Vincent T, Hermansson M, Bolton M, Wait R, Saklatvala J. Basic FGF mediates an immediate response of articular cartilage to mechanical injury. *Proc Natl Acad Sci U S A* 2002;99(12):8259–8264.

45. Wenham CYJ, Conaghan PG. Optimising pain control in osteoarthritis. *Practitioner* 2010;254(1735):23–26, 2–3.

46. Schroder K, Tschopp J. The inflammasomes. *Cell* 2010;140(6): 821–832.

47. Denoble AE, Huffman KM, Stabler TV et al. Uric acid is a danger signal of increasing risk for osteoarthritis through inflammasome activation. *Proc Natl Acad Sci U S A* 2011;108(5):2088–2093.

48. Gruber J, Vincent TL, Hermansson M et al. Induction of interleukin-1 in articular cartilage by explantation and cutting. *Arthritis Rheum* 2004;50(8):2539–2546.

49. Tschopp J. Mitochondria: Sovereign of inflammation? *Eur J Immunol* 2011;41(5):1196–1202.

50. Lotz M. Osteoarthritis year 2011 in review: biology. *Osteoarthritis Cartilage* 2012;20(3):192–196.

51. Loeser RF, Olex AL, McNulty MA et al. Microarray analysis reveals age-related differences in gene expression during the development of osteoarthritis in mice. *Arthritis Rheum* 2012;64(3):705–717.

52. Bayliss MT, Howat S, Davidson C, Dudhia J. The organization of aggrecan in human articular cartilage. Evidence for age-related changes in the rate of aggregation of newly synthesized molecules. *J Biol Chem* 2000;275(9):6321–6327.

53. Verzijl N, DeGroot J, Bank RA et al. Age-related accumulation of the advanced glycation endproduct pentosidine in human articular cartilage aggrecan: the use of pentosidine levels as a quantitative measure of protein turnover. *Matrix Biol* 2001;20(7):409–417.

54. Spector TD, Nandra D, Hart DJ, Doyle DV. Is hormone replacement therapy protective for hand and knee osteoarthritis in women?: The Chingford Study. *Ann Rheum Dis* 1997;56(7):432–434.

55. Ma H-L, Blanchet TJ, Peluso D et al. Osteoarthritis severity is sex dependent in a surgical mouse model. *Osteoarthritis Cartilage* 2007;15(6): 695–700.

56. Campbell L, Emmerson E, Davies F et al. Estrogen promotes cutaneous wound healing via estrogen receptor beta independent of its antiinflammatory activities. *J Exp Med* 2010;207(9):1825–1833.

57. Petrovska S, Dejanova B, Jurisic V. Estrogens: mechanisms of neuroprotective effects. *J Physiol Biochem* 2012;68(3):455–460.

58. Goldring MB, Marcu KB. Cartilage homeostasis in health and rheumatic diseases. *Arthritis Res Ther* 2009;11(3):224.

58a. arcOGEN Consortium; arcOGEN Collaborators. Identification of new susceptibility loci for osteoarthritis (arcOGEN): a genome-wide association study. *Lancet* 2012;380(9844):815–823.

59. Barter MJ, Bui C, Young DA. Epigenetic mechanisms in cartilage and osteoarthritis: DNA methylation, histone modifications and microRNAs. *Osteoarthritis Cartilage* 2012;20(5):339–349.

60. Hill CL, Hunter DJ, Niu J et al. Synovitis detected on magnetic resonance imaging and its relation to pain and cartilage loss in knee osteoarthritis. *Ann Rheum Dis* 2007;66(12):1599–1603.

61. Javaid MK, Lynch JA, Tolstykh I et al. Pre-radiographic MRI findings are associated with onset of knee symptoms: the most study. *Osteoarthritis Cartilage* 2010;18(3):323–328.

62. Walsh DA, McWilliams DF, Turley MJ et al. Angiogenesis and nerve growth factor at the osteochondral junction in rheumatoid arthritis and osteoarthritis. *Rheumatology* (Oxford) 2010;49(10):1852–1861.

63. Lane NE, Schnitzer TJ, Birbara CA et al. Tanezumab for the treatment of pain from osteoarthritis of the knee. *N Engl J Med* 2010;363(16): 1521–1531.

64. Schnitzer TJ, Lane NE, Birbara C et al. Long-term open-label study of tanezumab for moderate to severe osteoarthritic knee pain. *Osteoarthritis Cartilage* 2011;19(6):639–646.

65. McNamee KE, Burleigh A, Gompels LL et al. Treatment of murine osteoarthritis with TrkAd5 reveals a pivotal role for nerve growth factor in non-inflammatory joint pain. *Pain* 2010;149(2):386–392.

66. Tracey I. Can neuroimaging studies identify pain endophenotypes in humans? *Nat Rev Neurol* 2011;7(3):173–181.

67. Gwilym SE, Oag HCL, Tracey I, Carr AJ. Evidence that central sensitisation is present in patients with shoulder impingement syndrome and influences the outcome after surgery. *J Bone Joint Surg Br* 2011;93(4):498–502.

68. Cooper C, Reginster J-Y, Chapurlat R et al. Efficacy and safety of oral strontium ranelate for the treatment of knee osteoarthritis: rationale and design of randomised, double-blind, placebo-controlled trial. *Curr Med Res Opin* 2012;28(2):231–239.

69. Dell'accio F, Vincent TL. Joint surface defects: clinical course and cellular response in spontaneous and experimental lesions. *Eur Cell Mater* 2010;20:210–217.

Clinical features of osteoarthritis

Abhishek Abhishek and Michael Doherty

Introduction

Osteoarthritis (OA), the commonest of all arthropathies, is a leading cause of pain, disability, healthcare utilization, and economic loss. For example, in the United Kingdom symptomatic knee OA occurs in 15% of people over 55 years of age,[1] and approximately 2 million adults visit their GP each year with symptoms of OA. It is therefore important for healthcare professionals to diagnose and manage OA appropriately. In this chapter, we describe the symptoms and signs of OA, in general and for each of its clinical subsets.

Osteoarthritis in a clinical context—structural changes vs symptoms

There are several operational definitions of OA. These may be based on structural changes (e.g. Kellgren and Lawrence grade ≥2), irrespective of symptoms; symptoms (e.g. pain on most days of a month, regardless of structural changes); or require the presence of both. This is potentially confusing, as not all patients with radiographic structural changes have symptoms consistent with OA, and vice versa. Indeed, most patients with knee pain for more than 3 months who do not have radiographic knee OA, go on to develop radiographic changes over a 12 year period, suggesting that knee pain may be the first clinical manifestation of OA.[2] Thus, OA can be separated into two interrelated states:

◆ 'disease' OA—structural changes of OA at the joint level

◆ 'illness' OA—patient-reported symptoms and consequences of OA.[3]

Using this framework, it is clear that researchers studying structure modification target the 'disease' OA, and therefore define OA according to structural changes. However, until such interventions enter routine clinical practice, clinicians target the 'illness' OA. Therefore, in routine clinical practice, symptoms are more relevant when considering a diagnosis of OA than isolated structural changes alone.

Clinical presentations of osteoarthritis

Patients with OA may have

◆ symptoms and structural changes

◆ symptoms without apparent structural changes, or

◆ structural changes alone (incidentally identified on imaging or clinical examination).

The reason why a proportion of patients with structural changes of OA are asymptomatic is not well understood. Some of these may develop joint symptoms attributable to OA later in life. Symptomatic patients with OA have pain, stiffness, and locomotor restriction. These result in varying degrees of functional impairment, physical disability, and psychological distress. Though they are interrelated, there is often a marked discordance between symptoms, functional impairment, physical disability, and psychosocial impact.

Symptoms

Pain

Pain worsening with joint use and relieved by rest ('usage' or 'mechanical' pain) is often the chief complaint. It is insidious in onset, deep, aching, and frequently poorly localized, especially when chronic. For instance, diffuse knee pain may be present in just under one-quarter of symptomatic knee OA patients.[4] Pain in OA often progresses through three clinical stages[5]:

◆ **Stage 1 (early OA):** predictable sharp pain usually brought on by a mechanical insult that is intermittent but eventually limits some activities with relatively little effect on overall function.

◆ **Stage 2 (mild OA):** pain is more constant, begins to affect daily activities, and there may be unpredictable episodes of stiffness.

◆ **Stage 3 (advanced OA):** constant dull/aching pain, punctuated by short episodes of often unpredictable exhausting exacerbations.

Not all patients go through these three stages. Diurnal and seasonal variations in OA pain have been described. Pain due to OA may be worst on first rising, and subsequently improve over the next 2 hours.[6] It may then worsen during the late afternoon/early evening before lessening again later in the evening.[6] Night pain may also occur, and is regarded as a particularly poor prognostic factor indicating severe damage. Anecdotally, OA pain may be worse during damp, low-pressure weather.

The mechanism of pain in OA is incompletely understood. Hyaline cartilage is avascular and aneural,, therefore metabolic or structural alterations in this tissue are unlikely to be directly perceived as painful. Several mechanisms of OA related pain have been suggested (Figure 139.1).[5,7–11] These include:

♦ **Articular**:

– Synovial and capsular pain fibres and mechanoreceptors are stimulated by raised intra-articular pressure.

– Inflammatory mediators stimulate nociceptors in synovium and capsule.

♦ **Bony**:

– Denuded subchondral plate and subchondral microfractures stimulate nociceptors.

– Bone marrow lesions (areas of bone marrow necrosis, fibrosis, oedema, and trabecular abnormalities near subchondral plate on MRI) cause pain by intraosseous hypertension or by stimulating periosteal nerve fibres.

♦ **Periarticular**:Painful periarticular structures such as ligaments, entheses, periosteum (growing osteophytes may cause pain by this mechanism) and bursae possibly result from abnormal biomechanics and/or muscle weakness.

♦ **Neural**:

– Peripheral nociceptive system can become sensitized, resulting in hyperalgesia or allodynia.

– Adaptive changes in the spinal cord (central sensitization—persistent activation of the primary afferent neuron or 'wind-up') and brain can lead to intensified, and persistent pain perception.

It has been suggested that these different mechanisms may produce different pain characteristics.[5,7,9,12] It is suggested that pain:

♦ **on usage**—is principally due to mechanical or entheseal problems

♦ **after rest**—is inflammatory in origin

♦ **at night or at rest**—is due to intraosseous hypertension

♦ **burning (neuropathic) pain**, with associated hypersensitivity and paresthesia—is due to central sensitization.

Correlation between pain and radiographic change varies according to site. It is best at the hip and then the knee, with the poorest correlation occurring in the hands and intervertebral facet joints. Some people even with severe structural changes on radiographs may be asymptomatic. Joints with more severe radiographic changes are more likely to be symptomatic than those with mild change (Figure 139.2) but other factors are also important.[13] These include:

♦ **demographic factors** such as age, gender, socio-economic status, social support, racial and cultural background

♦ **constitutional factors** such as increasing body mass index (BMI), and pain at other sites[4,14]

♦ **psychological factors** including affect, cognitive state (e.g. pain beliefs, expectations, and memories), self-efficacy (individual's confidence in their abilities to accomplish a desired task e.g. control arthritis pain), and pain catastrophizing (the tendency to focus upon and feel helpless in the face of pain)

♦ **genetic factors** such as Val158Met single nucleotide polymorphism (SNP) in *COMT* (association with pain in hip OA),[15] and Ile585Ile SNP in *TRPV1* genes (negative association with pain in knee OA).[16]

Stiffness

Stiffness is the other chief complaint. It is of shorter duration than in inflammatory arthritis. Stiffness is difficulty or discomfort in movement due to a perceived inflexibility localized to the joint. This is sometimes described as 'gelling', i.e. short-lived joint stiffness after inactivity. Prolonged morning or inactivity stiffness, often taken as a reflection of inflammation, is uncommon but may occur in OA.

Aesthetic problems

Aesthetic problems such as swelling and deformity in hand OA and crepitus in knee OA may be prominent symptoms in some patients. Knee crepitus may be especially prominent when coming downstairs. At the knee, associated meniscal damage or loose body may result in other mechanical symptoms such as 'locking'. There may

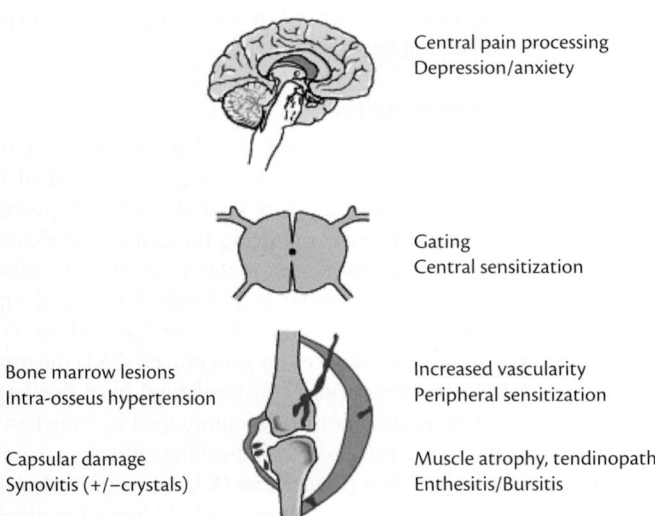

Fig. 139.1 Potential sites of pain perception and/or modification in osteoarthritis.
Reproduced from Jones AC, Doherty M, The treatment of Osteoarthritis. Br J Clin Pharmacol 1992 Apr;33(4):357–63 with permission of John Wiley & Son.

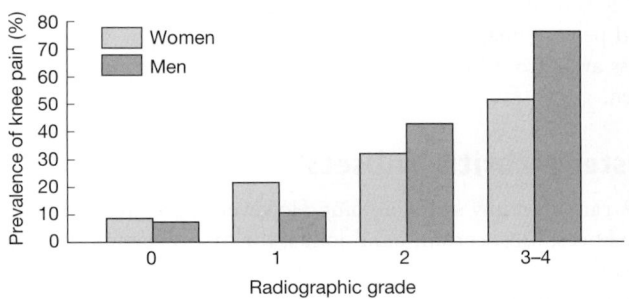

Fig. 139.2 Prevalence of knee pain by radiographic grade and gender in a United States community population.
Davis MA, Ettinger WH, Neuhaus JM, Barclay JD, Segal MR. Correlates of knee pain among US adults with and without radiographic knee osteoarthritis. J Rheumatol. 1992 Dec;19(12):1943–9.

be a feeling of instability or 'giving way'—especially at the knees or ankles.

Functional impairment

Disability is principally associated with pain. However, psychological factors and muscle weakness are also important and in most cases more important than radiographic change.[17–19] For an individual patient reduced range of movement (e.g. at the hip) may be associated with specific functional limitations, for instance during sexual intercourse or getting out of a car. Postural instability at the knee may impair mobility, and therefore restrict participation.[20]

Signs

Several features reflecting altered joint structure and function may be present.

- On inspection (**look**):

  - bony enlargement—due to remodelling and osteophytosis, seen at both large (e.g. knee), and small joints (e.g. interphalangeal joints)

  - deformity—occurs in late disease e.g. knee malalignment, and fixed flexion at the hip

  - muscle wasting around an affected joint—globally affecting all muscles acting over the joint.

- On palpation (**feel**):

  - palpable bony swelling and osteophyte

  - varying degrees of 'cool' joint effusion may be present, especially at the knee

  - joint line or periarticular tenderness

- During movement (**move**):

  - crepitus—a coarse crunching sensation or sound caused by friction between two articular surfaces, often more prominent during active movement and occurring throughout most of the range

  - restricted movement—equal for both active and passive movement

  - instability—may occur late in knee and thumb-base OA, but uncommon at other sites.

Signs of associated meniscal damage and 'loose body' can occur and periarticular sources of pain, demonstrated by point tenderness away from the joint line and by stress testing, are commonly seen.

Osteoarthritis 'subsets'

OA can affect any synovial joint. However, it preferentially targets the knees, hips, certain hand joints, the first metatarsophalangeal ('bunion') joint and apophyseal (facet) joints of the lower cervical and lower lumbar spine.[21] Since OA is a process that can potentially be triggered by diverse constitutional and environmental factors, a wide spectrum of clinical expression and outcome is expected. It is possible to look at OA as a single entity, or to try to classify

subgroups of patients with OA. Both strategies are fraught with difficulties.

OA was initially classified as primary (no cause identified) or secondary (an obvious cause identified, such as trauma or dysplasia). Indeed, such a distinction is still retained in the American College of Rheumatology (ACR) criteria.[22] However, such artificial separation has often proved unsatisfactory, for several reasons:

- frequent lack of an identifiable cause, resulting in a large heterogeneous primary group

- overlap between subsets, as shown, for example, by the influence of predisposition to 'primary' generalized OA in determining development of postmeniscectomy 'secondary' OA[23]

- lack of evidence to suggest that the underlying pathological features and processes differ.

Other, more objective, features have therefore often been used to define subsets:

- joint site involved (e.g. hip, knee, hand)

- site within a joint (e.g. medial tibiofemoral, lateral tibiofemoral, patellofemoral at the knee)

- number of joints involved (e.g. one, few, many)

- presence of associated calcium crystals

- presence of marked clinical inflammation

- radiographic bone response (e.g. atrophic, hypertrophic)

- age of onset (e.g. premature osteoarthritis under age 45)

- syndromal features (e.g. Stickler's syndrome or hereditary arthroophthalmopathy).

Although a number of 'subsets' have emerged it is important to note that sharp distinctions between subsets do not exist and many of the above characteristics represent different aspects of the OA process (e.g. the balance between damage and repair, the number of joints involved), and different characteristics may dominate the clinical picture at just one phase in the evolution of the condition. One 'subset' may thus evolve into another and different 'subsets' may exist at different sites within the same individual. The partitioning of OA may be revolutionized by the genetics of OA if specific genotypic subsetting becomes possible.

Generalized osteoarthritis

The concept of generalized OA, with hand involvement as the marker for a generalized predisposition, was first described by Haygarth in 1805 and is supported by several studies. A polyarticular subset of OA particularly involving the distal interphalangeal joints (DIPJs), thumb bases, first metatarsophalangeal joints (MTPJs), lower cervical and lumbar facet joints, knees, and hips was described by Kellgren, who coined the term 'generalized OA' for this subset.[24] The clinical marker for generalized OA is the presence of multiple Heberden's nodes (posterolateral hard swellings of DIPJs). Heberden's nodes are often accompanied by Bouchard's nodes—less well defined posterolateral swellings of the proximal interphalangeal joints (PIPJs) (Figure 139.3). Later on patients with identical targeting of joints as in generalized OA were identified, who did not have Heberden's nodes.[25,26] This led to the classification of generalized OA into two groups (although such a distinction is not supported by others):

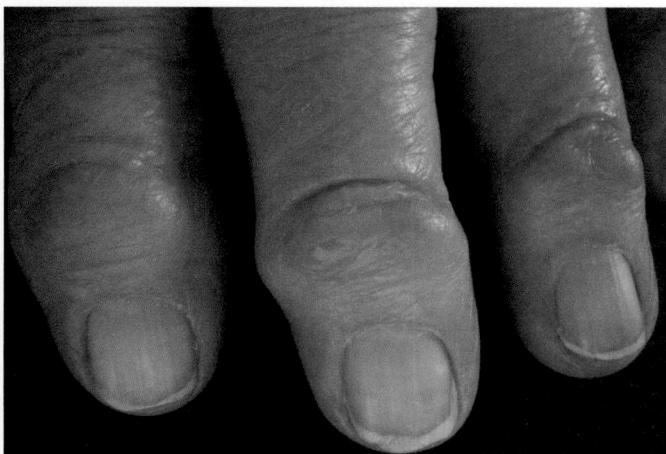

Fig. 139.3 Heberden's nodes: posterolateral hard swellings of distal interphalangeal joints.

- nodal generalized OA:
  - nodes
  - DIPJs involved more than PIPJs
  - marked female preponderance
  - familial aggregation
- non-nodal generalized OA:
  - PIPJs involved more than DIPJs
  - more equal sex distribution.

There is no single agreed definition for the number or location of joints that must be affected before a patient is regarded as having generalized OA. Expert panels constituted by ACR and the European League Against Rheumatism (EULAR) suggest that generalized OA is present if there is OA at the spine, or hand respectively, and in at least two other joint regions.[27,28]

Nodal generalized osteoarthritis

This is the best recognized subset and is characterized by:

- polyarticular finger IPJ involvement
- Heberden's and Bouchard's nodes
- female preponderance
- peak onset around the menopause
- predisposition to OA of the knee, hip, spine, and thumb base
- marked familial predisposition.

The typical patient is a woman aged 40–60 years who develops intermittent discomfort followed eventually by swelling of a single finger IPJ. A few months later another IPJ becomes painful, then another, producing a 'stuttering' onset polyarthritis of DIPJs and PIPJs. Affected IPJs may feel stiff and tender and show tight posterolateral swelling. Aspiration of early evolving swellings may reveal viscous, clear, hyaluronate-rich 'jelly'. These cysts are thought to represent mucoid transformation of periarticular fibro-adipose tissue and may communicate with the joint. Each IPJ tends to go through a symptomatic phase while the swelling and deformity becomes established, resulting in perhaps 1–3 years of episodic

discomfort and stiffness. Nodes most frequently appear at the index and middle finger[29] and thumb IPJs. The discrete radial and ulnar Heberden's nodes on one IPJ may eventually coalesce to form a single dorsal bar.

In almost all cases symptoms then subside, leaving the patient with:

- Heberden's and Bouchard's nodes
- characteristic ulnar/radial deviation of IPJs without instability
- underlying radiographic evidence of OA (Figure 139.4).

The functional prognosis for such hand OA seems to be good. A common classification problem is that one or just a few Heberden's nodes and limited IPJ OA are common often asymptomatic findings in elderly people and it is not always clear, therefore, when the title 'nodal generalized OA' should be applied. Although strict criteria for this have not been defined, some studies suggest that involvement of even a single IPJ may be relevant as a risk factor for OA elsewhere.[30]

Hand osteoarthritis

OA targets characteristic sites in hands, i.e. DIPJs (~50%), thumb bases (~35%), PIPJs (~20%), and metacarpophalangeal joints (MCPJs) (~10%), in descending order of frequency.[28,31] Symptoms in hand OA are usually bilateral and joint involvement is usually approximately symmetrical.[28,29] The clinical features of nodal OA have already been described. Thumb-base OA, the other common target site for OA in hands, involves the first carpometacarpal and/ or trapezioscaphoid joints and presents with mechanical joint pain maximal over the thumb base but often with distal or proximal radiation. There may be radial subluxation and adduction, giving the thumb a swollen 'squared' appearance.[28,29] Thumb-base OA commonly associates with persistent symptoms and functional impairment so the prognosis is more guarded than in IPJ OA.

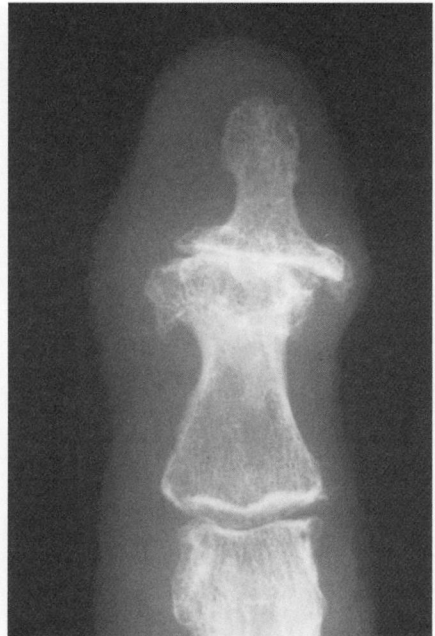

Fig. 139.4 Radiograph of distal interphalangeal joint showing many of the typical radiographic features of osteoarthritis (joint-space narrowing, sclerosis, osteophyte).

At the MCPJs, OA mainly targets the index, middle and thumb MCPJ in a descending order of frequency, often presenting with bony enlargement.[31] Relatively isolated MCPJ OA sometimes occurs, particularly in men with physically demanding occupations ('Missouri arthritis').[32] Widespread MCPJ OA with wrist arthropathy or chondrocalcinosis raises the possibility of haemochromatosis. The differential diagnosis for hand OA includes psoriatic arthritis (which targets DIPJs or commonly affects just one ray), rheumatoid arthritis (which targets wrists, MCPJs, PIPJs), gout (which may superimpose on pre-existing hand OA) and haemochromatosis.[28]

Erosive ('inflammatory') osteoarthritis

Erosive OA, an uncommon subset of OA is characterized by:

- finger IPJ involvement
- often florid inflammation
- lateral IPJ instability
- nodes that are not prominent (but may be present)
- radiographic subchondral erosive change
- tendency to IPJ ankylosis.

The condition clinically resembles nodal generalized OA in beginning as an additive polyarthritis of finger joints. However, multiple IPJs may be affected at the onset, i.e. synchronous polyarticular onset.[28,33] Inflammatory symptoms and signs are often marked although episodic. Pain, tenderness, and inflammation (warmth, soft tissue swelling—sometimes erythema) are more marked and prolonged in erosive OA than in nodal OA.[33,34] Erosive OA usually targets the IPJs, distal more often than proximal, and generally spares the thumb bases and MCPJs.[28,34] However, thumb base and MCPJ erosions have been identified in radiographic studies of hand OA. There is often no association with generalized OA.

IPJ instability, which is rare in nodal generalized OA, is common. The prognosis for hand function is less favourable in erosive OA.[35] Recent studies suggest that there may be individual and familial predispositions to this subset of OA.[36]

The radiographic hallmark feature of this condition is the presence of subchondral erosive change (Figure 139.5) which may lead to a 'gull's wing' appearance as remodelling occurs. Early, florid subchondral erosive change is easily recognized, but lesser degrees of erosion, particularly in established cases, may prove difficult to distinguish from the cysts and subchondral bony change of nodal generalized OA. It is unclear whether erosive OA is a distinct subset or one end of a spectrum of change.[37]

Radiographic subchondral erosion attributed to OA occurs in hands of 2.8% of people over 55 years of age, and in 7–10% of patients with symptomatic radiographic hand OA.[35,36] Whether this is 'erosive OA' in the classic context or not is open to debate. However, the presence of subchondral erosion in even a single joint may be significant as it associates with more disability and hand pain in radiographic hand OA.

Large-joint osteoarthritis

Knee osteoarthritis

Knee involvement is common in OA. It is usually bilateral unless there is predisposing trauma. Although OA may affect the knee as a mono- or pauci-articular problem, it often occurs in association with hand OA, especially in women.[24] Knee OA affects both the tibiofemoral (TFJ) and the patellofemoral joints (PFJ). In symptomatic knee OA, combined TFJ and PFJ involvement, isolated PFJ involvement, and isolated TFJ involvement occurred in 40%, 24% and 4% knees respectively.[38] Medial compartment TFJ OA is more common than lateral compartment TFJ OA (Figure 139.6).[39] Simultaneous involvement of medial TFJ compartment and of PFJ is the commonest distribution of OA in the knees, being present in 50% cases.[39] PFJ OA (lateral more than medial facet involvement), because of its intimate relationship with the quadriceps mechanism, is possibly associated with greater functional impairment.[1]

The location of pain points towards the affected knee compartment(s). Pain may be medial or generalized in medial compartment TFJ OA, and anterior in PFJ OA.[12] Pain from PFJ

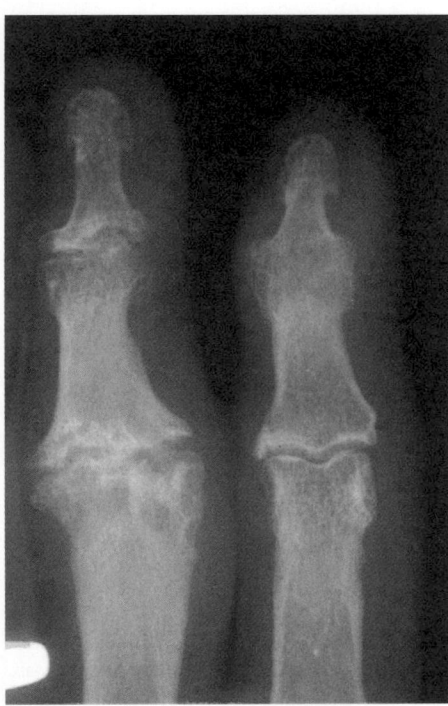

Fig. 139.5 Subchondral erosive change in erosive osteoarthritis.

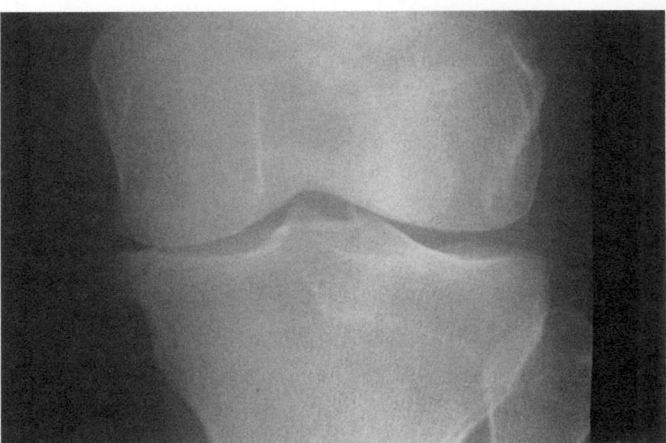

Fig. 139.6 Predominant medial compartment osteoarthritis at the knee (standing anteroposterior radiograph).

OA is typically exacerbated by prolonged sitting, standing from a low chair, and going up or downhill (coming down is more painful). Generalized knee pain with distal radiation suggests moderate to severe knee OA.[40] Knee OA usually does not cause posterior knee pain unless there is a complicating popliteal ('Baker's') cyst. Apart from pain, there may be a feeling of 'giving way' and instability, both of which may associate with falls.[41] This is particularly common with PFJ OA and associated lateral patellar subluxation. Medial compartment TFJ OA with severe bone and cartilage attrition results in a characteristic varus deformity (Fig. 139.7).

Mild to moderate knee effusion is common in patients attending hospitals, increasing in prevalence with the severity of OA.[42] Many painful periarticular soft tissue pathologies such as medial collateral ligament (inferior insertion) enthesopathy, anserine bursitis, semimembranosus-tibial collateral ligament bursitis, tender medial fat pad, and iliotibial band syndrome may coexist with knee OA.[43,44] Meniscal tears are common in knee OA but are not necessarily a cause of increased symptoms.[45]

Whether differing risk factors are important at different compartmental sites is unclear but some studies do suggest that this may be the case. For example, tibiofemoral disease may be more strongly associated with trauma whereas patellofemoral disease may be associated with coexisting calcium pyrophosphate (CPP) crystal deposition (CPPD), and female gender.

Hip osteoarthritis

Hip OA frequently occurs without OA at other joints, and is commonly unilateral.[46] Although several anatomic risk factors of hip OA have been described, e.g. reduced centre–edge angle (<20°), deep acetabular socket, and pistol grip deformity,[47,48] study of OA at this joint has been hampered by lack of a consistent definition and classification of pattern of involvement. Patients commonly present with pain—typically deep in the groin, aching, stiffness, and symptoms related to restricted movement. Pain in hip OA may be present in the anteromedial or upper lateral thigh, or may radiate to the knee, and occasionally to the shin and ankle. In some cases, hip OA presents with knee pain alone. Unlike knee-originated pain, such hip referred pain is usually more widespread and ill-defined, involves the distal thigh, and may improve on rubbing.

On examination, active and passive hip movements may be painful and/or restricted with internal rotation in flexion being the earliest movement to be affected. Impaired internal rotation in flexion is the most discriminating clinical sign for the presence of radiographic hip OA in those with hip pain.[49] Worsening restriction in hip movements in each plane, and increasing number of planes with restriction in movement, increases the probability of radiographic hip OA in those with hip pain.[49] Movements may be globally restricted in severe hip OA.[50] In advanced hip OA, the affected extremity may be shortened, with external rotation, adduction, and fixed flexion being the typical endstage deformity (Figure 139.8)

Hip OA should be distinguished from other causes of pain in the pelvic girdle. Anterior groin pain may result from avascular necrosis of the femoral head, femoro-acetabular impingement, iliopsoas bursitis, and transient osteoporosis; medial thigh pain may result from osteitis pubis and adductor enthesitis; lateral thigh pain may result from trochanteric bursitis/greater trochanter pain syndrome; while buttock pain may result from lumbar radiculopathy, sacroiliac joint pathology, iliolumbar ligament syndrome, and hip extensor muscle strain.[51]

Hip OA may be subclassified largely according to pattern of migration of the femoral head.[52,53] Differentiation of these patterns appears warranted since there may be implications for prognosis.[54] Two main patterns have been emphasized: superior pole OA and central (medial) OA.

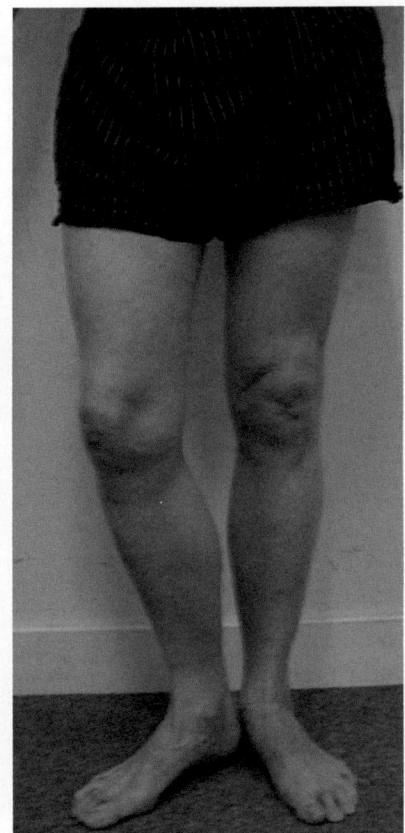

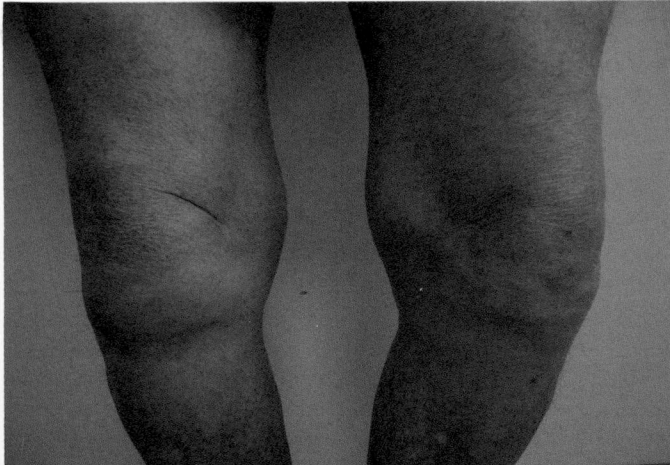

Fig. 139.7 Left knee showing genu varum. This suggests the presence of medial compartment tibiofemoral joint osteoarthritis in this knee.

Fig. 139.8 Posture in advanced right hip osteoarthritis: the affected extremity is shortened, with external rotation, adduction, and fixed flexion.

Superior pole OA

This is the commonest pattern, characterized by focal cartilage loss in the superior part of the joint (Figure 139.9). Further subdivision into supero-lateral, supero-intermediate or supero-medial is sometimes made. Osteophyte formation is most prominent at the lateral acetabular and medial femoral margins, often in combination with thickening (buttressing) of the cortex of the medial femoral neck by periosteal osteophyte (Figure 139.10). Subchondral sclerosis and cyst formation on both sides of the narrowed joint may be marked. Originally it was suggested that this pattern is:

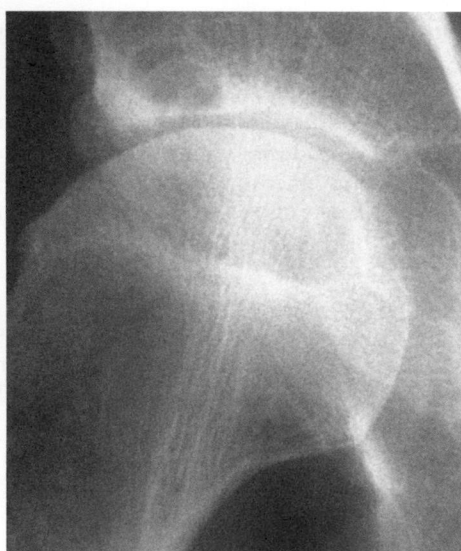

Fig. 139.9 Superior pole pattern of hip osteoarthritis (early) showing localized reduction in interosseous distance with focal sclerosis at the superior part of the joint, minor femoral osteophyte, and acetabular roof cyst.

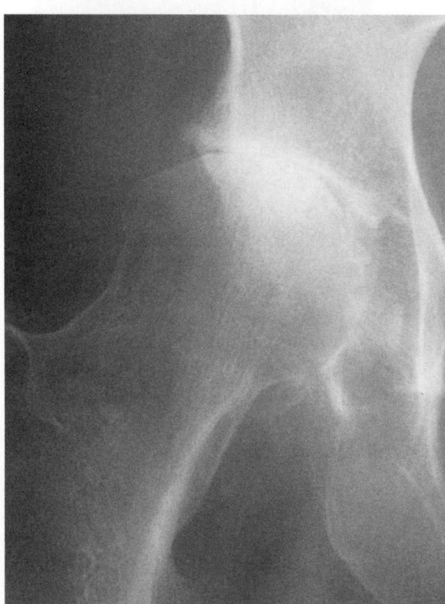

Fig. 139.10 Superior pole osteoarthritis (late) showing superolateral femoral head migration, bone attrition, and 'buttressing' medial periosteal osteophyte of the femoral neck.

◆ relatively more common in men
◆ mainly unilateral at presentation
◆ likely to progress, with superolateral (Figure 139.10) or supero-medial femoral migration
◆ commonly secondary to local structural abnormality.

Progression is more likely than with other patterns of hip migration.[54]

Central (medial) OA

This less common pattern shows more central joint-space loss, with less prominent femoral neck buttressing. It is suggested that this pattern is:

◆ relatively more common in women
◆ commonly bilateral at presentation
◆ more strongly associated with nodal generalized OA
◆ less likely to progress and when it does it is with axial or medial migration (Figure 139.11).

Other patterns are described (e.g. concentric) and many patients have 'indeterminate' radiographic patterns. Most disease is symmetrical unless there is a structural alteration in joint loading.[52]

Facet joint osteoarthritis

Facet joint OA usually coexists with degenerative disc disease (i.e.'spondylosis') and for this reason it can be difficult to attribute symptoms to each condition. Lumbar spine facet joint OA may result in localized pain which may radiate to the buttocks, groin, and thigh.[55] Symptoms are worse in the morning, during inactivity, when standing or sitting for a long time, and during exercise, e.g. lumbar spine extension or rotation, and are eased by lying flat and spinal flexion.[55] Similarly, cervical spine facet joint OA presents with ipsilateral neck pain radiating to the shoulder and worsened by neck rotation or extension.[56]

Osteoarthritis at other joint sites

Selection of OA for certain sites is striking. For example, involvement of the elbow, glenohumeral joint, or ankle is relatively

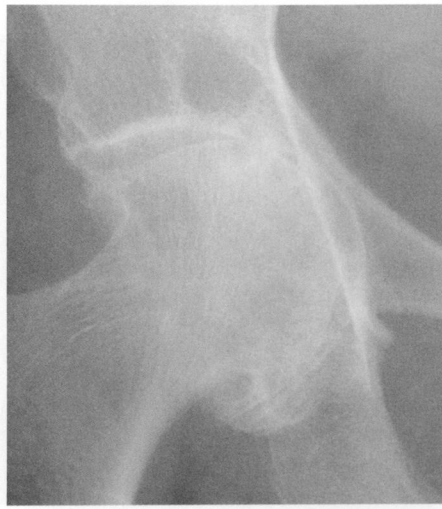

Fig. 139.11 Medial pole osteoarthritis, showing progression to a acetabular protrusion deformity.

uncommon and principally confined to elderly people. Especially in a younger person, bilateral ankle OA without preceding trauma, and widespread metacarpophalangeal OA, should both suggest haemochromatosis. As with other arthropathies, the predilection of OA for certain sites remains unexplained. One intriguing, unifying hypothesis is that in all species the joints most commonly affected by OA are in general those that have undergone the most rapid and recent evolutionary change. In humans these are the joints associated with bipedal locomotion and oppositional grip.[57] Such joints may not have had sufficient evolutionary time to fully adapt to the tasks demanded of them. They therefore have insufficient mechanical reserve, and thus 'fail' more commonly than joints that have had longer to adapt to their new function.

Crystal deposition in osteoarthritis

A number of particles are commonly identified in synovial fluid and other tissues from OA joints. These include CPP crystals and basic calcium phosphates (BCP)—mainly carbonate-substituted hydroxyapatite. By analogy with monosodium urate crystals in gout, it was initially assumed that such calcium crystals were always pathogenic and cause specific 'crystal deposition disease'. Shedding of CPP crystals into the joint cavity can certainly trigger florid synovitis—'acute CPP crystal arthritis'—but the possible role of CPP and BCP in chronic inflammation is unclear. In addition, being hard particles calcium crystals might also act as wear particles on the joint surface. However, the not uncommon occurrence of these crystals in asymptomatic, otherwise normal joints, and the lack of a clear association with specific clinical phenotypes other than acute CPP crystal arthritis have questioned such a direct pathogenic role. It currently seems that CPP and BCP in the context of common OA are epiphenomena possibly reflecting ageing and the underlying pathophysiological processes of OA respectively. Indeed, apatite is universally present in endstage knee and hip OA.[58,59] Apart from alerting the clinician to an underlying metabolic or genetic predisposition, their value in a clinical setting is unclear. Nevertheless the following OA phenotypes based on crystal deposition have been suggested.

Calcium pyrophosphate crystal deposition (CPPD) and osteoarthritis

CPPD is associated with a form of OA that may have several distinct features compared to common OA.[60] These characteristics include:

◆ predominance in older patients

◆ often florid inflammatory component, possibly with superimposed acute attacks

◆ particular involvement of the knee

◆ frequent involvement of joints and joint compartments uncommonly affected by 'sporadic OA' (e.g. glenohumeral, mid-tarsal, MCP);

◆ frequent 'hypertrophic' radiographic appearance.

Large and medium-sized joints are principally involved, with the knees being the most usual and severely affected site, followed by wrists, shoulders, elbows, hips, and mid-tarsal joints. In the hand, MCPJs (particularly index and middle) are often affected.

Symptoms are usually restricted to just a few joints, though single or multiple joint involvement also occurs.

Acute CPP crystal arthritis may be superimposed upon chronic symptoms. Affected joints show signs of OA (bony swelling, crepitus, restricted movement) and varying degrees of inflammation. Synovitis may be prominent and is usually most evident at the knee, radiocarpal, or glenohumeral joints (chronic CPP crystal inflammatory arthritis). In severe cases fixed flexion with either valgus or varus deformity may occur. Examination often reveals more widespread but asymptomatic joint abnormality.

In hospital-based studies, knees have been shown to have bi- or tricompartmental involvement, with marked, usually predominant patellofemoral disease. However, current evidence does not support the view that CPPD at the knee accelerates the progression of knee OA.[61] The radiographic changes of this arthropathy are basically those of OA, but characteristics which may suggest the presence of CPPD include:

◆ atypical joint and compartment involvement

◆ often prominent, exuberant osteophyte and cyst formation (particularly at the knee).

These features combine to produce a distinctive 'hypertrophic' appearance and distribution which suggests the presence of CPP crystals even in the absence of radiographic chondrocalcinosis (Figure 139.12). Many joints with CPPD + OA however, appear not dissimilar to 'uncomplicated' OA. Since nodal generalized OA often coexists in these patients, it is common to find otherwise typical OA changes in some joints, with more distinctive changes of CPPD + OA at other sites.

Apatite-associated destructive arthropathy (Milwaukee shoulder)

This uncommon condition[62,63] is usually:

◆ confined to elderly patients, particularly women

◆ localized to large joints

◆ associated with rapid progression with resultant joint instability

◆ associated with marked attrition of cartilage and bone

◆ characterized by abundant apatite deposition in synovial fluid and synovium.

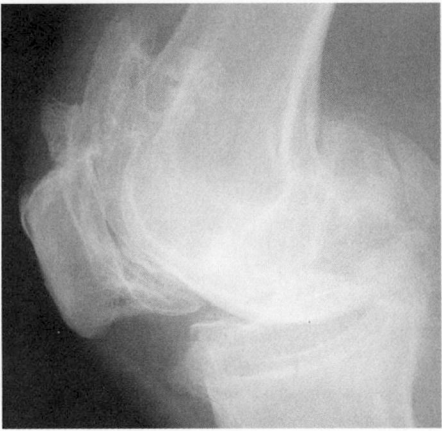

Fig. 139.12 Exuberant osteophytosis in patellofemoral compartment in CPPD-positive osteoarthritis.

Typical patients are elderly women with rapidly progressive arthropathy of the hip, shoulder, or knee. Usually only one or a few joints are affected. Onset is often quite sudden and within a few weeks or months the patient has severe rest and night pain, and the joint has a large, cool effusion, with gross instability. Aspirated synovial fluid is often bloodstained, highly viscous but with only a modest increased cellularity. Alazarin red S staining at acidic pH shows multiple calcium-containing aggregates which can be identified as BCP, most commonly carbonate-substituted hydroxyapatite, by more definitive means. The principal radiographic features are marked attrition of cartilage and bone, with a paucity of osteophyte and sclerosis, i.e. a markedly 'atrophic' appearance (Figure 139.13). Such rapidly progressive arthropathy may superimpose upon more typical chronic OA or present apparently de novo. The differential diagnosis includes sepsis, an atrophic neuropathic joint, and late avascular necrosis.

The pathogenesis of this condition, particularly as regards the role of the apatite aggregates, is controversial.[64] McCarty and colleagues emphasize the pathologic role of these crystals in causing structural damage. Others suggest that this is not the case, and that apatite primarily originates from subchondral and marginal bone, or that apatite deposition is just a manifestation of end stage OA. The speed of onset and progression, lack of overt inflammation, marked bone loss, specificity to certain anatomic sites, radiographic similarity to late avascular necrosis, and neuropathic joints support the contention that this arthropathy reflects a widespread nutritional catastrophe for the joint, possibly initiated by age-related compromise of subchondral bone blood flow. The large amount of observed apatite may thus simply reflect the rapidity of bone damage.

Mixed crystal deposition

Comparison of clinical and radiographic features of typical CPPD + OA and apatite-associated arthropathies shows marked contrasts, though each clearly falls within the spectrum of 'OA'. The finding of both CPP and BCP within the same OA joint is very common although there is little evidence that their combined presence is associated with particular clinical or radiographic characteristics.

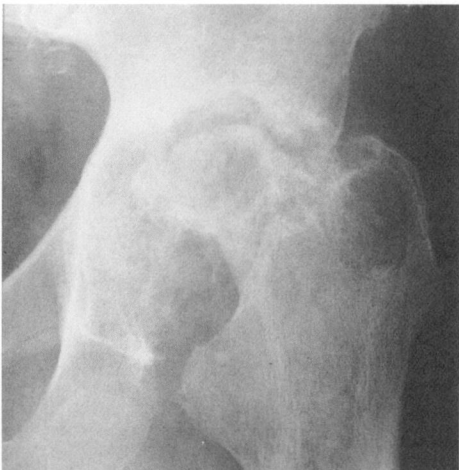

Fig. 139.13 Radiograph of apatite-associated destructive arthritis of the hip, showing apparent increase in joint space (non-loaded film), marked loss of bone (femoral and acetabular components), and minimal bone response.

Osteoarthritis as part of other diseases

If OA represents the inherent repair process of synovial joints, then it would be expected to occur during certain phases of other defined arthropathies. For example, in rheumatoid arthritis, osteophytosis, sclerosis, and remodelling often occur as a late feature once inflammation has largely been suppressed. In such instances, 'OA' can be viewed as an accompanying process of tissue response/repair rather than an acquired second condition. The same considerations pertain to other inflammatory, metabolic, or structural arthropathies. Ochronosis and spondyloepiphyseal dysplasia, for example, are sometimes included within the umbrella of OA since many of their radiographic features are typical of OA but of course many are not and are very distinctive. Similarly, endemic forms of OA need consideration in their own right. For clinical purposes, however, it may still be useful to consider together conditions that may result in a non-inflammatory arthropathy with radiographic changes predominantly of OA (Table 139.1) when an atypical presentation should lead one to search for a defined, possibly treatable underlying cause. In patients with 'OA' one should consider specific predisposing factors when there is:

- premature onset (<45 years) in the absence of preceding joint trauma/insult
- an atypical joint distribution for OA, for example, prominent MCPJ, radiocarpal or bilateral ankle involvement in haemochromatosis
- an atypical degree of clinical inflammation, or episodes of acute florid self-limiting synovitis at their worst within 24 hours (suspect CPPD or gout)
- premature onset of chondrocalcinosis (i.e. age <55 years)
- florid polyarticular chondrocalcinosis at any age.

Diagnosis of osteoarthritis

The diagnosis of OA is essentially clinical. It may be diagnosed without recourse to radiographic and/or laboratory investigations in the at-risk age group in the presence of typical symptoms and signs.[28,41,65] For example, NICE guidelines suggest that peripheral joint OA may be diagnosed on clinical grounds alone in the presence of persistent usage-related joint pain in one or few joints; age less than 45 years; and morning stiffness less than 30 minutes.[65] The presence of other clinical features adds to the diagnostic certainty.

The usefulness of radiography relates to exclusion of other diagnostic possibilities rather than confirmation of presence of OA. Appropriate imaging and laboratory assessments, should therefore be carried out in young individuals (i.e. <45 years of age), in the presence of atypical symptoms and signs (e.g. unusual site, clinically evident joint inflammation, marked rest and/or night pain, and rapidly progressive pain), if there is weight loss or constitutional upset, and at the knees if there is true mechanical 'locking'. Synovial fluid examination is not required to diagnose OA. However, joint aspiration and synovial fluid analysis are indicated if there is a suspicion of coexistent crystal deposition. OA encourages urate as well as CPP and BCP crystal deposition and synovial analysis should be undertaken in patients with peripheral joint OA who develop inflammatory features or episodes of acute synovitis.

Table 139.1 Principal conditions with presentations and radiographic changes that may simulate osteoarthritis

Generalized 'osteoarthritis'	Spondyloepiphyseal dysplasia
	Ochronosis
	Haemochromatosis
	Wilson's disease
	Endemic osteoarthritis (e.g. Kashin–Beck disease)
Pauciarticular (large joint) 'osteoarthritis'	Neuropathic joints:
	syringomyelia—shoulders, wrists, elbows
	diabetes—hindfoot, midfoot
	tabes—knees, spine
	Acromegaly
	Avascular necrosis (mainly proximal and distal femur, proximal humerus)

The commonest clinical situation is the patient presenting with joint pain. The priorities in this situation are to determine whether:

- 'OA' is the cause of the symptoms;
- there is an additional periarticular cause for the pain
- there are predisposing or adverse factors for the development or progression of OA
- there is another underlying arthropathy
- there are other factors that are modifying the pain experience.

Resolving these difficulties depends on a careful clinical history and examination; radiography and laboratory investigations play a relatively minor role. The clinical assessment aims to:

- localize the site of the pain—joint line or periarticular
- detect the presence of clinical signs of OA—crepitus, bony swelling, restricted range of motion
- define any adverse features—obesity, malalignment, reduced strength, abnormal usage (occupational or habitual)
- rule out features of other arthropathy—rheumatoid arthritis, gout, seronegative arthropathy
- determine factors which might influence pain experience—multiple regional pain, depression, sleep disturbance
- determine the existence of comorbidities like vestibular imbalance, postural instability, falls; and of polypharmacy, especially the use of sedatives, and opiate analgesics.

Radiographs merely help to confirm the presence of the structural change, but since the radiograph is relatively insensitive, particularly in early disease, a normal radiograph does not rule out a diagnosis of OA. Indeed, knee pain may be the first manifestation of OA, and predate radiographic changes of OA.[2] Conversely, abnormal radiographic changes may not be the cause of the patients' symptoms.

Neurological finding are important, particularly in the lumbar and cervical spine where osteophytosis of the facet or apophyseal joint may lead to foraminal encroachment and subsequent nerve root compression. Peripheral nerve entrapment may also occur as a result of osteophytosis or synovitis of peripheral joints. Possible sites for this are the ulnar nerve at the ulnar groove and the median nerve in the carpal tunnel. In such a situation, particularly in the spine, MRI and/or nerve conduction studies are required to fully elucidate the nature, site, and presence of nerve compression.

As well as direct pressure on a nerve, vascular claudication may also occur, particularly in the lumbar spine. In this situation, exercise results in neurological symptoms and signs in the legs. The diagnosis is essentially based on the history but evidence of canal and/or foraminal stenosis is sought, usually with MRI. In all situations, particularly in the spine, it is essential to ensure that there is a good match between clinical findings and demonstrated structural abnormalities.

Osteoarthritis prognosis

OA is a heterogeneous disease with diverse outcomes. For example, while one in six patients with peripheral joint OA referred to secondary care report a deterioration in their symptoms, 1 in 16 report an improvement during follow-up.[66] Progression of OA is modified not only by the severity of structural changes and symptoms, but also by coexistent risk factors (e.g. high BMI, gender, injury, occupation) and comorbidity (e.g. depression). From the available data one can be relatively optimistic about outcome for most patients, especially those with IPJ OA, and for many people with knee OA.

Knee or hip OA also shortens life expectancy (standardized mortality ratio (SMR) 1.55 (1.41–1.70).[67] This is predominantly due to excess cardiovascular deaths, but exists for other disease specific causes as well. Disability at baseline also associates with excess mortality (SMR 1.48 (1.17–1.86).[67,68] The mechanisms underlying this are unclear but may include:

- side effects of drugs, principally non-steroidal anti-inflammatory drugs
- increased cardiovascular morbidity due to either comorbidities (e.g. obesity, diabetes) or lack of aerobic fitness.

Knee

In a systematic review, risk factors of progression of knee OA included age, BMI, varus (or valgus) knee malalignment, OA at multiple sites, and severe radiographic changes.[69,70] There was not enough evidence to say if female gender, impaired function, and greater pain associated with progression of knee OA by themselves.[69] However, in previous studies female gender, young age of onset, and severity of knee symptoms have been associated with a poor outcome.[70,71] Moderate participation in physical activity is not associated with progression of knee OA.[69] However, intense sporting activity, chronic joint effusions, synovitis, and subchondral bone oedema have all been associated with progressive knee OA.[72] In one study of hospital-referred patients, only the presence of inflammation and CPPD was associated with progression.[73] However, in more recent studies chondrocalcinosis did not associate with radiographic progression of knee OA. In addition to increased morbidity, knee OA is also associated with increased mortality.[61]

Hip

Again the prognosis may be reasonably optimistic. Patients with radiographically severe OA are at a greater risk of structural progression. Over a 10 year period, Danielsson found deterioration in symptoms in only 17% of people with hip OA, while symptoms improved in 59% and completely resolved in 12%. Radiographic progression similarly occurred in only a minority of cases, principally those with an initial superolateral pattern of joint-space loss.[74] Occasional patients with apparently progressive OA which then improves with spontaneous 'healing' on radiographs (remodelling and partial restoration of joint space) are well described, although uncommon.[75] Possible risk factors for progression of hip OA include superior pole migration, atrophic bone response, chondrocalcinosis at other sites,[76] and possibly hip dysplasias.[54] Higher BMI does not associate with progressive hip OA.[54]

Hand

The prognosis for hand OA depends on the clinical subset. Generally speaking patients with nodal OA have better functional outlook than those with erosive OA or thumb-base OA. Prognosis for hand symptoms is worse in people with hand involvement as part of a generalized OA phenotype. Therefore, patients with generalized nodal OA may have a worse outlook for hand function than those with a few nodes, and underlying IPJ OA. For example, in those with hand OA, and OA at other sites, an increase in pain was reported by 40% whereas 26% reported improvement in pain at 6 years follow-up.[77] Over half of these patients reported worse hand function, while over one-quarter reported improvement in hand function at 6 years follow-up.[77]

Spine

Prognosis for OA of the spine is unclear. This is largely because of the difficulty of correlating symptoms with structural change. In cases with either cord or nerve root compression prognosis is unclear, but deterioration is often slow unless there is additional disc protrusion, vascular insult, or trauma.

Osteoarthritis with coexisting crystal deposition

The natural history of CPPD + OA is poorly documented. Despite often severe symptoms and structural change at presentation, one 5 year, hospital-based, prospective study suggests that most patients run a benign course. Symptomatic deterioration occurred mainly in large lower limb joints (i.e. knees and hips), but even in severely affected knees, two-thirds of patients showed stabilization or improvement of symptoms. The commonest radiographic change is an increase in osteophyte with bone remodelling, rather than progressive cartilage and bone attrition. A recent community-based prospective study of knee OA did not report any association between CC and progressive joint-space narrowing.[61] Nevertheless, severe, progressive 'destructive arthropathy' may occasionally occur, particularly at the knee, shoulder, and hip, especially in elderly women. The prognosis of apatite-associated destructive arthropathy is seemingly poor with the majority requiring joint replacement.

Conclusion

OA targets specific joints including the knees, interphalangeal joints, thumb bases, and hips. It presents with 'mechanical' joint pain, short-lived morning stiffness, and locomotor restriction. Clinical signs include bony enlargement, locomotor restriction, articular or periarticular tenderness, and muscle wasting.

Clinically severe OA is characterized by rest pain, night pain, and joint deformity. CPP or basic calcium phosphate crystals may coexist with OA.

References

1. McAlindon TE, Snow S, Cooper C, Dieppe PA. Radiographic patterns of osteoarthritis of the knee joint in the community: the importance of the patellofemoral joint. *Ann Rheum Dis* 1992;51(7):844–849.
2. Thorstensson CA, Andersson ML, Jonsson H, Saxne T, Petersson IF. Natural course of knee osteoarthritis in middle-aged subjects with knee pain: 12-year follow-up using clinical and radiographic criteria. *Ann Rheum Dis* 2009;68(12):1890–1893.
3. Lane NE, Brandt K, Hawker G et al. OARSI-FDA initiative: defining the disease state of osteoarthritis. *Osteoarthritis Cartilage* 2011;19(5):478–482.
4. Thompson LR, Boudreau R, Newman AB et al. The association of osteoarthritis risk factors with localized, regional and diffuse knee pain. *Osteoarthritis Cartilage* 2010;18(10):1244–1249.
5. Hawker GA, Stewart L, French MR et al. Understanding the pain experience in hip and knee osteoarthritis—an OARSI/OMERACT initiative. *Osteoarthritis Cartilage* 2008;16(4):415–422.
6. Allen KD, Coffman CJ, Golightly YM, Stechuchak KM, Keefe FJ. Daily pain variations among patients with hand, hip, and knee osteoarthritis. *Osteoarthritis Cartilage* 2009;17(10):1275–1282.
7. Arnoldi CC, Linderholm H, Mussbichler H. Venous engorgement and intraosseous hypertension in osteoarthritis of the hip. *J Bone Joint Surg Br* 1972;54(3):409–421.
8. Goddard NJ, Gosling PT. Intra-articular fluid pressure and pain in osteoarthritis of the hip. *J Bone Joint Surg Br* 1988;70(1):52–55.
9. Yusuf E, Kortekaas MC, Watt I, Huizinga TW, Kloppenburg M. Do knee abnormalities visualised on MRI explain knee pain in knee osteoarthritis? A systematic review. *Ann Rheum Dis* 2011;70(1):60–67.
10. Moisio K, Eckstein F, Chmiel JS et al. Denuded subchondral bone and knee pain in persons with knee osteoarthritis. *Arthritis Rheum* 2009;60(12):3703–3710.
11. Sofat N, Ejindu V, Kiely P. What makes osteoarthritis painful? The evidence for local and central pain processing. *Rheumatology* (Oxford) 2011;50(12):2157–2165.
12. Creamer P, Lethbridge-Cejku M, Hochberg MC. Where does it hurt? Pain localization in osteoarthritis of the knee. *Osteoarthritis Cartilage* 1998;6(5):318–323.
13. Hunter DJ, McDougall JJ, Keefe FJ. The symptoms of osteoarthritis and the genesis of pain. *Med Clin North Am* 2009;93(1):83–100, xi.
14. Suri P, Morgenroth DC, Kwoh CK et al. Low back pain and other musculoskeletal pain comorbidities in individuals with symptomatic osteoarthritis of the knee: data from the osteoarthritis initiative. *Arthritis Care Res* (Hoboken) 2010;62(12):1715–1723.
15. van Meurs JB, Uitterlinden AG, Stolk L et al. A functional polymorphism in the catechol-O-methyltransferase gene is associated with osteoarthritis-related pain. *Arthritis Rheum* 2009;60(2):628–629.
16. Valdes AM, De Wilde G, Doherty SA et al. The Ile585Val TRPV1 variant is involved in risk of painful knee osteoarthritis. *Ann Rheum Dis* 2011;70(9):1556–1561.
17. Davis MA, Ettinger WH, Neuhaus JM, Barclay JD, Segal MR. Correlates of knee pain among US adults with and without radiographic knee osteoarthritis. *J Rheumatol* 1992;19(12):1943–1949.
18. O'Reilly SC, Jones A, Muir KR, Doherty M. Quadriceps weakness in knee osteoarthritis: the effect on pain and disability. *Ann Rheum Dis* 1998;57(10):588–594.
19. Creamer P, Lethbridge-Cejku M, Hochberg MC. Factors associated with functional impairment in symptomatic knee osteoarthritis. *Rheumatology* (Oxford) 2000;39(5):490–496.
20. Tarigan TJ, Kasjmir YI, Atmakusuma D et al. The degree of radiographic abnormalities and postural instability in patients with knee osteoarthritis. *Acta Med Indones* 2009;41(1):15–19.

21. van Saase JL, van Romunde LK, Cats A, Vandenbroucke JP, Valkenburg HA. Epidemiology of osteoarthritis: Zoetermeer survey. Comparison of radiological osteoarthritis in a Dutch population with that in 10 other populations. *Ann Rheum Dis* 1989;48(4):271–280.

22. Altman RD. Classification of disease: osteoarthritis. *Semin Arthritis Rheum* 1991;20(6 Suppl 2):40–47.

23. Doherty M, Watt I, Dieppe P. Influence of primary generalised osteoarthritis on development of secondary osteoarthritis. *Lancet* 1983;2(8340):8–11.

24. Kellgren JH, Moore R. Generalized osteoarthritis and Heberden's nodes. *Br Med J* 1952;1(4751):181–187.

25. Kellgren JH, Lawrence JS, Bier F. Genetic factors in generalized osteo-arthrosis. *Ann Rheum Dis* 1963;22:237–255.

26. Lawrence JS. Generalized osteoarthrosis in a population sample. *Am J Epidemiol* 1969;90(5):381–389.

27. Altman R, Asch E, Bloch et al. Development of criteria for the classifica-tion and reporting of osteoarthritis. Classification of osteoarthritis of the knee. Diagnostic and Therapeutic Criteria Committee of the American Rheumatism Association. *Arthritis Rheum* 1986;29(8):1039–1049.

28. Zhang W, Doherty M, Leeb BF et al. EULAR evidence-based recom-mendations for the diagnosis of hand osteoarthritis: report of a task force of ESCISIT. *Ann Rheum Dis* 2009;68(1):8–17.

29. Altman R, Alarcon G, Appelrouth D et al. The American College of Rheumatology criteria for the classification and reporting of osteoar-thritis of the hand. *Arthritis Rheum* 1990;33(11):1601–1610.

30. Croft P, Cooper C, Wickham C, Coggon D. Is the hip involved in gener-alized osteoarthritis? *Br J Rheumatol* 1992;31(5):325–328.

31. Dahaghin S, Bierma-Zeinstra SM, Ginai AZ et al. Prevalence and pattern of radiographic hand osteoarthritis and association with pain and disability (the Rotterdam study). *Ann Rheum Dis* 2005;64(5):682–687.

32. Williams WV, Cope R, Gaunt WD et al. Metacarpophalangeal arthropa-thy associated with manual labor (Missouri metacarpal syndrome). Clinical radiographic, and pathologic characteristics of an unusual degeneration process. *Arthritis Rheum* 1987;30(12):1362–1371.

33. Punzi L, Ramonda R, Sfriso P. Erosive osteoarthritis. *Best Pract Res Clin Rheumatol* 2004;18(5):739–758.

34. Punzi L, Frigato M, Frallonardo P, Ramonda R. Inflammatory osteoar-thritis of the hand. *Best Pract Res Clin Rheumatol* 2010;24(3):301–312.

35. Kwok WY, Kloppenburg M, Rosendaal FR et al. Erosive hand osteoarthri-tis: its prevalence and clinical impact in the general population and symp-tomatic hand osteoarthritis. *Ann Rheum Dis* 2011;70(7):1238–1242.

36. Bijsterbosch J, van Bemmel JM, Watt I et al. Systemic and local factors are involved in the evolution of erosions in hand osteoarthritis. *Ann Rheum Dis* 2011;70(2):326–330.

37. Cobby M, Cushnaghan J, Creamer P, Dieppe P, Watt I. Erosive osteoar-thritis: is it a separate disease entity? *Clin Radiol* 1990;42(4):258–263.

38. Duncan RC, Hay EM, Saklatvala J, Croft PR. Prevalence of radiographic osteoarthritis—it all depends on your point of view. *Rheumatology* (Oxford) 2006;45(6):757–760.

39. Ledingham J, Regan M, Jones A, Doherty M. Radiographic patterns and associations of osteoarthritis of the knee in patients referred to hospital. *Ann Rheum Dis* 1993;52(7):520–526.

40. Wood LR, Peat G, Thomas E, Duncan R. Knee osteoarthritis in com-munity-dwelling older adults: are there characteristic patterns of pain location? *Osteoarthritis Cartilage* 2007;15(6):615–623.

41. Zhang W, Doherty M, Peat G et al. EULAR evidence-based recom-mendations for the diagnosis of knee osteoarthritis. *Ann Rheum Dis* 2010;69(3):483–489.

42. Cibere J, Zhang H, Thorne A et al. Association of clinical findings with pre-radiographic and radiographic knee osteoarthritis in a population-based study. *Arthritis Care Res* (Hoboken) 2010;62(12):1691–1698.

43. Hill CL, Gale DR, Chaisson CE et al. Periarticular lesions detected on magnetic resonance imaging: prevalence in knees with and without symptoms. *Arthritis Rheum* 2003;48(10):2836–2844.

44. O'Reilly S. Signs, symptoms, and laboratory tests. In: Brandt KD, Doherty M, Lohmander LS (eds) *Osteoarthritis*. Oxford University Press, Oxford, 2003:197–210.

45. Bhattacharyya T, Gale D, Dewire P et al. The clinical importance of meniscal tears demonstrated by magnetic resonance imaging in oste-oarthritis of the knee. *J Bone Joint Surg Am* 2003;85-A(1):4–9.

46. Gofton JP. Studies in osteoarthritis of the hip. I. Classification. *Can Med Assoc J* 1971;104(8):679–683.

47. Jacobsen S, Sonne-Holm S. Hip dysplasia: a significant risk factor for the development of hip osteoarthritis. A cross-sectional survey. *Rheumatology* (Oxford) 2005;44(2):211–218.

48. Gosvig KK, Jacobsen S, Sonne-Holm S, Palm H, Troelsen A. Prevalence of malformations of the hip joint and their relationship to sex, groin pain, and risk of osteoarthritis: a population-based survey. *J Bone Joint Surg Am* 2010;92(5):1162–1169.

49. Birrell F, Croft P, Cooper C et al. Predicting radiographic hip osteoarthritis from range of movement. *Rheumatology* (Oxford) 2001;40(5):506–512.

50. Altman R, Alarcon G, Appelrouth D et al. The American College of Rheumatology criteria for the classification and reporting of osteoar-thritis of the hip. *Arthritis Rheum* 1991;34(5):505–514.

51. Williams BS, Cohen SP. Greater trochanteric pain syndrome: a review of anatomy, diagnosis and treatment. *Anesth Analg* 2009;108(5):1662–1670.

52. Ledingham J, Dawson S, Preston B, Milligan G, Doherty M. Radiographic patterns and associations of osteoarthritis of the hip. *Ann Rheum Dis* 1992;51(10):1111–1116.

53. Lanyon P, Muir K, Doherty S, Doherty M. Influence of radiographic phenotype on risk of hip osteoarthritis within families. *Ann Rheum Dis* 2004;63(3):259–263.

54. Lievense AM, Bierma-Zeinstra SM, Verhagen AP, Verhaar JA, Koes BW. Prognostic factors of progress of hip osteoarthritis: a systematic review. *Arthritis Rheum* 2002;47(5):556–562.

55. Kalichman L, Hunter DJ. Lumbar facet joint osteoarthritis: a review. *Semin Arthritis Rheum* 2007;37(2):69–80.

56. van Eerd M, Patijn J, Lataster A et al. 5. Cervical facet pain. *Pain Pract* 2010;10(2):113–123.

57. Hutton CW. Generalised osteoarthritis: an evolutionary problem? *Lancet* 1987;1(8548):1463–1465.

58. Fuerst M, Bertrand J, Lammers L et al. Calcification of articular cartilage in human osteoarthritis. *Arthritis Rheum* 2009;60(9):2694–2703.

59. Fuerst M, Niggemeyer O, Lammers L et al. Articular cartilage min-eralization in osteoarthritis of the hip. *BMC Musculoskelet Disord* 2009;10:166.

60. Zhang W, Doherty M, Bardin T et al. European League Against Rheumatism recommendations for calcium pyrophosphate deposition. Part I: terminology and diagnosis. *Ann Rheum Dis* 2011;70(4):563–570.

61. Neogi T, Nevitt M, Niu J et al. Lack of association between chondrocal-cinosis and increased risk of cartilage loss in knees with osteoarthritis: results of two prospective longitudinal magnetic resonance imaging studies. *Arthritis Rheum* 2006;54(6):1822–1828.

62. McCarty DJ, Halverson PB, Carrera GF, Brewer BJ, Kozin F. 'Milwaukee shoulder'—association of microspheroids containing hydroxyapa-tite crystals, active collagenase, and neutral protease with rotator cuff defects. I. Clinical aspects. *Arthritis Rheum* 1981;24(3):464–473.

63. Dieppe PA, Doherty M, Macfarlane DG et al. Apatite associated destruc-tive arthritis. *Br J Rheumatol* 1984;23(2):84–91.

64. Halverson PB, McCarty DJ. Clinical aspects of basic calcium phosphate crystal deposition. *Rheum Dis Clin North Am* 1988;14(2):427–439.

65. NICE. *Osteoarthritis: national clinical guideline for care and management in adults. (CG59).* National Institute for Health and Clinical Excellence, London, 2008.

66. Dieppe P, Cushnaghan J, Tucker M, Browning S, Shepstone L. The Bristol 'OA500 study': progression and impact of the disease after 8 years. *Osteoarthritis Cartilage* 2000;8(2):63–68.

67. Nuesch E, Dieppe P, Reichenbach S, Williams S, Iff S, Juni P. All cause and disease specific mortality in patients with knee or hip osteoarthritis: population based cohort study. *BMJ* 2011;342:d1165.

68. Hochberg MC. Mortality in osteoarthritis. *Clin Exp Rheumatol* 2008;26(5 Suppl 51):S120–S124.

69. Chapple CM, Nicholson H, Baxter GD, Abbott JH. Patient characteristics that predict progression of knee osteoarthritis: a systematic review of prognostic studies. *Arthritis Care Res* (Hoboken) 2011;63(8):1115–1125.

70. Sharma L, Song J, Felson DT et al. The role of knee alignment in disease progression and functional decline in knee osteoarthritis. *JAMA* 2001;286(2):188–195.

71. Hernborg JS, Nilsson BE. The natural course of untreated osteoarthritis of the knee. *Clin Orthop Relat Res* 1977;123:130–137.

72. Bijlsma JW, Berenbaum F, Lafeber FP. Osteoarthritis: an update with relevance for clinical practice. *Lancet* 2011;377(9783):2115–2126.

73. Ledingham J, Regan M, Jones A, Doherty M. Factors affecting radiographic progression of knee osteoarthritis. *Ann Rheum Dis* 1995;54(1):53–58.

74. Danielsson LG. Incidence and prognosis of coxarthrosis. *Acta Orthop Scand Suppl* 1964;66:Suppl 66:1–114.

75. Perry GH, Smith MJ, Whiteside CG. Spontaneous recovery of the joint space in degenerative hip disease. *Ann Rheum Dis* 1972;31(6):440–448.

76. Menkes CJ, Decraemere W, Postel M, Forest M. Chondrocalcinosis and rapid destruction of the hip. *J Rheumatol* 1985;12(1):130–133.

77. Bijsterbosch J, Watt I, Meulenbelt I et al. Clinical and radiographic disease course of hand osteoarthritis and determinants of outcome after 6 years. *Ann Rheum Dis* 2011;70(1):68–73.

Sources of patient information

American College of Rheumatology: www.rheumatology.org

Arthritis Research UK: www.arthritisresearchuk.org/

CHAPTER 140

Osteoarthritis— management

Claire Y. J. Wenham and Philip G. Conaghan

Introduction

Osteoarthritis (OA) is the most common cause of disability in the United Kingdom. The resulting pain, stiffness, joint deformity, and loss of joint mobility can affect every aspect of a person's day-to-day activities, as well as their quality of life. The most common reason that people with OA present to their primary care physician is pain; over 50% of people with OA feel that pain is their worst problem.[1] The OA Nation survey of almost 2000 people with OA found that 81% with OA had constant pain or were limited in performing everyday tasks; when their OA pain was 'bad', over half struggled to get out of bed.[1] Management of OA has therefore focused around symptom management, although the concept of structural modification will also be included in this chapter.

Holistic assessment of osteoarthritis

All modern consensus guidelines recommend holistic assessment of people with OA as an essential part of a management strategy. A relationship in which treatment decisions are made jointly by both physician and patient will enhance a self-management approach. Each consultation should take into account a person's existing concerns and expectations and their available support network.

A typical evaluation of a person with OA would assess:

◆ Severity and extent of joint pain, including the number and pattern of joint involvement, as OA commonly involves multiple joints in the over 50s with differing impairment associations depending on pattern of joint involvement.[2] When are symptoms worse? For example, is knee pain worse at night time and preventing sleep?

◆ Impact of symptoms on daily living activities such as climbing steps or getting dressed.

◆ Impact on participation: what key activities have been prevented by the symptoms? OA is not just a disease of elderly people and many people affected by OA are still in employment. It is essential to judge any OA impact on the ability to perform their job, to determine if adjustments in the workplace necessary. This may be as simple as a new chair or forearm rests for a person with hand OA whose work involves a lot of keyboarding.

◆ Psychological effects of OA. This is very important and should not be underestimated. People with OA report loss of self-esteem, loss of independence and feeling old before their time.[3] Effects on sleep should be noted and if possible, management strategies altered to improve this. Depression is common and should be looked for and treated appropriately.[4]

◆ Previous treatments that a person may have tried. These include over-the-counter medications that a person is using. Note the types of medication that the person has used previously: which they found helpful and which were stopped because of side effects. The timing of analgesics is also important, for example a long-acting (e.g. modified-release) preparation may be more appropriate so that the analgesic effect is at its best during the most symptomatic period of the day or night.

Management of osteoarthritis symptoms

There are a number of recent excellent expert and evidence-based guidelines for the management of OA,[5,6] with some specific for site of OA—hip,[7–9] knee,[6,8–10] and hand.[11] It is of course important to understand the limitations of the published evidence which is used to underpin these guidelines. The majority of OA studies have focused on knee OA, with much fewer studies on the hip and only a small percentage involving the hand. The majority of studies have utilized pharmacological therapies and most are of short-term (typically 12 week) duration. The nature of clinical trials is such that many people with comorbidities are excluded. Taken together, all these factors influence the generalizability of the published evidence base.

The management options presented below are derived from all the major recommendations and where relevant, differences between treatment guidance will be discussed and specific examples cited; for example, the National Institute for Health and Clinical Excellence (NICE) guidance has a health economics perspective relevant to the United Kingdom. The management options for OA hand is considered separately to that of the knee and hip, and the management of OA of the foot is briefly discussed. Examples of the analgesic effect size (ES) of a treatment or intervention are included, with 95% confidence intervals presented in brackets. For

Table 140.1 Table demonstrating the effect size (ES) for pain relief dependent on the quality of clinical trials

	All trials ES (95% CI)	High-quality trials (Jaded = 5) ES (95% CI)
Acupuncture	0.35 (0.15–0.55)	0.22 (0.01–0.44)
Paracetamol	0.14 (0.05–0.23)	0.10 (0.03 to 0.23)
NSAIDs	0.29 (0.22–0.35)	0.39 (0.24–0.55)
Topical NSAIDs	0.44 (0.27–0.62)	0.42 (0.19–0.65)
Intra-articular HA	0.6 (0.37–0.83)	0.22 (0.11 to 0.54)
Glucosamine	0.58 (0.30–0.87)	0.29 (0.003–0.57)
Lavage/debridement	0.21 (−0.12 to 0.54)	−0.11 (−0.3 to 0.08)
Chondroitin	0.75 (0.5–1.01)	0.005 (−0.11 to 0.12)

HA, hyaluronic acid; NSAIDs, non-steroidal anti-inflammatory drugs.
From Zhang.[9]

clinical practice, an ES of 0.2 is considered small, 0.5 is moderate, and greater than 0.8 is large. A recent systematic review noted that the ES for many commonly used treatments is much smaller than previously thought, when only high-quality trials are included in the analysis. This is demonstrated in Table 140.1.[9]

Recent work has highlighted the importance and magnitude of the placebo effect in OA trials.[12] The non-drug-specific contextual effects of a therapy are highly important. This makes interpretation of trial data even more difficult and it is conceivable that many therapies with small ESs may be placebos.

All management guidelines agree that a combination of pharmacological and non-pharmacological treatment options should be considered for all people with OA and that several key or 'core' principles should be offered to all. These core management suggestions include patient education, exercise, and weight loss.

Patient education and information/encouraging self-management strategies

All treatment guidelines agree that everyone with OA should be offered information (e.g. an information booklet) and should be encouraged to take part in self-management programmes, to increase their understanding of the disease and the management options. Any misconceptions about OA, for example that it invariably progresses or that there are no helpful treatments, should be addressed as early as possible. Education may result in fewer visits to primary care, with one study of knee OA showing that 80% of the costs of delivering effective self-care education were offset within the first year by a reduced number of primary care visits.[13] Reliable websites such as those from arthritis societies can be another source of patient-friendly information. Although these interventions have a small ES in terms of analgesia, they improve other drivers of quality of life such as anxiety and self-efficacy.

Exercise

Exercise can be divided into joint-specific muscle strengthening and range of motion exercises, and general aerobic exercise. Generally, muscle strengthening is important before attempting aerobic exercise. For people with knee OA who cannot straight-leg raise, quadriceps exercises should be advised and forearm strengthening exercises advised for those with hand OA and weak grip. People should be encouraged to continue these exercises on a regular basis, setting personal achievement targets. It is important to consider analgesia at the time of exercise: this might mean taking medications prior to exercising or even intra-articular corticosteroid (see below). Exercise may be self-led or supervised in individual or group sessions, on land or in water. Exercise in water may be more comfortable for those with knee or hip OA and is effective for both hip and knee OA.[14] The benefits of exercise for knee OA are well known, with improvements in both knee pain and function, with a systematic review demonstrating the benefits of both aerobic walking and home-based quadriceps exercises for pain relief, with an ES of up to 0.52.[15] Although there is less available evidence for hip OA, exercise has also been shown to improve pain in hip OA (ES 0.38).[16] There is surprisingly little published evidence for exercises alone in hand OA so this recommendation is based on expert opinion.[11]

Weight loss (if overweight)

Weight loss, in order to maintain a body mass index (BMI) within normal range, (19–25) is advisable. Obesity is associated with the development and progression of knee OA[17] and weight loss reduces the adverse mechanical forces across a damaged joint. Weight loss can result in a small improvement in function and pain in knee OA[9,18] and although the evidence for the benefits of weight loss in hip OA is very limited, it is still recommended, as it will benefit the person's overall health.[7,9]

Once the core treatment options have been offered to all, a range of other treatments can be considered (Figure 140.1).

Non-pharmacological treatments

In addition to exercise and weight loss (if needed), additional non-drug treatments should be considered for all people with OA. These include simple therapies such as thermotherapy (applying heat or cold to the painful joint), an easy self-management therapy with good safety and very low cost, although there is little evidence for its effectiveness.

Acupuncture

Acupuncture is not a single intervention as it may applied in different ways (e.g. Western or traditional Chinese application) and

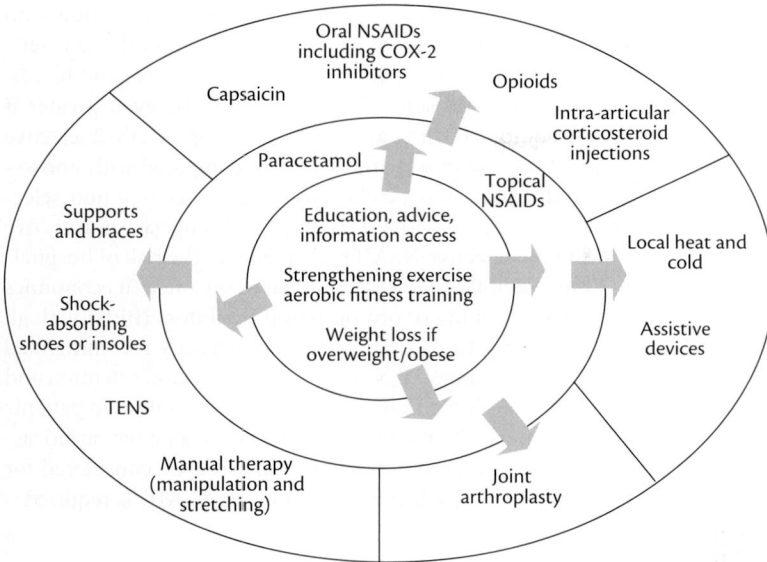

Fig. 140.1 Targeting osteoarthritis therapy.
Reproduced from BMJ Conaghan PG, Dickson J, Grant RL. Care and management of osteoarthritis in adults: summary of NICE guidance. 2008;336(7642):502–3 with permission from BMJ publishing group.

often in combination with other therapies. Acupuncture involves positioning fine needles around the site of pain and possibly in other sites, and the needles may be stimulated electrically (electroacupuncture). The neurophysiological mechanism of action of acupuncture is unclear but the release of endogenous opioids has been suggested; the contextual effect of application is important.[19] Courses of acupuncture may involve 6–12 sessions but repeat courses may be required. One difficulty of assessing trials which use acupuncture is that there is no adequate placebo—it is impossible to blind patient or therapist—and even 'sham' acupuncture, when the needles are put in the wrong site or not stimulated, is not thought to be an inactive placebo. Accepting this limitation, several systematic reviews and a recent meta-analysis have concluded that there is evidence for a short-term benefit of acupuncture for people with OA.[9] The ES for pain relief when compared to sham acupuncture is 0.35 (95% confidence interval 0.15–0.55). However, the benefit is usually short-lived, with the ES falling to 0.13 6 months after treatment.[9]

Transcutaneous electrical nerve stimulation

Transcutaneous electrical nerve stimulation (TENS) may stimulate specific nerve fibres via pulsed currents which are delivered through electrodes placed on the skin.[20] Only a few small studies have evaluated the use of TENS and suggest a minimal effect; however, it is a safe treatment that may provide some people with short-term pain relief.

Electromagnetic therapy

This is postulated to work by increasing blood flow to the stimulated area. However, as there is no good evidence for the benefit of electromagnetic therapy in OA,[9] it is not a recommended treatment.

Aids and devices

There is a surprising lack of good trial data in this area of OA treatment. There is no strong evidence to suggest that insoles (wedged or neutral) are of benefit in improving the symptoms of knee OA,[9] although they are recommended in recent management guidelines.[6] However, all people with lower limb OA should be advised

on sensible footwear, usually a flexible, shock-absorbing sole, broad fit, and with arch support.

A walking stick can provide some relief (when held in the contralateral hand to the affected knee or hip) and guidelines support their use if a person finds it helpful.[5,9,10] A knee brace, for those with OA knee with a varus or valgus deformity and instability, can reduce pain and improve function and may also reduce the risk of falls.[9] Specific referral to an orthotics department may be needed to provide a brace. Disability equipment assessment centres can provide expert advice for people struggling with activities of daily living. Likewise, a referral to occupational therapy may be useful for anyone whose joint disease results in significant impact on their day-to-day activities.

Pharmacological treatments for osteoarthritis

The potential side effects of pharmacological therapies must be considered before prescribing, particularly in elderly patients and those with other comorbidities, which are frequent in the OA population. After starting a pharmacological therapy, a person must be reviewed to judge the benefits and any potential side effects, so that treatment can be altered if needed.

Paracetamol

The mechanism of action of paracetamol (acetaminophen) is not completely understood, although it is known to be a weak inhibitor of the cyclo-oxygenase pathway,[21] thereby having anti-inflammatory effects; it also acts on the endogenous cannabinoid receptors.[22] The previous evidence from the few well conducted randomized, controlled trials (RCTs) for the effectiveness of paracetamol for the relief of pain in knee and hip OA[23] demonstrated a small overall ES of 0.21. However, updated management guidelines, which include clinical trials published up to 2009, have noted that the effect size is even smaller than previously thought at 0.14 and if only high-quality trials are assessed, the ES is minimal (0.109). Despite this, all current guidelines recommend that paracetamol should be a first-line treatment if additional analgesia is required after the core management options have been initiated. Regular dosing may be needed to achieve maximum analgesic effect. However there is some recent evidence of dose-dependent adverse gastrointestinal (GI) events,[12,24] and such data has led to the United States Food and Drug Administration (FDA) recently recommending that maximum adult daily dose of paracetamol should be less than 4 g daily.

Topical non-steroidal anti-inflammatory drugs

Topical non-steroidal anti-inflammatory drugs (NSAIDs) are effective analgesics for knee OA and they have a good safety record.[10] Most studies have evaluated diclofenac or ibuprofen. They are safer than oral NSAIDs as the plasma concentration is less than 15% of the equivalent dose of oral NSAID.[25] The ES (including high-quality trials) is moderate (0.42), although patients may need to be reminded that regular application may be required for the maximal benefit. Side effects from topical NSAIDs are uncommon but may include skin irritation at the site of application. Topical NSAIDs are not recommended for hip OA.

Topical capsaicin

Topical capsaicin cream (0.025% applied 4 times daily) reversibly desensitizes nociceptive C-fibres by acting on vanilloid receptors. This is an additional topical treatment that could be considered before prescribing oral treatments, although it may be relatively expensive. The data for the efficacy of capsaicin in knee OA is limited, hence it was not recommended in the recently published American College of Rheumatology (ACR) guidance.[6] Systemic side effects have not been reported although up to 40% of users will experience local redness or irritation.[9] Patients should be warned of this and advised to wash their hands after use. Patients should be advised that regular application is required for the maximum benefit, which may not be evident for several days.

Oral non-steroidal anti-inflammatory drugs

NSAIDs act by reducing the production of pain-inducing and proinflammatory prostaglandins. They can be broadly divided into selective and non-selective, depending on the differential inhibition of the cyclo-oxygenase (COX) enzymes COX-1 (important in maintaining a healthy GI mucosa) and COX-2 (unregulated at sites of inflammation; blocking this enzyme may alter the balance between pro- and anti-thrombotic mediators). Selective COX-2 inhibitor drugs have a lower incidence of GI side effects but, like all NSAIDs, a definite prothrombotic risk. NSAIDs are covered in detail in Chapter 77.

NSAIDs are effective analgesics in OA. However, there are difficulties with the current trial data in that detailed data is only available for the newer NSAIDs and the doses of drugs used in clinical trials may not represent the doses prescribed or used by patients on a day-to-day basis. Furthermore, the patients recruited to clinical trials of NSAIDs are not usually representative of the typical OA population, who tend to have other comorbidities. Head-to-head comparisons have demonstrated that NSAIDs are superior to paracetamol for pain relief in knee and hip OA, with the most recent review of trials demonstrating a greater ES (0.29) compared with paracetamol (0.149).[26] COX-2 selective drugs and non-selective NSAIDs demonstrate similar pain relief in clinical trials of knee OA.[5]

NSAIDs have potential renal, cardiovascular (CV), and GI side effects; these must be taken into account when prescribing and should be reviewed on a regular basis. NSAIDs should be used at the lowest effective dose for the shortest possible time, in order to minimize potential side effects. GI side effects are common with NSAID use, both gastric upset (discomfort or dyspepsia) and serious GI side effects such as peptic ulcers, perforations, and bleeds. The risk of serious GI side effects appears to be even greater if NSAIDs are combined with paracetamol.[24] Using a COX-2 selective drug reduces the risk of a serious GI event compared with non-selective NSAID,[24] and may be chosen in preference to a non-selective NSAID in a patient with GI risk factors. Using gastroprotective agents with non-selective NSAIDs also reduces the risk of hospitalization from a serious GI event[27] and based on a health economics analysis, the prescribing of proton pump inhibitors (PPIs) with all NSAIDs (including COX-2 inhibitors) is currently recommended in the United Kingdom.[5] All NSAIDs may cause fluid retention and aggravate hypertension and should be used with caution in patients with CV risk factors. Naproxen appears to have a better cardiovascular risk profile[28] than other NSAIDs and maybe considered for any patient with CV risk factors for whom an NSAID is required.

Opioids

Opioids work by acting on endogenous opioid receptors, although the differing opioid drugs may act on different receptor subtypes; they are also reviewed in Chapter 78. Opioids have a role in treating OA pain, and are recommended in evidence-based treatment guidelines, although their use is often limited by side effects, with around one-quarter of people treated with opioids in clinical trials withdrawing due to side effects. The most common reported side effects are nausea (30%), constipation (23%), dizziness (20%), drowsiness (18%), and vomiting (13%).[29] Opioids should be considered if paracetamol and topical NSAIDs have been ineffective in controlling symptoms, and if non-pharmacological treatments have also been instigated, but the side-effect profile must be born in mind when prescribing, particularly for elderly patients who are more prone to side effects.

A large meta-analysis[29] showed a moderate ES for pain relief with opioids in OA (0.78, 95% CI 0.59–0.98) and a small to moderate ES for improvement in function (0.31, 95% CI 0.24–0.39). There was a wide variety in the outcomes of the studies included in the analysis, which did not seem to be related to the type of opioid used. Oxycodone, fentanyl, and morphine sulphate were noted to be more likely to result in side effects which result in stopping the drug than tramadol or codeine. Opioids are available in different preparations. For example, fentanyl and buprenorphine are provided in transdermal patches which may improve patient compliance; and long-acting preparations, for example modified-release tramadol, may be useful for night pain.

Intra-articular corticosteroid

Corticosteroids (CS) have a potent anti-inflammatory action via a reduction in proinflammatory chemicals; they inhibit the production of interleukins (IL)-1 and IL-6 and tumour necrosis factor (TNFα) as well as decreasing the expression of COX-2. Intra-articular (IA) corticosteroid to the OA knee is not recommended for an isolated asymptomatic joint effusion but for the relief of moderate pain that has failed to respond to oral or topical analgesics. The period of pain relief post-injection is the ideal time to reinforce regular quadriceps strengthening exercises. IA CS is effective in the short-term (up to 4 weeks) for the relief of pain in knee OA,[30] although the evidence suggests a smaller effect on function. The ES is particularly high 1 week after injection (0.72,

95% CI 0.41–1.01) but falls to 0.28 after just 4 weeks.[9] One analysis assessing repeated IA corticosteroid injections every 3 months for 2 years noted a persistently high ES (0.67) for the first year of treatment but this had fallen to 0.25 by the second year.[30] There is no clear evidence on whether a particular preparation of CS is more effective than another[5]; an example of a CS used for the knee joint would be 80 mg methylprednisolone or 40 mg triamcinolone.

As yet, there are no current reliable predictors of response to IA steroid to the OA knee. Knees that have effusion may respond better,[31] but this has not been demonstrated in all studies.[32] IA CS is associated with few side effects and the risk of infection is very small.[5] Patients should be warned of potential fat atrophy, which can result in a cosmetic defect, and that symptoms may worsen transiently after injection. Although there have been concerns over potential cartilage toxicity with repeated CS injections, this remains controversial although as a general rule, IA CS should not be offered more than 4 times in a 12 month period.[8]

Although previous studies of IA corticosteroid to the OA hip demonstrated varying benefit,[33,34] a recent RCT demonstrated good pain relief at 8 weeks after IA CS[35]; IA CS could be used for patients with moderate to severe pain who are not responding to analgesics/NSAIDs.[9]

Intra-articular hyaluronan

Hyaluronic acid (also known as hyaluronan, HA) is a glycosaminoglycan (GAG) and a constituent of synovial fluid responsible for its viscous properties. In OA there is reduced HA quantity and quality and the theory of viscosupplementation is to restore good-quality HA in the joint. Several preparations are available with differing molecular weight and manufacturing sources and HA preparations may be administered as single or weekly injections over a period of 3–5 weeks. This heterogeneity of products and their applications makes the trial data complex to interpret. Although some studies suggest HA may give improved longer-term pain relief when compared with IA CS,[36] a recent analysis using only high-quality trials suggests a small ES of just 0.22 (−0.11 to 0.54).[9] There is even less evidence to support the use of HA in hip OA. Although some open-label studies noted an improvement in symptoms,[37] the only placebo-controlled RCT did not show a benefit of HA over CS or IA saline.[38]

IA HA may result in transient pain or swelling at the injection site, which is more likely with the higher molecular weight preparations.[9] There is disagreement among the OA treatment guidelines as to whether HA should be prescribed and it is not yet possible to predict which patients may show a better response.

Glucosamine/chondroitin

Glucosamine is an amino sugar that is a precursor in the production of glycosylated proteins, including GAGs. Chondroitin sulphate is a sulphated GAG. The rationale for these agents is that the limiting factor for the GAG component of cartilage may be the availability of substrates such as glucosamine and chondroitin sulphate. However, the mode of action of both of these agents remains controversial. Neither is licensed by the FDA so they are marketed in the United States as health food supplements. Analysis of previous trials is made difficult by the varying preparations of glucosamine and chondroitin, differing study populations, and differing analgesic use at the time of assessment. Trials of glucosamine sulphate for pain relief in knee OA have shown that the ES for pain is small

when only high-quality trials are considered, although there is very little evidence of harm. The analgesic efficacy of glucosamine hydrochloride is poor, with an ES of just 0.13 (0.02–0.259) Likewise the evidence for pain relief with chondroitin, when just high-quality trials are analysed, is very poor (ES 0.005).[9] The most recent meta-analysis, published in 2010, assessing the effectiveness of glucosamine and chondroitin at both symptom and structure modification for the OA joint concluded that neither has any benefit on pain or structure modification.[39] If patients remain keen to try glucosamine for symptomatic relief of OA, then a three-month trial of 1.5 g of glucosamine sulphate could be suggested as the drug is thought to be very safe, although patients should be advised to stop the treatment if no benefit is noted at 3 months.

Other nutritional supplements

Systematic reviews concluded that there were methodological flaws in the trials of methylsulphonylmethane (MSM), green-lipped muscle extract, and dimethyl sulphoxide (DMSO), so no definite evidence was available. However, the larger, better-designed RCTs of MSM do suggest a small benefit of 3 g MSM twice a day in decreasing pain and improving functional status.[40] The evidence for the efficacy of avocado soybean unsaponifiable (ASU) in trials combining hip and knee OA suggests a small symptomatic benefit in pain reduction (ES 0.39), although the ES reduces to 0.22 (−0.06 to 0.51) when only high-quality trials are assessed.[9] There is no good evidence for the symptomatic or structural benefit of ASU in the treatment of hip OA.[9]

Structure modification

Structure modification of OA with its potential for concomitant or subsequent reduction in symptoms remains an elusive goal of OA therapies. There are as yet no agents with regulatory approval as structure-modifying drugs. Current regulatory requirements mandate radiographic joint space width as the structural outcome of interest (as a surrogate measure of hyaline cartilage) and require an additional symptom-modifying component. The complexities of repositioning a given joint in longitudinal studies have made joint space width a difficult outcome measure to understand,[41] and in future MRI quantification of OA structural pathology may improve understanding in this area.

There is still controversy as to whether glucosamine or chondroitin may have structure-modifying effects in the OA joint. Trials of glucosamine are inconclusive,[9] but a recent meta-analysis suggests neither glucosamine nor chondroitin has structure-modifying effects.[39] Diacerhein is an anthraquinone derivative, thought to act via the inhibition of IL-1B. Its effect on symptoms is minimal (ES 0.24, 0.08–0.39), with considerable heterogeneity between trials. Diarrhoea is a significant side effect, especially at higher doses.[9] Diacerhein may slow the progression of joint space narrowing in the hip over a 3 year treatment period,[42] but because of its side effects it is not a widely accepted treatment for hip OA.

Bone as a target of structure modification?

Although historic studies have focused on hyaline cartilage as the main target of structure-modifying therapies, the subchondral bone may be a target for treatment in OA, as subchondral bone abnormalities seen on MRI have been associated with pain[43] and progression of cartilage loss. Histological studies have demonstrated altered trabecular structure within these areas[44,45] and there is also evidence of increased bone turnover in OA.[46] A large, multinational trial of a bisphosphonate, risedronate, noted that urinary levels of C-terminal cross-linking telopeptide of type II collagen (CTX-II), a marker of cartilage degradation, were reduced with risedronate but despite this, there was no reduction in radiographic structural progression or symptoms at 2 years.[47] However a recent trial using zoledronic acid (ZA) vs placebo infusion in people with MRI bone marrow lesions (BMLs) demonstrated that the ZA group had a reduction in total BML area and a small improvement in pain compared with the placebo group at 6 months. At 12 months, the total BML area was still significantly lower in the ZA group but this was not associated with any reduction in pain compared to the placebo group.[48]

There is evidence that oral salmon calcitonin, strontium ranelate, the selective oestrogen receptor modulator levomeloxifene, and oestrogen replacement therapy also lower CTX-II levels,[49–51] and preliminary results from recent trials have suggested structure modification for both strontium ranelate and calcitonin[52,53] in OA of the knee. Strontium demonstrated a reduction in joint space narrowing compared to placebo over a 3 year period, as well as an improvement in clinical symptoms.[53] Although the study using calcitonin in 1200 knees did not show a difference in reduction in joint space narrowing over 2 years, there was an increase in cartilage volume of 5% compared to 2.5% in the placebo group, suggesting potential structure-modifying effects of calcitonin.[52]

Treatment of hand osteoarthritis

Despite the high prevalence of symptomatic hand OA,[54] current therapies for hand OA are limited and there is a lack of high-quality RCTs for assessing treatments for hand OA.[55] As with the knee and hip, treatments can be divided into non-pharmacological and pharmacological, and general information and advice with regard to joint protection and exercises, both to improve range of motion and local strengthening exercises (forearm strengthening) should be provided to all people with hand OA. People with hand OA with hand pain and difficulty in performing everyday tasks should be referred to occupational therapy for assessment, advice and if needed, the provision of splints and devices to help with activities of daily living (e.g. tap turners). Simple treatments which the patient can initiate includes local application of heat (e.g. hot pack, paraffin wax); although there are no trials to support this, it may be effective and is very safe.

Aid and devices

The use of a splint for base of thumb (first carpometacarpal (CMC)) OA is a safe and effective therapy recommended in current management guidelines. A recent RCT assessed the use of a thumb base splint vs usual care and demonstrated that by 12 months, those using a splint had significantly reduced pain and disability.[56]

Oral analgesics

Paracetamol is the first oral pharmacological treatment of choice as recommended by current management guidelines; however, there are no placebo-controlled trials of paracetamol in hand OA, and paracetamol is recommended (at doses of up to 4 g per day) because of its previously good safety profile, low cost, and data showing some effectiveness (albeit small ES) in OA trials of other joints. There are few placebo-controlled trials of NSAIDs in the short-term treatment of hand OA, which show that oral NSAIDs are effective in the short-term at reducing pain in hand OA (ES 0.4, 0.2–0.6)[57] and could be used for those who have pain despite paracetamol and topical NSAIDs. However, potential side effects must be noted before prescribing, and NSAIDs should be used at the lowest effective dose and for the shortest possible time period. Opioids such as tramadol may be considered for those with persistent severe symptoms,[6] although side effects may limit its use, particularly in elderly people. There is very little data for the use of glucosamine, chondroitin, ASU, or diacerhein in hand OA. To date, there are no trials of diacerhein or ASU in hand OA.[57]

Topical therapies

Topical NSAIDs are an effective treatment for relieving pain in hand OA (ES 0.77, 0.32–1.22) and appear to have no more GI side effects than placebo.[57] Their effect size is higher than that for oral NSAIDs and the side-effect profile is much better. Topical NSAIDs could be used as an alternative or in addition to paracetamol for people who still have symptoms, although patients may need to be reminded that regular application may be required for the maximal effect. Two short-term (4 weeks) studies of topical capsaicin (0.025% four times a day) for hand OA have demonstrated that it is a useful treatment.[57] It may be a particularly useful therapy for those who are intolerant or at high risk of adverse events from oral analgesics, although it is relatively expensive. Patients should be warned of the potential redness or irritation, which occurs in around 40%, and that the drug must be used for several consecutive days to achieve maximum benefit.

Intra-articular therapies

There is one placebo-controlled RCT of IA corticosteroid to the first CMC joint in hand OA, which failed to show any benefit above placebo, although the study terminated early because of difficulty in recruitment.[58] Open-label studies have shown a short-term reduction (up to 6 weeks) in pain after IA corticosteroid to the first CMC joint[59–61]; the ACR management guidance did not support the use of IA corticosteroid due to the lack of clinical trials,[6] although other guidelines have supported the use of this therapy. IA CS to the base of thumb could be considered for those with persistent symptoms despite a trial of oral or topical analgesia. There is no well-designed RCT of HA in CMC OA.

Treatment of foot osteoarthritis

OA of the first metatarsophalangeal (MTP) joint is extremely common, but there is increasing evidence that midfoot OA is also common. Using a newly developed foot atlas, an Australian community cohort study (n = 197) showed radiographic OA was significantly more prevalent at the midfoot (60%) than the first MTP joint (42%) using anteroposterior and lateral foot views.[62]

Most of the available data for treatment of MTP OA pertains to surgical intervention and there is very little data for any other treatments. There is a lack of RCTs or systematic reviews that assess the effectiveness of either corticosteroid or HA injections to the OA foot. A recent trial noted that IA HA is no more effective than placebo in improving the symptoms of first MTP OA.[63] In clinical practice, injecting a small amount of corticosteroid into an osteoarthritic foot joint may provide some short-term relief but there is little evidence to support this.[64] A recent month-long investigation of functional foot orthoses highlighted that midfoot OA was associated with adverse biomechanics and that in-shoe orthoses have the potential to improve in foot pain and walking function in midfoot OA.[65] Further studies are needed to confirm this.

Surgical treatments for osteoarthritis

The wide variety of surgical interventions and their indication cannot be adequately covered in this chapter. Some common procedures are therefore briefly overviewed.

Joint replacement

Total knee arthroplasty involves the removal of the distal portion of the femur, proximal part of the tibia, and the anterior cruciate ligament and replacement of the damaged surfaces with metal prostheses, either with or without cement. Total hip arthroplasty involves replacing the acetabulum and the head and neck of the femur with prostheses. These operations are becoming increasingly common, with over 160 000 total hip and knee joint replacements performed in England and Wales last year. Hip resurfacing has been developed as an alternative to total hip replacement and consists of placing a metal cap over the head of the femur while a matching metal cup is placed in the acetabulum. This replaces the articulating surfaces of the hip but removes less bone than with a total joint replacement and may be considered for younger, active males.[66]

Total joint replacement is a safe and effective but irreversible treatment option for which a patient should be referred when a combination of non-pharmacological and pharmacological treatments has been tried and the patient still has significant symptoms that are substantially impacting on their life. Ideally, referral should be made before pain becomes severe or before an individual has longstanding functional difficulties, and patient factors such as obesity, smoking, or other comorbidities should not be a barrier to referral. A recent international study has demonstrated that there is no specific level of either pain or function that indicates the need for a joint replacement,[67] hence the decision for surgery should be made after discussion with the patient and clinician, and cannot rely on currently available scoring tools.

Studies note a significant reduction in pain and improvement in function after total joint replacement, with pain improving in particular in the first 3–6 months after surgery.[68] Revision rates at 10 years after total joint replacement have been reported as 7% for the hip and 10% for the knee.[69,70]

Unicompartmental knee replacement

This may be a treatment option for those with just one compartment of the knee affected (around 30% of those with knee OA), with similar outcomes for pain and function improvement.[9,71] The medial compartment is most commonly replaced, although the lateral compartment may also be suitable. In selected patients with patellofemoral compartment disease and no tibiofemoral OA, a patellofemoral replacement, although infrequently performed and usually only at specialist centres, may be an option.[71]

Arthroscopic lavage and debridement for knee osteoarthritis

A recent systematic review noted that there is no evidence for any benefit of arthroscopic lavage and debridement for the OA knee

above placebo.[9] Referral for arthroscopy should be reserved for those with a clear history of mechanical locking of the joint, suggestive of a meniscal tear or other loose body within the joint. The presence of loose bodies on imaging is not a reason to refer for an arthroscopy unless there is associated locking. Locking should not be confused with gelling of the joint, which is stiffening of a joint with rest (e.g. after sitting in a fixed position for a period of time).

Osteotomy

Osteotomy involves cutting and reshaping the tibia in order to alter the biomechanics of the knee joint in order to transfer the load-bearing area from the damaged to the normal compartment of the joint. The best evidence is for a high tibial osteotomy for medial knee OA, whereby a wedge of lateral tibia is removed. Although a systematic review noted that osteotomy results in improved pain and function, it is not known whether an osteotomy is better than no treatment at all, or which surgical technique is best.[72] Osteotomy may be considered for younger patients to delay the need for arthroplasty.[73]

Joint distraction

This is a technique whereby the bony ends of a joint are gradually separated over a period of time, using an external fixator to unload the joint. Preliminary studies of joint distraction have shown promising results, with improved pain scores and structural modification in both the ankle and knee,[74,75] but this technique is not yet in clinical use and needs further validation.

Surgery for hand osteoarthritis

Surgery should be considered for people with severe thumb base OA who are not responding to other treatments. Surgical options include arthrodesis, osteotomy, total joint replacement or trapeziectomy, with or without synthetic or biologic interpositions. A Cochrane review has shown that a combination of surgical procedures (e.g. trapeziectomy with ligament reconstruction) is no better than a single procedure (e.g. trapeziectomy) and single procedure was associated with fewer side effects. The ES for pain reduction was −0.17 (−0.57–0.24).[76]

Surgery for foot osteoarthritis

There are several new surgical techniques for minimally invasive correction of hallux valgus, which may have shorter recovery and rehabilitation times. However, at present, there is inadequate data (due to the heterogeneity of clinical trials) to be able recommend the use of minimally invasive techniques over routine management.[77]

Emerging treatments of osteoarthritis

The concept of targeting bone for symptom and structure modification has been mentioned above. As there is increasing evidence for inflammation within the OA joint,[78] other anti-inflammatory therapies have been trialled in OA. Case reports of anti-TNF medications note an improvement in symptoms in OA,[79,80] although this was not evident in a recent large study,[81] and methotrexate, a disease-modifying drug which is widely used in inflammatory arthritis, has also been trialled in OA to some effect, although data is limited.[82,83]

Increased nerve growth factor (NGF) expression has been noted in the OA joint, and a number of humanized monoclonal antibodies are in development that bind and inhibit NGF. One of these, tanezumab, showed good analgesic efficacy and an improvement in function in a study of 450 people with knee OA, compared to placebo.[84] However, despite this initial promising data, trials in OA were temporarily suspended due to concerns over accelerated rate of progression to total joint replacement. The anti-NGF FDA committee has recently voted to continue developing anti-NGF drugs as long as certain safety criteria are observed. Anti-NGF therapies may have a role in the future for reducing OA pain.

As well as peripheral sources of OA pain that may be targeted for analgesic treatments, there are new treatments for OA that target central pain in OA. Recently trialled therapies include centrally acting drugs such as duloxetine, a serotonin–noradrenaline reuptake inhibitor, for which there is growing evidence. Short-term (10 week) studies of duloxetine vs placebo, in over 500 people demonstrated a significant improvement in pain and function for people with painful knee OA (pain >4/10) already taking NSAIDs.[85] A 13 week, placebo-controlled study of 250 people also noted a significant reduction in pain and improvement in function scores in those taking duloxetine compared with placebo.[86] Side effects of duloxetine included nausea, dry mouth, and constipation, which may limit its use.

Novel opioid drugs are also in development, for example tapentadol, a centrally acting mu-opioid receptor agonist and noradrenaline reuptake inhibitor. A study of over 1000 people with chronic low back pain or OA pain, comparing tapentadol with the traditional opioid oxycodone, noted that both drugs provided sustained pain relief but that tapentadol was better tolerated with fewer side effects. Despite this, 22% of participants withdrew from the study due to side effects of tapentadol, although this was lower than the 37% who withdrew from the oxycodone group.[86a]

Side effects of opioids remain a major disadvantage of this class of drug. Opioid drugs formulated as extended-release preparations may have fewer side effects and these are undergoing phase 3 clinical trials, with two-thirds of patients noting good to excellent pain relief with extended-release oxycodone, with 22% discontinuing treatment due to adverse events.[87]

To date there are no studies assessing the use of pregabalin in people with OA, although one study has suggested decreased pain sensitivity in a rat model of OA.[88] The cannabinoid receptors, present in the central and peripheral nervous system, glutamate, a major central nervous system (CNS) neurotransmitter, the mu-opioid receptor, and the bradykinin-2 receptors[89] are also potential targets for pain relief and are under review.[90] As yet, these treatments remain in clinical trial stage.

Conclusion

OA is a common, painful and functionally limiting condition. All people with OA should be offered a combination of pharmacological and non-pharmacological treatments and the psychological effects of OA should also be considered. A range of treatments is available, although for many the ES is small, side effects limit the use of common pharmacological treatments, and there is very limited data to judge which people may respond better to a certain therapy than another. Ongoing research into optimal use of existing therapies and new treatments is needed to enable improved management of this common condition.

References

1. *Arthritis: the big picture*. Arthritis Research Campaign, London, 2002. Available from: www.ipsos-mori.com/_assets/polls/2002/pdf/arthritis.pdf.
2. Keenan AM, Tennant A, Fear J, Emery P, Conaghan PG. Impact of multiple joint problems on daily living tasks in people in the community over age fifty-five. *Arthritis Rheum* 2006;55(5):757–764.
3. Sale JE, Gignac M, Hawker G. The relationship between disease symptoms, life events, coping and treatment, and depression among older adults with osteoarthritis. *J Rheumatol* 2008;35(2):335–342.
4. Soares JJ, Jablonska B. Psychosocial experiences among primary care patients with and without musculoskeletal pain. *Eur J Pain* 2004;8(1):79–89.
5. Conaghan PG, Dickson J, Grant RL. Care and management of osteoarthritis in adults: summary of NICE guidance. *BMJ* 2008;336(7642):502–503.
6. Hochberg MC, Altman RD, April KT et al. American College of Rheumatology 2012 recommendations for the use of nonpharmacologic and pharmacologic therapies in osteoarthritis of the hand, hip, and knee. *Arthritis Care Res* (Hoboken) 2012;64(4):455–474.
7. Zhang W, Doherty M, Arden N et al. EULAR evidence based recommendations for the management of hip osteoarthritis: report of a task force of the EULAR Standing Committee for International Clinical Studies Including Therapeutics (ESCISIT). *Ann Rheum Dis* 2005;64(5):669–681.
8. Zhang W, Moskowitz RW, Nuki G et al. OARSI recommendations for the management of hip and knee osteoarthritis, Part II: OARSI evidence-based, expert consensus guidelines. *Osteoarthritis Cartilage* 2008;16(2):137–162.
9. Zhang W, Nuki G, Moskowitz RW et al. OARSI recommendations for the management of hip and knee osteoarthritis: part III: Changes in evidence following systematic cumulative update of research published through January 2009. *Osteoarthritis Cartilage* 2010;18(4):476–499.
10. Jordan KM, Arden NK, Doherty M et al. EULAR Recommendations 2003: an evidence based approach to the management of knee osteoarthritis: Report of a Task Force of the Standing Committee for International Clinical Studies Including Therapeutic Trials (ESCISIT). *Ann Rheum Dis* 2003;62(12):1145–1155.
11. Zhang W, Doherty M, Leeb BF et al. EULAR evidence based recommendations for the management of hand osteoarthritis: report of a Task Force of the EULAR Standing Committee for International Clinical Studies Including Therapeutics (ESCISIT). *Annals of the rheumatic diseases* 2007;66(3):377–388.
12. Doherty M, Dieppe P. The 'placebo' response in osteoarthritis and its implications for clinical practice. *Osteoarthritis and cartilage/OARS, Osteoarthritis Research Society* 2009;17(10):1255–1262.
13. Mazzuca SA, Brandt KD, Katz BP, Hanna MP, Melfi CA. Reduced utilization and cost of primary care clinic visits resulting from self-care education for patients with osteoarthritis of the knee. *Arthritis Rheum* 1999;42(6):1267–1273.
14. Bartels EM, Lund H, Hagen KB, Dagfinrud H, Christensen R, Danneskiold-Samsoe B. Aquatic exercise for the treatment of knee and hip osteoarthritis. *Cochrane Database Syst Revi* 2007;4:CD005523.
15. Roddy E, Zhang W, Doherty M. Aerobic walking or strengthening exercise for osteoarthritis of the knee? A systematic review. *Ann Rheum Dis* 2005;64(4):544–548.
16. Hernandez-Molina G, Reichenbach S, Zhang B, Lavalley M, Felson DT. Effect of therapeutic exercise for hip osteoarthritis pain: results of a meta-analysis. *Arthritis Rheum* 2008;59(9):1221–1228.
17. Niu J, Zhang YQ, Torner J et al. Is obesity a risk factor for progressive radiographic knee osteoarthritis? *Arthritis Rheum* 2009;61(3):329–335.
18. Christensen R, Bartels EM, Astrup A, Bliddal H. Effect of weight reduction in obese patients diagnosed with knee osteoarthritis: a systematic review and meta-analysis. *Annals of the rheumatic diseases* 2007;66(4):433–439.

19. White A, Foster NE, Cummings M, Barlas P. Acupuncture treatment for chronic knee pain: a systematic review. *Rheumatology* (Oxford) 2007;46(3):384–390.

20. Cheing GL, Hui-Chan CW. Would the addition of TENS to exercise training produce better physical performance outcomes in people with knee osteoarthritis than either intervention alone? *Clin Rehabil* 2004;18(5):487–497.

21. Hinz B, Cheremina O, Brune K. Acetaminophen (paracetamol) is a selective cyclooxygenase-2 inhibitor in man. *FASEB J* 2008;22(2):383–390.

22. Hogestatt ED, Jonsson BA, Ermund A et al. Conversion of acetaminophen to the bioactive N-acylphenolamine AM404 via fatty acid amide hydrolase-dependent arachidonic acid conjugation in the nervous system. *J Biol Chem* 2005;280(36):31405–31412.

23. Towheed TE, Maxwell L, Judd MG et al. Acetaminophen for osteoarthritis. *Cochrane Database Syst Rev* 2006;1:CD004257.

24. Rahme E, Barkun A, Nedjar H, Gaugris S, Watson D. Hospitalizations for upper and lower GI events associated with traditional NSAIDs and acetaminophen among the elderly in Quebec, Canada. *Am J Gastroenterol* 2008;103(4):872–882.

25. Dominkus M, Nicolakis M, Kotz R et al. Comparison of tissue and plasma levels of ibuprofen after oral and topical administration. *Arzneimittelforschung* 1996;46(12):1138–1143.

26. Zhang W, Jones A, Doherty M. Does paracetamol (acetaminophen) reduce the pain of osteoarthritis? A meta-analysis of randomised controlled trials. *Ann Rheum Dis* 2004;63(8):901–907.

27. Ray WA, Chung CP, Stein CM et al. Risk of peptic ulcer hospitalizations in users of NSAIDs with gastroprotective cotherapy versus coxibs. *Gastroenterology* 2007;133(3):790–798.

28. Conaghan PG. A turbulent decade for NSAIDs: update on current concepts of classification, epidemiology, comparative efficacy, and toxicity. *Rheumatol Int* 2012;32(6):1491–1502.

29. Avouac J, Gossec L, Dougados M. Efficacy and safety of opioids for osteoarthritis: a meta-analysis of randomized controlled trials. *Osteoarthritis Cartilage* 2007;15(8):957–965.

30. Bellamy N, Campbell J, Robinson V, Gee T, Bourne R, Wells G. Intraarticular corticosteroid for treatment of osteoarthritis of the knee. *Cochrane Database Syst Rev* 2006;2:CD005328.

31. Gaffney K, Ledingham J, Perry JD. Intra-articular triamcinolone hexacetonide in knee osteoarthritis: factors influencing the clinical response. *Ann Rheum Dis* 1995;54(5):379–381.

32. Jones A, Doherty M. Intra-articular corticosteroids are effective in osteoarthritis but there are no clinical predictors of response. *Ann Rheum Dis* 1996;55(11):829–832.

33. Kullenberg B, Runesson R, Tuvhag R, Olsson C, Resch S. Intraarticular corticosteroid injection: pain relief in osteoarthritis of the hip? *J Rheumatol* 2004;31(11):2265–2268.

34. Flanagan J, Casale FF, Thomas TL, Desai KB. Intra-articular injection for pain relief in patients awaiting hip replacement. *Ann R Coll Surg Engl* 1988;70(3):156–157.

35. Atchia I, Kane D, Reed MR, Isaacs JD, Birrell F. Efficacy of a single ultrasound-guided injection for the treatment of hip osteoarthritis. *Ann Rheum Dis* 2012;70(1):110–116.

36. Bannuru RR, Natov NS, Obadan IE et al. Therapeutic trajectory of hyaluronic acid versus corticosteroids in the treatment of knee osteoarthritis: a systematic review and meta-analysis. *Arthritis Rheum* 2009;61(12):1704–1711.

37. Fernandez Lopez JC, Ruano-Ravina A. Efficacy and safety of intraarticular hyaluronic acid in the treatment of hip osteoarthritis: a systematic review. *Osteoarthritis Cartilage* 2006;14(12):1306–1311.

38. Qvistgaard E, Christensen R, Torp-Pedersen S, Bliddal H. Intra-articular treatment of hip osteoarthritis: a randomized trial of hyaluronic acid, corticosteroid, and isotonic saline. *Osteoarthritis Cartilage* 2006;14(2):163–170.

39. Wandel S, Juni P, Tendal B et al. Effects of glucosamine, chondroitin, or placebo in patients with osteoarthritis of hip or knee: network meta-analysis. *BMJ* 2010;341:c4675.

40. Kim LS, Axelrod LJ, Howard P, Buratovich N, Waters RF. Efficacy of methylsulfonylmethane (MSM) in osteoarthritis pain of the knee: a pilot clinical trial. *OsteoarthritisCartilage* 2006;14(3):286–294.

41. Hellio Le Graverand-Gastineau MP. OA clinical trials: current targets and trials for OA. Choosing molecular targets: what have we learned and where we are headed? *Osteoarthritis Cartilage* 2009;17(11):1393–1401.

42. Dougados M, Nguyen M, Berdah L et al. Evaluation of the structure-modifying effects of diacerein in hip osteoarthritis: ECHODIAH, a three-year, placebo-controlled trial. Evaluation of the chondromodulating effect of diacerein in OA of the hip. *Arthritis Rheum* 2001;44(11):2539–2547.

43. Felson DT, Chaisson CE, Hill CL et al. The association of bone marrow lesions with pain in knee osteoarthritis. *Ann Intern Med* 2001;134(7):541–549.

44. Hunter DJ, Gerstenfeld L, Bishop G et al. Bone marrow lesions from osteoarthritis knees are characterized by sclerotic bone that is less well mineralized. *Arthritis Res Ther* 2009;11(1):R11.

45. Zanetti M, Bruder E, Romero J, Hodler J. Bone marrow edema pattern in osteoarthritic knees: correlation between MR imaging and histologic findings. *Radiology* 2000;215(3):835–840.

46. Dieppe P, Cushnaghan J, Young P, Kirwan J. Prediction of the progression of joint space narrowing in osteoarthritis of the knee by bone scintigraphy. *Ann Rheum Dis* 1993;52(8):557–563.

47. Bingham CO, 3rd, Buckland-Wright JC, Garnero P et al. Risedronate decreases biochemical markers of cartilage degradation but does not decrease symptoms or slow radiographic progression in patients with medial compartment osteoarthritis of the knee: results of the two-year multinational knee osteoarthritis structural arthritis study. *Arthritis Rheum* 2006;54(11):3494–3507.

48. Laslett LL, Dore DA, Quinn SJ et al. Zoledronic acid reduces bone marrow lesions and knee pain over one year. *Ann Rheum Dis* 2012;71(8):1322–1328.

49. Alexandersen P, Karsdal MA, Qvist P, Reginster JY, Christiansen C. Strontium ranelate reduces the urinary level of cartilage degradation biomarker CTX-II in postmenopausal women. *Bone* 2007;40(1):218–222.

50. Christgau S, Tanko LB, Cloos PA et al. Suppression of elevated cartilage turnover in postmenopausal women and in ovariectomized rats by estrogen and a selective estrogen-receptor modulator (SERM). *Menopause* 2004;11(5):508–518.

51. Ravn P, Warming L, Christgau S, Christiansen C. The effect on cartilage of different forms of application of postmenopausal estrogen therapy: comparison of oral and transdermal therapy. *Bone* 2004;35(5):1216–1221.

52. Karsdal M, Alexandersen P, John MR et al. Oral calcitonin demonstrated symptom-modifying efficacy and increased cartilage volume: results from a 2-year phase 3 trial in patients with osteoarthritis of the knee. *Osteoarthritis Cartilage* 2011;19S1:S35.

53. Reginster J, Chapurlat R, Christiansen C et al. Structure modifying effects of strontium ranelate in knee osteoarthritis. *Osteoporosis Int* 2012;23(Suppl 2):S58.

54. Haugen IK, Englund M, Aliabadi P et al. Prevalence, incidence and progression of hand osteoarthritis in the general population: the Framingham Osteoarthritis Study. *Ann Rheum Dis* 2011;70(9):1581–1586.

55. Towheed TE. Systematic review of therapies for osteoarthritis of the hand. *Osteoarthritis Cartilage* 2005;13(6):455–462.

56. Rannou F, Dimet J, Boutron I et al. Splint for base-of-thumb osteoarthritis: a randomized trial. *Ann Intern Med* 2009;150(10):661–669.

57. Zhang W, Doherty M, Leeb BF et al. EULAR evidence-based recommendations for the diagnosis of hand osteoarthritis: report of a task force of ESCISIT. *Ann Rheum Dis* 2009;68(1):8–17.

58. Meenagh GK, Patton J, Kynes C, Wright GD. A randomised controlled trial of intra-articular corticosteroid injection of the carpometacarpal joint of the thumb in osteoarthritis. *Ann Rheum Dis* 2004;63(10):1260–1263.

59. Joshi R. Intraarticular corticosteroid injection for first carpometacarpal osteoarthritis. *J Rheumatol* 2005;32(7):1305–1306.

60. Khan M, Waseem M, Raza A, Derham D. Quantitative assessment of improvement with single corticosteroid injection in thumb CMC joint osteoarthritis? *Open Orthop J* 2009;3:48–51.

61. Maarse W, Watts AC, Bain GI. Medium-term outcome following intra-articular corticosteroid injection in first CMC joint arthritis using fluoroscopy. *Hand Surg* 2009;14(2–3):99–104.

62. Menz HB, Munteanu SE, Landorf KB, Zammit GV, Cicuttini FM. Radiographic evaluation of foot osteoarthritis: sensitivity of radiographic variables and relationship to symptoms. *Osteoarthritis Cartilage* 2009;17(3):298–303.

63. Munteanu SE, Menz HB, Zammit GV et al. Efficacy of intra-articular hyaluronan (Synvisc(R)) for the treatment of osteoarthritis affecting the first metatarsophalangeal joint of the foot (hallux limitus): study protocol for a randomised placebo controlled trial. *J Foot Ankle Res* 2009;2:2.

64. Peterson CK, Buck F, Pfirrmann CW, Zanetti M, Hodler J. Fluoroscopically guided diagnostic and therapeutic injections into foot articulations: report of short-term patient responses and comparison of outcomes between various injection sites. *AJR Am J Roentgenol* 2011;197(4):949–953.

65. Rao S, Baumhauer JF, Becica L, Nawoczenski DA. Shoe inserts alter plantar loading and function in patients with midfoot arthritis. *J Orthop Sports Phys Ther* 2009;39(7):522–531.

66. Spencer RF. Evolution in hip resurfacing design and contemporary experience with an uncemented device. *J Bone Joint Surg Am* 2011;93 Suppl 2:84–88.

67. Gossec L, Paternotte S, Bingham CO et al. OARSI/OMERACT initiative to define states of severity and indication for joint replacement in hip and knee osteoarthritis. An OMERACT 10 Special Interest Group. *J Rheumatol* 2011;38(8):1765–1769.

68. Ethgen O, Bruyere O, Richy F, Dardennes C, Reginster JY. Health-related quality of life in total hip and total knee arthroplasty. A qualitative and systematic review of the literature. *J Bone Joint Surg Am* 2004;86-A(5):963–974.

69. Rand JA, Trousdale RT, Ilstrup DM, Harmsen WS. Factors affecting the durability of primary total knee prostheses. *J Bone Joint Surg Am* 2003;85-A(2):259–265.

70. Soderman P, Malchau H, Herberts P et al. Outcome after total hip arthroplasty: Part II. Disease-specific follow-up and the Swedish National Total Hip Arthroplasty Register. *Acta Orthop Scand* 2001;72(2):113–119.

71. Lutzner J, Kasten P, Gunther KP, Kirschner S. Surgical options for patients with osteoarthritis of the knee. *Nat Rev Rheumatol* 2009;5(6):309–316.

72. Brouwer RW, Raaij van TM, Bierma-Zeinstra SM et al. Osteotomy for treating knee osteoarthritis. *Cochrane Database Syst Rev* 2007;3:CD004019.

73. Gomoll AH. High tibial osteotomy for the treatment of unicompartmental knee osteoarthritis: a review of the literature, indications, and technique. *Phys Sports Med* 2011;39(3):45–54.

74. Intema F, Thomas TP, Anderson DD et al. Subchondral bone remodeling is related to clinical improvement after joint distraction in the treatment of ankle osteoarthritis. *Osteoarthritis Cartilage* 2011;19(6):668–675.

75. Intema F, Van Roermund PM, Marijnissen AC et al. Tissue structure modification in knee osteoarthritis by use of joint distraction: an open 1-year pilot study. *Ann Rheum Dis* 2011;70(8):1441–1446.

76. Wajon A, Ada L, Edmunds I. Surgery for thumb (trapeziometacarpal joint) osteoarthritis. *Cochrane Database Syst Rev* 2005;4:CD004631.

77. Maffulli N, Longo UG, Marinozzi A, Denaro V. Hallux valgus: effectiveness and safety of minimally invasive surgery. A systematic review. *Br Med Bull* 2010;97:149–167.

78. Sellam J, Berenbaum F. The role of synovitis in pathophysiology and clinical symptoms of osteoarthritis. *Nat Rev Rheumatol* 2010;6(11):625–635.

79. Fioravanti A, Fabbroni M, Cerase A, Galeazzi M. Treatment of erosive osteoarthritis of the hands by intra-articular infliximab injections: a pilot study. *Rheumatol Int* 2009;29(8):961–965.

80. Magnano MD, Chakravarty EF, Broudy C et al. A pilot study of tumor necrosis factor inhibition in erosive/inflammatory osteoarthritis of the hands. *J Rheumatol* 2007;34(6):1323–1327.

81. Verbruggen G, Wittoek R, Cruyssen BV, Elewaut D. Tumour necrosis factor blockade for the treatment of erosive osteoarthritis of the interphalangeal finger joints: a double blind, randomised trial on structure modification. *Ann Rheum Dis* 2012;71(6):891–898.

82. Holanda d. Baxia dose de methotrexate comparado a placebo em osteoartrite de joelho. *Rev Bras Reumatol* 2007;47:334–340.

83. Wenham CY, Grainger, AJ, Hensor EM, et al. Methotrexate for pain relief in knee osteo. arthritis- an open label study *Rheum (Oxford)* 2013;52:888–92.

84. Lane NE, Schnitzer TJ, Birbara CA et al. Tanezumab for the treatment of pain from osteoarthritis of the knee. *N Engl J Med* 2010;363(16):1521–1531.

85. Frakes EP, Risser RC, Ball TD, Hochberg MC, Wohlreich MM. Duloxetine added to oral nonsteroidal anti-inflammatory drugs for treatment of knee pain due to osteoarthritis: results of a randomized, double-blind, placebo-controlled trial. *Curr Med Res Opin* 2011;27(12):2361–2372.

86. Chappell AS, Desaiah D, Liu-Seifert H et al. A double-blind, randomized, placebo-controlled study of the efficacy and safety of duloxetine for the treatment of chronic pain due to osteoarthritis of the knee. *Pain Pract* 2011;11(1):33–41.

86a. Wild JE, Grond S, Kuperwasser B et al. Long-term safety and tolerability of tapentadol extended release for the management of chronic low back pain or osteoarthritis pain. *Pain Pract* 2010;10(5):416–427.

87. Friedmann N, Klutzaritz V, Webster L. Efficacy and safety of an extended-release oxycodone (Remoxy) formulation in patients with moderate to severe osteoarthritic pain. *J Opioid Manag* 2011;7(3):193–202.

88. Rahman W, Bauer CS, Bannister K et al. Descending serotonergic facilitation and the antinociceptive effects of pregabalin in a rat model of osteoarthritic pain. *Mol Pain* 2009;5:45.

89. Song IH, Althoff CE, Hermann KG et al. Contrast-enhanced ultrasound in monitoring the efficacy of a bradykinin receptor 2 antagonist in painful knee osteoarthritis compared with MRI. *Ann Rheum Dis* 2009;68(1):75–83.

90. Martel-Pelletier J, Wildi LM, Pelletier JP. Future therapeutics for osteoarthritis. *Bone* 2012;51(2):297–311.

SECTION 20

Crystal arthropathies

SECTION 141

Gout

Nicola Dalbeth

Introduction

Gout is the most common inflammatory arthritis affecting men. The central biochemical feature of gout is hyperuricaemia (elevated serum urate concentration) which leads to formation and deposition of monosodium urate monohydrate (MSU) crystals within the joint and soft tissues. Gout most often presents as recurrent, self-limiting episodes of severe acute arthritis. In the presence of prolonged hyperuricaemia, some patients also develop chronic tophaceous disease and joint damage. Gout is frequently associated with comorbid conditions such as chronic kidney disease, hypertension, diabetes, and dyslipidaemia; these comorbid conditions may add further complexity to the presentation and management of gout. Long-term management with urate-lowering therapy (ULT) using a treat-to-target approach is essential to promote dissolution of MSU crystals, suppression of acute gout attacks, and regression of tophi.

Definitions

The central feature of gout is deposition of MSU crystals. This crystal deposition may lead to acute inflammatory arthritis, chronic gouty synovitis, and/or chronic tophaceous disease. The gold standard for diagnosis of gout is identification of MSU crystals within tissue or synovial fluid (Figure 141.1). MSU crystals may be present in patients with gout and poorly controlled hyperuricaemia in previously unaffected joints.[1] Classification criteria that include clinical history, physical examination, laboratory tests, and radiography, exist for epidemiological studies of gout.[2] However, these criteria have relatively poor specificity and sensitivity for acute gout.[3] For this reason, crystal diagnosis should be attempted wherever possible for clinical diagnosis.

Epidemiology

In the United Kingdom adult population between 2000 and 2007, the incidence of gout per 1000 person-years was 2.68 (4.42 in men and 1.32 in women).[4] Most recent prevalence estimates of gout in the United States are 3.9% among adults in 2007–2008 (5.9% in men and 2.0% in women).[5] Similar prevalence data have been reported in the entire New Zealand population, with an estimated prevalence in the adult population in 2009 of 3.8% (6.0% in men and 1.8% in women).[6] The prevalence of gout in the United States has increased by 1.2% from the 1988–1994 period to the 2007–2008 period.[5]

Analysis of cross-sectional studies has demonstrated a number of factors associated with gout in the general population. These factors include male sex, increasing age, socio-economic deprivation, and ethnicity.[6] In particular, Polynesian ethnicity is associated with a 3–4-fold increased risk of gout.[6] Medical conditions associated with gout include obesity, chronic renal impairment, renal transplantation, cardiovascular disease, type 2 diabetes, hypertension, heart failure, hypertriglyceridaemia, and psoriasis.[5,7,8] Diuretic and cyclosporine use are also associated with gout.[7,9] The relationship between various comorbid conditions and gout is complex, and there is ongoing debate about the influence of hyperuricaemia and gout on development of comorbid conditions, and vice versa (Table 141.1). Nevertheless, in the general population, gout is associated with increased total mortality and cardiovascular mortality, even after adjusting for traditional cardiovascular risk factors.[10]

Analysis of large longitudinal cohort studies has shown that a number of dietary factors are associated with development of gout (Table 141.2); these factors include high intake of beer and spirits, sugar-sweetened soft drinks, fructose, meat, and seafood.[11–14]

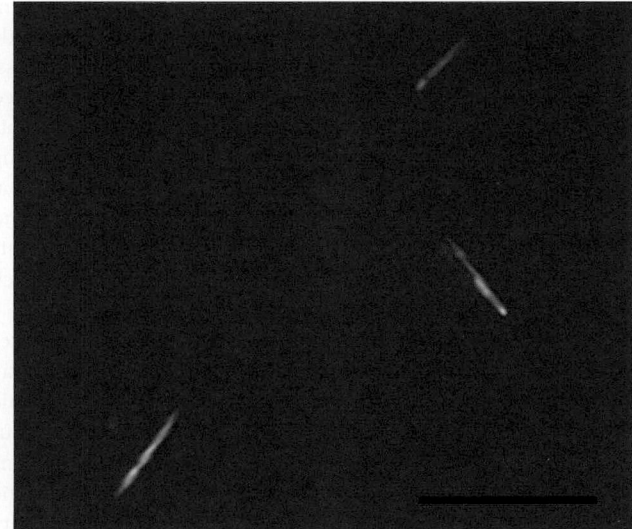

Fig. 141.1 Monosodium urate monohydrate crystals visualized under polarizing light microscopy. Scale bar indicates 20 μm.

Table 141.1 Relationship between development of gout and comorbid conditions

Comorbid condition	Prevalence in patients with gout	Refs	Risk of developing gout if comorbid condition is present	Refs	Risk of developing/ having comorbid condition if gout is present*	Refs
Obesity	22–67%	22,78	RR 2.33 for obesity RR 1.99 for weight gain	15	NA	–
Type 2 diabetes	29–33%	8,22	RR 0.67	90	RR 1.34	91
Hypertension	60–89%	8,22	RR 2.31	15	HR 1.81 (if hyperuricaemia present) NA for gout	92
Coronary artery disease	25–37%	8,22	NA		OR 1.26	93
Peripheral vascular disease	NA	–	NA	–	OR 1.33	94
Nephrolithiasis	27%	95	RR 1.05 (not significant)	96	RR 2.12	96
Chronic kidney disease	47%	8	RR 3.61 including those on diuretics RR 4.60 excluding those on diuretics	15	NA	–
Diuretic use	33%	7	RR 1.77	15	–	–

HR, multivariate adjusted hazard; NA, data not available; OR, multivariate adjusted odds ratio; RR, multivariate adjusted relative risk ratio.

Weight gain and obesity in younger life are strongly associated with development of gout.[15] Other dietary factors such as low-fat dairy products, coffee, and vitamin C are associated with reduced risk of developing gout.[11,16–18] Dietary intake of diet-sweetened soft drinks, wine, tea, high-fat dairy products, and vegetable purines does not appear to influence the development of gout.[11–13,16]

Clinical features

The first attack of gout most often presents as rapid onset of acute inflammation affecting the first metatarsophalangeal (MTP) joint or other joint in the lower limb. Triggers for gout flares include heavy alcohol intake, dehydration, joint trauma, medical illness, surgery, and intake of high-purine diet. In patients with established gout, commencement of ULT may also trigger a gout flare. Patients describe severe joint pain with difficulty walking and performing daily activities. Examination of the affected joint shows the cardinal features of inflammation; erythema, heat, tenderness, swelling, and loss of joint mobility. In the case of a severe gout attack, patients may also be systemically unwell with fever. The acute gout attack typically resolves spontaneously after 7–10 days.

In the presence of persistent hyperuricaemia, recurrent flares occur, with increasingly frequent and prolonged attacks which may affect numerous joints including those in the upper limbs. Chronic synovitis may also develop. In some patients, tophaceous gout develops, leading to cosmetic problems, ulceration and superimposed infection, mechanical obstruction of joint movement, bone and cartilage damage, and musculoskeletal disability. In a minority of patients, gouty tophi may be the initial manifestation of disease. This is particularly the case in elderly women with chronic kidney disease who are taking diuretics.[19] Chronic gout has an important impact on health-related quality of life and musculoskeletal function. In particular, recurrent gout flares, the presence of joint inflammation and tophi are associated with disability and poor health-related quality of life.[20] Work productivity is also reduced in patients of working age with severe gout, with an estimated mean work day loss of 25.1 days per year.[21]

In addition to the joint disease, patients with gout frequently have additional comorbid conditions such as type 2 diabetes, chronic kidney disease, hypertension, dyslipidaemia, and cardiovascular disease (CVD).[8] These comorbid conditions may impact on gout management; for example, thiazide diuretic use in patients with hypertension may increase serum urate concentrations and predispose individuals to gout, chronic kidney disease may limit the use of non-steroidal anti-inflammatory drugs (NSAIDs) and/or colchicine for management of acute flares, and blood sugar control may be difficult in patients with coexistent diabetes receiving corticosteroids for management of acute gout. The majority of patients with gout are at high risk for CVD events,[22] and a presentation with gout should be viewed as an opportunity to address musculoskeletal health, and also cardiovascular and metabolic risk factors.

Diagnosis of gout is confirmed by identification of MSU crystals in synovial fluid or tophus. MSU crystals may be present in joints previously unaffected by clinically apparent episodes of gout,[23] and crystal diagnosis should be attempted in all patients. In acute gout, synovial fluid analysis typically shows an inflammatory picture with high concentrations of neutrophils. During the acute flare, blood testing typically shows signs of acute inflammation with neutrophil leucocytosis and high acute phase reactants. Measurement of the serum urate concentration is essential in patients with gout. Most patients with untreated gout will have elevated serum urate concentration, above saturation concentrations (>0.41 mmol/L). However,

Table 141.2 Dietary factors and development of gout

Dietary factor	Risk of developing gout	Relative risk for developing gout[a]	References
All alcohol	Increased	2.53	12
Beer	Increased	2.51	12
Spirits	Increased	1.6	12
Wine	No effect	1.05	12
Meat	Increased	1.41	11
Seafood	Increased	1.51	11
Purine-rich vegetables	No effect	0.96	11
Low-fat dairy products	Reduced	0.58	11
High-fat dairy products	No effect	1.0	11
Coffee	Reduced	0.41 in men, 0.43 in women	16,18
Decaffeinated coffee	Reduced	0.73 in men, 0.77 in women	16,18
Tea	No effect	0.82 in men, 1.55 in women	16,18
Vitamin C	Reduced	0.55	17
Sugar-sweetened soft drinks	Increased	1.85 in men, 2.39 in women	13,14
Diet soft drinks	No effect	1.12 in men, 1.18 in women	13,14
Fructose-rich fruits	Increased	1.64 in men	13
Fruit juice	Increased	1.81 in men, 2.42 in women (orange juice)	13,14
Free fructose	Increased	2.02 in men, 1.62 in women	13,14

[a]Multivariate relative risk, typically comparing highest quintile of intake with referent group (no intake or lowest quintile of intake).

Adapted with permission from Dalbeth and So.[99]

during an acute gout flare, serum urate concentration drops into the normal range in approximately 40% of patients.[24] In this situation, repeat measurement of the serum urate concentration in the convalescent period is required.

Imaging has a role in diagnosis and assessment of disease severity and complications. Most often plain radiographs are normal, particularly in patients with recent presentation of gout. In patients with established disease, typical plain radiographic features are asymmetric soft-tissue masses (tophi) and well-corticated bone erosions with overhanging edges. Ultrasonography has the ability to detect erosion, synovitis, and tophi in affected joints. The 'double-contour' sign on ultrasonography—hyperechoic enhancement of the superficial margin of the hyaline cartilage—has high specificity for gout.[25] MRI is able to detect bone erosion, synovitis, and tophus deposition with high sensitivity, but is not usually required in clinical practice. MRI may have a particular role in detecting complications of gout, such as tendon rupture or superimposed infection; bone marrow oedema is not usually a major feature of uncomplicated gout, but is strongly suggestive of concurrent bone infection in patients with gout.[26] Conventional CT allows excellent visualization of tophi and bone erosion.[27] A further development in CT imaging of gout is dual-energy CT (DECT)—a system with two X-ray tubes scanning at 80 kbp and 140 kbp, which allows for colour identification of urate and calcium. DECT has the potential to allow non-invasive diagnosis of gout, and also measurement of total body urate burden, through three-dimensional volume assessment of tophi (Figure 141.2).[28] DECT scanners are not yet in widespread use,

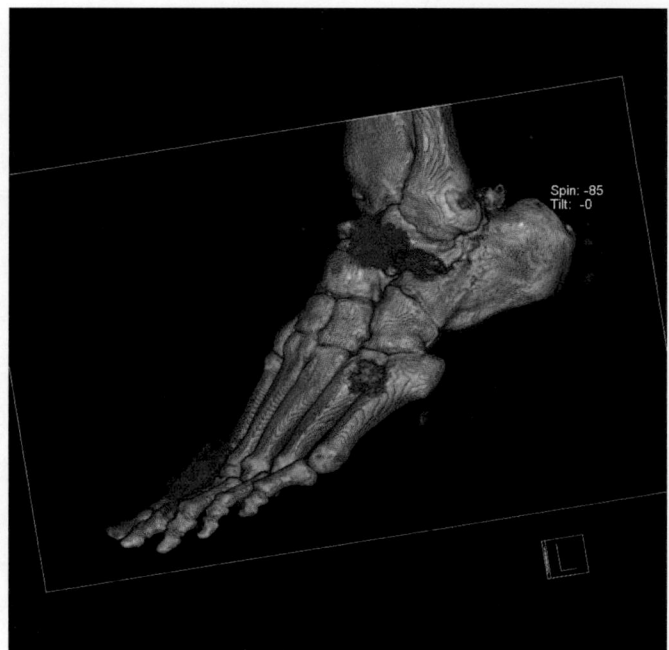

Fig. 141.2 Dual-energy CT scan of the foot affected by tophaceous gout, demonstrating collections of MSU crystals (shown in red)

and further information is required about the sensitivity and specificity of this method before it can be accepted as a tool for gout diagnosis.

Aetiopathogenesis

A number of key checkpoints exist for pathogenesis of gout (reviewed by Choi et al.[29]). The central biochemical feature of gout is hyperuricaemia. Urate is primarily derived from the catabolism of purines formed in the de-novo biosynthesis of nucleic acids and to a lesser extent from breakdown of dietary purines. Plasma urate is completely filtered at the glomerulus and almost totally reabsorbed by proximal tubule. Tubular secretion accounts for almost all urinary uric acid. Hyperuricaemia can be due to either an increase in endogenous biosynthesis of purines or reduction in renal excretion of uric acid or both.

Most dietary risk factors for gout are also associated with hyperuricaemia. Beer, red meat, and seafood have high purine content. Similarly, fructose increases urate production by increasing hepatic ATP degradation to AMP, a urate precursor, and high intake of fructose-sweetened beverages has been associated with hyperuricaemia.[30] Although genetic variants such as hypoxanthine-guanine phosphoribosyltransferase (HPRT) deficiency and PRPP synthetase (PRS) superactivity are been associated with urate overproduction and gout, these variants are rarely associated with gout in the general population.

Renal underexcretion of uric acid accounts for the majority of hyperuricaemia (90%). Renal underexcretion of uric acid may be present due to chronic kidney disease, diuretic use, and high circulating insulin concentrations.[31] Genetic variants in renal urate transporters also play an important role in development of hyperuricaemia and gout (Figure 141.3). Recent genome-wide association studies have identified that the majority of genes associated with hyperuricaemia are transporters implicated in renal transport of urate.[32] Variants in the *SLC2A9* gene contribute most to genetic risk for hyperuricaemia; in addition to its effects on renal uric acid transport, this transporter also transports glucose and fructose.[33] Variants in the *SLC2A9* gene have been associated with gout.[34,35] Other genes associated with both gout and hyperuricaemia in the general population are the renal transporters *ABCG2* and *NPT1*.[32,36]

MSU crystals form in vitro at physiological temperature and pH when urate concentrations rise above supersaturation concentrations of 0.41 mmol/litre (6.8 mg/dL).[37] The majority of individuals with serum urate concentrations above supersaturation concentrations do not develop gout.[38] Therefore, hyperuricaemia is necessary, but not sufficient, for development of gout. Other factors such as debris, proteins, local temperature, and pH within the joint may also influence whether crystal formation occurs.[37,39]

Histological examination of the synovium in acute gout shows lining-layer hyperplasia and intense infiltration of the membrane by neutrophils, monocyte-macrophages and lymphocytes.[40] Acute attacks of gout are often triggered by events such as joint trauma, dehydration, or sudden alterations in the serum urate concentration. These triggers may stimulate de-novo formation of MSU crystals or may promote release of crystals from preformed deposits within the joint.

A number of factors have been implicated in the initiation phase of the acute gout attack (reviewed by Dalbeth and Haskard[41]). These factors include signalling through the Toll-like receptors

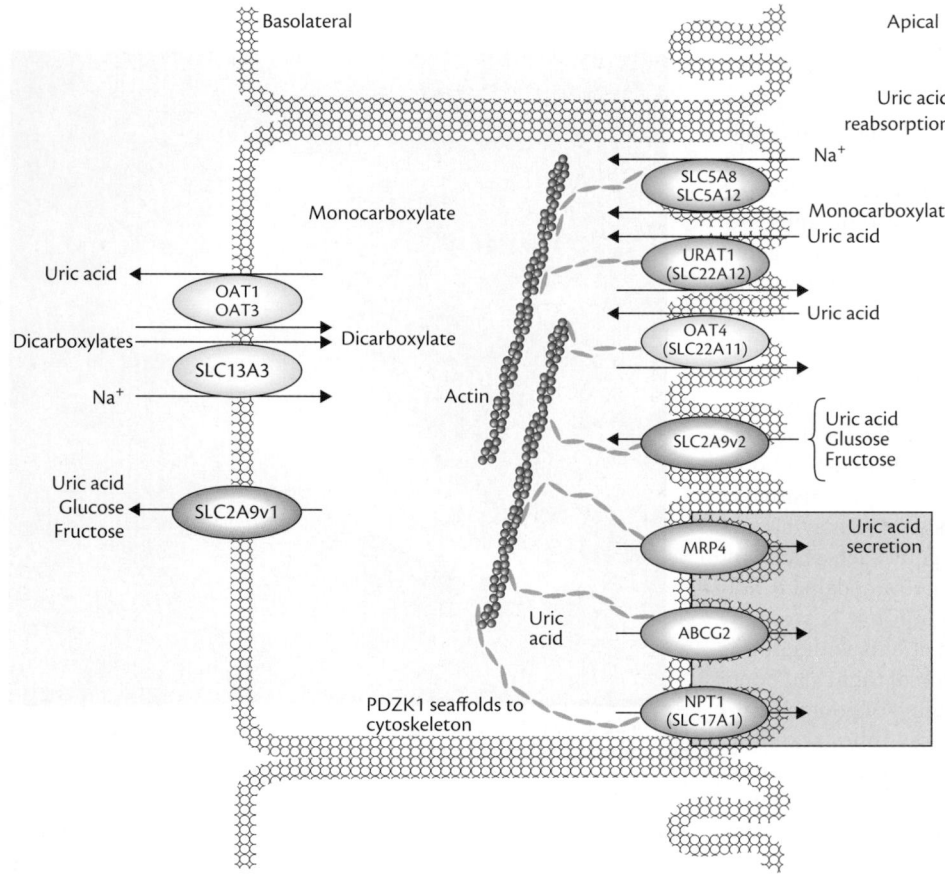

Fig. 141.3 Renal transport of uric acid within the proximal tubular cell.

Reprinted from Merriman TR, Dalbeth N. The genetic basis of hyperuricaemia and gout. Joint Bone Spine. 2011 Jan;78(1):35–40 with permission from Elsevier

TLR-2 and TLR-4, activation of the complement cascade, and mast cell degranulation. Activation of the NALP3 inflammasome within monocytes/macrophages is central in the initiation of the acute gout attack.[42] NALP3 inflammasome activation leads to release of mature interleukin (IL)-1β. IL-1β leads to endothelial activation and release of IL-8 from non-haematopoietic cells. These events, in turn, lead to an amplification phase with recruitment of neutrophils, monocytes, and other inflammatory cells. Leucocyte recruitment is likely to be enhanced by the local generation of other chemotactic factors such as leukotriene B4, C5a, and S100A8/A9.[41]

Intense infiltration of neutrophils into both synovial membrane and fluid is the central feature of acute gout, and these cells provide the main cellular mechanism of inflammatory amplification in acute gout.[43] The consequences of neutrophil interaction with MSU crystals include the synthesis and release of a large variety of mediators that promote vasodilatation, erythema and pain associated with the acute gout attack. These include reactive oxygen species, nitric oxide, arachadonic acid metabolites, enzymes, IL-1, and chemokines including S100A8, S100A9, and IL-8. Infiltrating monocytes also amplify the inflammatory response in acute gout.[44] Following exposure to MSU crystals, monocytes also become activated, resulting in expression of a number of proinflammatory genes, including IL-1, tumour necrosis factor (TNFα), IL-6, IL-8 and cyclooxygenase-2.[41]

Even in the absence of treatment, the acute inflammatory response in gout is typically self-limiting over 7–10 days. Factors contributing to the resolution phase of the acute gout attack are less well defined, but putative mechanisms include release of anti-inflammatory cytokines such as transforming growth factor (TGF)-β and IL-10, expression of melanocortin receptors, induction of anti-inflammatory signalling pathways such as PPARγ, and alterations in macrophage differentiation.[41]

In some individuals, persistent hyperuricaemia leads to the formation of tophaceous deposits of MSU crystals, typically in subcutaneous and periarticular areas. The tophus represents a complex and organized chronic inflammatory tissue response to MSU crystals involving both innate and adaptive immune cells.[45] Tophi may invade bone, leading to bone erosion and joint damage. Erosive gout is characterized by disturbance of normal bone turnover. Disordered osteoclastogenesis has been implicated, with numerous osteoclast-like cells within the tophus surrounding MSU crystal deposits at the tophus–bone interface.[46] MSU crystals have profound inhibitory effects on primary osteoblast viability, function and differentiation, and there is a relative paucity of osteoblasts at the tophus–bone interface.[47] Production of matrix metalloproteases and other degradative enzymes in response to MSU crystals may also lead to cartilage and bone matrix damage in tophaceous gout.[48]

Management

Gout management is separated into three key therapeutic goals: treatment of acute gout flares, prophylaxis against acute gout flares (usually at the time of initiating ULT), and long-term preventive treatment of chronic gout with ULT (Table 141.3). The European League Against Rhematism (EULAR) and the British Society for Rheumatology (BSR) have published gout treatment guidelines in the last decade,[49,50] and American College of Rheumatology (ACR) gout treatment guidelines were released in 2012.[51,52]

Treatment of acute gout

The goal of treating acute gout is resolution of pain and inflammation in the affected joint. Treatment should be commenced as soon as possible after development of symptoms. Management of the acute gout flare includes rest, icing of the affected joint, and analgesia. A number of pharmacological agents are effective in the management of acute gout. NSAIDs are first-line treatment in patients without contraindications. These drugs are most effective when used in a fast-acting preparation and at full dose (e.g. naproxen 500 mg twice daily, indomethacin 50 mg three times daily). Following treatment with NSAIDs, more than 50% patients

Table 141.3 Summary of gout management

Therapeutic goal	Pharmacological treatment options	Adjunctive treatment
Treatment of acute gout	NSAIDs	Rest
	Colchicine	Ice
	Prednisone/prednisolone	Analgesia
	Intra-articular corticosteroids	
	ACTH	
	IL-1 inhibitors[a]	
Prophylaxis against acute flares	NSAIDs	Gradual up-titration of urate-lowering therapy
	Colchicine	
	IL-1 inhibitors[a]	
Urate-lowering therapy	Xanthine oxidase inhibitors: allopurinol, febuxostat	Vitamin C
	Uricosuric agents: probenecid, sulphinpyrazone, benzbromarone	Losartan, fenofibrate, amlodipine, atorvastatin
		Dietary modification
	Recombinant uricase: pegloticase, rasburicase[a]	Weight loss

ACTH, adrenocorticotropic hormone; NSAIDs, non-steroidal anti-inflammatory drugs.

[a] In development/not currently approved for use in gout.

Adapted with permission from Dalbeth.[100]

experience a major clinical response within 2 days, and 80% after 5 days.[53] Compared with non-selective NSAIDs, COX-2 inhibitors such as etoricoxib (120 mg daily) and lumiracoxib (400 mg daily) have similar efficacy in treating acute gout, although COX-2 inhibitors are generally better tolerated.[53,54]

Colchicine has been used for centuries for treatment of acute gout. A recent clinical trial of oral colchicine showed that a low dose of colchicine (1.8 mg total over 1 hour) was as effective as a high dose (4.8 mg total over 6 hours), with substantially less toxicity.[55] In this study, clinical response (≥50% pain reduction at 24 hours without rescue medication) was observed in 38% of patients in the low-dose colchicine group, 33% in the high-dose colchicine group, and 15% in the placebo group. This study has led to United States Food and Drug Authority (FDA) recommendations that colchicine dosing for acute gout should be 1.2 mg stat followed by 0.6 mg in 1 hour (total 1.8 mg in the first 24 hours). Concomitant use of P-gp and moderate-strong CYP3A4 inhibitors (such as ciclosporin, clarithromycin, ketoconazole, ritonavir, verapamil, diltiazem, erythromycin) may cause severe drug interactions due to accumulation of colchicine, and dose reduction is recommended when these drugs are coadministered to avoid colchicine toxicity.[56] The dose of colchicine should also be reduced in patients with renal or liver disease.

Intra-articular corticosteroid injection of the affected joint leads to rapid improvement in pain and inflammation, and avoids the systemic complications of orally administered therapies. Oral prednisolone is particularly useful for treatment of acute gout in patients with medical comorbidities and/or concomitant medication that preclude the use of NSAIDs and colchicine. Two randomized controlled trials (RCTs) have demonstrated that oral prednisolone (30 mg or 35 mg daily for five days) is as effective as full-dose NSAIDs for treatment of acute gout.[57,58] This treatment protocol is at least as safe as NSAID therapy in patients with acute gout, with one study reporting fewer adverse events in the prednisone-treated group.[58] Adrenocorticotropic hormone (ACTH) injection is also effective in treatment of acute gout; typical doses are 40 IU.[59] The beneficial action of ACTH may occur through adrenal corticosteroid release and also activation of the melanocortin type 3 receptor (MC3R).[60]

The identification of the central role of IL-1β in initiation and amplification of the acute inflammatory response in gout has raised the possibility of cytokine-targeted treatment of acute gout. In an RCT of acute gout, a single 150 mg subcutaneous dose of canakinumab, a fully human anti-IL-1β monoclonal antibody, led to greater reduction in pain than 40 mg intramuscular triamcinolone.[61] At present, these therapies are not approved for treatment of acute gout.

Gout prophylaxis

Gout prophylaxis refers to the use of anti-inflammatory agents to prevent flares in patients with intercurrent or chronic gout. Prophylaxis is particularly relevant when commencing ULT, as this period is frequently associated with increased number and severity of flares. In the absence of prophylaxis, up to three-quarters of patients will have an acute flare following initiation of ULT.[62] Patients with high urate burden are at greater risk of recurrent gout flares, and prophylaxis may be required for longer in patients with tophi. Gout flares can be prevented, in part, by gradual up-titration of ULT.

Low-dose colchicine (0.5–1.5 mg daily) is the most frequently used prophylactic treatment for gout. Several RCTs have reported benefit of colchicine in patients commencing ULT, at doses of 0.6 mg twice daily and 0.5 mg three times daily.[62,63] Both of these studies reported increased adverse events in the colchicine group, most frequently diarrhoea which may limit the use of this medication particularly in patients with renal impairment. When used for gout prophylaxis, colchicine dose should be reduced in patients taking P-gp and moderate-strong CYP3A4 inhibitors and in those with renal impairment.[56]

Oral NSAIDs are frequently used in clinical practice and clinical trials for gout prophylaxis.[64] The role of NSAIDs specifically for gout prophylaxis has not been extensively studied. Renal impairment and poorly controlled hypertension are frequently present in patients with gout, and for this reason regular NSAIDs may be contraindicated.[7]

IL-1β inhibitors may also play a role in gout prophylaxis. In a clinical trial of patients commencing allopurinol, canakinumab at a single dose of ≥50 mg was superior to daily colchicine 0.5 mg daily for prevention of gout flares at 16 weeks.[65] Similar findings were observed in the RCT of canakinumab for treatment of acute gout, where canakinumab-treated patients experienced fewer gout flares 8 weeks after injection.[61] At present, anti-IL-1 therapies are not approved for gout prophylaxis.

Urate-lowering therapy for chronic gout

Long-term ULT is recommended for all patients with recurrent gout flares (more than one flare per year), gouty tophi, chronic gouty arthropathy, and/or radiographic erosions. A serum urate concentration below 0.36 mmol/litre (6 mg/dL) is recommended by EULAR as a treatment target for patients with gout.[49] This is the concentration that corresponds to that required to ultimately achieve resolution of MSU crystals within the joint, suppression of acute gout attacks and resolution of gouty tophi.[66–68] Lower serum urate concentrations lead to more rapid dissolution of tophi, and an even lower target of less than 0.30 mmol/L has been recommended by the BSR.[50] ULT should be tailored to each individual, in order to achieve this target. A number of urate-lowering agents are available. These agents can be separated into three main groups; the xanthine oxidase inhibitors, uricosuric agents, and recombinant uricase. The sites of action of these agents are shown in Figure 141.4.

Adjunctive therapies that have a modest urate-lowering effect include dietary modification (e.g. avoidance of beer, sugar-sweetened beverages, and large purine loads; increase in consumption of low-fat dairy, and coffee), and weight loss. Vitamin C at 500 mg-1000 mg daily has a modest urate-lowering effect and may a useful adjunct for those wishing to take supplementary therapies.[69] However, most patients with gout are unable to reduce their serum urate to target (<0.36 mmol/L) with adjunctive treatment alone, and in this situation, specific ULT is indicated.

Xanthine oxidase inhibitors

Xanthine oxidase is a critical enzyme in the metabolism of purines to urate, which catalyses the conversion of hypoxanthine to xanthine and xanthine to urate (Figure 141.4). Two agents that inhibit this enzyme currently used as ULT for patients with gout are allopurinol and febuxostat.

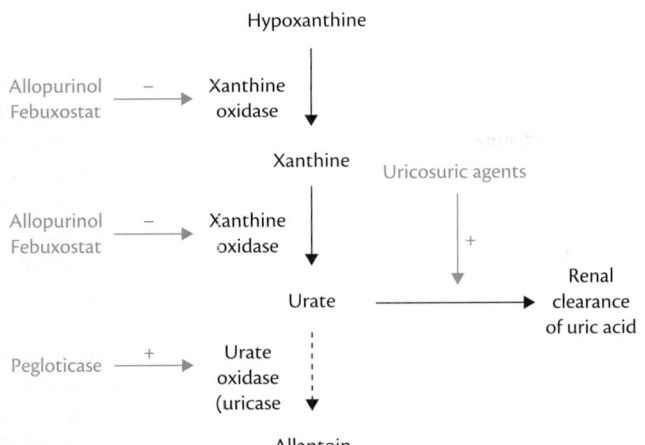

Hypoxanthine

Allopurinol Febuxostat — Xanthine oxidase

Xanthine

Allopurinol Febuxostat — Xanthine oxidase

Uricosuric agents +

Urate → Renal clearance of uric acid

Pegloticase + → Urate oxidase (uricase

Allantoin

Fig. 141.4 Summary of purine degradation and urate clearance, including sites of action of urate-lowering therapy.

Allopurinol

Allopurinol is first-line ULT. This drug inhibits xanthine oxidase, a critical enzyme in the metabolism of purines to urate, which catalyses the conversion of hypoxanthine to xanthine and xanthine to urate. Allopurinol is a structural analogue of hypoxanthine, and its active metabolite oxypurinol is a structural analogue of xanthine. Both allopurinol and oxypurinol inhibit xanthine oxidase, thereby reducing the production of urate. In comparison to allopurinol which has short half-life ($t_{1/2} \sim 1$ hour), oxypurinol has a much longer half-life ($t_{1/2} \sim 23$ hours). Oxypurinol is largely eliminated unchanged by the kidneys and thus its half-life is dependent on renal function. Allopurinol is effective in reducing serum urate, resorption of tophi, and reducing the number of gout flares. Allopurinol may also have a beneficial effect on renal function, CVD, hypertension and mortality.[70–73]

Although allopurinol is well tolerated in most patients, adverse events may occur. Approximately 2% of patients develop a mild rash. Allopurinol can be associated with a rare but potentially life-threatening allopurinol hypersensitivity syndrome (AHS) which is characterized by rash (e.g. toxic epidermal necrolysis, exfoliative dermatitis), eosinophilia, leucocytosis, fever, hepatitis, and progressive renal failure. The true incidence of AHS is unknown although it is estimated to be around 0.1%. Some cases of AHS occur as a result of T-cell-mediated immune reactions to oxypurinol. A number of studies have reported that renal impairment, diuretic use, and recent commencement of allopurinol therapy are risk factors for the development of severe AHS. *HLA B*5801* has been identified as an important risk factor for toxicity, particularly in Asian populations.[74] The mortality associated with AHS is as high as 27%. There is no cure for AHS and early recognition and drug withdrawal are important. Management consists of supportive care, and although corticosteroids and dialysis have been used, their role is controversial. Desensitization has been used successfully for patients with mild cutaneous hypersensitivity reactions, but is contraindicated for patients with life-threatening AHS.[75]

The role of allopurinol dosing in AHS was highlighted by Hande and colleagues who reported that most of the patients in their institution and literature review with AHS had pre-existing renal impairment and were treated with full doses of allopurinol ($\geq$300 mg daily).[76] This observation, together with studies of oxypurinol clearance in patients with renal impairment, lead to the development of dosing guidelines, recommending that allopurinol doses should be adjusted according to creatinine clearance. These guidelines are of great practical relevance, as renal impairment is a frequent finding in patients with gout.[7] However, adherence to these dosing guidelines for long-term prescribing of allopurinol results in suboptimal control of hyperuricaemia in the majority of patients with gout.[77] A recent report has described the safety and efficacy of gradual dose escalation of allopurinol in patients established on renally-adjusted doses.[78] Using this strategy, 89% of patients achieved a target serum urate concentration <0.36 mmol/L in 12 months, without serious toxicity.

Gout is common in solid organ transplant recipients and azathioprine is a commonly used immunosuppressive agent in these patients. 6-Mercaptopurine, the active metabolite of azathioprine, is partly inactivated by xanthine oxidase and therefore allopurinol may increase serum concentrations of 6-mercaptopurine with resultant myelosuppression. It is recommended that the dose of azathioprine be reduced by 50–75% before commencing allopurinol and that the starting dose of allopurinol be lower than normal. However, despite dose adjustment bone marrow suppression with this combination may occur after months or even years of therapy.[79] Therefore, azathioprine and allopurinol must be coprescribed with great caution and with careful blood monitoring for the duration of combination therapy.

Febuxostat

Febuxostat is a recently developed xanthine oxidase inhibitor that was approved by the European Medicines Agency in 2008 (at doses up to 120 mg daily) and by the FDA in 2009 (at doses up to 80 mg daily) for management of hyperuricaemia in patients with gout. Febuxostat is a potent and specific non-purine inhibitor of xanthine oxidase. Febuxostat is metabolized by hepatic conjugation and oxidation, and has at least three pharmacologically active metabolites: 67M-1, 67M-2, and 67M-4.

RCTs have demonstrated that febuxostat has superior urate-lowering efficacy compared with fixed-dose allopurinol. For example, in a phase 3 randomized, double-blind, 52 week trial of patients with gout and no significant renal impairment (as defined by creatinine clearance <50 mL/min), serum urate less than 0.36 mmol/litre (6 mg/dL) at the last three monthly measurements was achieved in 21% of those on 300 mg allopurinol, 53% of those on 80 mg febuxostat, and 62% of those on 120 mg febuxostat.[80] Gout flares were more common in the 120 mg febuxostat group in the first 8 weeks of treatment. However, other adverse event and serious adverse event rates was similar in the three treatment groups. The most common treatment-related adverse events for all groups were liver function test abnormalities, diarrhoea, headache, and musculoskeletal signs and symptoms. Similarly, in another large phase 3, randomized, double-blind, 28 week trial comparing the safety and efficacy of febuxostat with allopurinol, serum urate less than 0.36 mmol/litre (6 mg/dL) at the final visit was achieved in 42% of those on allopurinol (300 mg or 200 mg/day, based on renal function), 45% of patients treated with febuxostat 40 mg, and 67% of those on 80 mg febuxostat.[81] In those patients with mild/moderate renal impairment, serum urate less than 6 mg/dL was achieved in 50% of patients treated with febuxostat 40 mg, 72% of those on 80 mg febuxostat, and 42% of those on allopurinol. Rates of adverse events and serious adverse events did not differ across treatment groups. Long-term extension studies have shown that serum urate-lowering persists during treatment with febuxostat, with associated resolution of gout flares and tophi.[82]

In summary, febuxostat is an effective urate-lowering agent. A dose of 40 mg/day may be effective in achieving a target serum urate below 0.36 mmol/litre. However, a higher dose of 80 mg or 120 mg/day may be required to achieve this target. Febuxostat appears to be well tolerated and does not require dose adjustment in patients with mild–moderate renal or hepatic impairment. Liver function tests should be monitored while patients are taking febuxostat. Intensive prophylaxis against gout flares should be prescribed for up to 6 months when commencing febuxostat. To date, drug–drug interaction studies between febuxostat and azathioprine or 6-mercaptopurine have not been reported. This combination should be avoided because of the risk of significant toxicity.

Febuxostat should be considered for those patients with gout who have failed to achieve a target serum urate below0.36 mmol/litre on an adequate dose of allopurinol. Febuxostat may be particularly useful in the context of renal impairment, where allopurinol dosing is most complicated and carries the greatest risk of toxicity. However, clinical experience of febuxostat in patients with severe renal impairment, severe liver disease, and transplantation is very limited, and the safety of febuxostat in these situations is unknown. Similarly, the use of this drug in the paediatric context is not well recognized. While febuxostat has been shown to be more effective than fixed-dose allopurinol for reduction of serum urate, it is not yet known whether this drug is superior to allopurinol when a treat-to-target serum urate approach is employed with allopurinol. Although this agent has been recommended in the United Kingdom for patients who are intolerant to allopurinol or have contraindications to it,[83] the experience of this agent in patients with previous severe allopurinol reactions is limited; in a case series of 13 such patients treated with febuxostat, one patient developed a hypersensitivity-type cutaneous vasculitis early in febuxostat treatment.[84] Thus, use of febuxostat in such patients requires caution, careful dose escalation, and close monitoring.

Uricosuric drugs

Uricosuric drugs increase uric acid excretion through interactions with various urate transporters (Figure 141.3). Due to the higher uric acid concentrations in the renal tract, these drugs have the potential to promote urate stone formation, and should be avoided in patients with nephrolithiasis. Liberal fluid intake is recommended for patients taking uricosuric agents, and urine alkalinization should also be considered when commencing these agents, using sodium bicarbonate (3–7.5 g daily) or potassium citrate (7.5 g daily).

Probenecid has been used for more than 60 years as a uricosuric agent. This agent promotes urate excretion through interactions with various renal tubular urate transporters including URAT1, NPT4, the organic anion transporters OAT1, OAT2, and OAT4, and multidrug resistance protein MRP4 (Figure 141.3). In patients without severe chronic renal impairment (defined as CrCl <30 mL/min) who have not achieved normouricaemia (defined as serum urate ≤0.30 mmol/litre) with fixed-dose allopurinol, target serum urate below 0.36 mmol/litre was achieved in 68% patients treated with probenecid.[85] In additional to use as monotherapy, probenecid in combination with allopurinol leads to excellent serum urate lowering with up to 95% patients achieving serum urate concentrations of less than 0.30 mmol/litre.[86] Probenecid is typically commenced at 250 mg twice daily, increasing to 1 g twice daily depending on serum urate concentrations and tolerance. Patients with chronic kidney disease may have less response to probenecid, particularly those with CrCl <30 mL/min. Probenecid is generally well tolerated, but may cause gastrointestinal intolerance in up to 23% of patients.[85] Headache, hypersensitivity reactions, nephrotic syndrome, hepatitis, and anaemia are rare complications.

Sulphinpyrazone has similar urate-lowering efficacy to probenecid, and is also most effective in patients with normal renal function. This agent promotes uric acid excretion through interactions with renal tubular urate transporters such as OAT4 and MRP4. Typical starting doses are 100–200 mg daily, increasing up to 600 mg daily in divided doses as needed to achieve serum urate target. Sulphinpyrazone is contraindicated in patients with active peptic ulcer disease, severe renal disease, and severe liver disease. Sulphinpyrazone may potentiate the action of sulphonylureas, insulin, salicylates, and anticoagulants. Gastrointestinal intolerance is the most common adverse event, but other serious side effects are skin rash and blood dyscrasia such as anaemia, agranulocytosis, and thrmobocytopenia. Monitoring of the full blood count is essential throughout treatment.

Benzbromarone is a potent uricosuric agent with documented efficacy in patients with gout. It interacts with a number of renal urate transporters including SLC2A9 and URAT1. Benzbromarone is particularly beneficial for patients with renal impairment who are intolerant to allopurinol or have an insufficient response to recommended doses of allopurinol. RCTs have demonstrated that benzbromarone has superior efficacy over standard doses of allopurinol and is also more effective than probenecid in patients who have failed allopurinol treatment (due to inadequate serum urate lowering or intolerance). For example, in patients who had not achieved normouricaemia (defined as serum urate ≤0.30 mmol/litre) with fixed-dose allopurinol, target serum urate below 0.36 mmol/litre was achieved in 92% patients treated with benzbromarone.[85] Typical starting dose is 50 mg daily, increasing to 100 mg daily. Occasionally 200 mg daily is required to achieve normouricaemia. Benzbromarone was widely used in Europe until 2003 when it was withdrawn after reports of fulminant hepatitis leading to death in two patients. It appears that hepatotoxicity is extremely rare and was not reported in the clinical trials of benzbromarone. The EULAR gout treatment guidelines have endorsed the use of benzbromarone as an alternative to allopurinol, particularly in patients with renal impairment.[49] Close monitoring of liver function tests is required in patients receiving this drug.

Case history 1

A 78 year old woman presents with extensive gouty tophi affecting the hands and feet. These tophi are discharging and cause difficulty with gripping, toileting, and putting on shoes. She has treated heart failure and hypertension. Her medications include furosemide 80 mg twice daily. She is intolerant to allopurinol which caused blistering skin rash, eosinophilia, and raised creatinine. Examination shows extensive tophi but no synovitis.

Serum urate is 0.68 mmol/litre, creatinine 119 μmol/litre, and creatinine clearance 37 mL/min. Radiographs show gouty erosions. Swab of a discharging tophus confirms MSU crystals. What are the treatment options?

Comments: This patient has chronic tophaceous gout, likely due to chronic kidney disease and diuretic use. She has major musculoskeletal disability and radiographic damage due to her gout. Management is further complicated by intolerance to allopurinol. Serum urate lowering below 0.36 mmol/litre (and ideally lower) is required to achieve dissolution of MSU crystals and regression of tophi. Depending on drug availability, benzbromarone or cautious use of febuxostat would be appropriate first-line therapies. Probenecid could be trialled but may not be effective because of the degree of her chronic kidney disease. Allopurinol desensitization is contraindicated because of the severity of her allopurinol drug reaction.

Recombinant uricase

Uricase (urate oxidase) converts urate to 5-hydroxy isourate and H_2O_2, with subsequent formation of allantoin. Allantoin is soluble and is readily eliminated by the kidney. Unlike most other mammals, humans lack a functional uricase gene; the absence of uricase is a major contributor to elevated serum urate concentrations in humans compared with other species. Administration of recombinant uricase leads to profound reductions in serum urate concentrations, often to undetectable levels. Rasburicase, an agent used in the oncology setting for management of tumour lysis syndrome, has been described as a potent urate-lowering agent in patients with severe refractory gout.[87] Use of rasburicase for long-term management of gout is limited by the relatively short half-life, high cost, and risk of hypersensitivity reactions with repeated infusions.

Pegloticase is a recombinant mammalian uricase modified by polyethylene glycol which was approved in the United States in 2010 for treatment of chronic gout that is refractory to conventional therapy. In two phase 3 clinical trials, intravenous administration of 8 mg pegloticase every 2 or 4 weeks lead to higher numbers of patients achieving target plasma urate concentrations below 0.36 mmol/litre after 3 and 6 months of treatment; overall, this target was achieved in 42% of the fortnightly pegloticase group, 35% of the monthly pegloticase group, and 0% of the placebo group.[88] After 6 months of treatment, patients treated with pegloticase on a fortnightly basis had greater regression of tophi, fewer gout flares, fewer tender joints, less disability, improved physical function, and less pain compared with the placebo-treated group. Overall adverse event rates were similar between the pegloticase and placebo groups, but more serious adverse events were observed in the pegloticase groups, primarily due to greater frequency of infusion reactions in pegloticase-treated patients. Infusion reactions occur in up to one-quarter of patients treated with pegloticase, and may present as chest discomfort, chest pain, dyspnoea, erythema, flushing, rash, and urticaria. To reduce the risk of infusion reactions, premedication with antihistamines and corticosteroids is recommended, and patients should be closely monitored for infusion reactions during and after drug administration. Importantly, loss of urate-lowering efficacy precedes development of infusion reactions in most patients with infusion reactions, and should be viewed as an important warning sign of potential drug reaction. In those patients with loss of urate-lowering efficacy on two consecutive treatments, pegloticase should be discontinued. The recommended dose of pegloticase is 8 mg administered as an intravenous infusion over at least 2 hours, every 2 weeks.

Management of comorbid conditions

The high prevalence of comorbid conditions associated with gout (Table 141.1) necessitates consideration of these conditions when formulating a management plan for patients with gout. Gout may be considered a 'red flag' for future metabolic and CVD, and risk factors should be carefully addressed. This includes assessment of smoking status, BMI, blood pressure, serum creatinine, fasting glucose, and lipids. A focused, patient-centred approach to these risk factors is of benefit in patients with gout,[89] and includes weight loss strategies, promotion of physical activity, smoking cessation support (including nicotine replacement therapy), and pharmacological management of hypertension, dyslipidaemia, and diabetes. Despite its mild urate-elevating effects, low-dose aspirin should not be withheld in patients at high cardiovascular risk. Thiazide diuretics should be avoided for management of hypertension in patients with gout. Certain agents such as losartan, fenofibrate, amlodipine, and atorvastatin have modest urate-lowering effects and may be preferentially selected to manage relevant comorbidities in patients with gout.[9]

Case history 2

A 50 year old man has had recurrent gout flares for the last 15 years. He is currently experiencing gout flares every 2 months, usually in his feet or knees. He has had 2 weeks off work in the last year due to gout flares. He has a family history of gout affecting his father and paternal uncle. He is currently taking bendrofluazide, accupril, and felodipine for management of hypertension, and allopurinol 300 mg daily. He drinks 25 units of beer per week. Examination shows BMI 35 kg/m², blood pressure 150/90 mmHg, no tophi or synovitis. Serum urate is 0.45 mmol/litre (0.65 mmol/litre prior to starting allopurinol), creatinine 92 μmol/litre, eGFR 80 ml/min/1.73 m², total cholesterol/HDL ratio 8.2, fasting glucose 6.8 mmol/litre. Knee aspiration at the time of a previous gout flare has confirmed the presence of MSU crystals. What are the treatment options?

Comments: This man has recurrent gout flares with associated work disability. It is likely that his gout has occurred due to his genetic risk, obesity, diuretic use, and high purine intake. Serum urate-lowering below 0.36 mmol/litre is required to achieve dissolution of MSU crystals and suppression of acute gout attacks. Non-pharmacological therapy should include weight loss, avoidance of sugar-sweetened drinks, and reduction of beer intake. Prevention of gout flares can be achieved through low-dose colchicine prophylaxis (0.5 mg daily–twice daily), and intensification of his ULT. Adherence to allopurinol should be assessed. Provided adherence is assured, allopurinol dose should be gradually increased (by 100 mg monthly, to maximum dose 900 mg daily) to achieve a target serum urate. He also has poorly controlled hypertension, dyslipidaemia, and impaired fasting glucose. Management of these comorbid conditions includes screening for type 2 diabetes, stopping bendrofluazide, and commencing alternative anti-hypertensive agents such as losartan and amlodipine. Lipid-lowering therapy with atorvastatin should also be commenced.

Education and adherence

Despite the availability of effective therapies for gout management, this condition is often poorly managed, with low ULT prescription rates, infrequent monitoring of serum urate, poor adherence to ULT, and failure to achieve serum urate targets.[90] Suboptimal gout management leads to unnecessary pain, disability, and loss of productivity. Both practitioners and patients may contribute to poor gout management, and education of both groups is essential. A treat-to serum urate target is frequently effective in improving long-term gout management.[91] This approach allows both the health professional and the patient to determine the efficacy of treatment, which is particularly important in the early stages of ULT when the clinical benefits may not be immediately apparent. Practitioners need to provide appropriate education to patients, ensure continuity of ULT prescription, modify ULT according to serum urate results, and arrange careful monitoring of serum urate concentrations, to ensure that serum urate targets are achieved and maintained. Patients should also have an action plan to ensure prompt, safe, and effective management of flares. Patient education focusing on the central role of hyperuricaemia in MSU crystal formation, and the importance of serum urate reduction to a level below saturation levels is essential to ensure engagement and adherence to long-term ULT. Careful commencement of ULT at gradually increasing doses and with appropriate prophylaxis also plays an important role in ensuring that the patient continues with ULT long-term.

Conclusion

Gout is a common inflammatory arthritis caused by deposition of MSU crystals. This condition causes important musculoskeletal disability, and is frequently associated with major comorbid conditions. A number of treatments are available for effective management of gout, to manage and prevent acute flares, and to prevent the consequences of MSU crystal deposition. Long-term successful therapy of gout requires reduction of serum urate below saturation concentrations, at least below 0.36 mmol/litre.

Conflict of interest statement

Nicola Dalbeth has acted as a consultant to the following companies: Takeda, Ardea Biosciences, Novartis, Fonterra, Metabolex, Abbott Laboratories, Roche.

References

1. Pascual E. Persistence of monosodium urate crystals and low-grade inflammation in the synovial fluid of patients with untreated gout. *Arthritis Rheum* 1991;34:141–145.
2. Wallace SL, Robinson H, Masi AT et al. Preliminary criteria for the classification of the acute arthritis of primary gout. *Arthritis Rheum* 1977;20:895–900.
3. Harrold LR, Saag KG, Yood RA et al. Validity of gout diagnoses in administrative data. *Arthritis Rheum* 2007;57:103–108.
4. Cea Soriano L, Rothenbacher D, Choi HK, Garcia Rodriguez LA. Contemporary epidemiology of gout in the UK general population. *Arthritis Res Ther* 2011;13:R39.
5. Zhu Y, Pandya BJ, Choi HK. Prevalence of gout and hyperuricemia in the US general population: The National Health and Nutrition Examination Survey 2007–2008. *Arthritis Rheum* 2011;63:3136–3141.
6. Winnard D, Wright C, Taylor WJ et al. National prevalence of gout derived from administrative health data in Aotearoa New Zealand. *Rheumatology* (Oxford) 2012;51(5):901–909.
7. Mikuls TR, Farrar JT, Bilker WB et al. Gout epidemiology: results from the UK General Practice Research Database, 1990–1999. *Ann Rheum Dis* 2005;64:267–272.
8. Keenan RT, O'Brien WR, Lee KH et al. Prevalence of contraindications and prescription of pharmacologic therapies for gout. *Am J Med* 2011;124:155–163.
9. Choi HK, Soriano LC, Zhang Y, Rodriguez LA. Antihypertensive drugs and risk of incident gout among patients with hypertension: population based case-control study. *BMJ* 2012;344:d8190.
10. Choi HK, Curhan G. Independent impact of gout on mortality and risk for coronary heart disease. *Circulation* 2007;116:894–900.
11. Choi HK, Atkinson K, Karlson EW, Willett W, Curhan G. Purine-rich foods, dairy and protein intake, and the risk of gout in men. *N Engl J Med* 2004;350:1093–1103.
12. Choi HK, Atkinson K, Karlson EW, Willett W, Curhan G. Alcohol intake and risk of incident gout in men: a prospective study. *Lancet* 2004;363:1277–1281.
13. Choi HK, Curhan G. Soft drinks, fructose consumption, and the risk of gout in men: prospective cohort study. *BMJ* 2008;336:309–312.
14. Choi HK, Willett W, Curhan G. Fructose-rich beverages and risk of gout in women. *JAMA* 2010;304:2270–2278.
15. Choi HK, Atkinson K, Karlson EW, Curhan G. Obesity, weight change, hypertension, diuretic use, and risk of gout in men: the health professionals follow-up study. *Arch Intern Med* 2005;165:742–748.
16. Choi HK, Willett W, Curhan G. Coffee consumption and risk of incident gout in men: a prospective study. *Arthritis Rheum* 2007;56:2049–2055.
17. Choi HK, Gao X, Curhan G. Vitamin C intake and the risk of gout in men: a prospective study. *Arch Intern Med* 2009;169:502–507.
18. Choi HK, Curhan G. Coffee consumption and risk of incident gout in women: the Nurses' Health Study. *Am J Clin Nutr* 2010;92:922–927.
19. ter Borg EJ, Rasker JJ. Gout in the elderly, a separate entity? *Ann Rheum Dis* 1987;46:72–76.
20. Becker MA, Schumacher HR, Benjamin KL et al. Quality of life and disability in patients with treatment-failure gout. *J Rheumatol* 2009;36:1041–1048.
21. Edwards NL, Sundy JS, Forsythe A et al. Work productivity loss due to flares in patients with chronic gout refractory to conventional therapy. *J Med Econ* 2011;14:10–15.
22. Colvine K, Kerr AJ, McLachlan A et al. Cardiovascular disease risk factor assessment and management in gout: an analysis using guideline-based electronic clinical decision support. *N Z Med J* 2008;121:73–81.
23. Pascual E, Batlle-Gualda E, Martinez A, Rosas J, Vela P. Synovial fluid analysis for diagnosis of intercritical gout. *Ann Intern Med* 1999;131:756–759.
24. Logan JA, Morrison E, McGill PE. Serum uric acid in acute gout. *Ann Rheum Dis* 1997;56:696–697.
25. Thiele RG, Schlesinger N. Diagnosis of gout by ultrasound. *Rheumatology* (Oxford) 2007;46:1116–1121.
26. Poh YJ, Dalbeth N, Doyle A, McQueen FM. Magnetic resonance imaging bone oedema is not a major feature of gout unless there is concomitant osteomyelitis: ten year findings from a high prevalence population. *J Rheumatol* 2011;38(11):2475–2481.
27. Dalbeth N, Clark B, Gregory K et al. Mechanisms of bone erosion in gout: a quantitative analysis using plain radiography and computed tomography. *Ann Rheum Dis* 2009;68:1290–1295.
28. Choi HK, Al-Arfaj AM, Eftekhari A et al. Dual energy computed tomography in tophaceous gout. *Ann Rheum Dis* 2009;68:1609–1612.
29. Choi HK, Mount DB, Reginato AM. Pathogenesis of gout. *Ann Intern Med* 2005;143:499–516.
30. Choi JW, Ford ES, Gao X, Choi HK. Sugar-sweetened soft drinks, diet soft drinks, and serum uric acid level: the Third National Health and Nutrition Examination Survey. *Arthritis Rheum* 2008;59:109–116.
31. Facchini F, Chen YD, Hollenbeck CB, Reaven GM. Relationship between resistance to insulin-mediated glucose uptake, urinary uric acid clearance, and plasma uric acid concentration. *JAMA* 1991;266:3008–3011.

32. Kolz M, Johnson T, Sanna S et al. Meta-analysis of 28,141 individuals identifies common variants within five new loci that influence uric acid concentrations. *PLoS Genet* 2009;5:e1000504.

33. Caulfield MJ, Munroe PB, O'Neill D et al. SLC2A9 is a high-capacity urate transporter in humans. *PLoS Med* 2008;5:e197.

34. Vitart V, Rudan I, Hayward C et al. SLC2A9 is a newly identified urate transporter influencing serum urate concentration, urate excretion and gout. *Nat Genet* 2008;40:437–442.

35. Doring A, Gieger C, Mehta D et al. SLC2A9 influences uric acid concentrations with pronounced sex-specific effects. *Nat Genet* 2008;40:430–436.

36. Dehghan A, Kottgen A, Yang Q et al. Association of three genetic loci with uric acid concentration and risk of gout: a genome-wide association study. *Lancet* 2008;372:1953–1961.

37. Loeb JN. The influence of temperature on the solubility of monosodium urate. *Arthritis Rheum* 1972;15:189–192.

38. Campion EW, Glynn RJ, DeLabry LO. Asymptomatic hyperuricemia. Risks and consequences in the Normative Aging Study. *Am J Med* 1987;82:421–426.

39. McGill NW, Dieppe PA. Evidence for a promoter of urate crystal formation in gouty synovial fluid. *Ann Rheum Dis* 1991;50:558–561.

40. Schumacher HR. Pathology of the synovial membrane in gout. Light and electron microscopic studies. Interpretation of crystals in electron micrographs. *Arthritis Rheum* 1975;18:771–782.

41. Dalbeth N, Haskard DO. Mechanisms of inflammation in gout. *Rheumatology* (Oxford) 2005;44:1090–1096.

42. Martinon F, Petrilli V, Mayor A, Tardivel A, Tschopp J. Gout-associated uric acid crystals activate the NALP3 inflammasome. *Nature* 2006;440:237–241.

43. Naccache PH, Grimard M, Roberge CJ et al. Crystal-induced neutrophil activation. I. Initiation and modulation of calcium mobilization and superoxide production by microcrystals. *Arthritis Rheum* 1991;34:333–342.

44. Martin WJ, Shaw O, Liu X, Steiger S, Harper JL. Monosodium urate monohydrate crystal-recruited noninflammatory monocytes differentiate into M1-like proinflammatory macrophages in a peritoneal murine model of gout. *Arthritis Rheum* 2011;63:1322–1332.

45. Dalbeth N, Pool B, Gamble GD et al. Cellular characterization of the gouty tophus: a quantitative analysis. *Arthritis Rheum* 2010;62:1549–1556.

46. Dalbeth N, Smith T, Nicolson B et al. Enhanced osteoclastogenesis in patients with tophaceous gout: urate crystals promote osteoclast development through interactions with stromal cells. *Arthritis Rheum* 2008;58:1854–1865.

47. Chhana A, Callon KE, Pool B et al. Monosodium urate monohydrate crystals inhibit osteoblast viability and function: implications for development of bone erosion in gout. *Ann Rheum Dis* 2011;70:1684–1691.

48. Schweyer S, Hemmerlein B, Radzun HJ, Fayyazi A. Continuous recruitment, co-expression of tumour necrosis factor-alpha and matrix metalloproteinases, and apoptosis of macrophages in gout tophi. *Virchows Arch* 2000;437:534–539.

49. Zhang W, Doherty M, Bardin T et al. EULAR evidence based recommendations for gout. Part II: Management. Report of a task force of the EULAR Standing Committee for International Clinical Studies Including Therapeutics (ESCISIT). *Ann Rheum Dis* 2006;65:1312–1324.

50. Jordan KM, Cameron JS, Snaith M et al. British Society for Rheumatology and British Health Professionals in Rheumatology guideline for the management of gout. *Rheumatology* (Oxford) 2007;46:1372–1374.

51. Khanna D, Fitzgerald JD, Khanna PP et al. 2012 American College of Rheumatology guidelines for management of gout. Part 1: systematic nonpharmacologic and pharmacologic therapeutic approaches to hyperuricemia. *Arthritis Care Res* (Hoboken) 2012;64:1431–1446.

52. Khanna D, Khanna PP, Fitzgerald JD et al. 2012 American College of Rheumatology guidelines for management of gout. Part 2: therapy and antiinflammatory prophylaxis of acute gouty arthritis. *Arthritis Care Res* (Hoboken) 2012;64:1447–1461.

53. Schumacher HR, Jr., Boice JA, Daikh DI et al. Randomised double blind trial of etoricoxib and indometacin in treatment of acute gouty arthritis. *BMJ* 2002;324:1488–1492.

54. Willburger RE, Mysler E, Derbot J et al. Lumiracoxib 400 mg once daily is comparable to indomethacin 50 mg three times daily for the treatment of acute flares of gout. *Rheumatology* (Oxford) 2007;46:1126–1132.

55. Terkeltaub RA, Furst DE, Bennett K et al. High versus low dosing of oral colchicine for early acute gout flare: Twenty-four-hour outcome of the first multicenter, randomized, double-blind, placebo-controlled, parallel-group, dose-comparison colchicine study. *Arthritis Rheum* 2010;62:1060–1068.

56. Terkeltaub RA, Furst DE, Digiacinto JL, Kook KA, Davis MW. Novel evidence-based colchicine dose-reduction algorithm to predict and prevent colchicine toxicity in the presence of cytochrome P450 3A4/P-glycoprotein inhibitors. *Arthritis Rheum* 2011;63:2226–2237.

57. Janssens HJ, Janssen M, van de Lisdonk EH, van Riel PL, van Weel C. Use of oral prednisolone or naproxen for the treatment of gout arthritis: a double-blind, randomised equivalence trial. *Lancet* 2008;371:1854–1860.

58. Man CY, Cheung IT, Cameron PA, Rainer TH. Comparison of oral prednisolone/paracetamol and oral indomethacin/paracetamol combination therapy in the treatment of acute goutlike arthritis: a double-blind, randomized, controlled trial. *Ann Emerg Med* 2007;49:670–677.

59. Ritter J, Kerr LD, Valeriano-Marcet J, Spiera H. ACTH revisited: effective treatment for acute crystal induced synovitis in patients with multiple medical problems. *J Rheumatol* 1994;21:696–699.

60. Getting SJ, Christian HC, Flower RJ, Perretti M. Activation of melanocortin type 3 receptor as a molecular mechanism for adrenocorticotropic hormone efficacy in gouty arthritis. *Arthritis Rheum* 2002;46:2765–2775.

61. So A, De Meulemeester M, Pikhlak A et al. Canakinumab for the treatment of acute flares in difficult-to-treat gouty arthritis: Results of a multicenter, phase II, dose-ranging study. *Arthritis Rheum* 2010;62:3064–3076.

62. Borstad GC, Bryant LR, Abel MP et al. Colchicine for prophylaxis of acute flares when initiating allopurinol for chronic gouty arthritis. *J Rheumatol* 2004;31:2429–2432.

63. Paulus HE, Schlosstein LH, Godfrey RG, Klinenberg JR, Bluestone R. Prophylactic colchicine therapy of intercritical gout. A placebo-controlled study of probenecid-treated patients. *Arthritis Rheum* 1974;17:609–614.

64. Wortmann RL, Macdonald PA, Hunt B, Jackson RL. Effect of prophylaxis on gout flares after the initiation of urate-lowering therapy: analysis of data from three phase III trials. *Clin Ther* 2010;32:2386–2397.

65. Schlesinger N, Mysler E, Lin HY et al. Canakinumab reduces the risk of acute gouty arthritis flares during initiation of allopurinol treatment: results of a double-blind, randomised study. *Ann Rheum Dis* 2011;70:1264–1271.

66. Li-Yu J, Clayburne G, Sieck M et al. Treatment of chronic gout. Can we determine when urate stores are depleted enough to prevent attacks of gout? *J Rheumatol* 2001;28:577–580.

67. Shoji A, Yamanaka H, Kamatani N. A retrospective study of the relationship between serum urate level and recurrent attacks of gouty arthritis: evidence for reduction of recurrent gouty arthritis with antihyperuricemic therapy. *Arthritis Rheum* 2004;51:321–325.

68. Perez-Ruiz F, Calabozo M, Pijoan JI, Herrero-Beites AM, Ruibal A. Effect of urate-lowering therapy on the velocity of size reduction of tophi in chronic gout. *Arthritis Rheum* 2002;47:356–360.

69. Juraschek SP, Miller ER, 3rd, Gelber AC. Effect of oral vitamin C supplementation on serum uric acid: A meta-analysis of randomized controlled trials. *Arthritis Care Res* (Hoboken) 2011;63:1295–1306.

70. Siu YP, Leung KT, Tong MK, Kwan TH. Use of allopurinol in slowing the progression of renal disease through its ability to lower serum uric acid level. *Am J Kidney Dis* 2006;47:51–59.

71. Noman A, Ang DS, Ogston S, Lang CC, Struthers AD. Effect of high-dose allopurinol on exercise in patients with chronic stable angina: a randomised, placebo controlled crossover trial. *Lancet* 2010;375:2161–2167.

72. Feig DI, Soletsky B, Johnson RJ. Effect of allopurinol on blood pressure of adolescents with newly diagnosed essential hypertension: a randomized trial. *JAMA* 2008;300:924–932.

73. Luk AJ, Levin GP, Moore EE, Zhou XH, Kestenbaum BR, Choi HK. Allopurinol and mortality in hyperuricaemic patients. *Rheumatology* (Oxford) 2009;48:804–806.

74. Hung SI, Chung WH, Liou LB et al. HLA-B*5801 allele as a genetic marker for severe cutaneous adverse reactions caused by allopurinol. *Proc Natl Acad Sci U S A* 2005;102:4134–4139.

75. Fam AG, Dunne SM, Iazzetta J, Paton TW. Efficacy and safety of desensitization to allopurinol following cutaneous reactions. *Arthritis Rheum* 2001;44:231–238.

76. Hande KR, Noone RM, Stone WJ. Severe allopurinol toxicity. Description and guidelines for prevention in patients with renal insufficiency. *Am J Med* 1984;76:47–56.

77. Dalbeth N, Kumar S, Stamp L, Gow P. Dose adjustment of allopurinol according to creatinine clearance does not provide adequate control of hyperuricemia in patients with gout. *J Rheumatol* 2006;33:1646–1650.

78. Stamp LK, O'Donnell JL, Zhang M et al. Using allopurinol above the dose based on creatinine clearance is effective and safe in patients with chronic gout, including those with renal impairment. *Arthritis Rheum* 2011;63:412–421.

79. Cummins D, Sekar M, Halil O, Banner N. Myelosuppression associated with azathioprine-allopurinol interaction after heart and lung transplantation. *Transplantation* 1996;61:1661–1662.

80. Becker MA, Schumacher HR, Jr., Wortmann RL et al. Febuxostat compared with allopurinol in patients with hyperuricemia and gout. *N Engl J Med* 2005;353:2450–2461.

81. Becker MA, Schumacher HR, Espinoza LR et al. The urate-lowering efficacy and safety of febuxostat in the treatment of the hyperuricemia of gout: the CONFIRMS trial. *Arthritis Res Ther* 2010;12:R63.

82. Becker MA, Schumacher HR, MacDonald PA, Lloyd E, Lademacher C. Clinical efficacy and safety of successful longterm urate lowering with febuxostat or allopurinol in subjects with gout. *J Rheumatol* 2009;36:1273–1282.

83. Stevenson M, Pandor A. Febuxostat for the treatment of hyperuricaemia in people with gout: a single technology appraisal. *Health Technol Assess* 2009;13 Suppl 3:37–42.

84. Chohan S. Safety and efficacy of febuxostat treatment in subjects with gout and severe allopurinol adverse reactions. *J Rheumatol* 2011;38:1957–1959.

85. Reinders MK, van Roon EN, Jansen TL et al. Efficacy and tolerability of urate-lowering drugs in gout: a randomised controlled trial of benzbromarone versus probenecid after failure of allopurinol. *Ann Rheum Dis* 2009;68:51–56.

86. Stocker SL, Graham GG, McLachlan AJ, Williams KM, Day RO. Pharmacokinetic and pharmacodynamic interaction between allopurinol and probenecid in patients with gout. *J Rheumatol* 2011;38:904–910.

87. Richette P, Briere C, Hoenen-Clavert V, Loeuille D, Bardin T. Rasburicase for tophaceous gout not treatable with allopurinol: an exploratory study. *J Rheumatol* 2007;34:2093–2098.

88. Sundy JS, Baraf HS, Yood RA et al. Efficacy and tolerability of pegloticase for the treatment of chronic gout in patients refractory to conventional treatment: two randomized controlled trials. *JAMA* 2011;306:711–720.

89. McLachlan A, Kerr A, Lee M, Dalbeth N. Nurse-led cardiovascular disease risk management intervention for patients with gout. *Eur J Cardiovasc Nurs* 2011;10:94–100.

90. Harrold LR, Andrade SE, Briesacher BA et al. Adherence with urate-lowering therapies for the treatment of gout. *Arthritis Res Ther* 2009;11:R46.

91. Perez-Ruiz F. Treating to target: a strategy to cure gout. *Rheumatology* (Oxford) 2009;48 Suppl 2:ii9–ii14.

92. Rodriguez G, Soriano LC, Choi HK. Impact of diabetes against the future risk of developing gout. *Ann Rheum Dis* 2010;69:2090–2094.

93. Choi HK, De Vera MA, Krishnan E. Gout and the risk of type 2 diabetes among men with a high cardiovascular risk profile. *Rheumatology* (Oxford) 2008;47:1567–1570.

94. Krishnan E, Kwoh CK, Schumacher HR, Kuller L. Hyperuricemia and incidence of hypertension among men without metabolic syndrome. *Hypertension* 2007;49:298–303.

95. Krishnan E, Baker JF, Furst DE, Schumacher HR. Gout and the risk of acute myocardial infarction. *Arthritis Rheum* 2006;54:2688–2696.

96. Baker JF, Schumacher HR, Krishnan E. Serum uric acid level and risk for peripheral arterial disease: analysis of data from the multiple risk factor intervention trial. *Angiology* 2007;58:450–457.

97. Shimizu T, Hori H. The prevalence of nephrolithiasis in patients with primary gout: a cross-sectional study using helical computed tomography. *J Rheumatol* 2009;36:1958–1962.

98. Kramer HJ, Choi HK, Atkinson K, Stampfer M, Curhan GC. The association between gout and nephrolithiasis in men: The Health Professionals' Follow-Up Study. *Kidney Int* 2003;64:1022–1026.

99. Dalbeth N, So A. Hyperuricaemia and gout: state of the art and future perspectives. *Ann Rheum Dis* 2010;69:1738–1743.

100. Dalbeth N. Gout in 2010: progress and controversies in treatment. *Nat Rev Rheumatol* 2011;7:77–78.

101. Merriman TR, Dalbeth N. The genetic basis of hyperuricaemia and gout. *Joint Bone Spine* 2011;78:35–40.

Sources of patient information

American College of Rheumatology: www.rheumatology.org/practice/clinical/patients/diseases_and_conditions/gout.pdf

Arthritis Research UK: www.arthritisresearchuk.org/Files/2015-Gout.pdf

Health Navigator NZ: www.healthnavigator.org.nz/health-topics/gout/

UK Gout Society: www.ukgoutsociety.org/allabout.htm.

CHAPTER 142

Calcium pyrophosphate crystal deposition (CPPD)

Edward Roddy and Michael Doherty

Introduction

Calcium pyrophosphate (CPP) crystal deposition (CPPD) in articular cartilage is a common age-related phenomenon. CPP crystals deposit almost exclusively within articular tissues, preferentially fibrocartilage, and are the most common cause of cartilage calcification (chondrocalcinosis, CC). In 1961, Daniel McCarthy first identified CPP crystals in synovial fluid obtained from acutely inflamed knees of patients with CC, leading to introduction of the term 'pseudogout', because of its clinical similarity to acute gout.[1]

Definitions and classification criteria

After the identification of CPP crystals as the cause of acute pseudogout by McCarty and colleagues,[1] other clinical phenotypes were soon recognized. Their descriptions were also prefixed by 'pseudo' and included 'pseudo-rheumatoid arthritis', 'pseudo-osteoarthritis' (with or without inflammation) and 'pseudo-neuropathic' arthritis in addition to 'lanthanic' (asymptomatic) radiographic CC.[2] Furthermore, the term 'pyrophosphate arthropathy' became increasingly used to describe CPPD occurring with coexistent structural osteoarthritis (OA). This expanding complex nomenclature caused considerable confusion over subsequent years, leading to inconsistent application of these terms. Furthermore, it is unclear whether all these syndromes are distinct, mutually exclusive subsets and whether CPP crystals are the causative agents in all subsets or are merely innocent bystanders. Also the prefix 'pseudo-' arguably implies that CPPD is of less interest and importance than other crystal arthropathies, principally gout.[3]

The European League Against Rheumatism (EULAR) CPPD Task Force has recently suggested a simplified terminology (Table 142.1),[4] proposing that:

- 'Calcium pyrophosphate dihydrate' crystals be simplified to **calcium pyrophosphate (CPP)** crystals, analogous to gout where 'monosodium urate monohydrate' is abbreviated to monosodium urate.
- **Calcium pyrophosphate deposition (CPPD)** should be used as an umbrella term for all instances of CPP crystal occurrence.

- **Chondrocalcinosis (CC)** is used to describe cartilage calcification of any cause including CPPD or basic calcium phosphates (BCP) identified by imaging or histological examination.
- **Acute CPP crystal arthritis** is used to describe acute onset, self-limiting attacks of synovitis due to CPP crystals (formerly 'pseudogout').
- **OA with CPPD** refers to concurrence of CPPD in a joint with structural changes of OA (previously 'pyrophosphate arthropathy') whether symptomatic or asymptomatic.
- **Chronic CPP crystal inflammatory arthritis** describes the occurrence of a chronic inflammatory arthritis (often with changes of OA) with associated CPPD.

Epidemiology

CPPD is a common age-related phenomenon in the general population. Epidemiological studies report the prevalence of radiographic CC and/or OA with CPPD (formerly 'pyrophosphate arthropathy') (Table 142.2). The true prevalence of symptomatic CPPD is unknown. A community survey of 1727 adults (mean age 63.7 years) from Nottingham (United Kingdom) identified a crude prevalence of radiographic knee CC of 7.0% which equated to an age, gender, and knee pain standardized prevalence estimate of 4.5% in those aged 40 years and over.[5] In the Framingham survey, a similar prevalence estimate for radiographic knee CC of 8.1% was found in a population of 1425 adults aged over 63 years.[6] The prevalence of radiographic CC at the knee and/or wrist was 10% in a Spanish population of 261 general practice attenders aged over 60 years.[7] Similarly, a community survey of 1629 subjects aged 65 years and over from north-eastern Italy found the crude prevalence of radiographic CC at the knee and/or pelvis to be 10.4%, equating to a prevalence of 10.0% after adjustment for age and gender.[8] The prevalence of radiographic CC at the knee and wrist have been compared between white subjects from the Framingham population and a population of 2506 Chinese subjects aged 60 years and over from Beijing (China).[9] Radiographic CC at both sites was less prevalent in Chinese subjects than white subjects, with wrist CC being particularly uncommon in the Chinese population. A Swedish cross-sectional survey of three cohorts of adults aged 70,

Table 142.1 EULAR proposal for terminology

Term	Definition
Calcium pyrophosphate (CPP) crystals	Simplified name for calcium pyrophosphate dihydrate crystals
Calcium pyrophosphate deposition (CPPD)	Umbrella term for all instances of CPP crystal occurrence
Chondrocalcinosis (CC)	Cartilage calcification, identified by imaging or histological identification. Commonly but not always due to CPPD
Clinical presentations associated with CPPD	
Asymptomatic CPPD	CPPD with no apparent clinical consequence, either isolated CC or OA with CPPD
OA with CPPD	CPPD in a joint which also shows changes of OA, on imaging or histological examination
Acute CPP crystal arthritis	Acute onset, self-limiting synovitis with CPPD (replacing the term 'pseudogout')
Chronic CPP crystal inflammatory arthritis	Chronic inflammatory arthritis associated with CPPD

CPP, calcium pyrophosphate; CPPD; calcium pyrophosphate crystal deposition; EULAR, European League Against Rheumatism; OA, osteoarthritis.
From Zhang et al.[4]

Table 142.2 Prevalence of chondrocalcinosis (CC) by age and gender

Author	Study location	Study population	Joints examined	Prevalence of CC	Prevalence by gender		Prevalence by age group	
Bergström[10]	Göteborg, Sweden	352 adults aged 70, 75, and 79 years	Knees, wrists, fingers	11.5%	Women	14.7%	70 years	7.5%
					Men	5.5%	75 years	10.1%
							79 years	16.0%
Felson[6]	Framingham, USA	1425 adults aged 63–93 years	Knees	8.1%	Women	9.0%	<65 years	3.6%
					Men	6.9%	65–69 years	3.2%
					Age-adjusted RR 1.33 (95% CI 0.92, 1.92)		70–74 years	7.3%
							75–79 years	9.8%
							80–84 years	16.5%
							≥85 years	27.1%
Sanmarti[7]	Catalonia, Spain	261 GP attenders aged ≥60 years	Knees, hands	10%	Women	14%	60–69 years	7%
					Men	6%	70–79 years	13%
							≥80 years	43%
Neame[5]	Nottingham, UK	1727 adults aged ≥40 years	Knees	Crude 7.0% Standardized[a] 4.5%	Women	6.1%	Ranges from:	
					Men	8.2%	55–59 years	3.7%
					Age-adjusted OR 0.79 (95% CI 0.51, 1.12)		to	
							80–84 years	17.5%
Ramonda[8]	North-eastern Italy	1629 adults aged ≥65 years	Knees, pelvis	10.4%	Women	12.8%	65–74 years	7.8%
					Men	7.0%	75–84 years	9.4%
							≥85 years	21.1%

CI, confidence interval; GP, general practitioner; RR, relative risk.

[a]Standardized for age, gender, and knee pain.

75, and 79 years (352 participants) found that radiographic CC was most common at the knee (8.5%) followed by the wrist (5.1%) and then the fingers (1.7%).[10]

There is clear evidence that the prevalence of radiographic CC increase with age (Table 142.2).[5-10] The risk of CPPD doubles with every 10-year increase in age between 45 and 85 years (odds ratio (OR) 2.25, 95% confidence interval (CI) 1.79, 2.82).[11] However, the association of CPPD with gender is less clear. Radiographic CC was more prevalent in females than males in the Spanish (females 14%, males 6%), Italian (female 12.8%, males 7%), and Swedish (females 14.7%, males 5.6%) populations described above.[7,8,10] However, in the Nottingham and Framingham populations no difference in the prevalence of radiographic CC at the knee was seen between the genders after adjustment for age.[5,6]

In the Nottingham study,[11] OA with CPPD ('pyrophosphate arthropathy') at the knee was defined as the occurrence of radiographic CC with radiographic evidence of OA (Kellgren and Lawrence grade ≥2[12]). The crude prevalence of OA with CPPD at the knee was 3.4%, reducing slightly to 2.4% when standardized for age, gender, and knee pain.[11] There was an increased risk of OA with CPPD with increasing age (OR 2.88 per 10-year increase) but no association with gender.

Aetiopathogenesis

Pathophysiology

CPP crystals form in the extracellular compartment of cartilage from calcium ions and extracellular inorganic pyrophosphate (ePPi). The concentration of ePPi appears to be the most important factor determining formation of CPP crystals,[13] high calcium concentration alone being insufficient to increase CPP crystal formation.[14]

Inorganic pyrophosphate is not absorbed from the gut, so all PPi in humans is produced endogenously. PPi is an important regulator of normal mineralization in bones and teeth and inhibits calcium crystal formation elsewhere in the body. Modest concentrations of PPi stimulate BCP formation, but higher concentrations inhibit BCP crystal formation and growth. In cartilage, nucleotide triphosphates are released from resting chondrocytes and hydrolysed by nucleotide pyrophosphohydrolase (NTPPH) enzymes to produce PPi.[15,16] The ectoenzyme NTPPH plasma cell-membrane glycoprotein-1 (PC-1) on chondrocytes and matrix vesicles is the dominant source of cartilage matrix and synovial fluid PPi.[17,18] However, ePPi may also originate from the transport of intracellular PPi across the plasma membrane by the multipass transmembrane protein ANKH (Ankylosis human).[19,20] Once formed, ePPi is hydrolysed to orthophosphate by tissue non-specific alkaline phosphatase (TNAP),[21] requiring magnesium as a cofactor. High ePPi levels therefore can arise from reduced TNAP activity or increased activity of PC-1 or ANKH (Figure 142.1). Growth factors including transforming growth factor (TGF)-β, interleukin (IL)-1β, and insulin-like growth factor-1 (IGF-1) influence ePPi levels via their action on PC-1, TNAP, or ANKH.[3] Histologically, CPP crystals mainly occur in the mid-zone of cartilage and strongly coassociate with the hypertrophic chondrocyte phenotype. Such metabolically active cells associate with higher ePPi levels in cartilage and synovial fluid.[3]

A sufficiently high ionic product for (Ca × ePPi) is essential for CPP crystal formation, but additional characteristics of the cartilage

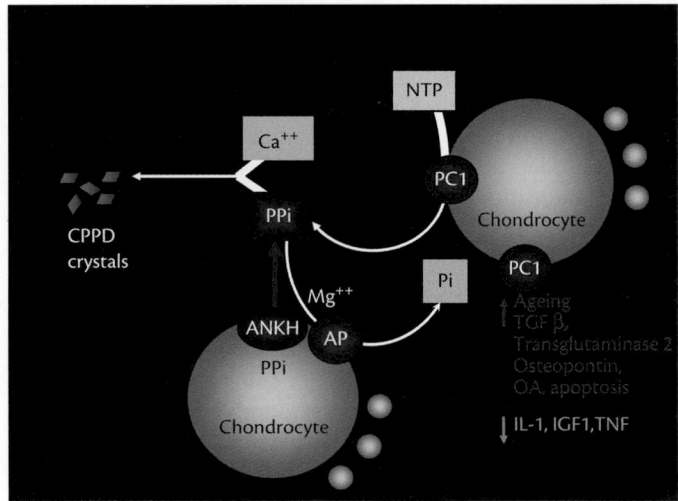

Fig. 142.1 Outline of metabolism of inorganic pyrophosphate. ANKH, ankylosis human multipass transmembrane protein; AP, alkaline phosphatase; Ca++, calcium ions; CPPD, Calcium pyrophosphate crystal deposition; IGF1, insulin-like growth factor-1; IL-1, interleukin-1; Mg2+, magnesium ions; NTP, nucleotide triphosphates; OA, osteoarthritis; PC1, plasma cell-membrane glycoprotein-1; Pi, orthophosphate; PPi, inorganic pyrophosphate; TGFβ, transforming growth factor-β; TNF, tumour necrosis factor.

extracellular matrix may either increase or inhibit the initial nucleation and subsequent growth of CPP crystals. We know very little about these tissue factors but there are data to support proteoglycan as an inhibitor and lipid, osteopontin and transglutaminases as promotors of CPPD.[3] In OA cartilage, the balance of these opposing factors is in favour of CPP crystal formation.

Acute CPP crystal arthritis is presumed to occur from 'shedding' of preformed CPP crystals from cartilage into the joint space, analogous to that in gout. Within cartilage the crystals are protected from interaction with inflammatory mediators, but inside the joint space CPP crystals trigger acute inflammation via activation of the NALP3 'inflammasome' with subsequent IL-1β driven neutrophilic inflammation.[3,22] Presumably low-grade chronic inflammation may be caused by more sustained release of smaller amounts of crystals. CPPD may also have detrimental biomechanical effects on load transmission through cartilage and shed CPP crystals may act as abrasives at the cartilage–cartilage interface.[3]

Risk factors for CPPD

Age

As discussed above, there is very strong evidence that age is an important risk factor for sporadic CC.

Prior joint damage and osteoarthritis

There is a clear, well-established association between OA and CPPD. Based on pooled data from nine epidemiological studies analysed by the EULAR Task Force, people with OA have between two and three times the risk of CPPD of people without OA (pooled OR 2.66; 95%CI 2.00, 3.54).[4] However, the role of CPP crystals in the pathogenesis of OA and vice versa is not completely understood.[23] Whereas BCP crystals are universally found in endstage OA, endstage articular cartilage specimens from knees and hips display CPP crystals in only 18% and 10% respectively.[24,25] Deposition of crystals, both monosodium urate and CPP, occurred predominantly at sites of cartilage damage in one cadaveric observational study, although 8% of crystal deposits occurred without gross evidence of cartilage damage, suggesting that damage is not essential for crystal deposition.[26] The presence of CPP crystals associates with greater radiographic OA severity.[27] CPP crystals exacerbate OA when directly introduced into mechanically stressed rabbit knee joints,[28] and promote expression of inflammatory cytokines and matrix metalloproteinases.[29] CPP crystals have therefore been assumed to promote cartilage damage in humans. The presence of synovial fluid CPP crystals or radiographic CC led to progression of radiographic knee OA in one prospective study of 350 participants.[30] A number of local mechanical factors including joint hypermobility, ligamentous laxity and instability,[31,32] trauma,[33] and joint damage from surgery including meniscectomy[34] have been suggested to predispose to localized secondary deposition of CPPD crystals in the context of joint damage. In contrast, other radiographic and MRI studies have not found an association between CPPD and OA progression. In one prospective study of 104 participants with CPPD at various joints, change in structural arthropathy was minimal over 4.6 years and unrelated to the presence, extent, or progression of radiographic CC.[35] In prospective studies of cartilage loss measured with serial MRI scans, radiographic CC was not predictive of cartilage loss in one cohort and even suggested to protect against cartilage loss in another.[36] To explain this latter finding, CC has been proposed to be a marker of hypertrophic chondrocyte differentiation and a reparative response of the chondrocyte matrix to cartilage damage.

One community-based case-control study found that the association between radiographic CC and patellofemoral and tibiofemoral OA occurs through a shared association with osteophyte,[5] although this finding is not supported by all studies including pooled data analysed by the EULAR Task Force.[4]

Familial CPPD

Familial CC due to CPPD, usually showing autosomal dominant inheritance, is rare but has been reported from many different countries. The commonest phenotype is early onset in the third to fourth decades of recurrent acute CPP crystal arthritis, florid polyarticular CC, and a variable severity of associated structural arthritis (radiographically identical to OA) ranging from absent to marked.[37-39] A less frequently reported phenotype is late onset presentation in the sixth to seventh decades of oligoarticular CC mainly confined to the knees, and arthritis resembling sporadic OA with CPPD.[40] However, this second, less dramatic form may be relatively under-recognized. In one United Kingdom family recurrent infantile seizures between the ages of 6 months and 6 years occurs in all affected individuals,[39] but extra-articular associations are not reported in other kindreds.

Two genetic associations have been identified in familial CC due to CPPD: the CC gene 1 (*CCAL1*) locus on chromosome 8q in one American family with premature OA and CPPD,[41] and CC gene 2 (*CCAL2*) on chromosome 5p15 in British, French, and Argentinian families with CC.[42,43] No responsible gene has been identified at the *CCAL1* locus but *CCAL2* has been identified as the *ANKH* gene. A mutation of the homologous *ANK* gene in mice was first studied as a cause of extensive intra-and extra-articular BCP deposition which results in progressive joint immobility (hence 'ankylosis'). The mouse mutation leads to reduced activity of ANK and thus low levels of ePPi; in the absence of normal

inhibition of BCP by ePPi there is uncontrolled widespread BCP crystal deposition.[44] However the *ANKH* mutation identified in human familial CC leads to a gain rather than a loss in function of ANKH with resulting very high levels of ePPi and predisposition to CPPD.

The heritability of common CC and CPPD remains unclear. One United Kingdom community-based sibling study found no significant genetic contribution to apparently sporadic CC or OA with CPPD,[11] but one case-control study found increased risk of apparently sporadic CC through inheritance of a −4 bp G-to-A *ANKH* 5⊠-untranslated region transition that upregulates expression of ANKH with subsequent elevation of ePPi.[45]

Metabolic diseases

Numerous metabolic conditions have been reported to associate with CC. However, the best evidence exists for primary hyperparathyroidism, haemochromatosis, hypomagnesaemia, and hypophosphatasia.[46,47]

Uncontrolled case series provide evidence of an association between CC and primary hyperparathyroidism. Whereas primary hyperparathyroidism is very uncommon in patients with CC (none out of 91 patients in one series[48]), as many as one in five patients with primary hyperparathyroidism exhibit radiographic CC.[49] Analysis of pooled data by the EULAR Task Force found patients with hyperparathyroidism to be three times more likely to have CPPD than controls (OR 3.03; 95%CI 1.15, 8.02).[4] Hyperparathyroidism potentially predisposes to CPP crystal formation by increasing ePPi levels (via inhibition of TNAP by calcium ions and parathyroid hormone (PTH) and stimulation of adenylate cyclase by PTH) and by increasing calcium and thus the (Ca × PPi) ionic product (Figure 142.1).

Like hyperparathyroidism, hereditary haemochromatosis has a very low prevalence in people with CC. In one study, the *C282Y* homozygous and *C282Y/H63D* heterozygous states were seen in 1.6% and 3.1% of people with CC and/or acute CPP crystal arthritis respectively.[50] In contrast, the prevalence of CC in untreated hereditary haemochromatosis was 30% in one study and CC appeared to correlate with age and ferritin levels.[51] Furthermore, the concentration of serum PTH 44–68 also correlates with the number of joints affected by CC in hereditary haemochromatosis and is increased in CPPD.[51,52] Hospital-based studies suggest that CPPD occurs at a younger age in patients with haemochromatosis than those without and that the presence of CC in haemochromatosis associates with structural arthropathy.[52,53] Iron has an inhibitory effect on TNAP activity and is also a nucleating factor for CPP crystals (Figure 142.1).

Hypomagnesaemia predisposes to CPPD in congenital magnesium-losing nephropathies (Gitelman's and Bartter's syndromes) and intestinal failure.[54,55] Diuretic-induced hypomagnesaemia is thought to explain the association of radiographic CC with diuretic use (OR 2.07; 95%CI 1.02, 4.19).[5] The breakdown of ePPi to inorganic phosphate by TNAP requires magnesium as a cofactor, hence hypomagnesaemia impairs this reaction allowing PPi to accumulate (Figure 142.1).

Case reports and case series also report an association between young-onset CC and severe hypophosphatasia which is characterized by skeletal deformities and marked underactivity of TNAP (Figure 142.1).[46,47] The very high ePPi levels inhibit BCP formation leading to poor bone mineralization and tendency to fracture.

Clinical features

Asymptomatic CPPD

CC due to CPPD, with or without changes of structural changes of OA, is a frequent incidental radiographic finding in elderly people. Although radiographic CC can be associated with clinical symptoms (mainly acute CPP crystal arthritis), a thorough clinical assessment is required as regional pain can easily be erroneously attributed to CPPD.

Osteoarthritis with CPPD

CPPD is commonly accompanied by OA, particularly in elderly women. Clinical presentation mimics OA and is characterized by chronic pain, stiffness, and functional impairment. The knee is the most frequent and severely affected joint.[56] Other commonly affected joints include the shoulder, wrist/hand, and ankle. Examination reveals physical signs of OA: bony swelling, crepitus, restricted movement, and deformity. However, there may also be superimposed attacks of acute CPP crystal arthritis (see below) or varying degrees of synovitis (often most marked at the knee, radiocarpal, or glenohumeral joint).

OA with CPPD can be difficult to distinguish from uncomplicated OA, particularly at the knee. However, several clinical clues can aid differentiation:

+ the distribution of affected joints; although both conditions commonly affect the knee, target joints for CPPD (shoulder, ankle, wrist) are uncommon sites for primary OA

+ superimposed acute attacks (NB: osteoarthritic joints also encourage urate crystal deposition)

+ the presence of more symptoms and signs of inflammation than in uncomplicated OA.

The prognosis of OA with CPPD is generally good. The course is usually benign, particularly with respect to small and medium-sized joints. In one prospective hospital-based study, only 27% of participants reported a decline in symptoms over a mean follow-up period of 4.6 years.[35] Progression, when it occurs, is usually slow and related to knees, hips, or shoulders although patients with OA and CPPD undergo total knee replacement surgery at an older age than patients with uncomplicated OA.[57] Occasionally severe, rapidly progressive, destructive arthropathy may occur at these sites, usually in very elderly women and is associated with severe pain, recurrent haemarthrosis (shoulder, knee), and occasional joint leakage. Mixed crystal deposition (CPP plus BCP) is often found on synovial fluid analysis.

Acute CPP crystal arthritis

Acute CPP crystal arthritis should be considered in the differential diagnosis of any acute hot swollen joint in the elderly. It usually presents with an acute attack of synovitis affecting a single peripheral joint. The most commonly affected joint is the knee followed by the wrist/hand, ankle, and shoulder.[56] Pain is usually severe and typically reaches peak intensity rapidly, within 6–24 hours of symptom onset. Signs of synovitis, namely swelling, warmth, exquisite tenderness to touch, and sometimes overlying erythema, are present on physical examination. EULAR recommendations for the diagnosis of CPPD state that rapid development of synovitis with pain, stiffness, swelling, and tenderness with or without erythema

are highly characteristic of acute crystal synovitis but are not specific to CPP crystals; however, involvement of the knee, wrist, or shoulder in a person aged over 65 years makes acute crystal CPP arthritis likely.[4]

Oligoarticular attacks are uncommon and polyarticular attacks rare. Systemic features such as fever or confusion are common in elderly people. Attacks are usually spontaneous, but may be provoked by intercurrent illness, local trauma, or surgery. Even without treatment, attacks are self-limiting and typically resolve within 1–2 weeks.

Chronic CPP crystal inflammatory arthritis

Chronic CPP crystal inflammatory arthritis presents with chronic inflammatory symptoms and signs such as morning stiffness and synovitis with occasional systemic upset. The pattern of joint involvement is most commonly mono- or oligoarticular (89%) but may be polyarticular (11%).[48] The differential diagnosis includes rheumatoid arthritis and polymyalgia rheumatica.

Rarer presentations

Although CPP crystals usually deposit within articular cartilage within synovial joints, soft tissue CPPD can cause acute tendinitis (triceps, Achilles),[58] tenosynovitis (hand flexors, extensors),[59] and bursitis (olecranon, infrapatellar, retrocalcaneal),[60] usually in patients with widespread CPP crystals. Flexor tenosynovitis at the wrist can cause median and ulnar nerve compression.[59] In contrast to gout, where tophi occur relatively commonly, tophaceous CPPD is rare and usually presents as solitary lesions in areas of chondroid metaplasia (usually benign cartilage tumours).

Spinal CPPD is uncommon with cervical spinal involvement particularly rare. Acute CPP crystal arthritis can present with acute severe posterior neck pain and systemic upset ('crowned dens' syndrome). Fever is present in up to 80% of patients.[61] CT imaging of the cervical spine demonstrates linear calcific deposits within the transverse ligament of the atlas and other periodontoid structures. Compressive cervical myelopathy due to CPPD involvement of the cervical spine is also described.[62]

Investigation and diagnosis

Synovial fluid analysis

Identification of CPP crystals by compensated polarized light microscopy of aspirated synovial fluid is the reference standard for the diagnosis of CPPD.[4] CPP crystals often exhibit no birefringence, or only weak (positive) birefringence, and are small (2–10 μm in length) and of varying morphology, most commonly rhomboid or rod-shaped (Figure 142.2). Identification of CPP crystals confirms the diagnosis of acute CPP crystal arthritis, OA with CPPD, and chronic CPP crystal inflammatory arthritis, and allows the important differential diagnoses of septic arthritis and gout to be excluded. CPP crystals can be seen in synovial fluid aspirated from asymptomatic knees that have never been affected by acute CPP crystal arthritis or in between attacks.[63] In acute CPP crystal arthritis, aspirated fluid is often turbid or bloodstained with an elevated cell count (more than 90% neutrophils). Acute CPP crystal arthritis and septic arthritis can coexist, so if joint sepsis is suspected on clinical grounds then microbiological examination of aspirated fluid must be performed even if CPP crystals are identified.[4]

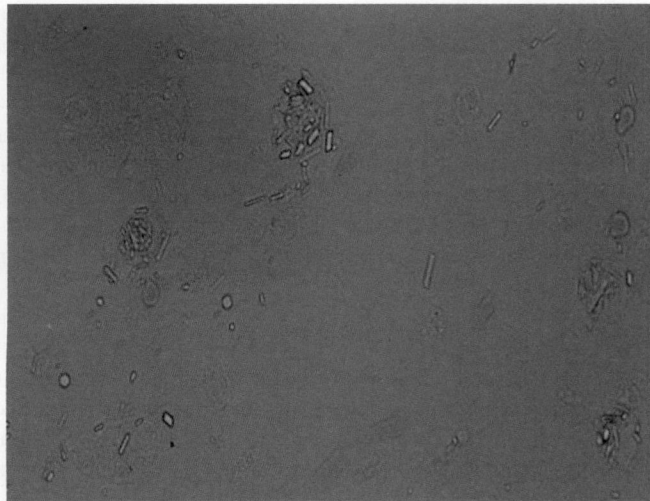

Fig. 142.2 Photograph of CPP crystals under compensated polarized light microscopy.

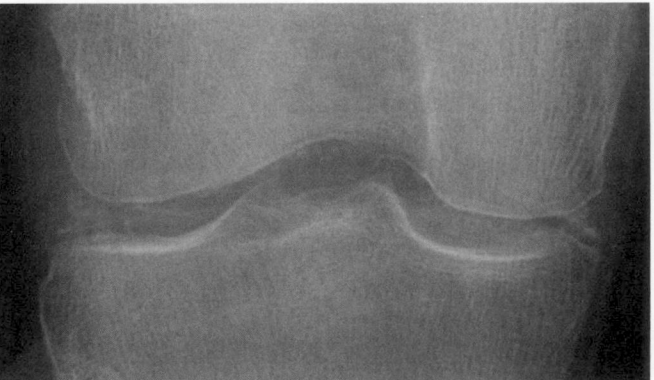

Fig. 142.3 Plain radiograph of the knee showing chondrocalcinosis (CC) of articular hyaline and fibrocartilage within the medial and lateral tibiofemoral compartments.

Plain radiographs

The cardinal radiographic feature of CPPD is CC—calcification of articular fibrocartilage or hyaline cartilage (Figure 142.3). This is most commonly seen at the menisci of the knees, wrist triangular cartilage, and symphysis pubis. Although radiographic CC of articular cartilage is often taken to be diagnostic of CPPD, other crystals, principally BCP, can also appear as linear calcification of articular cartilage. Furthermore, radiographs are insensitive and may fail to detect small crystal deposits. Radiographic CC is seen in only 29–93% of cases of proven CPPD.[4,48,63] Hence, although radiographic CC supports the diagnosis of CPPD, definitive diagnosis needs to be crystal proven.[4]

OA with CPPD is characterized by CC and features of OA: cartilage loss, subchondral cysts and sclerosis, and osteophytes (Figure 142.4). There are certain radiographic features which may help to distinguish OA with CPPD from uncomplicated OA:

◆ distribution of affected joints includes joints that are uncommonly affected by primary OA (eg wrist, shoulder, ankle)

◆ prominent osteophyte formation giving a distinctive hypertrophic OA appearance

◆ prominent osteochondral bodies.

In destructive arthropathy, marked cartilage and bone attrition with fragmentation and loose osseous bodies may resemble a Charcot joint.

Plain radiographs can also be helpful in distinguishing chronic CPP crystal inflammatory arthritis from other inflammatory arthropathies such as rheumatoid arthritis (RA). Wrist involvement is common in both RA and CPPD and rheumatoid factor more commonly positive in elderly people, which may make it difficult to tell them apart. In addition to radiographic CC and identification of CPP crystals, absence of marginal erosions is suggestive of chronic CPP crystal inflammatory arthritis.[23]

Ultrasound

Three patterns of ultrasonographic calcification have been proposed to represent CPPD[64,65]:

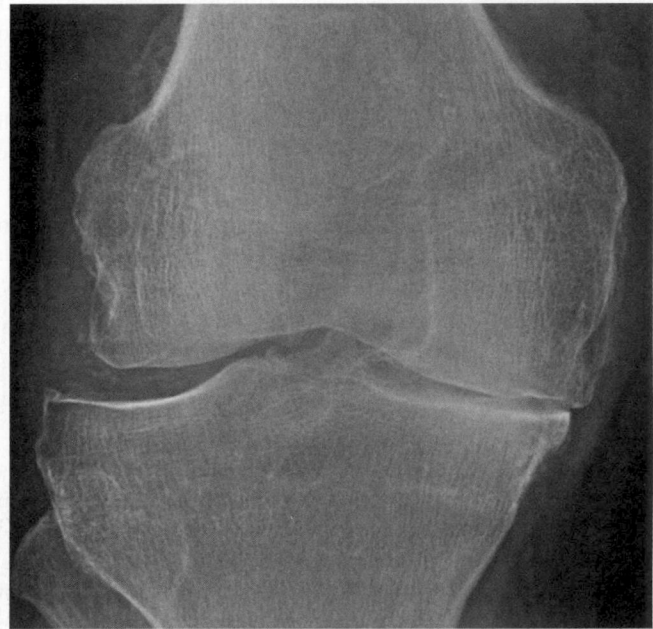

Fig. 142.4 Plain radiograph of the knee showing OA with CPPD: note chondrocalcinosis (CC) of articular fibrocartilage within the lateral tibiofemoral compartment and osteophyte and joint space narrowing at the medial tibiofemoral compartment.

1. thin hyperechoic bands, parallel to the surface of the hyaline cartilage (frequently observed in the knee)

2. a 'punctuate' pattern consisting of several thin hyperechoic spots, more common in fibrous cartilage and tendons

3. homogeneous hyperechoic nodular or oval deposits localized in bursae and articular recesses.

In a small study of 11 subjects with ultrasonographic evidence of CPPD at the knee, wrist and shoulder and 13 control subjects, pattern 2 was the most common, followed by pattern 1: pattern 3 was seen in only one participant.[65] Further analysis of the findings of this study by the EULAR Task Force found the sensitivity of ultrasound to detect CPPD using a gold standard of synovial fluid CPP crystal identification to be 100% compared to 82% for radiographs.[4] One further small study reported ultrasonography to be both sensitive (87%) and specific (96%) to detect CPPD at the knee, again compared to synovial fluid CPP crystal identification.[66] The EULAR Task Force conclude that positive ultrasound findings strongly support the diagnosis of CPPD (likelihood ratio 24.2).[4]

Ultrasound has the additional advantages of minimizing ionizing radiation exposure, providing 'real-time', dynamic, high-resolution images at low cost, identifying subclinical joint effusions which can be aspirated facilitating a crystal-proven diagnosis, and allowing differentiation between crystal arthropathies. The 'double contour sign'—thickening and hyperechogenecity of the superficial margin of the articular cartilage independent of the angle of insonation—is an ultrasonographic feature specific to gout.[64,67,68] Furthermore, CPPD calcification appears hyperechogenic on ultrasound and creates a posterior shadowing only with large lesions (>10 mm diameter) in contrast to BCP crystal deposits which are hypoechoic and present posterior shadowing even at an early stage.[65] However, although ultrasound has great potential as a diagnostic technique for CPPD further large studies are required to validate these preliminary findings.

Blood tests and screening for predisposing metabolic conditions

There are no specific diagnostic blood tests for CPPD. However, during attacks of acute CPP crystal arthritis a marked acute-phase response is usually seen, with high erythrocyte sedimentation rate (ESR), neutrophil leucocytosis, thrombocytosis, elevated C-reactive protein (CRP). Modest elevations of ESR and CRP may also accompany chronic CPP crystal inflammatory arthritis.

Metabolic predisposition is rare and routine screening of all patients is unwarranted. Nevertheless, CPPD can be the presenting feature of metabolic or familial disease, and screening for primary hyperparathyroidism, haemochromatosis, hypomagnesaemia and hypophosphatasia should be considered:

- in patients aged under 55 years with CC or acute CPP crystal arthritis
- if there is florid polyarticular CC[4]
- if there are additional clinical features to suggest metabolic disease.

Screening tests should include serum calcium, alkaline phosphatase, magnesium, ferritin, and liver function.

Management

Asymptomatic chondrocalcinosis

Asymptomatic CC does not require specific management other than screening for metabolic disorders as described above.

Osteoarthritis with CPPD

Treatment of OA with CPPD is very similar to the treatment of OA alone.[69] In contrast to gout, where urate-lowering therapy forms the mainstay of long-term management, there is no specific treatment to reduce and prevent deposition of CPP crystals. Optimal treatment combines non-pharmacological and pharmacological modalities and should include education and advice, local quadriceps strengthening and generalized aerobic fitness exercises,

weight loss if the patient is overweight or obese, and graded analgesia commencing with oral paracetamol and topical NSAID, as advocated in numerous clinical guidelines.[70-74] In some cases, joint replacement surgery may be required. Superimposed attacks of acute CPP crystal arthritis should be treated as outlined in the next section.

Acute CPP crystal arthritis

Treatment of acute CPP crystal arthritis aims to rapidly relieve associated pain and swelling. There are few high-quality research studies of interventions for acute CPP crystal arthritis and existing recommendations are based largely on clinical experience, expert consensus, and extrapolation of research evidence supporting treatments for acute gout.[69] Available treatments include local application of ice topically to an affected joint, oral non-steroidal anti-inflammatory drugs (NSAIDs) (with a proton pump inhibitor if indicated), colchicine, glucocorticosteroids (intra-articular, oral or parenteral), or adrenocorticotrophic hormone (ACTH).

There are no published research studies to date of topical ice therapy for acute CPP crystal arthritis. However, one small randomized controlled trial (RCT) demonstrates its efficacy for the treatment of acute gout,[75] and the use of topical ice therapy for acute CPP crystal arthritis, with temporary rest of the affected joint, was strongly supported by the EULAR Task Force.[69] Clinical experience suggests that both NSAID and oral colchicine are effective treatments for acute CPP crystal arthritis. However, robust studies are lacking and the recommendation for their use is extrapolated from studies of acute gout. Both treatments should be used with caution in elderly people because of the high incidence of side effects such as gastrointestinal bleeding, cardiovascular events, and renal failure with NSAIDs and diarrhoea, nausea, and vomiting with oral colchicine. Drug interactions between NSAIDs and other drugs such as aspirin and warfarin are also commonplace in elderly people. The EULAR Task Force advises that consideration should be given to coprescription of a gastroprotective agent with NSAIDs.[69] Traditional oral colchicine dosing regimes such as 1 mg loading followed by 0.5 mg every 2 hours very frequently result in gastrointestinal adverse events. The incidence of diarrhoea and vomiting was 100% in an RCT of a similar high-dose regime for acute gout.[76] A lower-dose regime (e.g. 0.5 mg two to four times daily) is therefore recommended by the EULAR Task Force,[69] based on expert consensus. Although the efficacy of intravenous colchicine is reported,[77] the intravenous route is no longer recommended because of the risk of serious, potentially life-threatening, toxicity.

In view of frequent comorbidity and contraindications to or poor tolerance of NSAIDs or oral colchicine in the older person with acute CPP crystal arthritis, management can be challenging. Glucocorticosteroids can be a particularly useful and effective treatment.[69] The EULAR Task Force strongly recommends joint aspiration and intra-articular injection of long-acting glucocorticosteroid as an effective and safe treatment for mono- or oligoarticular attacks of acute CPP crystal arthritis, although again research evidence for this is very weak.[69,78] In a hospital setting, especially in an elderly patient with an attack triggered by intercurrent illness or surgery, joint aspiration and injection should be considered best practice.

Case history

A 72-year woman is being treated in hospital following a fall. Her medical history includes knee osteoarthritis and hypertension. She develops acute onset of severe pain and swelling affecting her right knee which was extremely painful within just 6 hours. She feels unwell and has a low-grade fever. Examination reveals a hot, tender, tense effusion with restricted movement. There is wasting of the quadriceps and palpable coarse crepitus.

Because of the rapidity of development of her synovitis a diagnosis of acute crystal synovitis is made. She has no history of chronic diuretic use or renal impairment, and this together with her age and known knee OA suggest acute CPP crystal arthritis rather than acute gout. 80 mL of turbid synovial fluid is aspirated from the knee and she is injected with intra-articular triamcinolone acetonide and given local ice packs, resulting in rapid reduction in her pain. Compensated polarized light microscopy of the aspirated fluid reveals small predominantly intracellular rhomboid crystals exhibiting weak positive or no birefringence. ESR and CRP are both elevated at 66 mm/hour and 133 mg/dL respectively. Plain radiography of the knee reveals linear calcification of articular fibrocartilage, and features of osteoarthritis, namely medial joint space narrowing and osteophytosis. Gram stain and culture of the fluid at 48 hours does not reveal any organisms (sepsis is extremely unlikely given the rapidity of development of her tense effusion, but coexistent sepsis should be excluded in an unwell hospitalized patient). She is provided with verbal and written information about OA with CPPD and given advice on how to lose weight. She is also assessed and treated by a physiotherapist who prescribes a home exercise programme consisting of quadriceps strengthening exercises and aerobic exercise. Oral paracetamol and topical NSAIDs are recommended for long-term analgesia.

Intramuscular glucocorticosteroid is a useful treatment when monoarticular attacks occur at sites not amenable to injection, such as the midfoot, or attacks are oligo- or polyarticular. One small non-randomized trial demonstrates the superior efficacy of both intramuscular betamethasone 7 mg and intravenous methylprednisolone 125 mg compared to oral diclofenac in patients with acute crystal synovitis[79] (number needed to treat 3[69]). Intramuscular injection of triamcinolone acetonide 60 mg provided rapid relief from acute CPP crystal arthritis in one small prospective uncontrolled study.[80] Although there are no RCTs of oral glucocorticosteroids for acute CPP crystal arthritis, oral prednisolone 35 mg daily is as effective as NSAID for the treatment of acute gout,[81] and is an effective alternative to intra-articular glucocorticosteroid for polyarticular attacks.[69]

ACTH stimulates adrenal glucocorticosteroid release and has a direct anti-inflammatory effect via the melanocortin type 3 receptor.[82] Parenteral ACTH 40 or 80 units (three intravenous, intramuscular, or subcutaneous doses) provided rapid symptomatic relief in a retrospective study of 38 patients with acute crystal-induced synovitis.[83] Side effects included hypokalaemia, hyperglycaemia, fluid retention, and rebound arthritis although these were reported as mild and easily controlled. Although not widely used in routine clinical practice, ACTH may be a safe and effective treatment for acute CPP crystal arthritis, though further studies are required.

Recently, there has been interest in the use of IL-1 receptor antagonists to treat acute CPP crystal arthritis. Following phagocytosis by synovial cells, CPP crystals activate the NALP3 inflammasome, an intracellular receptor within monocytes.[22] Subsequently, secretion of IL-1β initiates a neutrophilic inflammatory reaction.[3,22] The efficacy of the IL-1 receptor antagonist anakinra (100 mg daily) to provide rapid symptomatic relief from resistant acute CPP crystal arthritis in which glucocorticosteroids, NSAIDs, and colchicine were either ineffective or contra-indicated is described.[84] Other IL-1 inhibitors such as rilonacept have been used to treat acute gout,[85] and may also be effective for the treatment of acute CPP crystal arthritis although further evaluation is required.

Prophylaxis against frequent recurrent attacks of acute CPP crystal arthritis can be attempted with low-dose oral colchicine (e.g. 0.5 mg once to twice daily) or low-dose oral NSAID (with gastroprotection if indicated).[69] There are no empirical research studies of NSAIDs in this setting. However, one small uncontrolled study followed 10 patients with acute CPP crystal arthritis for 1 year before and 1 year after receiving oral colchicine (0.6 mg twice daily), demonstrating a reduction in the number of acute attacks from 32 in the year preceding initiation of therapy to 10 while taking the drug.[86] These findings suggest that colchicine may be of benefit for prophylaxis against acute attacks. However, use of NSAID or colchicine needs to be considered carefully in elderly patients and further evidence is required.

Chronic CPP crystal inflammatory arthritis

There is no specific therapy for chronic CPP crystal inflammatory arthritis. The EULAR Task Force recommends, in order of preference, an oral NSAID (with gastroprotection if necessary), colchicine 0.5–1.0 mg daily, low-dose glucocorticosteroid, methotrexate, and hydroxychloroquine.[69] The recommendation of NSAID is based upon clinical experience and extrapolation from research studies in gout and OA. The Task Force commented that there is no evidence to support the use of low-dose glucocorticosteroids for chronic CPP crystal inflammatory arthritis.

Low-dose colchicine (0.5 mg twice daily for 8 weeks) has been shown to have additional benefit for pain and function to intraarticular methylprednisolone and oral piroxicam in a randomized double-blind placebo-controlled trial of 39 patients with OA of the knee and clinical signs of persistent inflammation, although only 74% and 38% of participants had a crystal-proven diagnosis of CPPD and radiographic CC respectively.[87] Colchicine was well tolerated and the incidence of gastrointestinal side effects in the colchicine group did not differ significantly from those given placebo.

A small case series of five patients with polyarticular chronic CPP crystal inflammatory arthritis reported improvements in pain, swollen and tender joint counts, and acute-phase reactants such as ESR and CRP with methotrexate at a doses of 5–20 mg weekly.[88] However, another series of just three patients with severe destructive monoarticular or oligoarticular CPPD treated with methotrexate at doses of 7.5–12.5 mg weekly did not report any benefit.[89] Hence further larger studies of methotrexate in CPPD are needed.

Hydroxychloroquine at doses of 200–400 mg daily brought about superior differences in joint swelling and tenderness to placebo in a small 6-month double-blind RCT of 36 participants with chronic CPP crystal inflammatory arthritis.[90] Treatment was well tolerated.

Since magnesium has an important role as a cofactor for TNAP in the metabolism of PPi and hypomagnesaemia is a recognized risk factor for CPPD, magnesium supplementation would appear to be a logical treatment approach for CPPD, although it was not recommended by the EULAR Task Force.[69] In a randomized placebo-controlled trial of 38 participants with chronic CPP crystal inflammatory arthritis, greater improvements in pain, stiffness, knee effusion and tenderness were seen at 6 months in those treated with magnesium carbonate (30 mEq per day) compared to placebo.[91] Improvement was unrelated to baseline magnesium level and there was no change in radiographic CC over the course of the study.

Although not specifically recommended by the EULAR Task Force, intra-articular injection of yttrium-90 (radiosynovectomy) may be of benefit for chronic CPP crystal inflammatory arthritis. In one small study of 15 patients with bilateral symmetrical CPPD of the knee, each participant underwent intra-articular injection of yttrium-90 plus triamcinolone hexacetonide into one knee and saline plus triamcinolone hexacetonide into the other knee.[92] At 6 months, improvements were seen in pain, stiffness, joint-line tenderness, effusion, and range of movement in the yttrium-90-injected knees compared to saline-injected knees. The EULAR Task Force concludes that the role of radiosynovectomy is unclear as this is the only published study.[69]

Given the reported success of IL-1 blockade of acute crystal synovitis with anakinra and rilonacept,[84,85] it would appear logical that such agents would be beneficial for chronic CPP crystal inflammatory arthritis. However, specific RCTs examining the use of these agents in chronic CPP crystal inflammatory arthritis are required.

Conclusion

CPPD is a common age-related phenomenon in the general population. Recent developments include: the proposal of a new uniform terminology and the first evidence-based recommendations for diagnosis and management of CPPD by the EULAR CPPD Task Force; advances in understanding of the pathophysiology of PPi metabolism and the mechanisms by which crystals invoke an inflammatory response via the NALP3 inflammasome and secretion of IL-1β; and the emergence of new diagnostic modalities such as ultrasound. However, although there is a great wealth of clinical experience of the treatment of this prevalent, painful and disabling condition, there is a paucity of large, high-quality research studies concerning its diagnosis and management. Existing recommendations for treatment are largely based on clinical experience, expert consensus and extrapolation from other crystal arthropathies such as gout. Further high-quality studies are much needed.

References

1. Hollander, Jessar RA, McCarty DJ. Synovianalysis: an aid in arthritis diagnosis. *Bull Rheum Dis* 1961;12:263–264.
2. McCarty DJ. Calcium pyrophosphate dihydrate crystal deposition disease—1975. *Arthritis Rheum* 1976;19Suppl:85.
3. Abhishek A, Doherty M. Pathophysiology of articular chondrocalcinosis—role of ANKH. *Nat Rev Rheumatol* 2011;7(2):96–104.
4. Zhang W, Doherty M, Bardin T et al. European League Against Rheumatism recommendations for calcium pyrophosphate deposition. Part I: terminology and diagnosis. *Ann Rheum Dis* 2011;70(4):563–570.
5. Neame RL, Carr AJ, Muir K, Doherty M. UK community prevalence of knee chondrocalcinosis: evidence that correlation with osteoarthritis is through a shared association with osteophyte. *Ann Rheum Dis* 2003;62(6):513–518.
6. Felson DT, Anderson JJ, Naimark A, Kannel W, Meenan RF. The prevalence of chondrocalcinosis in the elderly and its association with knee osteoarthritis: the Framingham Study. *J Rheumatol* 1989;16(9):1241–1245.
7. Sanmarti R, Panella D, Brancos MA et al. Prevalence of articular chondrocalcinosis in elderly subjects in a rural area of Catalonia. *Ann Rheum Dis* 1993;52(6):418–422.
8. Ramonda R, Musacchio E, Perissinotto E et al. Prevalence of chondrocalcinosis in Italian subjects from northeastern Italy. The Pro.V.A. (PROgetto Veneto Anziani) study. *Clin Exp Rheumatol* 2009;27(6):981–984.
9. Zhang Y, Terkeltaub R, Nevitt M et al. Lower prevalence of chondrocalcinosis in Chinese subjects in Beijing than in white subjects in the United States: the Beijing Osteoarthritis Study. *Arthritis Rheum* 2006;54(11):3508–3512.
10. Bergstrom G, Bjelle A, Sundh V, Svanborg A. Joint disorders at ages 70, 75 and 79 years—a cross-sectional comparison. *Br J Rheumatol* 1986;25(4):333–341.
11. Zhang W, Neame R, Doherty S, Doherty M. Relative risk of knee chondrocalcinosis in siblings of index cases with pyrophosphate arthropathy. *Ann Rheum Dis* 2004;63(8):969–973.
12. Kellgren JH, Lawrence JS. *The epidemiology of chronic rheumatism. Vol. II. Atlas of standard radiographs of arthritis.* Blackwell Scientific Publications, Oxford, 1963.
13. Terkeltaub RA. Inorganic pyrophosphate generation and disposition in pathophysiology. *Am J Physiol Cell Physiol* 2001;281(1):C1–C11.
14. Mandel NS, Mandel GS, Carroll DJ, Halverson PB. Calcium pyrophosphate crystal deposition. An in vitro study using a gelatin matrix model. *Arthritis Rheum* 1984;27(7):789–796.
15. Ryan LM, Kurup IV, Derfus BA, Kushnaryov VM. ATP-induced chondrocalcinosis. *Arthritis Rheum* 1992;35(12):1520–1525.
16. Graff RD, Lazarowski ER, Banes AJ, Lee GM. ATP release by mechanically loaded porcine chondrons in pellet culture. *Arthritis Rheum* 2000;43(7):1571–1579.
17. Lotz M, Rosen F, McCabe G et al. Interleukin 1 beta suppresses transforming growth factor-induced inorganic pyrophosphate (PPi) production and expression of the PPi-generating enzyme PC-1 in human chondrocytes. *Proc Natl Acad Sci U S A* 1995;92(22):10364–10368.
18. Johnson K, Vaingankar S, Chen Y et al. Differential mechanisms of inorganic pyrophosphate production by plasma cell membrane glycoprotein-1 and B10 in chondrocytes. *Arthritis Rheum* 1999;42(9):1986–1997.
19. Pendleton A, Johnson MD, Hughes A et al. Mutations in ANKH cause chondrocalcinosis. *Am J Hum Genet* 2002;71(4):933–940.
20. Gurley KA, Reimer RJ, Kingsley DM. Biochemical and genetic analysis of ANK in arthritis and bone disease. *Am J Hum Genet* 2006;79(6):1017–1029.
21. Caswell A, Guilland-Cumming DF, Hearn PR, McGuire MK, Russell RG. Pathogenesis of chondrocalcinosis and pseudogout. Metabolism of inorganic pyrophosphate and production of calcium pyrophosphate dihydrate crystals. *Ann Rheum Dis* 1983;42 Suppl 1:27–37.
22. Martinon F, Petrilli V, Mayor A, Tardivel A, Tschopp J. Gout-associated uric acid crystals activate the NALP3 inflammasome. *Nature* 2006;440(7081):237–241.
23. Wise CM. Crystal-associated arthritis in the elderly. *Rheum Dis Clin North Am* 2007;33(1):33–55.
24. Fuerst M, Bertrand J, Lammers L et al. Calcification of articular cartilage in human osteoarthritis. *Arthritis Rheum* 2009;60(9):2694–2703.
25. Fuerst M, Niggemeyer O, Lammers L et al. Articular cartilage mineralization in osteoarthritis of the hip. *BMC Musculoskelet Disord* 2009;10:166.
26. Muehleman C, Li J, Aigner T et al. Association between crystals and cartilage degeneration in the ankle. *J Rheumatol* 2008;35(6):1108–1117.

27. Nalbant S, Martinez JA, Kitumnuaypong T, Clayburne G, Sieck M, Schumacher HR,Jr. Synovial fluid features and their relations to osteoarthritis severity: new findings from sequential studies. *Osteoarthritis Cartilage* 2003;11(1):50–54.

28. Fam AG, Morava-Protzner I, Purcell C et al. Acceleration of experimental lapine osteoarthritis by calcium pyrophosphate microcrystalline synovitis. *Arthritis Rheum* 1995;38(2):201–210.

29. Liu R, O'Connell M, Johnson K et al. Extracellular signal-regulated kinase 1/extracellular signal-regulated kinase 2 mitogen-activated protein kinase signaling and activation of activator protein 1 and nuclear factor kappaB transcription factors play central roles in interleukin-8 expression stimulated by monosodium urate monohydrate and calcium pyrophosphate crystals in monocytic cells. *Arthritis Rheum* 2000;43(5):1145–1155.

30. Ledingham J, Regan M, Jones A, Doherty M. Factors affecting radiographic progression of knee osteoarthritis. *Ann Rheum Dis* 1995;54(1):53–58.

31. Bird HA, Tribe CR, Bacon PA. Joint hypermobility leading to osteoarthrosis and chondrocalcinosis. *Ann Rheum Dis* 1978;37(3):203–211.

32. Settas L, Doherty M, Dieppe P. Localised chondrocalcinosis in unstable joints. *Br Med J* (Clin Res Ed) 1982;285(6336):175–176.

33. de Lange EE, Keats TE. Localized chondrocalcinosis in traumatized joints. *Skeletal Radiol* 1985;14(4):249–256.

34. Doherty M, Watt I, Dieppe PA. Localised chondrocalcinosis in postmeniscectomy knees. *Lancet* 1982;1(8283):1207–1210.

35. Doherty M, Dieppe P, Watt I. Pyrophosphate arthropathy: a prospective study. *Br J Rheumatol* 1993;32(3):189–196.

36. Neogi T, Nevitt M, Niu J et al. Lack of association between chondrocalcinosis and increased risk of cartilage loss in knees with osteoarthritis: results of two prospective longitudinal magnetic resonance imaging studies. *Arthritis Rheum* 2006;54(6):1822–1828.

37. Bjelle AO. Morphological study of articular cartilage in pyrophosphate arthropathy. (Chondrocalcinosis articularis or calcium pyrophosphate dihydrate crystal deposition diseases). *Ann Rheum Dis* 1972;31(6):449–456.

38. Reginato AJ, Hollander JL, Martinez V et al. Familial chondrocalcinosis in the Chiloe Islands, Chile. *Ann Rheum Dis* 1975;34(3):260–268.

39. Doherty M, Hamilton E, Henderson J, Misra H, Dixey J. Familial chondrocalcinosis due to calcium pyrophosphate dihydrate crystal deposition in English families. *Br J Rheumatol* 1991;30(1):10–15.

40. Rodriguez-Valverde V, Tinture T et al. Familial chondrocalcinosis. Prevalence in Northern Spain and clinical features in five pedigrees. *Arthritis Rheum* 1980;23(4):471–478.

41. Baldwin CT, Farrer LA, Adair R et al. Linkage of early-onset osteoarthritis and chondrocalcinosis to human chromosome 8q. *Am J Hum Genet* 1995;56(3):692–697.

42. Hughes AE, McGibbon D, Woodward E, Dixey J, Doherty M. Localisation of a gene for chondrocalcinosis to chromosome 5p. *Hum Mol Genet* 1995;4(7):1225–1228.

43. Andrew LJ, Brancolini V, de la Pena LS et al. Refinement of the chromosome 5p locus for familial calcium pyrophosphate dihydrate deposition disease. *Am J Hum Genet* 1999;64(1):136–145.

44. Ho AM, Johnson MD, Kingsley DM. Role of the mouse ank gene in control of tissue calcification and arthritis. *Science* 2000;289(5477):265–270.

45. Zhang Y, Johnson K, Russell RG et al. Association of sporadic chondrocalcinosis with a -4-basepair G-to-A transition in the 5⊠-untranslated region of ANKH that promotes enhanced expression of ANKH protein and excess generation of extracellular inorganic pyrophosphate. *Arthritis Rheum* 2005;52(4):1110–1117.

46. Jones AC, Chuck AJ, Arie EA, Green DJ, Doherty M. Diseases associated with calcium pyrophosphate deposition disease. *Semin Arthritis Rheum* 1992;22(3):188–202.

47. Richette P, Bardin T, Doherty M. An update on the epidemiology of calcium pyrophosphate dihydrate crystal deposition disease. *Rheumatology* (Oxford) 2009;48(7):711–715.

48. Louthrenoo W, Sukitawut W. Calcium pyrophosphate dihydrate crystal deposition: a clinical and laboratory analysis of 91 Thai patients. *J Med Assoc Thai* 1999;82(6):569–576.

49. Huaux JP, Geubel A, Koch MC et al. The arthritis of hemochromatosis. A review of 25 cases with special reference to chondrocalcinosis, and a comparison with patients with primary hyperparathyroidism and controls. *Clin Rheumatol* 1986;5(3):317–324.

50. Timms AE, Sathananthan R, Bradbury L et al. Genetic testing for haemochromatosis in patients with chondrocalcinosis. *Ann Rheum Dis* 2002;61(8):745–747.

51. Pawlotsky Y, Le Dantec P, Moirand R et al. Elevated parathyroid hormone 44–68 and osteoarticular changes in patients with genetic hemochromatosis. *Arthritis Rheum* 1999;42(4):799–806.

52. Valenti L, Fracanzani AL, Rossi V et al. The hand arthropathy of hereditary hemochromatosis is strongly associated with iron overload. *J Rheumatol* 2008;35(1):153–158.

53. Dymock IW, Hamilton EB, Laws JW, Williams R. Arthropathy of haemochromatosis. Clinical and radiological analysis of 63 patients with iron overload. *Ann Rheum Dis* 1970;29(5):469–476.

54. Calo L, Punzi L, Semplicini A. Hypomagnesemia and chondrocalcinosis in Bartter's and Gitelman's syndrome: review of the pathogenetic mechanisms. *Am J Nephrol* 2000;20(5):347–350.

55. Richette P, Ayoub G, Lahalle S et al. Hypomagnesemia associated with chondrocalcinosis: a cross-sectional study. *Arthritis Rheum* 2007;57(8):1496–1501.

56. Dieppe PA, Alexander GJ, Jones HE et al. Pyrophosphate arthropathy: a clinical and radiological study of 105 cases. *Ann Rheum Dis* 1982;41(4):371–376.

57. Viriyavejkul P, Wilairatana V, Tanavalee A, Jaovisidha K. Comparison of characteristics of patients with and without calcium pyrophosphate dihydrate crystal deposition disease who underwent total knee replacement surgery for osteoarthritis. *Osteoarthritis Cartilage* 2007;15(2):232–235.

58. Gerster JC, Lagier R, Boivin G. Achilles tendinitis associated with chondrocalcinosis. *J Rheumatol* 1980;7(1):82–88.

59. Gerster JC, Lagier R. Upper limb pyrophosphate tenosynovitis outside the carpal tunnel. *Ann Rheum Dis* 1989;48(8):689–691.

60. Gerster JC, Lagier R, Boivin G. Olecranon bursitis related to calcium pyrophosphate dihydrate crystal deposition disease. *Arthritis Rheum* 1982;25(8):989–996.

61. Sekijima Y, Yoshida T, Ikeda S. CPPD crystal deposition disease of the cervical spine: a common cause of acute neck pain encountered in the neurology department. *J Neurol Sci* 2010;296(1–2):79–82.

62. Fye KH, Weinstein PR, Donald F. Compressive cervical myelopathy due to calcium pyrophosphate dihydrate deposition disease: report of a case and review of the literature. *Arch Intern Med* 1999;159(2):189–193.

63. Martinez Sanchis A, Pascual E. Intracellular and extracellular CPPD crystals are a regular feature in synovial fluid from uninflamed joints of patients with CPPD related arthropathy. *Ann Rheum Dis* 2005;64(12):1769–1772.

64. Filippucci E, Riveros MG, Georgescu D, Salaffi F, Grassi W. Hyaline cartilage involvement in patients with gout and calcium pyrophosphate deposition disease. An ultrasound study. *Osteoarthritis Cartilage* 2009;17(2):178–181.

65. Frediani B, Filippou G, Falsetti P et al. Diagnosis of calcium pyrophosphate dihydrate crystal deposition disease: ultrasonographic criteria proposed. *Ann Rheum Dis* 2005;64(4):638–640.

66. Filippou G, Frediani B, Gallo A et al. A 'new' technique for the diagnosis of chondrocalcinosis of the knee: sensitivity and specificity of high-frequency ultrasonography. *Ann Rheum Dis* 2007;66(8):1126–1128.

67. Filippucci E, Scire CA, Delle Sedie A et al. Ultrasound imaging for the rheumatologist. XXV. Sonographic assessment of the knee in patients with gout and calcium pyrophosphate deposition disease. *Clin Exp Rheumatol* 2010;28(1):2–5.

68. Thiele RG, Schlesinger N. Diagnosis of gout by ultrasound. *Rheumatology* (Oxford) 2007;46(7):1116–1121.

69. Zhang W, Doherty M, Pascual E et al. EULAR recommendations for calcium pyrophosphate deposition. Part II: management. *Ann Rheum Dis* 2011;70(4):571–575.

70. Jordan KM, Arden NK, Doherty M et al. EULAR Recommendations 2003: an evidence based approach to the management of knee osteoarthritis: Report of a Task Force of the Standing Committee for International Clinical Studies Including Therapeutic Trials (ESCISIT). *Ann Rheum Dis* 2003;62(12):1145–1155.

71. Zhang W, Doherty M, Arden N et al. EULAR evidence based recommendations for the management of hip osteoarthritis: report of a task force of the EULAR Standing Committee for International Clinical Studies Including Therapeutics (ESCISIT). *Ann Rheum Dis* 2005;64(5):669–681.

72. Zhang W, Doherty M, Leeb BF et al. EULAR evidence based recommendations for the management of hand osteoarthritis: report of a Task Force of the EULAR Standing Committee for International Clinical Studies Including Therapeutics (ESCISIT). *Ann Rheum Dis* 2007;66(3):377–388.

73. Zhang W, Nuki G, Moskowitz RW et al. OARSI recommendations for the management of hip and knee osteoarthritis: part III: Changes in evidence following systematic cumulative update of research published through January 2009. *Osteoarthritis Cartilage* 2010;18(4):476–499.

74. Conaghan PG, Dickson J, Grant RL, Guideline Development Group. Care and management of osteoarthritis in adults: summary of NICE guidance. *BMJ* 2008;336(7642):502–503.

75. Schlesinger N, Detry MA, Holland BK et al. Local ice therapy during bouts of acute gouty arthritis. *J Rheumatol* 2002;29(2):331–334.

76. Ahern MJ, Reid C, Gordon TP et al. Does colchicine work? The results of the first controlled study in acute gout. *Aust N Z J Med* 1987;17(3):301–304.

77. Tabatabai MR, Cummings NA. Intravenous colchicine in the treatment of acute pseudogout. *Arthritis Rheum* 1980;23(3):370–374.

78. Zhang W, Doherty M, Bardin T et al. EULAR evidence based recommendations for gout. Part II: Management. Report of a task force of the EULAR Standing Committee for International Clinical Studies Including Therapeutics (ESCISIT). *Ann Rheum Dis* 2006;65(10):1312–1324.

79. Werlen D, Gabay C, Vischer TL. Corticosteroid therapy for the treatment of acute attacks of crystal-induced arthritis: an effective alternative to nonsteroidal antiinflammatory drugs. *Rev Rhum Engl Ed* 1996;63(4):248–254.

80. Roane DW, Harris MD, Carpenter MT et al. Prospective use of intramuscular triamcinolone acetonide in pseudogout. *J Rheumatol* 1997;24(6):1168–1170.

81. Janssens HJ, Janssen M, van de Lisdonk EH, van Riel PL, van Weel C. Use of oral prednisolone or naproxen for the treatment of gout arthritis: a double-blind, randomised equivalence trial. *Lancet* 2008;371(9627):1854–1860.

82. Getting SJ, Christian HC, Flower RJ, Perretti M. Activation of melanocortin type 3 receptor as a molecular mechanism for adrenocorticotropic hormone efficacy in gouty arthritis. *Arthritis Rheum* 2002; 46(10):2765–2775.

83. Ritter J, Kerr LD, Valeriano-Marcet J, Spiera H. ACTH revisited: effective treatment for acute crystal induced synovitis in patients with multiple medical problems. *J Rheumatol* 1994;21(4):696–699.

84. McGonagle D, Tan AL, Madden J, Emery P, McDermott MF. Successful treatment of resistant pseudogout with anakinra. *Arthritis Rheum* 2008;58(2):631–633.

85. Terkeltaub R, Sundy JS, Schumacher HR et al. The interleukin 1 inhibitor rilonacept in treatment of chronic gouty arthritis: results of a placebo-controlled, monosequence crossover, non-randomised, single-blind pilot study. *Ann Rheum Dis* 2009;68(10):1613–1617.

86. Alvarellos A, Spilberg I. Colchicine prophylaxis in pseudogout. *J Rheumatol* 1986;13(4):804–805.

87. Das SK, Mishra K, Ramakrishnan S et al. A randomized controlled trial to evaluate the slow-acting symptom modifying effects of a regimen containing colchicine in a subset of patients with osteoarthritis of the knee. *Osteoarthritis Cartilage* 2002;10(4):247–252.

88. Chollet-Janin A, Finckh A, Dudler J, Guerne PA. Methotrexate as an alternative therapy for chronic calcium pyrophosphate deposition disease: an exploratory analysis. *Arthritis Rheum* 2007;56(2):688–692.

89. Doan TH, Chevalier X, Leparc JM et al. Premature enthusiasm for the use of methotrexate for refractory chondrocalcinosis: comment on the article by Chollet-Janin et al. *Arthritis Rheum* 2008;58(7):2210–2211.

90. Rothschild B, Yakubov LE. Prospective 6-month, double-blind trial of hydroxychloroquine treatment of CPDD. *Compr Ther* 1997;23(5):327–331.

91. Doherty M, Dieppe PA. Double-blind, placebo-controlled trial of magnesium carbonate in chronic pyrophosphate arthropathy. *Ann Rheum Dis* 1983;42:Suppl 1:106.

92. Doherty M, Dieppe PA. Effect of intra-articular yttrium-90 on chronic pyrophosphate arthropathy of the knee. *Lancet* 1981;2(8258): 1243–1246.

Sources of patient information

Arthritis Research UK Arthritis information leaflet. Calcium crystal diseases. Available at: www.arthritisresearchuk.org/Files/2051-Calcium-crystal-diseases.pdf

SECTION 21

Diseases of bone and cartilage

Diseases of bone and cartilage

CHAPTER 143

Osteoporosis

Kanako Yoshida, Rosemary J. Hollick, and David M. Reid

Introduction

The management of osteoporosis aims to prevent a first or subsequent fracture. Lifestyle changes are helpful but for individuals with a high fracture risk pharmacological intervention is necessary. Recent advances in our understanding of bone biology has expanded the number of drugs available for the prevention and treatment of postmenopausal osteoporosis to include oral and intravenous bisphosphonates, strontium ranelate, raloxifene, parathyroid hormone analogues and most recently denosumab. A few studies have also examined their efficacy in the treatment of osteoporosis in men, glucocorticoid-induced osteoporosis, and cancer treatment induced bone loss. As an increasing number of drugs becoming available for the management of osteoporosis, along with some emerging concerns regarding their long term safety, there is an increasing need for a more stratified approach, with individual fracture risk assessment targeting therapy to those most at risk of fracture.

Introduction

Osteoporosis is the most common metabolic bone disease and has been defined as 'a systemic bone disease characterized by low bone mass and microarchitectural deterioration of bone tissue, leading to enhanced fragility and a consequent increase in fracture risk'.[1–2]

Epidemiology

Osteoporosis is a silent disease and the consequent condition of fracture is serious with significant morbidity and mortality. The global burden of osteoporotic fractures is significant particularly in the developed countries, with fractures estimated to account for 1.75% of the burden of non-communicable diseases in Europe and 0.83% worldwide.[3] Nine million osteoporotic fractures were estimated to have occurred worldwide in 2000, with 1.6 million hip and 1.4 million clinical vertebral fractures, the greatest number of these occurring in Europe (34.8%).[3] A total of 2.7 million osteoporotic fractures were estimated in men and women in Europe with an estimated direct cost of € 36 billion. In the United Kingdom, the lifetime risk of having any fractures was estimated to be 53.2% in women and 20.7% in men who are 50 years old.[4] In Sweden, the remaining lifetime risk of hip fracture alone at age 50 years old is quoted as 22.9% for women and 10.7% for men, while for any common osteoporotic fracture, which additionally includes the spine, shoulder, and forearm, it is 46.4% in women and 22.4% in men. With the rapidly growing elderly population and the fracture incidence increasing exponentially in some countries with age, numbers are expected to rise to 6.3 million hip fractures (? worldwide) in 2050.[5]

Hip fractures are the most serious adverse outcome of osteoporotic fractures and the 1 year mortality rates have been reported as 18–31%.[6] Many studies have suggested that the mortality in elderly women sustaining a hip fracture is highest for the 6 months immediately after the fracture but the effect may remain for several years afterwards,[7] unexplained by pre-existing comorbidities. Although men are less at risk of fractures overall, morbidity and mortality, particularly for hip fractures, is graver in men than women,[8] with men being twice as likely to die as women.[9] Many survivors are left with significant morbidity,[10] with one-half of ambulatory patients requiring assistance with activities of daily living and up to one-third of older people become totally dependent or in a nursing home within a year of hip fracture.[7]

Diagnosis

Although microarchitectural structural composition can be seen using three-dimensional (3D) CT or scanning electron micrograph (SEM) to look for osteoporosis (Figure 143.1), it is not practical to use these techniques for diagnosis. Dual-energy X-ray absorptiometry (DXA) was developed as a non-invasive, reproducible, and acceptable method to measure the amount of bone, expressed as bone mineral density (BMD). Conventionally DXA measurements are undertaken at the proximal femur and lumbar spine. BMD has a normal distribution in the population, and the cut-off for 'osteoporosis' using DXA, as defined by a World Health Organization (WHO) report[2] for postmenopausal women, is more than 2.5 standard deviations (SD) below the young normal mean (defined as a T-score), with 'osteopenia' defined as T-score of 1–2.5 SD and 'normal' defined as T-score no more than 1 SD below the

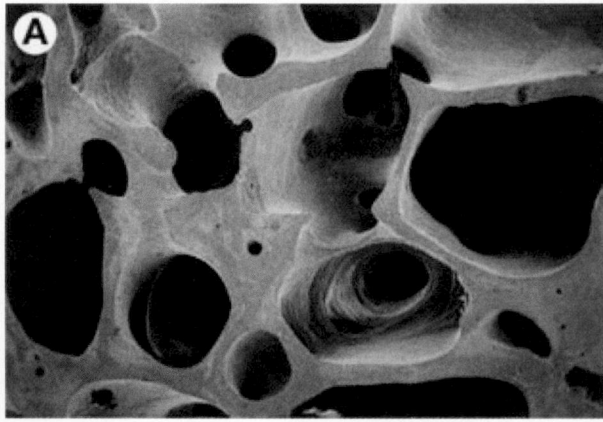
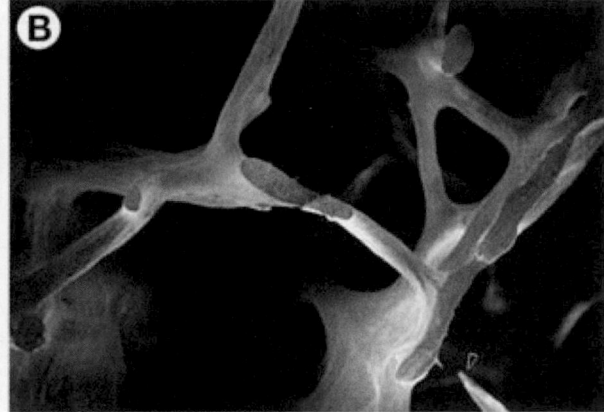

Fig. 143.1 Scanning electron micrograph of the trabecular structure of cancellous bone from a (A) normal subject and a patient with osteoporosis (B).
Reproduced with permission from Dempster, D.W., *The contribution of trabecular architecture to cancellous bone quality*. Journal of Bone and Mineral Research, 2000. 15(1): p. 20–23 © John Wiley and Sons.

young adult mean. However, the definition based on DXA only captures information on the amount of bone, with no information regarding its quality, architectural properties, or geometry. Furthermore, although BMD can be a useful measure of osteoporosis at the population level, it does not adequately predict fragility fractures in individuals when used alone. Accordingly, the focus has shifted recently to assess individual risk using a combination of risk factors, some of which are independent of BMD—the most commonly used technology at present is the FRAX tool.[12]

As a fracture occurs when the force of the impact is greater than the strength of the bone, risk factors for fracture can encompass both of these elements, as shown schematically in Figure 143.2. The relationship is complex, with many risk factors affecting both bone strength and force of impact to the bone.

Risk factors for osteoporosis and fracture

Age and sex

Epidemiological studies have shown the overall fracture incidence has a bimodal distribution with a peak in childhood and early adulthood and a secondary peak in later life, but it is the increased

fractures seen after the age of 50 which relate primarily to osteoporosis. Although vertebral fracture is the most common fragility fracture in both males and females, hip fracture is the most clinically important outcome of osteoporosis, requiring hospital admission and leading to major disability and excess mortality. The majority of hip fractures occur after a fall, with that risk increasing with age especially in women.[13] Although men have a higher mortality rate after hip fracture than women,[14] 80% of hip fractures occur in women and 90% in those over the age of 50. There is an exponential rise in hip fracture incidence after age 75 in women.[15] In contrast, only about 25% of vertebral fractures are related to falls and the prevalence of vertebral fractures in both sexes is much closer, perhaps as a result of a predominance of occupation-related trauma fractures in men. Wrist fracture pattern is similar to that of the hip with female predominance with estimated female to male ratio of 4:1.

Bone mineral density

Age and sex also influence bone strength and studies have focused on BMD as a measurable factor determining bone strength. Bone mass peaks around age 30, and starts to decline thereafter. Unlike

Fig. 143.2 Schematic diagram illustrating risk factors of fracture. Fracture occurs as a consequence of force of impact to the bone being greater than bone strength. *Drug use will contribute to the risk of fracture either as having an effect on bone strength such as with steroid use, or through increasing the falls risk, as seen with the use of benzodiazepines, or potentially via both mechanisms, as with anti-psychotic drug use.

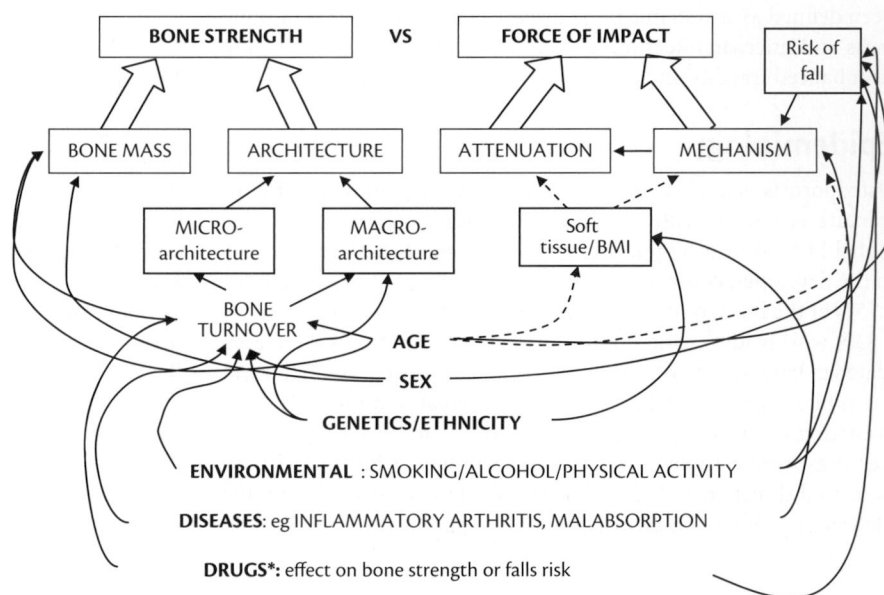

men who have a gradual and linear loss in bone mass after the age of 40, women have smaller bone size and lower peak bone mass and, in addition undergo accelerated bone loss immediately after the menopause. For each decrease in standard deviation of BMD, there is an estimated 1.5–3-fold increase in fracture risk.[16] When BMD is considered as the diagnostic marker of osteoporosis, its prevalence increases with age at the hip and other skeletal sites categorizing 30% of postmenopausal white women aged 50 or over as having osteoporosis.[2]

Genetics

Genetic factors have the strongest influence on BMD; it is estimated that 70–80% is heritable. Many genes have been implicated in association studies,[17] but increasingly genome-wide association studies (GWAS) are flagging up new genomic areas with influences on BMD and/or fracture. A recent meta-analysis showed 56 loci, of which 32 were new, associated with BMD at the hip and/or spine, and 14 of these also appeared to be associated with fracture risk.[18]

Previous fracture

Subsequent fracture risk is greatly increased by previous osteoporotic fracture especially at the same site, with a greater than 10-fold increased risk of subsequent vertebral fracture in those with an incident vertebral fracture.[19] In the multicentre United States Study of Osteoporotic Fractures (SOF) involving 9704 women aged 65 years or more, vertebral deformity was associated with a relative risk of 5.4 (95% CI 4.4–6.6) of future vertebral deformity, 2.8-fold risk (95% CI 2.3–3.4) of future hip fracture deformity, and 1.9-fold risk (95% CI 1.7–2.1) of non-vertebral deformity with significance remaining after adjustment for age and calcaneal BMD.[20] Similarly in a European study, European Prospective Osteoporosis Study (EPOS), the number and nature of vertebral deformity predicted not only future vertebral deformities[21] but also incident hip fracture with an age-adjusted rate ratio of 2.8 (95% CI 2.1–9.4).[22]

Geographical distribution and ethnicity

The incidence and prevalence of fractures also varies according to ethnicity and geographical location and this is most prominently seen in hip fracture. North American and Scandinavian countries have the highest age-adjusted rates, while Mediterranean countries, Latin America, and Asian populations have lower fracture rates. Many studies including the Women's Health Initiative have reported that black women have a lower risk of fracture than white women.[23] Vertebral fracture prevalence was 20–80% greater in Hiroshima[24] and 25% lower in Beijing[25] than for postmenopausal white women in Minnesota, despite the lower hip rates in both Asian cities. Geographical variation in fracture rates have also been observed within the same country, with people from rural regions having lower fracture rates than those from urban areas of the same country,[26,27] suggesting the importance of environmental factors.

Time trends

In many developed countries including the United States,[28] Canada,[29] Finland,[30] Norway,[31] England,[32] and Australia,[33] age-standardized fracture rates have started to plateau or decline, at least for hip fractures in women, although others have not reported this, including Germany[34] and Japan,[35] where age-adjusted rates continue to show an increase. Ethnicity and geographic variation may affect the findings; the incidence of hip fracture doubled in Hispanic women in California from 1983 to 2000,[36] and significant increases have been recently observed in the rapidly urbanizing city of Beijing, China.[37] The trend of increasing fractures in Asia contributes significantly to the estimated increasing global burden of fractures with over one-half of female hip fractures occurring in Asia by 2050.[5] Although hip fracture rates are not decreasing in all settings, inpatient mortality rates appear to be declining,[28,32] perhaps reflecting an improvement in hip fracture care.

Additional risk factors, some of which are independent of BMD, are shown in Table 143.1. In addition a number of both hereditary and non-hereditary diseases and drugs (Table 143.2) are linked to osteoporosis primarily by an influence on bone mass.

Table 143.1 Summary of risk factors for fracture

Female gender	Premature menopause
Age[a]	Primary or secondary amenorrhoea
	Primary and secondary hypogonadism in man
Asian or white ethnicity	Previous fragility fracture[a]
Low BMD	Glucocorticoid therapy[a]
High bone turnover[a]	Family history of hip fracture[a]
Poor visual acuity[a]	Low body weight[a]
Neuromuscular disorders[a]	Cigarette smoking[a]
	Excessive alcohol consumption[a]
	Prolonged immobilization
	Low dietary calcium intake
	Vitamin D deficiency

[a]Independent or partly independent of bone mineral density (BMD).
Reproduced with permission from Kanis.[38]

Table 143.2 Diseases and their drugs associated with osteoporosis

Diseases associated with osteoporosis	Drugs and associated diseases associated with osteoporosis
Hereditary	Exogenous glucocorticoids
Rickets and osteogenesis imperfecta	Cancer therapies
Endocrine and metabolic	Aromatase inhibitors
Hyogonadism, hyperparathyroidism, hyperthyroidism, Cushing's syndrome,	Gonadotrophin releasing hormone agonists
Gut diseases	Androgen deprivation therapies
Coeliac disease	Others
Bone marrow diseases	Warfarin?
Multiple myeloma, mastocytosis	Proton pump inhibitors (e.g. omeprazole)
Rheumatological diseases	Thyroid hormones in excess
Systemic lupus erythematosus, ankylosing spondylitis, rheumatoid arthritis	Medroxyprogesterone acetate

Management of osteoporosis

Goals of intervention

The management of postmenopausal osteoporosis aims to prevent a first or subsequent fracture by slowing/preventing bone loss, maintaining bone strength, and minimizing skeletal trauma. Changes in lifestyle are helpful but women with a high fracture risk will often also need pharmacological intervention. In primary care, specific goals are to:

◆ maximize peak bone mass

◆ identify patients at highest risk of fracture

◆ use investigations cost-effectively

◆ exclude secondary osteoporosis

◆ provide lifestyle advice to all those at risk

◆ provide appropriate drug treatment to those at highest risk and encourage compliance

◆ identify and manage those at increased risk of falls.

All women should be encouraged to take steps to prevent bone loss and fractures, such as eating a balanced diet (including adequate intake of calcium and vitamin D), participating in appropriate weightbearing exercise, not smoking, avoiding excessive alcohol consumption, and instituting measures to prevent falls. Some of these steps, such as smoking cessation and exercise, offer health benefits beyond their effects on osteoporosis.

Ensuring adequate 'intake' of vitamin D may be achieved by eating a healthy diet—oily fish and some eggs—and getting 10 minutes' exposure to the sun once or twice per day to the extremities in summer (between May and September in the Northern hemisphere). Falls prevention strategies include ensuring a safe and well-lit home environment, appropriate footwear/walking devices, optimizing medical conditions (e.g. Parkinson's disease), ensuring adequate visual correction, and minimizing iatrogenic causes such as postural hypotension or excessive sedation. Recent guidelines extol the virtue of exercise and vitamin D in fall prevention.[39]

Investigation of patients with osteoporosis or fracture

Before embarking on pharmaceutical therapy it is important to exclude secondary cause of osteoporosis, especially in those with pre-existing vertebral fractures (Table 143.3). The assessment of serum 25-hydroxyvitamin D is controversial but should be considered in those in whom deficiency may influence the choice of therapy, for example when using intravenous bisphosphonates, which may induce hypocalcaemia if the patients is not vitamin D replete.

Assessment and treatment

Who to treat with drugs?

Population screening for osteoporosis or risk of fracture is not yet considered cost-effective. However, in those with incident fracture, especially vertebral fracture, or in whom multiple clinical risk factors are detected, further assessment and treatment is recommended.[40] Increasingly the use of assessment tools based on 10-year assessment of fracture risk such as the online FRAX tool[12] are being used. An alternative approach for use in general

Table 143.3 Investigations to exclude secondary osteoporosis

Serum/plasma test	Secondary cause considered
ESR	Malignancy, inflammatory musculoskeletal disorders
FBC	Multiple myeloma
Calcium, phosphate, alkaline phosphatase	Osteomalacia, Paget's disease, hyperparathyroidism and other metabolic bone diseases
Liver function tests (AAT, γGT, etc)	Chronic liver disease
Proteins and electrophoresis	Multiple myeloma
Creatinine	Chronic renal disease
Endomyseal antibodies	Coeliac disease
T_4, TSH	Exclude thyrotoxicosis
25-OH vitamin D	Severe deficiency

ESR, erythrocyte sedimentation rate; FBC, full blood count; T_4, thyroxine; TSH, thyroid stimulating hormone.

practice, Qfracture,[41] does not allow the incorporation of BMD. In the United Kingdom, intervention thresholds have been published by the National Osteoporosis Guideline Group (NOGG)[42] (available via the UK version of the FRAX tool[12,43]).

Drug therapy

The main pharmacological therapies available for the prevention and treatment of osteoporosis are bisphosphonates, strontium ranelate, raloxifene, parathyroid hormone analogues, and more recently denosumab. All reduce the risk of vertebral fracture and some also reduce the risk of non-vertebral fracture, including hip fracture. In the United Kingdom, evidence based guidelines from the National Institute for Health and Clinical Excellence (NICE) for primary[44] and secondary[45] prevention of osteoporosis, the Scottish Intercollegiate Guidelines Network (SIGN),[46] and National Osteoporosis Guideline Group (NOGG)[47] all recommend oral bisphosphonates as first-line choice in the management of postmenopausal osteoporosis because of their efficacy and cost-effectiveness. For those who are intolerant of oral bisphosphonates or in whom their use is contraindicated, alternative options include intravenous bisphosphonate preparations such as ibandronate and zoledronic acid, strontium ranelate, raloxifene, and denosumab. Because of their high cost, use of parathyroid hormone analogues such as teriparatide is generally restricted to those with severe osteoporosis at very high risk of fracture. Table 143.4 summarizes the grading of evidence relating to the fracture reduction efficacy of drug therapies currently licensed for the management of osteoporosis. There is still a role for hormone replacement therapy (HRT) in the management of osteoporosis however it is no longer considered first-line treatment in the majority of women due to an increased risk of breast cancer.

Bisphosphonates

Bisphosphonates are synthetic analogues of pyrophosphate with a high affinity for hydroxyapatite crystals in bone, suppressing bone turnover and increasing BMD at the lumbar spine and other sites via inhibition of osteoclast-mediated bone resorption. First-generation

Table 143.4 Grade of evidence relating to fracture reduction of pharmacological interventions in postmenopausal women with osteoporosis

Drug	Vertebral fracture	Non-vertebral fracture	Hip fracture
Alendronate	A	A	A
Ibandronate	A	A[a]	nae
Risedronate	A	A	A
Zolendronate	A	A	A
Denosumab	A	A	A
Raloxifene	A	nae	nae
Strontium ranelate	A	A	A[a]
Teriparatide	A	A	nae
PTH (1–84)	A	nae	nae

nae, not adequately evaluated; PTH, recombinant parathyroid hormone.
[a]In subsets of patients (post-hoc analysis).
Adapted from National Osteoporosis Guideline Group Guideline for the diagnosis and management of osteoporosis in postmenopausal women and men from the age of 50 years in the UK.[48]

bisphosphonates such as etidronate induce apoptosis in osteoclasts, whereas newer nitrogen-containing bisphosphonates such as alendronate, risedronate, ibandronate, and zoledronate interfere with the mevalonate pathway and inhibit recruitment and function of osteoclasts.[49]

Alendronate and risedronate are usually administered once weekly for greater convenience. Ibandronate is a monthly therapy at a dose of 150 mg and is also available as a 3 mg intravenous injection every 3 months. Meta-analyses have demonstrated that alendronate and risedronate reduce the incidence of vertebral, non-vertebral, and hip fractures. Both etidronate and ibandronate have been shown to reduce the incidence of vertebral fractures, but their impact on non-vertebral and hip fractures is less clear.[50] Therapeutic equivalence has been demonstrated between oral and intravenous ibandronate.[51] Zoledronic acid is licensed for the treatment of osteoporosis in both men and women as a 5 mg intravenous infusion once yearly. It has been shown to significantly reduce the risk of vertebral, non-vertebral, and hip fractures in osteoporotic postmenopausal women,[52] and to reduce vertebral and non-vertebral fractures and mortality in both men and women following surgical repair of hip fracture.[53]

Tolerability and safety of bisphosphonates
Gastrointestinal side effects
Gastrointestinal (GI) side effects are common and include nausea, dyspepsia, diarrhoea, oesophageal and gastric irritation, erosions, and ulceration.[54] They are a major cause of poor compliance and discontinuation of therapy and are more common in patients with a history of upper GI disorders and those taking concomitant non-steroidal anti-inflammatory drugs (NSAIDs), proton pump inhibitors, or histamine receptor blockers.[55] The anatomical distribution of oesophageal and gastric damage is consistent with a topical irritant effect.[54] Oral bisphosphonates interact with food and drink and therefore must be taken on an empty stomach at least 30 minutes before eating and with plenty of water, with the patient remaining upright for at least 30 minutes after dosing to minimize side effects.[49] Intravenous preparations may circumvent the topical irritant effects of oral bisphosphonates.

Atrial fibrillation
Atrial fibrillation (AF) was first identified in a phase 3 zoledronic acid registration trial, but a subsequent meta-analysis of randomized controlled trials (RCTs) and observational studies found a non-significantly higher risk of AF in bisphosphonate users although registry-based studies suggest little or no increased risk of AF in bisphosphonate users.[56–59]

Subtrochanteric and femoral shaft fractures
The overall incidence of subtrochanteric and femoral shaft fractures is very low, accounting for less than 10% of all femoral fractures. The majority occur as a result of high-energy trauma, but almost 300 case series and reports of subtrochanteric/femoral shaft fractures occurring in patients treated with long-term bisphosphonate therapy have been identified (median duration 7 years; range 1.3–17 years). Recent studies have shown that the risk of atypical fracture appears to increase with increasing duration of bisphosphonate use, although the overall absolute risk of atypical fracture was extremely low. It is difficult to draw definitive conclusions regarding causality and further carefully adjudicated large scale clinical case-control studies are required.

Osteonecrosis of the jaw
Defined by the presence of exposed bone in the mouth which fails to heal after appropriate intervention over a period of 6–8 weeks, osteonecrosis of the jaw has been associated with bisphosphonate use, mainly in those receiving high-dose intravenous bisphosphonates for the management of malignant conditions. It is likely that bisphosphonate-induced osteonecrosis of the jaw (BONJ) results from direct toxicity to cells of the bone and soft tissue from high-potency bisphosphonates, probably acting through their effects on the mevalonate pathway. Incidence is rare, with estimates ranging from 1 in 10 000 to less than 1 in 100 000 persons per year of exposure. Patients should not be discouraged from taking bisphosphonates in the first instance, nor from undergoing dental treatment while taking them. There is no evidence that stopping ongoing bisphosphonate therapy prior to dental work is necessary as bisphosphonates persist in the skeletal system for years after discontinuation, although it is recommended that patients inform their dentist if they are taking a bisphosphonate and ensure regular dental check-ups.[57]

Oesophageal carcinoma
In 2009, the United States Food and Drug Administration (FDA) reported on 23 cases in the United States and 31 cases in Europe and Japan of oesophageal carcinoma in patients receiving oral bisphosphonates. Registry studies from Denmark and the United States found no increased incidence amongst oral bisphosphonate users compared to those receiving other osteoporosis medications, and two subsequent studies using data from the UK General Practice Research Database have produced conflicting results.[58,59] Conclusive evidence for a casual association between oesophageal cancer and bisphosphonate use is lacking.

Other side effects of treatment
Intravenous bisphosphonates are associated with an acute-phase reaction occurring to a variable degree in 10–50% of patients, comprising of fever, myalgia, arthralgia, and flu-like symptoms 1–3 days

post-infusion. It is much less likely to occur with second and subsequent infusions.[56] Bisphosphonates have also rarely been associated with ocular disturbances such as conjunctivitis, blurred vision, eye pain. and uveitis.[60] Zoledronic acid has been associated with reports of renal failure and impairment following its use, especially in patients with pre-existing renal impairment or concomitant use of nephrotoxic drugs. Zoledronate should not be used in patients with a creatinine clearance less than 35 mL/min,[61] although caution should also be exercised when using oral bisphosphonates in patients with significant renal impairment.

Strontium ranelate

Strontium ranelate is an orally active agent that appears to act by dissociating bone resorption from bone formation, thus increasing bone mass and strength, although its exact mechanism of action remains unclear.[62] In phase 2 trials strontium ranelate 2 g/day reduced the relative risk of new vertebral fractures by 41%[63] with a relative risk reduction of 16% for all non-vertebral fractures and 19% for major fragility fractures.[64] Subgroup analysis of women aged 74 years or more(mean age 80 years) with femoral neck BMD within the osteoporotic range, demonstrated a 36% relative risk reduction in hip fracture. Follow-up studies suggest that the antifracture efficacy of strontium ranelate is sustained over a period of 8 years.[65] The increases in BMD observed in all studies involving strontium ranelate were larger than expected. This partly reflects the uptake of strontium in bone, which has a higher X-ray absorption than calcium, resulting in artificially higher BMD values [66] that account for approximately 50% of the measured change in BMD over 3 years of treatment with strontium ranelate.

The majority of the fracture reduction efficacy with strontium ranelate comes from studies involving elderly osteoporotic patients over the age of 75 years, and it is a useful alternative in such patients who are intolerant or have a contraindication to bisphosphonate therapy or who struggle with the strict dosing instructions. It is administered daily as a 2 g sachet dissolved in water. Food, milk, and calcium-containing products reduce the bioavailability of strontium ranelate by up to 70%, therefore it should be taken at least 2 hours after eating, preferably at night.

Commonly noted side effects include nausea, diarrhoea, and headache, which were usually mild and transient. However, pooled results from the two major phase 3 trials[63,64] revealed that the annual incidence of venous thromboembolism (VTE) observed over 5 years in the strontium ranelate group was approximately 0.9% vs 0.6% in the placebo group. The European Medicines Agency recently recommended that strontium ranelate is contraindicated in patients with a current or previous history of VTE and those who are temporarily or permanently immobilized. Other side effects reported include hypersensitivity reactions such as drug rash with eosinophilia and systemic symptoms (DRESS), Stevens–Johnson syndrome, and toxic epidermal necrolysis.

Selective oestrogen receptor modulators

Selective oestrogen receptor modulators (SERMs) provide the skeletal benefits of oestrogen without its adverse effects on the endometrium and breast. Raloxifene is the only SERM currently available in the United Kingdom for use in the prevention and treatment of osteoporosis. Other SERMs with proven anti-fracture efficacy include bazedoxifene and lasofoxifene. Raloxifene acts as an agonist at the oestrogen receptor in bone, mimicking the actions of oestrogen by inhibiting bone resorption and increasing bone density, whereas in uterine and breast tissue it acts as an antagonist at the oestrogen receptor.[67] The main evidence for fracture reduction with raloxifene comes from the MORE (Multiple Outcomes of Raloxifene Evaluation) study,[68] where women with postmenopausal osteoporosis randomized to raloxifene 60 mg/day (the licensed dose) had a 30–50% relative risk reduction in vertebral fracture compared to placebo depending on the presence or absence of pre-existing vertebral fractures. No significant reduction in the risk of non-vertebral fractures was observed, a finding supported by the subsequent CORE (Continuing outcomes Relevant to Evista) study.[69]

SERMs are generally indicated for use in women who are within 10 years of the menopause as this period is associated with a marked increase in bone resorption and subsequent bone loss as a result of the reduction in oestrogen levels.

Common adverse effects of raloxifene include hot flushes, leg cramps, peripheral oedema, and influenza symptoms,[67,70] and a pooled 1.7-fold increase in the incidence of VTE (95% CI 0.93–3.14). SERMs should not therefore be prescribed to women with an active or past history of VTE, and treatment discontinued at least 72 hours before and during any periods of prolonged immobilization. Despite the beneficial effects of SERMs on lipid metabolism, studies have found no significant difference in the incidence of myocardial infarction or stroke and in the RUTH (Raloxifene Use for The Heart) study[71] there was an increased risk of fatal stroke (HR 1.49; 95% CI 1.00–2.24) The RUTH study also demonstrated a significant reduction in the risk of oestrogen receptor positive invasive breast cancer, consistent with observations from previous studies.

Denosumab

Denosumab is a fully human monoclonal immunoglobulin G2 (IgG2) antibody directed against receptor activator of NFκB ligand (RANKL).[72] Denosumab binds to RANKL, preventing interaction with its receptor RANK, located on osteoclasts and osteoclast precursors, thereby inhibiting osteoclast differentiation and reversibly inhibiting osteoclast-mediated bone resorption in cortical and trabecular bone.[73] Denosumab is recommended for use in postmenopausal women with osteoporosis who are unable to tolerate oral bisphosphonates, or comply with their strict dosing instructions, or have a contraindication to their use, at a dose of 60 mg by subcutaneous injection every 6 months.[74,75] In those patients with significant renal impairment, denosumab represents a useful alternative treatment option as renal impairment has no effect on the pharmacokinetics of denosumab.[72]

The main evidence for fracture reduction efficacy comes from the phase 3 Fracture Reduction Evaluation of Denosumab in Osteoporosis Every 6 Months (FREEDOM) trial,[76] which showed that 60 mg denosumab given subcutaneously every 6 months for 3 years significantly reduced the risk of new radiographic vertebral fracture by 68%, non-vertebral fracture by 20% (HR 0.80; 95% CI 0.67–0.95, p<0.01) and hip fracture by 40%. Denosumab was also associated with a relative increase in BMD at the lumbar spine and total hip, with significant reductions in bone turnover markers (BTMs) relative to placebo, an effect which appears rapidly reversible on stopping treatment. An extension study[77] has shown fracture incidence rates remaining low, with a progressive increase in BMD and sustained, but not progressive, reductions in BTMs in

The role of testosterone in older men at risk of fracture is controversial and there is no clear consensus regarding its use in this group. There is no clear evidence that testosterone prevents fractures and that fact that both bisphosphonates and teriparatide are effective in increasing BMD in men, regardless of gonadal function, suggests that it may be more appropriate to treat this group with an established osteoporotic drug.[99]

Glucocorticoid-induced osteoporosis

Drugs that have a European licence for the prevention of treatment of glucocorticoid-induced osteoporosis (GIO) include alendronate, risedronate, etidronate (postmenopausal women), zoledronic acid, and teriparatide (men and women). In practice the weekly bisphosphonates are the most tried and tested and have evidence of vertebral fracture prevention. The threshold for intervention for prevention is lower in GIO as fractures tend to occur at a higher level of BMD than is the case in postmenopausal women, and often treatment is advised in younger men and women at high risk of fracture.

Cancer-treatment-induced bone loss

Studies which determined the benefit of drugs that have specific effects in the prevention or management of osteoporosis associated with breast cancer treatments, especially the aromatase inhibitors, are limited but the best evidence to date is with the bisphosphonates, specifically intravenous zoledronic acid. Published guidance[104] suggests using any of the oral or intravenous bisphosphonates although subcutaneous denosumab may also prove valuable in the future.

With prostate cancer treatment in men, androgen deprivation produces a major excess fracture risk. Again evidence of bone loss protection is relatively scanty but zoledronic acid again seems to have a benefit and denosumab has a specific licence for use in this situation.

Duration of treatment

Emerging concerns regarding atypical fractures with prolonged bisphosphonate use have focused attention on initiating therapy in those patients who will benefit most in terms of the risk-benefit ratio of bisphosphonate therapy. The WHO FRAX model goes some way to addressing this. In patients currently receiving bisphosphonate therapy, the ongoing need for treatment should be regularly reviewed and formally reassessed after 5 years with a view to continuing therapy in those at highest risk of fracture. After 5–10 years of treatment, good clinical practice would suggest a drug-free period of 1–2 years before resuming treatment in those patients in whom ongoing fracture risk remains high. Although there is some evidence that anti-fracture efficacy persists for alendronate and perhaps risedronate following cessation of treatment, there is no evidence that a drug-free period reduces the risk of atypical fractures and the risks and benefits of stopping bisphosphonate therapy need to be considered on an individual basis.

Monitoring of treatment

The questions as to 'whether to monitor?' or 'how to monitor?' remain contentious. Increasingly, BTMs, especially serum CTX for bone resorption and serum P1NP for bone formation, are being used in specialist centres but they have not become freely available and suffer from the disadvantage of having to be measured in a fasting state. Classically, repeat BMD measurements are used and

have benefit in providing some reassurance to patients that their treatment is being effective. The best site to assess effectiveness of therapy is the lumbar spine but even here for most anti-resorptive therapies 2 years of treatment will be needed before real improvements in BMD will exceed the 'least significant change' measurement error. Changes in the lumbar spine site can be difficult to reliably assess, however, especially in elderly patients where preexisting fracture, lumbar spondylosis, or aortic calcification may interfere with the reproducibility of repeated measurements. In this situation the total hip site can be used but interpreted with care, recognizing that many treatments have lesser magnitude of effect at that site.

Conclusion

Osteoporosis and fractures are frequent in the community but there is increasing evidence that they can be prevented with judicious use of oral and parenteral drug therapy in particular. Slowly, guidance is emerging on 'who to treat' and 'how long to treat'. With increasing future availability of new drugs with effects on bone resorption and bone formation there will be an increasing need for a stratified medicine approach to target appropriate treatments to individual patients.

References

1. Anonymous. Consensus development conference: Diagnosis, prophylaxis, and treatment of osteoporosis. *Am J Med* 1993;94(6):646–650.
2. Assessment of fracture risk and its application to screening for postmenopausal osteoporosis. Report of a WHO Study Group. *World Health Organization Technical Report Series* 1994;843:1–129.
3. Johnell O, Kanis JA. An estimate of the worldwide prevalence and disability associated with osteoporotic fractures. *Osteoporosis Int* 2006;17(12):1726–1733.
4. Van Staa TP, Dennison EM, Leufkens HG et al. Epidemiology of fractures in England and Wales. *Bone* 2001;29(6):517–522.
5. Cooper C, Campion G, Melton LJ III. Hip fractures in the elderly: A world-wide projection. *Osteoporosis Int* 1992;2(6):285–289.
6. Bentler SE, Liu L, Obrizan M et al. The aftermath of hip fracture: Discharge placement, functional status change, and mortality. *Am J Epidemiol* 2009;170(10):1290–1299.
7. Cummings SR, Melton LJ III. Osteoporosis I: Epidemiology and outcomes of osteoporotic fractures. *Lancet* 2002;359(9319):1761–1767.
8. Myers AH, Robinson EG, Van Natta ML et al. Hip fractures among the elderly: Factors associated with in-hospital mortality. *Am J Epidemiol* 1991;134(10):1128–1137.
9. Wehren LE, Hawkes WG, Orwig DL et al. Gender differences in mortality after hip fracture: the role of infection. *J Bone Miner Res* 2003;18(12):2231–2237.
10. Leibson CL, Tosteson AN, Gabriel SE et al. Mortality, disability, and nursing home use for persons with and without hip fracture: A population-based study. *J Am Geriatr Soc* 2002;50(10):1644–1650.
11. Dempster DW. The contribution of trabecular architecture to cancellous bone quality. *J Bone Miner Res* 2000;15(1):20–23.
12. World Health Organization Collaborating Centre for Metabolic Bone Diseases, University of Sheffield, UK. FRAX: WHO Fracture Risk Assessment Tool, 2012. Available at: www.shef.ac.uk/frax.
13. Sattin RW, Lambert H, Devito C et al. The incidence of fall injury events among the elderly in a defined population. *Am J Epidemiol* 1990;131(6):1028–1037.
14. Johnell O, Kanis JA, Odén A et al. Mortality after osteoporotic fractures. *Osteoporosis Int* 2004;15(1):38–42.
15. Sambrook P, Cooper C. Osteoporosis. *Lancet* 2006;367(9527):2010–2018.

16. Marshall D, Johnell O, Wedel H. Meta-analysis of how well measures of bone mineral density predict occurrence of osteoporotic fractures. *BMJ* 1996;312(7041):1254–1259.

17. Ralston SH. Genetics of osteoporosis. *Ann N Y Acad Sci* 2010;1192: 181–189.

18. Estrada K, Styrkarsdottir U, Evangelou E et al. Genome-wide meta-analysis identifies 56 bone mineral density loci and reveals 14 loci associated with risk of fracture. *Nat Genet* 2012;44(5):491–501.

19. Melton LJ III, Atkinson EJ, Cooper C et al. Vertebral fractures predict subsequent fractures. *Osteoporosis Int* 1999;10(3):214–221.

20. Black DM, Arden NK, Palermo L et al. Prevalent vertebral deformities predict hip fractures and new vertebral deformities but not wrist fractures. *J Bone Miner Res* 1999;14(5):821–828.

21. Lunt M, O'Neill TW, Pye S et al. Characteristics of a prevalent vertebral deformity predict subsequent vertebral fracture: Results from the European Prospective Osteoporosis Study (EPOS). *Bone* 2003;33(4):505–513.

22. Ismail AA, Cockerill W, Cooper C et al. Prevalent vertebral deformity predicts incident hip though not distal forearm fracture: Results from the European prospective osteoporosis study. *Osteoporosis Int* 2001;12(2):85–90.

23. Cauley JA, Wu L, Wampler NS et al. Clinical risk factors for fractures in multi-ethnic women: The Women's Health Initiative. *J Bone Miner Res* 2007;22(11):1816–1826.

24. Ross PD, Fujiwara S, Huang C et al. Vertebral fracture prevalence in women in Hiroshima compared to Caucasians or Japanese in the US. *Int J Epidemiol* 1995;24(6):1171–1177.

25. Ling X, Cummings SR, Mingwei Q et al. Vertebral fractures in Beijing, China: The Beijing osteoporosis project. *J Bone Miner Res* 2000;15(10):2019–2025.

26. Melton LJ III, Crowson CS, O'Fallon WM. Fracture incidence in Olmsted County, Minnesota: Comparison of urban with rural rates and changes in urban rates over time. *Osteoporosis Int* 1999;9(1):29–37.

27. Omsland TK, Ahmed LA, Gronskag A et al. More forearm fractures among urban than rural women: The NOREPOS study based on the Tromsø study and the HUNT study. *J Bone Miner Res* 2011;26(4):850–856.

28. Brauer CA, Coca-Perraillon M, Cutler DM et al. Incidence and mortality of hip fractures in the United States. *JAMA* 2009;302(14): 1573–1579.

29. Leslie WD, O'Donnell S, Jean S et al. Trends in hip fracture rates in Canada. *JAMA* 2009;302(8):883–889.

30. Kannus P, Leiponen P, Parkkari J et al. Nationwide decline in incidence of hip fracture. *J Bone Miner Res* 2006;21(12):1836–1838.

31. Støen RO, Nordsletten L, Meyer HE et al. Hip fracture incidence is decreasing in the high incidence area of Oslo, Norway. *Osteoporosis Int* 2012;1–8.

32. Wu TY, Jen MH, Bottle A et al. Admission rates and in-hospital mortality for hip fractures in England 1998 to 2009: Time trends study. *J Publ Health* 2011;33(2):284–291.

33. Pasco JA, Brennan SL, Henry MJ et al. Changes in hip fracture rates in southeastern Australia spanning the period 1994–2007. *J Bone Miner Res* 2011;26(7):1648–1654.

34. Icks A, Haastert B, Wildner M et al. Trend of hip fracture incidence in Germany 1995–2004: A population-based study. *Osteoporosis Int* 2008;19(8):1139–1145.

35. Hagino H, Furukawa K, Fujiwara S et al. Recent trends in the incidence and lifetime risk of hip fracture in Tottori, Japan. *Osteoporosis Int* 2009;20(4):543–548.

36. Zingmond DS, Melton LJ III, Silverman SL. Increasing hip fracture incidence in California Hispanics 1983 to 2000. *Osteoporosis Int* 2004;15(8):603–610.

37. Xia WB, He SL, Xu L et al. Rapidly increasing rates of hip fracture in Beijing, China. *J Bone Miner Res* 2012;27(1):125–129.

38. Kanis JA. Diagnosis of osteoporosis and assessment of fracture risk. *Lancet* 2002;359(9321):1929–1936.

39. Moyer VA. Prevention of falls in community-dwelling older adults: U.S. Preventive Services Task Force Recommendation Statement. *Ann Intern Med* 2012;157(3):197–204.

40. Kanis J, Burlet N, Cooper C et al. European guidance for the diagnosis and management of osteoporosis in postmenopausal women. *Osteoporosis Int* 2008;19(4):399–428.

41. Hippisley-Cox J, Coupland C. Derivation and validation of updated QFracture algorithm to predict risk of osteoporotic fracture in primary care in the United Kingdom: prospective open cohort study. *BMJ* 2012;344: e3427.

42. Compston J, Cooper A, Cooper C et al. Guidelines for the diagnosis and management of osteoporosis in postmenopausal women and men from the age of 50 years in the UK. *Maturitas* 2009;62(2):105–108.

43. Johansson H, Kanis JA, Oden A et al. A comparison of case-finding strategies in the UK for the management of hip fractures. *Osteoporosis Int* 2012;23(3):907–915.

44. National Institute for Clinical Excellence (NICE). Osteoporosis—primary prevention: guidance (TA160), 2011 (cited 10 March 2012). Available at: www.guidance.nice.org.uk/TA160/Guidance/pdf/English.

45. National Institute for Clinical Excellence (NICE). Osteoporosis—secondary prevention including strontium ranelate (TA161), 2011 (cited 19 March 2012). Available at: www.nice.org.uk/TA161.

46. Scottish Intercollegiate Guidelines Network. Management of Osteoporosis: A national clinical guideline (cited 10 March 2012). Available at: www.sign.ac.uk/pdf/sign71.pdf.

47. National Osteoporosis Society. Guideline for the diagnosis and management of osteoporosis in postmenopausal women and men from the age of 50 years in the UK, 2010 (cited 10 March 2012). Available at: www.shef.ac.uk/NOGG/NOGG_Pocket_Guide_for_Healthcare_Professionals. pdf.

48. National Osteoporosis Guideline Group. Guideline for the diagnosis and management of osteoporosis in postmenopausal women and men from the age of 50 years in the UK, 2010 (cited 10 March 2012). Available at: www.shef.ac.uk/NOGG/NOGG_Pocket_Guide_for_Healthcare_Professionals. pdf.

49. Reid D. *Handbook of osteoporosis*. Springer Healthcare, London, 2010.

50. MacLean C, Newberry S, Maglione M et al. Systematic review: comparative effectiveness of treatments to prevent fractures in men and women with low bone density or osteoporosis. *Ann Intern Med* 2008;148(3): 197–213.

51. Delmas PD, Adami S, Strugala C et al. Intravenous ibandronate injections in postmenopausal women with osteoporosis—One-year results from the dosing intravenous administration study. *Arthritis Rheum* 2006;54(6):1838–1846.

52. Black DM, Delmas PD, Eastell R et al. Once-yearly zoledronic acid for treatment of postmenopausal osteoporosis. *N Engl J Med* 2007;356(18):1809–1822.

53. Lyles KW, Colon-Emeric CS, Magaziner JS et al. Zoledronic acid and clinical fractures and mortality after hip fracture. *N Engl J Med* 2007;357(18):1799–1809.

54. Graham DY. What the gastroenterologist should know about the gastrointestinal safety profiles of bisphosphonates. *Dig Dis Sci* 2002;47(8): 1665–1678.

55. Cramer JA, Silverman S. Persistence with bisphosphonate treatment for osteoporosis: finding the root of the problem. *Am J Med* 2006; 119(4 Suppl 1):S12–S17.

56. Hollick RJ, Reid DM. Role of bisphosphonates in the management of postmenopausal osteoporosis: an update on recent safety anxieties. *Menopause Int* 2011;17(2):66–72.

57. Scottish Dental Clinical Effectiveness Programme. Oral health management of patients prescribed bisphosphonates: dental clinical guidance, 2011 (cited 10 March 2012). Available at: www.sdcep.org.uk/index.aspx?o=3017.

58. Cardwell CR, Abnet CC, Cantwell MM et al. Exposure to oral bisphosphonates and risk of esophageal cancer. *JAMA* 2010;304(6): 657–663.

59. Green J, Czanner G, Reeves G et al. Oral bisphosphonates and risk of cancer of the oesophagus, stomach, and colorectum: case-control analysis within a UK primary care cohort. *BMJ* 2010;341:c4444.

60. Fraunfelder FW, Fraunfelder FT. Bisphosphonates and ocular inflammation. *N Engl J Med* 2003;348(12):1187–1188.

61. MHRA. Important safety information for bisphosphonates issued by the MHRA, September 2010 (cited 10 March 2012). Available at: www.mhra.gov.uk/Safetyinformation/Generalsafetyinformationandadvice/Product-specificinformationandadvice/Product-specificinformationandadvice-A-F/Bisphosphonates/index.htm#l22.

62. Marie PJ, Felsenberg D, Brandi ML. How strontium ranelate, via opposite effects on bone resorption and formation, prevents osteoporosis. *Osteoporosis Int* 2011;22(6):1659–1667.

63. Meunier PJ, Roux C, Seeman E et al. The effects of strontium ranelate on the risk of vertebral fracture in women with postmenopausal osteoporosis. *N Engl J Med* 2004;350(5):459–468.

64. Reginster JY, Seeman E, De Vernejoul MC et al. Strontium ranelate reduces the risk of nonvertebral fractures in postmenopausal women with osteoporosis: treatment of peripheral osteoporosis (TROPOS) Study. *J Clin Endocrinol Metab* 2005;90(5):2816–2822.

65. Reginster JY, Bruyère O, Sawicki A et al. Long-term treatment of postmenopausal osteoporosis with strontium ranelate: Results at 8 years. *Bone* 2009;45(6):1059–1064.

66. Blake GM, Fogelman I. Effect of bone strontium on BMD measurements. *J Clin Densitom* 2007;10(1):34–38.

67. European Medicines Agency. Raloxifene tiva: summary of product characteristics (cited 19 March 2012). Available at: www.ema.europa.eu/docs/en_GB/document_library/EPAR_-_Product_Information/human/001075/WC500091420.pdf.

68. Ettinger B, Black DM, Mitlak BH et al. Reduction of vertebral fracture risk in postmenopausal women with osteoporosis treated with raloxifene: results from a 3-year randomized clinical trial. Multiple Outcomes of Raloxifene Evaluation (MORE) Investigators. *JAMA* 1999;282(7):637–645.

69. Siris ES, Harris ST, Eastell R et al. Skeletal effects of raloxifene after 8 years: results from the continuing outcomes relevant to Evista (CORE) study. *J Bone Miner Res* 2005;20(9):1514–1524.

70. Martino S, Disch D, Dowsett SA et al. Safety assessment of raloxifene over eight years in a clinical trial setting. *Curr Med Res Opin* 2005;21(9):1441–1452.

71. Barrett-Connor E, Mosca L, Collins P et al. Effects of raloxifene on cardiovascular events and breast cancer in postmenopausal women. *N Engl J Med* 2006;355(2):125–137.

72. European Medicines Agency. Denosumab (Prolia): summary of product characteristics, 2011.

73. Delmas PD. Clinical potential of RANKL inhibition for the management of postmenopausal osteoporosis and other metabolic bone diseases. *J Clin Densitom* 2008;11(2):325–338.

74. Scottish Medicines Consortium. SMC advice denosumab (Prolia), 2010 (cited 12 March 2012). Available at: www.scottishmedicines.org.uk/files/advice/denosumab_Prolia_FINAL_November_2010_for_website.pdf.

75. NICE. Denosumab for the prevention of osteoporotic fractures in postmenopausal women, 2010. Available at: www.nice.org.uk/guidance/TA204.

76. Cummings SR, San Martin J, McClung MR et al. Denosumab for prevention of fractures in postmenopausal women with osteoporosis. *N Engl J Med* 2009;361(8):756–765.

77. Papapoulos S, Chapurlat R, Libanati C et al. Five years of denosumab exposure in women with postmenopausal osteoporosis: Results from the first two years of the FREEDOM extension. *J Bone Miner Res* 2012;27(3):694–701.

78. U.S. Food and Drug Administration. Background document for meeting of Advisory Committee for Reproductive Health Drugs. Denosumab (proposed trade name: PROLIA), Amgen Inc, 2009 (cited 17 March 2012). Available at: www.fda.gov/downloads/AdvisoryCommittees/CommitteesMeetingMaterials/Drugs/ReproductiveHealthDrugsAdvisoryCommittee/UCM176605.pdf.

79. Neer RM, Arnaud CD, Zanchetta JR et al. Effect of parathyroid hormone (1–34) on fractures and bone mineral density in postmenopausal women with osteoporosis. *N Engl J Med* 2001;344(19):1434–1441.

80. Fahrleitner-Pammer A, Langdahl BL, Marin F et al. Fracture rate and back pain during and after discontinuation of teriparatide: 36-month data from the European Forsteo Observational Study (EFOS). *Osteoporos Int* 2011;22(10):2709–2719.

81. Obermayer-Pietsch BM, Marin F, McCloskey EV. Effects of two years of daily teriparatide treatment on bone mineral density in postmenopausal women with severe osteoporosis with and without prior antiresorptive therapy. *J Bone Miner Res* 2008;23(10):1591–1600.

82. Torgerson DJ, Bell-Syer SE. Hormone replacement therapy and prevention of nonvertebral fractures: a meta-analysis of randomized trials. *JAMA* 2001;285(22):2891–2897.

83. Rossouw JE, Anderson GL, Prentice RL et al.; Writing Group for the Women's Health Initiative Investigators. Risks and benefits of estrogen plus progestin in healthy post-menopausal women: principal results from the Women's Health Initiative randomized controlled trial. *JAMA* 2002;288:321–333.

84. Beral V; Million Women Study Collaborators, Breast cancer and hormone-replacement therapy in the Million Women Study. *Lancet* 2003; 362:419–427.

85. Wasserheil-Smoller S, Hendrix SL, Limacher M et al. Effect of estrogen plus progestin on stroke in postmenopausal women. The Women's Health Initiative: a randomized trial. *JAMA* 2003;289(20):2673–2684.

86. CMDh. Core SPC for hormone replacement therapy products. December 2009. Available at: www.hma.eu/fileadmin/dateien/Human_Medicines/CMD_h_/Product_Information/Core_SPC_PL/Core_SPCs/CMDh_131_2003_Rev3_Clean_2010_01_Core_SmPC_for_HRT.pdf

87. National Osteoporosis Society. National Osteoporosis Society policy on hormone replacement for the treatment and prevention of osteoporosis, 2010 (cited 10 March 2012). Available at: www.nos.org.uk/page.aspx?pid=1075&srcid=1074.

88. Bolland MJ, Avenell A, Baron JA et al. Effect of calcium supplements on risk of myocardial infarction and cardiovascular events: meta-analysis. *BMJ* 2010;341:c3691–c3691.

89. Bolland MJ, Grey A, Avenell A. et al. Calcium supplements with or without vitamin D and risk of cardiovascular events: reanalysis of the Women's Health Initiative limited access dataset and meta-analysis. *BMJ* 2011;342:d2040.

90. Bischoff-Ferrari HA, Willett WC, Wong JB et al. Fracture prevention with vitamin D supplementation: a meta-analysis of randomized controlled trials. *JAMA* 2005;293(18):2257–2264.

91. Bergman GJ, Fan T, McFetridge JT et al. Efficacy of vitamin D3 supplementation in preventing fractures in elderly women: a meta-analysis. *Curr Med Res Opin* 2010;26(5):1193–1201.

92. Avenell A, Gillespie WJ, Gillespie LD et al. Vitamin D and vitamin D analogues for preventing fractures associated with involutional and post-menopausal osteoporosis. *Cochrane Database Syst Rev* 2009;2: CD000227.

93. Bischoff-Ferrari HA, Dawson-Hughes B, Willett WC et al. Effect of vitamin D on falls: a meta-analysis. *JAMA* 2004;291(16):1999–2006.

94. Murad MH, Elamin KB, Abu Elnour NO et al. Clinical review: The effect of vitamin D on falls: a systematic review and meta-analysis. *J Clin Endocrinol Metab* 2011;96(10):2997–3006.

95. Bischoff-Ferrari HA, Willett WC, Orav EJ et al. A pooled analysis of vitamin D dose requirements for fracture prevention. *N Engl J Med* 2012;367(1):40–49.

96. Rejnmark L, Mosekilde L. New and emerging antiresorptive treatments in osteoporosis. *Curr Drug Saf* 2011;6(2):75–88.

97. Binkley N, Bone H, Gilchrist N et al. Treatment with the cathepsin K inhibitor odanacatib in postmenopausal women with low BMD: 5 year results of a phase 2 trial. *J Bone Miner Res* 2011;26(Suppl 1).

98. Padhi D, Jang G, Stouch B et al. Single-dose, placebo-controlled, randomized study of AMG 785, a sclerostin monoclonal antibody. *J Bone Miner Res* 2011;26(1):19–26.

99. Khosla S, Amin S, Orwoll E. Osteoporosis in men. *Endocr Rev* 2008;29(4):441–464.

100. Orwoll E, Ettinger M, Weiss S et al. Alendronate for the treatment of osteoporosis in men. *N Engl J Med* 2000;343(9):604–610.

101. Boonen S, Delmas PD, Wenderoth DH et al. Risedronate shown to be safe and effective in men with osteoporosis in a 2-year, double-blind, randomized, placebo-controlled, multicentre study. *Osteoporos Int* 2006;17 (Suppl 2):S230–S231.

102. Orwoll ES, Scheele WH, Paul S et al. The effect of teriparatide (human parathyroid hormone (1–34)) therapy on bone density in men with osteoporosis. *J Bone Miner Res* 2003;18(1):9–17.

103. Kaufman JM, Orwoll E, Goemaere S et al. Teriparatide effects on vertebral fractures and bone mineral density in men with osteoporosis: treatment and discontinuation of therapy. *Osteoporos Int* 2005;16(5):510–516.

104. Reid DM, Doughty J, Eastell R et al. Guidance for the management of breast cancer treatment-induced bone loss: a consensus position statement from a UK Expert Group. *Cancer Treat Rev* 2008;34, Suppl 1: S3–S18.

CHAPTER 144

Paget's disease of bone

Stuart H. Ralston

Introduction

Paget's disease of bone (PDB) is a common metabolic bone disorder in people of European descent, characterized by focal abnormalities of increased and disorganized bone remodelling which can affect one or multiple bones throughout the skeleton. The characteristic clinical features of the disease were described by Sir James Paget in 1876 and the disease has borne his name ever since.

Epidemiology

Paget's disease predominantly affects older people, with an average age at diagnosis of about 65 years. The risk of developing Paget's disease is strongly age-dependent; the prevalence doubles each decade from the age of about 50 onwards to affect up to 7.5% of men and 5% of women by the eighth decade.[1] (Figure 144.1). Marked ethnic differences in susceptibility exist. The highest rates in the world are in the United Kingdom but the disease is also common in Spain, France, and Italy and in people from these countries who have migrated to other parts of the world such as Australia, New Zealand, the United States, and Canada. Conversely, Paget's is uncommon in Scandinavia and is extremely rare in the Indian subcontinent, China, Japan, and other Asian countries. These ethnic differences in disease susceptibility point to the importance of genetic factors in aetiology, but there is also evidence to suggest that environmental factors play a role. There have been significant reductions in prevalence and clinical severity of Paget's in the United Kingdom and New Zealand over the past 25 years.[2] However for reasons that remain unclear, no changes in prevalence or severity have been observed in Italy over recent years.[3] The reductions in prevalence of Paget's disease that have occurred in some countries because of changes in ethnic make-up of the population due to an influx of migrants from low-prevalence countries such as India and Pakistan and an efflux of members of the indigenous population to other parts of the world. It seems likely that there have also been changes in environmental triggers for the disease over the past 50–100 years. The nature of these triggers are unknown, but possible candidates include a reduced incidence of infections, improvements in nutrition, and reduced mechanical loading and fewer injuries to the skeleton.

Pathophysiology

Bone tissue is normally renewed and repaired throughout the skeleton through the process of bone remodelling. During the bone remodelling cycle, old and damaged bone is removed by osteoclasts and this is followed by infilling of the resorption space by osteoblasts which lay down new bone. This process is markedly accelerated within Pagetic bone lesions. Osteoclasts are increased in number and size and some contain nuclear inclusion bodies which are composed of microcylindrical structures organized into paracrystalline arrays (Figure 144.2). There is marrow fibrosis and increased vascularity of the bone marrow. Osteoblast numbers are also increased and bone formation is elevated, but the bone matrix is laid down in an irregular fashion, leading to the production of woven bone which has reduced mechanical strength. This in turn, impairs mechanical strength, predisposing to the development of deformities, especially when weightbearing bones of the lower limbs are affected. The risk of pathological fractures is also increased. Two factors contribute to the increased in bone turnover that occurs in Paget's disease. First, osteoclast precursors have increased sensitivity to the effects of bone resorbing factors such as calcitriol and the receptor activator of NFκB ligand (RANKL). Secondly, bone marrow stromal cells are better able to support osteoclast formation because of enhanced RANKL expression. There is increasing evidence to suggest that these cellular abnormalities are accounted for by mutations and polymorphisms in the genes that regulate osteoclast differentiation and function as discussed in more detail later in this chapter.

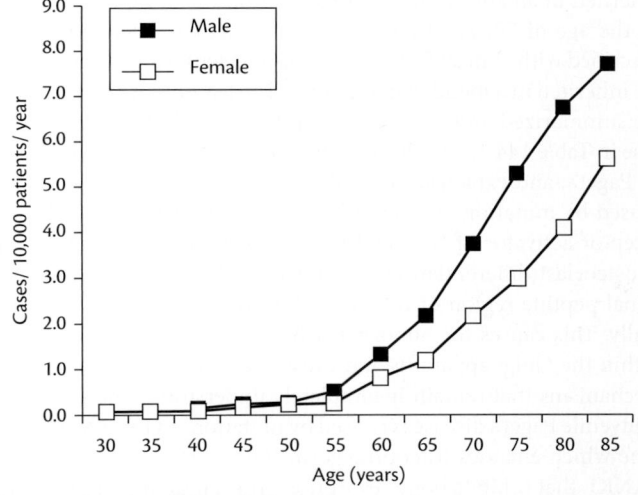

Fig. 144.1 Prevalence of Paget's disease in men and women.
Reproduced with permission from van Staa TP, Selby P, Leufkens HG, Lyles K, Sprafka JM, Cooper C. Incidence and natural history of Paget's disease of bone in England and Wales. J Bone Miner Res 2002; 17(3):465–471 © John Wiley & Sons.

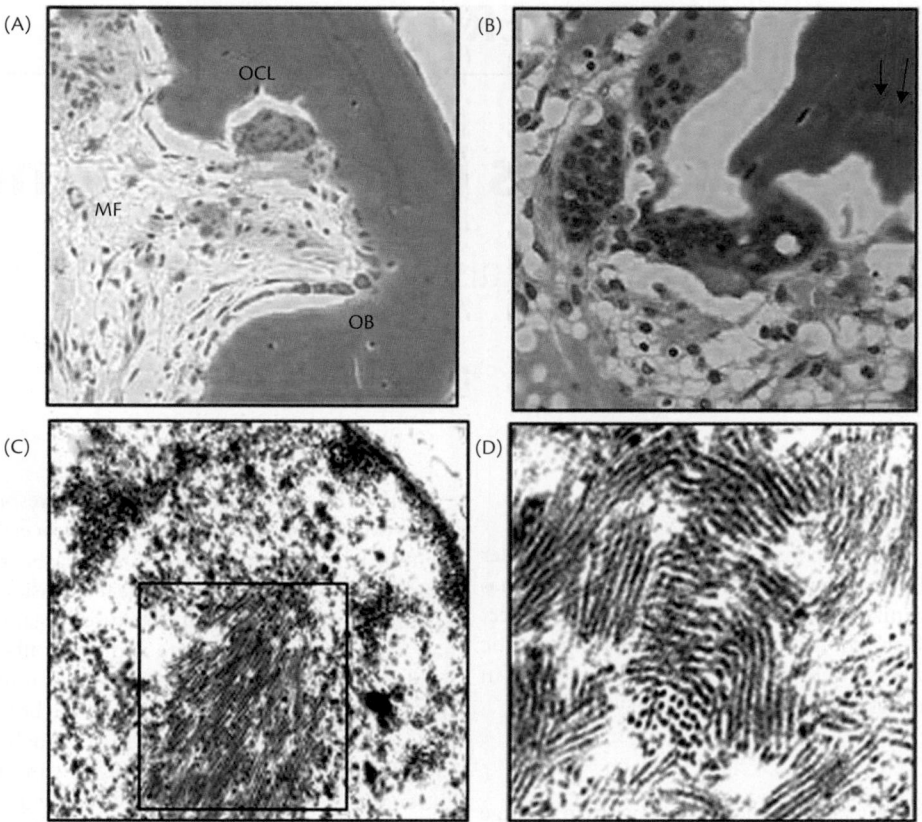

Fig. 144.2 Histological characteristics of Paget's bone lesions: (A) Histological section of a pagetic bone lesion stained with haematoxylin and eosin, The bone is stained pink. A large osteoclast is visible (OCL) next to a row of osteoblasts (OB). There is marked marrow fibrosis. (B) Higher-power image of a different area in the same lesion. Three large multinucleated osteoclasts are visible. Irregular cement lines are evident indicative of woven bone (arrows). (C) Scanning electron microscope image of a nuclear inclusion body in a Paget's osteoclasts (box). (D) The same inclusion body at higher magnification.

Aetiology

Genetic factors play a central role in regulating susceptibility to Paget's disease. Approximately 15% of patients have a positive family history and the risk of developing Paget's is about 7 times increased in first-degree relatives of patients compared with controls.[4] Many families have also been described where the disease is inherited in an autosomal dominant fashion with high penetrance by the age of 70. Furthermore, several rare disorders have been described with clinical features overlapping with Paget's disease that are inherited in a mendelian manner.[5] The features of these diseases are summarized and compared with those of classical Paget's disease in Table 144.1. Familial expansile osteolysis, early-onset familial Paget's, and expansile skeletal hyperplasia are related disorders caused by mutations of the *TNFRSF11A* gene which encodes the receptor activator of NFκB (RANK) which plays an essential role in osteoclast differentiation and function. All mutations affect the signal peptide region of RANK and prevent it being cleaved normally. This causes the abnormal RANK molecules to accumulate within the Golgi apparatus and causes activation of osteoclasts by mechanisms that remain incompletely understood. The syndrome of juvenile Paget's disease is caused by mutations in the *TNFRSF11B* gene which encodes osteoprotegerin (OPG), a decoy receptor for RANKL that inhibits bone resorption. The causal mutations either delete the gene in its entirety or impair the ability of OPG to inhibit RANK signalling. The syndrome of inclusion body myopathy, Paget's disease, and frontotemporal dementia (IBMPFD) is caused

by *VCP* gene mutations. These affect a conserved region of the VCP protein which is involved in ubiquitin binding, but the mechanisms by which this causes osteoclast activation are poorly understood. Classical Paget's disease is a polygenic disorder with at least eight known predisposing genes and loci, many of which are involved in regulating osteoclast differentiation and function through effects on the RANKL–RANK–OPG–NFκB pathway as illustrated in Figure 144.3.

The most important susceptibility gene for the development of classical PDB is sequestosome 1 (*SQSTM1*) which encodes p62, a scaffold protein that is involved in the RANK signalling pathway. Mutations of *SQSTM1* have been reported to occur in 20–50% of patients with a family history of PDB and 5–20% of cases of 'sporadic' PDB. Most causal mutations affect the ubiquitin-associated (UBA) domain of p62 and impair its ability to bind polyubiquitin chains and other molecules in the RANK signalling complex. An important consequence of the UBA domain mutations is that these prevent p62 binding to the deubiquitinating enzyme CYLD and recruiting it to the intracellular RANK receptor complex. The consequence of this is that CYLD can no longer fulfil its normal function of inhibiting RANK signalling by deubiquitinating TRAF6, leading to activation of NFκB signalling and enhanced osteoclastogenesis.[6] Recently, several other susceptibility loci for Paget's disease have identified by genome-wide association studies.[7] These have shown that genetic variants close to the *TNFRSF11A*, *CSF1*, *TM7SF4*, and *OPTN* genes all strongly predispose to Paget's disease. Additional strong susceptibility loci were identified on chromosomes 7q33,

Table 144.1 Features of Paget's disease and related syndromes

Disease	Age at diagnosis	Inheritance	Genes and loci implicated	Other features
Paget's disease	55–75	Autosomal dominant/ polygenic	SQSTM1 TNFRSF11A CSF1 TM7SF$ OPTN Chr 7q33 Chr 14 Chr 15	
Familial expansile osteolysis	15–20	Autosomal dominant	TNFRSF11A	Premature deafness, tooth loss
Expansile skeletal hyperplasia	15–20	Autosomal dominant	TNFRSF11A	Premature deafness, tooth loss, hypercalcaemia
Early-onset familial Paget's	15–20	Autosomal dominant	TNFRSF11A	Premature deafness, and tooth loss
Juvenile Paget's disease	1–5	Autosomal recessive	TNFRSF11B	Multiple fractures Vascular calcification
Inclusion body myopathy, Paget's disease, frontotemporal dementia	40–50	Autosomal dominant	VCP	Myopathy Dementia

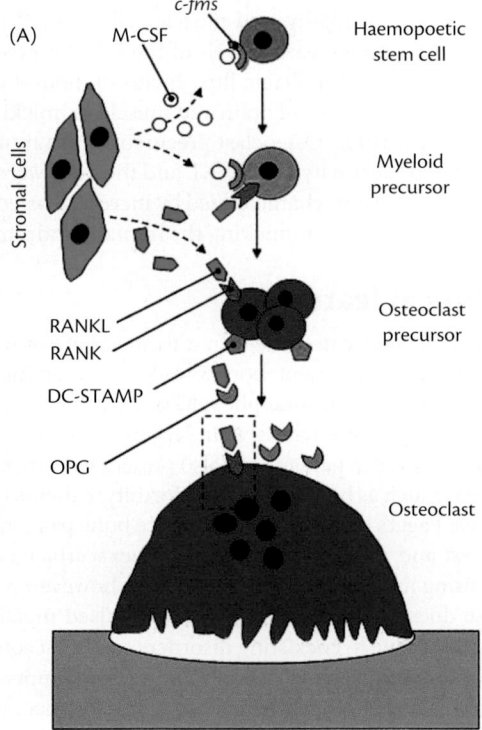

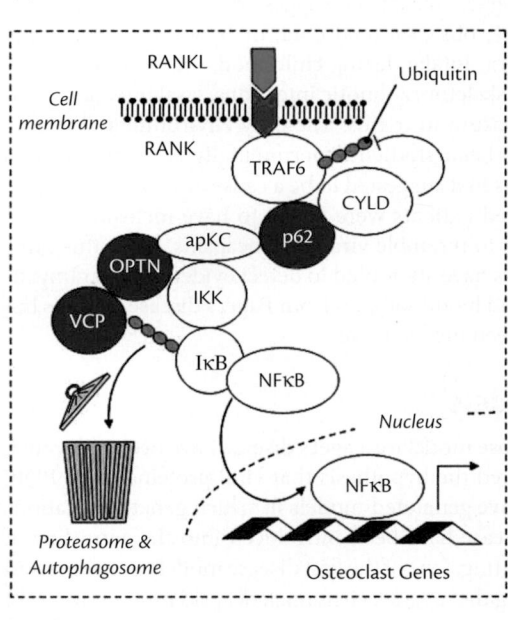

Fig. 144.3 Mediators of osteoclast differentiation and function: (A) Haemopoetic stem cells differentiate down the myeloid lineage in response to M-CSF which is secreted by bone marrow stromal cells and which activates the *c-fms* receptor. Further differentiation down the osteoclast lineage is dependent on both M-CSF and RANKL which by binding to its receptor RANK, promotes osteoclast differentiation and bone resorption by mature osteoclasts. This interaction is blocked by OPG which inhibits bone resorption. Fusion of osteoclast precursors to form mature multinucleated osteoclasts is dependent on DC-STAMP which is upregulated by RANKL. (B) Within the osteoclast, binding of RANKL to RANK activates the NFκB signalling pathway by recruiting TNF-receptor associated factor 6 (TRAF6) to the intracellular tail of the receptor complex. The *SQSTM1* gene product p62 recruits CYLD to the receptor complex by its UBA domain and CYLD negatively regulates NFκB signalling by deubiquinating TRAF6. Mutations affecting the UBA domain of p62 prevent this occurring, thereby activating NFκB signalling. In addition p62 promotes NFκB signalling by binding to atypical protein kinase C which activates IKK. The IKK protein phosphorylates inhibitor of kappa B (IκB) which becomes ubiquitinated and targeted for degradation by the proteasome and/or autophagosome. This allows the p65 component of NFκB to translocate to the nucleus, and activate expression of osteoclast specific genes. The VCP protein is involved in regulating degradation of IκB whereas the optineurin protein (OPTN) inhibits NFκB signalling by an effect on IKK. Both of these proteins also play a role in autophagy, although the relevance of this to osteoclast activation is unclear.

14q32, and 15q24 in which the causal genes are less clear. The *TNFRSF11A*, *CSF1*, and *TM7SF4* genes all play key roles in regulating osteoclast differentiation and function. The importance of *TNFRSF11A* in osteoclast activity has already been discussed. The *CSF1* gene encodes macrophage colony stimulating factor (M-CSF), which together with RANK, is required for osteoclast differentiation. The *TM7SF4* gene encodes dendritic cell specific membrane protein (DC-STAMP) which is required for mononuclear osteoclast precursors to fuse to form mature osteoclasts.[8] The *OPTN* gene is involved in regulating NFκB signalling by modulating inhibitor of kappa B kinase activity (IKK) and is also involved in regulating autophagy. This is the process by which cells dispose of unwanted proteins and organelles.[9] Since the *SQSMT1* and *VCP* genes also play important roles in regulating autophagy, it has been suggested that the osteoclast nuclear inclusions that occur in Paget's disease may be undegraded protein aggregates due to defects in autophagy.[10] It is at present unclear, however, whether abnormalities of autophagy contribute to osteoclast activation in Paget's disease or whether this is a bystander phenomenon. The inherited susceptibility to Paget's disease seems to be mediated by a combination of rare and common variants in genes that regulate osteoclast differentiation and function, although the mechanisms by which these variants cause Paget's remains incompletely understood.

The changes in prevalence and severity that have occurred in many countries over recent years indicate that environmental factors also play a key role in the pathogenesis of PDB. Several potential environmental triggers have been suggested on the basis of epidemiological studies, observational data, or hypotheses, including low dietary calcium intake during childhood, repetitive mechanical loading of the skeleton, zoonotic infections, viral infections, and occupational exposure to toxins. The only environmental trigger for PDB that has been studied experimentally is paramyxovirus infection. This was first suggested to be a cause of PDB when osteoclasts from affected patients were found to have inclusion bodies that were thought to resemble viral nucleocapsids. Since this time, many investigators have attempted to detect evidence of paramyxoviruses in bone and blood samples from Paget's disease patients but the results have been inconclusive.

Disease models

Two types of disease model for Paget's disease have been generated. Some have explored the hypothesis that viral proteins cause PDB, whereas others have generated models in which genetic mutations that cause the disease have been introduced into the germ-line of mice by gene targeting. One of the first disease models was generated by over-expressing the measles virus nucleocapsid protein (MVNP) in mice, driven by the tartrate-resistant acid phosphatase (TRAP) promoter which preferentially targets expression to osteoclasts. Histological analysis of vertebral bone from these mice showed evidence of increased bone turnover.[11] Osteoclast precursors had increased sensitivity to $1,25(OH)_2D_3$ and formed hypernucleated osteoclasts as compared with those generated from wild-type littermates. High levels of interleukin (IL)-6 were found in these cultures and the osteoclast formation was inhibited by antibodies to IL-6, indicating that osteoclast activation in this model was due in part to production of this cytokine. Models of *SQSTM1*-mediated PDB have also been generated. Two groups of investigators independently generated mice in which the proline residue at codon 394 of

the mouse p62 protein is replaced by a leucine residue, mimicking the human P392L mutation.[10,12] Both groups reported that osteoclast precursors from these mice were hypersensitive to RANKL and in one study stromal cells from the mutant mice were reported to support osteoclast formation more efficiently than wild type in association with increased RANKL production. While no evidence of focal bone lesions was detected in one study on the basis of histological analysis of the vertebrae,[13] the other study showed that the P394L mice developed a bone disease with remarkable similarity to Paget's disease.[10] In this model, the mice developed focal bone lesions characteristic of Paget's disease which mainly targeted the hindlimbs, but which seldom targeted the vertebrae. Histological analysis showed evidence of increased bone turnover within the lesions, large hypernucleated osteoclasts, and increased bone formation with production of woven bone. Nuclear inclusion bodies similar to those observed in human Paget's disease were found in some osteoclasts. The difference between studies was most probably due to the fact that microCT analysis was used to localize lesions in one study[10] but not in the other.[13] Targeted inactivation of the *TNFRSF11B* gene in mice results in a generalized state of increased bone turnover associated with multiple fractures, providing a model for juvenile Paget's disease.[14] A model of IBMPFD has also been generated in which the arginine at codon 155 of the VCP protein is substituted by a histidine (R155H), modelling one of the most common human mutations.[15] These mice were reported to develop myopathy, and muscle cells showed increased rates of apoptosis and increased levels of the LC3B protein consistent with an increase in autophagic flux. Inclusion bodies were observed on histological analysis of brain and muscle, mimicking the findings in human IBMPFD. Osteoclast precursors from mutant mice showed increased sensitivity to RANKL and the mice were reported to have focal bone lesions characterized by increased osteoclast and osteoblast activity, again mimicking the human syndrome.

Clinical features

Paget's disease can present in a wide variety of ways. Probably the most common presentation nowadays is as an incidental finding of a raised serum alkaline phosphatase (ALP) or an abnormal radiograph in patients who are undergoing investigation of other diseases. However, patients can also present with specific features of the disease such as bone pain and deformity. Patients with metabolically active Paget's disease may experience bone pain. This can be present at rest and at night but also may be exacerbated by weightbearing or using an affected limb. Frequently, however, pain in Paget's disease does not occur as the result of raised metabolic activity, but instead is due to coexisting disorders such as secondary osteoarthritis, degenerative disc disease, and nerve compression syndromes. Careful evaluation of the patient is therefore necessary to determine the underlying cause of pain so that it can be treated appropriately.

Physical examination is usually normal in Paget's disease but sometimes deformity may be apparent, especially when the disease affects the tibia, skull, or facial bones (Figure 144.4). The skin temperature may be increased over affected bones in patients with metabolically active Paget's disease, but this is usually detectable only over the tibia.

Paget's disease can be associated with several complications including deafness, pathological fracture, secondary osteoarthritis, cranial nerve compression syndromes, and spinal stenosis

(Table 144.2). Although many of these conditions are also common in elderly patients without PDB, epidemiological studies have shown that Paget's patients are 3.1 times more likely to need a hip replacement for osteoarthritis compared with aged matched controls and 1.7 times more likely to need a knee replacement.[1] Other complications that are significantly more common in Paget's disease when compared with controls include hearing loss (1.6-fold increase); tinnitus (1.5-fold); dizziness (1.3-fold), back pain (2.1-fold), osteoarthritis (1.7-fold), and fracture (1.2-fold). Osteosarcoma is a rare complication of PDB, which is estimated to occur in 0.01% to 0.1% of patients. However, most osteosarcomas that occur in adulthood are associated with PDB.[1] Hypercalcaemia can occur in PDB patients who are immobilized. The most common clinical scenario is as the result of dehydration when an affected patient is confined to bed because of an intercurrent illness or postoperatively. High-output cardiac failure can rarely occur as a complication of active PDB due to increased blood flow through affected bone, and a similar mechanism has been proposed to account at least in part, for the development of paraplegia which can occur as a complication of Paget's disease of the spine.

Table 144.2 Complications of Paget's disease of bone

Complication	Estimated frequency
Bone pain	4.6%
Deformity	2.5%
Pathological fracture	0.6%
Osteoarthritis	1.2%
Deafness	1.5%
Spinal stenosis	<0.1%
Nerve compression syndromes	<0.1%
Hydrocephalus	<0.1%
Paraplegia	<0.1%
High-output cardiac failure	<0.1%
Osteosarcoma	0.01%

The estimated frequency of complications is based on the assumption that about 7% of patients with Paget's disease come to medical attention and that the complications in those that do present clinically are similar to those recorded in the PRISM study which was representative of patients being treated by secondary care referral centres in the United Kingdom.

Investigations

The diagnosis of Paget's disease is usually straightforward. A radionuclide bone scan should be performed to localize sites of involvement followed by radiographs of affected bones or areas that are painful. The bone scan appearances in untreated Paget's disease are quite distinctive, showing a homogeneous increase in tracer uptake in affected bones (Figure 144.5). Radiographs show evidence of bone expansion with thickening of the cortex and disruption of the normal trabecular architecture by areas of osteolysis alternating with areas of osteosclerosis. Stress fractures may also be observed, especially when there is deformity of weightbearing lower limbs (Figure 144.5). A routine biochemical screen should be performed with measurement of urea and electrolytes, liver function tests, ALP, calcium and albumin. Serum total ALP levels provide a convenient and sensitive measure of metabolic activity in Paget's disease which is adequate for most patients. Serum total ALP values are raised in 95% of untreated patients with PDB but a normal value does not exclude the diagnosis since ALP can be within the normal range in patients with monostotic disease and in those with metabolically inactive disease. Bone-specific alkaline phosphatase (BSAP) levels track closely with those of total ALP except in patients with chronic liver disease where BSAP measurements would be the preferred method of assessing metabolic activity. Occasionally patients may be encountered where the results of the above investigations are inconclusive. In this situation, bone biopsy can sometimes be required to differentiate between Paget's disease and other causes of osteosclerosis such as prostate cancer metastatic to bone.

Management

The optimal management of Paget's disease requires a multidisciplinary approach. The elevated bone turnover in Paget's disease can be corrected in most cases by treatment with anti-resorptive therapy with one of the many potent bisphosphonates which are now available. Intravenous zoledronic acid in particular can induce biochemical remission of Paget's disease in a high proportion of patients for periods of up to 5 years.[16] In many patients, however, additional measures need to be adopted for pain management and to deal with other complications that respond poorly to bisphosphonates.

Anti-resorptive drugs

Inhibitors of osteoclastic bone resorption are widely used in the treatment of Paget's disease. The main indication is bone pain

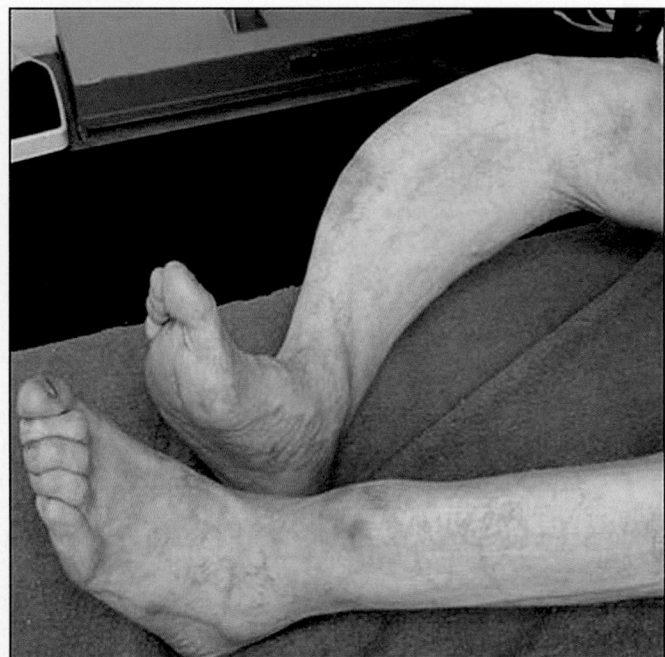

Fig. 144.4 Severe pagetic deformity of the tibia.

Table 144.3 Bisphosphonates used in the treatment of Paget's disease

Drug	Trade name	Dose
Etidronate	Didronel	400 mg/day for 3 months
Clodronate[a]	Loron, Bonefos	400–1600 mg/day orally for 3–6 months or 300 mg/day IV for 5 days
Pamidronate	Aredia	60 mg/day IV for 3 days
Alendronate[a]	Fosamax	40 mg/day for 6 months
Tiludronate	Skelid	400 mg/day for 3 months
Risedronate	Actonel	30 mg/day for 2 months
Zoledronate	Aclasta	5 mg IV

[a]Not licensed in the UK for Paget's disease.

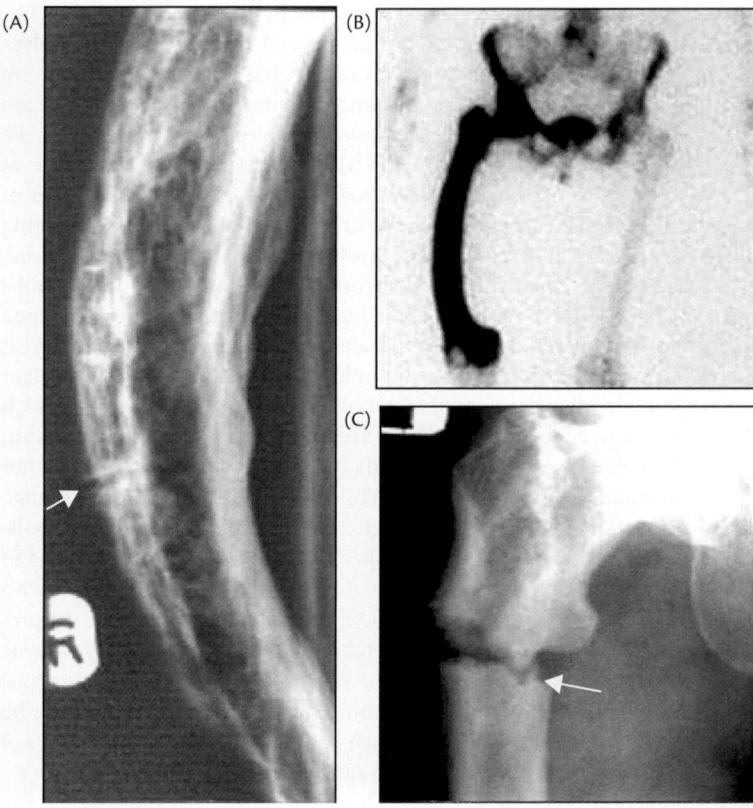

Fig. 144.5 Radiographic and scintigraphic features of Paget's disease: (A) Radiological appearances of advanced Paget's disease showing bone expansion, cortical thickening and loss of normal trabecular architecture, A pseudofracture is visible in the lateral cortex (white arrow). (B) Radionuclide bone scan showing intense tracer uptake in an aff ected femur. (C) Pathological subtrochanteric fracture in patient with Paget's disease. In this instance the fracture occurred at the site of a pre-existing pseudofracture.

caused by increased bone turnover at an affected site. Repeated courses of treatment can be given in patients who experience a recurrence of symptoms or if the initial course of treatment fails to give an adequate clinical or biochemical response.

Bisphosphonates are generally considered to be the anti-resorptive drugs of first choice in Paget's disease. Several bisphosphonates have been studied in PDB (Table 144.3) and most are effective at reducing the elevations in bone turnover that are characteristic of the disease. The nitrogen-containing bisphosphonates such as pamidronate, risedronate, and zoledronate are much more effective at inhibiting bone turnover in Paget's disease than older bisphosphonates such as etidronate and tiludronate. Despite this, randomized comparative trials have shown only

modest differences between different drugs and their effects on bone pain.[17] This is probably because pain in Paget's disease can arise as the result of many different reasons, and not just increased bone turnover. As a reflection of this bisphosphonate therapy has been found to have a limited little impact on quality of life in patients with long-standing Paget's disease who have pre-existing bone deformity.[18]

Bisphosphonates can either be given orally or intravenously. Oral bisphosphonate therapy is an effective treatment for Paget's, but the dosing instructions are complex. Oral bisphosphonates need be taken on an empty stomach with a large glass of water and subsequently the patient must fast for between 30 minutes (risedronate) and 120 minutes (etidronate and tiludronate) to ensure that intestinal absorption is adequate. The most common side effect with risedronate is dyspepsia, whereas diarrhoea is the most common side effect with tiludronate and etidronate. Pamidronate and zoledronic acid are administered by intravenous infusion. The most common side effect with these bisphosphonates is a transient flu-like illness which is characterized by fever, malaise, muscle, and joint pain lasting 2–3 days, known as the acute-phase response. In some patients these symptoms can be quite severe but they can be ameliorated by coadministration of paracetamol or non-steroidal anti-inflammatory drugs (NSAIDs). It is of interest that the acute-phase response is milder or absent after second and subsequent infusions of intravenous bisphosphonates, indicating that tolerance occurs. Hypocalcaemia can also occur after intravenous bisphosphonate therapy, especially in patients with active Paget's disease where ALP levels are elevated more than five times above normal. The risk of hypocalcaemia is increased in patients with vitamin D deficiency and it is important that this is corrected prior to administration of intravenous bisphosphonates. Some clinicians also prescribe calcium and vitamin D supplements for 1–2 weeks after intravenous bisphosphonates as a prophylactic measure. Bisphosphonates are contraindicated in patients with significant renal impairment and intravenous bisphosphonate therapy has been associated with the development of acute renal failure in patients with pre-existing renal dysfunction. The risk of this can be minimized by ensuring that the patient is properly hydrated at the time of the infusion; by ensuring that the infusion is given at the correct rate; and by avoiding coprescription with other potentially nephrotoxic drugs. Other rare side effects of bisphosphonates include uveitis, skin rashes, atrial fibrillation, osteonecrosis of the jaw, atypical subtrochanteric fractures, and bone and joint pain.

Some bisphosphonates have been reported to promote healing of osteolytic lesions and to restore normal bone histology in Paget's disease. Based on these observations, it has been suggested that bisphosphonate therapy should also be given to asymptomatic patients with the aim of preventing complications like bone deformity, deafness, and fractures. Unfortunately, there is no evidence as yet to show that long-term suppression of metabolic activity in Paget's disease prevents these complications. The only trial that has been performed in an attempt to address this issue is the PRISM study in which patients were treated with intensive bisphosphonate therapy or symptomatic treatment over a 3 year period. This showed no difference between the treatment groups in rates of fracture, requirement for orthopaedic surgery, progression of deafness or in quality of life.[18]

Calcitonin has inhibitory effects on bone turnover and has been successfully used in the treatment of bone pain associated with Paget's disease. It is rarely used nowadays however because of its weak anti-resorptive effects, high cost, and relatively short duration of action. The most common side effects are nausea and flushing.

Monitoring the response to anti-resorptive treatment

The response to anti-resorptive therapy can be conveniently monitored by measurements of total serum ALP activity. Following treatment, ALP levels fall progressively with a nadir at about 3–6 months. Treatment of Paget's disease with aminobisphosphonates such as risedronate and zoledronate is associated with prolonged suppression of ALP levels. In one study, a single infusion of zoledronic acid was reported to suppress ALP levels for periods of up to 6.5 years in some patients with Paget's disease.[16]

Other supportive treatments

Although anti-resorptive therapy can help bone pain, patients with established PDB often require analgesics and anti-inflammatory drugs for adequate symptom control, especially in the presence of complications such as arthritis.[18] Other non-pharmacological approaches such as acupuncture, physiotherapy, hydrotherapy, and transcutaneous electrical nerve stimulation (TENS) may also be used for pain control, and specific problems such as limb shortening and deformity can be helped by aids and devices such as walking sticks and shoe raises. The effectiveness of these strategies has not been specifically evaluated in PDB, but aids and devices were associated with significantly improved health-related quality of life indices participants of the PRISM study.[18]

Orthopaedic surgery

Surgical intervention is frequently required for the management of complications. The most common indication for surgical treatment is joint replacement for osteoarthritis, but others include fracture fixation, osteotomy to correct bone deformity, and surgery to correct spinal stenosis. The operative fixation of pagetic fractures can be technically challenging because of bony enlargement, deformity, hard bone, and increased vascularity, although in general operative treatment for PDB is very useful in improving quality of life for sufferers of the condition, particularly those with advanced osteoarthritis.[19] Bisphosphonate therapy is frequently given prior to elective orthopaedic surgery in the hope that this might reduce operative blood loss, but the effects of bisphosphonate therapy on blood loss have never been studied in a controlled trial. Orthopaedic surgery may also be required in patients who develop osteosarcoma, but the prognosis is poor even with aggressive operative treatment with an overall 5 year survival of about 6%.[20]

References

1. van Staa TP, Selby P, Leufkens HG et al Incidence and natural history of Paget's disease of bone in England and Wales. *J Bone Miner Res* 2002;17(3):465–471.
2. Cundy HR, Gamble G, Wattie D, Rutland M, Cundy T. Paget's disease of bone in New Zealand: continued decline in disease severity. *Calcif Tissue Int* 2004;75(5):358–364.
3. Gennari L, Di SM, Merlotti D et al. Prevalence of Paget's disease of bone in Italy. *J Bone Miner Res* 2005;20(10):1845–1850.
4. Siris ES, Ottman R, Flaster E, Kelsey JL. Familial aggregation of Paget's disease of bone. *J Bone Miner Res* 1991;6:495–500.
5. Lucas GJ, Daroszewska A, Ralston SH. Contribution of genetic factors to the pathogenesis of Paget's disease of bone and related disorders. *J Bone Miner Res* 2006;21 Suppl 2:31–37.
6. Jin W, Chang M, Paul EM et al. Deubiquitinating enzyme CYLD negatively regulates RANK signaling and osteoclastogenesis in mice. *J Clin Invest* 2008;118:1858–1866.
7. Albagha OME, Wani S, Visconti MR et al. Genome-wide association identifies three new susceptibility loci for Paget's disease of bone. *Nat Genet* 2011;43(7):685–689.
8. Yagi M, Miyamoto T, Sawatani Y et al. DC-STAMP is essential for cell-cell fusion in osteoclasts and foreign body giant cells. *J Exp Med* 2005;202(3):345–351.

9. Ravikumar B, Futter M, Jahreiss L et al. Mammalian macroautophagy at a glance. *J Cell Sci* 2009;122(Pt 11):1707–1711.

10. Daroszewska A, van't Hof RJ, Rojas JA et al. A point mutation in the ubiquitin associated domain of SQSMT1 is sufficient to cause a Paget's disease like disorder in mice. *Hum Mol Genet* 2011;20(14):2734–2744.

11. Kurihara N, Zhou H, Reddy SV et al. Expression of measles virus nucleocapsid protein in osteoclasts induces Paget's disease-like bone lesions in mice. *J Bone Miner Res* 2006;21(3):446–455.

12. Kurihara N, Hiruma Y, Zhou H et al. Mutation of the sequestosome 1 (p62) gene increases osteoclastogenesis but does not induce Paget disease. *J Clin Invest* 2007;117(1):133–142.

13. Hiruma Y, Kurihara N, Subler MA et al. A SQSTM1/p62 mutation linked to Paget's disease increases the osteoclastogenic potential of the bone microenvironment. Hum Mol Genet 2008;17(23):3708–3719.

14. Bucay N, Sarosi I, Dunstan CR et al. osteoprotegerin-deficient mice develop early onset osteoporosis and arterial calcification. *Genes Dev* 1998;12(9):1260–1268.

15. Badadani M, Nalbandian A, Watts GD et al. VCP associated inclusion body myopathy and Paget disease of bone knock-in mouse model exhibits tissue pathology typical of human disease. *PLoS One* 2010;5(10).

16. Reid IR, Lyles K, Su G et al. A single infusion of zoledronic acid produces sustained remissions in Paget's disease—data to 6.5 years. *J Bone Miner Res* 2011;26(9):2261–2270.

17. Ralston SH, Langston AL, Reid IR. Pathogenesis and management of Paget's disease of bone. *Lancet* 2008;372(9633):155–163.

18. Langston AL, Campbell MK, Fraser WD et al. Randomised trial of intensive bisphosphonate treatment versus symptomatic management in Paget's disease of bone. *J Bone Miner Res* 2010;25:20–31.

19. Kaplan FS. Surgical management of Paget's disease. *J Bone Miner Res* 1999;14 Suppl 2:34–38.

20. Sharma H, Jane MJ, Reid R. Scapulo-humeral Paget's sarcoma: Scottish Bone Tumour Registry experience. *Eur J Cancer Care* (Engl) 2005;14(4):367–372.

CHAPTER 145

Paediatric metabolic bone disease

Nick Bishop

Introduction

Childhood metabolic bone diseases typically present with fracture, bony deformity, bone pain, or short stature, either alone or in combination. To substantiate a diagnosis of osteoporosis, a child must be shown to have a low (more than two standard deviations below the mean) bone mass adjusted for body size with either one lower limb or vertebral fracture, or two upper limb fractures. The fractures should have resulted from low energy or no apparent trauma.[1]

Bone mass is usually assessed by dual energy X-ray absorptiometry (DXA). DXA measurements are significantly impacted by bone size; hence a larger child will have a higher measurement than a smaller child of the same age with the same true volumetric density.

There is evidence from studies of healthy children that supports the concept of body-size-adjusted bone mass being predictive of future fracture risk.[2] There are no prospective studies, however, that clearly link bone density measured by DXA to future fracture risk in the patient groups listed below .[3] There is no uniform method of adjusting for body size when assessing bone mass by DXA, and a large number of methods for undertaking such adjustments have been proposed.[4] Sequential measurements (usually twice yearly) assessed alongside a growth chart are helpful in evaluating bone mass trajectory in response to therapy. Indications for the use of DXA in primary and secondary osteoporosis in children, along with supporting evidence ranked by validity, are given on the International Society for Clinical Densitometry (ISCD) website (www.iscd.org/visitors/pdfs/ISCD2007OfficialPositions-Pediatric.pdf). These include all of the conditions listed in the following sections on primary and secondary osteoporosis, starting either from the age of first fracture, or from age 5 years when reliable measurements can be obtained.

Primary osteoporosis

Osteogenesis imperfecta

See Table 145.1 for classification of osteogenesis imperfecta (OI). The principal features are bone fragility, typically with low bone mass, leading to fractures and bone deformity with growth retardation.[5] Children often have delayed motor development, while ligamentous laxity, dentinogenesis imperfecta, hearing loss, hernias, heart valve defects, and blue scleral hue are variable features. In 90% of cases OI is dominantly inherited due to defects in the type I collagen genes COL1A1 and COL1A2. Mutations in the C-propeptide of COL1A1 can cause Caffey's disease, a segmental hyperostosis of infancy.[6] Recessively inherited OI is now reported for multiple genes that regulate collagen molecule folding (CRTAP, LEPRE1, PPIB),[7–10] chaperone the molecule intracellularly (FKBP10),[11] or have a stabilizing role (SERPINH1).[12] SERPINF1 encodes pigment epithelium-derived factor (PEDF), a secreted protein with multiple roles[13–14]; SERPINF1 is deficient in type VI OI,[15] allowing a biochemical diagnosis by serum measurement of PEDF and possible future treatment with infused recombinant protein. A single case of OI due to mutation in OSX/FP7 encoding osterix, a transcription factor in the osteoblast differentiation pathway, has been reported.[16] Type V OI is dominantly inherited but the gene defect is not known.[17] It is characterized by disordered control of endochondral bone formation in addition to low bone mass, resulting in a rachitic appearance to the growth plates in early infancy,[18] and later interosseous membrane calcification and hypertrophic callus formation at fracture and osteotomy sites. Surgeons need to be aware of this since perioperative therapy with indomethacin can reduce the risk of massive hyperplastic callus formation, a devastating condition. Approximately 5% of OI cases still have no clear genetic origin identified.

Idiopathic juvenile osteoporosis (IJO)

In idiopathic juvenile osteoporosis (IJO), 15–20% of cases are due to heterozygous mutations in the low -density lipoprotein receptor related protein 5 (LRP5) gene.[19] IJO typically presents precocious or early puberty with metaphyseal and vertebral crush fractures. Homozygous mutations result in the osteoporosis pseudoglioma syndrome[20]; affected children have tumour-like eye lesions that consist of non-malignant vitreous hyperplastic tissue. Bisphosphonate therapy can increase bone mass, reduce bone pain and improve vertebral size and shape, and may improve growth.[21–30] Early treatment in more severely affected individuals may reduce the risk of scoliosis which is otherwise reported in 100% of type III OI cases by age 7 years. Neridronate,[24] pamidronate,[25–26,31–34] and zoledronic acid[34] are all used for intravenous therapy. The most widely used bisphosphonate is pamidronate at a dose of 9–12 mg/kg per year,

Table 145.1 Classification of osteogenesis imperfecta

OI Type	Phenotype (during childhood)	Genetic origin
I	Mild motor delay. Bowing of long bones. Vertebral crush fractures. Ligamentous laxity, hernias, mixed conductive/sensorineural deafness, blue sclerae. Subdivided on the basis of the presence or absence of DI (A, absent; B, present)	Typically null allele of COL1A1, resulting from stop, frameshift, or splice site mutations
II	Lethal. Subdivided by appearance of ribs	Missense mutations in COL1A1 or COL1A2 Complete loss of CRTAP, PPIB, or LEPRE1
III	Severe, progressively deforming. Typically have fractures in utero, very poor post-=natal growth. Characteristic facies with small midface and pointed chin. Triangular facial appearance less noticeable with bisphosphonate treatment. Very delayed motor development. Almost all need intramedullary rodding. All have DI. Mutations in LEPRE1 are most often reported in families originating from West Africa, Pakistan, and Ireland	Missense mutations in COL1A1, COL1A2; null allele of COL1A2 Mutations in CRTAP, PPIB, or LEPRE1, SERPINH1, FKBP10, OSX/FP7
IV	Moderately severe. May have fractures in utero, but better post-natal growth than type III. Blue sclerae fade with age; may have DI	Missense mutations in COL1A1, COL1A2
V	Moderately severe. Metaphyseal changes that resemble rickets at birth, progressing to sclerosis in early life, followed by calcification of interosseous membranes in the forearm and lower leg. Characteristic bowing of the forearms. Hypertrophic callus formation following fractures and surgery	Unknown
VI	Severe, progressively deforming. Osteomalacic on bone biopsy, possibly as a result of abnormal matrix deposition—normal lamellar structure is disrupted	SERPINF1, encoding PEDF which can be measured in serum
Bruck 1	Contractures. White sclerae, mild DI. Moderately severe bone disease	FKBP10
Bruck 2	Clinical phenotype as for Bruck 1	PLOD2; bone-specific telopeptide lysyl hydroxylase
Cole–Carpenter	Normal at birth; develop craniosynostosis, ocular proptosis, hydrocephalus and diaphyseal fractures	Unknown

DI, dentinogenesis imperfect.

usually given in 3 monthly cycles. Oral therapy in milder OI cases with risedronate 1 mg/kg per week is safe and effective at increasing bone mass in line with the expected increase for age, but catch-up in moderate–severe cases may require higher doses (2 mg/kg per week).[23] Oral bisphosphonate therapy is less clearly effective than intravenous therapy in more severely affected children at both increasing bone mass and restoring the architecture of previously crush-fractured vertebrae, but has been reported to reduce fracture risk.[23,35]

Children receiving bisphosphonates should have bone densitometry and biochemical testing undertaken at 6 month intervals to ensure that they are responding appropriately to therapy, and to help guide therapy changes.[3] Some children can have their treatment dose reduced as they reconstruct their vertebrae and attain a normal bone mass for age. Others find that dose reduction leads to unacceptable levels of pain. Stopping therapy before growth ceases may increase fracture risk.[36] Serial monitoring of bone formation and resorption markers is used to detect evidence of oversuppression of bone remodelling activity. Vitamin D homeostasis and adequacy should be monitored, as vitamin D inadequacy impairs the skeletal response to bisphosphonate therapy.

Secondary osteoporosis

It is important to note that although fractures and in particular vertebral crush fractures are more common in the disease categories cited, vertebral crush fractures can resolve spontaneously if the underlying disease remits, or if treatment with glucocorticoids is withdrawn or replaced with a different disease-modifying agent.

Inflammatory conditions

Up to 7% of children with inflammatory joint disease of whatever cause—including but not limited to juvenile systemic lupus erythematosus, juvenile dermatomyositis and polyarticular juvenile idiopathic arthritis (JIA)—have one or more vertebral crush fracture prior to use of glucocorticoids.[37] These fractures are often silent. Vertebral crush fractures also occur during steroid therapy in these children and are not limited to those with crush fractures at presentation. Fractures are generally more common in these children.[38] Recent data from the STOPP consortium indicate an association between falling lumbar spine bone mineral density (BMD) Z-score (for age) and incident vertebral fracture during the first 12 months of glucocorticoid therapy.[39] Vertebral fractures are typically silent in children with rheumatological disease; detection requires imaging of the spine with radiographic or MRI-based techniques. Bone loss and fractures are more common in Crohn's disease than in ulcerative colitis, both prior to and after commencing glucocorticoids.[40–42] Bone mass loss occurs after the first decade in children with cystic fibrosis with a concomitant increase in fracture risk.[43]

Glucocorticoid effects

There is an increased risk of fracture when taking oral glucocorticoids, irrespective of the underlying condition; four courses of corticosteroids in a 12 month period increases incident fracture by 20%, but this risk appears to resolve 3–6 months after steroid cessation.[44] Corticosteroids reduce cortical bone turnover, resulting in retention of older, more heavily mineralized bone.[45] At a tissue level, corticosteroids increase apoptosis of osteoblast lineage cells, reducing bone formation and possibly impairing the skeletal response to mechanical stimulation. More rapid loss of trabecular bone leads to increased risk of vertebral fracture[39]; however, there has been no quantitation of this risk in relation to either dose or duration of glucocorticoid therapy.

Disuse

Long-bone fractures occur in children with cerebral palsy during handling; the bones are narrow, with thin cortices. In long bones, resistance to fracture is dependent on bone width—a tube that is twice as wide is eight times as strong under three-point bending.[46] Boys with Duchenne muscular dystrophy have low bone mass secondary to disuse and the early introduction of corticosteroids; fractures occur while they are still mobile, but increase in frequency once the patient becomes wheelchair dependent.[47] Intravenous bisphosphonate therapy has been reported to prevent further deterioration of vertebral crush fractures, restore some vertebral height, and relieve pain.[48] In children with epidermolysis bullosa, bone loss occurs due to immobility.

Endocrine disturbance

Low bone mass may not be apparent in children or adolescents with anorexia nervosa, but low bone mass is consistently reported in adult women who were anorexic as teenagers. The exact underlying mechanism is obscure. In Cushing's syndrome, low bone mass and fractures are reported; vertebral crush fractures have been shown to resolve on treatment of the underlying disorder.[49] There is no evidence of low bone mass or fractures during childhood in girls with Turner's syndrome.

Haematology and oncology

Children with acute leukaemia have an increased risk of fracture and bone loss both at diagnosis and during treatment. Up to 16% have one or more vertebral crush fractures at diagnosis, and in many of these children further crush fractures occur. Back pain is a cardinal feature in such children.[50] Studies suggest that chemotherapy alone does not lead to increased later fracture risk, but that the risk is increased in those receiving radiotherapy to the head and spine.

Children with thalassaemia are at increased risk of low bone mass and fracture.[51] Vertebral fractures are also seen post-transplantation, particularly following heart, lung, liver, and intestinal transplantation (infrequently following renal transplantation).[52]

Rare disorders presenting in the neonatal period with fractures

These disorders include:

♦ akinesia

♦ spinal muscular atrophy with arthrogryposis

♦ neurofibromatosis

♦ cytomegalovirus inclusion disease

♦ Caffey's disease

♦ I-cell disease (mucolipidosis II)

♦ Bruck's syndrome (OI with contractures)

♦ infantile hypophosphatasia

♦ severe neonatal hyperparathyroidism.

All of these rare disorders have other features that help distinguish them from OI.

Osteomalacia and rickets

See Table 145.2.

Vitamin D deficiency

The typical clinical features are bowed limbs presenting as genu varum, metaphyseal swelling, bossed forehead, and musculoskeletal pain. The vast majority of cases result from poor sunlight exposure or dietary inadequacy. In recent years the widespread use of sunscreen has increased the incidence of rickets among fair-skinned children, but rickets is still more common in darker-skinned individuals living in colder climates—more so when little skin is exposed because of cultural mores.[53] Vitamin D deficiency results in myopathy and musculoskeletal aches and pains; infants are usually miserable and have delayed motor development that improves quickly with treatment. Investigations should ideally be undertaken on a fasting sample: serum calcium (Ca), phosphate (PO_4), alkaline phosphatase (ALP), parathyroid hormone (PTH), and 25-hydroxy-vitamin D (25OHD); wrist and knee radiographs. Expect phosphate to be reduced and alkaline phosphatase increased in active disease; serum calcium is variable. PTH is typically elevated above the upper limit of the adult normal range; it is unusual to see rickets in an individual whose 25OH vitamin D is above 25 nmol/litre and in such cases the possibility of X-linked hypophosphataemic rickets should be considered (see below). The radiological changes in mild rickets can be subtle and limited to widening of the growth plates; such changes are often best seen at the ulna in the wrist, and at the knees. More florid rachitic changes are cupping, splaying and fraying of the metaphyses, with osteopenia (literally, thin-looking bones), and periosteal elevation. Fractures are uncommon without clear rachitic change in infants born at term; however, preterm infants may have fractures without clear rachitic change, reflecting the role of other factors in the genesis of their bone disease (see below).

The threshold for deficiency in asymptomatic individuals without radiological changes is debated widely; a typical cut-off is anywhere from 25 to 50 nmol/litre 25OH vitamin D. Above this, supplementation (200–400 IU/day) is given. Sufficiency is generally accepted as being in excess of 75 nmol/litre, based on the fact that further increases in 25OHD are not associated with a reduction in serum PTH.

Table 145.2 Inherited forms of rickets

Type	Phenotype	Investigations	Genotype
Vitamin D resistant rickets type 1a (VDDR1a)	Motor delay Severe rickets Poor growth Hypocalcaemia Seizures	Low serum Ca, PO$_4$ Raised serum ALP Raised serum PTH Absent 1,25OH2D	*CYP27B1* (vitamin D 1α-hydroxylase gene) -/-
Vitamin D resistant rickets type 1b (VDDR1b)	Rickets at age 2–7 years	Low serum PO$_4$ Normal serum Ca Raised serum ALP Low 25OHD Normal 1,25OH2D	Mutations in *CYP2R1* (vitamin D 25-hydroxylase gene) -/-
Hereditary vitamin D resistant rickets	Early-onset severe rickets Hypocalcaemia Alopecia in those with DNA-binding domain defect	Low serum Ca, PO4 Raised serum ALP Raised serum PTH Raised serum 1,25OH2D	*VDR* (vitamin D receptor gene) -/-
X-linked hypophosphataemic rickets (XLH)	Short stature Bone deformities Frontal bossing Craniosynostosis Root abscesses Rachitic change on radiographs	Low serum PO4 Raised serum ALP Normal PTH Inappropriately normal 1,25OH2D	*PHEX* -/-
Autosomal dominant hypophosphataemic rickets (ARHR)	Short stature Bone deformities Frontal bossing Rachitic change on radiographs	Low serum PO$_4$ Raised serum ALP Normal PTH Inappropriately normal 1,25OH2D	FGF-23 R179 mutation resulting in failure to degrade FGF-23
Autosomal recessive hypophosphataemic rickets (ARHR)	Short stature Bone deformities Frontal bossing Rachitic change on radiographs	Low serum PO4 Raised serum ALP Normal PTH Inappropriately normal 1,25OH2D	*DMP1* -/-
Hypophosphatasia Infantile form	Hypercalcaemia Failure to thrive Motor delay Severe rickets with osteopenia Death	Very low/absent ALP Raised serum calcium Nephrocalcinosis Raised serum pyridoxal-5-phosphate, pyrophosphate Raised urine phosphoethanolamine	*TNSALP* -/-
Hypophosphatasia childhood/adult form	Early tooth loss Small bone fractures in early adulthood Mild rickets Mild motor delay	Low serum ALP Raised urine phosphoethanolamine	*TNSALP* +/-

ALP, alkaline phosphatase; PTH, parathyroid hormone.

Treatment is with ergo/cholecalciferol daily for 2 months. Infants up to 24 months age receive 3000 IU/day (5 μg/day); 2–10 years 6000 IU/day (150 μg/day); 10+ years 10 000 IU/day (250 μg/day). Infants with severe vitamin D deficiency may present with seizures or in heart failure. In such cases, correction of hypocalcemia is needed and further calcium supplementation may be required. With the exception of the infant in heart failure, where calcitriol may improve cardiac function, there is no place for the use of active vitamin D metabolites in the treatment of 'simple' vitamin D deficiency.

Metabolic bone disease of prematurity

The rapidly growing premature infant can outstrip the supply of calcium and phosphate available from either oral or intravenous nutrition. Breast milk should be supplemented with at least

Table 145.3 High bone mass due to increased bone formation

Disorder	Phenotype	Investigations	Genotype
Sclerosteosis 1	High bone mass Gigantism Syndactyly Square jaw Nerve compression	Radiographs show high bone mass, thickened cortices	SOST (sclerostin gene) -/-
Sclerosteosis 2	As for sclerosteosis 1	Radiographs show high bone mass, thickened cortices	LRP4 -/- or +/-
Van Buchem disease	High bone mass Nerve compression	Radiographs show high bone mass, thickened cortices ALP elevated	Deletion of a SOST-specific regulatory element
Autosomal dominant osteopetrosis 1	High bone mass Torus palatinus	Radiographs show high bone mass, thickened cortices	LRP5 +/-

Table 145.4 High bone mass due to reduced bone resorption

Disorder	Phenotype	Investigations	Genotype
Malignant osteopetrosis	Early marrow failure Hepatosplenomegaly Cranial nerve compression Fractures more frequent, heal poorly Rickets	Radiographs show dense bones with failure of remodelling; bones are undertubulated, bone-in-bone appearance in long bones and vertebrae Low RBC, WBC, and platelets Bone biopsy shows increased numbers of multinucleated giant cells without associated resorption cavities Bone biopsy in children with osteoclast formation defects shows few/absent osteoclasts	Loss of factors creating acidification by osteoclasts: TCIRG1 -/- CLCN7 -/- Loss of factors leading to osteoclast formation and function: RANKL -/- RANK -/- PLEKHM1 -/- OSTM1 -/-
Intermediate osteopetrosis	Fractures more frequent, heal poorly Renal tubular acidosis, nephrocalcinosis, intracranial calcification,	Increased bone density	Carbonic anhydrase II -/-
Pycnodysostosis	Distal acrolysis Craniosynostosis, raised intracranial pressure. Persistent anterior fontanelle. Fractures more frequent, heal poorly. Growth failure	Growth hormone deficiency in some. Intracranial pressure monitoring, may require craniectomy	Cathepsin K -/-
Autosomal dominant osteopetrosis type 2	Generalized sclerosis Fractures more frequent, heal poorly	Increased bone mass	CLCN7 +/-

1 mmol/100 mL milk in order to provide sufficient phosphate. Calcium may also need to be added, but care should be taken not to cause coprecipitation. Immobilization adds to the failure to accrete adequate bone mass. Fractures may occur in infants up to 6 months old; particularly at risk are those who are slow (>30 days) to establish enteral feeds, those with conjugated hyperbilirubinaemia, chronic lung disease, or who receive diuretics, and those with clear rachitic changes on radiograph.[54] Vitamin D supplementation in excess of 800 U/day has not been shown to confer any short- or longer-term benefit. There is no place for the use of active vitamin D metabolites. Recent data suggests that despite its lower mineral content, early exposure to breast milk is associated with greater height at skeletal maturity, possibly due to anabolic factors in breast milk such as IGF-1.[55]

Inherited rickets

Rarely, defects of vitamin D metabolism occur; loss of renal 25-hdroxyvitamin D 1-α hydroxylase activity results in vitamin D resistant rickets type I; treatment is with 1-alfacalcidol or calcitriol. Loss of the vitamin D receptor requires treatment with overnight intravenous calcium infusions up to around the age of 2 years, followed by substantial oral calcium supplementation (7 g/day). Alopecia is seen in infants where the receptor DNA-binding domain is defective.[56-57]

The most common inherited form of rickets is X-linked hypophosphataemic rickets (see Table 145.2). Children usually present in the second year of life with bowed legs. In common with the rarer inherited rachitides, increased circulating FGF-23 is found, which promotes phosphaturia and inhibits renal production of the vitamin D metabolite 1,25-dihydroxyvitamin D. Autosomal dominant and recessive rickets as well as tumour-induced osteomalacia and McCune–Albright syndrome/polyostotic fibrous dysplasia also have raised circulating FGF-23 and the expected consequences thereof. Replacement therapy with oral phosphate in divided doses (40–50 mg/kg per day) and 1,25 dihydroxyvitamin D or 1-α calcidol (30–50 ng/kg per day) is currently used in those with rickets; the role of such intervention in McCune–Albright sufferers is unclear.[58] Trials of anti-FGF-23 antibody are under way.

Regular monitoring of serum calcium, alkaline phosphatase, PTH, and urine calcium:creatinine ratio are required. Excessive calcium losses can lead to nephrocalcinosis. Treatment needs to balance the effects of phosphate insufficiency on the growth plate with the effect on PTH production. Osteomalacic lesions contributing to bone softening and bowing deformity only heal when 1,25 dihydroxyvitamin D adequacy is attained, but excess 1-α calcidol can lead to excessive urine calcium losses.

High bone mass disorders

Increased bone formation

Autosomal dominant osteopetrosis type 1 is due to mutations in LRP5 that inhibit binding of inhibitors (SOST and DKK1) of the receptor. Some develop a torus palatinus (a protruding bone appearance on the roof of the mouth.[57] Sclerosteosis and Van Buchem's disease are due to mutations in the gene (*SOST*) encoding sclerostin (sclerosteosis) or in an upstream regulatory region that affects sclerostin production (van Buchem's disease). The main clinical problems result from cranial nerve compression.[59]

See Table 145.3.

Reduced bone resorption

In osteopetrosis[60-62] there is increased bone mass due to failure to resorb bone. Many cases result from mutations in genes that modulate the secretion of hydrogen and chloride ions into the subcellular space beneath the multinucleated giant cell's ruffled border or, less commonly, encode for the pathway resulting in osteoclast formation and activation, the RANK/RANKL pathway. Severe cases present early in life with bone marrow failure and incipient blindness: urgent decompression of the optic nerves may be required to maintain vision. Some respond well to bone marrow transplantation; those with neuropathic features or without osteoclasts generally do not. Milder forms present later in life, with nerve compression and poor fracture healing being significant problems.

Children with pycnodysostosis cases may develop raised intracranial pressure and require surgical intervention.

See Table 145.4.

References

1. Lewiecki EM, Gordon CM, Baim S et al. Special report on the 2007 adult and pediatric Position Development Conferences of the International Society for Clinical Densitometry. *Osteoporos Int* 2008;19:1369–1378.
2. Clark EM, Ness AR, Bishop NJ, Tobias JH. Association between bone mass and fractures in children: a prospective cohort study, *J Bone Miner Res* 2006;21:1489–1495.
3. Bishop N, Braillon P, Burnham J et al. Dual-energy X-ray aborptiometry assessment in children and adolescents with diseases that may affect the skeleton: the 2007 ISCD Pediatric Official Positions. *J Clin Densitom* 2008;11:29–42.
4. Dimitri P, Wales JK, Bishop N. Fat and bone in children: differential effects of obesity on bone size and mass according to fracture history, *J Bone Miner Res* 2010;25:527–536.
5. Bishop N. Characterising and treating osteogenesis imperfecta. *Early Hum Dev* 2010;86:743–746.
6. Glorieux FH. Caffey disease: an unlikely collagenopathy, *J Clin Invest* 2005;115:1142–1144.
7. Barnes AM, Chang W, Morello R et al. Deficiency of cartilage-associated protein in recessive lethal osteogenesis imperfecta. *N Engl J Med* 2006;355:2757–2764.
8. Cabral WA, Chang W, Barnes AM et al. Prolyl 3-hydroxylase 1 deficiency causes a recessive metabolic bone disorder resembling lethal/severe osteogenesis imperfecta, *Nat Genet* 2007;39:359–365.
9. Morello R, Bertin TK, Chen Y et al. CRTAP is required for prolyl 3-hydroxylation and mutations cause recessive osteogenesis imperfecta. *Cell* 2006;127:291–304.
10. van Dijk FS, Nesbitt IM, Zwikstra EH et al. PPIB mutations cause severe osteogenesis imperfecta. *Am J Hum Genet* 2009;85:521–527.
11. Alanay Y, Avaygan H, Camacho N et al. Mutations in the gene encoding the RER protein FKBP65 cause autosomal-recessive osteogenesis imperfecta. *Am J Hum Genet* 2010;86:551–559.
12. Christiansen HE, Schwarze U, Pyott SM et al. Homozygosity for a missense mutation in SERPINH1, which encodes the collagen chaperone protein HSP47, results in severe recessive osteogenesis imperfecta. *Am J Hum Genet* 2010;86:389–398.
13. Becker J, Semler O, Gilissen C et al. Exome sequencing identifies truncating mutations in human SERPINF1 in autosomal-recessive osteogenesis imperfecta. *Am J Hum Genet* 2011;88:362–371.
14. Homan EP, Rauch F, Grafe I et al. Mutations in SERPINF1 cause osteogenesis imperfecta type VI, *J Bone Miner Res* 2011;26:2798–2803.
15. Glorieux FH, Ward LM, Rauch F et al. Osteogenesis imperfecta type VI: a form of brittle bone disease with a mineralization defect. *J Bone Miner Res* 2002;17:30–38.
16. Lapunzina P, Aglan M, Temtamy S et al. Identification of a frameshift mutation in Osterix in a patient with recessive osteogenesis imperfecta. *Am J Hum Genet* 2010;87:110–114.
17. Glorieux FH, Rauch F, Plotkin H et al. Type V osteogenesis imperfecta: a new form of brittle bone disease. *J Bone Miner Res* 2000;15:1650–1658.
18. Arundel P, Offiah A, Bishop NJ. Evolution of the radiographic appearance of the metaphyses over the first year of life in type V osteogenesis imperfecta: clues to pathogenesis. *J Bone Miner Res* 2011;26:894–898.
19. Hartikka H, Makitie O, Mannikko M et al. Heterozygous mutations in the LDL receptor-related protein 5 (LRP5) gene are associated with primary osteoporosis in children. *J Bone Miner Res* 2005;20:783–789.
20. Gong Y, Slee RB, Fukai N et al. LDL receptor-related protein 5 (LRP5) affects bone accrual and eye development. *Cell* 2001;107:513–523.
21. Adami S, Gatti D, Colapietro F et al. Intravenous neridronate in adults with osteogenesis imperfecta. *J Bone Miner Res* 2003;18:126–130.

22. Astrom E, Soderhall S. Beneficial effect of bisphosphonate during five years of treatment of severe osteogenesis imperfecta. *Acta Paediatr* 1998;87:64–68.

23. Bishop N, Harrison R, Ahmed F et al. A randomized, controlled dose-ranging study of risedronate in children with moderate and severe osteogenesis imperfecta. *J Bone Miner Res* 2010;25:32–40.

24. Gatti D, Antoniazzi F, Prizzi R et al. Intravenous neridronate in children with osteogenesis imperfecta: a randomized controlled study. *J Bone Miner Res* 2005;20:758–763.

25. Glorieux FH, Bishop NJ, Plotkin H et al. Cyclic administration of pamidronate in children with severe osteogenesis imperfecta. *N Engl J Med* 1998;339:947–952.

26. Letocha AD, Cintas HL, Troendle JF et al. Controlled trial of pamidronate in children with types III and IV osteogenesis imperfecta confirms vertebral gains but not short-term functional improvement. *J Bone Miner Res* 2005;20:977–986.

27. Rauch F, Munns CF, Land C, Cheung M, Glorieux FH. Risedronate in the treatment of mild pediatric osteogenesis imperfecta: a randomized placebo-controlled study. *J Bone Miner Res* 2009;24:1282–1289.

28. Ward LM, Rauch F, Whyte MP et al. Alendronate for the treatment of pediatric osteogenesis imperfecta: a randomized placebo-controlled study. *J Clin Endocrinol Metab* 2011;96:355–364.

29. Zeitlin L, Rauch F, Plotkin H, Glorieux FH. Height and weight development during four years of therapy with cyclical intravenous pamidronate in children and adolescents with osteogenesis imperfecta types I, III, and IV. *Pediatrics* 2003;111:1030–1036.

30. Heino TJ, Astrom E, Laurencikas E, Savendahl L, Soderhall S. Intravenous pamidronate treatment improves growth in prepubertal osteogenesis imperfecta patients. *Horm Res Paediatr* 2011;75:354–361.

31. Arikoski P, Silverwood B, Tillmann V, Bishop NJ. Intravenous pamidronate treatment in children with moderate to severe osteogenesis imperfecta: assessment of indices of dual-energy X-ray absorptiometry and bone metabolic markers during the first year of therapy. *Bone* 2004;34:539–546.

32. Astrom E, Soderhall S. Beneficial effect of long term intravenous bisphosphonate treatment of osteogenesis imperfecta. *Arch Dis Child* 2002;86:356–364.

33. Rauch F, Munns C, Land C, Glorieux FH. Pamidronate in children and adolescents with osteogenesis imperfecta: effect of treatment discontinuation. *J Clin Endocrinol Metab* 2006;91:1268–1274.

34. Brown JJ, Zacharin MR. Safety and efficacy of intravenous zoledronic acid in paediatric osteoporosis. *J Pediatr Endocrinol Metab* 2009;22:55–63.

35. Sakkers R, Kok D, Engelbert R et al. Skeletal effects and functional outcome with olpadronate in children with osteogenesis imperfecta: a 2-year randomised placebo-controlled study. *Lancet* 2004;363:1427–1431.

36. Ward KA, Adams JE, Freemont TJ, Mughal MZ. Can bisphosphonate treatment be stopped in a growing child with skeletal fragility? *Osteoporos Int* 2007;18:1137–1140.

37. Huber AM, Gaboury I, Cabral DA et al. Prevalent vertebral fractures among children initiating glucocorticoid therapy for the treatment of rheumatic disorders, *Arthritis Care Res* (Hoboken) 2010;62:516–526.

38. Burnham JM, Shults J, Weinstein R, Lewis JD, Leonard MB. Childhood onset arthritis is associated with an increased risk of fracture: a population based study using the General Practice Research Database. *Ann Rheum Dis* 2006;65:1074–1079.

39. Rodd C, Lang B, Ramsay T et al. Incident vertebral fractures among children with rheumatic disorders 12 months after glucocorticoid initiation: a national observational study. *Arthritis Care Res* (Hoboken) 2012;64:122–131.

40. Loftus EV Jr, Achenbach SJ, Sandborn WJ et al. Risk of fracture in ulcerative colitis: a population-based study from Olmsted County, Minnesota. *Clin Gastroenterol Hepatol* 2003;1:465–473.

41. Loftus EV Jr, Crowson CS, Sandborn WJ et al. Long-term fracture risk in patients with Crohn's disease: a population-based study in Olmsted County, Minnesota. *Gastroenterology* 2002;123:468–475.

42. van Staa TP, Cooper C, Brusse LS et al. Inflammatory bowel disease and the risk of fracture. *Gastroenterology* 2003;125:1591–1597.

43. Buntain HM, Schluter PJ, Bell SC et al. Controlled longitudinal study of bone mass accrual in children and adolescents with cystic fibrosis. *Thorax* 2006;61:146–154.

44. van Staa TP, Cooper C, Leufkens HG, Bishop N. Children and the risk of fractures caused by oral corticosteroids, *J Bone Miner Res* 2003;18:913–918.

45. Burnham JM, Shults J, Petit MA et al. Alterations in proximal femur geometry in children treated with glucocorticoids for crohn disease or nephrotic syndrome: impact of the underlying disease. *J Bone Miner Res* 2007;22:551–559.

46. Henderson RC. Bone density and other possible predictors of fracture risk in children and adolescents with spastic quadriplegia, *Dev Med Child Neurol* 1997;39:224–227.

47. Bianchi ML, Morandi L, Andreucci E et al. Low bone density and bone metabolism alterations in Duchenne muscular dystrophy: response to calcium and vitamin D treatment. *Osteoporos Int* 2011;22:529–539.

48. Sbrocchi AM, Rauch F, Jacob P et al. The use of intravenous bisphosphonate therapy to treat vertebral fractures due to osteoporosis among boys with Duchenne muscular dystrophy. *Osteoporos Int* 2012;23:2703–2711.

49. Vestergaard P, Emborg C, Stoving RK et al. Fractures in patients with anorexia nervosa, bulimia nervosa, and other eating disorders—a nationwide register study. *Int J Eat Disord* 2002;32:301–308.

50. Halton J, Gaboury I, Grant R et al. Advanced vertebral fracture among newly diagnosed children with acute lymphoblastic leukemia: results of the Canadian Steroid-Associated Osteoporosis in the Pediatric Population (STOPP) research program. *J Bone Miner Res* 2009;24:1326–1334.

51. Vogiatzi MG, Macklin EA, Fung EB et al. Prevalence of fractures among the thalassemia syndromes in North America. *Bone* 2006;38:571–575.

52. Helenius I, Remes V, Salminen S et al. Incidence and predictors of fractures in children after solid organ transplantation: a 5-year prospective, population-based study. *J Bone Miner Res* 2006;21:380–387.

53. Wharton B, Bishop N. Rickets. *Lancet* 2003;362:1389–1400.

54. Bishop N, Sprigg A, Dalton A. Unexplained fractures in infancy: looking for fragile bones. *Arch Dis Child* 2007;92:251–256.

55. Fewtrell MS, Williams JE, Singhal A et al. Early diet and peak bone mass: 20 year follow-up of a randomized trial of early diet in infants born preterm. *Bone* 2009;45:142–149.

56. Malloy PJ, Wang J, Srivastava T, Feldman D. Hereditary 1,25-dihydroxyvitamin D-resistant rickets with alopecia resulting from a novel missense mutation in the DNA-binding domain of the vitamin D receptor. *Mol Genet Metab* 2010;99:72–79.

57. Little RD, Carulli JP, Del Mastro RG et al. A mutation in the LDL receptor-related protein 5 gene results in the autosomal dominant high-bone-mass trait. *Am J Hum Genet* 2002;70:11–19.

58. Pettifor JM. What's new in hypophosphataemic rickets? *Eur J Pediatr* 2008;167:493–499.

59. de Vernejoul MC, and Kornak, U. Heritable sclerosing bone disorders: presentation and new molecular mechanisms. *Ann N Y Acad Sci* 2010;1192:269–277.

60. Steward CG. Hematopoietic stem cell transplantation for osteopetrosis. *Pediatr Clin North Am* 2010;57:171–180.

61. Driessen GJ, Gerritsen EJ, Fischer A et al. Long-term outcome of haematopoietic stem cell transplantation in autosomal recessive osteopetrosis: an EBMT report. *Bone Marrow Transplant* 2003;32:657–663.

62. Villa A, Guerrini MM, Cassani B, Pangrazio A, Sobacchi C. Infantile malignant, autosomal recessive osteopetrosis: the rich and the poor. *Calcif Tissue Int* 2009;84:1–12.

CHAPTER 146

Disorders of bone mineralization—osteomalacia

Deepak R. Jadon, Tehseen Ahmed, and Ashok K. Bhalla

Introduction

Osteomalacia is a metabolic bone disorder characterized by impaired or defective mineralization of bone matrix following the closure of the growth plates. **Rickets** is a condition of deficient mineralization at the growth plate of long bones in children and adolescents. By comparison, in osteoporosis bone mineralization occurs in normal quantities but there is an overall lack of bone stock.

Epidemiology

Osteomalacia is endemic in some parts of the world such as southern Chile and Argentina due to the low sun exposure at southerly latitudes,[1] and in the Middle East and parts of Asia, secondary to the use of clothing that covers most of the body. In the United Kingdom, nutritional osteomalacia is uncommon among the white population but can be found in elderly housebound subjects.[2] In the Asian population of the United Kingdom, osteomalacia is relatively more prevalent secondary to dietary deficiency, lack of sun exposure, and skin pigmentation.[2] Osteomalacia is rarer in the United States as foodstuffs are commonly fortified with vitamin D. Vitamin D deficiency or insufficiency remains common in both children and adults throughout the world, especially those living in northern latitudes.

Homeostasis of vitamin D, calcium, and phosphate

Vitamin D maintains extracellular calcium ion levels by regulating intestinal calcium absorption, altering parathyroid hormone (PTH) secretion, and releasing calcium from bone (Figure 146.1). The majority of bodily vitamin D (80–90%) is endogenously derived and in the form vitamin D_3 (cholecalciferol). Cutaneous conversion of a cholesterol derivative (7-dehydrocholesterol) under the stimulus of the ultraviolet-B component of sunlight (wavelengths 290–315 nm) generates vitamin D_3. The amount of vitamin D_3 formed depends on the season, latitude, amount of skin exposed, and skin pigmentation. Exogenous dietary sources provide the remainder, as vitamin D_3 and vitamin D_2 (ergocalciferol).[3] Vitamin D_2 is synthesized by UV irradiation of the plant sterol, ergosterol.

Both vitamin D_3 and D_2 are further metabolized in the liver and kidney to 25-hydroxyvitamin D (25(OH)D; calcidiol) and 1,25 dihydroxyvitamin D (1,25(OH)$_2$D; calcitriol), the active metabolite which has properties more in keeping with a hormone than a vitamin. 1,25(OH)$_2$D increases calcium and phosphorous absorption from the small intestine, increases reabsorption of calcium and phosphate in the renal tubules, decreases PTH secretion, and promotes calcium and phosphate release from bone (resorption) into the extracellular compartment. Without vitamin D, only 10–15% of dietary calcium and approximately 60% of phosphorus is absorbed.[3] Increasing calcium and phosphorus concentrations in the extracellular fluid promotes calcification of osteoid to form bone. 1,25(OH)$_2$D synthesis is promoted by PTH, hypocalcaemia, and hypophosphataemia.[2] and suppressed by hypercalcaemia, hyperphosphataemia, impaired renal function, and fibroblast growth factor 23 (FGF23).[2,3] An individual's vitamin D status is reflected in the circulating levels of 25(OH)D, rather than its active metabolite 1,25(OH)$_2$D.

Aetiology and classification

Calcium and inorganic phosphate are the key precursors for bone mineralization and growth, and their deficiency forms the basis of rickets and osteomalacia classification: hypocalcaemic rickets is caused primarily by calcium deficiency; hypophosphataemic rickets/osteomalacia is caused primarily by phosphate deficiency. Rickets and osteomalacia have multiple aetiologies (Box 146.1) with much overlap, and these are discussed individually later in this chapter.

Clinical features

Detailed history-taking can give indications of poor calcium and vitamin D dietary habits, concurrent or previous illness, drug history, and family history. The key clinical features of osteomalacia

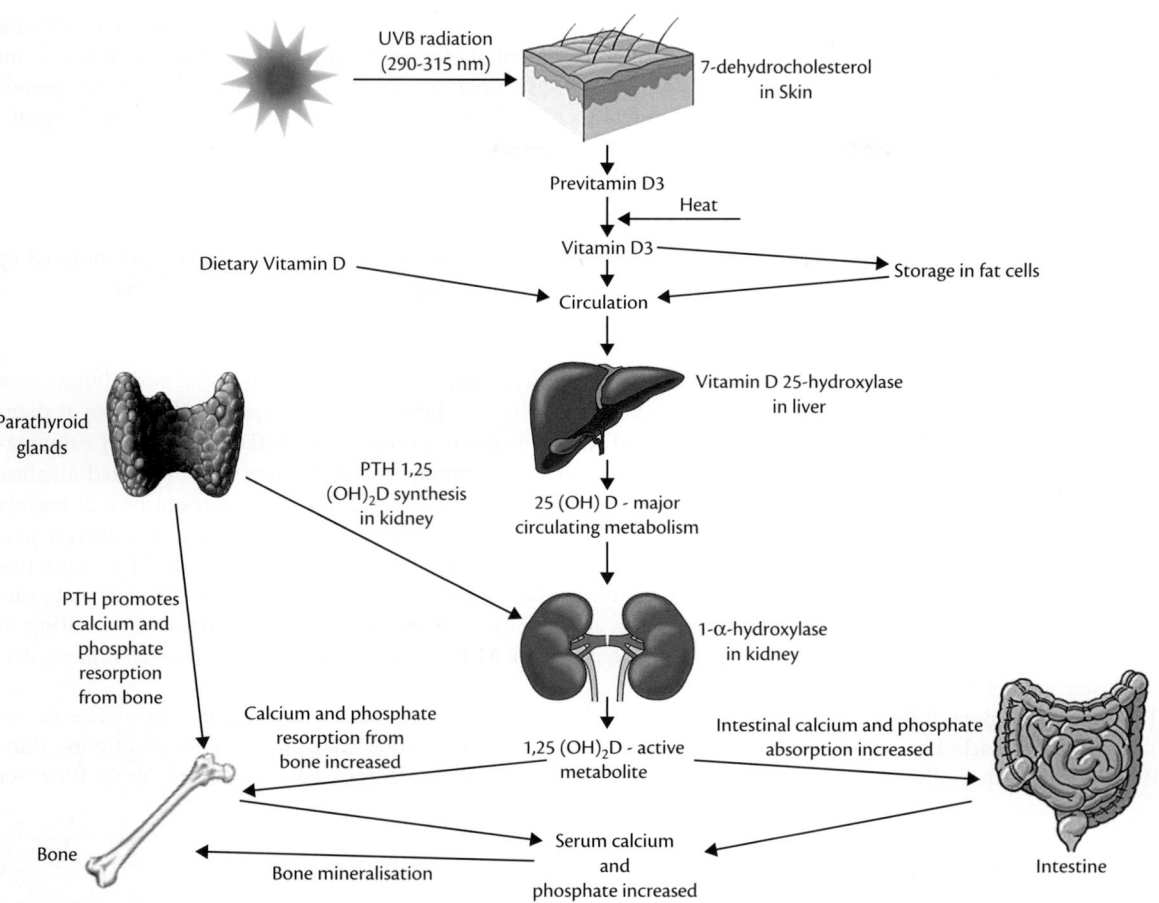

Fig. 146.1 Vitamin D metabolism.

Box 146.1 Causes of rickets and osteomalacia

Vitamin D related rickets/osteomalacia

- Nutritional: low dietary intake and/or sun exposure and skin pigmentation

- Gastrointestinal malabsorption: coeliac disease, gastric and small bowel surgery, inflammatory bowel disease and pancreatitis

- Defects in vitamin D metabolism: chronic liver disease, chronic renal failure, and abnormalities of vitamin D receptors (see below)

- Anti-epileptics

- Vitamin D receptor/enzyme deficiency:

  - Non-functioning 25 hydroxylase

  - Absent 1α-hydroxylase: pseudo-vitamin D deficiency (vitamin D dependent rickets type 1)

  - Non-functioning VDR: hereditary vitamin D resistant (vitamin D dependent rickets type 2)

Phosphate deficiency

- Hereditary hypophosphatemic rickets:

  - X-linked hypophosphataemic rickets (XLH)

  - Autosomal dominant hypophosphataemic rickets (ADHR)

  - Autosomal recessive hypophosphataemic rickets (ARHR)

  - Hypophosphataemic rickets with hypercalciuria (HHRH)

- Tumour-induced osteomalacia (TIO)/oncogenic osteomalacia

- Renal tubular phosphate wasting

- Fanconi's syndrome

- Distal renal tubular acidosis

- Dent's disease

- Lowe's syndrome

- Furosemide

- Renal tubular damage

Calcium deficiency

- Very low calcium intake in children

Miscellaneous

- Aluminium intoxication

- Cadmium intoxication

- Etidronate overdose

- Hypophosphatasia

are bone pain and tenderness, muscle pain and weakness, skeletal deformity, and fracture.

Presentation of osteomalacia

The bone pain of osteomalacia is diffuse, affects bone rather than joints, is exacerbated by weight bearing and use of local muscles, and affects the spine, rib cage, shoulder girdle, and pelvis.[1,4] Pain is usually symmetrical, starting in the lumbar spine and spreading to the pelvis, hips, upper thighs, ribs, and upper back. Percussion at these sites elicits tenderness. The localization of pain to the axial rather than the peripheral skeleton is thought to be due to the greater proportion of unmineralized osteoid that accumulates in trabecular bone *vs* cortical bone.[4] Pain is thought to occur due to unmineralized bone matrix becoming hydrated, resulting in stretching of the periosteum.[3] Deformities due to softening of the adult skeleton include kyphosis, scoliosis, coxa vara, pectus carinatum, protrusio acetabulae, and triradiate pelvis.[1]

Osteomalacia usually causes mild proximal weakness. More pronounced weakness in the hip girdle results in a waddling gait. In severe cases patients may be confined to a wheelchair or bed bound, and be more prone to falls. Muscle atrophy is often mild relative to the weakness. Muscle tone is often reduced, but reflexes tend to be preserved.[4] Patients may report difficulty rising from a sitting position or climbing stairs. Muscle strength demonstrates correlation with 25(OH)D levels, especially at lower levels of 25(OH)D.[5]

Oligoarticular joint effusions and joint pain occur rarely and raise the differential of a seronegative inflammatory arthritis. Joint effusions in osteomalacia are due to local microfractures or pseudofractures.[1] In adolescence, osteomalacia may present with significant hypocalcaemia manifesting as cramp or tetany.[2]

Investigation

The clinical diagnosis of osteomalacia should be corroborated by biochemical and radiological assessments (Figure 146.2).

Biochemistry

The biochemical picture varies according to the underlying cause and stage of disease (Table 146.1). Vitamin D deficiency is diagnosed when measuring serum 25(OH)D. Adults with osteomalacia secondary to vitamin D deficiency show elevated alkaline phosphatase (ALP) as one of the first manifestations, alongside low/normocalcaemia, hypophosphataemia, and reduced urinary calcium excretion. Serum ALP is produced by overactive osteoblasts during mineralization of bone and growth plate cartilage. It leaks into the extracellular compartment, resulting in elevated serum ALP concentration that accurately reflects disease activity.[6]

PTH levels increase as 25(OH)D levels decrease. The excess PTH leads to increased bone resorption and cortical bone thinning, resulting in an increased risk of fracture. Bone turnover markers rise.

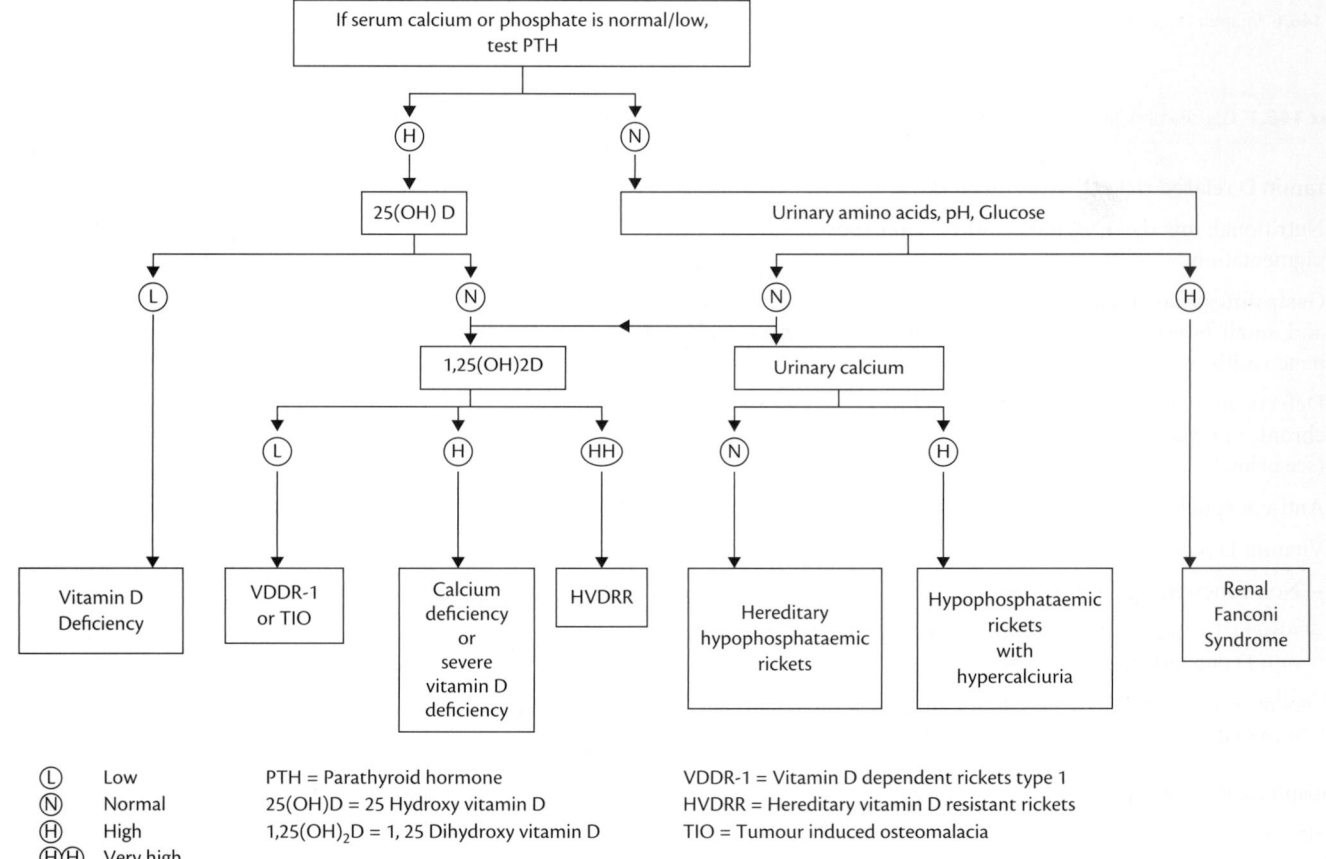

Fig. 146.2 Algorithm for investigating the cause of rickets and osteomalacia.

Table 146.1 Biochemical abnormalities seen in different aetiologies of rickets and osteomalacia

Type	Serum calcium	Serum phosphate	ALP	Serum PTH	25(OH)D	1,25(OH)₂D	Urine calcium	TmP/GFR	Intestinal calcium absorption	Intestinal phosphate absorption
Congenital										
VDDR-1	↓	↓/N	↑↑	↑	N	↓↓	↓	–	–	–
HVDRR	↓	↓/N	↑↑	↑	N	↑↑	↓	-	-	-
XLH	N	↓↓	↑	N	N	N/↓	↓	↓	↓	↓
HHRH	N	↓↓	N/↑	N	N	↑	↑	↓	↑	-
ADHR	N/↓	↓	N/↑	N	N	↓	↓	↓	↓	↓
Dent's disease	N	N/↓	N/↑	N/↓	N	↓	↓	N/↓	↓	↓
Hypophosphatasia	N	N	↓	N	N	N	N	N/↑	–	–
Acquired										
Vitamin D deficiency	↓/N	↓/N	↑	↑	↓	↓/N	↓/N	–	–	–
TIO	N/↓	↓	N/↑	N	N	↓	↓	↓	↓	↓
Tumoral calcinosis	N/↑	↑	N	N	N	↑	↑	↑	↑	N
Fanconi's syndrome type 1	N/↓	↓	N/↑	N	N	↓	↓	↓	↓	↓
Fanconi's syndrome type 2	N/↑	↓	N/↑	N/↑	N	↑	↑	↓	↑	–

ADHR, Autosomal dominant hypophosphataemic rickets; DD, Dent's disease (X-linked recessive hypophosphataemic rickets); HHRH, hereditary hypophosphataemic rickets with hypercalciuria; HVDRR, hereditary vitamin D resistant rickets; TIO, tumour-induced osteomalacia; VDDR1, vitamin D dependent rickets type 1; XLH, X-linked hypophosphataemic rickets.

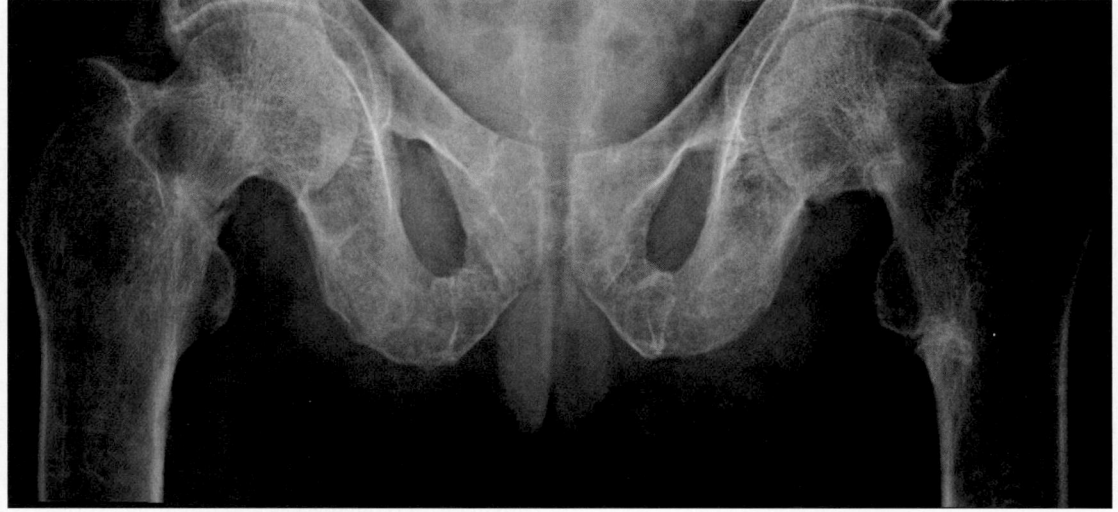

Fig. 146.3 Antero-posterior plain radiograph of the pelvis. A patient with osteomalacia demonstrates a Looser's zone just distal to the left lesser trochanter of the femur and bilateral superior pubic rami fractures.

Imaging

There may be osteopenia with poor definition of unmineralized trabecular osteoid. However, the best known radiographic feature of osteomalacia is the characteristic Looser's zone (see Figure 146.3), first described by Emil Looser in 1920. Looser's zones (pseudofractures) are narrow radiolucent lines 2–5 mm in width with sclerotic borders perpendicular to the cortex that mimic the appearance of a fracture. They most commonly occur in the ribs, pubic rami, and lateral scapula. In addition, they can be found on the inferior aspects of the femoral neck, lesser trochanters, metatarsals, and medial aspects of the shafts of long bones.[1] They can lead to complete fractures and significant bony deformities.

Secondary hyperparathyroidism causes cortical thinning and subperiosteal erosions involving the phalanges, distal ends of the clavicles, and pubic symphysis.[7] Secondary and tertiary hyperparathyroidism can manifest as the 'rugger jersey' sign; alternating bands of increased/decreased bone density of vertebral bodies on a lateral lumbar spine plain radiograph.[2] It occurs due to weakened trabecular bone being condensed adjacent to the vertebral endplates. Intervertebral discs compressing softened endplates in osteomalacia give rise to biconcave or 'codfish' vertebrae.[7]

Hypophosphatasia and hypophosphataemia can cause chondrocalcinosis and calcific enthesopathy that can mimic features of seronegative spondyloarthropathies.[1] In hypophosphatasia, Looser's zones tend to occur on the outer cortex of long bones.

Bone mineral density (BMD), assessed by DEXA, may show low values consistent with osteopenia or osteoporosis as the amount of unmineralized bone (osteoid bone) is high in osteomalacia. A rapid increase in BMD occurs after therapy has been started.[8]

Radioisotope bone scans can detect Looser's zones and fractures more reliably than plain radiographs.[9] When present at multiple sites, the uptake may mimic metastatic cancer. Bone scans may also show generalized increased uptake in the skeleton, particularly of the skull.

Bone biopsy is rarely needed, but remains the gold standard for diagnosis of osteomalacia, particularly in those patients whose biochemical and clinical picture is uncertain. The changes on biopsy include thickened osteoid seams and excessive osteoid volume.[2] However, these features can occur in other disorders with high turnover such as Paget's disease, thyrotoxicosis, and hyperparathyroidism.[4] Tetracycline bone labelling is helpful as it demonstrates reduced or absent mineralization activity in osteomalacia.

Vitamin D deficiency osteomalacia

Vitamin D deficiency is the commonest cause of osteomalacia. It results in impaired intestinal calcium absorption, with subsequent hypocalcaemia, normal phosphate, and elevated PTH. Later, the secondary hyperparathyroidism reduces renal phosphorus reabsorption leading to hyperphosphaturia, normalizing serum calcium levels and further reducing calcium deposition in bone, leading to rickets and osteomalacia. The final stage is of low calcium, low phosphate, and tertiary hyperparathyroidism.

The definition of vitamin D 'insufficiency' and 'deficiency' varies even among experts. In the United Kingdom the definition of vitamin D sufficiency in most centres is either 50 nmol/litre or more, or 75 nmol/litre or more. Levels below 25 nmol/litre in the United Kingdom generally reflect vitamin D deficiency and concentrations of 25–50 nmol/litre may indicate vitamin D insufficiency.

In winter months at latitudes of 52° or more (i.e. most of the United Kingdom), the ultraviolet (UV) light intensity is inadequate for the cutaneous synthesis of vitamin D; during the remainder of the year, effective UV light occurs mostly between 1100 and 1500 hours, when most people are indoors, at work, or at school. During the winter and spring, 16% of adults in the United Kingdom will have severe vitamin D deficiency (<25 nmol/litre).[10] In the United Kingdom's South Asian community the prevalence of severe vitamin D deficiency during the winter and spring has been estimated at 50%.[11] Causes of vitamin D deficiency leading to osteomalacia in adults are as follows.

- **Primary vitamin D deficiency**: Inadequate sun exposure, resulting from social, economic, cultural, and health-related factors, combined with reduced dietary intake is the most common cause. Housebound elderly patients and those with pigmented skin produce lower amounts of vitamin D.[12]

- **Secondary vitamin D deficiency**: Malabsorption disorders are the second most common cause of vitamin D deficiency and osteomalacia. Malabsorption is usually secondary to a reduced effective surface area for absorption as in small bowel and gastric surgery, or due to an abnormal absorptive surface, as in coeliac disease and inflammatory bowel diseases. Disorders causing fat malabsorption (e.g. pancreatic insufficiency) can also lead to vitamin D deficiency, as vitamin D is fat-soluble.

- **Defects of vitamin D metabolism**: Abnormal hepatic hydroxylation is a rare cause of vitamin D deficiency and osteomalacia. In comparison, impaired renal hydroxylation of 25-hydroxyvitamin D (secondary to reduced renal function, loss of renal mass, and renal tubular disorders) is the most common cause of osteomalacia after primary vitamin D deficiency and malabsorption disorders.

- **Iatrogenic causes**: Drugs such as phenobarbitone and phenytoin can induce cytochrome P450 enzymes and increase catabolism of 25(OH)D.

Management of vitamin D deficiency

The aims of management are to reduce symptoms, fracture risk, bone deformity, and sequelae. There are no universally agreed protocols for managing vitamin D deficiency. Deficiency can be prevented by adequate sun exposure to the face and arms for a mean of 15–30 minutes, between 1100 and 1500 hours, 2–3 times per week. Such a recommendation may not be effective at different times of the year and will depend upon both latitude and skin pigmentation. Patients with osteomalacia should be given vitamin D and calcium supplementation. One regime is to use 60 000 IU of cholecalciferol weekly for 8–12 weeks, followed by 1000–2000 IU daily as maintenance therapy.[13] Additionally, 1 g calcium should be given daily. 25(OH)D levels should be checked to monitor successful replacement. If necessary, 24 hour urinary calcium and serum PTH can be used to monitor treatment.[7] The aim should be to bring the 25(OH)D concentration to around 50 nmol/litre. In a very symptomatic patient calcitriol may be used in the short term in addition to vitamin D_2 or D_3.

In malabsorption-related osteomalacia, higher doses of vitamin D and calcium may be needed. Patients with liver disease and impaired synthesis of 25(OH)D can be treated with calcidiol supplements if they do not respond to vitamin D_2 or D_3 replacement. Patients with renal disease and impaired synthesis of $1,25(OH)_2D$ can be treated with calcitriol as well as vitamin D. Vitamin D intoxication is rare, with serum levels up to 220 nmol/litre having been reported as safe.[14] Preparations containing up to 1000 IU/pill of vitamin D_3 are available over the counter in many pharmacies and healthfood stores. High-strength preparations must be prescribed by a medical practitioner. Some studies suggest that treatment with vitamin D_2 is less efficient than vitamin D_3 and may require more frequent dosing. Symptoms improve within the first month of therapy and serum calcium improves after week 4. There may be an initial increase in ALP before reaching a steady state.[15]

Other presentations of osteomalacia

Phosphate deficiency is associated with a variety of disorders (listed in Box 146.1) of which X-linked hypophosphataemic rickets is the commonest form. They share many phenotypic features and often present in childhood (see Chapter 145). For differential diagnoses for osteomalacia see Box 146.2.

Tumour-induced osteomalacia

Tumour-induced osteomalacia (TIO; or oncogenic osteomalacia) is a rare acquired paraneoplastic syndrome of renal phosphate wasting that shares many features with genetic forms of hypophosphataemic rickets. It is most often caused by benign mesenchymal tumours but has also been noted in association with carcinomas, sarcomas, osteoblastomas, neurofibromatosis, fibrous dysplasia, and schwannomas among others.[7,16] The tumours have a predilection for the craniofacial region and extremities.[17] Tumour by-products impair phosphate transport in renal epithelial cells of the proximal renal tubule and may reduce calcitriol synthesis through altered 1-α-hydroxylase activity.[18] FGF23 is thought to have a critical pathogenic role since at least two studies have shown reduction in elevated FGF23 levels after surgical tumour resection.[19] Other proposed mediators of disease include MEPE and frizzled related protein-4 (FRP4).[20]

TIO may present at any age, although most patients are adults. Presentation is with similar symptoms to X-linked hypophosphataemic rickets (XLH) with longstanding progressive muscle and bone pain. Children with TIO present with rickets, gait disturbance, growth retardation, and skeletal deformities. TIO may be differentiated from other hypophosphataemic syndromes by the severe associated muscle weakness and lack of family history, given that this is an acquired rather than inherited disorder.

Biochemical testing demonstrates severe hypophosphataemia, phosphaturia, inappropriately low plasma $1,25(OH)_2D$ concentrations, and normocalcaemia.[16] Small tumours within bone can be difficult to localize and therefore the time from symptom onset to identification of the responsible tumour can be prolonged. MRI is the commonest imaging modality. Sensitivity can be improved by combining with indium-111-labelled octreotide scintigraphy, given that tumours usually express somatostatin receptors.[2] Selective venous sampling for FGF23 can identify target regions for imaging with MRI.

Tumour resection effectively normalizes biochemistry and allows bone healing. Pharmacological therapies are similar to those used in XLH and are given until the tumour is resected, or indefinitely if the tumour is unresectable or non-localizable. There is conflicting evidence for the use of octreotide, an anatagonist of the somatostatin receptors expressed by tumours, in patients with unlocalizable tumours.[21] Prognosis after tumour resection is good, with only a limited burden of nephrocalcinosis.

Vitamin D deficiency

See section above, 'Vitamin D deficiency osteomalacia'.

Hypophosphatasia

Hypophosphatasia is an inherited condition characterized by impaired mineralization of bones and teeth. It is caused by inactivating mutations of the *TNSALP* gene resulting in deficiencies of serum and bone ALP activity.[22] Consequently, inorganic pyrophosphate accumulates extracellularly and impairs skeletal mineralization. The prevalence of severe hypophosphatasia has been estimated to be 1/100,000; however, the prevalence of milder forms is likely to be much higher.[23] Six clinical forms are recognized[22,23]:

◆ The **perinatal form** is lethal and is characterized by markedly impaired mineralization of bone.

◆ In the **prenatal form**, in-utero mineralization defects are noted and can mimic osteogenesis imperfecta but then seem to spontaneously improve towards the end of pregnancy.

◆ The **infantile form** manifests during the first 6 months of life and often results in premature death.

◆ The **childhood form** manifests after the first year of life and presents with skull deformities, enlarged joints, short stature, delay in walking, and a waddling gait. Patients also exhibit premature loss of dentition.

◆ **Odontohypophosphatasia** is characterized by dental disease without features of skeletal disease.

◆ **Adult hypophosphatasia** presents in middle age with stress fractures, pseudofractures, osteomalacia, chondrocalcinosis, and osteoarthropathy. There is often a history of premature loss of teeth.

A diagnosis can be made by a combination of clinical features, radiological findings, biochemical assays (such as reduced serum activity of ALP, elevated urine levels of phosphoethanolamine and raised serum levels of pyridoxal-5-phosphate), and genetic screening. There is currently no curative treatment for hypophosphatasia and management therefore consists of symptomatic treatments such as non-steroidal anti-inflammatory drugs (NSAIDs). There have been reports of successful treatment with PTH as well as bone marrow cell transplantation and these represent avenues for further research.[23]

Hypophosphatasaemia

This is an acquired state of low ALP that can be readily differentiated from hypophosphatasia, and occurs under conditions of starvation, hypothyroidism, severe anaemia, Wilson's disease, coeliac disease, and glucocorticoid and chemotherapy exposure.

Renal osteodystrophy

Renal osteodystrophy is the result of two major processes: secondary hyperparathyroidism and rickets or osteomalacia from a deficiency of

---

Box 146.2 Differential diagnoses for osteomalacia

◆ Localized soft tissue disorders

◆ Fracture

◆ Seronegative arthritides

◆ Polymyalgia rheumatica

◆ Myositis

◆ Osteoporosis

◆ Paget's disease

◆ Metastatic disease

◆ Fibromyalgia syndrome

◆ Somatization disorders

1,25(OH)$_2$D. Kidneys play a central role in mineral metabolism and patients with renal failure may develop abnormalities in bone metabolism early in the course of their disease. These abnormalities may be linked to elevated levels of FGF23 that serve to work in a compensatory fashion to maintain normal serum phosphate levels.[24] FGF23 also acts to inhibit 1-α-hydroxylase reducing levels of 1,25(OH)$_2$D. This is thought to act as the initial step in the development of secondary hyperparathyroidism.[24] Later in the course of chronic renal failure, a hyperphosphataemic state occurs, further inhibiting renal 1-α-hydroxylase activity, resulting in further decreases of 1,25(OH)$_2$D and reduced intestinal calcium absorption. These changes exacerbate the secondary hyperparathyroidism. Rapid bone remodelling ensues and can manifest as osteitis fibrosa cystica.[7]

In addition to the above changes, some patients exhibit abnormal mineralization of bony matrix leading to osteomalacia. This has been seen with the excessive use of aluminium hydroxide as a phosphate binder, although alternative methods to reduce serum phosphate are now more commonly used.[7] Osteomalacia can also occur in patients receiving dialysis if supplies of vitamin D and calcium are inadequate. 25(OH)D levels should be checked regularly to help to ensure an adequate maintenance level. Patients with stage 4–5 chronic kidney disease require 1,25(OH)$_2$D supplementation as they are unable to make enough themselves. This helps to reduce PTH levels and the risk of renal osteodystrophy.[3]

Adult Fanconi's syndrome

Adult Fanconi's syndrome is a rare disorder characterized by generalized wasting of amino acids, glucose, phosphate, uric acid, and bicarbonate from the proximal renal tubules.[25] It can be inherited or acquired and can cause renal failure and bone disease as well as other metabolic changes. Anti-retroviral drugs have been recognized to cause renal tubular dysfunction and Fanconi's syndrome.[26] Patients present with typical clinical and radiological features of osteomalacia. Hypophosphataemia, low 1,25(OH)$_2$D levels (not universal), and acidosis (due to bicarbonate leak and uraemia) contribute to the development of osteomalacia.[27] Secondary hyperparathyroidism may also contribute in some cases.

Treatment involves correcting the biochemical defects by administering phosphate and 1,25(OH)$_2$D, while withdrawing any offending agent.

Conclusion

Osteomalacia is characterized by inadequate mineralization extending beyond the growth plate into the osteoid bone. Although common causes of osteomalacia such as vitamin D deficiency have been recognized since the 17th century, considerable advances have been made over the last decade in our knowledge of gene mutations responsible for inherited osteomalacia and the mechanisms underpinning TIO. In time, this may improve preventive and therapeutic choices. However, the vast majority of cases of osteomalacia continue to be caused by vitamin D deficiency. It is imperative that we all have a low threshold for investigating patients who present with typical features and suggestive risk factors, so they can be treated effectively.

References

1. Reginato AJ, Coquia JA. Musculoskeletal manifestations of osteomalacia and rickets. *Best Pract Res Clin Rheumatol* 2003;17:1063–1080.

2. Berry JL, Davies M, Mee AP. Vitamin D metabolism, rickets, and osteomalacia. *Semin Musculoskelet Radiol* 2002;6:173–182.

3. Holick MF. Vitamin D deficiency. *N Engl J Med* 2007;357:266–281.

4. Bhan A, Rao AD, Rao DS. Osteomalacia as a result of vitamin D deficiency. *Endocrinol Metab Clin North Am* 2010;39:321–331.

5. Bischoff-Ferrari HA, Dawson-Hughes B, Willett WC et al. Effect of vitamin D on falls: a meta-analysis. *JAMA* 2004;291:1999–2006.

6. Whyte MP. Hypophosphatasia and the role of alkaline phosphatase in skeletal mineralization. *Endocr Rev* 1994;15:439.

7. Whyte MP, Thakker RV. Rickets and osteomalacia. *Medicine* 2009;37:483–488.

8. Bhambri R, Naik V, Malhotra N et al. Changes in bone mineral density following treatment of osteomalacia. *J Clin Densitom* 2006;9:120–127.

9. Haugeberg G. Imaging of metabolic bone diseases. *Best Pract Res Clin Rheumatol* 2006;22:1127–1139.

10. Hypponen E, Power C. Hypovitaminosis D in British adults at age 45 y: nationwide cohort study of dietary and lifestyle predictors. *Am J Clin Nutr* 2007;85:860–868.

11. Pal BR, Marshall T, James C, Shaw NJ. Distribution analysis of vitamin D highlights differences in population subgroups: preliminary observations from a pilot study in UK adults. *J Endocrinol* 2003;179:119–129.

12. Russell LA. Osteoporosis and osteomalacia. *Rheum Dis Clin North Am* 2010;36:665–680.

13. Pearce SHS, Cheetham T. Diagnosis and management of vitamin D deficiency. *BMJ* 2010;340:142–147.

14. Hathcock JN, Shao A, Vieth R, Heany R. Risk assessment for vitamin D. *Am J Clin Nutr* 2007;85:6–18.

15. Allen SC, Raut S. Biochemical recovery time scales in elderly patients with osteomalacia. *J R Soc Med* 2004;97:527.

16. Lewiecki EM, Urig Jr. EJ, Williams Jr. RC. Tumor-induced osteomalacia: lessons learned. *Arthritis Rheum* 2008;58:773–777.

17. Sundaram M. Metabolic bone disease: what has changed in 30 years? *Skeletal Radiol* 2009;38:841–853.

18. Drezner MK. Tumor-induced osteomalacia. In: Favus MJ (ed) *Primer on the metabolic bone diseases and disorders of mineral metabolism*. Lippincott Williams & Wilkins, Philadelphia, 1999:331.

19. Jonsson KB, Zahradnik R, Larsson T et al. Fibroblast growth factor 23 in oncogenic osteomalacia and X-linked hypophosphatemia. *N Engl J Med* 2003;348:1656.

20. White KE, Larsson TE, Econs MJ. The roles of specific genes implicated as circulating factors involved in normal and disordered phosphate homeostasis: frizzled related protein-4, matrix extracellular phosphoglycoprotein, and fibroblast growth factor 23. *Endocr Rev* 2006;27:221–241.

21. Paglia F, Dionisi S, Minisola S. Octreotide for tumor-induced osteomalacia. *N Engl J Med* 2002;346:1748.

22. Barvencik F, Timo Beil F, Gebauer M et al. Skeletal mineralization defects in adult hypophosphatasia—a clinical and histological analysis. *Osteoporos Int* 2011;22:2667–2675.

23. Mornet E. Hypophosphatasia. *Orphanet J Rare Dis* 2007;2:40.

24. Wesseling-Perry K. FGF-23 in bone biology. *Pediatr Nephrol* 2010;25:603–608.

25. Ma CX, Lacy MQ, Rompala JF, et al. Acquired Fanconi syndrome is an indolent disorder in the absence of overt multiple myeloma. *Blood* 2004;104:40–42.

26. Wong T, Girgis CM, Ngu MC, et al. Hypophosphatemic osteomalacia after low-dose adefovir dipivoxil therapy for hepatitis B. *J Clin Endocrinol Metab* 2010;95:479–480.

27. Clarke BL, Wynne AG, Wilson DM, Fitzpatrick LA. Osteomalacia associated with adult Fanconi's syndrome: clinical and diagnostic features. *Clin Endocrinol* 1995;43:479–490.

Sources of patient information

Arthritis Research UK. Osteomalacia (soft bones): www.arthritisresearchuk.org/arthritis_information/arthritis_types__symptoms/osteomalacia_soft_bones.aspx

CHAPTER 147

Bone tumours

Thomas Beckingsale and Craig Gerrand

Introduction

Bone tumours comprise a heterogeneous mix of post-traumatic, developmental, benign, and malignant lesions. They can be sub-classified according to their histological matrix as bone-forming, cartilage-forming, or fibre-forming, although some do not produce a specific matrix (non-matrix-producing).[1] Perhaps the most important distinction is between malignant tumours, which have a predisposition to invasive and destructive local growth and distant metastasis, and benign tumours, which do not metastasize, although some can demonstrate locally aggressive behaviour (Table 147.1).

Primary malignant tumours of bone (bone sarcomas) are rare and so a high index of suspicion must be maintained to ensure timely diagnosis and avoid mismanagement.[2] Delays in diagnosis are common, and earlier diagnosis would undoubtedly lead to improved outcomes in terms both of survival and of less-damaging surgery being required.[2] Symptoms of bone pain should never be dismissed, especially unilateral 'growing pains' in children.

Radiographic investigation is mandatory to exclude bony malignancy, avoid delay in diagnosis, and prevent incorrect treatment such as arthroscopy or steroid injection when there is an underlying tumour. If radiography indicates that bone cancer is a possibility, an urgent referral should be made to a bone cancer multidisciplinary team (MDT).[3]

Guidance

In the United Kingdom, the National Institute for Health and Clinical Excellence (NICE) publishes guidelines for referral of suspected cancer, and informs the organization of cancer services, which are appointed by the National Commissioning Group (NCG).[2,3] In the United States of America, the National Comprehensive Cancer Network (NCCN) issues clinical practice guidelines for the treatment of bone sarcomas.[4]

Aetiology

Primary malignant tumours of bone are rare entities, with an incidence in England of around 0.85 per 100 000 for men, and 0.60 per 100 000 for women. They account for just 0.2% of all malignant tumours, but 4% of malignancies in children under the age of 14. Males are affected more than females, with a ratio of 13:10.[5] The three most common malignant tumours of bone are osteosarcoma, Ewing's sarcoma, and chondrosarcoma. The incidence of osteosarcoma has a bimodal distribution with the first (larger) peak in adolescence and a second peak in old age. The incidence of Ewing's sarcoma also peaks in adolescence but it is extremely rare after the age of 30 years. Chondrosarcoma increases in incidence with age. Absolute numbers of bone sarcomas are rising annually with the ageing population.[5] More than one-third (34%) of bone sarcomas occur in the long bones of the lower limbs, 14% occur in the bones of the pelvis, sacrum, and coccyx, and a further 10% occur in the scapula and long bones of the upper limb.[5] Relative survival from bone sarcomas has improved steadily over the last 30 years and is currently 58% for males and 59% for females in England.[5]

Presentation

Bone tumours, both benign and malignant, can present with unexplained pain and swelling. Swelling may initially be due to soft tissue oedema, but later can be from bony enlargement and soft tissue extension. Pain from bony lesions is typically worse at night and can often be mistaken for 'growing pains' in children. Patients often present after a coincidental injury, which, although not causative, draws attention to the swelling. Acute presentation can also follow pathological fracture through the lesion in 5–10% of cases. Occasionally, neuralgia or paraesthesiae may be the presenting complaint due to nerve compression from an enlarging lesion. Malignant tumours are associated with cachexia and weight loss, with acute pyrexia on occasion. Symptomatic metastasis to the lung can, rarely, lead to presenting complaints of shortness of breath, chest pain or haemoptysis. Unexplained bony pain mandates careful clinical examination and radiography to look for possible bony tumours. The following 'red flags' should raise suspicion:

- pain—worse at night
- swelling
- cachexia, weight loss, pyrexia
- pathological fracture
- respiratory symptoms from metastases to the lung.

Other than pathological fracture, these symptoms are all common in general rheumatological practice, and hence a high index of suspicion is required to prevent missed or delayed diagnoses.

Table 147.1 Bone tumours

	Bone-forming tumours	Cartilage-forming tumours	Fibre-forming tumours	Non-matrix-producing tumours
Reactive/post-traumatic	Florid reactive periostistis Subungal exostoses		Periosteal 'desmoid' tumour	Unicameral bone cyst Aneurysmal bone cyst
Developmental/hamartomatous	Bone island Osteopoikilosis Melorheostosis Osteopathia striata	Osteochondroma Hereditary multiple exostoses Dysplasia epiphysealis hemimelica Enchondromatosis	Non-ossifying fibroma Fibrous dysplasia	Haemangioma
Benign	Osteoid osteoma Osteoblastoma	Enchondroma Chondroblastoma Chondromyxoid fibroma Fibromyxoma	Osteofibrous dysplasia Desmoplastic fibroma	Eosinophilic granuloma Giant cell tumour Lipoma of bone
Malignant	Osteosarcoma (Paget's sarcoma) (radiation sarcoma)	Chondrosarcoma Chordoma	Fibrosarcoma Malignant fibrous histiocytoma Adamantinoma	Ewing's sarcoma Immunohaematopoietic tumours: myeloma lymphoma leukaemia Metastatic disease

Principles of investigation

Radiography

Radiography is used to make the initial diagnosis. The bone in which the lesion originates, the location within that bone (epiphyseal, metaphyseal, or diaphyseal), and the relationship to the medullary cavity or cortex (central or eccentric), give clues to the diagnosis. For example, unicameral bone cysts originate in the metaphysis of the proximal humerus in 50% of cases.

The effect of the lesion on the bone, and the response of the bone to that lesion, can give useful information about the local behaviour of the tumour. Benign lesions have a narrow zone of transition, which is well defined and 'geographic' (like the edge of a landmass on a map), indicating that the tumour is growing slowly enough to be walled off at its margins. Malignant tumours have a wider zone of transition, indicating aggressive and rapid enlargement, seen as a permeative lesion with poorly demarcated borders. Endosteal scalloping and cortical resorption may also be seen.

The periosteum reacts to the presence of tumour by forming reactive new bone at the edge of the tumour where it is elevated, seen as a Codman's triangle. New bone formation may also be seen as 'sunray spicules' perpendicular to the tumour, as in osteosarcoma, or may be seen in concentric layers, like 'onion-skin', reflecting phases of tumour growth, classically in Ewing's sarcoma.

MRI and CT

MRI is used to delineate the local extent, stage and relationships (with regard to neurovascular structures, compartments, and joints) of the tumour. Pathological detail is shown, as well as the presence or absence of skip lesions and lymphadenopathy. The extent of local oedema is also shown, allowing surgical planning for adequate margins.

CT scanning can be a useful adjunct to MRI, giving further local information about the tumour. This is particularly useful for bony tumours where, for instance, it may demonstrate the nidus of an osteoid osteoma, or endosteal scalloping and matrix formation in cartilaginous tumours. However, CT is primarily used for systemic staging, assessing for the presence of metastases, or looking for a primary tumour when indicated.

Isotope bone scan and positron emission tomography

Isotope bone scanning is used to screen the entire skeleton for the presence of bony metastases or multifocal disease (e.g. polyostotic fibrous dysplasia). PET scanning gives metabolic information and is often combined with a CT scan to provide anatomical detail. Currently it is rarely used in orthopaedic oncology as a primary investigation, but it can be useful to detect recurrent or metastatic disease.

Biopsy

Biopsies are performed to make a histological diagnosis, grade the tumour, and plan treatment. It is recommended that they be performed by the surgical team who will perform the definitive tumour resection because the biopsy track must be excised during the definitive procedure.

Staging

Local staging follows MRI scan to show local extent of the tumour, the size of an associated soft tissue mass, and the involvement of critical anatomical structures. MRI scanning allows biopsy planning and should precede it. Systemic staging involves CT chest (the most common site for metastases), and whole-body bone scan. Tumours are staged according to the American Joint Committee on Cancer (AJCC) system. They are staged depending on the histological grade of the tumour, the size of the tumour, and the presence or absence lymphatic spread or metastases.[4]

Principles of treatment for malignant tumours

The three most common primary malignant tumours of bone are osteosarcoma, chondrosarcoma, and Ewing's sarcoma. Because of the wide range of presentations and treatments and the need to carefully coordinate treatment, malignant bone tumours should be treated within the setting of a MDT comprising pathologists, radiologists, surgeons (orthopaedic, plastic, general, and thoracic), clinical and medical oncologists, paediatric oncologists, and specialist nurses. Wherever possible, patients should be entered into clinical trials. Some chemosensitive tumours (e.g. osteosarcoma or Ewing's tumours) require a combined approach to treatment, classically with adjuvant (preoperative) chemotherapy, local therapy (usually surgery), then adjuvant chemotherapy.

Reconstructive/limb-salvage surgery

The aim of surgery must be complete removal of the tumour with a surrounding cuff of normal tissue. Margins are defined as

- **intralesional**, where the resection passes through the tumour and macroscopic tumour deposits are left in the wound
- **marginal**, where the tumour is excised with an intact pseudo-capsule but the reactive zone around the tumour (an area of oedema and neo-vascularity characterized by the presence of inflammatory cells and micronodules of tumour) is violated, possibly leaving microscopic satellites of tumour within the wound
- **wide**, where the tumour is excised with a cuff of normal surrounding tissue
- **radical**, where the entire anatomical compartment in which the tumour resides is excised en bloc, in theory removing the entire tumour.[6]

As a rule, safe margins must not be compromised for a preferred functional or reconstructive outcome.

Patients who undergo limb salvage have a slightly higher local recurrence rate than those who have an amputation, but the overall survival of the two groups is indistinguishable. Hence, limb salvage has become the norm with rates of 90% in most centres.[7,8] Amputation is now generally reserved for tumours that extensively involve neurovascular structures, or where safe margins cannot be achieved.

The greatest experience of megaprosthesis use is in long bones, especially the femur, tibia, and humerus, and extendable prostheses are available to accommodate growth in children. The 10 year implant survival rates are around 75%, depending on anatomical site and length of resection. However, with revision procedures, durability of limb salvage can be as high as 90% at 20 years. The durability of implants has been improved by the use of hydroxyapatite collars, aiding long-term implant fixation to the bone, and the menace of infection, the most common reason for implant failure and secondary amputation, has been reduced by silver-coating the implants, rendering them resistant to bacterial adhesion and biofilm formation.[8]

Radiotherapy

Osteosarcomas and chondrosarcomas are poorly radiosensitive, and hence radiotherapy does not form part of their treatment protocol. On the other hand, Ewing's sarcoma is radiosensitive, and radiotherapy can occasionally form the mainstay of treatment for these tumours when they arise in areas where surgical access for resection is difficult, for example in the pelvis.

Chemotherapy

Survival from osteosarcoma and Ewing's sarcoma has, greatly improved since the advent of effective chemotherapy over the last 30 years. There is presently no widely available systemic agent for the treatment of chondrosarcoma, the treatment of which remains primarily surgical.

Radiologically detectable metastases are found in about 30% of patients at the time of diagnosis, but it is likely that a much greater percentage have clinically undetectable micrometastases. Neoadjuvant chemotherapy allows early and effective treatment of these micrometastases. Such neoadjuvant also has the added benefit of reducing the inflammation around the tumour, and sometimes in the size of the tumour itself, both of which ease and facilitate surgical resection.

Randomized trials have demonstrated increased disease-free and overall survival for osteosarcoma and Ewing's sarcoma with the use of multiagent chemotherapy. The treatment protocol for osteosarcoma includes doxorubicin, cisplatin, and high-dose methotrexate, whereas the standard treatment protocol for Ewing's sarcoma includes vincristine, doxorubicin, cyclofosfamide, ifosfamide, and etoposide.[9] The response of the tumour to neoadjuvant chemotherapy, measured in osteosarcomas as percentage necrosis on histology of the resected specimen, is prognostically significant. Greater than 90% histological necrosis is considered a good response and is associated with an improved survival rate. Osteosarcomas that respond well to neoadjuvant chemotherapy are treated with the same agents after surgery, but etoposide and ifosfamide are added for poor responders after surgery.

Bone-forming tumours

Post-traumatic lesions

Florid reactive periostitis

Florid reactive periostitis is a rare, reactive process that occurs most commonly in the hands and feet, and usually presents with progressive swelling, erythema, and pain around the metacarpophalangeal joints. Ossification occurs in the soft tissues around the short tubular bones, but in the early stages of the disease this may not be visible on radiographs. Treatment is with rest, non-steroidal anti-inflammatory drugs (NSAIDs), and corticosteroids, which may decrease the size of the lesion. Surgical excision is occasionally required with low rates of local recurrence.[10]

Developmental or hamartomatous lesions

Bone islands

These are solitary enostoses and are seen radiographically as small areas of increased density, 1–2 mm in diameter, within areas of cancellous bone.

Osteopoikilosis

Osteopoikilosis is a rare, clinically benign, and usually symptomless condition of multiple bone islands, which is inherited as an autosomal dominant trait. It sometimes presents with cutaneous nodules, suggesting a generalized mesenchymal defect. Histological examination of the cutaneous nodules reveals fibrous tissue, resembling scleroderma-like lesions.

Melorheostosis

Melorheostosis is a rare condition characterized by irregular cortical hyperostosis, described as looking like 'melting wax dripping down the sides of a candle'. Para-articular fibrosis and vascular malformations are common early manifestations and may precede the osseous abnormalities. The condition can lead to leg-length discrepancy and joint contractures, resulting in deformity and pain. Surgical management has generally proved disappointing.[11]

Benign tumours

Osteoid osteomas

Osteoid osteomas are benign, painful lesions, more than 50% of which present in the cortical diaphyses of the femur or tibia. Other common sites of presentation include the hands, feet, and spine. They are usually less than 1 cm in diameter, and are seen as a central, lucent nidus within an area of cortical sclerosis on radiographs and CT scans. An isotope bone scan shows markedly increased uptake. The classic history is of severe night pain, relieved dramatically by NSAIDs, which, on occasion, are the only treatment modality required. Traditional surgical treatment is by en-bloc excision or 'burr-down' technique, but CT-guided radioablation is the more modern approach.[12]

Osteoblastomas

These are very similar in appearance to osteoid osteomas but they are larger, usually greater than 1 cm, and present more commonly in the spine, usually in the vertebral arch, where they can lead to radicular or myelopathic symptoms. Treatment is by curettage and grafting or en-bloc excision.

Malignant tumours

Osteosarcoma

Osteosarcoma[13] is the second most common primary bone tumour, myeloma being the first, but the most common sarcomatous tumour of bone. It makes up 20% of all primary bone tumours, but 55% of all bone tumours in children and adolescents. Presentation is most common around the knee with 35% arising in the distal femur and 20% arising in the proximal tibia. The incidence has a bimodal distribution with a first large peak during the growth spurt in adolescence, and a second smaller peak after the fifth decade because of Paget's sarcoma and radiation sarcoma, which carry a poor prognosis. Osteosarcoma is associated with retinoblastoma and a number of progeroid and precancerous syndromes such as Li–Fraumeni, Rothmund–Thompson, and Bloom. Ninety-five per cent of osteosarcomas are intramedullary, of which 90% are high grade. The remaining 5% are surface lesions, of which 90% are low grade.

Radiographs of 'classic' osteoblastic, intramedullary osteosarcoma show a sclerotic, destructive lesion in the metaphysis of a long bone, invading the cortex and extending into the soft tissues with a 'sunburst' pattern. Elevated levels of alkaline phosphatase, in the absence of metastases, are suggestive of larger primary tumours, whereas elevated lactate dehydrogenase levels suggest a more biologically active tumour. Both are associated with a poorer prognosis.

Treatment of osteosarcoma is with neoadjuvant chemotherapy, involving an anthracycline (doxorubincin), a platinum (cisplatin), and high-dose methotrexate, surgical resection, and adjuvant chemotherapy. Etoposide and ifosfamide are added to the chemotherapeutic regime during adjuvant treatment for tumours that have responded poorly to the standard regime during the neoadjuvant period. Radiologically detectable metastasis is present at diagnosis in 30% of cases and is associated with a poorer prognosis. Another key factor in prognosis is the response of the tumour to chemotherapy, where a good response (>90% necrosis) carries a better prognosis.

Muramyl tripeptide (MTP) is a novel agent being trialled as an addition to the standard chemotherapy regime. MTP is not directly tumoricidal, but works by stimulating the immune system, causing macrophages to exhibit cytotoxic anti-tumour activity. A randomized trial showed that 6 year overall survival improved from 70% to 78% when MTP was added to the standard chemotherapy regime for osteosarcoma.[14]

Cartilage-forming tumours

Developmental or hamartomatous tumours

Solitary osteochondromas

These are osteocartilaginous exostoses, whose formation follows mutation within the *EXT* genes, leading to aberrant growth of a fragment of epiphyseal growth plate. The fragment continues to grow by enchondral ossification, resulting in a subperiosteal, cartilage-capped, bony projection. They most commonly present in the metaphyses of long bones around the knee, with more than one-quarter of them arising in the distal femur. They usually manifest clinically during the second decade due to symptoms secondary to local irritation, trauma, or fracture, and their growth usually ceases after physeal closure. Osteochondromas may, rarely, present in the epiphysis where the condition is known as dysplasia epiphsealis hemimelica, or Trevor's disease. Radiographs show either a flattened (sessile) or stalked (pedunculated) juxta-articular protuberance, the cortices of which are contiguous with the adjoining cortical bone, growing away from the adjacent joint. Malignant transformation to a chondrosarcoma is extremely rare in solitary osteochondromas. Symptomatic exostoses are treated by surgical excision through the base of the lesion. Recurrence is rare, but is more common if the cartilage cap is incompletely excised.

Multiple hereditary exostoses

Otherwise known as diaphyseal aclasia, multiple hereditary exostoses are an autosomal dominant trait, resulting in multiple osteocartilaginous exostoses secondary to mutation in the *EXT* genes. It is the most common skeletal dysplasia and it results in short stature, bony deformity, and disfigurement. The ulnae are often shortened, leading to Madelung-like deformities. Radiologically and macroscopically the resulting exostoses are similar to solitary osteochondromas but histology often reveals a more disorganized structure. Malignant change, too, is more common than in solitary osteochondromas and occurs in around 1–5%.

Enchondromatosis

Enchondromatosis or Ollier's disease is a non-familial condition of multiple intraosseous cartilaginous tumours, which is often unilateral and confined to a single limb. Histologically, tumours are more cellular and myxoid that solitary enchondromas. The risk of malignancy is high, with a 10% risk of developing a bony malignancy. However, the overall risk of malignancy is 25% if associated visceral and brain tumours are included. Enchondromatosis in conjunction with multiple soft tissue and visceral haemangiomas is known as Maffucci's syndrome and the risk of malignancy approaches 100%.

Benign tumours

Enchondromas

These are common, solitary, asymptomatic, intramedullary, cartilaginous tumours, which arise in the tubular bones of the hand in more than 50% of cases. They often present after pathological fracture, particularly in the bones of the hands and feet. Histologically lesions in long bones may be difficult to distinguish from low-grade chondrosarcomas, and malignant transformation, although very rare, can sometimes occur is such lesions. Radiographs show enchondromas as well-defined lucent lesions, with a short zone of transition and a matrix of stippled or 'popcorn' calcification. These lesions are usually treated by curettage with or without grafting.

Malignant tumours

Chondrosarcomas

These are malignant, cartilaginous tumours, the diagnosis of which critically depends on the clinical, radiological, and histological findings, as it can be difficult to distinguish enchondromas from low-grade chondrosarcomas on histological grounds alone. Incidence increases with age, most presenting after the fifth decade. Fifty per cent of lesions arise in the femur and pelvis, presenting with persistent pain and swelling. Radiographs show lucent metaphyseal or diaphyseal defects with endosteal scalloping and 'popcorn' calcification. T2 weighting on MRI scan reveals a bright lesion due to the high water content of the cartilaginous matrix.

Chondrosarcomas are resistant to radiotherapy and chemotherapy, and hence treatment is surgical. Low-grade tumours rarely metastasize and are often treated by intralesional curettage, whereas high-grade lesions require wide surgical excision. Prognosis is largely dependent on the grade of the tumour and the presence or absence of metastases. Low-grade (grade I) chondrosarcomas are distinguished from enchondromas by their location within long bone and the pelvis, and by microscopic evidence of haversian invasion. They are very rarely metastatic and have a greater than 90% 5 year survival. Grade II tumours histologically show definite increased cellularity and nuclear size, as well as focal myxoid change. They are metastatic in more than 10% of cases and have a 5 year survival of 80%. High-grade III tumours are distinguished by their marked hypercellularity, cellular atypia, and high mitotic activity. They are aggressive, rapidly enlarging lesions, which are metastatic in over 70% of cases, and have a 5 year survival of only 30%. Ten per cent of tumours undergo dedifferentiation in one area, becoming highly malignant sarcomas with spindle cells and bizarre giant cells, similar to fibrosarcoma

or malignant fibrous histiocytoma. Radiographs show an area of lucency within the classic 'popcorn' calcification. Presentation is often with pathological fracture in elderly patients, and prognosis is dismal.

Chordomas

These arise from remnants of the embryological notochord, and hence present exclusively in the axial skeleton, with around 50% arising in the sacrococcygeal region. They are a slow-growing lesion, presenting usually in the fifth decade, but are metastatic in around 50% of cases to lymph nodes, lung, liver, and bone.

Fibre-forming tumours

Developmental or hamartomatous tumours

Non-ossifying fibromas

These are very common, asymptomatic lesions, present in up to 35% of normal children. Radiographs show a well-demarcated, solitary, eccentrically placed, metaphyseal lucency with a sclerotic margin. Presentation is usually as an incidental finding, but may follow pathological fracture. Treatment is by observation unless there is a significant risk of pathological fracture, as these lesions usually resolve by adulthood.

Fibrous dysplasia

This is a common fibro-osseous lesion, usually arising monostotically in a long bone of the lower-limb. The lesion is often discovered as an incidental finding but can also present with swelling or pathological fracture, usually in adolescence. Radiographs show a well-demarcated lesion with fusiform expansion, ground-glass calcification, and cortical thinning. In the proximal femur, the lesion can sometimes lead to multiple, sequential pathological fractures, resulting in a 'shepherd's crook' deformity.

Malignant tumours

Fibrosarcomas

These are rare, malignant spindle cell tumours, arising in the ends of long bones around the knee 50% of the time. They present most commonly in the third to sixth decades. Radiographs show a poorly demarcated, lucent lesion with a mottled appearance, cortical destruction, and extension into the soft tissues. Treatment is by wide excision and reconstruction.

Malignant fibrous histiocytomas

Malignant fibrous histiocytomasare rare tumours, arising in the metaphyses of long bones around the knee in adults. Radiographs show a poorly demarcated, lucent lesion with cortical erosion but minimal periosteal new bone formation. Histology reveals a spindle cell tumour with a distinctive storiform or 'starry night' pattern. Treatment is as for osteosarcoma with chemotherapy, wide excision and reconstruction.

Adamantinomas

Adamantinomas are rare, slow-growing, low-grade spindle cell tumours arising in the tibia in over 90% of cases. Radiographs show a multicystic lucency with cortical thinning and bony expansion. The lesion is generally only locally aggressive but can metastasize in up to 20% of cases late in the disease process. Treatment is with wide excision and reconstruction.

Non-matrix-producing tumours

Reactive or post-traumatic lesions

Unicameral bone cysts

These are solitary, cystic lesions arising in the metaphyses of long bones in childhood and adolescence. The classic site is the proximal humerus, where 50% of such lesions arise. A further one-quarter arise in the proximal femur, where pathological fracture can be difficult to manage. Presentation is usually with fracture, pain (which usually indicates impending fracture), or as an incidental finding. Pathological fractures through these lesions usually heal well, but the cysts only partially resolve. Radiographs reveal a well-demarcated lucent area with a sclerotic margin. The classic 'fallen leaf' sign indicates a fracture, at least partially, through the lesion. Treatment is usually by observation for the majority, but surgical intervention is indicated for those at risk of pathological fracture. Options described include minimally invasive decompression and curettage (the authors' preferred method), curettage and grafting, surgical fixation through the cyst with an intramedullary nail, or corticosteroid injection.

Aneurysmal bone cysts

These are solitary, expansile, multiloculated, eccentrically placed, cystic lesions, usually arising in long bones or the spine and presenting with pain usually before the third decade. Radiographs show an expansile lesion, as described above, with a trabeculated appearance, and MRI shows multiple fluid levels. In many cases the lesion is a secondary, reactive lesion to another benign lesion such as an osteoblastoma, chondroblastoma, or giant cell tumour. It is important to distinguish this benign entity from telangiectatic osteosarcoma, which can have aneurysmal change within it. Treatment is with curettage and grafting, but recurrence rates can be high, approaching 50%.

Developmental or hamartomatous tumours

Haemangiomas of bone

These are solitary, asymptomatic lesions usually arising in the lumbar vertebral bodies and are comprised of thin-walled, cavernous blood vessels. Radiographs show accentuated, thickened vertical trabeculae, described as 'jail bar' striations. No treatment is required, but pathological collapse can occur. Widespread disease is occasionally seen as skeletal haemangiomatosis, which has no familial tendency and is self-limiting.

Benign tumours

Giant cell tumours of bone

These rare, solitary, locally aggressive lesions are seen at the epiphyseal ends of long bones, with 50% arising around the knee. The incidence is 1–2 per million of population per year. Radiographs show an aggressive, juxta-articular, lytic lesion. Frequently there is near-complete cortical destruction and an associated soft tissue mass. Histology reveals spindle-shaped tumour cells and multinucleated giant cells, which are indistinguishable from osteoclasts. It is essential to differentiate the lesion from a giant-cell-rich osteosarcoma. Treatment is by curettage and grafting with the use of a surgical adjuvant such as liquid nitrogen and/or polymethylmethacrylate cement. Agents that interfere with osteoclast recruitment, such as bisphosphonates and RANK-ligand inhibitors, can also play a useful role in difficult cases. Recurrence rate is high after surgical curettage alone. Malignant transformation and metastasis is another rare but well-recognized complication, which appears to be more likely in locally recurrent tumours.

Malignant tumours

Ewing's sarcoma

Ewing's sarcoma is a malignant, small, round blue cell tumour of bone, which can, very rarely, arise in the soft tissues. It presents most commonly in the metaphyses and diaphyses of the long bones either side of the knee or in the pelvis. Symptoms are of pain and swelling associated with the lesion, but erythema, pyrexia, a leucocytosis, and a raised erythrocyte sedimentation rate (ESR) can also be present at diagnosis, incorrectly leading the unwary to a diagnosis of infection. Radiographs show a lytic, moth-eaten appearance to the bone with a laminated, 'onion peel' periosteal bone reaction. MRI shows the extent of the tumour and the degree of soft tissue extension. Investigations for Ewing's sarcoma must also include a whole-body isotope bone scan and a bone marrow biopsy to rule out metastatic or multifocal disease, which is associated with a poorer prognosis. Genetically, reciprocal translation between chromosomes 11 and 22 is seen (t(11;22)(q24;q12). Systemic treatment by chemotherapy is with doxorubicin, vincristine, cyclofosfamide, ifosfamide, and etoposide. Local management is with radiation, surgery, or both. Overall 5 year survival is 66% but is as high as 75% if the tumour responds well to chemotherapy, and as low as 20% if the tumour responds poorly.

Immunohaematopoietic tumours and metastatic bone disease

It is beyond the scope of this chapter to describe all the haematological malignancies and secondary malignancies that may involve bone. These include plasmacytomas, multiple myeloma, lymphoma, and leukaemia. Treatment of immunohaematopoietic tumours usually involves chemotherapy and radiotherapy, but rarely involves surgery. Adjuvant treatment for metastatic bone disease depends largely on the sensitivities of the primary lesion. Surgery for immunohaematopoietic and metastatic tumours is generally reserved for the treatment of impending or completed pathological fractures.

References

1. Bullough PG. *Orthopaedic pathology*, 4th edn. Mosby, Edinburgh, 2007.
2. NICE. *Guidance on improving cancer services: improving outcomes for people with sarcoma. the manual*. National Institute for Health and Clinical Excellence, London, 2006.
3. NICE. *Referral guidelines for suspected cancer (clinical guidline 27)*. National Institute for Health and Clinical Excellence, London, 2005.
4. NCCN. *NCCN clinical practice guidelines in oncology. Bone cancer. V.1*, 2009. Avaialbe at: www.nccn.org/professionals/physician_gls/f_guidelines.asp#bone
5. NCIN. *Bone sarcomas: incidence and survival rates in England*. National Cancer Intelligence Network, London, 2010.
6. Enneking WF, Spanier SS, Malawer MM. The effect of the anatomic setting on the results of surgical procedures for soft parts sarcoma of the thigh. *Cancer* 1981;47(5):1005–1022.
7. Grimer RJ, Carter SR, Pynsent PB. The cost-effectiveness of limb-salvage for bone tumours. *J Bone Joint Surg Br* 1997;79-B:558–561.
8. Jeys L, Grimer R. The long-term risks of infection and amputation with limb salvage surgery using endoprostheses. *Recent Results Cancer Res* 2009;179:75–84.

9. Schuetze SM, Arbor A. Chemotherapy in the management of osteosarcoma and Ewing's sarcoma. *J Natl Comp Canc Netw* 2007;5(4):449–455.

10. Spjut HJ, Dorfman HD. Florid reactive periostitis of the tubular bones of the hands and feet. A benign lesion which may simulate osteosarcoma. *Am J Surg Pathol* 1981;5(5):423–433.

11. Gagliardi GG, Mahan KT. Melorheostosis: a literature review and case report with surgical considerations. *J Foot Ankle Surg* 2010;49(1):80–85.

12. Papathanassiou ZG, Megas P, Petsas T et al. Osteoid osteoma: diagnosis and treatment. *Orthopaedics* 2008;31(11):1118.

13. Beckingsale TB, Gerrand CH. Osteosarcoma. *Orthopaed Trauma* 2010;24(5):321–331.

14. Meyers PA, Schwartz CL, Krailo MD et al. Osteosarcoma: the addition of muramyl tripeptide to chemotherapy improves overall survival—a report from the Children's Oncology Group. *J Clin Oncol* 2008;26:633–638.

CHAPTER 148

Avascular necrosis

Stefan Rehart and Martina Henniger

Introduction

Avascular necroses are acquired skeletal diseases with typical development and localization. The actual frequency is unknown. The joint surface is not necessarily involved. There are three major forms: aseptic osteonecrosis, septic osteonecrosis, and post-traumatic osteonecrosis. Many bones may be affected by osteonecrosis, and many sites have eponyms associated (Table 148.1).

Table 148.1 Sites and names of the common eponymous osteonecroses

Site	Name
Vertebral body	Calvé
Vertebral plate	Scheuermann
Synchrondrosis ischiopubica	Van Neck
Sternal end of clavicle	Friedrich
Distal part of the ribs	Tietze
Caput humeri	Hass
Capitulum humeri	Panner
Trochlea humeri	Hegemann
Caput radii	Hegemann
Distal radial epiphysis	De Cuvelan
Os scaphoideum	Preiser
Os lunatum	Kienböck
Metacarpal head	Dietrich
Basis of the middle- and end phalanges	Thiemann
Femoral head and neck in early childhood	Calvé–Legg–Perthes
Apophysis of calcaneus	Haglund
Talus	Vogel
Os naviculare pedis	Köhler (I)
Metatarsal head II–V	Freiberg–Köhler (II)
Basis of the base phalanx of the great toe	Thiemann
Os cuneiforme laterale	Lance
Basis metatarsal V	Iselin

For various, often unknown, reasons there is direct or indirect damage of the bone vascularization. Certain diseases or factors facilitate the occurrence of aseptic osteonecroses. More than 50% of all commercial scuba divers, 30% of all patients with systemic lupus erythematosus (SLE) and 29% with type 1 Gaucher's disease develop osteonecrosis.[1,2] Ischaemia of bone cells leads to cell death of bone, cartilage, and bone marrow cells, which are subsequently destroyed. The defects may be without consequence or lead to severe, irreversible damage to bones and joints depending on the extent and localization. In general, every bone at any age can be affected.

Aetiology and epidemiology

Certain fractures and/or dislocations as well as infections can lead to arterial injury and to post-traumatic or septic osteonecrosis. However, the cause of aseptic osteonecrosis is less clear and its incidence seems to be very complex, including multifactorial causes. The most likely pathophysiological mechanism is an intravascular coagulation with spreading of the fibrin thrombus. Because the osteonecrotic lesions do not widen, but stay about the same size or shrink slightly, the osteonecrosis is apparently the result of only one ischaemic event, not of repeated ischaemic reinfarction.[3]

Risk factors for osteonecrosis are listed in Box 148.1.[4]

Pathogenesis

Osteonecrosis results from a direct or indirect injury, or damage to the vascular flow (injury/embolism/mechanical disturbance of arterial blood supply or venous backflow obstruction). Circulatory deficiency results in bone and bone marrow cell death (osteocytes, haematopoetic cells, adipocytes). Osteonecrosis develops only in the bone marrow, which consists mainly of adipocytes in patients with sickle cell anaemia and Gaucher's disease. The necrotic tissue triggers repair, during which necrotic parts may be resorbed by macrophages and osteoclasts. A reactive surface develops at the boundary with healthy bone. When there is a revitalization of the necrosis due to ingrowth of blood vessels and connective tissue from the healthy surroundings substituting for abnormal and biomechanically weak bones, smaller lesions can heal. If this healing remains incomplete, due to the anatomical position, the subchondral bone will break from repeated microtrauma and various significant defects will result.

Box 148.1 Risk factors for osteonecrosis

- Thrombophilia: APC resistance, protein C deficiency, protein S deficiency, anti-thrombin III deficiency, hyperhomocysteinemia

- Hyperlipoproteinemia and fat embolism: alcoholism, diabetes mellitus, hyperlipidaemia type I and IV, elevated C-reactive protein, obesity, pregnancy, decompression disease, haemoglobinopathies, burns, fractures

- Hypersensitization reactions: host-vs-graft disease, anaphylaxis, anti-phospholipid syndrome, immune complexes, serum sickness, SLE, transfusion incidents

- Hypofibronolysis: dysfibrinogenaemia, plasminogen deficiency, decreased tissue plasminogen activator, elevated plasminogen activator inhibitor type 1

- Infections: endotoxic bacterial reactions, bacterial lipopolysaccharides, bacterial mucopolysaccharides, 'Schwartzmann reaction', toxic shock syndrome, viral infections

- Proteolytic enzymes: pancreatitis, snake bites

- Tissue factor release: inflammatory intestinal diseases, malignancies, neural trauma, pregnancy

- Other prethrombotic conditions: acidosis, anorexia nervosa, oestrogen, smoking, Gaucher's disease, haemolytic uraemic syndrome, haemolysis, hyperfibrinogenaemia, hyperviscosity, shock, lipoprotein, nephrotic syndrome, polycythaemia, sickle cell crisis, thrombocytosis, thrombocytopenia purpura, vascular changes

The pathophysiological sequence is very flexible in time and takes weeks to years. The progression of the disease can be classified into five pathophysiologic stages, as described in the Association Research Circulation Osseous (ARCO) classification.[5]

Association Research Circulation Osseous (ARCO) classification

Initial stage (ARCO 0)

The initial stage is an ischaemic attack, which is still reversible and usually asymptomatic. At most, pathological perfusion can be shown by means of a dynamic contrast MRI scan. Histologically, only minimal changes can be found.

Reversible early stage (ARCO I)

Next comes an oedema of the bone marrow with extended medullary cavity necroses, the start of repair processes, and gradual replacement of necrosis through growth of fibrous vascular tissue. In the MRI scan a subchondral necrotic lesion with medullar cavity oedema and other unspecific signal changes of the repair process can be seen, but still without signs of a reactive interface.

Non-reversible early stage (ARCO II)

Histological transformation processes, in the sense of bone resorption and formation in the bone marrow and the trabecular, are found. Vascular granulation tissue attempts to repair the necrotic area on the inside of the sclerotic zone, which is directly opposed to the area of vital bone tissue. In the MRI scan the so-called 'MR double line sign', which is pathognomonic for osteonecrosis, appears in the T2-weighted image. It corresponds to the reactive interface. In plain radiographs only blotchy changes with sclerotic edges are visible.

Transitional stage (ARCO III)

Mechanical failure of the affected bone area leads to subchondral microfractures. It usually begins at the margin of the defect and is a consequence of insufficient repair. On radiographs, a small subchondral crescent sign is visible. If the fracture gap is filled with synovial fluid the subchondral fractures can also be seen as an MR crescent sign.

Late stage (ARCO IV)

In the late stage there are secondary arthritic lesions (calcification, resorptive cysts) and deformations, which can be detected by any imaging method.

Diagnosis

The diagnosis cannot be made on the basis of laboratory tests. Sometimes the erythrocyte sedimentation rate (ESR) can be increased. Laboratory examinations are used to exclude a septic event and detect risk factors (coagulation disorders, sickle cell anaemia, hyperlipoproteinaemia).

Several imaging techniques are available for diagnosing AVN.

Radiography

In plain radiography there may be minimal changes that are very difficult to make out. Here, the radiograph serves mainly to exclude other pathologies.

Later on, if the necrosis leads to perifocal osteoporosis or the vital bone surrounding the necrosis reacts with bone formation/sclerosis, changes also become perceptible on radiographs. Due to osteolysis of necrotic bone and sprouting of new blood vessels, bright spots and intensifications in the bone can be seen. Later, fractures and progressive collapse as well as increasing arthritic changes are seen.

Scintigraphy

In early stage (ARCO I), when conventional radiographs do not yet show lesions, a cold spot can be seen in 99 m-technetium scintigraphy. In due course, when repair processes begin (ARCO II), specific hot spots or cold in hot spots are found. Simultaneously, multifocal bone diseases can be excluded through scintigraphy.

MRI

Today MRI is the most sensitive and specific method for diagnosis and assessment in respect of lesion size and the stage of osteonecrosis (Figures 148.1 and 148.2). The characteristic image is a hypointense oval zone or a hypointense crescent sign in a subchondral position. In most cases the pathognomonic MR double line sign is found in T2-weighted images. This corresponds to the reactive interface between healthy and necrotic bone. A line of low signal intensity is found at the face of healthy bone, whereas at the interface with necrotic area there may be a line of high signal intensity.

CT

CT scanning has a higher sensitivity and specificity than conventional radiography, but it is inferior to MRI, particularly in the early stages. However, in the diagnosis of subchondral fractures,[6]

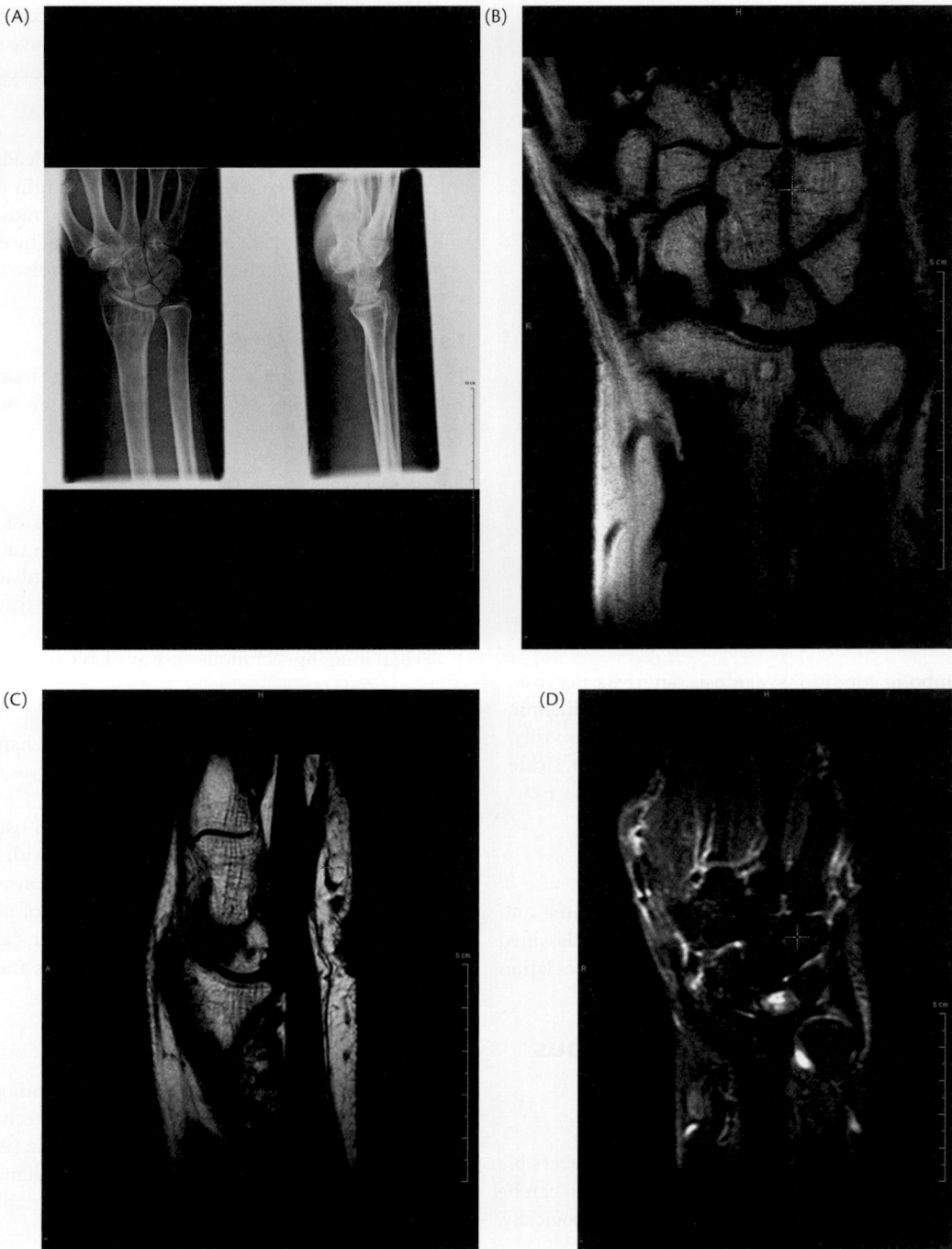

Fig. 148.1 Lunate malacia (Kienböck's disease): (a) Radiograph (secondary finding: former radius fracture). (b–d) MRI.

often the deciding factor for therapy, CT becomes increasingly important as it has a higher sensitivity than MRI and conventional radiography.

Common localizations

Humeral head necrosis

Occasionally humeral head necrosis occurs spontaneously, but far more commonly it is associated with the risk factors listed in Box 148.1. Usually, osteonecrosis of the humeral head becomes symptomatic later than a comparable finding in the hip and knee joint. This is easy to understand as it has less weight loading

and maybe decreased conformity of the glenoid in comparison to the acetabulum. Clinical signs are pain at rest and nocturnal pain, and later also an active and passive painful restriction of movement.

Staging will be done on the basis of conventional radiography and MRI (see above). The size and location of the osteonecrosis as seen in MRI allows a prognosis concerning the further clinical course.[7]

In ARCO stages I and II conservative therapy is used. This essentially consists of mechanical load reduction. To avoid stiffening of the joint, at least passive physiotherapeutic movement therapy should be applied.

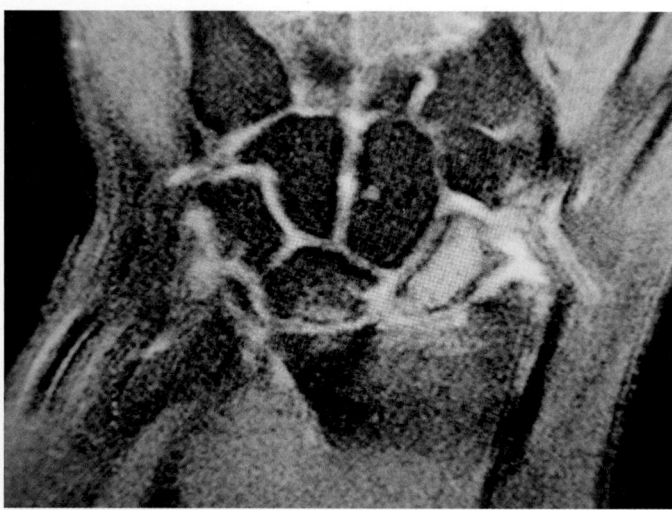

Fig. 148.2 MRI of scaphoid osteonecrosis (Preiser's disease).

When symptoms persist and there are signs of collapse of the humeral head, surgical therapy is indicated.[8] Joint-preserving and joint-replacing surgical techniques are available. In early stages decompression can be achieved by means of a core decompression. This leads to pain relief and possibly to revascularization. Further joint-preserving techniques are a vascular bone transplant or removal of necrosis with subsequent spongiosa transplant, similar to necrosis of the femoral head. However, there is not a large number of cases and re-examinations for the assessment of efficacy.

In more advanced stages with explicit joint destruction, joint replacement methods are used. The choice of implant depends on condition of the bone (bone quality, glenoid destruction), the state of the soft tissues (particularly the rotator cuff), and the individual requirements of the patient.

Lunate malacia—Kienböck's disease

Necrosis of the lunate bone was first described by Peste in 1843.[9] In 1910 the Viennese radiologist Kienböck published a paper focusing on lunate malacia and its subsequent results.[10] Even today its pathogenesis is not fully understood. Important aetiological factors may be vibration and microtraumatization, for example when working with compressed air apparatus and power saws; arterial injury; negative ulnar variance, and hence increased pressure stress; venous backflow obstruction due to wrist dorsal extension; systemic diseases; or corticosteroid therapy (for multiple sclerosis, rheumatoid arthritis, dermatomyositis, SLE, systemic sclerodermia or sickle cell anaemia). Single traumatic events with perilunar luxation or luxation-fracture are not a very likely cause.[11] Symptoms consist of pain that is difficult to localize—especially in the form of diffuse pain in the wrist in dorsal extension—as well as a loss of strength as time goes by. Clinically, synovitis and local swelling is found in combination with defined pain in palpation.

Diagnostically, in early stages specific changes in the MRI are detected At this point conventional radiology may still be completely without pathological findings. Only later are increased sclerosis and intraosseus cysts found; still later, the continuous collapse of the lunate as well as ongoing perilunar osteoarthritic defects are seen.

The stages are defined according to Lichtman and Ross or to Decoulx, modified after Martini and Schiltenwolf[12]:

+ **Stage I**: morphologically normal radiographic appearance; enhancement in the MRI scan; diffuse pain.

+ **Stage II**: radiology reveals increased sclerosis of the spongy trabecular structures and an inhomogenous appearance. The height of the lunate is still normal. If subchondral proximal fractures are detectable (CT) the findings are staged as IIb. The MRI shows homogeneity (oedema), inhomogeneity (partial necrosis), or lack of enhancement (complete necrosis) of the contrast fluid. Clinically, pain persists.

+ **Stage IIIA**: radiologically fractures and the progressive collapse of the lunate without rotational dislocation of the scaphoid and normal carpal height are seen.

+ **Stage IIIB**: fractures and the complete collapse of the lunate in combination with a rotational dislocation of the scaphoid, together with a positive ring sign, are seen on radiographs.

+ **Stage IV**: advanced collapse of the lunate and the entire carpus with massive osteoarthritis occurs.

Therapy depends on the stage of the disease:

+ In **stage I** immobilization is indicated. Should that not be sufficient, corrective interventions with regard to the length of the radius or the ulna are considered. In general, the technically easier radius shortening (rather than ulna lengthening) is preferred.

+ In **stage II** length-levelling operations are definitely indicated.[13] Alternatively, revascularizing interventions may be possible (arterial-vessel based bone transplants, e.g. os pisiforme). Unfortunately in many cases the collapse of the lunate cannot be prevented in this way.

+ In **stage IIIA** partial arthrodeses of the wrist are performed; length-levelling operations may still be possible.

+ In **stage IIIB** reconstruction of the wrist height with an STT arthrodesis (fusion of the scaphoid with the trapezium and the trapezoideum) or an SC arthrodesis (fusion of the scaphoid with the capitate) is chosen.

+ In **stage IV** partial arthrodeses, proximal row resection, or the total fusion of the wrist are performed.

Femoral head necrosis

Men are affected four times more than women in this context, especially in the third to the fifth decade. In 30–70% of cases the disease affects both sides. Without therapy the prognosis is poor; in more than 85% a collapse of the femoral head is noticed, in combination with severe secondary destruction of the joint.

Clinically, most of patients in early stages do not complain of any symptoms. Later in the course of this illness pain, limping, and increasing deficits in the function of the hip (range of motion) can be seen.

Conventional radiographs reveal the necrosis only in the advanced stages, when irreversible damage has occurred (ARCO II), but for reasons of differential diagnosis they are always to be done in any case. MRI is the method of choice in diagnosing the necrosis. Therapy and prognosis depend on the stage, dimension, and the location of the lesion. In the so-called precollapse stage

(ARCO 0–II), prevention of weightbearing of the hip in question by the use of crutches for several weeks may prove favourable. Further conservative therapy options are magnetic field, shock wave, or hyperbaric oxygen therapy as well as medication with cytokines, vasodilation with calcium antagonists, prostaglandin analogues, or osteoprotective bisphosphonates.[14] The efficacy of these measures is confirmed by case-reports only.[15] Should conservative measurements fail, or if the disease is at an advanced stage (>ARCO II), surgical interventions may be planned. The choice of these depends on the stage, the size, and location of the osteonecrotic area, as well as the diameter of the impression of the femoral head and the involvement of the acetabulum. Further dependencies are the individual perioperative risks of the patient (age, general condition, comorbidities, etc.).

Core Decompression

The most common operation is core decompression of the femoral head, an intervention introduced by Arlet and Ficat 30 years ago. The best results are achieved with small to medium-sized defects in the precollapse stage.[16] This procedure reduces the intraosseus pressure and improves the arterial blood supply.[5] The release of pressure provides immediate pain relief for the patient. The assumption that reparative power in the necrotic area is increased by the increase in regeneration of the vessels has not been proven by MRI and histomorphological findings, so this surgical intervention is considered controversial.[17] However, lack of success subsequently offers access to further operative procedures without severe disadvantages.

Corrective osteotomy

The principle of the osteotomies consists in the removal of the defective site from the main load transmission area. Most suitable for this are small, medially located lesions in the pre- and postcollapse stage. Most frequently varus osteotomies, combined flexion osteotomies, and technically very demanding high transtrochanteric rotation osteotomies are performed. As well as the possibly quite high complication rates for this kind of surgery, the deterioration of the background for the arthroplasties that are generally later indicated has to be taken into account.

Bone transplantation

This method may be discussed when joint-preserving interventions of large defects in the postcollapse stage are foreseen. It is important to differentiate between vascularized and non-vascularized bone transplants. Most commonly the arterial-blood-supplied fibula graft is used in the autologous bone marrow impaction technique, introduced via a transtrochanteric bone channel. The operation is time-consuming and technically very demanding. So far it is not clear whether any reparative capacity may be gained by it.

Arthroplasty

Joint replacement is indicated in ARCO stages III and IV, together with unfavourable factors such as additional risk factors, underlying disease, large defects, fast progression of the disease, or non-compliance of the patient in combination with high demands.[18]

Osteonecrosis of the femoral condyle—Ahlbäck's disease

Osteonecrosis of the femoral condyle was first described by Ahlbäck in the 1960s.[19] The aetiology is still not known. Generally the medial femur condyle is affected, but the lateral femur condyle as well as the medial tibia plateau may also be involved. The peak age is 60 years, and women are three times more affected than men. Patients usually complain about sudden, very intense knee pain in the medial or lateral joint space. Clinically, limping and pressure pain in the according area are found, but also intra-articular swelling or a reduction of the range of motion of the knee may be determined. Radiography, scintigraphy, and MRI may be of help in securing the diagnosis (Figure 148.3).

According to Aglietti, five stages may be differentiated in radiographs[20]:

- **Stage I**: normal radiograph.
- **Stage II**: flattening of the concerned femur condyle.
- **Stage III**: typical lesion with subchondral brightening of variable size and depth, surrounded by sclerosis.
- **Stage IV**: the brightening zone is demarcated by a sclerotic wall area. The subchondral bone collapses and is noted as a calcified plate.
- **Stage V**: secondarily osteoarthritic changes are diagnosed; a deviation of the axes of the leg may be present.

The prognosis as well as the choice of therapy depends on the size of the defect, the relation of the defect size to the width of the condyle, and the stage. For early stage disease with lesions less than 3.5 cm² in size affecting less than 40% of the femur condyles, the prognosis is reasonably good.[21]

Conservative treatment is suitable for lesions with a good prognosis. This includes physical therapy, painkillers, and anti-phlogistic medication and possibly raising the outer edge of the shoe by 4 mm for the discharge of the medial condyle.[21]

Poor prognosis qualifies for surgical interventions. These consist of arthroscopic cleaning, smoothing, and drilling out of the necrotic focus. Occasionally the lesions are emptied out and replaced with fresh or frozen grafts. Another possibility is replacement with tricortical iliac crest transplants with periosteum. Further operative treatment is tibial head correcting osteotomy, or unicompartmental medial joint arthroplasty. (Severe) secondary osteoarthritic destruction requires total joint arthroplasty.[21]

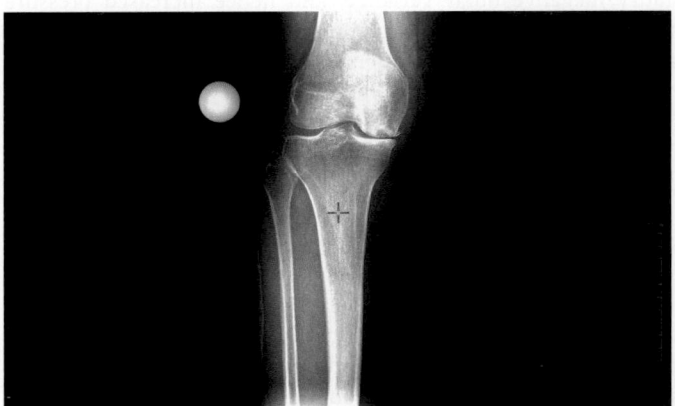

Fig. 148.3 Radiograph of osteonecrosis of the medial femoral condyle (Ahlbäck's disease).

Juvenile osteochondrosis and osteonecrosis

Osteochondrosis and osteonecrosis occur during growth in adolescence, in various locations at different ages. Affected areas are epiphyses, metaphyses and apophyses of the long bones, and enchondrally ossified bones of the wrist and foot. Here, too, the aetiology remains unknown. One hypothesis is that there is a transient mismatch between the arterial blood supply and the process of ossification during skeletal growth. In general, apart from aseptic osteonecrosis of the foot (Freiberg–Köhler and Köhler II disease) boys are more often affected than girls. The effects may be uni- or bilateral or occur simultaneously in different skeletal locations.[22] Pathophysiology, symptoms, and the course of the illness extend over months or years and—despite the various locations—are quite similar.

The disease occurs in four stages:

+ **Initial stage**: the necrosis of the osteocytes and the bony parts of the joints by means of disturbance of the blood supply may be noted. Relative to that, the further growth of the cartilage represents a mismatch in front of the concomitant joint swelling, which can be seen radiologically as an apparent widening of the joint space.

+ **Condensing stage**: radiologically the impaction of the bony parts of the joints can be seen because of the sintering of necrotic parts of the bones combined with hypermineralization.

+ **Fragmentation stage**: resorption of the necrotic parts occurs, while simultaneously reparative processes act with the formation of osteoid and fibrocartilage. Radiologically, flocculent resolution of the bone is noticed with osteolytic and sclerotic areas and the deformation of parts of the joint.

+ **Reparative stage**: new vital bone is formed and the fibrocartilage is remodelled to lamellar bone. The radiographs show aligned bone marrow structures.

Without therapy, various degrees of deformity occur after the healing process. The involvement of the joint surfaces represents a prearthrotic deformity. The destruction of the epiphyseal plate in children and adolescents leads to growth defects, which further increase the deformities. The most common osteonecroses of childhood and adolescence are localized in the lower extremity.

Juvenile osteochondrosis of the femoral head—Perthes' disease

The disease consist of the aseptic ischaemic necrosis of the ossification centre of the femoral head because of the perturbation of the blood supply in children of 4–8 years of age. Boys are four times more likely to be affected than girls. In terms of aetiology, disruption of the arterial blood supply, the intra-articular or intraosseus pressure increase, growth disturbance (retardation of the patient's skeletal age), coagulation defects, and genetic factors have all been proposed.

Clinically, from limping, pain, and a decrease in the range of motion of the hip joint (especially abduction and internal rotation) can be seen. The diagnosis is conformed by means of conventional radiographs and particularly by MRI.

The Caterall classification, which serves as a judgement tool for prognosis and therapy, divides the disease into four groups,

corresponding to the extent of the epiphyseal participation. The epiphysis is considered to be divided into four quadrants.

+ **Group I**: the anterolateral quadrant is affected.
+ **Group II**: the anterior one-third or one-half of the femoral head is affected.
+ **Group III**: up to 75% of the femoral head is affected; only the dorsal part remains intact.
+ **Group IV**: the entire femoral head is affected.

Groups I and II generally show a better prognosis, groups III and IV a poor one. Additionally the so-called 'head at risk signs' are considered:

+ lateral calcification of the epiphysis
+ metaphyseal involvement
+ Gage sign: a V-shaped brightening in the area of the lateral epiphysis and the adjacent metaphysis
+ horizontal positioning of the epiphyseal plate
+ lateral subluxation (of the femoral head out of the acetabulum).

Therapy depends on the clinical findings and the age of the child. The goal is to maintain the containment, the correct orientation of the femoral head in the acetabulum, and the spherical femoral head.

The onset of the disease before the age of 7 years is compatible with a reasonably good prognosis, and generally leads to conservative treatment. This usually means physiotherapy for many years. The orthoses used in the past did not lead to additional success. For groups III and IV, 'head at risk signs', children older than 7 years, or deterioration of the range of motion with physiotherapy, a surgical intervention should be considered. The best time for surgery is in the condensation or early fragmentation stage. Intertrochanteric osteotomy of the femur to centre the femoral head and to improve the abduction and adduction via the medialization of the femur with the resulting relaxation of the iliopsoas muscle is the usual choice. Alternatively pelvis osteotomies may be used for a better roof of the femoral head.

Osteochondrosis dissecans

Osteochondrosis dissecans is a subchondral osteonecrosis which in due course demarcates and may later show dissection with loose bodies in the joint. Mostly convex articular surfaces are affected, especially the femur condyles, the talus, and the capitulum of the humerus (Panner's disease) (Figure 148.4). Usually osteochondrosis dissecans occurs in older children, adolescents, or young adults. Boys and athletes are prone to the disease. In 30–40% the illness is bilateral. In general the symptoms consist of pain, limping (if a joint of the lower extremity is affected), and restricted range of motion. Should dissection already be present, entrapment may occur. Diagnostically, conventional radiographs and MRI are indicative.

In the knee joint the necrotic area is situated in the lateral part of the medial femur condyle in most cases. Scintigraphy is suited for the course of observation. Diagnostically, the chondral surfaces are best investigated by means of arthroscopy. Initial signs of a dissection beginning are changes of the colour (yellowish cartilage) or the findings when pressing the cartilage with a probe.

The aetiology remains unknown, although recurrent trauma may possibly play a key role.

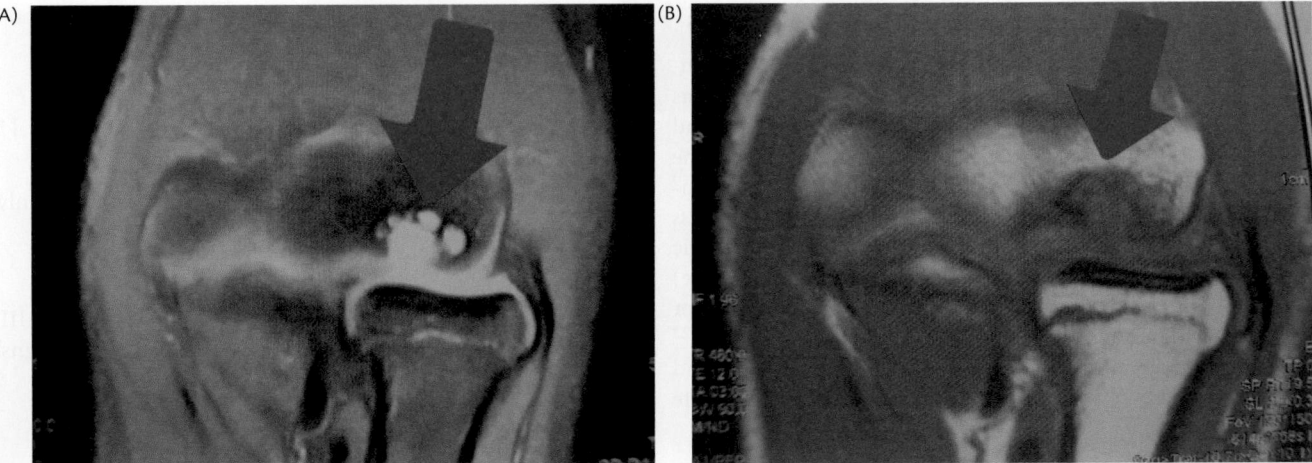

Fig. 148.4 MRI of osteochondrosis dissecans of the capitulum of the humerus (Panner's disease) in a 12 year old boy.

In the upper ankle joint most often the anterolateral surface of the talus, rarely the posteromedial part, is affected. The peak is found in the second decade of life, and boys are affected more often. In 10–25% the finding is bilateral. A common cause seem to be trauma (single events as well as repetitive microtrauma), but also deterioration of local blood supply, metabolic disorders, overweight, and family predisposition. Osteochondrosis dissecans increases the risk of developing osteoarthritis later. The prognosis depends on the age (the younger the better) and on the presence of a dissecate. In younger children with small necrotic areas and few complaints, the indication is for a conservative treatment with leg relief (crutches for 6–10 weeks/orthoses), physiotherapy, relative protection, and abstention from sports activities. Every 3 months a MRI reinvestigation is appropriate. In the presence of intact chondral surfaces, procedures for revascularization of the defect by means of retrograde bone marrow plastic or retrograde punching of the sclerotic area are indicated. In the case of a beginning dissection, debridement of the defect in combination with a solid refixation of the dissecate via screws, fibrin glue, or resorbable pins is appropriate. Autologous bone–cartilage grafting (dorsal femur condyle or lateral patella—alternatively, homologue from a cadaver) is necessary when large or non-vital defects are given. Older cartilage defects may benefit from Pridie drilling (anterograde for the ingrowth of vessels and the induction of surface-covering fibrocartilage). In case of deviation of the leg axes, osteotomies for the reduction of weightbearing by the knee may be considered.

Osteochondroses of the capitulum of the humerus (Panner's disease) generally affect boys in the 5–12 years age range. Here, too, repetitive microtrauma (frequent valgus loading of the elbow in tennis or throwing sports) and local disturbances of microcirculation seem to be the main reason for their development. The clinical signs are non-specific. Visible and palpable swelling of the joint, extension deficit, and rarely entrapment can be found. The diagnosis is normally confirmed by radiographs and MRI.

Therapy is mostly conservative. Temporary immobilization (dorsal cast of the arm) with the elbow situated in 90° flexion for a period of 3–4 weeks and anti-inflammatory medication are prescribed. Should more severe and persisting symptoms be demonstrated, arthroscopy may be indicated. The prognosis of the disease is benign, only rarely an extension lag of the elbow persists.

Bisphosphonate-associated osteonecrosis of the jaws

In recent years an increasing number of articles concerning bisphosphonate-associated osteonecrosis of the jaws have been published in the literature. The bisphosphonates are used mainly in the therapy of osteoporosis, Paget's disease, and tumour-induced hypercalcaemia, as well as skeletal metatases. The incidence of bisphosphonate-associated osteonecrosis of the jaws is estimated to be approximately 2–9%.[23–25] Risk factors are malignant disease, the relative potency of the medication in question (the highest risk for osteonecrosis of the jaws is represented by high-potency medications such as zoledronic acid) and the form of application, the duration of the therapy, extraction of teeth, or other oral surgical procedures such as root canal treatment.

Symptoms of a bisphosphonate-associated osteonecrosis of the jaws are non-specific and extend from non-symptomatic affections to extreme pain with loss of sensation. Clinically, signs similar to infections such as reddening, swelling, putrid secretion, and formation of abscesses may be seen, as well as exposed bone in the jaw with a yellow-brown colour and very hard composition. The surface of this may appear rough, typically in the area of extraction alveoli or in the alveolar crest, in the toothless jaw, or in the lateral area of the lower mandible teeth.

Diagnostically, in addition to panoramic radiographs to show the extent of the lesion and the accompanying infection, CT or MRI is indicated. A biopsy is recommended for a definite conformation of diagnosis and in order to exclude malignant tumours. The most important therapy concept, other than systemic antibiotics, is prevention. Before the use of bisphosphonates, dental presentation, with extraction of teeth not worthy of preservation, and the therapy of infectious sites, is imperative. Patients who are taking bisphosphonates regularly should see their dentist frequently.[26]

References

1. Rodrigue SW, Rosenthal DI, Barton NW, Zurakowski D, Mankin HJ. Risk factors for osteonecrosis in patients with type I Gaucher's disease. *Clin Orthop* 1999;362:201–207.
2. Yoo MC, Cho YJ, Lee SG. Bony lesions of professional divers in Korea. *J Korean Orthop Assoc* 1992;27:331–340.

3. Yamamoto T, DiCarlo EF, Bullough PG. The prevalence and clinico-pathological appearance of extension of osteonecrosis in the femoral head. *J Bone Joint Surg Br* 1999;81:328–332.

4. Jones JP. [Epidemiological risk factors for non-traumatic osteonecrosis]. *Orthopäde* 2000;29:370–379.

5. Mont MA, Hungerford DS. Non-traumatic avascular necrosis of the femoral head. *J Bone Joint Surg Am* 1995;77:459–474.

6. Stevens K, Tao C, Lee SU et al.. Subchondral fractures in osteonecrosis of the femoral head: comparison of radiography, CT, and MR imaging. *Am J Roentgenol* 2003;180:363–368.

7. Sakai T, Sugano N, Nishii T, Hananouchi T, Yoshikawa H. Extent of osteonecrosis on MRI predicts humeral head collapse. *Clin Orthop Relat Res* 2008;466:1074–1080.

8. Sarris I, Weiser R, Sotereanos DG. Pathogenesis and treatment of osteonecrosis of the shoulder. *Orthop Clin North Am* 2004;35(3):397–404.

9. Peste JL. Discussion. *Bull Soc Anat Paris* 1843;18:169.

10. Kienböck R. [Traumatic malacia of the lunate and its sequelae: compression fractures and degenerative forms.] *Fortschr Röntgenstrahlen* 1910;16:77–103.

11. Stahl S, Lotter O, Santos Stahl A et al. [100 years after Kienböck's description. Review of the etiology of Kienböck's disease from a historical perspective.] *Orthopäde* 2012;41(1):66–72.

12. Martini AK, Schiltenwolf M. A new classification of semilunar bone necrosis. *Handchir Mikrochir Plast Chir* 1998;30:151–157.

13. Rehart S. Shortening of the distal radius in Kienböcks's disease. In: DuParc J (ed.) *Surgical techniques in orthopaedics and traumatology Vol. 5, Wrist and hand*. Elsevier Masson, Paris, 2003.

14. Hofmann S, Mazieres B. [Osteonecrosis: natural course and conservative therapy] *Orthopäde* 2000;29:403–410.

15. Pape D, Kohn D. [Necrosis of the femoral head.] In: Scharf HP, Rüter A, Pohlemann T et al. (eds). *Orthopädie und Unfallchirurgie*. Elsevier, München, 2008:223–227.

16. Fairbank AC, Bhatiaw D, Jinnah RH, Hungerford DS. Long-term results of core decompression for ischemic necrosis of the femoral head. *J Bone Joint Surg Br* 1995;77:42–49.

17. Plenk H Jr, Hofmann S, Breitenseher M, Urban M. [Pathomorphological aspects and repair mechanisms of femur head necrosis.] *Orthopäde* 2000;29:389–402.

18. Hofmann S, Kramer J, Plank H. [Osteonecrosis of the hip (ON) in the adult.] *Orthopäde* 2005;34:171–184.

19. Ahlbäck S, Bauer GCH, Bohne WH. Spontaneous osteonecrosis of the knee. *Arthritis Rheum* 1968;11:705–733.

20. Aglietti P, Insall JN, Buzzi R, Dechamps G. Idiopathic osteonecrosis of the knee. *J Bone Joint Surg Am* 1983;65-B, 588–597.

21. Wirth CJ, Stukenborg-Colsman C, Wefer A. [Osteonecrosis of the femoral condyle]. *Orthopäde* 1998;27:501–507.

22. Petje G, Radler C, Aigner N, Kriegs-Au G, Ganger R, Grill F. [Aseptic osteonecrosis in childhood: diagnosis and treatment.] *Orthopäde* 2002;31:1027–1038.

23. Bamias A, Kastritis E, Bamia C et al.. Osteonecrosis of the jaw in cancer after treatment with bisphosphonates: incidence and risk factors. *J Clin Oncol* 2005;23:8580–8587.

24. Durie BG, Katz M, Crowley J. Osteonecrosis of the jaw and bisphosphonates. *N Engl J Med* 2005;353:99–102.

25. Mavrokokki T, Cheng A, Stein B, Goss A. Nature and frequency of bisphosphonate-associated osteonecrosis of the jaws in Australia. *J Oral Maxillofac Surg* 2007;65:415–423.

26. Dannemann C, Grätz KW, Zwahlen RA. [Bisphosphonate-associated osteonecrosis of the jaw.] *Schweiz Monatsschr Zahnmed* 2008;118:113–118.

CHAPTER 149

Renal osteodystrophy

Thomas Bardin and Tilman Drüeke

Introduction

Renal osteodystrophy (ROD) is a term that encompasses the various consequences of chronic kidney disease (CKD) for the bone. It has been divided into several entities based on bone histomorphometry observations. ROD is accompanied by several abnormalities of mineral metabolism: abnormal levels of serum calcium, phosphorus, parathyroid hormone (PTH), vitamin D metabolites, alkaline phosphatases, fibroblast growth factor-23 (FGF-23) and klotho, which all have been identified as cardiovascular risk factors in patients with CKD.[1,2] The term CKD mineral and bone disorder (CKD-MBD) has been proposed by the KDIGO group (Kidney Disease: Improving Global Outcome).[3] It is meant to describe the entire systemic disorder of mineral and bone metabolism associated with CKD manifested by either one or a combination of the following: (1) abnormalities of calcium, phosphorus, PTH, or vitamin D metabolism, (2) abnormalities in bone turnover, mineralization, volume, linear growth, or strength, (3) vascular or other soft tissue calcification.[3]

Renal osteodystrophy

ROD can presently be schematically divided into three main types by histology: (1) osteitis fibrosa as the bony expression of secondary hyperparathyroidism (sHP), which is a high bone turnover disease developing early in CKD; (2) adynamic bone disease (ABD), the most frequent type of ROD in dialysis patients,[4,5] which is at present most often observed in the absence of aluminium intoxication and develops mainly as a result of excessive PTH suppression; and (3) mixed ROD, a combination of osteitis fibrosa and osteomalacia whose prevalence has decreased in the last decade. Pure osteomalacia has become exceptional in CKD patients.

Skeletal resistance to PTH is an important and early feature of CKD, which has been evidenced by the lower than normal hypercalcaemic response to PTH infusions in CKD patients. It can be explained by several factors (Box 149.1).[6–7] As PTH is the main stimulant of bone turnover, higher than normal serum levels of PTH are required to maintain normal bone turnover in CKD patients with PTH resistance.[8]

Secondary hyperparathyroidism

Osteitis fibrosa due to sHP is a naturally occurring type of ROD and develops early on in the course of CKD. A cross-sectional study of a large unreferred CKD patient cohort in the United States found increased serum 'intact' PTH levels (>65 pg/mL; normal, 10–65 pg/mL) in 12% of patients with an eGFR greater than 80 mL/min, and 56% of those with an eGFR less than 60 mL/min.[9] The international KDIGO CKD-MBD guideline recommends starting serum PTH measurements when the creatinine clearance decreases below 60 mL/min (CKD stage 3) in order to avoid, by implementing appropriate measures, the deleterious consequences of a progressively worsening sHP.[10]

Pathophysiology of secondary hyperparathyroidism
Endstage chronic kidney disease

Numerous factors explain the development of sHP in most patients with advanced CKD when preventive measures are not undertaken (Figure 149.1). Classical aetiological factors, which have been the main therapeutic targets for many years, include hyperphosphataemia, insufficient 1,25-dihydroxyvitamin D (1,25 diOH D) production, and a negative calcium balance. Hyperphosphataemia plays an important part in advanced renal failure.[11] It induces hypocalcaemia by favouring soft tissue precipitation of calcium in the form of calcium phosphate, decreases the activity of renal 1α-OH-vitamin D hydroxylase and directly stimulates parathyroid cell proliferation and PTH secretion. Decreased renal synthesis of 1,25 diOH D is due to nephron reduction, hyperphosphataemia, metabolic acidosis, and the presence of uraemic toxins.[12] It leads to decreased intestinal calcium absorption, which favours hypocalcaemia and in turn enhanced PTH secretion. Reduced tissue expression of the vitamin D receptor (VDR) due to uraemic toxins and other mechanisms further contributes to enhanced parathyroid cell proliferation and

---

Box 149.1 Main mechanisms of uraemic bone resistance to PTH

- Decrease of 1,25-dihydroxyvitamin D production
- Decrease of osteoblast PTH receptors
- Progressive increase of serum osteoprotegerin, which impairs bone response to PTH (osteoprotegerin being very high in dialysis patients)
- Presence of PTH fragment 7–84 in uraemic serum, having opposite effects to those of PTH, i.e. lowering serum calcium and inhibiting bone resorption.

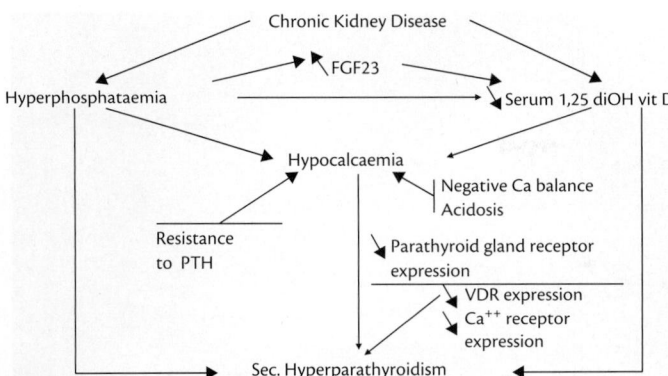

Fig. 149.1 Pathophysiology of secondary hyperparathyroidism in endstage kidney disease.

PTH oversecretion by a transcriptional mechanism.[13] The reduced VDR expression, together with reduced calcium sensing receptor (CaR) expression,[14] particularly in nodular areas of the hyperplastic parathyroid glands, is indicative of the presence of clonally growing, tumoural sHP,[15] which has escaped physiological control and become refractory to medical treatment. In 24% of parathyroid tumours removed from dialysis patients who underwent parathyroid surgery for refractory sHP, chromosomal abormalities were observed, characterized by both allelic losses and gains.[16]

Early stages of renal disease

In early CKD, a different sequence of mineral disturbances is involved in the pathophysiology of sHP. The predominant role of FGF-23 has been progressively recognized in recent years. It now appears that an increase in serum FGF-23 levels is the first reaction of the organism to prevent an increase in serum phosphate during the early stages of CKD, some time before the well-known increase in PTH secretion.[17] Owing to these two defence mechanisms, phosphate retention secondary to a progressively reduced renal excretory capacity is avoided until CKD stages 4–5 (corresponding to creatinine clearances <30 to <15 mL/min), and hyperphosphataemia becomes a late event. FGF-23 is secreted by osteoblasts and osteocytes and targets FGF receptor–α-klotho complexes in the kidney to inhibit both renal phosphate reabsorption and production of 1,25 diOH D. The latter effect favours sHP. A study of the disturbances of mineral metabolism in early CKD has suggested that inappropriate postprandial calciuria with episodic hypocalcaemia may represent an additional mechanism contributing to sHP.[18] Another important mechanism is the early decrease in renal 1,25 diOH D synthesis as a consequence of increased serum FGF-23 levels, reduced nephron mass, and impaired substrate availability.[19] Vitamin D deficiency is frequent in CKD patients and may also contribute to sHP via reduced 1,25 diOH D synthesis.[19] Last but not least, the occurrence of skeletal resistance to PTH also plays a role.[6,7] Of note, in CKD there is also a partial resistance to the action of FGF23, owing to downregulation of both FGF receptor-1 and α-klotho in various tissues, including the parathyroid gland and the kidney.[20,21]

Clinical, biochemical, imaging, and pathological features of secondary hyperparathyroidism

Clinically, sHP is most often asymptomatic although severe disease can cause mechanical bone pain, arthralgias, myalgias, and

an erosive enthesopathy which put the patient at risk of tendon rupture. Systemic features include asthenia, pruritus, pancreatitis hypertension, cardiac failure, and erythropoietin-resistant anaemia. Cardiovascular mortality is increased, even when sHP is moderate in predialysis CKD stages.[22]

Laboratory features include increased serum levels of PTH and bone turnover markers such as total and bone alkaline phosphatases, osteocalcin, and several products of type I collagen metabolism products.[23] Serum phosphorus is increased only in CKD stages 4–5.[9] Serum calcium levels are variable. They may be low initially, but hypercalcaemia develops in case of severe sHP. Serum 25-OH-vitamin D (25OHD) levels are generally below 30 ng/mL, indicating vitamin D insufficiency or deficiency.[24]

Radiography shows subperisostal bone resorption which is particularly well expressed at the radial border of the second phalanges of the second and third fingers (Figure 149.2) where radiographic and histological features are best correlated. Resorption of the third phalangeal ends is an early feature of severe sHP and can lead to distal osteolysis translating clinically into a pseudo-hippocratism (Figure 149.3). Subchondral bone resorption (Figure 149.4) causes widening of pubic symphysis and sacroiliac and acromioclavicular joint spaces. In the axial skeleton, bone resorption and formation frequently coexist, leading to a 'salt-and-pepper' appearance of the skull (Figure 149.5) and the so-called 'rugger jersey' vertebrae in which condensed plates contrast with low density of the central parts. In severe cases, bone condensation can result in a rare pseudo-pagetic aspect, which, in contrast to true Paget's disease, involves the whole axial skeleton. Brown tumours due to sHP should be differentiated from amyloid erosions which always involve articular areas. Soft tissue calcifications, in particular vascular (Figure 149.6), valvular, periarticular (Figure 149.7), cutaneous, and eye calcification, may develop and should be taken into account for management.

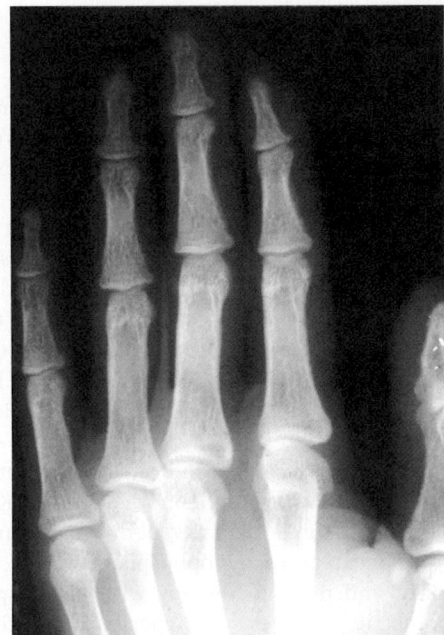

Fig. 149.2 Subperiosteal bone resorption at the radial aspect of the second phalanges in secondary hyperparathyroidism.

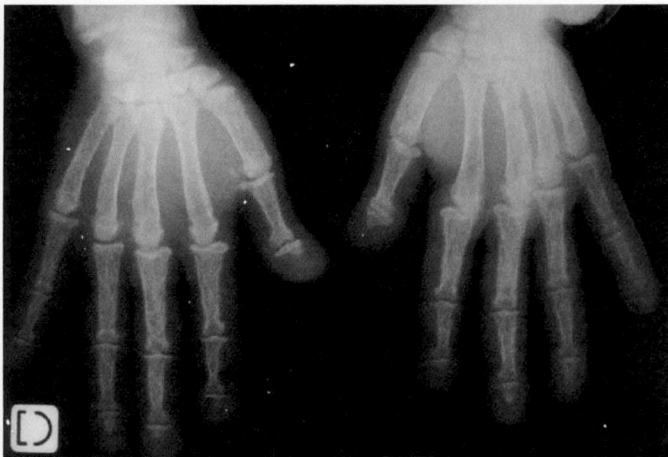

Fig. 149.3 Severe secondary hyperparathyroidism with massive lysis of third phalange.

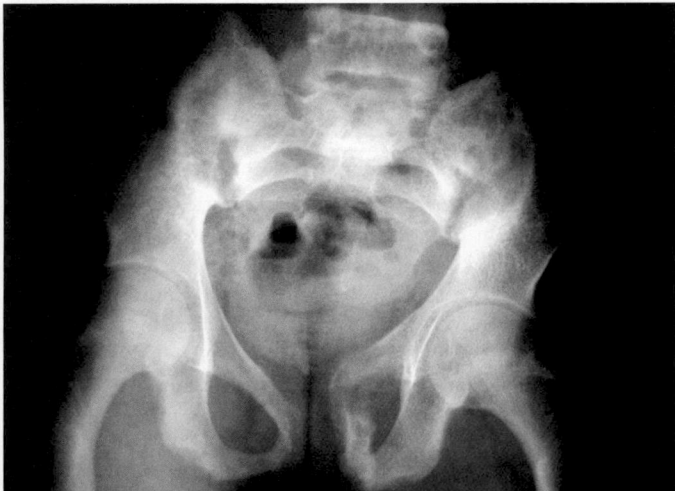

Fig. 149.4 Subchondral bone resorption at the sacro-iliac joint and pubic symphysis.

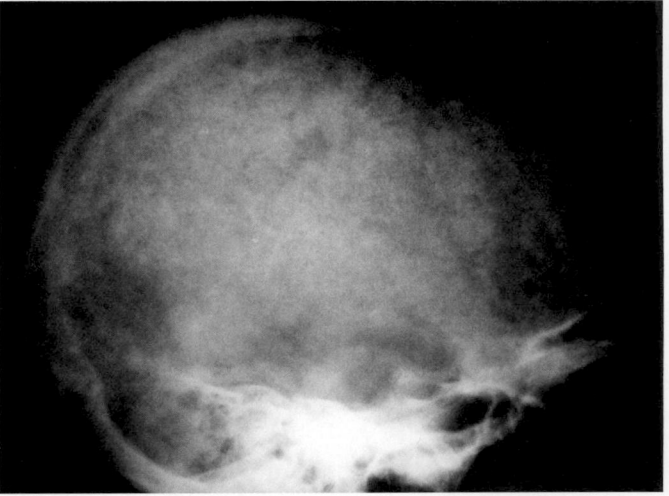

Fig. 149.5 Radiograph of the skull in chronic haemodialysis patient with secondary hyperparathyroidism.

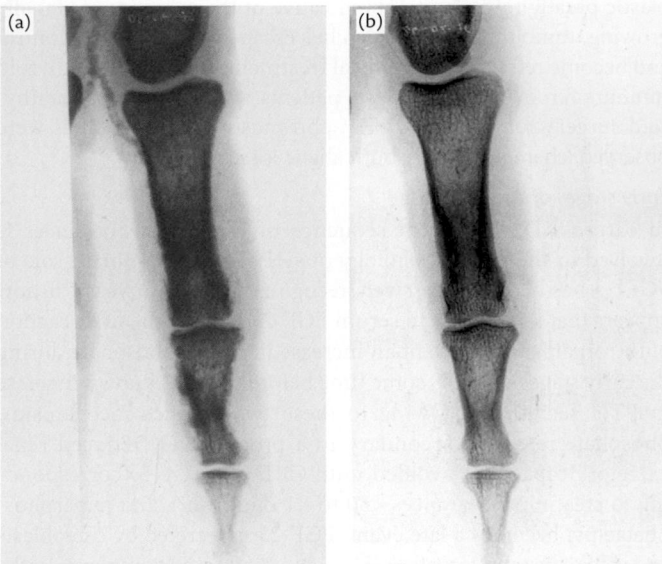

Fig. 149.6 Vascular calcification in female adult haemodialysis patient with severe secondary hyperparathyroidism: (a) before parathyroidectomy (PTX); (b) 12 months after PTX.

Bone scan demonstrates an increased uptake of technetium-99m pyrophosphate or bisphosphonate in the axial skeleton resulting for increased bone turnover.[25] It also can pick up large extraskeletal calcifications.

Parathyroid gland imaging is useful for the indication of parathyroidectomy, especially in the case of recurrent sHP. Ultrasound is the first-line technique but generally misses ectopic glands. CT and/MRI can be used to visualize ectopic glands but often cannot differentiate parathyroid tissue from lymph node or thyroid nodule. Scintigraphy using ^{99m}Tc sestamibi coupled with ^{123}I is the most specific technique. It allows detection of parathyroid tissue with a false-positive rate inferior to 5%.[26]

Transiliac bone biopsy is seldom indicated at present in clinical practice. It should, however, be done more often in CKD patients with unexplained fractures, persistent bone pain, unexplained hypercalcaemia, unexplained hypophosphataemia, possible aluminium toxicity, and prior to therapy with bisphosphonates.[10] Histomorphometric features of hyperparathyroidism (HP) (Figure 149.8) include increased bone resorption and formation and bone marrow fibrosis.[27]

Management of secondary hyperparathyroidism
Target PTH

Because of the skeletal resistance to PTH, greater than normal serum levels of PTH are required for normal bone turnover. In dialysis patients, the 2003 American KDOQI guidelines recommended serum 'intact' PTH to be maintained between 150 and 300 pg/mL.[8] The more recent (2009) international KDIGO guideline recommends serum PTH levels to be maintained in the range of approximately 2–9 times the upper normal normal limit of the assay and to intervene only in case of significant changes in PTH levels.[10] This wider PTH target range followed changes in the immunoassays used, the awareness of major interassay and intraindividual variability of PTH measurements,[28,29] and the demonstration that normal bone turnover was not accurately predicted by the KDOQI targeted values (see below).

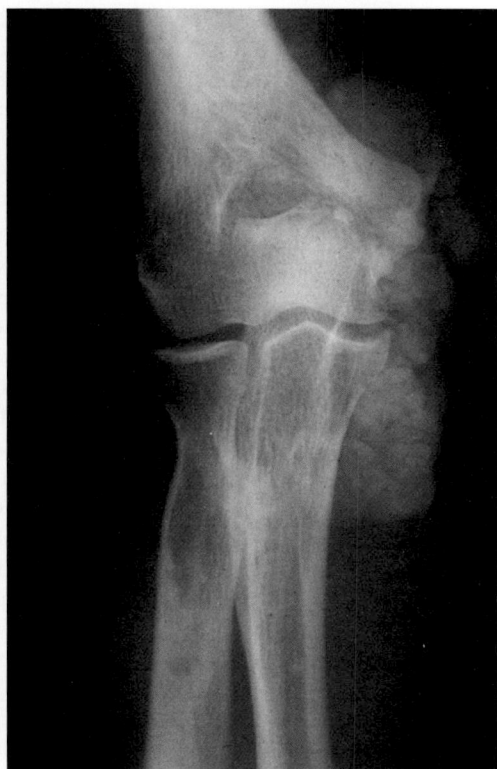

Fig. 149.7 Pericarticular calcification in a chronic haemodialysis patient.

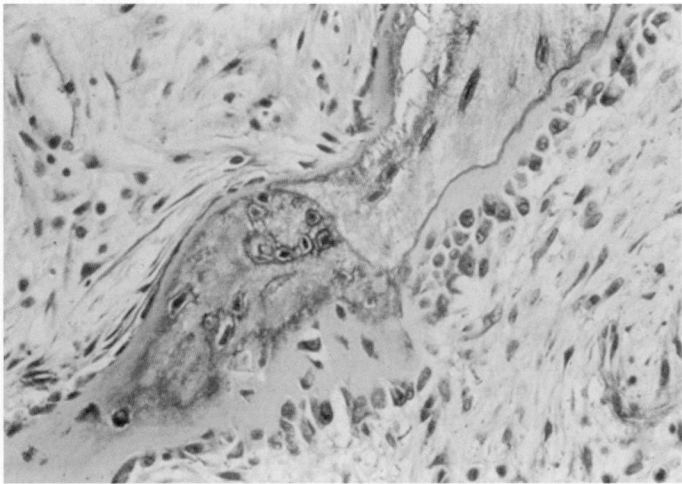

Fig. 149.8 Severe osteitis fibrosa (chronic haemodialysis patient).
Courtesy of Dr Giulia Cournot-Witmer.

Calcium intake

Because the most active form of vitamin D is reduced in CKD, intestinal calcium absorption is low. It is generally recommended that calcium intake should be up to 2 g per day including intake with food and administration of calcium supplements or calcium-containing phosphate binders. The KDIGO guideline suggests caution in prescribing the latter in presence of extraskeletal calcification and/or adynamic bone and strongly recommends refraining from their administration in the presence of hypercalcaemia [10]

Control of hyperphosphataemia

Reduction of serum phosphorus towards the normal range in patients with endstage kidney failure has become a major

objective.[10] Therapeutic means include a decrease in dietary phosphate intake to 800–1000 mg/day, but without inducing a protein deficiency state. It should be implemented as soon as hyperphosphataemia occurs. However, rigid dietary restriction is rarely followed in the long term and carries the risk of malnutrition. Renal replacement therapies allow elimination of phosphate, which can be improved by increasing dialysis performance. The most efficacious means remains the use of oral phosphate binders which reduce the availability of phosphate for intestinal absorption (Box 149.2). Aluminium-containing binders are a potential source of aluminium intoxication and are contraindicated except for short periods of time.[10] By the 1990s, they had been replaced by calcium-containing binders. When taken with meals, calcium salts have been said to form poorly absorbed complexes with dietary phosphorus, but much of the unbound calcium is nevertheless absorbed. Calcium carbonate provides bicarbonate, which is useful against metabolic acidosis, and has been widely used in France. Large doses, especially when prescribed together with vitamin D sterols, are a source of hypercalcaemia and extraskeletal calcification. KDOQI therefore recommended that doses of elemental calcium should not exceed 1.5 g/day. Aluminium-free, calcium-free phosphate binders should be preferentially used when calcium-containing chelators are not sufficient or contraindicated. Sevelamer hydrochloride (Renagel) was the first to be developed. It appears as effective as calcium carbonate, while inducing less hypercalcaemia and cardiovascular calcification.[30] Sevelamer carbonate has been introduced more recently in an attempt to increase serum bicarbonate. Lanthanum carbonate is an alternative which has shown similar efficacy in reducing hyperphosphataemia.[31] However, these new phosphate binders are costly and their superiority over calcium-containing binders in delaying the progression of vascular calcification and hard clinical outcomes remains a matter of debate.

Native vitamin D and vitamin D derivatives (Box 149.3)

Vitamin D depletion is found in about one-half of endstage renal disease patients.[24] It is associated with poor survival in CKD patients.[32] However, such associations based on retrospective, uncontrolled studies do not prove a causal relationship. The effect of native vitamin D supplements on hard patient outcomes remains so far uncertain. It seems nevertheless reasonable to correct vitamin D insufficiency/deficiency in CKD patients.[10] This may increase serum 1,25 diOH D even in dialysis patients with only minimal or no excretory kidney function,[33] suggesting that vitamin D depletion, together with poor renal or extrarenal 1-α-25OH vitamin D hydroxylase activity plays a role in the pathogenesis of sHP. Once sHP has developed, active vitamin D derivatives such as alfacalcidol or calcitriol are indicated in order to halt its progression. These drugs are generally given orally but the IV route during dialysis sessions is also possible. Note that excessive doses

---

Box 149.2 Oral phosphate binders used in patients with CKD

- Aluminium hydroxide
- Calcium carbonate and calcium acetate
- Magnesium hydroxide and magnesium carbonate
- Sevelamer hydrochloride and sevelamer carbonate
- Lanthanum carbonate

Box 149.3 Vitamin D sterols used in patients with CKD

- Cholecalciferol (vitamin D_3)
- Ergocalciferol (vitamin D_2)
- Calcidiol (25 hydroxy vitamin D_3)
- Calcitriol (1,25 dihydroxy vitamin D_3)
- Alfacalcidol (1α hydroxy vitamin D_3)
- Paricalcitol (19-nor-1α,25 dihydroxy vitamin D_2)
- Doxercalciferol (1α-hydroxy vitamin D_2)

---

of active vitamin D derivatives increase the serum Ca × P product and may induce ABD by oversuppression of PTH secretion. Serum calcium, phosphorus, and iPTH levels should be closely monitored and these compounds should be avoided in case of hypercalcaemia, extraskeletal calcification, and low PTH levels.[10] Vitamin D analogues such as paracalcitol (19-nor-1α,25 $(OH)_2D_2$), maxacalcitol (22-oxa-calcitriol), and doxercalciferol (1α-(OH)D2) can also be used and decrease PTH secretion to a similar degree. However, the claim that they are less hypercalcaemic and induce ABD less often remains unproven.[34]

Calcimimetics

The finding that the calcium sensing receptor (CaR) is expressed in parathyroid cells and the discovery of drugs able to activate this receptor (CaR agonists or calcimimetics) has opened a new avenue in the management of sHP. Cinacalcet-HCl (Mimpara) has been approved for the management of sHP in dialysis patients. Cinacalcet is administered orally. In most instances, a dose of 30–60 mg/day is sufficient. Randomized controlled trials (RCTs) have shown that cinacalcet allows to reach target PTH values in 56% of patients, compared with only 10% of control patients receiving optimal standard therapy.[35] In contrast to the latter, cinacalcet not only decreases serum PTH levels but also reduces serum calcium and phosphorus. The occurrence of transient hypocalcaemia is an indication for increased calcium and/or vitamin D sterol intake, thereby improving cinacalcet effectiveness. Cinacalcet use has been found to be associated with a lower frequency of parathyroidectomy, bone fractures, hospitalization rate for cardiovascular causes, and an improvement in quality of life. An RCT is under way aimed at confirming such beneficial effects prospectively. The most frequent side effects, in addition to hypocalcaemia, are nausea and vomiting. In the majority of patients, these adverse effects disappear after prolonged administration.

Parathyroidectomy

Parthyroidectomy (PTX) should be considered when facing sHP refractory to medical management. Before the availability of calcimimetic drugs, PTX, which is rarely performed in non-dialysis patients, was indicated in dialysis patients at a yearly rate of approximately 1–3%, which increased with dialysis vintage. The most frequent indications were the persistence of very high serum PTH level (>800 pg/mL) after a 6–8 week trial of active vitamin D sterol treatment or the coexistence of refractory hypercalcaemia and/or hyperphosphataemia with soft tissue calcifications contraindicating the use of vitamin D derivatives. The degree of parathyroid gland hyperplasia was also taken into accounts, as very large glands often contain areas of monoclonal growth and are less sensitive to medical

management.[15] Calcimimetics, which can now be prescribed in settings where vitamine D derivatives are contraindicated, appear to lower the rate of parathyroidectomy; however, this needs to be confirmed by long-term trials which should also evaluate the cost-effectivenes of calcimimetics as compared to PTX.

Aluminium-induced bone diseases

Aluminium osteopathy is a dramatic disease. It is associated with bone pain and frequently leads to fractures of various bones, including the upper ribs which are rarely affected by other causes of bone frailty. The elimination of aluminium contamination of the dialysis fluid and the avoidance of aluminium-containing phosphate binders has practically led to the disappearance of aluminium intoxication in developed countries. Classically, there were two types of aluminium-induced osteopathy: osteomalacia and ABD. They shared three pathological features, including (1) presence of aluminium deposits at the mineralized bone–osteoid interface, (2) a major decrease in osteoblast number along bone trabeculae, and (3) a massive slowdown of mineralization speed.[36] Aluminium-induced osteomalacia, characterized by an additional accummumation of non-mineralized osteoid (Figure 149.9), was the first recognized type. It was clinically the most severe form and arose after massive aluminium intoxication through contamination of the dialysate in a number of dialysis centres.[37] ABD, which differs from osteomalacia by the lack of excess osteoid, was identified later. It usually resulted from less severe aluminium intoxication following chronic ingestion of aluminium-containing phosphate binders. In general, it was clinically less severe although it could also be associated with proximal limb pain, myopathy and fractures. The main mechanism by which aluminium is involved in decreased bone turnover was believed to originate via aluminium deposits in the parathyroid glands. The resulting impairment of PTH production would then lead to low bone turnover. PTX has been shown to worsen the consequences of aluminium intoxication on bone and is contraindicated in the presence of significant aluminium intoxication.

The diagnosis of aluminium intoxication can be made by aluminium staining of a bone biopsy or by measuring excessive levels of aluminium in the blood, either spontaneously or after deferoxamine infusion. Management relies on the cessation of the intoxication and on regular infusions of deferoxamine.

Non-aluminium-associated adynamic bone disease

ABD, in the absence of aluminium intoxication, has become the most frequent type of renal osteodystrophy in both haemodialysis and peritoneal dialysis patients since the end of the 20th century.[5,38,39] The main aetiological factor appears to be excessive iatrogenic PTH suppression, resulting in serum PTH levels too low to maintain normal bone turnover. The disease should be preventable by targeting serum PTH levels at values 2–9 times above the normal range.[10] This should go along with a normal bone turnover despite the resistance of the uraemic skeleton to PTH. Other factors of ABD include diabetes mellitus and old age.

In dialysis patients, the diagnosis is suspected when serum 'intact' PTH levels are below 150 pg/mL and serum bone turnover markers are decreased.[10] However, levels of PTH within the target range have been observed in patients with histological evidence of ABD.[5] The imperfection and lack of standardization of presently available assays to measure PTH are probably one of the reasons for this failure.[28] The so-called 'intact' PTH assays not only recognize the whole

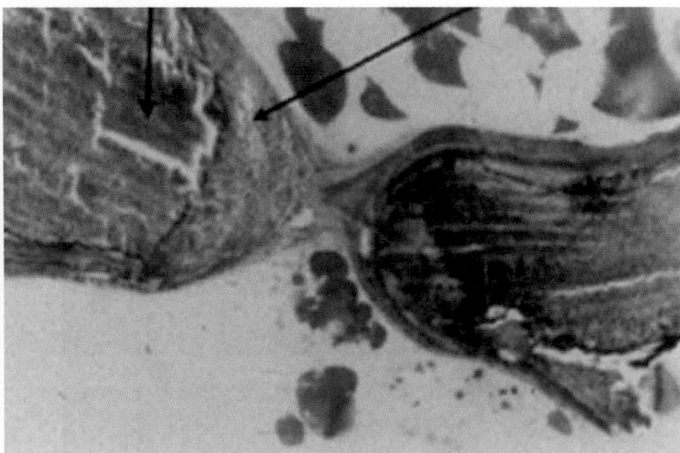

Fig. 149.9 Aluminium-associated osteomalacia.
Courtesy of Dr Giulia Cournot-Witmer.

hormone but also its 7–84 fragment and other fragments, which accumulate in renal failure and may contribute to the pathogenesis of ABD. The 7–84 fragment has been shown to exert an effect on serum calcium opposite to that of whole PTH and is believed to play a part in the skeletal resistance to the hormone in CKD. Reliable measurement methods of serum levels of the whole PTH molecule and of the 7–84 PTH fragment, respectively, are needed to improve the diagnosis, treatment, and prevention of ABD.

Its prevalence has been estimated to be 5–30% in non-dialysis CKD patients, and to reach even higher levels in dialysis patients, with variations according to dialysis technique: 32–40% in haemodialysis patients and 48–65% in those treated by peritoneal dialysis.[4,39] The latter difference can be explained by generally higher serum calcium levels in peritoneal dialysis patients with easier suppression of PTH secretion.

Non-aluminium-associated ABD is most frequently asymptomatic. The risk of hypercalcaemia and of extraskeletal calcifications is important in case of excessive prescription of oral calcium and/or vitamin D sterols, reflecting decreased bone buffering capacity. Consequences in terms of bone fragility remain debatable. In children, adynamic bone exposes to delayed skeletal growth. Management is difficult. Prescription of calcium-containing phosphate binders should be limited in patients with ABD to avoid a positive calcium balance and vascular calcifications. This favours the use of non-aluminium-, non-calcium-containing chelators to control hyperphosphataemia. Lowering the calcium concentration of the dialysate allows the stimulation of parathyroid gland activity.

Hyperphosphataemia

Hyperphosphataemia is a very frequent feature in CKD stages 4–5 and 5D (dialysis). It is observed in association with all types of renal osteodystrophy. A nationwide American study has shown that an increase of serum phosphorus above 5.0 mg/dL was associated with a significant increase in relative mortality risk, which was independent of serum PTH and calcium.[40] A recent review has concluded that the risk of death increased by 18% for every 1 mg/dL increase in serum phosphorus. Hyperphosphataemia is a source of sHP and a major contributor to extraskeletal, in particular vascular calcifications (see below). The control of hyperphosphataemia is a major objective of CKD patient management. The recent KDIGO guideline suggests lowering the serum phosphorus levels of CKD stage 5D patients towards the normal range.[10]

Extraskeletal calcification

Periarticular deposits of basic calcium phosphate are frequent in end stage kidney disease patients (Figure 149.7). They are favoured by hyperphosphataemia and hypercalcaemia, dialysis vintage, and high active vitamin D sterol doses. Deposits are frequently multiple and may induce acute inflammatory episodes.[41]

The prevalence and incidence of vascular and valvular calcification are also greatly increased in CKD patients. The calcification often appears at a much younger age than in the population at large. This has been well illustrated by several studies, including the one by Goodman et al.[42] who demonstrated an elevated frequency (21/39) and rapid progression of coronary artery calcification in children and young adults on dialysis, and by Shroff et al.[43] who observed an increase in arterial calcium load already in the predialysis stage of uraemic children. An increase in coronary calcification has also been observed in the earlier stages of adult CKD patients. This matter is a subject of considerable interest as vascular calcification has been shown to contribute to the poor cardiovascular outcome of patients wih CKD.[44]

Vascular calcification (Figure 149.10) most often involves the intima, where it associates with atherosclerotic plaques. It occurs at all stages of CKD and increases with the progression of CKD.[45] Atherosclerotic plaques have been shown to be more calcified in patients with CKD stages 4–5 and 5D than in age-matched controls. Vascular calcifications of CKD patients may also involve the media. They generally occur only at the stage of dialysis, with particularly high prevalence in CKD patients with diabetes. Medial calcification leads to arterial stiffness via the loss of vessel wall elasticity and associates with a marked increase in the relative risk of mortality, as does intimal calcification linked to atherosclerosis.[44]

A number of factors are associated with the development of vascular calcifications in CKD patients. Decreased concentrations of several inhibitors such as fetuin A and pyrophosphate, together with increased concentrations of promoters such as calcium, phosphate, vitamin D, and many others all play a role. Vitamin K deficiency has also been incriminated more recently. Vitamin K favours gamma-carboxylation and thus activation of matrix gla protein, another important inhibitor of vascular calcification. Arterial calcification is also a cell-mediated phenomenon involving the transformation of vascular smooth muscle cells into chondroblast- and osteoblast-like cells. In-vitro studies have shown that hyperphosphataemia plays a major role in this active process, as the elevation of phosphorus concentration in the culture medium resulted in the increase of various soluble mediators, appearance of osteoblasts, and calcification of the artery wall. Bone and mineral disorders including hyperphosphataemia, hypercalcaemia, renal osteodystrophy, and its management by calcium and vitamin D supplements play an important part. Of interest, studies have shown an inverse relationship between bone mineralization status and arterial calcification in patients with CKD, as has long been demonstrated in general population. A study pointed out the importance of bone activity in the occurrence of vascular calcification in association with a high calcium load which was shown to have a particularly important influence on aortic calcification in presence of ABD. A likely explanation was that the adynamic bone lost its buffering capacity

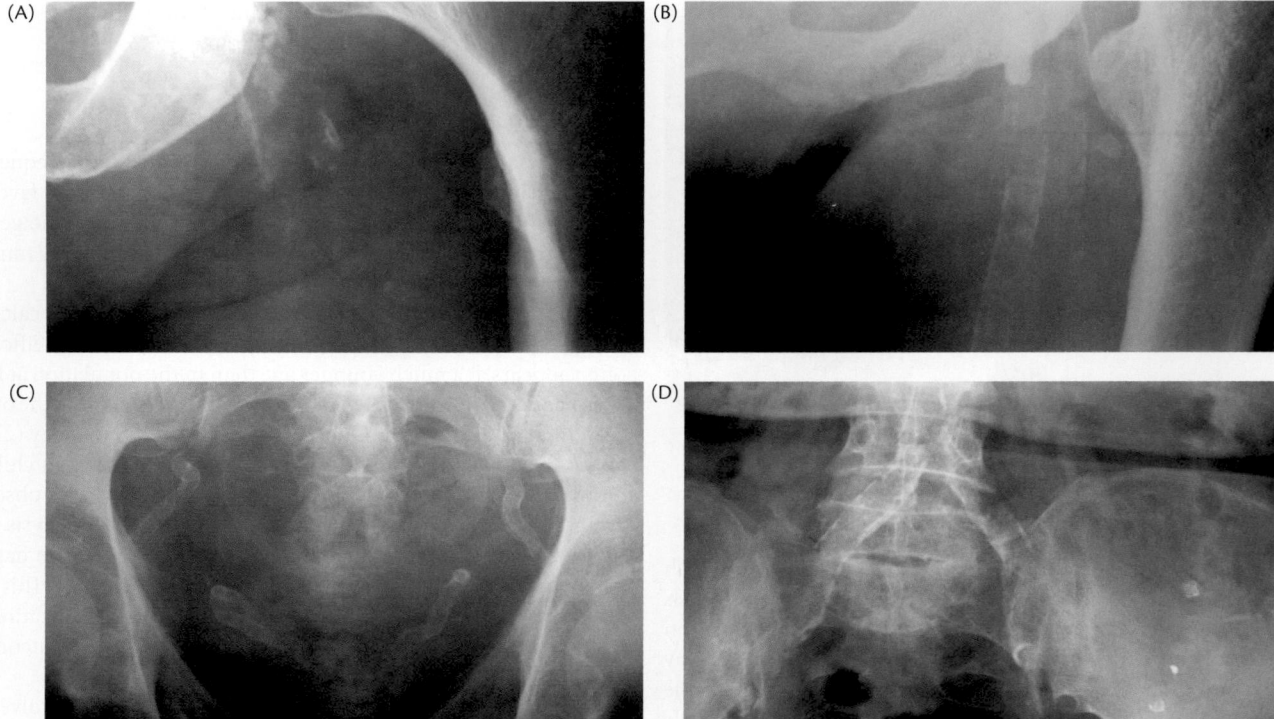

Fig. 149.10 Intima and media calcifications.

Reproduced from London GM et al, Arterial media calcification in end-stage renal disease: Impact on all-cause and cardiovascular mortality. Nephrol Dial Transplant. 2003;18:1731–40, by permission of Oxford University Press.

for calcium, therefore favouring hypercalcaemia and extraskeletal calcifications in response to large amounts of ingested calcium.

Osteoporosis

Bone mineral density (BMD) decreases in parallel with the progression of CKD.[46] Several transversal studies have shown a decrease of BMD in haemodialysis patients, in particular at the distal forearm as lumbar osteoarthritis and aorta calcification can lead to an overestimate of BMD at the lumbar spine. However, BMD imaging is not considered to be useful in patients with CKD stages 5–5D since a marked decrease in mineral density does not allow one to differentiate between severe ostitis fibrosa and ABD.[10] In difficult cases a bone biopsy is still recommended.

Fracture rate is increased in dialysis patients, as shown by a national American study which observed a relative risk of femoral neck fracture of 4.44 in men and 4.40 in women in dialysis patients as compared to an age- and sex- matched control population.[47]

Studies have identified various risk factors of fracture in dialysis patients.[48] These include duration of survival under dialysis, presence of peripheral arteriopathy, and, most importantly, factors known to play a role in the population at large: age, sex, white skin colour, impaired muscle strength, low body mass index, and cigarette smoking. Low BMD increased fracture risk in some, but not all studies. Early menopause, which is frequent in CKD, is another important factor of decreased BMD in women on maintenance dialysis. Steroid treatment that patients may have received for the management of their renal disease or during a previous kidney transplantation also plays an obvious role. Whereas aluminium-induced osteomalacia was clearly associated with an major fracture risk, the role of the two presently observed major types of renal osteodystrophy—sHP and non-aluminium-associated ABD—is more difficult to ascertain.

Some authors failed to observe an influence of serum PTH in their important American registry study, whereas other investigators observed an increased fracture rate in patients with low serum PTH levels, a negative correlation between serum PTH level and BMD, or an elevated fracture rate in patients with sHP. Vascular calcification is also associated with vertebral fractures.

Management of osteoporosis in endstage kidney disease patients is a difficult challenge. General measures such as exercise and satisfactory nutritional status are frequently difficult to implement. Excessive long-term phosphorus restriction through a low-protein diet may increase the risk of osteoporosis.[49] Vitamin D-deficient patients should be supplemented with vitamin D. Serum calcium levels should be maintained within the normal range according to KDOQI and KDIGO guidelines, and the KDOQI guidelines recommended a total elemental calcium intake of not more than 2 g/day to reduce the risk of extraskeletal calcification in patients with CKD stages 3–5.[10] Serum PTH levels should be kept in the target range.

Oestrogen replacement in young women with early menopause is usually advised, but the risk of breast cancer and cardiovascular toxicity should be carefully weighed against their use. Bisphosphonates, which may induce ABD, and strontium ranelate are not approved in these patients. Raloxifene has been found to improve BMD in postmenopausal women on haemodialysis therapy,[50] but is known to increase the risk of arteriovenous thromboembolism.

References

1. Floege J, Kim J, Ireland E, Chazot C et al.. Serum iPTH, calcium and phosphate, and the risk of mortality in a European haemodialysis population. *Nephrol Dial Transplant* 2011;26:1948–1955.
2. Isakova T, Xie H, Yang W et al. Fibroblast growth factor 23 and risks of mortality and end-stage renal disease in patients with chronic kidney disease. *JAMA* 2011;305:2432–2439.

3. Moe SM, Drueke T, Lameire N, Eknoyan G. Chronic kidney disease-mineral-bone disorder: a new paradigm. *Adv Chronic Kidney Dis* 2007;14:3–12.

4. Sherrard DJ, Hercz G, Pei Y et al. The spectrum of bone disease in end-stage renal failure—an evolving disorder. *Kidney Int* 1993;43:436–442.

5. Barreto FC, Barreto DV, Moyses RM et al. K/DOQI-recommended intact PTH levels do not prevent low-turnover bone disease in hemodialysis patients. *Kidney Int* 2008;73:771–777.

6. Urena P, Ferreira A, Morieux C, Drueke T, de Vernejoul MC. PTH/PTHrP receptor mRNA is down-regulated in epiphyseal cartilage growth plate of uraemic rats. *Nephrol Dial Transplant* 1996;11:2008–2016.

7. Kazama JJ, Shigematsu T, Yano K et al. Increased circulating levels of osteoclastogenesis inhibitory factor (osteoprotegerin) in patients with chronic renal failure. *Am J Kidney Dis* 2002;39:525–532.

8. K/DOQI clinical practice guidelines for bone metabolism and disease in chronic kidney disease. *Am J Kidney Dis* 2003;42:S1–S01.

9. Levin A, Bakris GL, Molitch M et al. Prevalence of abnormal serum vitamin D, PTH, calcium, and phosphorus in patients with chronic kidney disease: results of the study to evaluate early kidney disease. *Kidney Int* 2007;71:31–38.

10. KDIGO clinical practice guideline for the diagnosis, evaluation, prevention, and treatment of chronic kidney disease-mineral and bone disorder (CKD-MBD). *Kidney Int Suppl* 2009:S1–S130.

11. Roussanne MC, Lieberherr M, Souberbielle JC et al. Human parathyroid cell proliferation in response to calcium, NPS R-467, calcitriol and phosphate. *Eur J Clin Invest* 2001;31:610–616.

12. Patel SR, Ke HQ, Vanholder R, Koenig RJ, Hsu CH. Inhibition of calcitriol receptor binding to vitamin D response elements by uremic toxins. *J Clin Invest* 1995;96:50–59.

13. Fukuda N, Tanaka H, Tominaga Y et al. Decreased 1,25-dihydroxyvitamin D3 receptor density is associated with a more severe form of parathyroid hyperplasia in chronic uremic patients. *J Clin Invest* 1993;92:1436–1443.

14. Gogusev J, Duchambon P, Hory B et al. Depressed expression of calcium receptor in parathyroid gland tissue of patients with hyperparathyroidism. *Kidney Int* 1997;51(1):328–336.

15. Arnold A, Brown MF, Urena P et al. Monoclonality of parathyroid tumors in chronic renal failure and in primary parathyroid hyperplasia. *J Clin Invest* 1995;95:2047–2053.

16. Imanishi Y, Tahara H, Palanisamy N et al. Clonal chromosomal defects in the molecular pathogenesis of refractory hyperparathyroidism of uremia. *J Am Soc Nephrol* 2002;13:1490–1498.

17. Isakova T, Wahl P, Vargas GS et al. Fibroblast growth factor 23 is elevated before parathyroid hormone and phosphate in chronic kidney disease. *Kidney Int* 2011;79:1370–1378.

18. Isakova T, Gutierrez O, Shah A et al. Postprandial mineral metabolism and secondary hyperparathyroidism in early CKD. *J Am Soc Nephrol* 2008, 19:615–623.

19. Dusso AS, Tokumoto M: Defective renal maintenance of the vitamin D endocrine system impairs vitamin D renoprotection: a downward spiral in kidney disease. *Kidney Int* 2011;79:715–729.

20. Hu MC, Shi M, Zhang J et al. Klotho deficiency causes vascular calcification in chronic kidney disease. *J Am Soc Nephrol* 2011;22:124–136.

21. Komaba H, Goto S, Fujii H et al. Depressed expression of Klotho and FGF receptor 1 in hyperplastic parathyroid glands from uremic patients. *Kidney Int* 2010;77:232–238.

22. Kovesdy CP, Ahmadzadeh S, Anderson JE, Kalantar-Zadeh K. Secondary hyperparathyroidism is associated with higher mortality in men with moderate to severe chronic kidney disease. *Kidney Int* 2008;73:1296–1302.

23. Urena P, De Vernejoul MC. Circulating biochemical markers of bone remodeling in uremic patients. *Kidney Int* 1999;55:2141–2156.

24. Mehrotra R, Kermah DA, Salusky IB et al. Chronic kidney disease, hypovitaminosis D, and mortality in the United States. *Kidney Int* 2009;76:977–983.

25. Karsenty G, Vigneron N, Jorgetti V et al. Value of the 99 mTc-methylene diphosphonate bone scan in renal osteodystrophy. *Kidney Int* 1986;29:1058–1065.

26. Hindie E, Urena P, Jeanguillaume C et al. Preoperative imaging of parathyroid glands with technetium-99 m-labelled sestamibi and iodine-123 subtraction scanning in secondary hyperparathyroidism. *Lancet* 1999;353:2200–2204.

27. de Vernejoul MC, Kuntz D, Miravet L et al. Bone histomorphometry in hemodialysed patients. *Metab Bone Dis Relat Res* 1981;3:175–179.

28. Souberbielle JC, Boutten A, Carlier MC et al. Inter-method variability in PTH measurement: implication for the care of CKD patients. *Kidney Int* 2006;70:345–350.

29. Gardham C, Stevens PE, Delaney MP et al. Variability of parathyroid hormone and other markers of bone mineral metabolism in patients receiving hemodialysis. *Clin J Am Soc Nephrol* 2010; 5:1261–1267.

30. Chertow GM, Raggi P, McCarthy JT et al. The effects of sevelamer and calcium acetate on proxies of atherosclerotic and arteriosclerotic vascular disease in hemodialysis patients. *Am J Nephrol* 2003;23: 307–314.

31. Joy MS, Finn WF. Randomized, double-blind, placebo-controlled, dose-titration, phase III study assessing the efficacy and tolerability of lanthanum carbonate: a new phosphate binder for the treatment of hyperphosphatemia. *Am J Kidney Dis* 2003;42:96–107.

32. Jean G, Lataillade D, Genet L et al. Impact of hypovitaminosis D and alfacalcidol therapy on survival of hemodialysis patients: results from the French ARNOS study. *Nephron Clin Pract* 2011;118:c204–c210.

33. Jean G, Terrat JC, Vanel T et al. Evidence for persistent vitamin D 1-alpha-hydroxylation in hemodialysis patients: evolution of serum 1,25-dihydroxycholecalciferol after 6 months of 25-hydroxycholecalciferol treatment. *Nephron Clin Pract* 2008;110:c58–c65.

34. Drueke TB. Which vitamin D derivative to prescribe for renal patients. *Curr Opin Nephrol Hypertens* 2005;14:343–349.

35. Block GA, Martin KJ, de Francisco AL et al. Cinacalcet for secondary hyperparathyroidism in patients receiving hemodialysis. *N Engl J Med* 2004;350:1516–1525.

36. Hodsman AB, Sherrard DJ, Alfrey AC et al. Bone aluminum and histomorphometric features of renal osteodystrophy. *J Clin Endocrinol Metab* 1982;54:539–546.

37. Parkinson IS, Ward MK, Feest TG, Fawcett RW, Kerr DN. Fracturing dialysis osteodystrophy and dialysis encephalopathy. An epidemiological survey. *Lancet* 1979.1:406–409.

38. Cohen-Solal ME, Sebert JL, Boudailliez B et al. Non-aluminic adynamic bone disease in non-dialyzed uremic patients: a new type of osteopathy due to overtreatment? *Bone* 1992;13:1–5.

39. Rodriguez-Perez JC, Plaza C, Torres A et al. Low turnover bone disease is the more common form of bone disease in CAPD patients. *Adv Perit Dial* 1992;8:376–380.

40. Block GA, Hulbert-Shearon TE, Levin NW, Port FK. Association of serum phosphorus and calcium x phosphate product with mortality risk in chronic hemodialysis patients: a national study. *Am J Kidney Dis* 1998;31:607–617.

41. Bardin T, Vasseur M, de Vernejoul MC et al. [Prospective study of articular involvement in patients on hemodialysis for 10 years]. *Rev Rhum Mal Osteoartic* 1988;55:131–133.

42. Goodman WG, Goldin J, Kuizon BD et al. Coronary-artery calcification in young adults with end-stage renal disease who are undergoing dialysis. *N Engl J Med* 2000;342:1478–1483.

43. Shroff RC, McNair R, Figg N et al. Dialysis accelerates medial vascular calcification in part by triggering smooth muscle cell apoptosis. *Circulation* 2008;118:1748–1757.

44. London GM, Guerin AP, Marchais SJ et al. Arterial media calcification in end-stage renal disease: impact on all-cause and cardiovascular mortality. *Nephrol Dial Transplant* 2003;18:1731–1740.

45. Nakano T, Ninomiya T, Sumiyoshi S et al. Association of kidney function with coronary atherosclerosis and calcification in autopsy samples from Japanese elders: the Hisayama study. *Am J Kidney Dis* 2010;55:21–30.

46. Jassal SK, von Muhlen D, Barrett-Connor E. Measures of renal function, BMD, bone loss, and osteoporotic fracture in older adults: the Rancho Bernardo study. *J Bone Miner Res* 2007;22:203–210.

47. Alem AM, Sherrard DJ, Gillen DL et al. Increased risk of hip fracture among patients with end-stage renal disease. *Kidney Int* 2000;58:396–399.

48. Stehman-Breen CO, Sherrard DJ, Alem AM et al. Risk factors for hip fracture among patients with end-stage renal disease. *Kidney Int* 2000;58:2200–2205.

49. Lafage-Proust MH, Combe C, Barthe N, Aparicio M. Bone mass and dynamic parathyroid function according to bone histology in nondialyzed uremic patients after long-term protein and phosphorus restriction. *J Clin Endocrinol Metab* 1999;84:512–519.

50. Hernandez E, Valera R, Alonzo E et al. Effects of raloxifene on bone metabolism and serum lipids in postmenopausal women on chronic hemodialysis. *Kidney Int* 2003;63:2269–2274.

CHAPTER 150

Skeletal dysplasias

B. P. Wordsworth

Introduction

The human skeleton is not just a supporting frame for the rest of the body but also acts as an accessible mineral store. Bone is metabolically active throughout life and metabolic disturbances may have wide-ranging consequences that are not restricted to altering its mechanics. The study of some genetic bone diseases has already provided remarkable insights into the normal regulation of bone metabolism. In some cases this has been translated into new treatments for conditions, such as osteoporosis and Paget's disease.

Most of the conditions described in this chapter are monogenic disorders but only a small sample is covered here. For a fuller description of these and other related disorders the reader is directed not only to the references but also to the online compendium, Mendelian Inheritance in Man (www.ncbi.nlm.nih.gov/omim).[1–5] Some of these disorders are associated with abnormalities of bone mineral density while others cause abnormalities of stature which is often disproportionate. These changes may be quite subtle and have to be judged carefully against the range of the normal human phenotype.

Skeletal dysplasias are developmental disorders of the chondroosseous tissues commonly resulting in short stature, which is often disproportionate. The underlying mutations are often in the structural genes encoding components of the matrix but may also involve growth factors or cell signalling. In contrast, the dysostoses tend to affect single bones or groups of bones, reflecting the transient nature of the many different signalling factors to which they are responsive during development.

Abnormalities of bone density (high or low) may be due to primary deficiency of bone matrix synthesis (e.g. osteogenesis imperfecta and hypophosphatasia) but may also reflect an imbalance between bone formation and resorption. This may be caused by abnormalities of bone formation (e.g. hyperostosis/sclerosteosis and osteoporosis pseudoglioma syndrome) or bone resorption (e.g. classic osteopetrosis and fibrous dysplasia). Linear growth is often not affected by these conditions.

Deformity and short stature

Faced with the small child in clinic it can be a difficult task to decide who and when to investigate further. Short stature (defined as less than 0.4th centile) can be divided into proportionate and disproportionate forms, of which the most frequent is caused by short limbs. About three-quarters of children with short stature either have familial short stature or constitutional delay of growth and puberty; others have chronic disease (10%), syndromic short stature (6%), chromosomal abnormalities (5%), or hormone deficiencies (1–2%). It is important to recognize that only 1% have true skeletal dysplasias. Particular attention should be paid to children whose height progressively crosses the centile ranges. There may be associated deformities, including knock knees, bowed legs, enlarged epiphyses, and bossing of the skull, that may heighten suspicion of an underlying growth disorder. Particularly in the more severe cases, skeletal surveys may be very valuable so long as they are interpreted by experts.

Osteogenesis imperfecta: the brittle bone syndrome

Osteogenesis imperfecta (OI) affects about 1 in 20 000 births but exists in several quite distinct clinical forms. Type 2 OI is a leading cause of lethal short-limbed dwarfism. It was among the first of the skeletal dysplasias for which the underlying genetic mutation was found.

Pathophysiology

OI is a genetic disorder of type I collagen and affects those tissues which contain it. These include particularly bone and dentine but also the sclerae, joints, tendons, heart valves, and skin.

In the so-called 'mild' type 1 OI the quantity and quality of bone is reduced, typically by about 50%. In the extraskeletal tissues, the sclerae are thin (often blue or grey in colour), there is often a degree of ligmamentous laxity, some hyperextensibility of the skin, and occasionally incompetence of the heart valves. The teeth may also be affected (dentinogenesis imperfecta) in which case they tend to be brittle and opalescent.

Clinical features

Type 1 OI (OMIM 166200) is the most frequent form (60%) and least serious. Fractures, which usually heal without deformity, are not present at birth but typically start during childhood, becoming less frequent after adolescence as peak bone mass is achieved. In later life fractures tend to recur although in some unusual cases the initial fracture tendency may even be delayed until the early menopause. Life expectancy is near normal.

Type 2 OI (OMIM 166210) is one of the most common forms of lethal short-limbed dwarfism, but not all infants with fractures at birth succumb immediately. A few survive the perinatal period, later merging with type 3 OI (severe, progressively deforming).

Patients with type 3 OI (OMIM 259420) are likely to survive but present major management problems because their disability is severe and progressive. Although intramedullary rods may be tried in some cases such patients rarely walk, even after multiple operations, and have very short stature (Figure 150.1).

Type 4 OI (OMIM 166220) is intermediate in severity between types 1 and 3 but the sclerae are white, in contrast to type 1 disease. It is more commonly associated with dentinogenesis imperfecta and craniocervical abnormalities than type 1 OI, particularly in those with multiple wormian bones in the skull. Life expectancy is only modestly reduced in type 4 disease in contrast to more severe type 3 disease.

Diagnosis

In the first few years of life non-accidental injury is the main differential diagnosis. Although this may be suggested by multiple fractures at different sites and of different ages, there are no pathognomonic signs. Some fractures, such as metaphyseal 'corner' fractures and posterior rib fractures, are more often seen in non-accidental injury, but any type of fracture can also occur in OI. The distinction between OI and non-accidental injury is legally important and can be difficult. In adult life, mild OI may go unrecognized. Genetic testing is useful in some cases where the clinical diagnosis is in doubt since mutations in one or other of the type I collagen genes (*COL1A1* or *COL1A2*) can be detected in around 90% of cases. A small minority of cases of lethal or severe OI are caused not by collagen mutations but by recessive genes involved in the post-translational processing of collagen which can be identified in appropriate situations by serial DNA sequencing.

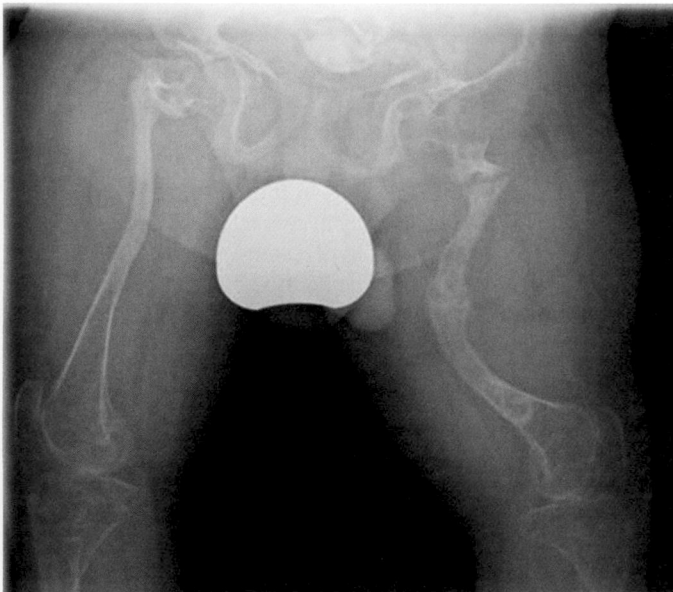

Fig. 150.1 Severe type 3 OI with profound pelvic deformity, slender deformed long bones and ununited fractures of the femur.

Treatment

Bisphosphonates have been increasingly used in the treatment of OI in recent years, particularly in infants with the more severe forms of OI in whom regular intravenous pamidronate has proved effective in increasing bone density although its effects on reducing fracture rates are somewhat less secure. Oral bisphosphonates should be considered in those with less severe disease, and vitamin D levels should be checked routinely given the high prevalence of insufficiency or even deficiency in those with OI. Fractures should heal normally in those with type 1 OI but non-union and malunion are relatively common in the more severe forms. Craniocervical surgery may be need in those with marked invagination of the foramen magnum to prevent hydrocephalus.

Chondrodysplasias

In these conditions the abnormalities of the bone are secondary to defects in endochondral ossification. Many of these conditions are due to mutations in collagens or other cartilage matrix components. Radiographs are essential to determine whether the metaphyses of the long bones or the epiphyses are primarily affected. The presence of spinal involvement in many of these disorders may be quite subtle. Most patients with skeletal dysplasias have some degree of restricted growth, and most are short-limbed. Achondroplasia is the best-known example but there are many different types, most of which are rare and require expert advice to be distinguished.

Achondroplasia

In achondroplasia (OMIM 100800), there are abnormalities in the epiphyseal growth cartilage. These reflect the underlying activating mutation in the *FGFR3* receptor that exerts a negative influence on longitudinal growth by inhibiting proliferation of chondrocytes in the growth plate. Radiological features include metaphyseal irregularity and flaring in the long bones, irregular and late-appearing epiphyses, a narrow pelvis in its anteroposterior diameter, with short iliac wings and deep sacroiliac notches. The spine shows progressive caudal narrowing of the interpedicular distance which is commonly associated with significant spinal stenosis. Spinal surgery for decompression of stenosis is commonly required, often at multiple levels. Eventual height can vary between about 80 and 150 cm. Significant increase in height can be achieved by limb lengthening procedures (often in several stages) but this should be carefully assessed in individual cases.

Epiphyseal dysplasias

These are characterized by prominent involvement of the growing end of the long bones (epiphyses) that typically results in reduced limb growth and variable short-limbed short stature. There are many different forms which vary considerably in their severity and the degree to which the spine is also involved (spondyloepiphyseal dysplasias). Many are caused by abnormalities in matrix components, including type II collagen (the most abundant cartilage matrix protein), type 9 collagen, COMP (cartilage oligomeric matrix protein), matrilin 3, and proteoglycans

Type II collagenopathies

These particularly illustrative examples of epiphyseal dysplasias exhibit a wide variety of phenotype, ranging from the lethal achondrogenesis type II (OMIM 200610), through intermediate forms, spondyloepiphyseal dysplasia congenita (OMIM 183900) and Kniest dysplasia (OMIM 156550), to milder variants, including classic Stickler's syndrome (OMIM 108300). The different underlying mutations in type II collagen illustrate the variation in effect of different mutations in the same gene (see 'Osteogenesis imperfecta' above). Abnormalities of linear growth may lead to angular limb deformity (Figure 150.2) and premature osteoarthritis occurs commonly in these disorders.

Other epiphyseal dysplasias

These conditions include various forms of multiple epiphyseal dysplasia, some of which have very characteristic radiographic appearances (Figure 150.3). Epiphyseal dysplasias have been linked to mutations in type 9 collagen (OMIM 600204 and 600969), type 11 collagen (OMIM 604841), and abnormal proteoglycan sulphation (OMIM 226900). The latter can also cause much more severe forms of dysplasia known as achondrogenesis type 1B (OMIM 600972) and diastrophic dysplasia (OMIM 222600), respectively.

Spondyloepiphyseal dysplasias

This heterogeneous group of disorders exhibits prominent spinal involvement and the short stature is partly due to shortness of the trunk. In the dominantly inherited pseudoachondroplasia (OMIM 1777170), short stature is pronounced in childhood and adult life but does not become apparent until about the second birthday. In contrast to achondroplasia the face appears normal. Hypermobility is marked and early osteoarthritis quite typical, particularly in the hips. Hip joint replacement is often required in early adult life.

Spondyloepiphyseal dysplasia (tarda) is most commonly an X-linked recessive condition (OMIM 313400) caused by mutations in *SEDLIN*, a gene which appears to play an intracellular role in trafficking from the endoplasmic reticulum to the Golgi apparatus. The spine is disproportionately short with a characteristic 'heaped up' appearance to the centre and posterior parts of the vertebral bodies (Figure 150.4). Premature arthritis in the hips is particularly troublesome in early to middle life.

Metaphyseal dysplasias

In these disorders the growth plate itself is involved, with variable restriction of growth. For example, in metaphyseal chondrodysplasia Schmid type (OMIM 156500) there are mutations in type X collagen, which is transiently expressed by chondrocytes in the hypertrophic zone. Varus deformities of the hip and knees are common and surgical procedures to correct deformity may be necessary. These may be coupled with some leg lengthening since staure is typically somewhat reduced (Figure 150.5). It can be distinguished from nutritional rickets by the normal vitamin D levels. Other more severe forms of metaphyseal chondrodysplasia include the Jansen type (OMIM 156400) in which hypercalcaemia and very short stature is caused by mutations in the parathyroid hormone (PTH) receptor, and the McKusick type (OMIM 250250) in which abnormalities also include sparse hair growth and immune deficiencies.

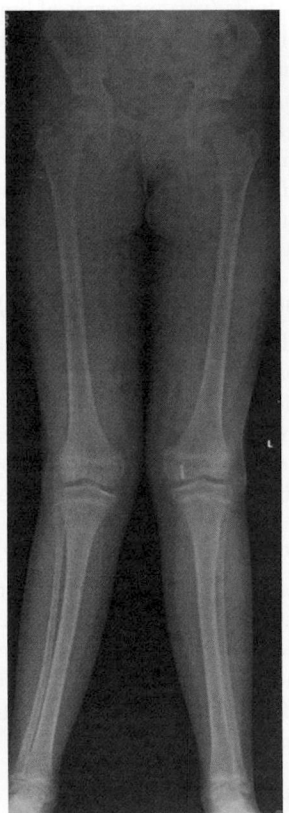

Fig. 150.2 Long leg views of a child with Stickler syndrome demonstrating repair of osteochondritis dissecans in the distal femoral epiphysis. Th bilateral valgus deformities of the knees were subsequently successfully corrected by medial distal femoral epiphysiodesis.

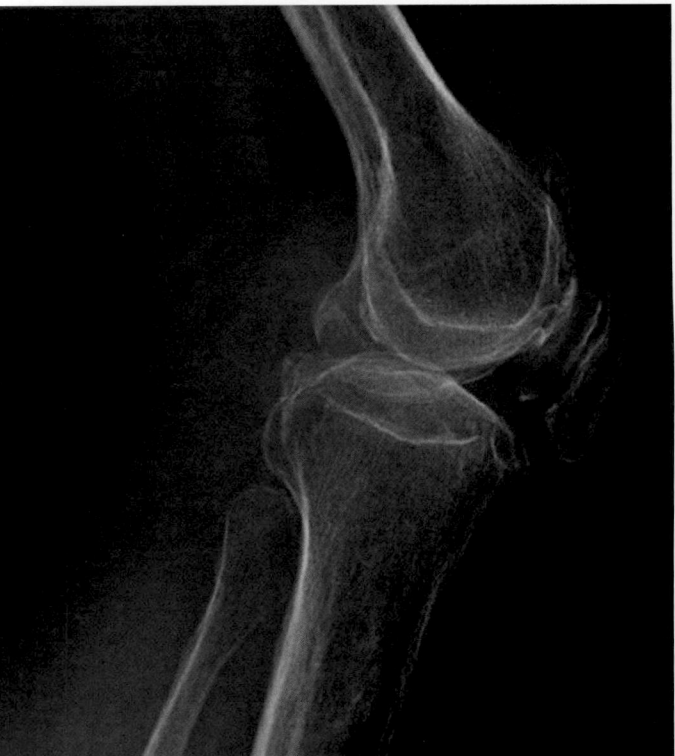

Fig. 150.3 The characteristic double layered patella characteristic of EDM4, a recessive form of multiple epiphyseal dysplasia caused by mutations in a solute carrier important in the sulfation of proteoglycan.

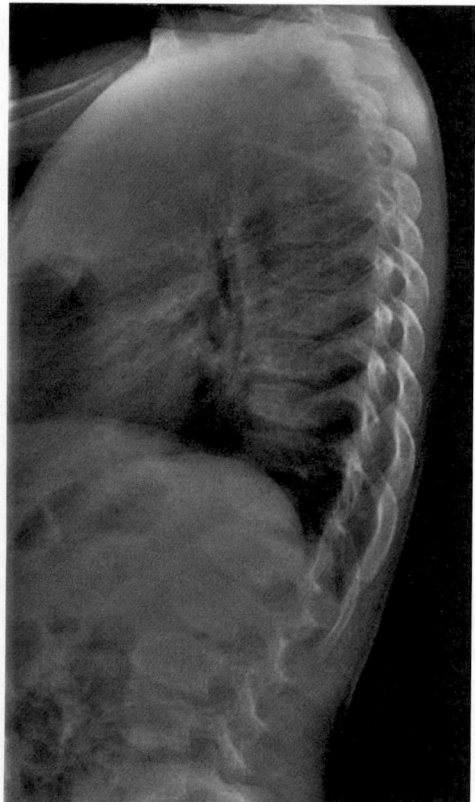

Fig. 150.4 Lateral thoracolumbar spine showing moderate flattening of the vertebrae (platyspondyly) and 'heaping up' of the posterior aspect of the vertebral bodies characteristic of the X-linked form of spondyloepiphyseal dysplasia tarda.

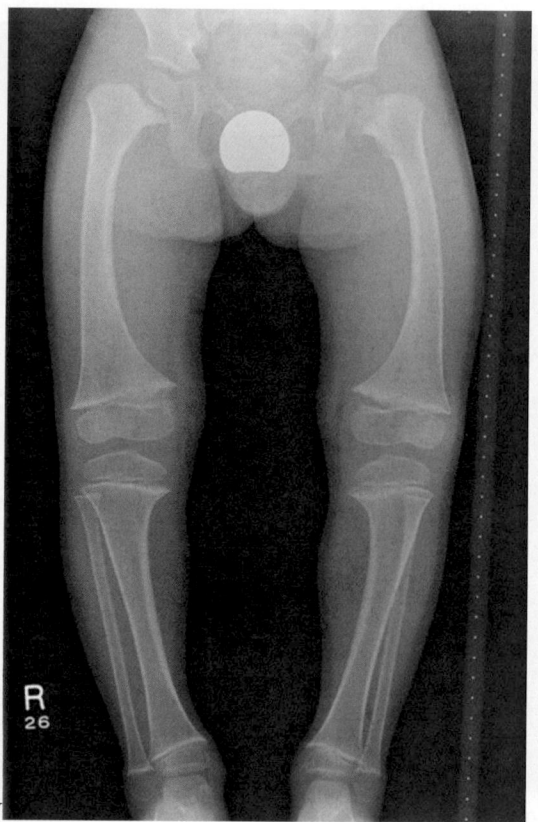

Fig. 150.5 Varus deformities of the hips and knees in a patient with Schmid type metaphyseal chondrodysplasia. The metaphyses are clearly widened and splayed at all the major large joints in the lower limbs.

Multiple hereditary exostoses

This condition (OMIM 133700) has also been referred to as diaphyseal aclasis in the past and is one of the more common abnormalities of bone structure. The mutant gene (exostosin) is involved in cell surface expression of heparan sulphate proteoglycan and appears to function as a tumour suppressor gene. Clinically it is characterized by a juxtaepiphyseal disorder of bone growth, limited to bones developed in cartilage, which gives rise to cartilage-capped exostoses that point away from the joint. Stature is usually normal. Surgical removal of large exostoses may be required if there is mechanical interference with joint function. After skeletal maturity is reached there is a significant risk of malignant change in these exostoses that has been estimated at around 1–5% (lifetime risk). Any increase in size should raise the suspicion of malignant change which can be most effectively screened using ultrasonography to measure the thickness of the cartilage cap on the exostosis.

Dysostoses

These disorders of skeletal development can be distinguished from the true skeletal dysplasias because of the distinct patterns of bone groups that are affected. Those with predominantly axial involvement include vertebral segmentation defects (Klippel–Feil anomalies) and spondylocostal dysostosis (OMIM 277300). Mild varieties tend to be inherited in dominant fashion while the more severe types are recessive. Other forms have more prominent involvement of the limbs. In some cases this may involve the hands with variably short digits (various forms of brachydactyly) and/or fusion of the phalanges (symphalangism). Webbing of the fingers (synphalangism) may also occur to a varying degree. In dyschondrosteosis (OMIM 127300) there is mesomelic shortening of the limb in which the radius and tibia appear relatively short, causing a Madelung deformity in the forearm. It is of particular interest that the mutant *SHOX* gene is in the pseudoautosomal region of the sex chromosomes and females are considerably worse affected than males.

Nail–patella syndrome (OMIM 277300)

This dominantly inherited condition is associated with dystrophic nails, hypoplastic patellae, iliac horns, and a tendency to progressive nephrosis which causes renal failure in 20% of cases. The mutant *LMX1B* gene is involved in dorsoventral patterning of the developing limb and in the processing of type 4 collagen found in the basement membrane of the renal glomerulus.

Cleidocranial dysplasia (OMIM 119600)

In this rare condition involvement of the membrane bones is prominent; the clavicles are hypoplastic or absent, the fontanelles remain open, there are supernumerary teeth and wormian bones may be apparent on skull radiographs. It is caused by mutations in *RUNX2*, a key transcription factor in osteoblast differentiation and cartilage hypertrophy at the growth plate.

Disorders of bone density

Bone density reflects the balance between bone formation and resorption. Consequently, disorders of either can result in quantitative and qualitative disturbances of bone. Wnt signalling pathways and bone morphogenetic proteins are involved in osteoblast activation but natural antagonists, including sclerostin, dickkopf, and noggin, modulate these effects. Mutations in many of these have now been described that affect bone density. Likewise abnormalities of osteoclast function are also implicated.

Osteopetrosis

Patients with osteopetrosis (Albers–Schönberg disease) have increased bone density and abnormal bony architecture. Pathological fractures are an important consequence. The classic forms of osteopetrosis reflect failure in the function of the osteoclasts, particularly relating to the generation of an acid milieu in the resorption pit. This can result from mutations in an osteoclast-specific proton pump, chloride channels or carbonic anhydrase that is necessary to generate hydrogen ions in the osteoclast (OMIM 259730). There is substantial variation in the severity of the condition; some forms are lethal in infancy from bone marrow failure (OMIM 259700) while others (Figure 150.6) may produce relatively few symptoms throughout life (OMIM 166600). The mild forms vary widely in severity. The bones are relatively fragile despite being dense since they lack the normal capacity for remodelling along lines of maximum stress. Pyknodysostosis (OMIM 265800) causes a particular form of osteopetrosis with short stature, homogeneous increased bone density, wormian bones and acro-osteolysis. In this disorder mutations of the proteolytic enzyme cathepsin K render osteoclasts inefficient at bone resorption.

Other causes of increased bone density

Other forms of increased bone density reflect increased bone formation by overactivity of osteoblasts induced by excess Wnt signalling through the LRP5 receptor. These include familial high bone mass and various types of endosteal hyperostosis (e.g. OMIM 144750). Sclerosteosis (OMIM 269500) is another hyperostosis in which there are inactivating mutations of the natural bone morphogenetic protein (BMP) inhibitor sclerostin. Diaphyseal dysplasia or Camurati–Englemann disease (OMIM 131300) is caused by activating mutations in TGFβ. It is characterized by enlarged long bones and proximal myopathy.

Melorheostosis (literally 'flowing limb') is a rare form of hyperostosis with a typically segmental distribution. It is thought to reflect local genetic mosaicism in the developing embryo and can cause severe soft tissue contractures as well as local enlargement of the affected bones (Figure 150.7).

Fibrodysplasia ossificans progressiva (OMIM 135100)

FOP is rare, with an incidence of less than 1 per million. Diagnosis depends on the combination of developmental abnormalities of the skeleton and progressive widespread myositis, leading to ossification in the major skeletal muscles. Initially there is oedema and cellular infiltration throughout the muscle, with myofibrillar breakdown. Later endochondral ossification leads to mature bone, within which is haemopoietic marrow. The upper paraspinal trunk is typically first affected, and the peripheral skeleton and associated

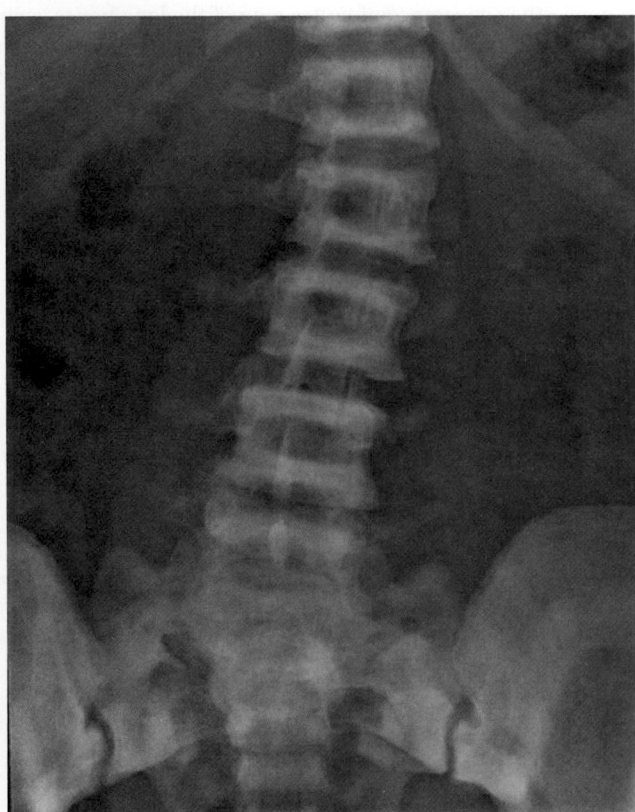

Fig. 150.6 Radiograph of the pelvis and lumbar spine of a young woman with typical dominantly inherited osteopetrosis caused by a CLCN7 chloride channel defect. There is obvious heterogeneous increased density of the bones with a classic endobone ('bone within bone') appearance in the iliac wings.

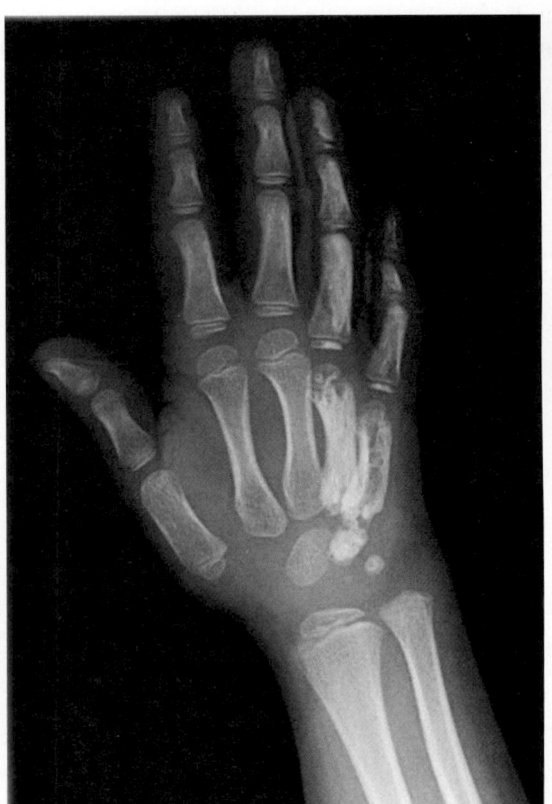

Fig. 150.7 Sclerosis and thickening of the bones of the fourth and fifth rays of the hand in a child with melorheostosis.

soft tissues are often spared. Typically, the affected muscle and/or associated fascia becomes swollen and hard, sometimes following injury; after a week or two these features subside, but the apparent improvement may be followed by ossification within the muscle and progressive joint fixation. Myositis usually begins in the upper paraspinal muscles in early childhood. By late childhood or adolescence ossification will have usually occurred widely in the trunk but also within the muscles around the shoulders, hips, and less commonly knees, to fix these joints and to complete the disability. The large, striated muscles are affected; ossification does not involve the small muscles of the hands and feet, the diaphragm, the cardiac, or the smooth muscles. Ossification in the muscles around the jaw may fix it almost completely. The diagnostic skeletal abnormalities affect the big toes, to a lesser extent the thumbs and the cervical spine (Figure 150.8). There is no effective treatment to prevent or reverse the abnormal ossification. Surgical removal of ectopic bone is technically difficult and may ultimately worsen the disability.

Reduced bone density

Various forms of inherited osteoporosis have been described in addition to OI. One of these is the osteoporosis pseudoglioma syndrome (OMIM 259770), in which reduced Wnt signalling as a result of inactivating mutations in the LRP5 receptor leads to reduced osteoblast activity and failure of the normal development of the eye. Of interest, LRP5 has also been shown to be a key regulator of bone mass in the genral population.

Hypophosphatasia

This rare disorder has similarities with rickets and osteomalacia. It is due to alkaline phosphatase deficiency which leads to defective mineralization of bone and varying degrees of fracture risk. In the adult form, progressive stiffness, pain in the bones, and apparent

'stress' fractures can occur (Figure 150.9). Approximately 50% of such patients have a childhood history of bone disease or premature loss of deciduous teeth. Recurrent poorly healing metatarsal fractures occur. Partial fractures of the long bones characteristically occur on the convex outer surface (in contrast to Looser's zones in osteomalacia). Calcium pyrophosphate chondrocalcinosis is also common and may be associated with arthropathy (pseudogout). More severe (lethal and childhood) variants are also described, reflecting correspondingly more severe deficiency of alkaline phosphatase.

Other conditions affecting the skeleton

Fibroblast growth factor 23 related disorders

FGF-23 is a crucial factor in determing phosphate excretion from the kidney. It may accumulate under certain circumstances to cause a renal phosphate leak and osteomalacia. This is exemplified by oncogenic osteomalacia where excess production of FGF-23 by a vascular tumour (eg. haemangiopericytoma). Widespread bone pain and pathological fractures may result.

Vitamin D-resistant rickets

Typically this is an X-linked dominant disorder (OMIM 307800) in which FGF-23 acclumulates as a result of mutations in the metalloproteinase PHEX which normally inactivates FGF-23. Affected individuals are short, develop angular limb deformities that often require corrective surgery, and may develop Looser's zones (cf. vitamin D deficient rickets). In adult life there is excessive bone deposition giving the appearance of buttressing of the long bones, spinal stenosis, and widespread enthesopathy (Figure 150.10). Treatment in the child is with regular phosphate supplementation and 1α-hydroxylated analogues of vitamin D. A rare form of autosomal dominant hypophosphataemia exists in which the cleavage site for

(A)

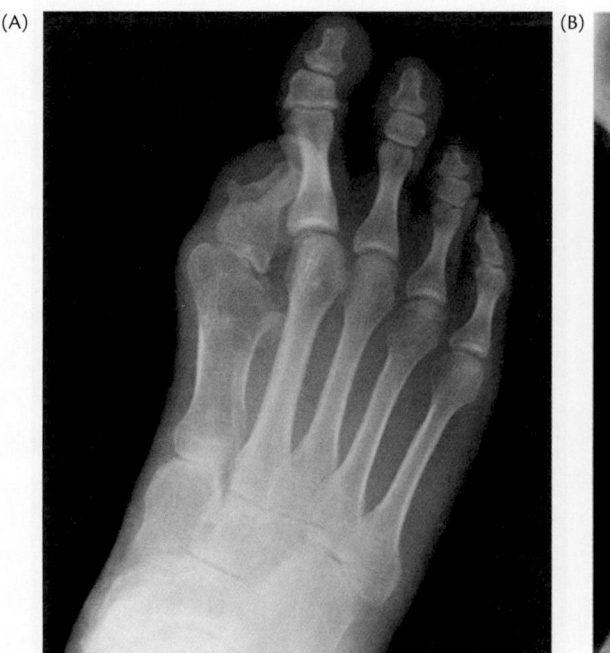

(B)

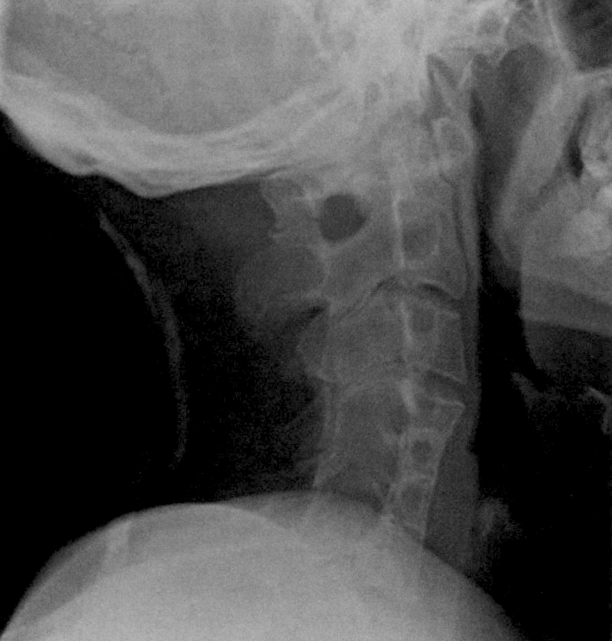

Fig. 150.8 Classic shortened monophalangic great toe in an adolescent with FOP (A). The cervical spine shows typical small vertebral bodies and poor develop of the intervertebral joints. There is extensive ossification in the soft tissues (B).

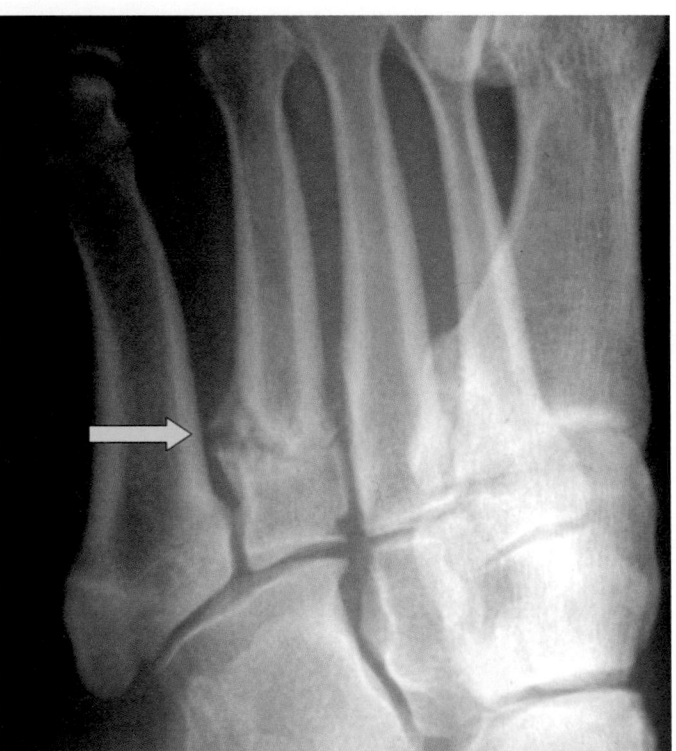

Fig. 150.9 Chronic fractures through base of the fourth metatarsal (arrowed) in a patient with the adult type of hypophosphatasia.

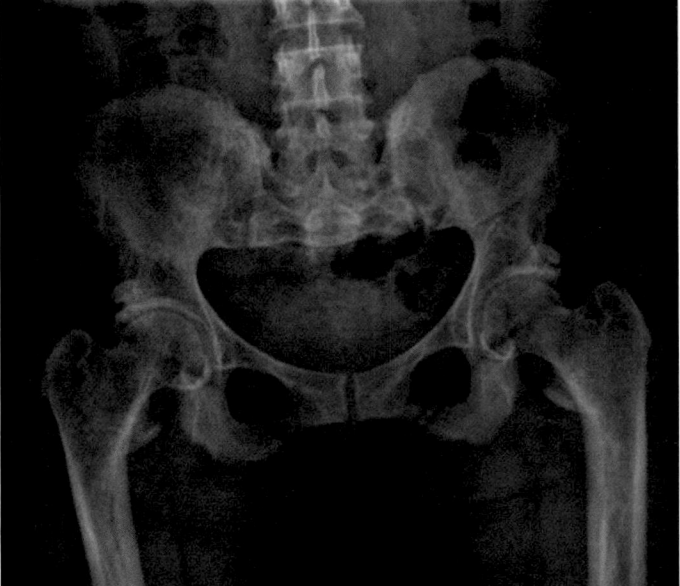

Fig. 150.10 Widespread enthesopathy in a patient with X-linked hypophosphataemia. There is extensive ossification of the hip joint capsule causing severe impingement syndrome.

PHEX in FGF-23 is missing, thereby also causing active FGF-23 to accumulate (OMIM 193100).

Marfan's syndrome

In Marfan syndrome the fundamental genetic defect lies in fibrillin, one of the key microfibrillar components of elastic tissues. Accurate diagnosis is dependent on the presence of major involvement of **at** **least two** organ systems and/or a definite history of the condition in a first-degree relative.[6]

Pathology

Deficiency of the microfibrillar architecture of elastic tissues is undoubtedly responsible for some of the clinical features of Marfan's syndrome. However, it is now recognized that dysregulated tissue growth factor beta (TGF-β) signalling also plays an important part. Latent TGF-β is normally sequestered in the connective tissue matrix bound to latent TGF-β binding protein, which itself binds to fibrillin in the matrix. Abnormal fibrillin microfibrillar architecture allows excessive amounts of activated TGF-β to be released with adverse consequences for organogenesis and growth. These effects can be neutralized in animal models by anti TGF-β antibodies and also angiotensin receptor antagonists, which are now entering clinical trials in humans.

Clinical features

Marfan's syndrome is dominantly inherited. Its main effects are on the skeleton, cardiovascular, and ocular systems. In the typical patient with Marfan's syndrome, overall height is increased and the limbs are long relative to the trunk. Long, thin fingers (arachnodactyly) are common. Scoliosis is common, may be severe, and worsens with the pre-adolescent growth spurt (Figure 150.11). Anterior chest-wall deformity (pectus carinatum/pectus excavatum) is often associated with scoliosis. Dislocation of the lens is the main ocular feature of Marfan's syndrome, but the most severe complication is

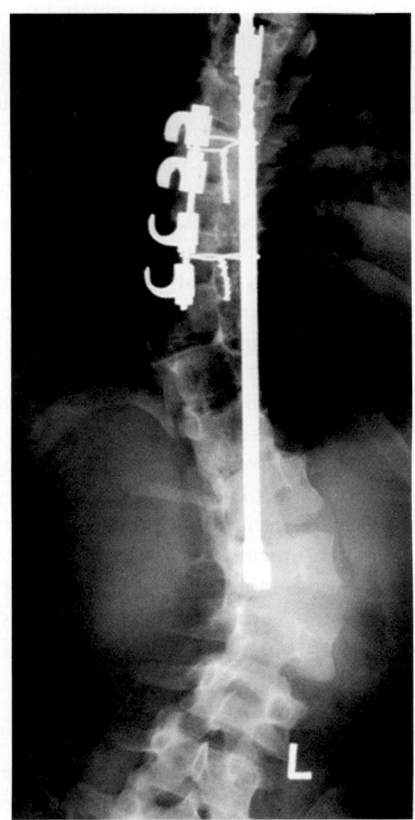

Fig. 150.11 Complex thoracolumbar scoliosis in a patient with Marfan's syndrome stabilized with spinal rods.

dilatation of the ascending aorta leading to aortic incompetence and/or dissection.

Treatment

There is no specific treatment yet for the underlying defect, but many of the clinical manifestations require attention. Once the diagnosis is established it is generally recommended that treatment with beta-blockers should be initiated to retard the rate of dilatation of the proximal aorta. Regular monitoring of the aortic root by echocardiography is desirable since dissection is much more likely to occur if it exceeds 5 cm in diameter, at which point aortic root/valve repair should be considered. Life expectancy is considerably reduced, although this depends on the severity of cardiac involvement. Earlier intervention and improvements in elective cardiac surgical techniques have had a significant impact on survival in those with more severe forms of the disease.

Scoliosis may be progressive and severe. Bracing is largely ineffective and operative stabilization, ideally in adolescence, may be necessary. Epiphysiodesis may be considered in either sex where predicted height is in excess of that deemed to be socially acceptable. Surgical correction of chest-wall deformities should be undertaken only in the most severe cases because of the possibility of complicating potential surgical field for later cardiac surgery. Milder chest-wall deformities often become less obvious with age because of the accumulation of subcutaneous fat. Tailored footwear is necessary for many individuals with foot deformities, but these will sometimes need surgical correction.

Ehlers–Danlos syndrome

This heterogeneous syndrome includes individuals with the common clinical features of abnormal velvety hyperelastic skin, easy bruising, hyperextensible joints, and lax ligaments (see also Chapter 170). The Villefranche nosology[7] lists seven types of Ehlers–Danlos syndrome (EDS) but many individuals do not accurately fit comfortably into any of these. Classic EDS is caused by mutations in type V collagen, vascular EDS by mutations in type III collagen, oculoscoliotic EDS by mutations in lysyl hydroxylase, which causes abnormal cross-linking of collagen trimers, and the arthrochalasia/dermatosparaxis forms of EDS result from abnormal processing of the N-terminal domain of type I collagen. Individuals with EDS are more susceptible to ligament rupture but the results of surgical repair are unpredictable. The vascular form of EDS (type 4) carries a particularly adverse prognosis; it is associated with catastrophic rupture of blood vessels and other hollow viscera (see further reading). Mortality and morbidity in pregnancy is particularly severe. The most commonly diagnosed form of EDS is type 3 (benign joint hypermobility syndrome) which is clinically and pathologically highly heterogeneous. It is sometimes, but by no means invariably, associated with widespread joint pains and should be carefully distinguished from the more severe variants (e.g. vascular and oculoscoliotic types) which carry an adverse prognosis. Genetic testing is only rarely required for EDS.

Alkaptonuria

In this rare condition (<1:150 000), enzyme deficiency causes accumulation of homogentisic acid in the tissues. The most important effects of this disease are on the spine and later on the larger joints. The intervertebral discs lose height and later calcify (Figure 150.12).

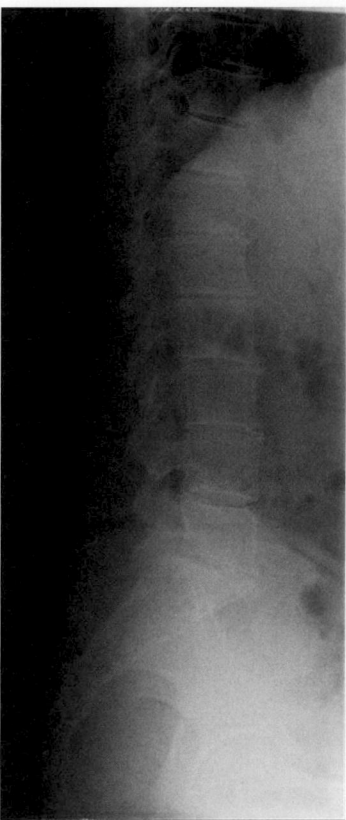

Fig. 150.12 The appearance of the thoracolumbar spine in a 40 year old woman with alkaptonuria. There is universal calcification of the intervertebral discs and gross loss of disc height throughout.

The spine becomes rigid and short and the lumbar lordosis is lost. In the large joints, such as the knees, shoulders, and hips, there are effusions and loose bodies. No effective medical treatment for the condition exists but monitoring of the heart valves is recommended as these may also be involved and become incompetent in later life.

Mucopolysaccharidoses

Failure of the normal lysosomal breakdown of complex carbohydrates or glycosaminoglycans leads to their accumulation in the tissues. Hurler's, Hunter's, and Morquio's syndromes are such examples. See also Chapter 170.

Hurler's syndrome (OMIM 607014)

This is the most severe type of mucopolysaccharidosis and causes death at an early age. The physical features include proportionate short stature, a typical facial appearance, a short neck with a lumbar gibbus and chest deformity, and a protuberant abdomen. Similar but less severe features are seen in Hunter's syndrome.

Morquio's syndrome (OMIM 253000)

In this disorder the orthopaedic manifestations are striking, but intelligence is normal. Characteristically the neck is short, the sternum is protuberant, and there may be a flexed stance with knock knees. Importantly, the odontoid may be hypoplastic, leading to atlantoaxial instability, compression of the long spinal tracts, and paraplegia.

Gaucher's disease

This is a rare lysosomal storage disorder in which glucocerebroside-containing macrophages accumulate in the bone marrow, spleen, liver, and other organs. The skeletal manifestations are often severe and disabling. They vary from a characteristic but clinically insignificant failure of remodelling in the lower femora (Erlenmeyer flask appearance) to diffuse and localized bone loss and osteosclerotic and osteonecrotic lesions, which cause pain and pathological fracture, often requiring precocious joint replacement surgery.

Fibrous dysplasia

Fibrous dysplasia of bone is a condition in which areas of immature fibrous tissue are found within the skeleton. Monostotic and polyostotic fibrous dysplasia are both caused by activating mutations in the *GNAS1* gene, encoding a component of the G-protein signalling system. However, these mutations are not in the germ-line (which would be lethal) but occur somatically in the developing embryo. The extent of involvement reflects the degree of mosaicism present in the affected individual.

Monostotic fibrous dysplasia

This disorder is relatively common in orthopaedic practice and reflects late postzygotic mosaicism. The lesions may occur in any bone and the most frequent presenting symptom at any age is a fracture, often of the upper end of the femur. There is a smooth-walled translucent area within the bone, often with thinning of the cortex and sometimes with associated deformity. The differential diagnosis is from other causes of bone cysts, including Paget's disease and hyperparathyroidism with osteitis fibrosa cystica. The large size of some of the defects in the shafts of the long bones may make conventional stabilization of fractures very difficult. Bisphosphonates may be effective in many cases where there is clear evidence of increased osteoclast activity.

Polyostotic fibrous dysplasia

The bone lesions tend to increase in size and number but less rapidly after growth has ceased. The skeletal lesions may cause complications such as spinal cord compression, and may be associated with hypophosphataemic osteomalacia. Radiologically, the bones are deformed, the cortex may be difficult to detect, and the medullary bone takes on a 'ground glass' or 'smoky' appearance (Figure 150.13). This variant of fibrous dysplasia is often associated with involvement of many additional tissues in the McCune–Albright syndrome. Classic features include skin pigmentation, precocious puberty, hyperthyroidism and, sometimes, pituitary gigantism. Of interest, diffuse idiopathic skeletal hyperostosis (DISH)-like new bone formation may also occur in disorders associated with inactivating mutations in *GNAS*, such asa pseudohypoparathyroidism (Figure 150.14).

Miscellaneous bone disorders

Vitamin C (ascorbic acid) deficiency (scurvy) is reflected in weakness of collagen-containing tissues, notably causing haemorrhage and fractures. Extensive subperiosteal haemorrhage leads to pain and immobility; the legs are held in a 'frog-like' position. Radiographs in infancy show a widened zone of provisional calcification in the metaphyses and failure of new bone formation.

Prolonged parenteral nutrition can produce a form of bone disease similar to osteomalacia. The main symptom is periarticular bone pain, particularly in the ankles. The radiographic appearances suggest osteoporosis.

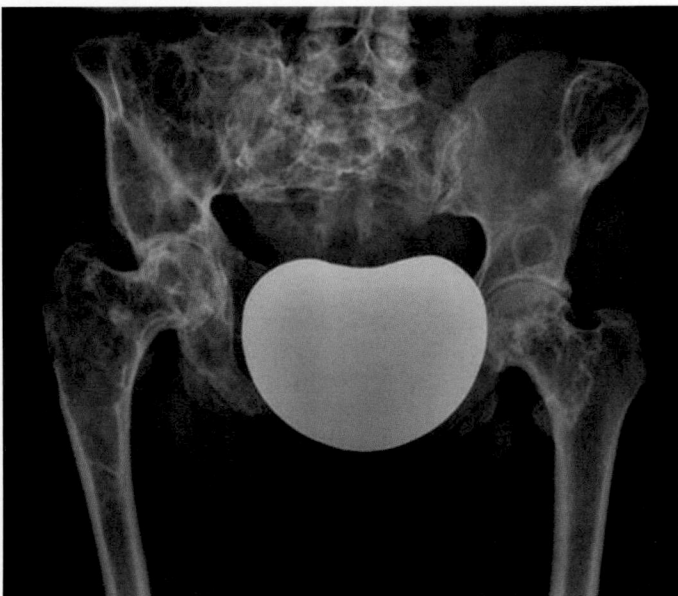

Fig. 150.13 Polyostotic fibrous dysplasia affecting the pelvis in a 65 year old woman. The cystic lesions are particularly obvious in the right hemipelvis and proximal femur.

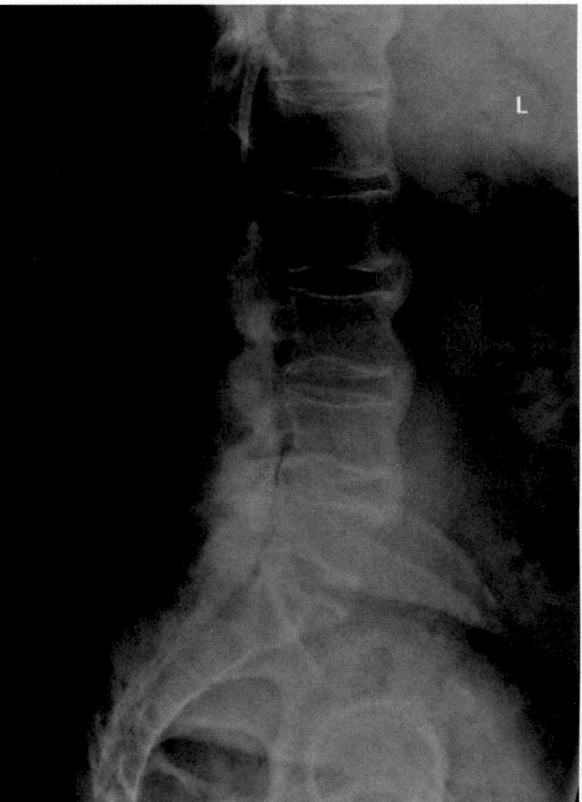

Fig. 150.14 DISH-like new bone formation bridging the lumbar vertebrae in a patient with pseudohypoparathyroidism.

Deposition of excess fluoride in the skeleton can result from an excess in the diet (endemic fluorosis), from industrial exposure (during the manufacture of aluminium, steel, and glass, and from exposure to the dust of fluoride-containing rock), and from the administration of sodium fluoride in treatment. There is a generalized increase in bone density (with loss of the normal corticomedullary junction), and the tendons, ligaments, and sometimes muscles may be mineralized. Compression of the spinal cord and its roots, with progressive neurological disability has been described.

The prolonged use of vitamin A (retinoids) for the treatment of skin disease, such as psoriasis and ichthyosis, leads particularly to calcification of the spinal ligaments, causing stiffness and reduced mobility. There is a resemblance to Forestier's disease (DISH).

Chronic vitamin D overdosage leads to soft tissue calcification, especially in the arteries and kidneys. After several years, progressive stiffness in the spine, major joints, and feet lead to difficulty in walking. Radiographs show ligamentous calcification. Lead poisoning in the growing skeleton produces a radiologically dense line near the growth plate.

References

1. Smith R, Wordsworth P. *Clinical and biochemical disorders of the skeleton*. Oxford University Press, Oxford, 2005.

2. Spranger JW, Brill PW, Poznanski A. *Bone dysplasias*, 2nd edn. Oxford University Press, Oxford 2002

3. Online Mendelian Inheritance In Man (OMIM). www.ncbi.nlm.nih.gov/omim/

4. Royce PM, Steinmann B. *Connective tissue and its heritable disorders*, 2nd edn. Wiley-Liss, New York, 2002.

5. Firth HV, Hurst JA. *Oxford desk reference clinical genetics*. Oxford University Press, Oxford, 2005.

6. De Paepe A, Devereux RB, Dietz HC, Hennekam RCM, Pyeritz RE. Revised diagnostic criteria for the Marfan syndrome *Am J Med Genet* 1996;62:417–426.

7. Beighton P, de Paepe A, Steinmann B, Tsipouras P, Wenstrup RJ. Ehlers Danlos syndromes: revised nosology, Villefranche 1997. *Am J Med Genet* 1998;77:31–37.

SECTION 22

Regional rheumatic disease

CHAPTER 151

Shoulder

Andrew J. K. Östör

Introduction

The shoulder is the most complex and enigmatic joint in the body and disorders in and around the joint are frequent. The prevalence of shoulder pain in the community approximates 30% and represents the second most common musculoskeletal complaint presenting to primary care after back pain.[1,2] Subacromial impingement syndrome is the commonest source of shoulder pain, with rotator cuff tendinopathy underlying this in the majority of cases.[3] The differential diagnosis of shoulder pain is vast, however, encompassing both intrinsic and extrinsic aetiologies, and thus an open mind must be maintained when assessing shoulder discomfort or dysfunction (Table 151.1).

The impact of shoulder pathology on the individual, including interference with work and leisure activities, is enormous, particularly in older people.[3,4] The resultant economic strain on society due to healthcare utilization and lost productivity is enormous.[5,6] Despite this the field is plagued by a poor understanding of the epidemiology, assessment, diagnosis, and management of shoulder conditions. This chapter deals with the more common disorders affecting the shoulder which are likely to be encountered in clinical practice.

Anatomy

The shoulder complex is a multiaxial spheroidal joint comprised of three articulations (glenohumeral, acromioclavicular (AC), sternoclavicular) and two virtual ones (subacromial, scapulothoracic) (Figures 151.1–151.3] The glenohumeral joint represents the 'true' shoulder joint and comprises the articulation between the glenoid of the scapula and the humeral head. In order to increase the surface area of the glenoid a cartilaginous cuff surrounds its margins, this having evolved to improve the stability of the joint. Mobility of the joint is maximized by an extensive synovial-lined joint capsule allowing up to 3 cm of separation of the bones. The majority of shoulder movement occurs at the glenohumeral joint, in particular the first 90° of abduction. The fibrocartilaginous AC joint, between the lateral end of the clavicle and the tip of the acromion, stabilizes the shoulder. The synovial sternoclavicular joint occurring between the superolateral facet of the sternum and the medial end of the clavicle allows increased mobility of the shoulder, particularly abduction.

The subacromial space lies between the superior aspect of the humeral head and the undersurface of the acromion. This virtual joint allows smooth movement of the joint, especially shoulder abduction. The subacromial bursa lies in this area to further facilitate mobility. The scapulothoracic 'joint' occurs between the posterior aspect of the thoracic wall and the undersurface of the scapula. This articulation allows abduction of the shoulder beyond 90°. A number of ligaments lend support to the shoulder including the glenohumeral, coracoacromial, coracohumeral, and transverse humeral ligaments.

The rotator cuff

The musculotendinous complex known as the rotator cuff is made up of the supraspinatus, infraspinatus, subscapularis, and teres minor muscles, and the honorary member, long head of biceps (Figure 151.4). The cuff is the predominant stabilizing structure of the joint as well as playing a role in shoulder movement (Table 151.2). The cuff also contributes up to 50% of the power of the shoulder in abduction and 80% in external rotation.

The supraspinatus muscle originates from the supraspinatus fossa of the scapula and inserts into the greater tuberosity of the humerus. Its main responsibility is to initiate shoulder abduction. The infraspinatus muscle arises from the posterior aspect of the scapula inferior to its spine and inserts into the posterosuperior aspect of the greater tuberosity of the humerus. Its chief action is to externally rotate the shoulder. The teres minor muscle arises from the axillary border of the scapula and inserts into the posterinferior aspect of the greater tuberosity of the humerus. This muscle aids the infraspinatus as a shoulder external rotator. The subscapularis originates from the subscapular fossa and inserts into the lesser tuberosity of the humerus lateral to the glenoid labrum. Subscapularis is separated from the rest of the cuff by the bicipital groove. Its predominant action is to internally rotate the adducted arm. The long head of biceps arises from the superior aspect of the glenoid labrum (the short head arising from the coracoid process) and inserts into the radial tuberosity. It may be considered part of the rotator cuff due to its position and role in shoulder stability. The action of the long head of biceps is to flex the elbow and to supinate the forearm.

A number of bursae are present around the shoulder. The most important of these is the subacromial bursa lying between the joint capsule and deltoid muscle laterally and inferior to the acromion and coracoacromial ligament medially. This bursa allows smooth

Table 151.1 Differential diagnosis of shoulder pain

Soft tissue/ periarticular lesions	Rotator cuff tendinopathy	Tendinosis
		Partial/full-thickness tear
		Tendon rupture
	Calcific tendonitis	
	Bicipital tendinopathy	Partial/full thickness tear
		Tendon rupture
		Tenosynovitis
	Subacromial bursitis	
	Adhesive capsulitis	
	Impingement syndromes	
	Subluxation/dislocation	
Arthritic lesions	Osteoarthritis	
	Rheumatoid arthritis	
	Spondyloarthritis	
	Gout	
	Pseudogout	
	Calcium hydroxyapatite deposition (Milwaukee shoulder)	
	Septic arthritis	
	Glenohumeral instability	
Neurological	Radicular pain from cervical root impingement	
	Neuralgic amyotrophy	
	Spinal cord lesions	Tumours
		Syringomyelia
	Thoracic outlet syndrome	
Neurovascular	Complex regional pain syndrome type 1 (CRPS 1]	
Thoracic pathology	Ischaemic heart disease	
	Tumours	Mediastinal
		Pancoast's tumour
Abdominal pathology	Cholecystitis	
	Subphrenic abscess	
Bone disorders	Tumours	
	Avascular necrosis	
	Paget's disease	
	Tuberculosis	
	Glenoid labral lesions	
	Fracture	
Systemic disorders	Polymyalgia rheumatica	
	Myopathies	
	Chronic pain syndromes	
	Inflammatory arthritides	

(a)

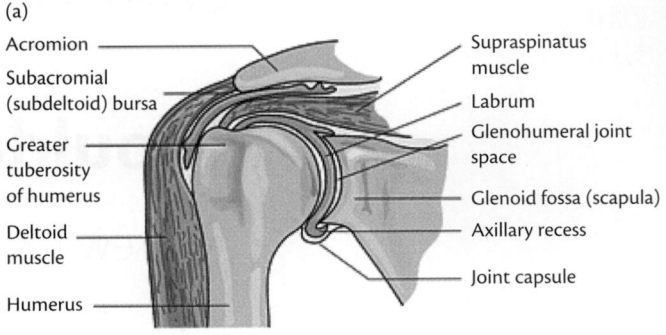

(b)

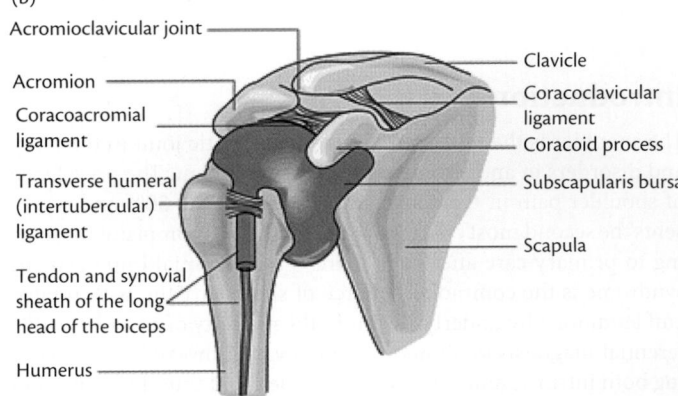

Fig. 151.1 Anatomy of the shoulder joint.

movement of the rotator cuff in the subacromial space. Other muscles involved with shoulder movement include the deltoid (flexion, abduction, and extension), pectoralis major (adductor and internal rotator), latissimus dorsi (adductor, internal rotator, and extensor) (Figure 151.4).

Disorders of the shoulder joint

The differential diagnosis of shoulder pain is extensive (Table 151.1). The primary question is whether the pathology is intrinsic to the shoulder itself or due to a cause outside the shoulder. A thorough history and examination is required to help define the abnormality followed by judicious use of imaging. The most commonly encountered intrinsic shoulder disorders are further discussed.

Subacromial impingement syndrome

Although it is strictly not a specific entity, the concept of subacromial impingement syndrome has emerged over the last decade as a system to help classify shoulder disease.[7,8] Subacromial impingement is said to occur when anatomical structures, most commonly the supraspinatus tendon and subacromial bursa, are trapped between the inferior surface of the acromion, AC joint, and coracoacromial ligament, and the superior aspect of the humeral head. Predisposing factors for impingement include a down-sloping or hook-like acromion, AC osteophytes, subacromial spur, muscle imbalance secondary to cuff weakness, joint instability, and manual work carried out overhead.

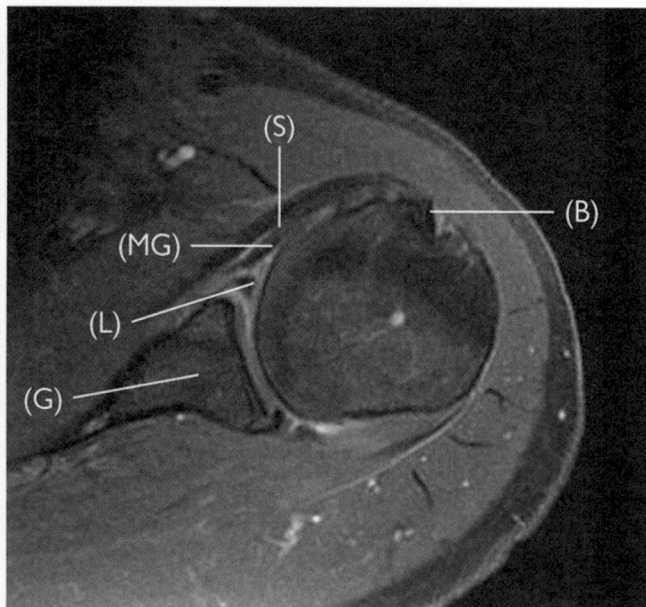

Fig. 151.2 Fat-saturated (FS) T1 arthrogram of the glenohumeral joint showing the subscapularis (S), the biceps tendon (B), the middle glenohumeral ligament (MG), the glenoid (G) and the labrum (L).

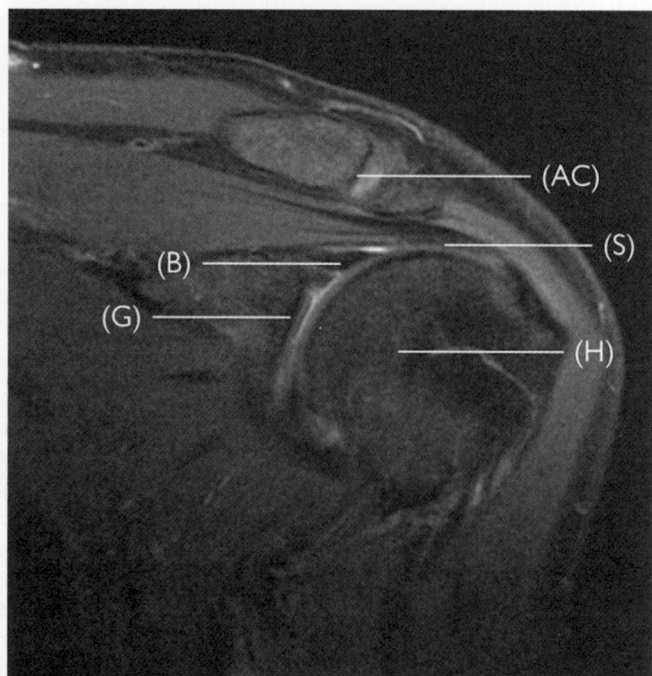

Fig. 151.3 Coronal oblique fat-saturated (FS) T1 MR arthrogram showing acromioclavicular joint (AC), biceps origin (B), supraspinatus tendon (S), glenoid (G), and humeral head (H).

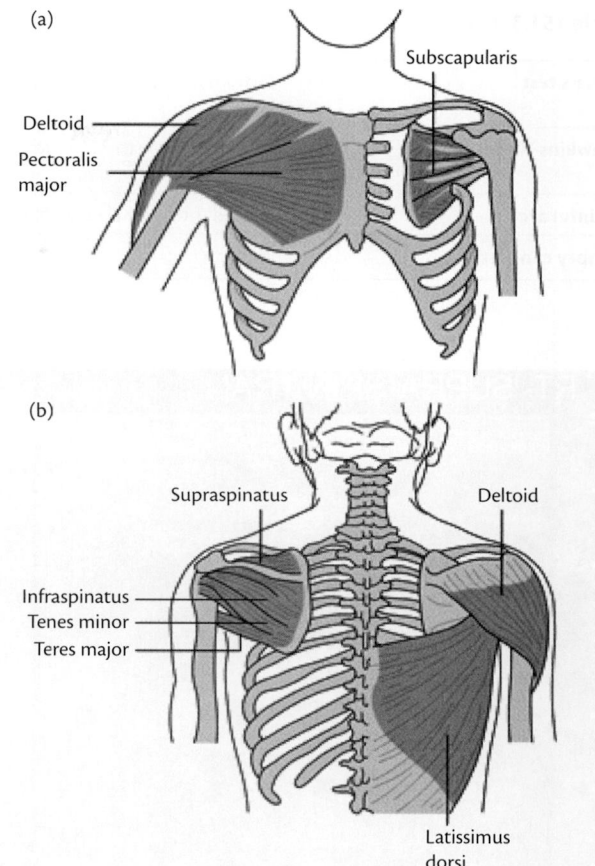

Fig. 151.4 Muscles of the shoulder girdle and rotator cuff.

Table 151.2 Main actions of the rotator cuff (other than shoulder stabilization)

Muscle	Action
Supraspinatus	Initiation of abduction (first 10°); active throughout range of movement
Infraspinatus	External rotation
Subscapularis	Internal rotation
Teres minor	External rotation (acting with infraspinatus)
Biceps (not strictly rotator cuff muscle but involved with it)	Elbow flexion; forearm supination

Clinical

Impingement is the most common clinical syndrome presenting with shoulder pain.[7] It may occur at any age but is usually found in those over 40 years of age. The onset may be acute or chronic, and pain is felt in the shoulder region and upper arm. Night pain may be prominent, especially following lying on the affected shoulder. Both active and passive movements may be limited and a painful arc is common. A number of tests have been developed to detect subacromial impingement (Table 151.3, Figure 151.5). Persistent impingement may lead to chronic subacromial bursitis and tendinopathy of the rotator cuff.

Imaging

Plain radiographs may show degenerative change of the AC joint, irregularity of the undersurface of the acromion, humeral greater tuberosity degenerative change, and elongation of the anterior process of the acromion. Ultrasound may be normal but frequently reveals degenerative change in the cuff tendons with or without subacromial bursitis. MRI mirrors the plain film findings, often showing a degenerative AC joint indenting the superior surface of

Table 151.3 Impingement tests

Neer's test	Passive forward flexion of arm fixing scapula	Pain develops during this action which is relieved following a subacromial injection of local anaesthetic
Hawkins-Kennedy test	Arm abducted to 90° with 30° flexion. Arm is then passively internally rotated	Pain develops during internal rotation of arm
Painful arc	Arm abducted through full range of movement	Classic painful arc occurs between 60–120° of abduction
Empty can test	(see table 3)	

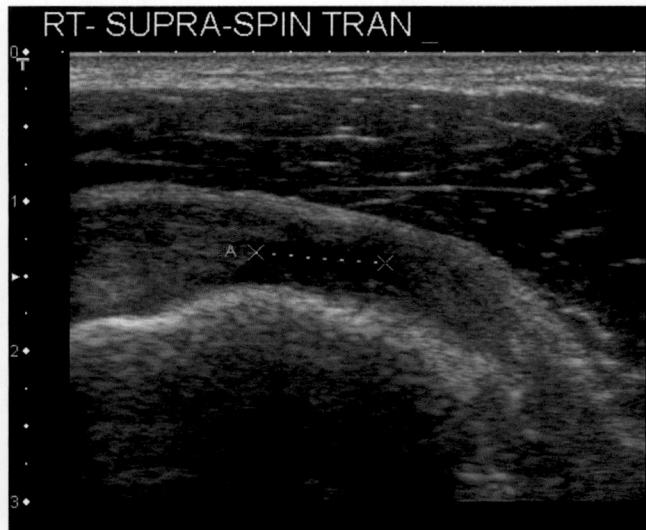

Fig. 151.5 Tests for subacromial impingement.

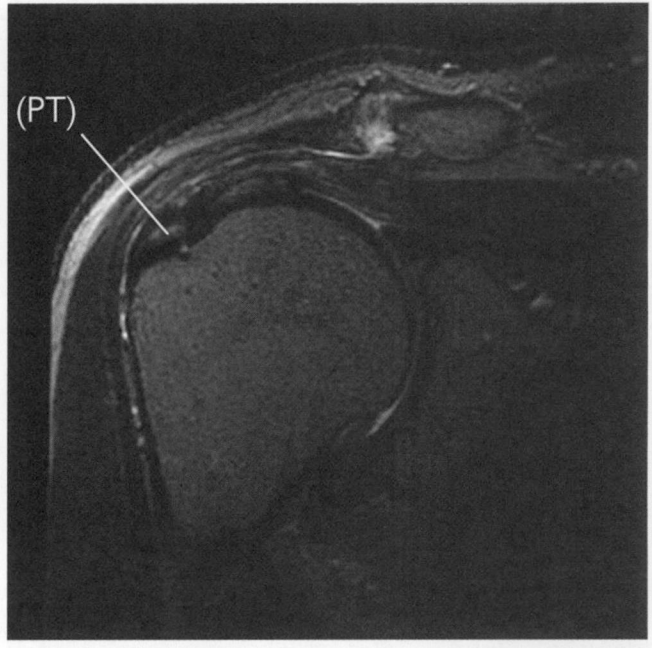

Fig. 151.6 Partial thickness tear of the supraspinatus tendon, on a background of severe tendonosis0020 (PT)?.

the supraspinatus tendon. Other features may include an os acromiale, an impingement cyst in the humeral head, rotator cuff tendinopathy and subacromial bursitis.

Management

The majority of patients settle with time following conservative treatment consisting of simple analgesia and non-steroidal anti-inflammatory drugs (NSAIDs), lifestyle modification, physiotherapy, and subacromial corticosteroid injections. The evidence for all of these modalities is limited, however. In a pragmatic randomized controlled trial (RCT) in the treatment of patients with subacromial impingement syndrome, injection plus exercise and exercise only were similarly effective at 12 weeks.[8] In a further study over the short term (3 months), a specific exercise strategy improved outcomes and reduced the subsequent need for surgery.[9] In a meta-analysis therapeutic exercise appeared to be effective for the treatment of painful shoulder conditions.[10] For patients who fail the above, surgical subacromial decompression is an option.

Rotator cuff disease

Although impingement is the most common clinical syndrome presenting with shoulder pain, the most common pathology underlying this is damage to the rotator cuff. The prevalence has been estimated to be 4.5% among men and 6.1% of women of working age; however, these figures vary as a consequence of difficulties with case definition estimates.[3,4,11] The socio-economic impact is substantial, with both direct and indirect costs including

those related to reduced productivity. The precise aetiology of rotator cuff disease has not been determined, but genetic factors, age-related degeneration with reduced blood supply, and inflammation appear to be intimately involved.[12] Not all rotator cuff damage is symptomatic, however, with studies showing full-thickness tears in up to 80% of individuals over 80 years of age without shoulder complaints.[13]

The rotator cuff may be affected by a number of defined lesions. Tendinosis refers to tendon degeneration; partial thickness tears (bursal and/or humeral aspects) refers to tendons which are frayed or torn but overall remain intact (Figure 151.6), full-thickness lesions refer to tears which have passed completely through the tendon substance although some fibres may remain intact (Figure 151.7). Complete tears describe total disruption of the tendon with resultant tendon retraction, and cuff rupture implies large complete tears. The tendon of supraspinatus is the most commonly affected, but combined lesions are common.[3]

Clinical features

Rotator cuff tears usually occur in individuals over 40 years of age and may either have an insidious onset or occur suddenly especially following trauma. Pain is often aching in nature, felt diffusely in

(a)

Painful arc
(active)

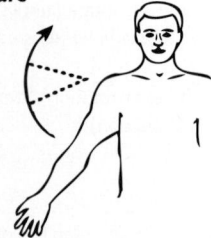

| Action: | Patient standing. Slow arm abduction (scapular plane). |
| Positive test: | Pain onset (maximal) at (variable) angular range |

(b)

Neer test
(passive)

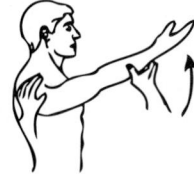

| Action: | Patient sitting/standing. Passive forward flexion. Scapula fixed. |
| Positive test: | Pain at (variable) angle of flexion. |

(c)

Empty can
(active)

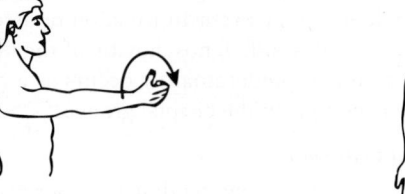

| Action: | Patient sitting/standing. Active forward flexion to 90° then internal rotation—'can empties'. |
| Positive test: | Pain with flexion or rotation of arm. |

(d)

Kennedy–Hawkins
(passive)

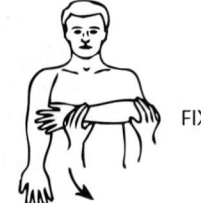

FIX

| Action: | Patient sitting/standing. Passive forward flexion (90°). Fix elbow with hand. Passive internal rotation. |
| Positive test: | Pain at some stage of elevation or rotation. |

Fig. 151.7 Ultrasound showing a supraspinatus full-thickness tear.

the shoulder region, with radiation into the upper arm. Night pain is common and sleep is affected when lying on the affected side. Performing activities above the head and behind the back are problematic. Work involving repetitive movements or lifting heavy loads may lead to the slow development of a tear and may exacerbate the symptoms. Muscle wasting around the shoulder can occur, especially the supraspinatus, and winging of the scapula may be present. A painful arc is frequently present (classically between 60–120° of abduction) as are signs of impingement (Tables 151.3 and 151.4, Figure 151.5). If weakness of the muscles develops, active shoulder movement is reduced but passive mobility is preserved. Complete tears and rupture will lead to total loss of movement, however. A number of tests have been developed to assess the rotator cuff more precisely, including eliciting impingement, although the true validity of all of these is unclear (Tables 151.3 and 151.4, Figure 151.5). Some experts suggest that weakness out of proportion to pain when assessing the rotator cuff implies tendon tear. Impingement testing relies on the ability to force the subacromial structures (e.g. bursa

and rotator cuff) between the inferior surface of the acromion and the humeral head.[14]

Imaging

Further investigation is not required in most cases of uncomplicated shoulder pain, but in persistent or severe cases radiological assessment is necessary. Plain radiographs may show degenerative change in the AC joint and impingement changes in the greater tuberosity with a narrowing of the subacromial space. Both ultrasound and MRI are extremely useful modalities for assessing the rotator cuff, with similar sensitivities and specificities.[15] Ultrasound has the advantage of being dynamic but the disadvantage of being operator dependent. MRI allows assessment of the entire shoulder complex, although cost and access are limiting factors.

Management

In the acute phase pain relief is necessary using simple analgesics and NSAIDs; ice, acupuncture, and laser therapy may be helpful.

Table 151.4 Special tests for rotator cuff tendinopathy

Supraspinatus	'Empty can' test	Arm abducted to 90° with 30° of flexion then internally rotated until thumbs facing ground. Pressure then applied from above by examiner (resisted abduction)
		Pain develops during the 'emptying of the can' (internal rotation). Weakness/pain upon downward pressure on arm (resisted abduction)
Infraspinatus and teres minor	External rotation of arm in neutral position, elbow flexed to 90°	Pain/weakness on resisted external rotation
Subscapularis	Lift-off test. Alternative is 'Napoleon' position with palm of hand placed against abdomen	Hand is placed behind back, palm facing outwards. Patient then lifts off hand away from back
		Alternative method is to then push hand into abdomen
		Pain/weakness upon resisted internal rotation
Biceps brachii	Speed's test	Resisted flexion of the shoulder with the arm in extension
	Yergeson's test	Resisted supination of the arm with the elbow at 90° of flexion

These modalities are utilized essentially to maintain passive joint movement to prevent secondary capsulitis. In latter stages physiotherapists may use a variety of modalities to improve the symptoms, including stretching and cuff-strengthening exercises, as well as muscle balance and re-education programmes especially for those patients with instability.[16] Education regarding avoidance of exacerbating activities is paramount.

The evidence regarding any treatment modality for shoulder pathology is limited: a systematic review of RCTs of physiotherapy for patients with soft tissue disorders concluded that ultrasound therapy was not effective and that the benefit of other interventions (low-level laser therapy, transcutaneous electrical stimulation, pulsed electromagnetic fields, cold therapy, thermotherapy, exercises, mobilizations, and manipulations) was inconclusive.[17] A randomized trial of the effectiveness of corticosteroid injections in comparison with physiotherapy for the treatment of painful stiff shoulder concluded that injections were superior to physiotherapy in the short term.[18] Although corticosteroid injections into the subacromial space are used extensively, the evidence for any long-term benefit is minimal. A Cochrane review concluded that the evidence from RCTs supports the administration of subacromial corticosteroid injections for rotator cuff disease although the effect may be small, short-lived, and no more effective than NSAIDS.[19] Injections should not be given in the acute setting and are generally undertaken if analgesia and physiotherapy fail.

Surgical intervention is appropriate for active patients who suffer from a full-thickness tear or rupture and for those where the above modalities have failed. This may be undertaken in an open fashion or increasingly via the arthroscopic route.[20] Surgery may involve subacromial decompression with or without repair of a torn tendon.

Prognosis

Although it was previously thought to have a favourable prognosis, reports vary as to the long-term outcome in patients with disorders of the rotator cuff. Studies in primary care have shown persist shoulder pain beyond 18 months in more than one-half of patients.[21,22] In another study, after 13 years' follow-up of patients with a rotator cuff tear diagnosed by MRI or arthrography, 90% of patients had no or only slight pain and 70% had no disturbance in activities of daily living.[23]

Biceps tendon lesions

Disorders of the biceps tendon include tendonitis/tenosynovitis, tendinosis, partial tear, full-thickness tear, complete rupture, and instability in the bicipital groove (subluxation or dislocation). Any of these lesions may occur in isolation or associated with damage to the rest of the cuff. Tenosynovitis of the long head of biceps is uncommon and predominantly occurs as a consequence of local friction over bone in the bicipital groove.

Clinical features

Pathology of the biceps tendon may occur at any age although rupture is uncommon in those under 40 years of age. Pain in the anterior shoulder may develop acutely or chronically, but tendon rupture may be painless. A history of trauma to the shoulder may be present. Tenderness is common over the tendon in the bicipital groove and weakness may occur following a tear. The 'Popeye' sign (prominent belly of biceps in the lower third of the arm) is characteristic following rupture of the long head of the biceps. A snapping sound may occur with subluxation and dislocation of the tendon.

Imaging

Ultrasound and MRI are the optimal modalities to evaluate the spectrum of biceps tendon disorders if required.

Management

The mainstay of treatment is analgesia and physiotherapy. Despite the deformity associated with tendon rupture functional limitation is usually minimal and thus patients should be reassured. Corticosteroid injections are not recommended for lesions of the biceps, including tenosynovitis, because of the potential for iatrogenic tendon rupture.

Rotator cuff calcification (calcific tendonitis)

Calcific tendonitis occurs following calcium hydroxyapatite deposition in the rotator cuff (most commonly the tendon of supraspinatus). The aetiology is unclear, although it has been suggested that injury leads to tendon calcification which is followed by variable degrees of resorption of the deposit. Inflammation associated with the resorptive phase (where calcium deposits are extravasated into the subacromial bursa) may be responsible for the severe pain which characterizes the condition.[24] Asymptomatic calcification within the cuff is not an infrequent finding and thus the association between this and the clinical presentation remains unclear.

Clinical features

Calcific tendonitis affects up to 10% of the population usually between 30 and 60 years of age. It often presents with rapid-onset severe, diffuse shoulder pain in the absence of trauma. The discomfort is constant and night pain is prominent. Systemic symptoms such as fever and anorexia may be present. The shoulder is often tender, and mobility (particularly abduction) is greatly reduced secondary to the pain. Wasting of the supraspinatus may be seen in chronic cases. The arm is usually held in internal rotation and a painful arc is frequent. Signs of impingement are invariable.

Imaging

Plain radiography is the best technique for demonstrating calcific tendonitis as calcium deposition is easily seen. This may be in discrete deposits, or fluffy in appearance, depending upon the stage of disease (Figure 151.8). It is worth noting that calcium deposition may be absent in the early phase. Ultrasound can also detect calcific deposits, but MRI does not as it is reliant on the presence of protons.

Management

The most important aspect of management is adequate pain relief starting with simple analgesics (paracetamol ± codeine) and NSAIDs. Gentle physiotherapy to maintain range of movement is important but is frequently limited by pain. Subacromial injections of corticosteroids and local anaesthetic have been used with variable success. Arthroscopy or ultrasound-guided needling of the calcium deposits has been advocated in severe cases.[25]

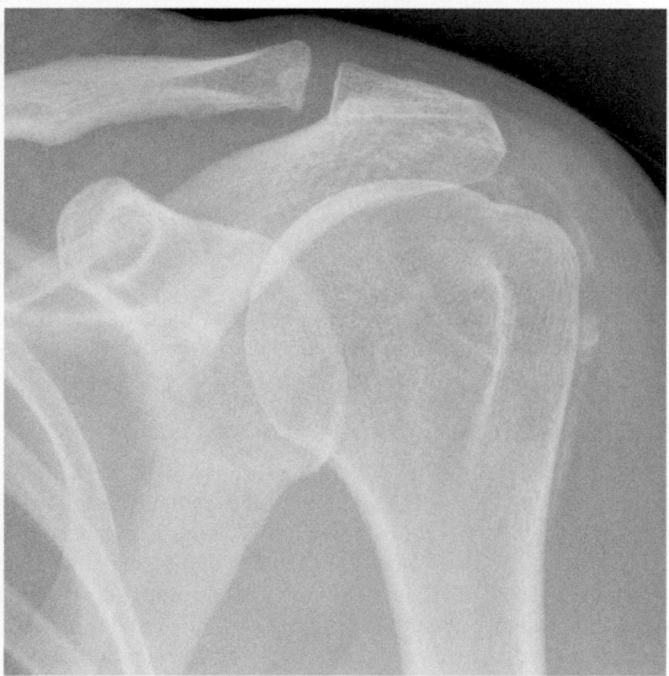

Fig. 151.8 Frontal plain film displaying calcium in the subacromial subdeltoid bursa. This has arisen from calcific tendonitis of the supraspinatus tendon which has burst into the bursa.

Adhesive capsulitis (frozen shoulder)

Adhesive capsulitis is one of the most perplexing conditions facing clinicians. It represents a common cause of shoulder pain and disability affecting up to 3% of the population predominantly in the 6th decade.[26] The incidence in diabetics is higher, having been estimated to be up to 38%.[26] The aetiology of adhesive capsulitis is unknown, although chronic inflammatory cell infiltration of the subsynovial capsule with fibrosis, and focal degeneration of collagen, has been described. As a consequence the capsule becomes thickened and contracted, leading to profound loss of movement. A number of conditions are associated with adhesive capsulitis (Box 151.1).

Three overlapping phases have been described for adhesive capsulitis:

- **freezing** phase where the shoulder becomes painful and mobility reduces (10–36 weeks)
- **frozen (adhesive)** phase where the shoulder is immobile and pain subsides (4–12 months)
- **thawing (resolution)** phase where pain resolves and movement returns (12–42 months).

United Kingdom consensus criteria have defined the condition as: symptoms of unilateral pain in the deltoid area with equal restriction of active and passive glenohumeral movement in a capsular pattern (external rotation > abduction > internal rotation).[27]

Clinical features

The onset may be acute, subacute, or chronic and a history of trauma is often described. Pain is felt deep in the shoulder, is poorly localized, and night pain may be severe. Bilateral disease either synchronously or metachronously occurs in up to 17% within 5 years. Following prolonged immobility, wasting of the shoulder muscles ensues. The cardinal feature of adhesive capsulitis is a globally reduced range of movement of the shoulder, especially external rotation and abduction. Assessment of other shoulder structures is generally not possible because of the pain and immobility. The diagnosis should be made on clinical grounds following exclusion of other causes of a painful, 'stiff' shoulder (e.g. glenohumeral osteoarthritis, inflammatory arthritis, crystal disease).

Box 151.1 Conditions associated with adhesive capsulitis

- Rotator cuff tendinopathy
- Diabetes mellitus (types 1 and 2)
- Thyroid disease (hyper- and hypothyroidism)
- Immobility (e.g. post stroke)
- Post myocardial infarction
- Chronic regional pain syndrome type 1
- Thoracotomy
- Dupytren's disease
- Shoulder surgery
- Parkinson's disease
- Pulmonary disease

Imaging

Plain radiographs, ultrasound, and MRI are usually normal. Arthrography is the only radiological way to diagnose adhesive capsulitis. Injection of contrast medium into the shoulder may lead to the following features: less than 5 mL can be injected, irregularity of the capsular attachment to the anatomical neck of the humerus, obliteration of the subscapular and axillary recesses, lymphatic filling, syringe refills once pressure is removed from the plunger, the injection is painful.

Management

The main therapeutic focus of adhesive capsulitis is adequate pain relief (simple analgesics and NSAIDs) in order to maintain and improve shoulder mobility. Physiotherapy is critical to this process and should be introduced early.[28] Oral and intra-articular steroids as well as arthroscopy (including manipulation under anaesthesia) have been advocated; however, the evidence for these is sparse and iatrogenic damage to shoulder structures may occur following surgery.[29,30] Hydrodilatation has been suggested as a useful treatment modality.[31] It is worth noting that no therapeutic intervention has been consistently successful for the condition and therefore an elixir of time coupled with adequate patient education regarding the prolonged course of the condition is the mainstay of management.

Prognosis

The natural history of adhesive capsulitis is of slow resolution which may take 3–4 years. Residual restriction of movement occurs in up to 15% of patients. Diabetics often have a more severe and prolonged course.[26]

Acute dislocation

Acute shoulder dislocation is a frequent presentation to the Emergency Department and usually follows forced abduction, external rotation, and extension of the shoulder. In 98% of cases the dislocation occurs anteriorly and recurrence is common (up to 80%). Posterior dislocation is rare and usually follows trauma, an epileptic seizure, or electrocution.

Clinical features

Shoulder dislocation is a disorder of teenagers and young adults. It is most frequent in females and those with hypermobility or ligamentous laxity. The patient presents with sudden-onset excruciating pain in the shoulder region with anterior bulging of the shoulder (rarely posteriorly). A 'square-shoulder' appearance, with prominence of the acromion, may be present with anterior dislocations. The arm is usually held in slight abduction and external rotation and movement is limited because of pain and anatomical derangement. Middle-aged patients may suffer from an associated rotator cuff tear. Dislocation can lead to humeral head damage, posing an increased risk for further instability and arthritis.

Imaging

Plain radiographs confirm the diagnosis as the head of the humerus is no longer located in the glenoid fossa (Figure 151.9). Two orthogonal views are required if the dislocation is subtle or subluxation has occurred.

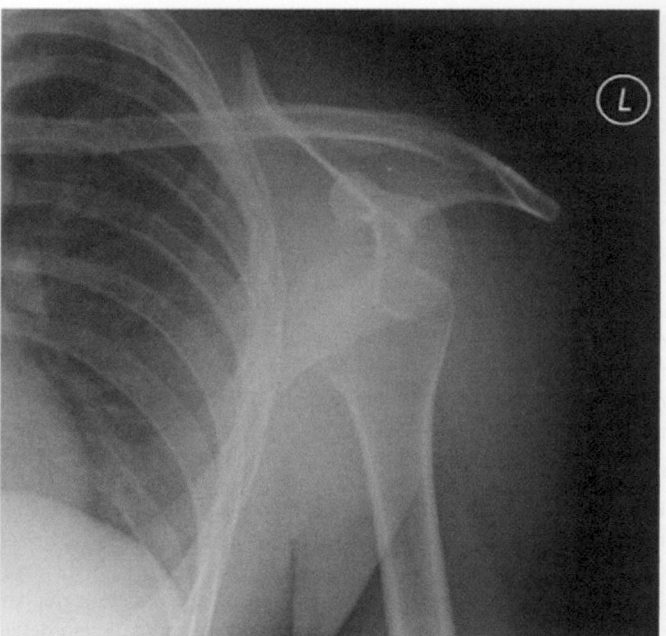

Fig. 151.9 Acute anterior dislocation of the right shoulder.

Management

Reduction of the dislocation should occur as soon as possible. Adequate analgesia is required and occasionally a general anaesthetic is necessary. Surgery is reserved for those with recurrent dislocations (to tighten the joint capsule) and for those with associated lesions (see below).[32]

Prognosis

Following dislocation the anteroinferior aspect of the joint capsule and the labrum may be torn off the glenoid, occasionally with a bony fragment (Bankart lesion). This may be accompanied by a compression fracture of the posterior surface of the humeral head (Hills–Sachs lesion) following impaction against the anterior glenoid rim. Recurrence of shoulder dislocation is common, occurring in up to 80%.

Shoulder instability

As the shoulder is the most mobile joint in the body, instability is not uncommon. Instability is defined as an inability to maintain the humeral head within the glenoid fossa and may be classified by the direction of the abnormal movement (anterior, posterior, multidirectional), as well as by its severity and causality.

Clinical features

In general anterior instability first presents in patients under 30 years of age. Pain is intermittent and may develop following specific movements such as throwing. Clicking is a subtle sign, but clucks are a feature of major instability. In a young athlete the development of rotator cuff tendinosis may point to underlying shoulder instability. A pathognomonic sign of shoulder instability/subluxation is 'dead arm syndrome' with transient numbness, tingling, pain, and weakness of the arm or hand followed by a dull ache occurring following certain activities. Often there is a history of throwing sports, swimming, gymnastics, or ballet. Full active and passive movement is retained and features of hypermobility may be present (see also Chapter 159). The humeral head may be rocked forward and backwards in the glenoid fossa when the patient is relaxed, the 'draw sign' (best appreciated in the supine position). Signs of impingement may also be present. The 'apprehension' test is specific for anterior instability. With the patient in the supine position, pain and anxiety may occur following abduction and external rotation of the arm ('javelin' position). Anterior pressure applied to the humeral head often relieves the discomfort, only to recur when the stabilizing force is removed.

Clinically posterior instability may be identified by noting a concavity below the acromion, anterior deltoid flattening, and a palpable humeral head posteriorly. The arm is usually held in adduction and internal rotation with reduced active and passive external rotation. Applying a downward pressure to the flexed, adducted, and internally rotated arm leads to pain or a feeling of joint dislocation in patients with posterior instability. Posterior instability may be a feature of congenital laxity.

Multidirectional instability is a feature of general laxity of the ligaments or hypermobility syndrome. Dislocation following minimal trauma may point to this predisposition. As with anterior instability, a painful arc may be present. Traction applied to the arm will lead to the shoulder subluxing inferiorly (sulcus sign) and the draw sign may be present. Individuals with multidirectional instability should be assessed for conditions such as Ehlers–Danlos syndrome, osteogenesis imperfect, and Marfan's syndrome.

Imaging

This is usually normal in uncomplicated instability, but plain radiography will show an abnormally placed humeral head if instability has led to dislocation. MR arthrography has 80–90% sensitivity and specificity for labral pathology.

Management

Physiotherapy to improve the strength of the rotator cuff muscles is imperative. Education regarding avoidance of activities leading to pain is mandatory, although difficult in those who pursue sport at a high level. Surgery is reserved for those with disabling symptoms or recurrent dislocations.[33]

Prognosis

The prognosis is good with appropriate management and education. Repeated paroxysms of instability may lead to rotator cuff tendinopathy and signs of impingement. A reverse Hills–Sacks lesion (fracture of the glenoid rim and proximal humerus) may occur following posterior dislocation. A superior labrum in the anterior-posterior (SLAP) lesion may occur in patients with underlying instability of the shoulder (Figure 151.10). Surgery is advocated for labral tears.

Shoulder arthritis

The shoulder is frequently involved in arthritic conditions which may affect the glenohumeral, AC, and/or sternoclavicular joints.

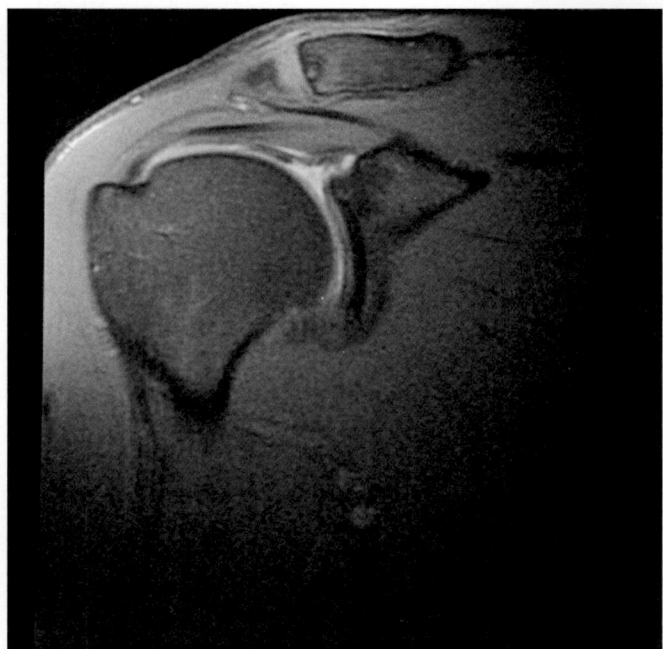

Fig. 151.10 Coronal oblique MR arthrogram showing tear and disruption of the anterior labrum anterosuperiorly (T).

Glenohumeral joint

Up to 90% of patients with rheumatoid arthritis (RA) have involvement of the glenohumeral joint and it is also a common site for gout and pseudogout. Degenerative disease occurs rarely here but may develop secondary to inflammatory arthritidies, avascular necrosis or after trauma.

Clinical features

Chronic, deep-seated pain affecting the whole shoulder in patients over 40 years of age characterizes shoulder arthritis. Degenerative disease is aggravated by activity and improved with rest, the opposite being true of inflammatory arthritis. Sleep is often disturbed and early-morning stiffness may be a feature (<30 minutes with degenerative disease, >30 minutes with inflammatory disease). Swelling is a feature of inflammatory and crystal arthritis and crepitus is a sign of bony surfaces grating. Both active and passive movement is significantly limited, especially external rotation and abduction. True glenohumeral movement only occurs up to 90° of abduction (further abduction allowed by the scapulothoracic articulation). Careful assessment is required as patients may 'cheat' and hunch the shoulder giving the impression of glenohumeral movement. If inflammatory arthritis is considered, a full musculoskeletal review of the patient is required.

Imaging

Radiographs may show narrowing of the joint space, irregularity of the joint surfaces, osteophytes, and soft tissue swelling (Figure 151.11). For inflammatory arthritis ultrasound and MRI allow further characterization of the pathology.

Management and prognosis

The treatment and prognosis of degenerative, inflammatory, and crystalline disorders are dealt with in other sections of the book. In

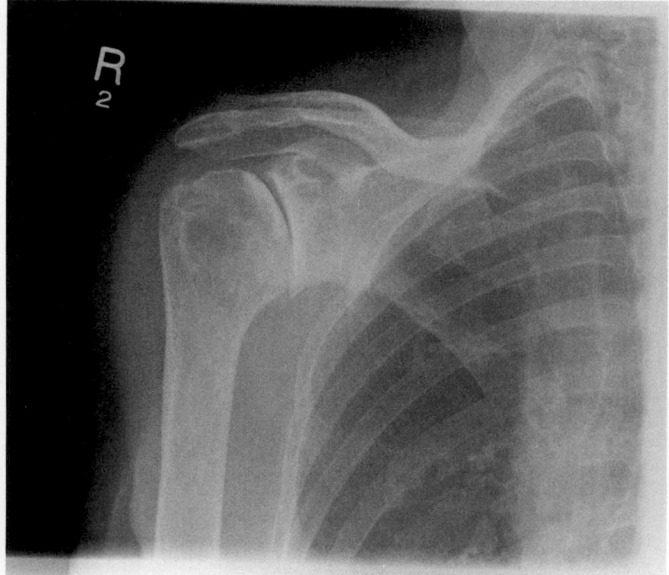

Fig. 151.11 Osteoarthritis of the glenohumeral joint.

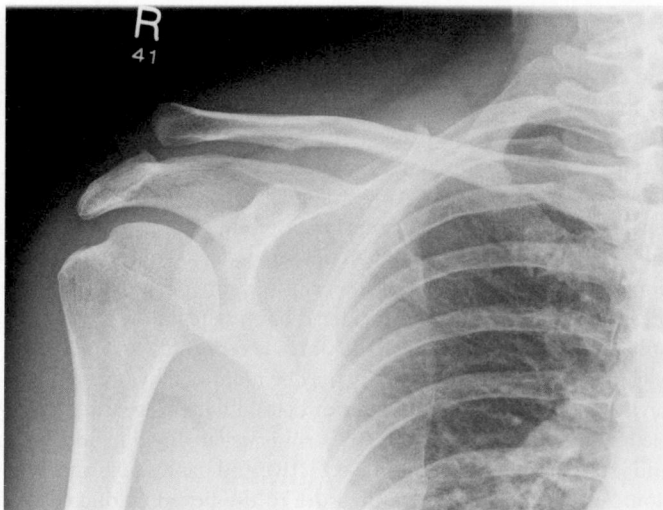

Fig. 151.12 Total dislocation of the right acromioclavicular joint.

principle analgesia is mandatory and corticosteroid injections may be useful in selected patients. Severe glenohumeral disease often requires hemiarthoplasty or total shoulder replacement. As up to 35% of patients who require arthroplasty have rotator cuff tear, these should be repaired simultaneously.

Acromioclavicular joint trauma

Trauma to the AC joint is common particularly among athletes undertaking contact sports. This may lead to sprain/strain, subluxation, or dislocation of the joint.

Clinical features

The onset of pain is acute following trauma and may occur at any age. Discomfort is worse with movement and activities such as carrying heavy loads and overhead work. The pain is well localized to the shoulder tip, and symptoms at night are common. Weakness is not a feature although shoulder instability may develop. Deformity of the AC joint implies subluxation or dislocation. A high arc of pain may be evident and full active and passive movement is often limited by discomfort.

Imaging

Plain radiographs will delineate AC joint subluxation or dislocation (Figure 151.12). The degree of damage can then be staged.[34]

Management

AC joint subluxation may be managed conservatively. Dislocation generally requires surgical intervention which should be undertaken early.

Acromioclavicular joint arthritis

This joint is commonly affected by osteoarthritic change, especially in older people.

Clinical features as for AC joint trauma. Features of rotator cuff tendinopathy may develop secondary to AC joint degenerative

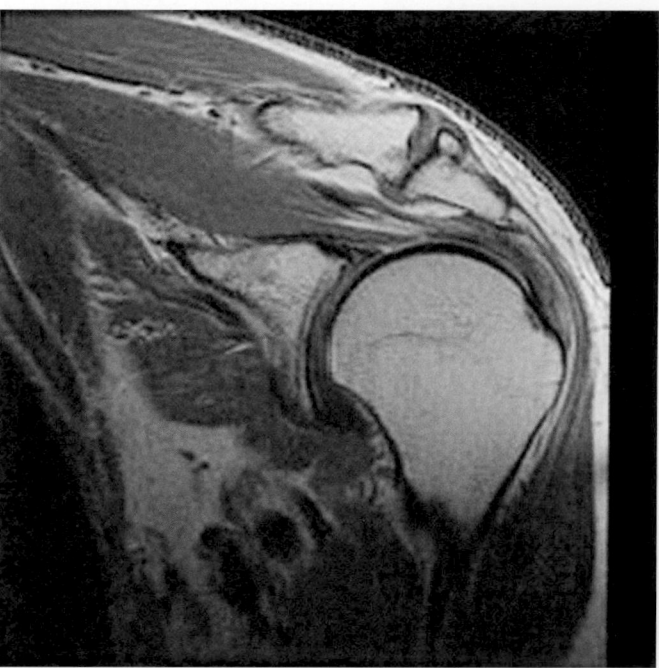

Fig. 151.13 Moderately severe degenerative change of the acromioclavicular joint (*).

disease. Plain films display degenerative disease of the bones with osteophyte development. MRI may also demonstrate associated rotator cuff damage (Figure 151.13).

Sternoclavicular joint

Degenerative disease occurs rarely in this area. Inflammatory disease occurs more commonly in this joint including RA, spondyloarthropathies, and SAPHO (synovitis, acne, pustulosis, hyperostosis, osteitis). The mainstay of therapy for osteoarthritis of the sternoclavicular joint is analgesia, education, and physiotherapy. Intraarticular corticosteroid injections may help but the effect is usually short lived. Surgery is rarely required.

References

1. Peter D, Davies P, Pietroni P. Musculoskeletal clinic in general practice: a study of one year's referrals. *Br J Gen Pract* 1994;44(378):25–29.

2. Linsell L, Dawson J, Zondervan K et al. Prevalence and incidence of adults consulting for shoulder conditions in UK primary care: patterns of diagnosis and referral. *Rheumatology* 2006;45(2):215–221.

3. Ostör AJ, Richards CA, Prevost AT, Speed CA, Hazleman BL. Diagnosis and relation to general health of shoulder disorders presenting to primary care. *Rheumatology* 2005;44:800–805.

4. Walker-Bone KE, Palmer KT, Reading I, Coggon D, Cooper C. Prevalence and impact of musculoskeletal disorders of the upper limb in the general population. *Arthritis Rheum* 2004;51:642–651.

5. Nygren A, Berlund A, von Koch M. Neck and shoulder pain, an increasing problem: strategies for using insurance material to follow trends. *Scand J Rehabil Med Suppl* 1995;32:107–112.

6. Van der Heijden GJ. Shoulder disorders: a state of the art review. *Baillieres Best Prac Res Clinic Rheumatol* 1999;13(2):287–309.

7. Lewis JS. Rotator cuff tendinopathy/subacromial impingement syndrome: is it time for a new method of assessment? *Br J Sports Med* 2009;43(4):259–264.

8. Crawshaw DP, Helliwell PS, Hensor EM et al. Exercise therapy after corticosteroid injection for moderate to severe shoulder pain: large pragmatic randomised trial. *BMJ* 2010;28;340:c3037.

9. Holmgren T, Hallgren HB, Oberg B, Adolfsson L, Johansson K. Effect of specific exercise strategy on need for surgery in patients with subacromial impingement syndrome: randomised controlled study. *BMJ* 2012;344:e787.

10. Marinko LN, Chacko JM, Dalton D, Chacko CC. The effectiveness of therapeutic exercise for painful shoulder conditions: a meta-analysis. *J Shoulder Elbow Surg* 2011;20:1351–1359.

11. Walker-Bone KE, Palmer KT, Reading I, Cooper C. Criteria for assessing pain and nonarticular soft-tissue rheumatic disorders of the neck and upper limb. *Semin Arthritis Rheum* 2003;33:168–184.

12. Benson RT, McDonnell SM, Knowles HJ et al. Tendinopathy and tears of the rotator cuff are associated with hypoxia and apoptosis. *J Bone Joint Surg Br* 2010;92:448–453.

13. Sher JS, Uribe JW, Posada A, Murphy BJ, Zlatkin MB. Abnormal findings on magnetic resonance images of asymptomatic shoulders. *J Bone Joint Surg Am* 1995;77:10–15.

14. Neer CS 2nd. Impingement lesions. *Clin Orthop Relat Res* 1983;173;70–77.

15. de Jesus JO, Parker L, Frangos AJ, Nazarian LN. Accuracy of MRI, MR arthrography, and ultrasound in the diangosis of rotator cuff tears: a meta-analysis. *Am J Roentgenol* 2009;192:1701–1707.

16. Kuhn JE. Exercise in the treatment of rotator cuff impingement: a systematic review and a synthesized evidence-based rehabilitation protocol. *J Shoulder Elbow Surg* 2009;18:138–160.

17. Van der Heijden GJ, van der Windt DA, de Winter AF. Physiotherapy for patients with soft tissue diorders: a systematic review of randomised controlled trials. *BMJ* 1997;315:25–30. .

18. Van der Windt DA, Koes BW, Deville W et al. Effectiveness of corticosteroid injections versus physiotherapy for treatment of painful stiff shoulder in primary care: randomised trial. *BMJ* 1998;317:1292–1296.

19. Buchbinder R, Green S, Youd JM. Corticosteroid injections for shoulder pain. *Cochrane Database Syst Rev* 2003;1:CD004016.

20. Severud E, Ruotolo C, Abbott D et al. All-arthroscopic versus mini-open rotator cuff repair: a long-term retrospective outcome comparison. *Arthroscopy* 2003;19:234–238.

21. Oh LS, Wolf BR, Hall MP, Levy BA, Marx RG. Indications for rotator cuff repair: a systematic review. *Clin Orthop Relat Res* 2007;455:52–63.

22. Croft P, Pope D, Silman A. The clinical course of shoulder pain: prospective cohort study in primary care. Primary Care Rheumatology Society Shoulder Study Group. *BMJ* 1996;313:601–602.

23. Kijima H, Minagawa H, Nishi T, Kikuchi K, Shimada Y. Long term follow-up of cases of rotator cuff tear treated conservatively. *J Shoulder Elbow Surg* 2012;21:491–494.

24. Oliva F, Via AG, Maffulli N. Calcific tendinopathy of the rotator cuff tendons. *Sports Med Arthrosc* 2011;19:237–243.

25. Sconfienza LM, Bandirali M, Serafini G et al. Rotator cuff calcific tendinitis: does warm saline solution improve the short-term outcome of double-needle US-guided treatment? *Radiology* 2012;262:560–566.

26. Tighe CB, Oakley WS Jr. The prevalence of a diabetic condition and adhesive capsulitis of the shoulder. *South Med J* 2008;101:591–595.

27. Harrington JM, Carter JT, Birrell L, Gompertz D. Surveillance case definitions for work related upper limb pain syndromes. *Occup Environ Med* 1998;55:264–271.

28. Tashjian RZ. The effectiveness of nonoperative treatment for frozen shoulder: a systematic review. *Clin J Sports Med* 2012;22:168–169.

29. Lorbach O, Anagnostakos K, Scherf C et al. Nonoperative management of adhesive capsulitis of the shoulder: oral cortisone application versus intra-articular cortisone injections. *J Shoulder Elbow Surg* 2010;19:172–179.

30. Robinson CM, Seah KT, Chee YH, Hindle P, Murray IR. Frozen shoulder. *J Bone Joint Surg Br* 2012;94(1):1–9.

31. Quraishi NA, Johnston P, Bayer J, Crowe M, Chakrabarti AJ. Thawing the frozen shoulder. A randomised trial comparing manipulation under anaesthesia with hydrodilatation. *J Bone Joint Surg Br* 2007;89:1197–1200.

32. Sileo MJ, Joseph S, Nelson CO, Botts JD, Penna J. Management of acute glenohumeral dislocations. *Am J Orthop* 2009;38:282–290.

33. Budoff JE, Wolf EM Arthroscopic treatment of glenohumeral instability. *J Hand Surg Am* 2006;31:1387–1396.

34. Macdonald PB, Lapointe P. Acromioclavicular and sternoclavicular joint injuries. *Orthop Clin North Am* 2008;39(4):535–545.

CHAPTER 152

Elbow

Karen Walker-Bone

Introduction

Elbow pain affects around 12% of adults at any point in time[1,2] and occurs at similar rates in both genders.[3] It may occur as part of a multisystem inflammatory arthropathy such as rheumatoid arthritis (RA) or gout or may be caused by degenerative changes, but it is uncommon for elbow symptoms to be the presenting feature in these conditions. The most common causes of elbow symptoms are soft tissue periarticular conditions such as epicondylitis, olecranon bursitis, and ulnar neuropathy.

Structure and function of the elbow joint

The elbow is a compound synovial joint involving articulation of the greater head of the distal humerus with the ulna, producing flexion/extension. Forearm pronation/supination results from two articulations: one between the lesser head of the humerus and the depression on the radial head and the other between the circumference of the radial head and the proximal ulna. All articular surfaces are covered with cartilage and combine in one capsule and joint cavity. Flexion/extension is stabilized by medial and lateral collateral ligaments. Additional stabilization of the proximal radioulnar joint is ensured by the annular ligament, a complex structure formed of joint capsule fibres and part of the lateral ligament complex and surrounding the radial head.[4]

The healthy elbow is capable of 150° of flexion/extension. In early and late flexion, the shape of the articulation between the distal humerus and the proximal ulna is oblique causing rotation and a valgus angle at full extension and supination (the carrying angle), which is typically greater among women (20–25°) than men (10–15°). Varus deformity of the elbow may result from any elbow joint pathology or from trauma (Figure 152.1). The healthy elbow can extend completely (0°), although healthy young women may achieve additional extension (5°) and patients with hypermobility syndrome or other ligamentous conditions frequently hyperextend further. Rotation of the forearm (typically around 160°) is achieved through pronation/supination at the proximal and distal radioulnar joints accompanied by a twisting movement between the shafts of both bones.

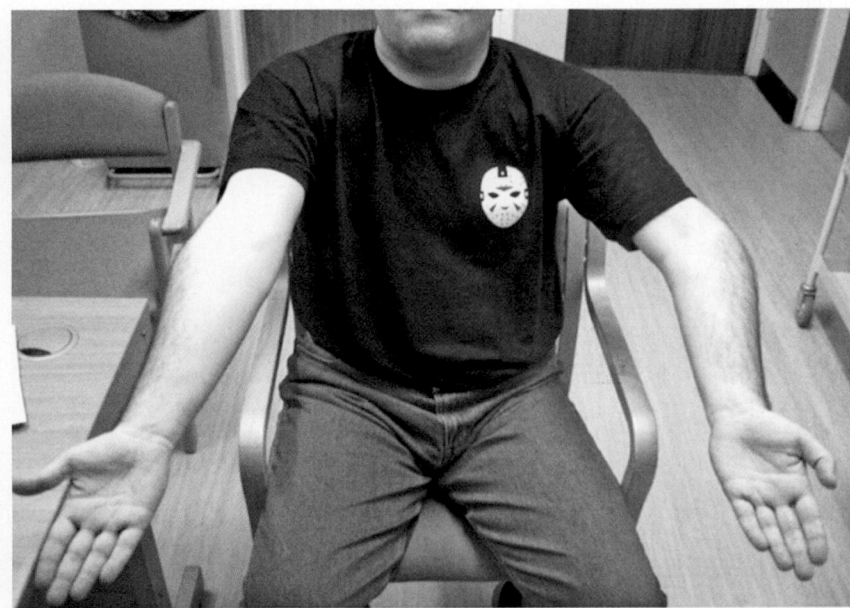

Fig. 152.1 Cubitus varus left elbow caused by trauma.

Differential diagnosis of elbow pain

In any patient with elbow pain, the clinician should consider if the symptom is a manifestation of a more generalized problem such as: a polyarthropathy (degenerative or inflammatory); referred pain from the cervical spine, peripheral nerves, nerve roots, brachial plexus, the shoulder or the wrist; a chronic widespread pain syndrome such as fibromyalgia; or another disease, e.g. metastasis from a primary malignancy.

History

The nature of onset of elbow symptoms is useful diagnostically (Table 152.1). Was there a preceding injury? Exactly what took place, and what were the immediate effects and subsequent progression? Enquire specifically about head/neck and shoulder injuries as well as elbow injury. Pain is the most common symptom: enquire about nature, site (articular, periarticular, regional), radiation (proximal and distal), variation over time, progression, exacerbating and relieving factors, therapies tried and response to those therapies. Has the patient ever had similar symptoms at the elbow or other sites? Enquire specifically about pain in the neck/shoulder and forearm, wrist/hand. Associated symptoms may include stiffness, swelling, heat, redness, dysaesthesiae, muscle weakness, crepitus, or locking. If the patient reports stiffness, enquire about distribution and effects on movements as well as timing and duration. Enquire specifically about functional impairment at home and in the workplace. In taking an occupational history, ask precisely what type and frequency of physical exposures are involved: for example, bending/straightening the elbow; lifting heavy weights; forceful and/or repetitive movements. It is important to establish the arrangements for rotation of tasks and the demands on the patient, e.g. if the patient is paid piecemeal based upon number of tasks completed. Establish which is the dominant arm and which exposures affect only the dominant side and which are bilateral.

Examination

The examiner should keep an open mind during the examination of a patient with elbow symptoms (Table 152.1). To do this, neck and both arms should be fully exposed. The examiner should also consider examining all other joints and a full clinical examination if there is any possibility of multisystem disease. Arms should be compared for wasting, scarring, or asymmetry, bearing in mind, however, that the dominant side may have better-developed musculature. Inspection should focus on the neck, thoracic spine, shoulders, and both hands/wrists as well as the elbows. Inspection of the elbow should include the antecubital fossa, posterior elbow and olecranon bursa and the distal insertion of the triceps, both epicondyles, and the proximal and distal musculature. The joint is continuous, so any inflammatory joint condition will affect all three joints, but swelling is usually best observed posteriorly and/or laterally where it may obliterate the paraolecranon grooves. With an acutely inflamed joint, the patient will often 'guard' the join in flexion but full flexion/extension may be restricted, as may pronation/supination. The bony landmarks should be palpated including the joint line medially and laterally over the distal humerus and the lateral and medial epicondyles. Active and passive range of motion of flexion–extension and pronation and supination should be evaluated and in suspected tendinitis, movement should be examined against resistance. Neurovascular function should also be assessed, including for

Table 152.1 Classification of elbow disorders

Articular	**Arthritis of the elbow joint and proximal** radioulnar joints
	Rheumatoid arthritis
	Psoriatic arthritis
	Gout
	Septic arthritis
	Osteoarthritis
	Traumatic
	Trauma to the joint capsule or ligaments
Periarticular	Lateral epicondylitis (tennis elbow)
	Medial epicondylitis (golfer's elbow)
	Tendinitis affecting the distal insertion of biceps brachii, triceps, or brachialis
Olecranon bursitis	Trauma or friction
	Inflammatory
	Septic
	Olecranon impingement syndrome
Bone disorder	Fracture
	Neoplasm (primary or secondary)
	Osteomyelitis
	Osteochondritis dissecans
Neurological	Cubital tunnel syndrome (ulnar nerve)
	Pronator teres syndrome (median nerve)
	Radial tunnel syndrome (posterior interosseous nerve)
	Spiral groove syndrome (radial nerve)
	Thoracic outlet syndrome (brachial plexus compression)
	Radiculopathy from cervical spine
	Syringomyelia
	Spinal cord tumours
Chronic widespread pain syndrome	Fibromyalgia syndrome
Regional pain syndrome	Complex regional pain syndrome type II (reflex sympathetic dystrophy)
	Somatoform pain syndrome
Vascular	Upper limb claudication
	Systemic vasculitis, e.g. Takayasu's arteritis
	Compartment syndrome

example Tinel's test for cubital tunnel syndrome (performed over the ulnar nerve in the ulnar groove) where appropriate. Comparison of the symmetry of upper limb pulse rate, volume, and character at each of the brachial and radial arteries may be indicated and blood pressure in both upper limbs may need to be compared.

Investigation and imaging of the elbow

Depending upon the working diagnosis, radiography, ultrasonography, diagnostic joint or bursa aspiration with microscopy, culture and sensitivities of the aspirate as well as polarizing light microscopy, CT scan, MRI scan, electromyography (EMG), and nerve conduction studies may be helpful diagnostically.

Elbow symptoms as the presenting feature of inflammatory polyarthritis

Gout, RA, reactive arthritis, psoriatic arthritis, and other types of inflammatory polyarthritis may all involve the elbow joint. It would be uncommon for patients with most of these conditions to present for the first time with symptoms confined to the elbow. Usually, therefore, a history of pain, swelling, and early-morning stiffness affecting other joints can be expected and the pattern and distribution of this will be helpful in diagnosis. Elbow involvement may occur in acute gout, often causing pain and inflammation in the olecranon bursa from where crystals may be aspirated. Most patients with gout (>80%) will have experienced at least one episode of podagra within the first 12 months of their gout, and enquiry should be made specifically about this.

Lateral epicondylitis (tennis elbow)

Lateral epicondylitis, thought to be synonymous with Morris's 1882 description of 'lawn tennis arm',[5] is associated with characteristic pain and sensitivity in the lateral elbow region, at or near the origin of the extensor carpi radialis brevis.

Epidemiology

The annual incidence of lateral epicondylitis was estimated in Sweden as 0.5–1%,[6] and one primary care survey in the United Kingdom found 0.4% of patients presented with a new episode annually.[7] Rates of point prevalence between 0.7–2.5% have been reported.[8,9] Higher rates of occurrence have been suggested among workers performing strenuous manual tasks, e.g. packers and sausage makers.[10] Despite its idiom, the epidemiology of epicondylitis among racket players has been poorly studied. Gruchow[11] reported an incidence rate of 9% among tennis players over a 2 month period but relied on self-reported symptoms rather than objective physical examination for diagnostic criteria. Rates of occurrence seemed

to be higher among men than women and rates peaked in the 45–54 year age group.[9]

Lateral epicondylitis is associated with the use of heavy tools and forceful, repetitive work, particularly when the wrist is in the non-neutral position, e.g. using power tools, saws, or jackhammers.[12] Repeated pronation and supination of the forearm, which may be an integral part of some jobs, aggravates the condition, but whether symptoms can arise ab initio from this action is more contentious. Even allowing for a clustering of the condition in families and a tendency for individuals to have more than one soft tissue lesion at other sites, not necessarily all simultaneously, the balance of probability is that this lesion can be induced in the workplace, particularly if the ergonomic insult corresponds with the use of the forearm muscles. In addition to physical factors, psychosocial risk factors can increase the occurrence of elbow disorders.[13]

Classification and diagnostic criteria

In their multidisciplinary Delphi investigation, Harrington and colleagues reached a consensus case definition of: pain and tenderness over the lateral epicondyle associated with exacerbation of lateral elbow pain on resisted wrist extension (Figure 152.2).[14] These diagnostic criteria have been used in a number of epidemiological studies,[15,16] although some investigators also use 'pain or weakness on gripping'. There is currently no gold standard for investigation of lateral epicondylitis. Radiographs may show evidence of a periostitis, but this is far from a consistent finding and radiographs would rarely be indicated. MRI or ultrasound may have a future role in the diagnosis of this disorder, but both techniques are currently only used as research tools. One clinical study suggested that thermography may have a role in detecting epicondylitis patients from controls.[17]

Aetiopathogenesis

Over 25 mechanisms of lateral epicondylitis have been proposed, but it is unclear how many of these are causes of non-specific lateral elbow pain, rather than 'true' epicondylitis. Few cases come

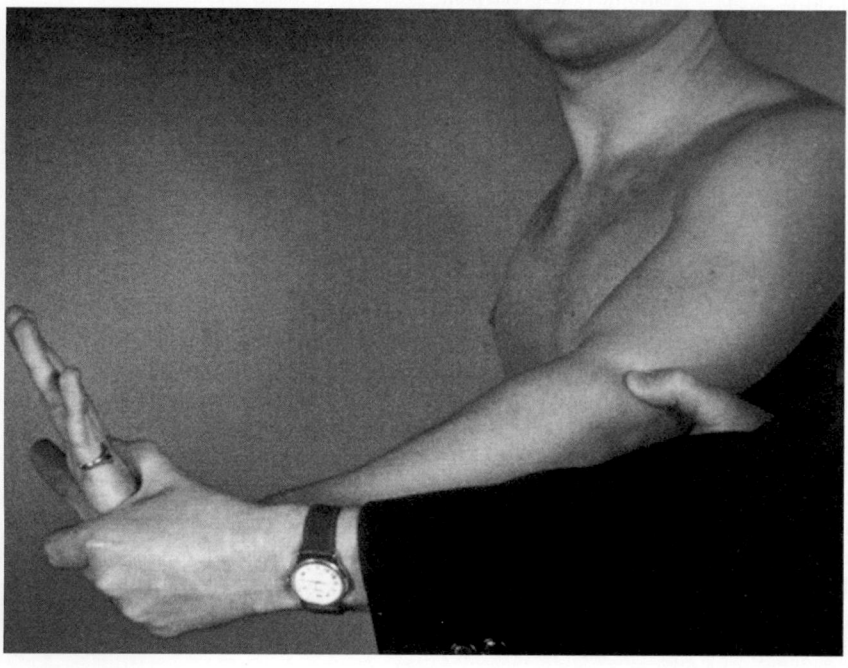

Fig. 152.2 Provocation test for lateral epicondylitis.

to surgery so that pathological material is rare and really only available in severe and chronic cases, but a number of pathological abnormalities have been described, including periostitis, infection, bursitis, radiohumeral joint disease, fibrillation of the radial head, proximal radioulnar joint disease, radial nerve entrapment, and annular ligament lesions. Despite this, the current consensus is that lateral epicondylitis is probably a tendinopathy of the common extensor-supinator tendon rather than an 'epicondylitis'. Ageing is associated with anatomical alteration at the enthesis, including changes in collagen content and increasing lipids, that may predispose to injury. Degenerative micro-tears can be demonstrated in the common extensor tendon origin and these are hypothesized to be due to cumulative or repetitive mechanical overload.

Clinical features

Patients present with lateral elbow pain and tenderness increased upon gripping, typically resulting in functional restrictions, e.g. in carrying shopping bags. There may be a history of an acute onset such as a wrenching injury, but more commonly the onset is gradual and insidious with no one particular trigger factor but rather longer-term overuse or strain especially with repeated flexion–extension or pronation–supination.

Management

In the acute phase, using ice over the lateral elbow, relative rest of exacerbating activities, analgesia, and use of non-steroidal anti-inflammatory drugs (NSAIDs) topically or orally may be helpful. In more prolonged symptoms, patients seek help from a variety of sources and may be offered local orthotics, local ultrasound, deep friction tissue massage, acupuncture, and extracorporeal shockwave therapy (ESWT). Unfortunately most of these approaches have to date rarely been studied in high-quality randomized controlled trials (RCTs).

Orthotics

In their recent Cochrane review, Striys et al. deduced that no definitive conclusions could be drawn concerning effectiveness of orthotic devices for lateral epicondylitis because there are not enough well-designed and well-conducted RCTs of sufficient power.[18]

Local ultrasound

Ultrasound has been evaluated as part of the treatment of lateral epicondylitis but usually as part of a 'package' of physical therapies including exercise or deep tissue massage, for example. As such, the authors of a Cochrane systematic review found insufficient evidence to conclude whether or not ultrasound alone was effective.[19]

Deep friction massage

One Cochrane review evaluated deep friction massage as a treatment for lateral epicondylitis but only two RCTs were found and the authors concluded that these showed no benefit of deep transverse friction massage combined with concurrent physiotherapy modalities, when compared to either a control group with the same physiotherapy modalities but without the massage, or other active therapies such as phonophoresis or therapeutic ultrasound combined with placebo ointment, for either improved functional performance or increased grip strength.[20] Their conclusions were limited by the lack of RCTs, the use of subjective and non-validated scales for measuring pain, the assessment of a combination of several physiotherapy modalities, and the small sample sizes.

Extracorporeal shockwave therapy

A Cochrane review of ESWT found that it had been evaluated in 1006 patients and that overall, there was 'platinum' evidence that it was of no benefit in reduction of pain or improvement of function from lateral epicondylitis and 'silver' evidence in 93 patients that steroid injection was superior to ESWT.[21] The National Institute for Health and Clinical Excellence (NICE) guidance on ESWT in the treatment of refractory tennis elbow suggested that there were no major safety concerns with this therapy, but found inconsistent evidence for the efficacy of this approach and recommended further research.[22]

Acupuncture

The evidence for acupuncture is conflicting. There have been few studies, including only small numbers of patients. As with evaluating the efficacy of acupuncture in most conditions, blinding of the patient and the assessor is difficult and rarely achieved. It is therefore currently unclear how effective acupuncture is in the treatment of lateral epicondylitis.[23]

Local steroid injections

Given its historically presumed inflammatory origin, local steroid injections have been used for lateral epicondylitis for many years.[24] Remarkably, however, there had been very little formal evaluation of the safety and efficacy of this approach until relatively recently. A 2002 systematic review using a highly sensitive search strategy found only 13 studies making 15 different comparisons (steroids vs placebo, n = 2; steroids vs. local anaesthetic, n = 5; steroids vs. another conservative treatment, n = 5; one type of steroids vs. another type of steroid injection, n = 3) with generally poor internal validity scores.[25] For short–term outcomes (≤6 weeks), including pain, grip strength and function, steroid injections produced better outcomes than placebo, local anaesthetic and conservative treatments. However, for intermediate (>6 weeks and ≤6 months) and longer outcomes (>6 months) there was no evidence for benefit of steroid injections in any 'clinically relevant' outcomes.[25] Another systematic review of corticosteroid injections (in the management of tendinopathy at different sites), again found significant effect sizes in favour of corticosteroid injections for lateral epicondylalgia in the short term (≤6 weeks) but no evidence of efficacy beyond this.[26] It can be generally concluded that although the available evidence is in favour of corticosteroid injections in the short term, it is impossible to draw firm conclusions on effectiveness given the absence of studies of good quality with intermediate and longer-term follow-up.[25]

Autologous blood injection

A small number of studies have been performed using autologous blood injection instead of corticosteroids injected over the lateral epicondyle. In their 2009 review of this procedure, NICE concluded that current evidence for this technique was inadequate in quantity and quality and that the procedure could not currently be recommended.[26]

Surgery

Surgical intervention is usually considered in severe, intractable cases after prolonged conservative therapy. Case series suggest reasonable benefit in some, but not all, study subjects and to date, surgical intervention has not been evaluated by RCTs.

Course and prognosis

Although it is generally described as a condition that is benign and self-limiting,[27] 5% of affected working-aged adults had taken sick leave because of their lateral epicondylitis, recording a median of 29 days' absence.[13] Up to 20% of those affected have symptoms persistent beyond 1 year, particularly if they have persevered with the activity that caused it.[28] Recurrence may be more common in manual workers where it may be attributable to repeated grasping or lifting activity.

Medial epicondylitis

The underlying disease process is thought to be similar in medial and lateral epicondylitis. Despite its misnomer, medial epicondylitis (golfer's elbow) too is probably a tendinopathy reflecting overuse or strain, affecting the flexor/pronator muscle group that inserts at the medial epicondyle.

Epidemiology

The epidemiology of medial epicondylitis has rarely been studied. Among those presenting with epicondylitis in primary care in the United Kingdom, lateral epicondylar symptoms were six times more common than medial.[7] Among a case series based in a hospital population (likely to represent a skewed sample), the incidence of medial epicondylitis was 1/100 000 person-years (nine times less common than lateral epicondylitis).[29] Using a standardized clinical examination and a predefined case definition,[14] one population survey found a prevalence of 0.6% among men and 1.1% among women with highest rates of occurrence among those aged 45–54 years.[9] The prevalence of medial and lateral epicondylitis was similar among women but lateral epicondylitis was twice as common as medial among men. Risk factors included repetitive bending/straightening the elbow for greater than 1 hour out of the working day (odds ratio 5.1, 95% confidence interval 1.8–14.3).[13] It is currently unclear what proportion of medial epicondylitis occurs among people who play golf.

Diagnostic and classification criteria

Few epidemiological surveys have included criteria for medial epicondylitis. Based upon consensus, Harrington and colleagues published a case definition of tenderness on/around the medial epicondyle associated with pain aggravated by resisted wrist flexion, with the forearm extended.[14] A recent radiographic study showed that diagnostic ultrasound was able to differentiate symptomatic elbows from those without symptoms among a study of 45 elbows, 21 with medial epicondylitis and 25 without elbow pain.[30]

Clinical features

Patients generally present with medial elbow pain radiating proximally or distally and associated with functional restriction. As with lateral epicondylitis, there will sometimes be an acute triggering factor or event but most cases tend to have a gradual and insidious onset. Grip strength may be reduced, predominantly because of the pain.

Management

In general, the same management strategies are applied to medial as to lateral epicondylitis including ice, rest, analgesia, physiotherapy, acupuncture, orthoses, and topical or oral NSAIDs. However, even fewer of these treatment modalities have undergone formal evaluation in medial epicondylitis and their recommendation for use is based mostly on extrapolation from those data available from lateral epicondylitis. Corticosteroid injections are advocated in most reviews but there are relatively few RCT data available. Stahl and Kaufman performed a double-blind RCT comparing the effect of corticosteroid (40 mg depomedrone) against saline in the treatment of 58 patients with a diagnosis of medial epicondylitis and found that both groups significantly improved at 3 months and 12 months of follow-up.[31] However, the depomedrone demonstrated marginally better results after 6 weeks when compared with the control saline injections (p <0.03). Ulnar nerve injury has been described as a consequence of medial epicondylar injection.[32] Surgical intervention is usually considered only after prolonged conservative treatment. In surgical series, it appears that concomitant ulnar neuritis is frequently identified and that surgical outcomes are less good when it is present.[33] This case series, and that of another surgical group, suggest improvement in pain may be achieved in the majority, but not all, cases of intractable medial epicondylitis.[34]

Course and prognosis

Most of the literature implies that medial epicondylitis is more resistant to treatment than lateral epicondylitis. However, few long-term follow-up studies are available for either condition and there are less data in medial epicondylitis. The results of the available surgical series suggest that 50–70% of patients obtain pain relief and functional improvement after surgery but it is likely that these cases represent a relatively small proportion of the overall numbers.[33–35]

Olecranon bursitis

The elbow is one of the anatomical sites most frequently affected by bursitis. In most cases, it is the superficial olecranon bursa that is affected. Olecranon bursitis can be an inflammatory phenomenon, occurring as part of a crystal arthropathy or RA or may be septic. Aseptic bursitis may also arise as a response to trauma, either a direct injury or chronic repetitive frictional trauma.

Epidemiology

There is very little published epidemiology regarding the occurrence of olecranon bursitis and almost nothing from general population samples. The available data come from hospital-based rates of presentation in Emergency Departments. Here, it has been estimated that olecranon bursitis and prepatellar bursitis together are responsible for 0.1–1.2/1000 Emergency Department visits per year.[36] Different hospital case series provide widely variable estimates of the proportion of cases of acute bursitis that occur at the olecranon (20–80%).[37,38] Predictably, the majority of cases presenting in Emergency Departments are caused by septic bursitis, with a small proportion only found to have acute gout, chondrocalcinosis or bleeding.[36] In acute bursitis presenting to Emergency Departments, risk factors are male gender, mean age 40–50 years, and a history of recent trauma to the affected limb or sustained (occupational) pressure on the elbow. Septic bursitis was also more common amongst those with diabetes mellitus, pre-existing nonseptic bursal disease, alcoholism, immunosuppression, and/or exposure to glucocorticoids.

Classification and diagnostic criteria

For aseptic olecranon bursitis, there are no diagnostic criteria that have been validated for use in general population studies. It has been proposed however that a suitable definition could include 'localized pain *and* a fluid-filled swelling over the posterior elbow'. Criteria have, however, been published for the differentiation of septic from aseptic acute bursitis based upon retrospective case series.[39]

Aetiopathogenesis

Septic bursitis

This may occur after direct inoculation through local skin lesions (often relatively trivial in nature) and local injections of corticosteroid precede up to 10% of cases. Commonly, more than 80% of cases are associated with *Staphylococcus aureus* and the next most common organism is streptococcus. However, many atypical organisms have been aspirated and reported in the literature.

Aseptic bursitis

Less is known about the aetiopathogenesis of aseptic bursitis. Acute or repetitive trauma appears to predispose to chronic pain and swelling of bursae at other anatomical sites (prominently the prepatellar bursa) and inflammation caused by proinflammatory cytokines has been postulated to occur (for example, RA) and bleeding onto the bursa has also been hypothesized to be responsible but the precise mechanism is yet to be understood.

Clinical features

The onset of symptoms can occur over hours or several days. The patient usually complains of posterior elbow pain associated with localized swelling but the severity at presentation may range from a relatively painless lump to acute, hot, red swelling with severe pain, pyrexia, and cellulitis. There may be features in the history to suggest gout or RA, which can help to differentiate these causes. Patients with septic bursitis usually seek help earlier and about 50% will have pyrexia,[37] but patients with acute gout may also have pyrexia and be systemically unwell. A swollen bursa without pain will almost always be aseptic. Pain, warmth and tenderness are generally worse in septic bursitis but these signs are poorly discriminative in the acute presentation. Erythema is common in septic bursitis (63–100% of cases) but also occurs in up to 25% of aseptic cases. An accompanying effusion of the elbow joint may be present in patients with gout or RA. If in any doubt, diagnosis must be made by aspiration of the bursa and the results of laboratory investigations.

Investigation

Laboratory investigation is mandatory when there is a possibility of septic bursitis. Microscopy can identify urate crystals and Gram stain may demonstrate bacteria in 53–100% of cases of septic bacterial bursitis. Bacterial culture will usually yield the causative organism providing that samples are taken before administration of antibiotics.

Other relevant investigations may include full blood count (total white blood cell count and differential); inflammatory markers (erythrocyte sedimentation rate and/or C-reactive protein); blood cultures; blood glucose; serum urate; rheumatoid factor; anti-cyclic citrullinated peptide antibodies; plain radiography of the elbow and/or ultrasonography or MRI scanning.

Management

Where there remains doubt about diagnosis, treatment with antibiotics may need to be commenced for 'presumed' septic bursitis while awaiting results of cultures. In confirmed septic bursitis, it may be necessary to aspirate the bursa to dryness on one or more occasions. Incision and drainage may be necessary if there is abscess formation or aspiration and antibiotics are failing to control progression. Advice should be sought from local microbiology colleagues as to the policy for treatment of septic bursitis while awaiting culture results, but penicillins and erythromycin penetrate the olecranon bursa effectively.

In established aseptic bursitis, management may be with ice, NSAIDs, and local support with a dressing or bandage. Aspiration may produce lasting benefit without any additional treatment but swelling will remain persistent in up to 10% of patients at 6 months. The results of one RCT showed that intrabursal injection of depomedrone produced more rapid resolution of swelling and reduced risk of recurrence,[40] but follow-up in this trial only took place for 6 months so long-term safety and effectiveness of this approach are not fully evaluated.

Course and prognosis

Where aspiration and antibiotics are commenced promptly for septic bursitis, resolution is usually prompt and long-lasting without the need for surgical treatment. Symptoms of pain and/or swelling may, however, persist for some weeks or even months after presentation. One retrospective case series of septic bursitis (severe enough to require hospital admission) found 343 episodes between 1996–2009 at a surgical unit in Geneva, 85% associated with *Staphylococcus aureus*, and mostly (91%) managed surgically.[41] They showed that total duration of adjuvant antibiotic therapy was not associated with cure and that amongst all other factors; only immunosuppression was a significant predictor of recurrence. Their results showed that neither 8–14 days nor more than 14 days of antibiotics was more effective than ≤7 days.[41]

After treatment in the acute phase, it may be wise to explore underlying risk factors for the original presentation, particularly if the causative organism is atypical or there is no clear history of preceding trauma. Aseptic bursitis may be associated with prolonged swelling (with or without aspiration) but pain will usually settle more rapidly. If pain recurs or fails to settle in an aseptic bursitis, it is important to review the diagnosis, particularly if aspiration or steroid injections have been performed. Rarely, chronic recurrent symptomatic aseptic bursitis may require surgical debridement.

Ulnar neuropathy

At the elbow, the ulnar nerve becomes relatively superficial on its passage through the cubital tunnel behind the medial epicondyle. At this point it becomes vulnerable to trauma, compression, and elbow dislocation. After carpal tunnel syndrome, ulnar neuropathy is the second most common entrapment neuropathy of the upper limb. Although this condition has been described in the literature for more than 100 years, and the ulnar nerve can be compressed at any point in its course, the most common site of compression is within the cubital tunnel and hence, the term 'cubital tunnel syndrome' was coined by Feindel and Stratford in 1958.[42,43]

Epidemiology

Although it is widely agreed to be the second most common nerve entrapment syndrome, there are few epidemiological data on this condition and none derived from general population studies. There is a growing literature on the occurrence of this condition among throwing athletes, particularly athletes who throw overhead.[44] A recent systematic review of work-related factors and elbow disorders concluded that the occurrence of cubital tunnel syndrome was associated with 'holding a tool in position' (odds ratio 3.53).[45]

Diagnostic and classification criteria

Cubital tunnel syndrome is often overlooked or misdiagnosed.[42] A multiplicity of different clinical tests of motor and sensory function can be utilized in practice,[46] but there is currently no widespread agreement on the gold standard method of diagnosis. In practice, most suspected cases are referred for electrophysiological testing although the sensitivity and specificity of sensory and motor neurophysiology for this condition are currently unknown. Imaging with MRI or ultrasonography is also sometimes used clinically and is thought to demonstrate morphological changes in the nerve in the cubital tunnel, but here also there are limited data as to the validity of the techniques for diagnosis and more research is required.[47]

Clinical features

Patients may complain of deep, aching pain at the medial elbow and proximal forearm which can radiate proximally or distally. Paraesthesiae radiate distally into the hand and/or wrist along the medial border, including the little finger and ulnar aspect of the ring finger. Paraesthesiae may be aggravated by activity (particularly elbow extension) and may be worse at night. Onset may be acute or insidious, depending upon underlying cause, and can progress over time from mild intermittent symptoms to contact anaesthesia. Ultimately, weakness may be detectable in the intrinsic muscles of the hand supplied by the ulnar nerve causing loss of dexterity and clumsiness and eventually wasting of the hand musculature accompanied by weakness and 'clawing' of the ring and little finger.

Management

Conservative management includes rest, splinting, ice, NSAIDs, physiotherapy, and simple analgesics. Unfortunately, few of these approaches have been evaluated formally in RCTs. The recent Cochrane review of the treatment of ulnar neuropathy at the elbow found only limited RCTs providing only moderate quality evidence.[48] The authors concluded that there was insufficient evidence to define the optimal treatment on the basis of clinical, neurophysiological and imaging characteristics,[48] nor whether to treat a patient conservatively or surgically. The results of their meta-analysis did, however, suggest that simple decompression and decompression with transposition were equally effective in the treatment when nerve impairment was severe.

Course and prognosis

Prognosis is likely to be poorer among patients with prolonged symptoms, motor and/or sensory loss, and instability of the elbow joint. In the absence of these adverse features, most patients (90%) are believed to improve with conservative measures only.[49] It is also stated that spontaneous improvement occurs in up to one-half of patients with cubital tunnel syndrome.[50] In severe cases, several surgical techniques are employed and it is difficult to find longer-term follow-up studies of patients treated with these different approaches.

Conclusion

Elbow pain affects around 12% of men and women at any point in time. It may occur as part of a generalized arthropathy, either inflammatory or degenerative and rarely will be the presenting feature of these conditions. Most elbow pain is caused by soft tissue conditions such as epicondylitis and bursitis.

References

1. Andersson HI, Ejlertsson G, Leden I, Rosenberg C. Chronic neck pain in a geographically defined general population: studies of differences in age, gender, social class and pain localisation. *Clin J Pain* 1993;9:174–182.
2. Walker-Bone K, Reading I, Coggon D, Cooper C, Palmer K. The anatomical pattern and determinants of pain in the neck and upper limbs: an epidemiologic study. *Pain* 2004;109:45–51.
3. Urwin M, Symmons D, Allison T et al. Estimating the burden of musculoskeletal disorders in the community: the comparative prevalence of symptoms at different anatomical sites. *Ann Rheum Dis* 1998;57:649–655.
4. Sanal HT, Chen L, Haghighi P, Trudell DJ, Resnick DL. Annular ligament of the elbow: MR arthrography appearance with anatomic and histologic correlation. *AJR* 2009;193(2):W122–W126.
5. Morris H. Rider's sprain. *Lancet* ii 1882;557.
6. Jacobsson L, Lindgarde F, Manthorpe R. The commonest rheumatic complaints of over six weeks' duration in a twelve month period in a defined Swedish population. *Scand J Rheumatol* 1989;18:353–360.
7. Hamilton PG. The prevalence of humeral epicondylitis: a survey in general practice. *J Royal Coll Gen Pract* 1986;36:464–465.
8. Allander E. Prevalence, incidence and remission rates of some rheumatic diseases and syndromes. *Scand J Rheumatol* 1974;3:145–153.
9. Walker-Bone K, Palmer K, Reading I, Coggon D, Cooper C. Prevalence and impact of soft tissue musculoskeletal disorders of the neck and upper limb in the general population. *Arthritis Rheum* 2004;51:642–651.
10. Kurppa K, Viikari-Juntura E, Kuosma E, Huuskonen M, Kivi P. Incidence of tenosynovitis or peritendinitis and epicondylitis in a meat-processing factory. *Scand J Work Environ Health* 1991;17:32–37.
11. Gruchow W, Pelletier D. An epidemiologic study of tennis elbow. *Am J Sports Med* 1979;7:234–238.
12. Haahr JP, Andersen JH. Physical and psychosocial risk factors for lateral epicondylitis: A population based case-referent study. *Occup Environ Med* 2003;60:322–329.
13. Walker-Bone K, Palmer KT, Reading I, Coggon DNMC, Cooper C. Occupation and epicondylitis: a population-based study. *Rheumatology (Oxford)* 2012;51(2):305–310.
14. Harrington JM, Carter TJ, Birrell L, Gompertz D. Surveillance case definitions for work related upper limb syndromes. *Occup Environ Med* 1998;55(4):264–271.
15. Waris P, Kuorinka I, Kurppa K, et al. Epidemiologic screening of occupational neck and upper limb disorders. *Scand J Work Environ Health* 1979;5(Suppl 3):25–38.
16. Walker-Bone K, Palmer KT, Reading I, Cooper C. Criteria for assessing pain and non-articular soft tissue rheumatic disorders of the neck and upper limb. *Semin Arthritis Rheum* 2003;33:168–184.
17. Binder AI, Patry L, Page Thomas P, Hazelman BL. A clinical and thermographic study of lateral epicondylitis. *Br J Rheumatol* 1983;22:77–81.
18. Struijs PAA, Smidt N, Arola H et al. Orthotic devices for the treatment of tennis elbow. *Cochrane Database Syst Rev* 2002;1:CD001821.
19. Smidt N, Assendelft WJJ, Arola H, et al. Physiotherapy and physiotherapeutical modalities for lateral epicondylitis. *Cochrane Database Syst Rev* 1999;2:CD001459.
20. Brosseau L, Casimiro L, Milne S et al. Deep transverse friction massage for treating tendinitis. *Cochrane Database Syst Rev* 2002;4:CD003528.
21. Buchbinder R, Green S, Youd JM et al. Shock wave therapy for lateral elbow pain. *Cochrane Database of Systematic Reviews* 2005;4:CD003524.

22. National Institute for Health and Clinical Excellence. Extracorporeal shockwave therapy for refractory tennis elbow. Available at www.nice.org.uk/nicemedia/live/12124/45249/45249.pdf (accessed Jan 2012).

23. Green S, Buchbinder R, Barnsley L et al. Acupuncture for lateral elbow pain. *Cochrane Database Syst Rev* 2002;1:CD003527.

24. Smidt N, Assendelft WJJ, van der Windt D et al. Corticosteroid injections for lateral epicondylitis. *Pain* 2002;96:23–40.

25. Coombes BK, Bisset L, Vicenzio B. Efficacy and safety of corticosteroid injections and other injections for management of tendinopathy: a systematic review of randomised controlled trials. *Lancet* 2010;376:9754:1751–1767.

26. National Institute for Health and Clinical Excellence. Autologous blood injection for tendinopathy, 2009. Available at www.nice.org.uk/nicemedia/live/11979/42918/42918.PDF (accessed Jan 2012).

27. Cyriax JH. The pathology and treatment of tennis elbow. *J Bone J Surg* 1936;XVIII:921–940.

28. Binder AI, Hazelman B. Lateral humeral epicondylitis—a study of the natural history and the effect on conservative therapy. *Br J Rheumatol* 1983;20:73–76.

29. O'Dwyer KJ, Howie CR. Medial epicondylitis of the elbow. *Int Orthop* 1995;19:69–71.

30. Park GY, Lee SM, Lee MY. Diagnostic value of ultrasonography for clinical medial epicondylitis. *Arch Phys Med Rehabil* 2008;89(4):738–742.

31. Stahl S, Kaufman T. The efficacy of an injection of steroids for medial epicondylitis. A prospective study of sixty elbows. *J Bone Joint Surg Am* 1997;79(11):1648–1652.

32. Stahl S, Kaufman T. Ulnar nerve injury at the elbow after steroid injection for medial epicondylitis. *J Hand Surg Br* 1997;22 (1):69–70.

33. Kurvers H, Verhaar J. The results of operative treatment of medial epicondylitis. *J Bone Joint Surg Am* 1995;77 (9):1374–1379.

34. Ollivierre CO, Nirschl RP, Pettrone FA. Resection and repair for medial tennis elbow. A prospective analysis. *Am J Sports Med* 1995;23(2):214–221.

35. Vangsness CT Jr, Jobe FW. Surgical treatment of medial epicondylitis. Results in 35 elbows. *J Bone Joint Surg Br* 1991;73(3):409–411.

36. Mathieu S, Prati C, Bossert M et al. Acute prepatellar and olecranon bursitis. Retrospective observational study in 46 patients. *Joint Bone Spine* 2011;78:423–424.

37. Ho G, Tice AD, Kaplan SR. Septic bursitis in the prepatellar and olecranon bursae: an analysis of 25 cases. *Ann Intern Med* 1978;89:21–27.

38. Soderquist B, Hedstrom SA. Predisposing factors, bacteriology and antibiotic therapy in 35 cases of septic bursitis. *Scand J Inf Dis* 1986;18(4):305–311.

39. Stell IM. Septic and non-septic olecranon bursitis in the accident and emergency department—an approach to management. *J Accid Emerg Med* 1996;13:351–353.

40. Smith DI, McAfee JH, Lucas LM, Kumar KL, Romney DM. Treatment of nonseptic olecranon bursitis, a controlled blinded prospective trial. *Arch Intern Med* 1989;149:2527–2530.

41. Perez C, Huttner A, Assal M, et al. Infectious olecranon and patellar bursitis: short-course adjuvant antibiotic therapy is not a risk factor for recurrence in adult hospitalized patients. *J Antimicrob Chemother* 2010;65:1008–1014.

42. Robertson C, Saratsiotis J. A review of compressive ulnar neuropathy at the elbow. *J Manipulative Physiol Ther* 2005;28(345):e1–e18.

43. Feindel W, Stratford J. Cubital tunnel syndrome in tardy ulnar palsy. *Can Med Assoc J* 1958;78:351–353.

44. Hariri S, McAdams TR. Nerve injuries about the elbow. *Clin Sports Med* 2010;29:655–675.

45. Van Rijn RM, Huisstede BM, Koes BW, Burdorf A. Associations between work-related factors and specific disorders at the elbow: a systematic literature review. *Rheumatology* 2009;48:528–536.

46. Folberg CR, Weiss APC, Akelman E. Cubital tunnel syndrome part I: presentation and diagnosis. *Orthop rev* 1994;23:136–144.

47. Beekman R, Visser LH, Verhagen WI. Ultrasonography in ulnar neuropathy at the elbow: a critical review. *Muscle Nerve* 2011;43:627–635.

48. Caliandro P, La Torre G, Padua R, Giannini F, Padua L. Treatment for ulnar neuropathy at the elbow. *Cochrane Database Syst Rev* 2011;2:CD006839.

49. Dellon AL, Hament W, Gittelshon A. Non-operative management of cubital tunnel syndrome. *Neurology* 1993;43:1673–1677.

50. Szabo RM, Kwak C. Natural history and conservative management of cubital tunnel syndrome. *Hand Clin* 2007;23:311–318.

CHAPTER 153

Forearm, hand, and wrist

Karen Walker-Bone and Benjamin Ellis

Structure and function of the forearm, hand, and wrist

Anatomy

The wrist joint is complex, consisting of 19 bones making a total of 17 articulations coordinated by 19 muscles and an array of tendons. The wrist (carpus) has a proximal (scaphoid, lunate, triquetrum, and pisiform) and distal (trapezium, trapezoid, capitate, and hamate) row of bones. The radius and ulna articulate distally with the proximal row of the carpus. The healthy wrist is capable of approximately 130° of total flexion/extension and 40° of radio/ulnar deviation. The ellipsoid shape of the radioulnar joint allows circumduction of approximately 150° (not true rotation) as the distal radius moves about the distal end of the ulna. The wrist is stabilized by ligaments (radial and ulnar collateral and radiocarpal ligaments).

The distal row of the carpus articulates with the proximal carpi at the carpometacarpal (CMC) joints. At the thumb, the first CMC joint allows an extensive range of motion (flexion/extension 40–50°, abduction and adduction 40–70°), facilitated by its saddle shape between the trapezium and base of the first metacarpal. The distal carpi articulate with the proximal phalanges at the metacarpophalangeal (MCP) joints, which are hinge joints but allow radial and ulnar deviation. The MCP joint of the thumb has two sesamoid bones on its palmar surface. The interphalangeal joints are hinge joints, tightly supported by collateral ligaments. Healthy proximal interphalangeal joints (PIPs) allow 100–120° palmar flexion and do not allow hyperextension. The distal interphalangeal joints (DIPs) allow approximately 50–80° palmar flexion and dorsiflex to a small extent (5–10°).

The majority of the hand musculature is on the palmar surface. Releasing grip is effected by the long extensor muscles of the forearm, connected to the hand by long tendons along the back of the hand. Movement of the hand is controlled by two main groups of muscles: one group are in the forearm and attach to bony prominences in the hand (extrinsic muscles) and the other group are the intrinsic muscles of the hand. The extrinsic muscles constitute the long flexor and extensor tendons of the forearm, which attach to the phalanges and metacarpals and some of the carpals and allow strong grip and control of gross motor functions of the hand. The intrinsic muscles include the thenar eminence which produces movement at the thumb, the hypothenar eminence which produces movement at the little finger, the palmar and dorsal interossei, and the lumbricals. The intrinsic muscles facilitate fine movements of the fingers and thumb such as opposition and pinch. The centre of the palm is covered by the thick palmar aponeurosis.

Anatomy of the carpal tunnel

On the palmar surface, the carpus forms a concave arch or tunnel (the carpal tunnel) with the pisiform and hook of the hamate as bony landmarks on the medial side and the tuberosities of the scaphoid and trapezium on the radial side. These four bony prominences are bridged by the flexor retinaculum, producing a natural ceiling over the carpal tunnel which functions to hold the long flexor tendons (flexor digitorum profundus, flexor digitorum superficialis, and flexor pollicis longus) in place during wrist flexion. The median nerve runs through this compartment (Figure 153.1).

Nerve supply to the forearm, hand, and wrist

From the brachial plexus, the important nerves for hand/wrist function are the median (C5–8), ulnar (C8, T1), and radial (C6–8) nerves. Radial nerve compression above the elbow causes wrist drop due to weakness of wrist extension, stiffness in the distal arm and forearm, and inability to extend the little finger. Ulnar nerve lesions in the forearm produce pain and dysaesthesia along the lateral forearm and wrist and into the ring and little fingers. Longer term, the intrinsic muscles of the ring and little fingers may become wasted and contracted into flexion. Median nerve entrapment may occur at the elbow within pronator teres, causing diffuse arm pain, weakness of wrist pronation, and paraesthesia in a median nerve distribution (palmar surface of thumb, index, middle and radial half of ring finger). More commonly, median nerve compression occurs at the carpal tunnel, resulting in the paraesthesia as described and longer term, weakness of thumb opposition, and wasting of the thenar eminence.

Differential diagnosis of hand/wrist pain

Hand and/or wrist pain are common early symptoms of a polyarthropathy, inflammatory or degenerative. Additionally, the physician must consider peripheral nerve lesions, referral from the cervical spine, nerve root lesions, brachial plexus involvement, disease of the shoulder or elbow, or whether the presenting symptoms

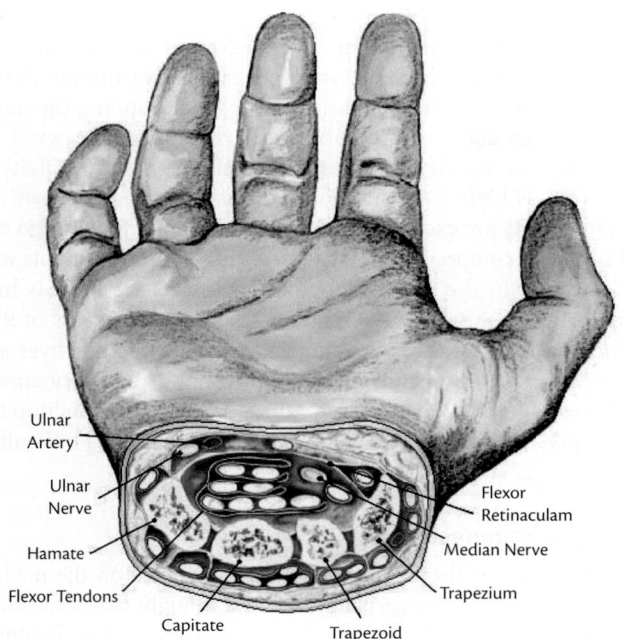

Fig. 153.1 Anatomy of the carpal tunnel.

Ulnar Artery

Ulnar Nerve

Hamate

Flexor Tendons

Capitate

Trapezoid

Flexor Retinaculam

Median Nerve

Trapezium

Table 153.1 Classification of hand and wrist disorders

Articular	Arthritis of the hand/wrist joints
	Rheumatoid arthritis or other inflammatory arthritis
	Psoriatic arthritis
	Gout
	Septic arthritis
	Osteoarthritis
	Traumatic
	Neoplasm (primary or secondary)
Periarticular	Jaccoud's arthropathy
	Hypermobility syndrome
	Rheumatoid nodules
	Calcinosis
	Tophus (gout)
	Dupuytren's contracture
	Ganglion
	Tenosynovitis (flexor or extensor)
	Trigger finger
	De Quervain's tenosynovitis
	Acute calcific periarthritis (wrist and MCP most commonly)
Bone disorder	Neoplasm (primary or secondary)
	Osteomyelitis
	Fractures
	Osteonecrosis (e.g. keinbock syndrome)
Neurological	Nerve entrapment syndromes in the upper limb
	Carpal tunnel syndrome (median nerve)
	Pronator teres syndrome (median nerve)
	Radial tunnel syndrome (posterior interosseous syndrome)
	Spiral groove syndrome (radial nerve)
	Cubital tunnel syndrome (ulnar nerve)
	Thoracic outlet syndrome (brachial plexus lesion)
	Nerve root lesions proximal to the upper limb
	Radiculopathy
	Syringomyelia
	Spinal cord tumours
Chronic widespread pain syndrome	Fibromyalgia syndrome
Regional pain syndrome	Complex regional pain syndrome type II
	Somatoform pain syndrome
Vascular	Upper limb claudication
	Systemic vasculitis
	Primary Raynaud's
	Secondary Raynaud's with connective tissue disease
	Compartment syndrome

may constitute part of another disease, e.g. metastasis or fibromyalgia syndrome (Table 153.1).

History

The history should enquire about dominant limb, nature of onset, precipitating injury, and involvement of the head/neck, shoulder, or elbow on the same and other sides. The duration and progression of symptoms is useful diagnostically. With pain, enquire about site, nature, variation with time, progression, exacerbating and relieving factors, therapies tried and response. Ask about symptoms of associated inflammation, dysaesthesia, and muscle weakness. A thorough functional assessment is essential to understand completely what home and workplace activities are being performed.

Examination

Examination should be comprehensive including exposure of the neck, shoulders, and upper limbs bilaterally at a minimum. Inspection should focus on the neck and both arms as well as the hand/wrist looking for asymmetry, wasting, or scarring. Specific deformities such as Dupuytren's contracture in the palmar aponeurosis, ganglia, congenital deformities, swelling, or thickening of tendon sheaths should be noted as should visible deformities of the wrist or any small joints of the hand/wrist, including Heberden's and Bouchard's nodes seen in osteoarthritis and the characteristic deformities of swelling of MCPs and PIPs, rheumatoid nodules, subluxation, ulnar deviation, swan neck, or boutonnière deformity seen in rheumatoid arthritis (RA). Signs of skin psoriasis, nail changes, and involvement of the DIPs with/without partial resorption of the phalanges may suggest psoriatic arthritis. Rarer but important abnormalities may be detected: e.g. sclerodactyly, Gottron's papules, calcinosis, telangiectasiae, capillary nailfold abnormalities, digital ulceration, nailfold infarcts, Jaccoud's arthropathy, or signs of an underlying connective tissue disease.

To detect wrist synovitis, place it in slight flexion and use your thumbs to examine carefully for dorsal synovial thickening while supporting the wrist with your fingers. A large effusion may produce fluctuance. The thickening associated with tenosynovitis is more linear along the line of the tendon and extends beyond the joint margins proximally and/or distally. Palpate the first CMC joint for tenderness, crepitus, and 'squaring' of the joint. Palpate each MCP joint dorsally either side of the extensor tendon using your thumbs while supporting the fingers in your own fingers. Palpate the PIPs and DIPs using your thumb while gently pinching the medial and lateral aspects of the same joint in your other hand so as to detect fluctuance.

Finger joints and thumb joints may be assessed actively and passively and cumulatively or in isolation. For example, extending the fingers, making a fist, testing grip strength, and touching each finger to the thumb are quick 'screening' tests which allow gross assessment of areas of dysfunction. Each small joint of the hand may be isolated and tested actively and passively if appropriate. At the thumb, flexion, extension, abduction, and adduction should all be assessed as well as strength of opposition to the little finger, using your own thumb opposed to test as a comparison.

Investigation of symptoms at the hand and wrist

Radiography, ultrasonography, diagnostic joint aspiration with microscopy, culture and sensitivities of the aspirate, as well as polarizing light microscopy, CT scan, MRI scan, radionuclide scanning, electromyography (EMG), and nerve conduction studies may all be useful for the investigation of hand/wrist symptoms.

Carpal tunnel syndrome

The most common entrapment neuropathy, carpal tunnel syndrome, has an estimated incidence of 99/100 000 per year[1] and prevalence as high as 7–19%, although prevalence estimates vary widely partly depending on case definition.[2] Carpal tunnel syndrome occurs more commonly in women, with an annual incidence of 1.5 per 1000 compared to 0.5 per 1000 for men.[3] Patterns of incidence also differ, such that the incidence among women peaks at age 45–54 years whereas the incidence in men continues to rise with age.

The difference in the pattern of occurrence between the genders may be explained at least partly by hormonal factors: pregnant and breastfeeding women have increased incidence,[4] as well as those taking the oral contraceptive pill and hormone replacement therapy.[5] Oophorectomy appears to reduce the incidence but there is an increased incidence in the first menopausal year.

Obesity is strongly associated with carpal tunnel syndrome, with every 1 unit increase in body mass index (BMI) increasing risk by 8%.[4] A relatively small number of cases are associated with endocrine conditions such as hypothyroidism, acromegaly, and diabetes mellitus. Damage and inflammation of the wrist itself due to wrist fractures and inflammatory rheumatic disorders, such as RA, also increase risk.[5]

There is an extensive body of evidence to suggest that occupational exposure to forceful or repetitive movements, or to hand–arm vibration, increases the risk of carpal tunnel syndrome,[6,7] particularly when these exposures are combined with adverse posture, such as bending or twisting of the wrist/hand.[7] Despite considerable interest, an association with keyboard use has not been convincingly demonstrated.

Classification and diagnostic criteria

Patients typically present with pain and/or dysaesthesia of the fingers (typically the lateral 3½ digits, although it can be diffuse throughout the hand). Symptoms are often worse at night or in the early morning. Pain may be diffuse and extend proximal to the hand. Examination in advanced cases may reveal wasting of the thenar eminence and/or weakness of thumb abduction. Provocation tests such as those of Tinel (tapping the flexor retinaculum) and Phalen (full passive flexion of the wrist for 1 minute) are widely used, but the sensitivity and specificity of these tests is highest in the more advanced cases and sensitivity and specificity are excellent among patients about to undergo carpal tunnel decompression but much reduced among patients with dysaesthesia in the general population.[2] EMG testing has high diagnostic sensitivity (60–84%) and specificity in excess of 95% among patients awaiting decompression, but false positives and negatives may still occur and again its diagnostic utility among the general population is poorer. A negative nerve conduction test in the presence of a positive clinical diagnosis is thus difficult to interpret.

Aetiopathogenesis

Carpal tunnel syndrome arises from any pressure on the median nerve as it traverses the carpal tunnel. It is thought that some families have a congenitally small carpal tunnel. In most individuals, though, compression arises from local pressure caused for example by obesity, wrist inflammation, repetitive occupational use, hormonal factors, or distortions to the median nerve.

Differential diagnosis

Cervical radiculopathies at C6–7 may mimic the sensory symptoms of carpal tunnel syndrome, although in such cases motor involvement will be in the distribution of the radial nerve, affecting wrist flexion and triceps. Pain itself may be difficult to localize and the possibility of an ulnar or small-fibre neuropathy should be considered for patients with neuropathic palmar digit pain, along with other causes of medial neuropathy. Wasting of the thenar muscles may also be caused by a T1 radiculopathy.

Management

Initial management is conservative, including nocturnal splinting to hold the wrist in a neutral position, along with analgesia and addressing any causative risk factors. The evidence does not support specific use of non-steroidal anti-inflammatory drugs (NSAIDs),[8] though oral steroids confer short-term benefit. A single local steroid injection is better than placebo at improving symptoms at 1 month[9] and, combined with splinting, is more effective than splinting alone.[10] Surgery to divide the flexor retinaculum and release the median nerve can be performed as an open procedure or endoscopically, and carries a long-term success rate of over 75%.[11]

De Quervain's tenosynovitis

The extensor retinaculum passes from the lateral radius to the medial carpal bones, and is divided into six compartments by fibrous septa passing to the radius and ulna, with each compartment having its own synovial lining. The tendons of extensor pollicis longus and brevis pass through the lateral or first, dorsal compartment in a single sheath and emerge to form the radial border of the anatomical snuffbox. De Quervain's tenosynovitis is a stenosing tenosynovitis of this first dorsal compartment of the wrist at the radial styloid.

Epidemiology

Few epidemiological studies have explored the occurrence of de Quervain's tenosynovitis in the general population. Where evaluated, it appears more common among women than men with an annual incidence rate of 2.8 cases/1000 women compared to 0.6/1000 men,[12] and point prevalence 1.3% among women and 0.5% among men.[13] Incidence increases with age, so that age over 40 years is a significant risk factor,[14] and there may be an increased rate among black people.[12]

No specific occupational determinants have been demonstrated, although cases have been attributed to repetitive thumb use in piano-playing, sewing, and knitting,[14] as well as text messaging.[15] Hormonal factors may play a role as cases have been described during pregnancy[16] and in the postpartum period.[17,18] Associations have also been reported between de Quervain's tenosynovitis and the inflammatory arthritides and local trauma.

Classification and diagnostic criteria

De Quervain's tenosynovitis typically presents as pain over the radial wrist associated with impaired thumb function. Clinical findings include swelling, crepitus, and tenderness over the first dorsal compartment along with a positive Finkelstein's provocation test (Figure 153.2). Imaging is not routinely required, though ultrasonography and MRI may detect thickening and inflammation of the extensor pollicis longus and brevis tendons. Thumb-base osteoarthritis may cause a similar distribution of pain but typically has different clinical findings on examination.

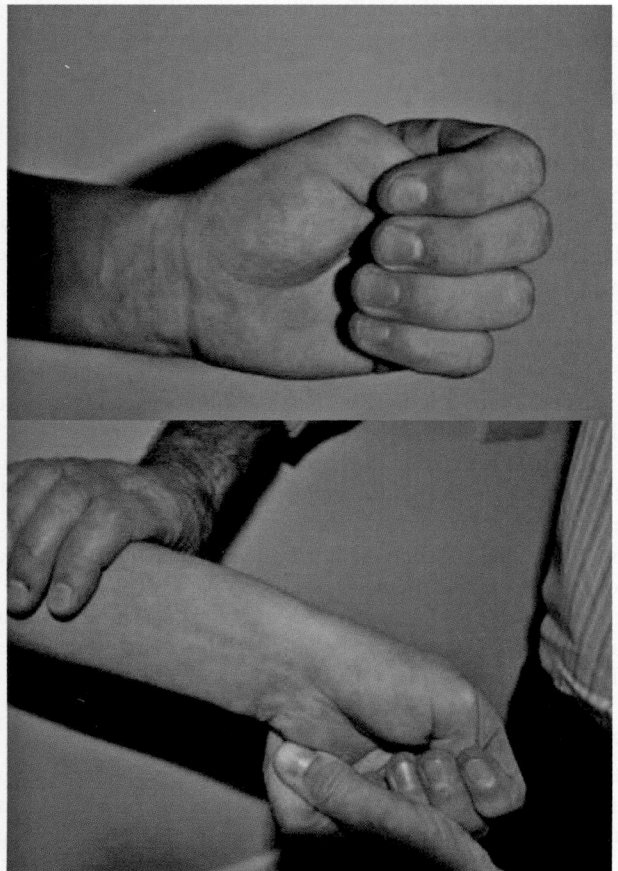

Fig. 153.2 Finkelstein's test.

Aetiopathogenesis

Repetitive radial and ulnar deviation of the wrist combined with gripping ('washerwoman's wrist') is thought to lead to friction and inflammation of the tendon sheath as it passes through the extensor retinaculum.

Management

Conservative treatment with thumb spica[19] splinting and NSAIDs is usually first-line treatment and this may be most effective for people with relatively mild symptoms.[20] Provoking or exacerbating activities at home or work, e.g. rowing, may need to be avoided. Local injections of glucocorticoid have been shown to be highly effective in the treatment of de Quervain's tenosynovitis, and have been suggested by some as first-line treatment.[21] Using ultrasound to guide injection may reduce side effects,[22] but both intrasynovial and extrafibrous injection appear to convey similar benefit.[23] Where conservative management has failed, there is evidence that surgical decompression to divide the extensor retinaculum can be effective.[24]

Flexor and extensor tenosynovitis of the wrist and fingers

Tenosynovitis occurs at sites where tendons are lined with synovium and occurs most frequently at the wrist (radial, flexor, and extensor compartment) and on the flexor tendons of the digits (trigger digits).

Epidemiology

Tenosynovitis appears more common among women than men, with population prevalence rates estimated at 1.1% among men and 2.2% among women.[13] Tenosynovitis is associated with repetitive hand movements, and some types of factory workers and machinists appear to be at increased risk.[25–27] Imaging of the tendon sheaths amongst patients with early RA shows that tenosynovitis is a frequent finding,[28] and this may predispose to tendon rupture.[29] Diabetics are at increased risk of stenosing flexor tenosynovitis.[30] Urate crystal deposition can also cause tenosynovitis. A rare but important cause of tenosynovitis is infection which may be caused by a penetrating injury, or haematogenous spread with organisms such as neisseria.

Classification and diagnostic criteria

The typical clinical findings of pain, tenderness, and swelling along the length of the tendon or tendon sheath, accompanied by pain increased by resisted movement of that individual tendon, is suggestive of tenosynovitis. Sometimes crepitus may also be demonstrated. Ultrasonography or MRI may confirm the diagnosis when there is uncertainty, but are not routinely required. In patients with RA, tendon rupture may be the first clinical sign of tenosynovitis, and should be suspected if there is painless loss of active movement. In infective flexor tendon tenosynovitis, in addition to pain there may also be a rapid onset of fusiform swelling of the digit, which will be guarded in flexion with pain on passive extension. It is important to remember that these signs may be absent in immunosuppressed patients, or those partially treated with antibiotics. Definitive diagnosis of infection or gouty tenosynovitis requires aspiration.

Aetiopathogenesis

Pathophysiologically, a distinction is made between the true synovial inflammation of tenosynovitis, inflammation of a tendon itself (tendinitis) and the degenerative process of tendinosis, where repetitive mechanical loading leads to collagen degradation with resultant pain and dysfunction. Some tendons are more prone to inflammation than others; for example, flexor carpi ulnaris tenosynovitis is said to be more common than flexor carpi radialis.

Management

Appropriate treatment depends on the cause. First-line therapy for tenosynovitis involves ice, rest, splinting, and NSAIDs. Local injections of glucocorticoid may be administered where needed. Because of the superficiality of the tendon sheath, it is wise to use short-acting steroid preparations such as hydrocortisone acetate and warn the patient of a risk of local steroid atrophy of the skin at the injection site. Where possible, the precipitating activity should be avoided. As with de Quervain's tenosynovitis, surgical release may occasionally be required. In gout or inflammatory arthritis, the management of the tenosynovitis relies upon control of the underlying condition.[31] Where infective tenosynovitis is suspected, empirical intravenous antibiotics should be started for those organisms most commonly involved (staphylococci and streptococci), taking advice from local microbiological colleagues. Although early infective tenosynovitis may respond to antibiotic therapy alone, surgical drainage is frequently recommended to prevent the complications of osteomyelitis, tendon necrosis, and skin loss.

Trigger digit (tenosynovitis of the flexor tendons of the thumb and digits)

At the level of the MCP joint, the superficial and deep finger flexors pass through the first annual (A1) pulley. 'Triggering' occurs as a mechanical catch when there is insufficient space for the tendon to traverse.

Epidemiology

The population prevalence of trigger digit has been estimated to be 2.6%, with women 2–3 times more commonly affected than men.[32] Incidence is greatest in the 40–50 years age group, but rarely can be congenital. The thumb of the dominant hand is the most common digit to be affected, with relative sparing of the index and little fingers.[33]

Chronic repetitive activities are implicated in the development of trigger digit, and there may be increased prevalence among some manual workers.[34,35] Activities such as knitting or sewing[33] may also increase risk. Risk of trigger finger is greatly increased amongst people with all types of diabetes mellitus,[36,37] where trigger digit may be multiple and bilateral. Other associations include hypothyroidism, Dupuytren's contracture, carpal tunnel syndrome, RA, and amyloidosis [33]

Classification and diagnostic criteria

Typically trigger digit presents as a painful catching or clicking/popping feeling when the affected digit is extended, sometimes associated with inability to actively extend the affected digit. There may also be a tender palpable nodule at the level of the metacarpal head. Acute onset of a trigger finger with associated severe pain and swelling should raise the suspicion of infective tenosynovitis or a gouty tenosynovitis and aspiration should be considered where this is the case.

Aetiopathogenesis

The mechanism is most commonly tenosynovitis, perhaps related to friction or overuse. The result is commonly chronic fibrous nodular enlargement of the flexor digitorum superficialis close to the metacarpal head.

Management

Initial management may consist of rest, ice and oral NSAIDs, and there may be a role for splinting. Local corticosteroid injections may be very effective whether or not they are placed intra-sheath.[38] The injections may be more effective in nodular, rather than diffuse disease.[39] Where symptoms have not resolved, repeat injections can be beneficial resulting in improvements of over 90% at 1 year.[40] A comparison of surgical release with local corticosteroid injection showed that after 1 month, patients with injections achieved greater range of motion than those treated by percutaneous release but that 6-month assessment showed a higher chance of recurrence in those treated with injections.[41] If possible, causative factors should be addressed and underlying inflammatory conditions aggressively treated.

Dupuytren's contracture

Characterized by nodular thickening and contracture of the palmar aponeurosis, Dupuytren's is a relatively common condition. The condition draws the MCP joints into flexion, usually at the ring finger and little finger, but occasionally involves other joints.

Epidemiology

The classical case, with flexion contractures, is easily recognized but more minor forms are more difficult to diagnose reliably so that the epidemiology is difficult to characterize. Dupuytren's contracture becomes more prevalent with increasing age.[42] and is up to sixfold more common among men than women.[43] The incidence of new Dupuytren's nodules in previously unaffected individuals aged over 66 years is around 3%.[44] Typically Dupuytren's is bilateral, but when it is unilateral the dominant hand is more frequently affected. A relationship with local repetitive and/or occupational trauma remains unproven but there is an association between Dupuytren's and vibration-induced white finger.[45]

Dupuytren's contracture is more common in people with elevated fasting blood glucose and diabetes mellitus,[44,46] and may be less common in people with RA.[47] Increased reported prevalence among people with epilepsy may be attributable to medication.[48] Heavy smokers (>25 cigarettes daily) are more likely to be affected,[49–51] but a relationship with excessive alcohol intake has not been clearly established. There appears to be familial clustering of Dupuytren's, with a possible autosomal dominant pattern of inheritance.[52]

Classification and diagnostic criteria

The diagnosis of Dupuytren's is based on the clinical findings of palmar nodularity, overlying skin tethering and puckering, and fixed flexion of the MCP joint distal to the affected area. Ultrasonography can confirm the structural changes, but is not usually required for diagnosis.

Aetiopathogenesis

The pathology is one of fibrous nodule formation within the palmar aponeurosis. Histopathologically, fibroblasts and myofibroblasts proliferate superficially in the palmar fascia and the dermis is infiltrated by fibroblastic cells, resulting in the contracture of the superficial layers which may ultimately be tethered.

Management

In early disease, management may be expectant. Repeated intralesional injections of triamcinolone may reduce nodularity which may in turn prevent contracture formation, but such injections do not reverse a contracture once present. Injectable collagenase clostridium histolyticum, however, has been shown to reduce contractures and improve range of motion in affected joints.[53] Once the affected digit is permanently flexed, surgery is usually offered. This is usually performed under local anaesthetic and consists of either needle aponeurotomy or percutaneous fasciotomy, but following both procedures recurrence rates may be as high as 50%.[54,55] A more extensive fasciectomy can also be performed to dissect away all affected fascia but recurrence rates remain high even with this procedure, with up to 15% of patients requiring repeat surgery.[56]

Raynaud's phenomenon

Raynaud's phenomenon is the name given to intermittent digital vasospasm occurring in response to stress or cold. There is usually a clear line of demarcation, distal to which the skin colour changes caused by vasoconstriction (white), cyanosis (blue), then hyperaemia (red), often accompanied by pain. Primary (benign) Raynaud's phenomenon (Raynaud's disease) occurs commonly with a family history, is usually symmetrical, and begins typically at the age of 15–25 years, in girls more commonly than boys. Secondary Raynaud's reflects endothelial, vascular structural, neural, and intravascular abnormalities; it may occur for the first time at any age and may be asymmetrical.

Epidemiology

The population prevalence varies between 4% and 15%, with higher rates among women.[57] The annualized incidence has been estimated at 2.2% in women and 1.5% in men,[58] with 80–90% of these being primary Raynaud's. The onset of primary Raynaud's is typically in the second or third decades of life, whereas the epidemiology of the secondary Raynaud's reflects that of the underlying disorder.

Primary Raynaud's may more common in people with a family history.[59] Occupational exposure to organic solvents,[60] particularly vinyl chloride,[61] increases the risk of secondary Raynaud's. Prevalence of Raynaud's is doubled among people exposed to hand-transmitted vibration.[62] Raynaud's is associated with a number of autoimmune diseases including systemic sclerosis, mixed connective tissue disease, systemic lupus erythematosus (SLE), vasculitis, RA, and myositis, as well as cryoglobulinaemia and systemic malignancies.

Classification and diagnostic criteria

Raynaud's is diagnosed clinically based upon intermittent painful, frequently bilateral, well-demarcated triphasic colour change of one or more digits (white to blue to red), often precipitated by cold. Primary Raynaud's is diagnosed when there is no history of digital ulceration, no clinical features suggestive of a connective tissue disorder, and negative immunological testing such as erythrocyte sedimentation rate (ESR) and nuclear antibodies. In secondary Raynaud's, capillaroscopy may reveal dilated nailfold capillaries.

Raynaud's should be discriminated from median or ulnar neuropathy or radiculopathy, which cause similar digital pain without colour change. Painful, hot, red fingers, usually in response to a heat stimulus, may be due to erythromelalgia. Acrocyanosis is a painless, persistent, non-paroxysmal bluish-red, symmetrical discoloration to hands and feet, but there is no initial pallor phase. Chilblains occur in response to cold and can cause erythema, pruritus, and ulceration, but lack the clearly demarcated triphasic colour change of Raynaud's.

Aetiopathogenesis

The typical aetiopathogenesis is vasospasm, which may be triggered by cold or stress. Whiteness is caused by restricted blood flow, cyanosis by local ischaemia and deoxygenation, and redness by the typical hyperaemia once blood flow is restored; this latter phase is typically painful.

Management

Initial management is with lifestyle modification, including avoiding triggers such as cold (wearing gloves and lined footwear, avoiding smoking, and addressing any apparent risk factors such as chemical or vibration exposure). Initial pharmacological treatment may include the dihydropyridine calcium channel blockers, including nifedipine,[63] which may be used regularly, or as required. Drugs inhibiting the renin–aldosterone axis, in particular losartan, may reduce the frequency and severity of attacks.[64] Topical nitroglycerin may be effective,[65] though headache is a frequent side effect which may restrict utility. Other treatment options include alpha-blockade[66] and fluoxetine.[67] In secondary Raynaud's, particularly with digital ulceration, treatment with parenteral prostaglandins, such as intravenous iloprost,[68] sildenafil, or bosentan[69] may be indicated.[70] In severe cases, surgical or chemical sympathectomy, including using botulinum toxin,[71] may be required when other treatments have failed.

Non-specific (diffuse) forearm pain

One of the differential diagnoses for hand/wrist tenosynovitis includes non-specific forearm pain. This diagnostic classification has been utilized in the United Kingdom since the publication of a consensus set of case definitions derived from a multidisciplinary workshop, sponsored by the UK Health and Safety Executive, employing a Delphi approach.[72] Prior to this, diagnostic labels such as 'repetitive strain injury', 'occupational cervicobrachial disorder', 'work-related upper limb disorder' had grown in use, with different terms in different countries and different diagnostic criteria, but with the obvious encumbrance of implied causation within their nomenclature which was hindering epidemiological research.

Epidemiology

It is difficult to be certain how commonly diffuse forearm pain occurs, because of the extraordinary diversity of diagnostic criteria that have been applied in epidemiological studies, some of which are likely to be different but overlapping. Using the UK case definition, a prevalence rate of 0.5% was reported among working-aged adults,[74] but in a prospective cohort study of 782 people from 12 different occupational groups, prevalence of new onset forearm pain over 12 months was 8.3% (7.2% in men and 10% in women).[75] Risk factors for diffuse forearm pain include lifting heavy loads, adverse postural factors (e.g. working with hands above shoulder height), repetitive movements, and psychosocial factors—psychological distress, monotonous work, low job satisfaction, and low levels of control in the workplace. A clear relationship between this condition and workplace keyboard use has not been established.[74]

Diagnostic and classification criteria

Non-specific forearm pain is essentially a diagnosis of exclusion. The published consensus case definition from Harrington et al. was: 'pain in the forearm in the absence of a specific diagnosis or pathology (sometimes includes loss of function, weakness, cramp, muscle tenderness, allodynia, slowing of fine movements).[72] There should be no clinical signs suggestive of specific pathology, and diagnostic testing for specific causes of forearm pain should by definition be negative.

Aetiopathogenesis

The aetiology of non-specific forearm pain may be complex. There is currently no agreement as to underlying cause, though mechanisms involving local tissue damage, peripheral neurological abnormality, referred pain from the neck, sensory cortical change, and pain amplification have all been proposed.[73] There may be overlap with conditions presumed to be predominantly neurological such as focal dystonia and 'writer's cramp'. Tenosynovitis is thought to be a separate entity. It remains to be established whether non-specific arm pain may sometimes constitute the prodromal phase of forearm tenosynovitis.

Clinical features

Patients describe their symptoms as aching, soreness, or tingling which may be diffuse in the forearm. Subjective swelling, dysaesthesia, focal tenderness, and abnormal pain sensitivity may be demonstrated. Sometimes symptoms become more widespread (shoulder–hand syndrome). There may be disturbance of sleep patterns, and generalized fatigue is common. There may be predisposing factors in the workplace, e.g. a change in technique or working practices. Typically, symptoms are relieved initially by a short period of rest, but as symptoms become more chronic not even 2–3 weeks of annual holiday provide relief.

Management

In the absence of consensus on causation, there is currently no specific treatment for this condition. Best practice is to offer an approach that is multimodal and multidisciplinary,[73] including pain management, occupational therapy, and physiotherapy. Occupational health services should be involved early and undertake a workplace ergonomic assessment and psychological support; treatment for anxiety or depression should be initiated where appropriate. The medical approach should be positive and reassuring, emphasizing the absence of local tissue damage, along with encouragement to remain active and if possible in the workplace.

Conclusion

Forearm, hand, and wrist symptoms are common. It should be borne in mind that these are common sites of onset of a polyarthropathy but, once such a condition has been excluded, careful history-taking and examination should facilitate a correct diagnosis and management plan.

References

1. Von Shroeder HP, Botte MJ. Carpal tunnel syndrome. *Hand Clin* 1996;12:643–655.
2. Ferry S, Pritchard T, Keenan J, Croft P, Silman A. Estimating the prevalence of delayed median nerve conduction in the general population. *Br J Rheumatol* 1998;37:630–635.
3. Stevens JC, Sun S, Beard CM, O'Fallon WM, Kurland LT. Carpal tunnel syndrome in Rochester, Minnesota, 1961 to 1980. *Neurology* 1988;38:134–138.
4. Nordstrom DL, Vierkant RA, DeStefano F, Layde PM. Risk factors for carpal tunnel syndrome in a general population. *Occup Environ Med* 1997;54:734–740.
5. Solomon DH, Katz JN, Bohn R, Mogun H, Avorn J. Nonoccupational risk factors for carpal tunnel syndrome. *J Gen Intern Med* 1999;14:310–314.
6. Abbas MEF, Abdelmonem AA, Zhang ZW, Kraus JF. Meta-analysis of published studies of work-related carpal tunnel syndrome. *Int J Occup Environ Health* 1998;4:160–167.
7. Bernard BP (ed.). *Musculoskeletal disorders (MSDs) and workplace factors*. U.S. Department of Health and Human Services. Cincinnati, OH, 1997.
8. Graham B. Nonsurgical treatment of carpal tunnel syndrome. *J Hand Surg Am* 2009;34(3):531–534.
9. Marshall S, Tardif G, Ashworth N. Local corticosteroid injection for carpal tunnel syndrome. *Cochrane Database Syst Rev* 2007;2:CD001554.
10. Ucan H, Yagci I, Yilmaz L et al. Comparison of splinting, splinting plus local steroid injection and open carpal tunnel release outcomes in idiopathic carpal tunnel syndrome. *Rheumatol Int* 2006;27(1):45–51.
11. Bland JD. Carpal tunnel syndrome. *BMJ* 2007;335(7615):343–346.
12. Wolf JM, Sturdivant RX, Owens BD. Incidence of de Quervain's tenosynovitis in a young, active population. *J Hand Surg Am* 2009;34(1):112–115.
13. Walker-Bone K, Palmer KT, Reading I, Coggon D, Cooper C. Prevalence and impact of musculoskeletal disorders of the upper limb in the general population. *Arthritis Rheum* 2004;51(4):642–651.
14. Moore JS. de Quervain's tenosynovitis. *J Occup Environ Med* 1997;39:990–1002.
15. Ashurst JV, Turco DA, Lieb BE. Tenosynovitis caused by texting: an emerging disease. *J Am Osteopath Assoc* 2010;110(5):294–296.
16. Schumacher HR, Dorwart BB, Korzeniowski OM. Occurrence of de Quervain's tendinitis during pregnancy. *Arch Intern Med* 1985;145:2083–2085.
17. Johnson CA. Occurrence of de Quervain's disease in postpartum women. *J Fam Pract* 1991;32:325–327.
18. Nygaard IE, Saltzman CL, Whitehose MB, Hankin FM. Hand problems in pregnancy. *Am Fam Physician* 1989;39:123–126.
19. Ilyas AM, Ast M, Schaffer AA et al. De Quervain tenosynovitis of the wrist. *J Am Acad Orthop Surg* 2007;15(12):757–764.
20. Lane LB, Boretz RS, Stuchin SA. J Treatment of de Quervain's disease: role of conservative management. *Hand Surg Br* 2001;26(3):258–260.
21. Peters-Veluthamaningal C, van der Windt D, Winters JC, Meyboom-de Jong B. Corticosteroid injection for de Quervain's tenosynovitis. Corticosteroid injection for de Quervain's tenosynovitis. *Cochrane Database Syst Rev* 2009;3:CD005616.

22. Jeyapalan K, Choudhary S. Ultrasound-guided injection of triamcinolone and bupivacaine in the management of De Quervain's disease. *Skeletal Radiol* 2009;38(11):1099–1103.

23. Apimonbutr P, Budhraja N. Suprafibrous injection with corticosteroid in de Quervain's disease. *J Med Assoc Thai* 2003;86(3):232–237.

24. Scheller A, Schuh R, Honle W, et al. Long-term results of surgical release of de Quervain's stenosing tenosynovitis. *Int Orthop* 2009;33(5):1301–1303.

25. Thompson AR, Plewes LW, Shaw EG. Peritendinitis crepitans and simple tenosynovitis: a clinical study of 544 cases in industry. *Br J Ind Med* 1951;8:150–160.

26. Luopajarvi T, Kuorinka I, Virolainen M, Holmberg M. Prevalence of tenosynovitis and other injuries of the upper extremities in repetitive work. *Scand J Work Environ Health* 1979;5(Suppl 3):48–55..

27. McCormack RR, Inman RD, Wells A, Berntsen C, Imbus HR. Prevalence of tendinitis and related disorders of the upper extremity in a manufacturing workforce. *J Rheumatol* 1990;17:958–964..

28. Eshed I, Feist E, Althoff CE, Hamm B, Konen E, Burmester GR, et al. Tenosynovitis of the flexor tendons of the hand detected by MRI: an early indicator of rheumatoid arthritis. *Rheumatology* (Oxford) 2009;48(8):887–891.

29. Ferlic DC. Rheumatoid flexor tenosynovitis and rupture. *Hand Clin* 1996;12(3):561–572.

30. Kameyama M, Meguro S, Funae O, Atsumi Y, Ikegami H. The presence of limited joint mobility is significantly associated with multiple digit involvement by stenosing flexor tenosynovitis in diabetics. *J Rheumatol* 2009;36(8):1686–1690.

31. Hammer HB, Kvien TK. Ultrasonography shows significant improvement in wrist and ankle tenosynovitis in rheumatoid arthritis patients treated with adalimumab. *Scand J Rheumatol* 2011;40(3):178–182.

32. Strom L. Trigger finger in diabetes. *J Med Soc NJ* 1977;74:951–954.

33. Moore JS. Flexor tendon entrapment of the digits (trigger finger and trigger thumb). *J Occup Environ Med* 2000;42:526–545.

34. Bonnici AV, Spencer JD. A survey of 'trigger finger' in adults. *J Hand Surg* 1988;21-B:244–245.

35. Gorsche R, Wiley JP, Renger R et al. Prevalence and incidence of stenosing flexor tenosynovitis (trigger finger) in a meat-packing plant. *J Occup Environ Med* 1998;40:556–560.

36. Yosipovitch G, Yosipovitch Z, Karp M, Mukamel M. Trigger finger in young patients with insulin dependent diabetes. *J Rheumatol* 1990;17:951–952.

37. Gamstedt A, Holm-Glad J, Ohlson CG, Sundstrom M. Hand abnormalities are strongly associated with the duration of diabetes mellitus. *J Intern Med* 1993;234:189–193.

38. Taras JS, Raphael JS, Pan WT, Movagharnia F, Sotereanos DG. Corticosteroid injections for trigger digits: is intra-sheath injection necessary? *J Hand Surg* 1998;23(4):717–722.

39. Freiberg A, Mulholland RS, Levine R. Nonoperative treatment of trigger fingers and thumbs. *J Hand Surg Am* 1989;14(3):553–558.

40. Marks MR, Gunther SF. Efficacy of cortisone injection in treatment of trigger fingers and thumbs. *J Hand Surg Am* 1989;14(4):722–727.

41. Zyluk A, Jagielski G. Percutaneous A1 pulley release vs. steroid injection for trigger digit: the results of a prospective, randomized trial. *J Hand Surg Eur* 2011;36(1):53–56.

42. Early PF. Population studies in Dupuytren's contracture. *J Bone Joint Surg* 1962;44:602–613.

43. Wilbrand S, Ekbom A, Gerdin B. The sex ratio and rate of re-operation and rate of reoperation for Dupuytren's contracture in men and women. *J Hand Surg [Br]* 1999;24(4):456–459.

44. Gudmundsson KG, Arngrimsson R, Jonsson T. Eighteen years follow-up study of the clinical manifestations and progression of Dupuytren's disease. *Scand J Rheumatol* 2001;30:31–34.

45. Thomas PR, Clarke D. Vibration white finger and Dupuytren's contracture: are they related? *J Soc Occup Med* 1992;42:155–158.

46. Noble J, Heathcote JG, Cohen H. Diabetes mellitus in the aetiology of Dupuytren's disease. *J Bone J Surg* 1984;66:322–325.

47. Arafa M, Steingold RF, Noble J. The incidence of Dupuytren's disease in patients with rheumatoid arthritis. *J Hand Surg* 1984;9-B:165–166.

48. Hart MG, Hooper G. Clinical associations of Dupuytren's disease. *Postgrad Med J* 2005;81:425–428.

49. Gudmundsson KG, Arngrimsson R, Sigfusson N, Bjornsson A JT. Epidemiology of Dupuytren's disease. Clinical, serological and social assessment. The Reykjavik Study. *J Clin Epidemiol* 2000;53: 291–296.

50. Brage S, Bjekedal T. Musculoskeletal pain and smoking in Norway. *J Epidemiol Community Health* 1996;50:166–169.

51. Howard S, Southworth SR, Jackson T, Russ B. Cigarette smoking and Dupuytren's contracture of the hand. *J Hand Surg* 1988;13:872–873.

52. Ling RSM. The genetic factor in Dupuytren's disease. *J Bone J Surg* 1963;45:709–718.

53. Hurst LC, Badalamente MA, Hentz VR, et al; CORD I Study Group. Injectable collagenase clostridium histolyticum for Dupuytren's contracture. *N Engl J Med* 2009;361:968–979.

54. van Rijssen AL, Gerbrandy FS, Ter Linden H et al. A comparison of the direct outcomes of percutaneous needle fasciotomy and limited fasciectomy for Dupuytren's disease: a 6-week follow-up study. *J Hand Surg Am* 2006;31:717–725.

55. Bryan AS, Ghorbal MS. The long-term results of closed palmar fasciotomy in the management of Dupuytren's contracture. *J Hand Surg Br* 1988;13:254–256.

56. Rodrigo JJ, Niebauer JJ, Brown RL, Doyle JR. Treatment of Dupuytren's contracture. Long-term results after fasciotomy and fascial excision. *J Bone Joint Surg Am* 1976;58(3):380–387.

57. Palmer KT, Griffin MJ, Syddall H et al. Prevalence of Raynaud's phenomenon in Great Britain and its relation to hand transmitted vibration: a national postal survey. *Occup Environ Med*. 2000;57(7):448–452.

58. Suter LG, Murabito JM, Felson DT, Fraenkel L. The incidence and natural history of Raynaud's phenomenon in the community. *Arthritis Rheum* 2005;52(4):1259–1263.

59. Freedman RR, Mayes MD. Familial aggregation of primary Raynaud's disease. *Arthritis Rheum* 1996;39:1189–1191.

60. Purdie GL, Purdie DJ, Harrison AA. Raynaud's phenomenon in medical laboratory workers who work with solvents. *J Rheumatol* 2011;38(9):1940–1946.

61. Laplanche A, Clavel F, Contassot JC, Lanouziere C. Exposure to vinyl chloride monomer: report on a cohort study. *Br J Ind Med*. 1987;44(10):711–715.

62. Palmer KT, Griffin MJ, Syddall H et al. Prevalence of Raynaud's phenomenon in Great Britain and its relation to hand transmitted vibration: a national postal survey. *Occup Environ Med*. 2000;57(7):448–452.

63. Thompson AE, Pope JE. Calcium channel blockers for primary Raynaud's phenomenon: a meta-analysis. *Rheumatology* (Oxford). 2005;44:145–150.

64. Wood HM, Ernst ME. Renin-angiotensin system mediators and Raynaud's phenomenon. *Ann Pharmacother* 2006;40(11):1998–2002.

65. Generali J, Cada D. Nitroglycerin (topical): Raynaud phenomenon. *Hosp Pharm* 2008;43:980–981.

66. Eliasson K, Danielson M, Hylander B et al. Raynaud's phenomenon caused by beta-receptor blocking drugs. Improvement after treatment with a combined alpha- and beta-blocker. *Acta Med Scand* 1984;215:333–339.

67. Coleiro B, Marshall SE, Denton CP et al. Treatment of Raynaud's phenomenon with the selective serotonin reuptake inhibitor fluoxetine. *Rheumatology* (Oxford) 2001;40(9):1038–1043.

68. Wigley FM, Wise RA, Seibold JR et al. Intravenous iloprost infusion in patients with Raynaud phenomenon secondary to systemic sclerosis. A multicenter, placebo-controlled, double-blind study. *Ann Intern Med* 1994;120:199–206.

69. Korn JH, Mayes M, Matucci-Cerinic M et al. Digital ulcers in systemic sclerosis: prevention by treatment with bosentan, an oral endothelin receptor antagonist. *Arthritis Rheum* 2004;50:3985–3993.

70. Fries R, Shariat K, von Wilmowsky H et al. Sildenafil in the treatment of Raynaud's phenomenon resistant to vasodilatory therapy. *Circulation* 2005;112:2980–2985.

71. Neumeister MW, Chambers CB, Herron MS et al. Botox therapy for ischemic digits. *Plast Reconstr Surg* 2009;124:191–201.

72. Harrington JM, Carter JT, Birrell L, Gompertz D. Surveillance case definitions for work related upper limb pain syndromes. *Occup Environ Med* 1998;55(4):264–271.

73. MacIver H, Smyth G, Bird HA. Occupational disorders: non-specific forearm pain. *Best Pract Res Clin Rheumatol* 2007;21(2):349–365.

74. Walker-Bone K, Reading I, Palmer KT, Coggon D, Cooper C. 'Repetitive strain injury' is rare among working-aged adults and is not associated with keyboard use [abstract]. *Rheumatology* (Oxford) 2004; 43(suppl 1):S19.

75. Macfarlane GJ, Hunt IM, Silman AJ. Role of mechanical and psychosocial factors in the onset of forearm pain: prospective population based study. *BMJ* 2000;321:1–5.

CHAPTER 154

Pelvis, groin, and thigh

Cathy Speed

Introduction

Conditions affecting the groin, hip, and thigh can result in significant pain and disability, and can affect those across all age ranges and activity levels. In this chapter, the clinical assessment, diagnosis, and treatment of common conditions in this region are reviewed.

Epidemiology

The overall incidence of problems around the hip, groin, and thigh is not known, but this region is a common source of pain and disability. For example, 4.4% of adults over the age of 55 years have symptomatic osteoarthritis (OA) of the hip.[1] Approximately 2.5% of all sport-related injuries are in the pelvic region. Most of these are soft tissue injuries, but articular complaints are increasingly recognized. Paediatric disorders are also common, and can be serious.

Causes of problems around the hip, groin, and thigh

Most problems of the hip, groin, and thigh cause pain. Complaints can be considered according to the principal site of pain (Table 154.1).

Pain in the anterior hip, groin, and thigh

Articular complaints

Clinical features

Most articular disorders of the hip present with pain that is typically focused in the groin, and aggravated by weightbearing and, in particular, impact-related activity. A mechanism of onset may be identified. As the condition progresses, the pain becomes more intrusive and pain at rest occurs. Posterior hip/buttock pain is variable. Pain may be noted in the thigh and/or knee. Night pain is a feature of more severe complaints.

Examination may reveal gluteal weakness (including a positive Trendelenburg sign), pain, and/or restriction on hip movement and in particular on rotation.

Additional features typical to specific complaints are described below.

Osteoarthritis

The prevalence of moderate to severe radiographic OA adults over the age of 55 years is 1.5% and the prevalence of symptomatic OA of the hip 4.4% (3.6% female; 5.5% male). The age and sex-standardized incidence rates of symptomatic OA of the hip is 88 per 100 000 person-years. Incidence rates increase with age, and level off around age 80. Women have higher rates than men, especially after age 50; men have a 36% reduced risk of hip OA than women. Fifty to sixty per cent of hip OA may be genetically determined.[1–3]

Established modifiable risk factors include excess body mass (though less than for knee OA), joint injury, excessive loadbearing physical activity,[4] occupation involving excessive mechanical stress, structural malalignment, and muscle weakness. Non-modifiable risk factors are female gender, increasing age until 75 years, race (e.g. lower risk in Asians), and genetics. Other risk factors that have been postulated are oestrogen deficiency, osteoporosis (inversely related to OA), and high C-reactive protein.[5,6]

Risk factors for disease progression in hip OA are patient age, baseline joint space width, femoral head migration, femoral osteophytes, bony sclerosis, a Kellgren Lawrence hip grade of 3, baseline hip pain, and a Lequesne index score (an algofunctional index that measures disease activity in the hip and knee) of at least 10.[7,8]

Diagnostic criteria for osteoarthritis of the hip

The American College of Rheumatology (ACR) criteria for hip OA classification offer several methods for diagnosis. The standard approach requires the presence of hip pain and at least two of the following three criteria: radiographic evidence of femoral or acetabular osteophytes, radiographic evidence of joint space narrowing (superior, axial, or medial), and an erythrocyte sedimentation rate (ESR) less than 20 mm/hour. This approach yields a sensitivity of 89% and a specificity of 91%.[9]

Additional diagnostic criteria that may be helpful for diagnosing OA of the hip include internal hip rotation of 15° or less, morning stiffness in the hip lasting 1 hour or less, and age of 50 years or older.

MRI and MR arthrography allow earlier imaging-based diagnosis of OA than plain radiographs, although further improvements in the technology are still required to accurately image early cartilage changes.[10]

Management

The major clinical guidelines for management of hip OA[11–15] show minor differences. All recommend patient education, weight loss, insoles and a variety of exercise orientated approaches. Paracetamol (acetaminophen) is the analgesic of first choice, moving on to oral

Table 154.1 Causes of pain in the hip, groin, and thigh

Anterior	Posterior	Lateral
Articular		
Osteoarthritis	Advanced hip pathologies	
Inflammatory arthritis	Sacroiliac disease and dysfunctions	
Septic arthritis	Referred facet joint pain	
Osteomyelitis	Sacral bone stress injuries	
Avascular necrosis		
Bone marrow oedema syndromes and transient osteoporosis of the hip		
Femeroacetabular impingement		
Labral injury		
Paget's disease		
Osteitis pubis		
Paediatric conditions: Perthes', slipped upper femoral epiphysis, dysplasias		
Fractures		
Referred pain from the spine		
Soft tissue		
Adductor tendinopathies	Hamstrings pathology	Gluteal tendinopathies
Iliopsoas tendinopathies	Piriformis syndrome	Trochanteric bursitis
Quadriceps/rectus femoris injuries		
Sportsman's abdominal wall syndromes		
Calcific tendinitis of the hip		
Capsulitis		
Neural		
Spinal nerve root compression	Sciatic pain	Spinal referred pain
Meralgia Paraesthetica (thigh pain)	Obturator nerve entrapment	
Ilioinguinal, genitofemoral neuropathy (groin pain)		

non-steroidal anti-inflammatory drugs (NSAIDs) at their lowest effective dose if necessary. Choice of a COX-2 inhibitor or standard NSAID + proton pump inhibitor (PPI) is made according to the patient's cardiac and gastroenterological risk factors. Guided intra-articular glucocorticoids are recommended for those who have ongoing pain. While viscosupplement injections are not included in the guidelines for hip OA, studies subsequent to published guidelines indicate benefit.[16,17] Unlike the ACR guidelines, those from the European League Against Rheumatism (EULAR) do not rule out the use of glucosamine sulfate, chondroitin sulfate, or diacerein.[12,13,15] Opioids, with or without paracetamol, may also be used should other oral analgesics fail in those with severe pain.

Total joint arthroplasty provides marked pain relief and functional improvement in the vast majority of patients with OA. Indications from the United States National Institutes of Health (NIH) for total hip replacement include 'radiographic evidence of joint damage and moderate to severe persistent pain or disability, or both, that is not substantially relieved by an extended course of nonsurgical management'.[18] The United Kingdom National Institute

for Health and Clinical Excellence (NICE) guidelines[14] adhere to clinical criteria, recommending that referral for joint replacement surgery should be considered for people with OA who experience joint symptoms (pain, stiffness, and reduced function) that have a substantial impact on their quality of life and are refractory to non-surgical treatment. Referral should be made before there is prolonged and established functional limitation and severe pain.

Inflammatory arthritis

Hip disease occurs infrequently in adult-onset RA. However, hip pathology in the form of fracture can occur due to osteoporosis, which has an increased incidence in RA, particularly those with severe disease. With such improvements in medical management of RA, total hip arthroplasties are less commonly needed.

Unlike adult RA, hip disease develops in 30–50% of children with juvenile RA and can result in significant long-term disability, emphasizing the need for aggressive management of such cases.

In ankylosing spondylitis, sacroiliitis typically causes buttock pain, but may refer to the groin. Hip involvement itself occurs in approximately 10–15% of those with AS after 10 years' disease duration in western Europeans. The incidence is up to 50% in other populations. Hip involvement is related to the degree of spinal involvement, and is considered a bad prognostic sign.[19]

Hip joint architecture and impingement syndromes

Several features of hip joint architecture, such as acetabular dysplasia, pistol grip deformity, wide femoral neck, and altered femoral neck–shaft angle have a strong genetic influence. These features can play an important role in the pathogenesis of osteoarthritis and hip (femoroacetabular) impingement syndromes.[20] The latter can be associated with labral tears and non-specific pain on hip flexion and rotation, typically in young people. Patients present with groin pain and have signs of pain on hip flexion and internal or (less commonly) external rotation. Plain radiography and CT show hip geometry best. In the absence of a labral tear, conservative management through activity modification and physiotherapy should be the first line of approach prior to consideration for surgical interventions.

Bone oedema syndromes of the hip

The hip is a common site of bone marrow oedema syndromes. Bone marrow oedema is an MRI-based diagnosis and is neither a specific MRI finding nor a specific diagnosis. It describes a pattern of signal change of bone on MRI (decreased on T1-weighted and increased on T2-weighted imaging). It may be seen in a number of hip disorders. Bone marrow oedema syndromes of the hip include transient osteoporosis of the hip (TOH), regional migratory osteoporosis (RMO), and complex regional pain syndrome (CRPS type 1). Such conditions are usually benign and self-limiting.

Patients present with non-specific hip/groin pain and a limp. Other symptoms and signs may be present, depending upon the underlying condition. MRI is used to confirm the diagnosis, help to exclude other pathologies, and monitor the condition. Scrutiny for more significant disorders is vital. These include other causes of hip pain, and conditions associated with bone marrow oedema on MRI: stress injury, avascular necrosis/osteonecrosis, osteomyelitis, articular pathologies, myeloproliferative diseases, sickle cell disease. Such conditions can usually be differentiated by their clinical pictures and further investigations as necessary.[21]

In TOH, MRI findings do not show focal changes that are seen in avascular necrosis (AVN); see next section. Plain radiograph shows osteopenia of the femoral head and in some cases into the femoral neck and acetabulum, typically after 4 weeks of symptoms, and in particular transient subchondral cortical thinning that resolves with time. Scintigraphy shows homogenous increased uptake throughout the femoral head, with an epicentre of uptake at the centre of the femoral head.

RMO is a rare condition characterized by a migrating arthralgia involving the weightbearing joints of the lower limb, and typically affecting men aged 40–60 years. There are also more rare intra-articular and spinal forms. The imaging findings on imaging are indistinguishable from TOH. TOH can occur in women in the third trimester of pregnancy. TOH and RMO are likely to be part of the same spectrum of disease. Systemic osteoporosis is seen more commonly in this group of patients.

Avascular necrosis

The reader is directed to a review of AVN elsewhere in this text (Chapter 148). A brief overview relating to the hip is provided here.

AVN of the femoral head is a potentially devastating disorder affecting young people between the third and fifth decades. The femoral head is particularly vulnerable, due to the patterns of its blood supply.

Higher-risk patients include those who have had corticosteroid therapy, particularly long term, alcoholism, myeloproliferative disease, caisson disease, venous outflow occlusion, arterial embolism or thrombosis, autoimmune disease (e.g. systemic lupus erythematosus), and those who have had local radiation therapy or a renal transplant. In those on steroids, reducing the dosage may help to reduce the size of the lesion. Bilateral AVN of the hip in pregnancy has also been described.

On MRI, there are focal subchondral signal changes. Lesions are circumscribed by a rim of low signal intensity on T1-weighted images or a double line consisting of concentric low- and high-signal intensity bands on T2-weighted imaging. Gadolinium fails to enhance areas of early osteonecrosis (ON), while surrounding uninvolved areas do enhance. ON can occasionally appear similar to TOH on initial MR. Plain radiographs may be normal initially but with time usually show collapse of subchondral bone. In 50% of all cases accompanying joint effusion may be found. In later stages calcification as well as new bone formation and microfractures are typically demonstrated and visualized best with plain radiographs and CT.

The prognosis depends on the location, size, stage of the lesion, and underlying risk factors. Those with diffuse involvement of the femoral head or lesions affecting the lateral third of the weightbearing portion of the femoral head have a 90% chance of femoral head collapse.[22]

Fifty per cent of patients develop bilateral disease. Many classification systems have been recommended, but all are associated with observer and/or technical errors.

Non-operative approaches, such as rest and crutches, hyperbaric therapy, statins, bisphosphonate therapy, iloprost infusions, and extracorporeal shock wave therapy (ESWT) have all been proposed. The evidence base for all is limited. Surgical intervention is reported to show superior outcomes to non-surgical. Core decompression is the most common initial surgical procedure, with a reported good outcome in 64% or patients compared to less than 30% of those managed conservatively.[23]

Pubic symphysis instability

Pubic symphysis instability typically occurs in postpartum women and male athletes. Associated symptoms may include local symphysis, groin, adductor, and perineal pain and clicking, all aggravated by activity and lifting. Radiographs may show signs of irregularity and sclerosis of the symphysis, but such changes are frequently seen in asymptomatic active individuals. MRI and bone scan will be more sensitive to active osteitis. Stork radiograph views of the symphysis may reveal instability (>0.2 mm movement).

Management involves lengthy rehabilitation to improve pelvic floor and core muscle strength. In postpartum women a sacroiliac belt and reassurance are particularly useful. Surgery is very rarely indicated.

Osteitis pubis

The term 'osteitis pubis' implies an inflammatory process affecting the pubic symphysis. True osteitis at this site can be related to osteomyelitis, hyperparathyroidism, sarcoidosis, inflammatory arthritis, and haemachromatosis. All such conditions are rare compared to activity-related 'osteitis', when the term is usually used to describe radiological changes at the symphysis, including widening, demineralization, resorption, periosteal reaction, and sclerosis. This is usually due to symphysis instability, and the symptoms are similar.

Scintigraphy will show increased uptake in the joint in active lesions, but MRI scanning has superseded this. MRI shows oedema within the pubic symphysis in patients with chronic groin pain. Nevertheless, the findings must be taken in the clinical context. The recommended treatment of mechanical osteitis pubis includes a long period of relative rest, analgesics, and stability work. Steroid injections should be discouraged, as they are rarely beneficial. In those rare cases with infective or metabolic causes the underlying condition should be managed accordingly.

Soft tissue injuries

In sport, intrinsic risk factors including increased age, female sex, previous injury and inadequate rehabilitation, and extremes of body mass index (BMI) have been reported to have some role in increasing tendency for injury. Extrinsic factors for injury include the athlete's skill level, the competitive nature of the sport, and the type of playing surface.

Acute or chronic adductor injuries may occur along the myotendinous junction, the tendon, or at the enthesis, and may be associated with osteitis pubis or symphysis instability. Adductor longus is most commonly involved. In young, growing athletes, an avulsion injury can occur. There is pain and tenderness of the adductors and pain on resisted adduction. MRI and ultrasound will demonstrate tendinopathies and myotendinous damage, but non-specific intra-tendinous alterations on imaging are common in asymptomatic active patients. Treatment is relative rest, stretching, and progressive strengthening. In chronic tendinopathy, peritendinuos infiltration with steroid may be helpful in achieving pain relief. Rarely, adductor tenotomy may be necessary.

Snapping hip syndrome

A 'snapping hip' may arise as a result of a number of intra- and extra- articular pathologies, including hip subluxation, labral tears, or soft tissue movement. Typically the source is the iliopsoas tendon; the tendon glides over the lesser trochanter or iliopectineal eminence and snaps as it does so. Usually this is due to tightness or a lack of lumbopelvic control. A bursitis may be present. Diagnostic ultrasound confirms the diagnosis and treatment is rehabilitation to strengthen the area and achieve balanced flexibility. Occasionally the iliopsoas tendon sheath or bursa may warrant injection to reduce the pain.

Iliopsoas bursitis

Iliopsoas bursitis can be related to underlying joint pathology or iliopsoas pathology, or may occur in isolation after overuse or trauma. Anterior groin pain with or without a clunk or snap and a deep ache occur. When sufficiently large, a bursitis may also present as a painful or painless inguinal mass, or with symptoms related to a compressive effect, such as femoral nerve irritation or femoral venous engorgement. A large bursa can even cause compression of the large bowel or bladder. An ultrasound scan will confirm the diagnosis. Further evaluation of the hip should be considered. Anti-inflammatories are usually required. If steroid injection is considered then the clinician should be mindful that communication with the joint is possible and the patient must be counselled in the same way as they would for an intra-articular injection.

Calcific tendinitis of the hip

Though rare, calcification of the hip soft tissues including the origins of one or more muscles of the thigh, most commonly the rectus femoris, gluteus maximus, or vastus lateralis, can occur. Acute groin pain and limitation of movement (due to pain), without a history of trauma, are presenting features. Management includes relative rest, analgesics or NSAIDs, ultrasound, ESWT, and if necessary imaging-guided local corticosteroid injection.

Paediatric and adolescent conditions

Regional problems in the paediatric patient are discussed elsewhere in this text (Chapter 158). Table 154.2 provides an overview of conditions specifically affecting the hip.

Lateral hip and thigh pain

Gluteal enthesopathy and trochanteric bursitis

Enthesopathy of the insertion of gluteus medius and minimus at the trochanter is a common condition, particularly in women, and

Table 154.2 Differential diagnosis of hip pain in the young patient

Condition	Age (years)	Clinical features	Frequency	Diagnosis
Apophyseal avulsion fracture	12–25	Pain after sudden forceful movement	Often	History of trauma; radiography
Hip apophysitis	12–25	Activity-related hip pain	Often	History of overuse; radiography to rule out fractures
Transient synovitis	<10	Limping or hip pain	Often	Radiography; laboratory testing; ultrasonography
Fracture	All	Pain after traumatic event	Occasionally	History of trauma; radiography
Slipped capital femoral epiphysis	10–15	Hip, groin, thigh, or knee pain; limping	Occasionally	Bilateral hip radiography (anteroposterior and lateral)
Legg–Calvé–Perthes disease	4–9	Vague hip pain, decreased internal rotation of hip	Infrequently	Hip radiography or MRI
Septic arthritis	All	Fever, limping, hip pain	Infrequently	Radiography; laboratory testing; joint aspiration

Reproduced with permission from Peck.[24]

often inappropriately termed 'trochanteric bursitis'. The enthesopathy arises as a result of a lack of gluteal strength and the patient may also have longstanding back pain and have weak gluteals and pelvic floor and poor core stability. Other factors include muscle imbalances, hip pathology (with limitation of internal rotation and reflex tightening of the external rotators), and leg length differences.

The aetiological and clinical features of trochanteric bursitis overlap with gluteal enthesopathy, but bursitis is much less common. There are four trochanteric bursae, situated deep to the soft tissues at the lateral hip, protecting them from the bony surface of the greater trochanter.

Ultrasound or MRI confirm the diagnosis. Treatment involves correction of underlying cases, strengthening, and in those with bursitis, guided injection of the bursa with corticosteroid.

Posterior hip, buttock, and thigh pain

Hamstring injuries

The hamstrings, and in particular the biceps femoris, are the most commonly injured muscle group in relation to sporting activities. Pain, swelling, and bruising are typical in an acute injury. Injuries to the tendon can also occur. Ultrasound and MRI are useful in confirming the site and extent of the injury. Avulsion injuries can occur, usually in those aged under 18 years. In all cases the principle of management is focused on pain management to allow rehabilitation to proceed. Myotendinous ruptures can be managed conservatively, but can take 18 months, and functional outcome may be poor. For this reason, some recommend early repair, particularly in proximal hamstring rupture in athletes. In avulsion injuries where there is a displacement of more than 3 cm, or in any patient where significant hamstrings weakness seems likely, surgical reattachment should be considered. Early surgery followed by hamstring rehabilitation is also recommended in adult athletes.

Piriformis and hamstring syndromes

Posterior thigh pain in the absence of identifiable hamstring pathology or lumbar nerve root compression is a challenge to any sports medicine team. The sciatic nerve can conceivably be compressed or irritated as it travels beneath the pelvic muscles, particularly the piriformis and hamstrings. The 'hamstring syndrome' is considered to be due to neural dysfunction, either as a result of functional 'compression' beneath semitendinosis and biceps femoris, pelvic rotation, or lumbar dysfunction. There may be a constricting band in the vicinity of the nerve deep to the associated muscles, although usually one is not identified.

Piriformis syndrome is considered to be present when there is sciatic nerve irritation in the absence of any spinal pathology, presumably due to a tight piriformis. Adverse neurodynamics are usually present, with a positive straight-leg raise and slump tests. Treatment is stretching, neurodynamic work, and acupuncture.

Ischial (ischiogluteal) bursitis

Ishcial bursitis is rare. It can occur after direct trauma, resulting in localized pain and tenderness. The diagnosis is confirmed on diagnostic ultrasound or MRI. Relative rest, ice, anti-inflammatories, and cushioning are usually effective but a local guided injection of corticosteroid may be necessary. Surgical excision of the bursa is rarely necessary.

References

1. Lawrence RC, Felson DT, Helmick CG et al. Estimates of the prevalence of arthritis and other rheumatic conditions in the United States. Part II. *Arthritis Rheum* 2008;58(1):26–35.
2. Felson DT. Risk factors for osteoarthritis. *Clin Orthoped Rel Res* 2004;427S:S16–S21.
3. Rossignol M, Leclerc A, Allaert FA et al. Primary osteoarthritis of hip, knee and hand in relation to occupational exposure. *Occup Environ Med* 2005;62:772–777.
4. Cooper C, Inskip H, Croft P et al. Individual risk factors for hip osteoarthritis: obesity, hip injury, and physical activity. *Am J Epidemiol* 1998;147(6):516–522.
5. Jordan JM, Helmick CG, Renner JB et al. Prevalence of knee symptoms and radiographic and symptomatic knee osteoarthritis in African Americans and Caucasians: The Johnston County Osteoarthritis Project. *J Rheumatol* 2007;34(1):172–180.
6. Felson DT, Zhang Y. An update on the epidemiology of knee and hip osteoarthritis with a view to prevention. *Arthritis Rheum* 1998;41(8): 1343–1355.
7. Wright AA, Cook C, Abbott JH. Variables associated with the progression of hip osteoarthritis: a systematic review. *Arthritis Rheum.* 2009;61(7):925–936.
8. Lequesne M. Indices of severity and disease activity for osteoarthritis. *Semin Arthritis Rheum* 1991;20(6 suppl 2):48–54.
9. Altman R, Alarcón G, Appelrouth D et al. The American College of Rheumatology criteria for the classification and reporting of osteoarthritis of the hip. *Arthritis Rheum* 1991;34(5):505–514.
10. Kilowsi R. Clinical cartilage imaging of the knee and hip joints. *Am J Roentgenol* 2010;195:618–628.
11. American College of Rheumatology Subcommittee on Osteoarthritis Guidelines. Recommendations for the medical management of osteoarthritis of the hip and knee: 2000 update. *Arthritis Rheum* 2000;43(9): 1905–1915.
12. Zhang W, Moskowitz RW, Nuki G et al. OARSI recommendations for the management of hip and knee osteoarthritis, part II: OARSI evidence-based, expert consensus guidelines. *Osteoarthritis Cartilage* 2008;16(2):137–162.
13. Zhang W, Doherty M, Leeb BF et al. EULAR evidence based recommendations for the management of hand osteoarthritis: report of a Task Force of the EULAR Standing Committee for International Clinical Studies Including Therapeutics (ESCISIT). *Ann Rheum Dis* 2007;66(3):377–388.
14. National Institute for Health and Clinical Excellence (NICE). *Osteoarthritis: the care and management of osteoarthritis in adults (CG59).* NICE, London, 2008.
15. Zhang W, Doherty M, Arden N et al. EULAR evidence based recommendations for the management of hip osteoarthritis: report of a Task Force of the EULAR Standing Committee for International Clinical Studies Including Therapeutics (ESCISIT). *Ann Rheum Dis* 2005;64(5): 669–681.
16. Migliore A, Granata M, Tormenta S et al. Hip viscosupplementation under ultra-sound guidance reduces NSAID consumption in symptomatic hip osteoarthritis patients in a long follow-up. Data from Italian registry. *Eur Rev Med Pharmacol Sci* 2011;15:25–43.
17. Migliore A, Massafra U, Bizzi E et al. Comparative, double-blind, controlled study of intra-articular hyaluronic acid (Hyalubrix) injections versus local anesthetic in osteoarthritis of the hip. *Arthritis Res Ther* 2009;11(6): R183.
18. National Institutes of Health. Total hip replacement. *NIH Consensus Statement* 1994;12:1.
19. Brophy S, Calin A. Ankylosing spondylitis: interaction between genes, joints, age at onset, and disease expression. *J Rheumatol.* 2001;28(10):2283–2288.
20. Baker-LePain JC, Lane NE. Relationship between joint shape and the development of osteoarthritis. *Curr Opin Rheumatol* 2010;22:538–543.

21. Korompilias AV, Karantanas AH, Lykissas MG, Beris AE. Bone marrow oedema syndrome. *Skeletal Radiol* 2009;38(5):425–436.

22. Ohzono K, Saito M, Sugano N, Takaoka K, Ono K. The fate of nontraumatic avascular necrosis of the femoral head. A radiologic classification to formulate prognosis. *Clin Orthop Relat Res* 1992;277:73–78.

23. Steinberg ME, Brighton CT, Corces A et al. Osteonecrosis of the femoral head. Results of core decompression and grafting with and without electrical stimulation. *Clin Orthop Relat Res* 1989;249:199–207.

24. Peck D. Slipped capital femoral epiphysis: diagnosis and management. *Am Fam Physician* 2010;82(3):258–262.

CHAPTER 155

Knee

Roger Wolman

Introduction

Knee pain is a common complaint affecting up to 20% of the adult population. In young adults it is most often caused by injury to the patellofemoral joint, menisci, ligaments, or the soft tissues surrounding the knee. In the older population osteoarthritis (OA) is the most common cause. Knee pain may also be the presenting symptom of disorders referred from elsewhere, in particular the hip and lower back.

Functional anatomy

The knee joint is the largest joint in the body. It is a synovial joint and a common source of symptoms in inflammatory arthritis. It is a hinge joint, predominantly moving in the anterior–posterior plane. There is also a small amount of gliding between the tibia and femur and a small rotatory component which can be a cause of injury. These additional movements are restricted by the two cruciate ligaments in the centre of the knee and the medial and lateral collateral ligaments.

The knee has two different articulations. The tibiofemoral joint consists of the medial and lateral femoral and tibial condyles with the medial and lateral menisci lying in between. The patellofemoral joint forms the articulation between the patella and the trochlear groove between the anterior aspect of the medial and lateral femoral condyles. The patella glides through the trochlear groove as the knee flexes and extends. On knee flexion of 90° or more the patella is in close contact with the groove while on full extension it predominantly sits above the groove. This explains why patellofemoral joint pain is often worse on sitting.

The patellofemoral joint is a common source of knee pain and some of this pain may arise from malalignment. Patella alignment within the groove is controlled by several factors. This includes the direction of pull of the quadriceps on the patella, the force of which follows a line from the centre of the patella to the anterior superior iliac spine. The Q angle is the angle formed by this line and a line drawn from the tibial tubercle to the centre of the patella. The Q angle is increased by having a wide pelvis, by femoral neck anteversion and external tibial torsion. A Q angle of greater than 20° is regarded as abnormal and can lead to maltracking of the patella and even dislocation. The quadriceps is made up of four muscle groups—the rectus femoris and the three vasti (medialis, intermedius, and lateralis). These are attached to the patella through the quadriceps tendon with fibrous expansions onto the medial and lateral borders of the patella (the medial and lateral patellar retinacula). The relative strength of the medialis compared to the lateralis influences the stability of the patella. The patella is connected to the tibial tuberosity through the patellar tendon. This can be a source of pain at either end of its attachments in the adolescent, and an overuse injury of the proximal patellar tendon is common, especially in jumping sports. Additional lateral stability of the knee is provided by the iliotibial band. This is a thick fibrous band that attaches into the lateral tibia and the lateral patellar retinaculum. Proximately it is attached to the tensor fascia lata muscle. This structure helps to stabilize the knee in full extension but can be a source of injury, especially in runners.

The three hamstrings are the main flexors of the knee and originate from the ischial tuberosity. The biceps femoris is inserted posterolaterally into the proximal tibia and fibula; the semimembranosus is inserted posteromedially into the tibia; the semitendinosus tendon combines with those of gracilis and sartorius to form the pes anserinus which inserts into the medial aspect of the proximal tibia.

There are several bursas surrounding the knee which can become the source of pain. These include the prepatellar and infrapatellar bursas which lie anterior to the patella and patellar tendon respectively. They can become inflamed as a result of kneeling or from a direct blow to the front of the knee. There are also bursas at the back of the knee, including one lying deep to the semimembranosus and another deep to the popliteus. On the medial aspect of the knee lies the pes anserinus bursa which separates the tendon of the same name from the medial collateral ligament.

Clinical assessment

The history is very important.[1] Pain is the most common presentation but swelling, giving way, or locking may also occur. It is important to know how the symptoms began—sudden onset or insidious. If the onset was acute then what was the mechanism—e.g. twisting, falling, or a direct blow to the knee. If the symptoms are related to activity then it is important to know what activities provoke it and what types of exercise was the person doing at the time of onset of the symptoms. Many overuse injuries around the knee are due to errors in training or the use of unsuitable equipment.

Swelling may be generalized due to an effusion or more localized due to an enlarged bursa. A joint effusion that develops within an

Table 155.1 Causes of knee pain classified by site of pain

Anterior	Posterior	Medial	Lateral	General
Patellofemoral pain syndrome	Baker's cyst (joint effusion)	OA	OA	OA
Patellar instability	Meniscal tear (posterior horn)	Meniscal tear	Meniscal tear	Referred pain (hip or lumbar spine)
Patellar tendinopathy	Hamstring tendinopathy	Medial ligament injury	Lateral ligament injury	Synovitis
Osgood–Schlatters disease		Chronic pain and fibromyalgia	Iliotibial band friction syndrome	Cruciate ligament tear
Pre- and infrapatellar bursitis				Osteochondritis dissecans
Quadriceps tendinopathy	Postero-lateral corner injury	Pes anserinus bursitis/tendinopathy	Proximal tibiofibular joint pain	PVNS
	Popliteus tendinopathy	Pellegrini–Stieda disease		Osteochondromatosis

OA, osteoarthritis; PVNS, pigmented villonodular synovitis.

hour of an acute injury is usually due to a haemarthrosis whereas one taking much longer to develop is due to synovial fluid. The sensation of 'giving way' is usually due to acute pain (such as a catching of the patellofemoral joint) but may be due to instability (as a result of ligament rupture). 'Locking' may be due to a meniscal tear or a loose body within the joint but can occur as a result of patellofemoral joint irritation (often referred to as pseudo-locking). The anatomical site of the pain can help to make the diagnosis—anterior, medial, posterior, lateral, and generalized (Table 155.1).

Anterior knee pain

Patellofemoral pain syndrome

This is a common disorder, often caused by maltracking of the patella in the trochlear groove leading to irritation on the joint surface.[2] As described above there are several factors which help to control patellar alignment. Additional factors in the upper thigh, such as excessive hip adduction and internal rotation (femoral neck anteversion), and in the lower leg, such as rearfoot eversion and overpronation on walking, will also adversely affect patellar alignment.

The patient presents with pain at the front of the knee which is aggravated by walking (especially on a slope), stairs, and prolonged sitting with the knee bent (described as a positive theatre/cinema sign). Wearing high-heeled shoes, by encouraging knee flexion, can cause further pain. Sporting activities such as running, cycling, and swimming (especially breast stroke) may also aggravate the symptoms. The knee may give way due to pain inhibition of the quadriceps. There may also be a sensation of locking in full extension due to pain (pseudo-locking).

Examination findings include patellofemoral joint tenderness and pain on patella grind. There may be a small effusion and quadriceps muscle wasting, especially affecting the vastus medialis. Examination should also include an assessment of the factors that affect patellofemoral alignment as described above.

Treatment will initially include decreasing or avoiding activities that provoke the symptoms (relative or absolute rest). The patient should be referred for physiotherapy[3] to address the biomechanical problems and provide muscle reconditioning for the quadriceps (vastus medialis especially) and glutei as well as flexibility training for the hamstrings. Techniques to loosen tight lateral knee structures such as the iliotibial band and the lateral retinaculum will

also help. Taping of the patella as well as the use of foot orthotics in patients with overpronated feet should be considered. It is important to treat this condition, as recent evidence suggests that prolonged symptoms related to this condition increase the risk of patellofemoral osteoarthritis (OA).[4]

Patella dislocation and instability

Patella dislocation and instability occurs most commonly in adolescent girls. The biomechanical risk factors, which are similar to those for patellofemoral pain syndrome, also include a shallow trochlear groove and a high-riding patella where the patellar tendon is relatively long (patella alta) and the patella may lie above the groove. Joint hypermobility also increases the risk.

An acute dislocation may be the first sign of the problem. This may occur as a result of trauma but can occur spontaneously. The patella dislocates laterally and will usually reduce spontaneously or with relatively little pressure. Traumatic dislocation will be associated with acute swelling due to a haemarthrosis. The swelling may be less following a spontaneous dislocation. There will be tenderness over the medial retinaculum as a result of the torn fibres. Investigations should include plain radiographs, in particular lateral and skyline views to look for patella alta and a shallow groove, and MRI will help to determine whether an osteochondral fracture has occurred.

Acute dislocation requires immobilization in extension in a leg cylinder for 4–6 weeks followed by physiotherapy. Recurrent dislocation or instability will require more extensive physiotherapy addressing the biomechanical issues that may have contributed to the injury. In cases that do not respond to conservative treatment, surgery should be considered. This includes a release of the lateral retinaculum or patella realignment procedures.[5]

Patellar tendinopathy

As this is seen in athletes doing jumping sports, such as basketball and volleyball, it is often referred as jumper's knee. However, it also occurs in other sports and in the non-sporting population. The abnormality occurs at the proximal end of the patellar tendon with degenerative changes, new vessel formation, and tears evident on histology. The patient will have infrapatellar tenderness and pain aggravated by weightbearing exercise and especially by squats. It may occur with patellofemoral joint pain, as they share similar biomechanical risk factors.

Diagnosis can usually be made clinically and confirmed on ultrasound scanning. This shows changes at the proximal end with enlargement of the tendon, new vessel formation, disruption of the fibres and areas of low echogenicity. Changes can also be seen on MRI (Figure 155.1).

Treatment involves relative rest to help offload the tendon. Biomechanical factors should be addressed. Rehabilitation should include slowly progressive quadriceps strengthening, including eccentric exercises. Image-guided injections of either whole blood or platelet-rich plasma have been advocated although at present there is no strong evidence-base for their use.[6] Resolution of the problem may take up to 6 months. If the problem persists beyond this time despite good conservative treatment then surgery should be considered. There are a range of surgical treatments but the outcomes are unpredictable.

Quadriceps tendinopathy

This occurs at the site of attachment of the quadriceps to the upper border of the patella. There is pain and localized tenderness over this site. It is far less common than patellar tendinopathy. Treatment principles are similar with relative rest, quadriceps reconditioning exercise, and possibly the use of injections.

Enthesial disorders in adolescence

Osgood–Schlatter disease

This occurs at the site of attachment of the patellar tendon to the tibial tuberosity apophysis (Figure 155.2). This is weaker during

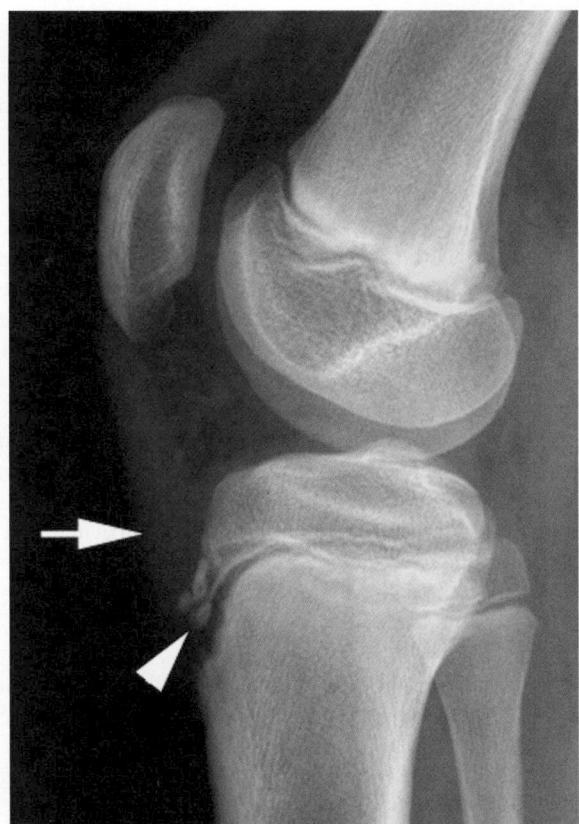

Fig. 155.2 Osgood–Schlatters disease: lateral radiograph of the knee showing swelling of the distal patellar tendon (arrow) and new bone formation (arrowhead) at the tendon insertion to the tibial tuberosity.
All the imaging has been provided by Dr A Saifuddin, Consultant Radiologist, Royal National Orthopaedic Hospital.

the adolescent growth spurt and therefore vulnerable to the intense traction that occurs with weightbearing sports. It tends to occur in girls between 11–13 years and in boys between 13–16 years. There will be a localized area of pain and tenderness and the tuberosity may become more prominent.[7] With mild symptoms the adolescent can continue to exercise through it. With more severe symptoms relative rest and physiotherapy may help. The symptoms usually resolve within a year.

Sinding–Larsen–Johansson syndrome

This occurs at the site of attachment of the patellar tendon to lower pole of the patella and occurs in a similar age group as seen in Osgood–Schlatter's, although it is far less common. Management is similar.

Prepatellar and infrapatellar bursitis

These can occur as a result of prolonged kneeling (housemaid's and clergyman's knee respectively). They may also occur as a result of a direct blow. They present with swelling at the front of the knee with relatively little pain. Examination reveals a well-circumscribed fluctuant mass with thickening of the adjacent soft tissues. Diagnosis can be confirmed on ultrasound which will demonstrate the fluid-filled sack and increased Doppler signal on the deep surface due to its good blood supply.

Treatment requires avoidance of kneeling and may require aspiration of the fluid and injection of steroid. This may need to be repeated. Very occasionally a surgical bursectomy is required.

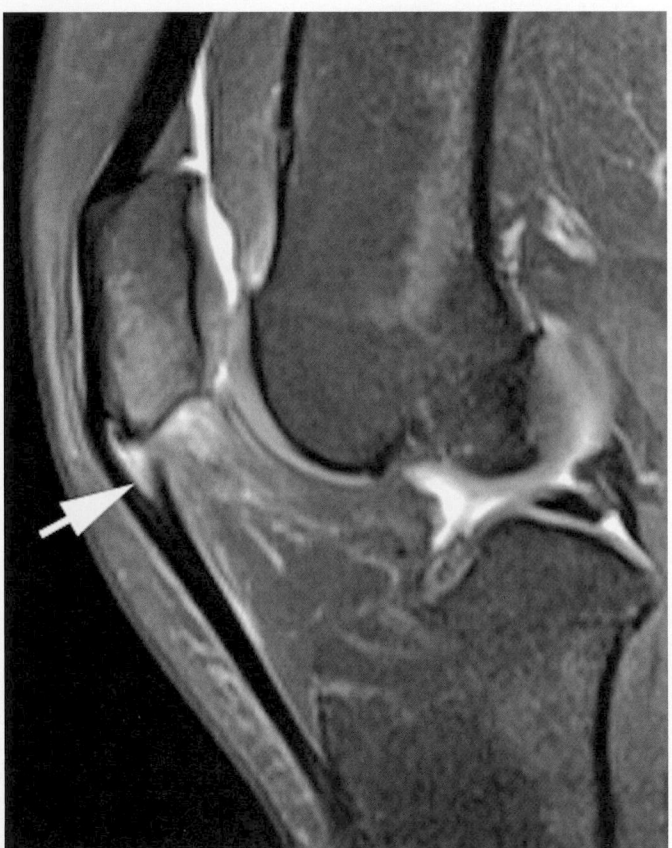

Fig. 155.1 Patellar tendinopathy: sagittal fat-suppressed PDW FSE MRI showing fluid signal intensity within the proximal patellar tendon, indicative of patellar tendinopathy.
All the imaging has been provided by Dr A Saifuddin, Consultant Radiologist, Royal National Orthopaedic Hospital.

Medial knee pain

The soft tissues on the medial aspect of the knee are a common trigger-spot site. It occurs in fibromyalgia and may be associated with vague pain.

Medial meniscus injury

An acute twisting injury to the knee can result in a tear to the medial meniscus with pain, joint effusion, and possibly locking. A small tear results in mild, more localized symptoms. In middle age, changes in the medial meniscus can result in symptomatic degenerative tears. These can produce pain along the medial joint line on weightbearing with associated joint-line tenderness, a positive McMurray's test, and pain on full flexion of the knee. The diagnosis can be confirmed on MRI. These tears usually respond to conservative management of rest and rehabilitation.[8] Occasionally an arthroscopic meniscectomy is indicated. However, the risk of partial meniscectomy is that it may expose the articular cartilage which, in a middle-aged patient, may itself be degenerate. This can sometimes make the pain worse.

Medial osteoarthritis

Medial tibiofemoral joint osteoarthritis and a degenerative meniscal tear can produce similar symptoms. They often occur together. Patients may have a varus deformity of the knee. Radiographs help to confirm the diagnosis of OA and MRI will help to distinguish between the two conditions.

Medial ligament injury (medial ligament syndrome)

Injury to the medial collateral ligament occurs as a result of valgus stress on the knee. This is more common in women, who are more likely to have a valgus alignment of the knee. It can also occur in breaststroke swimming, where there is a persistent valgus stress on the knee. This can produce a grade I injury (sprain without a tear). Acute knee injuries caused by sudden valgus stress, as in football, can cause more severe injuries including a partial (grade II) or complete tear (grade III) of the ligament. These can be diagnosed clinically by assessing for pain and/or laxity on applying a valgus stress to the knee. Conservative treatment with a combination of rest and immobilization followed by rehabilitation is usually successful.[9]

Pellegrini–Stieda disease

This occurs as a result of a tear to the femoral origin of the medial collateral ligament. Calcification forms at the site which can be seen on the radiograph (Figure 155.3). There will be pain, tenderness, and swelling on the medial aspect of the knee. This usually responds to rest, physical therapy, and non-steroidal anti-inflammatory drugs (NSAIDs). Occasionally a steroid injection can help.

Pes anserinus bursitis/tendinopathy

This tendon, as described above, inserts into the anteromedial upper tibia. The bursa lies between the tendon and the tibial surface (Figure 155.4). This can become symptomatic. It is associated with valgus deformity of the knee,[10] and occurs in runners and breaststroke swimmers. The features include localized swelling and tenderness with pain on activity. Treatment consists of rest and physical therapy. A corticosteroid injection will be helpful if there is a significant bursal swelling.

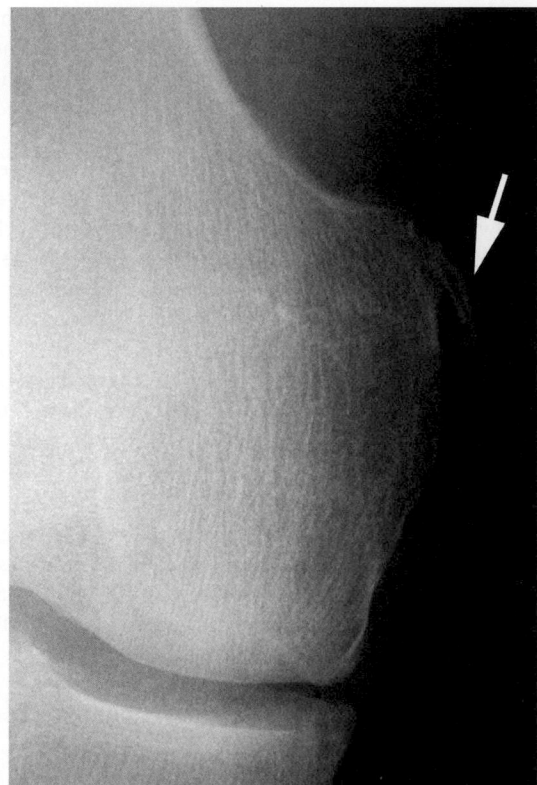

Fig. 155.3 Pelligrini–Stieda lesion: coned AP radiograph of the right knee showing ossification in the femoral attachment of the medial collateral ligament (arrow) indicative of a chronic Pelligrini–Stieda lesion.

All the imaging has been provided by Dr A Saifuddin, Consultant Radiologist, Royal National Orthopaedic Hospital.

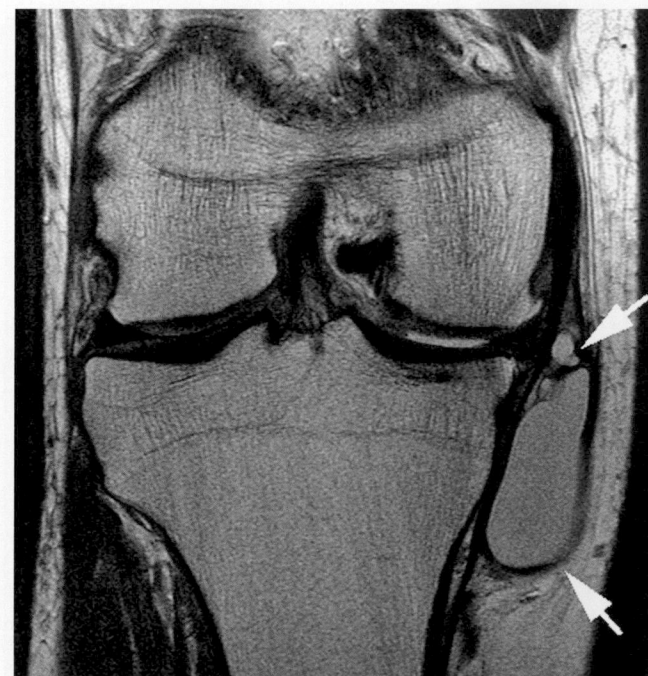

Fig. 155.4 Pes anserinus bursitis: coronal PDW FSE MRI showing a prominent bursa (arrows) overlying the medial collateral ligament and involving the distal pes anserinus tendons.

All the imaging has been provided by Dr A Saifuddin, Consultant Radiologist, Royal National Orthopaedic Hospital.

Posterior knee pain

The most common cause is a joint effusion which can stretch the posterior joint capsule to cause pain. It can cause a Baker's cyst where the capsule herniates between the two heads of gastrocnemius. It is important to address the cause of the effusion. Tears affecting the posterior aspect of either meniscus may also cause posterior pain.

Posterolateral corner injury

This refers to an injury of the structures that stabilize the posterolateral corner of the knee. It includes the lateral collateral ligament, the popliteus, the iliotibial band, and a series of small ligaments in this area. It is often combined with an injury to the lateral meniscus and posterior cruciate ligament, producing laxity to the lateral knee, a varus deformity, and ultimately medial joint arthritis. The injury occurs when a posterolateral force is directed onto the medial aspect of the tibia leading to varus stress. The patient complains of pain and instability. There are several clinical tests that help to point to the diagnosis which can be confirmed on stress radiographs, MRI (Figure 155.5), or diagnostic arthroscopy. Mild injuries can be treated conservatively but more severe injuries require surgical correction.[11]

Popliteus tendinopathy causes posterior knee pain. It rarely occurs in isolation,[12] usually being part of the above injury.

Hamstring injury

The biceps femoris is the hamstring tendon that is most commonly injured, causing posterolateral knee pain. Diagnosis can be made clinically by tenderness over the tendon and pain on resisted knee flexion and on stretching the tendon. It can be confirmed on ultrasound. It usually responds to rest and rehabilitation over a 3–6 week period.[13]

Lateral knee pain

Injuries to the lateral collateral ligament in isolation are relatively uncommon. They occur as a result of a varus stress applied to the knee and usually occur in association with other structures of the posterolateral corner as described above.

Iliotibial band friction syndrome

This occurs as a result of friction between the deep surface of the iliotibial band and the lateral epicondyle of the femur. It occurs in runners, especially on going downhill. It can occasionally be seen in downhill walkers. Biomechanical factors such as overpronated feet increase the risk. The patient typically complains of lateral knee pain brought on by running. If they continue to run through it the pain will tend to come on earlier in the run and will eventually prevent them from running. Examination reveals tenderness over the lateral femoral condyle and tightness of the iliotibial band on Ober's test, which may also provoke the pain. Diagnosis can be confirmed on ultrasound or MRI (Figure 155.6). Treatment consists of relative rest and the use of ice and NSAIDs to reduce the irritation. Occasionally

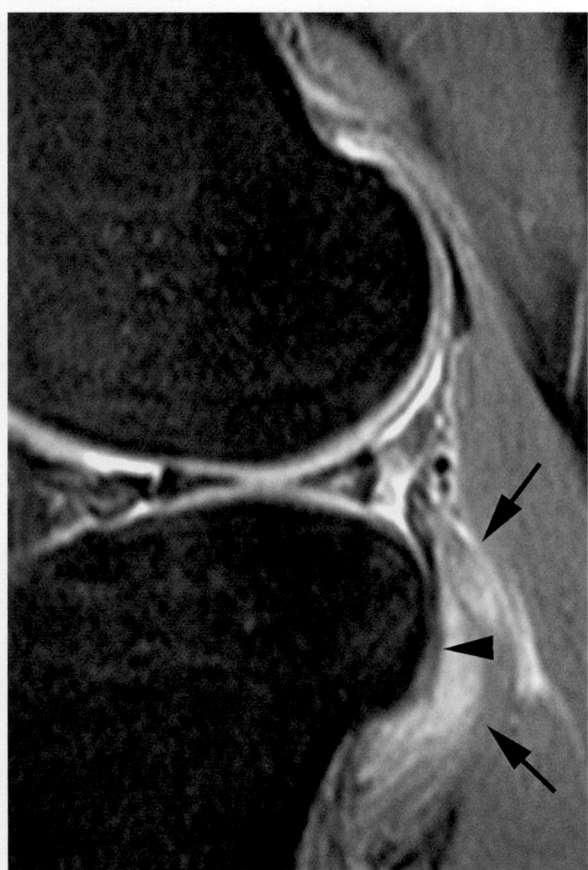

Fig. 155.5 Posterolateral corner injury: sagittal fat-suppressed PDW FSE MRI showing oedema (black arrows) at the popliteus musculotendinous junction (black arrowhead).

All the imaging has been provided by Dr A Saifuddin, Consultant Radiologist, Royal National Orthopaedic Hospital.

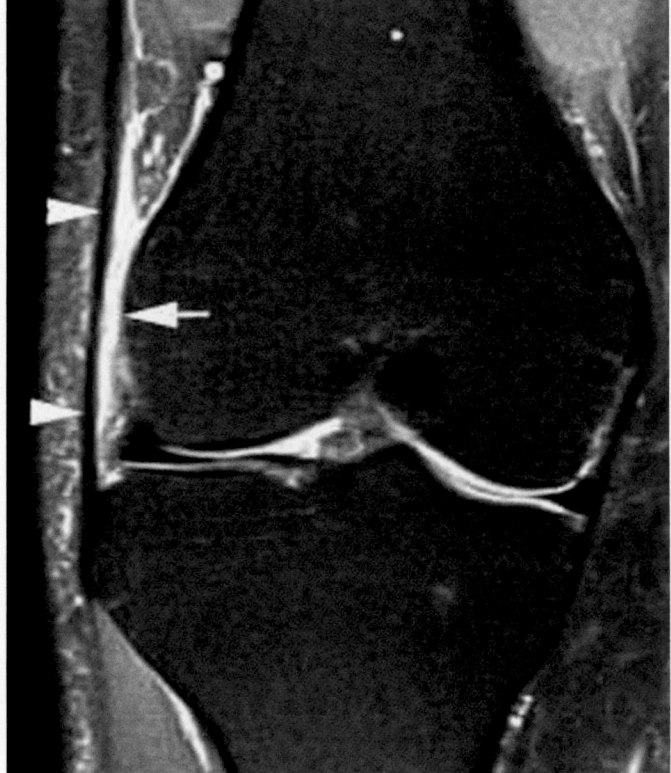

Fig. 155.6 Iliotibial band friction syndrome: coronal fat-suppressed PDW FSE MRI showing fluid (white arrow) deep to the iliotibial band (white arrowheads) consistent with iliotibial band friction syndrome.

All the imaging has been provided by Dr A Saifuddin, Consultant Radiologist, Royal National Orthopaedic Hospital.

a steroid injection is required. Rehabilitation consists of stretching exercises for the iliotibial band and addressing other biomechanical factors which may be contributing to the symptoms.[14]

Lateral meniscus injury

Tears to the lateral meniscus are less common than the medial meniscus. They also respond less well to surgery. Acute tears can occur in the young athlete, while chronic degenerative tears occur in middle age causing knee pain on weightbearing. Examination will demonstrate positive meniscal signs. Occasionally a lump is seen on the lateral joint due to subluxation of the meniscus or due to a meniscal cyst. Diagnosis can be confirmed on MRI. For chronic degenerative tears the treatment of choice is conservative with rest and rehabilitation. Surgery is reserved for those not responding to conservative treatment.[15]

Proximal tibiofibular joint pain

This joint can become symptomatic as a result of a direct blow or following a rotational injury to the knee. The joint may then become unstable causing lateral knee pain, especially on weightbearing. MRI may be helpful in demonstrating soft tissue damage around the joint. Treatment is usually conservative and may involve immobilization of the joint following an acute injury. Physiotherapy can be helpful. Surgery may be required for a persistently unstable symptomatic joint.[16]

Generalized knee pain

Intra-articular pathology may lead to a more generalized knee pain. Inflammatory arthritis often causes synovitis within the knee with associated pain and swelling.

Cruciate ligament ruptures

These injuries occur in weightbearing twisting sports and more commonly affect the anterior ligament (Figure 155.7). Once this injury has occurred the risk of developing OA in later life is high, even if surgical

reconstruction is performed. In the young adult who wants to get back to a similar level of sport, a reconstruction operation is usually required. In the middle-aged adult, or in an adult who is willing to make lifestyle changes, conservative treatment is usually successful.[17,18]

Osteochondritis dissecans

In this condition a piece of articular cartilage becomes detached from the subchondral bone probably as a result of avascular necrosis (AVN), possibly caused by trauma. It most commonly occurs in teenage males. The main symptoms are pain, swelling, limitation of movement, and possibly locking. Diagnosis can be made on imaging (plain radiograph, CT, and/or MRI; Figure 155.8). Treatment initially consists of rest and physiotherapy. If the fragment is stable this is likely to be successful but if the fragment is loose or has detached then arthroscopic surgery is usually required. This will include removal of the loose fragment or reattachment to the bone. If there is an area of exposed bone then drilling to encourage fibrotic healing or cartilage transplantation are treatment options. There is an increased risk of developing OA.[19]

Pigmented villonodular synovitis

This is a rare proliferative disorder of synovial tissue. The knee is the most common joint to be involved. Although it is locally invasive and has a high recurrence rate, it remains unclear whether this is an inflammatory or neoplastic condition.[20] It most commonly occurs between the ages of 20 and 50 years and presents with pain, swelling, and limitation of movement. Examination findings include a joint effusion and quadriceps wasting. Joint aspiration usually produces bloodstained synovial fluid which should raise the possibility of this diagnosis. MRI gives a very characteristic appearance (Figure 155.9) and is the investigation of choice for making the diagnosis. Aspiration and steroid injection only provides brief pain relief. Surgical synovectomy (either arthroscopic or open) is the treatment of choice although the recurrence rate is 40–60% at 5 years. Radiation (using a yttrium implant or external radiation)

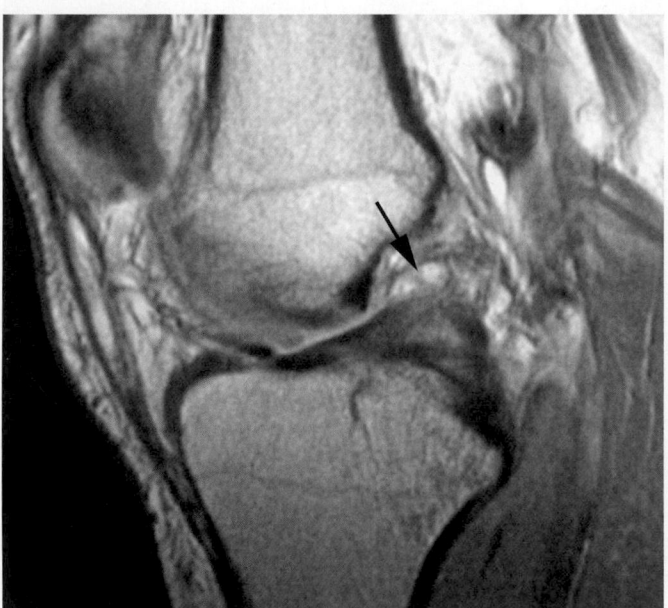

Fig. 155.7 Anterior cruciate ligament (ACL) rupture: sagittal PDW FSE MRI showing a complete rupture of the femoral attachment of the ACL (arrow).

All the imaging has been provided by Dr A Saifuddin, Consultant Radiologist, Royal National Orthopaedic Hospital.

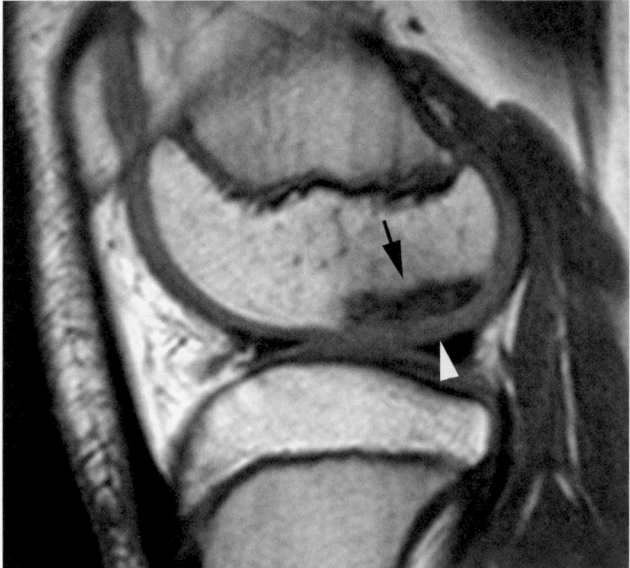

Fig. 155.8 Osteochrondritis dissecans: sagittal T1W MRI showing an osteochondral lesion (black arrow) of the posterior weightbearing surface of the lateral femoral condyle, with intact overlying cartilage (white arrowhead).

All the imaging has been provided by Dr A Saifuddin, Consultant Radiologist, Royal National Orthopaedic Hospital.

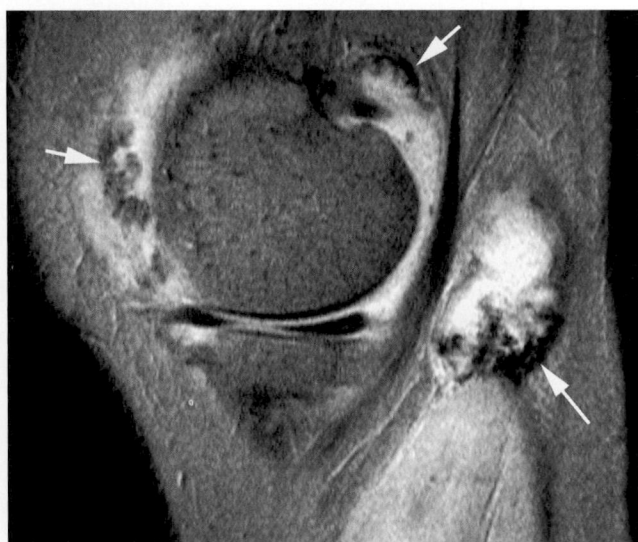

Fig. 155.9 Pigmented villonodular synovitis (PVNS): sagittal T2*W GE MRI showing a joint effusion with extensive hypointense synovitis (arrows) typical of diffuse PVNS. All the imaging has been provided by Dr A Saifuddin, Consultant Radiologist, Royal National Orthopaedic Hospital.

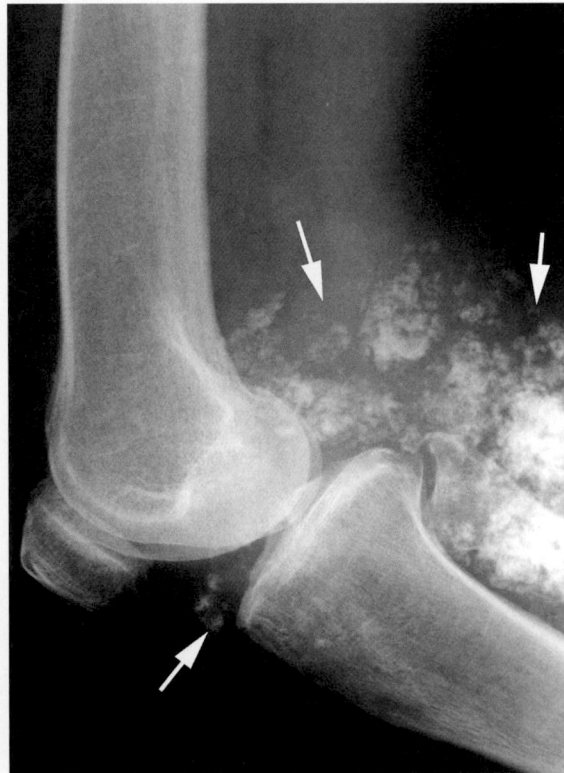

Fig. 155.10 Osteochondromatosis: lateral radiograph of the knee showing extensive periarticular chondral-type soft tissue calcifications (arrows) typical of synovial osteochondromatosis.
All the imaging has been provided by Dr A Saifuddin, Consultant Radiologist, Royal National Orthopaedic Hospital.

or chemical synovectomy (using osmic acid) offer alternative treatment strategies.[21]

Osteochondromatosis

The aetiology of this condition is poorly understood. It tends to occur between the ages of 30 and 50 years, more commonly in men. The knee is the most common joint to be affected. Synovial cells undergo chondroblastic metaplasia, which then produce deposits of cartilage in the synovial membrane. These grow, calcify, and eventually detach to become loose bodies within the joint. They then become symptomatic causing pain, swelling, and locking. Examination findings are non-specific. Diagnosis can be made on radiograph (Figure 155.10), CT, and/or MRI. Treatment is surgical and should include arthroscopic removal of the loose bodies together with synovectomy to reduce the risk of recurrence.[22] The prognosis is good with a recurrence rate of 5–10%. Malignant transformation is rare.

Lipoma arborescens

This is a very rare disorder of the synovium, of unknown aetiology. It most commonly affects the knee, in particular the suprapatellar pouch. Macroscopically there are numerous papillary villi containing mature adipose tissue with an overlying synovial membrane. The patient presents with pain, swelling, and restricted movement. MRI shows a characteristic appearance of the synovial tissue within the joint. Definitive treatment is with open or arthroscopic synovectomy. Alternative treatments include radiation or chemical synovectomy.[23]

Acknowledgement

All the imaging has been provided by Dr A. Saifuddin, Consultant Radiologist, Royal National Orthopaedic Hospital.

References

1. Spalding T. History and examination of the knee. In Bulstrode C, Wilson-MacDonald J, Eastwood D et al (eds). *Oxford Textbook of Trauma and Orthopaedics*, 2nd edn. Oxford University Press, Oxford, 2011:633–641.
2. Donell S. The patellofemoral joint. In: Bulstrode C, Wilson-MacDonald J, Eastwood D et al (eds). *Oxford Textbook of Trauma and Orthopaedics*, 2nd edn. Oxford University Press, Oxford, 2011:693–70.
3. Crossley K, Bennell K, Green S, McConnell J. A systematic review of physical interventions for patellofemoral pain syndrome. *Clin J Sport Med* 2001;11:103–110.
4. Utting MR, Davies G, Newman JH. Is anterior knee pain a predisposing factor to patellofemoral osteoarthritis? *Knee* 2005;12:362–365.
5. Stefancin J, Parker R, Spindler K, Wright R. First-time traumatic patellar dislocation: a systematic review. *Clin Orthop Relat Res* 2007;455:93–101.
6. Van Ark M, Zwerver J, Van den Akker-Scheek I. Injection treatments for patellar tendinopathy. *Br J Sports Med* 2011;45:1068–1076.
7. Weiler R, Ingram M, Wolman R. 10 minute consultation: Osgood Schlatter disease. *BMJ* 2011;343:d4534.
8. Herrlin S, Hallander M, Wange P, Weidenhielm, Werner S. Arthroscopic or conservative treatment of degenerative medial meniscal tears: a prospective randomised trial Arthroscopic or conservative treatment of degenerative medial meniscal tears: a prospective randomised trial. *Knee Surg Sports Traumatol Arthrosc* 2007;15:393–401.
9. Duffy PS, Miyamoto RG. Management of medial collateral ligament injuries in the knee: an update and review. *Phys Sportsmed* 2010;38:48–54.
10. Alvarez-Nemegyei J. Risk factors for pes anserinus tendinitis/bursitis syndrome: a case control study. *J Clin Rheumatol* 2007;13:63–65.
11. Jonathan M. Cooper JM, McAndrews PT, LaPrade RF. Posterolateral corner injuries of the knee: anatomy, diagnosis, and treatment. *Sports Med Arthrosc Rev* 2006;14:213–220.
12. Blake SM, Treble NJ. Popliteus tendon tenosynovitis. *Br J Sports Med* 2005;39:e42.
13. Linklater JM, Hamilton B, Carmichael J, Orchard J, Wood DG. Hamstring injuries: anatomy, imaging, and intervention. *Semin Musculoskelet Radiol* 2010; 14:131–161.
14. Lavine R. Iliotibial band friction syndrome. *Curr Rev Musculoskelet Med* 2010;3:18–22.

15. Salata MJ, Gibbs AE, Sekiya JK. A systematic review of clinical outcomes in patients undergoing meniscectomy. *Am J Sports Med* 2010; 38:1907–1916.

16. Sekiya JK, Kuhn JE. Instability of the proximal tibiofibular joint. *J Am Acad Orthop Surg* 2003;11:120–128.

17. Frobell RB, Roos EM, Roos HP, Ranstam J, Lohmander LS. A randomized trial of treatment for acute anterior cruciate ligament tears. *N Engl J Med* 2010;363:331–342.

18. Meuffels DE, Favejee MM, Vissers MM et al. Ten year follow-up study comparing conservative versus operative treatment of anterior cruciate ligament ruptures. A matched-pair analysis of high level athletes. *Br J Sports Med* 2009;43:347–351.

19. Edge A., Porter K. Osteochondritis dissecans: a review. *Trauma* 2011;13:23–33.

20. Kramer DE, Frassica FJ, Frassica DA, Cosgarea AJ. Pigmented villonodular synovitis of the knee: diagnosis and treatment. *J Knee Surgery* 2009;22:243–254.

21. Bessant R, Steuer A, Rigby, Gumpel M. Osmic acid revisited: factors that predict a favourable response. *Rheumatology* 2003;42:1036–1043.

22. Ogilvie-Harris DJ, Saleh K. Generalized synovial chondromatosis of the knee: A comparison of removal of the loose bodies alone with arthroscopic synovectomy. *Arthroscopy* 1994;10:166–170.

23. Azzouz D, Tekaya R, Hamdi R, Kchir M. Lipoma arborescens of the knee. *J Clin Rheumatol* 2008;14:370–372.

CHAPTER 156

Foot and ankle

Anthony C. Redmond and Philip S. Helliwell

Introduction

Foot problems are common, with approximately 10% of adults reporting significant foot pain at any given time. The prevalence increases with age such that one-half of people over 50 years of age have foot pain.[1,2] Foot problems are five times more common in females than males.[3,4] Foot problems impact significantly, interfering with daily activities,[5,6] and they rarely occur in isolation, usually presenting concomitantly with other musculoskeletal problems such as hip or knee pain.[7] The relevance of musculoskeletal foot pain is relatively well recognized in systemic diseases such as inflammatory arthritis, but the majority of foot pain occurs in otherwise healthy people[6] and foot problems should be considered in a context of local function as well as general health. Although the prevalence of foot symptoms is high in people attending rheumatology clinics, the foot and ankle remains relatively neglected. Possibly this is due to poor training in clinical examination techniques,[8] which is compounded by the inconvenience of accessing feet that may be considered unsightly or smelly. As a consequence foot problems are often ignored or may be referred on unseen to allied services such as podiatry.

Clinical assessment

A basic assessment need take no more than approximately one minute per foot as long as it is performed by an assessor with the requisite knowledge, skill and practice. A basic starting point for a lower limb assessment is the Regional Examination of the Musculoskeletal System (REMS),[8] supplemented by further foot-specific assessments as required (Box 156.1).

For more detailed foot evaluation, we have described extensively a Leeds foot assessment protocol which is a comprehensive assessment of foot problems developing the standard sequential approach of history → observation → examination. A thorough development of this can be found elsewhere.[9,10]

Foot and ankle pathology in rheumatology

The remainder of this chapter focuses on the conditions affecting the foot and ankle, as encountered in rheumatology practice. Much of the best evidence surrounding foot and ankle problems in rheumatology centres on rheumatoid arthritis (RA), and this, and the other systemic conditions, is be covered in detail. The chapter

---

Box 156.1 Regional Examination of the Musculoskeletal System: foot components

- Examine sole of patient's feet
- Recognize hallux valgus, claw and hammer toes
- Assess the patient's feet in standing
- Assess for flat feet (including patient standing on tiptoe)
- Recognize hindfoot/heel pathologies
- Assess plantar- and dorsiflexion of the ankle
- Assess movements of inversion and eversion of the foot
- Assess the subtalar joint
- Perform a lateral squeeze across the metatarsophalangeal joints
- Assess flexion/extension of the big toe
- Examine the patient's footwear

After Coady et al.[8]

---

starts, however, with a brief summary of the many foot conditions often encountered that are not the product of systemic disease and can be dealt with purely through their local effects.

Local foot and ankle problems

Flat feet (pes planus) and high-arched feet (pes cavus)

One of the more common non-specific foot complaints is so-called 'flat feet', which may or may not underlie symptoms resulting from 'overuse' type stresses and strains. Although some feet show frank flattening of the medial arch, the structural and functional variations are relatively complex. The presence of a flat foot (or indeed a high-arched foot) does not inherently imply pathology, as the range of normal foot postures is wide. It is unusual to initiate treatment of an asymptomatic flat foot and so therapy is directed at the combination of the symptoms and the underlying mechanics. Mechanical therapies can include footwear modifications, foot orthoses, taping, splints, and braces. Usually the goal is to limit excessive joint mobility and promote stability. Therapy for the cavoid foot is aimed at improving shock absorbency and stretching tight soft tissues. Treatments can include cushioning insoles, change in footwear, and stretching exercises.

Nerve entrapments

Nerve entrapments occur in the feet of rheumatology patients because of the complex anatomy and high prevalence of osteophytes and altered bony structures in this population. The most common nerve entrapment syndrome in the foot is Morton's neuroma, which affects the plantar digital nerve just proximal to the metatarsal heads. It is usually seen in the third and fourth metatarsal space, but can occur between any digits. Tight footwear and high-heeled shoes exacerbate the symptoms and the clinical diagnosis can be aided by squeezing the forefoot across the metatarsals, while exerting a pressure between the metatarsophalangeal (MTP) joints of the affected area to reproduce symptoms. Treatment may include advice to adopt wider-fitting shoes, orthoses, local steroid injection, or oral non-steroidal anti-inflammatory drugs (NSAIDs). Surgery may be required in severe cases. The other significant nerve entrapment found in rheumatology is tarsal tunnel syndrome, which arises when the tibial nerve is compressed as it passes around the medial aspect of the ankle in close association with the tendons under the flexor retinaculum. Tarsal tunnel syndrome may be caused by chronic inflammation of the medial tendons, or secondary to severe valgus position of the ankle, such as can occur in RA. The symptoms are tingling, numbness, and pain in the arch area, which can extend to the plantar surface and medial aspect of the ankle. Clinical diagnosis is made by percussion using Tinel's sign. If the compression arises from local inflammation (e.g. tenosynovitis), local injection of steroid may be helpful. Where heel position is the cause, short-term reduction of symptoms can sometimes be achieved by splinting, taping, or orthoses, although in severe cases referral for surgical assessment is required.

Tendinopathy

The two most common tendonopathies affect the Achilles tendon and the tendon of tibialis posterior. The Achilles tendon can be affected at the myotendinous junction, in the tendon substance, or at the insertion into the calcaneus. Acute, traumatic tears do not usually present in rheumatology outpatient clinics. Chronic lesions are picked up on clinical examination with symptoms of pain and swelling over the tendon exacerbated by weightbearing and dorsiflexion of the foot. Over time the tendon thickens and a fusiform swelling may be palpable and confirmed on MRI or ultrasound imaging (Figure 156.1). There are no definitive treatments,

but Alfredson and Cook[11] have proposed a treatment algorithm based on rest, ice, compression, and rehabilitation, combined with offloading of the Achilles through taping or a heel lift and careful eccentric strengthening.

Tibialis posterior dysfunction is a progressive tendinopathy which leads to an acquired flat foot. Patients (often postmenopausal women) experience pain and swelling on the medial aspect of the ankle and there may be progressive flattening of the arch. Characteristically, the patient is unable to stand on tiptoe on the affected side, unless stabilized by the contralateral limb. Definitive diagnosis is made with ultrasound or MRI[12] and early identification and treatment is important to prevent progression. Non-surgical treatment focuses on symptom relief symptoms and offloading the tendon using orthoses, footwear, ankle taping, or braces. Surgical treatment employs tendon transfer in the early stages with additional rearfoot osteotomy if required. Total reconstruction and arthrodesis of the rearfoot is required in severe cases.

Heel pain

Plantar heel pain affects one in ten of all people at some stage in their lives and is again more common in rheumatology patients.[13] The most common underlying pathology is plantar fasciitis, characterized by thickening of the plantar fascia at the proximal enthesis and sometimes extending along the fascia (Figure 156.2). The typical symptom is pain along the plantar surface of the heel or midfoot during activity or weightbearing. There may be focal tenderness at the origin, particularly first thing in the morning or after period of non-weightbearing. The clinical signs and symptoms are usually sufficient for diagnosis but ultrasound can be useful to confirming thickening. Treatment is change of footwear and weight loss where appropriate as a first option, with physical therapies sometimes helpful. There is some evidence for the efficacy of taping[14] and contoured foot orthoses,[15] and there is also limited evidence for the short-term efficacy of injection therapy with corticosteroid although the injections are painful and the long-term efficacy of injection is doubtful.[16,17]

Posterior to the heel are two sites sometimes affected by bursitis: the retrocalcaneal bursa, an anatomical bursa deep to the Achilles tendon, and the Achilles bursa which, when present, is adventitious and superficial to the tendon. The Achilles bursa is particularly prone to aggravation from footwear. The deeper, retrocalcaneal

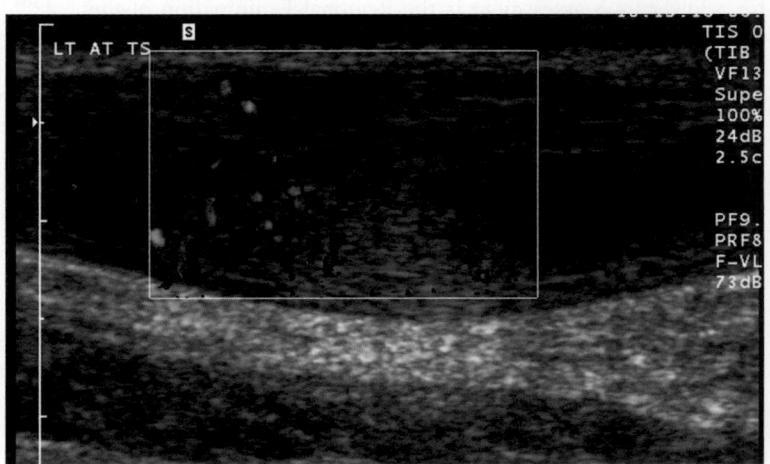

Fig. 156.1 Achilles tendonopathy: a fusiform swelling of the tendo Achilles with power Doppler signal indicating severe tendonopathy [a].
Reproduced with permission from: Redmond, Helliwell and Robinson. Investigating Foot and ankle problems, in Conaghan, O'Connor and Isenberg. Oxford specialist handbook in musculoskeletal imaging. Oxford University Press 2009.

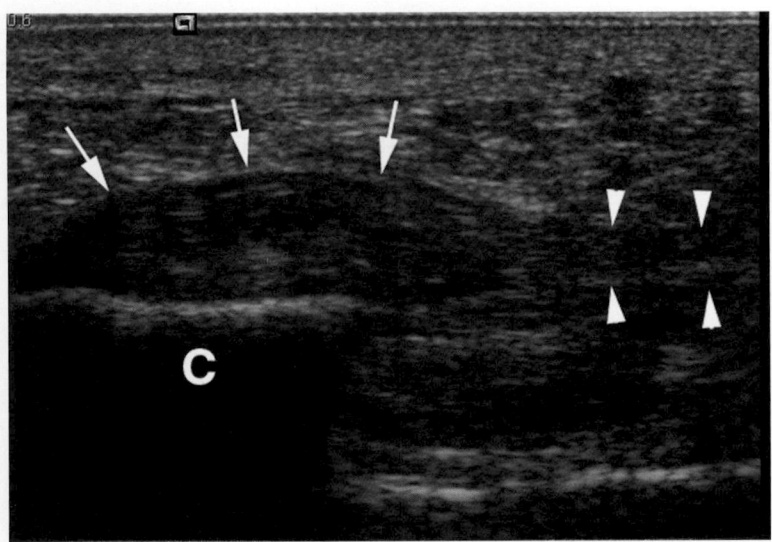

Fig. 156.2 Plantar fasciitis: at the origin from the calcaneus (c) there is thickening of the plantar fascia (white arrows) relative to the normal fascia (white arrowheads).

Reproduced with permission from: Redmond, Helliwell and Robinson. Investigating Foot and ankle problems, in Conaghan, O'Connor and Isenberg. Oxford specialist handbook in musculoskeletal imaging. Oxford University Press 2009.

bursa is more often associated with systemic inflammatory disease such as RA. MRI or ultrasound imaging is diagnostic.

Treatment of local, mechanical bursitis centres on physical therapies and NSAIDs. Modification to footwear is essential to prevent further irritation. Bursitis associated with inflammatory disease usually responds to corticosteroid injection.

Forefoot pain

In the forefoot, MTP joint mechanical overload can occur because of clawing/subluxation of the toes or loss of fat-pad protection. There may be low-grade discomfort, and associated thickening of the skin, pathological thickening of the skin (callus and corn formation), or bursitis overlying the MTP joints or inflammation of the intermetatarsal bursas. Intermetatarsal bursitis is a common manifestation of inflammatory arthritis and can also be seen in otherwise healthy individuals. Sharp pain will be elicited with a lateral squeeze test across the metatarsal heads. MRI and ultrasound is required for definitive diagnosis. Bursitis will respond well to local injection of corticosteroid.

The foot and ankle in rheumatoid arthritis

The foot has many synovial structures and so the foot is involved in about 80–90% of people with RA.[18–20] Even in early disease, estimates of foot involvement range from 32% to 75%,[21,22] and initial symptoms are reported in the foot almost as frequently as in the hands. The forefoot is the most commonly involved region,[21,23] and the subtalar joint is also involved in two-thirds to three-quarters of all people with longstanding RA. The ankle joint proper is relatively spared, being affected in only 10–20% of people with established RA. As many as one-quarter of patients experience soft tissue problems in the foot, such as plantar fasciitis, peroneal tendonitis, or bursitis.[19,24]

While the articular damage occurs primarily because of synovitis, the inflammatory damage is compounded by the mechanical stresses affecting weightbearing structures. The combination of damage drivers results in irreversible structural changes such as characteristic forefoot changes, flattening of the arch, valgus deformity of the heel, and tibialis posterior dysfunction (Figure 156.3).[24] With better disease-modifying anti-rheumatic

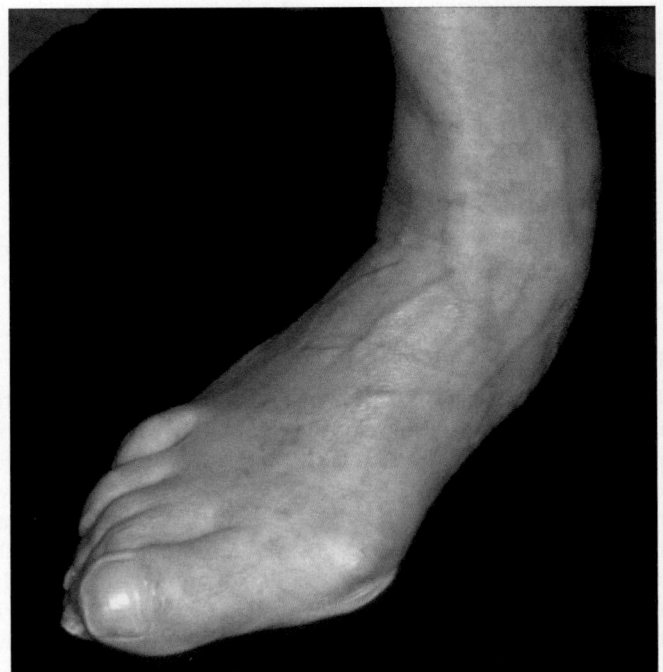

Fig. 156.3 The typical changes occurring in the feet of a person with rheumatoid arthritis.

Reproduced with permission from: Redmond and Helliwell. Musculoskeletal Disorders in Frowen et al, Neale's Disorders of the Foot (8th Ed). Elsevier 2010.

drug (DMARD) therapy and better early intervention, the presentation of the typical 'rheumatoid foot' appears to be less common, although not all patients do well, even on biologics. Synovitis in the MTP joints leads to stretching and weakening of the joint capsule and failure of the stabilizing structures in the forefoot.[25,26] When the MTP joint dislocates, the plantar fat pad is pulled distally, exposing the metatarsal heads.[27] DMARD therapy helps attenuate this process, although a recent study has indicated that the prevalence and severity of forefoot joint damage continues to accumulate in patients with RA even in the face of clinically effective DMARD treatment.[28]

Soft tissues involved in RA include tendon sheaths, bursas, and entheses.[29] Tenosynovitis of the tibialis posterior or peroneal tendons may be florid. Retrocalcaneal bursitis may present as swelling either side of the Achilles tendon. Nodules may occur, typically at the Achilles tendon, the heel pad, or over bony prominences.

Treatment approaches are set out in the National Institute for Health and Clinical Excellence (NICE) Clinical Guideline CG 79, which recommends that all patients with RA and foot problems should be referred for podiatry assessment,[30] and in the Podiatry Rheumatic Care Association (PRCA) Standards of Care for People with Musculoskeletal Foot Health Problems, which reinforce the need for assessment and management of foot problems in RA, particularly in early RA.[31] Foot health services for rheumatology patients remain highly variable, with large regional variation in the provision of services and a significant unmet need.[32]

There is reasonable evidence that foot orthoses reduce foot pain and improve functional ability in people with RA,[33] although a critical review of foot orthoses in patients with RA demonstrated a lack of consensus on the precise types of foot orthoses likely to do best.[34] Provision of footwear for patients with RA is supported by national guidelines and therapeutic footwear has been shown to provide good symptom relief and improvement in function in patients with RA. Compliance with prescribed footwear can be poor, however, due to dissatisfaction with fit, comfort, and style, particularly in women.

Finally, painful plantar callosities can build up over metatarsal heads and regular scalpel debridement has been the treatment of choice. Callus reduction appears ineffective if used in isolation, however, and should at least be combined with other interventions, such as provision of foot orthoses, to prevent recurrence of symptoms.[35]

Psoriatic arthritis and seronegative diseases

Dactylitis is the classic presenting feature for psoriatic arthritis in the foot, and involvement of the skin and nails completes the picture. Articular involvement varies from involvement of a single mid- or rearfoot joint, to a destructive polyarthritis with extensive bone loss. Bezza et al. reported foot symptoms including plantar heel pain, metatarsal pain, dactylitis, and involvement of the ankle and midfoot as a possible initial manifestation of disease.[36] In established disease, as many as 95% of people with psoriatic arthritis have forefoot involvement including hallux valgus and claw toes; rearfoot deformity in the form of pes planovalgus has been reported in 65%.[37]

Imaging studies have shown inflammation in the midfoot joints in psoriatic arthritis and, given the limitations of clinical examination in this area, appropriate imaging is necessary if midfoot involvement is suspected.

Enthesitis is the striking feature of seronegative disease in the foot, typically at the insertion of the Achilles tendon and origin of the plantar fascia. Even in early psoriatic arthritis, the prevalence of plantar fasciitis and Achilles insertional enthesitis has been reported as 12% and 6%, respectively.[38] On imaging, enthesitis may also be seen at the attachment of the tibialis posterior tendon and the insertion of peroneus brevis as well as other sites.[37] Prior to diagnosis, a presentation of isolated, recurrent, or bilateral Achilles enthesitis should suggest a diagnosis of spondyloarthropathy. There may be osteitis close to the affected entheses, although this is seldom appreciated clinically, and osteitis may also occur in the sesamoid bones. The management of enthesitis is largely empirical; steroids can be used with good effect at the insertions of the peroneus brevis, tibialis posterior, and plantar fascia. The Achilles insertion poses a particular challenge: the use of depot steroids in this locality is discouraged because of the catastrophic risk of rupture.

Dactylitis as a manifestation of all of the above features is more common in the feet than the hands, with the fourth toes most frequently involved.[39] Dactylitis is an adverse prognostic factor; and the presence of any dactylitis is associated with more severe disease, including arthritis mutilans. Plain radiography may show typical changes such as erosion of the terminal phalangeal tufts, juxta-articular and entheseal new bone formation, periostitis, and severe osteolysis. In dactylitis, determining a precise location for steroid injection can be difficult although it is likely that wherever the steroid is deposited, there will be some diffusion and (beneficial) effect in nearby tissues. There is currently no specific evidence to support the use of interventions such as the provision of footwear and orthoses in psoriatic arthritis, but drawing on the combination of evidence for RA and clinical experience, it is reasonable to conclude that the inflammatory and mechanical factors that affect the feet in psoriatic arthritis should be addressed in much the same way as in RA.

Crystal diseases

Acute gout may occur in any of the joints of the foot although it is most common in the first MTP joint. The presentation is of an acute, hot, swollen joint which is exquisitely tender, with rapid onset. The pain is severe enough to prevent weightbearing but acute episodes typically settle in 10–14 days. Chronic (tophaceous) gout usually occurs insidiously and is often involves large and small joints. The chronic form is likely to be associated with radiological abnormalities such as peri-articular erosions. Tophi may occur in the Achilles tendon and in juxta-articular positions, associated with deformity and swelling. Chronic discharging tophaceous gout is associated with severe pain and disability.

Osteoarthritis

Specific information about foot osteoarthritis (OA) is poor because of lack of consistency in definitions. Radiological definitions generally lead to higher estimates of prevalence, while clinical presentations (symptoms/pain) yield variable rates. Subclinical signs are noted in many older patients, with one cadaveric study reporting moderate or severe degeneration in onehalf of first MTP joints.[40] Beyond the first MTP joint, most cases of foot OA are secondary to mechanical damage, trauma, or systemic disease.[41] Joint pain is common in the feet of older adults and presents most commonly in combination with other joints such as knees, back, hands, and hips.[7]

Clinical signs are stiffness, aching, and/or crepitus in the affected region and degenerative joint disease is often noted during ultrasound examination of foot joints, although the finding is often incidental, reflecting the subclinical nature. The best-known manifestation of OA in the foot is at the first MTP joint where the joint damage presents as limitation, fixation, or deformity of the hallux joint (known as hallux limitus, hallux rigidus, or hallux valgus). Restorative therapies are not well developed for foot OA and so NSAIDs and rest remain the initial treatments of choice, along with advice on exercise, weight loss, and footwear. Insoles and therapeutic footwear may be of benefit and are recommended by NICE as adjunct therapies. Where conservative treatment fails, surgical intervention can be definitive. Arthrodesis remains the surgical option of choice for most foot OA although at the first MTP joint, where joint-preserving 'bunion' surgeries have become more sophisticated, the prognosis has improved markedly in recent years.

Connective tissue diseases

Vascular features are found in the feet of 90% of people with connective tissue diseases (CTDs) and include Raynaud's phenomenon, telangiectasia, and purpura. Vasculitis and ulceration occur in 10–20% of people with CTDs, in the hands and in the lower extremity.[42] Large-vessel vasculitis and accelerated atherosclerosis compound the effects of local vasculitis, leading to gangrene and increased risk of amputation.[43] Vasculitic ulcers are often intensely painful and the healing process can be lengthy. Patients with CTDs may have coincident inflammatory arthropathy in the feet although it is usually milder than seen in RA.

In systemic sclerosis, Raynaud's phenomenon is often the initial presentation with later oedema and fibrosis of hands or feet (Figure 156.4). Flexion contractures can impair mobility and calcified nodules may manifest on the digits or other areas of mechanical stress. Synovitis may be present, but tends to affect larger joints more than the feet.[44] Similarly, involvement of the foot is generally less common and less severe in the feet than in the hands.[45] Onycholysis and pitting of the nails may also be seen, similar to that occurring in psoriasis. Splinter haemorrhages may also be seen in the nail beds, reflecting the vascular involvement.

The effect of skin and subcutaneous fibrosis, combined with changes in the underlying skeletal structures has been reported to lead to difficulties with shoe fitting,[46] and although not mandated by NICE in the same way as for people with RA, it appears sensible that patients with systemic sclerosis should undergo regular foot checks and should have access to foot health services.

Hypermobility syndromes

In the opening section of this chapter, the local effects of foot posture were discussed and are compounded in the presence of systemic hypermobility. There is some evidence that people with joint hypermobility have greater foot impairment than matched controls, and that the severity of symptoms correlates with severity of systemic hypermobility.[47] Where there is laxity of foot joints, the midfoot appears more unstable than the hindfoot joints.[48] Treatments are aimed at improving mechanical stability, although there is minimal formal evidence. Building muscle strength may be advantageous, and Pilates-type approaches seem generally helpful. People with hypermobile joints may have pathological tightness of surrounding muscles and tendons, and gentle stretching can also be useful. Footwear choice is important, and a stable shoe combined with cushioning shock-absorbing materials may help to relieve symptoms. Some people with mechanical foot pain will benefit from foot orthoses which control joint function and stabilize specific foot joints.

Conclusion

The foot and ankle are often involved in rheumatic diseases but are often neglected in rheumatology practice. The presentations in the foot can reflect disease manifestations in general but, in addition to treating the systemic disease, particular local circumstances—e.g. the increased mechanical demands on weightbearing structures—dictate a targeted approach local to the foot. If the foot is not considered by the assessing clinician, and there may be a number of barriers to successful assessment of this region, implementation of appropriate therapies will not occur.

References

1. Peat G, Thomas E, Wilkie R, Croft P. Multiple joint pain and lower extremity disability in middle and old age. *Disabil Rehabil* 2006;28(24): 1543–1549.
2. Garrow AP, Silman AJ, Macfarlane GJ. The Cheshire Foot Pain and Disability Survey: a population survey assessing prevalence and associations. *Pain* 2004;110(1–2):378–384.
3. Dunn JE, Link CL, Felson DT et al. Prevalence of foot and ankle conditions in a multiethnic community sample of older adults. *Am J Epidemiol* 2004;159(5):491–498.
4. Benvenuti F, Ferrucci L, Guralnik JM, Gangemi S, Baroni A. Foot pain and disability in older persons: an epidemiologic survey. *J Am Geriatr Soc* 1995;43(5):479–484.
5. Chen J, Devine A, Dick IM, Dhaliwal SS, Prince RL. Prevalence of lower extremity pain and its association with functionality and quality of life in elderly women in Australia. *J Rheumatol* 2003;30(12):2689–2693.
6. Thomas E, Peat G, Harris L, Wilkie R, Croft P. The prevalence of pain and pain interference in a general population of older adults: cross-sectional findings from the North Staffordshire Osteoarthritis Project (NorStOP). *Pain* 2004;110:361–368.
7. Keenan AM, Tennant A, Fear J, Emery P, Conaghan PG. Impact of multiple joint problems on daily living tasks in people in the community over age fifty-five. *Arthritis Rheum* 2006;55(5):757–764.
8. Coady D, Walker D, Kay L. Regional Examination of the Musculoskeletal System (REMS): a core set of clinical skills for medical students. *Rheumatology* 2004;43(5):633–639.
9. Redmond AC, Helliwell PS. Musculoskeletal disorders. In: Frowen P, Lorimer D, O'Donnell M, Burrow G, eds. *Neale's disorders of the foot*, 8th edn. Churchill Livingstone, Edinburgh, 2010.
10. Helliwell P, Woodburn J, Redmond AC, Turner DE, Davys HJ. The foot and ankle. In: *Rheumatoid arthritis: a comprehensive guide*. Churchill Livingstone, Edinburgh, 2006.
11. Alfredson H, Cook J. A treatment algorithm for managing Achilles tendinopathy: new treatment options. *Br J Sports Med* 2007;41(4):211–216.
12. Miller SD, Van Holsbeeck M, Boruta PM, Wu KK, Katcherian DA. Ultrasound in the diagnosis of posterior tibial tendon pathology. *Foot Ankle Int* 1996;17(9):555–558.

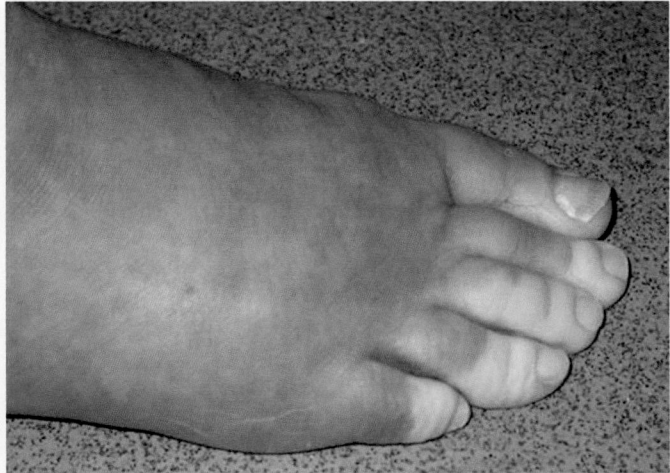

Fig. 156.4 Secondary Raynaud's associated with systemic sclerosis.

13. Crawford F, Atkins D, Edwards J. Interventions for treating plantar heel pain (Cochrane Review). *Cochrane Database Syst Rev* 2003(3): CD000416.

14. Radford JA, Landorf KB, Buchbinder R, Cook C. Effectiveness of low-Dye taping for the short-term treatment of plantar heel pain: a randomised trial. *BMC Musculoskelet Disord* 2006;7:64.

15. Landorf KB, Keenan AM, Herbert RD. Effectiveness of foot orthoses to treat plantar fasciitis: a randomized trial. *Arch Intern Med* 2006;166(12): 1305–1310.

16. Ball EMA, McKeeman HMA, Patterson C et al. Steroid injection for inferior heel pain: a randomised controlled trial. *Ann Rheum Dis* 2012 Jun 27. [Epub ahead of print]

17. McMillan AM, Landorf KB, Gilheany MF et al. Ultrasound guided corticosteroid injection for plantar fasciitis: randomised controlled trial. *BMJ* 2012;344:e3260.

18. Kerry RM, Holt GM, Stockley I. The foot in chronic rheumatoid arthritis: a continuing problem. *Foot* 1994;4(4):201–203.

19. Michelson J, Easley M, Wigley FM, Hellmann D. Foot and ankle problems in rheumatoid arthritis. *Foot Ankle Int* 1994;15(11):608–613.

20. Vainio K. The rheumatoid foot. A clinical study with pathological and roentgenological comments. *Clin Orthop Relat Res* 1991;265:4–8.

21. Grondal L, Tengstrand B, Nordmark B, Wretenberg P, Stark A. The foot: still the most important reason for walking incapacity in rheumatoid arthritis: distribution of symptomatic joints in 1000 RA patients. *Acta Orthop* 2008;79(2):257–261.

22. van der Leeden M, Steultjens M, Dekker JHM, Prins P, Dekker J. Is disease duration related to foot function, pain and disability in rheumatoid arthritis patients with foot complaints? *Clin Biomech* 2008;23(5):693.

23. Otter SJ, Lucas K, Springett K et al.. Foot pain in rheumatoid arthritis prevalence, risk factors and management: an epidemiological study. *Clin Rheumatol* 2010;29:255–271.

24. Bouysset M, Bonvoisin B, Lejeune E, Bouvier M. Flattening of the rheumatoid foot in tarsal arthritis on X-ray. *Scand J Rheumatol* 1987;16(2): 127–133.

25. Keenan MA, Peabody TD, Gronley JK, Perry J. Valgus deformities of the feet and characteristics of gait in patients who have rheumatoid arthritis. *J Bone Joint Surg* 1991;73(2):237–247.

26. Jaakkola JI, Mann RA. A review of rheumatoid arthritis affecting the foot and ankle. *Foot Ankle Int* 2004;25(12):866–874.

27. Klenerman L. The foot and ankle in rheumatoid arthritis. *Br J Rheumatol* 1995;34(5):443–448.

28. Van Der Leeden M, Steultjens MPM, Ursum J et al.. Prevalence and course of forefoot impairments and walking disability in the first eight years of rheumatoid arthritis. *Arthritis Rheum* 2008;59(11):1596–1602.

29. Boutry N, Larde A, Lapegue F et al. Magnetic resonance imaging appearance of the hands and feet in patients with early rheumatoid arthritis. *J Rheumatol* 2003;30(4):671–679.

30. National Institute for Health and Clinical Excellence. *The care and management of rheumatoid arthritis in adults (CG 79)*. NICE, London, 2009.

31. *Standards of care for people with musculoskeletal foot health problems*. Arthritis and Musculoskeletal Alliance, Podiatry Rheumatic Care Association, London, 2008.

32. Redmond AC, Waxman R, Helliwell PS. Provision of foot health services in rheumatology in the UK. *Rheumatology* 2006;45(5):571–576.

33. Woodburn J, Barker S, Helliwell PS. A randomized controlled trial of foot orthoses in rheumatoid arthritis. *J Rheumatol* 2002;29(7):1377–1383.

34. Clark H, Rome K, Plant M, O'Hare K, Gray J. A critical review of foot orthoses in the rheumatoid arthritic foot. *Rheumatology* 2006;45(2): 139–145.

35. Davys HJ, Turner DE, Helliwell PS et al.. Debridement of plantar callosities in rheumatoid arthritis: a randomized controlled trial. *Rheumatology* 2005;44(2):207–210.

36. Bezza A, Niamane R, Amine B et al. Involvement of the foot in patients with psoriatic arthritis. A review of 26 cases. *Joint Bone Spine* 2004;71(6): 546–549.

37. Hyslop E, McInnes IB, Woodburn J, Turner DE. Foot problems in psoriatic arthritis: high burden and low care provision. *Ann Rheum Dis* 2010;69(5):928.

38. Kane D. The role of ultrasound in the diagnosis and management of psoriatic arthritis. *Curr Rheumatol Rep* 2005;7(4):319–324.

39. Brockbank JE, Stein M, Schentag CT, Gladman DD. Dactylitis in psoriatic arthritis: a marker for disease severity? *Ann Rheum Dis* 2005;64(2):188–190.

40. Muehleman C, Bareither D, Huch K, Cole AA, Kuettner KE. Prevalence of degenerative morphological changes in the joints of the lower extremity. *Osteoarthritis Cartilage.* 1997;5(1):23–37.

41. Thomas RH, Daniels TR. Current concepts review. Ankle arthritis. *J Bone Joint Surg Am* 2003;85A(5):923–936.

42. Cawley MI. Vasculitis and ulceration in rheumatic diseases of the foot. *Baillieres Clin Rheumatol* 1987;1(2):315–333.

43. Theodoridou A, Bento L, D'Cruz DP, Khamashta MA, Hughes GRV. Prevalence and associations of an abnormal ankle-brachial index in systemic lupus erythematosus: a pilot study. *Ann Rheum Dis* 2003;62: 1199–1203.

44. Gold RH, Bassett LW, Seeger LL. The other arthritides. Roentgenologic features of osteoarthritis, erosive osteoarthritis, ankylosing spondylitis, psoriatic arthritis, Reiter's disease, multicentric reticulohistiocytosis, and progressive systemic sclerosis. *Radiol Clin North Am* 1988;26(6): 1195–1212.

45. La Montagna G, Baruffo A, Tirri R, Buono G, Valentini G. Foot involvement in systemic sclerosis: a longitudinal study of 100 patients. *Semin Arthritis Rheum* 2002;31(4):248–255.

46. Sari-Kouzel H, Hutchinson CE, Middleton A et al.. Foot problems in patients with systemic sclerosis. *Rheumatology* 2001;40(4):410–413.

47. Redmond AC, Helliwell PS, Bird HA et al.. Pain and health status in people with hypermobility syndrome are associated with overall joint mobility and selected local mechanical factors. *Rheumatology* 2006;45(1):108.

48. Redmond AC, Crosbie J, Ouvrier RA. Development and validation of a novel rating system for scoring standing foot posture: The Foot Posture Index. *Clin Biomech* 2006;21(1):89–98.

Sources of patient information

UK National Rheumatoid Arthritis Society: www.nras.org.uk/about_rheumatoid_arthritis/living_with_rheumatoid_arthritis/foot_health/default.aspx

Arthritis Research UK: www.arthritisresearchuk.org/arthritis-information/conditions/foot-pain.aspx, www.arthritisresearchuk.org/arthritis-information/conditions/foot-pain/footwear.aspx

Psoriasis and Psoriatic Arthritis Association: www.papaa.org/further-information/psoriatic-arthritis-feet

UK Scleroderma Society: www.sclerodermasociety.co.uk/Thefeetandsclerodermal.php

CHAPTER 157

Cervical and lumbar spine

David A. Walsh

Introduction

Axial pain is a major source of distress and disability. Mechanisms underlying the pain are often complex, and treatments may not always alter its natural history. Problems of the cervical and lumbar spine therefore place substantial demands on healthcare resources, and pose challenges to practicing clinicians. Chronic spinal pain is so common that it may be considered a normal, albeit undesirable, attribute of life.

Many different theoretical models have been developed in order to explain spinal pain, each supported by research evidence. These models inform diverse treatment strategies among different health care professionals. Some see spinal pain as a result of specific structural or pathological change, leading, for example, to diagnostic and therapeutic injections and surgery. Some see it as an abnormality of neuromuscular control, recommending to specific exercise therapies. Some see it as a result of abnormal processing of sensory signals by the central nervous system, and some see it as a consequence of various adverse psychosocial factors. These models are not mutually exclusive. Many patients are not 'cured' by any single treatment and, as they progress through often complex treatment pathways, they may experience diverse and apparently contradictory explanations and treatment recommendations.

The expert practitioner should provide a coherent explanation that is consistent with management advice, respecting and building upon the patient's prior understanding and experiences. Success in this requires a clear understanding of the mechanisms behind spinal pain, and the congruity between explanatory models. It also requires the ability to convey this understanding unambiguously to the patient.

Epidemiology

Low back pain is one of the commonest causes of pain and disability in Western populations, with a lifetime prevalence of up to 85%.[1] Nearly one-third of a United Kingdom population experienced back or neck pain in any month, nearly one-half of whom reported that their pain was disabling.[2] The problem of mechanical low back pain peaks in the sixth decade, and, although prevalence may remain stable at around 20% in later life, its impact may increase as general health declines.[2–4] Diverse factors may predict spinal pain, including female gender and adverse psychosocial factors.[2,5] Although slightly less common than low back pain, lifetime prevalence of neck pain may be up to 70% with 12 month prevalence up to 50%.[6] Back and neck pain often coincide with each other, and with other chronic musculoskeletal pain problems.[2,5]

Normal anatomy of the cervical and lumbar spine

The spine provides stability, a high degree of mobility, and protection of the spinal cord. To achieve this it has evolved a complex and highly specialized structure. Vertebrae undergo endochondral ossification during development with primary ossification centres in the centre of the vertebral body, one each side of the neural arch at the base of the transverse processes, and ring epiphyses around the outer boarders of each vertebral endplate. Secondary ossification centres are located in the transverse and spinous processes. During childhood and adolescence, coordinated growth around these multiple centres maintains into adulthood the normal resting cervical and lumbar lordoses and dorsal kyphosis, without rotation or lateral angulation (scoliosis).

Vertebrae articulate with each other through the intervertebral discs and facet joints (Figure 157.1). The disc comprises a highly hydrated nucleus pulposus enclosed by the annulus fibrosus that contains little water. These appear bright and dark respectively on T2-weighted MRI. The caudal and rostral disc surfaces interface with hyaline cartilage coating the vertebral endplate. Facet joints, unlike discs, are lined by synovium. The spinal canal is in close proximity to the facet joints and posterior region of the disc, and spinal nerve roots emerge through the spinal foramina whose borders (and therefore size) are determined by the disc, facet joint and ligamentum flavum.

Sources of axial pain are incompletely understood, although several spinal structures contain sensory nerves. Fine, unmyelinated nerves containing neuropeptides such as substance P and calcitonin gene-related peptide (CGRP) are localized to facet joint synovium, muscle, ligaments, tendons, bone, and the annulus fibrosus.[7] Unmyelinated sensory nerves may convey slow, ongoing pain, often described as burning. Faster-conducting, myelinated fibres in muscle, tendons, ligaments, and bone may be responsible for immediate, but again often continuing pain. By contrast, the nucleus pulposus and the hyaline cartilage coating the vertebral endplates and facet joints contain no sensory nerves in healthy adults and therefore cannot of themselves be sources of pain. These structures are

(A)

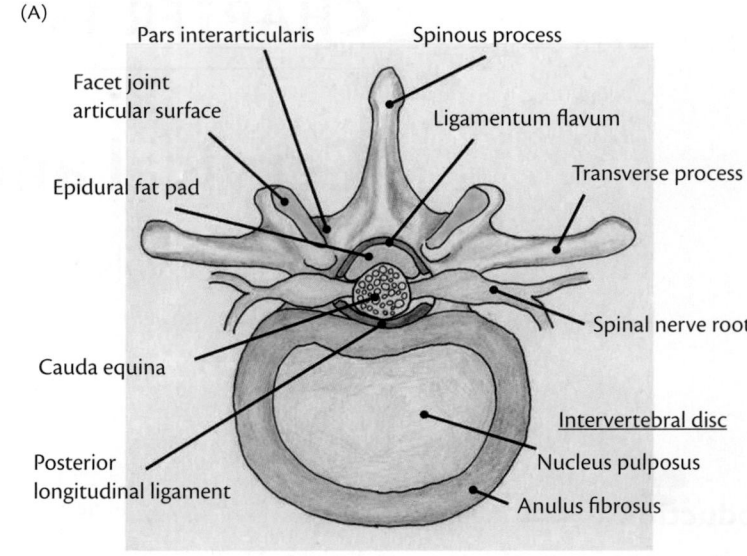

(B)

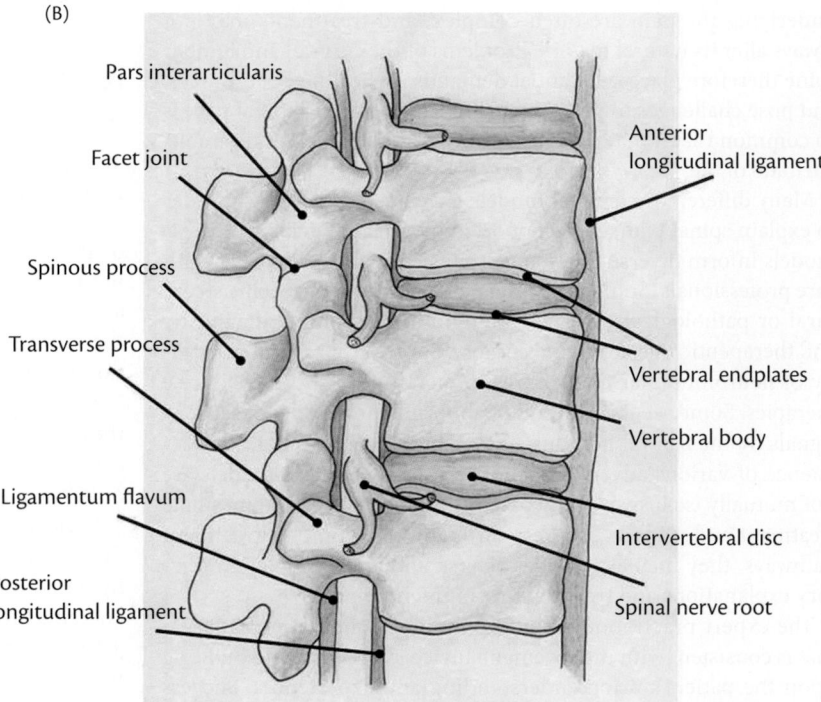

Fig. 157.1 Schematic diagram of the normal (lumbar) spine indicating close relationships of disc to spinal canal and foraminal contents. (A) Superior aspect. The transected intervertebral disc obscures the underlying vertebral endplate. Below approximately L2, lower motor neurons and sensory nerves of the cauda equina occupy the vertebral canal that at higher levels contains the spinal cord. (B) Lateral aspect.

Graphics by Harriet Walsh.

exposed to high compressive and shearing forces during normal back movements, and their lack of sensory innervation permits normal, pain-free activity. The site at which pain is experienced depends on the central mapping of pain pathways, and need not indicate directly the site of pathology. Radicular pain felt in the arm or leg originates from nerve root irritation in the spine.

Spinal pathology

Facet joint osteoarthritis

Facet joints, are subject to diseases that also affect other synovial joints such as osteoarthritis (OA). Radiological evidence of facet joint OA may be associated with chronic low back pain, and local anaesthetic injection into the facet joint may reduce back pain.[8] Facet joint OA may also contribute to symptoms of nerve root irritation.

Discogenic pain

Several lines of evidence indicate the disc as a source of low back pain. Radiological evidence of disc disease (Figure 157.2) is associated with low back pain.[9] Such evidence includes osteophytosis at the margins of the vertebral endplates and disc space narrowing, evident on plain radiographs, and reduced signal from the nucleus pulposus on T2-weighted MRI views, or tears in the annulus fibrosus. Discography, comprising fluid injection into the disc, can reproduce the specific qualities of back pain.[10] Surgery directed at

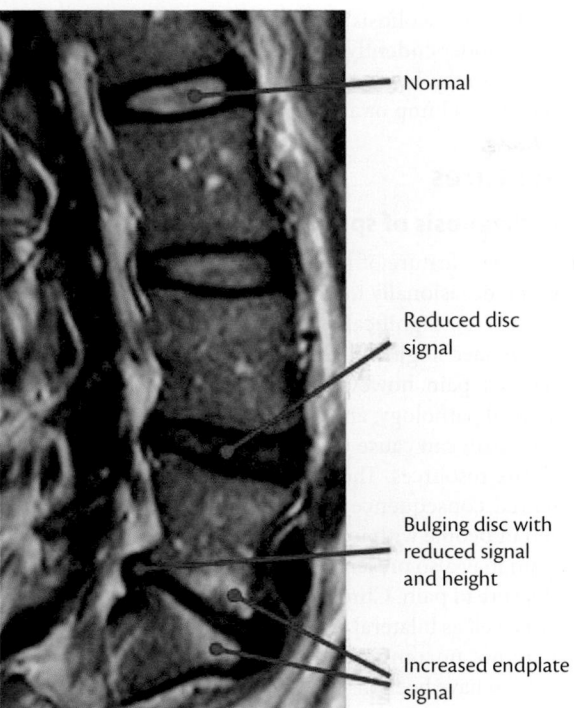

Normal

Reduced disc signal

Bulging disc with reduced signal and height

Increased endplate signal

Fig. 157.2 MRI from a patient experiencing low back pain. T2-weighted sagittal image showing normal appearances at L2/3 and evidence of disc disease at L4/5 and L5/S1. Disc changes are more commonly found in people with pain, but may be noted in pain-free individuals and should not be taken to indicate symptom severity.

reducing stresses on the disc by fusing adjacent vertebrae, or replacing the disc with an artificial implant, may each be successful in reducing pain in appropriately selected patients.[11,12]

The mechanisms by which discs cause pain remain unclear. More nerves were localized deeper within discs in which discography elicited pain, than in discs from non-painful levels, implicating the disc itself as a source of pain.[7] Loss of the mechanical and chemical barrier between disc and subchondral bone, and the altered biomechanical properties of diseased discs, may result in abnormal stimulation of subchondral nerves in the vertebral endplates. Episodes of spinal pain may be associated with annular tears at the edges of discs, or inflammatory activity in the subchondral bone. Genetic factors predispose, through unknown mechanisms, to both pain and radiographic changes.[13]

Spondylosis

Spondylosis indicates the commonly coexisting radiological features of disc space narrowing, osteophytosis, and facet joint OA. The association between radiographic spondylosis and pain and disability, although significant, is weak. The prevalence and extent of radiographic spondylosis, being irreversible, increases with age, whereas the problem of mechanical low back pain peaks in the sixth decade.[4]

Diagnostic terminology can be confusing for patients.[14] Healthcare professionals often use descriptive terms such as 'degenerative disc disease' or 'wear and tear arthritis'. This distinguishes these conditions from medically serious fractures, infection, or malignancy, but may also seem to contradict evidence-based recommendations that activities should be maintained and a graded

approach to increasing exercise should be adopted. Spondylotic change may be regarded as 'normal' or 'normal for age', and ageing and degeneration are closely linked concepts.[14] This may facilitate acceptance, but, alternatively, may seem to negate the patient's experience ('they don't believe I have a problem'), undermine confidence that the cause of their pain has been adequately investigated, and suggest that, as ageing is inevitable, so deteriorating symptoms must also be expected with time. Very few people become wheelchair bound due to low back pain, although many more fear that that is what the future holds for them.

Radiographic changes may alternatively be viewed as consequences of successful repair, rather than wear and tear.[14] Indeed, spondylosis is associated with new bone formation (osteophytes) and increased, rather than decreased, bone densities. Discs undergo fibrovascular repair, which may be likened to scarring of injured skin. Activity is required for the musculoskeletal system to repair most effectively, and fear of activity is a more important predictor of poor prognosis than is the nature of any initiating injury or the appearance of radiographs.[15]

Spondylolysthesis

Displacement between adjacent vertebrae (spondylolysthesis) may be due to defects in the pars articularis (spondylolysis), or to abnormalities of the facet joints. Spondylolysis occurs in up to 11% of the adult population,[16] and may be developmental, 'degenerative', or traumatic.[17] Fracture across the pars interarticularis may be either due to significant trauma, or to repetitive hyperextension, e.g. in athletes such as gymnasts. Developmental or degenerative spondylolysis or spondylolysthesis are not of themselves associated with low back pain,[16,17] and even spondylolysthesis with up to 50% loss of contact between adjacent vertebral endplates (grade 2) are typically managed conservatively. Degenerative spondylolysthesis, however, occurs in conjunction with other evidence of spondylosis, either because abnormal stresses necessitate enhanced repair, or because structural repair permits vertebral malalignment. Traumatic spondylolysis will commonly recover with conservative management, although response to surgical stabilization is more successful than for spondylosis-associated spondylolysthesis.

Intravertebral disc herniation

Intervertebral discs may herniate through insufficiencies in the vertebral endplate and produce localized back pain. Acute intravertebral herniation is associated with MRI evidence of inflammation in the adjacent bone marrow. This should not be confused with Schmorl's nodes, which have similar appearance on plain radiographs, but are longstanding, and not associated with local inflammation. Schmorl's nodes may be present in one-fifth of people without back pain.[18] Disc herniation under the ring epiphysis in childhood may be a cause of limbus vertebra. The triangular ossification centre remains visible at the anterosuperior angle of the vertebral body due to failed epiphyseal fusion, but this does not cause pain.

Radicular pain

Pain radiating into the leg or arm, or around the chest or abdomen, may either indicate nerve root pain (radicular), or represent imprecise somatotopic representation of deep structures (pseudoradicular). Sciatica (pain in the sciatic distribution extending below the knee), cruralgia (in the femoral distribution), and brachalgia (in the arm) classify radicular symptoms without defining underlying pathogenesis. Causes may include foraminal stenosis due to prolapsed intervertebral disc, osteophytosis, or hypetrophy of the ligamentum flavum, local inflammation, spondylolisthesis, or, rarely, space-occupying lesions, either benign (e.g. synovial cysts at the facet joint) or malignant. Rarely radicular pain may be due to other pathology involving the nerve, such as neuroma or infiltrating malignancy. Non-resolving symptoms should lead to further investigation.

Prolapsed ('slipped') intervertebral disc is a common cause of acute radicular pain. Symptoms classically follow a specific mechanical insult, for example during extension from the flexed position while twisting. Radicular pain may not be immediately apparent but evolve over days after injury, and, conversely, radicular pain may occur without significant axial pain. The prolapsed disc represents extrusion of nucleus pulposus through a tear in the annulus fibrosus. Unlike books on a shelf, discs do not slip back into place. Annular tears and extruded disc contents induce local inflammation. Prostaglandins, tumour necrosis factor alpha (TNFα), and nerve growth factor (NGF) facilitate tissue repair, but also activate and sensitize local nerves and adjacent nerve roots.[19] Extruded disc material and oedema can additionally compress the exiting nerve root.

Chronic radicular pain is commonly associated with foraminal stenosis due to facet joint hypertrophy with or without associated disc protrusion or spondylolysthesis. Foraminal stenosis may be associated with continuous pain, or with unilateral, sometimes dermatomal, claudicant symptoms. Sensitization leads to spontaneous or mechanically induced nerve activation that may be experienced as shooting pains and/or paraesthesiae, and neuronal dysfunction may lead to alteration or loss of sensation.

Spinal canal stenosis

Normal variability in spinal canal dimensions is genetically determined. Osteophytosis, hypertrophy of the ligamentum flavum, prolapsed intervertebral discs, spondylolysthesis, and, rarely, posterior longitudinal ligament ossification, epidural fat, or space-occupying lesions can further narrow the canal. Inflammatory arthritis can cause clinically important stenosis due to pannus or subluxation in the cervical spine. Acute cord or cauda equina compression, for example due to central disc prolapse, constitutes a surgical emergency as delay may result in permanent disability. Chronic lumbar spinal stenosis is often identified by imaging in the absence of symptoms or signs and its clinical relevance requires careful evaluation. MRI evidence of cord pathology such as inflammation, demyelination, or syringomyelia secondary to cord compression is of greater clinical significance than reduced canal dimensions alone.

Kyphosis and scoliosis

Abnormal kyphosis (forward curvature) or scoliosis (lateral curvature) may be developmental or acquired. Uncoordinated vertebral growth in childhood may cause scoliosis or exaggerated dorsal kyphosis (Scheuermann's disease), which, if severe, may contribute to restrictive lung impairment and psychosocial problems. Exaggerated dorsal kyphosis may develop in later life, for example following osteoporotic 'wedge' fractures. Scoliosis may also indicate structural deformity, or may represent postural compensation for pelvic asymmetry or leg length disparity. In acute back pain it may be due to paraspinal muscle spasm and therefore disappear as pain

improves. Kyphosis or scoliosis do not of themselves predict spinal pain in adults independently of other disc changes.[20] However, onset of back pain may be the factor that leads people to notice spinal asymmetry as a lump or abnormal bend.

Clinical features

Differential diagnosis of spinal symptoms

Spinal pain may be a feature of multisystem disease, referred from other organs, and occasionally indicative of a need for urgent intervention (Table 157.1). Significant pathology such as aortic aneurysm, renal or gynaecological disease can each present with back pain. Most low back pain, however, is not accompanied by treatable medical or surgical pathology, and overinvestigation of people with simple low back pain can cause unnecessary distress and consume limited healthcare resources. The clinician must balance probabilities and potential consequences, while being alert to alternative diagnoses even in people with longstanding symptoms.

Low back pain may also present as the primary focus for a patient with more widespread pain. Chronic widespread pain by definition includes axial as well as bilateral arm and leg pain,[21] and features of fibromyalgia are not uncommon in people with back and/or neck pain.[22] People who have been discharged from secondary care services following treatment for low back pain have a high likelihood of presenting again with pain at another location. Recognizing the interplay between axial and non-axial pain, and associated psychological distress (particularly depression and anxiety) is an important part of diagnosis, as exclusive focus on the presenting site of pain may fail to identify important treatable morbidity and barriers to recovery.

Rheumatoid arthritis (RA) and seronegative spondylarthritides are uncommon causes of spinal pain, and first presentation of RA with isolated spinal symptoms is extremely rare. Although spinal pain is common in people with inflammatory arthritis, it often has mechanical origins.[23] However, attribution of chronic pain to inflammatory rather than mechanical diagnoses may be associated with lower levels of psychological distress.[14]

Radicular pain and neuronal compromise

Radicular pain is classically localized to specific dermatomes, although variations between individuals in dermatomal topography, imprecise perception of sensory boundaries, and nociceptor recruitment from adjacent segments through central sensitization may confound interpretation of pain distribution. This is particularly the case where symptoms are intermittent or historical, as pain memory is thankfully imprecise.

Radicular pain often has characteristics in common with other neuropathic pain, described as burning or lancinating. Shooting pains may be spontaneous or triggered by movement. Dysaesthesiae can include abnormal spontaneous cutaneous or deep sensations. Allodynia, the experience of normally non-noxious stimuli such as the touch of bedclothes as painful, indicates central sensitization. Paraesthesiae (ongoing mechanoceptor afferent activity) or numbness, although not actually painful, may be unpleasant and distressing. Their bothersomeness can reduce with time even if symptoms persist.

Bilateral limb pain or weakness, or upper motor neuron signs in the lower limbs should raise suspicion of spinal cord compromise. Lower motor neuron signs may indicate the level of cervical canal

Table 157.1 Differential diagnosis of spinal pain

Conditions that may affect any spinal level

Spinal

Facet joint osteoarthritis

Discogenic pain

Muscle tension/spasm

Trauma

       disc prolapse

       fracture

Neoplasia (metastatic)

Osteomyelitis

Epidural abscess

Discitis (infective or sterile)

Ankylosing spondylitis

Paget's disease of the bone

Regional

Shingles

Diffuse

Fibromyalgia

Polymyalgia rheumatica

Myeloma

Region-specific conditions		
Neck	**Thoracic**	**Lumbar**
Spinal		
Whiplash		
Cervical dystonia		
Rheumatoid arthritis		
Regional		
Pharyngeal infection	Aortic aneurysm	Pancreatitis
Cervical lymphadenitis		Gynaecological pathology
Meningitis		Renal infection
Subarachnoid haemorrhage		Pregnancy
Occipital neuralgia		
Temporomandibular joint dysfunction		
Carotid artery dissection		
Posterior fossa lesions		
Referred		
Ischaemic heart disease		
Pancoast's tumour		
Bronchogenic carcinoma		
Diaphragmatic irritiation		
Gastric ulcer		

within minutes of resting, but recurs after walking a similar distance again. Spinal and vascular claudication can be difficult to distinguish. Clinical evidence of cardiovascular risk factors, abdominal bruits, and absent peripheral pulses suggest vascular causation, but can coincide with spinal pathology. Spinal claudication may be indicated by bilateral pain extending into the thighs, associated paraesthesiae or feelings of heaviness or weakness, or lack of symptoms walking upstairs or during forward flexion, positions which increase dimensions of the spinal canal.

Assessment of the patient with spinal pain

Assessment fulfils several purposes; evaluation of the nature and extent of the problem, diagnosis and exclusion of important (treatable) differential diagnoses, identifying comorbidities and factors that may limit response to treatment, and formulation and engagement of the patient in an appropriate treatment plan. Clinical assessment may also be used for other purposes, such as to support or defend litigation, or inform decisions on benefits or future employment. It is important that patients and clinicians share the same understanding of the purpose of an assessment, as this will influence its content.

A full history and examination is essential both to guide further investigations and management, and to create a productive working relationship with the patient. History should address symptom onset; previous episodes and how the current episode may be similar or different; the nature, severity, and functional impact of current symptoms; and evidence of possible underlying conditions that if left untreated may lead to significant harm. The clinician should also enquire about factors that may limit engagement with or response to treatment, such as fear avoidance, depression and anxiety. These are often referred to as psychosocial 'yellow flags', predict poor outcome in low back pain, and may be amenable to specific interventions such as cognitive behavioural therapy (CBT).

Examination is directed to the spine itself, and to evidence of neurological deficit (Figure 157.3, Table 157.2) and systemic disease. Important pathology can exist in the absence of hard examination findings. Spinal canal stenosis may produce no symptoms or signs at rest, despite seriously limiting walking. An L4/5 disc prolapse may cause significant L5 nerve root compression without impairment of tendon reflexes, because knee extensors and ankle flexors are innervated from multiple levels. Furthermore, an absence of signs does not indicate that symptoms are mild, nor should the patient be expected to see their problem as 'not serious'.

The concept of 'red flag' symptoms and signs has proved useful in guiding management of low back pain (Box 157.1). Surgical red flags focus on cauda equina syndrome, and medical red flags may indicate other pathology requiring specific intervention. Red flags have not been comprehensively tested for specificity and sensitivity, although some are more reliable than others. Difficulty in passing urine is common in people with low back pain, particularly during flares. Sleep disturbance is also common, and people are often uncertain as to whether they wake with or because of their pain.[24] Mechanical low back pain is not uncommon in older people, even though osteoporosis and malignancy are more likely with increasing age. However, the onset of bilateral lower motor neuron signs in the legs, loss of anal tone, and perineal sensory loss or incontinence should never be ignored as possible features of cauda equina syndrome. Acute cauda equina compression can rapidly lead to irreversible neuronal compromise and should precipitate immediate

stenosis, with upper motor neuron signs more caudally. The adult spinal cord terminates around the L1/2 vertebrae, below which the nerve roots of the cauda equina pass through the spinal canal to their exiting foramina. Lumbar canal stenosis produces lower, rather than upper motor neuron features.

Lumbar spinal canal stenosis can cause spinal claudication. Patients describe increasing leg pain during walking, which resolves

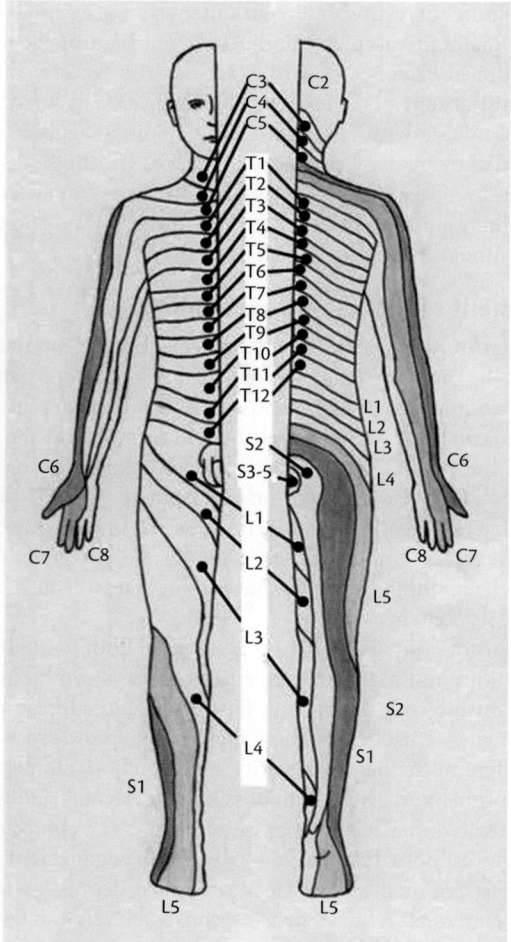

Fig. 157.3 Dermatomes affected by spinal problems. Schematic diagram of human dermatomes highlighting those nerve roots most commonly affected by prolapsed intervertebral discs; in the upper limb C6 (pink) and C7 (blue), and in the lower limb L5 (blue) and S1 (pink). Dermatome maps conceal overlap between dermatomes, and marked interindividual variations lead to diagnostic imprecision.

Graphics by Harriet Walsh.

admission for imaging and surgical decompression, irrespective of back pain. Fever, weight loss, history of malignancy, or an associated acute-phase response should similarly prompt further investigation to exclude treatable infection, malignancy, or inflammatory spinal disease.

Investigations should be instigated where there is a likelihood of underlying pathology that may influence treatment. Urinalysis may provide evidence of renal infection. Full blood count, acute-phase reactants, urea and electrolytes, liver function, and bone profile may reveal a need for further investigation, although abnormalities often prove to be coincidental rather than causes of spinal pain. Plain radiographs are not recommended for the investigation of simple mechanical back pain.[25] Spondylosis is common irrespective of the presence or absence of pain, whereas apparently normal disc spaces on radiographs may contain discs with reduced signal on T2-weighted MRI. Plain radiographs from a single time point have low sensitivity in detecting early inflammatory spinal disease or malignancy, are unable to identify or exclude significant disc prolapse or canal stenosis, and cannot distinguish between recent and longstanding osteoporotic fractures.

MRI is not indicated for all patients, nor for all episodes of spinal pain.[25] Where plain radiographs have already demonstrated multi-level spondylotic changes at multiple levels, further imaging is only indicated if additional treatable pathology is suspected. Undertaking MRI may improve patient satisfaction, but is not necessarily reassuring and may not be a cost-effective means of improving long-term outcomes.[25] MRI is the method of choice for detecting nerve root compression, spinal cord pathology, canal stenosis, or inflammatory and infective spinal disease.

Imaging lacks specificity in determining the source of pain. Discography or local anaesthetic injections may be used to further define the pain's anatomical origin. Discography aims to briefly reproduce symptoms during the injection of contrast medium into the nucleus pulposus. Facet joint injection with local anaesthetic may temporarily reduce pain if appropriately placed. However, there is little robust evidence that such techniques reliably predict response to more permanent nerve ablation or surgical procedures, and back pain rarely originates from a single structure.[26]

Table 157.2 Myotomes affected by spinal problems. Nerve roots most commonly affected by disc prolapse are highlighted in bold. Overlap between myotomes and marked interindividual variations lead to diagnostic imprecision

Disc	Root	Weakness	Reflex
C4/C5	C5	Shoulder abduction, elbow flexion	Biceps (brachoradialis)
C5/C6	**C6**	(Elbow flexion), **wrist extension**	(Biceps) **Brachoradialis**
C6/C7	**C7**	**Elbow extension, wrist flexion**	**Triceps**
C7/T1	C8	Finger flexors	None
L1/L2	L2	Hip flexion	(Knee)
L2/L3	L3	Hip flexion, knee extension	Knee
L3/L4	L4	Knee extension	Knee
L4/L5	**L5**	**Ankle dorsiflexion/eversion**	**None** (knee)
L5/S1	**S1**	**Ankle plantarflexion**	**Ankle**
Central protrusion below L2	Cauda equine (S2–4)	Anal/bladder sphincters	(Ankle/toe) None

Box 157.1 Red flag symptoms and signs that should raise suspicion of important and potentially treatable underlying surgical and medical conditions in people presenting with spinal pain

Significant neurological compromise (cauda equine syndrome or cord compression)

- Saddle anaesthesia around anus, perineum, or genitals
- Recent onset of bladder dysfunction or faecal incontinence
- Laxity of anal sphincter
- Widespread (>one nerve root) or progressive motor weakness in the legs or gait disturbance
- Sensory level

Spinal fracture

- Sudden-onset severe, localized pain, relieved by lying down
- Major trauma (e.g. fall from height, road traffic accident)
- Minor trauma (if osteoporosis or advanced ankylosing spondylitis)
- Structural deformity of the spine

Infection or cancer

- Onset >50 or <20 years of age
- Constitutional symptoms (fever, unexplained weight loss)
- Constant, progressive pain
- Pain disturbing sleep
- Thoracic pain
- Previous or current cancer
- Recent bacterial infection
- Intravenous drug use
- Immune suppression

Inflammatory spinal disease

- Gradual onset before age 40
- Pain disturbing sleep
- Thoracolumbar or sacroiliac pain
- Marked morning stiffness
- Persisting limitation spinal movements in all directions
- Peripheral joint involvement
- Iritis, psoriasis, colitis
- Preceding infective diarrhoea or sexually transmitted infection
- Family history of spondylitis

Assessment may differ in emphasis according to age, pain location, and comorbidities. Children not infrequently complain of back pain, but spondylosis and disc prolapse are rare under the age of 18, indicating a need for further investigation. Medical pathologies including osteoporosis are most common over the age of 50. A greater proportion of thoracic pain may be attributable to medical pathology, justifying a lower threshold for investigation. However, disc disease is not uncommon in the thoracic spine, particularly

when also present elsewhere. Osteoporotic fracture should be considered in those at risk, or with increasing spinal deformity or height loss. Recurrent episodes of back pain while on treatment for osteoporosis may indicate a need for further assessment of bone mineral density and consideration of treatment escalation.[27] Acute episodes of pain in patients whose spines are fused due to inflammatory spinal disease should be imaged by MRI or CT, as unstable fractures may not be apparent on plain radiographs. Instability in the cervical spine may have greater clinical significance than in the low back, and MRI is indicated if patients develop shooting pains or other neurological symptoms or upper motor neuron signs in the lower limbs. Cervical spine imaging should be considered in patients with RA to help assess general anaesthetic risk, and in those who go off their feet.[28]

Management

Principles of management

A large number of national guidelines have been produced regarding the treatment of spinal pain, particularly low back pain, and there is a high degree of consistency between countries.[25,29–32] For the majority of patients, spinal and radicular pain improve or resolve during the months after presentation, even when there is MRI evidence of substantial disc herniation and nerve root entrapment.[33] In the absence of evidence of cord or cauda equina compression, initial management is non-surgical. Management aims to reassure, minimize impact, and facilitate recovery, achieved through adequate explanation, analgesia and pain management, treating any specific pathology, and encouraging activity. However, spinal pain is often recurrent, with exacerbations of varying duration, and sometimes incomplete resolution before the onset of another flare. Management of the current episode should always be complemented with advice for the future.

Management should be proportional to severity and risk. The majority of episodes will respond well to non-specific treatments, and inappropriate investigation may delay appropriate management. Investigations, therefore, are not routinely recommended within 3 months of the onset of spinal pain in the absence of red flag symptoms or signs.[34] However, investigations may be justified if symptoms persist and the patient wishes to consider specific treatments such as surgery, or if suspicion is raised of underlying medical pathology.

More intensive non-surgical treatments may lead to better outcomes overall, but may not be cost-effective if offered to all patients. Initial screening determines the likelihood of pathology requiring specific treatment (detection of red flags), and likely prognosis. In general, those with worse prognosis gain most from intensive treatment. Prognosis is traditionally determined by early progress, whereby all patients are offered the same range of treatments in the first instance, and those who respond less well are subsequently offered more intensive therapy (see e.g. Savigny et al.[25]). However, questionnaires may help identify patients for whom intensive therapy should be offered early.[35,36]

Advice and education

Early advice should include an explanation of the likely cause of the pain, consistent both with the patient's own experience and with a recommendation to maintain or return to normal activities as far and as soon as possible. Advice should be reinforced by consistent written information, such as that provided in *The Back Book*.[37] Explanation alone, provided in a single consultation, has little impact on outcomes in controlled clinical trials. However, the initial consultation sets the context through which other interventions are delivered, and it is important that information provided by all members of the team remains consistent.

Patients bring to the consultation their own understanding of spinal pain, based on their experiences and information obtained from family, friends, media, and other professionals. Such beliefs may be barriers to rehabilitation,[14,15] and care must be taken not to reinforce unhelpful beliefs by a casual use of terminology. Noting coincidental findings such as scoliosis may focus attention away from modifiable factors that make more important contributions to pain.

Pharmacological analgesia

Patients should be advised to use both non-pharmacological and pharmacological therapies to help reduce pain in order to help maintain activity, and to reduce symptoms and distress. Emphasizing how movement and activity facilitate repair can help counter fears that masking symptoms will allow further injury. Pharmacological therapies include paracetamol, non-steroidal anti-inflammatory drugs, and opioids.[25] Tricyclic anti-depressants may reduce pain and improve sleep disturbance in people with chronic low back pain.[25,38] Clinical trials support starting at a low dosage and increasing up to the maximum recommended anti-depressant dosage until therapeutic benefit or unacceptable side effects. For patients with nerve root irritation, treatments effective for neuropathic pain such as tricyclic anti-depressants and/or gabapentin or pregabalin may be helpful.[38] Decisions on continuing analgesic medications should always be based on individual response.

Physical treatments

Physical treatments provide additional benefit to information alone for the management of low back pain.[25] Training in specific exercises aimed at muscle strengthening, postural control, movement instruction and stretching, and aerobic activity, and approaches based on cognitive behavioural principles each have shown similar beneficial effects in randomized controlled trials (RCTs).[25] Physiotherapy may be provided individually or in group settings. Group programmes are generally recommended because of their lower cost, with some evidence of equal efficacy to individual therapy.[25] Such programmes, however, require adequate throughput of patients to be efficient, and group work may not suit all patients. Yoga has also been found helpful for low back pain.[39] Passive physical therapies, such as manipulation or massage, may also provide relief from low back pain, although their clinical effect sizes may be small and short-lived.[40] Interventions that discourage movement and activity, including bed rest, traction, and surgical appliances such as corsets, are not recommended for low back pain. Cervical collars may facilitate temporary pain relief, but have not been associated in prospective trials with sustained benefit.

Fear-avoidance beliefs are associated with high levels of reported pain and disability, and are common barriers to rehabilitation in low back pain.[15] Muscle spasm or inflammation play greater roles in pain exacerbation than does structural damage, and imaging even during severe pain can be unremarkable. Similarly, patients often feel that their back is 'unstable' due to abnormal processing of nociceptive and proprioceptive inputs, but this is rarely associated with biomechanical instability. By contrast, graded, supervised exercise can reduce fear avoidance, and improves low back pain and function.[15] Fear avoidance and catastrophic beliefs should be addressed when they occur. For the back to repair itself fully requires normal activity. Effective rehabilitation aims to reintroduce rather than avoid valued activities.

Complementary therapies

As with other conditions that evade simple cure, a wide range of therapies for spinal pain are commonly accessed outside traditional healthcare. These may complement medical approaches or be offered as alternatives.

Acupuncture needling is commonly recommended for spinal pain due to evidence of efficacy and cost-effectiveness when provided as a course of limited duration.[25,41] Evidence of long-term benefit from ongoing acupuncture is less strong, and increased treatment duration escalates costs. A graded return to normal activity should be advised in conjunction with acupuncture. Transcutaneous electrical nerve stimulation (TENS) has been advocated, although systematic reviews of RCTs are inconclusive.[25]

Mechanisms by which complementary treatments help are incompletely understood, and context may be as important as any specific pathophysiological target. Acupuncture may be more beneficial than waiting list or 'usual care' controls, but similar to sham procedures.[25] Indeed, contextual factors may contribute much of the benefit of prescribing analgesic drugs,[42] and optimizing the context within which treatments are provided has considerable potential for improving patient wellbeing.

Multidisciplinary approaches

The multifaceted nature of spinal pain has led to complex interventions that bring together different and potentially synergistic treatments. Combined physical and psychological (CPP) programmes combine cognitive behavioural approaches and exercise.[25] CPP may be more effective than either component alone, and cost is minimized through group programmes, and selecting patients who continue to have high disability or significant psychological distress despite at least one less intensive treatment. Even programmes involving 100 hours contact over 8 weeks may be cost-effective. Interdisciplinary working, with cognitive behavioural approaches delivered by appropriately trained physiotherapists, may reduce costs and permit wider access to psychological interventions.[43] However, treatment fidelity can be difficult to maintain in routine health service practice, and physiotherapist-led interventions may still leave an important number of people with significant disability and distress from low back pain.

Full multidisciplinary pain management programmes (PMPs) are recommended for people with persistent spinal pain where there is no realistic prospect of cure.[44] PMPs facilitate self-management and reduce the impact of spinal pain on patients' lives. Such programmes combine expertise in clinical psychology and physiotherapy, often including medical and occupational therapy input, to provide a coherent intervention within a group setting. Effectiveness may improve with greater treatment intensity, either through increased contact time or using an inpatient context.[45] Best evidence is for PMPs using traditional CBT-based approaches, challenging unhelpful beliefs and helping patients achieve their goals.[46]

More recently acceptance and commitment therapy (ACT) and mindfulness approaches have focused on acceptance and patients' life values,[47] but RCTs are required.

Back pain disability has great impact on productivity and costs to employers, insurance agencies, and social care. Successful programmes resulting in return to work have typically combined physical therapies, education, and specialist employment advice.[32,48] Return to work is influenced by expectations of both patients and employers. Employment consultants, by helping match patients to opportunities, may facilitate return to work even after several years of disability.

Public health interventions

Social context influences the management and outcome of spinal pain, and different stakeholders—patients, employers, health professionals, insurers, and governments—view outcomes from different perspectives. Benefit thresholds balance costs to the taxpayer against the poverty that can accompany back pain disability. Individualized approaches are effective but costly when delivered for problems as common as spinal pain. Public information campaigns, addressing commonly held but unhelpful beliefs about exercise and activity, have had important benefits, both in the short and long term.[49] Key issues addressed by such campaigns may differ between countries and at different times.

Invasive interventions

Interventional therapies aim to reduce pain either directly (e.g. injection therapies), or by altering spinal structure. Testing such procedures by RCTs raises ethical and methodological difficulties, and trial data often seem inconsistent with cohort studies. This may indicate important contextual or placebo effects, but also the often complex and individualized nature of interventional therapies that is difficult to replicate in controlled trials.

Epidural injections of glucocorticosteroid and local anaesthetic may reduce inflammation around a nerve root, and alter central processing following temporary reduction in afferent barrage. They can reduce the duration or severity of nerve root pain, particularly if nucleus pulposus is extruded/sequestrated outside the annulus fibrosus.[50] The epidural space may be accessed by caudal, interlaminar, or foraminal approaches. Fluoroscopic guidance is recommended to optimize response and reduce adverse events. Although lower lumbar root irritation may be relieved by caudal injection, transforaminal injections may be favoured.[51] Epidural injection has low propensity for systemic adverse effects, and may permit engagement in physical therapy and reduce rates of subsequent surgery. However, pain relief may be temporary and health economic evidence of benefit is incomplete. There is little evidence to suggest that epidural injections provide benefit for symptoms of spinal claudication or back pain.[52] Facet joint injection with glucocorticosteroid and local anaesthetic, and more permanent nerve ablation procedures, have been advocated although evidence of efficacy remains inconclusive.[52]

Surgery aims to decompress, stabilize, and, more recently, replace discs. Surgical decompression of the cauda equina or spinal cord is a matter of immediate urgency if permanent neurological deficit is to be avoided after acute presentation. Decompression is also recommended if progressive muscle weakness follows acute disc prolapse. However, nerve root pain from even large disc protrusions may adequately resolve with conservative management,[53] and surgery does not obviate the need for intensive rehabilitation. Discectomy, either open or with perioperative microscopy (microdiscectomy), may improve outcomes at 1 year for leg pain due to disc prolapse compared with conservative management. However, in cases where natural recovery may occur, there is no long-term disadvantage in initially taking a conservative approach.[54] Decompression is not expected to reduce spinal pain itself, and the balance between axial and referred symptoms should be considered carefully before embarking on surgery.

Surgical decompression may relieve spinal claudication symptoms in people with canal stenosis associated with spondylosis, although the magnitude of benefit compared to conservative treatments remains uncertain.[55] Where canal stenosis is associated with spondylolisthesis, fusion may be combined with decompression.[56] In cases presenting with spinal claudication, imaging often reveals multilevel changes and surgical amelioration may be complex and not without its own risks.

Surgery for severe simple mechanical back pain should only be considered after completion of an optimal package of conservative care, including a CPP treatment programme.[25] Significant psychological distress should be optimally treated prior to surgical referral. Spinal stabilization can reduce back pain, particularly for patients with single-level disease. However, the precise anatomical origin of pain can be difficult to determine, and an immobilized spinal segment may place additional stresses on adjacent levels. This may explain the mixed outcomes observed after fusion surgery.[55] More recently, non-rigid surgical stabilization has been explored for low back pain although controlled trials have not yet consistently demonstrated improved benefit over rigid fusion.[57]

Discs may be replaced with artificial prostheses, which permit continued movement at the operated level and therefore minimize biomechanical stresses to adjacent levels. RCTs comparing cervical disc replacement with fusion suggest improved cervical disability and quality of life up to 12 months, and reduced need for further surgical intervention up to 2 years after disc replacement surgery.[12] RCTs comparing lumbar disc replacement with fusion also suggest improved disability and quality of life following disc replacement surgery, although evidence for maintenance of this benefit beyond 6 months is less strong.[11] Disc replacement surgery may be most suitable for patients with severe pain and disability from localized spinal disease.

Treatments for specific pathologies

Osteoporotic fractures are a common cause of acute spinal pain in older people, although may evade medical diagnosis by resolving with self-management. Differentiation from other forms of pathological fracture (e.g. metastatic or myeloma) requires further investigation and imaging where suspected. Osteoporosis typically results in wedge or endplate compression fractures in the thoracic or lumbar spine. These are inherently stable, and only rarely cause neuronal compression or require surgical fixation. Vertebroplasty, the introduction of cement into the fracture site, has been used to reduce symptoms and subsequent deformity, although clinically important benefit has not been universally found in RCTs.[58,59] Osteoporosis is exacerbated by bed rest, and primary management of osteoporotic fractures should be analgesia and early mobilization.[60] Spinal manipulation is not recommended. Optimizing bone mineral density by treatments such as bisophosphonates together with calcium and vitamin D, and reducing falls risk, are essential. Bone-strengthening treatments do not, however, reduce current spinal pain, and the distinction between analgesic and preventive therapies should be explained clearly.

Spinal infection is rare, but serious if not treated promptly. Infective discitis and spinal osteomyelitis typically affect a single level, often in the context of previous disease. Diagnosis depends on a combination of MRI, raised acute-phase response, and bacteriological confirmation, either from blood culture or from infected material obtained by aspiration or open surgery. A distant focus of infection may provide material for bacteriology, either as the primary source, or resulting from haematological spread. Bowel or urological foci should particularly be considered as these may influence antibiotic choice, and concurrent bacterial endocarditis requires involvement of the cardiology team. The commonest implicated organisms are staphylococci, especially *Staphylococcus aureus*, although enterobacteria may account for up to 30% of cases. The low levels of vascularization of the intervertebral disc and cartilage on the vertebral endplates compromise access of antibiotics to infected tissues, reducing efficacy and encouraging the development of resistant strains. Prolonged courses of antibiotic combinations are recommended, administered intravenously for at least 2 weeks and continued orally to complete at least 2 months. Paraspinal fluid collections may be present and require surgical drainage. Spinal pain often continues long after resolution of infection, for which management converges with spinal pain from other causes.

Recommendations for the treatment of inflammatory spinal pain are largely congruent with those for mechanical pain, although some aspects of inflammatory spinal pain may dictate specific therapeutic approaches. Discitis at presentation or in established spondylarthropathy may resemble bacterial infection, but can respond to systemic glucorticosteroids or anti-TNFα therapy. High leverage stresses due to spinal fusion in ankylosing spondylitis combine with associated osteoporosis to increase risk of spinal fracture. Vertebral fractures in ankylosing spondylitis are likely to result in spinal instability and spontaneous or surgical bony repair may be impaired by lack of compensatory movements at adjacent spinal levels. RA commonly affects the cervical spine, although lumbar symptoms are no more common in RA than in matched non-arthritic populations.[23] Cervical (particularly subaxial) instability and pannus each may cause significant cord compression. Pannus may decrease in volume during immunosuppressive therapy.[61] Therapeutic manipulation is not recommended in patients with inflammatory arthritis. Management of inflammatory spinal disease often requires close interaction between specialist rheumatological and surgical units.

Conclusion

Much progress has been made in understanding and treating spinal pain over recent years, but much remains unknown. Many approaches are supported by evidence from RCTs, and even more by cohort or anecdotal evidence. Offering multiple treatments either concurrently or in sequence may enhance benefit, but also increases healthcare costs. Diverse management plans can cause confusion, particularly when based on apparently contradictory explanatory models. Treatment failure can result in disengagement from healthcare services. Further research is required to optimize and definitively determine benefit from existing treatments.

References

1. WHO. The burden of musculoskeletal conditions at the start of the new millennium. *World Health Organ Tech Rep Ser* 2003;919:1–218.
2. Webb R, Brammah T, Lunt M, Urwin M, Allison T, Symmons D. Prevalence and predictors of intense, chronic, and disabling neck and back pain in the UK general population. *Spine* 2003;28(11):1195–1202.
3. Dionne CE, Dunn KM, Croft PR. Does back pain prevalence really decrease with increasing age? A systematic review. *Age Ageing* 2006;35(3):229–234.
4. Clermont DE, Dunn KM, Croft PR. Does back pain prevalence really decrease with increasing age? A systematic review. *Age Ageing* 2006;35(3):229–234.
5. Papageorgiou AC, Croft PR, Thomas E et al. Influence of previous pain experience on the episode incidence of low back pain: results from the South Manchester Back Pain Study. *Pain* 1996;66(2–3):181–185.
6. Hogg-Johnson S, van der Velde G, Carroll LJ et al. The burden and determinants of neck pain in the general population: results of the Bone and Joint Decade 2000–2010 Task Force on Neck Pain and Its Associated Disorders. *Spine* 2008;33(4 Suppl):S39–S51.
7. Freemont AJ, Peacock TE, Goupille P et al. Nerve ingrowth into diseased intervertebral disc in chronic back pain. *Lancet* 1997;350(9072):178–181.
8. Boswell MV, Colson JD, Sehgal N, Dunbar EE, Epter R. A systematic review of therapeutic facet joint interventions in chronic spinal pain. *Pain Physician* 2007;10(1):229–253.
9. Videman T, Battie MC, Gibbons LE et al. Associations between back pain history and lumbar MRI findings. *Spine* 2003;28(6):582–588.
10. Buenaventura RM, Shah RV, Patel V, Benyamin R, Singh V. Systematic review of discography as a diagnostic test for spinal pain: an update. *Pain Physician* 2007;10(1):147–164.
11. NICE. *Interventional procedures overview; prosthetic intervertebral disc replacement in the lumbar spine.* HMSO, London, 2009.
12. NICE. *Interventional procedures overview; prosthetic intervertebral disc replacement in the cervical spine.* HMSO, London, 2009.
13. Hartvigsen J, Nielsen J, Kyvik KO et al. Heritability of spinal pain and consequences of spinal pain: a comprehensive genetic epidemiologic analysis using a population-based sample of 15,328 twins ages 20–71 years. *Arthritis Rheum* 2009;61(10):1343–1351.
14. Sloan TJ, Walsh DA. Explanatory and diagnostic labels and perceived prognosis in chronic low back pain. *Spine* 2010;35(21):E1120–E1125.
15. Leeuw M, Goossens MEJB, Linton SJ et al. The fear-avoidance model of musculoskeletal pain: current state of scientific evidence. *J Behav Med* 2007 Feb;30(1):77–94.
16. Kalichman L, Kim DH, Li L, Guermazi A, Berkin V, Hunter DJ. Spondylolysis and spondylolisthesis: prevalence and association with low back pain in the adult community-based population. Spine 2009;34(2):199–205.
17. Hu SS, Tribus CB, Diab M, Ghanayem AJ. Spondylolisthesis and spondylolysis. *J Bone Joint Surg Am* 2008;90(3):656–671.
18. Williams FMK, Manek NJ, Sambrook PN, Spector TD, Macgregor AJ. Schmorl's nodes: common, highly heritable, and related to lumbar disc disease. *Arthritis Rheum* 2007;57(5):855–860.
19. Genevay S, Viatte S, Finckh A et al. Adalimumab in severe and acute sciatica: a multicenter, randomized, double-blind, placebo-controlled trial. *Arthritis Rheum* 2010;62(8):2339–2346.
20. Christensen ST, Hartvigsen J. Spinal curves and health: a systematic critical review of the epidemiological literature dealing with associations between sagittal spinal curves and health. *J Manipulative Physiol Ther* 2008;31(9):690–714.
21. Macfarlane GJ, Pye SR, Finn JD et al. Investigating the determinants of international differences in the prevalence of chronic widespread pain: evidence from the European Male Ageing Study. *Ann Rheum Dis* 2009;68(5):690–695.
22. Kindler LL, Jones KD, Perrin N, Bennett RM. Risk factors predicting the development of widespread pain from chronic back or neck pain. *J Pain* 2010;11(12):1320–1328.

23. Neva MH, Hakkinen A, Isomaki P, Sokka T. Chronic back pain in patients with rheumatoid arthritis and in a control population: prevalence and disability—a 5-year follow-up. *Rheumatology* (Oxford) 2011; 50(9):1635–1639.

24. Harding IJ, Davies E, Buchanan E, Fairbank JT. The symptom of night pain in a back pain triage clinic. *Spine* 2005;30(17):1985–1988.

25. Savigny P, Kuntze S, Watson P et al. *Low back pain: early management of persistent non-specific low back pain.* National Collaborating Centre for Primary Care and Royal College of General Practitioners, London, 2009.

26. Chou R, Atlas SJ, Stanos SP, Rosenquist RW. Nonsurgical interventional therapies for low back pain: a review of the evidence for an American Pain Society clinical practice guideline. *Spine* 2009;34(10): 1078–1093.

27. NICE. *Technology Appraisal Guidance TA161 (amended); Alendronate, etidronate, risedronate, raloxifene, strontium ranelate and teriparatide for the secondary prevention of osteoporotic fragility fractures in postmenopausal women.* HMSO, London, 2011.

28. Neva MH, Hakkinen A, Makinen H et al. High prevalence of asymptomatic cervical spine subluxation in patients with rheumatoid arthritis waiting for orthopaedic surgery. *Ann Rheum Dis* 2006;65(7):884–888.

29. Koes BW, van Tulder M, Lin C-WC et al. An updated overview of clinical guidelines for the management of non-specific low back pain in primary care. *Eur Spine J* 2010;19(12):2075–2094.

30. Chou R, Loeser JD, Owens DK et al. Interventional therapies, surgery, and interdisciplinary rehabilitation for low back pain: an evidence-based clinical practice guideline from the American Pain Society. *Spine* 2009;34(10):1066–1077.

31. Chou R, Qaseem A, Snow V et al. Diagnosis and treatment of low back pain: a joint clinical practice guideline from the American College of Physicians and the American Pain Society. *Ann Intern Med* 2007;147(7):478–491.

32. Airaksinen O, Brox JI, Cedraschi C et al. Chapter 4. European guidelines for the management of chronic nonspecific low back pain. *Eur Spine J* 2006;15 Suppl 2:S192–S300.

33. Benson RT, Tavares SP, Robertson SC, Sharp R, Marshall RW. Conservatively treated massive prolapsed discs: a 7-year follow-up. *Ann R Coll Surg Engl* 2010;92(2):147–153.

34. Koes B, van Tulder M. Low back pain (acute). *Clin Evid* 2006;15: 1619–1633.

35. Linton SJ, Hallden K. Can we screen for problematic back pain? A screening questionnaire for predicting outcome in acute and subacute back pain. *Clin J Pain* 1998;14(3):209–215.

36. Hill JC, Whitehurst DGT, Lewis M et al. Comparison of stratified primary care management for low back pain with current best practice (STarT Back): a randomised controlled trial. *Lancet* 2011;378:1560–1571.

37. Royal College of General Practitioners, NHS Executive. *The back book: the best way to deal with back pain; get back active.* The Stationery Office, Norwich, 2002.

38. Chou R, Huffman LH, American Pain Society, American College of Physicians. Medications for acute and chronic low back pain: a review of the evidence for an American Pain Society/American College of Physicians clinical practice guideline. *Ann Intern Med* 2007;147(7): 505–514.

39. Tilbrook HE, Cox H, Hewitt CE et al. Yoga for chronic low back pain: a randomized trial. *Ann Intern Med* 2011;155(9):569–578.

40. Rubinstein SM, van Middelkoop M, Assendelft WJJ, de Boer MR, van Tulder MW. Spinal manipulative therapy for chronic low-back pain. *Cochrane Database Syst Rev* 2011;2:CD008112.

41. Fu L-M, Li J-T, Wu W-S. Randomized controlled trials of acupuncture for neck pain: systematic review and meta-analysis. *J Altern Complement Med* 2009;15(2):133–145.

42. Zhang W, Robertson J, Jones AC, Dieppe PA, Doherty M. The placebo effect and its determinants in osteoarthritis: meta-analysis of randomised controlled trials. *Ann Rheum Dis* 2008;67(12):1716–1723.

43. Lamb SE, Hansen Z, Lall R et al. Group cognitive behavioural treatment for low-back pain in primary care: a randomised controlled trial and cost-effectiveness analysis. *Lancet* 2010;375(9718):916–923.

44. British Pain Society. *Recommended guidelines for pain management programmes for adults.* British Pain Society, London, 2007.

45. Williams AC, Richardson PH, Nicholas MK et al. Inpatient vs. outpatient pain management: results of a randomised controlled trial. *Pain* 1996;66(1):13–22.

46. Eccleston C, Williams ACdC, Morley S. Psychological therapies for the management of chronic pain (excluding headache) in adults. *Cochrane Database Syst Rev* 2009;2:CD007407.

47. Vowles KE, McCracken LM. Acceptance and values-based action in chronic pain: a study of treatment effectiveness and process. *J Consult Clin Psychol* 2008;76(3):397–407.

48. Meijer EM, Sluiter JK, Frings-Dresen MHW. Evaluation of effective return-to-work treatment programs for sick-listed patients with non-specific musculoskeletal complaints: a systematic review. *Int Arch Occup Environ Health* 2005;78(7):523–532.

49. Buchbinder R, Jolley D. Effects of a media campaign on back beliefs is sustained 3 years after its cessation. *Spine* 2005;30(11):1323–1330.

50. Buttermann GR. Treatment of lumbar disc herniation: epidural steroid injection compared with discectomy. A prospective, randomized study. *J Bone Joint Surg Am* 2004;86-A(4):670–679.

51. Thomas E, Cyteval C, Abiad L et al. Efficacy of transforaminal versus interspinous corticosteroid injection in discal radiculalgia—a prospective, randomised, double-blind study. *Clin Rheumatol* 2003;22(4–5): 299–304.

52. Staal JB, de Bie R, de Vet HCW, Hildebrandt J, Nelemans P. Injection therapy for subacute and chronic low-back pain. *Cochrane Database Syst Rev* 2008;3:CD001824.

53. Weber H, Holme I, Amlie E. The natural course of acute sciatica with nerve root symptoms in a double-blind placebo-controlled trial evaluating the effect of piroxicam. *Spine* 1993;18(11):1433–1438.

54. Gibson JA, Waddell G. Surgical interventions for lumbar disc prolapse. *Cochrane Database Syst Rev* 2007;1:CD001350.

55. Gibson JNA, Waddell G. Surgery for degenerative lumbar spondylosis. *Cochrane Database Syst Rev* 2005;4:CD001352.

56. North American Spine Society. *Diagnosis and treatment of degenerative lumbar spondylolisthesis.* NASS, Burr Ridge, IL, 2008.

57. NICE. *Interventional procedure guidance; Non-rigid stabilisation techniques for the treatment of low back pain.* HMSO, London, 2010.

58. Buchbinder R, Osborne RH, Ebeling PR et al. A randomized trial of vertebroplasty for painful osteoporotic vertebral fractures. *N Engl J Med* 2009;361(6):557–568.

59. Kallmes DF, Comstock BA, Heagerty PJ et al. A randomized trial of vertebroplasty for osteoporotic spinal fractures. *N Engl J Med* 2009;361(6): 569–579.

60. National Osteoporosis Guideline Group. *Osteoporosis; clinical guideline for treatment and prevention.* International Osteoporosis Foundation, Sheffield, 2010.

61. Robinson AJ, Taylor DH, Wright GD. Infliximab therapy reduces periodontoid rheumatoid pannus formation. *Rheumatology* (Oxford) 2008;47(2):225–226.

Sources of patient information

Arthritis Research UK: www.arthritisresearchuk.org/arthritis_information/arthritis_types_and_symptoms/back_pain.aspx

Backcare: www.backcare.org.uk/323/back-pain.html

British Pain Society: www.britishpainsociety.org/book_pmp_patients.pdf

NHS: www.nhs.uk/Conditions/Back-pain/Pages/Introduction.aspx

NICE: http://guidance.nice.org.uk/CG88/PublicInfo/pdf/English

Royal College of General Practitioners, NHS Executive. *The back book: the best way to deal with back pain; get back active.* The Stationery Office, Norwich.

CHAPTER 158

Childhood regional conditions

Kristin Houghton

Introduction

Musculoskeletal (MSK) pain is common in childhood and more frequent in adolescence.[1] The majority of causes are benign and self-limited, but musculoskeletal symptoms may be the presenting feature of infectious, inflammatory, and oncologic conditions, and amplified musculoskeletal pain syndromes. It is important to recognize 'red flags' on history and physical examination that warrant further investigations (Table 158.1). This chapter reviews common non-inflammatory regional pain conditions in childhood (Table 158.2).

Shoulder

Chronic shoulder pain is often due to an overuse injury. Rotator cuff tendinopathy affects skeletally mature adolescents who present with the insidious onset of localized pain coincident with increased activity.

Humeral epiphysitis affects skeletally immature children aged 11–16 years who present with shoulder pain associated with overhead activity. It is commonly referred to as Little League shoulder, as it typically affects baseball pitchers.[2] Tennis players, swimmers, and gymnasts may also be affected. Repetitive microtrauma to the proximal humeral physis causes tenderness over the physis and pain or weakness with internal and external rotation. Radiographs may show widening of the physis or separation of the epiphysis.

Table 158.1 Red flags for pain

Symptom	Differential diagnosis
Fever, weight loss, night sweats, malaise	Systemic disease (malignancy, infection, systemic inflammatory disease)
Night pain, discrete bone pain	Oncological disease
Morning stiffness, joint swelling	Inflammatory disease
Weakness, altered sensation, radiating pain, regression of developmental milestones	Neurological disease

Multidirectional instability (MDI) of the shoulder may be isolated or associated with generalized hypermobility. MDI may cause pain from related subacromial impingement or labral pathology.[3]

Treatment of tendinopathy, humeral epiphysitis, MDI, and secondary impingement includes ice, anti-inflammatory drugs, relative rest, and physiotherapy. Labral pathology requires orthopaedic referral and possible surgical repair.

Elbow

Chronic elbow pain is not common in childhood and causes are fairly specific to skeletal maturity. Skeletally mature adolescents with overuse injury or strain usually present with localized pain and a history of recent increased activity. Injury to the flexor pronator muscle group causes medial elbow pain (medial epicondylitis or 'golfer's elbow') and injury to the extensor supinator muscle group causes lateral elbow pain (lateral epicondylitis or 'tennis elbow'). As with other overuse injuries, pain is present during and after activity, which helps distinguish the pain from inflammatory enthesopathy that is classically present in the morning, at rest, and improves with activity.

Osteochondritis dissecans (OCD) of the capitellum affects skeletally immature children aged 11–16 years who present with progressive lateral elbow pain with activity. Microtrauma from chronic compression (throwing, gymnastics) combined with poor blood supply leads to injury to subchondral bone and its overlying articular cartilage.[4] On examination, there is tenderness over the anterolateral elbow, mild swelling, and lack of full extension. Mechanical symptoms of locking or catching may be present if there is a loose body. Radiographs of early lesions may be normal or show lucency of the capitellum and late radiographs may show sclerosis, joint collapse, or loose bodies. MRI may better evaluate the extent of the lesion.

Medial epicondyle apophysitis (Little League elbow in baseball pitchers) affects skeletally immature children aged 8–15 years who present with medial elbow pain associated with throwing.[5] Repetitive valgus stress on the elbow causes tenderness over the medial epicondyle and pain with valgus stress, and pain or weakness with resisted wrist flexion and forearm pronation. Radiographs are often normal and may show widening of the physis or avulsion fracture.

Table 158.2 Mechanical and developmental conditions presenting with regional pain

Region	Mechanical conditions and overuse injuries	Osteochondroses (eponym: site)	Developmental conditions and anatomical variants
Back	Spondylolysis	Scheuermann: thoracic spine epiphysis	Scoliosis
Shoulder	Tendinopathy Instability Impingement		Humeral epiphysitis
Elbow	Tendinopathy	Panner: capitellum	Pulled elbow Olecranon apophysitis Medial epicondyle apophysitis
Wrist and hand	Tendinopathy TFCC	Kienbock: lunate	
Hip and pelvis	Tendinopathy Apophyseal injuries	Legg–Calvé–Perthes: femoral head	SCFE
Knee	Patellofemoral pain	Osgood–Schlatter: tibial tuberosity	Patellofemoral dysplasia
	Iliotibial band syndrome	Sinding–Larsen–Johansson: inferior pole patella	Synovial plica
	Tendinopathy		Bipartite patella
	OCD—femoral condyles, patella		Discoid meniscus
	Fat pad irritation		
Ankle and foot	Tendinopathy	Frieberg: MT head (2nd, 3rd)	Pes planus
	Chronic lateral ligament instability	Sever: calcaneus	Tarsal coalition
	Plantar fascitis	Iselin: 5th MT tuberosity	Bipartite sesamoid
	Stress fracture		Os trigonum
	OCD—talus		Accessory navicular

MT, metatarsal; OCD, osteochondritis dissecans; SCFE, TFCC, triangular fibrocartilage complex injury.

Panner's disease, an osteochondrosis or idiopathic avascular necrosis of the capitellum, affects children aged 7–12 years who present with dull, aching pain over the lateral elbow, maximal tenderness over the radiocapitellar joint, and loss of extension.[6] Swelling is uncommon. Radiographs show early demineralization and/or fragmentation with eventual consolidation of the capitellum, although persistent flattening may be present. MRI is sensitive in detecting early disease. Panner's disease generally resolves with no long-term sequelae and can be distinguished from OCD by age, pain onset, and radiographic appearance of the lesion.

Treatment of medial and lateral epicondylitis, medial epicondyle apophysitis and Panner's disease includes ice, anti-inflammatory drugs, relative rest, and physiotherapy. OCD requires orthopaedic or sports medicine referral and possible surgical repair.

Wrist and hand

Acute injuries of the wrist and hand are common in childhood. The most common mechanism of injury is a fall on an outstretched hand, often resulting in sprain or fracture. Chronic pain following an acute injury should prompt assessment for physeal injury, distal radioulnar joint instability, non-union or avascular necrosis of scaphoid fracture, scapholunate ligament instability, or triangular fibrocartilage complex injury.

Chronic tendon injury typically occurs in children involved in sports requiring repetitive wrist motion such as rowing, throwing, and racquet sports. DeQuervain's tenosynovitis, extensor carpi ulnaris tendonitis, and intersection syndrome present with the insidious onset of localized pain coincident with increased activity.

Stress injury to the distal radial physis occurs in skeletally immature children involved in weightbearing activity such as gymnastics. Children present with dorsal wrist pain during weight-loading activities (handstands, handsprings) and tenderness over the dorsum of the distal radial physis.[7] Early radiographs may show widening and irregularity of the physis and late radiographs may show distal radius deformity or distal ulna overgrowth.[8] MRI may aid early diagnosis and show oedema on the metaphyseal and epiphyseal sides of the physis before radiographic changes are apparent.[9]

Kienbock's disease, an avascular necrosis of the lunate possibly due to repetitive trauma, affects skeletally mature adolescents and young adults.[10] Adolescents present with dorsal wrist pain, swelling, and loss of grip strength. Radiographs may show sclerosis, collapse, or fragmentation of the lunate. MRI is sensitive in detecting early disease. Some adolescents have progressive disease with eventual degenerative arthritis.

Treatment of chronic sequelae of acute wrist and hand injury requires orthopaedic or sports medicine referral and possible surgical repair. Treatment of chronic wrist and hand injury includes ice, anti-inflammatory drugs, bracing, relative rest, and physiotherapy. Adolescents with Kienbock's disease may be treated conservatively with immobilization; however, radial shortening may be indicated for persistent pain or advanced disease on imaging.[10]

Back

Back pain is common in childhood, with 1 year prevalence rates varying from 7% to 58%.[11] Paediatric doctrine states that children with back pain may have serious pathology, including malignancy and infection. However, most cases are non-specific and self limiting. A recent prospective study of 73 children under the age of 18 years, with back pain of greater than 3 months duration, found only 21% of the patients had positive findings after diagnostic evaluation or a minimum of 2 years follow-up. Spondylolysis with or without spondylolisthesis was the most common diagnosis.[12]

Spondylolysis is a defect in the pars interarticularis and most commonly affects the fifth and fourth lumbar vertebrae. The majority of cases in childhood represent a stress fracture in the pars interarticularis (Figure 158.1). It is more common in boys and in sports involving repetitive extension, flexion, and rotation (gymnastics, diving, wrestling). Acute and overuse injuries both occur, with overuse injuries being more common. Spondylolithesis occurs with bilateral pars defects and is defined by forward translation of one vertebra on the next caudal segment. Spondylolithesis is graded on the basis of the percentage of slip of one vertebral body on the vertebral body below: grade 1, 0–25% slip; grade 2, 25–50%; grade 3, 50–75%; grade 4, >75%.[13] Posterior element overuse syndrome—also referred to as spondylogenic back pain, hyperlordotic back pain, mechanical low back pain, and lumbar facet syndrome—should be considered if investigations are negative for

spondylolysis.[14] It includes injury to the muscle–tendon units, ligaments, joint capsules, and facet joints. Adolescents with spondylolysis, spondylolisthesis, and posterior element overuse syndrome present with insidious onset of low back pain, worsened by extension, activity, or prolonged standing. Radicular symptoms may be present if there is nerve root irritation. Adolescents may have exaggerated lumbar hyperlordosis, tight hamstrings, limited forward flexion and straight-leg raise, painful spinal extension (especially single leg extension on the affected side, 'stork test'), focal tenderness over the site of a pars lesion, and a step-off at the lumbosacral junction with spondylolisthesis. A neurological deficit affecting the L5 or S1 nerve roots may be present, with nerve root irritation and high-grade spondylolisthesis. Radiographs (standing lateral, anteroposterior) characterize gross bony abnormalities and stage spondylolisthesis and single-photon emission computed tomography (SPECT) bone scan confirms spondylolytic lesions and acuity.[15] Skeletally immature adolescents with bilateral spondylolysis or spondylolisthesis require standing lateral radiographs every 6–12 months until skeletal maturity to assess for slip progression. Treatment includes activity restriction until asymptomatic and physiotherapy focused on core strength and hamstring flexibility. The use of braces is controversial, with studies showing bony healing with the use of a rigid brace, a soft brace, or no brace.[15] Most adolescents return to activities by 6 months after diagnosis. Adolescents with greater than 50% slip (grade 3 or 4) warrant orthopaedic referral and possible surgical treatment.

Scheuermann's disease is the most common cause of kyphotic deformity in adolescence (Table 158.3), with onset just prior to puberty.[16] The thoracic pattern is more common than the thoracolumbar pattern. Adolescents usually present with cosmetic concerns but may have pain with prolonged sitting posture and exercise. The kyphosis is fixed, distinguishing Scheuermann's from postural kyphosis which disappears with forward flexion. Neurological deficits are rare.[17] Standing lateral and anterior-posterior (AP) radiographic features classically show anterior wedging of at least three adjacent vertebral bodies by 5° or more, end plate irregularities, loss of disc space height, Schmorl nodes and Cobb angle of at least 45°.[18] Treatment includes physiotherapy for minor curves and possible bracing for thoracic curves greater than 55° or thoracolumbar curves greater than 40°. Adolescents with curvature of 70° or greater, refractory pain, or neurological deficit may need surgical treatment.[19]

Idiopathic scoliosis affects 1–3% of children and adolescents.[20] Scoliosis is usually painless but one study reported pain in 32% with only 9% having an identifiable cause for pain.[21] Untreated scoliosis may also cause back pain.[20] On examination, forward flexion of the spine accentuates the curve (imbalanced rib cage with one side higher than the other). Standing coronal radiograph with Cobb

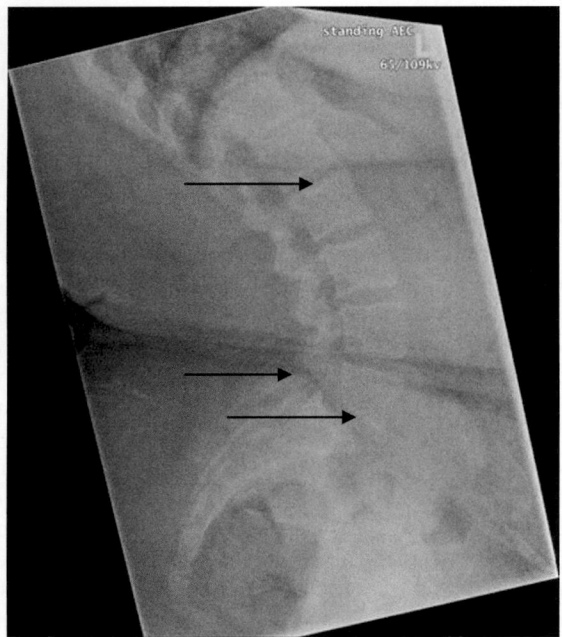

Fig. 158.1 Lateral radiograph of the lumbosacral spine in a 12 year old obese girl with bilateral spondylolysis (middle arrow) and grade I spondylolisthesis of L5 on S1 (bottom arrow). There is also evidence of Schmorl's nodes (top arrow) within the thoracic spine.

Radiograph courtesy of the Department of Radiology, British Columbia's Children's Hospital.

Table 158.3 Back pain in adolescence

Clinical presentation	Clinical condition
Pain with extension	Posterior element overuse syndrome, spondylolysis, spondylolisthesis
Pain with flexion ± neurological symptoms	Disc pathology
Kyphotic posture, occasionally pain	Scheuermann's disease

angle of at least 10° confirms the diagnosis.[22] Treatment is dependent on skeletal maturity and degree of curvature and includes observation, physiotherapy, orthoses, and surgery.

Lumbar disc herniation (primarily L4–5 or L5–S1) is uncommon in childhood.[23] Children present with low back, buttock, or hip pain worsened by bending forward, coughing, sneezing, or straining with bowel movements. Children may have limitation of forward flexion and positive straight-leg raise test. Neurological findings are uncommon. Radiographs and MRI help differentiate between spondylolysis with nerve root impingement or disc herniation with nerve root impingement.[24] Treatment includes rest, analgesics, and physical therapy. Adolescents do not fare as well with conservative therapy as do adults. Adolescents who fail to respond to conservative therapy and those with progressive neurological deficit warrant orthopaedic referral for possible surgical treatment.

Hip

Transient synovitis and septic arthritis are the most common diseases among young children with acute hip pain. Causes of chronic hip pain are often related to skeletal maturity and are fairly specific to the age of the child (Table 158.4).

Perthes' disease, an idiopathic avascular necrosis of the femoral epiphysis, affects children aged 4–10 years old (peak 5–7 years), is more common in boys (4:1) and is bilateral in 10%.[25] Children present with a limp or pain in the hip, thigh, or knee; limited and painful rotation and abduction of the hip; and Trendelenburg sign may be positive. Radiographs of early lesions may show decreased size or increased density of the proximal femoral epiphyses and crescent sign (a subchondral fracture that correlates with the extent of necrosis). Late radiographs may show fragmentation, reossification, remodelling, and healing. Perthes' disease generally resolves with no long-term sequelae but early osteoarthritis may occur. Age greater than 6 years is worse prognosis than younger children and femoral head involvement of more than 50% is the strongest predictor of poor outcome.[26] Treatment includes rest and range-of-motion exercises. Older children with greater femoral head involvement may require orthoses or surgery.

Slipped capital femoral epiphyses (SCFE), displacement of the proximal femoral epiphysis off the femoral neck, affects preadolescents (peak 11–14 years) is more common in boys and in obese children, and is bilateral in 20–40%.[27] Children present with a limp; hip, groin, or knee pain; decreased range of motion of the hip (active and passive internal rotation, flexion and abduction); and Trendelenburg sign may be positive. SCFE is classified as stable or unstable based on a child's ability to weightbear on the affected leg.[28] Radiographs of the hip may show widening and irregularity of the physis with posterior inferior displacement of the femoral head. On the AP view, a line drawn from the superior femoral neck (Klein's line) should intersect some portion of the femoral

head (Figure 158.2).[27] Treatment includes non-weightbearing, and surgery with epiphyseal fixation and possible osteotomy. Most children do well after surgical fixation but avascular necrosis and chondrolysis may occur. Unstable slips have worse prognosis. Children require long-term follow-up as SCFE may develop within 12–18 months in the contralateral hip, if prophylactic pinning is not done.[29] Children who do not fit the classic profile for SCFE (under age 10 or over age 16, thin) should undergo evaluation for associated endocrinopathies (thyroid disease, growth hormone abnormalities).[30]

Apophysitis and apophyseal avulsion fractures around the pelvis may occur in skeletally immature adolescents secondary to forceful or repetitive traction of the attached muscle. Apophysitis presents with dull, activity-related pain and avulsion fractures present with localized pain, swelling, and decreased active range of motion. Common sites of injury are the iliac crest (abdominal muscles), anterior superior iliac spine (sartorius), anterior inferior iliac spine (rectus femoris), ischial tuberosity (hamstrings), and lesser trochanter (iliopsoas). Radiographs may show widening of the apophyses in apophysitis and displacement of the apophyseal centre and bony reaction in apophyseal avulsion fracture. MRI is useful if radiographs are normal.[31] Treatment includes activity modification, and physiotherapy with the majority of adolescents recovering within 2 months. Surgical treatment is rarely required.

Idiopathic chondrolysis of the hip affects adolescents and is more common in girls. Adolescents present with pain, limp, and reduced range of motion of the hip. Investigations (haematological, microbiological, immunological, and acute-phase reactants) are normal. Early radiographs may be normal and late radiographs may show regional osteoporosis, premature closure of the femoral capital physis, joint space narrowing, and lateral overgrowth of the femoral head on the neck. MRI shows loss of articular cartilage with minimal synovial enhancement.[31] Many adolescents develop painful osteoarthritis of the hip. Treatment includes protective weightbearing, anti-inflammatories, physiotherapy, and orthopaedic intervention as necessary.

Snapping hip syndrome is a relatively common complaint in childhood. Anterior symptoms are caused by the iliopsoas tendon snapping under the inguinal ligament or over the iliopectineal eminence and lateral symptoms are caused by the iliotibial band snapping over the greater trochanter.[32] Pain may be present if there is an associated bursitis or if snapping is due to an acetabular labral tear. Children can usually reproduce their symptoms during examination. Treatment includes avoidance of aggravating activities and physiotherapy. Recalcitrant cases warrant orthopaedic referral for possible bursal excision and Z-plasty to lengthen the iliotibial band.[33]

Knee

Anterior knee pain is one of the most common musculoskeletal complaints seen in the paediatric population. Most causes involve the patellofemoral joint and the extensor mechanism of the knee.

Patellofemoral pain (PFP), secondary to excessive forces of compression and friction at the patellofemoral joint, affects active and inactive children, is more common in girls, and is most common during the adolescent growth spurt.[34] Children present with dull, achy peripatellar or retropatellar pain during and after weightbearing activity, stair use, and squatting. Stiffness may be present after

Table 158.4 Causes of hip pain during childhood and adolescence

Clinical condition	Age (years)
Toxic synovitis	2–10 (peak 5–6)
Legg–Calvé–Perthes	4–10 (peak 5–7)
Slipped capital femoral epiphyses	11–15

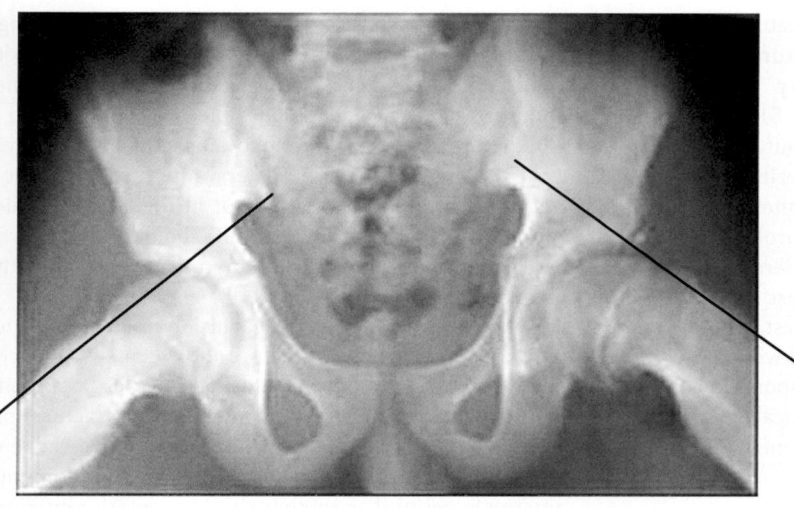

Fig. 158.2 Anterior posterior radiograph of the hips in a teenage boy with slipped capital femoral epiphyses on the right. Klein's line is drawn along the radiographic border of the neck of the femur. This line should intersect the epiphysis.
Radiograph courtesy of the Department of Radiology, British Columbia's Children's Hospital.

prolonged sitting with the knee in flexion ('theatre sign'). Symptoms usually affect both knees with one side more affected. On examination, children may have lower extremity malalignment (genu valgum, genu varum, genu recurvatum, leg length discrepancy, femoral anteversion, external tibial torsion, lateral displacement of the tibial tubercle, excessive pronation of the subtalar joint), vastus medialis wasting, patellar facet tenderness, tightness (hamstrings, quadriceps, iliotibial band, gastrocnemius) and weakness (quadriceps, hip external rotators, abductors, trunk muscles) of the lower extremity muscles. Painful quadriceps setting/grind test (Clarke's test; examiner applies pressure against the superior pole of the patient's patella during an isometric quadriceps contraction with knee in full extension) and patellar compression test (direct compression of the patella in to the trochlea) aid diagnosis.[35] Swelling is unusual. Treatment includes activity modification, ice, short-term anti-inflammatories, and physiotherapy focusing on patellar tracking exercises, strength, and flexibility. Shoe orthoses (subtalar pronation) and patellofemoral orthoses may reduce symptoms. Most children have gradual improvement and resolution of PFP.

Patellofemoral instability is more common in children with hypermobility and anatomic variants (patella alta, unifaceted or bipartite patella, shallow intercondylar groove, lateral attachment of the patellar ligament).[36] Children present with PFP, episodic giving way and locking, recurrent swelling, and positive patellar apprehension test. Treatment is the same as for PFP. Patellofemoral orthoses may prevent recurrent episodes of instability.

Children with recurrent patellar dislocation warrant orthopaedic referral.[36]

Patellar tendinopathy affects skeletally mature individuals who present with infrapatellar pain aggravated by jumping and maximal tenderness at the patellar attachment and proximal tendon. Patellar tendon thickening and nodules may be palpable.

Osgood–Schlatter disease (OSD) and Sinding–Larsen–Johansson disease (SLJD) are osteochondroses/traction apophysitis that affect skeletally immature children and present with pain at the attachments of the patellar tendon. OSD is more common than SLJD, affects 8–12 year old girls and 12–15 year old boys, and occurs at the growth plate of the tibial tuberosity. SLJD affects 10–12 year olds and occurs at the inferior pole of the patella.[37] Children present with localized pain during activity, focal tenderness, and soft tissue swelling. The presentation during growth and the temporal association

of pain during and after activity helps distinguish OSD and SJLD from inflammatory enthesopathy, which is classically present in the morning, at rest, and improves with activity. Radiographs are not required for diagnosis and typically show bony reaction and fragmentation. Treatment includes activity modification, ice, anti-inflammatories, physiotherapy, and infrapatellar strap. Recovery may be expedited by reduction of running and jumping sports, with the natural history being a resolution of symptoms over months to years at skeletal maturity.[38,39]

Osteochondritis dissecans of the knee classically affects the lateral aspect of the medial femoral condyle, but the lateral femoral condyle and patella may also be involved. Repetitive microtrauma combined with poor blood supply leads to injury to subchondral bone and its overlying articular cartilage.[40] Children present with activity-related knee pain and swelling. Mechanical symptoms of locking may be present if there is a loose body. On examination, there is focal bony tenderness and joint effusion, and extension block or palpable loose body may be noted. Radiographs may show a radiolucent lesion, subchondral fracture, separation with subchondral bone and a loose body (Figure 158.3).[40] MRI better evaluates the extent of the lesion. Skeletally immature children with smaller, stable, non-detached lesions have the best prognosis. Treatment includes protective weightbearing and immobilization with surgery reserved for recalcitrant symptoms and detached unstable lesions.[41]

Synovial plica syndrome presents with medial knee pain, and snapping and catching during flexion. There may be tenderness over the medial patellar retinaculum or anteromedial joint line and the plica may be palpable as a thickened band that is tender when pressed against the edge of the condyle. Treatment includes patellar mobilization and massage, anti-inflammatories, and physiotherapy. Recalcitrant cases warrant orthopaedic referral for possible surgical resection.

Fat pad impingement ('Hoffa's syndrome') presents with pain during knee extension, prolonged standing, and kneeling. On examination there is tenderness and swelling over the fat pad and painful knee extension. Treatment includes cryotherapy, anti-inflammatories, activity modification, and physiotherapy.

Discoid lateral meniscus is an anatomic variant that commonly presents in school-aged children and adolescents, with clicking and catching during knee extension. The abnormally shaped meniscus

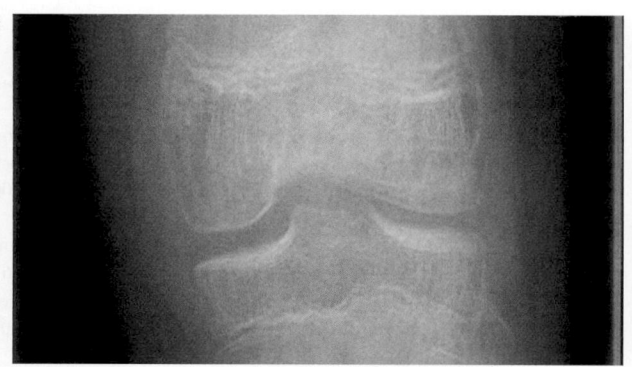
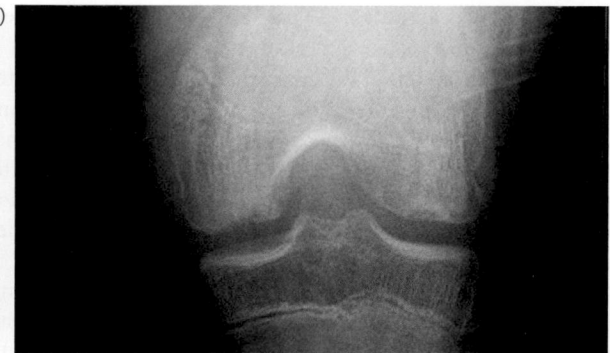

Fig. 158.3 Osteochondritis dissecans in a child with juvenile arthritis: (A) Anterior posterior view shows minimal cystic changes affecting the lateral femoral condyle. (B) Tunnel or notch view shows the lateral femoral condyle cystic changes with surrounding sclerosis more clearly. There is also irregularity of the medial femoral condyle suggesting an osteochondral lesion.
Radiograph courtesy of the Department of Radiology, British Columbia's Children's Hospital.

is easily torn, leading to swelling, instability, catching, and/or locking of the knee. Children may have painful clicking with extension, lateral joint line tenderness, and swelling. MRI confirms the diagnosis. Treatment includes activity modification and physiotherapy for intact discoid meniscus and orthopaedic referral for surgical management of torn discoid meniscus.[42]

Lower leg

'Shin splints'/medial tibial stress syndrome presents as activity-related shin pain and tenderness along the posteromedial border of the tibia due to periostitis and fascitis caused by repetitive stress. It is more common during the adolescent growth spurt, with subtalar pronation, and often presents after an increase in activity. Radiographs are normal and radionuclide bone scan shows diffuse increased uptake at the junction of the middle and distal thirds of the posteromedial tibia, differentiating it from focal uptake seen in stress fracture.[43] Treatment includes rest, ice, physiotherapy, and change in footwear or orthotic.

Foot and ankle

Foot and ankle pain is common in children and adolescents. Problems are usually related to skeletal maturity and are fairly specific to the age of the child.

Pes planus is common in children up to age 7 and occurs in 10–23% of the general population.[44,45] Flexible flat feet refers to the presence of an arch while toe-standing or sitting. Most children with flexible flat feet are asymptomatic; however, some children may have pain during or after activity. Painful flat feet should be imaged to rule out anatomic variants (tarsal coalition, vertical talus, or accessory navicular). Symptomatic children may benefit from a rigid medial arch support. Orthotics may decrease the risk of ankle or knee injury in young athletes with excessive pronation.

Sever's disease, a traction apophysitis of the os calcis at the insertion of the Achilles tendon, affects children aged 7–14 years, is more common in boys, and is bilateral in 60%.[46] Children present with heel pain during running and jumping activities, tenderness, and possible swelling over the posterior heel at the insertion of the Achilles tendon, pain with medial and lateral squeeze of the calcaneal apophysis, weakness of dorsiflexion, and contracture of the Achilles tendon. Radiographs show a normally irregular apophysis

and soft tissue swelling. The presentation during growth and the temporal association of pain with activity helps distinguish Sever's from inflammatory enthesopathy which is classically present in the morning, at rest, and improves with activity. Treatment includes ice, anti-inflammatories, activity modification, physiotherapy, and insertion of a heel lift or heel cup in footwear.

Iselin's disease, a traction apophysitis of the tuberosity of the fifth metatarsal at the insertion of the peroneus brevis tendon, affects 7–14 year olds, who present with lateral foot pain and point tenderness over the base of the fifth metatarsal. Radiographs differentiate Iselin's disease from avulsion fracture, as the apophysis is parallel to the long axis of the fifth metatarsal and fractures are usually transverse.[47] Treatment includes ice, anti-inflammatories, activity modification, immobilization, and physiotherapy.

Tarsal coalition, failure of complete segmentation between two or more tarsal bones, occurs in 3–5% of the population, affects boys twice as often as girls, and is often bilateral. Onset of symptoms usually occurs at the time of ossification; 8–12 years of age for calcaneonavicular and 12–16 years for talocalcaneal coalitions.[48] Children present with pain, a history of frequent 'ankle sprains' and a rigid flatfoot with restricted and possibly painful subtalar range of motion. Radiographs (oblique and axial views) may show calcaneonavicular coalitions but CT or MRI is needed for fibrous or cartilaginous coalition and other tarsal coalitions.[49] Treatment of symptomatic coalitions includes casting and/or orthoses, physiotherapy, and possible surgical management.

Kohler's disease, an osteochondroses of the tarsal navicular, affects children aged 5–9 years and is bilateral in up to 25% of cases.[50] Children present with midfoot pain with weightbearing activity and localized swelling and tenderness over the navicular. Radiographs show increased sclerosis of the navicular; however, irregular ossification is a normal growth variant and clinical correlation is required for diagnosis. Treatment includes anti-inflammatories, activity modification, and immobilization in a walking boot for severe cases.

Freiberg's disease, an osteonecrosis of the metatarsal head, affects the second and third metatarsals and is more common in athletic adolescent females.[50] Adolescents present with forefoot pain and focal tenderness over the affected metatarsal head. Radiographs show initial joint space widening, followed by collapse and eventual reossification of the metatarsal head.[50] Treatment includes anti-inflammatories, immobilization in a walking boot, and orthotics.

The healing process can take 2–3 years and surgical management may be required for persistent symptoms.

Osteochondral dissecans of the talar dome causes activity-related ankle pain and swelling. Mechanical symptoms of locking and catching may be present if there is a loose body. Radiographs may show a radiolucent lesion, bony defect, or loose body. MRI better characterizes the lesion. Treatment includes rest and immobilization with surgery reserved for recalcitrant symptoms and detached unstable lesions.[51]

Accessory ossification centres in the foot and ankle are normal growth variants and approximately 22% of children have at least one accessory ossicle.[48] Accessory bones are usually asymptomatic but may become painful with activity or may be confused with avulsion fractures. Symptomatic accessory navicular causes medial foot pain and focal tenderness over the bony prominence. Symptomatic os trigonum causes posterolateral ankle pain and focal tenderness over the posterior talus. Radiographs confirm the presence of accessory bones. Treatment includes physiotherapy and orthotics, with surgical excision reserved for recalcitrant cases.

Congenital talipes equinovarus (clubfoot) is a common musculoskeletal congenital anomaly, occurring in 1 in 1000 births.[52] Idiopathic clubfoot is most common, but it may occur in association with neurological disorders such as myelodysplasia and arthrogryposis or with multiple congenital anomalies. Untreated clubfoot leads to gait disturbance (weightbearing on sides and/or tops of the feet), potential pain due to callus formation, potential infection of skin and bone, and limited mobility. Optimal treatment for a pain-free and functional foot includes casting, bracing, and possible soft tissue release surgery.[53]

Growing pains

Growing pains, the most common cause of episodic childhood musculoskeletal pain, classically affect preschool and school-aged children.[54,55] Children present with non-articular leg aches at night that usually respond to massage and over-the-counter analgesics. Children report no pain during the day and are normally active. Increased daily activity may be associated with episodes of growing pains.

The physical examination is normal and there is no associated organic disease. However, growing pains may have a significant impact on a family due to school and work absences, daytime fatigue, and chronic analgesia use.

The cause of growing pains is not known and there are no diagnostic tests. Growing pains are a diagnosis of exclusion and it is important to rule out other causes. Investigations should be considered if there are atypical symptoms including unilateral pain, daytime pain, articular pain, daily pain (not episodic), systemic symptoms, or abnormalities on physical examination. Treatment includes education and reassurance that the pains are self-limited and benign. Over-the-counter analgesics and physiotherapy (flexibility exercises) may also be helpful for symptom management.[56]

References

1. De Inocencio J. Epidemiology of musculoskeletal pain in primary care. *Arch Dis Child* 2004;89(5):431–434.
2. Osbahr DC, Kim HJ, Dugas JR. Little league shoulder. *Curr Opin Pediatr* 2010;22(1):35–40.
3. Johnson SM, Robinson CM. Shoulder instability in patients with joint hyperlaxity. *J Bone Joint Surg Am* 2010;92(6):1545–1557.
4. Baker CL 3rd, Romeo AA, Baker CL Jr. Osteochondritis dissecans of the capitellum. *Am J Sports Med* 2010;38(9):1917–1928.
5. Benjamin HJ, Briner WW Jr. Little league elbow. *Clin J Sport Med* 2005;15(1):37–40.
6. Kobayashi K, Burton KJ, Rodner C, Smith B, Caputo AE.. Lateral compression injuries in the pediatric elbow: Panner's disease and osteochondritis dissecans of the capitellum. *J Am Acad Orthop Surg* 2004;12(4):246–254.
7. DiFiori JP. Overuse injury and the young athlete: the case of chronic wrist pain in gymnasts. *Curr Sports Med Rep* 2006;5(4):165–167.
8. DiFiori JP, Caine DJ, Malina RM. Wrist pain, distal radial physeal injury, and ulnar variance in the young gymnast. *Am J Sports Med* 2006;34(5):840–849.
9. Dwek JR, Cardoso F, Chung CB. MR imaging of overuse injuries in the skeletally immature gymnast: spectrum of soft-tissue and osseous lesions in the hand and wrist. *Pediatr Radiol* 2009;39(12):1310–1316.
10. Schuind F, Eslami S, Ledoux P. Kienbock's disease. *J Bone Joint Surg Br* 2008;90(2):133–139.
11. Smith DR, Leggat PA. Back pain in the young: a review of studies conducted among school children and university students. *Curr Pediatr Rev* 2007;3:69–77.
12. Bhatia NN, Chow G, Timon SJ, Watts HG. Diagnostic modalities for the evaluation of pediatric back pain: a prospective study. *J Pediatr Orthop* 2008;28(2):230–233.
13. Lonstein JE. Spondylolisthesis in children. Cause, natural history, and management. *Spine* 1999;24(24):2640–2648.
14. Purcell L, Micheli L. Low back pain in young athletes. *Sports Health* 2009;1(3):212–222.
15. Standaert CJ, Herring SA. Expert opinion and controversies in sports and musculoskeletal medicine: the diagnosis and treatment of spondylolysis in adolescent athletes. *Arch Phys Med Rehabil* 2007;88(4):537–540.
16. Lowe TG, Scheuermann's kyphosis. *Neurosurg Clin North Am* 2007;18(2):305–315.
17. Murray PM, Weinstein SL, Spratt KF. The natural history and long-term follow-up of Scheuermann kyphosis. *J Bone Joint Surg Am* 1993;75(2):236–248.
18. Sorenson KH. *Scheuermann's juvenile kyphosis. Clinical appearances, radiography, aetiology, and prognosis.* Munksgaard, Copenhagen, 1964.
19. Arlet V, Schlenzka D. Scheuermann's kyphosis: surgical management. *Eur Spine J* 2005;14(9):817–827.
20. Weinstein SL, Dolan LA, Cheng JC, Danielsson A, Morcuende JA. Adolescent idiopathic scoliosis. *Lancet* 2008;371(9623):1527–1537.
21. Ramirez N, Johnston CE, Browne RH. The prevalence of back pain in children who have idiopathic scoliosis. *J Bone Joint Surg Am* 1997;79(3):364–368.
22. Cobb JR. Outline for the study of scoliosis. *Am Acad Orthop Surg Inst Course Lect* 1948;5:261–275.
23. Kumar R, Kumar V, Das NK, Behari S, Mahapatra AK. Adolescent lumbar disc disease: findings and outcome. *Childs Nervous Syst* 2007;23(11):1295–1299.
24. Rodriguez DP, Poussaint TY. Imaging of back pain in children. *Am J Neuroradiol* 2010;31:787–802.
25. Catterall A. The natural history of Perthes' disease. *J Bone Joint Surg Br* 1971;53(1):37–53.
26. Wiig O, Terjesen T, and Svenningsen S. Prognostic factors and outcome of treatment in Perthes' disease: a prospective study of 368 patients with five-year follow-up. *J Bone Joint Surg Br* 2008;90(10):1364–1371.
27. Reynolds RA. Diagnosis and treatment of slipped capital femoral epiphysis. *Curr Opin Pediatr* 1999;11(1):80–83.
28. Loder RT, Richards BS, Shapiro PS, Reznick LR, Aronson DD. Acute slipped capital femoral epiphysis: the importance of physeal stability. *J Bone Joint Surg Am* 1993;75(8):1134–1140.
29. Castro FP Jr, Bennett JT, Doulens K. Epidemiological perspective on prophylactic pinning in patients with unilateral slipped capital femoral epiphysis. *J Pediatr Orthop* 2000;20(6):745–748.

30. Loder RT, Wittenberg B, DeSilva G. Slipped capital femoral epiphysis associated with endocrine disorders. *J Pediatr Orthop* 1995;15(3):349–356.

31. Sanders TG, Zlatkin MB. Avulsion injuries of the pelvis. *Semin Musculoskelet Radiol* 2008;12(1):42–53.

32. Allen WC, Cope R. Coxa saltans: the snapping hip revisited. *J Am Acad Orthop Surg* 1995;3(5):303–308.

33. Dobbs MB, Gordon JE, Luhmann SJ, Szymanski DA, Schoenecker PL. Surgical correction of the snapping iliopsoas tendon in adolescents. *J Bone Joint Surg Am* 2002;84(3):420–424.

34. LaBella C. Patellofemoral pain syndrome: evaluation and treatment. *Primary Care* 2004;31(4):977–1003.

35. Galanty HL, Matthews C, Hergenroeder AC. Anterior knee pain in adolescents. *Clin J Sport Med* 1994;4(4):176–181.

36. Hinton RY, Sharma KM. Acute and recurrent patellar instability in the young athlete. *Orthop Clin North Am* 2003;34(3):385–396.

37. Gholve PA, Scher DM, Khakharia S, Widmann RF, Green DW. Osgood Schlatter syndrome. *Curr Opin Pediatr* 2007;19(1):44–50.

38. Krause BL, Williams JP, Catterall A. Natural history of Osgood-Schlatter disease. *J Pediatr Orthop* 1990;10(1):65–68.

39. Bloom OJ, Mackler L, Barbee J. Clinical inquiries. What is the best treatment for Osgood-Schlatter disease? *J Family Pract* 2004;53(2):153–156.

40. Schenck RC Jr, Goodnight JM. Osteochondritis dissecans. *J Bone Joint Surg Am* 1996;78(3):439–456.

41. Wall E, Von Stein D. Juvenile osteochondritis dissecans. *Orthop Clin North Am* 2003;34(3):341–353.

42. Kelly BT, Green DW. Discoid lateral meniscus in children. *Curr Opin Pediatr* 2002;14(1):54–61.

43. Kortebein PM, et al. Medial tibial stress syndrome. *Med Science Sports Exerc* 2000;32(3 Suppl):S27–33.

44. Gould N, Moreland M, Alvarez R, Trevino S, Fenwick J.. Development of the child's arch. *Foot Ankle* 1989;9(5):241–245.

45. Barry RJ, Scranton PE Jr. Flat feet in children. *Clin Orthop Relat Res* 1983;181:68–75.

46. Manusov EG, Lillegard WA, Raspa RF, Epperly TD. Evaluation of pediatric foot problems: Part II. The hindfoot and the ankle. *Am Fam Physician,* 1996;54(3):1012–1026.

47. Canale ST, Williams KD. Iselin's disease. *J Pediatr Orthop* 1992;12(1):90–93.

48. Omey ML, Micheli LJ. Foot and ankle problems in the young athlete. *Med Sci Sports Exerc* 1999;31(7 Suppl):S470–486.

49. Newman JS, Newberg AH. Congenital tarsal coalition: multimodality evaluation with emphasis on CT and MR imaging. *Radiographics* 2000;20(2):321–332.

50. Manusov EG, Lillegard WA, Raspa RF, Epperly TD. Evaluation of pediatric foot problems: Part I. The forefoot and the midfoot. *Am Fam Physician* 1996;54(2):592–606.

51. Bruce EJ, Hamby T, Jones DG. Sports-related osteochondral injuries: clinical presentation, diagnosis, and treatment. *Primary Care,*2005;32(1):253–276.

52. Wynne-Davies R. Family studies and the cause of congenital club foot. Talipes equinovarus, talipes calcaneo-valgus and metatarsus varus. *J Bone Joint Surg Br* 1964;46:445–463.

53. Dobbs MB, Gurnett CA. Update on clubfoot: etiology and treatment. *Clin Orthop Relat Res* 2009;467(5):1146–1153.

54. Uziel Y, Hashkes PJ. Growing pains in children. *Pediatr Rheumatol Online J* 2007;5:5.

55. Evans AM, Scutter SD. Prevalence of 'growing pains' in young children. *J Pediatr* 2004;145(2):255–258.

56. Baxter MP, Dulberg C. 'Growing pains' in childhood—a proposal for treatment. *J Pediatr Orthop* 1988;8(4):402–406.

CHAPTER 159

Hypermobility syndromes

Alan J. Hakim and Rodney Grahame

Introduction

Hypermobility denotes an increased range in movement as a consequence of ligament and tendon laxity in an otherwise anatomically normal joint. The laxity may arise due to abnormalities of collagen or other connective tissue proteins.

Hypermobility may go unnoticed, confer advantage (e.g. for dancers, musicians, sports persons, and gymnasts), or lead to mechanical injury, tendonitis, dislocations, delayed recovery, and chronic myalgia and arthralgia. Equally, it may be the first clue as to the presence of heritable disorders of connective tissue (HDCT), including joint hypermobility syndrome (JHS), Ehlers–Danlos syndrome (EDS), and Marfan's syndrome (MFS).

Hypermobility can vary considerably between the HDCT and between individuals with the same disorder. In itself it should not make or break a diagnosis. Given the ubiquitous nature of connective tissue proteins, the clinical manifestations of the HDCT are varied. Further enquiry reveals skin abnormalities, vascular fragility, early-onset osteoarthritis and osteoporosis, abnormal stature, and cardiovascular, respiratory, visceral, ocular, auditory and dental pathologies. In addition, there is an association with chronic widespread pain, fatigue, bowel dysfunction, and neuromuscular and cardiovascular dysautonomia.

Osteogenesis imperfecta and Stickler's syndrome are two other discrete HDCT with certain clinical features that overlap with JHS, EDS, and MFS. These are discussed in Chapter 150. There are also many other very rare metabolic disorders associated with joint dysmorphism, joint laxity, and skin hyperextensibility. These usually present at birth or in early childhood and are beyond the scope of this chapter.

Epidemiology

Prevalence

Population studies show a wide variation in the prevalence of generalized joint hypermobility (JHM) with values of 10–30% in males and 20–40% in females in adolescence and adulthood. JHM diminishes with age, and is more common in people of African and Asian descent. Twin studies suggest that it is strongly heritable.[1]

The prevalence of JHS is unknown. Extrapolating from one study of JHM that recorded symptoms consistent with JHS, the prevalence of JHS may be high as 1 in 150 among white female adults.[2] Other evidence to infer JHS is common comes from surveys of general rheumatology clinics where it is identifiable in up to 40% of patients presenting to a rheumatologist with non-inflammatory widespread musculoskeletal pain.[3,4]

The combined prevalence of all types of EDS is approximately 1 in 10 000 worldwide. The hypermobility type (EDSHM) is the most common, but the true prevalence is unknown given that many cases are mild and may not present clinically. The classical type occurs in 1 in 15 000–20 000 of the population, and the vascular type approximately 1 in 200 000. The prevalence of the more rare variants of arthrochalasia, kyphoscoliosis, and dermatosparaxis is unknown.

At approximately 1 in 20 000–30 000, MFS has a similar prevalence to the classical variant of EDS, though, as the reader will learn below, defining true MFS can be challenging as several conditions mimic its features; the true prevalence may therefore be less.

Genetics

EDS arises as a consequence of mutations to genes encoding the assembly of collagens I, III, and V (e.g. *COL1A1*, *COL1A2*, *COL3A1*, *COL3A2*, *COL5A1*, and *COL5A2*), and enzymes (e.g. *ADAMTS2*, *PLOD1*) or extracellular matrix glycoproteins (e.g. *TNXB*) that process or interact with collagen. Mutations in genes encoding collagens I, III, and V, and collagen-modifying enzymes have been identified in most forms of EDS.[5] In many cases a gene defect is not found; the diagnosis is reliant on clinical features. Also, a gene mutation can occur sporadically, the individual presenting with no family history of the condition.

No molecular, biochemical, or ultrastructural defect has been identified in EDSHM other than approximately 5–10% of cases demonstrate diminished levels of tenascin-X, due to heterozygous mutations in the *TNXB* gene.[6] Similarly the genetics of JHS is not understood, anecdotal observation of large family pedigrees suggesting a dominant inheritance.

MFS arises as a result of mutations to the gene *FBN1* on chromosome 15q21. The *FBN1* gene encodes production of fibrillin-1, a key component of microfibrils that add strength and flexibility to connective tissue. In MFS the quality and quantity of fibrillin-1 is reduced, with excessive release of growth factors from the microfibrillar structure. MFS has an autosomal dominant pattern of inheritance; however, a new mutation of the *FBN1* gene may arise in up to 25% of cases.

In a small percentage of cases a Marfan-like disorder (classified by some experts as MFS type II) is caused by mutations of the

TGFBR2 gene that instructs the production of the transforming growth factor (TGF)-β type II receptor. Interference with receptor function results in aberrant intracellular signalling and production of growth factors. Several other conditions share clinical features of MFS. Their genetic markers are described in the next section.

Diagnostic criteria

JHS was originally defined as 'the occurrence of symptoms in otherwise healthy hypermobile individuals'. It is now considered more complex than this, is defined by the Brighton Criteria (see Box 159.1),[7] and shares similar clinical features to EDSHM. Most authorities consider JHS and EDSHM to be synonymous. Similarly, up to one-third of JHS cases have a marfanoid habitus (see Box 159.2) in the absence of MFS and over one-half have blue sclerae in the absence of osteogenesis imperfect (OI). The validation of the criteria for JHS is a subject of current international research amongst experts in the field.

The Villefranche 1997 nosology[8] classifies EDS based on clinical features, biochemical and genetic defect, and the pattern of inheritance (Table 159.1). Six main descriptions substitute for an earlier Roman numeral classification: classic type (EDS I and II), hypermobility type (EDS III), vascular type (EDS IV), kyphoscoliosis type (EDS VI), arthrochalasia type (EDS VIIA and VIIB),

---

Box 159.1 The Beighton diagnostic criteria for the joint hypermobility syndrome[7]

Major criteria

1. A Beighton score of 4/9 or greater (either currently or historically)

2. Arthralgia for longer than 3 months in four or more joints

Minor criteria

1. A Beighton score of 1, 2 or 3/9 (0, 1, 2 or 3 if aged 50+)

2. Arthralgia in 1–3 joints or back pain or spondylosis, spondylolysis/spondylolisthesis

3. Dislocation in more than one joint, or in one joint on more than one occasion

4. Three or more soft tissue lesions (e.g. epicondylitis, tenosynovitis, bursitis)

5. Marfanoid habitus (tall, slim, span > height upper segment:lower segment ratio less than 0.85, arachnodactyly)

6. Skin striae, hyperextensibility, thin skin, or abnormal scarring

7. Eye signs: drooping eyelids or myopia or anti-mongoloid slant

8. Varicose veins or hernia or uterine/rectal prolapse.

- JHS is diagnosed in the presence of **two** major criteria, or **one** major and **two** minor criteria, or **four** minor criteria. **Two** minor criteria will suffice where there is an unequivocally affected first-degree relative.

- JHS is excluded by presence of EDS (other than the EDS hypermobility type, formerly EDS III) or Marfan's syndrome.

Box 159.2 Features of the marfanoid habitus

- High arched palate

- Arachnodactyly:

  - 'wrist sign' (Walker): positive if able to wrap the thumb and fifth finger of one hand around the opposite wrist such that the nail bed of the digits overlap with each other, *and/or*

  - 'thumb sign' (Steinberg): positive if the adducted thumb across the palm projects beyond the ulnar border in the clenched hand

- Pectus excavatum or carinatum

- Scoliosis >20° is a major criteria in MFS. It is also a sign of EDS kyphoscoliotic type. In other EDSvariants, and in JHS it may be present to a milder degree.

- Arm span:height ratio > 1.05 (in adults)

- Tall stature with upper body (pubis to crown):lower limb length (floor to pubis) ratio <1 (aged 0–5 years) and <0.85 (aged ≥10 years)

- Foot length (heel to first toe):height ratio > 0.15

- Hand length (wrist crease to third finger):height ratio > 0.11

---

and dermatosparaxis type (EDS VIIC). Six other forms are listed, including types V, X, and the periodontitis type (EDS VIII), all of which are extremely rare, reported in a handful of cases.

The classification of MFS has been refined from the Ghent 1996 criteria[9] that defined a set of major and minor manifestations in the presence or absence of an associated *FBN1* mutation or family history. Several conditions share certain manifestations with the risk of inadvertent classification as MFS. The 2010 revised Ghent criteria[10] emphasize aortic root disease (dilatation and dissection) and ectopia lentis (EL) (lens dislocation) as cardinal features of MFS, separating it from other conditions on the basis of the following:

- Degree of aortic root dissection or dilatation recorded as the Z-score (a measure of the aortic root (sinus of Valsalva) diameter standardized for age and body size). A score of ≥2 is deemed pathological.

- Presence of EL.

- Presence of a genuine *FBN1* mutation or known linkage to an *FBN1* haplotype.

- A weighted score of systemic features described in the 1996 criteria.

Box 159.3 describes the criteria for a diagnosis, and Box 159.4 the weighted score for systemic features in MFS. The differential diagnosis of Marfan-like conditions is more clearly defined as a consequence of the 2010 MFS criteria and includes:

- Ectopia lentis syndrome (ELS)—EL associated with mutations of *FBN1* and *ADAMTsL4*, and systemic features of MFS, but not aortic root disease.

- A phenotype of mitral valve prolapse, myopia, borderline and non-progressive aortic enlargement, and skin/skeletal systemic

Table 159.1 Classification of Ehlers–Danlos syndromes[7]

Type (Previous number classification)	Clinical manifestations		IP	Protein	Gene and chromosome (Ch)
	Major criteria	Minor criteria			
Classic (type I/II)	Skin hyperextensibility Widened atrophic scarring Joint hypermobility	Easy bruising Smooth and velvety skin Molluscoid pseudotumours Subcutaneous spheroids Muscular hypotonia Complications of joint hypermobility Surgical complications Positive family history	AD	Type V procollagen (found in ~50%)	COL5A1 (Ch 9) COL5A2 (Ch 2)
Hypermobility (type III)	Generalized joint hypermobility Mild skin involvement	Recurring joint dislocations Chronic joint pain Positive family history Premature osteoarthritis Pitral valve prolapse	AD	Tenascin-X (found in ~5%)	TNXB
Vascular (type IV)	Excessive bruising Thin, translucent skin Arterial/intestinal/uterine fragility or rupture Characteristic facial appearance	Acrogeria Early-onset varicose veins Hypermobility of small joints Tendon and muscle rupture Arteriovenous or carotid-cavernous sinus fistula Pneumo (haemo)thorax Positive family history, sudden death in close relative(s)	AD	Type III procollagen	COL3A1 (Ch 2)
Kyphoscoliotic (type VI)	Severe muscular hypotonia at birth Generalized joint laxity Kyphoscoliosis at birth Scleral fragility and rupture of the globe	Tissue fragility, including atrophic scars Easy bruising Arterial rupture Marfanoid habitus Microcornea Osteopenia	AR	Type VIA: Lysyl hydroxylase 1 Type VIB: not known	PLOD1 (Ch 1)
Arthrochalasis (type VIIA&B)	Severe generalized joint hypermobility with recurrent subluxations Congenital bilateral hip dislocation	Skin hyperextensibility Tissue fragility, including atrophic scars Easy bruising Muscular hypotonia Kyphoscoliois Mild osteopenia	AD	Type I procollagen	COL1A1 (Ch 17) COL1A2 (Ch 7)
Dermatosparaxis (type VIIC)	Severe skin fragility Sagging, redundant skin Excessive bruising	Soft, doughy skin texture Premature rupture of membranes Large hernias	AR	Procollagen-N-proteinase	ADAMTS2 (Ch 5)

AD, autosomal dominant; AR, autosomal recessive; IP, inheritance pattern.

Box 159.3 The revised Ghent criteria for the diagnosis of Marfan's syndrome (MFS)[10]

In the absence of a family history of MFS a diagnosis is made in the presence of one of four situations:

1. Aortic root Z-score ≥ 2 (or dissection) *and* ectopia lentis (EL), irrespective of systemic features except where these are indicative of other conditions*, *or*

2. Aortic root Z-score ≥ 2 (or dissection) *and* a systemic feature (Box 159.4) score ≥ 7 except where these are indicative of other conditions*. EL is assumed absent otherwise classification reverts to (1) above, and FBN1 status may be unknown or negative, *or*

3. Aortic root Z-score ≥ 2 (or dissection) *and* a recognized *FBN1* mutation (or definite linkage to a predisposing *FBN1* haplotype), *or*

4. Ectopia lentis *and* an *FBN1* mutation unequivocally associated with aortic disease. Aortic root dilatation/dissection may be absent at the time.

With a positive family history (defined by any of the above), a diagnosis of MFS is made in the presence of one of the following three situations:

1. Ectopia lentis

2. A systemic features score ≥ 7 except where these are indicative of other conditions*, *or*

3. Aortic root Z-score ≥ 2 (or dissection) in an individual of 20 years of age and older, *or* aortic root Z-score ≥ 3 (or dissection) if under aged 20 years

* The following conditions should be excluded: vascular EDS (see Table 159.1), Shprintzen–Goldberg syndrome (*FBN1* mutation, craniosynostosis, and mental retardation), and Loeys–Dietz syndrome (*TGFBR1/2* mutations, bifid uvula, cleft palate, craniosynostosis, hypertelorism, cervical spine instability, thin velvety skin, easy bruising, and arterial tortuosity and aneurysms).

Box 159.4 Scores for systemic features of Marfan's syndrome[10]

One point is given for each one of the following eight features:

- At least three of the following five facial features: dolichocephaly, enophthalmus, downslanting palpebral fissures, malar hypoplasia, and retrognathia

- Reduced elbow extension

- Pectus excavatum or chest asymmetry (excluding carinatum which scores 2, as below)

- Reduced upper/lower segment and increased arm span/height ratio (see Box 159.2), in the absence of severe scoliosis

- Scoliosis or thoracolumbar kyphosis

- Skin striae

- Mitral valve prolapse

- Myopia greater than 3 dioptres

Two points are given for each of the following five features:

- Pectus carinatum

- Pneumothorax

- Dural ectasia

- Protrusio acetabulae

- Hindfoot deformity (if plain pes planus, only score 1)

Three points are given for:

- Wrist *and* thumb sign (see Box 159.2) (if only one of the two signs is present, only score 1).

The maximum score is 20. A score ≥7 is indicative of MFS with the caveats in Box 159.2.

Clinical signs, symptoms, and investigation in heritable disorders of connective tissue

The contents of Table 159.1 and Boxes 159.1–159.4 provide a concise picture of the breadth of clinical features found in EDS, JHS, and MFS respectively. In addition patients often present with chronic widespread pain, fatigue, and neuromuscular, cardiovascular, and bowel autonomic dysfunction. Table 159.2 links the signs and symptoms in HDCT to genetic and radiological testing in pursuit of a diagnosis.

Considerable clinical overlap occurs between the HDCT, particularly in relation to the degree of skin signs, presence of mitral valve prolapse, and the marfanoid habitus (see Box 159.2). It is essential the clinician appreciate the overlap and degree to which signs manifest, in addition to the cardinal features and genetic markers that define a specific condition.

Musculoskeletal

Hypermobility

The extent to which generalized hypermobility (JHM) is present is most often described by applying the Beighton 9-point scoring system (Figure 159.1),[11] a tool that was refined originally for the purposes of epidemiological research.

features (MASS), scoring ≥5 as defined in Box 159.1 with at least one skeletal feature, associated with mutations of *FBN1* but not with EL.

- Mitral valve prolapse syndrome—an *FBN1* mutation associated with systemic features of MFS with a score <5 (see Box 159.3), mild aortic root dilatation (Z-score <2), but not with EL.

- Congenital contractile arachnodactyly—joint contractures associated with mutation of *FBN2*.

- Familial thoracic aortic aneurysm syndrome—vascular pathology associated with mutations of *TGFBR1/2* and *ACTA2* but not with features of the marfanoid habitus.

- Homocystinuria—an autosomal recessive defect in methionine metabolism caused by deficiency in cystathionine beta-synthase (CBS), also associated with insufficient vitamin B_{12} synthesis, and a deficiency in methylene-tetrahydrofolate reductase. In relation to MFS characteristic features include arachnodactyly, EL, and myopia. The vascular pathology is thromboembolic, not dilatation/dissection.

Table 159.2 Differentiating the heritable disorders of connective tissue

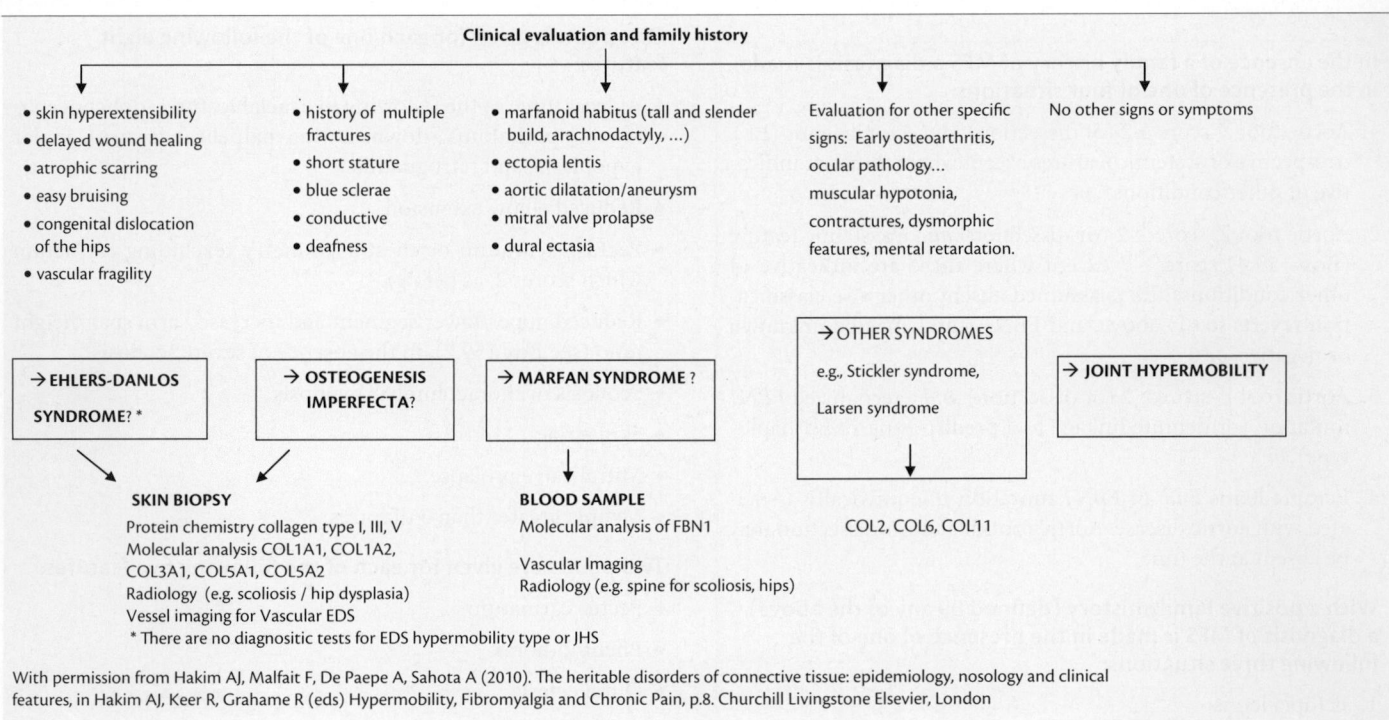

Clinical evaluation and family history

• skin hyperextensibility • delayed wound healing • atrophic scarring • easy bruising • congenital dislocation of the hips • vascular fragility	• history of multiple fractures • short stature • blue sclerae • conductive • deafness	• marfanoid habitus (tall and slender build, arachnodactyly, ...) • ectopia lentis • aortic dilatation/aneurysm • mitral valve prolapse • dural ectasia	Evaluation for other specific signs: Early osteoarthritis, ocular pathology... muscular hypotonia, contractures, dysmorphic features, mental retardation.	No other signs or symptoms

→ **EHLERS-DANLOS SYNDROME?** *

→ **OSTEOGENESIS IMPERFECTA?**

→ **MARFAN SYNDROME?**

→ OTHER SYNDROMES
e.g., Stickler syndrome, Larsen syndrome

→ **JOINT HYPERMOBILITY**

SKIN BIOPSY
Protein chemistry collagen type I, III, V
Molecular analysis COL1A1, COL1A2, COL3A1, COL5A1, COL5A2
Radiology (e.g. scoliosis / hip dysplasia)
Vessel imaging for Vascular EDS
* There are no diagnositic tests for EDS hypermobility type or JHS

BLOOD SAMPLE
Molecular analysis of FBN1

Vascular Imaging
Radiology (e.g. spine for scoliosis, hips)

COL2, COL6, COL11

With permission from Hakim AJ, Malfait F, De Paepe A, Sahota A (2010). The heritable disorders of connective tissue: epidemiology, nosology and clinical features, in Hakim AJ, Keer R, Grahame R (eds) Hypermobility, Fibromyalgia and Chronic Pain, p.8. Churchill Livingstone Elsevier, London

One point is given for each side of the body for the first four manoeuvres and one for spinal flexion. A value of 4 or more in males, and 5 or more in females, is considered suggestive of JHM. These figures are arbitrary cut-off points and the score ignores a number of joints that are often sites of injury and instability associated with hypermobility. These include the cervical and thoracic spine, shoulders, hips, ankles, midfoot, and first metatarsophalangeal (MTP) joint, and should be examined clinically to support the assertion of generalized JHM and determine sites of risk and pathology.

An alternative tool in screening for JHM is a simple five-part self-report questionnaire (Box 159.5).[12] It is a quick screen while taking the clinical history that may support the need for a detailed physical examination.

The presence and degree of hypermobility can vary considerably between the HDCT and between individuals with the same disorder. It is most pronounced in the variants of EDS and JHS and less common in MFS. Vascular EDS is typically associated with small-joint hypermobility affecting the digits.

Dislocation and subluxation

Joint dislocation or the lesser degree, subluxation, may be a recurrent in EDS and JHS. Sites often affected are the carpometacarpal and glenohumeral joint, and the patella. Congenital hip dislocation is a mark of arthrochalasia EDS, but may also be present in classic and hypermobility EDS. Severe joint hypermobility and multiple congenital joint dislocations of hips, elbows, and knees are the main features of Larsen's syndrome. Other symptoms of this condition include characteristic facial appearance of flat face, prominent forehead, widely spaced eyes, depressed nasal bridge, cleft palate

or uvula, dental abnormalities, short metacarpals and cylindrical fingers, equinovarus deformity of the foot, and cardiovascular lesions.

Tendinopathy and osteoarthritis

Abnormal tension forces and weightbearing at hypermobile joints can induce recurrent tendinosis and acute and chronic inflammation.

Population studies have not shown an association between JHM and local or generalized osteoarthritis. In EDS and JHS studies suggest an increased risk of articular dysfunction and premature osteoarthritis (OA) of the temporomandibular joint and or the knee where association with chondromalacia patellae is also reported and in the small joints of the hand (nodal OA).[13] At other sites such as the hip, premature secondary OA (see Chapter 139) might be accounted for by excessive prolonged weightbearing (e.g. dancers, athletes) or congenital anatomical abnormality including increased risk of recurrent dislocation.

Fractures

Low bone mineral density (BMD) is seen in EDS, MFS, and OI; it is especially common in OI. Osteopenia is a recognized feature of JHS. Aside from OI it is unknown whether the bone quality and low BMD in HDCT represents an independent risk for fragility fracture and there are no specific guidelines for managing osteoporosis associated with the HDCT. Assessment and treatment should be as per guidelines for the primary and secondary prevention of osteoporotic fracture in the general population (see Chapter 143).

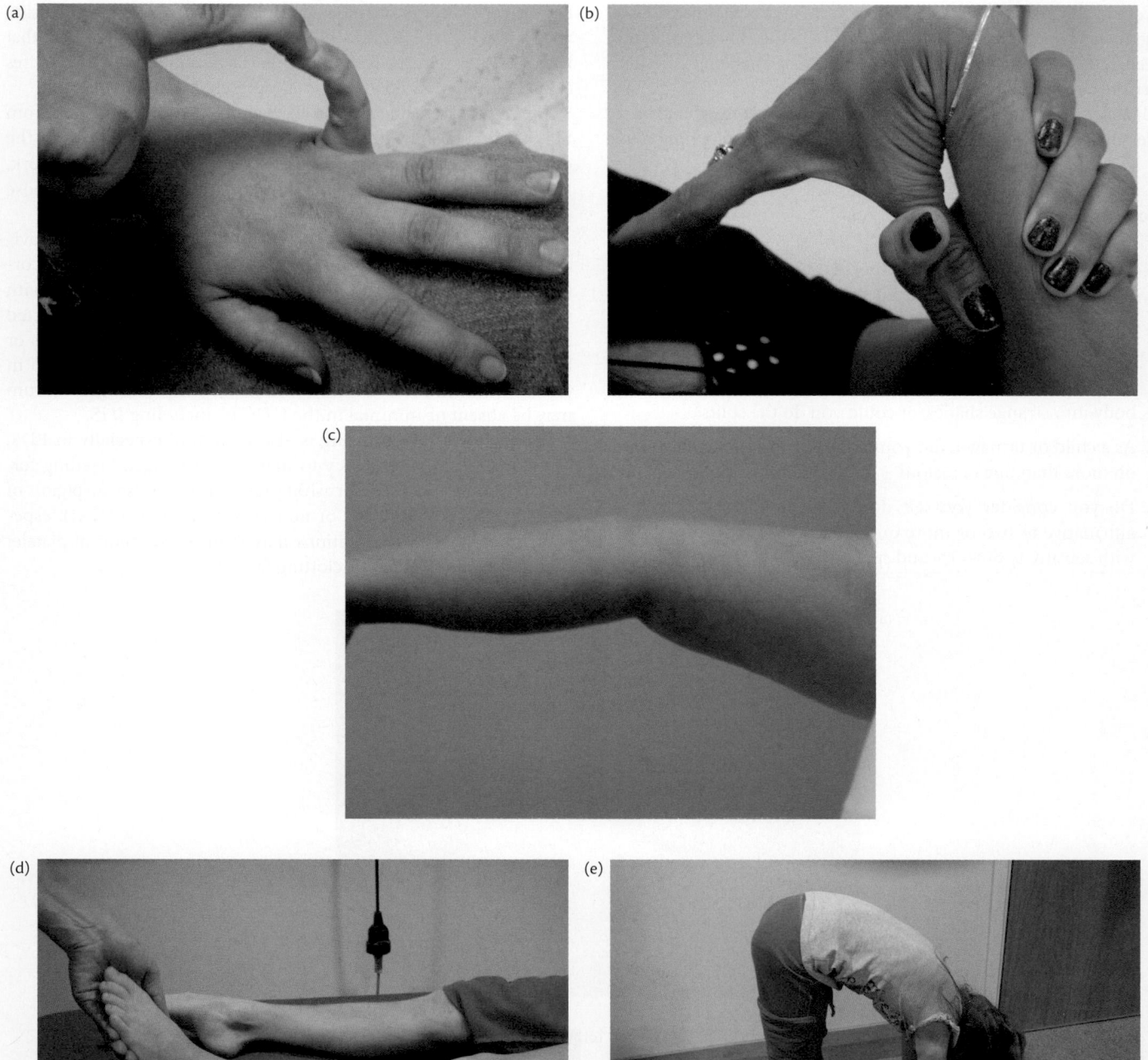

Fig. 159.1 The nine-point Beighton score for joint hypermobility.[11]

(a) Reproduced from Beighton PH, Solomon L, Soskolne CL (1973). Articular mobility in an African population. Ann Rheum Dis 32(5), 413–18 with permission of BMJ Ltd.

(b–e) Beighton PH, Solomon L, Soskolne CL (1973). Articular mobility in an African population. Ann Rheum Dis 32(5), 413–18

Skin, eyes, and dentition

Skin

Like the presence of JHM, skin signs are a valuable clue as to the presence of the HDCT. To varying degrees signs include soft and silky texture, semitransparency, hyperextensibility, easy bruising, abnormal scarring (such as atrophy or keloid), and early-onset stretch marks (striae atrophicae) at atypical sites (Figure 159.2).

Skin hyperextensibility is characteristic for all EDS subtypes, except for the vascular type. It is most prominent in classic EDS, severe in the rare dermatosparaxis variant, and evident to a lesser degree in EDSHM and JHS. In vascular EDS the skin is not hyperextensible, but thin and transparent, showing the venous pattern over the chest, abdomen, and extremities.

The skin overlying the dorsum of the hand is a convenient site for assessing extensibility. It is measured informally by pinching a fold between one's thumb and index finger and pulling the skin until resistance is felt (Figure 159.2A). The skin is hyperelastic, which means that it recoils after release. Testing in this way is subjective and requires experience. In MFS skin laxity is also present,[14] but infrequent.

The hyperextensible skin in EDS should be distinguished from that of cutis laxa syndromes, which result from mutations of the elastin gene and loss or fragmentation of the elastic fibre network. In the cutis laxa syndromes, the skin is redundant, hanging in loose folds, is not fragile, and heals normally.

Striae are common in the presence of pregnancy (striae gravidarum), obesity, Cushing's syndrome, or excess exogenous corticosteroids. In the HDCT there is often a different history with early-age onset of atrophic striae at body sites not usually affected by the other causes (e.g. extensor surfaces such as the elbows or knees, inner thigh, and across the chest). Striae are common in JHS and EDS, and to a lesser extent in MFS. Striae gravidarum may be absent or minimal in the HDCTs, including JHS.

Spontaneous easy bruising is also common, especially in EDS. The HDCT have a tendency to manifest prolonged bleeding following simple tasks, e.g. brushing teeth. It can raise suspicion of a haematological disorder, or non-accidental injury (NAI), especially in children. Investigations may require exclusion of platelet dysfunction and abnormal clotting factors.

Box 159.5 A brief questionnaire for identifying hypermobility[12]

1. Can you now (or could you ever) place your hands flat on the floor without bending your knees?

2. Can you now (or could you ever) bend your thumb to touch your forearm?

3. As a child, did you amuse your friends by contorting your body into strange shapes, *or* could you do the splits?

4. As a child or teenager, did your shoulder or kneecap dislocate on more than one occasion?

5. Do you consider yourself double-jointed?Answers in the affirmative to two or more questions suggests hypermobility with sensitivity 80–85% and specificity 80–90%.

(a)

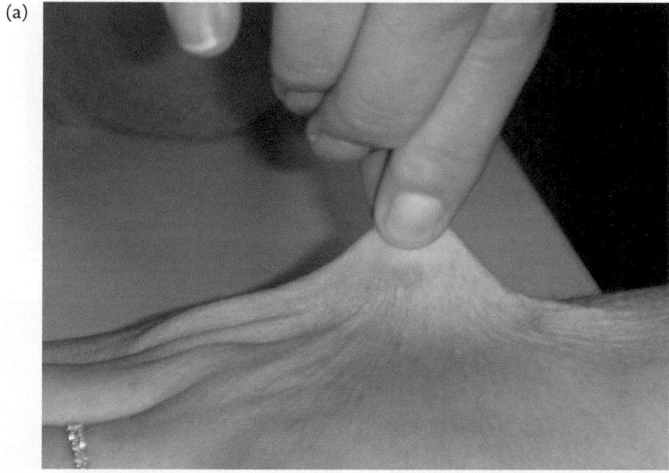

(b)

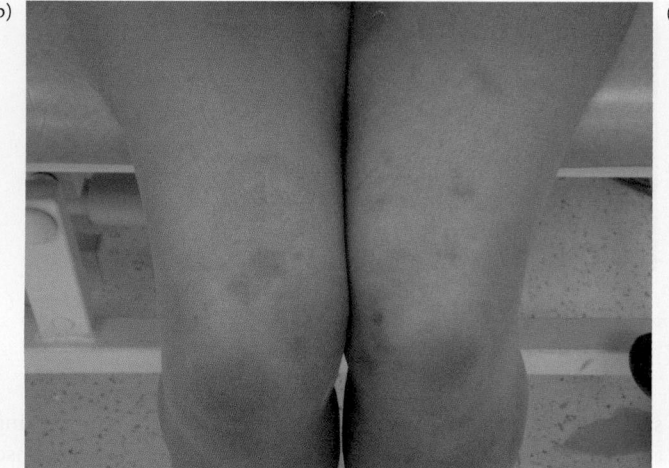

(c)

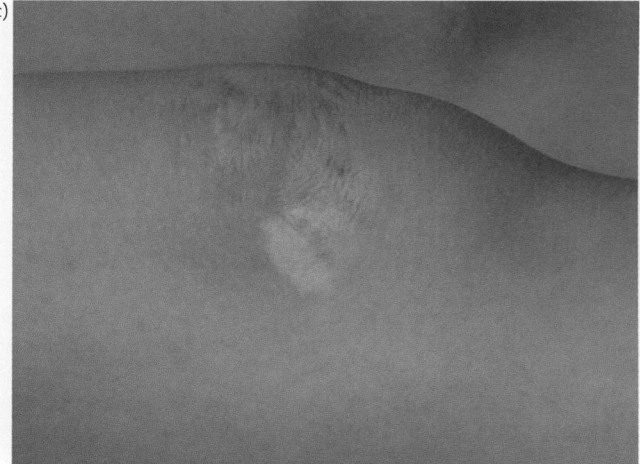

Fig. 159.2 Typical skin features in the heritable disorders of connective tissue.

With permission from Hakim AJ, Malfait F, De Paepe A, Sahota A (2010). The heritable disorders of connective tissue: epidemiology, nosology and clinical features, in Hakim AJ, Keer R, Grahame R (eds) Hypermobility, Fibromyalgia and Chronic Pain, p.14. Churchill Livingstone Elsevier, London.

Poor healing is another feature. Delayed wound healing and atrophic scarring is most prominent in classic, kyphoscoliotic, and arthrochalasia EDS. In JHS the pathology may be less obvious and something the patient may not have recognized as 'abnormal', only coming to light after surgery when the scar becomes atrophic.

Histological examination of the skin may assist in the diagnosis of EDS and OI (see Table 159.2) but may not be necessary where clinical signs are obvious, as in JHS, or when genetic markers are positive.

Eyes

Ocular pathologies in the HDCT range from the relatively benign and non-specific feature of blue sclera seen in OI or in a milder degree in JHS, to retinal detachments, keratoconus, scarring, and visual loss in MFS, Stickler's syndrome, and kyphoscoliotic EDS.

MFS is associated with EL (lens dislocation), early-onset cataract, glaucoma, severe myopia, and hypoplastic iris and ciliary muscles. Myopia is also a feature of JHS.

Formal assessment and treatment by an ophthalmologist is advised.

Dentition

Poor dentition (dentinogenesis imperfecta) is often present in OI. It is not specifically associated with JHS, EDS, or MFS, with the exception of the very rare variant of periodontitis EDS (type VIII). Potentially more problematic is the management of temporomandibular joint pain, sticking, and dislocation during normal dental care.

Visceral disorders

Abdomen and pelvis

Intrinsic weakness of supporting structures in JHS and EDS may lead to complications such as hiatus hernia, abdominal wall herniation, achalasia of the large bowel, and uterine or rectal prolapse.

There is growing recognition of functional gastrointestinal disorders (FGID) in JHS and EDS.[15] The symptoms are typical of irritable bowel syndrome, but may be a consequence of anatomical abnormalities as described above, autonomic dysfunction, or toxicity from analgesics such as non-steroidal anti-inflammatory drugs (NSAIDs) and opiates.

Upper and lower gastrointestinal (GI) endoscopy, tissue biopsy, and dynamic studies are necessary to delineate the nature of the FGID in patients who do not settle with simple remedies for irritable bowel.

The complications of pregnancy (Box 159.6) range from life-threatening (e.g. vascular collapse in MFS or EDS vascular type, or premature rupture of the fetal membranes and antepartum haemorrhage in the classical, vascular, and hypermobility types of EDS) to more benign but problematic. The latter include abdominal herniation, pelvic floor insufficiency, haemorrhoids, joint pain, trauma to the vaginal vault and surrounding soft tissues during labour with poor wound healing, and failure of anaesthetic nerve blocks.[16]

Pulmonary disease

Spontaneous pneumothorax occurs in approximately 5% of cases of MFS. Pneumothorax and asthma are also associated with EDS,[17]

Box 159.6 Potential complications of pregnancy and delivery in women with heritable disorders of connective tissue

- Life-threatening vascular rupture in MFS and vascular EDS
- Joint and spinal pains may increase during the course of pregnancy—typically in JHS and EDSHM
- Premature rupture of the membranes and thus of premature labour and delivery—typically classic or hypermobility types of EDS
- There is a tendency to rapid labour
- There is no absolute indication for caesarean section; the benefits and risks are a clinical judgement
- Positioning of the mother during labour should be done with caution, avoiding excessive force on overextended joints particularly at the hips and knees.
- Approximately two-thirds of patients with JHS/EDSHM report resistance to the effects of local anaesthetics.[15] This can complicate epidural anaesthesia or local infiltration for repair of soft tissue (e.g. episiotomy)
- Healing of wounds may be impaired and/or prolonged and surgical technique may need to be modified accordingly
- Care of the newborn baby more taxing than usual because of the degree of physical activity
- Pelvic floor problems (e.g. uterine prolapse) may occur in later life so that the practice of postnatal exercises is important
- Since many variants of the HDCT including JHS follow a dominant pattern of inheritance there is a high probability that offspring will manifest clinical features that may complicate delivery and the neonatal period, e.g. bruising, bleeding, dislocation, fracture

---

but are not specific to JHS. Investigation and treatment of asthma is the same as for the general population.

Cardiovascular disorders

Structural

Potentially life-threatening complications of MFS (see Box 159.3) include dilatation and dissection of the aortic root and ascending aorta. In vascular EDS there is an increased risk of rupture and/or dilatation/dissection of medium-sized vessels such as renal and splenic arteries. There is otherwise no significant arterial disease in other variants of EDS and JHS.

Mitral valve prolapse (MVP) is a common feature of MFS (and variants such as MASS) and less so of EDS and JHS. It may present with atypical chest pain or symptoms suggestive of extra/dropped beat and palpitations. More often in EDS and JHS it is a chance finding of no particular significance.

Concern over the possible presence of these pathologies should be investigated with echocardiography, Doppler ultrasound of the abdominal vasculature, and—if concerned as to the risk of aortic CT angiography or MRA of the aortic root, arch, and thoracic aorta. Annual echocardiography should be undertaken in the presence of aortic dilatation and MVP in MFS as both are progressive; in MFS individuals with normal aortic diameter repeat imaging is advisable every 2–3 years. The threshold for detailed imaging with MRA and preparation for surgical intervention is an aortic diameter of 4.5 cm or more, annual increases in aortic diameter in excess of 0.5cm, or a diameter of 5 cm or more at the sinus of Valsalva with or without aortic valve dysfunction.

Easy bruising is considered a consequence weakness of capillary connective tissue support structures. Varicose veins are also associated with EDS and JHS, potentially for the same reasons but also due to laxity of the vessel wall.

Autonomic

Patients with JHS and EDSHM often report fainting or feeling faint, palpitations, chest tightness, or shortness of breath in the absence of asthma or cardiac disease.

Often these symptoms are identifiable as autonomic disturbances of orthostatic hypotension, and postural orthostatic tachycardia syndrome (PoTS) is common in JHS. Hyperresponsiveness to α- and β-adrenoreceptor stimulation has been demonstrated.[18] Other postulated mechanisms for orthostasis include peripheral neuropathy and reduced vascular tone with lower-extremity pooling.

Autonomic dysfunction with orthostatic tachycardia and hypotension has also been documented in children with EDS. Similar atypical cardiac symptoms observed in adults with EDS, historically considered related to the presence of MVP, might also be secondary to cardiac dysautonomia.

These phenomena can be identified in clinic. Table 159.3 describes the typical features of each. More sophisticated testing using the facilities of an autonomic laboratory may be required if simple measures (see 'Management of heritable disorders of connective tissue' below) do not resolve the symptoms.

Pain

Musculoskeletal pain can occur in any of the HDCT. It can be severely disabling, as is often typical in JHS/EDSHM. It may be localized and acute, secondary to tendon or soft tissue inflammation or rupture, or to joint degeneration.

More often pain is widespread in the absence of significant mechanical damage to account for the symptoms. Axial, core and limb imbalance, poor proprioception, and poor recruitment within muscle groups, may account for the widespread nature of these symptoms. Neural tension related to peripheral nerve stretch in the presence of hypermobility may account for the neuropathic nature of the pain.

Often there is also an association with fatigue and disturbances of mood and psychosocial dysfunction similar to that of fibromyalgia and chronic fatigue syndrome.

Depending on the nature of the presentation, further investigation may require exclusion of a systemic inflammatory disorder, myopathy, nerve entrapment, or other causes of fatigue.

Management of the heritable disorders of connective tissue

There is no cure for HDCT. Management is multidisciplinary in the majority of cases, with a combination of symptom control and regression of deterioration through education, physical therapies, pharmacological interventions, and behavioural therapies (Figure 159.3).

Surgery

Surgical correction of structural problems such as intervertebral disc herniation, prolapse and, at its extreme, prevention of vascular rupture may be required. Surgery may be complicated by tissue fragility, bleeding, and scarring. These risks are of particular concern in classical and vascular EDS, and aortic involvement in MFS. To a lesser degree in JHS is associated with scarring and slow healing. Pregnancy and peripartum concerns are described in Box 159.6.

The surgical threshold for vascular intervention at the aorta is described above in the section on investigation. Beta-blockers remain the treatment of choice in preventing aortic complications.

Table 159.3 Definitions and associations with common cardiovascular autonomic disorders

Condition	Definition	Associations
Orthostatic hypotension (OH)	Rapid drop in blood pressure ≥20/10 mmHg in 3 min and up to 30 min (delayed reaction)	Dehydration
		Anaemia
		Extreme vasodilation, e.g. heat
		Congestive cardiac failure
		Drugs and substances associated with OH: diuretics, ACE inhibitors, alpha- and beta-blockers, tricyclic anti-depressants, nitrates, calcium channel blockers, opiates, sildenafil, phenothiazine, hydralazine, MAO inhibitors, bromocriptine, alcohol, illicit agents
Orthostatic intolerance	Delayed signs of OH	Deficiency of the renin–angiotensin–aldosterone system
Postural orthostatic tachycardia (PoTS)	>30 bpm rise in pulse, plus symptoms of OH, or>120 bpm within 10 min of head-up tilt or standing and usually without OH	Physical deconditioning

Adapted from Bravo J, Sanhueza G, Hakim AJ. Cardiovascular autonomic dysfunction and chronic fatigue in fibromyalgia and joint hypermobility syndrome. In: Hakim AJ, Keer R, Grahame R (eds) *Hypermobility, fibromyalgia and chronic pain*, Elsevier Churchill Livingstone, London, 2010:72.

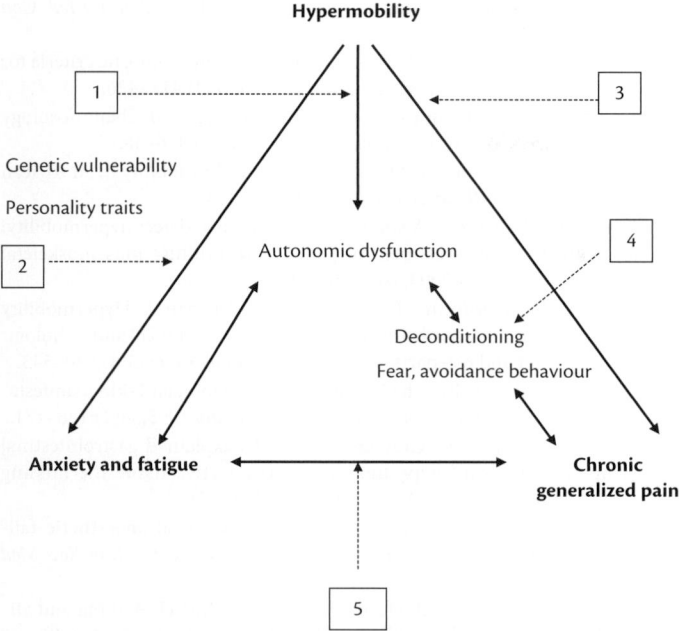

Hypermobility

1

Genetic vulnerability

Personality traits

2

Autonomic dysfunction

3

4

Deconditioning

Fear, avoidance behaviour

Anxiety and fatigue   Chronic generalized pain

5

1. Manage primary autonomic disturbance—beta-blockade, fluid balance etc
2. Treat primary and secondary anxiety/phobic syndromes
3. Analgesics
4. Physical rehabilitation
5. Behavioural therapies/clinical psychology/Antidepressants

Fig. 159.3 The association between hypermobility, autonomic disorders, anxiety syndromes, pain, physical pathologies and deconditioning, and the interplay of therapies.

Reproduced from Hakim AJ, Malfait F, De Paepe A, Sahota AThe heritable disorders of connective tissue: epidemiology, nosology and clinical features. In: Hakim AJ, Keer R, Grahame R (eds) Hypermobility, fibromyalgia and chronic pain, p.14. Churchill Livingstone Elsevier, London, 2010, with permission.

When they are not tolerated or are contraindicated, ACE inhibitors, calcium channel blockers, or angiotensin receptor blockers should be considered.

Intervention in aortic or mitral valve disease should be based on severity and speed of deterioration of valve and ventricular dysfunction. Acute dissection is a surgical emergency. Chronic dissection also warrants annual imaging. Indications for intervention include:

◆ sinus of Valsalva dilated more than 5 cm or the aorta at the site of dissection wider thanthan 5.5 cm

◆ annual increase in dilatation of the aorta in excess of 0.5 cm, or a strong family history of early dissection and rupture

◆ severe aortic regurgitation, or exacerbating ventricular dysfunction in the presence of severe mitral valve regurgitation

◆ intractable pain

◆ progressive limb and organ ischaemia

◆ planning pregnancy in high-risk individuals.

Orthopaedic intervention for recurrent dislocation and unstable joints is often unsuccessful in the long term and a last resort for severe cases when conservative measures have failed. Surgery for degenerative joint disorders is the same for hypermobile as non-hypermobile individuals, though rehabilitation needs to take account

of the individuals' general physical and cardiovascular well-being, as well as slow healing.

Pain relief

Analgesics are often helpful in acute and acute-on-chronic pain of soft tissue inflammation and joint degeneration. Widespread chronic pain tends not to respond to even the most potent analgesics. There are no randomized controlled trials of analgesics, neuropathic agents such as gabapentin and amitriptyline, or anti-depressants in the HDCT. Management is similar to that of fibromyalgia (see Chapter 160) and may incorporate the use of serotonergic and norepinephric agents that influence central pain processing as well as mood.[19] These agents may also assist in the symptom control of FGID.

The hormonal environment can also influence pain. Female patients report deterioration in their symptoms, including pain, clumsiness and reduced coordination, in the few days prior to menstruation when progesterone is at its highest. Progesterone-only contraceptive agents are more likely to exacerbate symptoms; this does not imply that oestrogen is specifically protective.

Cognitive behavioural therapies have also been shown to be of value in managing widespread pain, fatigue, and low mood in JHS.[20] This approach aims to:

◆ improve understanding of pain and communication with others over symptoms

◆ reduce pain related psychological distress

◆ improve sleep and reduce fatigue

◆ reduce dependency on opioid analgesics and other medication

◆ improve physical functioning with return to valued and enjoyable activities.

Interventions of autonomic dysfunction

The symptoms of cardiovascular autonomic dysfunction (CAD) can be reduced by ensuring good fluid balance and salt intake, physical conditioning to improve vascular return to the heart, intermittent use of elastic support stockings, and avoidance of very rapid changes in posture and environments that might cause rapid vasodilatation.[21] Pharmacological interventions should be used under the guidance of an autonomics specialist and usually after more detailed investigation including tilt-table testing. The aim is to either increase blood volume (fludrocortisone, clonidine, erythropoetin), increase vasoconstriction (midodrine, (pseudo)-ephidrine, etilefrine, selective serotonin re-uptake inhibitors, methylphenidate), or block the effect of (nor)epinephrine (adrenaline) (beta-blockers, disopyramide, ACE inhibitors).

Rehabilitation of patients with heritable disorders of connective tissue

In general rehabilitation/physiotherapy aims to improve function and enable individuals to self-manage their condition more effectively. A comprehensive assessment identifies postural abnormalities, movement faults, muscle imbalances, and weakness and balance deficits. A specific, individualized exercise programme is developed with the patient on the basis of the examination findings. The programme is usually focused on functional restoration through improvement of movement control, joint stability, stretching, muscle strength, and general fitness.[22]

Physiotherapy and occupational therapy methods need to be adapted to account of lax tissues with low tensile strength, a deconditioned musculature, poor proprioceptive acuity,[23] and age, with attention to specific needs (e.g. schooling, fitness) in childhood and adolescence.[24–26] Physical interventions aim to:

- build up muscles responsible for joint and core stability

- improve diminished proprioception

- mobilize to restore natural hypermobile range while avoiding harmful postures, weightbearing, or resting at the extremes of the hypermobile range

- improve general fitness by encouraging muscle-strengthening exercises

- educate in self-management

- support clinical psychology by enabling pacing, relaxation etc.

Occupational therapy (OT) and podiatry interventions include splints to protect unstable joints (e.g. small joints of the hands, wrist, elbow, knee, and ankle) and orthotics to correct midfoot pronation and hindfoot deformities that often induce discomfort when walking and encourage instability due to malalignment of the lower limbs. Hand therapy is invaluable in improving handwriting and other manual activities in hypermobile children and adults by means of improving hand strength and stamina.

Conclusion

The clinical manifestations of the HDCT are varied and as such individuals may present first to one of a number of clinicians. The challenge is to recognize each syndrome early and direct further investigation in the pursuit of cardinal signs and genetic markers accordingly. This requires a strong clinical acumen. While it is essential to exclude cardiovascular and ocular pathologies, even the more benign and non-life-threatening conditions can have a high morbidity. Interventions should be multidisciplinary, addressing the breadth of complications in a coordinated and holistic manner.

References

1. Hakim AJ, Cherkas LF, Grahame R, Spector T, MacGregor AJ. The genetic epidemiology of joint hypermobility: a female twin population study. *Arthritis Rheum* 2004;50(8):2640–2646.
2. Klemp P, Williams SM, Stansfield. Articular mobility in Maori and European New Zealanders. *Rheumatology* 2002;41(5):554–557.
3. Hakim AJ, Grahame R. High prevalence of joint hypermobility syndrome in clinic referrals to a North London community hospital. *Rheumatology* 2004;43(3 Suppl 1):198.
4. Bravo JF, Wolff C. Clinical study of hereditary disorders of connective tissues in a Chilean population: joint hypermobility syndrome and vascular Ehlers-Danlos syndrome. *Arthritis Rheum* 2006;54(2):515–523.
5. Pope FM, Burrows NP. Ehlers Danlos syndrome has varied molecular mechanisms. *J Med Genet* 1997;34(5):400–410.
6. Zweers M, Hakim AJ, Grahame R, Schalkwijk J. Tenascin-X deficiency and haploinsufficiency as a cause of generalized joint hypermobility. *Arthritis Rheum* 2004;50(9):2742–2749.
7. Grahame R, Bird HA, Dolan AL et al. The revised (Brighton 1998) criteria for the diagnosis of benign joint hypermobility syndrome. *J Rheumatol* 2000;27(7):1777–1779.
8. Beighton P, De Paepe A, Steinmann B et al. Ehlers Danlos syndromes: revised nosology, Villefranche 1997. Ehlers Danlos National Foundation

(USA) and Ehlers Danlos Support Group (UK). *Am J Med Gen* 1998;77(1):31–37.
9. De Paepe A, Devereux RB, Dietz HC et al. Revised diagnostic criteria for the Marfan syndrome. *Am J Med Genet* 1996;62(4):417–426.
10. Loeys BL, Dietz HC, Braverman AC et al. The revised Ghent nosology for the Marfan syndrome. *J Med Genet* 2010;47(7):476–485.
11. Beighton PH, Solomon L, Soskolne CL. Articular mobility in an African population. *Ann Rheum Dis* 1973;32(5):413–418.
12. Hakim AJ, Grahame R. A simple questionnaire to detect hypermobility: an adjunct to the assessment of patients with diffuse musculoskeletal pain. *Int J Clin Pract* 2003;57(2):163–166.
13. Jonnson H, Valtysdottir ST, Kjartansson O, Breddan A. Hypermobility associated with osteoarthritis of the thumb base: a clinical and radiological subset of hand osteoarthritis. *Ann Rheum Dis* 1996;55(8):540–543.
14. Grahame R, Pyeritz RE. The Marfan syndrome: joint and skin manifestations are prevalent and correlated. *Br J Rheumatol* 1995;34(2):126–131.
15. Zarate N, Farmer AD, Grahame R et al. Unexplained gastrointestinal symptoms and joint hypermobility: is connective tissue the missing link? *Neurogastroenterol Motil* 2010;22(3):252–e78.
16. Hakim AJ, Norris P, Hopper C, Grahame R. Local anaesthetic failure: does joint hypermobility provide the answer? *J Roy Soc Med* 2005;98(2):84–85.
17. Morgan AW, Pearson SB, Davies S, Gooi HC, Bird H. Asthma and airways collapse in two heritable disorders of connective tissue. *Ann Rheum Dis* 2007;66(10):1369–1373.
18. Gazit Y, Nahir AM, Grahame R, Jacob G. Dysautonomia in the joint hypermobility syndrome. *Am J Med* 2003;115(1):33–40.
19. Bird H. Pharmacotherapy in joint hypermobility syndrome. In: Hakim AJ, Keer R, Grahame R (eds) *Hypermobility, fibromyalgia and chronic pain*. Churchill Livingstone Elsevier, London, 2010:118–124.
20. Daniel HC. Pain management and cognitive behavioural therapy. In: Hakim AJ, Keer R, Grahame R (eds) *Hypermobility, fibromyalgia and chronic pain*. Churchill Livingstone Elsevier, London, 2010:125–141.
21. Bravo J, Sanhueza G, Hakim AJ. Cardiovascular autonomic dysfunction and chronic fatigue in fibromyalgia and joint hypermobility syndrome. In: Hakim AJ, Keer R, Grahame R (eds) *Hypermobility, fibromyalgia and chronic pain*. Churchill Livingstone Elsevier, London, 2010:69–82.
22. Keer R, Simmonds J. Joint protection and physical rehabilitation of the adult with hypermobility syndrome. *Curr Opin Rheumatol* 2010;23(2):131–136.
23. Ferrell WR, Tennant N, Sturrock RD et al. Proprioceptive enhancement ameliorates symptoms in the joint hypermobility syndrome. *Arthritis Rheum* 2004;50(10):3323–3328.
24. Keer R, Butler K. Physiotherapy and occupational therapy in the hypermobile adult. In: Hakim AJ, Keer R, Grahame R (eds) *Hypermobility, fibromyalgia and chronic pain*. Churchill Livingstone Elsevier, London, 2010:143–162.
25. Middleditch A. Physiotherapy and occupational therapy in the hypermobile adolescent. In: Hakim AJ, Keer R, Grahame R (eds) *Hypermobility, fibromyalgia and chronic pain*. Churchill Livingstone Elsevier, London, 2010:163–178.
26. Maillard SM, Payne J. Physiotherapy and occupational therapy in the hypermobile child. In: Hakim AJ, Keer R, Grahame R (eds) *Hypermobility, fibromyalgia and chronic pain*. Churchill Livingstone Elsevier, London, 2010:179–196.

Sources of patient information

Ehlers–Danlos syndrome: Ehlers-Danlos Support UK, PO Box 748, Borehamwood WD6 9HU www.ehlers-danlos.org

Hypermobility syndrome: Hypermobility Syndrome Association, 49 Orchard Crescent, Oreston, Plymouth PL9 7NF www.hypermobility.org/alert.htm

Marfan's syndrome: Marfan Association UK, Rochester House, 5 Aldershot Road, Fleet, Hants, GU51 3NG. www.marfan-association.org.uk

CHAPTER 160

Fibromyalgia and chronic widespread pain syndromes—adult onset

Anoop Kuttikat and Nicholas Shenker

Introduction

Pain and fatigue are the two most common symptoms of many musculoskeletal conditions. Chronic widespread pain and excessive fatigue have been reported in the Western medical literature since the 19th century. Sir William Gowers introduced the term 'fibrositis' in 1904 to describe this clinical constellation of symptoms believed to be caused by inflammation of fibrous tissue overlying muscles.[1] This term has been discarded since the understanding that there is no real inflammation in the tissues. Fibromyalgia syndrome (FMS) was adopted as the preferred name for this condition in the1970s and has gained international acceptance since the publication of American College of Rheumatology (ACR) classification criteria in 1990. The focus of this chapter is on FMS as the prototype disease manifesting with chronic widespread pain and fatigue.

Epidemiology

Chronic widespread pain is very common in the general population, with an estimated point prevalence of 11% in the United Kingdom.[2] The prevalence of FMS is 2–4% and increases with age, reaching a peak between 60 and 79 years. It is about six times more common in women.[3] Lower income, being disabled, divorced or separated, and having a lower educational status, are associated with FMS. Epidemiological studies in China have reported that FMS has rarely been seen there.[4] Genetic differences in pain processing and sociocultural attitudes to reporting chronic pain may explain this low prevalence. Investigation of FMS prevalence in migrant Chinese communities will help to delineate various factors underlying this phenomenon. FMS has a significant economic impact on society, in terms of both direct medical care costs and indirect costs related to work productivity loss. A study in the United States estimated that the annual costs per patient were $10 199 in 2005, nearly double that of matched controls.[5]

Classification and preliminary diagnostic criteria

The ACR classification criteria for FMS, published in 1990, are widely used in clinical trials (Box 160.1) These criteria have a sensitivity of 88.4% and a specificity of 81.1% in a population of patients with rheumatic disorders.[6]

Box 160.1 American College of Rheumatology 1990 classification criteria for fibromyalgia syndrome[a]

A. History of widespread pain for at least 3 months. Pain is considered widespread when it is present at all of the following sites:[b]

- the left side of the body
- the right side of the body
- above the waist
- below the waist
- in the axial skeletal (cervical spine *or* anterior chest *or* thoracic spine *or* low back)

B. Pain on digital palpation in at least 11 of the 18 tender point sites shown in Figure 160.1; all sites bilateral:[c]

[a]For purposes of classification, patients will be said to have FMS if both criteria A and B are satisfied. The presence of a second clinical disorder does not exclude the classification of FMS.

[b]Pain in a patient in for instance the left shoulder, right buttock, and cervical spine is generalized, according to these criteria.

[c]Digital palpation should be performed with an approximate force of 4 kg. For a tender point to be considered positive, the palpation has to be painful. 'Tender points' that are only tender are not tender points.

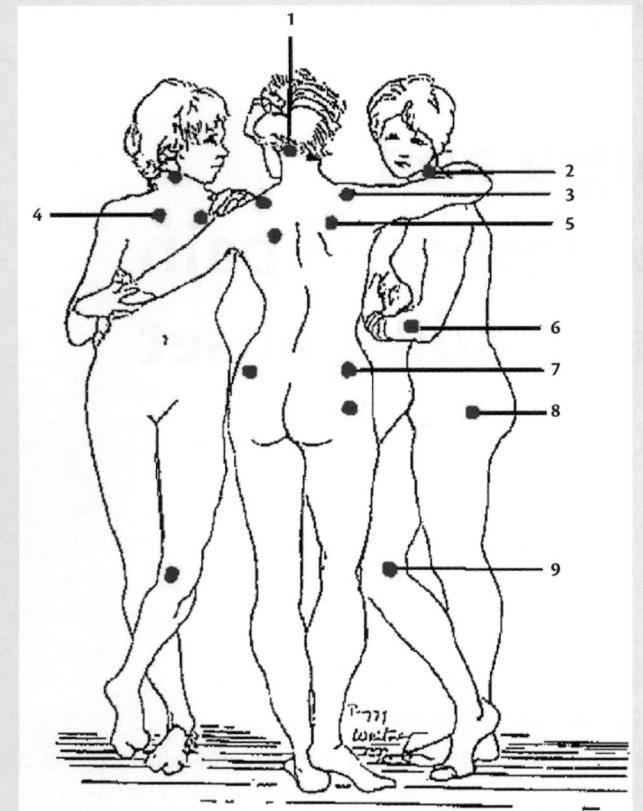

Fig. 160.1 Tender points in fibromyalgia syndrome: 1, occiput; 2, low cervical; 3, trapezius; 4, second rib; 5, supraspinatus; 6, lateral epicondyle; 7, gluteal; 8, greater trochanter; 9, knee. "Spinal irritation" and fibromyalgia: a Surgeon General and The Three Graces. Weissmann G. FASEB J. 2008 Feb;22(2):327–31.

The ACR has subsequently published preliminary diagnostic criteria in 2010 (Box 160.2), taking into account the importance of somatic symptoms such as fatigue and cognitive difficulties associated with FMS. These practical criteria developed for clinical use have a symptoms severity scale, making them useful for longitudinal use. They do not require a tender point count.[7]

Aetiopathogenesis

The precise aetiopathogenesis of FMS remains unclear. The current understanding is that the primary abnormality is in pain processing within the central nervous system. This dysfunctional pain processing results from the interplay between different factors including central sensitization, blunting of inhibitory pain pathways, altered neurotransmitters, and psychosocial stressors (Figure 160.2).[8]

FMS patients have augmented pain perception and decreased threshold to sensory stimuli such as heat, cold, electrical stimuli, and auditory tones.[9,10] Functional MRI studies have demonstrated that the insula is the part of the brain consistently hyperactive in FMS patients. The insula is critical in sensory integration and emotional processing of pain.[11] Decreased central μ-opioid receptor availability has been reported in FMS.[12] Substance P, an important neurotransmitter in pain, has been found to be increased threefold in the cerebrospinal fluid (CSF) of FMS patients compared to controls.[13] Excess levels of glutamate have been found in the posterior insula.[14] MRI studies have demonstrated significant loss of grey matter and accelerated age-related grey matter changes in FMS patients compared to controls.[15]

Box 160.2 American College of Rheumatology 2010 preliminary diagnostic criteria for fibromyalgia syndrome

Criteria

A patient satisfies diagnostic criteria for FMS if the following three conditions are met:

1. Widespread pain index (WPI) ≥7 and symptom severity (SS) scale score ≥5 or WPI 3–6 and SS scale score ≥9.

2. Symptoms have been present at a similar level for at least 3 months.

3. The patient does not have a disorder that would otherwise explain the pain.

Ascertainment

1. WPI

◆ Note the number of areas in which the patient has had pain over the last week. In how many areas has the patient had pain?

Shoulder girdle (left, right)	Hip (left, right)	Jaw (left, right)	Upper back
Upper arm (left, right)	Upper leg (left, right)	Chest	Lower back
Lower arm (left, right)	Lower leg (left, right)	Abdomen	Neck

◆ Score will be between 0 and 19.

2. **SS scale score**: fatigue, waking unrefreshed, cognitive symptoms

◆ For the each of the three symptoms above, indicate the level of severity over the past week using the following scale: 0 = no problem, 1 = slight or mild problems, generally mild or intermittent, 2 = moderate, considerable problems, often present and/or at a moderate level, 3 = severe: pervasive, continuous, life-disturbing problems

◆ Considering somatic symptoms in general*, indicate whether the patient has: 0 = no symptoms, 1 = few symptoms, 2 = a moderate number of symptoms, 3 = a great deal of symptoms

◆ The SS scale score is the sum of the severity of the three symptoms (fatigue, waking unrefreshed, cognitive symptoms) plus the extent (severity) of somatic symptoms in general.

◆ The final score is between 0 and 12.

* Somatic symptoms that might be considered
Muscle pain, irritable bowel syndrome, fatigue/tiredness, thinking or remembering problem, muscle weakness, headache, pain/cramps in the abdomen, numbness/tingling, dizziness, insomnia, depression, constipation, pain in the upper abdomen, nausea, nervousness, chest pain, blurred vision, fever, diarrhoea, dry mouth, itching, wheezing, Raynaud's phenomenon, hives/welts, ringing in ears, vomiting, heartburn, oral ulcers, loss of/change in taste, seizures, dry eyes, shortness of breath, loss of appetite, rash, sun sensitivity, hearing difficulties, easy bruising, hair loss, frequent urination, painful urination, and bladder spasms.

Sleep abnormalities

Disrupting slow wave sleep in healthy volunteers for three consecutive nights was found to be associated with decreased pain threshold and fatigue.[16] An increased cyclic alternating pattern, an

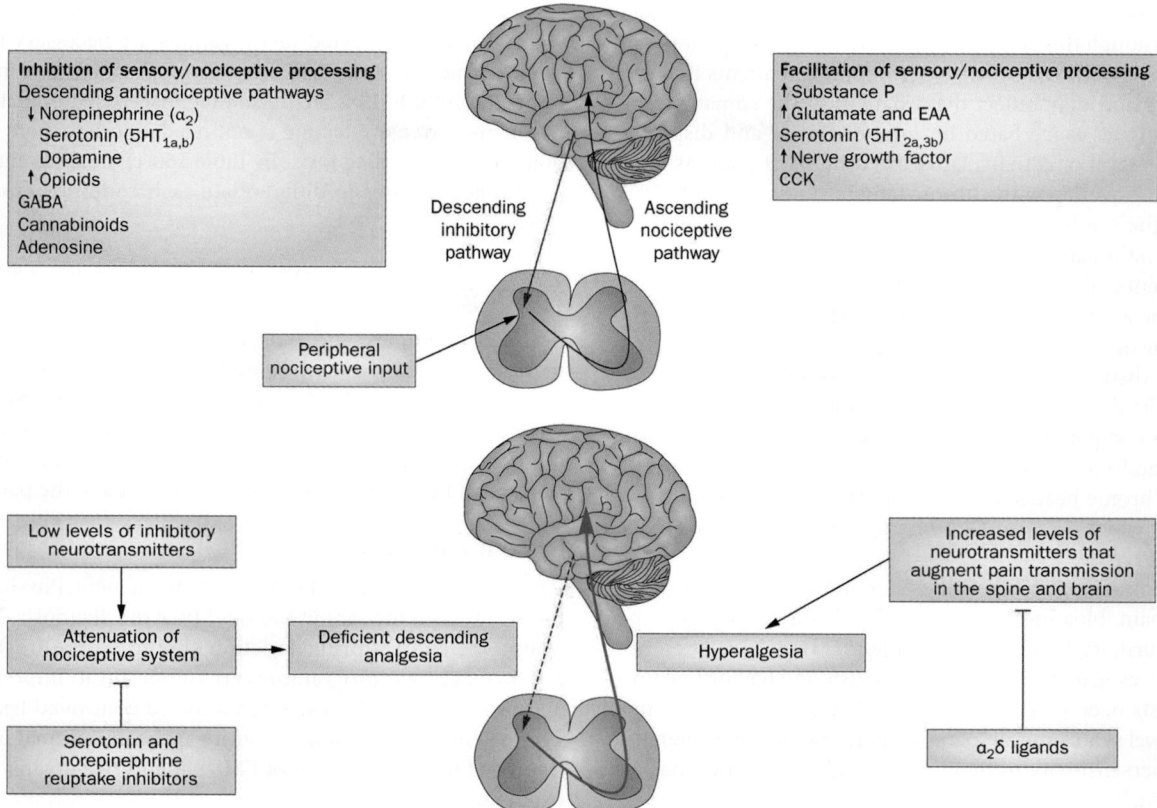

Fig. 160.2 Pathways of pain processing implicated in fibromyalgia syndrome: (a) Central nervous system neurotransmitters that either facilitate or inhibit pain transmission. (b) Low levels of inhibitory neurotransmitters lead to an attenuated anti-nociceptive system. Serotonin–noradrenaline (norepinephrine) reuptake inhibitors increase anti-nociceptive activity. Levels of neurotransmitters that augment pain transmission, such as substance P, glutamate/EAA and nerve growth factor, are increased in fibromyalgia, and probably contribute to increased activity in ascending pain transmission pathways. $\alpha_2\delta$ ligands might be working to decrease the release of excitatory neurotransmitters. 5-HT, 5-hydroxytryptamine (serotonin); CCK, cholecystokinin; CNS, central nervous system; DNIC, diffuse noxious inhibitory control; EAA, excitatory amino acids; GABA, γ-aminobutyric acid.

(Adapted from Schmidt-Wilcke T, Clauw DJ. Fibromyalgia: from pathophysiology to therapy. Nat Rev Rheumatol 2011, with permission.)

electroencephalographic marker of unstable sleep, was noted to be correlated to the severity of symptoms in FMS.[17] However, these changes are neither specific nor sensitive for FMS.

Hypothalamic–pituitary–adrenal axis dysfunction

Hyperactive stress response linked to altered hypothalamic–pituitary–adrenal (HPA) axis activity has been demonstrated in some patients. Corticotropin-releasing factor (CRF) is the principal central nervous system (CNS) mediator of the stress response. CRF concentration in the CSF was found to be associated with pain but not fatigue symptoms in FMS.[18]

Autonomic dysfunction

Dysautonomia has been documented in some patients using heart rate variability analysis and the tilt table test. Dysfunctional autonomic system is characterized as a sympathetic nervous system that is persistently hyperactive but is hyporeactive to stress. This could potentially explain many FMS symptoms including orthostatic hypotension causing dizziness, excessive arousal/awakening episodes, sicca symptoms, and pseudo-Raynaud's phenomenon.[19]

Genetics

Observational studies have shown familial aggregation of chronic pain disorders. A proband study showed that first-degree relatives

of FMS patients are 8.5 times more likely to have FMS than relatives of rheumatoid arthritis patients.[20] Family members of FMS patients are also much more likely to have irritable bowel syndrome, temporomandibular disorder, headaches, and other regional pain syndromes.[21] A Swedish twin registry study of 15 950 pairs of twins estimated that approximately 50% of the risk of developing chronic widespread pain is genetic or shared environmental influences.[22] A large candidate gene association study revealed that four genes—*TAAR1* (trace amine associated receptor 1), *CNRI* (cannabinoid receptor 1), *RGS4* (regulator of G protein signalling 4), and *GRIA4* (glutamate receptor, ionotrophic, AMPA 4)—were associated with FMS. These genes may contribute to the pathophysiology of FMS and represent potential therapeutic targets.[23]

Infection

Several infectious agents including hepatitis C, Epstein–Barr virus, borrelia, mycoplasma, and HIV have been postulated as potential triggers although none has conclusively been proven to be associated with FMS.[24]

Clinical features

FMS patients complain of generalized aches and pains affecting all four quadrants of the body. The pain is usually reported in the muscles and joints. They describe a feeling of joint swelling or 'puffiness', although this is not clinically evident. Poor spatiotemporal awareness is reported by many chronic pain patients including FMS patients and may reflect disturbances in the somatosensory system.[25] Fatigue, exacerbated by minor activity and disproportionate to the level of activity, is reported by most patients. There is considerable overlap with chronic fatigue syndrome and 55% of chronic fatigue syndrome patients fulfil the diagnostic criteria for FMS.[26] Paraesthesiae in arms and legs are reported in more than 80% of patients, although formal neurological testing is usually normal in the absence of a coexistent disorder such as carpal tunnel syndrome or cervical radiculopathy.[27]

Cognitive disturbances including short-term memory impairment and difficulties in concentrating are more common in fibromyalgia patients compared to patients with other rheumatic diseases.[28] Depression and/or anxiety have been reported in 30–50% of FMS patients.[29] Chronic headaches were reported in 76% of patients in one study, of which 63% were of the migraine type and 8% related to analgesic overuse.[30]

FMS patients may also have other symptoms such as chest pain, abdominal pain, bloating, alternating diarrhoea/constipation, pelvic pain, or urinary frequency and urgency. They have often been previously investigated by different specialists and having had unremarkable tests been given a diagnosis of 'non-cardiac chest pain', 'irritable bowel syndrome' or 'painful bladder syndrome/interstitial cystitis'. Hypersensitivity to light, noise, and temperature has also been reported.[31]

Differential diagnosis and investigations

FMS can coexist with other systemic diseases. Many systemic diseases can present with some of the fibromyalgia symptoms. FMS was found in 22% of systemic lupus erythematosus (SLE) and 17% of inflammatory arthritides patients in a cohort study of over 23 000

patients.[32] Careful history and physical examination combined with limited but targeted investigations are necessary to diagnose other mimics or coexisting conditions. However, it is important to remember that FMS is a clinical diagnosis based on pattern recognition and extensive testing is not needed unless there are specific pointers to other diagnosis. In Table 160.1, the differential diagnosis and key features to differentiate each condition from FMS are listed.

Management

FMS is a complex and heterogeneous condition and effective management should adopt a multidisciplinary approach. Careful assessment of pain, function, and psychosocial context is essential. Patient education, physical therapies, psychological therapies, and pharmacotherapy are the four pillars of management. The interventions must be tailored to the individual needs of the patient.

Patient education

Patient education plays a key part in management. Physicians should provide reassurance about the validity of the diagnosis. Minimizing symptoms and restoring function should be the treatment goal. Self-management programmes are important to improve function and promote self-efficacy. A randomized controlled trial (RCT) of 216 patients found that a 2 month psychoeducational intervention improved functional status of FMS patients to a greater extent than usual care.[33]

Physical therapies

Physical therapies have been investigated in over 90 clinical trials with more than 5000 patients with FMS in the last three decades. However, many of these trials have suffered from lack of quality and high attrition rates.[34] Balneotherapy or heated pool therapy was found to be effective in a small number of fairly high-quality studies.

Table 160.1 Differential diagnosis of fibromyalgia syndrome

Condition	Key differentiating features	Investigations
Rheumatoid arthritis	Symmetrical synovitis	ESR, CRP, RF, anti-CCP, radiography
SLE/Sjögren's	Systemic features (eye, skin, kidney involvement)	ANA, anti-dsDNA, ENA, ESR, Schirmer's test
Polymyalgia rheumatica	Age > 50, stiffness > pain, rapid response to prednisolone (dose < 15 mg/;day)	ESR, CRP
Polymyositis/;dermatomyositis	Muscle weakness, rash	CK, ANA
Hypothyroidism	Puffy facies, delayed relaxation of deep tendon reflexes	TFTs
Hyperparathyroidism	Renal stones, bone disease	Calcium, phosphate, 25(OH) D, PTH, AP
Vitamin D deficiency/osteomalacia	Presence of risk factors: lack of sunlight exposure, malabsorption, intestinal bypass surgery, coeliac disease, chronic liver or kidney disease	25(OH) D
Disseminated malignancy/;myeloma	Significant weight loss; rapidly progressive symptoms	CRP, ESR, radiography, isotope bone scan, serum and urine protein electrophoresis
Glucocorticoid withdrawal	Medication history	SST

25(OH) D, 25-hydroxy vitamin D; ANA, anti-nuclear antibodies; anti-CCP, anti-cyclic citrullinated peptide; anti-dsDNA, anti-double-stranded DNA; AP, alkaline phosphatase; CK, creatine kinase; CRP, C-reactive protein; ENA, extractable nuclear antigens; ESR, erythrocyte sedimentation rate; PTH, parathyroid hormone; RF, rheumatoid factor; SLE, systemic lupus erythematosis; SST, short synacthen test; TFTs, thyroid function tests.

Three out of the five studies also included exercise. Improvement in both pain and function was reported.[35,36]

Moderate to high-intensity aerobic exercise by means of Nordic walking twice a week for 15 weeks was found to improve functional capacity in an RCT of 67 patients. Pain severity, however, did not change over time during the exercise period.[37] Individually tailored exercise programmes are recommended, given their safety and benefit to general health.[38] T'ai chi, a Chinese mind–body practice, was found to produce significant improvement in pain and function in a randomized trial lasting 12 weeks when compared to a control group who had wellness education and stretching exercises. Longer and larger studies are needed to confirm the usefulness of t'ai chi.[39]

Psychological therapies

Psychological therapies including cognitive behavioural therapy (CBT), mindfulness-based treatments, relaxation, and biofeedback are used to treat FMS. CBT offers short-term, goal-orientated psychotherapy emphasizing changes in thought patterns and behaviours. CBT is incorporated into pain management programmes based on the physiological link between chronic pain and mood disorders. A meta-analysis of 23 trials involving nearly 1400 patients found a significant but small size effect for CBT and relaxation/biofeedback in reducing pain, improving sleep, and decreasing depression.[40]

Pharmacotherapy

Pregabalin, milnacipran, and duloxetine are approved by the United States Food and Drug Authority (FDA) for FMS. The European Medicines Agency, to date, has not authorized any drugs specifically for FMS. Milnacipran is currently not available in the United Kingdom. Several agents are recommended by the European League Against Rheumatism (EULAR) for treating FMS (Table 160.2). EULAR and the American Pain Society recommend the use of low-dose tricyclic anti-depressants, particularly amitriptyline, as initial

Table 160.2 Pharmacotherapy in fibromyalgia syndrome

Drug	Mechanism	Dose (mg/day)	Approval/ recommendation	NNT
Amitryptiline	Serotonin and/or norepinephrine reuptake inhibitor anti-cholinergic and anti-histaminergic	10–75	EULAR	3.54
Tramadol	Weak μ-opioid receptor agonist Norepinephrine reuptake inhibitor	50–400	EULAR	5.5
Milnacipran	SNRI	100–200	EULAR, FDA	10.96
Duloxetine	SNRI	30–120	EULAR, FDA	8.21
Pregabalin	$\alpha_2\delta$ ligand	75–450	EULAR, FDA	6.6
Gabapentin	$\alpha_2\delta$ ligand	900–2700	EULAR	5.8

$\alpha_2\delta$ ligand, blocks $\alpha_2\delta$ subunit of voltage-gated calcium channels; EULAR, European League Against Rheumatism; FDA, United States Food and Drug Authority; NNT, number needed to treat to improve pain by ≥30%; SNRI, serotonin norepinephrine (noradrenaline) reuptake inhibitor.

pharmacological management of patients with FMS.[41,42] Selective serotonin reuptake inhibitors (e.g. fluoxetine) were found to be less efficacious than the tricyclics or serotonin–norepinephrine (noradrenaline) reuptake inhibitors (e.g. duloxetine, milnacipran), suggesting a critical role for norepinephrine in the analgesic effect in FMS.[43]

A large meta-analysis that compared the efficacy and acceptability of amitriptyline, duloxetine, and milnacipran found that all three were superior to placebo except duloxetine for fatigue, milnacipran for sleep disturbance, and amitriptyline for health-related quality of life. The significant effects of amitriptyline and duloxetine were small and those of milnacipran not substantial. There were no significant differences in acceptability of these drugs.[44] Pregabalin and gabapentin were found to be safe and efficacious in large meta-analyses of RCTs. Dizziness, somnolence, and weight gain were the most frequently reported dose-related adverse effects.[45–47]

Expert opinion does not recommend corticosteroids or strong opiates for the treatment of FMS, as they have significant long-term side effects and there are no clinical trials data to support their use. Simple analgesics such as paracetamol (acetaminophen) and weak opiates may be considered as adjuncts for pain relief. Tramadol, alone and in combination with paracetamol, was found to be effective and well tolerated.[48] Combination of drugs with different mechanisms of action are useful in many patients. A randomized trial found that combining fluoxetine 20 mg in the morning with amitryptiline 25 mg in the evening was more effective than either medication alone.[49]

Case history

A 40 year old woman presented with a 1 year history of widespread pain, excessive fatigue, and unrefreshing sleep. She has noted 'puffiness' of her hands and paraesthesiae in her hands and legs. She reports alternating diarrhoea and constipation associated with abdominal cramps. She denies any bloody stools or weight loss. Past medical history includes irritable bowel syndrome and anxiety.

Physical examination reveals no signs of active synovitis or dactylitis. No skin rash or nail changes. Tinel's and Phalen's test are negative. No objective muscle weakness or sensory changes. There are multiple tender points in all four quadrants and along her spine.

This patient has a typical presentation of FMS. Initial tests include a full blood count, urea, electrolytes, CRP, ESR, thyroid function tests, liver function tests, bone profile, B$_{12}$, and folate to rule out coexisting conditions. Given her abdominal symptoms, screening for coeliac disease may be considered.

All laboratory tests were completely normal and she was given a diagnosis of FMS. She was relieved to know that all her symptoms can be explained by the diagnosis. She was given a patient information leaflet on FMS. She was started on amitriptiline 10 mg daily to be taken 2 hours before sleep and was advised that the dose can be gradually titrated up to 50 mg daily. She was also prescribed tramadol for breakthrough pain. She was enrolled in a holistic multidisciplinary programme incorporating physical and psychological therapies.

Prognosis and monitoring

A longitudinal study of 1500 FMS patients over 11 years found that 25% had at least moderate improvement of pain and 35% had worsening of symptoms.[50] In a 2007 cross-sectional study of an internet questionnaire in the United States, 51% of 1700 FMS patients in the working age group were working, with 70% of this group working more than 30 hours/week. Employment, higher income, and education were strongly associated with fewer symptoms.[51]

There is an increased risk of suicide and death from suicide among FMS patients.[52] An increased incidence of cancer and cardiovascular deaths in patients with chronic widespread pain has also been reported.[53] A British birth cohort study found that such individuals had unhealthy diet, increased rates of smoking, and higher body mass index compared to those without pain.[54] Physicians should emphasize the importance of improving lifestyle factors such as diet, smoking status, and body weight as part of the overall management plan.

The revised Fibromyalgia Impact Questionnaire (FIQR) is a validated tool useful for monitoring symptoms. It has good psychometric properties, can be completed in less than 2 minutes, and is easy to score.[55]

Conclusion

FMS is a common condition characterized by chronic widespread pain, unrefreshing sleep, excessive fatigue, and other somatic symptoms. There is altered pain processing in the CNS. Functional MRI studies have shown changes in neuronal circuitry responsible for sensory integration and emotional processing of pain. FMS can coexist with other systemic diseases. Careful history, detailed physical examination, and targeted investigations are needed to diagnose coexisting conditions. A multidisciplinary approach incorporating patient education, physical therapies, psychological therapies, and pharmacological agents can improve the quality of life of FMS patients. Improving lifestyle factors such as smoking status, diet, and weight can significantly extend their life expectancy.

References

1. Gowers WR. A lecture on lumbago: its lessons and analogues: delivered at the national hospital for the paralysed and epileptic. *Br Med J* 1904;1(2246):117–121.
2. Croft P, Rigby A, Boswell R, Schollum J, Silman A. The prevalence of chronic widespread pain in general population. *Rheumatol* 1993;20(4):710–713.
3. Wolfe F, Ross K, Anderson J, Russell IJ, Hebert L. The prevalence and characteristics of fibromyalgia in the general population. *Arthritis Rheum* 1995;38(1):19–28.
4. Zeng Q, Chen R, Darmanwan J et al. Rheumatic diseases in China. *Arthritis Res Ther* 2008;10(1):R17.
5. White LA, Birnbaum HG, Kaltenboeck A et al. Employees with fibromyalgia: medical comorbidity, healthcare costs, and work loss. *J Occup Environ Med* 2008;50(1):13–24.
6. Wolfe F, Smythe HA, Yunus MB et al. The American College of Rheumatology 1990 Criteria for the Classification of Fibromyalgia. Report of the Multicenter Criteria Committee. *Arthritis Rheum* 1990;33(2):160–172.
7. Wolfe F, Clauw DJ, Fitzcharles MA et al. The American College of Rheumatology preliminary diagnostic criteria for fibromyalgia and measurement of symptom severity. *Arthritis Care Res* 2010;62(5):600–610.
8. Abeles AM, Pillinger MH, Solitar BM, Abeles M. Narrative review: the pathophysiology of fibromyalgia. *Ann Intern Med* 2007;146(10):726–734.

9. Kosek E, Ekholm J, Hansson P. Sensory dysfunction in fibromyalgia patients with implications for pathogenic mechanisms. *Pain* 1996;68:375–383.
10. Gerster JC, Hadj-Djilani A. Hearing and vestibular abnormalities in primary Fibrositis syndrome. *J Rheumatol* 1984;11:678–680.
11. Smith HS, Harris R, Clauw D. Fibromyalgia: an afferent processing disorder leading to a complex pain generalized syndrome. *Pain Physician* 2011;14(2):E217–E245.
12. Harris RE, Clauw DJ, Scott DJ et al. Decreased central mu-opioid receptor availability in fibromyalgia. *J Neurosci* 2007;27(37):10000–10006.
13. Russell IJ, Orr MD, Littman B et al. Elevated cerebrospinal fluid levels of substance P in patients with the fibromyalgia syndrome. *Arthritis Rheum* 1994;37(11):1593–1601.
14. Harris RE, Sundgren PC, Craig AD et al. Elevated insular glutamate in fibromyalgia is associated with experimental pain. *Arthritis Rheum* 2009;60(10):3146–3152.
15. Kuchinad A, Schweinhardt P, Seminowicz DA et al. Accelerated brain gray matter loss in fibromyalgia patients: premature aging of the brain? *J Neurosci* 2007;27(15):4004–4007.
16. Lentz MJ, Landis CA, Rothermel J, Shaver JL. Effects of selective slow wave sleep disruption on musculoskeletal pain and fatigue in middle aged women. *J Rheumatol* 1999;26(7):1586–1592.
17. Rizzi M, Sarzi-Puttini P, Atzeni F et al. Cyclic alternating pattern: a new marker of sleep alteration in patients with fibromyalgia? *J Rheumatol* 2004;31(6):1193–1199.
18. McLean SA, Williams DA, Stein PK et al. Cerebrospinal fluid corticotropin-releasing factor concentration is associated with pain but not fatigue symptoms in patients with fibromyalgia. *Neuropsychopharmacology* 2006;31(12):2776–2782.
19. Martinez-Lavin M. Biology and therapy of fibromyalgia. Stress, the stress response system, and fibromyalgia. *Arthritis Res Ther* 2007;9(4):216.
20. Arnold LM, Hudson JI, Hess EV et al. Family study of fibromyalgia. *Arthritis Rheum* 2004;50(3):944–952.
21. Buskila D, Neumann L, Hazanov I, Carmi R. Familial aggregation in the fibromyalgia syndrome. *Semin Arthritis Rheum* 1996;26:605–611.
22. Kato K, Sullivan PF, Evengard B, Pedersen NL. Importance of genetic influences on chronic widespread pain. *Arthritis Rheum* 2006;54:1682–1686.
23. Smith SB, Maixner DW, Fillingim RB et al. Large candidate gene association study reveals genetic risk factors and therapeutic targets for fibromyalgia. *Arthritis Rheum* 2012;64(2):584–593.
24. Ablin JN, Shoenfeld Y, Buskila D.. Fibromyalgia, infection and vaccination: two more parts in the etiological puzzle. *J Autoimmun* 2006;27(3):145–152.
25. McCabe CS, Cohen H, Hall J et al. Somatosensory conflicts in complex regional pain syndrome type 1 and fibromyalgia syndrome. *Curr Rheumatol Rep* 2009;11(6):461–465.
26. Yunus MB. The prevalence of fibromyalgia in other chronic pain conditions. *Pain Res Treat* 2012;2012:584573.
27. Simms RW, Goldenberg DL. Symptoms mimicking neurologic disorders in fibromyalgia syndrome. *J Rheumatol* 1988;15(8):1271–1273.
28. Katz RS, Heard AR, Mills M, Leavitt F. The prevalence and clinical impact of reported cognitive difficulties (fibrofog) in patients with rheumatic disease with and without fibromyalgia. *J Clin Rheumatol* 2004;10(2):53–58.
29. Weir PT, Harlan GA, Nkoy FL et al. The incidence of fibromyalgia and its associated co-morbidities: a population-based retrospective cohort study based on International Classification of Diseases, 9th Revision codes. *J Clin Rheumatol* 2006;12(3):124–128.
30. Marcus DA, Bernstein C, Rudy TE. Fibromyalgia and headache: an epidemiological study supporting migraine as part of the fibromyalgia syndrome. *Clin Rheumatol* 2005;24(6):595–601.
31. Geisser ME, Glass JM, Rajcevska LD et al. A psychophysical study of auditory and pressure sensitivity in patients with fibromyalgia and healthy controls. *J Pain* 2008;9:417–422.
32. Wolfe F, Petri M, Alarcón GS et al. Fibromyalgia, systemic lupus erythematosus (SLE), and evaluation of SLE activity. *J Rheumatol* 2009;36(1):82–88.

33. Luciano JV, Martínez N, Peñarrubia-María MT et al. Effectiveness of a psychoeducational treatment program implemented in general practice for fibromyalgia patients: a randomized controlled trial. *Clin J Pain* 2011;27(5):383–391.

34. Häuser W, Klose P, Langhorst J et al. Efficacy of different types of aerobic exercise in fibromyalgia syndrome: a systematic review and meta-analysis of randomised controlled trials. *Arthritis Res Ther* 2010;12(3):R79.

35. Altan L, Bingol U, Aykac M, Koc Z, Yurtkuran M. Investigation of the effects of pool based exercise on fibromyalgia syndrome. *Rheumatol Int* 2004;24:272–277.

36. Evcik D, Kizilay B, Gokcen E. The effects of balneotherapy on fibromyalgia patients. *Rheumatol Int* 2002;22:56–59.

37. Mannerkorpi K, Nordeman L, Cider A, Jonsson G. Does moderate-to-high intensity Nordic walking improve functional capacity and pain in fibromyalgia? A prospective randomized controlled trial. *Arthritis Res Ther* 2010;12:R189.

38. Jones KD, Burckhardt CS, Clark SR, Bennett RM, Potempa KM. A randomized controlled trial of muscle strengthening versus flexibility training in fibromyalgia. *J Rheumatol* 2002;29:1041–1048.

39. Wang C, Schmid CH, Rones R et al.. A randomized trial of tai chi for fibromyalgia. *N Engl J Med* 2010;363(8):743–754.

40. Glombiewski JA, Sawyer AT, Gutermann J et al. Psychological treatments for fibromyalgia: a meta-analysis. *Pain* 2010;151(2):280–295.

41. Goldenberg DL. Pharmacologic treatment of fibromyalgia and other chronic musculoskeletal pain. *Best Pract Res Clin Rheumatol* 2007;21: 499–511.

42. Carville SF, Arendt-Nielsen S, Bliddal H et al. EULAR evidence based recommendations for the management of fibromyalgia syndrome. *Ann Rheum Dis* 2008;67:536–541.

43. Anderberg UM., Marteinsdottir I, von Knorring L. Citalopram in patients with fibromyalgia—a randomized, double-blind, placebo-controlled study. *Eur J Pain* 2000;4:27–35.

44. Häuser W, Petzke F, Üçeyler N, Sommer C. Comparative efficacy and acceptability of amitriptyline, duloxetine and milnacipran in fibromyalgia syndrome: a systematic review with meta-analysis. *Rheumatology* (Oxford) 2011;50(3):532–543.

45. Hauser W, Bernardy K, Uceyler N, Sommer C. Treatment of fibromyalgia syndrome with gabapentin and pregabalin—a meta-analysis of randomized controlled trials. *Pain* 2009;145:69–81.

46. Tzellos TG, Toulis KA, Goulis DG et al. Gabapentin and pregabalin in the treatment of fibromyalgia: A systematic review and a meta-analysis. *J Clin Pharm Ther* 2010;35:639–656.

47. Roskell NS, Beard SM, Zhao Y, Le TK. A meta-analysis of pain response in the treatment of fibromyalgia. *Pain Pract* 2011;11(6):516–527.

48. Bennett RM, Kamin M, Karim R, Rosenthal N. Tramadol and acetaminophen combination tablets in the treatment of fibromyalgia pain: a double-blind, randomized, placebo-controlled study. *Am J Med* 2003;114:537–545.

49. Goldenberg D, Mayskiy M, Mossey C, Ruthazer R, Schmid C. A randomized, double-blind crossover trial of fluoxetine and amitriptyline in the treatment of fibromyalgia. *Arthritis Rheum* 1996;39(11):1852–1859.

50. Walitt B, Fitzcharles MA, Hassett AL et al. The longitudinal outcome of fibromyalgia: a study of 1555 patients. *J Rheumatol* 2011;38(10): 2238–2246.

51. Rakovski C, Zettel-Watson L, Rutledge D. Association of employment and working conditions with physical and mental health symptoms for people with fibromyalgia. *Disabil Rehabil* 2012;34(15):1277–1283.

52. Wolfe F, Hassett AL, Walitt B, Michaud K. Mortality in fibromyalgia: a study of 8,186 patients over thirty-five years. *Arthritis Care Res,* 2011;63(1):94–101.

53. McBeth J, Symmons DP, Silman AJ et al. Musculoskeletal pain is associated with a long-term increased risk of cancer and cardiovascular-related mortality. *Rheumatology* 2009;48:74–77.

54. Vandenkerkhof EG, Macdonald HM, Jones GT, Power C, Macfarlane GJ. Diet, lifestyle and chronic widespread pain: results from the 1958 British Birth Cohort Study. *Pain Res Manag* 2011;16(2):87–92.

55. Bennett RM, Friend R, Jones KD et al. The revised fibromyalgia impact questionnaire (FIQR): validation and psychometric properties. *Arthritis Res Ther* 2009;11(4): R120.

Sources of patient information

Arthritis Care UK: 18 Stephenson Way, London NW1 2HD www.arthritis-care.org.uk

Arthritis Research UK: Copeman House, St Mary's Gate, Chesterfield, Derbyshire S41 7TD www.arthritisresearchuk.org

Fibromyalgia Association UK: PO Box 206, Stourbridge, West Midlands DY9 8YL. www.fibromyalgia-associationuk.org

CHAPTER 161

Chronic musculoskeletal pain in children and adolescents

Jacqui Clinch

Introduction

Paediatricians review a large number of children who have a wide variety of musculoskeletal pains.[1,2] The most common chronic pain conditions reviewed in paediatric rheumatology settings include diffuse idiopathic musculoskeletal pain (DIPs, also called juvenile fibromyalgia or chronic widespread pain), chronic pain related to childhood hypermobility, complex regional pain syndromes (CRPS), chronic back pain and persistent joint pain following previous or controlled inflammation, e.g. juvenile idiopathic arthritis (JIA). For most young people presenting to clinic the chronic experience of pain has often had a large and wholly negative impact on the physical and psychological well-being of the young person and their family.[1] Data has shown that chronic pain also has a serious negative impact on financial well-being, not only for each family but also for the economy as a whole. It is conservatively calculated that the annual financial burden of adolescent chronic pain on the United Kingdom economy is £3840 million.[3] Children who suffer persistent musculoskeletal pain and associated symptoms have a significant chance of developing chronic widespread pain and continuing to have pain and pain-associated disability in adult life.[4]

In this chapter, there is a review of the epidemiology of musculoskeletal pain in childhood; discussion of current theories of the aetiology of pain; evaluation of the impact of chronic pain, the clinical features of common pain presentations and their relevance to diagnosis and treatment planning and finally rehabilitation interventions aimed at the management of chronic pain.

Epidemiology

In a recent study up to 83% of the school-aged children had experienced an episode of pain during the preceding 3 months.[5] Pain is a normal sensation but becomes disabling when it persists and is associated with suffering. In this same study sample, 30.8% of the children and adolescents stated that the pains had been present for over 6 months. Musculoskeletal pains accounted for 64% of all the pains that were reported.[3] Other studies support this finding.[6,7]

Whether there is more chronic pain, or whether children with chronic pain are presenting more frequently, is not known.

The epidemiology of diffuse idiopathic pain (DIPs, also referred to as juvenile fibromyalgia or chronic widespread pain) is difficult to accurately assess.[8] The HUNT study[9] showed that 8.5% of a population of 7373 adolescents fulfilled the criteria for DIPs, whereas a United Kingdom study showed the prevalence of chronic widespread pain in over 6000 17 year old schoolchildren to be 4.3%.[10] Hypermobility, as currently defined, is present in 19.8% of the normal United Kingdom adolescent population.[11] We do not know the percentage of children who suffer pain as a direct consequence of their joint laxity. Undoubtedly some young people do have mechanical pain; whether this is directly due to a hypermobility syndrome is not currently evidenced in large studies.

Low back pain is common in adolescence; the HUNT study showed this to be 16.7% for girls and 11% for boys (one day a week for at least 3 months).[9]

The prevalence of CRPS in adults is 26 per 100 000 person-years.[12] In children the epidemiology has not been robustly evaluated but recent studies have demonstrated that, unlike the adult population, about 90% of the cases reported are females aged 8–16 years.[19–21] There tends to be delay in recognizing the diagnosis.[13] A complicating factor is the lack of clear diagnostic criteria for children; currently the adult International Association for the Study of Pain (IASP) criteria are used.

In JIA it is clear that persistent pain is a significant problem for many children.[14] Approximately 40% describe pain 5 years after diagnosis.[15] A significant minority progress to develop localized or diffuse musculoskeletal pain that is not directly related to the control of their inflammatory condition.[16]

There is a robust finding that girls experience more pain than boys[9,17] (although it should be noted that the incidence in boys may be increasing[5]). Children living in low-educated, low-income families have a 1.4-fold increase in the odds of having pain.[19] The incidence of chronic widespread musculoskeletal pain peaks in older adolescence.[17] Significantly, a large cohort study showed that multiple common symptoms in childhood are associated with a moderately increased risk of chronic widespread pain in adulthood.[4]

Clinical features of chronic musculoskeletal pain

General features

It is not unusual for pain to start in a localized area of the body and lead to a reluctance to mobilize. Discomfort and pain intensity increase and become constant and the young person may avoid contact with, or use of, an area of the body affected, which can lead to muscular spasms, abnormal posture and gait, and—with chronic avoidance—greatly reduced fitness. This can lead to fear of pain and movement, and a resultant amplification of the pain. In some circumstances pain has a direct effect on other systems, leading to symptoms that can be as disabling as the pain itself. Symptoms and signs frequently associated are listed in Box 161.1.

Box 161.1 Symptoms and signs frequently associated in chronic musculoskeletal pain

- **Hypervigilance and hypersensitivity**. Children often report a heightened awareness of pain and pain-associated cues.[2] It is unclear whether this is caused by fear of pain, or hypersensitivity of pain receptors in allodynic and hyperalgesic ranges. Clinically this presents as young people describing unbearable pain on minimal skin contact, and heightened fear of being touched, for example, on examination.

- **Perceived thermodysregulation**. This is more common in adolescent girls. Limbs are particularly cool and mottled. Occasionally there will be areas that are very red and hot to touch on a background of the mottled skin. There may also be an abnormal perception of temperature with an increase in thermal pain sensitivity.[18]

- **Autonomic dysfunction**. Pain is a powerful stressor. Continuous pain signals, immobility, and fatigue act directly on the autonomic system.[20] In an environment of physical and emotional anxiety, the sympathetic system is more active. This leads to tachycardia, hyperventilation (compounded with panic attacks), cold sweats, blurred vision, abdominal pain, and extreme pallor. Girls particularly complain of nausea, dizziness, and episodes of feeling faint. Children look unwell during these episodes of increased pain. It is not unusual for attending paediatricians to investigate cardiovascular, neurological, and gastrointestinal systems in an attempt to elicit pathology.

- **Musculoskeletal disequilibrium**. These young people are still growing, often in their peripubertal growth spurt, and this can have lasting effects on the final positioning. Proprioceptive signals from the joints are reduced and the limb held in a rigid, fixed position. Legs may 'give way'. Knees and hips are held flexed, feet are inverted, and hands are clenched with flexed wrists. These positions are often described as the most comfortable. Muscles and tendons quickly tighten and this complicates the pain and disability. The adaptive positioning of a young person with leg or abdominal pains particularly affects the gait and resting positions and thus alters the loads on the spine and pelvis.

Specific childhood musculoskeletal pain conditions commonly seen in a rheumatology setting

Diffuse idiopathic pain syndromes (juvenile fibromyalgia/chronic widespread pain)

This describes widespread pain, often located over muscles and joints, where there is significant pain-associated disability.[20,21] There are no current agreed criteria, although some authors have suggested the term juvenile fibromyalgia can be used and have recently proposed diagnostic criteria akin to the adult fibromyalgia criteria.[8]

The onset of pain in DIPs/juvenile fibromyalgia.[2,20] is often gradual. There may have been an initial insult or trauma but often there is no obvious trigger and only vague recollections of the time of onset. The pain is generalized. There may be areas of allodynia (profound hypersensitivity to light touch) and hyperalgesia, but there is often an absence of the autonomic changes that we see in more localized pain conditions.[1] What is striking in young people with diffuse pain is fatigue, poor sleep pattern, and extremely low mood. It is widely believed, however, that the low moods in adolescents are reactive (to the pain-associated disability) rather than a primary depression.[22] This is in contrast to adults with fibromyalgia where primary depression is frequently seen.[23]

Complex regional pain syndrome

The diagnosis of CRPS remains a clinical one.[24,25] There may be precipitating trauma. In children, the lower limb is much more commonly involved than the upper limb. The pain is usually out of proportion to the inciting event and accompanied by allodynia. The children most often describe the pain as burning and describe sensations akin to dysaesthesia. Autonomic changes are present; these include swelling, reduced cutaneous perfusion, and thermodynamic instability. As this is present on the background of a developing musculoskeletal system, limbs can become distorted and feet or hands held in seemingly fixed and often flexed positions. Cutaneous blood flow often reduces; the affected limb develops a purplish hue with other colour changes that can cause concern to the child and family (Figure 161.1). The skin takes on a shiny, stretched appearance, with coarse hairs developing in patches. In rare severe cases, trophic changes develop with ulceration and marked wasting. Figure 161.2 shows the marked changes on thermography (reduction in cutaneous blood flow represented by lack of heat detected) of the wasted, flexed, ulcerated foot that is shown in Figure 161.3. Although the pathophysiology is poorly understood, many features, particularly the neurological abnormalities, suggest both peripheral and central nervous system (CNS) involvement. Peripheral small-fibre neuropathy as an aetiology and inflammation involving small nerve fibres (neurogenic inflammatory pain) has been suggested. A tissue inflammatory aetiology has been investigated over the past 25 years. However, these inflammatory aspects differ from those seen in other conditions involving tissue inflammation. The suggestion that CRPS in children is a different clinical entity than that seen in the adult is probably incorrect, as recent evidence would suggest that the pathophysiology is most likely identical involving endocrine, behavioural, developmental, and environmental factors that distinguish clinical presentation in children from the adult.[13]

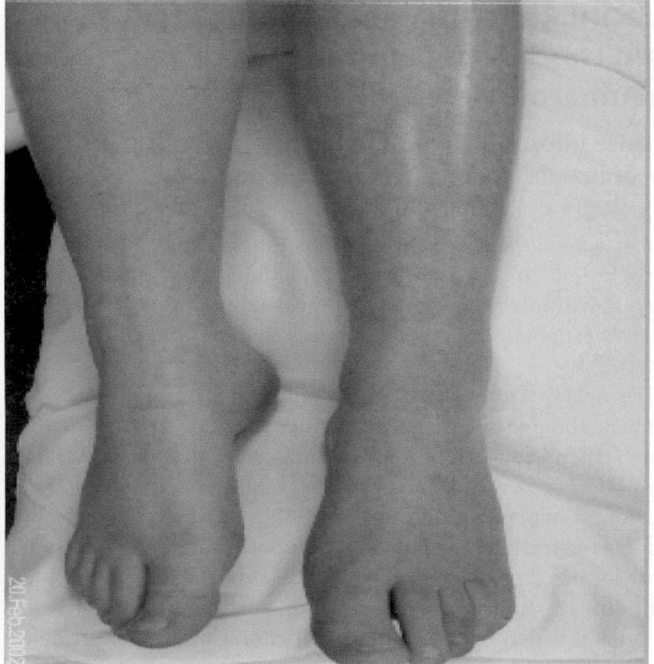

Fig. 161.1 Early changes in chronic regional pain syndrome; left leg.

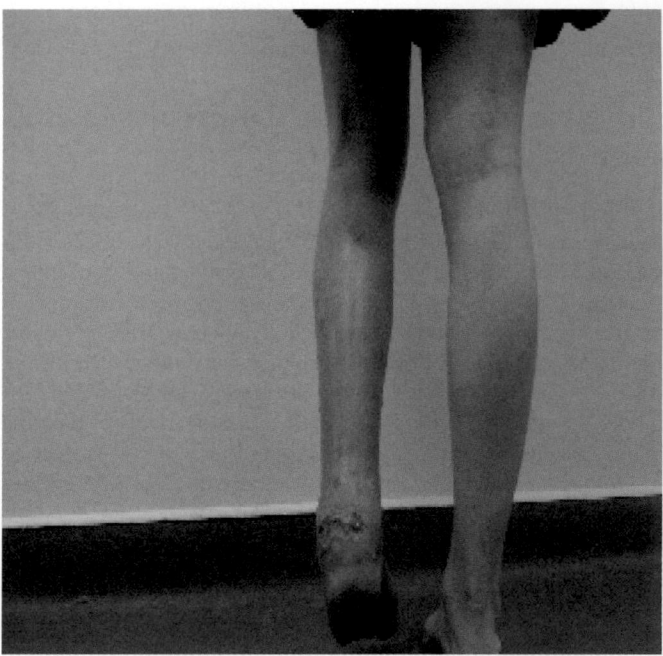

Fig. 161.3 Wasted, ulcerated left leg in advanced chronic regional pain syndrome.

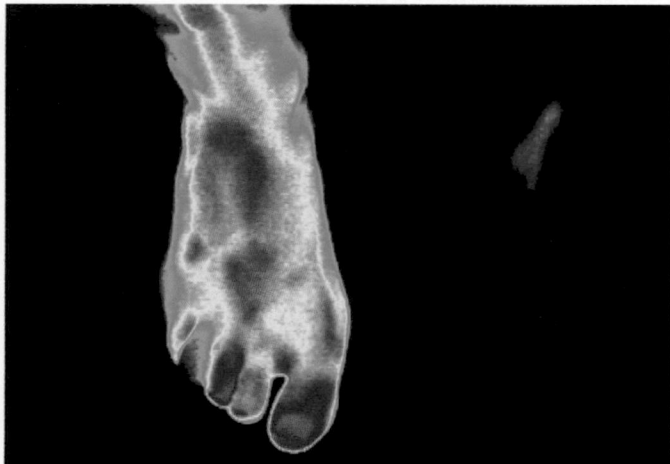

Fig. 161.2 Loss of cutaneous capillary blood flow in left foot on thermography. FASEB J. 2008 Feb;22(2):327–31.

The IASP has diagnostic criteria for adults with CRPS. Although these diagnostic criteria hold true for children and adolescents, it is widely believed that the dystrophic changes and long-term disability are less common than they are in adults.

Back pain

Adolescents commonly present with lower lumbar pain. Often this is thought to be related to lifestyle influences on a developing spine such as postural habit (slouching), load bearing on the back (e.g. schoolbags), or engagement in sedentary activity (e.g. computer use). There are insufficient data to bring clarity to these arguments although it is fair to say that there is no conclusive evidence for any one of these factors being significantly related to the increase in back pain.[26] Recent cross-sectional and prospective studies clearly indicate a role of psychological factors in the manifestation of chronic low back pain.[26] Red flags for pathology include nocturnal pain, presentation in young child, or long tract symptoms. These must be fully investigated to exclude inflammation, compression, and malignancy.

In some cases young people describe the back 'locking' or 'going in to spasm'. This causes a markedly altered gait and can lead to other generalized joint pains. For girls, menstruation can lead to an escalation in pain. A recent systematic review showed that idiopathic adolescent spinal pain is a risk factor for adult spinal pain.[27] A robust study from Denmark looked at 10 000 Danish twins and showed low back pain in adolescence to be a significant risk factor for low back pain in adulthood, with odds ratios as high as 4.[28]

Juvenile idiopathic arthritis and pain

The relationship between juvenile arthritis and chronic pain is well recognized.[14] Despite significant advances in medical treatments for children with JIA, persistent pain is a common complaint. Pain has been shown to be a primary determinant of the physical, emotional, and social functioning in these children.[14] As with other diseases, the degree of disabling pain does not always mirror inflammatory joint activity. A growing body of research in rheumatic diseases, such as JIA, highlights the importance of environmental and cognitive-behavioural influences in the pain experience of children, in addition to the contribution of disease activity.[29,30]

Idiopathic chronic limb pains

Many idiopathic pains are seen in paediatric settings that do not meet the criteria for DIPs/juvenile fibromyalgia or CRPS. These include the poorly understood 'growing pains'. These are described as recurrent bilateral non-articular pain in lower extremities that occur late in the evening or at night. They have been observed to coexist with vascular pain problems, including migraines; this has led to speculation that there may be a vascular component to the bone pain experienced. A recent small study challenged this theory.[31] Other describe growing pains as a form of overuse injury.[32] The jury remains out.

Juvenile hypermobility and pain

The association between joint hypermobility in children and diffuse pain[33] is poorly understood. A recent cross-sectional study of schoolchildren showed no association between joint laxity and pain.[34] Other authors of smaller studies suggested prevalence of pain among those children with generalized joint laxity ranging at around 30%.[35] A large cohort study has shown a positive association between generalized joint laxity and habitual levels of physical activity, body mass index (BMI), and maternal education in girls.[11] A proportion of children noted to be hypermobile can present with recurrent lower limb arthralgia, anterior knee pain syndromes, and back pain.[36] What seems clear is that the majority of hypermobile individuals will be not have pain or have any risk for specific musculoskeletal disorders in later life. Screening tools such as the Beighton score are likely to be inadequate in children, as they are generally more mobile than adults.[11] The challenge remains to interpret symptoms correctly as being related to the hypermobility and to predict why such children become symptomatic. The answer is likely to involve mechanical and psychosocial factors.

Possible aetiological factors

Over the past 10 years there has been significant advance in the understanding of pain processing in the developing brain. In adolescents there is a relationship, either singularly or in combination, to illness, injury, psychological distress, and environmental factors (Figure 161.4).[1] The neuroplasticity of the brain is key to understanding the possible effects of these factors on potential amplification or dampening of pain signals and the degree of pain-associated disability. The main topical aetiological factors are discussed below.

Psychological influences

There is no evidence for purely psychologically generated pain conditions in children. There are a few case reports of conversion neuroses manifesting as widespread pain complaints, but this is highly unusual. There is strong evidence for psychosocial influences as complicating factors and as being implicated in the maintenance of pain complaints,[4] but not their aetiology.[37]

Procedural pain

Although there is some evidence that early repeated exposure to invasive medical procedures that typically involve tissue cutting or puncture is a risk factor for lowered threshold to pain,[38] there is, to date, no evidence to suggest that any of the common childhood procedural pains, such as on immunization, is a risk factor for adult chronic pain. Recent research has shown a relationship between procedural pain in neonatal/early infancy and the potential centralization effect on pain pathways as the child gets older.[39] It is difficult to know whether a primary infectious or inflammatory condition (such as JIA) has an effect on the evolution of chronic pain or whether the pain is a consequence of the immobility, medical therapies, and environmental changes that are associated with these conditions, or a combination.

Injury

It is not unusual for a child with a localized chronic pain to recall a sporting injury, operation, or other trauma around the onset of chronic pain.[40] Hypermobility has also been associated with falls and subsequent pain problems. Altered proprioception that can accompany joint laxity, dyspraxia, and other musculoskeletal conditions frequently leads to falls and further pain escalation. There may be a period of enforced immobilization that can be an additional factor in the development of a localized chronic pain problem.

Genetic influences

There is emerging evidence that patients with CRPS may have a genetic predisposition[41] in Caucasian women, but the underlying genomics are far from clear. There have also been reports of chronic idiopathic musculoskeletal pains in siblings and parent–child pairs.[42]

Environmental influences

Although there is no strong evidence for the intergenerational transmission of pain and pain-related behaviour,[43] there is a lack

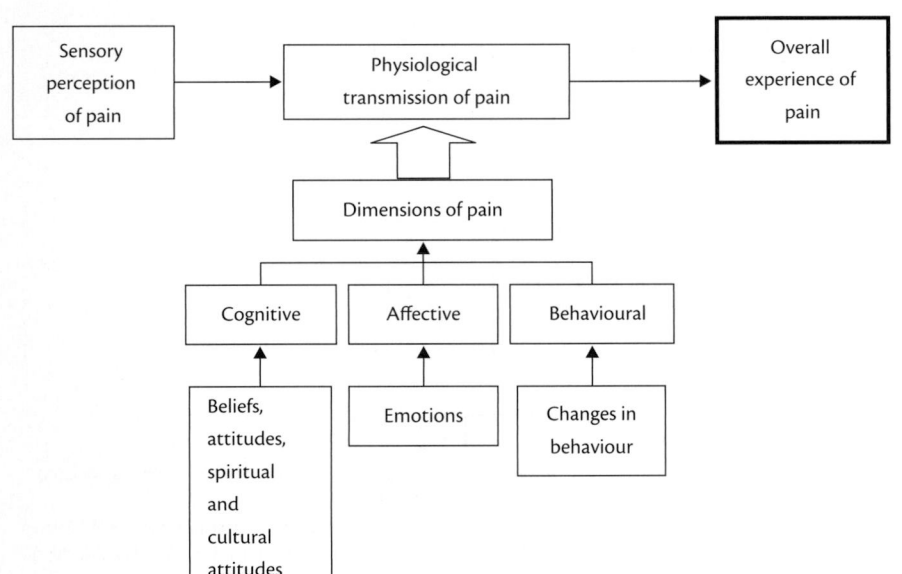

Fig. 161.4 Biopsychosocial model of complex pain. Irrespective of aetiology, pain is a multidimensional phenomenon with sensory, physiological, cognitive, affective, spiritual, and behavioural components.
Konijnenberg, A.Y., C.S Uiterwaal et al. (2005) "Children with Unexplained Chronic Pain" Arch Dis Child 90(7) 680–6

of study of common environmental risk factors other than social learning. Social history may show a recent life event (moving house/school, illness, or death in the family) that has relevance to the presentation.

Developmental influences

There is current interest in the neuropathic mechanisms of paediatric pain. Considerable postnatal development occurs within nociceptic pathways over the first few postnatal weeks.[39] Interruption of this development may have a direct role in the later susceptibility of a child to suffer neuropathic pain. Neonatal pain experience may also have a role in long-term alterations in pain processing and development, with a greater tendency to amplified pain behaviour as a child. There has been interest in the preliminary findings that pain sensitivity may be altered in adolescents who were born prematurely[44] and those exposed to early neonatal insult.

With functional MRI it has recently been shown that considerable CNS circuitry changes take place in young people with a diagnosis of CRPS.[45] Although a pathophysiological mechanism for CRPS remains unknown, a number of aetiologies have been proposed: a peripheral small-fibre neuropathy, an autonomic dysfunction, and an exaggerated regional inflammation.[15]

The impact of chronic pain on the child and family

Persistent or recurrent chronic pain, irrespective of the trigger(s), can bring persistent and recurrent distress, disability, adult attention, and widespread family disruption. Most families have relatively successful mechanisms for dealing with short-lived demands or disruption. However, a young person with chronic pain typically demands sustained physical, emotional, and financial resource.[3] Young people with chronic pain report sleep disturbance, disordered mood, appetite disruption, low feelings (depression is often masked in this population), social isolation, and unwelcome dependency on parents. It can be useful to graphically represent this with patients and others, as shown in Figure 161.5.

Children with chronic pain are commonly outside the formal education system, absent from normal schooling.[5] The routines of normal school, rigidly applied, are often unmanageable for children who experience severe pain when sitting, concentration and memory difficulties, interpersonal problems in explaining confusing problems to peers, frequent anxiety-provoking 'emergency events' associated with pain, and time away for hospital visits. Adolescence is by definition a time of change and experimentation. Adolescents with chronic pain report that they are less socially developed on virtually every metric than their peers.[46]

Levels of parental stress are clinically significant and parents experience severe distress and conflict in parenting their child. Typically they report struggling with the desire to cure their child's pain and comfort their child, while recognizing that the desire to protect may be counterproductive.

Managing chronic childhood musculoskeletal pain

Assessment

It is important to exclude significant disease. With serious medical causes excluded, one can then work to move on to de-medicalize and rehabilitate safely. In practice this is more difficult in paediatrics, as there can be a tendency to catastrophize about persistent pain by the family, and sometimes by the physician. The need to find a cause for the pain can be overwhelming and, in this way, the child may be overmedicalized.[47]

History

Table 161.1 summarizes the important areas that should be covered when taking a history from a child and their carers. For the physician, the goal of the history-taking is often to exclude serious possible causes, identify key problems, build a trusting relationship with the patient (and family), and identify a treatment plan. The child often has chronic experience of medical settings, feelings of being doubted, having the validity of their pain contested, and often

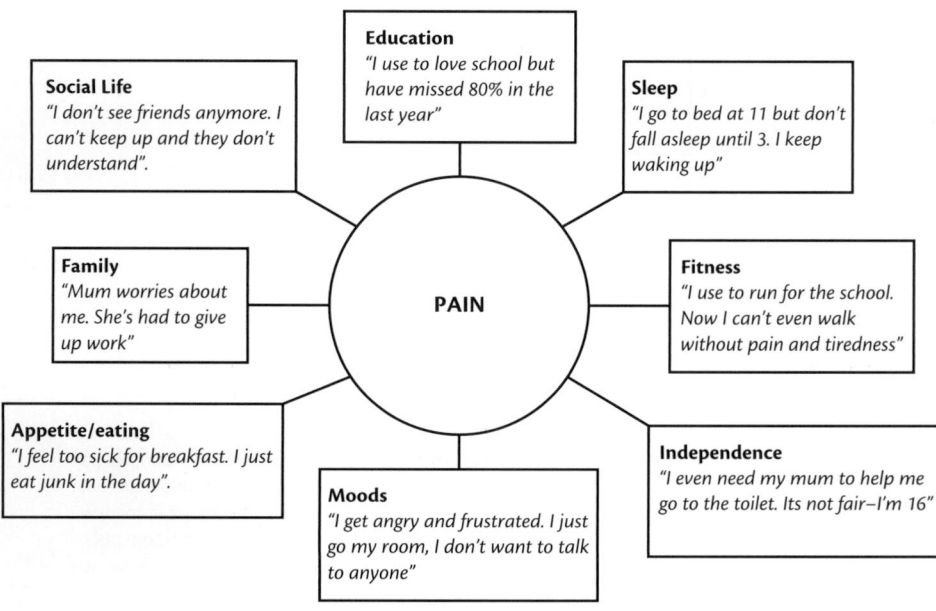

Fig. 161.5 Model illustrating pain associated disability in children.
Konijnenberg, A.Y., C.S Uiterwaal et al. (2005) "Children with Unexplained Chronic Pain" Arch Dis Child 90(7) 680–6.

Table 161.1 Outline of key areas to be addressed while taking a history

Questions	Reasons
Onset of pain	
When did the pain start?	Identify any nerve injury, muscular trauma or intercurrent infection that may have triggered pain
Where did it start?	
Was there a preceding infection, trauma or operation?	Therapeutic interventions that include long periods of immobilization, accelerated physical rehabilitation and repeat operative investigations may all be factors in pain amplification
How was it treated initially	
What was happening around the time the pain started	Environmental events (school, home, other medical episodes) may be factors in the onset of pain
Characteristics of the pain	
Has the pain spread from original place?	It is important to establish the nature of the pain episodes as this may direct management
How would you describe the pain?	
How severe is the pain on a good day and on a bad day?	
Is the pain constant?	
Has the pain got any better or worse?	
Do you suffer pins and needles?	Neuropathic pains are often described as burning, shooting, deep, electric and occasionally episodic. There may be pins and needles and areas of numbness
Is there variation in the pain during the day?	Erythromelalgia is usually worse at night, with painful burning sensations in hands and/or feet
Does the pain alter at night? Does it wake you up?	
What makes it worse?	Movement usually leads to an escalation of pain. Many young people avoid weightbearing or transferring for fear of a pain flare
What makes it better?	
Is it painful to lightly touch the area that is painful?	CRPS has neuropathic features and also extreme hypersensitivity (allodynia) over affected regions—'I cannot have a duvet on my leg at night'
Does that area look unusual?	The affected area may appear swollen and shiny. Young people often feel the limb is more swollen than it actually is
Other symptoms	
Is there a fever, rash or weight loss?	It is important to ensure there are no red flags indicating missed pathology. Nocturnal pain, extreme weight loss, hard neurological features are examples of symptoms and signs that need further paediatric work-up.
Has menstruation altered?	
Is there altered bowel habit?	
Do you have nausea?	Common pain-associated symptoms are included in this list on the left. On occasion these become as disabling as the pain and need to be included in the rehabilitation plan.
Do you suffer abdominal pain?	
Is there any muscle weakness?	
Do you have any areas that are numb?	
Do you suffer dizziness?	
Have you passed out or suddenly fallen to the floor?	
Is fatigue a problem?	
Do you suffer headaches/migraines?	
Do you feel colder/warmer than previously?	
Do you suffer from blurred vision?	
Has your mood been affected?	
Effect of pain on daily living	
Do you find it hard to get to sleep / stay asleep?	Pain can have a significant effect on sleep, mood, independence and general functioning. It is important to know how well a young person is sleeping (and where – it is not unusual for a previously independent teenager to go back into the parents' bed)
Do you 'catnap' in the day?	

(Continued)

Table 161. 1 (Continued)

Questions	Reasons
What can you do on a 'bad'/good day?	Establishing how catastrophic the effect on lifestyle has been is also key; children may have a history of lying on the sofa reading all day or they may have been competing for their country in hockey—by understanding expectations of quality of life you can tailor the rehabilitation process
How much school have you managed over the past 6 months?	
How is your concentration/memory?	
On 'bad/good days' how is your mood?	
How has the pain affected your fitness/hobbies?	
Do you need help in areas where you were previously independent?	
How has this affected your family?	
What do you think is causing this? Do you have fears about a particular illness?	
Do the parents have fears concerning the pain that they feel has not been addressed?	
Past and family history of illness	
Have you suffered painful conditions previously?	There is much recent research into past painful events on the developing nociceptive system. This is particularly relevant to children who have been premature and received intensive care
Have you suffered fatigue, sleeplessness or anxiety previously?	
Any operations or illnesses as a younger child?	
Any neonatal problems?	
Have any family members suffered illness?	Other family illness experience is relevant; there may be a direct genetic link with pain experienced and/or environmental aspects that are factors in the child developing a pain condition
Is there a family history of painful conditions?	
Family, emotional, and social circumstances	
Who currently lives at home?	Having an idea of the family environment is important. Parents often adapt their home life to care for the child and employment patterns change. Siblings' relationships and friendships may alter
What are the occupations of the main carers?	
Have one or both carers changed/stopped their job since the pain condition started?	
Can you identify any stressors in school, family or peer groups?	School often becomes challenging both physically and emotionally (previously able children may not know how to communicate their conditions to peers and have differing degrees of help from school staff)

a history of failed and pain-exacerbating interventions. Three key psychological features of this setting are worth keeping in mind:

- Both child and family are likely to be fearful, hoping for a cure, desperate to be helpful, but often 'on their best behaviour', so may not immediately appear to be distressed, and may have flat or neutral affect.

- Because of their history, any attempt to shift the treatment goal from one of cure to management or symptom control may be heard as blaming of patient and carer(s), and so should be done only after building trust.

- What matters is not necessarily what information has been given to the patient and carers, but what they believe to be true. Typically both patient and family will have heard a variety of stories about what may be happening to them.[47]

Physical examination

Time spent fully on examining at the beginning may prevent repetition and unnecessary, distressing investigations at a later date.[14] If there is concern regarding the diagnosis then this is the time to order all investigations and ensure that these are followed up. Undue delay leads to fear and often a worsening of pain symptoms and associated disability.

Psychometric instruments

There are some well-validated and commonly used tools, most notably the Varni/Thompson Paediatric Pain Questionnaire[48] focusing on pain, and the Functional Disability Index[49] focusing on disability. Pain intensity in children has long been measured using simple severity measurement tools, such as the visual analogue scale (VAS).[50] These give a subjective measure of the pain intensity according to the adolescent and/or that pain perceived by their carer. While these are useful measures, prospectively they give no indication of the impact of pain on the young person's life. For example, one adolescent with a pain score of 7 on the VAS may still get to school where another adolescent with the same score may not be getting out of bed.

Two multidisciplinary tools have recently been developed, one specifically for use in measuring the impact of pain on adolescents with chronic pain (Bath Adolescent Pain Questionnaire)[51] and one specifically for use in measuring the impact of adolescent chronic pain on parents (Bath Adolescent Pain Questionnaire for Parents).[52]

Physiological measures of pain-related indexes.

There are few data on the role or utility of measuring physiological processes in the context of childhood chronic pain. Functional

MRI has recently been shown to be a useful tool in evaluating the role of the CNS in childhood CRPS.[45] Quantitative Sensory Testing (QST) is a valuable tool for assessing sensory perception (including pain) in children.

Rehabilitation and self-management

A dedicated team that works consistently with the adolescent and family will facilitate communication, ensure effective delivery of therapy, reduce iatrogenic influences, and enable goals to be reached earlier.[20] Most approaches to rehabilitation share common features including education, symptom control, behavioural science, and physical therapy.

Education

Although the evidence for education alone as a treatment for behaviour change is wanting, the provision of a rationale for what are often counter-intuitive instructions in self-management is essential. Additionally, one should never underestimate that the average lay person's understanding of anatomy and physiology is at best partial, and more typically fantastic. A critical first step in all rehabilitation is to offer, re-offer, and reinforce an understanding of how one's body may be working to maintain pain. Children and their parents often have inflexible or rigid ideas not only about the cause of pain, but also of pain as an important signal of damage or disease. Rhetorical devices (metaphors, stories, examples, pictures) that counter this rigid thinking can be helpful. Back pain is extremely common but rarely related to malignancy or arthritis. Explaining the fascinating case of phantom limb experiences can also be helpful, to introduce flexibility to the idea that brain signals must signify peripheral damage.

Pharmacotherapy

The number of analgesics and interventions used is a sign that there are no well-controlled therapeutic trials in childhood chronic pain. It is becoming widely accepted, however, that any analgesic intervention should be used alongside multidisciplinary therapy.[53,54] Oral treatments that can be used, with variable success, include tricyclic anti-depressants, non-steroidal anti-inflammatory drugs (NSAIDs), opioids, anti-convulsants, and glucocorticoids.[55,56] Sympathetic blockade and botulinum toxin injections have been used in localized muscular pain.[55] Gabapentin and pregabalin may have a role in addressing neuropathic pain in CRPS. A Cochrane review in 2005 showed that tricyclic anti-depressants have a role in modifying aspects of neuropathic pain in some patients.[57]

The evidence supporting the efficacy of any of these therapies in children is lacking. In CRPS and neuropathic pain gabapentin and pregabalin have shown a small degree of promise but these have not been robustly studied in children. Some authors have shown effect of spinal cord stimulation, regional blocks, and epidural infusions in the small number of children with intractable CRPS[58]; it is widely accepted, however, that these more interventional techniques are only effective alongside active physical and psychological rehabilitation.

Medicine review is often an essential task in this population. Polypharmacy, risk of dosing and combination errors, and confusion over the utility of previously and currently prescribed medication is common. Drug withdrawal, detoxification, and replacement should be carefully managed.

Psychological therapies

A Cochrane systematic review of psychological therapy reported on the effectiveness of psychological treatments for pain control in common chronic pain problems.[59] Small studies using cognitive-behavioural therapy (CBT) in juvenile fibromyalgia show significant improvement in the child's confidence with managing the pain (but disappointing effect on functional disability and depressive symptoms).[8] For the complexly disabled patient there is evidence that an interdisciplinary programme for adolescents complexly disabled with chronic pain has a positive significant impact.[60] The role of the physician is often as an educator, to oversee analgesic withdrawal and to support the overall message that it is safe to increase activity despite pain and reduce reliance on medical support.[47]

Physical therapies

In conditions such as CRPS, early intensive physiotherapy (including desensitization) with behavioural support can provide dramatic reversal of the presenting signs and symptoms.[61] The aim of this is accelerated mobilization. This is complicated if the diagnosis is delayed and access to appropriate physical and psychological rehabilitation difficult. Many cases of diffuse pain will require a gentle, paced approach. Along with musculoskeletal pains, the more active the musculoskeletal system becomes the more likely the muscle spasms and tightening are to reduce. Proprioception improves and autonomic changes subside. Where possible, young people should work to devise their own 'fitness plan'. Using a local gym rather than a hospital physiotherapy gym allows them to start to return to a more normal environment.[60] Working in this consistent and paced manner can be extremely hard for the young person and their parents. The pain often continues at the beginning (if not throughout) and motivation is poor. Parental anxiety is high and there is a fear that damage will be done. Psychological support during this time is important. The young person will need help setting goals, learning how to communicate pain to peers and family, maintaining motivation on 'bad days', managing low mood, dealing with anger and frustration, and overcoming fears. Often they have not been at school for a long period of time and need help in preparing again for this difficult environment. In some cases, there may be other mental health needs that can be identified and appropriately treated.

There are ongoing studies that show promise, specifically with CRPS patients and visual counter-stimulation. Mirror therapy focusing on the hypothesis that incongruence between motor output and sensory input produces CRPS is under way with adults,[62] but there is no data for children.

Complementary therapies are commonly utilized by patients with chronic pain. The evidence supporting many of these therapies in children and adolescents is poor.[63]

Natural history and long-term outcomes

The natural history of chronic musculoskeletal pain in children shows that, in many cases, outcome is improved compared with that in adults.[64] Early, multidisciplinary input (including CBT) has favourable outcome.[60] CRPS in children generally has a favourable prognosis if early physiotherapy is initiated (with psychological support).[64] This is improved if the parents are involved in the rehabilitation process. However, a prolonged time to treatment and the presence of marked autonomic changes are not good prognostic indicators in this condition.

Practice points

1. Ensure an early, thorough history and physical musculoskeletal examination to rule out new or suboptimally treated pathology.

2. Evaluate the impact of the pain on the child and family (not just the level of pain) so that rehabilitation can be tailored.

3. Involve multidisciplinary team early (ideally in early clinics) to facilitate cohesive working and the introduction of psychological and physical therapies.

References

1. Malleson P, Clinch J. Pain syndromes in children. *Curr Opin Rheumatol* 2003;15:572–580.

2. O'Sullivan P, Beales D, Jensen L, Murray K, Myers T. Characteristics of chronic non-specific musculoskeletal pain in children and adolescents attending a rheumatology outpatients clinic: a cross-sectional study. *Pediatric Rheumatol Online J* 2011;9:3.

3. Sleed M, Eccelston C, Beecham J, Knapp M, Jordan A. The economic impact of chronic pain in adolescence: methodological considerations and a preliminary costs-of-illness study. *Pain* 2005;119:183–190.

4. Jones GT, Silman AJ, Power C, Macfarlane GJ. Are common symptoms in childhood associated with chronic widespread body pain in adulthood? Results from the 1958 British Birth Cohort Study. *Arthritis Rheum* 2007;56:1669–1675.

5. Roth-Isigkeit A. Pain among children and adolescents: restrictions in daily living and triggering factors. *Pediatrics* 2005;115:152–162.

6. Brattberg G. Do pain problems in young school children persist into early adulthood? A 13-year follow-up. *Eur J Pain* 2004;8:187–199.

7. Perquin CW, Hazebroek-Kampschreur AA, Hunfield JA et al. Pain in children and adolescents: a common experience. *Pain* 2000;87:51–58.

8. Kashikar-Zuck S. Treatment of children with unexplained chronic pain. *Lancet* 2006;367:380–382.

9. Hoftun GB, Romundstad PR, Zwart JA, Rygg M. Chronic idiopathic pain in adolescence—high prevalence and disability: The young HUNT study 2008. *Pain* 2011;152:2259–2266.

10. Deere K, Clinch J, Holliday K et al. Obesity is a risk factor for musculoskeletal pain in adolescents: findings from a population-based cohort. *Pain* 2012;153(9):1932–1938.

11. Clinch J, Deere K, Sayers A et al. Epidemiology of generalized joint laxity (hypermobility) in fourteen-year-old children from the UK. *Arthritis Rheum* 2011;63:2819–1827.

12. De Mos M, de Bruijn AGJ, Huygen FJPM et al. The incidence of complex regional pain syndrome:a population based study. *Pain* 2007;129:12–20.

13. Stanton Hicks M. Plasticity of complex regional pain syndrome (CRPS) in children. *Pain Med* 2010;11(8):1216–1223.

14. Anthony KK, Schanberg LE. Assessment and management of pain syndromes and arthritis pain in children and adolescents. *Rheum Dis Clin North Am* 2007;33: 625–660.

15. Lovell DJ, Walco GA Pain associated with juvenile rheumatoid arthritis. *Pediatr Clin North Am* 1989;36(4):1015–1027.

16. Haverman L, Grootenhuis MA, van den Berg JM et al. Predictors of health-related quality of life in children and adolescents with juvenile idiopathic arthritis: results from a web-based survey. *Arthritis Care Res* (Hoboken) 2012;64(5):694–703.

17. Groholt EK. Recurrent pain in children, socio-economic factors and accumulation in families. *Eur J Epidemiol* 2003;18:965–975; Brattberg G. The incidence of back pain and headache among Swedish school children. *Qual Life Res* 1994;3(Suppl.1):S27–S31.

18. Geisser ME, Casey KL, Brucksch CB et al. Perception of noxious and innocuous heat stimulation among healthy women and women with fibromyalgia: association with mood, somatic focus, and catastrophizing. *Pain* 2003;102:243–250.

19. Cohen H, Neumann L, Kotler K, Buskila D. Autonomic nervous system derangement in fibromyalgia syndrome and related disorders. *Isr Med Assoc J* 2001;3:755–760.

20. Malleson PN, Connell H, Bennett SM, Eccelston C. Chronic musculoskeletal and other idiopathic pain syndromes. *Arch Dis Child* 2001;84:189–192.

21. Wolfe F. New American College of Rheumatology criteria for fibromyalgia: a twenty-year journey. *Arthritis Care Res* (Hoboken) 2010;62(5):583–419.

22. Buskila D. Fibromyalgia in children—lessons from assessing nonarticular tenderness. *J Rheumatol* 1996;23:2017–2019.

23. Buskila D, Neumann L, Herschman E et al. Fibromyalgia syndrome in children—an outcome study. *J Rheumatol* 1995;22:525–528.

24. Berde CB, Lebel A. Complex regional pain syndrome in children and adolescents. *Anesthesiology* 2005;102(2):252–255.

25. Connelly M, Schanberg L. Latest developments in the assessment and management of chronic musculoskeletal pain syndromes in children. *Curr Opin Rheumatol* 2006;18:496–502.

26. Diepenmaat AC, van der Wal MF, de Vet HC, Hirasing RA. Neck/shoulder, low back, and arm pain in relation to computer use, physical activity, stress, and depression among Dutch adolescents. *Pediatrics* 2006;117:412–416.

27. Jeffries LJ, Milanese SF, Grimmer-Somers KA. Epidemiology of adolescent spinal pain: a systematic overview of the research literature. *Spine* 2007;32(23):2630–2637.

28. Hestbaek L, Leboeuf-Yde C, Kyvik KO, Manniche C. The course of low back pain from adolescence to adulthood: eight-year follow-up of 9600 twins. *Spine* 2006;31(4):468–472.

29. Vourimaa H, Tamm K, Honkanen V, Komulainen YT, Santavirta NL. Parents and children as agents of disease management in JIA. *Child Care Health Dev* 2009;35(4):578–585.

30. Connelly M, Anthony KK, Sarniak R et al. Parent pain responses as predictors of daily activities and mood in children with juvenile idiopathic arthritis: the utility of electronic diaries. *J Pain Symptom Manage* 2010;39(3):579–590.

31. Hashkes PJ, Gorenberg M, Oren V et al. Growing pains in children are not associated with changes in vascular perfusion patterns in painful regions. *Clin Rheumatol* 2005;24:342–345.

32. Friedland O, Hashkes PJ, Jaber et al. Decreased bone speed of sound in children with growing pains measured by quantitative ultrasound. *J Rheumatol* 2005;32:1354–1357.

33. Gedalia A, Press J, Klein M, Buskila D. Joint hypermobility and fibromyalgia in schoolchildren. *Ann Rheum Dis* 1993;52:494–496.

34. Leone V, Tornese G, Zerial M, Locatelli C, Ciambra R, Bensa M, et al. Joint hypermobility and its relationship to musculoskeletal pain in schoolchildren: a cross-sectional study. *Arch Dis Child* 2009;94:627–632.

35. El-Garf AK, Mahmoud GA, Mahgoub EH. Hypermobility among Egyptian children: prevalence and features. *J Rheumatol* 1998;25:1003–1005.

36. Adib N, Davies K, Grahame R, Woo P, Murray KJ. Joint hypermobility syndrome in childhood. A not so benign multisystem disorder? *Rheumatology* 2005;44:744–750.

37. Aasland A, Flato B, Vandvik IH. Psychosocial factors in children with idiopathic musculoskeletal pain: a prospective, longitudinal study. *Acta Paediatr* 1997;86:740–746.

38. Taddio A. The effects of early pain experience in neonates on pain responses in infancy and childhood. *Paediatr Drugs* 2005;7:245–257.

39. Fitzgerald M. The development of nociceptive circuits. *Nat Rev Neurosci* 2005;6:507–520.

40. Kristjansdottir G, Rhee H. Risk factors of back pain frequency in schoolchildren: a search for explanations to a public health problem. *Acta Paediatr* 2002;91:849–854.

41. Mailis A, Wade J. Profile of Caucasian women with possible genetic predisposition to reflex sympathetic dystrophy: a pilot study. *Clin J Pain* 1994;10:210–217.

42. Buskila D, Neumann L, Carmi R. Familial aggregation in the fibromyalgia syndrome. *Semin Arthritis Rheum* 1996;26:605–611.

43. Jones GT, Silman AJ, Macfarlane GJ. Parental pain is not associated with pain in the child: a population based study. *Ann Rheum Dis* 2004;63:1152–1154.

44. Walker SM, Franck LS, Fitzgerald M, Myles J, Stocks J, Marlow N. Long-term impact of neonatal intensive care and surgery on somatosensory perception in children born extremely preterm. *Pain* 2009;141(1–2):79–87.

45. Lebel A, Becerra L, Wallin D et al. fMRI reveals distinct CNS processing during symptomatic and recovered complex regional pain syndrome in children. *Brain* 2008;131(Pt 7):1854–1879.

46. Eccleston C, Wastell S, Crombez G, Jordan A. Adolescent social development and chronic pain. *Eur J Pain* 2008;12(6):765–774.

47. Clinch J, Eccleston C. Chronic musculoskeletal pain in children: assessment and management. *Rheumatology* (Oxford) 2009;48:466–474.

48. Varni JW, Thompson KL, Hanson V. The Varni/Thompson Pediatric Pain Questionnaire. I. Chronic musculoskeletal pain in juvenile rheumatoid arthritis. *Pain* 1987;28:27–38.

49. Walker LS, Greene JW. The functional disability inventory: measuring a neglected dimension of child health status. *J Pediatr Psychol* 1991;16:39–58.

50. Carlsson AM. Assessment of chronic pain. I. Aspects of the reliability and validity of the visual analogue scale. *Pain* 1983;16:87–101.

51. Eccleston C, Jordan A, McCracken LM, Connell H, Clinch J. The Bath Adolescent Pain Questionnaire (BAPQ): development and preliminary psychometric evaluation of an instrument to assess the impact of chronic pain on adolescents. *Pain* 2005;118:263–270.

52. Jordan A, Eccleston C, McCracken LM, Connell H, Clinch J. The Bath Adolescent Pain—Parental Impact Questionnaire (BAP-PIQ): development and preliminary psychometric evaluation of an instrument to assess the impact of parenting an adolescent with chronic pain. *Pain* 2008;137:478–487.

53. Stanton-Hicks M. Complex regional pain syndromes: guidelines for therapy. *Clin J Pain* 1998;14:155–166.

54. Kashikar-Zuck S. Treatment of children with unexplained chronic pain. *Lancet* 2006;367:380–382.

55. van de Vusse AC, Stomp-van den Berg SG, Kessels AH, Weber WE. Randomised controlled trial of gabapentin in complex regional pain syndrome type. *BMC Neurol* 2004;4:13.

56. Crofford LJ. Pain management in fibromyalgia. *Curr Opin Rheumatol* 2008;20:246–250.

57. Saarto T, Wiffen PJ. Antidepressants for neuropathic pain. *Cochrane Database Syst Rev* 2007;4:CD005454.

58. Olsson GL, Meyerson BA, Linderoth B. Spinal cord stimulation in adolescents with complex regional pain syndrome type 1. *Eur J Pain* 2008;12:53–59.

59. Eccleston C, Morley S, Williams A, Yorke L, Mastroyannopoulou A. Psychological therapies for the management of chronic and recurrent pain in children and adolescents. *Cochrane Database Syst Rev* 2009;2:CD003968.

60. Eccleston C, Malleson PM, Clinch J, Connell H, Sourbut C. Chronic pain in adolescents: evaluation of a programme of interdisciplinary cognitive behaviour therapy. *Arch Dis Child* 2003;88:881–858.

61. Lee BH, Schariff L, Sethna NF et al. Physical therapy and cognitive-behavioral treatment for complex regional pain syndromes. *J Pediatr* 2002;141(1):135–140.

62. McCabe CS, Haigh RC, Ring EF et al. A controlled pilot study of the utility of mirror visual feedback in the treatment of complex regional pain syndrome (type 1). *Rheumatology* 2003;42:97–101.

63. Tsao JC, Zeltzer LK. Complementary and alternative medicine approaches for pediatric pain: a review of the state-of-the-science. *Evid Based Complement Altern Med* 2005;2:149–159.

64. Bursch B, Walco GA, Zeltzer L. Clinical assessment and management of chronic pain and pain-associated disability syndrome. *Dev Behav Pediatr* 1998;1:45–53.

CHAPTER 162

Sports and exercise injuries

Nicola Maffulli and Angelo Del Buono

Introduction

Regular aerobic exercise has beneficial effects on the cardiovascular system, reduces the incidence of osteoporosis, increases the metabolic rate, and induces a general sense of well-being. However, injuries commonly occur in athletes: if not recognized or treated adequately, they may become recurrent or chronic. Different rates and patterns of injury are observed depending on the type of sport activity. Muscle, tendon, and ligaments are frequently injured acutely, and repeated sporting insults may result in strain, overuse, and fatigue. We describe the current evidence of clinical features and therapeutic aspects of muscle, ligament and tendon disorders.

Muscle injuries

Acute muscle strain injuries account for 10–55% of all acute sports injuries.[1,2] The hamstrings, rectus femoris, and medial head of the gastrocnemius are the most commonly injured muscles.[2] Most commonly occurring at the musculotendinous junction (MTJ), acute muscle injuries are classified as strains (grade i), partial tears (grade II), and complete tears (grade III),[3–5] can be intramuscular, proximal, or distal to the proximal and distal MTJ, and may extend to the osteotendinous junction.[6] Acute strains result from active contractions of muscles, or after indirect trauma and excessive tensile forces which disrupt the myofibres of the MTJ, as commonly happens in sprinting and jumping activities.[2,7] Indirect injuries may be active, usually resulting from eccentric overload, or passive, in response to tensile overstretching of the muscle, with no contraction.[8]

In grade I acute muscle injury (strain), changes are limited, less than 5% of fibres are disrupted, there is some swelling and discomfort, and strength and range of motion are not impaired. Ultrasonography (US) may show normal appearance, or focal or general increased echogenicity, but, given the difficulty of depicting the normal hyperechoic intramuscular portion of the tendon after injury, MRI is more accurate.[9]

Grade II injuries (partial tear) are partial thickness tears, with continuity of fibres at the injury site, involving from less than one-third (low-grade injuries) to more than two-thirds (high-grade) of the muscle fibres.[10] Strength may be reduced. Using US, muscle fibres appear discontinuous; the disruption site is hypervascular and altered in echogenicity in and around the lesion.[9] The appearance at MRI depends on the acuity and severity of the tear,

characterized by oedema and haemorrhage of the muscle or MTJ extending along the fascial planes between muscle groups, fibre disorganization, surrounding haematoma, and perifascial fluid.[11]

On US and MRI, grade III (complete tear) injuries show complete discontinuity of muscle fibres, associated hematoma, and retraction of the muscle ends.[9] If the tears are not treated, the ends of the muscle can become rounded and may tether to adjacent muscles or fascia.[12] However, both strains and complete tears occur most often at the MTJ, the weakest link within the muscle tendon unit, independently of the rate or direction of strain and differences in muscle architecture.[13] The pathophysiology of muscular strain is poorly understood, but any condition that diminishes the ability of a muscle to contract (e.g. fatigue, weakness) impairs the muscle's ability to absorb force, and exposes the muscle further risk of injury. Therefore, a weaker muscle is more predisposed to more deleterious injuries.

Management

Despite the high rate of muscle injuries, there is no consensus on their management, with a large number of different interventions being used. In acute injury, treatment includes ice and rest, followed by stretching, agility, and stability exercises. Even though non-steroidal anti-inflammatory drugs (NSAIDs) or manipulation have been commonly used, the evidence in support of their use is limited. Although platelet-rich plasma (PRP) injections are increasingly used, the evidence supporting their use is still scanty (see 'Regenerative therapies, below). Surgery is indicated in chronic tears unresponsive to conservative measures or in high-demand patients complaining of residual inability which impairs performance and requiring return to preinjury level of sport activity. Muscle reattachment is advocated as first line but when this is not possible, muscle release and removal of surrounding scar tissue and adhesions are recommended. Interestingly, from the analysis of risk and protective factors for recurrent hamstring injuries, it has emerged that athletes who follow agility/stabilization exercises rather than strength/stretching exercises have a lower risk of reinjury, whereas there is conflicting evidence that larger extent of initial trauma, a grade 1 hamstring injury, or a previous ipsilateral anterior cruciate ligament (ACL) reconstruction could predispose to recurrence.

Ligaments

Injuries to ligaments occur frequently in exercise. They can be graded from 1 to 3 (strain, partial tear, complete rupture). The most common injury sites are the lateral ligament complex in the ankle and the four main ligaments around the knee: the medial and lateral collateral, and the anterior and posterior cruciate (see also Chapter 155).

Anterior cruciate ligament

The management of an ACL tear continues to be the most studied area in sports medicine, and a recent debate concerns reconstruction using double-bundle or single-bundle techniques. Recent randomized clinical studies have demonstrated that the double-bundle technique is superior for pain scores and anterior knee laxity, with no significant differences in terms of rotational control and patient-reported pain and function scores.[14] However, the evidence is not convincing, and it appears that anatomical reconstruction of the ACL using a single-bundle technique is at least as good as a double-bundle technique, and less technically demanding.

From the comparison of ACL reconstructions with hamstring and patellar tendon autografts, no significant differences emerge in terms of patient-reported outcomes, osteoarthritis outcome scores, and laxity at 2, 8, and 10 years of follow-up;[15–17] however, patients undergoing patellar tendon reconstruction experience greater anterior knee pain. The best methods of fixation of the graft are still being investigated. Compared with other forms of fixation, biodegradable screws produce greater tunnel enlargement, but this is not clinically relevant.

New emerging areas are trying to elucidate the causes of development of osteoarthritis following ACL surgery, and evaluate the role of PRP in ACL primary repair and reconstruction.[18]

Posterior cruciate ligament

In posterior cruciate ligament (PCL) reconstruction, double- and single-bundle reconstruction, tibial inlay, and transtibial graft placement are increasingly compared. The comparison of transtibial single-bundle arthroscopic tibial inlay procedures and double-bundle arthroscopic tibial inlay procedures[19] has shown that the double-bundle arthroscopic tibial inlay procedure provides better posterior stability with no difference in terms of knee motion or Lysholm scores. The analysis of kinematics of single-bundle reconstruction has demonstrated that this procedure restores anteroposterior translation of the tibia, patellar flexion, and shift, with no effects on mediolateral translation, patellar rotation, and tilt.[20]

Posterolateral corner, posteromedial corner, and multiligamentous injury

The management of posterolateral corner injuries aims to restore normal knee kinematics. Anatomically based posterolateral corner reconstructions improve stability and clinical outcomes at intermediate follow-up,[21] and reconstruction is more reliable than repair.[22] Anatomical reconstruction of the medial collateral ligament and posteromedial corner injuries, including reconstruction of the posterior oblique ligament, is recommended.[21] A recent study on elite athletes with post-traumatic multiligamentous injury involving both cruciate ligaments and at least one collateral ligament suggests that early, single-stage procedures provide the best outcomes, but only one-third of patients return to preinjury activity levels.[23]

Patellofemoral joint

Stability of the patellofemoral articulation is complex and requires a thorough understanding of lower extremity alignment and soft tissue restraints. The medial patellofemoral ligament is the primary restraint to lateral patellar translation, but patella alta, trochlear dysplasia, systemic hyperlaxity, and malalignment also contribute to patellofemoral instability. There is still debate over the appropriate surgical intervention for patients with chronic patellar instability or malalignment. Important technical considerations for surgical correction regard appropriate tensioning of the medial soft tissue restraints and repair or reconstruction of the medial patellofemoral ligament. Medial patellofemoral ligament reconstructions provide good outcomes when indicated and if appropriately performed.[24] From a retrospective study comparing a novel derotational high tibial osteotomy and an Elmslie–Trillat–Fulkerson proximal–distal realignment, superior outcomes have been observed after derotational tibial osteotomy than in patients undergoing proximal–distal realignment, with significant improvement in gait patterns and functional scores.[25] Correction of tibial torsion reduces the valgus vector through more phases of the gait cycle than a proximal–distal realignment.

Lateral ankle injuries and instability

The lateral ligament complex of the ankle is commonly injured in recreational and professional athletes. Initial treatment is usually conservative, involving rest, ice, administration of anti-inflammatory drugs, brace wearing/plaster, partial weightbearing. Physical therapy and functional rehabilitation are also recommended. Although acute lateral ankle sprains usually respond to conservative management, chronic lateral instability resulting in reduced sport activity may occur in 15–20%, with an 80% reinjury rate in younger individuals.[26,27]

The anterior talofibular ligament (ATFL) is usually involved, whereas the calcaneofibular ligament (CFL) is insufficient in 15% of patients. With the aim of re-establishing stability and function without compromising ankle motion, high-demand patients with chronic lateral ankle instability are often candidates for surgery. Although anatomical and non-anatomical autologous tendon graft reconstructions using peroneus brevis, plantaris, semitendinosus, and gracilis tendons have been proposed,[28] arthroscopic and arthroscopically assisted plication and anchor fixation techniques may be used to reconstruct the lateral ligament complex of the ankle, attaching the anterior talofibular ligament to talus and/or fibula.[29] To date, better results have been reported with anatomical than non-anatomical techniques, and the anatomical Broström–Gould repair is considered a reliable alternative to more invasive and technically demanding reconstructions, which preserves ankle motion and provides functional stability.[29] The Brostrom procedure, repairing the ATFL and CFL, is thought to restore hindfoot kinematics, but the Gould modification aims to repair the ruptured lateral ligaments, and reinforces the construct with the inferior extensor retinaculum, providing additional support against inversion load, and similar biomechanical stability compared to the combined repair of the ATFL and CFL.[29]

Tendon ruptures

Tendon ruptures most frequently involve the Achilles tendon, the thickest and strongest tendon of the human body. Most (75%) acute ruptures occur during recreational activities in men 30–40 years of age.[30] There is no agreement on the best management. Recent well-conducted randomized controlled trials (RCTs) show that conservative and 'classical' (i.e. open) surgical management in an unselected population produce similar functional results, but operative management provides lower rerupture rate, early functional treatment, less calf atrophy, and stronger push-off, at the expense of long incisions, wound complications such as infections, and, occasionally, painful scars.[31]

In athletes, operative management followed by a short period of immobilization in a cast produces excellent results.[32] Minimally invasive repair techniques have been developed to reduce postoperative complications associated with open surgical procedures. These procedures provide accurate opposition of the tendon ends, improve cosmesis, and protect against wound breakdown, but reruptures and sural nerve damage have been reported.[33] Percutaneous techniques have comparable clinical effectiveness and lower complication rates than open procedures, are safe and effective in older individuals, in diabetic patients, and in high-performance athletes.

Tendinopathy

Tendinopathies are sport-related overuse injuries responsible for disability of most major tendons, including the Achilles, patellar, rotator cuff, and forearm extensor tendons. The term tendinopathy includes alterations of the tendon proper and, but is not limited to, the histopathological features of tendinosis, which presumes the presence of degenerative changes on histology, with no clinical or histological signs of intratendinous inflammation.[34] The essential lesion of tendinopathy includes a failed healing response, in which the healing process appears incomplete, with haphazard proliferation of tenocytes, intracellular abnormalities in tenocytes, disruption of collagen fibres, and increase in non-collagenous matrix.[35] What may appear clinically as an acute tendinopathy is actually an advanced failure of a chronic healing response with no histological nor biochemical evidence of inflammation.[36] These alterations lead to a mechanically less stable tendon, probably more susceptible to damage.[37] Inflammation is involved only in the initiation, but not in the propagation and progression of the disease process, whereas failed healing and tendinopathic features seem to be associated with chronic overload and exert a deleterious effect.[38] Although the diagnosis of tendinopathy is usually clinical, MRI and US should be used to better define and understand the location of the lesion.

Management

Different strategies have been proposed, but we have focused on the novel therapies emerging for management of tendinopathy.

Exercises

Eccentric exercises are thought to promote collagen fibre cross-link formation within the tendon, and facilitate tendon remodelling, protect the tendon from increased stresses, and thus prevent reinjury,[39] but the evidence of histological changes following a programme of eccentric exercise is lacking, and the mechanisms by which eccentric exercises may help to relieve the pain of tendinopathy remain unclear. It is possible that eccentric exercises do not just exert a beneficial mechanical effect, but also act on pain mediators, decreasing their presence in tendinopathic tendons. In general, eccentric exercises produce a positive effect, with no reported adverse effects.[39] Excellent clinical results have been reported in both athletic and sedentary patients, but these results have not been confirmed by other studies. The association of eccentric training with shock wave therapy produces higher success rates than those observed after eccentric loading alone or shock wave therapy alone.[40]

Extracorporeal shock wave therapy

Extracorporeal shock wave therapy (ESWT) is supposed to stimulate soft tissue healing and inhibit pain receptors. There is no agreement about using repetitive low-energy ESWT with no local anaesthesia, or high-energy ESWT with local or regional anaesthesia.[41] Low-energy ESWT has been proposed for tendinopathy to stimulate soft tissue healing and inhibit pain receptors.[41] In the scenario of Achilles tendinopathy, low-energy ESWT or eccentric exercises provided comparable results in an RCT, with outcomes superior to those observed after no intervention.[40] The results were disappointing in another study.[42]

Injections

The role of corticosteroids in the management of tendinopathy is still debated, and the evidence supporting the widespread use of intratendinous injections of corticosteroids is scanty, controversial, and disappointing. A meta-analysis of the effects of corticosteroid injections has showed little benefit. The use of ultrasound imaging needle guidance improves the safety of corticosteroid injections, keeping the needle outside the peritendinous space, to inject the fluid only in the Kager triangle, for the Achilles tendon, or in the Hoffa body, for the patellar tendon.

High-volume injections of normal saline solution, corticosteroids, and anaesthetics produce local mechanical effects of stretching, breaking, or occlusion of new blood vessels. This action on the vessels would induce either trauma or ischaemia on the accompanying nerve supply, reducing the pain in symptomatic patients with resistant Achilles tendinopathy. Preliminary studies have showed reduced pain and improved short- and long-term outcomes after management with high-volume injections of patients with Achilles[43] or patellar[44] tendinopathy, regardless of their symptoms. This modality of treatment is safe, relatively inexpensive, and allows a quick return to sports. The injection is performed under ultrasound guidance, so that corticosteroids have no direct action on the tendon itself.

Sclerosant therapy

Sclerosing treatment with polidocanol results in a moderate improvement of symptoms of tendinopathy, but the majority of athletes still have reduced function and substantial pain after 24 months of follow-up. Medium- or long-term outcomes still require investigation.

Surgery

Operative treatment aims to excise fibrotic adhesions, remove or debride areas of failed healing, restore vascularity, and stimulate viable cells to synthesize proteins to favour the healing process.[33] Multiple longitudinal tenotomies seem to trigger neoangiogenesis in the Achilles tendon and increase blood flow, promoting an environment which stimulates healing.[45] Percutaneous longitudinal tenotomies are suggested when conservative management fails in patients with isolated tendinopathy, a well-defined nodular lesion less than 2.5 cm long, and intact paratenon,[46] whereas they are ineffective in patients with pantendinopathy. This procedure is simple, can be performed in an ambulatory setting using local anaesthesia without tourniquet, with minimal complications and no long-term morbidity. Percutaneous longitudinal US-guided internal tenotomy of the Achilles tendon requires the use of high-resolution US to properly locate the tendinopathic area and to perform the initial stab incision.[46] Radiofrequency microtenotomy is safe and effective in managing patients with chronic tendinopathy. Technically, this procedure is simple to perform and allows a rapid and uncomplicated recovery. This management could induce acute degeneration and/or ablation of sensory nerve fibres, explaining the long-term pain relief.

In tendinopathic tendons, the pathological neovascularization and nerve ingrowth are considered as a possible cause of the pain. Endoscopy, electrocoagulation, and minimally invasive stripping have been proposed to disrupt the abnormal neoinnervation, and interfere with the pain sensation caused by tendinopathy. Tendoscopy allows endoscopic access to the posterior tibial tendon, peroneal tendons, and Achilles tendon, the posterior aspect of the ankle and subtalar joints, and extra-articular structures of the hindfoot such as the os trigonum, the flexor hallucis longus, and the deep portion of the deltoid ligament.[35]

Summary of management of tendinopathy

In general, physical therapy with a 12 week programme of eccentric exercises is the first approach to a patient with tendinopathy. If patients are unresponsive, ESWT is suggested, but the evidence on its efficacy is scanty. Otherwise, injections could be considered. Operative management is proposed after at least 3–6 months of non-operative management. However, patients should be informed that symptoms may recur after conservative and operative measures.

Regenerative therapies

There is increasing interest in the sports medicine community about providing endogenous growth factors directly to the injury site, using autologous blood products to potentially facilitate healing and earlier return to sport after injury. Despite this interest, and apparent widespread use, there is a lack of high-level evidence from RCTs assessing the efficacy of such products in treating ligament and tendon injuries.

PRP is an autologous concentrate of human platelets in a small volume of plasma, containing biologically active factors, responsible for haemostasis, synthesis of new connective tissue, and revascularization.[47] The term 'PRP' is used for two different liquid formulations: L-PRP contains 5–8 times more platelets and more leucocytes than peripheral blood; P-PRP, in which leucocytes are absent, has a moderate increase in platelet count (1.5–2.5-fold above baseline). Many questions about the best volume and frequency of the injections, the ideal period between multiple injections, mechanism of platelet activation, and degranulation are still unanswered.

First used in the 1980s to promote physiological wound healing of cutaneous ulcers, the use of PRP has spread to a wide range of specialist areas.[47] PRP has been used to enhance the healing of meniscus defects and muscle injuries, stimulate chondrocytes to engineer cartilaginous tissue, reduce pain and produce better and more balanced synovial fluid in arthritic knees, improve outcomes after total knee arthroplasty and subacromial decompression, accelerate bone formation, stimulate the healing of ACL injury central defects, improve the outcome of operated ruptured Achilles tendons, reduce pain in chronic tendinopathies, and prevent and reverse intervertebral disc degeneration. Although some trials report a positive effect, more recent well-designed studies report no beneficial effect, and possibly detrimental effects, of PRP.

In sports medicine, intramuscular PRP injections were initially prohibited, while all other routes of administration, such as peritendinous, were permitted. However, the different PRP formulations were not found to increase muscle growth beyond return to a normal physiological state. Although the prohibition for intramuscular injections of PRP was removed in the 2011 prohibited list, sporting authorities will continue to review PRP use as new medical and scientific information becomes available.[48] Because of the relative safety of these products, basic science, clinical discovery and patient-oriented research should be interdependent rather than successive steps.

References

1. Jarvinen MJ, Lehto MU. The effects of early mobilisation and immobilisation on the healing process following muscle injuries. *Sports Med* 1993;15:78–89.
2. Garrett WE. Muscle strain injuries. *Am J Sports Med* 1996;24:S2–S8.
3. Garrett WE, Safran MR, Seaber AV, Glisson RR, Ribbeck BM. Biomechanical comparison of stimulated and nonstimulated skeletal muscle pulled to failure. *Am J Sports Med* 1987;15:448–454.
4. Brandser EA, el-Khoury GY, Kathol MH, Callaghan JJ, Tearse DS. Hamstring injuries: radiographic, conventional tomographic, CT, and MR imaging characteristics. *Radiology* 1995;197:257–262.
5. Palmer WE, Kuong SJ, Elmadbouh HM. MR imaging of myotendinous strain. *AJR Am J Roentgenol* 1999;173:703–709.
6. De Smet AA, Best TM. MR imaging of the distribution and location of acute hamstring injuries in athletes. *AJR Am J Roentgenol* 2000;174:393–399.
7. Crisco JJ, Jokl P, Heinen GT, Connell MD, Panjabi MM. A muscle contusion injury model. Biomechanics, physiology, and histology. *Am J Sports Med* 1994;22:702–710.
8. Page P. Pathophysiology of acute exercise-induced muscular injury: clinical implications. *J Athl Train* 1995;30(1):29–34.
9. Malliaropoulos N, Isinkaye T, Tsitas K, Maffulli N. Reinjury after acute posterior thigh muscle injuries in elite track and field athletes. *Am J Sports Med* 2011;39:304–310.
10. Connell DA, Schneider-Kolsky ME, Hoving JL et al. Longitudinal study comparing sonographic and MRI assessments of acute and healing hamstring injuries. *AJR Am J Roentgenol* 2004;183:975–984.
11. Rubin SJ, Feldman F, Staron RB et al. Magnetic resonance imaging of muscle injury. *Clin Imaging* 1995;19:263–269.
12. Lee JC, Healy J. Sonography of lower limb muscle injury. *AJR Am J Roentgenol* 2004;182:341–351.
13. Hasselman CT, Best TM, Hughes C, Martinez S, Garrett WE. An explanation for various rectus femoris strain injuries using previously undescribed muscle architecture. *Am J Sports Med* 1995;23:493–499.
14. Aglietti P, Giron F, Losco M, Cuomo P, Ciardullo A, Mondanelli N. Comparison between single-and double-bundle anterior cruciate ligament reconstruction: a prospective, randomized, single-blinded clinical trial. *Am J Sports Med* 2010;38:25–34.
15. Barenius B, Nordlander M, Ponzer S, Tidermark J, Eriksson, K. Quality of life and clinical outcome after anterior cruciate ligament reconstruction using patellar tendon graft or quadrupled semitendinosus graft: an 8-year follow-up of a randomized controlled trial. *Am J Sports Med* 2010;38:1533–1541.
16. Holm I, Oiestad BE, Risberg MA, Aune AK. No difference in knee function or prevalence of osteoarthritis after reconstruction of the anterior cruciate ligament with 4-strand hamstring autograft versus patellar tendon-bone autograft: a randomized study with 10-year follow-up. *Am J Sports Med* 2010;38:448–454.
17. Taylor DC, DeBerardino TM, Nelson BJ et al. Patellar tendon versus hamstring tendon autografts for anterior cruciate ligament reconstruction: a randomized controlled trial using similar femoral and tibial fixation methods. *Am J Sports Med* 2009;37:1946–1957.

18. Nin JR, Gasque GM, Azcárate AV, Beola JD, Gonzalez MH. Has platelet-rich plasma any role in anterior cruciate ligament allograft healing? *Arthroscopy* 2009;25:1206–1213.

19. Kim SJ, Kim TE, Jo SB, Kung YP. Comparison of the clinical results of three posterior cruciate ligament reconstruction techniques. *J Bone Joint Surg Am* 2009;91:2543–2549.

20. Gill TJ, Van de Velde SK, Wing DW, Oh LS, Hosseini A, Li G. Tibiofemoral and patellofemoral kinematics after reconstruction of an isolated posterior cruciate ligament injury: in vivo analysis during lunge. *Am J Sports Med* 2009;37:2377–2385.

21. LaPrade RF, Johansen S, Agel J et al. Outcomes of an anatomic posterolateral knee reconstruction. *J Bone Joint Surg Am* 2010;92:16–22.

22. Levy BA, Dajani KA, Morgan JA et al. Repair versus reconstruction of the fibular collateral ligament and posterolateral corner in the multiligament-injured knee. *Am J Sports Med* 2010;38:804–809.

23. Hirschmann MT, Iranpour F, Müller W, Friederich NF. Surgical treatment of complex bicruciate knee ligament injuries in elite athletes: what long-term outcome can we expect? *Am J Sports Med* 2010;38:1103–1109.

24. Buckens CF, and Saris DB. Reconstruction of the medial patellofemoral ligament for treatment of patellofemoral instability: a systematic review. *Am J Sports Med* 2010;38:181–188.

25. Paulos L, Swanson SC, Stoddard GJ, Barber-Westin S. Surgical correction of limb malalignment for instability of the patella: a comparison of 2 techniques. *Am J Sports Med* 2009;37:1288–1300.

26. Ajis A, Younger AS, Maffulli N. Anatomic repair for chronic lateral ankle instability. *Foot Ankle Clin* 2006;11:539–545.

27. Ferran NA, and Maffulli N. Epidemiology of sprains of the lateral ankle ligament complex. *Foot Ankle Clin* 2006;11:659–662.

28. Baumhauer JF, and O'Brien T. Surgical considerations in the treatment of ankle instability. *J Athl Train* 2002;37:458–462.

29. Nery C, Raduan F, Del Buono A et al. Arthroscopic-assisted Broström-Gould for chronic ankle instability: a long-term follow-up. *Am J Sports Med* 2011;39(11):2381–2388.

30. Maffulli N, Ajis A, Longo UG, Denaro V. Chronic rupture of tendo Achilles. *Foot Ankle Clin* 2007;12:583–596.

31. Wong J, Barrass V, Maffulli N. Quantitative review of operative and nonoperative management of achilles tendon ruptures. *Am J Sports Med* 2002;30:565–575.

32. Maffulli N. Rupture of the Achilles tendon. *J Bone Joint Surg Am* 1999;81:1019–1036.

33. Longo UG, Ronga M, Maffulli N. Acute ruptures of the achilles tendon. *Sports Med Arthrosc* 2009;17:127–138.

34. Maffulli N, Khan KM, Puddu G. Overuse tendon conditions: time to change a confusing terminology. *Arthroscopy* 1998;14:840–843.

35. Maffulli N, Longo UG, Denaro V. Novel approaches for the management of tendinopathy. *J Bone Joint Surg Am* 2010;92:2604–2613.

36. Astrom M, Westlin N. No effect of piroxicam on achilles tendinopathy. A randomized study of 70 patients. *Acta Orthop Scand* 1992;63:631–634.

37. Arya S, Kulig K. Tendinopathy alters mechanical and material properties of the Achilles tendon. *J Appl Physiol* 2010;108:670–675.

38. Longo UG, Franceschi F, Ruzzini L et al. Light microscopic histology of supraspinatus tendon ruptures. *Knee Surg Sports Traumatol Arthrosc* 2007;15:1390–1394.

39. Maffulli N, Longo UG. How do eccentric exercises work in tendinopathy? *Rheumatology* (Oxford) 2008;47:1444–1445.

40. Rompe JD, Furia J, Maffulli N. Eccentric loading versus eccentric loading plus shock-wave treatment for midportion achilles tendinopathy: a randomized controlled trial. *Am J Sports Med* 2009;37:463–470.

41. Rompe JD, Maffulli N. Repetitive shock wave therapy for lateral elbow tendinopathy (tennis elbow): a systematic and qualitative analysis. *Br Med Bull* 2007;83:355–378.

42. Costa ML, Shepstone L, Donell ST, Thomas TL. Shock wave therapy for chronic Achilles tendon pain: a randomized placebo-controlled trial. *Clin Orthop Relat Res* 2005;440:199–204.

43. Chan O, O'Dowd D, Padhiar N et al. High volume image guided injections in chronic Achilles tendinopathy. *Disabil Rehabil* 2008;30:1697–1708.

44. Crisp T, Khan F, Padhiar N et al. High volume ultrasound guided injections at the interface between the patellar tendon and Hoffa's body are effective in chronic patellar tendinopathy: A pilot study. *Disabil Rehabil* 2008;30:1625–1634.

45. Maffulli N. Re: Etiologic factors associated with symptomatic Achilles tendinopathy. *Foot Ankle Int* 2007;28:660; author reply 660–661.

46. Maffulli N, Testa V, Capasso G, Bifulco G, Binfield, PM. Results of percutaneous longitudinal tenotomy for Achilles tendinopathy in middle- and long-distance runners. *Am J Sports Med* 1997;25:835–840.

47. Marx RE. Platelet-rich plasma (PRP): what is PRP and what is not PRP? *Implant Dent* 2001;10:225–228.

48. Engebretsen L, Steffen K, Alsousou, J. et al. IOC consensus paper on the use of platelet-rich plasma in sports medicine. *Br J Sports Med* 2010;44:1072–1081.

SECTION 23

Miscellaneous conditions

CHAPTER 163

Amyloidosis

Philip N. Hawkins

Introduction

Amyloidosis is a disorder of protein folding in which normally soluble proteins are deposited in the extracellular space as insoluble fibrils that progressively disrupt tissue structure and function.[1] More than 25 different unrelated proteins can form amyloid in vivo, and clinical amyloidosis is classified according to the fibril protein type (Table 163.1). The term amyloid is erroneously derived from the Greek for 'starch-like', and the term has been retained despite the protein nature of the deposits having been recognized well over 100 years ago. Protein misfolding and aggregation have increasingly been recognized in the pathogenesis of various other diseases, but amyloidosis—the disease directly caused by extracellular amyloid deposition—is a precise term with critical implications for patients with a specific group of life-threatening disorders.

Amyloid deposition is remarkable in its diversity; it can be systemic or localized, acquired or hereditary, life-threatening or merely an incidental finding. Clinical consequences occur when accumulation of amyloid is substantial enough to disrupt the structure of tissues or organs, leading to impairment of their function. The pattern of organ involvement varies within and between types of amyloidosis, but clinical phenotypes overlap greatly. In systemic amyloidosis, virtually any tissue may be involved and the disease is often fatal, although prognosis has improved as the result of increasingly effective treatments for many of the conditions that underlie it. Greater understanding of the pathogenesis of the disease allowing for improved diagnosis and clinical characterization, along with rational therapies and better supportive care including haemodialysis and solid organ transplantation have also favourably influenced the prognosis. Localized amyloid deposits are confined to a particular organ or tissue, and range from being clinically silent through to having serious consequences such as haemorrhage in the respiratory or urogenital tracts, or space-occupying effects. In addition to the disorders that are classified as a type of amyloidosis, local amyloid deposition is a pathological feature of uncertain significance in various other important diseases including Alzheimer's disease, the prion disorders, and type 2 diabetes mellitus, which are beyond the scope of this chapter.

Pathogenesis of amyloid

Amyloidosis defies the dogma that tertiary structure of proteins is determined solely by their primary amino acid sequence. Amyloid-forming proteins can adopt two completely different stable structures, the transformation involving massive refolding of the native form into one that predominantly consists of β-sheet and which can autoaggregate with like molecules in a highly ordered manner to produce characteristic, rigid, non-branching amyloid fibrils 10–15 nm in diameter and of indeterminate length.[2] Acquired biophysical properties that are common to all amyloid fibrils include insolubility in physiological solutions, relative resistance to proteolysis, and ability to bind Congo red dye in a spatially ordered manner that produces the diagnostic green birefringence under cross-polarized light.[3]

There are several circumstances in which amyloid deposition occurs. The first is a consequence of a sustained abnormally high concentration of certain proteins that are normally present at very low levels, such as serum amyloid A protein (SAA) in chronic inflammation and β_2-microglobulin in renal failure, which underlie susceptibility to AA and $A\beta_2M$ amyloidosis respectively. A second situation is when there is a normal concentration of a normal, but to some extent inherently amyloidogenic, protein over a very prolonged period, such as transthyretin in senile amyloidosis (ATTR) and β-protein in Alzheimer's disease. The third situation requires the presence of an acquired or inherited variant protein with an abnormal and markedly amyloidogenic structure, such as certain monoclonal immunoglobulin light chains in AL amyloidosis and the genetic amyloidogenic variants of transthyretin, lysozyme, apolipoprotein AI, fibrinogen Aα chain, etc., in hereditary amyloidosis. The genetic and/or environmental factors that influence individual susceptibility to and the timing of amyloid deposition remain unclear, but once the process has begun, further accumulation of amyloid is unremitting so long as the supply of the respective precursor protein continues. Although it is not clear why only the 20 or so known amyloidogenic proteins adopt the amyloid fold and persist as fibrils in vivo, a major unifying theme is that amyloid precursors are relatively unstable. Even under physiological conditions they populate partly unfolded states involving loss of tertiary structure but retention of β-sheet secondary structure, which can autoaggregate into protofilaments and thence mature amyloid fibrils. Seeding may play a facilitating role, consistent with observations that accumulation of amyloid can be remarkably rapid following its initiation.

Amyloid deposits consist mainly of these protein fibrils, but they also contain some common minor constituents, including certain

Table 163.1 Classification of amyloidosis[a]

Type	Fibril precursor protein	Clinical syndrome
AA	Serum amyloid A protein	Systemic amyloidosis usually with predominant renal involvement associated with acquired or hereditary chronic inflammatory diseases. Formerly known as secondary or reactive amyloidosis
AL	Monoclonal immunoglobulin light chains	Systemic amyloidosis potentially involving many organ systems associated with myeloma, monoclonal gammopathy, occult B-cell dyscrasias. Formerly known as primary amyloidosis
ATTR	Normal plasma transthyretin	Senile systemic amyloidosis with predominant cardiac involvement (senile cardiac amyloidosis)
ATTR	Genetic variants of TTR (e.g. ATTR Met30, Ala60, Ile122)	FAP, often with prominent amyloid cardiomyopathy. Predominant cardiac involvement without neuropathy with certain mutations, e.g. TTR Ile122
$A\beta_2M$	β_2-Microglobulin	DRA associated with renal failure and long-term dialysis. Predominant articular and periarticular involvement
$A\beta$	β-Protein precursor (and rare genetic variants)	Cerebrovascular and intracerebral plaque amyloid in Alzheimer's disease. Occasionally familial
AApoAI	Genetic variants of apolipoprotein AI (e.g. AApoAI Arg26, Arg60)	Autosomal dominant systemic amyloidosis. Predominantly non-neuropathic with prominent visceral involvement, especially nephropathy. Minor wild-type ApoAI amyloid deposits may occur in the aorta in aging individuals
AApoAII	Genetic variants of apolipoprotein AII	Autosomal dominant systemic amyloidosis with predominant renal involvement
AFib	Genetic variants of fibrinogen $A\alpha$ chain (e.g. AFib Val526)	Autosomal dominant systemic amyloidosis. Non-neuropathic with predominant nephropathy
ALys	Genetic variants of lysozyme (e.g. ALys His67)	Autosomal dominant systemic amyloidosis. Non-neuropathic with predominant renal and gastrointestinal involvement. Rarely presents with hepatic rupture
ACys	Genetic variant of cystatin C (ACys Gln68)	Hereditary cerebral haemorrhage with cerebral and systemic amyloidosis, in Icelandic subjects
AGel	Genetic variants of gelsolin (e.g. AGel Asn187)	Autosomal dominant systemic amyloidosis. Predominant cranial nerve involvement plus lattice corneal dystrophy. Described and most common in Finland

DRA, dialysis-related amyloidosis; FAP, familial amyloid polyneuropathy; TTR, transthyretin.

[a]Not exhaustive and amyloid composed of peptide hormones, prion protein, and unknown proteins not included.

glycosaminoglycans (GAGs) and the normal circulating plasma protein serum amyloid P component (SAP), as well as various other trace proteins. SAP binds in a specific calcium-dependent manner to a ligand that is present on all amyloid fibrils but not on their respective precursor proteins.[4] This phenomenon is the basis for the use of SAP scintigraphy in some centres for diagnostic imaging and quantitative monitoring of amyloid deposits. Studies in knockout mice indicate that SAP contributes to amyloidogenesis.

Amyloid fibril-associated GAGs mainly consist of heparan and dermatan sulphates.[5] Their universal presence, restricted heterogeneity, and intimate relationship with the fibrils suggest that they may also contribute to the development or stability of amyloid deposits, a possibility that has lately been supported by the inhibitory effect of low-molecular-weight GAG analogues on the experimental induction of AA amyloidosis in both mice and human patients.[6]

Many of the pathological effects of amyloid can be attributed to its physical presence. Extensive deposits, which may amount to kilograms, are structurally disruptive and incompatible with normal function, as are strategically located smaller deposits, for example in glomeruli or nerves. It remains possible that amyloid fibrils or prefibrillar aggregates may also be directly cytotoxic in some circumstances, but, curiously, amyloid deposits appear to evoke little or no local inflammatory reaction in the tissues. The relationship between the quantity of amyloid deposited and the degree of associated organ dysfunction differs greatly between individuals and

between different organs, and there is a strong impression that the rate of new amyloid deposition may be as important a determinant of progressive organ failure as the absolute amyloid load.

Treatments that substantially reduce the supply of amyloidogenic precursor proteins frequently result in stabilization or regression of existing amyloid deposits, and are often associated with preservation or improvement in the function of organs infiltrated by amyloid,[7,8] although the mechanisms by which amyloid deposits can be cleared are little understood at present.

Acquired amyloidosis

Acquired systemic amyloidosis is thought to be the cause of death in about 1 in 1300 patients in the United Kingdom, and is probably much underdiagnosed among elderly individuals, who are likely to be at greatest risk of developing it. Systemic AL amyloidosis is the most serious and commonly diagnosed type, and presently outnumbers referrals of AA amyloidosis to the United Kingdom National Amyloidosis Centre by a factor of 7:1. Although less serious, dialysis-related β_2-microglobulin amyloidosis affects about 1 million patients receiving long-term renal replacement therapy world wide, and causes much suffering. Senile transthyretin amyloidosis, which predominantly involves the heart, occurs in about one-quarter of individuals over the age of 80 years, a sector of the population that is ever rising.

Reactive systemic amyloidosis, AA amyloidosis

AA amyloidosis is a complication of chronic infections and inflammatory diseases, or indeed any condition that gives rise to overproduction of the acute-phase reactant, serum amyloid A protein (SAA). The amyloid fibrils are composed of AA protein, an N-terminal fragment of SAA, and AA amyloidosis occurs in up to about 1–5% of patients with rheumatoid arthritis, juvenile idiopathic arthritis, and Crohn's disease, and more frequently in those with lifelong autoinflammatory diseases such as familial Mediterranean fever.[9] Most patients present with proteinuric renal disease, and although liver and gastrointestinal involvement may occur at a later stage, clinically significant involvement of the heart and nerves is very rare.

The AA fibril protein is a single non-glycosylated polypeptide chain usually of mass 8000 Da comprising the 76-residue N-terminal portion of the 104-residue SAA. Smaller and larger AA fragments, even whole molecules, sometimes occur. SAA is an apolipoprotein of high-density lipoprotein particles and is the polymorphic product of a set of genes located on chromosome 11. SAA is highly conserved in evolution and is a major acute-phase reactant. Most of the SAA in plasma is produced by hepatocytes under transcriptional regulation by cytokines, especially interleukin 1 (IL-1), interleukin 6 (IL-6), and tumour necrosis factor (TNF). After secretion, SAA rapidly associates with high-density lipoproteins from which it displaces apolipoprotein AI. The circulating concentration can rise from normal levels of up to 3 mg/litre to over 1500 mg/litre within 24–48 hours of an acute stimulus, and can remain persistently high in the presence of chronic inflammation.

The AA protein is derived from circulating SAA by proteolytic cleavage, which can be produced by macrophages and by a variety of proteinases. However, it is not known whether cleavage of SAA occurs before and/or after aggregation of monomers during AA fibrillogenesis. Overproduction of SAA in the long term is a prerequisite for deposition of AA amyloid, but it is not known why the latter only occurs in some individuals in this situation. In mice, only one of the three major isoforms of murine SAA is the precursor of AA amyloid fibrils. Human SAA isoforms are more complex but homozygosity for particular types seems to favour amyloidogenesis, although there may also be ethnic differences in susceptibility.

The functions of SAA are not known, but may include modulating effects on reverse cholesterol transport and on lipid functions in the microenvironment of inflammatory foci. Regardless of its physiological role, the behaviour of SAA as an exquisitely sensitive acute-phase protein with an enormous dynamic range makes it an extremely valuable empirical clinical marker. It can be used to objectively monitor the extent and activity of all manner of infective, inflammatory, necrotic, and neoplastic diseases. Frequent long-term monitoring of SAA is vital in the management of all patients with AA amyloidosis since control of the primary inflammatory process sufficient to reduce SAA production is essential if amyloidosis is to be halted or enabled to regress. Automated immunoassay systems for SAA are available standardized on a World Health Organization International Reference Standard.[10]

AA amyloidosis occurs in association with chronic inflammatory disorders, chronic local or systemic microbial infections, and occasionally neoplasms, all of remarkable variety. In western Europe and the United States the most frequent predisposing conditions are idiopathic rheumatic diseases. The lifetime incidence of AA amyloidosis in patients with rheumatoid arthritis (RA) and juvenile idiopathic arthritis (JIA) in Europe is up to 1–5%, although for reasons that are not clear the incidence appears to be lower in the United States, and may generally be decreasing. Amyloidosis is exceptionally rare in systemic lupus erythematosus (SLE) and related connective tissue diseases, and in ulcerative colitis since these conditions provoke only a very modest acute-phase response. Tuberculosis and leprosy are important causes of AA amyloidosis in some parts of the world. Chronic osteomyelitis, bronchiectasis, chronically infected burns and decubitus ulcers, and the chronic pyelonephritis of paraplegia are other well-recognized associations. Hodgkin's disease and renal carcinoma, which often cause a major acute-phase response, are the malignancies most commonly associated with systemic AA amyloid. Curiously, about 7% of patients with AA amyloidosis do not have a clinically obvious chronic inflammatory disease, and these patients are prone to be assumed to have AL amyloidosis in error. Although it remains impossible to identify the aetiology of the causative acute-phase response in many such patients, the commonest identifiable pathologies in such cases in our own series have been hitherto undiagnosed inherited periodic fever syndromes and cytokine-secreting Castleman's disease tumours of the solitary plasma cell type, located in either the mediastinum or the gut mesentery.

The clinical features of AA amyloidosis are dominated by renal involvement, although histologically AA amyloid deposits are widely distributed. More than 90% of patients present with nonselective proteinuria due to glomerular deposition, and nephrotic syndrome may develop before progression to endstage renal failure. Haematuria, isolated tubular defects, nephrogenic diabetes insipidus, and diffuse renal calcification occur rarely. Kidney size is usually normal, but may be enlarged, or, in advanced cases, reduced. Endstage chronic renal failure is the cause of death in 40–60% of cases but acute renal failure may be precipitated by hypotension and/or salt and water depletion following surgery, excessive use of diuretics, or intercurrent infection, and may be associated with renal vein thrombosis. The second most common presentation is with organ enlargement, such as hepatosplenomegaly or occasionally thyroid goitre, with or without overt renal abnormality, but in all cases amyloid deposits are widespread at the time of presentation, which is the basis for diagnosis through random rectal and other biopsies. Histological involvement of the heart is frequent, but rarely results in cardiac failure. Gastrointestinal dysfunction is common in advanced disease, presenting predominantly with diarrhoea and occasional bleeding.

AA amyloidosis can present clinically early in the course of an associated inflammatory disease, but the incidence increases over time. The median duration of chronic inflammatory disease prior to diagnosis of amyloid is about 20 years, though it can be as little as just 1 year.[9] Prognosis is closely related to the degree of renal dysfunction and the effectiveness of treatment for the underlying inflammatory condition. In the presence of persistent, uncontrolled inflammation, 50% of patients with AA amyloidosis die within 10 years of diagnosis, whereas if the causative acute-phase response can be persistently suppressed proteinuria can resolve, renal function may be retained, and the prognosis is much better (see 'Treatment of amyloidosis' below). Availability of haemodialysis and renal transplantation prevents early death from uraemia per se, and despite amyloid deposition in extrarenal tissues the prognosis is quite similar to other causes of endstage renal failure.

Amyloidosis associated with immunocyte dyscrasia, AL amyloidosis

Systemic AL, formerly known as 'primary', amyloidosis occurs in about 2% of individuals with monoclonal B-cell dyscrasias.[11] AL fibrils are derived from monoclonal immunoglobulin light chains, which are unique in each patient and which explains the substantial heterogeneity of AL amyloidosis in terms of organ involvement and overall clinical course. Virtually any organ other than the brain may be directly affected, but involvement of the kidneys, heart, liver, or peripheral nervous system is most often associated with clinical consequences. Early symptoms are often non-specific, including marked fatigue. The underlying monoclonal gammopathy is often missed by routine screening techniques with potential to further delay the diagnosis, which even under favourable circumstances tends to be made at an advanced stage when the deposits are extensive. This emphasizes the need to consider AL amyloidosis as a potential diagnosis in a range of vague clinical presentations, and the need for prompt appropriate investigations, such as biopsy of affected organs and sensitive serum free light-chain analysis to identify associated subtle B-cell dyscrasias.[8]

AL amyloid fibrils are derived from the N-terminal region of monoclonal immunoglobulin light chains and consist of the whole or part of the variable (V_L) domain. The molecular mass of the fibril subunit protein therefore varies between about 8000 and 30 000 Da. Monoclonal light chains are unique to each individual, and the propensity for some to form amyloid fibrils is inherent to their particular structure. Only a small proportion of monoclonal light chains are amyloidogenic, but it is not possible to identify these with any certainty from their class or abundance.

The inherent 'amyloidogenicity' of certain monoclonal light chains has been demonstrated in an in-vivo model in which purified Bence Jones proteins were injected into mice.[12] Animals receiving light chains from patients with AL amyloid developed typical amyloid deposits composed of the human protein, whereas animals receiving light chains from myeloma patients without amyloid did not. AL fibrils are more commonly derived from λ than κ light chains, despite the fact that κ isotypes predominate among both normal immunoglobulins and monoclonal gammopathies. Some amyloidogenic light chains have distinctive amino acid replacements or insertions compared with non-amyloid monoclonal light chains, including replacement of hydrophilic framework residues by hydrophobic ones, changes that can promote aggregation and insolubility. Certain light-chain isotypes, notably $V\lambda_{VI}$, are especially amyloidogenic, and there is a degree of concordance between some isotypes and their tropism for being deposited as amyloid in particular organ systems. For example, the $V\lambda_{VI}$ isotype often presents with dominant renal involvement whereas the $V\lambda_{II}$ isotype frequently involves the heart.

The associated B-cell dyscrasias in systemic AL amyloidosis are heterogeneous and include almost any clonal proliferation of differentiated B lymphocytes, including multiple myeloma, Waldenström's macroglobulinaemia, and occasionally other malignant lymphomas or leukaemias. However, well over 80% of cases are associated with low-grade and otherwise 'benign' monoclonal gammopathies that are often difficult to demonstrate. Histological studies indicate that an element of minor and clinically insignificant amyloid deposition occurs in up to about 10% of patients with myeloma, and similarly in a much proportion of patients with monoclonal gammopathy of undetermined significance (MGUS). The cytogenetic abnormalities that commonly occur in multiple myeloma and MGUS, such as 14q translocations and 13q deletion, have also been observed in AL amyloidosis, but their prognostic significance has not been fully elucidated.

Systemic AL amyloidosis accounts for about 1 in 1500 deaths in the United Kingdom and occurs equally in men and women. The age-adjusted incidence of AL amyloidosis in the United States is estimated to be between 5.1 and 12.8 per million persons per year, which is equivalent to approximately 3000 new cases per year. The median age at presentation is 65 years, but it can sometimes occur in young adults and is probably underdiagnosed in older people, in whom monoclonal gammopathies have the highest prevalence.

The clinical features of AL amyloidosis are protean.[13] The heart is affected in 90% of AL patients, in 30% of whom restrictive cardiomyopathy is the presenting feature and in up to 50% of whom it is ultimately fatal. Other cardiac presentations include arrhythmias and angina. Renal AL amyloid has the same manifestations as renal AA amyloid, but the prognosis is worse. Gut involvement may cause motility disturbances (often secondary to autonomic neuropathy), malabsorption, perforation, haemorrhage, or obstruction. Macroglossia occurs rarely but is almost pathognomonic of AL type. Hyposplenism sometimes occurs in both AA and AL amyloidosis. Painful sensory polyneuropathy with early loss of pain and temperature sensation followed later by motor deficits is seen in 10–20% of cases and carpal tunnel syndrome in 20%. Autonomic neuropathy leading to orthostatic hypotension, impotence, and gastrointestinal disturbances may occur alone or together with the peripheral neuropathy, and has a very poor prognosis. Skin involvement takes the form of papules, nodules, and plaques usually on the face and upper trunk, and involvement of dermal blood vessels results in purpura occurring either spontaneously or after minimal trauma and is quite common. Articular amyloid is rare but may superficially mimic acute polyarticular RA, or it may present as asymmetrical arthritis affecting the hip or shoulder. Infiltration of the glenohumeral joint and surrounding soft tissues occasionally produces the characteristic 'shoulder pad' sign. A rare but serious manifestation of AL amyloid is an acquired bleeding diathesis that may be associated with deficiency of factor X and sometimes also factor IX, or with increased fibrinolysis. It does not occur in AA amyloidosis, although in all types of systemic amyloidosis there may be serious bleeding in the absence of any identifiable factor deficiency due to widespread vascular deposits.

Dialysis-related amyloidosis, β_2-microglobulin amyloidosis

β_2-microglobulin amyloid deposition occurs in patients with dialysis-dependent chronic renal failure, and predominantly in articular and periarticular structures.[14] The amyloid fibril precursor protein is β_2-microglobulin, which is the invariant chain of the MHC class I molecule, and is expressed by all nucleated cells. It is synthesized at an average rate of 150–200 mg per day and is normally filtered freely at the glomerulus and then reabsorbed and catabolized by the proximal tubular cells. Decreasing renal function causes a proportionate rise in concentration.

β_2-Microglobulin amyloidosis was first described in 1980 and occurs in patients who have been on dialysis for several years, or very occasionally those with longstanding severe chronic renal impairment. Dialysis-related amyloidosis (DRA) has mostly been recognized in the haemodialysis population but it also occurs in patients on continuous ambulatory peritoneal dialysis (CAPD). Relatively few patients are maintained on peritoneal dialysis for the 5–10 years required to develop symptomatic β_2-microglobulin amyloid, but histological studies of early subclinical deposits suggests that the incidence of DRA is similar among patients receiving the two modalities of dialysis. Indeed, β_2-microglobulin amyloid deposits are present in 20–30% of patients within 3 years of commencing dialysis for endstage renal failure.

The clinical features are largely confined to the locomotor system. Carpal tunnel syndrome is usually the first clinical manifestation of β_2-microglobulin amyloidosis. Some individuals develop symptoms within 3–5 years and by 20 years the prevalence is almost 100%. Older patients appear to be more susceptible to the disease, and tend to exhibit symptoms more rapidly. Amyloid arthropathy tends to occur a little later but eventually affects the most patients on dialysis. The arthralgia of β_2-microglobulin amyloidosis affects the shoulders, knees, wrists, and small joints of the hand and is associated with joint swelling, chronic tenosynovitis and, occasionally, haemarthroses. Spondylarthropathies are also recognized, as is cervical cord compression. β_2-Microglobulin amyloid deposition within the periarticular bone produces typical appearances of subchondral erosions and cysts which can contribute to pathological fractures particularly of the femoral neck, cervical vertebrae and scaphoid. Although β_2-microglobulin amyloidosis is a systemic form of amyloid, manifestations outside the musculoskeletal systemic are rare, but there have been reports of it causing congestive cardiac failure, gastrointestinal bleeding, perforation, and pseudo-obstruction.

Senile transthyretin (ATTR) amyloidosis

Microscopic, clinically silent systemic deposits of wild-type 'senile' transthyretin (TTR) amyloid are common in older people, involving the heart and blood vessel walls, smooth and striated muscle, fat tissue, renal papillae, and alveolar walls. In contrast to most other forms of systemic amyloidosis, including hereditary transthyretin amyloid caused by point mutations in the TTR gene, the spleen and renal glomeruli are rarely affected. The brain is not involved. Senile TTR amyloidosis almost always presents clinically with restrictive cardiomyopathy, and deposits in other tissues rarely ever attain clinical significance. About one-quarter of patients can be demonstrated to have gastrointestinal amyloid deposits on rectal biopsy. Most patients are at least 70 years of age, and there is very strong male preponderance.

Localized AL amyloidosis

Localized deposits of AL amyloid can occur almost anywhere in the body and are consequent on the presence of a focal monoclonal B-cell dyscrasia within the affected tissue, which is hard to demonstrate. Characteristic sites include the skin, airways, conjunctiva, and urogenital tract. They may be nodular or confluent and are associated with a usually inconspicuous focal infiltrate of clonal B cells producing amyloidogenic light chains. Progression of localized AL amyloid into a truly systemic disease is exceedingly rare, and conservative management is usually appropriate. It is also rare for the focal B-cell dyscrasia to become systemic and to require treatment in its own right.

Localized orbital AL amyloid presents as mass lesions which can disrupt eye movement and the structure of the orbit. Localized laryngeal AL amyloidosis is a well-recognized syndrome that is often amenable to direct or laser excision, but hereditary systemic ApoAI amyloidosis can also present in this manner. Amyloidosis presenting in the bronchial tree is virtually always localized AL type, as are solitary or multiple amyloid nodules within the lung tissue. If accessible, bronchoscopic lasering of stenotic lesions can relieve symptoms. In contrast, diffuse alveolar-septal parenchymal deposition is commonly a manifestation of systemic AL amyloidosis. There are anecdotal reports that inhaled steroids may benefit pulmonary symptoms. Breast amyloidosis is associated with Sjögren's syndrome in some cases, and MALT lymphoma should be excluded. Lichenoid and macular forms of cutaneous amyloid are distinct and are thought to be derived from keratin or related proteins, whereas nodular cutaneous amyloidosis deposits are generally localized AL type, but the latter can sometimes be a manifestation of systemic AL amyloidosis. Localized urogenital AL deposits are often incidental findings but may present with haematuria or, less commonly, obstruction. They can occur anywhere from the renal collecting system to the urethra, although are most usually identified within the bladder. Management is conservative or with transurethral laser resection when symptoms occur; cystectomy is rarely required.

Hereditary systemic amyloidosis

Hereditary systemic amyloidosis is caused by deposition of amyloid fibrils derived from genetically variant proteins, and is associated with mutations in the genes for TTR, cystatin C, gelsolin, lysozyme, fibrinogen A α-chain apolipoprotein AI, and, in just a few families, apolipoprotein AII. These diseases are all inherited in an autosomal dominant pattern with variable penetrance, and present clinically at various times from teenage to old age, though usually in mid-adult life. By far the commonest hereditary amyloidosis is caused by TTR variants, which usually presents as the syndrome of familial amyloid polyneuropathy with peripheral and autonomic neuropathy. Cystatin C amyloidosis presents as cerebral amyloid angiopathy with recurrent cerebral haemorrhage and clinically silent systemic deposits, and has been reported only in Icelandic families. Gelsolin amyloidosis presents with cranial neuropathy but is also extremely rare. Apolipoprotein AI, lysozyme and fibrinogen A α-chain amyloidosis present as non-neuropathic systemic amyloidosis that can affect any or all the major viscera, with renal involvement usually being prominent. Since a family history is quite often absent, these latter conditions are readily misdiagnosed as acquired 'primary' AL amyloidosis, and are less rare than previously thought. Indeed, recent routine use of DNA analysis suggests that 5–10% of patients presenting with systemic amyloidosis of non-AA type have hereditary forms of the disease.[15] It is imperative that hereditary amyloidosis is identified correctly, since prognosis, treatment, and implications for family members differ substantially as compared with acquired amyloidosis.

Familial amyloidotic polyneuropathy, variant transthyretin (ATTR) amyloidosis

Familial amyloidotic polyneuropathy (FAP) is associated with heterozygosity for point mutations in the gene for TTR. It is an autosomal dominant syndrome with peak onset between the third and seventh decades.[16] More than 100 variant forms of TTR are associated with FAP, and the amyloid fibrils are derived from a mixture of variant and wild-type TTR protein. There are probably several thousand patients with FAP in the world. The disease is characterized by progressive and disabling peripheral and autonomic neuropathy and varying degrees of visceral amyloid involvement, prominently including cardiac amyloidosis which can be the sole clinical feature in some cases. Deposits within the vitreous of the eye are well recognized, and are pathognomonic, whereas deposits in the kidneys, thyroid, spleen, and adrenals are usually asymptomatic. There are well-characterized foci of FAP associated with the most common variant, substitution of methionine for valine at residue 30 (TTR Met30), in Portugal, Japan, and Sweden, but FAP has been reported in most ethnic groups around the world. There is considerable phenotypic variation in the age of onset, rate of progression, involvement of different systems, and disease penetrance generally, even sometimes within a given family. Typically the disease progresses inexorably, causing death within 5–15 years.

Familial amyloid polyneuropathy with predominant cranial neuropathy

This is a very rare dominant form of hereditary amyloidosis that presents in mid to late adult life with cranial neuropathy, lattice corneal dystrophy and a mild distal peripheral neuropathy.[17] It was originally described in Finland but has since been reported in other ethnic groups. There may be skin, renal, and cardiac manifestations but these are usually covert and life expectancy approaches normal. There is no specific treatment and the disorder is progressively disfiguring and very distressing its late stages. The mutant gene responsible encodes a variant form of gelsolin, which is an actin-modulating protein. The functional role of circulating gelsolin is unknown but may be related to clearance of actin filaments released by apoptotic cells.

Non-neuropathic hereditary systemic amyloidosis

A physician in Germany named Ostertag first described the syndrome of hereditary systemic amyloidosis in 1932. He reported two families with dominantly inherited renal amyloidosis without neuropathy. This syndrome is now known to be caused by mutations in the genes for lysozyme, apolipoprotein AI and AII and fibrinogen A α-chain. Hitherto thought to be exceedingly rare, it has lately been demonstrated that many affected patients do not have a family history and up to 5% of patients presenting with systemic amyloidosis have a hereditary non-neuropathic type. This has led to widespread use of DNA screening in specialist amyloidosis centres.

Hereditary lysozyme systemic amyloidosis has been described in association with six lysozyme variants, all of which are extremely rare. Most patients present in middle age with proteinuria and very slowly progressive renal impairment.[18] There are usually substantial amyloid deposits in the liver, spleen, and upper gastrointestinal tract; dry eyes due to lacrimal gland involvement is an early diagnostic clue. Curiously some patients with the least rare histidine-67 variant present as young adults with hepatic rupture,[19] but most present later on with renal dysfunction. Cutaneous petechial haemorrhage from a young age is a peculiar feature in patients with the threonine-56 variant. Many patients suffer few symptoms despite substantial amyloid deposits, but acute gastrointestinal haemorrhage or perforation is a frequent cause of death.

Apolipoprotein AI is a major constituent of high-density lipoprotein. There are 14 known amyloidogenic variants, 11 of which are single amino acid substitutions, two are deletions, and one a deletion/insertion. The resulting clinical syndromes vary but are often associated with substantial amyloid deposits in the liver, spleen, and kidneys. Some mutations are associated with predominant cardiomyopathy and, in the case of the arginine-26 variant, a FAP-like syndrome.[20] Several C-terminal variants are associated with hoarseness due to laryngeal amyloid deposits. Other clinical consequences associated with particular mutations include male infertility and skin lesions. The majority of patients eventually develop renal failure but liver function usually remains well preserved despite extensive hepatic amyloid deposition. Normal wild-type apolipoprotein AI amyloid is itself weakly amyloidogenic, and is the precursor of small amyloid deposits that occur quite frequently in aortic atherosclerotic plaques.

Hereditary fibrinogen A α-chain amyloid was first identified in a family in 1993, since when eight further amyloidogenic mutations have been described. These include five single amino acid substitutions, three frame shifting deletion mutations, and a deletion–insertion mutation. Much the commonest mutation results in the substitution of valine for glutamic acid at position 526, which most often presents in the absence of a family history due to low penetrance. Indeed, nearly 5% of patients referred to the United Kingdom National Amyloidosis Centre with a presumed diagnosis of acquired AL amyloidosis have had hereditary fibrinogen A α-chain amyloidosis.[21] Most patients present in late middle age with proteinuria or hypertension and progress to endstage renal failure during the following 5 years or so. Amyloid deposition occurs in the kidneys, spleen, and sometimes the liver, but it is usually asymptomatic in the latter two sites. The majority of patients have an excellent outcome with renal replacement therapy.

Diagnosis and investigation of amyloidosis

The diagnosis of amyloidosis generally requires histological confirmation, although the mere demonstration of amyloid deposition does not by itself establish that it is clinically significant. While amyloidosis does not occur in the absence of amyloid deposits, the latter may be an incidental histological finding, especially in older subjects. The pathognomonic tinctorial property of amyloid deposits in tissue is apple green/red birefringence when stained with Congo red dye and viewed in intense light through cross-polarized filters. Immunohistochemical staining of amyloidotic tissue sections is the most accessible method for characterizing amyloid fibril protein type, but it does not always produce definitive results, especially in AL type. Amyloid deposits can be quite patchy and histology can never provide information about the overall whole body load or distribution of amyloid deposits, nor does it permit monitoring of the natural history of amyloidosis or its response to treatment. In order to overcome these problems we developed radiolabelled human SAP as a specific, non-invasive, quantitative in-vivo tracer for amyloid deposits, and have used it as a routine tool in our clinical practice for 20 years. We have performed some 10 000 studies, and scintigraphy and metabolic turnover studies with labelled SAP have contributed greatly to knowledge of amyloidosis and, especially its diagnosis, monitoring and response to treatment.

Histological diagnosis of amyloid

The diagnosis of amyloid is most frequently made following biopsy of the kidneys, liver, heart, gut, peripheral nerve, lymph node, skin, thyroid, or bone marrow. When a possible diagnosis of amyloidosis has already been considered, biopsy of subcutaneous fat or rectum is less invasive and is positive in about 50–80% of patients with systemic AA or AL types. Biopsies of affected organs have a higher yield but a greater risk of haemorrhage and other complications.

The Congo red stain, and its resultant green birefringence when viewed with high intensity polarized light, is the pathognomonic histochemical test for amyloidosis,[22] although other fluorochromes and metachromatic stains continue to be used quite widely. Congo red is unstable and must be freshly prepared every 2 months or less. Thick sections of 5–10 μm and inclusion in every staining run of a positive control tissue containing modest amounts of amyloid are critical.

Immunohistochemistry is the most accessible method for characterizing the type of amyloidosis, although its success varies with fibril type and it depends on availability of a suitable tissue sample that contains neither too little nor too much amyloid.[23] Antibodies to serum amyloid A protein are commercially available and virtually always stain AA deposits, as is the case with antibodies to β_2-microglobulin in haemodialysis-associated amyloid. In AL amyloid, the deposits in fixed specimens are stained convincingly with antibodies to κ or λ immunoglobulin light chains in only about two-thirds of cases, since the technique is hampered by abundant polyclonal immunoglobulin background and because the light-chain fragments in AL fibrils are chiefly variable domain and unique for each monoclonal protein. Immunohistochemical staining of TTR and other hereditary amyloid fibril proteins may require pretreatment of sections with formic acid, alkaline guanidine, or deglycosylation, and, even then, do not always yield definitive results.

Electron microscopy identifies amyloid as straight, rigid non-branching fibrils, of indeterminate length, and 10–15 nm in diameter. A diagnosis of amyloidosis made through electron microscopy alone should be regarded with caution since other fibrillar deposition diseases occur. Immunogold staining of amyloidotic biopsies can sometimes be diagnostic of fibril protein type when standard immunohistochemistry under light microscopy has not produced definitive results.

Problems of histological diagnosis include inadequate tissue samples, for example the failure to obtain submucosal vessels in a rectal biopsy, and indeed the failure to identify any amyloid in a target organ biopsy never completely excludes the diagnosis. The unavoidable sampling problem means that biopsies cannot reveal the extent or distribution of amyloid generally. Experience with Congo red staining is required if clinically important false-negative and false-positive results are to be avoided. Immunohistochemical staining requires positive and negative controls, including demonstration of specificity of staining by absorption of antisera with the respective antigens.

Non-histological investigations

Myocardial amyloid deposits cause a restrictive type of cardiomyopathy.[24] Two-dimensional echocardiography showing small,

concentrically thickened ventricles, diastolic dysfunction with or without various degrees of global systolic impairment, dilated atria, homogeneously echogenic valves, and 'sparkling' echodensity of ventricular walls is virtually diagnostic of cardiac amyloidosis (Figure 163.1). However, clinically significant diastolic impairment may be difficult to detect even by comprehensive Doppler and other functional studies, and can sometimes occur in the absence of left ventricular wall thickening. Newer echocardiographic techniques such as strain and strain rate measurements can be helpful. Cardiac MRI is emerging to be of value, including the peculiar phenomenon of diffuse subendocardial late gadolinium enhancement which appears to be strongly suggestive of amyloid. Electrocardiography characteristically shows reduced voltages, presumably reflecting replacement of myocardium by amyloid, although this finding is less common in cardiac amyloid of TTR type than AL type. Localization of isotope-labelled calcium-seeking tracers in the heart has poor sensitivity and specificity and is of no routine clinical value.

Elevation of serum N-terminal pro brain natriuretic peptide (NT-proBNP) and cardiac troponin concentrations occur in many types of cardiac dysfunction and in chronic kidney disease. However, significant cardiac AL amyloidosis is excluded by normal values of NT-proBNP.[25] Cardiac troponin and NT-proBNP concentrations appear to be powerful predictors of prognosis and survival after chemotherapy in AL amyloidosis, and a staging system for newly diagnosed AL amyloidosis patients using these two biomarkers has been proposed.

In cases of known or suspected hereditary amyloidosis the gene defect must be characterized. If amyloidotic tissue is available the fibril protein may be identified immunohistochemically and the corresponding gene can then be studied, but when no tissue is

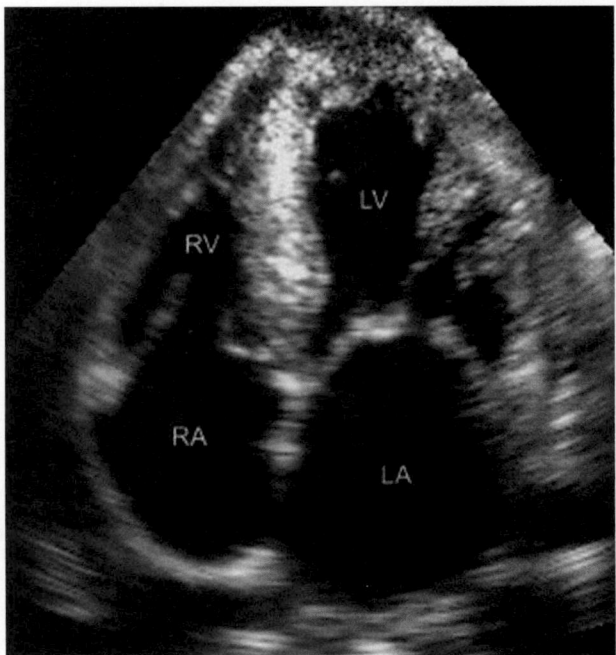

Fig. 163.1 Echocardiographic four-chamber view in a patient with cardiac AL amyloidosis showing concentric thickening of the ventricular walls, dilated atria, and thickened valves. Doppler flow studies demonstrated restrictive physiology, but systolic function was relatively well preserved.

available, screening of the genes for known amyloidogenic proteins must be undertaken.

Biochemical and immunochemical analyses for the presence in the plasma of genetically variant amyloidogenic variant proteins also exist, but DNA analysis is the most direct approach. However, it remains essential to corroborate DNA findings by confirming one way or another that the respective protein is indeed the main constituent of the amyloid.

Proteomic analyses of amyloidotic material are increasingly being used in specialist centres, enabling amyloid deposits in ever smaller samples to be characterized.[26]

Radiolabelled serum amyloid P component scintigraphy

The universal presence in amyloid deposits of SAP, derived from circulating SAP, is the basis for use of radioiodine-labelled SAP as a diagnostic tracer in amyloidosis.[27] No localization or retention of labelled SAP occurs in healthy subjects or in patients with diseases other than amyloidosis. Radioiodinated SAP has a short (24 hour) half-life in the plasma and is rapidly catabolized with complete excretion of the iodinated breakdown products in the urine. However, in patients with amyloidosis, the tracer rapidly and specifically localizes to the deposits, in proportion to the quantity of amyloid present, and persists there without breakdown or modification (Figure 163.2). Most experience has been gained with SAP labelled with the pure gamma emitter iodine-123. The associated dose of radioactivity is less than 4 mSv and well within accepted safety limits for diagnostic nuclear medicine imaging. The uptake of tracer into various organs can be precisely and repeatedly quantified.

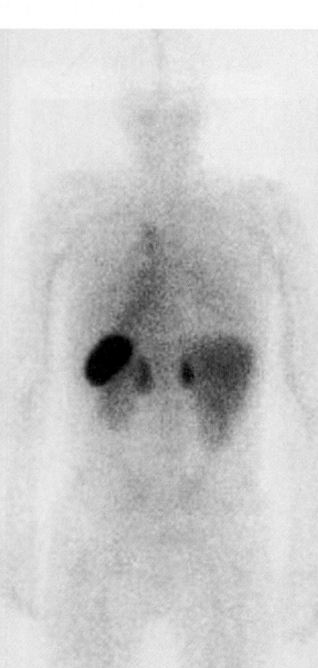
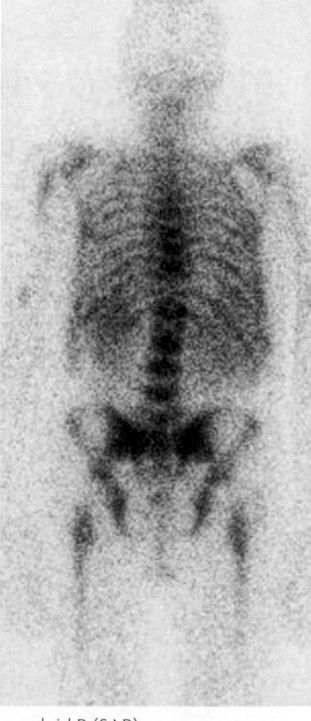

Fig. 163.2 Posterior whole body I^{123}-serum amyloid P (SAP) component scintigraphy demonstrating systemic amyloid deposits in the spleen, adrenal glands, and kidneys of a patient with AA amyloidosis (left), and throughout the bones of a patient with AL amyloidosis (right). Major uptake of I^{123}-SAP into bones only occurs in amyloidosis of AL type.

Important observations regarding amyloid, which have been made for the first time in vivo, include the following: the different distribution of amyloid in different forms of the disease; amyloid in anatomic sites not available for biopsy (adrenals, spleen); major systemic deposits in forms of amyloid previously thought to be organ-limited; a poor correlation between the quantity of amyloid present in a given organ and the level of organ dysfunction; a non-homogeneous distribution of amyloid within individual organs; and evidence for surprisingly rapid progression and regression of amyloid deposits with different rates in different organs. The long-held belief that amyloid deposition is irreversible and inexorably progressive is evidently incorrect, and simply reflects the persistent nature of the conditions that underlie it. Many case reports have described improvement in amyloidotic organ function when underlying conditions have been controlled, suggesting regression of amyloid, and serial SAP scintigraphy provided the means to prove this is indeed the case. Regression of amyloid has been observed when the supply of amyloid fibril precursor proteins has been reduced in AA amyloidosis by vigorous control of rheumatic inflammation, in AL amyloidosis by suppression of the clonal plasma cell disease by cytotoxic drugs, in haemodialysis-associated amyloidosis after renal transplantation, and in hereditary TTR and fibrinogen A α-chain amyloidosis following liver transplantation. It is now clear that amyloid deposits exist generally in a state of dynamic turnover, with encouraging implications for patient management. Labelled SAP studies thus make a valuable contribution to the diagnosis and management of patients with systemic amyloidosis, and are performed routinely at the NHS National Amyloidosis Centre at the Royal Free Hospital, London.

Assessment of organ involvement by amyloid

Internationally agreed consensus criteria for defining organ involvement in systemic amyloidosis were published in 2005 (Table 163.2).[28] Organ involvement by amyloid is variously defined clinically, histologically, and according to organ function and through other specialized investigations. ECG and two-dimensional Doppler echocardiography are the mainstays for assessing cardiac involvement, as are estimates of glomerular filtration and proteinuria for renal involvement. Liver size and serum alkaline phosphatase provide simple and accessible, but not overly sensitive, measures of liver involvement. In contrast, amyloid involvement of the gastrointestinal tract, lungs, soft tissues and nervous system are much less amenable to precise definitions and are even more challenging to monitor quantitatively over time.

Natural history and prognostic factors

Systemic amyloidosis is almost always a progressive disease which without successful treatment usually results in death within months to several years. Median survival of patients with AA amyloidosis whose underlying inflammatory disease is not well suppressed is in the order of 5–10 years. The prognosis in FAP is similar, but is usually much better in non-neuropathic hereditary types, i.e. those associated with mutations in apolipoprotein AI, fibrinogen A α-chain, and lysozyme. The prognosis of systemic AL amyloidosis is generally worse than AA and hereditary types, and median survival in some quite recent series was only 12–15 months. Important factors that influence prognosis are the extent and severity of organ involvement, availability of

Table 163.2 Diagnostic criteria for organ involvement by amyloid

Organ involvement	Consensus criteria[a]
Heart	Echocardiogram demonstrates a mean wall thickness >12 mm, no other cardiac cause found
Kidney	Proteinuria >0.5g/24 h, predominately albumin
Liver	Total liver span >15 cm in the absence of heart failure or alkaline phosphatase >1.5 times the institutional upper limit of normal
Nerve	Peripheral: clinical; symmetric lower extremity sensorimotor peripheral neuropathy
	Autonomic: gastric-emptying disorder, pseudo-obstruction, voiding dysfunction not related to direct organ infiltration
Gastrointestinal tract	Direct biopsy verification with symptoms
Lung	Direct biopsy verification with symptoms
	Interstitial radiographic pattern
Soft tissue	Tongue enlargement, clinical
	Arthropathy
	Claudication, presumed vascular amyloid
	Skin
	Myopathy by biopsy or psudohypertrophy
	Lymph node (may be localized)
	Carpal tunnel syndrome

[a]As reported by Gertz et al., *Am J Hematol* 2005;**79**:319–328.

Treatment of amyloidosis

Localized amyloid masses can only be treated surgically. The twin aims of management in systemic amyloidosis are reduction of the supply of amyloid fibril precursor proteins so that amyloid deposition diminishes and gradual regression of existing deposits may occur, and scrupulous general care, including dialysis and organ transplantation if necessary, to keep patients alive long enough for this to take effect. Awareness of the compromised functional reserve of amyloidotic organs and extreme care to protect renal function are critically important. Rational management has been greatly facilitated by the recent availability of routine assays for circulating SAA in AA amyloidosis, and serum free light chains in AL type, and outcomes are much better in centres with specialist expertise.

Treatment of AA amyloidosis

Treatment of the chronic inflammatory conditions responsible for AA amyloidosis, to reduce production of SAA, ideally to normal healthy baseline levels, dramatically improves survival and is associated with arrest of amyloid deposition and frequently regression of deposits (Figure 163.3). Plainly, treatment varies depending on the nature of the inflammatory disorder, but successful pharmacological approaches have ranged from non-specific immunosuppression in inflammatory arthritis using chlorambucil, to highly specific inhibition of IL-1 in patients with periodic fever syndromes.[9] Inflammatory arthritis underlies AA amyloidosis in two-thirds of cases, and biological agents targeting the key cytokine mediators of inflammation—TNFα, IL-1, and IL-6—potently

supportive measures including renal dialysis and organ transplantation, and the potential for and effectiveness of reducing the supply of the respective amyloid fibril precursor protein through intervention.

Systemic AL amyloidosis is not only the commonest type, but also the most heterogeneous in its organ involvement, presentation, and clinical course. One-half of deaths are due to cardiac involvement, and in patients in whom heart failure is evident at presentation, median survival is 6 months. There has been much recent effort to define prognostic factors in AL amyloidosis, and staging systems are in development. Symptomatic or substantial echocardiographic evidence of cardiac amyloid is associated with a prognosis of only 6–12 months. Patients with liver involvement and hyperbilirubinaemia above 35 μmol/litre rarely survive more than 4 months. Significant autonomic neuropathy, progressive clonal disease unresponsive to chemotherapy, and a bone marrow plasmacytosis of over 20% are also associated with poor outcomes. A large whole-body amyloid load on SAP scintigraphy and evidence of accumulation of amyloid on follow-up SAP scans are further poor prognostic features. A better prognosis is associated with proteinuria or peripheral neuropathy as the dominant clinical feature, substantial suppression of underlying clonal disease by chemotherapy, and regression of amyloid deposits on serial SAP scintigraphy. Elevated serum concentrations at diagnosis of the cardiac biomarkers troponin and B-natiuretic peptide (BNP) or its more stable precursor, NT-proBNP, are associated with a poor outcome, as is the absence of any early fall in their concentrations following chemotherapy.[29]

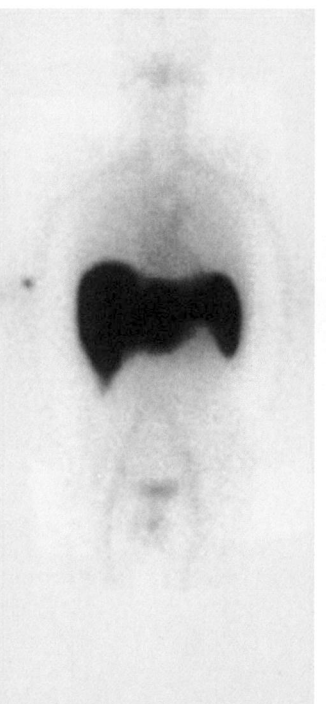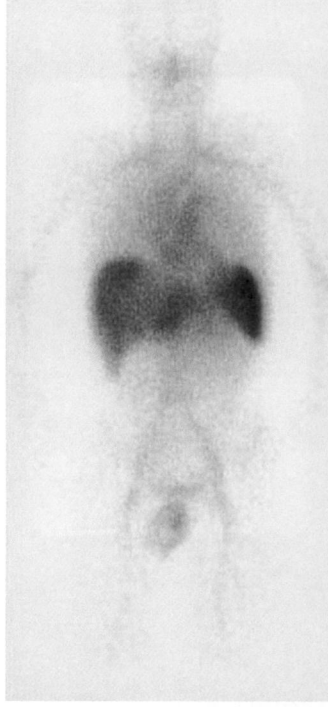

Fig. 163.3 Serial anterior I[123]-serum amyloid P (SAP) component scintigraphy demonstrating regression of hepatic and splenic AA amyloid deposits in a patient with rheumatoid arthritis, which remitted completely following treatment with oral chlorambucil. The scan on the left was obtained at presentation and the follow-up scan on the right was performed 2 years later.

suppress the acute-phase response in many patients with RA, JIA, and seronegative spondyloarthropathies. These drugs can also be effective in some patients with Crohn's disease. Regular prophylactic treatment with colchicine is highly effective in suppressing inflammatory disease activity in familial Mediterranean fever, in which it substantially prevents development and/or progression of AA amyloidosis.

Surgical treatments include excision of solitary cytokine-secreting Castleman's tumours and amputation of osteomyelitic limbs, and rarely excision of other inflammatory lesions.

A surprising finding among patients with AA amyloidosis is that of clinically covert inflammatory disease, which cannot be characterized, in about 7% of patients. Many such patients are presumed to have primary AL amyloidosis at presentation, emphasizing the need to perform confirmatory immunohistochemically in all cases. Anti-inflammatory treatment must be empiric in such cases but should be guided, as is the case in all patients with AA amyloidosis, by frequent SAA measurements.

Treatment of AL amyloidosis

The objective of treatment in AL amyloidosis is to suppress production of the amyloidogenic monoclonal light chains in the hope that progression of the disease will be slowed down, halted, or reversed (Figure 163.4). However, many patients have advanced multisystem disease at diagnosis and tolerate chemotherapy poorly. Quantitative measurements of serum free light chains using the robust, sensitive, Freelite immunoassay are usually the most effective means for evaluating the early effects of chemotherapy and the need for ongoing treatment.[8] Chemotherapy must be tailored to the individual patient, balancing the ideal for complete remission of the clonal disease with the need to minimize treatment toxicity and indeed

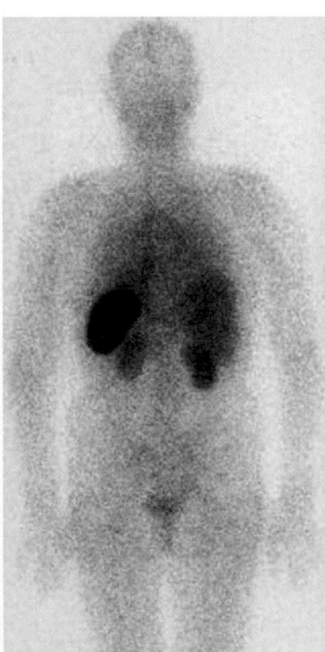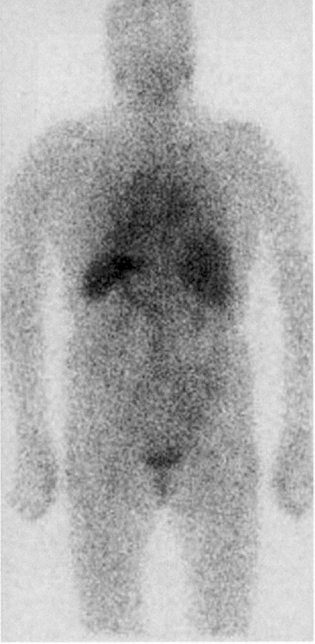

Fig. 163.4 Serial posterior I[123]-serum amyloid P component (SAP) scintigraphy demonstrating regression of splenic and renal AL amyloid deposits in a patient whose low-grade monoclonal gammopathy was suppressed by high-dose melphalan and stem cell rescue. The scan on the left was obtained at presentation in 1998 and the follow-up scan on the right was performed 3 years later.

treatment-related mortality. Certain organs affected by amyloid tend to fare better than others following treatment. Proteinuria and liver function often improve when the clonal disease is adequately suppressed, whereas cardiac disease, macroglossia, and peripheral nerve function tend to improve extremely slowly if at all.

Many different chemotherapy regimes are in current use, ranging from low-intensity oral melphalan and prednisolone through various intermediate dose drug combinations to high-dose chemotherapy with autologous peripheral stem cell rescue. The new agents bortezomib and lenalidomide, recently introduced for myeloma, are also showing great promise in AL. Some of the more commonly used regimes are reviewed briefly below.

Autologous peripheral blood stem cell transplantation (ASCT), also known as high-dose melphalan therapy, was first reported in AL amyloidosis in 1996, and several series have reported clinical benefit in up to 80% of patients who survived this arduous procedure. In the largest reported series, comprising 394 patients, complete clonal disease responses occurred in 41%, and median survival of such patients had not been reached after 10 years of follow-up.[30] However, treatment-related mortality associated with ASCT has been consistently problematic and substantially greater than in multiple myeloma, reflecting the compromised function of multiple organ systems by amyloid. Even just stem cell mobilization entails significant risks in patients with AL amyloidosis. Causes of death include cardiac arrhythmias, intractable hypotension, multiple organ failure, and gastrointestinal bleeding. Patient eligibility criteria for ASCT have been developed, favouring those without overt cardiac involvement, two or less vital organ systems clinically involved by amyloid, no history of gastrointestinal bleeding, and age less than 65 years, though despite this treatment-related mortality remains up to about 13% even in the most experienced centres. The role of ASCT in AL amyloidosis remains controversial and its apparently good outcome may reflect selection of fitter patients with good prognosis.[31] Only one randomized trial has been performed, in France using oral melpahalan and dexamethasone (Mel-Dex) as the comparator; no difference in response rates were demonstrated and treatment-related mortality (24%) was significantly higher within the ASCT arm.[32] This study was, however, relatively small.

Oral Mel-Dex has been used widely during the past 10 years, having been shown in open studies to be relatively well tolerated and associated with combined complete and partial clonal response rates of around 67% and median overall survival of about 5 years.[32] However, median time to haematological response is slow at over 4 months, and its potential for depleting bone marrow stem cell reserve is an issue in patients who may subsequently be considered for ASCT. Renal dose adjustment is required and long-term leukaemogenesis of this regimen has yet to be excluded.

Oral cyclophosphamide, thalidomide, and dexamethasone (CTD) has emerged as the most commonly used first-line treatment for AL amyloidosis in the United Kingdom.[33] Thalidomide has been used extensively in combination therapies for myeloma, but typical doses above 200 mg daily are poorly tolerated in AL amyloidosis, especially in patients with cardiac involvement or autonomic/peripheral neuropathy. However the CTD regimen comprising daily low-dose thalidomide, weekly oral cyclophosphamide, and intermittent pulses of dexamethasone, which can be risk-adapted utilizing still lower doses of thalidomide and dexamethasone in high-risk patients, is reasonably well tolerated and associated with a combined partial and complete clonal response rate of around

75%. Fatigue and fluid retention remain troublesome toxicities of this regimen. Patients with nephrotic syndrome are at particular risk of venous and arterial thrombosis, and should receive thromboprophylaxis. CTD has the advantages of being a stem-cell sparing oral regimen that does not require dose adjustment in renal impairment, and is more rapidly acting than Mel-Dex.

Bortezomib is a proteasome inhibitor developed for myeloma that is emerging as one of the most effective and rapidly acting therapies in the treatment of AL amyloidosis. Partial or complete clonal responses following bortezomib-based therapy were recently reported in 70% of 94 patients with relapsed or refractory haematological disease, including complete responses in 25%.[34] Furthermore, median time to clonal response was only 1 month and this subsequently translated into improved amyloidotic organ function in 30% of cases. Major toxicities included peripheral and autonomic neuropathy but, unlike myeloma cytopenias, were rare, most likely due to the smaller plasma cell burden in the bone marrow. Optimal dosing, long-term efficacy, and use of other agents in combination with bortezomib are being investigated.

Lenalidomide is a new thalidomide analogue that has lately also been investigated in several small studies in AL amyloidosis.[35] Maximum tolerated dose is typically about 15 mg daily. Efficacy is markedly improved when it is administered with dexamethasone, producing associated clonal response rates of about 67%, including complete responses in about 29%. Toxicity from infections, even without neutropenia, appears to be surprisingly high, especially in patients with severe renal or cardiac impairment. Time to haematological response is relatively slow, but lenalidomide remains an attractive treatment option in patients with severe neuropathy in whom thalidomide or bortezomib are relatively contraindicated. Use of lenalidomide in combination regimens and its potential as a maintenance therapy are currently being studied.

Melphalan and prednisolone given in oral cycles was the first treatment shown to have efficacy in AL amyloidosis,[36] but since responses are very slow and occur in only about 20% of cases this approach has generally been superseded. Other therapies that are occasionally used include intermediate dose intravenous melphalan ($12.5–25$ mg/m^2), principally in patients who cannot tolerate dexamethasone, and allogeneic bone marrow transplantation, which is associated with treatment-related mortality of 40% and for which there is little knowledge as yet regarding long-term benefit.[37]

Treatment of hereditary amyloidosis and organ transplantation

At present, other than transplantation to replace failed organs and in certain cases liver transplantation to remove the source of amyloidogenic proteins of hepatic origin, treatment of hereditary systemic amyloidosis is limited to managing symptoms. The liver is the source of plasma TTR and over 700 liver transplants have been performed for treatment of hereditary TTR amyloidosis since this 'surgical gene therapy' approach was introduced in 1991.[38] In younger patients carrying the common Met30Val amyloidogenic mutation the outcome is generally good, with arrest of neuropathy and regression of visceral amyloid, but vitreous amyloid may subsequently progresses, perhaps because some TTR is also produced within the eye. Cardiac amyloid may also progress, due to accumulation of wild-type TTR on the existing myocardial deposits. In some older Met30Val patients and in patients with other

amyloidogenic TTR mutations, liver transplantation has failed to arrest either amyloid deposition or progression of clinical disease. The livers of patients with hereditary TTR amyloidosis contain only microscopic amyloid deposits in the blood vessels and interstitial tissues, and retain normal liver function. A large number of domino liver transplants have therefore been conducted in recipients with various terminal liver diseases for whom normal livers were not available.[39] This has certainly prolonged their lives, but the first such recipient has now developed symptomatic systemic TTR amyloidosis 8 years after transplantation.[40]

In an AFib patient who had received two consecutive renal transplants and then developed amyloidotic liver failure, combined liver and kidney transplantation was dramatically successful,[41] and several more AFib patients have now received liver transplants. These operations have demonstrated that the liver is the sole site of synthesis of plasma fibrinogen, but clinical outcomes in the long term following the combined transplant approach have not yet been shown to be superior than solitary renal transplantation. Patients with apolipoprotein AI amyloidosis can develop kidney, liver, and cardiac amyloidosis, and various organ transplants have been performed, with generally excellent results in this particular type of amyloidosis.[42]

Supportive treatment

Supportive therapies remain a critical component of management of amyloidosis. For cardiac amyloidosis, the mainstay of treatment is diuretics coupled with fluid restriction, daily weighing, and a low-salt diet, while vasodilating drugs and beta-blockers are generally best avoided.[43] Refractory oedema may respond well to the addition of spironolactone and intermittent doses of metolozone. Salt-poor albumin infusions can also occasionally be helpful. Dysrhythmias may respond to amiodarone or to pacing. In renal amyloidosis, rigorous control of hypertension is vital, and ACE inhibition and/or angiotensin II blockade is often recommended in the context of proteinuria. Renal dialysis may be necessary, and is usually both feasible and acceptably tolerated. In autonomic neuropathy, fludrocortisone 100–200 μg/day can be helpful in some patients, but may simply exacerbate fluid retention. Midodrine is an effective pressor agent, starting at a dose range of 2.5 mg building up to 15 mg thrice daily. Midodrine exerts its actions via activation of the alphaadrenergic receptors of the arteriolar and venous vasculature, producing an increase in vascular tone and elevation of blood pressure. Its chief adverse effect is supine hypertension, and other pressor agents must be coadministered with caution. Gastroparesis causing symptoms of early satiety and nausea can be managed with prokinetic agents such as metaclopramide, along with advice about small, frequent meals of soft consistency. Diarrhoea due to amyloid gut involvement or autonomic neuropathy may respond to loperamide and codeine phosphate. Malnutrition is not uncommon and is often underestimated. Significant weight loss should be treated with protein and vitamin supplementation and the patient should be reviewed by an experienced dietitian. Feeding via gastrostomy may occasionally be required. Amyloid and chemotherapy-related peripheral neuropathy can be disabling and difficult to treat. Analgesia including opioids and non-steroidal anti-inflammatory drugs (NSAIDs), amitriptyline, venlafaxine, anti-epileptics, TENS, and/or gabapentin/pregabalin have all been used, although anecdotal reports suggest limited efficacy. Withdrawal or dose-reduction of any neurotoxic chemotherapies such as thalidomide or bortezomib should be considered.

New treatments and future directions

Elucidation of aspects of the molecular pathogenesis of amyloid and amyloidosis has led to the development of various novel approaches to therapy. These include treatments developed to stabilize and maintain circulating amyloid precursor proteins in their normal confirmation, agents that inhibit the interaction between amyloid fibrils and glycosaminglycans, immunotherapy approaches, and depletion of SAP. All of these potential new therapies have entered clinical testing, offering real promise that specific anti-amyloid therapies may become available within the next few years.

References

1. Pepys MB. Amyloidosis. *Annu Rev Med* 2006;57:223–241.
2. Booth DR, Sunde M, Bellotti V et al. Instability, unfolding and aggregation of human lysozyme variants underlying amyloid fibrillogenesis. *Nature* 1997;385:787–793.
3. Merlini G, Bellotti V. Molecular mechanisms of amyloidosis. *N Engl J Med* 2003;349:583–596.
4. Pepys MB, Rademacher TW, Amatayakul-Chantler S et al. Human serum amyloid P component is an invariant constituent of amyloid deposits and has a uniquely homogeneous glycostructure. *Proc Natl Acad Sci U S A* 1994;91:5602–5606.
5. Kisilevsky R, Fraser P. Proteoglycans and amyloid fibrillogenesis. *Ciba Found Symp* 1996;199:58–67.
6. Dember LM, Hawkins PN, Hazenberg BPC et al. Eprodisate for the treatment of renal disease in AA amyloidosis. *N Engl J Med* 2007;356:2349–2360.
7. Gillmore JD, Lovat LB, Persey MR et al. Amyloid load and clinical outcome in AA amyloidosis in relation to circulating concentration of serum amyloid A protein. *Lancet* 2001;358:24–29.
8. Lachmann HJ, Gallimore R, Gillmore JD et al. Outcome in systemic AL amyloidosis in relation to changes in concentration of circulating free immunoglobulin light chains following chemotherapy. *Br J Haematol* 2003;122:78–84.
9. Lachmann HJ, Goodman HJB, Gilbertson JA et al. Natural history and outcome in systemic AA amyloidosis. *N Engl J Med* 2007;356:2361–2371.
10. Wilkins J, Gallimore JR, Tennent GA et al. Rapid automated enzyme immunoassay of serum amyloid A. *Clin Chem* 1994;40:1284–1290.
11. Kyle RA, Therneau TM, Rajkumar SV et al. A long-term study of prognosis in monoclonal gammopathy of undetermined significance. *N Engl J Med* 2002;346:564–569.
12. Solomon A, Weiss DT, Kattine AA. Nephrotoxic potential of Bence Jones proteins. *N Engl J Med* 1991;324:1845–1851.
13. Kyle RA, Gertz MA. Primary systemic amyloidosis: clinical and laboratory features in 474 cases. *Semin Hematol* 1995;32:45–59.
14. Drüeke TB. Dialysis-related amyloidosis. *Nephrol Dial Transplant* 1998;13 (Suppl 1):58–64.
15. Lachmann HJ, Booth DR, Booth SE et al. Misdiagnosis of hereditary amyloidosis as AL (primary) amyloidosis. *N Engl J Med* 2002;346:1786–1791.
16. Benson MD, Uemichi T. Transthyretin amyloidosis. Amyloid. *Int J Exp Clin Invest* 1996;3:44–56.
17. Maury CPJ, Kere J, Tolvanen R et al. Finnish hereditary amyloidosis is caused by a single nucleotide substitution in the gelsolin gene. *FEBS Lett* 1990;276:75–77.
18. Gillmore JD, Booth DR, Madhoo S et al. Hereditary renal amyloidosis associated with variant lysozyme in a large English family. *Nephrol Dial Transplant* 1999;14:2639–2644.
19. Harrison RF, Hawkins PN, Roche WR et al. 'Fragile' liver and massive hepatic haemorrhage due to hereditary amyloidosis. *Gut* 1996;38:151–152.
20. Nichols WC, Gregg RE, Brewer HBJ et al. A mutation in apolipoprotein A-I in the Iowa type of familial amyloidotic polyneuropathy. *Genomics* 1990;8:318–323.
21. Gillmore JD, Lachmann HJ, Rowczenio D et al. Diagnosis, pathogenesis, treatment, and prognosis of hereditary fibrinogen A α-chain amyloidosis. *J Am Soc Nephrol* 2009;20:444–451.
22. Puchtler H, Sweat F, Levine M. On the binding of Congo red by amyloid. *J Histochem Cytochem* 1962;10:355–364.
23. Röcken C, Sletten K. Amyloid in surgical pathology. *Virchows Arch* 2003;443:3–16.
24. Selvanayagam JB, Hawkins PN, Paul B et al. Evaluation and management of the cardiac amyloidosis. *J Am Coll Cardiol* 2007;50:2101–2110.
25. Palladini G, Campana C, Klersy C et al. Serum N-terminal pro-brain natriuretic peptide is a sensitive marker of myocardial dysfunction in AL amyloidosis. *Circulation* 2003;107:2440–2445.
26. Rodriguez FJ, Gamez JD, Vrana JA et al. Immunoglobulin derived depositions in the nervous system: novel mass spectrometry application for protein characterization in formalin-fixed tissues. *Lab Invest* 2008;88:1024–1037.
27. Hawkins PN, Lavender JP, Pepys MB. Evaluation of systemic amyloidosis by scintigraphy with 123I-labeled serum amyloid P component. *N Engl J Med* 1990;323:508–513.
28. Gertz MA, Comenzo R, Falk RH et al. Definition of organ involvement and treatment response in immunoglobulin light chain amyloidosis (AL): A consensus opinion from the 10th International Symposium on Amyloid and Amyloidosis. *Am J Hematol* 2005;79:319–328.
29. Palladini G, Lavatelli F, Russo P et al. Circulating amyloidogenic free light chains and serum N-terminal natriuretic peptide type B decrease simultaneously in association with improvement of survival in AL. *Blood* 2006;107:3854–3858.
30. Skinner M, Sanchorawala V, Seldin DC et al. High-dose melphalan and autologous stem-cell transplantation in patients with AL amyloidosis: an 8-year study. *Ann Intern Med* 2004;140:85–93.
31. Dispenzieri A, Lacy MQ, Kyle RA et al. Eligibility for hematopoietic stem-cell transplantation for primary systemic amyloidosis is a favorable prognostic factor for survival. *J Clin Oncol* 2001;19:3350–3356.
32. Palladini G, Perfetti V, Obici L et al. Association of melphalan and high-dose dexamethasone is effective and well tolerated in patients with AL (primary) amyloidosis who are ineligible for stem cell transplantation. *Blood* 2004;103:2936–2938.
33. Wechalekar AD, Goodman HJ, Lachmann HJ et al. Safety and efficacy of risk-adapted cyclophosphamide, thalidomide, and dexamethasone in systemic AL amyloidosis. *Blood* 2007;109:457–464.
34. Wechalekar AD, Lachmann HJ, Offer M et al. Efficacy of bortezomib in systemic AL amyloidosis with relapsed/refractory clonal disease. *Haematologica* 2008;93:295–298.
35. Sanchorawala V, Wright DG, Rosenzweig M et al. Lenalidomide and dexamethasone in the treatment of AL amyloidosis: results of a phase 2 trial. *Blood* 2007;109:492–496.
36. Kyle RA, Gertz MA, Greipp PR et al. A trial of three regimens for primary amyloidosis: colchicine alone, melphalan and prednisone, and melphalan, prednisone, and colchicine. *N Engl J Med* 1997;336:1202–1207.
37. Schönland SO, Lokhorst H, Buzyn A et al. Allogeneic and syngeneic hematopoietic cell transplantation in patients with amyloid light-chain amyloidosis: a report from the European Group for Blood and Marrow Transplantation. *Blood* 2006;107:2578–2584.
38. Stangou AJ, Hawkins PN. Liver transplantation in transthyretin-related familial amyloid polyneuropathy. *Curr Opin Neurol* 2004;17:615–620.
39. Stangou AJ, Heaton ND, Rela M et al. Domino hepatic transplantation using the liver from a patient with familial amyloid polyneuropathy. *Transplantation* 1998;65:1496–1498.

40. Stangou AJ, Heaton ND, Hawkins PN: Transmission of systemic transthyretin amyloidosis by means of domino liver transplantation. *N Engl J Med* 2005;352:2356.

41. Gillmore JD, Booth DR, Rela M et al. Curative hepatorenal transplantation in systemic amyloidosis caused by the Glu526Val fibrinogen α-chain variant in an English family. *Q J Med* 2000;93:269–275.

42. Gillmore JD, Stangou AJ, Lachmann HJ et al. Organ transplantation in hereditary apolipoprotein AI amyloidosis. *Am J Transplant* 2006;6:2342–2347.

43. Falk RH: Diagnosis and management of the cardiac amyloidoses. *Circulation* 2005;112:2047–2060.

CHAPTER 164

Autoinflammatory diseases

Helen J. Lachmann and Philip N. Hawkins

Introduction

The concept of autoinflammatory disease, i.e. chronic multisystem inflammatory disorders without evidence of cell-mediated or humoral autoimmunity, began with the molecular characterization of monogenic inherited periodic fever syndromes. The term autoinflammatory was coined in 1999 but the concept has evolved to encompass a variety of acquired disorders that are broadly thought to be due to disturbances in the innate immune system (Table 164.1). Features of autoinflammatory disorders include recurrent episodes of fever and generalized inflammation affecting the eyes, joints, skin, and serosa, but many systems may be involved, and the rigid distinction between autoinflammatory and autoimmune disorders has become less clear as progress has been made in characterizing their pathogenesis.[1] Elucidation of the molecular basis of the cyropyrin-associated periodic syndrome (CAPS) has transformed understanding of regulation and importance of interleukin (IL)-1 in autoinflammatory disease. It now seems clear from both basic research and clinical studies that disordered regulation of IL-1 and nuclear factor-κB (NFκB) underlie the pathogenesis of the autoinflammatory syndromes. Clinical outcomes in autoinflammatory diseases have been transformed by the availability of IL-1-blocking drugs, and there is increasing interest in the role of autoinflammatory mechanisms in various common acquired diseases. These include diabetes types 1 and 2 and ischaemic heart disease, which are major scourges of the developed world (and increasingly of the developing world), and trials of IL-1 blockade are under way in both.

This article focuses on the inherited periodic fever syndromes (Table 164.2), and periodic fever, aphthous stomatitis, pharyngitis, and adenitis (PFAPA) and Schnizler's syndrome.

Inherited periodic fever syndromes

Familial Mediterranean fever

Familial Mediterranean fever (FMF) is much the commonest of the inherited syndromes. It was first described in 1945 and the term 'familial Mediterranean fever' was introduced in 1958.

Genetics and pathophysiology

The gene associated with FMF, *MEFV*, encodes a protein called pyrin. *MEFV* is constitutively expressed in neutrophils, eosinophils, monocytes, dendritic cells, and synovial and peritoneal fibroblasts, and is upregulated in response to inflammatory activators such as interferon-γ and tumour necrosis factor alpha (TNFα); 5′- and 3′- sequences are known to contribute to regulation of gene expression and polymorphisms may play a role in susceptibly to FMF. More than 200 coding variants have been reported, and 90 in association with FMF. These encode either single amino acid substitutions or deletions (Infevers registry database http://fmf.igh.cnrs.fr/ISSAID/infevers/).[2] Disease-causing mutations are clustered in exon 10, in the SPRY domain of pyrin, but are also found in exons 1, 2, 3, 5, and 9. Mutations in both *MEFV* alleles can be found in 80% of patients with FMF, and although the vast majority of individuals with a single mutated allele remain healthy, up to 20% of FMF patients have a single identified mutation.[3] The methionine residue at position 694 appears critical for pyrin's function: three different mutations involving M694 have been identified; homozygosity for M694V is associated with a severe phenotype; and heterozygous deletion of this residue has been associated with autosomal dominant FMF. Two or more mutations on a single allele can also cause dominant FMF, although pseudo-dominant inheritance due to consanguinity or a high prevalence of carriers is much commoner.

One particular variant, E148Q encoded in exon 2, has an allele frequency of 10–20% in Asian populations, and up to 1–2% in

Table 164.1 Examples of acquired diseases with a presumed autoinflammatory component

SoJIA and adult-onset Still's disease	Recurrent pericarditis	Granulomatous diseases: Crohn's disease and ulcerative colitis
		Sarcoidosis
		Giant cell arteritis
		Takayasu's arteritis
Behçet's syndrome	Recurrent uveitis	Crystal deposition diseases
		Gout
		Pseudo-gout
		Atherosclerosis
Psoriasis	Schnitzler's syndrome	Diabetes types 1 and 2
	PFAPA	Asbestosis and mesothelioma

PFAPA, periodic fever, aphthous stomatitis, pharyngitis, and adenitis; SoJIA, systemic-onset juvenile inflammatory arthritis.

Table 164.2 The autoinflammatory conditions of known genetic aetiology

Periodic fever syndrome	Gene	Mode of inheritance	Typical age at onset	Potential precipitants of attacks	Distinctive clinical features	Characteristic laboratory abnormalities	Treatment
FMF	*MEFV* Chromosome 16	Autosomal recessive (dominant in rare families)	Childhood/ early adult	Usually none Occasionally menstruation, fasting, stress, trauma	Short severe attacks Colchicine responsive Erysipelas-like erythema	Marked acute-phase response during attacks	Colchicine
TRAPS	*TNFRSF1A* Chromosome 12	Autosomal dominant, can be de novo	Childhood	Usually none. Sometimes travel, stress, fasting, menstrual cycle	Prolonged symptoms	Marked acute-phase response during attacks. Low levels of soluble TNFR1 when well	Anakinra, etanercept, high-dose corticosteroids
MKD	*MVK* Chromosome 12	Autosomal recessive	Infancy	Immunizations	Diarrhoea and lymphadenopathy	Elevated IgD and IgA, acute-phase response, and MVA during attacks	Anti-TNF and anti-IL-1 therapies
CAPS	*NLRP3* Chromosome 1	Autosomal dominant	Infancy	Exposure to cold environment, or none	Cold-induced fever, arthralgia, rash, eye inflammation, sensorineural deafness and conjunctivitis, chronic aseptic meningitis, deforming arthropathy	Varying but marked acute-phase response most of the time	Anti-IL-1 therapies
NALP12 associated periodic syndrome	*NALP12* Chromosome 19	Autosomal dominant	Infancy	Cold exposure or known	Cold-induced fever, urticarial rash, arthralgia and sensorineural deafness	Acute-phase response during attacks	None specific
DIRA	*IL1RN* Chromosome 2	Autosomal recessive	Infancy	None	Sterile multifocal osteomyelitis, periostitis, and pustulosis	Marked acute-phase response most of the time	Anti-IL-1 therapies
PAPA	*PSTPIP1 (CD2BP1)* Chromosome 15	Autosomal dominant	Childhood	None	Pyogenic arthritis, pyoderma gangrenosum, cystic acne	Acute-phase response during attacks	Anti-TNF therapy
Blau's syndrome	*NOD2 (CARD15)* Chromosome 16	Autosomal dominant	Childhood	None	Granulomatous polyarthritis, iritis, and dermatitis	Sustained modest acute-phase response	Corticosteroids, maybe biologicals
Majeed's syndrome	*LPIN2* Chromosome 18	Autosomal recessive	Neonatal	None	CRMO, dyserythropoietic anaemia, inflammatory dermatosis	Microcytic congenital dyserythropoietic anaemia	NSAIDS and corticosteroids
DITRA	*IL36RN* Chromosome 2	Autosomal recessive	Childhood to middle age	Sometimes stress, pregnancy, or drugs	Generalized sterile pustular rash and fever	Neutrophilia and raised acute-phase response	None specific
JMP and CANDLE syndromes	*PSMB8* Chromosome 6	Autosomal recessive	Neonatal to childhood	None	Erythematous rash, arthralgia/arthritis, joint contractures in JMP, progressive lipodystrophy	Raised acute-phase response, mixed myeloid, neutrophilic, and histiocytic infiltrate in affected skin	Partial response to IL-6 blockade has been reported

See text for abbreviations.

white Europeans. Although E148Q can cause FMF when an exon 10 mutation is also present, homozygosity for E148Q alone is not generally associated with FMF. There is however some evidence that carriers may have an augmented response to some types of non-FMF inflammation.[4]

The expression of *MEFV* is regulated in a very complex fashion at RNA and protein levels.[5] Neither the structure nor the function of pyrin has been fully characterized and its subcellular localization appears to vary according to cell type and isoform. The putative 781 amino acid protein has sequence homologies with proteins of apparently disparate function and cellular localization, and it appears to bind to several components of the inflammasome and modulate their activity. The pyrin SPRY domain appears to interact with NALP3, caspase-1m and its substrate pro-IL-1, and overexpression studies have shown inhibition of caspase 1 activation with reduced secretion of IL-1β.[6] Many of pyrin's interactions appear to involve its 100 amino acid N-terminal pyrin (PYD) death domain. The PYD domain occurs in more than 20 human proteins, including NLRP3 (the variant protein in CAPS), which all appear to be involved in the assembly and activation of apoptotic and inflammatory complexes through homotypic protein–protein interactions that regulate caspase 1 and thus modulate production of IL-1. Recent work suggests that pyrin may be cleaved by caspase 1 and that pyrin variants may serve as more efficient substrate than the wild-type protein.[7] The resulting N-terminal PYD cleavage fragments may be translocated to the nucleus where they could potentiate activation of NFκB through interaction with the adapter protein, apoptosis-associated speck-like protein with a caspase-recruitment domain (ASC) or with NFκB-p65.

Clinical features

FMF is commonest in Eastern Mediterranean populations but occurs worldwide. The prevalence of FMF is estimated to be 1/250 to 1/500 among Sephardic Jews and 1/1000 in the Turkish population. Carrier frequency exceeds 1 in 4 in some populations, prompting speculation that the FMF trait may have conferred survival benefit, possibly through enhanced resistance to microbial infection mediated via an upregulated innate immune response.[8] Sexes are affected equally and the disease usually presents in childhood.

Attacks of FMF occur irregularly and apparently spontaneously although some may be precipitated by minor physical or emotional stress, the menstrual cycle, or diet. Attacks evolve rapidly and symptoms resolve within 72 hours. Fever with serositis are the cardinal features, and diagnostic criteria for FMF have been validated in both adults and children.[9,10] Peritonitis that can mimic an acute surgical abdomen occurs in 85% of cases, and 40% of patients will have undergone surgery for a presumed acute surgical abdomen before diagnosis. Characteristically unilateral pleuritic chest pain occurs in 40%. Headache with meningitic features has been reported particularly in children, but the nervous system is not usually involved. Orchitis occurs in less than 5%, most commonly in early childhood. Joint involvement usually affects the lower limbs: arthralgia is common in acute attacks, usually subsiding within a couple of days; chronic destructive arthritis is rare. Erysipelas-like rash is seen in 20%, usually around the ankles. A degree of myalgia occurs with acute attacks, and up to 20% of patients complain of persistent calf muscle pain on exertion. Protracted febrile myalgia is a rare entity that presents with severe pain in the lower limbs or

abdominal musculature, persisting for weeks, and can be accompanied by a vasculitic rash; it usually responds to corticosteroids.

Acute attacks are accompanied by a neutrophil leucocytosis, raised erythrocyte sedimentation rate (ESR), very high calcitonin levels, and an intense acute-phase response.[11] Investigations may be required to exclude other diagnoses, but imaging during attacks is usually unrewarding.

Diagnosis is supported by DNA analysis but remains clinical, centring on the history of recurrent self-limiting attacks of fever and serositis that respond to prophylactic treatment with colchicine. Genetic results must be interpreted cautiously, given that some individuals with paired pathogenic *MEFV* mutations never develop FMF, and others with heterozygous 'carrier' status can do so.

Treatment

Supportive measures, particularly analgesia, are required during acute attacks. The mainstay of management is long-term prophylactic treatment with low-dose colchicine. This was discovered serendipitously in 1972,[12] and has transformed the outlook of the disease. Continuous treatment with colchicine at a dose of 1–2 mg daily in adults prevents or substantially reduces symptoms of FMF in at least 95%, and almost completely eliminates the risk of AA amyloidosis.

Colchicine was recently licensed by the United States Food and Drug Administration for the treatment of FMF from the age of 4 years upwards. Long-term treatment is advisable in all patients with FMF and mandatory in those who have AA amyloidosis. Although colchicine is very toxic in acute overdose, low doses are generally very well tolerated. Diarrhoea is the commonest side effect and can often be avoided by gradual introduction of the drug. Despite theoretical concerns, there is no evidence that colchicine causes infertility or birth defects, and it can be taken safely during breastfeeding.[13] Introduction or dose escalation of colchicine during an acute FMF attack is not generally effective. Genuine resistance to colchicine is probably very rare and may be associated with polymorphisms of the drug transporter gene *ABCB1*.[14] There have lately been reports of long-term benefit from treatment with IL-1 inhibitors, and to a lesser extent etanercept in 'refractory' patients.[15,16]

Tumour necrosis factor receptor-associated periodic syndrome

Genetics and pathophysiology

Tumour necrosis factor receptor-associated periodic syndrome (TRAPS), an autosomal dominant disease, is associated with mutations in the 10-exon gene tumour necrosis factor receptor superfamily 1A (*TNFRSF1A*).[17] TNF is a key mediator of inflammation with actions including induction of pyrexia, leucocyte activation, induction of cytokine secretion, and expression of adhesion molecules. Tumour necrosis factor receptor 1 (TNFR1) is a member of the death domain superfamily and consists of an extracellular region containing four cysteine-rich domains, a transmembrane domain, and an intracellular death domain. Binding of circulating TNF results in trimerization of the receptor and induction of NFκB with increased production of proinflammatory cytokines and potentially apoptosis via caspase 8, although activation of NFκB can also result in inhibition of apoptosis via cellular caspase 8-like inhibitory protein (cFLIP). The mechanism(s) by which heterozygous

TRFRSF1A mutations cause TRAPS remain unclear and probably differ between mutations.[18–20] Most TRAPS-associated mutations lie within exons 2–4 and about one-half are missense substitutions which disrupt structurally important cysteine–cysteine disulphide bonds in the extracellular domain. Under normal circumstances, TNF signalling is terminated by metalloproteinase-dependent cleavage of a proximal region of the extracellular domain. This also releases soluble TNFR1, which competes with cell-surface receptors in binding of circulating TNF. Cleavage of some TNFR1 variants is impaired, producing a 'shedding defect', but this is not the case in all TRAPS-causing mutations. It is thought that mutant misfolded receptors may give rise to enhanced or prolonged signalling, possibly through retention within the endoplasmic reticulum, resulting in mitochondrial stress and production of reactive oxygen species. Recent data suggest that cellular expression of mutant TNFR1 is itself an inflammatory signal, perhaps by activation of distinct intracellular signalling pathways with a proinflammatory outcome in a TNF-independent fashion.[21]

Clinical features

TRAPS was described in 1982 as familial Hibernian fever,[22] reflecting the Irish/Scottish ancestry of early patients, but the disease has subsequently been reported in many ethnic groups. The sexes are equally affected. Approximately 60% of patients report a family history of similar symptoms. Mean age at first symptoms is 7 years and the disease burden is high, with a median of 60 days of TRAPS-related illness per year.

Attacks in TRAPS are far less distinct than in FMF. Febrile episodes typically last more than 10 days and symptoms are near continuous in one-third of patients. The clinical picture varies: more than 95% experience fever and 90% have arthralgia or myalgia that typically follows a centripetal migratory path; abdominal pain occurs in 75%, and skin manifestations including migratory patches, erysepela-like erythema, oedematous plaques (often overlying areas of mylagic pain), urticaria, and discrete reticulate or serpiginous lesions occur in 60% of patients. Other features include headache, pleuritic pain, lymphadenopathy, periorbital oedema, and conjunctivitis. There are also reports of central nervous system (CNS) manifestations and imaging findings resembling multiple sclerosis.[23] Indeed the common polymorphism R92Q has been suggested as a susceptibility factor for multiple sclerosis.[24] Symptoms are almost universally accompanied by a marked acute-phase response, and genetic testing is central to diagnosis.

Two TNFRSF1A variants, P46L and R92Q, which may be associated with mild TRAPS,[25] are present in approximately 10% of healthy West Africans and 2% of healthy whites respectively. The vast majority of carriers of these variants are entirely well and the mechanisms by which they cause inflammatory disease in a minority remains obscure.

Treatment

Acute attacks respond to high-dose corticosteroids but in severe disease the cumulative doses required are considerable, necessitating addition of maintenance therapy. There is no evidence that conventional steroid-sparing immunosuppressant agents are of any benefit in TRAPS, and specific anti-cytokine agents are currently the only effective long-term treatment. Etanercept has been used for more than a decade and is effective in some patients, although responses are frequently partial and wane over time.[26] Paradoxically,

infliximab exacerbates disease and should be avoided.[27] Recent reports suggest that IL-1 blockade with anakinra is frequently extremely effective in TRAPS, and anti-IL-1 agents are now becoming the maintenance treatment of choice.[28]

Mevalonate kinase deficiency

Genetics and pathophysiology

Mevalonate kinase deficiency (MKD), also known as hyperimmunoglobulin D and periodic fever syndrome (HIDS), is an autosomal recessive disease caused by mutations in the mevalonate kinase (*MVK*) gene.[29] More than 100 mutations have been described, spanning the 11-exon gene, the commonest of which encode MVK variants V377I and I268T. MVK is the enzyme following HMG-CoA reductase in the pathway involved in cholesterol synthesis. This pathway is also responsible for farnasylation and geranylgerylation. Most HIDS-causing MVK mutations are missense variants that reduce enzyme activity by 90–99%.[30] Other mutations resulting in near complete absence of enzyme activity cause a much more severe disease, mevalonicaciduria (MVA), features of which include stillbirth, congenital malformations, psychomotor retardation, ataxia, myopathy, failure to thrive, and early death.

It is not yet known how MVK deficiency causes inflammation, though reduction in prenylation due to a relative deficiency of substrate for the geranylgeranyl pathway seems more likely to be responsible than accumulation of mevalonic acid. The relationship of the isoprenoid pathway to inflammation is of interest given the anti-inflammatory properties of drugs that are widely used to inhibit cholesterol synthesis. The RhoA and Rac1 GTPases require to be geranylgeranylated to function properly, and this has been demonstrated to be reduced both in MKD[31] and by HMG-CoA reductase inhibition with simvastatin. Various effects of statins on caspase-1 activation and IL-1 secretion have been postulated, and clinical studies have suggested conflicting results as a trial of simvastatin in six patients with MKD suggested minor benefit[32]; but two children with MVA were reported to have developed severe flares of inflammatory disease following statin treatment.[33]

Clinical features

MKD affects an estimated 200–600 individuals. It was described in the Netherlands in 1984 and the carriage rate of *MVK* V337I is 1 in 350 in the Dutch population,[34] but MKD has been reported in many other ethnic groups including Arabs and South-East Asians. The disease occurs equally in both sexes and usually presents in the first year of life.[35]

Attacks are irregular, typically lasting 4–7 days, and are characteristically provoked by vaccination, minor trauma, surgery, or stress, perhaps triggered by a reduction in MVK activity associated with increased body temperature. Attacks of MKD typically comprise fever, cervical lymphadenopathy, hepatomegaly and splenomegaly, and abdominal pain with vomiting and diarrhoea. Headache, eye inflammation causing conjunctivitis or keratitis, arthralgia, large-joint arthritis, erythematous macules and papules, and aphthous ulcers are also common. Retinitis pigmentosa has been reported, perhaps linked to the metabolic defect. MKD may partially ameliorate in adult life. Clinical criteria have recently been proposed to guide genetic testing.[36]

Diagnosis of MKD was thought to be supported by a high serum IgD concentration but this is non-specific, as it occurs in other fever syndromes, does not correlate with disease severity, and is not universal.[37] More accessibly, serum IgA concentration is elevated in 80%. Attacks are accompanied by an acute-phase response, leucocytosis and the transient presence of mevalonic acid in the urine. A mutation in both alleles of the *MVK* gene can be identified in most patients.

Treatment

Treatment is largely supportive, including non-steroidal anti-inflammatory drugs (NSAIDs), although responses to etanercept[38] and anakinra are reported.

Cryopyrin-associated periodic syndrome

CAPS comprises an overlapping severity spectrum of three separately described diseases: familial cold autoinflammatory syndrome (FCAS); Muckle–Wells syndrome (MWS); and chronic infantile neurological, cutaneous and articular syndrome (CINCA), known in the United States as neonatal onset multisystem inflammatory disease (NOMID).

Genetics and pathophysiology

CAPS is an autosomal dominant disease associated with mutations in *NLRP3/CIAS1*, a gene that encodes the death domain protein known as cryopyrin or NLRP3.[39] Approximately three-quarters of patients with FCAS and MWS have a family history of similar symptoms. CINCA is usually due to de-novo mutation. More than 100, mostly missense, mutations have been reported; the majority are in exon 3 but there are also variants in exon 4 and 6 and in a number of introns.

NLRP3 is expressed in granulocytes, dendritic cells, B and T lymphocytes, epithelial cells of the oral and genital tracts, and chondrocytes. It encodes a member of the death domain superfamily that has a pyrin (PYD) domain, a nucleotide-binding site (NBS) domain, and a leucine-rich repeat (LRR) motif. It is thought that recognition via the LRR of a variety of danger signals, including intracellular pathogen-associated molecular patterns (PAMPs), crystals such as uric acid and cholesterol, and fibres such as asbestos, results in conformational change and association of NLRP3 with other death domain superfamily proteins to form a multimeric cytosolic protein complex, known collectively as the inflammasome.[40,41] This brings molecules of pro-caspase-1 into close proximity, leading to proteolytic activation and release of the active catalytic domains p20 and p10. Active caspase-1 cleaves pro-IL-1β into its biologically active 17 kDa fragment, and also upregulates NFκB expression thereby increasing IL-1 gene expression.

Clinical features

Most known patients are of European descent but cases have been described from South Asia and elsewhere. Onset of disease is usually in early infancy, often from birth, and there is no sex bias.

The term FCAS, for the mildest form of CAPS, was coined recently, but the disorder was first described in 1940 as recurrent episodes of cold-induced fever, arthralgia, inflamed eyes, and rash. In 1962 a British kindred with what became called MWS was reported with almost daily attacks of urticarial rash, inflamed eyes, arthralgia, and fever, complicated by progressive sensorineural deafness, and a high incidence of AA amyloidosis. At the most severe end of the spectrum is CINCA. This presents neonatally with multisystem involvement including the skin, skeletal system, and CNS. Bony overgrowth and premature ossification may occur particularly in the skull and knees; chronic aseptic meningitis results in developmental retardation; blindness due to a combination of anterior chamber inflammation and optic atrophy and sensorineural deafness are common.

Clinical disease is accompanied by an acute-phase response, leucocytosis, thrombocytosis, and anaemia. When deafness occurs, it tends to progress in a stepwise fashion through childhood. Characteristic bony abnormalities may be evident radiologically. Anterior eye examination can show inflammatory changes ranging from conjunctivitis and acute anterior uveitis to keratitis and band keratopathy. Fundoscopy may show disc oedema, disc atrophy, and choroiditis. Brain MRI may show features consistent with chronic meningeal inflammation and elevated intracranial pressure. A mutation in *NLRP3* can be identified in almost all patients who can be characterized clinically as FCAS or MWS, but mutations are only found in about 50% of children with classical CINCA, in whom other genes may be implicated or there may be mosaicism.

Treatment

Inhibition of IL-1 produces rapid clinical and serological remission in CAPS. It is hoped that early anti-IL-1 therapy may prevent long-term complications, not only of AA amyloidosis in adults but potentially progressive neurological and physical disability in children. Daily injections of anakinra (recombinant receptor antagonist) have been reported to be effective in small case series, whereas two new longer-acting IL-1 inhibitors: canakinumab, a fully human anti-IL-1β antibody and rilonacept, an IL-1 Trap, have been tested in phase 3 trials, and are licensed for the treatment of CAPS with good safety to date.

NALP12-associated periodic fever syndrome

This autosomal dominant syndrome was described in 2008. Presentation is in infancy with features of cold induction, fever, arthralgia and myalgia, urticaria, and sensioneural deafness. The nonsense and splice site mutations identified in NALP12 appear to reduce the inhibitory effect of the protein on NFκB signalling.

Deficiency of the IL-1 receptor antagonist

Deficiency of the IL-1 receptor antagonist (DIRA) is an autosomal recessive disease described in 2009.[42] It is due to mutations in *IL1RN* that result in total deficiency of IL-1 receptor antagonist. The disease has been reported in a handful of families of various ethnic origins. The disease presents in the neonatal period with a pustular rash, joint swelling, multifocal osteitis of the ribs and long bones, heterotopic ossification, and periarticular soft tissue swelling.[43] Treatment is IL-1 blockade with anakinra.

Pyogenic sterile arthritis, pyoderma gangrenosum, and acne syndrome

Pyogenic sterile arthritis, pyoderma gangrenosum, and acne (PAPA) syndrome is an autosomal dominant disease caused by mutations in the proline serine threonine phosphatase-interacting protein 1 (*PTSTPIP*) gene that encodes a protein also known as CD2 binding protein 1 (CB2BP1). The underlying pathogenesis remains poorly understood although there is evidence that CD2BP1, an important component of cytoskeletal organization which interacts with actin, also interacts with pyrin and disease-associated mutations appear to potentiate this.[44] PAPA is characterized clinically by pyoderma gangrenosum, severe acne, and recurrent pustular sterile arthritis typically precipitated by minor trauma. Responses to corticosteroids are disappointing and case reports suggest that therapy with infliximab or anakinra may be effective.

Blau's syndrome

This syndrome is an autosomal dominant disorder characterized by non-caseating granulomatous infiltration[45] presenting in early childhood with a triad of a tan-coloured erythematous rash, polyarticular synovitis often causing camtodactyly, and uveitis. It is associated with missense mutations in NOD2/CARD15. This member of the death domain superfamily has also been implicated in familial Crohn's disease.

Majeed's syndrome

This autosomal recessive syndrome characterized by chronic recurrent multifocal osteomyelitis (CRMO), congenital dyserythropoietic anaemia, and inflammatory dermatosis was described in 1989. Disease onset is usually in the neonatal period and attacks consist of fever, pain, and the appearance of periarticular soft tissue swelling. Long-term complications of growth retardation and flexion contractures are well recognized. It is due to mutations in *LPIN2*, a gene of unknown function.[46]

Generalized pustular psoriasis or deficiency of IL-36 receptor antagonist

Generalized pustular psoriasis (GPP) or deficiency of IL-36 receptor antagonist (DITRA) is characterized by recurrent episodes of a generalized sterile pustular rash accompanied by neutrophilia, a marked acute-phase response, and fever. Age at onset varies from childhood to the sixth decade. Episodes may be precipitated by stress, pregnancy, or drugs and can be life threatening. GPP was found to be a recessively inherited autoinflammatory disease in 2011 when separate groups reported that it was due to recessive mutations in *IL36RN* on chromosome 2.[47] This encodes a member of the IL-1 superfamily, IL-36 receptor antagonist, which blocks the recruitment of the IL-1RL2 receptor complex, thus inhibiting downstream activation NFκB and MAP kinases.

Joint contractures, muscle atrophy, microcytic anaemia, and panniculitis-induced lipodystrophy; chronic atypical neutrophilic dermatosis with lipodystrophy and elevated temperature

Joint contractures, muscle atrophy, microcytic anaemia, and panniculitis-induced lipodystrophy (JMP syndrome) was first described in Japan in 1984 and subsequently in two white families. Affected patients are homozygous for the p.Thr75Met mutation in the proteasome subunit, β-type, 8 (*PSMB8*) gene.[48]

Chronic atypical neutrophilic dermatosis with lipodystrophy, and elevated temperature (CANDLE syndrome) seems to be a very similar disease characterized by a neonatal onset of intermittent fevers, erythematous rash with a mixed myeloid, neutrophilic, and histiocytic infiltrate, arthralgia/arthritis, and progressive lipodystrophy with raised inflammatory markers. Patients have also been found to carry *PSM8* mutations with evidence of dysregulation of the interferon signalling pathway.[49]

PSMB8 encodes a catalytic subunit of the 20S immunoproteasomes. These appear to be activated by interferon and are responsible for generation of antigenic epitopes presented by major histocompatibility complex (MHC) class I molecules as well as removing ubiquitinated intracellular proteins. It has been suggested that the mutations may disrupt antigen processing via reduced chymotrypsin-like proteasomal activity and/or increase intracellular stress and apotosis via accumulation of uubiquitin-rich cytoplasmic aggregates, although the mechanisms by which this causes the disease phenotype are unknown.

Autoinflammatory diseases of unknown aetiology

Periodic fever, aphthous stomatitis, pharyngitis, and adenitis

The diagnosis of PFAPA is suggested by the presence of a recurrent fever of early onset and at least one of: oral aphthous ulcers, cervical lymphadenopathy, or pharyngitis, in the absence of recurrent upper respiratory tract infections or cyclic neutropenia. Characteristically the children are entirely well between attacks. Median age at presentation is 2.5 years, and almost all present by their fifth birthday. The 'acronym' symptoms are frequently not all present during a single attack. In general the prognosis is good and most children will outgrow their symptoms within a decade.

A recent paper has shown that 16% of patients who fulfilled the diagnostic criteria for PFAPA in fact had an inherited periodic fever syndrome and another 18% carried a fever gene mutation or polymorphism.[50]

For many clinicians the strongest diagnostic pointers are the extreme regularity of attacks. Padeh et al. suggested that the dramatic response to a single oral dose of corticosteroids is sufficiently unique that it could be used as a diagnostic criterion.[51] Cimetidine and colchicine has been tried with variable reports of success. Tonsillectomy is the only treatment for which there is evidence from trials; more than 50% of children appear to have excellent long-term results. However, these data may be biased. Many centres selectively refer children with persistently enlarged tonsils for surgery, and it is possible that responses may occur preferentially in this subgroup.

Schnitzler's syndrome

This was described in 1974 and is characterized by a chronic urticarial rashes, a monoclonal immunoglobulin M (IgM) gammopathy, and systemic inflammation usually presenting as fever. The median age at onset is 51 years. There is a slight male preponderance and the majority of cases are of white European ethnicity.[52] The monoclonal protein appears central to the pathogenesis although the mechanism remains unclear, and is apparently unrelated to abundance of the paraprotein. About one-fifth of patients eventually progress to overt plasma cell malignancy. Chemotherapy does not appear to relieve the syndrome and should only be used for conventional haematological indications. The treatment of choice is IL-1 blockade, which completely abolishes symptoms although it has no effect on the paraprotein concentration.

References

1. McGonagle D, McDermott MF. A proposed classification of the immunological diseases. *PLoS Med* 2006;3:1242–1248.
2. Milhavet F, Cuisset L, Hoffman HM et al. The infevers autoinflammatory mutation online registry: update with new genes and functions. *Hum Mutat* 2008;29:803–808.

3. Kone-Paut I, Hentgen V, Guillaume-Czitrom S et al. The clinical spectrum of 94 patients carrying a single mutated MEFV allele. *Rheumatology* 2009;48:840–842.

4. Canete JD, Arostegui JI, Queiro R et al. An unexpectedly high frequency of MEFV mutations in patients with anti-citrullinated protein antibody-negative palindromic rheumatism. *Arthritis Rheum* 2007;56: 2784–2788.

5. Grandemange S, Aksentijevich I, Jeru I, Gul A, Touitou I. The regulation of MEFV expression and its role in health and familial Mediterranean fever. *Genes Immun* 2011;12:497–503.

6. Papin S, Cuenin S, Agostini L et al. The SPRY domain of Pyrin, mutated in familial Mediterranean fever patients, interacts with inflammasome components and inhibits proIL-1beta processing. *Cell Death Differ* 2007;14:1457–1466.

7. Chae JJ, Wood G, Richard K et al. The familial Mediterranean fever protein, pyrin, is cleaved by caspase-1 and activates NF-kappaB through its N-terminal fragment. *Blood* 2008;112:1794–1803.

8. Ross JJ. Goats, germs, and fever: Are the pyrin mutations responsible for familial Mediterranean fever protective against brucellosis? *Med Hypotheses* 2007;68:499–501.

9. Kondi A, Hentgen V, Piram M et al. Validation of the new paediatric criteria for the diagnosis of familial Mediterranean fever: data from a mixed population of 100 children from the French reference centre for auto-inflammatory disorders. *Rheumatology* (Oxford) 2010;49: 2200–2203.

10. Sohar E, Gafni G, Pras M. Tel Hashomer key to severity scores for FMF. In: Sohar E, Gafni J, Pras M (eds) *Proceedings of the First International Conference on FMF.* 1997; Freund Publishing House, London and Tel Aviv, 1997:208.

11. Kallinich T, Wittkowski H, Keitzer R, Roth J, Foell D. Neutrophil-derived S100A12 as novel biomarker of inflammation in familial Mediterranean fever. *Ann Rheum Dis* 2010;69:677–682.

12. Goldfinger SE. Colchicine for familial Mediterranean fever. *N Engl J Med* 1972;287:1302.

13. Ben-Chetrit E, Levy M. Reproductive system in familial Mediterranean fever: an overview. *Ann Rheum Dis* 2003;62:916–919.

14. Tufan A, Babaoglu MO, Akdogan A et al. Association of drug transporter gene ABCB1 (MDR1) 3435C to T polymorphism with colchicine response in familial Mediterranean fever. *J Rheumatol* 2007;34:1540–1544.

15. Mor A, Pillinger MH, Kishimoto M, Abeles AM, Livneh A. Familial Mediterranean fever successfully treated with etanercept. *J Clin Rheumatol* 2007;13:38–40.

16. Meinzer U, Quartier P, Alexandra JF et al. Interleukin-1 targeting drugs in familial Mediterranean fever: a case series and a review of the literature. *Semin Arthritis Rheum* 2011;41(2):265–271.

17. McDermott MF, Aksentijevich I, Galon J et al. Germline mutations in the extracellular domains of the 55 kDa TNF receptor, TNFR1, define a family of dominantly inherited autoinflammatory syndromes. *Cell* 1999;97:133–144.

18. Rebelo SL, Radford PM, Bainbridge SE, Todd I, Tighe PJ. Functional consequences of disease-associated mutations in TNFR1 elucidated by transcriptome analysis. *Adv Exp Med Biol* 2011;691:461–470.

19. Todd I, Radford PM, Daffa N et al. Mutant tumor necrosis factor receptor associated with tumor necrosis factor receptor-associated periodic syndrome is altered antigenically and is retained within patients' leukocytes. *Arthritis Rheum* 2007;56:2765–2773.

20. Nedjai B, Hitman GA, Yousaf N et al. Abnormal tumor necrosis factor receptor I cell surface expression and NF-kB activation in tumor necrosis factor receptor-associated periodic syndrome. *Arthritis Rheum* 2008;58:273–283.

21. Simon A, Park H, Maddipati R et al. Concerted action of wild-type and mutant TNF receptors enhances inflammation in TNF receptor 1-associated periodic fever syndrome. *Proc Natl Acad Sci U S A* 2010;107:9801–9806.

22. Williamson LM, Hull D, Mehta R et al. Familial Hibernian fever. *Q J Med* 1982;51:469–480.

23. Hoffmann LA, Lohse P, Konig FB et al. TNFRSF1A R92Q mutation in association with a multiple sclerosis-like demyelinating syndrome. *Neurology* 2008;70:1155–1156.

24. Kauffman MA, Gonzalez-Moron D, Garcea O, Villa AM. TNFSFR1A R92Q mutation, autoinflammatory symptoms and multiple sclerosis in a cohort from Argentina. *Mol Biol Rep* 2012;39:117–121.

25. Ravet N, Rouaghe S, Dode C et al. Clinical significance of P46L and R92Q substitutions in the tumour necrosis factor superfamily 1A gene. *Ann Rheum Dis* 2006;65:1158–1162.

26. Quillinan N, Mannion G, Mohammad A et al. Failure of sustained response to etanercept and refractoriness to anakinra in patients with T50M TNF-receptor-associated periodic syndrome. *Ann Rheum Dis* 2011;70:1692–1693.

27. Nedjai B, Quillinan N, Coughlan RJ et al. Lessons from anti-TNF biologics: infliximab failure in a TRAPS family with the T50M mutation in TNFRSF1A. *Adv Exp Med Biol* 2011;691:409–419.

28. Obici L, Meini A, Cattalini M et al. Favourable and sustained response to anakinra in tumour necrosis factor receptor-associated periodic syndrome (TRAPS) with or without AA amyloidosis. *Ann Rheum Dis* 2011;70:1511–1512.

29. van der Meer JW, Vossen JM, Radl J et al. Hyperimmunoglobulinaemia D and periodic fever: a new syndrome. *Lancet* 1984;1:1087–1090.

30. Cuisset L, Drenth JP, Simon A et al. Molecular analysis of MVK mutations and enzymatic activity in hyper-IgD and periodic fever syndrome. *Eur J Hum Genet* 2001;9:260–266.

31. Henneman L, Schneiders MS, Turkenburg M, Waterham HR. Compromized geranylgeranylation of RhoA and Rac1 in mevalonate kinase deficiency. *J Inherit Metab Dis* 2010;33:625–632.

32. Simon A, Drewe E, van der Meer JW et al. Simvastatin treatment for inflammatory attacks of the hyperimmunoglobulinemia D and periodic fever syndrome. *Clin Pharmacol Ther* 2004;75:476–483.

33. Hoffmann GF, Charpentier C, Mayatepek E et al. Clinical and biochemical phenotype in 11 patients with mevalonic aciduria. *Pediatrics* 1993;91:915–921.

34. Houten SM, van Woerden CS, Wijburg FA, Wanders RJ, Waterham HR. Carrier frequency of the V377I (1129G>A) MVK mutation, associated with Hyper-IgD and periodic fever syndrome, in the Netherlands. *Eur J Hum Genet* 2003;11:196–200.

35. Drenth JP, Haagsma CJ, van der Meer JW. Hyperimmunoglobulinemia D and periodic fever syndrome. The clinical spectrum in a series of 50 patients. International Hyper-IgD Study Group. *Medicine* (Baltimore) 1994;73:133–144.

36. Steichen O, van der Hilst J, Simon A, Cuisset L, Grateau G. A clinical criterion to exclude the hyperimmunoglobulin D syndrome (mild mevalonate kinase deficiency) in patients with recurrent fever. *J Rheumatol* 2009;36:1677–1681.

37. Ammouri W, Cuisset L, Rouaghe S et al. Diagnostic value of serum immunoglobulinaemia D level in patients with a clinical suspicion of hyper IgD syndrome. *Rheumatology* (Oxford) 2007;46:1597–1600.

38. Lachmann HJ, Goodman HJ, Andrews PA et al. AA amyloidosis complicating hyperimmunoglobulinemia D with periodic fever syndrome: a report of two cases. *Arthritis Rheum* 2006;54:2010–2014.

39. Hoffman HM, Mueller JL, Broide DH, Wanderer AA, Kolodner RD. Mutation of a new gene encoding a putative pyrin-like protein causes familial cold autoinflammatory syndrome and Muckle-Wells syndrome. *Nat Genet* 2001;29:301–305.

40. Tschopp J, Martinon F, Burns K. NALPs: a novel protein family involved in inflammation. *Nat Rev Mol Cell Biol* 2003;4:95–104.

41. Martinon F, Agostini L, Meylan E, Tschopp J. Identification of bacterial muramyl dipeptide as activator of the NALP3/cryopyrin inflammasome. *Curr Biol* 2004;14:1929–1934.

42. Aksentijevich I, Masters SL, Ferguson PJ et al. An autoinflammatory disease with deficiency of the interleukin-1-receptor antagonist. *N Engl J Med* 2009;360:2426–2437.

43. Thacker PG, Binkovitz LA, Thomas KB. Deficiency of interleukin-1-receptor antagonist syndrome: a rare auto-inflammatory

condition that mimics multiple classic radiographic findings. *Pediatr Radiol* 2012;42(4):495–498.

44. Wise CA, Gillum JD, Seidman CE et al. Mutations in CD2BP1 disrupt binding to PTP PEST and are responsible for PAPA syndrome, an autoinflammatory disorder. *Hum Mol Genet* 2002;11:961–969.

45. Rose CD, Martin TM, Wouters CH. Blau syndrome revisited. *Curr Opin Rheumatol* 2011;23:411–418.

46. Ferguson PJ, Chen S, Tayeh MK et al. Homozygous mutations in LPIN2 are responsible for the syndrome of chronic recurrent multifocal osteomyelitis and congenital dyserythropoietic anaemia (Majeed syndrome). *J Med Genet* 2005;42:551–557.

47. Onoufriadis A, Simpson MA, Pink AE et al. Mutations in IL36RN/IL1F5 are associated with the severe episodic inflammatory skin disease known as generalized pustular psoriasis. *Am J Hum Genet* 2011;89:432–437.

48. Agarwal AK, Xing C, DeMartino GN et al. PSMB8 encoding the beta5i proteasome subunit is mutated in joint contractures, muscle atrophy, microcytic anemia, and panniculitis-induced lipodystrophy syndrome. *Am J Hum Genet* 2010;87:866–872.

49. Liu Y, Ramot Y, Torrelo A et al. Mutations in PSMB8 cause chronic atypical neutrophilic dermatosis with lipodystrophy and elevated temperature with evidence of genetic and phenotypic heterogeneity. *Arthritis Rheum* 2012;64(3):895–907.

50. Gattorno M, Caorsi R, Meini A et al. Differentiating PFAPA syndrome from monogenic periodic fevers. *Pediatrics* 2009;124:e721–e728.

51. Padeh S, Brezniak N, Zemer D et al. Periodic fever, aphthous stomatitis, pharyngitis, and adenopathy syndrome: clinical characteristics and outcome. *J Pediatr* 1999;135:98–101.

52. Lipsker D. The Schnitzler syndrome. *Orphanet J Rare Dis* 2010;5:38.

CHAPTER 165

Panniculitides

Cord Sunderkötter and Luis Requena

Introduction

Panniculitis is a skin disorder which can be associated with rheumatological diseases (e.g. systemic lupus erythematosus, dermatomyositis or rheumatoid arthritis) (Table 165.1) as well as with adverse events secondary to rheumatological therapies (e.g. post-steroid panniculitis, erythema nodosum, infective panniculitis). The different forms of panniculitis have varying incidences and prevalences: Erythema nodosum is the most frequent one, having an annual incidence of at least 52 per million.[1]

The term panniculitis denotes inflammation that originates primarily in the panniculus adiposus, i.e. in the subcutaneous fatty tissue. The panniculitides are primarily classified according to histopathological criteria.[2–4] The subcutaneous fat or panniculus is organized into lobules, which consist of lipocytes (adipocytes), separated by thin septa of connective tissue. The septa are mostly composed of collagen fibres and elastic tissue, and contain vessels and nerves. Each individual lobule is supplied by a central arteriole or small artery. There are no anastomoses between adjacent lobules so that disrupted blood flow or obstruction of the central arteriole causes necrosis of the adipocytes with ensuing inflammatory reaction.

The panniculitides are first classified according to the denser localization of the inflammatory infiltrate in the panniculus. In a mostly septal panniculitis the infiltrate involves primarily the septa with small veins and arteries, while in a mostly lobular panniculitis it is mostly found in the lobules.[2] However, this is not a 'black and white' distinction, as an inflammatory infiltrate involves both the septa and lobules to some extent.

The second differentiation concerns the absence or presence of vasculitis (Box 165.1).[5–7] Polyarteritis nodosa (PAN) presents as septal panniculitis with vasculitis of the small arteries or arterioles within the septa while erythema nodosum is a septal panniculitis without vasculitis.[3,4] Additional criteria for classification involve the composition of the inflammatory infiltrate, the cause, and an underlying or associated disease (e.g. infections, lupus erythematosus).

Panniculitis generally results from an immunological or inflammatory response in the subcutis to different triggers, such as autoimmune diseases, foreign bodies, trauma, or infections.

The clinical hallmark of panniculitis is a subcutaneous nodule (a mass with a thickness of at least 1 cm), often, but not always located on the lower limb. The nodules are usually not sharply defined due to their location in the deep skin (explanation: the deeper an

Table 165.1 Association of certain forms of panniculitis with rheumatological diseases

Lupus erythematosus	Lupus panniculitis (LE profundus)
	Rheumatoid nodule
Dermatomyositis	Panniculitis in dermatomyositis
Rheumatoid arthritis	Rheumatoid nodule
	Neutrophilic lobular panniculitis associated with rheumatoid arthritis
	Lupus panniculitis
	Subcutaneous granuloma annulare (although no high degree of evidence)
Behçet's disease	Lobular neutrophilic panniculitis
	Erythema nodosum
Ankylosing spondylitis	Erythema nodosum
Anti-phospholipid antibody syndrome	Erythema nodosum
Recurrent polychondritis	Erythema nodosum,
Reactive arthritis	Erythema nodosum
Sjögren's syndrome	Erythema nodosum
	Lupus panniculitis
Takayasu's arteritis	Erythema nodosum
Granulomatosis with polyangiitis	Erythema nodosum
(Immune complex) vasculitis	Septal panniculitis with leukocytoclastic vasculitis

infiltrate is localized in the skin, the less well defined it appears on inspection or palpation, similar to an unknown object under a thick instead of a thin mattress). For clinical diagnosis the following qualities are helpful:

- **Colour**: the nodules usually take a red-violaceous hue. A bright erythema from dilated superficial vessels is a sign of early or acute panniculitis (e.g. in erythema nodosum); brown colour indicates deposition of haemosiderin engulfed by macrophages and is a sign of a non-acute lesion.

- **Consistency**: fluctuancy indicates fluid or pus (e.g. in infective or pancreatic panniculitis), calcification is seen in the panniculitis of dermatomyositis.

Box 165.1 Classification of panniculitides

Mostly septal panniculitides

With vasculitis

- Medium-sized vessels: (cutaneous and classical) polyarteritis nodosa

Without vasculitis

- Erythema nodosum
- Rheumatoid nodule
- Subcutaneous granuloma annulare
- Necrobiotic xanthogranuloma
- Necrobiosis lipoidica
- Deep morphoea

Mostly lobular panniculitides

With vasculitis

- Small vesssels in lobuli of panniculus: nodular vasculitis (erythema induratum of Bazin)
- Small vesssels in dermis and panniculus: erythema nodosum leprosum

Without vasculitis

- Calciphylaxis (with vascular calcification)
- Lupus panniculitis
- Panniculitis in dermatomyositis
- Cold panniculitis
- Pancreatic panniculitis
- α_1-Antitrypsin deficiency panniculitis
- Infective panniculitis
- Factitial panniculitis
- Traumatic panniculitis
- Subcutaneous sarcoidosis
- Poststeroid panniculitis
- Subcutaneous fat necrosis of the newborn
- Sclerema neonatorum
- Sclerosing panniculitis

Shortened version of the table by Requena and Yus.[3]

- **Location**: the involvement of areas other than lower legs is indicative for certain forms of panniculitis, e.g. in lupus panniculitis or cold-induced panniculitis.
- **Lipoatrophy**: deep, atrophy-forming gullies are a result of a preceding inflammation in the panniculus and when localized in the face or upper trunk they are characteristic for lupus panniculitis.
- **Scar**: indicative of previous ulceration.

- **Ulceration**: ulcers are a major secondary feature as they are indicators for panniculitides associated with vasculitis and subsequent ischaemic necrosis. They are also due to:
  - vasculopathy such as the calcified vessels found in calciphylaxis or arteriosclerotic vessels in necrobiosis lipoidica
  - caseous necrosis associated with *Mycobacterium tuberculosis*
  - trauma of exposed, pre-damaged tissue (e.g. in necrobiosis lipodica).

Once the clinical findings indicate a panniculitis, an appropriate biopsy is mandatory in most cases for exact determination of the type of panniculitis and for differential diagnosis. The biopsy must meet certain requirements for adequate histopathological analysis. It should:

- be taken from an early lesion, i.e. rather from brightly red than from brownish parts of nodules, and not from necrotic or ulcerated tissue
- include the subcutis.

Therefore an excisional biopsy should be performed down to the fascia. The sample should be sent to a pathologist or dermatopathologist with sufficient experience in panniculitis to avoid a laconic diagnosis of merely lobular, septal, or mixed panniculitis, which will not be of much diagnostic help given the often sparse and monotonous clinical criteria.

There are no clinical studies, guidelines, or National Institute for Health and Clinical Excellence (NICE) guidances for the panniculitides. When no underlying condition or cause can be identified, anti-inflammatory therapies often ameliorate panniculitides.

Mostly septal panniculitis, not associated with vasculitis

Erythema nodosum

Erythema nodosum (EN) is the most common form of panniculitis and a typical example of septal panniculitis. The incidence is highest between 20 and 30 years of age[8] and there is a female: male ratio of approximately 3–6: 1. EN is a cutaneous process in response to many different provoking factors. The aetiopathogenesis includes disturbed regulation of neutrophils with increased levels of reactive oxygen intermediates. In sarcoidosis, EN is associated with a nucleotide exchange (G→A) at position 308 of the gene promoter for tumour necrosis factor alpha (TNF).[9]

The number of triggers is large (Box 165.1).[10] The most common trigger in children is an infection of the upper respiratory tract with haemolytic *Streptococcus pyogenes*[8]; in adults it is sarcoidosis. The triad of EN, bilateral hilar adenopathy, and arthralgias with fever is an early manifestation of sarcoidosis (Löfgren's syndrome), but is also encountered in tuberculosis and infections with streptococci or *Coccidioides immitis*. In contrast, Behçet's disease, though sometimes described to be associated with EN, rather appears to be more often accompanied by EN-like lesions of a mostly lobular panniculitis with leucocytoclastic vasculitis.[11]

EN presents with a sudden symmetrical appearance of painful, tender, warm, erythematous nodes or plaques, usually on the shins (Figure 165.1). In children EN may present unilaterally on the palms and soles. The lesions show dynamic evolution from bright red to livid-red to purplish within a few days, then assume a characteristic

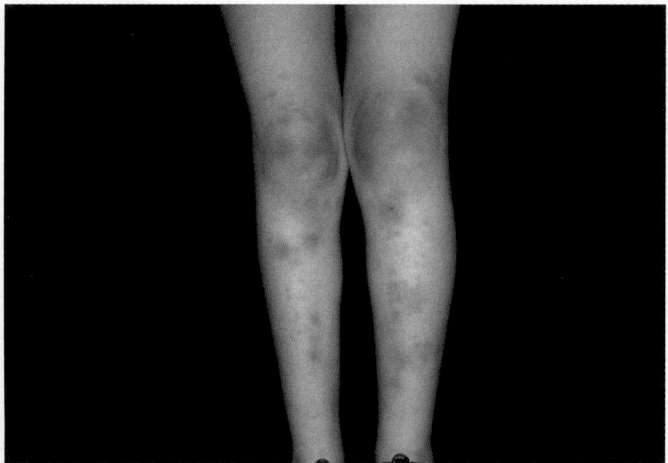

Fig. 165.1 Non-ulcerating nodes of erythema nodosum on the shins.

bruise-like appearance. They never ulcerate, but heal after about 2 weeks without scarring. New crops of lesions may arise for 3–8 weeks. Acute attacks of EN may be accompanied or preceded by fever, malaise, fatigue, headache, arthralgia, or gastrointestinal disturbances and even episcleral lesions. Clinical variants described under the name of erythema nodosum migrans and subacute nodular migratory panniculitis belong histopathologically to the spectrum of EN.

A biopsy is recommended when the differential diagnosis is not clear. The histopathological hallmark is the presence of Miescher's radial granulomas (small, well-defined nodular aggregations of small macrophages or other myeloid cells (immature neutrophils) around a central stellate or banana-shaped cleft) (Figure 165.2). The diagnostic procedure to search for triggers should include history, laboratory tests (complete white blood count, urine analysis, anti-streptolysin titres (optimally repeated after a 2 week interval to detect a rise of at least 30%), chest radiograph (to check for e.g. Löfgren's syndrome, *Chlamydia pneumoniae*, and in endemic areas for coccidioidomycosis or histoplasmosis) (Box 165.2). An intradermal tuberculin test or interferon (IFN) release assay is performed when tuberculosis cannot be ruled out.

Although usually EN regresses spontaneously within 2 months it may be painful and may reappear, warranting symptomatic therapy. This should be aimed at the causative agent or the underlying condition, if identified and treatable. The highest level of published evidence (e.g. uncontrolled study with 28 patients) is for potassium iodide.[12] If short bed rest is not sufficient, non-steroidal anti-inflammatory drugs (NSAIDs; aspirin, indomethacin, or naproxen) provide pain relief and even resolution. If the lesions persist longer, potassium iodide (3 × 150–300 mg daily) often improves symptoms after 2 weeks (saturated solution, preferably in orange juice or other soft drink to make it more palatable).[13] The mechanism of action of this therapy may include inhibition of neutrophil chemotaxis and reactive oxygen release.[13] Colchicine is helpful especially in presence of Behçet's disease, hydroxychloroquine in presence of lupus erythematosus (LE). Systemic corticosteroids are rarely indicated.

Rheumatoid nodule

The firm, usually asymptomatic subcutaneous nodules with a predilection for the elbows and fingers (size from a few millimeters to 3-4 cm) often indicate a more aggressive course of RA. Rarely, they also appear in systemic lupus erythematosus. Surgically excision is only indicated in case of ulceration or pain.

Subcutaneous variants of dermal disorders presenting as panniculitis

There are inflammatory disorders which (1) originate in the dermis, but frequently extend into the subcutis or (2) feature an exclusively subcutaneous form (panniculitis). None of them has a tight correlation to rheumatological disease, but they need to be considered in order to establish a differential diagnosis.

Profound (linear) morphoea

This variant of morphoea is completely situated in the subcutaneous fat. It leaves a linear depressed subcutaneous atrophy, sometimes accompanied by hyper- or hypopigmentation. It is not a subtype of systemic sclerosis and so does not present with sclerodactyly or vasculopathy.

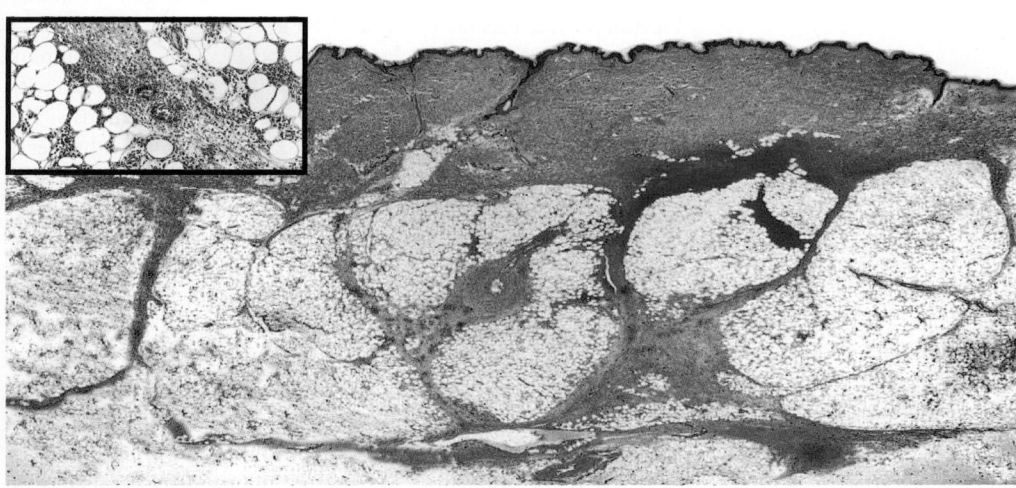

Fig. 165.2 Histology of erythema nodosum, showing an inflammatory infiltrate mostly in the septae of the subcutaneous tissue (pannus) (leading to a mostly septal panniculitis). The small insert depicts so-called Miescher's radial granulomas, i.e. small, well-defined nodular aggregations of small macrophages around a central stellate or banana-shaped cleft.

Box 165.2 Aetiological factors in erythema nodosum

1. Infections

- Bacterial infections: haemolytic streptococci, atypical and typical mycobacteria, *campylobacter*, chlamydia, *Mycoplasma pneumoniae*, shigella, yersinia
- Viral infections: Herpesviridae, hepatitis B and C, HIV
- Fungal infections: coccidioidmycosis and other systemic fungi
- Protozoal infections: amoebiasis, toxoplasmosis

2. Drugs

- Sulfonamides and many others

3. Malignant diseases

4. Miscellaneous conditions

- Sarcoidosis, adult Still's disease, ankylosing spondylitis, antiphospolipid antibody syndrome, Behçet's disease, granulomatosis with polyangiitis, IgA nephropathy, lupus erythematous, pregnancy, recurrent polychondritis, rheumatoid arthritis, Sjögren's syndrome, Sweet's syndrome, Takayasu's arteritis, ulcerative colitis (more often than Crohn's disease; occurrence of EN often signals a flare of the disease)

Shortened version of the table by Requena and Yus.[10]

Eosinophilic fasciitis (Shulman's syndrome)

Another variant of morphea, characterized by rapid onset of symmetric woody induration of the limbs and, less frequently, the trunk. The sclerotic process gives the connective tissue a homogeneously eosinophilic appearance. It may follow vigorous exercise or intake of simvastatin. Prednisone often is efficacious (40–60 mg daily until response, then tapering over the next months).[14] Without treatment complete recovery may take several years.

Subcutaneous granuloma annulare

Subcutaneous granuloma annulare presents with skin-coloured, rarely faintly violaceous subcutaneous nodules on shins, buttocks, hands and head with no visible inflammatory changes on the skin surface. It occurs more frequently in children.

Painful or cosmetically disturbing lesions may warrant treatment by cryotherapy, excision, intralesional injection or topical, occlusive application of corticosteroids.

It belongs to a spectrum of granulomatous diseases which are probably an immune-mediated reaction to a number of underlying, mostly rheumatological conditions and which encompass rheumatoid papules or interstitial granulomatous dermatitis with arthritis (includes palisaded neutrophilic dermatitis).

Necrobiosis lipoidica

This plaque-like panniculitis is often, but not exclusively found in patients with diabetes mellitus. The yellow-brown, firm plaques are usually located bilaterally on the shins. They show a slightly depressed atrophic centre, transparent for partially teleangiectatic vessels, and surrounded by a sharply defined, elevated erythematous margin. They enlarge gradually and may ulcerate, while resolution is rare. Progression may be halted by intralesional injection or by occlusive dressings with glucocorticoids.

Necrobiotic xanthogranuloma

This is rare and occurs in patients with IgG paraproteinemia, multiple myeloma, or other lymphoproliferative disorders. Clinical characteristics are several large, sharply demarcated, indurated plaques of yellow-orange to red-violaceous hue with telangiectasia and with a tendency to ulcerate spontaneously. Its predilection for the periorbital area makes the chronic progressive disease a cosmetic problem. It only rarely responds to treatments.

Mostly septal panniculitis, associated with vasculitis

Classical and cutaneous polyarteriitis nodosa (cutaneous arteritis)

PAN is a classic example of a vasculitis of medium-sized vessels (arterioles) and septal panniculitis.

Cutaneous PAN is a variant which is probably more common than classical PAN (referred to as cutaneous arteritis by the revised nomenclature of the Chapel Hill Consensus Conference).[6] The subcutaneous nodules in PAN are surrounded by livedo racemosa (often sparse) and some of them ulcerate due to stenotic occlusion of vessels. The livedo intermingles with postinflammatory hyperpigmentation to form the so-called 'starburst pattern'. Cutaneous PAN may be accompanied by elevated sedimentation rate, slight fever, arthralgia or myalgia, or even mononeuritis multiplex, but these symptoms remain restricted to the affected skin area (often the leg) and are not associated with involvement of systemic organs. It is sometimes associated with streptococcal infections or viral hepatitis.

Panniculitis with leucocytoclastic vasculitis

Leucocytoclastic vasculitis is a descriptive term for vasculitis of the small vessels referring to the degradation of neutrophils (leucocytoclasia, nuclear dust) which is always observed when there is a high number of neutrophils. Its most common occurrence is in vasculitis caused by immune complexes which usually affects postcapillary venules in the superficial dermis. In rare cases leucocytoclastic vasculitis is observed around postcapillary venules of the septa (leading to mostly septal panniculitis with vasculitis). It shows subcutaneous erythematous nodules due to a deeper infiltrate accompanied by extravasation of blood, but usually no ulceration.

Mostly lobular panniculitis not associated with vasculitis

Lupus panniculitis

Lupus panniculitis is a clinical variant of LE and synonymous with LE profundus. It presents as a recurrent panniculitis and may also be encountered in rheumatoid arthritis or Sjögren's syndrome.

About 1–3% of cutaneous LE cases present with lupus panniculitis. The female/male ratios vary from 2:1 to 9:1 (reviewed in Fraga and Garcia-Diez[15]).

The pathophysiological pathways are probably similar to those in other forms of cutaneous LE, but they do not include high UV sensitivity.

The nodules and/or plaques arise deep in the subcutaneous tissue. The overlying skin may be normal, but can also be affected by discoid lupus. Unlike most other forms of adult panniculitis, the lesions have a predilection for the face, shoulders, upper arms, and buttocks. In rare cases subcutaneous tissue is affected in the breast ('lupus mastitis', clinically and radiologically difficult to distinguish from breast cancer), the orbital (frequent in black South Africans), or the preauricular region.

Resolution of the nodules typically results in lipoatrophy (Figure 165.3). The ensuing depression of lesions on shoulders and upper arms are a hallmark of lupus panniculitis which allow diagnosis even without other cutaneous manifestations of LE.

Lupus panniculitis may be the only clinical manifestation of LE or appear before or after onset of discoid or systemic LE.[15]

However, patients with LE and lupus panniculitis usually have a mild disease course.[4] There may be an association with ensuing or simultaneous occurrence of subcutaneous panniculitis-like T-cell lymphoma. In contrast to lupus panniculitis it usually neither appears on the face nor resolves with lipatrophy.[16]

Local occlusive dressings with potent corticosteroids are helpful when applied early.

Treatment of first choice is hydroxychloroquine. Thalidomide is also effective, but potentially toxic.

Panniculitis in dermatomyositis

Panniculitis is less frequent in dermatomyositis than in LE,[17] but may occur subclinically with only histologically visible evidence.

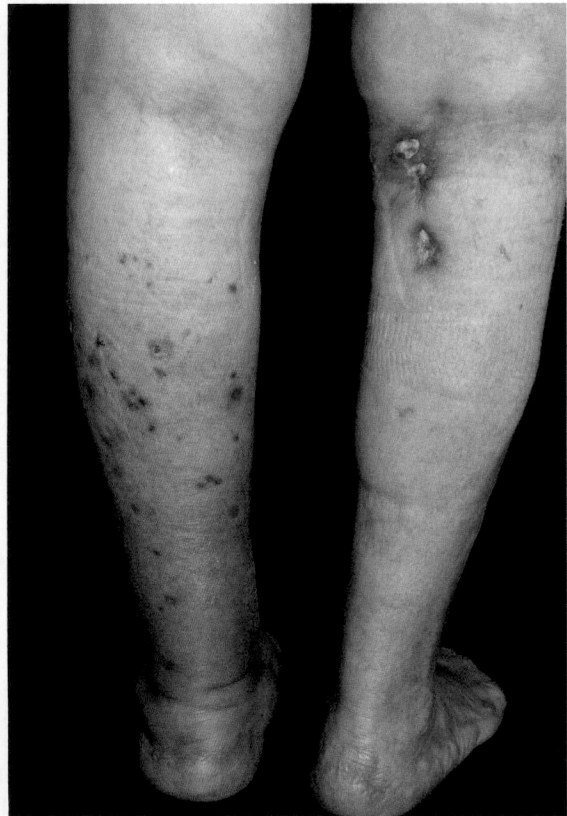

Fig. 165.3 Lipoatrophy in lupus panniculitis.

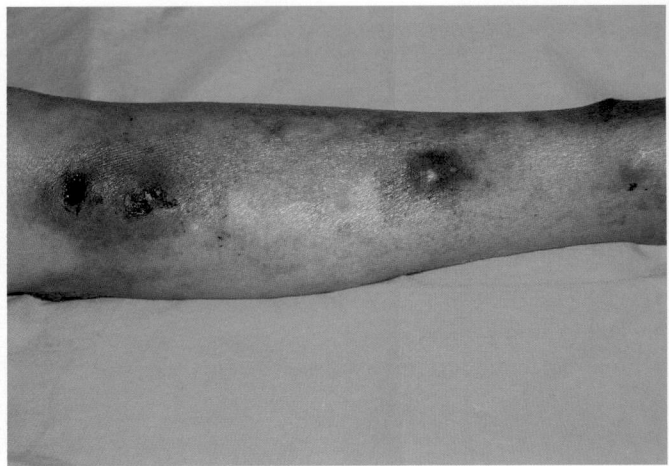

Fig. 165.4 Panniculitis in dermatomyositis.

As in lupus it may occur with or without the other cutaneous manifestations of dermatomyositis. It presents as an erythematous, tender nodule which often calcifies. It may be located on the thighs (Figure 165.4), arms, buttocks, and abdomen, and it may occur in juvenile dermatomyositis. It is responsive to the same systemic treatment as dermatomyositis, in particular to (high-dose) glucocorticoids with the accompanying use of steroid-sparing agents.

Cold panniculitis

Cold panniculitis is a form of panniculitis physically induced by cold exposure. There are two forms: (1) an apparently common response to cold exposure in infants and many children, induced on their cheeks or chins after prolonged cold exposure; (2) a response to cold exposure on the thighs and buttocks of (usually obese) young females wearing tight-fitting trousers, during riding or cycling.

Fat tissue in infants has a higher saturated fatty acid content, which gives it a higher solidification point and probably higher vulnerability to cooling. Cheeks and chins are areas in infants which are rich in subcutaneous fat and easily exposed to cold. In the adult form, tight clothing is supposed to obstruct blood supply and thermoregulation in areas rich in subcutaneous fat.

Clinical diagnosis is made by the appearance of indurated erythematous plaques or nodes with ill-defined margins 2–3 days after cold exposure (which may include sucking ice creams). Exposure to cold should be limited. Affected adults should wear protective and loose trousers.

Pancreatic panniculitis

This fairly characteristic form of panniculitis has been associated with primary or secondary pancreatitis, the latter due to e.g. carcinoma of pancreas (acinar cell carcinoma type), pseudocysts, or anatomical malformations (vasculopancreatic fistulas). It may be the presenting symptom of pancreatitis. The aetiology is unclear. Release of pancreatic lipase into the blood and its accumulation in the pannus may be the actual explanation.

Clinically, the erythematous subcutaneous nodules often ulcerate spontaneously and release an oily brown material, which results from liquefaction necrosis of adipocytes (Figure 165.5). The distal parts of the lower extremities, around the ankles and knees, are areas of predilection. It can be accompanied with panniculitis in periarticular fat tissue, manifesting as arthritis. In immunosuppressed

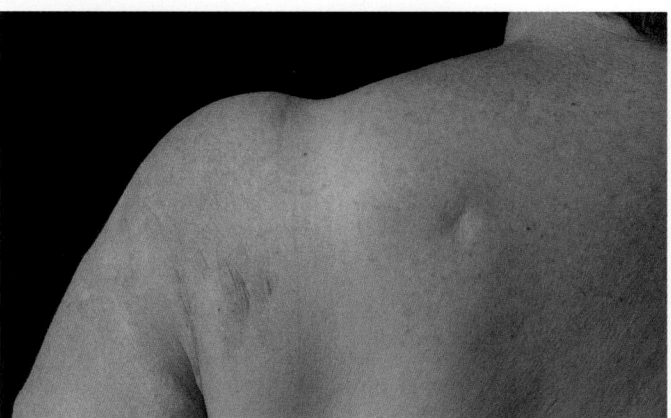

Fig. 165.5 Nodular vasculitis on the back of the lower legs with ulcerated nodes.

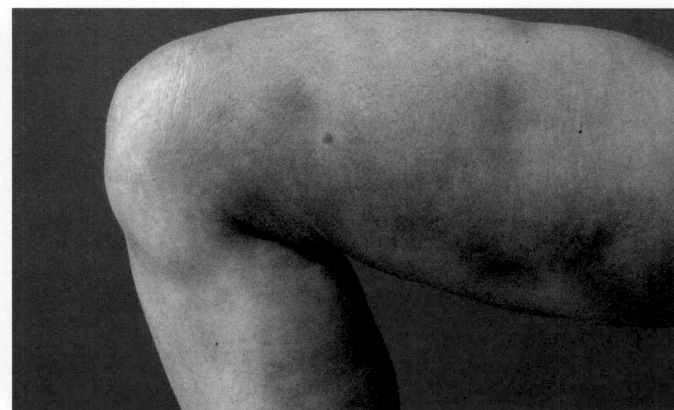

Fig. 165.6 Infective panniculitis by haematogeneous spread.

patients mucormycosis may cause panniculitis with similar histopathological features.[18] Pancreatic panniculitis improves with successful therapy of the underlying pancreatic disease.

α_1-Antitrypsin deficiency panniculitis

Patients with hereditary, homozygous α_1-antitrypsin or α_1-protease inhibitor deficiency develop emphysema, hepatitis, liver cirrhosis, vasculitis, angioedema, and panniculitis.

α_1-Antitrypsin is a serine protease inhibitor that inhibits activity of several proteases, most prominently of trypsin, but also of chymotrypsin, neutrophilic and pancreatic elastase, serine proteases, collagenase, thrombin, plasmin, factor VIII, and kallikrein. Consequently this deficiency results in disorders of innate immune response, blood coagulation, and fibrinolysis, and generally in abnormal activation of proenzymes and peptide hormones.

The subcutaneous nodules are mostly located in the skin of the lower abdomen and around the buttocks. They tend to ulcerate and to release an oily material from necrotic fat lobules similar to pancreatitic panniculitis.

Trauma and surgical debridement are precipitating factors and should be avoided. Dapsone is an effective treatment when panniculitis has developed. In severe forms of the disease (severe emphysema and liver failure), protease inhibitor concentrate should be supplemented.

Infective panniculitis

Soft tissue infection commonly involves the subcutaneous tissue and would therefore present as a form of panniculitis. This type of infective panniculitis occurs as a consequence of primary or direct inoculation of bacteria or certain fungi[19] due to trauma or also indwelling catheters. It therefore often begins in or involves the dermis.

A second type of infective panniculitis results from haematogenous dissemination of infectious microorganisms (mostly certain bacteria or fungi[19]; Figure 165.6) and presents as a panniculitis in the strict sense, both histologically (usually as lobular panniculitis, without relevant involvement of the dermis) and clinically with several nodules or subcutaneous abscesses on the legs or on the gluteal area, abdominal or thoracic wall, arms, or fingers. Fluctuation is present, but may not be palpable when the abscesses are deeply located.

Haematogenous dissemination is seen particularly, but not exclusively, in immunocompromised hosts. This includes patients treated for rheumatological diseases, while rheumatological diseases also tend to develop their own forms of panniculitis (e.g. lupus panniculitis). Therefore it is important to always take infective panniculitis into consideration in differential diagnosis of patients with rheumatic disease and panniculitis.

When in doubt, especially in presence of immunosuppression or signs of infection, a biopsy should be performed for both histology and for microbiological culture and/or detection of microbial nucleic acids. In immunocompromised patients infectious microorganisms are numerous in the tissue, thus facilitating diagnosis. Likewise, the presence of neutrophils in a lobular panniculitis should always prompt cultures of the biopsy specimen. Panniculitis due to hematogenous spread is more deeply seated than local infection, and the blood vessels are thrombosed and filled with infective organisms. Bacteraemia may in addition cause small-vessel vasculitis due to non-physiological local activation of endothelial cells and transmigrating neutrophils[20] (especially in infections with lipopolysaccharide-containing Gram-negative bacteria).

Therapy always encompasses systemic administration of antibiotics or antifungals.

Incision and drainage may be indicated depending on the extent of infection; early mycobacterial lesions (Buruli ulcer) can be excised.

Poststeroid panniculitis

Poststeroid panniculitis is a rare form which occurs in children in whom high doses of systemic corticosteroids were discontinued or decreased quickly. It is to be distinguished from glucocorticoid-induced lipoatrophy.

Clinically, erythematous subcutaneous nodules appear 1–10 days after discontinuation of high doses of gluocortiocids in those areas where the preceding glucocortiocid therapy has led to the highest accumulation of fat (e.g. cheeks). Its histopathology is indistinguishable from the subcutaneous fat necrosis of the newborn, showing necrotic adipocytes and histiocytes containing crystallized lipids.

Poststeroid panniculitis resolves after some weeks without residual lesion unless it has caused ulceration, which then leaves atrophic scars on the cheeks. Resuming high-dose systemic corticosteroid and moderate tapering is helpful.

Factitial panniculitis

Factitial or artifactual panniculitis is a response to mechanical, physical, or chemical injuries to the subcutaneous tissue. The injuries may be inflicted on purpose or by accident, or be iatrogenic. Iatrogenic injury is due to subcutaneous implantation of different materials for cosmetic or therapeutic reasons (e.g. paraffin, silicone, or polymethylsiloxane for augmentation of breasts or genitalia, or for correcting facial wrinkles)[21] or due to subcutaneously injected drugs (e.g. gold salts, pethidine (in the US meperidine), povidone iodine, vaccines), or due to extravasation of cytotoxic drugs such as antracyclines or taxanes.

In case of psychiatric disorders with personality aberrations some patients inject themselves with harmful substances such as acids, alkalis, mustard, milk, microbiologically contaminated material, urine, and faeces.

Oily materials (paraffin, vegetable oils, impurities e.g. in liquid silicone) cause a foreign body reaction in the subcutis, in some cases with a time lag of up to 30 years. In addition, immunological reactions and ischaemia by local drug-induced vasoconstriction may play a pathogenic role.

Self-induced panniculitis is usually localized in areas accessible to manipulation and often looks bizarre, without similarities to defined dermatoses. It is inherent to the disorder that patients may appear otherwise psychologically inconspicuous and are often not consciously aware of their manipulations, so that attempts to enforce the diagnosis are futile. However, occlusion of affected areas by bandages and ensuing lack of new lesions may help the physician's diagnosis.

A biopsy is recommended, as histopathology may provide hints for the cause, such as refractile foreign material seen on polarizing light microscopy.[22]

Patients with self-inflicted factitial panniculitis need psychiatric treatment. Materials implanted for cosmetic reasons should be removed and the reaction treated with glucocorticoids.

Traumatic panniculitis

Traumatic panniculitis may be considered a special form of facticial panniculitis, caused by accidental blunt trauma.

Calciphylaxis

Calciphylaxis is a disease in which calcification of the walls of cutaneous vessels results in livedo racemosa and often in large painful necrosis and ulceration. It is often, but not exclusively, associated with chronic renal failure. It occurs in about 4% of patients undergoing haemodialysis. The course in patients with calciphylaxis and renal failure show a high mortality of about 80% due to infection and sepsis.

There are two forms: (a) uraemic or renal calciphylaxis in patients with endstage renal failure undergoing haemodialysis or having received kidney transplantation; (2) non-renal form in patients without significant renal failure.

Both forms have features in common: (1) calcification of cutaneous small and medium-sized blood vessels (often arterioles, as seen in long-standing lesions of atherosclerosis) in the panniculus and parts of the dermis, (2) intimal hyperplasia with fibrosis, (3) intraluminal thrombi, and (4) mostly lobular panniculitis with necrosis and sometimes lobular calcifications.

Calciphylaxis should be distinguished from an entity called benign nodular calcification in which the course correlates more strongly with abnormalities of calcium–phosphorus metabolism.

Predispositions in non-renal calciphylaxis are primary hyperparathyroidism, collagen vascular diseases, malignant tumours, or hepatic cirrhosis. In the renal form they are hypercalcaemia, hyperphosphataemia, or hyperparathyroidism. Additional factors may be local trauma, arterial hypertension, posthemodialysis metabolic alkalosis, or intake of inorganic metal salts. Aetiopathogenesis involves a disturbed balance between procalcifying (calcium, phosphate, parathyroid hormone) and anticalcifying factors (fetuin A, pyrophosphate, matrix-Gla-protein). Reductions of the latter are caused e.g. by prolonged intake of vitamin K antagonists.[23–25]

There are two forms of independent aetiology : (1) ulcerating calciphylaxis, often located on areas rich in fat tissue such as trunk, buttocks, proximal thighs, more rarely on lower legs; the respective large, deep, non-healing ulcers are painful due to ischaemia; (2) non-ulcerating calciphylaxis is often located on distal legs and sometimes distal arms; it is often associated with violaceous, sometimes patchy or reticulated, livedo reticularis.

A biopsy confirms the diagnosis, but is only indicated when in doubt, as it can trigger an additional ulcer.

For therapy, the standard procedure is normalization of calcium and phosphorus serum levels by cinacalcet[9] (which is preferable to an irreversible parathyroidectomy), chelating agents (sodium thiosulfate often provides pain relief within 3 weeks and stimulates wound healing) and discontinuation of vitamin K antagonists or their replacement by heparin. A diet poor in calcium and phosphorus, and low-calcium haemodialysis, can also be helpful.

Sclerosing panniculitis (lipodermatosclerosis, hypodermitis sclerodermiformis)

This is a synonym and more appropriate term[26] for a complication of chronic venous insufficiency which, despite its common occurrence, causes diagnostic confusion. Most on the lower calf present as an indurated plaque with oedema, either with hyperpigmentation in the chronic forms or with bright erythema in the acute form (often confused with erysipelas). Often a marked reduction of the circumference of the distal lower leg occurs (like an inverted bottle), resulting from extensive deep sclerosis and ensuing atrophy of the subcutaneous fat.

Mostly lobular panniculitis associated with nodular (nodose) vasculitis (erythema induratum Bazin)

Nodular vasculitis is a lobular panniculitis with a primary vasculitis involving mostly the small blood vessels of the fat lobule (postcapillary venules) and only rarely small or medium sized vessels in the septae.[27] Vasculitis may not be visible in all histological sections, so that several sections need to be analysed, but it appears to be the primary event of this disease, as it is observed in biopsy sections of early lesions.[27]. In presence of tuberculosis (usually with hyperergic reaction) it has been referred to as erythema induratum Bazin.

Nodular vasculitis (like EN) appears to present a (hyper)reactive response to tuberculosis or other microbial antigens such as streptococci, candida, or *M. leprae*.[28] Exposure to cold and chronic venous insufficiency may provide additional or even the only eliciting factors.

Tender erythematous subcutaneous plaques and nodules arise on the posterior aspect of the calf. It occurs mostly in middle-aged women with lipoedema (column-like lower legs), livedo reticularis, or erythrocyanosis surrounding follicular pores. In the course of the disease most, but not all, nodules ulcerate. Healing is slow and leaves atrophic scars.

In cases where association with *M. tuberculosis* is suspected, INF-γ release assays are helpful for diagnosis and monitoring treatment.[29] Compression and NSAIDs or potassium iodide may alleviate symptoms when no cause can be detected or treated.[28,30]

Conclusion

The term panniculitis denotes an inflammation that originates primarily in the subcutaneous fatty tissue. It is characterized histopathologically according to the major or denser localization of the infiltrate as mostly septal panniculitis and mostly lobular panniculitis, and in those with and without vasculitis. The clinical hallmarks of panniculitis are subcutaneous nodules or plaques, often located on the lower limb. EN is the most common form of panniculitis and a typical example for septal panniculitis. It has multiple aetiological factors, the most frequent ones being infections and sarcoidosis.

References

1. Garcia-Porrua C, Gonzalez-Gay MA, Vazquez-Caruncho M et al. Erythema nodosum: etiologic and predictive factors in a defined population. *Arthritis Rheum* 2000;43(3):584–592.
2. Ackerman A, Chongchitnant N. *Histologic diagnosis of inflammatory skin diseases: an algorithmic method based on pattern analysis*. Williams & Wilkins, Baltimore, 1997.
3. Requena L, Sanchez Yus E. Panniculitis. Part I. Mostly septal panniculitis. *J Am Acad Dermatol* 2001;45(2):163–183; quiz 84–86.
4. Requena L, Sanchez Yus E. Panniculitis. Part II. Mostly lobular panniculitis. *J Am Acad Dermatol* 2001;45(3):325–361; quiz 62–64.
5. Basu N, Watts R, Bajema I et al. EULAR points to consider in the development of classification and diagnostic criteria in systemic vasculitis. *Ann Rheum Dis* 2010;69(10):1744–1750.
6. Jennette JC, Falk RJ, Bacon PA, et al. 2012 revised international chapel hill consensus conference nomenclature of vasculitides. *Arthritis Rheum* 2013 65(1):1–11.
7. Hunder GG, Arend WP, Bloch DA et al. The American College of Rheumatology 1990 criteria for the classification of vasculitis. Introduction. *Arthritis Rheum* 1990;33(8):1065–1067.
8. Cribier B, Caille A, Heid E, Grosshans E. Erythema nodosum and associated diseases. A study of 129 cases. *Int J Dermatol* 1998;37(9):667–672.
9. Labunski S, Posern G, Ludwig S et al. Tumour necrosis factor-alpha promoter polymorphism in erythema nodosum. *Acta Derm Venereol* 2001;81(1):18–21.
10. Requena L, Sanchez Yus E. Erythema nodosum. *Dermatol Clin* 2008; 26(4):425–438, v.
11. Kim B, LeBoit PE. Histopathologic features of erythema nodosum-like lesions in Behçet disease: a comparison with erythema nodosum focusing on the role of vasculitis. *Am J Dermatopathol* 2000;22(5): 379–390.
12. Schulz EJ, Whiting DA. Treatment of erythema nodosum and nodular vasculitis with potassium iodide. *Br J Dermatol* 1976;94(1):75–78.
13. Gilchrist H, Patterson JW. Erythema nodosum and erythema induratum (nodular vasculitis): diagnosis and management. *Dermatol Ther* 2010;23(4):320–327.
14. Lakhanpal S, Ginsburg WW, Michet CJ, Doyle JA, Moore SB. Eosinophilic fasciitis: clinical spectrum and therapeutic response in 52 cases. *Semin Arthritis Rheum* 1988;17(4):221–231.
15. Fraga J, Garcia-Diez A. Lupus erythematosus panniculitis. *Dermatol Clin* 2008;26(4):453–463, vi.
16. Pincus LB, LeBoit PE, McCalmont TH et al. Subcutaneous panniculitis-like T-cell lymphoma with overlapping clinicopathologic features of lupus erythematosus: coexistence of 2 entities? *Am J Dermatopathol* 2009;31(6):520–526.
17. Janis JF, Winkelmann RK. Histopathology of the skin in dermatomyositis. A histopathologic study of 55 cases. *Arch Dermatol* 1968;97(6): 640–650.
18. Requena L, Sitthinamsuwan P, Santonja C et al. Cutaneous and mucous mucormycosis mimicking pancreatic panniculitis and gouty panniculitis. *J Am Acad Dermatol* 2012;66(6):975–984.
19. Morrison LK, Rapini R, Willison CB, Tyring S. Infection and panniculitis. *Dermatol Ther* 2010;23(4):328–340.
20. Sunderkotter C, Seeliger S, Schonlau F et al. Different pathways leading to cutaneous leukocytoclastic vasculitis in mice. *Exp Dermatol* 2001;10(6):391–404.
21. Requena L, Requena C, Christensen L et al. Adverse reactions to injectable soft tissue fillers. *J Am Acad Dermatol* 2011;64(1):1–34; quiz 5–6.
22. Sanmartin O, Requena C, Requena L. Factitial panniculitis. *Dermatol Clin* 2008;26(4):519–527, viii.
23. Brandenburg VM, Cozzolino M, Ketteler M. Calciphylaxis: a still unmet challenge. *J Nephrol* 2011;24(2):142–148.
24. Rogers NM, Coates PT. Calcific uraemic arteriolopathy: an update. *Curr Opin Nephrol Hypertens* 2008;17(6):629–634.
25. Weenig RH. Pathogenesis of calciphylaxis: Hans Selye to nuclear factor kappa-B. *J Am Acad Dermatol* 2008;58(3):458–471.
26. Jorizzo JL, White WL, Zanolli MD et al. Sclerosing panniculitis. A clinicopathologic assessment. *Arch Dermatol* 1991;127(4):554–558.
27. Segura S, Pujol RM, Trindade F, Requena L. Vasculitis in erythema induratum of Bazin: a histopathologic study of 101 biopsy specimens from 86 patients. *J Am Acad Dermatol* 2008;59(5):839–851.
28. Mascaro JM Jr, Baselga E. Erythema induratum of Bazin. *Dermatol Clin* 2008;26(4):439–445, v.
29. Vera-Kellet C, Peters L, Elwood K, Dutz JP. Usefulness of Interferon-gamma release assays in the diagnosis of erythema induratum. *Arch Dermatol* 2011;147(8):949–952.
30. Sterling JB, Heymann WR. Potassium iodide in dermatology: a 19th century drug for the 21st century—uses, pharmacology, adverse effects, and contraindications. *J Am Acad Dermatol* 2000;43(4):691–697.

CHAPTER 166

Neutrophilic dermatoses

Pia Moinzadeh and Thomas Krieg

Introduction

The group of neutrophilic dermatoses (NDs) includes non-infectious skin diseases, which are characterized by a diffuse infiltrate of neutrophilic inflammatory cells throughout different layers of the skin. Patients suffering from NDs present with very heterogenous clinical features including either localized or generalized skin involvement as well as systemic symptoms. Depending on the localization of the inflammatory cells, i.e. subcorneal, intraepidermal, dermal, or subdermal, and the absence or presence of vessel damage, the group of ND can be subdivided into different subtypes (see Box 166.1).

Diagnosis of these disorders is based on clinical, laboratory and histopathological features (see Box 166.2) and requires a comprehensive assessment of all other possible conditions related to NDs. It is not uncommon that NDs are misdiagnosed due to mimicking other illnesses, which is risky for the patient because often inadequate treatment strategies are then used.

In this chapter we focus on those NDs in which the vessel wall is not affected; Behcet's disease and other vasculitides are discussed in other chapters (see Chapters 130–137).

Box 166.1 Neutrophilic dermatoses

- Sweet's syndrome
- Pyoderma gangrenosum
- Rheumatoid neutrophilic dermatitis
- Bowel-associated dermatosis–arthritis syndrome
- Subcorneal pustular dermatosis (Sneddon–Wilkinson syndrome)
- Behçet's disease
- Pustular psoriasis
- Acrodermatitis continua and palmoplantar pustulosis
- Acrodermatitis continua of Hallopeau
- Palmoplantar pustulosis
- Acute generalized exanthematous pustulosis
- Pustular bacterid (Andrew's disease)
- Neutrophilic eccrine hidradenitis

Sweet's syndrome—acute febrile neutrophilic dermatosis

Sweet's syndrome (SS), is one of the most frequently occurring entities of the group of NDs. It is defined by erythematous-livid, asymmetric, very painful plaques associated with non-specific systemic features, such as elevated temperature, arthralgias, weight loss, malaise, and elevated serum inflammation markers, such as

---

Box 166.2 Recommended diagnostic procedures for neutrophilic dermatoses

Medical history

- Clinical picture
- Pain
- Possible symptoms of further associated diseases
- Drug history

Physical examination

- Characteristics of skin lesions: efflorescence, type, size, location, extension
- General examination
- Inspection of the whole skin
- Inspection of lymph nodes

Laboratory investigations:

- Full blood count and biochemistry
- Erythrocyte sedimentation rate
- Serum protein electrophoresis
- Autoantibodies

Histopathological investigation of the skin

Clarification of associated systemic diseases:

- Chest radiograph/CT
- Vascular studies (venous and arterial)
- Endoscopy
- Bone marrow aspirate

neutrophilia, increased erythrocyte sedimentation rate (ESR) and C-reactive protein (CRP) levels.[1] Due to the abrupt onset of a combination of cardinal attributes, such as systemic symptoms, skin lesions as well as typical histological features, it is also known as acute febrile neutrophilic dermatosis. The classical histopathological features are dense dermal infiltrates of neutrophils without any signs of vasculitis.

Epidemiology

SS appears to be predominantly a female disease (4:1), without any racial predilection. Most of the patients are between 30 and 50 years old, but paediatric cases have also been reported without any gender predilection.[1–2] Patients developing SS may initially attract attention with symptoms suggestive of a febrile upper respiratory tract infection, which precede the onset of further symptoms. Different infectious agents such as yersinia, staphylococcus, streptococcus, mycobacteria, cytomegalovirus, HIV, and hepatitis A, B, and C infections have been considered to function as a trigger of this condition.[1–2] Malignancies with predominantly haematological origin (leukaemia) and also drugs, such as granulocyte colony-stimulating factor (G-CSF), and pregnancy can cause SS.[3]

- **Classical SS** occurs more frequently in female patients (80%), often associated with an infection, inflammatory bowel diseases or also pregnancy,[4] with a relapse of skin lesions in 33% of patients and an initial episode between the age of 30 and 60 years.[3]

- **Malignancy-associated SS** occurs in male and female patients, without definitive gender predilection. These patients usually suffer from haematological malignancies (acute myelogenous leukaemia) or solid tumours (genitourinary, breast, gastrointestinal cancer).[3–4] It is much less associated with an infection prior to the development of skin lesions and the relapse of skin lesions is positively and very closely correlated with the discovery, cure, or relapse of the cancer itself.[3]

- **Drug-induced SS** can be caused by several drugs (antibiotics, anti-epileptics, anti-hypertensives, anti-neoplastics, anti-psychotics, NSAIDS, diuretics, contraceptives, etc.), however, the most frequently drug triggering SS is G-CSF. Following discontinuation of the triggering drug, the skin lesions frequently heal completely without the need for systemic treatment and relapse if the causing drug is represcribed.[3]

Aetiopathogenesis

The aetiopathogenesis is still not fully elucidated, but it is thought to be a multifactorial interaction of a hypersensitivity reaction due to infections, autoimmune diseases with the production of autoantibodies, immune complexe formation, drugs (G-CSF), physical factors and genetic predisposition (specific HLA serotypes), proteases, and malignancies.[2] Also the fact that more women develop SS and contraceptives are a possible trigger imply that the endocrine system and/or hormonal changes also may play a role.[5] The genetic background of SS is uncertain. Twenty-eight Japanese patients with SS showed an increased frequency of HLA-Bw 54, while in 38 white women no significant association could be confirmed.[5] The appearance of perivascular leucocytoclasis has been suggested to be associated with the vascular deposition of immune complexes, as a kind of hypersensitivity reaction type III, but immunohistochemical studies showed controversial results.[5]

Several studies have suggested, that a dysregulation of cytokine cascades with an increased secretion of cytokines may be involved in the development of SS, including interleukin (IL)-1[5], IL-2,[6] IL-3,[5] IL-6,[5] and IL-8,[5] interferon (IFN)-γ,[6] granulocyte colony stimulating factor (G-CSF), and granulocyte-macrophage colony-stimulating factor (GM-CSF).[5] Increased serum levels of IL-1, IL-2, and IFN-γ suggest that helper Th1 cells are involved in the aetiopathogenesis.[6] IL-1, a neutrophil chemoattractant, seems to play the central role in the development of SS by stimulating macrophages to secrete GM-CSF and IL-8.[6] Going et al. hypothesized a release of IL-1 into the dermis[7] and there is evidence of elevated serum levels of IL-1α and IL-1β in comparison to normal controls.[6] Meng et al. showed that a mutation of *NLRP3* genes can induce a sudden skin inflammation in mice with a dense neutrophil infiltration of the dermis similar to SS, due to excessive production of IL-1β.[8]

Recent studies have also shown that neutrophil/NK cells are observable in SS skin lesions,[9] and that a defect in the transcriptional regulation of *PTPN6* seems to be involved in the pathogenesis of SS and pyoderma gangrenosum (PG).[10]

Clinical features

The cutaneous lesions in patients with SS are well defined, tender, purple-red, non-pruritic nodules, papules, or sharply bordered plaques of erythematous and/or violaceous colour, which can become very painful; they are preferentially localized asymmetrically as single or multiple lesions in the face, neck, upper trunk, and proximal extremities (Figure 166.1).[4] A small subgroup of patients also may develop a localized form of SS, which is known as 'neutrophilic dermatosis of the dorsal hands'.[11] Furthermore a positive cutaneous pathergy phenomenon has been reported with lesions occurring after skin biopsies, cat scratches, or sunburn.[12–13]

Secondary to the oedema in the upper dermis, the lesions may occasionally be misdiagnosed as bullae or vesicules (pseudovesicular appearance),[14] they can develop into pustules and also can become ulcerated (more common in malignancy-associated SS) or enlarge to large, irregular but sharply bordered plaques.[3] Patients appear often dramatically ill, due to fever, which can occur several days to weeks prior to skin lesions, leucocytosis, arthralgias, myalgia, malaise, nausea, vomiting, and headache.[4,13] But not all patients present with the entire spectrum of clinical features.

Extracutaneous manifestations

Patients can also develop subcutaneous lesions as well as extracutaneous lesions, involving the bones (sterile osteomyelitis), ears (SS nodules next to the tympanic membrane), eyes (conjunctivitis, episcleritis, iridocyclitis), renal system (mesangiocapillary glomerulonephritis, haematuria, proteinuria), central nervous system (acute benign encephalitis, neurologic symptoms, pareses, polyneuropathy), liver (hepatomegaly, elevated liver enzymes), cardiopulmponary system (aortitis, cardiomegaly, heart failure, alveolitis with cough or dyspnoea), mouth (oral ulcers, bullae, vesicles), muscles (myositis), and spleen (splenomegaly).[3] SS can also overlap with other autoimmune rheumatic diseases, such rheumatoid arthritis (RA), systemic lupus erythematosus (SLE), Sjögren's syndrome, sarcoidosis, Still's disease, or polychondritis.[2]

Histopathological features

Histopathology shows a dense diffusely distributed neutrophilic infiltrate in the superficial dermis, pronounced perivasculary with leucocytoclasia (fragmented neutrophil nuclei) and an oedema in

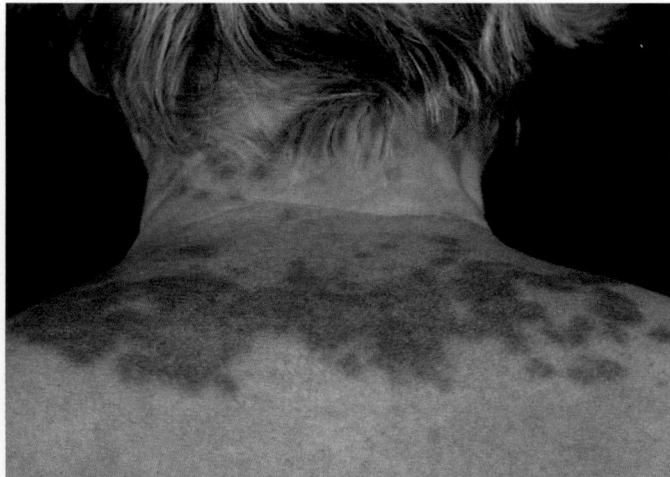

Fig. 166.1 Sweet's syndrome.

the papillary dermis, but without features of vasculitis. Besides the predominant cells, mature neutrophils and also eosinophils, lymphocytes, and/or histiocytes are occasionally present in the skin of SS patients. Patients with the subcutaneous form of SS show a very diffuse inflammatory infiltrate, involving the dermis but also the subcutaneous fat tissue.[15] These typical histopathological features in the skin, have also been reported in involved internal organs, with sterile neutrophilic inflammatory infiltrates.[3]

Diagnostic procedures

The diagnosis of classical and malignancy-associated SS is established, if patients meet two major and two of five minor criteria. The major criteria include (1) an abrupt onset of painful erythematous nodules, papules, or plaques and (2) typical histopathological findings, such as a dense neutrophilic infiltrate without evidence of leucocytoclastic vasculitis. The minor criteria are (1) elevated temperature; (2) an association with haematological or visceral malignancy, inflammatory, disease or pregnancy, or preceded by an upper respiratory tract infection, gastrointestinal infection, or a vaccination; (3) an excellent response to systemic steroid therapy or potassium iodide; and (4) abnormal laboratory tests (three of four) with an ESR in excess of 20 mm/hour, a high CRP, leucocytes in excess of 8000 with more than 70% of neutrophils.[2]

For the diagnosis of drug-induced SS all of the following criteria are required: (1) abrupt onset of painful erythematous plaques or nodules; (2) histopathological findings of dense neutrophilic infiltrates without the evidence of leucocytoclastic vasculitis; (3) fever above 38 °C; (4) a positive temporal relationship between the use of the drug and the clinical development of skin lesions or a relapse with readministration; and (5) a sudden disappearance of skin lesions after drug discontinuation or treatment with steroids.[2]

In malignancy-associated SS patients often present with leucopenia, lymphopenia, anaemia, and/or abnormal platelet counts.[1,5] In general it is very important to exclude infections with blood cultures, blood tests, urine analyses, and stool samples. Depending on the extracutaneous manifestations further investigations are necessary; patients with symptoms suggestive of central nervous system (CNS) involvement should be investigated, using brain SPECTs, CT scan, MRI, EEG, and/or cerebrospinal fluid (CSF) analysis. Urine analyses with evaluation of haematuria and/or proteinuria is helpful

to assess kidney involvement, while SS-associated liver involvement can be identified by elevation of liver enzymes. To exclude an underlying malignant process, patients should be investigated according to the recommendations of the American Cancer Society for the early identification of cancer in asymptomatic patients.[16]

Management

After approximately 6–8 weeks without treatment, most of the lesions resolve spontaneously, depending on the underlying disease, but very commonly patients develop new lesions recurrently. It is important to identify the underlying cause; if SS is triggered by a drug, the first step is to stop the drug and avoid similar (cognate) compounds. If the patient develops SS due to an infection, it is important to treat the infection, and if it is paraneoplastic, appropriate chemotherapy should be initiated.

Topical treatment options

In localized cases of SS topical and/or intralesional application of high-potency steroids can be effective.[3]

Systemic treatment options

SS shows a good response to systemic glucocorticoids (drug of first choice).[3] Skin and systemic symptoms tend to improve with glucocorticoids within 72 hours after starting therapy. Chronic relapsing disease may require the use of steroid-sparing immunosuppressive agents.

Alternative treatments include potassium iodide tablets or colchicine solution. Patients receiving potassium iodide therapy showed a resolution of symptoms and skin lesions within 3–5 days and patients who were initiated on colchicine therapy showed a resolution of skin and systemic symptoms after 2–5 days and normalization of the leucocytosis within 8–14 days.

Other treatments include indomethacin, clofazimine, dapsone, and ciclosporin. There have been reports of efficacy with mycophenolate mofetil, methotrexate, doxycycline, intravenous immunoglobulins, and etretinate.[2] The use of biologics such as infliximab or etanecept has been proposed for patients with SS and associated inflammatory bowel or rheumatic diseases.[17–18] Recent case reports support the use of anakinra in patients with SS because dysregulation of IL-1 secretion has been observed.[19]

Pyoderma gangrenosum

PG is a rare, non-infectious, chronic and relapsing, ulcerative skin disease. These skin lesions are defined as very painful, cutaneous ulcerations with a violaceous, undermined border surrounding a necrotic base (see figure 166.2).

Powell et al classified patients with PG into four different subtypes, such as ulcerative, pustular, bullous, and vegetative PG.[20] Many patients (50–70%) with PG suffer from concomitant diseases,[20–21] such as inflammatory bowel disease (ulcerative colitis, Crohn's disease), rheumatic disorders, monoclonal gammopathy, sarcoidosis or malignancies, mostly haematological background. Familial cases of PG have also been reported, especially a rare syndromic variant called PAPA (pyogenic sterile arthritis with PG and severe acne) syndrome.

Epidemiology

PG appears to be slightly more frequent in the female population in the age range 20–60 years.[20,22] A recently published retrospective study showed a female to male ratio of 3:1 and a mean age of onset of 51.6 years. The general incidence of PG is between 3 and 10 per million inhabitants per year.[23]

Aetiopathogenesis

The pathogenesis is not completely known, but it has been reported that patients with PG may have a hyper-reactive response to trauma, and internal diseases with a further dysfunction of their immune system, that results in the excessive release of leucocytes, and cytokines such as IL-1and IL-8.[24–26] The release of IL-1β by T lymphocytes is associated with a clonal expansion of those cells and a clonal expansion of neutrophils and a release of large amounts of anti-matrix metalloproteinases-9, -10 and tumour necrosis factor alpha (TNFα), which together cause ulceration and progression of the disease.[27–28] Bister et al. hypothesized that a lack of anti-matrix metalloproteinase 1 and 26 on the borders of PG wounds retards normal wound healing.[28] These findings were also confirmed by a recent study which showed immunoreactivities of CD3 (pan T cell marker), CD163 (macrophage marker), myeloperoxidase (neutrophil marker), TNFα, IL-8 (cytokine chemotactic for neutrophils), IL-17, MMP2, MMP9 (proteinase-mediating tissue damage), and vascular endothelial growth factor (VEGF) which were significantly higher expressed in skin of patients with PG than in healthy controls, especially in the bullous or ulcerative form.[29] Also the interplay between IL-6 (as an inducer of acute-phase response), IL-8, and anti-phosphatidylserine-prothrombin antibodies may be closely associated with the development of PG.[30] IL-23 may play a critical role in the pathogenesis of PG; after treatment with ustekinumab (anti-IL-12/IL-23p40 monoclonal antibody), IL-23 expression decreased significantly accompanying with the complete healing of PG skin lesions.[31]

Furthermore, an alteration in the gene encoding protein tyrosine phosphatase non-receptor type 6 (*PTPN6/SHP1*) has been suggested to be one candidate gene involved in the pathogenesis of ND (PG and SS).[10]

Recent findings in familial cases, such as the PAPA syndrome, have shown that the proline-rich, glutamic acid-rich, serine-rich, and threonine-rich (PEST) family of protein tyrosine phosphatases (regulator of adhesion and migration) is linked to a cytoskeleton-associated protein (PSTPIP1). A mutation in this protein, especially missense mutations, creating A230T or E250Q variants has been reported to alter its interplay with pyrin and inflammasomes. Consequently it has been hypothesized that the mutations in the *PSTPIP1* gene lead to a hyperphosphorylation of PSTPIP1 accompanying with an increased affinity to pyrin. Thus pyrin seems to lose its inhibitory effect within a proinflammatory signalling pathway, causing an uncontrolled cleavage of pro-IL-1β into active IL-1β.[32] These proteins seems to be involved in PG and other autoinflammatory diseases and specifically in the PAPA syndrome.[33]

Clinical features

PG is characterized by ulcerative skin lesions, which usually start with a small follicular pustule that might occur on nearly all sides of the body (preferentially pretibial) and which progress rapidly to necrotic ulceration (Figure 166.2). Powell et al. classified four different subtypes, depending on clinical and pathological features:[20]

♦ **Ulcerative PG** presents initially as a small pustule with a surrounding inflammatory erythematous halo. These small pustules

enlarge within a few days into large, very painful ulcers with well-defined violaceous undermined borders and a purulent base.[20] The centre of these lesions typically begins to necrose and spread centrifugally. They can occur everywhere, although predominantly on the lower limbs or the trunk.[22] Ulcerative PG can appear also (in 25% of patients) after surgery (pathergy phenomenon)[22] as well as at peristomal sites associated with inflammatory bowel disease (IBD).[34]

♦ **Malignant PG** is a rare but very aggressive variant, which typically appears in the neck and/or head region, predominantly in male patients and possibly associated with systemic vasculitis (granulomatosis with polyangiitis (Wegener's)).[20]

♦ **Pustular PG** is characterized by multiple sterile pustules, mainly located on the extensor sites of the extremities and upper trunk, which do not enlarge into ulcerative skin lesions.[20] There is a close correlation with ulcerative colitis but also with other IBDs. Usually the skin lesions clear if the underlying condition, such as the IBD, is therapeutically controlled.

♦ **Bullous PG** is a less destructive form with painful superficial bullae, erosions, or ulcerations, often associated with leukaemia. These skin lesions appear often as groups on the dorsum of the hands, extensor surface of the arms, or the scalp, showing a tendency to converge.[35] Patients with this form of PG sometimes also show overlapping features with bullous SS. Those patients are more frequently associated with myeloproliferative disorders.[35]

♦ **Vegetative PG** is defined as a solitary, mild, superficial limited, chronic erythematous-livid plaque without a typical lilaceous border. The skin lesions are non-purulent and not undermined in comparison to the classical ulcerative PG, and are usually located at the trunk, mainly in adults and are rarely associated with systemic diseases.[20]

The combination of sterile pyogenic arthritis, PG, and acne is called PAPA syndrome, which is a rare autosomal dominant disease (mutations in the *CD2BP1/PSTPIP1* gene).[36]

Extracutaneous manifestations

Extracutaneous manifestations are commonly in the lungs (pleural effusion, lung nodules, cavitation, bronchial pneumonia, and/or abscess), joints (RA, osteoarthritis), eye (sclerokeratitis), liver

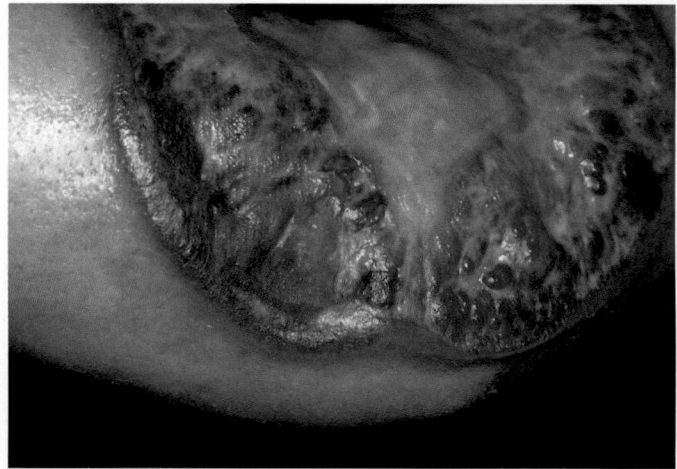

Fig. 166.2 Pyoderma gangrenosum.

(hepatitis, granulomas), and gastrointestinal tract, due to the inflammatory process.[2] Ulcerative and pustular PG forms are strongly associated with IBD. Many patients with ulcerative PG develop arthritis (up to 37%).[22] Immunosuppressed patients and patients with congenital and acquired hypogammaglobulinaemia may develop ulcerative PG lesions.[20] Patients with monoclonal gammopathy usually present ulcerative or bullous skin lesions, while in patients with malignant diseases bullous PG is most common.[20]

Histopathological features

Histopathological findings are diffuse neutrophilic infiltration involving the whole dermis, and also the follicular structures. Initially no vasculitic features are seen, in mature lesions focal vasculitic changes can be observed as a secondary phenomenon. In deeply ulcerated skin lesions a mixture of inflammatory cells and necrosis occur simultaneously.

Diagnostic procedures

A detailed medical history is essential and should include the development of skin lesion, severity of pain, progression, history of trauma or other causative factors, as well as symptoms of possible associated diseases. In addition to the physical examination of the patient, a biopsy and laboratory tests are required to exclude other diseases which may mimic PG. Depending on the type of skin lesion, other causes as well as other underlying systemic diseases should be ruled out by performing gastrointestinal tract studies, chest radiograph, and/or CT scans as well as bone marrow examinations.[35]

Management

The treatment in patients with PG is often very challenging for clinicians and patients.

Topical treatment options

Topical treatment of the wound is important for the therapeutic management of PG. Aggressive wound debridement should be avoided because of the risk of exacerbation (pathergy phenomenon).

There are different strategies to improve the PG lesions, such as the local injection of triamcinolone diacetate or the intralesional injection of ciclosporin. Topical tacrolimus 0.1%, and/or potent corticosteroids can be applied. Several studies and case reports have shown that hyperbaric oxygen,[37] topical sodium cromoglycate, topical 5-aminosalicylic acid, topical nitrogen mustard, or topical ciclosporin may improve PG lesions. In myelodysplastic syndromes the use of topical human platelet-derived growth factor (PDGF) has been reported.[20]

Systemic treatment options

Depending on the PG subtype it is necessary to use a combination of both local and systemic treatments. The drugs of choice, are oral or intravenous pulse glucocorticoids and ciclosporin.

Systemic glucocorticoids (prednisone) are usually used in a dosage of 1–2 mg/kg per day. In refractory cases it is also beneficial to use methylprednisolone in a dosage of 1 g daily for 1–5 days.

Vidal et al. showed that oral ciclosporin 5 mg/kg per day is probably the most effective treatment option, either as monotherapy or combined with systemic glucocorticoids. Other systemic steroid-sparing agents are azathioprine, methotrexate, sulfasalazine, and mycophenolate mofetil. In refractory cases cyclophosphamide may be helpful.[20] Skin grafting or skin substitution cell culture grafts in

combination with immunosuppressive treatment have been used to treat selected patients. In refractory cases, especially with an underlying IBD, infliximab can be beneficial but the risk of its use has to be balanced.[38–39]

Rheumatoid neutrophilic dermatitis

Rheumatoid neutrophilic dermatitis (RND) is a rare disease and occurs in patients with active and severe RA[40] or seronegative arthritis,[41–42] mostly in middle-aged women. Patients present slightly painful and tender, erythematous, symmetric distributed papules, nodules, or plaques, located symmetrically over the extensor surfaces of the joints, affecting predominantly the dorsal parts of the hands and/or arms[43] but also the trunk, shoulders and neck. Sometimes the skin lesions show an urticarial-like appearance but they can also ulcerate.

Histopathological examination show diffuse but dense superficial and dermal infiltrates of predominantly neutrophils with a papillary dermal oedema and occasionally focal epidermal ulcerations, again without any signs of vasculitis. The cutaneous lesions tend to resolve spontaneously without treatment or with control of the associated underlying disease,[44] but hydroxychloroquine, dapsone, cyclophosphamide and topical steroids have also been reported to be effective.[42]

Bowel-associated dermatosis–arthritis syndrome

Bowel-associated dermatosis–arthritis syndrome, also known as bowel bypass syndrome, is a complication that can occur after jejunoileal bypass surgery, biliopancreatic diversion, and Billroth II gastrectomy.[45–46] Initially it was considered to be an immune-complex disease caused by bacterial overgrowth, but it can also occur without bowel bypass, in IBDs, peptic ulceration, diverticulitis, and liver diseases.[1] When associated with surgical procedures and blind bowel loops it can appear up to 6 years after the surgical intervention.[47–48]

It may also involve the musculoskeletal system (polyarthritis, polyarthralgia, myalgia, and tenosynovitis) and the skin accompanied with elevated temperature and diarrhoea.[46] Patients usually suffer from symmetrical, non-deforming polyarthritis predominantly located at the small joints, such as the wrists, ankles, metacarpophalangeal, interphalangeal, and metatarsophalangeal joints. The skin lesions are characterized by widespread pustular eruptions on an erythematous base, evolving rapidly within hours or days. They can also resemble erythema nodosum, panniculitis, ecchymoses, and/or nodular erythematous plaques.[49]

Histopathologically it is very similar to SS. The pathogenesis is still unclear but it is thought that because of the blind loops patients develop bacterial overgrowth associated with an accumulation of peptidoglycan, a bacterial antigen, which then lead to an immune-complex disease.[50] This consideration is supported by the fact that antibiotic treatment has been used successfully.[1] Lesions may resolve after 2–4 weeks without treatment but may relapse at intervals.[1,50] A combination of antibiotics with non-steroidal anti-inflammatory drugs (NSAIDs), colchicines, dapsone, and systemic corticosteroids, especially in patients with systemic symptoms, is effective. In cases with only cutaneous lesions, it is also possible to treat with topical or intralesional steroids. However, the only

Table 166.1 Rare neutrophilic dermatoses

Neutrophilic dermatoses	Characteristics
Acute generalized exanthematous pustulosis (AGEP)[52]	AGEP is characterized by multiple, small, itchy, non-follicular, intraepidermal and/or subcorneal localized pustules, appearing with a sudden onset and based on an erythematous, oedematous, and/or exanthematous background. Usually the skin lesions are localized intertriginous or facial, but can also appear at the trunk or the upper limbs. Occasionally the development of pustules may be associated with elevated temperature, which begins at the same day (< = 1 day). It can be triggered by acute infection, mercury, and drugs. Because AGEP is a self-limiting disease, in most cases a specific treatment is not necessary
Acrodermatitis continua of Hallopeau (ACH)[51]	ACH is a variant of pustular psoriasis, localized ungula or periungual, with a chronic and recurrent appearance of erythematous and pustular lesions. It is often very painful and usually starts at the distal phalanges. Due to the relapsing of pustules it can be associated with onycholysis and onychodystrophy in later stages. It can be very therapy-resistant. Several different treatment strategies have been described in case reports, such as topical treatment with corticosteroids, calcipotriol, tacrolimus, UV therapy and systemic treatment with corticosteroids, colchicines, ciclosporin, dapsone, methotrexate, infliximab, retinoids, PUVA, etanercept, and tetracyclines
Palmoplantare pustulosis (PPP)[51]	PPP is a rare, chronic and recurrent dermatosis, characterized by multiple sterile pustules and erythematous scaly plaques, located in the stratum corneum of palms and soles. It appears predominantly in female patients, especially in those with a positive smoking history. There are still discussions whether PPP is just a variant of psoriasis. Topical anti-inflammatory drugs provide limited help while ciclosporin, PUVA, methotrexate and biologicals have been reported to be helpful, but placebo-controlled studies are required
Pustular bacterid (Andrew's disease; PB)	PB is characterized by pustules located at the hands and/or feet with small petechiae in between the pustules. Again there are discussions whether this condition is just a variant of PPP. It has been reported that PB is triggered by upper respiratory tract infections and that it is associated with sternoclavicular hyperostosis or Tietze's syndrome. It has been suggested to classify patients as having PB, when they develop isolated sterile pustules with an erythematous rim, without family history for psoriasis and without further psoriatic lesions and coincidence with an infection as well as good response to antibiotics
Neutrophilic eccrine hidradenitis[51]	The clinical presentation varies a lot between patients with infiltrated papules or plaques, varying in colour from erythematous and hyperpigmented. Furthermore the symptoms can also vary between completely asymptomatic and very pruritic. Pustules can be localized in the papules/plaques or can occur independently on normal skin. The lesions can be isolated but also grouped or diffuse extended. It has been reported to be associated with haematological malignancies, especially acute myelogenous leukaemia (AML) after receiving chemotherapy
Behçet's disease[2]	Patients present with recurrent oral and/or genital ulcerations as well as with ophthalmological manifestations such as uveitis, choroititis, and retinitis. In addition, articular manifestations in form of seronegative arthritis, usually monoarticular, are seen as well as vascular and cardiopulmonary involvement (deep or superficial thrombophlebitis, pericarditis, cardiomyopathy, pleural effusion, embolism, fibrosis), gastrointestinal involvement in form of ulcerative lesions, rarely renal and neurological/psychiatric manifestations. Depending on the clinical symptoms, patients with oral lesions are treated locally with anti-inflammatory, anaesthetic and anti-septic drugs. In case of extensive disease the combination with systemic drugs is necessary.
Subcorneal pustular dermatosis (SCPD)[51]	SCPD is defined as a rare, chronic skin condition, occurring with symmetrical, fragile pustular eruption, localized at the trunk, intertriginous and at flexor aspects of the limbs or palmoplantar, sparing face and mucous regions. It is predominantly a disease of women aged 40–50 years and may be associated with IgA and IgG monoclonal gammopathy as well as myeloproliferative disorders, such as multiple myeloma. The pustules are initially very small, arise on normal skin are flaccid and rupture very easily. They pustules contain a purulent and clear portion of ichor. After rupturing they leave superficial scaling causing annular, circinate lesions, superficial desquamation, crusts, and occasionally also faint hyperpigmentation. Topical treatment with corticosteroids is regularly used but sometimes not sufficient. Topical application can be combined with systemic therapies such as with dapsone (drug of first choice), acitretin, phototherapy (UVA and UVB), as well as biologicals

curative intervention is still the surgical correction of the blind bowel loop.[1]

Other neutrophilic dermatoses

There are several other ND, which are either very rare or restricted to the skin. They are not discussed in detail in this chapter but are mentioned in Box 166.1 and Table 166.1.

Conclusion

The ND are a group of diseases accompanied by typical histopathological features, such as diffuse epidermal and/or dermal inflammatory, neutrophilic infiltrations, without any signs of vasculitis. Depending on the form of disease and the localization of neutrophilic cells in the skin, patients usually present with a variety of skin lesions, ranging from papules, nodules, and plaques to pustules and ulcerations. It is also very common for them to develop further systemic clinical features with leucocytosis, arthralgia, and myalgia.

The pathogenesis is still not completely known, but ND can be caused and induced by underlying systemic inflammatory diseases, malignancies, pregnancy, and/or medications.

References

1. Saavedra AP, Kovacs SC, Moschella SL. Neutrophilic dermatoses. *Clin Dermatol* 2006;24(6):470–481.
2. Bonamigo RR, Razera F, Olm GS. Neutrophilic dermatoses: part I. *An Bras Dermatol* 2011;86(1):11–25; quiz 6–7.
3. Cohen PR. Sweet's syndrome—a comprehensive review of an acute febrile neutrophilic dermatosis. *Orphanet J Rare Dis* 2007;2:34.
4. Cohen PR, Kurzrock R. Sweet's syndrome revisited: a review of disease concepts. *Int J Dermatol* 2003;42(10):761–778.
5. von den Driesch P. Sweet's syndrome (acute febrile neutrophilic dermatosis). *J Am Acad Dermatol* 1994;31(4):535–556; quiz 57–60.
6. Giasuddin AS, El-Orfi AH, Ziu MM, El-Barnawi NY. Sweet's syndrome: is the pathogenesis mediated by helper T cell type 1 cytokines? *J Am Acad Dermatol* 1998;39(6):940–943.
7. Going JJ. Is the pathogenesis of Sweet's syndrome mediated by interleukin-1? *Br J Dermatol* 1987;116(2):282–283.
8. Meng G, Zhang F, Fuss I, Kitani A, Strober W. A mutation in the Nlrp3 gene causing inflammasome hyperactivation potentiates Th17 cell-dominant immune responses. *Immunity* 2009;30(6):860–874.
9. Costantini C, Micheletti A, Calzetti F, Perbellini O, Tamassia N, Albanesi C, et al. On the potential involvement of CD11d in co-stimulating the production of interferon-γ by natural killer cells upon interaction with neutrophils via intercellular adhesion molecule-3. *Haematologica* 2011;96(10):1543–1547.
10. Nesterovitch AB, Gyorfy Z, Hoffman MD et al. Alteration in the gene encoding protein tyrosine phosphatase nonreceptor type 6 (PTPN6/SHP1) may contribute to neutrophilic dermatoses. *Am J Pathol* 2011;178(4):1434–1441.
11. Larsen HK, Danielsen AG, Krustrup D, Weismann K. Neutrophil dermatosis of the dorsal hands. *J Eur Acad Dermatol Venereol* 2005;19(5):634–637.
12. Fett DL, Gibson LE, Su WP. Sweet's syndrome: systemic signs and symptoms and associated disorders. *Mayo Clin Proc* 1995;70(3):234–240.
13. Cohen PR, Kurzrock R. Sweet's syndrome: a neutrophilic dermatosis classically associated with acute onset and fever. *Clin Dermatol* 2000;18(3):265–282.
14. Neoh CY, Tan AW, Ng SK. Sweet's syndrome: a spectrum of unusual clinical presentations and associations. *Br J Dermatol* 2007;156(3):480–485.
15. Cohen PR. Subcutaneous Sweet's syndrome: a variant of acute febrile neutrophilic dermatosis that is included in the histopathologic differential diagnosis of neutrophilic panniculitis. *J Am Acad Dermatol* 2005;52(5):927–928.
16. Smith RA, Cokkinides V, Eyre HJ. Cancer screening in the United States, 2007: a review of current guidelines, practices, and prospects. *CA Cancer J Clin* 2007;57(2):90–104.
17. Vanbiervliet G, Anty R, Schneider S et al. [Sweet's syndrome and erythema nodosum associated with Crohn's disease treated by infliximab]. *Gastroenterol Clin Biol* 2002;26(3):295–297.
18. Yamauchi PS, Turner L, Lowe NJ, Gindi V, Jackson JM. Treatment of recurrent Sweet's syndrome with coexisting rheumatoid arthritis with the tumor necrosis factor antagonist etanercept. *J Am Acad Dermatol* 2006;54(3 Suppl 2):S122–S126.
19. Kluger N, Gil-Bistes D, Guillot B, Bessis D. Efficacy of anti-interleukin-1 receptor antagonist anakinra (Kineret(R)) in a case of refractory Sweet's syndrome. *Dermatology* 2011;222(2):123–127.
20. Powell FC, Su WP, Perry HO. Pyoderma gangrenosum: classification and management. *J Am Acad Dermatol* 1996;34(3):395–409; quiz 10–2.
21. Crowson AN, Mihm MC Jr, Magro C. Pyoderma gangrenosum: a review. *J Cutan Pathol* 2003;30(2):97–107.
22. Powell FC, Schroeter AL, Su WP, Perry HO. Pyoderma gangrenosum: a review of 86 patients. *Q J Med* 1985;55(217):173–186.
23. Binus AM, Qureshi AA, Li VW, Winterfield LS. Pyoderma gangrenosum: a retrospective review of patient characteristics, comorbidities, and therapy in 103 patients. *Br J Dermatol* 2011;165(6):1244–1250.
24. Adachi Y, Kindzelskii AL, Cookingham G et al. Aberrant neutrophil trafficking and metabolic oscillations in severe pyoderma gangrenosum. *J Invest Dermatol* 1998;111(2):259–268.
25. Oka M. Pyoderma gangrenosum and interleukin 8. *Br J Dermatol* 2007;157(6):1279–1281.
26. Oka M, Berking C, Nesbit M et al. Interleukin-8 overexpression is present in pyoderma gangrenosum ulcers and leads to ulcer formation in human skin xenografts. *Lab Invest* 2000;80(4):595–604.
27. Brooklyn TN, Williams AM, Dunnill MG, Probert CS. T-cell receptor repertoire in pyoderma gangrenosum: evidence for clonal expansions and trafficking. *Br J Dermatol* 2007;157(5):960–966.
28. Bister V, Makitalo L, Jeskanen L, Saarialho-Kere U. Expression of MMP-9, MMP-10 and TNF-alpha and lack of epithelial MMP-1 and MMP-26 characterize pyoderma gangrenosum. *J Cutan Pathol* 2007;34(12):889–898.
29. Marzano AV, Cugno M, Trevisan V et al. Role of inflammatory cells, cytokines and matrix metalloproteinases in neutrophil-mediated skin diseases. *Clin Exp Immunol* 2010;162(1):100–107.
30. Kawakami T, Yamazaki M, Soma Y. Reduction of interleukin-6, interleukin-8, and anti-phosphatidylserine-prothrombin complex antibody by granulocyte and monocyte adsorption apheresis in a patient with pyoderma gangrenosum and ulcerative colitis. *Am J Gastroenterol* 2009;104(9):2363–2364.
31. Guenova E, Teske A, Fehrenbacher B, et al. Interleukin 23 expression in pyoderma gangrenosum and targeted therapy with ustekinumab. *Arch Dermatol* 2011;147(10):1203–1205.
32. Smith EJ, Allantaz F, Bennett L et al. Clinical, molecular, and genetic characteristics of PAPA syndrome: a review. *Curr Genomics* 2010;11(7):519–527.
33. Wollina U, Haroske G. Pyoderma gangraenosum. *Curr Opin Rheumatol* 2011;23(1):50–56.
34. Cairns BA, Herbst CA, Sartor BR, Briggaman RA, Koruda MJ. Peristomal pyoderma gangrenosum and inflammatory bowel disease. *Arch Surg* 1994;129(7):769–772.
35. Conrad C, Trueb RM. Pyoderma gangrenosum. *J Dtsch Dermatol Ges* 2005;3(5):334–342.
36. Hong JB, Su YN, Chiu HC. Pyogenic arthritis, pyoderma gangrenosum, and acne syndrome (PAPA syndrome): report of a sporadic case without an identifiable mutation in the CD2BP1 gene. *J Am Acad Dermatol* 2009;61(3):533–535.

37. Mazokopakis EE, Kofteridis DP, Pateromihelaki AT, Vytiniotis SD, Karastergiou PG. Improvement of ulcerative pyoderma gangrenosum with hyperbaric oxygen therapy. *Dermatol Ther* 2011;24(1):134–136.

38. Tan MH, Gordon M, Lebwohl O, George J, Lebwohl MG. Improvement of pyoderma gangrenosum and psoriasis associated with Crohn disease with anti-tumor necrosis factor alpha monoclonal antibody. *Arch Dermatol* 2001;137(7):930–933.

39. Regueiro M, Valentine J, Plevy S, Fleisher MR, Lichtenstein GR. Infliximab for treatment of pyoderma gangrenosum associated with inflammatory bowel disease. *Am J Gastroenterol* 2003;98(8):1821–1826.

40. Sanchez JL, Cruz A. Rheumatoid neutrophilic dermatitis. *J Am Acad Dermatol* 1990;22(5 Pt 2):922–925.

41. Brown TS, Fearneyhough PK, Burruss JB, Callen JP. Rheumatoid neutrophilic dermatitis in a woman with seronegative rheumatoid arthritis. *J Am Acad Dermatol* 2001;45(4):596–600.

42. Lazarov A, Mor A, Cordoba M, Mekori YA. Rheumatoid neutrophilic dermatitis: an initial dermatological manifestation of seronegative rheumatoid arthritis. *J Eur Acad Dermatol Venereol* 2002;16(1):74–76.

43. Panopalis P, Stone M, Brassard A, Fitzcharles MA. Rheumatoid neutrophilic dermatitis: rare cutaneous manifestation of rheumatoid arthritis in a patient with palindromic rheumatism. *J Rheumatol* 2004;31(8):1666–1668.

44. Edgerton CC, Oglesby RJ, Bray D. Rheumatoid neutrophilic dermatitis. *J Clin Rheumatol.* 2006;12(5):266–267.

45. Slater GH, Kerlin P, Georghiou PR, Fielding GA. Bowel-associated dermatosis-arthritis syndrome after biliopancreatic diversion. *Obes Surg* 2004;14(1):133–135.

46. Tu J, Chan JJ, Yu LL. Bowel bypass syndrome/bowel-associated dermatosis arthritis syndrome post laparoscopic gastric bypass surgery. *Australas J Dermatol* 2011;52(1):e5–e7.

47. Kennedy C. The spectrum of inflammatory skin disease following jejuno-ileal bypass for morbid obesity. *Br J Dermatol* 1981;105(4):425–435.

48. Williams HJ, Samuelson CO, Zone JJ. Nodular nonsuppurative panniculitis associated with jejunoileal bypass surgery. *Arch Dermatol* 1979;115(9):1091–1093.

49. Delaney TA, Clay CD, Randell PL. The bowel-associated dermatosis–arthritis syndrome. *Australas J Dermatol* 1989;30(1):23–27.

50. Jorizzo JL, Apisarnthanarax P, Subrt P et al. Bowel-bypass syndrome without bowel bypass. Bowel-associated dermatosis-arthritis syndrome. *Arch Intern Med* 1983;143(3):457–461.

CHAPTER 167

Sarcoidosis

Joachim Müller-Quernheim,
Gernot Zissel, and Antje Prasse

Introduction

A number of the characteristics of the disease known as sarcoidosis—such as erythema nodosum, dermatological manifestations, giant cells, epitheloid cells, and granulomata—were first described in the 18th and 19th centuries. Today sarcoidosis is regarded as a systemic disorder which can affect virtually any organ of the body. This is based on the work of Jörgen Schaumann, a Swedish dermatologist, who recognized that Besnier's lupus pernio and Boeck's multiple sarcoids are manifestations of the same disease and suggested the term 'lymphogranulomatosis benigna' for the disease since it seemed to involve predominantly the lymphatic system. In 1915 the disease was recognized as a systemic disease with predominantly intrathoracic manifestations.[1]

Epidemiology

By definition sarcoidosis is a rare disorder with a prevalence of less than 50 per 100 000 population in most countries. In Sweden, Norway, and Denmark the prevalence is marginally above this level. Sarcoidosis can be found in any country and there is an evident north–south gradient in the northern hemisphere and a south–north gradient in the southern hemisphere. Close to the equator its prevalence is much higher in populations living at high altitudes in a climate with subpolar conditions than in populations living at sea level. African Americans suffer from more severe courses than white Americans and have a higher prevalence. Most interestingly, sarcoidosis is extremely rare in Japan but myocardial manifestations are more frequent in Japan than in Western countries.

Disease definition

Sarcoidosis is a systemic disorder, which is diagnosed by demonstrating non-necrotizing granulomata accompanied by a compatible pattern of symptoms and the exclusion of other granulomatous disorders of non-infectious or infectious origin. A wide spectrum of manifestations can be observed in any organ and at any age. About 50% of the cases are diagnosed at an age of 20–40 years. However, a second peak of primary manifestation for women is observed around the age of 60. This results in a slight preponderance of the female gender.[2]

On the basis of its wide clinical spectrum it can be assumed that sarcoidosis is a final pathological pathway of several aetiologies. Its cause or causes are elusive, but some pathophysiological contributions of infectious agents such as commensals may be assumed. In aggregate, it may be viewed as a hyper-reactivity elicited by one or several aetiological agents encountered by an individual with a genetic susceptibility.[3]

Aetiopathogenesis

Genetics

The influence of the individual genetic background, and in particular the MHC genes, on sarcoidosis manifestation and specific phenotypes has been known for many years and some distinct phenotypes such as acute and chronic disease have recently been attributed to a limited number of MHC alleles. Acute sarcoidosis and Löfgren's syndrome is associated with *DRB1*01* and *DRB1*03* and chronic disease with *DRB*07*, *DRB*14*, and *DRB*15*.[4]

Furthermore, by the use of genome-wide association studies a number of biallelic genes have been discovered of which the minor alleles contribute to the genetic susceptibility of sarcoidosis. Some of these susceptibility genes have already been reproduced in independent cohorts. In the butyrophylin-like-2 (*BTNL2*) gene on chromosome 6, a member of the B7 family of costimulatory molecules, a truncated variant encoded by the *A* allele is observed in about 30% of white populations. This truncation leads to the loss of the membrane anchor of the molecule which is necessary for its inhibitory function in inflammatory mechanisms. The *A* allele confers an increased sarcoidosis risk with an odds ratio of 1.7. Its presence in a haplotype with a *HLA-DR* risk allele increases the odds ratio from 1.3 due to *HLA-DR* to 2.3 resulting from this combination. More gene variants have been associated with an increased sarcoidosis risk, e.g. annexin A11, some tumour necrosis factor (TNF)-promoter polymorphisms, *RAB23*, *CCR2*, *CCR5*, *IL23R*, *CARD15*, and many others. Of note, many of the named genes need to be confirmed as a susceptibility factor in independent cohorts and their roles in inflammatory processes of sarcoidosis are still elusive. Nevertheless, they might serve as therapeutic targets in the near future.[5]

Histology

The human organism generates granulomata whenever an antigen cannot be degraded and completely eliminated by its macrophages. In these cases multinucleated giant cells and epithelioid cells emerge which are the building blocks of non-necrotizing granulomata characterizing sarcoidosis.[6]

Non-necrotizing granulomata, the histological hallmark of sarcoidosis, are found in any involved organ but they are not pathognomonic. Most interestingly, necrotizing granulomata can also be observed in sarcoidosis, which broadens the spectrum of differential diagnosis. Hypersensitivity pneumonitis, mycobacterial disorders, and chronic beryllium disease have to be considered. In general, granulomata caused by *Mycobacterium tuberculosis*, granulomatosus with polyangiitis (Wegener's), or silicosis can easily be distinguished by histological examination. In lymph nodes, however, cat scratch disease and brucellosis have to be considered as differential diagnoses in the presence of non-necrotizing granulomata. Sarcoid-like lesions can also be observed in lymph nodes draining areas harbouring neoplastic disorders and in lymph nodes involved in a reconstitution syndrome of AIDS or common variable immunodeficiency (CVID).[7,8]

Immunopathogenesis

Next to non-necrotizing granuloma, activated T cells and macrophages can be found in affected tissues. These inflammatory processes are compartmentalized, i.e. they are most obvious in the organ involved but cannot be found in the blood, or only to a limited extent. Sarcoid alveolar macrophages exhibit characteristics known from dendritic cells. Thus, in contrast to normal alveolar macrophages they are capable of presenting antigen and of stimulating T cells. Moreover, they secrete cytokines which are involved in the Th1 immune response and are chemotactic for Th1 lymphocytes, such as interleukin (IL)-1, IL-6, IL-12, CC-chemokine ligand (CCL)-10, and TNF.

In aggregate, the recent literature suggests the following immunopathogenetic concept: in acute and chronic sarcoidosis resident T cells and macrophages, of the lung in most cases, become activated by an antigen which is presented by alveolar macrophages. Accessory molecule interactions cause a strong stimulation in acute sarcoidosis (Figure 167.1) and a weak to moderate stimulation in chronic sarcoidosis due to missing accessory signals (Figure 167.1). In both cases additional stimulating signals are delivered by the recognition of pathogen-associated molecular patterns (PAMPs) or damage-associated molecular patterns (DAMPs) by pattern recognition receptors (PRRs). In acute disease the activated macrophages increase their expression of costimulatory molecules and release chemokines such as CXCL10, attracting additional T cells of CD4/TH1 phenotype (Figure 167.1). These T cells become activated by macrophages with exaggerated accessory function and proliferate by autocrine IL-2 production (Figure 167.1). IL-18 and IL-12 released by activated alveolar macrophages induce and maintain the differentiation of the lymphocytes into Th1 cells, which in turn release interferon-γ which upregulates the activation of alveolar macrophages. Within those aggregates TNF and granulocyte–macrophage colony stimulating factor (GM-CSF) induce the

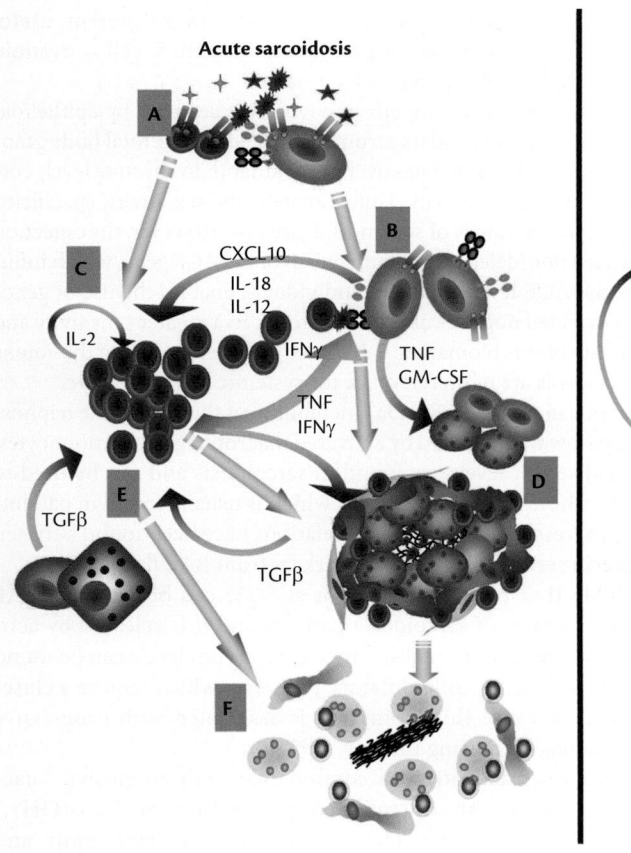

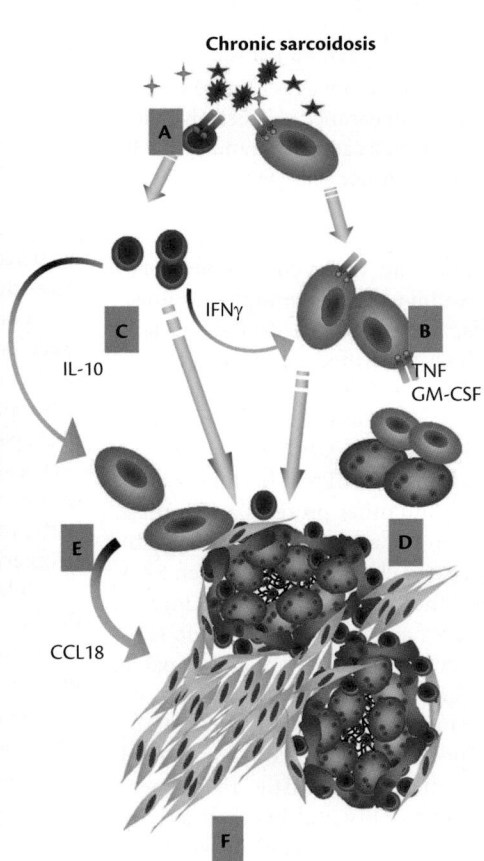

Fig. 167.1 Schematic depiction of immunopathological concepts for acute and chronic sarcoidosis: sufficient costimulatory signals and cytokine networking in acute disease allowing antigen elimination and complete resolution; low costimulation and strong cytokine networking towards scar formation in chronic disease. For further details see text.

fusion of these activated macrophages to multinucleated giant cells which build the non-necrotizing granuloma consisting of a core of multinucleated giant cells surrounded by epithelioid cells, fibroblasts, and T cells. The matrix within the granuloma or the giant cells binds and retains the granuloma-inducing agent (Figure 167.1.1D). These strong stimuli induce an extensive preponderance of TH1 lymphocytes and M1 macrophages in acute disease.

In marked contrast, in chronic disease the stimulatory processes result in low levels of TNF and other mediators. Noteworthy, CXCL10, IL-12 and IL-18 are found only at background levels which indicate a minor activation of alveolar macrophages (Figure 167.1). T-cell activation is also low due to lack of costimulation by alveolar macrophages and T-cell recruitment is minimal due to missing chemotactic factors. In this micromilieu the immigrating cells undergo only weak stimulation. Consequently, compared with acute disease the number of T cells in bronchoalveolar lavage (BAL) is reduced. Th1 commitment is incomplete because of insufficient levels of IL-12 and IL-18 (Figure 167.1). Nevertheless, activation of alveolar macrophages and release of TNF induce the generation of multinuclear giant cells and subsequently granuloma formation (Figure 167.1). IL-10 and the contact of alveolar macrophages with fibroblasts induce their differentiation into M2 macrophages releasing profibrotic CCL18 (Figure 167.1). CCL18 induces activation and matrix production by fibroblasts adjacent to granuloma, leading to fibrotic remodelling of the lung. Persistence of the disease-eliciting antigen or non-degradable remnants maintain inflammation with Th2 and M2 cells, which leads to a remodelling of the lower respiratory tract or any other involved tissue (Figure 167.1).

In acute disease however, the antigen contained in the granuloma is dissolved and eliminated. Consecutively, transforming growth factor beta (TGF-β) released by macrophages, epithelial cells, or cells of the granuloma itself leads to a downregulation of T-cell activation and TNF release of alveolar macrophages (Figure 167.1). This downregulation results in the disappearance of T-cell alveolitis and abrogates granuloma integrity. In most cases the granuloma will completely resolve or may leave only a minor scar (Figure 167.1).[6]

Aetiology

A number of recent studies demonstrate that a considerable percentage of sarcoidosis patients exhibit a specific immune response against mycobacterial antigens. Mycobacterial catalase G and propionibacterial DNA have been identified in sarcoid tissue. Interestingly, propionibacteria share a number of microbiological characteristics with mycobacteria. However, it is assumed that sarcoidosis is not of infectious aetiology but is based on an exaggerated immune response against PAMPs of harmless commensals. Serum amyloid A (SAA) and other proteins accumulate in the granuloma and serve to trap the aetiological agent, establishing a nidus which may give rise to chronicity. Moreover, SAA serves as a ligand for TLR2 and other receptors of innate immunity which stimulates macrophages and T cells. Inorganic substances such as beryllium and crystalline silica are also capable of inducing granulomatous immune responses which cannot be distinguished from sarcoidosis. Since sarcoidosis is a very heterogeneous disorder it can be assumed that not only one but several aetiological agents may induce the characteristic Th1 hyperreactivity. At present genetic susceptibility and hyper-reactivity against PAMPs of harmless commensals seem to be key factors of sarcoid aetiology.[9,10]

Immunological disturbances in affected organs

The lung is easily accessible by BAL. Therefore, the immunological changes in the context of sarcoid inflammation have been studied in great depth in this organ and there is evidence that similar mechanisms take place in other organs. Great numbers of mononuclear cells and small numbers of polymorph nuclear cells immigrate to the alveolar space and typical changes in the BAL differential cell count can be used to estimate sarcoid activity. An increased CD4/CD8 ratio is observed in acute sarcoidosis, and in patients with a ratio above 3.5 spontaneous resolution is frequently observed, which suggests just follow-up in those without mandatory treatment indication to allow spontaneous resolution to take place. A slight increase of polymorphnuclear cells above the background of 3% is associated with progressing disease requiring treatment in the near future.[11]

Immunological disturbances in peripheral blood

In acute sarcoidosis in particular, numerous alterations can be observed in peripheral blood. The immigration of CD4+ T cells to the organ manifestations causes a depletion of these cells which might be accompanied by lymphocytopenia.[12] In contrast to the exaggerated Th1 response in organ manifestations peripheral blood cells are in an immunosuppressed state, which can be demonstrated by their reduced or absent response to recall antigens. This is in accordance with the observation of increased numbers of regulatory T cells and increased concentrations of anti-inflammatory cytokines such as IL-10 in peripheral blood.[6]

In a routine setting sequential tests of T-cell function such as ex-vivo cytokine release are not practicable and serum markers are desired. Several molecules shed by activated immune cells or epithelioid cells give rise to elevated serum levels which may be used to probe the corresponding immune processes. At present, useful parameters are available for granuloma burden, T-cell activation, and macrophage/monocyte activation.

Angiotensin converting enzyme (ACE) is secreted by epithelioid cells of granulomata and its serum level indicates the total body granuloma burden.[13] Its changes over time rather than absolute levels correlate with disease activity. Unfortunately, the sensitivity, specificity, and prognostic values of serum ACE are low. However, the detection of an insertion/deletion polymorphism of the *ACE* gene, which influences the ACE level of healthy individuals, enables the use of genotype-corrected normal values which result in a greater sensitivity and specificity of this biomarker.[14] Elevated ACE levels during the course of sarcoidosis are of no relevance for systemic blood pressure.

Neopterin, a small (250 Da) metabolite of the guanosine triphosphate pathway, is released by activated macrophages and monocytes. Elevated serum levels are found in sarcoidosis and can be used to monitor the activity of these cells which is usually found in patients with progressing disease. No correlations have been found between neopterin serum levels and biomarkers from BAL fluid.[11,15]

Soluble IL-2 receptor (sL-2R or sCD25) can be found in BAL fluid and serum of sarcoidosis patients and it is released by activated alveolar immune cells.[16] Increased serum levels can be found in cases with active inflammatory processes which require a closer follow-up because this biomarker is associated with progressive organ damage requiring therapy.[11,15]

Macrophage activation in combination with an elusive cofactor may induce an upregulated production of 1,25-$(OH)_2$-cholecalciferol (vitamin D_3) which causes hypercalcemia and hypercalcuria in up to 10% and 50% of patients respectively.

Clinical features

Acute and chronic disease

The wide heterogeneity of sarcoidosis manifestations poses a diagnostic challenge. In about 95% of cases symptomatic pulmonary involvement is observed and diagnostic workup leads to the diagnosis of sarcoidosis. An acute, highly symptomatic course can be discriminated from a chronic one with unspecific symptoms such as fatigue, dry cough, and dyspnoea on exertion. A frequent subphenotype of acute disease is Löfgren's syndrome, characterized by acute onset, fever, erythema nodosum, arthralgia, and bihilar lymphadenopathy. Erythema nodosum and fever usually remit spontaneously within a few weeks and corticosteroid therapy is rarely needed. It is more frequent in white people of northern European descent and only rarely observed in Asians and African Americans with sarcoidosis. In typical cases a diagnosis can be made without demonstrating non-necrotizing granuloma in an involved organ. However, follow-up is required to confirm the diagnosis by observing a spontaneous resolution. In non-Löfgren's sarcoidosis it is suggested to support the clinical diagnosis by demonstrating non-necrotizing granulomata in a biopsy of an organ with abnormalities in imaging, most frequently lung parenchyma or paratracheal lymph nodes.[2]

Chronic sarcoidosis is observed in about one-third of the patients. Its onset is usually insidious and heralded by constitutional complaints. It may even be discovered in asymptomatic individuals by routine chest radiographs. Nevertheless, it occasionally manifests itself as a medical emergency. Involvement of the eye, the heart, the central nervous system, or the development of hypercalcaemia may require immediate action. More than 90% of sarcoid patients will eventually develop pulmonary abnormalities easily recognizable on chest radiographs or tests of pulmonary function. Organ involvement differs with ethnicity. An epidemiological study of 736 patients in the United States gives data which can be used in most countries with a white population with or without African admixture (Table 167.1).[17]

The natural course of sarcoidosis is unpredictable in an individual patient: patients with advanced pulmonary infiltrates and splenomegaly may have spontaneous recovery, whereas others with asymptomatic hilar lymphadenopathy may develop severe disease. Generally, the more severe the clinical findings at the time of diagnosis and the more organ systems are involved by the disease, the more frequent adverse outcomes have been observed. Cutaneous sarcoidosis frequently indicates chronic and disseminated involvement. In an epidemiological study from Denmark with a median follow-up of 27 years an excess mortality from sarcoidosis and sarcoidosis-related diseases in patients with advanced radiological findings and impaired lung function was observed in the first 20 years. Although the mortality of the sarcoid cohort was higher than that of the general population, the difference was not statistically significant.[18]

Patients with predominantly abdominal manifestations may exhibit an acute onset and laboratory findings of systemic inflammation. Exclusively pulmonary, neurological, or dermatological manifestations are primarily observed in chronic disease.

Thoracic manifestations

The chest radiograph is rarely normal and most commonly reveals bilateral hilar lymphadenopathy and/or diffuse reticulonodular infiltrates in the pulmonary parenchyma. Usually the basal areas

Table 167.1 Percentage of sarcoidosis patients with specified organ involvement[17]

Organ involvement[a]	Percentage
Lungs	95.0
Skin (excluding erythema nodosum)	15.9
Lymph node	15.2
Eye	11.8
Liver	11.5
Erythema nodosum	8.3
Spleen	6.7
Central nervous system	4.6
Salivary gland	3.9
Calcium metabolism	3.7
Ear, nose, and throat	3.0
Heart[b]	2.3
Kidney	0.7
Bone and joints[b]	0.5
Muscle[b]	0.4

[a]In white Americans hypercalcaemia was significantly more frequent than in African Americans. In African Americans, however, there were significantly more frequently involvements of the eye, liver, bone marrow, extrathoracic lymph node, and skin involvement other than erythema nodosum.
[b]These numbers may rise with a more frequent use of MRI.

of the lung are spared. Lung function tests reveal a decrease in lung volumes (vital capacity and total lung capacity), a reduced diffusing capacity, and a mildly reduced arterial oxygen tension that may decrease further with exercise. An obstructive pattern of pulmonary function test or unspecific bronchial hyper-reactivity may appear in up to 50% of patients. Bronchial hyper-reactivity and pulmonary hypertension due to obstruction of pulmonary vessels by lymphadenopathy or granulomata in the vessel walls are also manifestations of intrathoracic sarcoidosis.[2] The radiographic changes can be categorized into four types, I–IV. Unfortunately, there is a large intra- and interobserver variation using this system. Therefore, these chest radiographic types should only be used to give a rough estimate of the intrathoracic involvement. For therapy decisions a detailed evaluation of radiographic changes in the lung parenchyma and the adenopathy over a longer course of the disease is required. Nevertheless, these radiographic types are of prognostic usefulness (Table 167.2).

Uncommon pulmonary manifestations include cavities, lymph node calcifications, pleural thickening and calcification, pleural effusions, and in very rare cases pneumothorax. In many cases of obvious and severe radiographic changes there is only modest lung function impairment. This discrepancy is typical for sarcoidosis and not seen in any other parenchymal lung disease. Dyspnoea on exertion may be caused by pulmonary hypertension in sarcoidosis patients secondary to different pathomechanisms; it is frequently seen in those requiring lung transplantation and heralds poor outcome.[19,20]

Table 167.2 Radiographic types of sarcoidosis according to Scadding[2] and their prognostic usefulness[18]

Radiographic type	Radiographic characteristics	Prognosis
0	No visible findings	–
I	Bilateral hilar lymphadenopathy	Spontaneous resolution in most cases
II	Bilateral hilar lymphadenopathy and parenchymal infiltration	Spontaneous resolution possible
III	Parenchymal infiltration without hilar adenopathy in regular chest radiograph	Spontaneous resolution in rare cases
IV	Advanced fibrosis with evidence of honeycombing bronchiectasis, hilar retraction, bulla, and cysts	Permanent organ damage

Table 167.3 Differential diagnoses of intrathoracic sarcoidosis

Radiographic type	Differential diagnoses
I	Tuberculous lymphadenitis
	Malignancies (Hodgkin's disease, non-Hodgkin lymphoma, bronchial carcinoma)
	Salmonellosis
	Histoplasmosis
II and III	Miliary tuberculosis
	Hypersensitivity pneumonitis
	Pulmonary metastasis
	Chronic beryllium disease
	Lymphangiosis carcinomatosa
	Hodgkin's disease
	Pulmonary Langerhans cell histiocytosis
	Bronchoalveolar carcinoma
IV	Post tuberculosis syndrome
	Pneumoconiosis
	Pulmonary fibrosis (idiopathic, drug hypersensitivity, associated with extrapulmonary or systemic disorders)
	Hypersensitivity pneumonitis

Differential diagnosis of intrathoracic sarcoidosis differs with radiographic type (Table 167.3).

In general pulmonary manifestations are no indication of immediate therapy, but a follow-up is indicated to establish a progressive course requiring therapy. This clinical approach avoids unnecessary therapy of stable or regressing disease. In rare cases fulminant pulmonary symptoms accompanied by advanced function defects may require immediate initiation of therapy.

Unfortunately, clinically relevant inflammatory activity leading to organ malfunction or permanent damage may not be indicated by serum biomarkers. This activity can only be identified by a follow-up using functional tests. ^{18}F-FDG-PET-CT has recently

been introduced for the staging of sarcoid inflammatory activity. Hypermetabolism detected by this method correlates negatively with improvements in symptoms, lung function, or the above-mentioned serum markers in patients undergoing therapy, which generates interest in scanning for lung, heart or central nervous system (CNS) disease (Figure 167.2).[21,22]

Musculoskeletal manifestations

Many sarcoid patients report aching muscles, bones, and joints which are often accompanied by fatigue. However, sarcoid lesions can be clearly detected only in a minority of these patients. The exact percentage of patients with sarcoid musculoskeletal manifestations is unknown. In the past, clinicians did not search vigorously for musculoskeletal involvement because there was little clinical relevance. However, recent progress in PET and MRI techniques enables sensitive and non-invasive detection of sarcoid lesions in the musculoskeletal system.[23] Recent studies using these new techniques suggest a much higher frequency of sarcoid bone and muscle manifestations than previously thought.[23,24] Although acute sarcoid arthritis is often symptomatic, one-half of all patients with bone and muscle involvement are asymptomatic.

Blau's syndrome

Blau's syndrome, a monogenic disorder with systemic granulomatous manifestations, has to be distinguished from sarcoidosis. A mutation in the *NOD2* gene causes polyarticular lesions in about 95% of patients with a juvenile onset. In addition, cutaneous manifestations, eye disease, and phenotypes similar to Löfgren's syndrome, including erythema nodosum, were observed.[25]

Arthritis

Up to 70% of sarcoid patients report arthralgia.[26,27] There is an acute and a chronic arthritis form, of which the acute variant is far more common. Most often acute arthritis occurs within Löfgren's syndrome. Löfgren's syndrome includes acute arthritis of the ankles and sometimes also of the knees. In almost every patient with acute arthritis accompanying Löfgren's syndrome these manifestations

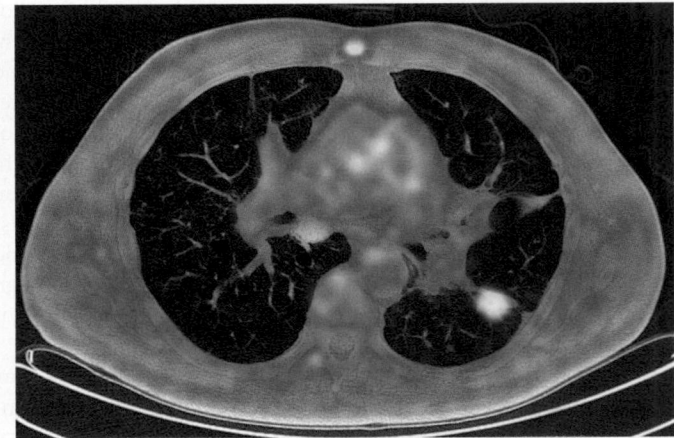

Fig. 167.2 In a patient with negative serum biomarkers but progressive pulmonary function defects ^{18}F-FDG-PET-CT fusion image shows hypermetabolism with increased standardized uptake value (SUV) which captures large areas of lung parenchyma (mottled yellow areas in the lung parenchyma, arrowheads). In the left lower lobe an intense uptake can be seen in a fibrotic area which did not change its configuration over an observation period of 24 months (arrow). In addition, an asymptomatic manifestation in the sternum is identified.

spontaneously resolve. Symptomatic treatment of acute arthritis with non-steroidal anti-inflammatory drugs (NSAIDs) is recommended. The chronic type of sarcoid arthritis is rare. Chronic granulomatous tendosynovitis, Jaccoud's type deformity, and dactylitis (sausage-like swelling of one or more digits) have been reported. Treatment options for chronic arthritis are prednisone, colchicine, hydrochloroquine, and infliximab.[27]

Bones

Osseous lesions are less common than arthritis.[26,27] Rough estimates assumed symptomatic osseous manifestations in less than 3% of all patients. However, modern techniques such as PET and MRI report a much higher incidence of asymptomatic lesions, which are detectable in approximately 13% of all patients, and severe courses are reported.[28] Osseous disease affects the proximal and middle phalanges and is associated with chronic disease. Typical findings are cystic lesions (osteitis cystoides Jüngling) of the proximal and middle phalanges, which are a sign of endstage disease. A nodular (focal) type of osseous lesions is rare and often accompanied with skin lesions (Figure 167.3). Osteoporosis can occur in the context of sarcoidosis but most often is associated with long-term prednisone treatment. Because of the disturbed vitamin D metabolism in sarcoidosis and the risk of hypercalcaemia it is recommended to treat sarcoid osteopenia using bisphosphonates; vitamin D and calcium supplementations are relatively contraindicated.

Muscle

Although many sarcoid patients suffer from diffuse muscle pain, fatigue, and reduced exercise capacity, the number of patients with detectable sarcoid muscle lesions is low (up to 13% in selected cohorts). Symptomatic muscle involvement in sarcoidosis can result in proximal muscle weakness, double vision, nystagmus (extraocular muscles), and dyspnoea due to diaphragm weakness. Muscle enzymes such as creatine kinase can be elevated.[29–31] A very important differential diagnosis is glucocorticoid-induced myopathy. Rarely, a painful nodular type of sarcoid lesion can be seen.

Hepatic manifestations

Hepatic involvement occurs in up to 50% of patients and CT imaging shows innumerable small hepatic nodules with low attenuation.

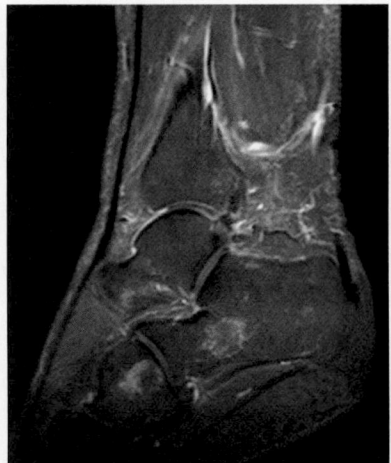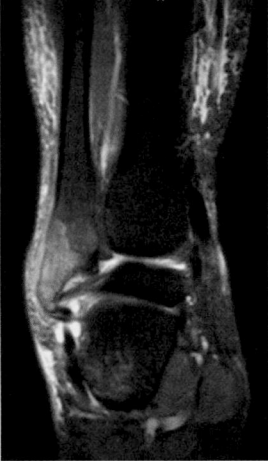

Fig. 167.3 MRI of sarcoid lesion of the right foot: hyperintense lesions in T2-weighted imaging.

The majority of hepatic manifestations are non-symptomatic. Patients presenting with symptoms complain about abdominal pain and pruritus. Abnormal liver function tests mandating therapy are rarely observed. Elevated alkaline phosphates and transaminases are frequently observed but elevated bilirubin levels occur only in cases progressing to cirrhosis. Differential diagnosis of sarcoid liver disease encompasses primary biliary cirrhosis, drug hypersensitivities, malignancies, and infectious disorders.

Myocardial manifestations

Cardiac sarcoidosis is a rare event which might be underdiagnosed because of the practical difficulties in demonstrating sarcoid inflammation within the myocardium. This might be overcome by the more frequent use of MRI and ^{18}F-FDG-PET-CT.[22,32] Myocardial involvement may cause sudden arrhythmias, brady-arrhythmias, heart failure, or even sudden death.

Neurosarcoidosis

The predilection sites of neurosarcoidosis are the base of the brain, resulting in cranial nerve palsy and neuroendocrine abnormalities with diabetes insipidus as the most frequent. Acute or chronic meningitis and peripheral neuropathy, including small-fibre neuropathy, are also observed and associate predominantly with a chronic course. Obstructive sleep apnoea syndrome (OSAS) is seen in patients with sarcoidosis not exhibiting the stigmata of metabolic syndrome and has to be distinguished from chronic fatigue which may result in sleepiness scores as high as in OSAS.[33]

Ophthalmologic manifestations

Ocular sarcoidosis can affect any part of the eye and manifestations range from asymptomatic to permanent vision loss. Anterior uveitis is the most common sarcoidosis lesion.

Dermatological manifestations

Specific sarcoid lesions exhibiting non-necrotizing granulomata include livid maculae, papules, nodules, infiltrated scars, and lupus pernio. They are mostly flesh coloured and asymptomatic. Lupus pernio may be disfiguring and requires corticosteroid therapy. Changes of papules and erythema in tattoos correlate well with systemic inflammatory activity of disease. Erythema nodosum and other lesions without granulomata are considered nonspecific lesions, with erythema nodosum being the most frequent.[34,35]

Therapy

Glucocorticoids are the mainstay of sarcoidosis therapy; however, studies on the long-term benefit, for prevention of pulmonary fibrosis, neurological defects, or increase survival, are inconclusive. United Kingdom guidelines on interstitial lung diseases, including sarcoidosis, were published in 2008 and describe an internationally accepted therapeutic approach.[36] A general rule is that therapy should be initiated when any organ function is threatened. Since sarcoidosis is not disabling in most patients treatment may be delayed in favour of careful monitoring to allow spontaneous resolution to take place, which is the case in about two-thirds of patients. In cases of highly symptomatic acute disease without mandatory indications for corticosteroid therapy, NSAIDs relieve symptoms and allow avoidance of corticosteroids.

Oral glucocorticoids are the first line in patients with progressive organ defects; inhaled corticosteroids cannot be used as a substitute or for sparing the systemic dose.[37] Treatment is initiated with 0.5-to 0.75 mg prednisolone/kg body weight per day for 4 weeks and tapered by 10 mg per 4 weeks depending on disease response. The above-mentioned biomarkers and pulmonary function tests can be used for monitoring. In most cases therapy can be terminated after 6 months when patients are asymptomatic and pulmonary function has improved, but refractory disease may need up to 24 months.[37] Whether a low-dose maintenance therapy for 6–12 months is of any benefit remains controversial. When glucocorticoids do not control the disease, intolerable side effects develop, or immediate relapse occurs, immunosuppressants can be used as corticosteroid-sparing additives. Azathioprine[38] and methotrexate[39] are generally accepted for this use. Mycophenolate mofetil and cyclophosphamide are alternatives but ciclosporin is of no benefit.[40] Lung transplantation should be considered in endstage disease and in particular in those with pulmonary hypertension.[41]

TNF has been identified as a pivotal mediator in refractory sarcoidosis,[6,42] which has led to clinical studies using a wide range of TNF inhibitors in monotherapy or as corticosparing agents. In this respect thalidomide and pentoxifylline have some potential.[43–45] Most interestingly, etanercept has no benefit in sarcoidosis[46] but even induces or exaggerates sarcoidosis, which may respond to monoclonal antibodies against TNF.[47] There are many case series demonstrating the usefulness of anti-TNF antibodies in sarcoidosis with much better benefit in extrathoracic than thoracic disease. A placebo-controlled trial with infliximab unequivocally showed a significant but small effect on restrictive lung function defect,[48] and a longer treatment period seems necessary.[49] The anti-inflammatory effects of infliximab correlated well with improvement in lung function and biomarkers including ^{18}F-FDG-PET-CT.[21]

Conclusion

Sarcoidosis is a systemic granulomatous disorder with predominant intrathoracic manifestations. However, in about 1% of patients musculoskeletal manifestations are observed and there is evidence that this number is a gross underestimation. There is a consensus that only symptomatic patients with organ malfunction due to disease activity receive prednisolone or immunosuppressive therapy, which is guided by biomarkers.

References

1. Zissel G, Müller-Quernheim J. Sarcoidosis, part I: Historical perspective and immunopathogenesis. *Respir Med* 1998;92:126–139.
2. Statement on sarcoidosis. Joint Statement of the American Thoracic Society (ATS), the European Respiratory Society (ERS) and the World Association of Sarcoidosis and Other Granulomatous Disorders (WASOG) adopted by the ATS Board of Directors and by the ERS Executive Committee, February 1999. *Am J Respir Crit Care Med* 1999;160(2):736–755.
3. Müller-Quernheim J. Sarcoidosis: immunopathogenetic concepts and their clinical application. *Eur Respir J* 1998;12(3):716–738.
4. Grunewald J. Review: role of genetics in susceptibility and outcome of sarcoidosis. *Semin Respir Crit Care Med* 2010;31(4):380–389.
5. Müller-Quernheim J, Schürmann M, Hofmann S, Gaede KI, Fischer A, Prasse A, Zissel G, Schreiber S. Genetics of sarcoidosis. *Clin Chest Med* 2008 Sep;29(3):391–414, viii.
6. Zissel G, Prasse A, Muller-Quernheim J. Immunologic response of sarcoidosis. *Semin Respir Crit Care Med* 2010;31(4):390–403.
7. El-Zammar OA, Katzenstein AL. Pathological diagnosis of granulomatous lung disease: a review. *Histopathology* 2007;50(3):289–310.
8. Rosen Y. Pathology of sarcoidosis. *Semin Respir Crit Care Med* 2007;28(1):36–52.
9. Chen ES, Moller DR. Sarcoidosis—scientific progress and clinical challenges. *Nat Rev Rheumatol* 2011;7(8):457–467.
10. Chen ES, Song Z, Willett MH et al. Serum amyloid A regulates granulomatous inflammation in sarcoidosis through Toll-like receptor-2. *Am J Respir Crit Care Med* 2010;181(4):360–373.
11. Ziegenhagen MW, Rothe ME, Schlaak M, Muller-Quernheim J. Bronchoalveolar and serological parameters reflecting the severity of sarcoidosis. *Eur Respir J* 2003;21(3):407–413.
12. Sweiss NJ, Salloum R, Gandhi S et al. Significant CD4, CD8, and CD19 lymphopenia in peripheral blood of sarcoidosis patients correlates with severe disease manifestations. *PLoS One* 2010;5(2):e9088.
13. Gilbert S, Steinbrech DS, Landas SK, Hunninghake GW. Amounts of angiotensin-converting enzyme mRNA reflect the burden of granulomas in granulomatous lung disease. *Am Rev Respir Dis* 1993;148:483–486.
14. Biller H, Zissel G, Ruprecht B et al. Genotype-corrected reference values for serum angiotensin-converting enzyme. *Eur Respir J* 2006;28(6):1085–1090.
15. Prasse A, Katic C, Germann M et al. Phenotyping sarcoidosis from a pulmonary perspective. *Am J Respir Crit Care Med* 2008;177(3):330–336.
16. Müller-Quernheim J, Pfeifer S, Strausz J, Ferlinz R. Correlation of clinical and immunological parameters of the inflammatory activity of pulmonary sarcoidosis. *Am Rev Respir Dis* 1991;144:1322–1329.
17. Baughman RP, Teirstein AS, Judson MA et al. Clinical characteristics of patients in a case control study of sarcoidosis. *Am J Respir Crit Care Med* 2001;164(10 Pt 1):1885–1889.
18. Viskum K, Vestbo J. Vital prognosis in intrathoracic sarcoidosis with special reference to pulmonary function and radiological stage. *Eur Respir J* 1993;6:349–353.
19. Palmero V, Sulica R. Sarcoidosis-associated pulmonary hypertension: assessment and management. *Semin Respir Crit Care Med* 2010;31(4):494–500.
20. Baughman RP, Engel PJ, Taylor L, Lower EE. Survival in sarcoidosis-associated pulmonary hypertension: the importance of hemodynamic evaluation. *Chest* 2010;138(5):1078–1085.
21. Keijsers RG, Verzijlbergen JF, van Diepen DM, van den Bosch JM, Grutters JC. 18F-FDG PET in sarcoidosis: an observational study in 12 patients treated with infliximab. *Sarcoidosis Vasc Diffuse Lung Dis* 2008;25(2):143–149.
22. Ohira H, Tsujino I, Sato T et al. Early detection of cardiac sarcoid lesions with (18)F-fluoro-2-deoxyglucose positron emission tomography. *Intern Med* 2011;50(11):1207–1209.
23. Blacksin MF, Acello AN, Kowalec J, Lyons MM. Osseous sarcoidosis of the foot: detection by MR imaging. *AJR Am J Roentgenol* 1994;163(6):1444–1445.
24. Marie I, Lahaxe L, Vera P, Edet-Samson A. Follow-up of muscular sarcoidosis using fluorodeoxyglucose positron emission tomography. *Q J Med* 2010;103(12):1000–1002.
25. Rose CD, Martin TM, Wouters CH. Blau syndrome revisited. *Curr Opin Rheumatol* 2011;23(5):411–418.
26. Judson MA. Extrapulmonary sarcoidosis. *Semin Respir Crit Care Med* 2007;28(1):83–101.
27. Sweiss NJ, Patterson K, Sawaqed R et al. Rheumatologic manifestations of sarcoidosis. *Semin Respir Crit Care Med* 2010 Aug;31(4):463–473.
28. Hyldgaard C, Bendstrup E, Hilberg O, Hjorthaug K, Lovgreen M. An unusual presentation of sarcoidosis with tetraplegia and severe osteolytic bone lesions. *Eur Respir J* 2011;37(4):964–966.
29. Baydur A, Alsalek M, Louie SG, Sharma OP. Respiratory muscle strength, lung function, and dyspnea in patients with sarcoidosis. *Chest* 2001;120(1):102–108.

30. Fayad F, Liote F, Berenbaum F, Orcel P, Bardin T. Muscle involvement in sarcoidosis: a retrospective and followup studies. *J Rheumatol* 2006;33(1):98–103.

31. Kabitz HJ, Lang F, Walterspacher S et al. Impact of impaired inspiratory muscle strength on dyspnea and walking capacity in sarcoidosis. *Chest* 2006;130(5):1496–1502.

32. Smedema JP, Snoep G, van Kroonenburgh MP et al. The additional value of gadolinium-enhanced MRI to standard assessment for cardiac involvement in patients with pulmonary sarcoidosis. *Chest* 2005;128(3): 1629–1637.

33. Nunes H, Freynet O, Naggara N et al. Cardiac sarcoidosis. *Semin Respir Crit Care Med* 2010;31(4):428–441.

34. Lodha S, Sanchez M, Prystowsky S. Sarcoidosis of the skin: a review for the pulmonologist. *Chest* 2009;136(2):583–596.

35. Marchell RM, Judson MA. Cutaneous sarcoidosis. *Semin Respir Crit Care Med* 2010;31(4):442–451.

36. Bradley B, Branley HM, Egan JJ et al. Interstitial lung disease guideline: the British Thoracic Society in collaboration with the Thoracic Society of Australia and New Zealand and the Irish Thoracic Society. *Thorax* 2008;63 Suppl 5:v1–v58.

37. Paramothayan S, Jones PW. Corticosteroid therapy in pulmonary sarcoidosis: a systematic review. *JAMA* 2002;287(10):1301–1307.

38. Müller-Quernheim J, Kienast K, Held M, Pfeifer S, Costabel U. Treatment of chronic sarcoidosis with an azathioprine/prednisolone regimen. *Eur Respir J* 1999;14(5):1117–1122.

39. Baughman RP, Winget DB, Lower EE. Methotrexate is steroid sparing in acute sarcoidosis: results of a double blind, randomized trial. *Sarcoidosis Vasc Diffuse Lung Dis* 2000;17(1):60–66.

40. Wyser CP, van Schalkwyk EM, Alheit B, Bardin PG, Joubert JR. Treatment of progressive pulmonary sarcoidosis with cyclosporin A. A randomized controlled trial. *Am J Respir Crit Care Med* 1997;156(5):1371–1376.

41. Shah L. Lung transplantation in sarcoidosis. *Semin Respir Crit Care Med* 2007;28(1):134–140.

42. Ziegenhagen MW, Rothe ME, Zissel G, Muller-Quernheim J. Exaggerated TNFalpha release of alveolar macrophages in corticosteroid resistant sarcoidosis. *Sarcoidosis Vasc Diffuse Lung Dis* 2002;19(3):185–190.

43. Judson MA, Silvestri J, Hartung C, Byars T, Cox CE. The effect of thalidomide on corticosteroid-dependent pulmonary sarcoidosis. *Sarcoidosis Vasc Diffuse Lung Dis* 2006;23(1):51–57.

44. Baughman RP, Judson MA, Teirstein AS, Moller DR, Lower EE. Thalidomide for chronic sarcoidosis. *Chest* 2002;122(1):227–232.

45. Park MK, Fontana Jr, Babaali H et al. Steroid-sparing effects of pentoxifylline in pulmonary sarcoidosis. *Sarcoidosis Vasc Diffuse Lung Dis* 2009;26(2):121–131.

46. Utz JP, Limper AH, Kalra S et al. Etanercept for the treatment of stage II and III progressive pulmonary sarcoidosis. *Chest* 2003;124(1):177–185.

47. Burns AM, Green PJ, Pasternak S. Etanercept-induced cutaneous and pulmonary sarcoid-like granulomas resolving with adalimumab. *J Cutan Pathol* 2012;39(2):289–293.

48. Baughman RP, Drent M, Kavuru M et al. Infliximab therapy in patients with chronic sarcoidosis and pulmonary involvement. *Am J Respir Crit Care Med* 2006;174(7):795–802.

49. Hostettler KE, Studler U, Tamm M, Brutsche MH. Long-term treatment with infliximab in patients with sarcoidosis. *Respiration* 2012;83(3):218–224.

Sources of patient information

International list of webpages: http://boeck.home.xs4all.nl/linkeng.html#

English language: www.nhlbi.nih.gov/health/health-topics/topics/sarc/

German language: www.sarkoidose.de/ (Germany), www.sarkoidose.ch/ (Switzerland)

Dutch language: www.sarcoidose.nl/, www.kuleuven.be/sarcoidose/

CHAPTER 168

Macrophage activation syndrome

Alexei A. Grom and Athimalaipet V. Ramanan

Introduction

Macrophage activation syndrome (MAS) is a potentially fatal complication of rheumatic diseases caused by excessive activation and expansion of T lymphocytes and macrophages characterized by the development of cytopenias, extreme hyperferritinaemia, liver dysfunction, and coagulopathy resembling disseminated intravascular coagulation (DIC).[1-5] The main pathognomonic feature of MAS is usually found in bone marrow: numerous well-differentiated macrophages actively phagocytosing normal haematopoietic elements. MAS is a life-threatening condition, and the reported mortality rates still reach 20–30%.[6,7]

Although MAS is increasingly reported in various inflammatory disorders, it is seen most frequently in systemic juvenile idiopathic arthritis (SJIA) and in its adult equivalent, adult-onset Still's disease.[6,8,9] About 10–15% of patients with SJIA develop overt MAS,[7] while mild 'subclinical' MAS may be seen in as many as one-third of patients with active systemic disease.[10,11] Systemic lupus erythematosus (SLE) and Kawasaki's disease are two other conditions in which MAS appears to occur more frequently than in other rheumatic diseases. MAS can occur during a flare of the underlying rheumatic disease or initial disease presentation, thus masking the clinical features of the underlying rheumatic disease.[12,13] In approximately one-half of cases, MAS is triggered by an infection,[6,14,15] but a change in drug therapy including introduction of biologics has also been reported in the literature as potential triggers.[2,16,17]

Macrophage activation syndrome and haemophagocytic lymphohistiocytosis

Since the predominant cell population in the inflammatory lesions in MAS are tissue macrophages, or histiocytes, exhibiting haemophagocytic activity, MAS is thought to be closely related to a group of histiocytic disorders collectively known as haemophagocytic lymphohistiocytosis (HLH).[18,19] HLH patients are often categorized as having either primary or secondary HLH.[20,21]

Patients in the primary category are those with clear familial inheritance or genetic causes. The term 'familial HLH' is often used to describe these patients. Familial haemophagocytic lymphohistiocytosis (FHLH) is a constellation of rare autosomal recessive immune disorders linked to defects in various genes all affecting the perforin-dependant cytolytic pathway (see later). The clinical symptoms of FHLH usually become evident within the first months of life. These patients have a clear risk of HLH recurrence and are not likely to survive long-term without haematopoietic stem cell transplantation. Though HLH in these patients can be associated with infections, the immunological trigger is often not apparent.

Secondary HLH tends to occur in older children and is more often associated with an identifiable infectious episode, most notably Epstein–Barr virus (EBV) or cytomegalovirus (CMV) infection. The group of secondary haemophagocytic disorders also includes malignancy-associated HLH. Patients with secondary HLH typically do not have a family history or known genetic cause of HLH. The exact relationship between HLH and MAS is an area of extensive investigations, and some rheumatologists believe that MAS should be categorized as secondary HLH occurring in a setting of a rheumatic disease.

In recent years, the distinction between primary and secondary HLH has become increasingly blurred as new genetic causes are identified, some of which are associated with less severe and somewhat distinct clinical presentations.[22] Some of these patients may present later in life due to heterozygous or compound heterozygous mutations in cytolytic pathway genes that confer a partial dominant negative effect on the cytolytic function.[23]

Pathophysiology

The main pathophysiologic feature of MAS is excessive activation and expansion of cytotoxic CD8+T cells and macrophages (or histiocytes). These activated immune cells produce large amounts of proinflammatory cytokines, creating a 'cytokine storm'. In clinically similar FHLH, the uncontrolled expansion of T cells and macrophages has been linked to decreased cytolytic activity of NK cells and cytotoxic CD8+T lymphocytes.[24-27] Although familial cases of MAS in SJIA have not been reported, as in FHLH, SJIA/MAS patients have functional defects in the cytolytic pathway[14] and these abnormalities are associated with specific polymorphisms in FHLH-associated genes.[28-30] Normally, NK cells and cytotoxic T lymphocytes induce apoptosis of cells infected with intracellular microbes or cells undergoing malignant transformation. In some circumstances, NK cells and cytotoxic T lymphocytes may also be involved in induction of apoptosis of activated macrophages and T cells during the contraction stage of the immune response.[31,32] It has been proposed that in both HLH and MAS, failure to induce apoptosis due to cytolytic dysfunction leads to prolonged expansion of T cells and macrophages and escalating production of proinflammatory cytokines.[22] As a result of chronic stimulation with mainly T-cell-derived cytokines such as interferon (IFN)-γ and macrophage colony-stimulating factor (M-CSF), macrophages become haemophagocytic. In addition to secreting multiple proinflammatory cytokines including interleukin (IL)-1, tumour necrosis factor alpha (TNFα), IL-6, and IL-18 responsible for many clinical manifestations of MAS,[33–35] the activated macrophages also produce a haemostatic tissue factor that contributes to the development of coagulopathy.

Clinical features

The clinical findings in MAS may evolve rapidly. Patients become acutely ill and develop high persistent fever, mental status changes, generalized lymphadenopathy, hepatosplenomegaly, and coagulopathy resembling DIC.[1–5] Haemorrhagic skin rashes from mild petechiae to extensive ecchymotic lesions are seen early in the course of MAS. At later stages, patients may develop epistaxis, haematemesis secondary to upper gastrointestinal bleeding, and rectal bleeding. Encephalopathy is another frequently reported clinical feature of MAS. Mental status changes, seizures, and coma are the most common manifestations of central nervous system (CNS) disease. Cerebrospinal fluid (CSF) pleiocytosis with mildly elevated protein has been noted in some studies.[2,3] Significant deterioration in renal function has been noted in several series, and was associated with particularly high mortality in one report.[7] Pulmonary infiltrates have been mentioned in several reports, and haemophagocytic macrophages can be found in bronchoalveolar lavage (BAL).[3,15]

The features that should raise immediate suspicion for MAS symptoms are typically found in laboratory evaluation. Sharp fall in at least two of three blood cell lines (leucocytes, erythrocytes, or platelets) is one of the early findings. The fall in platelet count is usually first to occur. Since bone marrow aspiration in these patients typically reveals significant hypercellularity and normal megakaryocytes,[3] such cytopenias are not likely to be due to inadequate production of cells. Increased destruction of the cells by phagocytosis and consumption at the inflammatory sites are more likely explanations.

Sharp fall in erythrocyte sedimentation rate (ESR) despite persistently high C-reactive protein (CRP) is another characteristic laboratory feature. Falling ESR probably reflects decreasing serum levels of fibrinogen secondary to fibrinogen consumption and liver dysfunction. Most patients with MAS develop marked hepatomegaly. Some develop mild jaundice. Liver function tests often reveal high serum transaminases activity but only mildly elevated levels of serum bilirubin. Moderate hypoalbuminaemia has been reported as well. Serum ammonia levels are typically normal or only mildly elevated, a feature that distinguishes MAS from Reye's syndrome.

One of the most striking laboratory findings in MAS is extreme hyperferritinaemia. Presumably, it occurs in response to the need to sequestrate free iron released during eryhtrophagocytosis. In MAS, increased release of free haemoglobin associated with erythrophagocytosis would require increased production of ferritin to sequestrate excessive amount of free iron. Indeed, strikingly high levels of serum ferritin (>10 000 ng/dL) is highly suggestive of MAS. A review of ferritin levels in paediatric patients showed a cut-off value of 10 000 μg/litre to be 90% sensitive and 96% specific for the diagnosis of HLH.[36]

Additional laboratory findings in MAS include highly elevated serum levels of triglycerides. Another laboratory test that may help with the diagnosis is highly elevated serum levels of SIL2Ra, chains presumably originating from overly activated T cells.[10] This test is, however, usually performed only in specialized laboratories.

Increasingly, MAS is being recognized in lupus patients as a secondary complication.[37] As fever, cytopenias, and raised liver enzymes can be seen as part of disease activity in lupus, diagnosis of MAS is harder in lupus patients. In any lupus patient with active or inactive disease, the development of fever, cytopenia, and raised liver enzymes, MAS must be considered in the differential diagnosis. Raised levels of serum ferritin could help discriminate between active lupus and MAS complicating lupus. As infections secondary to lupus or due to medications is also likely, infectious aetiologies must be considered before the diagnosis is made. In the clinical setting of an ill child with lupus and diagnostic uncertainty, IVIG might be a useful therapeutic agent.

Diagnosis

There are no validated diagnostic criteria for MAS and early diagnosis depends on a high level of vigilance in children with SJIA, lupus, and Kawasaki's disease. Diagnosis is often difficult because of the similarities to sepsis-like syndromes. As a general rule, in a patient with active underlying rheumatological disease, persistent fevers, a fall in the ESR and platelet count (acute drop in platelet count in SJIA from high levels), particularly in a combination with increase in serum D-dimer and ferritin levels, should raise a suspicion of impeding MAS (see Table 168.1). Although the diagnosis of MAS can confirmed by the demonstration of haemophagocytosis in the bone marrow, marrow involvement can by patchy and may require serial bone marrow aspirations.[38] In some cases, additional staining of the bone marrow with anti-CD163 antibodies may be helpful. This usually reveals massive expansion of highly activated histiocytes.

In contrast to MAS, the diagnosis of HLH is usually established based on the diagnostic criteria developed by the International Histiocyte Society.[39] The criteria include either:

◆ a molecular diagnosis based on specific mutations found in *PRF1*, *MUNC13–4*, *STX11*, *STXBP2*, *Rab27a*, *SH2D1A*, or *BIRC4*, *or*

◆ a clinical diagnosis based on the clinical criteria listed in Box 168.1.

The definite clinical diagnosis of HLH requires the presence of at least five of the eight criteria listed in Box 168.1.

When applied to SJIA patients with suspected MAS The HLH diagnostic criteria are highly specific but not sufficiently sensitive (sensitivity <30%).[38] Some of the HLH markers, such as lymphadenopathy, splenomegaly, and hyperferritinaemia, are common features of active SJIA itself and, therefore do not distinguish MAS from a conventional SJIA flare. Other HLH criteria, such as cytopenias and hypofibrinogenemia, become evident only at the late stages. This is related to the fact that SJIA patients often have increased white blood cell and platelet counts as well as serum levels

Table 168.1 Comparison of clinical and laboratory features of systemic juvenile idiopathic arthritis (SJIA) and macrophage activation syndrome (MAS)

	SJIA	MAS
Fever pattern	Quotidian	Unremitting
Rash	Evanescent, maculopapular	Petechial or purpuric
Hepatosplenomegaly	+	+
Lymphadenopathy	+	+
Arthritis	+	−
Serositis	+	−
Encephalopathy	±	
WC and neutrophil count	↑↑	↓
Haemoglobin	Normal or ↓	↓
Platelets	↑↑	↓
ESR	↑↑	Normal or sudden ↓
Bilirubin	Normal	Normal or ↑
ALT/AST	Normal or ↑	↑↑
PT	Normal	↑
PTT	Normal	↑
D-dimers	↑	↑↑
Fibrinogen	↑	↓
Ferritin	Normal or ↑	↑↑
SCD25	Normal or ↑	↑↑
CD163	Normal or ↑	↑↑

ALT, alanine aminotransferase; AST, asparate aminotransferase; MAS, macrophage activation syndrome; PT, prothrombin time, PTT, partial thromboplastin time; SJIA, systemic juvenile idiopathic arthritis; WCC, white cell count.

Box 168.1 HLH-2004: revised diagnostic guidelines for HLH[39] The diagnosis of HLH can be established if one of either 1 or 2 below is fulfilled:

1. A molecular diagnosis consistent with HLH (i.e. reported mutations found in either *PRF1* or *MUNC13–4*); *or*

2. Diagnostic criteria for HLH fulfilled (i.e. at least five of the eight criteria listed below present:

   ♦ Persistent fever

   ♦ Splenomegaly

   ♦ Cytopenias (affecting ≥2 of 3 lineages in the peripheral blood):

   – Haemoglobin <90 g/litre (in infants <4 weeks: <100 g/ litre)

   – Platelets <100 × 10⁹/ litre

   – Neutrophils <1.0 × 10⁹/ litre

   ♦ Hypertriglyceraemia and/or hypofibrinogaenemia:

   – Fasting triglycerides ≥3.0 mmol/litre (i.e. ≥265 mg/dL)

   – Fibrinogen ≤1.5 g/litre

   ♦ Haemophagocytosis in bone marrow* or spleen or lymph nodes, no evidence of malignancy

   ♦ Serum ferritin ≥ 500 μg/litre (i.e. 500 ng/mL)

   ♦ Low or absent NK cell activity (according to local laboratory reference)

   ♦ Increased serum sIL2Rα (according to local laboratory reference)

If haemophagocytic activity is not proven at the time of presentation, further search for haemophagocytic activity is encouraged. If the bone marrow specimen is not conclusive, material may be obtained from other organs.

of fibrinogen as a part of the inflammatory response seen in this disease. Therefore, when they develop MAS, they reach the degree of cytopenias and hypofibrinogenaemia seen in HLH only at the late stages of the syndrome. Attempts to modify the HLH criteria to increase their sensitivity and specificity for the diagnosis of MAS in rheumatic conditions have been initiated.[40] One consideration is that the relative decrease in white blood cell count, platelets, or fibrinogen rather than the low absolute numbers required by the HLH criteria may be more useful in making an early diagnosis. Another problem is that the minimum threshold level for hyperferritinaemia required for the diagnosis of HLH (500 μg/litre) is too low. It is well known that many patients with active SJIA, even in the absence of MAS, have ferritin levels above that threshold while in the acute phase of MAS, ferritin level generally peaks above 5000 μg/litre.

An international collaborative project has been started with the main aim of developing a new set of diagnostic criteria for MAS complicating SJIA.[40] As the first step in this project, the Delphi survey technique was used to identify the clinical features most pertinent to the diagnosis of MAS. The following 9 features were ranked most highly in the 232 respondents: (1) falling platelet count, (2) hyperferritinaemia, (3) presence of haemophagocytosis in the bone marrow, (4) increased liver enzymes, (5) falling leucocyte count, (6) persistent continuous fever of 38 °C or higher, (7) falling ESR, (8) hypofibrinogenaemia, and (9) hypertriglyceridaemia. Questionnaire respondents were intentionally not asked to indicate the threshold level for each laboratory test that they felt would be optimal for early identification of MAS. Instead, the threshold levels will be determined in the second part of the project, which will utilize real data from a large number of patients with and without MAS.

Treatment

MAS is a life-threatening condition still associated with high mortality rates. Therefore, early recognition and of this syndrome and immediate therapeutic intervention to produce a rapid response are critical. No clinical trials have been performed in MAS and treatment has developed mainly from anecdotal experience.

Early diagnosis and appropriate supportive care with corticosteroids will result in control of disease in almost one-half of the patients with MAS (Table 168.2). Most clinicians would start with intravenous methylprednisolone pulse therapy (30 mg/kg for three consecutive days) followed by 2 mg/kg per day in divided doses.

Table 168.2 Suggested management according to risk groups at initial diagnosis

Risk group	Suggested therapy
Low-risk group	
MAS in the absence of high-risk features	Corticosteroids
	IVIG (2 g/kg)
	Supportive care
High-risk group	
CNS involvement	Corticosteroids
Severe bleeding diathesis (DIC)	Ciclosporin, IVIG
Severe renal impairment	IVIG
Multiorgan failure	Consider etoposide
Failure to respond to initial therapy	Supportive care

DIC, disseminated intravascular coagulation; IVIG, intravenous immunoglobulin.

If response to steroids is not evident, addition of ciclosporin (2–7 mg/kg per day) should be considered.[3,16,41] IVIG (2 g/kg in a single dose) should be considered as well.

Intravenous immunoglobulin (IVIG) is a particularly useful agent when the differentiation between sepsis and MAS is uncertain in a clinically ill child. There are reports of effective use of IVIG alone in treatment of MAS, particularly secondary to SJIA or adult-onset Still's disease.[42]

Patients in whom MAS remains active despite the use of corticosteroids and ciclosporin present a serious challenge. In these patients, one might consider using the HLH-2004 treatment protocol developed by the International Histiocyte Society.[39] This protocol in addition to steroids and ciclosporin includes etoposide (or VP16), a podophyllatoxin derivative that inhibits DNA synthesis by forming a complex with topoisomerease II and DNA. Although, successful use of etoposide in MAS has been reported, the potential toxicity of the drug is a major concern, particularly in patients with hepatic impairment. Etoposide is metabolized by the liver, and then both unchanged drug and its metabolites are excreted through the kidneys. Since patients who may require the use of etoposide are very likely to have hepatic and renal involvement, caution should be exercised to adjust the dosage properly and thus limit the extent of potential side effects such as severe bone marrow suppression that may be detrimental. Reports describing deaths caused by severe bone marrow suppression and overwhelming infection have been published. In patients with MAS secondary to HLH it is not required to follow the entire of HLH-2004 protocol for administration of etoposide; if the patient recovers significantly after a few doses of etoposide then ongoing control of disease can be maintained with steroids and ciclosporin. This approach would limit the risks of etoposide such as infection and marrow suppression.

Recently it has been suggested that in patients unresponsive to the combination of steroids and ciclosporin, particularly in those with renal and hepatic impairment, anti-thymocyte globulin (ATG) might be an alternative to etoposide.[43,44] ATG depletes both CD4+ and CD8+ T cells through complement-dependent cell lysis. Mild depletion of monocytes is noted in some patients as well. Although in the reported cases this treatment was well tolerated, one must remember that infusion reactions are frequently reported with the use of ATG and adequate laboratory and supportive medical resources must be readily available if this treatment is used.

The utility of biological drugs in MAS treatment remains unclear. Although TNF inhibitors have been reported to be effective in occasional MAS patients, other reports describe patients in whom MAS developed while they were on TNF inhibitors. Since, at least in SJIA, MAS episodes are often triggered by the disease flare, biologics that neutralize either IL-1 or IL-6, two cytokines that play a pivotal role in SJIA pathogenesis,[45,46] have been tried by many authors. As with TNF inhibitors the results have, however, been conflicting.[47–52] If MAS is driven by EBV infection, one might also consider rituximab, a treatment that would eliminate B lymphocytes harbouring EBV.[53,54] This approach has been successfully used in EBV-induced lymphoproliferative disease.

Prognosis

MAS is a life-threatening condition with significant morbidity and mortality. Due to increasing awareness of this syndrome, early diagnosis and appropriate interventions have resulted in improved outcomes. A proportion of MAS patients may experience recurrent episodes and these patients may require closer monitoring. In future, the use of novel biomarkers to identify the children and adults with rheumatic disease who are at greatest risk of MAS will hopefully lead to better therapies and outcomes.

References

1. Silverman ED, Miller JJ, 3rd, Bernstein B et al. Consumption coagulopathy associated with systemic juvenile rheumatoid arthritis. *J Pediatr* 1983;103:872–876.
2. Hadchouel M, Prieur AM, Griscelli C. Acute hemorrhagic, hepatic, and neurologic manifestations in juvenile rheumatoid arthritis: possible relationship to drugs or infection. *J Pediatr* 1985;106:561–566.
3. Mouy R, Stephan JL, Pillet P et al. Efficacy of cyclosporine A in the treatment of macrophage activation syndrome in juvenile arthritis: report of five cases. *J Pediatr* 1996;129:750–754.
4. Grom AA, Passo MH. Macrophage activation syndrome in systemic juvenile idiopathic arthritis. *J Pediatr* 1996;129:630–632.
5. Ravelli A, De Benedetti F, Viola S et al. Macrophage activation syndrome in systemic juvenile rheumatoid arthritis successfully treated with cyclosporine. *J Pediatr* 1996;128:275–278.
6. Stephan JL, Kone-Paut I, Galambrun C et al. Reactive haemophagocytic syndrome in children with inflammatory disorders. A retrospective study of 24 patients. *Rheumatology* (Oxford) 2001;40(11):1285–1292.
7. Sawhney S, Woo P, Murray KJ. Macrophage activation syndrome: A potentially fatal complication of rheumatic disorders. *Arch Dis Child* 2001;85:421–426.
8. Grom AA. NK dysfunction: a common pathway in systemic onset juvenile rheumatoid arthritis, macrophage activation syndrome, and hemophagocytic lymphohistiocytosis. *Arthritis Rheum* 2004;50:689–698.
9. Ariet JB, Le Thi Huong D, Marinho A et al. Reactive haemophagocytic syndrome in adult-onset Still's disease: a report of six patients and a review of the literature. *Ann Rheum Dis* 2006;65:1596–1601.
10. Bleesing J, Prada A, Siegel DM et al. The diagnostic significance of soluble CD163 and soluble interleukin-2 receptor alpha-chain in macrophage activation syndrome and untreated new-onset systemic juvenile idiopathic arthritis. *Arthritis Rheum* 2007;56:965–971.
11. Behrens EM, Beukelman T, Paessler M et al. Occult macrophage activation syndrome in patients with systemic juvenile idiopathic arthritis. *J Rheumatol* 2007;34:1133–1138.
12. Prahalad S, Bove KE, Dickens D et al. Etanercept in the treatment of macrophage activation syndrome. *J Rheumatol* 2001;28:2120–2124.

13. Avcin T, Tse SML, Schneider R et al. Macrophage activation syndrome as the presenting manifestation of rheumatic diseases in childhood. *J Pediatr* 2006;148:683–686.

14. Grom, A.A., J. Villanueva, S. Lee et al. Natural killer cell dysfunction in patients with systemic-onset juvenile rheumatoid arthritis and macrophage activation syndrome. *J Pediatr* 2003;142:292–296.

15. Davies SV, Dean JD, Wardrop CA, Jones JH. Epstein-Barr virus-associated haemophagocytic syndrome in a patient with juvenile chronic arthritis. *Br J Rheumatol* 1994;33:495–497.

16. Ravelli A, Caria MC, Buratti S et al. Methotrexate as a possible trigger of macrophage activation syndrome in systemic juvenile idiopathic arthritis. *J Rheumatol* 2001;28:865.

17. Ramanan AV, Schneider R. Macrophage activation syndrome following initiation of etanercept in a child with systemic onset juvenile rheumatoid arthritis. *J Rheumatol* 2003;30(2):401–403.

18. Athreya BH. Is macrophage activation syndrome is a new entity? *Clin Exp Rheumatol* 2002;20:121–123.

19. Ramanan AV, Baildam EM. Macrophage activation syndrome is hemophagocytic lymphohistiocytosis—need for the right terminology. *J Rheumatol* 2002;29:1105.

20. Favara BE, Feller AC, Pauli M et al. Contemporary classification of histiocytic disorders. The WHO Committee On Histiocytic/Reticulum Cell Proliferations. Reclassification Working Group of the Histiocyte Society. *Med Pediatr Oncol* 1997;29:157–166.

21. Filipovich HA. Hemophagocytic lymphohistiocytosis. *Immunol Allergy Clin N Am* 2002;22:281–300.

22. Jordan MB, Allen CE, Weitzman S et al. How I treat hemophagocytic lymphohistiocytosis. *Blood* 2011;118:4041–4052.

23. Zhang K, Jordan MB, Marsh RA et al. Hypomorphic mutations in PRF1, MUNC13–4, and STXBP2 are associated with adult-onset familial HLH. *Blood* 2011;118:5794–5798.

24. Stepp SE, Dufourcq-Lagelouse R, Le Deist F et al. Perforin gene defects in familial hemophagocytic lymphohistiocytosis. *Science* 1999;286:1957–1959.

25. Feldmann J, Callebaut I, Raposo G et al. MUNC13–4 is essential for cytolytic granules fusion and is mutated in a form of familial hemophagocytic lymphohistiocytosis (FHL3). *Cell* 2003;115:461–473.

26. zur Stadt U, Schmidt S, Kasper B et al. Linkage of familial hemophagocytic lymphohistiocytosis (FHL) type-4 to chromosome 6q24 and identification of mutations in syntaxin 11. *Hum Mol Genet* 2005;14:827–834.

27. zur Stadt U, Rohr J, Seifert W et al. Familial hemophagocytic lymphohistiocytosis type 5 (FHL-5) is caused by mutations in Munc18–2 and impaired binding to syntaxin 11. *Am J Hum Genet* 2009;85:482–492.

28. Hazen MM, Woodward AL, Hofmann I et al. Mutations of the hemophagocytic lymphohistiocytosis-associated gene UNC13D in a patient with systemic juvenile idiopathic arthritis. *Arthritis Rheum* 2008;58:567–570.

29. Zhang K, Biroschak J, Glass DN et al. Macrophage activation syndrome in patients with systemic juvenile idiopathic arthritis is associated with MUNC13–4 polymorphisms. *Arthritis Rheum* 2008;58:2892–2896.

30. Vastert SJ, van Wijk R, D'Urbano LE et al. Mutations in the perforin gene can be linked to macrophage activation syndrome in patients with systemic onset juvenile idiopathic arthritis. *Rheumatology* (Oxford) 2010;49:441–449.

31. Kagi D, Odermatt B, Mak TW. Homeostatic regulation of CD8+ T cells by perforin. *Eur J Immunol* 1999;29:3262–3272.

32. Lykens JE, Terrell CE, Zoller EE, Risma K, Jordan MB. Perforin is a critical physiologic regulator of T-cell activation. *Blood* 2011;118:618–626.

33. Billiau AD, Roskams T, Van Damme-Lombaerts R et al.. Macrophage activation syndrome: characteristic findings on liver biopsy illustrating the key role of activated, IFN-gamma-producing lymphocytes and IL-6- and TNF-alpha-producing macrophages. *Blood* 2005;105:1648.

34. Mazodier K, Marin V, Novick D et al. Severe imbalance of IL-18/IL-18BP in patients with secondary hemophagocytic syndrome. *Blood* 2005;106:3483–3489.

35. Maeno N, Takei S, Imanaka H et al. Increased interleukin-18 expression in bone marrow of a patient with systemic juvenile idiopathic arthritis

and unrecognized macrophage-activation syndrome. *Arthritis Rheum* 2004;50:1935–1938.

36. Allen CE, Yu X, Kozinetz CA, McClain KL. Highly elevated ferritin levels and the diagnosis of hemophagocytic lymphohistiocytosis. *Pediatr Blood Cancer* 2008;50:1227–1235.

37. Parodi A, Davi S, Pringe AB et al. Macrophage activation syndrome in juvenile systemic lupus erythematosus: a multinational multicenter study of thirty-eight patients. *Arthritis Rheum* 2009;60:3388–3399.

38. Gupta A, Tyrrell P, Valani R et al. The role of the initial bone marrow aspirate in the diagnosis of hemophagocytic lymphohistiocytosis. *Pediatr Blood Cancer* 2008;51:402–404.

39. Henter JI, Horne A, Arico M et al. HLH-2004: Diagnostic and therapeutic guidelines for hemopagocytic lymphohistiocytosis. *Pediatr Blood Cancer* 2007;48:124–131.

40. Davi S, Consolaro A, Guseinova D et al. An international consensus survey of diagnostic criteria for macrophage activation syndrome in systemic juvenile idiopathic arthritis. *J Rheumatol* 2011;38:764–768.

41. Quesnel B, Catteau B, Aznar V, Bauters F, Fenaux P. Successful treatment of juvenile rheumatoid arthritis associated haemophagocytic syndrome by cyclosporin A with transient exacerbation by conventional-dose G-CSF. *Br J Haematol* 1997;97:508–510.

42. Tristano AG, Casanova-Escalona L, Torres A, Rodriguez MA. Macrophage activation syndrome in a patient with systemic onset rheumatoid arthritis: rescue with intravenous immunoglobulin therapy. *J Clin Rheumatol* 2003;9:253–258.

43. Mahlaoui N, Ouachee-Chardin M, de Saint Basile G et al. Immunotherapy of familial hemophagocytic lymphohistiocytosis with antithymocyte globulins: a single-center retrospective report of 38 patients. *Pediatrics* 2007;120:e622–e628.

44. Coca A, Bundy KW, Marston B et al. Macrophage activation syndrome: serological markers and treatment with anti-thymocyte globulin. *Clin Immunol* 2009;132:10–18.

45. Pascual V, Allantaz F, Arce E, Punaro M, Banchereau J. Role of interleukin-1 (IL-1) in the pathogenesis of systemic onset juvenile idiopathic arthritis and clinical response to IL-1 blockade. *J Exp Med* 2005;201:1479–1486.

46. Yokota S, Imagawa T, Mori M et al. Efficacy and safety of tocilizumab in patients with systemic-onset juvenile idiopathic arthritis: a randomised, double-blind, placebo-controlled, withdrawal phase III trial. *Lancet* 2008;371:998–1006.

47. Bruck N, Suttorp M, Kabus M et al. Rapid and sustained remission of systemic juvenile idiopathic arthritis-associated macrophage activation syndrome through treatment with anakinra and corticosteroids. *J Clin Rheumatol* 2011;17:23–27.

48. Fitzgerald AA, Leclercq SA, Yan A et al.. Rapid responses to anakinra in patients with refractory adult-onset Still's disease. *Arthritis Rheum* 2005;52:1794–1803.

49. Nigrovic PA, Mannion M, Prince FH et al. Anakinra as first-line disease-modifying therapy in systemic juvenile idiopathic arthritis: report of forty-six patients from an international multicenter series. *Arthritis Rheum* 2011;63:545–555.

50. Zeft A, Hollister R, LaFleur B et al. Anakinra for systemic juvenile arthritis: the Rocky Mountain experience. *J Clin Rheumatol* 2009;15:161–164.

51. Kobayashi M, Takahashi Y, Yamashita H et al. Benefit and a possible risk of tocilizumab therapy for adult-onset Still's disease accompanied by macrophage-activation syndrome. *Mod Rheumatol* 2011;21:92–96.

52. Kelly A, Ramanan AV. A case of macrophage activation syndrome successfully treated with anakinra. *Nat Clin Pract Rheumatol* 2008;4:615–620.

53. Balamuth NJ, Nichols KE, Paessler M, Teachey DT. Use of rituximab in conjunction with immunosuppressive chemotherapy as a novel therapy for Epstein Barr virus-associated hemophagocytic lymphohistiocytosis. *J Pediatr Hematol Oncol* 2007;29:569–573.

54. Bosman G, Langemeijer SM, Hebeda KM et al. The role of rituximab in a case of EBV-related lymphoproliferative disease presenting with haemophagocytosis. *Neth J Med* 2009;67:364–365.

CHAPTER 169

Multicentric reticulohistiocytosis

Hermann Einsele and Peter J. Maddison

Introduction

Multicentric reticulohistiocytosis (MRH) is a rare systemic disease that is recognized clinically by the combination of typical papular and nodular skin lesions and a severe and destructive polyarthritis, although virtually any organ system of the body can be involved. The term 'multicentric reticulohistiocytosis' was introduced by Goltz and Layman in 1954 to distinguish the disorder from solitary cutaneous nodules, termed reticulohistiocytomas, which have identical histological appearances but are not associated with systemic disease. There are a number of synonyms, including lipoid dermatoarthritis, reticulohistiocytosis, giant-cell reticulohistiocytosis, and normocholesterolaemic xanthomatosis. At one time it was thought to be a lipid storage disease but no consistent abnormality of serum or intracellular lipids has been identified. It is thought generally that the histiocytes and giant cells that characterize the lesions contain a non-specific accumulation of glycoprotein and lipids, and that this disease is a histiocytic granulomatous reaction to an unknown stimulus.[1] However, in one case, type VI collagen inclusions usually found in lymphohistiocytic neoplasms were demonstrated, supporting the concept of a proliferative rather than an inflammatory background for this condition.[2]

Clinical features

MRH is a characterized by mucocutaneous papulonodules and erosive arthritis. The cutaneous lesions consist of multiple reddish-brown papules and nodules, mainly involving the face and distal upper extremities. The arthritis preferentially involves the interphalangeal joints of the hands and can lead to joint destruction and deformities. All of these clinical symptoms are directly caused by the infiltration of reticulohistiocytes, which are histologically characterized by histiocytic multinucleated giant cells with eosinophilic ground-glass cytoplasm.[3]

MRH most commonly affects middle-aged white women. It is about three times more common in women than in men, with a mean age at onset in the fifth decade. MRH classically presents with reddish-brown nodules and papules, 1–2 mm to several centimetres in diameter, distributed acrally. The face (nose and paranasal areas) and hands (dorsum and lateral aspects of fingers and nailfolds) are affected. The ears, forearms, elbows, scalp, and muscosal surfaces can be affected as well. Patients may also present with fever, fatigue, and weight loss.[4] The differential diagnosis includes disseminated Langerhans cell histiocytosis, rheumatoid nodules, tuberous xanthomas, Gottron's papules, gout, progressive nodular histiocytomas, lipogranulomatosis, sarcoidosis, and psoriatic arthritis.[5] In up to 25% of cases, MRH has been found to occur in association with a wide range of underlying internal malignancies, suggesting that the disease may represent a paraneoplastic condition caused by reactive proliferative histiocytes.[6] This association with internal malignancy mandates that patients presenting with MRH should be investigated for an occult neoplastic disease.

The severe destructive arthropathy known as arthritis mutilans occurs in one-half of patients with joint involvement. Approximately 50% of patients with MRH initially develop polyarthritis, 25% initially develop the cutaneous nodules, and another 25% develop both skin and joint manifestations at the same time.[5] Periungual papules arranged around the nailfolds resemble 'coral beads' and have been noted in approximately 40% of cases. An estimated 50% of patients with MRH also develop papules and nodules of the oropharyngeal or nasopharyngeal mucosa; these may occasionally progress to histiocytomas. Rarely, patients develop visceral involvement resulting in serositis, gastric ulceration, and progressive heart failure.[5] Most patients have interphalangeal joint involvement of the hands, but there have also been sporadic cases of involvement of other joints including the knees, shoulders, wrists, hips, ankles, feet, and elbows, in decreasing frequency. The disabling arthritic process progresses rapidly in the early stage and then decreases in intensity to become less active over the ensuing 8–10 years.[1]

Laboratory, imaging, and histology findings

Laboratory results reveal elevated erythrocyte sedimentation rate (ESR) and anaemia in 50% of patients, and hypercholesterolaemia in 30%. The presence of cryoglobulinaemia and cold agglutinins, but not rheumatoid factor, is occasionally seen. The joint lesions of MRH are characterized by sharply circumscribed progressive erosions of the joint surfaces, often with concomitant separation of the bone ends.[5]

The diagnosis of MRH is based on the characteristic histopathological findings, presenting multinucleated giant cells of a foreign-body type, irregular in size and shape, reaching 50–100 µm in diameter. The cytoplasm of the giant cells is slightly eosinophilic and has a finely granulated ground-glass appearance or a foamy, vacuolated appearance. The pathogenesis of MRH is unknown; however, aberrant proliferation of the histiocytic population is postulated in response to monokines, cytokines, and other secretory products that promote macrophage proliferation and phagocytosis.[1] In addition, the biological nature and pathogenetic significance of the ground-glass-like multinucleated giant cells remain largely unknown.

Histochemically, the granular material in histiocytes and giant cells stains with periodic acid–Schiff and Sudan black, indicating the presence of glycolipids and/or glycoproteins and neutral fat.[5] CD68 staining is positive, and S-100 and CD1a are negative.

CD10 was demonstrated[7] to accumulate abundantly in the cytoplasm of ground-glass-like multinucleated giant cells in MRH. The feature was quite specific because in giant-cell tendon sheath tumour, pigmented villonodular synovitis, granuloma annulare, ruptured epidermoid cyst, sarcoidosis, and xanthogranuloma none of the multinucleated giant cells expressed CD10. The biological significance of CD10 in inflammatory and neoplastic disorders is largely unknown.

CD10 is a type 2 cell-surface neutral endopetidase. The CD10 positivity in tumour cells has been reported to correlate significantly with tumour progression and shorter survival in bladder cancer, diffuse large-cell lymphoma, renal pelvis transitional-cell carcinoma, and pancreatic endocrine tumours. The devastating osteolytic process of MRH may be related to the unfavourable biological effects of CD10+ ground-glass-like giant cells. Although the pathogenetic significance remains unknown, the aberrant expression of CD10 is a useful marker of ground-glass-like multinucleated giant cells in MRH and may be a potential target for treating intractable MRH.

Pathophysiology

The characteristic histiocytic proliferation MRH has been shown to result in the release of cytokines, including interleukin (IL)-12, IL-1, IL-6, and tumour necrosis factor alpha (TNFα).[8] Although almost any organ can be involved, the skin of the face and hands, and interphalangeal joints of the hands are most commonly affected. The stimulus for the histiocytic proliferation has not been fully elucidated, although there is an association with internal malignancies and abnormal immunological laboratory findings. Additionally, some patients with MRH are found to have a positive tuberculin skin test. In these patients, MRH will respond to anti-tuberculosis treatment. Additionally, patients with tuberculosis can also present with MRH.[8] This has led to the hypothesis that MRH is a paraneoplastic disease with chronic inflammatory and autoimmune features.

Associated conditions

MRH has been linked to a number of associated conditions, including hyperlipidaemia (30%), systemic vasculitis, tuberous sclerosis, a positive tuberculin test, and internal malignancy. A number of reports have identified a link between MRH and gynaecological malignancies. Two reports in the 1970s first described this association, with the appearance of MRH preceding the diagnosis of cervical carcinoma[9] and ovarian carcinoma[10] by 2 and 10 months, respectively. From 1980 to 2006, to our knowledge, there have been 20 cases of MRH reported in association with malignancy: 4 of these were associated with ovarian, cervical, or endometrial cancers and 5 were associated with breast cancer. In 4 of the 9 cases, MRH preceded the malignancy diagnosis. In 8 of the 9 cases, MRH followed a parallel course in response to the cancer treatment.[11–13] Breast, ovarian, endometrial, and cervical cancers are among the most commonly reported malignancies linked to MRH.

Diagnosis

The diagnosis is confirmed by skin or synovial biopsy. Solitary reticulohistiocytomas have identical histological findings but there is no evidence of systemic disease.[14] Diseases that may possibly be confused with multicentric reticulohistiocytosis on the basis of clinical or histological findings are:

- Rheumatoid or psoriatic arthritis; chronic gout
- Sarcoid dactylitis—associated with discrete tubercles that lack foam cells or giant cells typical of multicentric reticulohistiocytosis
- Xanthomas
- Fibroxanthoma
- Histiocytosis X—usually presents in childhood and proliferating cells are epidermotropic Langerhans cells rather than of true monocyte–macrophage lineage
- Generalized eruptive histiocytoma—not associated with arthritis and lesions do not exhibit the typical multinucleate giant cells
- Tendon sheath giant-cell tumours—solitary, well-circumscribed nodules in the hands
- Farber's disease—lipogranulomatosis, usually fatal in infancy.

Treatment and course

The disease often runs a waxing and waning course and sometimes stabilizes. It is difficult to predict the course in the individual case but as a rule the disease 'burns out' after 5–8 years, with regression of the cutaneous nodules, leaving the patient with severe joint deformities. Occasionally, systemic involvement can be severe enough to be life threatening but otherwise the prognosis is dominated by whether or not there is an associated malignancy. Various drug treatments have been proposed to suppress the condition, including corticosteroids, adrenocorticotropic hormone (ACT), salicylates, anti-malarials, cytotoxic agents, methotrexate (MTX), ciclosporin, and more recently TNFα blockers. There are no controlled trials, as the condition is so rare, and therefore reports of efficacy should be interpreted with caution. Up to 25% of cases have been associated with malignancy. There is no predominant type of cancer seen in this disorder and in most cases MRH does not run a parallel course to neoplasm. These observations have led several authors to avoid labelling MRH as a paraneoplastic disorder.[6,15] Nevertheless, several case reports emphasize the temporal association between MRH and underlying neoplasm, and stress the importance of treating the neoplasm to suppress the manifestations of MRH.[16–18] Regardless of whether MRH is a paraneoplastic disorder, work-up for underlying malignancy cannot be overemphasized.

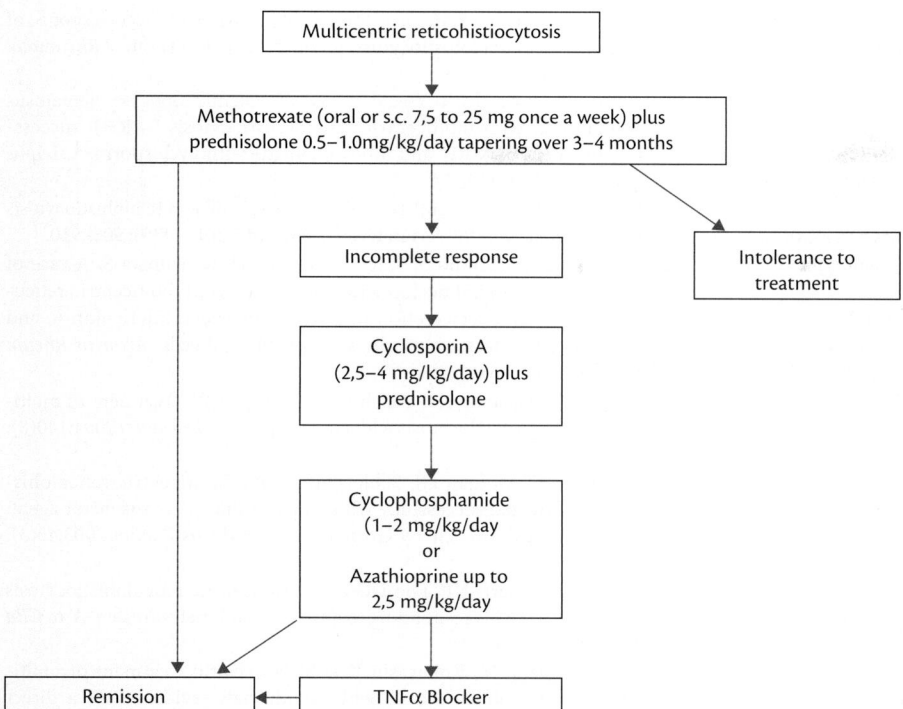

Fig. 169.1 An algorithm for treating multicentric histiocytosis.

Liang and Granston[19] reported 13 cases of complete or near complete remission. Medications utilized include alkylating agents (mainly cyclophosphamide), MTX, ACTH, hydroxychloroquine (HCQ), and corticosteroids. Cyclophosphamide alone induced complete remission in three patients, MTX in one, and chlorambucil in one. In their opinion the optimal treatment for MRH is oral MTX plus prednisone tapered gradually over 3–4 months. In case of treatment failure or intolerance, the authors recommended cyclophosphamide 0.5–2 mg/kg per day either alone or added to MTX.

Ciclosporin and azathioprine seem to be acceptable alternatives to MTX. MTX and ciclosporin were shown to be effective even after treatment failure with cyclophosphamide,[20–21] and induced (near) complete remission in five patients. Prednisone is always used in combination with other medications and does not usually induce complete remission when used alone. Of interest is the emerging role of TNFα blockers in the treatment of MRH. The presence of TNFα and IL-1β in the synovial tissue of MRH patients has been reported.[15,22–23] Indeed, two case reports of successful treatment of MRH with etanercept have been published.[24–25] In both cases etanercept was used after treatment failure with multiple immunosuppressive agents, including cyclophosphamide. Although no case reports of MRH responding to other biological agents have been identified, probably all biologics could be utilized to treat MRH. Treating MRH with TNFα-neutralizing drugs, one has to keep the possible association with malignancy in 15–30% of cases in mind and these products should thus be used with caution.[26] Recently Goto et al.[27] reported a case of MRH in a 44 year-old Japanese woman that responded to alendronate infusion. Immunohistochemical analysis showed that some of the mononuclear cells in the skin were positive for RANKL. The authors postulated that these cells may induce histiocytes to differentiate into osteoclast-like multinucleated giant cells locally in the skin. Alendronate may directly act on mononuclear cells, leading to inhibition of histiocyte differentiation and clinical remission. To the best of our knowledge this is the first case that reports a positive response to a bisphosphonate. This treatment modality deserves further study. Based on the above analysis, we propose an approach to the treatment of persistent MRH as shown in Figure 169.1.

References

1. Campbell DA, Edwards NL. Multicentric reticulohistiocytosis: systemic macrophage disorder. *Baillieres Clin Rheumatol* 1991;5(2):301–319.
2. Fortier-Beaulieu M, Thomine E, Boullie MC , Le Loët X, Lauret P, Hemet J. New electron microscopic findings in a case of multicentric reticulohistiocytosis. Long spacing collagen inclusions. *Am J Dermatopathol* 1993;15(6):587–589.
3. Barrow MV, Holubar K. Multicentric reticulohistiocytosis. A review of 33 patients. *Medicine* (Baltimore) 1969;48(4):287–305.
4. Tajirian AL, Malik MK, Robinson-Bostom L, Lally EV. Multicentric reticulohistiocytosis. *Clin Dermatol* 2006;24(6):486–492.
5. C, G. and C. R., Non-Langerhans cell histiocytosis. In: Freedburg IM, Eisen AZ, Wolff K et al. (eds) *Fitzpatrick's dermatology in general medicine*, 5th edn. McGraw-Hill, New York, 1999:1892–1900.
6. Luz FB, Gaspar TAP, Kalil-Gaspar N, Ramos-e-Silva M. Multicentric reticulohistiocytosis. *J Eur Acad Dermatol Venereol* 2001;15(6):524–531.
7. Tashiro A, Takeuchi S, Nakahara T , Oba J, Tsujita J, Fukushi J, Kiryu H, Oda Y, Xie L, Yan X, Takahara M, Moroi Y, Furue M. Aberrant expression of CD10 in ground-glass-like multinucleated giant cells of multicentric reticulohistiocytosis. *J Dermatol* 2010;37(11):995–997.
8. Trotta F, Castellino G, Lo Monaco A. Multicentric reticulohistiocytosis. *Best Pract Res Clin Rheumatol* 2004;18(5):759–772.
9. Hanauer LB. Reticulohistiocytosis: remission after cyclophosphamide therapy. *Arthritis Rheum* 1972;15(6):636–640.
10. Hall-Smith P. Multicentric reticulohistiocytosis with ovarian carcinoma. *Proc R Soc Med* 1976;69(5):380–381.
11. Catterall MD, White JE. Multicentric reticulohistiocytosis and malignant disease. *Br J Dermatol* 1978;98(2):221–224.

12. Kishikawa T, Miyashita T, Fujiwara E , Shimomura O, Yasuhi I, Niino D, Ito M, Amenomori M, Osumimoto H, Osumi M, Eguchi K, Migita K. Multicentric reticulohistiocytosis associated with ovarian cancer. *Mod Rheumatol* 2007;17(5):422–425.

13. Malik MK, Regan L, Robinson-Bostom L, Pan TD, McDonald CJ. Proliferating multicentric reticulohistiocytosis associated with papillary serous carcinoma of the endometrium. *J Am Acad Dermatol* 2005;53(6): 1075–1079.

14. Zelger B, Cerio R, Soyer HP et al. Reticulohistiocytoma and multicentric reticulohistiocytosis. Histopathologic and immunophenotypic distinct entities. *Am J Dermatopathol* 1994;16(6):577–584.

15. Gorman JD, Danning C, Schumacher HR, Klippel JH, Davis JC Jr. Multicentric reticulohistiocytosis: case report with immuno-histochemical analysis and literature review. *Arthritis Rheum* 2000;43(4):930–938.

16. Janssen BA, Kencian J, Brooks PM. Close temporal and anatomic relationship between multicentric reticulohistiocytosis and carcinoma of the breast. *J Rheumatol* 1992;19(2):322–324.

17. Nunnink JC, Krusinski PA, Yates JW. Multicentric reticulohistiocytosis and cancer: a case report and review of the literature. *Med Pediatr Oncol* 1985;13(5):273–279.

18. Snow JL, Muller SA. Malignancy-associated multicentric reticulohistiocytosis: a clinical, histological and immunophenotypic study. *Br J Dermatol* 1995;133(1):71–76.

19. Liang GC, GranstonAS. Complete remission of multicentric reticulohistiocytosis with combination therapy of steroid, cyclophosphamide, and low-dose pulse methotrexate. Case report, review of the literature, and proposal for treatment. *Arthritis Rheum* 1996;39(1):171–174.

20. Rentsch JL, Martin EM, Harrison LC, Wicks IP. Prolonged response of multicentric reticulohistiocytosis to low dose methotrexate. *J Rheumatol* 1998;25(5):1012–1015.

21. Saito K, Fujii K, Awazu Y et al. A case of systemic lupus erythematosus complicated with multicentric reticulohistiocytosis (MRH): successful treatment of MRH and lupus nephritis with cyclosporin A. *Lupus* 2001;10(2):129–132.

22. Bennassar A, Mas A, Guilabert A et al. Multicentric reticulohistiocytosis with elevated cytokine serum levels. *J Dermatol* 2011;38(9): 905–910.

23. Nakamura H, Yoshino S, Shiga H, Tanaka H, Katsumata S. A case of spontaneous femoral neck fracture associated with multicentric reticulohistiocytosis: oversecretion of interleukin-1beta, interleukin-6, and tumor necrosis factor alpha by affected synovial cells. *Arthritis Rheum* 1997;40(12):2266–2270.

24. Kovach BT, Calamia KT, Walsh JS, Ginsburg WW. Treatment of multicentric reticulohistiocytosis with etanercept. *Arch Dermatol* 2004;140(8): 919–921.

25. Matejicka C, Morgan GJ, Schlegelmilch JG. Multicentric reticulohistiocytosis treated successfully with an anti-tumor necrosis factor agent: comment on the article by Gorman et al. *Arthritis Rheum* 2003;48(3): 864–866.

26. De Knop KJ, Aerts NE, Ebo DG et al. Multicentric reticulohistiocytosis associated arthritis responding to anti-TNF and methotrexate. *Acta Clin Belg* 2011;66(1):66–69.

27. Goto H, Inaba M, Kobayashi K et al. Successful treatment of multicentric reticulohistiocytosis with alendronate: evidence for a direct effect of bisphosphonate on histiocytes. *Arthritis Rheum* 2003;48(12): 3538–3541.

CHAPTER 170

Inherited metabolic diseases

Bernhard Manger

Introduction

The term 'lysosomal storage diseases' (LSD) comprises a heterogeneous group of more than 40 hereditary diseases. They are all caused by a dysfunction of lysosomes. Lysosomal enzymes are necessary to metabolize various large molecules. Therefore, a genetic defect of such an enzyme usually leads to an accumulation of a non-degradable metabolite within the cell. The classification of LSD is based on the biochemical nature of this metabolite relevant for the pathogenesis of the disease. The most important subgroups are mucopolysaccharidoses (MPS), mucolipidoses, and sphingolipidoses (Table 170.1).[1] Glycogen storage diseases (except type 2—Pompe's disease) are not considered LSD. The first descriptions of LSD as separate disease entities date back to the late 19th century (Tay–Sachs disease 1881, Gaucher's disease 1882, Fabry's disease 1898). About 50 years later the role of lysosomal dysfunction was recognized and in 1963 the first underlying enzyme deficiency (α-glucosidase in Pompe's disease) was characterized. Most LSD are autosomal recessive disorders; the only exceptions are Fabry's disease and MPS type II (Hunter's disease) with an X-linked inheritance pattern.[2] The individual disease entities are very rare, most of them with a prevalence of less than 1 in 100 000. Considered as a group, however, one LSD occurs in about 8000 live births. The real prevalence might even be higher, because mild attenuated forms tend to be easily overlooked.[3] Enzyme replacement therapies (ERT) are currently available for Gaucher's, Fabry's, and Pompe's diseases as well as for several types of MPS.

Mucopolysaccharidoses

Pathogenesis

MPS are genetic, metabolic disorders caused by a deficiency of enzymes necessary for the degradation of glycosaminoglycans, such as dermatan, heparan, keratan, or chondroitin sulphates. Depending on the type of enzyme deficiency, the MPS are grouped into seven types (Table 170.1). The presenting symptoms of the various types, especially with respect to the musculoskeletal system, are fairly similar. The degree of the enzyme deficiency is responsible for the severity of the resulting disease. It can range from disability in early childhood with severe somatic and neurological manifestations to mild, attenuated forms with normal development and intelligence, which are frequently not diagnosed until adolescence or adulthood.

This is most evident in MPS I, the most frequent disorder in this group with an incidence of about 1 in 100 000. One of more than 100 known mutations of the gene for the enzyme α-L-iduronidase, located on chromosome 4, leads to an accumulation of heparan and dermatan sulphates in the lysosomes of various organs. Most involved are connective tissues, bone, airways, heart, kidneys, and in severe forms the central nervous system (CNS). The most severe manifestation is MPS I type Hurler, first described in 1919,[3] which presents within the first months of life with the typical phenotype (macrocephaly, broad nasal bridge, enlarged tongue and lips) and marked mental retardation. Without therapy these patients have a short life expectancy and will usually not be seen by a rheumatologist primarily.

A clinical presentation with much milder symptoms, MPS I type Scheie, is named after the ophthalmologist who first described this phenotype.[4] These patients have normal facial features and normal intellectual development, and may reach adulthood without having been diagnosed. Musculoskeletal and ocular symptoms are usually the reasons for the first consultation of a specialist. In 302 patients with MPS I type Scheie the diagnosis was made at a mean age of 9.3 years with a mean delay of 1.5 years after onset of symptoms.[5]

Between these two phenotypic presentations of MPS I exists a wide range of intermediate phenotypes, designated 'attenuated MPS I' or type Hurler/Scheie. The underlying genetic enzyme deficiencies of other MPS are summarized in Table 170.1.

Clinical manifestations

The musculoskeletal symptoms of MPS I, II, VI, and VII have many similar features and will be described together. They are frequently the first manifestation of the disease, especially in attenuated forms, and therefore the rheumatologist should be able to recognize them.[6,7] Joint stiffness or contractures are present in more than 80% of patients.[8] This is caused by a glycosaminoglycan (GAG) deposition in intra- and periarticular structures and is most prominent in the hands ('claw hands') (Figure 170.1), feet, and shoulders, but may involve any other joint. This reduced range of motion can cause considerable disability and a reduced quality of life. In contrast to other rheumatic disorders, which can cause reduced joint mobility, any signs of local or systemic inflammation are typically lacking in MPS.

Another frequent symptom is carpal tunnel syndrome, observed in 62% of MPS I type Scheie patients with a mean age of 12 years.[9] Since the overall frequency of carpal tunnel syndrome in children

Table 170.1 Lysosomal storage diseases

Disease	OMIM[a]	Enzyme deficiency
Mucopolysaccharidoses (MPS)		
MPS I		α-L-Iduronidase
Type Hurler	607014	
Type Scheie	607016	
Type Hurler/Scheie	607016	
MPS II (Hunter's syndrome)	309900	Iduronate sulphate sulphatase
MPS III (Sanfilippo's syndrome)		
Type III-A	252900	Heparan-S-sulphate-sulphaminidase
Type III-B	252920	
Type III-C	252930	N-Acetyl-D-glucosaminidase
Type III-D	252940	Acetyl-CoA-glucosaminide-N-acetyltransferase
		N-Acetylglucosaminine-6-sulphate-sulphatase
MPS IV (Morquio's syndrome)		
Type IV-A	253000	Galactosamine-6-sulphate-sulphatase
Type IV-B	253010	β-galactosidase
MPS VI (Maroteaux–Lamy syndrome)	253200	Arylsulfatase B
MPS VII (Sly's syndrome)	253220	β-Glucuronidase
MPS IX (Hyaluronidase deficiency)	601492	Hyaluronidase
Mucolipidoses (ML)		
ML II (I-cell disease)	252500	N-Acetylglucosaminyl-1-phosphotransferase
ML-III (Pseudo-Hurler's syndrome)		N-Acetylglucosaminyl-1-phosphotransferase
Type III-A	252600	
Type III-C	252605	
Sphingolipidoses		
GM1 Gangliosidosis		Ganglioside-β-galactosidase
Type I	230500	
Type II	230600	
Type III	230650	
GM2 Gangliosidosis		
Type I (Tay–Sachs disease)	272800	β-Hexosaminidase A
Type II (Sandhoff's disease)	268800	β-Hexosaminidase B
Type III (juvenile type)		β-Hexosaminidase A
GM2 activator protein deficiency	272750	GM2 activator protein
Niemann–Pick disease		Sphingomyelinase
Type A	257200	
Type B	607616	
Gaucher's disease		β-Glucocerebrosidase
Type I (adult form)	230800	
Type II (infantile form)	230900	
Type III (juvenile form)	231000	

Table 170.1 (Continued)

Lipogranulomatose (Farber's disease)	228000	Ceramidase
Fabry's disease	301500	α-Galactosidase A
Metachromatic leucodystrophy	250100	Arylsulpgatase A
Mucosulfatidosis	272200	Sulphatase-modifying factor 1
Krabbe's disease	245200	Galactosylceramide-β-galactosidase
Sphingolipid activatating protein deficiency	176801	Prosaposin, saposin B

[a]Online Mendelian Inheritance in Man, online database of the National Center for Biotechnology Information.

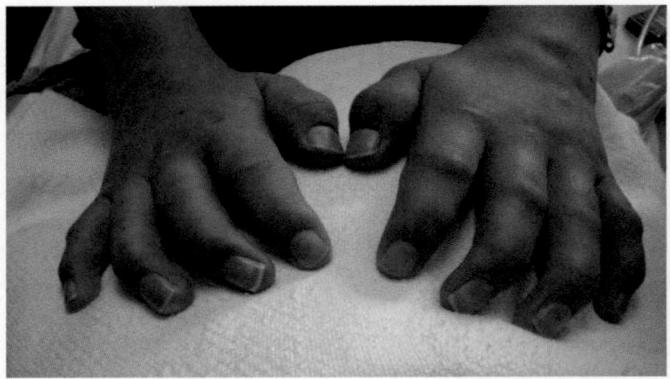

Fig. 170.1 Mild flexion contractures of the fingers in Hurler–Scheie syndrome. Reproduced with permission from Morishita K , Petty R E "Musculoskeletal manifestations of mucopolysaccharidoses" in Rheumatology 2011; Volume 50, Issue suppl 5Pp. v19–v25. © Oxford University Press.

is much lower than in adults, this symptom should raise the level of suspicion. More than one-half of all cases of carpal tunnel syndrome in children are caused by MPS.[10] Trigger fingers in MPS can be caused by glycosaminoglycan deposits within tendon sheaths.[11]

The characteristic bone involvement in MPS is described as dysostosis multiplex. This comprises skeletal abnormalities such as macrocephaly, odontoid hypoplasia, flattened vertebral bodies, thoracolumbar kyphosis, and thickening of ribs, clavicles, and phalanges. Lower limb abnormalities include flattened acetabula (Figure 170.2), dysplasia of femoral heads, coxa valga, and genu valgum. Growth retardation can be present but is usually not the leading symptom in attenuated MPS.

In contrast to the other variants, MPS type IV is characterized by significant joint hypermobility resulting from ligamentous laxity and bone hypoplasia or deformity. It is most obvious in hands and wrists and contrasts with proximal stiffness. MPS type III is mainly a neurological disorder with few or no musculoskeletal manifestations and for type IX there are only very few cases reported in the literature, with normal joint mobility.

Besides bone and joint manifestations, patients with attenuated forms of MPS frequently develop corneal clouding and thickening with dysfunction of mitral and aortic valves as leading symptoms. Other typical symptoms include frequent pulmonary and ear infections, obstructive sleep apnoea, hearing loss, abdominal hernias, hepatosplenomegaly, and spinal cord compression.[3]

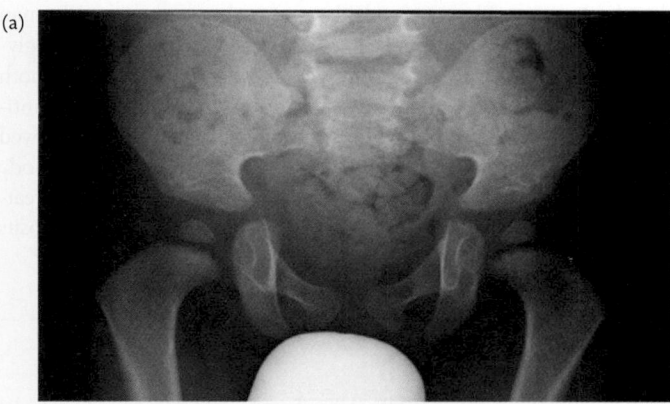

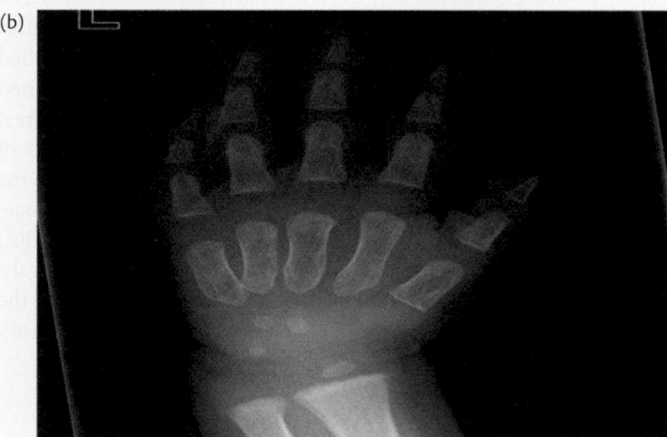

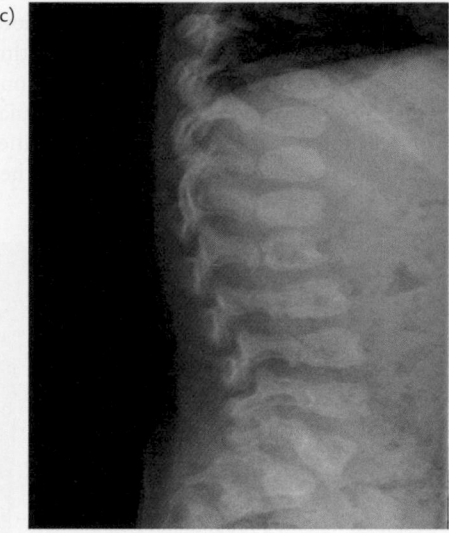

Fig. 170.2 Dysostosis multiplex. A 2 year old boy with Hunter's syndrome (MPS II): (A) Radiograph of the pelvis showing flared iliac bones with flattened acetabula. (B) Radiograph of the left hand showing bullet-shaped phalanges and short metacarpals with proximal pointing. (C) Radiograph of the thoracolumbar spine showing platyspondyly and inferior beaking of the second lumbar vertebra. Reproduced with permission from Morishita K , Petty R E "Musculoskeletal manifestations of mucopolysaccharidoses" in Rheumatology 2011;.Volume 50, Issue suppl 5Pp. v19-v25. © Oxford University Press.

Diagnosis

A recently published algorithm recommends a quantitative and qualitative analysis of GAG excretion in a specialized laboratory for all patients with joint contractures without clinical or laboratory signs of inflammation. Measuring an elevated GAG concentration in the urine is very suggestive for MPS, but a negative test does not rule out this diagnosis. The determination of specific enzyme activities in plasma or in cultured fibroblasts or leucocytes is the diagnostic gold standard for defined MPS disorders. Gene sequencing can then identify the underlying mutation.[8]

Therapy

The optimal treatment of all the comorbidities of MPS requires a multidisciplinary approach involving physiotherapists, cardiologists, otorhinolaryngologists, pneumologists, rheumatologists, neurosurgeons, and orthopaedic surgeons.[12]

Treatment of the underlying enzyme deficiency is possible by two different principles: haematopoietic stem cell transplantation and ERT. Haematopoietic stem cell transplantation within the first 2 years of life is indicated for severe MPS forms with neurological involvement, because stem cells can engraft and differentiate in the CNS. In contrast, infused enzymes are too large to cross the blood–brain barrier. Therefore, ERT is the treatment of choice for non-neurological types and attenuated forms of MPS. ERT with recombinant form of the deficient enzymes has been approved for MPS I (laronidase), MPS II (idursulfase), and MPS VI (galsufase), a therapy for MPS IV and VII, is in development. An improvement of hepatomegaly, walking ability, shoulder mobility, and enhanced quality of life has been demonstrated with ERT.[13,14]

Fabry's disease

Pathogenesis

Fabry's disease is a hereditary, X-linked LSD, caused by a reduced or absent activity of α-galactosidase A. More than 60 mutations of the gene for this enzyme, located on the long arm of the X chromosome, have been described. The reduced enzyme activity leads to an accumulation of the glycosphingolipid globotriaosylceramide in the lysosomes particularly of endothelial cells. The characteristic skin manifestations were first described in 1898, independently by two dermatologists, J. Fabry and W. Anderson.[12] The prevalence of the disease is about 1 in 40 000 males. Heterozygous women can also develop a form of Fabry's disease, but this is usually milder due to random X-chromosomal inactivation. The mean delay between the onset of symptoms and diagnosis is 14 years in men with Fabry's disease, in women even more than 16 years.[15]

Clinical manifestations

Normally, the first symptoms appear in schoolchildren or young adults. These consist of attacks of intense burning pain and paresthesias in the extremities (acroparesthesia). These attacks can be triggered by physical exercise, stress, rapid temperature changes, or infection. Such a disease flare itself can cause fever, adynamia, and elevation of inflammatory markers. For that reason, the pain in hands, wrists, feet, and ankles is sometimes misinterpreted as a symptom of juvenile idiopathic arthritis or rheumatic fever. The pathogenetic basis of these symptoms is a C-fibre neuropathy caused by globotriaosylceramide deposits in vasa nervorum, neurons, and spinal ganglia.[16] Crucial diagnostic information can be obtained from the medical history. Frequently patients report heat or exercise intolerance and the inability to sweat (hypohidrosis). When the patient reaches adulthood, the acroparesthesias slowly subside and symptoms from other organ systems arise. An early manifestation is also the appearance of non-blanching angiokeratomas at thighs, buttocks, and around the umbilicus (Figure 170.3). These

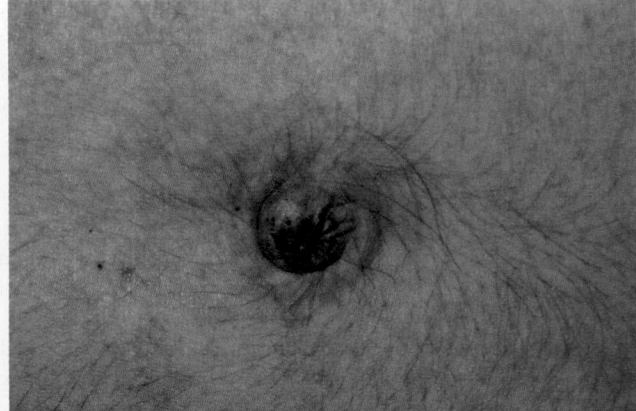

Fig. 170.3 Non-blanching angiokeratomas around the umbilicus in a patient with Fabry's disease.

are characteristic tiny, dark red, painless papules with a characteristic histology. Therefore, the initial diagnosis of Fabry's disease is frequently established by a dermatologist ('angiokeratoma corporis diffusum Fabry'). Another symptom is corneal clouding with a typical linear pattern of whorled opacities within the cornea (cornea verticillata). This finding is so characteristic on slit-lamp examination that the ophthalmologist also plays a key role in the diagnostic process. The only differential diagnoses of these corneal opacities are drug-induced alterations (e.g. amiodarone, chloroquine).

In adulthood, untreated Fabry's disease leads to various visceral manifestations: kidney involvement initially leads to proteinuria and slow loss of function progressing over the years to endstage renal failure. Typical cardiac manifestations are valvular abnormalities (most frequently mitral regurgitation), ventricular hypertrophy, congestive heart failure, atrial fibrillation, and other arrhythmias. Cerebrovascular symptoms include dizziness, tinnitus, hearing loss, transient ischaemic attacks, white matter lesions, and early stroke. Gastrointestinal involvement presents as diarrhoea, nausea, malabsorption, and abdominal pain. Affected women may experience acroparesthesias in adolescence and cardiac symptoms in adulthood, but a progression to endstage renal disease is very rare.

Diagnosis

The most important diagnostic clue is a detailed family history with a focus on renal, cardiac, or cerebrovascular disorders at a relatively young age in (male) relatives. In Fabry registers more than 90% of all patients had at least one diseased relative.[17] In males with the classic phenotype, the diagnosis is easily confirmed by measuring a reduced α-galactosidase A activity in plasma or leukocytes. In females the enzyme activity can be in the low normal range, so the direct detection of a mutation in at least one allele of the α-galactosidase A gene may be required.

Therapy

The infusion of α-galactosidase A can reverse globotriaosylceramide depositions in involved tissues and inhibit disease progression. Therefore, ERT is indicated in all affected men once the diagnosis is established. Women with substantial disease manifestations and children with severe acroparesthesia, fatigue, and exercise and heat intolerance should also receive this treatment. Two compounds have been approved for the treatment of Fabry's disease: a gene-activated

human α-galactosidase A (agalsidase α) and a recombinant human α-galactosidase A (agalsidase β). Despite slight differences in glycosylation patterns the specific activity and immunogenicity of both products appears similar, and infusion reactions caused by IgG antibodies to the protein moiety of the molecules can occur. The approved dosages are 0.2 mg/kg body weight for agalsidase α and 1 mg/kg body weight for agalsidase β as biweekly infusions.[18,19] After prolonged treatment with agalsidase β, a clearance of globotriaosylceramide deposits has been demonstrated histologically in kidneys, heart, and skin.[20]

Gaucher's disease

Pathogenesis

Gaucher's disease was initially described in 1882 and is considered the most frequent LSD with a prevalence of 1 in 60 000 live births. It is caused by a defect of the enzyme β-glucocerebrosidase encoded on chromosome 1. Because there are more than 200 described mutations the phenotype can be very heterogeneous. Of interest for the rheumatologist is mainly the non-neuronopathic type I of Gaucher's disease (about 85% of all cases). The underlying enzyme deficiency causes an accumulation of glucocerebrosides in tissue macrophages, causing them to increase in volume ('Gaucher cells') which leads to bone marrow replacement and hepatosplenomegaly. In addition, those macrophages become activated and influence the production of proinflammatory cytokines and immunoregulatory functions of B lymphocytes and neutrophils.[2,7]

Clinical manifestations

The musculoskeletal symptoms are mainly caused by the bone marrow infiltration and expansion by Gaucher cells. Vessel occlusions and elevated intraosseous pressure in combination with cytokine release lead to an increased bone turnover and defective bone remodelling. Consequences are osteopenia, bone pain, avascular necrosis, osteolytic lesions, pathologic fractures, and deformities (Figure 170.4). If these pathologies are located close to a joint, they

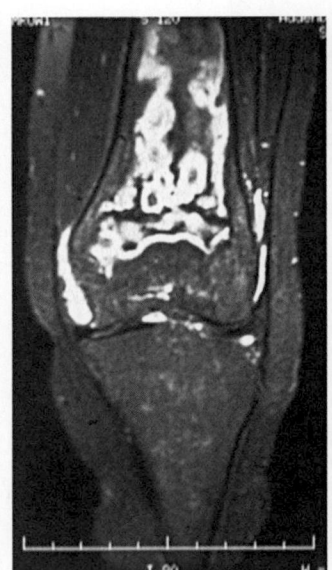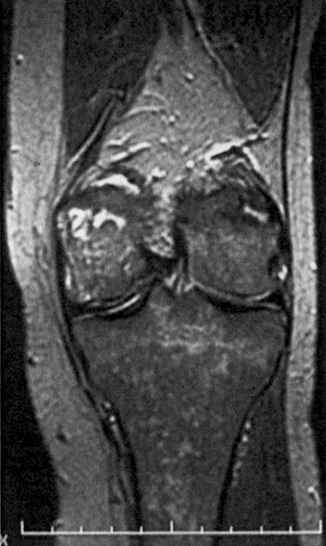

Fig. 170.4 T1 (left)- and T2 (right)-weighted MRI obtained from the lower femur and upper tibia of a 30 year old woman with non-neuronopathic Gaucher's disease experiencing pain due to acute avascular necrosis of bone.
P.B. Deegan, T.M. Cox Oxford Textbook of Medicine: Lysosomal disease

Table 170.2 Clinical and laboratory features of lysosomal storage diseases relevant for the rheumatologist

Disease	Musculoskeletal symptoms	General/visceral symptoms	Laboratory tests	Musculoskeletal imaging	Differential diagnosis
Mucopoly-saccharidoses	Joint contractures, carpal tunnel syndrome, trigger finger, dysostosis multiplex, hip dysplasia, spinal cord compression *In type IV:* ligamentous laxity/joint hypermobility	Corneal clouding, glaucoma, valvular heart disease, hernias, hepatosplenomegaly, pulmonary and ear infections, growth retardation	Inflammatory parameters normal, glucosaminoglycane excretion in urine ↑ (altered patterns of GAG excretion), enzyme activities in leukocytes ↓	Dysostosis multiplex, hip dysplasia, kyphosis, scoliosis, gibbus formation	Other causes for carpal tunnel syndrome, tenosynovitis, JIA, spondyloarthritis, fibromatoses
Fabry's disease	Painful attacks of acroparesthesia in hands and feet	Heat intolerance, hypohidrosis, fever, adynamia, cornea verticillata, angiokeratomas, proteinuria, renal failure, cardiac arrhythmias, ventricular hypertrophy, cardiomyopathy, cerebrovascular events, nausea, diarrhoea, malabsorption, abdominal pain	Inflammatory parameters ↑ (during flares), α-galactosidase in plasma or leucocytes ↓ or genotyping, *later:* creatinine ↑, proteinuria	Normal	Polyneuropathies, JIA, adult-onset Still's disease, autoinflammatory diseases, collagen vascular diseases, vasculitides, amyloidosis, 'growing pains'
Gaucher's disease	Bone pain, bone deformity, pathologic fracture, AVN	Splenomegaly, hepatomegaly, haemorrhagic diathesis, growth retardation	Pancytopenia, inflammatory parameters ↑, chitotriosidase ↑, β-glucocerebrosidase ↓	Osteopenia, osteolytic lesions, bone infarctions, AVN, bone marrow infiltration (MRI)	Other causes for AVN, oligoarthritis, autoinflammatory diseases, multiple myeloma, sickle cell anaemia, osteomyelitis

AVN, avascular necrosis; GAG, glycosaminoglycan; JIA, juvenile idiopathic arthritis.

can cause effusions and immobility. Because of the local and systemic inflammatory character a misinterpretation of the symptoms as chronic rheumatic condition is not uncommon.[21] The symptoms frequently present as flares or 'bone crises', therefore sickle cell anaemia or osteomyelitis also have to be considered in the differential diagnostic process. All symptomatic patients with Gaucher's disease present with splenomegaly and usually also hepatomegaly. The volume of the spleen can increase enormously and lead to pain, infarction, and replacement of abdominal or pelvic organs. The resulting hypersplenism results in anaemia, thrombocytopenia, and thus fatigue and bleeding diathesis. Less frequent organ manifestations are interstitial lung disease and pulmonary hypertension.

Diagnosis

In most cases, the bony deformities, osteolytic lesions, fractures, or avascular necroses are initially detected by conventional radiographs. In contrast, MRI is able to detect the underlying bone marrow infiltration already in early stages of the disease. Frequently, the initial diagnosis of Gaucher's disease is established when a bone marrow biopsy is performed because of cytopenias and the typical macrophages are found.

Confirmation of the diagnosis requires measurement of a reduced β-glucocerebrosidase activity in leucocytes. A helpful, but less specific test is the determination of plasma chitotriosidase activity. This parameter is markedly elevated in most Gaucher patients and can also be used for therapy monitoring.

Therapy

ERT is the treatment of choice in non-neuronopathic Gaucher's disease. Recombinant human glucocerebrosidase (imiglucerase,

velaglucerase α) is give as infusions of up to 60 U/kg body weight at 2 week intervals. Regular follow-up visits are required for dose adaptations depending on clinical and laboratory parameters. This treatment not only leads to a normalization of haematological parameters and reduction of liver and spleen size, but also an improvement of acute and chronic bone symptoms.[22]

Conclusion

LSD can cause a variety of musculoskeletal symptoms (Table 170.2). These are frequently the initial reason why children and young adults with these disorders seek medical advice. Because effective treatments are available for several of these disorders (MPS I, II, VI, Fabry's and Gaucher's disease), an early diagnosis has become crucial for the preservation of organ functions and quality of life. The rheumatologist may play a key role in the diagnostic process and should therefore be familiar with the typical clinical manifestations of these diseases.

References

1. *Lysosomal storage disorders.* The Merck Manuals Online Medical Library for Health Care Professionals. Available at: www.merck.com/media/mmpe/pdf/Table_296-4w.pdf (accessed 12 August 2011).
2. Manger B. Lysosomale Speicherkrankheiten. *Z Rheumatol* 2010;69: 527–538.
3. Aldenhoven M, Sakkers RJB, Boelens J, de Koning TJ, Wulffraat NM. Muskuloskelettal manifestations of lysosomal storage disorders. *Ann Rheum Dis* 2009;68:1659–1665.
4. Scheie H, Hambrick G, Barnes L. A newly recognized forme fruste of Hurler's disease (gargoylism). *Am J Ophthalmol* 1962;53:753–769.
5. Pastores GM, Arn P, Beck M *et al.* The MPS I registry: design, methodology, and early findings of a global disease registry for monitoring patients with mucopolysaccharidosis type I. *Mol Gen Metab* 2007;91:37–47.

6. Cimaz R, Vijay S, Haase C *et al.* Attenuated type I mucopolysaccharidosis in the differential diagnosis of juvenile idiopathic arthritis: a series of 13 patients with Scheie syndrome. *Clin Exp Rheumatol* 2006;24:196–202.

7. Manger B, Mengel E, Schaefer RM. Rheumatologic aspects of lysosomal storage diseases. *Clin Rheum* 2007;26:335–341.

8. Cimaz R, Coppa GV, Koné-Paut I *et al.* Joint contractures in the absence of inflammation may indicate mucopolysaccharidosis. *Pediatr Rheumatol Online J* 2009;7:18.

9. Manger B. Rheumatological manifestations are key in the early diagnosis of mucopolysaccharidosis type I. *Eur Musculoskelet Rev* 2008;3: 23–26.

10. VanMeir, de Smet L. Carpal tunnel syndrome in children. *Acta Orthop Belg* 2003;69:387–395.

11. Matsui Y, Kawabata H, Nakayama M et al. Scheie syndrome (MPS-IS) presented as bilateral trigger thumb. *Pediatr Int* 2003;45:91–92.

12. Michels H, Mengel E. Lysosomal storage diseases as differential diagnoses to rheumatic disorders. *Curr Opin Rheum* 2008;20:76–81.

13. Wraith JE, Clarke LA, Beck M, et al. Enzyme replacement therapy for mucopolysaccharidosis I: a randomized, double-blinded, placebo-controlled, multinational study of recombinant human alpha-L-iduronidase (laronidase). *J Pediatr* 2004;144:581–588.

14. Sifuentes M, Doroshow R, Hoft R. A follow-up study of MPS I patients treated with laronidase enzyme replacement therapy for 6 years. *Mol Genet Metab* 2007;90:171–180.

15. Mehta A, Ricci R, Widmer U *et al.* Fabry disease defined: baseline clinical manifestations of 366 patients in the Fabry Outcome Survey. *Eur J Clin Invest* 2004;34:236–242.

16. Clarke JT. Narrative review: Fabry disease. *Ann Intern Med* 2007;146: 425–433.

17. Eng CM, Fletcher J, Wilcox WR *et al.* Fabry disease: baseline medical characteristics of a cohort of 1756 males and females in the Fabry Registry. *J Inherit Metab Dis* 2007;30:184–192.

18. Schiffmann R, Koop JB, Austin HA III *et al.* Enzyme replacement therapy in Fabry disease: a randomized controlled trial. *JAMA* 2001;285: 2743–2749.

19. Eng CM, Guffon N, Wilcox WR *et al.* Safety and efficacy of recombinant human alpha-galactosidase A-replacement therapy in Fabry's disease. *New Engl J Med* 2001;345:9–16.

20. Thurberg BL, Rennke H, Colvin RB *et al.* Globotriaosylceramide accumulation in the Fabry kidney is cleared from multiple cell types after enzyme replacement therapy. *Kidney Int* 2002;62:1933–1946.

21. Weizman Z, Tennenbaum, Yatziv S. Interphalangeal joint involvement in Gaucher's disease, type I, resembling juvenile rheumatoid arthritis. *Arthritis Rheum* 1982;25:706–707.

22. Weinreb NJ, Charrow J, Andersson HC *et al.* Effectiveness of enzyme replacement therapy in 1028 patients with type I Gaucher disease after 2 to 5 years of treatment: a report from the Gaucher registry. *Am J Med* 2002;113:112–119.

CHAPTER 171

Rheumatological manifestations of endocrine disorders

Sanjeev Sharma and Gerry Rayman

Introduction

Involvement of the musculoskeletal and connective tissue systems is common in endocrine disorders, with many patients initially presenting to the rheumatologist. On the other hand patients, with established endocrine disease may later develop musculoskeletal-related complications. Therefore, to ensure that the associated condition is not missed or the diagnosis not delayed, both endocrinologists and rheumatologists need to be aware of these associations.

Endocrine disorders can involve a variety of tissues including bones, muscles, nerves, and joints. This chapter considers these associations from a rheumatologist's point of view and presents them in four categories: endocrine conditions that involve bones, joints, muscle, and supporting adnexa. A tabular classification of endocrine disorders with rheumatological complications has also been provided to complete the description from the endocrine perspective.

Disorders of bones

A large number of endocrine disorders can affect the skeletal system. The common skeletal disorders arising from or associated with endocrinopathies as now described.

Osteoporosis and osteomalacia

Osteoporosis results from bone loss due to age-related changes in bone remodelling as well as extrinsic and intrinsic factors that exaggerate this process, of which endocrinopathies constitute an important aggravating factor.[1] In contrast, osteomalacia refers to abnormal bone because of abnormal mineralization of the bone matrix. The following endocrine disorders are associated with these states.

Parathyroid disorders

Both hyperparathyroidism and hypoparathyroidism can worsen osteoporosis although the former is more commonly encountered in the clinical setting. Primary hyperparathyroidism (PHPT) results from parathyroid adenomas or hyperplasia of the parathyroids and is characterized by high levels of both calcium and parathyroid hormone (PTH; Table 171.1) or hypercalcaemia in the presence of detectable rather than suppressed PTH levels. It preferentially affects cortical bone as opposed to trabecular bone and therefore forearm bone mineral density (BMD) in comparison with vertebral BMD is helpful when assessing the extent of the involvement. Osteoporosis is one of the indications for parathyroidectomy. Silverberg et al.,[2] in a 10 year old prospective study, showed improvement of BMD and normalization of biochemical markers following surgical treatment of PHPT. Medical management of PHPT includes use of bisphophonates and correction of vitamin D deficiency.

Secondary hyperparathyroidism (SHPT) is encountered commonly in calcium and vitamin D deficiency and also in advanced chronic kidney disease. Rarely long-standing and untreated SHPT leads to autonomous activity of the parathyroid glands causing tertiary hyperparathyroidism (THPT).

Hypoparathyroidism is a relatively rare disorder, most commonly encountered following parathyroid and thyroid surgeries. Less common is primary hypoparathyroidism due to autoimmune destruction and very rarely hypoparathyroidism can follow neck radiation. Hypoparathyroidism is characterized by low calcium and high phosphate levels in the presence of a low PTH level. Rheumatological symptoms include bone pain, muscle cramps, and paraesthesiae. Untreated hypoparathyroidism can lead to entheseal

Table 171.1 Types of hyperparathyroidism

Type	Calcium	PTH	Management
Primary	↑	↑ (or normal)	Medical/surgical
Secondary	↓ (or normal)	↑	Correction of vitamin D deficiency, calcitriol, phosphate binders
Tertiary	↑	↑	Parathyroidectomy

PTH, parathyroid hormone.

and ligamentous ossifications. Replacement therapy with calcium and calcitriol is the cornerstone of treatment but care should be taken to prevent hypercalciuria since these patients are susceptible to nephrocalcinosis and urinary stone disease.

Hyperthyroidism

Hypothyroidism is defined as a state of excess circulatory thyroid hormones most commonly related to either overactivity of the thyroid gland (diffuse or nodular disease) or iatrogenic due to over-replacement of thyroid hormones. Hyperthyroidism leads to increased bone loss mainly affecting cortical than trabecular bone. Baqi et al.[3] showed that BMD and markers of bone turnover were significantly better when thyroid-stimulating hormone (TSH) was maintained between 0.35 mU/litre and 6.3 mU/litre compared to women with a TSH lower than 0.3 mU/;itre. While correction of the hyperthyroid state remains the cornerstone of management, use of bisphophonates can help to prevent bone loss in those in whom the hyperthyroid state is difficult to control[4] and in those who have already developed osteoporosis.

Vitamin D deficiency

In the United Kingdom, the prevalence of vitamin D deficiency in all adults is around 14.5%, but may be more than 30% in those over 65 years old, and as high as 94% in otherwise healthy South Asian adults.[5] UVB radiation mediates the majority of vitamin D production in the body by converting cutaneous 7-dehydrocholesterol to cholecalciferol (vitamin D_3), but this can be supplemented by ingestion of fatty fish (cod, salmon) and plant ergocalciferol (vitamin D_2).

Rickets, which is classically seen in children prior to the fusion of the epiphyses, is now uncommon in the developed world. Poor mineralization of bones leads to bowing of tibia, swelling of rib cartilages ('rachitic rosary'), widening of epiphyseal joints, and also causes developmental delay. Older people with reduced exposure to sunlight are susceptible to osteomalacia. Apart from bone pain, vitamin D deficiency may also cause proximal myopathy resulting in further restriction of daily activities. The Endocrine Society[6] recommends using the serum circulating 25-hydroxyvitamin D (25(OH) D) level, measured by a reliable assay, to evaluate vitamin D status in patients who are at risk of vitamin D deficiency.

Vitamin D *deficiency* is defined as a 25(OH) D level below 20 ng/mL (50 nmol/litre) and vitamin D *insufficiency* as a 25(OH) D of 21–29 ng/mL (50–72.5 nmol/litre). The Endocrine Practice Guidelines[6] recommended dietary intakes for patients at risk as given in (Table 171.2).

Table 171.2 Recommended intake of vitamin D[6]

Age group (years)		Daily requirement (IU)
Children	1–8	600–1000
Males	9–18	600–1000
	>19	1500–2000
Females	9–18	600–1000
	>19	1500–2000
Pregnancy		1500–2000
Lactation		1500–2000

Cushing's syndrome and use of glucocorticoids

Cushing's syndrome is caused by excessive endogenous production of steroids related to adrenal conditions (adenoma, hyperplasia, or malignancy) or less commonly due to a pituitary adenoma (Cushing's disease). The same phenotypical features of centripetal obesity, easy bruising, ecchymosis, and hypertension can also be caused iatrogenically by the use of glucocorticoid medications to treat other medical conditions. The rheumatological effects of glucocorticoid excess include increased bone resorption and acceleration of osteoporosis leading to increased risk of fractures, more in trabecular than cortical bone. In a study by Chiodiniet al.,[7] subclinical hypercortisolaemia was found in 4.8% among patients with osteoporosis.

All patients with Cushing's syndrome or on glucocorticoid therapy equivalent to 5 mg or more of prednisolone/day for 3 months should have modification of risk factors and BMD measured at baseline.[8] If the T-score is less than −1, then consider bone protection by treatment with bisphophonates along with calcium (total 1500 mg/day) and vitamin D (400–800 IU/day).[8]

Hyperprolactinaemia

Hyperprolactinaemia is the commonest of the pituitary disorders and can result from a variety of disorders that cause oversecretion of the peptide hormone prolactin by the lactotroph cells of the anterior pituitary gland. These are summarized in Box 171.1. Hyperprolactaemia commonly presents with one or a combination of galactorrhoea, amenorrhea, infertility, and loss of libido. Sustained elevation of prolactin levels results in hypoestrogenism with subsequent accelerated bone loss and osteoporotic fractures.[9] Hyperprolactinaemic patients should be screened for osteoporosis and treated on standard lines. Similarly, young patients with osteoporosis and amenorrhoea should be screened for hyperprolactinaemia.

Hypogonadal states

Age-related changes in skeletal architecture leading to osteoporosis in both sexes are due to diminution of sex steroids. The relationship of the female menopause with osteoporosis is well recognized, but male age-related osteoporosis is less well recognized; it is defined as the occurrence of osteoporosis in men over 70 years of age without any other known cause.[9] The rate of decline of both cortical and trabecular bone is similar in both sexes but men have a reduced fracture rate due to attainment of a higher peak bone density and unlike women, do not have the equivalent of a period of accelerated bone turnover as occurs during the perimenopausal period. While hypogonadal levels of total testosterone are clearly associated with osteoporosis and increased hip fractures,[10] across the testosterone range reduction of BMD has only been shown to be directly related to bioavailable testosterone and not total testosterone—the latter does not necessarily reflect bioactive testosterone, being influenced by the level of sex hormone binding globulin.[11]

Classical hypogonadal conditions such as Klinefelter's syndrome, Kallman's syndrome, and idiopathic hypogonadotrophic hypogonadism as well as secondary hypogonadism (e.g. pituitary adenomas, following hypophysectomy) are commonly associated with osteoporosis. Indeed, it is not unusual for these conditions to be discovered when the patient presents with a fragility fracture. Testosterone treatment in hypogonadal men is very effective and will increase BMD by approximately 7.5% in the lumbar region (L2–4) and by 5% in the femoral trochanteric area.[12] Such replacement

Box 171.1 Common causes of hyperprolactinaemia

Physiological hypersecretion

- Chest wall stimulation
- Sleep
- Stress
- Pregnancy
- Lactation

Systemic disorders

- Hypothyroidism
- Chronic renal failure
- Cirrhosis
- Epilepsy

Pituitary hypersecretion

- Prolactinoma
- Acromegaly

Hypothalamic–pituitary stalk damage

- Pituitary adenomas with stalk compression
- Non-pituitary tumours
  - Craniopharyngioma
  - Meningioma
  - Dysgerminoma
- Rathke's cyst
- Irradiation

Drug-induced secretion

- Dopamine synthesis inhibitors: α-methyl dopa
- Dopamine receptor blockers: chlorpromazine, haloperidol, metoclopramide
- Opiates
- H2 receptor antagonists: cimetidine, ranitidine
- Serotonin reuptake inhibitors: fluoxetine
- Calcium channel blockers: verapamil
- Oestrogens/androgens

has to be carefully instituted and the patient and spouse/partner counselled, as behavioural changes and increased libido can cause significant emotional and psychological distress to the patient and the relationship.

Hyperparathyroidism

Skeletal manifestations of hyperparathyroidism were common in the past but with increased awareness and earlier detection of asymptomatic cases, the overall incidence of skeletal-related compliactions is declining.

Osteitis fibrosa cystica

Osteitis fibrosa cystica (OFC), a distinctive feature of hyperparathyroidism, is now rare with a reported incidence of 3–4% in PHPT and 1.5% in SHPT in some series.[13] It is due to exaggerated osteoclast-mediated bony resorption with replacement of marrow and cellular elements with fibrosis. A classic example of OFC is the brown tumour commonly seen in the mandible and maxilla, but it can also involve ribs, clavicle and pelvis. Clinically, these are benign, soft, and painless but can lead to disfigurement. There is no specific treatment other than managing the hyperparathyroidism. Other associations of OFC include thinning of cortical bone leading to a 'salt-and-pepper' appearance and disappearance of lamina dura from the root of teeth.

'Rugger jersey' spine

This classic feature of SHPT associated with chronic renal failure (CRF) is characterized by alternate sclerotic bands on the upper and lower vertebral body margins sandwiching areas of lucency in the body, giving the striped appearance of a traditional rugby jersey. Some studies have reported an incidence as high as 27% in patients with CRF on haemodialysis.[14]

Subperiosteal resorption

This is now the commonest radiological feature of hyperparathyroidism. Resorption along the shaft of phalanges gives a 'sawtooth' appearance but can also affect the humerus, clavicles, and sacroiliac joints, leading to pseudo-widening of joints. Acroosteolysis is an extreme form of resorption of the tufts of terminal phalanges seen in radiographs of the hand.

Fragility fractures

One-half or more of patients with hyperparathyroidism are asymptomatic and diagnosed when screened for complications including fragility fractures, osteoporosis, and renal calculus. Although cortical bones are more affected, leading to involvement of the appendicular skeleton, the incidence of vertebral fractures is also increased. Involvement of sacroiliac joint causes deformities of the pelvic skeleton and gait problems.

Disorders of joints

Endocrine-associated arthropathies constitute an important differential in the diagnosis of arthritis associated with systemic disorders. Not uncommonly, the endocrine diagnosis only comes to light as a result of the investigations undertaken to evaluate the arthritic complaint.

Diabetes mellitus

This is the commonest of the endocrine conditions. In 2009, the estimated worldwide prevalence of diabetes was 285 million and this is expected to increase to 438 million by 2030.[15] In England in 2012, 2.9 million people have been diagnosed with diabetes with another 800 000 undiagnosed. It has been estimated that by 2025 there will be more than 4 million people with diabetes in the United Kingdom.[16] Broadly, type 1 diabetes is caused by absolute insulin deficiency mediated by an autoimmune destruction of the pancreatic beta cells, while type 2 diabetes is due to insulin resistance and relative insulin deficiency. Characterization of rheumatological manifestations in diabetes is mostly based on observational data,[17,18] although some conditions are classically seen in diabetes (Box 171.2).

Box 171.2 Rheumatological manifestations in diabetes mellitus

Manifestations specific to diabetes

- Diabetes muscle infarction (rare)

Manifestations more common in diabetes

- Limited joint mobility/diabetes cheiroarthropathy
- Charcot's osteoarthropathy
- Carpel tunnel syndrome
- Tarsal tunnel syndrome
- Dupuytren's disease
- Stenosing flexor tenosynovitis (trigger finger)
- Adhesive capsulitis of the shoulder (frozen shoulder syndrome)
- Calcific shoulder periarthritis
- Plantar faciitis
- Achilles tendonitis

Manifestations sharing risk factors of diabetes

- Diffuse idiopathic skeletal hypersostosis
- Crystal-induced arthropathies (gout and pseudogout)

Adapted from Lebiedz-Odrobina and Kay.[19]

Diabetes cheiroarthropathy (limited joint mobility)

First described by Lundbaek in 1957,[20] diabetes cheiroarthropathy is not a classical joint disorder since there is more involvement of periarticular structures. Different series have quoted its prevalence as 30–58% in type 1 diabetes and 45–76% in type 2 diabetes,[21] but common determinants in both groups include increased duration of diabetes and presence of microvascular complications including retinopathy and nephropathy.[22,23]

It is characterized by thick, tight, waxy skin on the dorsal aspect of the fingers and metacarpophalangeal joints and sclerosis of tendon sheaths resulting in limited joint mobility and characteristic flexion contractures (inability to fully flex or extend the fingers). The characteristic clinical finding is the so called 'prayer sign'—the inability to completely appose the palms without a gap remaining between opposed palms and fingers. The underlying cause is thought to be multifactorial and related to increased glycosylation of collagen in the skin and periarticular tissue. There is no specific therapy apart from physiotherapy and efforts to improve glycaemic control.

Charcot's osteoarthropathy

Although neuropathic osteoarthropathy was first described in 1868 by Jean-Martin Charcot as a complication of neurosyphilis,[24] diabetes is now its commonest cause, with an estimated prevalence of 0.15% which increases to 13% in specialized foot clinics. Pathophysiologically, its development is believed to be related to a combination of repetitive trauma or injury in an insensate foot *(neurotraumatic theory)* and autonomic neuropathy causing increased blood flow *(neurovascular theory)* leading to increased recruitment of osteoclasts causing release of proinflammatory cytokines which cause bone resorption and destruction. More recent evidence implicates the RANK/RANK-ligand/osteoprotegerin (OPG) system in the pathogenesis of the osteoclastic resorption and osteopaenia.[25] Although almost invariably associated with chronic painless diabetic neuropathy, acute Charcot's osteoarthropathy is often painful, but the degree of pain may be less than expected in relationship to the severity of the clinical and radiological findings, and indeed pain is frequently absent. The foot is the most commonly affected region, with a predilection to involve the ankle mortise, tarsometatarsal, metatarsophalangeal, and interphalageal joints. The area is characteristically warm, with overlying skin erythema and diffuse swelling. The diagnosis is mainly based on clinical features aided by radiological investigations (Figure 171.1) including MRI and indium-111-leucocyte (^{111}In-WBC); but even then distinction from osteomyelitis can remain difficult.

Immobilization with total contact cast for up to 12 months to support the joint and prevent further trauma is the cornerstone of treatment. Intravenous bisphophonates are commonly used as adjuvant therapy to inhibit osteoclast-mediated bone destruction but the evidence for their use is limited.[26]

Diffuse idiopathic skeletal hyperostosis—Forestier's disease

Diffuse idiopathic skeletal hyperostosis (DISH) was described in 1950 by Forestier and Rotes-Querol as an age-dependent condition characterized by calcification and ossification of ligament, tendon, and joint capsule (enthesial) insertions. The anterior and posterior longitudinal ligaments are commonly involved, resulting in restriction of a range of spinal movements. Its association with diabetes is probably related to hyperinsulinaemia as evidenced by prevalence

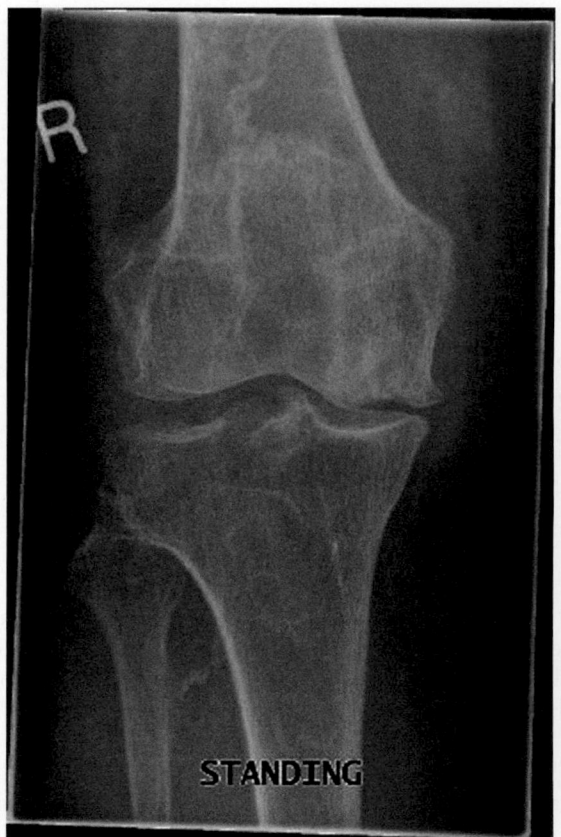

Fig. 171.1 Standing plain radiograph of knee showing early osteoarthritic changes and an increase in joint space

(13–40%)[27] when compared to the general population. Raised insulin and insulin-like growth factor (IGF)-1 levels have been postulated as contributory to accelerated ossification in DISH,[28] although this association has not been seen in patients with impaired glucose tolerance.[29]

Treatment is supportive with analgesia, local corticosteroid injections, and spinal physiotherapy.

Crystal-induced arthritis

Gout

Obesity, insulin resistance, and risk for type 2 diabetes as components of the metabolic syndrome have now been well documented in many population studies. Analysis of the NHANES III data showed that the prevalence of the metabolic syndrome increases substantially with increasing levels of serum urate.[30] After adjusting for age, gender, and risk factors for development of the metabolic syndrome, i.e. diabetes, hypertension, and body mass index (BMI), the likelihood of having the metabolic syndrome was found to be threefold greater if gout was present.[31] However the association between hyperuricaemia and diabetes remains an epidemiological observation and relative contributions of uric acid underexcretion and uric acid overproduction to the hyperuricemia of patients with the metabolic syndrome remain to be determined.

Pseudogout

The association between chondrocalcinosis (CC), i.e. deposition of calcium pyrophosphate dehydrate (CPP) crystals in hyaline and fibrous cartilage, remains debatable in the absence of any large population studies. In a study by Silveri and colleagues[32] no statistical difference was observed between the prevalence of diabetes mellitus and impaired glucose tolerance in CC patients vs controls.

Adhesive capsulitis of the shoulder (frozen shoulder syndrome)

Frozen shoulder syndrome is characterized by restricted shoulder joint movement especially affecting external rotation and abduction. It is more common in people with diabetes, with an estimated prevalence of around 10% in type 1 diabetes and 20% in type 2 diabetes.[33] There is no association with either glycaemic control or disease duration but it occurs more frequently in those with autonomic neuropathy and limited joint mobility.[34]

Pathophysiologically, it is believed to be related to increased expression of fibrogenic growth factors and proinflammatory cytokines including interleukin (IL)-1β and tumour necrosis factor (TNF)α and β leading to excessive accumulation of collagenous tissue. Analgesics, physiotherapy, and intra-articular corticosteroid injections form the cornerstone of treatment. The latter is very likely to cause deterioration in glycaemic control. It is therefore important to inform patients so that they can make appropriate changes to their diabetes medications or seek advice if they are not self-adjusting.

Acromegaly

Arthropathy is one of the most common complications of acromegaly affecting up to 75% of patients.[35] The condition is a relatively rare, insidious in onset, progressive, and potentially life-threatening endocrinopathy characterized by excessive and uncontrolled secretion of growth hormone (GH) and most commonly caused by a GH-secreting pituitary tumour. Other causes, all very rare, include increased growth hormone releasing hormone (GHRH) from hypothalamic tumours, ectopic GHRH from non-endocrine tumours, and ectopic GH secretion by non-endocrine tumours. Annual new patient incidence is estimated to be 3–4 cases per million population per year, with a mean age at presentation being 40–45 years. Excessive GH secretion leads to raised IGF-1 levels which act as the primary mediator of growth-promoting effects of GH. The pathogenesis of the arthropathy is a combination of early metabolic effects and subsequent mechanical changes. The direct effect of GH leads to growth of soft tissue and fibroblasts, causing excessive proliferation of connective tissue. Early treatment of the GH excess may reverse these changes, but if allowed to persist, altered joint geometry results in repeated intra-articular trauma resulting in scar, cyst, and osteophyte formation worsening the joint geometry. Box 171.3 provides a list of rheumatological manifestations of acromegaly.

Acromegalic arthropathy

Articular manifestations constitute an important and often presenting feature of acromegaly. Excessive and sustained GH levels, mediated by IGF-1, lead to proliferation of articular cartilage and periarticular supporting structures resulting in cartilage thickening and reduction of joint space. Initial changes including widening of joint spaces and periarticular soft tissue hypertrophy are partially reversible but continued GH secretion leads to irreversible changes which include and which in turn reduce joint mobility, laxity of joints and degenerative joint disease (Figure 171.2).[36]

Clinical features of acromegalic arthropathy include back pain due to involvement of the axial skeleton, especially the lumbar area. Large joints like hip, knee, and shoulder are also affected in 60–70% of patients. Permanent articular changes cause a considerable reduction of quality of life, which persists despite adequate medical or surgical treatment of the condition.

Box 171.3 Rheumatological manifestations of acromegaly

Phenotypical changes

- Prognathism
- Acral enlargement
- Macroglossia
- Acne
- Greasy skin
- Skin tags
- Gigantism (in childhood)

Musculoskeletal changes

- Arthralgia
- Arthropathy

Neurological changes

- Carpal tunnel syndrome
- Ulnar nerve compression
- Spinal stenosis

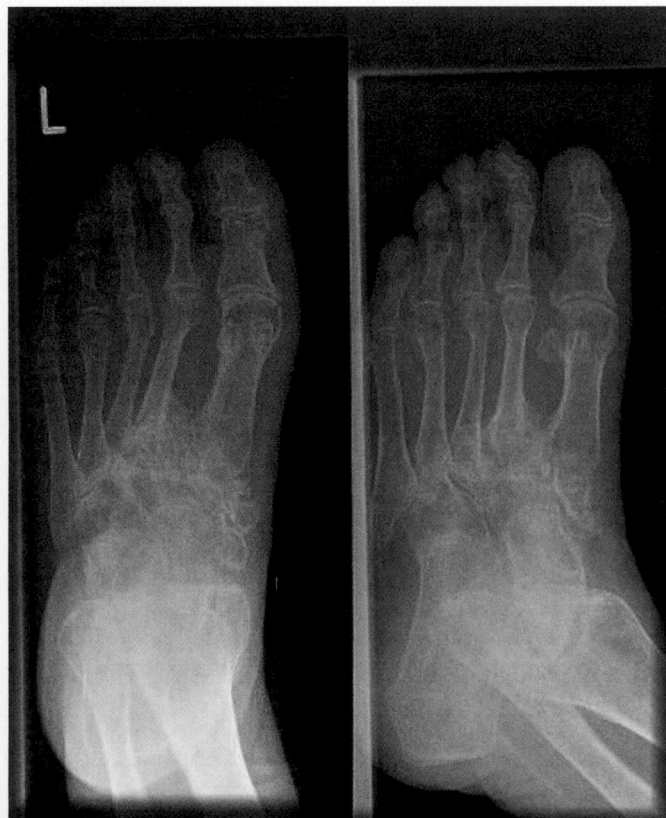

Fig. 171.2 Plain radiograph of ankle showing disrupted ankle mortise and midfoot due to a neuropathic joint.

Alterations of bone mineral density in acromegaly

There is conflicting data on whether acromegaly is a risk factor for osteoporosis. GH increase osteoblastic activity, an anabolic effect that is reflected in an increase in osteocalcin levels and an elevated BMD levels in cortical bone. When associated with reduced BMD this is related to the secondary hypogonadal state that is common in at least 50% of patients with acromegaly.[37] Importantly, the overall risk of fracture is not increased in acromegalics when compared with normal controls.[38]

Neuropathies

Acromegaly is also commonly associated with a variety of entrapment neuropathies which may present with classical symptoms such as paraesthesiae in the distribution of the median nerve in the hand, but not uncommonly non-classical features, e.g. aching in the forearm as in carpal tunnel syndrome. Spinal stenosis is a well-recognized complication of acromegaly and may present with lower back pain or lower limb ache and not necessarily as the classical intermittent claudication. Chronic GH and IGF-1 excess cause endochondral, marginal, and subligamentous growth of vertebral bone with resulting vertebral enlargement, and osteophyte formation and narrowing of the spinal canal. Early diagnosis and treatment are important in preventing this complication, which can progress to severely impair quality of life.

Endocrine conditions associated with calcium pyrophosphate deposition disease

Deposition of CPP crystals in found in a number of endocrine conditions, especially diabetes, hypothyroidism, and hyperparathyroidism.

It can lead to acute flare-ups of synovitis (pseudogout) or chronic degenerative disease (chondrocalcinosis).

Hyperparathyrodism

There is a strong association (18–25%) between CPP deposition disease and hyperparathyroidism,[39] and this was found to be a presenting feature in 7.5% of patients presenting with hyperparathyroidism for the first time.[40] Acute pseudogout attacks commonly involve the knees but can also involve the metacarpophalageal joints. This association could be due to the aggravating effects of sustained hypercalcaemia on age-related degenerative joint disease.

Hypothyroidism

There is a slightly increased prevalence of CC in hypothyroidism (odds ratio 1.94) but the mechanism is unclear. The joints commonly involved include knee, wrists, and metacarpals.

Disorders of muscles

Involvement of the muscular system is common in many endocrinopathies although their presentation can be non-specific. There are, however, some conditions such as diabetes muscle infarction (DMI) and diabetic amyotrophy that are specific to the endocrinopathy.

Diabetes muscle infarction

DMI is an unusual disorder of type 1 and type 2 diabetes patients with advanced microvascular damage including nephropathy. First described in Angervall in 1965,[41] more than 120 cases can be found in the literature,[42] and increasing awareness has led to prompt recognition of this previously underdiagnosed condition. Typically, acute presentation with atraumatic painful swelling, notably of the quadriceps or thigh muscles, is found in diabetic subjects with known microvascular complications including retinopathy and nephropathy. Laboratory investigations generally show high erythrocyte sedimentation rate (ESR), normal white cell count, and normal or mild elevation of creatine phosphokinase. MRI findings are invariably characterized by increased signal intensity of the diffusely enlarged muscle groups on T2-weighted sequences and gadolinium-enhanced images. Muscle biopsy is not necessary for diagnosis and should be reserved for patients with atypical presentations and lack of improvement. The disease is generally believed to be self-limiting, although recurrence occurs in one-half of the cases.[43] Treatment is usually supportive and consists of anti-inflammatory and anti-platelet agents.

Diabetic amyotrophy

Also known as proximal diabetic neuropathy, femoral neuropathy, or lumbosacral radioplexus neuropathy, this is due to an acute peripheral neuropathy usually affecting the thighs but occasionally the hips and buttocks. It is characterized by muscle pain with wasting and weakness and may present to the rheumatologist as pain in and around the hip with weakness. The cause is unclear but it is very commonly associated with symmetrical distal diabetic peripheral neuropathy. Characteristically it is accompanied by sudden weight loss and its resolution is accompanied by a return to former weight. It usually resolves after 6–12 months without specific treatment except supportive therapy, pain control, and maintaining good glycaemic control.

Myopathy

Myopathies are a group of conditions related to abnormal skeletal muscle state and present as muscle weakness, pain, cramps, muscle tenderness, and spasms in varying degrees. Although the exact pathophysiology remains incompletely understood, postulated mechanisms include disturbances in the function of the muscle fibres due to increased mitochondrial respiration, accelerated protein degradation, lipid oxidation and enhanced beta-adrenergic sensitivity to hormonal excess.[44] Common endocrinopathies that cause myopathies are the following:

- **Thyroid dysfunction**: both hypothyroidism and hyperthyroidism may cause a proximal myopathy.

- **Steroid myopathy**: Cushing's disease or the use of glucocorticoids may be associated with a proximal myopathy.

- **Parathyroid dysfunction**: both hyperparathyroidism and hypoparathyroidism, as previously described, can cause myopathy.

- **Hypoadrenalism and pituitary dysfunction**: when associated with secondary hypoadrenalism these may cause a variety of myopathic symptoms, but predominantly muscle weakness and symptoms of 'chronic fatigue'.

Disorders of supporting adnexa (ligaments, tendons, capsule, and retinacula)

Several important rheumatological manifestations of the adnexa are associated with endocrinopathies.

Carpal tunnel syndrome

Carpal tunnel syndrome (CTS) is an increasingly recognized neuromuscular disorder that has a prevalence of around 3.8% in the general population.[45] It is caused by entrapment of the median nerve within the carpal tunnel as it traverses the flexor retinaculum in the wrist, leading to pain and paraesthesia along the distribution of the median nerve in the hand. However, rheumatologists and other physicians should be aware of its increased occurrence in various endocrine disorders which include hypothyroidism (5–10%), acromegaly (30–50%), and diabetes mellitus (11–21%).

Dupuytren's disease

Dupuytren's disease (DD) is more common in diabetes (prevalence 16–42%) than in the general population (prevalence 7%).[46] It is a progressive but painless condition caused by hyperplastic contractures of the palmar aponeurosis (or palmar fascia). The ring and little finger are the fingers most commonly affected. The middle finger may be affected in advanced cases, but the index finger and the thumb are nearly always spared. Similar to diabetic cheiroarthropathy, the prevalence of DD among the diabetic population increases with age and duration of diabetes but is not associated with glycaemic control.[47]

Stenosing flexor tenosynovitis (trigger finger)

Compared to a prevalence of 2% in the general population, trigger finger is considerably commoner in the diabetic population with reported figures of 5–36%.[48] It is characterized by fixed flexion or extension contractures of the fingers due to fibrosis and thickening of the long flexor tendon sheaths. Similar to DD, it is more common in diabetics with a longer duration of disease and effects.

Lupus-like syndrome associated with anti-thyroid medications

Carbimazole and propylthiuracil are thionamide derivaties that are commonly used in the medical management of hyperthyroidism. Agranulocytosis is an uncommon but well-documented adverse effect of these drugs. Rarely, they have also been associated with lupus-like clinical states including rash, arthralgia, and positive

Table 171.3 Rheumatological manifestations of endocrine disorders

Endocrinopathy	Rheumatological manifestations affecting			
	Skeletal system	**Joints**	**Muscles**	**Supporting adnexa**
Hypothyroidism		CPPD	Hypothyroid myopathy	Carpal tunnel syndrome
Hyperthyroidism	Osteoporosis		Myopathy	Lupus-like syndrome
Hypoparathyroidism	DISH		Myopathy Neuromyotonia Rhabdomyolysis	
Hyperparathyroidism	Osteoporosis OFC Sub-perisoteal resorption Fragility fractures Rugger jersey spine	CPPD	Myopathy Proximal neuropathy	Tendon rupture and avulsions
Acromegaly		Arthropathy		Nerve compression syndromes
Diabetes mellitus		Charcot's osteoarthropathy Diabetic Cheiroarthropathy Crystal-induced arthritis	DMI	CTS Dupuytren's disease Trigger finger Adhesive capsulitis

CPPD, calcium pyrophosphate deposition; CTS, carpal tunnel syndrome; DISH, diffuse idiopathic skeletal hypersostosis; DMI, diabetic muscle infarction; OFC, osteitis fibrosa cystica.

antinuclear antibodies in 10–53% of patients.[49] However, they do not fulfil the diagnostic criteria for drug-induced systemic lupus erythematosus.[50]

Conclusion

Endocrine disorders are associated with a wide variety of conditions affecting the musculoskeletal system and as such the first presenting symptom may be rheumatological in nature. It is therefore important that general practitioners and rheumatologists are aware of these possible associations. Similarly, endocrinologists need to be aware of the rheumatological complications that may result from the endocrine disorder such as spinal stenosis in acromegaly and lupus-type syndrome complicating anti-thyroid therapy.

Table 171.3 provides a summary list of the various endocrinopathies and associated rheumatological manifestations.

References

1. Kelman A, Lane NE. The management of secondary osteoporosis. *Best Pract Res Clin Rheumatol* 2005;19(6):1021–1037.
2. Silverberg SJ, Shane E, Jacobs TP et al. A 10-year prospective study of primary hyperparathyroidism with or without parathyroid surgery. *N Engl J Med* 1999;341:1249–1255.
3. Baqi L, Player J, Killinger Z et al. Thyrotropin versus thyroid hormone in regulating bone density and turnover in premenopausal women. *Endocr Regul* 2010;44(2):57–63
4. Rosen HN, Moses AC, Gundberg C et al. Therapy with parenteral pamidronate prevents thyroid hormone-induced bone turnover in humans. *J Clin Endocrinol Metab* 1993;77(3):664–669.
5. Primary vitamin D deficiency in adults. *Drug Ther Bull* 2006;44:25–29.
6. Holick MF, Binkley NC, Heike A et al. Evaluation, treatment, and prevention of vitamin D deficiency: an Endocrine Society clinical practice guideline. *J Clin Endocrinol Metab* 2011;96(7):1911–1930.
7. Chiodini I, Mascia ML, Muscarella S et al. Subclinical hypercortisolism among outpatients referred for osteoporosis. *Ann Intern Med* 2007;147:541–548.
8. American College of Rheumatology Ad Hoc Committee on Glucocorticoid-Induced Osteoporosis. Recommendations for the prevention and treatment of glucocorticoid-induced osteoporosis: 2001 update. *Arthritis Rheum* 2001;44(7):1496–1503.
9. Melmed S, Casanueva FF, Hoffman AR et al. Diagnosis & treatment of hyperprolactinemia: an Endocrine Society clinical practice guideline. *J Clin Endocrinol Metab* 2011;96(2):273–288.
10. Boonen S, Vanderschueren D, Cheng XG et al. Age-related (type II) femoral neck osteoporosis in men: biochemical evidence for both hypovitaminosis D- and androgen deficiency-induced bone resorption. *J Bone Miner Res* 1997;12:2119–2126.
11. Kenny AM, Prestwood KM, Marcello KM et al. Determinants of bone density in healthy older men with low testosterone levels. *J Gerontol A Biol Sci Med Sci* 2000;55:492–497.
12. Snyder P, Peachey H, Berlin JA et al. Effect of testosterone treatment on body composition and muscle strength in men over 65 years of age. *J Clin Endocrinol Metab* 1999;84:2647–2653.
13. Takeshita T, Tanaka H, Harasawa A et al. Brown tumour of the sphenoid sinus in a patient with secondary hyperparathyroidism: CT and MR imaging findings. *Radiat Med* 2004;22:265–268.
14. Lacativa PH, Rranco FM, Pimentel JR et al. Prevalence of radiological finding among cases of severe secondary hyperparathyroidism. *San Paulo Med J* 2009;127:71–77.
15. International Diabetes Federation. *Diabetes atlas*, 4th edn (online), 2009 Available at: www.diabetesatlas.org. (Accessed 16 May 2012).
16. *Quality and Outcomes Framework (QOF), 2009: England* (online). Available at: www.ic.nhs.uk/statistics-and-data-collections/supporting-information/audits-andperformance/the-quality-and-outcomes-framework/qof-2008/09/data-tables/prevalence-data-tables. (Accessed 16 May 2012).
17. Crispin JC, Alcocer-Varela J Rheumatic manifestations of diabetes mellitus. *Am Med* 2003;114:753–757.
18. Cagliero E. Rheumatic manifestations of diabetes mellitus. *Curr Rheumatol Rep* 2003;5(3):189–194.
19. Lebiedz-Odrobina D, Kay J. Rheumatic manifestations of diabetes mellitus. In: Markenson JA (ed.) *Rheumatological manifestations of endocrine disease*. Rheumatic Clinics of North America, Philadelphia, 2010:681–682.
20. Lundbaek K. Stiff hands in long-term diabetes. *Acta Med Scand* 1957;158:447–451.
21. Pal N, Anderson J, Dick WC et al. Limitation of joint mobility and shoulder capsulitis in insulin- and non-insulin-dependent diabetes mellitus. *Br J Rheumatol* 1986;25(2):147–151.
22. Lawson PM, Maneschi F, Kohner EM. The relationship of hand abnormalities to diabetes and diabetic retinopathy. *Diabetes Care* 1983;6(2):140–143.
23. Arkkila PE, Kantola Im, Viikari JS. Limited joint mobility in type 1 diabetic patients: correlation to other diabetic complications. *J Intern Med* 1994;236(2):215–223.
24. Charcot JM. Sur quelques arthropathies qui paraissent dépendre d'une lésion du cerveau ou de la moelle épinière. *Arch Physiol Norm Pathol* 1868;1:161–171.
25. Jeffcoate W. The causes of the Charcot syndrome. *Clin Podiatr Med Surg* 2008;25(1):29–42, vi.
26. Rogers LC, Frykberg RG, Armstrong DA et al. The Charcot foot in diabetes. *Diabetes Care* 2011;34(9):2123–2129.
27. Julkunen H, Heinonen OP, Pyorala K. Hyperostosis of the spine in an adult population. Its relation to hyperglycaemia and obesity. *Ann Rheum Dis* 1971;30(6):605–612.
28. Kiss S, Szilagyi M, Paksy A et al. Risk factors for diffuse idiopathic skeletal hyperostosis: a case-control study. *Rheumatology* (Oxford) 2002; 41(1):27–30.
29. Mata S, Fortin P, Fitzcharles MA et al. A controlled study of diffuse idiopathic skeletal hyperostosis. Clinical features and functional status. *Medicine* (Baltimore) 1997;76(2):104–117.
30. Choi HK, Ford ES. Prevalence of the metabolic syndrome in individuals with hyperuricemia. *Am J Med* 2007;120:442–447.
31. Choi HK, Ford ES, Li C et al. Prevalence of the metabolic syndrome in patients with gout: the Third National Health and Nutrition Examination Survey. *Arthritis Rheum* 2007;57:109–115.
32. Silveri F, Adamo V, Corsi M et al. [Chondrocalcinosis and diabetes mellitus. The clinico-statistical data.] *Recenti Prog Med* 1994;85(2): 91–95.
33. Arkkila PE, Kantola IM, Viikari JS et al. Shoulder capsulitis in type I and type II diabetic patients: association with diabetic complications and related diseases. *Ann Rheum Dis* 1996;55(12):907–914.
34. Balci N, Balci MK, Tuzuner S. Shoulder adhesive capsulitis and shoulder range of movements in type II diabetes mellitus: association with diabetic complications. *J Diabetes Complications* 1999;13(3):135–140.
35. Harris AG. *Acromegaly and its management*. Lippincott-Raven, Philadelphia, 1996:24–35.
36. Chipman JJ, Attanasio AF, Birkett MA et al. The safety profile of GH therapy in adults. *Clin Endocrinol* 1997;46:473–481.
37. Guistina A, Mazzioti G, Canalis A. Growth hormone, insulin-like growth factors and the skeleton. *Endocr Rev* 2008;29:535–559.
38. Shane E. Osteoporosis associated with illness and medications. In: Marcus R, Feldman D, Reisey J (eds) *Osteoporosis*. Academic Press, San Diego, CA, 1996:925–946.

39. Dodds WJ, Steinbach HL. Primary hyperparathyroidism and articular cartilage calcification. *Am J Roentgenol Radium Ther Nucl Med* 1968;104:884–892.

40. Schumacher HR. Arthritis associated with endocrine and metabolic disease. In: Katz WA (ed.) *Rheumatic disease: diagnosis and management.* Lippincott, Philadelphia, 1977:682–697.

41. Angervall L, Stener B. Tumoriform focal muscular degeneration in two diabetic patients *Diabetologia* 1965;1:39–42.

42. Kattapuram TM, Suri R, Rosol MS et al. Idiopathic and diabetic skeletal muscle necrosis: evaluation by magnetic resonance imaging. *Skeletal Radiol* 2005;34(4):203–209.

43. Umpierrez GE, Stiles RG, Kleinbart J et al. Diabetic muscle infarction. *Am J Med* 1996;101:245–250.

44. Engel AG, Fransini-Armstrong C. Endocrine myopathies. In: *Myology,* vol 2. McGraw-Hill, New York, 1994:1726–1747.

45. Atroshi I, Gummesson C, Johnsson R et al. Prevalence of carpal tunnel syndrome in a general population. *JAMA* 1999;282(2):153–158.

46. Arduc F, Soyupek F, Karraman Y et al. The muscoskeletal complications seen in type II diabetics: predominance of hand involvement. *Clin Rheumatol* 2003;22(3):229–233.

47. Chammas M, Bousquet P, Renard E et al. Dupuytren's disease, carpal tunnel syndrome, trigger finger, and diabetes mellitus. *J Hand Surg Am* 1995;20(1):109–114.

48. Cagliero E, Appruzzese W, Perlmutter GS et al. Musculoskeletal disorders of the hand and shoulder in patients with diabetes mellitus. *Am J Med* 2001;112(6):487–490.

49. Hess EV. Introduction to drug-related lupus. *Arthritis Rheum* 1981;24(8):vi–ix.

50. Antonov D, Kazandjieva J, Etugov D et al. Drug-induced lupus erythematosus. *Clin Dermatol* 2004;22(2):157–166.

CHAPTER 172

Haemoglobinopathies

David Rees

Introduction

The haemoglobinopathies are a group of inherited disorders caused by mutations in one or more of the globin genes. They are the commonest single-gene disorders in the world, reaching polymorphic frequencies in most ethnic groups, apart from northern Europeans and the native populations of the Americas and Australia.[1] There are two main clinical syndromes caused by these mutations: thalassaemias and sickle cell disease. Other rarer phenotypes include haemolytic anaemia due to unstable haemoglobins, methaemoglobinaemia, and polycythaemia caused by mutations causing high oxygen affinity; none of these have significant rheumatological manifestations.

Thalassaemia syndromes

Thalassaemia is caused by a reduction in the rate of synthesis of one of the globin chains. The two main types are α thalassaemia and β thalassaemia.

α Thalassaemia

The α thalassaemias have relatively few rheumatological implications and are not considered in detail here. There are normally four functioning α globin genes, and α thalassaemia is usually caused by large deletions removing one or more of these, causing the following syndromes:

◆ **α Thalassaemia trait**: two or three functioning α globin genes cause this asymptomatic condition, associated with a reduction in the size and haemoglobin content of red cells.

◆ **Haemoglobin H disease**: if there is only one functioning α globin gene, mild to moderate haemolytic anaemia results, with the haemoglobin usually 70–100 g/L. Moderate splenomegaly is common and frequent blood transfusions rarely necessary. There is moderate erythroid bone marrow expansion, which is likely to result in some degree of osteopenia although this is rarely clinically significant.

◆ **Haemoglobin Bart's hydrops fetalis**: in this condition there are no functioning α globin genes, which causes severe fetal anaemia with almost inevitable fetal death in the third trimester.

β Thalassaemia

β Thalassaemia is caused by mutations in one or both of the β globin genes; these are typically point mutations or small deletions. There are more than 400 different β thalassaemia mutations, resulting in a full spectrum of clinical conditions from asymptomatic to transfusion dependence. Unlike α globin, β globin is not expressed in the fetus, and so the homozygous condition does not cause symptoms until three months of age at the earliest. The following syndromes occur:

◆ **β Thalassaemia trait**: inheriting one β thalassaemia allele causes mild, asymptomatic anaemia.

◆ **β Thalassaemia intermedia**: this condition involves significant anaemia and splenomegaly, which does not necessitate regular blood transfusions. Children are typically well for the first few years of life, but develop symptoms and require intermittent blood transfusions. It is caused by many different genotypes, most often when two mild β thalassaemia mutations are inherited.

◆ **β Thalassaemia major**: this occurs when two severe β thalassaemia mutations are inherited. Severe anaemia, failure to thrive, bony distortion, and massive splenomegaly occur in the first year of life; death occurs without the instigation of regular blood transfusions to maintain the haemoglobin above 95 g/L. These transfusions results in inevitable iron overload and chelation is started after about 12 transfusions, to prevent endocrinopathy and fatal cardiomyopathy. Haematopoietic stem cell transplantation is potentially curative if a suitable sibling donor is available.

Rheumatological complications of thalassaemia

Osteopenia

About 50% of adult patients with optimally treated thalassaemia major have severe reductions in bone mass with a Z-score of less than −2.5, with most of the remainder showing low bone mass, with a Z-score of −1 to −2.5.[2] This is multifactorial. Erythroid bone marrow expansion physically reduces the volume of bone cortex. Excess iron is directly deposited in bone, which impairs osteoid formation. Iron also causes endocrinopathy with low levels of sex hormones and delayed puberty. Iron chelators, particularly desferrioxamine, inhibit osteoblasts and collagen formation, and vitamin D deficiency is common in many non-tropical countries (Figure 172.1). Additionally, patients often have reduced levels of physical activity due to coexistent illness. About 40% thalassaemia major patients in the United States report a history of bone fracture, and the risk of fracture seems to increase with increasing endocrinopathy.[3] Bone

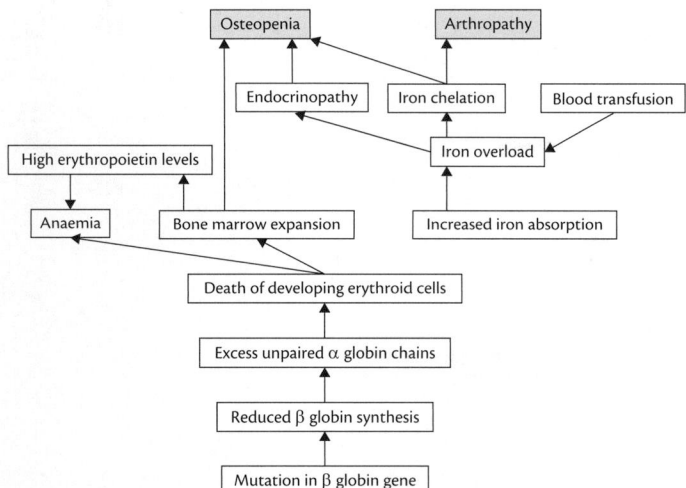

Fig. 172.1 Pathophysiology of osteopenia and arthropathy in β thalassaemia major.

pain is similarly a common symptom in thalassaemia major, often related to osteoporosis.

Management of osteopenia in thalassaemia major involves being aware of the risk and organising regular bone mineral density measurement from the age of about 10 years. Children and adults should be encouraged to be physically active, and vitamin D levels maintained in the optimal range with appropriate supplementation. Blood transfusion should be optimized to maintain the pre-transfusion haemoglobin above 95 g/L with the aim of limiting bone marrow expansion. Endocrinopathy should be prevented, by starting chelation early before significant iron accumulation occurs, usually after 10–12 transfusions. Overchelation can also cause bone damage, and care is needed once the serum ferritin is below 1000 µg/L. Several small studies suggest that bisphosphonates can reverse significant osteopenia, and this is probably the treatment of choice.[4]

Osteopenia is also a feature of thalassaemia intermedia, predominantly related to massive erythroid expansion. Significant osteopenia and pathological fractures suggest that regular blood transfusions should be started, although bone loss may then occur for other reasons. Bisphosphonates are also thought to be of therapeutic benefit.

Arthropathy

Before effective iron chelation was available, thalassaemia major patients with marked haemosiderosis sometimes developed osteoarthropathy, particularly affecting the ankles. It was probably related to hypoparathyroidism, bone marrow expansion, and iron deposition in the joints. Modern iron chelation has now made this rare in most countries.

About 15% patients using the oral iron chelator deferiprone (previously called L1) develop characteristic arthropathy as a side effect of the drug. This is often fairly mild and spontaneously recovers, although can result in severe and progressive joint damage, particularly in South Asian populations. The knees are most often affected, with joint effusions, irregularity of the subchondral bones, and cartilage damage on MRI.[5]

Other rheumatological complications

Massive erythroid expansion is seen in thalassaemia intermedia and undertransfused thalassaemia major, and results in the characteristic 'hair-on-end' appearance of skull radiograph. Related to this, thalassaemic facies can occur, with expansion of the maxillary bones and skull vault. Severe iron overload and chelation with desferrioxamine can result in calcification of intervertebral discs, which may contribute to back pain. Scoliosis and paraspinal extramedullary haematopoiesis are also fairly common.

Sickle cell disease

The term sickle cell disease (SCD) refers to a group of conditions, caused by the inheritance of mutated β globin, in which the sixth amino acid is changed from glutamic acid to valine. This sickle haemoglobin (HbS) forms polymers when deoxygenated, which damage the erythrocyte. Sickle cell anaemia (SCA) is the most common and severe form of the condition, in which HbS is inherited from both parents, although other compound heterozygous states cause similar syndromes (Table 172.1).[6] Pathological processes are complicated, involving an interrelated network, which starts with vaso-occlusion and includes infarction, vasculopathy, inflammation, haemolysis, reperfusion injury, nitric oxide deficiency, hypoxaemia, and hypercoagulability (Figure 172.2). It is a multisystem disorder with almost every tissue and organ involved, and rheumatological manifestations are common.

Clinical features include periods of apparent good health interspersed with unpredictable episodes of acute illness, usually involving acute pain and sometimes referred to as 'crises'. Acute lung complications and infection are also prevalent. These acute problems occur on a background of vasculopathy and progressive organ damage, resulting in an increased incidence of stroke, pulmonary hypertension, restrictive lung defects, retinopathy, renal impairment, cholelithiasis, priapism, leg ulcers, arthropathy, and bone damage. SCA is the commonest cause of paediatric stroke in the world.

Most complications are treated symptomatically. Penicillin prophylaxis in children has been shown to reduce morbidity and mortality from pneumococcal infection, and is recommended from about the age of 3 months in most countries. Randomized controlled trials have demonstrated that hydroxycarbamide improves the natural history of the condition; it reduces the frequency of acute pain and acute chest syndrome, and may delay organ damage and death.[6] Regular blood transfusions are used if there is evidence of severe, progressive vasculopathy, such as cerebrovascular disease. Haematopoietic stem cell transplantation is the only curative option, and the donor currently has to be an HLA-matched sibling; toxicity is still a significant issue, and only a minority of severely affected patients currently undergo this procedure.

Median life expectancy for SCA is probably about 50 years in the northern hemisphere, but considerably less in sub-Saharan Africa where most patients live, and the majority die in childhood. This increased mortality is probably primarily due to infections, including pneumococcus and malaria.[7]

Rheumatological complications of sickle cell disease

Acute bone pain

Acute bone pain is the commonest symptom in SCD, with severe episodes occurring on average about once per year, although this varies widely between individuals. The pain is thought to be due to vaso-occlusion of postcapillary venules, with infarction of the bone and subsequent inflammation. Most episodes are idiopathic,

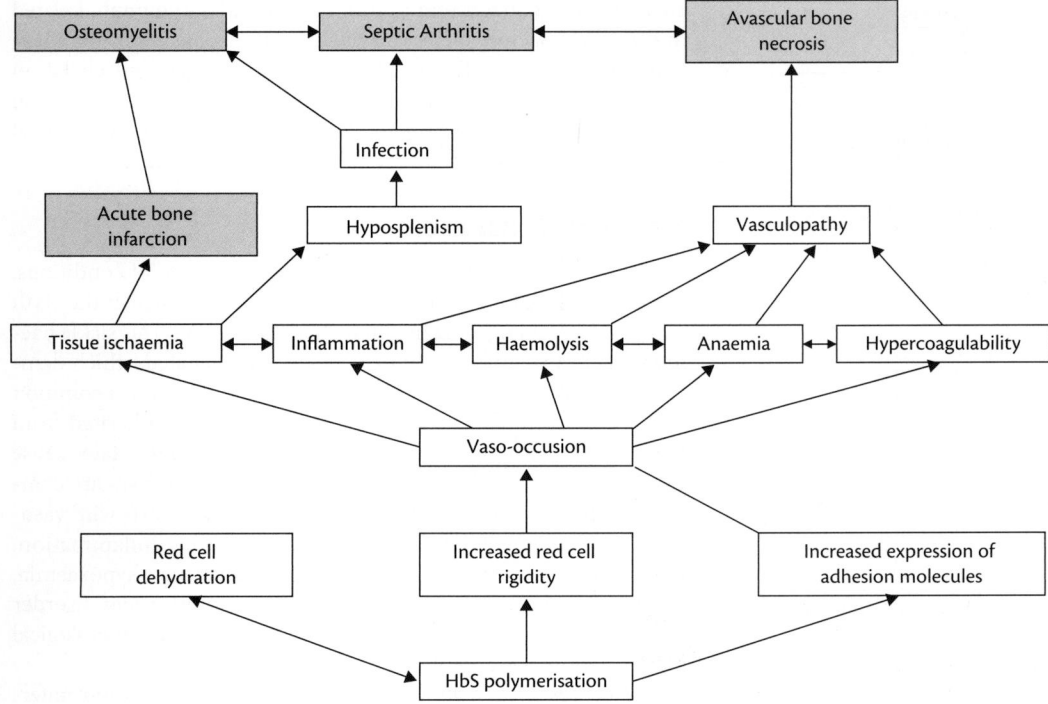

Fig. 172.2 Pathophysiology of rheumatological problems in sickle cell disease.

Table 172.1 Commoner types of sickle cell disease with ethnic distribution

Severe SCD	
HbS/S	SCA, the commonest form of SCD
HbS/β⁰thalassaemia	Most common in India, southern Europe
Severe HbS/β⁺thalassaemia	Most common in India, southern Europe
HbS/O^Arab	Rare but found in Middle East and Balkans
Moderate SCD	
HbS/C	25–30% cases of SCD in African populations
Moderate HbS/β⁺ thalassaemia	Most cases in Greece, Turkey. 6–15% HbA present
HbS/D^Punjab a	Found in India, Middle East but occurs all over the world
Mild SCD	
Mild HbS/β⁺⁺ thalassaemia	Mostly in people of African origin
HbS/E	HbE centred in South-East Asia and so HbSE uncommon, although increasing
HbS/hereditary persistence of fetal haemoglobin	High HbF levels protect against serious complications. Commonest in West Africa

SCA, sickle cell anaemia; SCD, sickle cell disease.
ªHbD^Punjab is also called HbD^Los Angeles.

although cold or windy weather, infection, dehydration, and stress may precipitate episodes. Pain typically involves the limbs and is often multifocal. The pain is described as deep-seated, like toothache, and the infarcted bones may be tender. Swelling of affected areas is common, particularly over the tibia.[8] In infants dactylitis, sometimes referred to as hand–foot syndrome, is the commonest

manifestation of bone infarction, in which painful swelling of the hands and feet occur for a few days (Figure 172.3).

There are no specific diagnostic tests. Plain radiographs are typically normal and should not be done unless to exclude fracture if there is a history of trauma; MRI may show evidence of bone infarction, although the appearances are not specific. Blood tests sometimes show neutrophilia, increased anaemia and increased bilirubin. C-reactive protein (CRP) and other inflammatory markers may be raised, although very high levels suggest coexistent infection. The erythrocyte sedimentation rate (ESR) is uninterpretable in SCD because of anaemia and the failure of sickle cells to form rouleaux.

There are no specific treatments for acute pain in SCD. Many episodes can be managed at home with paracetamol and non-steroidal anti-inflammatory drugs (NSAIDs), but severe pain requires hospital admission for treatment with opioids. These can be effective orally, although parenteral administration with nurse- or

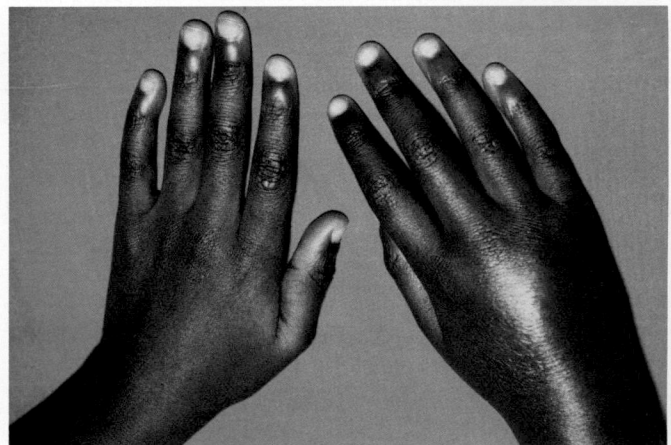

Fig. 172.3 Dactylitis of the right hand in a young child with sickle cell anaemia.

patient-controlled analgesia is sometimes necessary. Sedation levels should be monitored closely, as oversedation is one of the main causes of death during acute pain. Massage, distraction, and warmth are often helpful. Fluid balance should be monitored carefully, and intravenous hydration should only be used if the patient is unable to drink adequately. Antibiotics are usually given if the temperature is more than 38 °C.

Typical episodes of severe pain last several days before gradually resolving, although shorter episodes lasting only a few minutes also occur. Full recovery may take over a week and permanent bone or joint damage does not result from these acute episodes.

Osteomyelitis

Bone infarction and hyposplenism predispose people with SCD towards osteomyelitis. Approximately 10% patients with SCD develop this at some point, with the peak incidence in children and young adults. Salmonella and *Staphylococcus aureus* are most commonly isolated, but many other organisms have been implicated, including Gram-negative bacilli, tuberculosis, Klebsiella, and *Streptococcus pneumonia*. Any bone can be affected.

In the early stages, it is difficult to distinguish osteomyelitis from acute bony vaso-occlusion, although the latter is much more common. The diagnosis of osteomyelitis is suggested by high fevers, greater than 38.5 °C, marked bony swelling, and extreme tenderness, although all these can also be features of bone infarction. Very high CRP and other inflammatory markers also suggest osteomyelitis, but again are not diagnostic. Radiographs, MRI and bone scintigraphy cannot reliably distinguish infarction from infection for about the first week after onset. Ultrasound scans can be used to identify subperiosteal fluid, with larger volumes suggesting osteomyelitis.[9] Growth of organisms such as salmonella, together with a suggestive clinical picture, is usually sufficient to make the diagnosis. Definitive diagnosis relies on isolation of pus or bacteria from the affected bone, and is probably best achieved by early use of ultrasound, with drainage and culture of significant collections of periosteal fluid.

Treatment typically involves 6 weeks of antibiotics selected according to sensitivities of isolated bacteria. In general there is a trend to over diagnose osteomyelitis in SCD, and treatment should not be started unless an organism has been isolated, or there is a very strong index of clinical suspicion. If empirical antibiotics are started, they should cover salmonella and *S. aureus*; ceftriaxone or ciprofloxacin are often used, depending on local sensitivities. Surgery may be important to drain large collections of fluid. Incomplete or late diagnosis can result in chronic osteomyelitis requiring repeated surgery and course of antibiotics over many years.

Septic arthritis

As for osteomyelitis, septic arthritis is hard to distinguish from acute vaso-occlusion. It is much rarer than vaso-occlusion, and usually occurs as a consequence of infarction at the end of a long bone. Diagnosis relies on aspiration of synovial fluid when infection is suspected, and Salmonella and *S. aureus* are isolated most frequently. Treatment requires a prolonged course of antibiotics.

Avascular necrosis

Avascular necrosis (AVN) of the femoral and humeral heads is common in SCD, although the exact prevalence is uncertain and depends on methods of detection. Plain radiographs show changes of osteonecrosis of the femoral head in 10–15% of adults, whereas MRI changes are seen in about 40% of adults and 25% of children. AVN of the humeral head is present in about 10% of adults with SCD, although it often causes few symptoms. Typically AVN causes chronic pain of the affected joint with exacerbations, which can be difficult to distinguish from acute vaso-occlusive pain. There is no good evidence on how best to manage this condition. In children rest and simple analgesia can lead to a complete resolution of symptoms. Established osteonecrosis of the femoral head in SCD has been treated with osteotomy, core decompression, and autologous bone grafting, although there is not much evidence that any of these are better than physiotherapy.[10] Once AVN is established, collapse of the femoral head is almost inevitable, and hip replacement arthroplasty is necessary to relieve pain. As this often occurs in adolescents and young adults, repeat hip replacements are likely, and technically challenging. AVN of a wide range of other bones has been described in SCD, including the knee, skull, face, mandible, ribs, spine, and pelvis.

Coincidental rheumatological illness in sickle cell disease

SCD is a common condition and inevitably coincidental rheumatological disease occurs in some adults and children. Many patients with SCD in industrialized countries are now surviving into old age, with increasing numbers affected by degenerative diseases. Diagnosis of these conditions is often delayed because of the tendency to attribute all symptoms to SCD, and management is complicated by potential interactions between the different diseases and their medications. In particular, there is anecdotal evidence that long-term use of corticosteroids may increase the risk of complications in SCD, including severe acute pain, increased sepsis and stroke[11]; on this basis, it is probably sensible to start hydroxycarbamide or even long-term blood transfusions if rheumatological disease is also present which is likely to need long-term treatment with corticosteroids.

Systemic lupus erythematosus (SLE) is a particular problem in SCD. It is approximately five times more common in women of African origin living in Europe compared to native Europeans, making it relatively prevalent in SCD patients. Many of the symptoms overlap with SCD, including musculoskeletal pain, neurological and renal complications. Diagnosing SLE can therefore be difficult, as can identifying the cause of particular symptoms when both conditions are known to coexist. As mentioned earlier, corticosteroids can be problematic in SCD, and other immunosuppressive treatments increase infective complications. However, in general SLE treatment should be prioritized, with hydroxycarbamide or regular blood transfusions started if serious sickle complications occur.

References

1. Weatherall DJ. Hemoglobinopathies worldwide: present and future. *Curr Mol Med* 2008;8(7):592–599.
2. Wonke B. Bone disease in beta-thalassaemia major. *Br J Haematol* 1998;103(4):897–901.
3. Fung EB, Harmatz PR, Milet M et al. Fracture prevalence and relationship to endocrinopathy in iron overloaded patients with sickle cell disease and thalassemia. *Bone* 2008;43(1):162–168.
4. Haidar R, Musallam KM, Taher AT. Bone disease and skeletal complications in patients with beta thalassemia major. *Bone* 2011;48(3):425–432.

5. Kellenberger CJ, Schmugge M, Saurenmann T et al. Radiographic and MRI features of deferiprone-related arthropathy of the knees in patients with beta-thalassemia. *AJR Am J Roentgenol* 2004;183(4):989–994.

6. Rees DC, Williams TN, Gladwin MT. Sickle-cell disease. *Lancet* 2010;376(9757):2018–2031.

7. Williams TN, Uyoga S, Macharia A et al. Bacteraemia in Kenyan children with sickle-cell anaemia: a retrospective cohort and case-control study. *Lancet* 2009;374(9698):1364–1370.

8. Serjeant GR, Serjeant BE. *Sickle cell disease*, 3rd edn. Oxford University Press, Oxford, 2001.

9. William RR, Hussein SS, Jeans WD, Wali YA, Lamki ZA. A prospective study of soft-tissue ultrasonography in sickle cell disease patients with suspected osteomyelitis. *Clin Radiol* 2000;55(4):307–310.

10. Marti-Carvajal AJ, Sola I, Agreda-Perez LH. Treatment for avascular necrosis of bone in people with sickle cell disease. *Cochrane Database Syst Rev* 2009;3:CD004344.

11. Couillard S, Benkerrou M, Girot R et al. Steroid treatment in children with sickle-cell disease. *Haematologica* 2007;92(3):425–426.

CHAPTER 173

Haemochromatosis

Graeme J. Carroll, WIlliam H. Breidahl,
and John K. Olynyk

Introduction and history

Hereditary haemochromatosis (HH) is a common inherited metabolic disorder characterized by systemic iron overload.[1-2] HH affects approximately 1 in 200 people and is most common in persons of northern European origin. Organ damage in the pancreas, liver, heart, endocrine glands, skin, and joints has been described in HH. There is evidence that the frequency and extent of organ damage may be changing with time, perhaps due to earlier diagnosis and treatment.[3] In persons of northern European origin, homozygosity for the C282Y mutation in the *HFE* gene found on chromosome 6 is present in over 90% of patients with HH,[4] whereas in southern Europe as many as 30% of cases may be heterozygous or wild type for this mutation.[5] Individuals homozygous for the C282Y mutation in the *HFE* gene product have up to a 30% chance of developing significant disease as a result of iron overload.[1]

The clinical manifestations of the disorder were reviewed by Sheldon in 1935, but in his description an arthropathy is not recorded.[6] It was not until Schumacher described two cases and reported a peripheral arthritis in 5 of 23 hospital cases of idiopathic haemochromatosis in 1964 that arthropathy was identified in haemochromatosis.[7] Subsequent studies have confirmed the presence of a clinically recognizable arthropathy.[8-17] Although clinically and radiologically characteristic, the arthropathy is not specific for haemochromatosis, since it cannot be differentiated from monoarticular osteoarthritis in the same target joints or from the form of polyarticular osteoarthritis classified as type 2 polyarticular osteoarthritis (T2POA).[18,19] Moreover, differentiation from pyrophosphate deposition disease, diabetes with metacarpophalangeal (MCP) joint involvement and even rheumatoid arthritis (RA) can sometimes be difficult.[8,20,21]

Characteristics of the arthropathy

Frequency of arthropathy

Arthropathy in HH has been reported to range from 24% to 81% as can be seen in Table 173.1. The association observed between this arthropathy, homozygosity for C282Y, and total body iron burden determined by baseline ferritin concentrations, suggests that iron load is a major determinant of arthropathy in HH and more important than occupational factors.[16] Valenti et al. and others have also reported that arthropathy in HH is strongly associated with iron load.[15,17]

Considerable variation in the frequency of chondrocalcinosis has been reported, with estimates ranging from 5% to 49% of study participants as shown in Table 173.1.[9-11,13-15,17] Chondrocalcinosis is considered to be a late manifestation of the disease and by inference linked to disease chronicity. In one study, the incidence of chondrocalcinosis increased from 39% to 72% in 18 patients with known arthropathy who were undergoing regular venesection over a period of 10 years.[22] In no patient was diminution in size or disappearance of the chondrocalcinosis observed.

Joints affected—topography and course

The arthropathy of haemochromatosis is chronic and progressive. The index and middle finger metacarpophalangeal (MCP2,3) joints are most commonly affected. Importantly, from a pathogenetic perspective, these joints are also involved in some patients with juvenile HH, which has a different genetic basis.[23] The involvement of the MCP2,3 joints can be appreciated on clinical examination. Lack of flexion in these joints accounts for the 'iron fist' sign, an example of which is shown in Figure 173.1.[24]

Other joints in the hands can be affected in HH, but usually in association with the MCP2,3 joints. Coexistent interphalangeal (IP) joint disease due to osteoarthritis (OA) is not more frequent in HH than in population controls. Furthermore, primary idiopathic OA in the IP joints (type 1 polyarticular OA or T1POA) is also no more frequent in HH than in community controls.[17] A trend toward more frequent involvement of the triscaphe (scaphoid–trapezoid–trapezium) joint was noted by Valenti et al.[15] Occasionally the wrist and intercarpal joints can be affected as illustrated in the sentinel report by Schumacher[7] and the studies reported by Valenti et al.[15] However, in none of these other joints is there specificity for HH and even in the case of the MCP2,3 joints, there is a lack of disease specificity. Where chondrocalcinosis is present in either articular cartilage or fibrocartilage in association with a compatible MCP2,3 arthropathy, the specificity for the arthropathy of HH may be high, but to our knowledge this hypothesis has not been formally tested. The large joints such as the hip, ankle, radiocarpal, elbow, shoulder, and knee are also recognized sites in which the arthropathy of

Table 173.1 The frequency of arthropathy and chondrocalcinosis in reported series of patients with haemochromatosis and arthropathy

Study	Reference	Arthropathy [% frequency] (number studied)	Chondrocalcinosis % frequency (% of those with arthropathy)	% male in study
Dymock et al. 1970	9	57.4 (of 54 males)	49.2 (64.0)	93.1
Edwards et al. 1980	10	37.1 (n = 35)	17.1 (46.2)	60.0
Huaux et al. 1986	11	56.0 (n = 25)	20.0 (28) [n = 20]	72.0
Schumacher et al. 1988[b]	12	81.1 (n = 159)	NA	64.2
Faraawi et al. 1993	13	64 (n = 25)	36 [NA]	72.0
Sinigaglia et al. 1997	14	81.3 (n = 32)[a]	6.3 [NA]	
Valenti et al. 2007	15	36% for MCP disease (n = 88)	11% (100) [n = 10]	80.7
Richette et al. 2010	16	51% (OA in any of 7 regions) (n = 306)	NA	52.6
Carroll et al. 2011	17	24.4%[c] (n = 41)	4.9% (100%) [n = 2]	43.9

[a]31.2% had disease-specific arthropathy.
[b]Questionnaire study, frequency of arthralgias.
[c]14.6% with MCP arthropathy.

HH may manifest.[8,9,11,13,15] Joints such as the ankle and radiocarpal joints, which are usually spared in idiopathic or primary OA, may be involved in the arthropathy of HH. So far, no clinical criteria based on topography alone have been tested for diagnostic sensitivity and specificity for the arthropathy of HH.

Is the arthropathy inflammatory or non-inflammatory?

The arthropathy of HH is generally considered to be non-inflammatory. Despite the frequency of chondrocalcinosis, pseudogout presentations are uncommon. Case series draw attention to occasional cases where impressive clinical signs of synovitis have been observed and occasionally aspirates disclose numerous inflammatory cells and/or calcium pyrophosphate dihydrate (CPPD) crystals, but synovial fluids (SF) are mostly non-inflammatory. The observation that ferritin concentrations in the SF are higher in patients with OA who have *HFE* gene mutations raises the possibility that

SF ferritin may be a marker for an inflammatory component in the arthropathy of HH.[25]

Radiological findings in the arthropathy of hereditary haemochromatosis

The radiological features of the arthropathy of HH are similar to those in idiopathic osteoarthritis.[26,27] Subchondral sclerosis and joint space narrowing are typical. The latter can be rapidly progressive, with substantial deterioration within a matter of months.[11] More often however, the rate of progression is slow. Osteophytes may be present and can be prominent. In the MCP2,3 joints, hook-like osteophytes on the radial side of the metacarpal heads are characteristically seen. In one study, they were present in 17% of 41 definite or probable HH cases. The patients with hook-like osteophytes were all homozygous for the C282Y mutation.[17] Although regarded as a characteristic radiological feature of the arthropathy of HH, hook-like osteophytes do occur sometimes in OA and are thus not disease specific. The frequency with which subchondral lucencies, or geodes, are found in joints affected by the arthropathy accompanying HH is high, but has not been quantified. Dymock et al. described a strong correlation between subchondral lucencies and focal or eccentric chondral resorption and noted that cartilage loss occurred only occasionally in the absence of lucencies.[9] Lucencies may be prominent in the hip joint as depicted in Figure 173.2.[28] Erosions such as those seen in RA are not present, although infraction of marginal subchondral lucencies may be difficult to discriminate from rheumatoid erosions.

Pathology and aetiopathogenesis of arthropathy in hereditary haemochromatosis

Most of the information concerning joint pathology in HH has been obtained from surgical specimens derived at the time of joint

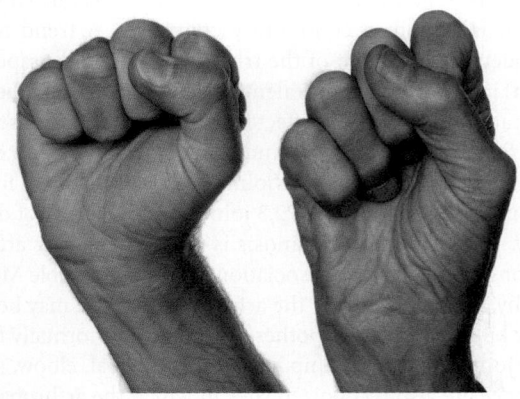

Fig. 173.1 Iron fist sign in hereditary haemochromatosis.

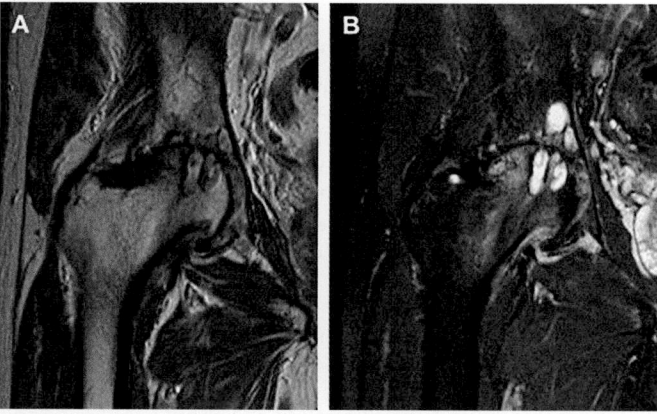

Fig. 173.2 MRI of the hip showing lucencies within the acetabulum and the femoral head.

replacement surgery and is therefore representative of advanced disease. Thinning or erosion of articular cartilage with exposure of eburnated bone is commonly described, but other findings such as iron deposition in cartilage, chondrocalcinosis, primary and secondary osteonecrosis, and articular cartilage avulsion at the tidemark in hip cartilage have been observed.[29,30] Cartilage avulsion is a very unusual finding in primary OA.[29] It is possible that dysregulated uptake of ferritin by osteocytes or chondrocytes may contribute to osteonecrosis and/or chondral damage.

In the synovium, deposits of iron have been observed, particularly in the synovial lining cells.[6,7,31–33] Indeed, deposition here as opposed to the sublining layers or synovial stroma is considered to be a point of differentiation between HH and secondary forms of haemochromatosis, such as occurs in thalassaemia major.[34] In the latter, sublining deposition is more marked.[31] Heiland et al. examined synovial tissue obtained from joint replacement specimens in patients with RA, OA, and HH,[32] and report many common features and very few differences overall. Importantly, haemosiderin deposits were found only in HH synovium and not in patients with RA or OA. Macrophage and neutrophil infiltration within the synovium was correlated with the extent of iron haemosiderin deposition. Interestingly, haemosiderin was still present in HH patients who had undergone regular venesection. In contrast, RA was easily distinguished from both OA and HH. The authors emphasize that HH arthropathy can be clearly differentiated from OA by the infiltration of cells of the innate immune response (macrophages, neutrophils) and also from RA by the lack of infiltrating specific immune cells (B cells, T cells). Thus in a number of respects the pathology of the arthropathy of HH is distinguishable and could perhaps be classified as 'intermediate' between that of RA and OA (Figure 173.3).

How iron is deposited and accumulates in the synovium in patients with HH is unclear, but the predominance of iron in the synovial lining layer raises the possibility that iron may be 'captured' from the synovial fluid as a result of persistently high serum ferritin concentrations and the phagocytic actions of synovial fibroblasts. Deposition may be effectively irreversible and accompanied by slowly progressive chondral resorption even in subjects who undergo regular venesection.[12,32] Iron deposition may of itself be seriously detrimental to the joint. Ferritin has recently been shown to act as a proinflammatory cytokine and could contribute directly to joint injury.[35] Importantly, in hepatic stellate cells, at nanomolar concentrations similar to those observed by one of the authors

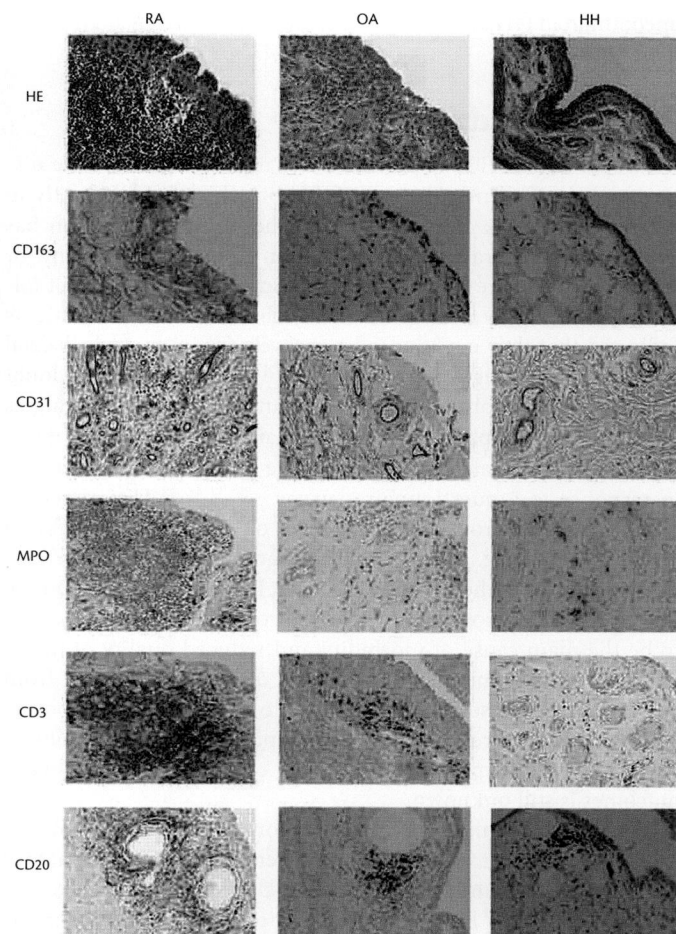

Fig. 173.3 Immunohistochemistry of synovium from RA, OA and hereditary haemochromatosis. Hereditary haemochromatosis can be differentiated from OA by the infiltration of cells of the innate immune response (macrophages, neutrophils) and also from RA by the lack of infiltrating specific immune cells (B cells, T cells).

(GJC) in SF in HH, ferritin was found to be a potent and rapid inducer of IL-1 gene expression.[35]

How excess iron contributes to the development of calcium pyrophosphate production and chondrocalcinosis is not well understood. In-vitro studies show that iron inhibits pyrophosphatase, suggesting that excess iron may promote pyrophosphate deposition in synovium or cartilage.[36] Additionally, accumulation of calcium pyrophosphate may be facilitated by reduced clearance in the setting of synovial siderosis.[37] While both ferric and ferrous iron influence CPPD formation, to date chondrocalcinosis has not been definitively linked to the level of iron overload.[38,39,40]

Osteoporosis in hereditary haemochromatosis

Osteoporosis (OP) is also a recognized feature of HH with a frequency estimated to range from 25% to 35%.[16,41,42] Indeed in a questionnaire-based study in which the frequency of OP in HH patients was compared to that in 'healthy blood donors', the odds ratio (OR) for OP was found to be 1.9 (confidence interval 1.1–3.5). The mechanism responsible for OP in HH is unknown. Possible contributory factors include reduced bone formation secondary to iron-mediated suppression of osteoblast activity[43–45] and increased bone resorption due to hypogonadism[45]; however, the latter is uncommon in HH and would not explain the relatively high prevalence of OP in HH.

Prognosis and treatment

Arthropathy in HH may predate other manifestations of the disease and is sometimes the manifestation which leads directly to diagnosis. There is conjecture as to whether iron depletion has any effect on arthralgia, other symptoms of the arthropathy, or its course. There are anecdotal descriptions of symptom relief following phlebotomy and in one survey about one-third of patients indicated that they experienced improvement in musculoskeletal symptoms following iron depletion.[7,46,47] Most authorities doubt that phlebotomy produces any substantial relief of arthralgias or other joint symptoms, but Harty et al. have described a mean reduction in arthralgia of 46% in those who reported arthralgia in response to a questionnaire survey.[8–12,31,46,48] It is generally accepted that 'de-ironing' has no effect on structural progression of the joint disease, although this has not been rigorously evaluated. In contrast, other manifestations of HH are clearly responsive to iron depletion, so much so that arthropathy is now considered to be the main cause of morbidity and reduced quality of life in treated disease. Whether 'tight control of iron metabolism' from an early age in those considered likely to manifest clinically overt HH or aggressive treatment to target approaches with phlebotomy could attenuate or prevent arthropathy or at least produce better outcomes is still unknown.

Other forms of medical treatment for the arthropathy of HH have been utilized. Analgesics, non-steroidal anti-inflammatory drugs (NSAIDs) and cyclooxygenase-2 inhibitors can produce symptomatic relief, but are not thought to have any disease-modifying effects, although no formal studies have been undertaken. Intra-articular steroids may be useful temporarily, but are generally unpredictable. In an open study, two patients with HH and in particular painful and disabling hand arthropathy responded temporarily to Anakinra 100 mg SC administered daily for 5 days and then regressed to baseline over the next 3 months.[49] Whether continuous treatment of HH with this or other IL-1 antagonists will provide sustained benefit remains to be determined. There is scope for major benefit from surgical interventions in HH arthropathy, not least from joint arthroplasties.

Conclusion

The arthropathy of haemochromatosis is relatively common even in patients with HH recruited from the community. It is a chronic, progressive arthropathy with a level of inflammatory activity that is both clinically and histopathologically intermediate between that of RA and OA. There is a predilection for the finger MCP joints and it is variably, but not commonly, accompanied by chondrocalcinosis. The precise mechanism responsible for tissue damage in affected joints remains unknown; however, there is growing evidence that iron load is a major determinant of the arthropathy. HH arthropathy is variably responsive to phlebotomy. Whether earlier diagnosis and treatment targeted to achieve tight control of iron metabolism from an early age or as soon as possible after diagnosis could produce better outcomes remains to be determined. Novel and more effective approaches to management with a view to prevention of structural joint damage still need to be developed.

References

1. Allen KJ, Gurrin LC, Constantine CC et al. Iron-overload-related disease in HFE hereditary hemochromatosis. *N Engl J Med* 2008;358:221–230.
2. Olynyk JK, Trinder D, Ramm GA, Britton RS, Bacon BR. Hereditary haemochromatosis in the post HFE-era. *Hepatology* 2008;48:991–1001.
3. Adams PC, Kertesz AE, Valberg LS. Clinical presentation of hemochromatosis: a changing scene. *Am J Med* 1991;4:445–449.
4. Feder JN, Gnirke A, Thomas W et al. A novel MHC class 1-like gene is mutated in patients with hereditary hemochromatosis. *Nat Genet* 1996;4:339–408.
5. Camashella C. Understanding iron homeostasis through genetic analysis of haemochromatosis and related disorders. *Blood* 2005;12:3710–3717.
6. Sheldon JH. *Haemochromatosis*. Oxford University Press, London, 1935.
7. Schumacher HR Jr. Hemochromatosis and arthritis. *Arthritis Rheum* 1964;7:41–50.
8. Hamilton E, Williams R, Barlow KA, Smith PM. The arthropathy of Idiopathic haemochromatosis. *Q J Med* 1968;145:171–182.
9. Dymock IW, Hamilton EBD, Laws JW, Williams R. Arthropathy of haemochromatosis. *Ann Rheum Dis* 1970; 29: 469–476.
10. Edwards CQ, Cartwright GE, Skolnick MH, Amos DB. Homozygosity for hemochromatosis: clinical manifestations. *Ann Intern Med* 1980;93: 519–525.
11. Huaux JP, Geubel A, Koch MC et al. The arthritis of Hemochromatosis. *Clin Rheumatol* 1986;5:317–324.
12. Schumacher HR, Straka PC, Krikker MA, Dudley AT. The arthropathy of hemochromatosis. *Ann N Y Acad Sci* 1988;526:522–533.
13. Farawi R, Harth M, Kertesz A, Bell D. Arthritis in haemochromatosis. *J Rheumatol* 1993;20:448.
14. Sinigaglia L, Fargion S, Fracanzani AL et al. Bone and joint involvement in genetic hemochromatosis: role of cirrhosis and iron overload. *J Rheumatol* 1997;9:1809–1813.
15. Valenti L, Fracanzani AL, Rossi V et al. The hand arthropathy of hereditary hemochromatosis is strongly associated with iron overload. *J Rheumatol* 2008;35:153–158.
16. Richette P, Ottaviani S, Vicaut E, Bardin T. Musculoskeletal complications of hereditary hemochromatosis: a case-control study. *J Rheumatol* 2010;37:2145–2150.
17. Carroll GJ, Breidahl WH, Bulsara MK, Olynyk JK. Hereditary hemochromatosis is characterised by a clinically definable arthropathy that correlates with iron load. *Arthritis Rheum* 2011;63:286–294.
18. Carroll GJ. Polyarticular osteoarthritis-two major phenotypes hypothesised. Med Hypotheses 2006;66:315–318.
19. Carroll GJ, Breidahl WH, Jazayeri J. Confirmation of two major polyarticular osteoarthritis (POA) phenotypes-differentiation on the basis of joint topography. *Osteoarthritis Cartilage* 2009;17:891–895.
20. Bensen WG, Laskin CA, Little HA, Fam AG. Hemochromatotic arthropathy mimicking rheumatoid arthritis. *Arthritis Rheum* 1978;21: 844–848.
21. Bulaj ZJ, Ajioka RS, Phillips JD et al. Disease-related conditions in relatives of patients with hemochromatosis. *N Engl J Med* 2000;343:1529–1535.
22. Hamilton EBD, Bomford AB, Laws JW, Williams R. The natural history of arthritis in idiopathic haemochromatosis: Progression of the clinical and radiological features over 10 years. *Q J Med* 1981;199:321–329.
23. Vaiopoulos G, Papanikolaou G, Politou M et al. Arthropathy in juvenile hemochromatosis. *Arthritis Rheum* 2003;48:227–230.
24. Cunnane G, O'Duffy JD. The iron salute: a sign of hemochromatosis. Arthritis Rheum 1995;38:558.
25. Carroll GJ, Sharma G, Upadhyay A, Jazayeri J. Ferritin concentrations in synovial fluid are higher in osteoarthritis (OA) patients with HFE gene mutations (C282Y or H63D) than in OA patients who are HFE wild type. *Scand J Rheum* 2010;39:413–420.
26. Axford JS. Rheumatic manifestations of haemochromatosis. *Bailliere's Clin Rheumatol* 1991;5:351–365.

27. Dallos T, Sahinbegovic E, Aigner E et al. Validation of a radiographic scoring system for haemochromatosis arthropathy. *Ann Rheum Dis* 2010;69:2145–2151.

28. Duval H, Lancien G, Marin F et al. Hip involvement in hereditary hemochromatosis: a clinical–pathologic study. *Joint Bone Spine* 2009;76:412–415.

29. Montgomery KD, Williams JR, Sculco TP, DiCarlo E. Clinical and pathological findings in haemochromatosis hip arthropathy. *Clin Orthop Relat Res* 1988;347:179–187.

30. Axford JS, Bomford A, Revell P et al. Hip arthropathy in hemochromatosis. *Arthritis Rheum* 1991;34:357–361.

31. Kra SJ, Hollingsworth JW, Finch SC. Arthritis with synovial iron deposition in a patient with hemochromatosis. *N Engl J Med* 1965;272:1268–1271.

32. Heiland GR, Aigner E, Dallos T et al. Synovial immunopathology in haemochromatosis arthropathy. *Ann Rheum Dis* 2010;69:1214–1219.

33. Schumacher HR. Articular cartilage in the degenerative arthropathy of hemochromatosis. *Arthritis Rheum* 1982;25:1460–1468.

34. Sella EJ, Goodman AH. Arthropathy secondary to transfusion hemochromatosis. *J Bone Joint Surg Am* 1973;55:1077–1081.

35. Ruddell RG, Hoang-Le D, Barwood JM et al. Ferritin functions as a proinflammatory cytokine via iron-independent protein kinase C zeta/nuclear factor kappa B-regulated signalling in rat hepatic stellate cells. *Hepatology* 2009;49:887–900.

36. McCarty DJ, Pepe PF. Erythrocyte neutral inorganic pyrophosphatase in pseudogout. *J Lab Clin Med* 1972;79:277–284.

37. McCarty DJ. Palmer DW, Garancis JC. Clearance of calcium pyrophosphate dihydrate crystals in vivo, III Effects of synovial hemosiderosis. *Arthritis Rheum* 1981;24:706–710.

38. Cheng PT, Pritzker KP. Ferrous, but not ferric ions inhibit de novo formation of calcium pyrophosphate dihydrate crystals: possible relationships to chondrocalcinosis and hemochromatosis. *J Rheumatol* 1988;15:321–324.

39. Mandel GS, Halverson PB, Mandel NS. Calcium pyrophosphate crystal deposition: the effect of soluble iron in a kinetic study using a gelatin matrix model. *Scanning Microsc* 1988;2(2):1177–1188.

40. Docquier Ch, Henrion J, Heller F, Tellier E, Lebacq E. L'arthropathie de l'hémochromatose idiopathique: à propos de 7 observations. *Acta Rhumatol* 1981;5:183–196.

41. Guggenbuhl P, Deugnier Y, Boisdet JF et al. Bone mineral density in men with genetic haemochromatosis. *Osteoporosis Int* 2005;16: 1809–1814.

42. Valenti L, Varenna M, Fracanzani AL et al. Association between iron overload and osteoporosis in patients with hereditary haemochromatosis *Osteoporosis Int* 2009;20:549–555.

43. de Vernejoul MC, Pointillart A, Golenzer CC et al. Effects of iron overload on bone remodelling in pigs. *Am J Pathol* 1984;116:377–384.

44. Diamond T, Stiel D, Posen S. Osteoporosis in haemochromatosis: iron excess, gonadal deficiency or other factors? *Ann Intern Med* 1989;110: 430–436.

45. Diamond T, Stiel D, Possen S. Effects of testosterone and venesection on spinal and peripheral bone mineral in six hypogonadal men with haemochromatosis *J Bone Miner Res* 1991;6:39–43.

46. Niederau C, Fischer R, Purschel A et al. Long-term survival in patients with hereditary haemochromatosis. *Gastroenterology* 1996;110:1107–1119.

47. Askari AD, Muir WA, Rosner IA et al. Arthritis of haemochromatosis: clinical spectrum, relation to histocompatibility antigens and effectiveness of early phlebotomy. *Am J Med* 1983;75:957–965.

48. Harty LC, Lai D, Connor S et al. Prevalence and progress of joint symptoms in hereditary haemochromatosis and symptomatic response to venesection. *J Clin Rheumatol* 2011;17:220–222.

49. Latourte A, Frazier A, Briere C, Ea H-K and Richette P. Interleukin-1 receptor antagonist in refractory haemochromatosis – related arthritis of the hands. *Ann Rheum Dis* 2013;1–2.

INDEX

Main index entries are given in **bold.** Entries in *italics* refer to figures, tables, and boxes.